ANESTHESIOLOGY & CRITICAL CARE DRUG HANDBOOK

Including Select Disease States & Perioperative Management

Senior Editors:
Verna L. Baughman, MD
Julie Golembiewski, PharmD
Jeffrey P. Gonzales, PharmD, BCPS
William Alvarez, Jr., PharmD, BCPS

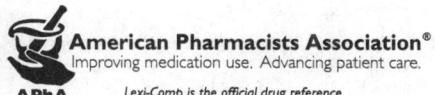

American Pharmacists Association®
Improving medication use. Advancing patient care.
APhA

Lexi-Comp is the official drug reference for the American Pharmacists Association

9th Edition

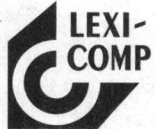

LEXI-COMP

ANESTHESIOLOGY & CRITICAL CARE DRUG HANDBOOK

Including Select Disease States & Perioperative Management

Verna L. Baughman, MD
Professor, Anesthesiology and Neurosurgery
University of Illinois
Chicago, Illinois

Jeffrey P. Gonzales, PharmD, BCPS
Assitant Professor, Critical Care
University of Maryland School of Pharmacy
Critical Care Clinical Pharmacy Specialist
Medical Intensive Care Unit
University of Maryland Medical Center
Baltimore, Maryland

Julie Golembiewski, PharmD
Clinical Pharmacist in Anesthesia/Pain
Departments of Pharmacy Service and Anesthesiology
University of Illinois Medical Center at Chicago
Clinical Associate Professor
Departments of Pharmacy Practice and Anesthesiology
University of Illinios at Chicago Colleges of Pharmacy and Medicine
Chicago, Illinois

William Alvarez Jr, PharmD, BCPS
*Pharmacotherapy Specialist,
Cardiology/Critical Care*
Lexi-Comp, Inc.
Hudson, Ohio

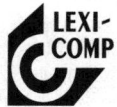

NOTICE

This data is intended to serve the user as a handy reference and not as a complete drug information resource. It does not include information on every therapeutic agent available. The publication covers over 580 commonly used drugs and is specifically designed to present important aspects of drug data in a more concise format than is typically found in medical literature or product material supplied by manufacturers.

The nature of drug information is that it is constantly evolving because of ongoing research and clinical experience and is often subject to interpretation. While great care has been taken to ensure the accuracy of the information and recommendations presented, the reader is advised that the authors, editors, reviewers, contributors, and publishers cannot be responsible for the continued currency of the information or for any errors, omissions, or the application of this information, or for any consequences arising therefrom. Therefore, the author(s) and/or the publisher shall have no liability to any person or entity with regard to claims, loss, or damage caused, or alleged to be caused, directly or indirectly, by the use of information contained herein. Because of the dynamic nature of drug information, readers are advised that decisions regarding drug therapy must be based on the independent judgment of the clinician, changing information about a drug (eg, as reflected in the literature and manufacturer's most current product information), and changing medical practices. Therefore, this data is designed to be used in conjunction with other necessary information and is not designed to be solely relied upon by any user. The user of this data hereby and forever releases the authors and publishers of this data from any and all liability of any kind that might arise out of the use of this data. The editors are not responsible for any inaccuracy of quotation or for any false or misleading implication that may arise due to the text or formulas as used or due to the quotation of revisions no longer official.

Certain of the authors, editors, and contributors have written this book in their private capacities. No official support or endorsement by any federal or state agency or pharmaceutical company is intended or inferred.

The publishers have made every effort to trace any third party copyright holders, if any, for borrowed material. If they have inadvertently overlooked any, they will be pleased to make the necessary arrangements at the first opportunity.

If you have any suggestions or questions regarding any information presented in this data, please contact our drug information pharmacists at (330) 650-6506.

This manual was produced using Lexi-Comp's Information Management System™ (LIMS) — A complete publishing service of Lexi-Comp, Inc.

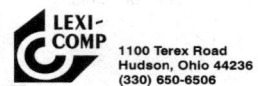

LEXI-COMP
1100 Terex Road
Hudson, Ohio 44236
(330) 650-6506

ISBN 978-1-59195-275-6

TABLE OF CONTENTS

ABOUT THE AUTHORS

Verna L. Baughman, MD

Dr Baughman is Professor of Anesthesiology and Neurosurgery at the University of Illinois at Chicago. She received her BA in 1968 from DePauw University, Greencastle, Indiana, with a major in both French and Biology. She then worked as a research editor/writer for the Encyclopaedia Britannica and as a hospital administrator. She attended Stritch School of Medicine at Loyola University, Chicago, receiving her medical degree in 1981. Following an internship and residency in Anesthesiology at Michael Reese Medical Center in Chicago, she spent a year as a Neuroanesthesia Research Fellow. Her interest in neuroanesthesia has dominated her laboratory and clinical research, with a focus on stroke and the effects of various drug therapies in ameliorating neuronal damage from ischemia. She is also interested in the effects of estrogen and menopause in relation to cerebral ischemia.

Dr Baughman has to her credit over 100 publications, including original research papers, textbook chapters, and editorials. She has been an active member of the editorial board for the Journal of Neurosurgical Anesthesia and Critical Care for 21 years. She currently reviews papers for *Anesthesiology, Anesthesia & Analgesia, Journal of Clinical Anesthesia, Stroke*, and *American Journal of Physiology*. She has been a visiting professor at many universities and a frequent lecturer at national meetings. Dr Baughman was cited in "Best Doctors in America" in 1995 and again in 1996.

Dr Baughman's interest in education is evidenced by consistently being voted by the resident staff as one of the best departmental teachers. She was selected to receive the 2001-2002 Excellence in Teaching Award, which recognizes quality teachers at the University of Illinois. In 2003 Dr Baughman was honored as the first Distinguished Teacher of the Year by the Society of Neurosurgical Anesthesia and Critical Care. She is active in the College of Medicine and Hospital communities involved in education and administration. She is also a consultant to the pharmaceutical industry, evaluating drugs and equipment. Dr Baughman is an active member of the American Society of Anesthesiologists, Society of Neuro-surgical Anesthesia and Critical Care, International Anesthesia Research Society, and Stroke Council of the American Heart Association.

Jeffrey P. Gonzales, PharmD, BCPS

Dr Gonzales is a Critical Care Assistant Professor at the University of Maryland School of Pharmacy. He is the course master of an elective course that emphasizes Critical Care Pharmacotherapy for the third-year pharmacy students. He also teaches critical care topics in a variety of courses throughout the School of Pharmacy curriculum. Dr Gonzales practices clinically as a Critical Care Clinical Pharmacy Specialist in the Medical Intensive Care Unit at the University of Maryland Medical Center, where he serves as a preceptor for residents and students. His areas of interest and research are sedation/delirium, sepsis, ARDS, pulmonary hypertension, and alterations in absorption in the critically ill.

Dr Gonzales received his Doctor of Pharmacy degree at Idaho State University in Pocatello, Idaho. He completed a Pharmacy Practice Residency at the University of Nebraska Medical Center, then completed his Critical Care training as a Critical Care Resident at Detroit Receiving Hospital-Detroit Medical Center. Following his residency training, Dr Gonzales completed a Postdoctoral Fellowship in Critical Care at The University of Michigan College of Pharmacy, where he was the recipient of the 1999 American College of Clinical Pharmacy-Bayer Critical Care Fellowship Award.

After completion of his postgraduate training, Dr Gonzales took a position as the Critical Care Clinical Specialist at The Cleveland Clinic Foundation and practiced in the Medical Intensive Care Unit for 6 years. During that time, he was awarded the Ohio College of Clinical Pharmacy Bayer Board Certification Award and became a Board Certified Pharmacotherapy Specialist (BCPS). At the Cleveland Clinic, he was involved with medical and pharmacy resident/student education and created the Critical Care Pharmacy Residency. He was a member of the Pharmacology

Curriculum Committee, Cleveland Clinic Lerner College of Medicine at Case Western Reserve University. He also received the 2004 Cleveland Clinic Foundation Department of Pharmacy Research and Education Award, as well as the 2005 Ohio College of Clinical Pharmacy-Pfizer Research Award.

Dr Gonzales is an active member of the Society of Critical Care Medicine (SCCM), the American College of Clinical Pharmacy (ACCP), and the American Society of Health-Systems Pharmacists (ASHP).

Julie Golembiewski, PharmD

Dr Golembiewski received her bachelor's degree in pharmacy and Doctor of Pharmacy degree from the University of Illinois at Chicago. She has over 20 years of active pharmacy experience, with the majority concentrated in the areas of operating room pharmacy and anesthesiology. She worked in the operating room pharmacy at the University of Illinois Medical Center at Chicago, then went on to manage an operating room pharmacy at Bergan Mercy Medical Center in Omaha, NE and The University of Michigan Health System in Ann Arbor, MI where she also held a faculty appointment of Clinical Associate Professor in the Clinical Sciences Department at the University of Michigan College of Pharmacy and Adjunct Assistant Professor of Anesthesiology at the University of Michigan Medical School.

Currently, Dr Golembiewski is a clinical pharmacist in anesthesia/pain at the University of Illinois Medical Center at Chicago (UIMCC) with a shared appointment in the Departments of Pharmacy Services and Anesthesiology. In addition, she holds the appointments of Clinical Associate Professor in the Departments of Pharmacy Practice and Anesthesiology at the University of Illinois at Chicago (UIC) College of Pharmacy and Medicine. At the UIMCC, Dr Golembiewski is a member of several committees, including the Pain Committee, Surgical Care Improvement Project Quality Improvement Team, the Department of Anesthesiology Quality Improvement Committees, the Pharmacy Resident and Department of Anesthesiology Research Committees, and Graduate Medical Education Committee for the Department of Anesthesiology. She is co-coordinator for the UIC Department of Anesthesiology for the Midwest Anesthesia Residents Conference. Dr Golembiewski teaches third-year pharmacy students at the UIC College of Pharmacy and serves as a clerkship preceptor for further pharmacy students and pharmacy residents.

Dr Golembiewski has published extensively in the areas of anesthesiology and operating room pharmacy and is often invited to speak at professional meetings on topics related to these areas. She is on the editorial advisory board of *Pharmacy Practice News* and writes a regular column for the *Journal of Preanesthesia Nursing*. Dr Golembiewski is an active member of the Illinois Society of Pharmacists, the American Society of Pharmacists, and the American Pharmacists Association.

William Alvarez, Jr, PharmD, BCPS

Dr Alvarez received his bachelor's degree in pharmacy and Doctor of Pharmacy degree from The Ohio State University (OSU) College of Pharmacy. After completing a specialized residency in Cardiology at The OSU Medical Center, he went on to hold a position at The Johns Hopkins Hospital (JHH) for 7 years as the Cardiovascular Clinical Specialist. His areas of practice included advanced cardiac life support, anticoagulation, cardiothoracic surgery, coronary care, critical care, and heart failure. He was actively involved with pharmacy resident training and cardiology fellowship training, and was the Program Director for the Pharmacotherapy Specialty Residency for 3 years while at JHH. He also served as a residency accreditation surveyor for the American Society of Pharmacists during his time as program director. He has been a Clinical Instructor for The OSU College of Pharmacy, the University of the Sciences in Philadelphia College of Pharmacy, and the University of Maryland School of Pharmacy. He has authored journal articles and has given numerous educational programs for JHH, the Maryland Society of Pharmacists, and the American Association of Critical Care Nurses Chesapeake Bay Chapter. He also has conducted numerous clinical research projects and has been a Board Certified Pharmacotherapy Specialist since 2002.

ABOUT THE AUTHORS

Dr Alvarez has been with Lexi-Comp, Inc since 2007. He is actively involved in the publication of the *Anesthesia and Critical Care Drug Handbook*, enhancing the database with particular focus on the areas of critical care and coronary care. He is an active participant in the Medical Science Division at Lexi-Comp, Inc.

Dr Alvarez is a member of the American College of Cardiology, the American College of Clinical Pharmacy, the Ohio College of Clinical Pharmacy, and the Society of Critical Care Medicine.

Larry D. Gray, PhD, ABMM
Director, Clinical Microbiology
TriHealth Laboratories
Bethesda and Good Samaritan
Hospitals
Cincinnati, Ohio

Tracy Hagemann, PharmD
Associate Professor
College of Pharmacy
The University of Oklahoma
Oklahoma City, Oklahoma

Martin D. Higbee, PharmD
Associate Professor
Department of Pharmacy Practice
and Science
The University of Arizona
Tucson, Arizona

Edward Horn, PharmD, BCPS
Clinical Specialist, Transplant Surgery
Allegheny General Hospital
Pittsburgh, Pennsylvania

Jane Hurlburt Hodding, PharmD
*Executive Director, Inpatient Pharmacy
Services and Clinical Nutrition Services*
Long Beach Memorial Medical Center
and Miller Children's Hospital
Long Beach, California

**Mark T. Holdsworth,
PharmD, BCOP**
*Associate Professor of
Pharmacy & Pediatrics
Pharmacy Practice Area Head*
College of Pharmacy
The University of New Mexico
Albuquerque, New Mexico

Collin A. Hovinga, PharmD
*Assistant Professor of Pharmacy
and Pediatrics*
College of Pharmacy
University of Tennessee
Health Science Center
Memphis, Tennessee

Darrell T. Hulisz, PharmD
Department of Family Medicine
Case Western Reserve University
Cleveland, Ohio

Michael A. Kahn, DDS
Professor and Chairman
Department of Oral and
Maxillofacial Pathology
Tufts University
School of Dental Medicine
Boston, Massachusetts

Jeannette Kaiser, MT, MBA
Medical Technologist
Akron General Medical Center
Akron, Ohio

**Polly E. Kintzel, PharmD,
BCPS, BCOP**
Clinical Pharmacy Specialist-Oncology
Spectrum Health
Grand Rapids, Michigan

Daren Knoell, PharmD
*Associate Professor of Pharmacy
Practice and Internal Medicine*
Davis Heart and Lung Research Institute
The Ohio State University
Columbus, Ohio

Sandra Knowles, RPh, BScPhm
Drug Safety Pharmacist
Sunnybrook and Women's College HSC
Toronto, Ontario

**Jill M. Kolesar, PharmD,
FCCP, BCPS**
Associate Professor
School of Pharmacy
Associate Professor
University of Wisconsin Paul P. Carbone
Comprehensive Cancer Center
University of Wisconsin
Madison, Wisconsin

**Donna M. Kraus,
PharmD, FAPhA**
*Associate Professor of
Pharmacy Practice*
Departments of Pharmacy Practice and
Pediatrics
Pediatric Clinical Pharmacist
University of Illinois
Chicago, Illinois

Daniel L. Krinsky RPh, MS
Manager, MTM Services
Giant Eagle Pharmacy
Ravenna, Ohio
Assistant Professor
Department of Pharmacy Practice
College of Pharmacy NEOUCOM
Rootstown, Ohio

Kay Kyllonen, PharmD
Clinical Specialist
The Cleveland Clinic Children's Hospital
Cleveland, Ohio

**Charles Lacy, MS, PharmD,
FCSHP**
*Vice President for Executive Affairs
Professor, Pharmacy Practice
Professor, Business Leadership*
University of Southern Nevada
Las Vegas, Nevada

8

Martha Sajatovic, MD
Professor of Psychiatry
Case Western Reserve University
Cleveland, Ohio
Department of Psychiatry
University Hospitals of Cleveland
Cleveland, Ohio

**Jennifer K. Sekeres,
PharmD, BCPS**
Infectious Diseases Clinical Specialist
The Cleveland Clinic Foundation
Cleveland, Ohio

**Todd P. Semla, MS, PharmD,
BCPS, FCCP, AGSF**
Clinical Pharmacy Specialist
Department of Veterans Affairs
Pharmacy Benefits
Management Services
Associate Professor, Clinical
Department of Medicine and Psychiatry
and Behavioral Health
Feinberg School of Medicine
Northwestern University
Chicago, Illinois

Joseph Snoke, RPh, BCPS
Manager
Core Pharmacology Group
Lexi-Comp, Inc
Hudson, Ohio

**Joni Lombardi Stahura, BS,
PharmD, RPh**
Pharmacotherapy Specialist
Lexi-Comp, Inc
Hudson, Ohio

**Stephen Marc Stout, PharmD,
MS, BCPS**
Pharmacotherapy Specialist
Lexi-Comp, Inc
Hudson, Ohio

Dan Streetman, PharmD, RPh
Pharmacotherapy Specialist
Lexi-Comp, Inc
Hudson, Ohio

**Darcie-Ann Streetman,
PharmD, RPh**
Clinical Pharmacist
University of Michigan Health System
Ann Arbor, Michigan

Carol K. Taketomo, PharmD
*Director of Pharmacy and
Nutrition Services*
Children's Hospital Los Angeles
Los Angeles, California

Mary Temple-Cooper, PharmD
Pediatric Clinical Research Specialist
Hillcrest Hospital
Mayfield Heights, Ohio

**Elizabeth A. Tomsik,
PharmD, BCPS**
Manager
Adverse Drug Reactions Group
Lexi-Comp, Inc
Hudson, Ohio

Dana Travis, RPh
Pharmacotherapy Specialist
Lexi-Comp, Inc
Hudson, Ohio

Jennifer Trofe-Clark, PharmD
Clinical Transplant Pharmacist
Hospital of The University
of Pennsylvania
Philadelphia, Pennsylvania

Beatrice B. Turkoski, RN, PhD
*Associate Professor, Graduate Faculty,
Pharmacology for Advanced
Practice Nurses*
College of Nursing
Kent State University
Kent, Ohio

Amy Van Orman, PharmD
Pharmacotherapy Specialist
Lexi-Comp, Inc
Hudson, Ohio

David M. Weinstein, PhD, RPh
Manager
Metabolism, Interactions,
and Genomics Group
Lexi-Comp, Inc
Hudson, Ohio

Anne Marie Whelan, PharmD
College of Pharmacy
Dalhousie University
Halifax, Nova Scotia

Nathan Wirick, PharmD
*Infectious Disease and Antibiotic
Management Clinical Specialist*
Hillcrest Hospital
Cleveland, Ohio

**Richard L. Wynn,
BSPharm, PhD**
Professor of Pharmacology
Baltimore College of Dental Surgery
Dental School
University of Maryland Baltimore
Baltimore, Maryland

PREFACE

Drug therapy in the perioperative and critical care settings continues to evolve as new medications are introduced into clinical practice and additional uses for existing medications are developed. Since patients undergoing surgery or admitted to an intensive care unit (ICU) are not confined to the operating room or ICU for the duration of their hospital stay, it is critical for all healthcare practitioners and students responsible for patient care to have a basic understanding of the medications used in these patient populations. The *Anesthesiology and Critical Care Drug Handbook* is designed to provide this information in a practical and convenient manner.

As in previous editions, special emphasis continues to be placed on medications used during the perioperative period (eg, neuromuscular blocking agents, antiemetic agents, volatile inhalation agents) and in critical care patients (eg, sedative agents, vasopressors), with comparative tables provided for the key drug classes. Monographs for other commonly prescribed medications in these patient populations are also contained in the handbook, which increases its usefulness as a drug reference. All of the monographs follow a standard format, with frequently used information (eg, use, mechanism of action, pharmacodynamics/kinetics, dosage, monitoring parameters, anesthesia and critical care concerns). In each of the monographs, special consideration has been given to including anesthetic drug interactions when applicable.

The Special Topics/Issues section of the handbook contains clear, concise summaries of frequently encountered patient conditions (eg, latex allergy), select uses of anesthesia-related medications (eg, conscious sedation), critical care issues (eg, sepsis guidelines), management of important clinical scenarios (eg, perioperative/periprocedural management of anticoagulant and antiplatelet therapies), and the management of various patient types (eg, critically-ill, morbidly obese patients; cardiac patients undergoing noncardiac surgery). This handbook presents recent literature related to specific treatments. The information will provide the practitioner with a quick overview of the most salient facts to consider for the particular condition or therapy being discussed.

The appendix contains information valuable to the anesthesia/critical care practitioner such as summaries of the various anesthesia discharge scoring systems, airway classification, stress replacement of glucocorticoids, treatment of malignant hyperthermia, and ACLS guidelines. Many useful comparative medication tables can also be found in the appendix. Pertinent references are included in each monograph.

DESCRIPTION OF SECTIONS AND FIELDS

The *Anesthesiology* & *Critical Care Drug Handbook* is divided into five sections.

The first section is a compilation of introductory text pertinent to the use of this book.

The drug information section of the handbook, in which all drugs are listed alphabetically, details information pertinent to each drug. Extensive cross-referencing is provided by brand names and index terms. Condensed monographs, containing limited fields of information, are included for drugs that are not anesthesia and critical care medications, but which may be encountered in surgery or the emergency room.

The third section is comprised of several text chapters dealing with various subjects and issues pertinent to perianesthetic patient management.

The fourth section is an invaluable appendix with charts, tables, nomograms, algorithms, management guidelines, and conversion information which can be helpful for patient care.

The last section of this handbook includes a pharmacologic category index.

Alphabetical Listing of Drugs

Drug information is presented in a consistent format and provides the following:

Generic Name	U.S. adopted name
Pronunciation	Phonetic pronunciation guide
Medication Safety Issue	In an effort to promote the safe use of medications, this field is intended to highlight possible sources of medication errors such as look-alike/sound-alike drugs or highly concentrated formulations which require vigilance on the part of healthcare professionals. In addition, medications which have been associated with severe consequences in the event of a medication error are also identified in this field.
Medication Guide	Information regarding the FDA-required distribution of patient Medication Guides for select drugs.
Related Information	Cross-reference to other pertinent drug information found elsewhere in this handbook
U.S. Brand Names	Trade names (manufacturer-specific) found in the United States. The symbol [DSC] appears after trade names that have been recently discontinued.
Canadian Brand Names	Trade names found in Canada
Index Terms	Includes names or accepted abbreviations of generic drug; may include common brand names no longer available; this field is used to create cross-references to monographs
Pharmacologic Category	Unique systematic classification of medications
Restrictions	The controlled substance classification from the Drug Enforcement Agency (DEA). U.S. schedules are I-V. Schedules vary by country and sometimes state (ie, Massachusetts uses I-VI). May also include restriced availability information.
Generic Available	Specifies whether a generic equivalent is available
Use	Information pertaining to appropriate FDA approved indications of the drug
Unlabeled/ Investigational Use	Information pertaining to non-FDA approved and investigational indications of the drug
Mechanism of Action	How the drug works in the body to elicit a response

Pharmacodynamics/ Kinetics	The magnitude of a drug's effect depends on the drug concentration at the site of action. The pharmacodynamics are expressed in terms of onset of action and duration of action. Pharmacokinetics are expressed in terms of absorption, distribution (including appearance in breast milk and crossing of the placenta), protein binding, metabolism, bioavailability, half-life, time to peak serum concentration, and elimination.
Dosage	The amount of the drug to be typically given or taken during therapy for children and adults; also includes any dosing adjustment/comments for renal impairment or hepatic impairment and other suggested dosing adjustments (eg, hematological toxicity)
Stability	Information regarding storage of product or steps for reconstitution. Provides the time and conditions for which a solution or mixture will maintain full potency. For example, some solutions may require refrigeration after reconstitution while stored at room temperature prior to preparation. Also includes compatibility information. **Note:** Professional judgment of the individual pharmacist in application of this information is imperative. While drug products may exhibit stability over longer durations of time, it may not be appropriate to utilize the drug product due to concerns in sterility.
Administration	Information regarding the recommended final concentrations, rates of administration for parenteral drugs, or other guidelines when giving the medication
Monitoring Parameters	Laboratory tests and patient physical parameters that should be monitored for safety and efficacy of drug therapy
Reference Range	Therapeutic and toxic serum concentrations listed including peak and trough levels
Anesthesia and Critical Care Concerns/Other Considerations	This field provides a focused summary of some of the important issues concerning anesthesia and critical care applications relevant to the drug; other additional information may be included
Pregnancy Risk Factor	Five categories established by the FDA to indicate the potential of a systemically absorbed drug for causing birth defects
Contraindications	Information pertaining to inappropriate use of the drug
Warnings/Precautions	Precautionary considerations, hazardous conditions related to use of the drug, and disease states or patient populations in which the drug should be cautiously used. Boxed warnings, when present, are clearly identified and are adapted from the FDA approved labeling. Consult the product labeling for the exact black box warning through the manufacturer's or the FDA website.
Adverse Reactions	Side effects are grouped by percentage of incidence and body system
Drug Interactions	
Metabolism/ Transport Effects	If a drug has demonstrated involvement with cytochrome P450 enzymes, or other metabolism or transport proteins, this field will identify the drug as an inhibitor, inducer, or substrate of the specific enzyme(s) (eg, CYP1A2 or UGT1A1). CYP450 isoenzymes are identified as substrates (minor or major), inhibitors (weak, moderate, or strong), and inducers (weak or strong).
Avoid Concomitant Use	Designates drug combinations which should not be used concomitantly, due to an unacceptable risk:benefit assessment. Frequently, the concurrent use of the agents is explicitly prohibited or contraindicated by the product labeling.
Increased Effect/ Toxicity	Drug combinations that result in a increased or toxic therapeutic effect between the drug listed in the monograph and other drugs or drug classes.
Decreased Effect	Drug combinations that result in a decreased therapeutic effect between the drug listed in the monograph and other drugs or drug classes.
Ethanol/Nutrition/Herb Interactions	Information regarding potential interactions with food, nutritionals (including herbal products or vitamins), or ethanol.
Test Interactions	Information regarding effect or implications of laboratory tests while taking the medication
Dietary Considerations	Includes information on how the medication should be taken relative to meals or food
Additional Information	Other data and facts about the drug are offered when appropriate

DESCRIPTION OF SECTIONS AND FIELDS

Product Availability	This field is utilized to provide availability information on products that have been approved by the FDA, but not yet available for use. Estimates for when a product may be available are included when this information is known. This field may also be used to provide any unique or critical drug availability issues (eg, drug shortage of a critical drug).
Dosage Forms	Information regarding form, strength, and availability of the drug. **Note:** Additional formulation information (eg, excipients, preservatives) is included when available. Please consult product labeling for further information.
References	Sources and literature used in the writing of the monograph

FDA PREGNANCY CATEGORIES

Throughout this book there is a field labeled Pregnancy Risk Factor and the letter A, B, C, D, or X immediately following which signifies a category. The FDA has established these five categories to indicate the potential of a systemically absorbed drug for causing birth defects. The key differentiation among the categories rests upon the reliability of documentation and the risk:benefit ratio. Pregnancy Category X is particularly notable in that if any data exists that may implicate a drug as a teratogen and the risk:benefit ratio is clearly negative, the drug is contraindicated during pregnancy.

These categories are summarized as follows:

A   Controlled studies in pregnant women fail to demonstrate a risk to the fetus in the first trimester with no evidence of risk in later trimesters. The possibility of fetal harm appears remote.

B   Either animal-reproduction studies have not demonstrated a fetal risk but there are no controlled studies in pregnant women, or animal-reproduction studies have shown an adverse effect (other than a decrease in fertility) that was not confirmed in controlled studies in women in the first trimester and there is no evidence of a risk in later trimesters.

C   Either studies in animals have revealed adverse effects on the fetus (teratogenic or embryocidal effects or other) and there are no controlled studies in women, or studies in women and animals are not available. Drugs should be given only if the potential benefits justify the potential risk to the fetus.

D   There is positive evidence of human fetal risk, but the benefits from use in pregnant women may be acceptable despite the risk (eg, if the drug is needed in a life-threatening situation or for a serious disease for which safer drugs cannot be used or are ineffective).

X   Studies in animals or human beings have demonstrated fetal abnormalities or there is evidence of fetal risk based on human experience, or both, and the risk of the use of the drug in pregnant women clearly outweighs any possible benefit. The drug is contraindicated in women who are or may become pregnant.

FDA NAME DIFFERENTIATION PROJECT THE USE OF TALL-MAN LETTERS

Confusion between similar drug names is an important cause of medication errors. For years, The Institute For Safe Medication Practices (ISMP), has urged generic manufacturers to use a combination of large and small letters as well as bolding (ie, chlorpro**MAZINE** and chlorpro**PAMIDE**) to help distinguish drugs with look-alike names, especially when they share similar strengths. Recently the FDA's Division of Generic Drugs began to issue recommendation letters to manufacturers suggesting this novel way to label their products to help reduce this drug name confusion. Although this project has had marginal success, the method has successfully eliminated problems with products such as diphenhydr**AMINE** and dimenhy**DRI-NATE**. Hospitals should also follow suit by making similar changes in their own labels, preprinted order forms, computer screens and printouts, and drug storage location labels.

Lexi-Comp Medical Publishing will use "Tall-Man" letters for the drugs suggested by the FDA or recommended by ISMP.

The following is a list of generic product names and recommended revisions.

Drug Product	Recommended Revision
acetazolamide	aceta**ZOLAMIDE**
acetohexamide	aceto**HEXAMIDE**
alprazolam	**ALPRAZ**olam
amiloride	a**MIL**oride
amlodipine	am**LODIP**ine
azacitidine	aza**CITID**ine
azathioprine	aza**THIO**prine
bupropion	bu**PROP**ion
buspirone	bus**PIR**one
carbamazepine	car**BAM**azepine
carboplatin	**CARBO**platin
cefazolin	ce**FAZ**olin
ceftriaxone	cef**TRIAX**one
chlordiazepoxide	chlordiaze**POXIDE**
chlorpromazine	chlorpro**MAZINE**
chlorpropamide	chlorpro**PAMIDE**
cisplatin	**CIS**platin
clomiphene	clomi**PHENE**
clomipramine	clomi**PRAMINE**
clonazepam	clonaze**PAM**
clonidine	clo**NID**ine
cycloserine	cyclo**SERINE**
cyclosporine	cyclo**SPORINE**
dactinomycin	**DACTIN**omycin
daptomycin	**DAPTO**mycin
daunorubicin	**DAUNO**rubicin
dimenhydrinate	dimenhy**DRINATE**
diphenhydramine	diphenhydr**AMINE**
dobutamine	**DOBUT**amine
dopamine	**DOP**amine

Drug Product	Recommended Revision
doxorubicin	**DOXO**rubicin
duloxetine	**DUL**oxetine
ephedrine	e**PHED**rine
epinephrine	**EPINEPH**rine
fentanyl	fenta**NYL**
fluoxetine	**FLU**oxetine
glipizide	glipi**ZIDE**
glyburide	gly**BURIDE**
guaifenesin	guai**FEN**esin
guanfacine	guan**FACINE**
hydralazine	hydr**ALAZINE**
hydrocodone	**HYDRO**codone
hydromorphone	**HYDRO**morphone
hydroxyzine	hydr**OXY**zine
idarubicin	**IDA**rubicin
infliximab	in**FLIX**imab
lamivudine	lami**VUD**ine
lamotrigine	lamo**TRI**gine
lorazepam	**LOR**azepam
medroxyprogesterone	medroxy**PROGESTER**one
metformin	met**FORMIN**
methylprednisolone	methyl**PREDNIS**olone
methyltestosterone	methyl**TESTOSTER**one
metronidazole	metro**NIDAZOLE**
nicardipine	ni**CAR**dipine
nifedipine	**NIFE**dipine
nimodipine	ni**MOD**ipine
olanzapine	**OLANZ**apine
oxcarbazepine	**OX**carbazepine
oxycodone	oxy**CODONE**
paroxetine	**PAR**oxetine
pentobarbital	**PENT**obarbital
phenobarbital	**PHEN**obarbital
prednisolone	predniso**LONE**
prednisone	predni**SONE**
quetiapine	**QUE**tiapine
quinidine	qui**NID**ine
quinine	qui**NINE**
rituximab	ri**TUX**imab
sitagliptin	sita**GLIP**tin
sufentanil	**SUF**entanil
sulfadiazine	sulf**ADIAZINE**
sulfisoxazole	sulfi**SOXAZOLE**
sumatriptan	**SUMA**triptan
tiagabine	tia**GAB**ine
tizanidine	ti**ZAN**idine
tolazamide	**TOLAZ**amide
tolbutamide	**TOLBUT**amide
tramadol	tra**MAD**ol
trazodone	tra**ZOD**one
valacyclovir	val**ACY**clovir

Drug Product	Recommended Revision
valganciclovir	val**GANCI**clovir
vinblastine	vin**BLAS**tine
vincristine	vin**CRIS**tine

Institute for Safe Medication Practices. "New Tall-Man Lettering Will Reduce Mix-Ups Due to Generic Drug Name Confusion," *ISMP Medication Safety Alert*, September 19, 2001. Available at: http://www.ismp.org.

Institute for Safe Medication Practices. "Prescription Mapping, Can Improve Efficiency While Minimizing Errors With Look-Alike Products," *ISMP Medication Safety Alert*, October 6, 1999. Available at: http://www.ismp.org.

Institute for Safe Medication Practices. "Use of Tall Man Letters Is Gaining Wide Acceptance," *ISMP Medication Safety Alert*, July 31, 2008. Available at: http://www.ismp.org.

U.S. Pharmacopeia, "USP Quality Review: Use Caution-Avoid Confusion," March 2001, No. 76. Available at: http://www.usp.org.

PREVENTING PRESCRIBING ERRORS

Prescribing errors account for the majority of reported medication errors and have prompted healthcare professionals to focus on the development of steps to make the prescribing process safer. Prescription legibility has been attributed to a portion of these errors and legislation has been enacted in several states to address prescription legibility. However, eliminating handwritten prescriptions and ordering medications through the use of technology [eg, computerized prescriber order entry (CPOE)] has been the primary recommendation. Whether a prescription is electronic, typed, or hand-printed, additional safe practices should be considered for implementation to maximize the safety of the prescribing process. Listed below are suggestions for safer prescribing:

- Ensure correct patient by using at least 2 patient identifiers on the prescription (eg, full name, birth date, or address). Review prescription with the patient or patient's caregiver.
- If pediatric patient, document patient's birth date or age and most recent weight. If geriatric patient, document patient's birth date or age.
- Prevent drug name confusion:
    - Use TALLman lettering (eg, buPROPion, busPIRone, predniSONE, prednisoLONE). For more information see: http://www.fda.gov/Drugs/DrugSafety/MedicationErrors/ucm164587.htm
    - Avoid abbreviated drug names (eg, MSO_4, $MgSO_4$, MS, HCT, 6MP, MTX), as they may be misinterpreted and cause error.
    - Avoid investigational names for drugs with FDA approval (eg, FK-506, CBDCA)
    - Avoid chemical names such as 6-mercaptopurine or 6-thioguanine, as sixfold overdoses have been given when these were not recognized as chemical names. The proper names of these drugs are mercaptopurine or thioguanine.
    - Use care when prescribing drugs that look or sound similar (eg, look-alike, sound-alike drugs). Common examples include: Celebrex® vs Celexa®, hydroxyzine vs hydralazine, Zyprexa® vs Zyrtec®.
- Avoid dangerous, error-prone abbreviations (eg, regardless of letter-case: U, IU, QD, QOD, μg, cc, @). Do not use apothecary system or symbols. Additionally, text messaging abbreviations (eg, "2Day") should never be used.
    - For more information see: http://www.ismp.org/Tools/errorproneabbreviations.pdf
- Always use a leading zero for numbers less than 1 (0.5 mg is correct and .5 mg is **incorrect**) and never use a trailing zero for whole numbers (2 mg is correct and 2.0 mg is **incorrect**)
- Always use a space between a number and its units as it is easier to read. There should be no periods after the abbreviations mg or mL (10 mg is correct and 10mg is **incorrect**)
- For doses that are greater than 1,000 dosing units, use properly placed commas to prevent 10-fold errors (100,000 units is correct and 100000 units is **incorrect**)
- Do not prescribe drug dosage by the type of container in which the drug is available (eg, do not prescribe "1 amp", "2 vials", etc).
- Do not write vague or ambiguous orders which have the potential for misinterpretation by other healthcare providers. Examples of vague orders to avoid: "resume pre-op medications," "give drug per protocol," or "continue home medications."
- Review each prescription with patient (or patient's caregiver) including the medication name, indication, and directions for use.

- Take extra precautions when prescribing *high alert drugs* (drugs that can cause significant patient harm when prescribed in error). Common examples of these drugs include: Anticoagulants, chemotherapy, insulins, opiates, and sedatives.

    - For more information see: http://www.ismp.org/Tools/highalert-medications.pdf

  To Err is Human: Building a Safer Health System, Kohn LT, Corrigan JM, and Donaldson MS, eds, Washington, D.C.: National Academy Press, 2000.

A Complete Outpatient Prescription[1]

A complete outpatient prescription can prevent the prescriber, the pharmacist, and/or the patient from making a mistake and can eliminate the need for further clarification. The complete outpatient prescription should contain:

- Patient's full name
- Medication indication
- Allergies
- Prescriber name and telephone or pager number
- For pediatric patients: Their birth date or age and current weight
- For geriatric patients: Their birth date or age
- Drug name, dosage form and strength
- For pediatric patients: Intended daily weight-based dose so that calculations can be checked by the pharmacist (ie, mg/kg/day or units/kg/day)
- Number or amount to be dispensed
- Complete instructions for the patient or caregiver, including the purpose of the medication, directions for use (including dose), dosing frequency, route of administration, duration of therapy, and number of refills.
- Dose should be expressed in convenient units of measure.
- When there are recognized contraindications for a prescribed drug, the prescriber should indicate knowledge of this fact to the pharmacist (ie, when prescribing a potassium salt for a patient receiving an ACE inhibitor, the prescriber should write "K serum leveling being monitored").

Upon dispensing of the final product, the pharmacist should ensure that the patient or caregiver can effectively demonstrate the appropriate administration technique. An appropriate measuring device should be provided or recommended. Household teaspoons and tablespoons should not be used to measure liquid medications due to their variability and inaccuracies in measurement; oral medication syringes are recommended.

For additional information see: http://www.ppag.org/attachments/files/111/Guidelines_Peds.pdf
[1]Levine SR, Cohen MR, Blanchard NR, et al, "Guidelines for Preventing Medication Errors in Pediatrics," *J Pediatr Pharmacol Ther*, 2001, 6:426-42.

ALPHABETICAL LISTING OF DRUGS

Abacavir (a BAK a veer)

U.S. Brand Names Ziagen®
Canadian Brand Names Ziagen®
Index Terms Abacavir Sulfate; ABC
Pharmacologic Category Antiretroviral Agent, Reverse Transcriptase Inhibitor (Nucleoside)
Use Treatment of HIV infections in combination with other antiretroviral agents
Pharmacodynamics/Kinetics
  Absorption: Rapid and extensive absorption
  Distribution: V_d: 0.86 L/kg
  Protein binding: 50%
  Metabolism: Hepatic via alcohol dehydrogenase and glucuronyl transferase to inactive carboxylate and glucuronide metabolites
  Bioavailability: 83%
  Half-life elimination: 1.5 hours
  Time to peak: 0.7-1.7 hours
  Excretion: Primarily urine (as metabolites, 1.2% as unchanged drug); feces (16% total dose)
Dosage Oral:
  Children: 3 months to 16 years: 8 mg/kg body weight twice daily (maximum: 300 mg twice daily) in combination with other antiretroviral agents
  Adults: 300 mg twice daily or 600 mg once daily in combination with other antiretroviral agents
  Dosage adjustment in hepatic impairment:
    Mild dysfunction (Child-Pugh score 5-6): 200 mg twice daily (oral solution is recommended)
    Moderate-to-severe dysfunction: Use is contraindicated by the manufacturer
Additional Information Complete prescribing information for this medication should be consulted for additional detail.
Dosage Forms Excipient information presented when available (limited, particularly for generics); consult specific product labeling.
  Solution, oral:
    Ziagen®: 20 mg/mL (240 mL) [strawberry-banana flavor]
  Tablet:
    Ziagen®: 300 mg
References
  Huang L, Quartin A, Jones D, et al, "Intensive Care of Patients With HIV Infection," *N Engl J Med*, 2006, 355(2):173-81.

◆ **Abacavir Sulfate** *see* Abacavir *on page 22*

◆ **Abbokinase** *see* Urokinase *on page 1438*

◆ **ABC** *see* Abacavir *on page 22*

◆ **ABCD** *see* Amphotericin B Cholesteryl Sulfate Complex *on page 102*

Abciximab (ab SIK si mab)

Related Information
  Regional Anesthesia in Patients Receiving Anticoagulant and Antiplatelet Therapy *on page 1642*
U.S. Brand Names ReoPro®
Canadian Brand Names ReoPro®
Index Terms 7E3; C7E3
Pharmacologic Category Antiplatelet Agent, Glycoprotein IIb/IIIa Inhibitor
Use Prevention of cardiac ischemic complications in patients undergoing percutaneous coronary intervention (PCI); prevention of cardiac ischemic complications in patients with unstable angina not responding to conventional therapy when PCI is scheduled within 24 hours

Note: Intended for use with aspirin and heparin, at a minimum.
Unlabeled/Investigational Use ST-elevation MI: Combination regimen of abciximab (full dose), tenecteplase (half dose), and heparin (unlabeled dose)

Pharmacodynamics/Kinetics Half-life elimination: ~30 minutes

Dosage

Percutaneous coronary intervention (PCI): I.V.: 0.25 mg/kg bolus administered 10-60 minutes prior to start of PCI followed by an infusion of 0.125 mcg/kg/minute (maximum: 10 mcg/minute) for 12 hours

Patients with unstable angina not responding to conventional medical therapy with planned PCI within 24 hours: 0.25 mg/kg bolus followed by an 18- to 24-hour infusion of 10 mcg/minute, concluding 1 hour after PCI.

ST-elevation MI combination regimen (unlabeled): Half-dose tenecteplase (15-25 mg based on weight), abciximab 0.25 mg/kg bolus then 0.125 mcg/kg/minute (maximum: 10 mcg/minute) for 12 hours and heparin dosing as follows: Concurrent bolus of 40 units/kg (maximum: 3000 units), then 7 units/kg/hour (maximum: 800 units/hour) as continuous infusion. Adjust to aPTT target of 50-70 seconds.

Anesthesia and Critical Care Concerns/Other Considerations Clinical Pearls/Comments: Platelet Effects: As an irreversible inhibitor of the platelet glycoprotein IIb/IIIa receptor, abciximab has a long duration of action and platelet effects reverse slowly. It can take 24-48 hours for platelet function to return to normal after discontinuation of infusion making it difficult to use in patients likely to need CABG. Antiplatelet effects can be reversed with platelet transfusions.

Platelet count monitoring is recommended 2-4 hours after initiation, and at 24 hours or prior to discharge, whichever is first. Profound thrombocytopenia occurs shortly after the initiation of abciximab therapy, generally between 2 and 31 hours (Jubelirer, 1999). Specific management guidelines for GP IIb/IIIa induced thrombocytopenia have been published (Berkovitz, 1997; Huxtable, 2006; Llevadot, 2000). Platelet counts should recover rapidly after discontinuation. Platelet transfusion may be necessary. The presence of active bleeding at any time, emergent invasive procedure, or a platelet level of <20,000 cells/microL should prompt the consideration of platelet transfusion.

Additional Information Complete prescribing information for this medication should be consulted for additional detail.

Dosage Forms Excipient information presented when available (limited, particularly for generics); consult specific product labeling.

Injection, solution:

ReoPro®: 2 mg/mL (5 mL)

References

Huxtable LM, Tafreshi MJ, and Rakkar AN, "Frequency and Management of Thrombocytopenia With the Glycoprotein IIb/IIIa Receptor Antagonists," *Am J Cardiol*, 2006, 97(3):426-9.

Jubelirer SJ, Koenig BA, and Bates MC, "Acute Profound Thrombocytopenia Following C7E3 Fab (Abciximab) Therapy: Case Reports, Review of the Literature and Implications for Therapy," *Am J Hematol*, 1999, 61(3):205-8.

Llevadot J, Coulter SA, and Giugliano RP, "A Practical Approach to the Diagnosis and Management of Thrombocytopenia Associated With Glycoprotein IIb/IIIa Receptor Inhibitors," *J Thromb Thrombolysis*, 2000, 9(2):175-80.

Acebutolol (a se BYOO toe lole)

Related Information
Beta-Blockers *on page 1669*
Hypertension *on page 1754*
Preoperative Evaluation of the Cardiac Patient for Noncardiac Surgery *on page 1598*

U.S. Brand Names Sectral®

Canadian Brand Names Apo-Acebutolol®; Gen-Acebutolol; Monitan®; Mylan-Acebutolol; Novo-Acebutolol; Nu-Acebutolol; Rhotral; Rhoxal-acebutolol; Sandoz-Acebutolol; Sectral®

Index Terms Acebutolol Hydrochloride

Pharmacologic Category Antiarrhythmic Agent, Class II; Beta Blocker With Intrinsic Sympathomimetic Activity

Use Treatment of hypertension; management of ventricular arrhythmias

Unlabeled/Investigational Use Treatment of chronic stable angina

Pharmacodynamics/Kinetics
Onset of action: 1-2 hours
Duration: 12-24 hours
Absorption: Oral: 40%
Distribution: V_d: 1.2 L/kg
Protein binding: ~26%
Metabolism: Extensive first-pass effect to equipotent and cardioselective diacetolol metabolite
Bioavailability: Acebutolol: 40%
Half-life elimination: Parent drug: 3-4 hours; Metabolite: 8-13 hours
Time to peak: 2-4 hours
Excretion: Feces (50% to 60%); urine (30% to 40%); diacetolol eliminated primarily in the urine

Dosage Oral:
Adults:
Ventricular arrhythmias: Initial: 400 mg/day in divided doses; maintenance: 600-1200 mg/day in divided doses; maximum: 1200 mg/day
Hypertension: 400-800 mg/day (larger doses may be divided); maximum: 1200 mg/day; usual dose range (JNC 7): 200-800 mg/day in 2 divided doses
Chronic stable angina (unlabeled use): 400 mg/day in divided doses; maintenance: 600-1200 mg/day in divided doses; maximum: 1200 mg/day
Elderly: Initial: 200-400 mg/day; dose reduction due to age-related decrease in Cl_{cr} will be necessary; do not exceed 800 mg/day

Dosing adjustment in renal impairment:
Cl_{cr} 25-49 mL/minute: Reduce dose by 50%.
Cl_{cr} <25 mL/minute: Reduce dose by 75%.

Dosing adjustment in hepatic impairment: Use with caution.

Additional Information Complete prescribing information for this medication should be consulted for additional detail.

Dosage Forms Excipient information presented when available (limited, particularly for generics); consult specific product labeling.
Capsule, as hydrochloride: 200 mg, 400 mg
Sectral®: 200 mg, 400 mg

References

Adams KF, Lindenfeld J, Arnold JMO, et al, "HFSA 2006 Comprehensive Heart Failure Practice Guideline," *J Card Fail*, 2006, 12(1):e1–122. Available at http://www.heartfailureguideline.org

"American Academy of Pediatrics Committee on Drugs. The Transfer of Drugs and Other Chemicals Into Human Milk," *Pediatrics*, 2001, 108(3):776-89.

Anderson JL, Adams CD, Antman EM, et al, "ACC/AHA 2007 Guidelines for the Management of Patients With Unstable Angina/Non ST-Elevation Myocardial Infarction: Executive Summary. A Report of the American College of Cardiology/American Heart Association Task Force on Practice Guidelines (Writing Committee to Revise the 2002 Guidelines for the Management of Patients with Unstable Angina/Non ST-Elevation Myocardial Infarction) Developed in Collaboration With the American College of Emergency Physicians, The Society of Cardiovascular Angiography and Interventions, and the Society of Thoracic Surgeons," *J Am Coll Cardiol*, 2007, 50(7):1-157. Available at http://content.onlinejacc.org/cgi/reprint/50/7/e1.

Antman EM, Anbe DT, Armstrong PW, et al. "ACC/AHA Guidelines for the Management of Patients With ST-Elevation Myocardial Infarction: A Report of the American College of Cardiology/American Heart Association Task Force on Practice Guidelines (Writing Committee to Revise the 1999 Guidelines for the Management of Patients With Acute Myocardial Infarction)," *J Am Coll Cardiol*, 2004, 44(3):671-719. Available at http://www.acc.org/qualityandscience/clinical/guidelines/stemi/Guideline1/index.htm

Boutroy MJ, Bianchetti G, Dubruc C, et al, "To Nurse When Receiving Acebutolol: Is It Dangerous for the Neonate?" *Eur J Clin Pharmacol*, 1986, 30(6):737-9.

Brauchli YB, Jick SS, Curtin F, et al, "Association Between Beta-Blockers, Other Antihypertensive Drugs and Psoriasis: Population-Based Case-Control Study," *Br J Dermatol*, 2008, 158 (6):1299-307.

Chobanian AV, Bakris GL, Black HR, et al, "The Seventh Report of the Joint National Committee on Prevention, Detection, Evaluation, and Treatment of High Blood Pressure: The JNC 7 Report," *JAMA*, 2003, 289(19):2560-71.

Dumez Y, Tchobroutsky C, Hornych H, et al, "Neonatal Effects of Maternal Administration of Acebutolol," *Br Med J (Clin Res Ed)*, 1981, 283(6299):1077-9.

Gibbons RJ, Abrams J, Chatterjee K, et al, "ACC/AHA 2002 Guideline Update for the Management of Patients With Chronic Stable Angina - Summary Article: A Report of the American College of Cardiology/American Heart Association Task Force on Practice Guidelines (Committee on the Management of Patients With Chronic Stable Angina)," *J Am Coll Cardiol*, 2003, 41(1):159-68. Available at http://www.acc.org/qualityandscience/clinical/guidelines/stable/stable_clean.pdf

Gibbons RJ, Chatterjee K, Daley J, et al, "ACC/AHA/ACP-ASIM Guidelines for the Management of Patients With Chronic Stable Angina: A Report of the American College of Cardiology/American Heart Association Task Force on Practice Guidelines," *J Am Coll Cardiol*, 1999, 33(7):2092-197.

Lang DM, "Anaphylactoid and Anaphylactic Reactions. Hazards of Beta-Blockers," *Drug Saf*, 1995, 12(5):299-304.

Mokhlesi B, Leikin JB, Murray P, et al, "Adult Toxicology in Critical Care: Part II: Specific Poisonings," *Chest*, 2003, 123(3):897-922.

Ryan TJ, Anderson JL, Antman EM, et al, "ACC/AHA Guidelines for the Management of Patients With Acute Myocardial Infarction. A Report of the American College of Cardiology/American Heart Association Task Force on Practice Guidelines (Committee on Management of Acute Myocardial Infarction)," *J Am Coll Cardiol*, 1996, 28(5):1328-428.

Schön MP and Boehncke WH, "Psoriasis," *N Eng J Med*, 2005, 352(18):1899-1912.

UK Prospective Diabetes Study Group, "Efficacy of Atenolol and Captopril in Reducing Risk of Macrovascular and Microvascular Complications in Type 2 Diabetes: UKPDS 39," *BMJ*, 1998, 317 (7160):713-20.

Vozeh S, Schmidlin O, and Taeschner W, "Pharmacokinetic Drug Data," *Clin Pharmacokinetics*, 1988, 15(4):254-82.

◆ **Acebutolol Hydrochloride** *see* Acebutolol *on page 24*

◆ **Aceon®** *see* Perindopril Erbumine *on page 1107*

◆ **Acephen™ [OTC]** *see* Acetaminophen *on page 25*

◆ **Acetadote®** *see* Acetylcysteine *on page 35*

Acetaminophen (a seet a MIN oh fen)

Medication Safety Issues

Sound-alike/look-alike issues:

Acephen® may be confused with AcipHex®

FeverALL® may be confused with Fiberall®

Tylenol® may be confused with atenolol, timolol, Tuinal®, Tylenol® PM, Tylox®

International issues:

Paralen® [Czech Republic] may be confused with Aralen® which is a brand name for chloroquine in the U.S.

Duorol® may be confused with Diuril® which is a brand name for chlorothiazide in the U.S.

Duplicate therapy issues: This product contains acetaminophen, which may be a component of combination products. Do not exceed the maximum recommended daily dose of acetaminophen.

Related Information

Acetaminophen and NSAIDS, Dosing in the Management of Pain *on page 1651*

Acute Postoperative Pain *on page 1502*

Anesthesia for Patients With Liver Disease *on page 1537*

Chronic Pain Management *on page 1546*

Porphyria: Safe and Unsafe Drugs *on page 1800*

U.S. Brand Names Acephen™ [OTC]; APAP 500 [OTC]; Apra [OTC] [DSC]; Aspirin Free Anacin® Extra Strength [OTC]; Cetafen® Extra [OTC]; Cetafen® [OTC]; Excedrin® Tension Headache [OTC]; FeverALL® [OTC]; Genapap™ Extra

Strength [OTC]; Genapap™ Infant [OTC] [DSC]; Genapap™ [OTC] [DSC]; Genebs Extra Strength [OTC]; Genebs [OTC] [DSC]; Infantaire [OTC]; Little Fevers™ [OTC]; Mapap Children's [OTC]; Mapap Extra Strength [OTC]; Mapap Infants [OTC]; Mapap Jr. Strength [OTC]; Mapap [OTC]; Nortemp Children's [OTC]; Pain Eze [OTC]; Silapap Children's [OTC]; Silapap Infant's [OTC]; Tycolene Maximum Strength [OTC]; Tycolene [OTC] [DSC]; Tylenol® 8 Hour [OTC]; Tylenol® Arthritis Pain Extended Relief [OTC]; Tylenol® Children's Meltaways [OTC]; Tylenol® Children's [OTC]; Tylenol® Extra Strength [OTC]; Tylenol® Infant's Concentrated [OTC]; Tylenol® Jr. Meltaways [OTC]; Tylenol® [OTC]; Valorin Extra [OTC]; Valorin [OTC]

Canadian Brand Names Abenol®; Apo-Acetaminophen®; Atasol®; Novo-Gesic; Pediatrix; Tempra®; Tylenol®

Index Terms APAP; N-Acetyl-P-Aminophenol; Paracetamol

Pharmacologic Category Analgesic, Miscellaneous

Generic Available Yes: Excludes extended release products

Use Treatment of mild-to-moderate pain and fever (analgesic/antipyretic); does not have antirheumatic or anti-inflammatory effects

Mechanism of Action Inhibits the synthesis of prostaglandins in the central nervous system and peripherally blocks pain impulse generation; produces antipyresis from inhibition of hypothalamic heat-regulating center

Pharmacodynamics/Kinetics

Onset of action: <1 hour

Duration: 4-6 hours

Absorption: Incomplete; varies by dosage form

Protein binding: 8% to 43% at toxic doses

Metabolism: At normal therapeutic dosages, hepatic to sulfate and glucuronide metabolites, while a small amount is metabolized by CYP to a highly reactive intermediate (acetylimidoquinone) which is conjugated with glutathione and inactivated; at toxic doses (as little as 4 g daily) glutathione conjugation becomes insufficient to meet the metabolic demand causing an increase in acetylimido-quinone concentration, which may cause hepatic cell necrosis

Half-life elimination: Prolonged following toxic doses

Neonates: 2-5 hours

Adults: 1-3 hours (may be increased in elderly; however, this should not affect dosing)

Time to peak, serum: Oral: 10-60 minutes; may be delayed in acute overdoses

Excretion: Urine (2% to 5% unchanged; 55% as glucuronide metabolites; 30% as sulphate metabolites)

Dosage Oral, rectal:

Children <12 years: 10-15 mg/kg/dose every 4-6 hours as needed; do **not** exceed 5 doses (2.6 g) in 24 hours; alternatively, the following age-based doses may be used; see table.

Acetaminophen Dosing

Age	Dosage (mg)	Age	Dosage (mg)
0-3 mo	40	4-5 y	240
4-11 mo	80	6-8 y	320
1-2 y	120	9-10 y	400
2-3 y	160	11 y	480

Note: Higher rectal doses have been studied for use in preoperative pain control in children. However, specific guidelines are not available and dosing may be product dependent. The safety and efficacy of alternating acetaminophen and ibuprofen dosing has not been established.

Adults: 325-650 mg every 4-6 hours or 1000 mg 3-4 times/day; do **not** exceed 4 g/day

Dosing interval in renal impairment:

Cl_{cr} 10-50 mL/minute: Administer every 6 hours

Cl_{cr} <10 mL/minute: Administer every 8 hours (metabolites accumulate)

Hemodialysis: Moderately dialyzable (20% to 50%)

Dosing adjustment/comments in hepatic impairment: Use with caution. Limited, low-dose therapy is usually well tolerated in hepatic disease/cirrhosis. However, cases of hepatotoxicity at daily acetaminophen dosages <4 g/day have been reported. Avoid chronic use in hepatic impairment.

Stability Do not freeze suppositories.

Administration Suspension, oral: Shake well before pouring a dose.

Monitoring Parameters Relief of pain or fever

Reference Range

Therapeutic concentration (analgesic/antipyretic): 10-30 mcg/mL

Toxic concentration (acute ingestion) with probable hepatotoxicity: >200 mcg/mL at 4 hours or 50 mcg/mL at 12 hours after ingestion

Anesthesia and Critical Care Concerns/Other Considerations

Evidence-Based Information: The 2002 ACCM/SCCM guidelines for analgesia (critically-ill adult) recommend prescribing <2 g/day for patients with a significant alcohol history or those with malnutrition. All other patients should be limited to ≤4 g/day when used for acute pain or fever (American Pain Society, 2008). If possible, long-term administration of acetaminophen should not exceed 3000 mg/day, based on evidence demonstrating an increased risk of hepatotoxicity compared to patients not receiving acetaminophen (Watkins, 2006). Susceptibility to acetaminophen hepatotoxicity may be due to induction of hepatic enzymes caused by chronic alcohol ingestion and/or concurrent use of cytochrome P450 1A2/2E1 inducers (eg, isoniazid), and impaired glucuronidation caused by fasting (American Pain Society, 2008; Brackett, 2000; Zenger, 2004).

Pregnancy Risk Factor B

Contraindications Hypersensitivity to acetaminophen or any component of the formulation

Warnings/Precautions Limit dose to <4 g/day. May cause severe hepatic toxicity on acute overdose; in addition, chronic daily dosing in adults has resulted in liver damage in some patients. Use with caution in patients with alcoholic liver disease; consuming ≥3 alcoholic drinks/day may increase the risk of liver damage. Use caution in patients with known G6PD deficiency.

OTC labeling: When used for self-medication, patients should be instructed to contact healthcare provider if used for fever lasting >3 days or for pain lasting >10 days in adults or >5 days in children.

Adverse Reactions Frequency not defined.

Dermatologic: Rash

Endocrine & metabolic: May increase chloride, uric acid, glucose; may decrease sodium, bicarbonate, calcium

Hematologic: Anemia, blood dyscrasias (neutropenia, pancytopenia, leukopenia)

Hepatic: Bilirubin increased, alkaline phosphatase increased

Renal: Ammonia increased, nephrotoxicity with chronic overdose, analgesic nephropathy

Miscellaneous: Hypersensitivity reactions (rare)

Drug Interactions

Metabolism/Transport Effects Substrate (minor) of CYP1A2, 2A6, 2C9, 2D6, 2E1, 3A4; **Inhibits** CYP3A4 (weak)

Avoid Concomitant Use There are no known interactions where it is recommended to avoid concomitant use.

Increased Effect/Toxicity

Acetaminophen may increase the levels/effects of: Vitamin K Antagonists

The levels/effects of Acetaminophen may be increased by: Imatinib; Isoniazid

Decreased Effect

The levels/effects of Acetaminophen may be decreased by: Anticonvulsants (Hydantoin); Barbiturates; CarBAMazepine; Cholestyramine Resin; Peginterferon Alfa-2b

Ethanol/Nutrition/Herb Interactions

Ethanol: Excessive intake of ethanol may increase the risk of acetaminophen-induced hepatotoxicity. Avoid ethanol or limit to <3 drinks/day.

Food: Rate of absorption may be decreased when given with food.

Herb/Nutraceutical: St John's wort may decrease acetaminophen levels.

Test Interactions Increased chloride, bilirubin, uric acid, glucose, ammonia (B), chloride (S), uric acid (S), alkaline phosphatase (S), chloride (S); decreased sodium, bicarbonate, calcium (S)

Dietary Considerations Chewable tablets may contain phenylalanine (amount varies, ranges between 3-12 mg/tablet); consult individual product labeling.

Dosage Forms Excipient information presented when available (limited, particularly for generics); consult specific product labeling. [DSC] = Discontinued product

Caplet, oral: 500 mg
　Cetafen® Extra: 500 mg
　Genapap™ Extra Strength: 500 mg [DSC]
　Genebs Extra Strength: 500 mg
　Mapap Extra Strength: 500 mg
　Pain Eze: 650 mg
　Tycolene Maximum Strength: 500 mg [DSC]
　Tylenol®: 325 mg
　Tylenol® Extra Strength: 500 mg
Caplet, extended release, oral:
　Tylenol® 8 Hour: 650 mg
　Tylenol® Arthritis Pain Extended Relief: 650 mg
Captab, oral: 500 mg
Elixir, oral:
　Apra: 160 mg/5 mL (118 mL) [ethanol free; contains benzoic acid, propylene glycol, sodium benzoate, sucrose; grape flavor] [DSC]
　Apra: 160 mg/5 mL (118 mL, 473 mL, 3785 mL) [ethanol free; contains propylene glycol, sodium benzoate, sucrose; cherry flavor] [DSC]
　Mapap Children's: 160 mg/5 mL (118 mL, 480 mL) [ethanol free; contains benzoic acid, propylene glycol, sodium benzoate; cherry flavor]
Gelcap, oral:
　Tylenol® Extra Strength: 500 mg [contains benzyl alcohol]
Geltab, oral:
　Excedrin® Tension Headache: 500 mg [contains caffeine 65 mg/geltab]
　Tylenol® Extra Strength: 500 mg [contains benzyl alcohol]
Liquid, oral:
　APAP 500: 500 mg/5 mL (237 mL) [ethanol free, sugar free; cherry flavor]
　Silapap Children's: 160 mg/5 mL (118 mL, 237 mL, 473 mL) [ethanol free, sugar free; contains propylene glycol, sodium benzoate; cherry flavor]
　Tylenol® Extra Strength: 500 mg/15 mL (240 mL) [ethanol free; contains propylene glycol, sodium benzoate; cherry flavor]
Solution, oral: 160 mg/5 mL (5 mL, 10 mL, 20 mL, 118 mL, 473 mL)
Solution, oral [drops]: 80 mg/0.8 mL (15 mL)
　Genapap™ Infant: 80 mg/0.8 mL (15 mL) [ethanol free; contains propylene glycol; fruit flavor] [DSC]
　Infantaire: 80 mg/0.8mL (15 mL, 30 mL)
　Little Fevers™: 80 mg/1 mL (30 mL) [dye free, ethanol free, gluten free; contains propylene glycol, sodium benzoate; berry flavor]
　Silapap Infant's: 80 mg/0.8 mL (15 mL, 30 mL) [ethanol free; contains propylene glycol, sodium benzoate; cherry flavor]
Suppository, rectal: 120 mg (12s, 50s, 100s); 325 mg (12s); 650 mg (12s, 50s, 100s)
　Acephen™: 120 mg (6s [DSC], 12s, 50s, 100s); 325 mg (6s, 12s, 50s, 100s); 650 mg (12s, 50s, 100s, 500s)
　FeverALL®: 120 mg (6s, 12s, 50s); 325 mg (6s, 12s, 50s); 650 mg (12s, 50s, 500s); 80 mg (6s, 50s)
　Mapap: 125 mg (12s)
Suspension, oral: 160 mg/5 mL (5 mL, 10 mL, 20 mL)
　Mapap Children's: 160 mg/5 mL (118 mL) [ethanol free; contains propylene glycol, sodium benzoate; cherry flavor]
　Nortemp Children's: 160 mg/5 mL (118 mL) [ethanol free; contains propylene glycol, sodium benzoate; cotton candy flavor]
　Tylenol® Children's Suspension: 160 mg/5 mL (120 mL) [ethanol free; contains propylene glycol, sodium benzoate; bubblegum, strawberry, grape flavors]
　Tylenol® Children's Suspension: 160 mg/5 mL (60 mL, 120 mL, 240 mL [DSC]) [ethanol free; contains propylene glycol, sodium benzoate; cherry flavor]

Tylenol® Children's Suspension: 160 mg/5 mL (120 mL) [dye free; ethanol free; contains propylene glycol, sodium benzoate; cherry flavor]

Suspension, oral [drops]:

Mapap Infant's: 80 mg/0.8 mL (15 mL, 30 mL) [ethanol free; contains propylene glycol, sodium benzoate; cherry flavor]

Tylenol® Infant's Concentrated: 80 mg/0.8 mL (15 mL, 30 mL) [ethanol free; contains sodium benzoate; cherry, grape flavors]

Tylenol® Infant's Concentrated: 80 mg/0.8 mL (30 mL) [dye free; ethanol free; contains propylene glycol; cherry flavor]

Tablet, oral: 325 mg, 500 mg

Aspirin Free Anacin® Extra Strength: 500 mg

Cetafen®: 325 mg

Genapap™: 325 mg [DSC]

Genapap™ Extra Strength: 500 mg

Genebs: 325 mg [DSC]

Genebs Extra Strength: 500 mg

Mapap: 325 mg

Tycolene: 325 mg [DSC]

Tylenol®: 325 mg

Valorin Extra®: 500 mg [sugar free]

Valorin®: 325 mg [sugar free]

Tablet, chewable, oral: 80 mg

Mapap Children's: 80 mg [bubblegum flavor] [DSC]

Mapap Children's: 80 mg [fruit flavor]

Mapap Children's: 80 mg [contains phenylalanine 3 mg/tablet; grape flavor] [DSC]

Mapap Junior Strength: 160 mg [contains phenylalanine 12 mg/tablet; grape flavor]

Tablet, orally disintegrating, oral: 80 mg, 160 mg, 325 mg, 500 mg

Tylenol® Children's Meltaways: 80 mg [bubblegum, grape flavors]

Tylenol® Jr. Meltaways: 160 mg [bubblegum, grape flavors]

References

"American Academy of Pediatrics Committee on Drugs. Acetaminophen Toxicity in Children," *Pediatrics*, 2001, 108(4):1020-4.

Brackett CC and Bloch JD, "Phenytoin as a Possible Cause of Acetaminophen Hepatotoxicity: Case Report and Review of the Literature," *Pharmacotherapy*, 2000, 20(2):229-33.

Bradley JD, Brandt KD, Katz BP, et al, "Comparison of an Antiinflammatory Dose of Ibuprofen, an Analgesic Dose of Ibuprofen, and Acetaminophen in the Treatment of Patients With Osteoarthritis of the Knee," *N Engl J Med*, 1991, 325(2):87-91.

Dionne RA, Campbell RA, Cooper SA, et al, "Suppression of Postoperative Pain by Preoperative Administration of Ibuprofen in Comparison to Placebo, Acetaminophen, and Acetaminophen Plus Codeine," *J Clin Pharmacol*, 1983, 23(1):37-43.

Jacobi J, Fraser GL, Coursin DB, et al, "Clinical Practice Guidelines for the Sustained Use of Sedatives and Analgesics in the Critically Ill Adult," *Crit Care Med*, 2002, 30(1):119-41. Available at: http://www.sccm.org/pdf/sedatives.pdf. Accessed August 2, 2003.

Mokhlesi B, Leikin JB, Murray P, et al, "Adult Toxicology in Critical Care: Part II: Specific Poisonings," *Chest*, 2003, 123(3):897-922.

"Principles of Analgesic Use in the Treatment of Acute Pain and Cancer Pain," 6th ed, Glenview, IL: American Pain Society, 2008.

Watkins PB, Kaplowitz N, Slattery JT, et al, "Aminotransferase Elevations in Healthy Adults Receiving 4 Grams of Acetaminophen Daily: A Randomized Controlled Trial," *JAMA*, 2006, 296(1):87-93.

Williams HJ, Ward JR, Egger MJ, et al, "Comparison of Naproxen and Acetaminophen in a Two-Year Study of Treatment of Osteoarthritis of the Knee," *Arthritis Rheum*, 1993, 36(9):1196-206.

Zenger F, Russmann S, Junker E, et al, "Decreased Glutathione in Patients With Anorexia Nervosa. Risk Factor for Toxic Liver Injury?" *Eur J Clin Nutr*, 2004, 58(2):238-43.

Acetaminophen and Codeine (a seet a MIN oh fen & KOE deen)

U.S. Brand Names Capital® and Codeine; Tylenol® with Codeine No. 3; Tylenol® with Codeine No. 4

Canadian Brand Names ratio-Emtec; ratio-Lenoltec; Triatec-30; Triatec-8; Triatec-8 Strong; Tylenol Elixir with Codeine; Tylenol No. 1; Tylenol No. 1 Forte; Tylenol No. 2 with Codeine; Tylenol No. 3 with Codeine; Tylenol No. 4 with Codeine

Index Terms Codeine and Acetaminophen; Tylenol #3

Pharmacologic Category Analgesic, Opioid

◀ **Restrictions** C-III; C-V

Note: In countries outside of the U.S., some formulations of Tylenol® with Codeine (eg, Tylenol® No. 3) include caffeine.

Use Relief of mild-to-moderate pain

Pharmacodynamics/Kinetics See individual agents.

Dosage Doses should be adjusted according to severity of pain and response of the patient. Adult doses ≥60 mg codeine fail to give commensurate relief of pain but merely prolong analgesia and are associated with an appreciably increased incidence of side effects. Oral:

Children: Analgesic:
Codeine: 0.5-1 mg codeine/kg/dose every 4-6 hours
Acetaminophen: 10-15 mg/kg/dose every 4 hours up to a maximum of 2.6 g/24 hours for children <12 years; **alternatively, the following can be used:**
3-6 years: 5 mL 3-4 times/day as needed of elixir
7-12 years: 10 mL 3-4 times/day as needed of elixir
>12 years: 15 mL every 4 hours as needed of elixir

Adults:
Antitussive: Based on codeine (15-30 mg/dose) every 4-6 hours (maximum: 360 mg/24 hours based on codeine component)
Analgesic: Based on codeine (30-60 mg/dose) every 4-6 hours (maximum: 4000 mg/24 hours based on acetaminophen component)
1-2 tablets every 4 hours to a maximum of 12 tablets/24 hours

Dosing adjustment in renal impairment: See individual agents.

Dosing adjustment in hepatic impairment: Use with caution. Limited, low-dose therapy is usually well tolerated in hepatic disease/cirrhosis; however, cases of hepatotoxicity at daily acetaminophen dosages <4 g/day have been reported. Avoid chronic use in hepatic impairment.

Additional Information Complete prescribing information for this medication should be consulted for additional detail.

Dosage Forms Excipient information presented when available (limited, particularly for generics); consult specific product labeling. [DSC] = Discontinued product; [CAN] = Canadian brand name

Caplet:
ratio-Lenoltec No. 1 [CAN], Tylenol No. 1 [CAN]: Acetaminophen 300 mg, codeine phosphate 8 mg, and caffeine 15 mg [not available in the U.S.]
Tylenol No. 1 Forte [CAN]: Acetaminophen 500 mg, codeine phosphate 8 mg, and caffeine 15 mg [not available in the U.S.]

Solution, oral [C-V]: Acetaminophen 120 mg and codeine phosphate 12 mg per 5 mL (5 mL, 10 mL, 12.5 mL, 15 mL, 120 mL, 480 mL) [contains alcohol 7%]
Tylenol Elixir with Codeine [CAN]: Acetaminophen 160 mg and codeine phosphate 8 mg per 5 mL (500 mL) [contains alcohol 7%, sucrose 31%; cherry flavor; not available in the U.S.]

Suspension, oral [C-V] (Capital® and Codeine): Acetaminophen 120 mg and codeine phosphate 12 mg per 5 mL (480 mL) [alcohol free; contains propylene glycol, sodium benzoate; fruit punch flavor]

Tablet [C-III]: Acetaminophen 300 mg and codeine phosphate 15 mg; acetaminophen 300 mg and codeine phosphate 30 mg; acetaminophen 300 mg and codeine phosphate 60 mg
ratio-Emtec [CAN], Triatec-30 [CAN]: Acetaminophen 300 mg and codeine phosphate 30 mg [not available in the U.S.]
ratio-Lenoltec No. 1 [CAN]: Acetaminophen 300 mg, codeine phosphate 8 mg, and caffeine 15 mg [not available in the U.S.]
ratio-Lenoltec No. 2 [CAN], Tylenol No. 2 with Codeine [CAN]: Acetaminophen 300 mg, codeine phosphate 15 mg, and caffeine 15 mg [not available in the U.S.]
ratio-Lenoltec No. 3 [CAN], Tylenol No. 3 with Codeine [CAN]: Acetaminophen 300 mg, codeine phosphate 30 mg, and caffeine 15 mg [not available in the U.S.]
ratio-Lenoltec No. 4 [CAN], Tylenol No. 4 with Codeine [CAN]: Acetaminophen 300 mg and codeine phosphate 60 mg [not available in the U.S.]
Triatec-8 [CAN]: Acetaminophen 325 mg, codeine phosphate 8 mg, and caffeine 30 mg [not available in the U.S.]

Triatec-8 Strong [CAN]: Acetaminophen 500 mg, codeine phosphate 8 mg, and caffeine 30 mg [not available in the U.S.]

Tylenol® with Codeine No. 3: Acetaminophen 300 mg and codeine phosphate 30 mg [contains sodium metabisulfite]

Tylenol® with Codeine No. 4: Acetaminophen 300 mg and codeine phosphate 60 mg [contains sodium metabisulfite]

♦ **Acetaminophen and Hydrocodone** *see* Hydrocodone and Acetaminophen *on page 697*

♦ **Acetaminophen and Oxycodone** *see* Oxycodone and Acetaminophen *on page 1072*

♦ **Acetaminophen and Propoxyphene** *see* Propoxyphene and Acetaminophen *on page 1197*

AcetaZOLAMIDE (a set a ZOLE a mide)

Medication Safety Issues
Sound-alike/look-alike issues:
AcetaZOLAMIDE may be confused with acetoHEXAMIDE
Diamox® Sequels® may be confused with Diabinese®, Dobutrex®, Trimox®
Related Information
Anesthesia Considerations for Neurosurgery *on page 1514*
U.S. Brand Names Diamox® Sequels®
Canadian Brand Names Apo-Acetazolamide®; Diamox®
Pharmacologic Category Anticonvulsant, Miscellaneous; Carbonic Anhydrase Inhibitor; Diuretic, Carbonic Anhydrase Inhibitor; Ophthalmic Agent, Antiglaucoma
Generic Available Yes
Use Treatment of glaucoma (chronic simple open-angle, secondary glaucoma, preoperatively in acute angle-closure); drug-induced edema or edema due to congestive heart failure (adjunctive therapy); centrencephalic epilepsies (immediate release dosage form); prevention or amelioration of symptoms associated with acute mountain sickness
Unlabeled/Investigational Use Metabolic alkalosis; respiratory stimulant in COPD; urine alkalinization
Mechanism of Action Reversible inhibition of the enzyme carbonic anhydrase resulting in reduction of hydrogen ion secretion at renal tubule and an increased renal excretion of sodium, potassium, bicarbonate, and water to decrease production of aqueous humor; also inhibits carbonic anhydrase in central nervous system to retard abnormal and excessive discharge from CNS neurons
Pharmacodynamics/Kinetics
Onset of action: Capsule, extended release: 2 hours; I.V.: 2 minutes
Peak effect: Capsule, extended release: 8-12 hours; I.V.: 15 minutes; Tablet: 2-4 hours
Duration: Inhibition of aqueous humor secretion: Capsule, extended release: 18-24 hours; I.V.: 4-5 hours; Tablet: 8-12 hours
Distribution: Erythrocytes, kidneys; blood-brain barrier and placenta; distributes into milk (~30% of plasma concentrations)
Excretion: Urine (70% to 100% as unchanged drug)
Dosage Note: I.M. administration is not recommended because of pain secondary to the alkaline pH

Children:
Glaucoma:
Oral: 8-30 mg/kg/day or 300-900 mg/m^2/day divided every 8 hours
I.V.: 20-40 mg/kg/24 hours divided every 6 hours, not to exceed 1 g/day
Edema: Oral, I.V.: 5 mg/kg or 150 mg/m^2 once every day
Epilepsy: Oral: 8-30 mg/kg/day in 1-4 divided doses, not to exceed 1 g/day; extended release capsule is not recommended for treatment of epilepsy
Adults:
Glaucoma:
Chronic simple (open-angle): Oral: 250 mg 1-4 times/day or 500 mg extended release capsule twice daily

Secondary, acute (closed-angle): I.V.: 250-500 mg, may repeat in 2-4 hours to a maximum of 1 g/day

Edema: Oral, I.V.: 250-375 mg once daily

Epilepsy: Oral: 8-30 mg/kg/day in 1-4 divided doses; not to exceed 1 g/day; **extended release capsule is not recommended for treatment of epilepsy**

Metabolic alkalosis (unlabeled use): I.V. 250 mg every 6 hours for 4 doses or 500 mg single dose; reassess need based upon acid-base status

Mountain sickness: Oral: 250 mg every 8-12 hours (or 500 mg extended release capsules every 12-24 hours)

Therapy should begin 24-48 hours before and continue during ascent and for at least 48 hours after arrival at the high altitude

Note: In situations of rapid ascent (such as rescue or military operations), 1000 mg/day is recommended.

Urine alkalinization (unlabeled use): Oral: 5 mg/kg/dose repeated 2-3 times over 24 hours

Respiratory stimulant in COPD (unlabeled use): Oral, I.V.: 250 mg twice daily

Elderly: Oral: Initial: 250 mg twice daily; use lowest effective dose

Dosing adjustment in renal impairment:

Cl_{cr} 10-50 mL/minute: Administer every 12 hours

Cl_{cr} <10 mL/minute: Avoid use (ineffective)

Hemodialysis: Moderately dialyzable (20% to 50%)

Peritoneal dialysis: Supplemental dose is not necessary

Stability

Capsules, tablets: Store at controlled room temperature.

Injection: Store vial for injection (prior to reconstitution) at controlled room temperature. Reconstitute with at least 5 mL sterile water to provide a solution containing not more than 100 mg/mL. Reconstituted solution may be refrigerated (2°C to 8°C) for 1 week, however, use within 12 hours is recommended. Further dilute in D_5W or NS for I.V. infusion. Stability of IVPB solution is 5 days at room temperature (25°C) and 44 days at refrigeration (5°C).

Administration

Oral: May be administered with food. May cause an alteration in taste, especially carbonated beverages. Short-acting tablets may be crushed and suspended in cherry or chocolate syrup to disguise the bitter taste of the drug; do not use fruit juices. Alternatively, submerge tablet in 10 mL of hot water and add 10 mL honey or syrup.

I.M.: I.M. administration is painful because of the alkaline pH of the drug; use by this route is not recommended.

I.V.: No specific guidance given by manufacturer, but I.V. push at a rate of up to 500 mg over 3 minutes has been reported in a clinical trial (Mazur, 1999); a study to assess cerebrovascular reserve has used rapid I.V. push of up to 1 g over ≤1 minute (Piepgras, 1990)

Monitoring Parameters Intraocular pressure, potassium, serum bicarbonate; serum electrolytes, periodic CBC with differential; monitor growth in pediatric patients

Pregnancy Risk Factor C

Contraindications Hypersensitivity to acetazolamide, sulfonamides, or any component of the formulation; hepatic disease or insufficiency; decreased sodium and/or potassium levels; adrenocortical insufficiency; cirrhosis; hyperchloremic acidosis; severe renal disease or dysfunction; severe pulmonary obstruction; long-term use in noncongestive angle-closure glaucoma

Warnings/Precautions Use with caution in patients with hepatic dysfunction; in cirrhosis, avoid electrolyte and acid/base imbalances that might lead to hepatic encephalopathy. Use with caution in patients with respiratory acidosis and diabetes mellitus (may change glucose control). Use with caution in the elderly; may be more sensitive to side effects. Impairment of mental alertness and/or physical coordination may occur. Chemical similarities are present among sulfonamides, sulfonylureas, carbonic anhydrase inhibitors, thiazides, and loop diuretics (except ethacrynic acid). Use in patients with sulfonamide allergy is specifically contraindicated in product labeling, however, a risk of cross-reaction exists in patients with allergy to any of these compounds; avoid use when previous reaction has been severe. Discontinue if signs of hypersensitivity are noted.

I.M. administration is painful because of the alkaline pH of the drug; use by this route is not recommended.

Adverse Reactions Frequency not defined.

Cardiovascular: Flushing

Central nervous system: Ataxia, confusion, convulsions, depression, dizziness, drowsiness, excitement, fatigue, fever, headache, malaise

Dermatologic: Allergic skin reactions, photosensitivity, Stevens-Johnson syndrome, toxic epidermal necrolysis, urticaria

Endocrine & metabolic: Electrolyte imbalance, growth retardation (children), hyperglycemia, hypoglycemia, hypokalemia, hyponatremia, metabolic acidosis

Gastrointestinal: Appetite decreased, diarrhea, melena, nausea, taste alteration, vomiting

Genitourinary: Crystalluria, glycosuria, hematuria, polyuria, renal failure

Hematologic: Agranulocytosis, aplastic anemia, leukopenia, thrombocytopenia, thrombocytopenic purpura

Hepatic: Cholestatic jaundice, fulminant hepatic necrosis, hepatic insufficiency, liver function tests abnormal

Local: Pain at injection site

Neuromuscular & skeletal: Flaccid paralysis, paresthesia

Ocular: Myopia

Otic: Hearing disturbance, tinnitus

Miscellaneous: Anaphylaxis

Drug Interactions

Metabolism/Transport Effects Inhibits CYP3A4 (weak)

Avoid Concomitant Use There are no known interactions where it is recommended to avoid concomitant use.

Increased Effect/Toxicity

AcetaZOLAMIDE may increase the levels/effects of: Alcohol (Ethyl); Alpha-/Beta-Agonists; Amifostine; Amphetamines; Anticonvulsants (Barbiturate); Anticonvulsants (Hydantoin); Antihypertensives; CarBAMazepine; CNS Depressants; Flecainide; Hypotensive Agents; Memantine; Methotrimeprazine; Primidone; QuiNIDine; RiTUXimab

The levels/effects of AcetaZOLAMIDE may be increased by: Diazoxide; Herbs (Hypotensive Properties); MAO Inhibitors; Methotrimeprazine; Pentoxifylline; Phosphodiesterase 5 Inhibitors; Prostacyclin Analogues; Salicylates

Decreased Effect

AcetaZOLAMIDE may decrease the levels/effects of: Methenamine; Primidone; Trientine

The levels/effects of AcetaZOLAMIDE may be decreased by: Herbs (Hypertensive Properties); Ketorolac; Mefloquine; Methylphenidate; Yohimbine

Test Interactions May cause false-positive results for urinary protein with Albustix®, Labstix®, Albutest®, Bumintest®; interferes with HPLC theophylline assay and serum uric acid levels

Dietary Considerations May be taken with food to decrease GI upset. May have additive effects with other folic acid antagonists. Sodium content of 500 mg injection: 47.2 mg (2.05 mEq).

Dosage Forms Excipient information presented when available (limited, particularly for generics); consult specific product labeling.

Capsule, extended release: 500 mg

Diamox® Sequels®: 500 mg

Injection, powder for reconstitution: 500 mg

Tablet: 125 mg, 250 mg

References

Marik PE, Kussman BD, Lipman J, et al, "Acetazolamide in the Treatment of Metabolic Alkalosis in Critically Ill Patients," *Heart Lung*, 1991, 20(5 Pt 1):455-9.

Mazur JE, Devlin JW, Peters MJ, et al, "Single Versus Multiple Doses of Acetazolamide for Metabolic Alkalosis in Critically Ill Medical Patients: A Randomized, Double-Blind Trial," *Crit Care Med*, 1999, 27(7):1257-61.

Acetylcholine (a se teel KOE leen)

Medication Safety Issues
Sound-alike/look-alike issues:
Acetylcholine may be confused with acetylcysteine
Related Information
Anesthesia for Geriatric Patients *on page 1523*
Management of Postoperative Arrhythmias *on page 1571*
U.S. Brand Names Miochol®-E
Canadian Brand Names Miochol®-E
Index Terms Acetylcholine Chloride
Pharmacologic Category Cholinergic Agonist; Ophthalmic Agent, Miotic
Generic Available No
Use Produces complete miosis in cataract surgery, keratoplasty, iridectomy, and other anterior segment surgery where rapid miosis is required
Mechanism of Action Causes contraction of the sphincter muscles of the iris, resulting in miosis and contraction of the ciliary muscle, leading to accommodation spasm
Pharmacodynamics/Kinetics
Onset of action: Rapid
Duration: ~10 minutes
Dosage Adults: Intraocular: 0.5-2 mL of 1% injection (5-20 mg) instilled into anterior chamber before or after securing one or more sutures
Stability Store unopened vial at 4°C to 25°C (39°F to 77°F); prevent from freezing. Prepare solution immediately before use and discard unused portion. Acetylcholine solutions are unstable; reconstitute immediately before use.
Administration Open under aseptic conditions only. Attach filter before irrigating eye.
Anesthesia and Critical Care Concerns/Other Considerations
Clinical Pearls/Comments: Systemic effects are rare after intraocular administration, but can occur. Caution should be used in patients with cardiovascular disease.
Pregnancy Risk Factor C
Contraindications Hypersensitivity to acetylcholine chloride or any component of the formulation; acute iritis and acute inflammatory disease of the anterior chamber
Warnings/Precautions During cataract surgery, use only after lens is in place. Systemic effects rarely occur but can cause problems for patients with acute cardiac failure, bronchial asthma, peptic ulcer, hyperthyroidism, GI spasm, urinary tract obstruction, and Parkinson's disease; open under aseptic conditions only. Safety and efficacy have not been established in children.
Adverse Reactions Frequency not defined.
Cardiovascular: Bradycardia, flushing, hypotension
Central nervous system: Headache
Ocular: Clouding, corneal edema, decompensation
Respiratory: Dyspnea
Miscellaneous: Diaphoresis
Drug Interactions
Avoid Concomitant Use There are no known interactions where it is recommended to avoid concomitant use.
Increased Effect/Toxicity
The levels/effects of Acetylcholine may be increased by: Acetylcholinesterase Inhibitors
Decreased Effect There are no known significant interactions involving a decrease in effect.
Dosage Forms Excipient information presented when available (limited, particularly for generics); consult specific product labeling.
Powder for solution, intraocular, as chloride:
Miochol®-E: 1:100 [20 mg; packaged with diluent (2 mL)]

◆ **Acetylcholine Chloride** *see* Acetylcholine *on page 34*

Acetylcysteine (a se teel SIS teen)

Medication Safety Issues
Sound-alike/look-alike issues:
Acetylcysteine may be confused with acetylcholine
Mucomyst® may be confused with Mucinex®

Related Information
Contrast Media Reactions, Premedication for Prophylaxis *on page 1735*

U.S. Brand Names Acetadote®

Canadian Brand Names Acetylcysteine Solution; Mucomyst®; Parvolex®

Index Terms *N*-Acetyl-L-cysteine; *N*-Acetylcysteine; Acetylcysteine Sodium; Mercapturic Acid; Mucomyst; NAC

Pharmacologic Category Antidote; Mucolytic Agent

Generic Available Yes: Solution for inhalation

Use Antidote for acute acetaminophen (APAP) poisoning; repeated supratherapeutic ingestion (RSTI) of APAP; adjunctive mucolytic therapy in patients with abnormal or viscid mucous secretions in acute and chronic bronchopulmonary diseases; pulmonary complications of surgery and cystic fibrosis; diagnostic bronchial studies

Unlabeled/Investigational Use Prevention of contrast-induced renal dysfunction (oral, I.V.); distal intestinal obstruction syndrome (DIOS, previously referred to as meconium ileus equivalent)

Mechanism of Action Exerts mucolytic action through its free sulfhydryl group which opens up the disulfide bonds in the mucoproteins thus lowering mucous viscosity.

In patients with APAP toxicity, acetylcysteine acts as a hepatoprotective agent by restoring hepatic glutathione, serving as a glutathione substitute, and enhancing the nontoxic sulfate conjugation of APAP.

The presumed mechanism in preventing contrast-induced nephropathy is its ability to scavenge oxygen-derived free radicals and improve endothelium-dependent vasodilation.

Pharmacodynamics/Kinetics
Onset of action: Inhalation: 5-10 minutes
Duration: Inhalation: >1 hour
Distribution: 0.47 L/kg
Protein binding: 83%
Half-life elimination:
Reduced acetylcysteine: 2 hours
Total acetylcysteine: Adults: 5.6 hours; Newborns: 11 hours
Time to peak, plasma: Oral: 1-2 hours
Excretion: Urine

Dosage
Acetaminophen poisoning: **Note:** Only the 72-hour oral and 21-hour I.V. regimens are FDA-approved. Ideally, in patients with an acute APAP ingestion, treatment should begin within 8 hours of ingestion. In patients who present following RSTI and treatment is deemed appropriate, acetylcysteine should be initiated immediately.

Children and Adults:
Oral: **Note:** Consultation with a poison control center or clinical toxicologist is highly recommended when considering the discontinuation of oral acetylcysteine prior to the conclusion of a full 18-dose course of therapy.
72-hour regimen: Consists of 18 doses; total dose delivered: 1330 mg/kg
Loading dose: 140 mg/kg
Maintenance dose: 70 mg/kg every 4 hours; repeat dose if emesis occurs within 1 hour of administration
I.V. (Acetadote®):
21-hour regimen: Consists of 3 doses; total dose delivered: 300 mg/kg
Loading dose: 150 mg/kg infused over 60 minutes
Second dose: 50 mg/kg infused over 4 hours
Third dose: 100 mg/kg infused over 16 hours

◀ **Note:** The fluid volume should be reduced in patients weighing <40 kg according to the following table:

Acetadote® Dosing / Fluid Volume Guidelines for Patients <40 kg

Body Weight (kg)	Loading Dose 150 mg/kg over 1 h		Second Dose 50 mg/kg over 4 h		Third Dose 100 mg/kg over 16 h	
	Acetadote® (mL)	D_5W (mL)	Acetadote® (mL)	D_5W (mL)	Acetadote® (mL)	D_5W (mL)
30	22.5	100	7.5	250	15	500
25	18.75	100	6.25	250	12.5	500
20	15	60	5	140	10	280
15	11.25	45	3.75	105	7.5	210
10	7.5	30	2.5	70	5	140

Adjuvant therapy in respiratory conditions: **Note:** Patients should receive an aerosolized bronchodilator 10-15 minutes prior to acetylcysteine.

Inhalation, nebulization (face mask, mouth piece, tracheostomy): Acetylcysteine 10% and 20% solution (dilute 20% solution with sodium chloride or sterile water for inhalation); 10% solution may be used undiluted

Infants: 1-2 mL of 20% solution or 2-4 mL of 10% solution until nebulized given 3-4 times/day

Children and Adults: 3-5 mL of 20% solution or 6-10 mL of 10% solution until nebulized given 3-4 times/day; dosing range: 1-10 mL of 20% solution or 2-20 mL of 10% solution every 2-6 hours

Inhalation, nebulization (tent, croupette): Children and Adults: Dose must be individualized; may require up to 300 mL solution/treatment

Direct instillation: Adults:

Into tracheostomy: 1-2 mL of 10% to 20% solution every 1-4 hours

Through percutaneous intratracheal catheter: 1-2 mL of 20% or 2-4 mL of 10% solution every 1-4 hours via syringe attached to catheter

Diagnostic bronchogram: Nebulization or intratracheal: Adults: 1-2 mL of 20% solution or 2-4 mL of 10% solution administered 2-3 times prior to procedure

Prevention of contrast-induced nephropathy (CIN) (unlabeled use): Adults: Oral: 600-1200 mg twice daily for 2 days (beginning the day before the procedure); may be given as powder in capsules (some centers use solution, diluted in cola beverage or juice)

Prevention of CIN in acute MI patients requiring emergent cardiac catheterization (unlabeled use): Adults: I.V.: 1200 mg over 5-10 minutes prior to cardiac catheterization, followed by 1200 mg **orally** twice daily for 48 hours

Stability

Solution for injection (Acetadote®): Store unopened vials at room temperature, 20°C to 25°C (68°F to 77°F). Following reconstitution with D_5W, solution is stable for 24 hours at room temperature. A color change may occur in opened vials (light purple) and does not affect the safety or efficacy.

Loading dose: Dilute 150 mg/kg in D_5W 200 mL.

Second dose: Dilute 50 mg/kg in D_5W 500 mL.

Third dose: Dilute 100 mg/kg in D_5W 1000 mL.

Note: To avoid fluid overload in patients <40 kg and those requiring fluid restriction, decrease volume of D_5W proportionally (see table in dosing section). Discard unused portion.

Solution for inhalation: Store unopened vials at room temperature; once opened, store under refrigeration and use within 96 hours. The 20% solution may be diluted with sodium chloride or sterile water; the 10% solution may be used undiluted. A color change may occur in opened vials (light purple) and does not affect the safety or efficacy.

Intravenous administration of solution for inhalation (unlabeled route): Using D_5W, dilute acetylcysteine 20% oral solution to a 3% solution.

Administration

Inhalation: Acetylcysteine is incompatible with tetracyclines, erythromycin, amphotericin B, iodized oil, chymotrypsin, trypsin, and hydrogen peroxide. Administer separately. Intermittent aerosol treatments are commonly given when patient arises, before meals, and just before retiring at bedtime.

Oral: Treatment of APAP poisoning, administer orally as a 5% solution. Dilute the 20% solution 1:3 with a cola, orange juice, or other soft drink. Use within 1 hour of preparation. Unpleasant odor becomes less noticeable as treatment progresses. If patient vomits within 1 hour of dose, readminister. (**Note:** It is helpful to put acetylcysteine on ice, in a cup with a cover, and drink through a straw; alternatively, administer via an NG tube).

I.V. (Acetadote®):

Acetaminophen poisoning:

Loading dose: Dilute in D_5W 200 mL; administer over 60 minutes.

Second dose: Dilute in D_5W 500 mL; administer over 4 hours.

Third dose: Dilute in D_5W 1000 mL; administer over 16 hours.

Note: To avoid fluid overload in patients <40 kg and those requiring fluid restriction, decrease volume of D_5W proportionally (see table in dosing section). Discard unused portion.

If the commercial I.V. form is unavailable, the solution for inhalation has been used; each dose should be infused through a 0.2 micron Millipore filter (in-line) over 60 minutes (Yip, 1998); intravenous administration of the solution for inhalation is not USP 797-compliant.

Prevention of CIN in acute MI patients requiring emergent cardiac catheterization (unlabeled use): Administer 1200 mg I.V. push over 5-10 minutes prior to contrast administration.

Monitoring Parameters Acetaminophen poisoning: Monitor patient for the development of anaphylaxis or anaphylactoid reactions; monitor serum APAP levels, AST, ALT, bilirubin, PT, INR, serum creatinine, BUN, serum glucose, hemoglobin, hematocrit, and electrolytes. Assess patient for nausea, vomiting, and skin rash following oral administration. Reassess LFTs for possible hepatotoxicity every 4-6 hours.

Acute ingestion: Obtain the first APAP level 4 hours postingestion (or as soon as possible thereafter); plot on the Rumack-Matthew nomogram. In patients who have ingested an extended release formulation of APAP or have coingested an agent known to delay gastric emptying, obtain a repeat serum APAP measurement 4-6 hours following the first measurement if the original level (taken at 4-8 hours postingestion) when plotted on the Rumack-Matthew nomogram indicated that treatment was not necessary.

Anesthesia and Critical Care Concerns/Other Considerations

Clinical Pearls/Comments: Intravenous acetylcysteine may be indicated over oral formulation in treatment of acetaminophen overdose for a restricted number of indications (oral cannot be tolerated, coingested toxin requires ongoing gastrointestinal decontamination, gastrointestinal tract nonfunctional, late presentation of acetaminophen overdose, neonatal toxicity from maternal overdose) (Yip, 1998). A commercially manufactured intravenous product is now available in the United States. If this formulation is unavailable, the product normally administered by inhalation can be administered intravenously. The inhalation preparation is sterile, but not labeled "pyrogen free."

Evidence-Based Information:

Adverse events related to administration: A retrospective case series was performed to determine adverse events associated with intravenous acetylcysteine. Adverse reactions occurred in four (~5%) cases. Flushing, pruritus, and phlebitis were reported; one was labeled as an "anaphylactic" reaction (Yip, 1998).

Another retrospective case series evaluated patients who received intravenous acetylcysteine and the literature to develop management guideline for anaphylactoid reactions (Bailey, 1998). Their recommendations for treatment of nonlife-threatening allergic reactions include administering diphenhydramine (1 mg/kg I.V.; maximum dose: 50 mg) and reassessing the need for intravenous acetylcysteine. If the acetylcysteine infusion was stopped initially and symptoms resolved, consider restarting infusion 1 hour after diphenhydramine's ▶

administration. Anaphylactoid reactions have also been reported with the commercial I.V. formulation. Monitor closely for allergic reactions. Be prepared to handle anaphylactoid reaction if it occurs.

Pregnancy Risk Factor B

Contraindications Hypersensitivity to acetylcysteine or any component of the formulation

Warnings/Precautions

Inhalation: Since increased bronchial secretions may develop after inhalation, percussion, postural drainage, and suctioning should follow. If bronchospasm occurs, administer a bronchodilator; discontinue acetylcysteine if bronchospasm progresses.

Intravenous: Acute flushing and erythema have been reported; usually occurs within 30-60 minutes and may resolve spontaneously. Serious anaphylactoid reactions have also been reported and are more commonly associated with I.V. administration. When used for APAP poisoning, the incidence is reduced when the initial loading dose is administered over 60 minutes. Acetylcysteine infusion may be interrupted until treatment of allergic symptoms is initiated; the infusion can then be carefully restarted. Treatment for anaphylactoid reactions should be immediately available. Use caution in patients with asthma or history of bronchospasm as these patients may be at increased risk. Conversely, patients with high APAP levels (>150 mg/dL) may be at a reduced risk for anaphylactoid reactions (Pakravan, 2008; Waring, 2008).

Acute APAP poisoning: Acetylcysteine is indicated in patients with a serum APAP level that indicates they are at "possible" risk or greater for hepatotoxicity when plotted on the Rumack-Matthew nomogram. There are several situations where the nomogram is of limited use. Serum acetaminophen levels obtained <4 hours postingestion are not interpretable; patients presenting late may have undetectable serum concentrations, despite having received a toxic dose. The nomogram is less predictive of hepatic injury following an acute overdose with an extended release APAP product or in patients who have coingested APAP with an agent known to delay gastric emptying. The nomogram also does not take into account patients who may be at higher risk of APAP toxicity (eg, alcoholics, malnourished patients). Nevertheless, acetylcysteine should be administered to any patient with signs of hepatotoxicity, even if the serum APAP level is low or undetectable. Patients who present >24 hours after an acute ingestion or patients who present following an acute ingestion at an unknown time may be candidates for acetylcysteine therapy; consultation with a poison control center or clinical toxicologist is highly recommended.

Repeated supratherapeutic ingestion (RSTI) of APAP: The Rumack-Matthew nomogram is not designed to be used following RSTIs. In general, an accurate past medical history, including a comprehensive APAP ingestion history, in conjunction with AST concentrations and serum APAP levels, may give the clinician insight as to the patient's risk of APAP toxicity. Some experts recommend that acetylcysteine be administered to any patient with "higher than expected" serum APAP levels or serum APAP level >10 mcg/mL, even in the absence of hepatic injury; others recommend treatment for patients with laboratory evidence and/or signs and symptoms of hepatotoxicity (Hendrickson, 2006; Jones, 2000). Consultation with a poison control center or a clinical toxicologist is highly recommended.

Adverse Reactions

Inhalation: Frequency not defined.

Central nervous system: Drowsiness, chills, fever

Gastrointestinal: Vomiting, nausea, stomatitis

Local: Irritation, stickiness on face following nebulization

Respiratory: Bronchospasm, rhinorrhea, hemoptysis

Miscellaneous: Acquired sensitization (rare), clamminess, unpleasant odor during administration

Intravenous:

>10%: Miscellaneous: Anaphylactoid reaction (8% to 18%; shorter infusion periods [eg, <60 minutes] associated with increased incidence)

1% to 10%:

Cardiovascular: Flushing (1% to 8%), tachycardia (1% to 4%), edema (1% to 2%)

Dermatologic: Urticaria (6% to 8%), rash (2% to 4%), pruritus (1% to 4%)

Gastrointestinal: Vomiting (2% to 10%), nausea (1% to 6%)

Respiratory: Pharyngitis (≤1%), rhinorrhea (≤1%), rhonchi (≤1%), throat tightness (≤1%)

<1% (Limited to important or life-threatening): Anaphylaxis, bronchospasm, chest tightness, cough, dyspnea, hypotension, respiratory distress, stridor, wheezing

Drug Interactions

Avoid Concomitant Use There are no known interactions where it is recommended to avoid concomitant use.

Increased Effect/Toxicity There are no known significant interactions involving an increase in effect.

Decreased Effect There are no known significant interactions involving a decrease in effect.

Dosage Forms Excipient information presented when available (limited, particularly for generics); consult specific product labeling.

Injection, solution:

Acetadote®: 20% (30 mL) [200 mg/mL; contains disodium edetate]

Solution, inhalation/oral: 10% (4 mL, 10 mL, 30 mL) [100 mg/mL]; 20% (4 mL, 10 mL, 30 mL) [200 mg/mL]

References

Allaqaband S, Tumuluri R, Malik AM, et al, "Prospective Randomized Study of N-Acetylcysteine, Fenoldopam, and Saline for Prevention of Radiocontrast-Induced Nephropathy," *Catheter Cardiovasc Interv*, 2002, 57(3):279-83.

Appelboam AV, Dargan PI, and Knighton J, "Fatal Anaphylactoid Reaction to N-Acetylcysteine: Caution in Patients With Asthma," *Emerg Med J*, 2002, 19(6):594-5.

Bailey B and McGuigan MA, "Management of Anaphylactoid Reactions to Intravenous N-Acetylcysteine," *Ann Emerg Med*, 1998, 31(6):710-5.

Curhan GC, "Prevention of Contrast Nephropathy," *JAMA*, 2003, 289(5):606-8.

Falk JL, "Oral N-Acetylcysteine Given Intravenously for Acetaminophen Overdose: We Shouldn't Have To, But We Must," *Crit Care Med*, 1998, 26(1):7.

Mokhlesi B, Leikin JB, Murray P, et al, "Adult Toxicology in Critical Care: Part II: Specific Poisonings," *Chest*, 2003, 123(3):897-922.

Prescott LF, Donovan JW, Jarvie DR, et al, "The Disposition and Kinetics of Intravenous N-Acetylcysteine in Patients With Paracetamol Overdosage," *Eur J Clin Pharmacol*, 1989, 37 (5):501-6.

Prescott LF, Illingworth RN, Critchley JA, et al, "Intravenous N-Acetylcysteine: The Treatment of Choice for Paracetamol Poisoning," *Br Med J*, 1979, 2(6198):1097-100.

Smilkstein MJ, Bronstein AC, Linden C, et al, "Acetaminophen Overdose: A 48-Hour Intravenous N-Acetylcysteine Treatment Protocol," *Ann Emerg Med*, 1991, 20(10):1058-63.

Tepel M, van der Giet M, Schwarzfeld C, et al, "Prevention of Radiographic-Contrast-Agent-Induced Reductions in Renal Function by Acetylcysteine," *N Engl J Med*, 2000, 343(3):180-4.

Woo OF, Mueller PD, Olson KR, et al, "Shorter Duration of Oral N-Acetylcysteine Therapy for Acute Acetaminophen Overdose," *Ann Emerg Med*, 2000, 35(4):363-8.

Yankaskas JR, Marshall BC, Sufian B, et al, "Cystic Fibrosis Adult Care: Consensus Conference Report," *Chest*, 2004, 125(1 Suppl):1-39.

Yip L, Dart RC, and Hurlbut KM, "Intravenous Administration of Oral N-Acetylcysteine," *Crit Care Med*, 1998, 26(1):40-3.

◆ **Acetylcysteine Sodium** *see* Acetylcysteine *on page 35*

◆ **Acetylcysteine Solution (Can)** *see* Acetylcysteine *on page 35*

◆ **Acetylsalicylic Acid** *see* Aspirin *on page 147*

◆ **Aciclovir** *see* Acyclovir *on page 40*

◆ **Acid Reducer (Can)** *see* Ranitidine *on page 1231*

◆ **Acid Reducer Maximum Strength Non Prescription (Can)** *see* Ranitidine *on page 1231*

◆ **Acilac (Can)** *see* Lactulose *on page 796*

◆ **AcipHex®** *see* Rabeprazole *on page 1221*

◆ **Actidose-Aqua® [OTC]** *see* Charcoal *on page 283*

◆ **Actidose® with Sorbitol [OTC]** *see* Charcoal *on page 283*

◆ **Actiq®** *see* FentaNYL *on page 587*

◆ **Activase®** *see* Alteplase *on page 67*

◆ **Activase® rt-PA (Can)** *see* Alteplase *on page 67*

◆ **Activated Carbon** *see* Charcoal *on page 283*

◆ **Activated Charcoal** *see* Charcoal *on page 283*

◆ **Activated Protein C, Human, Recombinant** *see* Drotrecogin Alfa *on page 466*

- ◆ **Actonel®** *see* Risedronate *on page 1250*
- ◆ **Actos®** *see* Pioglitazone *on page 1132*
- ◆ **Acular®** *see* Ketorolac *on page 784*
- ◆ **Acular LS®** *see* Ketorolac *on page 784*
- ◆ **Acular® PF [DSC]** *see* Ketorolac *on page 784*
- ◆ **ACV** *see* Acyclovir *on page 40*
- ◆ **Acycloguanosine** *see* Acyclovir *on page 40*

Acyclovir (ay SYE kloe veer)

Medication Safety Issues
Sound-alike/look-alike issues:
Acyclovir may be confused with ganciclovir, Retrovir®, valACYclovir
Zovirax® may be confused with Valtrex®, Zithromax®, Zostrix®, Zyloprim®, Zyvox®

International issues:
Opthavir® [Mexico] may be confused with Optivar® which is a brand name for azelastine in the U.S.

Related Information
Dosing Considerations for the Critically-Ill Patient With Morbid Obesity *on page 1561*

U.S. Brand Names Zovirax®

Canadian Brand Names Apo-Acyclovir®; Gen-Acyclovir; Mylan-Acyclovir; Novo-Acyclovir; Nu-Acyclovir; ratio-Acyclovir; Zovirax®

Index Terms Aciclovir; ACV; Acycloguanosine

Pharmacologic Category Antiviral Agent; Antiviral Agent, Topical

Generic Available Yes: Excludes cream, ointment

Use Treatment of genital herpes simplex virus (HSV), herpes labialis (cold sores), herpes zoster (shingles), HSV encephalitis, neonatal HSV, mucocutaneous HSV in immunocompromised patients, varicella-zoster (chickenpox)

Unlabeled/Investigational Use Prevention of HSV reactivation in HIV-positive patients; prevention of HSV reactivation in hematopoietic stem cell transplant (HSCT); prevention of HSV reactivation during periods of neutropenia in patients with cancer; prevention of varicella zoster virus (VZV) reactivation in allogenic HSCT; prevention of CMV reactivation in low-risk allogeneic HSCT; treatment of disseminated HSV or VZV in immunocompromised patients with cancer; empiric treatment of suspected encephalitis in immunocompromised patients with cancer

Mechanism of Action Acyclovir is converted to acyclovir monophosphate by virus-specific thymidine kinase then further converted to acyclovir triphosphate by other cellular enzymes. Acyclovir triphosphate inhibits DNA synthesis and viral replication by competing with deoxyguanosine triphosphate for viral DNA polymerase and being incorporated into viral DNA.

Pharmacodynamics/Kinetics
Absorption: Oral: 15% to 30%

Distribution: V_d: 0.8 L/kg (63.6 L): Widely (eg, brain, kidney, lungs, liver, spleen, muscle, uterus, vagina, CSF)

Protein binding: 9% to 33%

Metabolism: Converted by viral enzymes to acyclovir monophosphate, and further converted to diphosphate then triphosphate (active form) by cellular enzymes

Bioavailability: Oral: 10% to 20% with normal renal function (bioavailability decreases with increased dose)

Half-life elimination: Terminal: Neonates: 4 hours; Children 1-12 years: 2-3 hours; Adults: 3 hours

Time to peak, serum: Oral: Within 1.5-2 hours

Excretion: Urine (62% to 90% as unchanged drug and metabolite)

Dosage Note: Obese patients should be dosed using ideal body weight

Genital HSV:
I.V.: Children ≥12 years and Adults (immunocompetent): Initial episode, severe: 5 mg/kg/dose every 8 hours for 5-7 days

Oral:
  Children:
    Initial episode (unlabeled use): 40-80 mg/kg/day divided into 3-4 doses for 5-10 days (maximum: 1 g/day)
    Chronic suppression (unlabeled use; limited data): 80 mg/kg/day in 3 divided doses (maximum: 1 g/day), re-evaluate after 12 months of treatment
  Adults:
    Initial episode: 200 mg every 4 hours while awake (5 times/day) for 10 days (per manufacturer's labeling); 400 mg 3 times/day for 5-10 days has also been reported
    Recurrence: 200 mg every 4 hours while awake (5 times/day) for 5 days (per manufacturer's labeling; begin at earliest signs of disease); 400 mg 3 times/day for 5 days has also been reported
    Chronic suppression: 400 mg twice daily or 200 mg 3-5 times/day, for up to 12 months followed by re-evaluation (per manufacturer's labeling); 400-1200 mg/day in 2-3 divided doses has also been reported
Topical: Adults (immunocompromised): Ointment: Initial episode: $^{1}/_{2}$" ribbon of ointment for a 4" square surface area every 3 hours (6 times/day) for 7 days

Herpes labialis (cold sores): Topical: Children ≥12 years and Adults: Cream: Apply 5 times/day for 4 days

Herpes zoster (shingles):
Oral: Adults (immunocompetent): 800 mg every 4 hours (5 times/day) for 7-10 days
I.V.:
  Children <12 years (immunocompromised): 20 mg/kg/dose every 8 hours for 7 days
  Children ≥12 years and Adults (immunocompromised): 10 mg/kg/dose or 500 mg/m^2/dose every 8 hours for 7 days

HSV encephalitis: I.V.:
  Children 3 months to 12 years: 20 mg/kg/dose every 8 hours for 10 days (per manufacturer's labeling); dosing for 14-21 days also reported
  Children ≥12 years and Adults: 10 mg/kg/dose every 8 hours for 10 days (per manufacturer's labeling); 10-15 mg/kg/dose every 8 hours for 14-21 days also reported

Mucocutaneous HSV:
I.V.:
  Children <12 years (immunocompromised): 10 mg/kg/dose every 8 hours for 7 days
  Children ≥12 years and Adults (immunocompromised): 5 mg/kg/dose every 8 hours for 7 days (per manufacturer's labeling); dosing for up to 14 days also reported
Oral: Adults (immunocompromised, unlabeled use): 400 mg 5 times a day for 7-14 days
Topical: Ointment: Adults (nonlife-threatening, immunocompromised): $^{1}/_{2}$" ribbon of ointment for a 4" square surface area every 3 hours (6 times/day) for 7 days

Neonatal HSV: I.V.: Neonate: Birth to 3 months: 10 mg/kg/dose every 8 hours for 10 days (manufacturer's labeling); 15 mg/kg/dose or 20 mg/kg/dose every 8 hours for 14-21 days has also been reported

Varicella-zoster (chickenpox): Begin treatment within the first 24 hours of rash onset:
Oral: **Note:** The AIDS*info* guidelines recommended duration of therapy is 7-10 days or until no new lesions for 48 hours (for patients with mild varicella and no or moderate immune suppression).
  Children ≥2 years and ≤40 kg (immunocompetent): 20 mg/kg/dose (up to 800 mg/dose) 4 times/day for 5 days
  Children >40 kg and Adults (immunocompetent): 800 mg/dose 4 times a day for 5 days
I.V.:
  Manufacturer's labeling (immunocompromised):
    Children <12 years: 20 mg/kg/dose every 8 hours for 7 days
    Children ≥12 years and Adults: 10 mg/kg/dose every 8 hours for 7 days

AIDSinfo guidelines (immunocompromised):
   Children <1 year: 10 mg/kg/dose every 8 hours for 7-10 days or until no new lesions for 48 hours
   Children ≥1 year: 10 mg/kg/dose or 500 mg/m^2/dose every 8 hours for 7-10 days or until no new lesions for 48 hours
   Adolescents and Adults: 10-15 mg/kg/dose every 8 hours for 7-10 days

Prevention of HSV reactivation in HIV-positive patients, for use only when recurrences are frequent or severe (unlabeled use): Oral:
   Children: 80 mg/kg/day in 3-4 divided doses
   Adults: 200 mg 3 times/day or 400 mg 2 times/day

Prevention of HSV reactivation in HSCT (unlabeled use): *CDC recommendations:* **Note:** Start at the beginning of conditioning therapy and continue until engraftment or until mucositis resolves (~30 days)
Oral: Adults: 200 mg 3 times/day
I.V.:
   Children: 250 mg/m^2/dose every 8 hours or 125 mg/m^2/dose every 6 hours
   Adults: 250 mg/m^2/dose every 12 hours

Prevention of VZV reactivation in allogeneic HSCT (unlabeled use): *NCCN guidelines:* Oral: Adults: 800 mg twice a day

Prevention of CMV reactivation in low-risk allogeneic HSCT (unlabeled use): *NCCN guidelines:* **Note:** Requires close monitoring (due to weak activity); not for use in patients at high risk for CMV disease: Oral: Adults: 800 mg 4 times/day

Treatment of disseminated HSV or VZV or empiric treatment of suspected encephalitis in immunocompromised patients with cancer: (unlabeled use): *NCCN guidelines:* I.V.: Adults: 10-12 mg/kg/dose every 8 hours

Dosing adjustment in renal impairment:
   Oral:
      Cl_{cr} 10-25 mL/minute/1.73 m^2: Normal dosing regimen 800 mg every 4 hours: Administer 800 mg every 8 hours
      Cl_{cr} <10 mL/minute/1.73 m^2:
         Normal dosing regimen 200 mg every 4 hours or 400 mg every 12 hours: Administer 200 mg every 12 hours
         Normal dosing regimen 800 mg every 4 hours: Administer 800 mg every 12 hours
   I.V.:
      Cl_{cr} 25-50 mL/minute/1.73 m^2: Administer recommended dose every 12 hours
      Cl_{cr} 10-25 mL/minute/1.73 m^2: Administer recommended dose every 24 hours
      Cl_{cr} <10 mL/minute/1.73 m^2: Administer 50% of recommended dose every 24 hours
   Hemodialysis: Administer dose after dialysis
   Continuous ambulatory peritoneal dialysis (CAPD): Administer 50% of normal dose once daily; no supplemental dose needed
   Continuous renal replacement therapy (CRRT): Drug clearance is highly dependent on the method of renal replacement, filter type, and flow rate. Appropriate dosing requires close monitoring of pharmacologic response, signs of adverse reactions due to drug accumulation, as well as drug levels in relation to target trough (if appropriate). The following are general recommendations only (based on dialysate flow/ultrafiltration rates of 1 L/hour) and should not supersede clinical judgment:
   CVVH or CVVHD/CVVHDF: 5-7.5 mg/kg every 24 hours
   Note: The higher dose of 7.5 mg/kg is recommended for infections with CNS involvement (Trotman, 2005).

Stability
   Capsule, tablet: Store at controlled room temperature of 15°C to 25°C (59°F to 77°F). Protect from moisture.
   Cream, suspension: Store at controlled room temperature of 15°C to 25°C (59°F to 77°F).
   Ointment: Store at controlled room temperature of 15°C to 25°C (59°F to 77°F) in a dry place.
   Injection: Store powder at controlled room temperature of 15°C to 25°C (59°F to 77°F). Reconstitute acyclovir 500 mg powder with SWFI 10 mL; do not use

bacteriostatic water containing benzyl alcohol or parabens. For intravenous infusion, dilute in D_5W, D_5NS, $D_51/4NS$, $D_51/2NS$, LR, or NS to a final concentration ≤7 mg/mL. Concentrations >10 mg/mL increase the risk of phlebitis. Reconstituted solutions remain stable for 12 hours at room temperature. Do not refrigerate reconstituted solutions or solutions diluted for infusion as they may precipitate. Once diluted for infusion, use within 24 hours.

Administration
Oral: May be administered with or without food.

I.V.: Avoid rapid infusion; infuse over 1 hour to prevent renal damage; maintain adequate hydration of patient; check for phlebitis and rotate infusion sites. Avoid I.M. or SubQ administration.

Topical: Not for use in the eye. Apply using a finger cot or rubber glove to avoid transmission to other parts of the body or to other persons.

Monitoring Parameters Urinalysis, BUN, serum creatinine, liver enzymes, CBC

Pregnancy Risk Factor B

Contraindications Hypersensitivity to acyclovir, valacyclovir, or any component of the formulation

Warnings/Precautions Use with caution in immunocompromised patients; thrombocytopenic purpura/hemolytic uremic syndrome (TTP/HUS) has been reported. Use caution in the elderly, pre-existing renal disease (may require dosage modification), or in those receiving other nephrotoxic drugs. Renal failure (sometimes fatal) has been reported. Maintain adequate hydration during oral or intravenous therapy. Use I.V. preparation with caution in patients with underlying neurologic abnormalities, serious hepatic or electrolyte abnormalities, or substantial hypoxia.

Safety and efficacy of oral formulations have not been established in pediatric patients <2 years of age.

Varicella-zoster: Treatment should begin within 24 hours of appearance of rash; oral route not recommended for routine use in otherwise healthy children with varicella, but may be effective in patients at increased risk of moderate-to-severe infection (>12 years of age, chronic cutaneous or pulmonary disorders, long-term salicylate therapy, corticosteroid therapy).

Genital herpes: Physical contact should be avoided when lesions are present; transmission may also occur in the absence of symptoms. Treatment should begin with the first signs or symptoms.

Herpes labialis: For external use only to the lips and face; do not apply to eye or inside the mouth or nose. Treatment should begin with the first signs or symptoms.

Herpes zoster: Acyclovir should be started within 72 hours of appearance of rash to be effective.

Adverse Reactions
Systemic: Oral:
>10%: Central nervous system: Malaise (≤12%)

1% to 10%:
  Central nervous system: Headache (≤2%)
  Gastrointestinal: Nausea (2% to 5%), vomiting (≤3%), diarrhea (2% to 3%)

Systemic: Parenteral:
1% to 10%:
  Dermatologic: Hives (2%), itching (2%), rash (2%)
  Gastrointestinal: Nausea/vomiting (7%)
  Hepatic: Liver function tests increased (1% to 2%)
  Local: Inflammation at injection site or phlebitis (9%)
  Renal: BUN increased (5% to 10%), creatinine increased (5% to 10%), acute renal failure

Topical:
>10%: Dermatologic: Mild pain, burning, or stinging (ointment 30%)

1% to 10%: Dermatologic: Pruritus (ointment 4%), itching

All forms: <1% (Limited to important or life-threatening): Abdominal pain, aggression, agitation, alopecia, anaphylaxis, anemia, angioedema, anorexia, ataxia, coma, confusion, consciousness decreased, delirium, desquamation, disseminated intravascular coagulopathy (DIC), dizziness, dry lips, dysarthria, encephalopathy, erythema multiforme, fatigue, fever, gastrointestinal distress, hallucinations, hematuria, hemolysis, hepatitis, hyperbilirubinemia, hypotension, insomnia, jaundice, leukocytoclastic vasculitis, leukocytosis, leukopenia, local tissue necrosis (following extravasation), lymphadenopathy, mental depression, myalgia, neutrophilia, pain, paresthesia, peripheral edema, photosensitization, pruritus, psychosis, renal failure, renal pain, seizure, somnolence, sore throat, Stevens-Johnson syndrome, thrombocytopenia, thrombocytopenic purpura/ hemolytic uremic syndrome (TTP/HUS), thrombocytosis, toxic epidermal necrolysis, tremor, urticaria, visual disturbances

Drug Interactions

Avoid Concomitant Use

Avoid concomitant use of Acyclovir with any of the following: Zoster Vaccine

Increased Effect/Toxicity

Acyclovir may increase the levels/effects of: Mycophenolate; Tenofovir; Zidovudine

The levels/effects of Acyclovir may be increased by: Mycophenolate

Decreased Effect

Acyclovir may decrease the levels/effects of: Zoster Vaccine

Ethanol/Nutrition/Herb Interactions Food: Does not affect absorption of oral acyclovir.

Dietary Considerations May be taken with or without food. Acyclovir 500 mg injection contains sodium ~50 mg (~2 mEq).

Dosage Forms Excipient information presented when available (limited, particularly for generics); consult specific product labeling.

Capsule: 200 mg
   Zovirax®: 200 mg
Cream, topical:
   Zovirax®: 5% (2 g, 5 g)
Injection, powder for reconstitution, as sodium: 500 mg [base strength], 1000 mg [base strength]
Injection, solution, as sodium [preservative free]: 50 mg/mL (10 mL, 20 mL) [base strength]
Ointment, topical:
   Zovirax®: 5% (15 g)
Suspension, oral: 200 mg/5 mL (480 mL)
   Zovirax®: 200 mg/5 mL (480 mL) [banana flavor]
Tablet: 400 mg, 800 mg
   Zovirax®: 400 mg, 800 mg

◆ **Adalat® XL® (Can)** *see* NIFEdipine *on page 1006*

◆ **Adalat® CC** *see* NIFEdipine *on page 1006*

◆ **Adamantanamine Hydrochloride** *see* Amantadine *on page 77*

◆ **Adcirca™** *see* Tadalafil *on page 1345*

◆ **ADD 234037** *see* Lacosamide *on page 795*

◆ **Addaprin [OTC]** *see* Ibuprofen *on page 717*

◆ **Adderall®** *see* Dextroamphetamine and Amphetamine *on page 403*

◆ **Adderall XR®** *see* Dextroamphetamine and Amphetamine *on page 403*

◆ **Adenocard®** *see* Adenosine *on page 44*

◆ **Adenoscan®** *see* Adenosine *on page 44*

Adenosine (a DEN oh seen)

Related Information

Antiarrhythmic Drugs *on page 1656*
Dosing Considerations for the Critically-Ill Patient With Morbid Obesity *on page 1561*
Management of Postoperative Arrhythmias *on page 1571*

U.S. Brand Names Adenocard®; Adenoscan®

Canadian Brand Names Adenocard®; Adenoscan®; Adenosine Injection, USP

Index Terms 9-Beta-D-Ribofuranosyladenine

Pharmacologic Category Antiarrhythmic Agent, Class IV; Diagnostic Agent
Use
Adenocard®: Treatment of paroxysmal supraventricular tachycardia (PSVT) including that associated with accessory bypass tracts (Wolff-Parkinson-White syndrome); when clinically advisable, appropriate vagal maneuvers should be attempted prior to adenosine administration; **not effective for conversion of atrial fibrillation, atrial flutter, or ventricular tachycardia**
Adenoscan®: Pharmacologic stress agent used in myocardial perfusion thallium-201 scintigraphy

Unlabeled/Investigational Use
ACLS/PALS Guidelines (2005):
Stable, narrow-complex AV nodal or sinus nodal reentry tachycardias (eg, reentry SVT);
Unstable reentry SVT while preparations are made for synchronized direct-current cardioversion;
Undefined, stable, narrow-complex SVT as a combination therapeutic and diagnostic maneuver;
Stable, wide-complex tachycardias in patients with a recurrence of a known reentry pathway that has been previously defined
Adenoscan®: Acute vasodilator testing in pulmonary artery hypertension

Pharmacodynamics/Kinetics
Onset of action: Rapid
Duration: Very brief
Metabolism: Blood and tissue to inosine then to adenosine monophosphate (AMP) and hypoxanthine
Half-life elimination: <10 seconds

Dosage
Adenocard®: **Rapid I.V. push (over 1-2 seconds) via peripheral line:**
Infants and Children:
Paroxysmal supraventricular tachycardia: Manufacturer's recommendation:
<50 kg: Initial: 0.05-0.1 mg/kg (maximum initial dose: 6 mg). If conversion of PSVT does not occur within 1-2 minutes, may increase dose by 0.05-0.1 mg/kg. May repeat until sinus rhythm is established or to a maximum single dose of 0.3 mg/kg or 12 mg. Follow each dose with normal saline flush.
≥50 kg: Refer to Adult dosing
Pediatric advanced life support (PALS, 2005): Treatment of SVT: I.V., I.O.: Initial: 0.1 mg/kg (maximum initial dose: 6 mg); if not effective within 1-2 minutes, administer 0.2 mg/kg; may repeat 0.2 mg/kg if needed (maximum single dose: 12 mg). Follow each dose with normal saline flush.
Adults:
Paroxysmal supraventricular tachycardia: Initial: 6 mg; if not effective within 1-2 minutes, 12 mg may be given; may repeat 12 mg bolus if needed (maximum single dose: 12 mg). Follow each dose with normal saline flush.
Recommended dosage adjustment for adenosine when administered via central line or with concurrent carbamazepine or dipyridamole (ACLS, 2005): Initial dose: 3 mg

Adenoscan®:
Pharmacologic stress testing: Continuous I.V. infusion via peripheral line: 140 mcg/kg/minute for 6 minutes using syringe or columetric infusion pump; total dose: 0.84 mg/kg. Thallium-201 is injected at midpoint (3 minutes) of infusion.
Acute vasodilator testing in pulmonary artery hypertension (unlabeled use): I.V.: Initial: 50 mcg/kg/minute increased by 50 mcg/kg/minute every 2 minutes to a maximum dose of 500 mcg/kg/minute (Schrader, 1992) **or** to a maximum dose of 250 mcg/kg/minute (McLaughlin, 2009); acutely assess vasodilator response

Anesthesia and Critical Care Concerns/Other Considerations
Clinical Pearls/Comments: Short action is an advantage; has prolonged effects in patients taking dipyridamole or carbamazepine. In denervated transplanted hearts, the actions of adenosine are pronounced; adjust doses or choose alternative agent accordingly.

◄ Adenosine acts via interruption of AV-nodal conduction and, when used for this purpose, requires administration as rapid intravenous push in increasing doses followed by rapid administration of flushes. Because of more direct access when administered through a central line, lower doses of adenosine may be more appropriate. It is not uncommon to see heart block and sinus pause soon after adenosine administration. May aid in the identification of the arrhythmia by making the atrial fibrillation or flutter electrocardiographic morphology more apparent.

Additional Information Complete prescribing information for this medication should be consulted for additional detail.

Dosage Forms Excipient information presented when available (limited, particularly for generics); consult specific product labeling.

Injection, solution [preservative free]: 3 mg/mL (2 mL, 4 mL)

Adenocard®: 3 mg/mL (2 mL, 4 mL)

Adenoscan®: 3 mg/mL (20 mL, 30 mL)

◆ **Adenosine Injection, USP (Can)** *see* Adenosine *on page 44*

◆ **ADH** *see* Vasopressin *on page 1458*

◆ **ADL-2698** *see* Alvimopan *on page 75*

◆ **Adoxa®** *see* Doxycycline *on page 456*

◆ **Adrenalin®** *see* EPINEPHrine *on page 492*

◆ **Adrenaline** *see* EPINEPHrine *on page 492*

◆ **Adsorbent Charcoal** *see* Charcoal *on page 283*

◆ **Advagraf™ (Can)** *see* Tacrolimus *on page 1338*

◆ **Advate** *see* Antihemophilic Factor (Recombinant) *on page 124*

◆ **Advil® [OTC]** *see* Ibuprofen *on page 717*

◆ **Advil® (Can)** *see* Ibuprofen *on page 717*

◆ **Advil® Children's [OTC]** *see* Ibuprofen *on page 717*

◆ **Advil® Infants' [OTC]** *see* Ibuprofen *on page 717*

◆ **Advil® Migraine [OTC]** *see* Ibuprofen *on page 717*

◆ **Aerius® (Can)** *see* Desloratadine *on page 385*

◆ **Afeditab® CR** *see* NIFEdipine *on page 1006*

◆ **Aggrastat®** *see* Tirofiban *on page 1397*

◆ **Aggrenox®** *see* Aspirin and Dipyridamole *on page 152*

◆ **AGN 1135** *see* Rasagiline *on page 1236*

◆ **AgNO₃** *see* Silver Nitrate *on page 1291*

◆ **AHF (Recombinant)** *see* Antihemophilic Factor (Recombinant) *on page 124*

◆ **A-hydroCort** *see* Hydrocortisone *on page 699*

◆ **Airomir (Can)** *see* Albuterol *on page 49*

◆ **AK-Dilate®** *see* Phenylephrine *on page 1114*

◆ **Akne-Mycin®** *see* Erythromycin *on page 516*

◆ **Akten™** *see* Lidocaine *on page 836*

◆ **AKTob®** *see* Tobramycin *on page 1400*

◆ **Albert® Glyburide (Can)** *see* GlyBURIDE *on page 666*

Albumin (al BYOO min)

Medication Safety Issues

Sound-alike/look-alike issues:

Albutein® may be confused with albuterol

Buminate® may be confused with bumetanide

U.S. Brand Names Albuminar®; AlbuRx™; Albutein®; Buminate®; Flexbumin; Human Albumin Grifols®; Plasbumin®

Canadian Brand Names Plasbumin®-25; Plasbumin®-5

Index Terms Albumin (Human); Normal Human Serum Albumin; Normal Serum Albumin (Human); Salt Poor Albumin; SPA

Pharmacologic Category Blood Product Derivative; Plasma Volume Expander, Colloid

Generic Available Yes

Use Plasma volume expansion and maintenance of cardiac output in the treatment of certain types of shock or impending shock; may be useful for burn patients, ARDS, and cardiopulmonary bypass; other uses considered by some investigators (but not proven) are retroperitoneal surgery, peritonitis, and ascites; unless the condition responsible for hypoproteinemia can be corrected, albumin can provide only symptomatic relief or supportive treatment

Unlabeled/Investigational Use In cirrhotics, administered with diuretics to help facilitate diuresis; large volume paracentesis; volume expansion in dehydrated, mildly-hypotensive cirrhotics

Mechanism of Action Provides increase in intravascular oncotic pressure and causes mobilization of fluids from interstitial into intravascular space

Dosage I.V.:

5% should be used in hypovolemic patients or intravascularly-depleted patients

25% should be used in patients in whom fluid and sodium intake must be minimized

Dose depends on condition of patient:

Children: Hypovolemia: 0.5-1 g/kg/dose (10-20 mL/kg/dose of albumin 5%); maximum dose: 6 g/kg/day

Adults: Usual dose: 25 g; initial dose may be repeated in 15-30 minutes if response is inadequate; no more than 250 g should be administered within 48 hours

Hypoproteinemia: 0.5-1 g/kg/dose; repeat every 1-2 days as calculated to replace ongoing losses

Hypovolemia: 5% albumin: 0.5-1 g/kg/dose; repeat as needed. **Note:** May be considered after inadequate response to crystalloid therapy and when nonprotein colloids are contraindicated. The volume administered and the speed of infusion should be adapted to individual response.

Stability Store at a temperature ≤30°C (86°F); do not freeze. Do not use solution if it is turbid or contains a deposit; use within 4 hours after opening vial; discard unused portion.

If 5% human albumin is unavailable, it may be prepared by diluting 25% human albumin with 0.9% sodium chloride or 5% dextrose in water. Do not use sterile water to dilute albumin solutions, as this has been associated with hypotonic-associated hemolysis.

Administration For I.V. administration only. Use within 4 hours after opening vial; discard unused portion. In emergencies, may administer as rapidly as necessary to improve clinical condition. After initial volume replacement:

5%: Do not exceed 2-4 mL/minute in patients with normal plasma volume; 5-10 mL/minute in patients with hypoproteinemia

25%: Do not exceed 1 mL/minute in patients with normal plasma volume; 2-3 mL/minute in patients with hypoproteinemia

Do not dilute 5% solution. Rapid infusion may cause vascular overload. Albumin 25% may be given undiluted or diluted in normal saline. May give in combination or through the same administration set as saline or carbohydrates. Do not use with ethanol or protein hydrolysates, precipitation may form.

Monitoring Parameters Blood pressure, pulmonary edema, hematocrit

Anesthesia and Critical Care Concerns/Other Considerations

Clinical Pearls/Comments: The administration of 100 mL of 25% albumin will increase the intravascular volume approximately 3-5 times the amount infused, through the translocation of fluid from the interstitial compartment. In contrast, the administration of 500 mL of 5% albumin will increase the intravascular volume approximately 500 mL. However, in subjects with increased intravascular permeability (eg, critically ill, sepsis, trauma, burn), the translocation of fluid from the interstitial compartment to the intravascular compartment may decrease. Furthermore, in extreme intravascular permeability, albumin (or other colloids) may increase the interstitial space, pulling fluid from the intravascular compartment.

◀ **Evidence-Based Information:** An Australian/New Zealand critical care group published the SAFE (saline versus albumin fluid evaluation) study that evaluated 4% albumin versus normal saline for resuscitation in a heterogeneous intensive care population (Finfer, 2004). They conducted a multicenter, randomized, double-blind trial to compare the effects of resuscitation fluid on mortality from any cause during the 28-day period after randomization. Patients were eligible for inclusion if the treating clinician judged that fluid resuscitation was required for intravascular fluid depletion as supported by one of the following criteria:

Heart rate >90 bpm,

Systolic BP <100 mm Hg,

Mean arterial BP <75 mm Hg,

Decrease of 40 mm Hg in systolic or mean arterial BP (as compared with baseline),

CVP <10 mm Hg,

PCWP <12 mm Hg,

Respiratory variation in systolic or mean BP >5 mm Hg,

Capillary refill time >1 second, or

Urine output <0.5 mL/kg for 1 hour

Patients were excluded for a variety of reasons, including ICU transfer following cardiac or liver transplantation surgery, or burn treatment. Almost 7000 patients were randomized; 3497 to albumin and 3500 to saline. Baseline characteristics were similar between the groups, except CVP pressure was slightly higher in the albumin group (9.0 in albumin versus 8.6 in saline). There was no significant mortality difference between groups (726 deaths in albumin group; 729 deaths in saline group). There were no significant differences in secondary endpoints (length of stay in the ICU or hospital, days of mechanical ventilation, and days of renal replacement therapy). Similar outcomes resulted from use of either fluid for resuscitation in this patient population.

Pregnancy Risk Factor C

Contraindications Hypersensitivity to albumin or any component of the formulation; patients with severe anemia or cardiac failure

Warnings/Precautions Use with caution in patients with hepatic or renal failure because of added protein load; rapid infusion of albumin solutions may cause vascular overload. All patients should be observed for signs of hypervolemia such as pulmonary edema. Use with caution in those patients for whom sodium restriction is necessary. Avoid 25% concentration in preterm infants due to risk of intraventricular hemorrhage. Nutritional supplementation is not an appropriate indication for albumin.

Adverse Reactions Frequency not defined.

Cardiovascular: CHF precipitation, edema, hyper-/hypotension, hypervolemia, tachycardia

Central nervous system: Chills, fever, headache

Dermatologic: Pruritus, rash, urticaria

Gastrointestinal: Nausea, vomiting

Respiratory: Bronchospasm, pulmonary edema

Miscellaneous: Anaphylaxis

Drug Interactions

Avoid Concomitant Use There are no known interactions where it is recommended to avoid concomitant use.

Increased Effect/Toxicity There are no known significant interactions involving an increase in effect.

Decreased Effect There are no known significant interactions involving a decrease in effect.

Dietary Considerations Some products may contain sodium.

Dosage Forms Excipient information presented when available (limited, particularly for generics); consult specific product labeling.

Injection, solution [preservative free; human]: 5% (250 mL, 500 mL); 25% (50 mL, 100 mL)

Albuminar®: 5% (50 mL, 250 mL, 500 mL) [50 mg/mL; contains sodium 130-160 mEq/L and potassium ≤1 mEq/L; packaging contains dry natural rubber]; 25% (20 mL, 50 mL, 100 mL) [250 mg/mL; contains sodium 130-160 mEq/L and potassium ≤1 mEq/L; packaging contains dry natural rubber]

AlbuRx™: 5% (250 mL, 500 mL) [50 mg/mL; contains sodium 130-160 mEq/L and potassium ≤2 mEq/L]; 25% (50 mL, 100 mL) [250 mg/mL; contains sodium 130-160 mEq/L and potassium ≤2 mEq/L]

Albutein®: 5% (250 mL, 500 mL) [50 mg/mL; contains sodium 130-160 mEq/L and potassium ≤2 mEq/L]

Buminate®: 5% (250 mL, 500 mL) [50 mg/mL; contains sodium 130-160 mEq/L and potassium ≤2 mEq/L; packaging contains dry natural rubber]; 25% (20 mL, 50 mL, 100 mL) [250 mg/mL; contains sodium 130-160 mEq/L and potassium ≤2 mEq/L; packaging contains dry natural rubber]

Flexbumin: 25% (50 mL, 100 mL) [250 mg/mL; contains sodium 130-160 mEq/L and potassium ≤2 mEq/L]

Human Albumin Grifols®: 25% (50 mL, 100 mL) [250 mg/mL; contains sodium 130-160 mEq/L and potassium ≤2 mEq/L]

Plasbumin®: 5% (50 mL, 250 mL) [50 mg/mL; contains sodium ~145 mEq/L and potassium ≤2 mEq/L]; 25% (20 mL, 50 mL, 100 mL) [250 mg/mL; contains sodium ~145 mEq/L and potassium ≤2 mEq/L]

References

American Thoracic Society, "Evidence-Based Colloid Use in the Critically Ill: American Thoracic Society Consensus Statement," *Am J Respir Crit Care Med*, 2004, 170(11):1247-59.

Finfer S, Bellomo R, Boyce N, et al, "A Comparison of Albumin and Saline for Fluid Resuscitation in the Intensive Care Unit, SAFE Study Investigators," *N Engl J Med*, 2004, 350(22):2247-56.

◆ **Albuminar®** *see* Albumin *on page 46*

◆ **Albumin (Human)** *see* Albumin *on page 46*

◆ **AlbuRx™** *see* Albumin *on page 46*

◆ **Albutein®** *see* Albumin *on page 46*

Albuterol (al BYOO ter ole)

Medication Safety Issues

Sound-alike/look-alike issues:

Albuterol may be confused with Albutein®, atenolol

Proventil® may be confused with Bentyl®, Prilosec® Prinivil®

Salbutamol may be confused with salmeterol

Ventolin® may be confused with phentolamine, Benylin®, Vantin®

Related Information

Allergic Reactions *on page 1508*

Latex Allergy *on page 1511*

U.S. Brand Names AccuNeb®; ProAir® HFA; Proventil® HFA; Ventolin® HFA; VoSpire ER®

Canadian Brand Names Airomir; Alti-Salbutamol; Apo-Salvent®; Apo-Salvent® CFC Free; Apo-Salvent® Respirator Solution; Apo-Salvent® Sterules; Gen-Salbutamol; Mylan-Salbutamol Respirator Solution; Mylan-Salbutamol Sterinebs P.F.; PMS-Salbutamol; ratio-Inspra-Sal; ratio-Salbutamol; Rhoxal-salbutamol; Salbu-2; Salbu-4; Ventolin®; Ventolin® Diskus; Ventolin® HFA; Ventolin® I.V. Infusion; Ventrodisk

Index Terms Albuterol Sulfate; Salbutamol; Salbutamol Sulphate

Pharmacologic Category Beta$_2$-Adrenergic Agonist

Generic Available Yes

Use Bronchodilator in reversible airway obstruction due to asthma or COPD; prevention of exercise-induced bronchospasm

Unlabeled/Investigational Use As tocolytic agent (injectable form; not available in U.S.)

Mechanism of Action Relaxes bronchial smooth muscle by action on beta$_2$-receptors with little effect on heart rate

Pharmacodynamics/Kinetics

Onset of action: Peak effect:

Nebulization/oral inhalation: 0.5-2 hours

CFC-propelled albuterol: 10 minutes

Ventolin® HFA: 25 minutes

Oral: 2-3 hours

Duration: Nebulization/oral inhalation: 3-4 hours; Oral: 4-6 hours

Metabolism: Hepatic to an inactive sulfate

Half-life elimination: Inhalation: 3.8 hours; Oral: 3.7-5 hours
Excretion: Urine (30% as unchanged drug)

Dosage

Oral:

Children: Bronchospasm:

2-6 years: 0.1-0.2 mg/kg/dose 3 times/day; maximum dose not to exceed 12 mg/day (divided doses)

6-12 years: 2 mg/dose 3-4 times/day; maximum dose not to exceed 24 mg/day (divided doses)

Extended release: 4 mg every 12 hours; maximum dose not to exceed 24 mg/day (divided doses)

Children >12 years and Adults: Bronchospasm (treatment): 2-4 mg/dose 3-4 times/day; maximum dose not to exceed 32 mg/day (divided doses)

Extended release: 8 mg every 12 hours; maximum dose not to exceed 32 mg/day (divided doses). A 4 mg dose every 12 hours may be sufficient in some patients, such as adults of low body weight.

Elderly: Bronchospasm (treatment): 2 mg 3-4 times/day; maximum: 8 mg 4 times/day

Metered-dose inhaler (90 mcg/puff):

Children ≤4 years *(NIH Guidelines, 2007)*:

Quick relief: 1-2 puffs every 4-6 hours as needed

Exacerbation of asthma (acute, severe): 4-8 puffs every 20 minutes for 3 doses, then every 1-4 hours as needed

Exercise-induced bronchospasm (prevention): 1-2 puffs 5 minutes prior to exercise

Children 5-11 years *(NIH Guidelines, 2007)*:

Bronchospasm, quick relief: 2 puffs every 4-6 hours as needed

Exacerbation of asthma (acute, severe): 4-8 puffs every 20 minutes for 3 doses, then every 1-4 hours as needed

Exercise-induced bronchospasm (prevention): 2 puffs 5-30 minutes prior to exercise

Children ≥12 years and Adults:

Bronchospasm, quick relief *(NIH Guidelines, 2007)*: 2 puffs every 4-6 hours as needed

Exacerbation of asthma (acute, severe) *(NIH Guidelines, 2007)*: 4-8 puffs every 20 minutes for up to 4 hours, then every 1-4 hours as needed

Exercise-induced bronchospasm (prevention) *(NIH Guidelines, 2007)*: 2 puffs 5-30 minutes prior to exercise

Solution for nebulization:

Children 2-12 years (AccuNeb®): Bronchospasm: 0.63-1.25 mg every 4-6 hours as needed

Children ≤4 years *(NIH Guidelines, 2007)*:

Quick relief: 0.63-2.5 mg every 4-6 hours as needed

Exacerbation of asthma (acute, severe): 0.15 mg/kg (minimum: 2.5 mg) every 20 minutes for 3 doses, then 0.15-0.3 mg/kg (maximum: 10 mg) every 1-4 hours as needed **or** 0.5 mg/kg/hour by continuous nebulization

Children 5-11 years *(NIH Guidelines, 2007)*:

Quick relief: 1.25-5 mg every 4-8 hours as needed

Exacerbation of asthma (acute, severe): 0.15 mg/kg (minimum: 2.5 mg) every 20 minutes for 3 doses, then 0.15-0.3 mg/kg (maximum: 10 mg) every 1-4 hours as needed **or** 0.5 mg/kg/hour by continuous nebulization

Children ≥12 years and Adults:

Bronchospasm: 2.5 mg every 4-8 hours as needed

Quick relief *(NIH Guidelines, 2007)*: 1.25-5 mg every 4-8 hours as needed

Exacerbation of asthma (acute, severe) *(NIH Guidelines, 2007)*: 2.5-5 mg every 20 minutes for 3 doses then 2.5-10 mg every 1-4 hours as needed, **or** 10-15 mg/hour by continuous nebulization

I.V. continuous infusion: Adults (Ventolin® I.V. solution [not available in U.S.]): Severe bronchospasm and status asthmaticus: Initial: 5 mcg/minute; may increase up to 10-20 mcg/minute at 15- to 30-minute intervals if needed

Hemodialysis: Not removed

Peritoneal dialysis: Significant drug removal is unlikely based on physiochemical characteristics

Stability

HFA aerosols: Store at 15°C to 25°C (59°F to 77°F).

Ventolin® HFA: Discard after using 200 actuations or 3 months after removal from protective pouch, whichever comes first. Store with mouthpiece down.

Infusion solution (not available in U.S.): Ventolin® I.V.: Store at 15°C to 30°C (59°F to 86°F). Protect from light. After dilution, discard after 24 hours.

Inhalation solution: Solution for nebulization (0.5%): Store at 2°C to 30°C (36°F to 86°F). To prepare a 2.5 mg dose, dilute 0.5 mL of solution to a total of 3 mL with normal saline; also compatible with cromolyn or ipratropium nebulizer solutions.

AccuNeb®: Store at 2°C to 25°C (36°F to 77°F). Do not use if solution changes color or becomes cloudy. Use within 1 week of opening foil pouch.

Syrup: Store at 2°C to 30°C (36°F to 86°F).

Tablet: Store at 2°C to 30°C (36°F to 86°F).

Tablet, extended release: Store at 20°C to 25°C (68°F to 77°F)

Administration

Metered-dose inhaler: Shake well before use; prime prior to first use, and whenever inhaler has not been used for >2 weeks or when it has been dropped, by releasing 3-4 test sprays into the air (away from face). A spacer device or valved holding chamber is recommended for use with metered-dose inhalers.

Solution for nebulization: Concentrated solution should be diluted prior to use. Blow-by administration is not recommended, use a mask device if patient unable to hold mouthpiece in mouth for administration.

Infusion solution (Ventolin® I.V.): Do not inject undiluted. Reduce concentration by at least 50% before infusing. Administer as a continuous infusion via infusion pump. Discard unused portion of infusion within 24 hours of preparation.

Oral: Do not crush or chew extended release tablets. Administer with water 1 hour before or 2 hours after meals.

Monitoring Parameters FEV_1, peak flow, and/or other pulmonary function tests; blood pressure, heart rate; CNS stimulation; serum glucose, serum potassium; asthma symptoms; arterial or capillary blood gases (if patients condition warrants)

Anesthesia and Critical Care Concerns/Other Considerations

Clinical Pearls/Comments: High-dose inhaled beta-agonists may be used as part of a treatment regimen for the management of acute hyperkalemia by stimulating the sodium potassium (K) ATPase pump causing an intracellular shift of potassium. The hypokalemic effects typically have an onset of 30 minutes and may last several hours; however, the intracellular shift is temporary thus requiring the removal (ion-exchange resins or hemodialysis) of potassium from the body.

Frequent use of inhaled beta-agonists in patients with atrial fibrillation may counteract pharmacologic interventions directed at rate control.

Pregnancy Risk Factor C

Contraindications Hypersensitivity to albuterol, adrenergic amines, or any component of the formulation

Injection formulation (not available in U.S.): Patients with tachyarrhythmias; risk of abortion during first or second trimester

Warnings/Precautions Optimize anti-inflammatory treatment before initiating maintenance treatment with albuterol. Do not use as a component of chronic therapy without an anti-inflammatory agent. Only the mildest forms of asthma (Step 1 and/or exercise-induced) would not require concurrent use based upon asthma guidelines. Patient must be instructed to seek medical attention in cases where acute symptoms are not relieved or a previous level of response is diminished. The need to increase frequency of use may indicate deterioration of asthma, and treatment must not be delayed.

Use caution in patients with cardiovascular disease (arrhythmia or hypertension or HF), convulsive disorders, diabetes, glaucoma, hyperthyroidism, or hypokalemia. Beta-agonists may cause elevation in blood pressure, heart rate, and result in CNS stimulation/excitation. $Beta_2$-agonists may increase risk of arrhythmia, increase serum glucose, or decrease serum potassium.

Immediate hypersensitivity reactions (urticaria, angioedema, rash, broncho-spasm) have been reported. Do not exceed recommended dose; serious adverse events, including fatalities, have been associated with excessive use of inhaled sympathomimetics. Rarely, paradoxical bronchospasm may occur with use of inhaled bronchodilating agents; this should be distinguished from inadequate response. All patients should utilize a spacer device or valved holding chamber when using a metered-dose inhaler; in addition, face masks should be used in children <4 years of age.

Patient response may vary between inhalers that contain chlorofluorocarbons and those which are chlorofluorocarbon-free.

Adverse Reactions Incidence of adverse effects is dependent upon age of patient, dose, and route of administration.

Cardiovascular: Angina, atrial fibrillation, arrhythmias, chest discomfort, chest pain, extrasystoles, flushing, hyper-/hypotension, palpitation, supraventricular tachycardia, tachycardia

Central nervous system: CNS stimulation, dizziness, drowsiness, headache, insomnia, irritability, lightheadedness, migraine, nervousness, nightmares, restlessness, seizure

Dermatologic: Angioedema, rash, urticaria

Endocrine & metabolic: Hyperglycemia, hypokalemia, lactic acidosis

Gastrointestinal: Diarrhea, dry mouth, dyspepsia, gastroenteritis, nausea, unusual taste, vomiting

Genitourinary: Micturition difficulty

Local: Injection: Pain, stinging

Neuromuscular & skeletal: Muscle cramps, musculoskeletal pain, tremor, weakness

Otic: Otitis media, vertigo

Respiratory: Asthma exacerbation, bronchospasm, cough, epistaxis, laryngitis, oropharyngeal drying/irritation, oropharyngeal edema, pharyngitis, rhinitis, upper respiratory inflammation, viral respiratory infection

Miscellaneous: Allergic reaction, anaphylaxis, diaphoresis, lymphadenopathy

Postmarketing and/or case reports: Anxiety, glossitis, hoarseness, myocardial ischemia, pulmonary edema, throat irritation, tongue ulceration

Drug Interactions

Avoid Concomitant Use

Avoid concomitant use of Albuterol with any of the following: Iobenguane I 123

Increased Effect/Toxicity

Albuterol may increase the levels/effects of: Sympathomimetics

The levels/effects of Albuterol may be increased by: Atomoxetine; Cannabinoids; MAO Inhibitors; Tricyclic Antidepressants

Decreased Effect

Albuterol may decrease the levels/effects of: Iobenguane I 123

The levels/effects of Albuterol may be decreased by: Alpha-/Beta-Blockers; Beta-Blockers (Beta1 Selective); Beta-Blockers (Nonselective); Betahistine

Ethanol/Nutrition/Herb Interactions

Food: Avoid or limit caffeine (may cause CNS stimulation).

Herb/Nutraceutical: Avoid ephedra, yohimbe (may cause CNS stimulation). Avoid St John's wort (may decrease the levels/effects of albuterol).

Test Interactions Increased renin (S), increased aldosterone (S)

Dietary Considerations Oral forms should be taken with water 1 hour before or 2 hours after meals.

Dosage Forms Excipient information presented when available (limited, particularly for generics); consult specific product labeling. [DSC] = Discontinued product; [CAN] = Canadian brand name

Aerosol, for oral inhalation: 90 mcg/metered inhalation (17 g) [200 metered inhalations; contains chlorofluorocarbons] [DSC]

Aerosol, for oral inhalation:

ProAir® HFA: 90 mcg/metered inhalation (8.5 g) [200 metered inhalations; chlorofluorocarbon free]

Proventil® HFA: 90 mcg/metered inhalation (6.7 g) [200 metered inhalations; chlorofluorocarbon free]

Ventolin® HFA: 90 mcg/metered inhalation (8 g) [60 metered inhalation; chlorofluorocarbon free]; (18 g) [200 metered inhalations; chlorofluorocarbon free]

Injection, solution, as sulphate:
Ventolin® I.V. [CAN]: 1 mg/1mL (5 mL) [not available in U.S.]

Solution for nebulization [preservative free]: 0.021% (3 mL); 0.042% (3 mL); 0.083% (3 mL); 0.5% (0.5 mL, 20 mL)
AccuNeb®: 0.021% (3 mL); 0.042% (3 mL)

Syrup, oral: 2 mg/5 mL (480 mL)

Tablet, oral: 2 mg, 4 mg

Tablet, extended release, oral: 4 mg, 8 mg
VoSpire ER®: 4 mg, 8 mg

References

Expert Panel Report 3, "Guidelines for the Diagnosis and Management of Asthma," *Clinical Practice Guidelines*, National Institutes of Health, National Heart, Lung, and Blood Institute, NIH Publication No. 08-4051, prepublication 2007. Available at http://www.nhlbi.nih.gov/guidelines/asthma/asthgdln.htm

Katz RW, Kelly HW, Crowley MR, et al, "Safety of Continuous Nebulized Albuterol for Bronchospasm in Infants and Children," *Pediatrics*, 1993, 92(5):666-9.

Leikin JB, Linowiecki KA, Soglin DF, et al, "Hypokalemia After Pediatric Albuterol Overdose: A Case Series," *Am J Emerg Med*, 1994, 12(1):64-6.

Manthous CA, Chatila W, Schmidt GA, et al, "Treatment of Bronchospasm by Metered-Dose Inhaler Albuterol in Mechanically Ventilated Patients," *Chest*, 1995, 107(1):210-3.

Marik P, Hogan J, and Krikorian J, "A Comparison of Bronchodilator Therapy Delivered by Nebulization and Metered-Dose Inhaler in Mechanically Ventilated Patients," *Chest*, 1999, 115 (6):1653-7.

National Asthma Education and Prevention Program, "Expert Panel Report: Guidelines for the Diagnosis and Management of Asthma Update on Selected Topics - 2002," *J Allergy Clin Immunol*, 2002, 110(5 Suppl):141-219. Available at: www.nhlbi.nih.gov/guidelines/asthma/index.

Papo MC, Frank J, and Thompson AE, "A Prospective, Randomized Study of Continuous Versus Intermittent Nebulized Albuterol for Severe Status Asthmaticus in Children," *Crit Care Med*, 1993, 21(10):1479-86.

Schuh S, Parkin P, Rajan A, et al, "Bronchodilator Therapy With Metered Dose Inhaler Versus Nebulizer in Mechanically Ventilated Patients," *Respiratory Care*, (July) 2000, 817.

Schuh S, Parkin P, Rajan A, et al, "High- Versus Low-Dose, Frequently Administered, Nebulized Albuterol in Children With Severe, Acute Asthma," *Pediatrics*, 1989, 83(4):513-8.

Udezue E, D'Souza L, and Mahajan M, "Hypokalemia After Normal Doses of Nebulized Albuterol (Salbutamol)," *Am J Emerg Med*, 1995, 13(2):168-71.

♦ **Albuterol and Ipratropium** see Ipratropium and Albuterol *on page 762*

♦ **Albuterol Sulfate** see Albuterol *on page 49*

♦ **Alcohol, Absolute** see Alcohol (Ethyl) *on page 53*

♦ **Alcohol, Dehydrated** see Alcohol (Ethyl) *on page 53*

Alcohol (Ethyl) (AL koe hol, ETH il)

Medication Safety Issues
Sound-alike/look-alike issues:
Ethanol may be confused with Ethyol®, Ethamolin®

U.S. Brand Names EpiClenz™ [OTC]; Gel-Stat™ [OTC]; GelRite [OTC]; Isagel® [OTC]; Lavacol® [OTC]; Prevacare® [OTC]; Protection Plus® [OTC]; Purell® 2 in 1 [OTC]; Purell® Lasting Care [OTC]; Purell® Moisture Therapy [OTC]; Purell® with Aloe [OTC]; Purell® [OTC]

Canadian Brand Names Biobase-G™; Biobase™

Index Terms Alcohol, Absolute; Alcohol, Dehydrated; Ethanol; Ethyl Alcohol; EtOH

Pharmacologic Category Antidote; Pharmaceutical Aid

Generic Available Yes

Use Topical anti-infective; pharmaceutical aid; therapeutic neurolysis (nerve or ganglion block); replenishment of carbohydrate calories

Unlabeled/Investigational Use Antidote for ethylene glycol overdose; antidote for methanol overdose; treatment of fat occlusion of central venous catheters; septal ablation for hypertrophic obstructive cardiomyopathy (HOCM)

Mechanism of Action When used to treat ethylene glycol or methanol toxicity, ethyl alcohol competitively inhibits alcohol dehydrogenase, an enzyme which catalyzes the metabolism of ethylene glycol and methanol to their toxic metabolites.

Pharmacodynamics/Kinetics
Absorption: Oral: Rapid

Distribution: V_d: 0.6-0.7 L/kg; decreased in women

Metabolism: Hepatic (90% to 98%) to acetaldehyde or acetate

Half-life elimination: Rate: 15-20 mg/dL/hour (range: 10-34 mg/dL/hour); increased in alcoholics

Excretion: Kidneys and lungs (~2% unchanged)

Dosage
Antiseptic: Children and Adults: Liquid denatured alcohol: Topical: Apply 1-3 times/day as needed

Therapeutic neurolysis (nerve or ganglion block): Adults: Dehydrated alcohol injection 98%: Intraneural: Dosage variable depending upon the site of injection (eg, trigeminal neuralgia: 0.05-0.5 mL as a single injection per interspace vs subarachnoid injection: 0.5-1 mL as a single injection per interspace); single doses >1.5 mL are seldom required

Replenishment of fluid and carbohydrate calories: Adults: Dehydrated alcohol infusion: Alcohol 5% and dextrose 5%: 1-2 L/day by slow infusion

Septal ablation for HOCM (unlabeled use; Maron, 2003): Adults: Intracoronary (via balloon catheter): Dosage variable depending on septal anatomy and rate of contrast washout: 1-3 mL of at least 95% concentration infused slowly into septal perforator. **Note:** Smaller amounts may reduce the size of the septal infarct and incidence of complications (eg, complete heart block).

Treatment of methanol or ethylene glycol ingestion (unlabeled use): **Note:** I.V. administration is the preferred route; continue therapy until ethylene glycol and/ or methanol is no longer detected or levels are <20 mg/dL **and** the patient is asymptomatic **and** metabolic acidosis has been corrected. If ethylene glycol and/or methanol levels are not available in a timely manner, continue therapy until the estimated time of clearance of ethylene glycol and/or methanol has elapsed **and** the patient is asymptomatic with a normal pH. If patient has coingested ethanol, measure the baseline serum ethanol concentration and adjust the ethyl alcohol loading dose based on results to achieve a serum ethanol level of ~100 mg/dL.

Children and Adults: Absolute ethyl alcohol [98% (196 proof) = 77.4 g EtOH/dL]: I.V.:

Initial: 600-700 mg/kg [equivalent to 7.6-8.9 mL/kg using a **10% solution**]

Maintenance: Goal of therapy is to maintain serum ethanol levels >100 mg/dL.

Nondrinker: 66 mg/kg/hour [equivalent to 0.83 mL/kg/hour using a **10% solution**]

Chronic drinker: 154 mg/kg/hour [equivalent to 1.96 mL/kg/hour using a **10% solution**]

Dosage adjustment for hemodialysis: Maintenance dose:

Nondrinker: 169 mg/kg/hour [equivalent to 2.13 mL/kg/hour using a **10% solution**]

Chronic drinker: 257 mg/kg/hour [equivalent to 3.26 mL/kg/hour using a **10% solution**]

Oral: Solution must be diluted to a ≤20% concentration with water or juice and administered orally or via a nasogastric tube.

Initial: 600-700 mg/kg [equivalent to 0.78-0.9 mL/kg using a **98% solution**]

Maintenance: Goal of therapy is to maintain serum ethanol levels >100 mg/dL

Nondrinker: 66 mg/kg/hour [equivalent to 0.09 mL/kg/hour using a **98% solution**]

Chronic drinker: 154 mg/kg/hour [equivalent to 0.20 mL/kg/hour using a **98% solution**]

Dosage adjustment for hemodialysis: Maintenance dose:

Nondrinker: 169 mg/kg/hour [equivalent to 0.22 mL/kg/hour using a **98% solution**]

Chronic drinker: 257 mg/kg/hour [equivalent to 0.33 mL/kg/hour using a **98% solution**]

Treatment of fat occlusion of central venous catheters (unlabeled use): Children and Adults: Dehydrated alcohol injection: I.V. (see institutional-based protocol for catheter clearance assessment, the following assessment is a general methodology): Up to 3 mL of ethanol 70% (maximum: 0.55 mL/kg); the volume to instill is equal to the internal volume of the catheter

Administration

Oral: Ethylene glycol or methanol poisoning: Dilute ethyl alcohol to ≤20% solution with water or juice and administer hourly by mouth or via nasogastric tube. Out-of-hospital management with orally-administered ethanol is not recommended.

I.V.: Ethylene glycol or methanol poisoning: I.V. administration is the preferred route. Administer as a 10% solution in D_5W. Initial dose should be administered over 1 hour.

Treatment of occluded central venous catheter: Instill a 70% solution with a volume equal to the internal volume of the catheter. Assess patency at 30-60 minutes (or per institutional protocol).

Intraneural: Separate needles should be used for each of multiple injections or sites to prevent residual alcohol deposition at sites not intended for tissue destruction. Inject slowly after determining proper placement of needle. Since dehydrated alcohol is hypobaric when compared with spinal fluid, proper positioning of the patient is essential to control localization of injections into the subarachnoid space.

Monitoring Parameters Antidotal therapy: Blood ethanol levels every 1-2 hours until steady state, then every 2-4 hours; blood glucose, electrolytes (including serum magnesium), arterial pH, blood gases, methanol or ethylene glycol blood levels; heart rate, blood pressure

Reference Range Antidote for methanol/ethylene glycol: Blood ethanol level: Goal range: 100-150 mg/dL

Anesthesia and Critical Care Concerns/Other Considerations

Clinical Pearls/Comments: Neurolytic Block: Alcohol will destroy nerves and should be administered when pain is from malignant origin only. Pain will occur after initial injection for a short period of time and will subside when neurolysis occurs.

Evidence-Based Information: Methanol/Ethylene Glycol Poisoning: Treatment involves inhibiting the formation of toxic metabolites by inhibiting alcohol dehydrogenase and/or urgent dialytic removal of these alcohols and their metabolites. A target ethanol serum level is 100-150 mg/dL. Alcohol administration is continued until the serum levels of ethylene glycol/methanol are <20 mg/dL and patient is asymptomatic with normal pH or poison levels are undetectable. Currently, fomepizole is the drug of choice because of its ease of use and lack of CNS toxicity.

Pregnancy Risk Factor C (D per expert opinion)/X (prolonged use or high doses at term)

Contraindications Hypersensitivity to ethyl alcohol or any component of the formulation; seizure disorder and diabetic coma; subarachnoid injection of dehydrated alcohol in patients receiving anticoagulants; pregnancy (prolonged use or high doses at term)

Warnings/Precautions Ethyl alcohol is a flammable liquid and should be kept cool and away from any heat source. Proper positioning of the patient for neurolytic administration is essential to control localization of the injection of dehydrated alcohol (which is hypobaric) into the subarachnoid space; avoid extravasation. Not for SubQ administration. Do not administer simultaneously with blood due to the possibility of pseudoagglutination or hemolysis; may potentiate severe hypoprothrombic bleeding. Clinical evaluation and periodic lab determinations, including serum ethanol levels, are necessary to monitor effectiveness, changes in electrolyte concentrations, and acid-base balance (when used as an antidote).

Use with caution in patients with diabetes (ethyl alcohol may decrease blood sugar), hepatic impairment, patients with gout, shock, following cranial surgery, and in anticipated postpartum hemorrhage. Monitor blood glucose closely, particularly in children as treatment of ingestions is associated with hypoglycemia. Avoid extravasation during I.V. administration. Ethyl alcohol passes freely into breast milk at a level approximately equivalent to maternal serum level; minimize dermal exposure of ethyl alcohol in infants as significant systemic absorption and toxicity can occur.

Adverse Reactions Frequency not defined.

Cardiovascular: Flushing, hypotension

◄ Central nervous system: Disorientation, encephalopathy, sedation, seizure (rare), vertigo

Endocrine & metabolic: Hypoglycemia

Genitourinary: Urinary retention

Local: Nerve and tissue destruction

Miscellaneous: Intoxication

Drug Interactions

Avoid Concomitant Use

Avoid concomitant use of Alcohol (Ethyl) with any of the following: Acitretin; Amprenavir; CycloSERINE; Didanosine; Disulfiram

Increased Effect/Toxicity

Alcohol (Ethyl) may increase the levels/effects of: Acitretin; Amprenavir; CycloSERINE; Didanosine; Ethionamide; Isotretinoin; NIFEdipine; Propranolol; Thiazide Diuretics

The levels/effects of Alcohol (Ethyl) may be increased by: Cefamandole; Cefotetan; CNS Depressants; Disulfiram; Furazolidone; Griseofulvin; MetroNI-DAZOLE; Sulfonylureas; Tacrolimus; Verapamil

Decreased Effect

Alcohol (Ethyl) may decrease the levels/effects of: Propranolol

Dosage Forms Excipient information presented when available (limited, particularly for generics); consult specific product labeling. [DSC] = Discontinued product

Foam, topical:

Epi-Clenz™: 62% (240 mL, 480 mL) [instant hand sanitizer; contains aloe vera and vitamin E]

Gel, topical:

Epi-Clenz™: 70% (45 mL, 120 mL, 480 mL) [instant hand sanitizer; contains aloe vera and vitamin E]

GelRite: 67% (120 mL, 480 mL, 800 mL) [instant hand sanitizer; contains vitamin E]

Gel-Stat™: 62% (120 mL, 480 mL) [instant hand sanitizer]

Isagel®: 60% (59 mL, 118 mL, 621 mL, 800 mL) [instant hand sanitizer]

Prevacare®: 60% (120 mL, 240 mL, 960 mL, 1200 mL, 1500 mL) [instant hand sanitizer]

Protection Plus®: 62% (800 mL) [instant hand sanitizer]

Purell®: 62% (15 mL, 30 mL, 59 mL, 120 mL, 236 mL, 250 mL, 360 mL, 500 mL, 800 mL, 1000 mL, 2000 mL) [instant hand sanitizer; contains moisturizers and vitamin E]

Purell® Lasting Care: 62% (120 mL, 240 mL, 1000 mL) [contains moisturizers]

Purell® Moisture Therapy: 62% (75 mL) [instant hand sanitizer]

Purell® with Aloe: 62% (15 mL, 59 mL, 236 mL, 360 mL, 800 mL, 1000 mL, 2000 mL) [instant hand sanitizer; contains aloe and tartrazine]

Infusion [in D_5W, dehydrated]: Alcohol 5% (1000 mL) [DSC]

Injection, solution [dehydrated]: 98% (1 mL, 5 mL)

Liquid, topical [denatured]: 70% (3840 mL)

Lavacol®: 70% (473 mL)

Lotion, topical:

Purell® 2 in 1: 62% (60 mL, 360 mL, 1000 mL) [instant hand sanitizer]

Towelettes, topical:

Isagel®: 60% (50s, 300s) [instant hand sanitizer]

Purell®: 62% (35s, 175s) [instant hand sanitizer]

References

Barceloux DG, Bond GR, Krenzelok EP, et al, "American Academy of Clinical Toxicology Practice Guidelines on the Treatment of Methanol Poisoning. Ad Hoc Committee," *J Toxicol Clin Toxicol*, 2002, 40(4):415-46.

Barceloux DG, Krenzelok EP, Olson K, et al, "American Academy of Clinical Toxicology Practice Guidelines on the Treatment of Ethylene Glycol Poisoning. Ad Hoc Committee," *J Toxicol Clin Toxicol*, 1999, 37(5):537-60.

Maron BJ, McKenna WJ, Danielson GK, et al, "American College of Cardiology/European Society of Cardiology Clinical Expert Consensus Document on Hypertrophic Cardiomyopathy. A Report of the American College of Cardiology Foundation Task Force on Clinical Expert Consensus Documents and the European Society of Cardiology Committee for Practice Guidelines," *J Am Coll Cardiol*, 2003, 42(9):1687-713.

Mokhlesi B, Leikin JB, Murray P, et al, "Adult Toxicology in Critical Care. Part 11:Specific Poisonings," *Chest*, 2003, 123(3):897-922.

Seggewiss H, Gleichmann U, Faber L, et al, "Percutaneous Transluminal Septal Myocardial Ablation in Hypertrophic Obstructive Cardiomyopathy: Acute Results and 3-Month Follow-Up in 25 Patients," *J Am Coll Cardiol*, 1998, 31(2):252-8.

♦ **Alcomicin® (Can)** *see* Gentamicin *on page 658*

♦ **Aldomet** *see* Methyldopa *on page 901*

Alendronate (a LEN droe nate)

Related Information
Anesthesia for Geriatric Patients *on page 1523*

U.S. Brand Names Fosamax®

Canadian Brand Names
Apo-Alendronate®; CO Alendronate; Dom-Alendronate; Fosamax®; Gen-Alendronate; Mylan-Alendronate; Novo-Alendronate; PHL-Alendronate; PHL-Alendronate-FC; PMS-Alendronate; PMS-Alendronate-FC; ratio-Alendronate; Riva-Alendronate; Sandoz Alendronate

Index Terms
Alendronate Sodium; Alendronic Acid Monosodium Salt Trihydrate; MK-217

Pharmacologic Category
Bisphosphonate Derivative

Use
Treatment and prevention of osteoporosis in postmenopausal females; treatment of osteoporosis in males; Paget's disease of the bone in patients who are symptomatic, at risk for future complications, or with alkaline phosphatase ≥2 times the upper limit of normal; treatment of glucocorticoid-induced osteoporosis in males and females with low bone mineral density who are receiving a daily dosage ≥7.5 mg of prednisone (or equivalent)

Pharmacodynamics/Kinetics
Distribution: 28 L (exclusive of bone)
Protein binding: ~78%
Metabolism: None
Bioavailability: Fasting: 0.6%; reduced 60% with food or drink
Half-life elimination: Exceeds 10 years
Excretion: Urine; feces (as unabsorbed drug)

Dosage
Oral: Adults: **Note:** Patients treated with glucocorticoids and those with Paget's disease should receive adequate amounts of calcium and vitamin D.

Osteoporosis in postmenopausal females:
Prophylaxis: 5 mg once daily **or** 35 mg once weekly
Treatment: 10 mg once daily **or** 70 mg once weekly

Osteoporosis in males: 10 mg once daily **or** 70 mg once weekly

Osteoporosis secondary to glucocorticoids in males and females: Treatment: 5 mg once daily; a dose of 10 mg once daily should be used in postmenopausal females who are not receiving estrogen.

Paget's disease of bone in males and females: 40 mg once daily for 6 months
Retreatment: Relapses during the 12 months following therapy occurred in 9% of patients who responded to treatment. Specific retreatment data are not available. Following a 6-month post-treatment evaluation period, retreatment with alendronate may be considered in patients who have relapsed based on increases in serum alkaline phosphatase, which should be measured periodically. Retreatment may also be considered in those who failed to normalize their serum alkaline phosphatase.

Elderly: No dosage adjustment is necessary

Dosage adjustment in renal impairment:
Cl_{cr} 35-60 mL/minute: None necessary
Cl_{cr} <35 mL/minute: Alendronate is not recommended due to lack of experience

Dosage adjustment in hepatic impairment: None necessary

Additional Information
Complete prescribing information for this medication should be consulted for additional detail.

Dosage Forms
Excipient information presented when available (limited, particularly for generics); consult specific product labeling.
Solution, oral:
Fosamax®: 70 mg/75 mL (75 mL) [raspberry flavor]
Tablet: 5 mg, 10 mg, 35 mg, 40 mg, 70 mg
Fosamax®: 5 mg, 10 mg, 35 mg, 40 mg, 70 mg

References

Author Unknown, "Safety Update: Bone-Building Drugs: Risks Explained," *Consum Rep Health*, 2006, 18(5):3.

Chesnut CH 3rd, McClung MR, Ensrud KE, et al, "Alendronate Treatment of the Postmenopausal Osteoporatic Woman: Effect of Multiple Dosages on Bone Mass and Bone Remodeling," *Am J Med*, 1995, 99(2):144-52.

French AE, Kaplan N, Lishner M, et al, "Taking Bisphosphonates During Pregnancy," *Can Fam Physician*, 2003, 49:1281-2.

Orwoll E, Ettinger M, Weiss S, et al, "Alendronate for the Treatment of Osteoporosis in Men," *N Engl J Med*, 2000, 343(9):604-10.

Marx RE, Sawatari Y, Fortin M, et al, "Bisphosphonate-Induced Exposed Bone (Osteonecrosis/Osteopetrosis) of the Jaws: Risk Factors, Recognition, Prevention, and Treatment," *J Oral Maxillofac Surg*, 2005, 63(11):1567-75.

Mavrokokki T, Cheng A, Stein B, et al, "Nature and Frequency of Bisphosphonate-Associated Osteonecrosis of the Jaws in Australia," *J Oral Maxillofac Surg*, 2007, 65(3):415-23.

Watts NB, "Treatment of Osteoporosis With Bisphosphonates," *Rheum Dis Clin North Am*, 1994, 20 (3):717-34.

◆ **Alendronate Sodium** *see* Alendronate *on page 57*

◆ **Alendronic Acid Monosodium Salt Trihydrate** *see* Alendronate *on page 57*

◆ **Aler-Cap [OTC]** *see* DiphenhydrAMINE *on page 430*

◆ **Aler-Dryl [OTC]** *see* DiphenhydrAMINE *on page 430*

◆ **Aler-Tab [OTC]** *see* DiphenhydrAMINE *on page 430*

◆ **Alertec® (Can)** *see* Modafinil *on page 947*

◆ **Alesse®** *see* Ethinyl Estradiol and Levonorgestrel *on page 549*

◆ **Aleve® [OTC]** *see* Naproxen *on page 987*

◆ **Alfenta®** *see* Alfentanil *on page 58*

Alfentanil (al FEN ta nil)

Medication Safety Issues

Sound-alike/look-alike issues:

Alfentanil may be confused with Anafranil®, fentanyl, remifentanil, sufentanil

Alfenta® may be confused with Sufenta®

High alert medication: The Institute for Safe Medication Practices (ISMP) includes this medication among its list of drug classes which have a heightened risk of causing significant patient harm when used in error.

Related Information

Anesthesia Considerations for Neurosurgery *on page 1514*

Anesthesia for Patients With Liver Disease *on page 1537*

Chronic Renal Failure *on page 1552*

Opioids *on page 1641*

U.S. Brand Names Alfenta®

Canadian Brand Names Alfentanil Injection, USP; Alfenta®

Index Terms Alfentanil Hydrochloride

Pharmacologic Category Analgesic, Opioid; Anilidopiperidine Opioid

Restrictions C-II

Generic Available Yes

Use Analgesic adjunct for the induction and maintenance of general anesthesia; analgesic component for monitored anesthesia care (MAC)

Mechanism of Action Binds with stereospecific receptors at many sites within the CNS, increases pain threshold, alters pain perception, inhibits ascending pain pathways; is an ultra short-acting narcotic

Pharmacodynamics/Kinetics

Onset of action: Rapid

Duration (dose dependent): 30-60 minutes

Distribution: V_d: Newborns, premature: 1 L/kg; Children: 0.163-0.48 L/kg; Adults: 0.46 L/kg

Half-life elimination: Newborns, premature: 5.33-8.75 hours; Children: 40-60 minutes; Adults: 83-97 minutes

Dosage Doses should be titrated to appropriate effects; wide range of doses is dependent upon desired degree of analgesia/anesthesia

Children <12 years: Dose not established

Adults: Dose should be based on ideal body weight as follows (see table):

Alfentanil

Indication	Approx Duration of Anesthesia (min)	Induction Period (Initial Dose) (mcg/kg)	Maintenance Period (Increments/ Infusion)	Total Dose (mcg/kg)	Effects
Incremental injection	≤30	8-20	3-5 mcg/kg or 0.5-1 mcg/kg/min	8-40	Spontaneously breathing or assisted ventilation when required.
	30-60	20-50	5-15 mcg/kg	Up to 75	Assisted or controlled ventilation required. Attenuation of response to laryngoscopy and intubation.
Continuous infusion	>45	50-75	0.5-3 mcg/kg/ min; average infusion rate 1-1.5 mcg/kg/min	Dependent on duration of procedure	Assisted or controlled ventilation required. Some attenuation of response to intubation and incision, with intraoperative stability.
Anesthetic induction	>45	130-245	0.5-1.5 mcg/kg/min or general anesthetic	Dependent on duration of procedure	Assisted or controlled ventilation required. Administer slowly (over 3 minutes). Concentration of inhalation agents reduced by 30% to 50% for initial hour.

Stability Store unopened ampuls at 20°C to 25°C (68°F to 77°F). Protect from light. For infusion, dilute in D_5W, NS, LR, or D_5NS to a concentration of 25-80 mcg/mL.

Administration Administer I.V. slowly over 3-5 minutes or by I.V. continuous infusion.

Monitoring Parameters Respiratory rate, blood pressure, heart rate

Reference Range 100-340 ng/mL (depending upon procedure)

Anesthesia and Critical Care Concerns/Other Considerations

Clinical Pearls/Comments: Alfentanil may produce more muscle rigidity compared to fentanyl; therefore, be sure to administer slowly. Alfentanil demonstrates synergistic respiratory depression when combined with benzodiazepines.

Pregnancy Risk Factor C

Contraindications Hypersensitivity to alfentanil hydrochloride, to narcotics, or any component of the formulation; increased intracranial pressure, severe respiratory depression

Warnings/Precautions Use with caution in patients with drug dependence, head injury, morbid obesity, acute asthma and respiratory conditions; hypotension has occurred in neonates with respiratory distress syndrome; use caution when administering to patients with bradyarrhythmias; inject slowly over 3-5 minutes (apid I.V. infusion may result in skeletal muscle and chest wall rigidity, impaired ventilation, or respiratory distress/arrest); use of a nondepolarizing skeletal muscle relaxant may be required. Alfentanil may produce more hypotension compared to fentanyl, therefore, administer slowly and ensure patient has adequate hydration. Shares the toxic potentials of opiate agonists, and precautions of opiate agonist therapy should be observed. Should be administered by trained individuals. Safety and efficacy have not been established in children <12 years old.

Adverse Reactions

>10%:

Cardiovascular: Bradycardia, peripheral vasodilation

Central nervous system: Drowsiness, sedation, intracranial pressure increased

Endocrine & metabolic: Antidiuretic hormone release

Gastrointestinal: Nausea, vomiting, constipation

Ocular: Miosis

1% to 10%:

Cardiovascular: Cardiac arrhythmia, orthostatic hypotension

Central nervous system: Confusion, CNS depression

Ocular: Blurred vision

<1% (Limited to important or life-threatening): Convulsions, mental depression, paradoxical CNS excitation or delirium, dizziness, dysesthesia, rash, urticaria, itching, biliary tract spasm, urinary tract spasm, respiratory depression, bronchospasm, laryngospasm, physical and psychological dependence with prolonged use; cold, clammy skin

Drug Interactions

Metabolism/Transport Effects Substrate of CYP3A4 (major)

Avoid Concomitant Use

Avoid concomitant use of Alfentanil with any of the following: MAO Inhibitors

Increased Effect/Toxicity

Alfentanil may increase the levels/effects of: Alcohol (Ethyl); Alvimopan; Beta-Blockers; Calcium Channel Blockers (Nondihydropyridine); CNS Depressants; Desmopressin; Fospropofol; MAO Inhibitors; Propofol; Selective Serotonin Reuptake Inhibitors; Thiazide Diuretics

The levels/effects of Alfentanil may be increased by: Amphetamines; Antifungal Agents (Azole Derivatives, Systemic); Antipsychotic Agents (Phenothiazines); Cimetidine; CYP3A4 Inhibitors (Moderate); CYP3A4 Inhibitors (Strong); Dasatinib; Diltiazem; Fluconazole; Macrolide Antibiotics; MAO Inhibitors; Succinylcholine

Decreased Effect

Alfentanil may decrease the levels/effects of: Pegvisomant

The levels/effects of Alfentanil may be decreased by: Ammonium Chloride; Rifamycin Derivatives

Dosage Forms Excipient information presented when available (limited, particularly for generics); consult specific product labeling.

Injection, solution [preservative free]: 500 mcg/mL (2 mL, 5 mL)

Alfenta®: 500 mcg/mL (2 mL, 5 mL, 10 mL, 20 mL)

References

Bartkowski RR and McDonnell TE, "Prolonged Alfentanil Effect Following Erythromycin Administration," *Anesthesiology,* 1990, 73(3):566-8.

Bartkowski RR, Goldberg ME, Larijani GE, et al, "Inhibition of Alfentanil Metabolism by Erythromycin," *Clin Pharmacol Ther,* 1989, 46(1):99-102.

Bodenham A and Park GR, "Alfentanil Infusions in Patients Requiring Intensive Care," *Clin Pharmacokinet,* 1988, 15(4):216-26.

Davis PJ, Killian A, Stiller RL, et al, "Pharmacokinetics of Alfentanil in Newborn Premature Infants and Older Children," *Dev Pharmacol Ther,* 1989, 13(1):21-7.

Kirkham SR and Pugh R, "Opioid Analgesia in Uraemic Patients," *Lancet,* 1995, 345(8958):1185.

Marlow N, Weindling AM, Van Peer A, et al, "Alfentanil Pharmacokinetics in Preterm Infants," *Arch Dis Child,* 1990, 65(4 Spec No):349-51.

Meistelman C, Saint-Maurice C, Lepaul M, et al, "A Comparison of Alfentanil Pharmacokinetics in Children and Adults," *Anesthesiology,* 1987, 66(1):13-6.

Mokhlesi B, Leikin JB, Murray P, et al, "Adult Toxicology in Critical Care. Part 11: Specific Poisonings," *Chest,* 2003, 123(3):897-922.

Pokela ML, Ryhanen PT, Koivisto ME, et al, "Alfentanil-Induced Rigidity in Newborn Infants," *Anesth Analg,* 1992, 75(2):252-7.

Scholz J, Steinfath M, and Schulz M, "Clinical Pharmacokinetics of Alfentanil, Fentanyl, and Sufentanil. An Update," *Clin Pharmacokinet,* 1996, 31(4):275-92.

◆ **Alfentanil Hydrochloride** see Alfentanil *on page 58*

◆ **Alfentanil Injection, USP (Can)** see Alfentanil *on page 58*

Aliskiren (a lis KYE ren)

Related Information
Angiotensin Agents *on page 1652*
U.S. Brand Names Tekturna®
Canadian Brand Names Rasilez®
Index Terms Aliskiren Hemifumarate; SPP100
Pharmacologic Category Renin Inhibitor
Use Treatment of hypertension, alone or in combination with other antihypertensive agents
Unlabeled/Investigational Use Treatment of persistent proteinuria in patients with type 2 diabetes mellitus, hypertension, and nephropathy despite administration of optimized recommended renoprotective therapy (eg, angiotensin II receptor blocker)
Pharmacodynamics/Kinetics
Onset of action: Maximum antihypertensive effect: Within 2 weeks
Absorption: Poor; absorption decreased by high-fat meal. Aliskiren is a substrate of P-glycoprotein; concurrent use of P-glycoprotein inhibitors may increase absorption.
Metabolism: Extent of metabolism unknown; *in vitro* studies indicate metabolism via CYP3A4
Bioavailability: ~3%
Half-life elimination: ~24 hours (range: 16-32 hours)
Time to peak, plasma: 1-3 hours
Excretion: Urine (~25% of absorbed dose excreted unchanged in urine); feces (unchanged via biliary excretion)
Dosage Oral:
Adults: Initial: 150 mg once daily; may increase to 300 mg once daily (maximum: 300 mg/day). **Note:** Prior to initiation, correct hypovolemia and/or closely monitor volume status in patients on concurrent diuretics during treatment initiation.
Elderly: No initial dosage adjustment required

Dosage adjustment in renal impairment
Mild-to-moderate impairment [GFR >30 mL/minute and/or S_{cr} <1.7 mg/dL (women); S_{cr} <2 mg/dL (men)]: No dose adjustment required
Severe impairment [GFR<30 mL/minute and/or S_{cr} >1.7 mg/dL (women); S_{cr} >2 mg/dL (men)]: Use caution; not studied in severe renal impairment
Dosage adjustment in hepatic impairment No dosage adjustment required
Additional Information Complete prescribing information for this medication should be consulted for additional detail.
Dosage Forms Excipient information presented when available (limited, particularly for generics); consult specific product labeling.
Tablet:
Tekturna®: 150 mg, 300 mg
References
Straessen JA, Li Y, and Richart T, "Oral Renin Inhibitors," *Lancet*, 2006, 368(9545):1449-56.
Vaidyanathan S, Warren V, Yeh C, et al, "Pharmacokinetics, Safety, and Tolerability of the Oral Renin Inhibitor Aliskiren in Patients With Hepatic Impairment," *J Clin Pharmacol*, 2007, 47(2):192-200.

Allopurinol (al oh PURE i nole)

Related Information
Chronic Renal Failure *on page 1552*
Desensitization Protocols *on page 1692*

U.S. Brand Names Aloprim®; Zyloprim®

Canadian Brand Names Alloprin®; Apo-Allopurinol®; Novo-Purol; Zyloprim®

Index Terms Allopurinol Sodium

Pharmacologic Category Xanthine Oxidase Inhibitor

Use

Oral: Prevention of attack of gouty arthritis and nephropathy; treatment of secondary hyperuricemia which may occur during treatment of tumors or leukemia; prevention of recurrent calcium oxalate calculi

I.V.: Treatment of elevated serum and urinary uric acid levels when oral therapy is not tolerated in patients with leukemia, lymphoma, and solid tumor malignancies who are receiving cancer chemotherapy

Pharmacodynamics/Kinetics

Onset of action: Peak effect: 1-2 weeks

Absorption: Oral: ~80%; Rectal: Poor and erratic

Distribution: V_d: ~1.6 L/kg; V_{ss}: 0.84-0.87 L/kg; enters breast milk

Protein binding: <1%

Metabolism: ~75% to active metabolites, chiefly oxypurinol

Bioavailability: 49% to 53%

Half-life elimination:
  Normal renal function: Parent drug: 1-3 hours; Oxypurinol: 18-30 hours
  End-stage renal disease: Prolonged

Time to peak, plasma: Oral: 30-120 minutes

Excretion: Urine (76% as oxypurinol, 12% as unchanged drug)

Allopurinol and oxypurinol are dialyzable

Dosage

Oral: Doses >300 mg should be given in divided doses.

Children ≤10 years: Secondary hyperuricemia associated with chemotherapy: 10 mg/kg/day in 2-3 divided doses **or** 200-300 mg/m^2/day in 2-4 divided doses, maximum: 800 mg/24 hours

  Alternative (manufacturer labeling): <6 years: 150 mg/day in 3 divided doses; 6-10 years: 300 mg/day in 2-3 divided doses

Children >10 years and Adults:

  Secondary hyperuricemia associated with chemotherapy: 600-800 mg/day in 2-3 divided doses for prevention of acute uric acid nephropathy for 2-3 days starting 1-2 days before chemotherapy

  Gout: Mild: 200-300 mg/day; Severe: 400-600 mg/day; to reduce the possibility of acute gouty attacks, initiate dose at 100 mg/day and increase weekly to recommended dosage. Maximum daily dose: 800 mg/day.

  Recurrent calcium oxalate stones: 200-300 mg/day in single or divided doses

Elderly: Initial: 100 mg/day, increase until desired uric acid level is obtained

I.V.: Hyperuricemia secondary to chemotherapy: Intravenous daily dose can be given as a single infusion or in equally divided doses at 6-, 8-, or 12-hour intervals. A fluid intake sufficient to yield a daily urinary output of at least 2 L in adults and the maintenance of a neutral or, preferably, slightly alkaline urine are desirable.

Children ≤10 years: Starting dose: 200 mg/m^2/day

Children >10 years and Adults: 200-400 mg/m^2/day (maximum: 600 mg/day)

Dosing adjustment in renal impairment: Must be adjusted due to accumulation of allopurinol and metabolites:

Oral: Removed by hemodialysis; adult maintenance doses of allopurinol (mg) based on creatinine clearance (mL/minute): See table on next page.

Adult Maintenance Doses of Allopurinol[1]

Creatinine Clearance (mL/min)	Maintenance Dose of Allopurinol (mg)
140	400 daily
120	350 daily
100	300 daily
80	250 daily
60	200 daily
40	150 daily
20	100 daily
10	100 every 2 days
0	100 every 3 days

[1]This table is based on a standard maintenance dose of 300 mg of allopurinol per day for a patient with a creatinine clearance of 100 mL/min.

I.V.:
Cl_{cr} 10-20 mL/minute: 200 mg/day
Cl_{cr} 3-10 mL/minute: 100 mg/day
Cl_{cr} <3 mL/minute: 100 mg/day at extended intervals

Hemodialysis: Administer dose posthemodialysis or administer 50% supplemental dose

Additional Information Complete prescribing information for this medication should be consulted for additional detail.

Dosage Forms Excipient information presented when available (limited, particularly for generics); consult specific product labeling.

Injection, powder for reconstitution, as sodium: 500 mg (base)
Aloprim®: 500 mg (base)
Tablet: 100 mg, 300 mg
Zyloprim®: 100 mg, 300 mg

◆ **Allopurinol Sodium** see Allopurinol on page 62

Almotriptan (al moh TRIP tan)

U.S. Brand Names Axert®
Canadian Brand Names Axert®
Index Terms Almotriptan Malate
Pharmacologic Category Antimigraine Agent; Serotonin 5-HT$_{1B, 1D}$ Receptor Agonist
Use Acute treatment of migraine with or without aura in adults (with a history of migraine) and adolescents (with a history of migraine lasting ≥4 hours when left untreated)
Pharmacodynamics/Kinetics
Absorption: Well absorbed
Distribution: V_d: ~180-200 L
Protein binding: ~35%
Metabolism: Via MAO type A oxidative deamination (~27% of dose) and CYP3A4 and 2D6 (~12% of dose) to inactive metabolites
Bioavailability: ~70%
Half-life elimination: 3-4 hours
Time to peak, plasma: 1-3 hours
Excretion: Urine (~75%; ~40% of total dose as unchanged drug); feces (~13% of total dose as unchanged drug and metabolites)
Dosage Oral: Children ≥12 years and Adults: Migraine: Initial: 6.25-12.5 mg in a single dose; if the headache returns, repeat the dose after 2 hours (maximum daily dose: 25 mg)

◀ **Note:** The safety of treating more than 4 migraines/month has not been established.

Dosage adjustment with concomitant use of an enzyme inhibitor:
Patients receiving a potent CYP3A4 inhibitor: Initial: 6.25 mg in a single dose; maximum daily dose: 12.5 mg

Patients with renal impairment and concomitant use of a potent CYP3A4 inhibitor: Avoid use

Patients with hepatic impairment and concomitant use of a potent CYP3A4 inhibitor: Avoid use

Dosage adjustment in renal impairment: Severe renal impairment (Cl_{cr} ≤30 mL/minute): Initial: 6.25 mg in a single dose; maximum daily dose: 12.5 mg

Dosage adjustment in hepatic impairment: Initial: 6.25 mg in a single dose; maximum daily dose: 12.5 mg

Anesthesia and Critical Care Concerns/Other Considerations Almotriptan should not be used in patients with a history of vasospastic disease, Prinzmetal's angina, or any critical vascular disease.

Additional Information Complete prescribing information for this medication should be consulted for additional detail.

Dosage Forms Excipient information presented when available (limited, particularly for generics); consult specific product labeling.
Tablet, as malate:
Axert®: 6.25 mg, 12.5 mg

◆ **Almotriptan Malate** *see Almotriptan on page 63*
◆ **Alodox™** *see Doxycycline on page 456*
◆ **Aloprim®** *see Allopurinol on page 62*
◆ **Alora®** *see Estradiol on page 531*
◆ **Aloxi®** *see Palonosetron on page 1079*
◆ **AlphaNine® SD** *see Factor IX on page 570*

ALPRAZolam (al PRAY zoe lam)

Related Information
Antidepressant Agents *on page 1660*
Benzodiazepines *on page 1666*

U.S. Brand Names Alprazolam Intensol®; Niravam™; Xanax XR®; Xanax®

Canadian Brand Names Alti-Alprazolam; Apo-Alpraz®; Apo-Alpraz® TS; Gen-Alprazolam; Mylan-Alprazolam; Novo-Alprazol; Nu-Alprax; Xanax TS™; Xanax®

Pharmacologic Category Benzodiazepine

Restrictions C-IV

Use Treatment of anxiety disorder (GAD); panic disorder, with or without agoraphobia; anxiety associated with depression

Unlabeled/Investigational Use Anxiety in children

Pharmacodynamics/Kinetics
Onset of action: Immediate release and extended release formulations: 1 hour
Duration: Immediate release: 5.1 ± 1.7 hours; Extended release: 11.3 ± 4.2 hours
Absorption: Extended release: Slower relative to immediate release formulation resulting in a concentration that is maintained 5-11 hours after dosing
Distribution: V_d: 0.9-1.2 L/kg; enters breast milk
Protein binding: 80%; primarily to albumin
Metabolism: Hepatic via CYP3A4; forms two active metabolites (4-hydroxyalprazolam and α-hydroxyalprazolam)
Bioavailability: 90%
Half-life elimination:
Adults: 11.2 hours (immediate release range: 6.3-26.9; extended release range: 10.7-15.8)
Elderly: 16.3 hours (range: 9-26.9 hours)
Alcoholic liver disease: 19.7 hours (range: 5.8-65.3 hours)
Obesity: 21.8 hours (range: 9.9-40.4 hours)

Time to peak, serum: Immediate release: 1-2 hours; Extended release: ~9 hours; decreased by 1 hour following bedtime dosing compared to morning dosing

Excretion: Urine (as unchanged drug and metabolites)

Dosage Oral: **Note:** Treatment >4 months should be re-evaluated to determine the patient's continued need for the drug

Children: Anxiety (unlabeled use): Immediate release: Initial: 0.005 mg/kg/dose or 0.125 mg/dose 3 times/day; increase in increments of 0.125-0.25 mg, up to a maximum of 0.02 mg/kg/dose or 0.06 mg/kg/day (0.375-3 mg/day). See "Dose Reduction" comment below.

Adults:

Anxiety: Immediate release: Effective doses are 0.5-4 mg/day in divided doses; the manufacturer recommends starting at 0.25-0.5 mg 3 times/day; titrate dose upward; usual maximum: 4 mg/day. Patients requiring doses >4 mg/day should be increased cautiously. Periodic reassessment and consideration of dosage reduction is recommended.

Anxiety associated with depression: Immediate release: Average dose required: 2.5-3 mg/day in divided doses

Ethanol withdrawal (unlabeled use): Immediate release: Usual dose: 2-2.5 mg/day in divided doses

Panic disorder:

Immediate release: Initial: 0.5 mg 3 times/day; dose may be increased every 3-4 days in increments ≤1 mg/day. Mean effective dosage: 5-6 mg/day; many patients obtain relief at 2 mg/day, as much as 10 mg/day may be required

Extended release: 0.5-1 mg once daily; may increase dose every 3-4 days in increments ≤1 mg/day (range: 3-6 mg/day)

Switching from immediate release to extended release: Patients may be switched to extended release tablets by taking the total daily dose of the immediate release tablets and giving it once daily using the extended release preparation.

Preoperative sedation: 0.5 mg in evening at bedtime and 0.5 mg 1 hour before procedure

Dose reduction: Abrupt discontinuation should be avoided. Daily dose may be decreased by 0.5 mg every 3 days, however, some patients may require a slower reduction. If withdrawal symptoms occur, resume previous dose and discontinue on a less rapid schedule.

Elderly: Initial: 0.125-0.25 mg twice daily; increase by 0.125 mg/day as needed. The smallest effective dose should be used. **Note:** Elderly patients may be more sensitive to the effects of alprazolam including ataxia and oversedation. The elderly may also have impaired renal function leading to decreased clearance. Titrate gradually, if needed.

Immediate release: Initial: 0.25 mg 2-3 times/day

Extended release: Initial: 0.5 mg once daily

Dosing adjustment in renal impairment: No guidelines for adjustment; use caution

Dosing adjustment in hepatic impairment: Reduce dose by 50% to 60% or avoid in cirrhosis

Anesthesia and Critical Care Concerns/Other Considerations Chronic use of this agent may increase the perioperative benzodiazepine dose needed to achieve desired effect. Patients who become physically dependent on alprazolam tend to have a difficult time discontinuing it; withdrawal symptoms may be severe. To minimize withdrawal symptoms, taper dosage slowly; do not discontinue abruptly. Abrupt discontinuation after sustained use (generally >10 days) may cause withdrawal symptoms.

Additional Information Complete prescribing information for this medication should be consulted for additional detail.

Dosage Forms Excipient information presented when available (limited, particularly for generics); consult specific product labeling.

Solution, oral [concentrate]:

Alprazolam Intensol®: 1 mg/mL (30 mL) [alcohol free, dye free, sugar free; contains propylene glycol]

Tablet: 0.25 mg, 0.5 mg, 1 mg, 2 mg

Xanax®: 0.25 mg, 0.5 mg, 1 mg, 2 mg

Tablet, extended release: 0.5 mg, 1 mg, 2 mg, 3 mg

Xanax XR®: 0.5 mg, 1 mg, 2 mg, 3 mg

Tablet, orally disintegrating [scored]: 0.25 mg, 0.5 mg, 1 mg, 2 mg
Niravam™: 0.25 mg, 0.5 mg, 1 mg, 2 mg [orange flavor]

◆ **Alprazolam Intensol®** *see ALPRAZolam on page 64*

Alprostadil (al PROS ta dill)

U.S. Brand Names Caverject Impulse®; Caverject®; Edex®; Muse®; Prostin VR
Pediatric®
Canadian Brand Names Caverject®; Muse® Pellet; Prostin® VR
Index Terms PGE$_1$; Prostaglandin E$_1$
Pharmacologic Category Prostaglandin; Vasodilator
Use
Prostin VR Pediatric®: Temporary maintenance of patency of ductus arteriosus in
neonates with ductal-dependent congenital heart disease until surgery can be
performed. These defects include cyanotic (eg, pulmonary atresia, pulmonary
stenosis, tricuspid atresia, Fallot's tetralogy, transposition of the great vessels)
and acyanotic (eg, interruption of aortic arch, coarctation of aorta, hypoplastic
left ventricle) heart disease.
Caverject®: Treatment of erectile dysfunction of vasculogenic, psychogenic, or
neurogenic etiology; adjunct in the diagnosis of erectile dysfunction
Edex®, Muse®: Treatment of erectile dysfunction of vasculogenic, psychogenic,
or neurogenic etiology
Unlabeled/Investigational Use Investigational: Treatment of pulmonary hyper-
tension in infants and children with congenital heart defects with left-to-right
shunts
Pharmacodynamics/Kinetics
Onset of action: Rapid
Duration: <1 hour
Distribution: Insignificant following penile injection
Protein binding, plasma: 81% to albumin
Metabolism: ~75% by oxidation in one pass via lungs
Half-life elimination: 5-10 minutes
Excretion: Urine (90% as metabolites) within 24 hours
Dosage
Patent ductus arteriosus (Prostin VR Pediatric®):
I.V. continuous infusion into a large vein, or alternatively through an umbilical
artery catheter placed at the ductal opening: 0.05-0.1 mcg/kg/minute with
therapeutic response, rate is reduced to lowest effective dosage; with
unsatisfactory response, rate is increased gradually; maintenance: 0.01-0.4
mcg/kg/minute
PGE$_1$ is usually given at an infusion rate of 0.1 mcg/kg/minute, but it is often
possible to reduce the dosage to $1/2$ or even $1/10$ without losing the therapeutic
effect. The mixing schedule is as follows. See table.

Alprostadil

Add 1 Ampul (500 mcg) to:	Concentration (mcg/mL)	Infusion Rate	
		mL/min/kg Needed to Infuse 0.1 mcg/kg/min	mL/kg/24 h
250 mL	2	0.05	72
100 mL	5	0.02	28.8
50 mL	10	0.01	14.4
25 mL	20	0.005	7.2

Therapeutic response is indicated by increased pH in those with acidosis or by
an increase in oxygenation (PO$_2$) usually evident within 30 minutes
Erectile dysfunction:
Caverject®, Edex®: Intracavernous: Individualize dose by careful titration;
doses >40 mcg (Edex®) or >60 mcg (Caverject®) are not recommended: Initial
dose must be titrated in physician's office. Patient must stay in the physician's
office until complete detumescence occurs; if there is no response, then the
next higher dose may be given within 1 hour; if there is still no response, a

1-day interval before giving the next dose is recommended; increasing the dose or concentration in the treatment of impotence results in increasing pain and discomfort

Vasculogenic, psychogenic, or mixed etiology: Initiate dosage titration at 2.5 mcg, increasing by 2.5 mcg to a dose of 5 mcg and then in increments of 5-10 mcg depending on the erectile response until the dose produces an erection suitable for intercourse, not lasting >1 hour; if there is absolutely no response to initial 2.5 mcg dose, the second dose may be increased to 7.5 mcg, followed by increments of 5-10 mcg

Neurogenic etiology (eg, spinal cord injury): Initiate dosage titration at 1.25 mcg, increasing to a dose of 2.5 mcg and then 5 mcg; increase further in increments 5 mcg until the dose is reached that produces an erection suitable for intercourse, not lasting >1 hour

Maintenance: Once appropriate dose has been determined, patient may self-administer injections at a frequency of no more than 3 times/week with at least 24 hours between doses

Muse® Pellet: Intraurethral:

Initial: 125-250 mcg

Maintenance: Administer as needed to achieve an erection; duration of action is about 30-60 minutes; use only two systems per 24-hour period

Elderly: Elderly patients may have a greater frequency of renal dysfunction; lowest effective dose should be used. In clinical studies with Edex®, higher minimally effective doses and a higher rate of lack of effect were noted.

Additional Information Complete prescribing information for this medication should be consulted for additional detail.

Dosage Forms Excipient information presented when available (limited, particularly for generics); consult specific product labeling. [DSC] = Discontinued product

Injection, powder for reconstitution:

Caverject®: 20 mcg, 40 mcg [contains lactose; diluent contains benzyl alcohol]

Caverject Impulse®: 10 mcg, 20 mcg [prefilled injection system; contains lactose; diluent contains benzyl alcohol]

Edex®: 10 mcg, 20 mcg, 40 mcg [contains lactose; packaged in kits containing diluent, syringe, and alcohol swab]

Injection, solution: 500 mcg/mL (1 mL)

Prostin VR Pediatric®: 500 mcg/mL (1 mL) [contains dehydrated alcohol]

Pellet, urethral:

Muse®: 125 mcg (6s) [DSC], 250 mcg (6s), 500 mcg (6s), 1000 mcg (6s)

♦ **Alrex®** see Loteprednol on page 859

♦ **Altace®** see Ramipril on page 1229

♦ **Altachlore [OTC]** see Sodium Chloride on page 1304

♦ **Altafrin** see Phenylephrine on page 1114

♦ **Altamist [OTC]** see Sodium Chloride on page 1304

♦ **Altaryl [OTC]** see DiphenhydrAMINE on page 430

Alteplase (AL te plase)

Medication Safety Issues

Sound-alike/look-alike issues:

Activase® may be confused with Cathflo® Activase®, TNKase®

Alteplase may be confused with Altace®

"tPA" abbreviation should not be used when writing orders for this medication; has been misread as TNKase (tenecteplase)

High alert medication: The Institute for Safe Medication Practices (ISMP) includes this medication (I.V.) among its list of drugs which have a heightened risk of causing significant patient harm when used in error.

Related Information

Anesthesia Considerations for Neurosurgery on page 1514

U.S. Brand Names Activase®; Cathflo® Activase®

Canadian Brand Names Activase® rt-PA; Cathflo® Activase®

◀ **Index Terms** Alteplase, Recombinant; Alteplase, Tissue Plasminogen Activator, Recombinant; tPA

Pharmacologic Category Thrombolytic Agent

Generic Available No

Use Management of ST-elevation myocardial infarction (STEMI) for the lysis of thrombi in coronary arteries; management of acute ischemic stroke (AIS); management of acute pulmonary embolism

Recommended criteria for treatment:

STEMI: Chest pain ≥20 minutes duration, onset of chest pain within 12 hours of treatment (or within prior 12-24 hours in patients with continuing ischemic symptoms), and ST-segment elevation >0.1 mV in at least two contiguous precordial leads or two adjacent limb leads on ECG or new or presumably new left bundle branch block (LBBB)

AIS: Onset of stroke symptoms within 3 hours of treatment

Acute pulmonary embolism: Age ≤75 years: Documented massive pulmonary embolism by pulmonary angiography or echocardiography or high probability lung scan with clinical shock

Cathflo® Activase®: Restoration of central venous catheter function

Unlabeled/Investigational Use Acute ischemic stroke presenting 3-4.5 hours after symptom onset; acute peripheral arterial occlusive disease

Mechanism of Action Initiates local fibrinolysis by binding to fibrin in a thrombus (clot) and converts entrapped plasminogen to plasmin

Pharmacodynamics/Kinetics

Duration: >50% present in plasma cleared ~5 minutes after infusion terminated, ~80% cleared within 10 minutes

Excretion: Clearance: Rapidly from circulating plasma (550-650 mL/minute), primarily hepatic; >50% present in plasma is cleared within 5 minutes after the infusion is terminated, ~80% cleared within 10 minutes

Dosage

I.V. (Activase®):

ST-elevation myocardial infarction (STEMI): Front loading dose (weight-based):

Patients >67 kg: Total dose: 100 mg over 1.5 hours; infuse 15 mg over 1-2 minutes. Infuse 50 mg over 30 minutes. Infuse remaining 35 mg of alteplase over the next hour. See **"Note."**

Patients ≤67 kg: Infuse 15 mg I.V. bolus over 1-2 minutes, then infuse 0.75 mg/kg (not to exceed 50 mg) over next 30 minutes, followed by 0.5 mg/kg over next 60 minutes (not to exceed 35 mg). See **"Note."**

Note: All patients should receive 162-325 mg of chewable nonenteric coated aspirin as soon as possible and then daily. Administer concurrently with heparin 60 units/kg bolus (maximum: 4000 units) followed by continuous infusion of 12 units/kg/hour (maximum: 1000 units/hour) and adjust to aPTT target of 50-70 seconds (or 1.5-2 times the upper limit of control).

Acute pulmonary embolism: 100 mg over 2 hours.

Acute ischemic stroke: Within 3 hours of the onset of symptom onset (labeled use) **or** within 3-4.5 hours of symptom onset (unlabeled use; del Zoppo, 2009; Hacke, 2008): **Note:** Initiation of anticoagulants (eg, heparin) or antiplatelet agents (eg, aspirin) within 24 hours after starting alteplase is not recommended; however, initiation of aspirin between 24-48 hours after stroke onset is recommended (Adams, 2007). Initiation of SubQ heparin (≤10,000 units) or equivalent doses of low molecular weight heparin for prevention of DVT during the first 24 hours of the 3-4.5 hour window trial did not increase incidence of intracerebral hemorrhage (Hacke, 2008).

Recommended total dose: 0.9 mg/kg (maximum total dose: 90 mg)

Patients ≤100 kg: Load with 0.09 mg/kg (10% of 0.9 mg/kg dose) as an I.V. bolus over 1 minute, followed by 0.81 mg/kg (90% of 0.9 mg/kg dose) as a continuous infusion over 60 minutes.

Patients >100 kg: Load with 9 mg (10% of 90 mg) as an I.V. bolus over 1 minute, followed by 81 mg (90% of 90 mg) as a continuous infusion over 60 minutes.

Intracatheter: Central venous catheter clearance (Cathflo® Activase® 1 mg/mL):

Patients <30 kg: 110% of the internal lumen volume of the catheter, not to exceed 2 mg/2 mL; retain in catheter for 0.5-2 hours; may instill a second dose if catheter remains occluded

Patients ≥30 kg: 2 mg (2 mL); retain in catheter for 0.5-2 hours; may instill a second dose if catheter remains occluded

Intra-arterial: Acute peripheral arterial occlusive disease (unlabeled use): 0.02-0.1 mg/kg/hour for up to 36 hours

Advisory Panel to the Society for Cardiovascular and Interventional Radiology on Thrombolytic Therapy recommendation: ≤2 mg/hour and subtherapeutic heparin (aPTT <1.5 times baseline)

Stability

Activase®: The lyophilized product may be stored at room temperature (not to exceed 30°C/86°F), or under refrigeration. Once reconstituted it should be used within 8 hours. Reconstitution:

50 mg vial: Use accompanying diluent (50 mL sterile water for injection); do not shake. Final concentration: 1 mg/mL.

100 mg vial: Use transfer set with accompanying diluent (100 mL vial of sterile water for injection); no vacuum is present in 100 mg vial; final concentration: 1 mg/mL.

Cathflo® Activase®: Store lyophilized product under refrigeration. To reconstitute, add 2.2 mL SWFI to vial; do not shake. Final concentration: 1 mg/mL. Once reconstituted, store at 2°C to 30°C (36°F to 86°F) and use within 8 hours. Do not mix other medications into infusion solution.

Administration

Activase®: ST-elevation MI: Accelerated infusion: Bolus dose may be prepared by one of three methods:

1) Removal of 15 mL reconstituted (1 mg/mL) solution from vial

2) Removal of 15 mL from a port on the infusion line after priming

3) Programming an infusion pump to deliver a 15 mL bolus at the initiation of infusion

Activase®: Acute ischemic stroke: Bolus dose (10% of total dose) may be prepared by one of three methods:

1) Removal of the appropriate volume from reconstituted solution (1 mg/mL)

2) Removal of the appropriate volume from a port on the infusion line after priming

3) Programming an infusion pump to deliver the appropriate volume at the initiation of infusion

Note: Remaining dose for STEMI, AIS, or total dose for acute pulmonary embolism may be administered as follows: Any quantity of drug not to be administered to the patient must be removed from vial(s) prior to administration of remaining dose.

50 mg vial: Either PVC bag or glass vial and infusion set

100 mg vial: Insert spike end of the infusion set through the same puncture site created by transfer device and infuse from vial

If further dilution is desired, may be diluted in equal volume of 0.9% sodium chloride or D_5W to yield a final concentration of 0.5 mg/mL.

Cathflo® Activase®: Intracatheter: Instill dose into occluded catheter. Do not force solution into catheter. After a 30-minute dwell time, assess catheter function by attempting to aspirate blood. If catheter is functional, aspirate 4-5 mL of blood in patients ≥10 kg or 3 mL in patients <10 kg to remove Cathflo® Activase® and residual clots. Gently irrigate the catheter with NS. If catheter remains nonfunctional, let Cathflo® Activase® dwell for another 90 minutes (total dwell time: 120 minutes) and reassess function. If catheter function is not restored, a second dose may be instilled.

Monitoring Parameters

Acute ischemic stroke: In addition to monitoring for bleeding complications, the 2007 AHA/ASA Guidelines for the early management of acute ischemic stroke recommends the following:

Perform neurological assessments every 15 minutes during infusion and every 30 minutes thereafter for the next 6 hours, then hourly until 24 hours after treatment.

If severe headache, acute hypertension, nausea, or vomiting occurs, discontinue the infusion and obtain emergency CT scan.

Measure BP every 15 minutes for the first 2 hours then every 30 minutes for the next 6 hours, then hourly until 24 hours after initiation of alteplase. Increase frequency if a systolic BP is ≥180 mm Hg or if a diastolic BP is ≥105 mm Hg; ▶

administer antihypertensive medications to maintain BP at or below these levels.

Obtain a follow-up CT scan at 24 hours before starting anticoagulants or antiplatelet agents.

Central venous catheter clearance: Assess catheter function by attempting to aspirate blood.

ST-elevation MI: Assess for evidence of cardiac reperfusion through resolution of chest pain, resolution of baseline ECG changes, preserved left ventricular function, cardiac enzyme washout phenomenon, and/or the appearance of reperfusion arrhythmias; assess for bleeding potential through clinical evidence of GI bleeding, hematuria, gingival bleeding, fibrinogen levels, fibrinogen degradation products, prothrombin times, and partial thromboplastin times.

Reference Range

Not routinely measured; literature supports therapeutic levels of 0.52-1.8 mcg/mL
Fibrinogen: 200-400 mg/dL
Activated partial thromboplastin time (aPTT): 22.5-38.7 seconds
Prothrombin time (PT): 10.9-12.2 seconds

Anesthesia and Critical Care Concerns/Other Considerations
Evidence-Based Information:

Acute Ischemic Stroke (AIS):

Presentation within 0-3 hours of stroke onset (FDA approved): Based on the National Institute of Neurological Disorders and Stroke (NINDS) rt-PA stroke study, administration of alteplase within 0-3 hours after symptom onset is an established therapeutic modality in the treatment of AIS. The NINDS trial demonstrated significant neurological improvement at 24 hours and a greater number of patients experienced a favorable outcome (complete or nearly complete neurological recovery) at 90 days if they received alteplase compared to those receiving placebo. The decision to administer alteplase should be made after careful consideration of the patient's eligibility including level of neurological deficit, time of presentation, and existence of contraindications to alteplase (eg, intracranial hemorrhage). Since a powerful time-to-treatment effect exists with the administration of alteplase for AIS, any delay in treatment once a patient is identified to be a candidate for alteplase may compromise efficacy and possibly safety. With administration of alteplase for AIS, the clinician should be keenly aware of the potential serious side effect of bleeding especially intracranial hemorrhage (ICH) which occurs at a rate of approximately 6% in this population. Strict adherence to established protocols is necessary to prevent higher rates of ICH. Orolingual angioedema, a rare but serious complication, may also occur and compromise the airway.

Presentation within 3-4.5 hours of stroke onset (non-FDA approved): Administration of alteplase is currently recommended for patients with AIS who may be treated within 3 hours of symptom onset (2007 AHA/ASA guideline). However, more recently, the European Cooperative Acute Stroke Study III (ECASS III; Hacke, 2008), a double-blind, multicenter trial enrolled 821 patients with AIS presenting with onset of stroke symptoms between 3-4.5 hours. Patients were randomized to either placebo or standard-dose alteplase (total dose: 0.9 mg/kg over 60 minutes; maximum: 90 mg; with 10% of 0.9 mg/kg given as loading dose). Patients were excluded if they had evidence of brain hemorrhage or major infarction. Other notable exclusion criteria were age >80 years, oral anticoagulation regardless of INR, severe stroke as assessed clinically (eg, NIH Stroke Scale >25) and/or by appropriate imaging techniques, and history of prior stroke and concomitant diabetes. The primary endpoint was disability at 90 days, dichotomized as a favorable or unfavorable outcome (score of 0-1 or 2-6 on the modified Rankin scale, respectively). The secondary endpoint was a global outcome analysis that combined the outcomes at day 90 of four neurologic and disability scores (modified Rankin scale, Barthel Index, NIH Stroke Scale, and Glasgow Outcome Scale). Median time to alteplase treatment was 239 minutes (3.9 hours) after onset of stroke symptoms. Compared to those who received placebo, patients receiving alteplase experienced less disability at 90 days (219 [52.4%] vs 182 [45.2%], p=0.04). A favorable global outcome was statistically more frequent with alteplase compared to placebo. More cases of intracranial hemorrhage (ICH) occurred in the alteplase group compared to placebo (any ICH, 113 [27%] vs 71 [17.6%], p=0.001; symptomatic ICH 10 [2.4%] vs 1 [0.2%], p=0.008), a rate similar to that of previous clinical trials when used within 0-3 hours. Although not a primary endpoint of the trial, there was no difference in mortality between the two groups (32 [7.7%] vs 34 [8.4%], p=0.68). ECASS III suggests the extension of the time window for treatment with alteplase and is now recommended by the AHA/ASA (Class Ib recommendation; del Zoppo, 2009).

Acute Pulmonary Embolism (PE): The American College of Chest Physicians (Kearon, 2008) recommends the following:

All patients with acute PE: All patients with diagnosed PE should undergo rapid risk stratification based on risk of death from PE and bleeding. In general, the majority of patients with PE will not require treatment with thrombolytics; however, treatment with anticoagulation (eg, enoxaparin, heparin) will be necessary unless contraindicated.

Patients with acute PE without hemodynamic compromise: In general, patients without hemodynamic compromise should not receive thrombolytic therapy. However, patients without hemodynamic compromise but with poor prognostic indicators (elevated troponin, right ventricular dysfunction on echocardiogram, etc) are at high risk of an adverse outcome and may derive benefit from receiving systemic thrombolysis. Therefore, the most recent recommendation is to administer thrombolysis in these selected high-risk patients who have a low risk of bleeding. The use of regimens with short infusion times (eg, 2-hour infusion) is recommended over longer infusion times (eg, 12-hour infusions). The most widely used thrombolytic for this indication is alteplase which is administered as an infusion of 100 mg over 2 hours. Urokinase may also be used; however, the administration time for urokinase is 12 hours.

Patients with acute PE with hemodynamic compromise: Since thrombolytic therapy has been shown to accelerate thrombolysis resulting in more rapid resolution of perfusion scan abnormalities, decrement angiographic thrombus, reduction in elevated pulmonary artery pressures, and normalization of right ventricular dysfunction in patients with PE and hemodynamic compromise (usually defined as SBP <90 mm Hg requiring vasopressor therapy), the use of thrombolytic therapy via a peripheral vein is recommended unless major contraindications exist. The use of regimens with short infusion times (eg, 2-hour infusion) is recommended over longer infusion times (eg, 12-hour infusions). The most widely used thrombolytic for this indication is alteplase which is administered as an infusion of 100 mg over 2 hours. Urokinase may also be used; however, the administration time for urokinase is 12 hours.

Patients with PE experiencing cardiac arrest: According to the 2005 ACLS guidelines, when PE is responsible for cardiac arrest and the patient is unresponsive to cardiopulmonary resuscitation (CPR), it is reasonable to administer bolus thrombolytic therapy, specifically alteplase (Böttiger, 2001); however, routine use in cardiac arrest or undifferentiated pulseless electrical activity (PEA) is not recommended. Of note, ongoing CPR is not a contra-indication in this setting.

Intracerebral Hemorrhage (ICH) Due to Thrombolysis: Overall management of ICH is similar regardless of cause; however, iatrogenic spontaneous ICH may have specific treatments. According to the 2007 ACC/ASA Guidelines for the Management of Spontaneous Intracerebral Hemorrhage, fibrinolytic-related ICH should be treated with infusion of platelets (6-8 units) and cryoprecipitate which contains factor VIII (Class IIb recommendation).

Peripheral Arterial Occlusive Disease (PAOD) and Deep Venous Thrombosis (DVT): The Surgery Versus Thrombolysis for Ischemia of the Lower Extremity (STILE) trial (*Ann Surg*, 1994) compared surgery to intra-arterial thrombolytic therapy with either urokinase (250,000 units bolus, followed by 4000 units/minute for 4 hours, followed by 2000 units/minute for ≤36 hours) or alteplase (0.05 mg/kg/hour for ≤12 hours) in patients with acute (<14 days) or chronic PAOD. Patients with acute PAOD who received either fibrinolytic treatment had a shorter hospital stay and an improved amputation-free survival rate. There was no difference between alteplase or urokinase with regard to efficacy or bleeding events. A group from Stanford University recently did a retrospective comparison evaluating efficacy, safety, and cost of low-dose alteplase (<2 mg/hour) and subtherapeutic

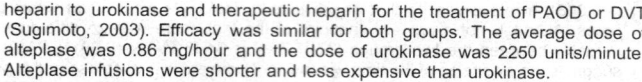

heparin to urokinase and therapeutic heparin for the treatment of PAOD or DVT (Sugimoto, 2003). Efficacy was similar for both groups. The average dose of alteplase was 0.86 mg/hour and the dose of urokinase was 2250 units/minute. Alteplase infusions were shorter and less expensive than urokinase.

Pregnancy Risk Factor C

Contraindications Hypersensitivity to alteplase or any component of the formulation

Treatment of STEMI or PE: Active internal bleeding; history of CVA; recent intracranial or intraspinal surgery or trauma; intracranial neoplasm; arteriovenous malformation or aneurysm; known bleeding diathesis; severe uncontrolled hypertension; suspected aortic dissection

Treatment of acute ischemic stroke: Evidence of intracranial hemorrhage or suspicion of subarachnoid hemorrhage on pretreatment evaluation; intracranial or intraspinal surgery within 3 months; stroke or serious head injury within 3 months; history of intracranial hemorrhage; uncontrolled hypertension at time of treatment (eg, >185 mm Hg systolic or >110 mm Hg diastolic); seizure at the onset of stroke; active internal bleeding; intracranial neoplasm; arteriovenous malformation or aneurysm; multilobar cerebral infarction (hypodensity >1/3 cerebral hemisphere; Adams, 2007); clinical presentation suggesting post-MI pericarditis; known bleeding diathesis including but not limited to current use of oral anticoagulants producing an INR >1.7, an INR >1.7, administration of heparin within 48 hours preceding the onset of stroke with an elevated aPTT at presentation, platelet count <100,000/mm^3.

Additional exclusion criteria within clinical trials:

Presentation <3 hours after initial symptoms (NINDS, 1995): Time of symptom onset unknown, rapidly improving or minor symptoms, major surgery within 2 weeks, GI or urinary tract hemorrhage within 3 weeks, aggressive treatment required to lower blood pressure, glucose level <50 or >400 mg/dL, and arterial puncture at a noncompressible site or lumbar puncture within 1 week.

Presentation 3-4.5 hours after initial symptoms (ECASS-III; Hacke, 2008): Age >80 years, time of symptom onset unknown, rapidly improving or minor symptoms, current use of anticoagulants regardless of INR, glucose level <50 or >400 mg/dL, aggressive intravenous treatment required to lower blood pressure, major surgery or severe trauma within 3 months, baseline National Institutes of Health Stroke Scale (NIHSS) score >25, and history of both stroke and diabetes.

Warnings/Precautions Concurrent heparin anticoagulation may contribute to bleeding. In the treatment of acute ischemic stroke, concurrent use of anticoagulants was not permitted during the initial 24 hours of the <3 hour window trial (NINDS, 1995). Initiation of SubQ heparin (≤10,000 units) or equivalent doses of low molecular weight heparin for prevention of DVT during the first 24 hours of the 3-4.5 hour window trial was permitted and did not increase the incidence of intracerebral hemorrhage (Hacke, 2008). Monitor all potential bleeding sites. Do not use doses >150 mg; associated with increased risk of intracranial hemorrhage. Intramuscular injections and nonessential handling of the patient should be avoided. Venipunctures should be performed carefully and only when necessary. If arterial puncture is necessary, use an upper extremity vessel that can be manually compressed. If serious bleeding occurs, the infusion of alteplase and heparin should be stopped. Avoid aspirin for 24 hours following administration of alteplase; administration within 24 hours increases the risk of hemorrhagic transformation.

For the following conditions, the risk of bleeding is higher with use of thrombolytics and should be weighed against the benefits of therapy: Recent major surgery (eg, CABG, obstetrical delivery, organ biopsy, pregnancy, previous puncture of noncompressible vessels), prolonged CPR with evidence of thoracic trauma, lumbar puncture within 1 week, cerebrovascular disease, recent gastrointestinal or genitourinary bleeding, recent trauma, hypertension (systolic BP >175 mm Hg and/or diastolic BP >110 mm Hg), high likelihood of left heart thrombus (eg, mitral stenosis with atrial fibrillation), acute pericarditis, subacute bacterial endocarditis, hemostatic defects including ones caused by severe renal or hepatic dysfunction, significant hepatic dysfunction, pregnancy, diabetic hemorrhagic retinopathy or other hemorrhagic ophthalmic conditions, septic thrombophlebitis or occluded AV cannula at seriously infected site, advanced age (eg, >75 years), any other condition in which bleeding constitutes a significant hazard or would be particularly difficult to manage because of location. When treating acute MI or pulmonary embolism, use with caution in patients receiving oral anticoagulants. In the treatment of acute ischemic stroke within 3 hours of stroke symptom onset, the current use of oral anticoagulants producing an INR >1.7 is contraindicated.

Coronary thrombolysis may result in reperfusion arrhythmias. Patients who present **within 3 hours** of stroke symptom onset should be treated with alteplase unless contraindications exist. A longer time window (**3-4.5 hours** after symptom onset) has now been formally evaluated and shown to be safe and efficacious for select individuals (del Zoppo, 2009; Hacke, 2008). Treatment of patients with minor neurological deficit or with rapidly improving symptoms is not recommended. Follow standard management for STEMI while infusing alteplase.

Cathflo® Activase®: When used to restore catheter function, use Cathflo® cautiously in those patients with known or suspected catheter infections. Evaluate catheter for other causes of dysfunction before use. Avoid excessive pressure when instilling into catheter.

Adverse Reactions As with all drugs which may affect hemostasis, bleeding is the major adverse effect associated with alteplase. Hemorrhage may occur at virtually any site. Risk is dependent on multiple variables, including the dosage administered, concurrent use of multiple agents which alter hemostasis, and patient predisposition. Rapid lysis of coronary artery thrombi by thrombolytic agents may be associated with reperfusion-related atrial and/or ventricular arrhythmia. **Note:** Lowest rate of bleeding complications expected with dose used to restore catheter function.

1% to 10%:
  Cardiovascular: Hypotension
  Central nervous system: Fever
  Dermatologic: Bruising (1%)
  Gastrointestinal: GI hemorrhage (5%), nausea, vomiting
  Genitourinary: GU hemorrhage (4%)
  Hematologic: Bleeding (0.5% major, 7% minor: GUSTO trial)
  Local: Bleeding at catheter puncture site (15.3%, accelerated administration)
<1% (Limited to important or life-threatening): Allergic reactions: Anaphylaxis, anaphylactoid reactions, laryngeal edema, rash, and urticaria (<0.02%); epistaxis; gingival hemorrhage; intracranial hemorrhage (0.4% to 0.87% when dose is ≤100 mg); pericardial hemorrhage; retroperitoneal hemorrhage
Additional cardiovascular events associated **with use in STEMI:** AV block, cardiogenic shock, heart failure, cardiac arrest, recurrent ischemia/infarction, myocardial rupture, electromechanical dissociation, pericardial effusion, pericarditis, mitral regurgitation, cardiac tamponade, thromboembolism, pulmonary edema, asystole, ventricular tachycardia, bradycardia, ruptured intracranial AV malformation, seizure, hemorrhagic bursitis, cholesterol crystal embolization
Additional events associated **with use in pulmonary embolism:** Pulmonary re-embolization, pulmonary edema, pleural effusion, thromboembolism
Additional events associated **with use in stroke:** Cerebral edema, cerebral herniation, seizure, new ischemic stroke
Drug Interactions
  Avoid Concomitant Use There are no known interactions where it is recommended to avoid concomitant use.
  Increased Effect/Toxicity
    Alteplase may increase the levels/effects of: Anticoagulants; Drotrecogin Alfa

    The levels/effects of Alteplase may be increased by: Antiplatelet Agents; Herbs (Anticoagulant/Antiplatelet Properties); Nonsteroidal Anti-Inflammatory Agents; Salicylates
  Decreased Effect
    The levels/effects of Alteplase may be decreased by: Aprotinin; Nitroglycerin
Ethanol/Nutrition/Herb Interactions Herb/Nutraceutical: Avoid cat's claw, dong quai, evening primrose, feverfew, red clover, horse chestnut, garlic, green tea, ginseng, ginkgo (all have additional antiplatelet activity).

◀ **Test Interactions** Altered results of coagulation and fibrinolytic agents

Dosage Forms Excipient information presented when available (limited, particularly for generics); consult specific product labeling.

Injection, powder for reconstitution, recombinant:

Activase®: 50 mg [29 million int. units; contains polysorbate 80; packaged with diluent]; 100 mg [58 million int. units; contains polysorbate 80; packaged with diluent and transfer device]

Cathflo® Activase®: 2 mg [contains polysorbate 80]

References

"A Comparison of Reteplase With Alteplase for Acute Myocardial Infarction. The Global Use of Strategies to Open Occluded Coronary Arteries (GUSTO III) Investigators," *N Engl J Med*, 1997, 337(16):1118-23.

Adams HP Jr, del Zoppo G, Alberts MJ, et al, "Guidelines for the Early Management of Adults With Ischemic Stroke: A Guideline From the American Heart Association/American Stroke Association Stroke Council, Clinical Cardiology Council, Cardiovascular Radiology and Intervention Council, and the Atherosclerotic Peripheral Vascular Disease and Quality of Care Outcomes in Research Interdisciplinary Working Groups: The American Academy of Neurology Affirms the Value of This Guideline as an Educational Tool for Neurologists," *Stroke*, 2007, 38(5):1655-711.

Böttiger BW, Bode C, Kern S, et al,"Efficacy and Safety of Thrombolytic Therapy After Initially Unsuccessful Cardiopulmonary Resuscitation: A Prospective Clinical Trial," *Lancet*, 2001, 357 (9268):1583-5.

Broderick J, Connolly S, Feldmann E, et al, "Guidelines for the Management of Spontaneous Intracerebral Hemorrhage in Adults: 2007 Update: A Guideline From the American Heart Association/American Stroke Association Stroke Council, High Blood Pressure Research Council, and the Quality of Care and Outcomes in Research Interdisciplinary Working Group," *Stroke*, 2007, 38(6):2001-23. Available at http://stroke.ahajournals.org/cgi/content/short/STROKEAHA.107.183689.

Comerota AJ and Schmieder FA, "Intraoperative Lytic Therapy: Agents and Methods of Administration," *Semin Vasc Surg*, 2001, 14(2):132-42.

del Zoppo GJ, Saver JL, Jauch EC, et al, "Expansion of the Time Window for Treatment of Acute Ischemic Stroke With Intravenous Tissue Plasminogen Activator: A Science Advisory From the American Heart Association/American Stroke Association," *Stroke*, 2009, [epub ahead of print]

ECC Committee, Subcommittees and Task Forces of the American Heart Association, "2005 American Heart Association Guidelines for Cardiopulmonary Resuscitation and Emergency Cardiovascular Care," *Circulation*, 2005, 112(24 Suppl):IV1-203.

Goodman SG, Menon V, Cannon CP, et al, "Acute ST-Segment Elevation Myocardial Infarction: American College of Chest Physicians Evidence-Based Clinical Practice," *Chest*, 2008, 133(6 Suppl):708-75.

Hacke W, Kaste M, Bluhmki E, et al, "Thrombolysis With Alteplase 3 to 4.5 Hours After Acute Ischemic Stroke," *N Engl J Med*, 2008, 359(13):1317-29.

Hirsh J, Guyatt G, Albers GW, et al, "Executive Summary: American College of Chest Physicians Evidence-Based Clinical Practice Guidelines (8th Edition)," *Chest*, 2008, 133(6 Suppl):71-109.

Kearon C, Kahn SR, Agnelli G, et al, "Antithrombotic Therapy for Venous Thromboembolic Disease: American College of Chest Physicians Evidence-Based Clinical Practice Guidelines (8th Edition)," *Chest*, 2008, 33(6 Suppl):454-545.

Konstantinides S, Geibel A, Heusel G, et al, "Heparin Plus Alteplase Compared With Heparin Alone in Patients With Submassive Pulmonary Embolism," *N Engl J Med*, 2002, 347(15):1143-50.

Leonard MC and Shermock KM, "Using Efficacy, Safety, and Cost Data to Support a Formulary Decision Regarding Thrombolytic Therapy," *Semin Vasc Surg*, 2001, 14(2):150-5.

Lundergan CF, Reiner JS, McCarthy WF, et al, "Clinical Predictors of Early Infarct-Related Artery Patency Following Thrombolytic Therapy: Importance of Body Weight, Smoking History, Infarct-Related Artery and Choice of Thrombolytic Regimen: The GUSTO-I Experience. Global Utilization of Streptokinase and t-PA for Occluded Coronary Arteries," *J Am Coll Cardiol*, 1998, 32(3):641-7.

Ouriel K, "Current Status of Thrombolysis for Peripheral Arterial Occlusive Disease," *Ann Vasc Surg*, 2002, 16(6):797-804.

Ponec D, Irwin D, Haire WD, et al, "Recombinant Tissue Plasminogen Activator (Alteplase) for Restoration of Flow in Occluded Central Venous Access Devices: A Double-Blind Placebo-Controlled Trial - The Cardiovascular Thrombolytic to Open Occluded Lines (COOL) Efficacy Trial," *J Vasc Interv Radiol*, 2001, 12(8):951-5.

"Results of a Prospective, Randomised Trial Evaluating Surgery Versus Thrombolysis for Ischemia of the Lower Extremity. The STILE Trial," *Ann Surg*, 1994, 220(3):251-66; discussion 266-8.

Semba CP, Murphy TP, Bakal CW, et al, "Thrombolytic Therapy With Use of Alteplase (rtPA) in Peripheral Arterial Occlusive Disease: Review of the Clinical Literature. The Advisory Panel," *J Vasc Interv Radiol*, 2000, 11(2 Pt 1):149-61.

Sugimoto K, Hofmann LV, Razavi MK, et al, "The Safety, Efficacy, and Pharmacoeconomics of Low-Dose Alteplase Compared With Urokinase for Catheter-Directed Thrombolysis of Arterial and Venous Occlusions," *J Vasc Surg*, 2003, 37(3):512-7.

The Gusto Angiographic Investigators, "The Effects of Tissue Plasminogen Activator, Streptokinase, or Both on Coronary-Artery Patency, Ventricular Function, and Survival After Acute Myocardial Infarction," *N Engl J Med*, 1993, 329(22):1615-22.

"Thrombolysis in the Management of Lower Limb Peripheral Arterial Occlusion - A Consensus Document. Working Party on Thrombolysis in the Management of Limb Ischemia," *Am J Cardiol*, 1998, 81(2):207-18.

"Tissue Plasminogen Activator for Acute Ischemic Stroke. The National Institute of Neurological Disorders and Stroke rt-PA Stroke Study Group," *N Engl J Med*, 1995, 333(24):1581-7.

Topol EJ, "Reperfusion Therapy for Acute Myocardial Infarction With Fibrinolytic Therapy or Combination Reduced Fibrinolytic Therapy and Platelet Glycoprotein IIb/IIIa Inhibition: The GUSTO V Randomized Trial. GUSTO V Investigators," *Lancet*, 2001, 357(9272):1905-14.

Zacharias JM, Weatherston CP, Spewak CR, et al, "Alteplase Versus Urokinase for Occluded Hemodialysis Catheters," *Ann Pharmacother*, 2003, 37(1):27-33.

◆ **Alteplase, Recombinant** *see* Alteplase *on page 67*

◆ **Alteplase, Tissue Plasminogen Activator, Recombinant** *see* Alteplase *on page 67*

◆ **Alti-Alprazolam (Can)** *see* ALPRAZolam *on page 64*

◆ **Alti-Amiodarone (Can)** *see* Amiodarone *on page 86*

◆ **Alti-Amoxi-Clav (Can)** *see* Amoxicillin and Clavulanate Potassium *on page 98*

◆ **Alti-Azathioprine (Can)** *see* AzaTHIOprine *on page 167*

◆ **Alti-Captopril (Can)** *see* Captopril *on page 239*

◆ **Alti-Clindamycin (Can)** *see* Clindamycin *on page 324*

◆ **Alti-Clonazepam (Can)** *see* ClonazePAM *on page 328*

◆ **Alti-Desipramine (Can)** *see* Desipramine *on page 384*

◆ **Alti-Divalproex (Can)** *see* Valproic Acid and Derivatives *on page 1445*

◆ **Alti-Flurbiprofen (Can)** *see* Flurbiprofen *on page 619*

◆ **Alti-Ipratropium (Can)** *see* Ipratropium *on page 760*

◆ **Alti-Nadolol (Can)** *see* Nadolol *on page 974*

◆ **Alti-Nortriptyline (Can)** *see* Nortriptyline *on page 1026*

◆ **Alti-Salbutamol (Can)** *see* Albuterol *on page 49*

◆ **Alti-Ticlopidine (Can)** *see* Ticlopidine *on page 1385*

◆ **Alti-Timolol (Can)** *see* Timolol *on page 1390*

◆ **Altoprev®** *see* Lovastatin *on page 859*

◆ **Aluminum Sucrose Sulfate, Basic** *see* Sucralfate *on page 1329*

◆ **Alupent® [DSC]** *see* Metaproterenol *on page 885*

Alvimopan (al vi MOE pan)

Medication Safety Issues
Sound-alike/look-alike issues:
Alvimopan may be confused with almotriptan

U.S. Brand Names Entereg®

Index Terms ADL-2698; LY246736

Pharmacologic Category Gastrointestinal Agent, Miscellaneous; Opioid Antagonist, Peripherally-Acting

Restrictions Only hospitals enrolled in the ENTEREG Access Support and Education (E.A.S.E.™) Program may administer this medication. Hospital staff must be educated on need to limit to short-term (no more than 15 doses) and inpatient use. Hospitals may contact the E.A.S.E.™ program at 1-866-423-6567 (1-866-4ADOLOR).

Generic Available No

Use Accelerate the time to upper and lower GI recovery following partial large or small bowel resection surgery with primary anastomosis

Mechanism of Action An opioid receptor antagonist which blocks opioid binding at the mu receptor; alvimopan has restricted ability to cross the blood-brain barrier at therapeutic doses. It selectively and competitively binds to the GI tract mu opioid receptors and antagonizes the peripheral effects of opioids on gastrointestinal motility and secretion. Does not affect opioid analgesic effects or induce opioid withdrawal symptoms.

Pharmacodynamics/Kinetics
Distribution: V_d: 20-40 L
Protein binding: Parent drug: 80%; metabolite: 94% (both primarily to albumin)
Metabolism: Hydrolyzed to an amide hydrolysis compound (active metabolite) by gut microflora; further metabolism of active metabolite to glucuronide conjugates and other minor metabolites.
Bioavailability: ~6% (range: 1% to 19%)

◀ Half-life elimination: 10-18 hours

Time to peak, plasma: ~2 hours

Excretion: Urine (35% as unchanged drug and metabolites); feces (via biliary excretion)

Dosage Note: For hospital use only

Oral: Adults:

Initial: 12 mg administered 30 minutes to 5 hours prior to surgery

Maintenance: 12 mg twice daily beginning the day after surgery for a maximum of 7 days or until discharged from hospital (maximum total treatment doses: 15 doses)

Dosage adjustment in renal impairment:

Mild-to-severe impairment: No adjustment needed; use caution

ESRD: Use not recommended

Dosage adjustment in hepatic impairment:

Mild-to-moderate impairment (Child-Pugh class A and B): No adjustment needed; use caution

Severe impairment (Child-Pugh class C): Use not recommended

Stability Store at controlled room temperature of 25°C (77°F).

Administration Patient must be hospitalized. Initial dose should be administered 30 minutes to 5 hours prior to surgery. May be administered with or without food.

Pregnancy Risk Factor B

Contraindications Patients who have taken therapeutic doses of opioids for more than 7 consecutive days immediately prior to alvimopan

Warnings/Precautions [U.S. Boxed Warning]: For short-term (≤15 doses) hospital use only. Only hospitals that have registered through the ENTEREG Access Support and Education (E.A.S.E.™) Program and met all requirements may use. It will not be dispensed to patients who have been discharged from the hospital. Use not recommended in patients with complete bowel obstruction. Use with caution in patients with hepatic or renal impairment; use not recommended in patients with severe hepatic impairment or ESRD. Use with caution is patients recently exposed to opioids; may be more sensitive to gastrointestinal adverse effects (eg, abdominal pain, diarrhea, nausea and vomiting). Contraindicated in patients who have received therapeutic opioids for >7 consecutive days immediately prior to use. A trend towards an increased incidence of MI was observed in alvimopan (low dose) treated patients compared to placebo in a 12-month study in patients treated with opioids for chronic pain. MI was generally observed more frequently in the initial 1-4 months of treatment. Other studies have not observed this trend and a causal relationship has not been found. Safety and efficacy have not been established in children.

Adverse Reactions Note: Incidence reported limited to bowel resection patients only. 1% to 10%:

Endocrine & metabolic: Hypokalemia (10%)

Gastrointestinal: Dyspepsia (7%)

Genitourinary: Urinary retention (3%)

Hematologic: Anemia (5%)

Neuromuscular & skeletal: Back pain (3%)

Drug Interactions

Metabolism/Transport Effects Substrate of P-glycoprotein

Avoid Concomitant Use There are no known interactions where it is recommended to avoid concomitant use.

Increased Effect/Toxicity

The levels/effects of Alvimopan may be increased by: Analgesics (Opioid)

Decreased Effect There are no known significant interactions involving a decrease in effect.

Ethanol/Nutrition/Herb Interactions Food: When administered with a high-fat meal, extent and rate of absorption may be reduced (C_{max} and AUC decreased by ~38% and 21%, respectively).

Dietary Considerations Take with or without food; high-fat meals may decrease the rate and extent of absorption

Dosage Forms Excipient information presented when available (limited, particularly for generics); consult specific product labeling.

Capsule:

Entereg®: 12 mg

References

Leslie JB, "Alvimopan for the Management of Postoperative Ileus," *Ann Pharmacother*, 2005, 39 (9):1502-10.

Taguchi A, Sharma N, Saleem RN, et al, "Selective Postoperative Inhibition of Gastrointestinal Opioid Receptors," *N Engl J Med*, 2001, 345(13):935-40.

Amantadine (a MAN ta deen)

U.S. Brand Names Symmetrel®

Canadian Brand Names Endantadine®; Mylan-Amantadine; PMS-Amantadine; Symmetrel®

Index Terms Adamantanamine Hydrochloride; Amantadine Hydrochloride

Pharmacologic Category Anti-Parkinson's Agent, Dopamine Agonist; Antiviral Agent; Antiviral Agent, Adamantane

Use Prophylaxis and treatment of influenza A viral infection (per manufacturer labeling; also refer to current ACIP guidelines for recommendations during current flu season); treatment of parkinsonism; treatment of drug-induced extrapyramidal symptoms

Note: In certain circumstances, the ACIP recommends use of amantadine in combination with oseltamivir for the treatment or prophylaxis of influenza A infection when resistance to oseltamivir is suspected.

Pharmacodynamics/Kinetics

Onset of action: Antidyskinetic: Within 48 hours

Absorption: Well absorbed

Distribution: V_d: Normal: 1.5-6.1 L/kg; Renal failure: 5.1 ± 0.2 L/kg; in saliva, tear film, and nasal secretions; in animals, tissue (especially lung) concentrations higher than serum concentrations; crosses blood-brain barrier

Protein binding: Normal renal function: ~67%; Hemodialysis: ~59%

Metabolism: Not appreciable; small amounts of an acetyl metabolite identified

Bioavailability: 86% to 90%

Half-life elimination: Normal renal function: 16 ± 6 hours (9-31 hours); Healthy, older (≥60 years) males: 29 hours (range: 20-41 hours); End-stage renal disease: 7-10 days

Time to peak, plasma: 2-4 hours

Excretion: Urine (80% to 90% unchanged) by glomerular filtration and tubular secretion

Dosage Oral:

Children: Influenza A treatment/prophylaxis: **Note:** Due to issues of resistance, amantadine is no longer recommended for the treatment or prophylaxis of influenza A. Please refer to the current ACIP recommendations. The following is based on the manufacturer's labeling and past ACIP dosing recommendations:

Influenza A treatment:

1-9 years: 5 mg/kg/day in 2 divided doses (manufacturers range: 4.4-8.8 mg/kg/day); maximum dose: 150 mg/day

≥10 years and <40 kg: 5 mg/kg/day in 2 divided doses; maximum dose: 150 mg/day (CDC, 2003)

≥10 years and ≥40 kg: 100 mg twice daily (CDC, 2003)

Note: Initiate within 24-48 hours after onset of symptoms; continue for 24-48 hours after symptom resolution (duration of therapy is generally 3-5 days)

Influenza A prophylaxis: Refer to "Influenza A treatment" dosing. **Note:** Continue prophylaxis throughout the peak influenza activity in the community or throughout the entire influenza season in patients who cannot be vaccinated. Development of immunity following vaccination takes ~2 weeks; amantadine therapy should be considered for high-risk patients from the time of vaccination until immunity has developed. For children <9 years receiving influenza vaccine for the first time, amantadine prophylaxis should continue for 6 weeks (4 weeks after the first dose and 2 weeks after the second dose).

Adults:

Drug-induced extrapyramidal symptoms: 100 mg twice daily; may increase to 300 mg/day in divided doses, if needed

Parkinson's disease: Usual dose: 100 mg twice daily as monotherapy; may increase to 400 mg/day in divided doses, if needed, with close monitoring. **Note:** Patients with a serious concomitant illness or those receiving high doses of other anti-parkinson drugs should be started at 100 mg/day; may increase to 100 mg twice daily, if needed, after one to several weeks.

Influenza A treatment/prophylaxis: **Note:** Due to issues of resistance, amantadine is no longer recommended for the treatment or prophylaxis of influenza A. Please refer to the current ACIP recommendations. The following is based on the manufacturer's labeling:

Influenza A treatment: 200 mg once daily **or** 100 mg twice daily (may be preferred to reduce CNS effects); **Note:** Initiate within 24-48 hours after onset of symptoms; continue for 24-48 hours after symptom resolution (duration of therapy is generally 3-5 days).

Influenza A prophylaxis: 200 mg once daily **or** 100 mg twice daily (may be preferred to reduce CNS effects). **Note:** Continue prophylaxis throughout the peak influenza activity in the community or throughout the entire influenza season in patients who cannot be vaccinated. Development of immunity following vaccination takes ~2 weeks; amantadine therapy should be considered for high-risk patients from the time of vaccination until immunity has developed.

Elderly (≥65 years): Adjust dose based on renal function; some patients tolerate the drug better when it is given in 2 divided daily doses (to avoid adverse neurologic reactions).

Influenza A treatment/prophylaxis: 100 mg once daily

Dosing interval in renal impairment:

Cl_{cr} 30-50 mL/minute: Administer 200 mg on day 1, then 100 mg/day

Cl_{cr} 15-29 mL/minute: Administer 200 mg on day 1, then 100 mg on alternate days

Cl_{cr} <15 mL/minute: Administer 200 mg every 7 days

Hemodialysis: Administer 200 mg every 7 days

Peritoneal dialysis: No supplemental dose is needed

Continuous arteriovenous or venous-venous hemofiltration: No supplemental dose is needed

Additional Information Complete prescribing information for this medication should be consulted for additional detail.

Dosage Forms Excipient information presented when available (limited, particularly for generics); consult specific product labeling.

Capsule, as hydrochloride: 100 mg

Capsule, softgel, as hydrochloride: 100 mg

Solution, oral, as hydrochloride: 50 mg/5 mL (473 mL)

Syrup, oral, as hydrochloride: 50 mg/5 mL (10 mL, 480 mL)

Tablet, as hydrochloride: 100 mg

Symmetrel®: 100 mg

◆ **Amantadine Hydrochloride** *see* Amantadine *on page 77*

◆ **Amatine® (Can)** *see* Midodrine *on page 939*

◆ **Ambien®** *see* Zolpidem *on page 1494*

◆ **Ambien CR®** *see* Zolpidem *on page 1494*

◆ **AmBisome®** *see* Amphotericin B (Liposomal) *on page 110*

◆ **Amerge®** *see* Naratriptan *on page 989*

◆ **A-Methapred** *see* MethylPREDNISolone *on page 911*

◆ **A-Methapred®** *see* MethylPREDNISolone *on page 911*

◆ **Amethocaine Hydrochloride** *see* Tetracaine *on page 1367*

◆ **Amethopterin** *see* Methotrexate *on page 898*

◆ **Ametop™ (Can)** *see* Tetracaine *on page 1367*

◆ **AMG 531** *see* Romiplostim *on page 1263*

◆ **Amicar®** *see* Aminocaproic Acid *on page 83*

◆ **Amidate®** *see* Etomidate *on page 564*

◆ **Amigesic® [DSC]** *see* Salsalate *on page 1275*

◆ **Amigesic® (Can)** *see* Salsalate *on page 1275*

Amikacin (am i KAY sin)

Medication Safety Issues
Sound-alike/look-alike issues:
Amikacin may be confused with Amicar®, anakinra
Amikin® may be confused with Amicar®, Kineret®
Canadian Brand Names Amikacin Sulfate Injection, USP; Amikin®
Index Terms Amikacin Sulfate
Pharmacologic Category Antibiotic, Aminoglycoside
Generic Available Yes
Use Treatment of serious infections (bone infections, respiratory tract infections, endocarditis, and septicemia) due to organisms resistant to gentamicin and tobramycin, including *Pseudomonas*, *Proteus*, *Serratia*, and other gram-negative bacilli; documented infection of mycobacterial organisms susceptible to amikacin
Unlabeled/Investigational Use Bacterial endophthalmitis
Mechanism of Action Inhibits protein synthesis in susceptible bacteria by binding to 30S ribosomal subunits

Pharmacodynamics/Kinetics
Absorption:
I.M.: Rapid
Oral: Poorly absorbed
Distribution: Primarily into extracellular fluid (highly hydrophilic); penetrates blood-brain barrier when meninges inflamed
Relative diffusion of antimicrobial agents from blood into CSF: Good only with inflammation (exceeds usual MICs)
CSF:blood level ratio: Normal meninges: 10% to 20%; Inflamed meninges: 15% to 24%
Protein-binding: 0% to 11%
Half-life elimination (renal function and age dependent):
Infants: Low birth weight (1-3 days): 7-9 hours; Full-term >7 days: 4-5 hours
Children: 1.6-2.5 hours
Adults: Normal renal function: 1.4-2.3 hours; Anuria/end-stage renal disease: 28-86 hours
Time to peak, serum: I.M.: 45-120 minutes
Excretion: Urine (94% to 98%)
Dosage Note: Individualization is critical because of the low therapeutic index
Use of ideal body weight (IBW) for determining the mg/kg/dose appears to be more accurate than dosing on the basis of total body weight (TBW)
In morbid obesity, dosage requirement may best be estimated using a dosing weight of IBW + 0.4 (TBW - IBW)
Initial and periodic peak and trough plasma drug levels should be determined, particularly in critically-ill patients with serious infections or in disease states known to significantly alter aminoglycoside pharmacokinetics (eg, cystic fibrosis, burns, or major surgery). Manufacturer recommends a maximum daily dose of 15 mg/kg/day (or 1.5 g/day in heavier patients). Higher doses may be warranted based on therapeutic drug monitoring or susceptibility information.

Usual dosage range:
Infants and Children: I.M., I.V.: 5-7.5 mg/kg/dose every 8 hours
Adults: I.M., I.V.: 5-7.5 mg/kg/dose every 8 hours
Note: Some clinicians suggest a daily dose of 15-20 mg/kg for all patients with normal renal function. This dose is at least as efficacious with similar, if not less, toxicity than conventional dosing.

Indication-specific dosing:
Adults:
Endophthalmitis, bacterial (unlabeled use): Intravitreal: 0.4 mg/0.1 mL NS in combination with vancomycin
Hospital-acquired pneumonia (HAP): I.V.: 20 mg/kg/day with antipseudomonal beta-lactam or carbapenem (American Thoracic Society/ATS guidelines)

◀ **Meningitis *(Pseudomonas aeruginosa):*** I.V.: 5 mg/kg every 8 hours (administered with another bacteriocidal drug)
Mycobacterium fortuitum, M. chelonae, or M. abscessus: I.V.: 10-15 mg/kg daily for at least 2 weeks with high dose cefoxitin

Dosing interval in renal impairment: Some patients may require larger or more frequent doses if serum levels document the need (ie, cystic fibrosis or febrile granulocytopenic patients).

Cl_{cr} ≥60 mL/minute: Administer every 8 hours

Cl_{cr} 40-60 mL/minute: Administer every 12 hours

Cl_{cr} 20-40 mL/minute: Administer every 24 hours

Cl_{cr} <20 mL/minute: Loading dose, then monitor levels

Hemodialysis: Dialyzable (50% to 100%); administer dose postdialysis or administer $2/3$ normal dose as a supplemental dose postdialysis and follow levels

Peritoneal dialysis: Dose as Cl_{cr} <20 mL/minute: Follow levels

Continuous arteriovenous or venovenous hemodiafiltration effects: Dose as for Cl_{cr} 10-40 mL/minute and follow levels

Stability Store at controlled room temperature. Following admixture at concentrations of 0.25-5 mg/mL, amikcain is stable for 24 hours at room temperature and 2 days at refrigeration when mixed in D_5W, NS, and LR.

Administration Administer around-the-clock to promote less variation in peak and trough serum levels. Do not mix with other drugs, administer separately.

I.M.: Administer I.M. injection in large muscle mass.

I.V.: Infuse over 30-60 minutes.

Some penicillins (eg, carbenicillin, ticarcillin, and piperacillin) have been shown to inactivate *in vitro*. This has been observed to a greater extent with tobramycin and gentamicin, while amikacin has shown greater stability against inactivation. Concurrent use of these agents may pose a risk of reduced antibacterial efficacy *in vivo*, particularly in the setting of profound renal impairment. However, definitive clinical evidence is lacking. If combination penicillin/aminoglycoside therapy is desired in a patient with renal dysfunction, separation of doses (if feasible), and routine monitoring of aminoglycoside levels, CBC, and clinical response should be considered.

Monitoring Parameters Urinalysis, BUN, serum creatinine, appropriately timed peak and trough concentrations, vital signs, temperature, weight, I & O, hearing parameters

Some penicillin derivatives may accelerate the degradation of aminoglycosides *in vitro*. This may be clinically-significant for certain penicillin (ticarcillin, piperacillin, carbenicillin) and aminoglycoside (gentamicin, tobramycin) combination therapy in patients with significant renal impairment. Close monitoring of aminoglycoside levels is warranted.

Reference Range

Sample size: 0.5-2 mL blood (red top tube) or 0.1-1 mL serum (separated)

Therapeutic levels:

Peak:

Life-threatening infections: 25-40 mcg/mL

Serious infections: 20-25 mcg/mL

Urinary tract infections: 15-20 mcg/mL

Trough: <8 mcg/mL

The American Thoracic Society (ATS) recommends trough levels of <4-5 mcg/mL for patients with hospital-acquired pneumonia.

Toxic concentration: Peak: >40 mcg/mL; Trough: >10 mcg/mL

Timing of serum samples: Draw peak 30 minutes after completion of 30-minute infusion or at 1 hour following initiation of infusion or I.M. injection; draw trough within 30 minutes prior to next dose

Pregnancy Risk Factor D

Contraindications Hypersensitivity to amikacin sulfate or any component of the formulation; cross-sensitivity may exist with other aminoglycosides

Warnings/Precautions [U.S. Boxed Warning]: Amikacin may cause neurotoxicity, nephrotoxicity, and/or neuromuscular blockade and respiratory paralysis; usual risk factors include pre-existing renal impairment, concomitant neuro-/nephrotoxic medications, advanced age and dehydration. Dose and/or frequency of administration must be monitored and modified in patients with renal impairment. Drug should be discontinued if signs of ototoxicity, nephrotoxicity, or hypersensitivity occur. Ototoxicity is proportional to the amount c *given and* the duration of treatment. Tinnitus or vertigo may be indications o ve *injury* and impending bilateral irreversible damage. Renal damage is us *ular injury* Use with caution in patients with neuromuscular disorders, hear *ersible.* hypocalcemia. Prolonged use may result in fungal or bacterial su *and ation,* including *C. difficile*-associated diarrhea (CDAD) and pseudomembra *us;* CDAD has been observed >2 months postantibiotic treatment. Solutic *is;* sodium metabisulfate; use caution in patients with sulfite allergy. *s*

Adverse Reactions

1% to 10%:
  Central nervous system: Neurotoxicity
  Otic: Ototoxicity (auditory), ototoxicity (vestibular)
  Renal: Nephrotoxicity
<1% (Limited to important or life-threatening): Allergic reaction, dy eosinophilia

Drug Interactions

Avoid Concomitant Use
  Avoid concomitant use of Amikacin with any of the following: Gallium Nitrate

Increased Effect/Toxicity
  Amikacin may increase the levels/effects of: AbobotulinumtoxinA; Bisphosphonate Derivatives; CARBOplatin; Colistimethate; CycloSPORINE; Gallium Nitrate; Neuromuscular-Blocking Agents; OnabotulinumtoxinA; RimabotulinumtoxinB

  The levels/effects of Amikacin may be increased by: Amphotericin B; Capreomycin; CISplatin; Loop Diuretics; Nonsteroidal Anti-Inflammatory Agents; Vancomycin

Decreased Effect
  Amikacin may decrease the levels/effects of: Typhoid Vaccine

  The levels/effects of Amikacin may be decreased by: Penicillins

Test Interactions Some penicillin derivatives may accelerate the degradation of aminoglycosides *in vitro*, leading to a potential underestimation of aminoglycoside serum concentration.

Dietary Considerations Sodium content of 1 g: 29.9 mg (1.3 mEq)

Dosage Forms Excipient information presented when available (limited, particularly for generics); consult specific product labeling.
Injection, solution, as sulfate: 50 mg/mL (2 mL); 250 mg/mL (2 mL, 4 mL)

References

American Thoracic Society and Infectious Diseases Society of America, "Guidelines for the Management of Adults With Hospital-Acquired, Ventilator-Associated, and Healthcare-Associated Pneumonia," *Am J Respir Crit Care Med*, 2005, 171(4):388-416.

Tunkel AR, Hartman BJ, Kaplan SL, et al, "Practice Guidelines for the Management of Bacterial Meningitis," *Clin Infect Dis*, 2004, 39(9):1267-84.

◆ **Amikacin Sulfate** *see* Amikacin *on page 79*

◆ **Amikacin Sulfate Injection, USP (Can)** *see* Amikacin *on page 79*

◆ **Amikin® (Can)** *see* Amikacin *on page 79*

Amino Acid Injection (a MEE noe AS id in JEK shun)

Medication Safety Issues
Sound-alike/look-alike issues:
  TrophAmine® may be confused with tromethamine

Related Information
  Dextrose *on page 406*
  Fat Emulsion *on page 578*
  Total Parenteral Nutrition *on page 1411*

U.S. Brand Names Aminosyn®; Aminosyn® II; Aminosyn®-HBC; Aminosyn®-PF; Aminosyn®-RF; BranchAmin®; Clinisol®; FreAmine® HBC®; FreAmine® III; HepatAmine®; Hepatasol®; NephrAmine®; PremaSol™; Prosol; Renamin®; Travasol®; TrophAmine®

Canadian Brand Names Aminosyn; Aminosyn-PF; Aminosyn-RF; Primene®

Pharmacologic Category Intravenous Nutritional Therapy

Use As part of parenteral nutrition to prevent nitrogen loss or treat negative nitrogen balance when alimentary tract cannot be used (eg, GI absorption is impaired, bowel rest is needed). Specialty amino acid formulas may be considered only in certain instances.

Usual dose Intravenous as a component of parenteral nutrition: Protein as amino acids: Children:

Preterm: Initial: 2.5 g/kg/day; Goal: 3 g/kg/day

Extremely (<1000 g) and very (<1500 g) low-birth-weight (stable): Initial: 1-1.5 g/kg/day; Goal: 3.5-3.85 g/kg/day to promote utero growth rates

Sepsis, hypoxia: Initial: 1 g/kg/day; goal: 3-3.85 g/kg/day

Adults:

Maintenance: 0.8-1 g/kg/day

Normal/mild stress level: 1-1.2 g/kg/day

Moderate stress level: 1.2-1.5 g/kg/day

Severe stress level: 1.5-2 g/kg/day

Burn patients (severe): Increase protein until significant wound healing achieved

Solid organ transplant: Perioperative: 1.5-2 g/kg/day

Renal failure:

Acute (severely malnourished or hypercatabolic): 1.5-1.8 g/kg/day

Chronic, with dialysis: 1.2-1.3 g/kg/day

Chronic, without dialysis: 0.6-0.8 g/kg/day

Continuous hemofiltration: ≥1 g/kg/day

Hepatic failure:

Acute management when other treatments have failed:

With encephalopathy: 0.6-1 g/kg/day

Without encephalopathy: 1-1.5 g/kg/day

Chronic encephalopathy: Use branch chain amino acid enriched diets only if unresponsive to pharmacotherapy

Pregnant women in second or third trimester: Add an additional 10-14 g/day

Stability Store at room temperature of 20°C to 25°C (68°F to 77°F); avoid excessive heat; do not freeze. Protect from light.

Administration Administered as a component of peripheral parenteral or total parenteral nutrition. Peripheral administration of nutrition is dependent upon osmolality of solution. Total parenteral nutrition must be administered via central venous access.

Monitoring Parameters General patient monitoring during I.V. nutritional therapy

Bone densitometry: Perform upon initiation of long-term therapy.

Efficacy: Nutrition and outcome parameters should be measured serially.

Electrolytes: Sodium, potassium, chloride, and bicarbonate should be monitored frequently upon initiation and until stable; phosphate should be monitored closely in patients with pulmonary disease.

Glucose: In patients with diabetes or patients with glucose intolerance risk factors, monitor closely. Monitor frequently upon initiation of therapy and with any changes in insulin dose or renal function.

Line site: Monitor for signs and symptoms of infection.

Liver function tests: Monitor periodically.

Neonates: Sodium, calcium, and phosphate should be monitored closely.

Refeeding syndrome: Patients at risk should have phosphorus, magnesium, potassium, and glucose levels monitored closely at initiation.

Triglycerides: Before initiation of lipid therapy and at least weekly during therapy.

Vitamin A status: Should be carefully monitored in patients with chronic renal failure.

Pregnancy Risk Factor C

Contraindications Inborn errors of amino acid metabolism

Warnings/Precautions Use with caution in patients sensitive to volume overload (eg, heart failure, hepatic failure); consider concentrated total parenteral nutrition formula. Use caution in protein delivery especially in patients with hepatic encephalopathy; dosage adjustments may be necessary. Use with caution in patients with severe renal impairment; dosage adjustments may be necessary depending upon renal replacement therapy options. It is essential to provide adequate calories in a minimal amount of fluid (monitor fluid balance closely). Solutions may contain aluminum; toxic levels may occur following prolonged administration in premature neonates or patients with renal impairment. Monitor fluid and electrolyte status. Some products contain sulfites as preservatives.

Adverse Reactions Frequency not defined.
Endocrine & metabolic: Fluid, electrolyte imbalance
Local: Erythema, phlebitis, thrombosis
Renal: Azotemia

Dosage Forms Excipient information presented when available (limited, particularly for generics); consult specific product labeling. Peripheral parenteral nutrition and total parenteral nutrition are usually compounded from optimal combinations of macronutrients (water, protein, dextrose, and lipids) and micronutrients (electrolytes, trace elements, and vitamins) to meet the specific nutritional requirements of a patient. Individual hospitals may have designated standard TPN formulas. There are a few commercially-available amino acids with electrolytes solutions; however, these products may not meet an individual's specific nutritional requirements. Consult with nutrition support service to determine adequate formula based upon patient specifics.

Injection, solution [branched chain]:
  Aminosyn®-HBC: 7% (500 mL, 1000 mL) [contains aluminum]
  BranchAmin®: 4% (500 mL) [contains alumnium]
  FreAmine® HBC: 6.9% (750 mL) [contains aluminum, sodium bisulfate]
Injection, solution [crystalline]:
  Aminosyn®: 3.5% (1000 mL) [contains aluminum]; 5% (500 mL, 1000 mL) [contains aluminum]; 7% (500 mL, 1000 mL) [contains aluminum]; 8.5% (500 mL, 1000 mL) [contains aluminum]; 10% (500 mL, 1000 mL) [contains aluminum]
  Aminosyn® II: 7% (500 mL) [contains aluminum]; 8.5% (500 mL, 1000 mL) [contains aluminum]; 10% (500 mL, 1000 mL) [contains aluminum]
  Aminosyn® II: 10% (2000 mL) [contains aluminum, sodium hydrosulfite]; 15% (2000 mL) [contains aluminum, sodium hydrosulfite]
  Clinisol®: 15% (500 mL, 2000 mL) [contains aluminum]
  FreAmine® III: 8.5% (500 mL) [contains aluminum]; 10% (500 mL, 1000 mL) [contains aluminum]
  PremaSol™: 6% (500 mL); 10% (500 mL, 1000 mL, 2000 mL)
  Prosol: 20% (2000 mL) [contains aluminum]
  Travasol®: 10% (500 mL, 1000 mL, 2000 mL)
Injection, solution [hepatic]:
  Aminosyn®-HF: 8% (500 mL) [contains aluminum, sodium hydrosulfite]
  HepatAmine®: 8% (500 mL) [contains aluminum, sodium hydrosulfite]
  Hepatasol®: 8% (500 mL) [contains aluminum]
Injection, solution [pediatric]:
  Aminosyn®-PF: 7% (500 mL) [contains aluminum]; 10% (1000 mL) [contains aluminum]
  TrophAmine®: 6% (500 mL); 10% (500 mL) [contains aluminum, sodium metabisulfate]
Injection, solution [renal]:
  Aminosyn®-RF: 5.2% (500 mL) [contains aluminum]
  NephrAmine®: 5.4% (250 mL) [contains aluminum, sodium hydrosulfite]
  Renamin®: 6.5% (500 mL) [contains aluminum, sodium hydrosulfite]

♦ **Aminobenzylpenicillin** see Ampicillin on page 115

Aminocaproic Acid (a mee noe ka PROE ik AS id)

Medication Safety Issues
Sound-alike/look-alike issues:
Amicar® may be confused with amikacin, Amikin®, Omacor®
Related Information
Perioperative / Periprocedural Management of Anticoagulant and Antiplatelet Therapy on page 1607
U.S. Brand Names Amicar®
Index Terms EACA; Epsilon Aminocaproic Acid
Pharmacologic Category Antifibrinolytic Agent; Antihemophilic Agent; Hemostatic Agent; Lysine Analog
Generic Available Yes

◀ **Use** To enhance hemostasis when fibrinolysis contributes to bleeding (causes may include cardiac surgery, hematologic disorders, neoplastic disorders, abruption placentae, hepatic cirrhosis, and urinary fibrinolysis)

Unlabeled/Investigational Use Treatment of traumatic hyphema; control bleeding in thrombocytopenia; control oral bleeding in congenital and acquired coagulation disorders; topical treatment (mouth rinse) of bleeding associated with dental procedures in patients on oral anticoagulant therapy; prevention of perioperative bleeding associated with cardiac surgery

Mechanism of Action Binds competitively to plasminogen; blocking the binding of plasminogen to fibrin and the subsequent conversion to plasmin, resulting in inhibition of fibrin degradation (fibrinolysis).

Pharmacodynamics/Kinetics

Onset of action: ~1-72 hours

Distribution: Widely through intravascular and extravascular compartments

V_d: Oral: 23 L, I.V.: 30 L

Metabolism: Minimally hepatic

Half-life elimination: ~2 hours

Time to peak: Oral: Within 2 hours

Excretion: Urine (65% as unchanged drug, 11% as metabolite)

Dosage

Acute bleeding syndrome:

Children (unlabeled use): Oral, I.V.: Loading dose: 100-200 mg/kg during the first hour, followed by continuous infusion at 33.3 mg/kg/hour (I.V.) or 100 mg/kg (oral or I.V.) every 6 hours

Adults: Oral, I.V.: Loading dose: 4-5 g during the first hour, followed by 1 g/hour (or 1.25 g/hour using oral solution) for 8 hours or until bleeding controlled (maximum daily dose: 30 g)

Control of bleeding in thrombocytopenia (unlabeled use): Adults:

Initial: I.V.: 100 mg/kg over 30-60 minutes

Maintenance: Oral: 1-3 g every 6 hours

Control of oral bleeding in congenital and acquired coagulation disorder (unlabeled use): Adults: Oral: 50-60 mg/kg every 4 hours

Prevention of dental procedure bleeding in patients on oral anticoagulant therapy (unlabeled use): Oral rinse: Hold 4 g/10 mL in mouth for 2 minutes then spit out. Repeat every 6 hours for 2 days after procedure (Souto, 1996). Concentration and frequency may vary by institution and product availability.

Prevention of perioperative bleeding associated with cardiac surgery (unlabeled use): I.V.:

Children: 100 mg/kg given over 20-30 minutes after induction and prior to incision, 100 mg/kg during cardiopulmonary bypass, and 100 mg/kg after protamine reversal of heparin

Adults: 10 g over 20-30 minutes prior to skin incision, followed by 1-2.5 g/hour (usual dose 2 g/hour) until the end of operation (may continue infusion for 4 hours after protamine reversal of heparin). May add 10 g to cardiopulmonary bypass circuit priming solution.

or

10 g over 20-30 minutes prior to skin incision, followed by 10 g after heparin administration then 10 g at discontinuation of cardiopulmonary bypass prior to protamine reversal of heparin

Traumatic hyphema (unlabeled use): Children and Adults: Oral: 100 mg/kg/dose every 4 hours (maximum daily dose: 30 g)

Dosing adjustment in renal impairment: May accumulate in patients with decreased renal function.

Stability Store intact vials, tablets, and syrup at 15°C to 30°C (59°F to 86°F). Do not freeze injection or syrup. Dilute I.V. solution in D_5W, 0.9% sodium chloride, or Ringer's injection. Solutions diluted for I.V. use in D_5W or NS to concentrations of 10-100 mg/mL are stable at 4°C (39°F) and 23°C (73°F) for 7 days (Zhang, 1997).

Administration Rapid I.V. injection (IVP) of undiluted solution is not recommended due to possible hypotension, bradycardia, and arrhythmia.

I.V.: Acute bleeding syndrome: Administer loading dose over 1 hour, followed by a continuous infusion

I.V.: Prevention of perioperative bleeding associated with cardiac surgery (unlabeled use): Administer loading dose over 20-30 minutes prior to skin incision, followed by a continuous infusion until the end of operation **or** as 2 additional bolus doses (over 20-30 minutes) given after heparin administration and at discontinuation of cardiopulmonary bypass prior to protamine reversal of heparin.

Monitoring Parameters Fibrinogen, fibrin split products, creatine phosphokinase (with long-term therapy), BUN, creatinine

Pregnancy Risk Factor C

Contraindications Disseminated intravascular coagulation (without heparin); evidence of an active intravascular clotting process

Warnings/Precautions Avoid rapid I.V. administration (may induce hypotension, bradycardia, or arrhythmia); rapid injection of undiluted solution is not recommended. Use with caution in patients with renal disease; aminocaproic acid may accumulate in patients with decreased renal function. Intrarenal obstruction may occur secondary to glomerular capillary thrombosis or clots in the renal pelvis and ureters. Do not use in hematuria of upper urinary tract origin unless possible benefits outweigh risks. Do not administer without a definite diagnosis of laboratory findings indicative of hyperfibrinolysis. Inhibition of fibrinolysis may promote clotting or thrombosis; more likely due to the presence of DIC. Skeletal muscle weakness ranging from mild myalgias and fatigue to severe myopathy with rhabdomyolysis and acute renal failure has been reported with prolonged use. Monitor CPK; discontinue treatment with a rise in CPK. Benzyl alcohol is used as a preservative in the injection; therefore, these products should not be used in the neonate. Do not administer with factor IX complex concentrates or anti-inhibitor coagulant complexes; may increase risk for thrombosis.

Adverse Reactions Frequency not defined.

Cardiovascular: Arrhythmia, bradycardia, edema, hypotension, intracranial hypertension, peripheral ischemia, syncope, thrombosis

Central nervous system: Confusion, delirium, dizziness, fatigue, hallucinations, headache, malaise, seizure, stroke

Dermatologic: Rash, pruritus

Gastrointestinal: Abdominal pain, anorexia, cramps, diarrhea, GI irritation, nausea, vomiting

Genitourinary: Dry ejaculation

Hematologic: Agranulocytosis, bleeding time increased, leukopenia, thrombocytopenia

Local: Injection site necrosis, injection site pain, injectionsite reactions

Neuromuscular & skeletal: CPK increased, myalgia, myositis, myopathy, rhabdomyolysis (rare), weakness

Ophthalmic: Vision decreased, watery eyes

Otic: Tinnitus

Renal: BUN increased, intrarenal obstruction (glomerular capillary thrombosis), myoglobinuria (rare), renal failure (rare)

Respiratory: Dyspnea, nasal congestion, pulmonary embolism

Miscellaneous: Allergic reaction, anaphylactoid reaction, anaphylaxis

Postmarketing and/or case reports: Hepatic lesion, myocardial lesion

Drug Interactions

Avoid Concomitant Use

Avoid concomitant use of Aminocaproic Acid with any of the following: Anti-inhibitor Coagulant Complex; Factor IX; Factor IX Complex (Human)

Increased Effect/Toxicity

Aminocaproic Acid may increase the levels/effects of: Anti-inhibitor Coagulant Complex; Factor IX; Factor IX Complex (Human); Fibrinogen Concentrate (Human)

The levels/effects of Aminocaproic Acid may be increased by: Fibrinogen Concentrate (Human); Tretinoin (Systemic)

Decreased Effect There are no known significant interactions involving a decrease in effect.

Dosage Forms Excipient information presented when available (limited, particularly for generics); consult specific product labeling.

Injection, solution: 250 mg/mL (20 mL)

Solution, oral: 1.25 g/5 mL (240 mL, 480 mL)
Syrup:
 Amicar®: 1.25 g/5 mL (480 mL) [raspberry flavor]
Tablet [scored]: 500 mg
 Amicar®: 500 mg, 1000 mg

♦ **5-Aminosalicylic Acid** *see* Mesalamine *on page 884*

♦ **Aminosyn®** *see* Amino Acid Injection *on page 81*

♦ **Aminosyn (Can)** *see* Amino Acid Injection *on page 81*

♦ **Aminosyn® II** *see* Amino Acid Injection *on page 81*

♦ **Aminosyn®-HBC** *see* Amino Acid Injection *on page 81*

♦ **Aminosyn®-PF** *see* Amino Acid Injection *on page 81*

♦ **Aminosyn-PF (Can)** *see* Amino Acid Injection *on page 81*

♦ **Aminosyn®-RF** *see* Amino Acid Injection *on page 81*

♦ **Aminosyn-RF (Can)** *see* Amino Acid Injection *on page 81*

Amiodarone (a MEE oh da rone)

Related Information
Antiarrhythmic Drugs *on page 1656*
Dosing Considerations for the Critically-Ill Patient With Morbid Obesity *on page 1561*
Heart Failure (Systolic) *on page 1739*
Management of Postoperative Arrhythmias *on page 1571*

U.S. Brand Names Cordarone®; Pacerone®

Canadian Brand Names Alti-Amiodarone; Amiodarone Hydrochloride for Injection®; Apo-Amiodarone®; Cordarone®; Dom-Amiodarone; Gen-Amiodarone; Mylan-Amiodarone; Novo-Amiodarone; PHL-Amiodarone; PMS-Amiodarone; PRO-Amiodarone; ratio-Amiodarone; ratio-Amiodarone I.V.; Riva-Amiodarone; Sandoz-Amiodarone

Index Terms Amiodarone Hydrochloride

Pharmacologic Category Antiarrhythmic Agent, Class III

Use Management of life-threatening recurrent ventricular fibrillation (VF) or hemodynamically-unstable ventricular tachycardia (VT) refractory to other antiarrhythmic agents or in patients intolerant of other agents used for these conditions

Unlabeled/Investigational Use
Cardiac arrest with persistent ventricular tachycardia (VT) or ventricular fibrillation (VF) if defibrillation, CPR, and vasopressor administration have failed (ACLS/PALS guidelines)

Control of hemodynamically-stable VT, polymorphic VT with a normal baseline QT interval, or wide-complex tachycardia of uncertain origin (ACLS/PALS guidelines)

Control of rapid ventricular rate due to accessory pathway conduction in pre-excited atrial arrhythmias (ACLS guidelines)

Heart rate control in patients with atrial fibrillation and heart failure [no accessory pathway] (ACC/AHA/ESC Practice Guidelines)

Paroxysmal supraventricular tachycardia (SVT)

Prevention of postoperative atrial fibrillation associated with cardiothoracic surgery

Pharmacologic adjunct to ICD therapy to suppress symptomatic ventricular tachyarrhythmias in otherwise optimally-treated patients with heart failure (ACC/AHA/ESC Practice Guidelines)

Pharmacologic conversion of atrial fibrillation to normal sinus rhythm; maintenance of normal sinus rhythm

Pharmacodynamics/Kinetics
Absorption: Slow and variable
Onset of action: Oral: 2 days to 3 weeks; I.V.: May be more rapid
 Peak effect: 1 week to 5 months

Duration after discontinuing therapy: 7-50 days
 Note: Mean onset of effect and duration after discontinuation may be shorter in children than adults
Distribution: V_d: 66 L/kg (range: 18-148 L/kg)
Protein binding: 96%
Metabolism: Hepatic via CYP2C8 and 3A4 to active N-desethylamiodarone metabolite; possible enterohepatic recirculation
Bioavailability: Oral: 35% to 65%
Half-life elimination: Terminal: 40-55 days (range: 26-107 days); shorter in children
Time to peak, serum: 3-7 hours
Excretion: Feces; urine (<1% as unchanged drug)

Dosage Note: Lower loading and maintenance doses are preferable in women and all patients with low body weight.

Oral:
 Children: Arrhythmias (unlabeled use):
  Loading dose: 10-20 mg/kg/day in 1-2 doses for 4-14 days or until adequate control of arrhythmia or prominent adverse effects occur; alternative loading dose in children <1 year: 600-800 mg/1.73 m^2/day in 1-2 divided doses/day
  Maintenance dose: Dose may be reduced to 5 mg/kg/day for several weeks (or 200-400 mg/1.73 m^2/day given once daily); if no recurrence of arrhythmia, dose may be further reduced to 2.5 mg/kg/day; maintenance doses may be given 5-7 days/week
 Adults:
  Ventricular arrhythmias: 800-1600 mg/day in 1-2 doses for 1-3 weeks, then when adequate arrhythmia control is achieved, decrease to 600-800 mg/day in 1-2 doses for 1 month; maintenance: 400 mg/day. Lower doses are recommended for supraventricular arrhythmias.
  Atrial fibrillation: Prophylaxis following open heart surgery (unlabeled use): Starting in postop recovery: 400 mg twice daily for up to 7 days. Alternative regimen of amiodarone: 600 mg/day for 7 days prior to surgery, followed by 200 mg/day until hospital discharge, has also been shown to decrease the risk of postoperative atrial fibrillation. **Note:** A variety of regimens have been used in clinical trials.
  Atrial fibrillation: Pharmacologic cardioversion (unlabeled use): ACC/AHA/ESC Practice Guidelines: Inpatient: 1.2-1.8 g/day in divided doses until 10 g total, then 200-400 mg/day maintenance. **Note:** Other regimens have been described and may be used clinically (Roy, 2000):
   400 mg 3 times/day for 5-7 days, then 400 mg/day for 1 month, then 200 mg/day
   or
   10 mg/kg/day for 14 days, followed by 300 mg/day for 4 weeks, followed by maintenance dosage of 100-200 mg/day
I.V.:
 Children:
  Arrhythmias (unlabeled use, dosing based on limited data): Loading dose: 5 mg/kg over 30 minutes; may repeat up to 3 times if no response. Maintenance dose: 2-20 mg/kg/day (5-15 mcg/kg/minute) by continuous infusion
  Note: I.V. administration at low flow rates (potentially associated with use in pediatrics) may result in leaching of plasticizers (DEHP) from intravenous tubing. DEHP may adversely affect male reproductive tract development. Alternative means of dosing and administration (1 mg/kg aliquots) may need to be considered.
  Pulseless VF or VT (PALS dosing): 5 mg/kg (maximum: 300 mg/dose) rapid I.V. bolus or I.O.; repeat up to a maximum daily dose of 15 mg/kg. (**Note:** Maximum recommended daily dose in adolescents is 2.2 g.)
  Perfusing tachycardias (PALS dosing): Loading dose: 5 mg/kg (maximum: 300 mg/dose) I.V. over 20-60 minutes or I.O.; may repeat up to maximum dose of 15 mg/kg/day. (**Note:** Maximum recommended daily dose in adolescents is 2.2 g.)
 Adults:
  Atrial fibrillation: Prophylaxis following open heart surgery (unlabeled use): Starting at postop recovery, 1000 mg infused over 24 hours for 2 days has

been shown to reduce the risk of postoperative atrial fibrillation. **Note:** A variety of regimens have been used in clinical trials.

Atrial fibrillation: Pharmacologic cardioversion (ACC/AHA/ESC Practice Guidelines) (unlabeled use): 5-7 mg/kg over 30-60 minutes, then 1.2-1.8 g/day continuous infusion or in divided oral doses until 10 g total. Maintenance: See oral dosing.

Ventricular arrhythmias:

Breakthrough VF or VT: 150 mg supplemental doses in 100 mL D_5W over 10 minutes

Pulseless VF or VT: I.V. push: Initial: 300 mg in 20-30 mL NS or D_5W; if VF or VT recurs, supplemental dose of 150 mg followed by infusion of 1 mg/minute for 6 hours, then 0.5 mg/minute (mean daily doses >2.1 g/day have been associated with hypotension)

Stable VT or SVT (unlabeled use): First 24 hours: 1050 mg according to following regimen

Step 1: 150 mg (100 mL) over first 10 minutes (mix 3 mL in 100 mL D_5W)

Step 2: 360 mg (200 mL) over next 6 hours (mix 18 mL in 500 mL D_5W): 1 mg/minute

Step 3: 540 mg (300 mL) over next 18 hours: 0.5 mg/minute

Note: After the first 24 hours: 0.5 mg/minute utilizing concentration of 1-6 mg/mL

I.V. to oral therapy conversion: Use the following as a guide:

<1 week I.V. infusion: 800-1600 mg/day

1- to 3-week I.V. infusion: 600-800 mg/day

>3-week I.V. infusion: 400 mg/day

Recommendations for conversion to intravenous amiodarone after oral administration: During long-term amiodarone therapy (ie, ≥4 months), the mean plasma-elimination half-life of the active metabolite of amiodarone is 61 days. Replacement therapy may not be necessary in such patients if oral therapy is discontinued for a period <2 weeks, since any changes in serum amiodarone concentrations during this period may **not** be clinically significant.

Elderly: No specific guidelines available. Dose selection should be cautious, at low end of dosage range, and titration should be slower to evaluate response.

Hemodialysis: Not dialyzable (0% to 5%); supplemental dose is not necessary.

Peritoneal dialysis effects: Not dialyzable (0% to 5%); supplemental dose is not necessary.

Dosing adjustment in hepatic impairment: Dosage adjustment is probably necessary in substantial hepatic impairment. No specific guidelines available. If hepatic enzymes exceed 3 times normal or double in a patient with an elevated baseline, consider decreasing the dose or discontinuing amiodarone.

Anesthesia and Critical Care Concerns/Other Considerations
Evidence-Based Information:

Cardiac Arrest: The ARREST trial was a randomized, placebo-controlled trial evaluating amiodarone's efficacy in patients who had an out-of-hospital cardiac arrest with pulseless ventricular tachycardia (VT) or ventricular fibrillation (VF). The primary endpoint was admission to the hospital with a spontaneous perfusing rhythm. Patients were randomized to receive 300 mg of intravenous amiodarone or placebo after being shocked ≥3 times, intubated, and receiving 1 mg of epinephrine. VF was the most common initial arrhythmia (88%). More patients in the amiodarone group were successfully resuscitated (44% amiodarone; 34% placebo; p=0.03) and admitted to the hospital, but mortality was similar in both groups (possibly due to sample size). The ALIVE trial, a randomized, double-blind, placebo controlled trial, compared amiodarone to lidocaine in 347 out-of-hospital cardiac arrest victims whose VF was resistant to 3 defibrillation attempts in addition to epinephrine and a fourth defibrillation attempt (Dorian, 2002). Other inclusion criteria included VF unrelated to trauma (or with other arrhythmias that converted to VF) and recurrent VF after successful initial defibrillation. The primary endpoint was the number of patients who were admitted to the hospital ICU alive. The initial amiodarone dose was 5 mg/kg and the lidocaine dose was 1.5 mg/kg. If VF persisted after another shock, then the study drug could be administered again (amiodarone 2.5 mg/kg, lidocaine 1.5 mg/kg). Significantly more amiodarone patients (~23%) were admitted to the hospital alive than lidocaine patients (12%). The majority (>90%) of patients in the ALIVE trial had VF as the initial arrhythmia. The authors concluded that intravenous amiodarone is superior to lidocaine in the treatment of shock-resistant, out-of-hospital VF.

Arrhythmias: In patients with severe left ventricular dysfunction, amiodarone is preferable over other antiarrhythmics due to its minimal negative inotropic effects.

Amiodarone injectable contains the emulsifier polysorbate 80 (also known as Tween 80) which is responsible for the transient hypotensive effects when administered too rapidly (Munoz, 1988). In patients with perfusing rhythms (eg, atrial fibrillation), the initial loading dose should be administered over at least 10 minutes.

Additional Information Complete prescribing information for this medication should be consulted for additional detail.

Dosage Forms Excipient information presented when available (limited, particularly for generics); consult specific product labeling.

Injection, solution, as hydrochloride: 50 mg/mL (3 mL, 9 mL, 18 mL) [contains benzyl alcohol and polysorbate 80]

Tablet, as hydrochloride [scored]: 200 mg, 400 mg

Cordarone®: 200 mg

Pacerone®: 100 mg [not scored], 200 mg, 400 mg

References

"2005 American Heart Association Guidelines for Cardiopulmonary Resuscitation and Emergency Cardiovascular Care," *Circulation*, 2005, 112(24 Suppl): 1-211.

Daoud EG, Strickberger SA, Man KC, et al, "Preoperative Amiodarone as Prophylaxis Against Atrial Fibrillation After Heart Surgery," *N Engl J Med*, 1997, 337(25):1785-91.

Dorian P, Cass D, Schwartz B, et al, "Amiodarone as Compared With Lidocaine for Shock-Resistant Ventricular Fibrillation," *N Engl J Med*, 2002, 346(12):884-90.

Goldschlager N, Epstein AE, Naccarelli G, et al, "Practical Guidelines for Clinicians Who Treat Patients With Amiodarone. Practice Guidelines Subcommittee, North American Society of Pacing and Electrophysiology," *Arch Intern Med*, 2000, 160(12):1741-8.

Guarnieri T, Nolan S, Gottlieb SO, et al, "Intravenous Amiodarone for the Prevention of Atrial Fibrillation After Open Heart Surgery: The Amiodarone Reduction in Coronary Heart (ARCH) Trial," *J Am Coll Cardiol*, 1999, 34(2):343-7.

Kudenchuk PJ, Cobb LA, Copass MK, et al, "Amiodarone for Resuscitation After Out-of-Hospital Cardiac Arrest Due to Ventricular Fibrillation," *N Engl J Med*, 1999, 341(12):871-8.

Munoz A, Karila P, Gallay P, et al, "A Randomized Hemodynamic Comparison of Intravenous Amiodarone With and Without Tween 80," *Eur Heart J*, 1988, 9(2):142-8.

Ott MC, Khoor A, Leventhal JP, et al, "Pulmonary Toxicity in Patients Receiving Low-Dose Amiodarone," *Chest*, 2003, 123:646-54.

Perry JC, Fenrich AL, Hulse JE, et al, "Pediatric Use of Intravenous Amiodarone: Efficacy and Safety in Critically Ill Patients From a Multicenter Protocol," *J Am Coll Cardiol*, 1996, 27(5):1246-50.

Stamou SC, Hill PC, Sample GA, et al, "Prevention of Atrial Fibrillation After Cardiac Surgery: The Significance of Postoperative Oral Amiodarone," *Chest*, 2001, 120(6):1936-41.

♦ **Amiodarone Hydrochloride** *see* Amiodarone *on page 86*

♦ **Amiodarone Hydrochloride for Injection® (Can)** *see* Amiodarone *on page 86*

Amitriptyline (a mee TRIP ti leen)

Medication Safety Issues

Sound-alike/look-alike issues:

Amitriptyline may be confused with aminophylline, imipramine, nortriptyline

Elavil® may be confused with Aldoril®, Eldepryl®, enalapril, Equanil®, Mellaril®, Oruvail®, Plavix®

Medication Guide An FDA-approved patient medication guide, which is available with the product information and at http://www.fda.gov/downloads/Drugs/DrugSafety/ucm088622.pdf, must be dispensed with this medication for each new outpatient prescription and refill.

Related Information

Antidepressant Agents *on page 1660*

Chronic Pain Management *on page 1546*

Canadian Brand Names Apo-Amitriptyline®; Levate®; Novo-Triptyn; PMS-Amitriptyline

Index Terms Amitriptyline Hydrochloride; Elavil

Pharmacologic Category Antidepressant, Tricyclic (Tertiary Amine)

Generic Available Yes

Use Relief of symptoms of depression

◄ **Unlabeled/Investigational Use** Analgesic for certain chronic and neuropathic pain; prophylaxis against migraine headaches; treatment of depressive disorders in children; post-traumatic stress disorder (PTSD)

Mechanism of Action Increases the synaptic concentration of serotonin and/or norepinephrine in the central nervous system by inhibition of their reuptake by the presynaptic neuronal membrane

Pharmacodynamics/Kinetics

Onset of action: Migraine prophylaxis: 6 weeks, higher dosage may be required in heavy smokers because of increased metabolism; Depression: 4-6 weeks, reduce dosage to lowest effective level

Distribution: Crosses placenta; enters breast milk

Metabolism: Hepatic to nortriptyline (active), hydroxy and conjugated derivatives; may be impaired in the elderly

Half-life elimination: Adults: 9-27 hours (average: 15 hours)

Time to peak, serum: ~4 hours

Excretion: Urine (18% as unchanged drug); feces (small amounts)

Dosage

Children:

Chronic pain management (unlabeled use): Oral: Initial: 0.1 mg/kg at bedtime, may advance as tolerated over 2-3 weeks to 0.5-2 mg/kg at bedtime

Depressive disorders (unlabeled use): Oral: Initial doses of 1 mg/kg/day given in 3 divided doses with increases to 1.5 mg/kg/day have been reported in a small number of children (n=9) 9-12 years of age; clinically, doses up to 3 mg/kg/day (5 mg/kg/day if monitored closely) have been proposed

Migraine prophylaxis (unlabeled use): Oral: Initial: 0.25 mg/kg/day, given at bedtime; increase dose by 0.25 mg/kg/day to maximum 1 mg/kg/day. Reported dosing ranges: 0.1-2 mg/kg/day; maximum suggested dose: 10 mg.

Adolescents: Depressive disorders: Oral: Initial: 25-50 mg/day; may administer in divided doses; increase gradually to 100 mg/day in divided doses

Adults:

Depression: Oral: 50-150 mg/day single dose at bedtime or in divided doses; dose may be gradually increased up to 300 mg/day

Chronic pain management (unlabeled use): Oral: Initial: 25 mg at bedtime; may increase as tolerated to 100 mg/day

Migraine prophylaxis (unlabeled use): Oral: Initial: 10-25 mg at bedtime; usual dose: 150 mg; reported dosing ranges: 10-400 mg/day

Post-traumatic stress disorder (PTSD) (unlabeled use): Oral: 75-200 mg/day

Elderly: Depression: Oral: Initial: 10-25 mg at bedtime; dose should be increased in 10-25 mg increments every week if tolerated; dose range: 25-150 mg/day

Dosing interval in hepatic impairment: Use with caution and monitor plasma levels and patient response

Hemodialysis: Nondialyzable

Monitoring Parameters Monitor blood pressure and pulse rate prior to and during initial therapy; evaluate mental status, suicidal ideation (especially at the beginning of therapy or when doses are increased or decreased); monitor weight; ECG in older adults and patients with cardiac disease

Reference Range Therapeutic: Amitriptyline and nortriptyline 100-250 ng/mL (SI: 360-900 nmol/L); nortriptyline 50-150 ng/mL (SI: 190-570 nmol/L); Toxic: >0.5 mcg/mL; plasma levels do not always correlate with clinical effectiveness

Anesthesia and Critical Care Concerns/Other Considerations Desired therapeutic effect (for analgesia) may take as long as 1-3 weeks. When used for migraine headache prophylaxis, therapeutic effect may take as long as 6 weeks.

Tricyclic antidepressants affect conduction and have anticholinergic effects and, therefore, should be used with caution in patients with underlying cardiovascular disease. Therapy is relatively contraindicated in patients with conduction abnormalities or in patients with symptomatic hypotension. Heart block may be precipitated in patients with pre-existing conduction system disease.

Pregnancy Risk Factor C

Contraindications Hypersensitivity to amitriptyline or any component of the formulation (cross-sensitivity with other tricyclics may occur); use of MAO inhibitors within past 14 days; acute recovery phase following myocardial infarction; concurrent use of cisapride

Warnings/Precautions [U.S. Boxed Warning]: Antidepressants increase the risk of suicidal thinking and behavior in children, adolescents, and young adults (18-24 years of age) with major depressive disorder (MDD) and other psychiatric disorders; consider risk prior to prescribing. Short-term studies did not show an increased risk in patients >24 years of age and showed a decreased risk in patients ≥65 years. Closely monitor for clinical worsening, suicidality, or unusual changes in behavior; the patient's family or caregiver should be instructed to closely observe the patient and communicate condition with healthcare provider. Such observation would generally include at least weekly face-to-face contact with patients or their family members or caregivers during the first 4 weeks of treatment, then every other week visits for the next 4 weeks, then at 12 weeks, and as clinically indicated beyond 12 weeks. Additional contact by telephone may be appropriate between face-to-face visits. Adults treated with antidepressants should be observed similarly for clinical worsening and suicidality, especially during the initial few months of a course of drug therapy, or at times of dose changes, either increases or decreases. A medication guide should be dispensed with each prescription. **Amitriptyline is not FDA-approved for use in children <12 years of age.**

The possibility of a suicide attempt is inherent in major depression and may persist until remission occurs. Monitor for worsening of depression or suicidality, especially during initiation of therapy (generally first 1-2 months) or with dose increases or decreases. Worsening depression and severe abrupt suicidality that are not part of the presenting symptoms may require discontinuation or modification of drug therapy. The patient's family or caregiver should be alerted to monitor patients for the emergence of suicidality and associated behaviors (such as agitation, irritability, hostility, impulsivity, and hypomania) and notify healthcare provider.

May worsen psychosis in some patients or precipitate a shift to mania or hypomania in patients with bipolar disorder. Patients presenting with depressive symptoms should be screened for bipolar disorder. Monotherapy in patients with bipolar disorder should be avoided. **Amitriptyline is not FDA approved for bipolar depression.**

The degree of sedation, anticholinergic effects, orthostasis, and conduction abnormalities are high relative to other antidepressants. Amitriptyline often causes drowsiness/sedation, resulting in impaired performance of tasks requiring alertness (eg, operating machinery or driving). Sedative effects may be additive with other CNS depressants and/or ethanol. Use with caution in patients with a history of cardiovascular disease (including previous MI, stroke, tachycardia, or conduction abnormalities). Use with caution in patients with urinary retention, benign prostatic hyperplasia, narrow-angle glaucoma, xerostomia, visual problems, constipation, or a history of bowel obstruction.

TCAs may rarely cause bone marrow suppression; monitor for any signs of infection and obtain CBC if symptoms (eg, fever, sore throat) evident. May alter glucose control - use with caution in patients with diabetes. Consider discontinuing, when possible, prior to elective surgery. Therapy should not be abruptly discontinued in patients receiving high doses for prolonged periods. May lower seizure threshold - use caution in patients with a previous seizure disorder or condition predisposing to seizures such as brain damage, alcoholism, or concurrent therapy with other drugs which lower the seizure threshold. Hyperpyrexia has been observed with TCAs in combination with anticholinergics and/or neuroleptics, particularly during hot weather. May increase the risks associated with electroconvulsive therapy. Use with caution in hyperthyroid patients or those receiving thyroid supplementation. Use with caution in patients with hepatic or renal dysfunction and in elderly patients.

Adverse Reactions Anticholinergic effects may be pronounced; moderate to marked sedation can occur (tolerance to these effects usually occurs).

Frequency not defined.

Cardiovascular: Orthostatic hypotension, tachycardia, ECG changes (non-specific), AV conduction changes, cardiomyopathy (rare), MI, stroke, heart block, arrhythmia, syncope, hypertension, palpitation

◀ Central nervous system: Restlessness, dizziness, insomnia, sedation, fatigue, anxiety, cognitive function impaired, seizure, extrapyramidal symptoms, coma, hallucinations, confusion, disorientation, coordination impaired, ataxia, headache, nightmares, hyperpyrexia

Dermatologic: Allergic rash, urticaria, photosensitivity, alopecia

Endocrine & metabolic: Syndrome of inappropriate ADH secretion

Gastrointestinal: Weight gain, xerostomia, constipation, paralytic ileus, nausea, vomiting, anorexia, stomatitis, peculiar taste, diarrhea, black tongue

Genitourinary: Urinary retention

Hematologic: Bone marrow depression, purpura, eosinophilia

Neuromuscular & skeletal: Numbness, paresthesia, peripheral neuropathy, tremor, weakness

Ocular: Blurred vision, mydriasis, ocular pressure increased

Otic: Tinnitus

Miscellaneous: Diaphoresis, withdrawal reactions (nausea, headache, malaise)

Postmarketing and/or case reports: Neuroleptic malignant syndrome (rare), serotonin syndrome (rare)

Drug Interactions

Metabolism/Transport Effects Substrate of CYP1A2 (minor), 2B6 (minor), 2C9 (minor), 2C19 (minor), 2D6 (major), 3A4 (minor); **Inhibits** CYP1A2 (weak), 2C9 (weak), 2C19 (weak), 2D6 (weak), 2E1 (weak)

Avoid Concomitant Use

Avoid concomitant use of Amitriptyline with any of the following: Artemether; Cisapride; Dronedarone; Iobenguane I 123; Lumefantrine; MAO Inhibitors; Nilotinib; Pimozide; QuiNINE; Sibutramine; Tetrabenazine; Thioridazine; Ziprasidone

Increased Effect/Toxicity

Amitriptyline may increase the levels/effects of: Alcohol (Ethyl); Alpha-/Beta-Agonists (Direct-Acting); Alpha1-Agonists; Amphetamines; Anticholinergics; Aspirin; Beta2-Agonists; Cisapride; CNS Depressants; Desmopressin; Dronedarone; NSAID (COX-2 Inhibitor); NSAID (Nonselective); Pimozide; QTc-Prolonging Agents; QuiNIDine; QuiNINE; Serotonin Modulators; Sulfonylureas; Tetrabenazine; Thioridazine; TraMADol; Vitamin K Antagonists; Yohimbine; Ziprasidone

The levels/effects of Amitriptyline may be increased by: Alfuzosin; Altretamine; Artemether; BuPROPion; Chloroquine; Cimetidine; Cinacalcet; Ciprofloxacin; CYP2D6 Inhibitors (Moderate); CYP2D6 Inhibitors (Strong); Dexmethylphenidate; DULoxetine; Gadobutrol; Lithium; Lumefantrine; MAO Inhibitors; Methylphenidate; Nilotinib; Pramlintide; Propoxyphene; Protease Inhibitors; QuiNIDine; QuiNINE; Selective Serotonin Reuptake Inhibitors; Sibutramine; Terbinafine; Valproic Acid

Decreased Effect

Amitriptyline may decrease the levels/effects of: Acetylcholinesterase Inhibitors (Central); Alpha2-Agonists; Iobenguane I 123

The levels/effects of Amitriptyline may be decreased by: Acetylcholinesterase Inhibitors (Central); Barbiturates; CarBAMazepine; Peginterferon Alfa-2b; St Johns Wort

Ethanol/Nutrition/Herb Interactions

Ethanol: Avoid ethanol (may increase CNS depression).

Food: Grapefruit juice may inhibit the metabolism of some TCAs and clinical toxicity may result.

Herb/Nutraceutical: St John's wort may decrease amitriptyline levels. Avoid valerian, St John's wort, kava kava, gotu kola (may increase CNS depression).

Test Interactions May cause false-positive reaction to EMIT immunoassay for imipramine

Dosage Forms Excipient information presented when available (limited, particularly for generics); consult specific product labeling.

Tablet, as hydrochloride: 10 mg, 25 mg, 50 mg, 75 mg, 100 mg, 150 mg

References

Mokhlesi B, Leikin JB, Murray P, et al, "Adult Toxicology in Critical Care. Part 11: Specific Poisonings," *Chest*, 2003, 123(3):897-922.

◆ **Amitriptyline Hydrochloride** *see* Amitriptyline *on page 89*

AmLODIPine (am LOE di peen)

Related Information
Calcium Channel Blockers *on page 1672*
Heart Failure (Systolic) *on page 1739*

U.S. Brand Names Norvasc®

Canadian Brand Names Apo-Amlodipine®; CO Amlodipine; GD-Amlodipine; Mylan-Amlodipine; Norvasc®; Novo-Amlodipine; PHL-Amlodipine; PMS-Amlodipine; Ran-Amlodipine; ratio-Amlodipine; Riva-Amlodipine; Sandoz-Amlodipine

Index Terms Amlodipine Besylate

Pharmacologic Category Calcium Channel Blocker; Calcium Channel Blocker, Dihydropyridine

Use Treatment of hypertension; treatment of symptomatic chronic stable angina, vasospastic (Prinzmetal's) angina (confirmed or suspected); prevention of hospitalization due to angina with documented CAD (limited to patients without heart failure or ejection fraction <40%)

Pharmacodynamics/Kinetics
Duration of antihypertensive effect: 24 hours
Absorption: Oral: Well absorbed
Distribution: V_d: 21 L/kg
Protein binding: 93% to 98%
Metabolism: Hepatic (>90%) to inactive metabolite
Bioavailability: 64% to 90%
Half-life elimination: 30-50 hours; increased with hepatic dysfunction
Time to peak, plasma: 6-12 hours
Excretion: Urine (10% as parent, 60% as metabolite)

Dosage Oral:
Children 6-17 years: Hypertension: 2.5-5 mg once daily
Adults:
 Hypertension: Initial dose: 5 mg once daily; maximum dose: 10 mg once daily. In general, titrate in 2.5 mg increments over 7-14 days. Usual dosage range (JNC 7): 2.5-10 mg once daily.
 Angina: Usual dose: 5-10 mg; lower dose suggested in elderly or hepatic impairment; most patients require 10 mg for adequate effect
 Elderly: Dosing should start at the lower end of dosing range due to possible increased incidence of hepatic, renal, or cardiac impairment. Elderly patients also show decreased clearance of amlodipine.
 Hypertension: 2.5 mg once daily
 Angina: 5 mg once daily

Dosage adjustmnent in renal impairment: Dialysis: Hemodialysis and peritoneal dialysis do not enhance elimination. Supplemental dose is not necessary.

Dosage adjustment in hepatic impairment:
Angina: Administer 5 mg once daily.
Hypertension: Administer 2.5 mg once daily.

Anesthesia and Critical Care Concerns/Other Considerations Amlodipine may be used safely to treat hypertension and/or angina in patients with heart failure.

Additional Information Complete prescribing information for this medication should be consulted for additional detail.

Dosage Forms Excipient information presented when available (limited, particularly for generics); consult specific product labeling.
Tablet: 2.5 mg, 5 mg, 10 mg
 Norvasc®: 2.5 mg, 5 mg, 10 mg

References
ALLHAT Officers and Coordinators for the ALLHAT Collaborative Research Group, "Major Outcomes in High-Risk Hypertensive Patients Randomized to Angiotensin-Converting Enzyme Inhibitor or Calcium Channel Blocker vs Diuretic: The Antihypertensive and Lipid-Lowering Treatment to Prevent Heart Attack Trial (ALLHAT)," *JAMA*, 2002, 288(23):2981-97.

Braunwald E, Antman EM, Beasley JW, et al, "ACC/AHA Guidelines for the Management of Patients With Unstable Angina and Non-ST-Segment Elevation Myocardial Infarction. A Report of the American College of Cardiology/American Heart Association Task Force on Practice Guidelines (Committee on the Management of Patients With Unstable Angina)," J Am Coll Cardiol, 2000, 36 (3):970-1062.

Chobanian AV, Bakris GL, Black HR, et al, "The Seventh Report of the Joint National Committee on Prevention, Detection, Evaluation, and Treatment of High Blood Pressure: The JNC 7 Report," JAMA, 2003, 289(19):2560-71.

Davies RF, Habibi H, Klinke WP, et al, "Effect of Amlodipine, Atenolol and Their Combination on Myocardial Ischemia During Treadmill Exercise and Ambulatory Monitoring. Canadian Amlodipine/Atenolol in Silent Ischemia Study (CASIS) Investigators," J Am Coll Cardiol, 1995, 25(3):619-25.

Grassi G, Spaziani D, Seravalle G, et al, "Effect of Amlodipine on Sympathetic Nerve Traffic and Baroreflex Control of Circulation in Heart Failure," Hypertension, 1999, 33(2):671-5.

Hall WD, Reed JW, Flack JM, et al, "Comparison of the Efficacy of Dihydropyridine Calcium Channel Blockers in African American Patients With Hypertension. ISHIB Investigators Group. International Society on Hypertension in Blacks," Arch Intern Med, 1998, 158(18):2029-34.

Hunt SA, Abraham WT, Chin MH, et al, "ACC/AHA 2005 Guideline Update for the Diagnosis and Management of Chronic Heart Failure in the Adult: A Report of the American College of Cardiology/American Heart Association Task Force on Practice Guidelines (Writing Committee to Update the 2001 Guidelines for the Evaluation and Management of Heart Failure)," available at http://www.acc.org/qualityandscience/clinical/guidelines/failure/update/index.pdf.

Joseffsson M, Zackrisson AL, and Ahlner J, "Effect of Grapefruit Juice on the Pharmacokinetics of Amlodipine in Healthy Volunteers," Eur J Clin Pharmacol, 1996, 51(2):189-93.

Meredith PA and Elliott HL, "Clinical Pharmacokinetics of Amlodipine," Clin Pharmacokinet , 1992, 22 (1):22-31.

National High Blood Pressure Education Program Working Group on High Blood Pressure in Children and Adolescents, "The Fourth Report on the Diagnosis, Evaluation, and Treatment of High Blood Pressure in Children and Adolescents," Pediatrics, 2004, 114(2 Suppl):555-76.

Neaton JD, Grimm RH Jr, Prineas RJ, et al, "Treatment of Mild Hypertension Study. Final Results. Treatment of Mild Hypertension Study Research Group," JAMA, 1993, 270(6):713-24.

Nissen SE, Tuzcu EM, Libby P, et al, "Effect of Antihypertensive Agents on Cardiovascular Events in Patients With Coronary Disease and Normal Blood Pressure: The CAMELOT Study: A Randomized Controlled Trial," JAMA, 2004, 292(18):2217-25.

Packer M, O'Connor CM, Ghali JK, et al, "Effect of Amlodipine on Morbidity and Mortality in Severe Chronic Heart Failure. Prospective Randomized Amlodipine Survival Evaluation Study Group," N Engl J Med, 1996, 335(15):1107-14.

Sever PS, Dahlof B, Poulter NR, et al, "Rationale, Design, Methods and Baseline Demography of Participants of the Anglo-Scandinavian Cardiac Outcomes Trial. ASCOT Investigators," J Hypertens, 2001, 19(6):1139-47.

Steele RM, Schuna AA, and Schreiber RT, "Calcium Antagonist-Induced Gingival Hyperplasia," Ann Intern Med, 1994, 120(8):663-4.

Vincent J, Harris SI, Foulds G, et al, "Lack of Effect of Grapefruit Juice on the Pharmacokinetics and Pharmacodynamics of Amlodipine," Br J Clin Pharmacol, 2000, 50(5):455-63.

Amlodipine and Olmesartan (am LOE di peen & olme SAR tan)

Related Information

AmLODIPine on page 93

Olmesartan on page 1045

U.S. Brand Names Azor™

Index Terms Amlodipine Besylate and Olmesartan Medoxomil; Olmesartan and Amlodipine

Pharmacologic Category Angiotensin II Receptor Blocker; Calcium Channel Blocker; Calcium Channel Blocker, Dihydropyridine

Use Treatment of hypertension, including initial treatment in patients who will require multiple antihypertensives for adequate control

Pharmacodynamics/Kinetics See individual agents.

Dosage Oral: Dose is individualized; combination product may be substituted for individual components in patients currently maintained on both agents separately or in patients not adequately controlled with monotherapy (using one of the agents or an agent the within same antihypertensive class). May also be used as initial therapy in patients who are likely to need >1 antihypertensive to control blood pressure.

Adults: Hypertension:

Initial therapy (antihypertensive naive): Amlodipine 5 mg/olmesartan 20 mg once daily; dose may be increased after 1-2 weeks of therapy. Maximum recommended dose: Amlodipine 10 mg/day; olmesartan 40 mg/day.

Add-on/replacement therapy: Amlodipine 5-10 mg and olmesartan 20-40 mg once daily depending upon previous doses, current control, and goals of therapy; dose may be titrated after 2 weeks of therapy. Maximum recommended doses: Amlodipine 10 mg/day; olmesartan 40 mg/day.

Elderly: Initial therapy is not recommended in patients ≥75 years of age.

Dosing adjustment in renal impairment: No specific guidelines for dosage adjustment

Dosing adjustment in hepatic impairment: Initial therapy is not recommended

Additional Information Complete prescribing information for this medication should be consulted for additional detail.

Dosage Forms Excipient information presented when available (limited, particularly for generics); consult specific product labeling.

Tablet:

Azor™ 5/20: Amlodipine besylate 5 mg and olmesartan medoxomil 20 mg

Azor™ 5/40: Amlodipine besylate 5 mg and olmesartan medoxomil 40 mg

Azor™ 10/20: Amlodipine besylate 10 mg and olmesartan medoxomil 20 mg

Azor™ 10/40: Amlodipine besylate 10 mg and olmesartan medoxomil 40 mg

◆ **Amlodipine Besylate** *see* AmLODIPine *on page 93*

◆ **Amlodipine Besylate and Olmesartan Medoxomil** *see* Amlodipine and Olmesartan *on page 94*

◆ **Amoclan** *see* Amoxicillin and Clavulanate Potassium *on page 98*

Amoxicillin (a moks i SIL in)

Related Information

Helicobacter pylori Treatment *on page 1746*

Prevention of Infective Endocarditis *on page 1718*

U.S. Brand Names Amoxil® [DSC]; Moxatag™

Canadian Brand Names Apo-Amoxi®; Gen-Amoxicillin; Lin-Amox; Mylan-Amoxicillin; Novamoxin®; Nu-Amoxi; PHL-Amoxicillin; PMS-Amoxicillin

Index Terms *p*-Hydroxyampicillin; Amoxicillin Trihydrate; Amoxycillin

Pharmacologic Category Antibiotic, Penicillin

Use Treatment of otitis media, sinusitis, and infections caused by susceptible organisms involving the upper and lower respiratory tract, skin, and urinary tract; prophylaxis of infective endocarditis in patients undergoing surgical or dental procedures; as part of a multidrug regimen for *H. pylori* eradication

Unlabeled/Investigational Use Postexposure prophylaxis for anthrax exposure with documented susceptible organisms

Pharmacodynamics/Kinetics

Absorption: Oral: Rapid and nearly complete; food does not interfere

Extended-release tablet: Rate of absorption is slower compared to immediate-release formulations; food decreases the rate but not extent of absorption

Distribution: Widely to most body fluids and bone; poor penetration into cells, eyes, and across normal meninges

Pleural fluids, lungs, and peritoneal fluid; high urine concentrations are attained; also into synovial fluid, liver, prostate, muscle, and gallbladder; penetrates into middle ear effusions, maxillary sinus secretions, tonsils, sputum, and bronchial secretions

CSF:blood level ratio: Normal meninges: <1%; Inflamed meninges: 8% to 90%

Protein binding: 17% to 20%

Metabolism: Partially hepatic

Half-life elimination:

Neonates, full-term: 3.7 hours

Infants and Children: 1-2 hours

Adults: Normal renal function: 0.7-1.4 hours

Cl_{cr} <10 mL/minute: 7-21 hours

Time to peak: Capsule: 2 hours; Extended-release tablet: 3.1 hours; Suspension: 1 hour

Excretion: Urine (60% as unchanged drug); lower in neonates; **Note:** Extended-release tablets: In healthy volunteers, serum drug concentrations were below 0.25 mcg/mL and undetectable at 16 hours following dosing.

Dosage

Usual dosage range:

Children ≤3 months: Oral: 20-30 mg/kg/day divided every 12 hours

Children >3 months and <40 kg: Oral: 20-50 mg/kg/day in divided doses every 8-12 hours

◄ Children ≥12 years: Oral: Extended-release tablet: 775 mg once daily
Adults: Oral: 250-500 mg every 8 hours or 500-875 mg twice daily
   Extended-release tablet: 775 mg once daily

Indication-specific dosing:

Children >3 months and <40 kg: Oral:

Acute otitis media: 80-90 mg/kg/day divided every 12 hours

Anthrax exposure (CDC guidelines): Note: Postexposure prophylaxis only with documented susceptible organisms: 80 mg/kg/day in divided doses every 8 hours (maximum: 500 mg/dose)

Community-acquired pneumonia:

4 months to <5 years: 80-100 mg/kg/day divided every 8 hours

5-15 years: 100 mg/kg/day divided every 8 hours; **Note:** Treatment with a macrolide or doxycycline (if age >8 years) is preferred due to higher prevalence of atypical pathogens in this age group

Ear, nose, throat, genitourinary tract, or skin/skin structure infections:

Mild-to-moderate: 25 mg/kg/day in divided doses every 12 hours **or** 20 mg/kg/day in divided doses every 8 hours

Severe: 45 mg/kg/day in divided doses every 12 hours **or** 40 mg/kg/day in divided doses every 8 hours

Tonsillitis and/or pharyngitis: Children ≥12 years: Extended-release tablet: 775 mg once daily

Lower respiratory tract infections: 45 mg/kg/day in divided doses every 12 hours **or** 40 mg/kg/day in divided doses every 8 hours

Lyme disease: 25-50 mg/kg/day divided every 8 hours (maximum: 500 mg)

Prophylaxis against infective endocarditis: 50 mg/kg 1 hour before procedure. **Note:** American Heart Association (AHA) guidelines now recommend prophylaxis only in patients undergoing invasive procedures and in whom underlying cardiac conditions may predispose to a higher risk of adverse outcomes should infection occur. As of April 2007, routine prophylaxis for GI/GU procedures is no longer recommended by the AHA.

Adults: Oral:

Anthrax exposure (CDC guidelines): Note: Postexposure prophylaxis in pregnant or nursing women only with documented susceptible organisms: 500 mg every 8 hours

Ear, nose, throat, genitourinary tract, or skin/skin structure infections:

Mild-to-moderate: 500 mg every 12 hours **or** 250 mg every 8 hours

Severe: 875 mg every 12 hours **or** 500 mg every 8 hours

Tonsillitis and/or pharyngitis: Extended-release tablet: 775 mg once daily

***Helicobacter pylori* eradication:** 1000 mg twice daily; requires combination therapy with at least one other antibiotic and an acid-suppressing agent (proton pump inhibitor or H_2 blocker)

Lower respiratory tract infections: 875 mg every 12 hours **or** 500 mg every 8 hours

Lyme disease: 500 mg every 6-8 hours (depending on size of patient) for 21-30 days

Prophylaxis against infective endocarditis: 2 g 30-60 minutes before procedure. **Note:** American Heart Association (AHA) guidelines now recommend prophylaxis only in patients undergoing invasive procedures and in whom underlying cardiac conditions may predispose to a higher risk of adverse outcomes should infection occur. As of April 2007, routine prophylaxis for GI/GU procedures is no longer recommended by the AHA.

Prophylaxis in total joint replacement patients undergoing dental procedures which produce bacteremia: 2 g 1 hour prior to procedure

Dosing interval in renal impairment: Use of certain dosage forms (eg, extended-release 775 mg tablet and immediate-release 875 mg tablet) should be avoided in patients with Cl_{cr} <30 mL/minute or patients requiring hemodialysis.

Cl_{cr} 10-30 mL/minute: 250-500 mg every 12 hours

Cl_{cr} <10 mL/minute: 250-500 mg every 24 hours

Dialysis: Moderately dialyzable (20% to 50%) by hemo- or peritoneal dialysis; approximately 50 mg of amoxicillin per liter of filtrate is removed by continuous arteriovenous or venovenous hemofiltration; dose as per Cl_{cr} <10 mL/minute guidelines

Additional Information Complete prescribing information for this medication should be consulted for additional detail.

Dosage Forms Excipient information presented when available (limited, particularly for generics); consult specific product labeling. [DSC] = Discontinued product

Capsule: 250 mg, 500 mg
Amoxil®: 500 mg [DSC]

Powder for suspension, oral: 125 mg/5 mL (80 mL, 100 mL, 150 mL); 200 mg/5 mL (50 mL, 75 mL, 100 mL); 250 mg/5 mL (80 mL, 100 mL, 150 mL); 400 mg/5 mL (50 mL, 75 mL, 100 mL)
Amoxil®: 250 mg/5 mL (100 mL, 150 mL) [contains sodium benzoate; bubble gum flavor] [DSC]; 400 mg/5 mL (100 mL) [contains sodium benzoate; bubble gum flavor] [DSC]

Powder for suspension, oral [drops]:
Amoxil®: 50 mg/mL (30 mL) [contains sodium benzoate; bubble gum flavor] [DSC]

Tablet: 500 mg, 875 mg

Tablet, chewable: 125 mg, 200 mg, 250 mg, 400 mg

Tablet, extended release:
Moxatag™: 775 mg

References

American Academy of Pediatrics Subcommittee on Management of Acute Otitis Media, "Diagnosis and Management of Acute Otitis Media," *Pediatrics*, 2004, 113(5):1451-65.

Boguniewicz M and Leung DY, "Hypersensitivity Reactions to Antibiotics Commonly Used in Children," *Pediatr Infect Dis J*, 1995, 14(3):221-31.

Bradley JS, "Management of Community-Acquired Pediatric Pneumonia in an Era of Increasing Antibiotic Resistance and Conjugate Vaccines," *Pediatr Infect Dis J*, 2002, 21:592-8.

Canafax DM, Yuan Z, Chonmaitree T, et al, "Amoxicillin Middle Ear Fluid Penetration and Pharmacokinetics in Children With Acute Otitis Media," *Pediatr Infect Dis J*, 1998, 17(2):149-56.

Chow MS, Quintiliani R, and Nightingale CH, "*In Vivo* Inactivation of Tobramycin by Ticarcillin. A Case Report," *JAMA*, 1982, 247(5):658-9.

Daly JS, Dodge RA, Glew RH, et al, "Effect of Time and Temperature on Inactivation of Aminoglycosides by Ampicillin at Neonatal Dosages," *J Perinatol*, 1997, 17(1):42-5.

Donowitz GR and Mandell GL, "Beta-Lactam Antibiotics," *N Engl J Med*, 1988, 318(7):419-26 and 318(8):490-500.

Dougall HT, Smith L, Duncan C, et al, "The Effect of Amoxicillin on Salivary Nitrite Concentrations: An Important Mechanism of Adverse Reactions?" *Br J Clin Pharmacol*, 1995, 39(4):460-2.

Dowell JA, Korth-Bradley J, Milisci M, et al, "Evaluating Possible Pharmacokinetic Interactions Between Tobramycin, Piperacillin, and a Combination of Piperacillin and Tazobactam in Patients With Various Degrees of Renal Impairment," *J Clin Pharmacol*, 2001, 41:979-86.

Farchione LA, "Inactivation of Aminoglycosides by Penicillins," *J Antimicrob Chemother*, 1982, 8 (Suppl A):27-36.

Fuchs PC, Stickel S, Anderson PH, et al, "*In Vitro* Inactivation of Aminoglycosides by Sulbactam, Other Beta-Lactams, and Sulbactam-Beta-Lactam Combinations," *Antimicrob Agents Chemother*, 1991, 35(1):182-4.

Halstenson CE, Wong MO, Herman CS, et al, "Effect of Concomitant Administration of Piperacillin on the Dispositions on Isepamicin and Gentamicin in Patients With End-Stage Renal Disease," *Antimicrob Agents Chemother*, 1992, 36(9):1832-36.

Hautekeete ML, Brenard R, Horsmans Y, et al, "Liver Injury Related to Amoxycillin-Clavulanic Acid: Interlobular Bile-Duct Lesions and Extrahepatic Manifestations," *J Hepatol*, 1995, 22(1):71-7.

Hill S, Yeates M, Pathy J, et al, "A Controlled Trial of Norfloxacin and Amoxicillin in the Treatment of Uncomplicated Urinary Tract Infection in the Elderly," *J Antimicrob Chemother*, 1985, 15(4):505-6.

Hitt CM, Patel KB, Nicolau DP, et al, "Influence of Piperacillin-Tazobactam on Pharmacokinetics of Gentamicin Given Once Daily," *Am J Health Syst Pharm*, 1997, 54(23):2704-8.

Jones KH and Hill SA, "The Toxicology, Absorption and Pharmacokinetics of Amoxicillin," *Adv Clin Pharmacol*, 1974, 7:20.

Konishi H, Goto M, Nakamoto Y, et al, "Tobramycin Inactivation by Carbenicillin, Ticarcillin, and Piperacillin," *Antimicrob Agents Chemother*, 1983, 23(5):653-57.

Korppi M, "Community-Acquired Pneumonia in Children. Issues in Optimizing Antibacterial Treatment," *Pediatr Drugs*, 2003, 5(12):821-32.

Lau A, Lee M, Flascha S, et al, "Effect of Piperacillin on Tobramycin Pharmacokinetics in Patients With Normal Renal Function," *Antimicrob Agents Chemother*, 1983, 24(4):533-37.

McIntosh K, "Community-Acquired Pneumonia in Children," *N Engl J Med*, 2002, 346(6):429-37.

Oe PL, Simonian S, Verhoef J, "Pharmacokinetics of the New Penicillins, Amoxicillin and Flucloxacillin in Patients With Terminal Renal Failure Undergoing Hemodialysis," *Chemotherapy*, 1973, 19:279.

Parry MF, "The Penicillins," *Med Clin North Am*, 1987, 71(6):1093-112.

Prignet JM, Galzin M, Duval JL, et al, "Amoxicillin-Induced Esophageal Ulcer With Intractable Hiccups as the Presenting Manifestation," *Sem Hop*, 1995, 71:186-7.

Russoe ME and Atkins-Thor E, "Gentamicin and Ticarcillin in Subjects With End-Stage Renal Disease. Comparison of Two Assay Methods and Evaluation of Inactivation Rate," *Clin Nephrol*, 1981, 15(4):175-80.

Swanson-Biearman B, Dean DS, Lopez G, et al, "The Effects of Penicillin and Cephalosporin Ingestions in Children Less Than Six Years of Age," *Vet Hum Toxicol*, 1988, 30(1):66-7.

Thompson MIB, Russo ME, Saxon BJ, et al, "Gentamicin Inactivation by Piperacillin or Carbenicillin in Patients With End-Stage Renal Disease," *Antimicrob Agents Chemother*, 1982, 21(2):268-73.

U.S. Food and Drug Administration, Center for Drug Evaluation and Research, "Commentary on Nonlabeled Dosing of Oral Amoxicillin in Adults and Pediatrics for Post-Exposure Inhalational Anthrax," December 10, 2001. Available at: http://www.fda.gov/cder/drugprepare/amox-anthrax.-htm. Accessed January 11, 2002.

Viollier AF, Standiford HC, Drusano GL, et al, "Comparative Pharmacokinetics and Serum Bactericidal Activity of Mezlocillin, Ticarcillin and Piperacillin, With and Without Gentamicin," *J Antimicrob Chemother*, 1985, 15(5):597-606.

Walterspiel JN, Feldman S, Van R, et al, "Comparative Inactivation of Isepamicin, Amikacin, and Gentamicin by Nine Beta-Lactams and Two Beta-Lactamase Inhibitors, Cilastatin and Heparin," *Antimicrob Agents Chemother*, 1991, 35(9):1875-8.

Westphal JF, Jehl F, Brogard JM, et al, "Amoxicillin Intestinal Absorption Reduction by Amiloride: Possible Role of the Na^+-H^+ Exchanger," *Clin Pharmacol Ther*, 1995, 57(3):257-64.

Wilson W, Taubert KA, Gewitz M, et al, "Prevention of Infective Endocarditis. Guidelines From the American Heart Association. A Guideline From the American Heart Association Rheumatic Fever, Endocarditis, and Kawasaki Disease Committee, Council on Cardiovascular Disease in the Young, and the Council on Clinical Cardiology, Council on Cardiovascular Surgery and Anesthesia, and the Quality of Care and Outcomes Research Interdisciplinary Working Group," *Circulation*, 2007, 115. Available at http://circ.ahajournals.org/cgi/reprint/CIRCULATIONAHA.106.183095v1; last accessed July 26, 2007.

Wright AJ, "The Penicillins," *Mayo Clin Proc*, 1999, 74(3):290-307.

Wynn RL, "Amoxicillin Update," *Gen Dent*, 1991, 39(5):322,4,6.

Amoxicillin and Clavulanate Potassium
(a moks i SIL in & klav yoo LAN ate poe TASS ee um)

U.S. Brand Names Amoclan; Augmentin ES-600®; Augmentin XR®; Augmentin®

Canadian Brand Names Alti-Amoxi-Clav; Apo-Amoxi-Clav®; Augmentin®; Clavulin®; Novo-Clavamoxin; ratio-Aclavulanate

Index Terms Amoxicillin and Clavulanic Acid; Clavulanic Acid and Amoxicillin

Pharmacologic Category Antibiotic, Penicillin

Use Treatment of otitis media, sinusitis, and infections caused by susceptible organisms involving the lower respiratory tract, skin and skin structure, and urinary tract; spectrum same as amoxicillin with additional coverage of beta-lactamase producing *B. catarrhalis*, *H. influenzae*, *N. gonorrhoeae*, and *S. aureus* (not MRSA). The expanded coverage of this combination makes it a useful alternative when amoxicillin resistance is present and patients cannot tolerate alternative treatments.

Pharmacodynamics/Kinetics Amoxicillin pharmacokinetics are not affected by clavulanic acid.
Amoxicillin: See Amoxicillin monograph.
Clavulanic acid:
  Protein binding: ~25%
  Metabolism: Hepatic
  Half-life elimination: 1 hour
  Time to peak: 1 hour
  Excretion: Urine (30% to 40% as unchanged drug)

Dosage Note: Dose is based on the amoxicillin component; see "Augmentin® Product-Specific Considerations" table on next page.
Usual dosage range:
  Infants <3 months: Oral: 30 mg/kg/day divided every 12 hours using the 125 mg/5 mL suspension
  Children ≥3 months and <40 kg: Oral: 20-90 mg/kg/day divided every 8-12 hours
  Children >40 kg and Adults: Oral: 250-500 mg every 8 hours or 875 mg every 12 hours
Indication-specific dosing:
  Children ≥3 months and <40 kg: Oral:
    Lower respiratory tract infections, severe infections, sinusitis: 45 mg/kg/day divided every 12 hours **or** 40 mg/kg/day divided every 8 hours
    Mild-to-moderate infections: 25 mg/kg/day divided every 12 hours or 20 mg/kg/day divided every 8 hours
    Otitis media (Augmentin ES-600®): 90 mg/kg/day divided every 12 hours for 10 days in children with severe illness and when coverage for β-lactamase-positive *H. influenzae* and *M. catarrhalis* is needed.

Children ≥16 years and Adults: Oral:

Acute bacterial sinusitis: Extended release tablet: Two 1000 mg tablets every 12 hours for 10 days

Bite wounds (animal/human): 875 mg every 12 hours **or** 500 mg every 8 hours

Chronic obstructive pulmonary disease: 875 mg every 12 hours **or** 500 mg every 8 hours

Diabetic foot: Extended release tablet: Two 1000 mg tablets every 12 hours for 7-14 days

Diverticulitis, perirectal abscess: Extended release tablet: Two 1000 mg tablets every 12 hours for 7-10 days

Erysipelas: 875 mg every 12 hours **or** 500 mg every 8 hours

Febrile neutropenia: 875 mg every 12 hours

Pneumonia:

Aspiration: 875 mg every 12 hours

Community-acquired: Extended release tablet: Two 1000 mg tablets every 12 hours for 7-10 days

Pyelonephritis (acute, uncomplicated): 875 mg every 12 hours **or** 500 mg every 8 hours

Skin abscess: 875 mg every 12 hours

Augmentin® Product-Specific Considerations

Strength	Form	Consideration
125 mg	CT, S	q8h dosing
	S	For adults having difficulty swallowing tablets, 125 mg/5 mL suspension may be substituted for 500 mg tablet.
200 mg	CT, S	q12h dosing
	CT	Contains phenylalanine
	S	For adults having difficulty swallowing tablets, 200 mg/5 mL suspension may be substituted for 875 mg tablet.
250 mg	CT, S, T	q8h dosing
	CT	Contains phenylalanine
	T	Not for use in patients <40 kg
	CT, T	Tablet and chewable tablet are not interchangeable due to differences in clavulanic acid.
	S	For adults having difficulty swallowing tablets, 250 mg/5 mL suspension may be substituted for 500 mg tablet.
400 mg	CT, S	q12h dosing
	CT	Contains phenylalanine
	S	For adults having difficulty swallowing tablets, 400 mg/5 mL suspension may be substituted for 875 mg tablet.
500 mg	T	q8h or q12h dosing
600 mg	S	q12h dosing
		Not for use in adults or children ≥40 kg
		600 mg/5 mL suspension is not equivalent to or interchangeable with 200 mg/5 mL or 400 mg/5 mL due to differences in clavulanic acid.
875 mg	T	q12h dosing; not for use in Cl_{cr} <30 mL/minute
1000 mg	XR	q12h dosing
		Not for use in children <16 years of age
		Not interchangeable with two 500 mg tablets
		Not for use if Cl_{cr} <30 mL/minute or hemodialysis

Legend: CT = chewable tablet, S = suspension, T = tablet, XR = extended release.

Dosing interval in renal impairment:

Cl_{cr} <30 mL/minute: Do not use 875 mg tablet or extended release tablets

Cl_{cr} 10-30 mL/minute: 250-500 mg every 12 hours

Cl_{cr} <10 mL/minute: 250-500 every 24 hours

◄ Hemodialysis: Moderately dialyzable (20% to 50%)

250-500 mg every 24 hours; administer dose during and after dialysis. Do not use extended release tablets.

Peritoneal dialysis: Moderately dialyzable (20% to 50%)

Amoxicillin: Administer 250 mg every 12 hours

Clavulanic acid: Dose for Cl$_{cr}$ <10 mL/minute

Continuous arteriovenous or venovenous hemofiltration effects:

Amoxicillin: ~50 mg of amoxicillin/L of filtrate is removed

Clavulanic acid: Dose for Cl$_{cr}$ <10 mL/minute

Additional Information Complete prescribing information for this medication should be consulted for additional detail.

Dosage Forms Excipient information presented when available (limited, particularly for generics); consult specific product labeling. [DSC] = Discontinued product

Powder for oral suspension: 200: Amoxicillin 200 mg and clavulanate potassium 28.5 mg per 5 mL (50 mL, 75 mL, 100 mL) [contains phenylalanine]; 400: Amoxicillin 400 mg and clavulanate potassium 57 mg per 5 mL (50 mL, 75 mL, 100 mL) [contains phenylalanine]; 600: Amoxicillin 600 mg and clavulanate potassium 42.9 mg per 5 mL (75 mL, 125 mL, 200 mL)

Amoclan:

200: Amoxicillin 200 mg and clavulanate potassium 28.5 mg per 5 mL (50 mL, 75 mL, 100 mL) [contains phenylalanine 7 mg/5 mL and potassium 0.14 mEq/ 5 mL; fruit flavor]

400: Amoxicillin 400 mg and clavulanate potassium 57 mg per 5 mL (50 mL, 75 mL, 100 mL) [contains phenylalanine 7 mg/5 mL and potassium 0.29 mEq/ 5 mL; fruit flavor]

600: Amoxicillin 600 mg and clavulanate potassium 42.9 mg per 5 mL (75 mL, 125 mL) [contains phenylalanine 7 mg/5 mL, potassium 0.248 mEq/5 mL; orange flavor]

Augmentin®:

125: Amoxicillin 125 mg and clavulanate potassium 31.25 mg per 5 mL (75 mL, 100 mL, 150 mL) [contains potassium 0.16 mEq/5 mL; banana flavor]

200: Amoxicillin 200 mg and clavulanate potassium 28.5 mg per 5 mL (50 mL, 75 mL, 100 mL) [contains phenylalanine 7 mg/5 mL and potassium 0.14 mEq/ 5 mL; orange flavor] [DSC]

250: Amoxicillin 250 mg and clavulanate potassium 62.5 mg per 5 mL (75 mL, 100 mL, 150 mL) [contains potassium 0.32 mEq/5 mL; orange flavor]

400: Amoxicillin 400 mg and clavulanate potassium 57 mg per 5 mL (50 mL, 75 mL, 100 mL) [contains phenylalanine 7 mg/5 mL and potassium 0.29 mEq/ 5 mL; orange flavor] [DSC]

Augmentin ES-600®: Amoxicillin 600 mg and clavulanate potassium 42.9 mg per 5 mL (75 mL, 125 mL, 200 mL) [contains phenylalanine 7 mg/5 mL and potassium 0.23 mEq/5 mL; strawberry cream flavor]

Tablet: 250: Amoxicillin 250 mg and clavulanate potassium 125 mg; 500: Amoxicillin 500 mg and clavulanate potassium 125 mg; 875: Amoxicillin 875 mg and clavulanate potassium 125 mg

Augmentin®:

250: Amoxicillin 250 mg and clavulanate potassium 125 mg [contains potassium 0.63 mEq/tablet]

500: Amoxicillin 500 mg and clavulanate potassium 125 mg [contains potassium 0.63 mEq/tablet]

875: Amoxicillin 875 mg and clavulanate potassium 125 mg [contains potassium 0.63 mEq/tablet]

Tablet, chewable: 200: Amoxicillin 200 mg and clavulanate potassium 28.5 mg [contains phenylalanine]; 400: Amoxicillin 400 mg and clavulanate potassium 57 mg [contains phenylalanine]

Tablet, extended release:

Augmentin XR®: 1000: Amoxicillin 1000 mg and clavulanate acid 62.5 mg [contains potassium 12.6 mg (0.32 mEq) and sodium 29.3 mg (1.27 mEq) per tablet; packaged in either a 7-day or 10-day package]

References

American Academy of Pediatrics Subcommittee on Management of Acute Otitis Media, "Diagnosis and Management of Acute Otitis Media," *Pediatrics*, 2004, 113(5):1451-65.

American Thoracic Society, "Guidelines for the Initial Management of Adults With Community-Acquired Pneumonia: Diagnosis, Assessment of Severity, and Initial Antimicrobial Therapy," *Am Rev Respir Dis*, 1993, 148(5):1418-26.

Ancill RJ, Ballard JH, and Capewell MA, "Urinary Tract Infections in Geriatric Inpatients: A Comparative Study of Amoxicillin-Clavulanic Acid and Co-trimoxazole," *Curr Ther Res Clin Exp*, 1987, 41(4):444-8.

Chow MS, Quintiliani R, and Nightingale CH, "*In Vivo* Inactivation of Tobramycin by Ticarcillin. A Case Report," *JAMA*, 1982, 247(5):658-9.

Daly JS, Dodge RA, Glew RH, et al, "Effect of Time and Temperature on Inactivation of Aminoglycosides by Ampicillin at Neonatal Dosages," *J Perinatol*, 1997, 17(1):42-5.

Donowitz GR and Mandell GL, "Beta-Lactam Antibiotics," *N Engl J Med*, 1988, 318(7):419-26 and 318(8):490-500.

Dowell JA, Korth-Bradley J, Milisci M, et al, "Evaluating Possible Pharmacokinetic Interactions Between Tobramycin, Piperacillin, and a Combination of Piperacillin and Tazobactam in Patients With Various Degrees of Renal Impairment," *J Clin Pharmacol*, 2001, 41:979-86.

Farchione LA, "Inactivation of Aminoglycosides by Penicillins," *J Antimicrob Chemother*, 1982, 8 (Suppl A):27-36.

Fuchs PC, Stickel S, Anderson PH, et al, "*In Vitro* Inactivation of Aminoglycosides by Sulbactam, Other Beta-Lactams, and Sulbactam-Beta-Lactam Combinations," *Antimicrob Agents Chemother*, 1991, 35(1):182-4.

Gan VN, Kusmiesz H, Shelton S, et al, "Comparative Evaluation of Loracarbef and Amoxicillin-Clavulanate for Acute Otitis Media," *Antimicrob Agents Chemother*, 1991, 35(5):967-71.

Halstenson CE, Wong MO, Herman CS, et al, "Effect of Concomitant Administration of Piperacillin on the Dispositions of Isepamicin and Gentamicin in Patients With End-Stage Renal Disease," *Antimicrob Agents Chemother*, 1992, 36(9):1832-36.

Hitt CM, Patel KB, Nicolau DP, et al, "Influence of Piperacillin-Tazobactam on Pharmacokinetics of Gentamicin Given Once Daily," *Am J Health Syst Pharm*, 1997, 54(23):2704-8.

Hoberman A, Paradise JL, Burch DJ, et al, "Equivalent Efficiency and Reduced Occurrence of Diarrhea From a New Formulation of Amoxicillin/Clavulanate Potassium (Augmentin®) for Treatment of Acute Otitis Media in Children," *Pediatr Infect Dis J*, 1997, 16(5):463-70.

Konishi M, Goto M, Nakamoto Y, et al, "Tobramycin Inactivation by Carbenicillin, Ticarcillin, and Piperacillin," *Antimicrob Agents Chemother*, 1983, 23(5):653-57.

Lau A, Lee M, Flascha S, et al, "Effect of Piperacillin on Tobramycin Pharmacokinetics in Patients With Normal Renal Function," *Antimicrob Agents Chemother*, 1983, 24(4):533-37.

Mandell LA, Bartlett JG, Dowell SF, et al, "Update of Practice Guidelines for the Management of Community-Acquired Pneumonia in Immunocompetent Adults," *Clin Infect Dis*, 2003, 37 (11):1405-33.

Reed MD, "Clinical Pharmacokinetics of Amoxicillin and Clavulanate," *Pediatr Infect Dis J*, 1996, 15 (10):949-54.

Russoe ME and Atkins-Thor E, "Gentamicin and Ticarcillin in Subjects With End-Stage Renal Disease. Comparison of Two Assay Methods and Evaluation of Inactivation Rate," *Clin Nephrol*, 1981, 15(4):175-80.

Swanson-Biearman B, Dean DS, Lopez G, et al, "The Effects of Penicillin and Cephalosporin Ingestions in Children Less Than Six Years of Age," *Vet Hum Toxicol*, 1988, 30(1):66-7.

Thoene DE and Johnson CE, "Pharmacotherapy of Otitis Media," *Pharmacotherapy*, 1991, 11 (3):212-21.

Thompson MIB, Russo ME, Saxon BJ, et al, "Gentamicin Inactivation by Piperacillin or Carbenicillin in Patients With End-Stage Renal Disease," *Antimicrob Agents Chemother*, 1982, 21(2):268-73.

Todd PA and Benfield P, "Amoxicillin/Clavulanic Acid. An Update of Its Antibacterial Activity, Pharmacokinetic Properties, and Therapeutic Use," *Drugs*, 1990, 39(2):264-307.

Viollier AF, Standiford HC, Drusano GL, et al, "Comparative Pharmacokinetics and Serum Bactericidal Activity of Mezlocillin, Ticarcillin and Piperacillin, With and Without Gentamicin," *J Antimicrob Chemother*, 1985, 15(5):597-606.

Walterspiel JN, Feldman S, Van R, et al, "Comparative Inactivation of Isepamicin, Amikacin, and Gentamicin by Nine Beta-Lactams and Two Beta-Lactamase Inhibitors, Cilastatin and Heparin," *Antimicrob Agents Chemother*, 1991, 35(9):1875-8.

Wright AJ, "The Penicillins," *Mayo Clin Proc*, 1999, 74(3):290-307.

Wynn RL and Bergman SA, "Antibiotics and Their Use in the Treatment of Orofacial Infections, Part I and Part II," *Gen Dent*, 1994, 42(5):398-402, 498-502.

Amphotericin B Cholesteryl Sulfate Complex
(am foe TER i sin bee kole LES te ril SUL fate KOM plecks)

Medication Safety Issues
Safety issues:

Lipid-based amphotericin formulations (Amphotec®) may be confused with conventional formulations (Amphocin®, Fungizone®)

Large overdoses have occurred when conventional formulations were dispensed inadvertently for lipid-based products. Single daily doses of conventional amphotericin formulation never exceed 1.5 mg/kg.

High alert medication: The Institute for Safe Medication Practices (ISMP) includes this medication among its list of drugs which have a heightened risk of causing significant patient harm when used in error.

Related Information
Antifungal Agents *on page 1664*
Desensitization Protocols *on page 1692*

U.S. Brand Names Amphotec®

Canadian Brand Names Amphotec®

Index Terms ABCD; Amphotericin B Colloidal Dispersion

Pharmacologic Category Antifungal Agent, Parenteral

Generic Available No

Use Treatment of invasive aspergillosis in patients who have failed amphotericin B deoxycholate treatment, or who have renal impairment or experience unacceptable toxicity which precludes treatment with amphotericin B deoxycholate in effective doses.

Unlabeled/Investigational Use Effective in patients with serious *Candida* species infections

Mechanism of Action Binds to ergosterol altering cell membrane permeability in susceptible fungi and causing leakage of cell components with subsequent cell death. Proposed mechanism suggests that amphotericin causes an oxidation-dependent stimulation of macrophages (Lyman, 1992).

Pharmacodynamics/Kinetics

Distribution: V_d: Total volume increases with higher doses, reflects increasing uptake by tissues (with 4 mg/kg/day = 4 L/kg); predominantly distributed in the liver; concentrations in kidneys and other tissues are lower than observed with conventional amphotericin B

Half-life elimination: 28-29 hours; prolonged with higher doses

Dosage Children and Adults: I.V.:

Premedication: For patients who experience chills, fever, hypotension, nausea, or other nonanaphylactic infusion-related immediate reactions, premedicate with the following drugs 30-60 minutes prior to drug administration: A nonsteroidal (eg, ibuprofen, choline magnesium trisalicylate) with or without diphenhydramine **or** acetaminophen with diphenhydramine **or** hydrocortisone 50-100 mg. If the patient experiences rigors during the infusion, meperidine may be administered.
Range: 3-4 mg/kg/day (infusion of 1 mg/kg/hour); maximum: 7.5 mg/kg/day

A regimen of 6 mg/kg/day has been used for treatment of life-threatening invasive mold infections in immunocompromised patients; maximum: 7.5 mg/kg/day

Initially infuse at 1 mg/kg/hour. Rate of infusion may be increased with subsequent doses to 3 mg/kg/hour as patient tolerance allows. Treatment should continue as patient tolerance allows, until complete resolution of microbiologic and clinical evidence of fungal disease.

Stability Store intact vials under refrigeration. Reconstitute 50 mg and 100 mg vials with 10 mL and 20 mL of SWI, respectively. The reconstituted vials contain 5 mg/mL of amphotericin B. Shake the vial gently by hand until all solid particles have dissolved. After reconstitution, the solution should be refrigerated at 2°C to 8°C (36°F to 46°F) and used within 24 hours.

Further dilute amphotericin B colloidal dispersion with dextrose 5% in water. Concentrations of 0.1-2 mg/mL in dextrose 5% in water are stable for 14 days at 4°C and 23°C if protected from light, however, due to the occasional formation of subvisual particles, solutions should be used within 48 hours.

Administration Avoid injection faster than 1 mg/kg/hour. For a patient who experiences chills, fever, hypotension, nausea, or other nonanaphylactic infusion-related reactions, premedicate with the following drugs 30-60 minutes prior to drug administration: A nonsteroidal (eg, ibuprofen, choline magnesium trisalicylate) with or without diphenhydramine **or** acetaminophen with diphenhydramine **or** hydrocortisone 50-100 mg. If the patient experiences rigors during the infusion, meperidine may be administered. If severe respiratory distress occurs, the infusion should be immediately discontinued.

Monitoring Parameters Liver function tests, electrolytes, BUN, Cr, temperature, CBC, I/O, signs of hypokalemia (muscle weakness, cramping, drowsiness, ECG changes)

Anesthesia and Critical Care Concerns/Other Considerations
Clinical Pearls/Comments:

Prevention of infusion-related reactions: Patients may be premedicated with acetaminophen 650 mg and diphenhydramine 25-50 mg 30 minutes prior to infusion. Hydrocortisone can be used if patient has experienced rigors with amphotericin in the past. Meperidine can also be used for the treatment of rigors during the infusion.

Controlled trials which compare the original formulation of amphotericin B to the newer liposomal formulations (ie, Amphotec®) are lacking. Thus, comparative data discussing differences among the formulations should be interpreted cautiously. Although the risk of nephrotoxicity and infusion-related adverse effects may be less with Amphotec®, the efficacy profiles of Amphotec® and the original amphotericin B formulation are comparable. Consequently, Amphotec® should be restricted to those patients who cannot tolerate or who fail a standard amphotericin B formulation. This product is significantly more expensive than conventional amphotericin B; infectious diseases consult is recommended.

Pregnancy Risk Factor B

Contraindications Hypersensitivity to amphotericin B or any component of the formulation

Warnings/Precautions Anaphylaxis has been reported with amphotericin B-containing drugs. If severe respiratory distress occurs, the infusion should be immediately discontinued. During the initial dosing, the drug should be administered under close clinical observation. Infusion reactions, sometimes severe, usually subside with continued therapy - manage with decreased rate of infusion and pretreatment with antihistamines/corticosteroids.

Adverse Reactions
>10%: Central nervous system: Chills, fever
1% to 10%:
    Cardiovascular: Hypotension, tachycardia
    Central nervous system: Headache
    Dermatologic: Rash
    Endocrine & metabolic: Hypokalemia, hypomagnesemia
    Gastrointestinal: Nausea, diarrhea, abdominal pain
    Hematologic: Thrombocytopenia
    Hepatic: LFT change
    Neuromuscular & skeletal: Rigors
    Renal: Creatinine increased
    Respiratory: Dyspnea

Note: Amphotericin B colloidal dispersion has an improved therapeutic index compared to conventional amphotericin B, and has been used safely in patients with amphotericin B-related nephrotoxicity; however, continued decline of renal function has occurred in some patients.

Drug Interactions
Avoid Concomitant Use
Avoid concomitant use of Amphotericin B Cholesteryl Sulfate Complex with any of the following: Gallium Nitrate

Increased Effect/Toxicity
Amphotericin B Cholesteryl Sulfate Complex may increase the levels/effects of: Aminoglycosides; Colistimethate; CycloSPORINE; Flucytosine; Gallium Nitrate

The levels/effects of Amphotericin B Cholesteryl Sulfate Complex may be increased by: Corticosteroids (Orally Inhaled); Corticosteroids (Systemic)

Decreased Effect

Amphotericin B Cholesteryl Sulfate Complex may decrease the levels/effects of: Saccharomyces boulardii

The levels/effects of Amphotericin B Cholesteryl Sulfate Complex may be decreased by: Antifungal Agents (Azole Derivatives, Systemic)

Dosage Forms Excipient information presented when available (limited, particularly for generics); consult specific product labeling.

Injection, powder for reconstitution:

Amphotec®: 50 mg, 100 mg

References

Lister J, "Amphotericin B Lipid Complex (Abelcet®) in the Treatment of Invasive Mycoses: The North American Experience," *Eur J Haematol Suppl*, 1996, 57:18-23.

Mora-Duarte J, Betts R, Rotstein C, et al, "Comparison of Caspofungin and Amphotericin B for Invasive Candidiasis," *N Engl J Med*, 2002, 347(25):2020-9.

Prentice HG, Hann IM, Herbrecht R, et al, "A Randomized Comparison of Liposomal Versus Conventional Amphotericin B for the Treatment of Pyrexia of Unknown Origin in Neutropenic Patients," *Br J Haematol*, 1997, 98(3):711-8.

Rex JH, Walsh TJ, Sobel JD, et al, "Practice Guidelines for the Treatment of Candidiasis. Infectious Diseases Society of America," *Clin Infect Dis*, 2000, 30(4):662-78.

Slain D, "Lipid-Based Amphotericin B for the Treatment of Fungal Infections," *Pharmacotherapy*, 1999, 19(3):306-23.

◆ **Amphotericin B Colloidal Dispersion** *see* Amphotericin B Cholesteryl Sulfate Complex *on page 102*

Amphotericin B (Conventional) (am foe TER i sin bee con VEN sha nal)

Medication Safety Issues

Safety issues:

Conventional amphotericin formulations (Amphocin®, Fungizone®) may be confused with lipid-based formulations (AmBisome®, Abelcet®, Amphotec®). Large overdoses have occurred when conventional formulations were dispensed inadvertently for lipid-based products. Single daily doses of conventional amphotericin formulation never exceed 1.5 mg/kg.

High alert medication: The Institute for Safe Medication Practices (ISMP) includes this medication (intrathecal administration) among its list of drugs which have a heightened risk of causing significant patient harm when used in error.

Related Information

Antifungal Agents *on page 1664*

Desensitization Protocols *on page 1692*

Canadian Brand Names Fungizone®

Index Terms Amphotericin B Desoxycholate

Pharmacologic Category Antifungal Agent, Parenteral

Generic Available Yes

Use Treatment of severe systemic and central nervous system infections caused by susceptible fungi such as *Candida* species, *Histoplasma capsulatum*, *Cryptococcus neoformans*, *Aspergillus* species, *Blastomyces dermatitidis*, *Torulopsis glabrata*, and *Coccidioides immitis*; fungal peritonitis; irrigant for bladder fungal infections; used in fungal infection in patients with bone marrow transplantation, amebic meningoencephalitis, ocular aspergillosis (intraocular injection), candidal cystitis (bladder irrigation), chemoprophylaxis (low-dose I.V.), immunocompromised patients at risk of aspergillosis (intranasal/nebulized), refractory meningitis (intrathecal), coccidioidal arthritis (intra-articular/I.M.).

Low-dose amphotericin B has been administered after bone marrow transplantation to reduce the risk of invasive fungal disease.

Mechanism of Action Binds to ergosterol altering cell membrane permeability in susceptible fungi and causing leakage of cell components with subsequent cell death. Proposed mechanism suggests that amphotericin causes an oxidation-dependent stimulation of macrophages (Lyman, 1992).

Pharmacodynamics/Kinetics

Distribution: Minimal amounts enter the aqueous humor, bile, CSF (inflamed or noninflamed meninges), amniotic fluid, pericardial fluid, pleural fluid, and synovial fluid

Protein binding, plasma: 90%

Half-life elimination: Biphasic: Initial: 15-48 hours; Terminal: 15 days

Time to peak: Within 1 hour following a 4- to 6-hour dose

Excretion: Urine (2% to 5% as biologically active form); ~40% eliminated over a 7-day period and may be detected in urine for at least 7 weeks after discontinued use

Dosage Premedication: For patients who experience infusion-related immediate reactions, premedicate with the following drugs 30-60 minutes prior to drug administration: NSAID (with or without diphenhydramine) **or** acetaminophen with diphenhydramine **or** hydrocortisone 50-100 mg. If the patient experiences rigors during the infusion, meperidine may be administered.

Usual dosage ranges:

Infants and Children:

Test dose: I.V.: 0.1 mg/kg/dose to a maximum of 1 mg; infuse over 30-60 minutes. Many clinicians believe a test dose is unnecessary.

Maintenance dose: 0.25-1 mg/kg/day given once daily; infuse over 2-6 hours. Once therapy has been established, amphotericin B can be administered on an every-other-day basis at 1-1.5 mg/kg/dose; cumulative dose: 1.5-2 g over 6-10 weeks.

Duration of therapy: Varies with nature of infection, usual duration is 4-12 weeks or cumulative dose of 1-4 g

Adults:

Test dose: 1 mg infused over 20-30 minutes. Many clinicians believe a test dose is unnecessary.

Maintenance dose: Usual: 0.05-1.5 mg/kg/day; 1-1.5 mg/kg over 4-6 hours every other day may be given once therapy is established; aspergillosis, rhinocerebral mucormycosis, often require 1-1.5 mg/kg/day; do not exceed 1.5 mg/kg/day

Indication-specific dosing:

Children: **Meningitis, coccidioidal or cryptococcal:** I.T.: 25-100 mcg every 48-72 hours; increase to 500 mcg as tolerated

Adults:

Aspergillosis, disseminated: I.V.: 0.6-0.7 mg/kg/day for 3-6 months

Bone marrow transplantation (prophylaxis): I.V.: Low-dose amphotericin B 0.1-0.25 mg/kg/day has been administered after bone marrow transplantation to reduce the risk of invasive fungal disease.

Candidemia (neutropenic or non-neutropenic): I.V.: 0.5-1 mg/kg/day until 14 days after last positive blood culture and resolution of signs and symptoms (Pappas, 2009)

Candidiasis, chronic, disseminated: I.V.: 0.5-0.7 mg/kg/day for 3-6 months and resolution of radiologic lesions (Pappas, 2009)

Dematiaceous fungi: I.V.: 0.7 mg/kg/day in combination with an azole

Endocarditis: I.V.: 0.6-1 mg/kg/day (with or without flucytosine) for 6 weeks after valve replacement; **Note:** If isolates susceptible and/or clearance demonstrated, guidelines recommend step-down to fluconazole; also for long-term suppression therapy if valve replacement is not possible (Pappas, 2009)

Endophthalmitis, fungal:

Intravitreal (unlabeled use): 10 mcg in 0.1 mL (in conjunction with systemic therapy)

I.V.: 0.7-1 mg/kg/day (with or without flucytosine) for at least 4-6 weeks (Pappas, 2009)

Esophageal: I.V.: 0.3-0.7 mg/kg/day for 14-21 days after clinical improvement

Histoplasmosis: Chronic, severe pulmonary or disseminated: I.V.: 0.5-1 mg/kg/day for 7 days, then 0.8 mg/kg every other day (or 3 times/week) until total dose of 10-15 mg/kg; may continue itraconazole as suppressive therapy (lifelong for immunocompromised patients)

Meningitis:

Candidal: I.V.: 0.7-1 mg/kg/day (with or without flucytosine) for at least 4 weeks; **Note:** Liposomal amphotericin favored by IDSA guidelines based on decreased risk of nephrotoxicity and potentially better CNS penetration (Pappas, 2009)

Cryptococcal or Coccidioides: I.T.: Initial: 25-300 mcg every 48-72 hours; increase to 500 mcg to 1 mg as tolerated; maximum total dose: 15 mg has been suggested

Histoplasma: I.V.: 0.5-1 mg/kg/day for 7 days, then 0.8 mg/kg every other day (or 3 times/week) for 3 months total duration; follow with fluconazole suppressive therapy for up to 12 months

Meningoencephalitis, cryptococcal: I.V.:

HIV positive: 0.7-1 mg/kg/day (plus flucytosine 100 mg/kg/day) for 2 weeks, then change to oral fluconazole for at least 10 weeks; alternatively, amphotericin and flucytosine may be continued uninterrupted for 6-10 weeks

HIV negative: 0.5-0.7 mg/kg/day (plus flucytosine) for 2 weeks

Oropharyngeal candidiasis: I.V.: 0.3 mg/kg/day for 7-14 days (Pappas, 2009)

Osteoarticular candidiasis: I.V.: 0.5-1 mg/kg/day for several weeks, followed by fluconazole for 6-12 months (osteomyelitis) or 6 weeks (septic arthritis)

Penicillium marneffei: I.V.: 0.6 mg/kg/day for 2 weeks

Pneumonia: Cryptococcal (mild-to-moderate): I.V.:

HIV positive: 0.5-1 mg/kg/day

HIV negative: 0.5-0.7 mg/kg/day (plus flucytosine) for 2 weeks

Sporotrichosis: Pulmonary, meningeal, osteoarticular, or disseminated: I.V.: Total dose of 1-2 g, then change to oral itraconazole or fluconazole for suppressive therapy

Urinary tract candidiasis (Pappas, 2009):

Fungus balls: I.V.: 0.5-0.7 mg/kg/day with or without flucytosine 25 mg/kg 4 times daily

Pyelonephritis: I.V.: 0.5-0.7 mg/kg/day with or without flucytosine 25 mg/kg 4 times daily for 2 weeks

Symptomatic cystitis: I.V.: 0.3-0.6 mg/kg/day for 1-7 days

Bladder irrigation: Irrigate with 50 mcg/mL solution instilled periodically or continuously for 5-10 days or until cultures are clear for fluconazole-resistant *Candida*

Dosing adjustment in renal impairment: If renal dysfunction is due to the drug, the daily total can be decreased by 50% or the dose can be given every other day; I.V. therapy may take several months

Dialysis: Poorly dialyzed; no supplemental dosage necessary when using hemo- or peritoneal dialysis or continuous renal replacement therapy (CRRT)

Administration in dialysate: Children and Adults: 1-2 mg/L of peritoneal dialysis fluid either with or without low-dose I.V. amphotericin B (a total dose of 2-10 mg/ kg given over 7-14 days). Precipitate may form in ionic dialysate solutions.

Stability Store intact vials under refrigeration. Protect from light. Add 10 mL of SWFI (without a bacteriostatic agent) to each vial of amphotericin B. Further dilute with 250-500 mL D$_5$W; final concentration should not exceed 0.1 mg/mL (peripheral infusion) or 0.25 mg/mL (central infusion).

Reconstituted vials are stable, protected from light, for 24 hours at room temperature and 1 week when refrigerated. Parenteral admixtures are stable, protected from light, for 24 hours at room temperature and 2 days under refrigeration. Short-term exposure (<24 hours) to light during I.V. infusion does **not** appreciably affect potency.

Administration May be infused over 4-6 hours. For a patient who experiences chills, fever, hypotension, nausea, or other nonanaphylactic infusion-related reactions, premedicate with the following drugs 30-60 minutes prior to drug administration: A nonsteroidal (eg, ibuprofen, choline magnesium trisalicylate) with or without diphenhydramine **or** acetaminophen with diphenhydramine **or** hydrocortisone 50-100 mg. If the patient experiences rigors during the infusion, meperidine may be administered. Bolus infusion of normal saline immediately preceding, or immediately preceding and following amphotericin B may reduce drug-induced nephrotoxicity. Risk of nephrotoxicity increases with amphotericin B doses >1 mg/kg/day. Infusion of admixtures more concentrated than 0.25 mg/mL should be limited to patients absolutely requiring volume contraction.

Monitoring Parameters Renal function (monitor frequently during therapy), electrolytes (especially potassium and magnesium), liver function tests, temperature, PT/PTT, CBC; monitor input and output; monitor for signs of hypokalemia (muscle weakness, cramping, drowsiness, ECG changes, etc)

Reference Range Therapeutic: 1-2 mcg/mL (SI: 1-2.2 μmol/L)

Anesthesia and Critical Care Concerns/Other Considerations

Clinical Pearls/Comments:

Prevention of infusion-related reactions: Patients may be premedicated with acetaminophen 650 mg and diphenhydramine 25-50 mg 30 minutes prior to infusion. Hydrocortisone can be used if patient has experienced rigors with amphotericin in the past. Meperidine can also be used for the treatment of rigors during the infusion.

Avoid rapid injection (usually 4- to 6-hour infusion required). Dosage adjustments are not necessary with renal impairment. If decreased renal function is due to amphotericin, the daily dose can be decreased by 50% or the dose can be given every other day.

Bolus infusion of normal saline immediately preceding, or immediately preceding and following amphotericin B may reduce drug-induced nephrotoxicity. Risk of nephrotoxicity increases with amphotericin B doses >1 mg/kg/day. Infusion of admixtures more concentrated than 0.25 mg/mL should be limited to patients absolutely requiring volume restriction. Amphotericin B does not have a bacteriostatic constituent, subsequently admixture expiration is determined by sterility more than chemical stability.

Pregnancy Risk Factor B

Contraindications Hypersensitivity to amphotericin or any component of the formulation

Warnings/Precautions Anaphylaxis has been reported with amphotericin B-containing drugs. During the initial dosing, the drug should be administered under close clinical observation. Avoid use with other nephrotoxic drugs; drug-induced renal toxicity usually improves with interrupting therapy, decreasing dosage, or increasing dosing interval. Infusion reactions are most common 1-3 hours after starting the infusion and diminish with continued therapy.

[U.S. Boxed Warning]: Should be used primarily for treatment of progressive, potentially life-threatening fungal infections, not noninvasive forms of infection. [U.S. Boxed warning]: Verify the product name and dosage if dose exceeds 1.5 mg/kg.

Adverse Reactions

Systemic:

>10%:

Cardiovascular: Hypotension, tachypnea

Central nervous system: Fever, chills, headache (less frequent with I.T.), malaise

Endocrine & metabolic: Hypokalemia, hypomagnesemia

Gastrointestinal: Anorexia, nausea (less frequent with I.T.), vomiting (less frequent with I.T.), diarrhea, heartburn, cramping epigastric pain

Hematologic: Normochromic-normocytic anemia

Local: Pain at injection site with or without phlebitis or thrombophlebitis (incidence may increase with peripheral infusion of admixtures)

Neuromuscular & skeletal: Generalized pain, including muscle and joint pains (less frequent with I.T.)

Renal: Decreased renal function and renal function abnormalities including azotemia, renal tubular acidosis, nephrocalcinosis (>0.1 mg/mL)

1% to 10%:

Cardiovascular: Hypertension, flushing

Central nervous system: Delirium, arachnoiditis, pain along lumbar nerves (especially I.T. therapy)

Genitourinary: Urinary retention

Hematologic: Leukocytosis

Neuromuscular & skeletal: Paresthesia (especially with I.T. therapy)

<1% (Limited to important or life-threatening): Acute liver failure, agranulocytosis, anuria, bone marrow suppression, cardiac arrest, coagulation defects, convulsions, dyspnea, hearing loss, leukopenia, maculopapular rash, renal failure, renal tubular acidosis, thrombocytopenia, vision changes

◄ **Drug Interactions**
Avoid Concomitant Use
Avoid concomitant use of Amphotericin B (Conventional) with any of the following: Gallium Nitrate
Increased Effect/Toxicity
Amphotericin B (Conventional) may increase the levels/effects of: Aminoglycosides; Colistimethate; CycloSPORINE; Flucytosine; Gallium Nitrate

The levels/effects of Amphotericin B (Conventional) may be increased by: Corticosteroids (Orally Inhaled); Corticosteroids (Systemic)
Decreased Effect
Amphotericin B (Conventional) may decrease the levels/effects of: Saccharomyces boulardii

The levels/effects of Amphotericin B (Conventional) may be decreased by: Antifungal Agents (Azole Derivatives, Systemic)
Test Interactions Increased BUN (S), serum creatinine, alkaline phosphate, bilirubin; decreased magnesium, potassium (S)
Dosage Forms Excipient information presented when available (limited, particularly for generics); consult specific product labeling.
Injection, powder for reconstitution, as desoxycholate: 50 mg
References
Branch RA, "Prevention of Amphotericin B-Induced Renal Impairment. A Review on the Use of Sodium Supplementation," *Arch Intern Med*, 1988, 148(11):2389-94.
Mora-Duarte J, Betts R, Rotstein C, et al, "Comparison of Caspofungin and Amphotericin B for Invasive Candidiasis," *N Engl J Med*, 2002, 347(25):2020-9.
Rex JH, Walsh TJ, Sobel JD, et al, "Practice Guidelines for the Treatment of Candidiasis. Infectious Diseases Society of America," *Clin Infect Dis*, 2000, 30(4):662-78.

♦ **Amphotericin B Desoxycholate** *see* Amphotericin B (Conventional) *on page 104*

Amphotericin B (Lipid Complex) (am foe TER i sin bee LIP id KOM pleks)

Medication Safety Issues
Safety issues:
Lipid-based amphotericin formulations (Abelcet®) may be confused with conventional formulations (Amphocin®, Fungizone®)
Large overdoses have occurred when conventional formulations were dispensed inadvertently for lipid-based products. Single daily doses of conventional amphotericin formulation never exceed 1.5 mg/kg.

High alert medication: The Institute for Safe Medication Practices (ISMP) includes this medication among its list of drugs which have a heightened risk of causing significant patient harm when used in error.
Related Information
Antifungal Agents *on page 1664*
Desensitization Protocols *on page 1692*
U.S. Brand Names Abelcet®
Canadian Brand Names Abelcet®
Index Terms ABLC
Pharmacologic Category Antifungal Agent, Parenteral
Generic Available No
Use Treatment of aspergillosis or any type of progressive fungal infection in patients who are refractory to or intolerant of conventional amphotericin B therapy
Unlabeled/Investigational Use Effective in patients with serious *Candida* species infections
Mechanism of Action Binds to ergosterol altering cell membrane permeability in susceptible fungi and causing leakage of cell components with subsequent cell death. Proposed mechanism suggests that amphotericin causes an oxidation-dependent stimulation of macrophages.
Pharmacodynamics/Kinetics
Distribution: V_d: Increases with higher doses; reflects increased uptake by tissues (131 L/kg with 5 mg/kg/day)
Half-life elimination: ~24 hours
Excretion: Clearance: Increases with higher doses (5 mg/kg/day): 400 mL/hour/kg

Dosage Children and Adults: I.V.:

Premedication: For patients who experience infusion-related immediate reactions, premedicate with the following drugs 30-60 minutes prior to drug administration: A nonsteroidal anti-inflammatory agent ± diphenhydramine **or** acetaminophen with diphenhydramine **or** hydrocortisone 50-100 mg. If the patient experiences rigors during the infusion, meperidine may be administered.

Range: 2.5-5 mg/kg/day as a single infusion

Dosing adjustment in renal impairment: None necessary; effects of renal impairment are not currently known

Hemodialysis: No supplemental dosage necessary

Peritoneal dialysis: No supplemental dosage necessary

Continuous renal replacement therapy (CRRT): No supplemental dosage necessary

Stability Intact vials should be stored at 2°C to 8°C (35°F to 46°F); do not freeze. Protect intact vials from exposure to light. Solutions for infusion are stable for 48 hours under refrigeration and for 6 hours at room temperature. Shake the vial gently until there is no evidence of any yellow sediment at the bottom. Dilute with D_5W to 1-2 mg/mL. Protect from light.

Do not dilute with saline solutions or mix with other drugs or electrolytes - compatibility has not been established

Do not use an in-line filter during administration.

Administration For patients who experience nonanaphylactic infusion-related reactions, premedicate 30-60 minutes prior to drug administration with a nonsteroidal anti-inflammatory agent ± diphenhydramine **or** acetaminophen with diphenhydramine **or** hydrocortisone 50-100 mg. If the patient experiences rigors during the infusion, meperidine may be administered.

Administer at an infusion rate of 2.5 mg/kg/hour (over 2 hours). Invert infusion container several times prior to administration and every 2 hours during infusion if it exceeds 2 hours.

Monitoring Parameters Renal function (monitor frequently during therapy), electrolytes (especially potassium and magnesium), liver function tests, temperature, PT/PTT, CBC; monitor input and output; monitor for signs of hypokalemia (muscle weakness, cramping, drowsiness, ECG changes, etc)

Anesthesia and Critical Care Concerns/Other Considerations
Clinical Pearls/Comments:

Prevention of infusion-related reactions: Patients may be premedicated with acetaminophen 650 mg and diphenhydramine 25-50 mg 30 minutes prior to infusion. Hydrocortisone can be used if patient has experienced rigors with amphotericin in the past. Meperidine can also be used for the treatment of rigors during the infusion.

This product is significantly more expensive than conventional amphotericin B. The incidence of nephrotoxicity with ABLC appears to be less when compared to conventional amphotericin B. The incidence of infusion-related reactions does not appear to be decreased with ABLC, but tolerance usually develops. Premedication may be considered to prevent/attenuate infusion-related adverse events. To prevent aggregation of the lipid products, it is important to shake the bag before hanging and once every 2 hours. *In vitro* experiments confirm that liposomal amphotericin B is at least as active as amphotericin B against clinical isolates of *Candida*, *Cryptococcus*, *Blastomyces*, and *Aspergillus*. Their activities also have appeared to be equal against *Fusarium*. Abelcet® may be restricted to patients who cannot tolerate or fail a standard amphotericin B formulation.

Pregnancy Risk Factor B

Contraindications Hypersensitivity to amphotericin or any component of the formulation

Warnings/Precautions Anaphylaxis has been reported with amphotericin B-containing drugs. If severe respiratory distress occurs, the infusion should be immediately discontinued. During the initial dosing, the drug should be administered under close clinical observation. Acute reactions (including fever and chills) may occur 1-2 hours after starting an intravenous infusion. These reactions are usually more common with the first few doses and generally diminish with subsequent doses.

◀ **Adverse Reactions** Nephrotoxicity and infusion-related hyperpyrexia, rigor, and chilling are reduced relative to amphotericin deoxycholate.

>10%:
  Central nervous system: Chills, fever
  Renal: Serum creatinine increased
  Miscellaneous: Multiple organ failure
1% to 10%:
  Cardiovascular: Hypotension, cardiac arrest
  Central nervous system: Headache, pain
  Dermatologic: Rash
  Endocrine & metabolic: Bilirubinemia, hypokalemia, acidosis
  Gastrointestinal: Nausea, vomiting, diarrhea, gastrointestinal hemorrhage, abdominal pain
  Renal: Renal failure
  Respiratory: Respiratory failure, dyspnea, pneumonia

Drug Interactions

Avoid Concomitant Use
  Avoid concomitant use of Amphotericin B (Lipid Complex) with any of the following: Gallium Nitrate

Increased Effect/Toxicity
  Amphotericin B (Lipid Complex) may increase the levels/effects of: Aminoglycosides; Colistimethate; CycloSPORINE; Flucytosine; Gallium Nitrate

  The levels/effects of Amphotericin B (Lipid Complex) may be increased by: Corticosteroids (Orally Inhaled); Corticosteroids (Systemic)

Decreased Effect
  Amphotericin B (Lipid Complex) may decrease the levels/effects of: Saccharomyces boulardii

  The levels/effects of Amphotericin B (Lipid Complex) may be decreased by: Antifungal Agents (Azole Derivatives, Systemic)

Test Interactions Increased BUN (S), serum creatinine, alkaline phosphate, bilirubin; decreased magnesium, potassium (S)

Dosage Forms Excipient information presented when available (limited, particularly for generics); consult specific product labeling.
Injection, suspension [preservative free]:
  Abelcet®: 5 mg/mL (20 mL)

References
Mora-Duarte J, Betts R, Rotstein C, et al, "Comparison of Caspofungin and Amphotericin B for Invasive Candidiasis," *N Engl J Med*, 2002, 347(25):2020-9.
Rex JH, Walsh TJ, Sobel JD, et al, "Practice Guidelines for the Treatment of Candidiasis. Infectious Diseases Society of America," *Clin Infect Dis*, 2000, 30(4):662-78.
Slain D, "Lipid-Based Amphotericin B for the Treatment of Fungal Infections," *Pharmacotherapy*, 1999, 19(3):306-23.

Amphotericin B (Liposomal) (am foe TER i sin bee lye po SO mal)

Medication Safety Issues
Safety issues:
  Lipid-based amphotericin formulations (AmBisome®) may be confused with conventional formulations (Amphocin®, Fungizone®) or with other lipid-based amphotericin formulations (Abelcet®, Amphotec®)
  Large overdoses have occurred when conventional formulations were dispensed inadvertently for lipid-based products. Single daily doses of conventional amphotericin formulation never exceed 1.5 mg/kg.

  High alert medication: The Institute for Safe Medication Practices (ISMP) includes this medication among its list of drugs which have a heightened risk of causing significant patient harm when used in error.

Related Information
  Antifungal Agents *on page 1664*
  Desensitization Protocols *on page 1692*

U.S. Brand Names AmBisome®
Canadian Brand Names AmBisome®
Index Terms L-AmB

Pharmacologic Category Antifungal Agent, Parenteral

Generic Available No

Use Empirical therapy for presumed fungal infection in febrile, neutropenic patients; treatment of patients with *Aspergillus* species, *Candida* species, and/or *Cryptococcus* species infections refractory to amphotericin B desoxycholate (conventional amphotericin), or in patients where renal impairment or unacceptable toxicity precludes the use of amphotericin B desoxycholate; treatment of cryptococcal meningitis in HIV-infected patients; treatment of visceral leishmaniasis

Unlabeled/Investigational Use Treatment of systemic *Histoplasmosis* infection

Mechanism of Action Binds to ergosterol altering cell membrane permeability in susceptible fungi and causing leakage of cell components with subsequent cell death. Proposed mechanism suggests that amphotericin causes an oxidation-dependent stimulation of macrophages (Lyman, 1992).

Pharmacodynamics/Kinetics

Distribution: V_d: 131 L/kg

Half-life elimination: Terminal: 174 hours

Dosage

Usual dosage range:

Children ≥1 month: I.V.: 3-6 mg/kg/day

Adults: I.V.: 3-6 mg/kg/day; **Note:** Higher doses (15 mg/kg/day) have been used clinically (Walsh, 2001)

Note: Premedication: For patients who experience nonanaphylactic infusion-related immediate reactions, premedicate with the following drugs 30-60 minutes prior to drug administration: A nonsteroidal anti-inflammatory agent ± diphenhydramine; **or** acetaminophen with diphenhydramine; **or** hydrocortisone 50-100 mg. If the patient experiences rigors during the infusion, meperidine may be administered.

Indication-specific dosing:

Children ≥1 month: I.V.:

Cryptococcal meningitis (HIV-positive): 6 mg/kg/day (may consider addition of oral flucytosine 25 mg/kg 4 times daily [unlabeled combination; AIDS*info* guidelines, 2008])

Empiric therapy: 3 mg/kg/day

Systemic fungal infections *(Aspergillus, Candida, Cryptococcus, Histoplasmosis)* : 3-5 mg/kg/day

General invasive Candidal disease: 3-5 mg/kg/day (may consider addition of oral flucytosine 25-37.5 mg/kg 4 times daily [unlabeled combination; AIDS*info* guidelines, 2008])

Candidal meningitis: 5 mg/kg/day; (may consider addition of oral flucytosine 25-37.5 mg/kg 4 times daily [unlabeled combination; AIDS*info* guidelines, 2008])

Histoplasmosis (unlabeled use): 3-5 mg/kg/day (AIDS*info* guidelines, 2008)

Visceral leishmaniasis:

Immunocompetent: 3 mg/kg/day on days 1-5, and 3 mg/kg/day on days 14 and 21; a repeat course may be given in patients who do not achieve parasitic clearance

Note: Alternate regimen of 10 mg/kg/day for 2 days has been reportedly effective.

Immunocompromised: 4 mg/kg/day on days 1-5, and 4 mg/kg/day on days 10, 17, 24, 31, and 38

Adults: I.V.:

Cryptococcal meningitis (HIV-positive): 6 mg/kg/day or 4-6 mg/kg/day in combination with addition of oral flucytosine 25 mg/kg 4 times daily (unlabeled combination; AIDS*info* guidelines, 2008)

Empiric candidiasis therapy: 3-5 mg/kg/day (Pappas, 2009)

Endocarditis: I.V.: 3-5 mg/kg/day (with or without flucytosine 25 mg/kg 4 times daily) for 6 weeks after valve replacement; **Note:** If isolates susceptible and/or clearance demonstrated, guidelines recommend step-down to fluconazole; also for long-term suppression therapy if valve replacement is not possible (Pappas, 2009)

Fungal sinusitis: Limited data in immunocompromised patients have shown efficacy with 3-10 mg/kg/day (Pagano, 2004; Rokicka, 2006; Barron, 2005). ▶

◄ **Note:** An azole antifungal is recommended if causative organism is *Aspergillus* spp or *Pseudallescheria boydii* (*Scedosporium* sp).

Osteoarticular candidiasis: I.V.: 3-5 mg/kg/day for several weeks, followed by fluconazole for 6-12 months (osteomyelitis) or 6 weeks (septic arthritis)

Systemic fungal infections *(Aspergillus, Candida, Cryptococcus, Histoplasmosis)*: 3-5 mg/kg/day

General invasive Candidal disease: 3-5 mg/kg/day with oral flucytosine 25 mg/kg 4 times daily (unlabeled combination; Pappas, 2009)

Candidal meningitis: 3-5 mg/kg/day with or without oral flucytosine 25 mg/kg 4 times daily (unlabeled combination; Pappas, 2009)

Histoplasmosis (unlabeled use): 3-5 mg/kg/day (AIDS*info* guidelines, 2008)

Visceral leishmaniasis:

Immunocompetent: 3 mg/kg/day on days 1-5, and 3 mg/kg/day on days 14 and 21; a repeat course may be given in patients who do not achieve parasitic clearance

Note: Alternate regimen of 2 mg/kg/day for 5 days has been reportedly effective.

Immunocompromised: 4 mg/kg/day on days 1-5, and 4 mg/kg/day on days 10, 17, 24, 31, and 38

Dosing adjustment in renal impairment: None necessary; effects of renal impairment are not currently known

Hemodialysis: No supplemental dosage necessary

Peritoneal dialysis effects: No supplemental dosage necessary

Continuous renal replacement therapy (CRRT): No supplemental dosage necessary

Stability Store intact vials at ≤25°C (≤77°F). Reconstituted vials are stable refrigerated at 2°C to 8°C (36°F to 46°F) for 24 hours. Do not freeze. Manufacturer's labeling states infusion should begin within 6 hours of dilution with D_5W; data on file with Astellas Pharma shows extended formulation stability when admixed in D_5W at 0.2-2 mg/mL (in polyolefin or PVC bags) for up to 11 days when stored refrigerated at 2°C to 8°C (36°F to 46°F).

Reconstitution: Reconstitute with 12 mL SWFI to a concentration of 4 mg/mL. The use of any solution other than those recommended, or the presence of a bacteriostatic agent in the solution, may cause precipitation. **Shake the vial vigorously** for 30 seconds, until dispersed into a translucent yellow suspension.

Filtration and dilution: The 5-micron filter should be on the syringe used to remove the reconstituted AmBisome®. Dilute to a final concentration of 1-2 mg/mL (0.2-0.5 mg/mL for infants and small children).

Administration Administer via intravenous infusion, over a period of approximately 2 hours. Infusion time may be reduced to approximately 1 hour in patients in whom the treatment is well-tolerated. If the patient experiences discomfort during infusion, the duration of infusion may be increased. Administer at a rate of 2.5 mg/kg/hour. Existing intravenous line should be flushed with D_5W prior to infusion (if not feasible, administer through a separate line). An in-line membrane filter (not less than 1 micron) may be used.

For a patient who experiences chills, fever, hypotension, nausea, or other nonanaphylactic infusion-related reactions, premedicate with the following drugs, 30-60 minutes prior to drug administration: A nonsteroidal (eg, ibuprofen, choline magnesium trisalicylate) with or without diphenhydramine **or** acetaminophen with diphenhydramine **or** hydrocortisone 50-100 mg. If the patient experiences rigors during the infusion, meperidine may be administered.

Monitoring Parameters Renal function (monitor frequently during therapy), electrolytes (especially potassium and magnesium), liver function tests, temperature, PT/PTT, CBC; monitor input and output; monitor for signs of hypokalemia (muscle weakness, cramping, drowsiness, ECG changes, etc); monitor cardiac function if used concurrently with corticosteroids

Anesthesia and Critical Care Concerns/Other Considerations

Clinical Pearls/Comments:

Prevention of infusion-related reactions: Patients may be premedicated with acetaminophen 650 mg and diphenhydramine 25-50 mg 30 minutes prior to infusion. Hydrocortisone can be used if patient has experienced rigors with amphotericin in the past. Meperidine can also be used for the treatment of rigors during the infusion.

This product is significantly more expensive than conventional amphotericin B; Infectious Disease consult is recommended. AmBisome® is a true single bilayer liposomal drug delivery system. Liposomes are closed, spherical vesicles created by mixing specific proportions of amphophilic substances such as phospholipids and cholesterol so that they arrange themselves into multiple concentric bilayer membranes when hydrated in aqueous solutions. Single bilayer liposomes are then formed by microemulsification of multilamellar vesicles using a homogenizer. AmBisome® consists of these unilamellar bilayer liposomes with amphotericin B intercalated within the membrane. Due to the nature and quantity of amphophilic substances used, and the lipophilic moiety in the amphotericin B molecule, the drug is an integral part of the overall structure of the AmBisome® liposomes. AmBisome® contains true liposomes that are <100 nm in diameter.

Pregnancy Risk Factor B

Contraindications Hypersensitivity to amphotericin B deoxycholate or any component of the formulation

Warnings/Precautions Patients should be under close clinical observation during initial dosing. As with other amphotericin B-containing products, anaphylaxis has been reported. Facilities for cardiopulmonary resuscitation should be available during administration. Acute infusion reactions (including fever and chills) may occur 1-2 hours after starting infusions; reactions are more common with the first few doses and generally diminish with subsequent doses. Immediately discontinue infusion if severe respiratory distress occurs; the patient should not receive further infusions. Concurrent use of amphotericin B with other nephrotoxic drugs may enhance the potential for drug-induced renal toxicity. Concurrent use with antineoplastic agents may enhance the potential for renal toxicity, bronchospasm or hypotension. Acute pulmonary toxicity has been reported in patients receiving simultaneous leukocyte transfusions and amphotericin B. Safety and efficacy have not been established in patients <1 month of age.

Adverse Reactions Percentage of adverse reactions is dependent upon population studied and may vary with respect to premedications and underlying illness. Incidence of decreased renal function and infusion-related events are lower than rates observed with amphotericin B deoxycholate.

>10%:

Cardiovascular: Peripheral edema (15%), edema (12% to 14%), tachycardia (9% to 19%), hypotension (7% to 14%), hypertension (8% to 20%), chest pain (8% to 12%), hypervolemia (8% to 12%)

Central nervous system: Chills (29% to 48%), insomnia (17% to 22%), headache (9% to 20%), anxiety (7% to 14%), pain (14%), confusion (9% to 13%)

Dermatologic: Rash (5% to 25%), pruritus (11%)

Endocrine & metabolic: Hypokalemia (31% to 51%), hypomagnesemia (15% to 50%), hyperglycemia (8% to 23%), hypocalcemia (5% to 18%), hyponatremia (9% to 12%)

Gastrointestinal: Nausea (16% to 40%), vomiting (11% to 32%), diarrhea (11% to 30%), abdominal pain (7% to 20%), constipation (15%), anorexia (10% to 14%)

Hematologic: Anemia (27% to 48%), blood transfusion reaction (9% to 18%), leukopenia (15% to 17%), thrombocytopenia (6% to 13%)

Hepatic: Alkaline phosphatase increased (7% to 22%), bilirubinemia (≤18%), ALT increased (15%), AST increased (13%), liver function tests abnormal (not specified) (4% to 13%)

Local: Phlebitis (9% to 11%)

Neuromuscular & skeletal: Weakness (6% to 13%), back pain (12%)

Renal: Nephrotoxicity (14% to 47%), creatinine increased (18% to 40%), BUN increased (7% to 21%), hematuria (14%)

Respiratory: Dyspnea (18% to 23%), lung disorder (14% to 18%), cough (2% to 18%), epistaxis (9% to 15%), pleural effusion (13%), rhinitis (11%)

Miscellaneous: Infusion reactions (4% to 21%), sepsis (7% to 14%), infection (11% to 13%)

2% to 10%:

Cardiovascular: Arrhythmia, atrial fibrillation, bradycardia, cardiac arrest, cardiomegaly, facial swelling, flushing, postural hypotension, valvular heart disease, vascular disorder, vasodilation

Central nervous system: Agitation, abnormal thinking, coma, depression, dysesthesia, dizziness (7% to 9%), hallucinations, malaise, nervousness, seizure, somnolence

Dermatologic: Alopecia, bruising, cellulitis, dry skin, maculopapular rash, petechia, purpura, skin discoloration, skin disorder, skin ulcer, urticaria, vesiculobullous rash

Endocrine & metabolic: Acidosis, fluid overload, hypernatremia (4%), hyperchloremia, hyperkalemia, hypermagnesemia, hyperphosphatemia, hypophosphatemia, hypoproteinemia, lactate dehydrogenase increased, nonprotein nitrogen increased

Gastrointestinal: Abdomen enlarged, amylase increased, dyspepsia, dysphagia, eructation, fecal incontinence, flatulence, gastrointestinal hemorrhage (10%), hematemesis, hemorrhoids, gum/oral hemorrhage, ileus, mucositis, rectal disorder, stomatitis, ulcerative stomatitis, xerostomia

Genitourinary: Vaginal hemorrhage

Hematologic: Coagulation disorder, hemorrhage, prothrombin decreased

Hepatic: Hepatocellular damage, hepatomegaly, veno-occlusive liver disease

Local: Injection site inflammation

Neuromuscular & skeletal: Arthralgia, bone pain, dystonia, myalgia, neck pain, paresthesia, rigors, tremor

Ocular: Conjunctivitis, dry eyes, eye hemorrhage

Renal: Abnormal renal function, acute renal failure, dysuria, renal failure, toxic nephropathy, urinary incontinence

Respiratory: Asthma, atelectasis, dry nose, hemoptysis, hyperventilation, pharyngitis, pneumonia, pulmonary edema, respiratory alkalosis, respiratory insufficiency, respiratory failure, sinusitis, hypoxia (6% to 8%)

Miscellaneous: Allergic reaction, cell-mediated immunological reaction, flu-like syndrome, graft-versus-host disease, herpes simplex, hiccup, procedural complication (8% to 10%), diaphoresis (7%)

Postmarketing and/or case reports: Agranulocytosis, angioedema, bronchospasm, cyanosis/hypoventilation, erythema, hemorrhagic cystitis

Drug Interactions

Avoid Concomitant Use

Avoid concomitant use of Amphotericin B (Liposomal) with any of the following: Gallium Nitrate

Increased Effect/Toxicity

Amphotericin B (Liposomal) may increase the levels/effects of: Aminoglycosides; Colistimethate; CycloSPORINE; Flucytosine; Gallium Nitrate

The levels/effects of Amphotericin B (Liposomal) may be increased by: Corticosteroids (Orally Inhaled); Corticosteroids (Systemic)

Decreased Effect

Amphotericin B (Liposomal) may decrease the levels/effects of: Saccharomyces boulardii

The levels/effects of Amphotericin B (Liposomal) may be decreased by: Antifungal Agents (Azole Derivatives, Systemic)

Dosage Forms Excipient information presented when available (limited, particularly for generics); consult specific product labeling.

Injection, powder for reconstitution:

AmBisome®: 50 mg [contains soy and sucrose]

References

Mora-Duarte J, Betts R, Rotstein C, et al, "Comparison of Caspofungin and Amphotericin B for Invasive Candidiasis," *N Engl J Med*, 2002, 347(25):2020-9.

Rex JH, Walsh TJ, Sobel JD, et al, "Practice Guidelines for the Treatment of Candidiasis. Infectious Diseases Society of America," *Clin Infect Dis*, 2000, 30(4):662-78.

Slain D, "Lipid-Based Amphotericin B for the Treatment of Fungal Infections," *Pharmacotherapy*, 1999, 19(3):306-23.

Ampicillin (am pi SIL in)

Medication Safety Issues
Sound-alike/look-alike issues:
Ampicillin may be confused with aminophylline

Related Information
Anesthesia for Patients With Liver Disease *on page 1537*
Desensitization Protocols *on page 1692*
Prevention of Infective Endocarditis *on page 1718*
Prevention of Wound Infection and Sepsis in Surgical Patients *on page 1721*
Skin Tests *on page 1707*

Canadian Brand Names Apo-Ampi®; Novo-Ampicillin; Nu-Ampi

Index Terms Aminobenzylpenicillin; Ampicillin Sodium; Ampicillin Trihydrate

Pharmacologic Category Antibiotic, Penicillin

Generic Available Yes

Use Treatment of susceptible bacterial infections (nonbeta-lactamase-producing organisms); treatment or prophylaxis of infective endocarditis; susceptible bacterial infections caused by streptococci, pneumococci, nonpenicillinase-producing staphylococci, *Listeria*, meningococci; some strains of *H. influenzae*, *Salmonella*, *Shigella*, *E. coli*, *Enterobacter*, and *Klebsiella*

Mechanism of Action Inhibits bacterial cell wall synthesis by binding to one or more of the penicillin-binding proteins (PBPs) which in turn inhibits the final transpeptidation step of peptidoglycan synthesis in bacterial cell walls, thus inhibiting cell wall biosynthesis. Bacteria eventually lyse due to ongoing activity of cell wall autolytic enzymes (autolysins and murein hydrolases) while cell wall assembly is arrested.

Pharmacodynamics/Kinetics
Absorption: Oral: 50%
Distribution: Bile, blister, and tissue fluids; penetration into CSF occurs with inflamed meninges only, good only with inflammation (exceeds usual MICs)
Normal meninges: Nil; Inflamed meninges: 5% to 10%
Protein binding: 15% to 25%
Half-life elimination:
Children and Adults: 1-1.8 hours
Anuria/end-stage renal disease: 7-20 hours
Time to peak: Oral: Within 1-2 hours
Excretion: Urine (~90% as unchanged drug) within 24 hours

Dosage
Usual dosage range:
Infants and Children:
Oral: 50-100 mg/kg/day in doses divided every 6 hours (maximum: 2-4 g/day)
I.M., I.V.: 100-400 mg/kg/day in divided doses every 6 hours (maximum: 12 g/day)
Adults: Oral, I.M., I.V.: 250-500 mg every 6 hours

Indication-specific dosing:
Infants and Children:
Prophylaxis against infective endocarditis:
Dental, oral, or respiratory tract procedures: I.M., I.V.: 50 mg/kg within 30-60 minutes prior to procedure in patients not allergic to penicillin and unable to take oral amoxicillin. Intramuscular injections should be avoided in patients who are receiving anticoagulant therapy. In these circumstances, orally administered regimens should be given whenever possible. Intravenously administered antibiotics should be used for patients who are unable to tolerate or absorb oral medications.
Note: American Heart Association (AHA) guidelines now recommend prophylaxis only in patients undergoing invasive procedures and in whom underlying cardiac conditions may predispose to a higher risk of adverse outcomes should infection occur.
Genitourinary and gastrointestinal tract procedures: I.M., I.V.:
High-risk patients: 50 mg/kg (maximum: 2 g) within 30 minutes prior to procedure, followed by ampicillin 25 mg/kg (or amoxicillin 25 mg/kg orally) 6 hours later; must be used in combination with gentamicin. **Note:** As of

April 2007, routine prophylaxis for GI/GU procedures is no longer recommended by the AHA.

Moderate-risk patients: 50 mg/kg within 30 minutes prior to procedure

Mild-to-moderate infections:
Oral: 50-100 mg/kg/day in doses divided every 6 hours (maximum: 2-4 g/day)
I.M., I.V.: 100-150 mg/kg/day in divided doses every 6 hours (maximum: 2-4 g/day)

Severe infections, meningitis: I.M., I.V.: 200-400 mg/kg/day in divided doses every 6 hours (maximum: 6-12 g/day)

Adults:

Actinomycosis: I.V.: 50 mg/kg/day for 4-6 weeks then oral amoxicillin

Cholangitis (acute): I.V.: 2 g every 4 hours with gentamicin

Diverticulitis: I.M., I.V.: 2 g every 6 hours with metronidazole

Endocarditis:
Infective: I.V.: 12 g/day via continuous infusion or divided every 4 hours

Prophylaxis: Dental, oral, or respiratory tract: I.M., I.V.: 2 g within 30-60 minutes prior to procedure in patients not allergic to penicillin and unable to take oral amoxicillin. Intramuscular injections should be avoided in patients who are receiving anticoagulant therapy. In these circumstances, orally administered regimens should be given whenever possible. Intravenously administered antibiotics should be used for patients who are unable to tolerate or absorb oral medications.

Note: American Heart Association (AHA) guidelines now recommend prophylaxis only in patients undergoing invasive procedures and in whom underlying cardiac conditions may predispose to a higher risk of adverse outcomes should infection occur.

Prophylaxis in total joint replacement patient: I.M., I.V.: 2 g 1 hour prior to the procedure

Genitourinary and gastrointestinal tract procedures:
High-risk patients: I.M., I.V.: 2 g within 30 minutes prior to procedure, followed by ampicillin 1 g (or amoxicillin 1g orally) 6 hours later; must be used in combination with gentamicin. **Note:** As of April 2007, routine prophylaxis for GI/GU procedures is no longer recommended by the AHA.
Moderate-risk patients: I.M., I.V.: 2 g within 30 minutes prior to procedure

Group B strep prophylaxis (intrapartum): I.V.: 2 g initial dose, then 1 g every 4 hours until delivery

Listeria **infections:** I.V.: 2 g every 4 hours (consider addition of aminoglycoside)

Sepsis/meningitis: I.M., I.V.: 150-250 mg/kg/day divided every 3-4 hours (range: 6-12 g/day)

Urinary tract infections (enterococcus suspected): I.V.: 1-2 g every 6 hours with gentamicin

Dosing interval in renal impairment:
Cl_{cr} >50 mL/minute: Administer every 6 hours
Cl_{cr} 10-50 mL/minute: Administer every 6-12 hours
Cl_{cr} <10 mL/minute: Administer every 12-24 hours
Hemodialysis: Moderately dialyzable (20% to 50%); administer dose after dialysis
Peritoneal dialysis: Moderately dialyzable (20% to 50%)
Administer 250 mg every 12 hours
Continuous arteriovenous or venovenous hemofiltration effects: Dose as for Cl_{cr} 10-50 mL/minute; ~50 mg of ampicillin per liter of filtrate is removed

Stability
Oral: Oral suspension is stable for 7 days at room temperature or for 14 days under refrigeration.
I.V.:
I.V. minimum volume: Concentration should not exceed 30 mg/mL due to concentration-dependent stability restrictions. Solutions for I.M. or direct I.V. should be used within 1 hour. Solutions for I.V. infusion will be inactivated by dextrose at room temperature. If dextrose-containing solutions are to be used, the resultant solution will only be stable for 2 hours versus 8 hours in the 0.9% sodium chloride injection. D_5W has limited stability.
Stability of parenteral admixture in NS at room temperature (25°C) is 8 hours.
Stability of parenteral admixture in NS at refrigeration temperature (4°C) is 2 days.
Standard diluent: 500 mg/50 mL NS; 1 g/50 mL NS; 2 g/100 mL NS

Administration Administer around-the-clock to promote less variation in peak and trough serum levels.

Oral: Administer on an empty stomach (ie, 1 hour prior to, or 2 hours after meals) to increase total absorption.

I.V.: Administer over 3-5 minutes (125-500 mg) or over 10-15 minutes (1-2 g). More rapid infusion may cause seizures. Ampicillin and gentamicin should not be mixed in the same I.V. tubing.

Some penicillins (eg, carbenicillin, ticarcillin, and piperacillin) have been shown to inactivate aminoglycosides *in vitro*. This has been observed to a greater extent with tobramycin and gentamicin, while amikacin has shown greater stability against inactivation. Concurrent use of these agents may pose a risk of reduced antibacterial efficacy *in vivo*, particularly in the setting of profound renal impairment. However, definitive clinical evidence is lacking. If combination penicillin/aminoglycoside therapy is desired in a patient with renal dysfunction, separation of doses (if feasible), and routine monitoring of aminoglycoside levels, CBC, and clinical response should be considered.

Monitoring Parameters With prolonged therapy, monitor renal, hepatic, and hematologic function periodically; observe signs and symptoms of anaphylaxis during first dose

Pregnancy Risk Factor B

Contraindications Hypersensitivity to ampicillin, any component of the formulation, or other penicillins

Warnings/Precautions Dosage adjustment may be necessary in patients with renal impairment. Serious and occasionally severe or fatal hypersensitivity (anaphylactoid) reactions have been reported in patients on penicillin therapy, especially with a history of beta-lactam hypersensitivity, history of sensitivity to multiple allergens, or previous IgE-mediated reactions (eg, anaphylaxis, angioedema, urticaria). Use with caution in asthmatic patients. High percentage of patients with infectious mononucleosis have developed rash during therapy with ampicillin; ampicillin-class antibiotics not recommended in these patients. Appearance of a rash should be carefully evaluated to differentiate a nonallergic ampicillin rash from a hypersensitivity reaction. Ampicillin rash occurs in 5% to 10% of children receiving ampicillin and is a generalized dull red, maculopapular rash, generally appearing 3-14 days after the start of therapy. It normally begins on the trunk and spreads over most of the body. It may be most intense at pressure areas, elbows, and knees. Prolonged use may result in fungal or bacterial superinfection, including *C. difficile*-associated diarrhea (CDAD) and pseudomembranous colitis; CDAD has been observed >2 months postantibiotic treatment.

Adverse Reactions Frequency not defined.

Central nervous system: Fever, penicillin encephalopathy, seizure

Dermatologic: Erythema multiforme, exfoliative dermatitis, rash, urticaria

Note: Appearance of a rash should be carefully evaluated to differentiate (if possible) nonallergic ampicillin rash from hypersensitivity reaction. Incidence is higher in patients with viral infection, *Salmonella* infection, lymphocytic leukemia, or patients that have hyperuricemia.

Gastrointestinal: Black hairy tongue, diarrhea, enterocolitis, glossitis, nausea, pseudomembranous colitis, sore mouth or tongue, stomatitis, vomiting, oral candidiasis

Hematologic: Agranulocytosis, anemia, hemolytic anemia, eosinophilia, leukopenia, thrombocytopenia purpura

Hepatic: AST increased

Renal: Interstitial nephritis (rare)

Respiratory: Laryngeal stridor

Miscellaneous: Anaphylaxis, serum sickness-like reaction

Drug Interactions

Avoid Concomitant Use There are no known interactions where it is recommended to avoid concomitant use.

Increased Effect/Toxicity

Ampicillin may increase the levels/effects of: Methotrexate

The levels/effects of Ampicillin may be increased by: Allopurinol; Uricosuric Agents

Decreased Effect
Ampicillin may decrease the levels/effects of: Atenolol; Mycophenolate; Typhoid Vaccine

The levels/effects of Ampicillin may be decreased by: Chloroquine; Fusidic Acid; Tetracycline Derivatives

Ethanol/Nutrition/Herb Interactions Food: Food decreases ampicillin absorption rate; may decrease ampicillin serum concentration.

Test Interactions May interfere with urinary glucose tests using cupric sulfate (Benedict's solution, Clinitest®)

Some penicillin derivatives may accelerate the degradation of aminoglycosides *in vitro*, leading to a potential underestimation of aminoglycoside serum concentration.

Dietary Considerations Take on an empty stomach 1 hour before or 2 hours after meals.

Sodium content of 5 mL suspension (250 mg/5 mL): 10 mg (0.4 mEq)
Sodium content of 1 g: 66.7 mg (3 mEq)

Dosage Forms Excipient information presented when available (limited, particularly for generics); consult specific product labeling.
Capsule: 250 mg, 500 mg
Injection, powder for reconstitution, as sodium: 125 mg, 250 mg, 500 mg, 1 g, 2 g, 10 g
Powder for oral suspension: 125 mg/5 mL (100 mL, 200 mL); 250 mg/5 mL (100 mL, 200 mL)

Ampicillin and Sulbactam (am pi SIL in & SUL bak tam)

U.S. Brand Names Unasyn®
Canadian Brand Names Unasyn®
Index Terms Sulbactam and Ampicillin
Pharmacologic Category Antibiotic, Penicillin
Generic Available Yes
Use Treatment of susceptible bacterial infections involved with skin and skin structure, intra-abdominal infections, gynecological infections; spectrum is that of ampicillin plus organisms producing beta-lactamases such as *S. aureus, H. influenzae, E. coli, Klebsiella, Acinetobacter, Enterobacter,* and anaerobes
Mechanism of Action The addition of sulbactam, a beta-lactamase inhibitor, to ampicillin extends the spectrum of ampicillin to include some beta-lactamase-producing organisms; inhibits bacterial cell wall synthesis by binding to one or more of the penicillin-binding proteins (PBPs) which in turn inhibits the final transpeptidation step of peptidoglycan synthesis in bacterial cell walls, thus inhibiting cell wall biosynthesis. Bacteria eventually lyse due to ongoing activity of cell wall autolytic enzymes (autolysins and murein hydrolases) while cell wall assembly is arrested.

Pharmacodynamics/Kinetics
Ampicillin: See Ampicillin.
Sulbactam:
Distribution: Bile, blister, and tissue fluids
Protein binding: 38%
Half-life elimination: Normal renal function: 1-1.3 hours
Excretion: Urine (~75% to 85% as unchanged drug) within 8 hours
Dosage Note: Unasyn® (ampicillin/sulbactam) is a combination product. Dosage recommendations for Unasyn® are based on the ampicillin component.
Usual dosage range:
Children ≥1 year: I.V.: 100-400 mg ampicillin/kg/day divided every 6 hours (maximum: 8 g ampicillin/day, 12 g Unasyn®). **Note:** The American Academy of Pediatrics recommends a dose of up to 300 mg/kg/day for severe infection in infants >1 month of age.
Adults: I.M., I.V.: 1-2 g ampicillin (1.5-3 g Unasyn®) every 6 hours (maximum: 8 g ampicillin/day, 12 g Unasyn®)

Indication-specific dosing:

Children: ≥1 year:

Epiglottitis: I.V.: 100-200 mg ampicillin/kg/day divided in 4 doses

Mild-to-moderate infections: I.V.: 100-200 mg ampicillin/kg/day (150-300 mg Unasyn®) divided every 6 hours (maximum: 8 g ampicillin/day, 12 g Unasyn®)

Peritonsillar and retropharyngeal abscess: I.V.: 50 mg ampicillin/kg/dose every 6 hours

Severe infections: I.V.: 200-400 mg ampicillin/kg/day divided every 6 hours (maximum: 8 g ampicillin/day, 12 g Unasyn®)

Adults: Doses expressed as ampicillin/sulbactam combination:

Amnionitis, cholangitis, diverticulitis, endometritis, endophthalmitis, epididymitis/orchitis, liver abscess, osteomyelitis (diabetic foot), peritonitis: I.V.: 3 g every 6 hours

Endocarditis: I.V.: 3 g every 6 hours with gentamicin or vancomycin for 4-6 weeks

Orbital cellulitis: I.V.: 1.5 g every 6 hours

Parapharyngeal space infections: I.V.: 3 g every 6 hours

Pasteurella multocida **(human, canine/feline bites):** I.V.: 1.5-3 g every 6 hours

Pelvic inflammatory disease: I.V.: 3 g every 6 hours with doxycycline

Peritonitis (CAPD): Intraperitoneal:

Anuric, intermittent: 3 g every 12 hours

Anuric, continuous: Loading dose: 1.5 g; maintenance dose: 150 mg

Pneumonia:

Aspiration, community-acquired: I.V.: 1.5-3 g every 6 hours

Hospital-acquired: I.V.: 3 g every 6 hours

Urinary tract infections, pyelonephritis: I.V.: 3 g every 6 hours for 14 days

Dosing interval in renal impairment:

Cl_{cr} 15-29 mL/minute: Administer every 12 hours

Cl_{cr} 5-14 mL/minute and hemodialysis: Administer every 24 hours; give dose after dialysis

Continuous ambulatory peritoneal dialysis (CAPD): 3 g every 24 hours

Continuous renal replacement therapy (CRRT): Drug clearance is highly dependent on the method of renal replacement, filter type, and flow rate. Appropriate dosing requires close monitoring of pharmacologic response, signs of adverse reactions due to drug accumulation, as well as drug levels in relation to target trough (if appropriate). The following are general recommendations only (based on dialysate flow/ultrafiltration rates of 1 L/hour) and should not supersede clinical judgment:

CVVH: 3 g every 12 hours

CVVHD/CVVHDF: 3 g every 8 hours

Stability Prior to reconstitution, store at ≤30°C (86°F).

I.M. and direct I.V. administration: Use within 1 hour after preparation. Reconstitute with sterile water for injection or 0.5% or 2% lidocaine hydrochloride injection (I.M.). Sodium chloride 0.9% (NS) is the diluent of choice for I.V. piggyback use. Solutions made in NS are stable up to 72 hours when refrigerated whereas dextrose solutions (same concentration) are stable for only 4 hours.

Administration Administer around-the-clock to promote less variation in peak and trough serum levels. Administer by slow injection over 10-15 minutes or I.V. over 15-30 minutes. Ampicillin and gentamicin should not be mixed in the same I.V. tubing.

Some penicillins (eg, carbenicillin, ticarcillin, and piperacillin) have been shown to inactivate aminoglycosides *in vitro*. This has been observed to a greater extent with tobramycin and gentamicin, while amikacin has shown greater stability against inactivation. Concurrent use of these agents may pose a risk of reduced antibacterial efficacy *in vivo*, particularly in the setting of profound renal impairment. However, definitive clinical evidence is lacking. If combination penicillin/aminoglycoside therapy is desired in a patient with renal dysfunction, separation of doses (if feasible), and routine monitoring of aminoglycoside levels, CBC, and clinical response should be considered.

◄ **Monitoring Parameters** With prolonged therapy, monitor hematologic, renal, and hepatic function; monitor for signs of anaphylaxis during first dose

Pregnancy Risk Factor B

Contraindications Hypersensitivity to ampicillin, sulbactam, penicillins, or any component of the formulations

Warnings/Precautions Dosage adjustment may be necessary in patients with renal impairment. Serious and occasionally severe or fatal hypersensitivity (anaphylactoid) reactions have been reported in patients on penicillin therapy, especially with a history of beta-lactam hypersensitivity, history of sensitivity to multiple allergens, or previous IgE-mediated reactions (eg, anaphylaxis, angioedema, urticaria). Use with caution in asthmatic patients. High percentage of patients with infectious mononucleosis have developed rash during therapy with ampicillin; ampicillin-class antibiotics not recommended in these patients. Appearance of a rash should be carefully evaluated to differentiate a nonallergic ampicillin rash from a hypersensitivity reaction. Prolonged use may result in fungal or bacterial superinfection, including *C. difficile*-associated diarrhea (CDAD) and pseudomembranous colitis; CDAD has been observed >2 months postantibiotic treatment. Safety and efficacy have not been established in children <1 year of age.

Adverse Reactions Also see Ampicillin.

>10%: Local: Pain at injection site (I.M.)

1% to 10%:
Dermatologic: Rash
Gastrointestinal: Diarrhea
Local: Pain at injection site (I.V.), thrombophlebitis
Miscellaneous: Allergic reaction (may include serum sickness, urticaria, bronchospasm, hypotension, etc)

<1% (Limited to important or life-threatening): Abdominal distension, candidiasis, chest pain, chills, dysuria, edema, epistaxis, erythema, facial swelling, fatigue, flatulence, glossitis, hairy tongue, headache, interstitial nephritis, itching, liver enzymes increased, malaise, mucosal bleeding, nausea, pseudomembranous colitis, seizure, substernal pain, throat tightness, thrombocytopenia, urine retention, vomiting

Drug Interactions

Avoid Concomitant Use There are no known interactions where it is recommended to avoid concomitant use.

Increased Effect/Toxicity

Ampicillin and Sulbactam may increase the levels/effects of: Methotrexate

The levels/effects of Ampicillin and Sulbactam may be increased by: Allopurinol; Uricosuric Agents

Decreased Effect

Ampicillin and Sulbactam may decrease the levels/effects of: Atenolol; Mycophenolate; Typhoid Vaccine

The levels/effects of Ampicillin and Sulbactam may be decreased by: Chloroquine; Fusidic Acid; Tetracycline Derivatives

Test Interactions May interfere with urinary glucose tests using cupric sulfate (Benedict's solution, Clinitest®).

Some penicillin derivatives may accelerate the degradation of aminoglycosides *in vitro*, leading to a potential underestimation of aminoglycoside serum concentration.

Dietary Considerations Sodium content of 1.5 g injection: 115 mg (5 mEq)

Dosage Forms Excipient information presented when available (limited, particularly for generics); consult specific product labeling.

Injection, powder for reconstitution: 1.5 g: Ampicillin 1 g and sulbactam 0.5 g [contains sodium 115 mg (5 mEq)/1.5 g]; 3 g: Ampicillin 2 g and sulbactam 1 g [contains sodium 115 mg (5 mEq)/1.5 g)]; 15 g: Ampicillin 10 g and sulbactam 5 g [bulk package; contains sodium 115 mg (5 mEq)/1.5 g]

Unasyn®:
1.5 g: Ampicillin 1 g and sulbactam 0.5 g [contains sodium 115 mg (5 mEq)/1.5 g)]
3 g: Ampicillin 2 g and sulbactam 1 g [contains sodium 115 mg (5 mEq)/1.5 g)]

15 g: Ampicillin 10 g and sulbactam 5 g [bulk package; contains sodium 115 mg (5 mEq)/1.5 g)]

♦ **Ampicillin Sodium** see Ampicillin on page 115

♦ **Ampicillin Trihydrate** see Ampicillin on page 115

♦ **Amrinone Lactate** see Inamrinone on page 737

Amyl Nitrite (AM il NYE trite)

Index Terms Isoamyl Nitrite

Pharmacologic Category Antidote; Vasodilator

Generic Available Yes

Use Coronary vasodilator in angina pectoris; adjunct in treatment of cyanide poisoning; produce changes in the intensity of heart murmurs

Mechanism of Action Relaxes vascular smooth muscle; decreased venous ratios and arterial blood pressure; reduces left ventricular work; decreases myocardial O_2 consumption; in cyanide poisoning, amyl nitrite converts hemoglobin to methemoglobin that binds with cyanide to form cyanate hemoglobin

Pharmacodynamics/Kinetics
Onset of action: Angina: Within 30 seconds
Duration: 3-15 minutes

Dosage Nasal inhalation:
Cyanide poisoning: Children and Adults: Inhale the vapor from a 0.3 mL crushed ampul every minute for 15-30 seconds until I.V. sodium nitrite infusion is available
Angina: Adults: 1-6 inhalations from 1 crushed ampul; may repeat in 3-5 minutes

Stability Store in cool place. Protect from light.

Administration Administer nasally. Patient should not be sitting. Crush ampul in woven covering between fingers and then hold under patient's nostrils.

Monitoring Parameters Monitor blood pressure during therapy

Anesthesia and Critical Care Concerns/Other Considerations
Clinical Pearls/Comments: Highly flammable; do not use where it might be ignited. Amyl nitrate is also used as a recreational drug during intercourse. However, when used in combination with phosphodiesterase-5 enzyme inhibitors, significant and profound hypotension may result.

Pregnancy Risk Factor C

Contraindications Hypersensitivity to nitrates; severe anemia; head injury; angle-closure glaucoma; postural hypotension; head trauma or cerebral hemorrhage; pregnancy

Warnings/Precautions Use with caution in patients with increased intracranial pressure, low systolic blood pressure, and coronary artery disease. Safety and efficacy have not been established in children.

Adverse Reactions Frequency not defined.
Cardiovascular: Postural hypotension, cutaneous flushing of head, neck, and clavicular area, palpitations, tachycardia, sinus tachycardia, vasodilation
Central nervous system: Headache, incoherent speech, restlessness
Dermatologic: Contact dermatitis
Gastrointestinal: Nausea, colitis, vomiting
Genitourinary: Penile erection enhanced, retarded ejaculation
Hematologic: Heinz body hemolysis/hemolytic anemia
Ocular: Increased intraocular pressure, blurred vision
Respiratory: Tracheobronchitis

Drug Interactions
Avoid Concomitant Use There are no known interactions where it is recommended to avoid concomitant use.
Increased Effect/Toxicity
Amyl Nitrite may increase the levels/effects of: Hypotensive Agents
Decreased Effect There are no known significant interactions involving a decrease in effect.

Dosage Forms Excipient information presented when available (limited, particularly for generics); consult specific product labeling.
Vapor for inhalation [crushable covered glass capsules]: Amyl nitrite USP (0.3 mL)

References
Dudley MJ and Solomon T, "A Case of Methaemoglobinaemia," *Arch Emerg Med*, 1993, 10(2):117-9.
Laaban JP, Bodenan P, and Rochemaure J, "Amyl Nitrate Poppers and Methemoglobinemia," *Ann Intern Med*, 1985, 103(5):804-5.
Mokhlesi B, Leikin JB, Murray P, et al, "Adult Toxicology in Critical Care. Part 11: Specific Poisonings," *Chest*, 2003, 123(3):897-922.
Osterloh J and Olson K, "Toxicities of Alkyl Nitrites," *Ann Intern Med*, 1986, 104(5):727.
Schwartz RH, "When to Suspect Inhalant Abuse," *Patient Care*, 1989, 23:39-64.

◆ **AN100226** *see* Natalizumab *on page 989*

◆ **Anaprox®** *see* Naproxen *on page 987*

◆ **Anaprox® DS** *see* Naproxen *on page 987*

Anastrozole (an AS troe zole)

U.S. Brand Names Arimidex®
Canadian Brand Names Arimidex®
Index Terms ICI-D1033; ZD1033
Pharmacologic Category Antineoplastic Agent, Aromatase Inhibitor
Use Treatment of locally-advanced or metastatic breast cancer (hormone receptor-positive or unknown) in postmenopausal women; treatment of advanced breast cancer in postmenopausal women with disease progression following tamoxifen therapy; adjuvant treatment of early hormone receptor-positive breast cancer in postmenopausal women
Unlabeled/Investigational Use Treatment of recurrent or metastatic endometrial or uterine cancers, treatment of recurrent ovarian cancer
Pharmacodynamics/Kinetics
Onset of estradiol reduction: 70% reduction after 24 hours; 80% after 2 weeks therapy
Duration of estradiol reduction: 6 days
Absorption: Well absorbed; extent of absorption not affected by food
Protein binding, plasma: 40%
Metabolism: Extensively hepatic (~85%) via N-dealkylation, hydroxylation, and glucuronidation; primary metabolite (triazole) inactive
Half-life elimination: ~40-50 hours
Time to peak, plasma: ~2 hours without food; 5 hours with food
Excretion: Feces; urine (urinary excretion accounts for ~11% of total elimination, mostly as metabolites)
Dosage Oral: Adults: Breast cancer: 1 mg once daily
Dosage adjustment in renal impairment: Dosage adjustment not necessary
Dosage adjustment in hepatic impairment:
Mild-to-moderate impairment or stable hepatic cirrhosis: Dosage adjustment is not required
Severe hepatic impairment: Has not been studied in this population
Additional Information Complete prescribing information for this medication should be consulted for additional detail.
Dosage Forms Excipient information presented when available (limited, particularly for generics); consult specific product labeling.
Tablet:
Arimidex®: 1 mg
References
Boeddinghaus IM and Dowsett M, "Comparative Clinical Pharmacology and Pharmacokinetic Interactions of Aromatase Inhibitors," *J Steroid Biochem Mol Biol*, 2001, 79(1-5):85-91.
Buzdar AU, Robertson JF, Eiermann W, et al, "An Overview of the Pharmacology and Pharmacokinetics of the Newer Generation Aromatase Inhibitors Anastrozole, Letrozole, and Exemestane," *Cancer*, 2002, 95(9):2006-16.
Higa GM and AlKhouri N, "Anastrozole: A Selective Aromatase Inhibitor for the Treatment of Breast Cancer," *Am J Health Syst Pharm*, 1998, 55(5):445-52.
Kendall A, Dowsett M, Folkerd E, et al, "Caution: Vaginal Estradiol Appears to be Contraindicated in Postmenopausal Women on Adjuvant Aromatase Inhibitors," *Ann Oncol*, 2006, 17(4):584-7.
Koberle D and Thurlimann B, "Anastrozole: Pharmacological and Clinical Profile in Postmenopausal Women With Breast Cancer," *Expert Rev Anticancer Ther*, 2001, 1(2):169-76.

Lonning PE, Geisler J, and Dowsett M, "Pharmacological and Clinical Profile of Anastrozole," *Breast Cancer Res Treat*, 1998, 49(Suppl 1):53-7.

Njar VC and Brodie AM, "Comprehensive Pharmacology and Clinical Efficacy of Aromatase Inhibitors," *Drugs*, 1999, 58(2):233-55.

◆ **Ancef** *see* CeFAZolin *on page 249*

◆ **Andriol® (Can)** *see* Testosterone *on page 1362*

◆ **Androderm®** *see* Testosterone *on page 1362*

◆ **AndroGel®** *see* Testosterone *on page 1362*

◆ **Andropository (Can)** *see* Testosterone *on page 1362*

◆ **Anectine®** *see* Succinylcholine *on page 1326*

◆ **Anestacon®** *see* Lidocaine *on page 836*

◆ **Anestafoam™ [OTC]** *see* Lidocaine *on page 836*

◆ **Anexate® (Can)** *see* Flumazenil *on page 613*

◆ **Angiomax®** *see* Bivalirudin *on page 193*

◆ **Anhydrous Glucose** *see* Dextrose *on page 406*

Anidulafungin (ay nid yoo la FUN jin)

Related Information
   Antifungal Agents *on page 1664*
U.S. Brand Names Eraxis™
Canadian Brand Names Eraxis™
Index Terms LY303366
Pharmacologic Category Antifungal Agent, Parenteral; Echinocandin
Generic Available No
Use Treatment of candidemia and other forms of *Candida* infections (including those of intra-abdominal, peritoneal, and esophageal locus)
Unlabeled/Investigational Use Treatment of infections due to *Aspergillus* spp.
Mechanism of Action Noncompetitive inhibitor of 1,3-beta-D-glucan synthase resulting in reduced formation of 1,3-beta-D-glucan, an essential polysaccharide comprising 30% to 60% of *Candida* cell walls (absent in mammalian cells); decreased glucan content leads to osmotic instability and cellular lysis
Pharmacodynamics/Kinetics
   Distribution: 30-50 L
   Protein binding: 84%
   Metabolism: No hepatic metabolism observed; undergoes slow chemical hydrolysis to open-ring peptide-lacking antifungal activity
   Half-life elimination: 27 hours
   Excretion: Feces (30%, 10% as unchanged drug); urine (<1%)
Dosage I.V.: Adults:
   Candidemia, intra-abdominal or peritoneal candidiasis: 200 mg loading dose on day 1, followed by 100 mg daily for at least 14 days after last positive culture
   Esophageal candidiasis: 100 mg loading dose on day 1, followed by 50 mg daily for at least 14 days and for at least 7 days after symptom resolution

Dosage adjustment in renal impairment: No adjustment necessary, including dialysis patients
Dosage adjustment in hepatic impairment: No adjustment necessary
Stability Store between 15°C to 30°C (59°F to 86°F). Aseptically add 15 mL (50 mg vial) or 30 mL (100 mg vial) of companion diluent (20% w/w dehydrated alcohol in water for injection) to each vial. Swirl to dissolve; do not shake. Further dilute 50 mg, 100 mg, or 200 mg in 100 mL, 250 mL, or 500 mL, respectively, of D₅W or NS. Reconstituted and diluted solutions are stable for 24 hours at room temperature. Do not refrigerate or freeze.
Administration For intravenous use only; infusion rate should not exceed 1.1 mg/minute
Monitoring Parameters Liver function tests
Pregnancy Risk Factor C
Contraindications Hypersensitivity to anidulafungin, other echinocandins, or any component of the formulation

Warnings/Precautions Histamine-mediated reactions (eg, urticaria, flushing, hypotension) have been observed; these may be related to infusion rate. Elevated liver function tests, hepatitis, and worsening hepatic failure have been reported. Monitor for progressive hepatic impairment if increased transaminase enzymes noted. Safety and efficacy in pediatric patients, neutropenic patients, or other *Candida* infections (eg, endocarditis, osteomyelitis, meningitis) have not been established.

Adverse Reactions

2% to 10%:
Endocrine & metabolic: Hypokalemia (3%)
Gastrointestinal: Diarrhea (3%)
Hepatic: Transaminase increased (<1% to 2%)
<2% (Limited to important or life-threatening): Abdominal pain, alkaline phosphatase increased, amylase increased, angioneurotic edema, atrial fibrillation, back pain, bilirubin increased, bundle branch block (right), candidiasis, cholestasis, clostridial infection, coagulopathy, constipation, cough, CPK increased, creatinine increased, diaphoresis, diarrhea, dizziness, DVT, dyspepsia, ECG abnormality (including QT prolongation), erythema, eye pain, fecal incontinence, flushing, fungemia, GGT increased, headache, hepatic necrosis, hepatitis, hepatic dysfunction, hot flushes, hypercalcemia, hyperglycemia, hyperkalemia, hypernatremia, hyper-/hypotension, hypomagnesemia, infusion-related reaction, leukopenia (0.7%), lipase increased, nausea, neutropenia (1%), peripheral edema, phlebitis, platelet count increased, prothrombin time prolonged, pruritus, pyrexia, rash, rigors, seizure, sinus arrhythmia, thrombocytopenia, thrombophlebitis, urea increased, urticaria, ventricular extrasystoles, vision blurred, visual disturbance, vomiting

Drug Interactions

Avoid Concomitant Use There are no known interactions where it is recommended to avoid concomitant use.

Increased Effect/Toxicity There are no known significant interactions involving an increase in effect.

Decreased Effect
Anidulafungin may decrease the levels/effects of: Saccharomyces boulardii

Dosage Forms Excipient information presented when available (limited, particularly for generics); consult specific product labeling.
Injection, powder for reconstitution:
Eraxis™: 50 mg [contains polysorbate 80; packaged with dehydrated alcohol as diluent]; 100 mg [contains polysorbate 80; packaged with dehydrated alcohol as diluent]

References

Trissel LA and Ogundele AB, "Compatibility of Anidulafungin With Other Drugs During Simulated Y-Site Administration," *Am J Health-Sys Pharm*, 2005, 62:834-7.
Vazquez JA, "Anidulafungin: A New Echinocandin With a Novel Profile," *Clin Ther*, 2005, 27 (6):657-73.
Walsh TJ, Anaissie EJ, Denning DW, et al, "Treatment of Aspergillosis: Clinical Practice Guidelines of the Infectious Diseases Society of America," *Clin Infect Dis*, 2008, 46(3):327-60.

◆ **Ansaid® (Can)** *see* Flurbiprofen *on page 619*

◆ **Antara®** *see* Fenofibrate *on page 582*

◆ **Anti-4 Alpha Integrin** *see* Natalizumab *on page 989*

◆ **Antidigoxin Fab Fragments, Ovine** *see* Digoxin Immune Fab *on page 422*

◆ **Antidiuretic Hormone** *see* Vasopressin *on page 1458*

Antihemophilic Factor (Recombinant)
(an tee hee moe FIL ik FAK tor ree KOM be nant)

Medication Safety Issues Confusion may occur due to the omitting of "Factor VIII" from some product labeling. Review product contents carefully prior to dispensing any antihemophilic factor.

U.S. Brand Names Advate; Helixate® FS; Kogenate® FS; Recombinate; ReFacto® [DSC]; Xyntha™

Canadian Brand Names Helixate® FS; Kogenate®; Kogenate® FS; Recombinate; ReFacto®

Index Terms AHF (Recombinant); Factor VIII (Recombinant); rAHF

Pharmacologic Category Antihemophilic Agent

Generic Available No

Use Prevention and treatment of hemorrhagic episodes in patients with hemophilia A (classic hemophilia or congenital factor VIII deficiency); perioperative management of hemophilia A; prophylaxis of joint bleeding and to reduce risk of joint damage in children with hemophilia A with no preexisting joint damage; can be of significant therapeutic value in patients with acquired factor VIII inhibitors ≤10 Bethesda units/mL

Mechanism of Action Factor VIII replacement, necessary for clot formation and maintenance of hemostasis. It activates factor X in conjunction with activated factor IX; activated factor X converts prothrombin to thrombin, which converts fibrinogen to fibrin, and with factor XIII forms a stable clot.

Pharmacodynamics/Kinetics

Distribution: V_{ss}: 0.36-0.57 dL/kg

Half-life elimination: Mean: 8-19 hours

Dosage I.V.:

Hemophilia: Children and Adults: Individualize dosage based on coagulation studies performed prior to treatment and at regular intervals during treatment. In general, administration of factor VIII 1 int. unit/kg will increase circulating factor VIII levels by ~2 int. units/dL. (General guidelines presented; consult individual product labeling for specific dosing recommendations.)

Joint bleeding prophylaxis (Helixate® FS, Kogenate® FS): Children: 25 int. units/kg every other day

Dosage based on desired factor VIII increase (%):

To calculate dosage needed based on desired factor VIII increase (%):

[Body weight (kg) x desired factor VIII increase (%)] divided by 2%/int. units/kg ≜ int. units factor VIII required

For example:

50 kg x 30 (% increase) divided by 2%/int. units/kg = 750 int. units factor VIII

Dosage based on expected factor VIII increase (%):

It is also possible to calculate the **expected** % factor VIII increase:

(# int. units administered x 2%/int. units/kg) divided by body weight (kg) = expected % factor VIII increase

For example:

(1400 int. units x 2%/int. units/kg) divided by 70 kg = 40%

General guidelines:

Minor hemorrhage: 10-20 int. units/kg as a single dose to achieve FVIII plasma level ~20% to 40% of normal. Mild superficial or early hemorrhages may respond to a single dose; may repeat dose every 12-24 hours for 1-3 days until bleeding is resolved or healing achieved.

Moderate hemorrhage/minor surgery: 15-30 int. units/kg to achieve FVIII plasma level 30% to 60% of normal. May repeat 1 dose at 12-24 hours if needed. Some products suggest continuing for ≥3 days until pain and disability are resolved.

Major to life-threatening hemorrhage: Initial dose 40-50 int. units/kg followed by a maintenance dose of 20-25 int. units/kg every 8-24 hours until threat is resolved, to achieve FVIII plasma level 60% to 100% of normal.

Major surgery: 50 int. units/kg given preoperatively to raise factor VIII level to 100% before surgery begins. May repeat as necessary after 6-12 hours initially and for a total of 10-14 days until healing is complete. Intensity of therapy may depend on type of surgery and postoperative regimen.

Bleeding prophylaxis: May be administered on a regular basis for bleeding prophylaxis. Doses of 24-40 int. units/kg 3 times/week have been reported in patients with severe hemophilia to prevent joint bleeding.

If bleeding is not controlled with adequate dose, test for presence of inhibitor. It may not be possible or practical to control bleeding if inhibitor titers >10 Bethesda units/mL.

Elderly: Response in the elderly is not expected to differ from that of younger patients; dosage should be individualized

Stability Store under refrigeration, 2°C to 8°C (36°F to 46°F); avoid freezing. Use within 3 hours of reconstitution. Gently agitate or rotate vial after adding diluent, do not shake vigorously. Do not refrigerate after reconstitution, a precipitation may occur.

Advate: May also be stored at room temperature for up to 6 months.

Helixate® FS, Kogenate® FS, ReFacto®, Xyntha™: May also be stored at room temperature (not to exceed 25°C [36°F]) up to 3 months. Avoid prolonged exposure to light during storage.

Recombinate: May also be stored at room temperature, not to exceed 30°C (86°F).

If refrigerated, the dried concentrate and diluent should be warmed to room temperature before reconstitution.

Administration I.V. infusion over 5-10 minutes (maximum: 10 mL/minute).

Advate: Infuse over ≤5 minutes (maximum: 10 mL/minute)

Helixate® FS, Kogenate® FS: Infuse over 1-15 minutes; based on patient tolerability

Xyntha™: Infuse over several minutes; adjust based on patient comfort. Do not admix or administer in same tubing as other medications.

Monitoring Parameters Heart rate and blood pressure (before and during I.V. administration); plasma factor VIII activity prior to and during treatment; development of factor VIII inhibitors; signs of bleeding

Reference Range Classification of hemophilia; normal is defined as 1 int. unit/mL of factor VIII

Severe: Factor level <1% of normal

Moderate: Factor level 1% to 5% of normal

Mild: Factor level >5% to <40% of normal

Pregnancy Risk Factor C

Contraindications Hypersensitivity to any component of the formulation

Warnings/Precautions Monitor for signs of formation of antibodies to factor VIII; may occur at anytime but more common in young children with severe hemophilia. The dosage requirement will vary in patients with factor VIII inhibitors; optimal treatment should be determined by clinical response. Allergic hypersensitivity reactions (including anaphylaxis) may occur; monitor. Products vary by preparation method. Recombinate is stabilized with human albumin. Helixate® FS and Kogenate® FS are stabilized with sucrose. Advate, Helixate® FS, Kogenate® FS, ReFacto®, and Xyntha™ may contain trace amounts of mouse or hamster protein. Recombinate may contain mouse, hamster or bovine protein. Products may contain von Willebrand factor for stabilization; however, efficacy has not been established for the treatment of von Willebrand's disease.

Adverse Reactions Actual frequency may vary by product.

>1%:

Central nervous system: Chills, dizziness, fever, headache, pain

Dermatologic: Pruritus, rash, urticaria

Gastrointestinal: Diarrhea, nausea, taste perversion, vomiting

Hematologic: Hemorrhage

Local: Injection site pain, injection site inflammation, infusion site reaction

Neuromuscular & skeletal: Arthralgia, weakness

Respiratory: Cough, dyspnea, nasopharyngitis, pharyngolaryngeal pain

Miscellaneous: Catheter thrombosis, factor VIII inhibitor formation

≤1% (Limited to important or life-threatening): Abdominal pain, adenopathy, allergic reactions, anaphylaxis, anemia, anorexia, arthralgia, AST increased, blood pressure decreased, chest discomfort, chest pain, constipation, depersonalization, diaphoresis, edema, epistaxis, facial edema, facial flushing, factor VIII decreased, fatigue, fever, GI hemorrhage, hives, hot flashes, hypersensitivity reaction, hyper-/hypotension (slight), infection, joint swelling, lethargy, otitis media, pallor, paresthesia, restlessness, rhinitis, rigors, somnolence, tachycardia, urinary tract infection, vasodilation, venous catheter access complications

Drug Interactions

Avoid Concomitant Use There are no known interactions where it is recommended to avoid concomitant use.

Increased Effect/Toxicity There are no known significant interactions involving an increase in effect.

Decreased Effect There are no known significant interactions involving a decrease in effect.

Dietary Considerations Some products may contain sodium and/or sucrose.

Product Availability Xyntha™: FDA approved February 2008; availability anticipated in September 2008

Wyeth is replacing ReFacto® with Xyntha™.

Dosage Forms Excipient information presented when available (limited, particularly for generics); consult specific product labeling. [DSC] = Discontinued product

Injection, powder for reconstitution, recombinant [preservative free]:

Advate: 250 int. units, 500 int. units, 1000 int. units, 1500 int. units, 2000 int. units, 3000 int. units [plasma/albumin free; contains polysorbate 80, sodium 108 mEq/L, mannitol; derived from hamster or mouse proteins]

Helixate® FS: 250 int. units, 500 int. units, 1000 int. units, 2000 int. unit, 3000 int. units [contains sucrose 28-52 mg/vial, sodium 26-36 mEq/L, polysorbate 80; derived from hamster or mouse protein]

Kogenate® FS: 250 int. units, 500 int. units, 1000 int. units, 2000 int. units, 3000 int. units [contains sucrose 28-56 mg/vial, sodium 27-36 mEq/L, polysorbate 80; derived from hamster or mouse protein]

Recombinate: 250 int. units, 500 int. units, 1000 int. units [contains human albumin, sodium 180 mEq/L, polysorbate 80; derived from bovine, hamster or mouse proteins; packaging contains natural rubber latex]

ReFacto®: 250 int. units, 500 int. units, 1000 int. units, 2000 int. units [contains polysorbate 80, sucrose; derived from hamster or mouse proteins] [DSC]

Xyntha™: 250 int. units, 500 int. units, 1000 int. units, 2000 int. units [albumin free; contains sucrose, polysorbate 80; derived from hamster proteins]

◆ **Anti-Hist [OTC]** *see* DiphenhydrAMINE *on page 430*

◆ **Antithrombin III** *see* Antithrombin III *on page 127*

Antithrombin III (an tee THROM bin)

Related Information

Anesthesia for Obstetric Patients in Nonobstetric Surgery *on page 1532*

Perioperative / Periprocedural Management of Anticoagulant and Antiplatelet Therapy *on page 1607*

U.S. Brand Names ATryn®; Thrombate III®

Canadian Brand Names Thrombate III®

Index Terms Antithrombin III; AT; AT-III; Heparin Cofactor I

Pharmacologic Category Anticoagulant; Blood Product Derivative

Use Treatment of hereditary antithrombin (AT or AT-III) deficiency in connection with surgical procedures, obstetrical procedures, or thromboembolism

Pharmacodynamics/Kinetics Half-life elimination: Biologic: 2.5 days (immunologic assay); 3.8 days (functional AT assay). Half-life may be decreased following surgery, with hemorrhage, acute thrombosis, and/or during heparin administration.

Dosage I.V.: Adults:

Initial loading dose: Dosing is individualized based on pretherapy antithrombin (AT) levels. The initial dose should raise AT levels to 120% and may be calculated based on the following formula:

[(desired AT level % - baseline AT level %) x body weight (kg)] **divided** by 1.4 = int. units of antithrombin required

For example, if a 70 kg adult patient had a baseline AT level of 57%, the initial dose would be

[(120% - 57%) x 70] divided by 1.4 = 3150 int. units

Maintenance dose: In general, subsequent dosing should be targeted to keep levels between 80% to 120% which may be achieved by administering 60% of the initial loading dose every 24 hours. Adjustments may be made by adjusting dose or interval. Maintain level within normal range for 2-8 days depending on type of procedure.

Additional Information Complete prescribing information for this medication should be consulted for additional detail.

◀ **Product Availability**
ATryn®: FDA approved February 2009; anticipated availability is currently undetermined

ATryn® is the first recombinant antithrombin product approved in the U.S.

Dosage Forms Excipient information presented when available (limited, particularly for generics); consult specific product labeling.

Injection, powder for reconstitution [preservative free]:

ATryn®: ~1750 int. units [exact potency labeled on each vial]

Thrombate III®: 500 int. units, 1000 int. units [contains heparin, sodium chloride 110-210 mEq/L; packaged with diluent]

♦ **Antizol®** see Fomepizole on page 625
♦ **Anucort-HC®** see Hydrocortisone on page 699
♦ **Anu-Med [OTC]** see Phenylephrine on page 1114
♦ **Anusol-HC®** see Hydrocortisone on page 699
♦ **Anusol® HC-1 [OTC]** see Hydrocortisone on page 699
♦ **Anzemet®** see Dolasetron on page 444
♦ **APAP** see Acetaminophen on page 25
♦ **APAP 500 [OTC]** see Acetaminophen on page 25
♦ **Apidra®** see Insulin Glulisine on page 745
♦ **Aplenzin™** see BuPROPion on page 217
♦ **Apo-Acebutolol® (Can)** see Acebutolol on page 24
♦ **Apo-Acetaminophen® (Can)** see Acetaminophen on page 25
♦ **Apo-Acetazolamide® (Can)** see AcetaZOLAMIDE on page 31
♦ **Apo-Acyclovir® (Can)** see Acyclovir on page 40
♦ **Apo-Alendronate® (Can)** see Alendronate on page 57
♦ **Apo-Allopurinol® (Can)** see Allopurinol on page 62
♦ **Apo-Alpraz® (Can)** see ALPRAZolam on page 64
♦ **Apo-Alpraz® TS (Can)** see ALPRAZolam on page 64
♦ **Apo-Amiodarone® (Can)** see Amiodarone on page 86
♦ **Apo-Amitriptyline® (Can)** see Amitriptyline on page 89
♦ **Apo-Amlodipine® (Can)** see AmLODIPine on page 93
♦ **Apo-Amoxi® (Can)** see Amoxicillin on page 95
♦ **Apo-Amoxi-Clav® (Can)** see Amoxicillin and Clavulanate Potassium on page 98
♦ **Apo-Ampi® (Can)** see Ampicillin on page 115
♦ **Apo-Atenol® (Can)** see Atenolol on page 155
♦ **Apo-Azathioprine® (Can)** see AzaTHIOprine on page 167
♦ **Apo-Azithromycin® (Can)** see Azithromycin on page 169
♦ **Apo-Baclofen® (Can)** see Baclofen on page 178
♦ **Apo-Benazepril® (Can)** see Benazepril on page 182
♦ **Apo-Benztropine® (Can)** see Benztropine on page 183
♦ **Apo-Benzydamine® (Can)** see Benzydamine on page 184
♦ **Apo-Bisoprolol® (Can)** see Bisoprolol on page 192
♦ **Apo-Bromocriptine® (Can)** see Bromocriptine on page 203
♦ **Apo-Buspirone® (Can)** see BusPIRone on page 219
♦ **Apo-Butorphanol® (Can)** see Butorphanol on page 220
♦ **Apo-Calcitonin® (Can)** see Calcitonin on page 226
♦ **Apo-Capto® (Can)** see Captopril on page 239
♦ **Apo-Carbamazepine® (Can)** see CarBAMazepine on page 241
♦ **Apo-Carvedilol® (Can)** see Carvedilol on page 244
♦ **Apo-Cefoxitin® (Can)** see Cefoxitin on page 261
♦ **Apo-Cefuroxime® (Can)** see Cefuroxime on page 272
♦ **Apo-Cetirizine® (Can)** see Cetirizine on page 282

- **Apo-Granisetron (Can)** *see* Granisetron *on page 669*
- **Apo-Haloperidol® (Can)** *see* Haloperidol *on page 672*
- **Apo-Haloperidol LA® (Can)** *see* Haloperidol *on page 672*
- **Apo-Hydralazine® (Can)** *see* HydrALAZINE *on page 694*
- **Apo-Hydro® (Can)** *see* Hydrochlorothiazide *on page 696*
- **Apo-Hydroxyurea® (Can)** *see* Hydroxyurea *on page 712*
- **Apo-Ibuprofen® (Can)** *see* Ibuprofen *on page 717*
- **Apo-Imipramine® (Can)** *see* Imipramine *on page 731*
- **Apo-Indomethacin® (Can)** *see* Indomethacin *on page 738*
- **Apo-Ipravent® (Can)** *see* Ipratropium *on page 760*
- **Apo-ISDN® (Can)** *see* Isosorbide Dinitrate *on page 772*
- **Apo-ISMN® (Can)** *see* Isosorbide Mononitrate *on page 774*
- **Apo-K® (Can)** *see* Potassium Chloride *on page 1151*
- **Apo-Keto® (Can)** *see* Ketoprofen *on page 783*
- **Apo-Ketoconazole® (Can)** *see* Ketoconazole *on page 780*
- **Apo-Keto-E® (Can)** *see* Ketoprofen *on page 783*
- **Apo-Ketorolac® (Can)** *see* Ketorolac *on page 784*
- **Apo-Ketorolac Injectable® (Can)** *see* Ketorolac *on page 784*
- **Apo-Keto SR® (Can)** *see* Ketoprofen *on page 783*
- **Apo-Labetalol® (Can)** *see* Labetalol *on page 791*
- **Apo-Lactulose® (Can)** *see* Lactulose *on page 796*
- **Apo-Lamotrigine® (Can)** *see* LamoTRIgine *on page 800*
- **Apo-Lansoprazole® (Can)** *see* Lansoprazole *on page 805*
- **Apo-Levetiracetam (Can)** *see* Levetiracetam *on page 816*
- **Apo-Levocarb® (Can)** *see* Levodopa and Carbidopa *on page 822*
- **Apo-Levocarb® CR (Can)** *see* Levodopa and Carbidopa *on page 822*
- **Apo-Levofloxacin® (Can)** *see* Levofloxacin *on page 823*
- **Apo-Lisinopril® (Can)** *see* Lisinopril *on page 849*
- **Apo-Lithium® Carbonate (Can)** *see* Lithium *on page 851*
- **Apo-Lithium® Carbonate SR (Can)** *see* Lithium *on page 851*
- **Apo-Lorazepam® (Can)** *see* LORazepam *on page 852*
- **Apo-Lovastatin® (Can)** *see* Lovastatin *on page 859*
- **Apo-Mefenamic® (Can)** *see* Mefenamic Acid *on page 870*
- **Apo-Meloxicam® (Can)** *see* Meloxicam *on page 870*
- **Apo-Metformin® (Can)** *see* MetFORMIN *on page 886*
- **Apo-Methotrexate® (Can)** *see* Methotrexate *on page 898*
- **Apo-Methyldopa® (Can)** *see* Methyldopa *on page 901*
- **Apo-Methylphenidate® (Can)** *see* Methylphenidate *on page 908*
- **Apo-Methylphenidate® SR (Can)** *see* Methylphenidate *on page 908*
- **Apo-Metoclop® (Can)** *see* Metoclopramide *on page 917*
- **Apo-Metoprolol® (Can)** *see* Metoprolol *on page 922*
- **Apo-Metronidazole® (Can)** *see* MetroNIDAZOLE *on page 928*
- **Apo-Midazolam® (Can)** *see* Midazolam *on page 935*
- **Apo-Midodrine® (Can)** *see* Midodrine *on page 939*
- **Apo-Misoprostol® (Can)** *see* Misoprostol *on page 945*
- **APO-Modafinil (Can)** *see* Modafinil *on page 947*
- **Apo-Nabumetone® (Can)** *see* Nabumetone *on page 973*
- **Apo-Nadol® (Can)** *see* Nadolol *on page 974*
- **Apo-Napro-Na® (Can)** *see* Naproxen *on page 987*
- **Apo-Napro-Na DS® (Can)** *see* Naproxen *on page 987*

- **Apo-Naproxen® (Can)** *see* Naproxen *on page 987*
- **Apo-Naproxen EC® (Can)** *see* Naproxen *on page 987*
- **Apo-Naproxen SR® (Can)** *see* Naproxen *on page 987*
- **Apo-Nifed® (Can)** *see* NIFEdipine *on page 1006*
- **Apo-Nifed PA® (Can)** *see* NIFEdipine *on page 1006*
- **Apo-Nizatidine® (Can)** *see* Nizatidine *on page 1022*
- **Apo-Nortriptyline® (Can)** *see* Nortriptyline *on page 1026*
- **Apo-Oflox® (Can)** *see* Ofloxacin *on page 1038*
- **Apo-Ofloxacin® (Can)** *see* Ofloxacin *on page 1038*
- **Apo-Omeprazole® (Can)** *see* Omeprazole *on page 1048*
- **Apo-Ondansetron® (Can)** *see* Ondansetron *on page 1057*
- **Apo-Orciprenaline® (Can)** *see* Metaproterenol *on page 885*
- **Apo-Oxaprozin® (Can)** *see* Oxaprozin *on page 1065*
- **Apo-Oxybutynin® (Can)** *see* Oxybutynin *on page 1068*
- **Apo-Pantoprazole® (Can)** *see* Pantoprazole *on page 1084*
- **Apo-Paroxetine® (Can)** *see* PARoxetine *on page 1089*
- **Apo-Perindopril® (Can)** *see* Perindopril Erbumine *on page 1107*
- **Apo-Pindol® (Can)** *see* Pindolol *on page 1130*
- **Apo-Pioglitazone (Can)** *see* Pioglitazone *on page 1132*
- **Apo-Piroxicam® (Can)** *see* Piroxicam *on page 1139*
- **Apo-Pramipexole (Can)** *see* Pramipexole *on page 1159*
- **Apo-Pravastatin® (Can)** *see* Pravastatin *on page 1162*
- **Apo-Prednisone® (Can)** *see* PredniSONE *on page 1166*
- **Apo-Procainamide® (Can)** *see* Procainamide *on page 1176*
- **Apo-Prochlorperazine® (Can)** *see* Prochlorperazine *on page 1180*
- **Apo-Propafenone® (Can)** *see* Propafenone *on page 1189*
- **Apo-Propranolol® (Can)** *see* Propranolol *on page 1198*
- **Apo-Quetiapine® (Can)** *see* QUEtiapine *on page 1212*
- **Apo-Quinidine® (Can)** *see* QuiNIDine *on page 1216*
- **Apo-Raloxifene (Can)** *see* Raloxifene *on page 1228*
- **Apo-Ramipril® (Can)** *see* Ramipril *on page 1229*
- **Apo-Ranitidine® (Can)** *see* Ranitidine *on page 1231*
- **Apo-Salvent® (Can)** *see* Albuterol *on page 49*
- **Apo-Salvent® CFC Free (Can)** *see* Albuterol *on page 49*
- **Apo-Salvent® Respirator Solution (Can)** *see* Albuterol *on page 49*
- **Apo-Salvent® Sterules (Can)** *see* Albuterol *on page 49*
- **Apo-Selegiline® (Can)** *see* Selegiline *on page 1282*
- **Apo-Simvastatin® (Can)** *see* Simvastatin *on page 1293*
- **Apo-Sotalol® (Can)** *see* Sotalol *on page 1321*
- **Apo-Sulfatrim® (Can)** *see* Sulfamethoxazole and Trimethoprim *on page 1333*
- **Apo-Sulfatrim® DS (Can)** *see* Sulfamethoxazole and Trimethoprim *on page 1333*
- **Apo-Sulfatrim® Pediatric (Can)** *see* Sulfamethoxazole and Trimethoprim *on page 1333*
- **Apo-Sulin® (Can)** *see* Sulindac *on page 1335*
- **Apo-Sumatriptan® (Can)** *see* SUMAtriptan *on page 1336*
- **Apo-Temazepam® (Can)** *see* Temazepam *on page 1357*
- **Apo-Theo LA® (Can)** *see* Theophylline *on page 1373*
- **Apo-Ticlopidine® (Can)** *see* Ticlopidine *on page 1385*
- **Apo-Timol® (Can)** *see* Timolol *on page 1390*
- **Apo-Timop® (Can)** *see* Timolol *on page 1390*
- **Apo-Topiramate® (Can)** *see* Topiramate *on page 1408*

◆ **Apo-Trazodone® (Can)** see TraZODone on page 1423

◆ **Apo-Trazodone D® (Can)** see TraZODone on page 1423

◆ **Apo-Triazo® (Can)** see Triazolam on page 1434

◆ **Apo-Valacyclovir® (Can)** see Valacyclovir on page 1441

◆ **Apo-Valproic® (Can)** see Valproic Acid and Derivatives on page 1445

◆ **Apo-Verap® (Can)** see Verapamil on page 1468

◆ **Apo-Verap® SR (Can)** see Verapamil on page 1468

◆ **Apo-Warfarin® (Can)** see Warfarin on page 1479

◆ **Apra [OTC] [DSC]** see Acetaminophen on page 25

Aprepitant (ap RE pi tant)

Medication Safety Issues
Sound-alike/look-alike issues:
Aprepitant may be confused with fosaprepitant
Emend® (aprepitant) oral capsule formulation may be confused with Emend® for injection (fosaprepitant).

Related Information
Postoperative Nausea and Vomiting on page 1593

U.S. Brand Names Emend®

Canadian Brand Names Emend®

Index Terms L 754030; MK 869

Pharmacologic Category Antiemetic; Substance P/Neurokinin 1 Receptor Antagonist

Generic Available No

Use Prevention of acute and delayed nausea and vomiting associated with moderately- and highly-emetogenic chemotherapy (in combination with other antiemetics); prevention of postoperative nausea and vomiting (PONV)

Mechanism of Action Prevents acute and delayed vomiting by inhibiting the substance P/neurokinin 1 (NK_1) receptor; augments the antiemetic activity of 5-HT_3 receptor antagonists and corticosteroids to inhibit acute and delayed phases of chemotherapy-induced emesis.

Pharmacodynamics/Kinetics
Distribution: V_d: ~70 L; crosses the blood brain barrier
Protein binding: >95%
Metabolism: Extensively hepatic via CYP3A4 (major); CYP1A2 and CYP2C19 (minor); forms 7 metabolites (weakly active)
Bioavailability: ~60% to 65%
Half-life elimination: Terminal: ~9-13 hours
Time to peak, plasma: ~3-4 hours

Dosage Oral: Adults:
Prevention of chemotherapy-induced nausea/vomiting: 125 mg 1 hour prior to chemotherapy on day 1, followed by 80 mg once daily on days 2 and 3 (in combination with a corticosteroid and 5-HT_3 antagonist antiemetic); **Note:** Fosaprepitant 115 mg 30 minutes prior to chemotherapy may be substituted for aprepitant 125 mg on day 1
Prevention of PONV: 40 mg within 3 hours prior to induction
Dosage adjustment in renal impairment: No dose adjustment necessary in patients with renal disease or end-stage renal disease maintained on hemodialysis.
Dosage adjustment in hepatic impairment:
Mild-to-moderate impairment (Child-Pugh classes A and B): No adjustment necessary
Severe impairment (Child-Pugh class C): Use caution; no data available

Stability Store at room temperature of 20°C to 25°C (68°F to 77°F).

Administration
Chemotherapy induced nausea/vomiting: Administer with or without food. First dose should be given 1 hour prior to antineoplastic therapy; subsequent doses should be given in the morning.
PONV: Administer within 3 hours prior to induction; follow healthcare providers instructions about food/drink restrictions prior to surgery.

Pregnancy Risk Factor B

Contraindications Hypersensitivity to aprepitant or any component of the formulation; concurrent use with cisapride or pimozide

Warnings/Precautions Use caution with agents primarily metabolized via CYP3A4; aprepitant is a 3A4 inhibitor. Effect on orally administered 3A4 substrates is greater than those administered intravenously. Chronic continuous use is not recommended; however, a single 40 mg aprepitant oral dose is not likely to alter plasma concentrations of CYP3A4 substrates. Use caution with severe hepatic impairment; has not been studied in patients with severe hepatic impairment (Child-Pugh class C). Not intended for treatment of existing nausea and vomiting or for chronic continuous therapy.

Adverse Reactions Note: Adverse reactions reported as part of a combination chemotherapy regimen or with general anesthesia.

>10%:
  Central nervous system: Fatigue (18% to 22%)
  Gastrointestinal: Nausea (7% to 13%), constipation (9% to 12%)
  Neuromuscular & skeletal: Weakness (3% to 18%)
  Miscellaneous: Hiccups (≤11%)

1% to 10%:
  Cardiovascular: Hypotension (≤6%), bradycardia (≤4%), flushing (≤3%)
  Central nervous system: Dizziness (≤7%)
  Endocrine & metabolic: Dehydration (≤6%)
  Gastrointestinal: Diarrhea (6% to 10%), dyspepsia (≤8%), abdominal pain (≤5%), stomatitis (≤5%), epigastric discomfort (≤4%), gastritis (≤4%), throat pain (≤3%)
  Hepatic: ALT increased (1% to 6%), AST increased (3%)
  Renal: Proteinuria (7%), BUN increased (5%)

>0.5% (Limited to important or life-threatening): Acid reflux, acne, albumin decreased, alkaline phosphatase increased, anaphylactic reaction, anemia, angioedema, anxiety, appetite decreased, arthralgia, back pain, bilirubin increased, candidiasis, confusion, conjunctivitis, cough, deglutition disorder, depression, diabetes mellitus, diaphoresis, disorientation, duodenal ulcer (perforating), DVT, dysarthria, dysphagia, dyspnea, dysuria, edema, enterocolitis, eructation, erythrocyturia, febrile neutropenia, flatulence, herpes simplex, hyperglycemia, hypersensitivity reaction, hypertension, hypoesthesia, hypokalemia, hyponatremia, hypothermia, hypovolemia, hypoxia, glucosuria, leukocytes increased, leukocyturia, malaise, MI, miosis, muscular weakness, musculoskeletal pain, myalgia, nasal secretion, neutropenic sepsis, obstipation, pain, palpitation, pelvic pain, peripheral neuropathy, pharyngitis, pneumonia, pneumonitis, pruritus, pulmonary embolism, rash, renal insufficiency, respiratory infection, respiratory insufficiency, rigors, salivation increased, sensory disturbance, sensory neuropathy, septic shock, Stevens-Johnson syndrome, syncope, tachycardia, taste disturbance, thrombocytopenia, tremor, urinary tract infection, urticaria, visual acuity decreased, vocal disturbance, weight loss, wheezing, xerostomia

Drug Interactions

Metabolism/Transport Effects Substrate of CYP1A2 (minor), 2C19 (minor), 3A4 (major); **Inhibits** CYP2C9 (weak), 2C19 (weak), 3A4 (moderate); **Induces** CYP2C9 (weak), 3A4 (weak)

Avoid Concomitant Use

Avoid concomitant use of Aprepitant with any of the following: Cisapride; Everolimus; Pimozide; Tolvaptan

Increased Effect/Toxicity

Aprepitant may increase the levels/effects of: Benzodiazepines (metabolized by oxidation); Cisapride; Colchicine; Corticosteroids (Systemic); CYP3A4 Substrates; Diltiazem; Eplerenone; Everolimus; FentaNYL; Halofantrine; Pimecrolimus; Pimozide; Ranolazine; Salmeterol; Saxagliptin; TOLBUTamide; Tolvaptan

The levels/effects of Aprepitant may be increased by: Antifungal Agents (Azole Derivatives, Systemic); CYP3A4 Inhibitors (Moderate); CYP3A4 Inhibitors (Strong); Dasatinib; Diltiazem

◄ **Decreased Effect**
Aprepitant may decrease the levels/effects of: Contraceptive (Progestins); CYP2C9 Substrates (High risk); Oral Contraceptive (Estrogens); Saxagliptin; Warfarin

The levels/effects of Aprepitant may be decreased by: CYP3A4 Inducers (Strong); Deferasirox; Herbs (CYP3A4 Inducers); Rifamycin Derivatives

Ethanol/Nutrition/Herb Interactions
Food: Aprepitant serum concentration may be increased when taken with grapefruit juice; avoid concurrent use.
Herb/Nutraceutical: Avoid St John's wort (may decrease aprepitant levels).

Dietary Considerations May be taken with or without food.

Dosage Forms Excipient information presented when available (limited, particularly for generics); consult specific product labeling.
Capsule:
Emend®: 40 mg, 80 mg, 125 mg
Combination package [each package contains]:
Emend®:
Capsule: 80 mg (2s)
Capsule: 125 mg (1s)

◆ **Apresoline [DSC]** *see* HydrALAZINE *on page 694*

◆ **Apresoline® (Can)** *see* HydrALAZINE *on page 694*

◆ **Apri®** *see* Ethinyl Estradiol and Desogestrel *on page 544*

◆ **Apriso™** *see* Mesalamine *on page 884*

Aprotinin (a proe TYE nin)

U.S. Brand Names Trasylol®
Canadian Brand Names Trasylol®
Pharmacologic Category Blood Product Derivative; Hemostatic Agent
Restrictions Available in U.S. under an investigational new drug (IND) process. The program will provide aprotinin for the treatment of adult patients undergoing coronary artery bypass graft (CABG) surgery requiring cardiopulmonary bypass (CPB) who are at increased risk of bleeding and transfusion during CABG surgery with no acceptable therapeutic alternative. Healthcare providers using aprotinin for this situation must also ensure that the benefits outweigh the risks for their patient. U.S. healthcare providers with patients who may qualify can access information and forms for enrollment at http://www.trasylol.com/main.htm or contact Bayer Medical Communications at (888) 842-2937.

Generic Available No

Use Prevention of perioperative blood loss in patients who are at increased risk for blood loss and blood transfusions in association with cardiopulmonary bypass in coronary artery bypass graft surgery

Mechanism of Action Bleeding from CABG surgery is thought to result from a systemic inflammatory response induced by the procedure. Contact of blood cells with the cardiopulmonary bypass (CPB) equipment leads to deregulated activation of the coagulation and fibrinolysis systems, with concurrent upregulation of proinflammatory cytokines. Aprotinin is a broad spectrum serine protease inhibitor that attenuates the coagulation, fibrinolytic and inflammatory pathways by interfering with the chemical mediators (thrombin, plasmin, kallikrein). Additionally, it protects platelet-expressed glycoproteins from mechanical shear forces. This preserves normal hemostatic activity through protease receptor-independent mechanisms (eg, via ADP, IIb/IIIa), while blocking CPB-induced thrombin-mediated aggregation.

Pharmacodynamics/Kinetics
Distribution: Extracellular space; renal phagolysosomes
Metabolism: Aprotinin is slowly degraded by lysosomal enzymes.
Half-life elimination: 2.5 hours (plasma); terminal: 10 hours
Excretion: Urine (25% to 40%; <10% as unchanged drug)

Dosage Adults: Test dose: **All** patients should receive a 1 mL (1.4 mg) I.V. test dose at least 10 minutes prior to the loading dose to assess the potential for allergic reactions.

Notes:
The loading dose should be given after induction of anesthesia but prior to sternotomy. In patients with previous exposure to aprotinin, administer loading dose just prior to cannulation. A constant infusion is continued until surgery is complete.

To avoid physical incompatibility with heparin when adding to pump-prime solution, each agent should be added during recirculation to assure adequate dilution.

Regimen A (standard dose):
2 million KIU (280 mg; 200 mL) loading dose I.V. over 20-30 minutes
2 million KIU (280 mg; 200 mL) into pump prime volume
500,000 KIU/hour (70 mg/hour; 50 mL/hour) I.V. during operation

Regimen B (low dose):
1 million KIU (140 mg; 100 mL) loading dose I.V. over 20-30 minutes
1 million KIU (140 mg; 100 mL) into pump prime volume
250,000 KIU/hour (35 mg/hour; 25 mL/hour) I.V. during operation

Dosage adjustment in renal impairment: No adjustment required, but increased risk of worsening renal dysfunction with use; monitor closely

Dosage adjustment in hepatic impairment: No information available

Stability Store at 2°C to 25°C (36°F to 77°F); protect from freezing.

Administration Administer through a central line. Infuse loading dose over 20-30 minutes, then continuous infusion at 50 mL/hour (regimen A) or 25 mL/hour (regimen B). Rapid infusion (<20 minutes) can cause transient blood pressure decrease; to avoid incompatibility with heparin, add while recirculating the prime fluid of the cardiac bypass circuit.

Monitoring Parameters Bleeding times, prothrombin time, activated clotting time, platelet count, red blood cell counts, hematocrit, hemoglobin and fibrinogen degradation products; for toxicity also include renal function tests and blood pressure

Because aPTT and ACT are difficult to interpret with aprotinin use, the manufacturer recommends two different ways to administer heparin:
1) Fixed heparin dosing where a standard loading dose of heparin plus the quantity of heparin added to the prime volume of the CPB circuit should total at least 350 units/kg. Additional heparin should be administered based on patient's weight and duration of CPB.
2) Heparin dosing based upon a protamine titration method. A heparin dose response, assessed by protamine titration, should be performed prior to administration of aprotinin to determine the heparin loading dose.

Reference Range Antiplasmin effects occur when plasma aprotinin concentrations are 125 KIU/mL and antikallikrein effects occur when plasma levels are 250-500 KIU/mL; it remains unknown if these plasma concentrations are required for clinical benefits to occur during cardiopulmonary bypass; **Note:** KIU = Kallikrein inhibitor unit

While institutional protocols may vary, a minimal celite ACT of 750 seconds or kaolin-ACT of 480 seconds is recommended in the presence of aprotinin. Consult the manufacturer's information on specific ACT test interpretation in the presence of aprotinin.

Anesthesia and Critical Care Concerns/Other Considerations In November, 2007, Bayer Pharmaceuticals Inc suspended the marketing of aprotinin (Trasylol) in the U.S. and Canada at the request of both the U.S. Food and Drug Administration (FDA) and Health Canada. Preliminary data from the now suspended *Blood Conservation Using Antifibrinolytics: A Randomized Trial in a Cardiac Surgery Population (BART)* study in Canada suggests an increased risk of death associated with aprotinin use when compared with other antifibrinolytic agents. In the study, hemorrhage-related deaths were observed more often in the aprotinin study population.

Aprotinin was also associated with an increased risk of long-term mortality (5 years of evaluation after CABG surgery) and serious end organ damage following use during surgery (Mangano, 2006).

Pregnancy Risk Factor B

Contraindications Hypersensitivity to aprotinin or any component of the formulation; known or suspected exposure (including through fibrin sealant products that contain aprotinin) within the past 12 months

◀ **Warnings/Precautions [U.S. Boxed Warning]: Anaphylactic reactions are possible.** Hypersensitivity reactions are more common with repeated use; the risk of fatal reactions appears to be greater upon re-exposure within 12 months of previous use. Patients with a history of allergic reactions may also be more likely to develop a reaction. All patients should receive a test dose at least 10 minutes before the loading dose, although the test dose does not fully predict a patient's risk. Fatal hypersensitivity reactions have occurred in patients who tolerated the test dose. Epinephrine, steroids, and facilities for cardiopulmonary resuscitation should be available in case such a reaction occurs. In order to administer in a more controlled setting, patients should be in the OR, intubated and ready for rapid cannulation and initiation of cardiopulmonary bypass before the test dose is administered. Delay adding aprotinin to the pump prime solution until after the loading dose has been safely administered. Hypotension is the most frequently reported sign of the hypersensitivity reaction.

Aprotinin has been linked to an increased risk of death, serious kidney damage, and heart failure in observational studies. Renal dysfunction (elevations of >0.5 mg/dL over baseline serum creatinine) may occur with use and may increase the need for dialysis in the perioperative period. Patients at greatest risk are those with pre-existing renal dysfunction (Cl_{cr} <60 mL/minute) or those receiving potential nephrotoxins (eg, aminoglycosides). Monitor renal function closely following administration. Safety and efficacy in children have not been established.

Adverse Reactions

>10%:

Central nervous system: Fever (15%)

Gastrointestinal: Nausea (11%)

1% to 10%:

Cardiovascular: Atrial flutter (6%), ventricular extrasystoles (6%), ventricular tachycardia (1% to 5%), heart failure (1% to 5%), arrhythmia (4%), supraventricular tachycardia (4%), bradycardia (1% to 2%), thrombosis (1% to 2%), bundle branch block (1% to 2%), cardiac arrest (1% to 2%), heart block (1% to 2%), hemorrhage (1% to 2%), myocardial ischemia (1% to 2%), pericardial effusion (1% to 2%), ventricular fibrillation (1% to 2%), shock (<1% to 2%)

Central nervous system: Agitation (1% to 2%), anxiety (1% to 2%), dizziness (1% to 2%), seizure (1% to 2%)

Endocrine & metabolic: Creatine phosphokinase increase (2%), acidosis (1% to 2%), hyperglycemia (1% to 2%), hypervolemia (1% to 2%), hypokalemia

Gastrointestinal: Diarrhea (3%), dyspepsia (1% to 2%), gastrointestinal hemorrhage (1% to 2%)

Hematologic: Disseminated intravascular coagulation (DIC), leukocytosis (1% to 2%), prothrombin decreased (1% to 2%), thrombocytopenia (1% to 2%)

Hepatic: Jaundice (1% to 2%), hepatic failure (1% to 2%)

Neuromuscular & skeletal: Arthralgia (1% to 2%)

Renal: Serum creatinine increase of >0.5 mg/dL above baseline (high dose: 9%), oliguria (1% to 2%), tubular necrosis (1% to 2%), kidney failure (1%)

Respiratory: Hypoxia (2%), pulmonary hypertension (1% to 2%), pneumonia (1% to 2%), apnea (1% to 2%), cough increased (1% to 2%)

Miscellaneous: Sepsis (1% to 2%), multisystem organ failure (1% to 2%)

<1% (Limited to important or life-threatening): Anaphylactic reaction/hypersensitivity (no prior exposure: <0.1%; re-exposure within 6 months 5%; re-exposure >6 months <1%), hemoperitoneum, skin discoloration

Drug Interactions

Avoid Concomitant Use There are no known interactions where it is recommended to avoid concomitant use.

Increased Effect/Toxicity There are no known significant interactions involving an increase in effect.

Decreased Effect

Aprotinin may decrease the levels/effects of: ACE Inhibitors; Thrombolytic Agents

Test Interactions Aprotinin significantly increases aPTT and celite Activated Clotting Time (ACT) which may not reflect the actual degree of anticoagulation by heparin. Kaolin-based ACTs are not affected by aprotinin to the same degree as celite ACTs.

Dosage Forms Excipient information presented when available (limited, particularly for generics); consult specific product labeling.
Injection, solution:
Trasylol®: 1.4 mg/mL [10,000 KIU/mL] (100 mL, 200 mL) [bovine derived]

References

Bidstrup BP, Royston D, Sapsford RN, et al, "Reduction in Blood Loss and Blood Use After Cardiovascular Bypass With High Dose Aprotinin," *J Thorac Cardiovasc Surg*, 1989, 97(3):364-72.

Boldt J, "Endothelial-Related Coagulation in Pediatric Surgery," *Ann Thorac Surg*, 1998, 65(6 Suppl):56-9.

Carrel TP, Schwanda M, Vogt P, et al, "Aprotinin in Pediatric Cardiac Operations: A Benefit in Complex Malformations and With High-Dose Regimen Only," *Ann Thorac Surg*, 1998, 66(1):153-8.

Cosgrove DM 3d, Heric B, Lytle BW, et al, "Aprotinin Therapy for Reoperative Myocardial Revascularization: A Placebo-Controlled Study," *Ann Thorac Surg*, 1992, 54(6):1031-6.

Huang H, Ding W, Su Z, et al, "Mechanism of the Preserving Effect of Aprotinin on Platelet Function and Its Use in Cardiac Surgery," *J Thorac Cardiovasc Surg*, 1993, 106(1):11-8.

Mangano DT, Miao Y, Vuylsteke A, et al, "Mortality Associated With Aprotinin During 5 Years Following Coronary Artery Bypass Graft Surgery," *JAMA*, 2007, 297(5):471-9.

Mangano DT, Tudor IC, Dietzel C, et al, "The Risk Associated With Aprotinin in Cardiac Surgery," *N Engl J Med*, 2006, 354(4):353-65.

Miller BE, Tosone SR, Tam VK, et al, "Hematologic and Economic Impact of Aprotinin in Reoperative Pediatric Cardiac Operations," *Ann Thorac Surg*, 1998, 66(2):535-41.

Penkoske P, Entwistle LM, Marchak BE, et al, "Aprotinin in Children Undergoing Repair of Congenital Heart Defects," *Ann Thorac Surg*, 1995, 60(6 Suppl):529-32.

Schulze K, Graeter T, Schaps D, et al, "Severe Anaphylactic Shock Due to Repeated Application of Aprotinin in Patients Following Intrathoracic Aortic Replacement," *Eur J Cardiothorac Surg*, 1993, 7 (9):495-6.

Spray TL, "Use of Aprotinin in Pediatric Organ Transplantation," *Ann Thorac Surg*, 1998, 65(6 Suppl):71-3.

Woodman RC and Harker LA, "Bleeding Complications Associated With Cardiopulmonary Bypass," *Blood*, 1990, 76(9):1680-97.

◆ **Aquachloral® Supprettes® [DSC]** *see* Chloral Hydrate *on page* 285

◆ **Aquacort® (Can)** *see* Hydrocortisone *on page* 699

◆ **AquaMEPHYTON® (Can)** *see* Phytonadione *on page* 1128

◆ **Aquanil™ HC [OTC]** *see* Hydrocortisone *on page* 699

◆ **Aquavan** *see* Fospropofol *on page* 642

◆ **Aranelle™** *see* Ethinyl Estradiol and Norethindrone *on page* 554

◆ **Aranesp®** *see* Darbepoetin Alfa *on page* 375

Arformoterol (ar for MOE ter ol)

Medication Guide An FDA-approved patient medication guide, which is available with the product information and at http://www.fda.gov/downloads/Drugs/DrugSafety/ucm088566.pdf, must be dispensed with this medication for each new outpatient prescription and refill.

U.S. Brand Names Brovana®

Index Terms (R,R)-Formoterol L-Tartrate; Arformoterol Tartrate

Pharmacologic Category Beta$_2$-Adrenergic Agonist; Beta$_2$-Adrenergic Agonist, Long-Acting

Generic Available No

Use Long-term maintenance treatment of bronchoconstriction in chronic obstructive pulmonary disease (COPD), including chronic bronchitis and emphysema

Mechanism of Action Arformoterol, the (R,R)-enantiomer of the racemic formoterol, is a long-acting beta$_2$-agonist that relaxes bronchial smooth muscle by selective action on beta$_2$-receptors with little effect on cardiovascular system.

Pharmacodynamics/Kinetics
Onset of action: 7-20 minutes
Peak effect: 1-3 hours
Absorption: A portion of inhaled dose is absorbed into systemic circulation
Protein binding: 52% to 65%

◄ Metabolism: Hepatic via direct glucuronidation and secondarily via O-demethylation; CYP2D6 and CYP2C19 (to a lesser extent) involved in O-demethylation

Half-life elimination: 26 hours

Time to peak: 0.5-3 hours

Dosage Nebulization: Adults: COPD: 15 mcg twice daily; maximum: 30 mcg/day

Dosage adjustment in renal impairment: No adjustment required

Dosage adjustment in hepatic impairment: No dosage adjustment required, but use caution; systemic drug exposure prolonged (1.3- to 2.4-fold)

Stability Prior to dispensing, store in protective foil pouch under refrigeration at 2°C to 8°C (36°F to 46°F). Protect from light and excessive heat. After dispensing, unopened foil pouches may be stored at room temperature at 20°C to 25°C (68°F to 77°F) for up to 6 weeks. Only remove vial from foil pouch immediately before use.

Administration Nebulization: Remove each vial from individually sealed foil pouch immediately before use. Use with standard jet nebulizer connected to an air compressor; administer with mouthpiece or face mask. Administer vial undiluted and do not mix with other medications in nebulizer.

Monitoring Parameters FEV_1, peak flow, and/or other pulmonary function tests; blood pressure, heart rate; CNS stimulation; serum glucose, serum potassium. Monitor for increased use of short-acting beta$_2$-agonist inhalers; may be marker of a deteriorating COPD condition.

Pregnancy Risk Factor C

Contraindications Hypersensitivity to arformoterol, racemic formoterol, or any component of the formulation

Warnings/Precautions [U.S. Boxed Warning]: Long-acting beta$_2$-agonists may increase the risk of asthma-related deaths. In a large, randomized clinical trial (SMART, 2006), salmeterol was associated with a small, but statistically significant increase in asthma-related deaths (when added to usual asthma therapy); risk may be greater in African-American patients versus Caucasians. Data is not available to determine whether rate of death is increased with long-acting beta$_2$-agonists in COPD setting. Rarely, paradoxical bronchospasm may occur with use of inhaled bronchodilating agents; this should be distinguished from inadequate response. Immediate hypersensitivity reactions (urticaria, angioedema, rash, bronchospasm) have been reported. Do not exceed recommended dose; serious adverse events, including fatalities, have been associated with excessive use of inhaled sympathomimetics.

Use with caution in patients with cardiovascular disease (eg, arrhythmia, hypertension, HF); beta-agonists may cause elevation in blood pressure, heart rate and result in CNS stimulation/excitation. Beta$_2$-agonists may also increase risk of arrhythmias and prolong QT_c interval. Arformoterol should only be used for long-term maintenance treatment and should not be used as rescue therapy in treatment of acute episodes. It should not be initiated in patients with acutely deteriorating COPD or combined with other long-acting beta$_2$-agonists. Use with caution in patients with diabetes mellitus; beta$_2$-agonists may increase serum glucose. Use caution in hepatic impairment; systemic clearance prolonged in hepatic dysfunction. Use with caution in hyperthyroidism; may stimulate thyroid activity. Use with caution in patients with hypokalemia; beta$_2$-agonists may decrease serum potassium. Use with caution in patients with seizure disorders; beta$_2$-agonists may result in CNS stimulation/excitation.

Tolerance/tachyphylaxis to the bronchodilator effect, measured by FEV_1, has been observed in studies. Patients using inhaled, short-acting beta$_2$-agonists should be instructed to discontinue routine use of these medications prior to beginning treatment; short-acting agents should be reserved for symptomatic relief of acute symptoms. Patients must be instructed to seek medical attention in cases where acute symptoms are not relieved or a previous level of response is diminished. The need to increase frequency of use may indicate deterioration of COPD, and treatment must not be delayed. Safety and efficacy have not been established in children.

Adverse Reactions

2% to 10%:

Cardiovascular: Chest pain (7%), peripheral edema (3%)

Central nervous system: Pain (8%)

Dermatologic: Rash (4%)

Gastrointestinal: Diarrhea (6%)

Neuromuscular & skeletal: Back pain (6%), leg cramps (4%)

Respiratory: Dyspnea (4%), sinusitis (5%), congestive conditions (2%)

Miscellaneous: Flu-like syndrome (3%)

<2% (Limited to important or life-threatening): Abscess, agitation, allergic reaction, arteriosclerosis, arthralgia, arthritis, atrial flutter, AV block, bone disorder, calcium crystalluria, cystitis, cerebral infarct, CHF, circumoral paresthesia, constipation, dehydration, dry skin, ECG changes, edema, fever, gastritis, glaucoma, glucose tolerance decreased, glycosuria, gout, heart block, hematuria, hyper-/hypoglycemia, hyperlipemia, hypokalemia, hypokinesia, inverted T-wave, kidney calculus, lung carcinoma, melena, MI, neck rigidity, neoplasm, nocturia, oral moniliasis, paradoxical bronchospasm, paralysis, pelvic pain, periodontal abscess, PSA increased, pyuria, QT interval increased, rectal hemorrhage, retroperitoneal hemorrhage, rheumatoid arthritis, skin discoloration, skin hypertrophy, somnolence, supraventricular tachycardia, tendinous contracture, tremor, urinary tract disorder, urine abnormality, viral infection, vision abnormalities, voice alteration

Drug Interactions

Metabolism/Transport Effects Substrate of CY2D6 (minor) and CYP2C19 (minor)

Avoid Concomitant Use

Avoid concomitant use of Arformoterol with any of the following: Iobenguane I 123

Increased Effect/Toxicity

Arformoterol may increase the levels/effects of: Sympathomimetics

The levels/effects of Arformoterol may be increased by: Atomoxetine; Cannabinoids; MAO Inhibitors; Tricyclic Antidepressants

Decreased Effect

Arformoterol may decrease the levels/effects of: Iobenguane I 123

The levels/effects of Arformoterol may be decreased by: Alpha-/Beta-Blockers; Beta-Blockers (Beta1 Selective); Beta-Blockers (Nonselective); Betahistine

Dosage Forms Excipient information presented when available (limited, particularly for generics); consult specific product labeling.

Solution for nebulization:

Brovana®: 15 mcg/2 mL (30s, 60s)

◆ **Arformoterol Tartrate** *see* Arformoterol *on page 137*

Argatroban (ar GA troh ban)

Medication Safety Issues

Sound-alike/look-alike issues:

Argatroban may be confused with Aggrastat®, Orgaran®

High alert medication: The Institute for Safe Medication Practices (ISMP) includes this medication among its list of drugs which have a heightened risk of causing significant patient harm when used in error.

Related Information

Continuous Renal Replacement Therapy *on page 1557*

Dosing Considerations for the Critically-Ill Patient With Morbid Obesity *on page 1561*

Pharmacologic Category Anticoagulant, Thrombin Inhibitor

Generic Available No

Use Prophylaxis or treatment of thrombosis in patients with heparin-induced thrombocytopenia (HIT); adjunct to percutaneous coronary intervention (PCI) in patients who have or are at risk of thrombosis associated with HIT

Unlabeled/Investigational Use To maintain extracorporeal circuit patency (prefilter administration) of continuous renal replacement therapy (CRRT) in critically-ill patients with HIT

◀ **Mechanism of Action** A direct, highly-selective thrombin inhibitor. Reversibly binds to the active thrombin site of free and clot-associated thrombin. Inhibits fibrin formation; activation of coagulation factors V, VIII, and XIII; activation of protein C; and platelet aggregation.

Pharmacodynamics/Kinetics

Onset of action: Immediate

Distribution: 174 mL/kg

Protein binding: Albumin: 20%; α_1-acid glycoprotein: 35%

Metabolism: Hepatic via hydroxylation and aromatization. Metabolism via CYP3A4/5 to four known metabolites plays a minor role. Unchanged argatroban is the major plasma component. Plasma concentration of metabolite M1 is 0% to 20% of the parent drug and is three- to fivefold weaker.

Half-life elimination: 39-51 minutes; Hepatic impairment: ≤181 minutes

Time to peak: Steady-state: 1-3 hours

Excretion: Feces (65%); urine (22%); low quantities of metabolites M2-4 in urine Clearance is decreased in critically-ill pediatric patients

Dosage I.V.:

Children: **Heparin-induced thrombocytopenia** (dosing based on limited data from critically-ill patients):

Initial dose: 0.75 mcg/kg/minute

Maintenance dose: Patient may not be at steady-state but measure aPTT after 2 hours; adjust dose until the steady-state aPTT is 1.5-3.0 times the initial baseline value, not exceeding 100 seconds; dosage may be adjusted in increments of 0.1-0.25 mcg/kg/minute. **Note:** Frequent dosage adjustments may be required to maintain desired anticoagulant activity.

Adults:

Heparin-induced thrombocytopenia:

Initial dose: 2 mcg/kg/minute; use actual body weight up to 130 kg (BMI up to 51 kg/m^2) (Rice, 2007)

Maintenance dose: Patient may not be at steady-state but measure aPTT after 2 hours; adjust dose until the steady-state aPTT is 1.5-3.0 times the initial baseline value, not exceeding 100 seconds; dosage should not exceed 10 mcg/kg/minute

Note: Critically-ill patients with normal hepatic function became excessively anticoagulated with FDA-approved or lower starting doses of argatroban. Doses between 0.15-1.3 mcg/kg/minute were required to maintain aPTTs in the target range (Reichert, 2003). In a prospective observational study of critically-ill patients with MODS and suspected or proven HIT, an initial infusion dose of 0.2 mcg/kg/minute was found to be sufficient and safe in this population (Beiderlinden, 2007). Consider reducing starting dose to 0.2 mcg/kg/minute in critically-ill patients with multiple organ dysfunction (MODS) defined as a minimum number of two organ failures. Another report of a cardiac patient with anasarca secondary to acute renal failure had a reduction in argatroban clearance similar to patients with hepatic dysfunction. Reduced clearance may have been due to reduced liver perfusion (de Denus, 2003). The American College of Chest Physicians has recommended an initial infusion rate of 0.5-1.2 mcg/kg/minute for patients with heart failure, MODS, severe anasarca, or postcardiac surgery (Hirsch, 2008).

Conversion to oral anticoagulant: Because there may be a combined effect on the INR when argatroban is combined with warfarin, loading doses of warfarin should not be used. Warfarin therapy should be started at the expected daily dose.

Patients receiving ≤2 mcg/kg/minute of argatroban: Argatroban therapy can be stopped when the combined INR on warfarin and argatroban is >4; repeat INR measurement in 4-6 hours; if INR is below therapeutic level, argatroban therapy may be restarted. Repeat procedure daily until desired INR on warfarin alone is obtained.

Patients receiving >2 mcg/kg/minute of argatroban: In order to predict the INR on warfarin alone, reduce dose of argatroban to 2 mcg/kg/minute; measure INR for argatroban and warfarin 4-6 hours after dose reduction; argatroban therapy can be stopped when the combined INR on warfarin and argatroban is >4. Repeat INR measurement in 4-6 hours; if INR is below therapeutic level, argatroban therapy may be restarted. Repeat procedure daily until desired INR on warfarin alone is obtained.

Note: The American College of Chest Physicians recommends monitoring chromogenic factor X assay when transitioning from argatroban to warfarin (Hirsh, 2008). Factor X levels <45% have been associated with INR values >2 after the effects of argatroban have been eliminated (Arpino, 2005).

Prefilter administration for continuous renal replacement therapy (CRRT) in critically-ill patients with HIT (unlabeled use; Link, 2008): 0.1-1.5 mcg/kg/minute. **Note:** Loading dose of 100 mcg/kg was administered during clinical trial; however, this may be unnecessary.

Percutaneous coronary intervention (PCI):

Initial: Begin infusion of 25 mcg/kg/minute and administer bolus dose of 350 mcg/kg (over 3-5 minutes). ACT should be checked 5-10 minutes after bolus infusion; proceed with procedure if ACT >300 seconds. Following initial bolus:

ACT <300 seconds: Give an additional 150 mcg/kg bolus, and increase infusion rate to 30 mcg/kg/minute (recheck ACT in 5-10 minutes)

ACT >450 seconds: Decrease infusion rate to 15 mcg/kg/minute (recheck ACT in 5-10 minutes)

Once a therapeutic ACT (300-450 seconds) is achieved, infusion should be continued at this dose for the duration of the procedure.

If dissection, impending abrupt closure, thrombus formation during PCI, or inability to achieve ACT >300 seconds: An additional bolus of 150 mcg/kg, followed by an increase in infusion rate to 40 mcg/kg/minute may be administered.

Note: Post-PCI anticoagulation, if required, may be achieved by continuing infusion at a reduced dose of 2-10 mcg/kg/minute, with close monitoring of aPTT.

Elderly: No adjustment is necessary for patients with normal liver function

Dosage adjustment in renal impairment: Removal during hemodialysis and continuous venovenous hemofiltration is clinically insignificant. No dosage adjustment required.

Dosage adjustment in hepatic impairment: Decreased clearance and increased elimination half-life are seen with hepatic impairment; dose should be reduced.

Children: Initial dose: 0.2 mcg/kg/minute; adjust dose in increments of ≤0.05 mcg/kg/minute

Adults: Initial dose for moderate hepatic impairment is 0.5 mcg/kg/minute. **Note:** During PCI, avoid use in patients with elevations of ALT/AST (>3 times ULN); the use of argatroban in these patients has not been evaluated.

Stability Prior to use, store at 15°C to 30°C (59°F to 86°F). Protect from light. The prepared solution is stable for 24 hours at 15°C to 30°C (59°F to 86°F) in ambient indoor light. Do not expose to direct sunlight. May be mixed with 0.9% sodium chloride injection, 5% dextrose injection, or lactated Ringer's injection. Do not mix with other medications.

To prepare solution for I.V. administration, dilute each 250 mg vial with 250 mL of diluent. Mix by repeated inversion for 1 minute. Once mixed, final concentration should be 1 mg/mL. A slight but brief haziness may occur prior to mixing. Prepared solutions that are protected from light and kept at controlled room temperature of 20°C to 25°C (68°F to 77°F) or under refrigeration at 2°C to 8°C (36°F to 46°F) are stable for up to 96 hours.

Administration Solution **must be diluted to 1 mg/mL** prior to administration.

Monitoring Parameters Obtain baseline aPTT prior to start of therapy. Patient may not be at steady-state but check aPTT 2 hours after start of therapy to adjust dose, keeping the steady-state aPTT 1.5-3 times the initial baseline value (not exceeding 100 seconds). Monitor hemoglobin, hematocrit, signs and symptoms of bleeding.

PCI: Monitor ACT before dosing, 5-10 minutes after bolus dosing, and after any change in infusion rate and at the end of the procedure. Additional ACT assessments should be made every 20-30 minutes during extended PCI procedures.

Anesthesia and Critical Care Concerns/Other Considerations

Clinical Pearls/Comments: Argatroban achieves steady state rapidly (4-5 hours after initiating therapy, with normal hepatic function) when administered I.V., with a predictable dose-response effect. PTTs generally remain stable at a given dose.

◀ Argatroban does not induce formation of antibodies that can alter its clearance, as is seen with lepirudin. Reduce initial dose (0.2-0.5 mcg/kg/minute) in critically-ill patients, particularly those who may have impaired hepatic perfusion and/or hepatic insufficiency.

Evidence-Based Information: In a prospective observational study of critically-ill patients with MODS and suspected or proven HIT, an initial infusion dose of 0.2 mcg/kg/minute was found to be sufficient and safe in this population (Beiderlindern, 2007). The American College of Chest Physicians Evidence Based Clinical Practice Guidelines (8th Edition, 2008) suggest reducing the initial argatroban dose (0.5-1.2 mcg/kg/minute) for the treatment of heparin-induced thrombocytopenia in patients with heart failure, multiple organ system failure, or severe anasarca or who are postcardiac surgery (Grade 2C).

Pregnancy Risk Factor B

Contraindications Hypersensitivity to argatroban or any component of the formulation; overt major bleeding

Warnings/Precautions Hemorrhage can occur at any site in the body. Extreme caution should be used when there is an increased danger of hemorrhage, such as severe hypertension, immediately following lumbar puncture, spinal anesthesia, major surgery (including brain, spinal cord, or eye surgery), congenital or acquired bleeding disorders, and gastrointestinal ulcers. Use caution in critically-ill patients; reduced clearance may require dosage reduction. Use caution with hepatic dysfunction. Argatroban prolongs the PT/INR. Concomitant use with warfarin will cause increased prolongation of the PT and INR greater than that of warfarin alone. If warfarin is initiated concurrently with argatroban, initial PT/INR goals while on argatroban may require modification; alternative guidelines for monitoring therapy should be followed. Safety and efficacy for use with other thrombolytic agents has not been established. Discontinue all parenteral anticoagulants prior to starting therapy. Allow reversal of heparin's effects before initiation. Patients with hepatic dysfunction may require >4 hours to achieve full reversal of argatroban's anticoagulant effect following treatment. Avoid use during PCI in patients with elevations of ALT/AST (>3 times ULN); the use of argatroban in these patients has not been evaluated. Limited pharmacokinetic and dosing information is available from use in critically-ill children with heparin-induced thrombocytopenia.

Adverse Reactions As with all anticoagulants, bleeding is the major adverse effect of argatroban. Hemorrhage may occur at virtually any site. Risk is dependent on multiple variables, including the intensity of anticoagulation and patient susceptibility.

>10%:
    Cardiovascular: Chest pain (PCI related: <1% to 15%), hypotension (7% to 11%)
    Gastrointestinal: Gastrointestinal bleed (major: <1% to 3%; minor: 3% to 14%)
    Genitourinary: Genitourinary bleed and hematuria (major: <1%; minor: 2% to 12%)
1% to 10%:
    Cardiovascular: Vasodilation (1% to 10%), cardiac arrest (6%), ventricular tachycardia (5%), bradycardia (5%), myocardial infarction (PCI: 4%), atrial fibrillation (3%), angina (2%), CABG-related bleeding (minor, 2%), myocardial ischemia (2%), cerebrovascular disorder (<1% to 2%), thrombosis (<1% to 2%)
    Central nervous system: Fever (<1% to 7%), headache (5%), pain (5%), intracranial bleeding (1% to 4%)
    Dermatologic: Skin reactions (bullous eruption, rash; 1% to <10%)
    Gastrointestinal: Nausea (5% to 7%), diarrhea (6%), vomiting (4% to 6%), abdominal pain (3% to 4%)
    Genitourinary: Urinary tract infection (5%)
    Hematologic: Hemoglobin decreased (<2 g/dL), hematocrit decreased (minor: 2% to 10%; major: <1%)
    Local: Bleeding at injection or access site (minor: 2% to 5%)
    Neuromuscular & skeletal: Back pain (PCI related: 8%)
    Renal: Abnormal renal function (3%)
    Respiratory: Dyspnea (8% to 10%), cough (3% to 10%), hemoptysis (minor: <1% to 3%), pneumonia (3%)
    Miscellaneous: Sepsis (6%), infection (4%)

<1% (Limited to important or life-threatening): Allergic reactions, GERD, limb and below-the-knee stump bleed, multisystem hemorrhage and DIC, pulmonary edema, retroperitoneal bleeding

Drug Interactions

Metabolism/Transport Effects Substrate of CYP3A4 (minor)

Avoid Concomitant Use There are no known interactions where it is recommended to avoid concomitant use.

Increased Effect/Toxicity

Argatroban may increase the levels/effects of: Anticoagulants; Ibritumomab; Tositumomab and Iodine I 131 Tositumomab

The levels/effects of Argatroban may be increased by: Antiplatelet Agents; Dasatinib; Herbs (Anticoagulant/Antiplatelet Properties); Nonsteroidal Anti-Inflammatory Agents; Pentosan Polysulfate Sodium; Prostacyclin Analogues; Salicylates; Thrombolytic Agents

Decreased Effect There are no known significant interactions involving a decrease in effect.

Test Interactions PT/INR levels may become elevated in the absence of warfarin. If warfarin is started, initial PT/INR goals while on argatroban may require modification.

Dosage Forms Excipient information presented when available (limited, particularly for generics); consult specific product labeling.

Injection, solution: 100 mg/mL (2.5 mL) [contains dehydrated alcohol 1000 mg/mL]

References

Arpino PA, Demirjian Z, and Van Cott EM, "Use of the Chromogenic Factor X Assay to Predict the International Normalized Ratio in Patients Transitioning from Argatroban to Warfarin," *Pharmacotherapy*, 2005, 25(2):157-64.

Beiderlinden M, Treschan TA, Gorlinger K, et al, "Argatroban Anticoagulation in Critically Ill Patients," *Ann Pharmacother*, 2007, 41(5):749-54.

Dager WE and White RH, "Pharmacotherapy of Heparin-Induced Thrombocytopenia," *Expert Opin Pharmacother*, 2003, 4(6):919-40.

de Denus S and Spinler SA, "Decreased Argatrogan Clearance Unaffected by Hemodialysis in Anasarca," *Ann Pharmacother*, 2003, 37(9):1237-40.

Hirsh J, Guyatt G, Albers GW, et al, "Executive Summary: American College of Chest Physicians Evidence-Based Clinical Practice Guidelines (8th Edition)," *Chest*, 2008, 133(6 Suppl):71-109.

Levine RL, Hursting MJ, and McCollum D, "Argatroban Therapy in Heparin-Induced Thrombocytopenia With Hepatic Dysfunction," *Chest*, 2006, 129(5):1167-75.

Lewis BE, Wallis DE, Berkowitz SD, et al, "Argatroban Anticoagulant Therapy in Patients With Heparin-Induced Thrombocytopenia," *Circulation*, 2001, 103(14):1838-43.

Link A, Girndt M, Selejan S, et al, "Argatroban for Anticoagulation in Continuous Renal Replacement Therapy," *Crit Care Med*, 2009 (epub ahead of print).

Reichert MG, MacGregor DA, Kincaid EH, et al, "Excessive Argatroban Anticoagulation for Heparin-Induced Thrombocytopenia," *Ann Pharmacother*, 2003, 37(5):652-4.

Tang IY, Cox DS, Patel K, et al, "Argatroban and Renal Replacement Therapy in Patients With Heparin-Induced Thrombocytopenia," *Ann Pharmacother*, 2005, 39(2):231-6.

Warkentin TE, Greinacher A, Koster A, et al, "Treatment and Prevention of Heparin-Induced Thrombocytopenia: American College of Chest Physicians Evidence-Based Clinical Practice Guidelines (8th Edition)," *Chest*, 2008, 133(6 Suppl):340S-380S.

◆ **8-Arginine Vasopressin** *see* Vasopressin *on page 1458*

◆ **Aricept®** *see* Donepezil *on page 447*

◆ **Aricept® ODT** *see* Donepezil *on page 447*

◆ **Aricept® RDT (Can)** *see* Donepezil *on page 447*

◆ **Arimidex®** *see* Anastrozole *on page 122*

Aripiprazole (ay ri PIP ray zole)

U.S. Brand Names Abilify Discmelt®; Abilify®
Canadian Brand Names Abilify®
Index Terms BMS 337039; OPC-14597
Pharmacologic Category Antipsychotic Agent, Atypical
Use

Oral: Acute and maintenance treatment of schizophrenia; stabilization, maintenance, and adjunctive therapy (to lithium or valproate) of bipolar disorder (with acute manic or mixed episodes); adjunctive treatment of major depressive disorder

Injection: Agitation associated with schizophrenia or bipolar mania

◀ **Unlabeled/Investigational Use** Depression with psychotic features; aggression (children); conduct disorder (children); Tourette syndrome (children); psychosis/agitation related to Alzheimer's dementia

Pharmacodynamics/Kinetics

Onset of action: Initial: 1-3 weeks

Absorption: Well absorbed

Distribution: V_d: 4.9 L/kg

Protein binding: ≥99%, primarily to albumin

Metabolism: Hepatic, via CYP2D6, CYP3A4 (dehydro-aripiprazole metabolite has affinity for D_2 receptors similar to the parent drug and represents 40% of the parent drug exposure in plasma)

Bioavailability: I.M.: 100%; Tablet: 87%

Half-life elimination: Aripiprazole: 75 hours; dehydro-aripiprazole: 94 hours
CYP2D6 poor metabolizers: Aripiprazole: 146 hours

Time to peak, plasma: I.M.: 1-3 hours; Tablet: 3-5 hours
With high-fat meal: Aripiprazole: Delayed by 3 hours; dehydro-aripiprazole: Delayed by 12 hours

Excretion: Feces (55%, ~18% unchanged drug); urine (25%, <1% unchanged drug)

Dosage Note: Oral solution may be substituted for the oral tablet on a mg-per-mg basis, up to 25 mg. Patients receiving 30 mg tablets should be given 25 mg oral solution. Orally disintegrating tablets (Abilify Discmelt®) are bioequivalent to the immediate release tablets (Abilify®).

Children: Oral: Aggression, conduct disorder, Tourette syndrome (unlabeled uses): 5-20 mg/day

Children ≥10 years: Oral: Bipolar I disorder (acute manic or mixed episodes): Initial: 2 mg daily for 2 days, followed by 5 mg daily for 2 days with a further increase to target dose of 10 mg daily as monotherapy or adjunctive therapy; subsequent dose increases may be made in 5 mg increments, up to a maximum of 30 mg/day

Adolescents ≥13 years: Oral: Schizophrenia: Initial: 2 mg daily for 2 days, followed by 5 mg daily for 2 days with a further increase to target dose of 10 mg daily; subsequent dose increases may be made in 5 mg increments up to a maximum of 30 mg/day (30 mg/day not shown to be more efficacious than 10 mg/day)

Adults:

Acute agitation (schizophrenia/bipolar mania): I.M.: 9.75 mg as a single dose (range: 5.25-15 mg); repeated doses may be given at ≥2-hour intervals to a maximum of 30 mg/day. **Note:** If ongoing therapy with aripiprazole is necessary, transition to oral therapy as soon as possible.

Bipolar disorder (acute manic or mixed episodes): Oral:

Stabilization: Initial: 15 mg once daily as monotherapy or adjunctive to lithium or valproic acid. May increase to 30 mg once daily if clinically indicated; safety of doses >30 mg/day has not been evaluated.

Maintenance: Continue stabilization dose for up to 6 weeks; efficacy of continued treatment >6 weeks has not been established

Depression (adjunctive with antidepressants): Oral: Initial: 2-5 mg/day (range: 2-15 mg/day); dose adjustments of up to 5 mg/day may be made in intervals of ≥1 week. **Note:** Dosing based on patients already receiving antidepressant therapy.

Schizophrenia: Oral: 10-15 mg once daily; may be increased to a maximum of 30 mg once daily (efficacy at dosages above 10-15 mg has not been shown to be increased). Dosage titration should not be more frequent than every 2 weeks.

Dosage adjustment with concurrent CYP450 inducer or inhibitor therapy: Oral:

CYP3A4 inducers (eg, carbamazepine): Aripiprazole dose should be doubled (20-30 mg/day); dose should be subsequently reduced (10-15 mg/day) if concurrent inducer agent discontinued.

CYP3A4 inhibitors (eg, ketoconazole): Aripiprazole dose should be reduced to $1/2$ of the usual dose, and proportionally increased upon discontinuation of the inhibitor agent.

CYP2D6 inhibitors (eg, fluoxetine, paroxetine): Aripiprazole dose should be reduced to $1/2$ of the usual dose, and proportionally increased upon discontinuation of the inhibitor agent.

Dosage adjustment in renal impairment: No dosage adjustment required

Dosage adjustment in hepatic impairment: No dosage adjustment required

Additional Information Complete prescribing information for this medication should be consulted for additional detail.

Dosage Forms Excipient information presented when available (limited, particularly for generics); consult specific product labeling.

Injection, solution:

Abilify®: 7.5 mg/mL (1.3 mL)

Solution, oral:

Abilify®: 1 mg/mL (150 mL) [contains propylene glycol, sucrose 400 mg/mL, and fructose 200 mg/mL; orange cream flavor]

Tablet:

Abilify®: 2 mg, 5 mg, 10 mg, 15 mg, 20 mg, 30 mg

Tablet, orally disintegrating:

Abilify Discmelt®: 10 mg [contains phenylalanine 1.12 mg; creme de vanilla flavor]; 15 mg [contains phenylalanine 1.68 mg; creme de vanilla flavor]

References

American Diabetes Association; American Psychiatric Association; American Association of Clinical Endocrinologists; North American Association for the Study of Obesity, "Consensus Development Conference on Antipsychotic Drugs and Obesity and Diabetes," *Diabetes Care*, 2004, 27 (2):596-601.

Barbee JG, Conrad EJ, and Jamhour NJ, "Aripiprazole Augmentation in Treatment-Resistant Depression," *Ann Clin Psychiatry*, 2004, 16(4):189-94.

Barzman DH, DelBello MP, Kowatch RA, et al "The Effectiveness and Tolerability of Aripiprazole for Pediatric Bipolar Disorders: A Retrospective Chart Review," *J Child Adolesc Psychopharmacol*, 2004, 14(4):593-600.

Biederman J, McDonnell MA, Wozniak, et al, "Aripiprazole in the Treatment of Pediatric Bipolar Disorder: A Systematic Chart Review," *CNS Spectr*, 2005, 10(2):141-8.

Burris KD, Molski TF, Xu C, et al, "Aripiprazole, A Novel Antipsychotic, Is a High-Affinity Partial Agonist at Human Dopamine D2 Receptors," *J Pharmacol Exp Ther*, 2002, 302(1):381-9.

Davis JM, Chen N, and Glick ID, "A Meta-Analysis of the Efficacy of Second-Generation Antipsychotics," *Arch Gen Psychiatry*, 2003, 60(6):553-64.

Duane DD, "Aripiprazole in Childhood and Adolescence for Tourette Syndrome," *J Child Neurol*, 2006, 21(4):358.

Durkin JP, "Aripiprazole in the Treatment of Bipolar Disorder in Children and Adolescents," *J Child Adolesc Psychopharmacol*, 2004, 14(4):505-6.

Hellerstein DJ, "Aripiprazole as an Adjunctive Treatment for Refractory Major Depression," *Prog Neuropsychopharmacol Biol Psychiatry*, 2004, 28(8):1347-8.

Inoue A, Miki S, Seto M, et al, "Aripiprazole, A Novel Antipsychotic Drug, Inhibits Quinpirole-Evoked GTPase Activity But Does Not Up-Regulate Dopamine D2 Receptor Following Repeated Treatment in the Rat Striatal Slices," *Eur J Pharmacol*, 1997, 321(1):105-11.

Jordan S, Koprivica V, Chen R, et al, "The Antipsychotic Aripiprazole Is a Potent, Partial Agonist at the Human 5-HT(1A) Receptor," *Eur J Pharmacol*, 2002, 441(3):137-40.

Kane JM, Carson WH, Saha AR, et al, "Efficacy and Safety of Aripiprazole and Haloperidol Versus Placebo in Patients With Schizophrenia and Schizoaffective Disorder," *J Clin Psychiatry*, 2002, 63 (9):763-71.

Ketter TA, Wang PW, Chandler RA, et al, "Adjunctive Aripiprazole in Treatment-Resistant Bipolar Depression," *Ann Clin Psychiatry*, 2006, 18(3):169-72.

Lawler CP, Prioleau C, Lewis MM, et al, "Interactions of the Novel Antipsychotic Aripiprazole (OPC-14597) With Dopamine and Serotonin Receptor Subtypes," *Neuropsychopharmacology*, 1999, 20 (6):612-27.

Matsubayashi H, Amano T, and Sasa M, "Inhibition by Aripiprazole of Dopaminergic Inputs to Striatal Neurons From Substantia Nigra," *Psychopharmacology* (Berl), 1999, 146(2):139-43.

McGavin JK and Goa KL, "Aripiprazole," *CNS Drugs*, 2002, 16(11):779-86.

Murphy TK, Bengtson MA, Soto O, et al, "Case Series on the Use Of Aripiprazole for Tourette Syndrome," *Int J Neuropsychopharmacol*, 2005, 8(3):489-90.

Papakostas GI, Petersen TJ, Kinrys G, et al, "Aripiprazole Augmentation of Selective Serotonin Reuptake Inhibitors for Treatment-Resistant Major Depressive Disorder," *J Clin Psychiatry*, 2005, 66(10):1326-30.

Patkar AA, Peindl K, Mago R, et al, "An Open-Label, Rater-Blinded, Augmentation Study of Aripiprazole in Treatment-Resistant Depression," *Prim Care Companion J Clin Psychiatry*, 2006, 8 (2):82-7.

Rugino TA and Janvier YM, "Aripiprazole in Children And Adolescents: Clinical Experience," *J Child Neurol*, 2005, 20(7):603-10.

Schneider LS, Tariot PN, Dagerman KS, et al, "Effectiveness of Atypical Antipsychotic Drugs in Patients With Alzheimer's Disease," *N Engl J Med*, 2006, 355(15):1525-38.

Simon JS and Nemeroff CB, "Aripiprazole Augmentation of Antidepressants for the Treatment of Partially Responding and Nonresponding Patients With Major Depressive Disorder," *J Clin Psychiatry*, 2005, 66(10):1216-20.

Stigler KA, Posey DJ, and McDougle CJ, "Aripiprazole for Maladaptive Behavior in Pervasive Developmental Disorders," *J Child Adolesc Psychopharmacol*, 2004, 14(3):455-63.

Worthington JJ 3rd, Kinrys G, Wygant LE, et al, "Aripiprazole as an Augmentor of Selective Serotonin Reuptake Inhibitors in Depression and Anxiety Disorder Patients," *Int Clin Psychopharmacol*, 2005, 20(1):9-11.

Yoo HK, Kim JY, Kim CY. "A Pilot Study of Aripiprazole in Children and Adolescents With Tourette's Disorder," *J Child Adolesc Psychopharmacol*, 2006, 16(4):505-6.

◆ **Aristospan®** *see* Triamcinolone *on page 1429*

◆ **Arixtra®** *see* Fondaparinux *on page 627*

Armodafinil (ar moe DAF i nil)

U.S. Brand Names Nuvigil™
Index Terms R-modafinil
Pharmacologic Category Stimulant
Restrictions C-IV
Use Improve wakefulness in patients with excessive daytime sleepiness associated with narcolepsy and shift work sleep disorder (SWSD); adjunctive therapy for obstructive sleep apnea/hypopnea syndrome (OSAHS)
Pharmacodynamics/Kinetics
Absorption: Readily absorbed
Distribution: V_d: 42 L
Protein binding: ~60% (based on modafinil; primarily albumin)
Metabolism: Hepatic, multiple pathways, including CYP3A4/5; metabolites include R-modafinil acid and modafinil sulfone
Clearance: 33 mL/minute, mainly via hepatic metabolism
Half-life elimination: 15 hours; Steady state: ~7 days
Time to peak, plasma: 2 hours (fasted)
Excretion: Urine (80% predominantly as metabolites; <10% as unchanged drug)
Dosage Oral:
Adults:
Narcolepsy: 150-250 mg once daily in the morning
Obstructive sleep apnea/hypopnea syndrome (OSAHS): 150-250 mg once daily in the morning; 250 mg was not shown to have any increased benefit over 150 mg
Shift work sleep disorder (SWSD): 150 mg given once daily ~1 hour prior to work shift
Elderly: Consider lower initial dosage. Concentrations were almost doubled in clinical trials (based on modafinil)
Dosage adjustment in renal impairment: Inadequate data to determine safety and efficacy in severe renal impairment.
Dosage adjustment in hepatic impairment: Severe hepatic impairment (Child-Pugh classes B and C): Based on modafinil, dose should be reduced by half
Additional Information Complete prescribing information for this medication should be consulted for additional detail.
Dosage Forms Excipient information presented when available (limited, particularly for generics); consult specific product labeling.
Tablet:
Nuvigil™: 50 mg, 150 mg, 250 mg
References
Hirshkowitz M, Black JE, Wesnes K, et al, "Adjunct Armodafinil Improves Wakefulness and Memory in Obstructive Sleep Apnea/Hypopnea Syndrome," *Respir Med*, 2007, 101(3):616-27.

Roth T, White D, Schmidt-Nowara W, et al, "Effects of Armodafinil in the Treatment of Residual Excessive Sleepiness Associated With Obstructive Sleep Apnea/Hypopnea Syndrome: A 12-week, Multicenter, Double-Blind, Randomized, Placebo-Controlled Study in nCPAP-AdherentAdults," *Clin Ther*, 2006, 28(5): 689-706.

◆ **Armour® Thyroid** *see* Thyroid, Desiccated *on page 1379*

◆ **ASA** *see* Aspirin *on page 147*

◆ **5-ASA** *see* Mesalamine *on page 884*

◆ **Asacol®** *see* Mesalamine *on page 884*

◆ **Asacol® 800 (Can)** *see* Mesalamine *on page 884*

◆ **Asacol® HD** *see* Mesalamine *on page 884*

- ♦ **Asaphen (Can)** *see* Aspirin *on page 147*
- ♦ **Asaphen E.C. (Can)** *see* Aspirin *on page 147*
- ♦ **Ascriptin® [OTC]** *see* Aspirin *on page 147*
- ♦ **Ascriptin® Maximum Strength [OTC]** *see* Aspirin *on page 147*
- ♦ **Aspart Insulin** *see* Insulin Aspart *on page 741*
- ♦ **Aspercin [OTC]** *see* Aspirin *on page 147*
- ♦ **Aspergum® [OTC]** *see* Aspirin *on page 147*

Aspirin (AS pir in)

Medication Safety Issues
Sound-alike/look-alike issues:
Aspirin may be confused with Afrin®, Asendin®
Ascriptin® may be confused with Aricept®
Ecotrin® may be confused with Akineton®, Edecrin®, Epogen®
Halfprin® may be confused with Halfan®, Haltran®
ZORprin® may be confused with Zyloprim®

International issues:
Cartia® [multiple international markets] may be confused with Cartia XT® which is a brand name for diltiazem in the U.S.

Related Information
Acetaminophen and NSAIDS, Dosing in the Management of Pain *on page 1651*
Acute Postoperative Pain *on page 1502*
Anesthesia Considerations for Neurosurgery *on page 1514*
Anesthesia for Geriatric Patients *on page 1523*
Chronic Pain Management *on page 1546*
Heart Failure (Systolic) *on page 1739*
Perioperative / Periprocedural Management of Anticoagulant and Antiplatelet Therapy *on page 1607*
Porphyria: Safe and Unsafe Drugs *on page 1800*
Preoperative Evaluation of the Cardiac Patient for Noncardiac Surgery *on page 1598*

U.S. Brand Names Ascriptin® Maximum Strength [OTC]; Ascriptin® [OTC]; Aspercin [OTC]; Aspergum® [OTC]; Aspirtab [OTC]; Bayer® Aspirin Extra Strength [OTC]; Bayer® Aspirin Regimen Adult Low Dose [OTC]; Bayer® Aspirin Regimen Children's [OTC]; Bayer® Aspirin Regimen Regular Strength [OTC]; Bayer® Genuine Aspirin [OTC]; Bayer® Plus Extra Strength [OTC]; Bayer® with Heart Advantage [OTC]; Bayer® Women's Aspirin Plus Calcium [OTC]; Buffasal [OTC]; Bufferin® Extra Strength [OTC]; Bufferin® [OTC]; Buffinol [OTC]; Easprin®; Ecotrin® Low Strength [OTC]; Ecotrin® Maximum Strength [OTC]; Ecotrin® [OTC]; Genacote™ [OTC]; Halfprin® [OTC]; St. Joseph® Adult Aspirin [OTC]; ZORprin®

Canadian Brand Names Asaphen; Asaphen E.C.; Entrophen®; Novasen; Praxis ASA EC 81 Mg Daily Dose

Index Terms Acetylsalicylic Acid; ASA; Baby Aspirin

Pharmacologic Category Antiplatelet Agent; Salicylate

Generic Available Yes: Excludes gum

Use Treatment of mild-to-moderate pain, inflammation, and fever; prevention and treatment of myocardial infarction (MI), acute ischemic stroke, and transient ischemic episodes; management of rheumatoid arthritis, rheumatic fever, osteoarthritis, and gout (high dose); adjunctive therapy in revascularization procedures (coronary artery bypass graft [CABG], percutaneous transluminal coronary angioplasty [PTCA], carotid endarterectomy), stent implantation

Unlabeled/Investigational Use Low doses have been used in the prevention of pre-eclampsia, complications associated with autoimmune disorders such as lupus or antiphospholipid syndrome; alternative therapy for prevention of thromboembolism associated with atrial fibrillation in patients not candidates for warfarin; pericarditis associated with MI; prosthetic valve thromboprophylaxis

◀ **Mechanism of Action** Irreversibly inhibits cyclooxygenase-1 and 2 (COX-1 and 2) enzymes, via acetylation, which results in decreased formation of prostaglandin precursors; irreversibly inhibits formation of prostaglandin derivative, thromboxane A_2, via acetylation of platelet cyclooxygenase, thus inhibiting platelet aggregation; has antipyretic, analgesic, and anti-inflammatory properties

Pharmacodynamics/Kinetics

Duration: 4-6 hours

Absorption: Rapid

Distribution: V_d: 10 L; readily into most body fluids and tissues

Metabolism: Hydrolyzed to salicylate (active) by esterases in GI mucosa, red blood cells, synovial fluid, and blood; metabolism of salicylate occurs primarily by hepatic conjugation; metabolic pathways are saturable

Bioavailability: 50% to 75% reaches systemic circulation

Half-life elimination: Parent drug: 15-20 minutes; Salicylates (dose dependent): 3 hours at lower doses (300-600 mg), 5-6 hours (after 1 g), 10 hours with higher doses

Time to peak, serum: ~1-2 hours

Excretion: Urine (75% as salicyluric acid, 10% as salicylic acid)

Dosage

Children:

Analgesic and antipyretic: Oral, rectal: 10-15 mg/kg/dose every 4-6 hours, up to a total of 4 g/day

Anti-inflammatory: Oral: Initial: 60-90 mg/kg/day in divided doses; usual maintenance: 80-100 mg/kg/day divided every 6-8 hours; monitor serum concentrations

Antiplatelet effects: Adequate pediatric studies have not been performed; pediatric dosage is derived from adult studies and clinical experience and is not well established; suggested doses have ranged from 3-5 mg/kg/day to 5-10 mg/kg/day given as a single daily dose. Doses are rounded to a convenient amount (eg, 1/2 of 81 mg tablet).

Mechanical prosthetic heart valves: 6-20 mg/kg/day given as a single daily dose (used in combination with an oral anticoagulant in children who have systemic embolism despite adequate oral anticoagulation therapy (INR 2.5-3.5) and used in combination with low-dose anticoagulation (INR 2-3) and dipyridamole when full-dose oral anticoagulation is contraindicated)

Blalock-Taussig shunts: 1-5 mg/kg/day given as a single daily dose

Kawasaki disease: Oral: 80-100 mg/kg/day divided every 6 hours; monitor serum concentrations; after fever resolves: 3-5 mg/kg/day once daily; in patients without coronary artery abnormalities, give lower dose for at least 6-8 weeks or until ESR and platelet count are normal; in patients with coronary artery abnormalities, low-dose aspirin should be continued indefinitely

Antirheumatic: Oral: 60-100 mg/kg/day in divided doses every 4 hours

Adults:

Acute ischemic stroke: Oral: 150-325 mg once daily, initiated within 48 hours (in patients who are not candidates for alteplase and not receiving systemic anticoagulation)

Analgesic and antipyretic:

Oral: 325-650 mg every 4-6 hours up to 4 g/day

Rectal: 300-600 mg every 4-6 hours up to 4 g/day

Anti-inflammatory: Oral: Initial: 2.4-3.6 g/day in divided doses; usual maintenance: 3.6-5.4 g/day; monitor serum concentrations

Atrial fibrillation (in patients not candidates for warfarin or at low risk of ischemic stroke): Oral: 75-325 mg once daily

Bioprosthetic aortic valve: Oral: 50-100 mg once daily; usual dose: 81 mg once daily

Bioprosthetic mitral valve (following 3 months of anticoagulation): Oral: 50-100 mg once daily; usual dose: 81 mg once daily

CABG: Oral: 75-100 mg once daily (usual dose: 81 mg) initiated 6 hours following surgery; if bleeding prevents administration at 6 hours after CABG, initiate as soon as possible

CABG (internal mammary bypass graft): Oral: 75-162 mg once daily

Carotid artery stenting: Oral: 81-325 mg once daily beginning at least 24 hours (preferably 4 days) prior to procedure with concomitant clopidogrel

Carotid endarterectomy: Oral: 50-100 mg once daily preoperatively and daily thereafter; usual dose: 81 mg once daily

Infrainguinal arterial reconstruction/bypass: Oral: 75-100 mg once daily (begin preoperatively); usual dose: 81 mg once daily

Mechanical heart valve (with additional risk factors for thromboembolism): Oral: 50-100 mg once daily (in addition to warfarin); usual dose: 81 mg once daily

Mitral annular calcification (with documented stroke, TIA, or systemic embolism): Oral: 50-100 mg once daily; usual dose: 81 mg once daily

Mitral valve prolapse (with documented stroke or TIA): Oral: 50-100 mg once daily; usual dose: 81 mg once daily

Myocardial infarction (primary prevention): Oral: 75-162 mg once daily (Antman, 2004) or 75-100 mg (usual dose: 81 mg) once daily (Hirsh, 2008)

Non-ST-segment elevation myocardial infarction (NSTEMI): Oral: Initial: 162-325 mg; Maintenance: 75-100 mg once daily indefinitely; usual maintenance dose: 81 mg once daily

PCI: Oral: Initial: 75-325 mg (300-325 mg in aspirin naive patients) starting at least 2 hours (preferably 24 hours) before procedure; post procedure: 162-325 mg once daily (dose and duration varies with type of stent implanted); **Note:** Dose may be reduced to 75-162 mg once daily after appropriate duration based on stent-type is complete

Pericarditis associated with myocardial infarction: Oral: 162-325 mg once daily; doses as high as 650 mg every 4-6 hours may be required

Peripheral arterial disease: Oral: 75-100 mg once daily; usual dose: 81 mg once daily

Pre-eclampsia prevention (unlabeled use): Oral: 60-81 mg once daily (usual dose: 81 mg) during gestational weeks 13-26 (patient selection criteria not established)

Prosthetic valve thromboprophylaxis in pregnancy: Oral:75-100 mg once daily; usual dose: 81 mg once daily

ST-segment elevation myocardial infarction (STEMI): Oral: Initial: 162-325 mg given on presentation (patient should chew nonenteric-coated aspirin especially if not taking before presentation); for patients unable to take oral, may use rectal suppository (300 mg). Maintenance (secondary prevention): 75-162 mg once daily indefinitely

Stroke (cardioembolic, anticoagulation contraindicated): Oral: 75-325 mg once daily

Stroke/TIA (noncardioembolic, secondary prevention): Oral: 50-325 mg once daily (Adams, 2008) or 50-100 mg once daily; usual dose: 81 mg once daily (Hirsh, 2008)

Dosing adjustment in renal impairment: Cl_{cr} <10 mL/minute: Avoid use.

Hemodialysis: Dialyzable (50% to 100%)

Dosing adjustment in hepatic disease: Avoid use in severe liver disease.

Stability Keep suppositories in refrigerator; do not freeze. Hydrolysis of aspirin occurs upon exposure to water or moist air, resulting in salicylate and acetate, which possess a vinegar-like odor. Do not use if a strong odor is present.

Administration Do not crush sustained release or enteric coated tablet. Administer with food or a full glass of water to minimize GI distress. For acute myocardial infarction, have patient chew tablet.

Reference Range Timing of serum samples: Peak levels usually occur 2 hours after ingestion. Salicylate serum concentrations correlate with the pharmacological actions and adverse effects observed. The serum salicylate concentration (mcg/mL) and the corresponding clinical correlations are as follows: See table on next page.

Serum Salicylate: Clinical Correlations

Serum Salicylate Concentration (mcg/mL)	Desired Effects	Adverse Effects / Intoxication
~100	Antiplatelet Antipyresis Analgesia	GI intolerance and bleeding, hypersensitivity, hemostatic defects
150-300	Anti-inflammatory	Mild salicylism
250-400	Treatment of rheumatic fever	Nausea/vomiting, hyperventilation, salicylism, flushing, sweating, thirst, headache, diarrhea, and tachycardia
>400-500		Respiratory alkalosis, hemorrhage, excitement, confusion, asterixis, pulmonary edema, convulsions, tetany, metabolic acidosis, fever, coma, cardiovascular collapse, renal and respiratory failure

Pregnancy Risk Factor C/D (full-dose aspirin in 3rd trimester - expert analysis)

Contraindications Hypersensitivity to salicylates, other NSAIDs, or any component of the formulation; asthma; rhinitis; nasal polyps; inherited or acquired bleeding disorders (including factor VII and factor IX deficiency); do not use in children (<16 years of age) for viral infections (chickenpox or flu symptoms), with or without fever, due to a potential association with Reye's syndrome; pregnancy (3rd trimester especially)

Warnings/Precautions Use with caution in patients with platelet and bleeding disorders, renal dysfunction, dehydration, erosive gastritis, or peptic ulcer disease. Heavy ethanol use (>3 drinks/day) can increase bleeding risks. Avoid use in severe renal failure or in severe hepatic failure. Low-dose aspirin for cardioprotective effects is associated with a two- to fourfold increase in UGI events (eg, symptomatic or complicated ulcers); risks of these events increase with increasing aspirin dose; during the chronic phase of aspirin dosing, doses >81 mg are not recommended unless indicated (Bhatt, 2008).

Discontinue use if tinnitus or impaired hearing occurs. Caution in mild-to-moderate renal failure (only at high dosages). Patients with sensitivity to tartrazine dyes, nasal polyps, and asthma may have an increased risk of salicylate sensitivity. In the treatment of acute ischemic stroke, avoid aspirin for 24 hours following administration of alteplase; administration within 24 hours increases the risk of hemorrhagic transformation. Surgical patients should avoid ASA if possible, for 1-2 weeks prior to surgery, to reduce the risk of excessive bleeding (except in patients with cardiac stents that have not completed their full course of dual antiplatelet therapy [aspirin, clopidogrel]; patient-specific situations need to be discussed with cardiologist; AHA/ACC/SCAI/ACS/ADA Science Advisory provides recommendations). When used concomitantly with ≤325 mg of aspirin, NSAIDs (including selective COX-2 inhibitors) substantially increase the risk of gastrointestinal complications (eg, ulcer); concomitant gastroprotective therapy (eg, proton pump inhibitors) is recommended (Bhatt, 2008).

When used for self-medication (OTC labeling): Children and teenagers who have or are recovering from chickenpox or flu-like symptoms should not use this product. Changes in behavior (along with nausea and vomiting) may be an early sign of Reye's syndrome; patients should be instructed to contact their healthcare provider if these occur.

Adverse Reactions As with all drugs which may affect hemostasis, bleeding is associated with aspirin. Hemorrhage may occur at virtually any site. Risk is dependent on multiple variables including dosage, concurrent use of multiple agents which alter hemostasis, and patient susceptibility. Many adverse effects of aspirin are dose related, and are extremely rare at low dosages. Other serious reactions are idiosyncratic, related to allergy or individual sensitivity. Accurate estimation of frequencies is not possible.

Cardiovascular: Hypotension, tachycardia, dysrhythmias, edema

Central nervous system: Fatigue, insomnia, nervousness, agitation, confusion, dizziness, headache, lethargy, cerebral edema, hyperthermia, coma

Dermatologic: Rash, angioedema, urticaria

Endocrine & metabolic: Acidosis, hyperkalemia, dehydration, hypoglycemia (children), hyperglycemia, hypernatremia (buffered forms)

Gastrointestinal: Nausea, vomiting, dyspepsia, epigastric discomfort, heartburn, stomach pain, gastrointestinal ulceration (6% to 31%), gastric erosions, gastric erythema, duodenal ulcers

Hematologic: Anemia, disseminated intravascular coagulation (DIC), prothrombin times prolonged, coagulopathy, thrombocytopenia, hemolytic anemia, bleeding, iron-deficiency anemia

Hepatic: Hepatotoxicity, transaminases increased, hepatitis (reversible)

Neuromuscular & skeletal: Rhabdomyolysis, weakness, acetabular bone destruction (OA)

Otic: Hearing loss, tinnitus

Renal: Interstitial nephritis, papillary necrosis, proteinuria, renal failure (including cases caused by rhabdomyolysis), BUN increased, serum creatinine increased

Respiratory: Asthma, bronchospasm, dyspnea, laryngeal edema, hyperpnea, tachypnea, respiratory alkalosis, noncardiogenic pulmonary edema

Miscellaneous: Anaphylaxis, prolonged pregnancy and labor, stillbirths, low birth weight, peripartum bleeding, Reye's syndrome

Postmarketing and/or case reports: Colonic ulceration, esophageal stricture, esophagitis with esophageal ulcer, esophageal hematoma, oral mucosal ulcers (aspirin-containing chewing gum), coronary artery spasm, conduction defect and atrial fibrillation (toxicity), delirium, ischemic brain infarction, colitis, rectal stenosis (suppository), cholestatic jaundice, periorbital edema, rhinosinusitis

Drug Interactions

Metabolism/Transport Effects Substrate of CYP2C9 (minor)

Avoid Concomitant Use

Avoid concomitant use of Aspirin with any of the following: Ketorolac

Increased Effect/Toxicity

Aspirin may increase the levels/effects of: Alendronate; Anticoagulants; Carbonic Anhydrase Inhibitors; Corticosteroids (Systemic); Drotrecogin Alfa; Heparin; Ibritumomab; Methotrexate; Pralatrexate; Salicylates; Sulfonylureas; Thrombolytic Agents; Tositumomab and Iodine I 131 Tositumomab; Valproic Acid; Varicella Virus-Containing Vaccines; Vitamin K Antagonists

The levels/effects of Aspirin may be increased by: Antidepressants (Tricyclic, Tertiary Amine); Antiplatelet Agents; Calcium Channel Blockers (Nondihydropyridine); Dasatinib; Ginkgo Biloba; Herbs (Anticoagulant/Antiplatelet Properties); Ketorolac; Loop Diuretics; Nonsteroidal Anti-Inflammatory Agents; NSAID (Nonselective); Omega-3-Acid Ethyl Esters; Pentosan Polysulfate Sodium; Pentoxifylline; Prostacyclin Analogues; Selective Serotonin Reuptake Inhibitors; Serotonin/Norepinephrine Reuptake Inhibitors; Treprostinil

Decreased Effect

Aspirin may decrease the levels/effects of: ACE Inhibitors; Loop Diuretics; NSAID (Nonselective); Tiludronate; Uricosuric Agents

The levels/effects of Aspirin may be decreased by: Corticosteroids (Systemic); Nonsteroidal Anti-Inflammatory Agents; NSAID (Nonselective)

Ethanol/Nutrition/Herb Interactions

Ethanol: Avoid ethanol (may enhance gastric mucosal damage).

Food: Food may decrease the rate but not the extent of oral absorption.

Folic acid: Hyperexcretion of folate; folic acid deficiency may result, leading to macrocytic anemia.

Iron: With chronic aspirin use and at doses of 3-4 g/day, iron-deficiency anemia may result.

Sodium: Hypernatremia resulting from buffered aspirin solutions or sodium salicylate containing high sodium content. Avoid or use with caution in CHF or any condition where hypernatremia would be detrimental.

Benedictine liqueur, prunes, raisins, tea, and gherkins: Potential salicylate accumulation.

Fresh fruits containing vitamin C: Displace drug from binding sites, resulting in increased urinary excretion of aspirin.

◀ Herb/Nutraceutical: Avoid cat's claw, dong quai, evening primrose, feverfew, garlic, ginger, ginkgo, red clover, horse chestnut, green tea, ginseng (all have additional antiplatelet activity). Limit curry powder, paprika, licorice; may cause salicylate accumulation. These foods contain 6 mg salicylate/100 g. An ordinary American diet contains 10-200 mg/day of salicylate.

Test Interactions False-negative results for glucose oxidase urinary glucose tests (Clinistix®); false-positives using the cupric sulfate method (Clinitest®); also, interferes with Gerhardt test, VMA determination; 5-HIAA, xylose tolerance test and T_3 and T_4

Dietary Considerations Take with food or large volume of water or milk to minimize GI upset.

Dosage Forms Excipient information presented when available (limited, particularly for generics); consult specific product labeling. [DSC] = Discontinued product
Caplet:
Bayer® Aspirin Extra Strength: 500 mg
Bayer® Aspirin Regimen Regular Strength: 325 mg
Bayer® Genuine Aspirin: 325 mg
Bayer® Plus Extra Strength: 500 mg [contains calcium carbonate]
Bayer® with Heart Advantage: 81 mg [contains phytosterols, tartrazine]
Bayer® Women's Aspirin Plus Calcium: 81 mg [contains elemental calcium 300 mg]
Caplet, buffered:
Ascriptin® Maximum Strength: 500 mg [contains aluminum hydroxide, calcium carbonate, and magnesium hydroxide]
Gum:
Aspergum®: 227 mg [cherry or orange flavor]
Suppository, rectal: 300 mg, 600 mg
Tablet: 325 mg
Aspercin, Aspirtab: 325 mg
Bayer® Genuine Aspirin: 325 mg
Tablet, buffered: 325 mg
Ascriptin®: 325 mg [contains aluminum hydroxide, calcium carbonate, and magnesium hydroxide]
Buffasal: 325 mg [contains magnesium oxide]
Bufferin®: 325 mg [contains calcium carbonate, magnesium oxide, and magnesium carbonate; contains calcium 65 mg/tablet, magnesium 50 mg/tablet]
Bufferin® Extra Strength: 500 mg [contains calcium carbonate, magnesium oxide, and magnesium carbonate; contains calcium 90 mg/tablet, magnesium 70 mg/tablet]
Buffinol: 325 mg [contains magnesium oxide]
Tablet, chewable: 81 mg
Bayer® Aspirin Regimen Children's: 81 mg [cherry or orange flavor]
St. Joseph® Adult Aspirin: 81 mg [orange flavor]
Tablet, controlled release:
ZORprin®: 800 mg
Tablet, delayed release, enteric coated:
Easprin®: 975 mg
Tablet, enteric coated: 81 mg, 325 mg, 500 mg, 650 mg, 975 mg [DSC]
Bayer® Aspirin Regimen Adult Low Dose, Ecotrin® Low Strength, St. Joseph Adult Aspirin: 81 mg
Ecotrin®, Genacote™: 325 mg
Ecotrin® Maximum Strength: 500 mg
Halfprin®: 81 mg, 162 mg

Aspirin and Dipyridamole (AS pir in & dye peer ID a mole)

Medication Safety Issues
Sound-alike/look-alike issues:
Aggrenox® may be confused with Aggrastat®
U.S. Brand Names Aggrenox®
Canadian Brand Names Aggrenox®

Index Terms Aspirin and Extended-Release Dipyridamole; Dipyridamole and Aspirin

Pharmacologic Category Antiplatelet Agent

Generic Available No

Use Reduction in the risk of stroke in patients who have had transient ischemia of the brain or ischemic stroke due to thrombosis

Unlabeled/Investigational Use Hemodialysis graft patency

Mechanism of Action The antithrombotic action results from additive antiplatelet effects. Dipyridamole inhibits the uptake of adenosine into platelets, endothelial cells, and erythrocytes. Aspirin inhibits platelet aggregation by irreversible inhibition of platelet cyclooxygenase and thus inhibits the generation of thromboxane A_2.

Pharmacodynamics/Kinetics See individual agents.

Dosage Oral: Adults:

Stroke prevention: One capsule (dipyridamole 200 mg, aspirin 25 mg) twice daily

Alternative regimen for patients with intolerable headache: One capsule at bedtime and low-dose aspirin in the morning. Return to usual dose (1 capsule twice daily) as soon as tolerance to headache develops (usually within a week).

Hemodialysis graft patency (unlabeled use): One capsule (dipyridamole 200 mg, aspirin 25 mg) twice daily

Dosage adjustment in renal impairment: Avoid use in patients with severe renal dysfunction (Cl_{cr} <10 mL/minute). Studies have not been done in patients with renal impairment.

Dosage adjustment in hepatic impairment: Avoid use in patients with severe hepatic impairment. Studies have not been done in patients with varying degrees of hepatic impairment.

Elderly: Plasma concentrations were 40% higher, but specific dosage adjustments have not been recommended.

Stability Store at 25°C (77°F); excursions permitted to 15°C to 30°C (59°F to 86°F). Protect from excessive moisture.

Administration Capsule should be swallowed whole; do not crush or chew. May be administered with or without food.

Monitoring Parameters Hemoglobin, hematocrit, signs or symptoms of bleeding, signs or symptoms of stroke or transient ischemic attack

Pregnancy Risk Factor D

Contraindications Hypersensitivity to dipyridamole, aspirin, or any component of the formulation; allergy to NSAIDs; patients with the syndrome of asthma, rhinitis, and nasal polyps; children <16 years of age with viral infections; pregnancy (third trimester; aspirin)

Additional Canadian contraindications (not in U.S. labeling): Patients with hereditary fructose and/or galactose intolerance

Warnings/Precautions Patients who consume ≥3 alcoholic drinks per day may be at risk of bleeding. Use cautiously use in patients with inherited or acquired bleeding disorders, renal impairment, hypotension, unstable angina, recent MI or hepatic dysfunction. Avoid use in patients with a history of active peptic ulcer disease, severe hepatic failure, or severe renal impairment (Cl_{cr} <10 mL/minute). Monitor for signs and symptoms of GI ulcers and bleeding. Discontinue use if dizziness, tinnitus, or impaired hearing occurs. Discontinue use 24 hours prior to pharmacologic (I.V. dipyridamole) stress testing. Discontinue 1-2 weeks before elective surgical procedures to reduce the risk of bleeding. Use caution in the elderly who are at high risk for adverse events. Dose of aspirin in this combination may not be adequate to prevent for cardiac indications (eg, MI prophylaxis). Avoid use in children due to risk of Reye's syndrome in certain viral illness associated with aspirin component. Formulation may contain lactose and/or sucrose. Use in patients with fructose and/or galactose intolerance is contraindicated in the Canadian labeling.

Adverse Reactions

>10%:

Central nervous system: Headache (39%; tolerance usually develops)

Gastrointestinal: Abdominal pain (18%), dyspepsia (18%), nausea (16%), diarrhea (13%)

◀ 1% to 10%:
Cardiovascular: Cardiac failure (2%), syncope (1%)
Central nervous system: Fatigue (6%), pain (6%), amnesia (2%), malaise (2%), seizure (2%), confusion (1%), somnolence (1%)
Dermatologic: Purpura (1%)
Gastrointestinal: Vomiting (8%), GI bleeding (4%), melena (2%), rectal bleeding (2%), hemorrhoids (1%), GI hemorrhage (1%), anorexia (1%)
Hematologic: Hemorrhage (3%), anemia (2%)
Neuromuscular & skeletal: Arthralgia (6%), back pain (5%), weakness (2%), arthritis (2%), arthrosis (1%), myalgia (1%)
Respiratory: Cough (2%), epistaxis (2%), upper respiratory tract infection (1%)
<1% (Limited to important or life-threatening): Agitation, allergic reaction, allergic vasculitis, alopecia, anaphylaxis, anemia (aplastic), angina pectoris, angioedema, antepartum and postpartum bleeding, arrhythmia, asthma, bronchospasm, bruising, cerebral edema, cerebral hemorrhage, chest pain, cholelithiasis, coagulopathy, coma, deafness, dehydration, disseminated intravascular coagulation (DIC), dizziness, dyspnea, ecchymosis, fever, flushing, gastritis, gastrointestinal perforation, gastrointestinal ulceration, gingival bleeding, hearing impairment, hematemesis, hematoma, hematuria, hemoptysis, hepatic function abnormality, hepatic failure, hepatitis, hyper-/hypoglycemia, hyper-/hypokalemia, hyperpnea, hypotension, hypothermia, interstitial nephritis, intracranial hemorrhage, jaundice, laryngeal edema, metabolic acidosis, migraine, palpitation, pancreatitis, pancytopenia, papillary necrosis, paresthesia, PT time prolonged, proteinuria, pruritus, pulmonary edema, rash, renal failure, renal insufficiency, respiratory alkalosis, Reye's syndrome, rhabdomyolysis, Stevens-Johnson syndrome, subarachnoid hemorrhage, supraventricular tachycardia, tachycardia, tachypnea, taste loss, thirst, thrombocytopenia, thrombocytosis, tinnitus, urticaria, uterine hemorrhage

Drug Interactions

Metabolism/Transport Effects Aspirin: **Substrate** of CYP2C9 (minor)

Avoid Concomitant Use

Avoid concomitant use of Aspirin and Dipyridamole with any of the following: Dabigatran Etexilate; Ketorolac; Silodosin

Increased Effect/Toxicity

Aspirin and Dipyridamole may increase the levels/effects of: Adenosine; Alendronate; Anticoagulants; Beta-Blockers; Carbonic Anhydrase Inhibitors; Colchicine; Corticosteroids (Systemic); Dabigatran Etexilate; Drotrecogin Alfa; Heparin; Hypotensive Agents; Ibritumomab; Methotrexate; P-Glycoprotein Substrates; Pralatrexate; Regadenoson; Rivaroxaban; Salicylates; Silodosin; Sulfonylureas; Thrombolytic Agents; Topotecan; Tositumomab and Iodine I 131 Tositumomab; Valproic Acid; Varicella Virus-Containing Vaccines; Vitamin K Antagonists

The levels/effects of Aspirin and Dipyridamole may be increased by: Antidepressants (Tricyclic, Tertiary Amine); Antiplatelet Agents; Calcium Channel Blockers (Nondihydropyridine); Dasatinib; Ginkgo Biloba; Herbs (Anticoagulant/Antiplatelet Properties); Ketorolac; Loop Diuretics; Nonsteroidal Anti-Inflammatory Agents; NSAID (Nonselective); Omega-3-Acid Ethyl Esters; Pentosan Polysulfate Sodium; Pentoxifylline; Prostacyclin Analogues; Selective Serotonin Reuptake Inhibitors; Serotonin/Norepinephrine Reuptake Inhibitors; Treprostinil

Decreased Effect

Aspirin and Dipyridamole may decrease the levels/effects of: ACE Inhibitors; Loop Diuretics; NSAID (Nonselective); Tiludronate; Uricosuric Agents

The levels/effects of Aspirin and Dipyridamole may be decreased by: Corticosteroids (Systemic); Nonsteroidal Anti-Inflammatory Agents; NSAID (Nonselective)

Ethanol/Nutrition/Herb Interactions Ethanol: Avoid ethanol (due to GI irritation).

Dietary Considerations May be taken with or without food.

Dosage Forms Excipient information presented when available (limited, particularly for generics); consult specific product labeling.

Capsule, variable release:
Aggrenox®: Aspirin 25 mg (immediate release) and dipyridamole 200 mg (extended release) [contains lactose, sucrose]

References

Albers GW, Amarenco P, Easton JD, et al, "Antithrombotic and Thrombolytic Therapy for Ischemic Stroke: American College of Chest Physicians Evidence-Based Clinical Practice Guidelines (8th Edition)," *Chest*, 2008, 133(6 Suppl):630-69.

◆ **Aspirin and Extended-Release Dipyridamole** *see* Aspirin and Dipyridamole *on page 152*

◆ **Aspirin Free Anacin® Extra Strength [OTC]** *see* Acetaminophen *on page 25*

◆ **Aspirtab [OTC]** *see* Aspirin *on page 147*

◆ **Astelin®** *see* Azelastine *on page 168*

◆ **Astepro®** *see* Azelastine *on page 168*

◆ **Astramorph/PF™** *see* Morphine Sulfate *on page 953*

◆ **AT** *see* Antithrombin III *on page 127*

◆ **AT-III** *see* Antithrombin III *on page 127*

◆ **Atacand®** *see* Candesartan *on page 237*

◆ **Atasol® (Can)** *see* Acetaminophen *on page 25*

Atenolol (a TEN oh lole)

Related Information

Antiarrhythmic Drugs *on page 1656*
Beta-Blockers *on page 1669*
Preoperative Evaluation of the Cardiac Patient for Noncardiac Surgery *on page 1598*

U.S. Brand Names Tenormin®

Canadian Brand Names Apo-Atenolol®; Gen-Atenolol; Mylan-Atenolol; Novo-Atenol; Nu-Atenol; PMS-Atenolol; RAN™-Atenolol; Rhoxal-atenolol; Riva-Atenolol; Sandoz-Atenolol; Tenolin; Tenormin®

Pharmacologic Category Beta Blocker, Beta$_1$ Selective

Use Treatment of hypertension, alone or in combination with other agents; management of angina pectoris; secondary prevention postmyocardial infarction

Unlabeled/Investigational Use Acute ethanol withdrawal, supraventricular and ventricular arrhythmias, and migraine headache prophylaxis

Pharmacodynamics/Kinetics

Onset of action: Peak effect: Oral: 2-4 hours
Duration: Normal renal function: 12-24 hours
Absorption: Oral: Rapid, incomplete (~50%)
Distribution: Low lipophilicity; does not cross blood-brain barrier
Protein binding: 6% to 16%
Metabolism: Limited hepatic
Half-life elimination: Beta:
Neonates: ≤35 hours; Mean: 16 hours
Children: 4.6 hours; children >10 years may have longer half-life (>5 hours) compared to children 5-10 years (<5 hours)
Adults: Normal renal function: 6-7 hours, prolonged with renal impairment; End-stage renal disease: 15-35 hours
Time to peak, plasma: Oral: 2-4 hours
Excretion: Feces (50%); urine (40% as unchanged drug)

Dosage Oral:

Children: Hypertension: 0.5-1 mg/kg/dose given daily; range of 0.5-1.5 mg/kg/day; maximum dose: 2 mg/kg/day up to 100 mg/day
Adults:
Hypertension: 25-50 mg once daily, may increase to 100 mg/day. Doses >100 mg are unlikely to produce any further benefit.
Angina pectoris: 50 mg once daily, may increase to 100 mg/day. Some patients may require 200 mg/day.
Postmyocardial infarction: 100 mg/day or 50 mg twice daily for 6-9 days postmyocardial infarction.

Dosing interval for oral atenolol in renal impairment:
Cl_{cr} 15-35 mL/minute: Administer 50 mg/day maximum.
Cl_{cr} <15 mL/minute: Administer 50 mg every other day maximum.
Hemodialysis: Moderately dialyzable (20% to 50%) via hemodialysis; administer dose postdialysis or administer 25-50 mg supplemental dose.
Peritoneal dialysis: Elimination is not enhanced; supplemental dose is not necessary.

Anesthesia and Critical Care Concerns/Other Considerations Atenolol may mask signs and symptoms of hypoglycemia; may potentiate hypoglycemia in patients with diabetes.

Evidence-Based Information:
Surgery: Based on available evidence, beta-blockers should be started days to weeks before elective surgery in selected patients when possible and titrated to a heart rate <65 beats per minute. Additional data suggest that long acting beta-blockers may be superior to short acting ones (Redelmeier, 2005). The ACC/AHA 2007 guidelines on perioperative cardiovascular evaluation and care for noncardiac surgery recommend beta-blockers be continued in patients undergoing surgery who are receiving beta-blockers to treat angina, symptomatic arrhythmias, hypertension, or other ACC/AHA Class I guideline indications (Class I recommendation). The guidelines also recommend that beta-blockers be given to patients undergoing vascular surgery who have myocardial ischemia demonstrated during preoperative testing (Class I recommendation).

The guidelines also state that beta-blockers are probably recommended in patients undergoing intermediate risk (eg, carotid endarterectomy, prostate surgery) or vascular surgery in whom preoperative assessment identifies coronary heart disease or high cardiac risk (Class IIa recommendation). High cardiac risk is defined as having >1 of the following clinical risk factors: History of ischemic heart disease, compensated or prior heart failure, cerebrovascular disease, diabetes mellitus, or renal insufficiency. The use of beta-blockers is uncertain in patients undergoing intermediate risk or vascular surgery with ≤1 clinical risk factor (Class IIb recommendation).

The majority of published trials suggest a benefit of perioperative beta-blocker use during noncardiac surgery especially in high-risk patients; however, more recent clinical trials have not shown a benefit to perioperative beta-blockade for noncardiac surgery (Juul, 2006; Yang, 2006).

Additional Information Complete prescribing information for this medication should be consulted for additional detail.

Dosage Forms Excipient information presented when available (limited, particularly for generics); consult specific product labeling.
Tablet: 25 mg, 50 mg, 100 mg
Tenormin®: 25 mg, 50 mg, 100 mg

References

Fleisher LA, Beckman JA, Brown KA, et al, "ACC/AHA 2006 Guideline Update on Perioperative Cardiovascular Evaluation for Noncardiac Surgery: Focused Update on Perioperative Beta-Blocker Therapy: A Report of the American College of Cardiology/American Heart Association Task Force on Practice Guidelines (Writing Committee to Update the 2002 Guidelines on Perioperative Cardiovascular Evaluation for Noncardiac Surgery) Developed in Collaboration With the American Society of Echocardiography, American Society of Nuclear Cardiology, Heart Rhythm Society, Society of Cardiovascular Anesthesiologists, Society for Cardiovascular Angiography and Interventions, and Society for Vascular Medicine and Biology," *J Am Coll Cardiol*, 2006, 47 (11):2343-55.

Juul AB, Wetterslev J, Gluud C, et al, "Effect of Perioperative Beta-Blockade in Patients With Diabetes Undergoing Major Noncardiac Surgery: Randomized Placebo Controlled, Blinded Multicentre Trial," *BMJ*, 2006, 332(7556):1482.

Lindenauer PK, Pekow P, Wang K, et al, "Perioperative Beta-Blocker Therapy and Mortality After Major Noncardiac Surgery," *N Engl J Med*, 2005, 353(4):349-61.

Mangano DT, Layug EL, Wallace A, et al, "Effect of Atenolol on Mortality and Cardiovascular Morbidity After Noncardiac Surgery. Multicenter Study of Perioperative Ischemia Research Group," *N Engl J Med*, 1996, 335(23):1713-20.

Radack K and Deck C, "Beta-Adrenergic Blocker Therapy Does Not Worsen Intermittent Claudication in Subjects With Peripheral Arterial Disease. A Meta-Analysis of Randomized Controlled Trials," *Arch Intern Med*, 1991, 151(9):1769-76.

Yang H, Raymer K, Butler R, et al, "The Effects of Perioperative Beta-Blockade: Results of the Metoprolol After Vascular Surgery (MaVS) Study, A Randomized Controlled Trial," *Am Heart J* 2006, 152(5):983-90.

♦ **Ativan®** *see* LORazepam *on page 852*

Atomoxetine (AT oh mox e teen)

U.S. Brand Names Strattera®

Canadian Brand Names Strattera®

Index Terms Atomoxetine Hydrochloride; LY139603; Methylphenoxy-Benzene Propanamine; Tomoxetine

Pharmacologic Category Norepinephrine Reuptake Inhibitor, Selective

Use Treatment of attention deficit/hyperactivity disorder (ADHD)

Pharmacodynamics/Kinetics
Absorption: Rapid
Distribution: V_d: I.V.: 0.85 L/kg
Protein binding: 98%, primarily albumin
Metabolism: Hepatic, via CYP2D6 and CYP2C19; forms metabolites (4-hydroxyatomoxetine, active, equipotent to atomoxetine; N-desmethylatomoxetine in poor metabolizers, limited activity)
Bioavailability: 63% in extensive metabolizers; 94% in poor metabolizers
Half-life elimination: Atomoxetine: 5 hours (up to 24 hours in poor metabolizers); Active metabolites: 4-hydroxyatomoxetine: 6-8 hours; N-desmethylatomoxetine: 6-8 hours (34-40 hours in poor metabolizers)
Time to peak, plasma: 1-2 hours
Excretion: Urine (80%, as conjugated 4-hydroxy metabolite); feces (17%)

Dosage Oral: **Note:** Atomoxetine may be discontinued without the need for tapering dose.
Children ≥6 years and ≤70 kg: ADHD: Initial: 0.5 mg/kg/day, increase after minimum of 3 days to ~1.2 mg/kg/day; may administer as either a single daily dose or 2 evenly divided doses in morning and late afternoon/early evening. Maximum daily dose: 1.4 mg/kg or 100 mg, whichever is less.
Dosage adjustment in patients receiving strong CYP2D6 inhibitors (eg, paroxetine, fluoxetine, quinidine) or patients known to be CYP2D6 poor metabolizers: Do not exceed 1.2 mg/kg/day; dose adjustments should occur only after 4 weeks.
Children ≥6 years and >70 kg and Adults: ADHD: Initial: 40 mg/day, increased after minimum of 3 days to ~80 mg/day; may administer as either a single daily dose or two evenly divided doses in morning and late afternoon/early evening. May increase to 100 mg/day in 2-4 additional weeks to achieve optimal response.
Dosage adjustment in patients receiving strong CYP2D6 inhibitors (eg, paroxetine, fluoxetine, quinidine) or patients known to be CYP2D6 poor metabolizers: Do not exceed 80 mg/day; dose adjustments should occur only after 4 weeks.
Elderly: Use has not been evaluated in the elderly

Dosage adjustment in renal impairment: No adjustment needed

Dosage adjustment in hepatic impairment:
Moderate hepatic insufficiency (Child-Pugh class B): All doses should be reduced to 50% of normal
Severe hepatic insufficiency (Child-Pugh class C): All doses should be reduced to 25% of normal

Additional Information Complete prescribing information for this medication should be consulted for additional detail.

Dosage Forms Excipient information presented when available (limited, particularly for generics); consult specific product labeling.
Capsule:
Strattera®: 10 mg, 18 mg, 25 mg, 40 mg, 60 mg, 80 mg, 100 mg

♦ **Atomoxetine Hydrochloride** *see* Atomoxetine *on page 157*

Atorvastatin (a TORE va sta tin)

Related Information
Hyperlipidemia Management *on page 1747*
Preoperative Evaluation of the Cardiac Patient for Noncardiac Surgery *on page 1598*

U.S. Brand Names Lipitor®
Canadian Brand Names Lipitor®
Index Terms Atorvastatin Calcium
Pharmacologic Category Antilipemic Agent, HMG-CoA Reductase Inhibitor
Use Treatment of dyslipidemias or primary prevention of cardiovascular disease (atherosclerotic) as detailed below:

Primary prevention of cardiovascular disease (high-risk for CVD): To reduce the risk of MI or stroke in patients without evidence of heart disease who have multiple CVD risk factors or type 2 diabetes. Treatment reduces the risk for angina or revascularization procedures in patients with multiple risk factors.

Secondary prevention of cardiovascular disease: To reduce the risk of MI, stroke, revascularization procedures, and angina in patients with evidence of coronary heart disease. To reduce the risk of hospitalization for heart failure.

Treatment of dyslipidemias: To reduce elevations in total cholesterol (C), LDL-C, apolipoprotein B, and triglycerides in patients with elevations of one or more components, and/or to increase low HDL-C as present in Fredrickson type IIa, IIb, III, and IV hyperlipidemias, heterozygous familial and nonfamilial hypercholesterolemia, and homozygous familial hypercholesterolemia

Treatment of heterozygous familial hypercholesterolemia (HeFH) in adolescent patients (10-17 years of age, females >1 year postmenarche) having LDL-C ≥190 mg/dL or LDL-C ≥160 mg/dL with positive family history of premature cardiovascular disease (CVD) or with two or more CVD risk factors.

Pharmacodynamics/Kinetics
Onset of action: Initial changes: 3-5 days; Maximal reduction in plasma cholesterol and triglycerides: 2 weeks

Absorption: Rapid

Distribution: V_d: ~381 L

Protein binding: ≥98%

Metabolism: Hepatic; forms active ortho- and parahydroxylated derivates and an inactive beta-oxidation product

Bioavailability: ~14% (parent drug); ~30% (parent drug and equipotent metabolites)

Half-life elimination: Parent drug: 14 hours; Equipotent metabolites: 20-30 hours
Time to peak, serum: 1-2 hours

Excretion: Bile; urine (<2% as unchanged drug)

Dosage Oral: **Note:** Doses should be individualized according to the baseline LDL-cholesterol levels, the recommended goal of therapy, and patient response; adjustments should be made at intervals of 2-4 weeks (4 weeks for children)

Children 10-17 years (females >1 year postmenarche): HeFH: 10 mg once daily (maximum: 20 mg/day)

Adults:

Hypercholesterolemia (heterozygous familial and nonfamilial) and mixed hyperlipidemia (Fredrickson types IIa and IIb): Initial: 10-20 mg once daily; patients requiring >45% reduction in LDL-C may be started at 40 mg once daily; range: 10-80 mg once daily

Homozygous familial hypercholesterolemia: 10-80 mg once daily

Dosage adjustment for atorvastatin with concomitant medications:

Cyclosporine: Atorvastatin dose should not exceed 10 mg/day

Clarithromycin, itraconazole, ritonavir plus saquinavir, or lopinavir plus ritonavir when atorvastatin dose >20 mg: Ensure that the lowest dose necessary of atorvastatin is used.

Dosing adjustment in renal impairment: No dosage adjustment is necessary.
Dosing adjustment in hepatic impairment: Contraindicated in active liver disease or in patients with unexplained persistent elevations of serum transaminases.

Anesthesia and Critical Care Concerns/Other Considerations
Evidence-Based Information:
Myopathy: Currently-marketed HMG-CoA reductase inhibitors appear to have a similar potential for causing myopathy. Incidence of severe myopathy is about 0.08% to 0.09%. The factors that increase risk include advanced age (especially >80 years), gender (occurs in women more frequently than men), small body frame, frailty, multisystem disease (eg, chronic renal insufficiency especially due to diabetes), multiple medications, and drug interactions (use with caution or avoid).

Perioperative use: Based on current research and clinical guidelines (Fleisher, 2007), HMG-CoA reductase inhibitors should be continued in the perioperative period. Postoperative discontinuation of statin therapy is associated with an increased risk of cardiac morbidity and mortality.

Additional Information Complete prescribing information for this medication should be consulted for additional detail.

Dosage Forms Excipient information presented when available (limited, particularly for generics); consult specific product labeling.
Tablet:
Lipitor®: 10 mg, 20 mg, 40 mg, 80 mg

References
Pasternak RC, Smith SC Jr, Bairey-Merz CN, et al, "ACC/AHA/NHLBI Clinical Advisory on the Use and Safety of Statins," *Stroke*, 2002, 33(9):2337-41. Available at: http://www.acc.org/clinical/alerts/statins_june02.htm. Accessed June 18, 2003.

◆ **Atorvastatin Calcium** *see* Atorvastatin *on page 158*

Atracurium (a tra KYOO ree um)

Medication Safety Issues
High alert medication: The Institute for Safe Medication Practices (ISMP) includes this medication among its list of drugs which have a heightened risk of causing significant patient harm when used in error.

United States Pharmacopeia (USP) 2006: The Interdisciplinary Safe Medication Use Expert Committee of the USP has recommended the following:
- Hospitals, clinics, and other practice sites should institute special safeguards in the storage, labeling, and use of these agents and should include these safeguards in staff orientation and competency training.
- Healthcare professionals should be on high alert (especially vigilant) whenever a neuromuscular-blocking agent (NMBA) is stocked, ordered, prepared, or administered.

Related Information
Allergic Reactions *on page 1508*
Anesthesia for Geriatric Patients *on page 1523*
Anesthesia for Patients With Liver Disease *on page 1537*
Chronic Renal Failure *on page 1552*
Dosing Considerations for the Critically-Ill Patient With Morbid Obesity *on page 1561*
Neuromuscular-Blocking Agents *on page 1684*

Canadian Brand Names Atracurium Besylate Injection

Index Terms Atracurium Besylate

Pharmacologic Category Neuromuscular Blocker Agent, Nondepolarizing

Generic Available Yes

Use Adjunct to general anesthesia to facilitate endotracheal intubation and to relax skeletal muscles during surgery; to facilitate mechanical ventilation in ICU patients; does not relieve pain or produce sedation

Mechanism of Action Blocks neural transmission at the myoneural junction by binding with cholinergic receptor sites

Pharmacodynamics/Kinetics
Onset of action (dose dependent): 2-3 minutes
Duration: Recovery begins in 20-35 minutes following initial dose of 0.4-0.5 mg/kg under balanced anesthesia; recovery to 95% of control takes 60-70 minutes
Metabolism: Undergoes ester hydrolysis and Hofmann elimination (nonbiologic process independent of renal, hepatic, or enzymatic function); metabolites have

no neuromuscular blocking properties; laudanosine, a product of Hofmann elimination, is a CNS stimulant and can accumulate with prolonged use. Laudanosine is hepatically metabolized.

Half-life elimination: Biphasic: Adults: Initial (distribution): 2 minutes; Terminal: 20 minutes

Excretion: Urine (<5%)

Dosage I.V. (not to be used I.M.): Dose to effect; doses must be individualized due to interpatient variability; use ideal body weight for obese patients

Children 1 month to 2 years: Initial: 0.3-0.4 mg/kg followed by maintenance doses as needed to maintain neuromuscular blockade

Children >2 years to Adults: 0.4-0.5 mg/kg, then 0.08-0.1 mg/kg 20-45 minutes after initial dose to maintain neuromuscular block, followed by repeat doses of 0.08-0.1 mg/kg at 15- to 25-minute intervals

Initial dose after succinylcholine for intubation (balanced anesthesia): Adults: 0.2-0.4 mg/kg

Pretreatment/priming: 10% of intubating dose given 3-5 minutes before initial dose

Continuous infusion:

Surgery: Initial: 9-10 mcg/kg/minute at initial signs of recovery from bolus dose; block usually maintained by a rate of 5-9 mcg/kg/minute under balanced anesthesia

ICU: Block usually maintained by rate of 11-13 mcg/kg/minute (rates for pediatric patients may be higher)

See table.

Atracurium Besylate Infusion Chart

Drug Delivery Rate (mcg/kg/min)	Infusion Rate (mL/kg/min) 0.2 mg/mL (20 mg/100 mL)	Infusion Rate (mL/kg/min) 0.5 mg/mL (50 mg/100 mL)
5	0.025	0.01
6	0.03	0.012
7	0.035	0.014
8	0.04	0.016
9	0.045	0.018
10	0.05	0.02

Dosage adjustment for hepatic or renal impairment is not necessary

Stability Refrigerate intact vials at 2°C to 8°C (36°F to 46°F); protect from freezing. Use vials within 14 days upon removal from the refrigerator to room temperature of 25°C (77°F). Dilutions of 0.2 mg/mL or 0.5 mg/mL in 0.9% sodium chloride, dextrose 5% in water, or 5% dextrose in sodium chloride 0.9% are stable for up to 24 hours at room temperature or under refrigeration. Atracurium should not be mixed with alkaline solutions.

Administration May be given undiluted as a bolus injection; not for I.M. injection due to tissue irritation; administration via infusion requires the use of an infusion pump; use infusion solutions within 24 hours of preparation

Monitoring Parameters Vital signs (heart rate, blood pressure, respiratory rate); degree of muscle relaxation (via peripheral nerve stimulator and presence of spontaneous movement); renal function (serum creatinine, BUN) and liver function when in ICU

In the ICU setting, prolonged paralysis and generalized myopathy, following discontinuation of agent, may be minimized by appropriately monitoring degree of blockade.

Anesthesia and Critical Care Concerns/Other Considerations

Evidence-Based Information: Atracurium is classified as an intermediate duration neuromuscular-blocking agent; does not appear to have a cumulative effect on the duration of blockade, synergistic effect when combined with steroidal-based nondepolarizing neuromuscular muscle relaxants (Meretoja, 1994).

Critically-Ill Adult Patients:

The 2008 Surviving Sepsis Campaign guidelines recommend avoiding use of neuromuscular blockers if at all possible in the septic patient due to the risk of prolonged neuromuscular blockade following discontinuation. If one is required, monitor the depth of blockade (Grade 1B).

The 2002 ACCM/SCCM/ASHP clinical practice guidelines for sustained neuro-muscular blockade in the adult critically-ill patient recommend:

Optimize sedatives and analgesics prior to initiation, and monitor and adjust accordingly during course. Neuromuscular blockers do not relieve pain or produce sedation.

Protect patient's eyes from development of keratitis and corneal abrasion by administering ophthalmic ointment and taping eyelids closed or using eye patches. Reposition patient routinely to protect pressure points from break-down. Address DVT prophylaxis.

Concurrent use of a neuromuscular blocker and corticosteroids appear to increase the risk of certain ICU myopathies; avoid or administer the corticosteroid at the lowest dose possible. Reassess need for neuromuscular blocker daily.

Using daily drug holidays (stopping neuromuscular-blocking agent until patient requires it again) may decrease the incidence of acute quadriplegic myopathy syndrome.

Tachyphylaxis can develop.

Acidosis and severe hypothermia may delay elimination.

Atracurium or cisatracurium is recommended for patients with significant hepatic or renal disease due to organ-independent Hofmann elimination and ester hydrolysis.

Monitor patients clinically and via "Train of Four" (TOF) testing with a goal of adjusting the degree of blockade to 1-2 twitches.

Pregnancy Risk Factor C

Contraindications Hypersensitivity to atracurium besylate or any component of the formulation

Warnings/Precautions Reduce initial dosage and inject slowly (over 1-2 minutes) in patients in whom substantial histamine release would be potentially hazardous (eg, patients with clinically-important cardiovascular disease). Maintenance of an adequate airway and respiratory support is critical. Certain clinical conditions may result in potentiation or antagonism of neuromuscular blockade:

Potentiation: Electrolyte abnormalities, severe hyponatremia, severe hypocalce-mia, severe hypokalemia, hypermagnesemia, neuromuscular diseases, acidosis, acute intermittent porphyria, renal failure, hepatic failure

Antagonism: Alkalosis, hypercalcemia, demyelinating lesions, peripheral neuro-pathies, diabetes mellitus

Increased sensitivity in patients with myasthenia gravis, Eaton-Lambert syndrome; resistance in burn patients (>30% of body) for period of 5-70 days postinjury; resistance in patients with muscle trauma, denervation, immobilization, infection, chronic treatment with atracurium. Cross-sensitivity with other neuro-muscular-blocking agents may occur; use extreme caution in patients with previous anaphylactic reactions. Use caution in the elderly. Bradycardia may be more common with atracurium than with other neuromuscular-blocking agents since it has no clinically-significant effects on heart rate to counteract the bradycardia produced by anesthetics. Should be administered by adequately trained individuals familiar with its use. Some dosage forms may contain benzyl alcohol which has been associated with "gasping syndrome" in neonates.

Adverse Reactions Mild, rare, and generally suggestive of histamine release

1% to 10%: Cardiovascular: Flushing

<1%: Bronchial secretions, erythema, hives, itching, wheezing

Postmarketing and/or case reports: Allergic reaction, bradycardia, bronchospasm, dyspnea, hypotension, injection site reaction, seizure, acute quadriplegic myopathy syndrome (prolonged use), laryngospasm, myositis ossificans (prolonged use), tachycardia, urticaria

Causes of prolonged neuromuscular blockade: Excessive drug administra-tion; cumulative drug effect, metabolism/excretion decreased (hepatic and/or renal impairment); accumulation of active metabolites; electrolyte imbalance (hypokalemia, hypocalcemia, hypermagnesemia, hypernatremia); hypothermia ▶

◄ **Drug Interactions**
  Avoid Concomitant Use
    Avoid concomitant use of Atracurium with any of the following: QuiNINE
  Increased Effect/Toxicity
    Atracurium may increase the levels/effects of: Cardiac Glycosides; Cortico-steroids (Systemic); OnabotulinumtoxinA; RimabotulinumtoxinB

    The levels/effects of Atracurium may be increased by: AbobotulinumtoxinA; Aminoglycosides; Calcium Channel Blockers; Capreomycin; Colistimethate; Inhalational Anesthetics; Ketorolac; Lincosamide Antibiotics; Lithium; Loop Diuretics; Magnesium Salts; Polymyxin B; Procainamide; QuiNIDine; QuiNINE; Spironolactone; Tetracycline Derivatives; Vancomycin
  Decreased Effect
    The levels/effects of Atracurium may be decreased by: Acetylcholinesterase Inhibitors; Loop Diuretics
Dosage Forms Excipient information presented when available (limited, particularly for generics); consult specific product labeling.
    Injection, as besylate: 10 mg/mL (10 mL) [contains benzyl alcohol]
    Injection, as besylate [preservative free]: 10 mg/mL (5 mL)
References
  Dellinger RP, Levy MM, Carlet JM, et al, "Surviving Sepsis Campaign: International Guidelines for Management of Severe Sepsis and Septic Shock: 2008," *Intensive Care Med*, 2008, 34(1): 17-60. Available at http://www.survivingsepsis.org/system/files/images/2008_20International_20SSC_20-Guidelines_1_.pdf.

  Meretoja OA, Taivainen T, Jalkanen L, et al, "Synergism Between Atracurium and Vecuronium in Infants and Children During Nitrous Oxide-Oxygen-Alfentanil Anaesthesia," *Br J Anaesth*, 1994, 73 (5):605-7.

  Murray MJ, Cowen J, DeBlock H, et al, "Clinical Practice Guidelines for Sustained Neuromuscular Blockade in the Adult Critically Ill Patient. Task Force of the American College of Critical Care Medicine (ACCM) of the Society of Critical Care Medicine (SCCM), American Society of Health-System Pharmacists, American College of Chest Physicians," *Crit Care Med*, 2002, 30(1):142-56. Available at: http://www.sccm.org/pdf/NeuromuscularBlockade.pdf. Accessed August 6, 2003.

  Peat SJ, Potter DR, and Hunter JM, "The Prolonged Use of Atracurium in a Patient With Tetanus," *Anaesthesia*, 1988, 43(11):962-3.

  Yate PM, Flynn PJ, Arnold RW, et al, "Clinical Experience and Plasma Laudanosine Concentrations During the Infusion of Atracurium in the Intensive Therapy Unit," *Br J Anaesth*, 1987, 59(2):211-7.

◆ **Atracurium Besylate** *see* Atracurium *on page* 159

◆ **Atracurium Besylate Injection (Can)** *see* Atracurium *on page* 159

◆ **AtroPen®** *see* Atropine *on page* 162

Atropine (A troe peen)

Medication Safety Issues
  International issues:
    Genatropine® [France] may be confused with Genotropin®
Related Information
  Anesthetic Considerations in the Substance-Abusing Patient *on page* 1613
  Cycloplegic Mydriatics *on page* 1679
  Management of Postoperative Arrhythmias *on page* 1571
  Porphyria: Safe and Unsafe Drugs *on page* 1800
U.S. Brand Names AtroPen®; Atropine-Care®; Isopto® Atropine; Sal-Tropine™
Canadian Brand Names Dioptic's Atropine Solution; Isopto® Atropine
Index Terms Atropine Sulfate
Pharmacologic Category Anticholinergic Agent; Anticholinergic Agent, Ophthalmic; Antidote; Antispasmodic Agent, Gastrointestinal; Ophthalmic Agent, Mydriatic
Restrictions The AtroPen® formulation is available for use primarily by the Department of Defense.
Generic Available Yes: Excludes tablet
Use
  Injection: Preoperative medication to inhibit salivation and secretions; treatment of symptomatic sinus bradycardia, AV block (nodal level); antidote for acetylcholinesterase inhibitor poisoning (carbamate insecticides, nerve agents, organophosphate insecticides); adjuvant use with anticholinesterases (eg, edrophonium, neostigmine) to decrease their side effects during reversal of neuromuscular blockade

Ophthalmic: Produce mydriasis and cycloplegia for examination of the retina and optic disc and accurate measurement of refractive errors; uveitis

Oral: Inhibit salivation and secretions

Unlabeled/Investigational Use Pulseless electric activity, asystole

Mechanism of Action Blocks the action of acetylcholine at parasympathetic sites in smooth muscle, secretory glands, and the CNS; increases cardiac output, dries secretions. Atropine reverses the muscarinic effects of cholinergic poisoning. The primary goal in cholinergic poisonings is reversal of bronchorrhea and bronchoconstriction. Atropine has no effect on the nicotinic receptors responsible for muscle weakness, fasciculations, and paralysis.

Pharmacodynamics/Kinetics

Onset of action: I.V.: Rapid

Absorption: Complete

Distribution: Widely throughout the body; crosses placenta; trace amounts enter breast milk; crosses blood-brain barrier

Metabolism: Hepatic

Half-life elimination: 2-3 hours

Excretion: Urine (30% to 50% as unchanged drug and metabolites)

Dosage

Neonates, Infants, and Children: Doses <0.1 mg have been associated with paradoxical bradycardia.

Inhibit salivation and secretions (preanesthesia): Oral, I.M., I.V., SubQ:

<5 kg: 0.02 mg/kg/dose 30-60 minutes preop then every 4-6 hours as needed. Use of a minimum dosage of 0.1 mg in neonates <5 kg will result in dosages >0.02 mg/kg. There is no documented minimum dosage in this age group.

>5 kg: 0.01-0.02 mg/kg/dose to a maximum 0.4 mg/dose 30-60 minutes preop; minimum dose: 0.1 mg

Alternate dosing:

3-7 kg (7-16 lb): 0.1 mg

8-11 kg (17-24 lb): 0.15 mg

11-18 kg (24-40 lb): 0.2 mg

18-29 kg (40-65 lb): 0.3 mg

>30 kg (>65 lb): 0.4 mg

Bradycardia: I.V., intratracheal: 0.02 mg/kg, minimum dose 0.1 mg, maximum single dose: 0.5 mg in children and 1 mg in adolescents; may repeat in 5-minute intervals to a maximum total dose of 1 mg in children or 2 mg in adolescents. (**Note:** For intratracheal administration, the dosage must be diluted with normal saline to a total volume of 1-5 mL). When treating bradycardia in neonates, reserve use for those patients unresponsive to improved oxygenation and epinephrine.

Infants and Children: Nerve agent toxicity management: See **Note** under adult dosing.

Prehospital ("in the field"): I.M.:

Birth to <2 years: Mild-to-moderate symptoms: 0.05 mg/kg; severe symptoms: 0.1 mg/kg

2-10 years: Mild-to-moderate symptoms: 1 mg; severe symptoms: 2 mg

>10 years: Mild-to-moderate symptoms: 2 mg; severe symptoms: 4 mg

Hospital/emergency department: I.M.:

Birth to <2 years: Mild-to-moderate symptoms: 0.05 mg/kg I.M. **or** 0.02 mg/kg I.V.; severe symptoms: 0.1 mg/kg I.M. **or** 0.02 mg/kg I.V.

2-10 years: Mild-to-moderate symptoms: 1 mg; severe symptoms: 2 mg

>10 years: Mild-to-moderate symptoms: 2 mg; severe symptoms: 4 mg

Note: Pralidoxime is a component of the management of nerve agent toxicity; consult Pralidoxime for specific route and dose. For prehospital ("in the field") management, repeat atropine I.M. (children: 0.05-0.1 mg/kg) at 5-10 minute intervals until secretions have diminished and breathing is comfortable or airway resistance has returned to near normal. For hospital management, repeat atropine I.M. (infants 1 mg; all others: 2 mg) at 5-10 minute intervals until secretions have diminished and breathing is comfortable or airway resistance has returned to near normal.

Children: Organophosphate or carbamate poisoning:

I.V.: 0.03-0.05 mg/kg every 10-20 minutes until atropine effect, then every 1-4 hours for at least 24 hours

I.M. (AtroPen®): Mild symptoms: Administer dose listed below as soon as exposure is known or suspected. If severe symptoms develop after first dose, 2 additional doses should be repeated in 10 minutes; do not administer more than 3 doses. Severe symptoms: Immediately administer 3 doses as follows:

<6.8 kg (15 lb): Use of **AtroPen® formulation not recommended;** administer atropine 0.05 mg/kg

6.8-18 kg (15-40 lb): 0.5 mg/dose

18-41 kg (40-90 lb): 1 mg/dose

>41 kg (>90 lb): 2 mg/dose

Adults (doses <0.5 mg have been associated with paradoxical bradycardia):

Asystole or pulseless electrical activity:

I.V.: 1 mg; repeat in 3-5 minutes if asystole persists; total dose of 0.04 mg/kg.

Intratracheal: Administer 2-2.5 times the recommended I.V. dose; dilute in 10 mL NS or distilled water. **Note:** Absorption is greater with distilled water, but causes more adverse effects on PaO_2.

Inhibit salivation and secretions (preanesthesia):

I.M., I.V., SubQ: 0.4-0.6 mg 30-60 minutes preop and repeat every 4-6 hours as needed

Oral: 0.4 mg; may repeat in 4 hours if necessary; 0.4 mg initial dose may be exceeded in certain cases and may repeat in 4 hours if necessary

Bradycardia: I.V.: 0.5-1 mg every 5 minutes, not to exceed a total of 3 mg or 0.04 mg/kg; may give intratracheally in 10 mL NS (intratracheal dose should be 2-2.5 times the I.V. dose)

Neuromuscular blockade reversal: I.V.: 25-30 mcg/kg 30-60 seconds before neostigmine or 7-10 mcg/kg 30-60 seconds before edrophonium

Organophosphate or carbamate poisoning: **Note:** The dose of atropine required varies considerably with the severity of poisoning. Total amount of atropine used in carbamate poisoning is usually less. Severely poisoned patients may exhibit significant tolerance to atropine; ≥2 times the suggested doses may be needed. Titrate to pulmonary status (decreased bronchial secretions). Once patient is stable for a period of time, the dose/dosing frequency may be decreased. If atropinization occurs after 1-2 mg of atropine then re-evaluate working diagnosis.

I.V.: Initial: 1-5 mg; doses should be doubled every 5 minutes until signs of muscarinic excess abate (clearing of bronchial secretions, bronchospasm, and adequate oxygenation). Overly aggressive dosing may cause anti-cholinergic toxicity (eg, delirium, hyperthermia, and muscle twitching).

I.V. Infusion: 0.5-1 mg/hour or 10% to 20% of loading dose/hour

I.M. (AtroPen®): Mild symptoms: Administer 2 mg as soon as exposure is known or suspected. If severe symptoms develop after first dose, 2 additional doses should be repeated in 10 minutes; do not administer more than 3 doses. Severe symptoms: Immediately administer three 2 mg doses.

Nerve agent toxicity management: I.M.: See **Note**. Prehospital ("in the field") or hospital/emergency department: Mild-to-moderate symptoms: 2-4 mg; severe symptoms: 6 mg

Note: Pralidoxime is a component of the management of nerve agent toxicity; consult Pralidoxime for specific route and dose. For prehospital ("in the field") management, repeat atropine I.M. (2 mg) at 5-10 minute intervals until secretions have diminished and breathing is comfortable or airway resistance has returned to near normal. For hospital management, repeat atropine I.M. (2 mg) at 5-10 minute intervals until secretions have diminished and breathing is comfortable or airway resistance has returned to near normal.

Mydriasis, cycloplegia (preprocedure): Ophthalmic (1% solution): Instill 1-2 drops 1 hour before procedure.

Uveitis: Ophthalmic:

1% solution: Instill 1-2 drops 4 times/day

Ointment: Apply a small amount in the conjunctival sac up to 3 times/day; compress the lacrimal sac by digital pressure for 1-3 minutes after instillation

Elderly, frail patients: Nerve agent toxicity management (unlabeled use): I.M.: See **Note** under adult dosing.

Prehospital ("in the field"): Mild-to-moderate symptoms: 1 mg; severe symptoms: 2-4 mg

Hospital/emergency department: Mild-to-moderate symptoms: 1 mg; severe symptoms: 2 mg

Stability Store injection at controlled room temperature of 15°C to 30°C (59°F to 86°F); avoid freezing. In addition, AtroPen® should be protected from light.

Administration

I.M.: AtroPen®: Administer to outer thigh. May be given through clothing as long as pockets at the injection site are empty. Hold autoinjector in place for 10 seconds following injection; massage the injection site.

I.V.: Administer undiluted by rapid I.V. injection; slow injection may result in paradoxical bradycardia.

Intratracheal: Dilute in NS or distilled water. Absorption is greater with distilled water, but causes more adverse effects on PaO_2. Pass catheter beyond tip of tracheal tube, stop compressions, spray drug quickly down tube. Follow immediately with several quick insufflations and continue chest compressions.

Monitoring Parameters Heart rate, blood pressure, pulse, mental status; intravenous administration requires a cardiac monitor

Anesthesia and Critical Care Concerns/Other Considerations Atropine, at usual recommended cardiovascular doses, causes blockade of muscarinic receptors at the cardiac SA-node and is parasympatholytic (ie, blocks vagal activity increasing heart rate). A dose 0.5-1 mg is recommended for the treatment of bradyarrhythmias. In administering atropine, it is important to recognize that lower doses (<0.5 mg) in adults may have vagalmimetic effects (ie, increase vagal tone causing paradoxical bradycardia). A total dose of 3 mg (0.04 mg/kg) results in full vagal blockade in adults. In the absence of vascular access, atropine can be administered intratracheally.

Pregnancy Risk Factor C

Contraindications Hypersensitivity to atropine or any component of the formulation; narrow-angle glaucoma; adhesions between the iris and lens; tachycardia; obstructive GI disease; paralytic ileus; intestinal atony of the elderly or debilitated patient; severe ulcerative colitis; toxic megacolon complicating ulcerative colitis; hepatic disease; obstructive uropathy; renal disease; myasthenia gravis (unless used to treat side effects of acetylcholinesterase inhibitor); asthma; thyrotoxicosis; Mobitz type II block

Warnings/Precautions Use with caution in children with spastic paralysis; use with caution in elderly patients. Low doses cause a paradoxical decrease in heart rates. Some commercial products contain sodium metabisulfite, which can cause allergic-type reactions. May accumulate with multiple inhalational administration, particularly in the elderly. Heat prostration may occur in hot weather. Use with caution in patients with autonomic neuropathy, prostatic hyperplasia, hyperthyroidism, HF, cardiac arrhythmias, chronic lung disease, biliary tract disease; anticholinergic agents are generally not well tolerated in the elderly and their use should be avoided when possible. Atropine is rarely used except as a preoperative agent or in the acute treatment of bradyarrhythmias.

AtroPen®: There are no absolute contraindications for the use of atropine in severe organophosphate poisonings, however in mild poisonings, use caution in those patients where the use of atropine would be otherwise contraindicated. Formulation for use by trained personnel only.

Adverse Reactions Severity and frequency of adverse reactions are dose related and vary greatly; listed reactions are limited to significant and/or life-threatening.

Cardiovascular: Arrhythmia, flushing, hypotension, palpitation, tachycardia

Central nervous system: Ataxia, coma, delirium, disorientation, dizziness, drowsiness, excitement, fever, hallucinations, headache, insomnia, nervousness

Dermatologic: Anhidrosis, urticaria, rash, scarlatiniform rash

Gastrointestinal: Bloating, constipation, delayed gastric emptying, loss of taste, nausea, paralytic ileus, vomiting, xerostomia, dry throat, nasal dryness

Genitourinary: Urinary hesitancy, urinary retention

Neuromuscular & skeletal: Weakness

Ocular: Angle-closure glaucoma, blurred vision, cycloplegia, dry eyes, mydriasis, ocular tension increased

Respiratory: Dyspnea, laryngospasm, pulmonary edema

Miscellaneous: Anaphylaxis

Drug Interactions

Avoid Concomitant Use There are no known interactions where it is recommended to avoid concomitant use.

Increased Effect/Toxicity

Atropine may increase the levels/effects of: Anticholinergics; Cannabinoids; Potassium Chloride

The levels/effects of Atropine may be increased by: Pramlintide

Decreased Effect

Atropine may decrease the levels/effects of: Acetylcholinesterase Inhibitors (Central); Secretin

The levels/effects of Atropine may be decreased by: Acetylcholinesterase Inhibitors (Central)

Dosage Forms Excipient information presented when available (limited, particularly for generics); consult specific product labeling.

Injection, solution, as sulfate: 0.05 mg/mL (5 mL); 0.1 mg/mL (5 mL, 10 mL); 0.4 mg/0.5 mL (0.5 mL); 0.4 mg/mL (0.5 mL, 1 mL, 20 mL); 1 mg/mL (1 mL)

AtroPen®: 0.25 mg/0.3 mL (0.3 mL); 0.5 mg/0.7 mL (0.7 mL); 1 mg/0.7 mL (0.7 mL); 2 mg/0.7 mL (0.7 mL) [prefilled autoinjector]

Ointment, ophthalmic, as sulfate: 1% (3.5 g)

Solution, ophthalmic, as sulfate: 1% (2 mL, 5 mL, 15 mL)

Atropine-Care®: 1% (2 mL) [contains benzalkonium chloride]

Isopto® Atropine: 1% (5 mL, 15 mL) [contains benzalkonium chloride]

Tablet, as sulfate:

Sal-Tropine™: 0.4 mg

References

American Heart Association, "2005 American Heart Association (AHA) Guidelines for Cardiopulmonary Resuscitation (CPR) and Emergency Cardiovascular Care (ECC) of Pediatric and Neonatal Patients: Pediatric Basic Life Support," *Pediatrics*, 2006, 117(5):e989-1004.

Eisenberg MS and Mengert TJ, "Cardiac Resuscitation," *N Engl J Med*, 2001, 344(17):1304-13.

Emergency Cardiac Care Committee and Subcommittees, "2005 American Heart Association Guidelines for Cardiopulmonary Resuscitation and Emergency Cardiac Care," *Circulation*, 2005, 112(24 Suppl):V1-203.

"Medical Management Guidelines (MMGs) for Nerve Agents: Tabun (GA); Sarin (GB); Soman (GD); and VX". Available at: www.atsdr.cdc.gov/MHMI/mmg166.html.

Mokhlesi B, Leikin JB, Murray P, et al, "Adult Toxicology in Critical Care. Part 11:Specific Poisonings," *Chest*, 2003, 123(3):897-922.

- **Axert®** *see Almotriptan on page 63*
- **Axid®** *see Nizatidine on page 1022*
- **Axid® AR [OTC]** *see Nizatidine on page 1022*
- **Ayr® Allergy Sinus [OTC]** *see Sodium Chloride on page 1304*
- **Ayr® Baby Saline [OTC]** *see Sodium Chloride on page 1304*
- **Ayr® Saline [OTC]** *see Sodium Chloride on page 1304*
- **Ayr® Saline No-Drip [OTC]** *see Sodium Chloride on page 1304*
- **Azactam®** *see Aztreonam on page 174*
- **Azasan®** *see AzaTHIOprine on page 167*
- **AzaSite®** *see Azithromycin on page 169*

AzaTHIOprine (ay za THYE oh preen)

U.S. Brand Names Azasan®; Imuran®
Canadian Brand Names Alti-Azathioprine; Apo-Azathioprine®; Gen-Azathioprine; Imuran®; Mylan-Azathioprine; Novo-Azathioprine
Index Terms Azathioprine Sodium
Pharmacologic Category Immunosuppressant Agent
Use Adjunctive therapy in prevention of rejection of kidney transplants; management of active rheumatoid arthritis (RA)
Unlabeled/Investigational Use Adjunct in prevention of rejection of solid organ (nonrenal) transplants; steroid-sparing agent for corticosteroid-dependent Crohn's disease (CD) and ulcerative colitis (UC); maintenance of remission in CD; fistulizing Crohn's disease

Pharmacodynamics/Kinetics
Absorption: Oral: Well absorbed
Distribution: Crosses placenta
Protein binding: ~30%
Metabolism: Hepatic, to 6-mercaptopurine (6-MP), possibly by glutathione S-transferase (GST). Further metabolism of 6-MP (in the liver and GI tract), via three major pathways: Hypoxanthine guanine phosphoribosyltransferase (to 6-thioguanine-nucleotides, or 6-TGN), xanthine oxidase (to 6-thiouric acid), and thiopurine methyltransferase (TPMT), which forms 6-methylmercapotpurine (6-MMP).
Half-life elimination: Parent drug: 12 minutes; mercaptopurine: 0.7-3 hours; End-stage renal disease: Slightly prolonged
Time to peak, plasma: 1-2 hours (including metabolites)
Excretion: Urine (primarily as metabolites)

Dosage Note: Patients with intermediate TPMT activity may be at risk for increased myelosuppression; those with low or absent TPMT activity receiving conventional azathioprine doses are at risk for developing severe, life-threatening myelotoxicity. Dosage reductions are recommended for patients with reduced TPMT activity.

I.V. dose is equivalent to oral dose (dosing should be transitioned from I.V. to oral as soon as tolerated):
Children (unlabeled) and Adults:
Renal transplantation (treatment usually started the day of transplant, however, has been initiated [rarely] 1-3 days prior to transplant): Oral, I.V.: Initial: 3-5 mg/kg/day usually given as a single daily dose, then 1-3 mg/kg/day maintenance
Rheumatoid arthritis: Oral:
Initial: 1 mg/kg/day given once daily or divided twice daily for 6-8 weeks; increase by 0.5 mg/kg every 4 weeks until response or up to 2.5 mg/kg/day; an adequate trial should be a minimum of 12 weeks
Maintenance dose: Reduce dose by 0.5 mg/kg every 4 weeks until lowest effective dose is reached; optimum duration of therapy not specified; may be discontinued abruptly
Adults: Oral:
Adjunctive management of severe recurrent aphthous stomatitis (unlabeled use): 50 mg once daily in conjunction with prednisone

Reduction of steroid use in CD or UC, maintenance of remission in CD or fistulizing disease (unlabeled uses): Initial: 50 mg once daily; may increase by 25 mg/day every 1-2 weeks as tolerated to target dose of 2-3 mg/kg/day

Dosage adjustment for concomitant use with allopurinol: Reduce azathioprine dose to one-third or one-fourth the usual dose when used concurrently with allopurinol. Patients with low or absent TPMT activity may require further dose reductions or discontinuation.

Dosage adjustment for toxicity:

Rapid WBC count decrease, persistently low WBC count, or serious infection: Reduce dose or temporarily withhold treatment

Severe toxicity in renal transplantation: May require discontinuation

Hepatic veno-occlusive disease: Permanently discontinue

Dosing adjustment in renal impairment: Although dosage reductions are recommended, specific guidelines are not available in the FDA-approved labeling; the following guidelines have been used by some clinicians (Aronoff, 2007):

Cl_{cr} >50 mL/minute: No adjustment recommended

Cl_{cr} 10-50 mL/minute: Administer 75% of normal dose

Cl_{cr} <10 mL/minute: Administer 50% of normal dose

Hemodialysis (dialyzable; ~45% removed in 8 hours): Children: Administer 50% of normal dose; Adults: Supplement: 0.25 mg/kg

CAPD: Children: Administer 50% of normal dose; Adults: Unknown

CRRT: Children and Adults: Administer 75% of normal dose

Additional Information Complete prescribing information for this medication should be consulted for additional detail.

Dosage Forms Excipient information presented when available (limited, particularly for generics); consult specific product labeling.

Injection, powder for reconstitution: 100 mg

Tablet [scored]: 50 mg

Azasan®: 75 mg, 100 mg

Imuran®: 50 mg

References

Baum D, Bernstein D, Starnes VA, et al, "Pediatric Heart Transplantation at Stanford: Results of a 15-Year Experience," *Pediatrics*, 1991, 88(2):203-14.

Lichtenstein GR, Abreu MT, Cohen R, et al, "American Gastroenterological Association Institute Medical Position Statement on Corticosteroids, Immunomodulators, and Infliximab in Inflammatory Bowel Disease," *Gastroenterology*, 2006, 130(3):935-9.

◆ **Azathioprine Sodium** *see* AzaTHIOprine *on page 167*

Azelastine (a ZEL as teen)

U.S. Brand Names Astelin®; Astepro®; Optivar®

Canadian Brand Names Astelin®

Index Terms Azelastine Hydrochloride

Pharmacologic Category Histamine H_1 Antagonist; Histamine H_1 Antagonist, Second Generation

Use

Nasal spray: Treatment of the symptoms of seasonal allergic rhinitis such as rhinorrhea, sneezing, and nasal pruritus; treatment of the symptoms of vasomotor rhinitis

Ophthalmic: Treatment of itching of the eye associated with seasonal allergic conjunctivitis

Pharmacodynamics/Kinetics

Onset of action: Peak effect: Nasal spray: 3 hours; Ophthalmic solution: 3 minutes

Duration: Nasal spray: 12 hours; Ophthalmic solution: 8 hours

Distribution: V_d: 14.5 L/kg

Protein binding: Azelastine: 88%; Desmethylazelastine: 97%

Metabolism: Hepatic via CYP; active metabolite, desmethylazelastine

Bioavailability: Intranasal: 40%

Half-life elimination: Intranasal: Azelastine: 22 hours; Desmethylazelastine: 52 hours

Time to peak, serum: 2-3 hours

Excretion: Feces (75 %, <10% as unchanged drug)

Dosage

Intranasal:

Seasonal allergic rhinitis:

Children 5-11 years (Astelin®): 1 spray in each nostril twice daily

Children ≥12 years and Adults (Astelin®, Astepro®): 1-2 sprays in each nostril twice daily

Vasomotor rhinitis: Children ≥12 years and Adults (Astelin®): 2 sprays in each nostril twice daily

Ophthalmic: Children ≥3 years and Adults: Instill 1 drop into affected eye(s) twice daily.

Additional Information Complete prescribing information for this medication should be consulted for additional detail.

Dosage Forms Excipient information presented when available (limited, particularly for generics); consult specific product labeling.

Solution, intranasal, as hydrochloride [spray]:

Astelin®: 1 mg/mL (30 mL) [contains benzalkonium chloride; 137 mcg/spray; 200 metered sprays]

Astepro®: 1 mg/mL (30 mL) [contains benzalkonium chloride; 137 mcg/spray; 200 metered sprays]

Astepro®: 1.5 mg/mL (30 mL) [contains benzalkonium chloride; 205.5 mcg/spray; 200 metered sprays]

Solution, ophthalmic, as hydrochloride:

Optivar®: 0.05% (6 mL) [contains benzalkonium chloride]

References

Dykewicz MS, Fineman S, Nicklas R, et al, "Diagnosis and Management of Rhinitis: Complete Guidelines of the Joint Task Force on Practice Parameters in Allergy, Asthma and Immunology. American Academy of Allergy, Asthma, and Immunology," *Ann Allergy Asthma Immunol*, 1998, 81(5 Pt 2):478-518.

♦ **Azelastine Hydrochloride** *see* Azelastine *on page 168*

♦ **Azilect®** *see* Rasagiline *on page 1236*

Azithromycin (az ith roe MYE sin)

Medication Safety Issues

Sound-alike/look-alike issues:

Azithromycin may be confused with azathioprine, erythromycin

Zithromax® may be confused with Fosamax®, Zinacef®, Zovirax®

Related Information

Prevention of Wound Infection and Sepsis in Surgical Patients *on page 1721*

U.S. Brand Names AzaSite®; Zithromax®; Zmax®

Canadian Brand Names Apo-Azithromycin®; CO Azithromycin; Dom-Azithromycin; GEN-Azithromycin; Mylan-Azithromycin; Novo-Azithromycin; PHL-Azithromycin; PMS-Azithromycin; PRO-Azithromycin; ratio-Azithromycin; Riva-Azithromycin; Sandoz-Azithromycin; Zithromax®

Index Terms Azithromycin Dihydrate; Azithromycin Hydrogencitrate; Azithromycin Monohydrate; Z-Pak; Zithromax® TRI-PAK™; Zithromax® Z-PAK®

Pharmacologic Category Antibiotic, Macrolide; Antibiotic, Ophthalmic

Generic Available Yes: Injection, powder for oral suspension (excludes extended release microspheres), tablet

Use

Oral, I.V.: Treatment of acute otitis media due to *H. influenzae*, *M. catarrhalis*, or *S. pneumoniae*; pharyngitis/tonsillitis due to *S. pyogenes*; treatment of mild-to-moderate upper and lower respiratory tract infections, infections of the skin and skin structure, community-acquired pneumonia, pelvic inflammatory disease (PID), sexually-transmitted diseases (urethritis/cervicitis); pharyngitis/tonsillitis (alternative to first-line therapy), and genital ulcer disease (chancroid) due to susceptible strains of *Chlamydophila pneumoniae, C. trachomatis, M. catarrhalis, H. influenzae, S. aureus, S. pneumoniae, Mycoplasma pneumoniae,* and *C. psittaci*; acute bacterial exacerbations of chronic obstructive pulmonary disease (COPD) due to *H. influenzae, M. catarrhalis,* or *S. pneumoniae*; acute bacterial sinusitis

Ophthalmic: Bacterial conjunctivitis

◀ **Unlabeled/Investigational Use** Prevention of (or to delay onset of) or treatment of MAC in patients with advanced HIV infection; prophylaxis of infective endocarditis in patients who are allergic to penicillin and undergoing surgical or dental procedures; pertussis

Mechanism of Action Inhibits RNA-dependent protein synthesis at the chain elongation step; binds to the 50S ribosomal subunit resulting in blockage of transpeptidation

Pharmacodynamics/Kinetics

Absorption: Oral: Rapid; Ophthalmic: Negligible

Distribution: Extensive tissue; distributes well into skin, lungs, sputum, tonsils, and cervix; penetration into CSF is poor; I.V.: 33.3 L/kg; Oral: 31.1 L/kg

Protein binding (concentration dependent): Oral, I.V.: 7% to 51%

Metabolism: Hepatic

Bioavailability: Oral: 38%, decreased by 17% with extended release suspension; variable effect with food (increased with immediate or delayed release oral suspension, unchanged with tablet)

Half-life elimination: Oral, I.V.: Terminal: Immediate release: 68-72 hours; Extended release: 59 hours

Time to peak, serum: Oral: Immediate release: 2-3 hours; Extended release: 5 hours

Excretion: Oral, I.V.: Biliary (major route); urine (6%)

Dosage Note: Extended release suspension (Zmax®) is not interchangeable with immediate release formulations. Use should be limited to approved indications. All doses are expressed as immediate release azithromycin unless otherwise specified.

Usual dosage range:

Children ≥6 months: Oral: 5-12 mg/kg given once daily (maximum: 500 mg/day) **or** 30 mg/kg as a single dose (maximum: 1500 mg)

Extended release suspension (Zmax®): 60 mg/kg as a single dose; **Note:** Extended release suspension (Zmax®): Dose in mL is equal to the weight in lbs for patients <75 lbs (34 kg). Pediatric patients ≥75 lbs should receive the adult dose.

Children ≥1 year and Adults: Ophthalmic: Instill 1 drop into affected eye(s) twice daily (8-12 hours apart) for 2 days, then 1 drop once daily for 5 days

Adolescents ≥16 years and Adults:

Oral: 250-600 mg once daily **or** 1-2 g as a single dose

Extended release suspension (Zmax®): 2 g as a single dose

I.V.: 250-500 mg once daily

Indication-specific dosing:

Children: Oral:

Bacterial sinusitis: 10 mg/kg once daily for 3 days (maximum: 500 mg/day)

Cat scratch disease (unlabeled use): <45.5 kg: 10 mg/kg as a single dose, then 5 mg/kg once daily for 4 days

Community-acquired pneumonia: 10 mg/kg on day 1 (maximum: 500 mg/day) followed by 5 mg/kg/day once daily on days 2-5 (maximum: 250 mg/day)

Extended release suspension (Zmax®):

<75 lbs (34 kg): 60 mg/kg as a single dose; dose in mL is equal to the weight in lbs for patients <75 lbs (34 kg)

≥75 lbs (34 kg): Refer to adult dose

Disseminated _M. avium_ (unlabeled use):

HIV-infected patients: 5 mg/kg/day once daily (maximum: 250 mg/day) or 20 mg/kg (maximum: 1200 mg) once weekly given alone or in combination with rifabutin

Treatment and secondary prevention in HIV-negative patients: 5 mg/kg/day once daily (maximum: 250 mg/day) in combination with ethambutol, with or without rifabutin

Prophylaxis against infective endocarditis (unlabeled use): 15 mg/kg 30-60 minutes before procedure (maximum: 500 mg). **Note:** American Heart Association (AHA) guidelines now recommend prophylaxis only in patients undergoing invasive procedures and in whom underlying cardiac conditions may predispose to a higher risk of adverse outcomes should infection occur.

As of April 2007, routine prophylaxis for GI/GU procedures is no longer recommended by the AHA.

Otitis media:

1-day regimen: 30 mg/kg as a single dose (maximum: 1500 mg)

3-day regimen: 10 mg/kg once daily for 3 days (maximum: 500 mg/day)

5-day regimen: 10 mg/kg on day 1 (maximum: 500 mg/day) followed by 5 mg/kg/day once daily on days 2-5 (maximum: 250 mg/day)

Pharyngitis, tonsillitis: Children ≥2 years: 12 mg/kg/day once daily for 5 days (maximum: 500 mg/day)

Pertussis (CDC guidelines):

Children <6 months: 10 mg/kg/day for 5 days

Children ≥6 months: 10 mg/kg on day 1 (maximum: 500 mg/day) followed by 5 mg/kg/day once daily on days 2-5 (maximum: 250 mg/day)

Uncomplicated chlamydial urethritis or cervicitis (unlabeled use): Children ≥45 kg: 1 g as a single dose

Children ≥1 year and Adults: Ophthalmic:

Bacterial conjunctivitis: Instill 1 drop into affected eye(s) twice daily (8-12 hours apart) for 2 days, then 1 drop once daily for 5 days

Adolescents ≥16 years and Adults:

Bacterial sinusitis: Oral: 500 mg/day for a total of 3 days

Extended release suspension (Zmax®): 2 g as a single dose

Cat scratch disease (unlabeled use): Oral: >45.5 kg: 500 mg as a single dose, then 250 mg once daily for 4 days

Chancroid due to *H. ducreyi*: Oral: 1 g as a single dose

Community-acquired pneumonia:

Oral: Extended release suspension (Zmax®): 2 g as a single dose

I.V.: 500 mg as a single dose for at least 2 days, follow I.V. therapy by the oral route with a single daily dose of 500 mg to complete a 7- to 10-day course of therapy.

Disseminated *M. avium* complex disease in patients with advanced HIV infection (unlabeled use): Oral:

Prophylaxis: 1200 mg once weekly (may be combined with rifabutin)

Treatment: 600 mg daily (in combination with ethambutol 15 mg/kg)

Prophylaxis against infective endocarditis (unlabeled use): Oral: 500 mg 30-60 minutes prior to the procedure. **Note:** American Heart Association (AHA) guidelines now recommend prophylaxis only in patients undergoing invasive procedures and in whom underlying cardiac conditions may predispose to a higher risk of adverse outcomes should infection occur. As of April 2007, routine prophylaxis for GI/GU procedures is no longer recommended by the AHA.

Mild-to-moderate respiratory tract, skin, and soft tissue infections: Oral: 500 mg in a single loading dose on day 1 followed by 250 mg/day as a single dose on days 2-5

Alternative regimen: Bacterial exacerbation of COPD: 500 mg/day for a total of 3 days

Pelvic inflammatory disease (PID): I.V.: 500 mg as a single dose for 1-2 days, follow I.V. therapy by the oral route with a single daily dose of 250 mg to complete a 7-day course of therapy

Pertussis (CDC guidelines): Oral: 500 mg on day 1 followed by 250 mg/day on days 2-5 (maximum: 500 mg/day)

Urethritis/cervicitis: Oral:

Due to C. trachomatis: 1 g as a single dose

Due to N. gonorrhoeae: 2 g as a single dose

Dosage adjustment in renal impairment: Use caution in patients with GFR <10 mL/minute

Dosage adjustment in hepatic impairment: Use with caution due to potential for hepatotoxicity (rare). Specific guidelines for dosing in hepatic impairment have not been established.

Stability

Injection (Zithromax®): Store intact vials of injection at room temperature. Reconstitute the 500 mg vial with 4.8 mL of sterile water for injection and shake until all of the drug is dissolved. Each mL contains 100 mg azithromycin. Reconstituted solution is stable for 24 hours when stored below 30°C (86°F).

Use of a standard syringe is recommended due to the vacuum in the vial (which may draw additional solution through an automated syringe).

The initial solution should be further diluted to a concentration of 1 mg/mL (500 mL) to 2 mg/mL (250 mL) in 0.9% sodium chloride, 5% dextrose in water, or lactated Ringer's. The diluted solution is stable for 24 hours at or below room temperature (30°C or 86°F) and for 7 days if stored under refrigeration (5°C or 41°F).

Ophthalmic solution: Prior to use, store unopened under refrigeration at 2°C to 8°C (36°F to 46°F). After opening, store at 2°C to 25°C (36°F to 77°F) for ≤14 days; discard any remaining solution after 14 days.

Suspension, immediate release (Zithromax®): Store dry powder below 30°C (86°F). Following reconstitution, store at 5°C to 30°C (41°F to 86°F).

Suspension, extended release (Zmax®): Store dry powder ≤30°C (86°F). Following reconstitution, store at 25°C (77°F); excursions permitted to 15°C to 30°C (59°F to 86°F); do not refrigerate or freeze. Should be consumed within 12 hours following reconstitution.

Tablet (Zithromax®): Store between 15°C to 30°C (59°F to 86°F).

Administration

I.V.: Infusate concentration and rate of infusion for azithromycin for injection should be either 1 mg/mL over 3 hours or 2 mg/mL over 1 hour. Other medications should not be infused simultaneously through the same I.V. line.

Ophthalmic: Shake bottle once prior to each administration. Wash hands before and after instillation.

Oral: Immediate release suspension and tablet may be taken without regard to food; extended release suspension should be taken on an empty stomach (at least 1 hour before or 2 hours following a meal), within 12 hours of reconstitution.

Monitoring Parameters Liver function tests, CBC with differential

Pregnancy Risk Factor B

Contraindications Hypersensitivity to azithromycin, other macrolide (eg, azalide or ketolide) antibiotics, or any component of the formulation

Warnings/Precautions Use with caution in patients with pre-existing liver disease; hepatic impairment, including hepatocellular and/or cholestatic hepatitis, with or without jaundice, has been observed. Discontinue if symptoms of malaise, nausea, vomiting, abdominal colic, and fever. Allergic reactions have been reported (rare); reappearance of allergic reaction may occur without further azithromycin exposure. May mask or delay symptoms of incubating gonorrhea or syphilis, so appropriate culture and susceptibility tests should be performed prior to initiating azithromycin. Prolonged use may result in fungal or bacterial superinfection, including *C. difficile*-associated diarrhea (CDAD) and pseudomembranous colitis; CDAD has been observed >2 months postantibiotic treatment. Use caution with renal dysfunction. Prolongation of the QT_c interval has been reported with macrolide antibiotics; use caution in patients at risk of prolonged cardiac repolarization. Use with caution in patients with myasthenia gravis. Safety and efficacy of systemically-administered azithromycin (oral, intravenous) have not been established in children <6 months of age with acute otitis media, acute bacterial sinusitis, or community-acquired pneumonia, or in children <2 years of age with pharyngitis/tonsillitis.

Ophthalmic solution should not be injected subconjunctivally or introduced directly into the anterior chamber of the eye. Ophthalmic solution contains benzalkonium chloride which may be absorbed by contact lenses; contact lens should not be worn during treatment of ophthalmic infections. Safety and efficacy for ophthalmic use have not been established in children <1 year of age.

Oral suspensions (immediate release and extended release) are not interchangeable.

Adverse Reactions

>10%: Gastrointestinal: Diarrhea (4% to 9%; high single-dose regimens 12% to 14%), nausea (≤7%; high single-dose regimens 18%)

2% to 10%:

Dermatologic: Pruritus, rash

Gastrointestinal: Abdominal pain, anorexia, cramping, vomiting (especially with high single-dose regimens)

Genitourinary: Vaginitis

Local: (with I.V. administration): Injection site pain, inflammation

Ocular (with ophthalmic solution use): Eye irritation (1% to 2%)

≤1% (Limited to important or life-threatening): Systemic therapy: Agitation, allergic reaction, anemia, angioedema, bronchospasm, candidiasis, chest pain, cholestatic jaundice, conjunctivitis, constipation, cough increased, dermatitis (fungal), diaphoresis, dizziness, dyspepsia, eczema, enteritis, facial edema, fatigue, fever, flatulence, fungal infection, gastritis, headache, hyperkinesia, insomnia, jaundice, leukopenia, malaise, melena, mucositis, nephritis, nervousness, oral moniliasis, pain, palpitation, pharyngitis, photosensitivity, pleural effusion, rhinitis, somnolence, taste perversion, urticaria, vertigo, vesiculobullous rash, weakness

1%: Ophthalmic solution: Contact dermatitis, corneal erosion, dysgeusia, nasal congestion, ocular discharge, ocular dryness; ocular stinging, burning, and irritation upon instillation; punctate keratitis, sinusitis

Postmarketing and/or case reports (all formulations): Acute renal failure, aggressive behavior, anaphylaxis, anxiety, arrhythmia (including ventricular tachycardia), arthralgia, deafness, dehydration, edema, erythema multiforme (rare), hearing disturbance, hearing loss, hepatic failure (rare), hepatic necrosis (rare), hepatitis, hyperactivity, hypertrophic pyloric stenosis, hypotension, interstitial nephritis, loss of smell, loss of taste, LFTs increased, neutropenia (mild), oral candidiasis, pancreatitis, paresthesia, pseudomembranous colitis, QT_c prolongation (rare), seizure, smell perversion, somnolence, Stevens-Johnson syndrome (rare), syncope, thrombocytopenia, tinnitus, tongue discoloration (rare), torsade de pointes (rare), toxic epidermal necrolysis (rare)

Drug Interactions

Metabolism/Transport Effects **Substrate** of CYP3A4 (minor); **Inhibits** CYP3A4 (weak)

Avoid Concomitant Use

Avoid concomitant use of Azithromycin with any of the following: Artemether; Dronedarone; Lumefantrine; Nilotinib; Pimozide; QuiNINE; Tetrabenazine; Thioridazine; Ziprasidone

Increased Effect/Toxicity

Azithromycin may increase the levels/effects of: Amiodarone; Cardiac Glycosides; CycloSPORINE; Dronedarone; Pimozide; QTc-Prolonging Agents; QuiNINE; Tacrolimus; Tetrabenazine; Thioridazine; Vitamin K Antagonists; Ziprasidone

The levels/effects of Azithromycin may be increased by: Alfuzosin; Artemether; Chloroquine; Ciprofloxacin; Gadobutrol; Lumefantrine; Nelfinavir; Nilotinib; QuiNINE

Decreased Effect

Azithromycin may decrease the levels/effects of: Typhoid Vaccine

Ethanol/Nutrition/Herb Interactions Food: Rate and extent of GI absorption may be altered depending upon the formulation. Azithromycin suspension, not tablet form, has significantly increased absorption (46%) with food.

Dietary Considerations Some products may contain sodium and/or sucrose.

Oral suspension, immediate release, may be administered with or without food.

Oral suspension, extended release, should be taken on an empty stomach (at least 1 hour before or 2 hours following a meal).

Tablet may be administered with food to decrease GI effects.

Dosage Forms Excipient information presented when available (limited, particularly for generics); consult specific product labeling.

Note: Strength expressed as base

Injection, powder for reconstitution, as dihydrate: 500 mg

Zithromax®: 500 mg [contains sodium 114 mg (4.96 mEq) per vial]

Injection, powder for reconstitution, as hydrogencitrate: 500 mg, 2.5 g

Injection, powder for reconstitution, as monohydrate: 500 mg

Microspheres for oral suspension, extended release, as dihydrate:

Zmax®: 2 g/bottle (60 mL) [contains sodium 148 mg per bottle, sucrose 19 g/bottle; cherry/banana flavor; product contains azithromycin 27 mg/mL after constitution]

Powder for oral suspension, as monohydrate: 100 mg/5 mL (15 mL); 200 mg/5 mL (15 mL, 22.5 mL, 30 mL); 1 g/packet (3s)

◀ Powder for oral suspension, as dihydrate:
   Zithromax®: 100 mg/5 mL (15 mL) [contains sodium 3.7 mg/ 5 mL; cherry creme de vanilla and banana flavor]; 200 mg/5 mL (15 mL, 22.5 mL, 30 mL) [contains sodium 7.4 mg/5 mL; cherry creme de vanilla and banana flavor]; 1 g/packet (3s, 10s) [single-dose packet; contains sodium 37 mg per packet; cherry creme de vanilla and banana flavor]
Solution, ophthalmic:
   AzaSite®: 1% (2.5 mL) [contains benzalkonium chloride]
Tablet, as dihydrate:
   Zithromax®: 250 mg [contains sodium 0.9 mg per tablet]; 500 mg [contains sodium 1.8 mg per tablet]; 600 mg [contains sodium 2.1 mg per tablet]
   Zithromax® TRI-PAK™ [unit-dose pack]: 500 mg (3s) [contains sodium 1.8 mg per tablet]
   Zithromax® Z-PAK® [unit-dose pack]: 250 mg (6s) [contains sodium 0.9 mg per tablet]
Tablet, as monohydrate: 250 mg, 500 mg, 600 mg

◆ **Azithromycin Dihydrate** see Azithromycin on page 169

◆ **Azithromycin Hydrogencitrate** see Azithromycin on page 169

◆ **Azithromycin Monohydrate** see Azithromycin on page 169

◆ **Azmacort®** see Triamcinolone on page 1429

◆ **Azor™** see Amlodipine and Olmesartan on page 94

◆ **Azthreonam** see Aztreonam on page 174

Aztreonam (AZ tree oh nam)

Medication Safety Issues
Sound-alike/look-alike issues:
   Aztreonam may be confused with azidothymidine
U.S. Brand Names Azactam®
Canadian Brand Names Azactam®
Index Terms Azthreonam
Pharmacologic Category Antibiotic, Miscellaneous
Generic Available No
Use Treatment of patients with urinary tract infections, lower respiratory tract infections, septicemia, skin/skin structure infections, intra-abdominal infections, and gynecological infections caused by susceptible gram-negative bacilli
Mechanism of Action Inhibits bacterial cell wall synthesis by binding to one or more of the penicillin binding proteins (PBPs) which in turn inhibits the final transpeptidation step of peptidoglycan synthesis in bacterial cell walls, thus inhibiting cell wall biosynthesis. Bacteria eventually lyse due to ongoing activity of cell wall autolytic enzymes (autolysins and murein hydrolases) while cell wall assembly is arrested. Monobactam structure makes cross-allergenicity with beta-lactams unlikely.

Pharmacodynamics/Kinetics
Absorption: I.M.: Well absorbed; I.M. and I.V. doses produce comparable serum concentrations; Oral: <1%
Distribution: Widely to most body fluids and tissues
   V_d: Children: 0.2-0.29 L/kg; Adults: 0.2 L/kg
   Relative diffusion of antimicrobial agents from blood into CSF: Good only with inflammation (exceeds usual MICs)
   CSF:blood level ratio: Meninges: Inflamed: 8% to 40%; Normal: ~1%
Protein binding: 56%
Metabolism: Hepatic (minor %)
Half-life elimination:
   Children 2 months to 12 years: 1.7 hours
   Adults: Normal renal function: 1.7-2.9 hours
   End-stage renal disease: 6-8 hours
Time to peak: I.M., I.V. push: Within 60 minutes; I.V. infusion: 1.5 hours
Excretion: Urine (60% to 70% as unchanged drug); feces (~13% to 15%)

Dosage

Children >1 month: I.M., I.V.:

Mild-to-moderate infections: I.M., I.V.: 30 mg/kg every 8 hours

Moderate-to-severe infections: I.M., I.V.: 30 mg/kg every 6-8 hours; maximum: 120 mg/kg/day (8 g/day)

Cystic fibrosis: I.V.: 50 mg/kg/dose every 6-8 hours (ie, up to 200 mg/kg/day); maximum: 8 g/day

Adults:

Urinary tract infection: I.M., I.V.: 500 mg to 1 g every 8-12 hours

Moderately-severe systemic infections: 1 g I.V. or I.M. or 2 g I.V. every 8-12 hours

Severe systemic or life-threatening infections (especially caused by *Pseudomonas aeruginosa*): I.V.: 2 g every 6-8 hours; maximum: 8 g/day

Meningitis (gram-negative): I.V.: 2 g every 6-8 hours

Dosing adjustment in renal impairment: Adults: Following initial dose, maintenance doses should be given as follows:

Cl_{cr} 10-30 mL/minute: 50% of usual dose at the usual interval

Cl_{cr} <10 mL/minute: 25% of usual dosage at the usual interval

Hemodialysis: Moderately dialyzable (20% to 50%); Loading dose of 500 mg, 1 g, or 2 g, followed by 25% of initial dose at usual interval; for serious/life-threatening infections, administer $1/8$ of initial dose after each hemodialysis session (given in addition to the maintenance doses)

Continuous ambulatory peritoneal dialysis (CAPD): Administer as for Cl_{cr} <10 mL/minute

Continuous renal replacement therapy (CRRT): Drug clearance is highly dependent on the method of renal replacement, filter type, and flow rate. Appropriate dosing requires close monitoring of pharmacologic response, signs of adverse reactions due to drug accumulation, as well as drug levels in relation to target trough (if appropriate). The following are general recommendations only (based on dialysate flow/ultrafiltration rates of 1 L/hour) and should not supersede clinical judgment:

CVVH: 1-2 g every 12 hours

CVVHD/CVVHDF: 2 g every 12 hours

Stability Prior to reconstitution, store at room temperature; avoid excessive heat. Reconstituted solutions are colorless to light yellow straw and may turn pink upon standing without affecting potency. Use reconstituted solutions and I.V. solutions (in NS and D_5W) within 48 hours if kept at room temperature (25°C) or 7 days under refrigeration (4°C).

I.M.: Reconstitute with at least 3 mL SWFI, sterile bacteriostatic water for injection, NS, or bacteriostatic sodium chloride.

I.V.:

Bolus injection: Reconstitute with 6-10 mL SWFI.

Infusion: Reconstitute to a final concentration ≤2%; the final concentration should not exceed 20 mg/mL. Solution for infusion may be frozen at less than -2°C (less than -4°F) for up to 3 months. Thawed solution should be used within 24 hours if thawed at room temperature or within 72 hours if thawed under refrigeration. **Do not refreeze.**

Administration Doses >1 g should be administered I.V.

I.M.: Administer by deep injection into large muscle mass, such as upper outer quadrant of gluteus maximus or the lateral part of the thigh

I.V.: Administer by slow I.V. push over 3-5 minutes or by intermittent infusion over 20-60 minutes.

Monitoring Parameters Periodic liver function test; monitor for signs of anaphylaxis during first dose

Anesthesia and Critical Care Concerns/Other Considerations

Clinical Pearls/Comments: Although marketed as an agent similar to aminoglycosides, aztreonam is a monobactam antimicrobial with almost pure gram-negative aerobic activity. It cannot be used for gram-positive infections, whereas aminoglycosides are often used for synergy in gram-positive infections.

Pregnancy Risk Factor B

Contraindications Hypersensitivity to aztreonam or any component of the formulation

Warnings/Precautions Rare cross-allergenicity to penicillins and cephalosporins has been reported. Use caution in renal impairment; dosing adjustment required. Prolonged use may result in fungal or bacterial superinfection, including *C. difficile*-associated diarrhea (CDAD) and pseudomembranous colitis; CDAD has been observed >2 months postantibiotic treatment.

Adverse Reactions As reported in adults:

1% to 10%:

Dermatologic: Rash

Gastrointestinal: Diarrhea, nausea, vomiting

Local: Thrombophlebitis, pain at injection site

<1% (Limited to important or life-threatening): Abdominal cramps, abnormal taste, anaphylaxis, anemia, angioedema, aphthous ulcer, breast tenderness, bronchospasm, *C. difficile*-associated diarrhea, chest pain, confusion, diaphoresis, diplopia, dizziness, dyspnea, eosinophilia, erythema multiforme, exfoliative dermatitis, fever, flushing, halitosis, headache, hepatitis, hypotension, insomnia, jaundice, leukopenia, liver enzymes increased, muscular aches myalgia, neutropenia, numb tongue, pancytopenia, paresthesia, petechiae, pruritus, pseudomembranous colitis, purpura, seizure, sneezing, thrombocytopenia, tinnitus, toxic epidermal necrolysis, urticaria, vaginitis, vertigo, weakness, wheezing

Drug Interactions

Avoid Concomitant Use There are no known interactions where it is recommended to avoid concomitant use.

Increased Effect/Toxicity There are no known significant interactions involving an increase in effect.

Decreased Effect

Aztreonam may decrease the levels/effects of: Typhoid Vaccine

Test Interactions May interfere with urine glucose tests containing cupric sulfate (Benedict's solution, Clinitest®); positive Coombs' test

Dosage Forms Excipient information presented when available (limited, particularly for generics); consult specific product labeling. [DSC] = Discontinued product

Infusion premixed iso-osmotic solution:

Azactam®: 1 g (50 mL); 2 g (50 mL)

Injection, powder for reconstitution:

Azactam®: 500 mg [DSC], 1 g, 2 g

References

Stutman HR, Chartrand SA, Tolentino T, et al, "Aztreonam Therapy for Serious Gram-Negative Infections in Children," *Am J Dis Child*, 1986, 140(11):1147-51.

Tunkel AR, Hartman BJ, Kaplan SL, et al, "Practice Guidelines for the Management of Bacterial Meningitis," *Clin Infect Dis*, 2004, 39(9):1267-84.

♦ **Baby Aspirin** *see* Aspirin *on page 147*

♦ **BabyBIG®** *see* Botulism Immune Globulin (Intravenous-Human) *on page 203*

♦ **Baciguent® [OTC]** *see* Bacitracin *on page 176*

♦ **Baciguent® (Can)** *see* Bacitracin *on page 176*

♦ **BaciIM®** *see* Bacitracin *on page 176*

♦ **Baciject® (Can)** *see* Bacitracin *on page 176*

♦ **Baci-Rx** *see* Bacitracin *on page 176*

Bacitracin (bas i TRAY sin)

Medication Safety Issues

Sound-alike/look-alike issues:

Bacitracin may be confused with Bactrim®, Bactroban®

U.S. Brand Names Baci-Rx; Baciguent® [OTC]; BaciIM®

Canadian Brand Names Baciguent®; Baciject®

Pharmacologic Category Antibiotic, Miscellaneous; Antibiotic, Ophthalmic; Antibiotic, Topical

Generic Available Yes

Use Treatment of susceptible bacterial infections mainly; has activity against grampositive bacilli; due to toxicity risks, systemic and irrigant uses of bacitracin should be limited to situations where less toxic alternatives would not be effective.

Unlabeled/Investigational Use Oral administration: Successful in antibiotic-associated colitis; has been used for enteric eradication of vancomycin-resistant enterococci (VRE)

Mechanism of Action Inhibits bacterial cell wall synthesis by preventing transfer of mucopeptides into the growing cell wall

Pharmacodynamics/Kinetics

Duration: 6-8 hours

Absorption: Poor from mucous membranes and intact or denuded skin; rapidly following I.M. administration; not absorbed by bladder irrigation, but absorption can occur from peritoneal or mediastinal lavage

Distribution: CSF: Nil even with inflammation

Protein binding, plasma: Minimal

Time to peak, serum: I.M.: 1-2 hours

Excretion: Urine (10% to 40%) within 24 hours

Dosage Do not administer I.V.:

Infants: I.M.:

≤2.5 kg: 900 units/kg/day in 2-3 divided doses

>2.5 kg: 1000 units/kg/day in 2-3 divided doses

Children: I.M.: 800-1200 units/kg/day divided every 8 hours

Adults: Oral:

Antibiotic-associated colitis: 25,000 units 4 times/day for 7-10 days

VRE eradication (unlabeled use): 25,000 units 4 times/day for 7-10 days

Children and Adults:

Topical: Apply 1-5 times/day

Ophthalmic, ointment: Instill 1/4" to 1/2" ribbon every 3-4 hours into conjunctival sac for acute infections, or 2-3 times/day for mild-to-moderate infections for 7-10 days

Irrigation, solution: 50-100 units/mL in normal saline, lactated Ringer's, or sterile water for irrigation; soak sponges in solution for topical compresses 1-5 times/day or as needed during surgical procedures

Stability For I.M. use. Bacitracin sterile powder should be dissolved in 0.9% sodium chloride injection containing 2% procaine hydrochloride. Once reconstituted, bacitracin is stable for 1 week under refrigeration (2°C to 8°C). Sterile powder should be stored in the refrigerator. Do not use diluents containing parabens.

Administration For I.M. administration only, **do not administer I.V.** Confirm any orders for parenteral use. pH of urine should be kept >6 by using sodium bicarbonate. Bacitracin sterile powder should be dissolved in 0.9% sodium chloride injection containing 2% procaine hydrochloride. Do not use diluents containing parabens.

Monitoring Parameters I.M.: Urinalysis, renal function tests

Contraindications Hypersensitivity to bacitracin or any component of the formulation; I.M. use is contraindicated in patients with renal impairment

Warnings/Precautions [U.S. Boxed Warning]: I.M. use may cause renal failure due to tubular and glomerular necrosis; monitor renal function daily. Avoid concurrent use with other nephrotoxic drugs; discontinue use if toxicity occurs. Prolonged use may result in fungal or bacterial superinfection, including *C. difficile*-associated diarrhea (CDAD) and pseudomembranous colitis; CDAD has been observed >2 months postantibiotic treatment. Do not administer intravenously because severe thrombophlebitis occurs.

Adverse Reactions

1% to 10%:

Cardiovascular: Hypotension, edema of the face/lips, chest tightness

Central nervous system: Pain

Dermatologic: Rash, itching

Gastrointestinal: Anorexia, nausea, vomiting, diarrhea, rectal itching

Hematologic: Blood dyscrasias

Miscellaneous: Diaphoresis

<1%: Rare cases of anaphylaxis have been reported in association with topical and intraoperative exposures.

Drug Interactions

Avoid Concomitant Use There are no known interactions where it is recommended to avoid concomitant use.

◀ **Increased Effect/Toxicity** There are no known significant interactions involving an increase in effect.

Decreased Effect There are no known significant interactions involving a decrease in effect.

Dosage Forms Excipient information presented when available (limited, particularly for generics); consult specific product labeling.

Injection, powder for reconstitution: 50,000 units
BaciiM®: 50,000 units

Ointment, ophthalmic: 500 units/g (3.5 g)

Ointment, topical: 500 units/g (0.9 g, 15 g, 30 g, 120 g, 454 g)
Baciguent®: 500 units/g (15 g, 30 g)

Powder, for prescription compounding [micronized]:
Baci-Rx: 5 million units

Baclofen (BAK loe fen)

Related Information
Chronic Pain Management *on page 1546*

U.S. Brand Names Lioresal®

Canadian Brand Names Apo-Baclofen®; Gen-Baclofen; Lioresal®; Liotec; Mylan-Baclofen; Nu-Baclo; PMS-Baclofen

Pharmacologic Category Skeletal Muscle Relaxant

Use Treatment of reversible spasticity associated with multiple sclerosis or spinal cord lesions

Orphan drug: Intrathecal: Treatment of intractable spasticity caused by spinal cord injury, multiple sclerosis, and other spinal disease (spinal ischemia or tumor, transverse myelitis, cervical spondylosis, degenerative myelopathy)

Unlabeled/Investigational Use Intractable hiccups, intractable pain relief, bladder spasticity, trigeminal neuralgia, cerebral palsy, Huntington's chorea

Pharmacodynamics/Kinetics
Onset of action: 3-4 days
Peak effect: 5-10 days
Absorption (dose dependent): Oral: Rapid
Protein binding: 30%
Metabolism: Hepatic (15% of dose)
Half-life elimination: 3.5 hours
Time to peak, serum: Oral: Within 2-3 hours
Excretion: Urine and feces (85% as unchanged drug)

Dosage
Oral (avoid abrupt withdrawal of drug):

Children (unlabeled use): Caution: Pediatric dosing expressed as a daily amount, and **NOT** in mg/kg. Limited published data in children; the following is a compilation of small prospective studies (Albright, 1996; Milla, 1977; Scheinberg, 2006) and one large retrospective study (Lubsch, 2006):

<2 years: 10-20 mg daily divided every 8 hours; titrate dose every 3 days in increments of 5-15mg/day to a maximum of 40 mg daily

2-7 years: Initial: 20-30 mg daily divided every 8 hours; titrate dose every 3 days in increments of 5-15 mg/day to a maximum of 60 mg daily

≥8 years: 30-40 mg daily divided every 8 hours; titrate dose every 3 days in increments of 5-15 mg/day to a maximum of 120 mg daily

Note: Baclofen dose may need to be increased over time. One retrospective analysis (Lubsch, 2006) suggested that increased doses were needed as the time increased from spasticity onset, as age increased, and as the number of concomitant antispasticity medications increased. A small number of patients required daily doses exceeding 200 mg.

Adults: 5 mg 3 times/day, may increase 5 mg/dose every 3 days to a maximum of 80 mg/day

Hiccups (unlabeled use): Usual effective dose: 10-20 mg 2-3 times/day

Intrathecal: Children and Adults:

Test dose: 50-100 mcg, doses >50 mcg should be given in 25 mcg increments, separated by 24 hours. A screening dose of 25 mcg may be considered in very small patients. Patients not responding to screening dose of 100 mcg should not be considered for chronic infusion/implanted pump.

Maintenance: After positive response to test dose, a maintenance intrathecal infusion can be administered via an implanted intrathecal pump. Initial dose via pump: Infusion at a 24-hour rate dosed at twice the test dose. Avoid abrupt discontinuation.

Elderly: Oral (the lowest effective dose is recommended): Initial: 5 mg 2-3 times/day, increasing gradually as needed; if benefits are not seen, withdraw the drug slowly.

Dosing adjustment in renal impairment: May be necessary to reduce dosage in renal impairment, but there are no specific guidelines available

Hemodialysis: Poor water solubility allows for accumulation during chronic hemodialysis. Low-dose therapy is recommended. There have been several case reports of accumulation of baclofen resulting in toxicity symptoms (organic brain syndrome, myoclonia, deceleration and steep potentials in EEG) in patients with renal failure who have received normal doses of baclofen.

Additional Information Complete prescribing information for this medication should be consulted for additional detail.

Dosage Forms Excipient information presented when available (limited, particularly for generics); consult specific product labeling.

Injection, solution, intrathecal [preservative free]:

Lioresal®: 50 mcg/mL (1 mL); 500 mcg/mL (20 mL); 2000 mcg/mL (5 mL, 20 mL)

Tablet: 10 mg, 20 mg

◆ **BactoShield® CHG [OTC]** *see* Chlorhexidine Gluconate *on page 291*

◆ **Bactrim™** *see* Sulfamethoxazole and Trimethoprim *on page 1333*

◆ **Bactrim™ DS** *see* Sulfamethoxazole and Trimethoprim *on page 1333*

◆ **Bactroban®** *see* Mupirocin *on page 965*

◆ **Bactroban Cream®** *see* Mupirocin *on page 965*

◆ **Bactroban Nasal®** *see* Mupirocin *on page 965*

◆ **Baking Soda** *see* Sodium Bicarbonate *on page 1301*

◆ **Balacet 325™** *see* Propoxyphene and Acetaminophen *on page 1197*

◆ **Balziva™** *see* Ethinyl Estradiol and Norethindrone *on page 554*

◆ **Band-Aid® Hurt-Free™ Antiseptic Wash [OTC]** *see* Lidocaine *on page 836*

◆ **Banophen™ [OTC]** *see* DiphenhydrAMINE *on page 430*

◆ **Banophen™ Anti-Itch [OTC]** *see* DiphenhydrAMINE *on page 430*

◆ **Banzel™** *see* Rufinamide *on page 1271*

Basiliximab (ba si LIK si mab)

U.S. Brand Names Simulect®
Canadian Brand Names Simulect®
Pharmacologic Category Monoclonal Antibody
Use Prophylaxis of acute organ rejection in renal transplantation
Pharmacodynamics/Kinetics

Duration: Mean: 36 days (determined by IL-2R alpha saturation)

Distribution: Mean: V_d: Children 1-11 years: 4.8 ± 2.1 L; Adolescents 12-16 years: 7.8 ± 5.1 L; Adults: 8.6 ± 4.1 L

Half-life elimination: Children 1-11 years: 9.5 days; Adolescents 12-16 years: 9.1 days; Adults: Mean: 7.2 days

Excretion: Clearance: Children 1-11 years: 17 mL/hour; Adolescents 12-16 years: 31 mL/hour; Adults: Mean: 41 mL/hour

Dosage Note: Patients previously administered basiliximab should only be re-exposed to a subsequent course of therapy with extreme caution.

I.V.:

Children <35 kg: Renal transplantation: 10 mg within 2 hours prior to transplant surgery, followed by a second 10 mg dose 4 days after transplantation; the second dose should be withheld if complications occur (including severe hypersensitivity reactions or graft loss)

Children ≥35 kg and Adults: Renal transplantation: 20 mg within 2 hours prior to transplant surgery, followed by a second 20 mg dose 4 days after transplantation; the second dose should be withheld if complications occur (including severe hypersensitivity reactions or graft loss)

Dosing adjustment/comments in renal or hepatic impairment: No specific dosing adjustment recommended

Additional Information Complete prescribing information for this medication should be consulted for additional detail.

Dosage Forms Excipient information presented when available (limited, particularly for generics); consult specific product labeling.

Injection, powder for reconstitution [preservative free]:

Simulect®: 10 mg, 20 mg

♦ **BAY 59-7939** *see* Rivaroxaban *on page* 1255

♦ **Baycadron™** *see* Dexamethasone *on page* 391

♦ **Bayer® Aspirin Extra Strength [OTC]** *see* Aspirin *on page* 147

♦ **Bayer® Aspirin Regimen Adult Low Dose [OTC]** *see* Aspirin *on page* 147

♦ **Bayer® Aspirin Regimen Children's [OTC]** *see* Aspirin *on page* 147

♦ **Bayer® Aspirin Regimen Regular Strength [OTC]** *see* Aspirin *on page* 147

♦ **Bayer® Genuine Aspirin [OTC]** *see* Aspirin *on page* 147

♦ **Bayer® Plus Extra Strength [OTC]** *see* Aspirin *on page* 147

♦ **Bayer® with Heart Advantage [OTC]** *see* Aspirin *on page* 147

♦ **Bayer® Women's Aspirin Plus Calcium [OTC]** *see* Aspirin *on page* 147

♦ **BCX-1812** *see* Peramivir *on page* 1104

♦ **BD™ Glucose [OTC]** *see* Dextrose *on page* 406

♦ **Bebulin® VH** *see* Factor IX Complex (Human) *on page* 573

Becaplermin (be KAP ler min)

Medication Safety Issues

Sound-alike/look-alike issues:

Regranex® may be confused with Granulex®, Repronex®

U.S. Brand Names Regranex®

Canadian Brand Names Regranex®

Index Terms Recombinant Human Platelet-Derived Growth Factor B; rPDGF-BB

Pharmacologic Category Growth Factor, Platelet-Derived; Topical Skin Product

Generic Available No

Use Adjunctive treatment of diabetic neuropathic ulcers occurring on the lower limbs and feet that extend into subcutaneous tissue (or beyond) and have adequate blood supply

Mechanism of Action Recombinant B-isoform homodimer of human platelet-derived growth factor (rPDGF-BB) which enhances formation of new granulation tissue, induces fibroblast proliferation and differentiation to promote wound healing; also promotes angiogenesis.

Pharmacodynamics/Kinetics

Onset of action: Complete healing: 15% of patients within 8 weeks, 25% at 10 weeks

Absorption: Minimal

Distribution: Binds to PDGF beta-receptors in normal skin and granulation tissue

Dosage Topical: Adults: Diabetic ulcers: Apply appropriate amount of gel once daily with a cotton swab or similar tool, as a coating over the ulcer. The amount of becaplermin to be applied will vary depending on the size of the ulcer area.

Note: If the ulcer does not decrease in size by ~30% after 10 weeks of treatment or complete healing has not occurred in 20 weeks, continued treatment with becaplermin gel should be reassessed.

To calculate the length of gel applied to the ulcer, measure the greatest length of the ulcer by the greatest width of the ulcer. Tube size and unit of measure will determine the formula used in the calculation. Recalculate amount of gel needed every 1-2 weeks, depending on the rate of change in ulcer area.

Centimeters:

15 g tube: [ulcer length (cm) x width (cm)] divided by 4 = length of gel (cm)

2 g tube: [ulcer length (cm) x width (cm)] divided by 2 = length of gel (cm)

Inches:
15 g tube: [length (in) x width (in)] x 0.6 = length of gel (in)
2 g tube: [length (in) x width (in)] x 1.3 = length of gel (in)

Stability Refrigerate at 2°C to 8°C (36°F to 46°F); do not freeze.

Administration For external use only. Squeeze appropriate amount of gel onto clean measuring surface (eg, wax paper), spread onto entire ulcer area in a thin, continuous layer ~1/16 inch thick. Cover with saline moistened dressing; leave dressing in place ~12 hours. After 12 hours, remove dressing, rinse with saline or water to remove residual becaplermin gel and cover with saline moistened dressing (without becaplermin gel) for remainder of the day. Continue use once daily until ulcer is completely healed.

Monitoring Parameters Ulcer volume (pressure ulcers); wound area; evidence of closure; drainage (diabetic ulcers); signs/symptoms of toxicity (erythema, local infections)

Pregnancy Risk Factor C

Contraindications Hypersensitivity to becaplermin or any component of the formulation; known neoplasm(s) at the site(s) of application

Warnings/Precautions For external use only; do not use in wounds that close by primary intention. Use with caution in ulcer wounds related to arterial or venous insufficiency and when there are thermal, electrical, or radiation burns at wound site. **[U.S. Boxed Warning]: In a retrospective study, an increase in mortality secondary to malignancy has been observed in patients treated with ≥3 tubes of becaplermin.** Malignancies of varying types have been reported; all were remote from the becaplermin treatment site; use with caution in patients with known malignancy. Effects on exposed joints, tendons, ligaments and bone have not been established. Safety and efficacy have not been established in children <16 years of age.

Adverse Reactions
1% to 10%: Dermatologic: Erythematous rash (2%)
<1% (Limited to important or life-threatening): Erythema with purulent discharge, ulcer infection, tunneling of ulcer, exuberant granulation tissue, local pain, skin ulceration

Drug Interactions
Avoid Concomitant Use There are no known interactions where it is recommended to avoid concomitant use.
Increased Effect/Toxicity There are no known significant interactions involving an increase in effect.
Decreased Effect There are no known significant interactions involving a decrease in effect.

Dosage Forms Excipient information presented when available (limited, particularly for generics); consult specific product labeling.
Gel, topical:
Regranex®: 0.01% (2 g, 15 g)

♦ **Benadryl® (Can)** *see* DiphenhydrAMINE *on page 430*

♦ **Benadryl® Allergy [OTC]** *see* DiphenhydrAMINE *on page 430*

♦ **Benadryl® Allergy Quick Dissolve [OTC]** *see* DiphenhydrAMINE *on page 430*

♦ **Benadryl® Children's Allergy [OTC]** *see* DiphenhydrAMINE *on page 430*

♦ **Benadryl® Children's Allergy Fastmelt® [OTC]** *see* DiphenhydrAMINE *on page 430*

♦ **Benadryl® Children's Allergy Perfect Measure™** *see* DiphenhydrAMINE *on page 430*

♦ **Benadryl® Children's Dye-Free Allergy [OTC]** *see* DiphenhydrAMINE *on page 430*

♦ **Benadryl® Children's Allergy Quick Dissolve [OTC] [DSC]** *see* DiphenhydrAMINE *on page 430*

♦ **Benadryl® Dye-Free Allergy [OTC]** *see* DiphenhydrAMINE *on page 430*

♦ **Benadryl® Itch Relief Extra Strength [OTC]** *see* DiphenhydrAMINE *on page 430*

♦ **Benadryl® Itch Stopping [OTC]** *see* DiphenhydrAMINE *on page 430*

♦ **Benadryl® Itch Stopping Extra Strength [OTC]** *see* DiphenhydrAMINE *on page 430*

Benazepril (ben AY ze pril)

Related Information
  Angiotensin Agents *on page 1652*
U.S. Brand Names Lotensin®
Canadian Brand Names Apo-Benazepril®; Lotensin®
Index Terms Benazepril Hydrochloride
Pharmacologic Category Angiotensin-Converting Enzyme (ACE) Inhibitor
Use Treatment of hypertension, either alone or in combination with other antihypertensive agents

Pharmacodynamics/Kinetics
  Reduction in plasma angiotensin-converting enzyme (ACE) activity:
    Onset of action: Peak effect: 1-2 hours after 2-20 mg dose
    Duration: >90% inhibition for 24 hours after 5-20 mg dose
  Reduction in blood pressure:
    Peak effect: Single dose: 2-4 hours; Continuous therapy: 2 weeks
  Absorption: Rapid (37%); food does not alter significantly; metabolite (benazeprilat) itself unsuitable for oral administration due to poor absorption
  Distribution: V_d: ~8.7 L
  Protein binding:
    Benazepril: ~97%
    Benazeprilat: ~95%
  Metabolism: Rapidly and extensively hepatic to its active metabolite, benazeprilat, via enzymatic hydrolysis; extensive first-pass effect
  Half-life elimination: Benazeprilat: Effective: 10-11 hours; Terminal: Children: 5 hours, Adults: 22 hours
  Time to peak: Parent drug: 0.5-1 hour
  Excretion:
    Urine (trace amounts as benazepril; 20% as benazeprilat; 12% as other metabolites)
    Clearance: Nonrenal clearance (ie, biliary, metabolic) appears to contribute to the elimination of benazeprilat (11% to 12%), particularly patients with severe renal impairment; hepatic clearance is the main elimination route of unchanged benazepril
    Dialysis: ~6% of metabolite removed within 4 hours of dialysis following 10 mg of benazepril administered 2 hours prior to procedure; parent compound not found in dialysate

Dosage Oral: Hypertension:
  Children ≥6 years: Initial: 0.2 mg/kg/day (up to 10 mg/day) as monotherapy; dosing range: 0.1-0.6 mg/kg/day (maximum dose: 40 mg/day)
  Adults: Initial: 10 mg/day in patients not receiving a diuretic; 20-80 mg/day as a single dose or 2 divided doses; the need for twice-daily dosing should be assessed by monitoring peak (2-6 hours after dosing) and trough responses.
    Note: Patients taking diuretics should have them discontinued 2-3 days prior to starting benazepril. If they cannot be discontinued, then initial dose should be 5 mg; restart after blood pressure is stabilized if needed.
  Elderly: Oral: Initial: 5-10 mg/day in single or divided doses; usual range: 20-40 mg/day; adjust for renal function; also see **Note** in adult dosing.
  Dosing interval in renal impairment: Cl_{cr} <30 mL/minute:
    Children: Use is not recommended.
    Adults: Administer 5 mg/day initially; maximum daily dose: 40 mg.
  Hemodialysis: Moderately dialyzable (20% to 50%); administer dose postdialysis or administer 25% to 35% supplemental dose.
  Peritoneal dialysis: Supplemental dose is not necessary.

Anesthesia and Critical Care Concerns/Other Considerations
  Clinical Pearls/Comments: In patients on chronic ACE inhibitor therapy, intraoperative hypotension may occur with induction and maintenance of general anesthesia; however, discontinuation of therapy prior to surgery is controversial. If continued preoperatively, avoidance of hypotensive agents during surgery is prudent. Episodes of intraoperative hypotension may be managed by fluid administration and/or modest doses of alpha-adrenergic agents. Severe hypotension may occur in patients who are sodium- and/or volume-depleted, initiate lower doses and monitor closely when starting therapy in these patients.

ACE inhibitor therapy may elicit an increase in potassium and creatinine, especially when used in patients with bilateral renal artery stenosis. In those patients experiencing cough on an ACE inhibitor, the ACE inhibitor may be discontinued and, if necessary, angiotensin-receptor blocker therapy instituted. Concomitant NSAID therapy may attenuate blood pressure control; use of NSAIDs should be avoided or limited, with monitoring of blood pressure control. In the setting of heart failure, NSAID use may be associated with an increased risk for fluid accumulation and edema. Because of the potent teratogenic effects of ACE inhibitors, these drugs should be avoided, if possible, when treating women of childbearing potential not on effective birth control measures. Aging patients with a decrease in glomerular filtration (also creatinine clearance), severe heart failure, and renal failure may experience an exaggerated response with administration of ACE inhibitors. Diabetic proteinuria is reduced and insulin sensitivity is enhanced.

Evidence-Based Information: ACE inhibitors decrease morbidity and mortality in patients with asymptomatic and symptomatic left ventricular dysfunction. In this situation, they decrease hospitalizations for, and retard progression to, decompensated heart failure. ACE inhibitors are also indicated in patients postmyocardial infarction in whom left ventricular ejection fraction is <40%. When used in patients with heart failure, the target dose or maximum tolerated dose should be achieved, if possible. Lower daily doses of ACE inhibitors have not demonstrated the same cardioprotective effects. ACE inhibitors have renal protective effects in patients with diabetic proteinuria. The HOPE trial examined the use of ramipril at a dose of between 2.5-10 mg daily in patients without heart failure at high risk for cardiovascular events and documented a significant improvement in cardiovascular outcome compared to placebo.

Additional Information Complete prescribing information for this medication should be consulted for additional detail.

Dosage Forms Excipient information presented when available (limited, particularly for generics); consult specific product labeling.
Tablet, as hydrochloride: 5 mg, 10 mg, 20 mg, 40 mg
  Lotensin®: 5 mg, 10 mg, 20 mg, 40 mg

◆ **Benazepril Hydrochloride** *see* Benazepril *on page* 182

◆ **BeneFix®** *see* Factor IX *on page* 570

◆ **Benemid [DSC]** *see* Probenecid *on page* 1175

◆ **Benicar®** *see* Olmesartan *on page* 1045

◆ **Ben-Tann [DSC]** *see* DiphenhydrAMINE *on page* 430

◆ **Benuryl™ (Can)** *see* Probenecid *on page* 1175

Benztropine (BENZ troe peen)

U.S. Brand Names Cogentin®
Canadian Brand Names Apo-Benztropine®
Index Terms Benztropine Mesylate
Pharmacologic Category Anti-Parkinson's Agent, Anticholinergic; Anticholinergic Agent
Use Adjunctive treatment of Parkinson's disease; treatment of drug-induced extrapyramidal symptoms (except tardive dyskinesia)
Pharmacodynamics/Kinetics
Onset of action: Oral: Within 1 hour; Parenteral: Within 15 minutes
Duration: 6-48 hours
Metabolism: Hepatic (N-oxidation, N-dealkylation, and ring hydroxylation)
Bioavailability: 29%
Dosage Use in children ≤3 years of age should be reserved for life-threatening emergencies
Drug-induced extrapyramidal symptom: Oral, I.M., I.V.:
  Children >3 years: 0.02-0.05 mg/kg/dose 1-2 times/day
  Adults: 1-4 mg/dose 1-2 times/day
Acute dystonia: Adults: I.M., I.V.: 1-2 mg

Parkinsonism: Oral:
Adults: 0.5-6 mg/day in 1-2 divided doses; if one dose is greater, administer at bedtime; titrate dose in 0.5 mg increments at 5- to 6-day intervals
Elderly: Initial: 0.5 mg once or twice daily; increase by 0.5 mg as needed at 5-6 days; maximum: 4 mg/day

Additional Information Complete prescribing information for this medication should be consulted for additional detail.

Dosage Forms Excipient information presented when available (limited, particularly for generics); consult specific product labeling.
Injection, solution, as mesylate (Cogentin®): 1 mg/mL (2 mL)
Tablet, as mesylate: 0.5 mg, 1 mg, 2 mg

◆ **Benztropine Mesylate** see Benztropine on page 183

Benzydamine (ben ZID a meen)

Canadian Brand Names Apo-Benzydamine®; Dom-Benzydamine; Novo-Benzydamine; PMS-Benzydamine; ratio-Benzydamine; Sun-Benz®; Tantum®

Index Terms Benzydamine Hydrochloride

Pharmacologic Category Local Anesthetic, Oral

Restrictions Not available in U.S.

Generic Available Yes

Use Symptomatic treatment of pain associated with acute pharyngitis; treatment of pain associated with radiation-induced oropharyngeal mucositis

Mechanism of Action Local anesthetic and anti-inflammatory, reduces local pain and inflammation. Does not interfere with arachidonic acid metabolism.

Pharmacodynamics/Kinetics
Absorption: Oral rinse may be absorbed, at least in part, through the oral mucosa
Excretion: Urine (primarily as unchanged drug)

Dosage Oral rinse: Adults:
Acute pharyngitis: Gargle with 15 mL of undiluted solution every $1^{1}/_{2}$-3 hours until symptoms resolve. Patient should expel solution from mouth following use; solution should not be swallowed.
Mucositis: 15 mL of undiluted solution as a gargle or rinse 3-4 times/day; contact should be maintained for at least 30 seconds, followed by expulsion from the mouth. Clinical studies maintained contact for ~2 minutes, up to 8 times/day. Patient should not swallow the liquid. Begin treatment 1 day prior to initiation of radiation therapy and continue daily during treatment. Continue oral rinse treatments after the completion of radiation therapy until desired result/healing is achieved.

Dosage adjustment in renal impairment: No adjustment required.

Stability Store at 15°C to 30°C; protect from freezing.

Contraindications Hypersensitivity to benzydamine or any component of the formulation

Warnings/Precautions May cause local irritation and/or burning sensation in patients with altered mucosal integrity. Dilution (1:1 in warm water) may attenuate this effect. Use caution in renal impairment. Safety and efficacy have not been established in children ≤5 years of age.

Adverse Reactions
Central nervous system: Drowsiness, headache
Gastrointestinal: Nausea and/or vomiting (2%), dry mouth
Local: Numbness (10%), burning/stinging sensation (8%)
Respiratory: Pharyngeal irritation, cough

Drug Interactions
Metabolism/Transport Effects Substrate (minor) of CYP1A2, 2C19, 2D6, 3A4
Avoid Concomitant Use There are no known interactions where it is recommended to avoid concomitant use.
Increased Effect/Toxicity There are no known significant interactions involving an increase in effect.
Decreased Effect There are no known significant interactions involving a decrease in effect.

Dosage Forms Excipient information presented when available (limited, particularly for generics); consult specific product labeling.
Oral rinse: 0.15% (100 mL, 250 mL) [not available in the U.S.]

◆ **Benzydamine Hydrochloride** *see* Benzydamine *on page 184*

◆ **Benzylpenicillin Potassium** *see* Penicillin G (Parenteral/Aqueous) *on page 1094*

◆ **Benzylpenicillin Sodium** *see* Penicillin G (Parenteral/Aqueous) *on page 1094*

Beractant (ber AKT ant)

Medication Safety Issues
Sound-alike/look-alike issues:
Survanta® may be confused with Sufenta®
U.S. Brand Names Survanta®
Canadian Brand Names Survanta®
Index Terms Bovine Lung Surfactant; Natural Lung Surfactant
Pharmacologic Category Lung Surfactant
Generic Available No
Use Prevention and treatment of respiratory distress syndrome (RDS) in premature infants

Prophylactic therapy: Body weight <1250 g in infants at risk for developing, or with evidence of, surfactant deficiency (administer within 15 minutes of birth)
Rescue therapy: Treatment of infants with RDS confirmed by x-ray and requiring mechanical ventilation (administer as soon as possible - within 8 hours of age)
Mechanism of Action Replaces deficient or ineffective endogenous lung surfactant in neonates with respiratory distress syndrome (RDS) or in neonates at risk of developing RDS. Surfactant prevents the alveoli from collapsing during expiration by lowering surface tension between air and alveolar surfaces.
Pharmacodynamics/Kinetics Excretion: Clearance: Alveolar clearance is rapid
Dosage
Prophylactic treatment: Administer 100 mg phospholipids (4 mL/kg) intratracheal as soon as possible; as many as 4 doses may be administered during the first 48 hours of life, no more frequently than 6 hours apart. The need for additional doses is determined by evidence of continuing respiratory distress; if the infant is still intubated and requiring at least 30% inspired oxygen to maintain a PaO_2 ≤80 torr.
Rescue treatment: Administer 100 mg phospholipids (4 mL/kg) as soon as the diagnosis of RDS is made; may repeat if needed, no more frequently than every 6 hours to a maximum of 4 doses
Stability Refrigerate; protect from light. Prior to administration, warm by standing at room temperature for 20 minutes or held in hand for 8 minutes. **Artificial warming methods should not be used.** Unused, unopened vials warmed to room temperature may be returned to the refrigerator within 8 hours of warming only once.
Administration
For intratracheal administration only
Suction infant prior to administration. Inspect solution to verify complete mixing of the suspension.
Administer intratracheally by instillation through a 5-French end-hole catheter inserted into the infant's endotracheal tube.
Administer the dose in four 1 mL/kg aliquots. Each quarter-dose is instilled over 2-3 seconds; each quarter-dose is administered with the infant in a different position. Slightly downward inclination with head turned to the right, then repeat with head turned to the left; then slightly upward inclination with head turned to the right, then repeat with head turned to the left.
Monitoring Parameters Continuous ECG and transcutaneous O_2 saturation should be monitored during administration; frequent arterial blood gases are necessary to prevent postdosing hyperoxia and hypocarbia
Warnings/Precautions For intratracheal administration only. Rapidly affects oxygenation and lung compliance; restrict use to a highly-supervised clinical setting with immediate availability of clinicians experienced in intubation and ventilatory management of premature infants. Transient episodes of bradycardia

◀ and decreased oxygen saturation occur. Discontinue dosing procedure and initiate measures to alleviate the condition; may reinstitute after the patient is stable. Produces rapid improvements in lung oxygenation and compliance that may require frequent adjustments to oxygen delivery and ventilator settings.

Adverse Reactions During the dosing procedure:
>10%: Cardiovascular: Transient bradycardia
1% to 10%: Respiratory: Oxygen desaturation
<1% (Limited to important or life-threatening): Apnea, endotracheal tube blockage, hypercarbia, hyper-/hypotension, post-treatment nosocomial sepsis probability increased, pulmonary air leaks, pulmonary interstitial emphysema, vasoconstriction

Drug Interactions
Avoid Concomitant Use There are no known interactions where it is recommended to avoid concomitant use.
Increased Effect/Toxicity There are no known significant interactions involving an increase in effect.
Decreased Effect There are no known significant interactions involving a decrease in effect.

Dosage Forms Excipient information presented when available (limited, particularly for generics); consult specific product labeling.
Suspension, intratracheal [preservative free; bovine derived]:
Survanta®: 25 mg/mL (4 mL, 8 mL)

♦ **9-Beta-D-Ribofuranosyladenine** see Adenosine on page 44

♦ **Betacaine® (Can)** see Lidocaine on page 836

♦ **Betaderm (Can)** see Betamethasone on page 186

♦ **Beta-HC®** see Hydrocortisone on page 699

♦ **Betaject™ (Can)** see Betamethasone on page 186

♦ **Betaloc® (Can)** see Metoprolol on page 922

♦ **Betaloc® Durules® (Can)** see Metoprolol on page 922

Betamethasone (bay ta METH a sone)

Medication Safety Issues
Sound-alike/look-alike issues:
Luxiq® may be confused with Lasix®

International issues:
Beta-Val® may be confused with Betanol® which is a brand name for metipranolol in Monaco

Related Information
Anesthesia for Obstetric Patients in Nonobstetric Surgery on page 1532
Corticosteroids on page 1676
Stress Replacement of Corticosteroids on page 1611

U.S. Brand Names Beta-Val®; Celestone®; Celestone® Soluspan®; Diprolene®; Diprolene® AF; Luxiq®

Canadian Brand Names Betaderm; Betaject™; Betnesol®; Betnovate®; Celestone® Soluspan®; Diprolene® Glycol; Diprosone®; Ectosone; Prevex® B; Taro-Sone®; Topilene®; Topisone®; Valisone® Scalp Lotion

Index Terms Betamethasone Dipropionate; Betamethasone Dipropionate, Augmented; Betamethasone Sodium Phosphate; Betamethasone Valerate; Flubenisolone

Pharmacologic Category Corticosteroid, Systemic; Corticosteroid, Topical

Generic Available Yes: Excludes aerosol, solution

Use Inflammatory dermatoses such as seborrheic or atopic dermatitis, neurodermatitis, anogenital pruritus, psoriasis, inflammatory phase of xerosis

Unlabeled/Investigational Use Accelerate fetal lung maturation in patients with preterm labor

Mechanism of Action Controls the rate of protein synthesis; depresses the migration of polymorphonuclear leukocytes, fibroblasts; reverses capillary permeability and lysosomal stabilization at the cellular level to prevent or control inflammation

Pharmacodynamics/Kinetics
Protein binding: 64%
Metabolism: Hepatic
Half-life elimination: 6.5 hours
Time to peak, serum: I.V.: 10-36 minutes
Excretion: Urine (<5% as unchanged drug)

Dosage Base dosage on severity of disease and patient response
Children: Use lowest dose listed as initial dose for adrenocortical insufficiency
(physiologic replacement)
    I.M.: ≤12 years: 0.0175-0.125 mg base/kg/day divided every 6-12 hours **or**
    0.5-7.5 mg base/m^2/day divided every 6-12 hours
    Oral: ≤12 years: 0.0175-0.25 mg/kg/day divided every 6-8 hours **or** 0.5-7.5 mg/
    m^2/day divided every 6-8 hours
    Topical:
      ≤12 years: Use is not recommended.
      ≥13 years: Use minimal amount for shortest period of time to avoid HPA axis
      suppression
        Gel, augmented formulation: Apply once or twice daily; rub in gently. **Note:** Do
        not exceed 2 weeks of treatment or 50 g/week.
        Lotion: Apply a few drops twice daily
          Augmented formulation: Apply a few drops once or twice daily; rub in gently.
          Note: Do not exceed 2 weeks of treatment or 50 mL/week.
        Cream/ointment: Apply once or twice daily.
          Augmented formulation: Apply once or twice daily. **Note:** Do not exceed 2
          weeks of treatment or 45 g/week.
Adolescents and Adults:
    Oral: 2.4-4.8 mg/day in 2-4 doses; range: 0.6-7.2 mg/day
    I.M.: Betamethasone sodium phosphate and betamethasone acetate: 0.6-9 mg/
    day (generally, $^1/_3$ to $^1/_2$ of oral dose) divided every 12-24 hours
Adults:
    Intrabursal, intra-articular, intradermal: 0.25-2 mL
    Intralesional: Rheumatoid arthritis/osteoarthritis:
      Very large joints: 1-2 mL
      Large joints: 1 mL
      Medium joints: 0.5-1 mL
      Small joints: 0.25-0.5 mL
    Topical:
      Foam: Apply to the scalp twice daily, once in the morning and once at night
      Gel, augmented formulation: Apply once or twice daily; rub in gently. **Note:** Do
      not exceed 2 weeks of treatment or 50 g/week.
      Lotion: Apply a few drops twice daily
        Augmented formulation: Apply a few drops once or twice daily; rub in gently.
        Note: Do not exceed 2 weeks of treatment or 50 mL/week.
      Cream/ointment: Apply once or twice daily
        Augmented formulation: Apply once or twice daily. **Note:** Do not exceed 2
        weeks of treatment or 45 g/week.

Dosing adjustment in hepatic impairment: Adjustments may be necessary in
patients with liver failure because betamethasone is extensively metabolized in
the liver

Administration
Oral: Not for alternate day therapy; once daily doses should be given in the
morning. May be administered with food to decrease GI distress.
I.M.: Do **not** give injectable sodium phosphate/acetate suspension I.V.
Topical: Apply topical sparingly to areas. Not for use on broken skin or in areas of
infection. Do not apply to wet skin unless directed; do not cover with occlusive
dressing. Do not apply very high potency agents to face, groin, axillae, or diaper
area.
    Foam: Invert can and dispense a small amount onto a saucer or other cool
    surface. Do not dispense directly into hands. Pick up small amounts of foam
    and gently massage into affected areas until foam disappears. Repeat until
    entire affected scalp area is treated.

Pregnancy Risk Factor C

Contraindications Hypersensitivity to betamethasone, other corticosteroids, or any component of the formulation; systemic fungal infections; I.M. administration contraindicated in idiopathic thrombocytopenia purpura

Warnings/Precautions Very high potency topical products are not for treatment of rosacea, perioral dermatitis; not for use on face, groin, or axillae; not for use in a diapered area. Avoid concurrent use of other corticosteroids.

May cause hypercorticism or suppression of hypothalamic-pituitary-adrenal (HPA) axis, particularly in younger children or in patients receiving high doses for prolonged periods. HPA axis suppression may lead to adrenal crisis. Withdrawal and discontinuation of a corticosteroid should be done slowly and carefully. Particular care is required when patients are transferred from systemic corticosteroids to inhaled products due to possible adrenal insufficiency or withdrawal from steroids, including an increase in allergic symptoms. Patients receiving >20 mg per day of prednisone (or equivalent) may be most susceptible. Fatalities have occurred due to adrenal insufficiency in asthmatic patients during and after transfer from systemic corticosteroids to aerosol steroids; aerosol steroids do not provide the systemic steroid needed to treat patients having trauma, surgery, or infections. In stressful situations, HPA axis-suppressed patients should receive adequate supplementation with natural glucocorticoids (hydrocortisone or cortisone) rather than betamethasone (due to lack of mineralocorticoid activity).

Acute myopathy has been reported with high dose corticosteroids, usually in patients with neuromuscular transmission disorders; may involve ocular and/or respiratory muscles; monitor creatine kinase; recovery may be delayed. Corticosteroid use may cause psychiatric disturbances, including depression, euphoria, insomnia, mood swings, and personality changes. Pre-existing psychiatric conditions may be exacerbated by corticosteroid use. Prolonged use of corticosteroids may also increase the incidence of secondary infection, mask acute infection (including fungal infections), prolong or exacerbate viral infections, or limit response to vaccines. Exposure to chickenpox should be avoided; corticosteroids should not be used to treat ocular herpes simplex. Corticosteroids should not be used for cerebral malaria or viral hepatitis. Close observation is required in patients with latent tuberculosis and/or TB reactivity; restrict use in active TB (only in conjunction with antituberculosis treatment). Prolonged treatment with corticosteroids has been associated with the development of Kaposi's sarcoma (case reports); if noted, discontinuation of therapy should be considered. High-dose corticosteroids should not be used to manage acute head injury.

Use with caution in patients with thyroid disease, hepatic impairment, renal impairment, cardiovascular disease, diabetes, glaucoma, cataracts, myasthenia gravis, patients at risk for osteoporosis, patients at risk for seizures, or GI diseases (diverticulitis, peptic ulcer, ulcerative colitis) due to perforation risk. Use caution following acute MI (corticosteroids have been associated with myocardial rupture). Because of the risk of adverse effects, systemic corticosteroids should be used cautiously in the elderly in the smallest possible effective dose for the shortest duration. Do not use occlusive dressings on weeping or exudative lesions and general caution with occlusive dressings should be observed; adverse effects may be increased. Discontinue if skin irritation or contact dermatitis should occur; do not use in patients with decreased skin circulation. Withdraw therapy with gradual tapering of dose. May affect growth velocity; growth should be routinely monitored in pediatric patients. Topical use in patients ≤12 years of age is not recommended.

Adverse Reactions
Systemic:
Cardiovascular: Congestive heart failure, edema, hyper-/hypotension

Central nervous system: Dizziness, headache, insomnia, intracranial pressure increased, lightheadedness, nervousness, pseudotumor cerebri, seizure, vertigo

Dermatologic: Ecchymoses, facial erythema, fragile skin, hirsutism, hyper-/hypopigmentation, perioral dermatitis (oral), petechiae, striae, wound healing impaired

Endocrine & metabolic: Amenorrhea, Cushing's syndrome, diabetes mellitus, growth suppression, hyperglycemia, hypokalemia, menstrual irregularities, pituitary-adrenal axis suppression, protein catabolism, sodium retention, water retention

Gastrointestinal: Abdominal distention, appetite increased, hiccups, indigestion, peptic ulcer, pancreatitis, ulcerative esophagitis

Local: Injection site reactions (intra-articular use), sterile abscess

Neuromuscular & skeletal: Arthralgia, muscle atrophy, fractures, muscle weakness, myopathy, osteoporosis, necrosis (femoral and humeral heads)

Ocular: Cataracts, glaucoma, intraocular pressure increased

Miscellaneous: Anaphylactoid reaction, diaphoresis, hypersensitivity, secondary infection

Topical:

Dermatologic: Acneiform eruptions, allergic dermatitis, burning, dry skin, erythema, folliculitis, hypertrichosis, irritation, miliaria, pruritus, skin atrophy, striae, vesiculation

Endocrine and metabolic effects have occasionally been reported with topical use.

Drug Interactions

Metabolism/Transport Effects Inhibits CYP3A4 (weak)

Avoid Concomitant Use

Avoid concomitant use of Betamethasone with any of the following: Natalizumab; Vaccines (Live)

Increased Effect/Toxicity

Betamethasone may increase the levels/effects of: Acetylcholinesterase Inhibitors; Amphotericin B; CycloSPORINE; Leflunomide; Loop Diuretics; Natalizumab; NSAID (COX-2 Inhibitor); NSAID (Nonselective); Thiazide Diuretics; Vaccines (Live); Warfarin

The levels/effects of Betamethasone may be increased by: Antifungal Agents (Azole Derivatives, Systemic); Aprepitant; Calcium Channel Blockers (Nondihydropyridine); CycloSPORINE; Estrogen Derivatives; Fluconazole; Fosaprepitant; Macrolide Antibiotics; Neuromuscular-Blocking Agents (Nondepolarizing); Quinolone Antibiotics; Salicylates; Trastuzumab

Decreased Effect

Betamethasone may decrease the levels/effects of: Antidiabetic Agents; Calcitriol; Corticorelin; Isoniazid; Salicylates; Vaccines (Inactivated); Vaccines (Live)

The levels/effects of Betamethasone may be decreased by: Aminoglutethimide; Antacids; Barbiturates; Bile Acid Sequestrants; Echinacea; Mitotane; Primidone; Rifamycin Derivatives

Ethanol/Nutrition/Herb Interactions

Ethanol: Avoid ethanol (may enhance gastric mucosal irritation).

Food: Betamethasone interferes with calcium absorption.

Herb/Nutraceutical: Avoid cat's claw, echinacea (have immunostimulant properties).

Dietary Considerations May be taken with food to decrease GI distress.

Dosage Forms Excipient information presented when available (limited, particularly for generics); consult specific product labeling.

Note: Potency expressed as betamethasone base.

Aerosol, topical, as valerate [foam]:

Luxiq®: 0.12% (50 g, 100 g, 150 g) [strength expressed as salt; contains ethanol 60.4%]

Cream, topical, as dipropionate: 0.05% (15 g, 45 g)

Cream, topical, as dipropionate augmented: 0.05% (15 g, 50 g)

Diprolene® AF: 0.05% (15 g, 50 g)

Cream, topical, as valerate (Beta-Val®): 0.1% (15 g, 45 g)

Beta-Val®: 0.1% (15 g, 45 g)

Gel, topical, as dipropionate augmented: 0.05% (15 g, 50 g)

Injection, suspension: Betamethasone sodium phosphate 3 mg and betamethasone acetate 3 mg per 1 mL (5 mL)

Celestone® Soluspan®: Betamethasone sodium phosphate 3 mg and betamethasone acetate 3 mg per 1 mL (5 mL) [6 mg/mL]

Lotion, topical, as dipropionate: 0.05% (60 mL)

Lotion, topical, as dipropionate augmented:

Diprolene®: 0.05% (30 mL, 60 mL)

◀ Lotion, topical, as valerate: 0.1% (60 mL)
  Beta-Val®: 0.1% (60 mL)
Ointment, topical, as dipropionate: 0.05% (15 g, 45 g)
Ointment, topical, as dipropionate augmented: 0.05% (15 g, 50 g)
  Diprolene®: 0.05% (15 g, 50 g)
Ointment, topical, as valerate: 0.1% (15 g, 45 g)
Solution, as base:
  Celestone®: 0.6 mg/5 mL (118 mL) [contains alcohol and sodium benzoate; cherry-orange flavor]

References

Abraham E and Evans T, "Corticosteroids and Septic Shock (editorial)," *JAMA*, 2002, 288(7):886-7.

Annane D, Sebille V, Charpentier C, et al, "Effect of Treatment With Low Doses of Hydrocortisone and Fludrocortisone on Mortality in Patients With Septic Shock," *JAMA*, 2002, 288(7):862-71.

Cooper MS and Stewart PM, "Corticosteroid Insufficiency in Acutely Ill Patients," *N Engl J Med*, 2003, 348(8):727-34.

Coursin DB and Wood KE, "Corticosteroid Supplementation for Adrenal Insufficiency," *JAMA*, 2002, 287(2):236-40.

de Jonghe B, Sharshar T, Lefaucheur JP, et al, "Paresis Acquired in the Intensive Care Unit. A Prospective Multicenter Study," *JAMA*, 2002, 288(22):2859-67.

Gamsu HR, Mullinger BM, Donnai P, et al, "Antenatal Administration of Betamethasone to Prevent Respiratory Distress Syndrome in Preterm Infants: Report of a UK Multicentre Trial," *Br J Obstet Gynaecol*, 1989, 96(4):401-10.

Hotchkiss RS and Karl IE, "The Pathophysiology and Treatment of Sepsis," *N Engl J Med*, 2003, 348(2):138-50.

Liggins GC and Howie RN, "A Controlled Trial of Antepartum Glucocorticoid Treatment of Respiratory Distress Syndrome in Premature Infants," *Pediatrics*, 1972, 50(4):515-25.

Salem M, Tainsh RE, Jr, Bromberg J, et al, "Perioperative Glucocorticoid Coverage: A Reassessment 42 Years After Emergence of a Problem," *Ann Surg*, 1994, 219(4):416-25.

◆ **Betamethasone Dipropionate** *see* Betamethasone *on page 186*

◆ **Betamethasone Dipropionate, Augmented** *see* Betamethasone *on page 186*

◆ **Betamethasone Sodium Phosphate** *see* Betamethasone *on page 186*

◆ **Betamethasone Valerate** *see* Betamethasone *on page 186*

◆ **Betapace®** *see* Sotalol *on page 1321*

◆ **Betapace AF®** *see* Sotalol *on page 1321*

◆ **Betasept® [OTC]** *see* Chlorhexidine Gluconate *on page 291*

◆ **Beta-Val®** *see* Betamethasone *on page 186*

Betaxolol (be TAKS oh lol)

Related Information
Beta-Blockers *on page 1669*

U.S. Brand Names Betoptic® S; Kerlone®

Canadian Brand Names Betoptic® S; Sandoz-Betaxolol

Index Terms Betaxolol Hydrochloride

Pharmacologic Category Beta Blocker, Beta$_1$ Selective; Ophthalmic Agent, Antiglaucoma

Use
Ophthalmic: Treatment of chronic open-angle glaucoma or ocular hypertension
Oral: Management of hypertension

Pharmacodynamics/Kinetics
Onset of action: Ophthalmic: 30 minutes; Oral: 1-1.5 hours
Duration: Ophthalmic: ≥12 hours
Absorption: Ophthalmic: Some systemic; Oral: ~100%
Metabolism: Hepatic to multiple metabolites
Protein binding: Oral: ~50%
Bioavailability: Oral: 89%
Half-life elimination: Oral: 14-22 hours; prolonged in hepatic disease and/or chronic renal failure
Time to peak: Ophthalmic: ~2 hours; Oral: 1.5-6 hours
Excretion: Urine (>80%; as unchanged drug [15%] and inactive metabolites)

Dosage
Children and Adults: Ophthalmic suspension (Betoptic® S): Instill 1 drop into affected eye(s) twice daily.

Adults:

Ophthalmic solution: Instill 1-2 drops into affected eye(s) twice daily.

Oral: 5-10 mg/day; may increase dose to 20 mg/day after 7-14 days if desired response is not achieved.

Elderly:

Ophthalmic: Refer to adult dosing.

Oral: Refer to adult dosing; initial dose: 5 mg/day

Dosage adjustment in renal impairment: Severe impairment: Initial dose: 5 mg/ day; may increase every 2 weeks up to a maximum of 20 mg/day

Hemodialysis: Initial dose: 5 mg/day; may increase every 2 weeks up to a maximum of 20 mg/day. Supplemental dose not required.

Anesthesia and Critical Care Concerns/Other Considerations

Surgery: Based on available evidence, beta-blockers should be started days to weeks before elective surgery in selected patients when possible and titrated to a heart rate <65 beats per minute. Additional data suggest that long acting beta-blockers may be superior to short acting ones (Redelmeier, 2005). The ACC/AHA 2007 guidelines on perioperative cardiovascular evaluation and care for noncardiac surgery recommend beta-blockers be continued in patients undergoing surgery who are receiving beta-blockers to treat angina, symptomatic arrhythmias, hypertension, and other ACC/AHA Class I guideline indications (Class I recommendation). The guidelines also recommend that beta-blockers be given to patients undergoing vascular surgery who have myocardial ischemia demonstrated during preoperative testing (Class I recommendation). Since the publication of these guidelines, there have been two large trials published regarding this issue.

The guidelines also state that beta-blockers are probably recommended in patients undergoing intermediate risk (eg, carotid endarterectomy, prostate surgery) or vascular surgery in whom preoperative assessment identifies coronary heart disease or high cardiac risk (Class IIa recommendation). High cardiac risk is defined as having >1 of the following clinical risk factors: History of ischemic heart disease, compensated or prior heart failure, cerebrovascular disease, diabetes mellitus, or renal insufficiency. The use of beta-blockers is uncertain in patients undergoing intermediate risk or vascular surgery with ≤1 clinical risk factor (Class IIb recommendation).

The majority of published trials suggest a benefit of perioperative beta-blocker use during noncardiac surgery especially in high-risk patients; however, more recent clinical trials have not shown a benefit to perioperative beta-blockade for noncardiac surgery (Juul, 2006; Yang, 2006).

Additional Information Complete prescribing information for this medication should be consulted for additional detail.

Dosage Forms Excipient information presented when available (limited, particularly for generics); consult specific product labeling. [DSC] = Discontinued product

Solution, ophthalmic: 0.5% (5 mL, 10 mL, 15 mL) [contains benzalkonium chloride]

Suspension, ophthalmic:

Betoptic® S: 0.25% (5 mL [DSC], 10 mL, 15 mL) [contains benzalkonium chloride]

Tablet, as hydrochloride: 10 mg, 20 mg

Kerlone®: 10 mg, 20 mg

References

Fleisher LA, Beckman JA, Brown KA, et al, "ACC/AHA 2006 Guideline Update on Perioperative Cardiovascular Evaluation for Noncardiac Surgery: Focused Update on Perioperative Beta-Blocker Therapy: A Report of the American College of Cardiology/American Heart Association Task Force on Practice Guidelines (Writing Committee to Update the 2002 Guidelines on Perioperative Cardiovascular Evaluation for Noncardiac Surgery) Developed in Collaboration With the American Society of Echocardiography, American Society of Nuclear Cardiology, Heart Rhythm Society, Society of Cardiovascular Anesthesiologists, Society for Cardiovascular Angiography and Interventions, and Society for Vascular Medicine and Biology," *J Am Coll Cardiol*, 2006, 47 (11):2343-55.

Juul AB, Wetterslev J, Gluud C, et al, "Effect of Perioperative Beta-Blockade in Patients With Diabetes Undergoing Major Noncardiac Surgery: Randomized Placebo Controlled, Blinded Multicentre Trial," *BMJ*, 2006, 332(7556):1482.

Yang H, Raymer K, Butler R, et al, "The Effects of Perioperative Beta-Blockade: Results of the Metoprolol After Vascular Surgery (MaVS) Study, A Randomized Controlled Trial," *Am Heart J* 2006, 152(5):983-90.

Bisoprolol (bis OH proe lol)

Related Information
Antiarrhythmic Drugs *on page 1656*
Beta-Blockers *on page 1669*
Heart Failure (Systolic) *on page 1739*

U.S. Brand Names Zebeta®

Canadian Brand Names Apo-Bisoprolol®; Monocor®; Novo-Bisoprolol; PMS-Bisoprolol; PRO-Bisoprolol; Sandoz-Bisoprolol; Zebeta®; ZYM-Bisoprolol

Index Terms Bisoprolol Fumarate

Pharmacologic Category Beta Blocker, Beta$_1$ Selective

Use Treatment of hypertension, alone or in combination with other agents

Unlabeled/Investigational Use Chronic stable angina, supraventricular arrhythmias, PVCs, heart failure (HF)

Pharmacodynamics/Kinetics
Onset of action: 1-2 hours

Absorption: Rapid and almost complete

Distribution: Widely; highest concentrations in heart, liver, lungs, and saliva; crosses blood-brain barrier

Protein binding: ~30%

Metabolism: Extensively hepatic; significant first-pass effect (~20%)

Bioavailability: ~80%

Half-life elimination: Normal renal function: 9-12 hours; Cl_{cr} <40 mL/minute: 27-36 hours; Hepatic cirrhosis: 8-22 hours

Time to peak: 2-4 hours

Excretion: Urine (50% as unchanged drug, remainder as inactive metabolites); feces (<2%)

Dosage
Oral:

Adults: 2.5-5 mg once daily; may be increased to 10 mg and then up to 20 mg once daily, if necessary

Hypertension (JNC 7): 2.5-10 mg once daily

HF (unlabeled use): Initial: 1.25 mg once daily; maximum recommended dose: 10 mg once daily. **Note:** Increase dose gradually and monitor for signs and symptoms of CHF.

Elderly: Initial dose: 2.5 mg/day; may be increased by 2.5-5 mg/day; maximum recommended dose: 20 mg/day

Dosing adjustment in renal impairment: Cl_{cr} <40 mL/minute: Initial: 2.5 mg/day; increase cautiously.

Hemodialysis: Not dialyzable

Anesthesia and Critical Care Concerns/Other Considerations

Surgery: Based on available evidence, beta-blockers should be started days to weeks before elective surgery in selected patients when possible and titrated to a heart rate <65 beats per minute. Additional data suggest that long acting beta-blockers may be superior to short acting ones (Redelmeier, 2005). The ACC/AHA 2007 guidelines on perioperative cardiovascular evaluation and care for noncardiac surgery recommend beta-blockers be continued in patients undergoing surgery who are receiving beta-blockers to treat angina, symptomatic arrhythmias, hypertension, or other ACC/AHA Class I guideline indications (Class I recommendation). The guidelines also recommend that beta-blockers be given to patients undergoing vascular surgery who have myocardial ischemia demonstrated during preoperative testing (Class I recommendation).

The guidelines also state that beta-blockers are probably recommended in patients undergoing intermediate risk (eg, carotid endarterectomy, prostate surgery) or vascular surgery in whom preoperative assessment identifies coronary heart disease or high cardiac risk (Class IIa recommendation). High cardiac risk is defined as having >1 of the following clinical risk factors: History of ischemic heart disease, compensated or prior heart failure, cerebrovascular disease, diabetes mellitus, or renal insufficiency. The use of beta-blockers is uncertain in patients undergoing intermediate risk or vascular surgery with ≤1 clinical risk factor (Class IIb recommendation).

The majority of published trials suggest a benefit of perioperative beta-blocker use during noncardiac surgery especially in high-risk patients; however, more recent clinical trials have not shown a benefit to perioperative beta-blockade for noncardiac surgery (Juul, 2006; Yang, 2006).

Additional Information Complete prescribing information for this medication should be consulted for additional detail.

Dosage Forms Excipient information presented when available (limited, particularly for generics); consult specific product labeling.

Tablet, as fumarate: 5 mg, 10 mg

References

Fleisher LA, Beckman JA, Brown KA, et al, "ACC/AHA 2006 Guideline Update on Perioperative Cardiovascular Evaluation for Noncardiac Surgery: Focused Update on Perioperative Beta-Blocker Therapy: A Report of the American College of Cardiology/American Heart Association Task Force on Practice Guidelines (Writing Committee to Update the 2002 Guidelines on Perioperative Cardiovascular Evaluation for Noncardiac Surgery) Developed in Collaboration With the American Society of Echocardiography, American Society of Nuclear Cardiology, Heart Rhythm Society, Society of Cardiovascular Anesthesiologists, Society for Cardiovascular Angiography and Interventions, and Society for Vascular Medicine and Biology," *J Am Coll Cardiol,* 2006, 47 (11):2343-55.

Juul AB, Wetterslev J, Gluud C, et al, "Effect of Perioperative Beta-Blockade in Patients With Diabetes Undergoing Major Noncardiac Surgery: Randomized Placebo Controlled, Blinded Multicentre Trial," *BMJ,* 2006, 332(7556):1482.

Yang H, Raymer K, Butler R, et al, "The Effects of Perioperative Beta-Blockade: Results of the Metoprolol After Vascular Surgery (MaVS) Study, A Randomized Controlled Trial," *Am Heart J* 2006, 152(5):983-90.

♦ **Bisoprolol Fumarate** *see* Bisoprolol *on page 192*

♦ **Bistropamide** *see* Tropicamide *on page 1437*

Bivalirudin (bye VAL i roo din)

Medication Safety Issues

High alert medication: The Institute for Safe Medication Practices (ISMP) includes this medication among its list of drugs which have a heightened risk of causing significant patient harm when used in error.

U.S. Brand Names Angiomax®

Canadian Brand Names Angiomax®

Index Terms Hirulog

Pharmacologic Category Anticoagulant, Thrombin Inhibitor

Generic Available No

Use Anticoagulant used in conjunction with aspirin for patients with unstable angina undergoing percutaneous transluminal coronary angioplasty (PTCA) or percutaneous coronary intervention (PCI) with provisional glycoprotein IIb/IIIa inhibitor; anticoagulant used in patients undergoing PCI with (or at risk of) heparin-induced thrombocytopenia (HIT) / thrombosis syndrome (HITTS)

Unlabeled/Investigational Use Heparin-induced thrombocytopenia (HIT); ST-elevation myocardial infarction (STEMI) undergoing primary PCI

Mechanism of Action Bivalirudin acts as a specific and reversible direct thrombin inhibitor; it binds to the catalytic and anionic exosite of both circulating and clot-bound thrombin. Catalytic binding site occupation functionally inhibits coagulant effects by preventing thrombin-mediated cleavage of fibrinogen to fibrin monomers, and activation of factors V, VIII, and XIII. Shows linear dose- and concentration-dependent prolongation of ACT, aPTT, PT, and TT.

Pharmacodynamics/Kinetics

Onset of action: Immediate

Duration: Coagulation times return to baseline ~1 hour following discontinuation of infusion

Distribution: 0.2 L/kg

Protein binding, plasma: Does not bind other than thrombin

Metabolism: Blood proteases

Half-life elimination: Normal renal function: 25 minutes; Cl_{cr} 10-29 mL/minute: 57 minutes; Dialysis-dependent patients (off dialysis): 3.5 hours

Excretion: Urine (20%), proteolytic cleavage

Dosage I.V.: Adults:

Unstable angina/non-ST-elevation myocardial infarction (UA/NSTEMI) (moderate-high risk) undergoing invasive strategy (unlabeled dose): Initial dose: 0.1 mg/kg bolus, followed by 0.25 mg/kg/hour. Prior to PCI, give an additional bolus of 0.5 mg/kg and increase infusion rate to 1.75 mg/kg/hour.

Anticoagulant in patients undergoing PTCA/PCI or PCI with HITS/HITTS (treatment should be started just prior to procedure): Initial: Bolus: 0.75 mg/kg, followed by continuous infusion: 1.75 mg/kg/hour for the duration of procedure and up to 4 hours postprocedure if needed; determine ACT 5 minutes after bolus dose; may administer additional bolus of 0.3 mg/kg if necessary.

A glycoprotein IIb/IIIa inhibitor may be administered concomitantly during the procedure.

If needed, infusion may be continued beyond initial 4 hours at 0.2 mg/kg/hour for up to 20 hours.

Cardiac surgery (unlabeled; Warkentin, 2008):

Off-pump: Initial bolus: 0.75 mg/kg, followed by continuous infusion 1.75 mg/kg/hour to maintain ACT >300 seconds

On-pump: Initial bolus: 1 mg/kg, followed by continuous infusion 2.5 mg/kg/hour; 50 mg bolus added to priming solution of cardiopulmonary bypass (CPB) circuit

Additional boluses of 0.1-0.5 mg may be given to maintain ACT >2.5 times baseline ACT. **Note:** Special maneuvers needed to prevent stasis and consequent clotting within CPB circuit during or after surgery.

HIT (unlabeled use; Warkentin, 2008): Normal renal function: Initial dose: ~0.15 mg/kg/hour; adjust to aPTT 1.5-2.5 times baseline value

STEMI undergoing primary PCI (unlabeled use; Stone, 2008): Initial: Bolus: 0.75 mg/kg, followed by continuous infusion: 1.75 mg/kg/hour for the duration of procedure

Dosage adjustment in renal impairment: Infusion dose should be reduced based on degree of renal impairment; initial bolus dose remains unchanged; monitor activated coagulation time (ACT) or aPTT depending on indication.

For use in PCI:

Cl_{cr} ≥30 mL/minute: No adjustment required

Cl_{cr} 10-29 mL/minute: Decrease infusion rate to 1 mg/kg/hour

Dialysis-dependent patients (off dialysis): Decrease infusion rate to 0.25 mg/kg/hour

Clearance of bivalirudin remains 1.8-fold greater than the glomerular filtration rate, regardless of the degree in renal impairment.

Hemodialysis: Approximately 25% removed during hemodialysis

Dosage adjustment in hepatic impairment: No dosage adjustment is needed

Elderly: No dosage adjustment is needed in elderly patients with normal renal function. Puncture site hemorrhage and catheterization site hemorrhage were seen in more patients ≥65 years of age than in patients <65 years of age

Stability Store unopened vials at 15°C to 30°C. Reconstitute each 250 mg with 5 mL SWFI. Gently swirl to dissolve. Further dilution in D_5W or NS (50 mL to make 5 mg/mL solution **or** 500 mL to make 0.5 mg/mL solution) is required prior to infusion. Do not administer in same line with other medications. Following reconstitution, vials should be stored at 2°C to 8°C. Do not freeze. Final dilutions of 0.5 mg/mL or 5 mg/mL are stable at room temperature for up to 24 hours.

Administration For I.V. administration only.

Monitoring Parameters Depends upon indication for use of bivalirudin: ACT or aPTT

Anesthesia and Critical Care Concerns/Other Considerations

Cardiac Surgery: Bivalirudin has been used as an anticoagulant in CABG surgery as documented by case reports, case series (Koster, 2003; 2004), and more recently larger clinical trials. Bivalirudin binds to both exosite 1 and the active site of thrombin, producing only transient inhibition of thrombin. This is because thrombin cleaves bivalirudin and allows the active site to function again. This may be problematic in cases where there is not continuous blood flow through catheters, autotransfusion machines (eg, cell-saver devices), or intravenous lines (eg, CABG).

A number of clinical trials have demonstrated effectiveness in cardiac surgery for patients **without** HIT/HITTS (Merry, 2004; Smedira, 2006; Dyke, 2006). However, higher rates of bleeding with the use of bivalirudin as an alternative to heparin/protamine during cardiac surgery preclude its routine use in this setting.

Two prospective, open-label, multicenter trials demonstrated the safety and efficacy of bivalirudin as an alternative to heparin in patients **with** HIT/HITTS requiring on pump (Koster, 2007) and off pump (Dyke, 2007) cardiac surgery.

On-Pump Trial (CHOOSE-ON): Forty-nine patients with HIT/HITTS requiring cardiac surgery (redo-CABG, single valve surgery, or CABG + single-valve surgery) were treated with bivalirudin during CPB. Patients were excluded if Cl_{cr} <30 mL/minute, dependent on dialysis, had an EF <30%, or required surgery on >1 heart valve. A bivalirudin bolus of 50 mg was added to the priming solution of the CPB circuit. The patient was administered a bivalirudin bolus of 1 mg/kg I.V., followed by a continuous infusion of 2.5 mg/kg/hour until ~15 minutes before end of CPB. Patients were considered adequately anticoagulated if the ACT was ≥2.5 times the baseline. The primary endpoint of the study was in-hospital acute procedural success (defined as absence of death, Q-wave MI, repeat coronary revascularization, or stroke). Mean ACT achieved was not reported. Twenty percent of the patients had a Cl_{cr} 30-60 mL/minute. Procedural success in hospital or at 7 days occurred in 46 (94%) of patients. Mean intraoperative and 24-hour blood loss was 575 ± 524 mL and 998 ± 595 mL, respectively. No differences in outcome were noted between patients overall versus patients with moderate renal impairment.

Off-Pump Trial (CHOOSE-OFF): Thirty-five patients with HIT/HITTS requiring off-pump coronary artery bypass (OPCAB) were treated with bivalirudin. Patients were excluded if Cl_{cr} <30 mL/minute, EF <30%, or recent stroke (within prior 6 months). A bivalirudin bolus of 0.75 mg/kg was administered to the patient upon the surgeon's request with a continuous infusion of 1.75 mg/kg/hour. The target ACT was >300 seconds. Additional boluses or infusion titration was discouraged. Mean maximum ACT post-baseline was 388.2 ± 53.2 seconds. Procedural success at 7 days/discharge occurred in 47 (92%) patients. Chest tube output within 24 hours after surgery was 936 ± 525 mL. Two patients required reexploration for persistent postoperative hemorrhage.

Hemofiltration during CPB can be used to reduce concentrations of bivalirudin at the end of the procedure if needed.

Heparin-Induced Thrombocytopenia (HIT): Because bivalirudin has no structural similarity to heparin, it may be safely administered to patients with HIT or heparin-induced thrombotic thrombocytopenia syndrome (HITTS) or a history of HIT or HITTS.

Pregnancy Risk Factor B

Contraindications Hypersensitivity to bivalirudin or any component of the formulation; active major bleeding

◀ **Warnings/Precautions** Not for intramuscular use. Safety and efficacy have not been established in patients with unstable angina or acute coronary syndromes who are not undergoing PTCA or PCI. Increased risk of thrombus formation (some fatal) has been reported with bivalirudin use in gamma brachytherapy. As with all anticoagulants, bleeding may occur at any site and should be considered following an unexplained fall in blood pressure or hematocrit, or any unexplained symptom. Use with caution in patients with disease states associated with increased risk of bleeding. Use with caution in patients with renal impairment; dosage reduction required. Safety and efficacy in pediatric patients have not been established.

Adverse Reactions As with all anticoagulants, bleeding is the major adverse effect of bivalirudin. Hemorrhage may occur at virtually any site. Risk is dependent on multiple variables, including the intensity of anticoagulation and patient susceptibility. Additional adverse effects are often related to idiosyncratic reactions, and the frequency is difficult to estimate. Adverse reactions reported were generally less than those seen with heparin.

>10%:
  Cardiovascular: Hypotension (3% to 12%)
  Central nervous system: Pain (15%), headache (3% to 12%)
  Gastrointestinal: Nausea (3% to 15%)
  Neuromuscular & skeletal: Back pain (9% to 42%)
1% to 10%:
  Cardiovascular: Hypertension (6%), bradycardia (5%), angina (up to 5%)
  Central nervous system: Insomnia (7%), anxiety (6%), fever (5%), nervousness (5%)
  Gastrointestinal: Vomiting (6%), dyspepsia (5%), abdominal pain (5%)
  Genitourinary: Urinary retention (4%)
  Hematologic: Major hemorrhage (2% to 4%, compared to 4% to 9% with heparin); transfusion required (1% to 2%, compared to 2% to 6% with heparin), thrombocytopenia (<1% to 4%)
  Local: Injection site pain (3% to 8%)
  Neuromuscular & skeletal: Pelvic pain (6%)
<1% (Limited to important or life-threatening): Allergic reaction (including anaphylaxis), cerebral ischemia, confusion, facial paralysis, fatal bleeding, intracranial bleeding, kidney failure, pulmonary edema, retroperitoneal bleeding, syncope, thrombus formation (during PCI, including intracoronary brachytherapy), ventricular fibrillation

Drug Interactions

Avoid Concomitant Use There are no known interactions where it is recommended to avoid concomitant use.

Increased Effect/Toxicity

Bivalirudin may increase the levels/effects of: Anticoagulants; Ibritumomab; Tositumomab and Iodine I 131 Tositumomab

The levels/effects of Bivalirudin may be increased by: Antiplatelet Agents; Dasatinib; Herbs (Anticoagulant/Antiplatelet Properties); Nonsteroidal Anti-Inflammatory Agents; Pentosan Polysulfate Sodium; Prostacyclin Analogues; Salicylates; Thrombolytic Agents

Decreased Effect There are no known significant interactions involving a decrease in effect.

Test Interactions PT/INR levels may become elevated in the absence of warfarin. If warfarin is initiated, initial PT/INR goals while on bivalirudin may require modification.

Dosage Forms Excipient information presented when available (limited, particularly for generics); consult specific product labeling.

Injection, powder for reconstitution: 250 mg

References

Davis Z, Anderson R, Short D, et al, "Favorable Outcome With Bivalirudin Anticoagulation During Cardiopulmonary Bypass," *Ann Thorac Surg*, 2003, 75(1):264-5.

Koster A, Chew D, Grundel M, et al, "Bivalirudin Monitored With the Ecarin Clotting Time for Anticoagulation During Cardiopulmonary Bypass," *Anesth Analg*, 2003, 96(2): 383-6.

Koster A, Spiess B, Chew DP, et al. "Effectiveness of Bivalirudin as a Replacement for Heparin During Cardiopulmonary Bypass in Patients Undergoing Coronary Artery Bypass Grafting," *Am J Cardiol*, 2004, 93(3):356-9.

Merry AF, Raudkivi PJ, Middleton NG, et al, "Bivalirudin Versus Heparin and Protamine in Off-Pump Coronary Artery Bypass Surgery," *Ann Thorac Surg*, 2004, 77:925-31.

Robson R, "The Use of Bivalirudin in Patients With Renal Impairment," *J Invasive Cardiol*, 2000, 12:33F-36F.

Vasquez JC, Vichiendilokkul A, Mahmood S, et al, "Anticoagulation With Bivalirudin During Cardiopulmonary Bypass in Cardiac Surgery," *Ann Thorac Surg*, 2002, 74(6):2177-9.

◆ **Blenoxane® [DSC]** *see* Bleomycin *on page* 197

◆ **Blenoxane® (Can)** *see* Bleomycin *on page* 197

◆ **Bleo** *see* Bleomycin *on page* 197

Bleomycin (blee oh MYE sin)

Medication Safety Issues

Sound-alike/look-alike issues:

Bleomycin may be confused with Cleocin®

High alert medication: The Institute for Safe Medication Practices (ISMP) includes this medication among its list of drugs which have a heightened risk of causing significant patient harm when used in error.

U.S. Brand Names Blenoxane® [DSC]

Canadian Brand Names Blenoxane®; Bleomycin Injection, USP

Index Terms Bleo; Bleomycin Sulfate; BLM; NSC-125066

Pharmacologic Category Antineoplastic Agent, Antibiotic

Generic Available Yes

Use Treatment of squamous cell carcinomas, melanomas, sarcomas, testicular carcinoma, Hodgkin's lymphoma, and non-Hodgkin's lymphoma; sclerosing agent for malignant pleural effusion

Mechanism of Action Inhibits synthesis of DNA; binds to DNA leading to single- and double-strand breaks

Pharmacodynamics/Kinetics

Absorption: I.M. and intrapleural administration: 30% to 50% of I.V. serum concentrations; intraperitoneal and SubQ routes produce serum concentrations equal to those of I.V.

Distribution: V_d: 22 L/m^2; highest concentrations in skin, kidney, lung, heart tissues; lowest in testes and GI tract; does not cross blood-brain barrier

Protein binding: 1%

Metabolism: Via several tissues including hepatic, GI tract, skin, pulmonary, renal, and serum

Half-life elimination: Biphasic (renal function dependent):

Normal renal function: Initial: 1.3 hours; Terminal: 9 hours

End-stage renal disease: Initial: 2 hours; Terminal: 30 hours

Time to peak, serum: I.M.: Within 30 minutes

Excretion: Urine (50% to 70% as active drug)

Dosage Maximum cumulative lifetime dose: 400 units; refer to individual protocols; 1 unit = 1 mg

May be administered I.M., I.V., SubQ, or intracavitary

Children and Adults:

Test dose for lymphoma patients: I.M., I.V., SubQ: Because of the possibility of an anaphylactoid reaction, administer 1-2 units of bleomycin before the first 1-2 doses; monitor vital signs every 15 minutes; wait a minimum of 1 hour before administering remainder of dose; if no acute reaction occurs, then the regular dosage schedule may be followed. **Note:** Test doses may produce false-negative results.

Single-agent therapy:

I.M./I.V./SubQ: Squamous cell carcinoma, lymphoma, testicular carcinoma: 0.25-0.5 units/kg (10-20 units/m^2) 1-2 times/week

CIV: 15 units/m^2 over 24 hours daily for 4 days

Pleural sclerosing: Intrapleural: 60 units as a single instillation (some recommend limiting the dose in the elderly to 40 units/m^2; usual maximum: 60 units). Dose may be repeated at intervals of several days if fluid continues to accumulate (mix in 50-100 mL of NS); may add lidocaine 100-200 mg to reduce local discomfort.

Dosing adjustment in renal impairment:
The FDA-approved labeling recommends the following adjustments:
Cl_{cr} 40-50 mL/minute: Administer 70% of normal dose
Cl_{cr} 30-40 mL/minute: Administer 60% of normal dose
Cl_{cr} 20-30 mL/minute: Administer 55% of normal dose
Cl_{cr} 10-20 mL/minute: Administer 45% of normal dose
Cl_{cr} 5-10 mL/minute: Administer 40% of normal dose
The following guidelines have been used by some clinicians:
Aronoff, 2007: Adults: Continuous renal replacement therapy (CRRT): Administer 75% of dose
Kintzel, 1995:
Cl_{cr} 46-60 mL/minute: Administer 70% of dose
Cl_{cr} 31-45 mL/minute: Administer 60% of dose
Cl_{cr} <30 mL/minute: Consider use of alternative drug
Dosing adjustment in hepatic impairment: Not studied in patients with hepatic impairment; adjustment for hepatic impairment may be needed.

Stability
Refrigerate intact vials of powder. Intact vials are stable for up to 1 month at 45°C. Solutions for infusion are stable for 96 hours at room temperature and 14 days under refrigeration.
Reconstitute powder with 1-5 mL BWFI or BNS which is stable at room temperature or under refrigeration for 28 days.
Standard I.V. dilution: Dose/50-1000 mL NS.

Administration
I.V. doses should be administered slowly (over 10-60 minutes).
I.M. or SubQ: May cause pain at injection site
Intrapleural: 60 units in 50-100 mL NS; use of topical anesthetics or narcotic analgesia is usually not necessary

Monitoring Parameters Pulmonary function tests (total lung volume, forced vital capacity, carbon monoxide diffusion), renal function, liver function, chest x-ray, temperature initially; check body weight at regular intervals

Anesthesia and Critical Care Concerns/Other Considerations
Clinical Pearls/Comments: The use of oxygen concentrations (>30%) in animals previously treated with bleomycin has been reported to promote pulmonary toxicity. Although this is still controversial, supplemental oxygen should be used judiciously in patients who have received bleomycin.

Pregnancy Risk Factor D
Contraindications Hypersensitivity to bleomycin or any component of the formulation; severe pulmonary disease; pregnancy
Warnings/Precautions Hazardous agent - use appropriate precautions for handling and disposal. **[U.S. Boxed Warnings]: Occurrence of pulmonary fibrosis (commonly presenting as pneumonitis) is higher in elderly patients, patients receiving >400 units total lifetime dose or single doses >30 units, smokers, and patients with prior radiation therapy or receiving concurrent oxygen. A severe idiosyncratic reaction consisting of hypotension, mental confusion, fever, chills, and wheezing (similar to anaphylaxis) has been reported in 1% of lymphoma patients treated with bleomycin.** Since these reactions usually occur after the first or second dose, careful monitoring is essential after these doses. Use caution when administering O_2 during surgery to patients who have received bleomycin. Use caution with renal impairment, may require dose adjustment. May cause renal or hepatic toxicity. **[U.S. Boxed Warning]: Should be administered under the supervision of an experienced cancer chemotherapy physician.**

Adverse Reactions
>10%:
Dermatologic: Pain at the tumor site, phlebitis. About 50% of patients develop erythema, rash, striae, induration, hyperkeratosis, vesiculation, and peeling of the skin, particularly on the palmar and plantar surfaces of the hands and feet. Hyperpigmentation (50%), alopecia, nailbed changes may also occur. These effects appear dose related and reversible with discontinuation.
Gastrointestinal: Stomatitis and mucositis (30%), anorexia, weight loss
Respiratory: Tachypnea, rales, acute or chronic interstitial pneumonitis, and pulmonary fibrosis (5% to 10%); hypoxia and death (1%). Symptoms include cough, dyspnea, and bilateral pulmonary infiltrates. The pathogenesis is not

certain, but may be due to damage of pulmonary, vascular, or connective tissue. Response to steroid therapy is variable and somewhat controversial.

Miscellaneous: Acute febrile reactions (25% to 50%)

1% to 10%:

Dermatologic: Skin thickening, diffuse scleroderma, onycholysis, pruritus

Miscellaneous: Anaphylactoid-like reactions (characterized by hypotension, confusion, fever, chills, and wheezing; onset may be immediate or delayed for several hours); idiosyncratic reactions (1% in lymphoma patients)

<1% (Limited to important or life-threatening): Angioedema, cerebrovascular accident, cerebral arteritis, hepatotoxicity, malaise, MI, nausea, Raynaud's phenomenon, renal toxicity, scleroderma-like skin changes, thrombotic micro-angiopathy, vomiting; Myelosuppression (rare); Onset: 7 days, Nadir: 14 days, Recovery: 21 days

Drug Interactions

Avoid Concomitant Use

Avoid concomitant use of Bleomycin with any of the following: Natalizumab; Vaccines (Live)

Increased Effect/Toxicity

Bleomycin may increase the levels/effects of: Leflunomide; Natalizumab; Vaccines (Live)

The levels/effects of Bleomycin may be increased by: Gemcitabine; Trastuzumab

Decreased Effect

Bleomycin may decrease the levels/effects of: Cardiac Glycosides; Vaccines (Inactivated); Vaccines (Live)

The levels/effects of Bleomycin may be decreased by: Echinacea

Dosage Forms Excipient information presented when available (limited, particularly for generics); consult specific product labeling. [DSC] = Discontinued product

Injection, powder for reconstitution, as sulfate: 15 units, 30 units

Blenoxane®: 30 units [DSC]

◆ **Bleomycin Injection, USP (Can)** *see Bleomycin on page 197*

◆ **Bleomycin Sulfate** *see Bleomycin on page 197*

◆ **BLM** *see Bleomycin on page 197*

◆ **Blocadren** *see Timolol on page 1390*

◆ **BMS 337039** *see Aripiprazole on page 143*

◆ **Bondronat® (Can)** *see Ibandronate on page 716*

◆ **Boniva®** *see Ibandronate on page 716*

Bosentan (boe SEN tan)

Medication Safety Issues

Sound-alike/look-alike issues:

Tracleer® may be confused with TriCor®

Medication Guide An FDA-approved patient medication guide, which is available with the product information and at http://www.fda.gov/downloads/Drugs/DrugSafety/ucm089801.pdf, must be dispensed with this medication for each new outpatient prescription and refill.

U.S. Brand Names Tracleer®

Canadian Brand Names Tracleer®

Pharmacologic Category Endothelin Antagonist; Vasodilator

Restrictions Bosentan (Tracleer®) is only available through a limited distribution program (Tracleer® Access Program [T.A.P.]). Only prescribers and pharmacies registered with T.A.P. may prescribe and dispense bosentan. Further information may be obtained from the manufacturer, Actelion Pharmaceuticals (1-866-228-3546).

Generic Available No

◄ **Use** Treatment of pulmonary artery hypertension (PAH) (WHO Group I) in patients with World Health Organization (WHO) Class II, III, or IV symptoms to improve exercise capacity and decrease the rate of clinical deterioration

Mechanism of Action Blocks endothelin receptors on vascular endothelium and smooth muscle. Stimulation of these receptors is associated with vasoconstriction. Although bosentan blocks both ET_A and ET_B receptors, the affinity is higher for the A subtype.

Pharmacodynamics/Kinetics

Distribution: V_d: ~18 L

Protein binding, plasma: >98% primarily to albumin

Metabolism: Hepatic via CYP2C9 and 3A4 to three primary metabolites (one contributing ~10% to 20% pharmacologic activity); autoinduction may occur with chronic dosing

Bioavailability: ~50%

Half-life elimination: 5 hours; prolonged with heart failure, possibly in PAH

Time to peak, plasma: 3-5 hours

Excretion: Feces (as metabolites); urine (<3% as unchanged drug)

Dosage Oral:

Children ≤12 years (unlabeled use):

10-20 kg: Initial: 31.25 mg once daily for 4 weeks; increase to maintenance dose of 31.25 mg twice daily

>20-40 kg: Initial: 31.25 mg twice daily for 4 weeks; increase to maintenance dose of 62.5 mg twice daily

>40 kg: Initial: 62.5 mg twice daily for 4 weeks; increase to maintenance dose of 125 mg twice daily

Adolescents >12 years and ≥40 kg and Adults: Initial: 62.5 mg twice daily for 4 weeks; increase to maintenance dose of 125 mg twice daily; patients <40 kg should be maintained at 62.5 mg twice daily. Doses >125 mg twice daily do not appear to confer additional clinical benefit but may increase risk of liver toxicity.

Note: When discontinuing treatment, consider a reduction in dosage to 62.5 mg twice daily for 3-7 days (to avoid clinical deterioration).

Dosage adjustment for concurrent use of ritonavir:

Coadministration of *bosentan* in patients currently receiving ritonavir: For patients receiving ritonavir for at least 10 days, begin with bosentan 62.5 mg once daily or every other day based on tolerability

Coadministration of *ritonavir* in patients currently receiving bosentan: Discontinue bosentan 36 hours prior to the initiation of ritonavir, after at least 10 days of ritonavir; resume bosentan 62.5 mg once daily or every other day based on tolerability

Dosage adjustment in renal impairment: No dosage adjustment required.

Dosage adjustment in hepatic impairment: Avoid use in patients with **pretreatment** moderate-to-severe hepatic insufficiency and/or transaminase increases >3 x ULN

Modification based on transaminase elevation:

If any elevation, regardless of degree, is accompanied by clinical symptoms of hepatic injury (unusual fatigue, nausea, vomiting, abdominal pain, fever, or jaundice) or a serum bilirubin ≥2 times the upper limit of normal, treatment should be stopped.

AST/ALT >3 times but ≤5 times upper limit of normal: Confirm with additional test; if confirmed, reduce dose or interrupt treatment. Monitor transaminase levels at least every 2 weeks. May continue or reintroduce treatment, as appropriate, following return to pretreatment values. Begin with initial dose (above) and recheck transaminases within 3 days

AST/ALT >5 times but ≤8 times upper limit of normal: Confirm with additional test; if confirmed, stop treatment. Monitor transaminase levels at least every 2 weeks. May reintroduce treatment, as appropriate, at starting dose, following return to pretreatment values. Recheck within 3 days and thereafter following reinitiation.

AST/ALT >8 times upper limit of normal: Stop treatment and do not reintroduce.

Stability Store at 20°C to 25°C (68°F to 77°F); excursions permitted to 15°C to 30°C (59°F to 86°F).

Administration May be administered with or without food, once in the morning and once in the evening. Women of childbearing potential should avoid excessive handling broken tablets.

Monitoring Parameters Serum transaminase (AST and ALT) and bilirubin should be determined prior to the initiation of therapy and at monthly intervals thereafter. Monitor for clinical signs and symptoms of liver injury (eg, abdominal pain, fatigue, fever, jaundice, nausea, vomiting).

A woman of childbearing potential must have a negative pregnancy test prior to the initiation of therapy and monthly thereafter (prior to shipment of monthly refill). Hemoglobin and hematocrit should be measured at baseline, at 1 month and 3 months of treatment, and every 3 months thereafter (generally stabilizes after 4-12 weeks of treatment).

Pregnancy Risk Factor X

Contraindications Hypersensitivity to bosentan or any component of the formulation; concurrent use of cyclosporine or glyburide; pregnancy

Warnings/Precautions Hazardous agent - use appropriate precautions for handling and disposal. **[U.S. Boxed Warning]: Avoid use in moderate-to-severe hepatic impairment.** Has been associated with a high incidence (11%) of significant transaminase elevations, and rare cases of unexplained hepatic cirrhosis have occurred, including after long-term therapy. Transaminase elevations are dose dependent, generally asymptomatic, occur both early and late in therapy, progress slowly, and are usually reversible after treatment interruption or discontinuation. Avoid use in patients with elevated serum transaminases (>3 times upper limit of normal [ULN]) at baseline. Monitor hepatic function closely (at least monthly) for the duration of treatment. Treatment should be stopped in patients who develop elevated transaminases (ALT or AST) in combination with symptoms of hepatic injury (unusual fatigue, jaundice, nausea, vomiting, abdominal pain, and/or fever) or elevated serum bilirubin ≥2 times upper limit of normal. Safety of reintroduction is unknown.

[U.S. Boxed Warning]: Use in pregnancy is contraindicated; may cause birth defects. Exclude pregnancy prior to initiation of therapy, monthly during therapy and 1 month after stopping bosentan. Two reliable methods of contraception must be used during therapy and for one month after stopping treatment except in patients with tubal ligation or an implanted IUD (Copper T 380A or LNg 20). No other contraceptive measures are required for these patients. A missed menses should be reported to healthcare provider and prompt immediate pregnancy testing. Women of childbearing potential should avoid excessive handling of broken tablets. Sperm counts may be reduced in men during treatment. No changes in sperm function or hormone levels have been noted.

[U.S. Boxed Warning]: Because of the risks of hepatic impairment and the high likelihood of teratogenic effects, bosentan is only available through the T.A.P. restricted distribution program. Patients, prescribers, and pharmacies must be registered with and meet conditions of T.A.P. Call 1-866-228-3546 for more information.

A reduction in hematocrit/hemoglobin may be observed within the first few weeks of therapy with subsequent stabilization of levels. Hemoglobin reductions >15% have been observed in some patients. Measure hemoglobin prior to initiating therapy, at 1 and 3 months, and every 3 months thereafter. Significant decreases in hemoglobin in the absence of other causes may warrant the discontinuation of therapy.

Development of peripheral edema due to treatment and/or disease state (pulmonary arterial hypertension) may occur. There have also been postmarketing reports of fluid retention requiring treatment (eg, diuretics, fluid management, hospitalization). Further evaluation may be necessary to determine cause and appropriate treatment or discontinuation of therapy. Bosentan should be discontinued in any patient with pulmonary edema suggestive of pulmonary veno-occlusive disease (PVOD). Dosage adjustment required for concurrent use of ritonavir.

Adverse Reactions
>10%:
    Cardiovascular: Edema (11%)

Central nervous system: Headache (15%)

Endocrine & metabolic: Spermatogenesis inhibition (25%)

Hematologic: Hemoglobin decreased (≥1 g/dL in up to 57%; <11 g/dL: 3% to 6%; typically in first 6 weeks of therapy)

Hepatic: Transaminases increased (>3 times upper limit of normal; up to 12%; dose-related)

Respiratory: Respiratory tract infection (22%)

1% to 10%:

Cardiovascular: Chest pain (5%), syncope (5%), flushing (4%), hypotension (4%), palpitation (4%)

Hematologic: Anemia (3%)

Hepatic: Abnormal hepatic function (4%)

Neuromuscular & skeletal: Arthralgia (4%)

Respiratory: Sinusitis (4%)

<1% (Limited to important or life-threatening): Angioneurotic edema, heart failure (exacerbation), cirrhosis (prolonged therapy), hyperbilirubinemia, hypersensitivity, jaundice, leukocytoclastic vasculitis, leukopenia, liver failure (rare), neutropenia, peripheral edema, rash, thrombocytopenia, weight gain

Drug Interactions

Metabolism/Transport Effects Substrate (major) of CYP2C9, 3A4; **Induces** CYP2C9 (strong), 3A4 (strong)

Avoid Concomitant Use

Avoid concomitant use of Bosentan with any of the following: CycloSPORINE; Dronedarone; Everolimus; GlyBURIDE; Nilotinib; Nisoldipine; Ranolazine; Tolvaptan

Increased Effect/Toxicity

The levels/effects of Bosentan may be increased by: Antifungal Agents (Azole Derivatives, Systemic); CycloSPORINE; CYP2C9 Inhibitors (Moderate); CYP2C9 Inhibitors (Strong); CYP3A4 Inhibitors (Moderate); CYP3A4 Inhibitors (Strong); Dasatinib; Eltrombopag; GlyBURIDE; Phosphodiesterase 5 Inhibitors; Ritonavir

Decreased Effect

Bosentan may decrease the levels/effects of: Contraceptive (Progestins); CycloSPORINE; CYP2C9 Substrates (High risk); CYP3A4 Substrates; Dronedarone; Everolimus; GlyBURIDE; HMG-CoA Reductase Inhibitors; Maraviroc; Nilotinib; Nisoldipine; Oral Contraceptive (Estrogens); Phosphodiesterase 5 Inhibitors; Ranolazine; Saxagliptin; Sorafenib; Tolvaptan; Vitamin K Antagonists

The levels/effects of Bosentan may be decreased by: CYP2C9 Inducers (Highly Effective); CYP3A4 Inducers (Strong); Deferasirox; GlyBURIDE; Herbs (CYP3A4 Inducers); Peginterferon Alfa-2b

Ethanol/Nutrition/Herb Interactions

Food: Bioavailability of bosentan is not affected by food. Bosentan serum concentrations may be increased by grapefruit juice.

Herb/Nutraceutical: Avoid St John's wort (may decrease serum concentrations of bosentan).

Dietary Considerations May be taken with or without food. Avoid grapefruit and grapefruit juice.

Dosage Forms Excipient information presented when available (limited, particularly for generics); consult specific product labeling.

Tablet:

Tracleer®: 62.5 mg, 125 mg

References

Badesch DB, Abman SH, Ahearn GS, et al, "Medical Therapy for Pulmonary Arterial Hypertension: ACCP Evidence-Based Clinical Practice Guidelines," *Chest*, 2004, 126(1 Suppl):35-62.

◆ **Botox®** *see* OnabotulinumtoxinA *on page 1053*

◆ **Botox® Cosmetic** *see* OnabotulinumtoxinA *on page 1053*

◆ **Botulinum Toxin Type A** *see* OnabotulinumtoxinA *on page 1053*

Botulism Immune Globulin (Intravenous-Human)
(BOT yoo lism i MYUN GLOB you lin, in tra VEE nus, YU man)

U.S. Brand Names BabyBIG®
Index Terms BIG-IV
Pharmacologic Category Blood Product Derivative; Immune Globulin
Restrictions Available from the California Department of Health
Use Treatment of infant botulism caused by toxin type A or B
Pharmacodynamics/Kinetics
  Duration: Protective neutralizing antibody levels: 6 months
  Half-life elimination: 28 days
Dosage I.V.: Children <1 year: Infant botulism: 1 mL/kg (50 mg/kg) as a single dose; infuse at 0.5 mL/kg/hour (25 mg/kg/hour) for the first 15 minutes; if well tolerated, may increase to 1 mL/kg/hour (50 mg/kg/hour)
Additional Information Complete prescribing information for this medication should be consulted for additional detail.
Dosage Forms Excipient information presented when available (limited, particularly for generics); consult specific product labeling.
  Injection, powder for reconstitution [preservative free]:
    BabyBIG®: ~100 mg [contains albumin and sucrose; packaged with SWFI]

- ◆ **Bovine Lung Surfactant** see Beractant on page 185
- ◆ **BranchAmin®** see Amino Acid Injection on page 81
- ◆ **Breathe Free® [OTC]** see Sodium Chloride on page 1304
- ◆ **Brethaire [DSC]** see Terbutaline on page 1360
- ◆ **Brethine** see Terbutaline on page 1360
- ◆ **Brevibloc®** see Esmolol on page 522
- ◆ **Brevicon®** see Ethinyl Estradiol and Norethindrone on page 554
- ◆ **Brevicon® 0.5/35 (Can)** see Ethinyl Estradiol and Norethindrone on page 554
- ◆ **Brevicon® 1/35 (Can)** see Ethinyl Estradiol and Norethindrone on page 554
- ◆ **Brevital® (Can)** see Methohexital on page 895
- ◆ **Brevital® Sodium** see Methohexital on page 895
- ◆ **Bricanyl [DSC]** see Terbutaline on page 1360
- ◆ **Bricanyl® (Can)** see Terbutaline on page 1360
- ◆ **Brioschi® [OTC]** see Sodium Bicarbonate on page 1301
- ◆ **BRL 43694** see Granisetron on page 669

Bromocriptine (broe moe KRIP teen)

Medication Safety Issues
  Sound-alike/look-alike issues:
    Bromocriptine may be confused with benztropine, brimonidine
    Cycloset® may be confused with Glyset®
    Parlodel® may be confused with pindolol, Provera®
U.S. Brand Names Cycloset®; Parlodel®; Parlodel® SnapTabs®
Canadian Brand Names Apo-Bromocriptine®; Parlodel®; PMS-Bromocriptine
Index Terms Bromocriptine Mesylate
Pharmacologic Category Anti-Parkinson's Agent, Dopamine Agonist; Ergot Derivative
Generic Available Yes
Use Treatment of hyperprolactinemia associated with amenorrhea with or without galactorrhea, infertility, or hypogonadism; treatment of prolactin-secreting adenomas; treatment of acromegaly; treatment of Parkinson's disease
Unlabeled/Investigational Use Neuroleptic malignant syndrome
Mechanism of Action Semisynthetic ergot alkaloid derivative and a dopamine receptor agonist which activates postsynaptic dopamine receptors in the tuberoinfundibular (inhibiting pituitary prolactin secretion) and nigrostriatal pathways (enhancing coordinated motor control).

Pharmacodynamics/Kinetics
Onset of action: Prolactin decreasing effect: 1-2 hours
Protein binding: 90% to 96%
Metabolism: Primarily hepatic via CYP3A; extensive first-pass biotransformation
Bioavailability: 28%
Half-life elimination: Biphasic: Terminal: 15 hours (range 8-20 hours)
Time to peak, serum: 1-3 hours
Excretion: Feces; urine (2% to 6% as unchanged drug and metabolites)

Dosage Oral:
Children: Hyperprolactinemia:
11-15 years (based on limited information): Initial: 1.25-2.5 mg daily; dosage may be increased as tolerated to achieve a therapeutic response (range: 2.5-10 mg daily).
≥16 years: Refer to adult dosing
Adults:
Parkinsonism: 1.25 mg twice daily, increased by 2.5 mg/day in 2- to 4-week intervals (usual dose range is 30-90 mg/day in 3 divided doses; maximum: 100 mg/day), though elderly patients can usually be managed on lower doses
Neuroleptic malignant syndrome (unlabeled use): 2.5-10 mg every 6-8 hours; continue therapy until NMS is controlled, then taper slowly
Acromegaly: Initial: 1.25-2.5 mg daily increasing by 1.25-2.5 mg daily as necessary every 3-7 days; usual dose: 20-30 mg/day (maximum: 100 mg/day)
Hyperprolactinemia: Initial: 1.25-2.5 mg/day; may be increased by 2.5 mg/day as tolerated every 2-7 days until optimal response (range: 2.5-15 mg/day)

Dosing adjustment in hepatic impairment: No guidelines are available, however, adjustment may be necessary

Administration May be administered with food to decrease GI distress.

Monitoring Parameters Monitor blood pressure closely as well as hepatic, hematopoietic, and cardiovascular function; visual field monitoring is recommended (prolactinoma); pregnancy test during amenorrheic period; growth hormone and prolactin levels.

Pregnancy Risk Factor B

Contraindications Hypersensitivity to bromocriptine, ergot alkaloids, or any component of the formulation; ergot alkaloids are contraindicated with potent inhibitors of CYP3A4 (includes protease inhibitors, azole antifungals, and some macrolide antibiotics); uncontrolled hypertension; severe ischemic heart disease or peripheral vascular disorders; pregnancy (risk to benefit evaluation must be performed in women who become pregnant during treatment for acromegaly, prolactinoma, or Parkinson's disease - hypertension during treatment should generally result in efforts to withdraw)

Warnings/Precautions Complete evaluation of pituitary function should be completed prior to initiation of treatment. Use caution in patients with a history of peptic ulcer disease, dementia, psychosis, or cardiovascular disease (myocardial infarction, arrhythmia). Symptomatic hypotension may occur in a significant number of patients. In addition, hypertension, seizures, MI, and stroke have been rarely associated with bromocriptine therapy. Severe headache or visual changes may precede events. The onset of reactions may be immediate or delayed (often may occur in the second week of therapy). Sudden sleep onset and somnolence have been reported with use, primarily in patients with Parkinson's disease. Patients must be cautioned about performing tasks which require mental alertness.

Concurrent antihypertensives or drugs which may alter blood pressure should be used with caution. Concurrent use with levodopa has been associated with an increased risk of hallucinations. Consider dosage reduction and/or discontinuation in patients with hallucinations. Hallucinations may require weeks to months before resolution.

Dopamine agonists have been associated with compulsive behaviors and/or loss of impulse control, which has manifested as pathological gambling, libido increases (hypersexuality), and/or binge eating. Causality has not been established, and controversy exists as to whether this phenomenon is related to the underlying disease, prior behaviors/addictions and/or drug therapy. Dose reduction or discontinuation of therapy has been reported to reverse these behaviors in some, but not all cases. Risk for melanoma development is increased in Parkinson's disease patients; drug causation or factors contributing to risk have not been established. Patients should be monitored closely and periodic skin examinations should be performed.

In the treatment of acromegaly, discontinuation is recommended if tumor expansion occurs during therapy. Digital vasospasm (cold sensitive) may occur in some patients with acromegaly; may require dosage reduction. Patients who receive bromocriptine during and immediately following pregnancy as a continuation of previous therapy (eg, acromegaly) should be closely monitored for cardiovascular effects. Should not be used postpartum in women with coronary artery disease or other cardiovascular disease. Use of bromocriptine to control or prevent lactation or in patients with uncontrolled hypertension is not recommended.

Monitoring and careful evaluation of visual changes during the treatment of hyperprolactinemia is recommended to differentiate between tumor shrinkage and traction on the optic chiasm; rapidly progressing visual field loss requires neurosurgical consultation. Discontinuation of bromocriptine in patients with macroadenomas has been associated with rapid regrowth of tumor and increased prolactin serum levels. Pleural and retroperitoneal fibrosis have been reported with prolonged daily use. Cardiac valvular fibrosis has also been associated with ergot alkaloids. Safety and efficacy have not been established in patients with hepatic or renal dysfunction. Safety and effectiveness in patients <11 years of age (for pituitary adenoma) have not been established. Safety has not been established for use >2 years in patients with Parkinson's disease.

Adverse Reactions Note: Frequency of adverse effects may vary by dose and/or indication.

>10%:
 Central nervous system: Dizziness, headache
 Gastrointestinal: Constipation, nausea

1% to 10%:
 Cardiovascular: Hypotension (including postural/orthostatic), Raynaud's syndrome exacerbation, syncope
 Central nervous system: Drowsiness, fatigue, lightheadedness
 Gastrointestinal: Abdominal cramps, anorexia, diarrhea, dyspepsia, GI bleeding, vomiting, xerostomia
 Neuromuscular & skeletal: Digital vasospasm
 Respiratory: Nasal congestion

Frequency not defined, postmarketing, and/or case reports: Abdominal discomfort, alcohol potentiation, alopecia, anxiety, arrhythmia, ataxia, blepharospasm, blurred vision, bradycardia, cerebrospinal fluid rhinorrhea, cold tolerance decreased, confusion, constrictive pericarditis, delusional psychosis, depression, dyskinesia, dysphagia, dyspnea, ear tingling, epileptiform seizure, ergotism, erythromelalgia, facial pallor, faintness, hallucinations, heavy headedness, insomnia, involuntary movements, lassitude, lethargy, lightheadedness, mottling of skin, muscle cramps, nervousness, nightmares, "on-off" phenomenon, paranoia, paresthesia, pericardial effusion, peripheral edema, pleural effusion, pleural/pulmonary fibrosis, psychomotor agitation/excitation, rash, sleep requirement decreased, sluggishness, urinary frequency, urinary retention, vasovagal attack, ventricular tachycardia, vertigo, visual disturbance, weakness

Withdrawal reactions: Abrupt discontinuation has resulted in rare cases of a withdrawal reaction with symptoms similar to neuroleptic malignant syndrome.

Reported with dopamine agonists: Impulsive/compulsive behaviors (eg, pathological gambling, hypersexuality, binge eating)

Drug Interactions

Metabolism/Transport Effects Substrate of CYP3A4 (major); **Inhibits** CYP1A2 (weak), 3A4 (weak)

Avoid Concomitant Use

Avoid concomitant use of Bromocriptine with any of the following: Efavirenz; Itraconazole; Posaconazole; Protease Inhibitors; Serotonin 5-HT1D Receptor Agonists; Sibutramine; Voriconazole

Increased Effect/Toxicity

Bromocriptine may increase the levels/effects of: CycloSPORINE; Serotonin 5-HT1D Receptor Agonists; Serotonin Modulators

The levels/effects of Bromocriptine may be increased by: Alpha-/Beta-Agonists; CYP3A4 Inhibitors (Moderate); CYP3A4 Inhibitors (Strong); Dasatinib; Efavirenz; Itraconazole; Macrolide Antibiotics; MAO Inhibitors; Posaconazole; Protease Inhibitors; Serotonin 5-HT1D Receptor Agonists; Sibutramine; Voriconazole

Decreased Effect
The levels/effects of Bromocriptine may be decreased by: Antipsychotics (Atypical); Antipsychotics (Typical); Metoclopramide

Ethanol/Nutrition/Herb Interactions
Ethanol: Avoid ethanol (may increase GI side effects or ethanol intolerance).
Herb/Nutraceutical: St John's wort may decrease bromocriptine levels.

Dietary Considerations May be taken with food to decrease GI distress.

Product Availability
Cycloset®: FDA approved May 2009; availability anticipated in the first quarter of 2010
Cycloset® has been approved for the treatment of type 2 diabetes.

Dosage Forms Excipient information presented when available (limited, particularly for generics); consult specific product labeling.
Capsule: 5 mg
Parlodel®: 5 mg
Tablet: 2.5 mg
Parlodel® SnapTabs®: 2.5 mg

References
Mueller PS, Vester JW, and Fermaglich J, "Neuroleptic Malignant Syndrome. Successful Treatment With Bromocriptine," *JAMA*, 1983, 249(3):386-8.
Strawn JR, Keck PE Jr, and Caroff SN, "Neuroleptic Malignant Syndrome," *Am J Psychiatry*, 2007, 164(6):870-6.

♦ **Bromocriptine Mesylate** *see* Bromocriptine *on page* 203

♦ **Brovana®** *see* Arformoterol *on page* 137

♦ **BTX-A** *see* OnabotulinumtoxinA *on page* 1053

♦ **B-type Natriuretic Peptide (Human)** *see* Nesiritide *on page* 999

♦ **Budeprion XL®** *see* BuPROPion *on page* 217

♦ **Budeprion SR®** *see* BuPROPion *on page* 217

Budesonide (byoo DES oh nide)

Related Information
Asthma *on page* 1728

U.S. Brand Names Entocort® EC; Pulmicort Flexhaler™; Pulmicort Respules®; Rhinocort® Aqua®

Canadian Brand Names Entocort®; Gen-Budesonide AQ; Mylan-Budesonide AQ; Pulmicort®; Rhinocort® Aqua™; Rhinocort® Turbuhaler®

Pharmacologic Category Corticosteroid, Inhalant (Oral); Corticosteroid, Nasal; Corticosteroid, Systemic

Use
Intranasal: Management of symptoms of seasonal or perennial rhinitis
Canadian labeling: Additional use (not in U.S. labeling): Prevention and treatment of nasal polyps
Nebulization: Maintenance and prophylactic treatment of asthma
Oral capsule: Treatment of active Crohn's disease (mild-to-moderate) involving the ileum and/or ascending colon; maintenance of remission (for up to 3 months) of Crohn's disease (mild-to-moderate) involving the ileum and/or ascending colon
Oral inhalation: Maintenance and prophylactic treatment of asthma; includes patients who require oral corticosteroids and those who may benefit from systemic dose reduction/elimination

Pharmacodynamics/Kinetics
Onset of action: Pulmicort Respules®: 2-8 days; Rhinocort® Aqua®: ~10 hours; Inhalation: 24 hours
Peak effect: Pulmicort Respules®: 4-6 weeks; Rhinocort® Aqua®: ~2 weeks; Inhalation: 1-2 weeks
Distribution: 2.2-3.9 L/kg

Protein binding: 85% to 90%

Metabolism: Hepatic via CYP3A4 to two metabolites: 16 alpha-hydroxyprednisolone and 6 beta-hydroxybudesonide; minor activity

Bioavailability: Limited by high first-pass effect; Capsule: 9% to 21%; Pulmicort Respules®: 6%; Inhalation: 6% to 13%; Nasal: 34%

Half-life elimination: 2-3.6 hours

Time to peak: Capsule: 0.5-10 hours (variable in Crohn's disease); Pulmicort Respules®: 10-30 minutes; Inhalation: 1-2 hours; Nasal: 1 hour

Excretion: Urine (60%) and feces as metabolites

Dosage

Nasal inhalation:

U.S. labeling (Rhinocort® Aqua®): Rhinitis: Children ≥6 years and Adults: 64 mcg/day as a single 32 mcg spray in each nostril. Some patients who do not achieve adequate control may benefit from increased dosage. A reduced dosage may be effective after initial control is achieved.

Maximum dose: Children <12 years: 128 mcg/day; Adults: 256 mcg/day

Canadian labeling:

Rhinocort® Aqua®: Children ≥6 years and Adults:

Nasal polyps: 256 mcg/day administered as a single 64 mcg spray in each nostril twice daily

Rhinitis: Initial: 256 mcg/day administered as two 64 mcg sprays in each nostril once daily or a single 64 mcg spray in each nostril twice daily; Maintenance: Individualize, lowest effective dose

Maximum dose: 256 mcg/day

Rhinocort® Turbuhaler®: Children ≥6 years and Adults:

Nasal polyps: 100 mcg into each nostril twice daily (maximum: 400 mcg/day)

Rhinitis: Initial: 200 mcg into each nostril once daily; Maintenance: Individualize, lowest effective dose (maximum: 400 mcg/day)

Nebulization: Children 12 months to 8 years: Asthma: Pulmicort Respules®: Titrate to lowest effective dose once patient is stable; start at 0.25 mg/day or use as follows:

Previous therapy of bronchodilators alone: 0.5 mg/day administered as a single dose or divided twice daily (maximum daily dose: 0.5 mg)

Previous therapy of inhaled corticosteroids: 0.5 mg/day administered as a single dose or divided twice daily (maximum daily dose: 1 mg)

Previous therapy of oral corticosteroids: 1 mg/day administered as a single dose or divided twice daily (maximum daily dose: 1 mg)

NIH Asthma Guidelines (NIH, 2007):

Children 0-4 years:

"Low" dose: 0.25-0.5 mg/day

"Medium" dose: >0.5-1 mg/day

"High" dose: >1 mg/day

Children 5-11 years:

"Low" dose: 0.5 mg/day

"Medium" dose: 1 mg/day

"High" dose: 2 mg/day

Oral inhalation: Asthma:

Children ≥6 years:

Pulmicort Flexhaler™: Initial: 180 mcg twice daily (some patients may be initiated at 360 mcg twice daily); maximum 360 mcg twice daily

NIH Asthma Guidelines (NIH, 2007) (administer in divided doses twice daily):

Children 5-11 years:

"Low" dose: 180-400 mcg/day

"Medium" dose: >400-800 mcg/day

"High" dose: >800 mcg/day

Children ≥12 years: Refer to adult dosing.

Pulmicort® Turbuhaler®: [CAN, not available in the U.S.]: Initial (during periods of severe asthma or when switching from oral corticosteroid therapy): 200-400 mcg daily in 2 divided doses; Maintenance: Individualized, lowest effective dose.

Adults:

Pulmicort Flexhaler™: Initial: 360 mcg twice daily (selected patients may be initiated at 180 mcg twice daily); maximum 720 mcg twice daily

NIH Asthma Guidelines (NIH, 2007) (administer in divided doses twice daily):
"Low" dose: 180-600 mcg/day
"Medium" dose: >600-1200 mcg/day
"High" dose: >1200 mcg/day

Pulmicort® Turbuhaler® [CAN, not available in the U.S.]: Initial (during periods of severe asthma or when switching from oral corticosteroid therapy): 400-2400 mcg daily in 2-4 divided doses; Maintenance: 200-400 mcg twice daily (higher doses may be needed for short periods of time). **Note:** Patients taking 400 mcg/day may take as a single daily dose

Oral: Crohn's disease (active): Adults: 9 mg once daily in the morning for up to 8 weeks; recurring episodes may be treated with a repeat 8-week course of treatment

Note: Patients receiving CYP3A4 inhibitors should be monitored closely for signs and symptoms of hypercorticism; dosage reduction may be required. If switching from oral prednisolone, prednisolone dosage should be tapered while budesonide (Entocort™ EC) treatment is initiated.

Maintenance of remission: Following treatment of active disease (control of symptoms with CDAI <150), treatment may be continued at a dosage of 6 mg once daily for up to 3 months. If symptom control is maintained for 3 months, tapering of the dosage to complete cessation is recommended. Continued dosing beyond 3 months has not been demonstrated to result in substantial benefit.

Dosage adjustment in hepatic impairment: Monitor closely for signs and symptoms of hypercorticism; dosage reduction may be required.

Anesthesia and Critical Care Concerns/Other Considerations

Surgery: For patients who have received oral systemic corticosteroids during the past 6 months and for selected patients on long-term, high-dose, inhaled corticosteroid (ICS), give stress doses of hydrocortisone intravenously during the surgical period and reduce the dose rapidly within 24 hours after surgery (Expert Panel Report 3, 2007). Clinically important adrenal suppression has been reported in patients receiving high doses of an ICS, particularly children.

Additional Information Complete prescribing information for this medication should be consulted for additional detail.

Dosage Forms Excipient information presented when available (limited, particularly for generics); consult specific product labeling. [CAN] = Canadian brand name; [DSC] = Discontinued product

Capsule, enteric coated:
Entocort® EC: 3 mg
Powder for nasal inhalation:
Rhinocort® Turbuhaler® [CAN]: 100 mcg/inhalation [delivers 200 metered actuations] [not available in the U.S.]
Powder for oral inhalation:
Pulmicort Flexhaler™: 90 mcg/inhalation (165 mg) [contains lactose; delivers ~80 mcg/inhalation; 60 actuations]
Pulmicort Flexhaler™: 180 mcg/inhalation (225 mg) [contains lactose; delivers ~160 mcg/inhalation; 120 actuations]
Pulmicort Turbuhaler® [CAN]: 100 mcg/inhalation [delivers 200 metered actuations]; 200 mcg/inhalation [delivers 200 metered actuations]; 400 mcg/inhalation [delivers 200 metered actuations] [not available in the U.S.]
Suspension, intranasal [spray]:
Rhinocort® Aqua®: 32 mcg/inhalation (8.6 g) [120 metered actuations]
Rhinocort® Aqua® [CAN]: 64 mcg/inhalation [120 metered actuations] [not available in the U.S.]
Suspension for nebulization:
Pulmicort Respules®: 0.25 mg/2 mL (2 mL); 0.5 mg/2 mL (2 mL); 1 mg/2 mL (2 mL)

References

Expert Panel Report 3, "Guidelines for the Diagnosis and Management of Asthma," *Clinical Practice Guidelines*, National Institutes of Health, National Heart, Lung, and Blood Institute, NIH Publication No. 08-4051, prepublication 2007. Available at http://www.nhlbi.nih.gov/guidelines/asthma/asthgdln.htm

Todd GR, Acerini CL, Buck JJ, et al, "Acute Adrenal Crisis in Asthmatics Treated With High-Dose Fluticasone Propionate," *Eur Respir J*, 2002, 19(6):1207-9.

Todd GR, Acerini CL, Ross-Russell R, et al, "Survey of Adrenal Crisis Associated With Inhaled Corticosteroids in the United Kingdom," *Arch Dis Child*, 2002, 87(6):457-61.

◆ **Buffasal [OTC]** *see* Aspirin *on page 147*

◆ **Bufferin® [OTC]** *see* Aspirin *on page 147*

◆ **Bufferin® Extra Strength [OTC]** *see* Aspirin *on page 147*

◆ **Buffinol [OTC]** *see* Aspirin *on page 147*

Bumetanide (byoo MET a nide)

Medication Safety Issues
Sound-alike/look-alike issues:
Bumetanide may be confused with Buminate®
Bumex® may be confused with Brevibloc®, Buprenex®, Permax®
Related Information
Diuretics, Loop *on page 1680*
Heart Failure (Systolic) *on page 1739*
U.S. Brand Names Bumex® [DSC]
Canadian Brand Names Bumex®; Burinex®
Pharmacologic Category Diuretic, Loop
Generic Available Yes

Use Management of edema secondary to heart failure or hepatic or renal disease including nephrotic syndrome; may be used alone or in combination with antihypertensives in the treatment of hypertension; can be used in furosemide-allergic patients

Mechanism of Action Inhibits reabsorption of sodium and chloride in the ascending loop of Henle and proximal renal tubule, interfering with the chloride-binding cotransport system, thus causing increased excretion of water, sodium, chloride, magnesium, phosphate, and calcium; it does not appear to act on the distal tubule

Pharmacodynamics/Kinetics
Onset of action: Oral, I.M.: 0.5-1 hour; I.V.: 2-3 minutes
Duration: 4-6 hours
Distribution: V_d: 13-25 L/kg
Protein binding: 95%
Metabolism: Partially hepatic
Half-life elimination: Neonates: ~6 hours; Infants (1 month): ~2.4 hours; Adults: 1-1.5 hours
Excretion: Primarily urine (as unchanged drug and metabolites)

Dosage
Oral, I.M., I.V.:
Neonates (see Warnings/Precautions): 0.01-0.05 mg/kg/dose every 24-48 hours
Infants and Children: 0.015-0.1 mg/kg/dose every 6-24 hours (maximum dose: 10 mg/day)
Adults:
Edema:
Oral: 0.5-2 mg/dose (maximum dose: 10 mg/day) 1-2 times/day
I.M., I.V.: 0.5-1 mg/dose; may repeat in 2-3 hours for up to 2 doses if needed (maximum dose: 10 mg/day)
Continuous I.V. infusion: Initial: 1 mg I.V. load then 0.5-2 mg/hour (ACC/AHA 2009 practice guidelines for heart failure)
Hypertension: Oral: 0.5 mg daily (maximum dose: 5 mg/day); usual dosage range (JNC 7): 0.5-2 mg/day in 2 divided doses

Stability
I.V.: Store vials at 15°C to 30°C (59°F to 86°F). Infusion solutions should be used within 24 hours after preparation. Light sensitive; discoloration may occur when exposed to light.
Tablet: Store at 15°C to 30°C (59°F to 86°F).

Administration Administer I.V. slowly, over 1-2 minutes. An alternate-day schedule or a 3-4 daily dosing regimen with rest periods of 1-2 days in between may be the most tolerable and effective regimen for the continued control of edema. Reserve I.V. administration for those unable to take oral medications.

Monitoring Parameters Blood pressure, serum electrolytes, renal function

◄ **Anesthesia and Critical Care Concerns/Other Considerations**
Clinical Pearls/Comments: If given the morning of surgery, it may render the patient volume depleted and blood pressure may be labile during general anesthesia.

Patients with impaired hepatic function must be monitored carefully due to increased risk of hepatic encephalopathy, often requiring reduced doses. Larger doses may be necessary in patients with impaired renal function to obtain the same therapeutic response.

Bumetanide may produce significant diuresis; it is important that patients are closely monitored for hypokalemia, hypomagnesemia, and volume depletion.

Dose equivalency (approximate): Bumetanide 1 mg = furosemide 40 mg = torsemide 10 mg
Pregnancy Risk Factor C (manufacturer); D (expert analysis)

Contraindications Hypersensitivity to bumetanide, any component of the formulation, or sulfonylureas; anuria; patients with hepatic coma or in states of severe electrolyte depletion until the condition improves or is corrected; pregnancy (based on expert analysis)

Warnings/Precautions [U.S. Boxed Warning]: Excessive amounts can lead to profound diuresis with fluid and electrolyte loss; close medical supervision and dose evaluation are required. In cirrhosis, avoid electrolyte and acid/base imbalances that might lead to hepatic encephalopathy. *In vitro* studies using pooled sera from critically-ill neonates have shown bumetanide to be a potent displacer of bilirubin; avoid use in neonates at risk for kernicterus. Coadministration of antihypertensives may increase the risk of hypotension.

Monitor fluid status and renal function in an attempt to prevent oliguria, azotemia, and reversible increases in BUN and creatinine; close medical supervision of aggressive diuresis required. Rapid I.V. administration, renal impairment, excessive doses, and concurrent use of other ototoxins is associated with ototoxicity. Asymptomatic hyperuricemia has been reported with use.

Chemical similarities are present among sulfonamides, sulfonylureas, carbonic anhydrase inhibitors, thiazides, and loop diuretics (except ethacrynic acid). Use in patients with sulfonylurea allergy is specifically contraindicated in product labeling, however, a risk of cross-reaction exists in patients with allergy to any of these compounds; avoid use when previous reaction has been severe. Discontinue if signs of hypersensitivity are noted.

Adverse Reactions
>10%:
Endocrine & metabolic: Hyperuricemia (18%), hypochloremia (15%), hypokalemia (15%)
Renal: Azotemia (11%)
1% to 10%:
Central nervous system: Dizziness (1%)
Endocrine & metabolic: Hyponatremia (9%); hyperglycemia (7%); variations in phosphorus (5%), CO_2 content (4%), bicarbonate (3%), and calcium (2%)
Neuromuscular & skeletal: Muscle cramps (1%)
Otic: Ototoxicity (1%)
Renal: Serum creatinine increased (7%)
<1% (Limited to important or life-threatening): Asterixis, dehydration, encephalopathy, hearing impaired, hypernatremia, hypotension, orthostatic hypotension, pruritus, rash, renal failure, vertigo, vomiting

Drug Interactions
Avoid Concomitant Use There are no known interactions where it is recommended to avoid concomitant use.
Increased Effect/Toxicity
Bumetanide may increase the levels/effects of: ACE Inhibitors; Allopurinol; Amifostine; Aminoglycosides; Antihypertensives; Dofetilide; Hypotensive Agents; Lithium; Neuromuscular-Blocking Agents; RiTUXimab; Salicylates

The levels/effects of Bumetanide may be increased by: Corticosteroids (Orally Inhaled); Corticosteroids (Systemic); Diazoxide; Herbs (Hypotensive

Properties); MAO Inhibitors; Pentoxifylline; Phosphodiesterase 5 Inhibitors; Prostacyclin Analogues

Decreased Effect

Bumetanide may decrease the levels/effects of: Lithium; Neuromuscular-Blocking Agents

The levels/effects of Bumetanide may be decreased by: Bile Acid Sequestrants; Herbs (Hypertensive Properties); Methylphenidate; Nonsteroidal Anti-Inflammatory Agents; Phenytoin; Salicylates; Yohimbine

Ethanol/Nutrition/Herb Interactions Herb/Nutraceutical: Avoid ephedra, yohimbe, ginseng (may worsen hypertension). Avoid dong quai if using for hypertension (has estrogenic activity). Avoid garlic (may have increased antihypertensive effect).

Dietary Considerations May require increased intake of potassium-rich foods.

Dosage Forms Excipient information presented when available (limited, particularly for generics); consult specific product labeling. [DSC] = Discontinued product

Injection, solution: 0.25 mg/mL (2 mL, 4 mL, 10 mL)
Tablet: 0.5 mg, 1 mg, 2 mg
Bumex®: 1 mg [DSC]

♦ **Bumex® [DSC]** *see* Bumetanide *on page 209*

♦ **Bumex® (Can)** *see* Bumetanide *on page 209*

♦ **Buminate®** *see* Albumin *on page 46*

Bupivacaine (byoo PIV a kane)

Medication Safety Issues
Sound-alike/look-alike issues:
Bupivacaine may be confused with mepivacaine, ropivacaine
Marcaine® may be confused with Narcan®

High alert medication: The Institute for Safe Medication Practices (ISMP) includes this medication (epidural administration) among its list of drug classes which have a heightened risk of causing significant patient harm when used in error.

Related Information
Acute Postoperative Pain *on page 1502*
Local Anesthetics *on page 1636*

U.S. Brand Names Marcaine®; Marcaine® Spinal; Sensorcaine®; Sensorcaine®-MPF; Sensorcaine®-MPF Spinal

Canadian Brand Names Marcaine®; Sensorcaine®

Index Terms Bupivacaine Hydrochloride

Pharmacologic Category Local Anesthetic

Generic Available Yes

Use Peripheral nerve block; infiltration; sympathetic block; spinal, caudal or epidural block; retrobulbar block

Mechanism of Action Blocks both the initiation and conduction of nerve impulses by decreasing the neuronal membrane's permeability to sodium ions, which results in inhibition of depolarization with resultant blockade of conduction

Pharmacodynamics/Kinetics
Onset of action: Anesthesia (route and dose dependent): 1-17 minutes
Duration (route and dose dependent): 2-9 hours
Protein binding: ~95%
Metabolism: Hepatic; forms metabolite (PPX)
Half-life elimination (age dependent): Neonates: 8.1 hours; Adults: 1.5-5.5 hours
Excretion: Urine (~6% unchanged)

Dosage Dose varies with procedure, depth of anesthesia, vascularity of tissues, duration of anesthesia, and condition of patient. Do not use solutions containing preservatives for caudal or epidural block.
Children >12 years and Adults:
Local anesthesia: Infiltration: 0.25% infiltrated locally; maximum: 175 mg
Caudal block (preservative free): 15-30 mL of 0.25% or 0.5%

Epidural block (other than caudal block; preservative free): Administer in 3-5 mL increments, allowing sufficient time to detect toxic manifestations of inadvertent I.V. or I.T. administration: 10-20 mL of 0.25% or 0.5%

Surgical procedures requiring a high degree of muscle relaxation and prolonged effects **only**: 10-20 mL of 0.75% (**Note:** Not to be used in obstetrical cases)

Peripheral nerve block: 5 mL of 0.25 or 0.5%; maximum: 400 mg/day

Sympathetic nerve block: 20-50 mL of 0.25%

Retrobulbar anesthesia: 2-4 mL of 0.75%

Adults: Spinal anesthesia: Preservative free solution of 0.75% bupivacaine in 8.25% dextrose:

Lower extremity and perineal procedures: 1 mL

Lower abdominal procedures: 1.6 mL

Normal vaginal delivery: 0.8 mL (higher doses may be required in some patients)

Cesarean section: 1-1.4 mL

Stability Store at controlled room temperature of 15°C to 30°C (59°F to 86°F).

Administration Solutions containing preservatives should not be used for epidural or caudal blocks.

Monitoring Parameters Vital signs, state of consciousness; signs of CNS toxicity; fetal heart rate during paracervical anesthesia

Anesthesia and Critical Care Concerns/Other Considerations

Local anesthetic toxicity: Cardiac arrest: Lipid infusion has been used in animal studies and several human cases (*Bupivacaine:* Rosenblatt, 2006; *Levobupivacaine:* Foxall, 2007; *Ropivacaine:* Litz, 2006) where cardiovascular toxicity, unresponsive to conventional resuscitation, resulted. Additional information is available at http://www.lipidrescue.org. The protocol from the website is: 20% Fat Emulsion: 1.5 mL/kg administered over 1 minute, followed immediately by an infusion of 0.25 mL/kg/minute. Continue chest compressions (lipid must circulate). Repeat bolus every 3-5 minutes up to 3 mL/kg total dose until circulation restored. Continue infusion until hemodynamic stability is restored. Increase the infusion rate to 0.5 mL/kg/minute if BP declines. A maximum total dose of 8 mL/kg is recommended.

Administration issue: The On-Q® infusion pump is used to slowly administer local anesthetics (eg, bupivacaine, lidocaine, ropivacaine) to or around surgical wound sites and/or in close proximity to nerves for pre- or postoperative regional anesthesia. When infused directly into the shoulder, destruction of articular cartilage (chondrolysis) has occurred. On-Q® pumps should never be placed directly into any joint (see https://www.ismp.org/Newsletters/acutecare/archives/May09.asp).

Pregnancy Risk Factor C

Contraindications Hypersensitivity to bupivacaine hydrochloride, amide-type local anesthetics, or any component of the formulation; obstetrical paracervical block anesthesia

Warnings/Precautions Use with caution in patients with hepatic impairment. Not recommended for use in children <12 years of age. The solution for spinal anesthesia should not be used in children <18 years of age. **Do not use solutions containing preservatives for caudal or epidural block.** Local anesthetics have been associated with rare occurrences of sudden respiratory arrest; convulsions due to systemic toxicity leading to cardiac arrest have also been reported, presumably following unintentional intravascular injection. **[U.S. Boxed Warning]: The 0.75% is not recommended for obstetrical anesthesia.** A test dose is recommended prior to epidural administration (prior to initial dose) and all reinforcing doses with continuous catheter technique. Use caution with cardiovascular dysfunction. Use caution in debilitated, elderly, or acutely ill patients; dose reduction may be required. Resuscitative equipment, oxygen, and other resuscitative drugs should be available for immediate use.

Adverse Reactions Note: Incidence of adverse reactions is difficult to define. Most effects are dose related, and are often due to accelerated absorption from the injection site, unintentional intravascular injection, or slow metabolic degradation. The development of any central nervous system symptoms may be an early indication of more significant toxicity (seizure).

Cardiovascular: Hypotension, bradycardia, palpitation, heart block, ventricular arrhythmia, cardiac arrest

Central nervous system: Restlessness, anxiety, dizziness, seizure (0.1%); rare symptoms (usually associated with unintentional subarachnoid injection during high spinal anesthesia) include persistent anesthesia, paresthesia, paralysis, headache, septic meningitis, and cranial nerve palsies

Gastrointestinal: Nausea, vomiting; rare symptoms (usually associated with unintentional subarachnoid injection during high spinal anesthesia) include fecal incontinence and loss of sphincter control

Genitourinary: Rare symptoms (usually associated with unintentional subarachnoid injection during high spinal anesthesia) include urinary incontinence, loss of perineal sensation, and loss of sexual function

Neuromuscular & skeletal: Weakness

Ocular: Blurred vision, pupillary constriction

Otic: Tinnitus

Respiratory: Apnea, hypoventilation (usually associated with unintentional subarachnoid injection during high spinal anesthesia)

Miscellaneous: Allergic reactions (urticaria, pruritus, angioedema), anaphylactoid reactions

Drug Interactions

Metabolism/Transport Effects Substrate (minor) of CYP1A2, 2C19, 2D6, 3A4

Avoid Concomitant Use There are no known interactions where it is recommended to avoid concomitant use.

Increased Effect/Toxicity There are no known significant interactions involving an increase in effect.

Decreased Effect

The levels/effects of Bupivacaine may be decreased by: Peginterferon Alfa-2b

Dosage Forms Excipient information presented when available (limited, particularly for generics); consult specific product labeling.

Injection, solution, as hydrochloride [preservative free]: 0.25% (10 mL, 20 mL, 30 mL, 50 mL); 0.5% (10 mL, 20 mL, 30 mL); 0.75% (10 mL, 20 mL, 30 mL)

Marcaine®: 0.25% (10 mL, 30 mL, 50 mL); 0.5% (10 mL, 30 mL); 0.75% (10 mL, 30 mL)

Sensorcaine®-MPF: 0.25% (10 mL, 30 mL); 0.5% (10 mL, 30 mL); 0.75% (10 mL, 30 mL)

Injection, solution, premixed in D8.25, as hydrochloride [preservative free]: 0.75% (2 mL)

Marcaine® Spinal: 0.75% (2 mL)

Sensorcaine®-MPF Spinal: 0.75% (2 mL)

Injection, solution, as hydrochloride: 0.25% (50 mL); 0.5% (50 mL)

Marcaine®: 0.5% (50 mL) [contains methylparaben]

Sensorcaine®: 0.25% (50 mL); 0.5% (50 mL) [contains methylparaben]

References

Corcoran W, Butterworth J, Weller RS, et al, "Local Anesthetic-Induced Cardiac Toxicity: A Survey of Contemporary Practice Strategies Among Academic Anesthesiology Departments," *Anesth Analg*, 2006, 103(5):1322-6.

Foxall G, McCahon R, Lamb J, et al, "Levobupivacaine-Induced Seizures and Cardiovascular Collapse Treated With Intralipid," *Anaesthesia*, 2007, 62(5):516-8.

Lehmann LJ and Pallares VS, "Subdural Injection of a Local Anesthetic With Steroids: Complication of Epidural Anesthesia," *South Med J*, 1995, 88(4):467-9.

Litz RJ, Popp M, Stehr SN, et al, "Successful Resuscitation of a Patient With Ropivacaine-Induced Asystole After Axillary Plexus Block Using lipid Infusion," *Anaesthesia*, 2006, 61(8):800-1.

Long WB, Rosenblum S, and Grady IP, "Successful Resuscitation of Bupivacaine-Induced Cardiac Arrest Using Cardiopulmonary Bypass," *Anesth Analg*, 1989, 69(3):403-6.

Rosenblatt MA, Abel M, Fischer GW, et al, "Successful Use of a 20% Lipid Emulsion to Resuscitate a Patient After a Presumed Bupivacaine-Related Cardiac Arrest," *Anesthesiology*, 2006, 105 (1):217-8.

Scott DB, Lee A, Fagan D, et al, "Acute Toxicity of Ropivacaine Compared With That of Bupivacaine," *Anesth Analg*, 1989, 69(5):563-9.

Sun KO, "Convulsion Following Spinal Anaesthesia," *Anaesth Intensive Care*, 1995, 23(4):520-1.

Tuominen MK, Pere P, and Rosenberg PH, "Unintentional Arterial Catheterization and Bupivacaine Toxicity Associated With Continuous Interscalene Brachial Plexus Block," *Anesthesiology*, 1991, 75 (2):356-8.

◆ **Bupivacaine Hydrochloride** see Bupivacaine on page 211

◆ **Buprenex®** see Buprenorphine on page 214

Buprenorphine (byoo pre NOR feen)

Medication Safety Issues
Sound-alike/look-alike issues:
Buprenex® may be confused with Brevibloc®, Bumex®

High alert medication: The Institute for Safe Medication Practices (ISMP) includes this medication among its list of drug classes which have a heightened risk of causing significant patient harm when used in error.

Related Information
Opioid Analgesics *on page 1688*
Opioids *on page 1641*

U.S. Brand Names Buprenex®; Subutex®

Canadian Brand Names Buprenex®; Subutex®

Index Terms Buprenorphine Hydrochloride

Pharmacologic Category Analgesic, Opioid

Restrictions Injection: C-V/C-III; Tablet: C-III
Prescribing of tablets for opioid dependence is limited to physicians who have met the qualification criteria and have received a DEA number specific to prescribing this product. Tablets will be available through pharmacies and wholesalers which normally provide controlled substances.

Generic Available Yes: Injection

Use
Injection: Management of moderate-to-severe pain
Tablet: Treatment of opioid dependence

Unlabeled/Investigational Use Injection: Heroin and opioid withdrawal

Mechanism of Action Buprenorphine exerts its analgesic effect via high affinity binding to μ opiate receptors in the CNS; displays partial mu agonist and weak kappa antagonist activity

Pharmacodynamics/Kinetics
Onset of action: Analgesic: 10-30 minutes
Duration: 6-8 hours
Absorption: I.M., SubQ: 30% to 40%
Distribution: V_d: 97-187 L/kg
Protein binding: High
Metabolism: Primarily hepatic; extensive first-pass effect
Half-life elimination: 2.2-3 hours
Excretion: Feces (70%); urine (20% as unchanged drug)

Dosage Long-term use is not recommended
Note: These are guidelines and do not represent the maximum doses that may be required in all patients. Doses should be titrated to pain relief/prevention. In high-risk patients (eg, elderly, debilitated, presence of respiratory disease) and/or concurrent CNS depressant use, reduce dose by one-half. Buprenorphine has an analgesic ceiling.

Acute pain (moderate-to-severe):
Children 2-12 years: I.M., slow I.V.: 2-6 mcg/kg every 4-6 hours
Children ≥13 years and Adults:
I.M.: Initial: Opiate-naive: 0.3 mg every 6-8 hours as needed; initial dose (up to 0.3 mg) may be repeated once in 30-60 minutes after the initial dose if needed; usual dosage range: 0.15-0.6 mg every 4-8 hours as needed
Slow I.V.: Initial: Opiate-naive: 0.3 mg every 6-8 hours as needed; initial dose (up to 0.3 mg) may be repeated once in 30-60 minutes after the initial dose if needed
Elderly: I.M., slow I.V.: 0.15 mg every 6 hours; elderly patients are more likely to suffer from confusion and drowsiness compared to younger patients
Heroin or opiate withdrawal (unlabeled use): Children ≥13 years and Adults: I.M., slow I.V.: Variable; 0.1-0.4 mg every 6 hours
Sublingual: Children ≥16 years and Adults: Opioid dependence:
Induction: Range: 12-16 mg/day (doses during an induction study used 8 mg on day 1, followed by 16 mg on day 2; induction continued over 3-4 days). Treatment should begin at least 4 hours after last use of heroin or short-acting opioid, preferably when first signs of withdrawal appear. Titrating dose to

clinical effectiveness should be done as rapidly as possible to prevent undue withdrawal symptoms and patient drop-out during the induction period.

Maintenance: Target dose: 16 mg/day; range: 4-24 mg/day; patients should be switched to the buprenorphine/naloxone combination product for maintenance and unsupervised therapy

Stability

Injection: Protect from excessive heat >40°C (>104°F). Protect from light.

Tablet: Store at room temperature of 25°C (77°F).

Administration

I.V.: Administer slowly, over at least 2 minutes.

Sublingual: Tablet should be placed under the tongue until dissolved; should not be swallowed. If two or more tablets are needed per dose, all may be placed under the tongue at once, or two at a time. To ensure consistent bioavailability, subsequent doses should always be taken the same way.

Monitoring Parameters Pain relief, respiratory and mental status, CNS depression, blood pressure; LFTs

Anesthesia and Critical Care Concerns/Other Considerations

Clinical Pearls/Comments: Buprenorphine has a longer duration of action than either morphine or meperidine. It may precipitate withdrawal in narcotic-dependent patients because the antagonist action at the kappa receptor prevails. Buprenorphine has a better safety profile than methadone because of its slow release from mu receptors, which limits withdrawal signs and symptoms. It is 25-40 times more potent than similar mg doses of morphine. Because it is a partial mu agonist, its analgesic effects plateau at higher doses and it then behaves like an antagonist. Buprenorphine is not readily reversed by naloxone.

Pregnancy Risk Factor C

Contraindications Hypersensitivity to buprenorphine or any component of the formulation

Warnings/Precautions An opioid-containing analgesic regimen should be tailored to each patient's needs and based upon the type of pain being treated (acute versus chronic), the route of administration, degree of tolerance for opioids (naive versus chronic user), age, weight, and medical condition. The optimal analgesic dose varies widely among patients. Doses should be titrated to pain relief/prevention.

May cause CNS depression, which may impair physical or mental abilities. Effects with other sedative drugs or ethanol may be potentiated. Elderly may be more sensitive to CNS depressant and constipating effects. May cause respiratory depression - use caution in patients with respiratory disease or pre-existing respiratory depression. Potential for drug dependency exists, abrupt cessation may precipitate withdrawal. Use caution in elderly, debilitated, pediatric patients, depression or suicidal tendencies. Tolerance, psychological and physical dependence may occur with prolonged use. Partial antagonist activity may precipitate acute narcotic withdrawal in opioid-dependent individuals.

Use with caution in patients with hepatic, pulmonary, or renal function impairment. Also use caution in patients with head injury or increased ICP, biliary tract dysfunction, patients with history of hyperthyroidism, morbid obesity, adrenal insufficiency, prostatic hyperplasia, urinary stricture, CNS depression, toxic psychosis, pancreatitis, alcoholism, delirium tremens, or kyphoscoliosis. May cause hypotension; use with caution in patients with hypovolemia, cardiovascular disease (including acute MI), or drugs which may exaggerate hypotensive effects (including phenothiazines or general anesthetics). May obscure diagnosis or clinical course of patients with acute abdominal conditions.

Tablets, which are used for induction treatment of opioid dependence, should not be started until effects of withdrawal are evident. Safety and efficacy of the tablet formulation have not been established in children <16 years of age; safety and efficacy of the injection formulation have not been established in children <2 years of age.

Adverse Reactions

Injection:

>10%: Central nervous system: Sedation

1% to 10%:

Cardiovascular: Hypotension

◀ Central nervous system: Respiratory depression, dizziness, headache
Gastrointestinal: Vomiting, nausea
Ocular: Miosis
Otic: Vertigo
Miscellaneous: Diaphoresis
<1% (Limited to important or life-threatening): Agitation, allergic reaction, apnea, appetite decreased, blurred vision, bradycardia, confusion, constipation, convulsion, coma, cyanosis, depersonalization, depression, diplopia, dyspnea, dysphoria, euphoria, fatigue, flatulence, flushing, hallucinations, hypertension, injection site reaction, malaise, nervousness, pallor, paresthesia, pruritus, psychosis, rash, slurred speech, tachycardia, tinnitus, tremor, urinary retention, urticaria, weakness, Wenckebach block, xerostomia

Tablet:

>10%:
Central nervous system: Headache (30%), pain (24%), insomnia (21% to 25%), anxiety (12%), depression (11%)
Gastrointestinal: Nausea (10% to 14%), abdominal pain (12%), constipation (8% to 11%)
Neuromuscular & skeletal: Back pain (14%), weakness (14%)
Respiratory: Rhinitis (11%)
Miscellaneous: Withdrawal syndrome (19%; placebo 37%), infection (12% to 20%), diaphoresis (12% to 13%)

1% to 10%:
Central nervous system: Chills (6%), nervousness (6%), somnolence (5%), dizziness (4%), fever (3%)
Gastrointestinal: Vomiting (5% to 8%), diarrhea (5%), dyspepsia (3%)
Ocular: Lacrimation (5%)
Respiratory: Cough (4%), pharyngitis (4%)
Miscellaneous: Flu-like syndrome (6%)

Drug Interactions

Metabolism/Transport Effects Substrate of CYP3A4 (major); **Inhibits** CYP1A2 (weak), 2A6 (weak), 2C19 (weak), 2D6 (weak)

Avoid Concomitant Use There are no known interactions where it is recommended to avoid concomitant use.

Increased Effect/Toxicity

Buprenorphine may increase the levels/effects of: Alcohol (Ethyl); Alvimopan; CNS Depressants; Desmopressin; Selective Serotonin Reuptake Inhibitors; Thiazide Diuretics

The levels/effects of Buprenorphine may be increased by: Amphetamines; Antipsychotic Agents (Phenothiazines); Atazanavir; CYP3A4 Inhibitors (Moderate); CYP3A4 Inhibitors (Strong); Dasatinib; Succinylcholine

Decreased Effect

Buprenorphine may decrease the levels/effects of: Pegvisomant

The levels/effects of Buprenorphine may be decreased by: Ammonium Chloride; CYP3A4 Inducers (Strong); Deferasirox; Herbs (CYP3A4 Inducers)

Ethanol/Nutrition/Herb Interactions

Ethanol: Avoid ethanol (may increase CNS depression).
Herb/Nutraceutical: Avoid valerian, St John's wort, kava kava, gotu kola (may increase CNS depression).

Dosage Forms Excipient information presented when available (limited, particularly for generics); consult specific product labeling.
Injection, solution: 0.3 mg/mL (1 mL) [C-III]
Buprenex®: 0.3 mg/mL (1 mL) [C-V]
Tablet, sublingual:
Subutex®: 2 mg, 8 mg

References

Carr DB, Jacox AK, Chapman RC, et al, "Acute Pain Management," Guideline Technical Report, No. 1. Rockville, MD: U.S. Department of Health and Human Services, Public Health Service, Agency for Health Care Policy and Research. AHCPR Publication No. 95-0034. February 1995.
"Drugs for Pain," *Treat Guidel Med Lett*, 2004, 2(23):47-54.
Gal TJ, "Naloxone Reversal of Buprenorphine-Induced Respiratory Depression," *Clin Pharmacol Ther*, 1989, 45(1):66-71.
Harcus AH, Ward AE, and Smith DW, "Buprenorphine: Experience in an Elderly Population of 975 Patients During a Year's Monitored Release," *Br J Clin Pract*, 1980, 34(5):144-6.

Jain PN and Shah SC, "Respiratory Depression Following Combination of Epidural Buprenorphine and Intramuscular Ketorolac," *Anaesthesia*, 1993, 48(10):898-9.

MacEvilly M and O'Carroll C, "Hallucinations After Epidural Buprenorphine," *Br Med J*, 1989, 298 (6678):928-9.

Mokhlesi B, Leikin JB, Murray P, et al, "Adult Toxicology in Critical Care. Part 11: Specific Poisonings," *Chest*, 2003, 123(3):897-922.

"Principles of Analgesic Use in the Treatment of Acute Pain and Cancer Pain," 6th ed, Glenview, IL: American Pain Society, 2008.

Sporer KA, "Buprenorphine: A Primer for Emergency Physicians," *Ann Emerg Med*, 2004, 43 (5):580-4.

♦ **Buprenorphine Hydrochloride** *see* Buprenorphine *on page 214*

♦ **Buproban®** *see* BuPROPion *on page 217*

BuPROPion (byoo PROE pee on)

Related Information
Antidepressant Agents *on page 1660*

U.S. Brand Names Aplenzin™; Budeprion SR®; Budeprion XL®; Buproban®; Wellbutrin SR®; Wellbutrin XL®; Wellbutrin®; Zyban®

Canadian Brand Names Bupropion SR®; Novo-Bupropion SR; PMS-Bupropion SR; ratio-Bupropion SR; SANDOZ-Bupropion SR; Wellbutrin XL®; Wellbutrin®; Zyban®

Index Terms Bupropion Hydrobromide; Bupropion Hydrochloride

Pharmacologic Category Antidepressant, Dopamine-Reuptake Inhibitor; Smoking Cessation Aid

Use Treatment of major depressive disorder, including seasonal affective disorder (SAD); adjunct in smoking cessation

Unlabeled/Investigational Use Attention-deficit/hyperactivity disorder (ADHD); depression associated with bipolar disorder

Pharmacodynamics/Kinetics
Absorption: Rapid

Distribution: V_d: ~20-47 L/kg (Laizure, 1985)

Protein binding: 84%

Metabolism: Extensively hepatic via CYP2B6 to hydroxybupropion; non-CYP-mediated metabolism to erythrohydrobupropion and threohydrobupropion. Metabolite activity ranges from 20% to 50% potency of bupropion.

Half-life:

Distribution: 3-4 hours

Elimination: 21 ± 9 hours; Metabolites: Hydroxybupropion: 20 ± 5 hours; Erythrohydrobupropion: 33 ± 10 hours; Threohydrobupropion: 37 ± 13 hours

Extended release (Aplenzin™): 21 ± 7 hours; Metabolites: Hydroxybupropion: 24 ± 5 hours; Erythrohydrobupropion: 31 ± 8 hours; Threohydrobupropion: 51 ± 9 hours

Time to peak, serum:

Bupropion: Immediate release: Within 2 hours; Sustained release: Within 3 hours; Extended release: ~5 hours

Metabolite: Hydroxybupropion: Immediate release: ~3 hours; Extended release, sustained release: ~6-7 hours

Excretion: Urine (87%, primarily as metabolites); feces (10%, primarily as metabolites)

Dosage Oral:
Children and Adolescents: ADHD (unlabeled use): Hydrochloride salt: 1.4-6 mg/kg/day

Adults:

Depression:

Immediate release hydrochloride salt: 100 mg 3 times/day; begin at 100 mg twice daily; may increase to a maximum dose of 450 mg/day

Sustained release hydrochloride salt: Initial: 150 mg/day in the morning; may increase to 150 mg twice daily by day 4 if tolerated; target dose: 300 mg/day given as 150 mg twice daily; maximum dose: 400 mg/day given as 200 mg twice daily

Extended release:

Hydrochloride salt: Initial: 150 mg/day in the morning; may increase as early as day 4 of dosing to 300 mg/day; maximum dose: 450 mg/day

◀ Hydrobromide salt (Aplenzin™): Target dose: 348 mg/day in the morning. Patients not previously on bupropion: Initial: 174 mg/day in the morning; may increase as early as day 4 of dosing to 348 mg/day; maximum dose: 522 mg/day. **Note:** 174 mg strength currently not available; 348 mg tablet cannot be split.

Switching from hydrochloride salt formulation (eg, Wellbutrin® immediate release, SR®, XL®) to hydrobromide salt formulation (Aplenzin™): **Note:** Patients being treated twice daily with bupropion hydrochloride would be switched to the equivalent once daily dose of bupropion hydrobromide.

Bupropion hydrochloride 150 mg is equivalent to bupropion hydrobromide 174 mg

Bupropion hydrochloride 300 mg is equivalent to bupropion hydrobromide 348 mg

Bupropion hydrochloride 450 mg is equivalent to bupropion hydrobromide 522 mg

SAD (Wellbutrin XL®): Initial: 150 mg/day in the morning; if tolerated, may increase after 1 week to 300 mg/day

Note: Prophylactic treatment should be reserved for those patients with frequent depressive episodes and/or significant impairment. Initiate treatment in the Autumn prior to symptom onset, and discontinue in early Spring with dose tapering to 150 mg/day for 2 weeks

Smoking cessation (Zyban®): Initiate with 150 mg once daily for 3 days; increase to 150 mg twice daily; treatment should continue for 7-12 weeks

Note: Therapy should begin at least 1 week before target quit date. Target quit dates are generally in the second week of treatment. If patient successfully quits smoking after 7-12 weeks, may consider ongoing maintenance therapy based on individual patient risk/benefit. Efficacy of maintenance therapy (300 mg/day) has been demonstrated for up to 6 months. Conversely, if significant progress has not been made by the seventh week of therapy, success is unlikely and treatment discontinuation should be considered.

Elderly: Depression: Hydrochloride salt: 50-100 mg/day, increase by 50-100 mg every 3-4 days as tolerated; there is evidence that the elderly respond at 150 mg/day in divided doses, but some may require a higher dose. **Note:** Patients with Alzheimer's dementia-related depression may require a lower starting dosage of 37.5 mg once or twice daily (100 mg/day sustained release), increased as needed up to 300 mg/day in divided doses (300 mg/day for sustained release)

Dosing conversion between hydrochloride salt (eg, Wellbutrin®) immediate, sustained, and extended release products: Convert using same total daily dose (up to the maximum recommended dose for a given dosage form), but adjust frequency as indicated for sustained (twice daily) or extended (once daily) release products.

Dosing adjustment/comments in renal impairment: Use with caution and consider a reduction in dosing frequency; limited pharmacokinetic information suggests elimination of bupropion and/or the active metabolites may be reduced.

Moderate-to-severe renal impairment: Bupropion exposure was approximately twofold higher compared to normal subjects following a 150 mg single dose administration.

End-stage renal failure: Per the manufacturer, the elimination of hydroxybupropion and threohydrobupropion are reduced in patients with end-stage renal failure.

Dosing adjustment in hepatic impairment:

Note: The mean AUC increased by ~1.5-fold for hydroxybupropion and ~2.5-fold for erythro/threohydrobupropion; median T_{max} was observed 19 hours later for hydroxybupropion, 31 hours later for erythro/threohydrobupropion; mean half-life for hydroxybupropion increased fivefold, and increased twofold for erythro/threohydrobupropion in patients with severe hepatic cirrhosis compared to healthy volunteers.

Mild-to-moderate hepatic impairment: Use with caution and/or reduced dose/frequency

Severe hepatic cirrhosis: Use with extreme caution; maximum dose:

Aplenzin™: 174 mg every other day

Wellbutrin®: 75 mg/day

Wellbutrin SR®: 100 mg/day or 150 mg every other day
Wellbutrin XL®: 150 mg every other day
Zyban®: 150 mg every other day

Anesthesia and Critical Care Concerns/Other Considerations

Clinical Pearls/Comments: There are relatively few cardiovascular side effects compared to tricyclic antidepressants. However, several case reports include cardiovascular complications, including hypotension and MI. Use with caution in patients with recent MI or unstable angina. Recent information suggests that hypertension, in some cases severe and requiring acute treatment, has been reported in patients receiving bupropion alone, and especially when bupropion is used in conjunction with nicotine replacement therapy. Monitoring of blood pressure is recommended in patients receiving the combination of bupropion and nicotine replacement, particularly in those with hypertension and/or significant coronary artery disease.

Additional Information Complete prescribing information for this medication should be consulted for additional detail.

Dosage Forms Excipient information presented when available (limited, particularly for generics); consult specific product labeling.

Tablet, as hydrochloride: 75 mg [generic for Wellbutrin®], 100 mg [generic for Wellbutrin®]
  Wellbutrin®: 75 mg, 100 mg
Tablet, extended release, as hydrobromide:
  Aplenzin™: 174 mg, 348 mg, 522 mg
Tablet, extended release, as hydrochloride: 100 mg [generic for Wellbutrin SR®], 150 mg [generic for Wellbutrin SR®], 150 mg [generic for Wellbutrin XL®], 150 mg [generic for Zyban®], 200 mg [generic for Wellbutrin SR®], 300 mg [generic for Wellbutrin XL®]
  Budeprion SR®: 100 mg [generic for Wellbutrin SR®; contains tartrazine], 150 mg [generic for Wellbutrin SR®]
  Budeprion XL®: 150 mg [generic for Wellbutrin XL®], 300 mg [contains tartrazine; generic for Wellbutrin XL®]
  Buproban®: 150 mg [generic for Zyban®]
  Wellbutrin XL®: 150 mg, 300 mg
Tablet, sustained release, as hydrochloride:
  Wellbutrin SR®: 100 mg, 150 mg, 200 mg
  Zyban®: 150 mg

◆ **Bupropion Hydrobromide** see BuPROPion on page 217

◆ **Bupropion Hydrochloride** see BuPROPion on page 217

◆ **Bupropion SR® (Can)** see BuPROPion on page 217

◆ **Burinex® (Can)** see Bumetanide on page 209

◆ **BurnaMycin [OTC]** see Lidocaine on page 836

◆ **Burn Jel® [OTC]** see Lidocaine on page 836

◆ **Burn-O-Jel [OTC]** see Lidocaine on page 836

◆ **Buscopan® (Can)** see Scopolamine Derivatives on page 1278

◆ **BuSpar®** see BusPIRone on page 219

◆ **Buspirex (Can)** see BusPIRone on page 219

BusPIRone (byoo SPYE rone)

U.S. Brand Names BuSpar®
Canadian Brand Names Apo-Buspirone®; BuSpar®; Buspirex; Bustab®; CO Buspirone; Dom-Buspirone; Gen-Buspirone; Lin-Buspirone; Mylan-Buspirone; Novo-Buspirone; Nu-Buspirone; PMS-Buspirone; ratio-Buspirone; Riva-Buspirone
Index Terms Buspirone Hydrochloride
Pharmacologic Category Antianxiety Agent, Miscellaneous
Use Management of generalized anxiety disorder (GAD)
Unlabeled/Investigational Use Management of aggression in mental retardation and secondary mental disorders; major depression; potential augmenting agent for antidepressants; premenstrual syndrome

◀ **Pharmacodynamics/Kinetics**
Absorption: Rapid
Distribution: V_d: 5.3 L/kg
Protein binding: 86% to 95%
Metabolism: Hepatic oxidation, primarily via CYP3A4; extensive first-pass effect
Bioavailability: ~4%
Half-life elimination: 2-3 hours
Time to peak, serum: 40-90 minutes
Excretion: Urine: 29% to 63% (<0.1% dose excreted unchanged); feces: 18% to 38%

Dosage Oral:
Generalized anxiety disorder:
Children ≥6 years and Adolescents: Initial: 5 mg daily; increase in increments of 5 mg/day at weekly intervals as needed, to a maximum dose of 60 mg/day divided into 2-3 doses
Adults: 15 mg/day (7.5 mg twice daily); may increase in increments of 5 mg/day every 2-3 days to a maximum of 60 mg/day; target dose for most people is 20-30 mg/day (10-15 mg twice daily)
Elderly: Initial: 5 mg twice daily, increase by 5 mg/day every 2-3 days as needed up to 20-30 mg/day; maximum daily dose: 60 mg/day.

Dosing adjustment in renal impairment: Patients with impaired renal function demonstrated increased plasma levels and a prolonged half-life of buspirone. Use in patients with severe renal impairment not recommended.

Dosing adjustment in hepatic impairment: Patients with impaired hepatic function demonstrated increased plasma levels and a prolonged half-life of buspirone. Use in patients with severe hepatic impairment not recommended.

Anesthesia and Critical Care Concerns/Other Considerations Takes 2-3 weeks for full effect. Because of slow onset, not appropriate for "as needed" (prn) use or for brief, situational anxiety; not effective for severe anxiety; does not show cross-tolerance with benzodiazepines or other sedatives; less sedating than other anxiolytics; has shown little potential for abuse; needs continuous use; ineffective for benzodiazepine or ethanol withdrawal

Additional Information Complete prescribing information for this medication should be consulted for additional detail.

Dosage Forms Excipient information presented when available (limited, particularly for generics); consult specific product labeling. [DSC] = Discontinued product
Tablet, as hydrochloride: 5 mg, 7.5 mg, 10 mg, 15 mg, 30 mg
BuSpar®: 5 mg, 10 mg, 15 mg; 30 mg [DSC]

◆ **Buspirone Hydrochloride** see BusPIRone on page 219
◆ **Bustab® (Can)** see BusPIRone on page 219

Butorphanol (byoo TOR fa nole)

Medication Safety Issues
Sound-alike/look-alike issues:
Stadol® may be confused with Haldol®, sotalol

High alert medication: The Institute for Safe Medication Practices (ISMP) includes this medication among its list of drug classes which have a heightened risk of causing significant patient harm when used in error.

Related Information
Opioid Analgesics on page 1688
Opioids on page 1641

Canadian Brand Names Apo-Butorphanol®; PMS-Butorphanol
Index Terms Butorphanol Tartrate; Stadol
Pharmacologic Category Analgesic, Opioid
Restrictions C-IV
Generic Available Yes
Use
Parenteral: Management of moderate-to-severe pain; preoperative medication; supplement to balanced anesthesia; management of pain during labor

Nasal spray: Management of moderate-to-severe pain, including migraine headache pain

Mechanism of Action Mixed narcotic agonist-antagonist with central analgesic actions; binds to opiate receptors in the CNS, causing inhibition of ascending pain pathways, altering the perception of and response to pain; produces generalized CNS depression

Pharmacodynamics/Kinetics

Onset of action: I.M.: 5-10 minutes; I.V.: <10 minutes; Nasal: Within 15 minutes

Peak effect: I.M.: 0.5-1 hour; I.V.: 4-5 minutes

Duration: I.M., I.V.: 3-4 hours; Nasal: 4-5 hours

Absorption: Rapid and well absorbed

Protein binding: 80%

Metabolism: Hepatic

Bioavailability: Nasal: 60% to 70%

Half-life elimination: 2.5-4 hours

Excretion: Primarily urine

Dosage Note: These are guidelines and do not represent the maximum doses that may be required in all patients. Doses should be titrated to pain relief/prevention. Butorphanol has an analgesic ceiling.

Adults:

Parenteral:

Acute pain (moderate-to-severe):

I.M.: Initial: 2 mg, may repeat every 3-4 hours as needed; usual range: 1-4 mg every 3-4 hours as needed

I.V.: Initial: 1 mg, may repeat every 3-4 hours as needed; usual range: 0.5-2 mg every 3-4 hours as needed

Preoperative medication: I.M.: 2 mg 60-90 minutes before surgery

Supplement to balanced anesthesia: I.V.: 2 mg shortly before induction and/or an incremental dose of 0.5-1 mg (up to 0.06 mg/kg), depending on previously administered sedative, analgesic, and hypnotic medications

Pain during labor (fetus >37 weeks gestation and no signs of fetal distress):

I.M., I.V.: 1-2 mg; may repeat in 4 hours

Note: Alternative analgesia should be used for pain associated with delivery or if delivery is anticipated within 4 hours

Nasal spray:

Moderate-to-severe pain (including migraine headache pain): Initial: 1 spray (~1 mg per spray) in 1 nostril; if adequate pain relief is not achieved within 60-90 minutes, an additional 1 spray in 1 nostril may be given; may repeat initial dose sequence in 3-4 hours after the last dose as needed

Alternatively, an initial dose of 2 mg (1 spray in each nostril) may be used in patients who will be able to remain recumbent (in the event drowsiness or dizziness occurs); additional 2 mg doses should not be given for 3-4 hours

Note: In some clinical trials, an initial dose of 2 mg (as 2 doses 1 hour apart or 2 mg initially - 1 spray in each nostril) has been used, followed by 1 mg in 1 hour; side effects were greater at these dosages

Elderly:

I.M., I.V.: Initial dosage should generally be 1/2 of the recommended dose; repeated dosing must be based on initial response rather than fixed intervals, but generally should be at least 6 hours apart

Nasal spray: Initial dose should not exceed 1 mg; a second dose may be given after 90-120 minutes

Dosage adjustment in renal impairment:

I.M., I.V.: Initial dosage should generally be 1/2 of the recommended dose; repeated dosing must be based on initial response rather than fixed intervals, but generally should be at least 6 hours apart

Nasal spray: Initial dose should not exceed 1 mg; a second dose may be given after 90-120 minutes

Dosage adjustment in hepatic impairment:

I.M., I.V.: Initial dosage should generally be 1/2 of the recommended dose; repeated dosing must be based on initial response rather than fixed intervals, but generally should be at least 6 hours apart

◀ Nasal spray: Initial dose should not exceed 1 mg; a second dose may be given after 90-120 minutes

Stability Store at room temperature; protect from freezing.

Administration Intranasal: Consider avoiding simultaneous intranasal migraine sprays; may want to separate by at least 30 minutes

Monitoring Parameters Pain relief, respiratory and mental status, blood pressure

Reference Range 0.7-1.5 ng/mL

Anesthesia and Critical Care Concerns/Other Considerations Butorphanol is a kappa agonist and a weak mu antagonist opioid. It is 5-8 times more potent than morphine (on a mg-to-mg basis). It may precipitate withdrawal in narcotic-dependent patients. Abrupt discontinuation after sustained use (generally >10 days) may cause withdrawal symptoms. This agent can potentially cause hallucinations.

Pregnancy Risk Factor C/D (prolonged use or high doses at term)

Contraindications Hypersensitivity to butorphanol or any component of the formulation; avoid use in opiate-dependent patients who have not been detoxified, may precipitate opiate withdrawal; pregnancy (prolonged use or high doses at term)

Warnings/Precautions An opioid-containing analgesic regimen should be tailored to each patient's needs and based upon the type of pain being treated (acute versus chronic), the route of administration, degree of tolerance for opioids (naive versus chronic user), age, weight, and medical condition. The optimal analgesic dose varies widely among patients. Doses should be titrated to pain relief/prevention. May cause CNS depression; use with caution in patients with head trauma, morbid obesity, thyroid dysfunction, hepatic/renal dysfunction, adrenal insufficiency, prostatic hyperplasia and/or urinary stricture, may elevate CSF pressure, may increase cardiac workload; tolerance of drug dependence may result from extended use. Use with caution in patients with biliary tract dysfunction; acute pancreatitis may cause constriction of sphincter of Oddi.

Partial antagonist activity may precipitate acute narcotic withdrawal in opioid-dependent individuals. Use with caution in patients with pre-existing respiratory compromise (hypoxia and/or hypercapnia), COPD or other obstructive pulmonary disease; critical respiratory depression may occur, even at therapeutic dosages. May cause hypotension; use with caution in patients with hypovolemia, cardiovascular disease (including acute MI), or drugs which may exaggerate hypotensive effects (including phenothiazines or general anesthetics). May obscure diagnosis or clinical course of patients with acute abdominal conditions.

Concurrent use of sumatriptan nasal spray and butorphanol nasal spray may increase risk of transient high blood pressure. Healthcare provider should be alert to problems of abuse, misuse, and diversion. Use with caution in the elderly and debilitated patients; may be more sensitive to adverse effects. Safety and efficacy have not been established in children.

Adverse Reactions
>10%:
Central nervous system: Drowsiness (43%), dizziness (19%), insomnia (Stadol® NS)
Gastrointestinal: Nausea/vomiting (13%)
Respiratory: Nasal congestion (Stadol® NS)
1% to 10%:
Cardiovascular: Vasodilation, palpitation
Central nervous system: Lightheadedness, headache, lethargy, anxiety, confusion, euphoria, somnolence
Dermatologic: Pruritus
Gastrointestinal: Anorexia, constipation, xerostomia, stomach pain, unpleasant aftertaste
Neuromuscular & skeletal: Tremor, paresthesia, weakness
Ocular: Blurred vision
Otic: Ear pain, tinnitus
Respiratory: Bronchitis, cough, dyspnea, epistaxis, nasal irritation, pharyngitis, rhinitis, sinus congestion, sinusitis, upper respiratory infection
Miscellaneous: Diaphoresis increased

<1% (Limited to important or life-threatening): Dependence (with prolonged use), depression, difficulty speaking (transient), dyspnea, hallucinations, hypertension, nightmares, paradoxical CNS stimulation, rash, respiratory depression, syncope, tinnitus, vertigo, withdrawal symptoms

Stadol® NS: Apnea, chest pain, convulsions, delusions, depressions, edema, hypertension, shallow breathing, tachycardia

Drug Interactions

Avoid Concomitant Use There are no known interactions where it is recommended to avoid concomitant use.

Increased Effect/Toxicity

Butorphanol may increase the levels/effects of: Alcohol (Ethyl); Alvimopan; CNS Depressants; Desmopressin; Selective Serotonin Reuptake Inhibitors; Thiazide Diuretics

The levels/effects of Butorphanol may be increased by: Amphetamines; Antipsychotic Agents (Phenothiazines); Succinylcholine

Decreased Effect

Butorphanol may decrease the levels/effects of: Pegvisomant

The levels/effects of Butorphanol may be decreased by: Ammonium Chloride

Ethanol/Nutrition/Herb Interactions

Ethanol: Avoid or limit ethanol (may increase CNS depression). Watch for sedation.

Herb/Nutraceutical: Avoid valerian, St John's wort, kava kava, gotu kola (may increase CNS depression).

Dosage Forms Excipient information presented when available (limited, particularly for generics); consult specific product labeling.

Injection, solution, as tartrate [preservative free]: 1 mg/mL (1 mL); 2 mg/mL (1 mL, 2 mL)

Injection, solution, as tartrate [with preservative]: 2 mg/mL (10 mL)

Solution, intranasal, as tartrate [spray]: 10 mg/mL (2.5 mL) [14-15 doses]

References

Bennie RE, Boehringer LA, Dierdorf SF, et al, "Transnasal Butorphanol Is Effective for Postoperative Pain Relief in Children Undergoing Myringotomy," *Anesthesiology*, 1998, 89(2):385-90.

Commiskey S, Fan LW, Ho IK, et al, "Butorphanol: Effects of a Prototypical Agonist-Antagonist Analgesic on Kappa-Opioid Receptors," *J Pharmacol Sci*, 2005, 98(2):109-16.

"Drugs for Pain," *Treat Guidel Med Lett*, 2004, 2(23):47-54.

Melanson SW, Morse JW, Pronchik DJ, et al, "Transnasal Butorphanol in the Emergency Department Management of Migraine Headache," *Am J Emerg Med*, 1997, 15(1):57-61.

Mokhlesi B, Leikin JB, Murray P, et al, "Adult Toxicology in Critical Care. Part 11: Specific Poisonings," *Chest*, 2003, 123(3):897-922.

Nelson KE and Eisenach JC, "Intravenous Butorphanol, Meperidine, and Their Combination Relieve Pain and Distress in Women in Labor," *Anesthesiology*, 2005, 102(5):1008-13.

"Principles of Analgesic Use in the Treatment of Acute Pain and Cancer Pain," 6th ed, Glenview, IL: American Pain Society, 2008.

Shyu WC, Morgenthien EA, and Barbhaiya RH, "Pharmacokinetics of Butorphanol Nasal Spray in Patients With Renal Impairment," *Br J Clin Pharmacol*, 1996, 41(5):397-402.

C1 Inhibitor (Human) (cee won in HIB i ter HYU man)

U.S. Brand Names Cinryze™

Index Terms C1 Esterase Inhibitor; C1-INH; C1-Inhibitor; C1INHRP; Human C1 Inhibitor

Pharmacologic Category Blood Product Derivative

Generic Available No

Use Routine prophylaxis against angioedema attacks in patients with hereditary angioedema (HAE) or inherited C1 inhibitor deficiency

Unlabeled/Investigational Use Treatment of acute or severe angioedema attacks (eg, laryngeal swelling) in patients with HAE

Mechanism of Action C1 inhibitor, one of the serine proteinase inhibitors found in human blood, plays a role in regulating the complement and intrinsic coagulation (contact system) pathway, and is also involved in the fibrinolytic and kinin pathways. C1 inhibitor therapy in patients with C1 inhibitor deficiency, such as HAE, is believed to suppress contact system activation via inactivation of plasma kallikrein and factor XIIa, thus preventing bradykinin production. Unregulated bradykinin production is thought to contribute to the increased vascular permeability and angioedema observed in HAE.

Pharmacodynamics/Kinetics

Onset of action: Increased plasma C1 inhibitor levels observed ~1 hour or less

Half-life elimination: 56 hours (range: 11-108 hours)

Time to peak: ~4 hours

Dosage I.V.: Adolescents and Adults: Routine prophylaxis against HAE attacks: 1000 units every 3-4 days

Stability Store under refrigeration at 2°C to 25°C (36°F to 77°F); do not freeze. **Protect from light** prior to reconstitution. Product should come to room temperature before combining with diluent (sterile water for injection). Reconstitute each vial with 5 mL of sterile water for injection using the double-ended transfer needle; do not use product if there is no vacuum in the vial. Use 2 reconstituted vials to make single 1000 unit dose. After combining with diluent, gently swirl vial to completely dissolve powder. Reconstituted product should be clear and colorless or slightly blue; do not use if turbid or discolored. The provided filter needle should be used to withdraw the reconstituted product. Remove filter needle and attach reconstituted solution to infusion set or appropriate needle for infusion and use within 3 hours of reconstitution.

Administration Administer intravenously at 1 mL/minute (over 10 minutes). Allow to warm to room temperature prior to administration and use within 3 hours of reconstitution.

Pregnancy Risk Factor C

Contraindications History of anaphylactic or life-threatening hypersensitivity reactions to human C1 inhibitor or any component of the formulation

Warnings/Precautions Severe hypersensitivity reactions (eg, urticaria, hives, wheezing, hypotension, anaphylaxis) may occur rarely during or after administration. Signs/symptoms of hypersensitivity reactions may be similar to the attacks associated with hereditary angioedema, therefore, consideration should be given to treatment methods. In the event of acute hypersensitivity reactions to C1 inhibitor therapy, treatment should be discontinued and epinephrine should be available. Consider potential risk of thrombosis with use; thrombotic events have been reported when used off-label at doses higher than recommended in product labeling. Product of human plasma; may potentially contain infectious agents which could transmit disease. Screening of donors, as well as testing and/or inactivation or removal of certain viruses, reduces the risk. Infections thought to be transmitted by this product should be reported to the manufacturer. Safety and efficacy have been established in adolescents and adults. Only a small number of children were included in clinical trials.

Adverse Reactions Reactions reported below were observed in a study involving 24 patients.

≥5%:

Central nervous system: Headache

Dermatologic: Pruritus, rash

Neuromuscular & skeletal: Back pain, extremity pain

Respiratory: Bronchitis, sinusitis, upper respiratory tract infection

Miscellaneous: Limb injury

Drug Interactions

Avoid Concomitant Use There are no known interactions where it is recommended to avoid concomitant use.

Increased Effect/Toxicity There are no known significant interactions involving an increase in effect.

Decreased Effect There are no known significant interactions involving a decrease in effect.

Dosage Forms

Injection, powder for reconstitution:

Cinryze™: 500 units [contains sucrose 21 mg/mL]

References

Cicardi M, Zingale L, "How Do We Treat Patients With Hereditary Angioedema," *Transfus Apher*, 2003, 29(3):221-7.

Farkas H, Jakab L, Temesszentandrasi G, et al, "Hereditary Angioedema: A Decade of Human C1-inhibitor Concentrate Therapy," *J Allergy Clin Immunol*, 2007, 120(4):941-7.

Frank M and Jiang H, "New Therapies for Hereditary Angioedema: Disease Outlook Changes Dramatically," *J Allergy Clin Immunol*, 2008, 121(1):272-80.

Hermans C, "Successful Management With C1-Inhibitor Concentrate of Hereditary Angioedema Attacks During Two Successive Pregnancies: A Case Report," *Arch Gynecol Obstet*, 2007, 276 (3):271-76.

◆ **Cafcit®** *see* Caffeine *on page 225*

Caffeine (KAF een)

U.S. Brand Names Cafcit®; Enerjets [OTC]; No Doz® Maximum Strength [OTC]; Vivarin® [OTC]

Index Terms Caffeine and Sodium Benzoate; Caffeine Citrate; Sodium Benzoate and Caffeine

Pharmacologic Category Stimulant

Use

Caffeine citrate: Treatment of idiopathic apnea of prematurity

Caffeine and sodium benzoate: Treatment of acute respiratory depression (not a preferred agent)

Caffeine [OTC labeling]: Restore mental alertness or wakefulness when experiencing fatigue

Unlabeled/Investigational Use Caffeine and sodium benzoate: Treatment of spinal puncture headache; CNS stimulant; diuretic; augmentation of seizure induction during electroconvulsive therapy (ECT)

Pharmacodynamics/Kinetics

Distribution: V_d:

Neonates: 0.8-0.9 L/kg

Children >9 months to Adults: 0.6 L/kg

Protein binding: 17% (children) to 36% (adults)

Metabolism: Hepatic, via demethylation by CYP1A2. **Note:** In neonates, interconversion between caffeine and theophylline has been reported (caffeine levels are ~25% of measured theophylline after theophylline administration and ~3% to 8% of caffeine would be expected to be converted to theophylline)

Half-life elimination:

Neonates: 72-96 hours (range: 40-230 hours)

Children >9 months and Adults: 5 hours

Time to peak, serum: Oral: Within 30 minutes to 2 hours

Excretion:

Neonates ≤1 month: 86% excreted unchanged in urine

Infants >1 month and Adults: In urine, as metabolites

Dosage Note: Caffeine citrate should not be interchanged with the caffeine sodium benzoate formulation.

Caffeine citrate: Neonates: Apnea of prematurity: Oral, I.V.:

Loading dose: 10-20 mg/kg as caffeine citrate (5-10 mg/kg as caffeine base). If theophylline has been administered to the patient within the previous 3 days, a full or modified loading dose (50% to 75% of a loading dose) may be given.

Maintenance dose: 5 mg/kg/day as caffeine citrate (2.5 mg/kg/day as caffeine base) once daily starting 24 hours after the loading dose. Maintenance dose is adjusted based on patient's response and serum caffeine concentrations.

Caffeine and sodium benzoate:

Children: Stimulant: I.M., I.V., SubQ: 8 mg/kg every 4 hours as needed

Children ≥12 years and Adults: OTC labeling (stimulant): Oral: 100-200 mg every 3-4 hours as needed

▶

Adults:
Electroconvulsive therapy: I.V.: 300-2000 mg
Respiratory depression: I.M., I.V.: 250 mg as a single dose; may repeat as needed. Maximum single dose should be limited to 500 mg; maximum amount in any 24-hour period should generally be limited to 2500 mg.
Spinal puncture headache (unlabeled use):
I.V.: 500 mg in 1000 mL NS infused over 1 hour, followed by 1000 mL NS infused over 1 hour; a second course of caffeine can be given for unrelieved headache pain in 4 hours.
Oral: 300 mg as a single dose
Stimulant/diuretic (unlabeled use): I.M., I.V.: 500 mg, maximum single dose: 1 g

Dosage adjustment in renal impairment: No dosage adjustment required.

Anesthesia and Critical Care Concerns/Other Considerations
Clinical Pearls/Comments: Caffeine has 40% of the bronchodilatory activity of theophylline. Lithium blood levels may increase during caffeine withdrawal. Analgesia from transcutaneous electrical nerve stimulation may be lessened with concomitant caffeine use.

Additional Information Complete prescribing information for this medication should be consulted for additional detail.

Dosage Forms Excipient information presented when available (limited, particularly for generics); consult specific product labeling. [DSC] = Discontinued product
Caplet:
NoDoz® Maximum Strength, Vivarin®: 200 mg
Injection, solution, as citrate [preservative free]: 20 mg/mL (3 mL) [equivalent to 10 mg/mL caffeine base]
Cafcit®: 20 mg/mL (3 mL) [equivalent to 10 mg/mL caffeine base]
Injection, solution [with sodium benzoate]: Caffeine 125 mg/mL and sodium benzoate 125 mg/mL (2 mL); caffeine 121 mg/mL and sodium benzoate 129 mg/mL (2 mL) [DSC]
Lozenge:
Enerjets®: 75 mg [classic coffee, hazelnut cream, or mochamint flavor]
Solution, oral, as citrate [preservative free]: 20 mg/mL (3 mL) [equivalent to 10 mg/mL caffeine base]
Cafcit®: 20 mg/mL (3 mL) [equivalent to 10 mg/mL caffeine base]
Tablet: 200 mg
Vivarin®: 200 mg

◆ **Caffeine and Sodium Benzoate** see Caffeine on page 225
◆ **Caffeine Citrate** see Caffeine on page 225
◆ **Calan®** see Verapamil on page 1468
◆ **Calan® SR** see Verapamil on page 1468
◆ **Calcimar® (Can)** see Calcitonin on page 226

Calcitonin (kal si TOE nin)

U.S. Brand Names Fortical®; Miacalcin®
Canadian Brand Names Apo-Calcitonin®; Calcimar®; Caltine®; Miacalcin® NS; Pro-Calcitonin
Index Terms Calcitonin (Salmon)
Pharmacologic Category Antidote; Hormone
Use Calcitonin (salmon): Treatment of Paget's disease of bone (osteitis deformans); adjunctive therapy for hypercalcemia; treatment of osteoporosis in women >5 years postmenopause
Pharmacodynamics/Kinetics
Hypercalcemia: I.M. or SubQ:
Onset of action: ~2 hours
Duration: 6-8 hours
Absorption: Nasal: ~3% of I.M. level (range: 0.3% to 31%)
Distribution: Does not cross placenta
Half-life elimination: SubQ: 1.2 hours; Nasal: 43 minutes

Time to peak: Nasal: ~30-40 minutes

Excretion: Urine (as inactive metabolites)

Dosage

Children: Dosage not established

Adults:

Paget's disease (Miacalcin®): I.M., SubQ: Initial: 100 units/day; maintenance: 50 units/day or 50-100 units every 1-3 days

Hypercalcemia (Miacalcin®): Initial: I.M., SubQ: 4 units/kg every 12 hours; may increase up to 8 units/kg every 12 hours to a maximum of every 6 hours

Postmenopausal osteoporosis:

I.M., SubQ: Miacalcin®: 100 units/every other day

Intranasal: Fortical®, Miacalcin®: 200 units (1 spray) in one nostril daily

Additional Information Complete prescribing information for this medication should be consulted for additional detail.

Dosage Forms Excipient information presented when available (limited, particularly for generics); consult specific product labeling.

Injection, solution [calcitonin-salmon]:

Miacalcin®: 200 int. units/mL (2 mL)

Solution, intranasal [spray, calcitonin-salmon]: 200 int. units/0.09 mL (3.7 mL, 3.8 mL)

Fortical®: 200 int. units/0.09 mL (3.7 mL) [rDNA origin; contains benzyl alcohol; delivers 30 doses, 200 int. units/actuation]

Miacalcin®: 200 int. units/0.09 mL (3.7 mL) [contains benzalkonium chloride; delivers 30 doses, 200 int. units/actuation]

References

Bauwens SF, "Osteomalacia and Osteoporosis," *Pharmacotherapy: A Pathophysiologic Approach*, 2nd ed, DiPiro JT, Talbert RL, Hayes PE, et al, eds, New York, NY, 1992, 1293-312.

Bergqvist E, Sjoberg HE, Hjern B, et al, "Calcitonin in the Treatment of Hypercalcaemic Crisis," *Acta Med Scand*, 1972, 192(5):385-9.

Lyritis GP, Tsakalakos N, Magiasis B, et al, "Analgesic Effect of Salmon Calcitonin in Osteoporotic Vertebral Fractures: A Double-Blind, Placebo-Controlled Clinical Study," *Calcif Tissue Int*, 1991, 49 (6):369-72.

Pontiroli AE, Pajetta E, Scaglia L, et al, "Analgesic Effect of Intranasal and Intramuscular Salmon Calcitonin in Postmenopausal Osteoporosis: A Double-Blind, Double-Placebo Study," *Aging (Milano)*, 1994, 6(6):459-63.

Reginster JY, Deroisy R, Lecart MP, et al, "A Double-Blind, Placebo-Controlled, Dose-Finding Trial of Intermittent Nasal Salmon Calcitonin for Prevention of Postmenopausal Lumbar Spine Bone Loss," *Am J Med*, 1995, 98(5):452-8.

Reginster JY, "Calcitonin for Prevention and Treatment of Osteoporosis," *Am J Med*, 1993, 95 (5A):44S-47S.

Stevenson JC, "Current Management of Malignant Hypercalcemia," *Drugs*, 1988, 36(2):229-30.

◆ **Calcitonin (Salmon)** *see* Calcitonin *on page 226*

Calcium Acetate (KAL see um AS e tate)

Medication Safety Issues

Sound-alike/look-alike issues:

PhosLo® may be confused with Phos-Flur®, ProSom™

U.S. Brand Names PhosLo®

Canadian Brand Names PhosLo®

Pharmacologic Category Antidote; Calcium Salt; Phosphate Binder

Generic Available Yes

Use Control of hyperphosphatemia in end-stage renal failure; does not promote aluminum absorption

Mechanism of Action Combines with dietary phosphate to form insoluble calcium phosphate which is excreted in feces

Pharmacodynamics/Kinetics

Absorption: Requires vitamin D; minimal unless chronic, high doses are given; calcium is absorbed in soluble, ionized form; solubility of calcium is increased in an acid environment

Distribution: Crosses placenta; enters breast milk

Excretion: Primarily feces (as unabsorbed calcium); urine (20%)

Dosage
Dietary Reference Intake:
0-6 months: 210 mg/day
7-12 months: 270 mg/day
1-3 years: 500 mg/day
4-8 years: 800 mg/day
Adults, Male/Female:
9-18 years: 1300 mg/day
19-50 years: 1000 mg/day
≥51 years: 1200 mg/day
Female: Pregnancy/lactating: Same as for Adults, Male/Female
Oral: Adults, on dialysis: Initial: 1334 mg with each meal, can be increased gradually to bring the serum phosphate value to <6 mg/dL as long as hypercalcemia does not develop (usual dose: 2001-2868 mg calcium acetate with each meal); do not give additional calcium supplements

Administration Administer with meals.

Monitoring Parameters Serum calcium, serum phosphate; for control of hypophosphatemia, serum calcium times phosphate should not exceed 66

Reference Range
Serum calcium: 8.4-10.2 mg/dL
Due to a poor correlation between the serum ionized calcium (free) and total serum calcium, particularly in states of low albumin or acid/base imbalances, direct measurement of ionized calcium is recommended.
In low albumin states, the corrected **total** serum calcium may be estimated by the following equation (assuming a normal albumin of 4 g/dL).
Corrected total calcium = total serum calcium + 0.8 (4.0 - measured serum albumin)
or
Corrected calcium = measured calcium - measured albumin + 4.0

Pregnancy Risk Factor C

Contraindications Hypersensitivity to any component of the formulation; hypercalcemia, renal calculi

Warnings/Precautions Constipation, bloating, and gas are common with calcium supplements. Hypercalcemia and hypercalciuria are most likely to occur in hypoparathyroid patients receiving high doses of vitamin D. Use with caution in patients who may be at risk of cardiac arrhythmias. Use with caution in digitalized patients; hypercalcemia may precipitate cardiac arrhythmias. Calcium administration interferes with absorption of some minerals and drugs; use with caution.

Adverse Reactions
Mild hypercalcemia (calcium: >10.5 mg/dL to ≤12 mg/dL) may be asymptomatic or manifest itself as constipation, anorexia, nausea, and vomiting
More severe hypercalcemia (calcium: >12 mg/dL) is associated with confusion, delirium, stupor, and coma
Postmarketing and/or case reports: Pruritus, allergic reaction

Drug Interactions
Avoid Concomitant Use There are no known interactions where it is recommended to avoid concomitant use.
Increased Effect/Toxicity
Calcium Acetate may increase the levels/effects of: CefTRIAXone

The levels/effects of Calcium Acetate may be increased by: Thiazide Diuretics
Decreased Effect
Calcium Acetate may decrease the levels/effects of: Bisphosphonate Derivatives; Calcium Channel Blockers; DOBUTamine; Eltrombopag; Estramustine; Phosphate Supplements; Quinolone Antibiotics; Thyroid Products; Trientine

The levels/effects of Calcium Acetate may be decreased by: Trientine
Dietary Considerations Oral dosage forms must be administered with meals to be effective.
Dosage Forms Excipient information presented when available (limited, particularly for generics); consult specific product labeling.
Gelcap: 667 mg
PhosLo®: 667 mg [equivalent to elemental calcium 169 mg (8.45 mEq)]

References
Kaiser W, Biesenbach G, Kramar R, et al, "Calcium Free Hemodialysis: An Effective Therapy in Hypercalcemic Crisis - Report of Four Cases," *Intensive Care Med*, 1989, 15(7):471-4.

Mokhlesi B, Leikin JB, Murray P, et al, "Adult Toxicology in Critical Care: Part II: Specific Poisonings," *Chest*, 2003, 123(3):897-922.

Texier D, Chevallier P, Perrotin D, et al, "Hypercalcemia Associated With Resorbable Haemostatic Compresses," *Lancet*, 1982, 1(8273):688-9.

Calcium Chloride (KAL see um KLOR ide)

Medication Safety Issues
Dosing issues:

Calcium chloride may be confused with calcium gluconate

Confusion with the different intravenous salt forms of calcium has occurred. There is a threefold difference in the primary cation concentration between calcium chloride (in which 1g = 13.6 mEq [270 mg] of elemental Ca++) and calcium gluconate (in which 1g = 4.65 mEq [90 mg] of elemental Ca++).

Prescribers should specify which salt form is desired. Dosages should be expressed either as mEq, mg, or grams of the salt form.

Pharmacologic Category Calcium Salt; Electrolyte Supplement, Parenteral

Generic Available Yes

Use Treatment of acute symptomatic hypocalcemia; cardiac disturbances of hyperkalemia or hypocalcemia; emergent treatment of hypocalcemic tetany; treatment of severe hypermagnesemia

Unlabeled/Investigational Use Calcium channel blocker overdose; severe hyperkalemia (K+ >7 mEq/L with toxic ECG changes) [ACLS guidelines]; malignant arrhythmias associated with hypermagnesemia [ACLS guidelines]

Mechanism of Action Moderates nerve and muscle performance via action potential excitation threshold regulation

Pharmacodynamics/Kinetics
Distribution: Crosses placenta; enters breast milk

Excretion: Primarily feces (80% as insoluble calcium); urine (20%)

Dosage Note: One gram of calcium chloride is equal to 270 mg of elemental calcium.

Dosages are expressed in terms of the <u>calcium chloride</u> **salt based on a solution concentration of 100 mg/mL (10%) containing 1.4 mEq (27.3 mg)/ mL elemental calcium.**

Acute, symptomatic ionized hypocalcemia, hyperkalemia, or magnesium toxicity: **Note:** Routine use in cardiac arrest is not recommended due to the lack of improved survival [PALS, ACLS 2005 Guidelines]: I.V.:

Neonates: 20 mg/kg; may repeat as necessary

Infants and Children: 20 mg/kg; may repeat as necessary [PALS 2005 Guidelines]

Adults: 500-1000 mg, may repeat as necessary [ACLS 2005 Guidelines]

Calcium channel blocker overdose (unlabeled use):

Neonates, Infants, and Children [PALS 2005 Guidelines]:

I.V., I.O.: 20 mg/kg (maximum: 1000 mg/dose) over 5-10 minutes; if favorable response obtained, consider I.V. infusion

I.V. infusion: 20-50 mg/kg/hour

Adults:

I.V.: 1000 mg every 10-20 minutes (total of 4 doses) **or** 1000 mg every 2-3 minutes until clinical effect is achieved; if favorable response obtained, consider I.V. infusion

I.V. infusion: 20-50 mg/kg/hour

Hypocalcemia secondary to citrated blood transfusion: I.V.: **Note:** Routine administration of calcium, in the absence of signs/symptoms of hypocalcemia, is generally not recommended. A number of recommendations have been published seeking to address potential hypocalcemia during massive transfusion of citrated blood; however, many practitioners recommend replacement only as guided by clinical evidence of hypocalcemia and/or serial monitoring of ionized calcium. In adults, clinically-significant hypocalcemia usually dose not occur until >5 units of packed red blood cells have been administered.

◀ Neonates, Infants, and Children: Give 32 mg (0.45 mEq elemental calcium) for each 100 mL citrated blood infused
Adults: 200-500 mg per 500 mL of citrated blood (infused into another vein)

Hypocalcemic tetany: I.V.:
Neonates: 40-60 mg/kg/dose repeated every 6-8 hours
Infants and Children: 10 mg/kg over 5-10 minutes; may repeat after 6-8 hours or follow with an infusion with a maximum dose of 200 mg/kg/day; alternatively, higher doses of 35-50 mg/kg/dose repeated every 6-8 hours have been used
Adults: 1000 mg over 10-30 minutes; may repeat after 6 hours

Dosing adjustment in renal impairment: Cl_{cr} <25 mL/minute: Dosage adjustments may be necessary depending on the serum calcium levels

Stability Do not refrigerate solutions; IVPB solutions/I.V. infusion solutions are stable for 24 hours at room temperature.
Although calcium chloride is not routinely used in the preparation of parenteral nutrition, it is important to note that phosphate salts may precipitate when mixed with calcium salts. Solubility is improved in amino acid parenteral nutrition solutions. Check with a pharmacist to determine compatibility.

Administration For I.V. administration only; avoid extravasation. Avoid rapid administration (do not exceed 100 mg/minute). May be given over 2-5 minutes if rapid increase in serum calcium concentration is required. For I.V. infusion, dilute to a maximum concentration of 20 mg/mL and infuse over 1 hour or no greater than 45-90 mg/kg/hour (0.6-1.2 mEq/kg/hour); administration via a central or deep vein is preferred; do not use scalp, small hand or foot veins for I.V. administration since severe necrosis and sloughing may occur. Monitor ECG if calcium is infused faster than 2.5 mEq/minute; **stop the infusion if the patient complains of pain or discomfort.** Warm to body temperature. **Do not infuse calcium chloride in the same I.V. line as phosphate-containing solutions.**

Monitoring Parameters Monitor infusion site, ECG when appropriate; serum calcium and ionized calcium (normal: 8.5-10.2 mg/dL [total]; 4.5-5.0 mg/dL [ionized]), albumin, serum phosphate

Reference Range
Serum calcium: 8.4-10.2 mg/dL
Due to a poor correlation between the serum ionized calcium (free) and total serum calcium, particularly in states of low albumin or acid/base imbalances, direct measurement of ionized calcium is recommended.
In low albumin states, the corrected **total** serum calcium may be estimated by the following equation (assuming a normal albumin of 4 g/dL).
Corrected total calcium = total serum calcium + 0.8 (4.0 - measured serum albumin)
or
Corrected calcium = measured calcium - measured albumin + 4.0
Serum/plasma chloride: 95-108 mEq/L

Anesthesia and Critical Care Concerns/Other Considerations
Clinical Pearls/Comments: One gram of calcium chloride is equal to 270 mg of elemental calcium.

Hypocalcemia in the Critically-Ill Patient: Treatment of patients with asymptomatic hypocalcemia, defined as a total serum calcium concentration <8.5 mg/dL (or ionized calcium <4.2 mg/dL; <1 mmol/L) with intravenous calcium salts is generally not recommended. Symptoms usually occur when ionized calcium levels fall to <2.5 mg/dL (<0.6 mmol/L). Symptoms include paresthesias of the extremities and face, muscle cramps, carpopedal spasm, stridor, tetany, and seizures. However, if the patient is experiencing hemodynamic compromise or life-threatening arrhythmias with any degree of hypocalcemia, treatment with intravenous calcium is warranted. Use of calcium chloride is preferred due to the higher bioavailability as compared with calcium gluconate. If the patient has concomitant hypomagnesemia, replacement with calcium may be ineffective until hypomagnesemia is corrected.

Calcium Channel Blocker (CCB) Overdose: Effects of CCB overdose vary depending on the type ingested. Dihydropyridine CCBs (eg, nifedipine) exhibit peripheral vasodilation primarily if large amounts are ingested, effects on the AV node may be seen. Nondihydropyridine CCBs (eg, verapamil) exhibit negative inotropic, chronotropic, and dromotropic actions although if large amounts are ingested, peripheral vasodilation effects may be present.

Calcium chloride may be an effective treatment for CCB overdose. In addition to the use of calcium chloride, other successful treatments include high-dose insulin with supplemental dextrose and potassium (HDIDK therapy), beta$_1$/alpha$_1$-agonists (eg, dopamine), and glucagon may be used.

Pregnancy Risk Factor C

Contraindications Hypercalcemia, known or suspected digoxin toxicity; not recommended as routine treatment in cardiac arrest (includes asystole, ventricular fibrillation, pulseless ventricular tachycardia, or pulseless electrical activity)

Warnings/Precautions For I.V. use only; do not inject SubQ or I.M.; avoid rapid I.V. administration (<100 mg/minute) unless being given emergently. Avoid extravasation. Use with caution in patients with hyperphosphatemia, respiratory acidosis, renal impairment, or respiratory failure; acidifying effect of calcium chloride may potentiate acidosis. Use with caution in patients with chronic renal failure to avoid hypercalcemia; frequent monitoring of serum calcium and phosphorus is necessary. Use with caution in hypokalemic or digitalized patients since acute rises in serum calcium levels may precipitate cardiac arrhythmias. Solutions may contain aluminum; toxic levels may occur following prolonged administration in premature neonates or patients with renal impairment. Avoid metabolic acidosis (ie, administer only 2-3 days then change to another calcium salt).

Adverse Reactions Frequency not defined. I.V.:

Cardiovascular: Arrhythmia, bradycardia, cardiac arrest, hypotension, syncope, vasodilation

Endocrine & metabolic: Hypercalcemia

Gastrointestinal: Irritation, chalky taste

Hepatic: Serum amylase increased

Neuromuscular & skeletal: Tingling sensation

Renal: Renal calculi

Miscellaneous: Hot flashes

Postmarketing and/or case reports: Calcinosis cutis

Drug Interactions

Avoid Concomitant Use There are no known interactions where it is recommended to avoid concomitant use.

Increased Effect/Toxicity

Calcium Chloride may increase the levels/effects of: CefTRIAXone

The levels/effects of Calcium Chloride may be increased by: Thiazide Diuretics

Decreased Effect

Calcium Chloride may decrease the levels/effects of: Bisphosphonate Derivatives; Calcium Channel Blockers; DOBUTamine; Eltrombopag; Phosphate Supplements; Thyroid Products; Trientine

The levels/effects of Calcium Chloride may be decreased by: Trientine

Test Interactions Increased calcium

Dosage Forms Excipient information presented when available (limited, particularly for generics); consult specific product labeling.

Injection, solution [preservative free]: 10% (10 mL) [equivalent to elemental calcium 27.2 mg (1.36 mEq)/mL]

Injection, solution: 10% (10 mL) [equivalent to elemental calcium 27.2 mg (1.36 mEq)/mL]

References

Ariyan CE and Sosa JA, "Assessment and Management of Patients With Abnormal Calcium," *Crit Care Med*, 2004, 32(4 Suppl):S146-54.

Bilezikian JP, "Management of Acute Hypercalcemia," *N Engl J Med*, 1992, 326(18):1196-215.

Binder LS, "Acute Arthropod Envenomation: Incidence, Clinical Features, and Management," *Med Toxicol Adverse Drug Exp*, 1989, 4(3):163-73.

Chin RL, Garmel GM, and Harter PM, "Development of Ventricular Fibrillation After Intravenous Calcium Chloride Administration in a Patient With Supraventricular Tachycardia," *Ann Emerg Med*, 1995, 25(3):416-9.

DeRoos F, "Calcium Channel Blockers," Goldfrank LG, et al, ed,*Goldfrank's Toxicologic Emergencies*, 7th ed, New York, (NY):McGraw-Hill Medical Publishing, 2002, 762-74.

Dickerson RN, "Treatment of Hypocalcemia in Critical Illness - Part 1," *Nutrition*, 2007, 23(4):358-61

Dickerson RN, "Treatment of Hypocalcemia in Critical Illness - Part 2," *Nutrition*, 2007, 23(5):436-7.

ECC Committee, Subcommittees and Task Forces of the American Heart Association, "2005 American Heart Association Guidelines for Cardiopulmonary Resuscitation and Emergency Cardiovascular Care," *Circulation*, 2005, 112(24 Suppl):IV1-203.

Howarth DM, Dawson AH, Smith AJ, et al, "Calcium Channel Blocking Drug Overdose: An Australian Series," *Hum Exp Toxicol*, 1994, 13(3):161-6.

Isbister GK, "Continuous Calcium Chloride Infusion for Massive Nifedipine Overdose," *Emerg Med J*, 2002, 19(4):355-7.

Lam YM, Tse HF, and Lau CP, "Delayed Asystolic Cardiac Arrest After Diltiazem Overdose: Resuscitation With High Dose Intravenous Calcium," *Chest*, 2001, 119(4):1280-2.

Luscher TF, Noll G, and Sturmer T, "Calcium Gluconate in Severe Verapamil Intoxication," *N Engl J Med*, 1994, 330(10):718-20.

McIvor ME, "Acute Fluoride Toxicity. Pathophysiology and Management," *Drug Saf*, 1990, 5(2):79-84.

Mokhlesi B, Leikin JB, Murray P, et al, "Adult Toxicology in Critical Care: Part II: Specific Poisonings," *Chest*, 2003, 123(3):897-922.

Pearigen PD and Benowitz NL, "Poisoning Due to Calcium Antagonists. Experience With Verapamil, Diltiazem, and Nifedipine," *Drug Saf*, 1991, 6(6):408-30.

Salhanick SD and Shannon MW, "Management of Calcium Channel Antagonist Overdose," *Drug Saf*, 2003, 26(2):65-79.

Shepherd G, "Treatment of Poisoning Caused by Beta-Adrenergic and Calcium-Channel Blockers," *Am J Health Syst Pharm*, 2006, 63(19):1828-35.

Slattery A, King WD, Nichols M, et al, "Hypercalcemia Following Damp-Rid™ Ingestion," *Clin Toxicol*, 1995, 33(5):487.

Worthley LI and Phillips PJ, "Intravenous Calcium Salts," *Lancet*, 1980, 2(8186):149.

Calcium Gluconate (KAL see um GLOO koe nate)

Medication Safety Issues

Sound-alike/look-alike issues:

Calcium gluconate may be confused with calcium glubionate

U.S. Brand Names Cal-G [OTC]; Cal-GLU™

Pharmacologic Category Calcium Salt; Electrolyte Supplement, Oral; Electrolyte Supplement, Parenteral

Generic Available Yes

Use Treatment and prevention of hypocalcemia; treatment of tetany, cardiac disturbances of hyperkalemia, cardiac resuscitation when epinephrine fails to improve myocardial contractions, hypocalcemia; calcium supplementation; hydrofluoric acid (HF) burns

Unlabeled/Investigational Use Calcium channel blocker overdose

Mechanism of Action As dietary supplement, used to prevent or treat negative calcium balance; in osteoporosis, it helps to prevent or decrease the rate of bone loss. The calcium in calcium salts moderates nerve and muscle performance and allows normal cardiac function.

Pharmacodynamics/Kinetics

Absorption: Requires vitamin D; calcium is absorbed in soluble, ionized form; solubility of calcium is increased in an acid environment

Distribution: Primarily in bones and teeth; crosses placenta; enters breast milk

Protein binding: Primarily albumin

Excretion: Primarily feces (as unabsorbed calcium); urine (20%)

Dosage

Adequate Intake (as elemental calcium):

0-6 months: 210 mg/day

7-12 months: 270 mg/day

1-3 years: 500 mg/day

4-8 years: 800 mg/day

9-18 years: 1300 mg/day

Adults, Male/Female:

19-50 years: 1000 mg/day

≥51 years: 1200 mg/day

Female: Pregnancy/Lactating: Same as for Adults, Male/Female

Dosage note: Calcium chloride has 3 times more elemental calcium than calcium gluconate. Calcium chloride is 27% elemental calcium; calcium gluconate is 9% elemental calcium. One gram of calcium chloride is equal to 270 mg of elemental calcium; 1 gram of calcium gluconate is equal to 90 mg of elemental calcium. The following dosages are expressed in terms of the calcium gluconate salt based on a solution concentration of 100 mg/mL (10%) containing 0.465 mEq (9.3 mg)/mL elemental calcium:

Hypocalcemia: I.V.:

Neonates: 200-800 mg/kg/day as a continuous infusion or in 4 divided doses (maximum: 1 g/dose)

Infants and Children: 200-500 mg/kg/day as a continuous infusion or in 4 divided doses (maximum: 2-3 g/dose)

Adults: 2-15 g/24 hours as a continuous infusion or in divided doses

Hypocalcemia: Oral:

Children: 200-500 mg/kg/day divided every 6 hours

Adults: 500 mg to 2 g 2-4 times/day

Hypocalcemia secondary to citrated blood infusion: I.V.: **Note:** Routine administration of calcium, in the absence of signs/symptoms of hypocalcemia, is generally not recommended. A number of recommendations have been published seeking to address potential hypocalcemia during massive transfusion of citrated blood; however, many practitioners recommend replacement only as guided by clinical evidence of hypocalcemia and/or serial monitoring of ionized calcium.

Neonates, Infants, and Children: Give 98 mg (0.45 mEq **elemental** calcium) for each 100 mL citrated blood infused

Adults: 500 mg to 1 g per 500 mL of citrated blood (infused into another vein). Single doses up to 2 g have also been recommended.

Hypocalcemic tetany: I.V.:

Neonates, Infants, and Children: 100-200 mg/kg/dose over 5-10 minutes; may repeat every 6-8 hours **or** follow with an infusion of 500 mg/kg/day

Adults: 1-3 g may be administered until therapeutic response occurs

Magnesium intoxication, cardiac arrest in the presence of hyperkalemia or hypocalcemia: I.V.:

Infants and Children: 60-100 mg/kg/dose (maximum: 3 g/dose)

Adults: 500-800 mg/dose (maximum: 3 g/dose)

Maintenance electrolyte requirements for total parenteral nutrition: I.V.: Daily requirements: Adults: 1.7-3.4 g/1000 kcal/24 hours

Calcium channel blocker overdose (unlabeled use): Adults: I.V. infusion: 10% solution: 0.6-1.2 mL/kg/hour or I.V. 0.2-0.5 ml/kg every 15-20 minutes for 4 doses (maximum: 2-3 g/dose). In life-threatening situations, 1 g has been given every 1-10 minutes until clinical effect is achieved (case reports of resistant hypotension reported use of 12-18 g total).

Dosing adjustment in renal impairment: Cl_{cr} <25 mL/minute: Dosage adjustments may be necessary depending on the serum calcium levels

Stability

Do not refrigerate solutions. IVPB solutions/I.V. infusion solutions are stable for 24 hours at room temperature.

Standard diluent: 1 g/100 mL D_5W or NS; 2 g/100 mL D_5W or NS.

Maximum concentration in parenteral nutrition solutions is variable depending upon concentration and solubility (consult detailed reference).

Administration Not for I.M. or SubQ administration. For I.V. administration only; administer slowly (~1.5 mL calcium gluconate 10% per minute) through a small needle into a large vein in order to avoid too rapid increased in serum calcium and extravasation.

Extravasation treatment example: Hyaluronidase: Add 1 mL NS to 150 unit vial to make 150 units/mL of concentration; mix 0.1 mL of above with 0.9 mL NS in 1 mL syringe to make final concentration = 15 units/mL

Reference Range

Serum calcium: 8.4-10.2 mg/dL: Monitor plasma calcium levels if using calcium salts as electrolyte supplements for deficiency

Due to a poor correlation between the serum ionized calcium (free) and total serum calcium, particularly in states of low albumin or acid/base imbalances, direct measurement of ionized calcium is recommended

In low albumin states, the corrected **total** serum calcium may be estimated by: Corrected total calcium = total serum calcium + 0.8 (4.0 - measured serum albumin)

Anesthesia and Critical Care Concerns/Other Considerations

Clinical Pearls/Comments: One gram of calcium gluconate is equal to 90 mg of elemental calcium.

Hypocalcemia in the Critically-Ill Patient: Treatment of patients with asymptomatic hypocalcemia, defined as a total serum calcium concentration <8.5 mg/dL (or ionized calcium <4.2 mg/dL; <1 mmol/L) with intravenous calcium salts is generally not recommended. Symptoms usually occur when ionized calcium levels fall to <2.5 mg/dL (<0.6 mmol/L). Symptoms include paresthesias of the extremities and face, muscle cramps, carpopedal spasm, stridor, tetany, and seizures. However, if the patient is experiencing hemodynamic compromise or life-threatening arrhythmias with any degree of hypocalcemia, treatment with intravenous calcium is warranted. Use of calcium chloride is preferred due to the higher bioavailability as compared with calcium gluconate. If the patient has concomitant hypomagnesemia, replacement with calcium may be ineffective until hypomagnesemia is corrected.

Calcium Channel Blocker (CCB) Overdose: Effects of CCB overdose vary depending on the type ingested. Dihydropyridine CCBs (eg, nifedipine) exhibit peripheral vasodilation primarily if large amounts are ingested, effects on the AV node may be seen. Nondihydropyridine CCBs (eg, verapamil) exhibit negative inotropic, chronotropic, and dromotropic actions although if large amounts are ingested, peripheral vasodilation effects may be present.

Calcium gluconate (or calcium chloride) may be an effective treatment for the CCB overdose. In addition to the use of calcium other successful treatments include high-dose insulin with supplemental dextrose and potassium (HDIDK therapy), beta$_1$/alpha$_1$-agonists (eg, dopamine), and glucagon may be used.

Pregnancy Risk Factor C

Contraindications Hypersensitivity to calcium gluconate or any component of the formulation; ventricular fibrillation during cardiac resuscitation; digitalis toxicity or suspected digoxin toxicity; hypercalcemia

Warnings/Precautions Injection solution is for I.V. use only; do not inject SubQ or I.M. Avoid too rapid I.V. administration and avoid extravasation. Use with caution in digitalized patients, severe hyperphosphatemia, respiratory failure, or acidosis. May produce cardiac arrest. Hypercalcemia may occur in patients with renal failure; frequent determination of serum calcium is necessary. Use caution with renal disease. Use caution when administering calcium supplements to patients with a history of kidney stones. Solutions may contain aluminum; toxic levels may occur following prolonged administration in premature neonates or patients with renal dysfunction. Oral: Constipation, bloating, and gas are common with oral calcium supplements (especially carbonate salt). Taking calcium (≤500 mg) with food improves absorption. Calcium administration interferes with absorption of some minerals and drugs; use with caution. It is recommended to concomitantly administer vitamin D for optimal calcium absorption.

Adverse Reactions Frequency not defined.

I.V.:

Cardiovascular: Arrhythmia, bradycardia, cardiac arrest, hypotension, vaso-dilation, and syncope may occur following rapid I.V. injection

Central nervous system: Sense of oppression

Gastrointestinal: Chalky taste

Local: Abscess and necrosis following I.M. administration

Neuromuscular & skeletal: Tingling sensation

Miscellaneous: Heat waves

Postmarketing and/or case reports: Calcinosis cutis

Oral: Gastrointestinal: Constipation

Drug Interactions

Avoid Concomitant Use There are no known interactions where it is recommended to avoid concomitant use.

Increased Effect/Toxicity
Calcium Gluconate may increase the levels/effects of: CefTRIAXone

The levels/effects of Calcium Gluconate may be increased by: Thiazide Diuretics
Decreased Effect
Calcium Gluconate may decrease the levels/effects of: Bisphosphonate Derivatives; Calcium Channel Blockers; DOBUTamine; Eltrombopag; Estramustine; Phosphate Supplements; Quinolone Antibiotics; Thyroid Products; Trientine

The levels/effects of Calcium Gluconate may be decreased by: Trientine
Test Interactions Increased calcium (S); decreased magnesium
Dosage Forms Excipient information presented when available (limited, particularly for generics); consult specific product labeling.
Capsule, oral:
Cal-G: 700 mg [gluten free, wheat free; equivalent to elemental calcium 65 mg]
Capsule, oral [preservative free]:
Cal-GLU™: 515 mg [dye free, sugar free; equivalent to elemental calcium 50 mg]
Injection, solution [preservative free]: 10% (10 mL, 50 mL, 100 mL, 200 mL) [100 mg/mL; equivalent to elemental calcium 9 mg/mL; calcium 0.46 mEq/mL]
Powder: 347 mg/tablespoonful (480 g)
Tablet: 500 mg [equivalent to elemental calcium 45 mg]; 650 mg [equivalent to elemental calcium 58.5 mg]; 975 mg [equivalent to elemental calcium 87.75 mg]
References

DeRoos F, "Calcium Channel Blockers," Goldfrank LG, et al, ed,*Goldfrank's Toxicologic Emergencies*, 7th ed, New York, (NY):McGraw-Hill Medical Publishing, 2002, 762-74.

Howarth DM, Dawson AH, Smith AJ, et al, "Calcium Channel Blocking Drug Overdose: An Australian Series," *Hum Exp Toxicol*, 1994, 13(3):161-6.

Isbister GK, "Continuous Calcium Chloride Infusion for Massive Nifedipine Overdose," *Emerg Med J*, 2002, 19(4):355-7.

Lam YM, Tse HF, and Lau CP, "Delayed Asystolic Cardiac Arrest After Diltiazem Overdose: Resuscitation With High Dose Intravenous Calcium," *Chest*, 2001, 119(4):1280-2.

Luscher TF, Noll G, and Sturmer T, "Calcium Gluconate in Severe Verapamil Intoxication," *N Engl J Med*, 1994, 330(10):718-20.

Mokhlesi B, Leikin JB, Murray P, et al, "Adult Toxicology in Critical Care: Part II: Specific Poisonings," *Chest*, 2003, 123(3):897-922.

Salhanick SD and Shannon MW, "Management of Calcium Channel Antagonist Overdose," *Drug Saf*, 2003, 26(2):65-79.

◆ **Calcium Leucovorin** *see* Leucovorin Calcium *on page 812*

◆ **Calcium Levoleucovorin** *see* LEVOleucovorin *on page 828*

◆ **Caldecort® [OTC]** *see* Hydrocortisone *on page 699*

◆ **Caldolor™** *see* Ibuprofen *on page 717*

Calfactant (kaf AKT ant)

U.S. Brand Names Infasurf®
Pharmacologic Category Lung Surfactant
Generic Available No
Use Prevention of respiratory distress syndrome (RDS) in premature infants at high risk for RDS and for the treatment ("rescue") of premature infants who develop RDS

Prophylaxis: Therapy at birth with calfactant is indicated for premature infants <29 weeks of gestational age at significant risk for RDS. Should be administered as soon as possible, preferably within 30 minutes after birth.
Treatment: For infants ≤72 hours of age with RDS (confirmed by clinical and radiologic findings) and requiring endotracheal intubation.
Mechanism of Action Endogenous lung surfactant is essential for effective ventilation because it modifies alveolar surface tension, thereby stabilizing the alveoli. Lung surfactant deficiency is the cause of respiratory distress syndrome (RDS) in premature infants and lung surfactant restores surface activity to the lungs of these infants.
Pharmacodynamics/Kinetics No human studies of absorption, biotransformation, or excretion have been performed

◄ **Dosage** Intratracheal administration **only**: Each dose is 3 mL/kg body weight at birth; should be administered every 12 hours for a total of up to 3 doses

Stability Gentle swirling or agitation of the vial of suspension is often necessary for redispersion. **Do not shake**. Visible flecks of the suspension and foaming under the surface are normal. Calfactant should be stored at refrigeration (2°C to 8°C/36°F to 46°F). Warming before administration is not necessary. Unopened and unused vials of calfactant that have been warmed to room temperature can be returned to the refrigeration storage within 24 hours for future use. Repeated warming to room temperature should be avoided. Each single-use vial should be entered only once and the vial with any unused material should be discarded after the initial entry.

Administration Gentle swirling or agitation of the vial is often necessary for redispersion as suspension settles during storage; do **not** shake; visible flecks in the suspension and foaming at the surface are normal; does not require reconstitution; do not dilute or sonicate.

Should be administered intratracheally through an endotracheal tube. Dose is drawn into a syringe from the single-use vial using a 20-gauge or larger needle with care taken to avoid excessive foaming. Should be administered in two aliquots of 1.5 mL/kg each. After each aliquot is instilled, the infant should be positioned with either the right or the left side dependent. Administration is made while ventilation is continued over 20-30 breaths for each aliquot, with small bursts timed only during the inspiratory cycles. A pause followed by evaluation of the respiratory status and repositioning should separate the two aliquots.

Monitoring Parameters Following administration, patients should be carefully monitored so that oxygen therapy and ventilatory support can be modified in response to changes in respiratory status.

Warnings/Precautions For intratracheal administration only. Rapidly affects oxygenation and lung compliance; restrict use to a highly-supervised clinical setting with immediate availability of clinicians experienced in intubation and ventilatory management of premature infants. Transient episodes of bradycardia, decreased oxygen saturation, endotracheal tube blockage or reflux of calfactant into endotracheal tube may occur. Discontinue dosing procedure and initiate measures to alleviate the condition; may reinstitute after the patient is stable. Produces rapid improvements in lung oxygenation and compliance that may require frequent adjustments to oxygen delivery and ventilator settings.

Adverse Reactions
Cardiovascular: Bradycardia (34%), cyanosis (65%)
Respiratory: Airway obstruction (39%), reflux (21%), requirement for manual ventilation (16%), reintubation (1% to 10%)

Drug Interactions
Avoid Concomitant Use There are no known interactions where it is recommended to avoid concomitant use.
Increased Effect/Toxicity There are no known significant interactions involving an increase in effect.
Decreased Effect There are no known significant interactions involving a decrease in effect.

Dosage Forms Excipient information presented when available (limited, particularly for generics); consult specific product labeling.
Suspension, intratracheal [preservative free; calf lung derived]:
Infasurf®: 35 mg/mL (3 mL, 6 mL)

◆ **Cal-G [OTC]** see Calcium Gluconate on page 232
◆ **Cal-GLU™** see Calcium Gluconate on page 232
◆ **Caltine® (Can)** see Calcitonin on page 226
◆ **Canasa®** see Mesalamine on page 884
◆ **Cancidas®** see Caspofungin on page 246

Candesartan (kan de SAR tan)

Related Information
Angiotensin Agents *on page 1652*
Heart Failure (Systolic) *on page 1739*
Preoperative Evaluation of the Cardiac Patient for Noncardiac Surgery *on page 1598*

U.S. Brand Names Atacand®
Canadian Brand Names Atacand®
Index Terms Candesartan Cilexetil
Pharmacologic Category Angiotensin II Receptor Blocker
Use Alone or in combination with other antihypertensive agents in treating essential hypertension; treatment of heart failure (NYHA class II-IV)

Pharmacodynamics/Kinetics
Onset of action: 2-3 hours
Peak effect: 6-8 hours
Duration: >24 hours
Distribution: V_d: 0.13 L/kg
Protein binding: 99%
Metabolism: To candesartan by the intestinal wall cells
Bioavailability: 15%
Half-life elimination (dose dependent): 5-9 hours
Time to peak: 3-4 hours
Excretion: Urine (26%)
Clearance: Total body: 0.37 mL/kg/minute; Renal: 0.19 mL/kg/minute

Dosage Adults: Oral:
Hypertension: Usual dose is 4-32 mg once daily; dosage must be individualized. Blood pressure response is dose related over the range of 2-32 mg. The usual recommended starting dose of 16 mg once daily when it is used as monotherapy in patients who are not volume depleted. It can be administered once or twice daily with total daily doses ranging from 8-32 mg. Larger doses do not appear to have a greater effect and there is relatively little experience with such doses.
Congestive heart failure: Initial: 4 mg once daily; double the dose at 2-week intervals, as tolerated; target dose: 32 mg
Note: In selected cases, concurrent therapy with an ACE inhibitor may provide additional benefit.
Elderly: No initial dosage adjustment is necessary for elderly patients (although higher concentrations (C_{max}) and AUC were observed in these populations), for patients with mildly impaired renal function, or for patients with mildly impaired hepatic function.

Dosage adjustment in hepatic impairment:
Mild hepatic impairment: No initial dosage adjustment required
Moderate hepatic impairment: Consider initiation at lower dosages (AUC increased by 145%).
Severe hepatic impairment and/or cholestasis: Contraindicated

Anesthesia and Critical Care Concerns/Other Considerations
Clinical Pearls/Comments: In patients on chronic angiotensin receptor blocker (ARB) therapy, intraoperative hypotension may occur with induction and maintenance of general anesthesia; however, discontinuation of therapy prior to surgery is controversial. If continued preoperatively, avoidance of hypotensive agents during surgery is prudent. Episodes of intraoperative hypotension may be managed by fluid administration and/or modest doses of alpha-adrenergic agents. Severe hypotension may occur in patients who are sodium- and/or volume-depleted; initiate lower doses and monitor closely when starting therapy in these patients. ARB therapy may elicit an increase in potassium and creatinine, especially when used in patients with bilateral renal artery stenosis. Concomitant NSAID therapy may attenuate blood pressure control; use of NSAIDs should be avoided or limited, with monitoring of blood pressure control. In the setting of heart failure, NSAID use may be associated with an increased risk for fluid accumulation and edema and therefore should be avoided.

Evidence-Based Information: The angiotensin II receptor antagonists have similar indications as ACE inhibitors. In heart failure, the angiotensin II antagonists

◀ are especially useful in providing an alternative therapy in those patients who have intractable cough due to ACE inhibitor therapy. Candesartan has been studied as an alternative therapy in chronic heart failure patients who cannot tolerate an ACE-I (CHARM-Alternative) and as an added therapy in heart failure patients who are maintained on an ACE-I (CHARM-Added). In both studies, the combined endpoint of cardiovascular death or heart failure hospitalizations was significantly improved over the placebo-treated group.

Additional Information May have an advantage over losartan due to minimal metabolism requirements and consequent use in mild-to-moderate hepatic impairment

Dosage Forms Excipient information presented when available (limited, particularly for generics); consult specific product labeling.

Tablet, as cilexetil:

Atacand®: 4 mg, 8 mg, 16 mg, 32 mg

References

Antman EM, Anbe SC, Alpert JS, et al, "ACC/AHA Guidelines for the Management of Patients With ST-Elevation Myocardial Infarction - Executive Summary: A Report of the American College of Cardiology/American Heart Association Task Force on Practice Guidelines (Writing Committee to Revise the 1999 Guidelines for the Management of Patients With Acute Myocardial Infarction)," *Circulation*, 2004, 110(5):588-636. Available at: http://www.circulationaha.org/cgi/content/full/110/5/588. Last accessed October 26, 2004. .

Chobanian AV, Bakris GL, Black HR, et al, "The Seventh Report of the Joint National Committee on Prevention, Detection, Evaluation, and Treatment of High Blood Pressure: The JNC 7 Report," *JAMA*, 2003, 289(19):2560-71.

Cohn JN and Tognoni G, "Valsartan Heart Failure Trial Investigators. A Randomized Trial of the Angiotensin-Receptor Blocker Valsartan in Chronic Heart Failure," *N Engl J Med*, 2001, 345 (23):1667-75.

Conlin P, Moore T, Swartz S, et al, "Effect of Indomethacin on Blood Pressure Lowering by Captopril and Losartan in Hypertensive Patients," *Hypertension*, 2000, 36(3):461-5.

"Consensus Recommendations for the Management of Chronic Heart Failure. On Behalf of the Membership of the Advisory Council to Improve Outcomes Nationwide in Heart Failure," *Am J Cardiol*, 1999, 83(2A):1A-38A.

Dahlof B, Devereux RB, Kjeldsen SE, et al, "Cardiovascular Morbidity and Mortality in the Losartan Intervention for Endpoint Reduction in Hypertension Study (LIFE): A Randomised Trial Against Atenolol," *Lancet*, 2002, 359(9311):995-1003.

Dickstein K and Kjekshus J, "Effects of Losartan and Captopril on Mortality and Morbidity in High-Risk Patients After Acute Myocardial Infarction: The OPTIMAAL Randomised Trial. Optimal Trial in Myocardial Infarction With Angiotensin II Antagonist Losartan," *Lancet* , 2002, 360(9335):752-60.

Epstein BJ and Gums JG, "Angiotensin Receptor Blockers Versus ACE Inhibitors: Prevention of Death and Myocardial Infarction in High-Risk Populations," *Ann Pharmacother*, 2005, 39(3):470-80.

Granger CB, McMurray JJ, Yusuf S, et al, "Effects of Candesartan in Patients With Chronic Heart Failure and Reduced Left-Ventricular Systolic Function Intolerant to Angiotensin-Converting-Enzyme Inhibitors: The CHARM-Alternative Trial," *Lancet*, 2003, 362(9386):772-6.

Hamroff G, Katz SD, Mancini D, et al, "Addition of Angiotensin II Receptor Blockade to Maximal Angiotensin-Converting Enzyme Inhibition Improves Exercise Capacity in Patients With Severe Congestive Heart Failure," *Circulation*, 1999, 99(8):990-2.

"K/DOQI Clinical Practice Guidelines for Chronic Kidney Disease: Evaluation, Classification, and Stratification. Kidney Disease Outcome Quality Initiative," *Am J Kidney Dis*, 2002, 39(2 Suppl 2):1-246. Available at: http://www.kidney.org/professionals/doqi/kdoqi/toc.htm. Last accessed August 1, 2003.

McInnes GT, O'Kane KP, Jonker J, et al, "The Efficacy and Tolerability of Candesartan Cilexetil in an Elderly Hypertensive Population," *J Hum Hypertens*, 1997, 11(Suppl 2):75-80.

McKelvie RS, Yusuf S, Pericak D, et al, "Comparison of Candesartan, Enalapril, and Their Combination in Congestive Heart Failure: Randomized Evaluation of Strategies for Left Ventricular Dysfunction (RESOLVD) Pilot Study: The RESOLVD Pilot Study Investigators," *Circulation*, 1999, 100(10):1056-64.

McMurray JJ, Ostergren J, Swedberg K, et al, "Effects of Candesartan in Patients With Chronic Heart Failure and Reduced Left-Ventricular Systolic Function Taking Angiotensin-Converting-Enzyme Inhibitors: The CHARM-Added Trial," *Lancet*, 2003, 362(9386):767-71.

Morsing P, Adler G, Brandt-Eliasson U, et al, "Mechanistic Differences of Various AT1-Receptor Blockers in Isolated Vessels of Different Origin," *Hypertension*, 1999, 33(6):1406-13.

Pfeffer MA, McMurray JJ, Velazquez EJ, et al, "Valsartan, Captopril, or Both in Myocardial Infarction Complicated by Heart Failure, Left Ventricular Dysfunction, or Both," *N Engl J Med*, 2004, 350 (2):203.

Pitt B, Poole-Wilson PA, Segal R, et al, "Effect of Losartan Compared With Captopril on Mortality in Patients With Symptomatic Heart Failure: Randomised Trial - The Losartan Heart Failure Survival Study ELITE II," *Lancet*, 2000, 355(9215):1582-7.

Reif M, White WB, Fagan TC, et al, "Effects of Candesartan Cilexetil in Patients With Systemic Hypertension. Candesartan Cilexetil Study Investigators," *Am J Cardiol*, 1998, 82(8):961-5.

Riegger GA, Bouzo H, Petr P, et al, "Improvement in Exercise Tolerance and Symptoms of Congestive Heart Failure During Treatment With Candesartan Cilexetil," *Circulation*, 1999, 100 (22):2224-30.

Swedberg K, Pfeffer M, Granger C, et al, "Candesartan in Heart Failure - Assessment of Reduction in Mortality and Morbidity (CHARM): Rationale and Design. Charm-Programme Investigators," *J Card Fail*, 1999, 5(3):276-82.

Yusuf S, Pfeffer MA, Swedberg K, et al, "Effects of Candesartan in Patients With Chronic Heart Failure and Preserved Left-Ventricular Ejection Fraction: The CHARM-Preserved Trial," *Lancet*, 2003, 362(9386):777-81.

♦ **Candesartan Cilexetil** *see* Candesartan *on page* 237

♦ **Candistatin® (Can)** *see* Nystatin *on page* 1032

♦ **Capital® and Codeine** *see* Acetaminophen and Codeine *on page* 29

♦ **Capoten® [DSC]** *see* Captopril *on page* 239

♦ **Capoten® (Can)** *see* Captopril *on page* 239

Captopril (KAP toe pril)

Related Information
Angiotensin Agents *on page* 1652
Heart Failure (Systolic) *on page* 1739
Hypertension *on page* 1754
Preoperative Evaluation of the Cardiac Patient for Noncardiac Surgery *on page* 1598

U.S. Brand Names Capoten® [DSC]

Canadian Brand Names Alti-Captopril; Apo-Capto®; Capoten®; Gen-Captopril; Mylan-Captopril; Novo-Captopril; Nu-Capto; PMS-Captopril

Index Terms ACE

Pharmacologic Category Angiotensin-Converting Enzyme (ACE) Inhibitor

Use Management of hypertension; treatment of heart failure, left ventricular dysfunction after myocardial infarction, diabetic nephropathy

Unlabeled/Investigational Use To delay the progression of nephropathy and reduce risks of cardiovascular events in hypertensive patients with type 1 or 2 diabetes mellitus; treatment of hypertensive crisis, rheumatoid arthritis; diagnosis of anatomic renal artery stenosis, hypertension secondary to scleroderma renal crisis; diagnosis of aldosteronism, idiopathic edema, Bartter's syndrome, postmyocardial infarction for prevention of ventricular failure; increase circulation in Raynaud's phenomenon, hypertension secondary to Takayasu's disease

Pharmacodynamics/Kinetics
Onset of action: Peak effect: Blood pressure reduction: 1-1.5 hours after dose

Duration: Dose related, may require several weeks of therapy before full hypotensive effect

Absorption: 60% to 75%; reduced 30% to 40% by food

Protein binding: 25% to 30%

Metabolism: 50%

Half-life elimination (renal and cardiac function dependent):
Adults, healthy volunteers: 1.9 hours; Heart failure: 2.06 hours; Anuria: 20-40 hours

Time to peak: 1 hour

Excretion: Urine (>95%) within 24 hours (40% to 50% as unchanged drug)

Dosage Note: Titrate dose according to patient's response; use lowest effective dose. Oral:

Infants: Initial: 0.15-0.3 mg/kg/dose; titrate dose upward to maximum of 6 mg/kg/day in 1-4 divided doses; usual required dose: 2.5-6 mg/kg/day

Children: Initial: 0.5 mg/kg/dose; titrate upward to maximum of 6 mg/kg/day in 2-4 divided doses

Older Children: Initial: 6.25-12.5 mg/dose every 12-24 hours; titrate upward to maximum of 6 mg/kg/day

Adolescents: Initial: 12.5-25 mg/dose given every 8-12 hours; increase by 25 mg/dose to maximum of 450 mg/day

Adults:
Acute hypertension (urgency/emergency): 12.5-25 mg, may repeat as needed (may be given sublingually, but no therapeutic advantage demonstrated)

Heart failure:
Initial dose: 6.25-12.5 mg 3 times/day in conjunction with cardiac glycoside and diuretic therapy; initial dose depends upon patient's fluid/electrolyte status
Target dose: 50 mg 3 times/day

Hypertension:
Initial dose: 12.5-25 mg 2-3 times/day; may increase by 12.5-25 mg/dose at 1- to 2-week intervals up to 50 mg 3 times/day; maximum dose: 150 mg 3 times/day; add diuretic before further dosage increases
Usual dose range (JNC 7): 25-100 mg/day in 2 divided doses

LV dysfunction after MI: Initial dose: 6.25 mg followed by 12.5 mg 3 times/day; then increase to 25 mg 3 times/day during next several days and then gradually increase over next several weeks to target dose of 50 mg 3 times/day (Some dose schedules are more aggressive to achieve an increased goal dose within the first few days of initiation.)

Diabetic nephropathy: 25 mg 3 times/day; other antihypertensives often given concurrently

Dosing adjustment in renal impairment:
Cl_{cr} 10-50 mL/minute: Administer at 75% of normal dose.
Cl_{cr} <10 mL/minute: Administer at 50% of normal dose.
Note: Smaller dosages given every 8-12 hours are indicated in patients with renal dysfunction; renal function and leukocyte count should be carefully monitored during therapy.

Hemodialysis: Moderately dialyzable (20% to 50%); administer dose postdialysis or administer 25% to 35% supplemental dose.

Peritoneal dialysis: Supplemental dose is not necessary.

Anesthesia and Critical Care Concerns/Other Considerations

Clinical Pearls/Comments: In patients on chronic ACE inhibitor therapy, intraoperative hypotension may occur with induction and maintenance of general anesthesia; however, discontinuation of therapy prior to surgery is controversial. If continued preoperatively, avoidance of hypotensive agents during surgery is prudent. Episodes of intraoperative hypotension may be managed by fluid administration and/or modest doses of alpha-adrenergic agents. Severe hypotension may occur in patients who are sodium- and/or volume-depleted, initiate lower doses and monitor closely when starting therapy in these patients. ACE inhibitor therapy may elicit an increase in potassium and creatinine, especially when used in patients with bilateral renal artery stenosis. In those patients experiencing cough on an ACE inhibitor, the ACE inhibitor may be discontinued and, if necessary, angiotensin-receptor blocker therapy instituted. Concomitant NSAID therapy may attenuate blood pressure control; use of NSAIDs should be avoided or limited, with monitoring of blood pressure control. In the setting of heart failure, NSAID use may be associated with an increased risk for fluid accumulation and edema. Because of the potent teratogenic effects of ACE inhibitors, these drugs should be avoided, if possible, when treating women of childbearing potential not on effective birth control measures. Aging patients with a decrease in glomerular filtration (also creatinine clearance), severe heart failure, and renal failure may experience an exaggerated response with administration of ACE inhibitors. Diabetic proteinuria is reduced and insulin sensitivity is enhanced.

Evidence-Based Information: ACE inhibitors decrease morbidity and mortality in patients with asymptomatic and symptomatic left ventricular dysfunction. In this situation, they decrease hospitalizations for, and retard progression to, decompensated heart failure. ACE inhibitors are also indicated in patients postmyocardial infarction in whom left ventricular ejection fraction is <40%. When used in patients with heart failure, the target dose or maximum tolerated dose should be achieved, if possible. Lower daily doses of ACE inhibitors have not demonstrated the same cardioprotective effects. ACE inhibitors have renal protective effects in patients with diabetic proteinuria. The HOPE trial examined the use of ramipril at a dose of between 2.5-10 mg daily in patients without heart failure at high risk for cardiovascular events and documented a significant improvement in cardiovascular outcome compared to placebo.

Additional Information Complete prescribing information for this medication should be consulted for additional detail.

Dosage Forms Excipient information presented when available (limited, particularly for generics); consult specific product labeling. [DSC] = Discontinued product
Tablet, oral: 12.5 mg, 25 mg, 50 mg, 100 mg
Capoten® [DSC]: 12.5 mg, 25 mg, 50 mg [scored], 100 mg

◆ **Carafate®** *see* Sucralfate *on page 1329*

◆ **Carapres® (Can)** *see* CloNIDine *on page 329*

Carbachol (KAR ba kole)

U.S. Brand Names Isopto® Carbachol; Miostat®
Canadian Brand Names Isopto® Carbachol; Miostat®
Index Terms Carbacholine; Carbamylcholine Chloride
Pharmacologic Category Cholinergic Agonist; Ophthalmic Agent, Antiglaucoma; Ophthalmic Agent, Miotic
Use Lowers intraocular pressure in the treatment of glaucoma; cause miosis during surgery
Pharmacodynamics/Kinetics
Ophthalmic instillation:
Onset of action: Miosis: 10-20 minutes
Duration: Reduction in intraocular pressure: 4-8 hours
Intraocular administration:
Onset of action: Miosis: 2-5 minutes
Duration: 24 hours
Dosage Adults:
Ophthalmic: Instill 1-2 drops up to 3 times/day
Intraocular: 0.5 mL instilled into anterior chamber before or after securing sutures
Additional Information Complete prescribing information for this medication should be consulted for additional detail.
Dosage Forms Excipient information presented when available (limited, particularly for generics); consult specific product labeling.
Solution, intraocular:
Miostat®: 0.01% (1.5 mL)
Solution, ophthalmic:
Isopto® Carbachol: 1.5% (15 mL); 3% (15 mL) [contains benzalkonium chloride]

◆ **Carbacholine** *see* Carbachol *on page 241*

CarBAMazepine (kar ba MAZ e peen)

Related Information
Antidepressant Agents *on page 1660*
Chronic Pain Management *on page 1546*
Perioperative Management of Patients on Antiseizure Medication *on page 1577*
Porphyria: Safe and Unsafe Drugs *on page 1800*
Status Epilepticus *on page 1737*
U.S. Brand Names Carbatrol®; Epitol®; Equetro®; Tegretol®; Tegretol®-XR
Canadian Brand Names Apo-Carbamazepine®; Bio-Carbamazepine; Carbamazepine; Dom-Carbamazepine; Gen-Carbamazepine CR; Mapezine®; Mylan-Carbamazepine CR; Novo-Carbamaz; Nu-Carbamazepine; PHL-Carbamazepine; PMS-Carbamazepine; Sandoz-Carbamazepine; Taro-Carbamazepine Chewable; Tegretol®
Index Terms CBZ; SPD417
Pharmacologic Category Anticonvulsant, Miscellaneous
Use
Carbatrol®, Tegretol®, Tegretol®-XR: Partial seizures with complex symptomatology (psychomotor, temporal lobe), generalized tonic-clonic seizures (grand mal), mixed seizure patterns, trigeminal neuralgia
Equetro®: Acute manic and mixed episodes associated with bipolar 1 disorder
Unlabeled/Investigational Use Treatment of resistant schizophrenia, ethanol withdrawal, restless leg syndrome, post-traumatic stress disorders

◄ **Pharmacodynamics/Kinetics**
Absorption: Slow
Distribution: V_d: Neonates: 1.5 L/kg; Children: 1.9 L/kg; Adults: 0.59-2 L/kg
Protein binding: Carbamazepine: 75% to 90%, may be decreased in newborns; Epoxide metabolite: 50%
Metabolism: Hepatic via CYP3A4 to active epoxide metabolite; induces hepatic enzymes to increase metabolism
Bioavailability: 85%
Half-life elimination: **Note:** Half-life is variable because of autoinduction which is usually complete 3-5 weeks after initiation of a fixed carbamazepine regimen.
Carbamazepine: Initial: 25-65 hours; Extended release: 35-40 hours; Multiple doses: Children: 8-14 hours; Adults: 12-17 hours
Epoxide metabolite: Initial: 25-43 hours
Time to peak, serum: Unpredictable:
Immediate release: Suspension: 1.5 hour; tablet: 4-5 hours
Extended release: Carbatrol®, Equetro®: 12-26 hours (single dose), 4-8 hours (multiple doses); Tegretol®-XR: 3-12 hours
Excretion: Urine 72% (1% to 3% as unchanged drug); feces (28%)
Dosage Dosage must be adjusted according to patient's response and serum concentrations. Administer tablets (chewable or conventional) in 2-3 divided doses daily and suspension in 4 divided doses daily. Oral:
Epilepsy:
Children:
<6 years: Initial: 10-20 mg/kg/day divided twice or 3 times daily as tablets or 4 times/day as suspension; increase dose every week until optimal response and therapeutic levels are achieved
Maintenance dose: Divide into 3-4 doses daily (tablets or suspension); maximum recommended dose: 35 mg/kg/day
6-12 years: Initial: 200 mg/day in 2 divided doses (tablets or extended release tablets) or 4 divided doses (oral suspension); increase by up to 100 mg/day at weekly intervals using a twice daily regimen of extended release tablets or 3-4 times daily regimen of other formulations until optimal response and therapeutic levels are achieved
Maintenance: Usual: 400-800 mg/day; maximum recommended dose: 1000 mg/day
Note: Children <12 years who receive ≥400 mg/day of carbamazepine may be converted to extended release capsules (Carbatrol®) using the same total daily dosage divided twice daily
Children >12 years and Adults: Initial: 400 mg/day in 2 divided doses (tablets or extended release tablets) or 4 divided doses (oral suspension); increase by up to 200 mg/day at weekly intervals using a twice daily regimen of extended release tablets or capsules, or a 3-4 times/day regimen of other formulations until optimal response and therapeutic levels are achieved; usual dose: 800-1200 mg/day
Maximum recommended doses:
Children 12-15 years: 1000 mg/day
Children >15 years: 1200 mg/day
Adults: 1600 mg/day; however, some patients have required up to 1.6-2.4 g/day
Trigeminal or glossopharyngeal neuralgia: Adults: Initial: 200 mg/day in 2 divided doses (tablets, extended release tablets, or extended release capsules) or 4 divided doses (oral suspension) with food, gradually increasing in increments of 200 mg/day as needed
Maintenance: Usual: 400-800 mg daily in 2 divided doses (tablets, extended release tablets, or extended release capsules) or 4 divided doses (oral suspension); maximum dose: 1200 mg/day
Bipolar disorder: Adults: Initial: 400 mg/day in 2 divided doses (tablets, extended release tablets, or extended release capsules) or 4 divided doses (oral suspension), may adjust by 200 mg/day increments; maximum dose: 1600 mg/day.
Note: Equetro® is the only formulation specifically approved by the FDA for the management of bipolar disorder.
Anesthesia and Critical Care Concerns/Other Considerations
Evidence-Based Information: Concurrent use with nondepolarizing Neuromuscular Blocking Agents (NMBAs): Patients on chronic carbamazepine therapy

(>7 days) require larger and more frequent doses of nondepolarizing NMBAs to attain the same degree of muscle relaxation. The most likely reason for this reduced sensitivity is increased clearance of the NMBA due to hepatic enzyme induction (Hans, 1997; Richard, 2005; Soriano, 2001).

Additional Information Complete prescribing information for this medication should be consulted for additional detail.

Dosage Forms Excipient information presented when available (limited, particularly for generics); consult specific product labeling.

Capsule, extended release:

Carbatrol®, Equetro®: 100 mg, 200 mg, 300 mg

Suspension, oral: 100 mg/5 mL (5 mL, 10 mL, 450 mL)

Tegretol®: 100 mg/5 mL (450 mL) [contains propylene glycol; citrus vanilla flavor]

Tablet: 200 mg

Epitol®, Tegretol®: 200 mg

Tablet, chewable: 100 mg

Tegretol®: 100 mg

Tablet, extended release:

Tegretol®-XR: 100 mg, 200 mg, 400 mg

References

Hans P, Brichant JF, Pieron F, et al, "Elevated Plasma Alpha 1-Acid Glycoprotein Levels: Lack of Connection to Resistance to Vecuronium Blockade Induced by Anticonvulsant Therapy," *J Neurosurg Anesthesiol*, 1997, 9(1):3-7.

Miles MV, Lawless ST, Tennison MB, et al, "Rapid Loading of Critically Ill Patients With Carbamazepine Suspension," *Pediatrics*, 1990, 86(2):263-6.

Richard A, Girard F, Girard DC, et al, "Cisatracurium-Induced Neuromuscular Blockade is Affected by Chronic Phenytoin or Carbamazepine Treatment in Neurosurgical Patients," *Anesth Analg*, 2005, 100(2):538-44.

Soriano SG, Sullivan LJ, Venkatakrishnan K, et al, "Pharmacokinetics and Pharmacodynamics of Vecuronium in Children Receiving Phenytoin or Carbamazepine for Chronic Anticonvulsant Therapy," *Br J Anaesth*, 2001, 86(2):223-9.

◆ **Carbamazepine (Can)** see CarBAMazepine on page 241

◆ **Carbamylcholine Chloride** see Carbachol on page 241

◆ **Carbatrol®** see CarBAMazepine on page 241

◆ **Carbocaine®** see Mepivacaine on page 878

◆ **Carbolith™ (Can)** see Lithium on page 851

◆ **Carbose D** see Carboxymethylcellulose on page 243

Carboxymethylcellulose (kar boks ee meth il SEL yoo lose)

Medication Safety Issues

Sound-alike/look-alike issues:

Optive™ may be confused with Optivar®

U.S. Brand Names Optive™ [OTC]; Refresh Liquigel® [OTC]; Refresh Plus® [OTC]; Refresh Tears® [OTC]; Tears Again® Gel Drops™ [OTC]; Tears Again® Night and Day™ [OTC]; Theratears® [OTC]

Canadian Brand Names Celluvisc™; Refresh Plus®; Refresh Tears®

Index Terms Carbose D; Carboxymethylcellulose Sodium

Pharmacologic Category Ophthalmic Agent, Miscellaneous

Generic Available Yes: Excludes gel

Use Artificial tear substitute

Dosage Ophthalmic: Adults: Instill 1-2 drops into eye(s) 3-4 times/day

Drug Interactions

Avoid Concomitant Use There are no known interactions where it is recommended to avoid concomitant use.

Increased Effect/Toxicity There are no known significant interactions involving an increase in effect.

Decreased Effect There are no known significant interactions involving a decrease in effect.

Dosage Forms Excipient information presented when available (limited, particularly for generics); consult specific product labeling.

◀ Gel, ophthalmic, as sodium:
Tears Again® Night and Day™: 1.5% (3.5 g)
Solution ophthalmic, as sodium [drops]:
Optive™: 0.5% (15 mL, 30 mL) [contains glycerin 0.9%]
Refresh Liquigel®: 1% (15 mL) [liquid gel formulation]
Refresh Tears®: 0.5% (15 mL)
Tears Again® Gel Drops™: 0.7% (15 mL)
Theratears®: 0.25% (15 mL)
Solution, ophthalmic, as sodium [drops; preservative free]:
Refresh Plus®: 0.5% (0.4 mL) [available in packages of 30 or 50]
Theratears®: 0.25% (0.6 mL)

◆ **Carboxymethylcellulose Sodium** *see* Carboxymethylcellulose *on page 243*

◆ **Cardene®** *see* NiCARdipine *on page 1002*

◆ **Cardene® I.V.** *see* NiCARdipine *on page 1002*

◆ **Cardene® SR** *see* NiCARdipine *on page 1002*

◆ **Cardizem®** *see* Diltiazem *on page 425*

◆ **Cardizem® CD** *see* Diltiazem *on page 425*

◆ **Cardizem® LA** *see* Diltiazem *on page 425*

◆ **Carimune® NF** *see* Immune Globulin (Intravenous) *on page 732*

◆ **Cartia XT®** *see* Diltiazem *on page 425*

Carvedilol (KAR ve dil ole)

Related Information
Antiarrhythmic Drugs *on page 1656*
Beta-Blockers *on page 1669*
Heart Failure (Systolic) *on page 1739*
Preoperative Evaluation of the Cardiac Patient for Noncardiac Surgery *on page 1598*

U.S. Brand Names Coreg CR®; Coreg®

Canadian Brand Names Apo-Carvedilol®; Coreg®; Dom-Carvedilol; Novo-Carvedilol; PHL-Carvedilol; PMS-Carvedilol; RAN™-Carvedilol; ratio-Carvedilol

Pharmacologic Category Beta Blocker With Alpha-Blocking Activity

Use Mild-to-severe heart failure of ischemic or cardiomyopathic origin (usually in addition to standard therapy); left ventricular dysfunction following myocardial infarction (MI) (clinically stable with LVEF ≤40%); management of hypertension

Unlabeled/Investigational Use Angina pectoris

Pharmacodynamics/Kinetics
Onset of action: 1-2 hours
Peak antihypertensive effect: ~1-2 hours
Absorption: Rapid and extensive
Distribution: V_d: 115 L
Protein binding: >98%, primarily to albumin
Metabolism: Extensively hepatic, via CYP2C9, 2D6, 3A4, and 2C19 (2% excreted unchanged); three active metabolites (4-hydroxyphenyl metabolite is 13 times more potent than parent drug for beta-blockade); first-pass effect; plasma concentrations in the elderly and those with cirrhotic liver disease are 50% and 4-7 times higher, respectively
Bioavailability: Immediate release: 25% to 35% (due to significant first-pass metabolism); Extended release: 85% of immediate release
Half-life elimination: 7-10 hours
Time to peak, plasma: Extended release: 5 hours
Excretion: Primarily feces

Dosage Oral: Adults: Reduce dosage if heart rate drops to <55 beats/minute.
Hypertension:
Immediate release: 6.25 mg twice daily; if tolerated, dose should be maintained for 1-2 weeks, then increased to 12.5 mg twice daily. If necessary, dosage may be increased to a maximum of 25 mg twice daily after 1-2 weeks.

Extended release: Initial: 20 mg once daily, if tolerated, dose should be maintained for 1-2 weeks then increased to 40 mg once daily if necessary; maximum dose: 80 mg once daily

Heart failure:

Immediate release: 3.125 mg twice daily for 2 weeks; if this dose is tolerated, may increase to 6.25 mg twice daily. Double the dose every 2 weeks to the highest dose tolerated by patient. (Prior to initiating therapy, other heart failure medications should be stabilized and fluid retention minimized.)

Maximum recommended dose:

Mild-to-moderate heart failure:
<85 kg: 25 mg twice daily
>85 kg: 50 mg twice daily

Severe heart failure: 25 mg twice daily

Extended release: Initial: 10 mg once daily for 2 weeks; if the dose is tolerated, increase dose to 20 mg, 40 mg, and 80 mg over successive intervals of at least 2 weeks. Maintain on lower dose if higher dose is not tolerated.

Left ventricular dysfunction following MI: **Note**: Should be initiated only after patient is hemodynamically stable and fluid retention has been minimized.

Immediate release: Initial 3.125-6.25 mg twice daily; increase dosage incrementally (ie, from 6.25-12.5 mg twice daily) at intervals of 3-10 days, based on tolerance, to a target dose of 25 mg twice daily.

Extended release: Initial: 10-20 mg once daily; increase dosage incrementally at intervals of 3-10 days, based on tolerance, to a target dose of 80 mg once daily.

Angina pectoris (unlabeled use): Immediate release: 25-50 mg twice daily

Conversion from immediate release to extended release (Coreg CR®):

Current dose immediate release tablets 3.125 mg twice daily: Convert to extended release capsules 10 mg once daily

Current dose immediate release tablets 6.25 mg twice daily: Convert to extended release capsules 20 mg once daily

Current dose immediate release tablets 12.5 mg twice daily: Convert to extended release capsules 40 mg once daily

Current dose immediate release tablets 25 mg twice daily: Convert to extended release capsules 80 mg once daily

Dosing adjustment in renal impairment: None necessary

Dosing adjustment in hepatic impairment: Use is contraindicated in severe liver dysfunction.

Anesthesia and Critical Care Concerns/Other Considerations
Evidence-Based Information:

Surgery: Based on available evidence, beta-blockers should be started days to weeks before elective surgery in selected patients when possible and titrated to a heart rate <65 beats per minute. Additional data suggest that long acting beta-blockers may be superior to short acting ones (Redelmeier, 2005). The ACC/AHA 2007 guidelines on perioperative cardiovascular evaluation and care for noncardiac surgery recommend beta-blockers be continued in patients undergoing surgery who are receiving beta-blockers to treat angina, symptomatic arrhythmias, hypertension, or other ACC/AHA Class I guideline indications (Class I recommendation). The guidelines also recommend that beta-blockers be given to patients undergoing vascular surgery who have myocardial ischemia demonstrated during preoperative testing (Class I recommendation).

The guidelines also state that beta-blockers are probably recommended in patients undergoing intermediate risk (eg, carotid endarterectomy, prostate surgery) or vascular surgery in whom preoperative assessment identifies coronary heart disease or high cardiac risk (Class IIa recommendation). High cardiac risk is defined as having >1 of the following clinical risk factors: History of ischemic heart disease, compensated or prior heart failure, cerebrovascular disease, diabetes mellitus, or renal insufficiency. The use of beta-blockers is uncertain in patients undergoing intermediate risk or vascular surgery with ≤1 clinical risk factor (Class IIb recommendation).

The majority of published trials suggest a benefit of perioperative beta-blocker use during noncardiac surgery especially in high-risk patients; however, more recent clinical trials have not shown a benefit to perioperative beta-blockade for noncardiac surgery (Juul, 2006; Yang, 2006).

Additional Information Complete prescribing information for this medication should be consulted for additional detail.

Dosage Forms Excipient information presented when available (limited, particularly for generics); consult specific product labeling.

Capsule, extended release; as phosphate:
Coreg CR®: 10 mg, 20 mg, 40 mg, 80 mg
Tablet: 3.125 mg, 6.25 mg, 12.5 mg, 25 mg
Coreg®: 3.125 mg, 6.25 mg, 12.5 mg, 25 mg

References

Fleisher LA, Beckman JA, Brown KA, et al, "ACC/AHA 2006 Guideline Update on Perioperative Cardiovascular Evaluation for Noncardiac Surgery: Focused Update on Perioperative Beta-Blocker Therapy: A Report of the American College of Cardiology/American Heart Association Task Force on Practice Guidelines (Writing Committee to Update the 2002 Guidelines on Perioperative Cardiovascular Evaluation for Noncardiac Surgery) Developed in Collaboration With the American Society of Echocardiography, American Society of Nuclear Cardiology, Heart Rhythm Society, Society of Cardiovascular Anesthesiologists, Society for Cardiovascular Angiography and Interventions, and Society for Vascular Medicine and Biology," *J Am Coll Cardiol*, 2006, 47 (11):2343-55.

Juul AB, Wetterslev J, Gluud C, et al, "Effect of Perioperative Beta-Blockade in Patients With Diabetes Undergoing Major Noncardiac Surgery: Randomized Placebo Controlled, Blinded Multicentre Trial," *BMJ*, 2006, 332(7556):1482.

Yang H, Raymer K, Butler R, et al, "The Effects of Perioperative Beta-Blockade: Results of the Metoprolol After Vascular Surgery (MaVS) Study, A Randomized Controlled Trial," *Am Heart J* 2006, 152(5):983-90.

Caspofungin (kas poe FUN jin)

Related Information
Antifungal Agents *on page 1664*

U.S. Brand Names Cancidas®

Canadian Brand Names Cancidas®

Index Terms Caspofungin Acetate

Pharmacologic Category Antifungal Agent, Parenteral; Echinocandin

Generic Available No

Use Treatment of invasive *Aspergillus* infections in patients who are refractory or intolerant of other therapy; treatment of candidemia and other *Candida* infections (intra-abdominal abscesses, esophageal, peritonitis, pleural space); empirical treatment for presumed fungal infections in febrile neutropenic patient

Mechanism of Action Inhibits synthesis of $\beta(1,3)$-D-glucan, an essential component of the cell wall of susceptible fungi. Highest activity in regions of active cell growth. Mammalian cells do not require $\beta(1,3)$-D-glucan, limiting potential toxicity.

Pharmacodynamics/Kinetics

Protein binding: ~97% to albumin

Metabolism: Slowly, via hydrolysis and *N*-acetylation as well as by spontaneous degradation, with subsequent metabolism to component amino acids. Overall metabolism is extensive.

Half-life elimination: Beta (distribution): 9-11 hours; Terminal: 40-50 hours

Excretion: Urine (41% as metabolites, 1% to 9% unchanged) and feces (35% as metabolites)

Dosage I.V.:

Children: 3 months to 17 years: Initial dose: 70 mg/m^2 on day 1, subsequent dosing: 50 mg/m^2 once daily, if clinical response inadequate, may increase to 70 mg/m^2 once daily if tolerated, but increased efficacy not demonstrated (maximum dose: 70 mg/day)

Adults: **Note:** Duration of caspofungin treatment should be determined by patient status and clinical response. Empiric therapy should be given until neutropenia resolves. In patients with positive cultures, treatment should continue until 14 days after last positive culture. In neutropenic patients, treatment should be given at least 7 days after both signs and symptoms of infection **and** neutropenia resolve.

Aspergillosis, invasive: Initial dose: 70 mg on day 1; subsequent dosing: 50 mg/day. If clinical response inadequate, may increase up to 70 mg/day if tolerated, but increased efficacy not demonstrated. **Note:** Duration of therapy should be a minimum of 6-12 weeks or throughout period of immunosuppression.

Candidiasis: Initial dose: 70 mg on day 1; subsequent dosing: 50 mg/day
Esophageal: 50 mg/day; **Note:** The majority of patients studied for this indication also had oropharyngeal involvement.

Empiric therapy: Initial dose: 70 mg on day 1; subsequent dosing: 50 mg/day; if clinical response inadequate, may increase up to 70 mg/day if tolerated, but increased efficacy not demonstrated

Concomitant use of an enzyme inducer:
Children: Patients receiving carbamazepine, dexamethasone, efavirenz, nevirapine, phenytoin, or rifampin (and possibly other enzyme inducers): Consider 70 mg/m^2 once daily (maximum: 70 mg/day)
Adults:
Patients receiving rifampin: 70 mg caspofungin daily
Patients receiving carbamazepine, dexamethasone, efavirenz, nevirapine, **or** phenytoin (and possibly other enzyme inducers) may require an increased daily dose of caspofungin (70 mg/day).
Elderly: The number of patients >65 years of age in clinical studies was not sufficient to establish whether a difference in response may be anticipated.

Dosage adjustment in renal impairment: No specific dosage adjustment is required; supplemental dose is not required following dialysis
Dosage adjustment in hepatic impairment:
Children: Mild-to-severe hepatic insufficiency: No clinical experience
Adults:
Mild hepatic insufficiency (Child-Pugh score 5-6): No adjustment necessary
Moderate hepatic insufficiency (Child-Pugh score 7-9): 35 mg/day; initial 70 mg loading dose should still be administered in treatment of invasive infections
Severe hepatic insufficiency (Child-Pugh score >9): No clinical experience

Stability Store vials at 2°C to 8°C (36°F to 46°F). Reconstituted solution may be stored at ≤25°C (≤77°F) for 1 hour prior to preparation of infusion solution. Infusion solutions may be stored at ≤25°C (≤77°F) and should be used within 24 hours; up to 48 hours if stored at 2°C to 8°C (36°F to 46°F).

Bring refrigerated vial to room temperature. Reconstitute vials using 0.9% sodium chloride for injection, SWFI, or bacteriostatic water for injection. Mix gently until clear solution is formed; do not use if cloudy or contains particles. Solution should be further diluted with 0.9%, 0.45%, or 0.225% sodium chloride or LR (do not exceed final concentration of 0.5 mg/mL).

Administration Infuse slowly, over 1 hour; monitor during infusion. Isolated cases of possible histamine-related reactions have occurred during clinical trials (rash, flushing, pruritus, facial edema).

Monitoring Parameters Liver function

Pregnancy Risk Factor C

Contraindications Hypersensitivity to caspofungin or any component of the formulation

Warnings/Precautions Concurrent use of cyclosporine should be limited to patients for whom benefit outweighs risk, due to a high frequency of hepatic transaminase elevations observed during concurrent use. Limited data are available concerning treatment durations longer than 4 weeks, however, treatment appears to be well tolerated. Use caution in hepatic impairment; dosage reduction required with moderate impairment. Safety and efficacy have not been established in children <3 months of age.

Adverse Reactions
>10%:
Cardiovascular: Hypotension (6% to 20%), peripheral edema (6% to 11%), tachycardia (4% to 11%)
Central nervous system: Fever (13% to 30%), chills (8% to 23%), headache (5% to 15%)
Dermatologic: Rash (4% to 23%)
Endocrine & metabolic: Hypokalemia (5% to 23%)
Gastrointestinal: Diarrhea (7% to 27%), vomiting (7% to 17%), nausea (4% to 15%)

Hematologic: Hemoglobin decreased (5% to 21%), hematocrit decreased (13% to 18%), WBC decreased (12%), anemia (2% to 11%)

Hepatic: Serum alkaline phosphatase increased (13% to 22%), transaminases increased (2% to 18%), bilirubin increased (5% to 13%)

Local: Phlebitis/thrombophlebitis (18%)

Renal: Serum creatinine increased (3% to 11%), urinary RBCs increased (10%)

Respiratory: Respiratory failure (11% to 20%), cough (6% to 11%), pneumonia (4% to 11%)

Miscellaneous: Infusion reactions (20% to 35%), septic shock (11%)

1% to 10%:

Cardiovascular: Hypertension (children 9% to 10%), edema (3% to 4%)

Dermatologic: Erythema (4% to 9%), pruritus (5% to 7%)

Endocrine & metabolic: Hypomagnesemia (7%), hyperglycemia (6%), hyperkalemia (3%)

Gastrointestinal: Mucosal inflammation (4% to 10%), abdominal pain (4% to 9%)

Hepatic: Albumin decreased (7%)

Local: Infection (1% to 9%, central line)

Neuromuscular & skeletal: Back pain (children up to 4%)

Renal: Nephrotoxicity (13%), blood urea nitrogen increased (4% to 9%)

Note: Nephrotoxicity defined as serum creatinine ≥2x baseline value or ≥1 mg/dL in patients with serum creatinine above ULN range (patients with Cl_{cr} <30 mL/minute were excluded)

Respiratory: Dyspnea (9%), pleural effusion (9%), respiratory distress (children up to 8%), rales (7%), tachypnea (1%)

<1% (Limited to important or life-threatening): Abdominal distention, anaphylaxis, anorexia, anxiety, appetite decrease, arrhythmia, arthralgia, atrial fibrillation, bradycardia, coagulopathy, confusion, constipation, depression, dizziness, dyspepsia, dystonia, epistaxis, erythema multiforme, fatigue, febrile neutropenia, fluid overload, flushing, hematuria, hepatic necrosis, hepatomegaly, hepatotoxicity, hypercalcemia, hypoxia, infusion site reactions (pain/pruritus/swelling), insomnia, jaundice, liver failure, MI, pain (extremities), pancreatitis, petechiae, pulmonary edema, renal failure/insufficiency, seizure, skin exfoliation, skin lesion, somnolence, stridor, Stevens-Johnson syndrome, tachypnea, thrombocytopenia, tremor, urinary tract infection, urticaria, weakness; histamine-mediated reactions (including facial swelling, bronchospasm, sensation of warmth) have been reported

Drug Interactions

Avoid Concomitant Use There are no known interactions where it is recommended to avoid concomitant use.

Increased Effect/Toxicity

The levels/effects of Caspofungin may be increased by: CycloSPORINE

Decreased Effect

Caspofungin may decrease the levels/effects of: Saccharomyces boulardii; Tacrolimus

The levels/effects of Caspofungin may be decreased by: Inducers of Drug Clearance; Rifampin

Dosage Forms Excipient information presented when available (limited, particularly for generics); consult specific product labeling.

Injection, powder for reconstitution, as acetate:

Cancidas®: 50 mg [contains sucrose 39 mg], 70 mg [contains sucrose 54 mg]

References

Mora-Duarte J, Betts R, Rotstein C, et al, "Comparison of Caspofungin and Amphotericin B for Invasive Candidiasis," *N Engl J Med*, 2002, 347(25):2020-9.

Pappas PG, Rex JH, Sobel JD, et al, "Guidelines for Treatment of Candidiasis," *Clin Infect Dis*, 2004, 38:161-89.

CeFAZolin (sef A zoe lin)

Medication Safety Issues
Sound-alike/look-alike issues:
CeFAZolin may be confused with cefprozil, cefTRIAXone, cephalexin, cephalothin
Kefzol® may be confused with Cefzil®

Related Information
Anesthesia for Patients With Liver Disease *on page* 1537
Dosing Considerations for the Critically-Ill Patient With Morbid Obesity *on page* 1561
Prevention of Infective Endocarditis *on page* 1718
Prevention of Wound Infection and Sepsis in Surgical Patients *on page* 1721

Index Terms Ancef; Cefazolin Sodium

Pharmacologic Category Antibiotic, Cephalosporin (First Generation)

Generic Available Yes

Use Treatment of respiratory tract, skin, genital, urinary tract, biliary tract, bone and joint infections, and septicemia due to susceptible gram-positive cocci (except enterococcus); some gram-negative bacilli including *E. coli*, *Proteus*, and *Klebsiella* may be susceptible; surgical prophylaxis

Unlabeled/Investigational Use Prophylaxis against infective endocarditis

Mechanism of Action Inhibits bacterial cell wall synthesis by binding to one or more of the penicillin-binding proteins (PBPs) which in turn inhibits the final transpeptidation step of peptidoglycan synthesis in bacterial cell walls, thus inhibiting cell wall biosynthesis. Bacteria eventually lyse due to ongoing activity of cell wall autolytic enzymes (autolysins and murein hydrolases) while cell wall assembly is arrested.

Pharmacodynamics/Kinetics
Distribution: Widely into most body tissues and fluids including gallbladder, liver, kidneys, bone, sputum, bile, pleural, and synovial; CSF penetration is poor
Protein binding: 74% to 86%
Metabolism: Minimally hepatic
Half-life elimination: 90-150 minutes; prolonged with renal impairment
Time to peak, serum: I.M.: 0.5-2 hours
Excretion: Urine (80% to 100% as unchanged drug)

Dosage
Usual dosage range: I.M., I.V.:
Children >1 month: 25-100 mg/kg/day divided every 6-8 hours; maximum: 6 g/day
Adults: 250 mg to 1.5 g every 6-12 (usually 8) hours, depending on severity of infection; maximum dose: 12 g/day

Indication-specific dosing:
Infants and Children: I.M., I.V.:
Prophylaxis against infective endocarditis (unlabeled use): 50 mg/kg 30-60 minutes before procedure; maximum dose: 1 g. Intramuscular injections should be avoided in patients who are receiving anticoagulant therapy. In these circumstances, orally administered regimens should be given whenever possible. Intravenously administered antibiotics should be used for patients who are unable to tolerate or absorb oral medications.
Note: American Heart Association (AHA) guidelines now recommend prophylaxis only in patients undergoing invasive procedures and in whom underlying cardiac conditions may predispose to a higher risk of adverse outcomes should infection occur. As of April 2007, routine prophylaxis for GI/GU procedures is no longer recommended by the AHA.

Adults: I.M., I.V.:

Endocarditis due to MSSA (without prosthesis) (unlabeled use): I.V.: 2 g every 8 hours; **Note:** Recommended for penicillin-allergic (non-anaphylactoid) patients (Baddour et al, 2005)

Prophylaxis against infective endocarditis (unlabeled use): 1 g 30-60 minutes before procedure. Intramuscular injections should be avoided in patients who are receiving anticoagulant therapy. In these circumstances, orally administered regimens should be given whenever possible. Intravenously administered antibiotics should be used for patients who are unable to tolerate or absorb oral medications.

> **Note:** American Heart Association (AHA) guidelines now recommend prophylaxis only in patients undergoing invasive procedures and in whom underlying cardiac conditions may predispose to a higher risk of adverse outcomes should infection occur. As of April 2007, routine prophylaxis for GI/GU procedures is no longer recommended by the AHA.

Moderate-to-severe infections: 500 mg to 1 g every 6-8 hours

Mild infection with gram-positive cocci: 250-500 mg every 8 hours

Perioperative prophylaxis: 1-2 g within 60 minutes prior to surgery (may repeat in 2-5 hours intraoperatively); followed by 500 mg to 1 g every 6-8 hours for 24 hours postoperatively

Cardiothoracic surgery: 1 g within 60 minutes prior to incision, followed by 1 g at sternotomy and 1 g after cardiopulmonary bypass; may continue 1 g every 6 hours for 24-48 hours postoperatively (Eagle, 2004)

Total joint replacement: 1 g 1 hour prior to the procedure

Pneumococcal pneumonia: 500 mg every 12 hours

Severe infection: 1-1.5 g every 6 hours

UTI (uncomplicated): 1 g every 12 hours

Dosing adjustment in renal impairment:

Cl_{cr} 35-54 mL/minute: Administer full dose in intervals of ≥8 hours

Cl_{cr} 11-34 mL/minute: Administer 1/2 usual dose every 12 hours

Cl_{cr} ≤10 mL/minute: Administer 1/2 usual dose every 18-24 hours

Hemodialysis: Moderately dialyzable (20% to 50%); administer dose postdialysis or administer supplemental dose of 0.5-1 g after dialysis

Continuous ambulatory peritoneal dialysis (CAPD): Administer 0.5 g every 12 hours

Continuous renal replacement therapy (CRRT): Drug clearance is highly dependent on the method of renal replacement, filter type, and flow rate. Appropriate dosing requires close monitoring of pharmacologic response, signs of adverse reactions due to drug accumulation, as well as drug levels in relation to target trough (if appropriate). The following are general recommendations only (based on dialysate flow/ultrafiltration rates of 1 L/hour) and should not supersede clinical judgment:

CVVH: 1-2 g every 12 hours

CVVHD/CVVHDF: 2 g every 12 hours

Stability Store intact vials at room temperature and protect from temperatures exceeding 40°C. Dilute large vial with 2.5 mL SWFI; 10 g vial may be diluted with 45 mL to yield 1 g/5 mL or 96 mL to yield 1 g/10 mL. May be injected or further dilution for I.V. administration in 50-100 mL compatible solution. Standard diluent is 1 g/50 mL D_5W or 2 g/50 mL D_5W.

Reconstituted solutions of cefazolin are light yellow to yellow. Protection from light is recommended for the powder and for the reconstituted solutions. Reconstituted solutions are stable for 24 hours at room temperature and for 10 days under refrigeration. Stability of parenteral admixture at room temperature (25°C) is 48 hours. Stability of parenteral admixture at refrigeration temperature (4°C) is 14 days.

DUPLEX™: Store at 20°C to 25°C (68°F to 77°F); excursions permitted to 15°C to 30°C (59°F to 86°F) prior to activation. Following activation, stable for 24 hours at room temperature and for 7 days under refrigeration.

Administration

I.M.: Inject deep I.M. into large muscle mass.

I.V.: Inject direct I.V. over 5 minutes. Infuse intermittent infusion over 30-60 minutes.

Some penicillins (eg, carbenicillin, ticarcillin, and piperacillin) have been shown to inactivate aminoglycosides *in vitro*. This has been observed to a greater extent with tobramycin and gentamicin, while amikacin has shown greater stability against inactivation. Concurrent use of these agents may pose a risk of reduced antibacterial efficacy *in vivo*, particularly in the setting of profound renal impairment. However, definitive clinical evidence is lacking. If combination penicillin/aminoglycoside therapy is desired in a patient with renal dysfunction, separation of doses (if feasible), and routine monitoring of aminoglycoside levels, CBC, and clinical response should be considered.

Monitoring Parameters Renal function periodically when used in combination with other nephrotoxic drugs, hepatic function tests, CBC; monitor for signs of anaphylaxis during first dose

Anesthesia and Critical Care Concerns/Other Considerations

Evidence-Based Information: Surgical Prophylaxis: Cefazolin should be avoided in patients with a history of serious beta-lactam allergy (eg, respiratory difficulty, angioedema, hives, hypotension). Examples of beta-lactam antibiotics include penicillin, ampicillin, piperacillin, and cephalosporins. In operations where prophylaxis is directed towards gram-positive cocci, vancomycin or clindamycin may be used depending on local susceptibility patterns (Bratzler, 2004).

Pregnancy Risk Factor B

Contraindications Hypersensitivity to cefazolin sodium, any component of the formulation, or other cephalosporins

Warnings/Precautions Modify dosage in patients with severe renal impairment. Use with caution in patients with a history of penicillin allergy, especially IgE-mediated reactions (eg, anaphylaxis, angioedema, urticaria). Prolonged use may result in fungal or bacterial superinfection, including *C. difficile*-associated diarrhea (CDAD) and pseudomembranous colitis; CDAD has been observed >2 months postantibiotic treatment. May be associated with increased INR, especially in nutritionally-deficient patients, prolonged treatment, hepatic or renal disease. Use with caution in patients with a history of seizure disorder; high levels, particularly in the presence of renal impairment, may increase risk of seizures.

Adverse Reactions Frequency not defined.

Central nervous system: Fever, seizure

Dermatologic: Rash, pruritus, Stevens-Johnson syndrome

Gastrointestinal: Diarrhea, nausea, vomiting, abdominal cramps, anorexia, pseudomembranous colitis, oral candidiasis

Genitourinary: Vaginitis

Hepatic: Transaminases increased, hepatitis

Hematologic: Eosinophilia, neutropenia, leukopenia, thrombocytopenia, thrombocytosis

Local: Pain at injection site, phlebitis

Renal: BUN increased, serum creatinine increased, renal failure

Miscellaneous: Anaphylaxis

Reactions reported with other cephalosporins: Toxic epidermal necrolysis, abdominal pain, cholestasis, superinfection, toxic nephropathy, aplastic anemia, hemolytic anemia, hemorrhage, prothrombin time prolonged, pancytopenia

Drug Interactions

Avoid Concomitant Use There are no known interactions where it is recommended to avoid concomitant use.

Increased Effect/Toxicity

CeFAZolin may increase the levels/effects of: Vitamin K Antagonists

The levels/effects of CeFAZolin may be increased by: Uricosuric Agents

Decreased Effect

CeFAZolin may decrease the levels/effects of: Typhoid Vaccine

Test Interactions Positive direct Coombs', false-positive urinary glucose test using cupric sulfate (Benedict's solution, Clinitest®, Fehling's solution), false-positive serum or urine creatinine with Jaffé reaction.

Some penicillin derivatives may accelerate the degradation of aminoglycosides *in vitro*, leading to a potential underestimation of aminoglycoside serum concentration.

Dietary Considerations Some products may contain sodium.

Dosage Forms Excipient information presented when available (limited, particularly for generics); consult specific product labeling.

Infusion [iso-osmotic dextrose solution]: 1 g (50 mL)

Injection, powder for reconstitution: 500 mg, 1 g, 10 g, 20 g

References

"Antimicrobial Prophylaxis for Surgery," *Treat Guidel Med Lett*, 2004, 2(20):27-32.

"ASHP Therapeutic Guidelines on Antimicrobial Prophylaxis in Surgery. American Society of Health-System Pharmacists," *Am J Health Syst Pharm*, 1999, 56(18):1839-88.

Bratzler DW, Houck PM, Surgical Infection Prevention Guidelines Writers Workgroup, et al, "Antimicrobial Prophylaxis for Surgery: An Advisory Statement From the National Surgical Infection Prevention Project," *Clin Infect Dis*, 2004, 38(12):1706-15.

Eagle KA, Guyton RA, Davidoff R, et al, "ACC/AHA 2004 Guideline Update for Coronary Artery Bypass Graft Surgery: A Report of the American College of Cardiology/American Heart Association Task Force on Practice Guidelines (Committee to Update the 1999 Guidelines for Coronary Artery Bypass Graft Surgery)," *Circulation*, 2004, 110(14):e340-437.

Gentry LO, Zeluff BJ, and Cooley DA, "Antibiotic Prophylaxis in Open-Heart Surgery: A Comparison of Cefamandole, Cefuroxime, and Cefazolin," *Ann Thorac Surg*, 1988, 46(2):167-71.

Wilson W, Taubert KA, Gewitz M, et al, "Prevention of Infective Endocarditis. Guidelines From the American Heart Association. A Guideline From the American Heart Association Rheumatic Fever, Endocarditis, and Kawasaki Disease Committee, Council on Cardiovascular Disease in the Young, and the Council on Clinical Cardiology, Council on Cardiovascular Surgery and Anesthesia, and the Quality of Care and Outcomes Research Interdisciplinary Working Group," *Circulation*, 2007, 115].

◆ **Cefazolin Sodium** *see* CeFAZolin *on page 249*

Cefdinir (SEF di ner)

U.S. Brand Names Omnicef®

Canadian Brand Names Omnicef®

Index Terms CFDN

Pharmacologic Category Antibiotic, Cephalosporin (Third Generation)

Use Treatment of community-acquired pneumonia, acute exacerbations of chronic bronchitis, acute bacterial otitis media, acute maxillary sinusitis, pharyngitis/tonsillitis, and uncomplicated skin and skin structure infections.

Pharmacodynamics/Kinetics

Distribution: V_d:

Children 6 months to 12 years: 0.29-1.05 L/kg

Adults: 0.06-0.64 L/kg

Protein binding: 60% to 70%

Metabolism: Minimal

Bioavailability: Capsule: 16% to 21%; suspension 25%

Half-life elimination: ~100 minutes

Time to peak, plasma: 3 hours

Excretion: Primarily urine (7% to 25% as unchanged drug)

Dosage

Usual dosage range:

Children 6 months to 12 years: Oral: 7 mg/kg/dose twice daily or 14 mg/kg/dose once daily (maximum: 600 mg/day)

Adolescents and Adults: Oral: 300 mg twice daily or 600 mg once daily

Indication-specific dosing:

Children 6 months to 12 years: Oral:

Acute bacterial otitis media, pharyngitis/tonsillitis: 7 mg/kg/dose twice daily for 5-10 days **or** 14 mg/kg/dose once daily for 10 days (maximum: 600 mg/day)

Acute maxillary sinusitis: 7 mg/kg/dose twice daily **or** 14 mg/kg/dose once daily for 10 days (maximum: 600 mg/day)

Uncomplicated skin and skin structure infections: 7 mg/kg/dose twice daily for 10 days (maximum: 600 mg/day)

Adolescents and Adults:

Acute exacerbations of chronic bronchitis, pharyngitis/tonsillitis: 300 mg twice daily for 5-10 days **or** 600 mg once daily for 10 days

Acute maxillary sinusitis: 300 mg twice daily **or** 600 mg once daily for 10 days

Community-acquired pneumonia, uncomplicated skin and skin structure infections: 300 mg twice daily for 10 days

Dosing adjustment in renal impairment: Cl$_{cr}$ <30 mL/minute:

Children: 7 mg/kg once daily (maximum: 300 mg/day)

Adults: 300 mg once daily

Hemodialysis removes cefdinir; recommended initial dose: 300 mg (or 7 mg/kg/ dose) every other day. At the conclusion of each hemodialysis session, 300 mg (or 7 mg/kg/dose) should be given. Subsequent doses (300 mg or 7 mg/kg/ dose) should be administered every other day.

Dosing adjustment in hepatic impairment: No adjustment necessary.

Additional Information Complete prescribing information for this medication should be consulted for additional detail.

Dosage Forms Excipient information presented when available (limited, particularly for generics); consult specific product labeling.

Capsule: 300 mg

Omnicef®: 300 mg

Powder for oral suspension: 125 mg/5 mL (60 mL, 100 mL); 250 mg/5 mL (60 mL, 100 mL)

Omnicef®: 125 mg/5 mL (60 mL, 100 mL) [contains sodium benzoate and sucrose 2.86 g/5 mL; strawberry flavor]; 250 mg/5 mL (60 mL, 100 mL) [contains sodium benzoate and sucrose 2.86 g/5 mL; strawberry flavor]

Cefepime (SEF e pim)

U.S. Brand Names Maxipime®

Canadian Brand Names Maxipime®

Index Terms Cefepime Hydrochloride

Pharmacologic Category Antibiotic, Cephalosporin (Fourth Generation)

Generic Available Yes

Use Treatment of uncomplicated and complicated urinary tract infections, including pyelonephritis caused by typical urinary tract pathogens; monotherapy for febrile neutropenia; uncomplicated skin and skin structure infections caused by *Streptococcus pyogenes*; moderate-to-severe pneumonia caused by pneumo-coccus, *Pseudomonas aeruginosa*, and other gram-negative organisms; complicated intra-abdominal infections (in combination with metronidazole). Also active against methicillin-susceptible staphylococci, *Enterobacter* sp, and many other gram-negative bacilli.

Children 2 months to 16 years: Empiric therapy of febrile neutropenia patients, uncomplicated skin/soft tissue infections, pneumonia, and uncomplicated/ complicated urinary tract infections.

Mechanism of Action Inhibits bacterial cell wall synthesis by binding to one or more of the penicillin-binding proteins (PBPs) which in turn inhibits the final transpeptidation step of peptidoglycan synthesis in bacterial cell walls, thus inhibiting cell wall biosynthesis. Bacteria eventually lyse due to ongoing activity of cell wall autolytic enzymes (autolysis and murein hydrolases) while cell wall assembly is arrested.

Pharmacodynamics/Kinetics

Absorption: I.M.: Rapid and complete

Distribution: V$_d$: Adults: 14-20 L; penetrates into inflammatory fluid at concentrations ~80% of serum levels and into bronchial mucosa at levels ~60% of those reached in the plasma; crosses blood-brain barrier

Protein binding, plasma: 16% to 19%

Metabolism: Minimally hepatic

Half-life elimination: 2 hours

Time to peak: 0.5-1.5 hours

Excretion: Urine (85% as unchanged drug)

Dosage

Usual dosage range:

Children: I.M., I.V.: 50 mg/kg every 8-12 hours (maximum not to exceed adult dosing)

Adults: I.V.: 1-2 g every 8-12 hours; I.M.: 500-1000 mg every 12 hours

Indication-specific dosing:

Children ≥2 months to 16 years (<40 kg):

Febrile neutropenia: I.V.: 50 mg/kg every 8 hours for 7 days or until neutropenia resolves

Skin and skin structure infections (uncomplicated) and pneumonia: I.V.: 50 mg/kg every 12 hours for 10 days

Urinary tract infections, complicated and uncomplicated: I.M., I.V.: 50 mg/kg every 12 hours for 7-10 days; **Note:** I.M. may be considered for mild-to-moderate infection only

Adults:

Brain abscess, postneurosurgical prevention (unlabeled use): I.V.: 2 g every 8 hours with vancomycin

Febrile neutropenia, monotherapy: I.V: 2 g every 8 hours for 7 days or until the neutropenia resolves

Intra-abdominal infections, complicated: I.V.: 2 g every 12 hours for 7-10 days with metronidazole

Otitis externa, malignant (unlabeled use): I.V.: 2 g every 12 hours

Pneumonia: I.V.:

Nosocomial (HAP/VAP): 1-2 g every 8-12 hours; **Note:** Duration of therapy may vary considerably (7-21 days); usually longer courses are required if *Pseudomonas*. In absence of *Pseudomonas*, and if appropriate empiric treatment used and patient responsive, it may be clinically appropriate to reduce duration of therapy to 7-10 days (American Thoracic Society Guidelines, 2005).

Community-acquired (including pseudomonal): 1-2 g every 12 hours for 10 days

Septic lateral/cavernous sinus thrombosis (unlabeled use): I.V.: 2 g every 8-12 hours; with metronidazole for lateral

Skin and skin structure, uncomplicated: I.V.: 2 g every 12 hours for 10 days

Urinary tract infections, complicated and uncomplicated:

Mild-to-moderate: I.M., I.V.: 500-1000 mg every 12 hours for 7-10 days

Severe: I.V.: 2 g every 12 hours for 10 days

Dosing adjustment in renal impairment: Adults: Recommended maintenance schedule based on creatinine clearance (mL/minute), compared to normal dosing schedule: See table.

Cefepime Hydrochloride

Creatinine Clearance (mL/minute)	Recommended Maintenance Schedule			
>60 (normal recommended dosing schedule)	500 mg every 12 hours	1 g every 12 hours	2 g every 12 hours	2 g every 8 hours
30-60	500 mg every 24 hours	1 g every 24 hours	2 g every 24 hours	2 g every 12 hours
11-29	500 mg every 24 hours	500 mg every 24 hours	1 g every 24 hours	2 g every 24 hours
<11	250 mg every 24 hours	250 mg every 24 hours	500 mg every 24 hours	1 g every 24 hours

Hemodialysis: Initial: 1 g (single dose) on day 1. Maintenance: 500 mg once daily (1 g once daily in febrile neutropenic patients). Dosage should be administered after dialysis on dialysis days.

Continuous ambulatory peritoneal dialysis (CAPD): Removed to a lesser extent than hemodialysis; administer normal recommended dose every 48 hours

Continuous renal replacement therapy (CRRT) (Trotman, 2005): Drug clearance is highly dependent on the method of renal replacement, filter type, and flow rate. Appropriate dosing requires close monitoring of pharmacologic response, signs of adverse reactions due to drug accumulation, as well as drug levels in relation to target trough (if appropriate). The following are general recommendations only (based on dialysate flow/ultrafiltration rates of 1 L/hour) and should not supersede clinical judgment:

CVVH: 1-2 g every 12 hours

CVVHDF: 2 g every 12 hours

Note: Consider higher dosage of 4 g/day if treating *Pseudomonas* or life-threatening infections in order to maximize time above MIC.

Stability

Vials: Store at 20°C to 25°C (68°F to 77°F). Protect from light. After reconstitution, stable in normal saline, D_5W, and a variety of other solutions for 24 hours at room temperature and 7 days refrigerated.

Premixed solution: Store frozen at -20°C (-4°F). Thawed solution is stable for 24 hours at room temperature or 7 days under refrigeration; do not refreeze.

Administration May be administered either I.M. or I.V.

Inject deep I.M. into large muscle mass. Inject direct I.V. over 5 minutes. Infuse intermittent infusion over 30 minutes.

Monitoring Parameters Obtain specimen for culture and sensitivity prior to the first dose. Monitor for signs of anaphylaxis during first dose.

Anesthesia and Critical Care Concerns/Other Considerations

Evidence-Based Information: The Food and Drug Administration (FDA) informed practitioners (November, 2007) of a review of new safety data and a request for additional data for cefepime after a recently published meta-analysis (Yahav, 2007) raised concerns of an increased risk of death in patients treated with cefepime. The authors of the meta-analysis reviewed the results from 57 randomized controlled trials comparing cefepime to other beta-lactams in a variety of infections. The primary outcome of the analysis was 30-day all-cause mortality; however, all-cause mortality data was only available in 41 of the trials. In addition, distribution of specific pathogens to infections in relation to all-cause mortality was not available, including patients with documented gram-negative and *Pseudomonas* infections. The authors reported an increase in all-cause mortality in the cefepime group relative to the comparator group (relative risk 1.26 [95% CI 1.08 to 1.40]; p=0.005). Only two subsets showed a significant difference in all cause mortality and include the group comparing cefepime to piperacillin-tazobactam (relative risk 2.14 [95% CI 1.17 to 3.89]; p=0.01) and the subset of patients with febrile neutropenia (relative risk 1.42 [95% CI 1.09 to 1.84]; p=0.009).

The FDA is currently evaluating the data, and in the interim, is reminding practitioners to consider the risks and benefits of cefepime prior to use. The FDA will provide additional communication and any recommendations, if necessary, following the conclusion of the evaluation.

Additional information may be found at http://www.fda.gov/Drugs/DrugSafety/PostmarketDrugSafetyInformationforPatientsandProviders/DrugSafetyInformationforHeathcareProfessionals/ucm070797.htm.

Pregnancy Risk Factor B

Contraindications Hypersensitivity to cefepime, any component of the formulation, or other cephalosporins

Warnings/Precautions Modify dosage in patients with severe renal impairment; use with caution in patients with a history of penicillin or cephalosporin allergy, especially IgE-mediated reactions (eg, anaphylaxis, urticaria). Prolonged use may result in fungal or bacterial superinfection, including *C. difficile*-associated diarrhea (CDAD) and pseudomembranous colitis; CDAD has been observed >2 months postantibiotic treatment. May be associated with increased INR, especially in nutritionally-deficient patients, prolonged treatment, hepatic or renal disease. Use with caution in patients with a history of seizure disorder; high levels, particularly in the presence of renal impairment, may increase risk of seizures.

Adverse Reactions

>10%: Hematologic: Positive Coombs' test without hemolysis

1% to 10%:

Central nervous system: Fever (1%), headache (1%)

◄ Dermatologic: Rash, pruritus

Gastrointestinal: Diarrhea, nausea, vomiting

Local: Pain, erythema at injection site

<1% (Limited to important or life-threatening): Agranulocytosis, anaphylactic shock, anaphylaxis, coma, encephalopathy, hallucinations, leukopenia, myoclonus, neuromuscular excitability, neutropenia, seizure, status epilepticus (nonconvulsive), thrombocytopenia

Reactions reported with other cephalosporins: Aplastic anemia, erythema multiforme, hemolytic anemia, hemorrhage, pancytopenia, PT prolonged, renal dysfunction, Stevens-Johnson syndrome, superinfection, toxic epidermal necrolysis, toxic nephropathy, vaginitis

Drug Interactions

Avoid Concomitant Use There are no known interactions where it is recommended to avoid concomitant use.

Increased Effect/Toxicity

The levels/effects of Cefepime may be increased by: Uricosuric Agents

Decreased Effect

Cefepime may decrease the levels/effects of: Typhoid Vaccine

Test Interactions Positive direct Coombs', false-positive urinary glucose test using cupric sulfate (Benedict's solution, Clinitest®, Fehling's solution), false-positive serum or urine creatinine with Jaffé reaction, false-positive urinary proteins and steroids

Dosage Forms Excipient information presented when available (limited, particularly for generics); consult specific product labeling.

Infusion, premixed iso-osmotic dextrose solution: 1 g (50 mL); 2 g (100 mL)

Injection, powder for reconstitution, as hydrochloride: 500 mg, 1 g, 2 g

Maxipime®: 500 mg, 1 g, 2 g

References

American Thoracic Society and Infectious Diseases Society of America, "Guidelines for the Management of Adults With Hospital-Acquired, Ventilator-Associated, and Healthcare-Associated Pneumonia," *Am J Respir Crit Care Med*, 2005, 171(4):388-416.

Tunkel AR, Hartman BJ, Kaplan SL, et al, "Practice Guidelines for the Management of Bacterial Meningitis," *Clin Infect Dis*, 2004, 39(9):1267-84.

Yahav D, Paul M, Fraser A, et al, "Efficacy and Safety of Cefepime: A Systematic Review and Meta-Analysis," *Lancet Infect Dis*, 2007, 7(5):338-48.

◆ **Cefepime Hydrochloride** *see* Cefepime *on page 253*

◆ **Cefizox®** *see* Ceftizoxime *on page 265*

Cefotaxime (sef oh TAKS eem)

Medication Safety Issues

Sound-alike/look-alike issues:

Cefotaxime may be confused with cefoxitin, ceftizoxime, cefuroxime

International issues:

Spectrocef® [Italy] may be confused with Spectracef® which is a brand name for cefditoren in the U.S.

U.S. Brand Names Claforan®

Canadian Brand Names Claforan®

Index Terms Cefotaxime Sodium

Pharmacologic Category Antibiotic, Cephalosporin (Third Generation)

Generic Available Yes: Powder

Use Treatment of susceptible infection in respiratory tract, skin and skin structure, bone and joint, urinary tract, gynecologic as well as septicemia, and documented or suspected meningitis. Active against most gram-negative bacilli (not *Pseudomonas*) and gram-positive cocci (not enterococcus). Active against many penicillin-resistant pneumococci.

Mechanism of Action Inhibits bacterial cell wall synthesis by binding to one or more of the penicillin-binding proteins (PBPs) which in turn inhibits the final transpeptidation step of peptidoglycan synthesis in bacterial cell walls, thus inhibiting cell wall biosynthesis. Bacteria eventually lyse due to ongoing activity of cell wall autolytic enzymes (autolysins and murein hydrolases) while cell wall assembly is arrested.

Pharmacodynamics/Kinetics

Distribution: Widely to body tissues and fluids including aqueous humor, ascitic and prostatic fluids, bone; penetrates CSF best when meninges are inflamed

Metabolism: Partially hepatic to active metabolite, desacetylcefotaxime

Half-life elimination:

Cefotaxime: Premature neonates <1 week: 5-6 hours; Full-term neonates <1 week: 2-3.4 hours; Adults: 1-1.5 hours; prolonged with renal and/or hepatic impairment

Desacetylcefotaxime: 1.5-1.9 hours; prolonged with renal impairment

Time to peak, serum: I.M.: Within 30 minutes

Excretion: Urine (as unchanged drug and metabolites)

Dosage

Usual dosage range:

Infants and Children 1 month to 12 years <50 kg: I.M., I.V.: 50-200 mg/kg/day in divided doses every 6-8 hours

Children >12 years and Adults: I.M., I.V.: 1-2 g every 4-12 hours

Indication-specific dosing:

Infants and Children 1 month to 12 years:

Epiglottitis: I.M., I.V.: 150-200 mg/kg/day in 4 divided doses with clindamycin for 7-10 days

Meningitis: I.M., I.V.: 200 mg/kg/day in divided doses every 6 hours

Pneumonia: I.V.: 200 mg/kg/day divided every 8 hours

Sepsis: I.V.: 150 mg/kg/day divided every 8 hours

Typhoid fever: I.M., I.V.: 150-200 mg/kg/day in 3-4 divided doses (maximum: 12 g/day); fluoroquinolone resistant: 80 mg/kg/day in 3-4 divided doses (maximum: 12 g/day)

Children >12 years and Adults:

Arthritis (septic): I.V.: 1 g every 8 hours

Brain abscess, meningitis: I.V.: 2 g every 4-6 hours

Caesarean section: I.M., I.V.: 1 g as soon as the umbilical cord is clamped, then 1 g at 6- and 12-hour intervals

Epiglottitis: I.V.: 2 g every 4-8 hours

Gonorrhea: I.M.: 1 g as a single dose

Disseminated: I.V.: 1 g every 8 hours

Life-threatening infections: I.V.: 2 g every 4 hours

Liver abscess: I.V.: 1-2 g every 6 hours

Lyme disease:

Cardiac manifestations: I.V.: 2 g every 4 hours

CNS manifestations: I.V.: 2 g every 8 hours for 14-28 days

Moderate-to-severe infections: I.M., I.V.: 1-2 g every 8 hours

Orbital cellulitis: I.V.: 2 g every 4 hours

Peritonitis (spontaneous): I.V.: 2 g every 8 hours, unless life-threatening then 2 g every 4 hours

Septicemia: I.V.: 2 g every 6-8 hours

Skin and soft tissue:

Mixed, necrotizing: I.V.: 2 g every 6 hours, with metronidazole or clindamycin

Bite wounds (animal): I.V.: 2 g every 6 hours

Surgical prophylaxis: I.M., I.V.: 1 g 30-90 minutes before surgery

Uncomplicated infections: I.M., I.V.: 1 g every 12 hours

Dosing interval in renal impairment:

Cl_{cr} 10-50 mL/minute: Administer every 8-12 hours

Cl_{cr} <10 mL/minute: Administer every 24 hours

Hemodialysis: Moderately dialyzable

Continuous ambulatory peritoneal dialysis (CAPD): Administer 0.5-1 g every 24 hours

Continuous renal replacement therapy (CRRT): Drug clearance is highly dependent on the method of renal replacement, filter type, and flow rate. Appropriate dosing requires close monitoring of pharmacologic response, signs of adverse reactions due to drug accumulation, as well as drug levels in relation to target trough (if appropriate). The following are general recommendations only (based on dialysate flow/ultrafiltration rates of 1 L/hour) and should not supersede clinical judgment:

CVVH: 1-2 g every 12 hours

CVVHD/CVVHDF: 2 g every 12 hours

Dosing adjustment in hepatic impairment: Moderate dosage reduction is recommended in severe liver disease

Continuous arteriovenous or venovenous hemodiafiltration effects: Administer 1 g every 12 hour

Stability Reconstituted solution is stable for 12-24 hours at room temperature and 7-10 days when refrigerated and for 13 weeks when frozen. For I.V. infusion in NS or D_5W, solution is stable for 24 hours at room temperature, 5 days when refrigerated, or 13 weeks when frozen in Viaflex® plastic containers. Thawed solutions previously of frozen premixed bags are stable for 24 hours at room temperature or 10 days when refrigerated.

Administration Can be administered IVP over 3-5 minutes or I.V. intermittent infusion over 15-30 minutes.

Monitoring Parameters Observe for signs and symptoms of anaphylaxis during first dose; CBC with differential (especially with long courses)

Pregnancy Risk Factor B

Contraindications Hypersensitivity to cefotaxime, any component of the formulation, or other cephalosporins

Warnings/Precautions Modify dosage in patients with severe renal impairment. Prolonged use may result in superinfection. A potentially life-threatening arrhythmia has been reported in patients who received a rapid bolus injection via central line. Granulocytopenia and more rarely agranulocytosis may develop during prolonged treatment (>10 days). Minimize tissue inflammation by changing infusion sites when needed. Use with caution in patients with a history of penicillin allergy, especially IgE-mediated reactions (eg, anaphylaxis, urticaria). Prolonged use may result in fungal or bacterial superinfection, including *C. difficile*-associated diarrhea (CDAD) and pseudomembranous colitis; CDAD has been observed >2 months postantibiotic treatment.

Adverse Reactions

1% to 10%:

Dermatologic: Rash, pruritus

Gastrointestinal: Diarrhea, nausea, vomiting, colitis

Local: Pain at injection site

<1% (Limited to important or life-threatening): Anaphylaxis, arrhythmia (after rapid I.V. injection via central catheter), BUN increased, candidiasis, creatinine increased, eosinophilia, erythema multiforme, fever, headache, interstitial nephritis, neutropenia, phlebitis, pseudomembranous colitis, Stevens-Johnson syndrome, thrombocytopenia, transaminases increased, toxic epidermal necrolysis, urticaria, vaginitis

Reactions reported with other cephalosporins: Agranulocytosis, aplastic anemia, cholestasis, hemolytic anemia, hemorrhage, pancytopenia, renal dysfunction, seizure, superinfection, toxic nephropathy.

Drug Interactions

Avoid Concomitant Use There are no known interactions where it is recommended to avoid concomitant use.

Increased Effect/Toxicity

The levels/effects of Cefotaxime may be increased by: Uricosuric Agents

Decreased Effect

Cefotaxime may decrease the levels/effects of: Typhoid Vaccine

Test Interactions Positive direct Coombs', false-positive urinary glucose test using cupric sulfate (Benedict's solution, Clinitest®, Fehling's solution), false-positive serum or urine creatinine with Jaffé reaction

Dietary Considerations Some products may contain sodium.

Dosage Forms Excipient information presented when available (limited, particularly for generics); consult specific product labeling.

Infusion [premixed iso-osmotic solution]:

Claforan®: 1 g (50 mL); 2 g (50 mL) [contains sodium 50.5 mg (2.2 mEq) per cefotaxime 1 g]

Injection, powder for reconstitution: 500 mg, 1 g, 2 g, 10 g, 20 g

Claforan®: 500 mg, 1 g, 2 g, 10 g [contains sodium 50.5 mg (2.2 mEq) per cefotaxime 1 g]

References
Tunkel AR, Hartman BJ, Kaplan SL, et al, "Practice Guidelines for the Management of Bacterial Meningitis," *Clin Infect Dis*, 2004, 39(9):1267-84.

◆ **Cefotaxime Sodium** *see* Cefotaxime *on page 256*

Cefotetan (SEF oh tee tan)

Medication Safety Issues
Sound-alike/look-alike issues:
Cefotetan may be confused with cefoxitin, Ceftin®
Cefotan® may be confused with Ceftin®

International issues:
Cefotan® may be confused with Lexotan® which is a brand name for bromazepam in multiple international markets
Cefotan® may be confused with Cefiton® which is a brand name for cefixime in Portugal

Related Information
Anesthesia for Patients With Liver Disease *on page 1537*

Index Terms Cefotetan Disodium

Pharmacologic Category Antibiotic, Cephalosporin (Second Generation)

Generic Available Yes

Use Surgical prophylaxis; intra-abdominal infections and other mixed infections; respiratory tract, skin and skin structure, bone and joint, urinary tract and gynecologic as well as septicemia; active against gram-negative enteric bacilli including *E. coli, Klebsiella,* and *Proteus*; less active against staphylococci and streptococci than first generation cephalosporins, but active against anaerobes including *Bacteroides fragilis*

Mechanism of Action Inhibits bacterial cell wall synthesis by binding to one or more of the penicillin-binding proteins (PBPs) which in turn inhibits the final transpeptidation step of peptidoglycan synthesis in bacterial cell walls, thus inhibiting cell wall biosynthesis. Bacteria eventually lyse due to ongoing activity of cell wall autolytic enzymes (autolysins and murein hydrolases) while cell wall assembly is arrested.

Pharmacodynamics/Kinetics
Distribution: Widely to body tissues and fluids including bile, sputum, prostatic, peritoneal; low concentrations enter CSF
Protein binding: 76% to 90%
Half-life elimination: 3-5 hours
Time to peak, serum: I.M.: 1.5-3 hours
Excretion: Primarily urine (as unchanged drug); feces (20%)

Dosage
Usual dosage range:
Children (unlabeled use): I.M., I.V.: 20-40 mg/kg/dose every 12 hours (maximum: 6 g/day)
Adults: I.M., I.V.: 1-6 g/day in divided doses every 12 hours
Indication-specific dosing:
Children (unlabeled use):
Preoperative prophylaxis: I.M., I.V.: 40 mg/kg 30-60 minutes prior to surgery
Adolescents and Adults:
Pelvic inflammatory disease: I.V.: 2 g every 12 hours; used in combination with doxycycline
Adults:
Orbital cellulitis, odontogenic infections: I.V.: 2 g every 12 hours
Preoperative prophylaxis: I.M., I.V.: 1-2 g 30-60 minutes prior to surgery; when used for cesarean section, dose should be given as soon as umbilical cord is clamped
Urinary tract infection: I.M., I.V.: 1-2 g may be given every 24 hours
Dosing interval in renal impairment:
Cl_{cr} 10-30 mL/minute: Administer every 24 hours
Cl_{cr} <10 mL/minute: Administer every 48 hours

◄ Hemodialysis: Dialyzable (5% to 20%); administer ¼ the usual dose every 24 hours on days between dialysis; administer ½ the usual dose on the day of dialysis.

Continuous arteriovenous or venovenous hemodiafiltration effects: Administer 750 mg every 12 hours

Stability Reconstituted solution is stable for 24 hours at room temperature and 96 hours when refrigerated. For I.V. infusion in NS or D_5W solution and after freezing, thawed solution is stable for 24 hours at room temperature or 96 hours when refrigerated. Frozen solution is stable for 12 weeks.

Administration

I.M.: Inject deep I.M. into large muscle mass.

I.V.: Inject direct I.V. over 3-5 minutes. Infuse intermittent infusion over 30 minutes.

Monitoring Parameters Observe for signs and symptoms of anaphylaxis during first dose; monitor for signs and symptoms of hemolytic anemia, including hematologic parameters where appropriate.

Pregnancy Risk Factor B

Contraindications Hypersensitivity to cefotetan, any component of the formulation, or other cephalosporins; previous cephalosporin-associated hemolytic anemia

Warnings/Precautions Modify dosage in patients with severe renal impairment. Although cefotetan contains the methyltetrazolethiol side chain, bleeding has not been a significant problem. Use with caution in patients with a history of penicillin allergy, especially IgE-mediated reactions (eg, anaphylaxis, urticaria). Cefotetan has been associated with a higher risk of hemolytic anemia relative to other cephalosporins (approximately threefold); monitor carefully during use and consider cephalosporin-associated immune anemia in patients who have received cefotetan within 2-3 weeks (either as treatment or prophylaxis). Prolonged use may result in fungal or bacterial superinfection, including *C. difficile*-associated diarrhea (CDAD) and pseudomembranous colitis; CDAD has been observed >2 months postantibiotic treatment. May be associated with increased INR, especially in nutritionally-deficient patients, prolonged treatment, hepatic or renal disease.

Adverse Reactions

1% to 10%:

Gastrointestinal: Diarrhea (1%)

Hepatic: Transaminases increased (1%)

Miscellaneous: Hypersensitivity reactions (1%)

<1%: Anaphylaxis, urticaria, rash, pruritus, pseudomembranous colitis, nausea, vomiting, eosinophilia, thrombocytosis, agranulocytosis, hemolytic anemia, leukopenia, thrombocytopenia, prolonged PT, bleeding, BUN increased, creatinine increased, nephrotoxicity, phlebitis, fever

Reactions reported with other cephalosporins: Seizure, Stevens-Johnson syndrome, toxic epidermal necrolysis, renal dysfunction, toxic nephropathy, cholestasis, aplastic anemia, hemolytic anemia, hemorrhage, pancytopenia, agranulocytosis, colitis, superinfection

Drug Interactions

Avoid Concomitant Use There are no known interactions where it is recommended to avoid concomitant use.

Increased Effect/Toxicity

Cefotetan may increase the levels/effects of: Alcohol (Ethyl); Vitamin K Antagonists

The levels/effects of Cefotetan may be increased by: Uricosuric Agents

Decreased Effect

Cefotetan may decrease the levels/effects of: Typhoid Vaccine

Ethanol/Nutrition/Herb Interactions Ethanol: Avoid ethanol (may cause a disulfiram-like reaction).

Test Interactions Positive direct Coombs', false-positive urinary glucose test using cupric sulfate (Benedict's solution, Clinitest®, Fehling's solution), false-positive serum or urine creatinine with Jaffé reaction

Dietary Considerations Some products may contain sodium.

Dosage Forms Excipient information presented when available (limited, particularly for generics); consult specific product labeling.
Injection, powder for reconstitution: 1 g, 2 g, 10 g [contains sodium 80 mg/g (3.5 mEq/g)]

References

Abramowicz M, "Antimicrobial Prophylaxis in Surgery," *Medical Letter on Drugs and Therapeutics, Handbook of Antimicrobial Therapy*, 16th ed, New York, NY: Medical Letter, 2002.

Centers for Disease Control and Prevention, "Sexually-Transmitted Diseases Treatment Guidelines - 2002," *MMWR Recomm Rep*, 2002, 51(RR-6):1-78.

Donowitz GR and Mandell GL, "Beta-Lactam Antibiotics," *N Engl J Med*, 1988, 318(7):419-26 and 318(8):490-500.

Marshall WF and Blair JE, "The Cephalosporins," *Mayo Clin Proc*, 1999, 74(2):187-95.

Martin C, Thomachot L, and Albanese J, "Clinical Pharmacokinetics of Cefotetan," *Clin Pharmacokinet*, 1994, 26(4):248-58.

◆ **Cefotetan Disodium** *see* Cefotetan *on page 259*

Cefoxitin (se FOKS i tin)

Medication Safety Issues

Sound-alike/look-alike issues:
Cefoxitin may be confused with cefotaxime, cefotetan, Cytoxan®
Mefoxin® may be confused with Lanoxin®

Related Information

Anesthesia for Patients With Liver Disease *on page 1537*
Prevention of Wound Infection and Sepsis in Surgical Patients *on page 1721*

Canadian Brand Names Apo-Cefoxitin®

Index Terms Cefoxitin Sodium

Pharmacologic Category Antibiotic, Cephalosporin (Second Generation)

Generic Available Yes

Use Less active against staphylococci and streptococci than first generation cephalosporins, but active against anaerobes including *Bacteroides fragilis*; active against gram-negative enteric bacilli including *E. coli*, *Klebsiella*, and *Proteus*; used predominantly for respiratory tract, skin, bone and joint, urinary tract and gynecologic as well as septicemia; surgical prophylaxis; intra-abdominal infections and other mixed infections; indicated for bacterial *Eikenella corrodens* infections

Mechanism of Action Inhibits bacterial cell wall synthesis by binding to one or more of the penicillin-binding proteins (PBPs) which in turn inhibits the final transpeptidation step of peptidoglycan synthesis in bacterial cell walls, thus inhibiting cell wall biosynthesis. Bacteria eventually lyse due to ongoing activity of cell wall autolytic enzymes (autolysins and murein hydrolases) while cell wall assembly is arrested.

Pharmacodynamics/Kinetics

Distribution: Widely to body tissues and fluids including pleural, synovial, ascitic, bile; poorly penetrates into CSF even with inflammation of the meninges
Protein binding: 65% to 79%
Half-life elimination: 45-60 minutes; significantly prolonged with renal impairment
Time to peak, serum: I.M.: 20-30 minutes
Excretion: Urine (85% as unchanged drug)

Dosage

Usual dosage range:
Infants >3 months and Children: I.M., I.V.: 80-160 mg/kg/day in divided doses every 4-6 hours (maximum dose: 12 g/day)
Adults: I.M., I.V.: 1-2 g every 6-8 hours (maximum dose: 12 g/day)
Note: I.M. injection is painful

Indication-specific dosing:
Infants >3 months and Children:
Mild-to-moderate infection: I.M., I.V.: 80-100 mg/kg/day in divided doses every 4-6 hours
Perioperative prophylaxis: I.V.: 30-40 mg/kg 30-60 minutes prior to surgery followed by 30-40 mg/kg/dose every 6 hours for no more than 24 hours after surgery depending on the procedure
Severe infection: I.M., I.V.: 100-160 mg/kg/day in divided doses every 4-6 hours

Adolescents and Adults:
Perioperative prophylaxis: I.M., I.V.: 1-2 g 30-60 minutes prior to surgery (may repeat in 2-5 hours intraoperatively) followed by 1-2 g every 6-8 hours for no more than 24 hours after surgery depending on the procedure

Adults:
Amnionitis, endomyometritis: I.M., I.V.: 2 g every 6-8 hours
Aspiration pneumonia, empyema, orbital cellulitis, parapharyngeal space, human bites: I.M., I.V.: 2 g every 8 hours
Liver abscess: I.V.: 1 g every 4 hours
Mycobacterium species, not MTB or MAI: I.V.: 12 g/day with amikacin
Pelvic inflammatory disease:
  Inpatients: I.V.: 2 g every 6 hours **plus** doxycycline 100 mg I.V. or 100 mg orally every 12 hours until improved, followed by doxycycline 100 mg orally twice daily to complete 14 days
  Outpatients: I.M.: 2 g **plus** probenecid 1 g orally as a single dose, followed by doxycycline 100 mg orally twice daily for 14 days
Dosing interval in renal impairment:
  Cl_{cr} 30-50 mL/minute: Administer 1-2 g every 8-12 hours
  Cl_{cr} 10-29 mL/minute: Administer 1-2 g every 12-24 hours
  Cl_{cr} 5-9 mL/minute: Administer 0.5-1 g every 12-24 hours
  Cl_{cr} <5 mL/minute: Administer 0.5-1 g every 24-48 hours
  Hemodialysis: Moderately dialyzable (20% to 50%); administer a loading dose of 1-2 g after each hemodialysis; maintenance dose as noted above based on Cl_{cr}
  Continuous arteriovenous or venovenous hemodiafiltration effects: Dose as for Cl_{cr} 10-50 mL/minute

Stability Reconstitute vials with SWFI, bacteriostatic water for injection, NS, or D_5W. For I.V. infusion, solutions may be further diluted in NS, $D_5^1/4NS$, $D_5^1/2NS$, D_5NS, D_5W, $D_{10}W$, LR, D_5LR, mannitol 10%, or sodium bicarbonate 5%. Reconstituted solution is stable for 6 hours at room temperature or 7 days when refrigerated; I.V. infusion in NS or D_5W solution is stable for 18 hours at room temperature or 48 hours when refrigerated. Premixed frozen solution, when thawed, is stable for 24 hours at room temperature or 21 days when refrigerated.

Administration
I.M.: Inject deep I.M. into large muscle mass.
I.V.: Can be administered IVP over 3-5 minutes at a maximum concentration of 100 mg/mL or I.V. intermittent infusion over 10-60 minutes at a final concentration for I.V. administration not to exceed 40 mg/mL

Monitoring Parameters Monitor renal function periodically when used in combination with other nephrotoxic drugs; observe for signs and symptoms of anaphylaxis during first dose

Anesthesia and Critical Care Concerns/Other Considerations
Evidence-Based Information: Surgical Prophylaxis: Cefoxitin should be avoided in patients with a history of serious beta-lactam allergy (eg, respiratory difficulty, angioedema, hives, hypotension). Examples of beta-lactam antibiotics include penicillin, ampicillin, piperacillin, and cephalosporins (Bratzler, 2004).

Pregnancy Risk Factor B

Contraindications Hypersensitivity to cefoxitin, any component of the formulation, or other cephalosporins

Warnings/Precautions Modify dosage in patients with severe renal impairment. Prolonged use may result in superinfection. Use with caution in patients with a history of penicillin allergy, especially IgE-mediated reactions (eg, anaphylaxis, urticaria). Prolonged use may result in fungal or bacterial superinfection, including *C. difficile*-associated diarrhea (CDAD) and pseudomembranous colitis; CDAD has been observed >2 months postantibiotic treatment.

Adverse Reactions
1% to 10%: Gastrointestinal: Diarrhea
<1% (Limited to important or life-threatening): Anaphylaxis, angioedema, bone marrow suppression, BUN increased, creatinine increased, dyspnea, eosinophilia, exacerbation of myasthenia gravis, exfoliative dermatitis, fever, hemolytic anemia, hypotension, interstitial nephritis, jaundice, leukopenia, nausea, nephrotoxicity (with aminoglycosides), phlebitis, prolonged PT, pruritus, pseudomembranous colitis, rash, thrombocytopenia, thrombophlebitis, toxic epidermal necrolysis, transaminases increased, urticaria, vomiting

Reactions reported with other cephalosporins: Agranulocytosis, aplastic anemia, cholestasis, colitis, erythema multiforme, hemolytic anemia, hemorrhage, pancytopenia, renal dysfunction, seizure, serum-sickness reactions, Stevens-Johnson syndrome, superinfection, toxic nephropathy, vaginitis

Drug Interactions

Avoid Concomitant Use There are no known interactions where it is recommended to avoid concomitant use.

Increased Effect/Toxicity
Cefoxitin may increase the levels/effects of: Vitamin K Antagonists

The levels/effects of Cefoxitin may be increased by: Uricosuric Agents

Decreased Effect
Cefoxitin may decrease the levels/effects of: Typhoid Vaccine

Test Interactions Positive direct Coombs', false-positive urinary glucose test using cupric sulfate (Benedict's solution, Clinitest®, Fehling's solution), false-positive serum or urine creatinine with Jaffé reaction

Dietary Considerations Some products may contain sodium.

Dosage Forms Excipient information presented when available (limited, particularly for generics); consult specific product labeling.

Injection, powder for reconstitution: 1 g, 2 g, 10 g [contains sodium 53.8 mg/g (2.3 mEq/g)]

Powder for prescription compounding: 100 g

References

"Antimicrobial Prophylaxis for Surgery," *Treat Guidel Med Lett*, 2004, 2(20):27-32.

Bratzler DW, Houck PM, Surgical Infection Prevention Guidelines Writers Workgroup, et al, "Antimicrobial Prophylaxis for Surgery: An Advisory Statement From the National Surgical Infection Prevention Project," *Clin Infect Dis*, 2004, 38(12):1706-15.

◆ **Cefoxitin Sodium** *see* Cefoxitin *on page 261*

Ceftazidime (SEF tay zi deem)

Medication Safety Issues
Sound-alike/look-alike issues:
Ceftazidime may be confused with ceftizoxime
Ceptaz® may be confused with Septra®
Tazicef® may be confused with Tazidime®
Tazidime® may be confused with Tazicef®

International issues:
Ceftim® [Italy] may be confused with Ceftin® which is a brand name for cefuroxime in the U.S.
Ceftim® [Italy] may be confused with Cefiton® which is a brand name for cefixime in Portugal
Ceftim® [Italy] may be confused with Ceftina® which is a brand name for cefalotin in Mexico

U.S. Brand Names Fortaz®; Tazicef®

Canadian Brand Names Fortaz®

Pharmacologic Category Antibiotic, Cephalosporin (Third Generation)

Generic Available Yes: Injection

Use Treatment of documented susceptible *Pseudomonas aeruginosa* infection and infections due to other susceptible aerobic gram-negative organisms; empiric therapy of a febrile, granulocytopenic patient

Unlabeled/Investigational Use Bacterial endophthalmitis

Mechanism of Action Inhibits bacterial cell wall synthesis by binding to one or more of the penicillin-binding proteins (PBPs) which in turn inhibits the final transpeptidation step of peptidoglycan synthesis in bacterial cell walls, thus inhibiting cell wall biosynthesis. Bacteria eventually lyse due to ongoing activity of cell wall autolytic enzymes (autolysins and murein hydrolases) while cell wall assembly is arrested.

Pharmacodynamics/Kinetics
Distribution: Widely throughout the body including bone, bile, skin, CSF (higher concentrations achieved when meninges are inflamed), endometrium, heart, pleural and lymphatic fluids

Protein binding: 17%

Half-life elimination: 1-2 hours, prolonged with renal impairment; Neonates <23 days: 2.2-4.7 hours

Time to peak, serum: I.M.: ~1 hour

Excretion: Urine (80% to 90% as unchanged drug)

Dosage

Usual dosage range:

Infants and Children 1 month to 12 years: I.V.: 30-50 mg/kg/dose every 8 hours (maximum dose: 6 g/day)

Adults: I.M., I.V.: 500 mg to 2 g every 8-12 hours

Indication-specific dosing:

Bacterial arthritis (gram-negative bacilli): I.V.: 1-2 g every 8 hours

Cystic fibrosis: I.V.: 30-50 mg/kg every 8 hours (maximum: 6 g/day)

Endophthalmitis, bacterial (unlabeled use): Intravitreal: 2.25 mg/0.1 mL NS in combination with vancomycin

Melioidosis: I.V.: 40 mg/kg every 8 hours for 10 days, followed by oral therapy with doxycycline or TMP/SMX

Otitis externa: I.V.: 2 g every 8 hours

Peritonitis (CAPD):

Anuric, intermittent: 1000-1500 mg/day

Anuric, continuous (per liter exchange): Loading dose: 250 mg; maintenance dose: 125 mg

Severe infections, including meningitis, complicated pneumonia, endoph-thalmitis, CNS infection, osteomyelitis, intra-abdominal and gynecological, skin and soft tissue: I.V.: 2 g every 8 hours

Dosing interval in renal impairment:

Cl_{cr} 30-50 mL/minute: Administer every 12 hours

Cl_{cr} 10-30 mL/minute: Administer every 24 hours

Cl_{cr} <10 mL/minute: Administer every 48-72 hours

Hemodialysis: Dialyzable (50% to 100%)

Continuous renal replacement therapy (CRRT): Drug clearance is highly dependent on the method of renal replacement, filter type, and flow rate. Appropriate dosing requires close monitoring of pharmacologic response, signs of adverse reactions due to drug accumulation, as well as drug levels in relation to target trough (if appropriate). The following are general recommendations only (based on dialysate flow/ultrafiltration rates of 1 L/hour) and should not supersede clinical judgment:

CVVH: 1-2 g every 12 hours

CVVHD/CVVHDF: 2 g every 12 hours

Stability

Vials: Reconstituted solution and solution further diluted for I.V. infusion are stable for 12 hours at room temperature, for 3 days when refrigerated, or for 12 weeks when frozen at -20°C (-4°F). After freezing, thawed solution in SWFI for I.M. administration is stable for 3 hours at room temperature or for 3 days when refrigerated, thawed solution in NS in a Viaflex® small volume container for I.V. administration is stable for 12 hours at room temperature or for 3 days when refrigerated, and thawed solution in SWFI in the original container is stable for 8 hours at room temperature or for 3 days when refrigerated.

Premixed frozen solution: Store frozen at -20°C (-4°F). Thawed solution is stable for 8 hours at room temperature or for 3 days under refrigeration; do not refreeze.

Administration Any carbon dioxide bubbles that may be present in the withdrawn solution should be expelled prior to injection. Administer around-the-clock to promote less variation in peak and trough serum levels. Ceftazidime can be administered deep I.M. into large mass muscle, IVP over 3-5 minutes, or I.V. intermittent infusion over 15-30 minutes. Do not admix with aminoglycosides in same bottle/bag. Final concentration for I.V. administration should not exceed 100 mg/mL.

Monitoring Parameters Observe for signs and symptoms of anaphylaxis during first dose

Pregnancy Risk Factor B

Contraindications Hypersensitivity to ceftazidime, any component of the formulation, or other cephalosporins

Warnings/Precautions Modify dosage in patients with severe renal impairment. Use with caution in patients with a history of penicillin allergy, especially IgE-mediated reactions (eg, anaphylaxis, urticaria). Prolonged use may result in fungal or bacterial superinfection, including *C. difficile*-associated diarrhea (CDAD) and pseudomembranous colitis; CDAD has been observed >2 months postantibiotic treatment. May be associated with increased INR, especially in nutritionally-deficient patients, prolonged treatment, hepatic or renal disease. Use with caution in patients with a history of seizure disorder; high levels, particularly in the presence of renal impairment, may increase risk of seizures.

Adverse Reactions
1% to 10%:
Gastrointestinal: Diarrhea (1%)
Local: Pain at injection site (1%)
Miscellaneous: Hypersensitivity reactions (2%)
<1% (Limited to important or life-threatening): Anaphylaxis, angioedema, asterixis, BUN increased, candidiasis, creatinine increased, dizziness, encephalopathy, eosinophilia, erythema multiforme, fever, headache, hemolytic anemia, hyperbilirubinemia, jaundice, leukopenia, myoclonus, nausea, neuromuscular excitability, paresthesia, phlebitis, pruritus, pseudomembranous colitis, rash, Stevens-Johnson syndrome, thrombocytosis, toxic epidermal necrolysis, transaminases increased, vaginitis, vomiting
Reactions reported with other cephalosporins: Agranulocytosis, aplastic anemia, cholestasis, colitis, hemolytic anemia, hemorrhage, interstitial nephritis, pancytopenia, prolonged PT, renal dysfunction, seizure, serum-sickness reactions, superinfection, toxic nephropathy, urticaria

Drug Interactions
Avoid Concomitant Use There are no known interactions where it is recommended to avoid concomitant use.
Increased Effect/Toxicity
The levels/effects of Ceftazidime may be increased by: Uricosuric Agents
Decreased Effect
Ceftazidime may decrease the levels/effects of: Typhoid Vaccine

Test Interactions Positive direct Coombs', false-positive urinary glucose test using cupric sulfate (Benedict's solution, Clinitest®, Fehling's solution), false-positive serum or urine creatinine with Jaffé reaction

Dietary Considerations Sodium content of 1 g: 2.3 mEq

Dosage Forms Excipient information presented when available (limited, particularly for generics); consult specific product labeling.
Infusion [premixed iso-osmotic solution, frozen]:
Fortaz®: 1 g (50 mL) [contains sodium carbonate, sodium ~54 mg (2.3 mEq)/g]; 2 g (50 mL) [contains sodium ~54 mg (2.3 mEq)/g]
Injection, powder for reconstitution: 1 g, 2 g, 6 g
Fortaz®: 500 mg, 1 g, 2 g, 6 g [contains sodium ~54 mg (2.3 mEq)/g]
Tazicef®: 1 g, 2 g, 6 g [contains sodium ~54 mg (2.3 mEq)/g]

References
American Thoracic Society and Infectious Diseases Society of America, "Guidelines for the Management of Adults With Hospital-Acquired, Ventilator-Associated, and Healthcare-Associated Pneumonia," *Am J Respir Crit Care Med*, 2005, 171(4):388-416.
Tunkel AR, Hartman BJ, Kaplan SL, et al, "Practice Guidelines for the Management of Bacterial Meningitis," *Clin Infect Dis*, 2004, 39(9):1267-84.

◆ **Ceftin®** see Cefuroxime on page 272

Ceftizoxime (sef ti ZOKS eem)

Medication Safety Issues
Sound-alike/look-alike issues:
Ceftizoxime may be confused with cefotaxime, ceftazidime, cefuroxime
U.S. Brand Names Cefizox®
Canadian Brand Names Cefizox®
Index Terms Ceftizoxime Sodium
Pharmacologic Category Antibiotic, Cephalosporin (Third Generation)
Generic Available No

Use Treatment of susceptible bacterial infections, mainly respiratory tract, skin and skin structure, bone and joint, urinary tract and gynecologic, as well as septicemia; active against many gram-negative bacilli (not *Pseudomonas*), some gram-positive cocci (not *Enterococcus*), and some anaerobes

Mechanism of Action Inhibits bacterial cell wall synthesis by binding to one or more of the penicillin-binding proteins (PBPs) which in turn inhibits the final transpeptidation step of peptidoglycan synthesis in bacterial cell walls, thus inhibiting cell wall biosynthesis. Bacteria eventually lyse due to ongoing activity of cell wall autolytic enzymes (autolysins and murein hydrolases) while cell wall assembly is arrested.

Pharmacodynamics/Kinetics

Distribution: V_d: 0.35-0.5 L/kg; widely into most body tissues and fluids including gallbladder, liver, kidneys, bone, sputum, bile, pleural and synovial fluids; has good CSF penetration

Protein binding: 30%

Half-life elimination: 1.6 hours; Cl_{cr} <10 mL/minute: 25 hours

Time to peak, serum: I.M.: 0.5-1 hour

Excretion: Urine (as unchanged drug)

Dosage

Usual dosage range:

Children ≥6 months: I.M., I.V.: 150-200 mg/kg/day divided every 6-8 hours (maximum: 12 g/24 hours)

Adults: I.M., I.V.: 1-4 g every 8-12 hours

Indication-specific dosing:

Adults:

Gonococcal:

Disseminated infection: I.M., I.V.: 1 g every 8 hours

Uncomplicated: I.M.: 1 g as single dose

Life-threatening infections: I.V.: 2 g every 4 hours or 4 g every 8 hours

Dosing adjustment in renal impairment: Adults:

Cl_{cr} 50-79 mL/minute: Administer 500-1500 mg every 8 hours.

Cl_{cr} 5-49 mL/minute: Administer 250-1000 mg every 12 hours.

Cl_{cr} 0-4 mL/minute: Administer 500-1000 mg every 48 hours or 250-500 mg every 24 hours.

Moderately dialyzable (20% to 50%)

Continuous arteriovenous hemofiltration: Dose as for Cl_{cr} 10-50 mL/minute.

Stability Reconstituted solution is stable for 24 hours at room temperature and 96 hours when refrigerated. For I.V. infusion in NS or D_5W solution is stable for 24 hours at room temperature, 96 hours when refrigerated, or 12 weeks when frozen. After freezing, thawed solution is stable for 24 hours at room temperature or 10 days when refrigerated.

Administration

I.M.: Inject deep I.M. into large muscle mass.

I.V.: Inject direct I.V. over 3-5 minutes. Infuse intermittent infusion over 30 minutes.

Monitoring Parameters Observe for signs and symptoms of anaphylaxis during first dose

Pregnancy Risk Factor B

Contraindications Hypersensitivity to ceftizoxime, any component of the formulation, or other cephalosporins

Warnings/Precautions Modify dosage in patients with severe renal impairment. Prolonged use may result in fungal or bacterial superinfection, including *C. difficile*-associated diarrhea (CDAD) and pseudomembranous colitis; CDAD has been observed >2 months postantibiotic treatment. Use with caution in patients with a history of penicillin allergy, especially IgE-mediated reactions (eg, anaphylaxis, urticaria).

Adverse Reactions

1% to 10%:

Central nervous system: Fever

Dermatologic: Rash, pruritus

Hematologic: Eosinophilia, thrombocytosis

Hepatic: Alkaline phosphatase increased, transaminases increased

Local: Pain, burning at injection site

<1% (Limited to important or life-threatening): Anaphylaxis, anemia, bilirubin increased, BUN increased, creatinine increased, diarrhea, injection site reactions, leukopenia, nausea, neutropenia, numbness, paresthesia, phlebitis, thrombocytopenia, vaginitis, vomiting

Reactions reported with other cephalosporins: Agranulocytosis, angioedema, aplastic anemia, asterixis, candidiasis, cholestasis, colitis, encephalopathy, erythema multiforme, hemolytic anemia, hemorrhage, interstitial nephritis, neuromuscular excitability, pancytopenia, prolonged PT, pseudomembranous colitis, renal dysfunction, seizure, serum-sickness reactions, Stevens-Johnson syndrome, superinfection, toxic epidermal necrolysis, toxic nephropathy

Drug Interactions

Avoid Concomitant Use There are no known interactions where it is recommended to avoid concomitant use.

Increased Effect/Toxicity

The levels/effects of Ceftizoxime may be increased by: Uricosuric Agents

Decreased Effect

Ceftizoxime may decrease the levels/effects of: Typhoid Vaccine

Test Interactions Positive direct Coombs', false-positive urinary glucose test using cupric sulfate (Benedict's solution, Clinitest®, Fehling's solution), false-positive serum or urine creatinine with Jaffé reaction

Dietary Considerations Sodium content of 1 g: 60 mg (2.6 mEq)

Dosage Forms Excipient information presented when available (limited, particularly for generics); consult specific product labeling.

Infusion [premixed iso-osmotic solution]:
  Cefizox®: 1 g (50 mL); 2 g (50 mL)
Injection, powder for reconstitution:
  Cefizox®: 1 g, 2 g, 10 g [DSC]

◆ **Ceftizoxime Sodium** *see* Ceftizoxime *on page 265*

CefTRIAXone (sef trye AKS one)

Medication Safety Issues
  Sound-alike/look-alike issues:
    CefTRIAXone may be confused with CeFAZolin, Cetraxal®
    Rocephin® may be confused with Roferon®

Related Information
  Desensitization Protocols *on page 1692*
  Prevention of Infective Endocarditis *on page 1718*

U.S. Brand Names Rocephin®

Canadian Brand Names Rocephin®

Index Terms Ceftriaxone Sodium

Pharmacologic Category Antibiotic, Cephalosporin (Third Generation)

Generic Available Yes

Use Treatment of lower respiratory tract infections, acute bacterial otitis media, skin and skin structure infections, bone and joint infections, intra-abdominal and urinary tract infections, pelvic inflammatory disease (PID), uncomplicated gonorrhea, bacterial septicemia, and meningitis; used in surgical prophylaxis

Unlabeled/Investigational Use Treatment of chancroid, epididymitis, complicated gonococcal infections; sexually-transmitted diseases (STD); periorbital or buccal cellulitis; salmonellosis or shigellosis; atypical community-acquired pneumonia; epiglottitis, Lyme disease; used in chemoprophylaxis for high-risk contacts and persons with invasive meningococcal disease; sexual assault; typhoid fever, Whipple's disease

Mechanism of Action Inhibits bacterial cell wall synthesis by binding to one or more of the penicillin-binding proteins (PBPs) which in turn inhibits the final transpeptidation step of peptidoglycan synthesis in bacterial cell walls, thus inhibiting cell wall biosynthesis. Bacteria eventually lyse due to ongoing activity of cell wall autolytic enzymes (autolysins and murein hydrolases) while cell wall assembly is arrested.

Pharmacodynamics/Kinetics
  Absorption: I.M.: Well absorbed

◀ Distribution: V_d: 6-14 L; widely throughout the body including gallbladder, lungs, bone, bile, CSF (higher concentrations achieved when meninges are inflamed)

Protein binding: 85% to 95%

Half-life elimination: Normal renal and hepatic function: 5-9 hours; Renal impairment (mild-to-severe): 12-16 hours

Time to peak, serum: I.M.: 2-3 hours

Excretion: Urine (33% to 67% as unchanged drug); feces (as inactive drug)

Dosage

Usual dosage range:

Infants and Children: I.M., I.V.: 50-100 mg/kg/day in 1-2 divided doses (maximum: 4 g/day [meningitis]; 2 g/day [nonmeningeal infections])

Adults: I.M., I.V.: 1-2 g every 12-24 hours

Indication-specific dosing:

Infants and Children:

Epiglottitis (unlabeled use): I.M., I.V.: 50-100 mg/kg once daily; reported duration of treatment ranged from 2-14 days

Gonococcal infections:

Conjunctivitis, complicated (unlabeled use): I.M.:

<45 kg: 50 mg/kg in a single dose (maximum: 1 g)

≥45 kg: 1 g in a single dose

Disseminated (unlabeled use): I.M., I.V.:

<45 kg: 25-50 mg/kg once daily (maximum: 1 g)

≥45 kg: 1 g once daily for 7 days

Endocarditis (unlabeled use):

<45 kg: I.M., I.V.: 50 mg/kg/day every 12 hours (maximum: 2 g/day) for at least 28 days

≥45 kg: I.V.: 1-2 g every 12 hours, for at least 28 days

Prophylaxis (due to maternal gonococcal infection): I.M., I.V.: 25-50 mg/kg as a single dose (maximum: 125 mg)

Uncomplicated: I.M.: 125 mg in a single dose

Infective endocarditis: I.M., I.V.:

Native valve: 100 mg/kg once daily for 2-4 weeks; **Note:** If using 2-week regimen, concurrent gentamicin is recommended

Prosthetic valve: 100 mg/kg once daily for 6 weeks (with or without 2 weeks of gentamicin [dependent on penicillin MIC]); **Note:** For HACEK organisms, duration of therapy is 4 weeks

Enterococcus faecalis (resistant to penicillin, aminoglycoside, and vancomycin), native or prosthetic valve: 100 mg/kg once daily for ≥8 weeks administered concurrently with ampicillin

Prophylaxis: 50 mg/kg 30-60 minutes before procedure; maximum dose: 1 g. Intramuscular injections should be avoided in patients who are receiving anticoagulant therapy. In these circumstances, orally administered regimens should be given whenever possible. Intravenously administered antibiotics should be used for patients who are unable to tolerate or absorb oral medications.

Note: American Heart Association (AHA) guidelines now recommend prophylaxis only in patients undergoing invasive procedures and in whom underlying cardiac conditions may predispose to a higher risk of adverse outcomes should infection occur. As of April 2007, routine prophylaxis for GI/GU procedures is no longer recommended by the AHA.

Lyme disease, persistent arthritis (unlabeled use): I.M., I.V.: 75-100 mg/kg (maximum: 2 g) for 2-4 weeks

Mild-to-moderate infections: I.M., I.V.: 50-75 mg/kg/day in 1-2 divided doses every 12-24 hours (maximum: 2 g/day); continue until at least 2 days after signs and symptoms of infection have resolved

Meningitis:

Gonococcal, complicated:

<45 kg: I.V.: 50 mg/kg/day given every 12 hours (maximum: 2 g/day); usual duration of treatment is 10-14 days

>45 kg: I.V.: 1-2 g every 12 hours; usual duration of treatment is 10-14 days

Uncomplicated: I.M., I.V.: Loading dose of 100 mg/kg (maximum: 4 g), followed by 100 mg/kg/day divided every 12-24 hours (maximum: 4 g/day); usual duration of treatment is 7-14 days

Otitis media:
Acute: I.M.: 50 mg/kg in a single dose (maximum: 1 g)
Persistent or relapsing (unlabeled use): I.M., I.V.: 50 mg/kg once daily for 3 days
Pneumonia: I.V.: 50-75 mg/kg once daily
Serious infections: I.V.: 80-100 mg/kg/day in 1-2 divided doses (maximum: 4 g/day)
Skin/skin structure infections: I.M., I.V.: 50-75 mg/kg/day in 1-2 divided doses (maximum: 2 g/day)
STD, sexual assault (unlabeled use): I.M.: 125 mg in a single dose
Typhoid fever (unlabeled use): I.V.: 75-80 mg/kg once daily for 5-14 days
Children >8 years (≥45 kg) and Adolescents:
Epididymitis, acute (unlabeled use): I.M.: 125 mg in a single dose

Children ≤15 years:
Chemoprophylaxis for high-risk contacts and persons with invasive meningococcal disease (unlabeled use): I.M.: 125 mg in a single dose. Children >15 years: Refer to adult dosing.

Adults:
Arthritis, septic (unlabeled use): I.V.: 1-2 g once daily
Brain abscess (unlabeled use): I.V.: 2 g every 12 hours with metronidazole
Cavernous sinus thrombosis (unlabeled use): I.V.: 2 g once daily with vancomycin or linezolid
Chancroid (unlabeled use): I.M.: 250 mg as single dose
Chemoprophylaxis for high-risk contacts and persons with invasive meningococcal disease (unlabeled use): I.M.: 250 mg in a single dose
Gonococcal infections:
Conjunctivitis, complicated (unlabeled use): I.M.: 1 g in a single dose
Disseminated (unlabeled use): I.M., I.V.: 1 g once daily for 7 days
Endocarditis (unlabeled use): I.M., I.V.: 1-2 g every 12 hours for at least 28 days
Epididymitis, acute (unlabeled use): I.M.: 250 mg in a single dose with doxycycline
Prostatitis (unlabeled use): I.M.: 125-250 mg in a single dose with doxycycline
Uncomplicated: I.M.: 125-250 mg in a single dose
Infective endocarditis: I.M., I.V.:
Native valve: 2 g once daily for 2-4 weeks; **Note:** If using 2-week regimen, concurrent gentamicin is recommended
Prosthetic valve: I.M., I.V.: 2 g once daily for 6 weeks (with or without 2 weeks of gentamicin [dependent on penicillin MIC]); **Note:** For HACEK organisms, duration of therapy is 4 weeks
Enterococcus faecalis (resistant to penicillin, aminoglycoside, and vancomycin), native or prosthetic valve: 2 g twice daily for ≥8 weeks administered concurrently with ampicillin
Prophylaxis: I.M., I.V.: 1 g 30-60 minutes before procedure. Intramuscular injections should be avoided in patients who are receiving anticoagulant therapy. In these circumstances, orally administered regimens should be given whenever possible. Intravenously administered antibiotics should be used for patients who are unable to tolerate or absorb oral medications.
Note: American Heart Association (AHA) guidelines now recommend prophylaxis only in patients undergoing invasive procedures and in whom underlying cardiac conditions may predispose to a higher risk of adverse outcomes should infection occur. As of April 2007, routine prophylaxis for GI/GU procedures is no longer recommended by the AHA.
Lyme disease (unlabeled use): I.V.: 2 g once daily for 14-28 days
Mastoiditis (hospitalized; unlabeled use): I.V.: 2 g once daily; >60 years old: 1 g once daily
Meningitis: I.V.: 2 g every 12 hours for 7-14 days (longer courses may be necessary for selected organisms)
Orbital cellulitis (unlabeled use) and endophthalmitis: I.V.: 2 g once daily
Pelvic inflammatory disease: I.M.: 250 mg in a single dose
Pneumonia, community-acquired: I.V.: 1 g once daily, usually in combination with a macrolide; consider 2 g/day for patients at risk for more severe infection

and/or resistant organisms (ICU status, age >65 years, disseminated infection)

Pyelonephritis (acute, uncomplicated): Females: I.V.: 1-2 g once daily (Stamm, 1993). Many physicians administer a single parenteral dose before initiating oral therapy (Warren, 1999).

Septic/toxic shock/necrotizing fasciitis (unlabeled use): I.V.: 2 g once daily; with clindamycin for toxic shock

STD prophylaxis in sexual assault victims: I.M.: 125 mg as a single dose

Surgical prophylaxis: I.V.: 1 g 30 minutes to 2 hours before surgery

Syphilis (unlabeled use): I.M., I.V.: 1 g once daily for 8-10 days

Typhoid fever (unlabeled use): I.V.: 2 g once daily for 14 days

Whipple's disease (unlabeled use): Initial: 2 g once daily for 10-14 days, then oral therapy for ~1 year.

Dosage adjustment in renal impairment: No adjustment is generally necessary;
  Note: Concurrent renal and hepatic dysfunction: Maximum dose ≤2 g/day
Hemodialysis: Not dialyzable (0% to 5%); administer dose postdialysis
Continuous ambulatory peritoneal dialysis (CAPD): Administer 1 g every 12 hours
Continuous renal replacement therapy (CRRT): Drug clearance is highly dependent on the method of renal replacement, filter type, and flow rate. Appropriate dosing requires close monitoring of pharmacologic response, signs of adverse reactions due to drug accumulation, as well as drug levels in relation to target trough (if appropriate). The following are general recommendations only (based on dialysate flow/ultrafiltration rates of 1 L/hour) and should not supersede clinical judgment:
  CVVH or CVVHD/CVVHDF: 2 g every 12-24 hours

Dosage adjustment in hepatic impairment: No adjustment necessary unless there is concurrent renal dysfunction (see dosage adjustment in renal impairment).

Stability

Powder for injection: Prior to reconstitution, store at room temperature ≤25°C (≤77°F). Protect from light.

Premixed solution (manufacturer premixed): Store at -20°C. Once thawed, solutions are stable for 3 days at room temperature of 25°C (77°F) or for 21 days refrigerated at 5°C (41°F). Do not refreeze.

Stability of reconstituted solutions:

10-40 mg/mL: Reconstituted in D_5W, $D_{10}W$, NS, or SWFI: Stable for 2 days at room temperature of 25°C (77°F) or for 10 days when refrigerated at 4°C (39°F). Stable for 26 weeks when frozen at -20°C when reconstituted with D_5W or NS. Once thawed (at room temperature), solutions are stable for 2 days at room temperature of 25°C (77°F) or for 10 days when refrigerated at 4°C (39°F); does not apply to manufacturer's premixed bags. Do not refreeze.

100 mg/mL:
  Reconstituted in D_5W, SWFI, or NS: Stable for 2 days at room temperature of 25°C (77°F) or for 10 days when refrigerated at 4°C (39°F).
  Reconstituted in lidocaine 1% solution or bacteriostatic water: Stable for 24 hours at room temperature of 25°C (77°F) or for 10 days when refrigerated at 4°C (39°F).

250-350 mg/mL: Reconstituted in D_5W, NS, lidocaine 1% solution, bacteriostatic water, or SWFI: Stable for 24 hours at room temperature of 25°C (77°F) or for 3 days when refrigerated at 4°C (39°F).

Reconstitution:

I.M. injection: Vials should be reconstituted with appropriate volume of diluent (including D_5W, NS, SWFI, bacteriostatic water, or 1% lidocaine) to make a final concentration of 250 mg/mL or 350 mg/mL.
  Volume to add to create a **250 mg/mL** solution:
    250 mg vial: 0.9 mL
    500 mg vial: 1.8 mL
    1 g vial: 3.6 mL
    2 g vial: 7.2 mL
  Volume to add to create a **350 mg/mL** solution:
    500 mg vial: 1.0 mL
    1 g vial: 2.1 mL
    2 g vial: 4.2 mL

I.V. infusion: Infusion is prepared in two stages: Initial reconstitution of powder, followed by dilution to final infusion solution.

Vials: Reconstitute powder with appropriate I.V. diluent (including SWFI, D_5W, $D_{10}W$, NS) to create an initial solution of ~100 mg/mL. Recommended volume to add:

250 mg vial: 2.4 mL
500 mg vial: 4.8 mL
1 g vial: 9.6 mL
2 g vial: 19.2 mL

Note: After reconstitution of powder, further dilution into a volume of compatible solution (eg, 50-100 mL of D_5W or NS) is recommended.

Piggyback bottle: Reconstitute powder with appropriate I.V. diluent (D_5W or NS) to create a resulting solution of ~100 mg/mL. Recommended initial volume to add:

1 g bottle:10 mL
2 g bottle: 20 mL

Note: After reconstitution, to prepare the final infusion solution, further dilution to 50 mL or 100 mL volumes with the appropriate I.V. diluent (including D_5W or NS) is recommended.

Administration Do not admix with aminoglycosides in same bottle/bag. Do not reconstitute, admix, or coadminister with calcium-containing solutions. Infuse intermittent infusion over 30 minutes.

I.M.: Inject deep I.M. into large muscle mass; a concentration of 250 mg/mL or 350 mg/mL is recommended for all vial sizes except the 250 mg size (250 mg/mL is suggested); can be diluted with 1:1 water and 1% lidocaine for I.M. administration.

I.V.: Infuse intermittent infusion over 30 minutes.

Monitoring Parameters Observe for signs and symptoms of anaphylaxis

Pregnancy Risk Factor B

Contraindications Hypersensitivity to ceftriaxone sodium, any component of the formulation, or other cephalosporins; **do not use in hyperbilirubinemic neonates**, particularly those who are premature since ceftriaxone is reported to displace bilirubin from albumin binding sites; concomitant use with intravenous calcium-containing solutions/products in neonates (≤28 days)

Warnings/Precautions Use with caution in patients with a history of penicillin allergy, especially IgE-mediated reactions (eg, anaphylaxis, urticaria). Abnormal gallbladder sonograms have been reported, possibly due to cetriaxone-calcium precipitates; discontinue in patients with signs and symptoms of gallbladder disease. Secondary to biliary obstruction, pancreatitis has been reported rarely. Use with caution in patients with a history of GI disease, especially colitis. Severe cases (including some fatalities) of immune-related hemolytic anemia have been reported in patients receiving cephalosporins, including ceftriaxone. Prolonged use may result in fungal or bacterial superinfection, including *C. difficile*-associated diarrhea (CDAD) and pseudomembranous colitis; CDAD has been observed >2 months postantibiotic treatment.

May be associated with increased INR (rarely), especially in nutritionally-deficient patients, prolonged treatment, hepatic or renal disease. No adjustment is generally necessary in patients with renal impairment; use with caution in patients with concurrent hepatic dysfunction and significant renal disease, dosage should not exceed 2 g/day. Ceftriaxone may complex with calcium causing precipitation. Fatal lung and kidney damage associated with calcium-ceftriaxone precipitates has been observed in premature and term neonates. Do not reconstitute, admix, or coadminister with calcium-containing solutions, even via separate infusion lines/sites or at different times in any neonatal patient. Ceftriaxone should not be diluted or administered simultaneously with any calcium-containing solution via a Y-site in any patient. However, ceftriaxone and calcium-containing solution may be administered sequentially of one another for use in patients **other than neonates** if infusion lines are thoroughly flushed, with a compatible fluid, between infusions

Adverse Reactions

>10%: Local: Induration (I.M. 5% to 17%), warmth (I.M.), tightness (I.M.)
1% to 10%:
Dermatologic: Rash (2%)

Gastrointestinal: Diarrhea (3%)
Hematologic: Eosinophilia (6%), thrombocytosis (5%), leukopenia (2%)
Hepatic: Transaminases increased (3%)
Local: Tenderness at injection site (I.V. 1%), pain
Renal: BUN increased (1%)
<1% (Limited to important or life-threatening): Abdominal pain, agranulocytosis, alkaline phosphatase increased, allergic dermatitis, allergic pneumonitis, anaphylaxis, anemia, basophilia, biliary lithiasis, bilirubin increased, broncho-spasm, chills, colitis, creatinine increased, diaphoresis, dizziness, dysgeusia, dyspepsia, edema, epistaxis, erythema multiforme, exanthema, fever, flatulence, flushing, gallbladder sludge, gallstones, glossitis, glycosuria, headache, hematuria, hemolytic anemia, jaundice, leukocytosis, Lyell's syndrome, lymphocytosis, lymphopenia, moniliasis, monocytosis, nausea, nephrolithiasis, neutropenia, oliguria, palpitation, pancreatitis, phlebitis, prolonged or decreased PT, pruritus, pseudomembranous colitis, renal and pulmonary ceftriaxone-calcium precipitations (neonates including some fatalities), seizure, serum sickness Stevens-Johnson syndrome, stomatitis, thrombocytopenia, toxic epidermal necrolysis, urinary casts, urticaria, vaginitis, vomiting

Reactions reported with other cephalosporins: Angioedema, allergic reaction, aplastic anemia, asterixis, cholestasis, encephalopathy, hemorrhage, hepatic dysfunction, hyperactivity (reversible), hypertonia, interstitial nephritis, LDH increased, neuromuscular excitability, pancytopenia, paresthesia, renal dys-function, superinfection, toxic nephropathy

Drug Interactions
Avoid Concomitant Use There are no known interactions where it is recommended to avoid concomitant use.
Increased Effect/Toxicity
CefTRIAXone may increase the levels/effects of: Vitamin K Antagonists

The levels/effects of CefTRIAXone may be increased by: Calcium Salts (Intravenous); Ringer's Injection (Lactated); Uricosuric Agents
Decreased Effect
CefTRIAXone may decrease the levels/effects of: Typhoid Vaccine
Test Interactions Positive direct Coombs', false-positive urinary glucose test using cupric sulfate (Benedict's solution, Clinitest®, Fehling's solution), false-positive serum or urine creatinine with Jaffé reaction
Dietary Considerations Some products may contain sodium.
Dosage Forms Excipient information presented when available (limited, particularly for generics); consult specific product labeling. [DSC] = Discontinued product
Infusion [premixed in dextrose]: 1 g (50 mL); 2 g (50 mL)
Injection, powder for reconstitution: 250 mg, 500 mg, 1 g, 2 g, 10 g
Rocephin®: 250 mg [DSC], 500 mg, 1 g, 2 g [DSC], 10 g [contains sodium ~83 mg (3.6 mEq) per ceftriaxone 1 g] [DSC]
References
Tunkel AR, Hartman BJ, Kaplan SL, et al, "Practice Guidelines for the Management of Bacterial Meningitis," *Clin Infect Dis*, 2004, 39(9):1267-84.
Wilson W, Taubert KA, Gewitz M, et al, "Prevention of Infective Endocarditis. Guidelines From the American Heart Association. A Guideline From the American Heart Association Rheumatic Fever, Endocarditis, and Kawasaki Disease Committee, Council on Cardiovascular Disease in the Young, and the Council on Clinical Cardiology, Council on Cardiovascular Surgery and Anesthesia, and the Quality of Care and Outcomes Research Interdisciplinary Working Group," *Circulation*, 2007, 115. Available at http://circ.ahajournals.org/cgi/reprint/CIRCULATIONAHA.106.183095v1; last accessed July 26, 2007.

◆ **Ceftriaxone Sodium** *see* CefTRIAXone *on page 267*

Cefuroxime (se fyoor OKS eem)

Medication Safety Issues
Sound-alike/look-alike issues:
Cefuroxime may be confused with cefotaxime, cefprozil, ceftizoxime, deferoxamine
Ceftin® may be confused with Cefzil®, Cipro®
Zinacef® may be confused with Zithromax®

International issues:
Ceftin® may be confused with Cefiton® which is a brand name for cefixime in Portugal
Ceftin® may be confused with Ceftina® which is a brand name for cefalotin in Mexico
Ceftin® may be confused with Ceftim® which is a brand name for ceftazidime in Italy

Related Information
Prevention of Wound Infection and Sepsis in Surgical Patients *on page 1721*

U.S. Brand Names Ceftin®; Zinacef®

Canadian Brand Names Apo-Cefuroxime®; Ceftin®; Cefuroxime For Injection; Pro-Cefuroxime; ratio-Cefuroxime; Zinacef®

Index Terms Cefuroxime Axetil; Cefuroxime Sodium

Pharmacologic Category Antibiotic, Cephalosporin (Second Generation)

Generic Available Yes

Use Treatment of infections caused by staphylococci, group B streptococci, *H. influenzae* (type A and B), *E. coli, Enterobacter, Salmonella*, and *Klebsiella*; treatment of susceptible infections of the upper and lower respiratory tract, otitis media, urinary tract, uncomplicated skin and soft tissue, bone and joint, sepsis, uncomplicated gonorrhea, and early Lyme disease; surgical prophylaxis

Mechanism of Action Inhibits bacterial cell wall synthesis by binding to one or more of the penicillin-binding proteins (PBPs) which in turn inhibits the final transpeptidation step of peptidoglycan synthesis in bacterial cell walls, thus inhibiting cell wall biosynthesis. Bacteria eventually lyse due to ongoing activity of cell wall autolytic enzymes (autolysins and murein hydrolases) while cell wall assembly is arrested.

Pharmacodynamics/Kinetics
Absorption: Oral (cefuroxime axetil): Increases with food
Distribution: Widely to body tissues and fluids; crosses blood-brain barrier; therapeutic concentrations achieved in CSF even when meninges are not inflamed
Protein binding: 33% to 50%
Bioavailability: Tablet: Fasting: 37%; Following food: 52%
Half-life elimination: Children 1-2 hours; Adults: 1-2 hours; prolonged with renal impairment
Time to peak, serum: I.M.: ~15-60 minutes; I.V.: 2-3 minutes; Oral: Children: 3-4 hours; Adults: 2-3 hours
Excretion: Urine (66% to 100% as unchanged drug)

Dosage Note: Cefuroxime axetil film-coated tablets and oral suspension are not bioequivalent and are not substitutable on a mg/mg basis

Usual dosage range:
Children 3 months to 12 years:
Oral: 20-30 mg/kg/day in 2 divided doses
I.M., I.V.: 75-150 mg/kg/day divided every 8 hours (maximum dose: 6 g/day)
Children ≥13 years and Adults:
Oral: 250-500 mg twice daily
I.M., I.V.: 750 mg to 1.5 g every 6-8 hours or 100-150 mg/kg/day in divided doses every 6-8 hours (maximum: 6 g/day)

Indication-specific dosing:
Children ≥3 months to 12 years:
Acute bacterial maxillary sinusitis, acute otitis media, and impetigo:
Oral: Suspension: 30 mg/kg/day in 2 divided doses for 10 days (maximum dose: 1 g/day); tablet: 250 mg twice daily for 10 days
I.M., I.V.: 75-150 mg/kg/day divided every 8 hours (maximum dose: 6 g/day)
Epiglottitis: Oral: 150 mg/kg/day in 3 divided doses for 7-10 days
Pharyngitis/tonsillitis:
Oral: Suspension: 20 mg/kg/day (maximum: 500 mg/day) in 2 divided doses for 10 days; tablet: 125 mg every 12 hours for 10 days
I.M., I.V.: 75-150 mg/kg/day divided every 8 hours (maximum: 6 g/day)
Children ≥13 years and Adults (all oral doses listed are for tablet formulation):
Bronchitis (acute and exacerbations of chronic bronchitis):
Oral: 250-500 mg every 12 hours for 10 days
I.V.: 500-750 mg every 8 hours (complete therapy with oral dosing)

◄ **Cellulitis, orbital:** I.V.: 1.5 g every 8 hours
Gonorrhea:
Disseminated: I.M., I.V.: 750 mg every 8 hours
Uncomplicated:
Oral: 1 g as a single dose
I.M.: 1.5 g as single dose (administer in 2 different sites with probenecid)
Lyme disease (early): Oral: 500 mg twice daily for 20 days
Pharyngitis/tonsillitis and sinusitis: Oral: 250 mg twice daily for 10 days
Pneumonia (uncomplicated): I.V.: 750 mg every 8 hours
Severe or complicated infections: I.M., I.V.: 1.5 g every 8 hours (up to 1.5 g every 6 hours in life-threatening infections)
Skin/skin structure infection (uncomplicated):
Oral: 250-500 mg every 12 hours for 10 days
I.M., I.V.: 750 mg every 8 hours
Surgical prophylaxis:
I.V.: 1.5 g 30 minutes to 1 hour prior to procedure (if procedure is prolonged can give 750 mg every 8 hours I.M.)
Open heart: I.V.: 1.5 g every 12 hours to a total of 6 g
Urinary tract infection (uncomplicated):
Oral: 125-250 mg every 12 hours for 7-10 days
I.M., I.V.: 750 mg every 8 hours
Dosing adjustment in renal impairment:
Cl_{cr} 10-20 mL/minute: Administer every 12 hours
Cl_{cr} <10 mL/minute: Administer every 24 hours
Hemodialysis: Dialyzable (25%)
Peritoneal dialysis: Dose every 24 hours
Continuous renal replacement therapy (CRRT): 1 g every 12 hours

Stability
Injection: Reconstituted solution is stable for 24 hours at room temperature and 48 hours when refrigerated. I.V. infusion in NS or D_5W solution is stable for 24 hours at room temperature, 7 days when refrigerated, or 26 weeks when frozen. After freezing, thawed solution is stable for 24 hours at room temperature or 21 days when refrigerated.
Oral suspension: Prior to reconstitution, store at 2°C to 30°C (36°F to 86°F). Reconstituted suspension is stable for 10 days at 2°C to 8°C (36°F to 46°F).
Tablet: Store at 15°C to 30°C (59°F to 86°F).

Administration
Oral suspension: Administer with food. Shake well before use.
I.M.: Inject deep I.M. into large muscle mass.
I.V.: Inject direct I.V. over 3-5 minutes. Infuse intermittent infusion over 15-30 minutes.

Monitoring Parameters Observe for signs and symptoms of anaphylaxis during first dose; with prolonged therapy, monitor renal, hepatic, and hematologic function periodically; monitor prothrombin time in patients at risk of prolongation during cephalosporin therapy (nutritionally-deficient, prolonged treatment, renal or hepatic disease)

Anesthesia and Critical Care Concerns/Other Considerations
Evidence-Based Information: Surgical prophylaxis: Cefuroxime should be avoided in patients with a history of serious beta-lactam allergy (eg, respiratory difficulty, angioedema, hives, hypotension). Examples of beta-lactam antibiotics include penicillin, ampicillin, piperacillin, and cephalosporins (Bratzler, 2004).

Pregnancy Risk Factor B

Contraindications Hypersensitivity to cefuroxime, any component of the formulation, or other cephalosporins

Warnings/Precautions Modify dosage in patients with severe renal impairment. Use with caution in patients with a history of penicillin allergy, especially IgE-mediated reactions (eg, anaphylaxis, urticaria). Prolonged use may result in fungal or bacterial superinfection, including *C. difficile*-associated diarrhea (CDAD) and pseudomembranous colitis; CDAD has been observed >2 months postantibiotic treatment. May be associated with increased INR, especially in nutritionally-deficient patients, prolonged treatment, hepatic or renal disease. Tablets and oral suspension are not bioequivalent (do not substitute on a mg-per-mg basis). Some products may contain phenylalanine.

Adverse Reactions

>10%: Gastrointestinal: Diarrhea (4% to 11%, duration-dependent)

1% to 10%:

Dermatologic: Diaper rash (3%)

Endocrine & metabolic: Alkaline phosphatase increased (2%), lactate dehydrogenase increased (1%)

Gastrointestinal: Nausea/vomiting (3% to 7%)

Genitourinary: Vaginitis (≤5%)

Hematologic: Eosinophilia (7%), hemoglobin and hematocrit decreased (10%)

Hepatic: Transaminases increased (2% to 4%)

Local: Thrombophlebitis (2%)

<1% (Limited to important or life-threatening): Anaphylaxis, angioedema, BUN increased, chest pain, cholestasis, colitis, creatinine increased, dyspnea, erythema multiforme, fever, GI bleeding, hemolytic anemia, hepatitis, hives, hyperbilirubinemia, hypersensitivity, interstitial nephritis, jaundice, leukopenia, neutropenia, pain at injection site, pancytopenia, positive Coombs test, prolonged PT/INR, pseudomembranous colitis, rash, renal dysfunction, seizure, Stevens-Johnson syndrome, stomach cramps, tachycardia, thrombocytopenia (rare), tongue swelling, toxic epidermal necrolysis, urticaria

Reactions reported with other cephalosporins: Agranulocytosis, aplastic anemia, asterixis, colitis, encephalopathy, hemorrhage, neuromuscular excitability, serum-sickness reactions, superinfection, toxic nephropathy

Drug Interactions

Avoid Concomitant Use There are no known interactions where it is recommended to avoid concomitant use.

Increased Effect/Toxicity

The levels/effects of Cefuroxime may be increased by: Uricosuric Agents

Decreased Effect

Cefuroxime may decrease the levels/effects of: Typhoid Vaccine

The levels/effects of Cefuroxime may be decreased by: Antacids; H2-Antagonists

Ethanol/Nutrition/Herb Interactions Food: Bioavailability is increased with food; cefuroxime serum levels may be increased if taken with food or dairy products.

Test Interactions Positive direct Coombs', false-positive urinary glucose test using cupric sulfate (Benedict's solution, Clinitest®, Fehling's solution); false-negative may occur with ferricyanide test. Glucose oxidase or hexokinase-based methods should be used.

Dietary Considerations Some products may contain phenylalanine and/or sodium.

Oral suspension: May be taken with food.

Dosage Forms Excipient information presented when available (limited, particularly for generics); consult specific product labeling.

Note: Strength expressed as base

Infusion, as sodium [premixed]: 750 mg (50 mL); 1.5 g (50 mL)

Zinacef®: 750 mg (50 mL); 1.5 g (50 mL) [contains sodium 4.8 mEq (111 mg) per 750 mg]

Injection, powder for reconstitution, as sodium: 750 mg, 1.5 g, 7.5 g, 75 g, 225 g

Zinacef®: 750 mg, 1.5 g, 7.5 g [contains sodium 1.8 mEq (41 mg) per 750 mg]

Powder for suspension, oral, as axetil: 125 mg/5 mL (100 mL); 250 mg/5 mL (50 mL, 100 mL)

Ceftin®: 125 mg/5 mL (100 mL) [contains phenylalanine 11.8 mg/5 mL; tutti-frutti flavor]; 250 mg/5 mL (50 mL, 100 mL) [contains phenylalanine 25.2 mg/5 mL; tutti-frutti flavor]

Tablet, as axetil: 250 mg, 500 mg

Ceftin®: 250 mg, 500 mg

References

Bratzler DW, Houck PM, Surgical Infection Prevention Guidelines Writers Workgroup, et al, "Antimicrobial Prophylaxis for Surgery: An Advisory Statement From the National Surgical Infection Prevention Project," *Clin Infect Dis*, 2004, 38(12):1706-15.

Mandell LA, Wunderink RG, Anzueto A, et al, "Infectious Diseases Society of America/American Thoracic Society Consensus Guidelines on the Management of Community-Acquired Pneumonia in Adults," *Clin Infect Dis*, 2007, 44(Suppl 2):27-72.

Celecoxib (se le KOKS ib)

Medication Safety Issues
Sound-alike/look-alike issues:
Celebrex® may be confused with Celexa®, cerebra, Cerebyx®, Cervarix®, Clarinex®

Medication Guide An FDA-approved patient medication guide, which is available with the product information and at http://www.fda.gov/downloads/Drugs/DrugSafety/ucm088567.pdf, must be dispensed with this medication for each new outpatient prescription and refill.

Related Information
Acetaminophen and NSAIDS, Dosing in the Management of Pain *on page 1651*
Acute Postoperative Pain *on page 1502*
Nonsteroidal Anti-Inflammatory Agents *on page 1687*

U.S. Brand Names Celebrex®

Canadian Brand Names Celebrex®; GD-Celecoxib

Pharmacologic Category Nonsteroidal Anti-inflammatory Drug (NSAID), COX-2 Selective

Generic Available No

Use Relief of the signs and symptoms of osteoarthritis, ankylosing spondylitis, juvenile rheumatoid arthritis (JRA), and rheumatoid arthritis; management of acute pain; treatment of primary dysmenorrhea; to reduce the number of intestinal polyps in familial adenomatous polyposis (FAP)

Canadian note: Celecoxib is only indicated for relief of symptoms of rheumatoid arthritis, osteoarthritis, and relief of acute pain in adults

Mechanism of Action Inhibits prostaglandin synthesis by decreasing the activity of the enzyme, cyclooxygenase-2 (COX-2), which results in decreased formation of prostaglandin precursors; has antipyretic, analgesic, and anti-inflammatory properties. Celecoxib does not inhibit cyclooxygenase-1 (COX-1) at therapeutic concentrations.

Pharmacodynamics/Kinetics
Distribution: V_d (apparent): ~400 L
Protein binding: ~97% primarily to albumin
Metabolism: Hepatic via CYP2C9; forms inactive metabolites
Bioavailability: Absolute: Unknown
Half-life elimination: ~11 hours (fasted)
Time to peak: ~3 hours
Excretion: Feces (~57% as metabolites, <3% as unchanged drug); urine (27% as metabolites, <3% as unchanged drug)

Dosage Note: Use the lowest effective dose for the shortest duration of time, consistent with individual patient goals. Oral:
Children ≥2 years: JRA
≥10 kg to ≤25 kg: 50 mg twice daily
>25 kg: 100 mg twice daily
Adults:
Acute pain or primary dysmenorrhea: Initial dose: 400 mg, followed by an additional 200 mg if needed on day 1; maintenance dose: 200 mg twice daily as needed
Ankylosing spondylitis: 200 mg/day as a single dose or in divided doses twice daily; if no effect after 6 weeks, may increase to 400 mg/day. If no response following 6 weeks of treatment with 400 mg/day, consider discontinuation and alternative treatment.
Familial adenomatous polyposis: 400 mg twice daily (with food)
Osteoarthritis: 200 mg/day as a single dose or in divided dose twice daily
Rheumatoid arthritis: 100-200 mg twice daily

Elderly: No specific adjustment based on age is recommended. However, the AUC in elderly patients may be increased by 50% as compared to younger subjects. Initiate at the lowest recommended dose in patients weighing <50 kg.

Dosing adjustment in poor CYP2C9 metabolizers: Consider reducing initial dose by 50%; consider alternative treatment in patients with JRA who are poor CYP2C9 metabolizers

Dosing adjustment in renal impairment:
Advanced renal disease: Use is not recommended, however, if celecoxib treatment cannot be avoided, monitor renal function closely
Severe renal insufficiency: Use is not recommended
Abnormal renal function tests (persistent or worsening): Discontinue use

Dosing adjustment in hepatic impairment:
Moderate hepatic impairment (Child-Pugh class B): Reduce dose by 50%
Severe hepatic impairment: Use is not recommended
Abnormal liver function tests (persistent or worsening): Discontinue use

Stability Store at controlled room temperature of 25°C (77°F); excursions permitted to 15°C to 30°C (59°F to 86°F).

Administration Lower doses (200 mg twice daily) may be taken without regard to meals. Larger doses (400 mg twice daily) should be taken with food to improve absorption. Capsules may be swallowed whole or the entire contents emptied onto a teaspoon of cool or room temperature applesauce. The contents of the capsules sprinkled onto applesauce may be stored under refrigeration for up to 6 hours.

Monitoring Parameters CBC; blood chemistry profile; occult blood loss and periodic liver function tests; monitor renal function (urine output, serum BUN and creatinine; monitor response (pain, range of motion, grip strength, mobility, ADL function), inflammation; observe for weight gain, edema; observe for bleeding, bruising; evaluate gastrointestinal effects (abdominal pain, bleeding, dyspepsia); blood pressure

FAP: Continue routine endoscopic exams
JRA: Monitor for development of abnormal coagulation tests with systemic onset JRA

Anesthesia and Critical Care Concerns/Other Considerations
Clinical Pearls/Comments: Celecoxib does not inhibit platelets or prolong bleeding time.

Pregnancy Risk Factor C (prior to 30 weeks gestation)/D (≥30 weeks gestation)

Contraindications Hypersensitivity to celecoxib, sulfonamides, aspirin, other NSAIDs, or any component of the formulation; perioperative pain in the setting of coronary artery bypass graft (CABG) surgery
Canadian labeling: Additional contraindications (not in U.S. labeling): Pregnancy (3rd trimester); women who are breast-feeding; severe, uncontrolled heart failure; active gastrointestinal ulcer (gastric, duodenal, peptic) or bleeding; inflammatory bowel disease; cerebrovascular bleeding; severe liver impairment or active hepatic disease; severe renal impairment (Cl_{cr} <30 mL/minute) or deteriorating renal disease; known hyperkalemia; use in children

Warnings/Precautions [U.S. Boxed Warning]: NSAIDs are associated with an increased risk of adverse cardiovascular thrombotic events, including MI and stroke. Risk may be increased with duration of use or pre-existing cardiovascular risk factors or disease. Carefully evaluate individual cardiovascular risk profiles prior to prescribing. New-onset or worsening of pre-existing hypertension may occur. May cause sodium and fluid retention; use with caution in patients with edema, cerebrovascular disease, or ischemic heart disease. Avoid use in heart failure. Long-term cardiovascular risk in children has not been evaluated.

[U.S. Boxed Warning]: Celecoxib is contraindicated for treatment of perioperative pain in the setting of coronary artery bypass graft (CABG) surgery. Risk of MI and stroke may be increased with use following CABG surgery.

[U.S. Boxed Warning]: NSAIDs may increase risk of gastrointestinal irritation, ulceration, bleeding, and perforation. These events may occur at any time during therapy and without warning. Use caution with a history of GI disease (bleeding or ulcers), concurrent therapy with aspirin, anticoagulants and/ or corticosteroids, smoking, use of alcohol, the elderly or debilitated patients. When used concomitantly with ≤325 mg of aspirin, a substantial increase in the risk of gastrointestinal complications (eg, ulcer) occurs; concomitant gastro-protective therapy (eg, proton pump inhibitors) is recommended (Bhatt, 2008).

Use the lowest effective dose for the shortest duration of time, consistent with individual patient goals, to reduce risk of cardiovascular or GI adverse events. Alternate therapies should be considered for patients at high risk.

NSAIDs may cause serious skin adverse events including exfoliative dermatitis, Stevens-Johnson syndrome (SJS), and toxic epidermal necrolysis (TEN). Anaphylactoid reactions may occur, even without prior exposure; patients with "aspirin triad" (bronchial asthma, aspirin intolerance, rhinitis) may be at increased risk. Do not use in patients who experience bronchospasm, asthma, rhinitis, or urticaria with NSAID or aspirin therapy. Use caution in other forms of asthma.

Use with caution in patients with decreased hepatic (dosage adjustments are recommended for moderate hepatic impairment; not recommended for patients with severe hepatic impairment) or renal function. Transaminase elevations have been reported with use; closely monitor patients with any abnormal LFT. Severe hepatic reactions (eg, fulminant hepatitis, liver failure) have occurred with NSAID use, rarely; discontinue if signs or symptoms of liver disease develop, if systemic manifestations occur, or with persistent or worsening abnormal hepatic function tests. NSAID use may compromise existing renal function; dose-dependent decreases in prostaglandin synthesis may result from NSAID use, causing a reduction in renal blood flow which may cause renal decompensation. Patients with impaired renal function, dehydration, heart failure, liver dysfunction, those taking diuretics and ACEI, and the elderly are at greater risk for renal toxicity. Rehydrate patient before starting therapy; monitor renal function closely. Not recommended for use in patients with advanced renal disease or severe renal insufficiency; discontinue use with persistent or worsening abnormal renal function tests. Long-term NSAID use may result in renal papillary necrosis.

Anaphylactoid reactions may occur, even with no prior exposure to celecoxib. Use with caution in patients with known or suspected deficiency of cytochrome P450 isoenzyme 2C9; poor metabolizers may have higher plasma levels due to reduced metabolism; consider reduced initial doses. Alternate therapies should be considered in patients with JRA who are poor metabolizers of CYP2C9.

Anemia may occur with use; monitor hemoglobin or hematocrit in patients on long-term treatment. Celecoxib does not affect PT, PTT or platelet counts; does not inhibit platelet aggregation at approved doses.

When used for the treatment of FAP, routine monitoring and care should be continued. When used for JRA, celecoxib is not FDA-approved in children <2 years of age or in children <10 kg. Use caution with systemic onset JRA (may be at risk for disseminated intravascular coagulation). Safety and efficacy have not been established for use in children for indications other than JRA.

Adverse Reactions

>10%:

Cardiovascular: Hypertension (≤13%)

Central nervous system: Headache (10% to 16%)

Gastrointestinal: Diarrhea (4% to 11%)

2% to 10%:

Cardiovascular: Peripheral edema (2%)

Central nervous system: Fever (≤9%), insomnia (2%), dizziness (1% to 2%)

Dermatologic: Skin rash (2%)

Gastrointestinal: Dyspepsia (9%), nausea (4% to 7%), gastroesophageal reflux (≤5%), abdominal pain (4% to 8%), vomiting (≤6%), flatulence (2%)

Neuromuscular & skeletal: Arthralgia (≤7%), back pain (3%)

Respiratory: Upper respiratory tract infection (8%), cough (≤7%), nasophar-yngitis (≤6%), sinusitis (5%), dyspnea (≤3%), pharyngitis (2%), rhinitis (2%)

Miscellaneous: Accidental injury (3%)

0.1% to 2%:

Cardiovascular: Angina, aortic valve incompetence, chest pain, coronary artery disorder, DVT, edema, facial edema, hypertension (aggravated), MI, palpitation, sinus bradycardia, tachycardia, ventricular hypertrophy

Central nervous system: Anxiety, cerebral infarction, depression, fatigue, hypoesthesia, migraine, nervousness, pain, somnolence, vertigo

Dermatologic: Alopecia, bruising, cellulitis, dermatitis, dry skin, nail disorder, photosensitivity, pruritus, rash (erythematous), rash (maculopapular), urticaria

Endocrine & metabolic: Breast fibroadenosis, breast neoplasm, breast pain, diabetes mellitus, dysmenorrhea, hot flashes, hypercholesterolemia, hyperglycemia, hyper-/hypokalemia, hypernatremia, menstrual disturbances, ovarian cyst, testosterone decreased

Gastrointestinal: Anorexia, appetite increased, constipation, diverticulitis, dysphagia, eructation, esophagitis, gastritis, gastroenteritis, gastrointestinal ulcer, hemorrhoids, hiatal hernia, melena, stomatitis, taste disturbance, tenesmus, tooth disorder, weight gain, xerostomia

Genitourinary: Cystitis, dysuria, incontinence, monilial vaginitis, prostate disorder, urinary frequency, urinary tract infection, vaginal bleeding, vaginitis

Hematologic: Anemia, thrombocytopenia

Hepatic: Alkaline phosphatase increased, transaminases increased

Neuromuscular & skeletal: Arthrosis, bone disorder, CPK increased, fracture, hypertonia, leg cramps, myalgia, neck stiffness, neuralgia, neuropathy, paresthesia, synovitis, tendon rupture, tendonitis, weakness

Ocular: Blurred vision, cataract, conjunctival hemorrhage, conjunctivitis, eye pain, glaucoma, vitreous floaters

Otic: Deafness, earache, labyrinthitis, otitis media, tinnitus

Renal: Albuminuria, BUN increased, creatinine increased, hematuria, nonprotein nitrogen increased, renal calculi

Respiratory: Bronchitis, bronchospasm, epistaxis, laryngitis, pneumonia

Miscellaneous: Allergic reactions, allergy aggravated, diaphoresis, flu-like syndrome, herpes infection, infection (bacterial, fungal, viral), moniliasis

<0.1% (Limited to important or life-threatening): Acute renal failure, agranulocytosis, anaphylactoid reactions, angioedema, aplastic anemia, aseptic meningitis, ataxia, cerebrovascular accident, CHF, cholelithiasis, colitis, erythema multiforme, esophageal perforation, exfoliative dermatitis, gangrene, gastrointestinal bleeding, hepatic failure, hepatic necrosis, hepatitis (including fulminant), hypoglycemia, hyponatremia, ileus, interstitial nephritis, intestinal obstruction, intestinal perforation, intracranial hemorrhage, jaundice, leukopenia, pancreatitis, pancytopenia, pulmonary embolism, renal papillary necrosis, sepsis, Stevens-Johnson syndrome, sudden death, suicide, syncope, thrombophlebitis, toxic epidermal necrolysis, vasculitis, ventricular fibrillation

Drug Interactions

Metabolism/Transport Effects Substrate of CYP2C9 (major), 3A4 (minor); Inhibits CYP2C8 (moderate), 2D6 (weak)

Avoid Concomitant Use

Avoid concomitant use of Celecoxib with any of the following: Ketorolac; Thioridazine

Increased Effect/Toxicity

Celecoxib may increase the levels/effects of: Aminoglycosides; Anticoagulants; Antiplatelet Agents; Bisphosphonate Derivatives; CycloSPORINE; CYP2C8 Substrates (High risk); CYP2D6 Substrates; Desmopressin; Eplerenone; Fesoterodine; Lithium; Methotrexate; Nebivolol; Nonsteroidal Anti-Inflammatory Agents; Potassium-Sparing Diuretics; Pralatrexate; Quinolone Antibiotics; Tamoxifen; Thioridazine; Thrombolytic Agents; Vancomycin; Vitamin K Antagonists

The levels/effects of Celecoxib may be increased by: Antidepressants (Tricyclic, Tertiary Amine); Corticosteroids (Systemic); CYP2C9 Inhibitors (Moderate); CYP2C9 Inhibitors (Strong); Herbs (Anticoagulant/Antiplatelet Properties); Ketorolac; Probenecid; Selective Serotonin Reuptake Inhibitors; Treprostinil

◄ **Decreased Effect**

Celecoxib may decrease the levels/effects of: ACE Inhibitors; Angiotensin II Receptor Blockers; Antiplatelet Agents; Beta-Blockers; Codeine; Eplerenone; HydrALAZINE; Loop Diuretics; Potassium-Sparing Diuretics; Thiazide Diuretics; TraMADol

The levels/effects of Celecoxib may be decreased by: Bile Acid Sequestrants; CYP2C9 Inducers (Highly Effective); Peginterferon Alfa-2b

Ethanol/Nutrition/Herb Interactions

Ethanol: Avoid ethanol (increased GI irritation).

Food: Peak concentrations are delayed and AUC is increased by 10% to 20% when taken with a high-fat meal.

Herb/Nutraceutical: Avoid concomitant use with herbs possessing anticoagulation/antiplatelet properties, including alfalfa, anise, bilberry, bladderwrack, bromelain, cat's claw, celery, chamomile, coleus, cordyceps, dong quai, evening primrose, fenugreek, feverfew, garlic, ginger, ginkgo biloba, ginseng (American, Panax, Siberian), grapeseed, green tea, guggul, horse chestnuts, horseradish, licorice, prickly ash, red clover, reishi, SAMe (S-adenosylmethionine), sweet clover, turmeric, white willow.

Dietary Considerations Lower doses (200 mg twice daily) may be taken without regard to meals. Larger doses (400 mg twice daily) should be taken with food to improve absorption.

Dosage Forms Excipient information presented when available (limited, particularly for generics); consult specific product labeling.

Capsule:

Celebrex®: 50 mg, 100 mg, 200 mg, 400 mg

References

Solomon SD, McMurray JJ, Pfeffer MA, et al, "Cardiovascular Risk Associated With Celecoxib in a Clinical Trial for Colorectal Adenoma Prevention," *N Engl J Med*, 2005, 352(11):1071-80.

◆ **Celestone®** see Betamethasone *on page 186*

◆ **Celestone® Soluspan®** see Betamethasone *on page 186*

◆ **CellCept®** see Mycophenolate *on page 966*

Cellulose (Oxidized Regenerated)
(SEL yoo lose, OKS i dyzed re JEN er aye ted)

Medication Safety Issues

Sound-alike/look-alike issues:

Surgicel® may be confused with Serentil®

U.S. Brand Names Surgicel®; Surgicel® Fibrillar; Surgicel® NuKnit

Index Terms Absorbable Cotton; Oxidized Regenerated Cellulose

Pharmacologic Category Hemostatic Agent

Generic Available No

Use Hemostatic; temporary packing for the control of capillary, venous, or small arterial hemorrhage

Mechanism of Action Cellulose, oxidized regenerated is saturated with blood at the bleeding site and swells into a brownish or black gelatinous mass which aids in the formation of a clot. When used in small amounts, it is absorbed from the sites of implantation with little or no tissue reaction. In addition to providing hemostasis, oxidized regenerated cellulose also has been shown *in vitro* to have bactericidal properties.

Pharmacodynamics/Kinetics Absorption: 7-14 days

Dosage Minimal amounts of the fabric strip are laid on the bleeding site or held firmly against the tissues until hemostasis occurs; remove excess material

Stability Store at controlled room temperature. Inactivated by autoclaving; do not resterilize. Do not use if package is damaged. Do not reuse after opening.

Pregnancy Risk Factor No data reported

Contraindications Hypersensitivity to any component of the formulation; implantation into bone defects; hemorrhage from large arteries; nonhemorrhagic oozing; use as an adhesion product

Warnings/Precautions Pain, numbness, or paralysis have been reported if used near a bony or neural space and left inside patient; use minimum amount necessary to achieve hemostasis. Remove as much of agent as possible after hemostasis is achieved. Do not leave in a contaminated or infected space. Always remove completely following hemostasis if applied in proximity to foramina in bone, areas of bony confine, the spinal cord or optic nerve and chasm; product may swell and exert unwanted pressure. The material should not be moistened before insertion since the hemostatic effect is greater when applied dry. The material should not be impregnated with anti-infective agents. Its hemostatic effect is not enhanced by the addition of thrombin.

Adverse Reactions Frequency not defined.

Central nervous system: Headache

Respiratory: Nasal burning or stinging, sneezing (rhinological procedures)

Miscellaneous: Encapsulation of fluid, foreign body reactions (with or without) infection

Postmarketing and/or case reports: Numbness, pain, paralysis

Drug Interactions

Avoid Concomitant Use There are no known interactions where it is recommended to avoid concomitant use.

Increased Effect/Toxicity There are no known significant interactions involving an increase in effect.

Decreased Effect There are no known significant interactions involving a decrease in effect.

Dosage Forms Excipient information presented when available (limited, particularly for generics); consult specific product labeling.

Fabric, fibrous (Surgicel® Fibrillar):
1" x 2" (10s)
2" x 4" (10s)
4" x 4" (10s)

Fabric, knitted (Surgicel® NuKnit):
1" x 1" (24s)
1" x 3½" (10s)
3" x 4" (24s)
6" x 9" (10s)

Fabric, sheer weave (Surgicel®):
½" x 2" (24s)
2" x 3" (24s)
2" x 14" (24s)
4" x 8" (24s)

◆ **Celluvisc™ (Can)** *see* Carboxymethylcellulose *on page 243*

◆ **Ceprotin** *see* Protein C Concentrate (Human) *on page 1208*

◆ **Cerebyx®** *see* Fosphenytoin *on page 638*

Certolizumab Pegol (cer to LIZ u mab PEG ol)

U.S. Brand Names Cimzia®
Canadian Brand Names Cimzia®
Index Terms CDP870

Pharmacologic Category Antirheumatic, Disease Modifying; Gastrointestinal Agent, Miscellaneous; Tumor Necrosis Factor (TNF) Blocking Agent

Use Treatment of moderately- to severely-active Crohn's disease in patients who have inadequate response to conventional therapy; moderately- to severely-active rheumatoid arthritis (as monotherapy or in combination with nonbiological disease-modifying antirheumatic drugs [DMARDS])

Pharmacodynamics/Kinetics
Distribution: V_{ss}: 6-8 L
Bioavailability: SubQ: ~80% (range: 76% to 88%)
Half-life elimination: ~14 days
Time to peak, plasma: 54-171 hours

◄ **Dosage Note:** Each 400 mg dose should be administered as 2 injections of 200 mg each

SubQ: Adults:

Crohn's disease: Initial: 400 mg, repeat dose 2 and 4 weeks after initial dose; Maintenance: 400 mg every 4 weeks

Rheumatoid arthritis: Initial: 400 mg, repeat dose 2 and 4 weeks after initial dose; Maintenance: 200 mg every other week. May consider maintenance dose of 400 mg every 4 weeks.

Dosing adjustment in renal impairment: Moderate-to-severe renal impairment: The pharmacokinetics of the pegylated (polyethylene glycol) component may be dependent on renal function; however, data is insufficient to provide a dosing recommendation.

Additional Information Complete prescribing information for this medication should be consulted for additional detail.

Dosage Forms Excipient information presented when available (limited, particularly for generics); consult specific product labeling.

Injection, powder for reconstitution [preservative free]:

Cimzia®: 200 mg [contains sucrose 100 mg]

Injection, solution [preservative-free]:

Cimzia®: 200 mg/mL (1 mL)

References

Rutgeerts P, Schreiber S, Feagan B, et al, "Certolizumab Pegol, a Monthly Subcutaneously Administered Fc-Free Anti-TNFalpha, Improves Health-Related Quality of Life in Patients With Moderate to Severe Crohn's Disease," *Int J Colorectal Dis*, 2008, 23(3):289-96.

Sandborn WJ, Feagan BG, Stoinov S, et al, "Certolizumab Pegol for the Treatment of Crohn's Disease," *N Engl J Med*, 2007, 357(3):228-38.

Schreiber S, Khaliq-Kareemi M, Lawrence IC, et al, "Maintenance Therapy With Certolizumab Pegol for Crohn's Disease," *N Engl J Med*, 2007, 357(3):239-50.

Schreiber S, Rutgeerts P, Fedorak RN, et al, "A Randomized, Placebo-Controlled Trial of Certolizumab Pegol (CDP870) for Treatment of Crohn's Disease," *Gastroenterology*, 2005, 129 (3):807-18.

◆ **C.E.S.** *see* Estrogens (Conjugated/Equine) *on page 534*

◆ **C.E.S.® (Can)** *see* Estrogens (Conjugated/Equine) *on page 534*

◆ **Cesia™** *see* Ethinyl Estradiol and Desogestrel *on page 544*

◆ **Cetacort® [DSC]** *see* Hydrocortisone *on page 699*

◆ **Cetafen® [OTC]** *see* Acetaminophen *on page 25*

◆ **Cetafen® Extra [OTC]** *see* Acetaminophen *on page 25*

Cetirizine (se TI ra zeen)

U.S. Brand Names All Day Allergy; Zyrtec® Allergy [OTC]; Zyrtec® Children's Allergy [OTC]; Zyrtec® Children's Hives Relief [OTC]

Canadian Brand Names Apo-Cetirizine®; PMS-Cetirizine; Reactine™

Index Terms Cetirizine Hydrochloride; P-071; UCB-P071

Pharmacologic Category Histamine H_1 Antagonist; Histamine H_1 Antagonist, Second Generation

Use Perennial and seasonal allergic rhinitis and other allergic symptoms including urticaria; chronic idiopathic urticaria

Pharmacodynamics/Kinetics

Onset of action: 15-30 minutes

Absorption: Rapid

Protein binding, plasma: Mean: 93%

Metabolism: Limited hepatic

Half-life elimination: 8 hours

Time to peak, serum: 1 hour

Excretion: Urine (70%); feces (10%)

Dosage Oral:

Children:

6-12 months: Chronic urticaria, perennial allergic rhinitis: 2.5 mg once daily

12 months to <2 years: Chronic urticaria, perennial allergic rhinitis: 2.5 mg once daily; may increase to 2.5 mg every 12 hours if needed

2-5 years: Chronic urticaria, perennial or seasonal allergic rhinitis: Initial: 2.5 mg once daily; may be increased to 2.5 mg every 12 hours **or** 5 mg once daily

Children ≥6 years and Adults: Chronic urticaria, perennial or seasonal allergic rhinitis: 5-10 mg once daily, depending upon symptom severity

Elderly: Initial: 5 mg once daily; may increase to 10 mg/day. **Note:** Manufacturer recommends 5 mg/day in patients ≥77 years of age.

Dosage adjustment in renal/hepatic impairment:
Children <6 years: Cetirizine use not recommended
Children 6-11 years: <2.5 mg once daily
Children ≥12 and Adults:
Cl_{cr} 11-31 mL/minute, hemodialysis, or hepatic impairment: Administer 5 mg once daily
Cl_{cr} <11 mL/minute, not on dialysis: Cetirizine use not recommended

Additional Information Complete prescribing information for this medication should be consulted for additional detail.

Dosage Forms Excipient information presented when available (limited, particularly for generics); consult specific product labeling. [DSC] = Discontinued product

Syrup, oral, as hydrochloride: 5 mg/5 mL (118 mL, 120 mL, 473 mL, 480 mL)
Zyrtec® Children's Allergy: 5 mg/5 mL (15 mL [DSC]; 118 mL) [contains propylene glycol; grape flavor]
Zyrtec® Children's Allergy: 5 mg/5 mL (118 mL) [dye free, sugar free; contains propylene glycol, sodium benzoate; bubblegum flavor]
Zyrtec® Children's Hives Relief: 5 mg/5 mL (118 mL) [contains propylene glycol; grape flavor]
Tablet, oral, as hydrochloride: 5 mg, 10 mg
All Day Allergy: 10 mg
Zyrtec® Allergy: 10 mg
Tablet, chewable, as hydrochloride:
Zyrtec® Children's Allergy: 5 mg, 10 mg [grape flavor]

References

Allegra L, Paupe J, Wieseman HG, et al, "Cetirizine for Seasonal Allergic Rhinitis in Children Aged 2-6 Years. A Double-Blind Comparison With Placebo," *Pediatr Allergy Immunol*, 1993; 4:157-61.
Barnes CL, McKenzie CA, Webster KD, et al, "Cetirizine: A New, Nonsedating Antihistamine," *Ann Pharmacother*, 1993; 27:464-70.
Kaiser HB, "Cetirizine in Allergic Rhinitis," *Pediatr Allergy Immunol*, 1993; 4(Suppl):44-6.
Ramaekers JG, Uiterwijk MM, and O'Hanlon J, "Effects of Loratadine and Cetirizine on Actual Driving and Psychometric Test Performance, and EEG During Driving," *Eur J Clin Pharmacol*, 1992; 42:363-9.

◆ **Cetirizine Hydrochloride** *see* Cetirizine *on page 282*

◆ **Cetraxal®** *see* Ciprofloxacin *on page 306*

◆ **CFDN** *see* Cefdinir *on page 252*

◆ **CG5503** *see* Tapentadol *on page 1350*

◆ **CGP 33101** *see* Rufinamide *on page 1271*

◆ **Charcadole® (Can)** *see* Charcoal *on page 283*

◆ **Charcadole®, Aqueous (Can)** *see* Charcoal *on page 283*

◆ **Charcadole® TFS (Can)** *see* Charcoal *on page 283*

◆ **Char-Caps [OTC]** *see* Charcoal *on page 283*

◆ **CharcoAid® G [OTC]** *see* Charcoal *on page 283*

Charcoal (CHAR kole AK tiv ay ted)

Medication Safety Issues
Sound-alike/look-alike issues:
Actidose® may be confused with Actos®

U.S. Brand Names Actidose-Aqua® [OTC]; Actidose® with Sorbitol [OTC]; Char-Caps [OTC]; CharcoAid® G [OTC]; Charcoal Plus® DS [OTC]; CharcoCaps® [OTC]; EZ-Char™ [OTC]; Kerr Insta-Char® [OTC]; Requa® Activated Charcoal [OTC]

Canadian Brand Names Charcadole®; Charcadole® TFS; Charcadole®, Aqueous

Index Terms Activated Carbon; Activated Charcoal; Adsorbent Charcoal; Liquid Antidote; Medicinal Carbon; Medicinal Charcoal

◀ **Pharmacologic Category** Antidote
Generic Available Yes: Powder
Use Emergency treatment in poisoning by drugs and chemicals; aids the elimination of certain drugs and improves decontamination of excessive ingestions of sustained-release products or in the presence of bezoars; repetitive doses have proven useful to enhance the elimination of certain drugs (eg, carbamazepine, dapsone, phenobarbital, quinine, or theophylline); repetitive doses for gastric dialysis in uremia to adsorb various waste products; dietary supplement (digestive aid)

Mechanism of Action Adsorbs toxic substances or irritants, thus inhibiting GI absorption; adsorbs intestinal gas; the addition of sorbitol results in hyperosmotic laxative action causing catharsis

Pharmacodynamics/Kinetics Excretion: Feces (as charcoal)

Dosage Oral:
Acute poisoning: **Note:** ~10 g of activated charcoal for each 1 g of toxin is considered adequate; this may require multiple doses. If sorbitol is also used, sorbitol dose should not exceed 1.5 g/kg. When using multiple doses of charcoal, sorbitol should be given with every other dose (not to exceed 2 doses/day).
Children:
<1 year: 0.5-1 g/kg (10-25 g) as a single dose; if multiple doses are needed, give as 0.25 g/kg/hour or equivalent (eg, 0.5 g/kg every 2 hours)
1-12 years: 0.5-1 g/kg (25-50 g) as a single dose; if multiple doses are needed, give as 0.25 g/kg/hour or equivalent (eg, 0.5 g/kg every 2 hours)
Children >12 years and Adults: 25-100 g as a single dose; if multiple doses are needed, additional doses may be given as 12.5 g/hour or equivalent (eg, 25 g every 2 hours)
Dietary supplement: Adult: 500-520 mg after meals; may repeat in 2 hours if needed (maximum: 10 g/day)

Stability Adsorbs gases from air, store in closed container. Dilute powder with at least 8 mL of water per 1 g of charcoal, or mix in a charcoal to water ratio of 1:4 to 1:8. Mix to form a slurry.

Administration Flavoring agents (eg, chocolate, concentrated fruit juice) or thickening agents (eg, bentonite, carboxymethylcellulose) can enhance charcoal's palatability. If treatment includes ipecac syrup, induce vomiting prior to administration of charcoal. Often given with a laxative or cathartic; check for presence of bowel sounds before administration. I.V. antiemetics may be required to reduce the risk of vomiting during multiple-dose therapy with charcoal.

Pregnancy Risk Factor C

Contraindications Hypersensitivity to charcoal or any component of the formulation; intestinal obstruction; GI tract not anatomically intact; patients at risk of hemorrhage or GI perforation; patients with an unprotected airway (eg, CNS depression without intubation); if use would increase risk and severity of aspiration

Warnings/Precautions When using ipecac with charcoal, ensure ipecac-induced vomiting has ceased prior to administering charcoal. Charcoal may cause vomiting; avoid in hydrocarbon and caustic ingestions. Use caution with decreased peristalsis. Coadministration of a cathartic (eg, sorbitol, mannitol, magnesium sulfate) is not recommended secondary to lack of compelling evidence and the increased morbidity associated with their use. If charcoal is administered with a cathartic, avoid excessive fluid and electrolyte losses, especially in children <1 year of age. Charcoal with sorbitol not recommended in children <1 year of age.

Not effective for cyanide, mineral acids, caustic alkalis, organic solvents, iron, ethanol, methanol, or lithium poisoning. Most effective when administered within 30-60 minutes of ingestion. Commercial charcoal products may contain propylene glycol.

Adverse Reactions Frequency not defined.
Endocrine & metabolic: Hypernatremia, hypokalemia, and hypermagnesemia may occur with coadministration of cathartics
Gastrointestinal: Vomiting (incidence may increase with sorbitol), diarrhea (with sorbitol), constipation, swelling of abdomen, bowel obstruction, appendicitis
Respiratory: Aspiration (both gastric contents and charcoal)
Miscellaneous: Fecal discoloration (black)

Drug Interactions

Avoid Concomitant Use There are no known interactions where it is recommended to avoid concomitant use.

Increased Effect/Toxicity There are no known significant interactions involving an increase in effect.

Decreased Effect

Charcoal, Activated may decrease the levels/effects of: Leflunomide

Ethanol/Nutrition/Herb Interactions Food: Do not mix with milk, ice cream, sherbet, or marmalade (may reduce charcoal's effectiveness).

Dosage Forms Excipient information presented when available (limited, particularly for generics); consult specific product labeling.

Capsule:
  Char-Caps, CharcoCaps®: 260 mg
Pellets, for suspension:
  EZ-Char™: 25 g
Powder for suspension: 30 g, 240 g
  CharcoAid® G: 15 g
Suspension:
  Actidose-Aqua®: 15 g (72 mL); 25 g (120 mL); 50 g (240 mL)
  Kerr Insta-Char®: 25 g (120 mL) [contains sodium benzoate; packaged with cherry flavor (cherry flavor contains propylene glycol and sodium benzoate)]; 50 g (240 mL) [contains sodium benzoate; unflavored or packaged with cherry flavor (cherry flavor contains propylene glycol and sodium benzoate)]
Suspension [with sorbitol]:
  Actidose® with Sorbitol: 25 g (120 mL); 50 g (240 mL)
  Kerr Insta-Char®: 25 g (120 mL) [contains sodium benzoate; packaged with cherry flavor (cherry flavor contains propylene glycol and sodium benzoate)]; 50 g (240 mL) [contains sodium benzoate; packaged with cherry flavor (cherry flavor contains propylene glycol and sodium benzoate)]
Tablet:
  Requa® Activated Charcoal: 250 mg
Tablet, enteric coated:
  Charcoal Plus® DS: 250 mg

References

Chyka PA, Seger D, Krenzelok EP, et al, American Academy of Clinical Toxicology; European Association of Poisons Centres and Clinical Toxicologists, "Position Paper: Single-Dose Activated Charcoal," *Clin Toxicol (Phila)*, 2005, 43(2):61-87 (review).

Vale JA, Krenzelok EP and Barceloux GD et al, American Academy of Clinical Toxicology; European Association of Poisons Centres and Clinical Toxicologists, "Position Statement and Practice Guidelines on the Use of Multiple-Dose Activated Charcoal in the Treatment of Acute Poisoning," *Clin Toxicol*, 1999, 37(6):731-51.

◆ **Charcoal Plus® DS [OTC]** *see* Charcoal *on page 283*

◆ **CharcoCaps® [OTC]** *see* Charcoal *on page 283*

◆ **CHG** *see* Chlorhexidine Gluconate *on page 291*

◆ **Chirocaine® [DSC]** *see* Levobupivacaine *on page 819*

◆ **Chirocaine® (Can)** *see* Levobupivacaine *on page 819*

◆ **Chloral** *see* Chloral Hydrate *on page 285*

Chloral Hydrate (KLOR al HYE drate)

Medication Safety Issues

High alert medication: The Institute for Safe Medication Practices (ISMP) includes this medication among its list of drugs which have a heightened risk of causing significant patient harm when used in error.

Related Information

Moderate Sedation *on page 1566*

U.S. Brand Names Aquachloral® Supprettes® [DSC]; Somnote®

Canadian Brand Names PMS-Chloral Hydrate

Index Terms Chloral; Hydrated Chloral; Trichloroacetaldehyde Monohydrate

Pharmacologic Category Hypnotic, Nonbenzodiazepine

Restrictions C-IV

◀ **Generic Available** Yes: Syrup and suppositories

Use Short-term sedative and hypnotic (<2 weeks); sedative/hypnotic for diagnostic procedures; sedative prior to EEG evaluations

Mechanism of Action Central nervous system depressant effects are due to its active metabolite trichloroethanol, mechanism unknown

Pharmacodynamics/Kinetics

Onset of action: Time to sleep: 0.5-1 hour

Duration: 4-8 hours

Absorption: Oral, rectal: Well absorbed

Distribution: Crosses placenta; negligible amounts enter breast milk

Metabolism: Rapidly hepatic to trichloroethanol (active metabolite); variable amounts hepatically and renally to trichloroacetic acid (inactive)

Half-life elimination: Active metabolite: 8-11 hours

Excretion: Urine (as metabolites); feces (small amounts)

Dosage

Children:

Sedation or anxiety: Oral, rectal: 5-15 mg/kg/dose every 8 hours (maximum: 500 mg/dose)

Prior to EEG: Oral, rectal: 20-25 mg/kg/dose, 30-60 minutes prior to EEG; may repeat in 30 minutes to maximum of 100 mg/kg or 2 g total

Hypnotic: Oral, rectal: 20-40 mg/kg/dose up to a maximum of 50 mg/kg/24 hours or 1 g/dose or 2 g/24 hours

Conscious sedation: Oral: 50-75 mg/kg/dose 30-60 minutes prior to procedure; may repeat 30 minutes after initial dose if needed, to a total maximum dose of 120 mg/kg or 1 g total

Adults: Oral, rectal:

Sedation, anxiety: 250 mg 3 times/day

Hypnotic: 500-1000 mg at bedtime or 30 minutes prior to procedure, not to exceed 2 g/24 hours

Discontinuation: Withdraw gradually over 2 weeks if patient has been maintained on high doses for prolonged period of time. Do not stop drug abruptly; sudden withdrawal may result in delirium.

Dosing adjustment/comments in renal impairment: Cl_{cr} <50 mL/minute: Avoid use

Hemodialysis: Dialyzable (50% to 100%); supplemental dose is not necessary

Dosing adjustment/comments in hepatic impairment: Avoid use in patients with severe hepatic impairment

Stability Sensitive to light. Exposure to air causes volatilization. Store in light-resistant, airtight container.

Administration Chilling the syrup may help to mask unpleasant taste. Do not crush capsule (contains drug in liquid form). Gastric irritation may be minimized by diluting dose in water or other oral liquid.

Monitoring Parameters Vital signs, O_2 saturation and blood pressure with doses used for conscious sedation

Pregnancy Risk Factor C

Contraindications Hypersensitivity to chloral hydrate or any component of the formulation; hepatic or renal impairment; gastritis or ulcers; severe cardiac disease

Warnings/Precautions Use with caution in patients with porphyria. Use with caution in neonates. Drug may accumulate with repeated use; prolonged use in neonates associated with hyperbilirubinemia. Tolerance to hypnotic effect develops, therefore, not recommended for use >2 weeks. Taper dosage to avoid withdrawal with prolonged use. Trichloroethanol (TCE), a metabolite of chloral hydrate, is a carcinogen in mice; there is no data in humans. Chloral hydrate is considered a second line hypnotic agent in the elderly. Recent interpretive guidelines from the Centers for Medicare and Medicaid Services (CMS) discourage the use of chloral hydrate in residents of long-term care facilities.

Adverse Reactions Frequency not defined.

Central nervous system: Ataxia, disorientation, sedation, excitement (paradoxical), dizziness, fever, headache, confusion, lightheadedness, nightmares, hallucinations, drowsiness, "hangover" effect

Dermatologic: Rash, urticaria

Gastrointestinal: Gastric irritation, nausea, vomiting, diarrhea, flatulence

Hematologic: Leukopenia, eosinophilia, acute intermittent porphyria

Miscellaneous: Physical and psychological dependence may occur with prolonged use of large doses

Drug Interactions

Avoid Concomitant Use There are no known interactions where it is recommended to avoid concomitant use.

Increased Effect/Toxicity

Chloral Hydrate may increase the levels/effects of: Alcohol (Ethyl); CNS Depressants; Methotrimeprazine

The levels/effects of Chloral Hydrate may be increased by: Methotrimeprazine

Decreased Effect

The levels/effects of Chloral Hydrate may be decreased by: Flumazenil

Ethanol/Nutrition/Herb Interactions

Ethanol: Avoid ethanol (may increase CNS depression).

Herb/Nutraceutical: Avoid valerian, St John's wort, kava kava, gotu kola (may increase CNS depression).

Test Interactions False-positive urine glucose using Clinitest® method; may interfere with fluorometric urine catecholamine and urinary 17-hydroxycorticosteroid tests

Dosage Forms Excipient information presented when available (limited, particularly for generics); consult specific product labeling. [DSC] = Discontinued product

Capsule:

Somnote®: 500 mg

Suppository, rectal: 500 mg

Aquachloral® Supprettes®: 325 mg [contains tartrazine] [DSC]

Syrup: 500 mg/5 mL (5 mL, 480 mL)

Chloramphenicol (klor am FEN i kole)

Medication Safety Issues

Sound-alike/look-alike issues:

Chloromycetin® may be confused with chlorambucil, Chlor-Trimeton®

Canadian Brand Names Chloromycetin®; Chloromycetin® Succinate; Diochloram®; Pentamycetin®

Pharmacologic Category Antibiotic, Miscellaneous

Generic Available Yes

Use Treatment of serious infections due to organisms resistant to other less toxic antibiotics or when its penetrability into the site of infection is clinically superior to other antibiotics to which the organism is sensitive; useful in infections caused by *Bacteroides*, *H. influenzae*, *Neisseria meningitidis*, *Salmonella*, and *Rickettsia*; active against many vancomycin-resistant enterococci

Mechanism of Action Reversibly binds to 50S ribosomal subunits of susceptible organisms preventing amino acids from being transferred to growing peptide chains thus inhibiting protein synthesis

Pharmacodynamics/Kinetics

Distribution: To most tissues and body fluids

Chloramphenicol: V_d: 0.5-1 L/kg

Chloramphenicol succinate: V_d: 0.2-3.1 L/kg; decreased with hepatic or renal dysfunction

Protein binding: Chloramphenicol: ~60%; decreased with hepatic or renal dysfunction and in newborn infants

Metabolism:

Chloramphenicol: Hepatic to metabolites (inactive)

Chloramphenicol succinate: Hydrolyzed in the liver, kidney and lungs to chloramphenicol (active)

Bioavailability:

Chloramphenicol: Oral: ~80%

Chloramphenicol succinate: I.V.: ~70%; highly variable, dependant upon rate and extent of metabolism to chloramphenicol

◄ Half-life elimination:
    Normal renal function:
        Chloramphenicol: Adults: ~4 hours; Children 4-6 hours; Infants: Significantly prolonged
        Chloramphenicol succinate: Adults: ~3 hours
    End-stage renal disease: Chloramphenicol: 3-7 hours
    Hepatic disease: Prolonged
Excretion: Urine (~30% as unchanged chloramphenicol succinate in adults, 6% to 80% in children; 5% to 15% as chloramphenicol)

Dosage
Neonates: Initial loading dose: I.V. (I.M. administration is not recommended): 20 mg/kg (the first maintenance dose should be given 12 hours after the loading dose)
    Maintenance dose: Postnatal age:
        ≤7 days: 25 mg/kg/day once every 24 hours
        >7 days, ≤2000 g: 25 mg/kg/day once every 24 hours
        >7 days, >2000 g: 50 mg/kg/day divided every 12 hours
Children: Usual dosing range: I.V.: 50-100 mg/kg/day in divided doses every 6 hours; maximum daily dose: 4 g/day
    Meningitis: I.V.: Infants >30 days and Children: 75-100 mg/kg/day divided every 6 hours
Adults: 50-100 mg/kg/day in divided doses every 6 hours; maximum daily dose: 4 g/day

Dosing adjustment in renal impairment: Use with caution; monitor serum concentrations

Dosing adjustment/comments in hepatic impairment: Use with caution; monitor serum concentrations

Stability Store at room temperature prior to reconstitution. Reconstituted solutions remain stable for 30 days. Use only clear solutions. Frozen solutions remain stable for 6 months.

Administration Do not administer I.M.; can be administered IVP over at least 1 minute at a concentration of 100 mg/mL, or I.V. intermittent infusion over 15-30 minutes at a final concentration for administration of ≤20 mg/mL.

Monitoring Parameters CBC with differential (baseline and every 2 days during therapy), periodic liver and renal function tests, serum drug concentration

Reference Range
Therapeutic levels:
    Meningitis:
        Peak: 15-25 mcg/mL; toxic concentration: >40 mcg/mL
        Trough: 5-15 mcg/mL
    Other infections:
        Peak: 10-20 mcg/mL
        Trough: 5-10 mcg/mL
Timing of serum samples: Draw levels 0.5-1.5 hours after completion of I.V. dose

Contraindications Hypersensitivity to chloramphenicol or any component of the formulation; treatment of trivial or viral infections; bacterial prophylaxis

Warnings/Precautions Gray syndrome characterized by circulatory collapse, cyanosis, acidosis, abdominal distention, myocardial depression, coma, and death has occurred. Use with caution in patients with impaired renal or hepatic function and in neonates. Reduce dose with impaired liver function. Use with care in patients with glucose 6-phosphate dehydrogenase deficiency. **[U.S. Boxed Warning]: Serious and fatal blood dyscrasias (aplastic anemia, hypoplastic anemia, thrombocytopenia, and granulocytopenia) have occurred after both short-term and prolonged therapy. Monitor CBC frequently in all patients;** discontinue if evidence of myelosuppression. Irreversible bone marrow suppression may occur weeks or months after therapy. Avoid repeated courses of treatment. Should not be used for minor infections or when less potentially toxic agents are effective. Prolonged use may result in fungal or bacterial super-infection, including *C. difficile*-associated diarrhea (CDAD) and pseudomembranous colitis; CDAD has been observed >2 months postantibiotic treatment.

Adverse Reactions Frequency not defined.
Central nervous system: Confusion, delirium, depression, fever, headache
Dermatologic: Angioedema, rash, urticaria
Gastrointestinal: Diarrhea, enterocolitis, glossitis, nausea, stomatitis, vomiting

Hematologic: Aplastic anemia, bone marrow suppression, granulocytopenia, hypoplastic anemia, pancytopenia, thrombocytopenia

Ocular: Optic neuritis

Miscellaneous: Anaphylaxis, hypersensitivity reactions, Gray syndrome

Drug Interactions

Metabolism/Transport Effects Inhibits CYP2C9 (weak), 3A4 (weak)

Avoid Concomitant Use There are no known interactions where it is recommended to avoid concomitant use.

Increased Effect/Toxicity

Chloramphenicol may increase the levels/effects of: Anticonvulsants (Hydantoin); Barbiturates; Sulfonylureas

Decreased Effect

Chloramphenicol may decrease the levels/effects of: Cyanocobalamin; Typhoid Vaccine

The levels/effects of Chloramphenicol may be decreased by: Anticonvulsants (Hydantoin); Barbiturates; Rifampin

Ethanol/Nutrition/Herb Interactions Food: May decrease intestinal absorption of vitamin B_{12} may have increased dietary need for riboflavin, pyridoxine, and vitamin B_{12}.

Test Interactions May cause false-positive results in urine glucose tests when using cupric sulfate (Benedict's solution, Clinitest®).

Dietary Considerations May have increased dietary need for riboflavin, pyridoxine, and vitamin B_{12}. Some products may contain sodium.

Dosage Forms Excipient information presented when available (limited, particularly for generics); consult specific product labeling.

Injection, powder for reconstitution: 1 g [contains sodium ~52 mg/g (2.25 mEq/g)]

References

Ambrose PJ, "Clinical Pharmacokinetics Of Chloramphenicol And Chloramphenicol Succinate," *Clin Pharmacokinet*, 1984, 9(3):222-38.

American Academy of Pediatrics Committee on Drugs, "The Transfer of Drugs and Other Chemicals Into Human Milk," *Pediatrics*, 2001, 108(3):776-89.

Aronoff GR, Bennett WM, Berns JS, et al, *Drug Prescribing in Renal Failure: Dosing Guidelines for Adults and Children*, 5th ed. Philadelphia, PA: American College of Physicians; 2007.

Cocke JG Jr, "Chloramphenicol Optic Neuritis. Apparent Protective Effects of Very High Daily Doses of Pyridoxine and Cyanocobalamin," *Am J Dis Child*, 1967, 114(4):424-6.

Doona M and Walsh JB, "Use of Chloramphenicol as Topical Eye Medication: Time to Cry Halt?" *BMJ*, 1995, 310(6989):1217-8.

Freundlich M, Cynamon H, Tamer A, et al, "Management of Chloramphenicol Intoxication in Infancy by Charcoal Hemoperfusion," *J Pediatr*, 1983, 103(3):485-7.

Hammett-Stabler CA and Johns T, "Laboratory Guidelines for Monitoring of Antimicrobial Drugs. National Academy of Clinical Biochemistry," *Clin Chem*, 1998, 44(5):1129-40.

Kunin CM, Glazko AJ, and Finland M, "Persistence of Antibiotics in Blood of Patients With Acute Renal Failure. II. Chloramphenicol and Its Metabolic Products in the Blood of Patients With Severe Renal Failure Disease or Hepatic Cirrhosis," *J Clin Invest*, 1959, 38(9):1498-508.

Messick CR and Pendland SL, "*In Vitro* Activity of Chloramphenicol Alone and in Combination With Vancomycin, Ampicillin, or RP 59500 (Quinupristin/Dalfopristin) Against Vancomycin-Resistant Enterococci," *Diagn Microbiol Infect Dis*, 1997, 29(3):203-5.

Montoro A, Cao A, Ordoqui E, et al, "Contact Sensitivity to Chloramphenicol," *J Allergy Clin Immunol*, 1995, 95:291.

Nahata MC and Powell DA, "Bioavailability and Clearance of Chloramphenicol After Intravenous Chloramphenicol Succinate," *Clin Pharmacol Ther*, 1981, 30(3):368-72.

Powell DA and Nahata MC, "Chloramphenicol: New Perspectives on an Old Drug," *Drug Intell Clin Pharm*, 1982, 16(4):295-300.

Ramilo O, Kinane BT, and McCracken GH Jr, "Chloramphenicol Neurotoxicity," *Pediatr Infect Dis J*, 1988, 7(5):358-9.

Smilack JD, Wilson WR, and Cockerill FR 3d, "Tetracyclines, Chloramphenicol, Erythromycin, Clindamycin, and Metronidazole," *Mayo Clin Proc*, 1991, 66(12):1270-80.

Tunkel AR, Wispelwey B, and Scheld M, "Bacterial Meningitis: Recent Advances in Pathophysiology and Treatment," *Ann Intern Med*, 1990, 112(8):610-23.

Vozeh S, Schmidlin O, and Taeschner W, "Pharmacokinetic Drug Data," *Clin Pharmacokinet*, 1988, 15(4):254-82.

Yoshikawa TT, "Antimicrobial Therapy for the Elderly Patient," *J Am Geriatr Soc*, 1990, 38 (12):1353-72.

Yunis AA, "Chloramphenicol: Relation of Structure to Activity and Toxicity," *Annu Rev Pharmacol Toxicol*, 1988, 28:83-100.

◆ **ChloraPrep® [OTC]** *see* Chlorhexidine Gluconate *on page 291*

◆ **ChloraPrep® Frepp® [OTC]** *see* Chlorhexidine Gluconate *on page 291*

◆ **ChloraPrep® Sepp® [OTC]** *see* Chlorhexidine Gluconate *on page 291*

◆ **Chlorascrub™ [OTC]** *see* Chlorhexidine Gluconate *on page 291*

◆ **Chlorascrub™ Maxi [OTC]** *see* Chlorhexidine Gluconate *on page 291*

ChlordiazePOXIDE (klor dye az e POKS ide)

Related Information
Benzodiazepines *on page 1666*

U.S. Brand Names Librium®

Canadian Brand Names Apo-Chlordiazepoxide®

Index Terms Methaminodiazepoxide Hydrochloride

Pharmacologic Category Benzodiazepine

Restrictions C-IV

Use Management of anxiety disorder or for the short-term relief of symptoms of anxiety; withdrawal symptoms of acute alcoholism; preoperative apprehension and anxiety

Pharmacodynamics/Kinetics
Distribution: V_d: 3.3 L/kg; crosses placenta; enters breast milk

Protein binding: 90% to 98%

Metabolism: Extensively hepatic to desmethyldiazepam (active and long-acting)

Half-life elimination: 6.6-25 hours; End-stage renal disease: 5-30 hours; Cirrhosis: 30-63 hours

Time to peak, serum: Oral: Within 2 hours; I.M.: Results in lower peak plasma levels than oral

Excretion: Urine (minimal as unchanged drug)

Dosage
Children:

  <6 years: Not recommended

  >6 years: Anxiety: Oral, I.M.: 0.5 mg/kg/24 hours divided every 6-8 hours

Adults:

  Anxiety:

    Oral: 15-100 mg divided 3-4 times/day

    I.M., I.V.: Initial: 50-100 mg followed by 25-50 mg 3-4 times/day as needed

  Preoperative anxiety: I.M.: 50-100 mg prior to surgery

  Ethanol withdrawal symptoms: Oral, I.V.: 50-100 mg to start, dose may be repeated in 2-4 hours as necessary to a maximum of 300 mg/24 hours

  Note: Up to 300 mg may be given I.M. or I.V. during a 6-hour period, but not more than this in any 24-hour period.

Dosing adjustment in renal impairment: Cl_{cr} <10 mL/minute: Administer 50% of dose

Hemodialysis: Not dialyzable (0% to 5%)

Dosing adjustment/comments in hepatic impairment: Avoid use

Anesthesia and Critical Care Concerns/Other Considerations Chronic use of this agent may increase the perioperative benzodiazepine dose needed to achieve desired effect. Abrupt discontinuation after sustained use (generally >10 days) may cause withdrawal symptoms.

Additional Information Abrupt discontinuation after sustained use (generally >10 days) may cause withdrawal symptoms.

Dosage Forms Excipient information presented when available (limited, particularly for generics); consult specific product labeling. [DSC] = Discontinued product

Capsule, oral, as hydrochloride: 5 mg, 10 mg, 25 mg

  Librium®: 5 mg [DSC]; 10 mg; 25 mg [DSC]

Injection, powder for reconstitution, as hydrochloride:

  Librium®: 100 mg [contains benzyl alcohol (in diluent), polysorbate 80 (in diluent), propylene glycol (in diluent)] [DSC]

References
Bailey DN, "Blood Concentrations and Clinical Findings Following Overdose of Chlordiazepoxide Alone and Chlordiazepoxide Plus Ethanol," *Clin Toxicol*, 1984, 22(5):433-46.

Burkhart KK and Kulig KW, "The Diagnostic Utility of Flumazenil (a Benzodiazepine Antagonist) in Coma of Unknown Etiology," *Ann Emerg Med*, 1990, 19(3):319-21.

Hicks R, Dysken MW, Davis JM, et al, "The Pharmacokinetics of Psychotropic Medication in the Elderly: A Review," *J Clin Psychiatry*, 1981, 42(10):374-85.

Minder EI, "Toxicity in a Case of Acute and Massive Overdose of Chlordiazepoxide and Its Correlation to Blood Concentration," *J Toxicol Clin Toxicol*, 1989, 27(1-2):117-27.

Mokhlesi B, Leikin JB, Murray P, et al, "Adult Toxicology in Critical Care: Part II: Specific Poisonings," *Chest*, 2003, 123(3):897-922.

Reidenberg MM, Levy M, Warner H, et al, "Relationship Between Diazepam Dose, Plasma Level, Age, and Central Nervous System Depression," *Clin Pharmacol Ther*, 1978, 23(4):371-4.

Chlorhexidine Gluconate (klor HEKS i deen GLOO koe nate)

Medication Safety Issues

Sound-alike/look-alike issues:

Peridex® may be confused with Precedex™

U.S. Brand Names Avagard™ [OTC]; BactoShield® CHG [OTC]; Betasept® [OTC]; ChloraPrep® Frepp® [OTC]; ChloraPrep® Sepp® [OTC]; ChloraPrep® [OTC]; Chlorascrub™ Maxi [OTC]; Chlorascrub™ [OTC]; Dyna-Hex® [OTC]; Hibiclens® [OTC]; Hibistat® [OTC]; Operand® Chlorhexidine Gluconate [OTC]; Peridex®; PerioChip®; PerioGard®

Canadian Brand Names Hibidil® 1:2000; ORO-Clense; Peridex® Oral Rinse

Index Terms 3M™ Avagard™ [OTC]; CHG

Pharmacologic Category Antibiotic, Oral Rinse; Antibiotic, Topical

Generic Available Yes: Oral liquid

Use Skin cleanser for line placement, skin wounds, preoperative skin preparation; germicidal hand rinse; antibacterial dental rinse. Chlorhexidine is active against gram-positive and gram-negative organisms, facultative anaerobes, aerobes, and yeast.

Orphan drug: Peridex®: Oral mucositis with cytoreductive therapy when used for patients undergoing bone marrow transplant

Mechanism of Action The bactericidal effect of chlorhexidine is a result of the binding of this cationic molecule to negatively charged bacterial cell walls and extramicrobial complexes. At low concentrations, this causes an alteration of bacterial cell osmotic equilibrium and leakage of potassium and phosphorous resulting in a bacteriostatic effect. At high concentrations of chlorhexidine, the cytoplasmic contents of the bacterial cell precipitate and result in cell death.

Pharmacodynamics/Kinetics

Topical hand sanitizer (Avagard™): Duration of antimicrobial protection: 6 hours

Oral rinse (Peridex®, PerioGard®):

Absorption: ~30% retained in the oral cavity following rinsing and slowly released into oral fluids; poorly absorbed

Time to peak, plasma: Oral rinse: Detectable levels not present after 12 hours

Excretion: Feces (~90%); urine (<1%)

Dosage Adults:

Oral rinse (Peridex®, PerioGard®):

Floss and brush teeth, completely rinse toothpaste from mouth and swish 15 mL (one capful) undiluted oral rinse around in mouth for 30 seconds, then expectorate. Caution patient not to swallow the medicine and instruct not to eat for 2-3 hours after treatment. (Cap on bottle measures 15 mL.)

Treatment of gingivitis: Oral prophylaxis: Swish for 30 seconds with 15 mL chlorhexidine, then expectorate; repeat twice daily (morning and evening). Patient should have a re-evaluation followed by a dental prophylaxis every 6 months.

Periodontal chip: One chip is inserted into a periodontal pocket with a probing pocket depth ≥5 mm. Up to 8 chips may be inserted in a single visit. Treatment is recommended every 3 months in pockets with a remaining depth ≥5 mm. If dislodgment occurs 7 days or more after placement, the subject is considered to have had the full course of treatment. If dislodgment occurs within 48 hours, a new chip should be inserted. The chip biodegrades completely and does not need to be removed. Patients should avoid dental floss at the site of PerioChip® insertion for 10 days after placement because flossing might dislodge the chip.

Insertion of periodontal chip: Pocket should be isolated and surrounding area dried prior to chip insertion. The chip should be grasped using forceps with the rounded edges away from the forceps. The chip should be inserted into the periodontal pocket to its maximum depth. It may be maneuvered into position using the tips of the forceps or a flat instrument.

Cleanser:

Surgical scrub: Scrub 3 minutes and rinse thoroughly, wash for an additional 3 minutes

◀ Hand sanitizer (Avagard™): Dispense 1 pumpful in palm of one hand; dip fingertips of opposite hand into solution and work it under nails. Spread remainder evenly over hand and just above elbow, covering all surfaces. Repeat on other hand. Dispense another pumpful in each hand and reapply to each hand up to the wrist. Allow to dry before gloving.

Hand wash: Wash for 15 seconds and rinse

Hand rinse: Rub 15 seconds and rinse

Stability Store at room temperature of 15°C to 30°C (59°F to 86°F).

Avagard™: Avoid excessive heat. Ethanol-containing products are flammable; keep away from flames or fire. Hand lotions and gel hand sanitizers are incompatible. The thickeners used in these products (eg, carbomer) react to form an insoluble salt and cause loss of antibacterial action.

Administration

Hand sanitizer (Avagard™): To facilitate drying, continue rubbing hand prep into hands until dry.

Periodontal chip insertion: Pocket should be isolated and surrounding area dried prior to chip insertion. The chip should be grasped using forceps with the rounded edges away from the forceps. The chip should be inserted into the periodontal pocket to its maximum depth. It may be maneuvered into position using the tips of the forceps or a flat instrument. The chip biodegrades completely and does not need to be removed. Patients should avoid dental floss at the site of PerioChip® insertion for 10 days after placement because flossing might dislodge the chip.

Topical: Keep out of eyes, ears, and mouth. Do not routinely apply to wounds which involve more than superficial layers of skin. Avoid contact with meninges (do not use on lumbar puncture sites). Solutions may be flammable (contain isopropyl alcohol); avoid exposure to open flame and/or ignition source (eg, electrocautery) until completely dry; avoid application to hairy areas which may significantly delay drying time.

Pregnancy Risk Factor B

Contraindications Hypersensitivity to chlorhexidine gluconate or any component of the formulation

Warnings/Precautions

Oral: Staining of oral surfaces (mucosa, teeth, tooth restorations, dorsum of tongue) may occur; may be visible as soon as 1 week after therapy begins and is more pronounced when there is a heavy accumulation of unremoved plaque and when teeth fillings have rough surfaces. Stain does not have a clinically adverse effect, but because removal may not be possible, patient with frontal restoration should be advised of the potential permanency of the stain.

Topical: For topical use only. Avoid application over large surfaces or into open wounds. Keep out of eyes and ears. May stain fabric. There have been case reports of anaphylaxis following chlorhexidine disinfection. Not for preoperative preparation of face or head; avoid contact with meninges (do not use on lumbar puncture sites). Solutions may be flammable (contain isopropyl alcohol); avoid exposure to open flame and/or ignition source (eg, electrocautery) until completely dry; avoid application to hairy areas which may significantly delay drying time. Avoid use in children <2 months of age due to increased absorption and/or irritation.

Adverse Reactions

Oral:

>10%: Tartar on teeth increased, taste changes. Staining of oral surfaces (mucosa, teeth, dorsum of tongue) may be visible as soon as 1 week after therapy begins and is more pronounced when there is a heavy accumulation of unremoved plaque and when teeth fillings have rough surfaces. Stain does not have a clinically adverse effect but because removal may not be possible, patient with frontal restoration should be advised of the potential permanency of the stain.

1% to 10%: Gastrointestinal: Tongue irritation, oral irritation

<1% (Limited to important or life-threatening): Dyspnea, facial edema, nasal congestion

Topical: Skin erythema and roughness, dryness, sensitization, allergic reactions

Drug Interactions

Avoid Concomitant Use There are no known interactions where it is recommended to avoid concomitant use.

Increased Effect/Toxicity There are no known significant interactions involving an increase in effect.

Decreased Effect There are no known significant interactions involving a decrease in effect.

Dosage Forms Excipient information presented when available (limited, particularly for generics); consult specific product labeling.

Chip, for periodontal pocket insertion:
    PerioChip®: 2.5 mg
Liquid, topical [surgical scrub]:
    BactoShield® CHG: 2% (120 mL, 480 mL, 750 mL, 960 mL, 3840 mL); 4% (120 mL, 480 mL, 960 mL, 3840 mL) [contains isopropyl alcohol]
    Betasept®: 4% (120 mL, 240 mL, 480 mL, 960 mL, 3840 mL) [contains isopropyl alcohol]
    ChloraPrep®: 2% (0.67 mL, 1.5 mL, 3 mL, 10.5 mL, 26 mL) [contains isopropyl alcohol 70%; prefilled applicator]
    Dyna-Hex®: 2% (120 mL, 480 mL, 960 mL, 3840 mL) [contains isopropyl alcohol]; 4% (120 mL, 480 mL, 960 mL, 3840 mL) [contains isopropyl alcohol]
    Hibiclens®: 4% (15 mL, 120 mL, 240 mL, 480 mL, 960 mL, 3840 mL) [contains isopropyl alcohol]
    Operand® Chlorhexidine Gluconate: 2% (120 mL); 4% (120 mL, 240 mL, 480 mL, 960 mL, 3840 mL) [contains isopropyl alcohol]
Liquid, oral [rinse]: 0.12% (480 mL)
    Peridex®: 0.12% (120 mL, 480 mL, 1920 mL) [contains alcohol 11.6%; mint flavor]
    PerioGard®: 0.12% (480 mL) [contains alcohol 11.6%; mint flavor]
Lotion, topical [surgical scrub]:
    Avagard™: 1% (500 mL) [contains ethyl alcohol and moisturizers]
Sponge/Brush, topical:
    BactoShield® CHG): 4% [contains isopropyl alcohol]
Sponge, topical [surgical scrub]:
    ChloraPrep® 3 mL: 2% (25s) [contains isopropyl alcohol; available in clear or Hi-Lite Orange™]
    ChloraPrep® 10.5 mL: 2% (25s) [contains isopropyl alcohol; available in clear, Hi-Lite Orange™, and Scrub Teal™]
    ChloraPrep® 26 mL: 2% (25s) [contains isopropyl alcohol; available in clear, Hi-Lite Orange™, and Scrub Teal™]
    ChloraPrep® Frepp 1.5 mL: 2% (20s) [contains isopropyl alcohol]
    ChloraPrep® Sepp 0.67 mL: 2% (200s) [contains isopropyl alcohol]
Swab, topical [prep pad]:
    Chlorascrub™: 3.15% (100s) [contains isopropyl alcohol]
Swabstick, topical [surgical scrub]:
    ChloraPrep® 1.75 mL: 2% (48s) [contains isopropyl alcohol]
    ChloraPrep® 5.25 mL: 2% (40s) [contains isopropyl alcohol]
    Chlorascrub™ 1.6 mL: 3.15% (50s) [contains isopropyl alcohol]
    Chlorascrub™ Maxi 5.1 mL: 3.15% (30s) [contains isopropyl alcohol]
Wipe, topical [towlette]:
    Hibistat®: 0.5% (50s) [contains isopropyl alcohol]

◆ **Chlormeprazine** *see Prochlorperazine on page 1180*

◆ **Chloromycetin® (Can)** *see Chloramphenicol on page 287*

◆ **Chloromycetin® Succinate (Can)** *see Chloramphenicol on page 287*

Chloroprocaine (klor oh PROE kane)

Medication Safety Issues

Sound-alike/look-alike issues:
    Nesacaine® may be confused with Neptazane®

High alert medication: The Institute for Safe Medication Practices (ISMP) includes this medication (epidural administration) among its list of drug classes

◀ which have a heightened risk of causing significant patient harm when used in error.

Related Information
Local Anesthetics *on page 1636*

U.S. Brand Names Nesacaine®; Nesacaine®-MPF

Canadian Brand Names Nesacaine®-CE

Index Terms Chloroprocaine Hydrochloride

Pharmacologic Category Local Anesthetic

Generic Available Yes

Use Infiltration anesthesia, peripheral nerve block, epidural anesthesia

Mechanism of Action Chloroprocaine HCl is benzoic acid, 4-amino-2-chloro-2-(diethylamino) ethyl ester monohydrochloride. Chloroprocaine is an ester-type local anesthetic, which stabilizes the neuronal membranes and prevents initiation and transmission of nerve impulses thereby affecting local anesthetic actions. Local anesthetics including chloroprocaine, reversibly prevent generation and conduction of electrical impulses in neurons by decreasing the transient increase in permeability to sodium. The differential sensitivity generally depends on the size of the fiber; small fibers are more sensitive than larger fibers and require a longer period for recovery. Sensory pain fibers are usually blocked first, followed by fibers that transmit sensations of temperature, touch, and deep pressure. High concentrations block sympathetic somatic sensory and somatic motor fibers. The spread of anesthesia depends upon the distribution of the solution. This is primarily dependent on the volume of drug injected.

Pharmacodynamics/Kinetics
Onset of action: 6-12 minutes
Duration: 30-60 minutes
Distribution: V_d: Depends upon route of administration; high concentrations found in highly perfused organs such as liver, lungs, heart, and brain
Metabolism: Plasma cholinesterases
Excretion: Urine

Dosage Dosage varies with anesthetic procedure, the area to be anesthetized, the vascularity of the tissues, depth of anesthesia required, degree of muscle relaxation required, and duration of anesthesia; range.

Children >3 years (normally developed): Maximum dose (without epinephrine): 11 mg/kg; for infiltration, concentrations of 0.5% to 1% are recommended; for nerve block, concentrations of 1% to 1.5% are recommended
Adults:
Maximum single dose (without epinephrine): 11 mg/kg; maximum dose: 800 mg
Maximum single dose (with epinephrine): 14 mg/kg; maximum dose: 1000 mg
Infiltration and peripheral nerve block:
Mandibular: 2%: 2-3 mL; total dose 40-60 mg
Infraorbital: 2%: 0.5-1 mL; total dose 10-20 mg
Brachial plexus: 2%; 30-40 mL; total dose 600-800 mg
Digital (without epinephrine): 1%; 3-4 mL; total dose: 30-40 mg
Pudendal: 2%; 10 mL each side; total dose: 400 mg
Paracervical: 1%; 3 mL per each of four sites
Caudal block: Preservative-free: 2% or 3%: 15-25 mL; may repeat at 40-60 minute intervals
Lumbar epidural block: Preservative-free: 2% or 3%: 2-2.5 mL per segment; usual total volume: 15-25 mL; may repeat with doses that are 2-6 mL less than initial dose every 40-50 minutes.

Stability Store at 15°C to 30°C (59°F to 86°F); protect from freezing. Protect from light. Dilute with NS. To prepare 1:200,000 epinephrine-chloroprocaine HCl injection, add 0.1 mL of a 1:1000 epinephrine injection to 20 mL of preservative free chloroprocaine. Discard Nesacaine®-MPF following single use.

Administration Before injecting, withdraw syringe plunger to ensure injection is not into vein or artery.

Monitoring Parameters Cardiovascular and respiratory status; mental status

Anesthesia and Critical Care Concerns/Other Considerations
Evidence-Based Information: Epidural administration of chloroprocaine can decrease the effectiveness of subsequent epidural opioid and bupivicaine administration (Coda, 1997; Corke, 1984).

Pregnancy Risk Factor C

Contraindications Hypersensitivity to chloroprocaine, other ester type anesthetics, or any component of the formulation; myasthenia gravis; do not use for subarachnoid administration

Warnings/Precautions Use with caution in patients with hepatic impairment or cardiovascular disease. Use with caution in the elderly, debilitated, acutely ill and pediatric patients. **Do not use solutions containing preservatives for caudal or epidural block.** Intravascular injections should be avoided. Careful and constant monitoring of the patient's state of consciousness should be done following each local anesthetic injection; at such times, restlessness, anxiety, tinnitus, dizziness, blurred vision, tremors, depression, or drowsiness may be early warning signs of CNS toxicity. Treatment is primarily symptomatic and supportive. Local anesthetics have been associated with rare occurrences of sudden respiratory arrest, seizures, and cardiac arrest. A test dose is recommended prior to epidural administration. Resuscitative equipment, oxygen, and other resuscitative drugs should be available for immediate use.

Adverse Reactions
Frequency not defined.
Cardiovascular: Bradycardia, cardiac arrest, hypotension, ventricular arrhythmia
Central nervous system: Anxiety, dizziness, restlessness, tinnitus, unconsciousness
Dermatologic: Angioneurotic edema, erythema, pruritus, urticaria
Ocular: Blurred vision
Respiratory: Respiratory arrest
Miscellaneous: Allergic reactions, anaphylactoid reactions
<1% (Limited to important or life-threatening): Seizure (0.1%)

Drug Interactions
Avoid Concomitant Use There are no known interactions where it is recommended to avoid concomitant use.
Increased Effect/Toxicity There are no known significant interactions involving an increase in effect.
Decreased Effect There are no known significant interactions involving a decrease in effect.

Dosage Forms Excipient information presented when available (limited, particularly for generics); consult specific product labeling.
Injection, solution, as hydrochloride:
Nesacaine®: 1% (30 mL); 2% (30 mL) [contains disodium EDTA and methylparaben]
Injection, solution, as hydrochloride [preservative free]: 2% (20 mL); 3% (20 mL)
Nesacaine®-MPF: 2% (20 mL); 3% (20 mL)

References
Coda B, Bausch S, Haas M, et al, "The Hypothesis That Antagonism of Fentanyl Analgesia by 2-Chloroprocaine Is Mediated by Direct Action on Opioid Receptors," *Reg Anesth*, 1997, 22(1):43-52.
Corke BC, Carlson CG, and Dettbarn WD, "The Influence of 2-Chloroprocaine on the Subsequent Analgesic Potency of Bupivacaine," *Anesthesiology*, 1984, 60(1):25-7.
Freeman DW and Arnold NI, "Paracervical Block With Low Doses of Chloroprocaine: Fetal and Maternal Effects," *JAMA*, 1975, 231(1):56-7.
Jankowsky EC, "Pharmacologic Aspects of Local Anesthetic Use," *Anesth Clin North Am*, 1990, 8:1-25.

◆ **Chloroprocaine Hydrochloride** *see* Chloroprocaine *on page 293*

Chlorothiazide (klor oh THYE a zide)

Medication Safety Issues
International issues:
Diuril® may be confused with Duorol® which is a brand name for acetaminophen in Spain
Related Information
Heart Failure (Systolic) *on page 1739*
U.S. Brand Names Diuril®; Sodium Diuril®
Canadian Brand Names Diuril®
Pharmacologic Category Diuretic, Thiazide
Generic Available Yes: Tablet

Use Management of mild-to-moderate hypertension; adjunctive treatment of edema

Mechanism of Action Inhibits sodium and chloride reabsorption in the distal tubules causing increased excretion of sodium, chloride, and water resulting in diuresis. Loss of potassium, hydrogen ions, magnesium, phosphate, and bicarbonate also occurs.

Pharmacodynamics/Kinetics
Onset of action: Diuresis: Oral: 2 hours; I.V.: 15 minutes
Duration of diuretic action: Oral: 6-12 hours; I.V.: ~2 hours
Absorption: Oral: Poor
Half-life elimination: 1-2 hours
Time to peak, serum: Oral: ~4 hours; I.V.: 30 minutes
Excretion: Urine (10% to 15% [oral], 96% [I.V.] as unchanged drug)

Dosage Note: The manufacturer states that I.V. and oral dosing are equivalent. Some clinicians may use lower I.V. doses; however, because of chlorothiazide's poor oral absorption. I.V. dosing in infants and children has not been well established.

Infants <6 months:
Oral: 10-30 mg/kg/day in 2 divided doses (maximum dose: 375 mg/day); anecdotal reports have used up to 40 mg/kg/day (unlabeled).
I.V. (unlabeled): 2-8 mg/kg/day in 2 divided doses; anecdotal reports have used up to 20 mg/kg/day

Infants >6 months and Children:
Oral: 10-20 mg/kg/day in 1-2 divided doses (maximum dose: 375 mg/day in children <2 years or 1 g/day in children 2-12 years)
I.V. (unlabeled route): 4 mg/kg/day in 1-2 divided doses; anecdotal reports have used up to 20 mg/kg/day

Adults:
Hypertension: Oral: 500-2000 mg/day divided in 1-2 doses (manufacturer labeling); doses of 125-500 mg/day have also been recommended (JNC 7)
Edema: Oral, I.V.: 500-1000 mg once or twice daily; intermittent treatment (eg, therapy on alternative days) may be appropriate for some patients
ACC/AHA 2009 Heart Failure guidelines:
Oral: 250-500 mg once or twice daily (maximum daily dose: 1000 mg)
I.V.: 500-1000 mg once or twice daily plus a loop diuretic

Dosage adjustment in renal impairment: Cl_{cr} <10 mL/minute: Avoid use. Ineffective with Cl_{cr} <30 mL/minute unless in combination with a loop diuretic (Aronoff, 2007)
Note: ACC/AHA 2009 Heart Failure guidelines suggest that thiazides lose their efficacy when Cl_{cr} <40 mL/minute

Stability
Powder for injection: Prior to reconstitution, store between 2°C to 25°C (36°F to 77°F). To reconstitute, add SWFI 18 mL to make 28 mg/mL. May be further diluted with dextrose or sodium chloride solutions. Reconstituted solution is stable for 24 hours at room temperature; precipitation will occur in <24 hours in pH <7.4. Single use only, discard any unused reconstituted solution.
Suspension, tablets: Store at room temperature 15°C to 30°C (59°F to 86°F); protect from freezing.

Administration Do **not** administer injection via I.M. or SubQ route.

Monitoring Parameters Serum electrolytes, renal function, blood pressure; assess weight, I & O reports daily to determine fluid loss

Anesthesia and Critical Care Concerns/Other Considerations Thiazide diuretics are effective first-line therapeutic agents in the management of hypertension and have proven to be of benefit in terms of cardiovascular outcome. If given the morning of surgery it may render the patient volume depleted and blood pressure may be labile during general anesthesia.

Pregnancy Risk Factor C (manufacturer); D (expert analysis)

Contraindications Hypersensitivity to chlorothiazide, any component of the formulation, thiazides, or sulfonamide-derived drugs; anuria

Warnings/Precautions Hypersensitivity reactions may occur. Use with caution in severe renal disease. Electrolyte disturbances (hypokalemia, hypochloremic alkalosis, hyponatremia, hypomagnesemia) can occur. Use with caution in severe hepatic dysfunction; hepatic encephalopathy can be caused by electrolyte disturbances. Gout can be precipitate in certain patients with a history of gout, a familial predisposition to gout, or chronic renal failure. Use caution in patients with diabetes; may see a change in glucose control. Can cause SLE exacerbation or activation. Use with caution in patients with moderate or high cholesterol concentrations. Photosensitization may occur. Correct hypokalemia before initiating therapy.

Chemical similarities are present among sulfonamides, sulfonylureas, carbonic anhydrase inhibitors, thiazides, and loop diuretics (except ethacrynic acid). Use in patients with thiazide or sulfonamide allergy is specifically contraindicated in product labeling. A risk of cross-reaction exists in patients with allergy to any of these compounds; avoid use when previous reaction has been severe. Discontinue if signs of hypersensitivity are noted.

Adverse Reactions Frequency not defined.
  Cardiovascular: Hypotension, orthostatic hypotension, necrotizing angiitis
  Central nervous system: Dizziness, fever, headache, restlessness, vertigo
  Dermatologic: Alopecia, erythema multiforme, exfoliative dermatitis, photosensitivity, purpura, rash, Stevens-Johnson syndrome, toxic epidermal necrolysis, urticaria
  Endocrine & metabolic: Cholesterol increased, hyperglycemia, hyperuricemia, hypochloremic alkalosis, hypokalemia, hyponatremia, hypomagnesemia, triglycerides increased
  Gastrointestinal: Abdominal cramping, anorexia, constipation, diarrhea, gastric irritation, nausea, pancreatitis, sialadenitis, vomiting
  Genitourinary: Impotence
  Hematologic: Agranulocytosis, aplastic anemia, hemolytic anemia, leukopenia, thrombocytopenia
  Hepatic: Jaundice
  Neuromuscular & skeletal: Muscle spasm, paresthesia, weakness
  Ocular: Blurred vision, xanthopsia
  Renal: Glycosuria, hematuria (I.V.), interstitial nephritis, renal failure, renal dysfunction
  Respiratory: Pneumonitis, pulmonary edema, respiratory distress
  Miscellaneous: Anaphylactic reactions, systemic lupus erythematosus

Drug Interactions
  Avoid Concomitant Use
    Avoid concomitant use of Chlorothiazide with any of the following: Dofetilide
  Increased Effect/Toxicity
    Chlorothiazide may increase the levels/effects of: ACE Inhibitors; Allopurinol; Amifostine; Antihypertensives; Calcitriol; Calcium Salts; Dofetilide; Hypotensive Agents; Lithium; RiTUXimab

    The levels/effects of Chlorothiazide may be increased by: Alcohol (Ethyl); Analgesics (Opioid); Barbiturates; Corticosteroids (Orally Inhaled); Corticosteroids (Systemic); Herbs (Hypotensive Properties); MAO Inhibitors; Pentoxifylline; Phosphodiesterase 5 Inhibitors; Prostacyclin Analogues
  Decreased Effect
    Chlorothiazide may decrease the levels/effects of: Antidiabetic Agents

    The levels/effects of Chlorothiazide may be decreased by: Bile Acid Sequestrants; Herbs (Hypertensive Properties); Methylphenidate; Nonsteroidal Anti-Inflammatory Agents; Yohimbine

Ethanol/Nutrition/Herb Interactions
  Ethanol: May increase risk of orthostatic hypotension.
  Food: Chlorothiazide serum levels may be increased if taken with food.
  Herb/Nutraceutical: Avoid bayberry, blue cohosh, cayenne, ephedra, ginger, ginseng (American), kola, licorice (may worsen hypertension). Avoid black cohosh, California poppy, coleus, golden seal, hawthorn, mistletoe, periwinkle, quinine, shepherd's purse (may have increased antihypertensive effect).

Test Interactions May interfere with tests for parathyroid function

Dietary Considerations May need to decrease sodium and calcium, may need to increase potassium, zinc, magnesium, and riboflavin in diet. Some products may contain sodium.

◀ **Dosage Forms** Excipient information presented when available (limited, particularly for generics); consult specific product labeling.

Injection, powder for reconstitution, as sodium:
Sodium Diuril®: 500 mg
Suspension, oral:
Diuril®: 250 mg/5 mL (237 mL) [contains alcohol 0.5% and benzoic acid]
Tablet: 250 mg, 500 mg

ChlorproMAZINE (klor PROE ma zeen)

Canadian Brand Names Largactil®; Novo-Chlorpromazine
Index Terms Chlorpromazine Hydrochloride; CPZ; Thorazine
Pharmacologic Category Antimanic Agent; Antipsychotic Agent, Typical, Phenothiazine
Use Control of mania; treatment of schizophrenia; control of nausea and vomiting; relief of restlessness and apprehension before surgery; acute intermittent porphyria; adjunct in the treatment of tetanus; intractable hiccups; combativeness and/or explosive hyperexcitable behavior in children 1-12 years of age and in short-term treatment of hyperactive children
Unlabeled/Investigational Use Management of psychotic disorders; behavioral symptoms associated with dementia (elderly); psychosis/agitation related to Alzheimer's dementia
Pharmacodynamics/Kinetics
Onset of action: I.M.: 15 minutes; Oral: 30-60 minutes
Absorption: Rapid
Distribution: V_d: 20 L/kg; crosses the placenta; enters breast milk
Protein binding: 92% to 97%
Metabolism: Extensively hepatic to active and inactive metabolites
Bioavailability: 20%
Half-life, biphasic: Initial: 2 hours; Terminal: 30 hours
Excretion: Urine (<1% as unchanged drug) within 24 hours
Dosage
Children ≥6 months:
Schizophrenia/psychoses:
Oral: 0.5-1 mg/kg/dose every 4-6 hours; older children may require 200 mg/day or higher
I.M., I.V.: 0.5-1 mg/kg/dose every 6-8 hours
<5 years (22.7 kg): Maximum: 40 mg/day
5-12 years (22.7-45.5 kg): Maximum: 75 mg/day
Nausea and vomiting:
Oral: 0.5-1 mg/kg/dose every 4-6 hours as needed
I.M., I.V.: 0.5-1 mg/kg/dose every 6-8 hours
<5 years (22.7 kg): Maximum: 40 mg/day
5-12 years (22.7-45.5 kg): Maximum: 75 mg/day
Adults:
Schizophrenia/psychoses:
Oral: Range: 30-800 mg/day in 1-4 divided doses, initiate at lower doses and titrate as needed; usual dose: 200-600 mg/day; some patients may require 1-2 g/day
I.M., I.V.: Initial: 25 mg, may repeat (25-50 mg) in 1-4 hours, gradually increase to a maximum of 400 mg/dose every 4-6 hours until patient is controlled; usual dose: 300-800 mg/day
Intractable hiccups: Oral, I.M.: 25-50 mg 3-4 times/day
Nausea and vomiting:
Oral: 10-25 mg every 4-6 hours
I.M., I.V.: 25-50 mg every 4-6 hours
Elderly: Behavioral symptoms associated with dementia (unlabeled use): Initial: 10-25 mg 1-2 times/day; increase at 4- to 7-day intervals by 10-25 mg/day. Increase dose intervals (bid, tid, etc) as necessary to control behavior response or side effects; maximum daily dose: 800 mg; gradual increases (titration) may prevent some side effects or decrease their severity.
Dosing comments in renal impairment: Hemodialysis: Not dialyzable (0% to 5%)

Dosing adjustment/comments in hepatic impairment: Avoid use in severe hepatic dysfunction

Additional Information Complete prescribing information for this medication should be consulted for additional detail.

Dosage Forms Excipient information presented when available (limited, particularly for generics); consult specific product labeling.
Injection, solution, as hydrochloride: 25 mg/mL (1 mL, 2 mL)
Tablet, as hydrochloride: 10 mg, 25 mg, 50 mg, 100 mg, 200 mg

◆ **Chlorpromazine Hydrochloride** *see* ChlorproMAZINE *on page 298*

◆ **Choline Fenofibrate** *see* Fenofibric Acid *on page 583*

Choline Magnesium Trisalicylate
(KOE leen mag NEE zhum trye sa LIS i late)

Related Information
Acetaminophen and NSAIDS, Dosing in the Management of Pain *on page 1651*

Index Terms Tricosal; Trilisate

Pharmacologic Category Salicylate

Generic Available Yes

Use Management of osteoarthritis, rheumatoid arthritis, and other arthritis; acute painful shoulder

Mechanism of Action Weakly inhibits cyclooxygenase enzymes, which results in decreased formation of prostaglandin precursors; antipyretic, analgesic, and anti-inflammatory properties.

Other proposed mechanisms not fully elucidated (and possibly contributing to the anti-inflammatory effect to varying degrees) include inhibiting chemotaxis, altering lymphocyte activity, inhibiting neutrophil aggregation/activation, and decreasing proinflammatory cytokine levels.

Pharmacodynamics/Kinetics
Onset of action: Peak effect: ~2 hours
Absorption: Stomach and small intestines
Distribution: Readily into most body fluids and tissues; crosses placenta; enters breast milk
Half-life elimination (dose dependent): Low dose: 2-3 hours; High dose: 30 hours
Time to peak, serum: ~2 hours

Dosage Oral (based on total salicylate content):
Children <37 kg: 50 mg/kg/day given in 2 divided doses; 2250 mg/day for heavier children
Adults: 500 mg to 1.5 g 2-3 times/day **or** 3 g at bedtime; usual maintenance dose: 1-4.5 g/day
Elderly: 750 mg 3 times/day
Dosing adjustment/comments in renal impairment: Avoid use in severe renal impairment

Stability Store at controlled room temperature of 15°C to 30°C (59°F to 86°F).

Administration Liquid may be mixed with fruit juice just before drinking. Do not administer with antacids. Take with a full glass of water and remain in an upright position for 15-30 minutes after administration.

Monitoring Parameters Serum magnesium with high dose therapy or in patients with impaired renal function; serum salicylate levels, renal function, hearing changes or tinnitus, abnormal bruising, weight gain and response (ie, pain)

Reference Range Salicylate blood levels for anti-inflammatory effect: 150-300 mcg/mL; analgesia and antipyretic effect: 30-50 mcg/mL

Anesthesia and Critical Care Concerns/Other Considerations
Clinical Pearls/Comments: This combination does not inhibit platelet aggregation at therapeutic levels and, therefore, should not be used for thromboprophylaxis.

Pregnancy Risk Factor C/D (3rd trimester)

Contraindications Hypersensitivity to salicylates, other nonacetylated salicylates, other NSAIDs, or any component of the formulation; bleeding disorders; pregnancy (3rd trimester)

Warnings/Precautions Salicylate salts may not inhibit platelet aggregation and, therefore, should not be substituted for aspirin in the prophylaxis of thrombosis. Use with caution in patients with impaired hepatic or renal function, dehydration, erosive gastritis, asthma, or peptic ulcer. Children and teenagers who have or are recovering from chickenpox or flu-like symptoms should not use this product. Changes in behavior (along with nausea and vomiting) may be an early sign of Reye's syndrome; patients should be instructed to contact their healthcare provider if these occur.

Elderly are a high-risk population for adverse effects from NSAIDs. As many as 60% of elderly can develop peptic ulceration and/or hemorrhage asymptomatically. Use lowest effective dose for shortest period possible. Tinnitus or impaired hearing may indicate toxicity. Tinnitus may be a difficult and unreliable indication of toxicity due to age-related hearing loss or eighth cranial nerve damage. CNS adverse effects may be observed in the elderly at lower doses than younger adults.

Adverse Reactions
<20%:
Gastrointestinal: Nausea, vomiting, diarrhea, heartburn, dyspepsia, epigastric pain, constipation
Otic: Tinnitus
<2%:
Central nervous system: Headache, lightheadedness, dizziness, drowsiness, lethargy
Otic: Hearing impairment
<1%: Anorexia, asthma, BUN and creatinine increased, bruising, confusion, duodenal ulceration, dysgeusia, edema, epistaxis, erythema multiforme, esophagitis, hallucinations, hearing loss (irreversible), hepatic enzymes increased, gastric ulceration, occult bleeding, pruritus, rash, weight gain

Drug Interactions
Avoid Concomitant Use There are no known interactions where it is recommended to avoid concomitant use.
Increased Effect/Toxicity
Choline Magnesium Trisalicylate may increase the levels/effects of: Anticoagulants; Carbonic Anhydrase Inhibitors; Corticosteroids (Systemic); Drotrecogin Alfa; Methotrexate; Pralatrexate; Salicylates; Sulfonylureas; Thrombolytic Agents; Valproic Acid; Varicella Virus-Containing Vaccines; Vitamin K Antagonists

The levels/effects of Choline Magnesium Trisalicylate may be increased by: Antiplatelet Agents; Calcium Channel Blockers (Nondihydropyridine); Ginkgo Biloba; Herbs (Anticoagulant/Antiplatelet Properties); Loop Diuretics; Treprostinil
Decreased Effect
Choline Magnesium Trisalicylate may decrease the levels/effects of: ACE Inhibitors; Loop Diuretics; Uricosuric Agents

The levels/effects of Choline Magnesium Trisalicylate may be decreased by: Corticosteroids (Systemic)
Ethanol/Nutrition/Herb Interactions
Ethanol: Avoid ethanol (may enhance gastric mucosal irritation).
Food: May decrease the rate but not the extent of oral absorption.
Herb/Nutraceutical: Avoid cat's claw, dong quai, evening primrose, feverfew, garlic, ginger, ginkgo, red clover, horse chestnut, green tea, ginseng (all have additional antiplatelet activity). Limit curry powder, paprika, licorice, Benedictine liqueur, prunes, raisins, tea, and gherkins; may cause salicylate accumulation. These foods contain 6 mg salicylate/100 g.
Test Interactions False-negative results for glucose oxidase urinary glucose tests (Clinistix®); false-positives using the cupric sulfate method (Clinitest®); also, interferes with Gerhardt test (urinary ketone analysis), VMA determination; 5-HIAA, xylose tolerance test, and T_3 and T_4; increased PBI
Dietary Considerations Take with food or large volume of water or milk to minimize GI upset. Liquid may be mixed with fruit juice just before drinking. Hypermagnesemia resulting from magnesium salicylate; avoid or use with caution in renal insufficiency.

Dosage Forms Excipient information presented when available (limited, particularly for generics); consult specific product labeling.

Liquid: 500 mg/5 mL (240 mL) [choline salicylate 293 mg and magnesium salicylate 362 mg per 5 mL; cherry cordial flavor]

Tablet: 500 mg [choline salicylate 293 mg and magnesium salicylate 362 mg]; 750 mg [choline salicylate 440 mg and magnesium salicylate 544 mg]; 1000 mg [choline salicylate 587 mg and magnesium salicylate 725 mg]

References

Danesh BJ, Saniabadi AR, Russell RI, et al, "Therapeutic Potential of Choline Magnesium Trisalicylate as an Alternative to Aspirin for Patients With Bleeding Tendencies," *Scott Med J*, 1987, 32(6):167-8.

- ◆ **Chronovera® (Can)** see Verapamil *on page 1468*
- ◆ **CI-1008** see Pregabalin *on page 1171*
- ◆ **Cialis®** see Tadalafil *on page 1345*
- ◆ **Cidecin** see DAPTOmycin *on page 372*

Cilazapril (sye LAY za pril)

Related Information

Angiotensin Agents *on page 1652*

Canadian Brand Names Apo-Cilazapril®; CO Cilazapril; Gen-Cilazapril; Inhibace®; Mylan-Cilazapril; Novo-Cilazapril; PHL-Cilazapril; PMS-Cilazapril

Index Terms Cilazapril Monohydrate

Pharmacologic Category Angiotensin-Converting Enzyme (ACE) Inhibitor

Restrictions Not available in U.S.

Use Management of hypertension; treatment of heart failure

Pharmacodynamics/Kinetics

Onset of action: Antihypertensive: ~1 hour

Duration: Therapeutic effect: 24 hours

Absorption: Rapid

Metabolism: To active form (cilazaprilat)

Bioavailability: 57%

Half-life elimination: Cilazaprilat: Terminal: 36-49 hours

Time to peak: 3-7 hours

Excretion: In urine (91%)

Dosage Oral:

Heart failure: Initial: 0.5 mg once daily; if tolerated, after 5 days increase to 1 mg/day (lowest maintenance dose); may increase to maximum of 2.5 mg once daily

Hypertension: 2.5-5 mg once daily (maximum dose: 10 mg/day)

Elderly: Initial: 1.25 mg once daily; titrate slowly as tolerated

Dosage adjustment in renal impairment:

Heart failure:

Cl_{cr} 10-40 mL/minute: Initial: 0.25-0.5 mg once daily (maximum dose: 2.5 mg once daily)

Cl_{cr} <10 mL/minute: 0.25-0.5 mg once or twice weekly

Hypertension:

Cl_{cr} 10-40 mL/minute: Initial: 0.5 mg once daily (maximum dose: 2.5 mg once daily)

Cl_{cr} <10 mL/minute: 0.25-0.5 mg once or twice weekly

Dosage adjustment in hepatic impairment: Initial: ≤0.5 mg once daily (with caution)

Anesthesia and Critical Care Concerns/Other Considerations

Clinical Pearls/Comments: In patients on chronic ACE inhibitor therapy, intraoperative hypotension may occur with induction and maintenance of general anesthesia; however, discontinuation of therapy prior to surgery is controversial. If continued preoperatively, avoidance of hypotensive agents during surgery is prudent. Episodes of intraoperative hypotension may be managed by fluid administration and/or modest doses of alpha-adrenergic agents. Severe hypotension may occur in patients who are sodium- and/or volume-depleted, initiate lower doses and monitor closely when starting therapy in these patients. ACE inhibitor therapy may elicit an increase in potassium and creatinine, especially when used in patients with bilateral renal artery stenosis. In those

◄ patients experiencing cough on an ACE inhibitor, the ACE inhibitor may be discontinued and, if necessary, angiotensin-receptor blocker therapy instituted. Concomitant NSAID therapy may attenuate blood pressure control; use of NSAIDs should be avoided or limited, with monitoring of blood pressure control. In the setting of heart failure, NSAID use may be associated with an increased risk for fluid accumulation and edema. Because of the potent teratogenic effects of ACE inhibitors, these drugs should be avoided, if possible, when treating women of childbearing potential not on effective birth control measures. Aging patients with a decrease in glomerular filtration (also creatinine clearance), severe heart failure, and renal failure may experience an exaggerated response with administration of ACE inhibitors. Diabetic proteinuria is reduced and insulin sensitivity is enhanced.

Evidence-Based Information: ACE inhibitors decrease morbidity and mortality in patients with asymptomatic and symptomatic left ventricular dysfunction. In this situation, they decrease hospitalizations for, and retard progression to, decompensated heart failure. ACE inhibitors are also indicated in patients postmyocardial infarction in whom left ventricular ejection fraction is <40%. When used in patients with heart failure, the target dose or maximum tolerated dose should be achieved, if possible. Lower daily doses of ACE inhibitors have not demonstrated the same cardioprotective effects. ACE inhibitors have renal protective effects in patients with diabetic proteinuria. The HOPE trial examined the use of ramipril at a dose of between 2.5-10 mg daily in patients without heart failure at high risk for cardiovascular events and documented a significant improvement in cardiovascular outcome compared to placebo.

Additional Information Not available in U.S.

Dosage Forms Excipient information presented when available (limited, particularly for generics); consult specific product labeling. [CAN] = Canadian brand name
Tablet:
Inhibace® [CAN], Novo-Cilazapril [CAN]: 1 mg, 2.5 mg, 5 mg [not available in the U.S.]

References

ALLHAT Officers and Coordinators for the ALLHAT Collaborative Research Group, "Major Outcomes in High-Risk Hypertensive Patients Randomized to Angiotensin-Converting Enzyme Inhibitor or Calcium Channel Blocker vs Diuretic: The Antihypertensive and Lipid-Lowering Treatment to Prevent Heart Attack Trial (ALLHAT)," *JAMA*, 2002, 288(23):2981-97.

American Diabetes Association, "Standards of Medical Care in Diabetes Mellitus – 2009," *Diabetes Care*, 2009, 32(Suppl 1):13-61.

Antman EM, Anbe SC, Alpert JS, et al, "ACC/AHA Guidelines for the Management of Patients With ST-Elevation Myocardial Infarction - Executive Summary: A Report of the American College of Cardiology/American Heart Association Task Force on Practice Guidelines (Writing Committee to Revise the 1999 Guidelines for the Management of Patients With Acute Myocardial Infarction)," *Circulation*, 2004, 110(5):588-636. Available at: http://www.circulationaha.org/cgi/content/full/110/5/588. Last accessed October 26, 2004.

Chase MP, Fiarman GS, Scholz FJ, et al, "Angioedema of the Small Bowel Due to an Angiotensin-Converting Enzyme Inhibitor," *J Clin Gastroenterol*, 2000, 31(3):254-7.

Chobanian AV, Bakris GL, Black HR, et al, "The Seventh Report of the Joint National Committee on Prevention, Detection, Evaluation, and Treatment of High Blood Pressure: The JNC 7 Report," *JAMA*, 2003, 289(19):2560-71.

Deget F and Brogden RN, "Cilazapril. A Review of Its Pharmacodynamic and Pharmacokinetic Properties, and Therapeutic Potential in Cardiovascular Disease," *Drugs*, 1991, 41(5):799-820.

Dossegger L, Nielsen T, Preston C, et al, "Heart Failure Therapy With Cilazapril: An Overview," *J Cardiovasc Pharmacol*, 1994, 24(Suppl 3):38-41.

Fox KM and EURopean Trial on Reduction of Cardiac Events With Perindopril in Stable Coronary Artery Disease Investigators, "Efficacy of Perindopril in Reduction of Cardiovascular Events Among Patients With Stable Coronary Artery Disease: Randomised, Double-Blind, Placebo-Controlled, Multicentre Trial (The EUROPA Study)," *Lancet*, 2003, 362(9386):782-8.

Hunt SA, Abraham WT, Chin MH, et al, "2009 Focused Update Incorporated into the ACC/AHA 2005 Guidelines for the Diagnosis and Management of Heart Failure in Adults: A Report of the American College of Cardiology Foundation/American Heart Association Task Force on Practice Guidelines Developed in Collaboration With the International Society for Heart and Lung Transplantation," *J Am Coll Cardiol*, 2009, 53(15):e1-e90.

Inhibace® product monograph, Hoffman-La Roche Ltd, Ontario, July 2001.

"K/DOQI Clinical Practice Guidelines for Chronic Kidney Disease: Evaluation, Classification, and Stratification. Kidney Disease Outcome Quality Initiative," *Am J Kidney Dis*, 2002, 39(2 Suppl 2):1-246. Available at: http://www.kidney.org/professionals/doqi/kdoqi/toc.htm. Accessed August 1, 2003.

Miller DR, Oliveria SA, Berlowitz DR, et al, "Angioedema Incidence in US Veterens Initiating Angiotensin-Converting Enzyme Inhibitors," *Hypertension*, 2008, 51(6):1-7.

Pfeffer MA, McMurray JJ, Velazquez EJ, et al, "Valsartan, Captopril, or Both in Myocardial Infarction Complicated by Heart Failure, Left Ventricular Dysfunction, or Both," *N Engl J Med*, 2003, 349 (20):1893-906.

Rosenthal JH, "Therapeutic Experience With Cilazapril," *J Cardiovasc Pharmacol*, 1994, 24 (Suppl2):65-9.

Smoger SH and Sayed MA, "Simultaneous Mucosal and Small Bowel Angioedema Due to Captopril," *South Med J*, 1998, 91(11):1060-3.

Song JC and White CM, "Clinical Pharmacokinetics and Selective Pharmacodynamics of New Angiotensin Converting Enzyme Inhibitors: An Update," *Clin Pharmacokinet*, 2002, 41(3):207-24.

Szues T, "Cilazapril. A Review," *Drugs*, 1991, 41(Suppl 1):18-24.

Yusuf S, Sleight P, Pogue J, et al, "Effects of an Angiotensin-Converting-Enzyme Inhibitor, Ramipril, on Cardiovascular Events in High-Risk Patients. The Heart Outcomes Prevention Evaluation Study Investigators," *N Engl J Med*, 2000, 342(3):145-53.

◆ **Cilazapril Monohydrate** *see* Cilazapril *on page 301*

Cilostazol (sil OH sta zol)

Medication Safety Issues
Sound-alike/look-alike issues:
Pletal® may be confused with Plendil®

Related Information
Heart Failure (Systolic) *on page 1739*

U.S. Brand Names Pletal®

Canadian Brand Names Pletal®

Index Terms OPC-13013

Pharmacologic Category Antiplatelet Agent; Phosphodiesterase Enzyme Inhibitor

Generic Available Yes

Use Symptomatic management of peripheral vascular disease, primarily intermittent claudication

Unlabeled/Investigational Use Adjunct with aspirin and clopidogrel for prevention of stent thrombosis and restenosis after coronary stent placement

Mechanism of Action Cilostazol and its metabolites are inhibitors of phosphodiesterase III. As a result, cyclic AMP is increased leading to reversible inhibition of platelet aggregation, vasodilation, and inhibition of vascular smooth muscle cell proliferation.

Pharmacodynamics/Kinetics
Onset of action: 2-4 weeks; may require up to 12 weeks

Protein binding: Cilostazol 95% to 98%; active metabolites 66% to 97%

Metabolism: Hepatic via CYP3A4 (primarily), 1A2, 2C19, and 2D6; at least one metabolite has significant activity

Half-life elimination: 11-13 hours

Excretion: Urine (74%) and feces (20%) as metabolites

Dosage Adults: Oral: 100 mg twice daily

Dosage adjustment for cilostazol with concomitant medications:
CYP2C19 inhibitors (see Drug Interactions): Dosage of cilostazol should be reduced to 50 mg twice daily

CYP3A4 inhibitors (see Drug Interactions): Dosage of cilostazol should be reduced to 50 mg twice daily

Stability Store at 25°C (77°F); excursions permitted to 15°C to 30°C (59°F to 86°F).

Administration Administer cilostazol 30 minutes before or 2 hours after meals.

Anesthesia and Critical Care Concerns/Other Considerations
Evidence-Based Information: Considered effective treatment in patients with lower extremity peripheral arterial disease (PAD) and is recommended for patients with moderate-to-severe disabling intermittent claudication (in the absence of heart failure) unresponsive to exercise therapy, and who are not candidates for surgical or catheter-based intervention (Sobel, 2008). A therapeutic trial should be considered in all patients with lifestyle-limiting claudication.

Pregnancy Risk Factor C

Contraindications Hypersensitivity to cilostazol or any component of the formulation; heart failure (HF) of any severity; hemostatic disorders or active bleeding

◀ **Warnings/Precautions [U.S. Boxed Warning]: The use of this drug is contraindicated in patients with heart failure.** Use with caution in severe underlying heart disease. Use with caution in patients receiving other platelet aggregation inhibitors or in patients with thrombocytopenia. Discontinue therapy if thrombocytopenia or leukopenia occur; progression to agranulocytosis (reversible) has been reported when cilostazol was not immediately stopped. When cilostazol and clopidogrel are used concurrently, manufacturer recommends checking bleeding times. Withhold for at least 4-6 half-lives prior to elective surgical procedures. Use with caution in patients receiving CYP3A4 inhibitors (eg, ketoconazole or erythromycin) or CYP2C19 inhibitors (eg, omeprazole). If concurrent use is warranted, consider dosage adjustment of cilostazol. Use caution in moderate-to-severe hepatic impairment. Use cautiously in severe renal impairment (Cl_{cr} <25 mL/minute). Safety and efficacy in pediatric patients have not been established.

Adverse Reactions

>10%:

Central nervous system: Headache (27% to 34%)

Gastrointestinal: Abnormal stools (12% to 15%), diarrhea (12% to 19%)

Respiratory: Rhinitis (7% to 12%)

Miscellaneous: Infection (10% to 14%)

2% to 10%:

Cardiovascular: Peripheral edema (7% to 9%), palpitation (5% to 10%), tachycardia (4%)

Central nervous system: Dizziness (9% to 10%), vertigo (up to 3%)

Gastrointestinal: Dyspepsia (6%), nausea (6% to 7%), abdominal pain (4% to 5%), flatulence (2% to 3%)

Neuromuscular & skeletal: Back pain (6% to 7%), myalgia (2% to 3%)

Respiratory: Pharyngitis (7% to 10%), cough (3% to 4%)

<2% (Limited to important or life-threatening): Agranulocytosis, anemia, aplastic anemia, asthma, atrial fibrillation, atrial flutter, blindness, blood pressure increased, bursitis, cardiac arrest, cerebral infarction/ischemia, cerebrovascular accident, chest pain, CHF, cholelithiasis, colitis, coronary stent thrombosis, cystitis, diabetes mellitus, duodenal ulcer, duodenitis, esophageal hemorrhage, esophagitis, extradural hematoma, gastrointestinal hemorrhage, gout, granulocytopenia, hemorrhage, hepatic dysfunction, hot flashes, hyperglycemia, hypotension, interstitial pneumonia, intracranial hemorrhage, jaundice, leukopenia, myocardial infarction/ischemia, neuralgia, nodal arrhythmia, pain, periodontal abscess, peptic ulcer, pneumonia, polycythemia, postural hypotension, pulmonary hemorrhage, pruritus, QT_c prolongation, rectal hemorrhage, retinal hemorrhage, retroperitoneal hemorrhage, Stevens-Johnson syndrome, subcutaneous hemorrhage, subdural hematoma, supraventricular tachycardia, syncope, thrombocytopenia, thrombosis, torsade de pointes, uric acid increased, ventricular tachycardia

Drug Interactions

Metabolism/Transport Effects Substrate of CYP1A2 (minor), 2C19 (minor), 2D6 (minor), 3A4 (major)

Avoid Concomitant Use There are no known interactions where it is recommended to avoid concomitant use.

Increased Effect/Toxicity

Cilostazol may increase the levels/effects of: Anticoagulants; Antiplatelet Agents; Drotrecogin Alfa; Ibritumomab; Salicylates; Thrombolytic Agents; Tositumomab and Iodine I 131 Tositumomab

The levels/effects of Cilostazol may be increased by: Antifungal Agents (Azole Derivatives, Systemic); CYP2C19 Inhibitors (Moderate); CYP2C19 Inhibitors (Strong); CYP3A4 Inhibitors (Moderate); CYP3A4 Inhibitors (Strong); Dasatinib; Herbs (Anticoagulant/Antiplatelet Properties); Macrolide Antibiotics; Nonsteroidal Anti-Inflammatory Agents; Omega-3-Acid Ethyl Esters; Omeprazole; Pentosan Polysulfate Sodium; Pentoxifylline; Prostacyclin Analogues

Decreased Effect

The levels/effects of Cilostazol may be decreased by: CYP3A4 Inducers (Strong); Deferasirox; Herbs (CYP3A4 Inducers); Nonsteroidal Anti-Inflammatory Agents; Peginterferon Alfa-2b

Ethanol/Nutrition/Herb Interactions

Food: Taking cilostazol with a high-fat meal may increase peak concentration by 90%. Avoid concurrent ingestion of grapefruit juice due to the potential to inhibit CYP3A4.

Herb/Nutraceutical: St John's wort may decrease the levels/effects of cilostazol. Avoid alfalfa, anise, bilberry, bladderwrack, bromelain, cat's claw, chamomile, coleus, cordyceps, dong quai, evening primrose oil, fenugreek, feverfew, garlic, ginger, ginkgo biloba, ginseng (American), ginseng (Panax), ginseng (Siberian), grape seed, green tea, guggul, horse chestnut seed, horseradish, licorice, prickly ash, red clover, reishi, SAMe (S-adenosylmethionine), sweet clover, turmeric, white willow (all have additional antiplatelet activity).

Dietary Considerations It is best to take cilostazol 30 minutes before or 2 hours after meals.

Dosage Forms Excipient information presented when available (limited, particularly for generics); consult specific product labeling.

Tablet: 50 mg, 100 mg

Pletal®: 50 mg, 100 mg

References

Hirsch AT, Haskal ZJ, Hertzer NR, et al, "ACC/AHA Guidelines for the Management of Patients With Peripheral Arterial Disease (Lower Extremity, Renal, Mesenteric, and Abdominal Aortic): A Collaborative Report from the American Association for Vascular Surgery/Society for Vascular Surgery, Society for Cardiovascular Angiography and Interventions, Society for Vascular Medicine and Biology, Society of Interventional Radiology, and the ACC/AHA Task Force on Practice Guidelines (Writing Committee to Develop Guidelines for the Management of Patients with Peripheral Arterial Disease). Available online at www.acc.org/clinical/guidelines/pad/index.pdf

Sobel M and Verhaeghe R, "Antithrombotic Therapy for Peripheral Artery Occlusive Disease: American College of Chest Physicians Evidence-Based Clinical Practice Guidelines (8th Edition), *Chest*, 2008, 133(6 Suppl):815S-43S.

◆ **Ciloxan®** *see* Ciprofloxacin *on page 306*

Cimetidine (sye MET i deen)

Related Information
Anesthesia for Obstetric Patients in Nonobstetric Surgery *on page 1532*

U.S. Brand Names Tagamet® HB 200 [OTC]

Canadian Brand Names Apo-Cimetidine®; Dom-Cimetidine; Mylan-Cimetidine; Novo-Cimetidine; Nu-Cimet; PMS-Cimetidine; Tagamet® HB

Pharmacologic Category Histamine H_2 Antagonist

Use Short-term treatment of active duodenal ulcers and benign gastric ulcers; long-term prophylaxis of duodenal ulcer; gastric hypersecretory states; gastroesophageal reflux; prevention of upper GI bleeding in critically-ill patients; labeled for OTC use for prevention or relief of heartburn, acid indigestion, or sour stomach

Unlabeled/Investigational Use Part of a multidrug regimen for *H. pylori* eradication to reduce the risk of duodenal ulcer recurrence

Pharmacodynamics/Kinetics
Onset of action: 1 hour

Duration: 4-8 hours

Absorption: Rapid

Distribution: Crosses placenta; enters breast milk

Protein binding: 20%

Metabolism: Partially hepatic, forms metabolites

Bioavailability: 60% to 70%

Half-life elimination: Neonates: 3.6 hours; Children: 1.4 hours; Adults: Normal renal function: 2 hours

Time to peak, serum: Oral: 1-2 hours

Excretion: Primarily urine (48% as unchanged drug); feces (some)

Dosage
Children: Oral, I.M., I.V.: 20-40 mg/kg/day in divided doses every 6 hours

Children ≥12 years and Adults: Oral: Heartburn, acid indigestion, sour stomach (OTC labeling): 200 mg up to twice daily; may take 30 minutes prior to eating foods or beverages expected to cause heartburn or indigestion

Adults:

Short-term treatment of active ulcers:

Oral: 300 mg 4 times/day or 800 mg at bedtime or 400 mg twice daily for up to 8 weeks

Note: Higher doses of 1600 mg at bedtime for 4 weeks may be beneficial for a subpopulation of patients with larger duodenal ulcers (>1 cm defined endoscopically) who are also heavy smokers (≥1 pack/day).

I.M., I.V.: 300 mg every 6 hours or 37.5 mg/hour by continuous infusion; I.V. dosage should be adjusted to maintain an intragastric pH ≥5

Prevention of upper GI bleed in critically-ill patients: 50 mg/hour by continuous infusion; I.V. dosage should be adjusted to maintain an intragastric pH ≥5

Note: Reduce dose by 50% if Cl_{cr} <30 mL/minute; treatment >7 days has not been evaluated.

Duodenal ulcer prophylaxis: Oral: 400 mg at bedtime

Gastric hypersecretory conditions: Oral, I.M., I.V.: 300-600 mg every 6 hours; dosage not to exceed 2.4 g/day

Gastroesophageal reflux disease: Oral: 400 mg 4 times/day or 800 mg twice daily for 12 weeks

Helicobacter pylori eradication (unlabeled use): 400 mg twice daily; requires combination therapy with antibiotics

Dosing adjustment/interval in renal impairment: Children and Adults:

Cl_{cr} 10-50 mL/minute: Administer 50% of normal dose

Cl_{cr} <10 mL/minute: Administer 25% of normal dose

Hemodialysis: Slightly dialyzable (5% to 20%); administer after dialysis

Dosing adjustment/comments in hepatic impairment: Usual dose is safe in mild liver disease but use with caution and in reduced dosage in severe liver disease; increased risk of CNS toxicity in cirrhosis suggested by enhanced penetration of CNS

Anesthesia and Critical Care Concerns/Other Considerations The 2008 Surviving Sepsis Campaign guidelines recommend that stress ulcer prophylaxis using an H_2 blocker (Grade 1A) or proton pump inhibitor (Grade 1B) be given to patients with severe sepsis to prevent upper GI bleed. Benefit of prevention of upper GI bleed must be weighed against potential effect of increased stomach pH on development of ventilator-associated pneumonia.

Additional Information Complete prescribing information for this medication should be consulted for additional detail.

Dosage Forms Excipient information presented when available (limited, particularly for generics); consult specific product labeling.

Note: Strength is expressed as base

Infusion, as hydrochloride [premixed in NS]: 300 mg (50 mL)

Injection, solution, as hydrochloride: 150 mg/mL (2 mL, 8 mL)

Solution, oral, as hydrochloride: 300 mg/5 mL (240 mL, 480 mL)

Tablet: 200 mg [OTC], 300 mg, 400 mg, 800 mg

Tagamet® HB 200: 200 mg

References

Dellinger RP, Levy MM, Carlet JM, et al, "Surviving Sepsis Campaign: International Guidelines for Management of Severe Sepsis and Septic Shock: 2008," *Intensive Care Med*, 2008, 34(1): 17-60. Available at http://www.survivingsepsis.org/system/files/images/2008_20International_20SSC_20-Guidelines_1_.pdf

◆ **Cimzia®** *see* Certolizumab Pegol *on page 281*

◆ **Cinryze™** *see* C1 Inhibitor (Human) *on page 223*

◆ **Cipralex® (Can)** *see* Escitalopram *on page 521*

◆ **Cipro®** *see* Ciprofloxacin *on page 306*

◆ **Cipro® XL (Can)** *see* Ciprofloxacin *on page 306*

Ciprofloxacin (sip roe FLOKS a sin)

Medication Safety Issues

Sound-alike/look-alike issues:

Cetraxal® may be confused with cefTRIAXone

Ciprofloxacin may be confused with cephalexin

Ciloxan® may be confused with cinoxacin, Cytoxan®

Cipro® may be confused with Ceftin®

Medication Guide An FDA-approved patient medication guide, which is available with the product information and as follows, must be dispensed with this medication for each new outpatient prescription and refill.

Cipro®: http://www.accessdata.fda.gov/drugsatfda_docs/label/2009/019537s701984744198575120780282147325L.pdf

Proquin® XR: http://www.accessdata.fda.gov/drugsatfda_docs/label/2009/021744s012lbl.pdf

Related Information

Desensitization Protocols *on page 1692*

Dosing Considerations for the Critically-Ill Patient With Morbid Obesity *on page 1561*

Prevention of Wound Infection and Sepsis in Surgical Patients *on page 1721*

U.S. Brand Names Cetraxal®; Ciloxan®; Cipro®; Cipro® I.V.; Cipro® XR; Proquin® XR

Canadian Brand Names Apo-Ciprofloxin®; Ciloxan®; Cipro®; Cipro® XL; CO Ciprofloxacin; Dom-Ciprofloxacin; Mint-Ciprofloxacin; Mylan-Ciprofloxacin; Novo-Ciprofloxacin; PHL-Ciprofloxacin; PMS-Ciprofloxacin; PRO-Ciprofloxacin; RAN-Ciprofloxacin; ratio-Ciprofloxacin; Riva-Ciprofloxacin; Sandoz-Ciprofloxacin; Taro-Ciprofloxacin

Index Terms Ciprofloxacin Hydrochloride

Pharmacologic Category Antibiotic, Ophthalmic; Antibiotic, Otic; Antibiotic, Quinolone

Generic Available Yes: Excludes ointment, otic solution, suspension

Use

Children: Complicated urinary tract infections and pyelonephritis due to *E. coli.* **Note:** Although effective, ciprofloxacin is not the drug of first choice in children.

Children and Adults: To reduce incidence or progression of disease following exposure to aerolized *Bacillus anthracis*. Ophthalmologically, for superficial ocular infections (corneal ulcers, conjunctivitis) due to susceptible strains. Auricularly, for acute otitis externa due to susceptible strains of *Pseudomonas aeruginosa* or *Staphylococcus aureus*

Adults: Treatment of the following infections when caused by susceptible bacteria: Urinary tract infections; acute uncomplicated cystitis in females; chronic bacterial prostatitis; lower respiratory tract infections (including acute exacerbations of chronic bronchitis); acute sinusitis; skin and skin structure infections; bone and joint infections; complicated intra-abdominal infections (in combination with metronidazole); infectious diarrhea; typhoid fever due to *Salmonella typhi* (eradication of chronic typhoid carrier state has not been proven); uncomplicated cervical and urethra gonorrhea (due to *N. gonorrhoeae*); nosocomial pneumonia; empirical therapy for febrile neutropenic patients (in combination with piperacillin)

Note: As of April 2007, the CDC no longer recommends the use of fluoroquinolones for the treatment of gonococcal disease.

Unlabeled/Investigational Use Acute pulmonary exacerbations in cystic fibrosis (children); cutaneous/gastrointestinal/oropharyngeal anthrax (treatment, children and adults); disseminated gonococcal infection (adults); chancroid (adults); prophylaxis to *Neisseria meningitidis* following close contact with an infected person; empirical therapy (oral) for febrile neutropenia in low-risk cancer patients; HACEK group endocarditis; infectious diarrhea (children)

Mechanism of Action Inhibits DNA-gyrase in susceptible organisms; inhibits relaxation of supercoiled DNA and promotes breakage of double-stranded DNA

Pharmacodynamics/Kinetics

Absorption: Oral: Immediate release tablet: Rapid (~50% to 85%)

Distribution: V_d: 2.1-2.7 L/kg; tissue concentrations often exceed serum concentrations especially in kidneys, gallbladder, liver, lungs, gynecological tissue, and prostatic tissue; CSF concentrations: 10% of serum concentrations (noninflamed meninges), 14% to 37% (inflamed meninges)

Protein binding: 20% to 40%

Metabolism: Partially hepatic; forms 4 metabolites (limited activity)

Half-life elimination: Children: 2.5 hours; Adults: Normal renal function: 3-5 hours

Time to peak: Oral:
  Immediate release tablet: 0.5-2 hours
  Extended release tablet: Cipro® XR: 1-2.5 hours, Proquin® XR: 3.5-8.7 hours
Excretion: Urine (30% to 50% as unchanged drug); feces (15% to 43%)
Dosage Note: Extended release tablets and immediate release formulations are not interchangeable. Unless otherwise specified, oral dosing reflects the use of immediate release formulations.
Usual dosage ranges:
  Children (see Warnings/Precautions):
    Oral: 20-30 mg/kg/day in 2 divided doses; maximum dose: 1.5 g/day
    I.V.: 20-30 mg/kg/day divided every 12 hours; maximum dose: 800 mg/day
  Adults:
    Oral: 250-750 mg every 12 hours
    I.V.: 200-400 mg every 12 hours
Indication-specific dosing:
  Children:
    Acute otitis externa: Children ≥1 year: Refer to adult dosing
    Anthrax:
      Inhalational (postexposure prophylaxis):
        Oral: 15 mg/kg/dose every 12 hours for 60 days; maximum: 500 mg/dose
        I.V.: 10 mg/kg/dose every 12 hours for 60 days; do **not** exceed 400 mg/dose (800 mg/day)
      Cutaneous (treatment, CDC guidelines): Oral: 10-15 mg/kg every 12 hours for 60 days (maximum: 1 g/day); amoxicillin 80 mg/kg/day divided every 8 hours is an option for completion of treatment after clinical improvement. **Note:** In the presence of systemic involvement, extensive edema, lesions on head/neck, refer to I.V. dosing for treatment of inhalational/gastrointestinal/oropharyngeal anthrax.
      Inhalational/gastrointestinal/oropharyngeal (treatment, CDC guidelines): I.V.: Initial: 10-15 mg/kg every 12 hours for 60 days (maximum: 500 mg/dose); switch to oral therapy when clinically appropriate; refer to adult dosing for notes on combined therapy and duration
    Bacterial conjunctivitis: See adult dosing
    Corneal ulcer: See adult dosing
    Cystic fibrosis (unlabeled use):
      Oral: 40 mg/kg/day divided every 12 hours administered following 1 week of I.V. therapy has been reported in a clinical trial; total duration of therapy: 10-21 days
      I.V.: 30 mg/kg/day divided every 8 hours for 1 week, followed by oral therapy, has been reported in a clinical trial
    Urinary tract infection (complicated) or pyelonephritis:
      Oral: 20-30 mg/kg/day in 2 divided doses (every 12 hours) for 10-21 days; maximum: 1.5 g/day
      I.V.: 6-10 mg/kg every 8 hours for 10-21 days (maximum: 400 mg/dose)
  Adults:
    Acute otitis externa: Otic solution: Instill 0.25 mL (contents of 1 single-dose container) into affected ear twice daily for 7 days
    Anthrax:
      Inhalational (postexposure prophylaxis):
        Oral: 500 mg every 12 hours for 60 days
        I.V.: 400 mg every 12 hours for 60 days
      Cutaneous (treatment, CDC guidelines): Oral: Immediate release formulation: 500 mg every 12 hours for 60 days. **Note:** In the presence of systemic involvement, extensive edema, lesions on head/neck, refer to I.V. dosing for treatment of inhalational/gastrointestinal/oropharyngeal anthrax
      Inhalational/gastrointestinal/oropharyngeal (treatment, CDC guidelines): I.V.: 400 mg every 12 hours. **Note:** Initial treatment should include two or more agents predicted to be effective (per CDC recommendations). Continue combined therapy for 60 days.
    Bacterial conjunctivitis:
      Ophthalmic solution: Instill 1-2 drops in eye(s) every 2 hours while awake for 2 days and 1-2 drops every 4 hours while awake for the next 5 days

Ophthalmic ointment: Apply a ¹/₂" ribbon into the conjunctival sac 3 times/day for the first 2 days, followed by a ¹/₂" ribbon applied twice daily for the next 5 days

Bone/joint infections:
Oral: 500-750 mg twice daily for 4-6 weeks
I.V.: Mild-to-moderate: 400 mg every 12 hours for 4-6 weeks; Severe/complicated: 400 mg every 8 hours for 4-6 weeks

Chancroid (CDC guidelines): Oral: 500 mg twice daily for 3 days

Corneal ulcer: Ophthalmic solution: Instill 2 drops into affected eye every 15 minutes for the first 6 hours, then 2 drops into the affected eye every 30 minutes for the remainder of the first day. On day 2, instill 2 drops into the affected eye hourly. On days 3-14, instill 2 drops into affected eye every 4 hours. Treatment may continue after day 14 if re-epithelialization has not occurred.

Endocarditis due to HACEK organisms (AHA guidelines, unlabeled use):
Note: Not first-line option; use only if intolerant of beta-lactam therapy:
Oral: 500 mg every 12 hours for 4 weeks
I.V.: 400 mg every 12 hours for 4 weeks

Febrile neutropenia*: I.V.: 400 mg every 8 hours for 7-14 days

Gonococcal infections:
Urethral/cervical gonococcal infections: Oral: 250-500 mg as a single dose (CDC recommends concomitant doxycycline or azithromycin due to possible coinfection with *Chlamydia*; **Note:** As of April 2007, the CDC no longer recommends the use of fluoroquinolones for the treatment of uncomplicated gonococcal disease.

Disseminated gonococcal infection (CDC guidelines): Oral: 500 mg twice daily to complete 7 days of therapy (initial treatment with ceftriaxone 1 g I.M./I.V. daily for 24-48 hours after improvement begins); **Note:** As of April 2007, the CDC no longer recommends the use of fluoroquinolones for the treatment of more serious gonococcal disease, unless no other options exist and susceptibility can be confirmed via culture.

Infectious diarrhea: Oral:
Salmonella: 500 mg twice daily for 5-7 days
Shigella: 500 mg twice daily for 3 days
Traveler's diarrhea: Mild: 750 mg for one dose; Severe: 500 mg twice daily for 3 days
Vibrio cholerae: 1 g for one dose

Intra-abdominal*:
Oral: 500 mg every 12 hours for 7-14 days
I.V.: 400 mg every 12 hours for 7-14 days

Lower respiratory tract, skin/skin structure infections:
Oral: 500-750 mg twice daily for 7-14 days
I.V.: Mild-to-moderate: 400 mg every 12 hours for 7-14 days; Severe/complicated: 400 mg every 8 hours for 7-14 days

Nosocomial pneumonia: I.V.: 400 mg every 8 hours for 10-14 days

Prostatitis (chronic, bacterial): Oral: 500 mg every 12 hours for 28 days

Sinusitis (acute): Oral: 500 mg every 12 hours for 10 days

Typhoid fever: Oral: 500 mg every 12 hours for 10 days

Urinary tract infection:
Acute uncomplicated, cystitis:
Oral:
Immediate release formulation: 250 mg every 12 hours for 3 days
Extended release formulation (Cipro® XR, Proquin® XR): 500 mg every 24 hours for 3 days
I.V.: 200 mg every 12 hours for 7-14 days
Complicated (including pyelonephritis):
Oral:
Immediate release formulation: 500 mg every 12 hours for 7-14 days
Extended release formulation (Cipro® XR): 1000 mg every 24 hours for 7-14 days
I.V.: 400 mg every 12 hours for 7-14 days
*Combination therapy generally recommended.
Elderly: No adjustment needed in patients with normal renal function

◀ **Dosing adjustment in renal impairment:** Adults:

Cl_{cr} 30-50 mL/minute: Oral: 250-500 mg every 12 hours

Cl_{cr} <30 mL/minute: Acute uncomplicated pyelonephritis or complicated UTI:
Oral: Extended release formulation: 500 mg every 24 hours

Cl_{cr} 5-29 mL/minute:
Oral: 250-500 mg every 18 hours
I.V.: 200-400 mg every 18-24 hours

Dialysis: Only small amounts of ciprofloxacin are removed by hemo- or peritoneal dialysis (<10%); usual dose: Oral: 250-500 mg every 24 hours following dialysis

Continuous renal replacement therapy (CRRT): I.V.:
CVVH: 200 mg every 12 hours
CVVHD or CVVHDF: 200-400 mg every 12 hours

Stability

Injection:

Premixed infusion: Store between 5°C to 25°C (41°F to 77°F); avoid freezing. Protect from light.

Vial: Store between 5°C to 30°C (41°F to 86°F); avoid freezing. Protect from light. May be diluted with NS, D_5W, SWFI, $D_{10}W$, $D_5^{1}/_4NS$, $D_5^{1}/_2NS$, LR. Diluted solutions of 0.5-2 mg/mL are stable for up to 14 days refrigerated or at room temperature.

Ophthalmic solution/ointment: Store at 2°C to 25°C (36°F to 77°F). Protect from light.

Otic solution: Store at 15°C to 25°C (59°F to 77°F). Protect from light. Store unused single-dose containers in foil overwrap pouch until immediately prior to use.

Microcapsules for oral suspension: Prior to reconstitution, store below 25°C (77°F); protect from freezing. Following reconstitution, store below 30°C (86°F) for up to 14 days; protect from freezing.

Tablet:

Immediate release: Store below 30°C (86°F).

Extended release: Store at room temperature of 15°C to 30°C (59°F to 86°F).

Administration

Ophthalmic ointment/solution: For topical ophthalmic use only; avoid touching tip of applicator to eye or other surfaces.

Oral: May administer with food to minimize GI upset; avoid antacid use; maintain proper hydration and urine output. Administer immediate release ciprofloxacin and Cipro® XR at least 2 hours before or 6 hours after, and Proquin® XR at least 4 hours before or 6 hours after antacids or other products containing calcium, iron, or zinc (including dairy products or calcium-fortified juices). Separate oral administration from drugs which may impair absorption (see Drug Interactions).

Oral suspension: Should not be administered through feeding tubes (suspension is oil-based and adheres to the feeding tube). Patients should avoid chewing on the microcapsules.

Nasogastric/orogastric tube: Crush immediate-release tablet and mix with water. Flush feeding tube before and after administration. Hold tube feedings at least 1 hour before and 2 hours after administration.

Tablet, extended release: Do not crush, split, or chew. May be administered with meals containing dairy products (calcium content <800 mg), but not with dairy products alone. Proquin® XR should be administered with a main meal of the day; evening meal is preferred.

Otic solution: For otic use only. Prior to use, warm solution by holding container in hands for at least 1 minute. Patient should lie down with affected ear upward and medication instilled. Patients should remain in the position for at least 1 minute to allow penetration of solution.

Parenteral: Administer by slow I.V. infusion over 60 minutes to reduce the risk of venous irritation (burning, pain, erythema, and swelling); final concentration for administration should not exceed 2 mg/mL.

Monitoring Parameters CBC, renal and hepatic function during prolonged therapy

Reference Range Therapeutic: 2.6-3 mcg/mL; Toxic: >5 mcg/mL

Pregnancy Risk Factor C

Contraindications Hypersensitivity to ciprofloxacin, any component of the formulation, or other quinolones; concurrent administration of tizanidine

Warnings/Precautions [U.S. Boxed Warning]: **There have been reports of tendon inflammation and/or rupture with quinolone antibiotics; risk may be increased with concurrent corticosteroids, organ transplant recipients, and in patients >60 years of age.** Rupture of the Achilles tendon sometimes requiring surgical repair has been reported most frequently; but other tendon sites (eg, rotator cuff, biceps) have also been reported. Strenuous physical activity, rheumatoid arthritis, and renal impairment may be an independent risk factor for tendonitis. Discontinue at first sign of tendon inflammation or pain. May occur even after discontinuation of therapy. Use with caution in patients with rheumatoid arthritis; may increase risk of tendon rupture. CNS stimulation may occur (tremor, restlessness, confusion, and very rarely hallucinations or seizures). Use with caution in patients with known or suspected CNS disorder. Potential for seizures, although very rare, may be increased with concomitant NSAID therapy. Use with caution in individuals at risk of seizures. Fluoroquinolones may prolong QT_c interval; avoid use in patients with a history of QT_c prolongation, uncorrected hypokalemia, hypomagnesemia, or concurrent administration of other medications known to prolong the QT interval (including Class Ia and Class III antiarrhythmics, cisapride, erythromycin, antipsychotics, and tricyclic antidepressants). Prolonged use may result in fungal or bacterial superinfection, including *C. difficile*-associated diarrhea (CDAD) and pseudomembranous colitis; CDAD has been observed >2 months postantibiotic treatment. Rarely crystalluria has occurred; urine alkalinity may increase the risk. Ensure adequate hydration during therapy. Adverse effects, including those related to joints and/or surrounding tissues, are increased in pediatric patients and therefore, ciprofloxacin should not be considered as drug of choice in children (exception is anthrax treatment). Rare cases of peripheral neuropathy may occur.

Fluoroquinolones have been associated with the development of serious, and sometimes fatal, hypoglycemia, most often in elderly diabetics but also in patients without diabetes. This occurred most frequently with gatifloxacin (no longer available systemically), but may occur at a lower frequency with other quinolones.

Severe hypersensitivity reactions, including anaphylaxis, have occurred with quinolone therapy. Reactions may present as typical allergic symptoms after a single dose, or may manifest as severe idiosyncratic dermatologic, vascular, pulmonary, renal, hepatic, and/or hematologic events, usually after multiple doses. Prompt discontinuation of drug should occur if skin rash or other symptoms arise. Quinolones may exacerbate myasthenia gravis, use with caution (rare, potentially life-threatening weakness of respiratory muscles may occur). Use caution in renal impairment. Avoid excessive sunlight and take precautions to limit exposure (eg, loose fitting clothing, sunscreen); may cause moderate-to-severe phototoxicity reactions. Discontinue use if photosensitivity occurs. Since ciprofloxacin is ineffective in the treatment of syphilis and may mask symptoms, all patients should be tested for syphilis at the time of gonorrheal diagnosis and 3 months later. Hemolytic reactions may (rarely) occur with quinolone use in patients with latent or actual G6PD deficiency.

Ciprofloxacin is a potent inhibitor of CYP1A2. Coadministration of drugs which depend on this pathway may lead to substantial increases in serum concentrations and adverse effects.

Adverse Reactions
Systemic:
1% to 10%:
  Central nervous system: Neurologic events (children 2%, includes dizziness, insomnia, nervousness, somnolence); fever (children 2%); headache (I.V. administration); restlessness (I.V. administration)
  Dermatologic: Rash (children 2%, adults 1%)
  Gastrointestinal: Nausea (children/adults 3%); diarrhea (children 5%, adults 2%); vomiting (children 5%, adults 1%); abdominal pain (children 3%, adults <1%); dyspepsia (children 3%)
  Hepatic: ALT increased, AST increased (adults 1%)
  Local: Injection site reactions (I.V. administration)
  Respiratory: Rhinitis (children 3%)
<1% (Limited to important or life-threatening): Abnormal gait, acute renal failure, agitation, agranulocytosis, albuminuria, allergic reactions, anaphylactic shock,

anaphylaxis, anemia, angina pectoris, angioedema, anorexia, anosmia, arthralgia, ataxia, atrial flutter, bone marrow depression (life-threatening), breast pain, bronchospasm, candidiasis, candiduria, cardiopulmonary arrest, cerebral thrombosis, chills, cholestatic jaundice, chromatopsia, confusion, constipation, crystalluria (particularly in alkaline urine), cylindruria, delirium, depersonalization, depression, dizziness, drowsiness, dyspepsia (adults), dysphagia, dyspnea, edema, eosinophilia, erythema multiforme, erythema nodosum, exfoliative dermatitis, fever (adults), fixed eruption, flatulence, gastrointestinal bleeding, hallucinations, headache (oral), hematuria, hemolytic anemia, hepatic failure (some fatal), hepatic necrosis, hyperesthesia, hyperglycemia, hyperpigmentation, hyper-/hypotension, hypertonia, insomnia, interstitial nephritis, intestinal perforation, irritability, jaundice, joint pain, laryngeal edema, light-headedness, lymphadenopathy, malaise, manic reaction, methemoglobinemia, MI, migraine, moniliasis, myalgia, myasthenia gravis, myoclonus, nephritis, nightmares, nystagmus, orthostatic hypotension, palpitation, pancreatitis, pancytopenia (life-threatening or fatal), paranoia, paresthesia, peripheral neuropathy, petechia, photosensitivity, pneumonitis, prolongation of PT/INR, pseudomembranous colitis, psychosis, pulmonary edema, renal calculi, seizure; serum cholesterol, glucose, triglycerides increased; serum sickness-like reactions, Stevens-Johnson syndrome, syncope, tachycardia, taste loss, tendon rupture, tendonitis, thrombophlebitis, tinnitus, torsade de pointes, toxic epidermal necrolysis (Lyell's syndrome), tremor, twitching, urethral bleeding, vaginal candidiasis, vaginitis, vasculitis, ventricular ectopy, visual disturbance, weakness

Otic:

1% to 10%:

Central nervous system: Headache (2% to 3%)

Local: Application site pain (2% to 3%), fungal superinfection (2% to 3%), pruritus (2% to 3%)

Drug Interactions

Metabolism/Transport Effects Inhibits CYP1A2 (strong), 3A4 (weak)

Avoid Concomitant Use

Avoid concomitant use of Ciprofloxacin with any of the following: TiZANidine

Increased Effect/Toxicity

Ciprofloxacin may increase the levels/effects of: Bendamustine; Caffeine; Corticosteroids (Systemic); CYP1A2 Substrates; Erlotinib; Methotrexate; Pentoxifylline; QTc-Prolonging Agents; Ropinirole; Ropivacaine; Sulfonylureas; Theophylline Derivatives; TiZANidine; Vitamin K Antagonists

The levels/effects of Ciprofloxacin may be increased by: Insulin; Nonsteroidal Anti-Inflammatory Agents; P-Glycoprotein Inhibitors; Probenecid

Decreased Effect

Ciprofloxacin may decrease the levels/effects of: Mycophenolate; Phenytoin; Sulfonylureas; Typhoid Vaccine

The levels/effects of Ciprofloxacin may be decreased by: Antacids; Calcium Salts; Didanosine; Iron Salts; Magnesium Salts; P-Glycoprotein Inducers; Quinapril; Sevelamer; Sucralfate; Zinc Salts

Ethanol/Nutrition/Herb Interactions

Food: Food decreases rate, but not extent, of absorption. Ciprofloxacin serum levels may be decreased if taken with dairy products or calcium-fortified juices. Ciprofloxacin may increase serum caffeine levels if taken with caffeine.

Enteral feedings may decrease plasma concentrations of ciprofloxacin probably by >30% inhibition of absorption. Ciprofloxacin should not be administered with enteral feedings. The feeding would need to be discontinued for 1-2 hours prior to and after ciprofloxacin administration. Nasogastric administration produces a greater loss of ciprofloxacin bioavailability than does nasoduodenal administration.

Herb/Nutraceutical: Avoid dong quai, St John's wort (may also cause photosensitization).

Test Interactions Some quinolones may produce a false-positive urine screening result for opiates using commercially-available immunoassay kits. This has been demonstrated most consistently for levofloxacin and ofloxacin, but other quinolones have shown cross-reactivity in certain assay kits. Confirmation of positive opiate screens by more specific methods should be considered.

Dietary Considerations

Food: Drug may cause GI upset; take without regard to meals (manufacturer prefers that immediate release tablet is taken 2 hours after meals). Extended release tablet may be taken with meals that contain dairy products (calcium content <800 mg), but not with dairy products alone.

Dairy products, calcium-fortified juices, oral multivitamins, and mineral supplements: Absorption of ciprofloxacin is decreased by divalent and trivalent cations. The manufacturer states that the usual dietary intake of calcium (including meals which include dairy products) has not been shown to interfere with ciprofloxacin absorption. Immediate release ciprofloxacin and Cipro® XR may be taken 2 hours before or 6 hours after, and Proquin® XR may be taken 4 hours before or 6 hours after, any of these products.

Caffeine: Patients consuming regular large quantities of caffeinated beverages may need to restrict caffeine intake if excessive cardiac or CNS stimulation occurs.

Dosage Forms Excipient information presented when available (limited, particularly for generics); consult specific product labeling.

Infusion [premixed in D_5W]: 200 mg (100 mL); 400 mg (200 mL)

Cipro® I.V.: 200 mg (100 mL); 400 mg (200 mL)

Injection, solution [concentrate]: 10 mg/mL (20 mL, 40 mL, 120 mL)

Cipro® I.V.: 10 mg/mL (20 mL, 40 mL [DSC])

Microcapsules for suspension, oral:

Cipro®: 250 mg/5 mL (100 mL); 500 mg/5 mL (100 mL) [strawberry flavor]

Ointment, ophthalmic, as hydrochloride:

Ciloxan®: 3.33 mg/g (3.5 g) [equivalent to ciprofloxacin base 0.3%]

Solution, ophthalmic, as hydrochloride: 3.5 mg/mL (2.5 mL, 5mL, 10 mL) [equivalent to ciprofloxacin base 0.3%]

Ciloxan®: 3.5 mg/mL (5 mL) [0.3% base; contains benzalkonium chloride]

Solution, otic, as hydrochloride [preservative free]:

Cetraxal®: 0.5 mg/0.25 mL (14s) [equivalent to ciprofloxacin base 0.2%]

Tablet, as hydrochloride: 100 mg [strength expressed as base], 250 mg [strength expressed as base], 500 mg [strength expressed as base], 750 mg [strength expressed as base]

Cipro®: 250 mg [strength expressed as base], 500 mg [strength expressed as base], 750 mg [strength expressed as base]

Tablet, extended release, as base and hydrochloride: 500 mg [strength expressed as base], 1000 mg [strength expressed as base]

Cipro® XR: 500 mg [strength expressed as base], 1000 mg [strength expressed as base]

Tablet, extended release, as hydrochloride:

Proquin® XR: 500 mg [strength expressed as base]

Tablet, extended release, as hydrochloride [dose pack]:

Proquin® XR: 500 mg (3s) [strength expressed as base]

References

American Thoracic Society and Infectious Diseases Society of America, "Guidelines for the Management of Adults With Hospital-Acquired, Ventilator-Associated, and Healthcare-Associated Pneumonia," *Am J Respir Crit Care Med*, 2005, 171(4):388-416.

"Antimicrobial Prophylaxis for Surgery," *Treat Guidel Med Lett*, 2004, 2(20):27-32.

Centers for Disease Control and Prevention, "Update: Investigation of Bioterrorism-Related Anthrax and Interim Guidelines for Exposure Management and Antimicrobial Therapy, October 2001," *MMWR Morb Mortal Wkly Rep*, October 26, 2001, 50(42):909-19. Available at: http://www.cdc.gov/mmwr/preview/mmwrhtml/mm5042a1.htm.

Fish DN, Bainbridge JL, and Peloquin CA, "Variable Disposition of Ciprofloxacin in Critically Ill Patients Undergoing Continuous Arteriovenous Hemodiafiltration," *Pharmacotherapy*, 1995, 15 (2):236-45.

Food and Drug Administration (FDA), "CIPRO (Ciprofloxacin) Use by Pregnant and Lactating Women." Available at http://www.fda.gov/cder/drug/infopage/cipro/cipropreg.htm. Last accessed August 9, 2004.

Trotman RL, Williamson JC, Shoemaker DM, et al, "Antibiotic Dosing in Critically Ill Adult Patients Receiving Continuous Renal Replacement Therapy," *Clin Infect Dis*, 2005, 41(8):1159-66.

◆ **Ciprofloxacin Hydrochloride** *see* Ciprofloxacin *on page 306*

◆ **Cipro® I.V.** *see* Ciprofloxacin *on page* 306
◆ **Cipro® XR** *see* Ciprofloxacin *on page* 306

Cisatracurium (sis a tra KYOO ree um)

Medication Safety Issues
Sound-alike/look-alike issues:
Nimbex® may be confused with Revex®

High alert medication: The Institute for Safe Medication Practices (ISMP) includes this medication among its list of drugs which have a heightened risk of causing significant patient harm when used in error.

United States Pharmacopeia (USP) 2006: The Interdisciplinary Safe Medication Use Expert Committee of the USP has recommended the following:
- Hospitals, clinics, and other practice sites should institute special safeguards in the storage, labeling, and use of these agents and should include these safeguards in staff orientation and competency training.
- Healthcare professionals should be on high alert (especially vigilant) whenever a neuromuscular-blocking agent (NMBA) is stocked, ordered, prepared, or administered.

Related Information
Allergic Reactions *on page* 1508
Anesthesia for Geriatric Patients *on page* 1523
Anesthesia for Patients With Liver Disease *on page* 1537
Chronic Renal Failure *on page* 1552
Neuromuscular-Blocking Agents *on page* 1684

U.S. Brand Names Nimbex®

Canadian Brand Names Nimbex®

Index Terms Cisatracurium Besylate

Pharmacologic Category Neuromuscular Blocker Agent, Nondepolarizing

Generic Available No

Use Adjunct to general anesthesia to facilitate endotracheal intubation and to relax skeletal muscles during surgery; to facilitate mechanical ventilation in ICU patients; does not relieve pain or produce sedation

Mechanism of Action Blocks neural transmission at the myoneural junction by binding with cholinergic receptor sites

Pharmacodynamics/Kinetics
Onset of action: I.V.: 2-3 minutes
Peak effect: 3-5 minutes
Duration: Recovery begins in 20-35 minutes when anesthesia is balanced; recovery is attained in 90% of patients in 25-93 minutes
Metabolism: Undergoes rapid nonenzymatic degradation in the bloodstream (Hofmann elimination) to laudanosine and inactive metabolites; laudanosine may cause CNS stimulation (association not established in humans) and has less accumulation with prolonged use than artracurium due to lower requirements for clinical effect
Half-life elimination: 22-29 minutes

Dosage I.V. (not to be used I.M.):
Operating room administration:
Infants 1-23 months: 0.15 mg/kg over 5-10 seconds during either halothane or opioid anesthesia
Children 2-12 years: Intubating doses: 0.1-0.15 mg/kg over 5-15 seconds during either halothane or opioid anesthesia. (**Note:** When given during stable opioid/nitrous oxide/oxygen anesthesia, 0.1 mg/kg produces maximum neuromuscular block in an average of 2.8 minutes and clinically effective block for 28 minutes.)
Adults: Intubating doses: 0.15-0.2 mg/kg as component of propofol/nitrous oxide/oxygen induction-intubation technique. (**Note:** May produce generally good or excellent conditions for tracheal intubation in 1.5-2 minutes with clinically effective duration of action during propofol anesthesia of 55-61 minutes.); initial dose after succinylcholine for intubation: 0.1 mg/kg; maintenance dose: 0.03 mg/kg 40-60 minutes after initial dose, then at ~20-minute intervals based on clinical criteria

Children ≥2 years and Adults: Continuous infusion: After an initial bolus, a diluted solution can be given by continuous infusion for maintenance of neuromuscular blockade during extended surgery; adjust the rate of administration according to the patient's response as determined by peripheral nerve stimulation. An initial infusion rate of 3 mcg/kg/minute may be required to rapidly counteract the spontaneous recovery of neuromuscular function; thereafter, a rate of 1-2 mcg/kg/minute should be adequate to maintain continuous neuromuscular block in the 89% to 99% range in most pediatric and adult patients. Consider reduction of the infusion rate by 30% to 40% when administering during stable isoflurane, enflurane, sevoflurane, or desflurane anesthesia. Spontaneous recovery from neuromuscular blockade following discontinuation of infusion of cisatracurium may be expected to proceed at a rate comparable to that following single bolus administration.

Intensive care unit administration: Follow the principles for infusion in the operating room. At initial signs of recovery from bolus dose, begin the infusion at a dose of 3 mcg/kg/minute and adjust rates accordingly; dosage ranges of 0.5-10 mcg/kg/minute have been reported. If patient is allowed to recover from neuromuscular blockade, readministration of a bolus dose may be necessary to quickly re-establish neuromuscular block prior to reinstituting the infusion. See table.

Cisatracurium Besylate Infusion Chart

Drug Delivery Rate (mcg/kg/min)	Infusion Rate (mL/kg/min) 0.1 mg/mL (10 mg/100 mL)	Infusion Rate (mL/kg/min) 0.4 mg/mL (40 mg/100 mL)
1	0.01	0.0025
1.5	0.015	0.00375
2	0.02	0.005
3	0.03	0.0075
5	0.05	0.0125

Dosing adjustment in renal impairment: Because slower times to onset of complete neuromuscular block were observed in renal dysfunction patients, extending the interval between the administration of cisatracurium and intubation attempt may be required to achieve adequate intubation conditions.

Stability Refrigerate intact vials at 2°C to 8°C (36°F to 46°F). Use vials within 21 days upon removal from the refrigerator to room temperature (25°C to 77°F). Per the manufacturer, dilutions of 0.1-0.2 mg/mL in 0.9% sodium chloride (NS) or dextrose 5% in water (D_5W) are stable for up to 24 hours at room temperature or under refrigeration and in D_5LR for up to 24 hours in the refrigerator. *Additional stability data:* Dilutions of 0.1, 2, and 5 mg/mL in D_5W or NS are stable in the refrigerator for up to 30 days; at room temperature (23°C), dilutions of 0.1 and 2 mg/mL began exhibiting substantial drug loss between 7-14 days; dilutions of 5 mg/mL in D_5W or NS are stable for up to 30 days at room temperature (23°C) (Xu, 1998). Usual concentration: 0.1-0.4 mg/mL.

Administration Administer I.V. only; the use of a peripheral nerve stimulator will permit the most advantageous use of cisatracurium, minimize the possibility of overdosage or underdosage and assist in the evaluation of recovery

Give undiluted as a bolus injection; not for I.M. injection, too much tissue irritation; continuous administration requires the use of an infusion pump

Monitoring Parameters Vital signs (heart rate, blood pressure, respiratory rate)

Anesthesia and Critical Care Concerns/Other Considerations

Clinical Pearls/Comments: Because cisatracurium does not cause histamine release, the associated problems of hypotension and bronchospasm are rare.

Evidence-Based Information: Cisatracurium is classified as an intermediate duration neuromuscular-blocking agent; does not appear to have a cumulative effect on the duration of blockade; synergistic effect when combined with steroidal-based nondepolarizing muscle relaxant (Breslin, 2004); neuromuscular-blocking potency is 3 times that of atracurium.

◀ **Critically-Ill Adult Patients:**

The 2008 Surviving Sepsis Campaign guidelines recommend avoiding use of neuromuscular blockers if at all possible in the septic patient due to the risk of prolonged neuromuscular blockade following discontinuation. If one is required, monitor the depth of blockade (Grade 1B).

The 2002 ACCM/SCCM/ASHP clinical practice guidelines for sustained neuromuscular blockade in the adult critically-ill patient recommend:

Optimize sedatives and analgesics prior to initiation and monitor and adjust accordingly during course. Neuromuscular blockers do not relieve pain or produce sedation.

Protect patient's eyes from development of keratitis and corneal abrasion by administering ophthalmic ointment and taping eyelids closed or using eye patches. Reposition patient routinely to protect pressure points from breakdown. Address DVT prophylaxis.

Concurrent use of a neuromuscular blocker and corticosteroids appear to increase the risk of certain ICU myopathies; avoid or administer the corticosteroid at the lowest dose possible. Reassess need for neuromuscular blocker daily.

Using daily drug holidays (stopping neuromuscular-blocking agent until patient requires it again) may decrease the incidence of acute quadriplegic myopathy syndrome.

Tachyphylaxis can develop.

Acidosis and severe hypothermia may delay elimination of cisatracurium.

Atracurium or cisatracurium is recommended for patients with significant hepatic or renal disease, due to organ-independent Hofmann elimination.

Monitor patients clinically and via "Train of Four" (TOF) testing with a goal of adjusting the degree of blockade to 1-2 twitches.

Pregnancy Risk Factor B

Contraindications Hypersensitivity to cisatracurium besylate or any component of the formulation

Warnings/Precautions Maintenance of an adequate airway and respiratory support is critical; certain clinical conditions may result in potentiation or antagonism of neuromuscular blockade:

Potentiation: Electrolyte abnormalities, severe hyponatremia, severe hypocalcemia, severe hypokalemia, hypermagnesemia, neuromuscular diseases, acidosis, acute intermittent porphyria, renal failure, hepatic failure

Antagonism: Alkalosis, hypercalcemia, demyelinating lesions, peripheral neuropathies, diabetes mellitus

Increased sensitivity in patients with myasthenia gravis, Eaton-Lambert syndrome; resistance in burn patients (>30% of body) for period of 5-70 days postinjury; resistance in patients with muscle trauma, denervation, immobilization, infection. Cross-sensitivity with other neuromuscular-blocking agents may occur; use extreme caution in patients with previous anaphylactic reactions. Bradycardia may be more common with cisatracurium than with other neuromuscular blocking agents since it has no clinically significant effects on heart rate to counteract the bradycardia produced by anesthetics. Use caution in the elderly. Should be administered by adequately trained individuals familiar with its use. Some dosage forms may contain benzyl alcohol which has been associated with "gasping syndrome" in neonates.

Adverse Reactions <1%: Effects are minimal and transient, bradycardia and hypotension, flushing, pruritus, rash, bronchospasm, acute quadriplegic myopathy syndrome (prolonged use), myositis ossificans (prolonged use)

Drug Interactions

Avoid Concomitant Use

Avoid concomitant use of Cisatracurium with any of the following: QuiNINE

Increased Effect/Toxicity

Cisatracurium may increase the levels/effects of: Cardiac Glycosides; Corticosteroids (Systemic); OnabotulinumtoxinA; RimabotulinumtoxinB

The levels/effects of Cisatracurium may be increased by: AbobotulinumtoxinA; Aminoglycosides; Calcium Channel Blockers; Capreomycin; Colistimethate; Inhalational Anesthetics; Ketorolac; Lincosamide Antibiotics; Lithium; Loop Diuretics; Magnesium Salts; Polymyxin B; Procainamide; QuiNIDine; QuiNINE; Spironolactone; Tetracycline Derivatives; Vancomycin

Decreased Effect

The levels/effects of Cisatracurium may be decreased by: Acetylcholinesterase Inhibitors; Loop Diuretics

Dosage Forms Excipient information presented when available (limited, particularly for generics); consult specific product labeling.

Injection, solution: 2 mg/mL (5 mL); 10 mg/mL (20 mL)

Injection, solution: 2 mg/mL (10 mL) [contains benzyl alcohol]

References

Belmont MR, Lien CA, Quessy S, et al, "The Clinical Neuromuscular Pharmacology of 51W89 in Patients Receiving Nitrous Oxide/Opioid/Barbiturate Anesthesia," *Anesthesiology*, 1995, 82 (5):1139-45.

Breslin DS, Jiao K, Habib AS, et al, "Pharmacodynamic Interactions Between Cisatracurium and Rocuronium," *Anesth Analg*, 2004, 98(1):107-10.

Dellinger RP, Levy MM, Carlet JM, et al, "Surviving Sepsis Campaign: International Guidelines for Management of Severe Sepsis and Septic Shock: 2008," *Intensive Care Med*, 2008, 34(1): 17-60. Available at http://www.survivingsepsis.org/system/files/images/2008_20International_20SSC_20-Guidelines_1_.pdf

Konstadt SN, Reich DL, Stanley TE 3d, et al, "A Two Center Comparison of the Cardiovascular Effects of Cisatracurium (Nimbex®) and Vecuronium in Patients With Coronary Artery Disease," *Anesth Analg*, 1995, 81(5):1010-4.

Lien CA, Belmont MR, "The Cardiovascular Effects and Histamine-Releasing Properties of 51W89 in Patients Receiving Nitrous Oxide/Opioid/Barbiturate Anesthesia," *Anesthesiology*, 1995, 82(5):1131-8.

Murray MJ, Cowen J, DeBlock H, et al, "Clinical Practice Guidelines for Sustained Neuromuscular Blockade in the Adult Critically Ill Patient. Task Force of the American College of Critical Care Medicine (ACCM) of the Society of Critical Care Medicine (SCCM), American Society of Health-System Pharmacists, American College of Chest Physicians," *Crit Care Med*, 2002, 30(1):142-56; viewable at http://www.sccm.org/pdf/NeuromuscularBlockade.pdf.

Prielipp RC, Coursin DB, Scuderi PE, et al, "Comparison of the Infusion Requirements and Recovery Profiles of Vecuronium and Cisatracurium 51W89 in Intensive Care Unit Patients," *Anesth Analg*, 1995, 81(1):3-12.

Sorooshian SS, Stafford MA, Eastwood NB, et al, "Pharmacokinetics and Pharmacodynamics of Cisatracurium in Young and Elderly Adult Patients," *Anesthesiology*, 1996, 84(5):1083-91.

◆ **Cisatracurium Besylate** *see* Cisatracurium *on page 314*

◆ **Citrovorum Factor** *see* Leucovorin Calcium *on page 812*

◆ **Claforan®** *see* Cefotaxime *on page 256*

◆ **Clarinex®** *see* Desloratadine *on page 385*

Clarithromycin (kla RITH roe mye sin)

Medication Safety Issues

Sound-alike/look-alike issues:

Clarithromycin may be confused with Claritin®, clindamycin, erythromycin

Related Information

Helicobacter pylori Treatment *on page 1746*

Prevention of Infective Endocarditis *on page 1718*

U.S. Brand Names Biaxin®; Biaxin® XL

Canadian Brand Names Apo-Clarithromycin; Biaxin®; Biaxin® XL; Gen-Clarithromycin; Mylan-Clarithromycin; PMS-Clarithromycin; ratio-Clarithromycin; Sandoz-Clarithromycin

Pharmacologic Category Antibiotic, Macrolide

Generic Available Yes

Use

Children:

Acute otitis media (*H. influenzae*, *M. catarrhalis*, or *S. pneumoniae*)

Community-acquired pneumonia due to susceptible *Mycoplasma pneumoniae*, *S. pneumoniae*, or *Chlamydia pneumoniae* (TWAR)

Pharyngitis/tonsillitis due to susceptible *S. pyogenes*, acute maxillary sinusitis due to susceptible *H. influenzae*, *S. pneumoniae*, or *Moraxella catarrhalis*, uncomplicated skin/skin structure infections due to susceptible *S. aureus*, *S. pyogenes*, and mycobacterial infections

Prevention of disseminated mycobacterial infections due to MAC disease in patients with advanced HIV infection

◀ Adults:

Pharyngitis/tonsillitis due to susceptible *S. pyogenes*

Acute maxillary sinusitis due to susceptible *H. influenzae, M. catarrhalis,* or *S. pneumoniae*

Acute exacerbation of chronic bronchitis due to susceptible *H. influenzae, H. parainfluenzae, M. catarrhalis,* or *S. pneumoniae*

Community-acquired pneumonia due to susceptible *H. influenzae, H. parainfluenzae, Mycoplasma pneumoniae, S. pneumoniae,* or *Chlamydia pneumoniae* (TWAR), *Moraxella catarrhalis*

Uncomplicated skin/skin structure infections due to susceptible *S. aureus, S. pyogenes*

Disseminated mycobacterial infections due to *M. avium* or *M. intracellulare*

Prevention of disseminated mycobacterial infections due to *M. avium* complex (MAC) disease (eg, patients with advanced HIV infection)

Duodenal ulcer disease due to *H. pylori* in regimens with other drugs including amoxicillin and lansoprazole or omeprazole, ranitidine bismuth citrate, bismuth subsalicylate, tetracycline, and/or an H_2 antagonist

Unlabeled/Investigational Use Pertussis (CDC guidelines); alternate antibiotic for prophylaxis of infective endocarditis in patients who are allergic to penicillin and undergoing surgical or dental procedures (ACC/AHA guidelines)

Mechanism of Action Exerts its antibacterial action by binding to 50S ribosomal subunit resulting in inhibition of protein synthesis. The 14-OH metabolite of clarithromycin is twice as active as the parent compound against certain organisms.

Pharmacodynamics/Kinetics

Absorption: Immediate release: Rapid; food delays rate, but not extent of absorption

Distribution: Widely into most body tissues except CNS

Protein binding: 42% to 50%

Metabolism: Partially hepatic via CYP3A4; converted to 14-OH clarithromycin (active metabolite)

Bioavailability: ~50%

Half-life elimination: Immediate release: Clarithromycin: 3-7 hours; 14-OH-clarithromycin: 5-9 hours

Time to peak: Immediate release: 2-3 hours

Excretion: Primarily urine (20% to 40% as unchanged drug; additional 10% to 15% as metabolite)

Clearance: Approximates normal GFR

Dosage

Usual dosage range:

Children ≥6 months: Oral: 7.5 mg/kg every 12 hours (maximum: 500 mg/dose) for 10 days

Adults: Oral: 250-500 mg every 12 hours **or** 1000 mg (two 500 mg extended release tablets) once daily for 7-14 days

Indication-specific dosing:

Children: Oral:

Community-acquired pneumonia, sinusitis, bronchitis, skin infections: 15 mg/kg/day divided every 12 hours for 10 days

Mycobacterial infection (prevention and treatment): 7.5 mg/kg (up to 500 mg) twice daily. **Note:** Safety of clarithromycin for MAC not studied in children <20 months.

Pertussis (unlabeled use; CDC guidelines):

Children 1-5 months: 15 mg/kg/day divided every 12 hours for 7 days

Children ≥6 months: 15 mg/kg/day divided every 12 hours for 7 days (maximum: 1 g/day)

Prophylaxis against infective endocarditis (unlabeled use): 15 mg/kg 30-60 minutes before procedure. **Note:** American Heart Association (AHA) guidelines now recommend prophylaxis only in patients undergoing invasive procedures and in whom underlying cardiac conditions may predispose to a higher risk of adverse outcomes should infection occur. As of April 2007, routine prophylaxis for GI/GU procedures is no longer recommended by the AHA.

Adults: Oral:

Acute exacerbation of chronic bronchitis:

M. catarrhalis and *S. pneumoniae*: 250 mg every 12 hours for 7-14 days **or** 1000 mg (two 500 mg extended release tablets) once daily for 7 days

H. influenzae: 500 mg every 12 hours for 7-14 days **or** 1000 mg (two 500 mg extended release tablets) once daily for 7 days

H. parainfluenzae: 500 mg every 12 hours for 7 days **or** 1000 mg (two 500 mg extended release tablets) once daily for 7 days

Acute maxillary sinusitis: 500 mg every 12 hours **or** 1000 mg (two 500 mg extended release tablets) once daily for 14 days .

Mycobacterial infection (prevention and treatment): 500 mg twice daily (use with other antimycobacterial drugs, eg, ethambutol or rifampin)

Peptic ulcer disease: Eradication of *Helicobacter pylori*: Dual or triple combination regimens with bismuth subsalicylate, amoxicillin, an H_2-receptor antagonist, or proton-pump inhibitor: 500 mg every 8-12 hours for 10-14 days

Pertussis (unlabeled use; CDC guidelines): 500 mg twice daily for 7 days

Pharyngitis, tonsillitis: 250 mg every 12 hours for 10 days

Pneumonia:

C. pneumoniae, *M. pneumoniae*, and *S. pneumoniae*: 250 mg every 12 hours for 7-14 days **or** 1000 mg (two 500 mg extended release tablets) once daily for 7 days

H. influenzae: 250 mg every 12 hours for 7 days **or** 1000 mg (two 500 mg extended release tablets) once daily for 7 days

H. parainfluenzae and *M. catarrhalis*: 1000 mg (two 500 mg extended release tablets) once daily for 7 days

Prophylaxis against infective endocarditis (unlabeled use): 500 mg 30-60 minutes prior to procedure. **Note:** American Heart Association (AHA) guidelines now recommend prophylaxis only in patients undergoing invasive procedures and in whom underlying cardiac conditions may predispose to a higher risk of adverse outcomes should infection occur. As of April 2007, routine prophylaxis for GI/GU procedures is no longer recommended by the AHA.

Skin and skin structure infection, uncomplicated: 250 mg every 12 hours for 7-14 days

Elderly: Pharmacokinetics are similar to those in younger adults; may have age-related reductions in renal function; monitor and adjust dose if necessary

Dosing adjustment in renal impairment:

Cl_{cr} <30 mL/minute: Half the normal dose or double the dosing interval

In combination with ritonavir:

Cl_{cr} 30-60 mL/minute: Decrease clarithromycin dose by 50%

Cl_{cr} <30 mL/minute: Decrease clarithromycin dose by 75%

Dosing adjustment in hepatic impairment: No dosing adjustment is needed as long as renal function is normal

Stability

Immediate release 250 mg tablets and granules for oral suspension: Store at controlled room temperature of 15°C to 30°C (59°F to 86°F). Reconstituted oral suspension should not be refrigerated because it might gel; microencapsulated particles of clarithromycin in suspension are stable for 14 days when stored at room temperature. Protect tablets from light.

Immediate release 500 mg tablets and Biaxin® XL: Store at controlled room temperature of 20°C to 25°C (68°F to 77°F); excursions permitted to 15°C to 30°C (59°F to 86°F).

Administration Clarithromycin immediate release tablets and oral suspension may be administered with or without meals. Give every 12 hours rather than twice daily to avoid peak and trough variation. Shake suspension well before each use.

Extended release tablets: Should be given with food. Do not crush or chew extended release tablet.

Monitoring Parameters CBC with differential, BUN, creatinine; perform culture and sensitivity studies prior to initiating drug therapy

Pregnancy Risk Factor C

Contraindications Hypersensitivity to clarithromycin, erythromycin, or any macrolide antibiotic; use with ergot derivatives, pimozide, cisapride

◀ **Warnings/Precautions** Dosage adjustment required with severe renal impairment; decreased dosage or prolonged dosing interval may be appropriate. Use with caution in patients with myasthenia gravis. Colchicine toxicity (including fatalities) has been reported with concomitant use. Prolonged use may result in fungal or bacterial superinfection, including *C. difficile*-associated diarrhea (CDAD) and pseudomembranous colitis; CDAD has been observed >2 months postantibiotic treatment. Macrolides (including clarithromycin) have been associated with rare QT prolongation and ventricular arrhythmias, including torsade de pointes. Use caution in patients with coronary artery disease. Avoid use of extended release tablets (Biaxin® XL) in patients with known stricture/narrowing of the GI tract.

Adverse Reactions

1% to 10%:

Central nervous system: Headache (adults and children 2%)

Dermatologic: Rash (children 3%)

Gastrointestinal: Abnormal taste (adults 3% to 7%), diarrhea (adults 3% to 6%; children 6%), vomiting (children 6%), nausea (adults 3%), abdominal pain (adults 2%; children 3%), dyspepsia (adults 2%)

Hepatic: Prothrombin time increased (adults 1%)

Renal: BUN increased (4%)

<1% (Limited to important or life-threatening): Alkaline phosphatase increased, ALT increased, anaphylaxis, anorexia, anxiety, AST increased, behavioral changes, bilirubin increased, cholestatic hepatitis, *Clostridium difficile* colitis, confusion, depersonalization, depression, disorientation, dizziness, GGT increased, glossitis, hallucinations, hearing loss (reversible), hepatic dysfunction, hepatic failure, hepatitis, hypoglycemia, insomnia, interstitial nephritis, jaundice, leukopenia, LDH increased, manic behavior, neutropenia, nightmares, oral moniliasis, pancreatitis, psychosis, QT prolongation, seizure, serum creatinine increased, smell loss, Stevens-Johnson syndrome, stomatitis, thrombocytopenia, tinnitus, tongue discoloration, tooth discoloration (reversible), torsade de pointes, toxic epidermal necrolysis, tremor, urticaria, ventricular tachycardia, ventricular arrhythmia, vertigo, white blood cell count decreased

Drug Interactions

Metabolism/Transport Effects Substrate of CYP3A4 (major); **Inhibits** CYP1A2 (weak), 3A4 (strong)

Avoid Concomitant Use

Avoid concomitant use of Clarithromycin with any of the following: Alfuzosin; Artemether; Cisapride; Dabigatran Etexilate; Disopyramide; Dronedarone; Eplerenone; Everolimus; Halofantrine; Lumefantrine; Nilotinib; Nisoldipine; Pimozide; QuiNINE; Ranolazine; Rivaroxaban; Salmeterol; Silodosin; Tetrabenazine; Thioridazine; Tolvaptan; Topotecan; Ziprasidone

Increased Effect/Toxicity

Clarithromycin may increase the levels/effects of: Alfentanil; Alfuzosin; Almotriptan; Alosetron; Antifungal Agents (Azole Derivatives, Systemic); Antineoplastic Agents (Vinca Alkaloids); Benzodiazepines (metabolized by oxidation); BusPIRone; Calcium Channel Blockers; CarBAMazepine; Cardiac Glycosides; Ciclesonide; Cilostazol; Cisapride; Clozapine; Colchicine; Corticosteroids (Systemic); CycloSPORINE; CYP3A4 Substrates; Dabigatran Etexilate; Disopyramide; Dronedarone; Dutasteride; Eletriptan; Eplerenone; Ergot Derivatives; Everolimus; FentaNYL; Fesoterodine; GlipiZIDE; GlyBURIDE; Halofantrine; HMG-CoA Reductase Inhibitors; Ixabepilone; Maraviroc; Nilotinib; Nisoldipine; Paricalcitol; P-Glycoprotein Substrates; Phosphodiesterase 5 Inhibitors; Pimecrolimus; Pimozide; Protease Inhibitors; QTc-Prolonging Agents; QuiNIDine; QuiNINE; Ranolazine; Repaglinide; Rifamycin Derivatives; Rivaroxaban; Salmeterol; Saxagliptin; Selective Serotonin Reuptake Inhibitors; Silodosin; Sirolimus; Sorafenib; Tacrolimus; Tadalafil; Temsirolimus; Tetrabenazine; Theophylline Derivatives; Thioridazine; Tolvaptan; Topotecan; Vitamin K Antagonists; Zidovudine; Ziprasidone; Zopiclone

The levels/effects of Clarithromycin may be increased by: Alfuzosin; Antifungal Agents (Azole Derivatives, Systemic); Artemether; Chloroquine; Ciprofloxacin; CYP3A4 Inhibitors (Moderate); CYP3A4 Inhibitors (Strong); Gadobutrol; Lumefantrine; Nilotinib; Protease Inhibitors; QuiNINE

Decreased Effect

Clarithromycin may decrease the levels/effects of: Clopidogrel; Prasugrel; Typhoid Vaccine; Zidovudine

The levels/effects of Clarithromycin may be decreased by: CYP3A4 Inducers (Strong); Deferasirox; Etravirine; Herbs (CYP3A4 Inducers); Protease Inhibitors

Ethanol/Nutrition/Herb Interactions

Food: Immediate release: Food delays rate, but not extent of absorption; Extended release: Food increases clarithromycin AUC by ~30% relative to fasting conditions.

Herb/Nutraceutical: St John's wort may decrease clarithromycin levels.

Dietary Considerations Clarithromycin immediate release tablets and oral suspension may be given with or without meals, and may be taken with milk. Extended release tablets should be taken with food.

Dosage Forms Excipient information presented when available (limited, particularly for generics); consult specific product labeling.

Granules for oral suspension: 125 mg/5 mL (50 mL, 100 mL); 250 mg/5 mL (50 mL, 100 mL)

Biaxin®: 125 mg/5 mL (50 mL, 100 mL); 250 mg/5 mL (50 mL, 100 mL) [fruit punch flavor]

Tablet: 250 mg, 500 mg

Biaxin®: 250 mg, 500 mg

Tablet, extended release: 500 mg

Biaxin® XL: 500 mg

References

Wilson W, Taubert KA, Gewitz M, et al, "Prevention of Infective Endocarditis. Guidelines From the American Heart Association. A Guideline From the American Heart Association Rheumatic Fever, Endocarditis, and Kawasaki Disease Committee, Council on Cardiovascular Disease in the Young, and the Council on Clinical Cardiology, Council on Cardiovascular Surgery and Anesthesia, and the Quality of Care and Outcomes Research Interdisciplinary Working Group," *Circulation*, 2007, 115. Available at http://circ.ahajournals.org/cgi/reprint/CIRCULATIONAHA.106.183095v1; last accessed July 26, 2007.

♦ **Clavulanic Acid and Amoxicillin** *see* Amoxicillin and Clavulanate Potassium *on page 98*

♦ **Clavulin® (Can)** *see* Amoxicillin and Clavulanate Potassium *on page 98*

♦ **Cleocin®** *see* Clindamycin *on page 324*

♦ **Cleocin HCl®** *see* Clindamycin *on page 324*

♦ **Cleocin Pediatric®** *see* Clindamycin *on page 324*

♦ **Cleocin Phosphate®** *see* Clindamycin *on page 324*

♦ **Cleocin T®** *see* Clindamycin *on page 324*

♦ **Cleocin® Vaginal Ovule** *see* Clindamycin *on page 324*

Clevidipine (klev ID i peen)

Medication Safety Issues

Sound-alike/look-alike issues:

Clevidipine may be confused with cladribine, clofarabine, clomiPRAMINE

Cleviprex™ may be confused with Claravis™

Related Information

Calcium Channel Blockers *on page 1672*

Hypertension *on page 1754*

Postoperative Hypertension *on page 1589*

U.S. Brand Names Cleviprex™

Index Terms Clevidipine Butyrate

Pharmacologic Category Calcium Channel Blocker; Calcium Channel Blocker, Dihydropyridine

Generic Available No

Use Management of hypertension when oral treatment is not feasible or not desirable

◀ **Mechanism of Action** Dihydropyridine calcium channel blocker with potent arterial vasodilating activity. Inhibits calcium ion influx through the L-type calcium channels during depolarization in arterial smooth muscle, producing a decrease in mean arterial pressure (MAP) by reducing systemic vascular resistance.

Pharmacodynamics/Kinetics

Onset of action: 2-4 minutes after start of infusion

Duration: I.V.: 5-15 minutes

Distribution: V_{dss}: 0.17 L/kg

Protein binding: >99.5%

Metabolism: Rapid hydrolysis primarily by esterases in blood and extravascular tissues to an inactive carboxylic acid metabolite and formaldehyde

Half-life elimination: Biphasic: Initial: 1 minute (predominant); Terminal: 15 minutes

Excretion: Urine (63% to 74% as metabolites); feces (7% to 22% as metabolites)

Dosage I.V.:

Adults: Initial: 1-2 mg/hour

Titration: Initial: dose may be doubled at 90-second intervals toward blood pressure goal. As blood pressure approaches goal, dose may be increased by less than double every 5-10 minutes. **Note:** For every 1-2 mg/hour increase in dose, an approximate reduction of 2-4 mm Hg in systolic blood pressure may occur.

Usual maintenance: 4-6 mg/hour; maximum: 21 mg/hour (1000 mL within a 24-hour period). There is limited short-term experience with doses up to 32 mg/hour. Data is limited beyond 72 hours.

Elderly: Initiate at the low end of the dosage range. Specific guidelines for adjustment of clevidipine are not available, but careful monitoring is warranted.

Dosing adjustment in renal impairment: No adjustment required with initial infusion rate

Dosing adjustment in hepatic impairment: No adjustment required with initial infusion rate

Stability Store in refrigerator at 2°C to 8°C (36°F to 46°F). Unopened vials are stable for 2 months at room temperature. Vials are stable for 4 hours once opened. Protect from light during storage. Do not freeze.

Administration I.V.: Maintain aseptic technique. Do not use if contamination is suspected. Do not dilute. Invert vial gently several times to ensure uniformity of emulsion prior to administration. Administer as a slow continuous infusion via central or peripheral line, using infusion device allowing for calibrated infusion rates. Use within 4 hours of puncturing vial; discard any tubing and unused portion, including that currently being infused.

Monitoring Parameters Blood pressure, heart rate; patients who receive prolonged infusions of clevidipine and are not transitioned to other antihypertensive therapy should be monitored for at least 8 hours after discontinuation

Pregnancy Risk Factor C

Contraindications Hypersensitivity to clevidipine or any component of the formulation (soybeans, soy products, eggs, egg products); hypertriglyceridemia or complications of hypertriglyceridemia (eg, acute pancreatitis); lipoid nephrosis; severe aortic stenosis

Warnings/Precautions Symptomatic hypotension with or without syncope and reflex tachycardia may rarely occur. Blood pressure must be lowered at a rate appropriate for the patient's clinical condition; dosage reductions may be necessary. Treatment of clevidipine-induced tachycardia with beta-blockers is **not** recommended. After prolonged use, discontinuation may cause rebound hypertension; monitor closely for ≥8 hours after discontinuation. Use with caution in patients with heart failure (may worsen symptoms). Clevidipine is formulated within a 20% fat emulsion (0.2 g/mL); hypertriglyceridemia is an expected side effect with high-dose or extended treatment periods; median infusion duration in clinical trials was approximately 6.5 hours (Aronson, 2008). Patients who develop hypertriglyceridemia (eg, >500 mg/dL) are at risk of developing pancreatitis. A reduction in the quantity of concurrently administered lipids may be necessary. Use is contraindicated in patients with hypertriglyceridemia or complications associated with hypertriglyceridemia (eg, acute pancreatitis) and lipoid nephrosis. Withdrawal from concomitant beta-blocker therapy should be done gradually. Initiate therapy at the low end of the dosage range in the elderly, with careful upward titration if needed. Vials may support microbial growth; maintain aseptic technique while handling.

Adverse Reactions

>10%:

Central nervous system: Fever (19%), insomnia (12%)

Gastrointestinal: Nausea (5% to 21%)

1% to 10%:

Central nervous system: Headache (6%)

Gastrointestinal: Vomiting (3%)

Hematologic: Postprocedural hemorrhage (3%)

Renal: Acute renal failure (9%)

Respiratory: Pneumonia (3%), respiratory failure (3%)

<1% (Limited to important or life-threatening): Cardiac arrest, dyspnea, MI, syncope, thrombophlebitis

Drug Interactions

Avoid Concomitant Use There are no known interactions where it is recommended to avoid concomitant use.

Increased Effect/Toxicity

Clevidipine may increase the levels/effects of: Amifostine; Antihypertensives; Hypotensive Agents; Magnesium Salts; Neuromuscular-Blocking Agents (Non-depolarizing); Nitroprusside; RiTUXimab

The levels/effects of Clevidipine may be increased by: Alpha1-Blockers; Diazoxide; Herbs (Hypotensive Properties); Magnesium Salts; MAO Inhibitors; Pentoxifylline; Phosphodiesterase 5 Inhibitors; Prostacyclin Analogues

Decreased Effect

Clevidipine may decrease the levels/effects of: QuiNIDine

The levels/effects of Clevidipine may be decreased by: Calcium Salts; Herbs (Hypertensive Properties); Methylphenidate; Yohimbine

Ethanol/Nutrition/Herb Interactions Herb/Nutraceutical: Avoid bayberry, blue cohosh, cayenne, ephedra, ginger, ginseng (American), kola, licorice (may worsen hypertension). Avoid black cohosh, California poppy, coleus, golden seal, hawthorn, mistletoe, periwinkle, quinine, shepherd's purse (may have increased antihypertensive effect).

Dietary Considerations Clevidipine is formulated in an oil-in-water emulsion containing 200 mg/mL of lipid (2 kcal/mL). If on parenteral nutrition, may need to adjust the amount of lipid infused. Emulsion contains soybean oil, egg yolk phospholipids, and glycerin.

Dosage Forms Excipient information presented when available (limited, particularly for generics); consult specific product labeling.

Injection, emulsion:

Cleviprex™: 0.5 mg/mL (50 mL, 100 mL) [contains egg yolk phospholipids, soy bean oil]

References

Chobanian AV, Bakris GL, Black HR, et al, "The Seventh Report of the Joint National Committee on Prevention, Detection, Evaluation, and Treatment of High Blood Pressure: The JNC 7 Report," *JAMA*, 2003, 289(19):2560-71.

Levy JH, Mancao MY, Gitter R, et al, "Clevidipine Effectively and Rapidly Controls Blood Pressure Preoperatively in Cardiac Surgery Patients: The Results of the Randomized, Placebo-Controlled Efficacy Study of Clevidipine Assessing Its Preoperative Antihypertensive Effect in Cardiac Surgery-1," *Anesth Analg*, 2007, 105(4):918-25.

Marik PE and Varon J, "Hypertensive Crises: Challenges and Management," *Chest*, 2007, 131(6); 1949-62. Available at http://chestjournal.org/cgi/content/abstract/131/6/1949

Peacock WF, Varon J, Garrison N, et al, "IV Clevidipine for Hypertension: Safety, Efficacy, and Transition to Oral Therapy," *Ann Emerg Med*, 2007, 50(3 Suppl 1):8-9.

Singla N, Warltier DC, Gandhi SD, et al, "Treatment of Acute Postoperative Hypertension in Cardiac Surgery Patients: An Efficacy Study of Clevidipine Assessing Its Postoperative Antihypertensive Effect in Cardiac Surgery-2 (ESCAPE-2), a Randomized, Double- Blind, Placebo-Controlled Trial," *Anesth Analg*, 2008, 107(1):59-67.

Varon J, "Treatment of Acute Severe Hypertension: Current and Newer Agents," *Drugs*, 2008, 68 (3):283-97.

Zhang JG, Dehal SS, Ho T, et al, "Human Cytochrome P450 Induction and Inhibition Potential of Clevidipine and Its Primary Metabolite H152/81," *Drug Metab Dispos*, 2006, 34(5):734-37.

◆ **Clevidipine Butyrate** *see* Clevidipine *on page 321*

◆ **Cleviprex™** *see* Clevidipine *on page 321*

◆ **Climara®** *see* Estradiol *on page 531*

◆ **Clindagel®** *see* Clindamycin *on page 324*

◆ **ClindaMax®** *see* Clindamycin *on page 324*

Clindamycin (klin da MYE sin)

Medication Safety Issues

Sound-alike/look-alike issues:

Cleocin® may be confused with bleomycin, Clinoril®, Cubicin®, Lincocin®

Clindamycin may be confused with clarithromycin, Claritin®, vancomycin

Related Information

Anesthesia for Patients With Liver Disease *on page 1537*

Prevention of Infective Endocarditis *on page 1718*

Prevention of Wound Infection and Sepsis in Surgical Patients *on page 1721*

U.S. Brand Names Cleocin HCl®; Cleocin Pediatric®; Cleocin Phosphate®; Cleocin T®; Cleocin®; Cleocin® Vaginal Ovule; Clindagel®; ClindaMax®; ClindaReach®; Clindesse®; Evoclin®

Canadian Brand Names Alti-Clindamycin; Apo-Clindamycin®; Clindamycin Injection, USP; Clindasol™; Dalacin® C; Dalacin® T; Dalacin® Vaginal; Gen-Clindamycin; Mylan-Clindamycin; Novo-Clindamycin; PMS-Clindamycin; ratio-Clindamycin; Riva-Clindamycin; Taro-Clindamycin

Index Terms Clindamycin Hydrochloride; Clindamycin Palmitate; Clindamycin Phosphate

Pharmacologic Category Antibiotic, Lincosamide; Topical Skin Product, Acne

Generic Available Yes: Excludes foam, granules, vaginal suppositories

Use Treatment of susceptible bacterial infections, mainly those caused by anaerobes, streptococci, pneumococci, and staphylococci; bacterial vaginosis (vaginal cream, vaginal suppository); pelvic inflammatory disease (I.V.); topically in treatment of severe acne; vaginally for *Gardnerella vaginalis*

Unlabeled/Investigational Use May be useful in PCP; alternate treatment for toxoplasmosis

Mechanism of Action Reversibly binds to 50S ribosomal subunits preventing peptide bond formation thus inhibiting bacterial protein synthesis; bacteriostatic or bactericidal depending on drug concentration, infection site, and organism

Pharmacodynamics/Kinetics

Absorption: Topical: Phosphate: Minimal; Oral, hydrochloride: Rapid (90%); Vaginal cream, phosphate: ~5%

Distribution: High concentrations in bone and urine; no significant levels in CSF, even with inflamed meninges

V_d: ~2 L/kg

Metabolism: Hepatic; forms metabolites (variable activity); Clindamycin phosphate is converted to clindamycin HCl (active)

Bioavailability: Topical: <1%

Half-life elimination: Neonates: Premature: 8.7 hours; Full-term: 3.6 hours; Children: ~2 hours; Adults: ~2-3 hours; Elderly 4 hours (range 3.4-5.1 hours)

Time to peak, serum: Oral: Within 60 minutes; I.M.: 1-3 hours; Vaginal cream: ~10-14 hours

Excretion: Urine (10%) and feces (~4%) as active drug and metabolites

Dosage

Usual dosage ranges:

Infants and Children:

Oral: 8-20 mg/kg/day as hydrochloride; 8-25 mg/kg/day as palmitate in 3-4 divided doses (minimum dose of palmitate: 37.5 mg 3 times/day)

I.M., I.V.:

<1 month: 15-20 mg/kg/day in 3-4 divided doses

>1 month: 20-40 mg/kg/day in 3-4 divided doses

Adults:

Oral: 150-450 mg/dose every 6-8 hours; maximum dose: 1.8 g/day

I.M., I.V.: 1.2-2.7 g/day in 2-4 divided doses; maximum dose: 4.8 g/day

Indication-specific dosing:
Children:
   Anthrax: I.V.: 7.5 mg/kg every 6 hours
   Babesiosis (unlabeled use): Oral: 20-40 mg/kg/day divided every 8 hours for 7 days plus quinine
   Orofacial infections:
      Oral: 10-20 mg/kg/day in 3-4 equally divided doses
      I.V.: 15-25 mg/kg/day in 3-4 equally divided doses
   Prophylaxis against infective endocarditis (unlabeled use):
      Oral: 20 mg/kg 30-60 minutes before procedure
      I.M., I.V.: 20 mg/kg 30-60 minutes before procedure. Intramuscular injections should be avoided in patients who are receiving anticoagulant therapy. In these circumstances, orally administered regimens should be given whenever possible. Intravenously administered antibiotics should be used for patients who are unable to tolerate or absorb oral medications.
      Note: American Heart Association (AHA) guidelines now recommend prophylaxis only in patients undergoing invasive procedures and in whom underlying cardiac conditions may predispose to a higher risk of adverse outcomes should infection occur. As of April 2007, routine prophylaxis for GI/GU procedures is no longer recommended by the AHA.
Children ≥12 years and Adults:
   Acne vulgaris: Topical:
      Gel, pledget, lotion, solution: Apply a thin film twice daily
      Foam (Evoclin®): Apply once daily
Adults:
   Amnionitis: I.V.: 450-900 mg every 8 hours
   Anthrax: I.V.: 900 mg every 8 hours with ciprofloxacin or doxycycline
   Babesiosis (unlabeled use):
      Oral: 600 mg 3 times/day for 7 days with quinine
      I.V.: 1.2 g twice daily for 7 days with quinine
   Bacterial vaginosis: Intravaginal:
      Suppositories: Insert one ovule (100 mg clindamycin) daily into vagina at bedtime for 3 days
      Cream:
         Cleocin®: One full applicator inserted intravaginally once daily before bedtime for 3 or 7 consecutive days in nonpregnant patients or for 7 consecutive days in pregnant patients
         Clindesse®: One full applicator inserted intravaginally as a single dose at anytime during the day in nonpregnant patients
   Bite wounds (canine): Oral: 300 mg 4 times/day with a fluoroquinolone
   Gangrenous pyomyositis: I.V.: 900 mg every 8 hours with penicillin G
   Group B streptococcus (neonatal prophylaxis): I.V.: 900 mg every 8 hours until delivery
   Orofacial/parapharyngeal space infections:
      Oral: 150-450 mg every 6 hours for 7 days, maximum 1.8 g/day
      I.V.: 600-900 mg every 8 hours
   Pelvic inflammatory disease: I.V.: 900 mg every 8 hours with gentamicin 2 mg/kg, then 1.5 mg/kg every 8 hours; continue after discharge with doxycycline 100 mg twice daily to complete 14 days of total therapy
   ***Pneumocystis jiroveci* pneumonia (unlabeled use):** I.V.: 600 mg every 8 hours with primaquine or pentamidine for 21 days
   Prophylaxis against infective endocarditis (unlabeled use):
      Oral: 600 mg 30-60 minutes before procedure
      I.M., I.V.: 600 mg 30-60 minutes before procedure. Intramuscular injections should be avoided in patients who are receiving anticoagulant therapy. In these circumstances, orally administered regimens should be given whenever possible. Intravenously administered antibiotics should be used for patients who are unable to tolerate or absorb oral medications.
      Note: American Heart Association (AHA) guidelines now recommend prophylaxis only in patients undergoing invasive procedures and in whom underlying cardiac conditions may predispose to a higher risk of adverse outcomes should infection occur. As of April 2007, routine prophylaxis for GI/GU procedures is no longer recommended by the AHA.

Prophylaxis in total joint replacement patients undergoing dental procedures which produce bacteremia:
Oral: 600 mg 1 hour prior to procedure
I.V.: 600 mg 1 hour prior to procedure (for patients unable to take oral medication)
Toxic shock syndrome: I.V.: 900 mg every 8 hours with penicillin G or ceftriaxone
Toxoplasmosis (unlabeled use): Oral, I.V.: 600 mg every 6 hours with pyrimethamine and folinic acid
Dosing adjustment in renal impairment: No adjustment required.
Dosing adjustment in hepatic impairment: Adjustment recommended in patients with severe hepatic disease

Stability
Capsule: Store at room temperature of 20°C to 25°C (68°F to 77°F).
Cream: Store at room temperature.
Foam: Store at room temperature of 20°C to 25°C (68°F to 77°F); avoid fire, flame, or smoking during or following application.
Gel: Store at room temperature.
Clindagel®: Do not store in direct sunlight.
I.V.: Infusion solution in NS or D$_5$W solution is stable for 16 days at room temperature, 32 days refrigerated, or 8 weeks frozen. Prior to use, store vials and premixed bags at controlled room temperature 20°C to 25°C (68°F to 77°F). After initial use, discard any unused portion of vial after 24 hours.
Lotion: Store at room temperature of 20°C to 25°C (68°F to 77°F).
Oral solution: Do not refrigerate reconstituted oral solution (it will thicken); following reconstitution, oral solution is stable for 2 weeks at room temperature of 20°C to 25°C (68°F to 77°F).
Ovule: Store at room temperature of 15°C to 30°C (68°F to 77°F).
Pledget: Store at room temperature.
Topical solution: Store at room temperature of 20°C to 25°C (68°F to 77°F).

Administration
I.M.: Deep I.M. sites, rotate sites; do not exceed 600 mg in a single injection.
Intravaginal:
Cream: Insertion should be as far as possible into the vagina without causing discomfort.
Ovule: The foil should be removed; if the applicator is used for insertion, it should be washed for additional use.
I.V.: **Never administer as bolus**; administer by I.V. intermittent infusion over at least 10-60 minutes, at a rate **not** to exceed 30 mg/minute (do not exceed 1200 mg/hour); final concentration for administration should not exceed 18 mg/mL.
Oral: Administer with a full glass of water to minimize esophageal ulceration; give around-the-clock to promote less variation in peak and trough serum levels.
Topical foam: Dispense directly into cap or onto a cool surface; do not dispense directly into hands.

Monitoring Parameters Observe for changes in bowel frequency. Monitor for colitis and resolution of symptoms. During prolonged therapy monitor CBC, liver and renal function tests periodically.

Anesthesia and Critical Care Concerns/Other Considerations
Clinical Pearls/Comments: Clindamycin may increase the duration of neuromuscular blockade after anesthesia. In adults, clindamycin injection can usually be dosed effectively on an every-8-hour basis.

Pregnancy Risk Factor B

Contraindications Hypersensitivity to clindamycin, lincomycin, or any component of the formulation
Topical and vaginal products: Additional contraindications: Previous pseudomembranous colitis, regional enteritis, ulcerative colitis

Warnings/Precautions Dosage adjustment may be necessary in patients with severe hepatic dysfunction. **[U.S. Boxed Warning]: Can cause severe and possibly fatal colitis.** Prolonged use may result in fungal or bacterial superinfection, including *C. difficile*-associated diarrhea (CDAD) and pseudomembranous colitis; CDAD has been observed >2 months postantibiotic treatment. Use with caution in patients with a history of gastrointestinal disease. Discontinue drug if significant diarrhea, abdominal cramps, or passage of blood and mucus occurs. Vaginal products may weaken condoms, or contraceptive diaphragms. Barrier contraceptives are not recommended concurrently or for 3-5 days (depending on the product) following treatment. Some dosage forms contain benzyl alcohol or tartrazine. Use caution in atopic patients.

Adverse Reactions

Systemic: Frequency not defined:

Cardiovascular: Cardiac arrest (rare; I.V. administration), hypotension (rare; I.V. administration)

Dermatologic: Erythema multiforme (rare), exfoliative dermatitis (rare), pruritus, rash, Stevens-Johnson syndrome (rare), urticaria

Gastrointestinal: Abdominal pain, diarrhea, esophagitis, nausea, pseudomembranous colitis, vomiting

Genitourinary: Vaginitis

Hematologic: Agranulocytosis, eosinophilia (transient), neutropenia (transient), thrombocytopenia

Hepatic: Jaundice, liver function test abnormal

Local: Induration/pain/sterile abscess (I.M.), thrombophlebitis (I.V.)

Neuromuscular & skeletal: Polyarthritis (rare)

Renal: Renal dysfunction (rare)

Miscellaneous: Anaphylactoid reactions (rare)

Topical:

>10%: Dermatologic: Dryness, burning, itching, scaliness, erythema, or peeling of skin (lotion, solution); oiliness (gel, lotion)

<1% (Limited to important or life-threatening): Pseudomembranous colitis, nausea, vomiting, diarrhea (severe), abdominal pain, folliculitis, hypersensitivity reactions

Vaginal:

>10%: Genitourinary: Vaginal candidiasis (≤13%), vulvovaginal pruritus (from *Candida albicans*)

1% to 10%:

Dermatologic: Pruritus (≤1%)

Genitourinary: Vulvovaginal disorder (3% to 7%), vulvovaginitis (4% to 6%), vaginal pain (≤2%), trichomonal vaginitis (1%)

Miscellaneous: Fungal infection (1% to 2%)

<1% (Limited to important or life-threatening): Abdominal cramps, allergic reaction, atrophic vaginitis, bacterial infection, diarrhea, dizziness, dysuria, endometriosis, epistaxis, erythema, fever, hypersensitivity, hyperthyroidism, local edema, menstrual disorder, metrorrhagia, nausea, pain, pruritus, pyelonephritis, rash, urinary tract infection, urticaria, vaginal burning, vertigo, vomiting

Drug Interactions

Avoid Concomitant Use

Avoid concomitant use of Clindamycin with any of the following: Erythromycin

Increased Effect/Toxicity

Clindamycin may increase the levels/effects of: Neuromuscular-Blocking Agents

Decreased Effect

Clindamycin may decrease the levels/effects of: Erythromycin; Typhoid Vaccine

The levels/effects of Clindamycin may be decreased by: Kaolin

Ethanol/Nutrition/Herb Interactions

Food: Peak concentrations may be delayed with food.

Herb/Nutraceutical: St John's wort may decrease clindamycin levels.

Dietary Considerations May be taken with food.

Dosage Forms Excipient information presented when available (limited, particularly for generics); consult specific product labeling. [DSC] = Discontinued product

Note: Strength is expressed as base

Aerosol, topical, as phosphate [foam]:

Evoclin®: 1% (50 g, 100 g) [contains ethanol 58%]

Capsule, as hydrochloride: 75 mg, 150 mg, 300 mg

Cleocin HCl®: 75 mg [contains tartrazine], 150 mg [contains tartrazine], 300 mg

Cream, vaginal, as phosphate: 2% (40 g)
  Cleocin®: 2% (40 g) [contains benzyl alcohol and mineral oil; packaged with 7 disposable applicators]
  ClindaMax®: 2% (40 g) [contains benzyl alcohol and mineral oil; packaged with 7 disposable applicators] [DSC]
  Clindesse®: 2% (5 g) [contains mineral oil; prefilled single disposable applicator]
Gel, topical, as phosphate: 1% (30 g, 60 g)
  Cleocin T®: 1% (30 g, 60 g)
  Clindagel®: 1% (40 mL, 75 mL)
  ClindaMax®: 1% (30 g, 60 g)
Granules for oral solution, as palmitate hydrochloride:
  Cleocin Pediatric®: 75 mg/5 mL (100 mL) [cherry flavor]
Infusion, as phosphate [premixed in D_5W]:
  Cleocin Phosphate®: 300 mg (50 mL); 600 mg (50 mL); 900 mg (50 mL) [contains edetate disodium]
Injection, solution, as phosphate: 150 mg/mL (2 mL, 4 mL, 6 mL, 60 mL)
  Cleocin Phosphate®: 150 mg/mL (2 mL, 4 mL, 6 mL, 60 mL) [contains benzyl alcohol and edetate disodium]
Lotion, as phosphate: 1% (60 mL)
  Cleocin T®, ClindaMax®: 1% (60 mL)
Pledgets, topical: 1% (60s, 69s)
  Cleocin T®: 1% (60s) [contains isopropyl alcohol 50%]
  ClindaReach®: 1% (120s) [contains isopropyl alcohol 50%; packaged as a kit containing 1 collapsible applicator, 64 appliques, and 64 unmedicated pads]
Solution, topical, as phosphate: 1% (30 mL, 60 mL)
  Cleocin T®: 1% (30 mL, 60 mL) [contains isopropyl alcohol 50%]
Suppository, vaginal, as phosphate:
  Cleocin® Vaginal Ovule: 100 mg (3s) [contains oleaginous base; single reusable applicator]

References

Wilson W, Taubert KA, Gewitz M, et al, "Prevention of Infective Endocarditis. Guidelines From the American Heart Association. A Guideline From the American Heart Association Rheumatic Fever, Endocarditis, and Kawasaki Disease Committee, Council on Cardiovascular Disease in the Young, and the Council on Clinical Cardiology, Council on Cardiovascular Surgery and Anesthesia, and the Quality of Care and Outcomes Research Interdisciplinary Working Group," *Circulation*, 2007, 115. Available at http://circ.ahajournals.org/cgi/reprint/CIRCULATIONAHA.106.183095v1; last accessed July 26, 2007.

◆ **Clindamycin Hydrochloride** *see* Clindamycin *on page 324*

◆ **Clindamycin Injection, USP (Can)** *see* Clindamycin *on page 324*

◆ **Clindamycin Palmitate** *see* Clindamycin *on page 324*

◆ **Clindamycin Phosphate** *see* Clindamycin *on page 324*

◆ **ClindaReach®** *see* Clindamycin *on page 324*

◆ **Clindasol™ (Can)** *see* Clindamycin *on page 324*

◆ **Clindesse®** *see* Clindamycin *on page 324*

◆ **Clinisol®** *see* Amino Acid Injection *on page 81*

◆ **Clinoril®** *see* Sulindac *on page 1335*

◆ **Clonapam (Can)** *see* ClonazePAM *on page 328*

ClonazePAM (kloe NA ze pam)

Related Information

  Benzodiazepines *on page 1666*
  Chronic Pain Management *on page 1546*
  Perioperative Management of Patients on Antiseizure Medication *on page 1577*

U.S. Brand Names Klonopin®; Klonopin® Wafers [DSC]

Canadian Brand Names Alti-Clonazepam; Apo-Clonazepam®; Clonapam; CO Clonazepam; Gen-Clonazepam; Klonopin®; Mylan-Clonazepam; Novo-Clonazepam; Nu-Clonazepam; PMS-Clonazepam; Pro-Clonazepam; Rho®-Clonazepam; Rivotril®; Sandoz-Clonazepam

Pharmacologic Category Benzodiazepine

Restrictions C-IV

Use Alone or as an adjunct in the treatment of petit mal variant (Lennox-Gastaut), akinetic, and myoclonic seizures; petit mal (absence) seizures unresponsive to succimides; panic disorder with or without agoraphobia

Unlabeled/Investigational Use Restless legs syndrome; neuralgia; multifocal tic disorder; parkinsonian dysarthria; bipolar disorder; adjunct therapy for schizophrenia

Pharmacodynamics/Kinetics

Onset of action: 20-60 minutes

Duration: Infants and young children: 6-8 hours; Adults: ≤12 hours

Absorption: Well absorbed

Distribution: Adults: V_d: 1.5-4.4 L/kg

Protein binding: 85%

Metabolism: Extensively hepatic via glucuronide and sulfate conjugation

Half-life elimination: Children: 22-33 hours; Adults: 19-50 hours

Time to peak, serum: 1-3 hours; Steady-state: 5-7 days

Excretion: Urine (<2% as unchanged drug); metabolites excreted as glucuronide or sulfate conjugates

Dosage Oral:

Children <10 years or 30 kg: Seizure disorders:

Initial daily dose: 0.01-0.03 mg/kg/day (maximum: 0.05 mg/kg/day) given in 2-3 divided doses; increase by no more than 0.5 mg every third day until seizures are controlled or adverse effects seen

Usual maintenance dose: 0.1-0.2 mg/kg/day divided 3 times/day, not to exceed 0.2 mg/kg/day

Adults:

Burning mouth syndrome (dental use): 0.25-3 mg/day in 2 divided doses, in morning and evening

Seizure disorders:

Initial daily dose not to exceed 1.5 mg given in 3 divided doses; may increase by 0.5-1 mg every third day until seizures are controlled or adverse effects seen (maximum: 20 mg/day)

Usual maintenance dose: 0.05-0.2 mg/kg; do not exceed 20 mg/day

Panic disorder: 0.25 mg twice daily; increase in increments of 0.125-0.25 mg twice daily every 3 days; target dose: 1 mg/day (maximum: 4 mg/day)

Discontinuation of treatment: To discontinue, treatment should be withdrawn gradually. Decrease dose by 0.125 mg twice daily every 3 days until medication is completely withdrawn.

Elderly: Initiate with low doses and observe closely

Hemodialysis: Supplemental dose is not necessary

Anesthesia and Critical Care Concerns/Other Considerations Flumazenil, a competitive benzodiazepine antagonist at the CNS receptor site, reverses benzodiazepine-induced CNS depression. Abrupt discontinuation after sustained use (generally >10 days) may cause withdrawal symptoms.

Additional Information Complete prescribing information for this medication should be consulted for additional detail.

Dosage Forms Excipient information presented when available (limited, particularly for generics); consult specific product labeling. [DSC] = Discontinued product

Tablet: 0.5 mg, 1 mg, 2 mg

Klonopin®: 0.5 mg, 1 mg, 2 mg

Tablet, orally disintegrating: 0.125 mg, 0.25 mg, 0.5 mg, 1 mg, 2 mg

Klonopin® Wafers: 0.125 mg, 0.25 mg, 0.5 mg, 1 mg, 2 mg [DSC]

CloNIDine (KLON i deen)

Medication Safety Issues

Sound-alike/look-alike issues:

CloNIDine may be confused with Clomid®, clomiPHENE, clonazePAM, clozapine, Klonopin®, quiNIDine

Catapres® may be confused with Cataflam®, Cetapred®, Combipres

◀ **High alert medication:** The Institute for Safe Medication Practices (ISMP) includes this medication (epidural administration) among its list of drug classes which have a heightened risk of causing significant patient harm when used in error.

Transdermal patch may contain conducting metal (eg, aluminum); remove patch prior to MRI.

Related Information
Anesthesia for Geriatric Patients *on page 1523*
Chronic Pain Management *on page 1546*
Hypertension *on page 1754*
Preoperative Evaluation of the Cardiac Patient for Noncardiac Surgery *on page 1598*

U.S. Brand Names Catapres-TTS®; Catapres®; Duraclon®

Canadian Brand Names Apo-Clonidine®; Carapres®; Dixarit®; Dom-Clonidine; Novo-Clonidine; Nu-Clonidine

Index Terms Clonidine Hydrochloride

Pharmacologic Category Alpha$_2$-Adrenergic Agonist

Generic Available Yes: Tablet

Use Management of mild-to-moderate hypertension; either used alone or in combination with other antihypertensives

Orphan drug: Duraclon®: For continuous epidural administration as adjunctive therapy with intraspinal opiates for treatment of cancer pain in patients tolerant to or unresponsive to intraspinal opiates

Unlabeled/Investigational Use Heroin or nicotine withdrawal; severe pain; dysmenorrhea; vasomotor symptoms associated with menopause; ethanol dependence; prophylaxis of migraines; glaucoma; diabetes-associated diarrhea; impulse control disorder, attention-deficit/hyperactivity disorder (ADHD), clozapine-induced sialorrhea

Mechanism of Action Stimulates alpha$_2$-adrenoceptors in the brain stem, thus activating an inhibitory neuron, resulting in reduced sympathetic outflow from the CNS, producing a decrease in peripheral resistance, renal vascular resistance, heart rate, and blood pressure; epidural clonidine may produce pain relief at spinal presynaptic and postjunctional alpha$_2$-adrenoceptors by preventing pain signal transmission; pain relief occurs only for the body regions innervated by the spinal segments where analgesic concentrations of clonidine exist

Pharmacodynamics/Kinetics
Onset of action: Oral: 0.5-1 hour; Transdermal: Initial application: 2-3 days
Duration: 6-10 hours
Distribution: V_d: Adults: 2.1 L/kg; highly lipid soluble; distributes readily into extravascular sites
Protein binding: 20% to 40%
Metabolism: Extensively hepatic to inactive metabolites; undergoes enterohepatic recirculation
Bioavailability: 75% to 95%
Half-life elimination: Adults: Normal renal function: 6-20 hours; Renal impairment: 18-41 hours
Time to peak: 2-4 hours
Excretion: Urine (65%, 32% as unchanged drug); feces (22%)

Dosage
Children:
Oral:
Hypertension: Children ≥12 years: Initial: 0.2 mg/day in 2 divided doses; increase gradually at 5- to 7-day intervals; usual maintenance dose: 0.2-0.6 mg/day in divided doses; maximum: 2.4 mg/day (rarely required)
Clonidine tolerance test (test of growth hormone release from pituitary): 0.15 mg/m^2 or 4 mcg/kg as single dose
ADHD (unlabeled use): Initial: 0.05 mg/day; increase every 3-7 days by 0.05 mg/day to 3-5 mcg/kg/day given in divided doses 3-4 times/day (maximum dose: 0.3-0.4 mg/day)
Epidural infusion: Pain management: Reserved for patients with severe intractable pain, unresponsive to other analgesics or epidural or spinal opiates: Initial: 0.5 mcg/kg/hour; adjust with caution, based on clinical effect

Adults:

Oral:

Acute hypertension (urgency): Initial 0.1-0.2 mg; may be followed by additional doses of 0.1 mg every hour, if necessary, to a maximum total dose of 0.6 mg
Unlabeled route of administration: Sublingual clonidine 0.1-0.2 mg twice daily may be effective in patients unable to take oral medication

Hypertension: Initial dose: 0.1 mg twice daily (maximum recommended dose: 2.4 mg/day); usual dose range (JNC 7): 0.1-0.8 mg/day in 2 divided doses

Nicotine withdrawal symptoms (unlabeled use; Fiore, 2008): Initial dose: Initial: 0.1 mg twice daily; dosage range used in clinical trials: 0.15-0.75 mg/day; duration of therapy ranged from 3-10 weeks in clinical trials

Transdermal:

Hypertension: Apply once every 7 days; for initial therapy start with 0.1 mg and increase by 0.1 mg at 1- to 2-week intervals (dosages >0.6 mg do not improve efficacy); usual dose range (JNC 7): 0.1-0.3 mg once weekly

Nicotine withdrawal symptoms (unlabeled use; Fiore, 2008): Initial: 0.1 mg/24 hour patch applied once every 7 days and increase by 0.1 mg at 1- to 2-week intervals if necessary; dosage range used in clinical trials: 0.1-0.2 mg/24 hours patch applied once every 7 days; duration of therapy ranged from 3-10 weeks in clinical trials

Note: If transitioning from oral to transdermal therapy, overlap oral regimen for 1-2 days; transdermal route takes 2-3 days to achieve therapeutic effects.

Conversion from oral to transdermal:

Day 1: Place Catapres-TTS® 1; administer 100% of oral dose.

Day 2: Administer 50% of oral dose.

Day 3: Administer 25% of oral dose.

Day 4: Patch remains, no further oral supplement necessary.

Epidural infusion: Pain management: Starting dose: 30 mcg/hour; titrate as required for relief of pain or presence of side effects; minimal experience with doses >40 mcg/hour; should be considered an adjunct to intraspinal opiate therapy

Elderly: Initial: 0.1 mg once daily at bedtime, increase gradually as needed

Dosing adjustment in renal impairment: Bradycardia may be more likely to occur in patients with renal failure; may consider using doses at the lower end of the dosing range and monitor closely

Not dialyzable (0% to 5%) via hemodialysis; supplemental dose is not necessary; unclear how much is removed via peritoneal dialysis (K/DOQI, 2005). Oral antihypertensive drugs given preferentially at night may reduce the nocturnal surge of blood pressure and minimize the intradialytic hypotension that may occur when taken the morning before a dialysis session.

Administration

Oral: Do not discontinue clonidine abruptly. If needed, gradually reduce dose over 2-4 days to avoid rebound hypertension

Transdermal patch: Patches should be applied weekly at bedtime to a clean, hairless area of the upper outer arm or chest. Rotate patch sites weekly. Redness under patch may be reduced if a topical corticosteroid spray is applied to the area before placement of the patch.

Monitoring Parameters Blood pressure, standing and sitting/supine, mental status, heart rate

When used for the treatment of ADHD, thoroughly evaluate for cardiovascular risk. Monitor heart rate, blood pressure (when started and weaned), and consider obtaining ECG prior to initiation (Vetter, 2008).

Reference Range Therapeutic: 1-2 ng/mL (SI: 4.4-8.7 nmol/L)

Anesthesia and Critical Care Concerns/Other Considerations Clinical Pearls/Comments: Abrupt withdrawal from clonidine therapy should be avoided. Clonidine patch has provided an important alternative to frequent daily dosing; may be used in patients unable to take oral medication. Transdermal therapy takes 2-3 days for therapeutic effects.

Pregnancy Risk Factor C

Contraindications Hypersensitivity to clonidine hydrochloride or any component of the formulation

◄ **Warnings/Precautions** Gradual withdrawal is needed (over 1 week for oral, 2-4 days with epidural) if drug needs to be stopped. Patients should be instructed about abrupt discontinuation (causes rapid increase in BP and symptoms of sympathetic overactivity). In patients on both a beta-blocker and clonidine where withdrawal of clonidine is necessary, withdraw the beta-blocker first and several days before clonidine. Then slowly decrease clonidine.

Use with caution in patients with severe coronary insufficiency; conduction disturbances; recent MI, CVA, or chronic renal insufficiency. Caution in sinus node dysfunction. Discontinue within 4 hours of surgery then restart as soon as possible after. Clonidine injection should be administered via a continuous epidural infusion device. **[U.S. Boxed Warning]: Epidural clonidine is not recommended for perioperative, obstetrical, or postpartum pain.** It is not recommended for use in patients with severe cardiovascular disease or hemodynamic instability. In all cases, the epidural may lead to cardiovascular instability (hypotension, bradycardia). Transdermal patch may contain conducting metal (eg, aluminum); remove patch prior to MRI. Due to the potential for altered electrical conductivity, remove transdermal patch before cardioversion or defibrillation. Clonidine cause significant CNS depression and xerostomia. Caution in patients with pre-existing CNS disease or depression. Elderly may be at greater risk for CNS depressive effects, favoring other agents in this population. Safety and efficacy of tablet and transdermal product have not been established in children <12 years of age. In pediatric patients, epidural clonidine should be reserved for cancer patients with severe intractable pain, unresponsive to other analgesics or epidural or spinal opiates.

Adverse Reactions Incidence of adverse events is not always reported.

>10%:
  Central nervous system: Drowsiness (35% oral, 12% transdermal), dizziness (16% oral, 2% transdermal)
  Dermatologic: Transient localized skin reactions characterized by pruritus, and erythema (15% to 50% transdermal)
  Gastrointestinal: Dry mouth (40% oral, 25% transdermal)
  Neuromuscular & skeletal: Weakness (10% transdermal)
1% to 10%:
  Cardiovascular: Orthostatic hypotension (3% oral)
  Central nervous system: Headache (1% oral, 5% transdermal), sedation (3% transdermal), fatigue (6% transdermal), lethargy (3% transdermal), insomnia (2% transdermal), nervousness (3% oral, 1% transdermal), mental depression (1% oral)
  Dermatologic: Rash (1% oral), allergic contact sensitivity (5% transdermal), localized vesiculation (7%), hyperpigmentation (5% at application site), edema (3%), excoriation (3%), burning (3%), throbbing, blanching (1%), papules (1%), and generalized macular rash (1%) has occurred in patients receiving transdermal clonidine.
  Endocrine & metabolic: Sodium and water retention, sexual dysfunction (3% oral, 2% transdermal), impotence (3% oral, 2% transdermal), weakness (10% transdermal)
  Gastrointestinal: Nausea (5% oral, 1% transdermal), vomiting (5% oral), anorexia and malaise (1% oral), constipation (10% oral, 1% transdermal), dry throat (2% transdermal), taste disturbance (1% transdermal), weight gain (1% oral)
  Genitourinary: Nocturia (1% oral)
  Hepatic: Liver function test (mild abnormalities, 1% oral)
  Miscellaneous: Withdrawal syndrome (1% oral)
<1% (Limited to important or life-threatening): Abdominal pain, agitation, alopecia, angioedema, AV block, behavioral changes, blurred vision, bradycardia, chest pain, CHF, contact dermatitis (transdermal), CVA, delirium, depression, dryness of eyes, ECG abnormalities, ethanol sensitivity increased, gynecomastia, hallucinations, hepatitis, localized hypo- or hyperpigmentation (transdermal), nightmares, orthostatic symptoms, pseudo-obstruction, rash, Raynaud's phenomenon, syncope, tachycardia, thrombocytopenia, urinary retention, urticaria, vomiting, withdrawal syndrome

Drug Interactions
Avoid Concomitant Use
Avoid concomitant use of CloNIDine with any of the following: Iobenguane I 123
Increased Effect/Toxicity
CloNIDine may increase the levels/effects of: Amifostine; Antihypertensives; Hypotensive Agents; RiTUXimab

The levels/effects of CloNIDine may be increased by: Beta-Blockers; Diazoxide; Herbs (Hypotensive Properties); MAO Inhibitors; Methylphenidate; Pentoxifylline; Phosphodiesterase 5 Inhibitors; Prostacyclin Analogues
Decreased Effect
CloNIDine may decrease the levels/effects of: Iobenguane I 123

The levels/effects of CloNIDine may be decreased by: Antidepressants (Alpha2-Antagonist); Herbs (Hypertensive Properties); Serotonin/Norepinephrine Reuptake Inhibitors; Tricyclic Antidepressants; Yohimbine
Ethanol/Nutrition/Herb Interactions
Ethanol: Avoid ethanol (may increase CNS depression).
Herb/Nutraceutical: Avoid dong quai if using for hypertension (has estrogenic activity). Avoid ephedra, yohimbe, ginseng (may worsen hypertension). Avoid valerian, St John's wort, kava kava, gotu kola (may increase CNS depression).
Dosage Forms Excipient information presented when available (limited, particularly for generics); consult specific product labeling.
Injection, solution, as hydrochloride [epidural; preservative free]:
Duraclon®: 100 mcg/mL (10 mL); 500 mcg/mL (10 mL)
Tablet, as hydrochloride: 0.1 mg, 0.2 mg, 0.3 mg
Catapres®: 0.1 mg, 0.2 mg, 0.3 mg
Transdermal system, topical [once-weekly patch]:
Catapres-TTS®-1: 0.1 mg/24 hours (4s)
Catapres-TTS®-2: 0.2 mg/24 hours (4s)
Catapres-TTS®-3: 0.3 mg/24 hours (4s)
References
Fiore MC, Jaen CR, Baker TB, et al, *Treating Tobacco Use and Dependence: 2008 Update.* Clinical Practice Guideline. Rockville, MD: U.S. Department of Health and Human Services. Public Health Service. May 2008. Available at http://www.surgeongeneral.gov/tobacco/treating_tobacco_use08.pdf.
"Principles of Analgesic Use in the Treatment of Acute Pain and Cancer Pain," 6th ed, Glenview, IL: American Pain Society, 2008.

◆ **Clonidine Hydrochloride** *see* CloNIDine *on page 329*

Clopidogrel (kloh PID oh grel)

Medication Safety Issues
Sound-alike/look-alike issues:
Plavix® may be confused with Elavil®, Paxil®
Related Information
Anesthesia for Geriatric Patients *on page 1523*
Perioperative / Periprocedural Management of Anticoagulant and Antiplatelet Therapy *on page 1607*
Preoperative Evaluation of the Cardiac Patient for Noncardiac Surgery *on page 1598*
Regional Anesthesia in Patients Receiving Anticoagulant and Antiplatelet Therapy *on page 1642*
U.S. Brand Names Plavix®
Canadian Brand Names Plavix®
Index Terms Clopidogrel Bisulfate
Pharmacologic Category Antiplatelet Agent; Antiplatelet Agent, Thienopyridine
Generic Available No
Use Reduces rate of atherothrombotic events (myocardial infarction, stroke, vascular deaths) in patients with recent MI or stroke, or established peripheral arterial disease; reduces rate of atherothrombotic events in patients with unstable angina or non-ST-segment elevation acute coronary syndromes (unstable angina and non-ST-segment elevation MI) managed medically or through percutaneous coronary intervention (PCI) (with or without stent) or CABG; reduces rate of death

◄ and atherothrombotic events in patients with ST-segment elevation MI (STEMI) managed medically

Unlabeled/Investigational Use In aspirin-allergic patients, initial treatment of acute coronary syndromes (ACS) or prevention of coronary artery bypass graft closure (saphenous vein)

Mechanism of Action Clopidogrel requires *in vivo* biotransformation to an active thiol metabolite. The active metabolite irreversibly blocks the $P2Y_{12}$ component of ADP receptors on the platelet surface, which prevents activation of the GPIIb/IIIa receptor complex, thereby reducing platelet aggregation. Platelets blocked by clopidogrel are affected for the remainder of their lifespan (~7-10 days).

Pharmacodynamics/Kinetics

Onset of action: Inhibition of platelet aggregation (IPA): Dose-dependent:

300-600 mg loading dose: Detected within 2 hours

50-100 mg/day: Detected by the second day of treatment

Peak effect: Time to maximal IPA: Dose-dependent: **Note:** Degree of IPA based on adenosine diphosphate (ADP) concentration used during light aggregometry: 300-600 mg loading dose:

ADP 5 µmol/L: 20% to 30% IPA at 6 hours post administration (Montelescot, 2006)

ADP 20 µmol/L: 30% to 37% IPA at 6 hours post administration (Montelescot, 2006)

50-100 mg/day: ADP 5 µmol/L: 50% to 60% IPA at 5-7 days (Herbert, 1993)

Absorption: Well absorbed

Protein binding: Parent drug: 98%; Inactive metabolite: 94%

Metabolism: Extensively hepatic via esterase-mediated hydrolysis to a carboxylic acid derivative (inactive) and via CYP450-mediated oxidation to a thiol metabolite (active)

Half-life elimination: Parent drug: ~6 hours; Inactive metabolite: ~8 hours

Time to peak, serum: ~0.75 hours

Excretion: Urine (50%); feces (46%)

Dosage Oral: Adults:

Recent MI, recent stroke, or established arterial disease: 75 mg once daily

Acute coronary syndrome (ACS):

Unstable angina, non-ST-segment elevation myocardial infarction (UA/NSTEMI): Initial: 300 mg loading dose, followed by 75 mg once daily (in combination with aspirin 75-325 mg once daily). **Note:** A loading dose of 600 mg given at least 2 hours (or 24 hours in patients unable to take aspirin) prior to PCI followed by 75 mg once daily is recommended (*Chest* guidelines, 2008)

ST-segment elevation myocardial infarction (STEMI): 75 mg once daily (in combination with aspirin 75-162 mg/day). CLARITY used a 300 mg loading dose of clopidogrel (with thrombolysis). The duration of therapy was <28 days (usually until hospital discharge) (Sabatine, 2005).

The American College of Chest Physicians (Goodman, 2008) recommends:

Patients ≤75 years: Initial: 300 mg loading dose, followed by 75 mg once daily for up to 28 days (in combination with aspirin)

Patients >75 years: 75 mg once daily for up to 28 days (with or without thrombolysis)

Note: *Coronary artery stents:* Duration of clopidogrel (in combination with aspirin): According to the ACC/AHA/SCAI guidelines, ideally 12 months following drug-eluting stent (DES) placement in patients not at high risk for bleeding; at a minimum, 1, 3, and 6 months for bare metal (BMS), sirolimus eluting, and paclitaxel eluting stents, respectively, for uninterrupted therapy (Smith, 2005). For newer drug-eluting stents (eg, everolimus [Xience™], zotarolimus [Endeavor®]), a minimum duration of 3 months is recommended. The 2008 *Chest* guidelines recommend for patients who undergo PCI and receive a BMS (with ongoing ACS) or a DES (with or without ongoing ACS) that clopidogrel be continued for at least 12 months. In patients receiving a BMS without ongoing ACS, clopidogrel may be continued for at least 1 month. In patients receiving a DES, therapy with clopidogrel beyond 12 months may be considered in patients without bleeding or tolerability issues (Becker, 2008). Premature interruption of therapy may result in stent thrombosis with subsequent fatal and nonfatal myocardial infarction.

Prevention of coronary artery bypass graft closure (saphenous vein) [*Chest* guidelines, 2008]: Aspirin-allergic patients (unlabeled use): Loading dose: 300 mg 6 hours following procedure; maintenance: 75 mg/day

Dosing adjustment in renal impairment and elderly: None necessary

Dosing adjustment in hepatic impairment: Use with caution; experience is limited. **Note:** Inhibition of ADP-induced platelet aggregation and mean bleeding time prolongation were similar in patients with severe hepatic impairment compared to healthy subjects after repeated doses of 75 mg once daily for 10 days.

Stability Store at 25°C (77°F); excursions permitted to 15°C to 30°C (59°F to 86°F).

Administration May be administered without regard to meals.

Monitoring Parameters Signs of bleeding; hemoglobin and hematocrit periodically

Anesthesia and Critical Care Concerns/Other Considerations
Evidence-Based Information:

Perioperative Management of Clopidogrel:
In patients with coronary stents, the risk of stent thrombosis becomes elevated depending on the type of stent deployed (bare metal vs drug-eluting stent) and the time from implantation. According to the American College of Chest Physicians (Becker, 2008), the recommended length of therapy for clopidogrel is at least 12 months in patients with ACS who undergo PCI with a bare metal stent (BMS) or drug-eluting stent (DES). In patients receiving a BMS without ongoing ACS, clopidogrel may be continued for at least 1 month. Early discontinuation of clopidogrel may result in stent thrombosis leading to nonfatal and fatal myocardial infarction. The perioperative recommendations for clopidogrel are below (Douketis, 2008):

Patients undergoing noncardiac surgery (low risk of cardiac event without coronary stent): Clopidogrel and other antiplatelet agents should be temporarily discontinued 5-10 days prior to surgery and resumed ~24 hours (or the next morning) after the procedure when adequate hemostasis is achieved.

Patients without coronary stent undergoing cardiac surgery (eg, CABG) or noncardiac surgery (high risk of cardiac event): Discontinue clopidogrel at least 5 days and, preferably, 10 days prior to surgery while continuing aspirin up to and beyond the time of surgery. If aspirin is interrupted, it should be reinitiated 6-48 hours after surgery; may resume clopidogrel ~24 hours (or the next morning) after the procedure when adequate hemostasis is achieved.

Patients undergoing cardiac surgery (eg, CABG) or noncardiac surgery (with coronary stent): Based on the risk of stent thrombosis, patients with a BMS who require surgery within 6 weeks of implantation or with a DES who require surgery within 12 months of implantation should continue on both aspirin and clopidogrel during the perioperative period.

The AHA/ACC/SCAI/ACS/ADA Science Advisory (2007) published recommendations (*Circulation*, February 13, 2007) to prevent premature discontinuation of dual antiplatelet therapy (clopidogrel and aspirin) in patients with coronary artery stents. The advisory panel agreed with the 2004 ACC/AHA guidelines stressing the importance of 12 months of dual antiplatelet therapy after placement of a drug-eluting stent (DES) in patients who are not at high risk of bleeding. The advisory panel included these recommendations. Minor surgery, teeth cleaning, and tooth extraction can usually be performed without increased bleeding on the dual antiplatelet regimen. If increased bleeding is anticipated, then the procedure should be delayed until the antiplatelet regimen is completed. Elective procedures with a significant risk of bleeding should be postponed until the antiplatelet regimen is completed. The advisory panel recommends healthcare providers who perform invasive or surgical procedures contact the patient's cardiologist before discontinuing antiplatelet therapy. For patients with drug-eluting stents who must undergo a procedure that requires discontinuation of thienopyridine therapy, aspirin should be continued if possible and the thienopyridine restarted as soon as possible after the procedure. "Bridging" stent patients with warfarin, other antithrombins, or glycoprotein IIb/IIIa agents is not supported by the Advisory Committee.

◀ For the complete review and additional recommendations available at http://www.acc.org/qualityandscience/clinical/pdfs/Final_Dual_Antiplatelet_Statement_010507.pdf

Pregnancy Risk Factor B

Contraindications Hypersensitivity to clopidogrel or any component of the formulation; active pathological bleeding such as peptic ulcer disease (PUD) or intracranial hemorrhage; coagulation disorders

Warnings/Precautions Use with caution in patients who may be at risk of increased bleeding, including patients with PUD, trauma, or surgery. Consider discontinuing 5 days before elective surgery (except in patients with cardiac stents that have not completed their full course of dual antiplatelet therapy; patient-specific situations need to be discussed with cardiologist; AHA/ACC/SCAI/ACS/ADA Science Advisory provides recommendations). Use caution in concurrent treatment with anticoagulants (eg, heparin, warfarin) or other antiplatelet drugs; bleeding risk is increased. Concurrent use with drugs known to inhibit CYP2C19 may reduce levels of active metabolite and subsequently reduce clinical efficacy; if possible, avoid concurrent use of CYP2C19 inhibitors. Use with caution in patients with severe liver or renal disease (experience is limited). Cases of thrombotic thrombocytopenic purpura (usually occurring within the first 2 weeks of therapy), resulting in some fatalities, have been reported; urgent plasmapheresis is required. Patients with one or more copies of the variant *CYP2C19*2* and/or *CYP2C19*3* alleles (and potentially other reduced-function variants) may have reduced conversion of clopidogrel to its active thiol metabolite. Lower metabolite exposure may result in reduced platelet inhibition and, thus, a higher rate of cardiovascular events following myocardial infarction or stent thrombosis following percutaneous coronary intervention. The optimal dose for these patients has yet to be determined. **Note:** Patients of Chinese ancestry have a higher incidence of *CYP2C19*2* and *CYP2C19*3* alleles compared to Caucasian or African-American patients. Safety and efficacy have not been established in pediatric patients.

Adverse Reactions As with all drugs which may affect hemostasis, bleeding is associated with clopidogrel. Hemorrhage may occur at virtually any site. Risk is dependent on multiple variables, including the concurrent use of multiple agents which alter hemostasis and patient susceptibility.

>10%: Gastrointestinal: The overall incidence of gastrointestinal events (including abdominal pain, vomiting, dyspepsia, gastritis, and constipation) has been documented to be 27% compared to 30% in patients receiving aspirin.

3% to 10%:
Cardiovascular: Chest pain (8%), edema (4%), hypertension (4%)
Central nervous system: Headache (3% to 8%), dizziness (2% to 6%), depression (4%), fatigue (3%), general pain (6%)
Dermatologic: Rash (4%), pruritus (3%)
Endocrine & metabolic: Hypercholesterolemia (4%)
Gastrointestinal: Abdominal pain (2% to 6%), dyspepsia (2% to 5%), diarrhea (2% to 5%), nausea (3%)
Genitourinary: Urinary tract infection (3%)
Hematologic: Bleeding (major 4%; minor 5%), purpura (5%), epistaxis (3%)
Hepatic: Liver function test abnormalities (<3%; discontinued in 0.11%)
Neuromuscular & skeletal: Arthralgia (6%), back pain (6%)
Respiratory: Dyspnea (5%), rhinitis (4%), bronchitis (4%), cough (3%), upper respiratory infection (9%)
Miscellaneous: Flu-like syndrome (8%)

1% to 3%:
Cardiovascular: Atrial fibrillation, cardiac failure, palpitation, syncope
Central nervous system: Fever, insomnia, vertigo, anxiety
Dermatologic: Eczema
Endocrine & metabolic: Gout, hyperuricemia
Gastrointestinal: Constipation, GI hemorrhage, vomiting
Genitourinary: Cystitis
Hematologic: Hematoma, anemia
Neuromuscular & skeletal: Arthritis, leg cramps, neuralgia, paresthesia, weakness
Ocular: Cataract, conjunctivitis

<1% (Limited to important or life-threatening): Acute liver failure, agranulocytosis, allergic reaction, anaphylactoid reaction, angioedema, aplastic anemia, bilirubinemia, bronchospasm, bullous eruption, confusion, erythema multiforme, fatty liver, fever, granulocytopenia, hallucination, hematuria, hemoptysis, hemothorax, hepatitis, hypersensitivity, hypochromic anemia, interstitial pneumonitis, intracranial hemorrhage (0.4%), ischemic necrosis, leukopenia, lichen planus, maculopapular rash, menorrhagia, neutropenia (0.05%), ocular hemorrhage, pancreatitis, pancytopenia, pulmonary hemorrhage, purpura, retroperitoneal bleeding, serum sickness, Stevens-Johnson syndrome, stomatitis, taste disorder, thrombocytopenia, thrombotic thrombocytopenic purpura (TTP), toxic epidermal necrolysis, urticaria, vasculitis

Drug Interactions
Metabolism/Transport Effects Substrate of CYP2C19, CYP3A4; CYP1A2 (minor) **Inhibits** CYP2C9 (weak)
Avoid Concomitant Use
Avoid concomitant use of Clopidogrel with any of the following: CYP2C19 Inhibitors (Moderate); CYP2C19 Inhibitors (Strong)
Increased Effect/Toxicity
Clopidogrel may increase the levels/effects of: Anticoagulants; Antiplatelet Agents; CYP2B6 Substrates; Drotrecogin Alfa; Ibritumomab; Salicylates; Thrombolytic Agents; Tositumomab and Iodine I 131 Tositumomab; Warfarin

The levels/effects of Clopidogrel may be increased by: Dasatinib; Herbs (Anticoagulant/Antiplatelet Properties); Nonsteroidal Anti-Inflammatory Agents; Omega-3-Acid Ethyl Esters; Pentosan Polysulfate Sodium; Pentoxifylline; Prostacyclin Analogues; Rifamycin Derivatives
Decreased Effect
The levels/effects of Clopidogrel may be decreased by: Calcium Channel Blockers; CYP2C19 Inhibitors (Moderate); CYP2C19 Inhibitors (Strong); Macrolide Antibiotics; Nonsteroidal Anti-Inflammatory Agents; Proton Pump Inhibitors

Ethanol/Nutrition/Herb Interactions Herb/Nutraceutical: Avoid alfalfa, anise, bilberry, bladderwrack, bromelain, cat's claw, chamomile, coleus, cordyceps, dong quai, evening primrose oil, fenugreek, feverfew, garlic, ginger, ginkgo biloba, ginseng (American), ginseng (Panax), ginseng (Siberian), grape seed, green tea, guggul, horse chestnut seed, horseradish, licorice, prickly ash, red clover, reishi, SAMe (S-adenosylmethionine), sweet clover, turmeric, white willow (all have additional antiplatelet activity).
Dietary Considerations May be taken without regard to meals.
Dosage Forms Excipient information presented when available (limited, particularly for generics); consult specific product labeling.
Tablet:
Plavix®: 75 mg, 300 mg
References
Grines CL, Bonow RO, Casey DE, et al, "AHA/ACC/SCAI/ACS/ADA Science Advisory, Prevention of Premature Discontinuation of Dual Antiplatelet Therapy in Patients With Coronary Artery Stents. A Science Advisory From the American Heart Association, American College of Cardiology, Society of Cardiovascular Angiography and Interventions, American College of Surgeons, and American Dental Association With Representation from the Amercian College of Physicians," *Circulation*, 2007, 115(6):813-8. Available at http://www.acc.org/qualityandscience/clinical/pdfs/Final_Dual_Antiplatelet_Statement_010507.pdf

◆ **Clopidogrel Bisulfate** see Clopidogrel on page 333

Clorazepate (klor AZ e pate)

Related Information
Benzodiazepines on page 1666
U.S. Brand Names Tranxene® SD™; Tranxene® SD™-Half Strength; Tranxene® T-Tab®
Canadian Brand Names Apo-Clorazepate®; Novo-Clopate
Index Terms Clorazepate Dipotassium; Tranxene T-Tab®
Pharmacologic Category Benzodiazepine
Restrictions C-IV

◀ **Use** Treatment of generalized anxiety disorder; management of ethanol withdrawal; adjunct anticonvulsant in management of partial seizures

Pharmacodynamics/Kinetics

Onset of action: 1-2 hours

Duration: Variable, 8-24 hours

Distribution: Crosses placenta; appears in urine

Metabolism: Rapidly decarboxylated to desmethyldiazepam (active) in acidic stomach prior to absorption; hepatically to oxazepam (active)

Half-life elimination: Adults: Desmethyldiazepam: 48-96 hours; Oxazepam: 6-8 hours

Time to peak, serum: ~1 hour

Excretion: Primarily urine

Dosage Oral:

Children 9-12 years: Anticonvulsant: Initial: 3.75-7.5 mg/dose twice daily; increase dose by 3.75 mg at weekly intervals, not to exceed 60 mg/day in 2-3 divided doses

Children >12 years and Adults: Anticonvulsant: Initial: Up to 7.5 mg/dose 2-3 times/day; increase dose by 7.5 mg at weekly intervals, not to exceed 90 mg/day

Adults:

Anxiety:

Regular release tablets (Tranxene® T-Tab®): 7.5-15 mg 2-4 times/day

Sustained release (Tranxene® SD™): 11.25 or 22.5 mg once daily at bedtime

Ethanol withdrawal: Initial: 30 mg, then 15 mg 2-4 times/day on first day; maximum daily dose: 90 mg; gradually decrease dose over subsequent days

Anesthesia and Critical Care Concerns/Other Considerations Abrupt discontinuation after sustained use (generally >10 days) may cause withdrawal symptoms.

Additional Information Complete prescribing information for this medication should be consulted for additional detail.

Dosage Forms Excipient information presented when available (limited, particularly for generics); consult specific product labeling.

Tablet, as dipotassium: 3.75 mg, 7.5 mg, 15 mg

Tranxene® SD™: 22.5 mg [once daily]

Tranxene® SD™-Half Strength: 11.25 mg [once daily]

Tranxene® T-Tab®: 3.75 mg, 7.5 mg, 15 mg

♦ **Clorazepate Dipotassium** *see* Clorazepate *on page* 337

♦ **Coagulation Factor I** *see* Fibrinogen Concentrate (Human) *on page* 600

♦ **Coagulation Factor VIIa** *see* Factor VIIa (Recombinant) *on page* 567

♦ **CO Alendronate (Can)** *see* Alendronate *on page* 57

♦ **CO Amlodipine (Can)** *see* AmLODIPine *on page* 93

♦ **CO Azithromycin (Can)** *see* Azithromycin *on page* 169

♦ **CO Buspirone (Can)** *see* BusPIRone *on page* 219

Cocaine (koe KANE)

Related Information

Anesthesia Considerations for Neurosurgery *on page* 1514

Anesthesia for Obstetric Patients in Nonobstetric Surgery *on page* 1532

Anesthetic Considerations in the Substance-Abusing Patient *on page* 1613

Inhalational Anesthetics *on page* 1632

Local Anesthetics *on page* 1636

Perioperative Management of Patients on Antiseizure Medication *on page* 1577

Index Terms Cocaine Hydrochloride

Pharmacologic Category Local Anesthetic

Restrictions C-II

Generic Available Yes

Use Topical anesthesia for mucous membranes

Mechanism of Action Ester local anesthetic blocks both the initiation and conduction of nerve impulses by decreasing the neuronal membrane's permeability to sodium ions, which results in inhibition of depolarization with resultant blockade of conduction; interferes with the uptake of norepinephrine by adrenergic nerve terminals producing vasoconstriction

Pharmacodynamics/Kinetics Following topical administration to mucosa:

Onset of action: ~1 minute
Peak effect: ~5 minutes
Duration (dose dependent): ≥30 minutes; cocaine metabolites may appear in urine of neonates up to 5 days after birth due to maternal cocaine use shortly before birth
Absorption: Well absorbed through mucous membranes; limited by drug-induced vasoconstriction; enhanced by inflammation
Distribution: Enters breast milk
Metabolism: Hepatic; major metabolites are ecgonine methyl ester and benzoyl ecgonine
Half-life elimination: 75 minutes
Excretion: Primarily urine (<10% as unchanged drug and metabolites)

Dosage Topical application (ear, nose, throat, bronchoscopy): Dosage depends on the area to be anesthetized, tissue vascularity, technique of anesthesia, and individual patient tolerance; the lowest dose necessary to produce adequate anesthesia should be used; concentrations of 1% to 10% are used (not to exceed 1 mg/kg). Use reduced dosages for children, elderly, or debilitated patients.

Stability Store in well closed, light-resistant containers.

Administration Topical: Use only on mucous membranes of the oral, laryngeal, and nasal cavities. Do not use on extensive areas of broken skin.

Monitoring Parameters Vital signs

Reference Range Therapeutic: 100-500 ng/mL (SI: 330 nmol/L); Toxic: >1000 ng/mL (SI: >3300 nmol/L)

Anesthesia and Critical Care Concerns/Other Considerations

Clinical Pearls/Comments: It is safe to anesthetize a cocaine-abusing patient when obvious signs of intoxication are not exhibited (eg, tachycardia, hypertension, hyperthermia, ECG changes including QRS and QT_c interval prolongation >500 msec) (Hill, 2006).

Evidence-Based Information: Due to the sympathomimetic actions of cocaine, the threshold for development of arrhythmias may be reduced increasing the risk of catecholamine-induced arrhythmias. Cocaine may also be associated with cerebral vascular accidents in patients without any previous risk factors.

Pregnancy Risk Factor C/X (nonmedicinal use)

Contraindications Hypersensitivity to cocaine or any component of the topical solution; ophthalmologic anesthesia (causing sloughing of the corneal epithelium); pregnancy (nonmedicinal use)

Warnings/Precautions For topical use only. Limit to office and surgical procedures only. Resuscitative equipment and drugs should be immediately available when any local anesthetic is used. Debilitated, elderly patients, acutely ill patients, and children should be given reduced doses consistent with their age and physical status. Use caution in patients with severely traumatized mucosa and sepsis in the region of the proposed application. Use with caution in patients with cardiovascular disease or a history of cocaine abuse. In patients being treated for cardiovascular complication of cocaine abuse, avoid beta-blockers for treatment.

Adverse Reactions

>10%:
Central nervous system: CNS stimulation
Gastrointestinal: Loss of taste perception
Respiratory: Rhinitis, nasal congestion
Miscellaneous: Loss of smell

1% to 10%:
Cardiovascular: Heart rate decreased with low doses, tachycardia with moderate doses, hypertension, cardiomyopathy, cardiac arrhythmia, myocarditis, QRS prolongation, Raynaud's phenomenon, cerebral vasculitis, thrombosis, fibrillation (atrial), flutter (atrial), sinus bradycardia, CHF, pulmonary hypertension, sinus tachycardia, tachycardia (supraventricular), arrhythmia (ventricular), vasoconstriction
Central nervous system: Fever, nervousness, restlessness, euphoria, excitation, headache, psychosis, hallucinations, agitation, seizure, slurred speech,

hyperthermia, dystonic reactions, cerebral vascular accident, vasculitis, clonic-tonic reactions, paranoia, sympathetic storm

Dermatologic: Skin infarction, pruritus, madarosis

Gastrointestinal: Nausea, anorexia, colonic ischemia, spontaneous bowel perforation

Genitourinary: Priapism, uterine rupture

Hematologic: Thrombocytopenia

Neuromuscular & skeletal: Chorea (extrapyramidal), paresthesia, tremor, fasciculations

Ocular: Mydriasis (peak effect at 45 minutes; may last up to 12 hours), sloughing of the corneal epithelium, ulceration of the cornea, iritis, chemosis

Renal: Myoglobinuria, necrotizing vasculitis

Respiratory: Tachypnea, nasal mucosa damage (when snorting), hyposmia, bronchiolitis obliterans organizing pneumonia

Miscellaneous: "Washed-out" syndrome

Drug Interactions

Metabolism/Transport Effects Substrate of CYP3A4 (major); **Inhibits** CYP2D6 (strong), 3A4 (weak)

Avoid Concomitant Use

Avoid concomitant use of Cocaine with any of the following: Iobenguane I 123; Tamoxifen; Thioridazine

Increased Effect/Toxicity

Cocaine may increase the levels/effects of: Atomoxetine; Cannabinoids; CYP2D6 Substrates; Fesoterodine; Nebivolol; Tamoxifen; Tetrabenazine; Thioridazine

The levels/effects of Cocaine may be increased by: CYP3A4 Inhibitors (Moderate); CYP3A4 Inhibitors (Strong); Dasatinib

Decreased Effect

Cocaine may decrease the levels/effects of: Codeine; Iobenguane I 123; TraMADol

Dosage Forms Excipient information presented when available (limited, particularly for generics); consult specific product labeling.

Powder, for prescription compounding, as hydrochloride: 1 g, 5 g, 25 g

Solution, topical, as hydrochloride: 4% (4 mL, 10 mL); 10% (4 mL, 10 mL)

References

Hill GE, Ogunnaike BO, and Johnson ER, "General Anaesthesia for the Cocaine Abusing Patient. Is it Safe?" *Br J Anaesth*, 2006, 97(5):654-7.

Kloner RA and Rezkalla SH, "Cocaine and the Heart," *N Engl J Med*, 2003, 348(6):487-8.

Lange RA and Hillis LD, "Cardiovascular Complications of Cocaine Use," *N Engl J Med*, 2001, 345 (5):351-8 (published erratum appears in *N Engl J Med*, 2001, 345[19]:1432).

Richards CF, Clark RF, Holbrook T, et al, "The Effect of Cocaine and Amphetamines on Vital Signs in Trauma Patients," *J Emerg Med*, 1995, 13(1):59-63.

◆ **Cocaine Hydrochloride** *see Cocaine on page 338*

◆ **CO Cilazapril (Can)** *see Cilazapril on page 301*

◆ **CO Ciprofloxacin (Can)** *see Ciprofloxacin on page 306*

◆ **CO Clonazepam (Can)** *see ClonazePAM on page 328*

Codeine (KOE deen)

Medication Safety Issues

Sound-alike/look-alike issues:

Codeine may be confused with Cardene®, Cophene®, Cordran®, iodine, Lodine®

High alert medication: The Institute for Safe Medication Practices (ISMP) includes this medication among its list of drug classes which have a heightened risk of causing significant patient harm when used in error.

Related Information
Acute Postoperative Pain *on page 1502*
Anesthetic Considerations in the Substance-Abusing Patient *on page 1613*
Chronic Pain Management *on page 1546*
Opioid Analgesics *on page 1688*
Skin Tests *on page 1707*

Canadian Brand Names Codeine Contin®

Index Terms Codeine Phosphate; Codeine Sulfate; Methylmorphine

Pharmacologic Category Analgesic, Opioid; Antitussive

Restrictions C-II

Generic Available Yes

Use Treatment of mild-to-moderate pain; antitussive in lower doses

Mechanism of Action Binds to opiate receptors in the CNS, causing inhibition of ascending pain pathways, altering the perception of and response to pain; causes cough supression by direct central action in the medulla; produces generalized CNS depression

Pharmacodynamics/Kinetics
Onset of action: Oral: 0.5-1 hour; I.M.: 10-30 minutes
  Peak effect: Oral: 1-1.5 hours; I.M.: 0.5-1 hour
Duration: 4-6 hours
Absorption: Oral: Adequate
Distribution: Crosses placenta; enters breast milk
Protein binding: 7%
Metabolism: Hepatic to morphine (active)
Half-life elimination: 2.5-3.5 hours
Excretion: Urine (3% to 16% as unchanged drug, norcodeine, and free and conjugated morphine)

Dosage Note: These are guidelines and do not represent the maximum doses that may be required in all patients. Doses should be titrated to pain relief/prevention. Doses >1.5 mg/kg body weight are not recommended.

Analgesic:
  Children: Oral, I.M., SubQ: 0.5-1 mg/kg/dose every 4-6 hours as needed; maximum: 60 mg/dose
  Adults:
    Oral: 30 mg every 4-6 hours as needed; patients with prior opiate exposure may require higher initial doses. Usual range: 15-120 mg every 4-6 hours as needed. **Note:** The American Pain Society recommends an initial dose of 30-60 mg for adults with moderate pain.
    Oral, controlled release formulation (Codeine Contin®, not available in U.S.): 50-300 mg every 12 hours. **Note:** A patient's codeine requirement should be established using prompt release formulations; conversion to long acting products may be considered when chronic, continuous treatment is required. Higher dosages should be reserved for use only in opioid-tolerant patients.
    I.M., SubQ: 30 mg every 4-6 hours as needed; patients with prior opiate exposure may require higher initial doses. Usual range: 15-120 mg every 4-6 hours as needed; more frequent dosing may be needed
Antitussive: Oral (for nonproductive cough):
  Children: 1-1.5 mg/kg/day in divided doses every 4-6 hours as needed; Alternative dose according to age:
    2-6 years: 2.5-5 mg every 4-6 hours as needed; maximum: 30 mg/day
    6-12 years: 5-10 mg every 4-6 hours as needed; maximum: 60 mg/day
  Adults: 10-20 mg/dose every 4-6 hours as needed; maximum: 120 mg/day

Dosing adjustment in renal impairment:
Cl$_{cr}$ 10-50 mL/minute: Administer 75% of dose
Cl$_{cr}$ <10 mL/minute: Administer 50% of dose

Dosing adjustment in hepatic impairment: Probably necessary in hepatic insufficiency

Stability Store injection between 15°C to 30°C; avoid freezing. Do not use if injection is discolored or contains a precipitate. Protect injection from light.

Administration Not approved for I.V. administration (although this route has been used clinically). If given intravenously, must be given slowly and the patient should be lying down. Rapid intravenous administration of narcotics may increase the incidence of serious adverse effects, in part due to limited opportunity to assess ▶

response prior to administration of the full dose. Access to respiratory support should be immediately available.

Monitoring Parameters Pain relief, respiratory and mental status, blood pressure, heart rate

Reference Range Therapeutic: Not established; Toxic: >1.1 mcg/mL

Anesthesia and Critical Care Concerns/Other Considerations

Clinical Pearls/Comments: May be administered to patients with chronic cough prior to surgical cases such as cataract extraction under MAC anesthesia to prevent movement during the procedure.

Evidence-Based Information: The 2002 ACCM/SCCM guidelines for analgesia (critically-ill adult) recommend against using codeine because of its lack of potency, histamine release (may cause hypotension), potential accumulation of active metabolites. The guidelines recommend fentanyl in patients who need immediate pain relief because of its rapid onset of action; fentanyl or hydromorphone is preferred in patients who are hypotensive or have renal dysfunction.

Pregnancy Risk Factor C/D (prolonged use or high doses at term)

Contraindications Hypersensitivity to codeine or any component of the formulation; pregnancy (prolonged use or high doses at term)

Warnings/Precautions Use with caution in patients with hypersensitivity reactions to other phenanthrene-derivative opioid agonists (morphine, hydro-codone, hydromorphone, levorphanol, oxycodone, oxymorphone); respiratory diseases including asthma, emphysema, COPD, adrenal insufficiency, biliary tract impairment, CNS depression/coma, head trauma, morbid obesity, prostatic hyperplasia, urinary stricture, thyroid dysfunction, or severe liver or renal insufficiency; some preparations contain sulfites which may cause allergic reactions; tolerance or drug dependence may result from extended use. May obscure diagnosis or clinical course of patients with acute abdominal conditions. May cause CNS depression, which may impair physical or mental abilities; patients must be cautioned about performing tasks which require mental alertness (eg, operating machinery or driving). May cause hypotension; use with caution in patients with hypovolemia, cardiovascular disease (including acute MI), or drugs which may exaggerate hypotensive effects (including phenothiazines or general anesthetics). Use caution in patients with two or more copies of the variant CYP2D6*2 allele; may have extensive conversion to morphine and thus increased opioid-mediated effects.

Not recommended for use for cough control in patients with a productive cough; not recommended as an antitussive for children <2 years of age; the elderly and debilitated patients may be particularly susceptible to adverse effects of narcotics

Not approved for I.V. administration (although this route has been used clinically). If given intravenously, must be given slowly and the patient should be lying down. Rapid intravenous administration of narcotics may increase the incidence of serious adverse effects, in part due to limited opportunity to assess response prior to administration of the full dose. Access to respiratory support should be immediately available.

Concurrent use of agonist/antagonist analgesics may precipitate withdrawal symptoms and/or reduced analgesic efficacy in patients following prolonged therapy with mu opioid agonists. Abrupt discontinuation following prolonged use may also lead to withdrawal symptoms.

Adverse Reactions

Frequency not defined: ALT increased, AST increased

>10%:

Central nervous system: Drowsiness

Gastrointestinal: Constipation

1% to 10%:

Cardiovascular: Hypotension, tachycardia or bradycardia

Central nervous system: Confusion, dizziness, false feeling of well being, headache, lightheadedness, malaise, paradoxical CNS stimulation, restlessness

Dermatologic: Rash, urticaria

Gastrointestinal: Anorexia, nausea, vomiting, xerostomia

Genitourinary: Ureteral spasm, urination decreased

Hepatic: LFTs increased

Local: Burning at injection site

Neuromuscular & skeletal: Weakness

Ocular: Blurred vision

Respiratory: Dyspnea

Miscellaneous: Histamine release

<1% (Limited to important or life-threatening): Biliary spasm, convulsions, hallucinations, insomnia, mental depression, muscle rigidity, nightmares, paralytic ileus, stomach cramps

Drug Interactions

Metabolism/Transport Effects Substrate of CYP2D6 (major), 3A4 (minor); **Inhibits** CYP2D6 (weak)

Avoid Concomitant Use There are no known interactions where it is recommended to avoid concomitant use.

Increased Effect/Toxicity

Codeine may increase the levels/effects of: Alcohol (Ethyl); Alvimopan; CNS Depressants; Desmopressin; Selective Serotonin Reuptake Inhibitors; Thiazide Diuretics

The levels/effects of Codeine may be increased by: Amphetamines; Antipsychotic Agents (Phenothiazines); Somatostatin Analogs; Succinylcholine

Decreased Effect

Codeine may decrease the levels/effects of: Pegvisomant

The levels/effects of Codeine may be decreased by: Ammonium Chloride; CYP2D6 Inhibitors (Moderate); CYP2D6 Inhibitors (Strong)

Ethanol/Nutrition/Herb Interactions

Ethanol: Avoid or limit ethanol (may increase CNS depression).

Herb/Nutraceutical: St John's wort may decrease codeine levels. Avoid valerian, St John's wort, kava kava, gotu kola (may increase CNS depression).

Test Interactions Some quinolones may produce a false-positive urine screening result for opiates using commercially-available immunoassay kits. This has been demonstrated most consistently for levofloxacin and ofloxacin, but other quinolones have shown cross-reactivity in certain assay kits. Confirmation of positive opiate screens by more specific methods should be considered.

Dosage Forms Excipient information presented when available (limited, particularly for generics); consult specific product labeling. [CAN] = Canadian brand name

Injection, as phosphate: 15 mg/mL (2 mL); 30 mg/mL (2 mL) [contains sodium metabisulfite]

Powder, for prescription compounding: 10 g, 25 g

Tablet, as phosphate: 30 mg, 60 mg

Tablet, as sulfate: 15 mg, 30 mg, 60 mg

Tablet, controlled release (Codeine Contin®) [CAN]: 50 mg, 100 mg, 150 mg, 200 mg [not available in U.S.]

References

"Clinical Practice Guidelines for the Sustained Use of Sedatives and Analgesics in the Critically Ill Adult. Task Force of the American College of Critical Care Medicine (ACCM) of the Society of Critical Care Medicine (SCCM), American Society of Health-System Pharmacists (ASHP), American College of Chest Physicians," *Am J Health Syst Pharm*, 2002, 59(2):150-78.

"Principles of Analgesic Use in the Treatment of Acute Pain and Cancer Pain," 6th ed, Glenview, IL: American Pain Society, 2008.

◆ **CO Ipra-Sal (Can)** *see* Ipratropium and Albuterol *on page 762*

Colchicine (KOL chi seen)

Medication Safety Issues
Sound-alike/look-alike issues:
  Colchicine may be confused with Cortrosyn®

Medication Guide An FDA-approved patient medication guide, which is available with the product information and at http://www.fda.gov/downloads/Drugs/DrugSafety/UCM176363.pdf, must be dispensed with this medication for each new outpatient prescription and refill.

U.S. Brand Names Colcrys™

Pharmacologic Category Colchicine

Generic Available Yes

Use Treatment of acute gout flares and familial Mediterranean fever (FMF)

Unlabeled/Investigational Use Primary biliary cirrhosis; pericarditis; prophylaxis of acute gout flares during initiation of antihyperuricemic therapy

Mechanism of Action Disrupts cytoskeletal functions by inhibiting β-tubulin polymerization into microtubules, preventing activation, degranulation, and migration of neutrophils associated with mediating some gout symptoms. In familial Mediterranean fever, may interfere with intracellular assembly of the inflammasome complex present in neutrophils and monocytes that mediate activation of interleukin-1β.

Pharmacodynamics/Kinetics
Onset of action: Oral: Pain relief: ~18-24 hours

Distribution: Concentrates in leukocytes, kidney, spleen, and liver; does not distribute in heart, skeletal muscle, and brain

V_d: 5-8 L/kg

Protein binding: ~39%

Metabolism: Hepatic via CYP3A4; 3 metabolites (2 primary, 1 minor)

Bioavailability: 45%

Half-life elimination: 27-31 hours (multiple oral doses; young, healthy volunteers)

Time to peak, serum: Oral: 0.5-3 hours

Excretion: Urine (40% to 65% as unchanged drug); enterohepatic recirculation and biliary excretion also possible

Dosage Oral:
Familial Mediterranean fever (FMF):
  Children:
    4-6 years: 0.3-1.8 mg/day in 1-2 divided doses
    6-12 years: 0.9-1.8 mg/day in 1-2 divided doses
  Children >12 years and Adults: 1.2-2.4 mg/day in 1-2 divided doses. Titration: Increase or decrease dose in 0.3 mg increments based on efficacy or adverse effects

Gout: Adults:
  Flares: Initial: 1.2 mg at the first sign of flare, followed in 1 hour with a single dose of 0.6 mg (maximum: 1.8 mg within 1 hour). **Note:** Current FDA-approved dose for gout flare is substantially lower than what has been historically used clinically. Doses larger than the currently recommended dosage for gout flare have not been proven to be more effective.
  Prophylaxis of acute attacks (unlabeled use): 0.6 mg twice daily; initial and/or subsequent dosage may be decreased (eg, 0.6 mg once daily) in patients who are intolerant (diarrhea) (Terkeltaub, 2009)

Pericarditis (unlabeled use): Adults: 0.6 mg twice daily (Antman, 2004)

Primary biliary cirrhosis (unlabeled use): Adults: 0.6 mg twice daily (Kaplan, 2005); **Note:** Use reserved for patients refractory to ursodiol.

Elderly: Use caution; reduce prophylactic daily dose by 50% in individuals >70 years (Terkeltaub, 2009)

Dosage adjustment for concomitant therapy with CYP3A4 or P-glycoprotein (P-gp) inhibitors: *Dosage adjustment also required in patients receiving CYP3A4 or P-gp inhibitors up to 14 days prior to initiation of colchicine.*

Coadministration of **strong** CYP3A4 inhibitor (eg, atazanavir, clarithromycin, indinavir, itraconazole, ketoconazole, nefazodone, nelfinavir, ritonavir, saquinavir, telithromycin):

FMF: Maximum dose: 0.6 mg/day (0.3 mg twice daily)

Gout flare: Initial: 0.6 mg, followed in 1 hour by a single dose of 0.3 mg; do not repeat for at least 3 days

Coadministration of **moderate** CYP3A4 inhibitor (eg, amprenavir, aprepitant, diltiazem, erythromycin, fluconazole, fosamprenavir, grapefruit juice, verapamil):

FMF: Maximum dose: 1.2 mg/day (0.6 mg twice daily)

Gout flare: 1.2 mg as a single dose; do not repeat for at least 3 days

Coadministration of P-gp inhibitor (eg, cyclosporine, ranolazine):

FMF: Maximum dose: 0.6 mg/day (0.3 mg twice daily)

Gout flare: Initial: 0.6 mg as a single dose; do not repeat for at least 3 days

Dosing adjustment in renal impairment: Concurrent use of colchicine and P-gp or strong CYP3A4 inhibitors is **contraindicated** in renal impairment. Fatal toxicity has been reported.

FMF:

Cl_{cr} 30-80 mL/minute: Monitor closely for adverse effects; dose reduction may be necessary

Cl_{cr} <30 mL/minute: Initial dose: 0.3 mg/day; use caution if dose titrated; monitor for adverse effects

Dialysis: 0.3 mg as a single dose; use caution if dose titrated; monitor for adverse effects. Not removed by dialysis.

Gout flares:

Cl_{cr} 30-80 mL/minute: Dosage adjustment not required; monitor closely for adverse effects

Cl_{cr} <30 mL/minute: Dosage reduction not required but may be considered; treatment course should not be repeated more frequently than every 14 days

Dialysis: 0.6 mg as a single dose; treatment course should not be repeated more frequently than every 14 days. Not removed by dialysis.

Gout prophylaxis (Terkeltaub, 2009):

Cl_{cr} 35-49 mL/minute: 0.6 mg once daily

Cl_{cr} 10-34 mL/minute: 0.6 mg every 2-3 days

Cl_{cr} <10 mL/minute: Avoid chronic use of colchicine.

Hemodialysis: Avoid chronic use of colchicine.

Dosage adjustment in hepatic impairment: Concurrent use of colchicine and P-gp or strong CYP3A4 inhibitors is **contraindicated** in hepatic impairment. Fatal toxicity has been reported.

FMF:

Mild-to-moderate impairment: Use caution; monitor closely for adverse effects

Severe impairment: Consider dosage reduction

Gout flares:

Mild-to-moderate impairment: Dosage adjustment not required; monitor closely for adverse effects

Severe impairment: Dosage reduction not required but may be considered; treatment course should not be repeated more frequently than every 14 days

Stability Store at 20°C to 25°C (68°F to 77°F). Protect from light.

Administration Administer orally with water and maintain adequate fluid intake.

Monitoring Parameters CBC, renal and hepatic function tests

Pregnancy Risk Factor C

Contraindications Concomitant use of a P-glycoprotein (P-gp) or strong CYP3A4 inhibitor in presence of renal or hepatic impairment

Warnings/Precautions Myelosuppression (eg, thrombocytopenia, leukopenia, granulocytopenia, pancytopenia) and aplastic anemia have been reported in patients receiving therapeutic doses. Neuromuscular toxicity (including rhabdomyolysis) has been reported in patients receiving therapeutic doses; patients with renal dysfunction and elderly patients are at increased risk. Concomitant use of cyclosporine, diltiazem, verapamil, fibrates, and statins may increase the risk of myopathy. Clearance is decreased in renal or hepatic impairment; monitor closely for adverse effects/toxicity. Dosage adjustments may be required depending on degree of impairment or indication, and may be affected by the use of concurrent medication (CYP3A4 or P-gp inhibitors). Concurrent use of P-gp or strong ▶

CYP3A4 inhibitors is contraindicated in renal impairment; fatal toxicity has been reported. Colchicine does not have analgesic activity and should not be used to treat pain from other causes.

Adverse Reactions

>10%: Gastrointestinal: Diarrhea (up to 23%), abdominal pain, cramping, nausea, vomiting

1% to 10%:
Central nervous system: Fatigue
Gastrointestinal: Anorexia
Respiratory: Pharyngolaryngeal pain

<1% (Limited to important or life-threatening): Alopecia, ALT increased, aplastic anemia, AST increased, azoospermia, bone marrow suppression, CPK increased, dermatosis, granulocytopenia, hepatotoxicity, hypersensitivity reaction, leukopenia, maculopapular rash, muscle weakness, myalgia, myopathy, myotonia, neuropathy, oligospermia, pancytopenia, peripheral neuritis, purpura, rash, rhabdomyolysis, thrombocytopenia

Drug Interactions

Metabolism/Transport Effects Substrate of CYP3A4 (major); **Induces** CYP2C8 (weak), 2C9 (weak), 2E1 (weak), 3A4 (weak)

Avoid Concomitant Use There are no known interactions where it is recommended to avoid concomitant use.

Increased Effect/Toxicity
Colchicine may increase the levels/effects of: HMG-CoA Reductase Inhibitors

The levels/effects of Colchicine may be increased by: CYP3A4 Inhibitors (Moderate); CYP3A4 Inhibitors (Strong); Dasatinib; Fibric Acid Derivatives; P-Glycoprotein Inhibitors

Decreased Effect
Colchicine may decrease the levels/effects of: Saxagliptin

The levels/effects of Colchicine may be decreased by: P-Glycoprotein Inducers

Ethanol/Nutrition/Herb Interactions

Ethanol: Avoid ethanol.
Food: Cyanocobalamin (vitamin B_{12}): Malabsorption of the substrate. May result in macrocytic anemia or neurologic dysfunction. Grapefruit juice may increase colchicine serum concentrations.
Herb/Nutraceutical: Vitamin B_{12} absorption may be decreased by colchicine.

Test Interactions May cause false-positive results in urine tests for erythrocytes or hemoglobin

Dietary Considerations May need to supplement with vitamin B_{12}. Avoid grapefruit juice.

Dosage Forms Excipient information presented when available (limited, particularly for generics); consult specific product labeling.
Tablet: 0.6 mg
Colcrys™: 0.6 mg

- ◆ **Colcrys™** *see* Colchicine *on page 344*
- ◆ **CO Levetiracetam (Can)** *see* Levetiracetam *on page 816*
- ◆ **CO Levofloxacin (Can)** *see* Levofloxacin *on page 823*
- ◆ **CO Lisinopril (Can)** *see* Lisinopril *on page 849*

Colistimethate (koe lis ti METH ate)

U.S. Brand Names Coly-Mycin® M
Canadian Brand Names Coly-Mycin® M
Index Terms Colistimethate Sodium; Colistin Methanesulfonate; Colistin Sulfomethate; Pentasodium Colistin Methanesulfonate
Pharmacologic Category Antibiotic, Miscellaneous
Generic Available Yes
Use Treatment of infections due to sensitive strains of certain gram-negative bacilli which are resistant to other antibacterials or in patients allergic to other antibacterials

Unlabeled/Investigational Use Used as nebulized inhalation in the prevention of *Pseudomonas aeruginosa* respiratory tract infections in immunocompromised patients, and used as nebulized inhalation adjunct agent for the treatment of *P. aeruginosa* infections in patients with cystic fibrosis and other seriously ill or chronically ill patients

Mechanism of Action Hydrolyzed to colistin, which acts as a cationic detergent which damages the bacterial cytoplasmic membrane causing leaking of intracellular substances and cell death

Pharmacodynamics/Kinetics

Distribution: Widely, except for CNS, synovial, pleural, and pericardial fluids

Metabolism: Colistimethate is hydrolyzed to colistin

Half-life elimination: I.M., I.V.: 2-3 hours; Anuria: ≤2-3 days

Time to peak: I.V.: 10 minutes

Excretion: Primarily urine (as unchanged drug)

Dosage Note: Doses should be based on ideal body weight in obese patients; dosage expressed in terms of colistin.

Children and Adults:

Susceptible infections:

I.M., I.V.: 2.5-5 mg/kg/day in 2-4 divided doses

Inhalation (unlabeled use): 50-75 mg in NS (3-4 mL total) via nebulizer 2-3 times/day

Cystic fibrosis (unlabeled use): I.V.:

Children: 3-8 mg/kg/day in 3 divided doses (maximum dose: 70 mg)

Adults: 3-8 mg/kg/day in 3 divided doses **or** 60-70 mg every 8 hours, if tolerated, may increase to 80-100 mg every 8 hours

Dosing interval in renal impairment: Adults:

S_{cr} 1.3-1.5 mg/dL: 75-115 mg twice daily (approximately 2.5-3.8 mg/kg/day)

S_{cr} 1.6-2.5 mg/dL: 66-150 mg once or twice daily (approximately 2.5 mg/kg/day)

S_{cr} 2.6-4 mg/dL: 100-150 mg every 36 hours (approximately 1.5 mg/kg/day)

Continuous renal replacement therapy (CRRT): Drug clearance is highly dependent on the method of renal replacement, filter type, and flow rate. Appropriate dosing requires close monitoring of pharmacologic response, signs of adverse reactions due to drug accumulation, as well as drug levels in relation to target trough (if appropriate). The following are general recommendations only (based on dialysate flow/ultrafiltration rates of 1 L/hour) and should not supersede clinical judgment:

CVVH or CVVHD/CVVHDF: 2.5 mg/kg every 48 hours

Note: A single case report has demonstrated that the use of 2.5 mg/kg every 48 hours with a dialysate flow rate of 1 L/hour may be inadequate and that dosing every 24 hours was well-tolerated. Based on pharmacokinetic analysis, the authors recommend dosing as frequent as every 12 hours in patients receiving CRRT (Li, 2005).

Stability Store intact vials (prior to reconstitution) at 20°C to 25°C (68°F to 77°F); reconstituted vials may be refrigerated at 2°C to 8°C (36°F to 46°F) or stored at 20°C to 25°C (68°F to 77°F) for up to 24 hours. Solutions for infusion should be freshly prepared; do not use beyond 24 hours. For I.V. use, reconstitute each vial with 2 mL of SWFI; swirl gently to avoid foaming. May further dilute in D_5W or NS for I.V. infusion. For nebulized inhalation (unlabeled use), reconstitute with NS; should be used promptly after preparation; do not use after 24 hours.

Administration

Parenteral: Reconstitute vial with 2 mL SWFI resulting in a concentration of 75 mg colistin/mL; swirl gently to avoid frothing. Administer by I.M., direct I.V. injection over 3-10 minutes, intermittent infusion over 30 minutes, or by continuous I.V. infusion. For continuous I.V. infusion, one-half of the total daily dose is administered by direct I.V. injection over 3-10 minutes followed 1-2 hours later by the remaining one-half of the total daily dose diluted in a compatible I.V. solution infused over 22-23 hours. The final concentration for administration should be based on the patient's fluid needs.

Inhalation (unlabeled): Further dilute dose to a total volume of 3-4 mL in NS and administer via nebulizer. If patient is on a ventilator, place medicine in a T-piece at the midinspiratory circuit of the ventilator. Administer solution promptly following preparation to decrease possibility of high concentrations of colistin from forming which may lead to potentially life-threatening lung toxicity.

Monitoring Parameters Serum creatinine, BUN; urine output; signs of neurotoxicity

Anesthesia and Critical Care Concerns/Other Considerations

Clinical Pearls/Comments:

Colistimethate for inhalation: Colistimethate, an inactive prodrug, is converted to the bioactive colistin by spontaneous hydrolysis once colistimethate is mixed into aqueous solution. Colistin is comprised of 2 components, colistin A (polymyxin E1) and colistin B (polymyxin E2). Polymyxin E1 has been shown to cause localized airway inflammation in animal studies and may result in lung toxicity in humans. Clinicians who continue to prescribe colistimethate for inhalation should be aware of this potentially life-threatening effect and should administer solutions for inhalation promptly following preparation of solution.

On June 12, 2007, the Cystic Fibrosis Foundation issued an alert recommending that patients not use colistimethate for inhalation premixed by pharmacies; patients should prepare their colistimethate nebulizer inhalation solutions immediately prior to use.

Pregnancy Risk Factor C

Contraindications Hypersensitivity to colistimethate, colistin, or any component of the formulation

Warnings/Precautions Nephrotoxicity has been reported; use with caution in patients with pre-existing renal disease; dosage adjustments may be required. Respiratory arrest has been reported with use; impaired renal function may increase the risk for neuromuscular blockade and apnea. Transient, reversible neurological disturbances (eg, dizziness, numbness, paresthesia, tingling, vertigo) may occur. Prolonged use may result in fungal or bacterial superinfection, including *C. difficile*-associated diarrhea (CDAD) and pseudomembranous colitis; CDAD has been observed >2 months postantibiotic treatment.

Adverse Reactions Frequency not defined.

Central nervous system: Dizziness, fever, headache, slurred speech, vertigo

Dermatologic: Pruritus, rash, urticaria

Gastrintestinal: GI upset

Neuromuscular & skeletal: Paresthesia (extremities, oral); weakness (lower limb)

Renal: BUN increased, creatinine increased, nephrotoxicity, proteinuria, urine output decreased

Respiratory: Apnea, respiratory arrest

Postmarketing, and/or case reports: Lung toxicity (bronchoconstriction, bronchospasm, chest tightness, respiratory distress, acute respiratory failure following inhalation)

Drug Interactions

Avoid Concomitant Use There are no known interactions where it is recommended to avoid concomitant use.

Increased Effect/Toxicity

Colistimethate may increase the levels/effects of: Neuromuscular-Blocking Agents

The levels/effects of Colistimethate may be increased by: Aminoglycosides; Amphotericin B; Capreomycin; Polymyxin B; Vancomycin

Decreased Effect

Colistimethate may decrease the levels/effects of: Typhoid Vaccine

Dosage Forms Excipient information presented when available (limited, particularly for generics); consult specific product labeling.

Injection, powder for reconstitution, as colistin base: 150 mg

Coly-Mycin® M: 150 mg

References

McCoy KS, "Compounded Colistimethate as Possible Cause of Fatal Acute Respiratory Distress Syndrome," *N Engl J Med*, 2007, 357(22):2310-1.

◆ **Colistimethate Sodium** *see* Colistimethate *on page 346*

◆ **Colistin Methanesulfonate** *see* Colistimethate *on page 346*

◆ **Colistin Sulfomethate** *see* Colistimethate *on page 346*

◆ **Colocort®** *see* Hydrocortisone *on page 699*

◆ **CO Lovastatin (Can)** *see* Lovastatin *on page 859*

♦ **Coly-Mycin® M** *see* Colistimethate *on page* 346

♦ **Combivent®** *see* Ipratropium and Albuterol *on page* 762

♦ **Combivent UDV (Can)** *see* Ipratropium and Albuterol *on page* 762

♦ **CO Meloxicam (Can)** *see* Meloxicam *on page* 870

♦ **CO Metformin (Can)** *see* MetFORMIN *on page* 886

♦ **Compazine** *see* Prochlorperazine *on page* 1180

♦ **Compound 347™** *see* Enflurane *on page* 483

♦ **Compound F** *see* Hydrocortisone *on page* 699

♦ **Compoz® Nighttime Sleep Aid [OTC]** *see* DiphenhydrAMINE *on page* 430

♦ **Compro™** *see* Prochlorperazine *on page* 1180

♦ **Concerta®** *see* Methylphenidate *on page* 908

Conivaptan (koe NYE vap tan)

U.S. Brand Names Vaprisol®

Index Terms Conivaptan Hydrochloride; YM087

Pharmacologic Category Vasopressin Antagonist

Generic Available No

Use Treatment of euvolemic and hypervolemic hyponatremia in hospitalized patients

Mechanism of Action Conivaptan is an arginine vasopressin (AVP) receptor antagonist with affinity for AVP receptor subtypes V_{1A} and V_2. The antidiuretic action of AVP is mediated through activation of the V_2 receptor, which functions to regulate water and electrolyte balance at the level of the collecting ducts in the kidney. Serum levels of AVP are commonly elevated in euvolemic or hypervolemic hyponatremia, which results in the dilution of serum sodium and the relative hyponatremic state. Antagonism of the V_2 receptor by conivaptan promotes the excretion of free water (without loss of serum electrolytes) resulting in net fluid loss, increased urine output, decreased urine osmolality, and subsequent restoration of normal serum sodium levels.

Pharmacodynamics/Kinetics

Protein binding: 99%

Metabolism: Hepatic via CYP3A4 to four minimally-active metabolites

Half-life elimination: ~5 hours

Excretion: Feces (83%); urine (12%, primarily as metabolites)

Dosage I.V.: Adults: 20 mg infused over 30 minutes as a loading dose, followed by a continuous infusion of 20 mg over 24 hours (0.83 mg/hour); may increase dose to 40 mg over 24 hours (1.7 mg/hour) if serum sodium not rising sufficiently; total duration of therapy not to exceed 4 days. **Note:** If patient requires 40 mg/24 hours and using manufacturer premixed solution, may administer two consecutive 20 mg/100 mL premixed solutions over 24 hours (ie, 20 mg over 12 hours followed by 20 mg over 12 hours).

Stability

Ampul: Store ampuls in original cardboard container at 25°C (77°F); excursions permitted to 15°C to 30°C (59°F to 86°F). Protect from light. Dilute loading dose of 20 mg in 100 mL D_5W and continuous infusion dose of 20-40 mg in 250 mL D_5W. After dilution, infusion bag (final concentration of 0.08-0.2 mg/mL) is stable at room temperature for 24 hours.

Premixed solution (manufacturer premixed): Store at 25°C (77°F); brief excursions permitted up to 40°C (104°F). Protect from light and freezing. Do not remove protective overwrap until ready for use.

Administration For intravenous use only; infuse into large veins and change infusion site every 24 hours to minimize vascular irritation. Do not administer ampuls undiluted (premixed solution does not require dilution).

Monitoring Parameters Rate of serum sodium increase, blood pressure, volume status, urine output

Pregnancy Risk Factor C

◄ **Contraindications** Hypersensitivity to conivaptan or any component of the formulation; use in hypovolemic hyponatremia; concurrent use with strong CYP3A4 inhibitors (eg, ketoconazole, itraconazole, ritonavir, indinavir, and clarithromycin)

Warnings/Precautions Monitor closely for rate of serum sodium increase and neurological status; overly rapid serum sodium correction (>12 mEq/L/24 hours) can lead to permanent neurological damage. Discontinue use if rate of serum sodium increase is undesirable; may reinitiate infusion (at reduced dose) if hyponatremia persists in the absence of neurological symptoms typically associated with rapid sodium rise. Discontinue if hypovolemia or hypotension occurs. Safety and efficacy in heart failure patients have not been established. Use in small numbers of hypervolemic, hyponatremic heart failure patients led to increased adverse events. In other heart failure studies, conivaptan did not show significant improvements in outcomes over placebo. Use with caution in patients with hepatic and renal impairment. May cause injection-site reactions. Safety and efficacy in pediatric patients have not been established.

Adverse Reactions

>10%:

Cardiovascular: Orthostatic hypotension (6% to 14%)

Central nervous system: Fever (5% to 11%)

Endocrine & metabolic: Hypokalemia (10% to 22%)

Local: Injection site reactions including pain, erythema, phlebitis, swelling (63% to 73%)

1% to 10%:

Cardiovascular: Hypertension (6% to 8%), hypotension (5% to 8%), peripheral edema (3% to 8%), phlebitis (5%), atrial fibrillation (2% to 5%), ECG abnormality (up to 5%)

Central nervous system: Headache (8% to 10%), insomnia (4% to 5%), confusion (up to 5%), pain (2%)

Dermatologic: Pruritus (1% to 5%), erythema (3%)

Endocrine & metabolic: Hyponatremia (6% to 8%), hypomagnesemia (2% to 5%), hyper-/hypoglycemia (3%)

Gastrointestinal: Constipation (6% to 8%), vomiting (5% to 7%), diarrhea (up to 7%), nausea (3% to 5%), dry mouth (4%), dehydration (2%), oral candidiasis (2%)

Genitourinary: Urinary tract infection (4% to 5%)

Hematologic: Anemia (5% to 6%)

Renal: Polyuria (5% to 6%), hematuria (2%)

Respiratory: Pneumonia (2% to 5%), pharyngolaryngeal pain (1% to 5%)

Miscellaneous: Thirst (3% to 6%)

<1%, postmarketing, and/or case reports (limited to important or life-threatening): Atrial arrhythmias, sepsis

Drug Interactions

Metabolism/Transport Effects Substrate of CYP3A4 (major); **Inhibits** CYP3A4 (strong)

Avoid Concomitant Use

Avoid concomitant use of Conivaptan with any of the following: Alfuzosin; Antifungal Agents (Azole Derivatives, Systemic); Dronedarone; Eplerenone; Everolimus; Halofantrine; Nilotinib; Nisoldipine; Ranolazine; Rivaroxaban; Salmeterol; Silodosin; Tolvaptan

Increased Effect/Toxicity

Conivaptan may increase the levels/effects of: Alfuzosin; Almotriptan; Alosetron; Ciclesonide; Colchicine; CYP3A4 Substrates; Digoxin; Dronedarone; Dutasteride; Eplerenone; Everolimus; FentaNYL; Fesoterodine; Halofantrine; Ixabepilone; Maraviroc; Nilotinib; Nisoldipine; Paricalcitol; Pimecrolimus; Ranolazine; Rivaroxaban; Salmeterol; Saxagliptin; Silodosin; Sorafenib; Tadalafil; Tolvaptan

The levels/effects of Conivaptan may be increased by: Antifungal Agents (Azole Derivatives, Systemic); CYP3A4 Inhibitors (Moderate); CYP3A4 Inhibitors (Strong); Dasatinib

Decreased Effect

Conivaptan may decrease the levels/effects of: Prasugrel

The levels/effects of Conivaptan may be decreased by: CYP3A4 Inducers (Strong); Deferasirox; Herbs (CYP3A4 Inducers)

Ethanol/Nutrition/Herb Interactions Herb/Nutraceutical: St John's wort may decrease the levels/effects of conivaptan.

Dosage Forms Excipient information presented when available (limited, particularly for generics); consult specific product labeling. [DSC] = Discontinued product

Infusion, premixed in D_5, as hydrochloride:
  Vaprisol®: 20 mg (100 mL)
Injection, solution, as hydrochloride:
  Vaprisol®: 5 mg/mL (4 mL) [single-use ampul; contains propylene glycol and ethanol] [DSC]

◆ **Conivaptan Hydrochloride** *see* Conivaptan *on page 349*

◆ **Conjugated Estrogen** *see* Estrogens (Conjugated/Equine) *on page 534*

◆ **Constulose** *see* Lactulose *on page 796*

◆ **CO Pantoprazole (Can)** *see* Pantoprazole *on page 1084*

◆ **CO Paroxetine (Can)** *see* PARoxetine *on page 1089*

◆ **CO Pioglitazone (Can)** *see* Pioglitazone *on page 1132*

◆ **CO Pramipexole (Can)** *see* Pramipexole *on page 1159*

◆ **CO Pravastatin (Can)** *see* Pravastatin *on page 1162*

◆ **CO Quetiapine (Can)** *see* QUEtiapine *on page 1212*

◆ **CO Ramipril (Can)** *see* Ramipril *on page 1229*

◆ **CO Ranitidine (Can)** *see* Ranitidine *on page 1231*

◆ **Cordarone®** *see* Amiodarone *on page 86*

◆ **Coreg®** *see* Carvedilol *on page 244*

◆ **Coreg CR®** *see* Carvedilol *on page 244*

◆ **Corgard®** *see* Nadolol *on page 974*

◆ **Corlopam®** *see* Fenoldopam *on page 584*

◆ **Coronex® (Can)** *see* Isosorbide Dinitrate *on page 772*

◆ **CO Ropinirole (Can)** *see* Ropinirole *on page 1265*

◆ **Cortaid® Intensive Therapy [OTC]** *see* Hydrocortisone *on page 699*

◆ **Cortaid® Maximum Strength [OTC]** *see* Hydrocortisone *on page 699*

◆ **Cortaid® Sensitive Skin [OTC]** *see* Hydrocortisone *on page 699*

◆ **Cortamed® (Can)** *see* Hydrocortisone *on page 699*

◆ **Cortef®** *see* Hydrocortisone *on page 699*

◆ **Cortenema®** *see* Hydrocortisone *on page 699*

◆ **Corticool® [OTC]** *see* Hydrocortisone *on page 699*

◆ **Cortifoam®** *see* Hydrocortisone *on page 699*

◆ **Cortifoam™ (Can)** *see* Hydrocortisone *on page 699*

◆ **Cortisol** *see* Hydrocortisone *on page 699*

◆ **Cortizone-10® Maximum Strength [OTC]** *see* Hydrocortisone *on page 699*

◆ **Cortizone-10® Maximum Strength Cooling Relief [OTC]** *see* Hydrocortisone *on page 699*

◆ **Cortizone-10® Maximum Strength Easy Relief [OTC]** *see* Hydrocortisone *on page 699*

◆ **Cortizone-10® Maximum Strength Intensive Healing Formula [OTC]** *see* Hydrocortisone *on page 699*

◆ **Cortizone-10® Plus Maximum Strength [OTC]** *see* Hydrocortisone *on page 699*

◆ **Cortizone-10® Quick Shot [OTC] [DSC]** *see* Hydrocortisone *on page 699*

◆ **Cortrosyn®** *see* Cosyntropin *on page 352*

◆ **Corvert®** *see* Ibutilide *on page 723*

◆ **CO Simvastatin (Can)** *see* Simvastatin *on page 1293*

◆ **CO Sotalol (Can)** *see* Sotalol *on page 1321*

♦ **CO Sumatriptan (Can)** *see* SUMAtriptan *on page 1336*

Cosyntropin (koe sin TROE pin)

Medication Safety Issues
Sound-alike/look-alike issues:
Cortrosyn® may be confused with colchicine, Cotazym®
U.S. Brand Names Cortrosyn®
Canadian Brand Names Cortrosyn®
Index Terms Synacthen; Tetracosactide
Pharmacologic Category Diagnostic Agent
Generic Available Yes
Use Diagnostic test to differentiate primary adrenal from secondary (pituitary) adrenocortical insufficiency
Mechanism of Action Stimulates the adrenal cortex to secrete adrenal steroids (including hydrocortisone, cortisone), androgenic substances, and a small amount of aldosterone
Pharmacodynamics/Kinetics Time to peak, serum: I.M., IVP: ~1 hour; plasma cortisol levels rise in healthy individuals within 5 minutes
Dosage
Adrenocortical insufficiency: I.M., I.V. (over 2 minutes): Peak plasma cortisol concentrations usually occur 45-60 minutes after cosyntropin administration
Children <2 years: 0.125 mg
Children >2 years and Adults: 0.25-0.75 mg
When greater cortisol stimulation is needed, an I.V. infusion may be used:
Children >2 years and Adults: 0.25 mg administered at 0.04 mg/hour over 6 hours
Stability Powder for injection: Store at controlled temperature of 15°C to 30°C (59°F to 86°F).

I.M.: Reconstitute cosyntropin 0.25 mg with NS 1 mL.
I.V. push: Reconstitute cosyntropin 0.25 mg with NS 2-5 mL.
I.V. infusion: Mix in NS or D_5W. Stable for 12 hours at room temperature; stable for 21 days under refrigeration.
Administration Administer I.V. doses over 2 minutes
Reference Range Normal baseline cortisol; increase in serum cortisol after cosyntropin injection of >7 mcg/dL or peak response >18 mcg/dL; plasma cortisol concentrations should be measured immediately before and exactly 30 minutes after a dose
Anesthesia and Critical Care Concerns/Other Considerations
Evidence-Based Information:

Septic Shock: Annane, et al (2002) randomized 300 septic shock patients to either hydrocortisone (50 mg I.V. push every 6 hours) and fludrocortisone (50 mcg tablet daily via nasogastric tube) or matching placebos for 7 days. The mean Simplified Acute Physiology Score II (SAPS II) was 57 ± 19 in the placebo group and 60 ± 19 in the active treatment group. The Logistic Organ Dysfunction score was 9 ± 3 in the placebo group and 9 ± 3 in the active treatment group. In patients who did not appropriately respond to cosyntropin (nonresponders), there were significantly fewer deaths in the active treatment group. Vasopressor therapy was withdrawn more frequently in this subset of the active treatment group. Adverse events were similar in both groups.

In the CORTICUS trial (Sprung, 2008), 484 septic shock patients were randomized within 72 hours of onset to receive either hydrocortisone (50 mg I.V. push every 6 hours) or placebo for 5 days followed by a 6-day taper. The primary endpoint was 28 day mortality in patients who did not respond to cosyntropin. The SAPS II score in the treatment group was 49.5 ± 17.8 and 48.6 ± 16.7 in the placebo group. The Sequential Organ Failure Assessment scores were 10.6 ± 3.4 in the treatment group and 10.6 ± 3.2 in the placebo group. Different than the Annane study, in the patients who did not respond to cosyntropin, there was no mortality difference at 28 days; 39.2% (95% CI 30.5-47.9) mortality in the hydrocortisone group and 36.1 % (95% CI 26.9-45.3, P=0.69) mortality in the placebo group. A trend towards increased incidence of superinfection was noted in hydrocortisone patients. New septic shock episodes, hyperglycemia, and hypernatremia were more frequent in the hydrocortisone group. Hydrocortisone did not improve survival in this population of septic shock patients regardless of corticotropin response.

The 2008 Surviving Sepsis Campaign Guidelines suggest the following: Intravenous hydrocortisone be given only to adult septic shock patients after blood pressure is identified to be poorly responsive to fluid resuscitation and vasopressor therapy (Grade 2C); ACTH stimulation test not be used to identify the subset of adults with septic shock who should receive hydrocortisone (Grade 2B); patients with septic shock should not receive dexamethasone if hydrocortisone is available (Grade 2B); the addition of fludrocortisone if hydrocortisone is not available and the steroid that is substituted does not have significant mineralocorticoid activity (Grade 2C); doses of corticosteroids comparable to >300 mg hydrocortisone daily **not** be used in severe sepsis or septic shock for the purpose of treating septic shock (Grade 1A). They also recommend corticosteroids **not** be administered for the treatment of sepsis in the absence of shock. There is, however, no contraindication to continuing maintenance steroid therapy or to using stress dose steroids if the patient's endocrine or corticosteroid administration history warrants (Grade 1D).

The 2008 Recommendations for the diagnosis and management of corticosteroid insufficiency in critically ill adult patients recommend a diagnosis of critical illness related corticosteroid insufficiency can be made by a delta cortisol level (after 250 mcg cosyntropin) of <9 mcg/dL or a random cortisol <10 mcg/dL (Grade 2B). However, they recommend **against** the use of ACTH stimulation test to determine if septic shock or ARDS patients should receive steroid therapy (Grade 2B). They recommend to consider using hydrocortisone in septic shock patients that have responded poorly to resuscitation and vasopressors (Grade 2B).

Pregnancy Risk Factor C

Contraindications Hypersensitivity to cosyntropin or any component of the formulation

Warnings/Precautions Use with caution in patients with pre-existing allergic disease or a history of allergic reactions to corticotropin.

Adverse Reactions Frequency not defined.
Cardiovascular: Bradycardia, hypertension, peripheral edema, tachycardia
Dermatologic: Rash
Local: Whealing with redness at the injection site
Miscellaneous: Anaphylaxis, hypersensitivity reaction

Drug Interactions

Avoid Concomitant Use There are no known interactions where it is recommended to avoid concomitant use.

Increased Effect/Toxicity There are no known significant interactions involving an increase in effect.

Decreased Effect There are no known significant interactions involving a decrease in effect.

Test Interactions Decreased effect: Spironolactone, hydrocortisone, cortisone, etomidate

Dosage Forms Excipient information presented when available (limited, particularly for generics); consult specific product labeling.
Injection, powder for reconstitution: 0.25 mg
Cortrosyn®: 0.25 mg

References

Annane D, Sebille V, Charpentier C, et al, "Effect of Treatment With Low Doses of Hydrocortisone and Fludrocortisone on Mortality in Patients With Septic Shock," *JAMA*, 2002, 288(7):862-71.

Dellinger RP, Levy MM, Carlet JM, et al, "Surviving Sepsis Campaign: International Guidelines for Management of Severe Sepsis and Septic Shock: 2008," *Intensive Care Med*, 2008, 34(1): 17-60. Available at http://www.survivingsepsis.org/system/files/images/2008_20International_20SSC_20-Guidelines_1_.pdf

Marik PE, Pastores SM, Annane D, et al, "Recommendations for the Diagnosis and Management of Corticosteroid Insufficiency in Critically Ill Adult Patients: Consensus Statements From an International Task Force by the American College of Critical Care Medicine," *Crit Care Med*, 2008, 36(6):1937-49.

Sprung CL, Annane D, Keh D, et al, "Hydrocortisone Therapy for Patients With Septic Shock," *N Engl J Med*, 2008, 358(2):111-24.

◆ **CO Temazepam (Can)** *see* Temazepam *on page 1357*

- ◆ **CO Topiramate (Can)** *see* Topiramate *on page 1408*
- ◆ **Co-Trimoxazole** *see* Sulfamethoxazole and Trimethoprim *on page 1333*
- ◆ **Coumadin®** *see* Warfarin *on page 1479*
- ◆ **CO Venlafaxine XR (Can)** *see* Venlafaxine *on page 1466*
- ◆ **Covera® (Can)** *see* Verapamil *on page 1468*
- ◆ **Covera-HS®** *see* Verapamil *on page 1468*
- ◆ **Coversyl® (Can)** *see* Perindopril Erbumine *on page 1107*
- ◆ **Cozaar®** *see* Losartan *on page 857*
- ◆ **CPM** *see* Cyclophosphamide *on page 354*
- ◆ **CPZ** *see* ChlorproMAZINE *on page 298*
- ◆ **Crestor®** *see* Rosuvastatin *on page 1270*
- ◆ **Crinone®** *see* Progesterone *on page 1184*
- ◆ **Cryselle® 28** *see* Ethinyl Estradiol and Norgestrel *on page 560*
- ◆ **Crystalline Penicillin** *see* Penicillin G (Parenteral/Aqueous) *on page 1094*
- ◆ **Crystapen® (Can)** *see* Penicillin G (Parenteral/Aqueous) *on page 1094*
- ◆ **CS-747** *see* Prasugrel *on page 1160*
- ◆ **CsA** *see* CycloSPORINE *on page 357*
- ◆ **CTX** *see* Cyclophosphamide *on page 354*
- ◆ **Cubicin®** *see* DAPTOmycin *on page 372*
- ◆ **Curosurf®** *see* Poractant Alfa *on page 1146*
- ◆ **Cutivate®** *see* Fluticasone *on page 620*
- ◆ **Cutivate™ (Can)** *see* Fluticasone *on page 620*
- ◆ **CyA** *see* CycloSPORINE *on page 357*
- ◆ **Cyanokit®** *see* Hydroxocobalamin *on page 711*
- ◆ **Cyclen® (Can)** *see* Ethinyl Estradiol and Norgestimate *on page 558*
- ◆ **Cyclessa®** *see* Ethinyl Estradiol and Desogestrel *on page 544*

Cyclophosphamide (sye kloe FOS fa mide)

Medication Safety Issues
Sound-alike/look-alike issues:
Cyclophosphamide may be confused with cycloSPORINE, ifosfamide
Cytoxan® may be confused with cefoxitin, Centoxin®, Ciloxan®, cytarabine, CytoGam®, Cytosar®, Cytosar-U®, Cytotec®

High alert medication: The Institute for Safe Medication Practices (ISMP) includes this medication among its list of drugs which have a heightened risk of causing significant patient harm when used in error.

U.S. Brand Names Cytoxan® [DSC]

Canadian Brand Names Cytoxan®; Procytox®

Index Terms CPM; CTX; CYT; Neosar

Pharmacologic Category Antineoplastic Agent, Alkylating Agent

Generic Available Yes

Use
Oncology-related uses: Treatment of Hodgkin's lymphoma, non-Hodgkin's lymphoma (including Burkitt's lymphoma), chronic lymphocytic leukemia (CLL), chronic myelocytic leukemia (CML), acute myelocytic leukemia (AML), acute lymphocytic leukemia (ALL), mycosis fungoides, multiple myeloma, neuroblastoma, retinoblastoma; breast cancer; ovarian adenocarcinoma
Nononcology uses: Treatment of nephrotic syndrome in children

Unlabeled/Investigational Use
Oncology-related uses: Ewing's sarcoma, rhabdomyosarcoma, Wilms tumor, ovarian germ cell tumors, small cell lung cancer, testicular cancer, pheochromocytoma, bone marrow transplantation conditioning regimen
Nononcology uses: Severe rheumatoid disorders, Wegener's granulomatosis, myasthenia gravis, multiple sclerosis, systemic lupus erythematosus, lupus

nephritis, autoimmune hemolytic anemia, idiopathic thrombocytic purpura (ITP), and antibody-induced pure red cell aplasia

Mechanism of Action Cyclophosphamide is an alkylating agent that prevents cell division by cross-linking DNA strands and decreasing DNA synthesis. It is a cell cycle phase nonspecific agent. Cyclophosphamide also possesses potent immunosuppressive activity. Cyclophosphamide is a prodrug that must be metabolized to active metabolites in the liver.

Pharmacodynamics/Kinetics

Absorption: Oral: Well absorbed

Distribution: V_d: 0.48-0.71 L/kg; crosses placenta; crosses into CSF (not in high enough concentrations to treat meningeal leukemia)

Protein binding: 10% to 60%

Metabolism: Hepatic to active metabolites acrolein, 4-aldophosphamide, 4-hydroperoxycyclophosphamide, and nor-nitrogen mustard

Bioavailability: >75%

Half-life elimination: 3-12 hours

Time to peak, serum: Oral: ~1 hour

Excretion: Urine (<30% as unchanged drug, 85% to 90% as metabolites)

Dosage Details concerns dosing in combination regimens should also be consulted.

Children:

Nephrotic syndrome: Oral: 2-3 mg/kg/day every day for up to 12 weeks when corticosteroids are unsuccessful

SLE (unlabeled use): I.V.: 500-750 mg/m^2 every month; maximum dose: 1 g/m^2

Children and Adults:

Oral: 50-100 mg/m^2/day as continuous therapy or 400-1000 mg/m^2 in divided doses over 4-5 days as intermittent therapy

I.V.:

Single doses: 400-1800 mg/m^2 (30-50 mg/kg) per treatment course (1-5 days) which can be repeated at 2-4 week intervals

Continuous daily doses: 60-120 mg/m^2 (1-2.5 mg/kg) per day

Autologous BMT (unlabeled use): IVPB: 50 mg/kg/dose x 4 days or 60 mg/kg/dose for 2 days; total dose is usually divided over 2-4 days

JRA/vasculitis (unlabeled use): 10 mg/kg every 2 weeks

Adults: Nephrotic syndrome (unlabeled use): Oral: 2-3 mg/kg/day every day for up to 12 weeks when corticosteroids are unsuccessful

Dosing adjustment in renal impairment: The FDA-approved labeling states there is insufficient evidence to recommend dosage adjustment and therefore, does not contain renal dosing adjustment guidelines. The following guidelines have been used by some clinicians (Aronoff, 2007): Children and Adults:

Cl_{cr} <10 mL/minute: Administer 75% of normal dose

Hemodialysis effects: Moderately dialyzable (20% to 50%)

Administer 50% of dose posthemodialysis

Continuous ambulatory peritoneal dialysis (CAPD): Administer 75% of normal dose

Continuous renal replacement therapy (CRRT): Administer 100% of normal dose

Dosing adjustment in hepatic impairment: The pharmacokinetics of cyclophosphamide are not significantly altered in the presence of hepatic insufficiency. The FDA-approved labeling does not contain hepatic dosing adjustment guidelines. The following guidelines have been used by some clinicians (Floyd, 2006):

Serum bilirubin 3.1-5 mg/dL or transaminases >3 times ULN: Administer 75% of dose

Serum bilirubin >5 mg/mL: Avoid use

Stability Store intact vials of powder at room temperature of 15°C to 30°C (59°F to 86°F). Reconstitute vials with sterile water, normal saline, or 5% dextrose to a concentration of 20 mg/mL. Reconstituted solutions are stable for 24 hours at room temperature and 6 days under refrigeration at 2°C to 8°C (36°F to 46°F). Further dilutions in D_5W or NS are stable for 24 hours at room temperature and 6 days at refrigeration.

◄ **Administration**

Injection: Administer I.P., intrapleurally, IVPB, or continuous I.V. infusion; may also be administered slow IVP in doses ≤1 g.

I.V. infusions may be administered over 1-24 hours

Doses >500 mg to approximately 2 g may be administered over 20-30 minutes

To minimize bladder toxicity, increase normal fluid intake during and for 1-2 days after cyclophosphamide dose. Most adult patients will require a fluid intake of at least 2 L/day. High-dose regimens should be accompanied by vigorous hydration with or without mesna therapy.

Oral: Tablets are not scored and should not be cut or crushed. To minimize the risk of bladder irritation, do not administer tablets at bedtime.

Monitoring Parameters CBC with differential and platelet count, BUN, UA, serum electrolytes, serum creatinine

Pregnancy Risk Factor D

Contraindications Hypersensitivity to cyclophosphamide or any component of the formulation; pregnancy

Warnings/Precautions Hazardous agent - use appropriate precautions for handling and disposal. Dosage adjustment may be needed for renal or hepatic failure. Hemorrhagic cystitis may occur; increased hydration and frequent voiding is recommended. Immunosuppression may occur; monitor for infections. May cause cardiotoxicity (HF, usually with higher doses); may potentiate the cardiotoxicity of anthracyclines. May impair fertility; interferes with oogenesis and spermatogenesis. Secondary malignancies (usually delayed) have been reported

Adverse Reactions

>10%:

Dermatologic: Alopecia (40% to 60%) but hair will usually regrow although it may be a different color and/or texture. Hair loss usually begins 3-6 weeks after the start of therapy.

Endocrine & metabolic: Fertility: May cause sterility; interferes with oogenesis and spermatogenesis; may be irreversible in some patients; gonadal suppression (amenorrhea)

Gastrointestinal: Nausea and vomiting, usually beginning 6-10 hours after administration; anorexia, diarrhea, mucositis, and stomatitis are also seen

Genitourinary: Severe, potentially fatal acute hemorrhagic cystitis (7% to 40%)

Hematologic: Thrombocytopenia and anemia are less common than leukopenia

Onset: 7 days

Nadir: 10-14 days

Recovery: 21 days

1% to 10%:

Cardiovascular: Facial flushing

Central nervous system: Headache

Dermatologic: Skin rash

Renal: SIADH may occur, usually with doses >50 mg/kg (or 1 g/m^2); renal tubular necrosis, which usually resolves with discontinuation of the drug, is also reported

Respiratory: Nasal congestion occurs when I.V. doses are administered too rapidly; patients experience runny eyes, rhinorrhea, sinus congestion, and sneezing during or immediately after the infusion.

<1% (Limited to important or life-threatening): High-dose therapy may cause cardiac dysfunction manifested as CHF; cardiac necrosis or hemorrhagic myocarditis has occurred rarely, but may be fatal. Interstitial pneumonitis and pulmonary fibrosis are occasionally seen with high doses. Cyclophosphamide may also potentiate the cardiac toxicity of anthracyclines. Other adverse reactions include anaphylactic reactions, darkening of skin/fingernails, dizziness, hemorrhagic colitis, hemorrhagic ureteritis, hepatotoxicity, hyperuricemia, hypokalemia, jaundice, malaise, neutrophilic eccrine hidradenitis, radiation recall, renal tubular necrosis, secondary malignancy (eg, bladder carcinoma), SAIDH, Stevens-Johnson syndrome, toxic epidermal necrolysis, weakness.

BMT:
Cardiovascular: Heart failure, cardiac necrosis, pericardial tamponade
Endocrine & metabolic: Hyponatremia
Hematologic: Methemoglobinemia
Gastrointestinal: Severe nausea and vomiting
Miscellaneous: Hemorrhagic cystitis, secondary malignancy

Drug Interactions

Metabolism/Transport Effects Substrate of CYP2A6 (minor), 2B6 (major), 2C9 (minor), 2C19 (minor), 3A4 (major); **Inhibits** CYP3A4 (weak); **Induces** CYP2B6 (weak), 2C8 (weak), 2C9 (weak)

Avoid Concomitant Use
Avoid concomitant use of Cyclophosphamide with any of the following: Natalizumab; Vaccines (Live)

Increased Effect/Toxicity
Cyclophosphamide may increase the levels/effects of: Leflunomide; Mivacurium [Off Market]; Natalizumab; Succinylcholine; Vaccines (Live); Vitamin K Antagonists

The levels/effects of Cyclophosphamide may be increased by: Allopurinol; CYP2B6 Inhibitors (Moderate); CYP2B6 Inhibitors (Strong); Etanercept; Pentostatin; Trastuzumab

Decreased Effect
Cyclophosphamide may decrease the levels/effects of: Cardiac Glycosides; Vaccines (Inactivated); Vaccines (Live); Vitamin K Antagonists

The levels/effects of Cyclophosphamide may be decreased by: CYP2B6 Inducers (Strong); Echinacea

Ethanol/Nutrition/Herb Interactions Herb/Nutraceutical: Avoid black cohosh, dong quai in estrogen-dependent tumors.

Dietary Considerations Tablets should be administered during or after meals.

Dosage Forms Excipient information presented when available (limited, particularly for generics); consult specific product labeling. [DSC] = Discontinued product
Injection, powder for reconstitution: 500 mg, 1 g, 2 g
  Cytoxan®: 500 mg, 1 g, 2 g [DSC]
Tablet: 25 mg, 50 mg
  Cytoxan®: 25 mg, 50 mg [DSC]

◆ **Cycloset®** *see* Bromocriptine *on page 203*

◆ **Cyclosporin A** *see* CycloSPORINE *on page 357*

CycloSPORINE (SYE kloe spor een)

Medication Safety Issues
Sound-alike/look-alike issues:
  CycloSPORINE may be confused with cyclophosphamide, Cyklokapron®, cycloSERINE
  CycloSPORINE modified (Neoral®, Gengraf®) may be confused with cyclo-SPORINE non-modified (Sandimmne®)
  Gengraf® may be confused with Prograf®
  Neoral® may be confused with Neurontin®, Nizoral®
  Sandimmune® may be confused with Sandostatin®

Related Information
  Dosing Considerations for the Critically-Ill Patient With Morbid Obesity *on page 1561*

U.S. Brand Names Gengraf®; Neoral®; Restasis®; Sandimmune®

Canadian Brand Names Apo-Cyclosporine; Neoral®; Rhoxal-cyclosporine; Sandimmune® I.V.; Sandoz-Cyclosporine

Index Terms CsA; CyA; Cyclosporin A

Pharmacologic Category Immunosuppressant Agent

Generic Available Yes: Excludes ophthalmic emulsion

Use Prophylaxis of organ rejection in kidney, liver, and heart transplants, has been used with azathioprine and/or corticosteroids; severe, active rheumatoid arthritis (RA) not responsive to methotrexate alone; severe, recalcitrant plaque psoriasis

◄ in nonimmunocompromised adults unresponsive to or unable to tolerate other systemic therapy

Ophthalmic emulsion (Restasis®): Increase tear production when suppressed tear production is presumed to be due to keratoconjunctivitis sicca-associated ocular inflammation (in patients not already using topical anti-inflammatory drugs or punctal plugs)

Unlabeled/Investigational Use Short-term, high-dose cyclosporine as a modulator of multidrug resistance in cancer treatment; allogenic bone marrow transplants for prevention and treatment of graft-versus-host disease; also used in some cases of severe autoimmune disease (eg, SLE, myasthenia gravis, inflammatory bowel disease) that are resistant to corticosteroids and other therapy; focal segmental glomerulosclerosis

Mechanism of Action Inhibition of production and release of interleukin II and inhibits interleukin II-induced activation of resting T-lymphocytes.

Pharmacodynamics/Kinetics

Absorption:
  Ophthalmic emulsion: Serum concentrations not detectable.
  Oral:
    Cyclosporine (non-modified): Erratic and incomplete; dependent on presence of food, bile acids, and GI motility; larger oral doses are needed in pediatrics due to shorter bowel length and limited intestinal absorption
    Cyclosporine (modified): Erratic and incomplete; increased absorption, up to 30% when compared to cyclosporine (non-modified); less dependent on food, bile acids, or GI motility when compared to cyclosporine (non-modified)

Distribution: Widely in tissues and body fluids including the liver, pancreas, and lungs; crosses placenta; enters breast milk
  V_{dss}: 4-6 L/kg in renal, liver, and marrow transplant recipients (slightly lower values in cardiac transplant patients; children <10 years have higher values)

Protein binding: 90% to 98% to lipoproteins

Metabolism: Extensively hepatic via CYP3A4; forms at least 25 metabolites; extensive first-pass effect following oral administration

Bioavailability: Oral:
  Cyclosporine (non-modified): Dependent on patient population and transplant type (<10% in adult liver transplant patients and as high as 89% in renal transplant patients); bioavailability of Sandimmune® capsules and oral solution are equivalent; bioavailability of oral solution is ~30% of the I.V. solution
    Children: 28% (range: 17% to 42%); gut dysfunction common in BMT patients and oral bioavailability is further reduced
  Cyclosporine (modified): Bioavailability of Neoral® capsules and oral solution are equivalent:
    Children: 43% (range: 30% to 68%)
    Adults: 23% greater than with cyclosporine (non-modified) in renal transplant patients; 50% greater in liver transplant patients

Half-life elimination: Oral: May be prolonged in patients with hepatic impairment and shorter in pediatric patients due to the higher metabolism rate
  Cyclosporine (non-modified): Biphasic: Alpha: 1.4 hours; Terminal: 19 hours (range: 10-27 hours)
  Cyclosporine (modified): Biphasic: Terminal: 8.4 hours (range: 5-18 hours)

Time to peak, serum: Oral:
  Cyclosporine (non-modified): 2-6 hours; some patients have a second peak at 5-6 hours
  Cyclosporine (modified): Renal transplant: 1.5-2 hours

Excretion: Primarily feces; urine (6%, 0.1% as unchanged drug and metabolites)

Dosage Neoral®/Genraf® and Sandimmune® are not bioequivalent and cannot be used interchangeably.

Children: Refer to adult dosing; children may require, and are able to tolerate, larger doses than adults.

Adults:
  Newly-transplanted patients: Adjunct therapy with corticosteroids is recommended. Initial dose should be given 4-12 hours prior to transplant or may be given postoperatively; adjust initial dose to achieve desired plasma concentration

Oral: Dose is dependent upon type of transplant and formulation:
Cyclosporine (modified):
Renal: 9 ± 3 mg/kg/day, divided twice daily
Liver: 8 ± 4 mg/kg/day, divided twice daily
Heart: 7 ± 3 mg/kg/day, divided twice daily
Cyclosporine (non-modified): Initial dose: 15 mg/kg/day as a single dose (range 14-18 mg/kg); lower doses of 10-14 mg/kg/day have been used for renal transplants. Continue initial dose daily for 1-2 weeks; taper by 5% per week to a maintenance dose of 5-10 mg/kg/day; some renal transplant patients may be dosed as low as 3 mg/kg/day

Note: When using the non-modified formulation, cyclosporine levels may increase in liver transplant patients when the T-tube is closed; dose may need decreased

I.V.: Cyclosporine (non-modified): Manufacturer's labeling: Initial dose: 5-6 mg/kg/day as a single dose ($1/3$ the oral dose), infused over 2-6 hours; use should be limited to patients unable to take capsules or oral solution; patients should be switched to an oral dosage form as soon as possible

Note: Many transplant centers administer cyclosporine as "divided dose" infusions (in 2-3 doses/day) or as a continuous (24-hour) infusion; dosages range from 3-7.5 mg/kg/day. Specific institutional protocols should be consulted.

Conversion to cyclosporine (modified) from cyclosporine (non-modified): Start with daily dose previously used and adjust to obtain preconversion cyclosporine trough concentration. Plasma concentrations should be monitored every 4-7 days and dose adjusted as necessary, until desired trough level is obtained. When transferring patients with previously poor absorption of cyclosporine (non-modified), monitor trough levels at least twice weekly (especially if initial dose exceeds 10 mg/kg/day); high plasma levels are likely to occur.

Rheumatoid arthritis: Oral: Cyclosporine (modified): Initial dose: 2.5 mg/kg/day, divided twice daily; salicylates, NSAIDs, and oral glucocorticoids may be continued (refer to Drug Interactions); dose may be increased by 0.5-0.75 mg/kg/day if insufficient response is seen after 8 weeks of treatment; additional dosage increases may be made again at 12 weeks (maximum dose: 4 mg/kg/day). Discontinue if no benefit is seen by 16 weeks of therapy.

Note: Increase the frequency of blood pressure monitoring after each alteration in dosage of cyclosporine. Cyclosporine dosage should be decreased by 25% to 50% in patients with no history of hypertension who develop sustained hypertension during therapy and, if hypertension persists, treatment with cyclosporine should be discontinued.

Psoriasis: Oral: Cyclosporine (modified): Initial dose: 2.5 mg/kg/day, divided twice daily; dose may be increased by 0.5 mg/kg/day if insufficient response is seen after 4 weeks of treatment. Additional dosage increases may be made every 2 weeks if needed (maximum dose: 4 mg/kg/day). Discontinue if no benefit is seen by 6 weeks of therapy. Once patients are adequately controlled, the dose should be decreased to the lowest effective dose. Doses lower than 2.5 mg/kg/day may be effective. Treatment longer than 1 year is not recommended.

Note: Increase the frequency of blood pressure monitoring after each alteration in dosage of cyclosporine. Cyclosporine dosage should be decreased by 25% to 50% in patients with no history of hypertension who develop sustained hypertension during therapy and, if hypertension persists, treatment with cyclosporine should be discontinued.

Focal segmental glomerulosclerosis (unlabeled use): Initial: 3 mg/kg/day divided every 12 hours

Autoimmune diseases (unlabeled use): 1-3 mg/kg/day

Keratoconjunctivitis sicca: Ophthalmic (Restasis®): Children ≥16 years and Adults: Instill 1 drop in each eye every 12 hours

Dosage adjustment in renal impairment: For severe psoriasis:
Serum creatinine levels ≥25% above pretreatment levels: Take another sample within 2 weeks; if the level remains ≥25% above pretreatment levels, decrease dosage of cyclosporine (modified) by 25% to 50%. If two dosage adjustments do not reverse the increase in serum creatinine levels, treatment should be discontinued.

◄ **Serum creatinine levels ≥50% above pretreatment levels:** Decrease cyclosporine dosage by 25% to 50%. If two dosage adjustments do not reverse the increase in serum creatinine levels, treatment should be discontinued.

Hemodialysis: Supplemental dose is not necessary.

Peritoneal dialysis: Supplemental dose is not necessary.

Dosage adjustment in hepatic impairment: Probably necessary; monitor levels closely

Stability

Capsule: Store at controlled room temperature.

Injection: Store at controlled room temperature; do not refrigerate. Ampuls should be protected from light. Stability of injection of parenteral admixture at room temperature (25°C) is 6 hours in PVC; 24 hours in Excel®, PAB® containers, or glass.

Sandimmune® injection: Injection should be further diluted [1 mL (50 mg) of concentrate in 20-100 mL of D_5W or NS] for administration by intravenous infusion.

Ophthalmic emulsion: Store at 15°C to 25°C (59°F to 77°F). Vials are single-use; discard immediately following administration.

Oral solution: Store at controlled room temperature; do not refrigerate. Use within 2 months after opening; should be mixed in glass containers.

Neoral® oral solution: Orange juice, apple juice; avoid changing diluents frequently; mix thoroughly and drink at once.

Sandimmune® oral solution: Milk, chocolate milk, orange juice; avoid changing diluents frequently; mix thoroughly and drink at once.

Administration

Oral solution: Do not administer liquid from plastic or styrofoam cup. May dilute Neoral® oral solution with orange juice or apple juice. May dilute Sandimmune® oral solution with milk, chocolate milk, or orange juice. Avoid changing diluents frequently. Mix thoroughly and drink at once. Use syringe provided to measure dose. Mix in a glass container and rinse container with more diluent to ensure total dose is taken. Do not rinse syringe before or after use (may cause dose variation).

I.V.: The manufacturer recommends that following dilution, intravenous admixture be administered over 2-6 hours. However, many transplant centers administer as divided doses (2-3 doses/day) or as a 24-hour continuous infusion. Discard solution after 24 hours. Anaphylaxis has been reported with I.V. use; reserve for patients who cannot take oral form. Patients should be under continuous observation for at least the first 30 minutes of the infusion, and should be monitored frequently thereafter. Maintain patent airway; other supportive measures and agents for treating anaphylaxis should be present when I.V. drug is given.

Ophthalmic emulsion: Prior to use, invert vial several times to obtain a uniform emulsion. Remove contact lenses prior to instillation of drops; may be reinserted 15 minutes after administration. May be used with artificial tears; allow 15 minute interval between products.

Monitoring Parameters Monitor blood pressure and serum creatinine after any cyclosporine dosage changes or addition, modification, or deletion of other medications. Monitor plasma concentrations periodically.

Transplant patients: Cyclosporine trough levels, serum electrolytes, renal function, hepatic function, blood pressure, lipid profile

Psoriasis therapy: Baseline blood pressure, serum creatinine (2 levels each), BUN, CBC, serum magnesium, potassium, uric acid, lipid profile. Biweekly monitoring of blood pressure, complete blood count, and levels of BUN, uric acid, potassium, lipids, and magnesium during the first 3 months of treatment for psoriasis. Monthly monitoring is recommended after this initial period. Also evaluate any atypical skin lesions prior to therapy. Increase the frequency of blood pressure monitoring after each alteration in dosage of cyclosporine. Cyclosporine dosage should be decreased by 25% to 50% in patients with no history of hypertension who develop sustained hypertension during therapy and, if hypertension persists, treatment with cyclosporine should be discontinued.

Rheumatoid arthritis: Baseline blood pressure, and serum creatinine (2 levels each); serum creatinine every 2 weeks for first 3 months, then monthly if patient is stable. Increase the frequency of blood pressure monitoring after each alteration in dosage of cyclosporine. Cyclosporine dosage should be decreased by 25% to 50% in patients with no history of hypertension who develop sustained hypertension during therapy and, if hypertension persists, treatment with cyclosporine should be discontinued.

Reference Range Reference ranges are method dependent and specimen dependent; use the same analytical method consistently

Method-dependent and specimen-dependent: Trough levels should be obtained:

Oral: 12-18 hours after dose (chronic usage)

I.V.: 12 hours after dose **or** immediately prior to next dose

Therapeutic range: Not absolutely defined, dependent on organ transplanted, time after transplant, organ function and CsA toxicity:

General range of 100-400 ng/mL

Toxic level: Not well defined, nephrotoxicity may occur at any level

Pregnancy Risk Factor C

Contraindications Hypersensitivity to cyclosporine or any component of the formulation. Rheumatoid arthritis and psoriasis: Abnormal renal function, uncontrolled hypertension, malignancies. Concomitant treatment with PUVA or UVB therapy, methotrexate, other immunosuppressive agents, coal tar, or radiation therapy are also contraindications for use in patients with psoriasis. Ophthalmic emulsion is contraindicated in patients with active ocular infections.

Warnings/Precautions [U.S. Boxed Warning]: Renal impairment, including structural kidney damage has occurred (when used at high doses); monitor renal function closely. Use caution with other potentially nephrotoxic drugs (eg, acyclovir, aminoglycoside antibiotics, amphotericin B, ciprofloxacin). **[U.S. Boxed Warning]: Increased risk of lymphomas and other malignancies, particularly those of the skin;** risk is related to intensity/duration of therapy and the use of >1 immunosuppressive agent; all patients should avoid excessive sun/UV light exposure. **[U.S. Boxed Warning]: Increased risk of infection; fatal infections have been reported. [U.S. Boxed Warning]: May cause hypertension.** Use caution when changing dosage forms. **[U.S. Boxed Warning]: Cyclosporine (modified) has increased bioavailability as compared to cyclosporine (nonmodified) and cannot be used interchangeably without close monitoring.** Monitor cyclosporine concentrations closely following the addition, modification, or deletion of other medications; live, attenuated vaccines may be less effective; use should be avoided. Increased hepatic enzymes and bilirubin have occurred (when used at high doses); improvement usually seen with dosage reduction.

Transplant patients: To be used initially with corticosteroids. May cause significant hyperkalemia and hyperuricemia, seizures (particularly if used with high dose corticosteroids), and encephalopathy. Make dose adjustments based on cyclosporine blood concentrations. **[U.S. Boxed Warning]: Adjustment of dose should only be made under the direct supervision of an experienced physician.** Anaphylaxis has been reported with I.V. use; reserve for patients who cannot take oral form. **[U.S. Boxed Warning]: Risk of skin cancer may be increased in transplant patients.**

Psoriasis: Patients should avoid excessive sun exposure; safety and efficacy in children <18 years of age have not been established. **[U.S. Boxed Warning]: Risk of skin cancer may be increased with a history of PUVA and possibly methotrexate or other immunosuppressants, UVB, coal tar, or radiation.**

Rheumatoid arthritis: Safety and efficacy for use in juvenile rheumatoid arthritis have not been established. If receiving other immunosuppressive agents, radiation or UV therapy, concurrent use of cyclosporine is not recommended.

Ophthalmic emulsion: Safety and efficacy have not been established in patients <16 years of age.

Products may contain corn oil, ethanol, or propylene glycol; injection also contains Cremophor® EL (polyoxyethylated castor oil), which has been associated with rare anaphylactic reactions.

◄ **Adverse Reactions** Adverse reactions reported with systemic use, including rheumatoid arthritis, psoriasis, and transplantation (kidney, liver, and heart). Percentages noted include the highest frequency regardless of indication/dosage. Frequencies may vary for specific conditions or formulation.

>10%:
  Cardiovascular: Hypertension (8% to 53%), edema (5% to 14%)
  Central nervous system: Headache (2% to 25%)
  Dermatologic: Hirsutism (21% to 45%), hypertrichosis (5% to 19%)
  Endocrine & metabolic: Triglycerides increased (15%), female reproductive disorder (9% to 11%)
  Gastrointestinal: Nausea (23%), diarrhea (3% to 13%), gum hyperplasia (2% to 16%), abdominal discomfort (<1% to 15%), dyspepsia (2% to 12%)
  Neuromuscular & skeletal: Tremor (7% to 55%), paresthesia (1% to 11%), leg cramps/muscle contractions (2% to 12%)
  Renal: Renal dysfunction/nephropathy (10% to 38%), creatinine increased (16% to ≥50%)
  Respiratory: Upper respiratory infection (1% to 14%)
  Miscellaneous: Infection (3% to 25%)
1% to 10%:
  Cardiovascular: Chest pain (4% to 6%), arrhythmia (2% to 5%), abnormal heart sounds, cardiac failure, flushes (<1% to 5%), MI, peripheral ischemia
  Central nervous system: Dizziness (8%), pain (6%), convulsions (1% to 5%), insomnia (4%), psychiatric events (4% to 5%), pain (3% to 4%), depression (1% to 6%), migraine (2% to 3%), anxiety, confusion, fever, hypoesthesia, emotional lability, impaired concentration, lethargy, malaise, nervousness, paranoia, somnolence, vertigo
  Dermatologic: Purpura (3% to 4%), acne (1% to 6%), brittle fingernails, hair breaking, abnormal pigmentation, angioedema, cellulitis, dermatitis, dry skin, eczema, folliculitis, keratosis, pruritus, rash, skin disorder, skin malignancies, urticaria
  Endocrine & metabolic: Gynecomastia (<1% to 4%), menstrual disorder (1% to 3%), breast fibroadenosis, breast pain, hyper-/hypoglycemia, diabetes mellitus, goiter, hot flashes, hyperkalemia, hyperuricemia, libido increased/decreased
  Gastrointestinal: Vomiting (2% to 10%), flatulence (5%), gingivitis (up to 4%), cramps (up to 4%), anorexia, constipation, dry mouth, dysphagia, enanthema, eructation, esophagitis, gastric ulcer, gastritis, gastroenteritis, gastrointestinal bleeding (upper), gingival bleeding, glossitis, mouth sores, peptic ulcer, pancreatitis, swallowing difficulty, salivary gland enlargement, taste perversion, tongue disorder, tooth disorder, weight loss/gain
  Genitourinary: Leukorrhea (1%), abnormal urine, micturition increased, micturition urgency, nocturia, polyuria, pyelonephritis, urinary incontinence, uterine hemorrhage
  Hematologic: Leukopenia (<1% to 6%), anemia, bleeding disorder, clotting disorder, platelet disorder, red blood cell disorder, thrombocytopenia
  Hepatic: Hepatotoxicity (<1% to 7%), hyperbilirubinemia
  Neuromuscular & skeletal: Arthralgia (1% to 6%), bone fracture, joint dislocation, joint pain, muscle pain, myalgia, neuropathy, stiffness, synovial cyst, tendon disorder, tingling, weakness
  Ocular: Abnormal vision, cataract, conjunctivitis, eye pain, visual disturbance
  Otic: Deafness, hearing loss, tinnitus, vestibular disorder
  Renal: BUN increased, hematuria, renal abscess
  Respiratory: Sinusitis (<1% to 7%), bronchospasm (up to 5%), cough (3% to 5%), pharyngitis (3% to 5%), dyspnea (1% to 5%), rhinitis (up to 5%), abnormal chest sounds, epistaxis, respiratory infection, pneumonia (up to 1%)
  Miscellaneous: Flu-like syndrome (8% to 10%), lymphoma (<1% to 6% reported in transplant), abscess, allergic reactions, bacterial infection, carcinoma, diaphoresis increased, fungal infection, herpes simplex, herpes zoster, hiccups, lymphadenopathy, moniliasis, night sweats, tonsillitis, viral infection
Postmarketing and/or case reports (any indication): Anaphylaxis/anaphylactoid reaction (possibly associated with Cremophor® EL vehicle in injection formulation), benign intracranial hypertension, cholesterol increased, death (due to renal deterioration), encephalopathy, gout, hyperbilirubinemia, hyperkalemia,

hypomagnesemia (mild), impaired consciousness, neurotoxicity, papilloedema, pulmonary edema (noncardiogenic), uric acid increased

Ophthalmic emulsion (Restasis®):

>10%: Ocular: Burning (17%)

1% to 10%: Ocular: Hyperemia (conjunctival 5%), eye pain, pruritus, stinging

Drug Interactions

Metabolism/Transport Effects Substrate of CYP3A4 (major); **Inhibits** CYP2C9 (weak), 3A4 (moderate)

Avoid Concomitant Use

Avoid concomitant use of CycloSPORINE with any of the following: Aliskiren; Bosentan; Dabigatran Etexilate; Dronedarone; Everolimus; Natalizumab; Pitavastatin; Silodosin; Sitaxsentan; Tacrolimus; Tolvaptan; Topotecan; Vaccines (Live)

Increased Effect/Toxicity

CycloSPORINE may increase the levels/effects of: Aliskiren; Ambrisentan; Bosentan; Calcium Channel Blockers (Dihydropyridine); Calcium Channel Blockers (Nondihydropyridine); Cardiac Glycosides; Caspofungin; Colchicine; Corticosteroids (Systemic); CYP3A4 Substrates; Dabigatran Etexilate; DOXOrubicin; Dronedarone; Eplerenone; Etoposide; Etoposide Phosphate; Everolimus; Ezetimibe; FentaNYL; Fibric Acid Derivatives; Halofantrine; HMG-CoA Reductase Inhibitors; Leflunomide; Methotrexate; Minoxidil; Natalizumab; P-Glycoprotein Substrates; Pimecrolimus; Pitavastatin; Protease Inhibitors; Ranolazine; Repaglinide; Rivaroxaban; Salmeterol; Saxagliptin; Silodosin; Sirolimus; Sitaxsentan; Tacrolimus; Tolvaptan; Topotecan; Vaccines (Live)

The levels/effects of CycloSPORINE may be increased by: ACE Inhibitors; Aminoglycosides; Amiodarone; Amphotericin B; Androgens; Antifungal Agents (Azole Derivatives, Systemic); Bromocriptine; Calcium Channel Blockers (Nondihydropyridine); Carvedilol; Corticosteroids (Systemic); CYP3A4 Inhibitors (Moderate); CYP3A4 Inhibitors (Strong); Dasatinib; Ezetimibe; Fluconazole; Grapefruit Juice; Imatinib; Macrolide Antibiotics; Melphalan; Methotrexate; Metoclopramide; MetroNIDAZOLE; Nonsteroidal Anti-Inflammatory Agents; Norfloxacin; Omeprazole; P-Glycoprotein Inhibitors; Protease Inhibitors; Quinupristin; Sirolimus; Sulfonamide Derivatives; Sulfonylureas; Tacrolimus; Temsirolimus; Trastuzumab

Decreased Effect

CycloSPORINE may decrease the levels/effects of: Mycophenolate; Vaccines (Inactivated); Vaccines (Live)

The levels/effects of CycloSPORINE may be decreased by: Antacids; Barbiturates; Bosentan; CarBAMazepine; CYP3A4 Inducers (Strong); Deferasirox; Echinacea; Fibric Acid Derivatives; Griseofulvin; Nafcillin; P-Glycoprotein Inducers; Phenytoin; Probucol; Pyrazinamide; Rifamycin Derivatives; Somatostatin Analogs; St Johns Wort; Sulfinpyrazone [Off Market]; Sulfonamide Derivatives; Terbinafine

Ethanol/Nutrition/Herb Interactions

Food: Grapefruit juice increases cyclosporine serum concentrations.

Herb/Nutraceutical: Avoid St John's wort; as an enzyme inducer, it may increase the metabolism of and decrease plasma levels of cyclosporine; organ rejection and graft loss have been reported. Avoid cat's claw, echinacea (have immunostimulant properties).

Test Interactions Specific whole blood, HPLC assay for cyclosporine may be falsely elevated if sample is drawn from the same line through which dose was administered (even if flush has been administered and/or dose was given hours before).

Dietary Considerations Administer this medication consistently with relation to time of day and meals. Avoid grapefruit juice with oral cyclosporine use.

Dosage Forms Excipient information presented when available (limited, particularly for generics); consult specific product labeling.

Capsule [modified]:

Gengraf®: 25 mg [contains alcohol 12.8%]; 100 mg [contains alcohol 12.8%]

Capsule [non-modified]: 25 mg, 100 mg

◄ Capsule, soft gel [modified]: 25 mg, 50 mg, 100 mg
  Neoral®: 25 mg [contains alcohol 11.9% and corn oil]; 100 mg [contains alcohol 11.9% and corn oil]
Capsule, soft gel [non-modified]:
  Sandimmune®: 25 mg [contains alcohol 12.7% and corn oil]; 100 mg [contains alcohol 12.7% and corn oil]
Emulsion, ophthalmic [preservative free]:
  Restasis®: 0.05% (0.4 mL) [contains 30 single-use vials/box]
Injection, solution [non-modified]: 50 mg/mL (5 mL)
  Sandimmune®: 50 mg/mL (5 mL) [contains Cremophor® EL (polyoxyethylated castor oil) and alcohol 32.9%]
Solution, oral [modified]: 100 mg/mL (50 mL)
  Gengraf®: 100 mg/mL (50 mL) [contains propylene glycol]
  Neoral®: 100 mg/mL (50 mL) [contains alcohol 11.9%, corn oil, and propylene glycol]
Solution, oral [non-modified]: 100 mg/mL (50 mL)
  Sandimmune®: 100 mg/mL (50 mL) [contains alcohol 12.5%]

- **Cymbalta®** *see* DULoxetine *on page 469*
- **CYT** *see* Cyclophosphamide *on page 354*
- **Cytomel®** *see* Liothyronine *on page 846*
- **Cytotec®** *see* Misoprostol *on page 945*
- **Cytovene®** *see* Ganciclovir *on page 654*
- **Cytoxan® [DSC]** *see* Cyclophosphamide *on page 354*
- **Cytoxan® (Can)** *see* Cyclophosphamide *on page 354*
- **D$_5$W** *see* Dextrose *on page 406*
- **D$_{10}$W** *see* Dextrose *on page 406*
- **D$_{25}$W** *see* Dextrose *on page 406*
- **D$_{30}$W** *see* Dextrose *on page 406*
- **D$_{40}$W** *see* Dextrose *on page 406*
- **D$_{50}$W** *see* Dextrose *on page 406*
- **D$_{60}$W** *see* Dextrose *on page 406*
- **D$_{70}$W** *see* Dextrose *on page 406*

Daclizumab (dac KLYE zue mab)

U.S. Brand Names Zenapax®
Canadian Brand Names Zenapax®
Pharmacologic Category Immunosuppressant Agent
Generic Available No
Use Part of an immunosuppressive regimen (including cyclosporine and corticosteroids) for the prophylaxis of acute organ rejection in patients receiving renal transplant
Unlabeled/Investigational Use Graft-versus-host disease; prevention of organ rejection after heart transplant
Mechanism of Action Daclizumab is a chimeric (90% human, 10% murine) monoclonal IgG antibody produced by recombinant DNA technology. Daclizumab inhibits immune reactions by binding and blocking the alpha-chain of the interleukin-2 receptor (CD25) located on the surface of activated lymphocytes.
Pharmacodynamics/Kinetics
Distribution: V_d:
  Adults: Central compartment: 0.031 L/kg; Peripheral compartment: 0.043 L/kg
  Children: Central compartment: 0.067 L/kg; Peripheral compartment: 0.047 L/kg
Half-life elimination (estimated): Adults: Terminal: 20 days; Children: 13 days
Dosage Daclizumab is used adjunctively with other immunosuppressants (eg, cyclosporine, corticosteroids, mycophenolate mofetil, and azathioprine): I.V.:
Children: Use same weight-based dose as adults
Adults:
  Immunoprophylaxis against acute renal allograft rejection: 1 mg/kg infused over 15 minutes within 24 hours before transplantation (day 0), then every 14 days for 4 additional doses

Treatment of graft-versus-host disease (unlabeled use, limited data): 0.5-1.5 mg/kg, repeat same dosage for transient response. Repeat doses have been administered 11-48 days following the initial dose.

Prevention of organ rejection after heart transplant (unlabeled use): 1 mg/kg up to a maximum of 100 mg; administer within 12 hours after heart transplant and on days 8, 22, 36, and 50 post-transplant

Dosage adjustment in renal impairment: No adjustment needed.

Dosage adjustment in hepatic impairment: No data available for patients with severe impairment.

Stability Refrigerate vials at 2°C to 8°C (36°F to 46°F). Do not shake or freeze; protect undiluted solution against direct sunlight. Dose should be further diluted in 50 mL 0.9% sodium chloride solution. When mixing, gently invert bag to avoid foaming; do not shake. Do not use if solution is discolored. Diluted solution is stable for 24 hours at 4°C or for 4 hours at room temperature. Do not mix with other medications or infuse other medications through same I.V. line.

Administration For I.V. administration following dilution. Daclizumab solution should be administered within 4 hours of preparation if stored at room temperature; infuse over a 15-minute period via a peripheral or central vein.

Pregnancy Risk Factor C

Contraindications Hypersensitivity to daclizumab or any component of the formulation

Warnings/Precautions Patients on immunosuppressive therapy are at increased risk for infectious complications and secondary malignancies. Long-term effects of daclizumab on immune function are unknown. Severe hypersensitivity reactions have been rarely reported; anaphylaxis has been observed on initial exposure and following re-exposure; medications for the management of severe allergic reaction should be available for immediate use. Anti-idiotype antibodies have been measured in patients who have received daclizumab (adults 14%; children 34%); detection of antibodies may be influenced by multiple factors and may therefore be misleading.

In cardiac transplant patients, the combined use of daclizumab, cyclosporine, mycophenolate mofetil, and corticosteroids has been associated with an increased mortality. Higher mortality may be associated with the use of antilymphocyte globulin and a higher incidence of severe infections. **[U.S. Boxed Warning]: Should be administered under the supervision of a physician experienced in immunosuppressive therapy.**

Adverse Reactions Although reported adverse events are frequent, when daclizumab is compared with placebo the incidence of adverse effects is similar between the two groups. Many of the adverse effects reported during clinical trial use of daclizumab may be related to the patient population, transplant procedure, and concurrent transplant medications. Diarrhea, fever, postoperative pain, pruritus, respiratory tract infection, urinary tract infection, and vomiting occurred more often in children than adults.

≥5%:
  Cardiovascular: Chest pain, edema, hyper-/hypotension, tachycardia, thrombosis
  Central nervous system: Dizziness, fatigue, fever, headache, insomnia, pain, post-traumatic pain, tremor
  Dermatologic: Acne, cellulitis, wound healing impaired
  Gastrointestinal: Abdominal distention, abdominal pain, constipation, diarrhea, dyspepsia, epigastric pain, nausea, pyrosis, vomiting
  Genitourinary: Dysuria
  Hematologic: Bleeding
  Neuromuscular & skeletal: Back pain, musculoskeletal pain
  Renal: Oliguria, renal tubular necrosis
  Respiratory: Cough, dyspnea, pulmonary edema
  Miscellaneous: Lymphocele, wound infection
≥2% to <5%:
  Central nervous system: Anxiety, depression, shivering
  Dermatologic: Hirsutism, pruritus, rash
  Endocrine & metabolic: Dehydration, diabetes mellitus, fluid overload
  Gastrointestinal: Flatulence, gastritis, hemorrhoids
  Genitourinary: Urinary retention, urinary tract bleeding

Local: Application site reaction

Neuromuscular & skeletal: Arthralgia, leg cramps, myalgia, weakness

Ocular: Vision blurred

Renal: Hydronephrosis, renal damage, renal insufficiency

Respiratory: Atelectasis, congestion, hypoxia, pharyngitis, pleural effusion, rales, rhinitis

Miscellaneous: Night sweats, prickly sensation, diaphoresis

<1% (Limited to important or life-threatening): Severe hypersensitivity reactions (rare): Anaphylaxis, bronchospasm, cardiac arrest, cytokine release syndrome, hypotension, laryngeal edema, pulmonary edema, pruritus, urticaria

Drug Interactions

Avoid Concomitant Use

Avoid concomitant use of Daclizumab with any of the following: Natalizumab; Vaccines (Live)

Increased Effect/Toxicity

Daclizumab may increase the levels/effects of: Leflunomide; Natalizumab; Vaccines (Live)

The levels/effects of Daclizumab may be increased by: Trastuzumab

Decreased Effect

Daclizumab may decrease the levels/effects of: Vaccines (Inactivated); Vaccines (Live)

The levels/effects of Daclizumab may be decreased by: Echinacea

Dosage Forms Excipient information presented when available (limited, particularly for generics); consult specific product labeling.

Injection, solution [concentrate; preservative free]:

Zenapax®: 5 mg/mL (5 mL) [contains polysorbate 80]

References

Hershberger RE, Starling RC, Eisen HJ, et al, "Daclizumab to Prevent Rejection After Cardiac Transplantation," *N Engl J Med*, 2005, 352(26):2705-13.

Vincenti F, Kirkman R, Light S, et al, "Interleukin-2 Receptor Blockade With Daclizumab to Prevent Acute Rejection in Renal Transplantation. Daclizumab Triple Therapy Study Group," *N Engl J Med*, 1998, 338(3):161-5.

◆ **Dalacin® C (Can)** *see* Clindamycin *on page 324*

◆ **Dalacin® T (Can)** *see* Clindamycin *on page 324*

◆ **Dalacin® Vaginal (Can)** *see* Clindamycin *on page 324*

◆ **Dalfopristin and Quinupristin** *see* Quinupristin and Dalfopristin *on page 1219*

◆ **Dalmane® [DSC]** *see* Flurazepam *on page 618*

◆ **Dalmane® (Can)** *see* Flurazepam *on page 618*

Dalteparin (dal TE pa rin)

Medication Safety Issues

High alert medication: The Institute for Safe Medication Practices (ISMP) includes this medication among its list of drugs which have a heightened risk of causing significant patient harm when used in error.

2009 National Patient Safety Goals: The Joint Commission on Accreditation of Healthcare Organizations requires healthcare organizations that provide anticoagulant therapy to have a process in place to reduce the risk of anticoagulant-associated patient harm. Patients receiving anticoagulants should receive individualized care through a defined process that includes standardized ordering, dispensing, administration, monitoring and education. This does not apply to routine short-term use of anticoagulants for prevention of venous thromboembolism when the expectation is that the patient's laboratory values will remain within or close to normal values (NPSG.03.05.01).

Related Information

Continuous Renal Replacement Therapy *on page 1557*

Regional Anesthesia in Patients Receiving Anticoagulant and Antiplatelet Therapy *on page 1642*

U.S. Brand Names Fragmin®

Canadian Brand Names Fragmin®

Index Terms Dalteparin Sodium; NSC-714371

Pharmacologic Category Low Molecular Weight Heparin

Generic Available No

Use Prevention of deep vein thrombosis which may lead to pulmonary embolism, in patients requiring abdominal surgery who are at risk for thromboembolism complications (eg, patients >40 years of age, obesity, patients with malignancy, history of deep vein thrombosis or pulmonary embolism, and surgical procedures requiring general anesthesia and lasting >30 minutes); prevention of DVT in patients undergoing hip-replacement surgery; patients immobile during an acute illness; acute treatment of unstable angina or non-Q-wave myocardial infarction; prevention of ischemic complications in patients on concurrent aspirin therapy; in patients with cancer, extended treatment (6 months) of acute symptomatic venous thromboembolism (DVT and/or PE) to reduce the recurrence of venous thromboembolism

Unlabeled/Investigational Use Active treatment of deep vein thrombosis (noncancer patients)

Mechanism of Action Low molecular weight heparin analog with a molecular weight of 4000-6000 daltons; the commercial product contains 3% to 15% heparin with a molecular weight <3000 daltons, 65% to 78% with a molecular weight of 3000-8000 daltons and 14% to 26% with a molecular weight >8000 daltons; while dalteparin has been shown to inhibit both factor Xa and factor IIa (thrombin), the antithrombotic effect of dalteparin is characterized by a higher ratio of antifactor Xa to antifactor IIa activity (ratio = 4)

Pharmacodynamics/Kinetics

Onset of action: 1-2 hours

Duration: >12 hours

Distribution: V_d: 40-60 mL/kg

Bioavailability: SubQ: 81% to 93%

Half-life elimination (route dependent): 2-5 hours

Time to peak, serum: 4 hours

Dosage Adults: SubQ:

Abdominal surgery:

Low-to-moderate DVT risk: 2500 int. units 1-2 hours prior to surgery, then once daily for 5-10 days postoperatively

High DVT risk: 5000 int. units the evening prior to surgery and then once daily for 5-10 days postoperatively. Alternatively in patients with malignancy: 2500 int. units 1-2 hours prior to surgery, 2500 int. units 12 hours later, then 5000 int. units once daily for 5-10 days postoperatively.

Patients undergoing total hip surgery: **Note:** Three treatment options are currently available. Dose is given for 5-10 days, although up to 14 days of treatment have been tolerated in clinical trials:

Postoperative start:

Initial: 2500 int. units 4-8 hours* after surgery

Maintenance: 5000 int. units once daily; start at least 6 hours after postsurgical dose

Preoperative (starting day of surgery):

Initial: 2500 int. units within 2 hours before surgery

Adjustment: 2500 int. units 4-8 hours* after surgery

Maintenance: 5000 int. units once daily; start at least 6 hours after postsurgical dose

Preoperative (starting evening prior to surgery):

Initial: 5000 int. units 10-14 hours before surgery

Adjustment: 5000 int. units 4-8 hours* after surgery

Maintenance: 5000 int. units once daily, allowing 24 hours between doses.

*Dose may be delayed if hemostasis is not yet achieved.

Unstable angina or non-Q-wave myocardial infarction: 120 int. units/kg body weight (maximum dose: 10,000 int. units) every 12 hours for 5-8 days with concurrent aspirin therapy. Discontinue dalteparin once patient is clinically stable.

Venous thromboembolism: Cancer patients:

Initial (month 1): 200 int. units/kg (maximum dose: 18,000 int. units) once daily for 30 days

◀ Maintenance (months 2-6): ~150 int. units/kg (maximum dose: 18,000 int. units) once daily. If platelet count between 50,000-100,000/mm³, reduce dose by 2,500 int. units until platelet count recovers to ≥100,000/mm³. If platelet count <50,000/mm³, discontinue dalteparin until platelet count recover to >50,000/mm³.

Immobility during acute illness: 5000 int. units once daily

Dosing adjustment in renal impairment: Half-life is increased in patients with chronic renal failure, use with caution, accumulation can be expected; specific dosage adjustments have not been recommended. In cancer patients, receiving treatment for venous thromboembolism, if Cl_{cr} <30 mL/minute, manufacturer recommends monitoring anti-Xa levels to determine appropriate dose.

Dosing adjustment in hepatic impairment: Use with caution in patients with hepatic insufficiency; specific dosage adjustments have not been recommended

Stability Store at temperatures of 20°C to 25°C (68°F to 77°F). Multidose vials may be stored for up to 2 weeks at room temperature after entering.

Administration Do not administer I.M.; for deep SubQ injection only. May be injected in a U-shape to the area surrounding the navel, the upper outer side of the thigh, or the upper outer quadrangle of the buttock. Use thumb and forefinger to lift a fold of skin when injecting dalteparin to the navel area or thigh. Insert needle at a 45- to 90-degree angle. The entire length of needle should be inserted. Do not expel air bubble from fixed-dose syringe prior to injection. Air bubble (and extra solution, if applicable) may be expelled from graduated syringes. In order to minimize bruising, do not rub injection site.

To convert from I.V. unfractionated heparin (UFH) infusion to SubQ dalteparin (Nutescu, 2007): Calculate specific dose for dalteparin based on indication, discontinue UFH and begin dalteparin within 1 hour

To convert from SubQ dalteparin to I.V. UFH infusion (Nutescu, 2007): Discontinue dalteparin; calculate specific dose for I.V. UFH infusion based on indication; omit heparin bolus/loading dose

Converting from SubQ dalteparin dosed every 12 hours: Start I.V. UFH infusion 10-11 hours after last dose of dalteparin

Converting from SubQ dalteparin dosed every 24 hours: Start I.V. UFH infusion 22-23 hours after last dose of dalteparin

Monitoring Parameters Periodic CBC including platelet count; stool occult blood tests; monitoring of PT and PTT is not necessary. Once patient has received 3-4 doses, anti-Xa levels, drawn 4-6 hours after dalteparin administration, may be used to monitor effect in patients with severe renal dysfunction or if abnormal coagulation parameters or bleeding should occur.

Reference Range Treatment: Venous thromboembolism: Target anti-Xa range: 0.5-1.5 int. units/mL

Anesthesia and Critical Care Concerns/Other Considerations

Evidence-Based Information: The American College of Chest Physicians Evidence Based Clinical Practice Guidelines (8th Edition, 2008) recommend for routine assessment and routine thromboprophylaxis in most critically ill patients (Grade 1A). For critically ill patients at a moderate risk (medically ill or postoperative) for VTE, they recommend using LMWH or low dose unfractionated heparin (Grade 1A). For critically ill patients at a high risk (major trauma or orthopedic surgery) for VTE, they recommend LMWH (Grade 1A). If bleeding risk prohibits the use of pharmacologic thromboprophylaxis, mechanical thromboprophylaxis is recommended until the risk decreases (Grade 1A).

Obesity/Renal Dysfunction: There is no consensus for adjusting/correcting the weight-based dosage of LMWH for patients who are morbidly obese. Monitoring of antifactor Xa concentration 4 hours after injection may be warranted. Patients who have a reduction in calculated creatinine clearance are at risk of accumulated anticoagulant effect when they are treated with certain LMWHs. All LMWHs may not behave the same in patients with renal dysfunction. Some clinicians monitor anti-Xa levels for patients with Cl_{cr} <30 mL/minute.

Pregnancy Risk Factor B

Contraindications Hypersensitivity to dalteparin or any component of the formulation; thrombocytopenia associated with a positive *in vitro* test for antiplatelet antibodies in the presence of dalteparin; hypersensitivity to heparin or pork products; patients with active major bleeding; patients with unstable angina, non-Q-wave MI, or acute venous thromboembolism undergoing regional anesthesia; not for I.M. or I.V. use

Warnings/Precautions [U.S. Boxed Warning]: Patients with recent or anticipated neuraxial anesthesia (epidural or spinal anesthesia) are at risk of spinal or epidural hematoma and subsequent paralysis. Consider risk versus benefit prior to neuraxial anesthesia. Risk is increased by concomitant agents which may alter hemostasis, as well as traumatic or repeated epidural or spinal puncture. Patient should be observed closely for bleeding if dalteparin is administered during or immediately following diagnostic lumbar puncture, epidural anesthesia, or spinal anesthesia.

Use with caution in patients with pre-existing thrombocytopenia, recent childbirth, subacute bacterial endocarditis, peptic ulcer disease, pericarditis or pericardial effusion, liver or renal function impairment, recent lumbar puncture, vasculitis, concurrent use of aspirin (increased bleeding risk), previous hypersensitivity to heparin, heparin-associated thrombocytopenia. Monitor platelet count closely. Rare thrombocytopenia may occur. Consider discontinuation of dalteparin in any patient developing significant thrombocytopenia related to initiation of dalteparin. Rare cases of thrombocytopenia with thrombosis have occurred. Use caution in patients with congenital or drug-induced thrombocytopenia or platelet defects. Cancer patients with thrombocytopenia may require dose adjustments for treatment of acute venous thromboembolism.

Use with caution in patients with known hypersensitivity to methylparaben or propylparaben. Monitor patient closely for signs or symptoms of bleeding. Certain patients are at increased risk of bleeding. Risk factors include bacterial endocarditis; congenital or acquired bleeding disorders; active ulcerative or angiodysplastic GI diseases; severe uncontrolled hypertension; hemorrhagic stroke; or use shortly after brain, spinal, or ophthalmology surgery; in patient treated concomitantly with platelet inhibitors; recent GI bleeding; thrombocytopenia or platelet defects; severe liver disease; hypertensive or diabetic retinopathy; or in patients undergoing invasive procedures.

Use with caution in patients with severe renal failure (has not been studied). Safety and efficacy in pediatric patients have not been established. Rare cases of thrombocytopenia with thrombosis have occurred. Multidose vials contain benzyl alcohol and should not be used in pregnant women. In neonates, large amounts of benzyl alcohol (>100 mg/kg/day) have been associated with fatal toxicity (gasping syndrome). Heparin can cause hyperkalemia by affecting aldosterone. Similar reactions could occur with dalteparin. Monitor for hyperkalemia. Do **not** administer intramuscularly. Not to be used interchangeably (unit for unit) with heparin or any other low molecular weight heparins.

There is no consensus for adjusting/correcting the weight-based dosage of LMWH for patients who are morbidly obese (BMI ≥40 kg/m^2). For patients undergoing inpatient bariatric surgery, the American College of Chest Physicians Practice Guidelines suggest using a higher thromboprophylaxis dose of LMWH for obese patients (Geerts, 2008).

Adverse Reactions

Note: As with all anticoagulants, bleeding is the major adverse effect of dalteparin. Hemorrhage may occur at virtually any site. Risk is dependent on multiple variables.

>10%:

Hematologic: Bleeding (3% to 14%)

1% to 10%:

Hematologic: Wound hematoma (up to 3%)

Hepatic: AST >3 times upper limit of normal (5% to 9%), ALT >3 times upper limit of normal (4% to 10%)

Local: Pain at injection site (up to 12%), injection site hematoma (up to 7%)

<1% (Limited to important or life-threatening): Thrombocytopenia (including heparin-induced thrombocytopenia), allergic reaction (fever, pruritus, rash, injections site reaction, bullous eruption), alopecia, anaphylactoid reaction, operative site bleeding, gastrointestinal bleeding, hemoptysis, skin necrosis, subdural hematoma, thrombosis (associated with heparin-induced thrombocytopenia). Spinal or epidural hematomas can occur following neuraxial anesthesia or spinal puncture, resulting in paralysis.

Drug Interactions

Avoid Concomitant Use There are no known interactions where it is recommended to avoid concomitant use.

Increased Effect/Toxicity

Dalteparin may increase the levels/effects of: Anticoagulants; Drotrecogin Alfa; Ibritumomab; Tositumomab and Iodine I 131 Tositumomab

The levels/effects of Dalteparin may be increased by: 5-ASA Derivatives; Antiplatelet Agents; Dasatinib; Herbs (Anticoagulant/Antiplatelet Properties); Nonsteroidal Anti-Inflammatory Agents; Pentosan Polysulfate Sodium; Pentoxifylline; Prostacyclin Analogues; Salicylates; Thrombolytic Agents

Decreased Effect There are no known significant interactions involving a decrease in effect.

Ethanol/Nutrition/Herb Interactions Herb/Nutraceutical: Alfalfa, anise, bilberry, bladderwrack, bromelain, cat's claw, celery, chamomile, coleus, cordyceps, dong quai, evening primrose oil, fenugreek, feverfew, garlic, ginger, ginkgo biloba, Ginseng (american), Ginseng (panax), Ginseng (siberian), grapeseed, green tea, guggul, horse chestnut seed, horseradish, licorice, prickly ash, red clover, reishi, SAMe (s-adenosylmethionine), sweet clover, turmeric, white willow (all have additional antiplatelet/anticoagulant activity)

Dosage Forms Excipient information presented when available (limited, particularly for generics); consult specific product labeling.

Injection, solution:

Fragmin®: Antifactor Xa 10,000 int. units per 1 mL (9.5 mL) [contains benzyl alcohol]; antifactor Xa 25,000 units per 1 mL (3.8 mL) [contains benzyl alcohol]

Injection, solution [preservative free]:

Fragmin®: Antifactor Xa 2500 int. units per 0.2 mL (0.2 mL); antifactor Xa 5000 int. units per 0.2 mL (0.2 mL); antifactor Xa 7500 int. units per 0.3 mL (0.3 mL); antifactor Xa 10,000 int. units per 1 mL (1 mL); antifactor Xa 12,500 int. units per 0.5 mL (0.5 mL); antifactor Xa 15,000 int. units per 0.6 mL (0.6 mL); antifactor Xa 18,000 int. units per 0.72 mL (0.72 mL)

References

Geerts WH, Bergqvist D, Pineo GF, et al, "Prevention of Venous Thromboembolism: American College of Chest Physicians Evidence-Based Clinical Practice Guidelines (8th Edition)," *Chest*, 2008, 133(6 Suppl):381S-453S.

Nagge J, Crowther M, and Hirsh J, "Is Impaired Renal Function a Contraindication to the Use of Low-Molecular Weight Heparin?" *Arch Intern Med*, 2002, 162(22):2605-9.

◆ **Dalteparin Sodium** *see* Dalteparin *on page 366*

◆ **Dantrium®** *see* Dantrolene *on page 370*

Dantrolene (DAN troe leen)

Medication Safety Issues

Sound-alike/look-alike issues:

Dantrium® may be confused with danazol, Daraprim®

Related Information

Malignant Hyperthermia *on page 1638*

U.S. Brand Names Dantrium®

Canadian Brand Names Dantrium®

Index Terms Dantrolene Sodium

Pharmacologic Category Skeletal Muscle Relaxant

Generic Available Yes: Capsule

Use Treatment of spasticity associated with upper motor neuron disorders (eg, spinal cord injury, stroke, cerebral palsy, or multiple sclerosis); management of malignant hyperthermia; prevention of malignant hyperthermia in susceptible individuals (preoperative/postoperative administration)

Unlabeled/Investigational Use Neuroleptic malignant syndrome (NMS)

Mechanism of Action Acts directly on skeletal muscle by interfering with release of calcium ion from the sarcoplasmic reticulum; prevents or reduces the increase in myoplasmic calcium ion concentration that activates the acute catabolic processes associated with malignant hyperthermia

Pharmacodynamics/Kinetics

Absorption: Oral: Slow and incomplete

Metabolism: Hepatic

Half-life elimination: 8.7 hours

Excretion: Feces (45% to 50%); urine (25% as unchanged drug and metabolites)

Dosage

Spasticity: Oral:

Children: Initial: 0.5 mg/kg/dose twice daily, increase frequency to 3-4 times/day at 4- to 7-day intervals, then increase dose by 0.5 mg/kg to a maximum of 3 mg/kg/dose 2-4 times/day up to 400 mg/day

Adults: 25 mg/day to start, increase frequency to 2-4 times/day, then increase dose by 25 mg every 4-7 days to a maximum of 100 mg 2-4 times/day or 400 mg/day

Malignant hyperthermia: Children and Adults:

Preoperative prophylaxis:

Oral: 4-8 mg/kg/day in 4 divided doses, begin 1-2 days prior to surgery with last dose 3-4 hours prior to surgery

I.V.: 2.5 mg/kg ~1 1/4 hours prior to anesthesia and infused over 1 hour with additional doses as needed and individualized

Crisis: I.V.: 2.5 mg/kg; may repeat dose up to cumulative dose of 10 mg/kg; if physiologic and metabolic abnormalities reappear, repeat regimen

Postcrisis follow-up: Oral: 4-8 mg/kg/day in 4 divided doses for 1-3 days; I.V. dantrolene may be used when oral therapy is not practical; individualize dosage beginning with 1 mg/kg or more as the clinical situation dictates

Neuroleptic malignant syndrome (unlabeled use): I.V.: 1 mg/kg; may repeat dose up to maximum cumulative dose of 10 mg/kg, then switch to oral dosage

Stability Reconstitute vial by adding 60 mL of sterile water for injection USP (**not bacteriostatic water for injection**). Protect from light. Use within 6 hours; avoid glass bottles for I.V. infusion.

Administration I.V.: Therapeutic or emergency dose can be administered with rapid continuous I.V. push. Follow-up doses should be administered over 2-3 minutes.

Monitoring Parameters Motor performance should be monitored for therapeutic outcomes; nausea, vomiting, and liver function tests should be monitored for potential hepatotoxicity; intravenous administration requires cardiac monitor and blood pressure monitor

Pregnancy Risk Factor C

Contraindications

I.V.: There are no contraindications listed within the manufacturers labeling.

Oral: Active hepatic disease; should not be used when spasticity is used to maintain posture/balance during locomotion or to obtain/maintain increased function

Warnings/Precautions [U.S. Boxed Warning]: Has potential for hepatotoxicity. Overt hepatitis has been most frequently observed between the third and twelfth month of therapy. Hepatic injury appears to be greater in females and in patients >35 years of age. Idiosyncratic and hypersensitivity reactions (sometimes fatal) of the liver have also occurred.

Use with caution in patients with impaired cardiac, hepatic, or pulmonary function. May cause photosensitivity. Patients should be cautioned about performing tasks which require mental alertness (eg, operating machinery or driving). The combination of I.V. dantrolene and calcium channel blockers is not recommended. Injection contains 3 g mannitol/vial; caution if additional mannitol required. Alkaline solution may cause tissue necrosis if extravasated. In addition to I.V. dantrolene, supportive measures must also be utilized for management of malignant hyperthermia. Long-term use in patients <5 years of age has not been established.

Adverse Reactions Frequency not defined.

Cardiovascular: Blood pressure (altered), heart failure, tachycardia

Central nervous system: Chills, confusion, dizziness, drowsiness, fatigue, fever, headache, insomnia, lightheadedness, malaise, mental depression, nervousness, seizure, speech disturbance

Dermatologic: Eczematoid eruption, hair growth (abnormal), pruritus, rash, urticaria

◀

Gastrointestinal: Abdominal cramps, anorexia, constipation, diarrhea, dysphagia, gastric irritation, gastrointestinal hemorrhage, nausea, taste change, vomiting

Genitourinary: Crystalluria, difficult erection, difficult urination, nocturia, polyuria, urinary frequency, urinary incontinence, urinary retention

Hematologic: Anemia (aplastic), leukopenia, thrombocytopenia

Hepatic: Hepatitis

Local: Injection site reaction, thrombophlebitis, tissue necrosis

Neuromuscular & skeletal: Back pain, muscle weakness, myalgia

Ocular: Blurred vision, diplopia, tearing (excessive)

Renal: Hematuria

Respiratory: Feeling of suffocation, pleural effusion (associated with pericarditis), pulmonary edema, respiratory depression

Miscellaneous: Anaphylaxis, diaphoresis, lymphocytic lymphoma, sialorrhea

Drug Interactions

Metabolism/Transport Effects Substrate of CYP3A4 (major)

Avoid Concomitant Use There are no known interactions where it is recommended to avoid concomitant use.

Increased Effect/Toxicity

Dantrolene may increase the levels/effects of: Alcohol (Ethyl); CNS Depressants; Methotrimeprazine

The levels/effects of Dantrolene may be increased by: CYP3A4 Inhibitors (Moderate); CYP3A4 Inhibitors (Strong); Dasatinib; Methotrimeprazine

Decreased Effect

The levels/effects of Dantrolene may be decreased by: CYP3A4 Inducers (Strong); Deferasirox; Herbs (CYP3A4 Inducers)

Ethanol/Nutrition/Herb Interactions

Ethanol: Avoid ethanol (may increase CNS depression).

Herb/Nutraceutical: Avoid valerian, St John's wort, kava kava, gotu kola (may increase CNS depression).

Dosage Forms Excipient information presented when available (limited, particularly for generics); consult specific product labeling.

Capsule, as sodium: 25 mg, 50 mg, 100 mg

Dantrium®: 25 mg, 50 mg, 100 mg

Injection, powder for reconstitution, as sodium:

Dantrium®: 20 mg [contains mannitol 3 g]

References

Guerrero RM and Shifrar KA, "Diagnosis and Treatment of Neuroleptic Malignant Syndrome," *Clin Pharm*, 1988, 7(9):697-701.

Rosenberg MR and Green M, "Neuroleptic Malignant Syndrome. Review of Response to Therapy," *Arch Intern Med*, 1989, 149(9):1927-31.

◆ **Dantrolene Sodium** *see* Dantrolene *on page 370*

◆ **Dapcin** *see* DAPTOmycin *on page 372*

DAPTOmycin (DAP toe mye sin)

Medication Safety Issues

Sound-alike/look-alike issues:

Cubicin® may be confused with Cleocin®

DAPTOmycin may be confused with DACTINomycin

Related Information

Dosing Considerations for the Critically-Ill Patient With Morbid Obesity *on page 1561*

U.S. Brand Names Cubicin®

Canadian Brand Names Cubicin®

Index Terms Cidecin; Dapcin; LY146032

Pharmacologic Category Antibiotic, Cyclic Lipopeptide

Generic Available No

Use Treatment of complicated skin and skin structure infections caused by susceptible aerobic gram-positive organisms; *Staphylococcus aureus* bacteremia, including right-sided infective endocarditis caused by MSSA or MRSA

Unlabeled/Investigational Use Treatment of severe infections caused by MRSA or VRE

Mechanism of Action Daptomycin binds to components of the cell membrane of susceptible organisms and causes rapid depolarization, inhibiting intracellular synthesis of DNA, RNA, and protein. Daptomycin is bactericidal in a concentration-dependent manner.

Pharmacodynamics/Kinetics

Distribution: 0.1 L/kg

Protein binding: 90% to 93%; 84% to 88% in patients with Cl_{cr}<30 mL/minute

Half-life elimination: 8-9 hours (up to 28 hours in renal impairment)

Excretion: Urine (78%; primarily as unchanged drug); feces (6%)

Dosage I.V.: Adults:

Skin and soft tissue: 4 mg/kg once daily for 7-14 days

Bacteremia, right-sided endocarditis caused by MSSA or MRSA: 6 mg/kg once daily for 2-6 weeks

Dosage adjustment in renal impairment: Cl_{cr} <30 mL/minute:

Skin and soft tissue infections: 4 mg/kg every 48 hours

Staphylococcal bacteremia: 6 mg/kg every 48 hours

Hemodialysis (administer after hemodialysis) and/or CAPD: Dose as in Cl_{cr} <30 mL/minute

Continuous renal replacement therapy (CRRT): Dose as in Cl_{cr} <30 mL/minute

Dosage adjustment in hepatic impairment: No adjustment required for mild-to-moderate impairment (Child-Pugh Class A or B); not evaluated in severe hepatic impairment

Stability Store under refrigeration at 2°C to 8°C (36°F to 46°F). Reconstitute vial with 10 mL NS. Add NS to vial and rotate gently to wet powder. Allow to stand for 10 minutes, then gently swirl to obtain completely reconstituted solution. Do not shake or agitate vial vigorously. Should be further diluted following reconstitution in an appropriate volume of NS. Reconstituted solution (either in vial or in infusion bag) is stable for a cumulative time of 12 hours at room temperature and 48 hours if refrigerated (2°C to 8°C). Incompatible with ReadyMED® elastomeric infusion pumps (Cardinal Health, Inc) due to an impurity (2-mercaptobenzothiazole) leaching from the pump system into the daptomycin solution.

Administration Infuse over 30 minutes. Do not use in conjunction with ReadyMED® elastomeric infusion pumps (Cardinal Health, Inc) due to an impurity (2-mercaptobenzothiazole) leaching from the pump system into the daptomycin solution.

Monitoring Parameters Monitor signs and symptoms of infection. CPK should be monitored at least weekly during therapy; more frequent monitoring if current or prior statin therapy, unexplained CPK increases, and/or renal impairment. Monitor for muscle pain or weakness, especially if noted in distal extremities.

Reference Range

Trough concentrations at steady-state:

4 mg/kg once daily: 5.9 ± 1.6 mcg/mL

6 mg/kg once daily: 6.7 ± 1.6 mcg/mL

Note: Trough concentrations are not predictive of efficacy/toxicity. Drug exhibits concentration-dependent bactericidal activity, so C_{max}:MIC ratios may be a more useful parameter.

Anesthesia and Critical Care Concerns/Other Considerations Clinical Pearls/Comments: Daptomycin should not be used for the treatment of pneumonia, due to the low volume of distribution and inactivation of the drug by surfactant.

Pregnancy Risk Factor B

Contraindications Hypersensitivity to daptomycin or any component of the formulation

Warnings/Precautions May be associated with an increased incidence of myopathy; discontinue in patients with signs and symptoms of myopathy in conjunction with an increase in CPK (>5 times ULN or 1000 units/L) or in asymptomatic patients with a CPK ≥10 times ULN. Myopathy may occur more frequently at dose and/or frequency in excess of recommended dosages. Use caution in patients receiving other drugs associated with myopathy (eg, HMG-CoA reductase inhibitors). Not indicated for the treatment of pneumonia (poor lung penetration). Use caution in renal impairment (dosage adjustment required). Symptoms suggestive of peripheral neuropathy have been observed with treatment; monitor for new-onset or worsening neuropathy. Prolonged use may result in fungal or bacterial superinfection, including *C. difficile*-associated diarrhea and pseudomembranous colitis. Safety and efficacy in patients <18 years of age have not been established.

Adverse Reactions

>10%:

Gastrointestinal: Diarrhea (5% to 12%), vomiting (3% to 12%), constipation (6% to 11%)

Hematologic: Anemia (2% to 13%)

1% to 10%:

Cardiovascular: Peripheral edema (7%), chest pain (7%), hypertension (1% to 6%), hypotension (2% to 5%)

Central nervous system: Insomnia (5% to 9%), headache (5% to7%), fever (2% to 7%), dizziness (2% to 6%), anxiety (5%)

Dermatologic: Rash (4% to 7%), pruritus (3% to 6%), erythema (5%)

Endocrine & metabolic: Hypokalemia (9%), hyperkalemia (5%), hyperphosphatemia (3%)

Gastrointestinal: Nausea (6% to 10%), abdominal pain (6%), dyspepsia (1% to 4%), loose stool (4%), GI hemorrhage (2%)

Genitourinary: Urinary tract infection (2% to 7%)

Hematologic: INR increased (2%), eosinophilia (2%)

Hepatic: Transaminases increased (2% to 3%), alkaline phosphatase increased (2%)

Local: Injection site reaction (3% to 6%)

Neuromuscular & skeletal: CPK increased (3% to 9%), limb pain (2% to 9%), back pain (7%), weakness (5%), arthralgia (1% to 3%)

Renal: Renal failure (2% to 3%)

Respiratory: Pharyngolaryngeal pain (8%), pleural effusion (6%), cough (3%), pneumonia (3%), dyspnea (2% to 3%)

Miscellaneous: Osteomyelitis (6%), bacteremia (5%), diaphoresis (5%), sepsis (5%), infection (fungal, 2% to 3%)

<1% (Limited to important or life-threatening): Anaphylaxis, appetite decreased, arthralgia, atrial fibrillation, atrial flutter, cardiac arrest, dyskinesia, dysphagia, eczema, electrolyte disturbance, eosinophilia, erythema (truncal), eye irritation, fatigue, flatulence, flushing, GI discomfort, gingival pain, hallucination, hives, hypomagnesemia, hypersensitivity, hypoesthesia, jaundice, jitteriness, LDH increased, leukocytosis, lymphadenopathy, mental status change, muscle cramps, muscle weakness, myalgia, myoglobin increased, osteomyelitis, paresthesia, peripheral neuropathy, proteinuria, prothrombin time prolonged, pulmonary eosinophilia, rhabdomyolysis, rigors, serum bicarbonate increased, shortness of breath, stomatitis, supraventricular arrhythmia, taste disturbance, thrombocytopenia, thrombocythemia, tinnitus, vertigo, vesiculobullous rash, vision blurred, xerostomia

Drug Interactions

Avoid Concomitant Use There are no known interactions where it is recommended to avoid concomitant use.

Increased Effect/Toxicity

The levels/effects of DAPTOmycin may be increased by: HMG-CoA Reductase Inhibitors

Decreased Effect There are no known significant interactions involving a decrease in effect.

Test Interactions Daptomycin may cause false prolongation of the PT and increase of INR with certain reagents. This appears to be a dose-dependent phenomenon. Therefore, it is recommended to obtain blood samples immediately prior to next daptomycin dose (eg, trough). If PT/INR elevated, clinicians should repeat PT/INR and evaluate for other causes of hypocoagulation.

Dosage Forms Excipient information presented when available (limited, particularly for generics); consult specific product labeling.

Injection, powder for reconstitution:

Cubicin®: 500 mg

References

Cha R, Grucz RG Jr, and Rybak MJ, "Daptomycin Dose-Effect Relationship Against Resistant Gram-Positive Organisms," *Antimicrob Agents Chemother*, 2003, 47(5):1598-603.

Lai JJ and Brodeur SK, "Physical and Chemical Compatibility of Daptomycin With Nine Medications," *Ann Pharmacother*, 2004, 38(10):1612-6.

Richter SS, Kealey DE, Murray CT, et al, "The *in vitro* Activity of Daptomycin Against *Staphylococcus aureus* and *Enterococcus* species," *J Antimicrob Chemother*, 2003, 52(1):123-7.

Silverman JA, Perlmutter NG, and Shapiro HM, "Correlation of Daptomycin Bactericidal Activity and Membrane Depolarization in *Staphylococcus aureus*," *Antimicrob Agents Chemother*, 2003, 47 (8):2538-44.

Darbepoetin Alfa (dar be POE e tin AL fa)

Medication Safety Issues

Sound-alike/look-alike issues:

Aranesp® may be confused with Aralast, Aricept®

Darbepoetin alfa may be confused with dalteparin, epoetin alfa, epoetin beta

Medication Guide An FDA-approved patient medication guide, which is available with the product information and at http://www.fda.gov/downloads/Drugs/DrugSafety/ucm085918.pdf, must be dispensed with this medication for each new outpatient prescription and refill.

U.S. Brand Names Aranesp®

Canadian Brand Names Aranesp®

Index Terms Erythropoiesis-Stimulating Agent (ESA); Erythropoiesis-Stimulating Protein; NSC-729969

Pharmacologic Category Colony Stimulating Factor; Growth Factor; Recombinant Human Erythropoietin

Generic Available No

Use Treatment of anemia (elevate/maintain red blood cell level and decrease the need for transfusions) associated with chronic renal failure (including patients on dialysis and not on dialysis); treatment of anemia due to concurrent chemotherapy in patients with metastatic cancer (nonmyeloid malignancies)

Note: Darbepoetin is **not** indicated for use in cancer patients under the following conditions:

- receiving hormonal therapy, therapeutic biologic products, or radiation therapy unless also receiving concurrent myelosuppressive chemotherapy
- receiving myelosuppressive therapy when the expected outcome is curative

Unlabeled/Investigational Use Treatment of symptomatic anemia in myelodysplastic syndrome (MDS)

Mechanism of Action Induces erythropoiesis by stimulating the division and differentiation of committed erythroid progenitor cells; induces the release of reticulocytes from the bone marrow into the bloodstream, where they mature to erythrocytes. There is a dose response relationship with this effect. This results in an increase in reticulocyte counts followed by a rise in hematocrit and hemoglobin levels. When administered SubQ or I.V., darbepoetin's half-life is ~3 times that of epoetin alfa concentrations.

Pharmacodynamics/Kinetics

Onset of action: Increased hemoglobin levels not generally observed until 2-6 weeks after initiating treatment

Absorption: SubQ: Slow

Distribution: V_d: 0.06 L/kg

Bioavailability: CRF: SubQ: Adults: ~37% (range: 30% to 50%); Children: 54% (range: 32% to 70%)

Half-life elimination:

CRF: Adults:

I.V.: 21 hours

SubQ: Nondialysis patients: 70 hours (range: 35-139 hours); Dialysis patients: 46 hours (range: 12-89 hours)

Cancer: Adults: SubQ: 74 hours (range: 24-144 hours); Children: 49 hours

Note: Darbepoetin half-life is approximately threefold longer than epoetin alfa following I.V. administration

Time to peak: SubQ:

CRF: Adults: 48 hours (range: 12-72 hours; independent of dialysis); Children: 36 hours (range: 10-58 hours)

Cancer: Adults: 71-90 hours (range: 28-123 hours); Children: 71 hours (range: 21-143 hours)

Dosage Note: Hemoglobin levels should not exceed 12 g/dL and should not rise >1 g/dL per 2-week time period during therapy in any patient.

◄ **Anemia associated with CRF:** Individualize dosing to achieve and maintain hemoglobin levels at a target range of 10-12 g/dL. Hemoglobin levels should not exceed 12 g/dL. **Note:** I.V. route is preferred in hemodialysis patients.

Children ≥1 year: Conversion from epoetin alfa: I.V., SubQ: Initial dose: Epoetin alfa doses of 1500 to ≥90,000 units per week may be converted to doses ranging from 6.25-200 mcg darbepoetin alfa per week (see pediatric column in conversion table).

Children 11-18 years: Initial treatment (unlabeled use): I.V., SubQ: Initial dose: 0.45 mcg/kg once weekly; titrate to hemoglobin response

Adults: I.V., SubQ: Initial: 0.45 mcg/kg once weekly; alternative dose for nondialysis patients: 0.75 mcg/kg once every 2 weeks; Maintenance: titrate to maintain hemoglobin levels between 10-12 g/dL as described below (may be administered once weekly or every 2 weeks; nondialysis patients may require lower maintenance doses)

Dosage adjustment:

Decrease dose by ~25%: If hemoglobin approaches 12 g/dL **or** hemoglobin increases >1 g/dL in any 2-week period. If hemoglobin continues to increase, temporarily discontinue therapy until hemoglobin begins to decrease, then resume therapy with a ~25% reduction from previous dose.

Increase dose by ~25%: If hemoglobin does not increase by 1 g/dL after 4 weeks of therapy (with adequate iron stores). Do not increase dose more frequently than at 4-week intervals.

Inadequate or lack of response: If patient does not attain target hemoglobin range of 10-12 g/dL after appropriate dose titrations over 12 weeks:

Do not continue to increase dose and use the minimum effective dose that will maintain a hemoglobin level sufficient to avoid red blood cell transfusions **and** evaluate patient for other causes of anemia.

Monitor hemoglobin closely thereafter, and if responsiveness improves, may resume making dosage adjustments as recommended above. If responsiveness does not improve and recurrent red blood cell transfusions continue to be needed, discontinue therapy.

Maintenance dose: Individualize to target hemoglobin range of 10-12 g/dL; limit additional dosage increase to every 4 weeks or longer. Patients generally require lower maintenance doses than initial doses to maintain target range.

Conversion from epoetin alfa: I.V., SubQ: Initial dose: Epoetin alfa doses may be converted to doses ranging from 6.25-200 mcg darbepoetin alfa per week (see conversion table).

Anemia associated with chemotherapy: Titrate dosage to use the minimum effective dose that will maintain a hemoglobin level sufficient to avoid red blood cell transfusions. Do not initiate therapy if hemoglobin ≥10 g/dL. Discontinue darbepoetin following completion of chemotherapy.

Children (unlabeled use): SubQ: 2.25 mcg/kg once weekly

Adults: SubQ: Initial: 2.25 mcg/kg once weekly **or** 500 mcg once every 3 weeks

Dosage adjustment:

Increase dose: If hemoglobin does not increase by 1 g/dL after 6 weeks of therapy (for patients receiving weekly therapy), the dose should be increased up to 4.5 mcg/kg once weekly.

Decrease dose by 40%: If hemoglobin increases >1g/dL in any 2-week period **or** hemoglobin reaches a level sufficient to avoid red blood cell transfusion.

Withhold dose: If hemoglobin exceeds a level needed to avoid red blood cell transfusion. Resume treatment with a dose 40% below the previous dose when hemoglobin approaches a level where transfusions may be required.

Discontinue: On completion of chemotherapy or if after 8 weeks of therapy there is no hemoglobin response or transfusions still required

Anemia associated with MDS (unlabeled use): Adults: SubQ: 150-300 mcg once weekly

Conversion from epoetin alfa to darbepoetin alfa: See table on next page.

Conversion From Epoetin Alfa to Darbepoetin Alfa (Initial Dose)

Previous Dosage of Epoetin Alfa (units/week)	Children Darbepoetin Alfa Dosage (mcg/week)	Adults Darbepoetin Alfa Dosage (mcg/week)
<1500	Not established	6.25
1500-2499	6.25	6.25
2500-4999	10	12.5
5000-10,999	20	25
11,000-17,999	40	40
18,000-33,999	60	60
34,000-89,999	100	100
≥90,000	200	200

Note: In patients receiving epoetin alfa 2-3 times per week, darbepoetin alfa is administered once weekly. In patients receiving epoetin alfa once weekly, darbepoetin alfa is administered once every 2 weeks. The darbepoetin dose to be administered every 2 weeks is derived by adding together 2 weekly epoetin alfa doses and then converting to the appropriate darbepoetin dose. Titrate dose to hemoglobin response thereafter (see dosage adjustment in renal impairment).

Dosage adjustment in renal impairment: Dosage requirements for patients with chronic renal failure who do not require dialysis may be lower than in dialysis patients. Monitor patients closely during the time period in which a dialysis regimen is initiated, dosage requirement may increase. The National Kidney Foundation Clinical Practice Guidelines for Anemia in Chronic Kidney Disease: 2007 Update of Hemoglobin Target (September, 2007) recommend hemoglobin levels in the range of 11-12 g/dL for dialysis and nondialysis patients receiving ESAs; hemoglobin levels should not be maintained >13 g/dL.
Hemodialysis: I.V. route is preferred in hemodialysis patients.

Stability Store at 2°C to 8°C (36°F to 46°F); do not freeze. Do not shake. Protect from light. Do not dilute or administer with other solutions.

Administration May be administered by SubQ or I.V. injection. The I.V. route is recommended in hemodialysis patients. Do not shake; vigorous shaking may denature darbepoetin alfa, rendering it biologically inactive. Do not dilute or administer in conjunction with other drug solutions. Discard any unused portion of the vial; do not pool unused portions.

Monitoring Parameters Hemoglobin (at least once per week until maintenance dose established and after dosage changes; monitor at regular intervals at least once per month once hemoglobin is stabilized); iron stores (transferrin saturation and ferritin) prior to and during therapy; serum chemistry (CRF patients); blood pressure

Anesthesia and Critical Care Concerns/Other Considerations
Evidence-Based Information:

Routine Use in Critically-Ill Patients: A prospective, randomized, double-blind, placebo-controlled, multicenter trial was performed with critically-ill patients assessing the efficacy of recombinant human erythropoietin in reducing red blood cell transfusions (Corwin, 2002). Patients were enrolled from December 1998 through June 2001. Over 1300 ICU (medical, surgical, or medical/surgical) patients were randomized to receive placebo or 40,000 units of erythropoietin subcutaneously on ICU day 3 and then weekly for a total of 3 doses for patients who remained in the hospital. Inclusion criteria included ICU stay for 3 days, age >18 years, and hematocrit <38%. Exclusion criteria were extensive and included acute ischemic heart disease, acute gastrointestinal bleed, and renal failure with hemodialysis. Each patient's physician determined the need for red blood cell transfusion. Results: The mean baseline hemoglobin was 9.97 g/dL in each group. Patients receiving erythropoietin were less likely to receive transfusions. The median number of units transfused per patient in the placebo group was 2 and in the erythropoietin group was 1 (p<0.001). The erythropoietin group had a 9.9% absolute reduction in RBC transfusions during 28 days (p<0.001, OR 0.67,

CI 0.54-0.83). Mortality and adverse clinical events were not significantly different between groups. The authors concluded that weekly administration of erythropoietin in critically-ill patients reduces red blood cell transfusions and increases hemoglobin. The authors also suggest that further study is needed to determine if use of erythropoietin results in improved clinical outcomes.

A restrictive transfusion trial was published after the above Corwin trial was underway (Hebert, 1999). Hebert and his group evaluated a restrictive transfusion strategy (transfuse if hemoglobin <7 g/dL to maintain between 7 and 9 g/dL) versus a liberal strategy (transfuse if hemoglobin <10 g/dL to maintain between 10 and 12 g/dL). Inclusion criteria included anticipated ICU stay >24 hours, hemoglobin ≤9 g/dL with 72 hours of ICU admission, and euvolemia after initial treatment. Exclusion criteria included chronic anemia, active bleeding, or admission after a routine cardiac surgical procedure. The restrictive approach to transfusion was at least as effective as and possibly superior to a liberal transfusion policy in critically-ill patients. The exception to this may be patients with acute myocardial infarction and unstable angina.

More recently, Corwin, et al (2007) once again evaluated the use of recombinant human erythropoietin in the critically ill. In this prospective, randomized, placebo-controlled trial, 1460 medical, surgical, or trauma patients were enrolled between December, 2003 and June, 2006. Patients received either subcutaneous erythropoietin 40,000 units or placebo once weekly for a maximum of 3 doses and were followed for 140 days. The primary endpoint of the study was the percentage of patients who received a red cell transfusion between days 1 and 29. Secondary endpoints included the number of red cell units transfused between days 1 and 29, mortality at day 29 and day 140, and the change in hemoglobin concentration from baseline to day 29. Patients were evaluated for inclusion into the study if they remained in that ICU for 2 days. Inclusion criteria were age >18 years and hemoglobin concentration <12 g/dL. Exclusion criteria were extensive and included acute ischemic heart disease during the ICU stay, acute gastrointestinal bleed, hemodialysis, and patients at risk for thrombosis (history of pulmonary embolism, deep venous thrombosis, ischemic stroke, other arterial or venous thrombosis). Red cell transfusions targeted hemoglobin concentrations between 7 and 9 g/dL, but the need for transfusion was determined by the treating physician (this is more consistent with clinical practice after the Hebert trial was published and different than the previous Corwin trial). Results: The mean baseline hemoglobin for each group was 9.6 g/dL. The use of erythropoietin did not significantly decrease the need for red cell transfusion (46.0% in the erythropoietin group transfused vs 48.3% in the placebo group, p=0.34). The hemoglobin concentration at day 29 increased more in the erythropoietin group compared to placebo (1.6 ± 2.0 g/dL vs 1.2 ± 1.8 g/dL, p<0.001); however, by day 42 the hemoglobin concentrations in both groups were similar. Mortality at day 29 was significantly lower in the group receiving erythropoietin (8.5% vs 11.4%, p=0.02) from the Kaplan-Meier estimate, but no difference was seen in the Cox model in the overall population. Only in the trauma subset was mortality at day 29 significantly lower in the erythropoietin group (3.5% vs 6.6%, p=0.04). At day 140, mortality was not significantly lower in the erythropoietin group. Thrombotic events (eg, DVT and myocardial infarction) were significantly higher in the erythropoietin group as compared to placebo and appeared to be dose-related (16.5% vs 11.5%, p=0.008, HR 1.41, CI 1.06-1.86). However, upon further analysis those patients who did not receive heparin at baseline developed these events more frequently. There was no difference in length of stay or the use of mechanical ventilation between groups. The authors concluded that although erythropoietin does not reduce the incidence of red cell transfusion in critically-ill patients, it may reduce mortality in trauma patients. Further investigation is required to define erythropoietin's role in this population. The routine use of erythropoietin in critically-ill, nontraumatic surgical or medical patients is not supported by this study.

The 2008 Surviving Sepsis Campaign guidelines do not recommend erythropoietin as a treatment for anemia associated with severe sepsis but suggest that it may be used when septic patients have other therapeutic indications (Grade 1B).

Pregnancy Risk Factor C

Contraindications Hypersensitivity to darbepoetin or any component of the formulation; uncontrolled hypertension

Warnings/Precautions [U.S. Boxed Warning]: ESAs increased the risk of serious cardiovascular events, thromboembolic events, mortality, and/or tumor progression in clinical studies; a rapid rise in hemoglobin (>1 g/dL over 2 weeks) or maintaining higher hemoglobin levels may contribute to these risks. **[U.S. Boxed Warning]: A shortened overall survival and/or increased risk of tumor progression or recurrence has been reported in studies with breast, cervical, head and neck, lymphoid, and non small cell lung cancer patients.** It is of note that in these studies, patients received ESAs to a target hemoglobin of ≥12 g/dL; although risk has not been excluded when dosed to achieve a target hemoglobin of <12 g/dL. **[U.S. Boxed Warnings]: To decrease these risks, and risk of cardio- and thrombovascular events, use ESAs in cancer patients only for the treatment of anemia related to concurrent chemotherapy and use the lowest dose needed to avoid red blood cell transfusions. Discontinue ESA following completion of the chemotherapy course. ESAs are not indicated for patients receiving myelosuppressive therapy when the anticipated outcome is curative. [U.S. Boxed Warning]: An increased risk of death and serious cardiovascular events was reported in chronic renal failure patients administered ESAs to target higher versus lower hemoglobin levels (13.5 vs 11.3 g/dL; 14 vs 10 g/dL) in two clinical studies; dosing should be individualized to achieve and maintain hemoglobin levels within 10-12 g/dL range.** Hemoglobin rising >1 g/dL in a 2-week period may contribute to the risk. Chronic renal failure patients who exhibit an inadequate hemoglobin response to ESA therapy may be at a higher risk for cardiovascular events and mortality compared to other patients. ESA therapy may reduce dialysis efficacy (due to increase in red blood cells and decrease in plasma volume); adjustments in dialysis parameters may be needed. An increased risk of DVT has been observed in patients treated with epoetin undergoing surgical orthopedic procedures. Darbepoetin is **not** approved for reduction in red blood cell transfusions in patients scheduled for surgical procedures. During therapy in any patient, hemoglobin levels should not exceed a target range of 10-12 g/dL and should not rise >1 g/dL per 2-week time period.

Use with caution in patients with hypertension or with a history of seizures; hypertensive encephalopathy and seizures have been reported. If hypertension is difficult to control, reduce or hold darbepoetin alfa. **Not** recommended for acute correction of severe anemia or as a substitute for transfusion. Consider discontinuing in patients who receive a renal transplant.

Prior to treatment, correct or exclude deficiencies of iron, vitamin B_{12}, and/or folate, as well as other factors which may impair erythropoiesis (aluminum toxicity, inflammatory conditions, infections). Prior to and during therapy, iron stores must be evaluated. Supplemental iron is recommended if serum ferritin <100 mcg/L or serum transferrin saturation <20%. Poor response should prompt evaluation of these potential factors, as well as possible malignant processes, occult blood loss, hemolysis, and/or bone marrow fibrosis. Severe anemia and pure red cell aplasia (PRCA) with associated neutralizing antibodies to erythropoietin has been reported, predominantly in patients with CRF receiving SubQ darbepoetin (the I.V. route is preferred for hemodialysis patients). Patients with loss of response to darbepoetin should be evaluated; discontinue treatment in patients with PRCA secondary to neutralizing antibodies to erythropoietin. Antibodies may cross-react; do not switch to another ESA in patients who develop antibody-mediated anemia.

Due to the delayed onset of erythropoiesis, darbepoetin is of no value in the acute treatment of anemia. Safety and efficacy in patients with underlying hematologic diseases have not been established, including porphyria, thalassemia, hemolytic anemia, and sickle cell disease. Potentially serious allergic reactions have been reported. Some products may contain albumin and the packaging of some formulations may contain latex. Safety and efficacy in children with cancer have not been established; children >1 year of age with CRF have been converted from epoetin alfa to darbepoetin.

◀ **Adverse Reactions**
>10%:
Cardiovascular: Edema (21%), hypertension (4% to 20%), hypotension (20%)
Central nervous system: Fatigue (9% to 33%), fever (4% to 19%), headache (12% to 16%), dizziness (7% to 14%)
Gastrointestinal: Diarrhea (14% to 22%), constipation (5% to 18%), vomiting (2% to 14%), nausea (11%)
Neuromuscular & skeletal: Muscle spasm (17%), arthralgia (9% to 13%)
Respiratory: Upper respiratory infection (15%)
Miscellaneous: Infection (24%)
1% to 10%:
Cardiovascular: Peripheral edema (10%), arrhythmia/arrest (8%), angina/chest pain (7% to 8%), fluid overload (6%), thrombosis (6%), CHF (5%), MI (2%)
Central nervous system: Stroke (2%), seizure (≤1%), TIA (≤1%)
Dermatologic: Rash (7%), pruritus (6%)
Endocrine & metabolic: Dehydration (3% to 5%)
Gastrointestinal: Abdominal pain (10%)
Local: Vascular access hemorrhage (7%), injection site pain (6%), vascular access infection (6%), vascular access thrombosis (6%)
Neuromuscular & skeletal: Limb pain (8%), myalgia (8%), back pain (7%), weakness (5%)
Respiratory: Dyspnea (2% to 10%), cough (9%), bronchitis (5%), pneumonia (3%), pulmonary embolism (1%)
Miscellaneous: Death (7% to 10 %; similar to placebo), flu-like syndrome (6%)
<1% (Limited to important or life-threatening): Abscess, allergic reaction, bacteremia, deep vein thrombosis, GI hemorrhage, hypertensive encephalopathy, peritonitis, pure red cell aplasia (PRCA), sepsis, severe anemia (with or without other cytopenias), thromboembolism, thrombophlebitis, thrombosis, tumor progression (cancer patients)

Drug Interactions
Avoid Concomitant Use There are no known interactions where it is recommended to avoid concomitant use.
Increased Effect/Toxicity There are no known significant interactions involving an increase in effect.
Decreased Effect There are no known significant interactions involving a decrease in effect.
Ethanol/Nutrition/Herb Interactions Ethanol: Should be avoided due to adverse effects on erythropoiesis.
Dietary Considerations Supplemental iron intake may be required in patients with low iron stores.
Dosage Forms Excipient information presented when available (limited, particularly for generics); consult specific product labeling.
Injection, solution [preservative free]:
Aranesp®: 25 mcg/0.42 mL (0.42 mL); 40 mcg/ 0.4 mL (0.4 mL); 60 mcg/0.3 mL (0.3 mL); 100 mcg/0.5 mL (0.5 mL); 150 mcg/0.3 mL (0.3 mL); 200 mcg/0.4 mL (0.4 mL); 300 mcg/0.6 mL (0.6 mL); 500 mcg/mL (1 mL) [contains polysorbate 80; prefilled syringe; needle cover contains latex]
Aranesp®: 25 mcg/mL (1 mL); 40 mcg/mL (1 mL); 60 mcg/mL (1 mL); 100 mcg/ mL (1 mL); 150 mcg/0.75 mL (0.75 mL); 200 mcg/mL (1 mL); 300 mcg/mL (1 mL) [contains polysorbate 80; single-dose vial]

References
Corwin HL, Gettinger A, Pearl RG, et al, "Efficacy of Recombinant Human Erythropoietin in Critically Ill Patients, A Randomized Controlled Trial," *JAMA*, 2002, 288:2827-35.
Dellinger RP, Levy MM, Carlet JM, et al, "Surviving Sepsis Campaign: International Guidelines for Management of Severe Sepsis and Septic Shock: 2008," *Intensive Care Med*, 2008, 34(1): 17-60. Available at http://www.survivingsepsis.org/system/files/images/2008_20International_20SSC_20-Guidelines_1_.pdf
Hebert PC, Wells G, Blajchman MA, et al, "A Multicenter, Randomized, Controlled Clinical Trial of Transfusion Requirements in Critical Care," *N Engl J Med*, 1999, 340(6):409-17.

◆ **Darvocet A500®** *see* Propoxyphene and Acetaminophen *on page 1197*

◆ **Darvocet-N® 50** *see* Propoxyphene and Acetaminophen *on page 1197*

◆ **Darvocet-N® 100** *see* Propoxyphene and Acetaminophen *on page 1197*

◆ **Darvon®** *see* Propoxyphene *on page 1194*

- **Darvon-N®** *see* Propoxyphene *on page 1194*
- **Daypro®** *see* Oxaprozin *on page 1065*
- **Daytrana™** *see* Methylphenidate *on page 908*
- **DDAVP®** *see* Desmopressin *on page 386*
- **DDAVP® Melt (Can)** *see* Desmopressin *on page 386*
- **1-Deamino-8-D-Arginine Vasopressin** *see* Desmopressin *on page 386*
- **Deep Sea [OTC]** *see* Sodium Chloride *on page 1304*
- **Dehydrobenzperidol** *see* Droperidol *on page 463*
- **Delatestryl®** *see* Testosterone *on page 1362*
- **Delestrogen®** *see* Estradiol *on page 531*
- **Delta-9-tetrahydro-cannabinol** *see* Dronabinol *on page 460*
- **Delta-9 THC** *see* Dronabinol *on page 460*
- **Deltacortisone** *see* PredniSONE *on page 1166*
- **Deltadehydrocortisone** *see* PredniSONE *on page 1166*
- **Deltahydrocortisone** *see* PrednisoLONE *on page 1164*
- **Demadex®** *see* Torsemide *on page 1409*
- **Demerol®** *see* Meperidine *on page 875*
- **Depacon®** *see* Valproic Acid and Derivatives *on page 1445*
- **Depade®** *see* Naltrexone *on page 985*
- **Depakene®** *see* Valproic Acid and Derivatives *on page 1445*
- **Depakote®** *see* Valproic Acid and Derivatives *on page 1445*
- **Depakote® ER** *see* Valproic Acid and Derivatives *on page 1445*
- **Depakote® Sprinkle** *see* Valproic Acid and Derivatives *on page 1445*
- **Deplin™** *see* Methylfolate *on page 906*
- **DepoDur®** *see* Morphine Sulfate *on page 953*
- **Depo®-Estradiol** *see* Estradiol *on page 531*
- **Depo-Medrol®** *see* MethylPREDNISolone *on page 911*
- **Depotest® 100 (Can)** *see* Testosterone *on page 1362*
- **Depo®-Testosterone** *see* Testosterone *on page 1362*
- **Deprenyl** *see* Selegiline *on page 1282*
- **Dermamycin® [OTC]** *see* DiphenhydrAMINE *on page 430*
- **Dermarest® Dricort® [OTC]** *see* Hydrocortisone *on page 699*
- **Dermtex® HC [OTC]** *see* Hydrocortisone *on page 699*

Desflurane (DES flure ane)

Medication Safety Issues
Sound-alike/look-alike issues:
Desflurane may be confused with Desferal®

High alert medication: The Institute for Safe Medication Practices (ISMP) includes this medication among its list of drug classes which have a heightened risk of causing significant patient harm when used in error.

Related Information
Anesthesia Considerations for Neurosurgery *on page 1514*
Anesthetic Considerations in the Substance-Abusing Patient *on page 1613*
Inhalational Anesthetics *on page 1632*

U.S. Brand Names Suprane®
Canadian Brand Names Suprane®
Pharmacologic Category General Anesthetic, Inhalation
Generic Available No

◄ **Use** Induction and/or maintenance of general anesthesia in adults; maintenance of anesthesia in intubated children; **Note:** Use of desflurane for induction of general anesthesia is not recommended due to its irritant properties and unpleasant odor which causes coughing, breath holding, laryngospasm, oxygen desaturation, increased secretions, hypertension, and tachycardia.

Unlabeled/Investigational Use Intraoperative cardio- and neuroprotection (ischemic preconditioning)

Mechanism of Action Although not completely defined, it is thought that desflurane enhances inhibitory postsynaptic channel activity and inhibits excitatory synaptic activity resulting in general anesthesia.

Pharmacodynamics/Kinetics

Onset of action: 1-2 minutes

Duration: Emergence time: Depends on blood concentration when desflurane is discontinued

The rate of change of anesthetic concentration in the lung is more rapid with desflurane because of its low blood/gas solubility (0.42), which is similar to nitrous oxide.

Metabolism: Hepatic (0.02%) to triflouroacetate (negligible) and inorganic fluoride

Excretion: Exhaled gases

Dosage

Note: Concurrent use with benzodiazepines, nitrous oxide, or opioids decreases the desflurane dose.

Children (intubated): Maintenance: Surgical levels of anesthesia range between 5.2% to 10%

Adults: The minimum alveolar concentration (MAC), the concentration at which 50% of patients do not respond to surgical incision, ranges from 6.0% (45 years of age) to 7.3% (25 years of age). The concentration at which amnesia and loss of awareness occur (MAC - awake) is 2.4%. Surgical levels of anesthesia are achieved with concentrations between 2.5% to 8.5%.

Elderly: MAC is reduced (5.2% at 70 years of age)

Note: Because of the higher vapor pressure of desflurane, its vaporizer is heated in order to deliver a constant concentration

Stability Store at room temperature of 15°C to 30°C (59°F to 86°F).

Administration Via desflurane-specific calibrated heated vaporizer

Monitoring Parameters Blood pressure, heart rate and rhythm, temperature, oxygen saturation, end-tidal CO_2 and end-tidal desflurane concentrations should be monitored prior to and throughout anesthesia

Anesthesia and Critical Care Concerns/Other Considerations

Evidence-Based Information: Acute, rapid increases in desflurane concentration can produce increased sympathetic cardiovascular stimulation which lasts for 2-4 minutes (Weiskopf, 1994). This can be blunted by concurrent use of nitrous oxide, opioids, beta-blockers, and alpha$_2$-agonists.

In animal studies, desflurane and other inhaled anesthetics have shown a protective effect (ischemic preconditioning) of the heart and brain. Human randomized controlled clinical trials have also been conducted and have supported this effect (Guarracino, 2006; Meco, 2007; Tritapepe, 2007).

Pregnancy Risk Factor B

Contraindications Hypersensitivity to desflurane, other halogenated anesthetic agents, or any component of the formulation; known or suspected susceptibility to malignant hyperthermia

Warnings/Precautions Desflurane may trigger malignant hyperthermia (MH); contraindicated in patients susceptible to MH. Due to higher incidences of airway irritation (eg, laryngospasm, coughing, breath-holding, increased secretions) in pediatric patients; do not use to induce and/or maintain anesthesia in nonintubated pediatric patients. Causes dose-dependent respiratory depression and blunted ventilatory response to hypoxia and hypercapnia. Hypoxic pulmonary vasoconstriction is blunted which may lead to increased pulmonary shunt. May produce elevated carbon monoxide levels in the presence of a dry carbon dioxide absorbent within the circle breathing system of an anesthetic machine; maintain fresh absorbent as per manufacturer guidelines regardless of state of colorimetric indicator.

Do not use desflurane as a single agent to induce anesthesia in patients with CAD or in whom an increase in heart rate or blood pressure should be avoided. Abrupt increases in inspired concentrations >1 MAC can produce a transient increase in blood pressure and heart rate due to increased plasma catecholamine levels. Hypotensive effect due to peripheral vasodilation is dose dependent and increases as anesthesia is deepened. May cause decrease in hepatic and/or renal blood flow. May dilate the cerebral vasculature and may, in certain conditions, increase intracranial pressure. In patients with intracranial space-occupying lesions, administer at ≤0.8 MAC in conjunction with a barbiturate induction and hyperventilation in the period before cranial decompression; maintain cerebral perfusion pressure. Use of other inhaled anesthetics has been associated with rare cases of perioperative hyperkalemia; concomitant use of succinylcholine was associated with many of the reported cases, but not all. Risk of hyperkalemia is increased in pediatric patients with underlying neuromuscular disease (eg, Duchenne muscular dystrophy). Other abnormalities may include elevation in CK and myoglobinuria. Monitor closely for arrhythmias. Aggressively identify and treat hyperkalemia. May cause sensitivity hepatitis in patients who have been sensitized by previous exposure to halogenated anesthetics.

Adverse Reactions
>10%:
  Gastrointestinal: Nausea (27%), vomiting (16%)
  Respiratory: Cough (3% to 34%), breath-holding (>1% to 30%), apnea (3% to 15%)
1% to 10%:
  Cardiovascular: Bradycardia, hypertension, nodal arrhythmia, tachycardia
  Central nervous system: Emergence delirium, headache
  Gastrointestinal: Salivation increased
  Ocular: Conjunctivitis
  Respiratory: Secretions increased (3% to 10%), laryngospasm (3% to 10%), oxyhemoglobin desaturation (3% to 10%), pharyngitis (>1% to 10%)
  Miscellaneous: Shivering
<1% (Limited to important or life-threatening): Abdominal pain, agitation, ALT increased, ammonia increased, arrhythmia, AST increased, asthma, bigeminy, bronchospasm, cardiac arrest, cholestasis, coagulopathy, CPK increased, cytolytic hepatitis, dizziness, dyspnea, ECG changes, erythema, hemoptysis, hemorrhage, hepatic failure, hepatic necrosis, hepatitis, hyperglycemia, hyper-/hypokalemia, hypotension, hypoxia, jaundice, malaise, malignant hypertension, malignant hyperthermia, metabolic acidosis, MI, myocardial ischemia, myalgia, ocular icterus, pancreatitis (acute), pruritus, respiratory arrest, respiratory distress, respiratory failure, rhabdomyolysis, seizure, shock, torsade de pointes, urticaria, vasodilation, ventricular failure, ventricular hypokinesia, WBC increased, weakness
Adverse reactions with accidental occupational exposure: Dizziness, encephalopathy, headache, migraine, ocular hyperpalpitations, tachyarrhythmia, unconsciousness

Drug Interactions
Avoid Concomitant Use
Avoid concomitant use of Desflurane with any of the following: Methylphenidate
Increased Effect/Toxicity
Desflurane may increase the levels/effects of: EPINEPHrine; Neuromuscular-Blocking Agents (Nondepolarizing)

The levels/effects of Desflurane may be increased by: Methylphenidate

Decreased Effect There are no known significant interactions involving a decrease in effect.

Dosage Forms Excipient information presented when available (limited, particularly for generics); consult specific product labeling.
Liquid, for inhalation:
  Suprane®: 100% (240 mL) [amber bottle]

References
Beck-Schimmer B, Breitenstein S, Urech S, et al, "A Randomized Controlled Trial on Pharmacological Preconditioning in Liver Surgery Using a Volatile Anesthetic," *Ann Surg*, 2008, 248(6):909-18.

Bein B, Renner J, Caliebe D, et al, "The Effects of Interrupted or Continuous Administration of Sevoflurane on Preconditioning Before Cardio-Pulmonary Bypass in Coronary Artery Surgery: Comparison With Continuous Propofol," *Anaesthesia*, 2008, 63(10):1046-55.

Campagna JA, Miller KW, and Forman SA, "Mechanisms of Action of Inhaled Anesthetics," *N Engl J Med*, 2003, 348(21):2110-23.

De Hert SG, Turani F, Mathur S, et al, "Cardioprotection With Volatile Anesthetics: Mechanisms and Clinical Implications," *Anesth Analg*, 2005, 100(6):1584-93.

Ebert TJ and Muzi M, "Sympathetic Hyperactivity During Desflurane Anesthesia in Healthy Volunteers. A Comparison With Isoflurane," *Anesthesiology*, 1993, 79(3):444-53.

Guarracino F, Landoni G, Tritapepe L, et al, "Myocardial Damage Prevented by Volatile Anesthetics: A Multicenter Randomized Controlled Study," *J Cardiothorac Vasc Anesth*, 2006, 20(4):477-83.

Lee MC, Chen CH, Kuo MC, et al, "Isoflurane Preconditioning-Induced Cardio-Protection in Patients Undergoing Coronary Artery Bypass Grafting," *Eur J Anaesthesiol*, 2006, 23(10):841-7.

Meco M, Cirri S, Gallazzi C, et al, "Desflurane Preconditioning in Coronary Artery Bypass Graft Surgery: A Double-Blinded, Randomised and Placebo-Controlled Study," *Eur J Cardiothorac Surg*, 2007, 32(2):319-25.

Sakai EM, Connolly LA, and Klauck J, "Inhalation Anesthesiology and Volatile Liquid Anesthetics: Focus on Isoflurane, Desflurane, and Sevoflurane," *Pharmacotherapy*, 2005, 25(12):1773-88.

Tritapepe L, Landoni G, Guarracino F, et al, "Cardiac Protection by Volatile Anaesthetics: A Multicentre Randomized Controlled Study in Patients Undergoing Coronary Artery Bypass Grafting With Cardiopulmonary Bypass," *Eur J Anaesthesiol*, 2007, 24(4):323-31.

Wang L, Traystman RJ, and Murphy SJ, "Inhalational Anesthetics as Preconditioning Agents in Ischemic Brain," *Curr Opin Pharmacol*, 2008, 8(1):104-10.

Weiskopf RB, Eger EI 2nd, Noorani M, et al, "Fentanyl, Esmolol, and Clonidine Blunt the Transient Cardiovascular Stimulation Induced by Desflurane in Humans," *Anesthesiology*, 1994, 81 (6):1350-5.

Weiskopf RB, Moore MA, Eger EI 2nd, et al, "Rapid Increase in Desflurane Concentration Is Associated With Greater Transient Cardiovascular Stimulation Than With Rapid Increase in Isoflurane Concentration in Humans," *Anesthesiology*, 1994, 80(5):1035-45.

Yasuda N, Lockhart SH, Eger EI 2nd, et al, "Kinetics of Desflurane, Isoflurane, and Halothane in Humans," *Anesthesiology*, 1991, 74(3):489-98.

◆ **Desiccated Thyroid** *see* Thyroid, Desiccated *on page 1379*

Desipramine (des IP ra meen)

Related Information
Antidepressant Agents *on page 1660*
Chronic Pain Management *on page 1546*
U.S. Brand Names Norpramin®
Canadian Brand Names Alti-Desipramine; Apo-Desipramine®; Norpramin®; Nu-Desipramine; PMS-Desipramine
Index Terms Desipramine Hydrochloride; Desmethylimipramine Hydrochloride
Pharmacologic Category Antidepressant, Tricyclic (Secondary Amine)
Use Treatment of depression
Unlabeled/Investigational Use Analgesic adjunct in chronic pain; peripheral neuropathies; substance-related disorders (eg, cocaine withdrawal); attention-deficit/hyperactivity disorder (ADHD); depression in children ≤12 years of age
Pharmacodynamics/Kinetics
Onset of action: 1-3 weeks; Maximum antidepressant effect: >2 weeks
Absorption: Well absorbed
Metabolism: Hepatic
Half-life elimination: Adults: 7-60 hours
Time to peak, plasma: 4-6 hours
Excretion: Urine (70%)
Dosage Oral (dose is generally administered at bedtime):
Children 6-12 years: Depression (unlabeled use): 10-30 mg/day or 1-3 mg/kg/day in divided doses; do not exceed 5 mg/kg/day
Adolescents: Depression: Initial: 25-50 mg/day; gradually increase to 100 mg/day in single or divided doses (maximum: 150 mg/day)
Adults:
Depression: Initial: 75 mg/day in divided doses; increase gradually to 150-200 mg/day in divided or single dose (maximum: 300 mg/day)
Cocaine withdrawal (unlabeled use): 50-200 mg/day in divided or single dose
Neuropathic pain (unlabeled use): Initial: 10-25 mg/day; increase dose every 3 days as necessary until the desired effect is obtained; usual effective dose: 50-150 mg/day (maximum dose: 150 mg/day)
Elderly: Depression: Initial dose: 10-25 mg/day; increase by 10-25 mg every 3 days for inpatients and every week for outpatients if tolerated; usual

maintenance dose: 75-100 mg/day, but doses up to 150 mg/day may be necessary

Hemodialysis/peritoneal dialysis: Supplemental dose is not necessary

Anesthesia and Critical Care Concerns/Other Considerations

Clinical Pearls/Comments: Desipramine causes less sedation and anticholinergic effects than with amitriptyline or imipramine.

Additional Information Complete prescribing information for this medication should be consulted for additional detail.

Dosage Forms Excipient information presented when available (limited, particularly for generics); consult specific product labeling.

Tablet, as hydrochloride: 10 mg, 25 mg, 50 mg, 75 mg, 100 mg, 150 mg

Norpramin®: 10 mg, 25 mg, 50 mg, 75 mg, 100 mg, 150 mg [contains soy oil]

References

American Pain Society, *Principles of Analgesic Use in the Treatment of Acute Pain and Cancer Pain*, 6th ed, Glenview, IL: American Pain Society, 2008.

◆ **Desipramine Hydrochloride** *see* Desipramine *on page 384*

Desloratadine (des lor AT a deen)

U.S. Brand Names Clarinex®

Canadian Brand Names Aerius®

Pharmacologic Category Histamine H$_1$ Antagonist; Histamine H$_1$ Antagonist, Second Generation

Use Relief of nasal and non-nasal symptoms of seasonal allergic rhinitis (SAR) and perennial allergic rhinitis (PAR); treatment of chronic idiopathic urticaria (CIU)

Pharmacodynamics/Kinetics

Protein binding: Desloratadine: 82% to 87%; 3-hydroxydesloratadine: 85% to 89%

Metabolism: Hepatic to active metabolite, 3-hydroxydesloratadine (specific enzymes not identified); undergoes glucuronidation. Decreased in slow metabolizers of desloratadine. Not expected to affect or be affected by medications metabolized by CYP with normal doses.

Half-life elimination: 27 hours

Time to peak: 3 hours

Excretion: Urine and feces (as metabolites)

Dosage Oral:

Children:

6-11 months: 1 mg once daily

12 months to 5 years: 1.25 mg once daily

6-11 years: 2.5 mg once daily

Children ≥12 years and Adults: 5 mg once daily

Dosage adjustment in renal/hepatic impairment:

Children: Not established

Adults: 5 mg every other day

Additional Information Complete prescribing information for this medication should be consulted for additional detail.

Dosage Forms Excipient information presented when available (limited, particularly for generics); consult specific product labeling.

Syrup:

Clarinex®: 0.5 mg/mL (480 mL) [contains propylene glycol, sodium benzoate; bubble gum flavor]

Tablet:

Clarinex®: 5 mg

Tablet, orally disintegrating:

Clarinex® RediTabs®: 2.5 mg [contains phenylalanine 1.4 mg/tablet; tutti-frutti flavor]; 5 mg [contains phenylalanine 2.9 mg/tablet; tutti-frutti flavor]

References

McClellan K and Jarvis B, "Desloratadine," *Drugs*, 2001, 61(6):789-96.

◆ **Desmethylimipramine Hydrochloride** *see* Desipramine *on page 384*

Desmopressin (des moe PRES in)

U.S. Brand Names DDAVP®; Stimate®

Canadian Brand Names Apo-Desmopressin®; DDAVP®; DDAVP® Melt; Minirin®; Novo-Desmopressin; Octostim®; PMS-Desmopressin

Index Terms 1-Deamino-8-D-Arginine Vasopressin; Desmopressin Acetate

Pharmacologic Category Antihemophilic Agent; Hemostatic Agent; Vasopressin Analog, Synthetic

Generic Available Yes

Use

Injection: Treatment of diabetes insipidus; maintenance of hemostasis and control of bleeding in hemophilia A with factor VIII coagulant activity levels >5% and mild-to-moderate classic von Willebrand's disease (type 1) with factor VIII coagulant activity levels >5%

Nasal solutions (DDAVP® Nasal Spray and DDAVP® Rhinal Tube): Treatment of central diabetes insipidus

Nasal spray (Stimate®): Maintenance of hemostasis and control of bleeding in hemophilia A with factor VIII coagulant activity levels >5% and mild-to-moderate classic von Willebrand's disease (type 1) with factor VIII coagulant activity levels >5%

Tablet: Treatment of central diabetes insipidus, temporary polyuria and polydipsia following pituitary surgery or head trauma, primary nocturnal enuresis

Unlabeled/Investigational Use Uremic bleeding associated with acute or chronic renal failure; prevention of surgical bleeding in patients with uremia

Mechanism of Action In a dose dependent manner, desmopressin increases cyclic adenosine monophosphate (cAMP) in renal tubular cells which increases water permeability resulting in decreased urine volume and increased urine osmolality; increases plasma levels of von Willebrand factor, factor VIII, and t-PA contributing to a shortened activated partial thromboplastin time (aPTT) and bleeding time.

Pharmacodynamics/Kinetics

Onset of action:

Intranasal: Antidiuretic: 15-30 minutes; Increased factor VIII and von Willebrand factor (vWF) activity (dose related): 30 minutes

Peak effect: Antidiuretic: 1 hour; Increased factor VIII and vWF activity: 1.5 hours

I.V. infusion: Increased factor VIII and vWF activity: 30 minutes (dose related)

Peak effect: 1.5-2 hours

Oral tablet: Antidiuretic: ~1 hour

Peak effect: 4-7 hours

Duration: Intranasal, I.V. infusion, Oral tablet: ~6-14 hours

Absorption: Sublingual: Rapid

Bioavailability: Intranasal: ~3.5%; Oral tablet: 5% compared to intranasal, 0.16% compared to I.V.

Half-life elimination: Intranasal: ~3.5 hours; I.V. infusion: 3 hours; Oral tablet: 2-3 hours

Renal impairment: ≤9 hours

Excretion: Urine

Dosage

Children:

Diabetes insipidus:

I.M., I.V., SubQ: Canadian labeling (not in U.S. labeling): ≥3 months: 0.4 mcg (0.1 mL) once daily or $^1/_{10}$ of the maintenance intranasal dose. Fluid restriction should be observed.

I.V., SubQ: Children <12 years: No definitive dosing available. Adult dosing should **not** be used in this age group; adverse events such as hyponatremia-induced seizures may occur. Dose should be reduced. Some have suggested an initial dosage range of 0.1-1 mcg in 1 or 2 divided doses (Cheetham, 2002). Initiate at low dose and increase as necessary. Closely monitor serum sodium levels and urine output; fluid restriction is recommended.

Intranasal (using 100 mcg/mL nasal solution): 3 months to 12 years: Initial: 5 mcg/day (0.05 mL/day) divided 1-2 times/day; range: 5-30 mcg/day (0.05-0.3 mL/day) divided 1-2 times/day; adjust morning and evening doses separately for an adequate diurnal rhythm of water turnover. **Note:** The nasal spray pump can only deliver doses of 10 mcg (0.1 mL) or multiples of 10 mcg (0.1 mL); if doses other than this are needed, the rhinal tube delivery system is preferred. Fluid restriction should be observed.

Oral:

U.S. labeling: ≥4 years: Initial: 0.05 mg twice daily; total daily dose should be increased or decreased as needed to obtain adequate antidiuresis (range: 0.1-1.2 mg divided 2-3 times/day). Fluid restriction should be observed.

Canadian labeling (not in U.S. labeling): ≥5 years: Initial: 0.1 mg 3 times/day; total daily dose should be increased or decreased as needed to obtain adequate antidiuresis (range: 0.3-1.2 mg divided 3 times/day). Divide daily doses so that the evening dose is 2 times higher than the morning or afternoon dose to ensure adequate antidiuresis during the night. Fluid restriction should be observed.

Sublingual formulation: Canadian labeling (not in U.S. labeling): ≥3 months: Initial: 60 mcg 3 times/day; total daily dose should be increased or decreased as needed to obtain adequate antidiuresis. Usual maintenance: 60-120 mcg 3 times/day (range: 120-720 mcg divided 2-3 times/day); divide daily doses so that the evening dose is 2 times higher than the morning or afternoon dose to ensure adequate antidiuresis during the night. Fluid restriction should be observed.

Hemophilia A and von Willebrand disease (type 1):

I.V.: ≥3 months: 0.3 mcg/kg by slow infusion; may repeat dose if needed; if used preoperatively, administer 30 minutes before procedure

Canadian labeling (not in U.S. labeling): Maximum I.V. dose: 20 mcg

Note: Adverse events such as hyponatremia-induced seizures have been reported especially in young children using this dosing regimen (Das, 2005; Molnar, 2005; Smith, 1989; Thumfart, 2005; Weinstein, 1989). Fluid restriction and careful monitoring of serum sodium levels and urine output are necessary.

Intranasal (using high concentration spray [1.5 mg/mL]): ≥11 months: Refer to adult dosing.

Nocturnal enuresis:

Oral: ≥6 years: 0.2 mg at bedtime; dose may be titrated up to 0.6 mg to achieve desired response. Fluid intake should be limited 1 hour prior to dose until the next morning, or at least 8 hours after administration. **Note:** In the Canadian labeling, use is approved for patients ≥5 years.

Sublingual formulation: Canadian labeling (not in U.S. labeling): ≥5 years: Initial: 120 mcg at bedtime; dose may be titrated up to 360 mcg to achieve desired response. Fluid intake should be limited 1 hour prior to dose until the next morning, or at least 8 hours after administration.

Children ≥12 years and Adults:

Diabetes insipidus:

I.V., SubQ: 2-4 mcg/day (0.5-1 mL) in 2 divided doses or 1/10 of the maintenance intranasal dose. Fluid restriction should be observed.

Intranasal (using 100 mcg/mL nasal solution): 10-40 mcg/day (0.1-0.4 mL) divided 1-3 times/day; adjust morning and evening doses separately for an adequate diurnal rhythm of water turnover. **Note:** The nasal spray pump can only deliver doses of 10 mcg (0.1 mL) or multiples of 10 mcg (0.1 mL); if doses other than this are needed, the rhinal tube delivery system is preferred. Fluid restriction should be observed.

Oral:

U.S. labeling: Initial: 0.05 mg twice daily; total daily dose should be increased or decreased as needed to obtain adequate antidiuresis (range: 0.1-1.2 mg divided 2-3 times/day). Fluid restriction should be observed.

Canadian labeling (not in U.S. labeling): Initial: 0.1 mg 3 times/day; total daily dose should be increased or decreased as needed to obtain adequate antidiuresis (range: 0.3-1.2 mg divided 3 times/day). Fluid restriction should be observed.

Sublingual formulation: Canadian labeling (not in U.S. labeling): Initial: 60 mcg 3 times/day; total daily dose should be increased or decreased as needed to

◀ obtain adequate antidiuresis. Usual maintenance: 60-120 mcg 3 times/day (range: 120-720 mcg divided 2-3 times/day). Fluid restriction should be observed.

Hemophilia A and mild-to-moderate von Willebrand disease (type 1):

I.V.: 0.3 mcg/kg by slow infusion; if used preoperatively, administer 30 minutes before procedure

Canadian labeling (not in U.S. labeling): Maximum I.V. dose: 20 mcg

Intranasal (using high concentration spray [1.5 mg/mL]): <50 kg: 150 mcg (1 spray); >50 kg: 300 mcg (1 spray each nostril); repeat use is determined by the patient's clinical condition and laboratory work; if using preoperatively, administer 2 hours before surgery

Adults:

Diabetes insipidus: I.M., I.V., SubQ: Canadian label (not in U.S. labeling): 1-4 mcg (0.25-1 mL) once daily or 1/10 of the maintenance intranasal dose. Fluid restriction should be observed.

Uremic bleeding associated with acute or chronic renal failure (unlabeled use; Watson, 1984): I.V.: 0.4 mcg/kg over 10 minutes

Prevention of surgical bleeding in patients with uremia (unlabeled use; Mannucci, 1983): I.V.: 0.3 mcg/kg over 30 minutes

Dosage adjustment in renal impairment: Cl_{cr} <50 mL/minute: Use is contraindicated according to the manufacturer; however, has been used in acute and chronic renal failure patients experiencing uremic bleeding or for prevention of surgical bleeding (unlabeled uses; Mannuccio, 1983; Watson, 1984)

Stability

DDAVP®:

Nasal spray: Store at controlled room temperature of 20°C to 25°C (68°F to 77°F). Keep nasal spray in upright position.

Rhinal Tube solution: Store refrigerated at 2°C to 8°C (36°F to 46°F). May store at controlled room temperature of 20°C to 25°C (68°F to 77°F) for up to 3 weeks.

Solution for injection: Store refrigerated at 2°C to 8°C (36°F to 46°F). Dilute solution for injection in 10-50 mL NS for I.V. infusion (10 mL for children ≤10 kg; 50 mL for adults and children >10 kg).

Tablet: Store at controlled room temperature of 20°C to 25°C (68°F to 77°F).

DDAVP® Melt (CAN; not available in U.S.): Store at 15°C to 25°C (59°F to 77°F) in original container. Protect from moisture.

Stimate® nasal spray: Store at controlled room temperature of 20°C to 25°C (68°F to 77°F). Keep nasal spray in upright position. Discard 6 months after opening.

Administration

I.M., I.V. push, SubQ injection: Central diabetes insipidus: Withdraw dose from ampul into appropriate syringe size (eg, insulin syringe). Further dilution is not required. Administer as direct injection.

I.V. infusion:

Hemophilia A, von Willebrand disease (type 1), and prevention of surgical bleeding in patients with uremia (unlabeled; Mannucci, 1983): Infuse over 15-30 minutes

Acute uremic bleeding (unlabeled; Watson, 1984): May infuse over 10 minutes

Intranasal:

DDAVP®: Nasal pump spray: Delivers 0.1 mL (10 mcg); for doses <10 mcg or for other doses which are not multiples, use rhinal tube. DDAVP® Nasal spray delivers fifty 10 mcg doses. For 10 mcg dose, administer in one nostril. Any solution remaining after 50 doses should be discarded. Pump must be primed prior to first use.

DDAVP® Rhinal tube: Insert top of dropper into tube (arrow marked end) in downward position. Squeeze dropper until solution reaches desired calibration mark. Disconnect dropper. Grasp the tube 3/4 inch from the end and insert tube into nostril until the fingertips reach the nostril. Place opposite end of tube into the mouth (holding breath). Tilt head back and blow with a strong, short puff into the nostril (for very young patients, an adult should blow solution into the child's nose). Reseal dropper after use.

Monitoring Parameters Blood pressure and pulse should be monitored during I.V. infusion

> **Note:** For all indications, fluid intake, urine volume, and signs and symptoms of hyponatremia should be closely monitored especially in high-risk patient subgroups (eg, young children, elderly, patients with heart failure).
>
> Diabetes insipidus: Urine specific gravity, plasma and urine osmolality, serum electrolytes
>
> Hemophilia A: Factor VIII coagulant activity, factor VIII ristocetin cofactor activity, and factor VIII antigen levels, aPTT
>
> von Willebrand disease: Factor VIII coagulant activity, factor VIII ristocetin cofactor activity, and factor VIII von Willebrand antigen levels, bleeding time
>
> Nocturnal enuresis: Serum electrolytes if used for >7 days

Anesthesia and Critical Care Concerns/Other Considerations Clinical Pearls/Comments: If desmopressin I.V. is given preoperatively, administer 30 minutes prior to surgery. If desmopressin intranasal is given preoperatively, administer 2 hours prior to surgery.

Pregnancy Risk Factor B

Contraindications Hypersensitivity to desmopressin or any component of the formulation; hyponatremia or a history of hyponatremia; moderate-to-severe renal impairment (Cl_{cr}<50 mL/minute)

> Canadian labeling: Additional contraindications (not in U.S. labeling): Type 2B or platelet-type (pseudo) von Willebrand's disease (injection, intranasal, oral, sublingual); known hyponatremia, habitual or psychogenic polydipsia, cardiac insufficiency or other conditions requiring diuretic therapy (intranasal, sublingual); nephrosis, severe hepatic dysfunction (sublingual); primary nocturnal enuresis (intranasal)

Warnings/Precautions Allergic reactions and anaphylaxis have been reported rarely with both the I.V. and intranasal formulations. Fluid intake should be adjusted downward in the elderly and very young patients to decrease the possibility of water intoxication and hyponatremia. Use may rarely lead to extreme decreases in plasma osmolality, resulting in seizures, coma, and death. Use caution with cystic fibrosis, heart failure, renal dysfunction, polydipsia (habitual or psychogenic [contraindicated in Canadian labeling]), or other conditions associated with fluid and electrolyte imbalance due to potential hyponatremia. Use caution with coronary artery insufficiency or hypertensive cardiovascular disease; may increase or decrease blood pressure leading to changes in heart rate. Consider switching from nasal to intravenous solution if changes in the nasal mucosa (scarring, edema) occur leading to unreliable absorption. Use caution in patients predisposed to thrombus formation; thrombotic events (acute cerebrovascular thrombosis, acute myocardial infarction) have occurred (rare).

Desmopressin (intranasal and I.V.), when used for hemostasis in hemophilia, is not for use in hemophilia B, type 2B von Willebrand disease, severe classic von Willebrand disease (type 1), or in patients with factor VIII antibodies. In general, desmopressin is also not recommended for use in patients with ≤5% factor VIII activity level, although it may be considered in selected patients with activity levels between 2% and 5%.

Consider switching from nasal to intravenous administration if changes in the nasal mucosa (scarring, edema) occur leading to unreliable absorption. Consider alternative rout of administration (I.V. or intranasal) with inadequate therapeutic response at maximum recommended oral doses. Therapy should be interrupted if patient experiences an acute illness (eg, fever, recurrent vomiting or diarrhea), vigorous exercise, or any condition associated with an increase in water consumption. Some patients may demonstrate a change in response after long-term therapy (>6 months) characterized as decreased response or a shorter duration of response.

Adverse Reactions Frequency may not be defined (may be dose or route related).

Cardiovascular: Blood pressure increased/decreased (I.V.), facial flushing

Central nervous system: Headache (2% to 5%), dizziness (intranasal; ≤3%), chills (intranasal; 2%)

Dermatologic: Rash

Endocrine & metabolic: Hyponatremia, water intoxication

◀ Gastrointestinal: Abdominal pain (intranasal; 2%), gastrointestinal disorder (intranasal; ≤2%), nausea (intranasal; ≤2%), abdominal cramps, sore throat

Hepatic: Transient increases in liver transaminases (associated primarily with tablets)

Local: Injection: Burning pain, erythema, and swelling at the injection site

Neuromuscular & Skeletal: Weakness (intranasal; ≤2%)

Ocular: Conjunctivitis (intranasal; ≤2%), eye edema (intranasal; ≤2%), lacrimation disorder (intranasal; ≤2%)

Respiratory: Rhinitis (intranasal; 3% to 8%), epistaxis (intranasal; ≤3%), nostril pain (intranasal; ≤2%), cough, nasal congestion, upper respiratory infection

<1% (Limited to important or life-threatening): Acute cerebrovascular thrombosis (I.V.), acute MI (I.V.), agitation, allergic reactions (rare), anaphylaxis (rare), balanitis, chest pain, coma, diarrhea, dyspepsia, edema, insomnia, itching eyes, light-sensitive eyes, pain, palpitation, seizure, somnolence, tachycardia, thinking abnormal, vomiting, vulval pain, warmth

Drug Interactions

Avoid Concomitant Use There are no known interactions where it is recommended to avoid concomitant use.

Increased Effect/Toxicity

Desmopressin may increase the levels/effects of: Lithium

The levels/effects of Desmopressin may be increased by: Analgesics (Opioid); CarBAMazepine; ChlorproMAZINE; LamoTRIgine; Nonsteroidal Anti-Inflammatory Agents; Selective Serotonin Reuptake Inhibitors; Tricyclic Antidepressants

Decreased Effect

The levels/effects of Desmopressin may be decreased by: Demeclocycline; Lithium

Ethanol/Nutrition/Herb Interactions Ethanol: Avoid ethanol (may decrease antidiuretic effect).

Dosage Forms Excipient information presented when available (limited, particularly for generics); consult specific product labeling. [CAN] = Canadian product

Injection, solution, as acetate: 4 mcg/mL (1 mL, 10 mL)

    DDAVP®: 5 mcg/mL (1 mL, 10 mL)

Solution, intranasal, as acetate: 100 mcg/mL (2.5 mL)

    DDAVP®: 100 mcg/mL (2.5 mL) [contains benzalkonium chloride; with rhinal tube]

Solution, as acetate, intranasal [spray]: 100 mcg/mL (5 mL)

    DDAVP®: 100 mcg/mL (5 mL) [contains benzalkonium chloride; delivers 10 mcg/spray]

    Stimate®: 1.5 mg/mL (2.5 mL) [delivers 150 mcg/spray]

Tablet, as acetate, oral: 0.1 mg, 0.2 mg

    DDAVP®: 0.1 mg, 0.2 mg [scored]

Tablet, as acetate, sublingual:

    DDAVP® Melt (CAN) [not available in U.S.]: 60 mcg, 120 mcg, 240 mcg

References

Cattaneo M, "Review of Clinical Experience of Desmopressin in Patients With Congenital and Acquired Bleeding Disorder," *Eur J Anesthesiol Suppl,* 1997, 14:10-4.

Chistolini A, Dragoni F, Ferrari A, et al, "Intranasal DDAVP®: Biological and Clinical Evaluation in Mild Factor VIII Deficiency," *Haemostasis,* 1991, 21(5):273-7.

Mannucci PM and Cattaneo M, "Desmopressin: A Nontransfusional Treatment of Hemophilia and von Willebrand Disease," *Haemostasis,* 1992, 22(5):276-80.

◆ **Desmopressin Acetate** *see* Desmopressin *on page 386*

◆ **Desogen®** *see* Ethinyl Estradiol and Desogestrel *on page 544*

◆ **Desogestrel and Ethinyl Estradiol** *see* Ethinyl Estradiol and Desogestrel *on page 544*

Desvenlafaxine (des ven la FAX een)

Related Information

    Antidepressant Agents *on page 1660*

U.S. Brand Names Pristiq®

Index Terms O-desmethylvenlafaxine; ODV

Pharmacologic Category Antidepressant, Serotonin/Norepinephrine Reuptake Inhibitor

Use Treatment of major depressive disorder

Pharmacodynamics/Kinetics

Distribution: V_d: 3.4 L/kg

Protein binding: 30%

Metabolism: Hepatic via conjugation, and oxidation via CYP3A4 (minor pathway)

Bioavailability: ~80%

Half-life elimination: ~11 hours; prolonged in renal failure

Time to peak, serum: ~7.5 hours

Excretion: Urine (45% as unchanged drug; ~24% as metabolites)

Dosage Oral: Adults: Depression: 50 mg once daily; doses up to 400 mg once daily have been studied; however, the manufacturer states there is no evidence that higher doses confer any additional benefit. A flat dose response curve for efficacy between 50-400 mg/day has been noted as well as an increase in adverse events.

Note: Gradually taper dose (by increasing dosing interval) if discontinuing.

Dosing adjustment in renal impairment:

Cl_{cr} ≥50 mL/minute: No dosage adjustment required

Cl_{cr} 30-50 mL/minute: 50 mg once daily (maximum)

Cl_{cr} <30 mL/minute: 50 mg every other day (maximum).

Hemodialysis: 50 mg every other day (maximum). Supplemental doses not required after HD.

Dosing adjustment in hepatic impairment: 50 mg once daily; maximum dose: 100 mg/day

Additional Information Complete prescribing information for this medication should be consulted for additional detail.

Dosage Forms Excipient information presented when available (limited, particularly for generics); consult specific product labeling.

Tablet, extended release:

Pristiq®: 50 mg, 100 mg

References

American College of Obstetricians and Gynecologists, "ACOG Committee Opinion No. 354: Treatment With Selective Serotonin Reuptake Inhibitors During Pregnancy," *Obstet Gynecol*, 2006, 108(6):1601-3.

American College of Obstetricians and Gynecologists, "ACOG Practice Bulletin No. 87 November 2007: Use of Psychiatric Medications During Pregnancy and Lactation," *Obstet Gynecol*, 2007, 110 (5):1179-98.

American Psychiatric Association, "Treatment Recommendations for Patients With Major Depressive Disorder," Second Edition, January 2000; http://www.psychiatryonline.com/pracGuide/pracGuide-Topic_7.aspx

Boyer EW and Shannon M, "The Serotonin Syndrome," *N Engl J Med*, 2005, 352(11):1112-20.

Chambers CD, Hernandez-Diaz S, Van Marter LJ, et al, "Selective Serotonin-Reuptake Inhibitors and Risk of Persistent Pulmonary Hypertension of the Newborn," *N Engl J Med*, 2006, 354(6):579-87.

DeMartinis NA, Yeung PP, Entsuah R, et al, "A Double-Blind, Placebo-Controlled Study of the Efficacy and Safety of Desvenlafaxine Succinate in the Treatment of Major Depressive Disorder," *J Clin Psychiatry*, 2007, 68(5):677-88.

Liebowitz MR, Yeung PP, and Entsuah R, "A Randomized, Double-Blind, Placebo-Controlled Trial of Desvenlavaxine Succinate in Adult Outpatients With Major Depressive Disorder," *J Clin Psychiatry*, 2007, 68(11):1663-72.

Septien-Velez L, Pitrosky B, Padmanabhan SK, et al, "A Randomized, Double-Blind, Placebo-Controlled Trial of Desvenlafaxine Succinate in The Treatment of Major Depressive Disorder," *Int Clin Psychopharmacol*, 2007, 22(6):338-47.

"Use of Psychoactive Medication During Pregnancy and Possible Effects on the Fetus and Newborn. Committee on Drugs. American Academy of Pediatrics," *Pediatrics*, 2000, 105(4 Pt 1):880-7.

◆ **Desyrel® (Can)** *see* TraZODone *on page 1423*

◆ **Detemir Insulin** *see* Insulin Detemir *on page 744*

◆ **Dex4® [OTC]** *see* Dextrose *on page 406*

Dexamethasone (deks a METH a sone)

Medication Safety Issues

Sound-alike/look-alike issues:

Dexamethasone may be confused with desoximetasone, dextroamphetamine

Decadron® may be confused with Percodan®

Maxidex® may be confused with Maxzide®

Related Information
Chronic Pain Management *on page 1546*
Corticosteroids *on page 1676*
Postoperative Nausea and Vomiting *on page 1593*
Stress Replacement of Corticosteroids *on page 1611*

U.S. Brand Names Baycadron™; Dexamethasone Intensol™; DexPak® 10 Day TaperPak®; DexPak® 13 Day TaperPak®; DexPak® 6 Day TaperPak®; DexPak® TaperPak® [DSC]; Maxidex®

Canadian Brand Names Apo-Dexamethasone®; Dexasone®; Diodex®; Maxidex®; PMS-Dexamethasone

Index Terms Dexamethasone Sodium Phosphate

Pharmacologic Category Anti-inflammatory Agent; Anti-inflammatory Agent, Ophthalmic; Antiemetic; Corticosteroid, Ophthalmic; Corticosteroid, Systemic

Generic Available Yes: Excludes ophthalmic suspension

Use

Systemic: Primarily as an anti-inflammatory or immunosuppressant agent in the treatment of a variety of diseases including those of allergic, dermatologic, endocrine, hematologic, inflammatory, neoplastic, nervous system, renal, respiratory, rheumatic, and autoimmune origin; may be used in management of cerebral edema, chronic swelling, as a diagnostic agent, diagnosis of Cushing's syndrome, antiemetic

Ophthalmic: Management of steroid responsive inflammatory conditions such as allergic conjunctivitis, iritis, or cyclitis; symptomatic treatment of corneal injury from chemical, radiation, or thermal burns, or penetration of foreign bodies.

Unlabeled/Investigational Use

Dexamethasone suppression test: General indicator consistent with depression and/or suicide

Accelerate fetal lung maturation in patients with preterm labor

Mechanism of Action Decreases inflammation by suppression of neutrophil migration, decreased production of inflammatory mediators, and reversal of increased capillary permeability; suppresses normal immune response. Dexamethasone's mechanism of antiemetic activity is unknown.

Pharmacodynamics/Kinetics

Onset of action: Acetate: Prompt

Duration of metabolic effect: 72 hours; acetate is a long-acting repository preparation

Metabolism: Hepatic

Half-life elimination: Normal renal function: 1.8-3.5 hours; Biological half-life: 36-54 hours

Time to peak, serum: Oral: 1-2 hours; I.M.: ~8 hours

Excretion: Urine and feces

Dosage Refer to individual protocols.

Children:

Antiemetic (prior to chemotherapy): I.V.: 10 mg/m^2 (initial dose) followed by 5 mg/m^2 every 6 hours as needed **or** 5-20 mg given 15-30 minutes before treatment

Anti-inflammatory immunosuppressant: Oral, I.M., I.V.: 0.08-0.3 mg/kg/day **or** 2.5-10 mg/m^2/day in divided doses every 6-12 hours

Extubation or airway edema: Oral, I.M., I.V.: 0.5-2 mg/kg/day in divided doses every 6 hours beginning 24 hours prior to extubation and continuing for 4-6 doses afterwards

Cerebral edema: I.V.: Loading dose: 1-2 mg/kg/dose as a single dose; maintenance: 1-1.5 mg/kg/day (maximum: 16 mg/day) in divided doses every 4-6 hours, taper off over 1-6 weeks

Bacterial meningitis in infants and children >2 months: I.V.: 0.6 mg/kg/day in 4 divided doses every 6 hours for the first 4 days of antibiotic treatment; start dexamethasone at the time of the first dose of antibiotic

Physiologic replacement: Oral, I.M., I.V.: 0.03-0.15 mg/kg/day **or** 0.6-0.75 mg/m^2/day in divided doses every 6-12 hours

Adults:

Antiemetic:

Prophylaxis: Oral, I.V.: 10-20 mg 15-30 minutes before treatment on each treatment day

Continuous infusion regimen: Oral or I.V.: 10 mg every 12 hours on each treatment day

Mildly emetogenic therapy: Oral, I.M., I.V.: 4 mg every 4-6 hours

Delayed nausea/vomiting: Oral: 4-10 mg 1-2 times/day for 2-4 days **or**

8 mg every 12 hours for 2 days; then

4 mg every 12 hours for 2 days **or**

20 mg 1 hour before chemotherapy; then

10 mg 12 hours after chemotherapy; then

8 mg every 12 hours for 4 doses; then

4 mg every 12 hours for 4 doses

Anti-inflammatory:

Oral, I.M., I.V. (injections should be given as sodium phosphate): 0.75-9 mg/day in divided doses every 6-12 hours

Intra-articular, intralesional, or soft tissue (as sodium phosphate): 0.4-6 mg/day

Ophthalmic:

Solution: Instill 1-2 drops into conjunctival sac every hour during the day and every other hour during the night; gradually reduce dose to every 3-4 hours, then to 3-4 times/day

Suspension: Instill 1-2 drops into conjunctival sac up to 4-6 times per day; may use hourly in severe disease; taper prior to discontinuation

Multiple myeloma: Oral, I.V.: 40 mg/day, days 1 to 4, 9 to 12, and 17 to 20, repeated every 4 weeks (alone or as part of a regimen)

Cerebral edema: I.V. 10 mg stat, 4 mg I.M./I.V. every 6 hours until response is maximized, then switch to oral regimen, then taper off if appropriate; dosage may be reduced after 24 days and gradually discontinued over 5-7 days

Extubation or airway edema: Oral, I.M., I.V. (injections should be given as sodium phosphate): 0.5-2 mg/day in divided doses every 6 hours beginning 24 hours prior to extubation and continuing for 4-6 doses afterwards

Dexamethasone suppression test (depression/suicide indicator) (unlabeled use): Oral: 1 mg at 11 PM, draw blood at 8 AM the following day for plasma cortisol determination

Cushing's syndrome, diagnostic: Oral: 1 mg at 11 PM, draw blood at 8 AM; greater accuracy for Cushing's syndrome may be achieved by the following:

Dexamethasone 0.5 mg by mouth every 6 hours for 48 hours (with 24-hour urine collection for 17-hydroxycorticosteroid excretion)

Differentiation of Cushing's syndrome due to ACTH excess from Cushing's due to other causes: Oral: Dexamethasone 2 mg every 6 hours for 48 hours (with 24-hour urine collection for 17-hydroxycorticosteroid excretion)

Multiple sclerosis (acute exacerbation): 30 mg/day for 1 week, followed by 4-12 mg/day for 1 month

Physiological replacement: Oral, I.M., I.V. (should be given as sodium phosphate): 0.03-0.15 mg/kg/day **or** 0.6-0.75 mg/m^2/day in divided doses every 6-12 hours

Treatment of shock:

Addisonian crisis/shock (ie, adrenal insufficiency/responsive to steroid therapy): I.V. (given as sodium phosphate): 4-10 mg as a single dose, which may be repeated if necessary

Unresponsive shock (ie, unresponsive to steroid therapy): I.V. (given as sodium phosphate): 1-6 mg/kg as a single I.V. dose or up to 40 mg initially followed by repeat doses every 2-6 hours while shock persists

Hemodialysis: Supplemental dose is not necessary

Peritoneal dialysis: Supplemental dose is not necessary

Stability

Injection solution: Store at room temperature; protect from light and freezing.

Stability of injection of parenteral admixture at room temperature (25°C): 24 hours

Stability of injection of parenteral admixture at refrigeration temperature (4°C): 2 days; protect from light and freezing.

Injection should be diluted in 50-100 mL NS or D$_5$W.

Administration

Oral: Administer with meals to decrease GI upset.

◄ I.V.: Administer as a 5-10 minute bolus; rapid injection is associated with a high incidence of perineal discomfort.

Ophthalmic: Remove soft contact lenses prior to using solutions containing benzalkonium chloride. Do not touch tip of container to eye.

Monitoring Parameters Hemoglobin, occult blood loss, serum potassium, and glucose; intraocular pressure (with use >6 weeks)

Reference Range Dexamethasone suppression test, overnight: 8 AM cortisol <6 mcg/100 mL (dexamethasone 1 mg); plasma cortisol determination should be made on the day after giving dose

Anesthesia and Critical Care Concerns/Other Considerations

Clinical Pearls/Comments: Dexamethasone is a long acting corticosteroid with minimal sodium-retaining potential. Corticosteroids and muscle relaxants appear to trigger some types of ICU myopathy; avoid or administer at the lowest dose possible.Patients will often have steroid-induced adverse effects on glucose tolerance and lipid profiles. In discontinuing steroid therapy in patients on long-term steroid supplementation, it is important that the steroid therapy be discontinued gradually. Abrupt withdrawal may result in adrenal insufficiency with hypotension and hyperkalemia. Patients on long-term steroid supplementation will require higher corticosteroid doses when subject to stress (ie, trauma, surgery, severe infection).Oral and intravenous steroid therapy in patients with heart failure should be administered cautiously with special attention given to signs and symptoms of fluid retention.

Evidence-Based Information:

The 2008 Surviving Sepsis Campaign Guidelines suggest the following: Intravenous hydrocortisone be given only to adult septic shock patients after blood pressure is identified to be poorly responsive to fluid resuscitation and vasopressor therapy (Grade 2C); ACTH stimulation test not be used to identify the subset of adults with septic shock who should receive hydrocortisone (Grade 2B); patients with septic shock should not receive dexamethasone if hydrocortisone is available (Grade 2B); the addition of fludrocortisone if hydrocortisone is not available and the steroid that is substituted does not have significant mineralocorticoid activity (Grade 2C); doses of corticosteroids comparable to >300 mg hydrocortisone daily **not** be used in severe sepsis or septic shock for the purpose of treating septic shock (Grade 1A). They also recommend corticosteroids **not** be administered for the treatment of sepsis in the absence of shock. There is, however, no contraindication to continuing maintenance steroid therapy or to using stress dose steroids if the patient's endocrine or corticosteroid administration history warrants (Grade 1D).

The 2008 Recommendations for the diagnosis and management of corticosteroid insufficiency in critically ill adult patients recommend a diagnosis of critical illness related corticosteroid insufficiency can be made by a delta cortisol level (after 250 mcg cosyntropin) of <9 mcg/dL or a random cortisol <10 mcg/dL (Grade 2B). However, they recommend **against** the use of ACTH stimulation test to determine if septic shock or ARDS patients should receive steroid therapy (Grade 2B). They recommend to consider using hydrocortisone in septic shock patients that have responded poorly to resuscitation and vasopressors (Grade 2B) and glucocorticoid treatment should be tapered slowly and not stopped abruptly (Grade 2B). Dexamethasone is **not** recommended for the treatment of septic shock or ARDS (Grade 1B). Fludrocortisone therapy is considered optional (Grade 2B).

Pregnancy Risk Factor C

Contraindications Hypersensitivity to dexamethasone or any component of the formulation; systemic fungal infections, cerebral malaria; ophthalmic use in viral (active ocular herpes simplex), fungal, or tuberculosis diseases of the eye

Warnings/Precautions Use with caution in patients with thyroid disease, hepatic impairment, renal impairment, cardiovascular disease, diabetes, glaucoma, cataracts, myasthenia gravis, patients at risk for osteoporosis, patients at risk for seizures, or GI diseases (diverticulitis, peptic ulcer, ulcerative colitis) due to perforation risk. Use caution following acute MI (corticosteroids have been associated with myocardial rupture). Because of the risk of adverse effects, systemic corticosteroids should be used cautiously in the elderly in the smallest possible effective dose for the shortest duration. May affect growth velocity; growth should be routinely monitored in pediatric patients. Withdraw therapy with gradual tapering of dose.

May cause hypercorticism or suppression of hypothalamic-pituitary-adrenal (HPA) axis, particularly in younger children or in patients receiving high doses for prolonged periods. HPA axis suppression may lead to adrenal crisis. Withdrawal and discontinuation of a corticosteroid should be done slowly and carefully. Particular care is required when patients are transferred from systemic corticosteroids to inhaled products due to possible adrenal insufficiency or withdrawal from steroids, including an increase in allergic symptoms. Patients receiving >20 mg per day of prednisone (or equivalent) may be most susceptible. Fatalities have occurred due to adrenal insufficiency in asthmatic patients during and after transfer from systemic corticosteroids to aerosol steroids; aerosol steroids do not provide the systemic steroid needed to treat patients having trauma, surgery, or infections. Dexamethasone does not provide adequate mineralocorticoid activity in adrenal insufficiency (may be employed as a single dose while cortisol assays are performed). The lowest possible dose should be used during treatment; discontinuation and/or dose reductions should be gradual.

Acute myopathy has been reported with high dose corticosteroids, usually in patients with neuromuscular transmission disorders; may involve ocular and/or respiratory muscles; monitor creatine kinase; recovery may be delayed. Corticosteroid use may cause psychiatric disturbances, including depression, euphoria, insomnia, mood swings, and personality changes. Pre-existing psychiatric conditions may be exacerbated by corticosteroid use. Prolonged use of corticosteroids may also increase the incidence of secondary infection, mask acute infection (including fungal infections), prolong or exacerbate viral infections, or limit response to vaccines. Exposure to chickenpox should be avoided; corticosteroids should not be used to treat ocular herpes simplex. Corticosteroids should not be used for cerebral malaria or viral hepatitis. Close observation is required in patients with latent tuberculosis and/or TB reactivity; restrict use in active TB (only in conjunction with antituberculosis treatment). Prolonged treatment with corticosteroids has been associated with the development of Kaposi's sarcoma (case reports); if noted, discontinuation of therapy should be considered. High-dose corticosteroids should not be used to manage acute head injury.

Adverse Reactions Frequency not defined.

Cardiovascular: Arrhythmia, bradycardia, cardiac arrest, cardiomyopathy, CHF, circulatory collapse, edema, hypertension, myocardial rupture (post-MI), syncope, thromboembolism, vasculitis

Central nervous system: Depression, emotional instability, euphoria, headache, intracranial pressure increased, insomnia, malaise, mood swings, neuritis, personality changes, pseudotumor cerebri (usually following discontinuation), psychic disorders, seizure, vertigo

Dermatologic: Acne, allergic dermatitis, alopecia, angioedema, bruising, dry skin, erythema, fragile skin, hirsutism, hyper-/hypopigmentation, hypertrichosis, perianal pruritus (following I.V. injection), petechiae, rash, skin atrophy, skin test reaction impaired, striae, urticaria, wound healing impaired

Endocrine & metabolic: Adrenal suppression, carbohydrate tolerance decreased, Cushing's syndrome, diabetes mellitus, glucose intolerance decreased, growth suppression (children), hyperglycemia, hypokalemic alkalosis, menstrual irregularities, negative nitrogen balance, pituitary-adrenal axis suppression, protein catabolism, sodium retention

Gastrointestinal: Abdominal distention, appetite increased, gastrointestinal hemorrhage, gastrointestinal perforation, nausea, pancreatitis, peptic ulcer, ulcerative esophagitis, weight gain

Genitourinary: Altered (increased or decreased) spermatogenesis

Hepatic: Hepatomegaly, transaminases increased

Local: Postinjection flare (intra-articular use), thrombophlebitis

Neuromuscular & skeletal: Arthropathy, aseptic necrosis (femoral and humoral heads), fractures, muscle mass loss, myopathy (particularly in conjunction with neuromuscular disease or neuromuscular-blocking agents), neuropathy, osteoporosis, parasthesia, tendon rupture, vertebral compression fractures, weakness

Ocular: Cataracts, exophthalmos, glaucoma, intraocular pressure increased

Renal: Glucosuria

Respiratory: Pulmonary edema

◄ Miscellaneous: Abnormal fat deposition, anaphylactoid reaction, anaphylaxis, avascular necrosis, diaphoresis, hiccups, hypersensitivity, impaired wound healing, infections, Kaposi's sarcoma, moon face, secondary malignancy

Drug Interactions

Metabolism/Transport Effects Substrate of CYP3A4 (major); **Induces** CYP2A6 (weak), 2B6 (weak), 2C8 (weak), 2C9 (weak), 3A4 (strong)

Avoid Concomitant Use

Avoid concomitant use of Dexamethasone with any of the following: Dronedarone; Everolimus; Natalizumab; Nilotinib; Nisoldipine; Ranolazine; Tolvaptan; Vaccines (Live)

Increased Effect/Toxicity

Dexamethasone may increase the levels/effects of: Acetylcholinesterase Inhibitors; Amphotericin B; CycloSPORINE; Leflunomide; Lenalidomide; Loop Diuretics; Natalizumab; NSAID (COX-2 Inhibitor); NSAID (Nonselective); Thalidomide; Thiazide Diuretics; Vaccines (Live); Warfarin

The levels/effects of Dexamethasone may be increased by: Antifungal Agents (Azole Derivatives, Systemic); Aprepitant; Asparaginase; Calcium Channel Blockers (Nondihydropyridine); CycloSPORINE; CYP3A4 Inhibitors (Moderate); CYP3A4 Inhibitors (Strong); Dasatinib; Estrogen Derivatives; Fluconazole; Fosaprepitant; Macrolide Antibiotics; Neuromuscular-Blocking Agents (Non-depolarizing); P-Glycoprotein Inhibitors; Quinolone Antibiotics; Salicylates; Trastuzumab

Decreased Effect

Dexamethasone may decrease the levels/effects of: Antidiabetic Agents; Calcitriol; Caspofungin; Corticorelin; CYP3A4 Substrates; Dabigatran Etexilate; Dronedarone; Everolimus; Isoniazid; Maraviroc; Nilotinib; Nisoldipine; P-Glycoprotein Substrates; Ranolazine; Salicylates; Sorafenib; Tadalafil; Tolvaptan; Vaccines (Inactivated); Vaccines (Live)

The levels/effects of Dexamethasone may be decreased by: Aminoglutethimide; Antacids; Barbiturates; Bile Acid Sequestrants; CYP3A4 Inducers (Strong); Deferasirox; Echinacea; Herbs (CYP3A4 Inducers); Mitotane; P-Glycoprotein Inducers; Primidone; Rifamycin Derivatives

Ethanol/Nutrition/Herb Interactions

Ethanol: Avoid ethanol (may enhance gastric mucosal irritation).

Food: Dexamethasone interferes with calcium absorption. Limit caffeine.

Herb/Nutraceutical: Avoid cat's claw, echinacea (have immunostimulant properties).

Dietary Considerations May be taken with meals to decrease GI upset. May need diet with increased potassium, pyridoxine, vitamin C, vitamin D, folate, calcium, and phosphorus.

Dosage Forms Excipient information presented when available (limited, particularly for generics); consult specific product labeling. [DSC] = Discontinued product

Elixir: 0.5 mg/5 mL (240 mL)

Baycadron™: 0.5 mg/5 mL (237 mL) [contains benzoic acid; ethanol 5.1%; propylene glycol; raspberry flavor]

Injection, solution, as sodium phosphate: 4 mg/mL (1 mL, 5 mL, 30 mL); 10 mg/mL (10 mL)

Injection, solution, as sodium phosphate [preservative free]: 10 mg/mL (1 mL)

Solution, ophthalmic, as sodium phosphate [drops]: 0.1% (5 mL)

Solution, oral: 0.5 mg/5 mL (500 mL)

Solution, oral [concentrate]:

Dexamethasone Intensol™: 1 mg/mL (30 mL) [dye free, sugar free; contains alcohol 30% and propylene glycol]

Suspension, ophthalmic [drops]:

Maxidex®: 0.1% (5 mL) [contains benzalkonium chloride]

Tablet [scored]: 0.5 mg, 0.75 mg, 1 mg, 1.5 mg, 2 mg, 4 mg, 6 mg

DexPak® 10 Day TaperPak®: 1.5 mg [35 tablets on taper dose card]

DexPak® 13 Day TaperPak®: 1.5 mg [51 tablets on taper dose card]

DexPak® 6 Day TaperPak®: 1.5 mg [21 tablets on taper dose card]

DexPak® TaperPak®: 1.5 mg [51 tablets on taper dose card] [DSC]

References

Coursin DB and Wood KE, "Corticosteroid Supplementation for Adrenal Insufficiency," *JAMA*, 2002, 287(2):236-40.

de Jonghe B, Sharshar T, Lefaucheur JP, et al, "Paresis Acquired in the Intensive Care Unit. A Prospective Multicenter Study," *JAMA*, 2002, 288(22):2859-67.

Dellinger RP, Levy MM, Carlet JM, et al, "Surviving Sepsis Campaign: International Guidelines for Management of Severe Sepsis and Septic Shock: 2008," *Intensive Care Med*, 2008, 34(1): 17-60. Available at http://www.survivingsepsis.org/system/files/images/2008_20International_20SSC_20-Guidelines_1_.pdf

Marik PE, Pastores SM, Annane D, et al, "Recommendations for the Diagnosis and Management of Corticosteroid Insufficiency in Critically Ill Adult Patients: Consensus Statements From an International Task Force by the American College of Critical Care Medicine," *Crit Care Med*, 2008, 36(6):1937-49.

Salem M, Tainsh RE Jr, Bromberg J, et al, "Perioperative Glucocorticoid Coverage. A Reassessment 42 Years After Emergence of a Problem," *Ann Surg*, 1994, 219(4):416-25.

Sprung CL, Annane D, Keh D, et al, "Hydrocortisone Therapy for Patients With Septic Shock," *N Engl J Med*, 2008, 358(2):111-24.

◆ **Dexamethasone Intensol™** *see* Dexamethasone *on page 391*

◆ **Dexamethasone Sodium Phosphate** *see* Dexamethasone *on page 391*

◆ **Dexasone® (Can)** *see* Dexamethasone *on page 391*

Dexmedetomidine (deks MED e toe mi deen)

Medication Safety Issues
Sound-alike/look-alike issues:
Precedex® may be confused with Peridex®

Related Information
Inhalational Anesthetics *on page 1632*
Moderate Sedation *on page 1566*
Preoperative Evaluation of the Cardiac Patient for Noncardiac Surgery *on page 1598*
Sedative Agents in the Intensive Care Unit *on page 1690*

U.S. Brand Names Precedex®

Canadian Brand Names Precedex®

Index Terms Dexmedetomidine Hydrochloride

Pharmacologic Category Alpha$_2$-Adrenergic Agonist; Sedative

Generic Available No

Use Sedation of initially intubated and mechanically ventilated patients during treatment in an intensive care setting; sedation prior to and/or during surgical or other procedures of nonintubated patients

Unlabeled/Investigational Use Unlabeled uses include premedication prior to anesthesia induction with thiopental; relief of pain and reduction of opioid dose following laparoscopic tubal ligation; as an adjunct anesthetic in ophthalmic surgery; treatment of shivering; premedication to attenuate the cardiostimulatory and postanesthetic delirium of ketamine; use in children

Mechanism of Action Selective alpha$_2$-adrenoceptor agonist with anesthetic and sedative properties thought to be due to activation of G-proteins by apha$_{2a}$-adrenoceptors in the brainstem resulting in inhibition of norepinephrine release; peripheral alpha$_{2b}$-adrenoceptors are activated at high doses or with rapid I.V. administration resulting in vasoconstriction.

Pharmacodynamics/Kinetics
Onset of action: I.V. Bolus: 5-10 minutes
  Peak effect: 15-30 minutes
Duration (dose dependent): 60-120 minutes
Distribution: V_{ss}: ~118 L; rapid
Protein binding: ~94%
Metabolism: Hepatic via N-glucuronidation, N-methylation, and CYP2A6
Half-life elimination: ~6 minutes; Terminal: ~2 hours
Excretion: Urine (95%); feces (4%)

Dosage Individualized and titrated to desired clinical effect. Manufacturer recommends duration of infusion should not exceed 24 hours; however, randomized clinical trials have demonstrated efficacy and safety comparable to lorazepam and midazolam with longer-term infusions of up to approximately 5 days. (Pandharipande, 2007; Riker, 2009).

◀ ICU sedation:

Adults: I.V.: Initial: Loading infusion (optional; see **"Note"**) of 1 mcg/kg over 10 minutes, followed by a maintenance infusion of 0.2-0.7 mcg/kg/hour; adjust rate to desired level of sedation; titration no more frequently than every 30 minutes may reduce the incidence of hypotension (Gerlach, 2009)

Note: *Loading infusion:* Administration of a loading infusion may increase the risk of hemodynamic compromise. For this indication, the loading dose may be omitted. *Maintenance infusion:* Dosing ranges between 0.2-1.4 mcg/kg/ hour have been reported during randomized controlled clinical trials (Pandharipande, 2007; Riker, 2009). Although infusion rates as high as 2.5 mcg/kg/hour have been used, it is thought that doses >1.5 mcg/kg/hour do not add to clinical efficacy (Venn, 2003).

Elderly (>65 years of age): Dosage reduction may need to be considered. No specific guidelines available. Dose selections should be cautious, at the low end of dosage range; titration should be slower, allowing adequate time to evaluate response.

Procedural sedation:

Adults: I.V.: Initial: Loading infusion of 1 mcg/kg (or 0.5 mcg/kg for less invasive procedures [eg, ophthalmic]) over 10 minutes, followed by a maintenance infusion of 0.6 mcg/kg/hour, titrate to desired effect; usual range: 0.2-1 mcg/kg/ hour

Elderly (>65 years of age): Initial: Loading infusion of 0.5 mcg/kg over 10 minutes; Maintenance infusion: Dosage reduction should be considered

Fiberoptic intubation (awake): I.V. Initial: Loading infusion of 1 mcg/kg over 10 minutes, followed by a maintenance infusion of 0.7 mcg/kg/hour until endotracheal tube is secured.

Dosage adjustment in renal impairment: Dosage reduction may need to be considered. No specific guidelines available.

Dosage adjustment in hepatic impairment: Dosage reduction may need to be considered. No specific guidelines available.

Stability Store at controlled room temperature of 25°C (77°F); excursions permitted to 15°C to 30°C (59°F to 86°F). Add 2 mL (200 mcg) of dexmedetomidine to 48 mL of 0.9% sodium chloride for a total volume of 50 mL (4 mcg/mL). Shake gently to mix.

Administration Administer using a controlled infusion device. Must be diluted in 0.9% sodium chloride solution to achieve the required concentration (4 mcg/mL) prior to administration. Advisable to use administration components made with synthetic or coated natural rubber gaskets. Parenteral products should be inspected visually for particulate matter and discoloration prior to administration. If loading dose used, administer over 10 minutes; may extend to 20 minutes to further reduce vasoconstrictive effects. Titration no more frequently than every 30 minutes may reduce the incidence of hypotension when used for ICU sedation (Gerlach, 2009).

Monitoring Parameters Level of sedation; heart rate, respiration, rhythm, blood pressure; pain control

Anesthesia and Critical Care Concerns/Other Considerations

Clinical Pearls/Comments: Dexmedetomidine causes minimal respiratory depression, inhibits salivation, and is analgesic-sparing. Assess the patient for pain during infusion; the sedation produced by this agent is not equivalent to analgesia. Adequate pain management should be addressed. Dexmedetomidine does not provide adequate and reliable amnesia; therefore, use of additional agents with amnestic properties may be necessary.

Hemodynamic effects: Dexmedetomidine is associated with hypotension and bradycardia due to inhibition of norepinephrine release from presynaptic neurons. Hypertension due to stimulation of peripheral vascular $alpha_{2b}$-adrenoceptors may also occur with rapid I.V. administration or high-dose infusion rates. In addition, rapid I.V. administration may also induce bradycardia. The loading infusion may be administered over a longer period of time (eg, 20-30 minutes) or may be omitted. Initiation of a maintenance infusion without administration of the loading infusion achieves similar levels of sedation without the undesirable hemodynamic effects (Ickeringill, 2004). When used for ICU sedation, a dosing protocol using a slower titration (≥ every 30 minutes) may reduce the incidence of hypotension associated with dexmedetomidine (Gerlach, 2009).

At low concentrations, mean arterial pressure (MAP) may be reduced without changes in other hemodynamic parameters (eg, pulmonary artery occlusion pressure [PAOP]); however, at higher concentrations (>1.9 ng/mL), MAP, CVP, PAOP, PVR, and SVR increase. An infusion rate of 0.7 mcg/kg/hour, the higher end of the manufacturer recommended dosing range, results in plasma concentrations of ~1.25 ng/mL.

Infusion duration: Infusion durations >24 hours are not recommended by the manufacturer due to the potential for the development of withdrawal symptoms (eg, hypertension, agitation). However, a study conducted in 20 critically ill patients with a mean APACHE II score of 23 (±9) demonstrated that although patients received prolonged infusions (median: 71.5 hours; range: 35-168 hours), dexmedetomidine did not produce cardiovascular rebound upon abrupt discontinuation. However, SBP and HR did increase by 7% and 11%, respectively. Patients were monitored for 24 hours after discontinuation (Shehabi, 2004).

Evidence-Based Information: In a prospective, observational study of 12 ventilator-dependent patients, dexmedetomidine was assessed as a sedative. Patients received a loading dose infusion of 1 mcg/kg over 10 minutes followed by the manufacturer's recommended infusion rate (0.2-0.7 mcg/kg/hour) for up to 7 days. Some patients required higher maintenance infusion rates than recommended by the manufacturer. Mean infusion rate was 1 ± 0.7 mcg/kg/hour. Although the maximum rate used in one patient was 2.5 mcg/kg/hour, the authors suggest that doses >1.5 mcg/kg/hour do not add to clinical efficacy. Adverse cardiovascular events were most frequently related to the initial loading infusion. These investigators suggested using a lower loading infusion; however, more recent clinical trials omit the loading infusion without compromising clinical efficacy (Pandharipande, 2007; Riker, 2009). Patients did not experience a withdrawal syndrome when the infusion was discontinued (Venn, 2003).

Double-blinded, randomized studies having enrolled a total of 481 mechanically-ventilated ICU patients have demonstrated that dexmedetomidine infusions of >24 hours duration were comparable to midazolam and lorazepam in terms of safety and efficacy. Riker et al (2009) showed that prolonged infusions (up to a maximum of 30 days) of dexmedetomidine (median duration: 3.5 days, n=224) and midazolam (median duration: 4.1 days, n=122) were not statistically different in their ability to maintain Richmond Agitation Sedation Scale (RASS) scores within a specified target range (light sedation). However, with secondary endpoints, dexmedetomidine treatment was associated with several statistically significant parameters (such as shorter time to extubation, less tachycardia, hypertension [requiring intervention], and delirium) compared to midazolam. Baseline delirium scores were high in both groups (~60%) and more patients in the dexmedetomidine group had sedation discontinued due to extubation (59% vs 45%). Dexmedetomidine treatment was associated with a significantly higher incidence of bradycardia (HR <40 beats/minute or 30% decrease from baseline), but the proportion of patients requiring intervention did not differ between the groups. The high baseline delirium rate, use of long term benzodiazepine infusions, and no standardized protocols for extubation, pain assessment, and stopping study drug may have affected the results. Previously, Pandharipande and colleagues (2007) had also shown patients sedated for up to 120 hours with dexmedetomidine (n=52) experienced a significantly lower incidence of coma and a longer percentage of time within RASS goal compared to lorazepam (n=51) sedation.

Although the overall role of dexmedetomidine for routine sedation still needs to be elucidated, it appears to be effective and safe for long term use. Comparative studies between nonbenzodiazepine regimens are in progress and will help clarify the role of dexmedetomidine for ICU sedation.

Pregnancy Risk Factor C

Contraindications There are no contraindications listed in the manufacturer's labeling.

Warnings/Precautions Should be administered only by persons skilled in management of patients in intensive care setting or operating room. Patients should be continuously monitored. Episodes of bradycardia, hypotension, and sinus arrest have been associated with dexmedetomidine. Use caution in patients with heart block, severe ventricular dysfunction, hypovolemia, diabetes, chronic ▶

hypertension, and elderly. Use with caution in patients with hepatic impairment; dosage reductions recommended. Use with caution in patients receiving vasodilators or drugs which decrease heart rate. If medical intervention is required, treatment may include stopping or decreasing the infusion; increasing the rate of I.V. fluid administration, use of pressor agents, and elevation of the lower extremities. Transient hypertension has been primarily observed during the loading dose administration and is associated with the initial peripheral vasoconstrictive effects of dexmedetomidine. Treatment of this is generally unnecessary; however, reduction of infusion rate may be required. Patients may be arousable and alert when stimulated. This alone should not be considered as lack of efficacy in the absence of other clinical signs/symptoms. When withdrawn abruptly in patients who have received >24 hours, withdrawal symptoms similar to clonidine withdrawal may result (eg, hypertension, nervousness, agitation, headaches). Use for >24 hours is not recommended by the manufacturer.

Adverse Reactions

>10%:

Cardiovascular: Hypotension (24% to 54%), bradycardia (5% to 14%)

Respiratory: Respiratory depression (37%; placebo 32%)

1% to 10%:

Cardiovascular: Atrial fibrillation (4% to 5%), hypovolemia (3%)

Endocrine & metabolic: Hypocalcemia (1%)

Gastrointestinal: Nausea (3% to 9%), xerostomia (3% to 4%)

Renal: Urine output decreased (1%)

Respiratory: Pleural effusion (32%), wheezing (≤1%)

Postmarketing and/or case reports: Abdominal pain, abnormal vision, acidosis, agitation, alkaline phosphatase increased, ALT increased, anemia, apnea, arrhythmia, AST increased, atrioventricular block, BUN increased, bronchospasm, cardiac arrest, confusion, delirium, diaphoresis, diarrhea, dizziness, dyspnea, extrasystoles, fever, GGT increased, hallucination, headache, heart block, hemorrhage, hepatic impairment, hyperbilirubinemia, hypercapnia, hyperkalemia, hypertension, hypoglycemia, hypoventilation, hypoxia, illusion, MI, neuralgia, neuritis, oliguria, pain, photopsia, pulmonary congestion, respiratory acidosis, rigors, seizure, speech disorder, supraventricular tachycardia, tachycardia, thirst, T-wave inversion, ventricular arrhythmia, ventricular tachycardia, vomiting

Drug Interactions

Metabolism/Transport Effects Substrate of CYP2A6 (major); **Inhibits** CYP1A2 (weak), 2C9 (weak), 2D6 (strong), 3A4 (weak)

Avoid Concomitant Use

Avoid concomitant use of Dexmedetomidine with any of the following: Iobenguane I 123

Increased Effect/Toxicity

Dexmedetomidine may increase the levels/effects of: Hypotensive Agents

The levels/effects of Dexmedetomidine may be increased by: Beta-Blockers; CYP2A6 Inhibitors (Moderate); CYP2A6 Inhibitors (Strong); MAO Inhibitors

Decreased Effect

Dexmedetomidine may decrease the levels/effects of: Iobenguane I 123

The levels/effects of Dexmedetomidine may be decreased by: Antidepressants (Alpha2-Antagonist); Serotonin/Norepinephrine Reuptake Inhibitors; Tricyclic Antidepressants

Dosage Forms Excipient information presented when available (limited, particularly for generics); consult specific product labeling.

Injection, solution [preservative free]:

Precedex®: 100 mcg/mL (2 mL)

References

Baddigam K, Russo P, Russo J, et al, "Dexmedetomidine in the Treatment of Withdrawal Syndromes in Cardiothoracic Surgery Patients," *J Intensive Care Med*, 2005, 20(2):118-23.

Gerlach AT and Dasta JF, "Dexmedetomidine: An Updated Review," *Ann Pharmacother*, 2007, 41 (2):245-52.

Ickeringill M, Shehabi Y, Adamson H, et al, "Dexmedetomidine Infusion Without Loading Dose in Surgical Patients Requiring Mechanical Ventilation: Haemodynamic Effects and Efficacy," *Anaesth Intensive Care*, 2004, 32(6):741-5.

Pandharipande PP, Pun BT, Herr DL, et al, "Effect of Sedation with Dexmedetomidine vs Lorazepam on Acute Brain Dysfunction in Mechanically Ventilated Patients. The MENDS Randomized Controlled Trial," *JAMA*, 2007, 298(22):2644-53.

Phan H and Nahata MC, "Clinical Uses of Dexmedetomidine in Pediatric Patients," *Paediatr Drugs*, 2008, 10(1):49-69.

Riker RR, Shehabi Y, Bokesch PM, et al, "Dexmedetomidine vs Midazolam for Sedation of Critically Ill Patients. A Randomized Trial," *JAMA*, 2009, 301(5):489-99.

Shehabi Y, Ruettimann U, Adamson H, et al, "Dexmedetomidine Infusion for More Than 24 Hours in Critically Ill Patients: Sedative and Cardiovascular Effects," *Intensive Care Med*, 2004, 30 (12):2188-96.

Venn M, Newman J, and Grounds M, "A Phase II Study To Evaluate the Efficacy of Dexmedetomidine for Sedation in the Medical Intensive Care Unit," *Intensive Care Med*, 2003, 29(2):201-7.

◆ **Dexmedetomidine Hydrochloride** see Dexmedetomidine on page 397

Dexmethylphenidate (dex meth il FEN i date)

U.S. Brand Names Focalin®; Focalin® XR
Index Terms Dexmethylphenidate Hydrochloride
Pharmacologic Category Central Nervous System Stimulant
Restrictions C-II
Use Treatment of attention-deficit/hyperactivity disorder (ADHD)
Pharmacodynamics/Kinetics
Onset of action: Extended release: ≥0.5 hours
Duration: Extended release: 12 hours
Absorption: Immediate release: Rapid; Extended release: Bimodal
Distribution: V_d: 1.54-3.76 L/kg
Protein binding: 12% to 15%
Metabolism: Via de-esterification to inactive metabolite, d-α-phenyl-piperidine acetate (d-ritalinic acid)
Bioavailability: 22% to 25%
Half-life elimination: Immediate release: Adults: 2-4.5 hours; Children: 2-3 hours
Time to peak: Fasting:
Immediate release: 1-1.5 hours
Extended release: First peak: 1.5 hours (range: 1-4 hours); Second peak: 6.5 hours (range: 4.5-7 hours)
Excretion: Urine (90%, primarily as inactive metabolite)
Dosage Treatment of ADHD: Oral:
Children ≥6 years: Patients not currently taking methylphenidate:
Immediate release: Initial: 2.5 mg twice daily; dosage may be adjusted in increments of 2.5-5 mg at weekly intervals (maximum dose: 20 mg/day); doses should be taken at least 4 hours apart
Extended release: Initial: 5 mg once daily; dosage may be adjusted in increments of 5 mg/day at weekly intervals (maximum dose: 20 mg/day)
Adults: Patients not currently taking methylphenidate:
Immediate release: Initial: 2.5 mg twice daily; dosage may be adjusted in increments of 2.5-5 mg at weekly intervals (maximum dose: 20 mg/day); doses should be taken at least 4 hours apart
Extended release: Initial: 10 mg once daily; dosage may be adjusted in increments of 10 mg/day at weekly intervals (maximum dose: 20 mg/day)
Conversion to dexmethylphenidate from methylphenidate: Immediate release, extended release: Initial: Half the total daily dose of racemic methylphenidate (maximum dexmethylphenidate dose: 20 mg/day)
Conversion from dexmethylphenidate immediate release to dexmethylphenidate extended release: When changing from Focalin® tablets to Focalin® XR capsules, patients may be switched to the same daily dose using Focalin® XR (maximum dose: 20 mg/day)
Dose reductions and discontinuation: Reduce dose or discontinue in patients with paradoxical aggravation of symptoms. Discontinue if no improvement is seen after one month of treatment.

Dosage adjustment in renal impairment: No data available. However, considering extensive metabolism to inactive compounds, renal insufficiency expected to have minimal effect on kinetics of dexmethylphenidate.
Dosage adjustment in hepatic impairment: No data available.

◀ **Additional Information** Complete prescribing information for this medication should be consulted for additional detail.

Dosage Forms Excipient information presented when available (limited, particularly for generics); consult specific product labeling.

Capsule, extended release:

Focalin® XR: 5 mg, 10 mg, 15 mg, 20 mg [bimodal release]

Tablet, as hydrochloride: 2.5 mg, 5 mg, 10 mg

Focalin®: 2.5 mg, 5 mg; 10 mg [dye free]

References

Nissen SE, "ADHD and Cardiovascular Risk," *N Engl J Med*, 2006, 354:1445-8.

◆ **Dexmethylphenidate Hydrochloride** *see* Dexmethylphenidate *on page 401*

◆ **DexPak® 6 Day TaperPak®** *see* Dexamethasone *on page 391*

◆ **DexPak® 10 Day TaperPak®** *see* Dexamethasone *on page 391*

◆ **DexPak® 13 Day TaperPak®** *see* Dexamethasone *on page 391*

◆ **DexPak® TaperPak® [DSC]** *see* Dexamethasone *on page 391*

Dextran (DEKS tran)

Medication Safety Issues

Sound-alike/look-alike issues:

Dextran may be confused with Dexatrim®, Dexedrine®

Related Information

Allergic Reactions *on page 1508*

U.S. Brand Names Gentran® [DSC]; LMD®

Canadian Brand Names Gentran®

Index Terms Dextran 40; Dextran 70; Dextran, High Molecular Weight; Dextran, Low Molecular Weight

Pharmacologic Category Plasma Volume Expander

Generic Available No

Use Blood volume expander used in treatment of shock or impending shock when blood or blood products are not available; dextran 40 is also used as a priming fluid in cardiopulmonary bypass and for prophylaxis of venous thrombosis and pulmonary embolism in surgical procedures associated with a high risk of thromboembolic complications

Mechanism of Action Produces plasma volume expansion by virtue of its highly colloidal starch structure, similar to albumin

Pharmacodynamics/Kinetics

Onset of action: Minutes to 1 hour (depending upon the molecular weight polysaccharide administered)

Excretion: Urine (~75%) within 24 hours

Dosage I.V. (requires an infusion pump): Dose and infusion rate are dependent upon the patient's fluid status and must be individualized:

Volume expansion/shock:

Children (Dextran 40 or 70): Total dose should not exceed 20 mL/kg during first 24 hours

Adults:

Dextran 40: 500-1000 mL at a rate of 20-40 mL/minute (maximum: 20 mL/kg/day for first 24 hours); 10 mL/kg/day thereafter; therapy should not be continued beyond 5 days

Dextran 70: 500-1000 mL at a rate of 20-40 mL/minute (maximum: 20 mL/kg/day for first 24 hours)

Pump prime (Dextran 40): Varies with the volume of the pump oxygenator; generally, the 10% solution is added in a dose of 1-2 g/kg

Prophylaxis of venous thrombosis/pulmonary embolism (Dextran 40): Begin during surgical procedure and give 50-100 g on the day of surgery; an additional 50 g (500 mL) should be administered every 2-3 days during the period of risk (up to 2 weeks postoperatively); usual maximum infusion rate for nonemergency use: 4 mL/minute

Dosing in renal and/or hepatic impairment: Use with extreme caution

Stability Store at room temperature. Discard partially used containers.

Administration For I.V. infusion only (use an infusion pump). Infuse initial 500 mL at a rate of 20-40 mL/minute if hypervolemic. Reduce rate for additional infusion to 4 mL/minute. **Observe patients closely for anaphylactic reaction.**

Monitoring Parameters Observe patient for signs of circulatory overload and/or monitor central venous pressure; observe patients closely during the first minute of infusion and have other means of maintaining circulation should dextran therapy result in an anaphylactoid reaction; monitor hemoglobin and hematocrit, electrolytes, serum protein

Anesthesia and Critical Care Concerns/Other Considerations Dextran should be used with extreme caution in patients with restrictive cardiovascular disease and renal or hepatic impairment. Patients should be observed closely during the first several minutes of the infusion in case anaphylactoid reaction occurs.

Dextran 40 is known as low molecular weight dextran (LMD®) and has an average molecular weight of 40,000.
Dextran 75 has an average molecular weight of 75,000.
Dextran 70 has an average molecular weight of 70,000.

Pregnancy Risk Factor C

Contraindications Hypersensitivity to dextran or any component of the formulation; marked hemostatic defects (thrombocytopenia, hypofibrinogenemia) of all types including those caused by drugs; marked cardiac decompensation; renal disease with severe oliguria or anuria

Warnings/Precautions Hypersensitivity reactions have been reported (dextran 40 rarely causes a reaction), usually early in the infusion. Monitor closely during infusion initiation for signs or symptoms of a hypersensitivity reaction. Administration can cause fluid or solute overload. Use caution in patients with fluid overload. Use with caution in patients with active hemorrhage. Renal failure has been reported. Fluid status including urine output should be monitored closely. Exercise care to prevent a depression of hematocrit <30% (can cause hemodilution). Observe for signs of bleeding.

Adverse Reactions <1% (Limited to important or life-threatening): Mild hypotension, tightness of chest, wheezing

Drug Interactions
Avoid Concomitant Use
Avoid concomitant use of Dextran with any of the following: Abciximab
Increased Effect/Toxicity
Dextran may increase the levels/effects of: Abciximab
Decreased Effect There are no known significant interactions involving a decrease in effect.

Dosage Forms Excipient information presented when available (limited, particularly for generics); consult specific product labeling. [DSC] = Discontinued product
Infusion [premixed in D_5W; low molecular weight]:
  LMD®: 10% Dextran 40 (500 mL)
Infusion [premixed in NS; high molecular weight]:
  Gentran®: 6% Dextran 70 (500 mL) [DSC]
Infusion [premixed in NS; low molecular weight]:
  LMD®: 10% Dextran (500 mL)

◆ **Dextran 40** *see Dextran on page* 402
◆ **Dextran 70** *see Dextran on page* 402
◆ **Dextran, High Molecular Weight** *see Dextran on page* 402
◆ **Dextran, Low Molecular Weight** *see Dextran on page* 402

Dextroamphetamine and Amphetamine
(deks troe am FET a meen & am FET a meen)

U.S. Brand Names Adderall XR®; Adderall®
Canadian Brand Names Adderall XR®
Index Terms Amphetamine and Dextroamphetamine
Pharmacologic Category Stimulant
Restrictions C-II

◀ **Use** Attention-deficit/hyperactivity disorder (ADHD); narcolepsy

Pharmacodynamics/Kinetics

Onset of action: 30-60 minutes

Duration: 4-6 hours

Absorption: Well-absorbed

Distribution: V_d: Adults: 3.5-4.6 L/kg; concentrates in breast milk (avoid breast-feeding); distributes into CNS, mean CSF concentrations are 80% of plasma

Half-life elimination:

Children 6-12 years: d-amphetamine: 9 hours; l-amphetamine: 11 hours

Adolescents 13-17 years: d-amphetamine: 11 hours; l-amphetamine: 13-14 hours

Adults: d-amphetamine: 10 hours; l-amphetamine: 13 hours

Metabolism: Hepatic via cytochrome P450 monooxygenase and glucuronidation

Time to peak: T_{max}: Adderall®: 3 hours; Adderall XR®: 7 hours

Excretion: Urine (highly dependent on urinary pH); 70% of a single dose is eliminated within 24 hours; excreted as unchanged amphetamine (30%, may range from ~1% in alkaline urine to ~75% in acidic urine), benzoic acid, hydroxyamphetamine, hippuric acid, norephedrine, and p-hydroxynorephedrine

Dosage Oral: **Note:** Use lowest effective individualized dose; administer first dose as soon as awake

ADHD:

Children: <3 years: Not recommended

Children: 3-5 years (Adderall®): Initial 2.5 mg/day given every morning; increase daily dose in 2.5 mg increments at weekly intervals until optimal response is obtained (maximum dose: 40 mg/day given in 1-3 divided doses); use intervals of 4-6 hours between additional doses

Children: ≥6 years:

Adderall®: Initial: 5 mg 1-2 times/day; increase daily dose in 5 mg increments at weekly intervals until optimal response is obtained (usual maximum dose: 40 mg/day given in 1-3 divided doses); use intervals of 4-6 hours between additional doses

Adderall XR®: 5-10 mg once daily in the morning; if needed, may increase daily dose in 5-10 mg increments at weekly intervals (maximum dose: 30 mg/day)

Adolescents 13-17 years (Adderall XR®): 10 mg once daily in the morning; maybe increased to 20 mg/day after 1 week if symptoms are not controlled; higher doses (up to 60 mg/day) have been evaluated; however, there is not adequate evidence that higher doses afford additional benefit.

Adults (Adderall XR®): Initial: 20 mg once daily in the morning; higher doses (up to 60 mg once daily) have been evaluated; however, there is not adequate evidence that higher doses afforded additional benefit

Narcolepsy (Adderall®):

Children: 6-12 years: Initial: 5 mg/day; increase daily dose in 5 mg at weekly intervals until optimal response is obtained (maximum dose: 60 mg/day given in 1-3 divided doses with intervals of 4-6 hours between doses)

Children >12 years and Adults: Initial: 10 mg/day; increase daily dose in 10 mg increments at weekly intervals until optimal response is obtained (maximum dose: 60 mg/day given in 1-3 divided doses with intervals of 4-6 hours between doses)

Additional Information Complete prescribing information for this medication should be consulted for additional detail.

Dosage Forms Excipient information presented when available (limited, particularly for generics); consult specific product labeling.

Capsule, extended release:

5 mg [dextroamphetamine sulfate 1.25 mg, dextroamphetamine saccharate 1.25 mg, amphetamine aspartate monohydrate 1.25 mg, amphetamine sulfate 1.25 mg (equivalent to amphetamine base 3.1 mg)]

10 mg [dextroamphetamine sulfate 2.5 mg, dextroamphetamine saccharate 2.5 mg, amphetamine aspartate monohydrate 2.5 mg, amphetamine sulfate 2.5 mg (equivalent to amphetamine base 6.3 mg)]

15 mg [dextroamphetamine sulfate 3.75 mg, dextroamphetamine saccharate 3.75 mg, amphetamine aspartate monohydrate 3.75 mg, amphetamine sulfate 3.75 mg (equivalent to amphetamine base 9.4 mg)]

20 mg [dextroamphetamine sulfate 5 mg, dextroamphetamine saccharate 5 mg, amphetamine aspartate monohydrate 5 mg, amphetamine sulfate 5 mg (equivalent to amphetamine base 12.5 mg)]

25 mg [dextroamphetamine sulfate 6.25 mg, dextroamphetamine saccharate 6.25 mg, amphetamine aspartate monohydrate 6.25 mg, amphetamine sulfate 6.25 mg (equivalent to amphetamine base 15.6 mg)]

30 mg [dextroamphetamine sulfate 7.5 mg, dextroamphetamine saccharate 7.5 mg, amphetamine aspartate monohydrate 7.5 mg, amphetamine sulfate 7.5 mg (equivalent to amphetamine base 18.8 mg)]

Adderall XR®

5 mg [dextroamphetamine sulfate 1.25 mg, dextroamphetamine saccharate 1.25 mg, amphetamine aspartate monohydrate 1.25 mg, amphetamine sulfate 1.25 mg (equivalent to amphetamine base 3.1 mg)]

10 mg [dextroamphetamine sulfate 2.5 mg, dextroamphetamine saccharate 2.5 mg, amphetamine aspartate monohydrate 2.5 mg, amphetamine sulfate 2.5 mg (equivalent to amphetamine base 6.3 mg)]

15 mg [dextroamphetamine sulfate 3.75 mg, dextroamphetamine saccharate 3.75 mg, amphetamine aspartate monohydrate 3.75 mg, amphetamine sulfate 3.75 mg (equivalent to amphetamine base 9.4 mg)]

20 mg [dextroamphetamine sulfate 5 mg, dextroamphetamine saccharate 5 mg, amphetamine aspartate monohydrate 5 mg, amphetamine sulfate 5 mg (equivalent to amphetamine base 12.5 mg)]

25 mg [dextroamphetamine sulfate 6.25 mg, dextroamphetamine saccharate 6.25 mg, amphetamine aspartate monohydrate 6.25 mg, amphetamine sulfate 6.25 mg (equivalent to amphetamine base 15.6 mg)]

30 mg [dextroamphetamine sulfate 7.5 mg, dextroamphetamine saccharate 7.5 mg, amphetamine aspartate monohydrate 7.5 mg, amphetamine sulfate 7.5 mg (equivalent to amphetamine base 18.8 mg)]

Tablet:

5 mg [dextroamphetamine sulfate 1.25 mg, dextroamphetamine saccharate 1.25 mg, amphetamine aspartate monohydrate 1.25 mg, amphetamine sulfate 1.25 mg (equivalent to amphetamine base 3.13 mg)]

7.5 mg [dextroamphetamine 1.875 mg, dextroamphetamine saccharate 1.875 mg, amphetamine aspartate monohydrate 1.875 mg, amphetamine sulfate 1.875 mg (equivalent to amphetamine base 4.7 mg)]

10 mg [dextroamphetamine sulfate 2.5 mg, dextroamphetamine saccharate 2.5 mg, amphetamine aspartate monohydrate 2.5 mg, amphetamine sulfate 2.5 mg (equivalent to amphetamine base 6.3 mg)]

12.5 mg [dextroamphetamine sulfate 3.125 mg, dextroamphetamine saccharate 3.125 mg, amphetamine aspartate monohydrate 3.125 mg, amphetamine sulfate 3.125 mg (equivalent to amphetamine base 7.8 mg)]

15 mg [dextroamphetamine sulfate 3.75 mg, dextroamphetamine saccharate 3.75 mg, amphetamine aspartate monohydrate 3.75 mg, amphetamine sulfate 3.75 mg (equivalent to amphetamine base 9.4 mg)]

20 mg [dextroamphetamine sulfate 5 mg, dextroamphetamine saccharate 5 mg, amphetamine aspartate monohydrate 5 mg, amphetamine sulfate 5 mg (equivalent to amphetamine base 12.6 mg)]

30 mg [dextroamphetamine sulfate 7.5 mg, dextroamphetamine saccharate 7.5 mg, amphetamine aspartate monohydrate 7.5 mg, amphetamine sulfate 7.5 mg (equivalent to amphetamine base 18.8 mg)]

Adderall®:

5 mg [dextroamphetamine sulfate 1.25 mg, dextroamphetamine saccharate 1.25 mg, amphetamine aspartate monohydrate 1.25 mg, amphetamine sulfate 1.25 mg (equivalent to amphetamine base 3.13 mg)]

7.5 mg [dextroamphetamine sulfate 1.875 mg, dextroamphetamine saccharate 1.875 mg, amphetamine aspartate monohydrate 1.875 mg, amphetamine sulfate 1.875 mg (equivalent to amphetamine base 4.7 mg)]

10 mg [dextroamphetamine sulfate 2.5 mg, dextroamphetamine saccharate 2.5 mg, amphetamine aspartate monohydrate 2.5 mg, amphetamine sulfate 2.5 mg (equivalent to amphetamine base 6.3 mg)]

12.5 mg [dextroamphetamine sulfate 3.125 mg, dextroamphetamine saccharate 3.125 mg, amphetamine aspartate monohydrate 3.125 mg, amphetamine sulfate 3.125 mg (equivalent to amphetamine base 7.8 mg)]

15 mg [dextroamphetamine sulfate 3.75 mg, dextroamphetamine saccharate 3.75 mg, amphetamine aspartate monohydrate 3.75 mg, amphetamine sulfate 3.75 mg (equivalent to amphetamine base 9.4 mg)]

20 mg [dextroamphetamine sulfate 5 mg, dextroamphetamine saccharate 5 mg, amphetamine aspartate monohydrate 5 mg, amphetamine sulfate 5 mg (equivalent to amphetamine base 12.6 mg)]

30 mg [dextroamphetamine sulfate 7.5 mg, dextroamphetamine saccharate 7.5 mg, amphetamine aspartate monohydrate 7.5 mg, amphetamine sulfate 7.5 mg (equivalent to amphetamine base 18.8 mg)]

References

Gandhi PJ, Ezeala GU, Luyen TT, et al, "Myocardial Infarction in an Adolescent Taking Adderall," *Am J Health Syst Pharm*, 2005, 62(14):1494-7.

Manos MJ, Short EJ, and Findling RL, "Differential Effectiveness of Methylphenidate and Adderall® in School-Age Youths With Attention-Deficit/Hyperactivity Disorder," *J Am Acad Child Adolesc Psychiatry*, 1999, 38(7):813-9.

Pelham WE, Aronoff HR, Midlam JK, et al, "A Comparison of Ritalin® and Adderall®: Efficacy and Time-Course in Children With Attention-Deficit/Hyperactivity Disorder," *Pediatrics*, 1999, 103(4):e43. Available at: http://www.pediatrics.org/cgi/content/full/103/4/e43.

Pelham WE, Gnagy EM, Chronis AM, et al, "A Comparison of Morning-Only and Morning/Late Afternoon Adderall® to Morning-Only, Twice-Daily, and Three Times-Daily Methylphenidate in Children With Attention-Deficit/Hyperactivity Disorder," *Pediatrics*, 1999, 104(6):1300-11.

Pliszka SR, Browne RG, Olvera RL, et al, "A Double-Blind, Placebo-Controlled Study of Adderall® and Methylphenidate in the Treatment of Attention-Deficit/Hyperactivity Disorder," *J Am Acad Child Adolesc Psychiatry*, 2000, 39(5):619-26.

Swanson JM, Wigal S, Greenhill LL, et al, "Analog Classroom Assessment of Adderall® in Children With ADHD," *J Am Acad Child Adolesc Psychiatry*, 1998, 37(5):519-26.

◆ **Dextropropoxyphene** *see* Propoxyphene *on page 1194*

Dextrose (DEKS trose)

Medication Safety Issues

Sound-alike/look-alike issues:

Glutose™ may be confused with Glutofac®

High alert medication: The Institute for Safe Medication Practices (ISMP) includes this medication (hypertonic solutions ≥20%) among its list of drugs which have a heightened risk of causing significant patient harm when used in error.

Inappropriate use of low sodium or sodium-free intravenous fluids (eg D5W, hypotonic saline) in pediatric patients can lead to significant morbidity and mortality due to hyponatremia (ISMP, 2009).

Related Information

Anesthesia for Geriatric Patients *on page 1523*
Desensitization Protocols *on page 1692*
Extravasation Treatment of Drugs *on page 1789*
Malignant Hyperthermia *on page 1638*
Perioperative Management of the Diabetic Patient *on page 1584*
Status Epilepticus *on page 1737*

U.S. Brand Names BD™ Glucose [OTC]; Dex4® [OTC]; Enfamil® Glucose; GlucoBurst® [OTC]; Glutol™ [OTC]; Glutose 15™ [OTC]; Glutose 45™ [OTC]; Insta-Glucose® [OTC]; Similac® Glucose

Index Terms Anhydrous Glucose; $D_{10}W$; $D_{25}W$; $D_{30}W$; $D_{40}W$; $D_{50}W$; D_5W; $D_{60}W$; $D_{70}W$; Dextrose Monohydrate; Glucose; Glucose Monohydrate; Glycosum

Pharmacologic Category Antidote, Hypoglycemia; Intravenous Nutritional Therapy

Generic Available Yes

Use

Oral: Treatment of hypoglycemia

5% and 10% solutions: Peripheral infusion to provide calories and fluid replacement

25% (hypertonic) solution: Treatment of acute symptomatic episodes of hypoglycemia in infants and children to restore depressed blood glucose levels; adjunctive treatment of hyperkalemia when combined with insulin

50% (hypertonic) solution: Treatment of insulin-induced hypoglycemia (hyperinsulinemia or insulin shock) and adjunctive treatment of hyperkalemia in adolescents and adults

≥10% solutions: Infusion after admixture with amino acids for nutritional support

Mechanism of Action Dextrose, a monosaccharide, is a source of calories and fluid for patients unable to obtain an adequate oral intake; may decrease body protein and nitrogen losses; promotes glycogen deposition in the liver. When used in the treatment of hyperkalemia (combined with insulin), dextrose stimulates the uptake of potassium by cells, especially in muscle tissue, lowering serum potassium.

Pharmacodynamics/Kinetics

Onset of action: Treatment of hypoglycemia: Oral: 10 minutes

Maximum effect: Treatment of hyperkalemia: I.V.: 30 minutes

Absorption: Oral: Rapidly from the small intestine by an active mechanism

Metabolism: Metabolized to carbon dioxide and water

Time to peak, serum: Oral: 40 minutes

Dosage

Hypoglycemia: Doses may be repeated in severe cases

I.V.:

Infants ≤6 months: 0.25-0.5 g/kg/dose (1-2 mL/kg/dose of 25% solution); maximum: 25 g/dose

Infants >6 months and Children: 0.5-1 g/kg/dose (2-4 mL/kg/dose of 25% solution); maximum: 25 g/dose

Adolescents and Adults: 10-25 g (40-100 mL of 25% solution or 20-50 mL of 50% solution)

Oral: Children >2 years and Adults: 10-20 g as single dose; repeat in 10 minutes if necessary

Treatment of Hyperkalemia: I.V. (in combination with insulin):

Infants and Children: 0.5-1 g/kg (using 25% or 50% solution) combined with regular insulin 1 unit for every 4-5 g dextrose given; infuse over 2 hours (infusions as short as 30 minutes have been recommended); repeat as needed

Adolescents and Adults: 25-50 g dextrose (250-500 mL D_{10}W) combined with 10 units regular insulin administered over 30-60 minutes; repeat as needed or as an alternative 25 g dextrose (50 mL D_{50}W) combined with 5-10 units regular insulin infused over 5 minutes; repeat as needed

Note: More rapid infusions (<30 minutes) may be associated with hyperglycemia and hyperosmolality and will exacerbate hyperkalemia; avoid use in patients who are already hyperglycemic

Stability Stable at room temperature; protect from freezing and extreme heat. Store oral dextrose in airtight containers.

Administration

Oral: Must be swallowed to be absorbed (see Warnings/Precautions)

Parenteral: Not for SubQ or I.M. administration; dilute concentrated dextrose solutions for peripheral venous administration to a maximum concentration of 12.5%; in emergency situations, 25% dextrose has been used peripherally; for direct I.V. infusion, infuse at a maximum rate of 200 mg/kg over 1 minute; continuous infusion rates very with tolerance and range from 4.5-15 mg/kg/minute; hyperinsulinemic neonates may require up to 15-25 mg/kg/minute infusion rates

Monitoring Parameters Blood and urine sugar, serum electrolytes, I & O, caloric intake

Reference Range Normal blood sugar:

Children 0-2 years: 60-105 mg/dL

Children >2 years and Adults: 70-110 mg/dL

Pregnancy Risk Factor C/A (oral)

Contraindications Hypersensitivity to corn or corn products; diabetic coma with hyperglycemia; hypertonic solutions in patients with intracranial or intraspinal hemorrhage; patients with delirium tremens and dehydration; patients with anuria, hepatic coma, or glucose-galactose malabsorption syndrome

Warnings/Precautions Hypertonic solutions (>10%) may cause thrombosis if infused via peripheral veins; administer hypertonic solutions via a central venous catheter. Rapid administration of hypertonic solutions may produce significant hyperglycemia, glycosuria, and shifts in electrolytes; this may result in ▶

dehydration, hyperosmolar syndrome, coma, and death especially in patients with chronic uremia or carbohydrate intolerance. Excessive or rapid dextrose administration in very low birth weight infants has been associated with increased serum osmolality and possible intracerebral hemorrhage.

Use with caution in patients with diabetes. Hyperglycemia and glycosuria may be functions of the rate of administration of dextrose; to minimize these effects, reduce the rate of infusion; addition of insulin may be necessary. Administration of potassium free I.V. dextrose solutions may result in significant hypokalemia, particularly if highly concentrated dextrose solutions are used; monitor closely and/or add potassium to dextrose solutions for patients with adequate renal function. Administration of low sodium or sodium-free I.V. dextrose solutions may result in significant hyponatremia or water intoxication in pediatric patients; monitor serum sodium concentration. Abrupt withdrawal of dextrose solution may be associated with rebound hypoglycemia. An unexpected rise in blood glucose level in an otherwise stable patient may be an early symptom of infection. Do not use oral forms in unconscious patients.

Parenteral dextrose solutions contain aluminum which may accumulate to toxic levels with prolonged administration particularly in patients with impaired renal function. Patients with impaired renal function including premature neonates who receive aluminum at >4-5 mcg/kg/day accumulate aluminum at levels associated with CNS and bone toxicity.

Adverse Reactions Frequency not defined. **Note:** Most adverse effects are associated with excessive dosage or rate of infusion.

Cardiovascular: Venous thrombosis, phlebitis, hypovolemia, hypervolemia, dehydration, edema

Central nervous system: Fever, mental confusion, unconsciousness, hyperosmolar syndrome

Endocrine & metabolic: Hyperglycemia, hypokalemia, acidosis, hypophosphatemia, hypomagnesemia

Genitourinary: Polyuria, glycosuria, ketonuria

Gastrointestinal: Polydipsia, nausea, diarrhea (oral)

Local: Pain, vein irritation, tissue necrosis

Respiratory: Tachypnea, pulmonary edema

Drug Interactions

Avoid Concomitant Use There are no known interactions where it is recommended to avoid concomitant use.

Increased Effect/Toxicity There are no known significant interactions involving an increase in effect.

Decreased Effect There are no known significant interactions involving a decrease in effect.

Dosage Forms Excipient information presented when available (limited, particularly for generics); consult specific product labeling.

Gel, oral:

Dex4®: 40% (38 g) [provides 15 g/tube; tropical fruit flavor]

GlucoBurst®: 40% (375 g) [provides 15 g/packet; contains potassium 10 mg/packet, sodium 30 mg/packet, and sodium benzoate; arctic cherry flavor; gluten free]

Glutose 15™: 40% (37.5 g) [provides dextrose 15 g/tube; lemon or grape flavor; dye free]

Glutose 45™: 40% (112.5 g) [provides dextrose 45 g/tube; lemon flavor]

Insta-Glucose®: 40% (30 g) [provides dextrose 12 g and additional carbohydrates 12 g/tube; cherry flavor]

Infusion:

Generics:

2.5% (1000 mL)

5% (25 mL, 50 mL, 100 mL, 150 mL, 250 mL, 500 mL, 1000 mL)

10% (250 mL, 500 mL, 1000 mL)

20% (500 mL)

30% (500 mL)

40% (500 mL)

50% (500 mL, 1000 mL, 2000 mL)

60% (500 mL, 1000 mL)

70% (500 mL, 1000 mL, 2000 mL)
Injection, solution: 10% (5 mL); 25% (10 mL); 50% (50 mL)
Injection, solution: 5% (10 mL) [for measurement of cardiac output]
Liquid, oral:
Dex4®: 15 g/60 mL (60 mL) [gluten free; berry burst and lemon-lime flavor]
Solution, oral:
Enfamil® Glucose: 5% (89 mL) [provides dextrose 4 g/bottle]; 10% (89 mL)
[provides dextrose 9 g/bottle]
Glutol™: 55% (180 mL) [provides dextrose 100 g/180 mL]
Similac® Glucose: 5% (60 mL); 10% (60 mL)
Tablet, chewable:
BD™ Glucose: 5 g [orange flavor]
Dex4®: 4 g [assorted fruit, grape, raspberry, orange, sour apple, and watermelon
flavor]
GlucoBurst®: 5 g [sour apple and sour cherry flavor; gluten free]

References

AACE Diabetes Mellitus Clinical Practice Guidelines Task Force, "American Association of Clinical
Endocrinologists Medical Guidelines for Clinical Practice for the Management of Diabetes Mellitus,"
Endocr Pract, 2007, 13(Suppl 1):1-68.
American Diabetes Association, "Standards of Medical Care in Diabetes Mellitus - 2008," *Diabetes
Care*, 2008, 30(Suppl 1):12-54.

◆ **Dextrose Monohydrate** *see* Dextrose *on page 406*

◆ **DHPG Sodium** *see* Ganciclovir *on page 654*

◆ **Diabeta** *see* GlyBURIDE *on page 666*

◆ **Diaβeta®** *see* GlyBURIDE *on page 666*

◆ **Diamox® (Can)** *see* AcetaZOLAMIDE *on page 31*

◆ **Diamox® Sequels®** *see* AcetaZOLAMIDE *on page 31*

◆ **Diastat®** *see* Diazepam *on page 409*

◆ **Diastat® AcuDial™** *see* Diazepam *on page 409*

◆ **Diastat® Rectal Delivery System (Can)** *see* Diazepam *on page 409*

◆ **Diazemuls® (Can)** *see* Diazepam *on page 409*

Diazepam (dye AZ e pam)

Medication Safety Issues
Sound-alike/look-alike issues:
Diazepam may be confused with diazoxide, diltiazem, Ditropan®, LORazepam
Valium® may be confused with Valcyte®

Related Information
Anesthesia Considerations for Neurosurgery *on page 1514*
Anesthesia for Patients With Liver Disease *on page 1537*
Anesthetic Considerations in the Substance-Abusing Patient *on page 1613*
Benzodiazepines *on page 1666*
Dosing Considerations for the Critically-Ill Patient With Morbid Obesity *on page 1561*
Intravenous Anesthetic Agents *on page 1635*
Moderate Sedation *on page 1566*
Perioperative Management of Patients on Antiseizure Medication *on page 1577*
Sedative Agents in the Intensive Care Unit *on page 1690*
Status Epilepticus *on page 1737*

U.S. Brand Names Diastat®; Diastat® AcuDial™; Diazepam Intensol™; Valium®

Canadian Brand Names Apo-Diazepam®; Diastat®; Diastat® Rectal Delivery
System; Diazemuls®; Novo-Dipam; Valium®

Pharmacologic Category Benzodiazepine

Restrictions C-IV

Generic Available Yes: Injection, tablet, solution only

Use Management of anxiety disorders, ethanol withdrawal symptoms; skeletal
muscle relaxant; treatment of convulsive disorders; preoperative or preprocedural
sedation and amnesia

◀ Rectal gel: Management of selected, refractory epilepsy patients on stable regimens of antiepileptic drugs requiring intermittent use of diazepam to control episodes of increased seizure activity

Unlabeled/Investigational Use Panic disorders

Mechanism of Action Binds to stereospecific benzodiazepine receptors on the postsynaptic GABA neuron at several sites within the central nervous system, including the limbic system, reticular formation. Enhancement of the inhibitory effect of GABA on neuronal excitability results by increased neuronal membrane permeability to chloride ions. This shift in chloride ions results in hyperpolarization (a less excitable state) and stabilization.

Pharmacodynamics/Kinetics

I.V.: Status epilepticus:

Onset of action: Almost immediate

Duration: 20-30 minutes

Absorption: Oral: 85% to 100%, more reliable than I.M.

Protein binding: 98%

Metabolism: Hepatic

Half-life elimination: Parent drug: Adults: 20-50 hours; increased half-life in neonates, elderly, and those with severe hepatic disorders; Active major metabolite (desmethyldiazepam): 50-100 hours; may be prolonged in neonates

Dosage Oral absorption is more reliable than I.M.

Children:

Conscious sedation for procedures: Oral: 0.2-0.3 mg/kg (maximum: 10 mg) 45-60 minutes prior to procedure

Muscle spasm associated with tetanus: I.V., I.M.:

Infants >30 days: 1-2 mg/dose every 3-4 hours as needed

Children ≥5 years: 5-10 mg/dose every 3-4 hours as needed

Sedation/muscle relaxant/anxiety:

Oral: 0.12-0.8 mg/kg/day in divided doses every 6-8 hours

I.M., I.V.: 0.04-0.3 mg/kg/dose every 2-4 hours to a maximum of 0.6 mg/kg within an 8-hour period if needed

Status epilepticus:

I.V.: Infants >30 days and Children: 0.1-0.3 mg/kg given over ≤5 mg/minute; may repeat dose after 5-10 minutes; maximum: 10 mg/dose (Hegenbarth, 2008)

Rectal gel: 0.5 mg/kg, then 0.25 mg/kg in 10 minutes if needed

Anticonvulsant (acute treatment): Rectal gel:

Children <2 years: Safety and efficacy have not been studied

Children 2-5 years: 0.5 mg/kg

Children 6-11 years: 0.3 mg/kg

Children ≥12 years: 0.2 mg/kg

Note: Dosage should be rounded upward to the next available dose, 2.5, 5, 7.5, 10, 12.5, 15, 17.5, and 20 mg/dose; dose may be repeated in 4-12 hours if needed; do not use for more than 5 episodes per month or more than one episode every 5 days

Adolescents: Conscious sedation for procedures:

Oral: 10 mg

I.V.: 5 mg, may repeat with 1/2 dose if needed

Adults:

Acute ethanol withdrawal: Oral: 10 mg 3-4 times during first 24 hours, then decrease to 5 mg 3-4 times/day as needed

Anticonvulsant (acute treatment): Rectal gel: 0.2 mg/kg

Note: Dosage should be rounded upward to the next available dose, 2.5, 5, 7.5, 10, 12.5, 15, 17.5, and 20 mg/dose; dose may be repeated in 4-12 hours if needed; do not use for more than 5 episodes per month or more than one episode every 5 days.

Anxiety (symptoms/disorders):

Oral: 2-10 mg 2-4 times/day

I.M., I.V.: 2-10 mg, may repeat in 3-4 hours if needed

Muscle spasm: I.V., I.M.: Initial: 5-10 mg; then 5-10 mg in 3-4 hours, if necessary. Larger doses may be required if associated with tetanus.

Sedation in the ICU patient: I.V.: 0.03-0.1 mg/kg every 30 minutes to 6 hours

Skeletal muscle relaxant (adjunct therapy): Oral: 2-10 mg 3-4 times/day

Status epilepticus:

I.V.: 5-10 mg every 5-10 minutes given over ≤5 mg/minute; maximum dose: 30 mg

Rectal gel: Premonitory/out-of-hospital treatment: 10 mg once; may repeat once if necessary

Rapid tranquilization of agitated patient (administer every 30-60 minutes): Oral: 5-10 mg; average total dose for tranquilization: 20-60 mg

Elderly/debilitated patients:

Oral: 2-2.5 mg 1-2 times/day initially; increase gradually as needed and tolerated

Rectal gel: Due to the increased half-life in elderly and debilitated patients, consider reducing dose.

Dosing adjustment in renal impairment: No dose adjustment recommended; decrease dose if administered for prolonged periods.

I.V.: Risk of propylene glycol toxicity; monitor closely if using for prolonged periods or at high doses

Hemodialysis: Not dialyzable (0% to 5%); supplemental dose is not necessary

Dosing adjustment in hepatic impairment: Use with caution

Stability

Injection: Store at 20° to 25°C (68° to 77°F); excursions permitted to 15°C to 30°C (59°F to 86°F). Protect from light. Potency is retained for up to 3 months when kept at room temperature. Most stable at pH 4-8; hydrolysis occurs at pH <3. Per manufacturer, do not mix I.V. product with other medications.

Rectal gel: Store at 25°C (77°F); excursion permitted to 15°C to 30°C (59°F to 86°F).

Tablet: Store at 15°C to 30°C (59°F to 86°F).

Administration Intensol™ should be diluted before use.

Continuous infusion is not recommended because of precipitation in I.V. fluids and absorption of drug into infusion bags and tubing. In children, do not exceed 1-2 mg/minute IVP; adults 5 mg/minute.

Rectal gel: Prior to administration, confirm that prescribed dose is visible and correct, and that the green "ready" band is visible. Patient should be positioned on side (facing person responsible for monitoring), with top leg bent forward. Insert rectal tip (lubricated) into rectum and push in plunger gently over 3 seconds. Remove tip of rectal syringe after 3 additional seconds. Buttocks should be held together for 3 seconds after removal. Dispose of syringe appropriately.

Monitoring Parameters Respiratory, cardiovascular, and mental status; check for orthostasis

Reference Range Therapeutic: Diazepam: 0.2-1.5 mcg/mL (SI: 0.7-5.3 µmol/L); N-desmethyldiazepam (nordiazepam): 0.1-0.5 mcg/mL (SI: 0.35-1.8 µmol/L)

Anesthesia and Critical Care Concerns/Other Considerations

Clinical Pearls/Comments: Oral absorption is more reliable than intramuscular, which is unpredictable. Intravenous administration is associated with thrombophlebitis. Diazepam does not have any analgesic effects and, in some patients, may cause paradoxical excitation. Chronic use of this agent may increase the perioperative benzodiazepine dose needed to achieve desired effect. Abrupt discontinuation after sustained use (generally >10 days) may cause withdrawal symptoms.

Evidence-Based Information: The 2002 ACCM/SCCM guidelines for the sustained use of sedatives and analgesics in critically-ill adults recommend diazepam or midazolam for rapid sedation of acutely agitated patients.

Pregnancy Risk Factor D

Contraindications Hypersensitivity to diazepam or any component of the formulation (cross-sensitivity with other benzodiazepines may exist); myasthenia gravis; severe respiratory insufficiency; severe hepatic insufficiency; sleep apnea syndrome; acute narrow-angle glaucoma; not for use in children <6 months of age (oral)

Warnings/Precautions Withdrawal has also been associated with an increase in the seizure frequency. Use with caution with drugs which may decrease diazepam metabolism. Use with caution in elderly or debilitated patients, obese patients, patients with hepatic disease (including alcoholics), or renal impairment. Active metabolites with extended half-lives may lead to delayed accumulation and adverse effects. Use with caution in patients with respiratory disease or impaired gag reflex.

Acute hypotension, muscle weakness, apnea, and cardiac arrest have occurred with parenteral administration. Acute effects may be more prevalent in patients receiving concurrent barbiturates, narcotics, or ethanol. Appropriate resuscitative equipment and qualified personnel should be available during administration and monitoring. Avoid use of the injection in patients with shock, coma, or acute ethanol intoxication. Intra-arterial injection or extravasation of the parenteral formulation should be avoided. Parenteral formulation contains propylene glycol, which has been associated with toxicity when administered in high dosages. Administration of rectal gel should only be performed by individuals trained to recognize characteristic seizure activity and monitor response.

Causes CNS depression (dose-related) resulting in sedation, dizziness, confusion, or ataxia which may impair physical and mental capabilities. Patients must be cautioned about performing tasks which require mental alertness (eg, operating machinery or driving). Use with caution in patients receiving other CNS depressants or psychoactive agents. Effects with other sedative drugs or ethanol may be potentiated. The dosage of narcotics should be reduced by approximately 1/3 when diazepam is added. Benzodiazepines have been associated with falls and traumatic injury and should be used with extreme caution in patients who are at risk of these events (especially the elderly). Use with caution in patients taking strong CYP3A4 inhibitors, moderate or strong CYP3A4 and CYP2C19 inducers and major CYP3A4 substrates.

Use caution in patients with depression or anxiety associated with depression, particularly if suicidal risk may be present. Use with caution in patients with a history of drug dependence. Benzodiazepines have been associated with dependence and acute withdrawal symptoms on discontinuation or reduction in dose. Acute withdrawal, including seizures, may be precipitated in patients after administration of flumazenil to patients receiving long-term benzodiazepine therapy.

Diazepam has been associated with anterograde amnesia. Psychiatric and paradoxical reactions, including hyperactive or aggressive behavior, have been reported with benzodiazepines, particularly in adolescent/pediatric or elderly patients. Does not have analgesic, antidepressant, or antipsychotic properties.

Rectal gel: Safety and efficacy have not been established in children <2 years of age.

Oral: Safety and efficacy have not been established in children <6 months of age.

Injection: Safety and efficacy have not been established in children <30 days of age. Solution for injection may contain sodium benzoate, benzyl alcohol, or benzoic acid. Large amounts have been associated with "gasping syndrome" in neonates.

Adverse Reactions Frequency not defined. Adverse reactions may vary by route of administration.

Cardiovascular: Hypotension, vasodilatation

Central nervous system: Amnesia, ataxia, confusion, depression, drowsiness, fatigue, headache, slurred speech, paradoxical reactions (eg, aggressiveness, agitation, anxiety, delusions, hallucinations, inappropriate behavior, increased muscle spasms, insomnia, irritability, psychoses, rage, restlessness, sleep disturbances, stimulation), vertigo

Dermatologic: Rash

Endocrine & metabolic: Libido changes

Gastrointestinal: Constipation, diarrhea, nausea, salivation changes (dry mouth or hypersalivation)

Genitourinary: Incontinence, urinary retention

Hepatic: Jaundice

Local: Phlebitis, pain with injection

Neuromuscular & skeletal: Dysarthria, tremor, weakness

Ocular: Blurred vision, diplopia

Respiratory: Apnea, asthma, respiratory rate decreased

Drug Interactions

Metabolism/Transport Effects Substrate of CYP1A2 (minor), 2B6 (minor), 2C9 (minor), 2C19 (major), 3A4 (major); **Inhibits** CYP2C19 (weak), 3A4 (weak)

Avoid Concomitant Use There are no known interactions where it is recommended to avoid concomitant use.

Increased Effect/Toxicity

Diazepam may increase the levels/effects of: Alcohol (Ethyl); Clozapine; CNS Depressants; Methotrimeprazine; Phenytoin

The levels/effects of Diazepam may be increased by: Antifungal Agents (Azole Derivatives, Systemic); Aprepitant; Calcium Channel Blockers (Nondihydropyridine); Cimetidine; CYP2C19 Inhibitors (Moderate); CYP2C19 Inhibitors (Strong); CYP3A4 Inhibitors (Moderate); CYP3A4 Inhibitors (Strong); Dasatinib; Disulfiram; Fluconazole; Fosaprepitant; Grapefruit Juice; Isoniazid; Macrolide Antibiotics; Methotrimeprazine; Nefazodone; Oral Contraceptive (Estrogens); Oral Contraceptive (Progestins); Protease Inhibitors; Proton Pump Inhibitors; Selective Serotonin Reuptake Inhibitors

Decreased Effect

The levels/effects of Diazepam may be decreased by: CarBAMazepine; CYP2C19 Inducers (Strong); CYP3A4 Inducers (Strong); Deferasirox; Rifamycin Derivatives; St Johns Wort; Theophylline Derivatives; Yohimbine

Ethanol/Nutrition/Herb Interactions

Ethanol: Avoid ethanol (may increase CNS depression).

Food: Diazepam serum concentrations may be increased if taken with food. Grapefruit juice may increase diazepam serum concentrations; avoid concurrent use.

Herb/Nutraceutical: St John's wort may decrease diazepam levels. Avoid valerian, St John's wort, kava kava, gotu kola (may increase CNS depression).

Test Interactions False-negative urinary glucose determinations when using Clinistix® or Diastix®

Dosage Forms Excipient information presented when available (limited, particularly for generics); consult specific product labeling.

Gel, rectal [adult rectal tip (6 cm)]:
  Diastat® AcuDial™: 20 mg (4 mL) [contains benzoic acid, benzyl alcohol, ethanol 10%, propylene glycol, and sodium benzoate; delivers set doses of 12.5 mg, 15 mg, 17.5 mg, and 20 mg]

Gel, rectal [pediatric rectal tip (4.4 cm)]:
  Diastat®: 5 mg/mL (0.5 mL) [contains benzoic acid, benzyl alcohol, ethanol 10%, propylene glycol, and sodium benzoate]

Gel, rectal [pediatric/adult rectal tip (4.4 cm)]:
  Diastat® AcuDial™: 10 mg (2 mL) [contains benzoic acid, benzyl alcohol, ethanol 10%, propylene glycol, sodium benzoate; delivers set doses of 5 mg, 7.5 mg, and 10 mg]

Injection, solution: 5 mg/mL (2 mL, 10 mL)

Solution, oral: 5 mg/5 mL (5 mL, 500 mL)

Solution, oral [concentrate]:
  Diazepam Intensol™: 5 mg/mL (30 mL) [contains ethanol 19%, propylene glycol]

Tablet: 2 mg, 5 mg, 10 mg

Valium®: 2 mg, 5 mg, 10 mg

References

Bleck TB, "Seizures, Stroke, and Other Neurologic Emergencies," In: Zimmerman JL, Roberts PR, eds. *Multidisciplinary Critical Care Review*, Des Plains, IL: Society of Critical Care Medicine; 2003, 325-34.

"Clinical Practice Guidelines for the Sustained Use of Sedatives and Analgesics in the Critically Ill Adult. Task Force of the American College of Critical Care Medicine (ACCM) of the Society of Critical Care Medicine (SCCM), American Society of Health-System Pharmacists (ASHP), American College of Chest Physicians," *Am J Health Syst Pharm*, 2002, 59(2):150-78.

Jacobi J, Fraser GL, Coursin DB, et al, "Clinical Practice Guidelines for the Sustained Use of Sedatives and Analgesics in the Critically Ill Adult," *Crit Care Med*, 2002, 30(1):119-41. Available at: http://www.sccm.org/pdf/sedatives.pdf. Accessed August 2, 2003.

"Treatment of Convulsive Status Epilepticus. Recommendations of the Epilepsy Foundation of America's Working Group on Status Epilepticus." *JAMA*, 1993, 270(7):854-9.

◆ **Diazepam Intensol™** *see* Diazepam *on page 409*

Diclofenac (dye KLOE fen ak)

Related Information

Acetaminophen and NSAIDS, Dosing in the Management of Pain *on page 1651*
Chronic Pain Management *on page 1546*
Nonsteroidal Anti-Inflammatory Agents *on page 1687*

U.S. Brand Names Cataflam®; Flector®; Solaraze®; Voltaren Ophthalmic®; Voltaren®; Voltaren® Gel; Voltaren®-XR; Zipsor™

Canadian Brand Names Apo-Diclo Rapide®; Apo-Diclo SR®; Apo-Diclo®; Cataflam®; Diclofenac ECT; Diclofenac SR; Dom-Diclofenac; Dom-Diclofenac SR; Novo-Difenac ECT; Novo-Difenac K; Novo-Difenac Suppositories; Novo-Difenac-SR; Nu-Diclo; Nu-Diclo-SR; Pennsaid®; PMS-Diclofenac; PMS-Diclofenac SR; PMS-Diclofenac-K; Pro-Diclo-Rapide; Sandoz-Diclofenac; Sandoz-Diclofenac Rapide; Sandoz-Diclofenac SR; Voltaren Ophtha®; Voltaren Rapide®; Voltaren SR®; Voltaren®; Voltaren® Emulgel™

Index Terms Diclofenac Diethylamine [CAN]; Diclofenac Epolamine; Diclofenac Potassium; Diclofenac Sodium

Pharmacologic Category Nonsteroidal Anti-inflammatory Drug (NSAID); Nonsteroidal Anti-inflammatory Drug (NSAID), Ophthalmic; Nonsteroidal Anti-inflammatory Drug (NSAID), Oral; Nonsteroidal Anti-inflammatory Drug (NSAID), Topical

Use

Capsule: Relief of mild-to-moderate acute pain

Immediate-release tablet: Ankylosing spondylitis; primary dysmenorrhea; acute and chronic treatment of rheumatoid arthritis, osteoarthritis

Delayed-release tablet: Acute and chronic treatment of rheumatoid arthritis, osteoarthritis, ankylosing spondylitis

Extended-release tablet: Chronic treatment of osteoarthritis, rheumatoid arthritis

Ophthalmic solution: Postoperative inflammation following cataract extraction; temporary relief of pain and photophobia in patients undergoing corneal refractive surgery

Suppository (CAN; not available in U.S.): Symptomatic treatment of rheumatoid arthritis and osteoarthritis (including degenerative joint disease of hip)

Topical gel 1%: Relief of osteoarthritis pain in joints amenable to topical therapy (eg, ankle, elbow, foot, hand, knee, wrist)

Canadian labeling (not in U.S. labeling): Relief of pain associated with acute, localized joint/muscle injuries (eg, sports injuries, strains) in patients ≥16 years of age

Topical gel 3%: Actinic keratosis (AK) in conjunction with sun avoidance

Topical patch: Acute pain due to minor strains, sprains, and contusions

Unlabeled/Investigational Use Juvenile rheumatoid arthritis

Pharmacodynamics/Kinetics

Onset of action:

Cataflam® is more rapid than sodium salt (Voltaren®) because it dissolves in the stomach instead of the duodenum

Suppository: More rapid onset, but slower rate of absorption when compared to enteric coated tablet

Absorption: Topical gel: 6% to 10%

Distribution: ~1.4 L/kg

Protein binding: 99%, primarily to albumin

Metabolism: Hepatic; undergoes first-pass metabolism; forms several metabolites (1 with weak activity)

Bioavailability: Voltaren®, Cataflam®: 55%

Half-life elimination: Voltaren®, Cataflam®: ~2 hours; Patch: ~12 hours

Time to peak, serum: Cataflam®: ~1 hour; Flector®: 10-20 hours; Solaraze® Gel: ~5 hours; Voltaren®: ~2 hours; Voltaren® Gel: 10-14 hours; Voltaren® XR ~5 hours; Zipsor™: ~0.5 hour; Suppository: ≤1 hour. **Note:** Suppository: C_{max}: Approximately two-thirds of that observed with enteric coated tablet (equivalent 50 mg dose).

Excretion: Urine (65%); feces (35%)

Dosage Adults:
Oral:
Analgesia:
Immediate release tablet: Starting dose: 50 mg 3 times/day (maximum dose: 150 mg/day); may administer 100 mg loading dose, followed by 50 mg every 8 hours (maximum dose day 1: 200 mg/day; maximum dose day 2 and thereafter: 150 mg/day)
Immediate release capsule: 25 mg 4 times/day
Primary dysmenorrhea: Immediate release tablet: Starting dose: 50 mg 3 times/day (maximum dose: 150 mg/day); may administer 100 mg loading dose, followed by 50 mg every 8 hours (maximum dose day 1: 200 mg/day; maximum dose day 2 and thereafter: 150 mg/day)
Rheumatoid arthritis: Immediate or delayed release tablet: 150-200 mg/day in 2-4 divided doses; Extended release tablet: 100-200 mg/day
Canadian labeling: 150 mg/day in 3 divided doses (75-150 mg/day of slow release tablet)
Osteoarthritis: Immediate or delayed release tablet: 100-150 mg/day in 2-3 divided doses; Extended release tablet: 100 mg/day
Canadian labeling: 150 mg/day in 3 divided doses (75-150 mg/day of slow release tablet)
Ankylosing spondylitis: Delayed release tablet: 100-125 mg/day in 4-5 divided doses
Ophthalmic:
Cataract surgery: Instill 1 drop into affected eye 4 times/day beginning 24 hours after cataract surgery and continuing for 2 weeks
Corneal refractive surgery: Instill 1-2 drops into affected eye within the hour prior to surgery, within 15 minutes following surgery, and then continue for 4 times/day, up to 3 days
Rectal suppository (not available in U.S.):
Osteoarthritis: *Canadian labeling:* Insert 50 mg or 100 mg suppository rectally as single dose to substitute for final (third) oral daily dose; maximum combined dose (rectal and oral): 150 mg/day
Rheumatoid arthritis: *Canadian labeling:* Insert 50 mg or 100 mg suppository rectally as single dose to substitute for final (third) oral daily dose (maximum combined dose [rectal and oral]: 150 mg/day
Topical gel:
Actinic keratoses (Solaraze® Gel): Apply 3% gel to lesion area twice daily for 60-90 days
Acute pain (strains, sprains, contusions) (Voltaren® Emulgel™ [CAN; not available in U.S.]): Apply to affected area(s) of skin 3 or 4 times daily for up to 7 days
Osteoarthritis (Voltaren® Gel): **Note:** Maximum total body dose of 1% gel should not exceed 32 g per day
Lower extremities: Apply 4 g of 1% gel to affected area 4 times daily (maximum: 16 g per joint per day)
Upper extremities: Apply 2 g of 1% gel to affected area 4 times daily (maximum: 8 g per joint per day)
Transdermal patch: Acute pain (strains, sprains, contusions): Apply 1 patch twice daily to most painful area of skin

Dosage adjustment in renal impairment: Not recommended in patients with advanced renal disease or significant renal impairment
Dosage adjustment in hepatic impairment: May require dosage adjustment.
Elderly: No specific dosing recommendations; elderly may demonstrate adverse effects at lower doses than younger adults, and >60% may develop asymptomatic peptic ulceration with or without hemorrhage; monitor renal function

Anesthesia and Critical Care Concerns/Other Considerations The 2002 ACCM/SCCM guidelines for analgesia (critically-ill adult) suggest that NSAIDs may be used in combination with opioids in select patients for pain management. Concern about adverse events (increased risk of renal dysfunction, altered platelet function and gastrointestinal irritation) limits its use in patients who have other underlying risks for these events.

In short-term use, NSAIDs vary considerably in their effect on blood pressure. When NSAIDs are used in patients with hypertension, appropriate monitoring of blood pressure responses should be completed and the duration of therapy, when possible, kept short. The use of NSAIDs in the treatment of patients with congestive heart failure may be associated with an increased risk for fluid accumulation and edema; may precipitate renal failure in dehydrated patients.

Additional Information Complete prescribing information for this medication should be consulted for additional detail.

Dosage Forms Excipient information presented when available (limited, particularly for generics); consult specific product labeling. [DSC] = Discontinued product; [CAN] = Canadian product [not available in U.S]

Capsule, liquid filled, as potassium:
  Zipsor™: 25 mg [contains gelatin]
Gel, as diethylamine:
  Voltaren® Emulgel™ [CAN]: 1.16% (20 g, 50 g, 100 g)
Gel, as sodium:
  Solaraze®: 3% (50 g, 100 g)
  Voltaren® Gel: 1% (100 g)
Solution, ophthalmic, as sodium [drops]: 0.1% (2.5 mL, 5 mL)
  Voltaren Ophthalmic®: 0.1% (2.5 mL, 5 mL)
Suppository, as sodium [CAN]:
  Voltaren®: 50 mg, 100 mg
Tablet, as potassium: 50 mg
  Cataflam®: 50 mg
Tablet, delayed release, enteric coated, as sodium: 50 mg, 75 mg
  Voltaren®: 25 mg [DSC], 50 mg [DSC], 75 mg
Tablet, extended release, as sodium: 100 mg
  Voltaren®-XR: 100 mg
Transdermal system, topical, as epolamine:
  Flector®: 1.3% (30s) [180 mg]

References
"Clinical Practice Guidelines for the Sustained Use of Sedatives and Analgesics in the Critically Ill Adult. Task Force of the American College of Critical Care Medicine (ACCM) of the Society of Critical Care Medicine (SCCM), American Society of Health-System Pharmacists (ASHP), American College of Chest Physicians," *Am J Health Syst Pharm*, 2002, 59(2):150-78.

Diflunisal (dye FLOO ni sal)

Related Information

Canadian Brand Names Apo-Diflunisal®; Novo-Diflunisal; Nu-Diflunisal

Index Terms Dolobid

Pharmacologic Category Nonsteroidal Anti-inflammatory Drug (NSAID), Oral

Use Management of inflammatory disorders usually including rheumatoid arthritis and osteoarthritis; can be used as an analgesic for treatment of mild-to-moderate pain

Pharmacodynamics/Kinetics

Onset of action: Analgesic: ~1 hour; maximal effect: 2-3 hours
Duration: 8-12 hours
Absorption: Well absorbed
Protein binding: >99%
Distribution: 0.11 L/kg
Metabolism: Extensively hepatic; metabolic pathways are saturable

Half-life elimination: 8-12 hours; prolonged with renal impairment

Time to peak, serum: 2-3 hours

Excretion: Urine (~3% as unchanged drug, 90% as glucuronide conjugates) within 72-96 hours

Dosage Adults: Oral:

Mild-to-moderate pain: Initial: 500-1000 mg followed by 250-500 mg every 8-12 hours; maximum daily dose: 1.5 g

Arthritis: 500-1000 mg/day in 2 divided doses; maximum daily dose: 1.5 g

Dosing adjustment in renal impairment: Use with caution; Cl_{cr} <50 mL/minute: Administer 50% of normal dose (Aronoff, 1998)

Hemodialysis: No supplement required

CAPD: No supplement require

CAVH: Dose for GFR 10-50

Anesthesia and Critical Care Concerns/Other Considerations The 2002 ACCM/SCCM guidelines for analgesia (critically-ill adult) suggest that NSAIDs may be used in combination with opioids in select patients for pain management. Concern about adverse events (increased risk of renal dysfunction, altered platelet function and gastrointestinal irritation) limits its use in patients who have other underlying risks for these events.

In short-term use, NSAIDs vary considerably in their effect on blood pressure. When NSAIDs are used in patients with hypertension, appropriate monitoring of blood pressure responses should be completed and the duration of therapy, when possible, kept short. The use of NSAIDs in the treatment of patients with congestive heart failure may be associated with an increased risk for fluid accumulation and edema; may precipitate renal failure in dehydrated patients.

Diflunisal is a salicylic acid derivative which is chemically different than aspirin and is not metabolized to salicylic acid. Diflunisal 500 mg is equal in analgesic efficacy to aspirin 650 mg, acetaminophen 650 mg, and acetaminophen 650 mg/ propoxyphene napsylate 100 mg, but has a longer duration of effect (8-12 hours). It is not recommended as an antipyretic. At doses ≥2 g/day, platelets are reversibly inhibited in function. Diflunisal is uricosuric at 500-750 mg/day. It causes less GI and renal toxicity than aspirin and other NSAIDs. Fecal blood loss is 1/2 that of aspirin at 2.6 g/day.

Additional Information Complete prescribing information for this medication should be consulted for additional detail.

Dosage Forms Excipient information presented when available (limited, particularly for generics); consult specific product labeling.

Tablet: 500 mg

♦ **Digibind®** see Digoxin Immune Fab on page 422

♦ **DigiFab™** see Digoxin Immune Fab on page 422

Digoxin (di JOKS in)

Medication Safety Issues

Sound-alike/look-alike issues:

Digoxin may be confused with Desoxyn®, doxepin

Lanoxin® may be confused with Lasix®, levothyroxine, Levoxyl®, Levsinex®, Lomotil®, Lonox®, Mefoxin®, naloxone, Xanax®

High alert medication: The Institute for Safe Medication Practices (ISMP) includes this medication among its list of drugs which have a heightened risk of causing significant patient harm when used in error.

International issues:

Dilacor®: Brand name for diltiazem in the U.S.; brand name for verapamil in Brazil; brand name for barnidipine in Argentina

Lanoxin® may be confused with Lemoxin® which is a brand bane for cefuroxime in Mexico

Lanoxin® may be confused with Limoxin® which is a brand name for amoxicillin in Mexico

▶

◀ **Related Information**
  Anesthesia for Patients With Liver Disease *on page 1537*
  Antiarrhythmic Drugs *on page 1656*
  Commonly Used Herbal Medicines *on page 1713*
  Dosing Considerations for the Critically-Ill Patient With Morbid Obesity *on page 1561*
  Heart Failure (Systolic) *on page 1739*
  Management of Postoperative Arrhythmias *on page 1571*
U.S. Brand Names Lanoxicaps® [DSC]; Lanoxin®

Canadian Brand Names Apo-Digoxin®; Digoxin CSD; Lanoxicaps®; Lanoxin®; Novo-Digoxin; Pediatric Digoxin CSD

Pharmacologic Category Antiarrhythmic Agent, Class IV; Cardiac Glycoside

Generic Available Yes: Excludes capsule

Use Treatment of congestive heart failure and to slow the ventricular rate in tachyarrhythmias such as atrial fibrillation, atrial flutter, and supraventricular tachycardia (paroxysmal atrial tachycardia); cardiogenic shock

Mechanism of Action
  Congestive heart failure: Inhibition of the sodium/potassium ATPase pump which acts to increase the intracellular sodium-calcium exchange to increase intracellular calcium leading to increased contractility

  Supraventricular arrhythmias: Direct suppression of the AV node conduction to increase effective refractory period and decrease conduction velocity - positive inotropic effect, enhanced vagal tone, and decreased ventricular rate to fast atrial arrhythmias. Atrial fibrillation may decrease sensitivity and increase tolerance to higher serum digoxin concentrations.

Pharmacodynamics/Kinetics
  Onset of action: Oral: 1-2 hours; I.V.: 5-30 minutes
    Peak effect: Oral: 2-8 hours; I.V.: 1-4 hours
  Duration: Adults: 3-4 days both forms
  Absorption: By passive nonsaturable diffusion in the upper small intestine; food may delay, but does not affect extent of absorption
  Distribution:
    Normal renal function: 6-7 L/kg
    V_d: Extensive to peripheral tissues, with a distinct distribution phase which lasts 6-8 hours; concentrates in heart, liver, kidney, skeletal muscle, and intestines. Heart/serum concentration is 70:1. Pharmacologic effects are delayed and do not correlate well with serum concentrations during distribution phase.
    Hyperthyroidism: Increased V_d
    Hyperkalemia, hyponatremia: Decreased digoxin distribution to heart and muscle
    Hypokalemia: Increased digoxin distribution to heart and muscles
    Concomitant quinidine therapy: Decreased V_d
    Chronic renal failure: 4-6 L/kg
    Decreased sodium/potassium ATPase activity - decreased tissue binding
    Neonates, full-term: 7.5-10 L/kg
    Children: 16 L/kg
    Adults: 7 L/kg, decreased with renal disease
  Protein binding: 30%; in uremic patients, digoxin is displaced from plasma protein binding sites
  Metabolism: Via sequential sugar hydrolysis in the stomach or by reduction of lactone ring by intestinal bacteria (in ~10% of population, gut bacteria may metabolize up to 40% of digoxin dose); metabolites may contribute to therapeutic and toxic effects of digoxin; metabolism is reduced with CHF
  Bioavailability: Oral (formulation dependent): Elixir: 75% to 85%; Tablet: 70% to 80%
  Half-life elimination (age, renal and cardiac function dependent):
    Neonates: Premature: 61-170 hours; Full-term: 35-45 hours
    Infants: 18-25 hours
    Children: 35 hours
    Adults: 38-48 hours
    Adults, anephric: 4-6 days
  Half-life elimination: Parent drug: 38 hours; Metabolites: Digoxigenin: 4 hours; Monodigitoxoside: 3-12 hours

Time to peak, serum: Oral: ~1 hour
Excretion: Urine (50% to 70% as unchanged drug)
Dosage When changing from oral (tablets or liquid) or I.M. to I.V. therapy, dosage should be reduced by 20% to 25%. See table.

Dosage Recommendations for Digoxin

Age	Total Digitalizing Dose[2] (mcg/kg[1])		Daily Maintenance Dose[3] (mcg/kg[1])	
	P.O.	I.V. or I.M.	P.O.	I.V. or I.M.
Preterm infant[1]	20-30	15-25	5-7.5	4-6
Full-term infant[1]	25-35	20-30	6-10	5-8
1 mo - 2 y[1]	35-60	30-50	10-15	7.5-12
2-5 y[1]	30-40	25-35	7.5-10	6-9
5-10 y[1]	20-35	15-30	5-10	4-8
>10 y[1]	10-15	8-12	2.5-5	2-3
Adults	0.75-1.5 mg	0.5-1 mg	0.125-0.5 mg	0.1-0.4 mg

[1]Based on lean body weight and normal renal function for age. Decrease dose in patients with ↓ renal function; digitalizing dose often not recommended in infants and children.

[2]Give one-half of the total digitalizing dose (TDD) in the initial dose, then give one-quarter of the TDD in each of two subsequent doses at 6- to 8-hour intervals. Obtain ECG 6 hours after each dose to assess potential toxicity.

[3]Divided every 12 hours in infants and children <10 years of age. Given once daily to children >10 years of age and adults.

Dosing adjustment/interval in renal impairment:
Cl_{cr} 10-50 mL/minute: Administer 25% to 75% of dose or every 36 hours
Cl_{cr} <10 mL/minute: Administer 10% to 25% of dose or every 48 hours
Reduce loading dose by 50% in ESRD
Hemodialysis: Not dialyzable (0% to 5%)
Stability Protect elixir and injection from light.
Administration
I.M.: Inject no more than 2 mL per injection site. May cause intense pain.
I.V.: May be administered undiluted or diluted fourfold in D_5W, NS, or SWFI for direct injection. Less than fourfold dilution may lead to drug precipitation. Inject slowly over ≥5 minutes.
Monitoring Parameters
When to draw serum digoxin concentrations: Digoxin serum concentrations are monitored because digoxin possesses a narrow therapeutic serum range; the therapeutic endpoint is difficult to quantify and digoxin toxicity may be life-threatening. Digoxin serum levels should be drawn **at least 4 hours after an intravenous dose** and **at least 6 hours after an oral dose (optimally 12-24 hours after a dose).**
Initiation of therapy:
If a loading dose is given: Digoxin serum concentration may be drawn within 12-24 hours after the initial loading dose administration. Levels drawn this early may confirm the relationship of digoxin plasma levels and response but are of little value in determining maintenance doses.
If a loading dose is not given: Digoxin serum concentration should be obtained after 3-5 days of therapy.
Maintenance therapy:
Trough concentrations should be followed just prior to the next dose or at a minimum of 4 hours after an I.V. dose and at least 6 hours after an oral dose.
Digoxin serum concentrations should be obtained within 5-7 days (approximate time to steady-state) after any dosage changes. Continue to obtain digoxin serum concentrations 7-14 days after any change in maintenance dose. **Note:** In patients with end-stage renal disease, it may take 15-20 days to reach steady-state.
Additionally, patients who are receiving potassium-depleting medications such as diuretics, should be monitored for potassium, magnesium, and calcium levels.

Digoxin serum concentrations should be obtained whenever any of the following conditions occur:

Questionable patient compliance or to evaluate clinical deterioration following an initial good response

Changing renal function

Suspected digoxin toxicity

Initiation or discontinuation of therapy with drugs (amiodarone, quinidine, verapamil) which potentially interact with digoxin; if quinidine therapy is started, the digoxin dose should be reduced by 25% to 50% and digoxin levels should be monitored closely. Any disease changes (hypothyroidism)

Any disease changes (hypothyroidism)

Heart rate and rhythm should be monitored along with periodic ECGs to assess both desired effects and signs of toxicity

Follow closely (especially in patients receiving diuretics or amphotericin) for decreased serum potassium and magnesium or increased calcium, all of which predispose to digoxin toxicity

Assess renal function

Be aware of drug interactions

Observe patients for noncardiac signs of toxicity, confusion, and depression

Reference Range

Digoxin therapeutic serum concentrations:

Congestive heart failure: 0.5-0.8 ng/mL

Arrhythmias: 0.8-2 ng/mL

Adults: <0.5 ng/mL; probably indicates underdigitalization unless there are special circumstances

Toxic: >2.5 ng/mL

Digoxin-like immunoreactive substance (DLIS) may cross-react with digoxin immunoassay. DLIS has been found in patients with renal and liver disease, congestive heart failure, neonates, and pregnant women (3rd trimester).

Anesthesia and Critical Care Concerns/Other Considerations

Clinical Pearls/Comments: Elderly are at risk for toxicity due to age-related changes; volume of distribution is diminished significantly; half-life is increased as a result of decreased total body clearance. Digoxin toxicity may be potentiated in patients with hypokalemia, hypomagnesemia, and hypercalcemia. Digoxin may also rapidly approach toxic levels in patients with renal failure. Signs of digoxin toxicity include both brady- and tachyarrhythmias. Bidirectional VT induced by digoxin indicates imminent development of ventricular fibrillation.

Digoxin has been used for many years in treatment of heart failure. Digoxin therapy is associated with a decrease in frequency in hospitalizations for exacerbations of heart failure. Digoxin use for ventricular rate control in patients with atrial fibrillation is a particularly useful strategy in those patients with coexisting systolic dysfunction. While digoxin may control ventricular response rate for atrial fibrillation at rest, the medication is less effective for rate control during exercise.

Pregnancy Risk Factor C

Contraindications Hypersensitivity to digoxin or any component of the formulation; hypersensitivity to cardiac glycosides (another may be tried); history of toxicity; ventricular tachycardia or fibrillation; idiopathic hypertrophic subaortic stenosis; constrictive pericarditis; amyloid disease; second- or third-degree heart block (except in patients with a functioning artificial pacemaker); Wolff-Parkinson-White syndrome and atrial fibrillation concurrently

Warnings/Precautions Watch for proarrhythmic effects (especially with digoxin toxicity). Withdrawal in HF patients may lead to recurrence of HF symptoms. Use with caution in patients with hypoxia, myxedema, hypothyroidism, acute myocarditis; patients with incomplete AV block (Stokes-Adams attack) may progress to complete block with digitalis drug administration; use with caution in patients with acute myocardial infarction, severe pulmonary disease, advanced heart failure, idiopathic hypertrophic subaortic stenosis, Wolff-Parkinson-White syndrome, sick-sinus syndrome (bradyarrhythmias), amyloid heart disease, and constrictive cardiomyopathies; adjust dose with renal impairment and when verapamil, quinidine or amiodarone are added to a patient on digoxin; elderly and neonates may develop exaggerated serum/tissue concentrations due to age-related alterations in clearance and pharmacodynamic differences; exercise will reduce serum concentrations of digoxin due to increased skeletal muscle uptake; recent studies indicate photopsia, chromatopsia and decreased visual acuity may occur even with therapeutic serum drug levels; reduce or hold dose 1-2 days before elective electrical cardioversion. In the Cardiac Arrhythmia Suppression Trial (CAST), recent (>6 days but <2 years ago) myocardial infarction patients with asymptomatic, non-life-threatening ventricular arrhythmias did not benefit and may have been harmed by attempts to suppress the arrhythmia with flecainide or encainide. An increased mortality or nonfatal cardiac arrest rate (7.7%) was seen in the active treatment group compared with patients in the placebo group (3%). The applicability of the CAST results to other populations is unknown. Antiarrhythmic agents should be reserved for patients with life-threatening ventricular arrhythmias.

Adverse Reactions Incidence not always reported.

Cardiovascular: Heart block; first-, second- (Wenckebach), or third-degree heart block; asystole; atrial tachycardia with block; AV dissociation; accelerated junctional rhythm; ventricular tachycardia or ventricular fibrillation; PR prolongation; ST segment depression

Central nervous system: Visual disturbances (blurred or yellow vision), headache (3.2%), dizziness (4.9%), apathy, confusion, mental disturbances (4.1%), anxiety, depression, delirium, hallucinations, fever

Dermatologic: Maculopapular rash (1.6%); erythematous, scarlatiniform, papular, vesicular, or bullous rash; urticaria; pruritus; facial, angioneurotic, or laryngeal edema; shedding of fingernails or toenails

Gastrointestinal: Nausea (3.2%), vomiting (1.6%), diarrhea (3.2%), abdominal pain

Neuromuscular & skeletal: Weakness

<1% (Limited to important or life-threatening): Abdominal pain, anorexia, eosinophilia, gynecomastia, hemorrhagic necrosis of the intestines, increased plasma estrogen and decreased serum luteinizing hormone in men and postmenopausal women and decreased plasma testosterone in men, intestinal ischemia, palpitation, sexual dysfunction, thrombocytopenia, unifocal or multi-form ventricular premature contractions (especially bigeminy or trigeminy), vaginal cornification

Any arrhythmia seen in a child on digoxin should be considered as digoxin toxicity. The gastrointestinal and central nervous system symptoms are not frequently seen in children.

Drug Interactions

Metabolism/Transport Effects Substrate of CYP3A4 (minor)

Avoid Concomitant Use There are no known interactions where it is recommended to avoid concomitant use.

Increased Effect/Toxicity

Digoxin may increase the levels/effects of: Dronedarone; Midodrine

The levels/effects of Digoxin may be increased by: Aminoquinolines (Antimalarial); Amiodarone; Antifungal Agents (Azole Derivatives, Systemic); Atorvastatin; Beta-Blockers; Calcitriol; Calcium Channel Blockers (Nondihydropyridine); Carvedilol; Conivaptan; CycloSPORINE; Dronedarone; Macrolide Antibiotics; Milnacipran; Nefazodone; Neuromuscular-Blocking Agents; P-Glycoprotein Inhibitors; Potassium-Sparing Diuretics; Propafenone; Protease Inhibitors; QuiNIDine; QuiNINE; Ranolazine; Spironolactone; Telmisartan

Decreased Effect

Digoxin may decrease the levels/effects of: Antineoplastic Agents (Anthracycline)

The levels/effects of Digoxin may be decreased by: 5-ASA Derivatives; Acarbose; Aminoglycosides; Antineoplastic Agents; Antineoplastic Agents (Anthracycline); Bile Acid Sequestrants; Kaolin; Penicillamine; P-Glycoprotein Inducers; Potassium-Sparing Diuretics; St Johns Wort; Sucralfate

Ethanol/Nutrition/Herb Interactions

Food: Digoxin peak serum levels may be decreased if taken with food. Meals containing increased fiber (bran) or foods high in pectin may decrease oral absorption of digoxin.

Herb/Nutraceutical: Avoid ephedra (risk of cardiac stimulation). Avoid natural licorice (causes sodium and water retention and increases potassium loss).

◀ **Dietary Considerations** Maintain adequate amounts of potassium in diet to decrease risk of hypokalemia (hypokalemia may increase risk of digoxin toxicity).

Dosage Forms Excipient information presented when available (limited, particularly for generics); consult specific product labeling. [CAN] = Canadian brand name; [DSC] = Discontinued product

Capsule:
  Lanoxicaps®: 100 mcg [contains ethanol; DSC]; 200 mcg [contains ethanol; DSC]
Injection, solution: 250 mcg/mL (1 mL, 2 mL)
  Lanoxin®: 250 mcg/mL (2 mL) [contains ethanol 10% and propylene glycol 40%]
Injection, solution [pediatric]: 100 mcg/mL (1 mL)
Solution, oral: 50 mcg/mL (2.5 mL, 5 mL [DSC], 60 mL)
Tablet: 125 mcg, 250 mcg
  Lanoxin®: 125 mcg, 250 mcg
  Apo-Digoxin® [CAN]: 62.5 mcg, 125 mcg, 250 mcg

◆ **Digoxin CSD (Can)** *see* Digoxin *on page* 417

Digoxin Immune Fab (di JOKS in i MYUN fab)

U.S. Brand Names Digibind®; DigiFab™
Canadian Brand Names Digibind®
Index Terms Antidigoxin Fab Fragments, Ovine
Pharmacologic Category Antidote
Generic Available No
Use Treatment of life-threatening or potentially life-threatening digoxin intoxication, including:
• acute digoxin ingestion (ie, >10 mg in adults or >4 mg in children)
• chronic ingestions leading to steady-state digoxin concentrations >6 ng/mL in adults or >4 ng/mL in children
• manifestations of digoxin toxicity due to overdose (life-threatening ventricular arrhythmias, progressive bradycardia, second- or third-degree heart block not responsive to atropine, serum potassium >5 mEq/L in adults or >6 mEq in children)

Mechanism of Action Digoxin immune antigen-binding fragments (Fab) are specific antibodies for the treatment of digitalis intoxication in carefully selected patients; binds with molecules of digoxin or digitoxin and then is excreted by the kidneys and removed from the body

Pharmacodynamics/Kinetics
Onset of action: I.V.: Improvement in 2-30 minutes for toxicity
Half-life elimination: 15-20 hours; prolonged with renal impairment
Excretion: Urine; undetectable amounts within 5-7 days

Dosage Each vial of Digibind® 38 mg or DigiFab™ 40 mg will bind ~0.5 mg of digoxin or digitoxin.
Note: Estimation of the dose is based on the body burden of digitalis. This may be calculated if the amount ingested is known or the postdistribution serum drug level is known (round dose to the nearest whole vial). If the amount of ingestion is unknown, general dosing guidelines should be used.
Acute ingestion of *unknown* amount: I.V.: Children and Adults: 20 vials is adequate to treat most life-threatening ingestions. May give as a single dose or give 10 vials, observe response, and give a second 10-vial dose if indicated.
Acute ingestion of *known* amount: I.V.:
Based on number of tablets/capsules ingested: Children and Adults:
  Step 1:
  Total body load (mg) = Amount (mg) digoxin capsules/digitoxin ingested
  Step 2:
  Dose (vials) = Total body load (mg) / (0.5 mg digitalis bound/vial)
  Alternatively, the table on the next page gives an estimation of the number of vials needed based on the number of digoxin tablets or capsules ingested.

Number of Digoxin Tablets or Capsules Ingested[1]	Dose of Digoxin Immune Fab (# of Vials)
25	10
50	20
75	30
100	40
150	60
200	80

[1]250 mcg tablets with 80% bioavailability or 200 mcg Lanoxicaps® capsules with 100% bioavailability.

Based on steady-state serum digoxin concentration:

Infants and Children ≤20 kg: May require smaller doses; calculate dose in milligrams, reconstitute with NS, and administer dose via tuberculin syringe

Step 1:

Dose (mg) = [(serum digoxin concentration [ng/mL] x weight [kg]) / 10] x (mg/vial)[1]

[1]Digibind® 38 mg/vial or DigiFab™ 40 mg/vial

Alternatively, the following table gives an estimation of the amount of **Digibind®** needed based on the steady-state serum digoxin concentration.

Infants and Small Children Dose Estimates of Digibind® (in mg) From Steady-State Serum Digoxin Concentration

Patient Weight (kg)	Serum Digoxin Concentration (ng/mL)						
	1	2	4	8	12	16	20
1	0.4 mg[1]	1 mg[1]	1.5 mg[1]	3 mg[1]	5 mg	6 mg	8 mg
3	1 mg[1]	2 mg[1]	5 mg	9 mg	14 mg	18 mg	23 mg
5	2 mg[1]	4 mg	8 mg	15 mg	23 mg	30 mg	38 mg
10	4 mg	8 mg	15 mg	30 mg	46 mg	61 mg	76 mg
20	8 mg	15 mg	30 mg	61 mg	91 mg	122 mg	152 mg

[1]Dilution of reconstituted vial to 1 mg/mL may be desirable.

Alternatively, the following table gives an estimation of the amount of **DigiFab™** needed based on the steady-state serum digoxin concentration.

Infants and Small Children Dose Estimates of DigiFab™ (in mg) From Steady-State Serum Digoxin Concentration

Patient Weight (kg)	Serum Digoxin Concentration (ng/mL)						
	1	2	4	8	12	16	20
1	0.4 mg[1]	1 mg[1]	1.5 mg[1]	3 mg[1]	5 mg	6.5 mg	8 mg
3	1 mg[1]	2.5 mg[1]	5 mg	10 mg	14 mg	19 mg	24 mg
5	2 mg[1]	4 mg	8 mg	16 mg	24 mg	32 mg	40 mg
10	4 mg	8 mg	16 mg	32 mg	48 mg	64 mg	80 mg
20	8 mg	16 mg	32 mg	64 mg	96 mg	128 mg	160 mg

[1]Dilution of reconstituted vial to 1 mg/mL may be desirable.

◀ Adults:
Step 1:
Dose (vials) = [(serum digoxin concentration [ng/mL] x weight [kg]) / 100]
Alternatively, the following table gives an estimation of the number of vials needed based on the steady-state serum digoxin concentration.

Adult Dose Estimates of Digibind® (in # of Vials)
From Steady-State Serum Digoxin Concentration

Patient Weight (kg)	Serum Digoxin Concentration (ng/mL)						
	1	2	4	8	12	16	20
40	0.5 v	1 v	2 v	3 v	5 v	7 v	8 v
60	0.5 v	1 v	3 v	5 v	7 v	10 v	12 v
70	1 v	2 v	3 v	6 v	9 v	11 v	14 v
80	1 v	2 v	3 v	7 v	10 v	13 v	16 v
100	1 v	2 v	4 v	8 v	12 v	16 v	20 v

v = vials.

Based on steady-state digitoxin concentration: Children and Adults: If the calculated dose based on the **digitoxin** concentration is different than that for the digoxin concentration, use the higher dose.
Step 1:
Dose (vials) = [serum **digitoxin** concentration (ng/mL) x weight (kg)] / 1000

Chronic toxicity (serum digoxin concentration unavailable): I.V.:
Infants and Children ≤20 kg: 1 vial is adequate to reverse most cases of toxicity
Adults: 6 vials is adequate to reverse most cases of toxicity
Stability Should be refrigerated (2°C to 8°C).
Digibind®: Reconstitute by adding 4 mL sterile water, resulting in 9.5 mg/mL for I.V. infusion. Reconstituted solutions should be used within 4 hours if refrigerated. For very small doses, reconstituted vial can be further diluted by adding an additional 34 mL of sterile isotonic saline to achieve a final concentration of 1 mg/mL.
DigiFab™: Reconstitute by adding 4 mL sterile water, resulting in 10 mg/mL for I.V. infusion. Reconstituted solutions should be used within 4 hours if refrigerated. For very small doses, reconstituted vial can be further diluted by adding an additional 36 mL of sterile isotonic saline to achieve a final concentration of 1 mg/mL.
Administration Continuous I.V. infusion over ≥30 minutes is preferred. May give by bolus injection if cardiac arrest is imminent. Small doses (infants/small children) may be administered using tuberculin syringe. Stopping the infusion and restarting at a slower rate may help if infusion-related reactions occur.
Monitoring Parameters Serum potassium, serum digoxin concentration prior to first dose of digoxin immune Fab; **digoxin levels will greatly increase with digoxin immune Fab use and are not an accurate determination of body stores** (has no clinical meaning; avoid monitoring serum concentrations); standard digoxin concentration measurements may be misleading until Fab fragments are eliminated from the body.

Patients with renal failure should be monitored for a prolonged period for reintoxication with digoxin following the rerelease of bound digoxin into the blood.
Pregnancy Risk Factor C
Contraindications Hypersensitivity to digoxin immune Fab, sheep products, or any component of the formulation
Warnings/Precautions Suicidal attempts often involve multiple drugs; consider other drug toxicities as well. Hypersensitivity reactions can occur. Epinephrine should be immediately available. Serum potassium levels should be monitored, especially during the first few hours after administration. Total serum digoxin concentrations will rise precipitously following administration of this drug (has no clinical meaning; avoid monitoring serum concentrations). If digoxin was being used to treat heart failure, may see exacerbation of symptoms as digoxin level is reduced. Use with caution in renal failure (experience limited); the complex will be removed from the body more slowly. Monitor for reoccurrence of digoxin toxicity.

Failure of response to adequate treatment may call diagnosis of digitalis toxicity into question. Digoxin immune Fab is processed with papain and may cause hypersensitivity reactions in patients allergic to papaya, other papaya extracts, papain, chymopapain, or the pineapple enzyme bromelain. There may also be cross allergy with dust mite and latex allergens.

Adverse Reactions Frequency not defined.

Cardiovascular: Effects (due to withdrawal of digitalis) include exacerbation of heart failure, rapid ventricular response in patients with atrial fibrillation; postural hypotension

Endocrine & metabolic: Hypokalemia

Local: Phlebitis

Miscellaneous: Allergic reactions, serum sickness

Drug Interactions

Avoid Concomitant Use There are no known interactions where it is recommended to avoid concomitant use.

Increased Effect/Toxicity There are no known significant interactions involving an increase in effect.

Decreased Effect There are no known significant interactions involving a decrease in effect.

Test Interactions Digibind® will interfere with digitalis immunoassay measurements - this will result in clinically misleading serum digoxin concentrations fragment is eliminated from the body (several days to >1 week after Digibind® administration).

Dosage Forms Excipient information presented when available (limited, particularly for generics); consult specific product labeling.

Injection, powder for reconstitution [ovine derived]:

Digibind®: 38 mg [derived from or manufactured using papain]

DigiFab™: 40 mg [derived from or manufactured using papain]

References

Bateman DN, "Digoxin-Specific Antibody Fragments: How Much and When?" *Toxicol Rev*, 2004, 23 (3):135-43.

◆ **Dihydrohydroxycodeinone** *see* OxyCODONE *on page 1069*

◆ **Dihydromorphinone** *see* HYDROmorphone *on page 707*

◆ **Dilacor XR®** *see* Diltiazem *on page 425*

◆ **Dilantin®** *see* Phenytoin *on page 1119*

◆ **Dilatrate®-SR** *see* Isosorbide Dinitrate *on page 772*

◆ **Dilaudid®** *see* HYDROmorphone *on page 707*

◆ **Dilaudid-HP®** *see* HYDROmorphone *on page 707*

◆ **Dilaudid-HP-Plus® (Can)** *see* HYDROmorphone *on page 707*

◆ **Dilaudid® Sterile Powder (Can)** *see* HYDROmorphone *on page 707*

◆ **Dilaudid-XP® (Can)** *see* HYDROmorphone *on page 707*

◆ **Dilt-CD** *see* Diltiazem *on page 425*

◆ **Diltia XT®** *see* Diltiazem *on page 425*

Diltiazem (dil TYE a zem)

Medication Safety Issues

Sound-alike/look-alike issues:

Cardizem® may be confused with Cardene®, Cardene SR®, Cardizem CD®, Cardizem SR®, cardiem, cortisone

Cartia XT® may be confused with Procardia XL®

Diltiazem may be confused with Calan®, diazepam, Dilantin®

Tiazac® may be confused with Tigan®, Tiazac® XC [CAN], Ziac®

High alert medication: The Institute for Safe Medication Practices (ISMP) includes this medication (I.V. formulation) among its list of drug classes which have a heightened risk of causing significant patient harm when used in error.

Significant differences exist between oral and I.V. dosing. Use caution when converting from one route of administration to another.

◀ International issues:

    Cardizem® may be confused with Cardem® which is a brand name for celiprolol in Spain

    Cartia XT® may be confused with Cartia® which is a brand name for aspirin in multiple international markets

    Dilacor®: Brand name for digoxin in Serbia, a brand name for verapamil in Brazil, and a brand name for barnidipine in Argentina

    Tiazac® may be confused with Tazac® which is a brand name for nizatidine in Australia

    Tiazac® may be confused with Tiazac® XC which is a brand name for diltiazem available in Canada (not available in U.S.)

Related Information

    Antiarrhythmic Drugs *on page 1656*
    Calcium Channel Blockers *on page 1672*
    Dosing Considerations for the Critically-Ill Patient With Morbid Obesity *on page 1561*
    Management of Postoperative Arrhythmias *on page 1571*

U.S. Brand Names Cardizem®; Cardizem® CD; Cardizem® LA; Cartia XT®; Dilacor XR®; Dilt-CD; Dilt-XR; Diltia XT®; Diltzac; Taztia XT®; Tiazac®

Canadian Brand Names Apo-Diltiaz CD®; Apo-Diltiaz SR®; Apo-Diltiaz TZ®; Apo-Diltiaz®; Apo-Diltiaz® Injectable; Cardizem® CD; Diltiazem HCl ER®; Diltiazem Hydrochloride Injection; Diltiazem TZ; Gen-Diltiazem; Gen-Diltiazem CD; Gen-Diltiazem SR; Med-Diltiazem; Novo-Diltazem; Novo-Diltazem-CD; Novo-Diltiazem HCl ER; Nu-Diltiaz; Nu-Diltiaz-CD; ratio-Diltiazem CD; Sandoz-Diltiazem CD; Sandoz-Diltiazem T; Tiazac® ; Tiazac® XC

Index Terms Diltiazem Hydrochloride

Pharmacologic Category Antiarrhythmic Agent, Class IV; Calcium Channel Blocker; Calcium Channel Blocker, Nondihydropyridine

Generic Available Yes: Excludes extended release tablet

Use

    Oral: Essential hypertension; chronic stable angina or angina from coronary artery spasm

    Injection: Atrial fibrillation or atrial flutter; paroxysmal supraventricular tachycardia (PSVT)

Unlabeled/Investigational Use Pediatric hypertension

Mechanism of Action Nondihydropyridine calcium channel blocker which inhibits calcium ion from entering the "slow channels" or select voltage-sensitive areas of vascular smooth muscle and myocardium during depolarization, producing a relaxation of coronary vascular smooth muscle and coronary vasodilation; increases myocardial oxygen delivery in patients with vasospastic angina

Pharmacodynamics/Kinetics

    Onset of action: Oral: Immediate release tablet: 30-60 minutes

    Absorption: Immediate release tablet: >90%; Extended release capsule: ~93%

    Distribution: V_d: 3-13 L/kg

    Protein binding: 70% to 80%

    Metabolism: Hepatic (extensive first-pass effect); following single I.V. injection, plasma concentrations of N-monodesmethyldiltiazem and desacetyldiltiazem are typically undetectable; however, these metabolites accumulate to detectable concentrations following 24-hour constant rate infusion. N-monodesmethyldiltiazem appears to have 20% of the potency of diltiazem; desacetyldiltiazem is about 25% to 50% as potent as the parent compound.

    Bioavailability: Oral: ~40% (undergoes extensive first-pass metabolism)

    Half-life elimination: Immediate release tablet: 3-4.5 hours, may be prolonged with renal impairment; Extended release tablet: 6-9 hours; Extended release capsules: 5-10 hours; I.V.: single dose: ~3.4 hours; continuous infusion: 4-5 hours

    Time to peak, serum: Immediate release tablet: 2-4 hours; Extended release tablet: 11-18 hours; Extended release capsule: 10-14 hours

    Excretion: Urine (2% to 4% as unchanged drug; 6% to 7% as metabolites); feces

Dosage

Children (unlabeled use): Minimal information available; some centers use the following: Oral: Hypertension: Immediate release tablets: Initial: 1.5-2 mg/kg/day divided in 3 doses/day (maximum dose 6 mg/kg/day up to 360 mg/day) (Flynn, 2000)

Adults:

Oral:

Angina:

Capsule, extended release:

Dilacor XR®, Dilt-XR, Diltia XT®: Initial: 120 mg once daily; titrate over 7-14 days; usual dose range: 120-320 mg/day: maximum: 480 mg/day

Cardizem® CD, Cartia XT®, Dilt-CD: Initial: 120-180 mg once daily; titrate over 7-14 days; usual dose range: 120-320 mg/day; maximum: 480 mg/day

Tiazac®, Taztia XT®: Initial: 120-180 mg once daily; titrate over 7-14 days; usual dose range: 120-320 mg/day; maximum: 540 mg/day

Tablet, extended release (Cardizem® LA, Tiazac® XC [CAN; not available in U.S.]): 180 mg once daily; may increase at 7- to 14-day intervals; usual dose range: 120-320 mg/day; maximum: 360 mg/day

Tablet, immediate release (Cardizem®): Usual starting dose: 30 mg 4 times/day; titrate dose gradually at 1- to 2-day intervals; usual dose range: 120-320 mg/day

Hypertension:

Capsule, extended release (once-daily dosing):

Cardizem® CD, Cartia XT®, Dilt-CD: Initial: 180-240 mg once daily; dose adjustment may be made after 14 days; usual dose range (JNC 7): 180-420 mg/day; maximum: 480 mg/day

Dilacor® XR, Diltia XT®, Dilt-XR: Initial: 180-240 mg once daily; dose adjustment may be made after 14 days; usual dose range (JNC 7): 180-420 mg/day; maximum: 540 mg/day

Tiazac®, Taztia XT®: Initial: 120-240 mg once daily; dose adjustment may be made after 14 days; usual dose range (JNC 7): 180-420 mg/day; maximum: 540 mg/day

Capsule, extended release (twice-daily dosing): Initial: 60-120 mg twice daily; dose adjustment may be made after 14 days; usual range: 240-360 mg/day

Note: Diltiazem is available as a generic intended for either once- or twice-daily dosing, depending on the formulation; verify appropriate extended release capsule formulation is administered.

Tablet, extended release (Cardizem® LA, Tiazac® XC [CAN; not available in U.S.]): Initial: 180-240 mg once daily; dose adjustment may be made after 14 days; usual dose range (JNC 7): 120-540 mg/day

Note: Elderly: Patients ≥60 years may respond to a lower initial dose (ie, 120 mg once daily using extended release capsule)

I.V.: *Atrial fibrillation, atrial flutter, PSVT:*

Initial bolus dose: 0.25 mg/kg actual body weight over 2 minutes (average adult dose: 20 mg)

Repeat bolus dose (may be administered after 15 minutes if the response is inadequate): 0.35 mg/kg actual body weight over 2 minutes (average adult dose: 25 mg)

Continuous infusion (infusions >24 hours or infusion rates >15 mg/hour are not recommended): Initial infusion rate of 10 mg/hour; rate may be increased in 5 mg/hour increments up to 15 mg/hour as needed; some patients may respond to an initial rate of 5 mg/hour.

If diltiazem injection is administered by continuous infusion for >24 hours, the possibility of decreased diltiazem clearance, prolonged elimination half-life, and increased diltiazem and/or diltiazem metabolite plasma concentrations should be considered.

Conversion from I.V. diltiazem to oral diltiazem:

Oral dose (mg/day) is approximately equal to [rate (mg/hour) x 3 + 3] x 10.

3 mg/hour = 120 mg/day

5 mg/hour = 180 mg/day

7 mg/hour = 240 mg/day

11 mg/hour = 360 mg/day

◀ **Dosing adjustment in renal impairment:** Use with caution; no dosing adjustments recommended

Dialysis: Not removed by hemo- or peritoneal dialysis; supplemental dose is not necessary.

Dosing adjustment in hepatic impairment: Use with caution; no specific dosing recommendations available; extensively metabolized by the liver; half-life is increased in patients with cirrhosis

Stability

Capsule, tablet: Store at room temperature. Protect from light.

Solution for injection: Store in refrigerator at 2°C to 8°C (36°F to 46°F); do not freeze. May be stored at room temperature for up to 1 month. Following dilution to ≤1 mg/mL with $D_5$1/2NS, D_5W, or NS, solution is stable for 24 hours at room temperature or under refrigeration.

Administration

Oral:

Immediate release tablet (Cardizem®): Administer before meals and at bedtime.

Long acting dosage forms: Do not open, chew, or crush; swallow whole.

Cardizem® CD, Cardizem® LA, Cartia XT®, Dilt-CD: May be administered without regards to meals.

Dilacor XR®, Dilt-XR, Diltia XT®: Administer on an empty stomach.

Taztia XT™, Tiazac®: Capsules may be opened and sprinkled on a spoonful of applesauce. Applesauce should not be hot and should be swallowed without chewing, followed by drinking a glass of water.

Tiazac® XC [CAN; not available in U.S.]: Administer at bedtime

I.V.: Bolus doses given over 2 minutes with continuous ECG and blood pressure monitoring. Continuous infusion should be via infusion pump.

Monitoring Parameters Liver function tests, blood pressure, ECG, heart rate

Anesthesia and Critical Care Concerns/Other Considerations Clinical **Pearls/Comments:** Diltiazem may be administered intravenously in the acute setting to attain ventricular rate control in patients with atrial fibrillation or flutter. Patients who respond, defined in general as at least a 20% decrease in ventricular response rate or attaining a rate <100 beats/minute, can be continued on oral therapy to maintain control.

Pregnancy Risk Factor C

Contraindications

Oral: Hypersensitivity to diltiazem or any component of the formulation; sick sinus syndrome (except in patients with a functioning artificial pacemaker); second- or third-degree AV block (except in patients with a functioning artificial pacemaker); severe hypotension (systolic <90 mm Hg); acute MI and pulmonary congestion

Intravenous (I.V.): Hypersensitivity to diltiazem or any component of the formulation; sick sinus syndrome (except in patients with a functioning artificial pacemaker); second- or third-degree AV block (except in patients with a functioning artificial pacemaker); severe hypotension (systolic <90 mm Hg); cardiogenic shock; administration concomitantly or within a few hours of the administration of I.V. beta-blockers; atrial fibrillation or flutter associated with accessory bypass tract (eg, Wolff-Parkinson-White syndrome); ventricular tachycardia (with wide-complex tachycardia, must determine whether origin is supraventricular or ventricular)

Canadian labeling: Additional contraindications (not in U.S. labeling): I.V. and oral: Pregnancy; use in women of childbearing potential

Warnings/Precautions Can cause first-, second-, and third-degree AV block or sinus bradycardia and risk increases with agents known to slow cardiac conduction. The most common side effect is peripheral edema; occurs within 2-3 weeks of starting therapy. Symptomatic hypotension with or without syncope can rarely occur; blood pressure must be lowered at a rate appropriate for the patient's clinical condition. Concomitant use with beta-blockers or digoxin can result in conduction disturbances. I.V. administration concomitantly or within a few hours of I.V. beta-blockers is contraindicated. Use caution in left ventricular dysfunction (may exacerbate condition). Avoid use of diltiazem in patients with heart failure and reduced ejection fraction (Hunt, 2009). Use with caution with hypertrophic obstructive cardiomyopathy; routine use is currently not recommended due to insufficient evidence (Maron, 2003). Use with caution in hepatic or renal dysfunction. Transient dermatologic reactions have been observed with use; if reaction persists, discontinue. May (rarely) progress to erythema multiforme or exfoliative dermatitis.

Adverse Reactions Note: Frequencies represent ranges for various dosage forms. Patients with impaired ventricular function and/or conduction abnormalities may have higher incidence of adverse reactions.

>10%:
  Cardiovascular: Edema (2% to 15%)
  Central nervous system: Headache (5% to 12%)
2% to 10%:
  Cardiovascular: AV block (first degree 2% to 8%), edema (lower limb, 2% to 8%), pain (6%), bradycardia (2% to 6%), hypotension (<2% to 4%), vasodilation (2% to 3%), extrasystoles (2%), flushing (1% to 2%), palpitation (1% to 2%)
  Central nervous system: Dizziness (3% to 10%), nervousness (2%)
  Dermatologic: Rash (1% to 4%)
  Endocrine & metabolic: Gout (1% to 2%)
  Gastrointestinal: Dyspepsia (1% to 6%), constipation (<2% to 4%), vomiting (2%), diarrhea (1% to 2%)
  Local: Injection site reactions: Burning, itching (4%)
  Neuromuscular & skeletal: Weakness (1% to 4%), myalgia (2%)
  Respiratory: Rhinitis (<2% to 10%), pharyngitis (2% to 6%), dyspnea (1% to 6%), bronchitis (1% to 4%), cough (≤3%), sinus congestion (1% to 2%)
<2% (Limited to important or life-threatening): Alkaline phosphatase increased, allergic reaction, ALT increased, AST increased, amblyopia, amnesia, arrhythmia, AV block (second or third degree), bundle branch block, CHF, depression, dysgeusia, extrapyramidal symptoms, gingival hyperplasia, hemolytic anemia, petechiae, photosensitivity, Stevens-Johnson syndrome, syncope, tachycardia, thrombocytopenia, tremor, toxic epidermal necrolysis

Drug Interactions

Metabolism/Transport Effects Substrate of CYP2C9 (minor), 2D6 (minor), 3A4 (major); **Inhibits** CYP2C9 (weak), 2D6 (weak), 3A4 (moderate)

Avoid Concomitant Use

Avoid concomitant use of Diltiazem with any of the following: Everolimus; Ranolazine; Tolvaptan

Increased Effect/Toxicity

Diltiazem may increase the levels/effects of: Alfentanil; Amifostine; Amiodarone; Antihypertensives; Aprepitant; Atorvastatin; Benzodiazepines (metabolized by oxidation); Beta-Blockers; BusPIRone; Calcium Channel Blockers (Dihydropyridine); CarBAMazepine; Cardiac Glycosides; Colchicine; Corticosteroids (Systemic); CycloSPORINE; CYP3A4 Substrates; Dronedarone; Eletriptan; Eplerenone; Everolimus; Fosaprepitant; Halofantrine; Hypotensive Agents; Lithium; Lovastatin; Magnesium Salts; Midodrine; Neuromuscular-Blocking Agents (Nondepolarizing); Nitroprusside; Phenytoin; Pimecrolimus; QuiNIDine; Ranolazine; Red Yeast Rice; RiTUXimab; Salicylates; Salmeterol; Saxagliptin; Simvastatin; Tacrolimus; Tolvaptan

The levels/effects of Diltiazem may be increased by: Alpha1-Blockers; Anilidopiperidine Opioids; Antifungal Agents (Azole Derivatives, Systemic); Aprepitant; Atorvastatin; Cimetidine; CycloSPORINE; CYP3A4 Inhibitors (Moderate); CYP3A4 Inhibitors (Strong); Dasatinib; Diazoxide; Dronedarone; Fluconazole; Fosaprepitant; Grapefruit Juice; Herbs (Hypotensive Properties); Lovastatin; Macrolide Antibiotics; Magnesium Salts; MAO Inhibitors; Pentoxifylline; P-Glycoprotein Inhibitors; Phosphodiesterase 5 Inhibitors; Prostacyclin Analogues; Protease Inhibitors; Quinupristin; Simvastatin

Decreased Effect

Diltiazem may decrease the levels/effects of: Clopidogrel

The levels/effects of Diltiazem may be decreased by: Barbiturates; Calcium Salts; CarBAMazepine; Colestipol; CYP3A4 Inducers (Strong); Deferasirox; Herbs (CYP3A4 Inducers); Herbs (Hypertensive Properties); Methylphenidate; Nafcillin; Peginterferon Alfa-2b; P-Glycoprotein Inducers; Rifamycin Derivatives; Yohimbine

Ethanol/Nutrition/Herb Interactions

Ethanol: Avoid ethanol (may increase risk of hypotension or vasodilation).
Food: Diltiazem serum levels may be elevated if taken with food. Serum concentrations were not altered by grapefruit juice in small clinical trials.

◀ Herb/Nutraceutical: St John's wort may decrease diltiazem levels. Avoid bayberry, blue cohosh, cayenne, ephedra, ginger, ginseng (American), kola, licorice, yohimbe (may worsen hypertension). Avoid black cohosh, California poppy, coleus, garlic, golden seal, hawthorn, mistletoe, periwinkle, quinine, shepherd's purse (may have increased antihypertensive effect).

Dosage Forms Excipient information presented when available (limited, particularly for generics); consult specific product labeling. [CAN] = Canadian brand name

Capsule, extended release, as hydrochloride [once-daily dosing]: 120 mg, 180 mg, 240 mg, 300 mg, 360 mg, 420 mg
    Cardizem® CD: 120 mg, 180 mg, 240 mg, 300 mg, 360 mg
    Cartia XT®: 120 mg, 180 mg, 240 mg, 300 mg
    Dilacor XR®: 120 mg, 180 mg, 240 mg
    Dilt-CD: 120 mg, 180 mg, 240 mg, 300 mg
    Dilt-XR: 120 mg, 180 mg, 240 mg
    Diltia XT®: 120 mg, 180 mg, 240 mg
    Diltzac: 120 mg, 180 mg, 240 mg, 300 mg, 360 mg
    Taztia XT®: 120 mg, 180 mg, 240 mg, 300 mg, 360 mg
    Tiazac®: 120 mg, 180 mg, 240 mg, 300 mg, 360 mg, 420 mg
Capsule, extended release, as hydrochloride [twice-daily dosing]: 60 mg, 90 mg, 120 mg
Injection, solution, as hydrochloride: 5 mg/mL (5 mL, 10 mL, 25 mL)
Injection, powder for reconstitution, as hydrochloride: 100 mg
Tablet, as hydrochloride: 30 mg, 60 mg, 90 mg, 120 mg
    Cardizem®: 30 mg, 60 mg, 90 mg, 120 mg
Tablet, extended release, as hydrochloride:
    Cardizem® LA: 120 mg, 180 mg, 240 mg, 300 mg, 360 mg, 420 mg
    Tiazac® XC [CAN; not available in U.S.]: 120 mg, 180 mg, 240 mg, 300 mg, 360 mg

References

Karth GD, Geppert A, Neunteufl T, et al, "Amiodarone vs. Diltiazem for Rate Control in Critically Ill Patients With Atrial Tachyarrhythmias," *Crit Care Med*, 2001, 29(6):1149-53.

◆ **Diltiazem HCl ER® (Can)** *see* Diltiazem *on page 425*

◆ **Diltiazem Hydrochloride** *see* Diltiazem *on page 425*

◆ **Diltiazem Hydrochloride Injection (Can)** *see* Diltiazem *on page 425*

◆ **Diltiazem TZ (Can)** *see* Diltiazem *on page 425*

◆ **Dilt-XR** *see* Diltiazem *on page 425*

◆ **Diltzac** *see* Diltiazem *on page 425*

◆ **Dimetapp® Toddler's [OTC]** *see* Phenylephrine *on page 1114*

◆ **Diochloram® (Can)** *see* Chloramphenicol *on page 287*

◆ **Diodex® (Can)** *see* Dexamethasone *on page 391*

◆ **Diogent® (Can)** *see* Gentamicin *on page 658*

◆ **Diomycin® (Can)** *see* Erythromycin *on page 516*

◆ **Dionephrine® (Can)** *see* Phenylephrine *on page 1114*

◆ **Diopred® (Can)** *see* PrednisoLONE *on page 1164*

◆ **Dioptic's Atropine Solution (Can)** *see* Atropine *on page 162*

◆ **Diotrope® (Can)** *see* Tropicamide *on page 1437*

◆ **Diovan®** *see* Valsartan *on page 1452*

◆ **Diphen [OTC]** *see* DiphenhydrAMINE *on page 430*

◆ **Diphenhist® [OTC]** *see* DiphenhydrAMINE *on page 430*

DiphenhydrAMINE (dye fen HYE dra meen)

Medication Safety Issues

Institute for Safe Medication Practices (ISMP) has reported cases of patients mistakenly *swallowing* Benadryl® Itch Stopping [OTC] gel intended for topical application. Unclear labeling and similar packaging of the topical gel in containers resembling an oral liquid are factors believed to be contributing to the administration errors. The topical gel contains camphor which can be toxic if swallowed. ISMP has requested the manufacturer to make the necessary changes to prevent further confusion.

Sound-alike/look-alike issues:

DiphenhydrAMINE may be confused with desipramine, dicyclomine, dimenhyDRINATE

Benadryl® may be confused with benazepril, Bentyl®, Benylin®, Caladryl®

Related Information
Allergic Reactions *on page 1508*
Contrast Media Reactions, Premedication for Prophylaxis *on page 1735*
Desensitization Protocols *on page 1692*
Latex Allergy *on page 1511*
Postoperative Nausea and Vomiting *on page 1593*
Skin Tests *on page 1707*

U.S. Brand Names Aler-Cap [OTC]; Aler-Dryl [OTC]; Aler-Tab [OTC]; AllerMax® [OTC]; Altaryl [OTC]; Anti-Hist [OTC]; Banophen™ Anti-Itch [OTC]; Banophen™ [OTC]; Ben-Tann [DSC]; Benadryl® Allergy Quick Dissolve [OTC]; Benadryl® Allergy [OTC]; Benadryl® Children's Allergy Fastmelt® [OTC]; Benadryl® Children's Allergy Perfect Measure™; Benadryl® Children's Allergy [OTC]; Benadryl® Children's Dye-Free Allergy [OTC]; Benadryl® Children's Allergy Quick Dissolve [OTC] [DSC]; Benadryl® Dye-Free Allergy [OTC]; Benadryl® Itch Relief Extra Strength [OTC]; Benadryl® Itch Stopping Extra Strength [OTC]; Benadryl® Itch Stopping [OTC]; Compoz® Nighttime Sleep Aid [OTC]; Dermamycin® [OTC]; Diphen [OTC]; Diphenhist® [OTC]; Dytan™; Genahist™ [OTC]; Histaprin [OTC]; Hydramine [OTC]; Nytol® Quick Caps [OTC]; Nytol® Quick Gels [OTC]; PediaCare® Children's Allergy [OTC]; PediaCare® Children's NightTime Cough [OTC]; Siladryl Allergy [OTC]; Silphen Cough [OTC]; Simply Sleep™ [OTC]; Sleep-ettes D [OTC]; Sleep-Tabs [OTC]; Sleepinal® [OTC]; Sominex® Maximum Strength [OTC]; Sominex® [OTC]; Theraflu® Thin Strips® Multi Symptom [OTC]; Triaminic Thin Strips® Children's Cough and Runny Nose [OTC]; Twilite® [OTC]; Unisom® SleepGels® Maximum Strength [OTC]; Unisom® SleepMelts™ [OTC]

Canadian Brand Names Allerdryl®; Allernix; Benadryl®; Nytol®; Nytol® Extra Strength; PMS-Diphenhydramine; Simply Sleep®

Index Terms Diphenhydramine Citrate; Diphenhydramine Hydrochloride; Diphenhydramine Tannate

Pharmacologic Category Histamine H_1 Antagonist; Histamine H_1 Antagonist, First Generation

Generic Available Yes: Excludes chewable tablet, gel, liquid stick, orally-disintegrating tablet, strip

Use Symptomatic relief of allergic symptoms caused by histamine release including nasal allergies and allergic dermatosis; adjunct to epinephrine in the treatment of anaphylaxis; nighttime sleep aid; prevention or treatment of motion sickness; antitussive; management of Parkinsonian syndrome including drug-induced extrapyramidal symptoms; topically for relief of pain and itching associated with insect bites, minor cuts and burns, or rashes due to poison ivy, poison oak, and poison sumac

Mechanism of Action Competes with histamine for H_1-receptor sites on effector cells in the gastrointestinal tract, blood vessels, and respiratory tract; anticholinergic and sedative effects are also seen

Pharmacodynamics/Kinetics
Onset of action: Maximum sedative effect: 1-3 hours
Duration: 4-7 hours
Distribution: V_d: 3-22 L/kg
Protein binding: 78%
Metabolism: Extensively hepatic n-demethylation via CYP2D6; minor demethylation via CYP1A2, 2C9 and 2C19; smaller degrees in pulmonary and renal systems; significant first-pass effect
Bioavailability: Oral: ~40% to 70%
Half-life elimination: 2-10 hours; Elderly: 13.5 hours
Time to peak, serum: 2-4 hours
Excretion: Urine (as unchanged drug)

◀ **Dosage Note:** Dosages are expressed as the hydrochloride salt.
Children:
    Allergic reactions or motion sickness: Oral, I.M., I.V.: 5 mg/kg/day or 150 mg/m^2/day in divided doses every 6-8 hours, not to exceed 300 mg/day
      Alternate dosing by age: Oral:
        2 to <6 years: 6.25 mg every 4-6 hours; maximum: 37.5 mg/day
        6 to <12 years: 12.5-25 mg every 4-6 hours; maximum: 150 mg/day
        ≥12 years: 25-50 mg every 4-6 hours; maximum: 300 mg/day
    Night-time sleep aid: Oral: Children ≥12 years: 50 mg at bedtime
    Antitussive: Oral:
      2 to <6 years: 6.25 mg every 4 hours; maximum 37.5 mg/day
      6 to <12 years: 12.5 mg every 4 hours; maximum 75 mg/day
      ≥12 years: 25 mg every 4 hours; maximum 150 mg/day
    Treatment of dystonic reactions: I.M., I.V.: 0.5-1 mg/kg/dose
    Relief of pain and itching: Topical: Children ≥2 years: Apply 1% or 2% to affected area up to 3-4 times/day
Adults:
    Allergic reactions or motion sickness: Oral: 25-50 mg every 6-8 hours
    Antitussive: Oral: 25 mg every 4 hours; maximum 150 mg/24 hours
    Nighttime sleep aid: Oral: 50 mg at bedtime
    Allergic reactions or motion sickness: I.M., I.V.: 10-50 mg per dose; single doses up to 100 mg may be used if needed; not to exceed 400 mg/day
    Dystonic reaction: I.M., I.V.: 50 mg in a single dose; may repeat in 20-30 minutes if necessary
    Relief of pain and itching: Topical: Apply 1% or 2% to affected area up to 3-4 times/day

    Elderly: Initial: 25 mg 2-3 times/day increasing as needed
Stability Injection: Store at room temperature of 15°C to 30°C (59°F to 86°F); protect from freezing. Protect from light.
Administration When used to prevent motion sickness, first dose should be given 30 minutes prior to exposure. Injection solution is for I.V. or I.M. administration only; local necrosis may result with SubQ or intradermal use. For I.V. administration, inject at a rate ≤25 mg/minute.
Monitoring Parameters Relief of symptoms, mental alertness
Reference Range
    Antihistamine effects at levels >25 ng/mL
    Drowsiness at levels 30-40 ng/mL
    Mental impairment at levels >60 ng/mL
    Therapeutic: Not established
    Toxic: >0.1 mcg/mL
Anesthesia and Critical Care Concerns/Other Considerations
    Clinical Pearls/Comments: Diphenhydramine's use as a sleep aid is discouraged due to its anticholinergic effects.
Pregnancy Risk Factor B
Contraindications Hypersensitivity to diphenhydramine or any component of the formulation; acute asthma; neonates or premature infants; breast-feeding; use as a local anesthetic (injection)
Warnings/Precautions Causes sedation, caution must be used in performing tasks which require alertness (eg, operating machinery or driving). Sedative effects of CNS depressants or ethanol are potentiated. Use with caution in the elderly; may be more sensitive to adverse effects. Antihistamines may cause excitation in young children. Use with caution in patients with angle-closure glaucoma, pyloroduodenal obstruction (including stenotic peptic ulcer), urinary tract obstruction (including bladder neck obstruction and symptomatic prostatic hyperplasia), asthma, hyperthyroidism, increased intraocular pressure, and cardiovascular disease (including hypertension and tachycardia). Some preparations contain soy protein; avoid use in patients with soy protein or peanut allergies. Some products may contain phenylalanine.

Self-medication (OTC use): Do not use with other products containing diphenhydramine, even ones used on the skin. Oral products are not for OTC use in children <6 years of age. Topical products should not be used on large areas of the body, or on chicken pox or measles. Healthcare provider should be contacted if topical use is needed for >7 days. Topical products are not for OTC use in children <2 years of age.

Adverse Reactions Frequency not defined.

Cardiovascular: Chest tightness, extrasystoles, hypotension, palpitation, tachycardia

Central nervous system: Chills, confusion, convulsion, disturbed coordination, dizziness, euphoria, excitation, fatigue, headache, insomnia, irritability, nervousness, paradoxical excitement, restlessness, sedation, sleepiness, vertigo

Dermatologic: Photosensitivity, rash, urticaria

Endocrine & metabolic: Menstrual irregularities (early menses)

Gastrointestinal: Anorexia, constipation, diarrhea, dry mucous membranes, epigastric distress, nausea, throat tightness, vomiting, xerostomia

Genitourinary: Difficult urination, urinary frequency, urinary retention

Hematologic: Agranulocytosis, hemolytic anemia, thrombocytopenia

Neuromuscular & skeletal: Neuritis, paresthesia, tremor

Ocular: Blurred vision, diplopia

Otic: Labyrinthitis (acute), tinnitus

Respiratory: Nasal stuffiness, thickening of bronchial secretions, wheezing

Miscellaneous: Anaphylactic shock, diaphoresis

Drug Interactions

Metabolism/Transport Effects Inhibits CYP2D6 (moderate)

Avoid Concomitant Use There are no known interactions where it is recommended to avoid concomitant use.

Increased Effect/Toxicity

DiphenhydrAMINE may increase the levels/effects of: Alcohol (Ethyl); Anticholinergics; CNS Depressants; CYP2D6 Substrates; Fesoterodine; Nebivolol; Tamoxifen

The levels/effects of DiphenhydrAMINE may be increased by: Pramlintide

Decreased Effect

DiphenhydrAMINE may decrease the levels/effects of: Acetylcholinesterase Inhibitors (Central); Betahistine; Codeine; TraMADol

The levels/effects of DiphenhydrAMINE may be decreased by: Acetylcholinesterase Inhibitors (Central); Amphetamines

Ethanol/Nutrition/Herb Interactions

Ethanol: Avoid ethanol (may increase CNS depression).

Herb/Nutraceutical: Avoid valerian, St John's wort, kava kava, gotu kola (may increase CNS depression).

Test Interactions May suppress the wheal and flare reactions to skin test antigens

Dietary Considerations Some products may contain sodium and/or phenylalanine.

Benadryl® Children's Allergy Fastmelt® contains and soy protein isolate (contraindicated in patients with soy protein allergies; use caution in peanut allergic individuals, ~10% are estimated to also have soy protein allergies).

Dosage Forms Excipient information presented when available (limited, particularly for generics); consult specific product labeling. [DSC] = Discontinued product

Caplet, as hydrochloride: 25 mg, 50 mg

Aler-Dryl, AllerMax®, Compoz® Nighttime Sleep Aid, Sleep-ettes D, Sominex® Maximum Strength, Twilite®: 50 mg

Anti-Hist, Histaprin, Nytol® Quick Caps: 25 mg

Simply Sleep™: 25 mg [contains calcium 20 mg/caplet]

Capsule, as hydrochloride: 25 mg, 50 mg

Aler-Cap, Banophen™, Diphen, Diphenhist®, Genahist™: 25 mg

Benadryl® Allergy: 25 mg [contains calcium 35 mg/capsule]

Sleepinal®: 50 mg

Capsule, softgel, as hydrochloride: 50 mg

Benadryl® Dye-Free Allergy: 25 mg [dye-free]

Compoz® Nighttime Sleep Aid, Nytol® Quick Gels, Unisom® SleepGels® Maximum Strength: 50 mg

Captab, as hydrochloride:

Diphenhist®: 25 mg

Cream, as hydrochloride: 2% (30 g)
  Banophen™ Anti-Itch: 2% (30 g) [contains zinc acetate 0.1%]
  Benadryl® Itch Stopping: 1% (15 g, 30 g) [contains zinc acetate 0.1%]
  Benadryl® Itch Stopping Extra Strength: 2% (15 g, 30 g) [contains zinc acetate 0.1%]
  Diphenhist®: 2% (30 g) [contains zinc acetate 0.1%]
Elixir, as hydrochloride: 12.5 mg/5 mL
  Altaryl: 12.5 mg/5 mL (120 mL, 480 mL, 3840 mL) [ethanol free; cherry flavor]
  Banophen™: 12.5 mg/5 mL (120 mL)
Gel, topical, as hydrochloride:
  Benadryl® Itch Stopping Extra Strength: 2% (120 mL)
Injection, solution, as hydrochloride: 50 mg/mL (1 mL, 10 mL)
Liquid, oral, as hydrochloride:
  AllerMax®: 12.5 mg/5 mL (120 mL)
  Benadryl® Children's Allergy: 12.5 mg/5 mL (120 mL, 240 mL) [ethanol free; contains sodium 14 mg/5 mL, sodium benzoate; cherry flavor]
  Benadryl® Children's Allergy Perfect Measure™: 12.5 mg/5 mL (5 mL) [ethanol free; contains sodium 14 mg/5 mL, sodium benzoate; cherry flavor]
  Benadryl® Children's Dye-Free Allergy: 12.5 mg/5 mL (120 mL) [ethanol free, dye free, sugar free; contains sodium 11 mg/5 mL, sodium benzoate; bubble gum flavor]
  Genahist™: 12.5 mg/5 mL (120 mL) [ethanol free, sugar free; contains sodium benzoate; cherry flavor]
  Hydramine: 12.5 mg/5 mL (120 mL, 480 mL) [ethanol free]
  Siladryl Allergy: 12.5 mg/5 mL (120 mL, 240 mL, 480 mL) [ethanol free, sugar free; black cherry flavor]
Liquid, topical, as hydrochloride [spray]:
  Benadryl® Itch Stopping Extra Strength: 2% (60 mL) [contains zinc acetate 0.1% and ethanol]
  Dermamycin®: 2% (60 mL) [contains menthol 1%]
Liquid, topical, as hydrochloride [stick]:
  Benadryl® Itch Relief Extra Strength: 2% (14 mL) [contains zinc acetate 0.1% and ethanol]
Solution, oral, as hydrochloride:
  Diphenhist®: 12.5 mg/5 mL (120 mL, 480 mL) [ethanol free; contains sodium benzoate]
Strips, orally disintegrating, as hydrochloride:
  Benadryl® Allergy Quick Dissolve: 25 mg (10s) [contains sodium 4 mg/strip; vanilla mint flavor]
  Benadryl® Children's Allergy Quick Dissolve: 12.5 mg (10s) [vanilla mint flavor] [DSC]
  Theraflu® Thin Strips® Multi Symptom: 25 mg (12s) [contains ethanol; cherry flavor]
  Triaminic Thin Strips® Children's Cough and Runny Nose: 12.5 mg (14s) [contains ethanol; grape flavor]
Suspension, as tannate:
  Ben-Tann: 25 mg/5 mL (120 ml) [contains sodium benzoate; strawberry flavor] [DSC]
Syrup, as hydrochloride:
  PediaCare® Children's Allergy: 12.5 mg/5 mL (120 mL) [contains sodium 14 mg/5 mL, sodium benzoate; cherry flavor]
  PediaCare® Children's NightTime Cough: 12.5 mg/5 mL (120 mL) [ethanol free; contains sodium 15 mg/5 mL, sodium benzoate; cherry flavor]
  Silphen Cough: 12.5 mg/5 mL (120 mL, 240 mL, 480 mL) [contains ethanol 5%; strawberry flavor]
Tablet, as hydrochloride: 25 mg, 50 mg
  Aler-Tab, Banophen™, Benadryl® Allergy, Genahist™, Sominex®, Sleep-Tabs: 25 mg
Tablet, chewable, as hydrochloride:
  Benadryl® Children's Allergy: 12.5 mg [contains phenylalanine 4.2 mg, magnesium 15 mg, and sodium 2 mg per tablet; grape flavor] [DSC]
Tablet, chewable, as tannate:
  Dytan™: 25 mg [contains phenylalanine; strawberry flavor]

Tablet, orally disintegrating, as citrate:

Benadryl® Children's Allergy Fastmelt®: 19 mg [equivalent to diphenhydramine hydrochloride 12.5 mg; contains phenylalanine 4.5 mg/tablet and soy protein isolate; cherry flavor] [DSC]

Tablet, orally dissolving, as hydrochloride:

Benadryl® Children's Allergy Fastmelt®: 12.5 mg [cherry and grape flavors]
Unisom® SleepMelts™: 25 mg [cherry flavor]

References

Sampson HA, Munoz-Furtong A, Campbell RL, et al, "Second Symposium on the Definition and Management of Anaphylaxis: Summary Report - Second National Institute of Allergy and Infectious Disease/Food Allergy and Anaphylaxis Network Symposium," *Ann Emerg Med*, 2006, 7(4):373-80.

◆ **Diphenhydramine Citrate** *see* DiphenhydrAMINE *on page 430*

◆ **Diphenhydramine Hydrochloride** *see* DiphenhydrAMINE *on page 430*

◆ **Diphenhydramine Tannate** *see* DiphenhydrAMINE *on page 430*

◆ **Diphenylhydantoin** *see* Phenytoin *on page 1119*

◆ **Diprivan®** *see* Propofol *on page 1190*

◆ **Diprolene®** *see* Betamethasone *on page 186*

◆ **Diprolene® AF** *see* Betamethasone *on page 186*

◆ **Diprolene® Glycol (Can)** *see* Betamethasone *on page 186*

◆ **Dipropylacetic Acid** *see* Valproic Acid and Derivatives *on page 1445*

◆ **Diprosone® (Can)** *see* Betamethasone *on page 186*

Dipyridamole (dye peer ID a mole)

Medication Safety Issues

Sound-alike/look-alike issues:

Dipyridamole may be confused with disopyramide

Persantine® may be confused with Periactin®, Permitil®

U.S. Brand Names Persantine®

Canadian Brand Names Apo-Dipyridamole FC®; Dipyridamole For Injection; Persantine®

Pharmacologic Category Antiplatelet Agent; Vasodilator

Generic Available Yes

Use

Oral: Used with warfarin to decrease thrombosis in patients after artificial heart valve replacement

I.V.: Diagnostic agent in CAD

Unlabeled/Investigational Use Stroke prevention (in combination with aspirin)

Mechanism of Action Inhibits the activity of adenosine deaminase and phosphodiesterase, which causes an accumulation of adenosine, adenine nucleotides, and cyclic AMP; these mediators then inhibit platelet aggregation and may cause vasodilation; may also stimulate release of prostacyclin or PGD_2; causes coronary vasodilation

Pharmacodynamics/Kinetics

Absorption: Readily, but variable

Distribution: Adults: V_d: 2-3 L/kg

Protein binding: 91% to 99%

Metabolism: Hepatic

Half-life elimination: Terminal: 10-12 hours

Time to peak, serum: 2-2.5 hours

Excretion: Feces (as glucuronide conjugates and unchanged drug)

Dosage

Oral: Children ≥12 years and Adults: Adjunctive therapy for prophylaxis of thromboembolism with cardiac valve replacement: 75-100 mg 4 times/day

I.V.: Adults: Evaluation of coronary artery disease: 0.14 mg/kg/minute for 4 minutes; maximum dose: 60 mg

Following dipyridamole infusion, inject thallium-201 within 5 minutes. **Note:** Aminophylline should be available for urgent/emergent use; dosing of 50-100 mg (range: 50-250 mg) I.V. push over 30-60 seconds.

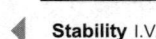 **Stability** I.V.: Store between 15°C to 25°C (59°F to 77°F); do not freeze. Protect from light. Prior to administration, dilute to a ≥1:2 ratio in NS, 1/2NS, or D$_5$W. Total volume should be ~20-50 mL.

Administration

I.V.: Infuse diluted solution over 4 minutes.

Tablet: Administer with water 1 hour before meals.

Monitoring Parameters Blood pressure, heart rate, ECG (stress test)

Anesthesia and Critical Care Concerns/Other Considerations

Clinical Pearls/Comments: For patients undergoing CABG, the 8th American College of Chest Physicians Consensus Conference recommends against the addition of dipyridamole to aspirin therapy for prevention of graft thrombosis (Becker, 2008).

Due to variable dipyridamole gastric absorption, a reformulated product (modified release dipyridamole/low-dose aspirin) provides improved bioavailability and is FDA-approved for stroke prevention (Patrono, 2008).

Pregnancy Risk Factor B

Contraindications Hypersensitivity to dipyridamole or any component of the formulation

Warnings/Precautions Use with in patients with hypotension, unstable angina, and/or recent MI. Use with caution in hepatic impairment. Use caution in patients on other antiplatelet agents or anticoagulation. Severe adverse reactions have occurred with I.V. administration (rarely); use the I.V. form with caution in patients with bronchospastic disease or unstable angina. Aminophylline should be available in case of urgency or emergency with I.V. use. Safety and efficacy in children <12 years of age have not been established.

Adverse Reactions

Oral:

>10%: Dizziness (14%)

1% to 10%:

Central nervous system: Headache (2%)

Dermatologic: Rash (2%)

Gastrointestinal: Abdominal distress (6%)

Frequency not defined: Diarrhea, vomiting, flushing, pruritus, angina pectoris, liver dysfunction

Postmarketing and/or case reports: Alopecia, arthritis, cholelithiasis, dyspepsia, fatigue, hepatitis, hypersensitivity reaction, hypotension, larynx edema, malaise, myalgia, nausea, palpitation, paresthesia, tachycardia, thrombocytopenia

I.V.:

>10%:

Cardiovascular: Exacerbation of angina pectoris (20%)

Central nervous system: Dizziness (12%), headache (12%)

1% to 10%:

Cardiovascular: Hypotension (5%), hypertension (2%), blood pressure lability (2%), ECG abnormalities (ST-T changes, extrasystoles; 5% to 8%), pain (3%), tachycardia (3%)

Central nervous system: Flushing (3%), fatigue (1%)

Gastrointestinal: Nausea (5%)

Neuromuscular & skeletal: Paresthesia (1%)

Respiratory: Dyspnea (3%)

<1% (Limited to important or life-threatening): Abdominal pain, abnormal coordination, allergic reaction (pruritus, rash, urticaria), appetite increased, arrhythmia (ventricular tachycardia, bradycardia, AV block, SVT, atrial fibrillation, asystole), arthralgia, asthenia, back pain, breast pain, bronchospasm, cardiomyopathy, cough, depersonalization, diaphoresis, dry mouth, dysgeusia, dyspepsia, dysphagia, earache, ECG abnormalities (unspecified), edema, eructation, flatulence, hypertonia, hyperventilation, injection site reaction, intermittent claudication leg cramping, malaise, MI, myalgia, orthostatic hypotension, palpitation, perineal pain, pharyngitis, pleural pain, renal pain, rhinitis, rigor, syncope, tenesmus, thirst, tinnitus, tremor, vertigo, vision abnormalities, vomiting

Drug Interactions

Avoid Concomitant Use
Avoid concomitant use of Dipyridamole with any of the following: Dabigatran Etexilate; Silodosin

Increased Effect/Toxicity
Dipyridamole may increase the levels/effects of: Adenosine; Anticoagulants; Antiplatelet Agents; Beta-Blockers; Colchicine; Dabigatran Etexilate; Drotrecogin Alfa; Hypotensive Agents; Ibritumomab; P-Glycoprotein Substrates; Regadenoson; Rivaroxaban; Salicylates; Silodosin; Thrombolytic Agents; Topotecan; Tositumomab and Iodine I 131 Tositumomab

The levels/effects of Dipyridamole may be increased by: Dasatinib; Herbs (Anticoagulant/Antiplatelet Properties); Nonsteroidal Anti-Inflammatory Agents; Omega-3-Acid Ethyl Esters; Pentosan Polysulfate Sodium; Pentoxifylline; Prostacyclin Analogues

Decreased Effect
The levels/effects of Dipyridamole may be decreased by: Nonsteroidal Anti-Inflammatory Agents

Ethanol/Nutrition/Herb Interactions Herb/Nutraceutical: Avoid cat's claw, dong quai, evening primrose, feverfew, garlic, ginger, ginkgo, red clover, horse chestnut, green tea, ginseng (all have additional antiplatelet activity).

Dietary Considerations Should be taken with water 1 hour before meals.

Dosage Forms Excipient information presented when available (limited, particularly for generics); consult specific product labeling.
Injection, solution: 5 mg/mL (2 mL, 10 mL)
Tablet: 25 mg, 50 mg, 75 mg
Persantine®: 25 mg, 50 mg, 75 mg

References
Becker RC, Meade TW, Berger PB, et al, "The Primary and Secondary Prevention of Coronary Artery Disease: American College of Chest Physicians Evidence-Based Clinical Practice Guidelines (8th Edition)," *Chest,* 2008, 133(6 Suppl):776S-814S.

Patrono C, Baigent C, Hirsh J, et al, "Antiplatelet Drugs: American College of Chest Physicians Evidence-Based Clinical Practice Guidelines (8th Edition)," *Chest,* 2008, 133(6 Suppl):199S-233S.

◆ **Dipyridamole and Aspirin** *see* Aspirin and Dipyridamole *on page 152*

◆ **Dipyridamole For Injection (Can)** *see* Dipyridamole *on page 435*

◆ **Disalicylic Acid** *see* Salsalate *on page 1275*

◆ **Disodium Thiosulfate Pentahydrate** *see* Sodium Thiosulfate *on page 1316*

Disopyramide (dye soe PEER a mide)

Related Information
Antiarrhythmic Drugs *on page 1656*

U.S. Brand Names Norpace®; Norpace® CR

Canadian Brand Names Norpace®; Rythmodan®; Rythmodan®-LA

Index Terms Disopyramide Phosphate

Pharmacologic Category Antiarrhythmic Agent, Class Ia

Use Suppression and prevention of unifocal and multifocal atrial and premature, ventricular premature complexes, coupled ventricular tachycardia; effective in the conversion of atrial fibrillation, atrial flutter, and paroxysmal atrial tachycardia to normal sinus rhythm and prevention of the recurrence of these arrhythmias after conversion by other methods

Unlabeled/Investigational Use Hypertrophic obstructive cardiomyopathy (HOCM)

Pharmacodynamics/Kinetics
Onset of action: 0.5-3.5 hours
Duration: 1.5-8.5 hours
Absorption: 60% to 83%
Distribution: V_d: 0.8-2 L/kg
Protein binding (concentration dependent): 20% to 60%
Metabolism: Hepatic to inactive metabolites
Half-life elimination: Adults: 4-10 hours; prolonged with hepatic or renal impairment

Time to peak, serum: Within 2 hours

Excretion: Urine (40% to 60% as unchanged drug); feces (10% to 15%)

Dosage Oral:

Children:

<1 year: 10-30 mg/kg/24 hours in 4 divided doses

1-4 years: 10-20 mg/kg/24 hours in 4 divided doses

4-12 years: 10-15 mg/kg/24 hours in 4 divided doses

12-18 years: 6-15 mg/kg/24 hours in 4 divided doses

Adults:

<50 kg: 100 mg every 6 hours or 200 mg every 12 hours (controlled release)

>50 kg: 150 mg every 6 hours or 300 mg every 12 hours (controlled release); if no response, increase to 200 mg every 6 hours. Maximum dose required for patients with severe refractory ventricular tachycardia is 400 mg every 6 hours.

Hypertrophic obstructive cardiomyopathy (unlabeled use): Initial: Controlled release: 200 mg twice daily. If symptoms do not improve, increase by 100 mg/ day at 2-week intervals to a maximum daily dose of 600 mg.

Elderly: Dose with caution, starting at the lower end of dosing range

Dosing adjustment in renal impairment: 100 mg (nonsustained release) given at the following intervals, based on creatinine clearance (mL/minute):

Cl_{cr} 30-40 mL/minute: Administer every 8 hours

Cl_{cr} 15-30 mL/minute: Administer every 12 hours

Cl_{cr} <15 mL/minute: Administer every 24 hours

or alter the dose as follows:

Cl_{cr} 30-<40 mL/minute: Reduce dose 50%

Cl_{cr} 15-30 mL/minute: Reduce dose 75%

Dialysis: Not dialyzable (0% to 5%) by hemo- or peritoneal methods; supplemental dose is not necessary.

Dosing interval in hepatic impairment: 100 mg every 6 hours or 200 mg every 12 hours (controlled release)

Anesthesia and Critical Care Concerns/Other Considerations In patients with pre-existing cardiovascular disease, the incidence of proarrhythmic effects and mortality may be increased with Class Ia antiarrhythmic agents. Disopyramide has significant anticholinergic effects which also limits its role in patients with cardiovascular disease.

Additional Information Complete prescribing information for this medication should be consulted for additional detail.

Dosage Forms Excipient information presented when available (limited, particularly for generics); consult specific product labeling.

Capsule (Norpace®): 100 mg, 150 mg

Capsule, controlled release (Norpace® CR): 100 mg, 150 mg

◆ **Disopyramide Phosphate** *see* Disopyramide *on page 437*

◆ **Ditropan®** *see* Oxybutynin *on page 1068*

◆ **Ditropan XL®** *see* Oxybutynin *on page 1068*

◆ **Diuril®** *see* Chlorothiazide *on page 295*

◆ **Divalproex Sodium** *see* Valproic Acid and Derivatives *on page 1445*

◆ **Divigel®** *see* Estradiol *on page 531*

◆ **Dixarit® (Can)** *see* CloNIDine *on page 329*

◆ ***D*-Mannitol** *see* Mannitol *on page 866*

DOBUTamine (doe BYOO ta meen)

Medication Safety Issues

Sound-alike/look-alike issues:

DOBUTamine may be confused with DOPamine

High alert medication: The Institute for Safe Medication Practices (ISMP) includes this medication among its list of drugs which have a heightened risk of causing significant patient harm when used in error.

Related Information

Heart Failure (Systolic) *on page 1739*
Hemodynamic Support, Intravenous *on page 1681*

Canadian Brand Names Dobutamine Injection, USP; Dobutrex®

Index Terms Dobutamine Hydrochloride

Pharmacologic Category Adrenergic Agonist Agent

Generic Available Yes

Use Short-term management of patients with cardiac decompensation

Unlabeled/Investigational Use Positive inotropic agent for use in myocardial dysfunction related to sepsis; stress echocardiography

Mechanism of Action Stimulates beta$_1$-adrenergic receptors, causing increased contractility and heart rate, with little effect on beta$_2$- or alpha-receptors

Pharmacodynamics/Kinetics

Onset of action: I.V.: 1-10 minutes
Peak effect: 10-20 minutes
Metabolism: In tissues and hepatically to inactive metabolites
Half-life elimination: 2 minutes
Excretion: Urine (as metabolites)

Dosage Administration requires the use of an infusion pump; I.V. infusion:
Neonates: 2-15 mcg/kg/minute, titrate to desired response
Children and Adults: 2.5-20 mcg/kg/minute; maximum: 40 mcg/kg/minute, titrate to desired response. See table.

Infusion Rates of Various Dilutions of Dobutamine

Desired Delivery Rate (mcg/kg/min)	Infusion Rate (mL/kg/min)	
	500 mcg/mL[1]	1000 mcg/mL[2]
2.5	0.005	0.0025
5	0.01	0.005
7.5	0.015	0.0075
10	0.02	0.01
12.5	0.025	0.0125
15	0.03	0.015

[1]500 mg per liter or 250 mg per 500 mL of diluent.
[2]1000 mg per liter or 250 mg per 250 mL of diluent.

Stability Remix solution every 24 hours. Store reconstituted solution under refrigeration for 48 hours or 6 hours at room temperature. Pink discoloration of solution indicates slight oxidation but **no** significant loss of potency.

Stability of parenteral admixture at room temperature (25°C): 48 hours; at refrigeration (4°C): 7 days.
Standard adult diluent: 250 mg/500 mL D$_5$W; 500 mg/500 mL D$_5$W.

Administration Use infusion device to control rate of flow; administer into large vein. Do not administer through same I.V. line as heparin, hydrocortisone sodium succinate, cefazolin, or penicillin.

To prepare for infusion:

$$\frac{6 \times weight\ (kg) \times desired\ dose\ (mcg/kg/min)}{I.V.\ infusion\ rate\ (mL/h)} = \begin{array}{c} mg\ of\ drug\ to\ be\ added\ to \\ 100\ mL\ of\ I.V.\ fluid \end{array}$$

Monitoring Parameters Blood pressure, ECG, heart rate, CVP, RAP, MAP, urine output; if pulmonary artery catheter is in place, monitor CI, PCWP, and SVR; also monitor serum potassium

Anesthesia and Critical Care Concerns/Other Considerations
Evidence-Based Information:

Septic Shock: Septic patients who have been adequately fluid resuscitated and have an adequate mean arterial pressure but low cardiac index (<2.5 L/minute/m^2) may require dobutamine. Dobutamine may help reverse tissue hypoperfusion

◀ by increasing cardiac output. Increasing cardiac output beyond the normal range has not been shown in clinical trials to improve patient outcome. The 2008 Surviving Sepsis Campaign guidelines recommend the use of dobutamine infusion when myocardial dysfunction is present with the goal of normalizing cardiac output. Avoid trying to increase cardiac index to supranormal levels (Grade 1C).

Early goal-directed therapy in the treatment of severe sepsis and septic shock provides significant survival benefits to this subset of patients. About 14% of the patients in the early goal-directed group received dobutamine. The early goal-directed patients received significantly more fluid, red-cell transfusions, and inotropic support during the initial 6 hours of their visit (Rivers, 2001). The 2008 Surviving Sepsis Campaign guidelines suggest that if central venous (superior vena cava) or mixed venous oxygen saturation of ≥70% or ≥65%, respectively, is not achieved (central venous pressure 8-12 mm Hg) within the first 6 hours of resuscitation, then transfuse packed red blood cells to a hematocrit of ≥30% and/or administer dobutamine (up to 20 mcg/kg/minute) to achieve this goal (Grade 2C).

Pregnancy Risk Factor B

Contraindications Hypersensitivity to dobutamine or sulfites (some contain sodium metabisulfate), or any component of the formulation; idiopathic hypertrophic subaortic stenosis (IHSS)

Warnings/Precautions May increase heart rate. Patients with atrial fibrillation may experience an increase in ventricular response. An increase in blood pressure is more common, but occasionally a patient may become hypotensive. May exacerbate ventricular ectopy. If needed, correct hypovolemia first to optimize hemodynamics. Ineffective therapeutically in the presence of mechanical obstruction such as severe aortic stenosis. Use caution post-MI (can increase myocardial oxygen demand). Use cautiously in the elderly starting at lower end of the dosage range. Use with extreme caution in patients taking MAO inhibitors. Dobutamine in combination with stress echo may be used diagnostically. Product may contain sodium sulfite.

Adverse Reactions Incidence of adverse events is not always reported.

Cardiovascular: Increased heart rate, increased blood pressure, increased ventricular ectopic activity, hypotension, premature ventricular beats (5%, dose related), anginal pain (1% to 3%), nonspecific chest pain (1% to 3%), palpitation (1% to 3%)

Central nervous system: Fever (1% to 3%), headache (1% to 3%), paresthesia

Endocrine & metabolic: Slight decrease in serum potassium

Gastrointestinal: Nausea (1% to 3%)

Hematologic: Thrombocytopenia (isolated cases)

Local: Phlebitis, local inflammatory changes and pain from infiltration, cutaneous necrosis (isolated cases)

Neuromuscular & skeletal: Mild leg cramps

Respiratory: Dyspnea (1% to 3%)

Drug Interactions

Avoid Concomitant Use

Avoid concomitant use of DOBUTamine with any of the following: Iobenguane I 123

Increased Effect/Toxicity

DOBUTamine may increase the levels/effects of: Sympathomimetics

The levels/effects of DOBUTamine may be increased by: Atomoxetine; Cannabinoids; COMT Inhibitors

Decreased Effect

DOBUTamine may decrease the levels/effects of: Iobenguane I 123

The levels/effects of DOBUTamine may be decreased by: Calcium Salts

Dosage Forms Excipient information presented when available (limited, particularly for generics); consult specific product labeling.

Infusion, as hydrochloride [premixed in dextrose]: 1 mg/mL (250 mL, 500 mL); 2 mg/mL (250 mL); 4 mg/mL (250 mL)

Injection, solution, as hydrochloride: 12.5 mg/mL (20 mL, 40 mL, 100 mL) [contains sodium bisulfite]

References

Dellinger RP, Levy MM, Carlet JM, et al, "Surviving Sepsis Campaign: International Guidelines for Management of Severe Sepsis and Septic Shock: 2008," *Intensive Care Med*, 2008, 34(1): 17-60. Available at http://www.survivingsepsis.org/system/files/images/2008_20International_20SSC_20-Guidelines_1_.pdf.

"Practice Parameters for Hemodynamic Support of Sepsis in Adult Patients. Task Force of the American College of Critical Care Medicine, Society of Critical Care Medicine," *Crit Care Med*, 1999, 27(3):639-60. Available at: http://www.sccm.org/pdf/Hemodynamic%20Support.pdf. Accessed August 13, 2003.

Rivers E, Nguyen B, Havstad S, et al, "Early Goal-Directed Therapy in the Treatment of Severe Sepsis and Septic Shock," *N Engl J Med*, 2001, 345(19):1368-77.

◆ **Dobutamine Hydrochloride** *see* DOBUTamine *on page* 438

◆ **Dobutamine Injection, USP (Can)** *see* DOBUTamine *on page* 438

◆ **Dobutrex® (Can)** *see* DOBUTamine *on page* 438

Dofetilide (doe FET il ide)

Related Information

Antiarrhythmic Drugs *on page* 1656
Heart Failure (Systolic) *on page* 1739

U.S. Brand Names Tikosyn®

Canadian Brand Names Tikosyn®

Pharmacologic Category Antiarrhythmic Agent, Class III

Restrictions Tikosyn® is only available to prescribers and hospitals that have confirmed their participation in a designated Tikosyn® Education Program. The program provides comprehensive education about the importance of in-hospital treatment initiation and individualized dosing.

T.I.P.S. is the Tikosyn® In Pharmacy System designated to allow retail pharmacies to stock and dispense Tikosyn® once they have been enrolled. A participating pharmacy must confirm receipt of the T.I.P.S. program materials and educate its pharmacy staff about the procedures required to fill an outpatient prescription for Tikosyn®. The T.I.P.S. enrollment form is available at www.tikosyn.com. Tikosyn® is only available from a special mail order pharmacy, and enrolled retail pharmacies. Pharmacists must verify that the hospital/prescriber is a confirmed participant before Tikosyn® is provided. For participant verification, the pharmacist may call 1-800-788-7353 or use the web site located at www.-tikosynlist.com. Further details and directions on the program are provided at www.tikosyn.com.

Dofetilide therapy must be initiated/adjusted in a hospital setting with proper monitoring under the guidance of experienced personnel.

Generic Available No

Use Maintenance of normal sinus rhythm in patients with chronic atrial fibrillation/atrial flutter of longer than 1-week duration who have been converted to normal sinus rhythm; conversion of atrial fibrillation and atrial flutter to normal sinus rhythm

Mechanism of Action Vaughan Williams Class III antiarrhythmic activity. Blockade of the cardiac ion channel carrying the rapid component of the delayed rectifier potassium current. Dofetilide has no effect on sodium channels, adrenergic alpha-receptors, or adrenergic beta-receptors. It increases the monophasic action potential duration due to delayed repolarization. The increase in the QT interval is a function of prolongation of both effective and functional refractory periods in the His-Purkinje system and the ventricles. Changes in cardiac conduction velocity and sinus node function have not been observed in patients with or without structural heart disease. PR and QRS width remain the same in patients with pre-existing heart block and or sick sinus syndrome.

Pharmacodynamics/Kinetics

Absorption: Well absorbed

Distribution: V_d: 3 L/kg

Protein binding: 60% to 70%

Metabolism: Hepatic via CYP3A4, but low affinity for it; metabolites formed by N-dealkylation and N-oxidation

Bioavailability: >90%

Half-life elimination: 10 hours

Time to peak, serum: Fasting: 2-3 hours

Excretion: Urine (80%; 80% as unchanged drug, 20% as inactive or minimally active metabolites); renal elimination consists of glomerular filtration and active tubular secretion via cationic transport system

Dosage Adults: Oral:

Note: QT or QT_c must be determined prior to first dose. If QT_c >440 msec (>500 msec in patients with ventricular conduction abnormalities), dofetilide is contraindicated (see Contraindications and Warnings/Precautions).

Initial: 500 mcg orally twice daily. Initial dosage must be adjusted in patients with estimated Cl_{cr} <60 mL/minute (see Dosage Adjustment in Renal Impairment). Dofetilide may be initiated at lower doses than recommended based on physician discretion.

Modification of dosage in response to initial dose: QT_c interval should be measured 2-3 hours after the initial dose. If the QT_c >15% of baseline, or if the QT_c is >500 msec (550 msec in patients with ventricular conduction abnormalities) dofetilide should be adjusted. If the starting dose is 500 mcg twice daily, then adjust to 250 mcg twice daily. If the starting dose was 250 mcg twice daily, then adjust to 125 mcg twice daily. If the starting dose was 125 mcg twice daily then adjust to 125 mcg every day.

Continued monitoring for doses 2-5: QT_c interval must be determined 2-3 hours after each subsequent dose of dofetilide for in-hospital doses 2-5. If the measured QT_c is >500 msec (550 msec in patients with ventricular conduction abnormalities) at any time, dofetilide should be discontinued.

Chronic therapy (following the 5th dose):

QT or QT_c and creatinine clearance should be evaluated every 3 months. If QT_c >500 msec (>550 msec in patients with ventricular conduction abnormalities), dofetilide should be discontinued.

Dosage adjustment in renal impairment: Note: The manufacturer recommends using actual body weight when using the Cockcroft-Gault equation to calculate creatinine clearance.

Cl_{cr} >60 mL/minute: Administer 500 mcg twice daily.

Cl_{cr} 40-60 mL/minute: Administer 250 mcg twice daily.

Cl_{cr} 20-39 mL/minute: Administer 125 mcg twice daily.

Cl_{cr} <20 mL/minute: Contraindicated in this group.

Dosage adjustment in hepatic impairment: No dosage adjustments required in Child-Pugh Class A and B. Patients with severe hepatic impairment were not studied.

Elderly: No specific dosage adjustments are recommended based on age, however, careful assessment of renal function is particularly important in this population.

Administration Do not open capsules.

Monitoring Parameters ECG monitoring with attention to QT_c and occurrence of ventricular arrhythmias, baseline serum creatinine and changes in serum creatinine. Check serum potassium and magnesium levels if on medications where these electrolyte disturbances can occur, or if patient has a history of hypokalemia or hypomagnesemia. QT or QT_c must be monitored at specific times prior to the first dose and during the first 3 days of therapy. Thereafter, QT or QT_c and creatinine clearance must be evaluated at 3-month intervals.

Anesthesia and Critical Care Concerns/Other Considerations

Clinical Pearl/Comments: Since dofetilide is ~80% renally eliminated and the QT interval is sensitive to changes in heart rate and electrolyte disturbances, the critically-ill patient continued on dofetilide should be closely monitored for QT_c prolongation, hypomagnesemia, hypokalemia, and hypocalcemia. Dosage adjustments should be made based on Cl_{cr} (Cockcroft-Gault method). Dofetilide should be discontinued if QT_c-prolongation exceeds 500 msec (or 550 msec in patients with ventricular conduction abnormalities) or if Cl_{cr} is <20 mL/minute given the elevated risk of torsade de pointes. QT_c should be determined using Bazett's formula if heart rate exceeds 60 bpm. The QT interval should be used to guide dosage adjustment if heart rate is <60 bpm.

Pregnancy Risk Factor C

Contraindications Hypersensitivity to dofetilide or any component of the formulation; patients with congenital or acquired long QT syndromes, do not use if a baseline QT interval or QT_c is >440 msec (500 msec in patients with ventricular conduction abnormalities); severe renal impairment (estimated Cl_{cr} <20 mL/minute); concurrent use with verapamil, cimetidine, hydrochlorothiazide (alone or in combinations), trimethoprim (alone or in combination with sulfamethoxazole), itraconazole, ketoconazole, prochlorperazine, or megestrol; baseline heart rate <50 beats/minute; other drugs that prolong QT intervals (phenothiazines, cisapride, bepridil, tricyclic antidepressants, moxifloxacin; hypokalemia or hypomagnesemia; concurrent amiodarone, clarithromycin, or erythromycin

Warnings/Precautions [U.S. Boxed Warning]: Must be initiated (or reinitiated) in a setting with continuous monitoring and staff familiar with the recognition and treatment of life-threatening arrhythmias. Patients must be monitored with continuous ECG for a minimum of 3 days, or for a minimum of 12 hours after electrical or pharmacological cardioversion to normal sinus rhythm, whichever is greater. Patients should be readmitted for continuous monitoring if dosage is later increased.

Reserve for patients who are highly symptomatic with atrial fibrillation/atrial flutter; torsade de pointes significantly increases with doses >500 mcg twice daily; hold Class Ia or Class II antiarrhythmics for at least three half-lives prior to starting dofetilide; use in patients on amiodarone therapy only if serum amiodarone level is <0.3 mg/L or if amiodarone was stopped for >3 months previously; correct hypokalemia or hypomagnesemia before initiating dofetilide and maintain within normal limits during treatment. Risk of hypokalemia and/or hypomagnesemia may be increased by potassium-depleting diuretics, increasing the risk of torsade de pointes. Concurrent use with other drugs known to prolong QT_c interval is not recommended.

Patients with sick sinus syndrome or with second or third-degree heart block should not receive dofetilide unless a functional pacemaker is in place. Defibrillation threshold is reduced in patients with ventricular tachycardia or ventricular fibrillation undergoing implantation of a cardioverter-defibrillator device. Safety and efficacy in children (<18 years of age) have not been established. Use with caution in renal impairment; not recommended in patients receiving drugs which may compete for renal secretion via cationic transport. Use with caution in patients with severe hepatic impairment.

In the Cardiac Arrhythmia Suppression Trial (CAST), recent (>6 days but <2 years ago) myocardial infarction patients with asymptomatic, non-life-threatening ventricular arrhythmias did not benefit and may have been harmed by attempts to suppress the arrhythmia with flecainide or encainide. An increased mortality or nonfatal cardiac arrest rate (7.7%) was seen in the active treatment group compared with patients in the placebo group (3%). The applicability of the CAST results to other populations is unknown. Antiarrhythmic agents should be reserved for patients with life-threatening ventricular arrhythmias.

Adverse Reactions
Supraventricular arrhythmia patients (incidence > placebo)
>10%: Central nervous system: Headache (11%)
2% to 10%:
  Central nervous system: Dizziness (8%), insomnia (4%)
  Cardiovascular: Ventricular tachycardia (2.6% to 3.7%), chest pain (10%), torsade de pointes (3.3% in CHF patients and 0.9% in patients with a recent MI; up to 10.5% in patients receiving doses in excess of those recommended). Torsade de pointes occurs most frequently within the first 3 days of therapy.
  Dermatologic: Rash (3%)
  Gastrointestinal: Nausea (5%), diarrhea (3%), abdominal pain (3%)
  Neuromuscular & skeletal: Back pain (3%)
  Respiratory: Respiratory tract infection (7%), dyspnea (6%)
  Miscellaneous: Flu syndrome (4%)
<2% (Limited to important or life-threatening): Angioedema, AV block (0.4% to 1.5%), bundle branch block, cardiac arrest, facial paralysis, flaccid paralysis, heart block, hepatotoxicity, MI, paralysis, paresthesia, stroke, syncope, ventricular fibrillation (0% to 0.4%)

Drug Interactions
Metabolism/Transport Effects Substrate of CYP3A4 (minor)

◀ **Avoid Concomitant Use**
Avoid concomitant use of Dofetilide with any of the following: Antifungal Agents (Azole Derivatives, Systemic); Artemether; Cimetidine; Dronedarone; Lumefantrine; Megestrol; Nilotinib; Pimozide; Prochlorperazine; QuiNINE; Tetrabenazine; Thiazide Diuretics; Thioridazine; Trimethoprim; Verapamil; Ziprasidone

Increased Effect/Toxicity
Dofetilide may increase the levels/effects of: Dronedarone; Pimozide; QTc-Prolonging Agents; QuiNINE; Tetrabenazine; Thioridazine; Ziprasidone

The levels/effects of Dofetilide may be increased by: Alfuzosin; Antifungal Agents (Azole Derivatives, Systemic); Artemether; Chloroquine; Cimetidine; Ciprofloxacin; Gadobutrol; Loop Diuretics; Lumefantrine; Megestrol; Nilotinib; Prochlorperazine; QuiNINE; Thiazide Diuretics; Trimethoprim; Verapamil

Decreased Effect There are no known significant interactions involving a decrease in effect.

Ethanol/Nutrition/Herb Interactions Herb/Nutraceutical: St John's wort may decrease dofetilide levels. Avoid ephedra (may worsen arrhythmia).

Dosage Forms Excipient information presented when available (limited, particularly for generics); consult specific product labeling.
Capsule: 125 mcg, 250 mcg, 500 mcg

References
Fuster V, Rydén LE, Asinger RW, et al, "ACC/AHA/ESC Guidelines for the Management of Patients with Atrial Fibrillation: A Report of the American College of Cardiology/American Heart Association Task Force on Practice Guidelines and the European Society of Cardiology Committee for Practice Guidelines and Policy Conferences," *J Am Coll Cardiol*, 2001, 38(4):1231-66.

Dolasetron (dol A se tron)

Medication Safety Issues
Sound-alike/look-alike issues:
Anzemet® may be confused with Aldomet®, Avandamet®
Dolasetron may be confused with granisetron, ondansetron, palonosetron

Related Information
Postoperative Nausea and Vomiting *on page 1593*

U.S. Brand Names Anzemet®

Canadian Brand Names Anzemet®

Index Terms Dolasetron Mesylate; MDL 73,147EF

Pharmacologic Category Antiemetic; Selective 5-HT$_3$ Receptor Antagonist

Generic Available No

Use Prevention of nausea and vomiting associated with emetogenic cancer chemotherapy; prevention of postoperative nausea and vomiting; treatment of postoperative nausea and vomiting (injectable form only).

Note: In Canada, the use of dolasetron is contraindicated in children <18 years of age and for the prevention and treatment of postoperative nausea and vomiting in adults. These are not labeled contraindications in the U.S.

Unlabeled/Investigational Use Breakthrough treatment of nausea and vomiting associated with chemotherapy

Mechanism of Action Selective serotonin receptor (5-HT$_3$) antagonist, blocking serotonin both peripherally (primary site of action) and centrally at the chemoreceptor trigger zone

Pharmacodynamics/Kinetics
Absorption: Rapid and complete
Distribution: Hydrodolasetron: 5.8 L/kg
Protein binding: Hydrodolasetron: 69% to 77% (50% bound to alpha$_1$-acid glycoprotein)
Metabolism: Hepatic; reduction by carbonyl reductase to hydrodolasetron (active metabolite); further metabolized by CYP2D6, CYP3A, and flavin monooxygenase
Bioavailability: 75%
Half-life elimination: Dolasetron: 10 minutes; hydrodolasetron: Adults: 6-8 hours; Children: 4-6 hours
Time to peak, plasma: Hydrodolasetron: I.V.: 0.6 hours; Oral: 1 hour

Excretion: Urine ~67% (53% to 61% as active metabolite hydrodolasetron); feces ~33%

Dosage

Prevention of chemotherapy-associated nausea and vomiting (including initial and repeat courses):

Children 2-16 years:

Oral: 1.8 mg/kg within 1 hour before chemotherapy; maximum: 100 mg/dose

I.V.: 1.8 mg/kg ~30 minutes before chemotherapy; maximum: 100 mg/dose

Adults:

Oral:100 mg single dose 1 hour prior to chemotherapy

I.V.: 1.8 mg/kg or 100 mg 30 minutes prior to chemotherapy

Prevention of postoperative nausea and vomiting:

Children 2-16 years:

Oral: 1.2 mg/kg within 2 hours before surgery; maximum: 100 mg/dose

I.V.: 0.35 mg/kg (maximum: 12.5 mg) ~15 minutes before stopping anesthesia

Adults:

Oral: 100 mg within 2 hours before surgery

I.V.: 12.5 mg ~15 minutes before stopping anesthesia

Treatment of postoperative nausea and vomiting: I.V. (only):

Children: 0.35 mg/kg (maximum: 12.5 mg) as soon as needed

Adults: 12.5 mg as soon as needed

Dosing adjustment for elderly, renal/hepatic impairment: No dosage adjustment is recommended

Stability Store intact vials and tablets at room temperature. Protect from light. A 20 mg/mL solution in syringes is stable for 8 months at room temperature. Dilute in 50-100 mL of a compatible solution (ie, 0.9% NS, D_5W, $D_5^{1}/_2NS$, D_5LR, LR, and 10% mannitol injection). Solutions diluted for infusion are stable at room temperature for 24 hours or under refrigeration for 48 hours.

Administration I.V. injection may be given either undiluted IVP over 30 seconds or diluted in 50 mL of compatible fluid and infused over 15 minutes. Line should be flushed, prior to and after, dolasetron administration. Dolasetron injection may be diluted in apple or apple-grape juice and taken orally; this dilution is stable for 2 hours at room temperature.

Monitoring Parameters Liver function tests, blood pressure and pulse, and ECG in patients with cardiovascular disease

Anesthesia and Critical Care Concerns/Other Considerations

Clinical Pearls/Comments: Oral administration of the intravenous solution is equivalent to tablets.

Pregnancy Risk Factor B

Contraindications Hypersensitivity to dolasetron or any component of the formulation

Note: In Canada, the use of dolasetron is contraindicated for all uses in children <18 years of age or in the treatment of postoperative nausea and vomiting in adults. These are not labeled contraindications in the U.S.

Warnings/Precautions Dolasetron should be administered with caution in patients with congenital long QT syndrome or other risk factors for QT prolongation (eg, medications known to prolong QT interval, electrolyte abnormalities, and cumulative high-dose anthracycline therapy). Dolasetron has been associated with a number of dose-dependent increases in ECG intervals (eg, PR, QRS duration, QT/QT_c, JT), usually occurring 1-2 hours after I.V. administration and usually lasting 6-8 hours; however, may last ≥24 hours and rarely lead to heart block or arrhythmia. Clinically relevant QT interval prolongation may occur resulting in torsade de pointes, when used in conjunction with other agents that prolong the QT interval (eg, Class I and III antiarrhythmics). Use with caution in patients at risk of QT prolongation and/or ventricular arrhythmia. Reduction in heart rate may also occur with the $5-HT_3$ antagonists. I.V. formulations of $5-HT_3$ antagonists have more association with ECG interval changes, compared to oral formulations. Use with caution in children and adolescents who have or may develop QT_c prolongation; rare cases of supraventricular and ventricular arrhythmias, cardiac arrest, and MI have been reported in this population.

Use with caution in patients allergic to other 5-HT$_3$ receptor antagonists; cross-reactivity has been reported. **For chemotherapy, should be used on a scheduled basis, not on an "as needed" (PRN) basis,** since data support the use of this drug only in the prevention of nausea and vomiting (due to antineoplastic therapy) and not in the rescue of nausea and vomiting. Not intended for treatment of nausea and vomiting or for chronic continuous therapy. Safety and efficacy in children <2 years of age have not been established.

Adverse Reactions Adverse events may vary according to indication

>10%:

Central nervous system: Headache (7% to 24%)

Gastrointestinal: Diarrhea (2% to 12%)

1% to 10%:

Cardiovascular: Bradycardia (4% to 5%), hypotension (5%), hypertension (2% to 3%), tachycardia (2% to 3%)

Central nervous system: Dizziness (1% to 6%), fatigue (3% to 6%), fever (4% to 5%), pain (≤3%), chills/shivering (1% to 2%), sedation (2%)

Dermatological: Pruritus (3% to 4%)

Gastrointestinal: Dyspepsia (2% to 3%), abdominal pain (≤3%)

Hepatic: Abnormal hepatic function (4%)

Neuromuscular & skeletal: Pain (3%)

Renal: Oliguria (1% to 3%)

<1% (Limited to important or life-threatening): Abnormal vision, abnormal dreaming, acute renal failure, alkaline phosphatase increased, ALT increased, anaphylactic reaction, anemia, anorexia, anxiety, arrhythmia (supraventricular and ventricular), AST increased, ataxia, AV block, bronchospasm, cardiac arrest, cardiac conduction abnormalities, chest pain, confusion, constipation, diaphoresis, dyspnea, dysuria, edema, epistaxis, facial edema, flushing, GGT increased, heart block, hematuria, hyperbilirubinemia, ischemia (peripheral), local injection site reaction, MI, myocardial ischemia, orthostatic hypotension, palpitation, pancreatitis, paresthesia, peripheral edema, photophobia, polyuria; prolonged PR, QRS, JT, and QT$_c$ intervals; prothrombin time increased, PTT increased, purpura/hematoma, rash, sleep disorder, syncope, taste perversion, thrombocytopenia, thrombophlebitis/phlebitis, tinnitus, tremor, twitching, urticaria, vertigo

Drug Interactions

Metabolism/Transport Effects Substrate (minor) of CYP2C9, 3A4; **Inhibits** CYP2D6 (weak)

Avoid Concomitant Use

Avoid concomitant use of Dolasetron with any of the following: Apomorphine; Artemether; Dronedarone; Lumefantrine; Nilotinib; Pimozide; QuiNINE; Tetrabenazine; Thioridazine; Ziprasidone

Increased Effect/Toxicity

Dolasetron may increase the levels/effects of: Apomorphine; Dronedarone; Pimozide; QTc-Prolonging Agents; QuiNINE; Tetrabenazine; Thioridazine; Ziprasidone

The levels/effects of Dolasetron may be increased by: Alfuzosin; Artemether; Chloroquine; Ciprofloxacin; Gadobutrol; Lumefantrine; Nilotinib; QuiNINE

Decreased Effect There are no known significant interactions involving a decrease in effect.

Dosage Forms Excipient information presented when available (limited, particularly for generics); consult specific product labeling.

Injection, solution, as mesylate:

Anzemet®: 20 mg/mL (0.625 mL) [single-use Carpuject® or vial; contains mannitol 38.2 mg/mL]; 20 mg/mL (5 mL) [single-use vial; contains mannitol 38.2 mg/mL]; 20 mg/mL (25 mL) [multidose vial; contains mannitol 29 mg/mL]

Tablet, as mesylate:

Anzemet®: 50 mg, 100 mg

References

Diemunsch P, Lesser J, Feiss P, et al, "Intravenous Dolasetron Mesilate Ameliorates Postoperative Nausea and Vomiting," *Can J Anaesth,* 1997, 44(2):173-81.

Gan TJ, Meyer TA, Apfel CC, et al, "Society for Ambulatory Anesthesia Guidelines for the Management of Postoperative Nausea and Vomiting," *Anesth Analg,* 2007, 105(6):1615-28.

Graczyk SG, McKenzie R, et al, "Intravenous Dolasetron for the Prevention of Postoperative Nausea and Vomiting After Outpatient Laparoscopic Gynecologic Surgery," *Anesth Analg*, 1997, 84 (2):325-30.

Kovac AI, Scuderi PE, et al, "Treatment of Postoperative Nausea and Vomiting With Single Intravenous Doses of Dolasetron Mesylate: A Multicenter Trial," *Anesth Analg*, 1997, 85(3):546-52.

- ◆ **Dolasetron Mesylate** *see* Dolasetron *on page 444*
- ◆ **Dolobid** *see* Diflunisal *on page 416*
- ◆ **Dolophine®** *see* Methadone *on page 888*
- ◆ **Doloral (Can)** *see* Morphine Sulfate *on page 953*
- ◆ **Dom-Alendronate (Can)** *see* Alendronate *on page 57*
- ◆ **Dom-Amiodarone (Can)** *see* Amiodarone *on page 86*
- ◆ **Dom-Azithromycin (Can)** *see* Azithromycin *on page 169*
- ◆ **Dom-Benzydamine (Can)** *see* Benzydamine *on page 184*
- ◆ **Dom-Buspirone (Can)** *see* BusPIRone *on page 219*
- ◆ **Dom-Carbamazepine (Can)** *see* CarBAMazepine *on page 241*
- ◆ **Dom-Carvedilol (Can)** *see* Carvedilol *on page 244*
- ◆ **Dom-Cimetidine (Can)** *see* Cimetidine *on page 305*
- ◆ **Dom-Ciprofloxacin (Can)** *see* Ciprofloxacin *on page 306*
- ◆ **Dom-Clonidine (Can)** *see* CloNIDine *on page 329*
- ◆ **Dom-Diclofenac (Can)** *see* Diclofenac *on page 414*
- ◆ **Dom-Diclofenac SR (Can)** *see* Diclofenac *on page 414*
- ◆ **Dom-Divalproex (Can)** *see* Valproic Acid and Derivatives *on page 1445*
- ◆ **Dom-Fenofibrate Supra (Can)** *see* Fenofibrate *on page 582*
- ◆ **Dom-Fluconazole (Can)** *see* Fluconazole *on page 607*
- ◆ **Dom-Fluoxetine (Can)** *see* FLUoxetine *on page 616*
- ◆ **Dom-Furosemide (Can)** *see* Furosemide *on page 645*
- ◆ **Dom-Gabapentin (Can)** *see* Gabapentin *on page 650*
- ◆ **DOM-Levetiracetam (Can)** *see* Levetiracetam *on page 816*
- ◆ **DOM-Lovastatin (Can)** *see* Lovastatin *on page 859*
- ◆ **Dom-Mefenamic Acid (Can)** *see* Mefenamic Acid *on page 870*
- ◆ **Dom-Metformin (Can)** *see* MetFORMIN *on page 886*
- ◆ **Dom-Methimazole (Can)** *see* Methimazole *on page 893*
- ◆ **Dom-Metoprolol (Can)** *see* Metoprolol *on page 922*
- ◆ **DOM-Ondansetron (Can)** *see* Ondansetron *on page 1057*
- ◆ **Dom-Oxybutynin (Can)** *see* Oxybutynin *on page 1068*
- ◆ **Dom-Piroxicam (Can)** *see* Piroxicam *on page 1139*
- ◆ **DOM-Pravastatin (Can)** *see* Pravastatin *on page 1162*
- ◆ **Dom-Propranolol (Can)** *see* Propranolol *on page 1198*
- ◆ **Dom-Ranitidine (Can)** *see* Ranitidine *on page 1231*
- ◆ **Dom-Simvastatin (Can)** *see* Simvastatin *on page 1293*
- ◆ **DOM-Sotalol (Can)** *see* Sotalol *on page 1321*
- ◆ **Dom-Sumatriptan (Can)** *see* SUMAtriptan *on page 1336*
- ◆ **Dom-Temazepam (Can)** *see* Temazepam *on page 1357*
- ◆ **Dom-Topiramate (Can)** *see* Topiramate *on page 1408*
- ◆ **Dom-Trazodone (Can)** *see* TraZODone *on page 1423*
- ◆ **Dom-Verapamil SR (Can)** *see* Verapamil *on page 1468*

Donepezil (doh NEP e zil)

U.S. Brand Names Aricept®; Aricept® ODT
Canadian Brand Names Aricept®; Aricept® RDT
Index Terms E2020
Pharmacologic Category Acetylcholinesterase Inhibitor (Central)

Use Treatment of mild, moderate, or severe dementia of the Alzheimer's type
Unlabeled/Investigational Use Attention-deficit/hyperactivity disorder (ADHD); behavioral syndromes in dementia; mild-to-moderate dementia associated with Parkinson's disease; Lewy body dementia
Pharmacodynamics/Kinetics
Absorption: Well absorbed
Protein binding: 96%, primarily to albumin (75%) and α_1-acid glycoprotein (21%)
Metabolism: Extensively to four major metabolites (two are active) via CYP2D6 and 3A4; undergoes glucuronidation
Bioavailability: 100%
Half-life elimination: 70 hours; time to steady-state: 15 days
Time to peak, plasma: 3-4 hours
Excretion: Urine 57% (17% as unchanged drug); feces 15%
Dosage Oral:
Children: ADHD (unlabeled use): 5 mg/day
Adults: Dementia of Alzheimer's type: Initial: 5 mg/day at bedtime; may increase to 10 mg/day at bedtime after 4-6 weeks
Additional Information Complete prescribing information for this medication should be consulted for additional detail.
Dosage Forms Excipient information presented when available (limited, particularly for generics); consult specific product labeling.
Tablet, as hydrochloride:
Aricept®: 5 mg, 10 mg
Tablet, orally disintegrating, as hydrochloride:
Aricept® ODT: 5 mg, 10 mg
References
Hardan AY and Handen BL, "A Retrospective Open Trial of Adjunctive Donepezil in Children and Adolescents With Autistic Disorder," *J Child Adolesc Psychopharmacol*, 2002, 12(3):237-41.
Hoopes SP, "Donepezil for Tourette's Disorder and ADHD," *J Clin Psychopharmacol*, 1999, 19 (4):381-2.
Rogers SL and Friedhoff LT, "The Efficacy and Safety of Donepezil in Patients With Alzheimer's Disease: Results of a U.S. Multicentre, Randomized, Double-Blind, Placebo-Controlled Trial," *Dementia*, 1996, 7(6):293-303.
Wilens TE, Biederman J, Wong J, et al, "Adjunctive Donepezil in Attention Deficit Hyperactivity Disorder Youth: Case Series," *J Child Adolesc Psychopharmacol*, 2000, 10(3):217-22.

DOPamine (DOE pa meen)

Medication Safety Issues
Sound-alike/look-alike issues:
DOPamine may be confused with DOBUTamine, Dopram®

High alert medication: The Institute for Safe Medication Practices (ISMP) includes this medication among its list of drugs which have a heightened risk of causing significant patient harm when used in error.
Related Information
Extravasation Treatment of Drugs *on page 1789*
Heart Failure (Systolic) *on page 1739*
Hemodynamic Support, Intravenous *on page 1681*
Postoperative Nausea and Vomiting *on page 1593*
Index Terms Dopamine Hydrochloride; Intropin
Pharmacologic Category Adrenergic Agonist Agent
Generic Available Yes
Use Adjunct in the treatment of shock (eg, MI, open heart surgery, renal failure, cardiac decompensation) which persists after adequate fluid volume replacement
Unlabeled/Investigational Use Symptomatic bradycardia or heart block unresponsive to atropine or pacing
Mechanism of Action Stimulates both adrenergic and dopaminergic receptors, lower doses are mainly dopaminergic stimulating and produce renal and mesenteric vasodilation, higher doses also are both dopaminergic and beta$_1$-adrenergic stimulating and produce cardiac stimulation and renal vasodilation; large doses stimulate alpha-adrenergic receptors
Pharmacodynamics/Kinetics
Children: Dopamine has exhibited nonlinear kinetics in children; with medication changes, may not achieve steady-state for ~1 hour rather than 20 minutes

Onset of action: Adults: 5 minutes

Duration: Adults: <10 minutes

Metabolism: Renal, hepatic, plasma; 75% to inactive metabolites by monoamine oxidase and 25% to norepinephrine

Half-life elimination: 2 minutes

Excretion: Urine (as metabolites)

Clearance: Neonates: Varies and appears to be age related; clearance is more prolonged with combined hepatic and renal dysfunction

Dosage I.V. infusion (administration requires the use of an infusion pump):

Neonates: 1-20 mcg/kg/minute continuous infusion, titrate to desired response.

Children: 1-20 mcg/kg/minute, maximum: 50 mcg/kg/minute continuous infusion, titrate to desired response.

Adults: 1-5 mcg/kg/minute up to 20 mcg/kg/minute, titrate to desired response (maximum: 50 mcg/kg/minute). Infusion may be increased by 1-4 mcg/kg/minute at 10- to 30-minute intervals until optimal response is obtained.

If dosages >20-30 mcg/kg/minute are needed, a more direct-acting pressor may be more beneficial (ie, epinephrine, norepinephrine).

The hemodynamic effects of dopamine are dose dependent:

Low-dose: 1-3 mcg/kg/minute, increased renal blood flow and urine output

Intermediate-dose: 3-10 mcg/kg/minute, increased renal blood flow, heart rate, cardiac contractility, and cardiac output

High-dose: >10 mcg/kg/minute, alpha-adrenergic effects begin to predominate, vasoconstriction, increased blood pressure

Stability Protect from light; solutions that are darker than slightly yellow should not be used.

Administration Administer into large vein to prevent the possibility of extravasation (central line administration); monitor continuously for free flow; use infusion device to control rate of flow; administration into an umbilical arterial catheter is not recommended; when discontinuing the infusion, gradually decrease the dose of dopamine (sudden discontinuation may cause hypotension).

To prepare for infusion:

$$\frac{6 \times \text{weight (kg)} \times \text{desired dose (mcg/kg/min)}}{\text{I.V. infusion rate (mL/h)}} = \frac{\text{mg of drug to be added to}}{100 \text{ mL of I.V. fluid}}$$

Extravasation management: Due to short half-life, withdrawal of drug is often only necessary treatment. Use phentolamine as antidote. Mix 5 mg with 9 mL of NS; inject a small amount of this dilution into extravasated area. Blanching should reverse immediately. Monitor site. If blanching should recur, additional injections of phentolamine may be needed.

Monitoring Parameters Blood pressure, ECG, heart rate, CVP, RAP, MAP, urine output; if pulmonary artery catheter is in place, monitor CI, PCWP, SVR, and PVR

Anesthesia and Critical Care Concerns/Other Considerations

Clinical Pearls/Comments:

Extravasation Management: Antidote for peripheral ischemia caused by dopamine extravasation: To prevent sloughing and necrosis in ischemic areas, the area should be infiltrated as soon as possible with 5-10 mg of Regitine® (phentolamine), an adrenergic-blocking agent, diluted in 10-15 mL of saline. A syringe with a fine hypodermic needle should be used, and the solution liberally infiltrated throughout the ischemic area. Sympathetic blockade with phentolamine causes immediate and conspicuous local hyperemic changes if the area is infiltrated within 12 hours. Therefore, phentolamine should be given as soon as possible after the extravasation is noted, as phentolamine may be ineffective if given >12 hours after extravasation.

Evidence-Based Information:

Low-Dose Dopamine: There is no clear evidence that low-dose dopamine confers any renal benefit. The 2004 ACCM/SCCM Practice Parameters for Hemodynamic Support of Sepsis in Adult Patients recommends against the use of low doses of dopamine to maintain renal function. Low-dose dopamine may ▶

increase renal blood flow in some patients requiring norepinephrine. Kellum and Decker (2001) reviewed 58 studies in a meta-analysis focused on determining if low-dose dopamine reduced the severity of acute renal failure, the need for dialysis, or mortality in critically-ill patients. They concluded that the use of low-dose dopamine for the treatment or prevention of acute renal failure cannot be justified. A more recent randomized, double-blind, placebo-controlled trial came to a similar conclusion (Australian and New Zealand Intensive Care Society Clinical Trials Group, 2000). This study enrolled over 300 ICU patients with clinical evidence of renal dysfunction. They were randomized to low-dose dopamine (2 mcg/kg/minute) or placebo. The investigators found no difference in serum creatinine, renal replacement therapy, intensive care length of stay, hospital stay, or mortality between the groups. The 2008 Surviving Sepsis Campaign guidelines also recommend against the use of low-dose dopamine for renal protection (Grade 1A).

Septic Shock: In septic shock, dopamine is effective in increasing mean arterial pressure in patients who remain hypotensive after adequate volume expansion. Undesirable effects include tachycardia, increased pulmonary shunt, and decreased P_aO_2. As catecholamine stores are depleted, tachyphylaxis may occur. The 2004 ACCM/SCCM Practice Parameters for Hemodynamic Support of Sepsis in Adult Patients recommend either norepinephrine or dopamine as vasopressor therapy. Norepinephrine has a wider dosage range than dopamine.

The 2008 Surviving Sepsis Campaign guidelines recommend using either norepinephrine or dopamine as the first-choice vasopressor agent in adult patients (Grade 1C). Norepinephrine is more potent than dopamine and may be more effective at reversing hypotension in septic shock. In pediatric patients with hypotension refractory to fluid resuscitation, the Surviving Sepsis Campaign guidelines suggest dopamine as the first choice of support (Grade 2C).

Pregnancy Risk Factor C

Contraindications Hypersensitivity to sulfites (commercial preparation contains sodium bisulfite); pheochromocytoma; ventricular fibrillation

Warnings/Precautions Use with caution in patients with cardiovascular disease or cardiac arrhythmias or patients with occlusive vascular disease. Correct hypovolemia and electrolytes when used in hemodynamic support. May cause increases in HR and arrhythmia. Use with caution in post-MI patients. Use with extreme caution in patients taking MAO inhibitors. Avoid extravasation; infuse into a large vein if possible. Avoid infusion into leg veins. Watch I.V. site closely. **[U.S. Boxed Warning]: If extravasation occurs, infiltrate the area with diluted phentolamine (5-10 mg in 10-15 mL of saline) with a fine hypodermic needle. Phentolamine should be administered as soon as possible after extravasation is noted.** Product may contain sodium metabisulfite.

Adverse Reactions Frequency not defined.

Most frequent:

Cardiovascular: Ectopic beats, tachycardia, anginal pain, palpitation, hypotension, vasoconstriction

Central nervous system: Headache

Gastrointestinal: Nausea and vomiting

Respiratory: Dyspnea

Infrequent:

Cardiovascular: Aberrant conduction, bradycardia, widened QRS complex, ventricular arrhythmia (high dose), gangrene (high dose), hypertension

Central nervous system: Anxiety

Endocrine & metabolic: Piloerection, serum glucose increased (usually not above normal limits)

Local: Extravasation of dopamine can cause tissue necrosis and sloughing of surrounding tissues

Ocular: Intraocular pressure increased, dilated pupils

Renal: Azotemia, polyuria

Drug Interactions

Avoid Concomitant Use

Avoid concomitant use of DOPamine with any of the following: Iobenguane I 123

Increased Effect/Toxicity

DOPamine may increase the levels/effects of: Sympathomimetics

The levels/effects of DOPamine may be increased by: Atomoxetine; Cannabinoids; COMT Inhibitors

Decreased Effect

DOPamine may decrease the levels/effects of: Iobenguane I 123

Dosage Forms Excipient information presented when available (limited, particularly for generics); consult specific product labeling.

Infusion, as hydrochloride [premixed in D_5W]: 0.8 mg/mL (250 mL, 500 mL); 1.6 mg/mL (250 mL, 500 mL); 3.2 mg/mL (250 mL)

Injection, solution, as hydrochloride: 40 mg/mL (5 mL, 10 mL); 80 mg/mL (5 mL); 160 mg/mL (5 mL) [contains sodium metabisulfite]

References

Bellomo R, Chapman M, Finfer S, et al, "Low-Dose Dopamine in Patients With Early Renal Dysfunction: A Placebo-Controlled Randomised Trial. Australian and New Zealand Intensive Care Society (ANZICS) Clinical Trials Group," *Lancet*, 2000, 356(9248):2139-43.

Dellinger RP, Carlet JM, Masur H, et al, "Surviving Sepsis Campaign Guidelines for Management of Severe Sepsis and Septic Shock," *Crit Care Med*, 2004, 32(3):858-73.

Dellinger RP, Levy MM, Carlet JM, et al, "Surviving Sepsis Campaign: International Guidelines for Management of Severe Sepsis and Septic Shock: 2008," *Intensive Care Med*, 2008, 34(1): 17-60. Available at http://www.survivingsepsis.org/system/files/images/2008_20International_20SSC_20-Guidelines_1_.pdf

Johnson RL Jr, "Low-Dose Dopamine and Oxygen Transport by the Lung," *Circulation*, 1998, 98 (2):97-9.

Kellum JA and Decker JM, "Use of Dopamine in Acute Renal Failure: A Meta-analysis," *Crit Care Med*, 2001, 29(8):1526-31.

Martin C, Papazian L, Perrin G, et al, "Norepinephrine or Dopamine for the Treatment of Hyperdynamic Septic Shock?" *Chest*, 1993, 103(6):1826-31.

"Practice Parameters for Hemodynamic Support of Sepsis in Adult Patients. Task Force of the American College of Critical Care Medicine, Society of Critical Care Medicine," *Crit Care Med*, 1999, 27(3):639-60. Available at: http://www.sccm.org/pdf/Hemodynamic%20Support.pdf. Accessed August 13, 2003.

van de Borne P, Oren R, and Somers VK, "Dopamine Depresses Minute Ventilation in Patients With Heart Failure," *Circulation*, 1998, 98(2):126-31.

◆ **Dopamine Hydrochloride** *see* DOPamine *on page 448*

◆ **Dopram®** *see* Doxapram *on page 453*

◆ **Doribax™** *see* Doripenem *on page 451*

Doripenem (dore i PEN em)

U.S. Brand Names Doribax™
Canadian Brand Names Doribax™
Index Terms S-4661
Pharmacologic Category Antibiotic, Carbapenem
Generic Available No

Use Treatment of complicated intra-abdominal infections and complicated urinary tract infections (including pyelonephritis) due to susceptible gram-positive, gram-negative (including *Pseudomonas aeruginosa*), and anaerobic bacteria

Unlabeled/Investigational Use Treatment of nosocomial pneumonia

Mechanism of Action Inhibits bacterial cell wall synthesis by binding to several of the penicillin-binding proteins, which in turn inhibits the final transpeptidation step of peptidoglycan synthesis in bacterial cell walls, thus inhibiting cell wall biosynthesis; bacteria eventually lyse due to ongoing activity of cell wall autolytic enzymes (autolysins and murein hydrolases) while cell wall assembly is arrested.

Pharmacodynamics/Kinetics

Distribution: V_d: 16.8 L

Protein binding: 8% to 9%

Metabolism: Non-CYP-mediated metabolism via dehydropeptidase-I to doripenem-M1 (inactive metabolite)

Half-life elimination: ~1 hour

Excretion: Urine (70% as unchanged drug; 15% as doripenem-M1 metabolite); feces (<1%)

◀ **Dosage**
  Usual dosage: Adults: I.V.: 500 mg every 8 hours
    Indication-specific dosing: Adults: I.V.:
      Intra-abdominal infection (complicated): 500 mg every 8 hours for 5-14 days
      Urinary tract infection (complicated) or pyelonephritis: 500 mg every 8 hours for 10-14 days
  Dosing adjustment in renal impairment:
    Cl_{cr} 30-50 mL/minute: 250 mg every 8 hours
    Cl_{cr} 11-29 mL/minute: 250 mg every 12 hours
  Hemodialysis: Dialyzable (~52% of dose removed during 4-hour session in ESRD patients)

Stability Store dry powder vials at 15°C to 30°C (59°F to 86°F). Reconstitute 500 mg vial with 10 mL of SWFI or NS. Further dilute for infusion with 100 mL of NS or D_5W. Shake gently until clear. Reconstituted vial may be stored for up to 1 hour prior to preparation of infusion solution. Stability of solution (concentration: 4.5 mg/mL) when diluted in NS is 12 hours at room temperature or 72 hours under refrigeration; stability in D_5W is 4 hours at room temperature and 24 hours under refrigeration.

Renal impairment: For preparation of a 250 mg dose in renal impairment, reconstitute 500 mg vial with 10 mL of SWFI or NS and further dilute with 100 mL of compatible solution as above, but remove and discard 55 mL from the infusion bag to leave the remaining solution containing the 250 mg dose (concentration: 4.5 mg/mL).

Administration Administer by I.V. infusion over 1 hour

Monitoring Parameters Monitor for signs of anaphylaxis during first dose; periodic renal assessment; consider hematologic monitoring during prolonged therapy

Pregnancy Risk Factor B

Contraindications Known serious hypersensitivity to doripenem or other carbapenems (eg, imipenem, ertapenem, meropenem); anaphylactic reactions to beta-lactam antibiotics

Warnings/Precautions Serious hypersensitivity reactions, including anaphylaxis, and skin reactions have been reported in patients receiving beta-lactams. Prolonged use may result in fungal or bacterial superinfection, including *C. difficile*-associated diarrhea (CDAD) and pseudomembranous colitis; CDAD has been observed >2 months postantibiotic treatment. Use with caution in patients with renal impairment; dosage adjustment required in patients with moderate-to-severe renal dysfunction. Levels of valproic acid may be decreased during concomitant use to subtherapeutic levels, increasing potential for breakthrough seizures. Administer via intravenous infusion only. Per manufacturer's labeling, investigational experience of doripenem via inhalation resulted in pneumonitis. Safety and efficacy have not been established in children <18 years of age.

Adverse Reactions
  >10%:
    Central nervous system: Headache (4% to 16%)
    Gastrointestinal: Nausea (4% to 12%), diarrhea (6% to 11%)
  1% to 10%:
    Dermatologic: Rash (1% to 5%; includes allergic/bullous dermatitis, erythema, macular/papular eruptions, urticaria, and erythema multiforme), pruritus (≤3%)
    Gastrointestinal: Oral candidiasis (1%)
    Hematologic: Anemia (2% to 10%)
    Hepatic: Transaminases increased (1% to 2%)
    Local: Phlebitis (4% to 8%)
    Renal: Renal impairment/failure (≤1%)
    Miscellaneous: Vulvomycotic infection (1% to 2%)
  Postmarketing and/or case reports: Anaphylaxis, interstitial pneumonia, leukopenia, neutropenia, Stevens-Johnson syndrome, seizure, toxic epidermal necrolysis

Drug Interactions
  Avoid Concomitant Use There are no known interactions where it is recommended to avoid concomitant use.

Increased Effect/Toxicity
The levels/effects of Doripenem may be increased by: Probenecid; Uricosuric Agents

Decreased Effect
Doripenem may decrease the levels/effects of: Typhoid Vaccine; Valproic Acid

Dosage Forms Excipient information presented when available (limited, particularly for generics); consult specific product labeling.
Injection, powder for reconstitution:
  Doribax™: 500 mg

References
Mesaros N, Nordmann P, Plésiat P, et al, "Pseudomonas aeruginosa: Resistance and Therapeutic Options at the Turn of the New Millennium," *Clin Microbiol Infect*, 2007, 13(6): 560-78.
Zhanel GG, Wiebe R, Dilay L, et al, "Comparative Review of the Carbapenems," *Drugs*, 2007, 67(7): 1027-52.

◆ **Doryx®** *see* Doxycycline *on page 456*

Doxapram (DOKS a pram)

Medication Safety Issues
Sound-alike/look-alike issues:
  Doxapram may be confused with doxacurium, doxazosin, doxepin, Doxinate®, DOXOrubicin
  Dopram® may be confused with DOPamine

U.S. Brand Names Dopram®

Index Terms Doxapram Hydrochloride

Pharmacologic Category Respiratory Stimulant; Stimulant

Generic Available Yes

Use Respiratory and CNS stimulant for respiratory depression secondary to anesthesia, drug-induced CNS depression; acute hypercapnia secondary to COPD

Mechanism of Action Stimulates respiration through action on respiratory center in medulla or indirectly on peripheral carotid chemoreceptors

Pharmacodynamics/Kinetics
Onset of action: Respiratory stimulation: I.V.: 20-40 seconds
  Peak effect: 1-2 minutes
Duration: 5-12 minutes
Half-life elimination, serum: Adults: Mean: 3.4 hours

Dosage
Respiratory depression following anesthesia:
  Intermittent injection: Initial: 0.5-1 mg/kg; may repeat at 5-minute intervals (only in patients who demonstrate initial response); maximum total dose: 2 mg/kg
  I.V. infusion: Initial: 5 mg/minute until adequate response or adverse effects seen; decrease to 1-3 mg/minute; maximum total dose: 4 mg/kg
Drug-induced CNS depression:
  Intermittent injection: Initial: Priming dose of 1-2 mg/kg, repeat after 5 minutes; may repeat at 1-2 hour intervals (until sustained consciousness); maximum: 3 g/day. May repeat in 24 hours if necessary.
  I.V. infusion: Initial: Priming dose of 1-2 mg/kg, repeat after 5 minutes. If no response, wait 1-2 hours and repeat. If some stimulation is noted, initiate infusion at 1-3 mg/minute (depending on size of patient/depth of CNS depression); suspend infusion if patient begins to awaken. Infusion should not be continued for >2 hours. May reinstitute infusion as described above, including bolus, after rest interval of 30 minutes to 2 hours; maximum: 3 g/day
Acute hypercapnia secondary to COPD: I.V. infusion: Initial: Initiate infusion at 1-2 mg/minute (depending on size of patient/depth of CNS depression); may increase to maximum rate of 3 mg/minute; infusion should not be continued for >2 hours. Monitor arterial blood gases prior to initiation of infusion and at 30-minute intervals during the infusion (to identify possible development of acidosis/CO_2 retention). Additional infusions are not recommended (per manufacturer).

Stability Store at 20°C to 25°C (68°F to 77°F).
Drug-induced CNS depression or postanesthesia: Mix doxapram 250 mg in 250 mL of D_5W, $D_{10}W$, or NS.

COPD-associated hypercapnia: Mix doxapram 400 mg in 180 mL of D_5W, $D_{10}W$, or NS (final concentration: 2 mg/mL).

Administration Avoid rapid infusion.

Monitoring Parameters Monitor heart rate, blood pressure, reflexes, CNS status, ECG, arterial blood gases (COPD)

Anesthesia and Critical Care Concerns/Other Considerations

Clinical Pearls/Comments: Doxapram should not be used as a drug of choice to treat anesthesia-induced respiratory depression due to its transient effect.

Pregnancy Risk Factor B

Contraindications Hypersensitivity to doxapram or any component of the formulation; cardiovascular disease, cerebral edema, cerebral vascular accident, epilepsy, head injury, hyperthyroidism, mechanical disorders of ventilation, mechanical ventilation or neuromuscular blockade, pheochromocytoma, pulmonary embolism, or severe hypertension

Warnings/Precautions Adequate airway required; consider airway protection in case of vomiting. Rapid infusion may result in hemolysis. Solution contains benzyl alcohol; not for use in neonates. If patient has received anesthesia with a volatile agent known to sensitize the myocardium to catecholamines, avoid use of doxapram until anesthetic has been eliminated. Use with caution in hepatic or renal dysfunction. Use with caution in patients with cerebral disease; lowered pCO_2 induced by hyperventilation produces cerebral vasoconstriction and decreased circulation. Use with caution in treating pulmonary disease; a pressor effect on pulmonary circulation may result in a fall in arterial pO_2. May cause severe CNS toxicity, seizures. Doxapram is neither a nonspecific CNS depressant antagonist nor an opiate antagonist. Resuscitative equipment (in addition to anticonvulsants and oxygen) should be readily available. Safety and efficacy have not been established in children <12 years of age.

Adverse Reactions Frequency not defined.

Cardiovascular: Arrhythmia, blood pressure increased, chest pain, chest tightness, flushing, heart rate changes, T waves lowered, ventricular tachycardia, ventricular fibrillation

Central nervous system: Apprehension, Babinski turns positive, disorientation, dizziness, hallucinations, headache, hyperactivity, pyrexia, seizure

Dermatologic: Burning sensation, pruritus

Gastrointestinal: Defecation urge, diarrhea, nausea, vomiting

Genitourinary: Spontaneous voiding, urinary retention

Hematologic: Hematocrit decreased, hemoglobin decreased, hemolysis, red blood cell count decreased

Local: Phlebitis

Neuromuscular & skeletal: Clonus, deep tendon reflexes increase, fasciculations, involuntary muscle movement, muscle spasm, paresthesia

Ocular: Pupillary dilatation

Renal: Albuminuria, BUN increased

Respiratory: Bronchospasm, cough, dyspnea, hiccups, hyperventilation, laryngospasm, rebound hypoventilation, tachypnea

Miscellaneous: Diaphoresis

Drug Interactions

Avoid Concomitant Use

Avoid concomitant use of Doxapram with any of the following: Iobenguane I 123

Increased Effect/Toxicity

Doxapram may increase the levels/effects of: Sympathomimetics

The levels/effects of Doxapram may be increased by: Atomoxetine; Cannabinoids

Decreased Effect

Doxapram may decrease the levels/effects of: Iobenguane I 123

Dosage Forms Excipient information presented when available (limited, particularly for generics); consult specific product labeling.

Injection, solution, as hydrochloride: 20 mg/mL (20 mL) [contains benzyl alcohol]

◆ **Doxapram Hydrochloride** *see* Doxapram *on page 453*

Doxepin (DOKS e pin)

Related Information
Antidepressant Agents *on page 1660*
U.S. Brand Names Prudoxin™; Sinequan® [DSC]; Zonalon®
Canadian Brand Names Apo-Doxepin®; Novo-Doxepin; Sinequan®; Zonalon®
Index Terms Doxepin Hydrochloride
Pharmacologic Category Antidepressant, Tricyclic (Tertiary Amine); Topical Skin Product

Use

Oral: Depression
Topical: Short-term (<8 days) management of moderate pruritus in adults with atopic dermatitis or lichen simplex chronicus
Unlabeled/Investigational Use Analgesic for certain chronic and neuropathic pain; anxiety

Pharmacodynamics/Kinetics

Onset of action: Peak effect: Antidepressant: Usually >2 weeks; Anxiolytic: may occur sooner
Absorption: Following topical application, plasma levels may be similar to those achieved with oral administration
Distribution: Crosses placenta; enters breast milk
Protein binding: 80% to 85%
Metabolism: Hepatic; metabolites include desmethyldoxepin (active)
Half-life elimination: Adults: 6-8 hours
Excretion: Urine

Dosage

Oral: Topical: Burning mouth syndrome (dental use): Cream: Apply 3-4 times daily
Oral (entire daily dose may be given at bedtime):
Depression or anxiety:
Children (unlabeled use): 1-3 mg/kg/day in single or divided doses
Adolescents: Initial: 25-50 mg/day in single or divided doses; gradually increase to 100 mg/day
Adults: Initial: 25-150 mg/day at bedtime or in 2-3 divided doses; may gradually increase up to 300 mg/day; single dose should not exceed 150 mg; select patients may respond to 25-50 mg/day
Elderly: Use a lower dose and adjust gradually
Chronic urticaria, angioedema, nocturnal pruritus: Adults and Elderly: 10-30 mg/day
Dosing adjustment in hepatic impairment: Use a lower dose and adjust gradually

Topical: Pruritus: Adults and Elderly: Apply a thin film 4 times/day with at least 3- to 4-hour interval between applications; not recommended for use >8 days. **Note:** Low-dose (25-50 mg) oral administration has also been used to treat pruritus, but systemic effects are increased.
Additional Information Complete prescribing information for this medication should be consulted for additional detail.
Dosage Forms Excipient information presented when available (limited, particularly for generics); consult specific product labeling. [DSC] = Discontinued product
Capsule, as hydrochloride: 10 mg, 25 mg, 50 mg, 75 mg, 100 mg, 150 mg
Sinequan®: 10 mg, 25 mg, 50 mg, 75 mg, 100 mg, 150 mg [DSC]
Cream, as hydrochloride:
Prudoxin™: 5% (45 g) [contains benzyl alcohol]
Zonalon®: 5% (30 g, 45 g) [contains benzyl alcohol]
Solution, oral concentrate, as hydrochloride: 10 mg/mL (120 mL)
Sinequan®: 10 mg/mL (120 mL) [DSC]

References

Mokhlesi B, Leikin JB, Murray P, et al, "Adult Toxicology in Critical Care: Part II: Specific Poisonings," *Chest*, 2003, 123(3):897-922.

◆ **Doxepin Hydrochloride** *see* Doxepin *on page 455*

◆ **Doxy100™** *see* Doxycycline *on page 456*

♦ **Doxycin (Can)** *see* Doxycycline *on page 456*

Doxycycline (doks i SYE kleen)

Medication Safety Issues
Sound-alike/look-alike issues:
Doxycycline may be confused with dicyclomine, doxepin, doxylamine
Doxy100™ may be confused with Doxil®
Monodox® may be confused with Maalox®
Oracea™ may be confused with Orencia®
Vibramycin® may be confused with vancomycin, Vibativ™
Vibra-Tabs® may be confused with Vibativ™

Related Information
Prevention of Wound Infection and Sepsis in Surgical Patients *on page 1721*

U.S. Brand Names Adoxa®; Alodox™; Doryx®; Doxy100™; Monodox®; Oracea™; Oraxyl™; Periostat®; Vibra-Tabs®; Vibramycin®

Canadian Brand Names Apo-Doxy Tabs®; Apo-Doxy®; Doxycin; Doxytec; Novo-Doxylin; Nu-Doxycycline; Periostat®; Vibra-Tabs®

Index Terms Doxycycline Calcium; Doxycycline Hyclate; Doxycycline Monohydrate

Pharmacologic Category Antibiotic, Tetracycline Derivative

Generic Available Yes: Excludes capsule (variable release), syrup, tablet (delayed release)

Use Principally in the treatment of infections caused by susceptible *Rickettsia*, *Chlamydia*, and *Mycoplasma*; alternative to mefloquine for malaria prophylaxis; treatment for syphilis, uncomplicated *Neisseria gonorrhoeae*, *Listeria*, *Actinomyces israelii*, and *Clostridium* infections in penicillin-allergic patients; used for community-acquired pneumonia and other common infections due to susceptible organisms; anthrax due to *Bacillus anthracis*, including inhalational anthrax (postexposure); treatment of infections caused by uncommon susceptible gram-negative and gram-positive organisms including *Borrelia recurrentis*, *Ureaplasma urealyticum*, *Haemophilus ducreyi*, *Yersinia pestis*, *Francisella tularensis*, *Vibrio cholerae*, *Campylobacter fetus*, *Brucella* spp, *Bartonella bacilliformis*, and *Calymmatobacterium granulomatis*, Q fever, Lyme disease; treatment of inflammatory lesions associated with rosacea; intestinal amebiasis; severe acne

Unlabeled/Investigational Use Sclerosing agent for pleural effusion injection; vancomycin-resistant enterococci (VRE)

Mechanism of Action Inhibits protein synthesis by binding with the 30S and possibly the 50S ribosomal subunit(s) of susceptible bacteria; may also cause alterations in the cytoplasmic membrane

Periostat® capsules (proposed mechanism): Has been shown to inhibit collagenase activity *in vitro*. Also has been noted to reduce elevated collagenase activity in the gingival crevicular fluid of patients with periodontal disease. Systemic levels do not reach inhibitory concentrations against bacteria.

Pharmacodynamics/Kinetics
Absorption: Oral: Almost complete
Distribution: Widely into body tissues and fluids including synovial, pleural, prostatic, seminal fluids, and bronchial secretions; saliva, aqueous humor, and CSF penetration is poor
Protein binding: 90%
Metabolism: Not hepatic; partially inactivated in GI tract by chelate formation
Half-life elimination: 12-15 hours (usually increases to 22-24 hours with multiple doses); End-stage renal disease: 18-25 hours
Time to peak, serum: 1.5-4 hours
Excretion: Feces (30%); urine (23%)

Dosage
Usual dosage range:
Children >8 years (<45 kg): Oral, I.V.: 2-5 mg/kg/day in 1-2 divided doses, not to exceed 200 mg/day
Children >8 years (>45 kg) and Adults: Oral, I.V.: 100-200 mg/day in 1-2 divided doses

Indication-specific dosing:

Children:

Anthrax: Doxycycline should be used in children if antibiotic susceptibility testing, exhaustion of drug supplies, or allergic reaction preclude use of penicillin or ciprofloxacin. For treatment, the consensus recommendation does not include a loading dose for doxycycline.

Inhalational (postexposure prophylaxis) (*MMWR*, 2001, 50:889-893): Oral, I.V. (use oral route when possible):

≤8 years: 2.2 mg/kg every 12 hours for 60 days
>8 years and ≤45 kg: 2.2 mg/kg every 12 hours for 60 days
>8 years and >45 kg: 100 mg every 12 hours for 60 days

Cutaneous (treatment): Oral: See dosing for "Inhalational (postexposure prophylaxis)"

Note: In the presence of systemic involvement, extensive edema, and/or lesions on head/neck, doxycycline should initially be administered I.V.

Inhalational/gastrointestinal/oropharyngeal (treatment): I.V.: Refer to dosing for inhalational anthrax (postexposure prophylaxis); switch to oral therapy when clinically appropriate

Note: Initial treatment should include two or more agents predicted to be effective (per CDC recommendations). Agents suggested for use in conjunction with doxycycline or ciprofloxacin include rifampin, vancomycin, imipenem, penicillin, ampicillin, chloramphenicol, clindamycin, and clarithromycin. May switch to oral antimicrobial therapy when clinically appropriate. Continue combined therapy for 60 days

Children ≥8 years:

Malaria prophylaxis: Oral: 2 mg/kg/day (maximum 100 mg/day). Start 1-2 days prior to travel to endemic area; continue daily during travel and for 4 weeks after leaving endemic area

Children ≥8 years (and >45 kg) and Adults:

Chlamydial infections, uncomplicated: Oral: 100 mg twice daily for ≥7 days
Lyme disease, Q fever, or tularemia: Oral: 100 mg twice daily for 14-21 days
Rickettsial disease or ehrlichiosis: Oral, I.V.: 100 mg twice daily for 7-14 days

Adults:

Anthrax:

Inhalational (postexposure prophylaxis): Oral, I.V. (use oral route when possible): 100 mg every 12 hours for 60 days (*MMWR*, 2001, 50:889-93)

Cutaneous (treatment): Oral: 100 mg every 12 hours for 60 days. **Note:** In the presence of systemic involvement, extensive edema, lesions on head/neck, refer to I.V. dosing for treatment of inhalational/gastrointestinal/oropharyngeal anthrax

Inhalational/gastrointestinal/oropharyngeal (treatment): I.V.: Initial: 100 mg every 12 hours; switch to oral therapy when clinically appropriate; some recommend initial loading dose of 200 mg, followed by 100 mg every 8-12 hours (*JAMA*, 1997, 278:399-411). **Note:** Initial treatment should include two or more agents predicted to be effective (per CDC recommendations). Agents suggested for use in conjunction with doxycycline or ciprofloxacin include rifampin, vancomycin, imipenem, penicillin, ampicillin, chloramphenicol, clindamycin, and clarithromycin. May switch to oral antimicrobial therapy when clinically appropriate. Continue combined therapy for 60 days

Brucellosis: Oral: 100 mg twice daily for 6 weeks with rifampin or streptomycin

Community-acquired pneumonia, bronchitis: Oral, I.V.: 100 mg twice daily

Endometritis, salpingitis, parametritis, or peritonitis: I.V.: 100 mg twice daily with cefoxitin 2 g every 6 hours for 4 days and for ≥48 hours after patient improves; then continue with oral therapy 100 mg twice daily to complete a 10- to 14-day course of therapy

Gonococcal infection, acute (PID) in combination with another antibiotic: I.V.: 100 mg every 12 hours until improved, followed by 100 mg orally twice daily to complete 14 days

Malaria prophylaxis: 100 mg/day. Start 1-2 days prior to travel to endemic area; continue daily during travel and for 4 weeks after leaving endemic area

Nongonococcal urethritis: Oral: 100 mg twice daily for 7 days

Periodontitis: Oral (Periostat®): 20 mg twice daily as an adjunct following scaling and root planing; may be administered for up to 9 months. Safety

◀

beyond 12 months of treatment and efficacy beyond 9 months of treatment have not been established.

Rosacea: (Oracea™): Oral: 40 mg once daily in the morning

Sclerosing agent for pleural effusion injection (unlabeled use): Irrigation: 500 mg as a single dose in 30-50 mL of NS or SWI

Syphilis:

Early syphilis: Oral, I.V.: 200 mg/day in divided doses for 14 days

Late syphilis: Oral, I.V.: 200 mg/day in divided doses for 28 days

Yersinia pestis (plague): Oral: 100 mg twice daily for 7 days

Vibrio cholerae: Oral: 300 mg as a single dose

Dosing adjustment in renal impairment: No adjustment necessary

Dialysis: Not dialyzable; 0% to 5% by hemo- and peritoneal methods or by continuous arteriovenous or venovenous hemofiltration: No supplemental dosage necessary

Stability

Capsule, tablet: Store at controlled room temperature of 25°C (77°F); excursions permitted to 15°C to 30°C (59°F to 86°F). Protect from light.

I.V. infusion: Following reconstitution with sterile water for injection, dilute to a final concentration of 0.1-1 mg/mL using a compatible solution. Solutions for I.V. infusion may be prepared using 0.9% sodium chloride, D_5W, Ringer's injection, lactated Ringer's, D_5LR. Protect from light. Stability varies based on solution.

Administration

Oral: May give with meals to decrease GI upset. Capsule and tablet: Administer with at least 8 ounces of water and have patient sit up for at least 30 minutes after taking to reduce the risk of esophageal irritation and ulceration.

Oracea™: Take on an empty stomach 1 hour before or 2 hours after meals.

Doryx®: May be administered by carefully breaking up the tablet and sprinkling tablet contents on a spoonful of cold applesauce. The delayed release pellets must not be crushed or damaged when breaking up tablet. Should be administered immediately after preparation and without chewing.

I.V.: Infuse I.V. doxycycline over 1-4 hours; avoid extravasation

Monitoring Parameters Perform culture and sensitivity testing prior to initiating therapy. CBC, renal and liver function tests periodically with prolonged therapy.

Pregnancy Risk Factor D

Contraindications Hypersensitivity to doxycycline, tetracycline or any component of the formulation; children ≤8 years of age, except in treatment of anthrax (including inhalational anthrax postexposure prophylaxis)

Warnings/Precautions Photosensitivity reaction may occur with this drug; avoid prolonged exposure to sunlight or tanning equipment. Antianabolic effects of tetracyclines can increase BUN (dose-related). Autoimmune syndromes have been reported. Hepatotoxicity rarely occurs: if symptomatic, conduct LFT and discontinue drug. Pseudotumor cerebri has been (rarely) reported with tetracycline use; usually resolves with discontinuation. Prolonged use may result in fungal or bacterial superinfection, including *C. difficile*-associated diarrhea (CDAD) and pseudomembranous colitis; CDAD has been observed >2 months postantibiotic treatment. May cause tissue hyperpigmentation, enamel hypoplasia, or permanent tooth discoloration; use of tetracyclines should be avoided during tooth development (children ≤8 years of age) unless other drugs are not likely to be effective or are contraindicated. However, recommended in treatment of anthrax exposure. Do not use during pregnancy. In addition to affecting tooth development, tetracycline use has been associated with retardation of skeletal development and reduced bone growth.

Additional specific warnings: Periostat®: Effectiveness has not been established in patients with coexistent oral candidiasis; use with caution in patients with a history or predisposition to oral candidiasis. Oracea™: Should not be used for the treatment or prophylaxis of bacterial infections, since the lower dose of drug per capsule may be subefficacious and promote resistance. Syrup contains sodium metabisulfite.

Adverse Reactions Frequency not defined.

Cardiovascular: Intracranial hypertension, pericarditis

Dermatologic: Angioneurotic edema, exfoliative dermatitis (rare), photosensitivity, rash, skin hyperpigmentation, urticaria

Endocrine & metabolic: Brown/black discoloration of thyroid gland (no dysfunction reported), hypoglycemia

Gastrointestinal: Anorexia, diarrhea, dysphagia, enterocolitis, esophagitis (rare), esophageal ulcerations (rare), glossitis, inflammatory lesions in anogenital region, nausea, oral (mucosal) pigmentation, pseudomembranous colitis, tooth discoloration (children), vomiting

Hematologic: Eosinophilia, hemolytic anemia, neutropenia, thrombocytopenia

Hepatic: Hepatotoxicity (rare)

Renal: BUN increased (dose related)

Miscellaneous: Anaphylactoid purpura, anaphylaxis, bulging fontanels (infants), serum sickness, SLE exacerbation

Note: Adverse effects in clinical trials with Periostat® occurring at a frequency more than 1% greater than placebo included nausea, dyspepsia, joint pain, diarrhea, menstrual cramp, and pain.

Drug Interactions

Metabolism/Transport Effects Inhibits CYP3A4 (moderate)

Avoid Concomitant Use

Avoid concomitant use of Doxycycline with any of the following: Retinoic Acid Derivatives

Increased Effect/Toxicity

Doxycycline may increase the levels/effects of: Neuromuscular-Blocking Agents; Retinoic Acid Derivatives; Vitamin K Antagonists

Decreased Effect

Doxycycline may decrease the levels/effects of: Penicillins; Typhoid Vaccine

The levels/effects of Doxycycline may be decreased by: Antacids; Barbiturates; Bile Acid Sequestrants; Bismuth; Bismuth Subsalicylate; CarBAMazepine; Iron Salts; Magnesium Salts; Phenytoin; Quinapril; Sucralfate

Ethanol/Nutrition/Herb Interactions

Ethanol: Chronic ethanol ingestion may reduce the serum concentration of doxycycline.

Food: Doxycycline serum levels may be slightly decreased if taken with food or milk. Administration with iron or calcium may decrease doxycycline absorption. May decrease absorption of calcium, iron, magnesium, zinc, and amino acids.

Herb/Nutraceutical: St John's wort may decrease doxycycline levels. Avoid dong quai, St John's wort (may also cause photosensitization).

Test Interactions False elevations of urine catecholamine levels; false-negative urine glucose using Clinistix®, Tes-Tape®

Dietary Considerations

Tetracyclines (in general): Take with food if gastric irritation occurs. While administration with food may decrease GI absorption of doxycycline by up to 20%, administration on an empty stomach is not recommended due to GI intolerance. Of currently available tetracyclines, doxycycline has the least affinity for calcium.

Oracea™: Take on an empty stomach 1 hour before or 2 hours after meals.

Doryx®: 75 mg, 100 mg, and 150 mg tablets contain sodium 4.5 mg, 6 mg, and 9 mg respectively.

Dosage Forms Excipient information presented when available (limited, particularly for generics); consult specific product labeling. [DSC] = Discontinued product

Note: Strength expressed as base.

Capsule, as hyclate: 50 mg, 100 mg
  Oraxyl™: 20 mg
  Vibramycin®: 100 mg
Capsule, as monohydrate: 50 mg, 100 mg
  Adoxa®: 150 mg
  Monodox®: 50 mg, 75 mg, 100 mg
Capsule, variable release:
  Oracea™: 40 mg [30 mg (immediate-release) and 10 mg (delayed-release)]
Injection, powder for reconstitution, as hyclate: 100 mg
  Doxy100™: 100 mg
Powder for oral suspension, as monohydrate: 25 mg/5 mL (60 mL)
  Vibramycin®: 25 mg/5 mL (60 mL) [raspberry flavor]

Syrup, as calcium:
Vibramycin®: 50 mg/5 mL (480 mL) [contains propylene glycol, sodium metabisulfite; raspberry-apple flavor]
Tablet, as hyclate: 20 mg, 100 mg
Alodox™: 20 mg [kit includes Alodox™ tablets (60s), Ocusoft® Lid Scrub™ pads, eyelid cleanser, and goggles]
Periostat®: 20 mg
Vibra-Tabs®: 100 mg
Tablet, as monohydrate: 50 mg, 75 mg, 100 mg, 150 mg
Adoxa®: 50 mg, 75 mg, 100 mg
Adoxa® Pak™ 1/75 [unit-dose pack]: 75 mg (31s)
Adoxa® Pak™ 1/100 [unit-dose pack]: 100 mg (31s) [DSC]
Adoxa® Pak™ 1/150 [unit-dose pack]: 150 mg (30s)
Adoxa® Pak™ 2/100 [unit-dose pack]: 100 mg (60s) [DSC]
Tablet, delayed-release coated pellets, as hyclate:
Doryx®: 75 mg [scored; contains sodium 4.5 mg (0.196 mEq); 100 mg [scored; contains sodium 6 mg (0.261 mEq)]; 150 mg [scored; contains sodium 9 mg (0.392 mEq)]

References

Centers for Disease Control and Prevention, "Update: Investigation of Anthrax Associated With Intentional Exposure and Interim Public Health Guidelines, October 2001," *MMWR*, 2001, 50 (41):889-93, accessed October 19, 2001. Available at: http://www.cdc.gov/mmwr/preview/mmwrhtml/mm5041a1.htm.

Centers for Disease Control and Prevention, "Update: Investigation of Bioterrorism-Related Anthrax and Interim Guidelines for Exposure Management and Antimicrobial Therapy, October 2001," *MMWR*, October 26, 2001, 50(42):909-19. http://www.cdc.gov/mmwr/preview/mmwrhtml/mm5042a1.htm. Accessed October 26, 2001.

◆ **Doxycycline Calcium** *see* Doxycycline *on page 456*

◆ **Doxycycline Hyclate** *see* Doxycycline *on page 456*

◆ **Doxycycline Monohydrate** *see* Doxycycline *on page 456*

◆ **Doxytec (Can)** *see* Doxycycline *on page 456*

◆ **DPA** *see* Valproic Acid and Derivatives *on page 1445*

◆ **DPH** *see* Phenytoin *on page 1119*

Dronabinol (droe NAB i nol)

U.S. Brand Names Marinol®
Canadian Brand Names Marinol®
Index Terms Delta-9 THC; Delta-9-tetrahydro-cannabinol; Tetrahydrocannabinol; THC
Pharmacologic Category Antiemetic; Appetite Stimulant
Restrictions C-III
Use Chemotherapy-associated nausea and vomiting refractory to other antiemetic(s); AIDS-related anorexia
Unlabeled/Investigational Use Cancer-related anorexia
Pharmacodynamics/Kinetics
Onset of action: Within 1 hour
Peak effect: 2-4 hours
Duration: 24 hours (appetite stimulation)
Absorption: Oral: 90% to 95%; 10% to 20% of dose gets into systemic circulation
Distribution: V_d: 10 L/kg; dronabinol is highly lipophilic and distributes to adipose tissue
Protein binding: 97% to 99%
Metabolism: Hepatic to at least 50 metabolites, some of which are active; 11-hydroxy-delta-9-tetrahydrocannabinol (11-OH-THC) is the major metabolite; extensive first-pass effect
Half-life elimination: Dronabinol: 25-36 hours (terminal); Dronabinol metabolites: 44-59 hours
Time to peak, serum: 0.5-4 hours
Excretion: Feces (50% as unconjugated metabolites, 5% as unchanged drug); urine (10% to 15% as acid metabolites and conjugates)

Dosage Refer to individual protocols. Oral:

Antiemetic: Children and Adults: 5 mg/m^2 1-3 hours before chemotherapy, then 5 mg/m^2/dose every 2-4 hours after chemotherapy for a total of 4-6 doses/day; increase doses in increments of 2.5 mg/m^2 to a maximum of 15 mg/m^2/dose.

Appetite stimulant: Adults: Initial: 2.5 mg twice daily (before lunch and dinner); titrate up to a maximum of 20 mg/day.

Additional Information Complete prescribing information for this medication should be consulted for additional detail.

Dosage Forms Excipient information presented when available (limited, particularly for generics); consult specific product labeling.

Capsule, soft gelatin: 2.5 mg, 5 mg, 10 mg

Marinol®: 2.5 mg, 5 mg, 10 mg [contains sesame oil]

Dronedarone (droe NE da rone)

Medication Guide An FDA-approved patient medication guide, which is available with the product information and at http://www.fda.gov/downloads/Drugs/DrugSafety/UCM171764.pdf, must be dispensed with this medication for each new outpatient prescription and refill.

Related Information

Antiarrhythmic Drugs *on page 1656*

Heart Failure (Systolic) *on page 1739*

U.S. Brand Names Multaq®

Canadian Brand Names Multaq®

Index Terms Dronedarone Hydrochloride; SR33589

Pharmacologic Category Antiarrhythmic Agent, Miscellaneous

Generic Available No

Use To reduce the risk of hospitalization related to paroxysmal or persistent atrial fibrillation (AF) or atrial flutter (AFl) in patients with a recent episode of AF/AFl and associated cardiovascular risk factors (eg, age >70 years, hypertension, diabetes, prior cerebrovascular accident, left atrial diameter ≥50 mm or left ventricular ejection fraction <40%), who are in normal sinus rhythm or will be cardioverted

Mechanism of Action A noniodinated antiarrhythmic agent structurally related to amiodarone exhibiting properties of all 4 antiarrhythmic classes. Dronedarone inhibits sodium (I_{Na}) and potassium (I_{Kr}, I_{KS}, I_{k1}, and I_{k-ACh}) channels resulting in prolongation of the action potential and refractory period in myocardial tissue without reverse-use dependent effects; decreases AV conduction and sinus node function through inhibition of calcium (I_{Ca-L}) channels and beta$_1$-receptor blocking activity. Similar to amiodarone, dronedarone also inhibits alpha$_1$-receptor mediated increases in blood pressure.

Pharmacodynamics/Kinetics

Distribution: V_d: ~20 L/kg (based on a 70 kg patient)

Protein binding: >98%

Metabolism: Hepatic via CYP3A4 to active N-debutyl metabolite ($^1/_{10}$ to $^1/_3$ as potent as dronedarone) and other inactive metabolites

Bioavailability: Oral: Without food: 4%; With high-fat meal: 15%

Half-life elimination: 13-19 hours

Time to peak, plasma: 3-6 hours

Excretion: Feces (84% mainly as metabolites); urine (~6% mainly as metabolites)

Dosage Oral: Adults: Atrial fibrillation/atrial flutter: 400 mg twice daily with morning and evening meals

Dosing adjustment in renal impairment: No dosage adjustment necessary.

Dosing adjustment in hepatic impairment: No dosage adjustment necessary for moderate hepatic impairment. Contraindicated with severe hepatic impairment.

Stability Store at room temperature of 25°C (77°F); excursions permitted to 15°C to 30°C (59°F to 86°F).

Administration Administer with a meal.

Monitoring Parameters Blood pressure, heart rate (ECG) and rhythm throughout therapy; assess patient for signs of lethargy, edema of the hands or feet; monitor serum electrolytes, especially potassium and magnesium

◀ Patients with implantable cardiac devices: Monitor pacing or defibrillation thresholds with initiation of dronedarone and during treatment.

Pregnancy Risk Factor X

Contraindications NYHA Class IV heart failure (HF); NYHA Class II-III HF with recent decompensation requiring hospitalization or referral to a specialized HF clinic; second- or third-degree heart block, or sick sinus syndrome (except in patients with a functioning artificial pacemaker); bradycardia <50 bpm; concomitant use of strong CYP3A4 inhibitors (eg, ketoconazole, itraconazole, voriconazole, cyclosporine, telithromycin, clarithromycin, nefazodone, or ritonavir); concomitant use of drugs or herbal products known to prolong the QT interval increasing the risk for torsade de pointes (eg, phenothiazine antipsychotics, tricyclic antidepressants, certain oral macrolide antibiotics, or class I and III antiarrhythmics); QT_c (Bazett) interval ≥500 msec or PR interval >280 msec; severe hepatic impairment; pregnancy; breast-feeding

Warnings/Precautions [U.S. Boxed Warning]: In patients with severe HF requiring recent hospitalization or referral to a specialized HF clinic for worsening symptoms, patients receiving dronedarone had a greater than twofold increase in mortality; use is contraindicated in patients with NYHA Class IV HF or NYHA Class II-III HF with recent decompensation requiring hospitalization or referral to a specialized HF clinic. If patients develop new or worsening HF symptoms (eg, weight gain, dependent edema, or increasing shortness of breath) while on therapy, consider suspension or discontinuation of dronedarone.

Dronedarone induces a moderate prolongation of the QT interval (average ~10 msec); much greater effects have been observed. Use in patients with QT_c (Bazett) interval ≥500 msec is contraindicated; discontinue use of dronedarone if this occurs during therapy. Following initiation, dronedarone may produce a slight increase in serum creatinine (~0.1 mg/dL) due to inhibition of tubular secretion; glomerular filtration rate is not affected; effect is reversible upon discontinuation.

Chronic administration of antiarrhythmic drugs may affect defibrillation or pacing thresholds; assess when initiating dronedarone and during therapy. Correct electrolyte disturbances, especially hypokalemia or hypomagnesemia, prior to use and throughout therapy. Use with caution in patients with mild to moderate hepatic impairment; use is contraindicated in severe hepatic impairment. Dronedarone is a moderate inhibitor of CYP3A4 and CYP2D6 enzymes and has potential to inhibit p-glycoprotein, which may lead to increased serum concentrations/toxicity of a number of medications. Safety and efficacy have not been established in children. Women of childbearing potential should use effective contraceptive methods during treatment.

Adverse Reactions

>10%:

Cardiovascular: QT_c (Bazett) prolongation (28% [placebo: 19%]; defined as >450 msec in males or >470 msec in females)

Renal: Serum creatinine increased ≥10% (51%; occurred 5 days after initiation)

1% to 10%:

Cardiovascular: Bradycardia (3%)

Dermatologic: Allergic dermatitis (≤5%), dermatitis (≤5%), eczema (≤5%), pruritus (≤5%), rash (≤5%; described as generalized, macular, maculopapular, erythematous)

Gastrointestinal: Diarrhea (9%), nausea (5%), abdominal pain (4%), dyspepsia (2%), vomiting (2%)

Neuromuscular & skeletal: Weakness (7%)

<1% (Limited to important or life-threatening): Dysgeusia, photosensitivity reaction

Drug Interactions

Avoid Concomitant Use

Avoid concomitant use of Dronedarone with any of the following: Artemether; CycloSPORINE; CYP3A4 Inducers (Strong); CYP3A4 Inhibitors (Strong); Dabigatran Etexilate; Everolimus; Grapefruit Juice; Lumefantrine; Nilotinib; Pimozide; QTc-Prolonging Agents; QuiNINE; Silodosin; St Johns Wort; Tetrabenazine; Thioridazine; Tolvaptan; Topotecan; Ziprasidone

Increased Effect/Toxicity

Dronedarone may increase the levels/effects of: Atorvastatin; Beta-Blockers; Calcium Channel Blockers (Nondihydropyridine); Colchicine; CYP2D6 Substrates; CYP3A4 Substrates; Dabigatran Etexilate; Digoxin; Eplerenone; Everolimus; FentaNYL; Fesoterodine; Lovastatin; P-Glycoprotein Substrates; Pimecrolimus; Pimozide; QTc-Prolonging Agents; QuiNINE; Red Yeast Rice; Rivaroxaban; Salmeterol; Saxagliptin; Silodosin; Simvastatin; Tamoxifen; Tetrabenazine; Thioridazine; Tolvaptan; Topotecan; Vitamin K Antagonists; Ziprasidone

The levels/effects of Dronedarone may be increased by: Alfuzosin; Artemether; Calcium Channel Blockers (Nondihydropyridine); Chloroquine; Ciprofloxacin; CycloSPORINE; CYP3A4 Inhibitors (Moderate); CYP3A4 Inhibitors (Strong); Digoxin; Gadobutrol; Grapefruit Juice; Lumefantrine; Nilotinib; QTc-Prolonging Agents; QuiNINE

Decreased Effect

Dronedarone may decrease the levels/effects of: Codeine; TraMADol

The levels/effects of Dronedarone may be decreased by: CYP3A4 Inducers (Strong); Deferasirox; St Johns Wort

Ethanol/Nutrition/Herb Interactions

Food: Increases the rate and extent of absorption of dronedarone. Grapefruit juice increases bioavailability of dronedarone threefold; altered effects are possible; use should be avoided during therapy.

Herb/Nutraceutical: St John's wort may decrease dronedarone levels. Avoid ephedra (may worsen arrhythmia). Avoid dong quai.

Dietary Considerations Take with a meal. Grapefruit juice is not recommended.

Dosage Forms Excipient information presented when available (limited, particularly for generics); consult specific product labeling.

Tablet:

Multaq®: 400 mg

References

Hohnloser SH, Crijns HJ, van Eickels M, et al, "Effect of Dronedarone on Cardiovascular Events in Atrial Fibrillation," *N Engl J Med*, 2009, 360(7):668-78.

Kober L, Torp-Pedersen C, McMurray JJV, et al, "Increased Mortality After Dronedarone Therapy for Severe Heart Failure," *N Engl J Med*, 2008, 358(25):2678-87.

Singh BN, Connolly SJ, Crijns HJ, et al, "Dronedarone for Maintenance of Sinus Rhythm in Atrial Fibrillation or Flutter," *N Engl J Med*, 2007, 357(10):987-99.

Tschuppert Y, Buclin T, Rothuizen LE, et al, "Effect of Dronedarone on Renal Function in Healthy Subjects," *Br J Clin Pharmacol*, 2007, 64(6):785-91.

Wegener FT, Ehrlich JR, and Hohnloser SH, "Dronedarone: An Emerging Agent With Rhythm- and Rate-Controlling Effects," *J Cardiovasc Electrolphysiol*, 2006, 17(Suppl 2):17-20.

◆ **Dronedarone Hydrochloride** *see* Dronedarone *on page 461*

Droperidol (droe PER i dole)

Medication Safety Issues

Sound-alike/look-alike issues:

Droperidol may be confused with dronabinol

Inapsine® may be confused with asenapine, Nebcin®

Related Information

Anesthesia Considerations for Neurosurgery *on page 1514*

Postoperative Nausea and Vomiting *on page 1593*

U.S. Brand Names Inapsine® [DSC]

Canadian Brand Names Droperidol Injection, USP

Index Terms Dehydrobenzperidol

Pharmacologic Category Antiemetic; Antipsychotic Agent, Typical

Generic Available Yes

Use Prevention and/or treatment of nausea and vomiting from surgical and diagnostic procedures

Mechanism of Action Droperidol is a butyrophenone antipsychotic; antiemetic effect is a result of blockade of dopamine stimulation of the chemoreceptor trigger zone. Other effects include alpha-adrenergic blockade, peripheral vascular dilation, and reduction of the pressor effect of epinephrine resulting in hypotension and decreased peripheral vascular resistance; may also reduce pulmonary artery pressure

◀ **Pharmacodynamics/Kinetics**

Onset of action: Peak effect: Parenteral:~30 minutes

Duration: Parenteral: 2-4 hours, may extend to 12 hours

Absorption: I.M.: Rapid

Distribution: Crosses blood-brain barrier and placenta

V_d: Children: ~0.25-0.9 L/kg; Adults: ~2 L/kg

Protein binding: Extensive

Metabolism: Hepatic, to *p*-fluorophenylacetic acid, benzimidazolone, *p*-hydroxypiperidine

Half-life elimination: Adults: 2.3 hours

Excretion: Urine (75%, <1% as unchanged drug); feces (22%, 11% to 50% as unchanged drug)

Dosage Titrate carefully to desired effect

Children 2-12 years: Nausea and vomiting: I.M., I.V.: 0.05-0.06 mg/kg (maximum initial dose: 0.1 mg/kg); additional doses may be repeated to achieve effect; administer additional doses with caution

Adults: Prevention of postoperative nausea and vomiting (PONV): I.M., I.V.: Initial: 0.625-2.5 mg; additional doses of 1.25 mg may be administered to achieve desired effect; administer additional doses with caution. Consensus guidelines recommend 0.625-1.25 mg I.V. administered after surgery (Gan, 2003).

Stability Droperidol ampuls/vials should be stored at room temperature and protected from light. Solutions diluted in NS or D_5W are stable at room temperature for up to 7 days.

Administration Administer I.M. or I.V.; according to the manufacturer, I.V. push administration should be slow (generally regarded as 2-5 minutes); however, many clinicians administer I.V. doses rapidly (over 30-60 seconds) in an effort to reduce the incidence of EPS. The effect, if any, of rapid administration on QT prolongation is unclear. For I.V. infusion, dilute in 50-100 mL NS or D_5W; ECG monitoring for 2-3 hours after administration is recommended regardless of rate of infusion.

Monitoring Parameters To identify QT prolongation, a 12-lead ECG prior to use is recommended; continued ECG monitoring for 2-3 hours following administration is recommended. Vital signs; lipid profile, fasting blood glucose/Hgb A_{1c}, serum magnesium and potassium; BMI; mental status, abnormal involuntary movement scale (AIMS); observe for dystonias, extrapyramidal side effects, and temperature changes

Anesthesia and Critical Care Concerns/Other Considerations

Clinical Pearls/Comments: May cause hypotension and reflex tachycardia; this is more pronounced when the drug is given intravenously. Droperidol does not possess analgesic effects and has little or no amnesic properties.

Evidence-Based Information: An FDA "black box" warning concerning QT prolongation has altered recommendations concerning perioperative use and monitoring. Baseline 12-lead ECG screening is recommended and continued ECG monitoring for 2-3 hours postadministration is advised. However, a large, statistically well-controlled study found that despite nearly 17,000 patient exposures to low-dose droperidol (<1.25 mg) before the FDA warning, no patient had documented torsade de pointes. The authors concluded that the FDA black box warning is excessive and unnecessary (Nuttall, 2007).

Pregnancy Risk Factor C

Contraindications Hypersensitivity to droperidol or any component of the formulation; known or suspected QT prolongation, including congenital long QT syndrome (prolonged QT_c is defined as >440 msec in males or >450 msec in females)

Warnings/Precautions May alter cardiac conduction. **[U.S. Boxed Warning]: Cases of QT prolongation and torsade de pointes, including some fatal cases, have been reported.** Use extreme caution in patients with bradycardia (<50 bpm), cardiac disease, concurrent MAO inhibitor therapy, Class I and Class III antiarrhythmics or other drugs known to prolong QT interval, and electrolyte disturbances (hypokalemia or hypomagnesemia), including concomitant drugs which may alter electrolytes (diuretics).

Use with caution in patients with seizures or severe liver disease. May be sedating, use with caution in disorders where CNS depression is a feature. Caution in patients with hemodynamic instability, predisposition to seizures, subcortical brain damage, pheochromocytoma or renal disease. Esophageal dysmotility and aspiration have been associated with antipsychotic use - use with caution in patients at risk of pneumonia (ie, Alzheimer's disease). Caution in breast cancer or other prolactin-dependent tumors (may elevate prolactin levels). May alter temperature regulation or mask toxicity of other drugs due to antiemetic effects. May cause orthostatic hypotension - use with caution in patients at risk of this effect or those who would tolerate transient hypotensive episodes (cerebrovascular disease, cardiovascular disease, or other medications which may predispose). Significant hypotension may occur.

May cause anticholinergic effects (confusion, agitation, constipation, xerostomia, blurred vision, urinary retention). Therefore, they should be used with caution in patients with decreased gastrointestinal motility, urinary retention, BPH, xerostomia, or visual problems. Conditions which also may be exacerbated by cholinergic blockade include narrow-angle glaucoma (screening is recommended) and worsening of myasthenia gravis. Relative to other neuroleptics, droperidol has a low potency of cholinergic blockade.

May cause extrapyramidal symptoms (EPS), including pseudoparkinsonism, acute dystonic reactions, akathisia, and tardive dyskinesia (risk of these reactions is high relative to other neuroleptics). Risk of dystonia (and possibly other EPS) may be greater with increased doses, use of conventional antipsychotics, males, and younger patients. May be associated with neuroleptic malignant syndrome (NMS) or pigmentary retinopathy. May mask toxicity of other drugs or conditions (eg, intestinal obstruction, Reye's syndrome, brain tumor) due to antiemetic effects. Use with caution in the elderly; reduce initial dose. Safety in children <2 years of age has not been established.

Adverse Reactions
>10%:
  Cardiovascular: QT_c prolongation (dose dependent)
  Central nervous system: Restlessness, anxiety, extrapyramidal symptoms, dystonic reactions, pseudoparkinsonian signs and symptoms, tardive dyskinesia, seizure, altered central temperature regulation, sedation, drowsiness
  Endocrine & metabolic: Swelling of breasts
  Gastrointestinal: Weight gain, constipation
1% to 10%:
  Cardiovascular: Hypotension (especially orthostatic), tachycardia, abnormal T waves with prolonged ventricular repolarization, hypertension
  Central nervous system: Hallucinations, persistent tardive dyskinesia, akathisia
  Gastrointestinal: Nausea, vomiting
  Genitourinary: Dysuria
<1% (Limited to important or life-threatening): Adynamic ileus, agranulocytosis, alopecia, arrhythmia, cholestatic jaundice, heat stroke, hyperpigmentation, laryngospasm, leukopenia, neuroleptic malignant syndrome (NMS), obstructive jaundice, photosensitivity (rare), priapism, rash, respiratory depression, retinal pigmentation, tardive dystonia, torsade de pointes, urinary retention, ventricular tachycardia, visual acuity decreased (may be irreversible)

Drug Interactions
Avoid Concomitant Use
  Avoid concomitant use of Droperidol with any of the following: Artemether; Dronedarone; Lumefantrine; Nilotinib; Pimozide; QuiNINE; Tetrabenazine; Thioridazine; Ziprasidone
Increased Effect/Toxicity
  Droperidol may increase the levels/effects of: Alcohol (Ethyl); Anticholinergics; CNS Depressants; Dronedarone; Pimozide; QTc-Prolonging Agents; QuiNINE; Tetrabenazine; Thioridazine; Ziprasidone

  The levels/effects of Droperidol may be increased by: Acetylcholinesterase Inhibitors (Central); Alfuzosin; Artemether; Chloroquine; Ciprofloxacin; Gadobutrol; Lithium formulations; Lumefantrine; MAO Inhibitors; Nilotinib; Pramlintide; QuiNINE; Tetrabenazine

◄ **Decreased Effect**
Droperidol may decrease the levels/effects of: Amphetamines; Anti-Parkinson's Agents (Dopamine Agonist)

The levels/effects of Droperidol may be decreased by: Lithium formulations

Dosage Forms Excipient information presented when available (limited, particularly for generics); consult specific product labeling. [DSC] = Discontinued product

Injection, solution [preservative free]: 2.5 mg/mL (1 mL, 2 mL)

Inapsine®: 2.5 mg/mL (1 mL, 2 mL) [DSC]

References

Gan TJ, Meyer T, Apfel CC, et al, "Consensus Guidelines for Managing Postoperative Nausea and Vomiting," *Anesth Analg*, 2003, 97(1):62-71.

Jackson CW, Sheehan AH, and Reddan JG, " Evidence-Based Review of the Black-Box Warning for Droperidol," *Am J Health Syst Pharm*, 2007, 64(11):1174-86.

Kao LW, Kirk MA, Evers SJ, et al, "Droperidol, QT Prolongation and Sudden Death: What Is the Evidence," *Ann Emerg Med*, 2003, 41(4):546-58.

Leslie JB and Gan TJ, "Meta-Analysis of the Safety of 5-HT3 Antagonists With Dexamethasone or Droperidol for Prevention of PONV," *Ann Pharmacother*, 2006, 40(5):856-72.

Nuttall GA, Eckerman KM, Jacob KA, et al, "Does Low-Dose Droperidol Administration Increase the Risk of Drug-Induced QT Prolongation and Torsade de Pointes in the General Surgical Population?" *Anesthesiology*, 2007, 107(4):531-6.

Wilhelm SM, Dehoorne-Smith ML, and Kale-Pradhan PB, "Prevention of Postoperative Nausea and Vomiting," *Ann Pharmacother*, 2007, 41(1):68-78.

◆ **Droperidol Injection, USP (Can)** *see* Droperidol *on page 463*

◆ **Drospirenone and Ethinyl Estradiol** *see* Ethinyl Estradiol and Drospirenone *on page 546*

Drotrecogin Alfa (dro TRE coe jin AL fa)

Related Information
Dosing Considerations for the Critically-Ill Patient With Morbid Obesity *on page 1561*

U.S. Brand Names Xigris®

Canadian Brand Names Xigris®

Index Terms Activated Protein C, Human, Recombinant; Drotrecogin Alfa, Activated; Protein C (Activated), Human, Recombinant; rhAPC

Pharmacologic Category Protein C (Activated)

Generic Available No

Use Reduction of mortality from severe sepsis (associated with organ dysfunction) in adults at high risk of death (eg, APACHE II score ≥25)

Unlabeled/Investigational Use Purpura fulminans

Mechanism of Action Inhibits factors Va and VIIIa, limiting thrombotic effects. Additional *in vitro* data suggest inhibition of plasminogen activator inhibitor-1 (PAF-1) resulting in profibrinolytic activity, inhibition of macrophage production of tumor necrosis factor, blocking of leukocyte adhesion, and limitation of thrombin-induced inflammatory responses. Relative contribution of effects on the reduction of mortality from sepsis is not completely understood.

Pharmacodynamics/Kinetics
Duration: Plasma nondetectable within 2 hours of discontinuation
Metabolism: Inactivated by endogenous plasma protease inhibitors; mean clearance: 40 L/hour; increased with severe sepsis (~50%)
Half-life elimination: 1.6 hours

Dosage I.V.:
Children and Adults: Purpura fulminans (unlabeled use): 24 mcg/kg/hour
Adults: Sepsis: 24 mcg/kg/hour for a total of 96 hours; stop infusion **immediately** if clinically-important bleeding is identified. **Note:** Use actual body weight for dosing.
For patient eligibility, may utilize the APACHE II scoring system (http://www.sfar.org/scores2/apache22.html).
Dosage adjustment in renal impairment: No specific adjustment recommended.

Stability Store vials under refrigeration at 2°C to 8°C (36°F to 46°F); do not freeze. Protect from light. Reconstitute 5 mg vials with 2.5 mL and 20 mg vials with 10 mL sterile water for injection (resultant solution ~2 mg/mL). Must be further diluted (within 3 hours of reconstitution) in 0.9% sodium chloride, typically to a concentration between 100 mcg/mL and 200 mcg/mL when using infusion pump and between 100 mcg/mL and 1000 mcg/mL when infused via syringe pump. Although product information states administration must be completed within 12 hours of preparation, additional studies (data on file, Lilly Research Laboratories) show that the final solution is stable for 14 hours at 15°C to 30°C (59°F to 86°F). If not used immediately, a prepared solution may be stored in the refrigerator for up to 12 hours. The total expiration time (refrigeration and administration) should be ≤24 hours from time of preparation.

Administration Infuse separately from all other medications. Only dextrose, normal saline, dextrose/saline combinations, and lactated Ringer's solution may be infused through the same line. May administer via infusion pump. Administration of prepared solution must be completed within 12 hours of preparation. Suspend administration for 2 hours prior to invasive procedures or other procedure with significant bleeding risk; may continue treatment immediately following uncomplicated, minimally-invasive procedures, but delay for 12 hours after major invasive procedures/surgery.

Monitoring Parameters Monitor for signs and symptoms of bleeding, hemoglobin/hematocrit, PT/INR, platelet count

Anesthesia and Critical Care Concerns/Other Considerations
Evidence-Based Information:

The 2008 Surviving Sepsis Campaign guidelines suggest that adult patients with sepsis-induced organ dysfunction (APACHE II ≥25 or multiple organ failure) receive drotrecogin alfa if there are no contraindications (Grade 2B except for patients within 30 days of surgery [Grade 2C]). Relative contraindications need to be considered also. The guidelines recommend that adult patients with severe sepsis and low risk of death (APACHE II <20) or one organ failure should not receive drotrecogin alfa (Grade 1A).

PROWESS trial: The inclusion criteria for the PROWESS trial (Bernard, 2001) may help in patient selection since it is the first clinical trial evaluating a fixed dose of drotrecogin alfa in severe sepsis. The patients included had a known or suspected infection, three or more signs of systemic inflammatory syndrome (SIRS), and sepsis-induced acute organ dysfunction. Indicators of infection included: White cells in a normally sterile body fluid, perforated viscus, radiographic evidence of pneumonia in association with purulent sputum, a syndrome associated with a high risk of infection (eg, ascending cholangitis). Modified (SIRS) criteria (needed ≥3 criteria): A core temperature of ≥38°C (100.4°F) or ≤36°C (96.8°F); heart rate ≥90 bpm except in patients with a medical condition known to increase the heart rate or those receiving treatment that would prevent tachycardia; respiratory rate ≥20 breaths/minute, a $PaCO_2$ ≤32 mm Hg, or the use of mechanical ventilation; WBC count ≥12,000/mm^3, ≤4000/mm^3, or a differential count with >10% immature neutrophils. Criteria for organ dysfunction included arterial blood pressure ≤90 mm Hg or a MAP ≤70 mm Hg for at least 1 hour despite adequate fluid resuscitation, adequate intravascular volume status, or the use of vasopressors; urine output <0.5 mL/kg/hour for 1 hour despite adequate fluid resuscitation; PaO_2/FiO_2 ≤250 in the presence of other dysfunctional organ systems or ≤200 if the lung is the only dysfunctional organ; platelet count <80,000/mm^3 or acute decrease by 50%; unexplained metabolic acidosis with a high plasma lactate level.

Severe sepsis and a low risk of death: Recently a randomized, double-blind, placebo-controlled, multicenter, international trial (Abraham, 2005) was conducted to evaluate the safety and efficacy of drotrecogin alfa in adult patients with severe sepsis and a low risk of death (APACHE II score <25 or single-organ failure). Patients were randomized to a 96 hour infusion of normal saline or drotrecogin alfa at the FDA approved dose; 2640 patients were enrolled in the study. There was no statistical difference between the groups in 28-day mortality. Hemorrhage accounted for 2 deaths (0.9%) in the placebo group and 7 deaths (2.9%) in the drotrecogin alfa group (p = 0.02) during the infusion. Drotrecogin alfa should not be used in patients with severe sepsis who are at low risk of death because of a lack of efficacy and an increased incidence of bleeding. There was no difference in mortality between active treatment and placebo in these-low risk patients after one year of follow up (Laterre, 2007).

Pregnancy Risk Factor C

Contraindications Hypersensitivity to drotrecogin alfa or any component of the formulation; active internal bleeding; recent hemorrhagic stroke (within 3 months); severe head trauma (within 2 months); recent intracranial or intraspinal surgery (within 2 months); intracranial neoplasm or mass lesion; evidence of cerebral herniation; presence of an epidural catheter; trauma with an increased risk of life-threatening bleeding

Warnings/Precautions Increases risk of bleeding; careful evaluation of risks and benefit is required prior to initiation. Bleeding risk is increased in patients receiving concurrent therapeutic heparin, oral anticoagulants, glycoprotein IIb/IIIa antagonists, platelet aggregation inhibitors, or aspirin at a dosage of >650 mg/day (within 7 days). In addition, an increased bleeding risk is associated with prolonged INR (>3), gastrointestinal bleeding (within 6 weeks), decreased platelet count (<30,000/mm^3), thrombolytic therapy (within 3 days), recent ischemic stroke (within 3 months), intracranial AV malformation or aneurysm, known bleeding diathesis, severe hepatic disease (chronic), or other condition where bleeding is a significant hazard or difficult to manage due to its location. Discontinue if significant bleeding occurs (may consider continued use after stabilization). Treatment interruption required for invasive procedures. During treatment, aPTT cannot be used to assess coagulopathy (PT/INR not affected).

Efficacy not established in adult patients at a low risk of death. Patients with pre-existing nonsepsis-related medical conditions with a poor prognosis (anticipated survival <28 days), patients with acute pancreatitis (no established source of infection), HIV-infected patients with a CD4 count ≤50 cells/mm^3, chronic dialysis patients, pre-existing hypercoagulable conditions, and patients who had received bone marrow, liver, lung, pancreas, or small bowel transplants were excluded from the clinical trial which established benefit. In addition, patients weighing >135 kg were not evaluated. Safety and efficacy have not been established in pediatric patients.

Adverse Reactions As with all drugs which may affect hemostasis, bleeding is the major adverse effect associated with drotrecogin alfa. Hemorrhage may occur at virtually any site. Risk is dependent on multiple variables, including the dosage administered, concurrent use of multiple agents which alter hemostasis, and patient predisposition.

>10%:

Dermatologic: Bruising

Gastrointestinal: Gastrointestinal bleeding

1% to 10%: Hematologic: Bleeding (serious 2.4% during infusion vs 3.5% during 28-day study period; individual events listed as <1%)

<1% (Limited to important or life-threatening): Gastrointestinal hemorrhage, genitourinary bleeding, immune reaction (antibody production), intracranial hemorrhage (0.2%; frequencies up to 2% noted in a previous trial without placebo control), intrathoracic hemorrhage, retroperitoneal bleeding, skin/soft tissue bleeding

Drug Interactions

Avoid Concomitant Use There are no known interactions where it is recommended to avoid concomitant use.

Increased Effect/Toxicity

Drotrecogin Alfa may increase the levels/effects of: Anticoagulants; Fondaparinux; Ibritumomab; Tositumomab and Iodine I 131 Tositumomab

The levels/effects of Drotrecogin Alfa may be increased by: Antiplatelet Agents; Antithrombin; Danaparoid; Dasatinib; Heparin; Heparin (Low Molecular Weight); Herbs (Anticoagulant/Antiplatelet Properties); Nonsteroidal Anti-Inflammatory Agents; Pentosan Polysulfate Sodium; Prostacyclin Analogues; Salicylates; Thrombolytic Agents; Vitamin K Antagonists

Decreased Effect There are no known significant interactions involving a decrease in effect.

Ethanol/Nutrition/Herb Interactions Herb/Nutraceutical: Recent use/intake of herbs with anticoagulant or antiplatelet activity (including cat's claw, feverfew, garlic, ginkgo, ginseng, and horse chestnut seed) may increase the risk of bleeding.

Test Interactions May interfere with one-stage coagulation assays based on the aPTT (such as factor VIII, IX, and XI assays).

Dosage Forms Excipient information presented when available (limited, particularly for generics); consult specific product labeling.

Injection, powder for reconstitution [preservative free]: 5 mg [contains sucrose 31.8 mg], 20 mg [contains sucrose 124.9 mg]

References

Abraham E, Laterre PF, Garg R, et al, "Drotrecogin Alfa (Activated) for Adults With Severe Sepsis and a Low Risk of Death," *N Engl J Med*, 2005, 353(13):1332-1400.

Bachli EB, Vavricka SR, Walter RB, et al, "Drotecogin Alfa (Activated) for the Treatment of Meningococcal Purpura Fulminans," *Intensive Care Med*, 2003, 29(2):337.

Barton P, Kalil AC, Nadel S, et al, "Safety, Pharmacokinetics, and Pharmacodynamics of Drotrecogin Alfa (Activated) in Children With Severe Sepsis, " *Pediatrics*, 2004, 113(1 Pt 1):7-17.

Bernard GR, Ely EW, Wright TJ, et al, "Safety and Dose Relationship of Recombinant Human Activated Protein C for Coagulopathy in Severe Sepsis," *Crit Care Med*, 2001, 29(11):2051-9.

Bernard GR, Vincent JL, Laterre PF, et al, "Efficacy and Safety of Recombinant Human Activated Protein C for Severe Sepsis," *N Engl J Med*, 2001, 344(10):699-709.

Cone LA, B Waterbor R, Sofonio MV, "Purpura Fulminans Due to *Streptococcus pneumoniae* Sepsis Following Gastric Bypass," *Obes Surg*, 2004, 14(5):690-4.

Dellinger RP, Levy MM, Carlet JM, et al, "Surviving Sepsis Campaign: International Guidelines for Management of Severe Sepsis and Septic Shock: 2008," *Intensive Care Med*, 2008, 34(1): 17-60. Available at http://www.survivingsepsis.org/system/files/images/2008_20International_20SSC_20-Guidelines_1_.pdf

Hasin T, Leibowitz D, Rot D, et al, "Early Treatment With Activated Protein C for Meningococcal Septic Shock: Case Report and Literature Review," *Intensive Care Med*, 2005, 31(7):1002-3.

Laterre PF, Abraham E, Janes JM, et al, "ADDRESS (ADministration of DRotrecogin Alfa [Activated] in Early Stage Severe Sepsis) Long-Term Follow-Up: One-Year Safety and Efficacy Evaluation," *Crit Care Med*, 2007, 35(6):1457-63.

Levy H, Small D, Heiselman DE, et al, "Obesity Does Not Alter the Pharmacokinetics of Drotrecogin Alfa (Activated) in Severe Sepsis," *Ann Pharmacother*, 2005, 39(2):262-7.

Mann HJ, Demmon SL, Boelk DA, et al, "Physical and Chemical Compatibility of Drotrecogin Alfa (Activated) With 34 Drugs During Simulated Y-Site Administration," *Am J Health Syst Pharm*, 2004, 61(24):2664-71.

◆ **Drotrecogin Alfa, Activated** see Drotrecogin Alfa on page 466

◆ **Droxia®** see Hydroxyurea on page 712

DULoxetine (doo LOX e teen)

Medication Safety Issues
Sound-alike/look-alike issues:
Cymbalta® may be confused with Symbyax®
DULoxetine may be confused with FLUoxetine

Medication Guide An FDA-approved patient medication guide, which is available with the product information and at http://www.fda.gov/downloads/Drugs/DrugSafety/ucm088579.pdf, must be dispensed with this medication for each new outpatient prescription and refill.

Related Information
Antidepressant Agents on page 1660
Chronic Pain Management on page 1546

U.S. Brand Names Cymbalta®

Canadian Brand Names Cymbalta®

Index Terms (+)-(S)-N-Methyl-γ-(1-naphthyloxy)-2-thiophenepropylamine Hydrochloride; Duloxetine Hydrochloride; LY248686

Pharmacologic Category Antidepressant, Serotonin/Norepinephrine Reuptake Inhibitor

Generic Available No

Use Acute and maintenance treatment of major depressive disorder (MDD); treatment of generalized anxiety disorder (GAD); management of pain associated with diabetic neuropathy; management of fibromyalgia

Unlabeled/Investigational Use Treatment of stress incontinence; management of chronic pain syndromes

◄ **Mechanism of Action** Duloxetine is a potent inhibitor of neuronal serotonin and norepinephrine reuptake and a weak inhibitor of dopamine reuptake. Duloxetine has no significant activity for muscarinic cholinergic, H_1-histaminergic, or alpha$_2$-adrenergic receptors. Duloxetine does not possess MAO-inhibitory activity.

Pharmacodynamics/Kinetics

Absorption: Well absorbed, 2-hour delay in absorption after ingestion; food decreases extent of absorption ~10% (no effect on C_{max})

Distribution: 1640 L (range: 701-3800 L)

Protein binding: >90%; primarily to albumin and α_1-acid glycoprotein

Metabolism: Hepatic, via CYP1A2 and CYP2D6; forms multiple metabolites (inactive)

Half-life elimination: 12 hours (range 8-17 hours)

Time to peak: 6 hours; 10 hours when ingested with food

Excretion: As metabolites; urine (72%), feces (19%)

Dosage Oral:

Adults:

Major depressive disorder: Initial: 40-60 mg/day; dose may be divided (ie, 20 or 30 mg twice daily) or given as a single daily dose of 60 mg; maintenance: 60 mg once daily; for doses >60 mg/day, titrate dose in increments of 30 mg/day over 1 week as tolerated to a maximum dose: 120 mg/day. **Note:** Doses >60 mg/day have not been demonstrated to be more effective.

Diabetic neuropathy: 60 mg once daily; lower initial doses may be considered in patients where tolerability is a concern and/or renal impairment is present. **Note:** Doses up to 120 mg/day administered in clinical trials offered no additional benefit and were less well tolerated than dose of 60 mg/day.

Fibromyalgia: Initial: 30 mg/day for 1 week, then increase to 60 mg/day as tolerated. **Note:** Doses up to 120 mg/day administered in clinical trials offered no additional benefit and were less well tolerated than dose of 60 mg/day.

Generalized anxiety disorder: Initial: 30-60 mg/day as a single daily dose; patients initiated at 30 mg/day should be titrated to 60 mg/day after 1 week; maximum dose: 120 mg/day. **Note:** Doses >60 mg/day have not been demonstrated to be more effective than 60 mg/day.

Chronic pain syndromes (unlabeled use): 60 mg once daily

Stress incontinence (unlabeled use): 40 mg twice daily

Elderly:

Major depressive disorder: Manufacturer does not recommend specific dosage adjustment. Conservatively, may initiate at a dose of 20 mg 1-2 times/day; increase to 40-60 mg/day as a single daily dose or in divided doses **or** initiate therapy at 30 mg/day for 1 week then increase to 60 mg/day as tolerated.

Other indications: Refer to adult dosing

Dosage adjustment in renal impairment: Not recommended for use in Cl_{cr} <30 mL/minute or ESRD (contraindicated in Canadian labeling); in mild-moderate impairment, lower initial doses may be considered with titration guided by response and tolerability

Dosage adjustment in hepatic impairment: Not recommended for use in hepatic impairment (contraindicated in Canadian labeling)

Stability Store at 25°C (77°F); excursions permitted to 15°C to 30°C (59°F to 86°F)

Administration Capsule should be swallowed whole; do not break open or crush. Administer without regard to meals.

Monitoring Parameters Blood pressure should be checked prior to initiating therapy and then regularly monitored, especially in patients with a high baseline blood pressure; mental status for depression, suicidal ideation (especially at the beginning of therapy or when doses are increased or decreased), anxiety, social functioning, mania, panic attacks; glucose levels and Hb A_{1c} levels in diabetic patients, creatinine, BUN, transaminases

Pregnancy Risk Factor C

Contraindications Concomitant use or within 2 weeks of MAO inhibitors; uncontrolled narrow-angle glaucoma

Canadian labeling: Additional contraindications (not in U.S. labeling): Hypersensitivity to duloxetine or any component of the formulation; hepatic impairment; severe renal impairment (eg, Cl_{cr} <30 mL/minute) or end-stage renal disease (ESRD); concomitant use with thioridazine or with CYP1A2 inhibitors

Warnings/Precautions [U.S. Boxed Warning]: Antidepressants increase the risk of suicidal thinking and behavior in children, adolescents, and young adults (18-24 years of age) with major depressive disorder (MDD) and other psychiatric disorders; consider risk prior to prescribing. Short-term studies did not show an increased risk in patients >24 years of age and showed a decreased risk in patients ≥65 years. Closely monitor for clinical worsening, suicidality, or unusual changes in behavior; the patient's family or caregiver should be instructed to closely observe the patient and communicate condition with healthcare provider. A medication guide concerning the use of antidepressants in children and teenagers should be dispensed with each prescription. **Duloxetine is not FDA approved for use in children.**

The possibility of a suicide attempt is inherent in major depression and may persist until remission occurs. Patients treated with antidepressants should be observed for clinical worsening and suicidality, especially during the initial (generally first 1-2 months) few months of a course of drug therapy, or at times of dose changes, either increases or decreases. Use caution in high-risk patients. Worsening depression and severe abrupt suicidality that are not part of the presenting symptoms may require discontinuation or modification of drug therapy. The patient's family or caregiver should be alerted to monitor patients for the emergence of suicidality and associated behaviors (such as agitation, irritability, hostility, impulsivity, and hypomania) and call healthcare provider.

May worsen psychosis in some patients or precipitate a shift to mania or hypomania in patients with bipolar disorder. Patients presenting with depressive symptoms should be screened for bipolar disorder. Monotherapy in patients with bipolar disorder should be avoided. **Duloxetine is not FDA approved for the treatment of bipolar depression.**

May cause orthostatic hypotension/syncope at therapeutic doses especially within the first week of therapy and after dose increases. Monitor blood pressure with initiation of therapy, dose increases (especially in patients receiving >60 mg/day), or with concomitant use of vasodilators or CYP1A2 inhibitors. Use caution in patients with hypertension. May increase blood pressure. Rare cases of hypertensive crisis have been reported in patients with pre-existing hypertension; evaluate blood pressure prior to initiating therapy and periodically thereafter; consider dose reduction or gradual discontinuation of therapy in individuals with sustained hypertension during therapy.

Modest increases in serum glucose and hemoglobin A_{1c} (Hb A_{1c}) levels have been observed in some diabetic patients receiving duloxetine therapy for diabetic peripheral neuropathy (DPN). Duloxetine may cause increased urinary resistance; advise patient to report symptoms of urinary hesitation/difficulty. Has a low potential to impair cognitive or motor performance. Use caution with a previous seizure disorder or condition predisposing to seizures such as brain damage or alcoholism. Avoid use in patients with substantial ethanol intake, evidence of chronic liver disease, or hepatic impairment (contraindicated in Canadian labeling). Rare cases of hepatic failure (including fatalities) have been reported with use. Hepatitis with abdominal pain, hepatomegaly, elevated transaminase levels >20 times the upper limit of normal (ULN) with and without jaundice have all been observed. Discontinue therapy with the presentation of jaundice or other signs of hepatic dysfunction and do not reinitiate therapy unless another source or cause is identified.

May cause hyponatremia/SIADH (elderly at increased risk); volume depletion (diuretics may increase risk). Use with caution in patients with controlled narrow angle glaucoma. May cause or exacerbate sexual dysfunction. Use caution with renal impairment (contraindicated in Canadian labeling for severe renal impairment or ESRD). Use caution with concomitant CNS depressants. May impair platelet aggregation; use caution with concomitant use of NSAIDs, ASA, or other drugs that affect coagulation; the risk of bleeding may be potentiated.

Serotonin syndrome and neuroleptic malignant syndrome (NMS)-like reactions have occurred with serotonin/norepinephrine reuptake inhibitors (SNRIs) and selective serotonin reuptake inhibitors (SSRIs) when used alone, and particularly when used in combination with serotonergic agents (eg, triptans) or antidopaminergic agents (eg, antipsychotics). Concurrent use with MAO inhibitors is contraindicated. Use caution during concurrent therapy with other drugs which lower the seizure threshold. To discontinue therapy with duloxetine, gradually taper dose. If intolerable symptoms occur following a decrease in dosage or upon discontinuation of therapy, then resuming the previous dose with a more gradual taper should be considered. May increase the risks associated with electroconvulsive therapy. Consider discontinuing, when possible, prior to elective surgery. Formulation contains sucrose; patients with fructose intolerance, glucose-galactose malabsorption, or sucrose-isomaltase deficiency should avoid use. Safety and efficacy have not been established in patients <18 years of age.

Adverse Reactions

>10%:

Central nervous system: Somnolence (7% to 21%), headache (13% to 20%), dizziness (6% to 17%), insomnia (8% to 16%), fatigue (2% to 15%)

Gastrointestinal: Nausea (14% to 30%), xerostomia (5% to 18%), constipation (5% to 15%), diarrhea (7% to 13%), appetite decreased (3% to 11%)

1% to 10%:

Cardiovascular: Palpitation (1% to 2%)

Central nervous system: Agitation (5% to 6%), anxiety (3%), sleep disorder (3%), dreams abnormal (2% to 3%), fever (1% to 3%), yawning (1% to 2%), hypoesthesia (1%), lethargy (1%), nightmares (1%), vertigo (1%)

Dermatologic: Hyperhydrosis (6% to 8%), rash (4%), pruritus (3%)

Endocrine & metabolic: Libido decreased (2% to 4%), orgasm abnormality (3%), hot flushes (2% to 3%), anorgasmia (1%)

Gastrointestinal: Vomiting (5% to 6%), dyspepsia (4% to 5%), anorexia (3% to 5%), loose stools (2% to 3%), taste abnormal (1% to 3%), weight gain/loss (2%), flatulence (1%)

Genitourinary: Erectile dysfunction (1% to 5%), pollakiuria (1% to 5%), ejaculatory dysfunction (2% to 4%), ejaculation delayed (3%), penis disorder (2%)

Hepatic: ALT >3x ULN (1%)

Neuromuscular & skeletal: Weakness (2% to 8%), muscle cramp (4% to 5%), musculoskeletal pain (1% to 5%), muscle spasms (4%), tremor (3% to 4%), myalgia (1% to 4%), paresthesia (1%), rigors (1%)

Ocular: Blurred vision (1% to 3%)

Respiratory: Nasopharyngitis (7% to 9%), upper respiratory infection (7%), cough (3% to 6%), pharyngolaryngeal pain (1% to 6%)

Miscellaneous: Diaphoresis increased (6%), seasonal allergies (3%)

<1% (Limited to important or life-threatening): Abdominal pain, acne, agitation, aggression, alkaline phosphatase increased, alopecia, anaphylactic reaction, anger, anemia, angioneurotic edema, aphthous stomatitis, ataxia, atrial fibrillation, bloody stools, bundle branch block, CHF, colitis, CPK increased, dehydration, dermatitis, diastolic blood pressure increased, diplopia, disorientation, diverticulitis, dysarthria, dyskinesia, dyslipidemia, dysphagia, dysuria, ecchymosis, eczema, edema (peripheral), erythema, erythema multiforme, esophageal stenosis, EPS, facial edema, flu-like syndrome, flushing, gait instability, gastric emptying impaired, gastric ulcer, gastritis, gastroenteritis, GI bleeding, gingivitis, glaucoma, hallucinations, Hb A_{1c} increased, hematochezia, hepatic failure, hepatic steatosis, hepatitis, hepatomegaly, hyperbilirubinemia, hypercholesterolemia, hyperglycemia, hyperlipidemia, hypersensitivity, hypertensive crisis, hyponatremia, hypothyroidism, irritability, irritable bowel syndrome, jaundice, keroconjunctivitis sicca, laryngitis, leukopenia, lymphadenopathy, macular degeneration, maculopathy, malaise, mania, melena, MI, micturition urgency, mood swings, muscle spasm, muscle tightness, muscle twitching, nephropathy, night sweats, nocturia, oropharyngeal edema, orthostatic hypotension, peripheral coldness, phlebitis, photosensitivity, polyuria, restless leg syndrome, retinal detachment, seizure, serotonin syndrome, sexual dysfunction, SIADH, Stevens-Johnson syndrome, stomatitis, suicide, supraventricular arrhythmia, syncope, systolic blood pressure increased, tachycardia, thirst, throat tightness, thrombocytopenia, tinnitus, transaminases increased, trismus, urinary retention, urticaria, vaginal bleeding, visual disturbance; withdrawal syndrome (including headache, dizziness, nightmares, irritability, paresthesia, and/or vomiting)

Drug Interactions

Metabolism/Transport Effects Substrate (major) of CYP1A2, 2D6; **inhibits** CYP2D6 (moderate)

Avoid Concomitant Use

Avoid concomitant use of DULoxetine with any of the following: Iobenguane I 123; MAO Inhibitors; Sibutramine; Thioridazine

Increased Effect/Toxicity

DULoxetine may increase the levels/effects of: Alcohol (Ethyl); Alpha-/Beta-Agonists; Aspirin; CNS Depressants; CYP2D6 Substrates; Fesoterodine; Methotrimeprazine; Nebivolol; NSAID (Nonselective); Serotonin Modulators; Tamoxifen; Thioridazine; Tricyclic Antidepressants

The levels/effects of DULoxetine may be increased by: CYP1A2 Inhibitors (Moderate); CYP1A2 Inhibitors (Strong); CYP2D6 Inhibitors (Moderate); CYP2D6 Inhibitors (Strong); Darunavir; Fluvoxamine; MAO Inhibitors; Methotrimeprazine; PARoxetine; Sibutramine

Decreased Effect

DULoxetine may decrease the levels/effects of: Alpha2-Agonists; Codeine; Iobenguane I 123

The levels/effects of DULoxetine may be decreased by: CYP1A2 Inducers (Strong); Peginterferon Alfa-2b

Ethanol/Nutrition/Herb Interactions

Ethanol: Avoid ethanol (may increase CNS depression and/or hepatotoxic potential of duloxetine).

Herb/Nutraceutical: Avoid valerian, St John's wort, SAMe, kava kava, and gotu kola (may increase CNS depression).

Dietary Considerations May be taken without regard to meals.

Dosage Forms Excipient information presented when available (limited, particularly for generics); consult specific product labeling.

Capsule, delayed release, enteric coated pellets:

Cymbalta®: 20 mg, 30 mg, 60 mg

References

Arnold LM, Lu Y, Crofford LJ, et al, "A Double-Blind, Multicenter Trial Comparing Duloxetine With Placebo in the Treatment of Fibromyalgia Patients With or Without Major Depressive Disorder," *Arthritis Rheum*, 2004, 50(9):2974-84.

Boyer EW and Shannon M, "The Serotonin Syndrome," *N Engl J Med*, 2005, 352:1112-20.

Chambers CD, Hernandez-Diaz S, Van Marter LJ, et al, "Selective Serotonin-Reuptake Inhibitors and Risk of Persistent Pulmonary Hypertension of the Newborn," *N Engl J Med*, 2006, 354(6):579-87.

Dmochowski RR, Miklos JR, Norton PA, et al, "Duloxetine Versus Placebo for the Treatment of North American Women With Stress Urinary Incontinence," *J Urol*, 2003, 170(4 Pt 1):1259-63.

Fava M, Mallinckrodt CH, Detke MJ, et al, "The Effect of Duloxetine on Painful Physical Symptoms in Depressed Patients: Do Improvements in These Symptoms Result in Higher Remission Rates?" *J Clin Psychiatry*, 2004, 65(4):521-30.

Goldstein DJ, Lu Y, Detke MJ, et al, "Duloxetine in the Treatment of Depression: A Double-Blind Placebo-Controlled Comparison With Paroxetine," *J Clin Psychopharmacol*, 2004, 24(4):389-99.

Millard RJ, Moore K, Rencken R, et al, "Duloxetine vs Placebo in the Treatment of Stress Urinary Incontinence: A Four-Continent Randomized Clinical Trial," *BJU Int*, 2004, 93(3):311-8.

Pass SE and Simpson RW, "Discontinuation and Reinstitution of Medications During the Perioperative Period," *Am J Health Syst Pharm*, 2004, 61(9):899-912.

Raskin J, Wiltse CG, Siegal A, et al, "Efficacy of Duloxetine on Cognition, Depression, and Pain in Elderly Patients With Major Depressive Disorder: An 8-Week, Double-Blind, Placebo-Controlled Trial," *Am J Psychiatry*, 2007, 164(6):900-9.

van Kerrebroeck P, Abrams P, Lange R, et al, "Duloxetine Versus Placebo in the Treatment of European and Canadian Women With Stress Urinary Incontinence," *BJOG*, 2004, 111(3):249-57.

- ◆ **7E3** *see* Abciximab *on page 22*
- ◆ **E2020** *see* Donepezil *on page 447*
- ◆ **E 2080** *see* Rufinamide *on page 1271*
- ◆ **EACA** *see* Aminocaproic Acid *on page 83*
- ◆ **Easprin®** *see* Aspirin *on page 147*
- ◆ **Ebixa® (Can)** *see* Memantine *on page 874*
- ◆ **EC-Naprosyn®** *see* Naproxen *on page 987*
- ◆ **Econopred® Plus [DSC]** *see* PrednisoLONE *on page 1164*
- ◆ **Ecotrin® [OTC]** *see* Aspirin *on page 147*
- ◆ **Ecotrin® Low Strength [OTC]** *see* Aspirin *on page 147*
- ◆ **Ecotrin® Maximum Strength [OTC]** *see* Aspirin *on page 147*
- ◆ **Ectosone (Can)** *see* Betamethasone *on page 186*
- ◆ **Edecrin®** *see* Ethacrynic Acid *on page 541*
- ◆ **Edex®** *see* Alprostadil *on page 66*
- ◆ **Edluar™** *see* Zolpidem *on page 1494*

Edrophonium (ed roe FOE nee um)

Related Information
Chronic Renal Failure *on page 1552*
U.S. Brand Names Enlon®
Canadian Brand Names Enlon®; Tensilon®
Index Terms Edrophonium Chloride
Pharmacologic Category Acetylcholinesterase Inhibitor; Antidote; Diagnostic Agent
Generic Available No
Use Diagnosis of myasthenia gravis; differentiation of cholinergic crises from myasthenia crises; reversal of nondepolarizing neuromuscular blockers
Mechanism of Action Inhibits destruction of acetylcholine by acetylcholinesterase. This facilitates transmission of impulses across myoneural junction and results in increased cholinergic responses such as miosis, increased tonus of intestinal and skeletal muscles, bronchial and ureteral constriction, bradycardia, and increased salivary and sweat gland secretions.
Pharmacodynamics/Kinetics
Onset of action: I.M.: 2-10 minutes; I.V.: 30-60 seconds
Duration: I.M.: 5-30 minutes; I.V.: 10 minutes
Distribution: V_d: Adults: 1.1 L/kg
Half-life elimination: Adults: 1.2-2.4 hours; Anephric patients: 2.4-4.4 hours
Excretion: Adults: Primarily urine (67%)
Dosage Usually administered I.V., however, if not possible, I.M. or SubQ may be used:
Infants:
I.M.: 0.5-1 mg
I.V.: Initial: 0.1 mg, followed by 0.4 mg if no response; total dose = 0.5 mg
Children:
Diagnosis: Initial: 0.04 mg/kg over 1 minute followed by 0.16 mg/kg if no response, to a maximum total dose of 5 mg for children <34 kg, or 10 mg for children >34 kg **or**
Alternative dosing (manufacturer's recommendation):
≤34 kg: 1 mg; if no response after 45 seconds, repeat dosage in 1 mg increments every 30-45 seconds, up to a total of 5 mg
>34 kg: 2 mg; if no response after 45 seconds, repeat dosage in 1 mg increments every 30-45 seconds, up to a total of 10 mg
I.M.:
<34 kg: 1 mg
>34 kg: 5 mg
Titration of oral anticholinesterase therapy: 0.04 mg/kg once given 1 hour after oral intake of the drug being used in treatment; if strength improves, an increase in neostigmine or pyridostigmine dose is indicated

Adults:

Diagnosis:

I.V.: 2 mg test dose administered over 15-30 seconds; 8 mg given 45 seconds later if no response is seen; test dose may be repeated after 30 minutes

I.M.: Initial: 10 mg; if no cholinergic reaction occurs, administer 2 mg 30 minutes later to rule out false-negative reaction

Titration of oral anticholinesterase therapy: 1-2 mg given 1 hour after oral dose of anticholinesterase; if strength improves, an increase in neostigmine or pyridostigmine dose is indicated

Reversal of nondepolarizing neuromuscular blocking agents (neostigmine with atropine usually preferred): I.V.: 10 mg over 30-45 seconds; may repeat every 5-10 minutes up to 40 mg

Termination of paroxysmal atrial tachycardia: I.V. rapid injection: 5-10 mg

Differentiation of cholinergic from myasthenic crisis: I.V.: 1 mg; may repeat after 1 minute. **Note:** Intubation and controlled ventilation may be required if patient has cholinergic crisis

Dosing adjustment in renal impairment: Dose may need to be reduced in patients with chronic renal failure

Administration Edrophonium is administered by direct I.V. injection; see Dosage

Monitoring Parameters Pre- and postinjection strength (cranial musculature is most useful); heart rate, respiratory rate, blood pressure

Anesthesia and Critical Care Concerns/Other Considerations

Clinical Pearls/Comments: Atropine or glycopyrrolate should be administered along with edrophonium when reversing the effects of nondepolarizing neuromuscular blocking agents to antagonize the cholinergic effects at the muscarinic receptors. It is important to recognize the difference in dose for diagnosis of myasthenia gravis versus reversal of muscle relaxant; a much larger dose is needed for desired effect of reversal of muscle paralysis.

Pregnancy Risk Factor C

Contraindications Hypersensitivity to edrophonium, sulfites, or any component of the formulation; GI or GU obstruction

Warnings/Precautions Use with caution in patients with bronchial asthma and those receiving a cardiac glycoside; atropine sulfate should always be readily available as an antagonist. Overdosage can cause cholinergic crisis which may be fatal. I.V. atropine should be readily available for treatment of cholinergic reactions. Use with caution in patients with cardiac arrhythmias (eg, bradyarrhythmias). Avoid use in myasthenia gravis; may exacerbate muscular weakness. Products may contain sodium sulfite.

Adverse Reactions Frequency not defined.

Cardiovascular: Arrhythmias (especially bradycardia), AV block, carbon monoxide decreased, cardiac arrest, ECG changes (nonspecific), flushing, hypotension, nodal rhythm, syncope, tachycardia

Central nervous system: Convulsions, dizziness, drowsiness, dysarthria, dysphonia, headache, loss of consciousness

Dermatologic: Skin rash, thrombophlebitis (I.V.), urticaria

Gastrointestinal: Diarrhea, dysphagia, flatulence, hyperperistalsis, nausea, salivation, stomach cramps, vomiting

Genitourinary: Urinary urgency

Neuromuscular & skeletal: Arthralgias, fasciculations, muscle cramps, spasms, weakness

Ocular: Lacrimation, small pupils

Respiratory: Bronchiolar constriction, bronchospasm, dyspnea, bronchial secretions increased, laryngospasm, respiratory arrest, respiratory depression, respiratory muscle paralysis

Miscellaneous: Allergic reactions, anaphylaxis, diaphoresis increased

Drug Interactions

Avoid Concomitant Use There are no known interactions where it is recommended to avoid concomitant use.

Increased Effect/Toxicity

Edrophonium may increase the levels/effects of: Beta-Blockers; Cholinergic Agonists; Succinylcholine

The levels/effects of Edrophonium may be increased by: Corticosteroids (Systemic); Ginkgo Biloba

Decreased Effect

Edrophonium may decrease the levels/effects of: Neuromuscular-Blocking Agents (Nondepolarizing)

Test Interactions Increased aminotransferase [ALT/AST] (S), amylase (S)

Dosage Forms Excipient information presented when available (limited, particularly for generics); consult specific product labeling.

Injection, solution, as chloride:

Enlon®: 10 mg/mL (15 mL) [contains natural rubber/natural latex in packaging; sodium sulfite]

References

Mokhlesi B, Leikin JB, Murray P, et al, "Adult Toxicology in Critical Care: Part II: Specific Poisonings," *Chest*, 2003, 123(3):897-922.

Edrophonium and Atropine (ed roe FOE nee um & A troe peen)

Related Information

Atropine *on page 162*

Edrophonium *on page 474*

U.S. Brand Names Enlon-Plus®

Index Terms Atropine Sulfate and Edrophonium Chloride; Edrophonium Chloride and Atropine Sulfate

Pharmacologic Category Acetylcholinesterase Inhibitor; Anticholinergic Agent; Antidote

Use Reversal of nondepolarizing neuromuscular blockers; adjunct treatment of respiratory depression caused by curare overdose

Pharmacodynamics/Kinetics See individual agents.

Onset of action: Edrophonium: Antagonism of nondepolarizing muscle relaxants: 3 minutes; Atropine: Heart rate: Immediate

Duration: Edrophonium: Antagonism of nondepolarizing muscle relaxants: 70 minutes; Atropine: Heart rate: 170 minutes

Protein binding: Atropine: 14%

Half-life elimination: Edrophonium: Adults: 1.2-2.4 hours; Anephric patients: 2.4-4.4 hours

Time to peak, plasma: Edrophonium: Antagonism of nondepolarizing muscle relaxants: 1.2 minutes; Atropine: Heart rate: 2-16 minutes

Excretion: Edrophonium: Primarily urine (67%)

Dosage I.V.: Adults: Reversal of neuromuscular blockade: 0.05-0.1 mL/kg given over 45-60 seconds. The dose delivered is 0.5-1 mg/kg of edrophonium and 0.007-0.014 mg/kg of atropine. An edrophonium dose of 1 mg/kg should rarely be exceeded. **Note:** Monitor closely for bradyarrhythmias.

Dosage adjustment in renal impairment: Adjustment not required.

Dosage adjustment in hepatic impairment: Adjustment not required.

Additional Information Complete prescribing information for this medication should be consulted for additional detail.

Dosage Forms Excipient information presented when available (limited, particularly for generics); consult specific product labeling.

Injection, solution:

Enlon-Plus®: Edrophonium chloride 10 mg/mL and atropine sulfate 0.14 mg/mL (5 mL, 15 mL) [contains sodium sulfite; packaging may contain natural rubber latex]

◆ **Edrophonium Chloride** *see* Edrophonium *on page 474*

◆ **Edrophonium Chloride and Atropine Sulfate** *see* Edrophonium and Atropine *on page 476*

◆ **E.E.S.®** *see* Erythromycin *on page 516*

◆ **EES® (Can)** *see* Erythromycin *on page 516*

◆ **Effexor®** *see* Venlafaxine *on page 1466*

◆ **Effexor XR®** *see* Venlafaxine *on page 1466*

◆ **Effexor® XR (Can)** *see* Venlafaxine *on page 1466*

◆ **Effient™** *see* Prasugrel *on page 1160*

◆ **Elavil** *see* Amitriptyline *on page 89*

◆ **Eldepryl®** *see* Selegiline *on page 1282*

◆ **Elestrin™** *see* Estradiol *on page 531*

Eletriptan (el e TRIP tan)

U.S. Brand Names Relpax®
Canadian Brand Names Relpax®
Index Terms Eletriptan Hydrobromide
Pharmacologic Category Antimigraine Agent; Serotonin 5-HT$_{1B, 1D}$ Receptor Agonist
Use Acute treatment of migraine, with or without aura
Pharmacodynamics/Kinetics
  Absorption: Well absorbed
  Distribution: V$_d$: 138 L
  Protein binding: ~85%
  Metabolism: Hepatic via CYP3A4; forms one metabolite (active)
  Bioavailability: ~50%, increased with high-fat meal
  Half-life elimination: 4 hours (Elderly: 4.4-5.7 hours); Metabolite: ~13 hours
  Time to peak, plasma: 1.5-2 hours
Dosage Oral: Adults: Acute migraine: 20-40 mg; if the headache improves but returns, dose may be repeated after 2 hours have elapsed since first dose; maximum 80 mg/day.

  Note: If the first dose is ineffective, diagnosis needs to be re-evaluated. Safety of treating >3 headaches/month has not been established.
  Dosage adjustment in renal impairment: No dosing adjustment needed; monitor for increased blood pressure
  Dosage adjustment in hepatic impairment:
    Mild-to-moderate impairment: No adjustment necessary
    Severe impairment: Use is contraindicated
Additional Information Complete prescribing information for this medication should be consulted for additional detail.
Dosage Forms Excipient information presented when available (limited, particularly for generics); consult specific product labeling.
  Tablet:
    Relpax®: 20 mg, 40 mg

◆ **Eletriptan Hydrobromide** *see* Eletriptan *on page 477*

◆ **Elixophyllin®** *see* Theophylline *on page 1373*

Eltrombopag (el TROM boe pag)

U.S. Brand Names Promacta®
Index Terms Eltrombopag Olamine; Revolade®; SB-497115; SB-497115-GR
Pharmacologic Category Colony Stimulating Factor; Thrombopoietic Agent
Restrictions Eltrombopag is approved for marketing under a Food and Drug Administration (FDA) approved, risk management, and restricted distribution program called Promacta® Cares™ (1-877-977-6622). Patients, prescribers, and pharmacies must be enrolled in the program.
Use Treatment of thrombocytopenia in patients with chronic immune (idiopathic) thrombocytopenic purpura (ITP) at risk for bleeding who have had insufficient response to corticosteroids, immune globulin, or splenectomy
Pharmacodynamics/Kinetics
  Onset of action: Platelet count increase: Within 1-2 weeks
    Peak platelet count increase: 14-16 days
  Duration: Platelets return to baseline: 1-2 weeks after last dose
  Protein binding: >99%
  Metabolism: Extensive hepatic metabolism; via CYP 1A2, 2C8 oxidation and UGT 1A1, 1A3 glucuronidation
  Bioavailability: ~52%
  Half-life elimination: ~21-32 hours in healthy individuals; ~26-35 hours in patients with ITP
  Time to peak, plasma: 2-6 hours

◄ Excretion: Feces (~59%, 20% as unchanged drug, 21% glutathione-related conjugates); urine (31%, 20% glucuronide of the phenypyrazole moiety)

Dosage Note: Discontinue if platelet count does not respond to a level that avoids clinically important bleeding after 4 weeks at the maximum daily dose of 75 mg.

Oral: Adults: ITP: Initial: 50 mg once daily; adjust dose to achieve and maintain platelet count ≥50,000/mm^3 to reduce the risk of bleeding; Maximum dose: 75 mg once daily

Dosage adjustment recommendations:

Platelet count <50,000/mm^3 (after at least 2 weeks): Increase daily dose by 25 mg; maximum dose: 75 mg/day

Platelet count >200,000/mm^3 (at any time): Reduce daily dose by 25 mg; reassess in 2 weeks

Platelet count >400,000/mm^3: Withhold dose; assess platelet count twice weekly; when platelet count <150,000/mm^3, resume with the daily dose reduced by 25 mg

Platelet count >400,000/mm^3 after 2 weeks at the lowest dose: Permanently discontinue

Dosage adjustment for patients of East-Asian ethnicity (eg, Chinese, Japanese, Korean, Taiwanese): Initial dose: 25 mg once daily

Dosage adjustment for toxicity:

ALT levels ≥3 times the upper limit of normal (ULN) **and** which are progressive, or persistent (≥4 weeks), or accompanied by increased direct bilirubin, or accompanied by clinical signs of liver injury or evidence of hepatic decompensation: Discontinue treatment

New or worsening cellular abnormalities or cytopenias: Discontinue treatment

Dosage adjustment in renal impairment: Has not been evaluated in patients with renal impairment; monitor closely

Dosage adjustment in hepatic impairment:

Mild impairment: No adjustment required

Moderate-to-severe impairment: Initial dose: 25 mg once daily

Additional Information Complete prescribing information for this medication should be consulted for additional detail.

Dosage Forms Excipient information presented when available (limited, particularly for generics); consult specific product labeling.

Tablet:

Promacta®: 25 mg, 50 mg

References

Bussel JB, Cheng G, Saleh MN, et al, "Eltrombopag for the Treatment of Chronic Idiopathic Thrombocytopenic Purpura," *N Engl J Med*, 2007, 357(22):2237-47.

Jenkins JM, Williams D, Deng Y, et al, "Phase 1 Clinical Study of Eltrombopag, An Oral, Nonpeptide Thrombopoietin Receptor Agonist," *Blood*, 2007, 109(11):4739-41.

Kuter DJ, "New Thrombopoietic Growth Factors," *Blood*, 2007, 109(11):4607-16.

McHutchison JG, Dusheiko G, Schiffman ML, et al, "Eltrombopag for Thrombocytopenia in Patients With Cirrhosis Associated With Hepatitis C," *N Engl J Med*, 2007, 357(22):2227-36.

◆ **Eltrombopag Olamine** *see* Eltrombopag *on page* 477

◆ **Eltroxin® (Can)** *see* Levothyroxine *on page* 831

◆ **Embeda™** *see* Morphine and Naltrexone *on page* 949

◆ **Emend®** *see* Aprepitant *on page* 132

◆ **Emo-Cort® (Can)** *see* Hydrocortisone *on page* 699

◆ **Emsam®** *see* Selegiline *on page* 1282

Enalapril (e NAL a pril)

Medication Safety Issues

Sound-alike/look-alike issues:

Enalapril may be confused with Anafranil®, Elavil®, Eldepryl®, ramipril

Significant differences exist between oral and I.V. dosing. Use caution when converting from one route of administration to another.

International issues:

Acepril® [Hungary, Switzerland] may be confused with Accupril® which is a brand name for quinapril in the U.S.

Acepril®: Brand name for lisinopril in Denmark; brand name for captopril in Great Britain

Nacor® [Spain] may be confused with Niacor® which is a brand name for niacin in the U.S.

Related Information

Angiotensin Agents *on page 1652*

Heart Failure (Systolic) *on page 1739*

Hypertension *on page 1754*

Postoperative Hypertension *on page 1589*

Preoperative Evaluation of the Cardiac Patient for Noncardiac Surgery *on page 1598*

U.S. Brand Names Vasotec®

Canadian Brand Names Apo-Enalapril®; CO Enalapril; Gen-Enalapril; Mylan-Enalapril; Novo-Enalapril; PMS-Enalapril; Pro-Enalapril; ratio-Enalapril; Riva-Enalapril; Sandoz-Enalapril; Taro-Enalapril; Vasotec®; Vasotec® I.V.

Index Terms Enalapril Maleate; Enalaprilat

Pharmacologic Category Angiotensin-Converting Enzyme (ACE) Inhibitor

Generic Available Yes

Use Treatment of hypertension; treatment of symptomatic heart failure; treatment of asymptomatic left ventricular dysfunction

Unlabeled/Investigational Use

Unlabeled: To delay the progression of nephropathy and reduce risks of cardiovascular events in hypertensive patients with type 1 or 2 diabetes mellitus; hypertensive crisis, diabetic nephropathy, hypertension secondary to scleroderma renal crisis, diagnosis of aldosteronism, idiopathic edema, Bartter's syndrome, postmyocardial infarction for prevention of ventricular failure

Investigational: Severe congestive heart failure in infants, neonatal hypertension, acute cardiogenic pulmonary edema (enalaprilat)

Mechanism of Action Competitive inhibitor of angiotensin-converting enzyme (ACE); prevents conversion of angiotensin I to angiotensin II, a potent vasoconstrictor; results in lower levels of angiotensin II which causes an increase in plasma renin activity and a reduction in aldosterone secretion

Pharmacodynamics/Kinetics

Onset of action: Oral: ~1 hour

Duration: Oral: 12-24 hours

Absorption: Oral: 55% to 75%

Protein binding: 50% to 60%

Metabolism: Prodrug, undergoes hepatic biotransformation to enalaprilat

Half-life elimination:

Enalapril: Adults: Healthy: 2 hours; Congestive heart failure: 3.4-5.8 hours

Enalaprilat: Infants 6 weeks to 8 months of age: 6-10 hours; Adults: 35-38 hours

Time to peak, serum: Oral: Enalapril: 0.5-1.5 hours; Enalaprilat (active): 3-4.5 hours

Excretion: Urine (60% to 80%); some feces

Dosage Use lower listed initial dose in patients with hyponatremia, hypovolemia, severe congestive heart failure, decreased renal function, or in those receiving diuretics.

Oral: **Enalapril**: Children 1 month to 17 years: Hypertension: Initial: 0.08 mg/kg/day (up to 5 mg) in 1-2 divided doses; adjust dosage based on patient response; doses >0.58 mg/kg (40 mg) have not been evaluated in pediatric patients

Investigational: Congestive heart failure: Initial oral doses of **enalapril**: 0.1 mg/kg/day increasing as needed over 2 weeks to 0.5 mg/kg/day have been used in infants

Investigational: Neonatal hypertension: I.V. doses of **enalaprilat**: 5-10 mcg/kg/dose administered every 8-24 hours have been used; monitor patients carefully; select patients may require higher doses

Adults:

Oral: **Enalapril**:

Asymptomatic left ventricular dysfunction: 2.5 mg twice daily, titrated as tolerated to 20 mg/day

Heart failure: Initial: 2.5 mg once or twice daily (usual range: 5-40 mg/day in 2 divided doses); titrate slowly at 1- to 2-week intervals. Target dose: 10-20 mg twice daily (ACC/AHA 2009 Heart Failure Guidelines)

◄ Hypertension: 2.5-5 mg/day then increase as required, usually at 1- to 2-week intervals; usual dose range (JNC 7): 2.5-40 mg/day in 1-2 divided doses. **Note:** Initiate with 2.5 mg if patient is taking a diuretic which cannot be discontinued. May add a diuretic if blood pressure cannot be controlled with enalapril alone.

I.V.: **Enalaprilat:**

Heart failure: Avoid I.V. administration in patients with unstable heart failure or those suffering acute myocardial infarction.

Hypertension: 1.25 mg/dose, given over 5 minutes every 6 hours; doses as high as 5 mg/dose every 6 hours have been tolerated for up to 36 hours. **Note:** If patients are concomitantly receiving diuretic therapy, begin with 0.625 mg I.V. over 5 minutes; if the effect is not adequate after 1 hour, repeat the dose and administer 1.25 mg at 6-hour intervals thereafter; if adequate, administer 0.625 mg I.V. every 6 hours.

Conversion from I.V. to oral therapy if not concurrently on diuretics: 5 mg once daily; subsequent titration as needed; if concurrently receiving diuretics and responding to 0.625 mg I.V. every 6 hours, initiate with 2.5 mg/day.

Dosing adjustment in renal impairment:

Oral: Enalapril:

Cl_{cr} 30-80 mL/minute: Administer 5 mg/day titrated upwards to maximum of 40 mg.

Cl_{cr} <30 mL/minute: Administer 2.5 mg day; titrated upward until blood pressure is controlled.

For heart failure patients with sodium <130 mEq/L or serum creatinine >1.6 mg/dL, initiate dosage with 2.5 mg/day, increasing to twice daily as needed. Increase further in increments of 2.5 mg/dose at >4-day intervals to a maximum daily dose of 40 mg.

I.V.: Enalaprilat:

Cl_{cr} >30 mL/minute: Initiate with 1.25 mg every 6 hours and increase dose based on response.

Cl_{cr} <30 mL/minute: Initiate with 0.625 mg every 6 hours and increase dose based on response.

Hemodialysis: Moderately dialyzable (20% to 50%); administer dose postdialysis (eg, 0.625 mg I.V. every 6 hours) or administer 20% to 25% supplemental dose following dialysis; Clearance: 62 mL/minute.

Peritoneal dialysis: Supplemental dose is not necessary, although some removal of drug occurs.

Dosing adjustment in hepatic impairment: Hydrolysis of enalapril to enalaprilat may be delayed and/or impaired in patients with severe hepatic impairment, but the pharmacodynamic effects of the drug do not appear to be significantly altered; no dosage adjustment.

Stability Enalaprilat: Clear, colorless solution which should be stored at <30°C. I.V. is 24 hours at room temperature in D_5W or NS.

Administration Injection solution: Administer direct IVP over at least 5 minutes or dilute up to 50 mL and infuse; discontinue diuretic, if possible, for 2-3 days before beginning enalapril therapy

Monitoring Parameters Blood pressure; serum creatinine and potassium; if patient has collagen vascular disease and/or renal impairment, periodically monitor CBC with differential

Anesthesia and Critical Care Concerns/Other Considerations

Clinical Pearls/Comments: In patients on chronic ACE inhibitor therapy, intraoperative hypotension may occur with induction and maintenance of general anesthesia; however, discontinuation of therapy prior to surgery is controversial. If continued preoperatively, avoidance of hypotensive agents during surgery is prudent. Episodes of intraoperative hypotension may be managed by fluid administration and/or modest doses of alpha-adrenergic agents. Severe hypotension may occur in patients who are sodium- and/or volume-depleted, initiate lower doses and monitor closely when starting therapy in these patients. ACE inhibitor therapy may elicit an increase in potassium and creatinine, especially when used in patients with bilateral renal artery stenosis. In those patients experiencing cough on an ACE inhibitor, the ACE inhibitor may be discontinued and, if necessary, angiotensin-receptor blocker therapy instituted. Concomitant NSAID therapy may attenuate blood pressure control; use of NSAIDs should be avoided or limited, with monitoring of blood pressure control. In the setting of heart failure, NSAID use may be associated with an increased risk for fluid accumulation and edema. Because of the potent teratogenic effects of ACE inhibitors, these drugs should be avoided, if possible, when treating women of childbearing potential not on effective birth control measures. Aging patients with a decrease in glomerular filtration (also creatinine clearance), severe heart failure, and renal failure may experience an exaggerated response with administration of ACE inhibitors. Diabetic proteinuria is reduced and insulin sensitivity is enhanced.

Evidence-Based Information: ACE inhibitors decrease morbidity and mortality in patients with asymptomatic and symptomatic left ventricular dysfunction. In this situation, they decrease hospitalizations for, and retard progression to, decompensated heart failure. ACE inhibitors are also indicated in patients postmyocardial infarction in whom left ventricular ejection fraction is <40%. When used in patients with heart failure, the target dose or maximum tolerated dose should be achieved, if possible. Lower daily doses of ACE inhibitors have not demonstrated the same cardioprotective effects. ACE inhibitors have renal protective effects in patients with diabetic proteinuria. The HOPE trial examined the use of ramipril at a dose of between 2.5-10 mg daily in patients without heart failure at high risk for cardiovascular events and documented a significant improvement in cardiovascular outcome compared to placebo.

Pregnancy Risk Factor C (1st trimester); D (2nd and 3rd trimesters)

Contraindications Hypersensitivity to enalapril or enalaprilat; angioedema related to previous treatment with an ACE inhibitor; patients with idiopathic or hereditary angioedema

Warnings/Precautions Anaphylactic reactions may occur rarely with ACE inhibitors. At any time during treatment (especially following first dose) angioedema may occur rarely with ACE inhibitors; it may involve the head and neck (potentially compromising airway) or the intestine (presenting with abdominal pain). African-Americans may be at an increased risk. Prolonged frequent monitoring may be required especially if tongue, glottis, or larynx are involved as they are associated with airway obstruction. Patients with a history of airway surgery may have a higher risk of airway obstruction. Aggressive early and appropriate management is critical. Use in patients with idiopathic or hereditary angioedema or previous angioedema associated with ACE inhibitor therapy is contraindicated. Severe anaphylactoid reactions may be seen during hemodialysis (eg, CVVHD) with high-flux dialysis membranes (eg, AN69), and rarely, during low density lipoprotein apheresis with dextran sulfate cellulose. Rare cases of anaphylactoid reactions have been reported in patients undergoing sensitization treatment with hymenoptera (bee, wasp) venom while receiving ACE inhibitors.

Symptomatic hypotension with or without syncope can occur with ACE inhibitors (usually with the first several doses); effects are most often observed in volume depleted patients; correct volume depletion prior to initiation; close monitoring of patient is required especially with initial dosing and dosing increases; blood pressure must be lowered at a rate appropriate for the patient's clinical condition. Initiation of therapy in patients with ischemic heart disease or cerebrovascular disease warrants close observation due to the potential consequences posed by falling blood pressure (eg, MI, stroke). Use with caution in hypertrophic cardiomyopathy with outflow tract obstruction, severe aortic stenosis, or before, during, or immediately after major surgery. **[U.S. Boxed Warning]: Based on human data, ACEIs can cause injury and death to the developing fetus when used in the second and third trimesters. ACEIs should be discontinued as soon as possible once pregnancy is detected.** Injection contains benzyl alcohol which has been associated with "gasping syndrome" in neonates.

Hyperkalemia may occur with ACE inhibitors; risk factors include renal dysfunction, diabetes mellitus, concomitant use of potassium-sparing diuretics, potassium supplements, and/or potassium-containing salts. Use cautiously, if at all, with these agents and monitor potassium closely. Cough may occur with ACE inhibitors. Other causes of cough should be considered (eg, pulmonary congestion in patients with heart failure) and excluded prior to discontinuation.

May be associated with deterioration of renal function and/or increases in serum creatinine, particularly in patients with low renal blood flow (eg, renal artery ▶

stenosis, heart failure) whose glomerular filtration rate (GFR) is dependent on efferent arteriolar vasoconstriction by angiotensin II; deterioration may result in oliguria, acute renal failure, and progressive azotemia. Small increases in serum creatinine may occur following initiation; consider discontinuation only in patients with progressive and/or significant deterioration in renal function. Use with caution in patients with unstented unilateral/bilateral renal artery stenosis. When unstented bilateral renal artery stenosis is present, use is generally avoided due to the elevated risk of deterioration in renal function unless possible benefits outweigh risks.

Rare toxicities associated with ACE inhibitors include cholestatic jaundice (which may progress to fulminant hepatic necrosis), agranulocytosis, neutropenia or leukopenia with myeloid hypoplasia. Patients with collagen vascular diseases (especially with concomitant renal impairment) or renal impairment alone may be at increased risk for hematologic toxicity; periodically monitor CBC with differential in these patients.

Adverse Reactions Note: Frequency ranges include data from hypertension and heart failure trials. Higher rates of adverse reactions have generally been noted in patients with CHF. However, the frequency of adverse effects associated with placebo is also increased in this population.

1% to 10%:

Cardiovascular: Hypotension (0.9% to 6.7%), chest pain (2%), syncope (0.5% to 2%), orthostasis (2%), orthostatic hypotension (2%)

Central nervous system: Headache (2% to 5%), dizziness (4% to 8%), fatigue (2% to 3%)

Dermatologic: Rash (1.5%)

Gastrointestinal: Abnormal taste, abdominal pain, vomiting, nausea, diarrhea, anorexia, constipation

Neuromuscular & skeletal: Weakness

Renal: Serum creatinine increased (0.2% to 20%), worsening of renal function (in patients with bilateral renal artery stenosis or hypovolemia)

Respiratory (1% to 2%): Bronchitis, cough, dyspnea

<1% (Limited to important or life-threatening): Agranulocytosis, alopecia, anaphylactoid reaction, angina pectoris, angioedema, ataxia, atrial fibrillation, atrial tachycardia, bone marrow suppression, bradycardia, bronchospasm, cardiac arrest, cerebral vascular accident, cholestatic jaundice, depression, eosinophilic pneumonitis, erythema multiforme, exfoliative dermatitis, flushing, giant cell arteritis, gynecomastia, hallucinations, hemolysis with G6PD, Henoch-Schönlein purpura, hepatitis, ileus, impotence, jaundice, lichen-form reaction, melena, MI, neutropenia, ototoxicity, pancreatitis, paresthesia, pemphigus, pemphigus foliaceus, peripheral neuropathy, photosensitivity, psychosis, pulmonary edema, pulmonary embolism, pulmonary infiltrates, Raynaud's phenomenon, sicca syndrome, somnolence, Stevens-Johnson syndrome, systemic lupus erythematosus, thrombocytopenia, toxic epidermal necrolysis, toxic pustuloderma, vertigo.

A syndrome which may include arthralgia, elevated ESR, eosinophilia and positive ANA, fever, interstitial nephritis, myalgia, rash, and vasculitis has been reported for enalapril and other ACE inhibitors.

Drug Interactions

Metabolism/Transport Effects Substrate of CYP3A4 (minor)

Avoid Concomitant Use There are no known interactions where it is recommended to avoid concomitant use.

Increased Effect/Toxicity

Enalapril may increase the levels/effects of: Allopurinol; Amifostine; Antihypertensives; AzaTHIOprine; CycloSPORINE; Ferric Gluconate; Gold Sodium Thiomalate; Hypotensive Agents; Iron Dextran Complex; Lithium; RiTUXimab

The levels/effects of Enalapril may be increased by: Angiotensin II Receptor Blockers; Diazoxide; Eplerenone; Herbs (Hypotensive Properties); Loop Diuretics; MAO Inhibitors; Pentoxifylline; Phosphodiesterase 5 Inhibitors; Potassium Salts; Potassium-Sparing Diuretics; Prostacyclin Analogues; Sirolimus; Temsirolimus; Thiazide Diuretics; Tolvaptan; Trimethoprim

Decreased Effect

The levels/effects of Enalapril may be decreased by: Antacids; Aprotinin; CYP3A4 Inducers (Strong); Deferasirox; Herbs (CYP3A4 Inducers); Herbs (Hypertensive Properties); Methylphenidate; Nonsteroidal Anti-Inflammatory Agents; Salicylates; Yohimbine

Ethanol/Nutrition/Herb Interactions Herb/Nutraceutical: Avoid bayberry, blue cohosh, cayenne, ephedra, ginger, ginseng (American), kola, licorice (may worsen hypertension). Avoid black cohosh, california poppy, coleus, golden seal, hawthorn, mistletoe, periwinkle, quinine, shepherd's purse (may have increased antihypertensive effect).

Test Interactions Positive Coombs' [direct]; may cause false-positive results in urine acetone determinations using sodium nitroprusside reagent

Dietary Considerations Limit salt substitutes or potassium-rich diet.

Dosage Forms Excipient information presented when available (limited, particularly for generics); consult specific product labeling.

Injection, solution, as enalaprilat: 1.25 mg/mL (1 mL, 2 mL) [contains benzyl alcohol]

Tablet, as maleate: 2.5 mg, 5 mg, 10 mg, 20 mg

Vasotec®: 2.5 mg, 5 mg, 10 mg, 20 mg

References

Erstad BL and Barletta JF, "Treatment of Hypertension in the Perioperative Patient," *Ann Pharmacother*, 2000, 34(1):66-79.

◆ **Enalaprilat** *see* Enalapril *on page 478*

◆ **Enalapril Maleate** *see* Enalapril *on page 478*

◆ **Encort™** *see* Hydrocortisone *on page 699*

◆ **Endantadine® (Can)** *see* Amantadine *on page 77*

◆ **Endocet®** *see* Oxycodone and Acetaminophen *on page 1072*

◆ **Endo®-Levodopa/Carbidopa (Can)** *see* Levodopa and Carbidopa *on page 822*

◆ **Endometrin®** *see* Progesterone *on page 1184*

◆ **Enerjets [OTC]** *see* Caffeine *on page 225*

◆ **Enfamil® Glucose** *see* Dextrose *on page 406*

Enflurane (EN floo rane)

Medication Safety Issues

Sound-alike/look-alike issues:

Enflurane may be confused with isoflurane

High alert medication: The Institute for Safe Medication Practices (ISMP) includes this medication among its list of drug classes which have a heightened risk of causing significant patient harm when used in error.

Related Information

Anesthesia Considerations for Neurosurgery *on page 1514*

Chronic Renal Failure *on page 1552*

Inhalational Anesthetics *on page 1632*

Perioperative Management of Patients on Antiseizure Medication *on page 1577*

U.S. Brand Names Compound 347™; Ethrane®

Pharmacologic Category General Anesthetic, Inhalation

Generic Available No

Use Induction and maintenance of general anesthesia; **Note:** Use for induction of general anesthesia is not recommended due to its irritant properties and unpleasant odor which causes breath-holding and coughing.

Pharmacodynamics/Kinetics

Onset of action: 7-10 minutes

Duration: Emergence time: Depends on blood concentration when enflurane is discontinued

Metabolism: Hepatic (2% to 10%)

Excretion: Exhaled gases

Dosage Minimum alveolar concentration (MAC), the concentration at which 50% of patients do not respond to surgical incision, is 1.6% for enflurane. The concentration at which amnesia and loss of awareness occur (MAC - awake) is

◀ 0.4%. Surgical levels of anesthesia are achieved with concentrations between 0.5% to 3%. MAC is reduced in the elderly.

Administration Via enflurane-specific calibrated vaporizers

Monitoring Parameters Blood pressure, heart rate and rhythm, temperature, oxygen saturation, end-tidal CO_2 and end-tidal enflurane concentrations should be monitored prior to and throughout anesthesia

Contraindications Hypersensitivity to enflurane, other halogenated anesthetics, or any component of the formulation; known or suspected genetic susceptibility to malignant hyperthermia; seizure disorder

Warnings/Precautions Decrease in blood pressure is dose dependent, primarily due to peripheral vasodilation. Enflurane does not depress cardiac conduction nor does it sensitize the myocardium to catecholamine-induced arrhythmias like halothane. Respiration is depressed with a $PaCO_2$ of 55 mm Hg at 1 MAC. Hypoxic pulmonary vasoconstriction is blunted. EEG seizure complexes have been seen with higher doses especially associated with hypocarbia; therefore, it is not recommended for use in patients with seizure history. Hypoxia induced increase in ventilation is abolished at low enflurane concentration. Enflurane dilates the cerebral vasculature and may, in certain conditions, increase intracranial pressure. Renal, splenic, and hepatic blood flow are reduced.

May trigger malignant hyperthermia; avoid use in patients susceptible to malignant hyperthermia. Risk of hyperkalemia is increased in pediatric patients with underlying neuromucular disease (eg, Duchenne muscular dystrophy).

Adverse Reactions Frequency not defined.

Cardiovascular: Hypotension, myocardial depression, tachycardia

Central nervous system: Seizure activity during or after emergence from enflurane anesthesia; motor activity and/or seizure, especially with hypocapnia, malignant hyperthermia

Gastrointestinal: Nausea, vomiting

Hepatic: Hepatic injury, hepatic failure (rare), necrosis

Renal: Renal dysfunction, nephrotoxicity

Respiratory: Respiratory depression/arrest, hypoxemia, breath holding, cough

Miscellaneous: Shivering

Drug Interactions

Metabolism/Transport Effects Substrate of CYP2E1 (major)

Avoid Concomitant Use

Avoid concomitant use of Enflurane with any of the following: Methylphenidate

Increased Effect/Toxicity

Enflurane may increase the levels/effects of: EPINEPHrine; Neuromuscular-Blocking Agents (Nondepolarizing)

The levels/effects of Enflurane may be increased by: CYP2E1 Inhibitors (Moderate); CYP2E1 Inhibitors (Strong); Methylphenidate

Decreased Effect There are no known significant interactions involving a decrease in effect.

Dosage Forms Excipient information presented when available (limited, particularly for generics); consult specific product labeling.

Liquid, for inhalation: >99.9% (250 mL)

References

Campagna JA, Miller KW, and Forman SA, "Mechanisms of Action of Inhaled Anesthetics," *N Engl J Med*, 2003, 348(21):2110-24.

Cousins MJ, Greenstein LR, Hitt BA, et al, "Metabolism and Renal Effects of Enflurane in Man," *Anesthesiology*, 1976, 44(1):44-53.

Gion H and Saidman LJ, "The Minimum Alveolar Concentration of Enflurane in Man," *Anesthesiology*, 1971, 35(4):361-4.

◆ **Engerix-B®** *see* Hepatitis B Vaccine *on page 686*

◆ **Engerix-B® and Havrix®** *see* Hepatitis A Inactivated and Hepatitis B (Recombinant) Vaccine *on page 684*

◆ **Enlon®** *see* Edrophonium *on page 474*

◆ **Enlon-Plus®** *see* Edrophonium and Atropine *on page 476*

Enoxaparin (ee noks a PA rin)

Medication Safety Issues

Sound-alike/look-alike issues:

Lovenox® may be confused with Lasix®, Levaquin®, Lotronex®, Protonix®

High alert medication: The Institute for Safe Medication Practices (ISMP) includes this medication among its list of drugs which have a heightened risk of causing significant patient harm when used in error.

International issues:

Lovenox® may be confused with Lotanax® which is a brand name for terfenadine in the Czech Republic

2009 National Patient Safety Goals: The Joint Commission on Accreditation of Healthcare Organizations requires healthcare organizations that provide anticoagulant therapy to have a process in place to reduce the risk of anticoagulant-associated patient harm. Patients receiving anticoagulants should receive individualized care through a defined process that includes standardized ordering, dispensing, administration, monitoring and education. This does not apply to routine short-term use of anticoagulants for prevention of venous thromboembolism when the expectation is that the patient's laboratory values will remain within or close to normal values (NPSG.03.05.01).

Related Information

Dosing Considerations for the Critically-Ill Patient With Morbid Obesity *on page 1561*

Regional Anesthesia in Patients Receiving Anticoagulant and Antiplatelet Therapy *on page 1642*

U.S. Brand Names Lovenox®

Canadian Brand Names Enoxaparin Injection; Lovenox®; Lovenox® HP

Index Terms Enoxaparin Sodium

Pharmacologic Category Low Molecular Weight Heparin

Generic Available No

Use

Acute coronary syndromes: Unstable angina (UA), non-ST-elevation (NSTEMI), and ST-elevation myocardial infarction (STEMI)

DVT prophylaxis: Following hip or knee replacement surgery, abdominal surgery, or in medical patients with severely-restricted mobility during acute illness who are at risk for thromboembolic complications

DVT treatment (acute): Inpatient treatment (patients with and without pulmonary embolism) and outpatient treatment (patients without pulmonary embolism)

Note: High-risk patients include those with one or more of the following risk factors: >40 years of age, obesity, general anesthesia lasting >30 minutes, malignancy, history of deep vein thrombosis or pulmonary embolism

Unlabeled/Investigational Use Prophylaxis and treatment of thromboembolism in children; anticoagulant bridge therapy during temporary interruption of vitamin K antagonist therapy in patients at high risk for thromboembolism; DVT prophylaxis following moderate-risk general surgery, major gynecologic surgery and following higher-risk general surgery for cancer; management of venous thromboembolism (VTE) during pregnancy (Hirsh, 2008)

Mechanism of Action Standard heparin consists of components with molecular weights ranging from 4000-30,000 daltons with a mean of 16,000 daltons. Heparin acts as an anticoagulant by enhancing the inhibition rate of clotting proteases by antithrombin III impairing normal hemostasis and inhibition of factor Xa. Low molecular weight heparins have a small effect on the activated partial thromboplastin time and strongly inhibit factor Xa. Enoxaparin is derived from porcine heparin that undergoes benzylation followed by alkaline depolymerization. The average molecular weight of enoxaparin is 4500 daltons which is distributed as (≤20%) 2000 daltons (≥68%) 2000-8000 daltons, and (≤15%) >8000 daltons. Enoxaparin has a higher ratio of antifactor Xa to antifactor IIa activity than unfractionated heparin.

Pharmacodynamics/Kinetics

Onset of action: Peak effect: SubQ: Antifactor Xa and antithrombin (antifactor IIa): 3-5 hours

485

◀ Duration: 40 mg dose: Antifactor Xa activity: ~12 hours
Distribution: 4.3 L (based on antifactor Xa activity)
Metabolism: Hepatic, to lower molecular weight fragments (little activity)
Protein binding: Does not bind to heparin binding proteins
Half-life elimination, plasma: 2-4 times longer than standard heparin, independent of dose; based on anti-Xa activity: 4.5-7 hours
Excretion: Urine (40% of dose; 10% as active fragments)

Dosage SubQ:
Infants and Children (unlabeled use; Monagle, 2008):
Infants <2 months: Initial:
Prophylaxis: 0.75 mg/kg every 12 hours
Treatment: 1.5 mg/kg every 12 hours
Infants >2 months and Children ≤18 years: Initial:
Prophylaxis: 0.5 mg/kg every 12 hours
Treatment: 1 mg/kg every 12 hours
Maintenance: See **Dosage Titration** table:

Enoxaparin Pediatric Dosage Titration

Antifactor Xa	Dose Titration	Time to Repeat Antifactor Xa Level
<0.35 units/mL	Increase dose by 25%	4 h after next dose
0.35-0.49 units/mL	Increase dose by 10%	4 h after next dose
0.5-1 unit/mL	Keep same dosage	Next day, then 1 wk later, then monthly (4 h after dose)
1.1-1.5 units/mL	Decrease dose by 20%	Before next dose
1.6-2 units/mL	Hold dose for 3 h and decrease dose by 30%	Before next dose, then 4 h after next dose
>2 units/mL	Hold all doses until antifactor Xa is 0.5 units/mL, then decrease dose by 40%	Before next dose and every 12 h until antifactor Xa <0.5 units/mL

Modified from Monagle P, Michelson AD, Bovill E, et al, "Antithrombotic Therapy in Children," *Chest*, 2001, 119:344S-70S.

Adults:
DVT prophylaxis:
Hip replacement surgery:
Twice-daily dosing: 30 mg every 12 hours, with initial dose within 12-24 hours after surgery, and every 12 hours for at least 10 days or until risk of DVT has diminished or the patient is adequately anticoagulated on warfarin.
Once-daily dosing: 40 mg once daily, with initial dose within 9-15 hours before surgery, and daily for at least 10 days (or up to 35 days postoperatively) or until risk of DVT has diminished or the patient is adequately anticoagulated on warfarin.
Knee replacement surgery: 30 mg every 12 hours, with initial dose within 12-24 hours after surgery, and every 12 hours for at least 10 days or until risk of DVT has diminished or the patient is adequately anticoagulated on warfarin.
Abdominal surgery: 40 mg once daily, with initial dose given 2 hours prior to surgery; continue until risk of DVT has diminished (usually 7-10 days).
Bariatric surgery: Roux-en-Y gastric bypass: Appropriate dosing strategies have not been clearly defined (Borkgren-Okonek, 2008; Scholten, 2002):
BMI ≤50 kg/m^2: 40 mg every 12 hours
BMI >50 kg/m^2: 60 mg every 12 hours
Note: Bariatric surgery guidelines suggest initiation 30-120 minutes before surgery and postoperatively until patient is fully mobile (Mechanick, 2009). Alternatively, limiting administration to the postoperative period may reduce perioperative bleeding.
Medical patients with severely-restricted mobility during acute illness: 40 mg once daily; continue until risk of DVT has diminished (usually 6-11 days).
DVT treatment (acute): **Note:** Start warfarin on the first treatment day and continue enoxaparin until INR is between 2 and 3 (usually 5-7 days).
Inpatient treatment (with or without pulmonary embolism): 1 mg/kg/dose every 12 hours or 1.5 mg/kg once daily.

Outpatient treatment (without pulmonary embolism): 1 mg/kg/dose every 12 hours.

Percutaneous coronary intervention (PCI), adjunctive therapy: In enoxaparin-treated patients undergoing PCI, if balloon inflation occurs ≤8 hours after the last SubQ enoxaparin dose, no additional dosing is needed. If balloon inflation occurs 8-12 hours after the last SubQ enoxaparin dose, a single I.V. dose of 0.3 mg/kg should be administered (Hirsh, 2008; King, 2007)

ST-elevation myocardial infarction (STEMI):

Patients <75 years of age: Initial: 30 mg I.V. single bolus plus 1 mg/kg (maximum 100 mg for the first 2 doses only) SubQ every 12 hours. The first SubQ dose should be administered with the I.V. bolus. Maintenance: After first 2 doses, administer 1 mg/kg SubQ every 12 hours.

Patients ≥75 years of age: Initial: SubQ: 0.75 mg/kg every 12 hours (**Note:** No I.V. bolus is administered in this population); a maximum dose of 75 mg is recommended for the first 2 doses. Maintenance: After first 2 doses, administer 0.75 mg/kg SubQ every 12 hours

Obesity: Use weight-based dosing; a maximum dose of 100 mg is recommended for the first 2 doses (Nutescu, 2009)

Additional notes on STEMI treatment: Therapy was continued for 8 days or until hospital discharge; optimal duration not defined. Unless contraindicated, all patients received aspirin (75-325 mg daily) in clinical trials. In patients with STEMI receiving thrombolytics, initiate enoxaparin dosing between 15 minutes before and 30 minutes after fibrinolytic therapy. In patients undergoing PCI, if balloon inflation occurs ≤8 hours after the last SubQ enoxaparin dose, no additional dosing is needed. If balloon inflation occurs 8-12 hours after last SubQ enoxaparin dose, a single I.V. dose of 0.3 mg/kg should be administered (Hirsh, 2008; King, 2007).

Unstable angina or non-ST-elevation myocardial infarction (NSTEMI): 1 mg/kg every 12 hours in conjunction with oral aspirin therapy (100-325 mg once daily); continue until clinical stabilization (a minimum of at least 2 days)

Elderly: Refer to adult dosing. Increased incidence of bleeding with doses of 1.5 mg/kg/day or 1 mg/kg every 12 hours; injection-associated bleeding and serious adverse reactions are also increased in the elderly. Careful attention should be paid to elderly patients, particularly those <45 kg. **Note:** Dosage alteration/adjustment may be required.

Dosing adjustment in renal impairment: SubQ:

Cl_{cr} ≥30 mL/minute: No specific adjustment recommended (per manufacturer); monitor closely for bleeding

Cl_{cr} <30 mL/minute:

DVT prophylaxis in abdominal surgery, hip replacement, knee replacement, or in medical patients during acute illness: 30 mg once daily

DVT treatment (inpatient or outpatient treatment in conjunction with warfarin): 1 mg/kg once daily

STEMI:

<75 years: Initial: I.V.: 30 mg as a single dose with the first dose of the SubQ maintenance regimen administered at the same time as the I.V. bolus

≥75 years of age: Omit I.V. bolus; Maintenance: SubQ: 1 mg/kg every 24 hours in all patients

Unstable angina, NSTEMI: SubQ: 1 mg/kg once daily

Dialysis: Enoxaparin has not been FDA approved for use in dialysis patients. It's elimination is primarily via the renal route. Serious bleeding complications have been reported with use in patients who are dialysis dependent or have severe renal failure. LMWH administration at fixed doses without monitoring has greater unpredictable anticoagulant effects in patients with chronic kidney disease. If used, dosages should be reduced and anti-Xa levels frequently monitored, as accumulation may occur with repeated doses. Many clinicians would not use enoxaparin in this population especially without timely anti-Xa levels.

Hemodialysis: Supplemental dose is not necessary.

Peritoneal dialysis: Significant drug removal is unlikely based on physiochemical characteristics.

Stability Store at 25°C (77°F); excursions permitted to 15°C to 30°C (59°F to 86°F); do not freeze.

◄ **Administration** Do **not** administer I.M.; should be administered by deep SubQ injection to the left or right anterolateral and left or right posterolateral abdominal wall. A single dose may be administered I.V. as part of treatment for ST-elevation myocardial infarction (STEMI) to patients <75 years of age; no I.V. bolus is given to patients ≥75 years of age. To avoid loss of drug from the 30 mg and 40 mg syringes, do not expel the air bubble from the syringe prior to injection. In order to minimize bruising, do not rub injection site. An automatic injector (Lovenox EasyInjector™) is available with the 30 mg and 40 mg syringes to aid the patient with self-injections. **Note:** Enoxaparin is available in 100 mg/mL and 150 mg/mL concentrations.

To convert from I.V. unfractionated heparin (UFH) infusion to SubQ enoxaparin (Nutescu, 2007): Calculate specific dose for enoxaparin based on indication, discontinue UFH and begin enoxaparin within 1 hour.

To convert from SubQ enoxaparin to I.V. UFH infusion (Nutescu, 2007): Discontinue enoxaparin, calculate specific dose for I.V. UFH infusion based on indication, omit heparin bolus/loading dose:

Converting from SubQ enoxaparin dosed every 12 hours: Start I.V. UFH infusion 10-11 hours after last dose of enoxaparin

Converting from SubQ enoxaparin dosed every 24 hours: Start I.V. UFH infusion 22-23 hours after last dose of enoxaparin

Monitoring Parameters Platelets, occult blood, anti-Xa levels, serum creatinine; monitoring of PT and/or aPTT is not necessary. Routine monitoring of anti-Xa levels is not required, but has been utilized in patients with obesity and/or renal insufficiency. Monitoring anti-Xa levels is recommended in pregnant women receiving therapeutic doses of enoxaparin (Hirsh, 2008).

Reference Range The following therapeutic ranges for anti-Xa levels have been suggested, but have not been validated in a controlled trial. Anti-Xa level measured 4 hours postdose.

DVT treatment (every-12-hour dosing): 0.6-1 units/mL

DVT treatment (once-daily dosing): 1-2 units/mL

Anesthesia and Critical Care Concerns/Other Considerations
Evidence-Based Information:

The American College of Chest Physicians Evidence Based Clinical Practice Guidelines (Geerts, 2008) recommend routine assessment for venous thromboembolism (VTE) risk and routine thromboprophylaxis in most critically ill patients (Grade 1A). For critically ill patients at a moderate risk (medically ill or postoperative) for VTE, they recommend using LMWH or low-dose unfractionated heparin (Grade 1A). For critically ill patients at a high risk (major trauma or orthopedic surgery) for VTE, they recommend LMWH (Grade 1A). If bleeding risk prohibits the use of pharmacologic thromboprophylaxis, mechanical thromboprophylaxis is recommended until risk decreases (Grade 1A).

Obesity/Renal Dysfunction: There is no consensus for adjusting/correcting the weight-based dosage of LMWH for patients who are morbidly obese. Anti-Xa levels are increased to appropriate levels when enoxaparin is dosed on actual body weight in obese patients weighing up to 144 kg (Sanderink, 2002). Monitoring of anti-Xa levels 4 hours after injection may be warranted. Patients who have a reduction in calculated creatinine clearance are at risk of accumulated anticoagulant effect when they are treated with certain LMWHs. All LMWHs may not behave the same in patients with renal dysfunction. Some clinicians monitor anti-Xa levels in patients with Cl_{cr} <30 mL/minute if assay results are readily available. Patients requiring dialysis should not receive enoxaparin due to an increased risk of bleeding resulting from drug accumulation.

Pregnancy Risk Factor B

Contraindications Hypersensitivity to enoxaparin, heparin, or any component of the formulation; thrombocytopenia associated with a positive *in vitro* test for antiplatelet antibodies in the presence of enoxaparin; hypersensitivity to pork products; active major bleeding; not for I.M. use

Warnings/Precautions [U.S. Boxed Warning]: Patients with recent or anticipated neuraxial anesthesia (epidural or spinal anesthesia) are at risk of spinal or epidural hematoma and subsequent paralysis. Consider risk versus benefit prior to neuraxial anesthesia; risk is increased by concomitant agents which may alter hemostasis or by the use of indwelling epidural catheters for analgesia, as well as traumatic or repeated epidural or spinal puncture. Patient should be observed closely for bleeding if enoxaparin is administered during or immediately following diagnostic lumbar puncture, epidural anesthesia, or spinal anesthesia.

Do not administer intramuscularly. Not recommended for thromboprophylaxis in patients with prosthetic heart valves (especially pregnant women). Not to be used interchangeably (unit for unit) with heparin or any other low molecular weight heparins. Use caution in patients with history of heparin-induced thrombocytopenia. Monitor patient closely for signs or symptoms of bleeding. Certain patients are at increased risk of bleeding. Risk factors include bacterial endocarditis; congenital or acquired bleeding disorders; active ulcerative or angiodysplastic GI diseases; severe uncontrolled hypertension; history of hemorrhagic stroke; use shortly after brain, spinal, or ophthalmic surgery; patients treated concomitantly with platelet inhibitors; recent GI bleeding; thrombocytopenia or platelet defects; severe liver disease; hypertensive or diabetic retinopathy; or in patients undergoing invasive procedures. Monitor platelet count closely. Rare cases of thrombocytopenia have occurred. Discontinue therapy and consider alternative treatment if platelets are <100,000/mm^3 and/or thrombosis develops. Rare cases of thrombocytopenia with thrombosis have occurred. Use caution in patients with congenital or drug-induced thrombocytopenia or platelet defects. Risk of bleeding may be increased in women <45 kg and in men <57 kg. Use caution in patients with renal failure; dosage adjustment needed if Cl$_{cr}$ <30 mL/minute. Use with caution in the elderly (delayed elimination may occur); dosage alteration/adjustment may be required (eg, omission of I.V. bolus in acute STEMI in patients ≥75 years of age). Monitor for hyperkalemia; can cause hyperkalemia possibly by suppressing aldosterone production. Multiple-dose vials contain benzyl alcohol (use caution in pregnant women). In neonates, large amounts of benzyl alcohol (>100 mg/kg/day) have been associated with fatal toxicity (gasping syndrome).

There is no consensus for adjusting/correcting the weight-based dosage of LMWH for patients who are morbidly obese (BMI ≥40 kg/m^2). For patients undergoing inpatient bariatric surgery, the American College of Chest Physicians Practice Guidelines suggest using a higher thromboprophylaxis dose of LMWH for obese patients (Geerts, 2008).

Adverse Reactions As with all anticoagulants, bleeding is the major adverse effect of enoxaparin. Hemorrhage may occur at virtually any site. Risk is dependent on multiple variables. At the recommended doses, single injections of enoxaparin do not significantly influence platelet aggregation or affect global clotting time (ie, PT or aPTT).

1% to 10%:

Central nervous system: Fever (5% to 8%), confusion, pain

Dermatologic: Erythema, bruising

Gastrointestinal: Nausea (3%), diarrhea

Hematologic: Hemorrhage (major, <1% to 4%; includes cases of intracranial, retroperitoneal, or intraocular hemorrhage; incidence varies with indication/population), thrombocytopenia (moderate 1%; severe 0.1% - see **"Note"**), anemia (<2%)

Hepatic: ALT increased, AST increased

Local: Injection site hematoma (9%), local reactions (irritation, pain, ecchymosis, erythema)

Renal: Hematuria (<2%)

<1% (Limited to important or life-threatening): Allergic reaction, anaphylactoid reaction, cutaneous vasculitis (hypersensitive), eczematous plaques, hematoma (see note on "Spinal or epidural hematomas"), hyperkalemia, hyperlipidemia, hypertriglyceridemia, intracranial hemorrhage (up to 0.8%), erythematous pruritic patches, pruritus, purpura, retroperitoneal bleeding, skin necrosis, thrombocytopenia with thrombosis, thrombocytosis, urticaria, vesicobullous rash

Notes:

Spinal or epidural hematomas: Can occur following neuraxial anesthesia or spinal puncture, resulting in paralysis. Risk is increased in patients with indwelling epidural catheters or concomitant use of other drugs affecting ▶

hemostasis. Prosthetic valve thrombosis, including fatal cases, has been reported in pregnant women receiving enoxaparin as thromboprophylaxis.

Thrombocytopenia with thrombosis: Cases of heparin-induced thrombocytopenia (some complicated by organ infarction, limb ischemia, or death) have been reported.

Drug Interactions

Avoid Concomitant Use There are no known interactions where it is recommended to avoid concomitant use.

Increased Effect/Toxicity

Enoxaparin may increase the levels/effects of: Anticoagulants; Drotrecogin Alfa; Ibritumomab; Tositumomab and Iodine I 131 Tositumomab

The levels/effects of Enoxaparin may be increased by: 5-ASA Derivatives; Antiplatelet Agents; Dasatinib; Herbs (Anticoagulant/Antiplatelet Properties); Nonsteroidal Anti-Inflammatory Agents; Pentosan Polysulfate Sodium; Pentoxifylline; Prostacyclin Analogues; Salicylates; Thrombolytic Agents

Decreased Effect There are no known significant interactions involving a decrease in effect.

Ethanol/Nutrition/Herb Interactions Herb/Nutraceutical: Avoid cat's claw, dong quai, evening primrose, feverfew, garlic, ginger, ginkgo, red clover, horse chestnut, green tea, ginseng (all have additional antiplatelet activity).

Dosage Forms Excipient information presented when available (limited, particularly for generics); consult specific product labeling.

Injection, solution, as sodium [graduated prefilled syringe; preservative free]:

Lovenox®: 60 mg/0.6 mL (0.6 mL); 80 mg/0.8 mL (0.8 mL); 100 mg/1 mL (1 mL); 120 mg/0.8 mL (0.8 mL); 150 mg/mL (1 mL)

Injection, solution, as sodium [multidose vial]:

Lovenox®: 100 mg/mL (3 mL) [contains benzyl alcohol]

Injection, solution, as sodium [prefilled syringe; preservative free]:

Lovenox®: 30 mg/0.3 mL (0.3 mL); 40 mg/0.4 mL (0.4 mL)

References

Farooq V, Hegarty J, Chandrasekar T, et al, "Serious Adverse Incidents With the Usage of Low Molecular Weight Heparins in Patients With Chronic Kidney Disease," *Am J Kidney Dis,* 2004, 43 (3):531-7.

Geerts WH, Bergqvist D, Pineo GF, et al, "Prevention of Venous Thromboembolism: American College of Chest Physicians Evidence-Based Clinical Practice Guidelines (8th Edition)," *Chest,* 2008, 133(6 Suppl):381S-453S.

Hirsh J, Guyatt G, Albers GW, et al, "Executive Summary: American College of Chest Physicians Evidence-Based Clinical Practice Guidelines (8th Edition)," *Chest,* 2008, 133(6 Suppl):71-109.

King SB 3rd, Smith SC Jr, Hirshfeld JW JR, et al, "2007 Focused Update of the ACC/AHA/SCAI 2005 Guideline Update for Percutaneous Coronary Intervention. A Report of the American College of Cardiology/American Heart Association Task Force on Practice Guidelines: 2007 Writing Group to Review New Evidence and Update the ACC/AHA/SCAI 2005 Guideline Update for Percutaneous Coronary Intervention, Writing on Behalf of the 2005 Writing Committee," *Circulation,* 2008, 117 (2):261-95.

Nagge J, Crowther M, and Hirsh J, "Is Impaired Renal Function a Contraindication to the Use of Low-Molecular Weight Heparin?" *Arch Intern Med,* 2002, 162(22):2605-9.

EPHEDrine (e FED rin)

Medication Safety Issues

Sound-alike/look-alike issues:

EPHEDrine may be confused with Epifrin®, EPINEPHrine

Related Information

Contrast Media Reactions, Premedication for Prophylaxis *on page 1735*
Inhalational Anesthetics *on page 1632*
Postoperative Nausea and Vomiting *on page 1593*

Index Terms Ephedrine Sulfate

Pharmacologic Category Alpha/Beta Agonist

Generic Available Yes

Use Treatment of bronchial asthma, acute bronchospasm, idiopathic orthostatic hypotension, anesthesia-induced hypotension

Unlabeled/Investigational Use Postoperative nausea and vomiting (PONV)

Mechanism of Action Releases tissue stores of norepinephrine and thereby produces an alpha- and beta-adrenergic stimulation; longer-acting and less potent than epinephrine

Pharmacodynamics/Kinetics

Onset of action: Oral: Bronchodilation: 0.25-1 hour
Duration: Oral: 3-6 hours
Distribution: Crosses placenta; enters breast milk
Metabolism: Minimally hepatic
Half-life elimination: 2.5-3.6 hours
Excretion: Urine (60% to 77% as unchanged drug) within 24 hours

Dosage

Children:

Oral, SubQ: 3 mg/kg/day or 25-100 mg/m^2/day in 4-6 divided doses every 4-6 hours

I.M., slow I.V. push: 0.2-0.3 mg/kg/dose every 4-6 hours

Adults:

Oral: 25-50 mg every 3-4 hours as needed

I.M., SubQ: 25-50 mg, parenteral adult dose should not exceed 150 mg in 24 hours

I.V.: 5-25 mg/dose slow I.V. push repeated after 5-10 minutes as needed, then every 3-4 hours not to exceed 150 mg/24 hours

Stability Protect all dosage forms from light.

Administration Dilute to 5 or 10 mg/mL. Administer as a slow I.V. push. Do not administer unless solution is clear.

Monitoring Parameters Injection solution: Monitor blood pressure, pulse

Anesthesia and Critical Care Concerns/Other Considerations

Clinical Pearls/Comments: May administer I.M. (0.5 mg/kg) to treat post-operative nausea nad vomiting in adults who failed traditional antiemetic therapy (Gan, 2003).

Pregnancy Risk Factor C

Contraindications Hypersensitivity to ephedrine or any component of the formulation; cardiac arrhythmias; angle-closure glaucoma; concurrent use of other sympathomimetic agents

Warnings/Precautions Blood volume depletion should be corrected before injectable ephedrine therapy is instituted; use caution in patients with unstable vasomotor symptoms, diabetes, hyperthyroidism, prostatic hyperplasia or a history of seizures; also use caution in the elderly and those patients with cardiovascular disorders such as coronary artery disease, arrhythmias, and hypertension. Ephedrine may cause hypertension. Long-term use may cause anxiety and symptoms of paranoid schizophrenia. Use with caution in the elderly, since it crosses the blood-brain barrier and may cause confusion. Use with extreme caution in patients taking MAO inhibitors.

Adverse Reactions Frequency not defined.

Cardiovascular: Arrhythmias, chest pain, elevation or depression of blood pressure, hypertension, palpitation, tachycardia, unusual pallor

Central nervous system: Agitation, anxiety, apprehension, CNS stimulating effects, dizziness, excitation, fear, headache hyperactivity, insomnia, irritability, nervousness, restlessness, tension

Gastrointestinal: Anorexia, GI upset, nausea, vomiting, xerostomia

Genitourinary: Painful urination

Neuromuscular & skeletal: Trembling, tremor (more common in the elderly), weakness

Respiratory: Dyspnea

Miscellaneous: Diaphoresis increased

Drug Interactions

Avoid Concomitant Use

Avoid concomitant use of EPHEDrine with any of the following: Iobenguane I 123; MAO Inhibitors

Increased Effect/Toxicity

EPHEDrine may increase the levels/effects of: Bromocriptine; Sympathomimetics

The levels/effects of EPHEDrine may be increased by: Antacids; Atomoxetine; Cannabinoids; Carbonic Anhydrase Inhibitors; MAO Inhibitors; Serotonin/Norepinephrine Reuptake Inhibitors

Decreased Effect

EPHEDrine may decrease the levels/effects of: Iobenguane I 123

The levels/effects of EPHEDrine may be decreased by: Spironolactone

Ethanol/Nutrition/Herb Interactions Herb/Nutraceutical: Avoid ephedra, yohimbe (may cause CNS stimulation).

Test Interactions Can cause a false-positive amphetamine EMIT assay

Dosage Forms Excipient information presented when available (limited, particularly for generics); consult specific product labeling.

Capsule, as sulfate: 25 mg

Injection, solution, as sulfate: 50 mg/mL (1 mL, 10 mL)

References

Gan TJ, Meyer T, Apfel CC, et al, "Consensus Guidelines for Managing Postoperative Nausea and Vomiting," *Anesth Analg*, 2003, 97(1):62-71.

Stein GC, "Requirements for Pharmacists Dispensing Ephedrine Products," *Am J Health Syst Pharm*, 1995, 52(15):1630.

◆ **Ephedrine Sulfate** *see* EPHEDrine *on page 490*

◆ **EpiClenz™ [OTC]** *see* Alcohol (Ethyl) *on page 53*

EPINEPHrine (ep i NEF rin)

Medication Safety Issues

Sound-alike/look-alike issues:

EPINEPHrine may be confused with ePHEDrine

Epifrin® may be confused with ephedrine, EpiPen®

EpiPen® may be confused with Epifrin®

High alert medication: The Institute for Safe Medication Practices (ISMP) includes this medication among its list of drugs which have a heightened risk of causing significant patient harm when used in error.

Medication errors have occurred due to confusion with epinephrine products expressed as ratio strengths (eg, 1:1000 vs 1:10,000).

Epinephrine 1:1000 = 1 mg/mL and is most commonly used I.M.

Epinephrine 1:10,000 = 0.1 mg/mL and is used I.V.

Medication errors have occurred when topical epinephrine 1 mg/mL (1:1000) has been inadvertently injected. Vials of injectable and topical epinephrine look very similar. Epinephrine should always be appropriately labeled with the intended administration.

International issues:

EpiPen® may be confused with Epigen® which is a brand name for glycyrrhizinic acid in Mexico

EpiPen® may be confused with Epopen® which is a brand name for epoetin alfa in Spain

Related Information

U.S. Brand Names Adrenalin®; EpiPen®; EpiPen® Jr; Primatene® Mist [OTC]; Raphon [OTC] [DSC]; S2® [OTC]; Twinject®

Canadian Brand Names Adrenalin®; EpiPen®; EpiPen® Jr; Twinject®

Index Terms Adrenaline; Epinephrine Bitartrate; Epinephrine Hydrochloride; Racemic Epinephrine; Racepinephrine

Pharmacologic Category Alpha/Beta Agonist

Generic Available Yes: Solution for injection

Use Treatment of bronchospasms, bronchial asthma, nasal congestion, viral croup, anaphylactic reactions, cardiac arrest; added to local anesthetics to decrease systemic absorption of intraspinal and local anesthetics and increase duration of action; decrease superficial hemorrhage

Unlabeled/Investigational Use ACLS guidelines: Ventricular fibrillation (VF) or pulseless ventricular tachycardia (VT) unresponsive to initial defibrillatory shocks; pulseless electrical activity; asystole; hypotension/shock unresponsive to volume resuscitation; symptomatic bradycardia unresponsive to atropine or pacing; inotropic support

Mechanism of Action Stimulates alpha-, beta$_1$-, and beta$_2$-adrenergic receptors resulting in relaxation of smooth muscle of the bronchial tree, cardiac stimulation (increasing myocardial oxygen consumption), and dilation of skeletal muscle vasculature; small doses can cause vasodilation via beta$_2$-vascular receptors; large doses may produce constriction of skeletal and vascular smooth muscle

Pharmacodynamics/Kinetics

Onset of action: Bronchodilation: SubQ: ~5-10 minutes; Inhalation: ~1 minute

Distribution: Crosses placenta

Metabolism: Taken up into the adrenergic neuron and metabolized by monoamine oxidase and catechol-o-methyltransferase; circulating drug hepatically metabolized

Excretion: Urine (as inactive metabolites, metanephrine, and sulfate and hydroxy derivatives of mandelic acid, small amounts as unchanged drug)

Dosage

Neonates: Cardiac arrest:

I.V.: 0.01-0.03 mg/kg (0.1-0.3 mL/kg of **1:10,000** solution) every 3-5 minutes until return of spontaneous circulation

Intratracheal: Although I.V. route is preferred, may consider administration of doses up to 0.1 mg/kg (1 mL/kg of **1:10,000** solution) every 3-5 minutes until I.V. access established or return of spontaneous circulation

Infants and Children:

Asystole/pulseless arrest, pulseless VT/VF (after failed defibrillations):

I.V., I.O.: 0.01 mg/kg (0.1 mL/kg of **1:10,000** solution) (maximum single dose: 1 mg) every 3-5 minutes until return of spontaneous circulation

Intratracheal: 0.1 mg/kg (0.1 mL/kg of **1:1000** solution) (maximum single dose: 10 mg) every 3-5 minutes until I.V./I.O access established or return of spontaneous circulation

Bradycardia (symptomatic; unresponsive to atropine or pacing):

I.V., I.O.: 0.01 mg/kg (0.1 mL/kg of **1:10,000** solution) (maximum single dose: 1 mg) every 3-5 minutes as needed

Intratracheal: 0.1 mg/kg or (0.1 mL/kg of **1:1000** solution) (maximum single dose: 10 mg) every 3-5 minutes as needed until I.V./I.O access established

Continuous I.V. infusion: 0.1-1 mcg/kg/minute; doses <0.3 mcg/kg/minute generally produce beta-adrenergic effects and higher doses generally produce alpha-adrenergic vasoconstriction; titrate dosage to desired effect

Bronchodilator:
  SubQ: 0.01 mg/kg (0.01 mL/kg of **1:1000** solution) (maximum single dose: 0.5 mg) every 20 minutes for 3 doses
  Nebulization: S2® (racepinephrine, OTC labeling):
    Children <4 years: Jet nebulizer: Croup: 0.05 mL/kg (maximum dose: 0.5 mL); dilute in 3 mL of NS. Administer over ~15 minutes; do not administer more frequently than every 2 hours
    Children ≥4 years: Refer to adult dosing.
  Inhalation: Children ≥4 years: Primatene® Mist: Refer to adult dosing.
Decongestant: Children ≥6 years: Refer to adult dosing
Hypersensitivity reaction: **Note:** SubQ administration results in slower absorption and is less reliable. I.M. administration in the anterolateral aspect of the thigh is preferred in the setting of anaphylaxis (ACLS guidelines, 2005; Kemp, 2008).
  I.M., SubQ: 0.01 mg/kg (0.01 mL/kg of **1:1000** solution) (maximum single dose: 0.5 mg) every 5-20 minutes; larger I.M. or SubQ doses, use of I.V. route, or continuous infusion may be needed for severe anaphylactic reactions
  Self-administration following severe allergic reactions (eg, insect stings, food): **Note:** World Health Organization (WHO) and Anaphylaxis Canada recommend the availability of 1 dose for every 10-20 minutes of travel time to a medical emergency facility:
    EpiPen® Jr: I.M., SubQ: Children 15-29 kg: 0.15 mg; if anaphylactic symptoms persist, dose may be repeated in 5-15 minutes using an additional EpiPen® Jr
    EpiPen®: I.M., SubQ: Children ≥30 kg: 0.3 mg; if anaphylactic symptoms persist, dose may be repeated in 5-15 minutes using an additional EpiPen®
    Twinject®: I.M. SubQ:
      Children 15-29 kg: 0.15 mg; if anaphylactic symptoms persist, dose may be repeated in 5-15 minutes using the same device after partial disassembly
      Children ≥30 kg: 0.3 mg; if anaphylactic symptoms persist, dose may be repeated in 5-15 minutes using the same device after partial disassembly
Hypotension/shock, fluid-resistant (unlabeled use): Continuous I.V. infusion: 0.1-1 mcg/kg/minute; doses up to 5 mcg/kg/minute may rarely be necessary (Hegenbarth, 2008)

Adults:
  Asystole/pulseless arrest, pulseless VT/VF:
    I.V., I.O.: 1 mg every 3-5 minutes until return of spontaneous circulation; if this approach fails, higher doses of epinephrine (up to 0.2 mg/kg) have been used for treatment of specific problems (eg, beta-blocker or calcium channel blocker overdose)
    Intratracheal: 2-2.5 mg every 3-5 minutes until I.V./I.O access established or return of spontaneous circulation; dilute in 5-10 mL NS or distilled water. **Note:** Absorption is greater with distilled water, but causes more adverse effects on PaO_2.
  Bradycardia (symptomatic; unresponsive to atropine or pacing): I.V. infusion: 1-10 mcg/minute; titrate to desired effect
  Bronchodilator:
    SubQ: 0.3-0.5 mg (**1:1000** solution) every 20 minutes for 3 doses
    Nebulization: S2® (racepinephrine, OTC labeling):
      Hand-bulb nebulizer: Add 0.5 mL (~10 drops) to nebulizer; 1-3 inhalations up to every 3 hours if needed
      Jet nebulizer: Add 0.5 mL (~10 drops) to nebulizer and dilute with 3 mL of NS; administer over ~15 minutes every 3-4 hours as needed
    Inhalation: Primatene® Mist (OTC labeling): One inhalation, wait at least 1 minute; if not relieved, may use once more. Do not use again for at least 3 hours.
  Decongestant: Intranasal: Apply **1:1000** solution locally as drops or spray or with sterile swab
  Hypersensitivity reaction: **Note:** SubQ administration results in slower absorption and is less reliable. I.M. administration in the anterolateral aspect of the thigh is preferred in the setting of anaphylaxis (ACLS guidelines, 2005; Kemp, 2008).
    I.M., SubQ: 0.3-0.5 mg (**1:1000** solution) every 15-20 minutes if condition requires

I.V.: 0.1 mg (**1:10,000** solution) over 5 minutes; may infuse at 1-4 mcg/minute to prevent the need to repeat injections frequently

Self-administration following severe allergic reactions (eg, insect stings, food):
Note: The World Health Organization (WHO) and Anaphylaxis Canada recommend the availability of one dose for every 10-20 minutes of travel time to a medical emergency facility. More than 2 doses should only be administered under direct medical supervision.
Twinject®: I.M., SubQ: 0.3 mg; if anaphylactic symptoms persist, dose may be repeated in 5-15 minutes using the same device after partial disassembly
EpiPen®: I.M., SubQ: 0.3 mg; if anaphylactic symptoms persist, dose may be repeated in 5-15 minutes using an additional EpiPen®

Hypotension/shock, severe and fluid resistant (unlabeled use): I.V. infusion: Initial: 1 mcg/minute; titrate to desired response; usual range: 2-10 mcg/minute (AHA, 2005)

Stability
Epinephrine is sensitive to light and air; protection from light is recommended. Oxidation turns drug pink, then a brown color. **Solutions should not be used if they are discolored or contain a precipitate.**
Adrenalin®: Store between 15°C to 25°C (59°F to 77°F); do not freeze. Protect from light. The 1:1000 solution should be discarded 30 days after initial use.
EpiPen® and EpiPen® Jr: Store at 25°C (77°F); excursions permitted to 15°C to 30°C (59°F to 86°F); do not freeze or refrigerate. Protect from light by storing in carrier tube provided.
Primatene® Mist: Store between 20°C to 25°C (68°F to 77°F).
Raphon: Store between 2°C to 25°C (36°F to 77°F). Refrigerate after opening.
S2®: Store between 2°C to 20°C (36°F to 68°F). Protect from light.
Twinject®: Store between 20°C to 25°C (68°F to 77°F); excursions permitted to 15°C to 30°C (59°F to 86°F); do not freeze or refrigerate. Protect from light.
Stability of injection of parenteral admixture at room temperature (25°C) or refrigeration (4°C) is 24 hours.
Standard I.V. diluent: 1 mg/250 mL NS.
Preparation of adult I.V. infusion: Dilute 1 mg in 250 mL of D_5W or NS (4 mcg/mL).
S2®: Dilution not required when administered via hand-bulb nebulizer; dilute with NS 3-5 mL if using jet nebulizer

Administration When administering as a continuous infusion, central line administration is preferred. I.V. infusions require an infusion pump. Epinephrine solutions for injection can be administered I.M., I.O., intratracheally, I.V., or SubQ.
Note: EpiPen® and EpiPen® Jr Auto-Injectors contain a single, fixed-dose of epinephrine. Twinject® Auto-Injectors contain two doses; the first fixed-dose is available for auto-injection; the second dose is available for manual injection following partial disassembly of device.

Subcutaneous: SubQ administration results in slower absorption and is less reliable.
I.M.: I.M. administration into the buttocks should be avoided. I.M. administration in the anterolateral aspect of the thigh is preferred in the setting of anaphylaxis (ACLS guidelines, 2005; Kemp, 2008). EpiPen®, EpiPen® Jr, and Twinject® Auto-Injectors should only be injected into the anterolateral aspect of the thigh, through clothing if necessary.
Inhalation: S2®: If using jet nebulizer: Administer over ~15 minutes; must be diluted.
Intratracheal: Dilute in NS or distilled water. Absorption is greater with distilled water, but causes more adverse effects on PaO_2. Pass catheter beyond tip of tracheal tube, stop compressions, spray drug quickly down tube. Follow immediately with several quick insufflations and continue chest compressions.

Extravasation management: Use phentolamine as antidote. Mix 5 mg with 9 mL of NS. Inject a small amount of this dilution into extravasated area. Blanching should reverse immediately. Monitor site. If blanching should recur, additional injections of phentolamine may be needed.
Monitoring Parameters Pulmonary function, heart rate, blood pressure, site of infusion for blanching, extravasation; cardiac monitor and blood pressure monitor required during continuous infusion. If using to treat hypotension, assess intravascular volume and support as needed.

Anesthesia and Critical Care Concerns/Other Considerations
Clinical Pearls/Comments:

Extravasation Management: Antidote for peripheral ischemia caused by epinephrine extravasation: To prevent sloughing and necrosis in ischemic areas, the area should be infiltrated as soon as possible with 5-10 mg of Regitine® (phentolamine), an adrenergic blocking agent, diluted in 10-15 mL of saline. A syringe with a fine hypodermic needle should be used, and the solution liberally infiltrated throughout the ischemic area. Sympathetic blockade with phentolamine causes immediate and conspicuous local hyperemic changes if the area is infiltrated within 12 hours. Therefore, phentolamine should be given as soon as possible after the extravasation is noted, as phentolamine may be ineffective if given >12 hours after extravasation.

Evidence Based Information:
Septic Shock: Epinephrine's use may be limited by its effects on renal and gastric blood flow and its propensity to increase lactic acid concentrations.

The 2008 Surviving Sepsis Campaign Guidelines (Dellinger, 2008) state that epinephrine should **not** be administered as the initial vasopressor in septic shock (Grade 2C) and should **only** be used as an alternative when blood pressure is poorly responsive to norepinephrine or dopamine (Grade 2B).

Cardiac Arrest: Epinephrine can be given by endotracheal route during cardiac resuscitation. High-intravenous dose epinephrine (0.1 mg/kg) has not shown to improve survival or neurological outcomes. May have more postresuscitation complications than survivors who receive standard dose epinephrine. Eight randomized clinical studies (>9000 patients) have found no improvement in survival to hospital discharge or neurological outcomes compared with standard epinephrine.

Out-of-hospital cardiac arrest: A prospective, multicenter, double-blind randomized, controlled trial evaluated the efficacy of vasopressin or epinephrine when administered to adult patients who suffered an out-of-hospital cardiac arrest (Wenzel, 2004). For inclusions, patients presented with ventricular fibrillation, pulseless electrical activity, or asystole. They were excluded if they were successfully defibrillated without the administration of a vasopressor, had a terminal illness or had a "do not resuscitate" (DNR) order, a lack of intravenous access, hemorrhagic shock, pregnancy, cardiac arrest due to trauma, or were <18 years of age. Eligible patients were randomized to intravenous vasopressin (40 units, n=589) or epinephrine (1 mg, n=597). Each patient received an injection of the study drug, if spontaneous circulation was not restored in 3 minutes they received a second dose (same amount) of the same study drug. If there was no response, the managing physician had the option of giving epinephrine. Patients with ventricular fibrillation were randomized after the first three attempts at defibrillation failed; all others were randomized immediately. The primary endpoint was survival to hospital admission; the secondary endpoint was survival to hospital discharge. Five hundred and eighty-nine patients were randomized to vasopressin and five hundred and ninety-seven patients were randomized to epinephrine. There was no significant difference in the rate of hospital admission between the vasopressin group and the epinephrine group if they had ventricular fibrillation (46.2% vs 43% respectively, p: 0.48) or pulseless electrical activity (33.7% vs 30.5% respectively, p: 0.65). Patients with asystole responded significantly better to vasopressin; having higher rates of hospital admission (29% vs 20.3% in the epinephrine group, p: 0.02) and hospital discharge (4.7% vs 1.5% in the epinephrine group, p: 0.04). Patients who failed vasopressin therapy and received additional epinephrine had significant improvement in survival to hospital admission (25.7% vs 16.4% in the epinephrine group, p: 0.002) and discharge (6.2% vs 1.7%, p: 0.002). Similar patients who were randomized to epinephrine and failed to respond did not improve with additional epinephrine. Cerebral performance among all patients who survived to discharge was similar in both groups. In this trial, vasopressin was superior to epinephrine in patients with asystole. Vasopressin followed by epinephrine may be more effective than epinephrine alone in refractory out-of-hospital cardiac arrest.

More recently, Gueugniaud, et al evaluated the combination of vasopressin and epinephrine compared to epinephrine alone in the treatment of out-of-hospital cardiac arrest (Gueugniaud, 2008). This multicenter, double-blind, randomized, controlled trial enrolled 2894 adult patients with out-of-hosptial cardiac arrest with either ventricular fibrillation, pulseless electrical activity, or asystole. Patients were exluded if <18 years of age, successfully defibrillated without vasopressors, traumatic cardiac arrest, pregnant, documented terminal illness, and DNR orders or irreversible cardiac arrest. Patients were randomized to either intravenous vasopressin (40 units) and epinephrine (1 mg) or epinephrine (1 mg) and a placebo. The medications/placebo were given within 10 seconds of each other and followed by a saline flush. Patients with ventricular fibrillation received defibrillation before the administration of study drug. The primary endpoint was survival to hospital admission; secondary endpoints were return of spontaneous circulation, survival to hospital discharge, good neurologic recovery, and 1-year survival. Similar to the previous study, there was no significant difference in the rate of hospital admission between the two groups (20.7% vs 21.3%, p=0.69). Also, return of spontaneous circulation, survival to hospital discharge, good neurologic recovery, and 1-year survival were all similar between groups. In contrast to the previous study, patients with asystole had no benefit from the combination of vasopressin and epinephrine when compared to epinephrine/ placebo. In this study, asystole was the most common initial cardiac rhythm, presenting in 82.8% of the patients. Based on the results of the most recent study, it appears that vasopressin plus epinephrine has no benefit over epinephrine in out-of-hospital cardiac arrest.

In-hospital cardiac arrest: A small in-hospital cardiac arrest study evaluated the efficacy of vasopressin or epinephrine in 200 patients. The investigators did not find any differences between the two treatment groups with regard to survival, hospital discharge, or cerebral performance (Stiell, 2001).

Pregnancy Risk Factor C

Contraindications There are no absolute contraindications to the use of injectable epinephrine (including EpiPen®, EpiPen® Jr, and Twinject®) in a life-threatening situation.

Injectable solution: Per the manufacturer, contraindicated in narrow-angle glaucoma; shock; during general anesthesia with halogenated hydrocarbons or cyclopropane (currently not available); individuals with organic brain damage; with local anesthesia of the digits; during labor; heart failure; coronary insufficiency

Primatene Mist®, S2®: concurrent use or within 2 weeks of MAO inhibitors

Raphon: Hypersensitivity to epinephrine or any component of the formulation

Warnings/Precautions Use with caution in elderly patients, patients with diabetes mellitus, cardiovascular diseases (eg, coronary artery disease, hypertension), thyroid disease, cerebrovascular disease, Parkinson's disease, or patients taking tricyclic antidepressants. Some products contain sulfites as preservatives; the presence of sulfites in some products (eg, EpiPen® and Twinject®) should not deter administration during a serious allergic or other emergency situation even if the patient is sulfite-sensitive. Use with caution in patients taking MAO inhibitors; the concomitant use with some formulations (eg, Primatene Mist®, S2®) of epinephrine is contraindicated. Accidental injection into digits, hands, or feet may result in local reactions including injection site pallor, coldness and hypoesthesia or injury resulting in bruising, bleeding, discoloration, erythema or skeletal injury; patient should seek immediate medical attention if this occurs. Rapid I.V. administration may cause death from cerebrovascular hemorrhage or cardiac arrhythmias; however, rapid I.V. administration during pulseless arrest is necessary. Avoid topical application where reduced perfusion could lead to ischemic tissue damage (eg, penis, ears, digits).

Adverse Reactions Frequency not defined.

Cardiovascular: Angina, cardiac arrhythmia, chest pain, flushing, hypertension, pallor, palpitation, sudden death, tachycardia (parenteral), vasoconstriction, ventricular ectopy

Central nervous system: Anxiety (transient), apprehensiveness, cerebral hemorrhage, dizziness, headache, insomnia, lightheadedness, nervousness, restlessness

Gastrointestinal: Dry throat, loss of appetite, nausea, vomiting, xerostomia

Genitourinary: Acute urinary retention in patients with bladder outflow obstruction

Neuromuscular & skeletal: Tremor, weakness

◀ Ocular: Allergic lid reaction, burning, eye pain, ocular irritation, precipitation of or exacerbation of narrow-angle glaucoma, transient stinging

Respiratory: Dyspnea, pulmonary edema

Miscellaneous: Diaphoresis

Drug Interactions

Avoid Concomitant Use

Avoid concomitant use of EPINEPHrine with any of the following: Iobenguane I 123

Increased Effect/Toxicity

EPINEPHrine may increase the levels/effects of: Bromocriptine; Sympathomimetics

The levels/effects of EPINEPHrine may be increased by: Antacids; Atomoxetine; Beta-Blockers; Cannabinoids; Carbonic Anhydrase Inhibitors; COMT Inhibitors; Inhalational Anesthetics; MAO Inhibitors; Serotonin/Norepinephrine Reuptake Inhibitors; Tricyclic Antidepressants

Decreased Effect

EPINEPHrine may decrease the levels/effects of: Iobenguane I 123

The levels/effects of EPINEPHrine may be decreased by: Spironolactone

Ethanol/Nutrition/Herb Interactions Herb/Nutraceutical: Avoid ephedra, yohimbe (may cause CNS stimulation).

Dosage Forms Excipient information presented when available (limited, particularly for generics); consult specific product labeling. [DSC] = Discontinued product

Aerosol for oral inhalation:

Primatene® Mist: 0.22 mg/inhalation (15 mL, 22.5 mL [DSC]) [contains CFCs]

Injection, solution [prefilled auto injector]:

EpiPen®: 0.3 mg/0.3 mL (2 mL) [1:1000 solution; delivers 0.3 mg per injection; contains sodium metabisulfite; available as single unit or in double-unit pack with training unit]

EpiPen® Jr: 0.15 mg/0.3 mL (2 mL) [1:2000 solution; delivers 0.15 mg per injection; contains sodium metabisulfite; available as single unit or in double-unit pack with training unit]

Twinject®: 0.15 mg/0.15 mL (1.1 mL) [1:1000 solution; delivers 0.15 mg per injection; contains sodium bisulfite; two 0.15 mg doses per injector]; 0.3 mg/0.3 mL (1.1 mL) [1:1000 solution; delivers 0.3 mg per injection; contains sodium bisulfite; two 0.3 mg doses per injector]

Injection, solution, as hydrochloride: 0.1 mg/mL (10 mL) [1:10,000 solution]; 1 mg/mL (1 mL) [1:1000 solution]

Adrenalin®: 1 mg/mL (1 mL) [1:1000 solution; contains sodium bisulfite]

Adrenalin®: 1 mg/mL (30 mL) [1:1000 solution; contains chlorobutanol, sodium bisulfite]

Solution for oral inhalation [racepinephrine; preservative free]:

S2®: 2.25% (0.5 mL) [as d-epinephrine 1.125% and l-epinephrine 1.125%]

Solution, intranasal, as hydrochloride [drops, spray]:

Adrenalin®: 1 mg/mL (30 mL) [1:1000 solution; contains sodium bisulfite]

Solution, topical [racepinephrine]:

Raphon: 2.25% (15 mL) [as d-epinephrine 1.125% and l-epinephrine 1.125%; contains benzoic acid, metabisulfites] [DSC]

References

"2005 American Heart Association Guidelines for Cardiopulmonary Resuscitation and Emergency Cardiovascular Care," *Circulation*, 2005, 112(24 Suppl): 1-211.

Dellinger RP, Levy MM, Carlet JM, et al, "Surviving Sepsis Campaign: International Guidelines for Management of Severe Sepsis and Septic Shock: 2008," *Intensive Care Med*, 2008, 34(1):17-60. Available at http://www.survivingsepsis.org/system/files/images/2008_20International_20SSC_20-Guidelines_1_.pdf.

Expert Panel Report 3, "Guidelines for the Diagnosis and Management of Asthma," *Clinical Practice Guidelines*, National Institutes of Health, National Heart, Lung, and Blood Institute, NIH Publication No. 08-4051, prepublication 2007. Available at http://www.nhlbi.nih.gov/guidelines/asthma/asthgdln.htm.

Gueugniaud PY, David JS, Chanzy E, et al, "Vasopressin and Epinephrine vs. Epinephrine Alone in Cardiopulmonary Resuscitation," *N Engl J Med*, 2008, 359(1):21-30.

Mokhlesi B, Leikin JB, Murray P, et al, "Adult Toxicology in Critical Care. Part 11: Specific Poisonings," *Chest*, 2003, 123(3):897-922.

Murphy FT, Manowk TJ, Knutson SW, et al, "Epinephrine-Induced Lactic Acidosis in the Setting of Status Asthmaticus," *South Med J*, 1995, 88(5):577-9.

Russell JA, Walley KR, Singer J, et al, "Vasopressin Versus Norepinephrine Infusion in Patients With Septic Shock," *N Engl J Med*, 2008, 358(9):877-87.

Stiell IG, Hebert PC, Wells GA, et al, "Vasopressin Versus Epinephrine for in Hospital Cardiac Arrest: A Randomised Controlled Trial," *Lancet*, 2001, 358(9276):105-9.

Wenzel V, Krismer AC, Arntz HR, et al, "A Comparison of Vasopressin and Epinephrine for Out-of-Hospital Cardiopulmonary Resuscitation," *N Engl J Med*, 2004, 350(2):105-13.

♦ **Epinephrine Bitartrate** *see* EPINEPHrine *on page* 492

♦ **Epinephrine Hydrochloride** *see* EPINEPHrine *on page* 492

♦ **EpiPen®** *see* EPINEPHrine *on page* 492

♦ **EpiPen® Jr** *see* EPINEPHrine *on page* 492

♦ **Epitol®** *see* CarBAMazepine *on page* 241

♦ **Epival® I.V. (Can)** *see* Valproic Acid and Derivatives *on page* 1445

♦ **Epivir®** *see* LamiVUDine *on page* 797

♦ **Epivir-HBV®** *see* LamiVUDine *on page* 797

Eplerenone (e PLER en one)

Related Information
Heart Failure (Systolic) *on page* 1739

U.S. Brand Names Inspra™

Pharmacologic Category Diuretic, Potassium-Sparing; Selective Aldosterone Blocker

Use Treatment of hypertension (may be used alone or in combination with other antihypertensive agents); treatment of heart failure (HF) following acute MI

Pharmacodynamics/Kinetics
Distribution: V_d: 43-90 L
Protein binding: ~50%; primarily to alpha$_1$-acid glycoproteins
Metabolism: Primarily hepatic via CYP3A4; metabolites inactive
Bioavailability: 69%
Half-life elimination: 4-6 hours
Time to peak, plasma: ~1.5 hours; may take up to 4 weeks for full antihypertensive effect
Excretion: Urine (~67%); feces (32%); <5% as unchanged drug in urine and feces

Dosage Oral: Adults:
Hypertension: Initial: 50 mg once daily; may increase to 50 mg twice daily if response is not adequate; may take up to 4 weeks for full therapeutic response. Doses >100 mg/day are associated with increased risk of hyperkalemia and no greater therapeutic effect.
Concurrent use with moderate CYP3A4 inhibitors: Initial: 25 mg once daily
Heart failure (post-MI): Initial: 25 mg once daily; dosage goal: Titrate to 50 mg once daily within 4 weeks, as tolerated
Dosage adjustment per serum potassium concentrations for HF (post-MI):
<5.0 mEq/L:
Increase dose from 25 mg every other day to 25 mg daily **or**
Increase dose from 25 mg daily to 50 mg daily
5.0-5.4 mEq/L: No adjustment needed
5.5-5.9 mEq/L:
Decrease dose from 50 mg daily to 25 mg daily **or**
Decrease dose from 25 mg daily to 25 mg every other day **or**
Decrease dose from 25 mg every other day to withhold medication
≥6.0 mEq/L: Withhold medication until potassium <5.5 mEq/L, then restart at 25 mg every other day

Dosage adjustment in renal impairment:
Hypertension: Cl_{cr} <50 mL/minute or serum creatinine >2.0 mg/dL in males or >1.8 mg/dL in females: Use is contraindicated; risk of hyperkalemia increases with declining renal function
All other indications: Cl_{cr} ≤30 mL/minute: Use is contraindicated.

Dosage adjustment in hepatic impairment: No dosage adjustment needed for mild-to-moderate impairment; safety and efficacy not established for severe impairment

Additional Information Complete prescribing information for this medication should be consulted for additional detail.

◄ **Dosage Forms** Excipient information presented when available (limited, particularly for generics); consult specific product labeling.
Tablet: 25 mg, 50 mg
Inspra™: 25 mg, 50 mg

◆ **EPO** *see* Epoetin Alfa *on page 500*

Epoetin Alfa (e POE e tin AL fa)

Medication Safety Issues
Sound-alike/look-alike issues:
Epoetin alfa may be confused with darbepoetin alfa, epoetin beta
Epogen® may be confused with Neupogen®

International issues:
Epopen® [Spain] may be confused with EpiPen® which is a brand name for epinephrine in the U.S.

Medication Guide An FDA-approved patient medication guide, which is available with the product information and as follows, must be dispensed with this medication for each new outpatient prescription and refill.
Epogen®: http://www.fda.gov/downloads/Drugs/DrugSafety/ucm088591.pdf
Procrit®: http://www.fda.gov/downloads/Drugs/DrugSafety/ucm088988.pdf

U.S. Brand Names Epogen®; Procrit®

Canadian Brand Names Eprex®

Index Terms rHuEPO-α; EPO; Erythropoiesis-Stimulating Agent (ESA); Erythropoietin; NSC-724223

Pharmacologic Category Colony Stimulating Factor

Generic Available No

Use Treatment of anemia (elevate/maintain red blood cell level and decrease the need for transfusions) associated with HIV (zidovudine) therapy, chronic renal failure (including patients on dialysis and not on dialysis); reduction of allogeneic blood transfusion for elective, noncardiac, nonvascular surgery; treatment of anemia due to concurrent chemotherapy in patients with metastatic cancer (nonmyeloid malignancies)

Note: Erythropoietin is **not** indicated for use in cancer patients under the following conditions:
• receiving hormonal therapy, therapeutic biologic products, or radiation therapy unless also receiving concurrent myelosuppressive chemotherapy
• receiving myelosuppressive therapy when the expected outcome is curative
• anemia due to other factors (eg, iron deficiency, folate deficiency, or gastrointestinal bleed)

Unlabeled/Investigational Use Treatment of anemia associated with critical illness; anemia of prematurity; symptomatic anemia in myelodysplastic syndrome (MDS)

Mechanism of Action Induces erythropoiesis by stimulating the division and differentiation of committed erythroid progenitor cells; induces the release of reticulocytes from the bone marrow into the bloodstream, where they mature to erythrocytes. There is a dose response relationship with this effect. This results in an increase in reticulocyte counts followed by a rise in hematocrit and hemoglobin levels.

Pharmacodynamics/Kinetics
Onset of action: Several days
Peak effect: 2-3 weeks
Distribution: V_d: 9 L; rapid in the plasma compartment; concentrated in liver, kidneys, and bone marrow
Metabolism: Some degradation does occur
Bioavailability: SubQ: ~21% to 31%; intraperitoneal epoetin: 3% (a few patients)
Half-life elimination: Cancer: SubQ: 16-67 hours; Chronic renal failure: I.V.: 4-13 hours
Time to peak, serum: Chronic renal failure: SubQ: 5-24 hours
Excretion: Feces (majority); urine (small amounts, 10% unchanged in normal volunteers)

Dosage Note: Hemoglobin levels should not exceed 12 g/dL and should not rise >1 g/dL per 2-week time period during therapy in any patient.

Chronic renal failure patients: Individualize dosing to achieve and maintain hemoglobin levels between 10-12 g/dL. Hemoglobin levels should not exceed 12 g/dL. **Note:** I.V. route is preferred for hemodialysis patients.

Children: I.V., SubQ: Initial dose: 50 units/kg 3 times/week

Adults: I.V., SubQ: Initial dose: 50-100 units/kg 3 times/week

Dosage adjustment in Children and Adults: SubQ, I.V.:

Decrease dose by 25%: If hemoglobin approaches 12 g/dL **or** hemoglobin increases >1 g/dL in any 2-week period. If hemoglobin continues to increase, temporarily discontinue therapy until hemoglobin begins to decrease, then resume therapy with a ~25% reduction from previous dose.

Increase dose by 25%: If hemoglobin <10 g/dL and does not increase by 1 g/dL after 4 weeks of therapy (with adequate iron stores) **or** hemoglobin decreases below 10 g/dL. If transferrin saturation >20%, may increase epoetin dose. Do not increase dose more frequently than at 4-week intervals, unless clinically indicated (hemoglobin response time for dose increases may be 2-6 weeks).

Inadequate or lack of response: If patient does not attain target hemoglobin range of 10-12 g/dL after appropriate dose titrations over 12 weeks:

Do not continue to increase dose and use the minimum effective dose that will maintain a hemoglobin level sufficient to avoid red blood cell transfusions **and** evaluate patient for other causes of anemia.

Monitor hemoglobin closely thereafter, and if responsiveness improves, may resume making dosage adjustments as recommended above. If responsiveness does not improve and recurrent red blood cell transfusions continue to be needed, discontinue therapy.

Maintenance dose: Individualize to target hemoglobin range of 10-12 g/dL; limit additional dosage increases to every 4 weeks (or longer)

Dialysis patients: Median dose:

Children: 167 units/kg/week (hemodialysis) **or** 76 units/kg/week (peritoneal dialysis), in 2-3 divided doses per week

Adults: 75 units/kg 3 times/week

Nondialysis patients:

Children: Dosing range: 50-250 units/kg 1-3 times/week

Adults: Dosing range: 75-150 units/kg/week

Zidovudine-treated, HIV-infected patients (patients with erythropoietin levels >500 mU/mL are **unlikely** to respond): Titrate dosage to use the minimum effective dose that will maintain a hemoglobin level sufficient to avoid red blood cell transfusions. Hemoglobin levels should not exceed 12 g/dL.

Children: SubQ, I.V.: Limited data available; reported dosing range: 50-400 units/kg 2-3 times/week

Adults (with serum erythropoietin levels ≤500 and zidovudine doses ≤4200 mg/week): SubQ, I.V.: 100 units/kg 3 times/week for 8 weeks

Dosage adjustment:

Increase dose by 50-100 units/kg 3 times/week: If response is not satisfactory in terms of reducing transfusion requirements **or** increasing hemoglobin after 8 weeks of therapy. Evaluate response every 4-8 weeks thereafter, and adjust the dose accordingly by 50-100 units/kg increments 3 times/week. If patients has not responded satisfactorily to 300 units/kg/dose 3 times/week, a response to higher doses is unlikely.

Withhold dose: If hemoglobin exceeds 12 g/dL. Resume treatment with a 25% dose reduction when hemoglobin drops below 11 g/dL

Cancer patient on chemotherapy: Treatment of patients with erythropoietin levels >200 mU/mL is **not recommended by the manufacturer.** Titrate dosage to use the minimum effective dose that will maintain a hemoglobin level sufficient to avoid red blood cell transfusions. Do not initiate therapy if hemoglobin ≥10 g/dL. Discontinue erythropoietin following completion of chemotherapy.

Children: I.V.: 600 units/kg once weekly (maximum: 40,000 units)

Dosage adjustment:

Increase dose: If response is not satisfactory after a sufficient period of evaluation (no increase in hemoglobin by ≥1 g/dL after 4 weeks of once-weekly therapy), the dose may be increased every 4 weeks (or longer) to

900 units/kg/week; maximum 60,000 units. If patient does not respond, a response to higher doses is unlikely.

Withhold dose: If hemoglobin exceeds a level needed to avoid red blood cell transfusion. Resume treatment with a 25% dose reduction when hemoglobin approaches a level where transfusions may be required.

Reduce dose by 25%: If hemoglobin increases >1 g/dL in any 2-week period **or** hemoglobin reaches a level sufficient to avoid red blood cell transfusion.

Discontinue: If after 8 weeks of therapy there is no response (ie, increased hemoglobin levels) or transfusions still required.

Adults: SubQ: Initial dose: 150 units/kg 3 times/week or 40,000 units once weekly; commonly used doses range from 10,000 units 3 times/week to 40,000-60,000 units once weekly.

Dosage adjustment:

Increase dose: If response is not satisfactory after a sufficient period of evaluation (no reduction in transfusion requirements or increase in hemoglobin after 8 weeks of 3 times/week therapy) **or** (no increase in hemoglobin by ≥1 g/dL after 4 weeks of once-weekly therapy), the dose may be increased every 4 weeks (or longer) to 300 units/kg 3 times/week, **or** when dosed weekly, increased all at once to 60,000 units weekly. If patient does not respond, a response to higher doses is unlikely.

Withhold dose: If hemoglobin exceeds a level needed to avoid red blood cell transfusion. Resume treatment with a 25% dose reduction when hemoglobin approaches a level where transfusions may be required.

Reduce dose by 25%: If hemoglobin increases >1 g/dL in any 2-week period **or** hemoglobin reaches a level sufficient to avoid red blood cell transfusion.

Discontinue: If after 8 weeks of therapy there is no response (ie, increased hemoglobin levels) or transfusions still required.

Surgery patients: Prior to initiating treatment, obtain a hemoglobin to establish that it is >10 g/dL and ≤13 g/dL: Adults: SubQ: Initial dose: 300 units/kg/day for 10 days before surgery, on the day of surgery, and for 4 days after surgery

Alternative dose: 600 units/kg in once weekly doses (21, 14, and 7 days before surgery) plus a fourth dose on the day of surgery

Anemia of critical illness (unlabeled use): Adults: SubQ: 40,000 units once weekly

Symptomatic anemia associated with MDS (unlabeled use): Adults: SubQ: 40,000-60,000 units 1-3 times/week

Anemia of prematurity (unlabeled use): Infants: I.V., SubQ: Dosing range: 500-1250 units/kg/week; commonly used dose: 250 units/kg 3 times/week; supplement with oral iron therapy 3-8 mg/kg/day

Dosage adjustment in renal impairment: The National Kidney Foundation Clinical Practice Guideline for Anemia in Chronic Kidney Disease: 2007 Update of Hemoglobin Target (September, 2007) recommend hemoglobin levels in the range of 11-12 g/dL for dialysis and nondialysis patients receiving ESAs; hemoglobin levels should not be >13 g/dL.

Hemodialysis: Supplemental dose is not necessary. I.V. route is preferred for hemodialysis patients.

Peritoneal dialysis: Supplemental dose is not necessary.

Stability

Vials should be stored at 2°C to 8°C (36°F to 46°F); **do not freeze or shake.** Protect from light.

Single-dose 1 mL vial contains no preservative: Use one dose per vial. Do not re-enter vial; discard unused portions.

Single-dose vials (except 40,000 units/mL vial) are stable for 2 weeks at room temperature. Single-dose 40,000 units/mL vial is stable for 1 week at room temperature.

Multidose 1 mL or 2 mL vial contains preservative. Store at 2°C to 8°C after initial entry and between doses. Discard 21 days after initial entry.

Multidose vials (with preservative) are stable for 1 week at room temperature.

Prefilled syringes containing the 20,000 units/mL formulation with preservative are stable for 6 weeks refrigerated (2°C to 8°C).

Dilutions of 1:10 and 1:20 (1 part epoetin:19 parts sodium chloride) are stable for 18 hours at room temperature.

Prior to SubQ administration, preservative free solutions may be mixed with bacteriostatic NS containing benzyl alcohol 0.9% in a 1:1 ratio. Dilutions of 1:10 in $D_{10}W$ with human albumin 0.05% or 0.1% are stable for 24 hours.

Administration SubQ, I.V.:

Patients with CRF on dialysis: I.V. route preferred; may be administered I.V. bolus into the venous line after dialysis.

Patients with CRF not on dialysis: May be administered I.V. or SubQ

Monitoring Parameters Blood pressure; hemoglobin, CBC with differential and platelets, transferrin saturation and ferritin, serum chemistry (CRF patients)

Suggested tests to be monitored and their frequency: See table.

Test	Initial Phase Frequency	Maintenance Phase Frequency
Hemoglobin	1-2 x/week	2-4 x/month
Blood pressure	3 x/week	3 x/week
Serum ferritin	Monthly	Quarterly
Transferrin saturation	Monthly	Quarterly
Serum chemistries including CBC with differential, creatinine, blood urea nitrogen, potassium, phosphorous	Regularly per routine	Regularly per routine

Reference Range

Zidovudine-treated HIV patients: Available evidence indicates patients with endogenous serum erythropoietin levels >500 mU/mL are unlikely to respond

Cancer chemotherapy patients: Measurement of endogenous serum erythropoietin levels in patients with cancer is generally not recommended (NCCN Cancer- and Chemotherapy-Induced Anemia Guidelines, v2.2009). Treatment of patients with endogenous serum erythropoietin levels >200 mU/mL is not recommended according to the manufacturer.

Anesthesia and Critical Care Concerns/Other Considerations
Evidence-Based Information:

Routine Use in Critically-Ill Patients: A prospective, randomized, double-blind, placebo-controlled, multicenter trial was performed with critically-ill patients assessing the efficacy of recombinant human erythropoietin in reducing red blood cell transfusions (Corwin, 2002). Patients were enrolled from December,1998 through June, 2001. Over 1300 ICU (medical, surgical, or medical/ surgical) patients were randomized to receive placebo or 40,000 units of erythropoietin subcutaneously on ICU day 3 and then weekly for a total of 3 doses for patients who remained in the hospital. Inclusion criteria included ICU stay for 3 days, age >18 years, and hematocrit <38%. Exclusion criteria were extensive and included acute ischemic heart disease, acute gastrointestinal bleed, and renal failure with hemodialysis. Each patient's physician determined the need for red blood cell transfusion. Results: The mean baseline hemoglobin was 9.97 g/dL in each group. Patients receiving erythropoietin were less likely to receive transfusions. The median number of units transfused per patient in the placebo group was 2 and in the erythropoietin group was 1 (p<0.001). The erythropoietin group had a 9.9% absolute reduction in RBC transfusions during 28 days (p<0.001, OR 0.67, CI 0.54-0.83). Mortality and adverse clinical events were not significantly different between groups. The authors concluded that weekly administration of erythropoietin in critically-ill patients reduces red blood cell transfusions and increases hemoglobin. The authors also suggest that further study is needed to determine if use of erythropoietin results in improved clinical outcomes.

A restrictive transfusion trial was published after the above Corwin trial was underway (Hebert, 1999). Hebert and his group evaluated a restrictive transfusion strategy (transfuse if hemoglobin <7 g/dL to maintain between 7 and 9 g/dL) versus a liberal strategy (transfuse if hemoglobin <10 g/dL to maintain between 10 and 12 g/dL). Inclusion criteria included anticipated ICU stay >24 hours, hemoglobin ≤9 g/dL with 72 hours of ICU admission, and euvolemia after initial treatment. Exclusion criteria included chronic anemia, active bleeding, or admission after a routine cardiac surgical procedure. The restrictive approach to transfusion was at least as effective as and possibly superior to a liberal transfusion policy in critically-ill patients. The exception to this may be patients with acute myocardial infarction and unstable angina.

More recently, Corwin, et al (2007) once again evaluated the use of recombinant human erythropoietin in the critically ill. In this prospective, randomized, placebo-controlled trial, 1460 medical, surgical, or trauma patients were enrolled between December, 2003 and June, 2006. Patients received either subcutaneous erythropoietin 40,000 units or placebo once weekly for a maximum of 3 doses and were followed for 140 days. The primary endpoint of the study was the percentage of patients who received a red cell transfusion between days 1 and 29. Secondary endpoints included the number of red cell units transfused between days 1 and 29, mortality at day 29 and day 140, and the change in hemoglobin concentration from baseline to day 29. Patients were evaluated for inclusion into the study if they remained in that ICU for 2 days. Inclusion criteria were age >18 years and hemoglobin concentration <12 g/dL. Exclusion criteria were extensive and included acute ischemic heart disease during the ICU stay, acute gastrointestinal bleed, hemodialysis, and patients at risk for thrombosis (history of pulmonary embolism, deep venous thrombosis, ischemic stroke, other arterial or venous thrombosis). Red cell transfusions targeted hemoglobin concentrations between 7 and 9 g/dL, but the need for transfusion was determined by the treating physician (this is more consistent with clinical practice after the Hebert trial was published and different than the previous Corwin trial). Results: The mean baseline hemoglobin for each group was 9.6 g/dL. The use of erythropoietin did not significantly decrease the need for red cell transfusion (46.0% in the erythropoietin group transfused vs 48.3% in the placebo group, p=0.34). The hemoglobin concentration at day 29 increased more in the erythropoietin group compared to placebo (1.6 ± 2.0 g/dL vs 1.2 ± 1.8 g/dL, p<0.001); however, by day 42 the hemoglobin concentrations in both groups were similar. Mortality at day 29 was significantly lower in the group receiving erythropoietin (8.5% vs 11.4%, p=0.02) from the Kaplan-Meier estimate, but no difference was seen in the Cox model in the overall population. Only in the trauma subset was mortality at day 29 significantly lower in the erythropoietin group (3.5% vs 6.6%, p=0.04). At day 140, mortality was not significantly lower in the erythropoietin group. Thrombotic events (eg, DVT and myocardial infarction) were significantly higher in the erythropoietin group as compared to placebo and appeared to be dose-related (16.5% vs 11.5%, p=0.008, HR 1.41, CI 1.06-1.86). However, upon further analysis those patients who did not receive heparin at baseline developed these events more frequently. There was no difference in length of stay or the use of mechanical ventilation between groups. The authors concluded that although erythropoietin does not reduce the incidence of red cell transfusion in critically-ill patients, it may reduce mortality in trauma patients. Further investigation is required to define erythropoietin's role in this population. The routine use of erythropoietin in critically-ill, nontraumatic surgical or medical patients is not supported by this study.

The 2008 Surviving Sepsis Campaign guidelines do not recommend erythropoietin as a treatment for anemia associated with severe sepsis, but suggest that it may be used when septic patients have other therapeutic indications (Grade 1B).

Pregnancy Risk Factor C

Contraindications Hypersensitivity to albumin (human) or mammalian cell-derived products; uncontrolled hypertension

Warnings/Precautions [U.S. Boxed Warning]: ESAs increased the risk of serious cardiovascular events, thromboembolic events, mortality, and/or tumor progression in clinical studies; a rapid rise in hemoglobin (>1 g/dL over 2 weeks) or maintaining higher hemoglobin levels may contribute to these risks. **[U.S. Boxed Warning]: A shortened overall survival and/or increased risk of tumor progression or recurrence has been reported in studies with breast, cervical, head and neck, lymphoid, and non small cell lung cancer patients.** It is of note that in these studies, patients received ESAs to a target hemoglobin of ≥12 g/dL; although risk has not been excluded when dosed to achieve a target hemoglobin of <12 g/dL. **[U.S. Boxed Warnings]: To decrease these risks, and risk of cardio- and thrombovascular events, use the lowest dose needed to avoid red blood cell transfusions. Use ESAs in cancer patients only for the treatment of anemia related to concurrent chemotherapy; discontinue ESA following completion of the chemotherapy course. ESAs are not indicated for patients receiving myelosuppressive therapy when the anticipated outcome is curative. [U.S. Boxed Warning]: An increased risk of death and serious cardiovascular events was reported in chronic renal failure patients administered ESAs to target higher versus lower hemoglobin levels (13.5 vs 11.3 g/dL; 14 vs 10 g/dL) in two clinical studies; dosing should be individualized to achieve and maintain hemoglobin levels within 10-12 g/ dL range.** Hemoglobin rising >1 g/dL in a 2-week period may contribute to the risk. Chronic renal failure patients who exhibit an inadequate hemoglobin response to ESA therapy may be at a higher risk for cardiovascular events and mortality compared to other patients. ESA therapy may reduce dialysis efficacy (due to increase in red blood cells and decrease in plasma volume); adjustments in dialysis parameters may be needed. Patients treated with epoetin may require increased heparinization during dialysis to prevent clotting of the artificial kidney. **[U.S. Boxed Warning]: Epoetin alfa increased the rate of DVT in perisurgery patients not receiving anticoagulant prophylaxis; consider DVT prophylaxis.** Increased mortality was also observed in patients undergoing coronary artery bypass surgery who received epoetin alfa; these deaths were associated with thrombotic events. Epoetin is not approved for reduction of red blood cell transfusion in patients undergoing cardiac or vascular surgery. During therapy in any patient, hemoglobin levels should not exceed a target range of 10-12 g/dL and should not rise >1 g/dL per 2-week time period.

Use with caution in patients with hypertension or with a history of seizures; hypertensive encephalopathy and seizures have been reported. If hypertension is difficult to control, reduce or hold epoetin alfa. An excessive rate of rise of hemoglobin is associated with hypertension or exacerbation of hypertension; decrease the epoetin dose if the hemoglobin increase exceeds 1 g/dL in any 2-week period. Blood pressure should be controlled prior to start of therapy and monitored closely throughout treatment. **Not** recommended for acute correction of severe anemia or as a substitute for transfusion.

Prior to treatment, correct or exclude deficiencies of iron, vitamin B_{12}, and/or folate, as well as other factors which may impair erythropoiesis (aluminum toxicity, inflammatory conditions, infections). Prior to and periodically during therapy, iron stores must be evaluated. Supplemental iron is recommended if serum ferritin <100 mcg/L or serum transferrin saturation <20%. Poor response should prompt evaluation of these potential factors, as well as possible malignant processes, occult blood loss, hemolysis, and/or bone marrow fibrosis. Severe anemia and pure red cell aplasia (PRCA) with associated neutralizing antibodies to erythropoietin has been reported, predominantly in patients with CRF receiving SubQ epoetin (the I.V. route is preferred for hemodialysis patients). Patients with loss of response to epoetin alfa should be evaluated; discontinue treatment in patients with PRCA secondary to neutralizing antibodies to epoetin. Antibodies may cross-react; do not switch to another ESA in patients who develop antibody-mediated anemia.

Due to the delayed onset of erythropoiesis, epoetin is of no value in the acute treatment of anemia. Safety and efficacy in patients with underlying hematologic diseases have not been established, including hypercoagulation disorders and sickle cell disease. Potentially serious allergic reactions have been reported. Use caution with porphyria, exacerbation of porphyria has been reported (rarely) in patients with chronic renal failure. Some products may contain albumin. Multidose vials contain benzyl alcohol; do not use in premature infants. Safety and efficacy in children <1 month of age have not been established.

Adverse Reactions

>10%:

Cardiovascular: Hypertension (5% to 24%), thrombotic/vascular events (coronary artery bypass graft surgery: 23%), edema (6% to 17%), deep vein thrombosis (3% to 11%)

Central nervous system: Fever (29% to 51%), dizziness (<7% to 21%), insomnia (13% to 21%), headache (10% to 19%)

Dermatologic: Pruritus (14% to 22%), skin pain (4% to 18%), rash (≤16%)

Gastrointestinal: Nausea (11% to 58%), constipation (42% to 53%), vomiting (8% to 29%), diarrhea (9% to 21%), dyspepsia (7% to 11%)

Genitourinary: Urinary tract infection (3% to 12%)

Local: Injection site reaction (<10% to 29%)

Neuromuscular & skeletal: Arthralgia (11%), paresthesia (11%)

Respiratory: Cough (18%), congestion (15%), dyspnea (13% to 14%), upper respiratory infection (11%)

1% to 10%:

Central nervous system: Seizure (1% to 3%)

Local: Clotted vascular access (7%)

<1% (Limited to important or life-threatening): Allergic reaction, anemia (severe; with or without other cytopenias), CVA, flu-like syndrome, hyperkalemia, hypersensitivity reactions, hypertensive encephalopathy, microvascular thrombosis, MI, myalgia, neutralizing antibodies, pulmonary embolism, pure red cell aplasia (PRCA), renal vein thrombosis, retinal artery thrombosis, tachycardia, temporal vein thrombosis, thrombophlebitis, thrombosis, TIA, urticaria

Drug Interactions

Avoid Concomitant Use There are no known interactions where it is recommended to avoid concomitant use.

Increased Effect/Toxicity There are no known significant interactions involving an increase in effect.

Decreased Effect There are no known significant interactions involving a decrease in effect.

Dosage Forms Excipient information presented when available (limited, particularly for generics); consult specific product labeling.

Injection, solution [preservative free]:

Epogen®, Procrit®: 2000 units/mL (1 mL); 3000 units/mL (1 mL); 4000 units/mL (1 mL); 10,000 units/mL (1 mL); 40,000 units/mL (1 mL) [contains human albumin]

Injection, solution [with preservative]:

Epogen®, Procrit®: 10,000 units/mL (2 mL); 20,000 units/mL (1 mL) [contains human albumin and benzyl alcohol]

References

Corwin HL, Gettinger A, Pearl RG, et al, "Efficacy of Recombinant Human Erythropoietin in Critically Ill Patients, A Randomized Controlled Trial," *JAMA*, 2002, 288:2827-35.

Dellinger RP, Levy MM, Carlet JM, et al, "Surviving Sepsis Campaign: International Guidelines for Management of Severe Sepsis and Septic Shock: 2008," *Intensive Care Med*, 2008, 34(1): 17-60. Available at http://www.survivingsepsis.org/system/files/images/2008_20International_20SSC_20-Guidelines_1_.pdf

Hebert PC, Wells G, Blajchman MA, et al, "A Multicenter, Randomized, Controlled Clinical Trial of Transfusion Requirements in Critical Care," *N Engl J Med*, 1999, 340(6):409-17.

National Kidney Foundation, "KDOQI Clinical Practice Guidelines and Clinical Practice Recommentaions for Anemia in Chronic Kidney Disease," *Am J Kidney Dis*, 2006, 47(5 Suppl 3):1-145. Available at http://www.kidney.org/professionals/KDOQI/guidelines_anemia/cpr31.htm. Accessed March 13, 2007.

◆ **Epogen®** *see* Epoetin Alfa *on page 500*

Epoprostenol (e poe PROST en ole)

Medication Safety Issues

High alert medication: The Institute for Safe Medication Practices (ISMP) includes this medication among its list of drugs which have a heightened risk of causing significant patient harm when used in error.

Related Information

Continuous Renal Replacement Therapy *on page 1557*

U.S. Brand Names Flolan®

Canadian Brand Names Flolan®

Index Terms Epoprostenol Sodium; PGI_2; PGX; Prostacyclin

Pharmacologic Category Prostacyclin; Prostaglandin; Vasodilator

Restrictions Orders for epoprostenol are distributed by two sources in the United States. Information on orders or reimbursement assistance may be obtained from either Accredo Health, Inc (1-800-935-6526) or TheraCom, Inc (1-877-356-5264).

Generic Available Yes

Use Treatment of idiopathic pulmonary arterial hypertension (IPAH); pulmonary hypertension associated with the scleroderma spectrum of disease (SSD) in NYHA Class III and Class IV patients who do not respond adequately to conventional therapy

Unlabeled/Investigational Use Acute vasodilator testing in pulmonary arterial hypertension (PAH)

Mechanism of Action Epoprostenol is also known as prostacyclin and PGI_2. It is a strong vasodilator of all vascular beds. In addition, it is a potent endogenous inhibitor of platelet aggregation. The reduction in platelet aggregation results from epoprostenol's activation of intracellular adenylate cyclase and the resultant increase in cyclic adenosine monophosphate concentrations within the platelets. Additionally, it is capable of decreasing thrombogenesis and platelet clumping in the lungs by inhibiting platelet aggregation.

Pharmacodynamics/Kinetics

Metabolism: Rapidly hydrolyzed; subject to some enzymatic degradation; forms one active metabolite and 13 inactive metabolites

Half-life elimination: 6 minutes

Excretion: Urine (84%); feces (4%)

Dosage I.V.: Children (unlabeled use) and Adults:

Pulmonary arterial hypertension (PAH): Initial: 1-2 ng/kg/minute, increase dose in increments of 1-2 ng/kg/minute every 15 minutes or longer until dose-limiting side effects are noted or tolerance limit to epoprostenol is observed. Significant patient variability in optimal dose exists. Maximum dose with chronic therapy has not been defined; however, doses as high as 195 ng/kg/minute have been described in children (Rosenzweig, 1999).

Note: The need for increased doses should be expected with chronic use; incremental increases occur more frequently during the first few months after the drug is initiated.

Dose adjustment:

Increase dose in 1-2 ng/kg/minute increments at intervals of at least 15 minutes if symptoms persist or recur following improvement. In clinical trials, dosing increases occurred at intervals of 24-48 hours.

Decrease dose in 2 ng/kg/minute decrements at intervals of at least 15 minutes in case of dose-limiting pharmacologic events. Avoid abrupt withdrawal or sudden large dose reductions.

Lung transplant: In patients receiving lung transplants, epoprostenol may be tapered after the initiation of cardiopulmonary bypass.

Acute vasodilator testing (unlabeled use; McLaughlin, 2009): Adults: Initial: 2 ng/kg/minute; increase dose in increments of 2 ng/kg/minute every 10-15 minutes; dosing range: 2-10 ng/kg/minute

Stability Prior to use, store vials at 15°C to 25°C (59°F to 77°F); do not freeze. Protect from light. Reconstitute only with provided sterile diluent. Following reconstitution, solution must be stored under refrigeration at 2°C to 8°C (36°F to 46°F) if not used immediately; do not freeze. Protect from light. Discard if refrigerated for >48 hours. See table on next page. During use, a single reservoir of solution may be used at room temperature for a total duration of 8 hours, or used with a cold pouch for administration up to 24 hours. Cold packs should be changed every 12 hours.

Preparation of Epoprostenol Infusion

Note: Only prepare with sterile diluent provided.	
To make 100 mL of solution with concentration:	**Directions**
3000 ng/mL	Dissolve one 0.5 mg vial with 5 mL supplied diluent, withdraw 3 mL, and add to a sufficient volume of supplied diluent to make a total of 100 mL.
5000 ng/mL	Dissolve one 0.5 mg vial with 5 mL supplied diluent, withdraw entire vial contents, and add to a sufficient volume of supplied diluent to make a total of 100 mL.
10,000 ng/mL	Dissolve two 0.5 mg vials each with 5 mL supplied diluent, withdraw entire vial contents, and add to a sufficient volume of supplied diluent to make a total of 100 mL.
15,000 ng/mL	Dissolve one 1.5 mg vial with 5 mL supplied diluent, withdraw entire vial contents, and add to a sufficient volume of supplied diluent to make a total of 100 mL.

Administration The ambulatory infusion pump should be small and lightweight, be able to adjust infusion rates in 2 ng/kg/minute increments, have occlusion, end of infusion, and low battery alarms, have ± 6% accuracy of the programmed rate, and have positive continuous or pulsatile pressure with intervals ≤3 minutes between pulses. The reservoir should be made of polyvinyl chloride, polypropylene, or glass. The infusion pump used in the most recent clinical trial was CADD-1 HFX 5100 (Pharmacia Deltec). Immediate access to back up pump, infusion sets and medication is essential to prevent treatment interruptions. Assess patient's and family's ability to manage a central venous catheter in the home setting. Clinicians should routinely review with patient the importance of infection control practices for the management of a central venous catheter (CVC). Guidelines related to the prevention of CVC-related blood stream infections have been published (Doran, 2008).

Monitoring Parameters Monitor for improvements in pulmonary function, decreased exertional dyspnea, fatigue, syncope and chest pain, pulmonary vascular resistance, pulmonary arterial pressure and quality of life. In addition, the pump device and catheters should be monitored frequently to avoid "system" related failure. Monitor arterial pressure; assess all vital functions. Hypoxia, flushing, and tachycardia may indicate overdose.

Pregnancy Risk Factor B

Contraindications Hypersensitivity to epoprostenol or to structurally-related compounds; chronic use in patients with heart failure due to severe left ventricular systolic dysfunction; patients who develop pulmonary edema during dose initiation

Warnings/Precautions Abrupt interruptions or large sudden reductions in dosage may result in rebound pulmonary hypertension; some patients with PAH have developed pulmonary edema during dosing adjustment and acute vasodilator testing (not an approved use), which may be associated with concomitant heart failure (LV systolic dysfunction with significantly elevated left heart filling pressures) or pulmonary veno-occlusive disease/pulmonary capillary hemangiomatosis. During chronic use, unless contraindicated, anticoagulants should be coadministered to reduce the risk of thromboembolism. Use cautiously in patients who have conditions that increase bleeding risk (inhibits platelet aggregation). Use with caution in patients receiving anticoagulants and antiplatelet agents. Chronic continuous I.V. infusion of epoprostenol via a chronic indwelling central venous catheter (CVC) has been associated with local infections and serious blood stream infections. Guidelines related to the prevention of CVC-related blood stream infections have been published (Doran, 2008). Clinical studies of epoprostenol in pulmonary hypertension did not include sufficient numbers of patients ≥65 years of age to substantiate its safety and efficacy in the geriatric population. As a result, in general, dose selection for an elderly patient should be cautious usually starting at the low end of the dosing range.

Adverse Reactions Note: Adverse events reported during dose initiation and escalation include flushing (58%), headache (49%), nausea/vomiting (32%), hypotension (16%), anxiety/nervousness/agitation (11%), chest pain (11%), dizziness, abdominal pain, bradycardia, musculoskeletal pain, dyspnea, back pain, diaphoresis, dyspepsia, hypoesthesia/paresthesia, and tachycardia are also reported. The following adverse events have been reported during chronic administration for IPAH. Although some may be related to the underlying disease state, anxiety, diarrhea, flu-like syndrome, flushing, headache, jaw pain, nausea, nervousness, and vomiting are clearly contributed to epoprostenol.

>10%:
  Cardiovascular: Chest pain (52% to 67%), palpitation (63%), tachycardia (35% to 43%), flushing (23% to 42%), arrhythmia (27%), bradycardia (15%), hypotension (13%)
  Central nervous system: Dizziness (83%), headache (46% to 83%), chills/fever/ sepsis/flu-like syndrome (13% to 25%), anxiety/nervousness/tremor (7% to 21%), depression/depression psychotic (13%)
  Dermatologic: Skin ulcer (39%), eczema/rash/urticaria (25%)
  Gastrointestinal: Nausea/vomiting (41% to 67%), anorexia (66%), diarrhea (37% to 50%), weight loss (27%)
  Hematologic: Hemorrhage (11% to 19%)
  Hepatic: Ascites (23%)
  Local: Injection site reactions: Infection (21%), pain (13%)
  Neuromuscular & skeletal: Weakness (87% to 100%), pain/neck pain/arthralgia (84%), jaw pain (54% to 75%), arthritis (52%), myalgia (44%), musculoskeletal pain (35%; predominantly involving legs and feet), back pain (13%), hypoesthesia/hyperparesthesia/paresthesia (5% to 12%)
  Respiratory: Dyspnea (90%)
  Miscellaneous: Diaphoresis (41%)
1% to 10%:
  Cardiovascular: Supraventricular tachycardia (8%), cerebrovascular accident (4%), MI (4%)
  Central nervous system: Insomnia (9%), seizure (4%), somnolence (4%)
  Dermatologic: Rash (10%), pruritus (4%)
  Endocrine & metabolic: Hypokalemia (6%), hyperkalemia (4%)
  Gastrointestinal: Abdominal pain (14%), constipation (4% to 6%), weight gain (6%), flatulence (5%), abdominal enlargement (4%)
  Genitourinary: Urinary tract infection (7%)
  Hematologic: Thrombocytopenia (4%)
  Ocular: Amblyopia (8%), vision abnormality (4%)
  Renal: Hematuria (5%)
  Respiratory: Epistaxis (4% to 9%), pleural effusion (4% to 7%), pharyngitis (5%), pneumonia (5%), pneumothorax (4%), pulmonary edema (4%)
<1% (Limited to important or life-threatening): Anemia, hepatic failure, hyper- splenism, hyperthyroidism, pancytopenia, pulmonary embolism, splenomegaly

Drug Interactions

Avoid Concomitant Use There are no known interactions where it is recommended to avoid concomitant use.

Increased Effect/Toxicity
Epoprostenol may increase the levels/effects of: Anticoagulants; Antihyperten- sives; Antiplatelet Agents

Decreased Effect There are no known significant interactions involving a decrease in effect.

Dosage Forms Excipient information presented when available (limited, particularly for generics); consult specific product labeling.
Injection, powder for reconstitution: 0.5 mg, 1.5 mg [provided with 50 mL sterile diluent]
  Flolan®: 0.5 mg, 1.5 mg

References
Badesch DB, Abman SH, Ahearn GS, et al, "Medical Therapy for Pulmonary Arterial Hypertension: ACCP Evidence-Based Clinical Practice Guideline," *Chest*, 2004, 126(1 Suppl):35-62.
Rosenzweig EB and Barst RJ, "Idiopathic Pulmonary Arterial Hypertension in Children," *Curr Opin Pediatr*, 2005, 17(3):372-80.

◆ **Epoprostenol Sodium** *see* Epoprostenol *on page 506*

◆ **Eprex® (Can)** *see* Epoetin Alfa *on page 500*

Eprosartan (ep roe SAR tan)

Related Information
Angiotensin Agents *on page 1652*
Heart Failure (Systolic) *on page 1739*
Preoperative Evaluation of the Cardiac Patient for Noncardiac Surgery *on page 1598*

U.S. Brand Names Teveten®
Canadian Brand Names Teveten®
Pharmacologic Category Angiotensin II Receptor Blocker
Use Treatment of hypertension; may be used alone or in combination with other antihypertensives

Pharmacodynamics/Kinetics
Protein binding: 98%
Metabolism: Minimally hepatic
Bioavailability: 300 mg dose: 13%
Half-life elimination: Terminal: 5-9 hours
Time to peak, serum: Fasting: 1-2 hours
Excretion: Feces (90%); urine (7%, mostly as unchanged drug)
Clearance: 7.9 L/hour

Dosage Adults: Oral: Dosage must be individualized; can administer once or twice daily with total daily doses of 400-800 mg. Usual starting dose is 600 mg once daily as monotherapy in patients who are euvolemic. Limited clinical experience with doses >800 mg.

Dosage adjustment in renal impairment: No starting dosage adjustment is necessary; however, carefully monitor the patient

Dosage adjustment in hepatic impairment: No starting dosage adjustment is necessary; however, carefully monitor the patient

Elderly: No starting dosage adjustment is necessary; however, carefully monitor the patient

Anesthesia and Critical Care Concerns/Other Considerations
Clinical Pearls/Comments: In patients on chronic angiotensin receptor blocker (ARB) therapy, intraoperative hypotension may occur with induction and maintenance of general anesthesia; however, discontinuation of therapy prior to surgery is controversial. If continued preoperatively, avoidance of hypotensive agents during surgery is prudent. Episodes of intraoperative hypotension may be managed by fluid administration and/or modest doses of alpha-adrenergic agents. Severe hypotension may occur in patients who are sodium- and/or volume-depleted; initiate lower doses and monitor closely when starting therapy in these patients. ARB therapy may elicit an increase in potassium and creatinine, especially when used in patients with bilateral renal artery stenosis. Concomitant NSAID therapy may attenuate blood pressure control; use of NSAIDs should be avoided or limited, with monitoring of blood pressure control. In the setting of heart failure, NSAID use may be associated with an increased risk for fluid accumulation and edema and therefore should be avoided.

Evidence-Based Information: The angiotensin II receptor antagonists appear to have similar indications as the ACE inhibitors. In heart failure, the angiotensin II antagonists are especially useful in providing an alternative therapy in those patients who have intractable cough in response to ACE inhibitor therapy. Candesartan has been studied as an alternative therapy in chronic heart failure patients who cannot tolerate an ACE-I (CHARM-Alternative) and as an added therapy in heart failure patients who are maintained on an ACE-I (CHARM-Added). In both studies, the combined endpoint of cardiovascular death or heart failure hospitalizations was significantly improved over the placebo-treated group.

Additional Information Complete prescribing information for this medication should be consulted for additional detail.

Dosage Forms Excipient information presented when available (limited, particularly for generics); consult specific product labeling.
Tablet: 400 mg, 600 mg

♦ **Epsilon Aminocaproic Acid** *see* Aminocaproic Acid *on page 83*
♦ **Epsom Salts** *see* Magnesium Sulfate *on page 863*

◆ **Eptacog Alfa (Activated)** *see* Factor VIIa (Recombinant) *on page 567*

Eptifibatide (ep TIF i ba tide)

Medication Safety Issues
High alert medication: The Institute for Safe Medication Practices (ISMP) includes this medication among its list of drugs which have a heightened risk of causing significant patient harm when used in error.

Related Information
Regional Anesthesia in Patients Receiving Anticoagulant and Antiplatelet Therapy *on page 1642*

U.S. Brand Names Integrilin®

Canadian Brand Names Integrilin®

Index Terms Intrifiban

Pharmacologic Category Antiplatelet Agent, Glycoprotein IIb/IIIa Inhibitor

Generic Available No

Use Treatment of patients with acute coronary syndrome (unstable angina/non-Q wave myocardial infarction [UA/NQMI]), including patients who are to be managed medically and those undergoing percutaneous coronary intervention (PCI including angioplasty, intracoronary stenting)

Mechanism of Action Eptifibatide is a cyclic heptapeptide which blocks the platelet glycoprotein IIb/IIIa receptor, the binding site for fibrinogen, von Willebrand factor, and other ligands. Inhibition of binding at this final common receptor reversibly blocks platelet aggregation and prevents thrombosis.

Pharmacodynamics/Kinetics
Onset of action: Within 1 hour

Duration: Platelet function restored ~4 hours following discontinuation

Protein binding: ~25%

Half-life elimination: 2.5 hours

Excretion: Primarily urine (as eptifibatide and metabolites); significant renal impairment may alter disposition of this compound

Clearance: Total body: 55-58 mL/kg/hour; Renal: ~50% of total in healthy subjects

Dosage I.V.: Adults:

Acute coronary syndrome: Bolus of 180 mcg/kg (maximum: 22.6 mg) over 1-2 minutes, begun as soon as possible following diagnosis, followed by a continuous infusion of 2 mcg/kg/minute (maximum: 15 mg/hour) until hospital discharge or initiation of CABG surgery, up to 72 hours. Concurrent aspirin and heparin therapy (target aPTT 50-70 seconds) are recommended.

Percutaneous coronary intervention (PCI) with or without stenting: Bolus of 180 mcg/kg (maximum: 22.6 mg) administered immediately before the initiation of PCI, followed by a continuous infusion of 2 mcg/kg/minute (maximum: 15 mg/hour). A second 180 mcg/kg bolus (maximum: 22.6 mg) should be administered 10 minutes after the first bolus. Infusion should be continued until hospital discharge or for up to 18-24 hours, whichever comes first. Concurrent aspirin (160-325 mg 1-24 hours before PCI and daily thereafter) and heparin therapy (ACT 200-300 seconds during PCI) are recommended. Heparin infusion after PCI is discouraged. In patients who undergo coronary artery bypass graft surgery, discontinue infusion prior to surgery.

Elderly: No dosing adjustment for the elderly appears to be necessary; adjust carefully to renal function.

Dosing adjustment in renal impairment: Dialysis is a contraindication to use.

Note: The Cockcroft-Gault equation using actual body weight should be used to estimate renal function.

Acute coronary syndrome: Cl_{cr} <50 mL/minute: Use 180 mcg/kg bolus (maximum: 22.6 mg) and 1 mcg/kg/minute infusion (maximum: 7.5 mg/hour)

Percutaneous coronary intervention (PCI) with or without stenting: Cl_{cr} <50 mL/minute: Use 180 mcg/kg bolus (maximum: 22.6 mg) administered immediately before the initiation of PCI and followed by a continuous infusion of 1 mcg/kg/minute (maximum: 7.5 mg/hour). A second 180 mcg/kg (maximum: 22.6 mg) bolus should be administered 10 minutes after the first bolus.

Stability Vials should be stored refrigerated at 2°C to 8°C (36°F to 46°F). Vials can ▶

be kept at room temperature for 2 months. Protect from light until administration. Do not use beyond the expiration date. Discard any unused portion left in the vial.

Administration Do not shake vial. Visually inspect for discoloration or particulate matter prior to administration. The bolus dose should be withdrawn from the 10 mL vial into a syringe and administered by I.V. push over 1-2 minutes. Begin continuous infusion immediately following bolus administration, administered directly from the 100 mL vial. The 100 mL vial should be spiked with a vented infusion set.

Monitoring Parameters Coagulation parameters, signs/symptoms of excessive bleeding. Laboratory tests at baseline and monitoring during therapy: hematocrit and hemoglobin, platelet count, serum creatinine, PT/aPTT (maintain aPTT between 50-70 seconds unless PCI is to be performed), and ACT with PCI (maintain ACT between 200-300 seconds during PCI).

Assess sheath insertion site and distal pulses of affected leg every 15 minutes for the first hour and then every 1 hour for the next 6 hours. Arterial access site care is important to prevent bleeding. Care should be taken when attempting vascular access that only the anterior wall of the femoral artery is punctured, avoiding a Seldinger (through and through) technique for obtaining sheath access. Femoral vein sheath placement should be avoided unless needed. While the vascular sheath is in place, patients should be maintained on complete bedrest with the head of the bed at a 30° angle and the affected limb restrained in a straight position.

Observe patient for mental status changes, hemorrhage, assess nose and mouth mucous membranes, puncture sites for oozing, ecchymosis and hematoma formation, and examine urine, stool and emesis for presence of occult or frank blood; gentle care should be provided when removing dressings.

Anesthesia and Critical Care Concerns/Other Considerations

Clinical Pearls/Comments: As a reversible inhibitor of the platelet glycoprotein (GP) IIb/IIIa receptor, eptifibatide has a short duration of action and hemostasis is restored within about 4 hours after discontinuation in patients with normal renal function.

Epifibatide-induced thrombocytopenia: Acute profound thrombocytopenia has been associated with eptifibatide use and may occur within 24 hours of initiation (Cheema, 2006; Coons, 2005; Nagge, 2003; Rezkalla, 2003; Salengro, 2003).

Platelet count monitoring is recommended 2-4 hours after initiation, and at 24 hours or prior to discharge, whichever is first. Specific management guidelines for GP IIb/IIIa induced thrombocytopenia have been published (Huxtable, 2006; Llevadot, 2000). Platelet counts should recover rapidly (within 1-5 days) after discontinuation of eptifibatide. Although sustained thrombocytopenia is less of a risk with eptifibatide compared to abciximab, the presence of active bleeding at any time, emergent invasive procedure, or a platelet level of <20,000 cells/microL should prompt the consideration of platelet transfusion.

Pregnancy Risk Factor B

Contraindications Hypersensitivity to eptifibatide or any component of the product; active abnormal bleeding or a history of bleeding diathesis within the previous 30 days; history of CVA within 30 days or a history of hemorrhagic stroke; severe hypertension (systolic blood pressure >200 mm Hg or diastolic blood pressure >110 mm Hg) not adequately controlled on antihypertensive therapy; major surgery within the preceding 6 weeks; current or planned administration of another parenteral GP IIb/IIIa inhibitor; thrombocytopenia; dependency on renal dialysis

Warnings/Precautions Bleeding is the most common complication. Most major bleeding occurs at the arterial access site where the cardiac catheterization was done. When bleeding can not be controlled with pressure, discontinue infusion and heparin. Use caution in patients with hemorrhagic retinopathy or with other drugs that affect hemostasis. Concurrent use with thrombolytics has not been established as safe. Minimize other procedures including arterial and venous punctures, I.M. injections, nasogastric tubes, etc. Prior to sheath removal, the aPTT or ACT should be checked (do not remove unless aPTT is <45 seconds or the ACT <150 seconds). Use caution in renal dysfunction (estimated Cl$_{cr}$ <50 mL/ minute); dosage adjustment required. Safety and efficacy in pediatric patients have not been determined.

Adverse Reactions Bleeding is the major drug-related adverse effect. Access site is often primary source of bleeding complications. Incidence of bleeding is also related to heparin intensity. Patients weighing <70 kg may have an increased risk of major bleeding.

>10%: Hematologic: Bleeding (major: 1% to 11%; minor: 3% to 14%; transfusion required: 2% to 13%)

1% to 10%:
Cardiovascular: Hypotension (up to 7%)
Hematologic: Thrombocytopenia (1% to 3%)
Local: Injection site reaction

<1% (Limited to important or life-threatening): Acute profound thrombocytopenia, anaphylaxis, fatal bleeding events, GI hemorrhage, intracranial hemorrhage (0.5% to 0.7%), pulmonary hemorrhage, stroke

Drug Interactions

Avoid Concomitant Use There are no known interactions where it is recommended to avoid concomitant use.

Increased Effect/Toxicity
Eptifibatide may increase the levels/effects of: Anticoagulants; Antiplatelet Agents; Drotrecogin Alfa; Ibritumomab; Salicylates; Thrombolytic Agents; Tositumomab and Iodine I 131 Tositumomab

The levels/effects of Eptifibatide may be increased by: Dasatinib; Herbs (Anticoagulant/Antiplatelet Properties); Nonsteroidal Anti-Inflammatory Agents; Omega-3-Acid Ethyl Esters; Pentosan Polysulfate Sodium; Pentoxifylline; Prostacyclin Analogues

Decreased Effect
The levels/effects of Eptifibatide may be decreased by: Nonsteroidal Anti-Inflammatory Agents

Ethanol/Nutrition/Herb Interactions Herb/Nutraceutical: Avoid alfalfa, anise, bilberry, bladderwrack, bromelain, cat's claw, celery, coleus, cordyceps, dong quai, evening primrose oil, fenugreek, feverfew, garlic, ginger, ginkgo biloba, ginseng (American), ginseng (Panax), ginseng (Siberian), grapeseed, green tea, guggul, horse chestnut seed, horseradish, licorice, prickly ash, red clover, reishi, same (s-adenosylmethionine), sweet clover, turmeric, and white willow (all have additional antiplatelet activity).

Dosage Forms Excipient information presented when available (limited, particularly for generics); consult specific product labeling.
Injection, solution: 0.75 mg/mL (100 mL); 2 mg/mL (10 mL, 100 mL)

References
Cheema AA, Teklinski AH, Maria V, et al, "Recurrent Acute Profound Thrombocytopenia Related to Readministration of Eptifibatide," *J Interv Cardiol*, 2006, 19(1):99-103.
Coons JC, Barcelona RA, Freedy T, et al, "Eptifibatide-Associated Acute, Profound Thrombocytopenia," *Ann Pharmacother*, 2005, 39(2):368-72.
Huxtable LM, Tafreshi MJ, and Rakkar AN, "Frequency and Management of Thrombocytopenia With the Glycoprotein IIb/IIIa Receptor Antagonists," *Am J Cardiol*, 2006, 97(3):426-9.
Llevadot J, Coulter SA, and Giugliano RP, "A Practical Approach to the Diagnosis and Management of Thrombocytopenia Associated With Glycoprotein IIb/IIIa Receptor Inhibitors," *J Thromb Thrombolysis*, 2000, 9(2):175-80.

◆ **Equetro®** *see* CarBAMazepine *on page 241*

◆ **Eraxis™** *see* Anidulafungin *on page 123*

Ertapenem (er ta PEN em)

Medication Safety Issues
Sound-alike/look-alike issues:
Ertapenem may be confused with imipenem, meropenem
Invanz® may be confused with Avinza™
U.S. Brand Names Invanz®
Canadian Brand Names Invanz®
Index Terms Ertapenem Sodium; L-749,345; MK0826

◀ **Pharmacologic Category** Antibiotic, Carbapenem
Generic Available No
Use Treatment of the following moderate-severe infections: Complicated intra-abdominal infections, complicated skin and skin structure infections (including diabetic foot infections without osteomyelitis), complicated UTI (including pyelonephritis), acute pelvic infections (including postpartum endomyometritis, septic abortion, post surgical gynecologic infections), and community-acquired pneumonia. Prophylaxis of surgical site infection following elective colorectal surgery. Antibacterial coverage includes aerobic gram-positive organisms, aerobic gram-negative organisms, anaerobic organisms.

Note: Methicillin-resistant *Staphylococcus*, *Enterococcus* spp, penicillin-resistant strains of *Streptococcus pneumoniae*, beta-lactamase-positive strains of *Haemophilus influenzae* are **resistant** to ertapenem, as are most *Pseudomonas aeruginosa*.

Mechanism of Action Inhibits bacterial cell wall synthesis by binding to one or more of the penicillin binding proteins; which in turn inhibits the final transpeptidation step of peptidoglycan synthesis in bacterial cell walls, thus inhibiting cell wall biosynthesis. Bacteria eventually lyse due to ongoing activity of cell wall autolytic enzymes (autolysins and murein hydrolases) while cell wall assembly is arrested.

Pharmacodynamics/Kinetics
Absorption: I.M.: Almost complete
Distribution: V_{dss}:
  Children 3 months to 12 years: ~0.2 L/kg
  Children 13-17 years: ~0.16 L/kg
  Adults: ~0.12 L/kg
Protein binding (concentration dependent, primarily to albumin): 85% at 300 mcg/mL, 95% at <100 mcg/mL
Metabolism: Non-CYP-mediated hydrolysis to inactive metabolite
Bioavailability: I.M.: ~90%
Half-life elimination:
  Children 3 months to 12 years: ~2.5 hours
  Children ≥13 years and Adults: ~4 hours
Time to peak: I.M.: ~2.3 hours
Excretion: Urine (~80% as unchanged drug and metabolite); feces (~10%)

Dosage Note: I.V. therapy may be administered for up to 14 days; I.M. therapy for up to 7 days

Usual dosage ranges:
  Children 3 months to 12 years: I.M., I.V.: 15 mg/kg twice daily (maximum: 1 g/day)
  Children ≥13 years and Adults: I.M., I.V.: 1 g/day

Indication-specific dosing:
  Children 3 months to 12 years: I.M., I.V.:
    Community-acquired pneumonia, complicated urinary tract infections (including pyelonephritis): 15 mg/kg twice daily (maximum: 1 g/day); duration of total antibiotic treatment: 10-14 days (**Note:** Duration includes possible switch to appropriate oral therapy after at least 3 days of parenteral treatment, once clinical improvement demonstrated.)
    Intra-abdominal infection: 15 mg/kg twice daily (maximum: 1 g/day) for 5-14 days
    Pelvic infections (acute): 15 mg/kg twice daily (maximum: 1 g/day) for 3-10 days
    Skin and skin structure infections: 15 mg/kg twice daily (maximum: 1 g/day) for 7-14 days
  Children ≥13 years and Adults: I.M., I.V.:
    Community-acquired pneumonia, complicated urinary tract infections (including pyelonephritis): 1 g/day; duration of total antibiotic treatment: 10-14 days (**Note:** Duration includes possible switch to appropriate oral therapy after at least 3 days of parenteral treatment, once clinical improvement demonstrated.)
    Intra-abdominal infection: 1 g/day for 5-14 days
    Pelvic infections (acute): 1 g/day for 3-10 days

Skin and skin structure infections (including diabetic foot infections): 1 g/ day for 7-14 days

Adults: I.V.: **Prophylaxis of surgical site following colorectal surgery:** 1 g given 1 hour preoperatively

Dosage adjustment in renal impairment:

Children: No data available for pediatric patients with renal insufficiency.

Adults:

Cl_{cr} >30 mL/minute/1.73 m^2: No adjustment required

Cl_{cr} ≤30 mL/minute/1.73 m^2 and ESRD: 500 mg/day

Hemodialysis: Adults: When the daily dose is given within 6 hours prior to hemodialysis, a supplementary dose of 150 mg is required following hemodialysis.

Dosage adjustment in hepatic impairment: Adjustments cannot be recommended (lack of experience and research in this patient population).

Stability Before reconstitution store at ≤25°C (77°F).

I.M.: Reconstitute 1 g vial with 3.2 mL of 1% lidocaine HCl injection (without epinephrine). Shake well. Use within 1 hour after preparation.

I.V.: Reconstitute 1 g vial with 10 mL of water for injection, 0.9% sodium chloride injection, or bacteriostatic water for injection. Shake well. For adults, transfer dose to 50 mL of 0.9% sodium chloride injection; for children, dilute dose with NS to a final concentration ≤20 mg/mL. Reconstituted I.V. solution may be stored at room temperature and must be used within 6 hours **or** refrigerated, stored for up to 24 hours and used within 4 hours after removal from refrigerator. Do not freeze.

Administration

I.M.: Avoid injection into a blood vessel. Make sure patient does not have an allergy to lidocaine or another anesthetic of the amide type. Administer by deep I.M. injection into a large muscle mass (eg, gluteal muscle or lateral part of the thigh). Do not administer I.M. preparation or drug reconstituted for I.M. administration intravenously.

I.V.: Infuse over 30 minutes

Monitoring Parameters Periodic renal, hepatic, and hematopoietic assessment during prolonged therapy; neurological assessment

Pregnancy Risk Factor B

Contraindications Hypersensitivity to ertapenem, other carbapenems, or any component of the formulation; anaphylactic reactions to beta-lactam antibiotics. If using intramuscularly, known hypersensitivity to local anesthetics of the amide type (lidocaine is the diluent).

Warnings/Precautions Use caution with renal impairment. Dosage adjustment required in patients with moderate-to-severe renal dysfunction; elderly patients often require lower doses (based upon renal function). Prolonged use may result in superinfection, including pseudomembranous colitis. Has been associated with CNS adverse effects, including confusional states and seizures; use caution with CNS disorders (eg, brain lesions, history of seizures, or renal impairment). Serious hypersensitivity reactions, including anaphylaxis, have been reported (some without a history of previous allergic reactions to beta-lactams). Doses for I.M. administration are mixed with lidocaine; consult Lidocaine on page 836 information for associated Warnings/Precautions. Safety and efficacy have not been established in children <3 months of age.

Adverse Reactions Note: Percentages reported in adults.

1% to 10%:

Cardiovascular: Swelling/edema (3%), chest pain (1% to 2%), hypertension (1% to 2%), hypotension (1% to 2%), tachycardia (1% to 2%)

Central nervous system: Headache (6% to 7%); altered mental status (eg, agitation, confusion, disorientation, decreased mental acuity, changed mental status, somnolence, stupor) (3% to 5%); fever (2% to 5%), insomnia (3%), dizziness (2%), fatigue (1%), anxiety (1%)

Dermatologic: Rash (2% to 3%), pruritus (1% to 2%), erythema (1% to 2%)

Endocrine & metabolic: Hypokalemia (2%), hyperglycemia (1% to 2%), hyperkalemia (≤1%)

Gastrointestinal: Diarrhea (9% to 10%), nausea (6% to 9%), abdominal pain (4%), vomiting (4%), constipation (3% to 4%), acid regurgitation (1% to 2%), dyspepsia (1%), oral candidiasis (≤1%)

◀ Genitourinary: Urine WBCs increased (2% to 3%), urine RBCs increased (1% to 3%), vaginitis (1% to 3%)

Hematologic: Platelet count increased (3% to 7%), hematocrit/hemoglobin decreased (3% to 5%), eosinophils increased (1% to 2%), leukopenia (1% to 2%), neutrophils decreased (1% to 2%), platelet count decreased (1%), prothrombin time increased (<1%)

Hepatic: Hepatic enzyme increased (5% to 9%), alkaline phosphatase increase (3% to 7%), albumin decreased (1% to 2%), bilirubin (total) increased (1% to 2%)

Local: Infused vein complications (5% to 7%), phlebitis/thrombophlebitis (2%), extravasation (1% to 2%)

Neuromuscular & skeletal: Weakness (1%), leg pain (≤1%)

Renal: Serum creatinine increased (1%)

Respiratory: Dyspnea (1% to 3%), cough (1% to 2%), pharyngitis (1%), rales/rhonchi (1%), respiratory distress (≤1%)

<1% (Limited to important or life-threatening): Abdominal distention, aggressive behavior, anaphylactoid reactions, anaphylaxis, anorexia, arrhythmia, asthma, asystole, atrial fibrillation, bicarbonate (serum) decreased, bilirubin (direct and indirect) increased, bladder dysfunction, bradycardia, bronchoconstriction, BUN increased, *C. difficile*-associated diarrhea, candidiasis, cardiac arrest, chills, cholelithiasis, dehydration, depression, dermatitis, desquamation, diaphoresis, duodenitis, dysphagia, epistaxis, epithelial (urine) cells increased, esophagitis, facial edema, flank pain, flatulence, flushing, gastritis, gastrointestinal hemorrhage, gout, hallucinations, heart failure, heart murmur, hematoma, hematuria, hemoptysis, hemorrhoids, hiccups, hypoesthesia, hypoxemia, ileus, injection site induration, injection site pain, jaundice, malaise, monocytes increased, mouth ulcer, muscle spasm, necrosis, nervousness, oliguria/anuria, pain, pancreatitis, paresthesia, pharyngeal discomfort, pleural effusion, pleuritic pain, pseudomembranous colitis, PTT increased, pyloric stenosis, renal insufficiency, seizure (0.5%), septicemia, septic shock, sodium (serum) increased, spasm, stomatitis, subdural hemorrhage, syncope, taste perversion, tremor, urinary retention, urticaria, vaginal candidiasis, vaginal pruritus, ventricular tachycardia, vertigo, voice disturbance, vulvovaginitis, weight loss

Drug Interactions

Avoid Concomitant Use There are no known interactions where it is recommended to avoid concomitant use.

Increased Effect/Toxicity

The levels/effects of Ertapenem may be increased by: Uricosuric Agents

Decreased Effect

Ertapenem may decrease the levels/effects of: Typhoid Vaccine; Valproic Acid

Dietary Considerations Some products may contain sodium.

Dosage Forms Excipient information presented when available (limited, particularly for generics); consult specific product labeling.

Injection, powder for reconstitution:

Invanz®: 1 g [contains sodium 137 mg/g (~6 mEq/g)]

◆ **Ertapenem Sodium** *see* Ertapenem *on page 513*

◆ **Erybid™ (Can)** *see* Erythromycin *on page 516*

◆ **Eryc® [DSC]** *see* Erythromycin *on page 516*

◆ **Eryc® (Can)** *see* Erythromycin *on page 516*

◆ **Eryderm® [DSC]** *see* Erythromycin *on page 516*

◆ **Erygel® [DSC]** *see* Erythromycin *on page 516*

◆ **EryPed®** *see* Erythromycin *on page 516*

◆ **Ery-Tab®** *see* Erythromycin *on page 516*

◆ **Erythrocin®** *see* Erythromycin *on page 516*

Erythromycin (er ith roe MYE sin)

Medication Safety Issues

Sound-alike/look-alike issues:

Erythromycin may be confused with azithromycin, clarithromycin, Ethmozine®

Akne-Mycin® may be confused with AK-Mycin®
E.E.S.® may be confused with DES®
Eryc® may be confused with Emcyt®, Ery-Tab®
Ery-Tab® may be confused with Eryc®
Erythrocin® may be confused with Ethmozine®

Related Information
Anesthesia for Patients With Liver Disease *on page 1537*
Management of Postoperative Arrhythmias *on page 1571*
Prevention of Wound Infection and Sepsis in Surgical Patients *on page 1721*

U.S. Brand Names Akne-Mycin®; E.E.S.®; Ery-Tab®; Eryc® [DSC]; Eryderm® [DSC]; Erygel® [DSC]; EryPed®; Erythro-RX; Erythrocin®; PCE®; Romycin®

Canadian Brand Names Apo-Erythro Base®; Apo-Erythro E-C®; Apo-Erythro-ES®; Apo-Erythro-S®; Diomycin®; EES®; Erybid™; Eryc®; Novo-Rythro Estolate; Novo-Rythro Ethylsuccinate; Nu-Erythromycin-S; PCE®; PMS-Erythromycin; Sans Acne®

Index Terms Erythromycin Base; Erythromycin Ethylsuccinate; Erythromycin Lactobionate; Erythromycin Stearate

Pharmacologic Category Acne Products; Antibiotic, Macrolide; Antibiotic, Ophthalmic; Antibiotic, Topical; Topical Skin Product; Topical Skin Product, Acne

Generic Available Yes: Capsule, gel, ophthalmic ointment, topical solution, suspension (as ethylsuccinate), swab, tablet (as base, ethylsuccinate, and stearate)

Use
Systemic: Treatment of susceptible bacterial infections including *S. pyogenes*, some *S. pneumoniae*, some *S. aureus*, *M. pneumoniae*, *Legionella pneumophila*, diphtheria, pertussis, *Chlamydia*, erythrasma, *N. gonorrhoeae*, *E. histolytica*, syphilis and nongonococcal urethritis, and *Campylobacter* gastroenteritis; used in conjunction with neomycin for decontaminating the bowel
Ophthalmic: Treatment of superficial eye infections involving the conjunctiva or cornea; neonatal ophthalmia
Topical: Treatment of acne vulgaris

Unlabeled/Investigational Use Systemic: Treatment of gastroparesis, chancroid; preoperative gut sterilization

Mechanism of Action Inhibits RNA-dependent protein synthesis at the chain elongation step; binds to the 50S ribosomal subunit resulting in blockage of transpeptidation

Pharmacodynamics/Kinetics
Absorption: Oral: Variable but better with salt forms than with base form; 18% to 45%; ethylsuccinate may be better absorbed with food
Distribution:
  Relative diffusion from blood into CSF: Minimal even with inflammation
  CSF:blood level ratio: Normal meninges: 2% to 13%; Inflamed meninges: 7% to 25%
Protein binding: Base: 73% to 81%
Metabolism: Demethylation primarily via hepatic CYP3A4
Half-life elimination: Peak: 1.5-2 hours; End-stage renal disease: 5-6 hours
Time to peak, serum: Base: 4 hours; Ethylsuccinate: 0.5-2.5 hours; delayed with food due to differences in absorption
Excretion: Primarily feces; urine (2% to 15% as unchanged drug)

Dosage Note: Due to differences in absorption, 400 mg erythromycin ethylsuccinate produces the same serum levels as 250 mg erythromycin base or stearate.

Usual dosage range:
Neonates: Ophthalmic: Prophylaxis of neonatal gonococcal or chlamydial conjunctivitis: 0.5-1 cm ribbon of ointment should be instilled into each conjunctival sac
Infants and Children:
  Oral:
    Base: 30-50 mg/kg/day in 2-4 divided doses; maximum: 2 g/day
    Ethylsuccinate: 30-50 mg/kg/day in 2-4 divided doses; maximum: 3.2 g/day
    Stearate: 30-50 mg/kg/day in 2-4 divided doses; maximum: 2 g/day
  I.V.: Lactobionate: 15-50 mg/kg/day divided every 6 hours, not to exceed 4 g/day

Children and Adults:
    Ophthalmic: Instill 1/2" (1.25 cm) 2-6 times/day depending on the severity of the infection
    Topical: Acne: Apply over the affected area twice daily after the skin has been thoroughly washed and patted dry
Adults:
    Oral:
        Base: 250-500 mg every 6-12 hours; maximum 4 g/day
        Ethylsuccinate: 400-800 mg every 6-12 hours; maximum: 4 g/day
    I.V.: Lactobionate: 15-20 mg/kg/day divided every 6 hours or 500 mg to 1 g every 6 hours, or given as a continuous infusion over 24 hours; maximum: 4 g/24 hours

Indication-specific dosing:
Children:
    ***Bartonella sp* infections (bacillary angiomatosis [BA], peliosis hepatis [PH]) (unlabeled use):** Oral: 40 mg/kg/day (ethylsuccinate) in 4 divided doses (maximum: 2 g/day) for 3 months (BA) or 4 months (PH)
    Conjunctivitis, neonatal *(C. trachomatis):* Oral: 50 mg/kg/day (base or ethylsuccinate) in 4 divided doses for 14 days
    Mild/moderate infection: Oral: 30-50 mg/kg/day in divided doses every 6-12 hours
    Pertussis: Oral: 40-50 mg/kg/day in 4 divided doses for 14 days; maximum 2 g/day (not preferred agent for infants <1 month due to IHPS)
    Pharyngitis, tonsillitis (streptococcal): Oral: 20 mg (base)/kg/day or 40 mg (ethylsuccinate)/kg/day in 2 divided doses for 10 days. **Note:** No longer preferred therapy due to increased organism resistance.
    Pneumonia *(C. trachomatis):* Oral: 50 mg/kg/day (base or ethylsuccinate) in 4 divided doses for 14-21 days
    Preop bowel preparation: Oral: 20 mg (base)/kg at 1, 2, and 11 PM on the day before surgery combined with mechanical cleansing of the large intestine and oral neomycin
    Severe infection: I.V.: 15-50 mg/kg/day; maximum: 4 g/day
Adults:
    ***Bartonella sp* infections (bacillary angiomatosis [BA], peliosis hepatis [PH]) (unlabeled use):** Oral: 500 mg (base) 4 times/day for 3 months (BA) or 4 months (PH)
    Chancroid (unlabeled use): Oral: 500 mg (base) 3 times/day for 7 days; Note: Not a preferred agent; isolates with intermediate resistance have been documented
    Gastrointestinal prokinetic (unlabeled use): I.V.: 200 mg initially followed by 250 mg (base) orally 3 times/day 30 minutes before meals. Lower dosages have been used in some trials.
    Granuloma inguinale *(K. granulomatis)* (unlabeled use): Oral: 500 mg (base) 4 times/day for 21 days
    Legionnaires' disease: Oral: 1.6-4 g (ethylsuccinate)/day or 1-4 g (base)/day in divided doses for 21 days. **Note:** No longer preferred therapy and only used in nonhospitalized patients.
    Lymphogranuloma venereum: Oral: 500 mg (base) 4 times/day for 21 days
    Nongonococcal urethritis (including coinfection with *C. trachomatis):* Oral: 500 mg (base) 4 times/day for 7 days or 800 mg (ethylsuccinate) 4 times/day for 7 days. **Note:** May use 250 mg (base) or 400 mg (ethylsuccinate) 4 times/day for 14 days if gastrointestinal intolerance.
    Pelvic inflammatory disease: I.V.: 500 mg every 6 hours for 3 days, followed by 1000 mg (base)/day orally in 2-4 divided doses for 7 days. **Note:** Not recommended therapy per current treatment guidelines.
    Pertussis: Oral: 500 mg (base) every 6 hours for 14 days
    Preop bowel preparation (unlabeled use): Oral: 1 g erythromycin base at 1, 2, and 11 PM on the day before surgery combined with mechanical cleansing of the large intestine and oral neomycin
    Syphilis, primary: Oral: 48-64 g (ethylsuccinate) or 30-40 g (base) in divided doses over 10-15 days. **Note:** Not recommended therapy per current treatment guidelines.

Dosage adjustment in renal impairment: Dialysis: Slightly dialyzable (5% to 20%); no supplemental dosage necessary in hemo- or peritoneal dialysis or in continuous arteriovenous or venovenous hemofiltration

Stability

Injection:

Store unreconstituted vials at 15°C to 30°C (59°F to 86°F). Erythromycin lactobionate should be reconstituted with sterile water for injection without preservatives to avoid gel formation. The reconstituted solution is stable for 2 weeks when refrigerated or for 8 hours at room temperature.

Erythromycin I.V. infusion solution is stable at pH 6-8. Stability of lactobionate is pH dependent. I.V. form has the longest stability in 0.9% sodium chloride (NS) and should be prepared in this base solution whenever possible. Do not use D_5W as a diluent unless sodium bicarbonate is added to solution. If I.V. must be prepared in D_5W, 0.5 mL of the 8.4% sodium bicarbonate solution should be added per each 100 mL of D_5W.

Stability of parenteral admixture at room temperature (25°C) and at refrigeration temperature (4°C) is 24 hours.

Standard diluent: 500 mg/250 mL D_5W/NS; 750 mg/250 mL D_5W/NS; 1 g/250 mL D_5W/NS.

Oral suspension:

Granules: Prior to mixing, store at <30°C (<86°F). After mixing, store under refrigeration and use within 10 days.

Powder: Refrigerate to preserve taste. Erythromycin ethylsuccinate may be stored at room temperature if used within 14 days. EryPed® drops should be used within 35 days following reconstitution. May store at room temperature or under refrigeration.

Tablet and capsule formulations: Store at <30°C (<86°F).

Topical and ophthalmic formulations: Store at room temperature.

Administration

Oral: Do not crush enteric coated drug product. GI upset, including diarrhea, is common. May be administered with food to decrease GI upset. Do not give with milk or acidic beverages.

I.V.: Infuse 1 g over 20-60 minutes. I.V. infusion may be very irritating to the vein. If phlebitis/pain occurs with used dilution, consider diluting further (eg, 1:5) if fluid status of the patient will tolerate, or consider administering in larger available vein. The addition of lidocaine or bicarbonate does not decrease the irritation of erythromycin infusions.

Ophthalmic: Avoid contact of tip of ophthalmic ointment tube with affected eye

Anesthesia and Critical Care Concerns/Other Considerations

Clinical Pearls/Comments: Erythromycin, when used with drugs that affect the QT interval (eg, cisapride, ergot derivatives, pimozide) or when administered to patients with a prolonged QT interval, may further increase the QT interval and the risk of torsade de pointes (proarrhythmias).

Pregnancy Risk Factor B

Contraindications Hypersensitivity to erythromycin or any component of the formulation

Systemic: Concomitant use with pimozide or cisapride

Warnings/Precautions Systemic: Use caution with hepatic impairment with or without jaundice has occurred, it may be accompanied by malaise, nausea, vomiting, abdominal colic, and fever; discontinue use if these occur. Use caution with other medication relying on CYP3A4 metabolism; high potential for drug interactions exists. Prolonged use may result in fungal or bacterial superinfection, including *C. difficile*-associated diarrhea (CDAD) and pseudomembranous colitis; CDAD has been observed >2 months postantibiotic treatment. Use in infants has been associated with infantile hypertrophic pyloric stenosis (IHPS). Macrolides have been associated with rare QT_c prolongation and ventricular arrhythmias, including torsade de pointes. Use caution in elderly patients, as risk of adverse events may be increased. Use caution in myasthenia gravis patients; erythromycin may aggravate muscular weakness.

Adverse Reactions Frequency not defined. Incidence may vary with formulation.

Systemic:

Cardiovascular: QT_c prolongation, torsade de pointes, ventricular arrhythmia, ventricular tachycardia

Central nervous system: Seizure

◀

Dermatitis: Pruritus, rash

Gastrointestinal: Abdominal pain, anorexia, diarrhea, infantile hypertrophic pyloric stenosis, nausea, oral candidiasis, pancreatitis, pseudomembranous colitis, vomiting

Hepatic: Cholestatic jaundice (most common with estolate), hepatitis, liver function tests abnormal

Local: Phlebitis at the injection site, thrombophlebitis

Neuromuscular & skeletal: Weakness

Otic: Hearing loss

Miscellaneous: Allergic reactions, anaphylaxis, hypersensitivity reactions, urticaria

Topical: 1% to 10%: Dermatologic: Erythema, desquamation, dryness, pruritus

Drug Interactions

Metabolism/Transport Effects Substrate of CYP2B6 (minor), 3A4 (major); **Inhibits** CYP1A2 (weak), 3A4 (moderate)

Avoid Concomitant Use

Avoid concomitant use of Erythromycin with any of the following: Artemether; Cisapride; Dabigatran Etexilate; Disopyramide; Dronedarone; Everolimus; Lincosamide Antibiotics; Lumefantrine; Nilotinib; Pimozide; QuiNINE; Silodosin; Tetrabenazine; Thioridazine; Tolvaptan; Topotecan; Ziprasidone

Increased Effect/Toxicity

Erythromycin may increase the levels/effects of: Alfentanil; Antifungal Agents (Azole Derivatives, Systemic); Antineoplastic Agents (Vinca Alkaloids); Benzodiazepines (metabolized by oxidation); BusPIRone; Calcium Channel Blockers; CarBAMazepine; Cardiac Glycosides; Cilostazol; Cisapride; Clozapine; Colchicine; Corticosteroids (Systemic); CycloSPORINE; CYP3A4 Substrates; Dabigatran Etexilate; Disopyramide; Dronedarone; Eletriptan; Eplerenone; Ergot Derivatives; Everolimus; FentaNYL; Fexofenadine; HMG-CoA Reductase Inhibitors; P-Glycoprotein Substrates; Phosphodiesterase 5 Inhibitors; Pimecrolimus; Pimozide; QTc-Prolonging Agents; QuiNIDine; QuiNINE; Repaglinide; Rifamycin Derivatives; Rivaroxaban; Salmeterol; Saxagliptin; Selective Serotonin Reuptake Inhibitors; Silodosin; Sirolimus; Tacrolimus; Temsirolimus; Tetrabenazine; Theophylline Derivatives; Thioridazine; Tolvaptan; Topotecan; Vitamin K Antagonists; Ziprasidone; Zopiclone

The levels/effects of Erythromycin may be increased by: Alfuzosin; Antifungal Agents (Azole Derivatives, Systemic); Artemether; Chloroquine; Ciprofloxacin; CYP3A4 Inhibitors (Moderate); CYP3A4 Inhibitors (Strong); Gadobutrol; Lumefantrine; Nilotinib; P-Glycoprotein Inhibitors; QuiNINE

Decreased Effect

Erythromycin may decrease the levels/effects of: Clopidogrel; Typhoid Vaccine; Zafirlukast

The levels/effects of Erythromycin may be decreased by: CYP3A4 Inducers (Strong); Deferasirox; Etravirine; Herbs (CYP3A4 Inducers); Lincosamide Antibiotics; P-Glycoprotein Inducers

Ethanol/Nutrition/Herb Interactions

Ethanol: Avoid ethanol (may decrease absorption of erythromycin or enhance ethanol effects).

Food: Erythromycin serum levels may be altered if taken with food (formulation-dependent).

Herb/Nutraceutical: St John's wort may decrease erythromycin levels.

Test Interactions False-positive urinary catecholamines

Dietary Considerations

Systemic: Drug may cause GI upset; may take with food.

Some products may contain sodium.

Dosage Forms Excipient information presented when available (limited, particularly for generics); consult specific product labeling. [DSC] = Discontinued product; [CAN] = Canadian brand name

Note: Strength expressed as base

Capsule, delayed release, enteric-coated pellets, as base: 250 mg

Eryc® 250 mg [DSC]

Gel, topical: 2% (30 g, 60 g)

Erygel® 2% (30 g, 60 g) [DSC] [contains alcohol 92%]

Granules for oral suspension, as ethylsuccinate:
E.E.S.®: 200 mg/5 mL (100 mL, 200 mL) [contains sodium 25.9 mg (1.1 mEq)/5 mL; cherry flavor]
Injection, powder for reconstitution, as lactobionate:
Erythrocin®: 500 mg, 1 g
Ointment, ophthalmic: 0.5% [5 mg/g] (1 g, 3.5 g)
Romycin®: 0.5% [5 mg/g] (3.5 g)
Ointment, topical:
Akne-Mycin®: 2% (25 g)
Powder for oral suspension, as ethylsuccinate:
EryPed®: 200 mg/5 mL (100 mL, 200 mL [DSC]) [contains sodium 117.5 mg (5.1 mEq)/5 mL; fruit flavor]; 400 mg/5 mL (100 mL, 200 mL [DSC]) [contains sodium 117.5 mg (5.1 mEq)/5 mL; banana flavor]
Powder for oral suspension, as ethylsuccinate [drops]:
EryPed®: 100 mg/2.5 mL (50 mL) [DSC] [contains sodium 58.8 mg (2.6 mEq)/dropperful; fruit flavor]
Powder, for prescription compounding:
Erythro-RX: USP (50 g)
Solution, topical: 2% (60 mL)
Eryderm®: 2% (60 mL) [contain alcohol] [DSC]
Sans acne [CAN]: 2% (60 mL) [contains ethyl alcohol 44%; not available in U.S.]
Suspension, oral, as ethylsuccinate: 200 mg/5 mL (480 mL) [DSC]; 400 mg/5 mL (480 mL) [DSC]
E.E.S.®: 200 mg/5 mL (100 mL, 480 mL) [fruit flavor] [DSC]; 400 mg/5 mL (100 mL, 480 mL) [orange flavor]
Tablet, as base: 250 mg, 500 mg
Tablet, as base [polymer-coated particles]:
PCE®: 333 mg, 500 mg
Tablet, as ethylsuccinate: 400 mg
E.E.S.®: 400 mg [DSC]
Tablet, as stearate: 250 mg, 500 mg
Erythrocin®: 250 mg, 500 mg
Tablet, delayed release, enteric coated, as base:
Ery-Tab®: 250 mg, 333 mg, 500 mg

References

"Antimicrobial Prophylaxis for Surgery," *Treat Guidel Med Lett*, 2004, 2(20):27-32.

MacLaren R, Kiser TH, Fish DN, et al, "Erythromycin vs Metoclopramide for Facilitating Gastric Emptying and Tolerance to Intragastric Nutrition in Critically Ill Patients," *JPEN J Parenter Enteral Nutr*, 2008, 32(4):412-9.

Nguyen NQ, Chapman MJ, Fraser RJ, et al, "Erythromycin Is More Effective Than Metoclopramide in the Treatment of Feed Intolerance in Critical Illness," *Crit Care Med*, 2007, 35(2):483-9.

Nguyen NQ, Chapman M, Fraser RJ, et al, "Prokinetic Therapy for Feed Intolerance in Critical Illness: One Drug or Two?" *Crit Care Med*, 2007, 35(11):2561-7.

◆ **Erythromycin Base** *see Erythromycin on page 516*

◆ **Erythromycin Ethylsuccinate** *see Erythromycin on page 516*

◆ **Erythromycin Lactobionate** *see Erythromycin on page 516*

◆ **Erythromycin Stearate** *see Erythromycin on page 516*

◆ **Erythropoiesis-Stimulating Agent (ESA)** *see Darbepoetin Alfa on page 375*

◆ **Erythropoiesis-Stimulating Agent (ESA)** *see Epoetin Alfa on page 500*

◆ **Erythropoiesis-Stimulating Protein** *see Darbepoetin Alfa on page 375*

◆ **Erythropoietin** *see Epoetin Alfa on page 500*

◆ **Erythro-RX** *see Erythromycin on page 516*

Escitalopram (es sye TAL oh pram)

Related Information
Antidepressant Agents *on page 1660*
U.S. Brand Names Lexapro®
Canadian Brand Names Cipralex®
Index Terms Escitalopram Oxalate; Lu-26-054; S-Citalopram
Pharmacologic Category Antidepressant, Selective Serotonin Reuptake Inhibitor

◄ **Use** Treatment of major depressive disorder; generalized anxiety disorders (GAD)

Unlabeled/Investigational Use Treatment of mild dementia-associated agitation in nonpsychotic patients

Pharmacodynamics/Kinetics

Onset of action: Depression: The onset of action is within a week; however, individual response varies greatly and full response may not be seen until 8-12 weeks after initiation of treatment.

Protein binding: ~56% to plasma proteins

Metabolism: Hepatic via CYP2C19 and 3A4 to an active metabolite, S-desmethylcitalopram (S-DCT; 1/7 the activity of escitalopram); S-DCT is metabolized to S-didesmethylcitalopram (S-DDCT; active; 1/27 the activity of escitalopram) via CYP2D6

Half-life elimination: Escitalopram: 27-32 hours; S-DCT: 59 hours

Time to peak: Escitalopram: ~5 hours; S-DCT: 14 hours

Excretion: Urine (Escitalopram: 8%; S-DCT: 10%)

Dosage Oral:

Children ≥12 years: Major depressive disorder: Initial: 10 mg once daily; dose may be increased to 20 mg once daily after at least 3 weeks

Adults: Major depressive disorder, generalized anxiety disorder: Initial: 10 mg once daily; dose may be increased to 20 mg once daily after at least 1 week

Elderly: 10 mg once daily

Dosage adjustment in renal impairment:

Mild-to-moderate impairment: No dosage adjustment needed

Severe impairment: Cl_{cr} <20 mL/minute: Use with caution

Dosage adjustment in hepatic impairment: 10 mg once daily

Additional Information Complete prescribing information for this medication should be consulted for additional detail.

Dosage Forms Excipient information presented when available (limited, particularly for generics); consult specific product labeling.

Solution, oral:

Lexapro®: 1 mg/mL (240 mL) [contains propylene glycol; peppermint flavor]

Tablet:

Lexapro®: 5 mg, 10 mg, 20 mg

Note: Cipralex® [CAN] is available only in 10 mg and 20 mg strengths.

References

Bernard L, Stern R, Lew D, et al, "Serotonin Syndrome After Concomitant Treatment With Linezolid and Citalopram," *Clin Infect Dis*, 2003, 36(9):1197.

Boyer EW and Shannon M, "The Serotonin Syndrome," *N Engl J Med*, 2005, 352:1112-20.

Chambers CD, Hernandez-Diaz S, Van Marter LJ, et al, "Selective Serotonin-Reuptake Inhibitors and Risk of Persistent Pulmonary Hypertension of the Newborn," *N Engl J Med*, 2006, 354(6):579-87.

Mahlberg R, Kunz D, Sasse J, et al, "Serotonin Syndrome With Tramadol and Citalopram," *Am J Psychiatry*, 2004, 161(6):1129.

Mokhlesi B, Leikin JB, Murray P, et al, "Adult Toxicology in Critical Care: Part II: Specific Poisonings," *Chest*, 2003, 123(3):897-922.

Montgomery SA, Loft H, Sanchez C, et al, "Escitalopram (S-Enantiomer of Citalopram): Clinical Efficacy and Onset of Action Predicted From a Rat Model," *Pharmacol Toxicol*, 2001, 88(5):282-6.

Pass SE and Simpson RW, "Discontinuation and Reinstitution of Medications During the Perioperative Period," *Am J Health Syst Pharm*, 2004, 61(9):899-912.

Tahir N, "Serotonin Syndrome as a Consequence of Drug-Resistant Infections: An Interaction Between Linezolid and Citalopram, *J Am Med Dir Assoc*, 2004, 5(2):111-3.

Von Moltke LL, Greenblatt DJ, Giancarlo GM, et al, "Escitalopram (S-Citalopram) and its Metabolites *in vitro*: Cytochromes Mediating Biotransformation, Inhibitory Effects, and Comparison to R-Citalopram," *Drug Metab Dispos*, 2001, 29(8):1102-9.

◆ **Escitalopram Oxalate** *see* Escitalopram *on page 521*

◆ **Eserine® (Can)** *see* Physostigmine *on page 1127*

◆ **Eserine Salicylate** *see* Physostigmine *on page 1127*

◆ **Eskalith** *see* Lithium *on page 851*

Esmolol (ES moe lol)

Medication Safety Issues

Sound-alike/look-alike issues:

Esmolol may be confused with Osmitrol®

Brevibloc® may be confused with bretylium, Brevital®, Bumex®, Buprenex®

High alert medication: The Institute for Safe Medication Practices (ISMP) includes this medication among its list of drugs which have a heightened risk of causing significant patient harm when used in error.

Related Information

Anesthesia Considerations for Neurosurgery *on page 1514*
Anesthesia for Patients With Liver Disease *on page 1537*
Anesthetic Considerations in the Substance-Abusing Patient *on page 1613*
Antiarrhythmic Drugs *on page 1656*
Beta-Blockers *on page 1669*
Chronic Renal Failure *on page 1552*
Dosing Considerations for the Critically-Ill Patient With Morbid Obesity *on page 1561*
Extravasation Treatment of Drugs *on page 1789*
Hypertension *on page 1754*
Management of Postoperative Arrhythmias *on page 1571*
Postoperative Hypertension *on page 1589*

U.S. Brand Names Brevibloc®

Canadian Brand Names Brevibloc®

Index Terms Esmolol Hydrochloride

Pharmacologic Category Antiarrhythmic Agent, Class II; Beta Blocker, Beta$_1$ Selective

Generic Available Yes: Excludes infusion

Use Treatment of supraventricular tachycardia (SVT) and atrial fibrillation/flutter (control ventricular rate); treatment of tachycardia and/or hypertension; treatment of noncompensatory sinus tachycardia

Unlabeled/Investigational Use In children, for SVT and postoperative hypertension

Mechanism of Action Class II antiarrhythmic: Competitively blocks response to beta$_1$-adrenergic stimulation with little or no effect of beta$_2$-receptors except at high doses, no intrinsic sympathomimetic activity, no membrane stabilizing activity

Pharmacodynamics/Kinetics

Onset of action: Beta-blockade: I.V.: 2-10 minutes (quickest when loading doses are administered)

Duration of hemodynamic effects: 10-30 minutes; prolonged following higher cumulative doses, extended duration of use

Distribution: V_d: Esmolol ~3.4 L/kg; Acid metabolite ~0.4 L/kg

Protein binding: Esmolol 55%; Acid metabolite 10%

Metabolism: In blood by red blood cell esterases; forms acid metabolite (negligible activity; produces no clinically important effects) and methanol (does not achieve concentrations associated with methanol toxicity)

Half-life elimination: Adults: Esmolol: 9 minutes; Acid metabolite: 3.7 hours; elimination of metabolite decreases with end-stage renal disease

Excretion: Urine (~69% as metabolites, 2% unchanged drug)

Dosage I.V. infusion requires an infusion pump (must be adjusted to individual response and tolerance):

Children:

SVT (unlabeled use): A limited amount of information regarding esmolol use in pediatric patients is currently available. Some centers have utilized doses of 100-500 mcg/kg given over 1 minute for control of supraventricular tachycardias.

Postoperative hypertension (unlabeled use): Loading doses of 500 mcg/kg/minute over 1 minute with maximal doses of 50-250 mcg/kg/minute (mean = 173) have been used in addition to nitroprusside to treat postoperative hypertension after coarctation of aorta repair.

Adults:

Intraoperative tachycardia and/or hypertension (immediate control): Initial bolus: 80 mg (~1 mg/kg) over 30 seconds, followed by a 150 mcg/kg/minute infusion, if necessary. Adjust infusion rate as needed to maintain desired heart rate and/or blood pressure, up to 300 mcg/kg/minute.

For control of postoperative hypertension, as many as one-third of patients may require higher doses (250-300 mcg/kg/minute) to control blood pressure; the safety of doses >300 mcg/kg/minute has not been studied.

◀ Supraventricular tachycardia or gradual control of postoperative tachycardia/ hypertension: Loading dose: 500 mcg/kg over 1 minute; follow with a 50 mcg/ kg/minute infusion for 4 minutes; response to this initial infusion rate may be a rough indication of the responsiveness of the ventricular rate.

Infusion may be continued at 50 mcg/kg/minute or, if the response is inadequate, titrated upward in 50 mcg/kg/minute increments (increased no more frequently than every 4 minutes) to a maximum of 200 mcg/kg/minute.

To achieve more rapid response, following the initial loading dose and 50 mcg/ kg/minute infusion, rebolus with a second 500 mcg/kg loading dose over 1 minute, and increase the maintenance infusion to 100 mcg/kg/minute for 4 minutes. If necessary, a third (and final) 500 mcg/kg loading dose may be administered, prior to increasing to an infusion rate of 150 mcg/kg/minute. After 4 minutes of the 150 mcg/kg/minute infusion, the infusion rate may be increased to a maximum rate of 200 mcg/kg/minute (without a bolus dose).

Usual dosage range (SVT): 50-200 mcg/kg/minute with average dose of 100 mcg/kg/minute.

Guidelines for transfer to oral therapy (beta-blocker, calcium channel blocker):

Infusion should be reduced by 50% 30 minutes following the first dose of the alternative agent

Manufacturer suggests following the second dose of the alternative drug, patient's response should be monitored and if control is adequate for the first hours, esmolol may be discontinued.

Dialysis: Not removed by hemo- or peritoneal dialysis; supplemental dose is not necessary.

Stability Clear, colorless to light yellow solution which should be stored at 25°C (77°F); do not freeze. Protect from excessive heat.

Stability of parenteral admixture at room temperature (25°C) is 24 hours.

Administration Infusions must be administered with an infusion pump. Concentrations >10 mg/mL or infusion into small veins or through a butterfly catheter should be avoided (can cause thrombophlebitis). Decrease or discontinue infusion if hypotension or congestive heart failure occur. Medication port of premixed bags should be used to withdraw only the initial bolus, if necessary (not to be used for withdrawal of additional bolus doses).

Monitoring Parameters Blood pressure, heart rate, MAP, ECG, respiratory rate, I.V. site; cardiac monitor and blood pressure monitor required

Anesthesia and Critical Care Concerns/Other Considerations

This agent is also used to blunt sympathetic response during intubation, in "at-risk" patients such as those with coronary artery disease (CAD), angina, uncontrolled hypertension, and hyperthyroidism. Esmolol may lose cardio-selection (beta$_1$ specificity) at higher doses. It should be used with caution in patients with bronchospastic pulmonary disease and diabetes. Esmolol may mask the signs of light anesthesia.

Esmolol provides an important mechanism for close titration of rate control in patients with atrial fibrillation; may also be useful in achieving blood pressure control. Esmolol should only be administered with hemodynamic monitoring. Potential adverse effects include hypotension and bradyarrhythmias (usually short-lived due to short half-life of 9 minutes).

Pregnancy Risk Factor C (manufacturer); D (2nd and 3rd trimesters - expert analysis)

Contraindications Hypersensitivity to esmolol or any component of the formulation; sinus bradycardia; heart block greater than first degree (except in patients with a functioning artificial pacemaker); cardiogenic shock; bronchial asthma (relative); uncompensated cardiac failure; hypotension; pregnancy (2nd and 3rd trimesters)

Warnings/Precautions Consider pre-existing conditions such as sick sinus syndrome before initiating. Hypotension is common; patients need close blood pressure monitoring. Administer cautiously in compensated heart failure and monitor for a worsening of the condition. Use caution in patients with PVD (can aggravate arterial insufficiency). Use caution with concurrent use of beta-blockers and either verapamil or diltiazem; bradycardia or heart block can occur. Use beta-blockers cautiously in patients with bronchospastic disease; monitor pulmonary status closely. Use cautiously in patients with diabetes because it can mask prominent hypoglycemic symptoms. Use with caution in patients with myasthenia gravis and psychiatric disease (may cause CNS depression). Use caution in patients with renal dysfunction (active metabolite retained). Adequate alpha-blockade is required prior to use of any beta-blocker for patients with untreated pheochromocytoma. Use caution with history of severe anaphylaxis to allergens; patients taking beta-blockers may become more sensitive to repeated challenges. Treatment of anaphylaxis (eg, epinephrine) in patients taking beta-blockers may be ineffective or promote undesirable effects. Beta-blocker therapy should not be withdrawn abruptly (particularly in patients with CAD), but gradually tapered to avoid acute tachycardia, hypertension, and/or ischemia. Do not use in the treatment of hypertension associated with vasoconstriction related to hypo-thermia. Concentrations >10 mg/mL or infusion into small veins or through a butterfly catheter should be avoided (can cause thrombophlebitis). Extravasation can lead to skin necrosis and sloughing. Safety and efficacy have not been established in children.

Adverse Reactions

>10%:

Cardiovascular: Asymptomatic hypotension (dose related: 25% to 38%), symptomatic hypotension (dose related: 12%)

Miscellaneous: Diaphoresis (10%)

1% to 10%:

Cardiovascular: Peripheral ischemia (1%)

Central nervous system: Dizziness (3%), somnolence (3%), confusion (2%), headache (2%), agitation (2%), fatigue (1%)

Gastrointestinal: Nausea (7%), vomiting (1%)

Local: Pain on injection (8%), infusion site reaction

<1% (Limited to important or life-threatening): Alopecia, bronchospasm, chest pain, CHF, depression, dyspnea, edema, exfoliative dermatitis, heart block, infusion site reactions, paresthesia, pruritus, pulmonary edema, rigors, seizure, severe bradycardia/asystole (rare), skin necrosis (from extravasation), syncope, thrombophlebitis, urinary retention

Drug Interactions

Avoid Concomitant Use

Avoid concomitant use of Esmolol with any of the following: Methacholine

Increased Effect/Toxicity

Esmolol may increase the levels/effects of: Alpha-/Beta-Agonists (Direct-Acting); Alpha1-Blockers; Alpha2-Agonists; Amifostine; Antihypertensives; Antipsychotic Agents (Phenothiazines); Cardiac Glycosides; Hypotensive Agents; Insulin; Lidocaine; Methacholine; Midodrine; RiTUXimab; Sulfonylureas

The levels/effects of Esmolol may be increased by: Acetylcholinesterase Inhibitors; Aminoquinolines (Antimalarial); Amiodarone; Anilidopiperidine Opioids; Antipsychotic Agents (Phenothiazines); Calcium Channel Blockers (Nondihydropyridine); Diazoxide; Dipyridamole; Disopyramide; Dronedarone; Herbs (Hypotensive Properties); MAO Inhibitors; Pentoxifylline; Phosphodiester-ase 5 Inhibitors; Propafenone; Propoxyphene; Prostacyclin Analogues; QuiNIDine; Reserpine

Decreased Effect

Esmolol may decrease the levels/effects of: Beta2-Agonists; Theophylline Derivatives

The levels/effects of Esmolol may be decreased by: Barbiturates; Herbs (Hypertensive Properties); Methylphenidate; Nonsteroidal Anti-Inflammatory Agents; Rifamycin Derivatives; Yohimbine

Test Interactions Increases cholesterol (S), glucose

Dosage Forms Excipient information presented when available (limited, particularly for generics); consult specific product labeling.

Infusion [premixed in sodium chloride; preservative free]:

Brevibloc®: 2000 mg (100 mL) [20 mg/mL; double strength]; 2500 mg (250 mL) [10 mg/mL]

Injection, solution, as hydrochloride: 10 mg/mL (10 mL)
Brevibloc®:
10 mg/mL (10 mL) [alcohol free; premixed in sodium chloride]
20 mg/mL (5 mL, 100 mL) [alcohol free; double strength; premixed in sodium chloride]

References

Antman EM, Anbe SC, Alpert JS, et al, "ACC/AHA Guidelines for the Management of Patients With ST-Elevation Myocardial Infarction - Executive Summary: A Report of the American College of Cardiology/American Heart Association Task Force on Practice Guidelines (Writing Committee to Revise the 1999 Guidelines for the Management of Patients With Acute Myocardial Infarction)," *Circulation*, 2004, 110:588-636. Available at: http://www.circulationaha.org/cgi/content/full/110/5/588. Last accessed August 26, 2004.

Braunwald E, Antman EM, Beasley JW, et al, "ACC/AHA 2002 Guideline Update for the Management of Patients With Unstable Angina and Non-ST-Segment Elevation Myocardial Infarction - Summary Article: A Report of the American College of Cardiology/American Heart Association Task Force on Practice Guidelines (Committee on the Management of Patients With Unstable Angina)," *J Am Coll Cardiol*, 2002, 40(7):1366-74. Available at: http://www.acc.org/clinical/guidelines/unstable/incorporated/index.htm. Accessed May 20, 2003.

Chobanian AV, Bakris GL, Black HR, et al, "The Seventh Report of the Joint National Committee on Prevention, Detection, Evaluation, and Treatment of High Blood Pressure," *JAMA*, 2003, 289 (19):2560-72.

Erstad BL and Barletta JF, "Treatment of Hypertension in the Perioperative Patient," *Ann Pharmacother*, 2000, 34(1):66-79.

Mokhlesi B, Leikin JB, Murray P, et al, "Adult Toxicology in Critical Care. Part 11: Specific Poisonings," *Chest*, 2003, 123(3):897-922.

◆ **Esmolol Hydrochloride** see Esmolol *on page 522*

Esomeprazole (es oh ME pray zol)

Medication Safety Issues
Sound-alike/look-alike issues:
Esomeprazole may be confused with aripiprazole
Nexium® may be confused with Nexavar®

Related Information
Helicobacter pylori Treatment *on page 1746*

U.S. Brand Names Nexium®

Canadian Brand Names Nexium®

Index Terms Esomeprazole Magnesium; Esomeprazole Sodium

Pharmacologic Category Proton Pump Inhibitor; Substituted Benzimidazole

Generic Available No

Use
Oral: Short-term (4-8 weeks) treatment of erosive esophagitis; maintaining symptom resolution and healing of erosive esophagitis; treatment of symptomatic gastroesophageal reflux disease (GERD); as part of a multidrug regimen for *Helicobacter pylori* eradication in patients with duodenal ulcer disease (active or history of within the past 5 years); prevention of gastric ulcers in patients at risk (age ≥60 years and/or history of gastric ulcer) associated with continuous NSAID therapy; long-term treatment of pathological hypersecretory conditions including Zollinger-Ellison syndrome
Canadian labeling: Additional use (not in U.S. labeling): Oral: Treatment of nonerosive reflux disease (NERD)
I.V.: Short-term (≤10 days) treatment of gastroesophageal reflux disease (GERD) when oral therapy is not possible or appropriate

Unlabeled/Investigational Use I.V.: Prevention of recurrent peptic ulcer bleeding postendoscopy

Mechanism of Action Proton pump inhibitor suppresses gastric acid secretion by inhibition of the H^+/K^+-ATPase in the gastric parietal cell

Pharmacodynamics/Kinetics
Distribution: V_{dss}: 16 L
Protein binding: 97%
Metabolism: Hepatic via CYP2C19 and 3A4 enzymes to hydroxy, desmethyl, and sulfone metabolites (all inactive)
Bioavailability: Oral: 90% with repeat dosing
Half-life elimination: ~1-1.5 hours
Time to peak: Oral: 1.5-2 hours

Excretion: Urine (80%, primarily as inactive metabolites; <1% as active drug); feces (20%)

Dosage

Children 1-11 years: Oral: **Note:** Safety and efficacy of doses >1 mg/kg/day and/ or therapy beyond 8 weeks have not been established.

Symptomatic GERD: 10 mg once daily for up to 8 weeks

Erosive esophagitis (healing):

<20 kg: 10 mg once daily for 8 weeks

≥20 kg: 10-20 mg once daily for 8 weeks

Nonerosive reflux disease (NERD) (Canadian labeling): 10 mg once daily for up to 8 weeks

Adolescents 12-17 years: Oral:

GERD: 20-40 mg once daily for up to 8 weeks

NERD (Canadian labeling): 20 mg once daily for 2-4 weeks; lack of symptom control after 4 weeks warrants further evaluation

Adults:

Oral:

Erosive esophagitis (healing): Initial: 20-40 mg once daily for 4-8 weeks; if incomplete healing, may continue for an additional 4-8 weeks; maintenance: 20 mg once daily (controlled studies did not extend beyond 6 months)

NERD (Canadian labeling): Initial: 20 mg once daily for 2-4 weeks; lack of symptom control after 4 weeks warrants further evaluation; maintenance (in patients with successful initial therapy): 20 mg once daily as needed

Symptomatic GERD: 20 mg once daily for 4 weeks; may continue an additional 4 weeks if symptoms persist

Helicobacter pylori eradication:

Manufacturer labeling: 40 mg once daily administered with amoxicillin 1000 mg *and* clarithromycin 500 mg twice daily for 10 days

American College of Gastroenterology guidelines (Chey, 2007):

Nonpenicillin allergy: 40 mg once daily administered with amoxicillin 1000 mg *and* clarithromycin 500 mg twice daily for 10-14 days

Penicillin allergy: 40 mg once daily administered with clarithromycin 500 mg *and* metronidazole 500 mg twice daily for 10-14 days **or** 40 mg once daily administered with bismuth subsalicylate 525 mg *and* metronidazole 250 mg *plus* tetracycline 500 mg 4 times/day for 10-14 days

Canadian labeling: 20 mg twice daily for 7 days; requires combination therapy

Prevention of NSAID-induced gastric ulcers: 20-40 mg once daily for up to 6 months

Treatment of NSAID-induced gastric ulcers (Canadian labeling): 20 mg once daily for 4-8 weeks.

Pathological hypersecretory conditions (Zollinger-Ellison syndrome): 40 mg twice daily; adjust regimen to individual patient needs; doses up to 240 mg/ day have been administered

I.V.:

Prevention of recurrent peptic ulcer bleeding postendoscopy (unlabeled use; Sung, 2009): I.V.: 80 mg over 30 minutes, followed by 8 mg/hour infusion for 72 hours, then 40 mg *orally* once daily for 27 additional days

Treatment of GERD (short-term): 20 mg or 40 mg once daily for ≤10 days; change to oral therapy as soon as appropriate

Elderly: No dosage adjustment needed.

Dosage adjustment in renal impairment: No dosage adjustment needed
Dosage adjustment in hepatic impairment:

Safety and efficacy not established in children with hepatic impairment.

Mild-to-moderate hepatic impairment (Child-Pugh class A or B): No dosage adjustment needed

Severe hepatic impairment (Child-Pugh class C): Dose should not exceed 20 mg/day

Stability

Capsule, granules: Store at 15°C to 30°C (59°F to 86°F). Keep container tightly closed.

Powder for injection: Store at 25°C (77°F); excursions permitted to 15°C to 30°C (59°F to 86°F). Protect from light.

For I.V. injection: Reconstitute powder with 5 mL NS.

◄ For I.V. infusion: Initially reconstitute powder with 5 mL of NS, LR, or D_5W, then further dilute to a final volume of 50 mL.

Per the manufacturer, following reconstitution, solution for injection prepared in NS, and solution for infusion prepared in NS or LR should be used within 12 hours. Following reconstitution, solution for infusion prepared in D_5W should be used within 6 hours. Refrigeration is not required following reconstitution.

Additional stability data: Following reconstitution, solutions for infusion prepared in D_5W, NS, or LR in PVC bags are chemically and physically stable for 48 hours at room temperature (25°C) and for at least 120 hours under refrigeration (4°C) (Kupiec, 2008).

Administration

Oral:

Capsule: Should be swallowed whole and taken at least 1 hour before eating (best if taken before breakfast). Capsule can be opened and contents mixed with 1 tablespoon of applesauce. Swallow immediately; mixture should not be chewed or warmed. For patients with difficulty swallowing, use of granules may be easiest.

Granules: Empty into container with 1 tablespoon of water and stir; leave 2-3 minutes to thicken. Stir and drink within 30 minutes. If any medicine remains after drinking, add more water, stir and drink immediately.

Tablet (Canadian formulation, not available in U.S.): Swallow whole or may be dispersed in a half a glass of noncarbonated water. Stir until tablets disintegrate, leaving a liquid containing pellets. Drink contents within 30 minutes. Do not chew or crush pellets. After drinking, rinse glass with water and drink.

I.V.: May be administered by injection (≥3 minutes), intermittent infusion (10-30 minutes), or continuous infusion for up to 72 hours (Sung, 2009). Flush line prior to and after administration with NS, LR, or D_5W.

Nasogastric tube:

Capsule: Open capsule and place intact granules into a 60 mL syringe; mix with 50 mL of water. Replace plunger and shake vigorously for 15 seconds. Ensure that no granules remain in syringe tip. Do not administer if pellets dissolve or disintegrate. Use immediately after preparation. After administration, flush nasogastric tube with additional water.

Granules: Delayed release oral suspension granules can also be given by nasogastric or gastric tube. Add 15 mL of water to a syringe, add granules from packet. Shake the syringe, leave 2-3 minutes to thicken. Shake the syringe and administer through nasogastric or gastric tube (French size 6 or greater) within 30 minutes. Refill the syringe with 15 mL of water, shake and flush nasogastric/gastric tube.

Tablet (Canadian formulation, not available in U.S.): Disperse tablets in 50 mL of noncarbonated water. Stir until tablets disintegrate leaving a liquid containing pellets. After administration, flush with additional 25-50 mL of water to clear the syringe and tube.

Monitoring Parameters Susceptibility testing recommended in patients who fail *H. pylori* eradication regimen (esomeprazole, clarithromycin, and amoxicillin). Monitor for rebleeding in patients with peptic ulcer bleed.

Anesthesia and Critical Care Concerns/Other Considerations

Evidence-Based Information:

Acute ulcer: Postendoscopy therapy: In a multicenter, double-blind trial conducted in 16 countries, 767 patients with peptic ulcer bleeding from a single gastric or duodenal source with high-risk features were randomized to intravenous esomeprazole (80 mg bolus over 30 minutes, followed by a continuous infusion of 8 mg/hour for a total of 72 hours) or placebo. After completion of intravenous therapy, all patients were administered oral esomeprazole 40 mg once daily for an additional 27 days. The use of intravenous esomeprazole demonstrated a significant reduction in the primary end point of clinically significant rebleeding within 72 hours (5.9% vs 10.3%, p=0.026). Although endoscopic therapy was not standardized, the efficacy of esomeprazole was not affected (Sung, 2009).

Intravenous omeprazole has also been studied in prevention of rebleeding in ulcer patients who are at high risk for rebleeding (endoscopic findings of active bleeding or nonbleeding visible vessel) after successful hemostasis (Lau, 2000; Lin, 1998).

Lin and his group treated 100 ulcer patients (actively bleeding ulcers or ulcers with nonbleeding visible vessels) endoscopically and then randomized them to cimetidine (300 mg bolus followed by 50 mg/hour infusion) or omeprazole (40 mg bolus, ~7 mg/hour infusion) for 72 hours. Patients were discharged on the oral form of the drug arm they were assigned to. The omeprazole group maintained an intragastric pH >6 for about 84% of the infusion duration, while the cimetidine group maintained their pH >6 only about 50% of the time. Rebleeding occurred significantly more often in the cimetidine group.

Lau and his colleagues treated patients with actively bleeding ulcers or ulcers with nonbleeding visible vessels with an epinephrine infusion followed by thermocoagulation. They were then randomized to omeprazole (80 mg bolus followed by a continuous infusion of 8 mg/hour for 72 hours) or placebo. All patients were discharged on oral omeprazole (20 mg/day) for 8 weeks and received *H. pylori* treatment if indicated. The primary goal was to evaluate the rate of rebleeding during the first 30 days after endoscopy. Two hundred and forty patients were enrolled with randomization of 120 into each group. Bleeding recurred in significantly more patients receiving placebo than omeprazole infusion. The authors concluded that after endoscopic therapy, omeprazole reduces the risk of rebleeding in patients with actively bleeding ulcers or ulcers with nonbleeding visible vessels.

Acute ulcer: Pre-endoscopy therapy: Lau and associates (2007) evaluated the effects of preemptive infusion of omeprazole before endoscopy in upper gastrointestinal bleeding. Consecutive patients (638) were stabilized and then randomly assigned to intravenous omeprazole (80 mg bolus followed by a continuous infusion of 8 mg/hour) or placebo infusion before endoscopy the next morning. The primary endpoint was the need for endoscopic therapy (eg, epinephrine, thermocoagulation). Seven patients were excluded from the analysis. The need for endoscopic treatment was significantly lower in the omeprazole group (60/314 patients; 19%) than in the placebo group (90/317; 28%). The active treatment group had a significantly shorter hospital stay. Duration of infusion before endoscopy was similar in both groups (~8-21 hours).

Stress ulcer prophylaxis: The 2008 Surviving Sepsis Campaign guidelines recommend that stress ulcer prophylaxis using an H_2 blocker (Grade 1A) or proton pump inhibitor (Grade 1B) be given to patients with severe sepsis to prevent upper GI bleed. Benefit of prevention of upper GI bleed must be weighed against potential effect of increased stomach pH on development of ventilator-associated pneumonia.

Pregnancy Risk Factor B

Contraindications Hypersensitivity to esomeprazole, substituted benzimidazoles (ie, lansoprazole, omeprazole, pantoprazole, rabeprazole), or any component of the formulation

Warnings/Precautions Use of proton pump inhibitors may increase the risk of gastrointestinal infections (eg, *Salmonella, Campylobacter*). Relief of symptoms does not preclude the presence of a gastric malignancy. Atrophic gastritis (by biopsy) has been noted with long-term omeprazole therapy; this may also occur with esomeprazole. No reports of enterochromaffin-like (ECL) cell carcinoids, dysplasia, or neoplasia have occurred. Severe liver dysfunction may require dosage reductions. Safety and efficacy of I.V. therapy >10 days have not been established; transition from I.V. to oral therapy as soon possible. Decreased *H. pylori* eradication rates have been observed with short-term (≤7 days) combination therapy. The American College of Gastroenterology recommends 10-14 days of therapy (triple or quadruple) for eradication of *H. pylori* (Chey, 2007).

Adverse Reactions Unless otherwise specified, percentages represent adverse reactions identified in clinical trials evaluating the oral formulation.

>10%: Central nervous system: Headache (I.V. 11%; oral ≤8%)
1% to 10%:
  Cardiovascular: Hypertension (≤3%), chest pain (>1%)
  Central nervous system: Pain (4%), dizziness (oral >1%; I.V. 3%), anxiety (2%), insomnia (2%), pyrexia (2%), fatigue (>1%)
  Dermatologic: Rash (>1%), pruritus (I.V. ≤1%)
  Endocrine & metabolic: Hypercholesterolemia (2%)

Gastrointestinal: Flatulence (oral ≤5%; I.V. 10%), diarrhea (oral ≤7%; I.V. 4%), abdominal pain (oral ≤6%; I.V. 6%), nausea (oral 5%; I.V. 6%), dyspepsia (oral > 1%; I.V. 6%), gastritis (≤6%), constipation (oral 2%; I.V. 3%), vomiting (≤3%), benign GI neoplasm (>1%), dyspepsia (>1%), duodenitis (>1%), epigastric pain (>1%), esophageal disorder (>1%), gastroenteritis (>1%), GI mucosal discoloration (>1%), serum gastrin increased (>1%), tooth disorder (>1%), xerostomia (1%)

Genitourinary: Urinary tract infection (4%)

Hematologic: Anemia (>1%)

Hepatic: Transaminases increased (>1%)

Local: Injection site reaction (I.V. 2%)

Neuromuscular & skeletal: Arthralgia (3%), back pain (>1%), fracture (>1%), arthropathy (1%), myalgia (1%)

Respiratory: Respiratory infection (oral ≤9%; I.V. 1%), bronchitis (4%), sinusitis (oral ≤4%; I.V. 2%), coughing (>1%), rhinitis (>1%), dyspnea (1%)

Miscellaneous: Accident/injury (≤8%), viral infection (4%), allergy (2%), ear infection (2%), hernia (>1%), flu-like syndrome (1%)

<1% (Limited to important or life-threatening): Abdominal rigidity, aggression, agitation, agranulocytosis, albuminuria, alkaline phosphatase increased, alopecia, anaphylactic reaction/shock, angioedema, anorexia, arthritis exacerbation, asthma exacerbation, benign polyps/nodules, bilirubinemia, blurred vision, bronchospasm, candidiasis (GI and genital), carcinoid tumor of stomach, cervical lymphadenopathy, conjunctivitis, cramps, creatinine increased, cystitis, dehydration, depression, dermatitis, dysmenorrhea, dysphagia, dysuria, edema (including facial, peripheral and tongue), epigastric pain, epistaxis, erythema multiforme, esophageal varices, fibromyalgia syndrome, flushing, fungal infection, gastric retention, GI dysplasia, glycosuria, goiter, gynecomastia, hallucinations, hematuria, hepatic encephalopathy, hepatic failure, hepatitis, hyperhidrosis, hyperparathyroidism, hypertonia, hyperuricemia, hypoesthesia, hypokalemia, hypomagnesemia, hyponatremia, impotence, infusion site reaction (eg, erythema, edema), interstitial nephritis, jaundice, larynx edema, leukocytosis, leukopenia, malaise, micturition increased, migraine, muscular weakness, nervousness, osteoporosis, otitis media, pancreatitis, pancytopenia, paresthesia, pharyngolaryngeal pain, pharyngitis, phlebitis, photosensitivity, polymyalgia rheumatica, polyuria, proteinuria, pruritus ani, rhinorrhea, rigors, sleep disorder, somnolence, Stevens-Johnson syndrome, stomatitis, tachycardia, taste disturbances, thrombocytopenia, thrombophlebitis, thyroid-stimulating hormone increased, tinnitus, total bilirubin increased, toxic epidermal necrolysis, tremor, urticaria, vaginitis, vertigo, vitamin B_{12} deficiency, weight changes

Drug Interactions

Metabolism/Transport Effects Substrate of CYP2C19 (major), 3A4 (major); **Inhibits** CYP2C19 (moderate)

Avoid Concomitant Use

Avoid concomitant use of Esomeprazole with any of the following: Delavirdine; Erlotinib; Nelfinavir; Posaconazole

Increased Effect/Toxicity

Esomeprazole may increase the levels/effects of: Benzodiazepines (metabolized by oxidation); CYP2C19 Substrates; Methotrexate; Raltegravir; Saquinavir; Tacrolimus; Vitamin K Antagonists; Voriconazole

The levels/effects of Esomeprazole may be increased by: Fluconazole; Ketoconazole

Decreased Effect

Esomeprazole may decrease the levels/effects of: Atazanavir; Clopidogrel; Dabigatran Etexilate; Dasatinib; Delavirdine; Erlotinib; Indinavir; Iron Salts; Itraconazole; Ketoconazole; Mesalamine; Mycophenolate; Nelfinavir; Posaconazole

The levels/effects of Esomeprazole may be decreased by: CYP2C19 Inducers (Strong); Tipranavir

Ethanol/Nutrition/Herb Interactions Food: Absorption is decreased by 43% to 53% when taken with food.

Dietary Considerations Take at least 1 hour before meals; best if taken before breakfast. The contents of the capsule may be mixed in applesauce or water; pellets also remain intact when exposed to orange juice, apple juice, and yogurt.

Dosage Forms Excipient information presented when available (limited, particularly for generics); consult specific product labeling. [CAN] = Canadian availability

Note: Strength expressed as base

Capsule, delayed release, as magnesium:
    Nexium®: 20 mg, 40 mg
Granules, for oral suspension, delayed release, as magnesium:
    Nexium®: 10 mg/packet (30s); 20 mg/packet (30s); 40 mg/packet (30s)
    Nexium® [CAN]: 10 mg/packet (28s)
Injection, powder for reconstitution, as sodium:
    Nexium®: 20 mg, 40 mg [contains edetate sodium]
Tablet, extended release, as magnesium:
    Nexium® [CAN]: 20 mg, 40 mg [not available in U.S.]

References

Lau JY, Leung WK, Wu JC, et al, "Omeprazole Before Endoscopy in Patients With Gastrointestinal Bleeding," *N Engl J Med*, 2007, 356(16):1631-40.

Lau JY, Sung JJ, Lee KK, et al, "Effect of Intravenous Omeprazole on Recurrent Bleeding After Endoscopic Treatment of Bleeding Peptic Ulcers," *N Engl J Med*, 2000, 343(5):310-6.

Lin HJ, Lo WC, Lee FY, et al, "A Prospective Randomized Comparative Trial Showing That Omeprazole Prevents Rebleeding in Patients With Bleeding Peptic Ulcer After Successful Endoscopic Therapy," *Arch Intern Med*, 1998, 158(1):54-8.

Natsch S, Vinks MH, Voogt AK, et al, "Anaphylactic Reactions to Proton-Pump Inhibitors," *Ann Pharmacother*, 2000, 34(4):474-6.

◆ **Esomeprazole Magnesium** *see* Esomeprazole *on page 526*

◆ **Esomeprazole Sodium** *see* Esomeprazole *on page 526*

◆ **Estrace®** *see* Estradiol *on page 531*

◆ **Estraderm®** *see* Estradiol *on page 531*

Estradiol (es tra DYE ole)

U.S. Brand Names Alora®; Climara®; Delestrogen®; Depo®-Estradiol; Divigel®; Elestrin™; Estrace®; Estraderm®; Estrasorb™; Estring®; EstroGel®; Evamist™; Femring®; Femtrace®; Gynodiol® [DSC]; Menostar®; Vagifem®; Vivelle-Dot®; Vivelle® [DSC]

Canadian Brand Names Climara®; Depo®-Estradiol; Estrace®; Estraderm®; Estradot®; Estring®; EstroGel®; Menostar®; Oesclim®; Sandoz-Estradiol Derm 100; Sandoz-Estradiol Derm 50; Sandoz-Estradiol Derm 75; Vagifem®

Index Terms Estradiol Acetate; Estradiol Cypionate; Estradiol Hemihydrate; Estradiol Transdermal; Estradiol Valerate

Pharmacologic Category Estrogen Derivative

Use Treatment of moderate-to-severe vasomotor symptoms associated with menopause; treatment of vulvar and vaginal atrophy; hypoestrogenism (due to hypogonadism, castration, or primary ovarian failure); prostatic cancer (palliation), breast cancer (palliation), osteoporosis (prophylaxis); abnormal uterine bleeding due to hormonal imbalance; postmenopausal urogenital symptoms of the lower urinary tract (urinary urgency, dysuria)

Pharmacodynamics/Kinetics

Absorption: Oral, topical: Well absorbed

Protein binding: 37% to sex hormone-binding globulin; 61% to albumin

Metabolism: Hepatic via oxidation and conjugation in GI tract; hydroxylated via CYP3A4 to metabolites; first-pass effect; enterohepatic recirculation; reversibly converted to estrone and estriol

Excretion: Primarily urine (as metabolites estrone and estriol); feces (small amounts)

Dosage All dosage needs to be adjusted based upon the patient's response

Oral:

Prostate cancer (androgen-dependent, inoperable, progressing): 10 mg 3 times/ day for at least 3 months

Breast cancer (inoperable, progressing in appropriately selected patients): 10 mg 3 times/day for at least 3 months

◄ Osteoporosis prophylaxis in postmenopausal females: 0.5 mg/day in a cyclic regimen (3 weeks on and 1 week off)

Female hypoestrogenism (due to hypogonadism, castration, or primary ovarian failure): 1-2 mg/day; titrate as necessary to control symptoms using minimal effective dose for maintenance therapy

Moderate-to-severe vasomotor symptoms associated with menopause: 1-2 mg/day, adjusted as necessary to limit symptoms; administration should be cyclic (3 weeks on, 1 week off). Patients should be re-evaluated at 3- to 6-month intervals to determine if treatment is still necessary.

I.M.:

Prostate cancer: Valerate: ≥30 mg or more every 1-2 weeks

Moderate-to-severe vasomotor symptoms associated with menopause:
Cypionate: 1-5 mg every 3-4 weeks
Valerate: 10-20 mg every 4 weeks

Female hypoestrogenism (due to hypogonadism):
Cypionate: 1.5-2 mg monthly
Valerate: 10-20 mg every 4 weeks

Topical:

Emulsion: Moderate-to-severe vasomotor symptoms associated with menopause: 3.84 g applied once daily in the morning

Gel:

Moderate-to-severe vasomotor symptoms associated with menopause:
Divigel®: 0.25 g/day; adjust dose based on patient response. Dosing range: 0.25-1 g/day
Elestrin™: 0.87g/day applied at the same time each day
EstroGel®: 1.25 g/day applied at the same time each day

Vulvar and vaginal atrophy:
Elestrin™: 0.87g/day applied at the same time each day
EstroGel®: 1.25 g/day applied at the same time each day

Spray: Moderate-to-severe vasomotor symptoms associated with menopause (Evamist™): Initial: One spray (1.53 mg) per day. Adjust dose based on patient response. Dosing range: 1-3 sprays per day.

Transdermal: Indicated dose may be used continuously in patients without an intact uterus. May be given continuously or cyclically (3 weeks on, 1 week off) in patients with an intact uterus **(exception - Menostar®, see specific dosing instructions)**. When changing patients from oral to transdermal therapy, start transdermal patch 1 week after discontinuing oral hormone (may begin sooner if symptoms reappear within 1 week):

Once-weekly patch:

Moderate-to-severe vasomotor symptoms associated with menopause, vulvar and vaginal atrophy associated with menopause, female hypoestrogenism (Climara®): Apply 0.025 mg/day patch once weekly. Adjust dose as necessary to control symptoms. Patients should be re-evaluated at 3- to 6-month intervals to determine if treatment is still necessary.

Osteoporosis prophylaxis in postmenopausal women:
Climara®: Apply patch once weekly; minimum effective dose 0.025 mg/day; adjust response to therapy by biochemical markers and bone mineral density
Menostar®: Apply patch once weekly. In women with a uterus, also administer a progestin for 14 days every 6-12 months

Twice-weekly patch:

Moderate-to-severe vasomotor symptoms associated with menopause, vulvar/vaginal atrophy, female hypogonadism: Titrate to lowest dose possible to control symptoms, adjusting initial dose after the first month of therapy; re-evaluate therapy at 3- to 6-month intervals to taper or discontinue medication:
Alora®, Estraderm®, Vivelle-Dot®: Apply 0.05 mg patch twice weekly
Vivelle®: Apply 0.0375 mg patch twice weekly

Prevention of osteoporosis in postmenopausal women:
Alora®, Vivelle®, Vivelle-Dot®: Apply 0.025 mg patch twice weekly, increase dose as necessary
Estraderm®: Apply 0.05 mg patch twice weekly

Vaginal cream: Vulvar and vaginal atrophy: Insert 2-4 g/day intravaginally for 2 weeks, then gradually reduce to 1/2 the initial dose for 2 weeks, followed by a maintenance dose of 1 g 1-3 times/week

Vaginal ring:

Postmenopausal vaginal atrophy, urogenital symptoms: Estring®: 2 mg intra-vaginally; following insertion, ring should remain in place for 90 days

Moderate-to-severe vasomotor symptoms associated with menopause; vulvar/vaginal atrophy: Femring®: 0.05 mg intravaginally; following insertion, ring should remain in place for 3 months; dose may be increased to 0.1 mg if needed

Vaginal tablets: Atrophic vaginitis: Vagifem®: Initial: Insert 1 tablet once daily for 2 weeks; maintenance: Insert 1 tablet twice weekly; attempts to discontinue or taper medication should be made at 3- to 6-month intervals

Dosing adjustment in hepatic impairment:

Mild-to-moderate liver impairment: Dosage reduction of estrogens is recommended

Severe liver impairment: **Not recommended**

Additional Information Complete prescribing information for this medication should be consulted for additional detail.

Dosage Forms Excipient information presented when available (limited, particularly for generics); consult specific product labeling. [DSC] = Discontinued product

Cream, vaginal:

Estrace®: 0.1 mg/g (42.5 g)

Emulsion, topical, as hemihydrate:

Estrasorb™: 2.5 mg/g (56s) [each pouch contains 4.35 mg estradiol hemihydrate; contents of two pouches delivers estradiol 0.05 mg/day]

Gel, topical:

Divigel®: 0.1% (0.25 g) [delivers estradiol 0.25 mg/packet]; (0.5 g) [delivers 0.5 mg estradiol/packet]; (1 g) [delivers estradiol 1 mg/packet]

Elestrin™: 0.06% (144 g) [delivers estradiol 0.52 mg/0.87 g; 100 actuations]

EstroGel®: 0.06% (50 g) [delivers estradiol 0.75 mg/1.25 g; 32 actuations; contains ethanol]

Injection, oil, as cypionate:

Depo®-Estradiol: 5 mg/mL (5 mL) [contains chlorobutanol, cottonseed oil]

Injection, oil, as valerate: 10 mg/mL (5 mL); 20 mg/mL (5 mL); 40 mg/mL (5 mL)

Delestrogen®:

10 mg/mL (5 mL) [contains chlorobutanol, sesame oil]

20 mg/mL (5 mL) [contains benzyl alcohol, castor oil]

40 mg/mL (5 mL) [contains benzyl alcohol, castor oil]

Ring, vaginal, as base:

Estring®: 2 mg (1s) [total estradiol 2 mg; releases 7.5 mcg/day over 90 days]

Ring, vaginal, as acetate:

Femring®: 0.05 mg/day (1s) [total estradiol 12.4 mg; releases 0.05 mg/day over 3 months]; 0.1 mg/day (1s) [total estradiol 24.8 mg; releases 0.1 mg/day over 3 months]

Solution, topical [spray]:

Evamist™: 1.53 mg/spray (8.1 mL) [contains 56 sprays after priming; contains ethanol]

Tablet, oral, as acetate:

Femtrace®: 0.45 mg, 0.9 mg, 1.8 mg

Tablet, oral, micronized: 0.5 mg, 1 mg, 2 mg

Estrace®: 0.5 mg, 1 mg, 2 mg [2 mg tablets contain tartrazine]

Gynodiol®: 0.5 mg [DSC], 1 mg [DSC], 1.5 mg [DSC], 2 mg [DSC]

Tablet, vaginal, as base:

Vagifem®: 25 mcg

Transdermal system: 0.025 mg/24 hours (4s) [once-weekly patch]; 0.0375 mg/24 hours (4s) [once-weekly patch]; 0.05 mg/24 hours (4s) [once-weekly patch]; 0.06 mg/24 hours (4s) [once-weekly patch]; 0.075 mg/24 hours [once-weekly patch]; 0.1 mg/24 hours (4s) [once-weekly patch]

Alora® [twice-weekly patch]:

0.025 mg/24 hours (8s) [9 cm^2, total estradiol 0.77 mg]

0.05 mg/24 hours (8s, 24s [DSC]) [18 cm^2, total estradiol 1.5 mg]

0.075 mg/24 hours (8s) [27 cm^2, total estradiol 2.3 mg]

0.1 mg/24 hours (8s) [36 cm^2, total estradiol 3.1 mg]

Climara® [once-weekly patch]:
  0.025 mg/24 hours (4s) [6.5 cm^2, total estradiol 2.04 mg]
  0.0375 mg/24 hours (4s) [9.375 cm^2, total estradiol 2.85 mg]
  0.05 mg/24 hours (4s) [12.5 cm^2, total estradiol 3.8 mg]
  0.06 mg/24 hours (4s) [15 cm^2, total estradiol 4.55 mg]
  0.075 mg/24 hours (4s) [18.75 cm^2, total estradiol 5.7 mg]
  0.1 mg/24 hours (4s) [25 cm^2, total estradiol 7.6 mg]
Estraderm® [twice-weekly patch]:
  0.05 mg/24 hours (8s) [10 cm^2, total estradiol 4 mg]
  0.1 mg/24 hours (8s) [20 cm^2, total estradiol 8 mg]
Menostar® [once-weekly patch]: 0.014 mg/24 hours (4s) [3.25 cm^2, total estradiol 1 mg]
Vivelle® [twice-weekly patch]:
  0.05 mg/24 hours (8s) [14.5 cm^2, total estradiol 4.33 mg] [DSC]
  0.1 mg/24 hours (8s) [29 cm^2, total estradiol 8.66 mg] [DSC]
Vivelle-Dot® [twice-weekly patch]:
  0.025 mg/day (24s) [2.5 cm^2, total estradiol 0.39 mg]
  0.0375 mg/day (24s) [3.75 cm^2, total estradiol 0.585 mg]
  0.05 mg/day (24s) [5 cm^2, total estradiol 0.78 mg]
  0.075 mg/day (24s) [7.5 cm^2, total estradiol 1.17 mg]
  0.1 mg/day (24s) [10 cm^2, total estradiol 1.56 mg]

References

American College of Physicians, "Guidelines for Counseling Postmenopausal Women About Preventive Hormone Therapy," *Ann Intern Med*, 1992, 117(12):1038-41.

Belchetz PE, "Hormone Treatment for Postmenopausal Women," *N Engl J Med*, 1994, 330 (15):1062-71.

Ettinger B, Friedman GD, Bush T, et al, "Reduced Mortality Associated With Long-Term Postmenopausal Estrogen Therapy," *Obstet Gynecol*, 1996, 87(1):6-12.

Grodstein F, Stampfer MJ, Colditz GA, et al, "Postmenopausal Hormone Therapy and Mortality," *N Engl J Med*, 1997, 336(25):1769-75.

Hulley S, Grady D, Bush T, et al, "Randomized Trial of Estrogen Plus Progestin for Secondary Prevention of Coronary Heart Disease in Postmenopausal Women. Heart and Estrogen/Progestin Replacement Study (HERS) Research Group," *JAMA*, 1998, 280(7):605-13.

Rossouw JE, Anderson GL, Prentice RL, et al, "Risks and Benefits of Estrogen Plus Progestin in Healthy Postmenopausal Women: Principle Results From the Women's Health Initiative Randomized Controlled Trial,"*JAMA*, 2002, 288(3):321-33.

Shumaker SA, Legault C, Rapp SR, et al, "WHIMS Investigators. Estrogen Plus Progestin and the Incidence of Dementia and Mild Cognitive Impairment in Postmenopausal Women: The Women's Health Initiative Memory Study: A Randomized Controlled Trial," *JAMA*, 2003, 289(20):2651-62.

Stallard S, Litherland JC, Cordiner CM, et al, "Effect of Hormone Replacement Therapy on the Pathological Stage of Breast Cancer: Population Based, Cross Sectional Study," *BMJ*, 2000, 320 (7231):348-9.

U.S. Food and Drug Administration, Department of Health and Human Services, "FDA Approves New Labels for Estrogen and Estrogen With Progestin Therapies for Postmenopausal Women Following Review of Women's Health Initiative Data," January 8, 2003. Available at: http://www.fda.gov/medwatch/SAFETY/2003/safety03.htm#prempr. Accessed April 17, 2003.

- ♦ **Estradiol Acetate** *see* Estradiol *on page 531*

- ♦ **Estradiol Cypionate** *see* Estradiol *on page 531*

- ♦ **Estradiol Hemihydrate** *see* Estradiol *on page 531*

- ♦ **Estradiol Transdermal** *see* Estradiol *on page 531*

- ♦ **Estradiol Valerate** *see* Estradiol *on page 531*

- ♦ **Estradot® (Can)** *see* Estradiol *on page 531*

- ♦ **Estrasorb™** *see* Estradiol *on page 531*

- ♦ **Estring®** *see* Estradiol *on page 531*

- ♦ **EstroGel®** *see* Estradiol *on page 531*

- ♦ **Estrogenic Substances, Conjugated** *see* Estrogens (Conjugated/Equine) *on page 534*

Estrogens (Conjugated/Equine)

jenz KON joo gate ed, EE kwine)

on Safety Issues

ike/look-alike issues:
  ı® may be confused with Primaxin®, Provera®, Remeron®
Names Premarin®

Canadian Brand Names C.E.S.®; Premarin®

Index Terms C.E.S.; CE; CEE; Conjugated Estrogen; Estrogenic Substances, Conjugated

Pharmacologic Category Estrogen Derivative

Generic Available No

Use Treatment of moderate-to-severe vasomotor symptoms associated with menopause; treatment of vulvar and vaginal atrophy; hypoestrogenism (due to hypogonadism, castration, or primary ovarian failure); prostatic cancer (palliation); breast cancer (palliation); osteoporosis (prophylaxis, postmenopausal women at significant risk only); abnormal uterine bleeding; moderate-to-severe dyspareunia (pain during intercourse) due to vaginal/vulvar atrophy of menopause

Unlabeled/Investigational Use Uremic bleeding

Mechanism of Action Conjugated estrogens contain a mixture of estrone sulfate, equilin sulfate, 17 alpha-dihydroequilin, 17 alpha-estradiol and 17 beta-dihydroequilin. Estrogens are responsible for the development and maintenance of the female reproductive system and secondary sexual characteristics. Estradiol is the principle intracellular human estrogen and is more potent than estrone and estriol at the receptor level; it is the primary estrogen secreted prior to menopause. Following menopause, estrone and estrone sulfate are more highly produced. Estrogens modulate the pituitary secretion of gonadotropins, luteinizing hormone, and follicle-stimulating hormone through a negative feedback system; estrogen replacement reduces elevated levels of these hormones in post-menopausal women.

Pharmacodynamics/Kinetics

Absorption: Well absorbed

Protein binding: Binds to sex-hormone-binding globulin and albumin

Metabolism: Hepatic via CYP3A4; estradiol is converted to estrone and estriol; also undergoes enterohepatic recirculation (avoided with vaginal administration); estrone sulfite is the main metabolite in postmenopausal women

Half-life elimination: Total estrone: 27 hours

Time to peak, plasma: Total estrone: 7 hours

Excretion: Urine (primarily estriol, also as estradiol, estrone, and conjugates

Dosage Adults:

Male: Androgen-dependent prostate cancer palliation: Oral: 1.25-2.5 mg 3 times/ day

Female:

Prevention of postmenopausal osteoporosis: Oral: Initial: 0.3 mg/day cyclically* or daily, depending on medical assessment of patient. Dose may be adjusted based on bone mineral density and clinical response. The lowest effective dose should be used.

Moderate-to-severe vasomotor symptoms associated with menopause: Oral: Initial: 0.3 mg/day, cyclically* or daily, depending on medical assessment of patient. The lowest dose that will control symptoms should be used. Medication should be discontinued as soon as possible.

Moderate-to-severe dyspareunia: Intravaginal: Vaginal cream: 0.5 g twice weekly (eg, Monday and Thursday) or once daily cyclically*

Vulvar and vaginal atrophy:

Oral: Initial: 0.3 mg/day; the lowest dose that will control symptoms should be used. May be given cyclically* or daily, depending on medical assessment of patient. Medication should be discontinued as soon as possible.

Vaginal cream: Intravaginal: 0.5-2 g/day given cyclically*

Abnormal uterine bleeding:

Acute/heavy bleeding:

Oral (unlabeled route): 1.25 mg, may repeat every 4 hours for 24 hours, followed by 1.25 mg once daily for 7-10 days

I.M., I.V.: 25 mg, may repeat in 6-12 hours if needed

Note: Treatment should be followed by a low-dose oral contraceptive; medroxyprogesterone acetate along with or following estrogen therapy can also be given

Nonacute/lesser bleeding: Oral (unlabeled route): 1.25 mg once daily for 7-10 days

Female hypogonadism: Oral: 0.3-0.625 mg/day given cyclically*; dose may be titrated in 6- to 12-month intervals; progestin treatment should be added to maintain bone mineral density once skeletal maturity is achieved.

Female castration, primary ovarian failure: Oral: 1.25 mg/day given cyclically*; adjust according to severity of symptoms and patient response. For maintenance, adjust to the lowest effective dose.

*Cyclic administration: Either 3 weeks on, 1 week off **or** 25 days on, 5 days off

Male and Female:
Breast cancer palliation, metastatic disease in selected patients: Oral: 10 mg 3 times/day for at least 3 months
Uremic bleeding (unlabeled use): I.V.: 0.6 mg/kg/day for 5 days

Elderly: Refer to adult dosing; a higher incidence of stroke and invasive breast cancer was observed in women >75 years in a WHI substudy.

Stability
Injection: Refrigerate at 2°C to 8°C (36°F to 46°F) prior to reconstitution. Reconstitute with sterile water for injection; slowly inject diluent against side wall of the vial. Agitate gently; do not shake violently. Use immediately following reconstitution.
Tablets, vaginal cream: Store at room temperature 20°C to 25°C (68°F to 77°F).

Administration
Injection: May also be administered intramuscularly; when administered I.V., drug should be administered slowly to avoid the occurrence of a flushing reaction
Oral tablet: Administer at bedtime to minimize adverse effects. May be administered without regard to meals.
Vaginal cream: Administer at bedtime to minimize adverse effects. To clean applicator, remove plunger from barrel. Wash with mild soap and warm water; do not boil or use hot water.

Monitoring Parameters Routine physical examination that includes blood pressure and Papanicolaou smear, breast exam, mammogram. Monitor for signs of endometrial cancer in female patients with uterus. Adequate diagnostic measures, including endometrial sampling, if indicated, should be performed to rule out malignancy in all cases of undiagnosed abnormal vaginal bleeding. Monitor for loss of vision, sudden onset of proptosis, diplopia, migraine; signs and symptoms of thromboembolic disorders; glycemic control in patients with diabetes; lipid profiles in patients being treated for hyperlipidemias; thyroid function in patients on thyroid hormone replacement therapy.
Menopausal symptoms: Assess need for therapy at 3- to 6-month intervals
Prevention of osteoporosis: Bone density measurement
Uremic bleeding: Bleeding time

Reference Range
Children: <10 mcg/24 hours (SI: <35 μmol/day) (values at Mayo Medical Laboratories)
Adults:
Male: 15-40 mcg/24 hours (SI: 52-139 μmol/day)
Female:
Menstruating: 15-80 mcg/24 hours (SI: 52-277 μmol/day)
Postmenopausal: <20 mcg/24 hours (SI: <69 μmol/day)

Contraindications Hypersensitivity to estrogens or any component of the formulation; undiagnosed abnormal vaginal bleeding; history of or current thrombophlebitis or venous thromboembolic disorders (including DVT, PE); active or recent (within 1 year) arterial thromboembolic disease (eg, stroke, MI); carcinoma of the breast (except in appropriately selected patients being treated for metastatic disease); estrogen-dependent tumor; hepatic dysfunction or disease; pregnancy

Warnings/Precautions
Cardiovascular-related considerations: **[U.S. Boxed Warning]: Estrogens with or without progestin should not be used to prevent cardiovascular disease.** Use caution with cardiovascular disease or dysfunction. May increase the risks of hypertension, myocardial infarction (MI), stroke, pulmonary emboli (PE), and deep vein thrombosis; incidence of these effects was shown to be significantly increased in postmenopausal women using conjugated estrogens (CE) alone or in combination with medroxyprogesterone acetate (MPA). Nonfatal MI, PE, and thrombophlebitis have also been reported in males taking high doses of CE

(eg, for prostate cancer). Estrogen compounds are generally associated with lipid effects such as increased HDL-cholesterol and decreased LDL-cholesterol. Triglycerides may also be increased; use with caution in patients with familial defects of lipoprotein metabolism. Whenever possible, estrogens should be discontinued at least 4 weeks prior to and for 2 weeks following elective surgery associated with an increased risk of thromboembolism or during periods of prolonged immobilization.

Neurological considerations: **[U.S. Boxed Warning]: The risk of dementia may be increased in postmenopausal women;** increased incidence was observed in women ≥65 years of age taking CE alone or in combination with MPA.

Cancer-related considerations: **[U.S. Boxed Warning]: Adequate diagnostic measures, including endometrial sampling, if indicated, should be performed to rule out malignancy in all cases of undiagnosed abnormal vaginal bleeding. Unopposed estrogens may increase the risk of endometrial carcinoma in postmenopausal women with an intact uterus.** Risk appears to be associated with long-term use The use of a progestin should be considered when administering estrogens to postmenopausal women with an intact uterus. Estrogens may exacerbate endometriosis. Malignant transformation of residual endometrial implants has been reported posthysterectomy with estrogen only therapy. Consider adding a progestin in women with residual endometriosis posthysterectomy. Presentation of irregular, unresolving vaginal bleeding warrants further evaluation including endometrial sampling, if indicated, to rule out malignancy. Estrogens may increase the risk of breast cancer. An increased risk of invasive breast cancer was observed in postmenopausal women using CE in combination with MPA; a smaller increase in risk was seen with estrogen therapy alone in observational studies. An increase in abnormal mammograms has also been reported with estrogen and progestin therapy. Estrogen use may lead to severe hypercalcemia in patients with breast cancer and bone metastases; discontinue estrogen if hypercalcemia occurs. Post-menopausal estrogen therapy and combined estrogen/progesterone therapy may increase the risk of ovarian cancer; however, the absolute risk to an individual woman is small. Although results from various studies are not consistent, risk does not appear to be significantly associated with the duration, route, or dose of therapy. In one study, the risk decreased after 2 years following discontinuation of therapy.

Estrogens may cause retinal vascular thrombosis; discontinue permanently if papilledema or retinal vascular lesions are observed on examination. Use with caution in patients with diseases which may be exacerbated by fluid retention, including asthma, epilepsy, migraine, diabetes, heart failure, or renal dysfunction. Use with caution in patients with a history of severe hypocalcemia, SLE, hepatic hemangiomas, porphyria, endometriosis, and gallbladder disease. Use caution with history of cholestatic jaundice associated with past estrogen use or pregnancy. Safety and efficacy in pediatric patients have not been established. Prior to puberty, estrogens may cause premature closure of the epiphyses, premature breast development in girls or gynecomastia in boys. Vaginal bleeding and vaginal cornification may also be induced in girls.

[U.S. Boxed Warning]: Estrogens with or without progestin should be used for shortest duration possible at the lowest effective dose consistent with treatment goals. Before prescribing estrogen therapy to postmenopausal women, the risks and benefits must be weighed for each patient. Women should be informed of these risks and benefits, as well as possible effects of progestin when added to estrogen therapy. Estrogens with or without progestin should be used for shortest duration possible consistent with treatment goals. Conduct periodic risk:benefit assessments.

When used solely for prevention of osteoporosis in women at significant risk, nonestrogen treatment options should be considered. When used solely for the treatment of vulvar and vaginal atrophy, topical vaginal products should be considered. Use caution applying topical products to severely atrophic vaginal mucosa. Use of the vaginal cream may weaken latex found in condoms, diaphragms or cervical caps.

▶

◄ **Adverse Reactions**

Note: Percentages reported in postmenopausal women following oral use.

>10%:

Central nervous system: Headache (26% to 32%; placebo 28%)

Endocrine & metabolic: Breast pain (7% to 12%; placebo 9%)

Gastrointestinal: Abdominal pain (15% to 17%)

Genitourinary: Vaginal hemorrhage (2% to 14%)

Neuromuscular & skeletal: Back pain (13% to 14%)

1% to 10%:

Central nervous system: Nervousness (2% to 5%)

Dermatologic: Pruritus (4% to 5%)

Gastrointestinal: Flatulence (6% to 7%)

Genitourinary: Vaginitis (5% to 7%), leukorrhea (4% to 7%), vaginal moniliasis (5% to 6%)

Neuromuscular & skeletal: Weakness (7% to 8%), leg cramps (3% to 7%)

Additional adverse reactions reported with injection or vaginal cream; frequency not defined:

Genitourinary: Cystis-like syndrome, genital pruritus, vulvovaginal discomfort

Local: injection site: Edema, pain, phlebitis

In addition, the following have been reported with estrogen and/or progestin therapy:

Cardiovascular: DVT, edema, hypertension, MI, stroke, superficial venous thrombosis

Central nervous system: Dementia, dizziness, epilepsy exacerbation, headache, irritability, mental depression, migraine, mood disturbances, nervousness

Dermatologic: Angioedema, chloasma, erythema multiforme, erythema nodosum, hemorrhagic eruption, hirsutism, loss of scalp hair, melasma, pruritus, rash, urticaria

Endocrine & metabolic: Breast cancer, breast discharge, breast enlargement, breast tenderness, dysmenorrhea, fibrocystic breast changes, galactorrhea, glucose intolerance, HDL-cholesterol increased, hyper-/hypocalcemia, LDL-cholesterol decreased, libido (changes in), ovarian cancer, serum triglycerides/phospholipids increased, thyroid-binding globulin increased, total thyroid hormone (T_4) increased

Gastrointestinal: Abdominal cramps, bloating, cholecystitis, cholelithiasis, gallbladder disease, ischemic colitis, nausea, pancreatitis, vomiting, weight gain/loss

Genitourinary: Abnormal uterine bleeding/spotting, changes in cervical ectropion, changes in cervical secretions, endometrial cancer, endometrial hyperplasia, increased size of uterine leiomyomata, vaginal candidiasis

Hematologic: Aggravation of porphyria, antithrombin III and antifactor Xa decreased; factors II, II-VII-X complex, VII, VIII, VII-X complex, IX, X, and XII increased; increased beta-thromboglobulin, fibrinogen levels, plasminogen/plasminogen activity, platelet aggregability, platelet count, and prothrombin

Hepatic: Cholestatic jaundice, hepatic hemangiomas enlarged

Neuromuscular & skeletal: Arthralgias, chorea, leg cramps

Local: Thrombophlebitis

Ocular: Contact lens intolerance, corneal curvature steepening, retinal vascular thrombosis

Respiratory: Asthma exacerbation, pulmonary thromboembolism

Miscellaneous: Anaphylactoid/anaphylactic reactions, benign meningioma growth potentiation

Drug Interactions

Metabolism/Transport Effects

Based on estradiol and estrone: **Substrate** of CYP1A2 (major), 2A6 (minor), 2B6 (minor), 2C9 (minor), 2C19 (minor), 2D6 (minor), 2E1 (minor), 3A4 (major); Inhibits CYP1A2 (weak), 2C8 (weak); Induces CYP3A4 (weak)

Avoid Concomitant Use

Avoid concomitant use of Estrogens (Conjugated/Equine) with any of the following: Anastrozole

Increased Effect/Toxicity

Estrogens (Conjugated/Equine) may increase the levels/effects of: Corticosteroids (Systemic); Ropinirole; Tipranavir

The levels/effects of Estrogens (Conjugated/Equine) may be increased by: Herbs (Estrogenic Properties)

Decreased Effect

Estrogens (Conjugated/Equine) may decrease the levels/effects of: Anastrozole; Saxagliptin; Somatropin; Thyroid Products

The levels/effects of Estrogens (Conjugated/Equine) may be decreased by: CYP1A2 Inducers (Strong); CYP3A4 Inducers (Strong); Deferasirox; Herbs (CYP3A4 Inducers); Peginterferon Alfa-2b; Tipranavir

Ethanol/Nutrition/Herb Interactions

Ethanol: Avoid ethanol (routine use increases estrogenplasma concentrations and risk of breast cancer). Ethanol may also increase the risk of osteoporosis.

Food: Folic acid absorption may be decreased.

Herb/Nutraceutical: St John's wort may decrease levels. Herbs with estrogenic properties may enhance the adverse/toxic effect of estrogen derivatives; examples include alfalfa, black cohosh, bloodroot, hops, kudzu, licorice, red clover, saw palmetto, soybean, thyme, wild yam, yucca.

Test Interactions Pathologist should be advised of estrogen/progesterone therapy when specimens are submitted. Reduced response to metyrapone test.

Dietary Considerations Ensure adequate calcium and vitamin D intake when used for the prevention of osteoporosis. Powder for reconstitution for injection (25 mg) contains lactose 200 mg.

Dosage Forms Excipient information presented when available (limited, particularly for generics); consult specific product labeling.

Cream, vaginal:
Premarin®: 0.625 mg/g (42.5 g)
Injection, powder for reconstitution:
Premarin®: 25 mg [contains benzyl alcohol (in diluent), lactose 200 mg]
Tablet:
Premarin®: 0.3 mg, 0.45 mg, 0.625 mg, 0.9 mg, 1.25 mg

Estrogens (Conjugated/Equine) and Medroxyprogesterone

(ES troe jenz KON joo gate ed/EE kwine & me DROKS ee proe JES te rone)

U.S. Brand Names Premphase®; Prempro™

Canadian Brand Names Premphase®; Premplus®; Prempro™

Index Terms Medroxyprogesterone and Estrogens (Conjugated); MPA and Estrogens (Conjugated)

Pharmacologic Category Estrogen and Progestin Combination

Use Women with an intact uterus: Treatment of moderate-to-severe vasomotor symptoms associated with menopause; treatment of atrophic vaginitis; osteoporosis (prophylaxis)

Pharmacodynamics/Kinetics See individual agents.

Dosage Oral: Adults:

Treatment of moderate-to-severe vasomotor symptoms associated with menopause or treatment of atrophic vaginitis in females with an intact uterus. (The lowest dose that will control symptoms should be used; medication should be discontinued as soon as possible):

Premphase®: One maroon conjugated estrogen 0.625 mg tablet daily on days 1 through 14 and one light blue conjugated estrogen 0.625 mg/MPA 5 mg tablet daily on days 15 through 28; re-evaluate patients at 3- and 6-month intervals to determine if treatment is still necessary; monitor patients for signs of endometrial cancer; rule out malignancy if unexplained vaginal bleeding occurs

Prempro™: One conjugated estrogen 0.3 mg/MPA 1.5 mg tablet daily; re-evaluate at 3-and 6-month intervals to determine if therapy is still needed; dose may be increased to a maximum of one conjugated estrogen 0.625 mg/MPA 5 mg tablet daily in patients with bleeding or spotting, once malignancy has been ruled out

Osteoporosis prophylaxis in females with an intact uterus:

Premphase®: One maroon conjugated estrogen 0.625 tablet daily on days 1 through 14 and one light blue conjugated estrogen 0.625 mg/MPA 5 mg tablet

◀

daily on days 15 through 28; monitor patients for signs of endometrial cancer; rule out malignancy if unexplained vaginal bleeding occurs

Prempro™: One conjugated estrogen 0.3 mg/MPA 1.5 mg tablet daily; dose may be increased to one conjugated estrogen 0.625 mg/MPA 5 mg tablet daily; in patients with bleeding or spotting, once malignancy has been ruled out

Elderly: Refer to adult dosing; a higher incidence of stroke and invasive breast cancer was observed in women >75 years in a WHI substudy.

Additional Information Complete prescribing information for this medication should be consulted for additional detail.

Dosage Forms Excipient information presented when available (limited, particularly for generics); consult specific product labeling.

Tablet:

Premphase® [therapy pack contains 2 separate tablet formulations]: Conjugated estrogens 0.625 mg [14 maroon tablets] and conjugated estrogen 0.625 mg/medroxyprogesterone acetate 5 mg [14 light blue tablets] (28s)

Prempro™:

0.3/1.5: Conjugated estrogens 0.3 mg and medroxyprogesterone acetate 1.5 mg (28s)

0.45/1.5: Conjugated estrogens 0.45 mg and medroxyprogesterone acetate 1.5 mg (28s)

0.625/2.5: Conjugated estrogens 0.625 mg and medroxyprogesterone acetate 2.5 mg (28s)

0.625/5: Conjugated estrogens 0.625 mg and medroxyprogesterone acetate 5 mg (28s)

References

Grodstein F, Stampfer MJ, Colditz GA, et al, "Postmenopausal Hormone Therapy and Mortality," *N Engl J Med*, 1997, 336(25):1769-75.

Hulley S, Grady D, Bush T, et al, "Randomized Trial of Estrogen Plus Progestin for Secondary Prevention of Coronary Heart Disease in Postmenopausal Women. Heart and Estrogen/Progestin Replacement Study (HERS) Research Group," *JAMA*, 1998, 280(7):605-13.

Rossouw JE, Anderson GL, Prentice RL, et al, "Risks and Benefits of Estrogen Plus Progestin in Healthy Postmenopausal Women: Principle Results From the Women's Health Initiative Randomized Controlled Trial,"*JAMA*, 2002, 288(3):321-33.

Shumaker S, Legault C, Thal L, et al, "Estrogen Plus Progestin and the Incidence of Dementia and Mild Cognitive Impairment in Postmenopausal Women: The Women's Health Initiative Memory Study: A Randomized Controlled Trial," *JAMA*, 2003, 289:2651-62.

U.S. Food and Drug Administration, Department of Health and Human Services, "FDA Approves New Labels for Estrogen and Estrogen with Progestin Therapies for Postmenopausal Women Following Review of Women's Health Initiative Data," January 8, 2003. Available at: http://www.fda.gov/medwatch/SAFETY/2003/safety03.htm#prempr. Accessed January 9, 2003.

U.S. Food and Drug Administration, Department of Health and Human Services, "WHIMS Study on Estrogen/Progestin," May 27, 2003. Available at: http://www.fda.gov/bbs/topics/ANSWERS/2003/ANS01226.html. Accessed May 29, 2003.

Wassertheil-Smoller S, Hendrix S, Limacher M, et al, "Effect of Estrogen Plus Progestin on Stroke in Postmenopausal Women: The Women's Health Initiative: A Randomized Trial," *JAMA*, 2003, 289:2673-84.

◆ **Estrogen® Fe** *see* Ethinyl Estradiol and Norethindrone *on page 554*

Eszopiclone (es zoe PIK lone)

U.S. Brand Names Lunesta®

Pharmacologic Category Hypnotic, Nonbenzodiazepine

Restrictions C-IV

Use Treatment of insomnia

Pharmacodynamics/Kinetics

Absorption: Rapid; high-fat/heavy meal may delay absorption

Protein binding: 52% to 59%

Metabolism: Hepatic via oxidation and demethylation (CYP2E1, 3A4); 2 primary metabolites; one with activity less than parent.

Half-life elimination: ~6 hours; Elderly (≥65 years): ~9 hours

Time to peak, plasma: ~1 hour

Excretion: Urine (up to 75%, primarily as metabolites; <10% as parent drug)

Dosage Oral:

Adults: Insomnia: Initial: 2 mg immediately before bedtime (maximum dose: 3 mg)
Concurrent use with strong CYP3A4 inhibitor: 1 mg immediately before bedtime; if needed, dose may be increased to 2 mg

Elderly:

Difficulty **falling** asleep: Initial: 1 mg immediately before bedtime; maximum dose: 2 mg

Difficulty **staying** asleep: 2 mg immediately before bedtime

Dosage adjustment in renal impairment: None required

Dosage adjustment in hepatic impairment:

Mild-to-moderate: Use with caution; dosage adjustment unnecessary

Severe: Initial dose: 1 mg; maximum dose: 2 mg

Additional Information Complete prescribing information for this medication should be consulted for additional detail.

Dosage Forms Excipient information presented when available (limited, particularly for generics); consult specific product labeling.

Tablet: 1 mg, 2 mg, 3 mg

References

Krystal AD, Walsh JK, Laska E, et al, "Sustained Efficacy of Eszopiclone Over 6 Months of Nightly Treatment: Results of a Randomized, Double-Blind, Placebo-Controlled Study in Adults With Chronic Insomnia," *Sleep*, 2003, 26(7):793-9.

◆ **Ethacrynate Sodium** *see* Ethacrynic Acid *on page 541*

Ethacrynic Acid (eth a KRIN ik AS id)

Medication Safety Issues

Sound-alike/look-alike issues:

Edecrin® may be confused with Eulexin®, Ecotrin®

Related Information

Diuretics, Loop *on page 1680*

Heart Failure (Systolic) *on page 1739*

U.S. Brand Names Edecrin®; Sodium Edecrin®

Canadian Brand Names Edecrin®

Index Terms Ethacrynate Sodium

Pharmacologic Category Diuretic, Loop

Generic Available No

Use Management of edema associated with congestive heart failure; hepatic cirrhosis or renal disease; short-term management of ascites due to malignancy, idiopathic edema, and lymphedema

Mechanism of Action Inhibits reabsorption of sodium and chloride in the ascending loop of Henle and distal renal tubule, interfering with the chloride-binding cotransport system, thus causing increased excretion of water, sodium, chloride, magnesium, and calcium

Pharmacodynamics/Kinetics

Onset of action: Diuresis: Oral: ~30 minutes; I.V.: 5 minutes

Peak effect: Oral: 2 hours; I.V.: 30 minutes

Duration: Oral: 12 hours; I.V.: 2 hours

Absorption: Oral: Rapid

Protein binding: >90%

Metabolism: Hepatic (35% to 40%) to active cysteine conjugate

Half-life elimination: Normal renal function: 2-4 hours

Excretion: Feces and urine (30% to 60% as unchanged drug)

Dosage I.V. formulation should be diluted in D_5W or NS (1 mg/mL) and infused over several minutes.

Children: Oral: 1 mg/kg/dose once daily; increase at intervals of 2-3 days as needed, to a maximum of 3 mg/kg/day.

Adults:

Oral: 50-200 mg/day in 1-2 divided doses; may increase in increments of 25-50 mg at intervals of several days; doses up to 200 mg twice daily may be required with severe, refractory edema.

I.V.: 0.5-1 mg/kg/dose (maximum: 100 mg/dose); repeat doses not routinely recommended; however, if indicated, repeat doses every 8-12 hours.

Dosing adjustment/comments in renal impairment: Cl_{cr} <10 mL/minute: Avoid use.

Dialysis: Not removed by hemo- or peritoneal dialysis; supplemental dose is not necessary.

Administration Injection should **not** be given SubQ or I.M. due to local pain and irritation; single I.V. doses should not exceed 100 mg; if a second dose is needed, use a new injection site to avoid possible thrombophlebitis

Monitoring Parameters Blood pressure, renal function, serum electrolytes, and fluid status closely, including weight and I & O daily; hearing

Anesthesia and Critical Care Concerns/Other Considerations

Clinical Pearls/Comments: Ethacrynic acid has limited use over other loop diuretics because of increased risk of ototoxicity. If given the morning of surgery, it may render the patient volume depleted and blood pressure may be labile during general anesthesia.

Pregnancy Risk Factor B

Contraindications Hypersensitivity to ethacrynic acid or any component of the formulation; anuria; history of severe watery diarrhea caused by this product; infants

Warnings/Precautions Loop diuretics are potent diuretics; excess amounts can lead to profound diuresis with fluid and electrolyte loss; close medical supervision and dose evaluation are required. Watch for and correct electrolyte disturbances; adjust dose to avoid dehydration. In cirrhosis, avoid electrolyte and acid/base imbalances that might lead to hepatic encephalopathy. Monitor fluid status and renal function in an attempt to prevent oliguria, azotemia, and reversible increases in BUN and creatinine; close medical supervision of aggressive diuresis required. Rapid I.V. administration, renal impairment, excessive doses, and concurrent use of other ototoxins is associated with ototoxicity; has been associated with a higher incidence of ototoxicity than other loop diuretics. Hypersensitivity reactions can rarely occur, however, ethacrynic acid has no cross-reactivity to sulfonamides or sulfonylureas. Coadministration of antihypertensives may increase the risk of hypotension.

Adverse Reactions Frequency not defined.

Central nervous system: Headache, fatigue, apprehension, confusion, fever, chills, encephalopathy (patients with pre-existing liver disease); vertigo

Dermatologic: Skin rash, Henoch-Schönlein purpura (in patient with rheumatic heart disease)

Endocrine & metabolic: Hyponatremia, hyperglycemia, variations in phosphorus, CO_2 content, bicarbonate, and calcium; reversible hyperuricemia, gout, hyperglycemia, hypoglycemia (occurred in two uremic patients who received doses above those recommended)

Gastrointestinal: Anorexia, malaise, abdominal discomfort or pain, dysphagia, nausea, vomiting, and diarrhea, gastrointestinal bleeding, acute pancreatitis (rare)

Genitourinary: Hematuria

Hepatic: Jaundice, abnormal liver function tests

Hematology: Agranulocytosis, severe neutropenia, thrombocytopenia

Local: Thrombophlebitis (with intravenous use), local irritation and pain

Ocular: Blurred vision

Otic: Tinnitus, temporary or permanent deafness

Renal: Increased serum creatinine

Drug Interactions

Avoid Concomitant Use

Avoid concomitant use of Ethacrynic Acid with any of the following: Furosemide

Increased Effect/Toxicity

Ethacrynic Acid may increase the levels/effects of: ACE Inhibitors; Allopurinol; Amifostine; Aminoglycosides; Antihypertensives; Dofetilide; Hypotensive Agents; Lithium; Neuromuscular-Blocking Agents; RiTUXimab; Salicylates

The levels/effects of Ethacrynic Acid may be increased by: Corticosteroids (Orally Inhaled); Corticosteroids (Systemic); Diazoxide; Furosemide; Herbs (Hypotensive Properties); MAO Inhibitors; Pentoxifylline; Phosphodiesterase 5 Inhibitors; Prostacyclin Analogues

Decreased Effect

Ethacrynic Acid may decrease the levels/effects of: Lithium; Neuromuscular-Blocking Agents

The levels/effects of Ethacrynic Acid may be decreased by: Bile Acid Sequestrants; Herbs (Hypertensive Properties); Methylphenidate; Nonsteroidal Anti-Inflammatory Agents; Phenytoin; Salicylates; Yohimbine

Dietary Considerations This product may cause a potassium loss. Your healthcare provider may prescribe a potassium supplement, another medication to help prevent the potassium loss, or recommend that you eat foods high in potassium, especially citrus fruits. Do not change your diet on your own while taking this medication, especially if you are taking potassium supplements or medications to reduce potassium loss. Too much potassium can be as harmful as too little.

Dosage Forms Excipient information presented when available (limited, particularly for generics); consult specific product labeling.
Injection, powder for reconstitution, as ethacrynate sodium:
  Sodium Edecrin®: 50 mg
Tablet:
  Edecrin®: 25 mg [scored]

◆ **Ethamolin®** *see* Ethanolamine Oleate *on page 543*
◆ **Ethanol** *see* Alcohol (Ethyl) *on page 53*

Ethanolamine Oleate (ETH a nol a meen OH lee ate)

Medication Safety Issues
Sound-alike/look-alike issues:
  Ethamolin® may be confused with ethanol
U.S. Brand Names Ethamolin®
Index Terms Monoethanolamine
Pharmacologic Category Sclerosing Agent
Generic Available No
Use Orphan drug: Sclerosing agent used for bleeding esophageal varices
Mechanism of Action Derived from oleic acid and similar in physical properties to sodium morrhuate; however, the exact mechanism of the hemostatic effect used in endoscopic injection sclerotherapy is not known. Intravenously injected ethanolamine oleate produces a sterile inflammatory response resulting in fibrosis and occlusion of the vein; a dose-related extravascular inflammatory reaction occurs when the drug diffuses through the venous wall. Autopsy results indicate that variceal obliteration occurs secondary to mural necrosis and fibrosis. Thrombosis appears to be a transient reaction.
Dosage Adults: 1.5-5 mL per varix, up to 20 mL total or 0.4 mL/kg for a 50 kg patient; doses should be decreased in patients with severe hepatic dysfunction and should receive less than recommended maximum dose
Administration Use care to use acceptable technique to avoid necrosis
Pregnancy Risk Factor C
Contraindications Hypersensitivity to agent or oleic acid
Warnings/Precautions Fatal anaphylactic shock has been reported following administration; fatal aspiration pneumonia has occurred; use with caution and decrease doses in patients with significant liver dysfunction (Child class C), with concomitant cardiorespiratory disease, or in the elderly or critically-ill. Safety and efficacy have not been established in children.
Adverse Reactions
1% to 10%:
  Central nervous system: Pyrexia (1.8%)
  Gastrointestinal: Esophageal ulcer (2%), esophageal stricture (1.3%)
  Respiratory: Pleural effusion (2%), pneumonia (1.2%)
  Miscellaneous: Retrosternal pain (1.6%)
<1% (Limited to important or life-threatening): Acute renal failure, anaphylaxis, esophagitis, injection necrosis, perforation

◀ **Drug Interactions**

Avoid Concomitant Use There are no known interactions where it is recommended to avoid concomitant use.

Increased Effect/Toxicity There are no known significant interactions involving an increase in effect.

Decreased Effect There are no known significant interactions involving a decrease in effect.

Dosage Forms Excipient information presented when available (limited, particularly for generics); consult specific product labeling.

Injection, solution: 5% [50 mg/mL] (2 mL) [contains benzyl alcohol]

Ethinyl Estradiol and Desogestrel
(ETH in il es tra DYE ole & des oh JES trel)

U.S. Brand Names Apri®; Cesia™; Cyclessa®; Desogen®; Kariva™; Mircette®; Ortho-Cept®; Reclipsen™; Solia™; Velivet™

Canadian Brand Names Cyclessa®; Linessa®; Marvelon®; Ortho-Cept®

Index Terms Desogestrel and Ethinyl Estradiol; Ortho Cept

Pharmacologic Category Contraceptive; Estrogen and Progestin Combination

Use Prevention of pregnancy

Unlabeled/Investigational Use Treatment of hypermenorrhea (menorrhagia); pain associated with endometriosis; dysmenorrhea; dysfunctional uterine bleeding

Pharmacodynamics/Kinetics

Absorption: Desogestrel and ethinyl estradiol: Rapid and complete

Protein binding: Etonogestrel (active metabolite): 98%, primarily to sex hormone-binding globulin; Ethinyl estradiol: primarily bound to albumin

Metabolism:

Desogestrel: Hepatic via CYP2C9 to active metabolite etonogestrel (3-keto-desogestrel); etonogestrel metabolized via CYP3A4

Ethinyl estradiol: Hepatic; forms metabolites

Half-life elimination: Etonogestrel: ~38 hours; Ethinyl estradiol: ~26 hours

Excretion: Etonogestrel and ethinyl estradiol: Urine and feces (as metabolites)

Dosage Oral: Adults: Females: Contraception:

Schedule 1 (Sunday starter): Dose begins on first Sunday after onset of menstruation; if the menstrual period starts on Sunday, take first tablet that very same day. **With a Sunday start, an additional method of contraception should be used until after the first 7 days of consecutive administration.**

For 21-tablet package: Dosage is 1 tablet daily for 21 consecutive days, followed by 7 days off of the medication; a new course begins on the 8th day after the last tablet is taken.

For 28-tablet package: Dosage is 1 tablet daily without interruption.

Schedule 2 (Day 1 starter): Dose starts on first day of menstrual cycle taking 1 tablet daily.

For 21-tablet package: Dosage is 1 tablet daily for 21 consecutive days, followed by 7 days off of the medication; a new course begins on the 8th day after the last tablet is taken.

For 28-tablet package: Dosage is 1 tablet daily without interruption.

If all doses have been taken on schedule and one menstrual period is missed, continue dosing cycle. If two consecutive menstrual periods are missed, pregnancy test is required before new dosing cycle is started.

Missed doses **monophasic formulations** (refer to package insert for complete information):

One dose missed: Take as soon as remembered or take 2 tablets next day

Two consecutive doses missed in the first 2 weeks: Take 2 tablets as soon as remembered or 2 tablets next 2 days. **An additional method of contraception should be used for 7 days after missed dose.**

Two consecutive doses missed in week 3 or three consecutive doses missed at any time:

Schedule 1 (Sunday starter): Continue to take 1 tablet daily until Sunday, then discard the rest of the pack, and a new pack is started that same day.

Schedule 2 (Day 1 starter): Current pack should be discarded, and a new pack started that same day. **An additional method of contraception should be used for 7 days after missed dose.**

Missed doses **biphasic/triphasic formulations** (refer to package insert for complete information):

One dose missed: Take as soon as remembered or take 2 tablets next day.

Two consecutive doses missed in week 1 or week 2 of the pack: Take 2 tablets as soon as remembered and 2 tablets the next day. Resume taking 1 tablet daily until the pack is empty. **An additional method of contraception should be used for 7 days after a missed dose.**

Two consecutive doses missed in week 3 of the pack; **an additional method of contraception must be used for 7 days after a missed dose**:

Schedule 1 (Sunday starter): Take 1 tablet every day until Sunday. Discard the remaining pack and start a new pack of pills on the same day.

Schedule 2 (Day 1 starter): Discard the remaining pack and start a new pack the same day.

Three or more consecutive doses missed; **an additional method of contraception must be used for 7 days after a missed dose**:

Schedule 1 (Sunday starter): Take 1 tablet every day until Sunday; on Sunday, discard the pack and start a new pack.

Schedule 2 (Day 1 starter): Discard the remaining pack and begin new pack of tablets starting on the same day.

Dosage adjustment in renal impairment: Specific guidelines not available; use with caution and monitor blood pressure closely. Consider other forms of contraception.

Dosage adjustment in hepatic impairment: Contraindicated in patients with hepatic impairment

Additional Information Complete prescribing information for this medication should be consulted for additional detail.

Dosage Forms Excipient information presented when available (limited, particularly for generics); consult specific product labeling.

Tablet, low-dose formulations:

Kariva™:

Day 1-21: Ethinyl estradiol 0.02 mg and desogestrel 0.15 mg [21 white tablets]

Day 22-23: 2 inactive light green tablets

Day 24-28: Ethinyl estradiol 0.01 mg [5 light blue tablets] (28s)

Mircette®:

Day 1-21: Ethinyl estradiol 0.02 mg and desogestrel 0.15 mg [21 white tablets]

Day 22-23: 2 inactive green tablets

Day 24-28: Ethinyl estradiol 0.01 mg [5 yellow tablets] (28s)

Tablet, monophasic formulations:

Apri® 28: Ethinyl estradiol 0.03 mg and desogestrel 0.15 mg (28s) [21 rose tablets and 7 white inactive tablets]

Desogen®, Reclipsen™, Solia™: Ethinyl estradiol 0.03 mg and desogestrel 0.15 mg (28s) [21 white tablets and 7 green inactive tablets]

Ortho-Cept® 28: Ethinyl estradiol 0.03 mg and desogestrel 0.15 mg (28s) [21 orange tablets and 7 green inactive tablets]

Tablet, triphasic formulations:

Cesia™, Cyclessa®:

Day 1-7: Ethinyl estradiol 0.025 mg and desogestrel 0.1 mg [7 light yellow tablets]

Day 8-14: Ethinyl estradiol 0.025 mg and desogestrel 0.125 mg [7 orange tablets]

Day 14-21: Ethinyl estradiol 0.025 mg and desogestrel 0.15 mg [7 red tablets]

Day 21-28: 7 green inactive tablets (28s)

Velivet™:

Day 1-7: Ethinyl estradiol 0.025 mg and desogestrel 0.1 mg [7 beige tablets]

Day 8-14: Ethinyl estradiol 0.025 mg and desogestrel 0.125 mg [7 orange tablets]

Day 14-21: Ethinyl estradiol 0.025 mg and desogestrel 0.15 mg [7 pink tablets]

Day 21-28: 7 white inactive tablets (28s)

References

"American Academy of Pediatrics Committee on Drugs. The Transfer of Drugs and Other Chemicals Into Human Milk," *Pediatrics*, 2001, 108(3):776-89.

"An Open-Label, Multicenter, Noncomparative Safety and Efficacy Study of Mircette, a Low-Dose Estrogen-Progestin Oral Contraceptive. The Mircette Study Group," *Am J Obstet Gynecol*, 1998, 179(1):S2-8.

Burkman R, Schlesselman JJ, and Zieman M, "Safety Concerns and Health Benefits Associated With Oral Contraception," *Am J Obstet Gynecol*, 2004, 190(4 Suppl):5-22

"Guidelines for the Use of Antiretroviral Agents in HIV-infected Adults and Adolescents. Panel on Clinical Practices for Treatment of HIV Infection," August 13, 2001. Available at: http://www.aidsinfo. nih.gov. Accessed September 5, 2001.

Holt VL, Scholes D, Wicklund KG, et al, "Body Mass Index, Weight, and Oral Contraceptive Failure Risk," *Obstet Gynecol*, 2005, 105(1):46-52.

Orme ML, Back DJ, and Breckenridge AM, "Clinical Pharmacokinetics of Oral Contraceptive Steroids," *Clin Pharmacokinet*, 1983, 8(2):95-136.

Shenfield GM and Griffin JM, "Clinical Pharmacokinetics of Contraceptive Steroids. An Update," *Clin Pharmacokinet*, 1991, 20(1):15-37.

Ethinyl Estradiol and Drospirenone
(ETH in il es tra DYE ole & droh SPYE re none)

U.S. Brand Names Ocella™; Yasmin®; Yaz®

Canadian Brand Names Yasmin®; Yaz®

Index Terms Drospirenone and Ethinyl Estradiol

Pharmacologic Category Contraceptive; Estrogen and Progestin Combination

Use Females: Prevention of pregnancy; treatment of premenstrual dysphoric disorder (PMDD); treatment of acne

Unlabeled/Investigational Use Treatment of hypermenorrhea (menorrhagia); pain associated with endometriosis; dysmenorrhea; dysfunctional uterine bleeding

Pharmacodynamics/Kinetics

Distribution: Drospirenone: 4 L/kg; Ethinyl estradiol: 4-5 L/kg

Protein binding: Drospirenone: Serum proteins (excluding sex hormone-binding globulin and corticosteroid-binding globulin): 97%; Ethinyl estradiol: ~98%

Metabolism: Drospirenone: To inactive metabolites, minor metabolism hepatically via CYP3A4; Ethinyl estradiol: Hepatic via CYP3A4; forms metabolites; undergoes enterohepatic circulation

Bioavailability: Drospirenone: 76%; Ethinyl estradiol: 40%

Half-life elimination: Drospirenone: 30 hours; Ethinyl estradiol: ~24 hours

Time to peak: 1-3 hours

Excretion: Drospirenone, ethinyl estradiol: Urine and feces

Dosage Oral:

Children ≥14 years and Adults: Females: Acne (Yaz®): Refer to dosing for contraception

Adults: Females: Contraception (Yasmin®, Yaz®), PMDD (Yaz®): Dosage is 1 tablet daily for 28 consecutive days. Dose should be taken at the same time each day, either after the evening meal or at bedtime. Dosing may be started on the first day of menstrual period (Day 1 starter) or on the first Sunday after the onset of the menstrual period (Sunday starter).

Day 1 starter: Dose starts on first day of menstrual cycle taking 1 tablet daily.

Sunday starter: Dose begins on first Sunday after onset of menstruation; if the menstrual period starts on Sunday, take first tablet that very same day. **With a Sunday start, an additional method of contraception should be used until after the first 7 days of consecutive administration.**

If all doses have been taken on schedule and one menstrual period is missed, continue dosing cycle. If two consecutive menstrual periods are missed, pregnancy test is required before new dosing cycle is started.

If doses have been missed during the first 3 weeks and the menstrual period is missed, pregnancy should be ruled out prior to continuing treatment.

Missed doses (monophasic formulations) (refer to package insert for complete information):

One dose missed: Take as soon as remembered or take 2 tablets next day

Two consecutive doses missed in the first 2 weeks: Take 2 tablets as soon as remembered or 2 tablets next 2 days. **An additional method of contraception should be used for 7 days after missed dose.**

Two consecutive doses missed in week 3 or three consecutive doses missed at any time: **An additional method of contraception must be used for 7 days after a missed dose.**
Day 1 starter: Current pack should be discarded, and a new pack should be started that same day.
Sunday starter: Continue dose of 1 tablet daily until Sunday, then discard the rest of the pack, and a new pack should be started that same day.
Any number of doses missed in week 4: Continue taking one pill each day until pack is empty; no back-up method of contraception is needed

Dosage adjustment in renal impairment: Contraindicated in patients with renal dysfunction (Cl_{cr} ≤50 mL/minute)
Dosage adjustment in hepatic impairment: Contraindicated in patients with hepatic dysfunction
Additional Information Complete prescribing information for this medication should be consulted for additional detail.
Dosage Forms Excipient information presented when available (limited, particularly for generics); consult specific product labeling.
Tablet:
Ocella™: Ethinyl estradiol 0.03 mg and drospirenone 3 mg (28s) [21 yellow active tablets and 7 white inactive tablets]
Yasmin®: Ethinyl estradiol 0.03 mg and drospirenone 3 mg (28s) [21 yellow active tablets and 7 white inactive tablets]
Yaz®: Ethinyl estradiol 0.02 mg and drospirenone 3 mg (28s) [24 light pink tablets and 4 white inactive tablets]

References
Burkman R, Schlesselman JJ, and Zieman M, "Safety Concerns and Health Benefits Associated With Oral Contraception," *Am J Obstet Gynecol*, 2004, 190(4 Suppl):5-22.
Holt VL, Scholes D, Wicklund KG, et al, "Body Mass Index, Weight, and Oral Contraceptive Failure Risk," *Obstet Gynecol*, 2005, 105(1):46-52.
Pearlstein TB, Bachmann GA, Zacur HA, et al, "Treatment of Premenstrual Dysphoric Disorder With a New Drospirenone-Containing Oral Contraceptive Formulation," *Contraception*, 2005, 72 (6):414-21.

Ethinyl Estradiol and Etonogestrel
(ETH in il es tra DYE ole & et oh noe JES trel)

U.S. Brand Names NuvaRing®
Canadian Brand Names NuvaRing®
Index Terms Etonogestrel and Ethinyl Estradiol
Pharmacologic Category Contraceptive; Estrogen and Progestin Combination
Use Prevention of pregnancy
Unlabeled/Investigational Use Treatment of hypermenorrhea (menorrhagia); pain associated with endometriosis; dysmenorrhea; dysfunctional uterine bleeding
Pharmacodynamics/Kinetics
Duration: Serum levels (contraceptive effectiveness) decrease after 3 weeks of continuous use
Absorption: Ethinyl estradiol and etonogestrel: Rapid
Tampons do not interfere with absorption.
Protein binding:
Ethinyl estradiol: 98%, primarily to albumin
Etonogestrel: 32% to sex hormone-binding globulin (SHBG) and 66% to albumin; SHBG capacity is affected by plasma ethinyl estradiol levels
Metabolism:
Ethinyl estradiol: Hepatic via CYP3A4; forms metabolites (weak estrogenic activity)
Etonogestrel: Hepatic via CYP3A4; forms metabolites (activity not known)
Bioavailability: Vaginal: Ethinyl estradiol: ~56% Etonogestrel: 100%
Half-life elimination: Ethinyl estradiol: 45 hours; Etonogestrel: 29 hours
Time to peak: Vaginal: Ethinyl estradiol: 60 hours; Etonogestrel: 200 hours
Excretion: Ethinyl estradiol and etonogestrel: Urine, bile, and feces
Dosage Vaginal: Adults: Females: Contraception: One ring, inserted vaginally and left in place for 3 consecutive weeks, then removed for 1 week. A new ring is inserted 7 days after the last was removed (even if bleeding is not complete) and

should be inserted at approximately the same time of day the ring was removed the previous week.

Initial treatment should begin as follows (pregnancy should always be ruled out first):

No hormonal contraceptive use in the past month: Insert ring on the first day of menstrual cycle ("Day 1"). May also insert on days 2-5 even if bleeding is not complete, however, **a spermicide or barrier method of contraception should be used for the following 7 days.**[*]

Switching from combination oral contraceptive: Ring can be inserted on any day within 7 days after the last **active** tablet in the cycle was taken and no later than the first day a new cycle of tablets would begin. Additional forms of contraception are not needed.

Switching from progestin-only contraceptive: **A spermicide or barrier method of contraception should be used for the following 7 days with any of the following.**[*]

If previously using a progestin-only mini-pill, insert the ring on any day of the month; do not skip days between the last pill and insertion of the ring.

If previously using an implant, insert the ring on the same day of implant removal.

If previously using a progestin-containing IUD, insert the ring on day of IUD removal.

If previously using a progestin injection, insert the ring on the day the next injection would be given.

Following complete 1st trimester abortion: Insert ring within the first 5 days of abortion. If not inserted within 5 days, follow instructions for "No hormonal contraceptive use within the past month" and instruct patient to use a nonhormonal contraceptive in the interim.

Following delivery or 2nd trimester abortion: Insert ring 4 weeks postpartum (in women who are not breast-feeding) or following 2nd trimester abortion. **A spermicide or barrier method of contraception should be used for the following 7 days.**[*]

If the ring is accidentally removed from the vagina at anytime during the 3-week period of use, it may be rinsed with cool or lukewarm water (not hot) and reinserted as soon as possible. If the ring is not reinserted within 3 hours, contraceptive effectiveness will be decreased. **A spermicide or barrier method of contraception should be used until the ring has been in place for 7 consecutive days.**[*]

If the ring has been removed for longer than 1 week, pregnancy must be ruled out prior to restarting therapy. **A spermicide or barrier method of contraception should be used for the following 7 days.**[*]

If the ring has been left in place for >3 weeks, a new ring should be inserted following a 1-week (ring-free) interval. Protection continues during week 4, however, if the ring is left in place >4 weeks, pregnancy must be ruled out prior to insertion and **a spermicide or barrier method of contraception should be used for the following 7 days.**[*]

Disconnected ring: In the event the ring disconnects at the weld joint, discard and replace with a new ring.

[*]Note: Diaphragms may interfere with proper ring placement, and therefore, are not recommended for use as an additional form of contraception.

Dosage adjustment in renal impairment: Specific guidelines not available; use with caution and monitor blood pressure closely. Consider other forms of contraception.

Dosage adjustment in hepatic impairment: Contraindicated in patients with hepatic impairment

Additional Information Complete prescribing information for this medication should be consulted for additional detail.

Dosage Forms Excipient information presented when available (limited, particularly for generics); consult specific product labeling.

Ring, vaginal:

NuvaRing®: Ethinyl estradiol 0.015 mg/day and etonogestrel 0.12 mg/day (1s) [3-week duration]

References

Burkman R, Schlesselman JJ, and Zieman M, "Safety Concerns and Health Benefits Associated With Oral Contraception," *Am J Obstet Gynecol*, 2004, 190(4 Suppl):5-22.

"Guidelines for the Use of Antiretroviral Agents in HIV-infected Adults and Adolescents. Panel on Clinical Practices for Treatment of HIV Infection," August 13, 2001. Available at: http://www.aidsinfo. nih.gov. Accessed September 5, 2001.

Holt VL, Scholes D, Wicklund KG, et al, "Body Mass Index, Weight, and Oral Contraceptive Failure Risk," *Obstet Gynecol*, 2005, 105(1):46-52.

Orme ML, Back DJ, and Breckenridge AM, "Clinical Pharmacokinetics of Oral Contraceptive Steroids," *Clin Pharmacokinet*, 1983, 8(2):95-136.

Shenfield GM and Griffin JM, "Clinical Pharmacokinetics of Contraceptive Steroids. An Update," *Clin Pharmacokinet*, 1991, 20(1):15-37.

Ethinyl Estradiol and Levonorgestrel

(ETH in il es tra DYE ole & LEE voe nor jes trel)

U.S. Brand Names Alesse®; Aviane™; Enpresse™; Jolessa™; Lessina™; Levlen®; Levlite™; Levora®; LoSeasonique™; Lutera™; Lybrel™; Nordette®; Portia™; Quasense™; Seasonale®; Seasonique™; Sronyx™; Triphasil®; Trivora®

Canadian Brand Names Alesse®; Aviane®; Min-Ovral®; Seasonale®; Triphasil®; Triquilar®

Index Terms Levonorgestrel and Ethinyl Estradiol

Pharmacologic Category Contraceptive; Estrogen and Progestin Combination

Use Prevention of pregnancy; postcoital contraception

Unlabeled/Investigational Use Treatment of hypermenorrhea (menorrhagia); pain associated with endometriosis; dysmenorrhea; dysfunctional uterine bleeding

Pharmacodynamics/Kinetics

Absorption: Rapid

Distribution: Ethinyl estradiol: 4.3 L/kg; Levonorgestrel: 1.8 L/kg

Protein binding:

Ethinyl estradiol: 95% to 97% to albumin

Levonorgestrel: 97% to 99% primarily to sex hormone binding globulin (SHBG), lesser amounts to albumin

Metabolism:

Ethinyl estradiol: Hepatic via CYP3A4; undergoes first-pass metabolism; forms metabolites

Levonorgestrel: Forms conjugated in unconjugated metabolites

Bioavailability: Ethinyl estradiol: 38% to 48%; Levonorgestrel: 100%

Half-life elimination: Ethinyl estradiol: 12-23 hours; Levonorgestrel: 22-49 hours

Excretion:

Ethinyl estradiol: Urine and feces

Levonorgestrel: Urine (40% to 68%, parent drug and metabolites); feces (16% to 48% as metabolites)

Dosage Oral: Adults: Females:

Contraception, 28-day cycle:

Schedule 1 (Sunday starter): Dose begins on first Sunday after onset of menstruation; if the menstrual period starts on Sunday, take first tablet that very same day. With a Sunday start, an additional method of contraception should be used until after the first 7 days of consecutive administration:

For 21-tablet package: 1 tablet/day for 21 consecutive days, followed by 7 days off of the medication; a new course begins on the 8th day after the last tablet is taken

For 28-tablet package: 1 tablet/day without interruption

Schedule 2 (Day 1 starter): Dose starts on first day of menstrual cycle taking 1 tablet/day:

For 21-tablet package: 1 tablet/day for 21 consecutive days, followed by 7 days off of the medication; a new course begins on the 8th day after the last tablet is taken

For 28-tablet package: 1 tablet/day without interruption

If all doses have been taken on schedule and one menstrual period is missed, continue dosing cycle. If two consecutive menstrual periods are missed, pregnancy test is required before new dosing cycle is started.

Missed doses **monophasic formulations** (refer to package insert for complete information):

One dose missed: Take as soon as remembered or take 2 tablets next day

Two consecutive doses missed in the first 2 weeks: Take 2 tablets as soon as remembered or 2 tablets next 2 days. An additional method of contraception should be used for 7 days after missed dose.

Two consecutive doses missed in week 3 or three consecutive doses missed at any time: An additional method of contraception must be used for 7 days after a missed dose:

Schedule 1 (Sunday starter): Continue dose of 1 tablet daily until Sunday, then discard the rest of the pack, and a new pack should be started that same day.

Schedule 2 (Day 1 starter): Current pack should be discarded, and a new pack should be started that same day.

Missed doses **biphasic/triphasic formulations** (refer to package insert for complete information):

One dose missed: Take as soon as remembered or take 2 tablets next day.

Two consecutive doses missed in week 1 or week 2 of the pack: Take 2 tablets as soon as remembered and 2 tablets the next day. Resume taking 1 tablet daily until the pack is empty. An additional method of contraception should be used for 7 days after a missed dose.

Two consecutive doses missed in week 3 of the pack: An additional method of contraception must be used for 7 days after a missed dose.

Schedule 1 (Sunday starter): Take 1 tablet every day until Sunday. Discard the remaining pack and start a new pack of pills on the same day.

Schedule 2 (Day 1 starter): Discard the remaining pack and start a new pack the same day.

Three or more consecutive doses missed: An additional method of contraception must be used for 7 days after a missed dose.

Schedule 1 (Sunday starter): Take 1 tablet every day until Sunday; on Sunday, discard the pack and start a new pack.

Schedule 2 (Day 1 starter): Discard the remaining pack and begin new pack of tablets starting on the same day.

Contraception, 91-day cycle (extended cycle regimen): Dose begins on first Sunday after onset of menstruation; if the menstrual period starts on Sunday, take first tablet that very same day. An additional method of contraception should be used until after the first 7 days of consecutive administration:

Seasonale®: One active tablet/day for 84 consecutive days, followed by 1 inactive tablet/day for 7 days; if all doses have been taken on schedule and one menstrual period is missed, pregnancy should be ruled out prior to continuing therapy.

Seasonique™, LoSeasonique™: One active tablet/day for 84 consecutive days, followed by 1 low dose estrogen tablet/day for 7 days; if all doses have been taken on schedule and one menstrual period is missed, pregnancy should be ruled out prior to continuing therapy.

Missed doses:

One dose missed: Take as soon as remembered or take 2 tablets the next day

Two consecutive doses missed: Take 2 tablets as soon as remembered or 2 tablets the next 2 days. An additional nonhormonal method of contraception should be used for 7 consecutive days after the missed dose.

Three or more consecutive doses missed: Do not take the missed doses; continue taking 1 tablet/day until pack is complete. Bleeding may occur during the following week. An additional nonhormonal method of contraception should be used for 7 consecutive days after the missed dose.

Any number of pills during week 13: Throw away the missed pills and keep taking scheduled pills until the pack is finished. A back-up method of contraception is not needed

Contraception, continuous use (extended cycle regimen): Lybrel™: Take one tablet daily, at the same time each day, without a tablet-free interval. Therapy should be initiated as follows:

No previous contraception: Begin on the first day of menstrual cycle. Back-up contraception is not needed.

Previously taking a 21-day or 28-day combination hormonal contraceptive: Begin on day 1 of the withdrawal bleed (at the latest, 7 days after the last active tablet). Back-up contraception is not needed.

Previously using a progestin-only pill: Begin the day after taking a progestin only pill. Back-up contraception is needed for the first 7 days of therapy.

Previously using contraceptive implant: Begin the day of implant removal. Back-up contraception is needed for the first 7 days of therapy.

Previously using contraceptive injection: Begin when the next injection is due. Back-up contraception is needed for the first 7 days of therapy.

Missed doses:

One dose missed: Take as soon as remembered then take the next tablet at the regular time (2 tablets in 1 day). An additional nonhormonal method of contraception should also be used for 7 consecutive days.

Two consecutive doses missed: If remembered the day of the second missed tablet, take 2 tablets as soon as remembered, then 1 tablet the next day. If remembered the day after the second tablet is missed, take 2 tablets the day remembered, then 2 tablets the next day. An additional nonhormonal method of contraception should also be used for 7 consecutive days.

Three or more consecutive doses missed: Take 1 tablet daily and contact healthcare provider; do not take the missed pills. An additional nonhormonal method of contraception should also be used for 7 consecutive days.

Dosage adjustment in renal impairment: Specific guidelines not available; use with caution and monitor blood pressure closely. Consider other forms of contraception.

Dosage adjustment in hepatic impairment: Contraindicated in patients with hepatic impairment

Additional Information Complete prescribing information for this medication should be consulted for additional detail.

Dosage Forms Excipient information presented when available (limited, particularly for generics); consult specific product labeling. [DSC] = Discontinued product

Tablet, oral [low-dose formulation]:

Alesse® 28: Ethinyl estradiol 0.02 mg and levonorgestrel 0.1 mg (28s) [21 pink tablets and 7 light green inactive tablets]

Aviane™ 28: Ethinyl estradiol 0.02 mg and levonorgestrel 0.1 mg (28s) [21 orange tablets and 7 light green inactive tablets]

Lessina™ 28, Levlite™ 28: Ethinyl estradiol 0.02 mg and levonorgestrel 0.1 mg (28s) [21 pink tablets and 7 white inactive tablets]

Lutera™, Sronyx™: Ethinyl estradiol 0.02 mg and levonorgestrel 0.1 mg (28s) [21 white tablets and 7 peach inactive tablets]

Tablet, oral [monophasic formulation]:

Levlen® 28: Ethinyl estradiol 0.03 mg and levonorgestrel 0.15 mg (28s) [21 light orange tablets and 7 pink inactive tablets]

Levora® 28: Ethinyl estradiol 0.03 mg and levonorgestrel 0.15 mg (28s) [21 white tablets and 7 peach inactive tablets]

Nordette® 28: Ethinyl estradiol 0.03 mg and levonorgestrel 0.15 mg (28s) [21 light orange tablets and 7 pink inactive tablets]

Portia™ 28: Ethinyl estradiol 0.03 mg and levonorgestrel 0.15 mg (28s) [21 pink tablets and 7 white inactive tablets]

Tablet, oral [extended cycle regimen]:

Jolessa™, Seasonale®: Ethinyl estradiol 0.03 mg and levonorgestrel 0.15 mg (91s) [84 pink tablets and 7 white inactive tablets]

LoSeasonique™: Ethinyl estradiol 0.02 mg and levonorgestrel 0.1 mg (91s) [84 orange tablets] and ethinyl estradiol 0.01 mg [7 yellow tablets]

Quasense™: Ethinyl estradiol 0.03 mg and levonorgestrel 0.15 mg (91s) [84 white tablets and 7 peach inactive tablets]

Seasonique™: Ethinyl estradiol 0.03 mg and levonorgestrel 0.15 mg (91s) [84 light blue-green tablets] and ethinyl estradiol 0.01 mg [7 yellow tablets]

Tablet, oral [noncyclic regimen]:

Lybrel™: Ethinyl estradiol 0.02 mg and levonorgestrel 0.09 mg (28s) [28 yellow tablets]

◄ Tablet, oral [triphasic formulation]:

Enpresse™ 28:

Day 1-6: Ethinyl estradiol 0.03 mg and levonorgestrel 0.05 mg [6 pink tablets]

Day 7-11: Ethinyl estradiol 0.04 mg and levonorgestrel 0.075 mg [5 white tablets]

Day 12-21: Ethinyl estradiol 0.03 mg and levonorgestrel 0.125 mg [10 orange tablets]

Day 22-28: 7 light green inactive tablets (28s)

Triphasil® 28:

Day 1-6: Ethinyl estradiol 0.03 mg and levonorgestrel 0.05 mg [6 brown tablets]

Day 7-11: Ethinyl estradiol 0.04 mg and levonorgestrel 0.075 mg [5 white tablets]

Day 12-21: Ethinyl estradiol 0.03 mg and levonorgestrel 0.125 mg [10 light yellow tablets]

Day 22-28: 7 light green inactive tablets (28s)

Trivora® 28:

Day 1-6: Ethinyl estradiol 0.03 mg and levonorgestrel 0.05 mg [6 blue tablets]

Day 7-11: Ethinyl estradiol 0.04 mg and levonorgestrel 0.075 mg [5 white tablets]

Day 12-21: Ethinyl estradiol 0.03 mg and levonorgestrel 0.125 mg [10 pink tablets]

Day 22-28: 7 peach inactive tablets (28s)

References

Anderson FD, Gibbons W, and Portman D, "Safety and Efficacy of an Extended-Regimen Oral Contraceptive Utilizing Continuous Low-Dose Ethinyl Estradiol," *Contraception*, 2006, 73 (3):229-234.

Archer DF, Jensen JT, Johnson JV, et al, "Evaluation of a continuous Regimen of Levonorgestrel/ Ethinyl Estradiol: Phase 3 Study Results," *Contraception*, 2006 74(6):439-45.

Burkman R, Schlesselman JJ, and Zieman M, "Safety Concerns and Health Benefits Associated With Oral Contraception," *Am J Obstet Gynecol*, 2004, 190(4 Suppl):5-22.

"Guidelines for the Use of Antiretroviral Agents in HIV-infected Adults and Adolescents. Panel on Clinical Practices for Treatment of HIV Infection," August 13, 2001. Available at: http://www.aidsinfo. nih.gov. Accessed September 5, 2001.

Holt VL, Scholes D, Wicklund KG, et al, "Body Mass Index, Weight, and Oral Contraceptive Failure Risk," *Obstet Gynecol*, 2005, 105(1):46-52.

Orme ML, Back DJ, and Breckenridge AM, "Clinical Pharmacokinetics of Oral Contraceptive Steroids," *Clin Pharmacokinet*, 1983, 8(2):95-136.

Shenfield GM and Griffin JM, "Clinical Pharmacokinetics of Contraceptive Steroids. An Update," *Clin Pharmacokinet*, 1991, 20(1):15-37.

◆ **Ethinyl Estradiol and NGM** *see* Ethinyl Estradiol and Norgestimate *on page 558*

Ethinyl Estradiol and Norelgestromin
(ETH in il es tra DYE ole & nor el JES troe min)

U.S. Brand Names Ortho Evra®

Canadian Brand Names Evra®

Index Terms Norelgestromin and Ethinyl Estradiol; Ortho-Evra

Pharmacologic Category Contraceptive; Estrogen and Progestin Combination

Use Prevention of pregnancy

Pharmacodynamics/Kinetics

Ortho Evra®:

Absorption: Topical: Equivalent when applied to abdomen, buttock, upper outer arm, and upper torso

Ethinyl estradiol and norelgestromin: Rapid; reaches plateau by ~48 hours. Absorption of ethinyl estradiol may be increased with heat exposure due to sauna, whirlpool, or treadmill.

The amount of ethinyl estradiol absorbed is 20 mcg/day and results in greater exposure than produced by oral ethinyl estradiol 20 mcg. In contrast, peak levels of ethinyl estradiol are higher in women taking oral tablets.

Protein binding:

Ethinyl estradiol: Albumin

Norelgestromin and norgestrel: >97%; norelgestromin to albumin and norgestrel to sex-hormone-binding globulin

Metabolism: Topical:
Ethinyl estradiol: First-pass effect avoided; forms metabolites
Norelgestromin: Hepatic to norgestrel and others; first-pass effect avoided
Bioavailability: Ethinyl estradiol: ~60% greater using the topical patch when compared to oral tablets.
Half-life elimination: Topical:
Ethinyl estradiol: 17 hours
Norelgestromin: 28 hours
Excretion: Metabolites of ethinyl estradiol and norelgestromin: Urine and feces

Dosage Topical: Adults: Females:

Contraception: Apply one patch each week for 3 weeks (21 total days); followed by one week that is patch-free. Each patch should be applied on the same day each week ("patch change day") and only one patch should be worn at a time. No more than 7 days should pass during the patch-free interval.

Schedule 1 (Sunday starter): Dose begins on first Sunday after onset of menstruation; if the menstrual period starts on Sunday, apply one patch that very same day. **With a Sunday start, an additional method of contraception (nonhormonal) should be used until after the first 7 days of consecutive administration.** Each patch change will then occur on Sunday.

Schedule 2 (Day 1 starter): Dose starts on first day of menstrual cycle, applying one patch during the first 24 hours of menstrual cycle. No back-up method of contraception is needed as long as the patch is applied on the first day of cycle. Each patch change will then occur on that same day of the week.

Additional dosing considerations:

No bleeding during patch-free week/missed menstrual period: If patch has been applied as directed, continue treatment on usual "patch change day". If used correctly, no bleeding during patch-free week does not necessarily indicate pregnancy. However, if no withdrawal bleeding occurs for 2 consecutive cycles, pregnancy should be ruled out. If patch has not been applied as directed, and one menstrual period is missed, pregnancy should be ruled out prior to continuing treatment.

If a patch becomes partially or completely detached for <24 hours: Try to reapply to same place, or replace with a new patch immediately. Do not reapply if patch is no longer sticky, if it is sticking to itself or another surface, or if it has material sticking to it.

If a patch becomes partially or completely detached for >24 hours (or time period is unknown): Apply a new patch and use this day of the week as the new "patch change day" from this point on. **An additional method of contraception (nonhormonal) should be used until after the first 7 days of consecutive administration.**

Switching from oral contraceptives: Apply first patch on the first day of withdrawal bleeding. If there is no bleeding within 5 days of taking the last active tablet, pregnancy must first be ruled out. If patch is applied later than the first day of bleeding, **an additional method of contraception (nonhormonal) should be used until after the first 7 days of consecutive administration**

Use after childbirth: Therapy should not be started <4 weeks after childbirth. Pregnancy should be ruled out prior to treatment if menstrual periods have not restarted. **An additional method of contraception (nonhormonal) should be used until after the first 7 days of consecutive administration.**

Use after abortion or miscarriage: Therapy may be started immediately if abortion/miscarriage occur within the first trimester. If therapy is not started within 5 days, follow instructions for first time use. If abortion/miscarriage occur during the second trimester, therapy should not be started for at least 4 weeks. Follow directions for use after childbirth.

Dosage adjustment in renal impairment: Specific guidelines not available; use with caution and monitor blood pressure closely. Consider other forms of contraception.

Dosage adjustment in hepatic impairment: Contraindicated in patients with hepatic impairment

Additional Information Complete prescribing information for this medication should be consulted for additional detail.

◀ **Dosage Forms** Excipient information presented when available (limited, particularly for generics); consult specific product labeling. [CAN] = Canadian brand name

Note: The formulation available in Canada differs from the U.S. product in both composition and the manufacturing process (although delivery rates appear similar).

Patch, transdermal:

Ortho Evra®: Ethinyl estradiol 0.75 mg and norelgestromin 6 mg [releases ethinyl estradiol 20 mcg and norelgestromin 150 mcg per day] (1s, 3s)

Evra® [CAN]: Ethinyl estradiol 0.6 mg and norelgestromin 6 mg [releases ethinyl estradiol 20 mcg and norelgestromin 150 mcg per day] (1s, 3s) [Not available in U.S.]

References

"American Academy of Pediatrics Committee on Drugs. The Transfer of Drugs and Other Chemicals Into Human Milk," *Pediatrics*, 2001, 108(3):776-89.

"Guidelines for the Use of Antiretroviral Agents in HIV-infected Adults and Adolescents. Panel on Clinical Practices for Treatment of HIV Infection," August 13, 2001. Available at: http://www.aidsinfo. nih.gov. Accessed September 5, 2001.

Hendeles S, Galand N, Schwers J, "Metabolism of Orally-Administered D-norgestrel in Women," *Acta Endocrinol (Copenh)*, 1972, 71(3):557-68.

Orme ML, Back DJ, and Breckenridge AM, "Clinical Pharmacokinetics of Oral Contraceptive Steroids," *Clin Pharmacokinet*, 1983, 8(2):95-136.

Ethinyl Estradiol and Norethindrone
(ETH in il es tra DYE ole & nor eth IN drone)

U.S. Brand Names Aranelle™; Balziva™; Brevicon®; Estrostep® Fe; Femcon® Fe; femhrt®; Junel™; Junel™ Fe; Leena™; Loestrin®; Loestrin® 24 Fe; Loestrin® Fe; Microgestin™; Microgestin™ Fe; Modicon®; Necon® 0.5/35; Necon® 1/35; Necon® 10/11; Necon® 7/7/7; Norinyl® 1+35; Nortrel™; Nortrel™ 7/7/7; Ortho-Novum®; Ortho-Novum® 7/7/7; Ovcon®; Tilia™ Fe; Tri-Legest™ Fe; Tri-Norinyl®; Zenchent™

Canadian Brand Names Brevicon® 0.5/35; Brevicon® 1/35; FemHRT®; Loestrin™ 1.5/30; Minestrin™ 1/20; Ortho® 0.5/35; Ortho® 1/35; Ortho® 7/7/7; Select™ 1/35; Synphasic®

Index Terms Norethindrone Acetate and Ethinyl Estradiol; Ortho Novum

Pharmacologic Category Contraceptive; Estrogen and Progestin Combination

Use Prevention of pregnancy; treatment of acne; moderate-to-severe vasomotor symptoms associated with menopause; prevention of osteoporosis (in women at significant risk only)

Unlabeled/Investigational Use Treatment of hypermenorrhea (menorrhagia); pain associated with endometriosis, dysmenorrhea; dysfunctional uterine bleeding

Pharmacodynamics/Kinetics

Ethinyl estradiol:

Absorption: Rapid

Bioavailability: 43% to 55%

Distribution: V_d: 2-4 L/kg

Protein binding: >95% to albumin

Metabolism: Hepatic via oxidation and conjugation in GI tract; hydroxylated via CYP3A4 to metabolites; first-pass effect; enterohepatic recirculation; reversibly converted to estrone and estriol

Half-life elimination: 19-24 hours

Excretion: Urine (as estradiol, estrone, and estriol); feces

Dosage Oral:

Adolescents ≥15 years and Adults: Females: Acne: Estrostep® Fe: Refer to dosing for contraception

Adults: Females:

Moderate-to-severe vasomotor symptoms associated with menopause: Initial: femhrt® 0.5/2.5: 1 tablet daily; patient should be re-evaluated at 3- to 6-month intervals to determine if treatment is still necessary; patient should be maintained at the lowest effective dose

Prevention of osteoporosis: Initial: femhrt® 0.5/2.5: 1 tablet daily; patient should be maintained on the lowest effective dose

Contraception:

Schedule 1 (Sunday starter): Dose begins on first Sunday after onset of menstruation; if the menstrual period starts on Sunday, take first tablet that very same day. With a Sunday start, an additional method of contraception should be used until after the first 7 days of consecutive administration.

For 21-tablet package: Dosage is 1 tablet daily for 21 consecutive days, followed by 7 days off of the medication; a new course begins on the 8th day after the last tablet is taken.

For 28-tablet package: Dosage is 1 tablet daily without interruption.

Schedule 2 (Day 1 starter): Dose starts on first day of menstrual cycle taking 1 tablet daily.

For 21-tablet package: Dosage is 1 tablet daily for 21 consecutive days, followed by 7 days off of the medication; a new course begins on the 8th day after the last tablet is taken.

For 28-tablet package: Dosage is 1 tablet daily without interruption.

If all doses have been taken on schedule and one menstrual period is missed, continue dosing cycle. If two consecutive menstrual periods are missed, pregnancy test is required before new dosing cycle is started.

Missed doses **monophasic formulations** (refer to package insert for complete information):

One dose missed: Take as soon as remembered or take 2 tablets next day Two consecutive doses missed in the first 2 weeks: Take 2 tablets as soon as remembered or 2 tablets next 2 days. An additional method of contraception should be used for 7 days after missed dose.

Two consecutive doses missed in week 3 or three consecutive doses missed at any time: An additional method of contraception must be used for 7 days after a missed dose.

Schedule 1 (Sunday starter): Continue dose of 1 tablet daily until Sunday, then discard the rest of the pack, and a new pack should be started that same day.

Schedule 2 (Day 1 starter): Current pack should be discarded, and a new pack should be started that same day.

Missed doses **biphasic/triphasic formulations** (refer to package insert for complete information):

One dose missed: Take as soon as remembered or take 2 tablets next day.

Two consecutive doses missed in week 1 or week 2 of the pack: Take 2 tablets as soon as remembered and 2 tablets the next day. Resume taking 1 tablet daily until the pack is empty. An additional method of contraception should be used for 7 days after a missed dose.

Two consecutive doses missed in week 3 of the pack: An additional method of contraception must be used for 7 days after a missed dose.

Schedule 1 (Sunday Starter): Take 1 tablet every day until Sunday. Discard the remaining pack and start a new pack of pills on the same day.

Schedule 2 (Day 1 starter): Discard the remaining pack and start a new pack the same day.

Three or more consecutive doses missed: An additional method of contraception must be used for 7 days after a missed dose.

Schedule 1 (Sunday Starter): Take 1 tablet every day until Sunday; on Sunday, discard the pack and start a new pack.

Schedule 2 (Day 1 Starter): Discard the remaining pack and begin new pack of tablets starting on the same day.

Dosage adjustment in renal impairment: Specific guidelines not available; use with caution and monitor blood pressure closely. Consider other forms of contraception.

Dosage adjustment in hepatic impairment: Contraindicated in patients with hepatic impairment.

Additional Information Complete prescribing information for this medication should be consulted for additional detail.

Dosage Forms Excipient information presented when available (limited, particularly for generics); consult specific product labeling.

Tablet:

femhrt® 1/5: Ethinyl estradiol 5 mcg and norethindrone acetate 1 mg [white tablets] femhrt® 0.5/2.5: Ethinyl estradiol 2.5 mcg and norethindrone acetate 0.5 mg [white tablets]

Tablet, monophasic formulations:

Balziva™: Ethinyl estradiol 0.035 mg and norethindrone 0.4 mg (28s) [21 light peach tablets and 7 white inactive tablets]

Brevicon®: Ethinyl estradiol 0.035 mg and norethindrone 0.5 mg (28s) [21 blue tablets and 7 orange inactive tablets]

Junel™ 21 1/20: Ethinyl estradiol 0.02 mg and norethindrone acetate 1 mg (21s) [yellow tablets]

Junel™ 21 1.5/30: Ethinyl estradiol 0.03 mg and norethindrone acetate 1.5 mg (21s) [pink tablets]

Junel™ Fe 1/20: Ethinyl estradiol 0.02 mg and norethindrone acetate 1 mg (28s) [21 yellow tablets] and ferrous fumarate 75 mg [7 brown tablets]

Junel™ Fe 1.5/30: Ethinyl estradiol 0.03 mg and norethindrone acetate 1.5 mg (28s) [21 pink tablets] and ferrous fumarate 75 mg [7 brown tablets]

Loestrin® 21 1/20, Microgestin™ 1/20: Ethinyl estradiol 0.02 mg and norethindrone acetate 1 mg (21s) [white tablets]

Loestrin® 21 1.5/30, Microgestin™ 1.5/30: Ethinyl estradiol 0.03 mg and norethindrone acetate 1.5 mg (21s) [green tablets]

Loestrin® 24 Fe: 1/20: Ethinyl estradiol 0.02 mg and norethindrone acetate 1 mg (28s) [24 white tablets] and ferrous fumarate 75 mg [4 brown tablets]

Loestrin® Fe 1/20, Microgestin™ Fe 1/20: Ethinyl estradiol 0.02 mg and norethindrone acetate 1 mg (28s) [21 white tablets] and ferrous fumarate 75 mg [7 brown tablets]

Loestrin® Fe 1.5/30, Microgestin™ Fe 1.5/30: Ethinyl estradiol 0.03 mg and norethindrone acetate 1.5 mg (28s) [21 green tablets] and ferrous fumarate 75 mg [7 brown tablets]

Modicon® 28: Ethinyl estradiol 0.035 mg and norethindrone 0.5 mg (28s) [21 white tablets and 7 green inactive tablets]

Necon® 0.5/35-28: Ethinyl estradiol 0.035 mg and norethindrone 0.5 mg (28s) [21 light yellow tablets and 7 white inactive tablets]

Necon® 1/35-28: Ethinyl estradiol 0.035 mg and norethindrone 1 mg (28s) [21 dark yellow tablets and 7 white inactive tablets]

Norinyl® 1+35: Ethinyl estradiol 0.035 mg and norethindrone 1 mg (28s) [21 yellow-green tablets and 7 orange inactive tablets]

Nortrel™ 0.5/35 mg:
  Ethinyl estradiol 0.035 mg and norethindrone 0.5 mg (21s) [light yellow tablets]
  Ethinyl estradiol 0.035 mg and norethindrone 0.5 mg (28s) [21 light yellow tablets and 7 white inactive tablets]

Nortrel™ 1/35 mg:
  Ethinyl estradiol 0.035 mg and norethindrone 1 mg (21s) [yellow tablets]
  Ethinyl estradiol 0.035 mg and norethindrone 1 mg (28s) [21 yellow tablets and 7 white inactive tablets]

Ortho-Novum® 1/35 28: Ethinyl estradiol 0.035 mg and norethindrone 1 mg (28s) [21 peach tablets and 7 green inactive tablets]

Ovcon® 35 28-day: Ethinyl estradiol 0.035 mg and norethindrone 0.4 mg (28s) [21 peach tablets and 7 green inactive tablets]

Ovcon® 50: Ethinyl estradiol 0.05 mg and norethindrone 1 mg (28s) [21 yellow tablets and 7 green inactive tablets]

Zenchent™: Ethinyl estradiol 0.035 mg and norethindrone 0.4 mg (28s) [21 light peach tablets and 7 white inactive tablets]

Tablet, chewable, monophasic formulations:

Femcon® Fe: Ethinyl estradiol 0.035 mg and norethindrone 0.4 mg (28s) [21 white tablets and 7 brown ferrous fumarate 75 mg tablets] [spearmint flavor]

Tablet, biphasic formulations:

Necon® 10/11-28:
  Day 1-10: Ethinyl estradiol 0.035 mg and norethindrone 0.5 mg [10 light yellow tablets]
  Day 11-21: Ethinyl estradiol 0.035 mg and norethindrone 1 mg [11 dark yellow tablets]
  Day 22-28: 7 white inactive tablets (28s)

556

Ortho-Novum® 10/11-28:

Day 1-10: Ethinyl estradiol 0.035 mg and norethindrone 0.5 mg [10 white tablets]

Day 11-21: Ethinyl estradiol 0.035 mg and norethindrone 1 mg [11 peach tablets]

Day 22-28: 7 green inactive tablets (28s)

Tablet, triphasic formulations:

Aranelle™:

Day 1-7: Ethinyl estradiol 0.035 mg and norethindrone 0.5 mg [7 light yellow tablets]

Day 8-16: Ethinyl estradiol 0.035 mg and norethindrone 1 mg [9 white tablets]

Day 17-21: Ethinyl estradiol 0.035 mg and norethindrone 0.5 mg [5 light yellow tablets]

Day 22-28: 7 peach inactive tablets (28s)

Estrostep® Fe:

Day 1-5: Ethinyl estradiol 0.02 mg and norethindrone acetate 1 mg [5 white triangular tablets]

Day 6-12: Ethinyl estradiol 0.03 mg and norethindrone acetate 1 mg [7 white square tablets]

Day 13-21: Ethinyl estradiol 0.035 mg and norethindrone acetate 1 mg [9 white round tablets]

Day 22-28: Ferrous fumarate 75 mg [7 brown tablets] (28s)

Leena™:

Day 1-7: Ethinyl estradiol 0.035 mg and norethindrone 0.5 mg [7 light blue tablets]

Day 8-16: Ethinyl estradiol 0.035 mg and norethindrone 1 mg [9 light yellow-green tablets]

Day 17-21: Ethinyl estradiol 0.035 mg and norethindrone 0.5 mg [5 light blue tablets]

Day 22-28: 7 orange inactive tablets (28s)

Necon® 7/7/7, Ortho-Novum® 7/7/7 28:

Day 1-7: Ethinyl estradiol 0.035 mg and norethindrone 0.5 mg [7 white tablets]

Day 8-14: Ethinyl estradiol 0.035 mg and norethindrone 0.75 mg [7 light peach tablets]

Day 15-21: Ethinyl estradiol 0.035 mg and norethindrone 1 mg [7 peach tablets]

Day 22-28: 7 green inactive tablets (28s)

Nortrel™ 7/7/7 28:

Day 1-7: Ethinyl estradiol 0.035 mg and norethindrone 0.5 mg [7 light yellow tablets]

Day 8-14: Ethinyl estradiol 0.035 mg and norethindrone 0.75 mg [7 blue tablets]

Day 15-21: Ethinyl estradiol 0.035 mg and norethindrone 1 mg [7 peach tablets]

Day 22-28: 7 white inactive tablets (28s)

Ortho-Novum® 7/7/7 28:

Day 1-7: Ethinyl estradiol 0.035 mg and norethindrone 0.5 mg [7 white tablets]

Day 8-14: Ethinyl estradiol 0.035 mg and norethindrone 0.75 mg [7 light peach tablets]

Day 15-21: Ethinyl estradiol 0.035 mg and norethindrone 1 mg [7 peach tablets]

Day 22-28: 7 green inactive tablets (28s)

Tilia™ Fe:

Day 1-5: Ethinyl estradiol 0.02 mg and norethindrone acetate 1 mg [5 white triangular tablets]

Day 6-12: Ethinyl estradiol 0.03 mg and norethindrone acetate 1 mg [7 white square tablets]

Day 13-21: Ethinyl estradiol 0.035 mg and norethindrone acetate 1 mg [9 white round tablets]

Day 22-28: Ferrous fumarate 75 mg [7 brown tablets] (28s)

Tri-Legest™ Fe:

Day 1-5: Ethinyl estradiol 0.02 mg and norethindrone acetate 1 mg [5 light pink tablets]

◄
Day 6-12: Ethinyl estradiol 0.03 mg and norethindrone acetate 1 mg [7 light yellow tablets]

Day 13-21: Ethinyl estradiol 0.035 mg and norethindrone acetate 1 mg [9 light blue tablets]

Day 22-28: Ferrous fumarate 75 mg [7 brown tablets] (28s)

Tri-Norinyl® 28:

Day 1-7: Ethinyl estradiol 0.035 mg and norethindrone 0.5 mg [7 blue tablets]

Day 8-16: Ethinyl estradiol 0.035 mg and norethindrone 1 mg [9 yellow-green tablets]

Day 17-21: Ethinyl estradiol 0.035 mg and norethindrone 0.5 mg [5 blue tablets]

Day 22-28: 7 orange inactive tablets (28s)

References

Burkman R, Schlesselman JJ, and Zieman M, "Safety Concerns and Health Benefits Associated With Oral Contraception," *Am J Obstet Gynecol*, 2004, 190(4 Suppl):5-22.

"Guidelines for the Use of Antiretroviral Agents in HIV-infected Adults and Adolescents. Panel on Clinical Practices for Treatment of HIV Infection," August 13, 2001. Available at: http://www.aidsinfo.nih.gov. Accessed September 5, 2001.

Holt VL, Scholes D, Wicklund KG, et al, "Body Mass Index, Weight, and Oral Contraceptive Failure Risk," *Obstet Gynecol*, 2005, 105(1):46-52.

Orme ML, Back DJ, and Breckenridge AM, "Clinical Pharmacokinetics of Oral Contraceptive Steroids," *Clin Pharmacokinet*, 1983, 8(2):95-136.

Rossouw JE, Anderson GL, Prentice RL, et al, "Risks and Benefits of Estrogen Plus Progestin in Healthy Postmenopausal Women: Principle Results From the Women's Health Initiative Randomized Controlled Trial,"*JAMA*, 2002, 288(3):321-33.

Shenfield GM and Griffin JM, "Clinical Pharmacokinetics of Contraceptive Steroids. An Update," *Clin Pharmacokinet*, 1991, 20(1):15-37.

U.S. Food and Drug Administration, Department of Health and Human Services, "FDA Approves New Labels for Estrogen and Estrogen with Progestin Therapies for Postmenopausal Women Following Review of Women's Health Initiative Data," January 8, 2003. Available at: http://www.fda.gov/medwatch/SAFETY/2003/safety03.htm#prempr. Accessed January 9, 2003.

Ethinyl Estradiol and Norgestimate

(ETH in il es tra DYE ole & nor JES ti mate)

U.S. Brand Names MonoNessa®; Ortho Tri-Cyclen®; Ortho Tri-Cyclen® Lo; Ortho-Cyclen®; Previfem®; Sprintec®; Tri-Lo-Sprintec™; Tri-Previfem®; Tri-Sprintec®; TriNessa®

Canadian Brand Names Cyclen®; Tri-Cyclen® ; Tri-Cyclen® Lo

Index Terms Ethinyl Estradiol and NGM; Norgestimate and Ethinyl Estradiol; Ortho Cyclen; Ortho Tri Cyclen

Pharmacologic Category Contraceptive; Estrogen and Progestin Combination

Use Prevention of pregnancy; treatment of acne

Unlabeled/Investigational Use Treatment of hypermenorrhea (menorrhagia); pain associated with endometriosis; dysmenorrhea; dysfunctional uterine bleeding

Pharmacodynamics/Kinetics

Absorption: Ethinyl estradiol (EE) and norgestimate (NGM): Rapid and well absorbed

Protein binding:

EE: >97% to albumin

Norelgestromin (NGMN): >97% to albumin

Norgestrel (NG): >97% to sex hormone-binding globulin (SHBG); SHBG capacity is affected by plasma ethinyl estradiol levels

Metabolism:

EE: Hepatic; forms metabolites

NGM: Hepatic; forms NGMN (major active metabolite) which is further metabolized to NG (active) and other metabolites

Half-life elimination:

EE: 10-16 hours

NGMN: 18-25 hours

NG: 38-45 hours

Time to peak, plasma: EE and NGM: ~2 hours

Excretion:

EE: Urine and feces

NGM: Urine (~47%) and feces (~37%) as metabolites

Dosage Oral:

Children ≥15 years and Adults: Females: Acne (Ortho Tri-Cyclen®): Refer to dosing for contraception

Adults: Females:

Contraception:

Schedule 1 (Sunday starter): Dose begins on first Sunday after onset of menstruation; if the menstrual period starts on Sunday, take first tablet that very same day. **With a Sunday start, an additional method of contraception should be used until after the first 7 days of consecutive administration.**

For 21-tablet package: Dosage is 1 tablet daily for 21 consecutive days, followed by 7 days off of the medication; a new course begins on the 8th day after the last tablet is taken.

For 28-tablet package: Dosage is 1 tablet daily without interruption.

Schedule 2 (Day 1 starter): Dose starts on first day of menstrual cycle taking 1 tablet daily.

For 21-tablet package: Dosage is 1 tablet daily for 21 consecutive days, followed by 7 days off of the medication; a new course begins on the 8th day after the last tablet is taken.

For 28-tablet package: Dosage is 1 tablet daily without interruption.

If all doses have been taken on schedule and one menstrual period is missed, continue dosing cycle. If two consecutive menstrual periods are missed, pregnancy test is required before new dosing cycle is started.

Missed doses **monophasic formulations** (refer to package insert for complete information):

One dose missed: Take as soon as remembered or take 2 tablets next day

Two consecutive doses missed in the first 2 weeks: Take 2 tablets as soon as remembered or 2 tablets next 2 days. **An additional method of contraception should be used for 7 days after missed dose.**

Two consecutive doses missed in week 3 or three consecutive doses missed at any time: **An additional method of contraception must be used for 7 days after a missed dose:**

Schedule 1 (Sunday starter): Continue dose of 1 tablet daily until Sunday, then discard the rest of the pack, and a new pack should be started that same day.

Schedule 2 (Day 1 starter): Current pack should be discarded, and a new pack should be started that same day.

Missed doses **biphasic/triphasic formulations** (refer to package insert for complete information):

One dose missed: Take as soon as remembered or take 2 tablets next day.

Two consecutive doses missed in week 1 or week 2 of the pack: Take 2 tablets as soon as remembered and 2 tablets the next day. Resume taking 1 tablet daily until the pack is empty. **An additional method of contraception must be used for 7 days after a missed dose.**

Two consecutive doses missed in week 3 of the pack. **An additional method of contraception must be used for 7 days after a missed dose.**

Schedule 1 (Sunday starter): Take 1 tablet every day until Sunday. Discard the remaining pack and start a new pack of pills on the same day.

Schedule 2 (Day 1 starter): Discard the remaining pack and start a new pack the same day.

Three or more consecutive doses missed. **An additional method of contraception must be used for 7 days after a missed dose.**

Schedule 1 (Sunday starter): Take 1 tablet every day until Sunday; on Sunday, discard the pack and start a new pack.

Schedule 2 (Day 1 starter): Discard the remaining pack and begin new pack of tablets starting on the same day.

Dosage adjustment in renal impairment: Specific guidelines not available; use with caution and monitor blood pressure closely. Consider other forms of contraception.

Dosage adjustment in hepatic impairment: Contraindicated in patients with hepatic impairment.

Additional Information Complete prescribing information for this medication should be consulted for additional detail.

◄ **Dosage Forms** Excipient information presented when available (limited, particularly for generics); consult specific product labeling.

Tablet, monophasic formulations:

MonoNessa®, Ortho-Cyclen®: Ethinyl estradiol 0.035 mg and norgestimate 0.25 mg (28s) [21 blue tablets and 7 green inactive tablets]

Previfem®: Ethinyl estradiol 0.035 mg and norgestimate 0.25 mg (28s) [21 blue tablets and 7 teal inactive tablets]

Sprintec®: Ethinyl estradiol 0.035 mg and norgestimate 0.25 mg (28s) [21 blue tablets and 7 white inactive tablets]

Tablet, triphasic formulations:

Ortho Tri-Cyclen®, TriNessa®:

Day 1-7: Ethinyl estradiol 0.035 mg and norgestimate 0.18 mg [7 white tablets]

Day 8-14: Ethinyl estradiol 0.035 mg and norgestimate 0.215 mg [7 light blue tablets]

Day 15-21: Ethinyl estradiol 0.035 mg and norgestimate 0.25 mg [7 blue tablets]

Day 22-28: 7 green inactive tablets (28s)

Tri-Lo-Sprintec™:

Day 1-7: Ethinyl estradiol 0.025 mg and norgestimate 0.18 mg [7 white tablets]

Day 8-14: Ethinyl estradiol 0.025 mg and norgestimate 0.215 mg [7 light blue tablets]

Day 15-21: Ethinyl estradiol 0.025 mg and norgestimate 0.25 mg [7 blue tablets]

Day 22-28: 7 white inactive tablets (28s)

Tri-Previfem®:

Day 1-7: Ethinyl estradiol 0.035 mg and norgestimate 0.18 mg [7 white tablets]

Day 8-14: Ethinyl estradiol 0.035 mg and norgestimate 0.215 mg [7 light blue tablets]

Day 15-21: Ethinyl estradiol 0.035 mg and norgestimate 0.25 mg [7 blue tablets]

Day 22-28: 7 teal inactive tablets (28s)

Tri-Sprintec®:

Day 1-7: Ethinyl estradiol 0.035 mg and norgestimate 0.18 mg [7 gray tablets]

Day 8-14: Ethinyl estradiol 0.035 mg and norgestimate 0.215 mg [7 light blue tablets]

Day 15-21: Ethinyl estradiol 0.035 mg and norgestimate 0.25 mg [7 blue tablets]

Day 22-28: 7 white inactive tablets (28s)

Ortho Tri-Cyclen® Lo:

Day 1-7: Ethinyl estradiol 0.025 mg and norgestimate 0.18 mg [7 white tablets]

Day 8-14: Ethinyl estradiol 0.025 mg and norgestimate 0.215 mg [7 light blue tablets]

Day 15-21: Ethinyl estradiol 0.025 mg and norgestimate 0.25 mg [7 dark blue tablets]

Day 22-28: 7 green inactive tablets (28s)

References

Burkman R, Schlesselman JJ, and Zieman M, "Safety Concerns and Health Benefits Associated With Oral Contraception," *Am J Obstet Gynecol*, 2004, 190(4 Suppl):5-22.

"Guidelines for the Use of Antiretroviral Agents in HIV-infected Adults and Adolescents. Panel on Clinical Practices for Treatment of HIV Infection," August 13, 2001. Available at: http://www.aidsinfo.nih.gov. Accessed September 5, 2001.

Holt VL, Scholes D, Wicklund KG, et al, "Body Mass Index, Weight, and Oral Contraceptive Failure Risk," *Obstet Gynecol*, 2005, 105(1):46-52.

Orme ML, Back DJ, and Breckenridge AM, "Clinical Pharmacokinetics of Oral Contraceptive Steroids," *Clin Pharmacokinet*, 1983, 8(2):95-136.

Shenfield GM and Griffin JM, "Clinical Pharmacokinetics of Contraceptive Steroids. An Update," *Clin Pharmacokinet*, 1991, 20(1):15-37.

Ethinyl Estradiol and Norgestrel (ETH in il es tra DYE ole & nor JES trel)

U.S. Brand Names Cryselle® 28; Lo/Ovral®-28; Low-Ogestrel®; Ogestrel®

Canadian Brand Names Ovral®

Index Terms Morning After Pill; Norgestrel and Ethinyl Estradiol

Pharmacologic Category Contraceptive; Estrogen and Progestin Combination

Use Prevention of pregnancy; postcoital contraceptive or "morning after" pill

Unlabeled/Investigational Use Treatment of hypermenorrhea (menorrhagia); pain associated with endometriosis; dysmenorrhea; dysfunctional uterine bleeding

Dosage Oral: Adults: Females:

Contraception:

Schedule 1 (Sunday starter): Dose begins on first Sunday after onset of menstruation; if the menstrual period starts on Sunday, take first tablet that very same day. **With a Sunday start, an additional method of contraception should be used until after the first 7 days of consecutive administration.**

For 21-tablet package: Dosage is 1 tablet daily for 21 consecutive days, followed by 7 days off of the medication; a new course begins on the 8th day after the last tablet is taken.

For 28-tablet package: Dosage is 1 tablet daily without interruption.

Schedule 2 (Day 1 starter): Dose starts on first day of menstrual cycle taking 1 tablet daily.

For 21-tablet package: Dosage is 1 tablet daily for 21 consecutive days, followed by 7 days off of the medication; a new course begins on the 8th day after the last tablet is taken.

For 28-tablet package: Dosage is 1 tablet daily without interruption.

If all doses have been taken on schedule and one menstrual period is missed, continue dosing cycle. If two consecutive menstrual periods are missed, pregnancy test is required before new dosing cycle is started.

Missed doses **monophasic formulations** (refer to package insert for complete information):

One dose missed: Take as soon as remembered or take 2 tablets next day

Two consecutive doses missed in the first 2 weeks: Take 2 tablets as soon as remembered or 2 tablets next 2 days. **An additional method of contraception should be used for 7 days after missed dose.**

Two consecutive doses missed in week 3 or three consecutive doses missed at any time:

Schedule 1 (Sunday starter): Continue to take 1 tablet daily until Sunday, then discard the rest of the pack, and a new pack is started that same day.

Schedule 2 (Day 1 starter): Current pack should be discarded, and a new pack started that same day. **An additional method of contraception should be used for 7 days after missed dose.**

Postcoital contraception:

Ethinyl estradiol 0.03 mg and norgestrel 0.3 mg formulation: 4 tablets within 72 hours of unprotected intercourse and 4 tablets 12 hours after first dose

Ethinyl estradiol 0.05 mg and norgestrel 0.5 mg formulation: 2 tablets within 72 hours of unprotected intercourse and 2 tablets 12 hours after first dose

Dosage adjustment in renal impairment: Specific guidelines not available; use with caution and monitor blood pressure closely. Consider other forms of contraception.

Dosage adjustment in hepatic impairment: Contraindicated in patients with hepatic impairment.

Additional Information Complete prescribing information for this medication should be consulted for additional detail.

Dosage Forms Excipient information presented when available (limited, particularly for generics); consult specific product labeling.

Tablet, monophasic formulations:

Cryselle® 28: Ethinyl estradiol 0.03 mg and norgestrel 0.3 mg [21 white tablets and 7 light green inactive tablets] (28s)

Low-Ogestrel®: Ethinyl estradiol 0.03 mg and norgestrel 0.3 mg [21 white tablets and 7 peach inactive tablets] (28s)

Lo/Ovral®-28: Ethinyl estradiol 0.03 mg and norgestrel 0.3 mg [21 white tablets and 7 pink inactive tablets] (28s)

Ogestrel®: Ethinyl estradiol 0.05 mg and norgestrel 0.5 mg [21 white tablets and 7 peach inactive tablets] (28s)

References

"American Academy of Pediatrics Committee on Drugs, The Transfer of Drugs and Other Chemicals Into Human Milk," *Pediatrics*, 2001, 108(3):776-89.

Burkman R, Schlesselman JJ, and Zieman M, "Safety Concerns and Health Benefits Associated With Oral Contraception," *Am J Obstet Gynecol*, 2004, 190(4 Suppl):5-22.

"Guidelines for the Use of Antiretroviral Agents in HIV-infected Adults and Adolescents. Panel on Clinical Practices for Treatment of HIV Infection," August 13, 2001. Available at: http://www.aidsinfo. nih.gov. Accessed September 5, 2001.

Hendeles SM, Galand N, and Schwers J, "Metabolism of Orally Administered D-norgestrel in Women," *Acta Endocrinol (Copenh)*, 1972, 71(3):557-68.

Holt VL, Scholes D, Wicklund KG, et al, "Body Mass Index, Weight, and Oral Contraceptive Failure Risk," *Obstet Gynecol*, 2005, 105(1):46-52.

Orme ML, Back DJ, and Breckenridge AM, "Clinical Pharmacokinetics of Oral Contraceptive Steroids," *Clin Pharmacokinet*, 1983, 8(2):95-136.

"Prescription Drug Products; Certain Combined Oral Contraceptives for Use as Postcoital Emergency Contraception," *Fed Regist*, 1997, 62(37):8610-12 (Notice).

Shenfield GM and Griffin JM, "Clinical Pharmacokinetics of Contraceptive Steroids. An Update," *Clin Pharmacokinet*, 1991, 20(1):15-37.

Ethosuximide (eth oh SUKS i mide)

Related Information
Perioperative Management of Patients on Antiseizure Medication *on page 1577*

U.S. Brand Names Zarontin®

Canadian Brand Names Zarontin®

Pharmacologic Category Anticonvulsant, Succinimide

Use Management of absence (petit mal) seizures

Pharmacodynamics/Kinetics
Distribution: Adults: V_d: 0.62-0.72 L/kg

Metabolism: Hepatic (~80% to 3 inactive metabolites)

Half-life elimination, serum: Children: 30 hours; Adults: 50-60 hours

Time to peak, serum: Capsule: ~2-4 hours; Syrup: <2-4 hours

Excretion: Urine, slowly (50% as metabolites, 10% to 20% as unchanged drug); feces (small amounts)

Dosage Oral:
Children 3-6 years: Initial: 250 mg/day; increase every 4-7 days; usual maintenance dose: 20 mg/kg/day; maximum dose: 1.5 g/day in divided doses

Children ≥6 years and Adults: Initial: 500 mg/day; increase by 250 mg as needed every 4-7 days, up to 1.5 g/day in divided doses; usual maintenance dose for most pediatric patients is 20 mg/kg/day.

Dosing comment in renal/hepatic dysfunction: Use with caution.

Additional Information Complete prescribing information for this medication should be consulted for additional detail.

Dosage Forms Excipient information presented when available (limited, particularly for generics); consult specific product labeling.

Capsule: 250 mg

    Zarontin®: 250 mg

Solution, oral: 250 mg/5 mL (473 mL)

    Zarontin®: 250 mg/5 mL [contains sodium benzoate; raspberry flavor]

Syrup: 250 mg/5 mL (473 mL)

References
Marbury TC, Lee CS, Perchalski RJ, et al, "Hemodialysis Clearance of Ethosuximide in Patients With Chronic Renal Disease," *Am J Hosp Pharm*, 1981, 38(11):1757-60.

Marquardt ED, Ishisaka DY, Batra KK, et al, "Removal of Ethosuximide and Phenobarbital by Peritoneal Dialysis in a Child," *Clin Pharm*, 1992, 11(12):1030-1.

♦ **ETH-Oxydose™ [DSC]** *see* OxyCODONE *on page 1069*

♦ **Ethoxynaphthamido Penicillin Sodium** *see* Nafcillin *on page 975*

♦ **Ethrane®** *see* Enflurane *on page 483*

♦ **Ethyl Alcohol** *see* Alcohol (Ethyl) *on page 53*

Etodolac (ee toe DOE lak)

Related Information
Acetaminophen and NSAIDS, Dosing in the Management of Pain *on page 1651*

Chronic Pain Management *on page 1546*

Nonsteroidal Anti-Inflammatory Agents *on page 1687*

Canadian Brand Names Apo-Etodolac®; Utradol™

Index Terms Etodolic Acid; Lodine

Pharmacologic Category Nonsteroidal Anti-inflammatory Drug (NSAID), Oral

Use Acute and long-term use in the management of signs and symptoms of osteoarthritis; rheumatoid arthritis and juvenile rheumatoid arthritis; management of acute pain

Pharmacodynamics/Kinetics

Onset of action: Analgesic: 2-4 hours; Maximum anti-inflammatory effect: A few days

Absorption: ≥80%

Distribution: V_d:

Immediate release: Adults:0.4 L/kg

Extended release: Adults: 0.57 L/kg; Children (6-16 years): 0.08 L/kg

Protein binding: ≥99%, primarily albumin

Metabolism: Hepatic

Half-life elimination: Terminal: Adults: 5-8 hours

Extended release: Children (6-16 years): 12 hours

Time to peak, serum:

Immediate release: Adults: 1-2 hours

Extended release: Extended release: 5-7 hours, increased 1.4-3.8 hours with food

Excretion: Urine 73% (1% unchanged); feces 16%

Dosage Note: For chronic conditions, response is usually observed within 2 weeks.

Children 6-16 years: Oral: Juvenile rheumatoid arthritis: Extended release formulation:

20-30 kg: 400 mg once daily

31-45 kg: 600 mg once daily

46-60 kg: 800 mg once daily

>60 kg: 1000 mg once daily

Adults: Oral:

Acute pain: Immediate release formulation: 200-400 mg every 6-8 hours, as needed, not to exceed total daily doses of 1000 mg

Rheumatoid arthritis, osteoarthritis:

Immediate release formulation: 400 mg 2 times/day **or** 300 mg 2-3 times/day **or** 500 mg 2 times/day (doses >1000 mg/day have not been evaluated)

Extended release formulation: 400-1000 mg once daily

Elderly: Refer to adult dosing; in patients ≥65 years, no dosage adjustment required based on pharmacokinetics. The elderly are more sensitive to antiprostaglandin effects and may need dosage adjustments.

Dosage adjustment in renal impairment:

Mild-to-moderate: No adjustment required

Severe: Use not recommended; use with caution

Hemodialysis: Not removed

Dosage adjustment in hepatic impairment: No adjustment required.

Anesthesia and Critical Care Concerns/Other Considerations The 2002 ACCM/SCCM guidelines for analgesia (critically-ill adult) suggest that NSAIDs may be used in combination with opioids in select patients for pain management. Concern about adverse events (increased risk of renal dysfunction, altered platelet function and gastrointestinal irritation) limits its use in patients who have other underlying risks for these events.

In short-term use, NSAIDs vary considerably in their effect on blood pressure. When NSAIDs are used in patients with hypertension, appropriate monitoring of blood pressure responses should be completed and the duration of therapy, when possible, kept short. The use of NSAIDs in the treatment of patients with congestive heart failure may be associated with an increased risk for fluid accumulation and edema. May precipitate renal failure in dehydrated patients.

Additional Information Complete prescribing information for this medication should be consulted for additional detail.

Dosage Forms Excipient information presented when available (limited, particularly for generics); consult specific product labeling.

Capsule: 200 mg, 300 mg

Tablet: 400 mg, 500 mg

Tablet, extended release: 400 mg, 500 mg, 600 mg

◆ **Etodolic Acid** see Etodolac on page 562

◆ **EtOH** *see* Alcohol (Ethyl) *on page 53*

Etomidate (e TOM i date)

Medication Safety Issues
Sound-alike/look-alike issues:
Etomidate may be confused with etidronate

High alert medication: The Institute for Safe Medication Practices (ISMP) includes this medication among its list of drugs which have a heightened risk of causing significant patient harm when used in error.

Related Information
Anesthesia Considerations for Neurosurgery *on page 1514*
Anesthesia for Patients With Liver Disease *on page 1537*
Anesthetic Considerations in the Substance-Abusing Patient *on page 1613*
Dosing Considerations for the Critically-Ill Patient With Morbid Obesity *on page 1561*
Inhalational Anesthetics *on page 1632*
Intravenous Anesthetic Agents *on page 1635*
Perioperative Management of Patients on Antiseizure Medication *on page 1577*

U.S. Brand Names Amidate®

Canadian Brand Names Amidate®

Pharmacologic Category General Anesthetic

Generic Available Yes

Use Induction and maintenance of general anesthesia

Unlabeled/Investigational Use Sedation for diagnosis of seizure foci

Mechanism of Action Ultrashort-acting nonbarbiturate hypnotic (benzylimidazole) used for the induction of anesthesia; chemically, it is a carboxylated imidazole which produces a rapid induction of anesthesia with minimal cardiovascular effects; produces EEG burst suppression at high doses

Pharmacodynamics/Kinetics
Onset of action: 30-60 seconds
Peak effect: 1 minute
Duration: 3-5 minutes; terminated by redistribution
Distribution: V_d: 2-4.5 L/kg
Protein binding: 76%;
Metabolism: Hepatic and plasma esterases
Half-life elimination: Terminal: 2.6 hours

Dosage Children >10 years and Adults: I.V.: Initial: 0.2-0.6 mg/kg over 30-60 seconds for induction of anesthesia; maintenance: 5-20 mcg/kg/minute

Stability Store at room temperature.

Administration Administer I.V. push over 30-60 seconds. Solution is highly irritating; avoid administration into small vessels; in some cases, preadministration of lidocaine may be considered.

Monitoring Parameters Cardiac monitoring and blood pressure required

Anesthesia and Critical Care Concerns/Other Considerations Etomidate 2 mg/mL contains propylene glycol 362.6 mg/mL (35% v/v).

Clinical Pearls/Comments: In critically-ill patients, a single dose of etomidate will produce adrenal insufficiency, which may contribute to increased hospital and ICU lengths of stay and an increased number of ventilator days (Dellinger, 2008; Hildreth, 2008). During electroconvulsive therapy, etomidate prolongs seizure duration but is associated with increased postprocedure side effects (confusion, nausea, vomiting) (Ding, 2002).

Evidence-Based Information: Etomidate decreases cerebral metabolism and cerebral blood flow while maintaining perfusion pressure; can enhance somatosensory and motor-evoked potential recordings. Premedication with opioids or benzodiazepines can decrease myoclonus.

Pregnancy Risk Factor C

Contraindications Hypersensitivity to etomidate or any component of the formulation

Warnings/Precautions Etomidate inhibits 11-B-hydroxylase, an enzyme important in adrenal steroid production. A single induction dose blocks the normal stress-induced increase in adrenal cortisol production for 4-8 hours, up to 24 hours in elderly and debilitated patients. Continuous infusion of etomidate for sedation in the ICU may increase mortality because patients may not be able to respond to stress. No increase in mortality has been identified with a single dose for induction of anesthesia. Consider exogenous corticosteroid replacement in patients undergoing severe stress. Safety and efficacy have not been established in children <10 years of age.

Adverse Reactions

>10%:

Gastrointestinal: Nausea, vomiting on emergence from anesthesia

Local: Pain at injection site (30% to 80%)

Neuromuscular & skeletal: Myoclonus (33%), transient skeletal movements, uncontrolled eye movements

1% to 10%: Hiccups

<1% (Limited to important or life-threatening): Apnea, arrhythmia, bradycardia, decreased cortisol synthesis, hypertension, hyperventilation, hypotension, hypoventilation, laryngospasm, tachycardia

Drug Interactions

Avoid Concomitant Use There are no known interactions where it is recommended to avoid concomitant use.

Increased Effect/Toxicity There are no known significant interactions involving an increase in effect. Fentanyl w/ it ↑ elim 1/2 lifc ↓ plasma concent

Decreased Effect There are no known significant interactions involving a decrease in effect.

Dosage Forms Excipient information presented when available (limited, particularly for generics); consult specific product labeling.

Injection, solution: 2 mg/mL (10 mL, 20 mL) [contains propylene glycol 35% v/v]

References

Dellinger RP, Levy MM, Carlet JM, et al, "Surviving Sepsis Campaign: International Guidelines for Management of Severe Sepsis and Septic Shock: 2008," *Intensive Care Med*, 2008, 34(1):17-60.

Ding Z and White PF, "Anesthesia for Electroconvulsive Therapy," *Anesth Analg*, 2002, 94 (5):1351-64.

Hildreth AN, Mejia VA, Maxwell RA, et al, "Adrenal Suppression Following a Single Dose of Etomidate for Rapid Sequence Induction: A Prospective Randomized Study," *J Trauma*, 2008, 65(3):573-9.

♦ **Etonogestrel and Ethinyl Estradiol** see Ethinyl Estradiol and Etonogestrel on page 547

Etravirine (et ra VIR een)

U.S. Brand Names Intelence™

Canadian Brand Names Intelence™

Index Terms TMC125

Pharmacologic Category Antiretroviral Agent, Reverse Transcriptase Inhibitor (Non-nucleoside)

Use Treatment of HIV-1 infection in combination with at least two additional antiretroviral agents in treatment-experienced patients exhibiting viral replication with documented non-nucleoside reverse transcriptase inhibitor (NNRTI) resistance

Pharmacodynamics/Kinetics

Absorption: Increased 50% with food

Protein binding: 99.9%

Metabolism: Hepatic, primarily by CYP3A4, 2C9, and 2C19; major metabolites exhibit ~10% of parent drug activity against HIV

Half-life elimination: 41 hours (± 20 hours)

Time to peak, plasma: 2.5-4 hours

Excretion: Feces (94%, up to 86% as unchanged drug); urine (1%)

Dosage Oral: Adults: 200 mg twice daily after meals

Dosage adjustment in renal impairment: Due to minimal renal clearance, dose adjustment likely unnecessary in renal impairment.

Dosage adjustment in hepatic impairment: No adjustment required for mild-to-moderate (Child-Pugh class A/B) impairment; no data in severe impairment.

Additional Information Complete prescribing information for this medication should be consulted for additional detail.

◄ **Dosage Forms** Excipient information presented when available (limited, particularly for generics); consult specific product labeling.
Tablet:
Intelence™: 100 mg

References
Lazzarin A, Campbell T, Clotet B, et al, "Efficacy and Safety of TMC125 (Etravirine) in Treatment-Experienced HIV-1-Infected Patients in DUET-1: 24-Week Results From a Randomised, Double-Blind, Placebo-Controlled Trial," *Lancet*, 2007, 370(9581):39-48.
Madruga JV, Cahn P, Grinsztejn B, et al, "Efficacy and Safety of TMC125 (Etravirine) in Treatment-Experienced HIV-1-Infected Patients in DUET-1: 24-Week Results From a Randomised, Double-Blind, Placebo-Controlled Trial," *Lancet*, 2007, 370(9581):29-38.

◆ **Euglucon® (Can)** *see* GlyBURIDE *on page 666*

◆ **Euro-Lithium (Can)** *see* Lithium *on page 851*

◆ **Euthyrox (Can)** *see* Levothyroxine *on page 831*

◆ **Evamist™** *see* Estradiol *on page 531*

◆ **Everone® 200 (Can)** *see* Testosterone *on page 1362*

◆ **Evista®** *see* Raloxifene *on page 1228*

◆ **Evoclin®** *see* Clindamycin *on page 324*

◆ **Evra® (Can)** *see* Ethinyl Estradiol and Norelgestromin *on page 552*

◆ **Excedrin® Tension Headache [OTC]** *see* Acetaminophen *on page 25*

Exenatide (ex EN a tide)

U.S. Brand Names Byetta®
Index Terms AC 2993; AC002993; Exendin-4; LY2148568
Pharmacologic Category Antidiabetic Agent, Incretin Mimetic
Use Management (adjunctive) of type 2 diabetes mellitus (noninsulin dependent, NIDDM) in patients receiving a sulfonylurea, thiazolidinedione, or metformin (or a combination of these agents)
Pharmacodynamics/Kinetics
Distribution: V_d: 28.3 L
Metabolism: Minimal systemic metabolism; proteolytic degradation may occur following glomerular filtration
Half-life elimination: 2.4 hours
Time to peak, plasma: SubQ: 2.1 hours
Excretion: Urine (majority of dose)
Dosage SubQ: Adults: Initial: 5 mcg twice daily within 60 minutes prior to a meal; after 1 month, may be increased to 10 mcg twice daily (based on response)
Dosage adjustment in renal impairment:
Cl_{cr} ≥30 mL/minute: No adjustment necessary
Cl_{cr} <30 mL/minute: Not recommended
Additional Information Complete prescribing information for this medication should be consulted for additional detail.
Dosage Forms Excipient information presented when available (limited, particularly for generics); consult specific product labeling.
Injection, solution:
Byetta®: 250 mcg/mL (1.2 mL [5 mcg/0.02 mL; 60-dose pen]); (2.4 mL [10 mcg/0.04 mL; 60-dose pen])

References
Buse JB, Henry RR, Han J, et al, "Effects of Exenatide (Exendin-4) on Glycemic Control Over 30 Weeks in Sulfonylurea-Treated Patients With Type-2 Diabetes," *Diabetes Care*, 2004, 27 (11):2628-35.
Defronzo RA, Ratner RE, Han J, et al, "Effects of Exenatide (Exendin-4) on Glycemic Control and Weight Over 30 Weeks in Metformin-Treated Patients With Type-2 Diabetes," *Diabetes Care*, 2005, 28(5):1092-1100.
Fineman MS, Shen LZ, Taylor K, et al, "Effectiveness of Progressive Dose-Escalation of Exenatide (Exendin-4) in Reducing Dose-Limiting Side Effects in Subjects With Type 2 Diabetes," *Diabetes Metab Res Rev*, 2004, 20(5):411-7.
Joy SV, Rodgers PT, and Scates AC, "Incretin Mimetics as Emerging Treatments for Type 2 Diabetes," *Ann Pharmacother*, 2005, 39(1):110-8.
Kendall DM, Riddle MC, Rosenstock J, et al, "Effects of Exenatide (Exendin-4) on Glycemic Control Over 30 Weeks in Patients With Type 2 Diabetes Treated With Metformin and a Sulfonylurea," *Diabetes Care*, 2005, 28(5):1083-91.

Movassat J, Beattie GM, Lopez AD, et al, "Exendin 4 Up-Regulates Expression of PDX 1 and Hastens Differentiation and Maturation of Human Fetal Pancreatic Cells," *J Clin Endocrinol Metab*, 2002, 87(10):4775-8.

Ogawa N, List JF, Habener JF, et al, "Cure of Overt Diabetes in NOD Mice by Transient Treatment With Anti-Lymphocyte Serum and Exendin-4," *Diabetes*, 2004, 53(7):1700-5.

◆ **Exendin-4** *see* Exenatide *on page 566*

◆ **Extina®** *see* Ketoconazole *on page 780*

◆ **EZ-Char™ [OTC]** *see* Charcoal *on page 283*

Ezetimibe (ez ET i mibe)

Related Information
Hyperlipidemia Management *on page 1747*
U.S. Brand Names Zetia®
Canadian Brand Names Ezetrol®
Pharmacologic Category Antilipemic Agent, 2-Azetidinone
Use Use in combination with dietary therapy for the treatment of primary hypercholesterolemia (as monotherapy or in combination with HMG-CoA reductase inhibitors); homozygous sitosterolemia; homozygous familial hypercholesterolemia (in combination with atorvastatin or simvastatin); mixed hyperlipidemia (in combination with fenofibrate)
Pharmacodynamics/Kinetics
Protein binding: >90% to plasma proteins
Metabolism: Undergoes glucuronide conjugation in the small intestine and liver; forms metabolite (active); may undergo enterohepatic recycling
Bioavailability: Variable
Half-life elimination: 22 hours (ezetimibe and metabolite)
Time to peak, plasma: 4-12 hours
Excretion: Feces (78%, 69% as ezetimibe); urine (11%, 9% as metabolite)
Dosage Oral:
Children ≥10 years and Adults: 10 mg/day
Elderly: Refer to adult dosing

Dosage adjustment in renal impairment: AUC increased with severe impairment (Cl_{cr} <30 mL/minute); no dosing adjustment recommended
Dosage adjustment in hepatic impairment: AUC increased with hepatic impairment
Mild impairment (Child-Pugh class A): No dosing adjustment necessary
Moderate-to-severe impairment (Child-Pugh classes B and C): Use of ezetimibe not recommended
Additional Information Complete prescribing information for this medication should be consulted for additional detail.
Dosage Forms Excipient information presented when available (limited, particularly for generics); consult specific product labeling.
Tablet:
Zetia®: 10 mg
References
Gustavson LE, Schweitzer SM, Burt DA, et al, "Evaluation of the Potential for Pharmacokinetic Interaction Between Fenofibrate and Ezetimibe: A Phase I, Open-Label, Multiple-Dose, Three-Period Crossover Study in Healthy Subjects," *Clin Ther*, 2006, 28 (3):373-87.

Mauro VF and Tuckerman CE, "Ezetimibe for Management of Hypercholesterolemia," *Ann Pharmacother*, 2003, 37(6):839-48.

"Three New Drugs for Hyperlipidemia," *Med Lett Drugs Ther*, 2003, 45(1151):17-9.

von Bergmann K, Salen G, Lutjohann D, et al, "Ezetimibe Effectively Reduces Serum Plant Sterols in Patients With Sitosterolemia (abstract). 73rd European Atherosclerosis Society Congress, 2002. Available at: www.kenes.com/73eas/program/abstracts/405.doc. Accessed July 7, 2003.

◆ **Ezetrol® (Can)** *see* Ezetimibe *on page 567*

Factor VIIa (Recombinant) (FAK ter SEV en aye ree KOM be nant)

Medication Safety Issues
Sound-alike/look-alike issues:
NovoSeven® may be confused with Novacet®

◄ **Related Information**
Perioperative / Periprocedural Management of Anticoagulant and Antiplatelet Therapy *on page 1607*

U.S. Brand Names NovoSeven [DSC]; NovoSeven® RT

Canadian Brand Names Niastase®

Index Terms Coagulation Factor VIIa; Eptacog Alfa (Activated); rFVIIa

Pharmacologic Category Antihemophilic Agent; Blood Product

Generic Available No

Use Treatment of bleeding episodes and prevention of bleeding in surgical interventions in patients with hemophilia A or B with inhibitors to factor VIII or factor IX, acquired hemophilia, and in patients with congenital factor VII deficiency

Unlabeled/Investigational Use Reduction of hematoma growth in patients with acute intracerebral hemorrhage, warfarin-related intracerebral hemorrhage

Mechanism of Action Recombinant factor VIIa, a vitamin K-dependent glycoprotein, promotes hemostasis by activating the extrinsic pathway of the coagulation cascade. It replaces deficient activated coagulation factor VII, which complexes with tissue factor and may activate coagulation factor X to Xa and factor IX to IXa. When complexed with other factors, coagulation factor Xa converts prothrombin to thrombin, a key step in the formation of a fibrin-platelet hemostatic plug.

Pharmacodynamics/Kinetics

Distribution: V_d: 103 mL/kg (78-139)

Half-life elimination: 2.3 hours (1.7-2.7)

Excretion: Clearance: 33 mL/kg/hour (27-49)

Dosage Children and Adults: I.V. administration only:

Hemophilia A or B with inhibitors:

Bleeding episodes: 90 mcg/kg every 2 hours until hemostasis is achieved or until the treatment is judged ineffective. The dose and interval may be adjusted based upon the severity of bleeding and the degree of hemostasis achieved. For patients experiencing severe bleeds, dosing should be continued at 3- to 6-hour intervals after hemostasis has been achieved and the duration of dosing should be minimized.

Surgical interventions: 90 mcg/kg immediately before surgery; repeat at 2-hour intervals for the duration of surgery. Continue every 2 hours for 48 hours, then every 2-6 hours until healed for minor surgery; continue every 2 hours for 5 days, then every 4 hours until healed for major surgery.

Congenital factor VII deficiency: Bleeding episodes and surgical interventions: 15-30 mcg/kg every 4-6 hours until hemostasis. Doses as low as 10 mcg/kg have been effective.

Acquired hemophilia: 70-90 mcg/kg every 2-3 hours until hemostasis is achieved

Intracerebral hemorrhage (warfarin-related) (unlabeled use; Freeman, 2004; Ilyas, 2008): 10-100 mcg/kg (see **"Note"**) administered concurrently with I.V. vitamin K (to correct the non-factor VII coagulation factors).

Note: Lower doses (10-20 mcg/kg) are generally preferred given the higher risk of thromboembolic complications with higher doses; response is highly variable; monitor INR frequently after administration since rebound increases in INR occur quickly given the short half-life of rFVIIa; duration of INR correction is dose dependent.

Stability Prior to reconstitution, bring vials to room temperature.

NovoSeven®: Store under refrigeration at 2°C to 8°C (36°F to 46°F). Protect from light. Add recommended diluent along wall of vial; do not inject directly onto powder. Gently swirl until dissolved. Reconstitute each vial to a final concentration of 0.6 mg/mL as follows:

1.2 mg vial: 2.2 mL sterile water

2.4 mg vial: 4.3 mL sterile water

4.8 mg vial: 8.5 mL sterile water

Reconstituted solutions may be stored at room temperature or under refrigeration, but must be infused within 3 hours of reconstitution. Do not freeze reconstituted solutions. Do not store reconstituted solutions in syringes.

NovoSeven® RT: Prior to reconstitution, store under refrigeration or between 2°C to 25°C (36°F to 77°F). Protect from light. Add recommended diluent along wall of vial; do not inject directly onto powder. Gently swirl until dissolved. Reconstitute each vial to a final concentration of 1 mg/mL using the provided histidine diluent as follows:

1 mg vial: 1.1 mL histidine diluent

2 mg vial: 2.1 mL histidine diluent

5 mg vial: 5.2 mL histidine diluent

Reconstituted solutions may be stored at room temperature or under refrigeration, but must be infused within 3 hours of reconstitution. Do not freeze reconstituted solutions. Do not store reconstituted solutions in syringes.

Administration I.V. administration only; bolus over 2-5 minutes. Administer within 3 hours after reconstitution.

Monitoring Parameters Monitor for evidence of hemostasis; although the prothrombin time, aPTT, and factor VII clotting activity have no correlation with achieving hemostasis, these parameters may be useful as adjunct tests to evaluate efficacy and guide dose or interval adjustments

Anesthesia and Critical Care Concerns/Other Considerations Evidence-Based Information: Factor VIIa exerts its mechanism of action at the site of vascular injury where tissue factor is expressed and activated platelets are found. Factor VIIa binds directly to the surface of activated platelets and activates factor X to Xa and generates thrombin as a result. Adequate platelets and fibrinogen are required for factor VIIa to properly induce coagulation. A number of factors influence the efficacy of factor VIIa including hypothermia, thrombocytopenia, acidosis, and the amount of blood products transfused prior to administration.

Management of Intracerebral Hemorrhage (ICH): The 2007 AHA/ASA Guidelines for the Management of Spontaneous Intracerebral Hemorrhage in Adults state that treatment with recombinant factor VIIa (rFVIIa) within the first 3-4 hours after onset to slow progression of bleeding has shown promise; however, it cannot be routinely recommended (Class IIb recommendation).

The FAST trial demonstrated a statistically significant reduction in the growth of hematoma volume with the use of rFVIIa 80 mcg/kg (-3.8 mL vs placebo, p=0.009) compared to 20 mcg/kg (-2.6 mL vs placebo, p=0.08) given within 4 hours of onset of ICH; however, rFVIIa did not improve survival or functional outcome and therefore cannot be routinely recommended. Of note, arterial thromboembolic events occurred more frequently in the 80 mcg/kg group (Mayer, 2008).

Use of rFVIIa (with I.V. vitamin K) has shown promise for warfarin-related ICH (Freeman, 2004; Ilyas, 2008). Advantages include lower volume and faster onset of action compared to FFP and vitamin K. Disadvantages include a short half-life (~2.6 hours) requiring multiple doses to maintain a normalized INR and an increased risk of thromboembolic complications.

Pregnancy Risk Factor C

Contraindications There are no contraindications listed within the FDA-approved labeling.

Warnings/Precautions Use with caution in patients with known hypersensitivity to mouse, hamster, or bovine proteins, or factor VIIa, or any components of the product. Patients should be monitored for signs and symptoms of activation of the coagulation system or thrombosis. Thrombotic events may be increased in patients with disseminated intravascular coagulation (DIC), advanced athero-sclerotic disease, sepsis, crush injury, or concomitant treatment with prothrombin complex concentrates. Decreased dosage or discontinuation is warranted in confirmed DIC. Efficacy with prolonged infusions and data evaluating this agent's long-term adverse effects are limited.

Adverse Reactions

1% to 10%:

Cardiovascular: Hypertension

Central nervous system: Fever

Hematologic: Hemorrhage, plasma fibrinogen decreased

Neuromuscular & skeletal: Hemarthrosis

<1% (Limited to important or life-threatening): Abnormal renal function, allergic reaction, anaphylactic reaction, arterial thrombosis, arthrosis, bradycardia, cerebral infarction and/or ischemia, coagulation disorder, consumptive

coagulopathy, deep vein thrombosis, disseminated intravascular coagulation (DIC), edema, fibrinolysis increased, gastrointestinal bleeding, headache, hypersensitivity, hypotension, injection site reactions, intracranial hemorrhage, localized phlebitis, MI, myocardial ischemia, pain, pneumonia, prothrombin decreased, pruritus, pulmonary embolism, purpura, rash, splenic hematoma, therapeutic response decreased, thrombophlebitis, thrombosis, vomiting

Drug Interactions

Avoid Concomitant Use There are no known interactions where it is recommended to avoid concomitant use.

Increased Effect/Toxicity There are no known significant interactions involving an increase in effect.

Decreased Effect There are no known significant interactions involving a decrease in effect.

Dietary Considerations Some products may contain sodium.

Product Availability

Novoseven® RT: FDA approved May 2008; formulation is currently available.

Novo Nordisk® is replacing Novoseven® with Novoseven® RT, a room temperature formulation that allows the product to be stored either refrigerated or at room temperature (2°C to 25°C/36°F to 77°F) prior to reconstitution. The previously available Novoseven® required refrigeration prior to reconstitution.

Dosage Forms Excipient information presented when available (limited, particularly for generics); consult specific product labeling. [DSC] = Discontinued product

Injection, powder for reconstitution [preservative free]:

NovoSeven®: 1.2 mg, 2.4 mg, 4.8 mg [contains sodium 0.44 mEq/mg rFVIIa, polysorbate 80] [DSC]

NovoSeven® RT:

1 mg [contains polysorbate 80, sodium 0.4 mEq/mg rFVIIa, sucrose 10 mg/vial]

2 mg [contains polysorbate 80, sodium 0.4 mEq/mg rFVIIa, sucrose 20 mg/vial]

5 mg [contains polysorbate 80, sodium 0.4 mEq/mg rFVIIa, sucrose 50 mg/vial]

References

Broderick J, Connolly S, Feldmann E, et al, "Guidelines for the Management of Spontaneous Intracerebral Hemorrhage in Adults: 2007 Update: A Guideline From the American Heart Association/American Stroke Association Stroke Council, High Blood Pressure Research Council, and the Quality of Care and Outcomes in Research Interdisciplinary Working Group," *Stroke*, 2007, 38(6):2001-23. Available at http://stroke.ahajournals.org/cgi/content/short/STROKEAHA.107.183689.

Freeman WD, Brott TG, Barrett KM, et al, "Recombinant Factor VIIa for Rapid Reversal of Warfarin Anticoagulation in Acute Intracranial Hemorrhage," *Mayo Clin Proc*, 2004, 79(12):1495-500.

Ilyas C, Beyer GM, Dutton RP, et al, "Recombinant Factor VIIa for Warfarin-Associated Intracranial Bleeding," *J Clin Anesth*, 2008, 20(4):276-9.

Mayer SA, Brun NC, Begtrup K, et al, "Efficacy and Safety of Recombinant Activated Factor VII for Acute Intracerebral Hemorrhage," *N Engl J Med*, 2008, 358(20):2127-37.

Mayer SA, Brun NC, Begtrup K, et al, "Recombinant Activated Factor VII for Acute Intracerebral Hemorrhage," *N Engl J Med*, 2005, 352(8):777-85.

Mohr AM, Holcomb JB, Dutton RP, et al, "Recombinant Activated Factor VIIa and Hemostasis in Critical Care: A Focus on Trauma," *Crit Care*, 2005, 9 (Suppl 5):37-42.

◆ **Factor VIII (Recombinant)** *see* Antihemophilic Factor (Recombinant) *on page 124*

Factor IX (FAK ter nyne)

U.S. Brand Names AlphaNine® SD; BeneFix®; Mononine®

Canadian Brand Names BeneFix®; Immunine® VH; Mononine®

Index Terms Factor IX Concentrate

Pharmacologic Category Antihemophilic Agent; Blood Product Derivative

Generic Available No

Use Control bleeding in patients with factor IX deficiency (hemophilia B or Christmas disease)

Mechanism of Action Replaces deficient clotting factor IX. Hemophilia B, or Christmas disease, is an X-linked inherited disorder of blood coagulation characterized by insufficient or abnormal synthesis of the clotting protein factor IX. Factor IX is a vitamin K-dependent coagulation factor which is synthesized in the liver. Factor IX is activated by factor XIa in the intrinsic coagulation pathway. Activated factor IX (IXa), in combination with factor VII:C activates factor X to Xa, resulting ultimately in the conversion of prothrombin to thrombin and the formation of a fibrin clot. The infusion of exogenous factor IX to replace the deficiency present in hemophilia B temporarily restores hemostasis.

Pharmacodynamics/Kinetics Half-life elimination: IX component: Adults: 21-31 hours; children: 14-28 hours

Dosage Dosage is expressed in int. units of factor IX activity; dosing must be individualized based on severity of factor IX deficiency, extent and location of bleeding, and clinical status of patient. I.V.:

Formula for int. units required to raise blood level %:

AlphaNine® SD, Mononine®: Children and Adults:

Number of factor IX int. units required = body weight (in kg) x desired factor IX level increase (int. units/dL or % of normal) x 1 int. unit/kg

For example, for a 100% level a 70 kg patient who has an actual level of 20%: Number of factor IX int. units needed = 70 kg x 80% x 1 int. unit/kg = 5600 int. units

BeneFix®:

Children <15 years:

Number of factor IX int. units required = body weight (in kg) x desired factor IX level increase (int. units/dL or % of normal) x 1.4 int. units/kg

Children ≥15 years and Adults:

Number of factor IX int. units required = body weight (in kg) x desired factor IX level increase (int. units/dL or % of normal) x 1.3 int. units/kg

Guidelines: As a general rule, the level of factor IX required for treatment of different conditions is listed below:

Minor spontaneous hemorrhage, prophylaxis:

Desired levels of factor IX for hemostasis: 15% to 25%

Initial loading dose to achieve desired level: 20-30 int. units/kg

Frequency of dosing: Every 12-24 hours if necessary

Duration of treatment: 1-2 days

Moderate hemorrhage:

Desired levels of factor IX for hemostasis: 25% to 50%

Initial loading dose to achieve desired level: 25-50 int. units/kg

Frequency of dosing: Every 12-24 hours

Duration of treatment: 2-7 days

Major hemorrhage:

Desired levels of factor IX for hemostasis: >50%

Initial loading dose to achieve desired level: 30-50 int. units/kg

Frequency of dosing: Every 12-24 hours, depending on half-life and measured factor IX levels (after 3-5 days, maintain at least 20% activity)

Duration of treatment: 7-10 days, depending upon nature of insult

Surgery or major trauma:

Desired levels of factor IX for hemostasis: 50% to 100%

Initial loading dose to achieve desired level: 50-100 int. units/kg

Frequency of dosing: Every 12-24 hours or every 18-30 hours, depending on half-life and measured factor IX levels

Duration of treatment: 7-10 days, depending upon nature of insult

Stability When stored at refrigerator temperature, 2°C to 8°C (36°F to 46°F), coagulation factor IX is stable for the period indicated by the expiration date on its label. Avoid freezing which may damage container for the diluent.

AlphaNine® SD: May also be stored at room temperature not to exceed 30°C (86°F) for up to 1 month,

BeneFix®: May also be stored at room temperature not to exceed 25°C (77°F) for up to 6 months. Reconstituted solution at room temperature should be used within 3 hours.

Mononine®: May also be stored at room temperature not to exceed 25°C (77°F) for up to 1 month.

Reconstitution: Refer to instructions for individual products. Diluent and factor IX complex should come to room temperature before combining.

Administration Solution should be infused at room temperature

I.V. administration only: Should be infused **slowly**: The rate of administration should be determined by the response and comfort of the patient.

◀   AlphaNine® SD: Administer I.V. at a rate not exceeding 10 mL/minute

BeneFix®: Administer I.V. over several minutes

Mononine®: Administer I.V. at a rate of ~2 mL/minute. Administration rates of up to 225 int. units/minute have been regularly tolerated without incident (when reconstituted as directed to ~100 int. units/mL).

Monitoring Parameters Levels of factors IX, PTT, BP, HR, signs of hypersensitivity reactions

Reference Range Average normal factor IX levels are 50% to 150%; patients with severe hemophilia will have levels <1%, often undetectable. Moderate forms of the disease have levels of 1% to 10% while some mild cases may have 11% to 49% of normal factor IX.

Maintain factor IX plasma level at least 20% until hemostasis achieved after acute joint or muscle bleeding.

In preparation for and following surgery:

Level to prevent spontaneous hemorrhage: 5%

Minimum level for hemostasis following trauma and surgery: 30% to 50%

Severe hemorrhage: >50%

Major surgery: ≥50% prior to procedure and for 48 hours after surgery, and 30% to 50% for 10 days thereafter

Pregnancy Risk Factor C

Contraindications Hypersensitivity to mouse protein (Mononine®) or hamster protein (BeneFix®)

Warnings/Precautions Hypersensitivity and anaphylactic reactions have been reported with use. Delayed reactions (up to 20 days after infusion) in previously untreated patients may also occur. Due to potential for allergic reactions, the initial ~10-20 administrations should be performed under appropriate medical supervision. The development of factor IX antibodies (or inhibitors) has been reported with factor IX therapy; the risk of severe hypersensitivity reactions occurring may be greater in these patients. Patients experiencing allergic reactions should be evaluated for factor IX inhibitors.

Observe closely for signs or symptoms of intravascular coagulation or thrombosis; risk is generally associated with the use of factor IX complex concentrates (containing therapeutic amounts of additional factors); however, potential risk exists with use of factor IX products (containing only factor IX). Use with caution when administering to patients with liver disease, postoperatively, neonates, or patients at risk of thromboembolic phenomena, disseminated intravascular coagulation or patients with signs of fibrinolysis due to the potential risk of thromboembolic complications.

Factor IX is **NOT INDICATED** for the treatment or reversal of coumarin-induced anticoagulation, hemophilia A patients with factor VIII inhibitors, or patients in a hemorrhagic state caused by reduced production of liver-dependent coagulation factors (eg, hepatitis, cirrhosis). AlphaNine® SD and Mononine® contain **nondetectable levels of factors II, VII, and X** and are, therefore, **NOT INDICATED** for replacement therapy of any of these clotting factors. AlphaNine® SD and Mononine® are products of human plasma and may potentially contain infectious agents which could transmit disease. Screening of donors, as well as testing and/or inactivation or removal of certain viruses, reduces the risk. Infections thought to be transmitted by this product should be reported to the manufacturer. Safety and efficacy have not been established with factor IX products in immune tolerance induction. Nephrotic syndrome has occurred following immune tolerance induction in patients with factor IX inhibitors and a history of allergic reactions to therapy.

Adverse Reactions Frequency not defined.

Cardiovascular: Cyanosis, flushing, hypotension, chest tightness, thrombosis

Central nervous system: Chills, dizziness, drowsiness, fever (including transient fever following rapid administration), headache, lethargy, lightheadedness, somnolence

Dermatologic: Angioedema, photosensitivity reaction, rash, urticaria

Gastrointestinal: Abnormal taste, diarrhea, nausea, vomiting

Hematologic: Disseminated intravascular coagulation (DIC)

Hepatic: Alkaline phosphatase increased, ALT increased, AST increased

Local: Injection site reactions: Cellulitis, discomfort, pain, phlebitis, stinging

Neuromuscular & skeletal: Neck tightness, paresthesia, rigors

Ocular: Visual disturbance

Respiratory: Allergic rhinitis, asthma, cough, dyspnea, hypoxia, laryngeal edema, lung disorder

Miscellaneous: Allergic reaction, anaphylaxis, burning sensation in jaw/skull, factor IX inhibitor development, hypersensitivity reaction

Postmarketing and/or case reports: HAV seroconversion, inadequate response/recovery, nephrotic syndrome (associated with immune tolerance induction), parvovirus B19 seroconversion, renal infarction

Drug Interactions

Avoid Concomitant Use

Avoid concomitant use of Factor IX with any of the following: Aminocaproic Acid

Increased Effect/Toxicity

The levels/effects of Factor IX may be increased by: Aminocaproic Acid

Decreased Effect There are no known significant interactions involving a decrease in effect.

Dosage Forms Excipient information presented when available (limited, particularly for generics); consult specific product labeling.

Injection, powder for reconstitution (**Note:** Exact potency labeled on each vial):

BeneFix® [contains polysorbate 80; sucrose 0.8%; recombinant formulation; supplied with diluent]

Injection, powder for reconstitution [human derived] (**Note:** Exact potency labeled on each vial):

AlphaNine® SD [contains polysorbate 80; solvent detergent treated; virus filtered; contains nondetectable levels of factors II, VII, X; supplied with diluent]

Mononine® [contains polysorbate 80; monoclonal antibody purified; contains nondetectable levels of factors II, VII, X; supplied with diluent]

Factor IX Complex (Human) (FAK ter nyne KOM pleks HYU man)

U.S. Brand Names Bebulin® VH; Profilnine® SD

Index Terms Prothrombin Complex Concentrate

Pharmacologic Category Antihemophilic Agent; Blood Product Derivative; Prothrombin Complex Concentrate (PCC)

Generic Available No

Use Prevention and control of bleeding in patients with factor IX deficiency (hemophilia B or Christmas disease)

Unlabeled/Investigational Use Emergency correction of the coagulopathy of warfarin excess in critical situations. **Note:** Products contain low or nontherapeutic levels of factor VII component.

Mechanism of Action Replaces deficient clotting factor including factor X; hemophilia B, or Christmas disease, is an X-linked recessively inherited disorder of blood coagulation characterized by insufficient or abnormal synthesis of the clotting protein factor IX. Factor IX is a vitamin K-dependent coagulation factor which is synthesized in the liver. Factor IX is activated by factor XIa in the intrinsic coagulation pathway. Activated factor IX (IXa), in combination with factor VII:C, activates factor X to Xa, resulting ultimately in the conversion of prothrombin to thrombin and the formation of a fibrin clot. The infusion of exogenous factor IX to replace the deficiency present in hemophilia B temporarily restores hemostasis.

Pharmacodynamics/Kinetics Half-life elimination: IX component: ~24 hours

Dosage Children and Adults: Dosage is expressed in units of factor IX activity and must be individualized. When multiple doses are required, administer at 24-hour intervals unless otherwise specified. Administer I.V. only:

Formula for units required to raise blood level %:

Bebulin® VH: In general, Factor IX 1 int. unit/kg will increase the plasma factor IX level by 0.8%:

Number of Factor IX int. units required = body weight (kg) x desired factor IX increase (% of normal) x 1.2 int. units/kg

Profilnine® SD: In general, Factor IX 1 int. unit/kg will increase the plasma factor IX level by 1%:

Number of Factor IX int. units required = bodyweight (kg) x desired factor IX increase (% of normal) x 1 int. unit/kg

▶

◀ **As a general rule, the level of factor IX required for treatment of different conditions is listed below:**

Minor bleeding (early hemarthrosis, minor epistaxis, gingival bleeding, mild hematuria: Raise Factor IX level to 20% of normal; generally a single dose required.

Moderate bleeding (severe joint bleeding, early hematoma, major open bleeding, minor trauma, minor hemoptysis, hematemesis, melena, major hematuria): Raise Factor IX level to 40% of normal; average duration of treatment is 2 days or until adequate wound healing.

Major bleeding (severe hematoma, major trauma, severe hemoptysis, hematemesis, melena): Raise Factor IX level to 50 to ≥60% of normal; average duration of treatment is 2-3 days or until adequate wound healing. Do not raise ≥50% in patients who may be predisposed to thrombosis.

Minor surgery: Raise Factor IX level to 40% to 60% of normal on day of surgery then decrease from 40% of normal to 20% of normal during initial postoperative period (1-2 weeks or until adequate wound healing). The preoperative dose should be given 1 hour prior to surgery. The average dosing interval may be every 12 hours initially, then every 24 hours later in the postoperative period.

Dental surgery: Raise Factor IX level to 40% to 60% of normal on day of surgery. One infusion is generally sufficient for the extraction of one tooth; for the extraction of multiple teeth replacement therapy may be required for up to 1 week (See dosing guidelines for Minor Surgery).

Major surgery: Raise Factor IX level to ≥60% of normal on day of surgery; do not raise ≥50% in patients who may be predisposed to thrombosis. Decrease from 60% of normal to 20% of normal during initial post operative period (1-2 weeks), and late postoperative period (≥3 weeks) continuing until adequate wound healing is achieved. The preoperative dose should be given 1 hour prior to surgery. The average dosing interval may be every 12 hours initially, then every 24 hours later in the postoperative period.

Long-term prophylactic treatment: 20-30 int. units/kg once or twice a week may reduce frequency of spontaneous hemorrhage; dosing should be individualized.

Warfarin associated hemorrhage (unlabeled use): I.V.: **Note:** Administer vitamin K (phytonadione) 10 mg by slow I.V. infusion; vitamin K may be repeated every 12 hours if INR is persistently elevated (Ansell, 2008)

Fixed-dose regimen (Yasaka, 2005): INR ≤5: 500 int. units

Adjusted-dose regimen, weight based (Makris, 2001):

INR 2-3.9: 25 int. units/kg

INR 4-5.9: 35 int. units/kg

INR ≥6: 50 int. units/kg

Stability

Bebulin® VH: Prior to use, store under refrigeration at 2°C to 8°C (36°F to 46°F); avoid freezing. Bring diluent and concentrate to room temperature; gently rotate or agitate to dissolve. Following reconstitution, do not refrigerate and use within 3 hours.

Profilnine® SD: Prior to use, store under refrigeration at 2°C to 8°C (36°F to 46°F); avoid freezing; may also stored at room temperature (not to exceed 30°C) for up to 3 months. Bring diluent and concentrate to room temperature; gently rotate or agitate to dissolve. Following reconstitution, do not refrigerate and use within 3 hours.

Administration I.V. administration only; should be infused **slowly**. Rate should not exceed 2 mL/minute for Bebulin® VH or 10 mL/minute for Profilnine® SD. Slowing the rate of infusion, changing the lot of medication, or administering antihistamines may relieve some adverse reactions

Monitoring Parameters Levels of factor IX; PT, PTT; signs and symptoms of hypersensitivity reactions, DIC, thrombosis

Reference Range Patients with severe hemophilia will have levels <1%, often undetectable. Moderate forms of the disease have levels of 1% to 10% while some mild cases may have 5% to 49% of normal factor IX.

Anesthesia and Critical Care Concerns/Other Considerations

Evidence-Based Information: Management of Intracerebral Hemorrhage (ICH) Due to Warfarin: The 2007 AHA/ASA Guidelines for the Management of Spontaneous Intracerebral Hemorrhage in Adults state that factor IX complex can be used but with greater risk of thromboembolism (Class IIB) or with intravenous vitamin K and fresh forzen plasma (Class I).

Pregnancy Risk Factor C

Contraindications There are no contraindications listed in the manufacturer's labeling.

Warnings/Precautions Thrombosis or disseminated intravascular coagulation (DIC) may occur with use, particularly following surgery. Use with caution in patients with liver dysfunction; may be at increased risk of developing thrombosis or DIC. Products do not contain therapeutic levels of factor VII and should not be used for the treatment of factor VII deficiency. Product of human plasma; may potentially contain infectious agents which could transmit disease. Screening of donors, as well as testing and/or inactivation or removal of certain viruses, reduces the risk. Infections thought to be transmitted by this product should be reported to the manufacturer. Some products may contain heparin. Use with caution in patients with a history of heparin-induced thrombocytopenia type II. Some product packaging may contain natural rubber latex.

Adverse Reactions Frequency not defined.

Cardiovascular: Fatal intracardiac thrombosis (INR reversal [Warren, 2009]), flushing, thrombosis

Central nervous system: Chills, fever, headache, lethargy, somnolence

Dermatologic: Rash, urticaria

Gastrointestinal: Nausea, vomiting

Hematologic: DIC

Neuromuscular & skeletal: Paresthesia

Respiratory: Dyspnea

Miscellaneous: Anaphylactic shock, clotting factor antibodies (development of), heparin-induced thrombocytopenia type II (with products containing heparin)

Drug Interactions

Avoid Concomitant Use

Avoid concomitant use of Factor IX Complex (Human) with any of the following:
Aminocaproic Acid

Increased Effect/Toxicity

The levels/effects of Factor IX Complex (Human) may be increased by:
Aminocaproic Acid

Decreased Effect There are no known significant interactions involving a decrease in effect.

Dosage Forms Excipient information presented when available (limited, particularly for generics); consult specific product labeling. [DSC] = Discontinued product

Injection, powder for reconstitution (**Note:** Exact potency labeled on each vial):

Bebulin® VH [single-dose vial; vapor heated; supplied with sterile water for injection; contains heparin; packaging contains latex]

Profilnine® SD [single-dose vial; solvent detergent treated]

References

Broderick J, Connolly S, Feldmann E, et al, "Guidelines for the Management of Spontaneous Intracerebral Hemorrhage in Adults: 2007 Update: A Guideline From the American Heart Association/American Stroke Association Stroke Council, High Blood Pressure Research Council, and the Quality of Care and Outcomes in Research Interdisciplinary Working Group," *Stroke*, 2007, 38(6):2001-23. Available at http://stroke.ahajournals.org/cgi/content/short/STROKEAHA.107.183689.

◆ **Factor IX Concentrate** see Factor IX *on page 570*

Famotidine (fa MOE ti deen)

Medication Safety Issues

Sound-alike/look-alike issues:

Famotidine may be confused with FLUoxetine, furosemide

U.S. Brand Names Pepcid®; Pepcid® AC Maximum Strength [OTC]; Pepcid® AC [OTC]

Canadian Brand Names Apo-Famotidine®; Apo-Famotidine® Injectable; Famotidine Omega; Gen-Famotidine; Mylan-Famotidine; Novo-Famotidine; Nu-Famotidine; Pepcid®; Pepcid® AC; Pepcid® I.V.; ratio-Famotidine; Riva-Famotidine; Ulcidine

◀ **Pharmacologic Category** Histamine H_2 Antagonist
Generic Available Yes: Injection, tablet
Use Maintenance therapy and treatment of duodenal ulcer; treatment of gastroesophageal reflux, active benign gastric ulcer, and pathological hyper-secretory conditions

OTC labeling: Relief of heartburn, acid indigestion, and sour stomach
Unlabeled/Investigational Use Part of a multidrug regimen for *H. pylori* eradication to reduce the risk of duodenal ulcer recurrence; stress ulcer prophylaxis in critically-ill patients; symptomatic relief in gastritis
Mechanism of Action Competitive inhibition of histamine at H_2 receptors of the gastric parietal cells, which inhibits gastric acid secretion

Pharmacodynamics/Kinetics
Onset of action: GI: Oral: Within 1-3 hour; I.V.: 30 minutes

Duration: 10-12 hours

Protein binding: 15% to 20%

Bioavailability: Oral: 40% to 45%

Half-life elimination: Injection, oral suspension, tablet: 2.5-3.5 hours; prolonged with renal impairment; Oliguria: >20 hours

Time to peak, serum: Oral: ~1-3 hours

Excretion: Urine (25% to 30% [oral], 65% to 70% [I.V.] as unchanged drug)

Dosage
Children: Treatment duration and dose should be individualized

Peptic ulcer: 1-16 years:

Oral: 0.5 mg/kg/day at bedtime or divided twice daily (maximum dose: 40 mg/day); doses of up to 1 mg/kg/day have been used in clinical studies

I.V.: 0.25 mg/kg every 12 hours (maximum dose: 40 mg/day); doses of up to 0.5 mg/kg have been used in clinical studies

GERD: Oral:

<3 months: 0.5 mg/kg once daily

3-12 months: 0.5 mg/kg twice daily

1-16 years: 1 mg/kg/day divided twice daily (maximum dose: 40 mg twice daily); doses of up to 2 mg/kg/day have been used in clinical studies

Children ≥12 years and Adults: Heartburn, indigestion, sour stomach: OTC labeling: Oral: 10-20 mg every 12 hours; dose may be taken 15-60 minutes before eating foods known to cause heartburn

Adults:

Duodenal ulcer: Oral: Acute therapy: 40 mg/day at bedtime for 4-8 weeks; maintenance therapy: 20 mg/day at bedtime

Helicobacter pylori eradication (unlabeled use): 40 mg once daily; requires combination therapy with antibiotics

Gastric ulcer: Oral: Acute therapy: 40 mg/day at bedtime

Hypersecretory conditions: Oral: Initial: 20 mg every 6 hours, may increase in increments up to 160 mg every 6 hours

GERD: Oral: 20 mg twice daily for 6 weeks

Esophagitis and accompanying symptoms due to GERD: Oral: 20 mg or 40 mg twice daily for up to 12 weeks

Patients unable to take oral medication: I.V.: 20 mg every 12 hours

Dosing adjustment in renal impairment: Cl_{cr} <50 mL/minute: Manufacturer recommendation: Administer 50% of dose **or** increase the dosing interval to every 36-48 hours (to limit potential CNS adverse effects).

Stability
Oral:

Powder for oral suspension: Prior to mixing, dry powder should be stored at controlled room temperature of 25°C (77°F). Reconstituted oral suspension is stable for 30 days at room temperature; do not freeze.

Tablet: Store at controlled room temperature. Protect from moisture.

I.V.:

Solution for injection: Prior to use, store at 2°C to 8°C (36°F to 46°F). If solution freezes, allow to solubilize at controlled room temperature.

I.V. push: Dilute famotidine with NS (or another compatible solution) to a total of 5-10 mL (some centers also administer undiluted). Following preparation, solutions for I.V. push should be used immediately, or may be stored in refrigerator and used within 48 hours.

Infusion: Dilute with D_5W 100 mL or another compatible solution. Following preparation, the manufacturer states may be stored for up to 48 hours under refrigeration; however, solutions for infusion have been found to be physically and chemically stable for 7 days at room temperature.

Solution for injection, premixed bags: Store at controlled room temperature of 25°C (77°F); avoid excessive heat.

Administration

Oral:

Suspension: Shake vigorously before use. May be taken without regard to meals.

Tablet: May be taken without regard to meals.

I.V.:

I.V. push: Inject over at least 2 minutes.

Solution for infusion: Administer over 15-30 minutes.

Anesthesia and Critical Care Concerns/Other Considerations

Evidence-Based Information: The 2008 Surviving Sepsis Campaign guidelines recommend that stress ulcer prophylaxis using an H_2 blocker (Grade 1A) or proton pump inhibitor (Grade 1B) be given to patients with severe sepsis to prevent upper GI bleed. Benefit of prevention of upper GI bleed must be weighed against potential effect of increased stomach pH on development of ventilator-associated pneumonia.

Pregnancy Risk Factor B

Contraindications Hypersensitivity to famotidine, other H_2 antagonists, or any component of the formulation

Warnings/Precautions Modify dose in patients with moderate-to-severe renal impairment. Relief of symptoms does not preclude the presence of a gastric malignancy. Reversible confusional states, usually clearing within 3-4 days after discontinuation, have been linked to use. Increased age (>50 years) and renal or hepatic impairment are thought to be associated. Multidose vials for injection contain benzyl alcohol.

OTC labeling: When used for self-medication, patients should be instructed not to use if they have difficulty swallowing, are vomiting blood, or have bloody or black stools. Not for use with other acid reducers.

Adverse Reactions

Note: Agitation and vomiting have been reported in up to 14% of pediatric patients <1 year of age.

1% to 10%:

Central nervous system: Headache (5%), dizziness (1%)

Gastrointestinal: Diarrhea (2%), constipation (1%)

<1% (Limited to important or life-threatening): Abdominal discomfort, acne, agitation, agranulocytosis, allergic reaction, alopecia, anaphylaxis, angioedema, anorexia, anxiety, arrhythmia, arthralgia, AV block, bradycardia, bronchospasm, BUN/creatinine increased, cholestatic jaundice, confusion, depression, drowsiness, facial edema, fatigue, fever, flushing, hallucinations, injection site reactions, insomnia, interstitial pneumonia, jaundice, leukopenia, libido decreased, liver function tests increased, muscle cramps, nausea, palpitation, pancytopenia, paresthesia, proteinuria, pruritus, rash, seizure, somnolence, Stevens-Johnson syndrome, tinnitus, thrombocytopenia, toxic epidermal necrolysis, urticaria, vomiting, weakness, xerostomia

Drug Interactions

Avoid Concomitant Use

Avoid concomitant use of Famotidine with any of the following: Delavirdine; Erlotinib

Increased Effect/Toxicity

Famotidine may increase the levels/effects of: Saquinavir

Decreased Effect

Famotidine may decrease the levels/effects of: Antifungal Agents (Azole Derivatives, Systemic); Atazanavir; Cefpodoxime; Cefuroxime; Dasatinib; Delavirdine; Erlotinib; Fosamprenavir; Indinavir; Iron Salts; Mesalamine; Nelfinavir

◄ Ethanol/Nutrition/Herb Interactions
Ethanol: Avoid ethanol (may cause gastric mucosal irritation).
Food: Famotidine bioavailability may be increased if taken with food.

Dietary Considerations May be taken without regard to meals.

Dosage Forms Excipient information presented when available (limited, particularly for generics); consult specific product labeling. [DSC] = Discontinued product

Gelcap:
  Pepcid® AC: 10 mg [DSC]
Infusion [premixed in NS]: 20 mg (50 mL)
Injection, solution: 10 mg/mL (4 mL, 20 mL, 50 mL)
Injection, solution [preservative free]: 10 mg/mL (2 mL)
Powder for oral suspension:
  Pepcid®: 40 mg/5 mL (50 mL) [contains sodium benzoate; cherry-banana-mint flavor]
Tablet: 10 mg [OTC], 20 mg, 40 mg
  Pepcid®: 20 mg, 40 mg
  Pepcid® AC: 10 mg, 20 mg
  Pepcid® AC Maximum Strength: 20 mg

References
Dellinger RP, Levy MM, Carlet JM, et al, "Surviving Sepsis Campaign: International Guidelines for Management of Severe Sepsis and Septic Shock: 2008," *Intensive Care Med*, 2008, 34(1): 17-60. Available at http://www.survivingsepsis.org/system/files/images/2008_20International_20SSC_20-Guidelines_1_.pdf

◆ **Famotidine Omega (Can)** *see* Famotidine *on page* 575

◆ **Fanapt™** *see* Iloperidone *on page* 725

Fat Emulsion (fat e MUL shun)

U.S. Brand Names Intralipid®; Liposyn® II; Liposyn® III
Canadian Brand Names Intralipid®; Liposyn® II
Index Terms Intravenous Fat Emulsion
Pharmacologic Category Caloric Agent
Generic Available No

Use Source of calories and essential fatty acids for patients requiring parenteral nutrition of extended duration; prevention and treatment of essential fatty acid deficiency (EFAD)

Unlabeled/Investigational Use Local anesthetic-induced cardiac arrest unresponsive to conventional resuscitation

Mechanism of Action Fat emulsion is metabolized and utilized as an energy source; provides the essential fatty acids, linoleic acid, and alpha linolenic acid necessary for normal structure and function of cell membranes; in local anesthetic toxicity, lipid emulsion probably extracts lipophilic local anesthesia from cardiac muscle

Pharmacodynamics/Kinetics
Metabolism: Undergoes lipolysis to free fatty acids which are utilized by reticuloendothelial cells
Half-life elimination: 0.5-1 hour

Dosage I.V.: **Note:** At the onset of therapy, the patient should be observed for any immediate allergic reactions.
Nutrition:
  Premature infants: Initial dose: 0.25-0.5 g/kg/day, increase by 0.25-0.5 g/kg/day to a maximum of 3 g/kg/day depending on needs/nutritional goals; limit to 1 g/kg/day if on phototherapy; should be administered over 24 hours (A.S.P.E.N. guidelines)
  Infants and Children: Initial dose: 0.5-1 g/kg/day, increase by 0.5 g/kg/day to a maximum of 3 g/kg/day depending on needs/nutritional goals; may administer over 24 hours (A.S.P.E.N. guidelines)
  Note: Pediatric patients: Monitor triglycerides while receiving intralipids. If serum triglyceride levels >200 mg/dL, stop infusion and restart at 0.5-1 g/kg/day. Intravenous heparin (1 unit/mL of parenteral nutrition) may enhance the clearance of lipid emulsions.

Adults: Initial dose: 1 g/kg/day, increase by 0.5-1 g/kg/day to a maximum of 2.5-3 g/kg/day

Prevention of essential fatty acid deficiency (EFAD): Adults: Administer 8% to 10% of total caloric intake as fat emulsion (may be higher in stressed patients with EFAD); may be given 2-3 times weekly to meet essential fatty acid requirements

Local anesthetic toxicity (unlabeled use): Adults: 20%: 1.5 mL/kg administered over 1 minute, followed immediately by an infusion of 0.25 mL/kg/minute. Continue chest compressions (lipid must circulate). Repeat bolus every 3-5 minutes up to 3 mL/kg total dose until circulation restored. Continue infusion until hemodynamic stability is restored. Increase the infusion rate to 0.5 mL/kg/minute if BP declines. A maximum total dose of 8 mL/kg is recommended.

Stability Do not freeze. Do not store partly used containers; fat emulsion can support the growth of various organisms. Do not use if emulsion appears to be oiling out.

Intralipid®: Store below 25°C (77°F).

Liposyn®: Store below 30°C (86°F).

Administration Can be administered in a peripheral line or by central venous infusion. At the onset of therapy, the patient should be observed for any immediate allergic reactions such as dyspnea, cyanosis, and fever. Change tubing after each infusion. May be simultaneously infused with amino acid dextrose mixtures by means of Y-connector located near infusion site or administered in total nutrient mixtures (3-in-1) with amino acids, dextrose, and other nutrients. Hang fat emulsion higher than other fluids (has low specific gravity and could run up into other lines). Infuse via pump using either peripheral or central venous line.

Intralipid®, Liposyn® II: Do not use <1.2 micron filter

Liposyn® III: Do not use a filter.

Children: Infuse for 10-15 minutes at a slower rate. Infuse 10% at ≤0.1 mL/minute; can increase to 1 mL/kg/hour if tolerated. Infuse 20% at ≤0.05 mL/minute; can increase to 0.5 mL/kg/hour if tolerated. **Note:** Premature and/or septic infants may need to reduce infusion rate. Do not exceed 1 g fat/kg in 4 hours in this population.

Adults: Infuse for 15-30 minutes at a slower rate. Infuse 10% at 1 mL/minute. If no untoward effects, can double rate. Infuse 20% at 0.5 mL/minute initially; can double rate if tolerated.

Monitoring Parameters Monitor line site for signs and symptoms of infection.

Monitor liver function tests periodically. Monitor triglycerides before initiation of lipid therapy and at least weekly during therapy; monitor especially closely in premature infants, septic infants, and patients with pancreatitis or liver disease.

Neonates: Frequent (some advise daily) platelet counts should be performed in neonatal patients receiving parenteral lipids.

Anesthesia and Critical Care Concerns/Other Considerations

Evidence-Based Information:

Local anesthetic toxicity: Cardiac arrest: Lipid infusion has been used in animal studies and several human cases (*Bupivacaine:* Rosenblatt, 2006; *Levobupivacaine:* Foxall, 2007; *Ropivacaine:* Litz, 2006) where cardiovascular toxicity, unresponsive to conventional resuscitation, resulted. Additional information is available at http://www.lipidrescue.org.

Pregnancy Risk Factor C

Contraindications Hypersensitivity to fat emulsion or any component of the formulation; severe egg or legume (soybean) allergies; pathologic hyperlipidemia, lipoid nephrosis, acute pancreatitis associated with hyperlipemia

Warnings/Precautions Premature and small for gestational age infants clear intravenous fat emulsion poorly; Serious and sometimes fatal reactions have occurred. **[U.S. Boxed Warning]: Strict adherence to proper infusion rates, dosing, and monitoring are necessary;** infusion rate should not exceed 1g fat/kg in 4 hours; strict monitoring of metabolic tolerance and elimination of infused fat from the circulation must occur.

Some formulations may contain aluminum which may accumulate following prolonged administration in renally-impaired patients. Due to immature renal function, premature neonates are at higher risk of accumulation/toxicity from aluminum. Use caution in patients with severe liver damage. To avoid ▶

hyperlipidemia and/or fat deposition, do not exceed recommended daily doses. Monitor by appropriate laboratory evaluation (eg, triglycerides). Use caution in patients with pancreatitis without hyperlipidemia; ensure triglyceride levels remain <400 mg/dL. Lipid emulsion in a three-in-one mixture may obscure the presence of a precipitate; follow compounding guidelines, especially for calcium and phosphate additions.

Adverse Reactions <1% (Limited to important or life-threatening): Allergic reactions, brown pigment deposition in the reticuloendothelial system ("intravenous fat pigment"), cholestasis, cyanosis, hepatomegaly, hypercoagulability, hyperlipidemia, infusion site irritation, jaundice, leukopenia, liver function tests increased, pancreatitis, overloading syndrome (focal seizures, fever, leukocytosis, hepatomegaly, splenomegaly, shock), thrombocytopenia

Dietary Considerations

Phosphorus: ~1.5 mMol /100 mL of emulsion

Caloric content: 10% fat emulsion = 1.1 kcal/mL; 20% fat emulsion = 2 kcal/mL; 30% fat emulsion = 3 kcal/mL

Fat emulsion should not exceed 60% of the total daily calories.

Dosage Forms Excipient information presented when available (limited, particularly for generics); consult specific product labeling.

Injection, emulsion:

Intralipid®: 20% (100 mL, 250 mL, 500 mL, 1000 mL) [contains aluminum, egg yolk phospholipids, and soybean oil]; 30% (500 mL) [contains aluminum, egg yolk phospholipids, and soybean oil]

Liposyn® II: 10% (500 mL) [contains aluminum, egg yolk phospholipids, safflower oil, and soybean oil]; 20% (500 mL) [contains aluminum, egg yolk phospholipids, safflower oil, and soybean oil]

Liposyn® III: 10% (200 mL, 500 mL) [contains aluminum, egg yolk phospholipids, and soybean oil]; 20% (200 mL, 500 mL) [contains aluminum, egg yolk phospholipids, and soybean oil]; 30% (500 mL) [contains aluminum, egg yolk phospholipids, and soybean oil]

References

ASPEN Board of Directors and the Clinical Guidelines Task Force, "Guidelines for the Use of Parenteral and Enteral Nutrition in Adult and Pediatric Patients," *JPEN J Parenter Enteral Nutr*, 2002, 26(1 Suppl):1-138.

Corcoran W, Butterworth J, Weller RS, et al, "Local Anesthetic-Induced Cardiac Toxicity: A Survey of Contemporary Practice Strategies Among Academic Anesthesiology Departments," *Anesth Analg*, 2006, 103(5):1322-26.

Foxall G, McCahon R, Lamb J, et al, "Levobupivacaine-Induced Seizures and Cardiovascular Collapse Treated With Intralipid," *Anaesthesia*, 2007, 62(5):516-8.

Litz RJ, Popp M, Stehr SN, et al, "Successful Resuscitation of a Patient With Ropivacaine-Induced Asystole After Axillary Plexus Block Using Lipid Infusion," *Anaesthesia*, 2006, 61(8):800-1.

Mirtallo J, Canada T, Johnson D, et al, "Safe Practices for Parenteral Nutrition. Task Force for the Revision of Safe Practices for Parenteral Nutrition," *JPEN J Parenter Enteral Nutr*, 2004, 28(6): S39-70.

Rosenblatt MA, Abel M, Fischer GW, et al, "Successful Use of a 20% Lipid Emulsion to Resuscitate a Patient After a Presumed Bupivacaine-Related Cardiac Arrest," *Anesthesiology*, 2006, 105 (1):217-8.

Felbamate (FEL ba mate)

Related Information

Perioperative Management of Patients on Antiseizure Medication *on page 1577*

U.S. Brand Names Felbatol®

Pharmacologic Category Anticonvulsant, Miscellaneous

Restrictions A patient "informed consent" form should be completed and signed by the patient and physician. Copies are available from Wallace Pharmaceuticals by calling 800-526-3840 or 609-655-6147.

Use Not as a first-line antiepileptic treatment; only in those patients who respond inadequately to alternative treatments and whose epilepsy is so severe that a substantial risk of aplastic anemia and/or liver failure is deemed acceptable in light of the benefits conferred by its use. Patient must be fully advised of risk and provide signed written informed consent. Felbamate can be used as either monotherapy or adjunctive therapy in the treatment of partial seizures (with and without generalization) and in adults with epilepsy. Used as adjunctive therapy in the treatment of partial and generalized seizures associated with Lennox-Gastaut syndrome in children.

Pharmacodynamics/Kinetics

Absorption: Rapid and almost complete; food has no effect upon the tablet's absorption

Distribution: V_d: 0.7-0.8 L/kg

Protein binding: 22% to 25%, primarily to albumin

Half-life elimination: 20-23 hours (average); prolonged in renal dysfunction

Time to peak, serum: 3-5 hours

Excretion: Urine (40% to 50% as unchanged drug, 40% as inactive metabolites)

Dosage Anticonvulsant:

Monotherapy: Children >14 years and Adults:

Initial: 1200 mg/day in divided doses 3 or 4 times/day; titrate previously untreated patients under close clinical supervision, increasing the dosage in 600 mg increments every 2 weeks to 2400 mg/day based on clinical response and thereafter to 3600 mg/day as clinically indicated

Conversion to monotherapy: Initiate at 1200 mg/day in divided doses 3 or 4 times/day, reduce the dosage of the concomitant anticonvulsant(s) by 20% to 33% at the initiation of felbamate therapy; at week 2, increase the felbamate dosage to 2400 mg/day while reducing the dosage of the other anticonvulsant(s) up to an additional 33% of their original dosage; at week 3, increase the felbamate dosage up to 3600 mg/day and continue to reduce the dosage of the other anticonvulsant(s) as clinically indicated

Adjunctive therapy: **Note:** Dose of concomitant carbamazepine, phenobarbital, phenytoin, or valproic acid should be decreased by 20% to 33% when initiating felbamate therapy. Further dosage reductions may be necessary as dose of felbamate is increased.

Children 2-14 years with Lennox-Gastaut syndrome: Initial: 15 mg/kg/day in divided doses 3 or 4 times/day; may increase once per week by 15 mg/kg/day increments up to 45 mg/kg/day in divided doses 3 or 4 times/day.

Children >14 years and Adults: Initial: 1200 mg/day in divided doses 3 or 4 times/day; may increase once per week by 1200 mg/day increments up to 3600 mg/day in divided doses 3 or 4 times/day.

Dosage adjustment in renal impairment: Use caution; reduce initial and maintenance doses by 50% (half-life prolonged by 9-15 hours)

Anesthesia and Critical Care Concerns/Other Considerations Monotherapy has not been associated with gingival hyperplasia, impaired concentration, weight gain, or abnormal thinking. Because felbamate is the only drug shown effective in Lennox-Gastaut syndrome, it is considered an orphan drug.

Additional Information Monotherapy has not been associated with gingival hyperplasia, impaired concentration, weight gain, or abnormal thinking. Because felbamate is the only drug shown effective in Lennox-Gastaut syndrome, it is considered an orphan drug for this indication.

Dosage Forms Excipient information presented when available (limited, particularly for generics); consult specific product labeling.

Suspension, oral:

Felbatol®: 600 mg/5 mL (240 mL, 960 mL)

Tablet:

Felbatol®: 400 mg; 600 mg

Fenofibrate (fen oh FYE brate)

Related Information

Hyperlipidemia Management *on page 1747*

U.S. Brand Names Antara®; Fenoglide™; Lipofen®; Lofibra®; TriCor®; Triglide™

Canadian Brand Names Apo-Feno-Micro®; Apo-Fenofibrate®; Dom-Fenofibrate Supra; Feno-Micro-200; Fenomax; Gen-Fenofibrate Micro; Lipidil EZ®; Lipidil Micro®; Lipidil Supra®; Mylan-Fenofibrate Micro; Novo-Fenofibrate; Novo-Fenofibrate-S; Nu-Fenofibrate; PHL-Fenofibrate Supra; PMS-Fenofibrate Micro; Pro-Feno-Super; ratio-Fenofibrate MC; Riva-Fenofibrate Micro; Sandoz Fenofibrate S

Index Terms Procetofene; Proctofene

Pharmacologic Category Antilipemic Agent, Fibric Acid

Use Adjunct to dietary therapy for the treatment of adults with elevations of serum triglyceride levels (types IV and V hyperlipidemia); adjunct to dietary therapy for the reduction of low density lipoprotein cholesterol (LDL-C), total cholesterol (total-C), triglycerides, and apolipoprotein B (apo B) in adult patients with primary hypercholesterolemia or mixed dyslipidemia (Fredrickson types IIa and IIb)

Pharmacodynamics/Kinetics

Absorption: Increased when taken with meals

Distribution: Widely to most tissues

Protein binding: >99%

Metabolism: Tissue and plasma via esterases to active form, fenofibric acid; undergoes inactivation by glucuronidation hepatically or renally

Half-life elimination: Fenofibric acid: Mean: 20 hours (range: 10-35 hours)

Time to peak: 3-8 hours

Excretion: Urine (60% as metabolites); feces (25%); hemodialysis has no effect on removal of fenofibric acid from plasma

Dosage Oral:

Adults:

Hypertriglyceridemia: Initial:

Antara® (micronized): 43-130 mg/day; maximum dose: 130 mg/day

Fenoglide™: 40-120 mg/day; maximum dose: 120 mg/day

Lipidil EZ® [CAN; not available in U.S.]: 145 mg/day; maximum dose: 145 mg/day

Lipidil Micro® [CAN; not available in U.S.]: 200 mg/day; maximum dose: 200 mg/day

Lipidil Supra® [CAN; not available in U.S.]: 160 mg/day; maximum dose: 200 mg/day

Lipofen®: 50-150 mg/day; maximum dose: 150 mg/day

Lofibra® (micronized): 67-200 mg/day with meals; maximum dose: 200 mg/day

Lofibra® (tablets): 54-160 mg/day; maximum dose: 160 mg/day

TriCor®: 48-145 mg/day; maximum dose: 145 mg/day

Triglide™: 50-160 mg/day; maximum dose: 160 mg/day

Hypercholesterolemia or mixed hyperlipidemia:

Antara® (micronized): 130 mg/day

Fenoglide™: 120 mg/day

Lipidil EZ® [CAN; not available in U.S.]: 145 mg/day; maximum dose: 145 mg/day

Lipidil Micro® [CAN; not available in U.S.]: 200 mg/day; maximum dose: 200 mg/day

Lipidil Supra® [CAN; not available in U.S.]: 160 mg/day; maximum dose: 200 mg/day

Lipofen®: 150 mg/day

Lofibra® (micronized): 200 mg/day

Lofibra® (tablets): 160 mg/day

TriCor®: 145 mg/day

Triglide™: 160 mg/day

Elderly: Initial:

Antara® (micronized): 43 mg/day

Fenoglide™: Adjust dosage based on creatinine clearance

Lipidil EZ® [CAN; not available in U.S.]: 48 mg/day
Lipidil Micro® [CAN; not available in U.S.]: Adjust dosage based on creatinine clearance
Lipidil Supra® [CAN; not available in U.S.]: Adjust dosage based on creatinine clearance
Lipofen®: 50 mg/day
Lofibra® (micronized): 67 mg/day
Lofibra® (tablets): 54 mg/day
TriCor®: Adjust dosage based on creatinine clearance
Triglide™: 50 mg/day

Dosage adjustment/interval in renal impairment: Monitor renal function and lipid panel before adjusting. Decrease dose or increase dosing interval for patients with renal failure: **Note:** Use in severe renal impairment is contra-indicated (see specific product labeling):
Antara® (micronized): 43 mg/day
Fenoglide™: Cl_{cr} 31-80 mL/minute: 40 mg/day
Lipidil EZ® [CAN; not available in U.S.]: Cl_{cr} ≥20-50 mL/minute: 48 mg/day
Lipidil Micro® [CAN; not available in U.S.]: Cl_{cr} ≥20-100 mL/minute: 67 mg/day; **Note:** Lipidil Micro® 67 mg capsules are discontinued in Canada. Micronized formulation at this dosage strength is available through other manufacturers in Canada.
Lipidil Supra® [CAN; not available in U.S.]: Cl_{cr} ≥20-100 mL/minute: 100 mg/day
Lipofen®: 50 mg/day
Lofibra® (micronized): 67 mg/day
Lofibra® (tablets): 54 mg/day
TriCor®: Cl_{cr} 31-80 mL/minute: 48 mg/day
Triglide™: 50 mg/day

Additional Information Complete prescribing information for this medication should be consulted for additional detail.

Dosage Forms Excipient information presented when available (limited, particularly for generics); consult specific product labeling. [DSC] = Discontinued product
Capsule:
Lipofen®: 50 mg; 100 mg [DSC]; 150 mg
Capsule [micronized]: 67 mg, 134 mg, 200 mg
Antara®: 43 mg, 130 mg
Lofibra®: 67 mg, 134 mg, 200 mg
Tablet: 54 mg, 160 mg
Fenoglide™: 40 mg, 120 mg
Lofibra®: 54 mg, 160 mg
TriCor®: 48 mg, 145 mg [contains soybean lecithin]
Triglide™: 50 mg, 160 mg [contains egg lecithin]

References
de Lorgeril M, Salen O, Paillard F, et al, "Lipid-Lowering Drugs and Homocyst(e)ine," *Lancet*, 1999, 353(9148):209-10.
"Executive Summary of The Third Report of The National Cholesterol Education Program (NCEP) Expert Panel on Detection, Evaluation, and Treatment of High Blood Cholesterol in Adults (Adult Treatment Panel III)," *JAMA*, 2001, 285(19):2486-97.
Farnier M, Bonnefous F, Debbas N, et al, "Comparative Efficacy and Safety of Micronized Fenofibrate and Simvastatin in Patients With Primary Type IIa or IIb Hyperlipidemia," *Arch Intern Med*, 1994, 154(4):441-9.
Mahley RW and Bersot TP, "Drug Therapy for Hypercholesterolemia and Dyslipidemia," *Goodman and Gilman's The Pharmacological Basis of Therapeutics*, 10th ed, Hardman JE and Limbird LE, eds, New York, NY: McGraw-Hill, 2001, 993-5.
Sitori CR, Montanari G, Gianfranceschi G, et al, "Correlation Between Plasma Levels of Fenofibrate and Lipoprotein Changes in Hyperlipidaemic Patients," *Eur J Clin Pharmacol*, 1985, 28(6):619-24.

Fenofibric Acid (fen oh FYE brik AS id)

U.S. Brand Names Fibricor™; TriLipix™
Index Terms ABT-335; Choline Fenofibrate
Pharmacologic Category Antilipemic Agent, Fibric Acid
Use Adjunct to dietary therapy for the treatment of severely elevated serum triglyceride levels; adjunct to dietary therapy for the reduction of low density

◄ lipoprotein cholesterol (LDL-C), total cholesterol (total-C), triglycerides, and apolipoprotein B (apo B) and to increase high density lipoprotein cholesterol (HDL-C) in patients with primary hypercholesterolemia or mixed dyslipidemia

TriLipix™ is also indicated as adjunct to dietary therapy concomitantly with a statin to reduce triglyceride levels and increase HDL-C levels in patients with mixed dyslipidemia and coronary heart disease (CHD) or at risk for CHD

Pharmacodynamics/Kinetics
Absorption: Well absorbed
Protein binding: ~99%
Metabolism: Fenofibric acid (active form) undergoes inactivation by glucuronidation. The choline salt dissociates in the GI tract to form fenofibric acid (free acid)
Bioavailability: TriLipix™: ~81%
Half-life elimination: ~20 hours
Time to peak, plasma: Fibricor™: ~2.5 hours; TriLipix™: 4-5 hours
Excretion: Urine (as fenofibric acid and fenofibric acid glucuronide)

Dosage Oral:
Adults:
Mixed dyslipidemia (coadministered with a statin): TriLipix™: 135 mg once daily (maximum: 135 mg/day)
Hypertriglyceridemia:
Fibricor™: Initial: 35-105 mg once daily; Maintenance: Individualize according to patient response (maximum: 105 mg/day)
TriLipix™: Initial: 45-135 mg once daily; Maintenance: Individualize according to patient response (maximum: 135 mg/day)
Primary hypercholesterolemia or mixed dyslipidemia:
Fibricor™: 105 mg once daily (maximum: 105 mg/day)
TriLipix™: 135 mg once daily (maximum: 135 mg/day)
Elderly: Dosage based on renal function

Dosage adjustment/interval in renal impairment:
Mild-to-moderate impairment (Cl_{cr} 30-80 mL/minute): Initial: Fibricor™: 35 mg once daily or TriLipix™: 45 mg once daily; only increase once effects on lipids and renal function evaluated
Severe impairment (Cl_{cr} <30 mL/minute; with or without dialysis): Contraindicated
Additional Information Complete prescribing information for this medication should be consulted for additional detail.
Dosage Forms Excipient information presented when available (limited, particularly for generics); consult specific product labeling.
Capsule, delayed release:
TriLipix™: 45 mg, 135 mg
Tablet: 35 mg, 105 mg
Fibricor™: 35 mg, 105 mg

References
Mohiuddin SM, Pepine CJ, Kelly MT, et al, "Efficacy and Safety of ABT-335 (Fenofibric Acid) in Combination With Simvastatin In Patients With Mixed Dyslipidemia: A Phase 3, Randomized, Controlled Study," Am Heart J, 2009, 157(1):195-203.

◆ **Fenoglide™** see Fenofibrate on page 582

Fenoldopam (fe NOL doe pam)

Related Information
Chronic Renal Failure on page 1552
Hypertension on page 1754
Postoperative Hypertension on page 1589
U.S. Brand Names Corlopam®
Canadian Brand Names Corlopam®
Index Terms Fenoldopam Mesylate
Pharmacologic Category Dopamine Agonist
Generic Available Yes
Use Treatment of severe hypertension (up to 48 hours in adults), including in patients with renal compromise; short-term (up to 4 hours) blood pressure reduction in pediatric patients

Mechanism of Action A selective postsynaptic dopamine agonist (D_1-receptors) which exerts hypotensive effects by decreasing peripheral vasculature resistance with increased renal blood flow, diuresis, and natriuresis; 6 times as potent as dopamine in producing renal vasodilitation; has minimal adrenergic effects

Pharmacodynamics/Kinetics
Onset of action: I.V.: 10 minutes
Duration: I.V.: 1 hour
Distribution: V_d: 0.6 L/kg
Half-life elimination: I.V.: Children: 3-5 minutes; Adults: ~5 minutes
Metabolism: Hepatic via methylation, glucuronidation, and sulfation; the 8-sulfate metabolite may have some activity; extensive first-pass effect
Excretion: Urine (90%); feces (10%)

Dosage I.V.: Hypertension, severe:
Children: Initial: 0.2 mcg/kg/minute; may be increased to dosages of 0.3-0.5 mcg/kg/minute every 20-30 minutes (maximum dose: 0.8 mcg/kg/minute); limited to short-term (4 hours) use
Adults: Initial: 0.1-0.3 mcg/kg/minute (lower initial doses may be associated with less reflex tachycardia); may be increased in increments of 0.05-0.1 mcg/kg/minute every 15 minutes until target blood pressure is reached; the maximal infusion rate reported in clinical studies was 1.6 mcg/kg/minute

Dosing adjustment in renal impairment: None required
Dosing adjustment in hepatic impairment: None published
Stability Store at 2°C to 30°C (35°F to 86°F). Must be diluted prior to infusion. Final dilution for children is 60 mcg/mL and for adults is 40 mcg/mL. Following dilution, store at room temperature and use solution within 24 hours.
Administration For I.V. infusion using an infusion pump.
Monitoring Parameters Blood pressure, heart rate, ECG, renal/hepatic function tests
Reference Range Mean plasma fenoldopam levels after a 2 hour infusion (at 0.5 mcg/kg/minute) and a 100 mg dose is approximately 13 ng/mL and 50 ng/mL
Anesthesia and Critical Care Concerns/Other Considerations Suitable for use in patients whose condition is unstable or rapidly changing because the effects of the drug are predictable and easily reversible; it has been found to safely control blood pressure in patients with a variety of pre-existing conditions including kidney disease, liver disease, and heart failure. (Clinical benefit other than blood pressure reduction has not been established.) Dosage adjustment is not required in any of these situations. The drug is quickly metabolized into inactive substances before it is excreted. Unlike the situation with some other intravenous antihypertensives, the patient does not need an arterial line for blood pressure monitoring; a blood pressure cuff is sufficient. Since the drug induces natriuresis, diuresis, and increased creatinine clearance, it may have an advantage over nitroprusside, especially in patients with severe renal insufficiency and in volume-overloaded patients.

Contrast Nephropathy: Fenoldopam is ineffective in the prevention of contrast-induced nephropathy.
Pregnancy Risk Factor B
Contraindications Hypersensitivity of fenoldopam or any component of the formulation
Warnings/Precautions Use caution in patients with glaucoma or intraocular hypertension. A dose-related tachycardia can occur, especially at infusion rates >0.1 mcg/kg/minute. Use caution in angina patients (can increase myocardial oxygen demand with tachycardia). Close monitoring of blood pressure is necessary (hypotension can occur). Monitor for hypokalemia at intervals of 6 hours during infusion. For continuous infusion only (no bolus doses). The effects of hemodialysis on the pharmacokinetics of fenoldopam have not been evaluated. Use caution with increased intracranial pressure. Contains sulfites; may cause allergic reaction in susceptible individuals.
Adverse Reactions Frequency not always defined.
Cardiovascular: Angina, asymptomatic T wave flattening on ECG, chest pain, edema, facial flushing (>5%), fibrillation (atrial), flutter (atrial), hypotension (>5%), tachycardia
Central nervous system: Dizziness, headache (>5%)

▶

Endocrine & metabolic: Hypokalemia

Gastrointestinal: Abdominal pain/fullness, diarrhea, nausea (>5%), vomiting, xerostomia

Local: Injection site reactions

Ocular: Intraocular pressure increased, blurred vision

Hepatic: Increases in portal pressure in cirrhotic patients

Drug Interactions

Avoid Concomitant Use There are no known interactions where it is recommended to avoid concomitant use.

Increased Effect/Toxicity There are no known significant interactions involving an increase in effect.

Decreased Effect There are no known significant interactions involving a decrease in effect.

Dosage Forms Excipient information presented when available (limited, particularly for generics); consult specific product labeling.

Injection, solution: 10 mg/mL (1 mL, 2 mL)

Corlopam®: 10 mg/mL (1 mL, 2 mL) [contains propylene glycol, sodium metabisulfite]

References

Allaqaband S, Tumuluri R, Malik AM, et al, "Prospective Randomized Study of N-acetylcysteine, Fenoldopam, and Saline for Prevention of Radiocontrast-Induced Nephropathy," *Catheter Cardiovascular Interv*, 2002, 57(3):279-83.

Erstad BL and Barletta JF, "Treatment of Hypertension in the Perioperative Patient," *Ann Pharmacother*, 2000, 34(1):66-79.

Stone GW, McCullough PA, Tumlin JA, et al, "Fenoldopam Mesylate for the Prevention of Contrast-Induced Nephropathy: A Randomized Controlled Trial," *JAMA*, 2003, 290(17):2284-91.

◆ **Fenoldopam Mesylate** *see* Fenoldopam *on page 584*

◆ **Fenomax (Can)** *see* Fenofibrate *on page 582*

◆ **Feno-Micro-200 (Can)** *see* Fenofibrate *on page 582*

Fenoprofen (fen oh PROE fen)

Related Information

Acetaminophen and NSAIDS, Dosing in the Management of Pain *on page 1651*

Chronic Pain Management *on page 1546*

Nonsteroidal Anti-Inflammatory Agents *on page 1687*

U.S. Brand Names Nalfon®

Canadian Brand Names Nalfon®

Index Terms Fenoprofen Calcium

Pharmacologic Category Nonsteroidal Anti-inflammatory Drug (NSAID), Oral

Use Symptomatic treatment of acute and chronic rheumatoid arthritis and osteoarthritis; relief of mild-to-moderate pain

Pharmacodynamics/Kinetics

Onset of action: A few days; full benefit: up to 2-3 weeks

Absorption: Rapid, 80%

Protein binding: 99%; to albumin

Metabolism: Extensively hepatic

Half-life elimination: 2.5-3 hours

Time to peak, serum: ~2 hours

Excretion: Urine (2% to 5% as unchanged drug); feces (small amounts)

Dosage Adults: Oral:

Rheumatoid arthritis, osteoarthritis: 300-600 mg 3-4 times/day; maximum dose: 3.2 g/day

Mild-to-moderate pain: 200 mg every 4-6 hours as needed; maximum dose: 3.2 g/day

Dosage adjustment in renal impairment: Not recommended in patients with advanced renal disease

Anesthesia and Critical Care Concerns/Other Considerations The 2002 ACCM/SCCM guidelines for analgesia (critically-ill adult) suggest that NSAIDs may be used in combination with opioids in select patients for pain management. Concern about adverse events (increased risk of renal dysfunction, altered platelet function and gastrointestinal irritation) limits its use in patients who have other underlying risks for these events.

in short-term use, NSAIDs vary considerably in their effect on blood pressure. When NSAIDs are used in patients with hypertension, appropriate monitoring of blood pressure responses should be completed and the duration of therapy, when possible, kept short. The use of NSAIDs in the treatment of patients with congestive heart failure may be associated with an increased risk for fluid accumulation and edema. May precipitate renal failure in dehydrated patients.

Additional Information Complete prescribing information for this medication should be consulted for additional detail.

Dosage Forms Excipient information presented when available (limited, particularly for generics); consult specific product labeling.
Capsule, as calcium:
  Nalfon®: 200 mg
Tablet, as calcium: 600 mg

◆ **Fenoprofen Calcium** *see* Fenoprofen *on page 586*

FentaNYL (FEN ta nil)

Medication Safety Issues
Sound-alike/look-alike issues:
  FentaNYL may be confused with alfentanil, SUFentanil

Dosing of transdermal fentanyl patches may be confusing. Transdermal fentanyl patches should always be prescribed in mcg/hour, not size. Patch dosage form of Duragesic®-12 actually delivers 12.5 mcg/hour of fentanyl. Use caution, as orders may be written as "Duragesic 12.5" which can be erroneously interpreted as a 125 mcg dose.

Fentora®, Onsolis™, and Actiq® are not interchangeable; do not substitute doses on a mcg-per-mcg basis.

High alert medication: The Institute for Safe Medication Practices (ISMP) includes this medication among its list of drug classes which have a heightened risk of causing significant patient harm when used in error.
  Fentanyl transdermal system patches: Leakage of fentanyl gel from the patch has been reported; patch may be less effective; do not use. Thoroughly wash any skin surfaces coming into direct contact with gel with water (do not use soap).

Medication Guide An FDA-approved patient medication guide, which is available with the product information and as follows, must be dispensed with each new outpatient prescription and refill.
  Actiq®: http://www.fda.gov/downloads/Drugs/DrugSafety/ucm085817.pdf
  Duragesic®: http://www.fda.gov/downloads/Drugs/DrugSafety/ucm088584.pdf
  Fentora®: http://www.fda.gov/downloads/Drugs/DrugSafety/ucm088597.pdf
  Onsolis™ http://www.accessdata.fda.gov/drugsatfda_docs/label/2009/022266s000MedGuide.pdf

Related Information
  Acute Postoperative Pain *on page 1502*
  Anesthesia Considerations for Neurosurgery *on page 1514*
  Anesthesia for Geriatric Patients *on page 1523*
  Anesthesia for Obstetric Patients in Nonobstetric Surgery *on page 1532*
  Anesthesia for Patients With Liver Disease *on page 1537*
  Anesthetic Considerations in the Substance-Abusing Patient *on page 1613*
  Chronic Pain Management *on page 1546*
  Chronic Renal Failure *on page 1552*
  Dosing Considerations for the Critically-Ill Patient With Morbid Obesity *on page 1561*
  Moderate Sedation *on page 1566*
  Opioid Analgesics *on page 1688*
  Opioids *on page 1641*

U.S. Brand Names Actiq®; Duragesic®; Fentora®; Onsolis™; Sublimaze®

Canadian Brand Names Actiq®; Duragesic MAT; Duragesic®; Fentanyl Citrate Injection, USP; Novo-Fentanyl; RAN™-Fentanyl Transdermal System; ratio-Fentanyl

Index Terms Fentanyl Citrate; Fentanyl Hydrochloride; OTFC (Oral Transmucosal Fentanyl Citrate)

Pharmacologic Category Analgesic, Opioid; Anilidopiperidine Opioid; General Anesthetic

Restrictions C-II

Onsolis™ (fentanyl buccal film) is only available through the restricted distribution program (FOCUS™). Enrollment in the FOCUS™ program is required for prescribers, pharmacies, and patients. Further information may be obtained from the manufacturer, Meda Pharmaceuticals, Inc (1-877-466-7654).

Generic Available Yes: Excludes buccal film, buccal tablet

Use

Injection: Relief of pain, preoperative medication, adjunct to general or regional anesthesia

Iontophoretic transdermal system (Ionsys™): Short-term, in-hospital management of acute postoperative pain

Transdermal patch (eg, Duragesic®): Management of persistent moderate-to-severe chronic pain

Transmucosal lozenge (eg, Actiq®), buccal tablet (Fentora®), buccal film (Onsolis™): Management of breakthrough cancer pain in opioid-tolerant patients

Mechanism of Action Binds with stereospecific receptors at many sites within the CNS, increases pain threshold, alters pain reception, inhibits ascending pain pathways

Pharmacodynamics/Kinetics

Onset of action: Analgesic: I.M.: 7-8 minutes; I.V.: Almost immediate; Transmucosal: 5-15 minutes

Peak effect: Transmucosal: Analgesic: 15-30 minutes

Duration: I.M.: 1-2 hours; I.V.: 0.5-1 hour; Transmucosal: Related to blood level; respiratory depressant effect may last longer than analgesic effect

Absorption:

Transdermal: Initial application: Gradually absorbed for the first 12-24 hours, followed by a constant absorption for the remainder of the dosing interval. Absorption is decreased in cachectic patients (compared to normal size patients).

Transmucosal, buccal tablet and buccal film: Rapid, ~50% from the buccal mucosa; remaining 50% swallowed with saliva and slowly absorbed from GI tract.

Transmucosal, lozenge: Rapid, ~25% from the buccal mucosa; 75% swallowed with saliva and slowly absorbed from GI tract

Distribution: 4-6 L/kg; Highly lipophilic, redistributes into muscle and fat

Protein binding: 80% to 85%

Metabolism: Hepatic, primarily via CYP3A4

Bioavailability:

Buccal film: 71% (mucositis did not have a clinically significant effect on C_{max} and AUC; however, bioavailability is expected to decrease if film is inappropriately chewed and swallowed)

Buccal tablet: 65% (range: 45% to 85%)

Lozenge: 47% (range: 37% to 57%)

Half-life elimination:

I.V.: 2-4 hours

Transdermal patch: 17 hours (13-22 hours, half-life is influenced by absorption rate)

Transmucosal: Lozenge: 7 hours; Buccal film: ~14 hours; Buccal tablet: 100-200 mcg: 3-4 hours, 400-800 mcg: 11-12 hours

Time to peak:

Buccal film: 0.75-4 hours (median: 1 hour)

Buccal tablet: 20-240 minutes (median: 47 minutes)

Lozenge: 20-480 minutes (median: 20-40 minutes)

Transdermal patch: 24-72 hours, after several sequential 72-hour applications, steady state serum concentrations are reached

Excretion: Urine 75% (primarily as metabolites, <7% to 10% as unchanged drug); feces ~9%

Dosage Note: These are guidelines and do not represent the maximum doses that may be required in all patients. Doses and dosage intervals should be titrated to pain relief/prevention. Monitor vital signs routinely. Single I.M. doses have a duration of 1-2 hours, single I.V. doses last 0.5-1 hour.

Minor procedures/analgesia (unlabeled use): I.V.:

Children 1-12 years: 0.5-2 mcg/kg/dose given 3 minutes prior to procedure; may repeat every 1-2 hours

Children >12 years: 0.5-2 mcg/kg/dose (maximum 50 mcg/dose) given 3 minutes prior to procedure; may repeat in 5 minutes if necessary; if more than 2 doses are needed, repeat with a maximum of 25 mcg/dose up to 5 times

Surgery:

Children ≥2 years: Adjunct to anesthesia (induction and maintenance): Slow I.V.: 2-3 mcg/kg/dose every 1-2 hours as needed

Adults:

Premedication: I.M., slow I.V.: 50-100 mcg/dose 30-60 minutes prior to surgery

Adjunct to regional anesthesia: Slow I.V.: 25-100 mcg/dose over 1-2 minutes. **Note:** An I.V. should be in place with regional anesthesia so the I.M. route is rarely used but still maintained as an option in the package labeling.

Adjunct to general anesthesia: Slow I.V.:

Low dose: 0.5-2 mcg/kg/dose depending on the indication

Moderate dose: Initial: 2-20 mcg/kg/dose; Maintenance (bolus or infusion): 1-2 mcg/kg/hour. Discontinuing fentanyl infusion 30-60 minutes prior to the end of surgery will usually allow adequate ventilation upon emergence from anesthesia. For "fast-tracking" and early extubation following major surgery, total fentanyl doses are limited to 10-15 mcg/kg.

High dose: 20-50 mcg/kg/dose; **Note:** Fentanyl is rarely used, but is still maintained in the package labeling.

Pain management:

Children (unlabeled use): I.V.: 0.5-2 mcg/kg/dose given every 1-2 hours as needed; continuous infusion: 0.5-2 mcg/kg/hour; titrate to desired effects

Patient-controlled analgesia (PCA) (unlabeled use; American Pain Society, 2008): Children <50 kg: **Note:** Opiate-naive: Consider lower end of dosing range:

Usual concentration: 10 mcg/mL

Demand dose: 0.5-1 mcg/kg/dose

Lockout interval: 6-8 minutes

Usual basal rate: 0-0.5 mcg/kg/hour

Adults:

I.V. (unlabeled use): Bolus at start of infusion: 1-2 mcg/kg **or** 25-100 mcg/dose; continuous infusion rate: 1-2 mcg/kg/hour **or** 25-200 mcg/hour

Severe pain: I.M, I.V. (unlabeled): 50-100 mcg/dose every 1-2 hours as needed; patients with prior opiate exposure may tolerate higher initial doses

Patient-controlled analgesia (PCA) (unlabeled use): I.V.:

Usual concentration: 10 mcg/mL

Demand dose: Usual: 20 mcg; range: 10-50 mcg

Lockout interval: 5-8 minutes

Usual basal rate: ≤50 mcg/hour

Critically-ill patients (unlabeled dose): Slow I.V.: 25-100 mcg (based on ~70 kg patient) **or** 0.35-1.5 mcg/kg every 30-60 minutes as needed. **Note:** More frequent dosing may be needed (eg, mechanically-ventilated patients).

Continuous infusion: 50-700 mcg/hour (based on ~70 kg patient) **or** 0.7-10 mcg/kg/hour

Intrathecal (I.T.) (unlabeled use; American Pain Society, 2008): **Must be preservative-free.** Doses must be adjusted for age, injection site, and patient's medical condition and degree of opioid tolerance.

Single dose: 5-25 mcg/dose; may provide adequate relief for up to 6 hours

Continuous infusion: Not recommended in acute pain management due to risk of excessive accumulation. For chronic cancer pain, infusion of very small doses may be practical (American Pain Society, 2008).

Epidural (unlabeled use; American Pain Society, 2008): **Must be preservative-free.** Doses must be adjusted for age, injection site, and patient's medical condition and degree of opioid tolerance

Single dose: 25-100 mcg/dose; may provide adequate relief for up to 8 hours

Continuous infusion: 25-100 mcg/hour

Breakthrough cancer pain: For patients who are tolerant to and currently receiving opioid therapy for persistent cancer pain; dosing should be individually titrated to provide adequate analgesia with minimal side effects. Dose titration should be done if patient requires more than 1 dose/breakthrough pain episode for several consecutive episodes. Patients experiencing >4 breakthrough pain episodes/day should have the dose of their long-term opioid re-evaluated.

Children ≥16 years and Adults: Lozenge: Initial dose: 200 mcg; the second dose may be started 15 minutes after completion of the first dose. Consumption should be limited to ≤4 units/day. Additional requirements suggest need for improved baseline therapy.

Adults:

Buccal film (Onsolis™): Initial dose: 200 mcg for all patients **Note:** Patients previously using another transmucosal product should be initiated at doses of 200 mcg; do **not** switch patients using any other fentanyl product on a mcg-per-mcg basis.

Dose titration: If titration required, increase dose in 200 mcg increments once per episode using multiples of the 200 mcg film; do not redose within a single episode of breakthrough pain and separate single doses by ≥2 hours. During titration, do not exceed 4 simultaneous applications of the 200 mcg films (800 mcg). If >800 mcg required, treat next episode with one 1200 mcg film (maximum dose: 1200 mcg). Once maintenance dose is determined, all other unused films should be disposed of and that strength (using a single film) should be used. During any pain episode, if adequate relief is not achieved after 30 minutes following buccal film application, a rescue medication (as determined by healthcare provider) may be used.

Maintenance: Determined dose applied as a single film once per episode and separated by ≥2 hours (dose range: 200-1200 mcg); limit to 4 applications/day. Consider increasing the around-the-clock opioid therapy in patients experiencing >4 breakthrough pain episodes/day.

Buccal tablet (Fentora®): Initial dose: 100 mcg; a second 100 mcg dose, if needed, may be started 30 minutes after the start of the first dose. **Note:** For patients previously using the transmucosal lozenge (Actiq®), the initial dose should be selected using the conversions listed below (maximum: 2 doses per breakthrough pain episode every 4 hours).

Dose titration, if required, should be done using multiples of the 100 mcg tablets. Patient can take two 100 mcg tablets (one on each side of mouth). If that dose is not successful, can use four 100 mcg tablets (two on each side of mouth). If titration requires >400 mcg/dose, then use 200 mcg tablets.

Conversion from lozenge to buccal tablet (Fentora®):

Lozenge dose 200-400 mcg, then buccal tablet 100 mcg

Lozenge dose 600-800 mcg, then buccal tablet 200 mcg

Lozenge dose 1200-1600 mcg, then buccal tablet 400 mcg

Note: Four 100 mcg buccal tablets deliver approximately 12% and 13% higher values of C_{max} and AUC, respectively, compared to one 400 mcg buccal tablet. To prevent confusion, patient should only have one strength available at a time. Using more than four buccal tablets at a time has not been studied.

Elderly >65 years: Transmucosal lozenge (eg, Actiq®): In clinical trials, patients who were >65 years of age were titrated to a mean dose that was 200 mcg less than that of younger patients.

Chronic pain management: Children ≥2 years and Adults (opioid-tolerant patients): Transdermal patch (eg, Duragesic®):

Initial: To convert patients from oral or parenteral opioids to transdermal patch, a 24-hour analgesic requirement should be calculated (based on prior opiate use). Using the tables, the appropriate initial dose can be determined. The initial fentanyl dosage may be approximated from the 24-hour morphine dosage equivalent and titrated to minimize adverse effects and provide analgesia. With the initial application, the absorption of transdermal fentanyl requires several hours to reach plateau; therefore transdermal fentanyl is inappropriate for management of acute pain. Change patch every 72 hours.

Conversion from continuous infusion of fentanyl: In patients who have adequate pain relief with a fentanyl infusion, fentanyl may be converted to transdermal dosing at a rate equivalent to the intravenous rate. A two-step taper of the infusion to be completed over 12 hours has been recommended (Kornick, 2001) after the patch is applied. The infusion is decreased to 50% of the original rate six hours after the application of the first patch, and subsequently discontinued twelve hours after application.

Titration: Short-acting agents may be required until analgesic efficacy is established and/or as supplements for "breakthrough" pain. The amount of supplemental doses should be closely monitored. Appropriate dosage increases may be based on daily supplemental dosage using the ratio of 45 mg/24 hours of oral morphine to a 12.5 mcg/hour increase in fentanyl dosage.

Frequency of adjustment: The dosage should not be titrated more frequently than every 3 days after the initial dose or every 6 days thereafter. Patients should wear a consistent fentanyl dosage through two applications (6 days) before dosage increase based on supplemental opiate dosages can be estimated. **Note:** Upon discontinuation, ~17 hours are required for a 50% decrease in fentanyl levels.

Frequency of application: The majority of patients may be controlled on every 72-hour administration; however, a small number of patients require every 48-hour administration.

Dose conversion guidelines for transdermal fentanyl[1] (see tables below and on next page).

Recommended Initial Duragesic® Dose Based Upon Daily Oral Morphine Dose[1]

Oral 24-Hour Morphine (mg/d)	Duragesic® Dose (mcg/h)
60-134[2]	25
135-224	50
225-314	75
315-404	100
405-494	125
495-584	150
585-674	175
675-764	200
765-854	225
855-944	250
945-1034	275
1035-1124	300

[1]The table should NOT be used to convert from transdermal fentanyl (eg, Duragesic®) to other opioid analgesics. Rather, following removal of the patch, titrate the dose of the new opioid until adequate analgesia is achieved.

[2]Pediatric patients initiating therapy on a 25 mcg/hour Duragesic® system should be opioid-tolerant and receiving at least 60 mg oral morphine equivalents per day.

Dosing Conversion Guidelines[1,2]

Current Analgesic	Daily Dosage (mg/day)			
Morphine (I.M./I.V.)	10-22	23-37	38-52	53-67
Oxycodone (oral)	30-67	67.5-112	112.5-157	157.5-202
Oxycodone (I.M./I.V.)	15-33	33.1-56	56.1-78	78.1-101
Codeine (oral)	150-447	448-747	748-1047	1048-1347
Hydromorphone (oral)	8-17	17.1-28	28.1-39	39.1-51
Hydromorphone (I.V.)	1.5-3.4	3.5-5.6	5.7-7.9	8-10
Meperidine (I.M.)	75-165	166-278	279-390	391-503
Methadone (oral)	20-44	45-74	75-104	105-134
Methadone (I.M.)	10-22	23-37	38-52	53-67
Fentanyl transdermal recommended dose (mcg/h)	25 mcg/h	50 mcg/h	75 mcg/h	100 mcg/h

[1]The table should NOT be used to convert from transdermal fentanyl (eg, Duragesic®) to other opioid analgesics. Rather, following removal of the patch, titrate the dose of the new opioid until adequate analgesia is achieved.

[2]Duragesic® product insert, Janssen Pharmaceutica, Feb 2008.

Opioid Analgesics Initial Oral Dosing Commonly Used for Severe Pain

Drug	Equianalgesic Dose (mg)		Initial Oral Dose	
	Oral[1]	Parenteral[2]	Children (mg/kg)	Adults (mg)
Buprenorphine	—	0.4	—	—
Butorphanol	—	2	—	—
Hydromorphone	7.5	1.5	0.06	4-8
Levorphanol	Acute: 4 Chronic: 1	Acute: 2 Chronic: 1	0.04	2-4
Meperidine	300	75	Not recommended	
Methadone	Acute: 10 Chronic: Varies depending upon opioid dose[3]	Acute: 5	0.2	5-10
Morphine	30	10	0.3	15-30
Nalbuphine	—	10	—	—
Pentazocine	50	30	—	—
Oxycodone	20	—	0.2	10-20
Oxymorphone	10	1	—	5-10

From "Principles of Analgesic Use in the Treatment of Acute Pain and Cancer Pain," *Am Pain Soc*, Sixth Ed.

[1]Elderly: Starting dose should be lower for this population group

[2]Standard parenteral doses for acute pain in adults; can be used to convert doses for I.V. infusions and repeated small I.V. boluses. For single I.V. boluses, use half the I.M. dose. Children >6 months: I.V. dose = parenteral equianalgesic dose x weight (kg)/100

[3]Conversion of higher doses may be guided by the following (consult a pain or palliative care specialist if unfamiliar with methadone prescribing): As the total daily dose of morphine increases, the equianalgesic dose ratio (methadone:morphine) increases in adults with ongoing cancer pain. (American Pain Society, 2008; National Comprehensive Cancer Network®, 2009). Applicability to pediatric patients is unknown.

Dosing adjustment in hepatic impairment: Actiq®: Although fentanyl kinetics may be altered in hepatic disease, Actiq® can be used successfully in the management of breakthrough cancer pain. Doses should be titrated to reach clinical effect with careful monitoring of patients with severe hepatic disease.

Stability

Injection formulation: Store at controlled room temperature of 20°C to 25°C (68°F to 77°F). Protect from light.

Transdermal patch: Do not store above 25°C (77°F).

Transmucosal (buccal film, buccal tablet, lozenge): Store at controlled room temperature of 20°C to 25°C (68°F to 77°F). Protect from freezing and moisture.

Administration

I.V.: Administer as slow I.V. infusion over 1-2 minutes. May also be administered as continuous infusion or PCA (unlabeled use) routes. Muscular rigidity may occur with rapid I.V. administration.

Transdermal patch (eg, Duragesic®): Apply to nonirritated and nonirradiated skin, such as chest, back, flank, or upper arm. Do not shave skin; hair at application site should be clipped. Prior to application, clean site with clear water and allow to dry completely. Do not use damaged, cut or leaking patches; patch may be less effective. Skin exposure from fentanyl gel leaking from patch may lead to serious adverse effects; thoroughly wash affected skin surfaces with water (do not use soap). Firmly press in place and hold for 30 seconds. Change patch every 72 hours. Do **not** use soap, alcohol, or other solvents to remove transdermal gel if it accidentally touches skin; use copious amounts of water. Avoid exposing application site to external heat sources (eg, heating pad, electric blanket, heat lamp, hot tub). If there is difficulty with patch adhesion, the edges of the system may be taped in place with first-aid tape. If there is continued difficulty with adhesion, an adhesive film dressing (eg, Bioclusive®, Tegaderm®) may be applied over the system.

Lozenge: Foil overwrap should be removed just prior to administration. Place the unit in mouth and allow it to dissolve. Do not chew. Lozenge may be moved from one side of the mouth to the other. The unit should be consumed over a period of 15 minutes. Handle should be removed after it is consumed or if patient has achieved an adequate response and/or shows signs of respiratory depression.

Buccal film: Foil overwrap should be removed just prior to administration. Prior to placing film, wet inside of cheek using tongue or by rinsing with water. Place film inside mouth with the pink side of the unit against the inside of the moistened cheek. With finger, press the film against cheek and hold for 5 seconds. The film should stick to the inside of cheek after 5 seconds. The film should be left in place until it dissolves (usually within 15-30 minutes after application). Liquids may be consumed after 5 minutes of application. Food can be eaten after film dissolves. If using more than 1 film simultaneously (during titration period), apply films on either side of mouth (do not apply on top of each other). Do not chew or swallow film. Do not cut or tear the film. All patients must initiate therapy using the 200 mcg film.

Buccal tablet: Patient should not open blister until ready to administer. The blister backing should be peeled back to expose the tablet; tablet should not be pushed out through the blister. Immediately use tablet once removed from blister. Place entire tablet in the buccal cavity (above a rear molar, between the upper cheek and gum). Tablet should not be broken, sucked, chewed, or swallowed. Should dissolve in about 14-25 minutes when left between the cheek and the gum. If remnants remain they may be swallowed with water.

Monitoring Parameters Respiratory and cardiovascular status, blood pressure, heart rate; signs of misuse, abuse, or addiction

Transdermal patch: Monitor for 24 hours after application of first dose

Anesthesia and Critical Care Concerns/Other Considerations

Clinical Pearls/Comments: Fentanyl or hydromorphone is preferred in patients who are hypotensive or have renal dysfunction. Morphine or hydromorphone is recommended for intermittent, scheduled therapy. Both have a longer duration of action requiring less frequent administration. Fentanyl is useful in preventing pain during a procedure and can be dosed intermittently for such an application. Prolonged analgesia requires an infusion.

Fentanyl has less hypotensive effects than morphine due to lack of histamine release; however, fentanyl may cause rigidity with high doses. If the patient has ▶

required high-dose analgesia or has used for a prolonged period (~7 days), taper dose to prevent withdrawal.

Pretreatment with fentanyl may reduce pain on injection from propofol (Pang, 1997). Fentanyl demonstrates synergistic respiratory depression when combined with benzodiazepines. In healthy volunteers, the combination of midazolam (0.05 mg/kg) with fentanyl (2 mcg/kg) produces synergistic respiratory depression (92% incidence of hypoxemia [SaO_2 <90%] and 50% incidence of apnea) (Bailey, 1990).

Evidence-Based Information: The 2002 ACCM/SCCM guidelines for analgesia (critically-ill adult) recommend fentanyl in patients who need immediate pain relief because of its rapid onset of action. Repeated doses or a continuous infusion of fentanyl may cause accumulation.

Pregnancy Risk Factor C/D (prolonged use or high doses at term)

Contraindications Hypersensitivity to fentanyl or any component of the formulation

Transdermal system: Severe respiratory disease or depression including acute asthma (unless patient is mechanically ventilated); paralytic ileus; patients requiring short-term therapy, management of intermittent pain

Transmucosal buccal tablets (Fentora®), buccal films (Onsolis™), lozenges (eg, Actiq®), and/or transdermal patches (eg, Duragesic®): Contraindicated in the management of acute or postoperative pain (including headache, migraine, dental pain or use in emergency room), and in patients who are not opioid tolerant

Warnings/Precautions An opioid-containing analgesic regimen should be tailored to each patient's needs and based upon the type of pain being treated (acute versus chronic), the route of administration, degree of tolerance for opioids (naive versus chronic user), age, weight, and medical condition. The optimal analgesic dose varies widely among patients. Doses should be titrated to pain relief/prevention. May cause CNS depression, which may impair physical or mental abilities; patients must be cautioned about performing tasks which require mental alertness (eg, operating machinery or driving). When using with other CNS depressants, reduce dose of one or both agents. Fentanyl shares the toxic potentials of opiate agonists, and precautions of opiate agonist therapy should be observed; use with caution in patients with bradycardia or bradyarrhythmias; rapid I.V. infusion may result in skeletal muscle and chest wall rigidity leading to respiratory distress and/or apnea, bronchoconstriction, laryngospasm; inject slowly over 3-5 minutes. **[U.S. Boxed Warning]: Healthcare provider should be alert to problems of abuse, misuse, and diversion.** Tolerance or drug dependence may result from extended use. The elderly may be particularly susceptible to the CNS depressant and constipating effects of narcotics. Use extreme caution in patients with COPD or other chronic respiratory conditions. Use caution with head injuries, morbid obesity, renal impairment, or hepatic dysfunction. **[U.S. Boxed Warning]: Use with strong or moderate CYP3A4 inhibitors may result in increased effects and potentially fatal respiratory depression.** Concurrent use of agonist/antagonist analgesics may precipitate withdrawal symptoms and/or reduced analgesic efficacy in patients following prolonged therapy with mu opioid agonists. Abrupt discontinuation following prolonged use may also lead to withdrawal symptoms. Safety and efficacy have not been established in children <16 years of age for the lozenge and <18 years of age for the buccal tablet. **[U.S. Boxed Warning]: Safety and efficacy of the transdermal patch have been limited to children ≥2 years of age who are opioid-tolerant. [U.S. Boxed Warning]: Buccal film (Onsolis™): Not indicated for use in opioid-tolerant cancer patients <18 years of age.**

[U.S. Boxed Warning] Actiq®, Duragesic®, Fentora®, Onsolis™: May cause potentially life-threatening hypoventilation, respiratory depression, and/or death; Actiq®, Duragesic®, Fentora®, or Onsolis™ should only be prescribed for opioid-tolerant patients. Risk of respiratory depression increased in elderly patients, debilitated patients, and patients with conditions associated with hypoxia or hypercapnia; usually occurs after administration of initial dose in nontolerant patients or when given with other drugs that depress respiratory function.

Transmucosal: Lozenge (eg, Actiq®), buccal tablet (Fentora®), buccal film (Onsolis™): **[U.S. Boxed Warning]: Should be used only for the care of** opioid-tolerant cancer patients with breakthrough pain and is intended for use by specialists who are knowledgeable in treating cancer pain. Not approved for use in management of acute or postoperative pain. **[U.S. Boxed Warning]: Buccal film, buccal tablet and lozenge preparations contain an amount of medication that can be fatal to children. Keep all units out of the reach of children and discard any open units properly.** Patients and caregivers should be counseled on the dangers to children including the risk of exposure to partially-consumed units.

Transmucosal: Buccal film (eg, Onsolis™): **[U.S. Boxed Warning]: Available only through the FOCUS Program, a restricted distribution program with prescriber, pharmacy, and patient required enrollment. [U.S. Boxed Warning]: Onsolis™ is contraindicated in the management of acute or postoperative pain, including headache/migraine. [U.S. Boxed Warning]: Due to higher bioavailability of fentanyl in the buccal film formulation, do not substitute Onsolis™ on a mcg-per-mcg basis for any other fentanyl product. Serious adverse events, including death, may occur when used inappropriately (improper dose or patient selection). All patients must begin therapy with a 200 mcg dose and titrate, if needed. During therapy, patients must wait at least 2 hours before taking another dose.**

Transmucosal: Buccal tablet (Fentora®): **[U.S. Boxed Warning]: Due to the higher bioavailability of fentanyl in Fentora®, when converting patients from oral transmucosal fentanyl citrate (OTFC, Actiq®) to Fentora®, do not substitute Fentora®: on a mcg-per-mcg basis for any other fentanyl product. [U.S. Boxed Warning]: Fentora® is contraindicated in the management of acute or postoperative pain, including headache/migraine. Serious adverse events, including death, have been reported when used inappropriately (improper dose or patient selection). [U.S. Boxed Warning]: Patients using Fentora® who experience breakthrough pain may only take one additional dose using the same strength and must wait four hours before taking another dose.**

Transdermal patches (eg, Duragesic®): **[U.S. Boxed Warning]: Indicated for the management of persistent moderate-to-severe pain when around the clock pain control is needed for an extended time period. Should only be used in patients who are already receiving opioid therapy, are opioid tolerant, and who require a total daily dose equivalent to 25 mcg/hour transdermal patch. Contraindicated in patients who are not opioid tolerant, in the management of short-term analgesia, or in the management of postoperative pain. Should be applied only to intact skin. Use of a patch that has been cut, damaged, or altered in any way may result in overdosage.** Serum fentanyl concentrations may increase approximately one-third for patients with a body temperature of 40°C secondary to a temperature-dependent increase in fentanyl release from the patch and increased skin permeability. **[U.S. Boxed Warning]: Avoid exposure of application site and surrounding area to direct external heat sources.** Patients who experience fever or increase in core temperature should be monitored closely. Patients who experience adverse reactions should be monitored for at least 24 hours after removal of the patch.

Adverse Reactions

>10%:

Cardiovascular: Bradycardia, edema

Central nervous system: CNS depression, confusion, dizziness, drowsiness, fatigue, headache, sedation

Endocrine & metabolic: Dehydration

Gastrointestinal: Nausea, vomiting, constipation, xerostomia

Local: Application-site reaction erythema

Neuromuscular & skeletal: Chest wall rigidity (high dose I.V.), muscle rigidity, weakness

Ocular: Miosis

Respiratory: Dyspnea, respiratory depression

Miscellaneous: Diaphoresis

◄ 1% to 10%:
Cardiovascular: Cardiac arrhythmia, chest pain, DVT, flushing, hyper-/hypotension, orthostatic hypotension, pallor, palpitation, peripheral edema, somnolence, syncope, tachycardia, vasodilation

Central nervous system: Abnormal dreams, abnormal thinking, agitation, amnesia, anxiety, depression, euphoria, fever, hallucinations, hypoesthesia, insomnia, lethargy, malaise, mental status change, migraine, nervousness, paranoid reaction, stupor, vertigo

Dermatologic: Alopecia, bruising, cellulitis, erythema, hyperhidrosis, papules, pruritus, rash

Endocrine & metabolic: Breast pain, hot flashes, hyper-/hypocalcemia, hyper-/hypoglycemia, hypoalbuminemia, hypokalemia, hypomagnesemia

Gastrointestinal: Abdominal pain, abnormal taste, anorexia, appetite decreased, biliary tract spasm, diarrhea, dyspepsia, dysphagia (buccal tablet/film), flatulence, GI hemorrhage, gingival pain (buccal tablet), gingivitis (lozenge), glossitis (lozenge), ileus, intestinal obstruction (buccal film), periodontal abscess (lozenge/buccal tablet), stomatitis (lozenge/buccal tablet), weight loss

Genitourinary: Dysuria, urinary incontinence, urinary retention, vaginitis, vaginal hemorrhage

Hematologic: Anemia, leukopenia, neutropenia, thrombocytopenia

Hepatic: Ascites, jaundice

Local: Application site pain, application site irritation

Neuromuscular & skeletal: Abnormal coordination, abnormal gait, arthralgia, back pain, myalgia, neuropathy, paresthesia, rigors, tremor

Ocular: Blurred vision, diplopia

Renal: Renal failure

Respiratory: Apnea, asthma, bronchitis, cough, epistaxis, hemoptysis, hypoventilation, hypoxia, nasopharyngitis, pharyngolaryngeal pain, pharyngitis, pneumonia, rhinitis, sinusitis, upper respiratory infection, wheezing

Miscellaneous: Hiccups, flu-like syndrome, lymphadenopathy, speech disorder

<1% (Limited to important or life-threatening): Abdominal distention, amblyopia, allergic reaction, anaphylaxis, angina, anorgasmia, aphasia, bladder pain, bronchospasm, CNS excitation or delirium, cold/clammy skin, dental caries (lozenge), depersonalization, dysesthesia, ejaculatory difficulty, emotional lability, eructation, esophageal stenosis, exfoliative dermatitis, fecal impaction, flank pain, gum line erosion (lozenge), gum hemorrhage (lozenge), hematuria, hostility, hyper-/hypotonia, laryngospasm, libido decreased, moniliasis (lozenge/buccal tablet), mouth ulceration (lozenge/buccal tablet), myasthenia, nocturia, oliguria, pancytopenia, paradoxical dizziness, physical and psychological dependence with prolonged use, pleural effusion, polyuria, pustules, speech disorder, stertorous breathing, seizure, sputum increased, tooth loss (lozenge), urinary tract spasm, urticaria, vertigo

Drug Interactions

Metabolism/Transport Effects Substrate of CYP3A4 (major); **Inhibits** CYP3A4 (weak)

Avoid Concomitant Use

Avoid concomitant use of FentaNYL with any of the following: MAO Inhibitors

Increased Effect/Toxicity

FentaNYL may increase the levels/effects of: Alcohol (Ethyl); Alvimopan; Beta-Blockers; Calcium Channel Blockers (Nondihydropyridine); CNS Depressants; Desmopressin; MAO Inhibitors; Selective Serotonin Reuptake Inhibitors; Thiazide Diuretics

The levels/effects of FentaNYL may be increased by: Amphetamines; Antipsychotic Agents (Phenothiazines); CYP3A4 Inhibitors (Moderate); CYP3A4 Inhibitors (Strong); Dasatinib; MAO Inhibitors; Protease Inhibitors; Succinylcholine

Decreased Effect

FentaNYL may decrease the levels/effects of: Pegvisomant

The levels/effects of FentaNYL may be decreased by: Ammonium Chloride; Rifamycin Derivatives

Ethanol/Nutrition/Herb Interactions

Ethanol: Avoid ethanol (may increase CNS depression).

Herb/Nutraceutical: St John's wort may decrease fentanyl levels. Avoid valerian, St John's wort, kava kava, gotu kola (may increase CNS depression).

Dietary Considerations Transmucosal lozenge contains 2 g sugar per unit.

Dosage Forms Excipient information presented when available (limited, particularly for generics); consult specific product labeling.

Note: Strengths expressed as base.

Film, for buccal application, as citrate:
Onsolis™: 200 mcg, 400 mcg, 600 mcg, 800 mcg, 1200 mcg

Injection, solution, as citrate [preservative free]: 0.05 mg/mL (2 mL, 5 mL, 10 mL, 20 mL; 30 mL [DSC]; 50 mL)
Sublimaze®: 0.05 mg/mL (2 mL, 5 mL, 10 mL [DSC], 20 mL)

Lozenge, oral, as citrate [transmucosal]: 200 mcg, 400 mcg, 600 mcg, 800 mcg, 1200 mcg, 1600 mcg
Actiq®: 200 mcg, 400 mcg, 600 mcg, 800 mcg, 1200 mcg, 1600 mcg [contains sugar 2 g/lozenge; berry flavor]

Powder, for prescription compounding, as citrate: USP (1 g)

Tablet, for buccal application, as citrate:
Fentora®: 100 mcg, 200 mcg, 300 mcg, 400 mcg, 600 mcg, 800 mcg

Transdermal system, topical, as base: 12 (5s) [delivers 12.5 mcg/hour; 3.13 cm^2]; 12 (5s) [delivers 12.5 mcg/hour; 5 cm^2]; 25 (5s) [delivers 25 mcg/hour; 10 cm^2]; 25 (5s) [delivers 25 mcg/hour; 6.25 cm^2]; 50 (5s) [delivers 50 mcg/hour; 12.5 cm^2]; 50 (5s) [delivers 50 mcg/hour; 20 cm^2]; 75 (5s) [delivers 75 mcg/hour; 18.75 cm^2]; 75 (5s) [delivers 75 mcg/hour; 30 cm^2]; 75 (5s) [delivers 75 mcg/hour; 32.1 cm^2]; 100 (5s) [delivers 100 mcg/hour; 25 cm^2]; 100 (5s) [delivers 100 mcg/hour; 40 cm^2]; 100 (5s) [delivers 100 mcg/hour; 42.8 cm^2]

Duragesic®: 12 (5s) [delivers 12.5 mcg/hour; 5 cm^2; contains ethanol 0.1 mL/10 cm^2]; 25 (5s) [delivers 25 mcg/hour; 10 cm^2; contains ethanol 0.1 mL/10 cm^2]; 50 (5s) [delivers 50 mcg/hour; 20 cm^2; contains ethanol 0.1 mL/10 cm^2]; 75 (5s) [delivers 75 mcg/hour; 30 cm^2; contains ethanol 0.1 mL/10 cm^2]; 100 (5s) [delivers 100 mcg/hour; 40 cm^2; contains ethanol 0.1 mL/10 cm^2]

References

Bailey PL, Pace NL, Ashburn MA, et al, "Frequent Hypoxemia and Apnea After Sedation With Midazolam and Fentanyl," *Anesthesiology*, 1990, 73(5):826-30.

Bedforth NM and Lockey DJ, "Raynaud's Syndrome Following Intravenous Induction of Anaesthesia," *Anaesthesia*, 1995, 50(3):248-9.

Bennett MR and Adams AP, "Postoperative Respiratory Complications of Opiates," *Clin Anaesthesiol*, 1983, 1:41-56.

Furuya H and Okumura F, "Hemolysis After Administration of High Dose Fentanyl," *Anesth Analg*, 1986, 65(2):207-8.

Jacobi J, Fraser GL, Coursin DB, et al, "Clinical Practice Guidelines for the Sustained Use of Sedatives and Analgesics in the Critically Ill Adult," *Crit Care Med*, 2002, 30(1):119-41. Available at: http://www.sccm.org/pdf/sedatives.pdf.

Katz R, Kelly HW, and Hsi A, "Prospective Study on the Occurrence of Withdrawal in Critically Ill Children Who Receive Fentanyl by Continuous Infusion," *Crit Care Med*, 1994, 22(5):763-7.

Mokhlesi B, Leikin JB, Murray P, et al, "Adult Toxicology in Critical Care. Part 11: Specific Poisonings," *Chest*, 2003, 123(3):897-922.

Pang WW, Huang S, Chung YT, et al, "Comparison of Intravenous Retention of Fentanyl and Lidocaine on Local Analgesia in Propofol Injection Pain," *Acta Anaesthesiol Sin*, 1997, 35 (4):217-21.

"Principles of Analgesic Use in the Treatment of Acute Pain and Cancer Pain," 6th ed, Glenview, IL: American Pain Society, 2008.

◆ **Fentanyl Citrate** *see* FentaNYL *on page* 587

◆ **Fentanyl Citrate Injection, USP (Can)** *see* FentaNYL *on page* 587

◆ **Fentanyl Hydrochloride** *see* FentaNYL *on page* 587

◆ **Fentora®** *see* FentaNYL *on page* 587

◆ **Feraheme™** *see* Ferumoxytol *on page* 597

Ferumoxytol (fer ue MOX i tol)

Medication Safety Issues

Sound-alike/look-alike issues:

Ferumoxytol may be confused with ferric gluconate, iron dextran complex, iron sucrose

U.S. Brand Names Feraheme™

Pharmacologic Category Iron Salt

◀ **Generic Available** No

Use Treatment of iron-deficiency anemia in chronic kidney disease

Mechanism of Action Superparamagnetic iron oxide coated with a low molecular weight semisynthetic carbohydrate; iron-carbohydrate complex enters the reticuloendothelial system macrophages of the liver, spleen, and bone marrow where the iron is released from the complex. The released iron is either transported into storage pools or is transported via plasma transferrin for incorporation into hemoglobin.

Pharmacodynamics/Kinetics

Distribution: V_d: 3.16 L

Metabolism: Iron released from iron-carbohydrate complex after uptake in the reticuloendothelial system macrophages of the liver, spleen, and bone marrow

Half-life elimination: ~15 hours

Dialysis: Ferumoxytol is not removed by hemodialysis

Dosage Doses expressed in mg of **elemental** iron. **Note:** Test dose: Product labeling does not indicate need for a test dose.

I.V.: Adults: Iron-deficiency anemia in chronic kidney disease: 510 mg (17 mL) as a single dose, followed by a second 510 mg dose 3-8 days after initial dose. Recommended dose may be readministered in patients with persistent or recurrent iron deficiency anemia.

Dosage adjustment in renal impairment: Hemodialysis patients should receive injection after at least 1 hour of hemodialysis has been completed and once blood pressure has stabilized.

Stability Store vials at controlled room temperature of 20°C to 25°C (68°F to 77°F); do not freeze.

Administration Administer intravenously as an undiluted injection at a rate ≤1 mL/second (30 mg of elemental iron/second). Do not administer if solution has particulate matter or is discolored (solution is black to reddish-brown).

Hemodialysis patients should receive injection after at least 1 hour of hemodialysis has been completed and once blood pressure has stabilized.

Monitoring Parameters Hemoglobin, serum ferritin, serum iron, transferrin saturation (for at least 1 month following second injection and periodically); signs/symptoms of hypotension following administration; signs/symptoms of hypersensitivity reactions (≥30 minutes following administration)

Reference Range

Hemoglobin: Adults:

Males: 13.5-16.5 g/dL

Females: 12.0-15.0 g/dL

Serum iron: 40-160 mcg/dL

Total iron-binding capacity: 230-430 mcg/dL

Transferrin: 204-360 mg/dL

Percent transferrin saturation: 20% to 50%

Pregnancy Risk Factor C

Contraindications Hypersensitivity to ferumoxytol or any component of the formulation; evidence of iron overload; anemia not caused by iron deficiency

Warnings/Precautions Hypersensitivity reactions, including rare anaphylactic and anaphylactoid reactions, may occur; equipment for resuscitation and trained personnel experienced in handling emergencies should be immediately available during use. Monitor patients for signs/symptoms of hypersensitivity reactions for ≥30 minutes after administration. Hypotension, including serious hypotensive reactions, may occur; monitor patients for hypotension following administration.

Withhold iron in the presence of tissue iron overload; periodic monitoring of hemoglobin, serum ferritin, serum iron, and transferrin saturation is recommended. Serum iron and transferrin-bound iron may be overestimated in laboratory assays if level is drawn during the first 24 hours following administration. Administration may alter magnetic resonance (MR) imaging; conduct anticipated MRI studies prior to use. MR imaging alterations may persist for ≤3 months following use, with peak alterations anticipated in the first 2 days following administration. If MR imaging is required within 3 months after administration, use T1- or proton density-weighted MR pulse sequences to decrease effect on imagining. Do not use T2-weighted sequence MR imaging prior to 4 weeks following ferumoxytol administration. Ferumoxytol does not interfere with X-ray, computed tomography (CT), positron emission tomography (PET), single photon emission computed tomography (SPECT), ultrasound or nuclear medicine imaging.

Not FDA-approved for use in children.

Adverse Reactions

1% to 10%:

Cardiovascular: Hypotension (≤3%), edema (2%), peripheral edema (2%), chest pain (1%), hypertension (1%)

Central nervous system: Dizziness (3%), headache (2%), fever (1%)

Dermatologic: Pruritus (1%), rash (1%)

Gastrointestinal: Diarrhea (4%), nausea (3%), constipation (2%), vomiting (2%), abdominal pain (1%)

Neuromuscular & skeletal: Back pain (1%), muscle spasms (1%)

Respiratory: Cough (1%), dyspnea (1%)

Miscellaneous: Hypersensitivity reactions (≤4%; serious reactions: <1%)

<1% (Limited to important or life-threatening): Fatigue; infusion site reactions (including bruising, burning, erythema, irritation, pain, swelling, warmth); urticaria, wheezing

Drug Interactions

Avoid Concomitant Use

Avoid concomitant use of Ferumoxytol with any of the following: Dimercaprol

Increased Effect/Toxicity

The levels/effects of Ferumoxytol may be increased by: Dimercaprol

Decreased Effect There are no known significant interactions involving a decrease in effect.

Test Interactions May interfere with MR imaging; alterations may persist for ≤3 months following use, with peak alterations anticipated in the first 2 days following administration. If MR imaging is required within 3 months after administration, use T1- or proton density-weighted MR pulse sequences to decrease effect on imaging. Do not use T2-weighted sequence MR imaging prior to 4 weeks following administration.

Serum iron and transferrin-bound iron may be overestimated in laboratory assays if level is drawn during the first 24 hours following administration (due to contribution of iron in feruxomytol).

Dosage Forms Excipient information presented when available (limited, particularly for generics); consult specific product labeling.

Injection, solution:

Feraheme™: Elemental iron 30 mg/mL (17 mL)

References

American College of Obstetricians and Gynecologists, "ACOG Practice Bulletin No. 95: Anemia in Pregnancy," *Obstet Gynecol*, 2008, 112(1):201-7.

Auerbach M, "Ferumoxytol as a New, Safer, Easier-to-Administer Intravenous Iron: Yes or No", *Am J of Kidney Dis*, 2008, 52(5):826-9 [editorial].

Baker WF Jr, "Iron Deficiency in Pregnancy, Obstetrics, and Gynecology," *Hematol Oncol Clin North Am*, 2000, 14(5):1061-77.

"Nutrition During Lactation." Subcommittee on Nutrition During Lactation, Committee on Nutritional Status During Pregnancy and Lactation, Food and Nutrition Board Institute of Medicine, National Academy of Sciences Washington, DC: National Academy Press, 1991. Available at http://www.nap.edu.

"Recommendations to Prevent and Control Iron Deficiency in the United States. Centers for Disease Control and Prevention," *MMWR Recomm Rep*, 1998, 47(RR-3):1-29.

"Routine Iron Supplementation During Pregnancy. Review Article. US Preventive Services Task Force," *JAMA*, 1993, 270(23):2848-54.

Singh A, Patel T, Hertel J, et al, "Safety of Ferumoxytol in Patients With Anemia and CKD", *Am J of Kidney Dis*, 2008, 52(5):907-15.

◆ **FESO** *see* Fesoterodine *on page 599*

Fesoterodine (fes oh TER oh deen)

U.S. Brand Names Toviaz™
Index Terms FESO; Fesoterodine Fumarate
Pharmacologic Category Anticholinergic Agent
Use Treatment of patients with an overactive bladder with symptoms of urinary frequency, urgency, or urge incontinence.

◀ **Pharmacodynamics/Kinetics**
Absorption: Well absorbed
Distribution: I.V.: 5-HMT: V_d: 169 L
Protein binding: 5-HMT: ~50% (primarily to albumin and alpha$_1$-acid glycoprotein)
Metabolism: Fesoterodine is rapidly and extensively metabolized to its active metabolite (5-hydroxymethyl tolterodine; 5-HMT) by nonspecific esterases; 5-HMT is further metabolized via CYP2D6 and CYP3A4 to inactive metabolites.
Bioavailability: 5-HMT: 52%
Half-life elimination: ~7 hours
Time to peak, plasma: 5-HMT: ~5 hours; C_{max} higher in poor CYP2D6 metabolizers
Excretion: Urine (~70%; 16% as 5-HMT, ~53% as inactive metabolites); feces (7%)

Dosage Oral: Adults: Overactive bladder: 4 mg once daily; dose may be increased to 8 mg once daily based on individual response and tolerability
Dosing adjustment for concomitant CYP3A4 inhibitors: Maximum dose: 4 mg/day when administered concomitantly with potent CYP3A4 inhibitors including (but not limited to) ketoconazole, itraconazole, and clarithromycin. Concurrent therapy of weak or moderate CYP3A4 inhibitors and fesoterodine should be limited to 4 mg/day and increased to 8 mg/day after assessing tolerability.

Dosing adjustment in renal impairment:
Mild-to-moderate renal impairment (Cl_{cr} 30-80 mL/minute): No dose adjustment is recommended
Severe renal impairment (Cl_{cr} <30 mL/minute): Maximum dose: 4 mg
Dosing adjustment in hepatic impairment:
Moderate hepatic impairment (Child-Pugh class B): No dose adjustment is recommended
Severe hepatic impairment (Child-Pugh class C): Use is not recommended; not studied in severe impairment
Additional Information Complete prescribing information for this medication should be consulted for additional detail.
Dosage Forms Excipient information presented when available (limited, particularly for generics); consult specific product labeling.
Tablet, extended release, oral, as fumarate:
Toviaz™: 4 mg, 8 mg [contains soya lecithin]

References
Chapple C, Van Kerrebroeck P, Tubaro A, et al, "Clinical Efficacy, Safety, and Tolerability of Once-Daily Fesoterodine in Subjects With Overactive Bladder," *Eur Urol*, 2007, 52(4):1204-12.
Khullar V, Rovner ES, Dmochowski R, et al, "Fesoterodine Dose Response in Subjects With Overactive Bladder Syndrome," *Urology*, 2008, 71(5):839-43.
Michel M, "Fesoterodine: A Novel Muscarinic Receptor Antagonist for the Treatment of Overactive Bladder Syndrome," *Expert Opin Pharmacother*, 2008, 9(10):1787-96.
Nitti VW, Dmochowski R, Sand PK, et al, "Efficacy, Safety and Tolerability of Fesoterodine for Overactive Bladder Syndrome," *J Urol*, 2007, 178(5):2488-94.

◆ **Fesoterodine Fumarate** *see* Fesoterodine *on page 599*

◆ **FeverALL® [OTC]** *see* Acetaminophen *on page 25*

◆ **Fibricor™** *see* Fenofibric Acid *on page 583*

Fibrinogen Concentrate (Human)
(fi BRIN o gin KON suhn trate HYU man)

U.S. Brand Names RiaSTAP™
Index Terms Coagulation Factor I
Pharmacologic Category Blood Product Derivative
Use Treatment of acute bleeding episodes in patients with congenital fibrinogen deficiency (afibrinogenemia and hypofibrinogenemia)
Pharmacodynamics/Kinetics
Distribution: V_d: 45-60 mL/kg (range 36-68 mL/kg)
Half-life elimination: 61-97 hours (range 56-117 hours); may be decreased in children <16 years of age
Dosage I.V.: Children and Adults: Congenital fibrinogen deficiency: **Note:** Adjust dose based on laboratory values and condition of patient. Maintain a target fibrinogen level of 100 mg/dL until hemostasis is achieved.

When baseline fibrinogen level is known:

Dose (mg/kg) = [Target level (mg/dL) - measured level (mg/dL)] **divided by** 1.7 (mg/dL per mg/kg body weight)

When baseline fibrinogen level is not known: 70 mg/kg

Additional Information Complete prescribing information for this medication should be consulted for additional detail.

Dosage Forms Excipient information presented when available (limited, particularly for generics); consult specific product labeling. [DSC] = Discontinued product

Injection, powder for reconstitution:

RiaSTAP™: 900-1300 mg [contains albumin (human); exact potency labeled on vial]

References

Acharya SS and Dimichele DM, "Rare Inherited Disorders of Fibrinogen," *Haemophilia*, 2008, 14 (6):1151-8.

Kreuz W, Meili E, Peter-Salonen K, et al. "Efficacy and Tolerability of a Pasteurised Human Fibrinogen Concentrate in Patients With Congenital Fibrinogen Deficiency," *Transfus Apher Sci*, 2005, 32(3):247-53.

Filgrastim (fil GRA stim)

Medication Safety Issues

Sound-alike/look-alike issues:

Neupogen® may be confused with Epogen®, Neulasta®, Neumega®, Neupro®, Nutramigen®

U.S. Brand Names Neupogen®

Canadian Brand Names Neupogen®

Index Terms G-CSF; Granulocyte Colony Stimulating Factor; NSC-614629

Pharmacologic Category Colony Stimulating Factor

Generic Available No

Use Stimulation of granulocyte production in chemotherapy-induced neutropenia (nonmyeloid malignancies, acute myeloid leukemia, and bone marrow transplantation); severe chronic neutropenia (SCN); mobilization of hematopoietic progenitor cells in patients undergoing peripheral blood progenitor cell (PBPC) collection

Unlabeled/Investigational Use Treatment of anemia in myelodysplastic syndrome; treatment of drug-induced (nonchemotherapy) agranulocytosis in the elderly

Mechanism of Action Stimulates the production, maturation, and activation of neutrophils; filgrastim activates neutrophils to increase both their migration and cytotoxicity.

Pharmacodynamics/Kinetics

Onset of action: ~24 hours; plateaus in 3-5 days

Duration: ANC decreases by 50% within 2 days after discontinuing filgrastim; white counts return to the normal range in 4-7 days; peak plasma levels can be maintained for up to 12 hours

Absorption: SubQ: 100%

Distribution: V_d: 150 mL/kg; no evidence of drug accumulation over a 11- to 20-day period

Metabolism: Systemically degraded

Half-life elimination: 1.8-3.5 hours

Time to peak, serum: SubQ: 2-8 hours

Dosage Details concerning dosing in combination regimens and institution protocols should also be consulted.

Dosing, even in morbidly obese patients, should be based on actual body weight. Rounding doses to the nearest vial size often enhances patient convenience and reduces costs without compromising clinical response.

Children and Adults:

Chemotherapy-induced neutropenia: SubQ, I.V.: 5 mcg/kg/day; doses may be increased by 5 mcg/kg according to the duration and severity of the neutropenia; continue for up to 14 days or until the ANC reaches 10,000/mm^3

◀ Bone marrow transplantation: SubQ, I.V.: 10 mcg/kg/day; adjust the dose according to the duration and severity of neutropenia; recommended steps based on neutrophil response:

When ANC >1000/mm^3 for 3 consecutive days: Reduce filgrastim dose to 5 mcg/kg/day

If ANC remains >1000/mm^3 for 3 more consecutive days: Discontinue filgrastim

If ANC decreases to <1000/mm^3: Resume at 5 mcg/kg/day

If ANC decreases <1000/mm^3 during the 5 mcg/kg/day dose, increase filgrastim to 10 mcg/kg/day and follow the above steps

Peripheral blood progenitor cell (PBPC) collection: SubQ: 10 mcg/kg daily in donors, usually for 6-7 days. Begin at least 4 days before the first leukopheresis and continue until the last leukopheresis; consider dose adjustment for WBC >100,000/mm^3

Hematopoietic stem cell mobilization (in combination with plerixafor, for autologous transplantation in patients with non-Hodgkin's lymphoma and multiple myeloma): SubQ: 10 mcg/kg once daily; begin 4 days before initiation of plerixafor; continue G-CSF on each day prior to apheresis

Severe chronic neutropenia: SubQ:

Congenital: 6 mcg/kg twice daily; adjust the dose based on ANC and clinical response

Idiopathic/cyclic: 5 mcg/kg/day; adjust the dose based on ANC and clinical response

Anemia in myelodysplastic syndrome (unlabeled use - in combination with epoetin): SubQ: 0.3-3 mcg/kg daily **or** 30-150 mcg daily **or** 1-2 mcg/kg 2-3 times weekly

Elderly: Refer to adult dosing.

Drug-induced agranulocytosis (nonchemotherapy) in the elderly (unlabeled use): SubQ: 300 mcg daily until ANC >1500/mm^3

Stability Intact vials and prefilled syringes should be stored under refrigeration at 2°C to 8°C (36°F to 46°F) and protected from direct sunlight. Filgrastim should be protected from freezing and temperatures >30°C to avoid aggregation. If inadvertently frozen, thaw in a refrigerator and use within 24 hours; do not use if frozen >24 hours or frozen more than once. Do not shake.

Filgrastim vials and prefilled syringes are stable for 24 hours at 9°C to 30°C (47°F to 86°F).

Undiluted filgrastim is stable for 24 hours at 15°C to 30°C (59°F to 86°F) and for up to 14 days at 2°C to 8°C (36°F to 46°F) (data on file, Amgen Medical Information) in BD tuberculin syringes; however, sterility has only been assessed and maintained for up to 7 days when prepared under strict aseptic conditions (Singh, 1994; Jacobson, 1996). The manufacturer recommends using syringes within 24 hours due to the potential for bacterial contamination.

Do not dilute with saline at any time; product may precipitate. Filgrastim may be diluted with D_5W or with D_5W with albumin for I.V. infusion administration (5-15 mcg/mL; minimum concentration is 5 mcg/mL). This diluted solution is stable for 7 days at 2°C to 8°C (36°F to 46°F), however, should be used within 24 hours due to the possibility for bacterial contamination. Dilution to <5 mcg/mL is not recommended. Concentrations 5-15 mcg/mL require addition of albumin (final concentration of 2 mg/mL) to prevent adsorption to plastics.

Administration May be administered undiluted by SubQ injection. May also be administered by I.V. bolus over 15-30 minutes in D_5W, or by continuous SubQ or I.V. infusion. Do not administer earlier than 24 hours after or in the 24 hours prior to cytotoxic chemotherapy.

Monitoring Parameters CBC with differential prior to treatment and twice weekly during filgrastim treatment for chemotherapy-induced neutropenia (3 times a week following marrow transplantation). For severe chronic neutropenia, monitor CBC with differential twice weekly during the first month of therapy and for 2 weeks following dose adjustments; monthly thereafter. In PBPC mobilization, monitor platelets.

Reference Range No clinical benefit seen with ANC >10,000/mm^3

Pregnancy Risk Factor C

Contraindications Hypersensitivity to filgrastim, *E. coli*-derived proteins, or any component of the formulation

Warnings/Precautions Do not use filgrastim in the period 24 hours before to 24 hours after administration of cytotoxic chemotherapy because of the potential sensitivity of rapidly dividing myeloid cells to cytotoxic chemotherapy. May potentially act as a growth factor for any tumor type, particularly myeloid malignancies; precaution should be exercised in the usage of filgrastim in any malignancy with myeloid characteristics. Increases circulating leukocytes when used in conjunction with plerixafor for stem cell mobilization; monitor WBC; use with caution in patients with neutrophil count >50,000/mm^3; tumor cells released from marrow could be collected in leukapheresis product; potential effect of tumor cell re-infusion is unknown. Reports of alveolar hemorrhage, manifested as pulmonary infiltrates and hemoptysis, have occurred in healthy donors undergoing PBPC collection (not FDA approved for use in healthy donors); hemoptysis resolved upon discontinuation. Safety and efficacy have not been established with patients receiving radiation therapy, or with chemotherapy associated with delayed myelosuppression (eg, nitrosoureas, mitomycin C).

Allergic-type reactions (rash, urticaria, wheezing, dyspnea, tachycardia and/or hypotension) have occurred with first or later doses. Reactions tended to occur more frequently with intravenous administration and within 30 minutes of administration. Rare cases of splenic rupture or acute respiratory distress syndrome have been reported in association with filgrastim; patients must be instructed to report left upper quadrant pain or shoulder tip pain or respiratory distress. Cutaneous vasculitis has been reported, generally occurring in SCN patients on long-term therapy; dose reductions may improve symptoms to allow for continued therapy. Use caution in patients with sickle cell diseases; sickle cell crises have been reported following filgrastim therapy. Cytogenetic abnormalities, transformation to AML and MDS have been observed in patients treated with filgrastim for congenital neutropenia; a longer duration of treatment and poorer ANC response appear to increase the risk. The packaging of some forms may contain latex.

Adverse Reactions

>10%:

Central nervous system: Fever (12%)

Dermatologic: Petechiae (17%), rash (12%)

Gastrointestinal: Splenomegaly (severe chronic neutropenia: 30%; rare in other patients)

Hepatic: Alkaline phosphatase increased (21%)

Neuromuscular & skeletal: Bone pain (22% to 33%), commonly in the lower back, posterior iliac crest, and sternum

Respiratory: Epistaxis (9% to 15%)

1% to 10%:

Cardiovascular: Hyper-/hypotension (4%), S-T segment depression (3%), myocardial infarction/arrhythmias (3%)

Central nervous system: Headache (7%)

Gastrointestinal: Nausea (10%), vomiting (7%), peritonitis (2%)

Hematologic: Leukocytosis (2%)

Miscellaneous: Transfusion reaction (10%)

<1% (Limited to important or life-threatening): Acute respiratory distress syndrome, allergic reactions, alopecia, alveolar hemorrhage, arthralgia, capillary leak syndrome, cerebral hemorrhage, cutaneous vasculitis, dyspnea, edema (facial), erythema nodosum, hematuria, hemoptysis, hepatomegaly, hypersensitivity reaction, injection site reaction, osteoporosis, pericarditis, proteinuria, psoriasis exacerbation, pulmonary infiltrates, renal insufficiency, sickle cell crisis, splenic rupture, Sweet's syndrome (acute febrile dermatosis), tachycardia, thrombocytopenia (in PBPC mobilization), thrombophlebitis, transient supraventricular arrhythmia, urticaria, wheezing

Drug Interactions

Avoid Concomitant Use There are no known interactions where it is recommended to avoid concomitant use.

Increased Effect/Toxicity

Filgrastim may increase the levels/effects of: Topotecan

▶

Decreased Effect There are no known significant interactions involving a decrease in effect.

Test Interactions May interfere with bone imaging studies; increased hematopoietic activity of the bone marrow may appear as transient positive bone imaging changes

Dietary Considerations Solution for injection contains sodium 0.035 mg/mL and sorbitol.

Dosage Forms Excipient information presented when available (limited, particularly for generics); consult specific product labeling.

Injection, solution [preservative free]:

Neupogen®: 300 mcg/mL (1 mL, 1.6 mL) [vial; contains sodium 0.035 mg/mL and sorbitol]

Injection, solution [preservative free]:

Neupogen®: 600 mcg/mL (0.5 mL, 0.8 mL) [prefilled Singleject® syringe; contains sodium 0.035 mg/mL and sorbitol; needle cover contains latex]

References

Smith TJ, Khatcheressian J, Lyman GH, et al, "2006 Update of Recommendations for the Use of White Blood Cell Growth Factors: An Evidence-Based Clinical Practice Guideline," *J Clin Oncol*, 2006, 24(19):3187-205.

Finasteride (fi NAS teer ide)

U.S. Brand Names Propecia®; Proscar®
Canadian Brand Names Propecia®; Proscar®
Pharmacologic Category 5 Alpha-Reductase Inhibitor
Use

Propecia®: Treatment of male pattern hair loss in **men only**. Safety and efficacy were demonstrated in men between 18-41 years of age.

Proscar®: Treatment of symptomatic benign prostatic hyperplasia (BPH); can be used in combination with an alpha-blocker, doxazosin

Unlabeled/Investigational Use Prostate cancer prevention (to reduce the incidence); treatment of female hirsutism

Pharmacodynamics/Kinetics

Onset of action: 3-6 months of ongoing therapy

Duration:

After a single oral dose as small as 0.5 mg: 65% depression of plasma dihydrotestosterone levels persists 5-7 days

After 6 months of treatment with 5 mg/day: Circulating dihydrotestosterone levels are reduced to castrate levels without significant effects on circulating testosterone; levels return to normal within 14 days of discontinuation of treatment

Distribution: V_{dss}: 76 L

Protein binding: 90%

Metabolism: Hepatic via CYP3A4; two active metabolites (<20% activity of finasteride)

Bioavailability: Mean: 63%

Half-life elimination, serum: Elderly: 8 hours; Adults: 6 hours (3-16)

Time to peak, serum: 2-6 hours

Excretion: Feces (57%) and urine (39%) as metabolites

Dosage Oral: Adults:

Male:

Benign prostatic hyperplasia (Proscar®): 5 mg once daily as a single dose; clinical responses occur within 12 weeks to 6 months of initiation of therapy; long-term administration is recommended for maximal response

Male pattern baldness (Propecia®): 1 mg daily

Prostate cancer prevention (unlabeled use): 5 mg once daily; planned duration of treatment was 7 years (Kramer, 2009; Thompson, 2003)

Female hirsutism (unlabeled use): 5 mg/day

Dosing adjustment in renal impairment: No dosage adjustment is necessary

Dosing adjustment in hepatic impairment: Use with caution in patients with liver function abnormalities because finasteride is metabolized extensively in the liver

Anesthesia and Critical Care Concerns/Other Considerations Finasteride may be useful in men with moderately symptomatic BPH who either refuse prostatectomy or are poor surgical candidates. Currently, there is no way to predict which men will respond to finasteride. Treatment with finasteride does not alter the ratio of free to total PSA, which is used to detect prostatic cancer.

Additional Information Complete prescribing information for this medication should be consulted for additional detail.

Dosage Forms Excipient information presented when available (limited, particularly for generics); consult specific product labeling.
Tablet: 5 mg
Propecia®: 1 mg
Proscar®: 5 mg

References

Lepor H, Williford WO, Barry MJ, et al, "The Efficacy of Terazosin, Finasteride, or Both in Benign Prostatic Hyperplasia," N Engl J Med, 1996, 335(8):533-9.

McConnell JD, Roehrborn CG, Bautista OM, et al, "The Long-Term Effect of Doxazosin, Finasteride, and Combination Therapy on the Clinical Progression of Benign Prostatic Hyperplasia. Medical Therapy of Prostatic Symptoms (MTOPS) Research Group," N Engl J Med, 2003, 349(25):2387-98.

Pole M and Koren G, "Finasteride. Does It Affect Spermatogenesis and Pregnancy," Can Fam Physician, 2001, 47:2469-70.

Thompson IM, Goodman PJ, Tangen CM, et al, "The Influence of Finasteride on the Development of Prostate Cancer," N Engl J Med, 2003, Jul 349(3):215-24.

♦ **First™-Progesterone VGS** *see* Progesterone *on page 1184*

♦ **First®-Testosterone** *see* Testosterone *on page 1362*

♦ **First®-Testosterone MC** *see* Testosterone *on page 1362*

♦ **Fisalamine** *see* Mesalamine *on page 884*

♦ **FK506** *see* Tacrolimus *on page 1338*

♦ **Flagyl®** *see* MetroNIDAZOLE *on page 928*

♦ **Flagyl® 375** *see* MetroNIDAZOLE *on page 928*

♦ **Flagyl® ER** *see* MetroNIDAZOLE *on page 928*

♦ **Flamazine® (Can)** *see* Silver Sulfadiazine *on page 1292*

♦ **Flebogamma®** *see* Immune Globulin (Intravenous) *on page 732*

Flecainide (fle KAY nide)

Related Information
Antiarrhythmic Drugs *on page 1656*

U.S. Brand Names Tambocor™

Canadian Brand Names Apo-Flecainide®; Tambocor™

Index Terms Flecainide Acetate

Pharmacologic Category Antiarrhythmic Agent, Class Ic

Use Prevention and suppression of documented life-threatening ventricular arrhythmias (eg, sustained ventricular tachycardia); controlling symptomatic, disabling supraventricular tachycardias in patients without structural heart disease in whom other agents fail

Pharmacodynamics/Kinetics
Absorption: Oral: Rapid
Distribution: Adults: V_d: 5-13.4 L/kg
Protein binding: Alpha$_1$ acid glycoprotein: 40% to 50%
Metabolism: Hepatic
Bioavailability: 85% to 90%
Half-life elimination: Infants: 11-12 hours; Children: 8 hours; Adults: 7-22 hours, increased with congestive heart failure or renal dysfunction; End-stage renal disease: 19-26 hours
Time to peak, serum: ~1.5-3 hours
Excretion: Urine (80% to 90%, 10% to 50% as unchanged drug and metabolites)

Dosage Oral:
Children:
Initial: 3 mg/kg/day or 50-100 mg/m^2/day in 3 divided doses
Usual: 3-6 mg/kg/day or 100-150 mg/m^2/day in 3 divided doses; up to 11 mg/kg/day or 200 mg/m^2/day for uncontrolled patients with subtherapeutic levels

Adults:
Life-threatening ventricular arrhythmias:
Initial: 100 mg every 12 hours
Increase by 50-100 mg/day (given in 2 doses/day) every 4 days; maximum: 400 mg/day.

Use of higher initial doses and more rapid dosage adjustments have resulted in an increased incidence of proarrhythmic events and congestive heart failure, particularly during the first few days. Do not use a loading dose. Use very cautiously in patients with history of congestive heart failure or myocardial infarction.

Prevention of paroxysmal supraventricular arrhythmias in patients with disabling symptoms but no structural heart disease: Initial: 50 mg every 12 hours; increase by 50 mg twice daily at 4-day intervals; maximum: 300 mg/day

Paroxysmal atrial fibrillation: Outpatient: "Pill-in-the-pocket" dose (unlabeled dose): 200 mg (weight <70 kg), 300 mg (weight ≥70 kg). May not repeat in ≤24 hours. **Note:** An initial inpatient conversion trial should have been successful before sending patient home on this approach. Patient must be taking an AV nodal-blocking agent (eg, beta-blocker, nondihydropyridine calcium channel blocker) prior to initiation of antiarrhythmic.

Dosing adjustment in severe renal impairment: GFR ≤50 mL/minute: Decrease dose by 50%; dose increases should be made cautiously at intervals >4 days and serum levels monitored frequently.

Hemodialysis: No supplemental dose recommended.

Peritoneal dialysis: No supplemental dose recommended.

Dosing adjustment/comments in hepatic impairment: Monitoring of plasma levels is recommended because of significantly increased half-life.

When transferring from another antiarrhythmic agent, allow for 2-4 half-lives of the agent to pass before initiating flecainide therapy.

Anesthesia and Critical Care Concerns/Other Considerations Based on adverse outcomes noted with flecainide in the CAST trial, the FDA recommends that use of flecainide be limited to patients with life-threatening ventricular arrhythmias.

Additional Information Complete prescribing information for this medication should be consulted for additional detail.

Dosage Forms Excipient information presented when available (limited, particularly for generics); consult specific product labeling.

Tablet, as acetate: 50 mg, 100 mg, 150 mg

Fluconazole (floo KOE na zole)

Medication Safety Issues

Sound-alike/look-alike issues:

Fluconazole may be confused with flecainide, FLUoxetine, furosemide, itraconazole

Diflucan® may be confused with diclofenac, Diprivan®, disulfiram

International issues:

Canesten® [Great Britain]: Brand name for clotrimazole in multiple international markets

Related Information

Antifungal Agents *on page 1664*

Dosing Considerations for the Critically-Ill Patient With Morbid Obesity *on page 1561*

U.S. Brand Names Diflucan®

Canadian Brand Names Apo-Fluconazole®; CO Fluconazole; Diflucan®; Dom-Fluconazole; Fluconazole Injection; Fluconazole Omega; Gen-Fluconazole; GMD-Fluconazole; Mylan-Fluconazole; Novo-Fluconazole; PHL-Fluconazole; PMS-Fluconazole; Pro-Fluconazole; Riva-Fluconazole; Taro-Fluconazole; Zym-Fluconazole

Pharmacologic Category Antifungal Agent, Oral; Antifungal Agent, Parenteral

Generic Available Yes

Use Treatment of candidiasis (vaginal, oropharyngeal, esophageal, urinary tract infections, peritonitis, pneumonia, and systemic infections); cryptococcal meningitis; antifungal prophylaxis in allogeneic bone marrow transplant recipients

Mechanism of Action Interferes with fungal cytochrome P450 activity (lanosterol 14-α-demethylase), decreasing ergosterol synthesis (principal sterol in fungal cell membrane) and inhibiting cell membrane formation

Pharmacodynamics/Kinetics

Distribution: Widely throughout body with good penetration into CSF, eye, peritoneal fluid, sputum, skin, and urine

Relative diffusion blood into CSF: Adequate with or without inflammation (exceeds usual MICs)

CSF:blood level ratio: Normal meninges: 70% to 80%; Inflamed meninges: >70% to 80%

Protein binding, plasma: 11% to 12%

Bioavailability: Oral: >90%

Half-life elimination: Normal renal function: ~30 hours

Time to peak, serum: Oral: 1-2 hours

Excretion: Urine (80% as unchanged drug)

Dosage The daily dose of fluconazole is the same for oral and I.V. administration

Usual dosage ranges:

Neonates: First 2 weeks of life, especially premature neonates: Same dose as older children every 72 hours

Children: Loading dose: 6-12 mg/kg; maintenance: 3-12 mg/kg/day; duration and dosage depends on severity of infection

Adults: 200-800 mg/day; duration and dosage depends on severity of infection

Indication-specific dosing:

Children:

Candidiasis:

Oropharyngeal: Loading dose: 6 mg/kg; maintenance: 3 mg/kg/day for 2 weeks

Esophageal: Loading dose: 6 mg/kg; maintenance: 3-12 mg/kg/day for 21 days and at least 2 weeks following resolution of symptoms

Systemic infection: 6 mg/kg every 12 hours for 28 days

Meningitis, cryptococcal: Loading dose: 12 mg/kg; maintenance: 6-12 mg/kg/day for 10-12 weeks following negative CSF culture; relapse suppression (HIV-positive): 6 mg/kg/day

Adults:

Candidiasis (Pappas, 2009):

Candidemia (neutropenic and non-neutropenic): Loading dose: 800 mg on first day, then 400 mg/day for 14 days after last positive blood culture and resolution of signs/symptoms; **Note:** Not recommended for neutropenic patients with recent azole exposure and critical illness

Chronic, disseminated: 400 mg/day until calcification or lesion resolution

CNS candidemia: 400-800 mg/day until CSF/radiological abnormalities resolved; **Note:** Recommended as alternative therapy in patients intolerant of amphotericin B

Oropharyngeal (long-term suppression): 100-200 mg/day for 7-14 days; chronic therapy of 100 mg 3 times weekly is recommended in immunocompromised patients with history of oropharyngeal candidiasis (OPC)

Osteoarticular: 400 mg/day for 6-12 months (osteomyelitis) or 6 weeks (septic arthritis)

Esophageal: 200-400 mg/day for 14-21 days

Prophylaxis:

Solid organ: 200-400 mg/day for 7-14 days

Neutropenic patients: 400 mg/day for duration of neutropenia

Urinary tract:

Fungus balls: 200-400 mg/day

Pyelonephritis: 200-400 mg/day for 2 weeks

Symptomatic cystitis: 200 mg/day for 2 weeks

Vaginal: 150 mg as a single dose

Coccidiomycosis (unlabeled use, IDSA guideline): 400 mg/day; doses of 800-1000 mg/day have been used for meningeal disease; usual duration of therapy ranges from 3-6 months for primary uncomplicated infections and up to 1 year for pulmonary (chronic and diffuse) infection

Endocarditis, prosthetic valve, early (unlabeled use, IDSA guideline): 400-800 mg/day for 6 weeks after valve replacement (as step-down in stable, culture-negative patients); long-term suppression in absence of valve replacement: 400-800 mg/day

Endophthalmitis: 400-800 mg/day for 4-6 weeks until examination indicates resolution

Meningitis, cryptococcal: Amphotericin 0.7-1 mg/kg +/- 5-FC for 2 weeks then fluconazole 400 mg/day for at least 10 weeks (consider life-long in HIV-positive); maintenance (HIV-positive): 200-400 mg/day life-long

Pericarditis or myocarditis: 400-800 mg/day

Pneumonia, cryptococcal (mild-to-moderate) (unlabeled use, IDSA guideline): 200-400 mg/day for 6-12 months (consider life-long in HIV-positive patients)

Dosing adjustment/interval in renal impairment:

No adjustment for vaginal candidiasis single-dose therapy

For multiple dosing, administer usual load then adjust daily doses as follows:

Cl_{cr} ≤50 mL/minute (no dialysis): Administer 50% of recommended dose or administer every 48 hours.

Hemodialysis: 50% is removed by hemodialysis; administer 100% of daily dose (according to indication) after each dialysis treatment.

Continuous renal replacement therapy (CRRT): Drug clearance is highly dependent on the method of renal replacement, filter type, and flow rate. Appropriate dosing requires close monitoring of pharmacologic response, signs of adverse reactions due to drug accumulation, as well as drug levels in relation to target trough (if appropriate). The following are general recommendations only (based on dialysate flow/ultrafiltration rates of 1 L/hour) and should not supersede clinical judgment:

CVVH: 200-400 mg every 24 hours

CVVHD/CVVHDF: 400-800 mg every 24 hours

Note: Higher daily doses of 400 mg (CVVH) and 800 mg (CVVHD/CVVHDF) should be considered when treating resistant organisms and/or when employing combined ultrafiltration and dialysis flow rates of ≥2 L/hour for CVVHD/CVVHDF (Trotman, 2005).

Stability

Powder for oral suspension: Store dry powder at ≤30°C (86°F). Following reconstitution, store at 5°C to 30°C (41°F to 86°F). Discard unused portion after 2 weeks. Do not freeze.

Injection: Store injection in glass at 5°C to 30°C (41°F to 86°F). Store injection in Viaflex® at 5°C to 25°C (41°F to 77°F). Do not freeze. Do not unwrap unit until ready for use.

Administration

I.V.: Infuse over approximately 1-2 hours; do not exceed 200 mg/hour

Oral: May be administered without regard to meals.

Monitoring Parameters Periodic liver function tests (AST, ALT, alkaline phosphatase) and renal function tests, potassium

Pregnancy Risk Factor C

Contraindications Hypersensitivity to fluconazole, other azoles, or any component of the formulation; concomitant administration with cisapride

Warnings/Precautions Should be used with caution in patients with renal and hepatic dysfunction or previous hepatotoxicity from other azole derivatives. Patients who develop abnormal liver function tests during fluconazole therapy should be monitored closely and discontinued if symptoms consistent with liver disease develop. Rare exfoliative skin disorders have been observed; monitor closely if rash develops. The manufacturer reports rare cases of QT_c prolongation and TdP associated with fluconazole use and advises caution in patients with concomitant medications or conditions which are arrhythmogenic. However, given the limited number of cases and the presence of multiple confounding variables, the likelihood that fluconazole causes conduction abnormalities appears remote.

Adverse Reactions Frequency not always defined.

Cardiovascular: Angioedema, pallor, QT prolongation (rare, case reports), torsade de pointes(rare, case reports)

Central nervous system: Headache (2% to 13%), seizure, dizziness

Dermatologic: Rash (2%), alopecia, toxic epidermal necrolysis, Stevens-Johnson syndrome

Endocrine & metabolic: Hypercholesterolemia, hypertriglyceridemia, hypokalemia

Gastrointestinal: Nausea (4% to 7%), abdominal pain (2% to 6%), diarrhea (2% to 3%), vomiting (2%), dyspepsia, taste perversion

Hematologic: Agranulocytosis, leukopenia, neutropenia, thrombocytopenia

Hepatic: Alkaline phosphatase increased, ALT increased, AST increased, cholestasis, hepatic failure (rare), hepatitis, jaundice

Respiratory: Dyspnea

Miscellaneous: Anaphylactic reactions (rare)

Drug Interactions

Metabolism/Transport Effects Inhibits CYP1A2 (weak), 2C9 (strong), 2C19 (strong), 3A4 (moderate)

Avoid Concomitant Use

Avoid concomitant use of Fluconazole with any of the following: Artemether; Cisapride; Clopidogrel; Conivaptan; Dofetilide; Dronedarone; Everolimus; Lumefantrine; Nilotinib; Pimozide; QuiNIDine; QuiNINE; Ranolazine; Tetrabenazine; Thioridazine; Tolvaptan; Ziprasidone

Increased Effect/Toxicity

Fluconazole may increase the levels/effects of: Alfentanil; Aprepitant; Benzodiazepines (metabolized by oxidation); Bosentan; BusPIRone; Busulfan; Calcium Channel Blockers; CarBAMazepine; Cardiac Glycosides; Carvedilol; Cilostazol; Cinacalcet; Cisapride; Citalopram; Colchicine; Conivaptan; Corticosteroids (Orally Inhaled); Corticosteroids (Systemic); CycloSPORINE; CYP2C19 Substrates; CYP2C9 Substrates (High risk); CYP3A4 Substrates; Docetaxel; Dofetilide; Dronedarone; Eletriptan; Eplerenone; Erlotinib; Eszopiclone; Everolimus; FentaNYL; Fosaprepitant; Gefitinib; HMG-CoA Reductase Inhibitors; Imatinib; Irbesartan; Irinotecan; Losartan; Macrolide Antibiotics; Methadone; Phenytoin; Phosphodiesterase 5 Inhibitors; Pimecrolimus; Pimozide; Protease Inhibitors; Proton Pump Inhibitors; QTc-Prolonging Agents; QuiNIDine; QuiNINE; Ramelteon; Ranolazine; Repaglinide; Rifamycin Derivatives; Salmeterol; Saxagliptin; Sirolimus; Solifenacin; Sulfonylureas; Sunitinib; Tacrolimus; Temsirolimus; Tetrabenazine; Thioridazine; Tolterodine; Tolvaptan; Trimetrexate; Vitamin K Antagonists; Zidovudine; Ziprasidone; Zolpidem

The levels/effects of Fluconazole may be increased by: Alfuzosin; Artemether; Chloroquine; Ciprofloxacin; Gadobutrol; Grapefruit Juice; Lumefantrine; Macrolide Antibiotics; Nilotinib; Protease Inhibitors; QuiNINE

◀ **Decreased Effect**

Fluconazole may decrease the levels/effects of: Amphotericin B; Clopidogrel; Saccharomyces boulardii

The levels/effects of Fluconazole may be decreased by: Didanosine; Phenytoin; Rifamycin Derivatives; Sucralfate

Dietary Considerations Take without regard to meals.

Dosage Forms Excipient information presented when available (limited, particularly for generics); consult specific product labeling.

Infusion [premixed in sodium chloride or dextrose]: 200 mg (100 mL); 400 mg (200 mL)

Diflucan® [premixed in sodium chloride or dextrose]: 200 mg (100 mL); 400 mg (200 mL)

Powder for oral suspension: 10 mg/mL (35 mL); 40 mg/mL (35 mL)

Diflucan®: 10 mg/mL (35 mL); 40 mg/mL (35 mL) [contains sodium benzoate; orange flavor]

Tablet: 50 mg, 100 mg, 150 mg, 200 mg

Diflucan®: 50 mg, 100 mg, 150 mg, 200 mg

References

Pappas PG, Rex JH, Sobel JD, et al, "Guidelines for Treatment of Candidiasis," *Clin Infect Dis*, 2004, 38(2):161-89.

Pelz RK, Hendrix CW, Swoboda SM, et al, "Double-Blind Placebo-Controlled Trial of Fluconazole to Prevent Candidal Infections in Critically Ill Surgical Patients," *Ann Surg*, 2001, 233(4):542-8.

Valtonen M, Tiula E, and Neuvonen PJ, "Effect of Continuous Veno-Venous Haemofiltration and Haemodiafiltration on the Elimination of Fluconazole in Patients With Acute Renal Failure," *J Antimicrob Chemother*, 1997, 40(5):695-700.

◆ **Fluconazole Injection (Can)** *see* Fluconazole *on page 607*

◆ **Fluconazole Omega (Can)** *see* Fluconazole *on page 607*

Fludrocortisone (floo droe KOR ti sone)

Medication Safety Issues

Sound-alike/look-alike issues:

Florinef® may be confused with Fioricet®, Fiorinal®

Related Information

Corticosteroids *on page 1676*

Stress Replacement of Corticosteroids *on page 1611*

Canadian Brand Names Florinef®

Index Terms 9α-Fluorohydrocortisone Acetate; Florinef; Fludrocortisone Acetate; Fluohydrisone Acetate; Fluohydrocortisone Acetate

Pharmacologic Category Corticosteroid, Systemic

Generic Available Yes

Use Partial replacement therapy for primary and secondary adrenocortical insufficiency in Addison's disease; treatment of salt-losing adrenogenital syndrome

Mechanism of Action Promotes increased reabsorption of sodium and loss of potassium from renal distal tubules

Pharmacodynamics/Kinetics

Absorption: Rapid and complete

Protein binding: 42%

Metabolism: Hepatic

Half-life elimination, plasma: 30-35 minutes; Biological: 18-36 hours

Time to peak, serum: ~1.7 hours

Dosage Oral:

Infants and Children: 0.05-0.1 mg/day

Adults: 0.1-0.2 mg/day with ranges of 0.1 mg 3 times/week to 0.2 mg/day

Addison's disease: Initial: 0.1 mg/day; if transient hypertension develops, reduce the dose to 0.05 mg/day. Preferred administration with cortisone (10-37.5 mg/day) or hydrocortisone (10-30 mg/day).

Salt-losing adrenogenital syndrome: 0.1-0.2 mg/day

Administration Administration in conjunction with a glucocorticoid is preferable

Monitoring Parameters Monitor blood pressure and signs of edema when patient is on chronic therapy; very potent mineralocorticoid with high glucocorticoid activity; monitor serum electrolytes, serum renin activity, and blood pressure; monitor for evidence of infection; stop treatment if a significant increase in weight or blood pressure, edema, or cardiac enlargement occurs

Anesthesia and Critical Care Concerns/Other Considerations

Clinical Pearls/Comments: In patients with salt-losing forms of congenital adrenogenital syndrome, use along with cortisone or hydrocortisone. Fludrocortisone 0.1 mg has sodium retention activity equal to DOCA® 1 mg.

Evidence-Based Information:

Adrenal Insufficiency: Patients on long-term steroid supplementation will require higher corticosteroid doses when subject to stress (ie, trauma, surgery, severe infection). This agent has significant mineralocorticoid activity with consequent hemodynamic effects. Fludrocortisone has been used to treat severe orthostatic hypotension. Abrupt withdrawal may result in adrenal insufficiency with hypotension and hyperkalemia. Guidelines for glucocorticoid replacement during various surgical procedures have been published (Coursin, 2002; Salem, 1994).

Septic Shock: Annane, et al (2002) randomized 300 septic shock patients to either hydrocortisone (50 mg I.V. push every 6 hours) and fludrocortisone (50 mcg tablet daily via nasogastric tube) or matching placebos for 7 days. The mean Simplified Acute Physiology Score II (SAPS II) was 57 ± 19 in the placebo group and 60 ± 19 in the active treatment group. The Logistic Organ Dysfunction score was 9 ± 3 in the placebo group and 9 ± 3 in the active treatment group. In patients who did not appropriately respond to cosyntropin (nonresponders), there were significantly fewer deaths in the active treatment group. Vasopressor therapy was withdrawn more frequently in this subset of the active treatment group. Adverse events were similar in both groups.

In the CORTICUS trial (Sprung, 2008), 484 septic shock patients were randomized within 72 hours of onset to receive either hydrocortisone (50 mg I.V. push every 6 hours) or placebo for 5 days followed by a 6-day taper. The primary endpoint was 28-day mortality in patients who did not respond to cosyntropin. The SAPS II score in the treatment group was 49.5 ± 17.8 and 48.6 ± 16.7 in the placebo group. The Sequential Organ Failure Assessment scores were 10.6 ± 3.4 in the treatment group and 10.6 ± 3.2 in the placebo group. Different than the Annane study, in the patients who did not respond to cosyntropin, there was no mortality difference at 28 days; 39.2% (95% CI: 30.5-47.9) mortality in the hydrocortisone group and 36.1% (95% CI: 26.9-45.3, p=0.69) mortality in the placebo group. A trend towards increased incidence of superinfection was noted in hydrocortisone patients. New septic shock episodes, hyperglycemia, and hypernatremia were more frequent in the hydrocortisone group. Hydrocortisone did not improve survival in this population of septic shock patients regardless of corticotropin response.

The 2008 Surviving Sepsis Campaign Guidelines suggest the following: Intravenous hydrocortisone be given only to adult septic shock patients after blood pressure is identified to be poorly responsive to fluid resuscitation and vasopressor therapy (Grade 2C); ACTH stimulation test not be used to identify the subset of adults with septic shock who should receive hydrocortisone (Grade 2B); patients with septic shock should not receive dexamethasone if hydrocortisone is available (Grade 2B); the addition of fludrocortisone if hydrocortisone is not available and the steroid that is substituted does not have significant mineralocorticoid activity (Grade 2C); doses of corticosteroids comparable to >300 mg hydrocortisone daily **not** be used in severe sepsis or septic shock for the purpose of treating septic shock (Grade 1A). They also recommend corticosteroids **not** be administered for the treatment of sepsis in the absence of shock. There is, however, no contraindication to continuing maintenance steroid therapy or to using stress dose steroids if the patient's endocrine or corticosteroid administration history warrants (Grade 1D).

The 2008 Recommendations for the diagnosis and management of corticosteroid insufficiency in critically ill adult patients recommend a diagnosis of critical illness related corticosteroid insufficiency can be made by a delta cortisol level (after 250 mcg cosyntropin) of <9 mcg/dL or a random cortisol <10 mcg/dL (Grade 2B). However, they recommend **against** the use of ACTH stimulation test to determine if septic shock or ARDS patients should receive steroid therapy (Grade 2B). They

◀ recommend to consider using hydrocortisone in septic shock patients who have responded poorly to resuscitation and vasopressors (Grade 2B) and glucocorticoid treatment should be tapered slowly and not stopped abruptly (Grade 2B). Dexamethasone is **not** recommended for the treatment of septic shock or ARDS (Grade 1B). Fludrocortisone therapy is considered optional (Grade 2B).

Pregnancy Risk Factor C

Contraindications Hypersensitivity to fludrocortisone or any component of the formulation; systemic fungal infections

Warnings/Precautions May cause hypercorticism or suppression of hypothalamic-pituitary-adrenal (HPA) axis, particularly in younger children or in patients receiving high doses for prolonged periods. HPA axis suppression may lead to adrenal crisis. Withdrawal and discontinuation of a corticosteroid should be done slowly and carefully. Fludrocortisone is primarily a mineralocorticoid agonist, but may also inhibit the HPA axis. May increase risk of infection and/or limit response to vaccinations; close observation is required in patients with latent tuberculosis and/or TB reactivity. Restrict use in active TB (only in conjunction with antituberculosis treatment). Use with caution in patients with sodium retention and potassium loss, hepatic impairment, myocardial infarction, osteoporosis, and/or renal impairment. Use with caution in the elderly. Withdraw therapy with gradual tapering of dose. Safety and efficacy have not been established in children.

Adverse Reactions Frequency not defined.
Cardiovascular: CHF, edema, hypertension
Central nervous system: Dizziness, headache, seizures
Dermatologic: Acne, bruising, rash
Endocrine & metabolic: HPA suppression, hyperglycemia, hypokalemic alkalosis, suppression of growth
Gastrointestinal: Peptic ulcer
Neuromuscular & skeletal: Muscle weakness
Ocular: Cataracts
Miscellaneous: Anaphylaxis (generalized), diaphoresis

Drug Interactions

Avoid Concomitant Use
Avoid concomitant use of Fludrocortisone with any of the following: Natalizumab; Vaccines (Live)

Increased Effect/Toxicity
Fludrocortisone may increase the levels/effects of: Acetylcholinesterase Inhibitors; Amphotericin B; CycloSPORINE; Leflunomide; Loop Diuretics; Natalizumab; NSAID (COX-2 Inhibitor); NSAID (Nonselective); Thiazide Diuretics; Vaccines (Live); Warfarin

The levels/effects of Fludrocortisone may be increased by: Antifungal Agents (Azole Derivatives, Systemic); Aprepitant; Calcium Channel Blockers (Non-dihydropyridine); CycloSPORINE; Estrogen Derivatives; Fluconazole; Fosaprepitant; Macrolide Antibiotics; Neuromuscular-Blocking Agents (Nondepolarizing); Quinolone Antibiotics; Salicylates; Trastuzumab

Decreased Effect
Fludrocortisone may decrease the levels/effects of: Antidiabetic Agents; Calcitriol; Corticorelin; Isoniazid; Salicylates; Vaccines (Inactivated); Vaccines (Live)

The levels/effects of Fludrocortisone may be decreased by: Aminoglutethimide; Antacids; Barbiturates; Bile Acid Sequestrants; Echinacea; Mitotane; Primidone; Rifamycin Derivatives

Dietary Considerations Systemic use of mineralocorticoids/corticosteroids may require a diet with increased potassium, vitamins A, B_6, C, D, folate, calcium, zinc, and phosphorus, and decreased sodium. With fludrocortisone, a decrease in dietary sodium is often not required as the increased retention of sodium is usually the desired therapeutic effect.

Dosage Forms Excipient information presented when available (limited, particularly for generics); consult specific product labeling.
Tablet, as acetate: 0.1 mg

References

Abraham E and Evans T, "Corticosteroids and Septic Shock (editorial)," *JAMA*, 2002, 288(7):886-7.
Annane D, Sebille V, Charpentier C, et al, "Effect of Treatment With Low Doses of Hydrocortisone and Fludrocortisone on Mortality in Patients With Septic Shock," *JAMA*, 2002, 288(7):862-71.

Coursin DB and Wood KE, "Corticosteroid Supplementation for Adrenal Insufficiency," *JAMA*, 2002, 287(2):236-40.

Cooper MS and Stewart PM, "Corticosteroid Insufficiency in Acutely Ill Patients," *N Engl J Med*, 2003, 348(8):727-34.

Dellinger RP, Levy MM, Carlet JM, et al, "Surviving Sepsis Campaign: International Guidelines for Management of Severe Sepsis and Septic Shock: 2008," *Intensive Care Med*, 2008, 34(1): 17-60. Available at http://www.survivingsepsis.org/system/files/images/2008_20International_20SSC_20-Guidelines_1_.pdf

Hotchkiss RS and Karl IE, "The Pathophysiology and Treatment of Sepsis," *N Engl J Med*, 2003, 348 (2):138-50.

Marik PE, Pastores SM, Annane D, et al, "Recommendations for the Diagnosis and Management of Corticosteroid Insufficiency in Critically Ill Adult Patients: Consensus Statements From an International Task Force by the American College of Critical Care Medicine," *Crit Care Med*, 2008, 36(6):1937-49.

Salem M, Tainsh RE Jr, Bromberg J, et al, "Perioperative Glucocorticoid Coverage. A Reassessment 42 Years After Emergence of a Problem," *Ann Surg*, 1994, 219(4):416-25.

Sprung CL, Annane D, Keh D, et al, "Hydrocortisone Therapy for Patients With Septic Shock," *N Engl J Med*, 2008, 358(2):111-24.

◆ **Fludrocortisone Acetate** *see* Fludrocortisone *on page 610*

◆ **Flumadine®** *see* Rimantadine *on page 1249*

Flumazenil (FLOO may ze nil)

Medication Safety Issues

Sound-alike/look-alike issues:

Flumazenil may be confused with influenza virus vaccine

Related Information

Moderate Sedation *on page 1566*

U.S. Brand Names Romazicon®

Canadian Brand Names Anexate®; Flumazenil Injection; Flumazenil Injection, USP; Romazicon®

Pharmacologic Category Antidote

Generic Available Yes

Use Benzodiazepine antagonist; reverses sedative effects of benzodiazepines used in conscious sedation and general anesthesia; treatment of benzodiazepine overdose

Mechanism of Action Competitively inhibits the activity at the benzodiazepine receptor site on the GABA/benzodiazepine receptor complex. Flumazenil does not antagonize the CNS effect of drugs affecting GABA-ergic neurons by means other than the benzodiazepine receptor (ethanol, barbiturates, general anesthetics) and does not reverse the effects of opioids

Pharmacodynamics/Kinetics

Onset of action: 1-3 minutes; 80% response within 3 minutes

Peak effect: 6-10 minutes

Duration: Resedation: ~1 hour; duration related to dose given and benzodiazepine plasma concentrations; reversal effects of flumazenil may wear off before effects of benzodiazepine

Distribution: Initial V_d: 0.5 L/kg; V_{dss} 0.77-1.6 L/kg

Protein binding: 40% to 50%

Metabolism: Hepatic; dependent upon hepatic blood flow

Half-life elimination: Adults: Alpha: 7-15 minutes; Terminal: 41-79 minutes; Moderate hepatic dysfunction: 1.3 hours; severe hepatic impairment: 2.4 hours

Excretion: Feces; urine (0.2% as unchanged drug)

Dosage

Children and Adults: I.V.: See table on next page.

Flumazenil

Pediatric Dosage	
Pediatric dosage for **reversal of conscious sedation and general anesthesia:**	
Initial dose	0.01 mg/kg over 15 seconds (maximum: 0.2 mg)
Repeat doses (maximum: 4 doses)	0.005-0.01 mg/kg (maximum: 0.2 mg) repeated at 1-minute intervals
Maximum total cumulative dose	1 mg or 0.05 mg/kg (whichever is lower)
Adult Dosage	
Adult dosage for **reversal of conscious sedation and general anesthesia:**	
Initial dose	0.2 mg intravenously over 15 seconds
Repeat doses (maximum: 4 doses)	If desired level of consciousness is not obtained, 0.2 mg may be repeated at 1-minute intervals.
Maximum total cumulative dose	1 mg (usual dose: 0.6-1 mg) **In the event of resedation:** Repeat doses may be given at 20-minute intervals with maximum of 1 mg/dose and 3 mg/hour.
Adult dosage for **suspected benzodiazepine overdose:**	
Initial dose	0.2 mg intravenously over 30 seconds; if the desired level of consciousness is not obtained, 0.3 mg can be given over 30 seconds
Repeat doses	0.5 mg over 30 seconds repeated at 1-minute intervals
Maximum total cumulative dose	3 mg (usual dose 1-3 mg) Patients with a partial response at 3 mg may require additional titration up to a total dose of 5 mg. If a patient has not responded 5 minutes after cumulative dose of 5 mg, the major cause of sedation is not likely due to benzodiazepines. **In the event of resedation:** May repeat doses at 20-minute intervals with maximum of 1 mg/dose and 3 mg/hour.

Resedation: Repeated doses may be given at 20-minute intervals as needed; repeat treatment doses of 1 mg (at a rate of 0.5 mg/minute) should be given at any time and no more than 3 mg should be given in any hour. After intoxication with high doses of benzodiazepines, the duration of a single dose of flumazenil is not expected to exceed 1 hour; if desired, the period of wakefulness may be prolonged with repeated low intravenous doses of flumazenil, or by an infusion of 0.1-0.4 mg/hour. Most patients with benzodiazepine overdose will respond to a cumulative dose of 1-3 mg and doses >3 mg do not reliably produce additional effects. Rarely, patients with a partial response at 3 mg may require additional titration up to a total dose of 5 mg. **If a patient has not responded 5 minutes after receiving a cumulative dose of 5 mg, the major cause of sedation is not likely to be due to benzodiazepines.**

Elderly: No differences in safety or efficacy have been reported. However, increased sensitivity may occur in some elderly patients.

Dosing in renal impairment: Not significantly affected by renal failure (Cl_{cr} <10 mL/minute) or hemodialysis beginning 1 hour after drug administration

Dosing in hepatic impairment: Use caution with initial and/or repeat doses in patients with liver disease

Stability Store at 15°C to 30°C (59°F to 86°F). For I.V. use only. Once drawn up in the syringe or mixed with solution use within 24 hours. Discard any unused solution after 24 hours.

Administration I.V.: Administer in freely-running I.V. into large vein. Inject over 15 seconds for conscious sedation and general anesthesia and over 30 seconds for overdose.

Monitoring Parameters Monitor patients for return of sedation or respiratory depression

Anesthesia and Critical Care Concerns/Other Considerations

Clinical Pearls/Comments: Flumazenil does **not** antagonize the CNS effects of other GABA agonists (such as ethanol, barbiturates, or general anesthetics), nor does it reverse narcotics. See Warnings/Precautions section for additional concerns.

Pregnancy Risk Factor C

Contraindications Hypersensitivity to flumazenil, benzodiazepines, or any component of the formulation; patients given benzodiazepines for control of potentially life-threatening conditions (eg, control of intracranial pressure or status epilepticus); patients who are showing signs of serious cyclic-antidepressant overdosage

Warnings/Precautions [U.S. Boxed Warning]: Benzodiazepine reversal may result in seizures in some patients. Patients who may develop seizures include patients on benzodiazepines for long-term sedation, tricyclic antidepressant overdose patients, concurrent major sedative-hypnotic drug withdrawal, recent therapy with repeated doses of parenteral benzodiazepines, myoclonic jerking or seizure activity prior to flumazenil administration. Flumazenil may not reliably reverse respiratory depression/hypoventilation. Flumazenil is not a substitute for evaluation of oxygenation; establishing an airway and assisting ventilation, as necessary, is always the initial step in overdose management. Resedation occurs more frequently in patients where a large single dose or cumulative dose of a benzodiazepine is administered along with a neuromuscular-blocking agent and multiple anesthetic agents. Flumazenil should be used with caution in the intensive care unit because of increased risk of unrecognized benzodiazepine dependence in such settings. Should not be used to diagnose benzodiazepine-induced sedation. Reverse neuromuscular blockade before considering use. Flumazenil does not antagonize the CNS effects of other GABA agonists (such as ethanol, barbiturates, or general anesthetics); nor does it reverse narcotics. Flumazenil does not consistently reverse amnesia; patient may not recall verbal instructions after procedure.

Use with caution in patients with a history of panic disorder; may provoke panic attacks. Use caution in drug and ethanol-dependent patients; these patients may also be dependent on benzodiazepines. Not recommended for treatment of benzodiazepine dependence. Use with caution in head injury patients. Use caution in patients with mixed drug overdoses; toxic effects of other drugs taken may emerge once benzodiazepine effects are reversed. Use caution in hepatic dysfunction and in patients relying on a benzodiazepine for seizure control. Safety and efficacy have not been established in children <1 year of age.

Adverse Reactions

>10%: Gastrointestinal: Vomiting, nausea

1% to 10%:

Cardiovascular: Vasodilation (1% to 3%), palpitation

Central nervous system: Dizziness (10%), agitation (3% to 9%), emotional lability (1% to 3%), fatigue (1% to 3%), headache (1% to 3%)

Gastrointestinal: Xerostomia

Local: Pain at injection site (3% to 9%)

Neuromuscular & skeletal: Tremor, weakness, paresthesia (1% to 3%)

Ocular: Abnormal vision, blurred vision (3% to 9%)

Respiratory: Dyspnea, hyperventilation (3% to 9%)

Miscellaneous: Diaphoresis

<1%: Abnormal hearing, altered blood pressure increased/decreased, confusion, sensation of coldness, bradycardia, chest pain, generalized seizure, hiccups, hypertension, junctional tachycardia, shivering, somnolence, tachycardia, thick tongue, ventricular tachycardia, withdrawal syndrome

Drug Interactions

Avoid Concomitant Use There are no known interactions where it is recommended to avoid concomitant use.

Increased Effect/Toxicity There are no known significant interactions involving an increase in effect.

Decreased Effect

Flumazenil may decrease the levels/effects of: Hypnotics (Nonbenzodiazepine)

Dosage Forms Excipient information presented when available (limited, particularly for generics); consult specific product labeling.

Injection, solution: 0.1 mg/mL (5 mL, 10 mL)

Romazicon®: 0.1 mg/mL (5 mL, 10 mL) [contains edetate disodium]

◄ **References**

Mokhlesi B, Leikin JB, Murray P, et al, "Adult Toxicology in Critical Care. Part 11: Specific Poisonings," *Chest*, 2003, 123(3):897-922.

Trujillo MH, Guerrero J, Fragachan C, et al, "Pharmacologic Antidotes in Critical Care Medicine: A Practical Guide for Administration," *Crit Care Med*, 1998, 26(2):377-91.

◆ **Flumazenil Injection (Can)** *see* Flumazenil *on page 613*

◆ **Flumazenil Injection, USP (Can)** *see* Flumazenil *on page 613*

◆ **Fluohydrisone Acetate** *see* Fludrocortisone *on page 610*

◆ **Fluohydrocortisone Acetate** *see* Fludrocortisone *on page 610*

◆ **9α-Fluorohydrocortisone Acetate** *see* Fludrocortisone *on page 610*

FLUoxetine (floo OKS e teen)

Related Information
   Antidepressant Agents *on page 1660*
   Chronic Pain Management *on page 1546*

U.S. Brand Names Prozac®; Prozac® Weekly™; Sarafem®; Selfemra™

Canadian Brand Names Apo-Fluoxetine®; CO Fluoxetine; Dom-Fluoxetine; Fluoxetine; FXT 40; Gen-Fluoxetine; Mylan-Fluoxetine; Novo-Fluoxetine; Nu-Fluoxetine; PHL-Fluoxetine; PMS-Fluoxetine; PRO-Fluoxetine; Prozac®; ratio-Fluoxetine; Riva-Fluoxetine; Sandoz-Fluoxetine; ZYM-Fluoxetine

Index Terms Fluoxetine Hydrochloride

Pharmacologic Category Antidepressant, Selective Serotonin Reuptake Inhibitor

Use Treatment of major depressive disorder (MDD); treatment of binge-eating and vomiting in patients with moderate-to-severe bulimia nervosa; obsessive-compulsive disorder (OCD); premenstrual dysphoric disorder (PMDD); panic disorder with or without agoraphobia; in combination with olanzapine for treatment-resistant or bipolar I depression

Unlabeled/Investigational Use Selective mutism; treatment of mild dementia-associated agitation in nonpsychotic patients; post-traumatic stress disorder (PTSD)

Pharmacodynamics/Kinetics
   Onset of action: Depression: The onset of action is within a week; however, individual response varies greatly and full response may not be seen until 8-12 weeks after initiation of treatment.
   Absorption: Well absorbed; delayed 1-2 hours with weekly formulation
   Distribution: V_d: 12-43 L/kg
   Protein binding: 95% to albumin and alpha$_1$ glycoprotein
   Metabolism: Hepatic, via CYP2C19 and 2D6, to norfluoxetine (activity equal to fluoxetine)
   Half-life elimination: Adults:
      Parent drug: 1-3 days (acute), 4-6 days (chronic), 7.6 days (cirrhosis)
      Metabolite (norfluoxetine): 9.3 days (range: 4-16 days), 12 days (cirrhosis)
   Time to peak, serum: 6-8 hours
   Excretion: Urine (10% as norfluoxetine, 2.5% to 5% as fluoxetine)

   Note: Weekly formulation results in greater fluctuations between peak and trough concentrations of fluoxetine and norfluoxetine compared to once-daily dosing (24% daily/164% weekly; 17% daily/43% weekly, respectively). Trough concentrations are 76% lower for fluoxetine and 47% lower for norfluoxetine than the concentrations maintained by 20 mg once-daily dosing. Steady-state fluoxetine concentrations are ~50% lower following the once-weekly regimen compared to 20 mg once daily. Average steady-state concentrations of once-daily dosing were highest in children ages 6 to <13 (fluoxetine 171 ng/mL; norfluoxetine 195 ng/mL), followed by adolescents ages 13 to <18 (fluoxetine 86 ng/mL; norfluoxetine 113 ng/mL); concentrations were considered to be within the ranges reported in adults (fluoxetine 91-302 ng/mL; norfluoxetine 72-258 ng/mL).

   Dosage Oral: **Note:** Upon discontinuation of fluoxetine therapy, gradually taper dose. If intolerable symptoms occur following a dose reduction, consider resuming the previously prescribed dose and/or decrease dose at a more gradual rate.

Children:

Depression: 8-18 years: 10-20 mg/day; lower-weight children can be started at 10 mg/day, may increase to 20 mg/day after 1 week if needed

Obsessive-compulsive disorder: 7-17 years: Initial: 10 mg/day; may increase after 2 weeks if inadequate clinical response to 20 mg/day; further increases may be considered after several weeks to recommended range of 20-30 mg/day (lower weight children) or 20-60 mg/day (adolescents and higher weight children)

Selective mutism (unlabeled use): 5-18 years: Initial: 5-10 mg/day; titrate upwards as needed (usual maximum dose: 60 mg/day)

Adults: 20 mg/day in the morning; may increase after several weeks by 20 mg/day increments; maximum: 80 mg/day; doses >20 mg may be given once daily or divided twice daily. **Note:** Lower doses of 5-10 mg/day have been used for initial treatment.

Indication-specific dosing:

Bulimia nervosa: 60 mg/day

Depression: Initial: 20 mg/day; may increase after several weeks if inadequate response (maximum: 80 mg/day). Patients maintained on Prozac® 20 mg/day may be changed to Prozac® Weekly™ 90 mg/week, starting dose 7 days after the last 20 mg/day dose

Depression associated with bipolar disorder (in combination with olanzapine): Initial: 20 mg in the evening; adjust as tolerated to usual range of 20-50 mg/day. See "Note."

Obsessive-compulsive disorder: Initial: 20 mg/day; may increase after several weeks if inadequate response; recommended range: 20-60 mg/day (maximum: 80 mg/day)

Panic disorder: Initial: 10 mg/day; after 1 week, increase to 20 mg/day; may increase after several weeks; doses >60 mg/day have not been evaluated

Post-traumatic stress disorder (PTSD) (unlabeled use): 20-40 mg/day

Premenstrual dysphoric disorder (Sarafem®): 20 mg/day continuously, **or** 20 mg/day starting 14 days prior to menstruation and through first full day of menses (repeat with each cycle)

Treatment-resistant depression (in combination with olanzapine): Initial: 20 mg in the evening; adjust as tolerated to usual range of 20-50 mg/day. See "Note."

Note: When using individual components of fluoxetine with olanzapine rather than fixed dose combination product (Symbyax®), approximate dosage correspondence is as follows:

Olanzapine 2.5 mg + fluoxetine 20 mg = Symbyax® 3/25

Olanzapine 5 mg + fluoxetine 20 mg = Symbyax® 6/25

Olanzapine 12.5 mg + fluoxetine 20 mg = Symbyax® 12/25

Olanzapine 5 mg + fluoxetine 50 mg = Symbyax® 6/50

Olanzapine 12.5 mg + fluoxetine 50 mg = Symbyax® 12/50

Elderly: Depression: Some patients may require an initial dose of 10 mg/day with dosage increases of 10 and 20 mg every several weeks as tolerated; should not be taken at night unless patient experiences sedation

Dosing adjustment in renal impairment:

Single dose studies: Pharmacokinetics of fluoxetine and norfluoxetine were similar among subjects with all levels of impaired renal function, including anephric patients on chronic hemodialysis

Chronic administration: Additional accumulation of fluoxetine or norfluoxetine may occur in patients with severely impaired renal function

Hemodialysis: Not removed by hemodialysis; use of lower dose or less frequent dosing is not usually necessary.

Dosing adjustment in hepatic impairment: Elimination half-life of fluoxetine is prolonged in patients with hepatic impairment; a lower or less frequent dose of fluoxetine should be used in these patients

Cirrhosis patients: Administer a lower dose or less frequent dosing interval

Compensated cirrhosis without ascites: Administer 50% of normal dose

Anesthesia and Critical Care Concerns/Other Considerations

Clinical Pearls/Comments: SSRIs are relatively safe compared to other antidepressants in patients with cardiovascular disease.

◀ **Additional Information** Complete prescribing information for this medication should be consulted for additional detail.

Dosage Forms Excipient information presented when available (limited, particularly for generics); consult specific product labeling. **Note:** Strength expressed as base unless otherwise noted. [DSC] = Discontinued product

Capsule: 10 mg, 20 mg, 40 mg
  Prozac®: 10 mg, 20 mg, 40 mg
  Sarafem®: 10 mg, 20 mg [DSC]
  Selfemra™: 10 mg, 20 mg [contains soya lecithin]
Capsule, delayed release, enteric coated pellets:
  Prozac® Weekly™: 90 mg
Solution, oral: 20 mg/5 mL (5 mL, 120 mL) [contains ethanol 0.23% and benzoic acid; mint flavor]
  Prozac®: 20 mg/5 mL (120 mL) [contains ethanol 0.23% and benzoic acid; mint flavor]
Tablet: 10 mg, 20 mg
  Sarafem®: 10 mg, 20 mg

References
Mokhlesi B, Leikin JB, Murray P, et al, "Adult Toxicology in Critical Care: Part II: Specific Poisonings," *Chest*, 2003, 123(3):897-922.

◆ **Fluoxetine (Can)** *see* FLUoxetine *on page 616*
◆ **Fluoxetine Hydrochloride** *see* FLUoxetine *on page 616*

Flurazepam (flure AZ e pam)

Related Information
  Benzodiazepines *on page 1666*
U.S. Brand Names Dalmane® [DSC]
Canadian Brand Names Apo-Flurazepam®; Dalmane®; Som Pam
Index Terms Flurazepam Hydrochloride
Pharmacologic Category Hypnotic, Benzodiazepine
Restrictions C-IV
Use Short-term treatment of insomnia
Pharmacodynamics/Kinetics
  Onset of action: Hypnotic: 15-20 minutes
  Peak effect: 3-6 hours
  Duration: 7-8 hours
  Distribution: V_d: 3.4 L/kg
  Protein binding: ~97%
  Metabolism: Hepatic to N-desalkylflurazepam (active) and N-hydroxy-ethylflurazepam
  Half-life elimination:
    Flurazepam: 2.3 hours
    N-desalkylflurazepam:
      Adults: Single dose: 74-90 hours; Multiple doses: 111-113 hours
      Elderly (61-85 years): Single dose: 120-160 hours; Multiple doses: 126-158 hours
  Time to peak, serum:
    N-desalkylflurazepam: 10.6 hours (range: 7.6-13.6 hours)
    N-hydroxyethylflurazepam: ~1 hour
  Excretion: Urine: N-hydroxyethylflurazepam (22% to 55%); N-desalkylflurazepam (<1%)
Dosage Oral:
  Children: Insomnia:
    <15 years: Dose not established
    ≥15 years: 15 mg at bedtime
  Adults: Insomnia: 15-30 mg at bedtime
  Elderly: Insomnia: Oral: 15 mg at bedtime; avoid use if possible
Anesthesia and Critical Care Concerns/Other Considerations Chronic use of this agent may increase the perioperative benzodiazepine dose needed to achieve desired effect. Abrupt discontinuation after sustained use (generally >10 days) may cause withdrawal symptoms.

Additional Information Complete prescribing information for this medication should be consulted for additional detail.

Dosage Forms Excipient information presented when available (limited, particularly for generics); consult specific product labeling. [DSC] = Discontinued product

Capsule, as hydrochloride: 15 mg, 30 mg
  Dalmane®: 15 mg, 30 mg [DSC]

◆ **Flurazepam Hydrochloride** see Flurazepam on page 618

Flurbiprofen (flure BI proe fen)

Related Information
  Acetaminophen and NSAIDS, Dosing in the Management of Pain on page 1651
  Chronic Pain Management on page 1546
  Nonsteroidal Anti-Inflammatory Agents on page 1687
U.S. Brand Names Ocufen®
Canadian Brand Names Alti-Flurbiprofen; Ansaid®; Apo-Flurbiprofen®; Froben-SR®; Froben®; Novo-Flurprofen; Nu-Flurprofen; Ocufen®
Index Terms Flurbiprofen Sodium
Pharmacologic Category Nonsteroidal Anti-inflammatory Drug (NSAID), Ophthalmic; Nonsteroidal Anti-inflammatory Drug (NSAID), Oral
Use
  Oral: Treatment of rheumatoid arthritis and osteoarthritis
  Ophthalmic: Inhibition of intraoperative miosis
Pharmacodynamics/Kinetics
  Onset of action: ~1-2 hours
  Distribution: V_d: 0.12 L/kg
  Protein binding: 99%, primarily albumin
  Metabolism: Hepatic via CYP2C9; forms metabolites such as 4-hydroxy-flurbiprofen (inactive)
  Half-life elimination: 5.7 hours
  Time to peak: 1.5 hours
  Excretion: Urine (primarily as metabolites)
Dosage
  Oral:
    Rheumatoid arthritis and osteoarthritis: 200-300 mg/day in 2, 3, or 4 divided doses; do not administer more than 100 mg for any single dose; maximum: 300 mg/day
    Dental: Management of postoperative pain: 100 mg every 12 hours
  Ophthalmic: Instill 1 drop every 30 minutes, beginning 2 hours prior to surgery (total of 4 drops in each affected eye)
  Dosage adjustment in renal impairment: Not recommended in patients with advanced renal disease
Anesthesia and Critical Care Concerns/Other Considerations The 2002 ACCM/SCCM guidelines for analgesia (critically-ill adult) suggest that NSAIDs may be used in combination with opioids in select patients for pain management. Concern about adverse events (increased risk of renal dysfunction, altered platelet function, and gastrointestinal irritation) limits its use in patients who have other underlying risks for these events.

In short-term use, NSAIDs vary considerably in their effect on blood pressure. When NSAIDs are used in patients with hypertension, appropriate monitoring of blood pressure responses should be completed and the duration of therapy, when possible, kept short. The use of NSAIDs in the treatment of patients with congestive heart failure may be associated with an increased risk for fluid accumulation and edema; may precipitate renal failure in dehydrated patients.
Additional Information Complete prescribing information for this medication should be consulted for additional detail.
Dosage Forms Excipient information presented when available (limited, particularly for generics); consult specific product labeling.
  Solution, ophthalmic, as sodium: 0.03% (2.5 mL)
    Ocufen®: 0.03% (2.5 mL)
  Tablet: 50 mg, 100 mg

◆ **Flurbiprofen Sodium** *see* Flurbiprofen *on page 619*

Fluticasone (floo TIK a sone)

Related Information
Asthma *on page 1728*
Corticosteroids *on page 1676*

U.S. Brand Names Cutivate®; Flonase®; Flovent® Diskus®; Flovent® HFA; Veramyst®

Canadian Brand Names Apo-Fluticasone; Avamys™; Cutivate™; Flonase®; Flovent® Diskus®; Flovent® HFA; ratio-Fluticasone

Index Terms Fluticasone Furoate; Fluticasone Propionate

Pharmacologic Category Corticosteroid, Inhalant (Oral); Corticosteroid, Nasal; Corticosteroid, Topical

Use
Oral inhalation: Maintenance treatment of asthma as prophylactic therapy; also indicated for patients requiring oral corticosteroid therapy for asthma to assist in total discontinuation or reduction of total oral dose

Intranasal:
Flonase®: Management of seasonal and perennial allergic rhinitis and nonallergic rhinitis
Veramyst®: Management of seasonal and perennial allergic rhinitis
Avamys™ [CAN]: Management of seasonal allergic rhinitis

Topical: Relief of inflammation and pruritus associated with corticosteroid-responsive dermatoses; atopic dermatitis

Pharmacodynamics/Kinetics
Onset of action: Intranasal: Maximal benefit may take several days
Flovent® HFA, Flovent® Diskus®: Maximal benefit may take 1-2 weeks or longer

Absorption:
Topical cream: 5% (increased with inflammation)
Oral inhalation: Absorbed systemically (Flovent® Diskus®: ~18%) primarily via lungs, minimal GI absorption (<1%) due to presystemic metabolism

Distribution: Propionate: 4.2 L/kg

Protein binding: 91% to >99%

Metabolism: Hepatic via CYP3A4 to 17β-carboxylic acid (negligible activity)

Bioavailability: Nasal: ≤2%; Oral inhalation: (~18% to 21%)

Excretion: Feces (as parent drug and metabolites); urine (<5% as metabolites)

Dosage
Children:

Asthma: Inhalation, oral:
Flovent® HFA:
Children 4-11 years: 88 mcg twice daily
Children ≥12 years: Refer to adult dosing.
NIH Asthma Guidelines (NIH, 2007) (administer in divided doses twice daily):
"Low" dose:
0-4 years: 176 mcg/day
5-11 years: 88-176 mcg/day
≥12 years: 88-264 mcg/day
"Medium" dose:
0-4 years: >176-352 mcg/day
5-11 years: >176-352 mcg/day
≥12 years: >264-440 mcg/day
"High" dose:
0-4 years: >352 mcg/day
5-11 years: >352 mcg/day
≥12 years: >440 mcg/day
Flovent® Diskus® *(U.S. labeling)*:
Children 4-11 years: Usual starting dose: 50 mcg twice daily; may increase to 100 mcg twice daily in patients not adequately controlled after 2 weeks of therapy. Higher starting doses may be considered in patients with poorer asthma control or those requiring high ranges of inhaled corticosteroids.

Titrate to the lowest effective dose once asthma stability is achieved (maximum dose: 100 mcg twice daily)

Children >11 years: Refer to adult dosing.

Flovent® Diskus® *(Canadian labeling)*:

Children 4-16 years: Usual starting dose: 50-100 mcg twice daily; may increase to 200 mcg twice daily in patients not adequately controlled; titrate to the lowest effective dose once asthma stability is achieved

Children ≥16 years: Refer to adult dosing.

Corticosteroid-responsive dermatoses: Topical: Children ≥3 months: Cream: Apply sparingly to affected area twice daily. If no improvement is seen within 2 weeks, reassessment of diagnosis may be necessary. **Note:** Safety and efficacy of treatment >4 weeks duration have not been established.

Atopic dermatitis: Topical:

Children ≥3 months: Cream: Apply sparingly to affected area 1-2 times/day. If no improvement is seen within 2 weeks, reassessment of diagnosis may be necessary.

Children ≥1 year: Lotion: Apply sparingly to affected area once daily

Note: Safety and efficacy of treatment >4 weeks duration have not been established.

Rhinitis: Intranasal:

Flonase® (fluticasone propionate): Children ≥4 years and Adolescents: Initial: 1 spray (50 mcg/spray) per nostril once daily; patients not adequately responding or patients with more severe symptoms may use 2 sprays (100 mcg) per nostril. Depending on response, dosage may be reduced to 100 mcg daily. Total daily dosage should not exceed 2 sprays in each nostril (200 mcg)/day. Dosing should be at regular intervals.

Veramyst® (fluticasone furoate):

Children 2-11 years: Initial: 1 spray (27.5 mcg/spray) per nostril once daily (55 mcg/day); patients not adequately responding may use 2 sprays per nostril once daily (110 mcg/day). Once symptoms are controlled, dosage may be reduced to 55 mcg once daily. Total daily dosage should not exceed 2 sprays in each nostril (110 mcg)/day.

Children ≥12 years and Adolescents: Initial: 2 sprays (27.5 mcg/spray) per nostril once daily (110 mcg/day). Once symptoms are controlled, dosage may be reduced to 1 spray per nostril once daily (55 mcg/day). Total daily dosage should not exceed 2 sprays in each nostril (110 mcg)/day.

Avamys™ [CAN] (fluticasone furoate): Children ≥12 years: 2 sprays (27.5 mcg/spray) in each nostril once daily (110 mcg/day). Total daily dosage should not exceed 2 sprays in each nostril (110 mcg)/day.

Adults:

Asthma: Inhalation, oral: **Note:** Titrate to the lowest effective dose once asthma stability is achieved

Flovent® HFA: Manufacturers labeling: Dosing based on previous therapy

Bronchodilator alone: Recommended starting dose: 88 mcg twice daily; highest recommended dose: 440 mcg twice daily

Inhaled corticosteroids: Recommended starting dose: 88-220 mcg twice daily; highest recommended dose: 440 mcg twice daily; a higher starting dose may be considered in patients previously requiring higher doses of inhaled corticosteroids

Oral corticosteroids: Recommended starting dose: 440 mcg twice daily

Highest recommended dose: 880 mcg twice daily; starting dose is patient dependent. In patients on chronic oral corticosteroids therapy, reduce prednisone dose no faster than 2.5-5 mg/day on a weekly basis; begin taper after 1 week of fluticasone therapy.

NIH Asthma Guidelines (NIH, 2007) (administer in divided doses twice daily):

"Low" dose: 88-264 mcg/day

"Medium" dose: >264-440 mcg/day

"High" dose: >440 mcg/day

Flovent® Diskus® *(U.S. labeling)*: **Note:** May increase dose after 2 weeks of therapy in patients not adequately controlled. Higher starting doses may be considered in patients with poorer asthma control or those requiring high ranges of inhaled corticosteroids. Titrate to the lowest effective dose once asthma stability is achieved.

◀ Bronchodilator alone: Recommended starting dose: 100 mcg twice daily; maximum recommended dose: 500 mcg twice daily

Inhaled corticosteroids: Recommended starting dose: 100-250 mcg twice daily; maximum recommended dose: 500 mcg twice daily

Oral corticosteroids: Recommended starting dose: 500-1000 mcg twice daily; maximum recommended dose: 1000 mcg twice daily. Starting dose is patient dependent. In patients on chronic oral corticosteroids therapy, reduce prednisone dose no faster than 2.5 mg/day on a weekly basis; begin taper after 1 week of fluticasone therapy.

Flovent® Diskus® *(Canadian labeling)*:

Mild asthma: 100-250 mcg twice daily

Moderate asthma: 250-500 mcg twice daily

Severe asthma: 500 mcg twice daily; may increase to 1000 mcg twice daily in very severe patients requiring high doses of corticosteroids

Corticosteroid-responsive dermatoses: Topical: Cream, lotion, ointment: Apply sparingly to affected area twice daily. If no improvement is seen within 2 weeks, reassessment of diagnosis may be necessary.

Atopic dermatitis: Topical: Cream, lotion: Apply sparingly to affected area once or twice daily. If no improvement is seen within 2 weeks, reassessment of diagnosis may be necessary.

Rhinitis: Intranasal:

Flonase® (fluticasone propionate): Initial: 2 sprays (50 mcg/spray) per nostril once daily; may also be divided into 100 mcg twice a day. After the first few days, dosage may be reduced to 1 spray per nostril once daily for maintenance therapy.

Veramyst® (fluticasone furoate): Initial: 2 sprays (27.5 mcg/spray) per nostril once daily (110 mcg/day). Once symptoms are controlled, may reduce dosage to 1 spray per nostril once daily (55 mcg/day) for maintenance therapy.

Avamys™ [CAN] (fluticasone furoate): 2 sprays (27.5 mcg/spray) in each nostril once daily (110 mcg/day). Total daily dosage should not exceed 2 sprays in each nostril (110 mcg)/day.

Elderly: No differences in safety have been observed in the elderly when compared to younger patients. Based on current data, no dosage adjustment is needed based on age.

Dosage adjustment in hepatic impairment: Fluticasone is primarily cleared in the liver. Fluticasone plasma levels may be increased in patients with hepatic impairment, use with caution; monitor.

Anesthesia and Critical Care Concerns/Other Considerations

Surgery: For patients who have received oral systemic corticosteroids during the past 6 months and for selected patients on long-term, high-dose, inhaled corticosteroid (ICS), give stress doses of hydrocortisone intravenously during the surgical period and reduce the dose rapidly within 24 hours after surgery (Expert Panel Report 3, 2007). Clinically important adrenal suppression has been reported in patients receiving high doses of an ICS, particularly children.

Additional Information Complete prescribing information for this medication should be consulted for additional detail.

Dosage Forms Excipient information presented when available (limited, particularly for generics); consult specific product labeling. [CAN] = Canadian brand name

Aerosol for oral inhalation, as propionate [CFC free]:

Flovent® HFA: 44 mcg/inhalation (10.6 g) [120 metered actuations]

Flovent® HFA: 110 mcg/inhalation (12 g) [120 metered actuations]

Flovent® HFA: 220 mcg/inhalation (12 g) [120 metered actuations]

Cream, as propionate: 0.05% (15 g, 30 g, 60 g)

Cutivate®: 0.05% (30 g, 60 g)

Lotion, as propionate:

Cutivate®: 0.05% (120 mL)

Ointment, as propionate: 0.005% (15 g, 30 g, 60 g)

Cutivate®: 0.005% (30 g, 60 g)

Powder for oral inhalation, as propionate:

Flovent® Diskus® [U.S.]: 50 mcg (60s) [contains lactose; prefilled blister pack]

Flovent® Diskus® [CAN]: 50 mcg (28s, 60s) [contains lactose; prefilled blister pack] [not available in the U.S.]

Flovent® Diskus® [CAN]: 100 mcg (28s, 60s) [contains lactose; prefilled blister pack] [not available in the U.S.]

Flovent® Diskus® [CAN]: 250 mcg (28s, 60s) [contains lactose; prefilled blister pack] [not available in the U.S.]

Flovent® Diskus® [CAN]: 500 mcg (28s, 60s) [contains lactose; prefilled blister pack] [not available in the U.S.]

Suspension, intranasal, as furoate [spray]:

Avamys™ [CAN]: 27.5 mcg/inhalation (4.5 g) [30 metered actuations; contains benzalkonium chloride]; (10 g) [120 metered actuations; contains benzalkonium chloride] [not available in the U.S.]

Veramyst®: 27.5 mcg/inhalation (10 g) [120 metered actuations; contains benzalkonium chloride]

Suspension, intranasal, as propionate [spray]: 50 mcg/inhalation (16 g) [120 metered actuations]

Flonase®: 50 mcg/inhalation (16 g) [120 metered actuations; contains benzalkonium chloride]

References

Expert Panel Report 3, "Guidelines for the Diagnosis and Management of Asthma," *Clinical Practice Guidelines*, National Institutes of Health, National Heart, Lung, and Blood Institute, NIH Publication No. 08-4051, prepublication 2007. Available at http://www.nhlbi.nih.gov/guidelines/asthma/asthgdln.htm

Goedert JJ, Vitale F, Lauria C, et al, "Risk Factors for Classical Kaposi's Sarcoma," *J Natl Cancer Inst*, 2002, 94(22):1712-8.

Todd GR, Acerini CL, Buck JJ, et al, "Acute Adrenal Crisis in Asthmatics Treated With High-Dose Fluticasone Propionate," *Eur Respir J*, 2002, 19(6):1207-9.

Todd GR, Acerini CL, Ross-Russell R, et al, "Survey of Adrenal Crisis Associated With Inhaled Corticosteroids in the United Kingdom," *Arch Dis Child*, 2002, 87(6):457-61.

◆ **Fluticasone Furoate** *see* Fluticasone *on page 620*

◆ **Fluticasone Propionate** *see* Fluticasone *on page 620*

Fluvastatin (FLOO va sta tin)

Related Information

Hyperlipidemia Management *on page 1747*
Preoperative Evaluation of the Cardiac Patient for Noncardiac Surgery *on page 1598*

U.S. Brand Names Lescol®; Lescol® XL

Canadian Brand Names Lescol®; Lescol® XL

Pharmacologic Category Antilipemic Agent, HMG-CoA Reductase Inhibitor

Use To be used as a component of multiple risk factor intervention in patients at risk for atherosclerosis vascular disease due to hypercholesterolemia

Adjunct to dietary therapy to reduce elevated total cholesterol (total-C), LDL-C, triglyceride, and apolipoprotein B (apo-B) levels and to increase HDL-C in primary hypercholesterolemia and mixed dyslipidemia (Fredrickson types IIa and IIb); to slow the progression of coronary atherosclerosis in patients with coronary heart disease; reduce risk of coronary revascularization procedures in patients with coronary heart disease

Pharmacodynamics/Kinetics

Onset of action: Peak effect: Maximal LDL-C reductions achieved within 4 weeks

Distribution: V_d: 0.35 L/kg

Protein binding: >98%

Metabolism: To inactive and active metabolites (oxidative metabolism via CYP2C9 [75%], 2C8 [~5%], and 3A4 [~20%] isoenzymes); active forms do not circulate systemically; extensive (saturable) first-pass hepatic extraction

Bioavailability: Absolute: Capsule: 24%; Extended release tablet: 29%

Half-life elimination: Capsule: <3 hours; Extended release tablet: 9 hours

Time to peak: Capsule: 1 hour; Extended release tablet: 3 hours

Excretion: Feces (90%): urine (5%)

◄ **Dosage**

Adolescents 10-16 years: Oral: Heterozygous familial hypercholesterolemia: Initial: 20 mg once daily; may increase every 6 weeks based on tolerability and response to a maximum recommended dose of 80 mg/day, given in 2 divided doses (immediate release capsule) or as a single daily dose (extended release tablet)

Note: Indicated only for adjunctive therapy when diet alone cannot reduce LDL-C below 190 mg/dL, or 160 mg/dL (with cardiovascular risk factors). Female patients must be 1 year postmenarche.

Adults: Oral:

Patients requiring ≥25% decrease in LDL-C: 40 mg capsule once daily in the evening, 80 mg extended release tablet once daily (anytime), or 40 mg capsule twice daily

Patients requiring <25% decrease in LDL-C: Initial: 20 mg capsule once daily in the evening; may increase based on tolerability and response to a maximum recommended dose of 80 mg/day, given in 2 divided doses (immediate release capsule) or as a single daily dose (extended release tablet)

Dosage adjustment in renal impairment: Less than 6% excreted renally; no dosage adjustment needed with mild-to-moderate renal impairment; use with caution in severe impairment

Dosage adjustment in hepatic impairment: Levels may accumulate in patients with liver disease (increased AUC and C_{max}); use caution with severe hepatic impairment or heavy ethanol ingestion; contraindicated in active liver disease or unexplained transaminase elevations; decrease dose and monitor effects carefully in patients with hepatic insufficiency

Elderly: No dosage adjustment necessary based on age

Anesthesia and Critical Care Concerns/Other Considerations

Clinical Pearls/Comments: Myopathy: Currently-marketed HMG-CoA reductase inhibitors appear to have a similar potential for causing myopathy. Incidence of severe myopathy is about 0.08% to 0.09%. The factors that increase risk include advanced age (especially >80 years), gender (occurs in women more frequently than men), small body frame, frailty, multisystem disease (eg, chronic renal insufficiency especially due to diabetes), multiple medications, and drug interactions (use with caution or avoid).

Based on current research and clinical guidelines (Fleisher, 2007), HMG-CoA reductase inhibitors should be continued in the perioperative period. Postoperative discontinuation of statin therapy is associated with an increased risk of cardiac morbidity and mortality.

Additional Information Complete prescribing information for this medication should be consulted for additional detail.

Dosage Forms Excipient information presented when available (limited, particularly for generics); consult specific product labeling.

Capsule (Lescol®): 20 mg, 40 mg

Tablet, extended release (Lescol® XL): 80 mg

References

de Denus S and Spinler SA, "Early Statin Therapy for Acute Coronary Syndromes," *Ann Pharmacother*, 2002, 36(11):1749-58.

"Executive Summary of The Third Report of The National Cholesterol Education Program (NCEP) Expert Panel on Detection, Evaluation, and Treatment of High Blood Cholesterol in Adults (Adult Treatment Panel III)," *JAMA*, 2001, 285(19):2486-97.

Fleisher LA, Beckman JA, Brown KA, et al, "ACC/AHA 2007 Guidelines on Perioperative Cardiovascular Evaluation and Care for Noncardiac Surgery: A Report of the American College of Cardiology/American Heart Association Task Force on Practice Guidelines (Writing Committee to Revise the 2002 Guidelines on Perioperative Cardiovascular Evaluation for Noncardiac Surgery) Developed in Collaboration With the American Society of Echocardiography, American Society of Nuclear Cardiology, Heart Rhythm Society, Society of Cardiovascular Anesthesiologists, Society for Cardiovascular Angiography and Interventions, Society for Vascular Medicine and Biology, and Society for Vascular Surgery," *J Am Coll Cardiol*, 2007, 50(17):e159-241.

Fonarow GC, French WJ, Parsons LS, et al, "Use of Lipid-Lowering Medications at Discharge in Patients With Acute Myocardial Infarction: Data From the National Registry of Myocardial Infarction 3," *Circulation*, 2001, 103(1):38-44.

Heeschen C, Hamm CW, Laufs U, et al, "Withdrawal of Statins Increases Event Rates in Patients With Acute Coronary Syndromes," *Circulation*, 2002, 105(12):1446-52.

Koren MJ, Smith DG, Hunninghake DB, et al, "The Cost of Reaching National Cholesterol Education Program (NCEP) Goals in Hypercholesterolaemic Patients. A Comparison of Atorvastatin, Simvastatin, Lovastatin, and Fluvastatin," *Pharmacoeconomics*, 1998, 14(1):59-70.

LaRosa JC, Grundy SM, Waters DD, et al, "Intensive Lipid Lowering With Atorvastatin in Patients With Stable Coronary Disease," *N Engl J Med*, 2005, 352(14):1425-35.

LeManach Y, Godet G, Coriat P, et al, "The Impact of Postoperative Discontinuation or Continuation of Chronic Statin Therapy on Cardiac Outcome After Major Vascular Surgery," *Anesth Analg*, 2007, 104(6):1326-33.

"MRC/BHF Heart Protection Study of Cholesterol Lowering With Simvastatin in 20,536 High-Risk Individuals: A Randomised Placebo-Controlled Trial. Heart Protection Study Collaborative Group," *Lancet*, 2002, 360(9326):7-22.

Pasternak RC, Smith SC Jr, Bairey-Merz CN, et al, "ACC/AHA/NHLBI Clinical Advisory on the Use and Safety of Statins," *Stroke*, 2002, 33(9):2337-41. Available at: http://www.acc.org/clinical/alerts/statins_june02.htm. Accessed June 18, 2003.

Pearson TA, Mensah GA, Alexander RW, et al, "Markers of Inflammation and Cardiovascular Disease: Application to Clinical and Public Health Practice: A Statement for Healthcare Professionals From the Centers for Disease Control and Prevention and the American Heart Association," *Circulation*, 2003, 107(3):499-511.

Phillips BG, Yim JM, Brown EJ Jr, et al, "Pharmacologic Profile of Survivors of Acute Myocardial Infarction at United States Academic Hospitals," *Am Heart J*, 1996, 131(5):872-8.

Poldermans D, Bax JJ, Kertai MD, et al, "Statins Are Associated With a Reduced Incidence of Perioperative Mortality in Patients Undergoing Major Noncardiac Vascular Surgery," *Circulation*, 2003, 107(14):1848-51.

Ridker PM, Danielson E, Fonseca FAH, et al, "Rosuvastatin to Prevent Vascular Events in Men and Women With Elevated C-Reactive Protein," *N Engl J Med*, 2008, 359(21):2195-207.

Sever PS, Dahlof B, Poulter NR, et al, "Prevention of Coronary and Stroke Events With Atorvastatin in Hypertensive Patients Who Have Average or Lower-Than-Average Cholesterol Concentrations, in the Anglo-Scandinavian Cardiac Outcomes Trial - Lipid Lowering Arm (ASCOT-LLA): A Multicentre Randomised Controlled Trial," *Lancet*, 2003, 361(9364):1149-58.

Shepherd J, Cobbe SM, Ford I, et al, "Prevention of Coronary Heart Disease With Pravastatin in Men With Hypercholesterolemia. West of Scotland Coronary Prevention Study Group," *N Engl J Med*, 1995, 333(20):1301-7.

◆ **Focalin®** *see* Dexmethylphenidate *on page 401*

◆ **Focalin® XR** *see* Dexmethylphenidate *on page 401*

◆ **Folinic Acid (error prone synonym)** *see* Leucovorin Calcium *on page 812*

Fomepizole (foe ME pi zole)

Medication Safety Issues
Sound-alike/look-alike issues:
Fomepizole may be confused with omeprazole

U.S. Brand Names Antizol®

Index Terms 4-Methylpyrazole; 4-MP

Pharmacologic Category Antidote

Generic Available Yes

Use Treatment of methanol or ethylene glycol poisoning alone or in combination with hemodialysis

Unlabeled/Investigational Use Pediatric administration; treatment of propylene glycol toxicity

Mechanism of Action Fomepizole competitively inhibits alcohol dehydrogenase, an enzyme which catalyzes the metabolism of ethanol, ethylene glycol, and methanol to their toxic metabolites. Ethylene glycol is metabolized to glycoaldehyde, then oxidized to glycolate, glyoxylate, and oxalate. Glycolate and oxalate are responsible for metabolic acidosis and renal damage. Methanol is metabolized to formaldehyde, then oxidized to formic acid. Formic acid is responsible for metabolic acidosis and visual disturbances.

Pharmacodynamics/Kinetics
Onset of effect: Peak effect: Maximum: 1.5-2 hours

Absorption: Oral: Readily absorbed

Distribution: V_d: 0.6-1.02 L/kg; rapidly into total body water

Protein binding: Negligible

Metabolism: Hepatic to 4-carboxypyrazole (80% to 85% of dose), 4-hydroxymethylpyrazole, and their N-glucuronide conjugates; following multiple doses, induces its own metabolism via CYP oxidases after 30-40 hours

Half-life elimination: Has not been calculated; varies with dose

Excretion: Urine (1% to 3.5% as unchanged drug and metabolites)

Dosage Note: Fomepizole therapy should begin immediately upon suspicion of ethylene glycol or methanol ingestion.

◄ Children (unlabeled use) and Adults: Ethylene glycol and methanol toxicity: I.V.: A loading dose of 15 mg/kg should be administered, followed by doses of 10 mg/kg every 12 hours for 4 doses, then 15 mg/kg every 12 hours thereafter until ethylene glycol levels have been reduced <20 mg/dL and patient is asymptomatic with normal pH

Dosage adjustment in renal impairment: I.V.: The manufacturer provides the following dosage recommendations:
Dose at the beginning of hemodialysis:
If <6 hours since last fomepizole dose: Do not administer dose
If ≥6 hours since last fomepizole dose: Administer next scheduled dose
Dosing during hemodialysis: Dose every 4 hours
Dosing at the time hemodialysis is complete, based on time between last dose and the end of hemodialysis:
<1 hour: Do not administer dose at the end of hemodialysis
1-3 hours: Administer 1/2 of next scheduled dose
>3 hours: Administer next scheduled dose
Maintenance dose when off hemodialysis: Give next scheduled dose 12 hours from last dose administered.
Alternatively, a loading dose of 10-20 mg/kg followed by 1-1.5 mg/kg/hour continuous infusion during hemodialysis has been described in case reports (Jobard, 1996).

Dosage adjustment in hepatic impairment: Fomepizole is metabolized in the liver; specific dosage adjustments have not been determined in patients with hepatic impairment
Stability Store at controlled room temperature, 20°C to 25°C (68°F to 77°F); fomepizole solidifies at temperatures <25°C (77°F). If solution becomes solid in the vial, it be should be carefully warmed by running the vial under warm water or by holding in the hand. Solidification does not affect the efficacy, safety, or stability of the drug.
Prior to administration, dilute in at least 100 mL 0.9% sodium chloride or dextrose 5% water for injection; diluted solution is stable for at least 24 hours when stored refrigerated or at room temperature. Although, it is chemically and physically stable when diluted as recommended, sterile precautions should be observed because diluents generally do not contain preservatives.
Administration The appropriate dose of fomepizole should be drawn from the vial with a syringe and injected into at least 100 mL of sterile 0.9% sodium chloride injection or dextrose 5% injection. All doses should be administered as a slow intravenous infusion (IVPB) over 30 minutes.
Monitoring Parameters Fomepizole plasma levels should be monitored; response to fomepizole; monitor plasma/urinary ethylene glycol or methanol levels, urinary oxalate (ethylene glycol), plasma/urinary osmolality, renal/hepatic function, serum electrolytes, arterial blood gases; anion and osmolar gaps, resolution of clinical signs and symptoms of ethylene glycol or methanol intoxication
Reference Range The manufacturer recommends concentrations 100-300 µmol/L (8.2-24.6 mg/L) to achieve enzyme inhibition of alcohol dehydrogenase; according to practice guidelines, serum fomepizole concentrations of ≥0.8 mg/L provide constant inhibition of alcohol dehydrogenase
Anesthesia and Critical Care Concerns/Other Considerations
Clinical Pearls/Comments: Alternate therapies, including ethanol and hemodialysis, are difficult to use in children. Fomepizole's affinity for alcohol dehydrogenase is 8000 times greater than ethanol.
Pregnancy Risk Factor C
Contraindications Hypersensitivity to fomepizole, other pyrazoles, or any component of the formulation
Warnings/Precautions Should not be given undiluted or by bolus injection. Fomepizole is metabolized in the liver and excreted in the urine; use caution with hepatic or renal impairment. Hemodialysis should be used in patients with renal failure, significant or worsening metabolic acidosis, or ethylene glycol/methanol levels ≥50 mg/dL. Pediatric administration is not FDA approved; however, safe and efficacious use in this patient population for ethylene glycol and methanol intoxication has been reported (Baum, 2000; Benitez, 2000; Boyer, 2001;

Brown, 2001; De Brabander, 2005; Detaille, 2004; Fisher, 1998); consider consultation with a clinical toxicologist or poison control center.

Adverse Reactions

>10%:

Central nervous system: Headache (14%)

Gastrointestinal: Nausea (11%)

1% to 10% (≤3% unless otherwise noted):

Cardiovascular: Bradycardia, facial flush, hypotension, shock, tachycardia

Central nervous system: Dizziness (6%), drowsiness increased (6%), agitation, anxiety, fever, lightheadedness, seizure, vertigo

Dermatologic: Rash

Endocrine & metabolic: Liver function tests increased

Gastrointestinal: Bad/metallic taste (6%), abdominal pain, appetite decreased, diarrhea, heartburn, vomiting

Hematologic: Anemia, disseminated intravascular coagulation (DIC), eosinophilia, lymphangitis

Local: Application site reaction, injection site inflammation, pain during injection, phlebitis

Neuromuscular & skeletal: Backache

Ocular: Nystagmus, transient blurred vision, visual disturbances

Renal: Anuria

Respiratory: Abnormal smell, hiccups, pharyngitis

Miscellaneous: Multiorgan failure, speech disturbances

<1% (Limited to important or life-threatening): Mild allergic reactions (mild rash, eosinophilia)

Drug Interactions

Avoid Concomitant Use There are no known interactions where it is recommended to avoid concomitant use.

Increased Effect/Toxicity There are no known significant interactions involving an increase in effect.

Decreased Effect There are no known significant interactions involving a decrease in effect.

Ethanol/Nutrition/Herb Interactions Ethanol: Ethanol decreases the rate of fomepizole elimination by ~50%; conversely, fomepizole decreases the rate of elimination of ethanol by ~40%.

Dosage Forms Excipient information presented when available (limited, particularly for generics); consult specific product labeling.

Injection, solution [preservative free]: 1 g/mL (1.5 mL)

Antizol®: 1 g/mL (1.5 mL)

References

Barceloux DG, Bond GR, Krenzelok EP, et al, "American Academy of Clinical Toxicology Practice Guidelines on the Treatment of Methanol Poisoning," *J Toxicol Clin Toxicol*, 2002, 40(4):415-46.

Barceloux DG, Krenzelok EP, Olson K, et al, "American Academy of Clinical Toxicology Practice Guidelines on the Treatment of Ethylene Glycol Poisoning. Ad Hoc Committee," *J Toxicol Clin Toxicol*, 1999, 37(5):537-60.

Brent J, McMartin K, Phillips S, et al, "Fomepizole for the Treatment of Methanol Poisoning," *N Engl J Med*, 2001, 344(6):424-9.

Mokhlesi B, Leikin JB, Murray P, et al, "Adult Toxicology in Critical Care. Part II: Specific Poisonings," *Chest*, 2003, 123(3):897-922.

Fondaparinux (fon da PARE i nuks)

Medication Safety Issues

High alert medication: The Institute for Safe Medication Practices (ISMP) includes this medication among its list of drugs which have a heightened risk of causing significant patient harm when used in error.

U.S. Brand Names Arixtra®

Canadian Brand Names Arixtra®

Index Terms Fondaparinux Sodium

Pharmacologic Category Factor Xa Inhibitor

Generic Available No

Use Prophylaxis of deep vein thrombosis (DVT) in patients undergoing surgery for hip replacement, knee replacement, hip fracture (including extended prophylaxis following hip fracture surgery), or abdominal surgery (in patients at risk for thromboembolic complications); treatment of acute pulmonary embolism (PE); treatment of acute DVT without PE

Note: Additional Canadian approvals (not approved in U.S.): Unstable angina or non-ST segment elevation myocardial infarction (UA/NSTEMI) for the prevention of death and subsequent MI; ST segment elevation MI (STEMI) for the prevention of death and myocardial reinfarction

Unlabeled/Investigational Use Prophylaxis of DVT in patients with a history of heparin-induced thrombocytopenia (HIT)

Mechanism of Action Fondaparinux is a synthetic pentasaccharide that causes an antithrombin III-mediated selective inhibition of factor Xa. Neutralization of factor Xa interrupts the blood coagulation cascade and inhibits thrombin formation and thrombus development.

Pharmacodynamics/Kinetics

Absorption: SubQ: Rapid and complete

Distribution: V_d: 7-11 L; mainly in blood

Protein binding: ≥94% to antithrombin III

Bioavailability: SubQ: 100%

Half-life elimination: 17-21 hours; prolonged with renal impairment

Time to peak: SubQ: 2-3 hours

Excretion: Urine (~77%, unchanged drug)

Dosage SubQ: Adults:

DVT prophylaxis: Adults ≥50 kg: 2.5 mg once daily. **Note:** Initiate dose after hemostasis has been established, 6-8 hours postoperatively.

DVT prophylaxis with history of HIT (unlabeled use): 2.5 mg once daily

Usual duration: 5-9 days (up to 10 days following abdominal surgery or up to 11 days following hip replacement or knee replacement)

Extended prophylaxis is recommended following hip fracture surgery (has been tolerated for up to 32 days total).

Acute DVT/PE treatment: **Note:** Start warfarin on the first treatment day and continue fondaparinux until INR is between 2 and 3 (usually 5-7 days) (Hirsh, 2008):

<50 kg: 5 mg once daily

50-100 kg: 7.5 mg once daily

>100 kg: 10 mg once daily

Usual duration: 5-9 days (has been administered up to 26 days)

Canadian labeling only: Adults:

UA/NSTEMI: SubQ: 2.5 mg once daily; initiate as soon as possible after diagnosis; treat for up to 8 days or until hospital discharge.

STEMI: I.V.: 2.5 mg once; subsequent doses: SubQ: 2.5 mg once daily; treat for up to 8 days or until hospital discharge

Dosage adjustment in renal impairment:

Cl_{cr} 30-50 mL/minute: Use caution

Cl_{cr} <30 mL/minute: Contraindicated

Dosage adjustment in hepatic impairment:

Mild-to-moderate impairment: Dosage adjustment not required; monitor for signs of bleeding

Severe impairment: No data

Stability Store at 25°C (77°F); excursions permitted to 15°C to 30°C (59°F to 86°F).

Canadian labeling: For I.V. administration: May mix with 25 mL or 50 mL NS; manufacturer recommends immediate use once diluted in NS, but is stable for up to 24 hours at 15°C to 30°C (59°F to 86°F).

Administration Do **not** administer I.M.; for SubQ administration only. Do not mix with other injections or infusions. Do not expel air bubble from syringe before injection. Administer according to recommended regimen; early initiation (before 6 hours after surgery) has been associated with increased bleeding.

To convert from I.V. unfractionated heparin (UFH) infusion to SubQ fondaparinux (Nutescu, 2007): Calculate specific dose for fondaparinux based on indication, discontinue UFH, and begin fondaparinux within 1 hour

To convert from SubQ fondaparinux to I.V. UFH infusion (Nutescu, 2007): Discontinue fondaparinux; calculate specific dose for I.V. UFH infusion based on indication; omit heparin bolus/loading dose

For subQ fondaparinux dosed every 24 hours: Start I.V. UFH infusion 22-23 hours after last dose of fondaparinux

Canadian labeling only: STEMI patients: I.V. push or mixed in 25-50 mL of NS and infused over 2 minutes. Flush tubing with NS after infusion to ensure complete administration of fondaparinux. Infusion bag should not be mixed with other agents.

Monitoring Parameters Periodic monitoring of CBC, serum creatinine, occult blood testing of stools recommended. Anti-Xa activity of fondaparinux can be measured by the assay if fondaparinux is used as the calibrator. PT and aPTT are insensitive measures of fondaparinux activity. If unexpected changes in coagulation parameters or major bleeding occur, discontinue fondaparinux (elevated aPTT associated with bleeding events have been reported in postmarketing data).

Pregnancy Risk Factor B

Contraindications Hypersensitivity to fondaparinux or any component of the formulation; severe renal impairment (Cl_{cr} <30 mL/minute); body weight <50 kg (prophylaxis); active major bleeding; bacterial endocarditis; thrombocytopenia associated with a positive *in vitro* test for antiplatelet antibody in the presence of fondaparinux

Warnings/Precautions [U.S. Boxed Warning]: Patients with recent or anticipated neuraxial anesthesia (epidural or spinal anesthesia) are at risk of spinal or epidural hematoma and subsequent paralysis. Not to be used interchangeably (unit-for-unit) with heparin, low molecular weight heparins (LMWHs), or heparinoids. Use caution in patients with moderate renal dysfunction (Cl_{cr} 30-50 mL/minute); contraindicated in patients with Cl_{cr} <30 mL/minute. Discontinue if severe dysfunction or labile function develops.

Use caution in congenital or acquired bleeding disorders; bacterial endocarditis; renal impairment; hepatic impairment; active ulcerative or angiodysplastic gastrointestinal disease; hemorrhagic stroke; shortly after brain, spinal, or ophthalmologic surgery; or in patients taking platelet inhibitors. Risk of major bleeding may be increased if initial dose is administered earlier than recommended (initiation recommended at 6-8 hours following surgery). Discontinue agents that may enhance the risk of hemorrhage if possible. Although considered an insensitive measure of fondaparinux activity, there have been postmarketing reports of bleeding associated with elevated aPTT. Thrombocytopenia has occurred with administration, including reports of thrombocytopenia with thrombosis similar to heparin-induced thrombocytopenia. Monitor patients closely and discontinue therapy if platelets fall to <100,000/mm^3.

For subcutaneous administration; not for I.M. administration. Do not use interchangeably (unit for unit) with low molecular weight heparins, heparin, or heparinoids. Use caution in patients <50 kg who are being treated for DVT/PE; dosage reduction recommended. Contraindicated in patients <50 kg when used for prophylactic therapy. Use with caution in the elderly. The needle guard contains natural latex rubber.

The administration of fondaparinux is **not recommended** prior to and during primary PCI in patients with STEMI, due to an increased risk for guiding-catheter thrombosis. Patients with UA/NSTEMI or STEMI undergoing any PCI should not receive fondaparinux as the sole anticoagulant. Use of an anticoagulant with antithrombin activity (eg, unfractionated heparin) is recommended as adjunctive therapy to PCI even if prior treatment with fondaparinux (must take into account whether GP IIb/IIIa antagonists have been administered) (King, 2008). Do not administer with other agents that increase the risk of hemorrhage unless they are essential for the management of the underlying condition (eg, warfarin for treatment of VTE).

Additional Canadian labeling warnings: Following sheath removal, fondaparinux therapy should not resume for at least 2 hours in patients with UA/NSTEMI and 3 hours in patients with STEMI. Avoid administration 24 hours before and 48 hours after coronary artery bypass graft (CABG) surgery.

◀ **Adverse Reactions** As with all anticoagulants, bleeding is the major adverse effect. Hemorrhage may occur at any site. Risk appears increased by a number of factors including renal dysfunction, age (>75 years), and weight (<50 kg).

>10%:
  Central nervous system: Fever (4% to 14%)
  Gastrointestinal: Nausea (3% to 11%)
  Hematologic: Anemia (1% to 20%)

1% to 10%:
  Cardiovascular: Edema (9%), hypotension (4%), hypertension (2%), chest pain (1%), thrombosis PCI catheter (without heparin 1%)
  Central nervous system: Insomnia (4% to 5%), headache (2% to 5%), dizziness (4%), confusion (3%), pain (2%), anxiety (1%)
  Dermatologic: Rash (8%), purpura (4%), bullous eruption (3%), bruising (1%)
  Endocrine & metabolic: Hypokalemia (1% to 4%)
  Gastrointestinal: Constipation (5% to 9%), vomiting (1% to 6%), diarrhea (2% to 3%), dyspepsia (2%), abdominal pain (1%)
  Genitourinary: Urinary tract infection (2% to 4%), urinary retention (3%)
  Hematologic: Minor bleeding (2% to 4%), moderate thrombocytopenia (50,000-100,000/mm^3: 3%), hematoma (3%), major bleeding (1% to 3%), prothrombin decreased (1%), risk of major bleeding increased as high as 5% in patients receiving initial dose <6 hours following surgery
  Hepatic: ALT increased (≤3%), AST increased (≤2%)
  Local: Injection site reaction (bleeding, rash, pruritus)
  Neuromuscular & skeletal: Back pain (1%), leg pain (1%)
  Respiratory: Cough (2%), pneumonia (2%), epistaxis (1%)
  Miscellaneous: Wound drainage increased (5%)

<1% (Limited to important or life-threatening): aPTT increased (associated with bleeding), heparin-induced thrombocytopenia (1 case report), hepatic dysfunction, severe thrombocytopenia (<50,000/mm^3)

Drug Interactions
  Avoid Concomitant Use There are no known interactions where it is recommended to avoid concomitant use.
  Increased Effect/Toxicity
  Fondaparinux may increase the levels/effects of: Anticoagulants; Ibritumomab; Tositumomab and Iodine I 131 Tositumomab

  The levels/effects of Fondaparinux may be increased by: Antiplatelet Agents; Dasatinib; Drotrecogin Alfa; Herbs (Anticoagulant/Antiplatelet Properties); Nonsteroidal Anti-Inflammatory Agents; Pentosan Polysulfate Sodium; Prostacyclin Analogues; Salicylates; Thrombolytic Agents
  Decreased Effect There are no known significant interactions involving a decrease in effect.

Ethanol/Nutrition/Herb Interactions Herb/Nutraceutical: Avoid alfalfa, anise, bilberry, bladderwrack, bromelain, cat's claw, celery, coleus, cordyceps, dong quai, evening primrose oil, fenugreek, feverfew, garlic, ginger, ginkgo biloba, ginseng (American/Panax/Siberian), grapeseed, green tea, guggul, horse chestnut seed, horseradish, licorice, prickly ash, red clover, reishi, sweet clover, turmeric, white willow (all possess anticoagulant or antiplatelet activity and as such, may enhance the anticoagulant effects of fondaparinux).

Test Interactions International standards of heparin or LMWH are not the appropriate calibrators for antifactor Xa activity of fondaparinux.

Dosage Forms Excipient information presented when available (limited, particularly for generics); consult specific product labeling.
  Injection, solution, as sodium [preservative free]: 2.5 mg/0.5 mL (0.5 mL); 5 mg/0.4 mL (0.4 mL); 7.5 mg/0.6 mL (0.6 mL); 10 mg/0.8 mL (0.8 mL) [prefilled syringe]

References
Bauer KA, "Fondaparinux Sodium: A Selective Inhibitor of Factor Xa," *Am J Health-Syst Pharm*, 2001, 58(Suppl 2):14-7.

Bauer KA, Eriksson BI, Lassen MR, et al, "Fondaparinux Compared With Enoxaparin for the Prevention of Venous Thromboembolism After Elective Major Knee Surgery," *N Engl J Med*, 2001, 345(18):1305-10.

Eriksson BI, Bauer KA, Lassen MR, et al, "Fondaparinux Compared With Enoxaparin for the Prevention of Venous Thromboembolism After Hip-Fracture Surgery," *N Engl J Med*, 2001, 345 (18):1298-304.

Warkentin TE, Maurer BT, and Aster RH, "Heparin-Induced Thrombocytopenia Associated With Fondaparinux," *N Engl J Med*, 2007, 356(25):2653-55.

◆ **Fondaparinux Sodium** *see* Fondaparinux *on page 627*

◆ **Foradil® (Can)** *see* Formoterol *on page 631*

◆ **Foradil® Aerolizer®** *see* Formoterol *on page 631*

◆ **Forane®** *see* Isoflurane *on page 765*

Formoterol (for MOH te rol)

U.S. Brand Names Foradil® Aerolizer®; Perforomist™
Canadian Brand Names Foradil®; Oxeze® Turbuhaler®
Index Terms Formoterol Fumarate; Formoterol Fumarate Dihydrate
Pharmacologic Category Beta$_2$-Adrenergic Agonist; Beta$_2$-Adrenergic Agonist, Long-Acting
Use Maintenance treatment of asthma and prevention of bronchospasm in patients ≥5 years of age with reversible obstructive airway disease, including patients with symptoms of nocturnal asthma, who require regular treatment with inhaled, short-acting beta$_2$-agonists; maintenance treatment of bronchoconstriction in patients with COPD; prevention of exercise-induced bronchospasm in patients ≥5 years of age

Note:
Oxeze® is also approved in Canada for acute relief of symptoms ("on demand" treatment) in patients ≥6 years of age.
Perforomist™ is only indicated for maintenance treatment of bronchoconstriction in patients with COPD.

Pharmacodynamics/Kinetics
Onset of action: Within 3 minutes
Peak effect: 80% of peak effect within 15 minutes
Duration: Improvement in FEV$_1$ observed for 12 hours in most patients
Absorption: Rapidly into plasma
Protein binding: 61% to 64% *in vitro* at higher concentrations than achieved with usual dosing
Metabolism: Hepatic via direct glucuronidation and O-demethylation; CYP2D6, CYP2C8/9, CYP2C19, CYP2A6 involved in O-demethylation
Half-life elimination: Powder: ~10-14 hours; Nebulized solution: ~7 hours
Time to peak: Maximum improvement in FEV$_1$ in 1-3 hours
Excretion:
Children 5-12 years: Urine (7% to 9% as direct glucuronide metabolites, 6% as unchanged drug)
Adults: Urine (15% to 18% as direct glucuronide metabolites, 2% to 10% as unchanged drug)

Dosage
Asthma maintenance treatment: Children ≥5 years and Adults: Inhalation: **Note:** For long-term asthma control, long-acting beta$_2$-agonists (LABAs) should be used in combination with inhaled corticosteroids and **not** as monotherapy
Foradil®: 12 mcg capsule inhaled every 12 hours via Aerolizer™ device
Oxeze® (CAN): **Note:** Not labeled for use in the U.S.: Children ≥6 years and Adults: Inhalation: 6 mcg or 12 mcg every 12 hours. Maximum dose: Children: 24 mcg/day; Adults: 48 mcg/day
Prevention of exercise-induced bronchospasm: Children ≥5 years and Adults: Inhalation:
Foradil®:12 mcg capsule inhaled via Aerolizer™ device at least 15 minutes before exercise on an "as needed" basis; additional doses should not be used for another 12 hours. **Note:** If already using for asthma maintenance, then should not use additional doses for exercise-induced bronchospasm. Because LABAs may disguise poorly controlled persistent asthma, frequent or chronic use of LABAs for exercise-induced bronchospasm is discouraged by the NIH Asthma Guidelines (NIH, 2007).
Oxeze® (CAN): **Note:** Not labeled for use in the U.S.: Children ≥6 years and Adults: Inhalation: 6 mcg or 12 mcg at least 15 minutes before exercise.
COPD maintenance treatment: Adults: Inhalation:
Foradil®: 12 mcg capsule inhaled every 12 hours via Aerolizer™ device

◄ Perforomist™: 20 mcg unit-dose vial twice daily (maximum dose: 40 mcg/day)

Additional indication for Oxeze® (approved in Canada): Acute ("on demand") relief of bronchoconstriction: Children ≥12 years and Adults: 6 mcg or 12 mcg as a single dose (maximum dose: 72 mcg in any 24-hour period). The prolonged use of high dosages (48 mcg/day for ≥3 consecutive days) may be a sign of suboptimal control, and should prompt the re-evaluation of therapy.

Additional Information Complete prescribing information for this medication should be consulted for additional detail.

Dosage Forms Excipient information presented when available (limited, particularly for generics); consult specific product labeling. [CAN] = Canadian brand name

Powder for oral inhalation, as fumarate:
   Foradil® Aerolizer™ [capsule]: 12 mcg (12s, 60s) [contains lactose 25 mg]
   Oxeze® Turbuhaler® [CAN]: 6 mcg/inhalation [delivers 60 metered doses; contains lactose 600 mcg/dose]; 12 mcg/inhalation [delivers 60 metered doses; contains lactose 600 mcg/dose] [not available in the U.S.]
Solution for nebulization, as fumarate dihydrate:
   Perforomist™: 20 mcg/2 mL (2 mL)

◆ **Formoterol Fumarate** *see Formoterol on page 631*

◆ **Formoterol Fumarate Dihydrate** *see Formoterol on page 631*

◆ **Formulation R™ [OTC]** *see Phenylephrine on page 1114*

◆ **5-Formyl Tetrahydrofolate** *see Leucovorin Calcium on page 812*

◆ **Fortamet®** *see MetFORMIN on page 886*

◆ **Fortaz®** *see Ceftazidime on page 263*

◆ **Fortical®** *see Calcitonin on page 226*

◆ **Fosamax®** *see Alendronate on page 57*

Foscarnet (fos KAR net)

U.S. Brand Names Foscavir® [DSC]
Canadian Brand Names Foscavir®
Index Terms PFA; Phosphonoformate; Phosphonoformic Acid
Pharmacologic Category Antiviral Agent
Generic Available Yes
Use Treatment of acyclovir-resistant mucocutaneous herpes simplex virus (HSV) infections in immunocompromised persons (eg, with advanced AIDS); treatment of CMV retinitis in persons with HIV
Unlabeled/Investigational Use Other CMV infections (eg, colitis, esophagitis, neurological disease); CMV prophylaxis for cancer patients receiving alemtuzumab therapy or allogeneic stem cell transplant
Mechanism of Action Pyrophosphate analogue which acts as a noncompetitive inhibitor of many viral RNA and DNA polymerases as well as HIV reverse transcriptase. Similar to ganciclovir, foscarnet is a virostatic agent. Foscarnet does not require activation by thymidine kinase.
Pharmacodynamics/Kinetics
   Distribution: V_d: ~0.5 L/kg; up to 28% of cumulative I.V. dose may be deposited in bone
   Protein binding: 14% to 17%
   Metabolism: Biotransformation does not occur
   Half-life elimination: Elimination: ~3-4 hours; terminal: ~88 hours (due to bone deposition)
   Excretion: Urine (≤28% as unchanged drug)
Dosage
   CMV retinitis: I.V.:
      Induction treatment: 60 mg/kg/dose every 8 hours **or** 90 mg/kg every 12 hours for 14-21 days
      Maintenance therapy: 90-120 mg/kg/day as a single daily infusion
   Herpes simplex infections (acyclovir-resistant): Induction: I.V.: 40 mg/kg/dose every 8-12 hours for 14-21 days

Therapy of CMV infection in cancer patients (unlabeled use): I.V.:

Prophylaxis: 60 mg/kg every 8-12 hours for 7 days, followed by 90-120 mg/kg daily until day 100 after HSCT

Pre-emptive treatment: 60 mg/kg every 12 hours for 14 days; if CMV still detectable, continue with 90 mg/kg daily for 5 days/week for 2 additional weeks

Treatment: 90 mg/kg every 12 hours for 2 weeks, followed by 120 mg/kg daily for ≥2 weeks

Dosage adjustment in renal impairment: Induction and maintenance dosing schedules based on creatinine clearance (mL/minute/kg): See tables.

Induction Dosing of Foscarnet in Patients With Abnormal Renal Function

Cl_{cr} (mL/min/kg)	HSV Equivalent to 40 mg/kg q12h	HSV Equivalent to 40 mg/kg q8h	CMV Equivalent to 60 mg/kg q8h	CMV Equivalent to 90 mg/kg q12h
<0.4	Not recommended	Not recommended	Not recommended	Not recommended
≥0.4-0.5	20 mg/kg every 24 hours	35 mg/kg every 24 hours	50 mg/kg every 24 hours	50 mg/kg every 24 hours
>0.5-0.6	25 mg/kg every 24 hours	40 mg/kg every 24 hours	60 mg/kg every 24 hours	60 mg/kg every 24 hours
>0.6-0.8	35 mg/kg every 24 hours	25 mg/kg every 12 hours	40 mg/kg every 12 hours	80 mg/kg every 24 hours
>0.8-1.0	20 mg/kg every 12 hours	35 mg/kg every 12 hours	50 mg/kg every 12 hours	50 mg/kg every 12 hours
>1.0-1.4	30 mg/kg every 12 hours	30 mg/kg every 8 hours	45 mg/kg every 8 hours	70 mg/kg every 12 hours
>1.4	40 mg/kg every 12 hours	40 mg/kg every 8 hours	60 mg/kg every 8 hours	90 mg/kg every 12 hours

Maintenance Dosing of Foscarnet in Patients With Abnormal Renal Function

Cl_{cr} (mL/min/kg)	CMV Equivalent to 90 mg/kg q24h	CMV Equivalent to 120 mg/kg q24h
<0.4	Not recommended	Not recommended
≥0.4-0.5	50 mg/kg every 48 hours	65 mg/kg every 48 hours
>0.5-0.6	60 mg/kg every 48 hours	80 mg/kg every 48 hours
>0.6-0.8	80 mg/kg every 48 hours	105 mg/kg every 48 hours
>0.8-1.0	50 mg/kg every 24 hours	65 mg/kg every 24 hours
>1.0-1.4	70 mg/kg every 24 hours	90 mg/kg every 24 hours
>1.4	90 mg/kg every 24 hours	120 mg/kg every 24 hours

Hemodialysis:

Foscarnet is highly removed by hemodialysis (up to ~38% in 2.5 hours HD with high-flux membrane)

Doses of 50 mg/kg/dose posthemodialysis have been found to produce similar serum concentrations as doses of 90 mg/kg twice daily in patients with normal renal function

Doses of 60-90 mg/kg/dose loading dose (posthemodialysis) followed by 45-60 mg/kg/dose posthemodialysis (3 times/week) with the monitoring of weekly plasma concentrations to maintain peak plasma concentrations in the range of 400-800 µMolar have been recommended by some clinicians

Continuous arteriovenous or venovenous hemodiafiltration effects: Dose as for Cl_{cr} 10-50 mL/minute

Stability Foscarnet injection is a clear, colorless solution. Store intact bottles at room temperature of 15°C to 30°C (59°F to 86°F) and protect from temperatures >40°C and from freezing. Diluted solution is stable for 24 hours at room temperature or under refrigeration. ▶

Foscarnet should be diluted in D₅W or NS. For peripheral line administration, foscarnet **must** be diluted to ≤12 mg/mL with D₅W or NS. For central line administration, foscarnet may be administered undiluted.

Administration Foscarnet is administered by intravenous infusion, using an infusion pump, at a rate not exceeding 1 mg/kg/minute. Undiluted (24 mg/mL) solution can be administered without further dilution when using a central venous catheter for infusion. For peripheral vein administration, the solution **must** be diluted to a final concentration **not to exceed** 12 mg/mL. The manufacturer recommends 750-1000 mL of NS or D₅W be administered prior to first infusion to establish diuresis. With subsequent infusions of 90-120 mg/kg, this volume would be repeated. If the dose were 40-60 mg/kg, then the volume could be reduced to 500 mL. After the first dose, the hydration fluid should be administered concurrently with foscarnet.

Monitoring Parameters 24-hour creatinine clearance at baseline and periodically thereafter. During induction therapy: Obtain complete blood counts, and electrolytes (including serum creatinine, calcium, magnesium, potassium and phosphorus) twice weekly and then one weekly during maintenance therapy. More frequent monitoring may be required in some patients. Check hydration status before and after infusion.

Pregnancy Risk Factor C

Contraindications Hypersensitivity to foscarnet or any component of the formulation

Warnings/Precautions Hazardous agent - use appropriate precautions for handling and disposal. **[U.S. Boxed Warning]: Indicated only for immunocompromised patients with CMV retinitis and mucocutaneous acyclovir-resistant HSV infection. [U.S. Boxed Warning]: Renal impairment occurs to some degree in the majority of patients treated with foscarnet;** renal impairment may occur at any time and is usually reversible within 1 week following dose adjustment or discontinuation of therapy, however, several patients have died with renal failure within 4 weeks of stopping foscarnet; therefore, renal function should be closely monitored. To reduce the risk of nephrotoxicity and the potential to administer a relative overdose, always calculate the creatine clearance even if serum creatinine is within the normal range. Adequate hydration may reduce the risk of nephrotoxicity; the manufacturer makes specific recommendations regarding this (see Administration).

Imbalance of serum electrolytes or minerals occurs in at least 15% of patients (hypocalcemia, low ionized calcium, hyper/hypophosphatemia, hypomagnesemia, or hypokalemia). Correct electrolytes before initiating therapy. Use caution when administering other medications that cause electrolyte imbalances. Patients who experience signs or symptoms of an electrolyte imbalance should be assessed immediately. **[U.S. Boxed Warning]: Seizures related to plasma electrolyte/mineral imbalance may occur;** incidence has been reported in up to 10% of HIV patients. Risk factors for seizures include impaired baseline renal function, low total serum calcium, and underlying CNS conditions. May cause anemia and granulocytopenia. May cause genital/vascular tissue irritation/ulceration; adequately hydrate and administer only into vein with adequate blood flow to minimize risk. Foscarnet is deposited in teeth and bone of young, growing animals; it has adversely affected tooth enamel development in rats.

Adverse Reactions

>10%:

Central nervous system: Fever (65%), headache (26%)

Endocrine & metabolic: Hypokalemia (16% to 48%), hypocalcemia (15% to 30%), hypomagnesemia (15% to 30%), hypophosphatemia (8% to 26%)

Gastrointestinal: Nausea (47%), diarrhea (30%), vomiting (26%)

Hematologic: Anemia (33%), granulocytopenia (17%)

Renal: Abnormal renal function/decreased creatinine clearance (12%; without adequate hydration 33%)

1% to 10%:

Cardiovascular: Chest pain (1% to 5%), edema (1% to 5%), facial edema (1% to 5%), flushing (1% to 5%), hyper-/hypotension (1% to 5%), palpitation (1% to 5%), ECG changes (1% to 5%)

Central nervous system: Seizure (includes grand mal; 8%), anxiety (≥5%), confusion (≥5%), depression (≥5%), dizziness (≥5%), fatigue (≥5%), hypoesthesia (≥5%), malaise (≥5%), pain (≥5%), aggressiveness (1% to 5%), agitation (1% to 5%), amnesia (1% to 5%), aphasia (1% to 5%), ataxia (1% to 5%), coordination abnormal (1% to 5%), dementia (1% to 5%), EEG abnormal (1% to 5%), hallucination (1% to 5%), insomnia (1% to 5%), meningitis (1% to 5%), nervousness (1% to 5%), somnolence (1% to 5%), stupor (1% to 5%)

Dermatologic: Rash (≥5%), erythematous rash (1% to 5%), maculopapular rash (1% to 5%), pruritus (1% to 5%), seborrhea (1% to 5%), skin discoloration (1% to 5%), skin ulceration (1% to 5%)

Endocrine & metabolic: Hyperphosphatemia (6%), acidosis (1% to 5%), hyponatremia (1% to 5%)

Gastrointestinal: Abdominal pain (≥5%), anorexia (≥5%), constipation (1% to 5%), dyspepsia (1% to 5%), dysphasia (1% to 5%), flatulence (1% to 5%), melena (1% to 5%), pancreatitis (1% to 5%), rectal hemorrhage (1% to 5%), taste perversion (1% to 5%), ulcerative stomatitis (1% to 5%), weight loss (1% to 5%), xerostomia (1% to 5%)

Genitourinary: Dysuria (1% to 5%), nocturia (1% to 5%), urinary retention (1% to 5%)

Hematologic: Leukopenia (≥5%), lymphadenopathy (1% to 5%), thrombocytopenia (1% to 5%), thrombosis (1% to 5%)

Hepatic: Alkaline phosphatase increased (1% to 5%), ALT increased (1% to 5%), AST increased (1% to 5%), hepatic function abnormal (1% to 5%), LDH increased (1% to 5%)

Local: Injection site pain/inflammation (1% to 5%)

Neuromuscular & skeletal: Paresthesia (≥5%), involuntary muscle contractions (≥5%), rigors (≥5%), neuropathy (peripheral; ≥5%), weakness (≥5%), arthralgia (1% to 5%), back pain (1% to 5%), leg cramps (1% to 5%), myalgia (1% to 5%), tremor (1% to 5%)

Ocular: Vision abnormalities (≥5%), conjunctivitis (1% to 5%), eye pain (1% to 5%)

Renal: Acute renal failure (1% to 5%), albuminuria (1% to 5%), BUN increased (1% to 5%), polyuria (1% to 5%), urinary tract infection (1% to 5%)

Respiratory: Cough (≥5%), dyspnea (≥5%), bronchospasm (1% to 5%), hemoptysis (1% to 5%), pharyngitis (1% to 5%), pneumonia (1% to 5%), pneumothorax (1% to 5%), rhinitis (1% to 5%), sinusitis (1% to 5%), stridor (1% to 5%)

Miscellaneous: Diaphoresis (≥5%), sepsis (≥5%), infection (includes bacterial and fungal; ≥5%), flu-like syndrome (1% to 5%), malignancies (lymphoma/sarcoma 1% to 5%), thirst (1% to 5%)

<1% (Limited to important or life-threatening): Amylase increased, cardiac arrest, coma, creatine phosphokinase increased, dehydration, diabetes insipidus (usually nephrogenic), erythema multiforme, GGT increased muscle weakness, hematuria, hypoproteinemia, myopathy, myositis, neutropenia, pancytopenia, QT_c prolongation, renal calculus, rhabdomyolysis, Stevens-Johnson syndrome, syndrome of inappropriate antidiuretic hormone (SIADH), toxic epidermal necrolysis, ventricular arrhythmia, vesiculobullous eruptions

Drug Interactions

Avoid Concomitant Use

Avoid concomitant use of Foscarnet with any of the following: Artemether; Dronedarone; Lumefantrine; Nilotinib; Pimozide; QuiNINE; Tetrabenazine; Thioridazine; Ziprasidone

Increased Effect/Toxicity

Foscarnet may increase the levels/effects of: Dronedarone; Pimozide; QTc-Prolonging Agents; QuiNINE; Tetrabenazine; Thioridazine; Ziprasidone

The levels/effects of Foscarnet may be increased by: Alfuzosin; Artemether; Chloroquine; Ciprofloxacin; Gadobutrol; Lumefantrine; Nilotinib; QuiNINE

Decreased Effect There are no known significant interactions involving a decrease in effect.

Dosage Forms Excipient information presented when available (limited, particularly for generics); consult specific product labeling. [DSC] = Discontinued product

Injection, solution, as sodium [preservative-free]: 24 mg/mL (250 mL, 500 mL)
Foscavir®: 24 mg/mL (500 mL) [DSC]

◀ **References**

Aweeka FT, Jacobson MA, Martin-Munley S, et al, "Effect of Renal Disease and Hemodialysis on Foscarnet Pharmacokinetics and Dosing Recommendations," *J Acquir Immune Def Syndr Hum Retrovirol*, 1999, 20(4):350-7.

Benson CA, Kaplan JE, Masur H, et al, "Treating Opportunistic Infections Among HIV-Exposed and Infected Adults and Adolescents: Recommendations from CDC, the National Institutes of Health and the HIV Medicine Association/IDSA," *MMWR Recomm Rep* 2004, 53(RR-15):1-112.

Butler KM, DeSmet MD, Husson RN, et al, "Treatment of Aggressive Cytomegalovirus Retinitis With Ganciclovir in Combination With Foscarnet in a Child Infected With Human Immunodeficiency Virus," *J Pediatr*, 1992, 120(3):483-6.

Calligaro KD, Stern J, and DeLaurentis DA, "Foscarnet: A Possible Cause of Ulnar Artery Thrombosis in a Patient With AIDS," *J Vasc Surg*, 1994, 20(6):1007-8.

Chilukuri S and Rosen T, "Management of Acycovir-Resistant Herpes Simplex Virus," *Dermatol Clin*, 2003, 21(2):311-20.

Chrisp P and Clissold SP, "Foscarnet. A Review of Its Antiviral Activity, Pharmacokinetic Properties and Therapeutic Use in Immunocompromised Patients With Cytomegalovirus Retinitis," *Drugs*, 1991, 41(1):104-29.

Deray G, Martinez F, Katlama C, et al, "Foscarnet Nephrotoxicity: Mechanism, Incidence and Prevention," *Am J Nephrol*, 1989, 9:316-21.

"Drugs for Non-HIV Viral Infections," *Med Lett Drugs Ther*, 1994, 36(919):27.

Jacobson MA, "Review of the Toxicities of Foscarnet," *J Acquir Immune Defic Syndr*, 1992, 5(Suppl 1):11-7.

Jayaweera DT, "Minimizing the Dosage-Limiting Toxicities of Foscarnet Induction Therapy," *Drug Saf*, 1997, 16(4):258-66.

Keating MR, "Antiviral Agents," *Mayo Clin Proc*, 1992, 67(2):160-78.

Mofenson LM, Oleske J, Serchuck L, et al, "Treating Opportunistic Infections Among HIV-Exposed and Infected Children: Recommendations from CDC, the National Institutes of Health, and the Infectious Diseases Society of America," *Clin Infect Dis*, 2005, 40 (Suppl 1):1-84.

Morales JM, Munoz MA, Fernandez Zatarain G, et al, "Reversible Acute Renal Failure Caused by the Combined Use of Foscarnet and Cyclosporin in Organ Transplanted Patients," *Nephrol Dial Transplant*, 1995, 10(6):882-3.

National Comprehensive Cancer Network (NCCN), "Clinical Practice Guidelines in Oncology™: Prevention and Treatment of Cancer-Related Infections," Version 1, 2008. Available at http://www.nccn.org/professionals/physician_gls/PDF/infections.pdf.

Polis MA, "Foscarnet and Ganciclovir in the Treatment of Cytomegalovirus Retinitis," *J Acquir Immune Defic Syndr*, 1992, 5(Suppl 1):3-10.

Whitley RJ, Jacobson MA, Friedberg DN, et al, "Guidelines for the Treatment of Cytomegalovirus Diseases in Patients With AIDS in the Era of Potent Antiretroviral Therapy: Recommendations of an International Panel. International AIDS Society-USA," *Arch Intern Med*, 1998, 158(9):957-69.

◆ **Foscavir® [DSC]** see Foscarnet *on page 632*

◆ **Foscavir® (Can)** see Foscarnet *on page 632*

Fosinopril (foe SIN oh pril)

Related Information

Angiotensin Agents *on page 1652*
Heart Failure (Systolic) *on page 1739*
Preoperative Evaluation of the Cardiac Patient for Noncardiac Surgery *on page 1598*

U.S. Brand Names Monopril®

Canadian Brand Names Apo-Fosinopril®; Gen-Fosinopril; Monopril®; Mylan-Fosinopril; Novo-Fosinopril; PMS-Fosinopril; RAN-Fosinopril; Riva-Fosinopril

Index Terms Fosinopril Sodium

Pharmacologic Category Angiotensin-Converting Enzyme (ACE) Inhibitor

Use Treatment of hypertension, either alone or in combination with other antihypertensive agents; treatment of heart failure (HF)

Pharmacodynamics/Kinetics

Onset of action: 1 hour

Duration: 24 hours

Absorption: 36%

Protein binding: 95%

Metabolism: Prodrug, hydrolyzed to its active metabolite fosinoprilat by intestinal wall and hepatic esterases

Bioavailability: 36%

Half-life elimination, serum (fosinoprilat): 12 hours

Time to peak, serum: ~3 hours

Excretion: Urine and feces (as fosinoprilat and other metabolites in roughly equal proportions, 45% to 50%)

Dosage Oral:

Children ≥6 years and >50 kg: Hypertension: Initial: 5-10 mg once daily (maximum: 40 mg/day)

Adults:

Heart failure: Initial: 10 mg/day (5 mg if renal dysfunction present) and increase, as needed, to a maximum of 40 mg once daily over several weeks; usual dose: 20-40 mg/day. If hypotension, orthostasis, or azotemia occur during titration, consider decreasing concomitant diuretic dose, if any.

Hypertension: Initial: 10 mg/day; most patients are maintained on 20-40 mg/day (maximum: 80 mg/day). May need to divide the dose into two if trough effect is inadequate; discontinue the diuretic, if possible 2-3 days before initiation of therapy; resume diuretic therapy carefully, if needed.

Dosing adjustment/comments in renal impairment: None needed since hepatobiliary elimination compensates adequately diminished renal elimination.

Hemodialysis: Moderately dialyzable (20% to 50%)

Anesthesia and Critical Care Concerns/Other Considerations

Clinical Pearls/Comments: In patients on chronic ACE inhibitor therapy, intraoperative hypotension may occur with induction and maintenance of general anesthesia; however, discontinuation of therapy prior to surgery is controversial. If continued preoperatively, avoidance of hypotensive agents during surgery is prudent. Episodes of intraoperative hypotension may be managed by fluid administration and/or modest doses of alpha-adrenergic agents. Severe hypotension may occur in patients who are sodium- and/or volume-depleted, initiate lower doses and monitor closely when starting therapy in these patients. ACE inhibitor therapy may elicit an increase in potassium and creatinine, especially when used in patients with bilateral renal artery stenosis. In those patients experiencing cough on an ACE inhibitor, the ACE inhibitor may be discontinued and, if necessary, angiotensin-receptor blocker therapy instituted. Concomitant NSAID therapy may attenuate blood pressure control; use of NSAIDs should be avoided or limited, with monitoring of blood pressure control. In the setting of heart failure, NSAID use may be associated with an increased risk for fluid accumulation and edema. Because of the potent teratogenic effects of ACE inhibitors, these drugs should be avoided, if possible, when treating women of childbearing potential not on effective birth control measures. Aging patients with a decrease in glomerular filtration (also creatinine clearance), severe heart failure, and renal failure may experience an exaggerated response with administration of ACE inhibitors. Diabetic proteinuria is reduced and insulin sensitivity is enhanced.

Evidence-Based Information: ACE inhibitors decrease morbidity and mortality in patients with asymptomatic and symptomatic left ventricular dysfunction. In this situation, they decrease hospitalizations for, and retard progression to, decompensated heart failure. ACE inhibitors are also indicated in patients postmyocardial infarction in whom left ventricular ejection fraction is <40%. When used in patients with heart failure, the target dose or maximum tolerated dose should be achieved, if possible. Lower daily doses of ACE inhibitors have not demonstrated the same cardioprotective effects. ACE inhibitors have renal protective effects in patients with diabetic proteinuria. The HOPE trial examined the use of ramipril at a dose of between 2.5-10 mg daily in patients without heart failure at high risk for cardiovascular events and documented a significant improvement in cardiovascular outcome compared to placebo.

Additional Information Complete prescribing information for this medication should be consulted for additional detail.

Dosage Forms Excipient information presented when available (limited, particularly for generics); consult specific product labeling. [DSC] = Discontinued product

Tablet, as sodium: 10 mg, 20 mg, 40 mg

Monopril®: 10 mg [DSC]; 20 mg [DSC]; 40 mg

◆ **Fosinopril Sodium** *see* Fosinopril *on page 636*

Fosphenytoin (FOS fen i toyn)

Medication Safety Issues

Sound-alike/look-alike issues:

Cerebyx® may be confused with Celebrex®, Celexa™, Cerezyme®, Cervarix®

Fosphenytoin may be confused with fospropofol

Overdoses have occurred due to confusion between the **mg per mL concentration** of fosphenytoin (50 mg PE/mL) and **total drug content per vial** (either 100 mg PE/2 mL vial or 500 mg PE/10 mL vial). ISMP recommends that the total drug content per container is identified instead of the concentration in mg per mL to avoid confusion and potential overdosages. Additionally, since most errors have occurred with overdoses in children, they recommend that pediatric hospitals should consider stocking only the 2 mL vial.

Related Information

Perioperative Management of Patients on Antiseizure Medication *on page 1577*

Status Epilepticus *on page 1737*

U.S. Brand Names Cerebyx®

Canadian Brand Names Cerebyx®

Index Terms Fosphenytoin Sodium

Pharmacologic Category Anticonvulsant, Hydantoin

Generic Available Yes

Use Used for the control of generalized convulsive status epilepticus and prevention and treatment of seizures occurring during neurosurgery; indicated for short-term parenteral administration when other means of phenytoin administration are unavailable, inappropriate, or deemed less advantageous (the safety and effectiveness of fosphenytoin use for more than 5 days has not been systematically evaluated)

Mechanism of Action Diphosphate ester salt of phenytoin which acts as a water soluble prodrug of phenytoin; after administration, plasma esterases convert fosphenytoin to phosphate, formaldehyde, and phenytoin as the active moiety; phenytoin works by stabilizing neuronal membranes and decreasing seizure activity by increasing efflux or decreasing influx of sodium ions across cell membranes in the motor cortex during generation of nerve impulses

Pharmacodynamics/Kinetics Also refer to Phenytoin monograph for additional information.

Protein binding: Fosphenytoin: 95% to 99% to albumin; can displace phenytoin and increase free fraction (up to 30% unbound) during the period required for conversion of fosphenytoin to phenytoin

Metabolism: Fosphenytoin is rapidly converted via hydrolysis to phenytoin; phenytoin is metabolized in the liver and forms metabolites

Bioavailability: I.M.: Fosphenytoin: 100%

Half-life elimination:

Fosphenytoin: 15 minutes

Phenytoin: Variable (mean: 12-29 hours); kinetics of phenytoin are saturable

Time to peak: Conversion to phenytoin: Following I.V. administration (maximum rate of administration): 15 minutes; following I.M. administration, peak phenytoin levels are reached in 3 hours

Excretion: Phenytoin: Urine (as inactive metabolites)

Dosage The dose, concentration in solutions, and infusion rates for fosphenytoin are expressed as phenytoin sodium equivalents (PE); fosphenytoin should always be prescribed and dispensed in phenytoin sodium equivalents (PE)

Infants and Children (unlabeled use): I.V.:

Loading dose: 10-20 mg PE/kg for the treatment of generalized convulsive status epilepticus

Maintenance dosing: Phenytoin dosing guidelines in pediatric patients are used when dosing fosphenytoin using doses in PE equal to the phenytoin doses (ie, phenytoin 1 mg = fosphenytoin 1 PE); maintenance doses may be started 8-12 hours after a loading dose

Adults:

Status epilepticus: I.V.: Loading dose: 15-20 mg PE/kg I.V. administered at 100-150 mg PE/minute

Nonemergent loading and maintenance dosing: I.V. or I.M.:

Loading dose: 10-20 mg PE/kg I.V. or I.M. (maximum I.V. rate: 150 mg PE/minute)

Initial daily maintenance dose: 4-6 mg PE/kg/day I.V. or I.M.

I.M. or I.V. substitution for oral phenytoin therapy: May be substituted for oral phenytoin sodium at the same total daily dose; however, Dilantin® capsules are ~90% bioavailable by the oral route; phenytoin, supplied as fosphenytoin, is 100% bioavailable by both the I.M. and I.V. routes; for this reason, plasma phenytoin concentrations may increase when I.M. or I.V. fosphenytoin is substituted for oral phenytoin sodium therapy; in clinical trials, I.M. fosphenytoin was administered as a single daily dose utilizing either 1 or 2 injection sites; some patients may require more frequent dosing

Dosing adjustments in renal/hepatic impairment: Phenytoin clearance may be substantially reduced in cirrhosis and plasma level monitoring with dose adjustment advisable; free phenytoin levels should be monitored closely in patients with renal or hepatic disease or in those with hypoalbuminemia; furthermore, fosphenytoin clearance to phenytoin may be increased without a similar increase in phenytoin in these patients leading to increased frequency and severity of adverse events

Stability Refrigerate at 2°C to 8°C (36°F to 46°F). Do not store at room temperature for more than 48 hours. Do not use vials that develop particulate matter. Must be diluted to concentrations of 1.5-25 mg PE/mL, in normal saline or D_5W, for I.V. infusion.

Administration

I.M.: May be administered as a single daily dose using either 1 or 2 injection sites.

I.V.: Rates of infusion:

Children: 1-3 mg PE/kg/minute

Adults: Should not exceed 150 mg PE/minute

Monitoring Parameters Continuous blood pressure, ECG, and respiratory function monitoring with loading dose and for 10-20 minutes following infusion; vital signs, CBC, liver function tests, plasma level monitoring (plasma levels should not be measured until conversion to phenytoin is complete, ~2 hours after an I.V. infusion or ~4 hours after an I.M. injection)

Reference Range

Therapeutic: 10-20 mcg/mL (SI: 40-79 μmol/L); toxicity is measured clinically, and some patients require levels outside the suggested therapeutic range

Toxic: 30-50 mcg/mL (SI: 120-200 μmol/L)

Lethal: >100 mcg/mL (SI: >400 μmol/L)

Manifestations of toxicity:

Nystagmus: 20 mcg/mL (SI: 79 μmol/L)

Ataxia: 30 mcg/mL (SI: 118.9 μmol/L)

Decreased mental status: 40 mcg/mL (SI: 159 μmol/L)

Coma: 50 mcg/mL (SI: 200 μmol/L)

Peak serum phenytoin level after a 375 mg I.M. fosphenytoin dose in healthy males: 5.7 mcg/mL

Peak serum fosphenytoin levels and phenytoin levels after a 1.2 g infusion (I.V.) in healthy subjects over 30 minutes were 129 mcg/mL and 17.2 mcg/mL, respectively

Anesthesia and Critical Care Concerns/Other Considerations

Clinical Pearls/Comments: Fosphenytoin 1.5 mg is approximately equivalent to phenytoin 1 mg.

Fosphenytoin is compatible with all diluents; does not require propylene glycol or ethanol for solubility. Since there is no precipitation problem with fosphenytoin, no I.V. filter is required. Formaldehyde production is not expected to be clinically consequential (about 200 mg) if used for 1 week. As with phenytoin, fosphenytoin, when given I.V., especially when high doses are given too rapidly, may cause marked and dramatic hypotension and reflex tachycardia. Fosphenytoin administration is safer, in that the risk of hypotension may be somewhat less, and there are no adverse effects of extravasation. Avoid rapid I.V. infusion of

◀ fosphenytoin (infusion rates >150 mg of phenytoin equivalent per minute). Pruritus can be severe, requiring discontinuation of infusion.

Pregnancy Risk Factor D

Contraindications Hypersensitivity to phenytoin, other hydantoins, or any component of the formulation; patients with sinus bradycardia, sinoatrial block, second- and third-degree AV block, or Adams-Stokes syndrome; occurrence of rash during treatment (should not be resumed if rash is exfoliative, purpuric, or bullous); treatment of absence seizures

Warnings/Precautions Doses of fosphenytoin are expressed as their phenytoin sodium equivalent (PE). Antiepileptic drugs should not be abruptly discontinued. Hypotension may occur, especially after I.V. administration at high doses and high rates of administration. Administration of phenytoin has been associated with atrial and ventricular conduction depression and ventricular fibrillation. Careful cardiac monitoring is needed when administering I.V. loading doses of fosphenytoin. Acute hepatotoxicity associated with a hypersensitivity syndrome characterized by fever, skin eruptions, and lymphadenopathy has been reported to occur within the first 2 months of treatment. Discontinue if skin rash or lymphadenopathy occurs. A spectrum of hematologic effects have been reported with use (eg, neutropenia, leukopenia, thrombocytopenia, pancytopenia, and anemias). Use with caution in patients with hypotension, severe myocardial insufficiency, diabetes mellitus, porphyria, hypoalbuminemia, hypothyroidism, fever, or hepatic or renal dysfunction. Effects with other sedative drugs or ethanol may be potentiated. Safety and efficacy have not been established in children. Severe reactions, including toxic epidermal necrolysis and Stevens-Johnson syndromes, although rarely reported, have resulted in fatalities; drug should be discontinued if there are any signs of rash. Patients of Asian descent with the variant *HLA-B*1502* may be at an increased risk of developing Stevens-Johnson syndrome and/or toxic epidermal necrolysis.

Adverse Reactions The more important adverse clinical events caused by the I.V. use of fosphenytoin or phenytoin are cardiovascular collapse and/or central nervous system depression. Hypotension can occur when either drug is administered rapidly by the I.V. route. Do not exceed a rate of 150 mg phenytoin equivalent/minute when administering fosphenytoin.

The adverse clinical events most commonly observed with the use of fosphenytoin in clinical trials were nystagmus, dizziness, pruritus, paresthesia, headache, somnolence, and ataxia. Paresthesia and pruritus were seen more often following fosphenytoin (versus phenytoin) administration and occurred more often with I.V. fosphenytoin than with I.M. administration. These events were dose and rate related (doses ≥15 mg/kg at a rate of 150 mg/minute). These sensations, generally described as itching, burning, or tingling are usually not at the infusion site. The location of the discomfort varied with the groin mentioned most frequently. The paresthesia and pruritus were transient events that occurred within several minutes of the start of infusion and generally resolved within 10 minutes after completion of infusion.

Transient pruritus, tinnitus, nystagmus, somnolence, and ataxia occurred 2-3 times more often at doses ≥15 mg/kg and rates ≥150 mg/minute.

I.V. administration (maximum dose/rate):
>10%:
    Central nervous system: Nystagmus, dizziness, somnolence, ataxia
    Dermatologic: Pruritus
1% to 10%:
    Cardiovascular: Hypotension, vasodilation, tachycardia
    Central nervous system: Stupor, incoordination, paresthesia, extrapyramidal syndrome, tremor, agitation, hypoesthesia, dysarthria, vertigo, brain edema, headache
    Gastrointestinal: Nausea, tongue disorder, dry mouth, vomiting
    Neuromuscular & skeletal: Pelvic pain, muscle weakness, back pain
    Ocular: Diplopia, amblyopia
    Otic: Tinnitus, deafness
    Miscellaneous: Taste perversion

I.M. administration (substitute for oral phenytoin):
1% to 10%:
Central nervous system: Nystagmus, tremor, ataxia, headache, incoordination, somnolence, dizziness, paresthesia, reflexes decreased
Dermatologic: Pruritus
Gastrointestinal: Nausea, vomiting
Hematologic/lymphatic: Ecchymosis
Neuromuscular & skeletal: Muscle weakness
<1% (Limited to important or life-threatening): Acidosis, acute hepatic failure, acute hepatotoxicity, alkalosis, anemia, atrial flutter, bundle branch block, cardiac arrest, cardiomegaly, cerebral hemorrhage, cerebral infarct, CHF, cyanosis, dehydration, hyperglycemia, hyperkalemia, hypertension, hypochromic anemia, hypokalemia, hypophosphatemia, ketosis, leukocytosis, leukopenia, lymphadenopathy, palpitation, postural hypotension, pulmonary embolus, QT interval prolongation, sinus bradycardia, syncope, Stevens-Johnson syndrome, thrombocytopenia, thrombophlebitis, toxic epidermal necrolysis, ventricular extrasystoles

Drug Interactions
Metabolism/Transport Effects As phenytoin: **Substrate** of CYP2C9 (major), 2C19 (major), 3A4 (minor); **Induces** CYP2B6 (strong), 2C8 (strong), 2C9 (strong), 2C19 (strong), 3A4 (strong)

Avoid Concomitant Use
Avoid concomitant use of Fosphenytoin with any of the following: Dronedarone; Everolimus; Nilotinib; Nisoldipine; Ranolazine; Tolvaptan

Increased Effect/Toxicity
Fosphenytoin may increase the levels/effects of: Alcohol (Ethyl); CNS Depressants; Methotrimeprazine

The levels/effects of Fosphenytoin may be increased by: Carbonic Anhydrase Inhibitors; Chloramphenicol; Cimetidine; CYP2C19 Inhibitors (Moderate); CYP2C19 Inhibitors (Strong); CYP2C9 Inhibitors (Moderate); CYP2C9 Inhibitors (Strong); Methotrimeprazine

Decreased Effect
Fosphenytoin may decrease the levels/effects of: Acetaminophen; Chloramphenicol; CYP2B6 Substrates; CYP2C19 Substrates; CYP2C8 Substrates (High risk); CYP2C9 Substrates (High risk); CYP3A4 Substrates; Dronedarone; Everolimus; Maraviroc; Nilotinib; Nisoldipine; Ranolazine; Saxagliptin; Sorafenib; Tadalafil; Tolvaptan; Treprostinil

The levels/effects of Fosphenytoin may be decreased by: Antacids; CYP2C19 Inducers (Strong); CYP2C9 Inducers (Highly Effective); Ketorolac; Mefloquine; Peginterferon Alfa-2b

Ethanol/Nutrition/Herb Interactions
Ethanol:
Acute use: Avoid or limit ethanol (inhibits metabolism of phenytoin); watch for sedation.
Chronic use: Avoid or limit ethanol (stimulates metabolism of phenytoin).

Test Interactions Increased glucose, alkaline phosphatase (S); decreased thyroxine (S), calcium (S); serum sodium increased in overdose setting

Dietary Considerations Provides phosphate 0.0037 mmol/mg PE fosphenytoin

Dosage Forms Excipient information presented when available (limited, particularly for generics); consult specific product labeling.
Injection, solution, as sodium: 75 mg/mL (2 mL, 10 mL) [equivalent to phenytoin sodium 50 mg/mL]
Cerebyx®: 75 mg/mL (2 mL, 10 mL) [equivalent to phenytoin sodium 50 mg/mL]

References
Chapman MG, Smith M, and Hirsch NP, "Status Epilepticus," *Anaesthesia*, 2001, 56(7):648-59.
Manno EM, "New Management Strategies in the Treatment of Status Epilepticus," *Mayo Clin Proc*, 2003, 78(4):508-18.

♦ **Fosphenytoin Sodium** *see* Fosphenytoin *on page 638*

Fospropofol (fos PROE po fole)

Medication Safety Issues
Sound-alike/look-alike issues:
Fospropofol may be confused with fosaprepitant, fosphenytoin, propofol

High alert medication: The Institute for Safe Medication Practices (ISMP) includes this medication among its list of drugs which have a heightened risk of causing significant patient harm when used in error.

Onset of action: The onset of action will be delayed due to need for conversion to the active metabolite, propofol. If supplemental doses are administered before full effect occurs, the risk of dose-stacking may be elevated resulting in deeper sedation than intended.

U.S. Brand Names Lusedra™

Index Terms Aquavan; Fospropofol Disodium; GPI 15715

Pharmacologic Category Sedative

Restrictions Pending information: The Drug Enforcement Agency has proposed that fospropofol be placed into schedule C-IV

Generic Available No

Use Monitored anesthesia care (MAC) sedation in patients undergoing diagnostic or therapeutic procedures

Mechanism of Action Fospropofol disodium is a prodrug of propofol. Propofol interacts with the GABA$_A$ receptor, which is the presumed mechanism of action whereby it produces a sedative/hypnotic effect. Propofol is an alkyl-phenolic compound with intravenous general anesthetic properties.

Pharmacodynamics/Kinetics
Onset of action: Bolus (dose dependent): Attainment of adequate sedation was achieved between 2-28 minutes (median: 8 minutes)

Duration of sedation: Time to fully alert: ≤1 hour (median: 5 minutes)

Distribution:
Fospropofol: V_d: 0.26-0.4 L/kg
Propofol: V_d: ~6 L/kg; decreased in the elderly

Protein binding: Fospropofol: ~98% to albumin; does not affect protein binding of propofol (also ~98% bound to albumin)

Metabolism: Fospropofol is completely metabolized by plasma alkaline phosphatases to propofol, formaldehyde (rapidly converted to formate), and phosphate. Propofol is further metabolized hepatically to water-soluble sulfate and glucuronide conjugates (~50%).

Half-life elimination:
Fospropofol: 0.8-0.96 hours
Propofol: 0.85-1.41 hours

Time to peak: Propofol (from fospropofol): Median: 12 minutes

Excretion:
Fospropofol: Urine (<0.02% unchanged)
Propofol: Urine (~88% as metabolites, 40% as glucuronide metabolite); feces (<2%)

Dosage Monitored anesthesia care (MAC) sedation: I.V.: **Note: Onset of effect is delayed as compared to propofol-emulsion due to need for conversion to active component.** If <60 kg, base dosing on 60 kg; however, lower doses may be used to achieve lower levels of sedation. If >90 kg, base dosing on 90 kg.

Healthy adults <65 years or with mild systemic disease (ASA-PS1 or -PS2): *Standard dosing regimen:* Initial: 6.5 mg/kg (maximum initial dose: 577.5 mg or 16.5 mL), followed by supplemental doses of 1.6 mg/kg (maximum supplemental dose: 140 mg or 4 mL) no more frequently than every 4 minutes as needed to achieve desired level of sedation.

Elderly patients ≥65 years or patients with severe systemic disease (ASA-PS3 or -PS4): *Modified dosing regimen:* Initial: 4.9 mg/kg (maximum initial dose: 437.5 mg or 12.5 mL), followed by supplemental doses of 1.2 mg/kg (maximum supplemental dose: 105 mg or 3 mL) no more frequently than every 4 minutes as needed to achieve desired level of sedation.

Dosage adjustment in renal impairment: No dosage adjustment recommended. Use with caution in patients with severe renal impairment (Cl_{cr} <30 mL/minute); limited safety and efficacy data available in these patients.

Dosage adjustment in hepatic impairment: No dosage adjustment recommended. Use with caution in patients with hepatic impairment; has not been adequately studied in this population.

Stability Store at controlled room temperature of 25°C (77°F); excursions permitted between 15°C and 30°C (59°F and 86°F). Single-use vials do not need to be diluted prior to administration. Draw into sterile syringes immediately after opening vials. Discard any unused portion at the end of procedure.

Administration Administer as an I.V. bolus (no recommendations on rate of administration provided by manufacturer) via via a secure, freely flowing, peripheral I.V. line. Flush I.V. line with NS or other compatible fluid before and after administration. Strict aseptic technique must be maintained in handling. Discard any unused portion at the end of the procedure. Do not filter.

Monitoring Parameters ECG, blood pressure, respiration, oxygen saturation; patient responsiveness

Pregnancy Risk Factor B

Contraindications There are no contraindications in the manufacturer's FDA approved labeling.

Note: Applicable contraindications to propofol include: Hypersensitivity to propofol; when general anesthesia or sedation is contraindicated

Warnings/Precautions The major cardiovascular effect is hypotension; use with caution in patients who are hemodynamically unstable, hypovolemic, have abnormally low vascular tone (eg, sepsis) or compromised myocardial function (eg, heart failure). The **onset of action will be delayed** due to need for conversion to the active metabolite, propofol. If supplemental doses are administered before full effect occurs, the risk of dose-stacking may be elevated resulting in deeper sedation than intended.

Use requires careful patient monitoring; should only be administered by persons trained in the administration of general anesthesia and not involved in the conduct of the diagnostic or therapeutic procedure. Sedated patients should be continuously monitored, and facilities for maintenance of a patent airway, providing artificial ventilation, administering supplemental oxygen, and instituting cardiovascular resuscitation must be immediately available. Patients should be continuously monitored during sedation and through the recovery process for early signs of hypotension, apnea, airway obstruction, and/or oxygen desaturation. Use to induce moderate (conscious) sedation in patients warrants monitoring equivalent to that seen with general anesthesia. May cause loss of spontaneous respiration and/or hypoxemia; supplemental oxygen is recommended for all patients receiving fospropofol; monitor patient closely. The risk of these effects may be increased with the concomitant use of opioids and/or other sedatives. May cause patients to become unresponsive or minimally responsive to vigorous tactile or painful stimuli.

Use lower doses in patients ≥65 years and/or ASA-PS 3/4 patients to reduce the incidence of unwanted cardiorespiratory and neurologic depressive events. Use with caution in patients with hepatic impairment or severe renal impairment (Cl_{cr} <30 mL/minute). Use with caution in patients with respiratory disease; risk of cardiorespiratory depression may be increased. Use with caution in patients with a history of epilepsy or seizures; seizure may occur during recovery phase.

Concomitant use of opioids/sedative-hypnotics may lead to increased sedative or respiratory depressant effects of fospropofol, more pronounced decreases in systolic, diastolic, and mean arterial pressures, heart rate, and cardiac output. Fospropofol lacks analgesic properties; pain management requires specific use of analgesic agents. Fospropofol should only be used in pregnancy if clearly needed. Not recommended for use in obstetrics, including cesarean section deliveries. Safety and efficacy have not been established in patients <18 years of age.

Adverse Reactions

>10%:

Dermatologic: Pruritus (see "Note"; 8% to 28%)

Neuromuscular & skeletal: Paresthesia (see "Note"; 52% to 74%)
Respiratory: Hypoxemia (1% to 11%)
1% to 10%:
Cardiovascular: Hypotension (2% to 7%)
Central nervous system: Headache (1% to 2%)
Gastrointestinal: Nausea (≤4%), vomiting (≤3%)
Miscellaneous: Procedural pain (≤2%)
<1% (Limited to important or life-threatening): Apnea, myoclonus, systolic blood pressure increased, heart rate increased
Note: Paresthesias (including perineal discomfort or burning sensation) and pruritus (including genital, perineal, and generalized pruritus) are mostly limited to the first 5 minutes of administration and usually described as mild-moderate in intensity. No pretreatments are helpful in reducing the incidence of these adverse effects.

Drug Interactions

Metabolism/Transport Effects Substrate of CYP1A2 (minor), 2A6 (minor), 2B6 (major), 2C9 (major), 2C19 (minor), 2D6 (minor), 2E1 (minor), 3A4 (minor); **Inhibits** CYP1A2 (moderate), 2C9 (weak), 2C19 (moderate), 2D6 (weak), 2E1 (weak), 3A4 (strong)

Avoid Concomitant Use There are no known interactions where it is recommended to avoid concomitant use.

Increased Effect/Toxicity

Fospropofol may increase the levels/effects of: Ropivacaine

The levels/effects of Fospropofol may be increased by: Alfentanil; CYP2B6 Inhibitors (Moderate); CYP2B6 Inhibitors (Strong)

Decreased Effect There are no known significant interactions involving a decrease in effect.

Product Availability Lusedra™: FDA approved December 2008; anticipated availability is currently undetermined

Dosage Forms Excipient information presented when available (limited, particularly for generics); consult specific product labeling.
Injection [preservative-free]:
Lusedra™: 35 mg/mL (30 mL)

References

Cohen LB, "Clinical Trial: a dose-response study of fospropofol disodium for moderate sedation during colonoscopy," *Aliment Pharmacol Ther*, 2008, 27(7):597-608.
Silvestri GA, Vincent BD, Wahidi MM, et al, "A Phase 3, Randomized, Double-blind, Study to Assess the Efficacy and Safety of Fospropofol Disodium Injection for Moderate Sedation in Patients Undergoing Flexible Bronchoscopy," *Chest*, 2009, 135(1):41-7.

Frovatriptan (froe va TRIP tan)

U.S. Brand Names Frova®
Canadian Brand Names Frova®
Index Terms Frovatriptan Succinate
Pharmacologic Category Antimigraine Agent; Serotonin 5-HT$_{1B,\ 1D}$ Receptor Agonist
Use Acute treatment of migraine with or without aura
Pharmacodynamics/Kinetics
Distribution: Male: 4.2 L/kg; Female: 3.0 L/kg
Protein binding: ~15%
Metabolism: Primarily hepatic via CYP1A2
Bioavailability: Male: ~20%; Female: ~30%
Half-life elimination: ~26 hours

Time to peak: 2-4 hours
Excretion: Feces (62%); urine (32%; <10% as unchanged drug)

Dosage Oral: Adults: Migraine:

U.S. labeling: 2.5 mg; if headache recurs, a second dose may be given if first dose provided relief and at least 2 hours have elapsed since the first dose (maximum daily dose: 7.5 mg)

Canadian labeling: 2.5 mg; if headache recurs, a second dose may be given if first dose provided relief and at least 4 hours have elapsed since the first dose (maximum daily dose: 5 mg)

Note: The safety of treating more than 4 migraines/month has not been established.

Dosage adjustment in renal impairment: No adjustment necessary

Dosage adjustment in hepatic impairment: No adjustment necessary in mild-to-moderate hepatic impairment; use with caution in severe impairment (has not been studied in severe impairment).

Canadian labeling (not in U.S. labeling): Use is contraindicated in severe hepatic impairment.

Additional Information Complete prescribing information for this medication should be consulted for additional detail.

Dosage Forms Excipient information presented when available (limited, particularly for generics); consult specific product labeling.
Tablet:
Frova®: 2.5 mg

♦ **Frovatriptan Succinate** *see Frovatriptan on page 644*

♦ **Frusemide** *see Furosemide on page 645*

♦ **Fucidin® (Can)** *see Fusidic Acid on page 649*

♦ **Fucithalmic® (Can)** *see Fusidic Acid on page 649*

♦ **Fungizone® (Can)** *see Amphotericin B (Conventional) on page 104*

Furosemide (fyoor OH se mide)

Medication Safety Issues
Sound-alike/look-alike issues:
Furosemide may be confused with famotidine, finasteride, fluconazole, FLUoxetine, fosinopril, loperamide, torsemide
Lasix® may be confused with Esidrix®, Lanoxin®, Lidex®, Lomotil®, Lovenox®, Luvox®, Luxiq®

International issues:
Urex® [Australia] may be confused with Eurax® which is a brand name for crotamiton in the U.S.
Urex® [Australia]: Brand name for methenamine in the U.S.

Related Information
Anesthesia Considerations for Neurosurgery *on page 1514*
Diuretics, Loop *on page 1680*
Heart Failure (Systolic) *on page 1739*

U.S. Brand Names Lasix®

Canadian Brand Names Apo-Furosemide®; Dom-Furosemide; Furosemide Injection, USP; Furosemide Special; Lasix®; Lasix® Special; Novo-Semide; Nu-Furosemide; PMS-Furosemide

Index Terms Frusemide

Pharmacologic Category Diuretic, Loop

Generic Available Yes

Use Management of edema associated with heart failure and hepatic or renal disease; acute pulmonary edema; treatment of hypertension (alone or in combination with other antihypertensives)

Mechanism of Action Inhibits reabsorption of sodium and chloride in the ascending loop of Henle and distal renal tubule, interfering with the chloride-binding cotransport system, thus causing increased excretion of water, sodium, chloride, magnesium, and calcium

◀ **Pharmacodynamics/Kinetics**

Onset of action: Diuresis: Oral, S.L.: 30-60 minutes; I.M.: 30 minutes; I.V.: ~5 minutes

Symptomatic improvement with acute pulmonary edema: Within 15-20 minutes; occurs prior to diuretic effect

Peak effect: Oral, S.L.: 1-2 hours

Duration: Oral, S.L.: 6-8 hours; I.V.: 2 hours

Protein binding: 91% to 99%; primarily to albumin

Metabolism: Minimally hepatic

Bioavailability: Oral tablet: 47% to 64%; Oral solution: 50%; S.L. administration of oral tablet: ~60%; results of a small comparative study (n=11) showed bioavailability of S.L. administration of tablet was ~12% higher than oral administration of tablet (Haegeli, 2007)

Half-life elimination: Normal renal function: 0.5-2 hours; End-stage renal disease: 9 hours

Excretion: Urine (Oral: 50%, I.V.: 80%) within 24 hours; feces (as unchanged drug); nonrenal clearance prolonged in renal impairment

Dosage

Infants and Children: Edema, heart failure:

Oral: Initial: 2 mg/kg/dose increased in increments of 1-2 mg/kg/dose with each succeeding dose at intervals of 6-8 hours until a satisfactory response is achieved; maximum dose: 6 mg/kg/dose

I.M., I.V.: Initial: 1 mg/kg/dose; if response not adequate, may increase dose in increments of 1 mg/kg/dose and administer not sooner than 2 hours after previous dose, until a satisfactory response is achieved; may administer maintenance dose at intervals of every 6-12 hours; maximum dose: 6 mg/kg/dose

Children 1-17 years: Hypertension, resistant (unlabeled; AAP, 2004): Oral: Initial: 0.5-2 mg/kg/dose once or twice daily; maximum dose: 6 mg/kg/dose

Adults:

Edema, heart failure:

Oral: Initial: 20-80 mg/dose; if response not adequate, may repeat the same dose or increase dose in increments of 20-40 mg/dose at intervals of 6-8 hours; usual maintenance dose interval is once or twice daily; may be titrated up to 600 mg/day with severe edematous states. **Note:** May also be given on 2-4 consecutive days every week.

I.M., I.V.: Initial: 20-40 mg/dose; if response not adequate, may repeat the same dose or increase dose in increments of 20 mg/dose and administer 1-2 hours after previous dose (maximum dose: 200 mg/dose). Individually determined dose should then be given once or twice daily although some patients may initially require dosing as frequent as every 6 hours. **Note:** ACC/AHA 2009 guidelines for heart failure recommend a maximum single dose of 160-200 mg.

Continuous I.V. infusion (Howard, 2001; Hunt, 2009): Initial: I.V. bolus dose 20-40 mg over 1-2 minutes, followed by continuous I.V. infusion doses of 10-40 mg/hour. If urine output is <1 mL/kg/hour, double as necessary to a maximum of 80-160 mg/hour. The risk associated with higher infusion rates (80-160 mg/hour) must be weighed against alternative strategies. **Note:** ACC/AHA 2009 guidelines for heart failure recommend 40 mg I.V. load, then 10-40 mg/hour infusion.

Acute pulmonary edema: I.V.: 40 mg over 1-2 minutes. If response not adequate within 1 hour, may increase dose to 80 mg. **Note:** ACC/AHA 2009 guidelines for heart failure recommend a maximum single dose of 160-200 mg.

Hypertension, resistant (Chobanian, 2003; JNC 7): Oral: 20-80 mg/day in 2 divided doses

Refractory heart failure: Oral, I.V.: Doses up to 8 g/day have been used.

Elderly: Oral, I.M., I.V.: Initial: 20 mg/day; increase slowly to desired response.

Dosing adjustment/comments in renal impairment: Acute renal failure: High doses (up to 1-3 g/day - oral/I.V.) have been used to initiate desired response; avoid use in oliguric states.

Dialysis: Not removed by hemo- or peritoneal dialysis; supplemental dose is not necessary.

Dosing adjustment/comments in hepatic disease: Diminished natriuretic effect with increased sensitivity to hypokalemia and volume depletion in cirrhosis; monitor effects, particularly with high doses.

Stability

Injection: Store at room temperature of 15°C to 30°C (59°F to 86°F). Protect from light. Exposure to light may cause discoloration; do not use furosemide solutions if they have a yellow color. Furosemide solutions are unstable in acidic media, but very stable in basic media. Refrigeration may result in precipitation or crystallization; however, resolubilization at room temperature or warming may be performed without affecting the drug's stability.

I.V. infusion solution mixed in NS or D_5W solution is stable for 24 hours at room temperature. May also be diluted for infusion to 1-2 mg/mL (maximum: 10 mg/mL).

Tablet: Store at 25°C (77°F); excursions permitted to 15°C to 30°C (59°F to 89°F). Protect from light.

Administration

I.V.: I.V. injections should be given slowly. In adults, undiluted direct I.V. injections may be administered at a rate of 20-40 mg per minute; maximum rate of administration for short-term intermittent infusion is 4 mg/minute; exceeding this rate increases the risk of ototoxicity. In children, a maximum rate of 0.5 mg/kg/minute has been recommended.

Oral: Administer on an empty stomach (Bard, 2004). May be administered with food or milk if GI distress occurs; however, this may reduce diuretic efficacy.

Note: When I.V. or oral administration is not possible, the sublingual route may be used. Place 1 tablet under tongue for at least 5 minutes to allow for maximal absorption. Patients should be advised not to swallow during disintegration time (Haegeli, 2007).

Monitoring Parameters Monitor weight and I & O daily; blood pressure, orthostasis; serum electrolytes, renal function; monitor hearing with high doses or rapid I.V. administration

Anesthesia and Critical Care Concerns/Other Considerations

Clinical Pearls/Comments: It is important that patients be closely followed for hypokalemia, hypomagnesemia, and volume depletion because of significant diuresis. If given the morning of surgery, it may render the patient volume depleted and blood pressure may be labile during general anesthesia.

Dose equivalency (approximate): Bumetanide 1 mg = furosemide 40 mg = torsemide 10 mg = ethacrynic acid 50 mg

Pregnancy Risk Factor C

Contraindications Hypersensitivity to furosemide or any component of the formulation; anuria

Warnings/Precautions [U.S. Boxed Warning]: If given in excessive amounts, furosemide, similar to other loop diuretics, can lead to profound diuresis, resulting in fluid and electrolyte depletion; close medical supervision and dose evaluation are required. Watch for and correct electrolyte disturbances; adjust dose to avoid dehydration. When electrolyte depletion is present, therapy should not be initiated unless serum electrolytes, especially potassium, are normalized. In cirrhosis, avoid electrolyte and acid/base imbalances that might lead to hepatic encephalopathy; correct electrolyte and acid/base imbalances prior to initiation when hepatic coma is present. Coadministration of antihypertensives may increase the risk of hypotension.

Monitor fluid status and renal function in an attempt to prevent oliguria, azotemia, and reversible increases in BUN and creatinine; close medical supervision of aggressive diuresis is required. Rapid I.V. administration, renal impairment, excessive doses, and concurrent use of other ototoxins is associated with ototoxicity. Asymptomatic hyperuricemia has been reported with use; rarely, gout may precipitate. Photosensitization may occur.

Use with caution in patients with prediabetes or diabetes mellitus; may see a change in glucose control. Use with caution in patients with systemic lupus erythematosus (SLE); may cause SLE exacerbation or activation. Chemical similarities are present among sulfonamides, sulfonylureas, carbonic anhydrase inhibitors, thiazides, and loop diuretics (except ethacrynic acid). A risk of cross-reaction exists in patients with allergy to any of these compounds; avoid use when previous reaction has been severe. Discontinue if signs of hypersensitivity are noted.

Adverse Reactions Frequency not defined.

Cardiovascular: Acute hypotension, chronic aortitis, necrotizing angiitis, orthostatic hypotension, vasculitis

Central nervous system: Dizziness, fever, headache, hepatic encephalopathy, lightheadedness, restlessness, vertigo

Dermatologic: Bullous pemphigoid, cutaneous vasculitis, erythema multiforme, exfoliative dermatitis, photosensitivity, pruritus, purpura, rash, urticaria

Endocrine & metabolic: Glucose tolerance test altered, gout, hyperglycemia, hyperuricemia, hypocalcemia, hypochloremia, hypokalemia, hypomagnesemia, hyponatremia, metabolic alkalosis

Gastrointestinal: Anorexia, constipation, cramping, diarrhea, nausea, oral and gastric irritation, pancreatitis, vomiting

Genitourinary: Urinary bladder spasm, urinary frequency

Hematological: Agranulocytosis (rare), anemia, aplastic anemia (rare), hemolytic anemia, leukopenia, thrombocytopenia

Hepatic: Intrahepatic cholestatic jaundice, ischemic hepatitis

Local: Injection site pain (following I.M. injection), thrombophlebitis

Neuromuscular & skeletal: Muscle spasm, paresthesia, weakness

Ocular: Blurred vision, xanthopsia

Otic: Hearing impairment (reversible or permanent with rapid I.V. or I.M. administration), tinnitus

Renal: Allergic interstitial nephritis, fall in glomerular filtration rate and renal blood flow (due to overdiuresis), glycosuria, transient rise in BUN

Miscellaneous: Anaphylaxis (rare), exacerbate or activate systemic lupus erythematosus

Drug Interactions

Avoid Concomitant Use

Avoid concomitant use of Furosemide with any of the following: Ethacrynic Acid

Increased Effect/Toxicity

Furosemide may increase the levels/effects of: ACE Inhibitors; Allopurinol; Amifostine; Aminoglycosides; Antihypertensives; Dofetilide; Ethacrynic Acid; Hypotensive Agents; Lithium; Neuromuscular-Blocking Agents; RiTUXimab; Salicylates

The levels/effects of Furosemide may be increased by: Corticosteroids (Orally Inhaled); Corticosteroids (Systemic); Diazoxide; Herbs (Hypotensive Properties); MAO Inhibitors; Pentoxifylline; Phosphodiesterase 5 Inhibitors; Prostacyclin Analogues

Decreased Effect

Furosemide may decrease the levels/effects of: Lithium; Neuromuscular-Blocking Agents

The levels/effects of Furosemide may be decreased by: Aliskiren; Bile Acid Sequestrants; Herbs (Hypertensive Properties); Methylphenidate; Nonsteroidal Anti-Inflammatory Agents; Phenytoin; Salicylates; Yohimbine

Ethanol/Nutrition/Herb Interactions

Food: Furosemide serum levels may be decreased if taken with food.

Herb/Nutraceutical: Avoid bayberry, blue cohosh, cayenne, ephedra, ginger, ginseng (American), kola, licorice (may worsen hypertension). Avoid black cohosh, California poppy, coleus, golden seal, hawthorn, mistletoe, periwinkle, quinine, shepherd's purse (may increase antihypertensive effect).

Dietary Considerations May cause potassium loss; potassium supplement or dietary changes may be required.

Dosage Forms Excipient information presented when available (limited, particularly for generics); consult specific product labeling.

Injection, solution: 10 mg/mL (2 mL, 4 mL, 10 mL)

Injection, solution [preservative free]: 10 mg/mL (2 mL, 4 mL, 10 mL)

Solution, oral: 10 mg/mL (60 mL, 120 mL) [orange flavor]; 40 mg/5 mL (5 mL, 500 mL) [pineapple-peach flavor]

Tablet: 20 mg, 40 mg, 80 mg

Lasix®: 20 mg

Lasix®: 40 mg, 80 mg [scored]

♦ **Furosemide Injection, USP (Can)** *see* Furosemide *on page 645*

♦ **Furosemide Special (Can)** *see* Furosemide *on page 645*

Fusidic Acid (fyoo SI dik AS id)

Canadian Brand Names Fucidin®; Fucithalmic®
Index Terms Sodium Fusidate
Pharmacologic Category Antibiotic, Miscellaneous
Restrictions Not available in U.S.
Generic Available No
Use

Systemic: Treatment of skin and soft tissue infections, or osteomyelitis, caused by susceptible organisms, including *Staphylococcus aureus* (penicillinase-producing or nonpenicillinase strains); may be used in the treatment of pneumonia, septicemia, endocarditis, burns, and cystic fibrosis caused by susceptible organisms when other antibiotics have failed

Topical: Treatment of primary and secondary skin infections caused by susceptible organisms

Ophthalmic: Treatment of superficial infections of the eye and conjunctiva caused by susceptible organisms

Mechanism of Action Inhibits protein synthesis by blocking aminoacyl-sRNA transfer to protein in susceptible bacteria.
Pharmacodynamics/Kinetics

Protein binding: 97%
Metabolism: Hepatic, to multiple metabolites
Half-life elimination: 5-6 hours
Time to peak, serum: Oral: 2-4 hours
Excretion: Feces (~100%, via bile)

Dosage

I.V.:
  Children ≤12 years: 20 mg/kg/day in 3 divided doses
  Children >12 years and Adults: 500 mg sodium fusidate 3 times/day
Ophthalmic: Children ≥2 years and Adults: Instill 1 drop in each eye every 12 hours for 7 days
Topical: Children and Adults: Apply to affected area 3-4 times/day until favorable results are achieved. If a gauze dressing is used, frequency of application may be reduced to 1-2 times/day.
Oral: Adults: 500 mg sodium fusidate 3 times/day. (**Note:** Oral dosage may be increased to 1000 mg 3 times/day in fulminating infections.)

Dosage adjustment in renal impairment: No dosage adjustment required
Dosage adjustment in hepatic impairment: Oral, I.V.: Use with extreme caution in patients with hepatic impairment; monitor liver function periodically during therapy
Stability

Cream: Store below 25°C.
Injection, powder for reconstitution: Store below 25°C. Reconstitute 500 mg vial of powder for injection by adding 10 mL of supplied diluent containing phosphate/citrate buffer. Reconstituted solution may be further diluted with NS or D$_5$W; should be used within 24 hours. Add to NS or D$_5$W to produce a final concentration of 1-2 mg/mL. For patients weighing <50 kg, reconstituted drug should be diluted at least 10-fold in a compatible solution. Discard solution if opalescence is observed.
Ointment: Store below 30°C.
Ophthalmic suspension: Store at 2°C to 25°C. Discard multidose vials 1 month after opening.

Administration I.V.: Should not be administered I.M. or SubQ. Intravenous administration should be via a large bore vein with good blood flow. Administer over 2 hours or more. Do not administer with whole blood or amino acid solutions.
Monitoring Parameters Monitor liver function tests, including bilirubin periodically during systemic therapy
Contraindications Hypersensitivity to fusidic acid or any component of the formulation

◄ **Warnings/Precautions** Use with extreme caution in hepatic impairment; monitor liver function regularly during treatment. Intravenous formulation contains phosphate/citrate buffer; excessive amounts may lead to hypocalcemia. Use with extreme caution in patients with pre-existing hypocalcemia. Should not be administered I.M. or SubQ; local tissue injury may occur.

Adverse Reactions
Cardiovascular: Edema (leg), thrombophlebitis, venospasm
Central nervous system: Dizziness, headache, psychic disturbance
Dermatologic: Pruritus, rash
Gastrointestinal: Anorexia, dyspepsia, diarrhea, epigastric distress, nausea, vomiting
Hepatic: Jaundice
Local: Injection site reaction (redness, irritation)
Ocular: Blurred vision

Ophthalmic suspension: Ocular: Transient stinging, tearing, eyelid edema, temporary blurred vision

Drug Interactions
Avoid Concomitant Use There are no known interactions where it is recommended to avoid concomitant use.
Increased Effect/Toxicity
Fusidic Acid may increase the levels/effects of: Atorvastatin; Protease Inhibitors; Simvastatin

The levels/effects of Fusidic Acid may be increased by: Protease Inhibitors
Decreased Effect
Fusidic Acid may decrease the levels/effects of: Penicillins
Dietary Considerations May take tablets with food to minimize gastrointestinal upset.
Dosage Forms Excipient information presented when available (limited, particularly for generics); consult specific product labeling. [CAN] = Canadian brand name
Cream, as fusidic acid:
Fucidin®: 2% (15 g, 30 g)
Injection, powder for reconstitution, as sodium fusidate:
Fucidin®: 500 mg [packaged with 10 mL diluent/buffer solution]
Ointment, topical, as sodium fusidate:
Fucidin®: 2% (15 g, 30 g) [contains lanolin]
Suspension, ophthalmic, as fusidic acid:
Fucithalmic®: 10 mg/g [1%] (0.2 g) [unit-dose, without preservative]; (3 g, 5 g) [multidose, contains benzalkonium chloride]
Tablet, as sodium fusidate:
Fucidin®: 250 mg

◆ **Fusilev™** *see* LEVOleucovorin *on page* 828
◆ **FXT 40 (Can)** *see* FLUoxetine *on page* 616

Gabapentin (GA ba pen tin)

Medication Safety Issues
Sound-alike/look-alike issues:
Neurontin® may be confused with Motrin®, Neoral®, nitrofurantoin, Noroxin®, Zarontin®
Related Information
Acute Postoperative Pain *on page* 1502
Chronic Pain Management *on page* 1546
Perioperative Management of Patients on Antiseizure Medication *on page* 1577
U.S. Brand Names Neurontin®
Canadian Brand Names Apo-Gabapentin®; CO Gabapentin; Dom-Gabapentin; Mylan-Gabapentin; Neurontin®; Novo-Gabapentin; PHL-Gabapentin; PMS-Gabapentin; PRO-Gabapentin; Ran-Gabapentin; ratio-Gabapentin; Riva-Gabapentin; ZYM-Gabapentin
Pharmacologic Category Anticonvulsant, Miscellaneous
Generic Available Yes: Capsule, tablet

Use Adjunct for treatment of partial seizures with and without secondary generalized seizures in patients >12 years of age with epilepsy; adjunct for treatment of partial seizures in pediatric patients 3-12 years of age; management of postherpetic neuralgia (PHN) in adults

Unlabeled/Investigational Use Neuropathic pain, diabetic peripheral neuropathy, fibromyalgia, postoperative pain, bipolar disorder, social phobia, vasomotor symptoms

Mechanism of Action Gabapentin is structurally related to GABA. However, it does not bind to $GABA_A$ or $GABA_B$ receptors, and it does not appear to influence synthesis or uptake of GABA. High affinity gabapentin binding sites have been located throughout the brain; these sites correspond to the presence of voltage-gated calcium channels specifically possessing the alpha-2-delta-1 subunit. This channel appears to be located presynaptically, and may modulate the release of excitatory neurotransmitters which participate in epileptogenesis and nociception.

Pharmacodynamics/Kinetics

Absorption: 50% to 60% from proximal small bowel by L-amino transport system

Distribution: V_d: 0.6-0.8 L/kg

Protein binding: <3%

Bioavailability: Inversely proportional to dose due to saturable absorption:

900 mg/day: 60%

1200 mg/day: 47%

2400 mg/day: 34%

3600 mg/day: 33%

4800 mg/day: 27%

Half-life elimination: 5-7 hours; anuria 132 hours; during dialysis 3.8 hours

Excretion: Proportional to renal function; urine (as unchanged drug)

Dosage Oral:

Children: Anticonvulsant:

3-12 years: Initial: 10-15 mg/kg/day in 3 divided doses; titrate to effective dose over ~3 days; dosages of up to 50 mg/kg/day have been tolerated in clinical studies

3-4 years: Effective dose: 40 mg/kg/day in 3 divided doses

≥5-12 years: Effective dose: 25-35 mg/kg/day in 3 divided doses

See **"Note"** in adult dosing.

Children >12 years and Adults:

Anticonvulsant: Initial: 300 mg 3 times/day; if necessary the dose may be increased up to 1800 mg/day. Doses of up to 2400 mg/day have been tolerated in long-term clinical studies; up to 3600 mg/day has been tolerated in short-term studies.

Note: If gabapentin is discontinued or if another anticonvulsant is added to therapy, it should be done slowly over a minimum of 1 week

Pain (unlabeled use): 300-1800 mg/day given in 3 divided doses has been the most common dosage range

Adults:

Postherpetic neuralgia or neuropathic pain: Day 1: 300 mg, Day 2: 300 mg twice daily, Day 3: 300 mg 3 times/day; dose may be titrated as needed for pain relief (range: 1800-3600 mg/day, daily doses >1800 mg do not generally show greater benefit)

Vasomotor symptoms associated with menopause (unlabeled use; Butt, 2008): 300 mg 3 times/day

Elderly: Studies in elderly patients have shown a decrease in clearance as age increases. This is most likely due to age-related decreases in renal function; dose reductions may be needed.

Dosing adjustment in renal impairment: Children ≥12 years and Adults: See table on next page.

Hemodialysis: Dialyzable

Gabapentin Dosing Adjustments in Renal Impairment

Creatinine Clearance (mL/min)	Daily Dose Range
≥60	300-1200 mg tid
>30-59	200-700 mg bid
>15-29	200-700 mg daily
15[1]	100-300 mg daily
Hemodialysis[2]	125-350 mg

[1]Cl_{cr}<15 mL/minute: Reduce daily dose in proportion to creatinine clearance.
[2]Single supplemental dose administered after each 4 hours of hemodialysis.

Stability Store at 25°C (77°F); excursions permitted to 15°C to 30°C (59°F to 86°F).

Administration Administer first dose on first day at bedtime to avoid somnolence and dizziness. Dosage must be adjusted for renal function; when given 3 times daily, the maximum time between doses should not exceed 12 hours.

Monitoring Parameters Monitor serum levels of concomitant anticonvulsant therapy; suicidality (eg, suicidal thoughts, depression, behavioral changes)

Pregnancy Risk Factor C

Contraindications Hypersensitivity to gabapentin or any component of the formulation

Warnings/Precautions Antiepileptics are associated with an increased risk of suicidal behavior/thoughts with use (regardless of indication); patients should be monitored for signs/symptoms of depression, suicidal tendencies, and other unusual behavior changes during therapy and instructed to inform their healthcare provider immediately if symptoms occur. Avoid abrupt withdrawal, may precipitate seizures; use cautiously in patients with severe renal dysfunction; male rat studies demonstrated an association with pancreatic adenocarcinoma (clinical implication unknown). May cause CNS depression, which may impair physical or mental abilities. Patients must be cautioned about performing tasks which require mental alertness (eg, operating machinery or driving). Effects with other sedative drugs or ethanol may be potentiated. Pediatric patients (3-12 years of age) have shown increased incidence of CNS-related adverse effects, including emotional lability, hostility, thought disorder, and hyperkinesia. Safety and efficacy in children <3 years of age have not been established.

Adverse Reactions As reported in patients >12 years of age, unless otherwise noted in children (3-12 years)
>10%:
  Central nervous system: Somnolence (20%; children 8%), dizziness (17% to 28%; children 3%), ataxia (13%), fatigue (11%)
  Miscellaneous: Viral infection (children 11%)
1% to 10%:
  Cardiovascular: Peripheral edema (2% to 8%), vasodilatation (1%)
  Central nervous system: Fever (children 10%), hostility (children 8%), emotional lability (children 4%), fatigue (children 3%), headache (3%), ataxia (3%), abnormal thinking (2% to 3%; children 2%), amnesia (2%), depression (2%), dysarthria (2%), nervousness (2%), abnormal coordination (1% to 2%), twitching (1%), hyperesthesia (1%)
  Dermatologic: Pruritus (1%), rash (1%)
  Endocrine & metabolic: Hyperglycemia (1%)
  Gastrointestinal: Diarrhea (6%), nausea/vomiting (3% to 4%; children 8%), abdominal pain (3%), weight gain (adults and children 2% to 3%), dyspepsia (2%), flatulence (2%), dry throat (2%), xerostomia (2% to 5%), constipation (2% to 4%), dental abnormalities (2%), appetite stimulation (1%)
  Genitourinary: Impotence (2%)
  Hematologic: Leukopenia (1%), decreased WBC (1%)
  Neuromuscular & skeletal: Tremor (7%), weakness (6%), hyperkinesia (children 3%), abnormal gait (2%), back pain (2%), myalgia (2%), fracture (1%)

Ocular: Nystagmus (8%), diplopia (1% to 6%), blurred vision (3% to 4%), conjunctivitis (1%)

Otic: Otitis media (1%)

Respiratory: Rhinitis (4%), bronchitis (children 3%), respiratory infection (children 3%), pharyngitis (1% to 3%), cough (2%)

Miscellaneous: Infection (5%)

Postmarketing and additional clinical reports (limited to important or life-threatening): Acute renal failure, anemia, angina, angioedema, aphasia, arrhythmias (various), aspiration pneumonia, blindness, bradycardia, bronchospasm, cerebrovascular accident, CNS tumors, coagulation defect, colitis, Cushingoid appearance, dyspnea, encephalopathy, facial paralysis, fecal incontinence, glaucoma, glycosuria, heart block, hearing loss, hematemesis, hematuria, hemiplegia, hemorrhage, hepatitis, hepatomegaly, hyper-/hypotension, hyperlipidemia, hyper-/hypothyroidism, hyper-/hypoventilation, gastroenteritis, heart failure, leukocytosis, liver function tests increased, local myoclonus, lymphadenopathy, lymphocytosis, meningismus, MI, migraine, nephrosis, nerve palsy, non-Hodgkin's lymphoma, ovarian failure, pulmonary thrombosis, pericardial rub, pulmonary embolus, pericardial effusion, pericarditis, pancreatitis, peptic ulcer, purpura, paresthesia, palpitation, peripheral vascular disorder, pneumonia, psychosis, renal stone, retinopathy, skin necrosis, status epilepticus, subdural hematoma, suicidal behavior/ideation, syncope, tachycardia, thrombocytopenia, thrombophlebitis

Drug Interactions

Avoid Concomitant Use There are no known interactions where it is recommended to avoid concomitant use.

Increased Effect/Toxicity

Gabapentin may increase the levels/effects of: Alcohol (Ethyl); CNS Depressants; Methotrimeprazine

The levels/effects of Gabapentin may be increased by: Methotrimeprazine

Decreased Effect

The levels/effects of Gabapentin may be decreased by: Ketorolac; Mefloquine

Ethanol/Nutrition/Herb Interactions

Ethanol: Avoid ethanol (may increase CNS depression).

Food: Does not change rate or extent of absorption.

Herb/Nutraceutical: Avoid evening primrose (seizure threshold decreased). Avoid valerian, St John's wort, kava kava, gotu kola (may increase CNS depression).

Test Interactions False positives have been reported with the Ames N-Multistix SG® dipstick test for urine protein

Dietary Considerations May be taken without regard to meals.

Dosage Forms Excipient information presented when available (limited, particularly for generics); consult specific product labeling.

Capsule: 100 mg, 300 mg, 400 mg

Neurontin®: 100 mg, 300 mg, 400 mg

Solution, oral:

Neurontin®: 250 mg/5 mL (480 mL) [cool strawberry anise flavor]

Tablet: 100 mg, 300 mg, 400 mg, 600 mg, 800 mg

Neurontin®: 600 mg, 800 mg

References

Butt DA, Lock M, Lewis JE, et al, "Gabapentin for the Treatment of Menopausal Hot Flashes: A Randomized Controlled Trial," *Menopause*, 2008, 15(2):310-8.

Dierking G, Duedahl TH, Rasmussen ML, et al, "Effects of Gabapentin on Postoperative Morphine Consumption and Pain After Abdominal Hysterectomy: A Randomized, Double-Blind Trial," *Acta Anaesthesiol Scand*, 2004, 48(3):322-7.

Dirks J, Fredensborg BB, Christensen D, et al, "A Randomized Study of the Effects of Single-Dose Gabapentin Versus Placebo on Postoperative Pain and Morphine Consumption After Mastectomy," *Anesthesiology*, 2002, 97(3):560-4.

Pandey CK, Priye S, Singh S, et al, "Preemptive Use of Gabapentin Significantly Decreases Postoperative Pain and Rescue Analgesic Requirements in Laparoscopic Cholecystectomy," *Can J Anaesth*, 2004, 51(4):358-63.

Rorarius MG, Mennander S, Suominen P, et al, "Gabapentin for the Prevention of Postoperative Pain After Vaginal Hysterectomy," *Pain*, 2004, 110(1-2):175-81.

Turan A, Memis D, Karamanlioglu B, et al, "The Analgesic Effects of Gabapentin in Monitored Anesthesia Care for Ear-Nose-Throat Surgery," *Anesth Analg*, 2004, 99(2):375-8, table of contents.

◆ **Gabitril®** *see* TiaGABine *on page 1381*

Gallium Nitrate (GAL ee um NYE trate)

U.S. Brand Names Ganite™
Index Terms NSC-15200
Pharmacologic Category Calcium-Lowering Agent
Use Treatment of symptomatic cancer-related hypercalcemia
Pharmacodynamics/Kinetics

Onset of calcium lowering: Seen within 24-48 hours of beginning therapy, with normocalcemia achieved within 4-7 days of beginning therapy

Duration: Normocalcemia: 7-10 days

Bioavailability: Oral: 5%

Distribution: Tissue concentrations were determined postmortem in one patient and concentrations were higher in liver and kidney than in lung, skin, muscle, heart, and cervix tumor; in dogs, tissue gallium concentrations were higher in renal cortex, bone, bone marrow, small intestine, and liver than in skeletal muscle and brain

Half-life elimination: Alpha: 1.25 hours; Beta: ~24 hours

Elimination half-life varies with method of administration (72-115 hours with prolonged intravenous infusion versus 24 hours with bolus administration); long elimination half-life may be related to slow release from tissue such as bone

Excretion: Primarily renal with no prior metabolism in the liver or kidney

Dosage Note: Initiate I.V. hydration prior to treatment; maintain throughout treatment.

I.V.: Adults: 200 mg/m^2/day for 5 days; duration may be shortened during a course if normocalcemia is achieved. If hypercalcemia is mild and with very few symptoms, 100 mg/m^2/day may be used.

Dosage adjustment in renal impairment:

Serum creatinine >2.5 mg/dL: Contraindicated

Serum creatinine 2 to ≤2.5 mg/dL: No guidelines exist; frequent monitoring is recommended

Additional Information Complete prescribing information for this medication should be consulted for additional detail.

Dosage Forms Excipient information presented when available (limited, particularly for generics); consult specific product labeling.

Injection, solution [preservative free]:

Ganite™: 25 mg/mL (20 mL)

♦ **Gamimune® N (Can)** see Immune Globulin (Intravenous) *on page 732*

♦ **Gammagard Liquid** see Immune Globulin (Intravenous) *on page 732*

♦ **Gammagard S/D** see Immune Globulin (Intravenous) *on page 732*

♦ **Gamunex®** see Immune Globulin (Intravenous) *on page 732*

Ganciclovir (gan SYE kloe veer)

Medication Safety Issues

Sound-alike/look-alike issues:

Cytovene® may be confused with Cytosar®, Cytosar-U®

Ganciclovir may be confused with acyclovir

U.S. Brand Names Cytovene®; Vitrasert®; Zirgan™
Canadian Brand Names Cytovene®; Vitrasert®
Index Terms DHPG Sodium; GCV Sodium; Nordeoxyguanosine
Pharmacologic Category Antiviral Agent
Generic Available Yes: Capsule
Use

Parenteral: Treatment of CMV retinitis in immunocompromised individuals, including patients with acquired immunodeficiency syndrome; prophylaxis of CMV infection in transplant patients

Oral: Alternative to the I.V. formulation for maintenance treatment of CMV retinitis in immunocompromised patients, including patients with AIDS, in whom retinitis is stable following appropriate induction therapy and for whom the risk of more rapid progression is balanced by the benefit associated with avoiding daily I.V. infusions.

Implant: Treatment of CMV retinitis

Unlabeled/Investigational Use May be given in combination with foscarnet in patients who relapse after monotherapy with either drug

Mechanism of Action Ganciclovir is phosphorylated to a substrate which competitively inhibits the binding of deoxyguanosine triphosphate to DNA polymerase resulting in inhibition of viral DNA synthesis

Pharmacodynamics/Kinetics

Distribution: V_d: 15.26 L/1.73 m^2; widely to all tissues including CSF and ocular tissue

Protein binding: 1% to 2%

Bioavailability: Oral: Fasting: 5%; Following food: 6% to 9%; Following fatty meal: 28% to 31%

Half-life elimination: 1.7-5.8 hours; prolonged with renal impairment; End-stage renal disease: 5-28 hours

Excretion: Urine (80% to 99% as unchanged drug)

Dosage

CMV retinitis: Slow I.V. infusion (dosing is based on total body weight):

Children >3 months and Adults:

Induction therapy: 5 mg/kg/dose every 12 hours for 14-21 days followed by maintenance therapy

Maintenance therapy: 5 mg/kg/day as a single daily dose for 7 days/week or 6 mg/kg/day for 5 days/week

CMV retinitis: Oral: 1000 mg 3 times/day with food **or** 500 mg 6 times/day with food

Prevention of CMV disease in patients with advanced HIV infection and normal renal function: Oral: 1000 mg 3 times/day with food

Prevention of CMV disease in transplant patients: Same initial and maintenance dose as CMV retinitis except duration of initial course is 7-14 days, duration of maintenance therapy is dependent on clinical condition and degree of immunosuppression

Intravitreal implant: One implant for 5- to 8-month period; following depletion of ganciclovir, as evidenced by progression of retinitis, implant may be removed and replaced

Elderly: Refer to adult dosing; in general, dose selection should be cautious, reflecting greater frequency of organ impairment

Dosing adjustment in renal impairment:

I.V. (Induction):

Cl_{cr} 50-69 mL/minute: Administer 2.5 mg/kg/dose every 12 hours

Cl_{cr} 25-49 mL/minute: Administer 2.5 mg/kg/dose every 24 hours

Cl_{cr} 10-24 mL/minute: Administer 1.25 mg/kg/dose every 24 hours

Cl_{cr} <10 mL/minute: Administer 1.25 mg/kg/dose 3 times/week following hemodialysis

I.V. (Maintenance):

Cl_{cr} 50-69 mL/minute: Administer 2.5 mg/kg/dose every 24 hours

Cl_{cr} 25-49 mL/minute: Administer 1.25 mg/kg/dose every 24 hours

Cl_{cr} 10-24 mL/minute: Administer 0.625 mg/kg/dose every 24 hours

Cl_{cr} <10 mL/minute: Administer 0.625 mg/kg/dose 3 times/week following hemodialysis

Oral:

Cl_{cr} 50-69 mL/minute: Administer 1500 mg/day or 500 mg 3 times/day

Cl_{cr} 25-49 mL/minute: Administer 1000 mg/day or 500 mg twice daily

Cl_{cr} 10-24 mL/minute: Administer 500 mg/day

Cl_{cr} <10 mL/minute: Administer 500 mg 3 times/week following hemodialysis

Hemodialysis effects: Dialyzable (50%) following hemodialysis; administer dose postdialysis. During peritoneal dialysis, dose as for Cl_{cr} <10 mL/minute. During continuous arteriovenous or venovenous hemofiltration, administer 2.5 mg/kg/dose every 24 hours.

Stability Intact vials should be stored at room temperature and protected from temperatures >40°C Reconstitute powder with unpreserved sterile water **not** bacteriostatic water because parabens may cause precipitation; dilute in 250-1000 mL D$_5$W or NS to a concentration ≤10 mg/mL for infusion.

Reconstituted solution is stable for 12 hours at room temperature, however, conflicting data indicates that reconstituted solution is stable for 60 days under refrigeration (4°C). Stability of parenteral admixture at room temperature (25°C) and at refrigeration temperature (4°C) is 5 days.

Administration

Oral: Should be administered with food.

I.V.: Should not be administered by I.M., SubQ, or rapid IVP; administer by slow I.V. infusion over at least 1 hour

Monitoring Parameters CBC with differential and platelet count, serum creatinine, ophthalmologic exams

Pregnancy Risk Factor C

Contraindications Hypersensitivity to ganciclovir, acyclovir, or any component of the formulation; absolute neutrophil count <500/mm^3; platelet count <25,000/mm^3

Warnings/Precautions Hazardous agent - use appropriate precautions for handling and disposal. **[U.S. Boxed Warning]: Granulocytopenia (neutropenia), anemia, and thrombocytopenia may occur.** Dosage adjustment or interruption of ganciclovir therapy may be necessary in patients with neutropenia and/or thrombocytopenia and patients with impaired renal function. **[U.S. Boxed Warning]: Animal studies have demonstrated carcinogenic and teratogenic effects, and inhibition of spermatogenesis;** contraceptive precautions for female and male patients need to be followed during and for at least 90 days after therapy with the drug; take care to administer only into veins with good blood flow. **[U.S. Boxed Warning]: Indicated only for treatment of CMV retinitis in the immunocompromised patient and CMV prevention in transplant patients at risk.**

Adverse Reactions

>10%:

Central nervous system: Fever (38% to 48%)

Dermatologic: Rash (15% oral, 10% I.V.)

Gastrointestinal: Diarrhea (40%), nausea (25%), abdominal pain (17% to 19%), anorexia (15%), vomiting (13%)

Hematologic: Leukopenia (30% to 40%), anemia (20% to 25%)

1% to 10%:

Central nervous system: Neuropathy (8% to 9%), headache (4%), confusion

Dermatologic: Pruritus (5%)

Hematologic: Thrombocytopenia (6%), neutropenia with ANC <500/mm^3 (5% oral, 14% I.V.)

Neuromuscular & skeletal: Paresthesia (6% to 10%), weakness (6%)

Ocular: Retinal detachment (8% oral, 11% I.V.; relationship to ganciclovir not established)

Miscellaneous: Sepsis (4% oral, 15% I.V.)

<1% (Limited to important or life-threatening): Alopecia, arrhythmia, ataxia, bronchospasm, coma, dyspnea, encephalopathy, eosinophilia, exfoliative dermatitis, extrapyramidal symptoms, hemorrhage, nervousness, pancytopenia, psychosis, renal failure, seizure, SIADH, Stevens-Johnson syndrome, torsade de pointes, urticaria, visual loss

Drug Interactions

Avoid Concomitant Use

Avoid concomitant use of Ganciclovir with any of the following: Imipenem

Increased Effect/Toxicity

Ganciclovir may increase the levels/effects of: Imipenem; Mycophenolate; Reverse Transcriptase Inhibitors (Nucleoside); Tenofovir

The levels/effects of Ganciclovir may be increased by: Mycophenolate

Decreased Effect There are no known significant interactions involving a decrease in effect.

Dietary Considerations Capsule should be taken with food. Some products may contain sodium.

Product Availability

Zirgan™: FDA approved September 2009; availability expected in early 2010

Zirgan™ is an ophthalmic gel indicated for the treatment of acute herpetic keratitis.

Dosage Forms Excipient information presented when available (limited, particularly for generics); consult specific product labeling.

Capsule: 250 mg, 500 mg
Implant, intravitreal:
   Vitrasert®: 4.5 mg [released gradually over 5-8 months]
Injection, powder for reconstitution, as sodium:
   Cytovene®: 500 mg

◆ **Ganite™** *see* Gallium Nitrate *on page 654*
◆ **GAR-936** *see* Tigecycline *on page 1388*
◆ **Garamycin® (Can)** *see* Gentamicin *on page 658*
◆ **G-CSF** *see* Filgrastim *on page 601*
◆ **GCV Sodium** *see* Ganciclovir *on page 654*
◆ **GD-Amlodipine (Can)** *see* AmLODIPine *on page 93*
◆ **GD-Celecoxib (Can)** *see* Celecoxib *on page 276*
◆ **GD-Quinapril (Can)** *see* Quinapril *on page 1214*
◆ **Gelnique™** *see* Oxybutynin *on page 1068*
◆ **GelRite [OTC]** *see* Alcohol (Ethyl) *on page 53*
◆ **Gel-Stat™ [OTC]** *see* Alcohol (Ethyl) *on page 53*
◆ **Gen-Acebutolol (Can)** *see* Acebutolol *on page 24*
◆ **Genacote™ [OTC]** *see* Aspirin *on page 147*
◆ **Gen-Acyclovir (Can)** *see* Acyclovir *on page 40*
◆ **Genahist™ [OTC]** *see* DiphenhydrAMINE *on page 430*
◆ **Gen-Alendronate (Can)** *see* Alendronate *on page 57*
◆ **Gen-Alprazolam (Can)** *see* ALPRAZolam *on page 64*
◆ **Gen-Amiodarone (Can)** *see* Amiodarone *on page 86*
◆ **Gen-Amoxicillin (Can)** *see* Amoxicillin *on page 95*
◆ **Genapap™ [OTC] [DSC]** *see* Acetaminophen *on page 25*
◆ **Genapap™ Extra Strength [OTC]** *see* Acetaminophen *on page 25*
◆ **Genapap™ Infant [OTC] [DSC]** *see* Acetaminophen *on page 25*
◆ **Gen-Atenolol (Can)** *see* Atenolol *on page 155*
◆ **Gen-Azathioprine (Can)** *see* AzaTHIOprine *on page 167*
◆ **GEN-Azithromycin (Can)** *see* Azithromycin *on page 169*
◆ **Gen-Baclofen (Can)** *see* Baclofen *on page 178*
◆ **Gen-Budesonide AQ (Can)** *see* Budesonide *on page 206*
◆ **Gen-Buspirone (Can)** *see* BusPIRone *on page 219*
◆ **Gen-Captopril (Can)** *see* Captopril *on page 239*
◆ **Gen-Carbamazepine CR (Can)** *see* CarBAMazepine *on page 241*
◆ **Gen-Cilazapril (Can)** *see* Cilazapril *on page 301*
◆ **Gen-Clarithromycin (Can)** *see* Clarithromycin *on page 317*
◆ **Gen-Clindamycin (Can)** *see* Clindamycin *on page 324*
◆ **Gen-Clonazepam (Can)** *see* ClonazePAM *on page 328*
◆ **Gen-Combo Sterinebs (Can)** *see* Ipratropium and Albuterol *on page 762*
◆ **Gen-Diltiazem (Can)** *see* Diltiazem *on page 425*
◆ **Gen-Diltiazem CD (Can)** *see* Diltiazem *on page 425*
◆ **Gen-Diltiazem SR (Can)** *see* Diltiazem *on page 425*
◆ **Gen-Divalproex (Can)** *see* Valproic Acid and Derivatives *on page 1445*
◆ **Genebs [OTC] [DSC]** *see* Acetaminophen *on page 25*
◆ **Genebs Extra Strength [OTC]** *see* Acetaminophen *on page 25*
◆ **Gen-Enalapril (Can)** *see* Enalapril *on page 478*
◆ **Generlac** *see* Lactulose *on page 796*
◆ **Gen-Famotidine (Can)** *see* Famotidine *on page 575*
◆ **Gen-Fenofibrate Micro (Can)** *see* Fenofibrate *on page 582*
◆ **Gen-Fluconazole (Can)** *see* Fluconazole *on page 607*

- ◆ **Gen-Fluoxetine (Can)** *see* FLUoxetine *on page 616*
- ◆ **Gen-Fosinopril (Can)** *see* Fosinopril *on page 636*
- ◆ **Gen-Glybe (Can)** *see* GlyBURIDE *on page 666*
- ◆ **Gengraf®** *see* CycloSPORINE *on page 357*
- ◆ **Gen-Hydroxyurea (Can)** *see* Hydroxyurea *on page 712*
- ◆ **Gen-Ipratropium (Can)** *see* Ipratropium *on page 760*
- ◆ **Gen-Lisinopril (Can)** *see* Lisinopril *on page 849*
- ◆ **Gen-Lovastatin (Can)** *see* Lovastatin *on page 859*
- ◆ **Gen-Meloxicam (Can)** *see* Meloxicam *on page 870*
- ◆ **Gen-Metformin (Can)** *see* MetFORMIN *on page 886*
- ◆ **Gen-Metoprolol (Can)** *see* Metoprolol *on page 922*
- ◆ **Gen-Nabumetone (Can)** *see* Nabumetone *on page 973*
- ◆ **Gen-Naproxen EC (Can)** *see* Naproxen *on page 987*
- ◆ **GEN-Nifedipine XL (Can)** *see* NIFEdipine *on page 1006*
- ◆ **Gen-Nitro (Can)** *see* Nitroglycerin *on page 1014*
- ◆ **Gen-Nizatidine (Can)** *see* Nizatidine *on page 1022*
- ◆ **Gen-Nortriptyline (Can)** *see* Nortriptyline *on page 1026*
- ◆ **Gen-Ondansetron (Can)** *see* Ondansetron *on page 1057*
- ◆ **Genotropin®** *see* Somatropin *on page 1318*
- ◆ **Genotropin Miniquick®** *see* Somatropin *on page 1318*
- ◆ **Gen-Pantoprazole (Can)** *see* Pantoprazole *on page 1084*
- ◆ **Gen-Pindolol (Can)** *see* Pindolol *on page 1130*
- ◆ **Gen-Pioglitazone (Can)** *see* Pioglitazone *on page 1132*
- ◆ **Gen-Piroxicam (Can)** *see* Piroxicam *on page 1139*
- ◆ **GEN-Pravastatin (Can)** *see* Pravastatin *on page 1162*
- ◆ **Genpril® [OTC] [DSC]** *see* Ibuprofen *on page 717*
- ◆ **Gen-Quetiapine (Can)** *see* QUEtiapine *on page 1212*
- ◆ **Gen-Ranidine (Can)** *see* Ranitidine *on page 1231*
- ◆ **Gen-Salbutamol (Can)** *see* Albuterol *on page 49*
- ◆ **Gen-Selegiline (Can)** *see* Selegiline *on page 1282*
- ◆ **Gen-Simvastatin (Can)** *see* Simvastatin *on page 1293*
- ◆ **Gen-Sotalol (Can)** *see* Sotalol *on page 1321*
- ◆ **Gen-Sumatriptan (Can)** *see* SUMAtriptan *on page 1336*
- ◆ **Gentak®** *see* Gentamicin *on page 658*

Gentamicin (jen ta MYE sin)

Medication Safety Issues
Sound-alike/look-alike issues:
Garamycin® may be confused with kanamycin, Terramycin®
Gentamicin may be confused with gentian violet, kanamycin, vancomycin

High alert medication: The Institute for Safe Medication Practices (ISMP) includes this medication (intrathecal administration) among its list of drug classes which have a heightened risk of causing significant patient harm when used in error.

Related Information
Anesthesia for Patients With Liver Disease *on page 1537*
Prevention of Wound Infection and Sepsis in Surgical Patients *on page 1721*

U.S. Brand Names Gentak®; Gentasol™

Canadian Brand Names Alcomicin®; Diogent®; Garamycin®; Gentamicin Injection, USP; SAB-Gentamicin

Index Terms Gentamicin Sulfate

Pharmacologic Category Antibiotic, Aminoglycoside; Antibiotic, Ophthalmic; Antibiotic, Topical

Generic Available Yes

Use Treatment of susceptible bacterial infections, normally gram-negative organisms, including *Pseudomonas, Proteus, Serratia,* and gram-positive *Staphylococcus*; treatment of bone infections, respiratory tract infections, skin and soft tissue infections, as well as abdominal and urinary tract infections, and septicemia; treatment of infective endocarditis; used topically to treat superficial infections of the skin or ophthalmic infections caused by susceptible bacteria

Mechanism of Action Interferes with bacterial protein synthesis by binding to 30S and 50S ribosomal subunits resulting in a defective bacterial cell membrane

Pharmacodynamics/Kinetics

Absorption:

Intramuscular: Rapid and complete

Oral: None

Distribution: Primarily into extracellular fluid (highly hydrophilic); high concentration in the renal cortex; minimal penetration to ocular tissues via I.V. route

V_d: Increased by edema, ascites, fluid overload; decreased with dehydration

Neonates: 0.4-0.6 L/kg

Children: 0.3-0.35 L/kg

Adults: 0.2-0.3 L/kg

Relative diffusion from blood into CSF: Minimal even with inflammation

CSF:blood level ratio: Normal meninges: Nil; Inflamed meninges: 10% to 30%

Protein binding: <30%

Half-life elimination:

Infants: <1 week: 3-11.5 hours; 1 week to 6 months: 3-3.5 hours

Adults: 1.5-3 hours; End-stage renal disease: 36-70 hours

Time to peak, serum: I.M.: 30-90 minutes; I.V.: 30 minutes after 30-minute infusion

Excretion: Urine (as unchanged drug)

Clearance: Directly related to renal function

Dosage Note: Dosage Individualization is **critical** because of the low therapeutic index.

Use of ideal body weight (IBW) for determining the mg/kg/dose appears to be more accurate than dosing on the basis of total body weight (TBW). In morbid obesity, dosage requirement may best be estimated using a dosing weight of IBW + 0.4 (TBW - IBW).

Initial and periodic plasma drug levels (eg, peak and trough with conventional dosing) should be determined, particularly in critically-ill patients with serious infections or in disease states known to significantly alter aminoglycoside pharmacokinetics (eg, cystic fibrosis, burns, or major surgery).

Usual dosage ranges:

Infants and Children <5 years: I.M., I.V.: 2.5 mg/kg/dose every 8 hours*

Children ≥5 years: I.M., I.V.: 2-2.5 mg/kg/dose every 8 hours*

*Note: Higher individual doses and/or more frequent intervals (eg, every 6 hours) may be required in selected clinical situations (cystic fibrosis) or serum levels document the need

Children and Adults:

Ophthalmic:

Ointment: Instill 1/2" (1.25 cm) 2-3 times/day to every 3-4 hours

Solution: Instill 1-2 drops every 2-4 hours, up to 2 drops every hour for severe infections

Topical: Apply 3-4 times/day to affected area

Adults:

I.M., I.V.:

Conventional: 1-2.5 mg/kg/dose every 8-12 hours; to ensure adequate peak concentrations early in therapy, higher initial dosage may be considered in selected patients when extracellular water is increased (edema, septic shock, postsurgical, or trauma)

Once daily: 4-7 mg/kg/dose once daily; some clinicians recommend this approach for all patients with normal renal function; this dose is at least as efficacious with similar, if not less, toxicity than conventional dosing

Intrathecal: 4-8 mg/day

◀ **Indication-specific dosing:**

Neonates: I.V.:

Meningitis:

0-7 days of age: <2000 g: 2.5 mg/kg every 18-24 hours; >2000 g: 2.5 mg/kg every 12 hours

8-28 days of age: <2000 g: 2.5 mg/kg every 8-12 hours; >2000 g: 2.5 mg/kg every 8 hours

Children and Adults: I.M., I.V.:

Brucellosis: 240 mg (I.M.) daily or 5 mg/kg (I.V.) daily for 7 days; either regimen recommended in combination with doxycycline

Cholangitis: 4-6 mg/kg once daily with ampicillin

Diverticulitis (complicated): 1.5-2 mg/kg every 8 hours (with ampicillin and metronidazole)

Endocarditis: Treatment: 3 mg/kg/day in 1-3 divided doses

Meningitis:

Enterococcus sp or *Pseudomonas aeruginosa*: Loading dose 2 mg/kg, then 1.7 mg/kg/dose every 8 hours (administered with another bacteriocidal drug)

Listeria: 5-7 mg/kg/day (with penicillin) for 1 week

Pelvic inflammatory disease: Loading dose: 2 mg/kg, then 1.5 mg/kg every 8 hours

Alternate therapy: 4.5 mg/kg once daily

Plague *(Yersinia pestis):* Treatment: 5 mg/kg/day, followed by postexposure prophylaxis with doxycycline

Pneumonia, hospital- or ventilator-associated: 7 mg/kg/day (with anti-pseudomonal beta-lactam or carbapenem)

Synergy (for gram-positive infections): 3 mg/kg/day in 1-3 divided doses (with ampicillin)

Tularemia: 5 mg/kg/day divided every 8 hours for 1-2 weeks

Urinary tract infection: 1.5 mg/kg/dose every 8 hours

Dosing interval in renal impairment:

Conventional dosing:

Cl_{cr} ≥60 mL/minute: Administer every 8 hours

Cl_{cr} 40-60 mL/minute: Administer every 12 hours

Cl_{cr} 20-40 mL/minute: Administer every 24 hours

Cl_{cr} <20 mL/minute: Loading dose, then monitor levels

High-dose therapy: Interval may be extended (eg, every 48 hours) in patients with moderate renal impairment (Cl_{cr} 30-59 mL/minute) and/or adjusted based on serum level determinations.

Hemodialysis: Dialyzable; removal by hemodialysis: 30% removal of aminoglycosides occurs during 4 hours of HD; administer dose after dialysis and follow levels

Removal by continuous ambulatory peritoneal dialysis (CAPD):

Administration via CAPD fluid:

Gram-negative infection: 4-8 mg/L (4-8 mcg/mL) of CAPD fluid

Gram-positive infection (eg, synergy): 3-4 mg/L (3-4 mcg/mL) of CAPD fluid

Administration via I.V., I.M. route during CAPD: Dose as for Cl_{cr} <10 mL/minute and follow levels

Removal via continuous arteriovenous or venovenous hemofiltration: Dose as for Cl_{cr} 10-40 mL/minute and follow levels

Dosing adjustment/comments in hepatic disease: Monitor plasma concentrations

Stability

Gentamicin is a colorless to slightly yellow solution which should be stored between 2°C to 30°C, but refrigeration is not recommended.

I.V. infusion solutions mixed in NS or D_5W solution are stable for 24 hours at room temperature and refrigeration.

Premixed bag: Manufacturer expiration date.

Out of overwrap stability: 30 days.

Administration

I.M.: Administer by deep I.M. route if possible. Slower absorption and lower peak concentrations, probably due to poor circulation in the atrophic muscle, may occur following I.M. injection; in paralyzed patients, suggest I.V. route.

Ophthalmic: Administer any other ophthalmics 10 minutes before or after gentamicin preparations.

Some penicillins (eg, carbenicillin, ticarcillin, and piperacillin) have been shown to inactivate aminoglycosides *in vitro*. This has been observed to a greater extent with tobramycin and gentamicin, while amikacin has shown greater stability against inactivation. Concurrent use of these agents may pose a risk of reduced antibacterial efficacy *in vivo*, particularly in the setting of profound renal impairment. However, definitive clinical evidence is lacking. If combination penicillin/aminoglycoside therapy is desired in a patient with renal dysfunction, separation of doses (if feasible), and routine monitoring of aminoglycoside levels, CBC, and clinical response should be considered.

Monitoring Parameters Urinalysis, urine output, BUN, serum creatinine; hearing should be tested before, during, and after treatment; particularly in those at risk for ototoxicity or who will be receiving prolonged therapy (>2 weeks)

Some penicillin derivatives may accelerate the degradation of aminoglycosides *in vitro*. This may be clinically-significant for certain penicillin (ticarcillin, piperacillin, carbenicillin) and aminoglycoside (gentamicin, tobramycin) combination therapy in patients with significant renal impairment. Close monitoring of aminoglycoside levels is warranted.

Reference Range

Timing of serum samples: Draw peak 30 minutes after 30-minute infusion has been completed or 1 hour after I.M. injection; draw trough immediately before next dose

Sample size: 0.5-2 mL blood (red top tube) or 0.1-1 mL serum (separated)

Therapeutic levels:

Peak:

Serious infections: 6-8 mcg/mL (12-17 µmol/L)

Life-threatening infections: 8-10 mcg/mL (17-21 µmol/L)

Urinary tract infections: 4-6 mcg/mL

Synergy against gram-positive organisms: 3-5 mcg/mL

Trough:

Serious infections: 0.5-1 mcg/mL

Life-threatening infections: 1-2 mcg/mL

The American Thoracic Society (ATS) recommends trough levels of <1 mcg/mL for patients with hospital-acquired pneumonia.

Obtain drug levels after the third dose unless renal dysfunction/toxicity suspected

Anesthesia and Critical Care Concerns/Other Considerations

Clinical Pearls/Comments: Gentamicin and tobramycin (lyophilized powder) are the only injectable aminoglycosides that are commercially available as preservative-free.

Pregnancy Risk Factor C (ophthalmic, topical); D (injection)

Contraindications Hypersensitivity to gentamicin or other aminoglycosides

Warnings/Precautions [U.S. Boxed Warning]: Aminoglycosides may cause neurotoxicity and/or nephrotoxicity; usual risk factors include pre-existing renal impairment, concomitant neuro-/nephrotoxic medications, advanced age and dehydration. Ototoxicity may be directly proportional to the amount of drug given and the duration of treatment; tinnitus or vertigo are indications of vestibular injury and impending hearing loss; renal damage is usually reversible. May cause neuromuscular blockade and respiratory paralysis; especially when given soon after anesthesia or muscle relaxants.

Not intended for long-term therapy due to toxic hazards associated with extended administration; use caution in pre-existing renal insufficiency, vestibular or cochlear impairment, myasthenia gravis, hypocalcemia, conditions which depress neuromuscular transmission. Dosage modification required in patients with impaired renal function. Prolonged use may result in fungal or bacterial superinfection, including *C. difficile*-associated diarrhea (CDAD) and pseudomembranous colitis; CDAD has been observed >2 months postantibiotic treatment.

Adverse Reactions

>10%:

Central nervous system: Neurotoxicity (vertigo, ataxia)

Neuromuscular & skeletal: Gait instability

Otic: Ototoxicity (auditory), ototoxicity (vestibular)

◄ Renal: Nephrotoxicity, decreased creatinine clearance

1% to 10%:

Cardiovascular: Edema

Dermatologic: Skin itching, reddening of skin, rash

<1% (Limited to important or life-threatening): Agranulocytosis allergic reaction, anorexia, burning, drowsiness, dyspnea, enterocolitis erythema, granulocytopenia headache, LFTs increased, muscle cramps, nausea, photosensitivity, pseudomotor cerebri, salivation increased, stinging, thrombocytopenia, tremor, vomiting, weakness, weight loss

Drug Interactions

Avoid Concomitant Use

Avoid concomitant use of Gentamicin with any of the following: Gallium Nitrate

Increased Effect/Toxicity

Gentamicin may increase the levels/effects of: AbobotulinumtoxinA; Bisphosphonate Derivatives; CARBOplatin; Colistimethate; CycloSPORINE; Gallium Nitrate; Neuromuscular-Blocking Agents; OnabotulinumtoxinA; RimabotulinumtoxinB

The levels/effects of Gentamicin may be increased by: Amphotericin B; Capreomycin; CISplatin; Loop Diuretics; Nonsteroidal Anti-Inflammatory Agents; Vancomycin

Decreased Effect

Gentamicin may decrease the levels/effects of: Typhoid Vaccine

The levels/effects of Gentamicin may be decreased by: Penicillins

Test Interactions

Some penicillin derivatives may accelerate the degradation of aminoglycosides *in vitro*, leading to a potential underestimation of aminoglycoside serum concentration.

Dietary Considerations Calcium, magnesium, potassium: Renal wasting may cause hypocalcemia, hypomagnesemia, and/or hypokalemia.

Dosage Forms Excipient information presented when available (limited, particularly for generics); consult specific product labeling. [DSC] = Discontinued product

Cream, topical: 0.1% (15 g, 30 g)

Infusion [premixed in NS]: 40 mg (50 mL); 60 mg (50 mL, 100 mL); 70 mg (50 mL); 80 mg (50 mL, 100 mL); 90 mg (100 mL); 100 mg (50 mL, 100 mL); 120 mg (100 mL)

Injection, solution: 10 mg/mL (6 mL, 8 mL, 10 mL)

Injection, solution: 40 mg/mL (2 mL, 20 mL)

Injection, solution [pediatric]: 10 mg/mL (2 mL)

Injection, solution [pediatric] [preservative free]: 10 mg/mL (2 mL)

Ointment, ophthalmic:

Gentak®: 0.3% [3 mg/g] (3.5 g)

Ointment, topical: 0.1% (15 g, 30 g)

Solution, ophthalmic: 0.3% (5 mL, 15 mL) [contains benzalkonium chloride]

Gentak®: 0.3% (5 mL; 15 mL [DSC]) [contains benzalkonium chloride]

Gentasol™: 0.3% (5 mL) [contains benzalkonium chloride]

References

American Thoracic Society and Infectious Diseases Society of America, "Guidelines for the Management of Adults With Hospital-Acquired, Ventilator-Associated, and Healthcare-Associated Pneumonia," *Am J Respir Crit Care Med*, 2005, 171(4):388-416.

Gilbert DN, Moellering RC, Eliopoulos GM, et al, eds, *The Sanford Guide To Antimicrobial Therapy*, 2006, 36th ed, Hyde Park, VT: Antimicrobial Therapy, Inc, 2006, 6-7.

Mann HJ, Fuhs DW, Awang R, et al, "Altered Aminoglycoside Pharmacokinetics in Critically Ill Patients With Sepsis," *Clin Pharm*, 1987, 6(2):148-53.

Tunkel AR, Hartman BJ, Kaplan SL, et al, "Practice Guidelines for the Management of Bacterial Meningitis," *Clin Infect Dis*, 2004, 39(9):1267-84.

Watling SM and Dasta JF, "Aminoglycoside Dosing Considerations in Intensive Care Unit Patients," *Ann Pharmacother*, 1993, 27(3):351-7.

Wilson W, Taubert KA, Gewitz M, et al, "Prevention of Infective Endocarditis. Guidelines From the American Heart Association. A Guideline From the American Heart Association Rheumatic Fever, Endocarditis, and Kawasaki Disease Committee, Council on Cardiovascular Disease in the Young, and the Council on Clinical Cardiology, Council on Cardiovascular Surgery and Anesthesia, and the Quality of Care and Outcomes Research Interdisciplinary Working Group," *Circulation*, 2007, 115. Available at http://circ.ahajournals.org/cgi/reprint/CIRCULATIONAHA.106.183095v1; last accessed July 26, 2007.

- ◆ **Gentamicin Injection, USP (Can)** *see* Gentamicin *on page* 658
- ◆ **Gentamicin Sulfate** *see* Gentamicin *on page* 658
- ◆ **Gentasol™** *see* Gentamicin *on page* 658
- ◆ **Gen-Temazepam (Can)** *see* Temazepam *on page* 1357
- ◆ **Gen-Ticlopidine (Can)** *see* Ticlopidine *on page* 1385
- ◆ **Gen-Timolol (Can)** *see* Timolol *on page* 1390
- ◆ **Gentran® [DSC]** *see* Dextran *on page* 402
- ◆ **Gentran® (Can)** *see* Dextran *on page* 402
- ◆ **Gen-Triazolam (Can)** *see* Triazolam *on page* 1434
- ◆ **GEN-Venlafaxine XR (Can)** *see* Venlafaxine *on page* 1466
- ◆ **Gen-Verapamil (Can)** *see* Verapamil *on page* 1468
- ◆ **Gen-Verapamil SR (Can)** *see* Verapamil *on page* 1468
- ◆ **Gen-Warfarin (Can)** *see* Warfarin *on page* 1479
- ◆ **Geodon®** *see* Ziprasidone *on page* 1490
- ◆ **GF196960** *see* Tadalafil *on page* 1345
- ◆ **GI87084B** *see* Remifentanil *on page* 1239
- ◆ **Glargine Insulin** *see* Insulin Glargine *on page* 744
- ◆ **Glibenclamide** *see* GlyBURIDE *on page* 666

GlipiZIDE (GLIP i zide)

U.S. Brand Names Glucotrol XL®; Glucotrol®
Index Terms Glydiazinamide
Pharmacologic Category Antidiabetic Agent, Sulfonylurea
Use Management of type 2 diabetes mellitus (noninsulin dependent, NIDDM)
Pharmacodynamics/Kinetics
Duration: 12-24 hours
Absorption: Rapid and complete; delayed with food
Distribution: 10-11 L
Protein binding: 98% to 99%; primarily to albumin
Bioavailability: 90% to 100%
Metabolism: Hepatic via CYP2C9; forms metabolites (inactive)
Half-life elimination: 2-5 hours
Time to peak: 1-3 hours; extended release tablets: 6-12 hours
Excretion: Urine (60% to 80%, 91% to 97% as metabolites); feces (11%)
Dosage Oral (allow several days between dose titrations): Adults: Initial: 5 mg/
day; adjust dosage at 2.5-5 mg daily increments as determined by blood glucose
response at intervals of several days.
Immediate release tablet: Maximum recommended once-daily dose: 15 mg;
maximum recommended total daily dose: 40 mg. Doses >15 mg/day should be
administered in divided doses.
Extended release tablet (Glucotrol XL®): Maximum recommended dose: 20 mg
When transferring from insulin to glipizide:
Current insulin requirement ≤20 units: Discontinue insulin and initiate glipizide at
usual dose
Current insulin requirement >20 units: Decrease insulin by 50% and initiate
glipizide at usual dose; gradually decrease insulin dose based on patient
response. Several days should elapse between dosage changes.
Elderly: Initial: 2.5 mg/day; increase by 2.5-5 mg/day at 1- to 2-week intervals

Dosing adjustment/comments in renal impairment: Cl_{cr} <10 mL/minute: Some
investigators recommend not using
Dosing adjustment in hepatic impairment: Initial dosage should be 2.5 mg/day
Anesthesia and Critical Care Concerns/Other Considerations
Clinical Pearls/Comments: The possibility of higher doses of sulfonylureas
eliciting an increase in cardiovascular events, because of their effects on blocking
potassium-sensitive ATP channels, has been raised. Longer-term prospective
trials of sulfonylurea therapy, such as the UKPDS and ADVANCE, do not reveal
any increased cardiovascular mortality.

◄ **Additional Information** Complete prescribing information for this medication should be consulted for additional detail.

Dosage Forms Excipient information presented when available (limited, particularly for generics); consult specific product labeling.

Tablet: 5 mg, 10 mg
Glucotrol®: 5 mg, 10 mg
Tablet, extended release: 2.5 mg, 5 mg, 10 mg
Glucotrol XL®: 2.5 mg, 5 mg, 10 mg

References
"Standards of Medical Care for Patients With Diabetes Mellitus. American Diabetes Association," *Diabetes Care*, 2007, 30(Suppl 1):4-41.

◆ **GlucaGen®** *see* Glucagon *on page* 664
◆ **GlucaGen® Diagnostic Kit** *see* Glucagon *on page* 664
◆ **GlucaGen® HypoKit™** *see* Glucagon *on page* 664

Glucagon (GLOO ka gon)

Medication Safety Issues
Sound-alike/look-alike issues:
Glucagon may be confused with Glaucon®

Related Information
Perioperative Management of the Diabetic Patient *on page* 1584

U.S. Brand Names GlucaGen®; GlucaGen® Diagnostic Kit; GlucaGen® HypoKit™; Glucagon Emergency Kit

Index Terms Glucagon Hydrochloride

Pharmacologic Category Antidote; Diagnostic Agent

Generic Available No

Use Management of hypoglycemia; diagnostic aid in radiologic examinations to temporarily inhibit GI tract movement

Unlabeled/Investigational Use Used with some success as a cardiac stimulant in management of severe cases of beta-adrenergic blocking agent overdosage; treatment of myocardial depression due to calcium channel blocker overdose

Mechanism of Action Stimulates adenylate cyclase to produce increased cyclic AMP, which promotes hepatic glycogenolysis and gluconeogenesis, causing a raise in blood glucose levels

Pharmacodynamics/Kinetics
Onset of action: Peak effect: Blood glucose levels: Parenteral:
I.V.: 5-20 minutes
I.M.: 30 minutes
SubQ: 30-45 minutes
Duration: Glucose elevation:
SubQ: 60-90 minutes
I.V.: 30 minutes
Metabolism: Primarily hepatic; some inactivation occurring renally and in plasma
Half-life elimination, plasma: 8-18 minutes

Dosage
Hypoglycemia or insulin shock therapy: I.M., I.V., SubQ:
Children <20 kg: 0.5 mg or 20-30 mcg/kg/dose; repeated in 20 minutes as needed
Children ≥20 kg and Adults: 1 mg; may repeat in 20 minutes as needed
Note: I.V. dextrose should be administered as soon as it is available; if patient fails to respond to glucagon, I.V. dextrose must be given.
Beta-blocker overdose, calcium channel blocker overdose (unlabeled use): Adults: I.V.: 5-10 mg over 1 minutes followed by an infusion of 1-10 mg/hour. The following has also been reported for beta-blocker overdose: 3-10 mg or initially 0.5-5 mg bolus followed by continuous infusion 1-5 mg/hour
Diagnostic aid: Adults: I.M., I.V.: 0.25-2 mg 10 minutes prior to procedure

Stability Prior to reconstitution, store at controlled room temperature of 20°C to 25°C (69°F to 77°F); do not freeze. Reconstitute powder for injection by adding 1 mL of sterile diluent to a vial containing 1 unit of the drug, to provide solutions containing 1 mg of glucagon/mL. Gently roll vial to dissolve. Use immediately after reconstitution. May be kept at 5°C for up to 48 hours if necessary.

Administration I.V.: Bolus may be associated with nausea and vomiting. Continuous infusions may be used in beta-blocker overdose/toxicity.

Monitoring Parameters Blood pressure, blood glucose, ECG, heart rate, mentation

Pregnancy Risk Factor B

Contraindications Hypersensitivity to glucagon or any component of the formulation; insulinoma; pheochromocytoma

Warnings/Precautions Use of glucagon is contraindicated in insulinoma; exogenous glucagon may cause an initial rise in blood glucose followed by rebound hypoglycemia. Use of glucagon is contraindicated in pheochromocytoma; exogenous glucagon may cause the release of catecholamines, resulting in an increase in blood pressure. Use caution with prolonged fasting, starvation, adrenal insufficiency or chronic hypoglycemia; levels of glucose stores in liver may be decreased. Supplemental carbohydrates should be given to patients who respond to glucagon for severe hypoglycemia to prevent secondary hypoglycemia. Monitor blood glucose levels closely. May contain lactose; avoid administration in hereditary galactose intolerance, Lapp lactase deficiency, or glucose-galactose malabsorption.

Adverse Reactions Frequency not defined.
Cardiovascular: Hypotension (up to 2 hours after GI procedures), hypertension, tachycardia
Gastrointestinal: Nausea, vomiting (high incidence with rapid administration of high doses)
Miscellaneous: Hypersensitivity reactions, anaphylaxis

Drug Interactions
Avoid Concomitant Use There are no known interactions where it is recommended to avoid concomitant use.
Increased Effect/Toxicity
Glucagon may increase the levels/effects of: Vitamin K Antagonists
Decreased Effect There are no known significant interactions involving a decrease in effect.

Ethanol/Nutrition/Herb Interactions Glucagon depletes glycogen stores.

Dietary Considerations Administer carbohydrates to patient as soon as possible after response to treatment.

Dosage Forms Excipient information presented when available (limited, particularly for generics); consult specific product labeling.
Injection, powder for reconstitution, as hydrochloride:
GlucaGen®: 1 mg [equivalent to 1 unit; contains lactose 107 mg]
GlucaGen® Diagnostic Kit: 1 mg [equivalent to 1 unit; contains lactose 107 mg; packaged with sterile water]
GlucaGen® HypoKit™: 1 mg [equivalent to 1 unit; contains lactose 107 mg; packaged with prefilled syringe containing sterile water]
Glucagon Emergency Kit: 1 mg [equivalent to 1 unit; contains lactose 49 mg; packaged with diluent syringe containing glycerin 12 mg/mL and water for injection]

References
American Heart Association Emergency Cardiovascular Care Committee," 2005 American Heart Association (AHA) Guidelines for Cardiopulmonary Resuscitation (CPR) and Emergency Cardiovascular Care (ECC)," *Circulation,* 2005, 112(24 Suppl):IV-67-77.
Bailey B, "Glucagon in Beta-Blocker and Calcium Channel Blocker Overdoses: A Systematic Review," *J Toxicol Clin Toxicol,* 2003, 41(5):595-602.
Mokhlesi B, Leikin JB, Murray P, et al, "Adult Toxicology in Critical Care. Part 11: Specific Poisonings," *Chest,* 2003, 123(3):897-922.

◆ **Glucagon Emergency Kit** *see* Glucagon *on page 664*

◆ **Glucagon Hydrochloride** *see* Glucagon *on page 664*

◆ **GlucoBurst® [OTC]** *see* Dextrose *on page 406*

◆ **Glucophage®** *see* MetFORMIN *on page 886*

◆ **Glucophage® XR** *see* MetFORMIN *on page 886*

◆ **Glucose** *see* Dextrose *on page 406*

◆ **Glucose Monohydrate** *see* Dextrose *on page 406*

◆ **Glucotrol®** *see* GlipiZIDE *on page 663*

♦ **Glucotrol XL®** *see* GlipiZIDE *on page* 663

♦ **Glulisine Insulin** *see* Insulin Glulisine *on page* 745

♦ **Glumetza™** *see* MetFORMIN *on page* 886

♦ **Glutol™ [OTC]** *see* Dextrose *on page* 406

♦ **Glutose 15™ [OTC]** *see* Dextrose *on page* 406

♦ **Glutose 45™ [OTC]** *see* Dextrose *on page* 406

♦ **Glybenclamide** *see* GlyBURIDE *on page* 666

♦ **Glybenzcyclamide** *see* GlyBURIDE *on page* 666

GlyBURIDE (GLYE byoor ide)

U.S. Brand Names Diaβeta®; Glynase® PresTab®; Micronase® [DSC]

Canadian Brand Names Albert® Glyburide; Apo-Glyburide®; Diaβeta®; Euglucon®; Gen-Glybe; Mylan-Glybe; Novo-Glyburide; Nu-Glyburide; PMS-Glyburide; PRO-Glyburide; ratio-Glyburide; Sandoz-Glyburide

Index Terms Diabeta; Glibenclamide; Glybenclamide; Glybenzcyclamide

Pharmacologic Category Antidiabetic Agent, Sulfonylurea

Use Adjunct to diet and exercise for the management of type 2 diabetes mellitus (noninsulin dependent, NIDDM)

Unlabeled/Investigational Use Alternative to insulin in women for the treatment of gestational diabetes mellitus (GDM) (11-33 weeks gestation)

Pharmacodynamics/Kinetics

Onset of action: Serum insulin levels begin to increase 15-60 minutes after a single dose

Duration: ≤24 hours

Absorption: Significant within 1 hour

Distribution: 9-10 L

Protein binding, plasma: >99% primarily to albumin

Metabolism: Hepatic; forms metabolites (weakly active)

Bioavailability: Variable among oral dosage forms

Half-life elimination: Diabeta®, Micronase®: 10 hours; Glynase® PresTab®: ~4 hours; may be prolonged with renal or hepatic impairment

Time to peak, serum: Adults: 2-4 hours

Excretion: Feces (50%) and urine (50%) as metabolites

Dosage Oral: Micronized glyburide tablets are **not** bioequivalent to conventional glyburide tablets; retitration should occur if patients are being transferred to a different glyburide formulation (eg, micronized-to-conventional or vice versa) or from other hypoglycemic agents.

Diaβeta®, Micronase®: Adults:

Initial: 2.5-5 mg/day, administered with breakfast or the first main meal of the day. In patients who are more sensitive to hypoglycemic drugs, start at 1.25 mg/day.

Increase in increments of no more than 2.5 mg/day at weekly intervals based on the patient's blood glucose response

Maintenance: 1.25-20 mg/day given as single or divided doses. Some patients (especially those receiving >10 mg/day) may have a more satisfactory response with twice-daily dosing. Maximum: 20 mg/day

Elderly: Initial: 1.25-2.5 mg/day, increase by 1.25-2.5 mg/day every 1-3 weeks

Micronized tablets (Glynase® PresTab®): Adults:

Initial: 1.5-3 mg/day, administered with breakfast or the first main meal of the day in patients who are more sensitive to hypoglycemic drugs, start at 0.75 mg/day. Increase in increments of no more than 1.5 mg/day in weekly intervals based on the patient's blood glucose response.

Maintenance: 0.75-12 mg/day given as a single dose or in divided doses. Some patients (especially those receiving >6 mg/day) may have a more satisfactory response with twice-daily dosing. Maximum: 12 mg/day

Management of noninsulin-dependent diabetes mellitus in patients previously maintained on insulin: Initial dosage dependent upon previous insulin dosage, see table on next page.

Dose Conversion: Insulin to Glyburide

Previous Daily Insulin Dosage (units/day)	Initial Glyburide Dosage *Conventional Formulation* (mg/day)	Initial Glyburide Dosage *Micronized Formulation* (mg/day)	Insulin Dosage Change (after glyburide started)
<20	2.5-5	1.5-3	Discontinue
20-40	5	3	Discontinue
>40	5 (increase in increments of 1.25-2.5 mg every 2-10 days)	3 (increase in increments of 0.75-1.5 mg every 2-10 days)	Reduce insulin dosage by 50% (gradually taper off insulin as glyburide dosage increased)

Dosing adjustment/comments in renal impairment: Cl_{cr} <50 mL/minute: **Not recommended**

Dosing adjustment in hepatic impairment: Use conservative initial and maintenance doses and avoid use in severe disease

Anesthesia and Critical Care Concerns/Other Considerations

Clinical Pearls/Comments: The possibility of higher doses of sulfonylureas eliciting an increase in cardiovascular events, because of their effects on blocking potassium-sensitive ATP channels, has been raised. Longer-term prospective trials of sulfonylurea therapy, such as the UKPDS and ADVANCE, do not reveal any increased cardiovascular mortality.

Additional Information Complete prescribing information for this medication should be consulted for additional detail.

Dosage Forms Excipient information presented when available (limited, particularly for generics); consult specific product labeling. [DSC] = Discontinued product

Tablet: 1.25 mg, 2.5 mg, 5 mg
  Diaβeta®: 1.25 mg, 2.5 mg, 5 mg
  Micronase® [DSC]: 1.25 mg, 2.5 mg, 5 mg
Tablet, micronized: 1.5 mg, 3 mg, 6 mg
  Glynase® PresTab®: 1.5 mg, 3 mg, 6 mg

References
"Standards of Medical Care for Patients With Diabetes Mellitus. American Diabetes Association," *Diabetes Care*, 2007, 30(Suppl 1):4-41.

♦ **Glyceryl Trinitrate** *see* Nitroglycerin *on page 1014*
♦ **Glycon (Can)** *see* MetFORMIN *on page 886*

Glycopyrrolate (glye koe PYE roe late)

Medication Safety Issues
Sound-alike/look-alike issues:
  Robinul® may be confused with Reminyl®

U.S. Brand Names Robinul®; Robinul® Forte

Canadian Brand Names Glycopyrrolate Injection, USP

Index Terms Glycopyrronium Bromide

Pharmacologic Category Anticholinergic Agent

Generic Available Yes

Use Inhibit salivation and excessive secretions of the respiratory tract preoperatively; control of upper airway secretions; adjunct in treatment of peptic ulcer (currently replaced by more effective agents); prevention and treatment of bradycardia

Unlabeled/Investigational Use Adjunct with acetylcholinesterase inhibitors (eg, neostigmine, edrophonium, pyridostigmine) to antagonize cholinergic effects

Mechanism of Action Blocks the action of acetylcholine at parasympathetic sites in smooth muscle, secretory glands, and the CNS

Pharmacodynamics/Kinetics
Onset of action: Oral: 50 minutes; I.M.: 15-30 minutes; I.V.: ~1 minute
  Peak effect: Oral: ~1 hour; I.M.: 30-45 minutes
Duration: Vagal effect: 2-3 hours; Inhibition of salivation: Up to 7 hours; Anticholinergic: Oral: 8-12 hours

Absorption: Oral: Poor and erratic

Distribution: V_d: 0.2-0.62 L/kg

Metabolism: Hepatic (minimal)

Bioavailability: ~10%

Half-life elimination: Infants: 22-130 minutes; Children 19-99 minutes; Adults: ~30-75 minutes

Excretion: Urine (as unchanged drug, I.M.: 80%, I.V.: 85%); bile (as unchanged drug)

Dosage

Children:

Reduction of secretions (preanesthetic):

Oral: 40-100 mcg/kg/dose 3-4 times/day

I.M., I.V.: 4-10 mcg/kg/dose every 3-4 hours; maximum: 0.2 mg/dose or 0.8 mg/24 hours

Intraoperative: I.V.: 4 mcg/kg not to exceed 0.1 mg; repeat at 2- to 3-minute intervals as needed

Preoperative: I.M.:

<2 years: 4-9 mcg/kg 30-60 minutes before procedure

>2 years: 4 mcg/kg 30-60 minutes before procedure

Children and Adults: Reverse neuromuscular blockade: I.V.: 0.2 mg for each 1 mg of neostigmine or 5 mg of pyridostigmine administered or 5-15 mcg/kg glycopyrrolate with 25-70 mcg/kg of neostigmine or 0.1-0.3 mg/kg of pyridostigmine (agents usually administered simultaneously, but glycopyrrolate may be administered first if bradycardia is present)

Adults:

Reduction of secretions:

Intraoperative: I.V.: 0.1 mg repeated as needed at 2- to 3-minute intervals

Preoperative: I.M.: 4 mcg/kg 30-60 minutes before procedure

Peptic ulcer:

Oral: 1-2 mg 2-3 times/day

I.M., I.V.: 0.1-0.2 mg 3-4 times/day

Stability Store at 20°C to 25°C (68°F to 77°F).

Administration For I.V. administration, glycopyrrolate may also be administered via the tubing of a running I.V. infusion of a compatible solution; may be administered in the same syringe with neostigmine or pyridostigmine.

Monitoring Parameters Heart rate; anticholinergic effects; bowel sounds

Pregnancy Risk Factor B

Contraindications Hypersensitivity to glycopyrrolate or any component of the formulation; severe ulcerative colitis, toxic megacolon complicating ulcerative colitis, paralytic ileus, obstructive disease of GI tract (eg, pyloric stenosis), intestinal atony in the elderly or debilitated patient; unstable cardiovascular status in acute hemorrhage; narrow-angle glaucoma; acute hemorrhage; tachycardia; obstructive uropathy; myasthenia gravis

Warnings/Precautions Diarrhea may be a sign of incomplete intestinal obstruction, treatment should be discontinued if this occurs. Use caution in elderly and in patients with autonomic neuropathy, hepatic or renal disease, or ulcerative colitis; may precipitate/aggravate toxic megacolon, hyperthyroidism, CAD, CHF, arrhythmias, tachycardia, BPH, or hiatal hernia with reflux. Use of anticholinergics in gastric ulcer treatment may cause a delay in gastric emptying due to antral statis. Caution should be used in individuals demonstrating decreased pigmentation (skin and iris coloration, dark versus light) since there has been some evidence that these individuals have an enhanced sensitivity to the anticholinergic response. May cause drowsiness, eye sensitivity to light, or blurred vision; caution should be used when performing tasks which require mental alertness, such as driving. Thr risk of heat stroke with this medication may be increased during exercise or hot weather. Infants, patients with Down syndrome, and children with spastic paralysis or brain damage may be hypersensitive to antimuscarine effects. Injection contains benzyl alcohol (associated with gasping syndrome in neonates). Not recommended for use in children <12 years of age for the management of peptic ulcer or <16 years for preanesthetic use.

Adverse Reactions Frequency not defined. **Note:** Includes adverse effects which may occur as an extension of the pharmacologic action of anticholinergics (including glycopyrrolate) and adverse effects reported postmarketing with glycopyrrolate.

Cardiovascular: Arrhythmias, cardiac arrest, heart block, hyper-/hypotension, malignant hyperthermia, palpitation, QT_c interval prolongation, tachycardia

Central nervous system: Confusion, dizziness, drowsiness, excitement, headache, insomnia, nervousness, seizure

Dermatologic: Dry skin, pruritus, sensitivity to light increased

Endocrine & metabolic: Lactation suppression

Gastrointestinal: Bloated feeling, constipation, loss of taste, nausea, vomiting, xerostomia

Genitourinary: Impotence, urinary hesitancy, urinary retention

Local: Irritation at injection site

Neuromuscular & skeletal: Weakness

Ocular: Blurred vision, cycloplegia, mydriasis, ocular tension increased, photophobia, sensitivity to light increased

Respiratory: Respiratory depression

Miscellaneous: Anaphylactoid reactions, diaphoresis decreased, hypersensitivity reactions

Drug Interactions

Avoid Concomitant Use There are no known interactions where it is recommended to avoid concomitant use.

Increased Effect/Toxicity

Glycopyrrolate may increase the levels/effects of: Anticholinergics; Cannabinoids; Potassium Chloride

The levels/effects of Glycopyrrolate may be increased by: MAO Inhibitors; Pramlintide

Decreased Effect

Glycopyrrolate may decrease the levels/effects of: Acetylcholinesterase Inhibitors (Central); Secretin

The levels/effects of Glycopyrrolate may be decreased by: Acetylcholinesterase Inhibitors (Central)

Dosage Forms Excipient information presented when available (limited, particularly for generics); consult specific product labeling. [DSC] = Discontinued product

Injection, solution: 0.2 mg/mL (1 mL, 2 mL, 5 mL, 20 mL)

  Robinul®: 0.2 mg/mL (1 mL, 2 mL, 5 mL; 20 mL [DSC]) [contains benzyl alcohol]

Tablet: 1 mg, 2 mg

  Robinul®: 1 mg

  Robinul® Forte: 2 mg

◆ **Glycopyrrolate Injection, USP (Can)** *see* Glycopyrrolate *on page 667*

◆ **Glycopyrronium Bromide** *see* Glycopyrrolate *on page 667*

◆ **Glycosum** *see* Dextrose *on page 406*

◆ **Glydiazinamide** *see* GlipiZIDE *on page 663*

◆ **Glynase® PresTab®** *see* GlyBURIDE *on page 666*

◆ **GMD-Fluconazole (Can)** *see* Fluconazole *on page 607*

◆ **GP 47680** *see* OXcarbazepine *on page 1066*

◆ **GPI 15715** *see* Fospropofol *on page 642*

◆ **GR38032R** *see* Ondansetron *on page 1057*

Granisetron (gra NI se tron)

Medication Safety Issues

Sound-alike/look-alike issues:

  Granisetron may be confused with dolasetron, ondansetron, palonosetron

Related Information

  Postoperative Nausea and Vomiting *on page 1593*

U.S. Brand Names Granisol™; Kytril®; Sancuso®

◄ **Canadian Brand Names** Apo-Granisetron; Kytril®
Index Terms BRL 43694
Pharmacologic Category Antiemetic; Selective 5-HT$_3$ Receptor Antagonist
Generic Available Yes

Use Prophylaxis of nausea and vomiting associated with emetogenic chemotherapy and radiation therapy; prophylaxis and treatment of postoperative nausea and vomiting (PONV)

Unlabeled/Investigational Use Breakthrough treatment of nausea and vomiting associated with chemotherapy

Mechanism of Action Selective 5-HT$_3$-receptor antagonist, blocking serotonin, both peripherally on vagal nerve terminals and centrally in the chemoreceptor trigger zone

Pharmacodynamics/Kinetics

Duration: Oral, I.V.: Generally up to 24 hours

Absorption: Oral: Tablets and oral solution are bioequivalent; Transdermal patch: ~66% over 7 days

Distribution: V$_d$: 2-4 L/kg; widely throughout body

Protein binding: 65%

Metabolism: Hepatic via N-demethylation, oxidation, and conjugation; some metabolites may have 5-HT$_3$ antagonist activity

Half-life elimination: Oral: 6 hours; I.V.: 9 hours

Time to peak, plasma: Transdermal patch: Maximum systemic concentrations: ~48 hours after application (range: 24-168 hours)

Excretion: Urine (12% as unchanged drug, 48% to 49% as metabolites); feces (34% to 38% as metabolites)

Dosage

Oral: Adults:

Prophylaxis of chemotherapy-related emesis: 2 mg once daily up to 1 hour before chemotherapy or 1 mg twice daily; the first 1 mg dose should be given up to 1 hour before chemotherapy.

Prophylaxis of radiation therapy-associated emesis: 2 mg once daily given 1 hour before radiation therapy.

I.V.:

Children ≥2 years and Adults: Prophylaxis of chemotherapy-related emesis:

Within U.S.: 10 mcg/kg/dose (maximum: 1 mg/dose) given 30 minutes prior to chemotherapy; for some drugs (eg, carboplatin, cyclophosphamide) with a later onset of emetic action, 10 mcg/kg every 12 hours may be necessary

Outside U.S.: 40 mcg/kg/dose (or 3 mg/dose); maximum: 9 mg/24 hours

Breakthrough: Granisetron has not been shown to be effective in terminating nausea or vomiting once it occurs and should not be used for this purpose.

Adults: PONV:

Prevention: 1 mg given undiluted over 30 seconds; the manufacturer recommends administration before induction of anesthesia or immediately before reversal of anesthesia. **Note:** The Society for Ambulatory Anesthesia (SAMBA) Guidelines recommend a dosage range of 0.35-1.5 mg administered at the end of surgery (Gan, 2007). However, doses ≤1 mg are generally used since doses >1 mg are not more effective. Of note, 5 mcg/kg (~0.35 mg in a 70 kg adult) has been shown to be effective; doses >5 mcg/kg were not more effective (Mikawa, 1997).

Treatment: 1 mg given undiluted over 30 seconds

Transdermal patch: Adults: Prophylaxis of chemotherapy-related emesis: Apply 1 patch at least 24 hours prior to chemotherapy; do not apply ≥48 hours before chemotherapy. Remove patch a minimum of 24 hours after chemotherapy completion. Maximum duration: Patch may be worn up to 7 days, depending on chemotherapy regimen duration.

Dosing interval in renal impairment: No dosage adjustment required.

Dosing interval in hepatic impairment: Kinetic studies in patients with hepatic impairment showed that total clearance was approximately halved, however, standard doses were very well tolerated, and dose adjustments are not necessary.

Stability

I.V.: Store at 15°C to 30°C (59°F to 86°F). Stable when mixed in NS or D_5W for 7 days under refrigeration and for 3 days at room temperature. Protect from light. Do not freeze vials.

Oral: Store tablet or oral solution at 15°C to 30°C (59°F to 86°F). Protect from light.

Transdermal patch: Store at 20°C to 25°C (68°F to 77°F). Keep patch in original packaging until immediately prior to use.

Administration

Oral: Doses should be given up to 1 hour prior to initiation of chemotherapy/radiation

I.V.: Administer I.V. push over 30 seconds or as a 5-10 minute-infusion

Prevention of PONV: Administer before induction of anesthesia or immediately before reversal of anesthesia.

Treatment of PONV: Administer undiluted over 30 seconds.

Transdermal (Sancuso®): Apply patch to clean, dry, intact skin on upper outer arm. Do not use on red, irritated or damaged skin. Remove patch from pouch immediately before application. Do not cut patch.

Anesthesia and Critical Care Concerns/Other Considerations

Clinical Pearls/Comments: For prevention of postoperative nausea and vomiting (PONV), granisetron has been shown effective in lower doses of 5 mcg/kg (~0.35 mg) (Mikawa, 1997).

Pregnancy Risk Factor B

Contraindications Hypersensitivity to granisetron or any component of the formulation

Warnings/Precautions Use with caution in patients with congenital long QT syndrome or other risk factors for QT prolongation (eg, medications known to prolong QT interval, electrolyte abnormalities, and cumulative high-dose anthracycline therapy). $5-HT_3$ antagonists have been associated with a number of dose-dependent increases in ECG intervals (eg, PR, QRS duration, QT/QT_c, JT), usually occurring 1-2 hours after I.V. administration. In general, these changes are not clinically relevant, however, when used in conjunction with other agents that prolong these intervals, arrhythmia may occur. When used with agents that prolong the QT interval (eg, Class I and III antiarrhythmics), clinically relevant QT interval prolongation may occur resulting in torsade de pointes. I.V. formulations of $5-HT_3$ antagonists have more association with ECG interval changes, compared to oral formulations.

For chemotherapy-related emesis, **granisetron should be used on a scheduled basis, not on an "as needed" (PRN) basis**, since data support the use of this drug in the prevention of nausea and vomiting and not in the rescue of nausea and vomiting. Granisetron should be used only in the first 24-48 hours of receiving chemotherapy or radiation. Data do not support any increased efficacy of granisetron in delayed nausea and vomiting.

Use with caution in patients allergic to other $5-HT_3$ receptor antagonists; cross-reactivity has been reported. Routine prophylaxis for PONV is not recommended in patients where there is little expectation of nausea and vomiting post-operatively. In patients where nausea and vomiting must be avoided post-operatively, administer to all patients even when expected incidence of nausea and vomiting is low. Use caution following abdominal surgery or in chemotherapy-induced nausea and vomiting; may mask progressive ileus or gastric distention. Application site reactions, generally mild, have occurred with transdermal patch use; if skin reaction is severe or generalized, remove patch. Cover patch application site with clothing to protect from natural or artificial sunlight exposure while patch is applied and for 10 days following removal; granisetron may potentially be affected by natural or artificial sunlight. Do not apply patch to red, irritated, or damaged skin. Injection contains benzyl alcohol (1 mg/mL) and should not be used in neonates.

Adverse Reactions

>10%:

Central nervous system: Headache (3% to 21%; transdermal patch: 1%)

Gastrointestinal: Constipation (3% to 18%)

Neuromuscular & skeletal: Weakness (5% to 18%)

◄ 1% to 10%:
Cardiovascular: QT_c prolongation (1% to 3%), hypertension (1% to 2%)
Central nervous system: Pain (10%), fever (3% to 9%), dizziness (4% to 5%), insomnia (<2% to 5%), somnolence (1% to 4%), anxiety (2%), agitation (<2%), CNS stimulation (<2%)
Dermatologic: Rash (1%)
Gastrointestinal: Diarrhea (3% to 9%), abdominal pain (4% to 6%), dyspepsia (3% to 6%), taste perversion (2%)
Hepatic: Liver enzymes increased (5% to 6%)
Renal: Oliguria (2%)
Respiratory: Cough (2%)
Miscellaneous: Infection (3%)
<1% (Limited to important or life-threatening): Agitation, allergic reactions; anaphylaxis (including hypotension, dyspnea, urticaria); angina, application site reactions (transdermal patch), arrhythmias, atrial fibrillation, extrapyramidal syndrome, hot flashes, hypotension, hypersensitivity, syncope

Drug Interactions
Metabolism/Transport Effects Substrate of CYP3A4 (minor)
Avoid Concomitant Use
Avoid concomitant use of Granisetron with any of the following: Apomorphine
Increased Effect/Toxicity
Granisetron may increase the levels/effects of: Apomorphine
Decreased Effect There are no known significant interactions involving a decrease in effect.

Dosage Forms Excipient information presented when available (limited, particularly for generics); consult specific product labeling. [DSC] = Discontinued product
Injection, solution: 1 mg/mL (1 mL, 4 mL)
Kytril®: 1 mg/mL (1 mL, 4 mL) [contains benzyl alcohol]
Injection, solution [preservative free]: 0.1 mg/mL (1 mL); 1 mg/mL (1 mL)
Kytril®: 0.1 mg/mL (1 mL)
Solution, oral:
Granisol™: 2 mg/10 mL (30 mL) [contains sodium benzoate; orange flavor]
Kytril®: 2 mg/10 mL (30 mL) [contains sodium benzoate; orange flavor] [DSC]
Tablet: 1 mg
Kytril®: 1 mg
Transdermal system, topical:
Sancuso®: 3.1 mg/24 hours (1s) [52 cm^2, total granisetron 34.3 mg]

References
Gan TJ, Meyer TA, Apfel CC, et al, "Society for Ambulatory Anesthesia Guidelines for the Management of Postoperative Nausea and Vomiting," *Anesth Analg*, 2007, 105(6):1615-28.
Mikawa K, Takao Y, Nishina K, et al, "Optimal Dose of Granisetron for Prophylaxis Against Postoperative Emesis After Gynecological Surgery," *Anesth Analg*, 1997, 85(3):652-6.

◆ **Granisol™** *see* Granisetron *on page 669*

◆ **Granulocyte Colony Stimulating Factor** *see* Filgrastim *on page 601*

◆ **Growth Hormone, Human** *see* Somatropin *on page 1318*

◆ **Gynodiol® [DSC]** *see* Estradiol *on page 531*

◆ **Halcion®** *see* Triazolam *on page 1434*

◆ **Haldol®** *see* Haloperidol *on page 672*

◆ **Haldol® Decanoate** *see* Haloperidol *on page 672*

◆ **Halfprin® [OTC]** *see* Aspirin *on page 147*

Haloperidol (ha loe PER i dole)

Medication Safety Issues
Sound-alike/look-alike issues:
Haloperidol may be confused Halotestin®
Haldol® may be confused with Halcion®, Halenol®, Halog®, Halotestin®, Stadol®

Related Information
  Sedative Agents in the Intensive Care Unit *on page 1690*
U.S. Brand Names Haldol®; Haldol® Decanoate
Canadian Brand Names Apo-Haloperidol LA®; Apo-Haloperidol®; Haloperidol Injection, USP; Haloperidol Long Acting; Haloperidol-LA; Haloperidol-LA Omega; Novo-Peridol; Peridol; PMS-Haloperidol LA
Index Terms Haloperidol Decanoate; Haloperidol Lactate
Pharmacologic Category Antipsychotic Agent, Typical
Generic Available Yes
Use Management of schizophrenia; control of tics and vocal utterances of Tourette's disorder in children and adults; severe behavioral problems in children
Unlabeled/Investigational Use Treatment of non-schizophrenia psychosis; may be used for the emergency sedation of severely-agitated or delirious patients; adjunctive treatment of ethanol dependence; antiemetic; psychosis/agitation related to Alzheimer's dementia
Mechanism of Action Haloperidol is a butyrophenone antipsychotic which blocks postsynaptic mesolimbic dopaminergic D_1 and D_2 receptors in the brain; depresses the release of hypothalamic and hypophyseal hormones; believed to depress the reticular activating system thus affecting basal metabolism, body temperature, wakefulness, vasomotor tone, and emesis
Pharmacodynamics/Kinetics
  Onset of action: Sedation: I.M., I.V.: 30-60 minutes
  Duration: Decanoate: 2-4 weeks
  Distribution: V_d: 8-18 L/kg; crosses placenta; enters breast milk
  Protein binding: 90%
  Metabolism: Hepatic to inactive compounds
  Bioavailability: Oral: 60%
  Half-life elimination: 18 hours; Decanoate: ~1 day
  Time to peak, serum: Oral: 2-6 hours; I.M.: 20 minutes; Decanoate: 7 days
  Excretion: Urine (33% to 40% as metabolites) within 5 days; feces (15%)
    Clearance: 550 ± 133 mL/minute
Dosage
  Children: 3-12 years (15-40 kg): Oral:
    Initial: 0.05 mg/kg/day or 0.25-0.5 mg/day given in 2-3 divided doses; increase by 0.25-0.5 mg every 5-7 days; maximum: 0.15 mg/kg/day
    Usual maintenance:
      Agitation or hyperkinesia: 0.01-0.03 mg/kg/day once daily
      Nonpsychotic disorders: 0.05-0.075 mg/kg/day in 2-3 divided doses
      Psychotic disorders: 0.05-0.15 mg/kg/day in 2-3 divided doses
  Children 6-12 years: Sedation/psychotic disorders: I.M. (as lactate): 1-3 mg/dose every 4-8 hours to a maximum of 0.15 mg/kg/day; change over to oral therapy as soon as able
  Adults:
    Psychosis:
      Oral: 0.5-5 mg 2-3 times/day; usual maximum: 30 mg/day
      I.M. (as lactate): 2-5 mg every 4-8 hours as needed
      I.M. (as decanoate): Initial: 10-20 times the daily oral dose administered at 4-week intervals
      Maintenance dose: 10-15 times initial oral dose; used to stabilize psychiatric symptoms
    Delirium in the intensive care unit (unlabeled use, unlabeled route):
      I.V.: 2-10 mg; may repeat bolus doses every 20-30 minutes until calm achieved then administer 25% of the maximum dose every 6 hours; monitor ECG and QT_c interval
      Intermittent I.V.: 0.03-0.15 mg/kg every 30 minutes to 6 hours
      Oral: Agitation: 5-10 mg
      Continuous intravenous infusion (100 mg/100 mL D_5W): Rates of 3-25 mg/hour have been used
    Rapid tranquilization of severely-agitated patient (unlabeled use): Administer every 30-60 minutes:
      Oral: 5-10 mg
      I.M. (as lactate): 5 mg
      Average total dose (oral or I.M.) for tranquilization: 10-20 mg

▶

Elderly: Nonpsychotic patient, dementia behavior (unlabeled use): Initial: Oral: 0.25-0.5 mg 1-2 times/day; increase dose at 4- to 7-day intervals by 0.25-0.5 mg/day; increase dosing intervals (twice daily, 3 times/day, etc) as necessary to control response or side effects

Hemodialysis/peritoneal dialysis: Supplemental dose is not necessary

Stability

Protect oral dosage forms from light.

Haloperidol lactate injection should be stored at controlled room temperature; do not freeze or expose to temperatures >40°C. Protect from light; exposure to light may cause discoloration and the development of a grayish-red precipitate over several weeks.

Haloperidol lactate may be administered IVPB or I.V. infusion in D_5W solutions. NS solutions should not be used due to reports of decreased stability and incompatibility.

Standardized dose: 0.5-100 mg/50-100 mL D_5W.

Stability of standardized solutions is 38 days at room temperature (24°C).

Administration The decanoate injectable formulation should be administered I.M. only, **do not administer decanoate I.V.** Dilute the oral concentrate with water or juice before administration. Avoid skin contact with oral suspension or solution; may cause contact dermatitis.

Monitoring Parameters Vital signs; lipid profile, fasting blood glucose/Hgb A_{1c}; BMI; mental status, abnormal involuntary movement scale (AIMS), extrapyramidal symptoms (EPS); ECG (with off-label intravenous administration)

Reference Range

Therapeutic: 5-20 ng/mL (SI: 10-40 nmol/L) (psychotic disorders - less for Tourette's and mania)

Toxic: >42 ng/mL (SI: >84 nmol/L)

Anesthesia and Critical Care Concerns/Other Considerations

Clinical Pearls/Comments:

Delirium in the ICU Patient: Set goals for control of delirium. Haloperidol has not been studied in well-controlled trials enrolling ICU patients with acute delirium or agitation. In September 2007, the FDA and Johnson and Johnson informed healthcare providers about an increased risk of QT prolongation, torsade de pointes (TdP), and sudden death associated with haloperidol use, particularly high dose, intravenous administration (unlabeled use). Case-control studies indicate a dose-response between intravenous haloperidol and TdP. Even when used at recommended doses, cardiac arrhythmias have occurred. Caution or avoidance of haloperidol is advised in patients with predisposing risk factors including electrolyte abnormalities (eg, hypokalemia, hypomagnesemia), hypothyroidism, familial long QT syndrome, concomitant medications which may augment QT prolongation, or any underlying cardiac abnormality which may also potentiate risk. In addition, ECG monitoring is recommended with off-label intravenous use of haloperidol.

Haloperidol may cause extrapyramidal symptoms. It is the most frequently implicated antipsychotic associated with neuroleptic malignant syndrome.

Pregnancy Risk Factor C

Contraindications Hypersensitivity to haloperidol or any component of the formulation; Parkinson's disease; severe CNS depression; coma

Warnings/Precautions [U.S. Boxed Warning]: Elderly patients with dementia-related psychosis treated with antipsychotics are at an increased risk of death compared to placebo. Most deaths appeared to be either cardiovascular (eg, heart failure, sudden death) or infectious (eg, pneumonia) in nature. Haloperidol is not approved for the treatment of dementia-related psychosis. Hypotension may occur, particularly with parenteral administration. Although the short-acting form (lactate) is used clinically, the I.V. use of the injection is not an FDA-approved route of administration; the decanoate form should never be administered intravenously.

May alter cardiac conduction and prolong QT interval; life-threatening arrhythmias have occurred with therapeutic doses of antipsychotics but risk may be increased with doses exceeding recommendations and/or intravenous administration (unlabeled route). Use caution or avoid use in patients with electrolyte abnormalities (eg, hypokalemia, hypomagnesemia), hypothyroidism, familial long

QT syndrome, concomitant medications which may augment QT prolongation, or any underlying cardiac abnormality which may also potentiate risk. Monitor ECG closely for dose-related QT effects. Adverse effects of decanoate may be prolonged. Avoid in thyrotoxicosis.

Leukopenia, neutropenia, and agranulocytosis (sometimes fatal) have been reported in clinical trials and postmarketing reports with antipsychotic use; presence of risk factors (eg, pre-existing low WBC or history of drug-induced leuko-/neutropenia) should prompt periodic blood count assessment. Discontinue therapy at first signs of blood dyscrasias or if absolute neutrophil count <1000/ mm^3.

May be sedating, use with caution in disorders where CNS depression is a feature. Effects may be potentiated when used with other sedative drugs or ethanol. Caution in patients with severe cardiovascular disease, predisposition to seizures, subcortical brain damage, or renal disease. Esophageal dysmotility and aspiration have been associated with antipsychotic use - use with caution in patients at risk of pneumonia (eg, Alzheimer's disease). Use associated with increased prolactin levels; clinical significance of hyperprolactinemia in patients with breast cancer or other prolactin-dependent tumors is unknown. May alter temperature regulation or mask toxicity of other drugs due to antiemetic effects. May cause orthostatic hypotension; use with caution in patients at risk of this effect or those who would tolerate transient hypotensive episodes (cerebrovascular disease, cardiovascular disease, or other medications which may predispose). Some tablets contain tartrazine. Antipsychotics have been associated with pigmentary retinopathy.

May cause anticholinergic effects (confusion, agitation, constipation, xerostomia, blurred vision, urinary retention). Therefore, they should be used with caution in patients with decreased gastrointestinal motility, urinary retention, BPH, xerostomia, or visual problems. Conditions which also may be exacerbated by cholinergic blockade include narrow-angle glaucoma and worsening of myasthenia gravis. Relative to other neuroleptics, haloperidol has a low potency of cholinergic blockade.

May cause extrapyramidal symptoms (EPS), including pseudoparkinsonism, acute dystonic reactions, akathisia, and tardive dyskinesia (risk of these reactions is high relative to other neuroleptics). Risk of dystonia (and possibly other EPS) may be greater with increased doses, use of conventional antipsychotics, males, and younger patients. May be associated with neuroleptic malignant syndrome (NMS). Use with caution in the elderly.

Adverse Reactions Frequency not defined.

Cardiovascular: Abnormal T waves with prolonged ventricular repolarization, arrhythmia, hyper-/hypotension, QT prolongation, sudden death, tachycardia, torsade de pointes

Central nervous system: Agitation, akathisia, altered central temperature regulation, anxiety, confusion, depression, drowsiness, dystonic reactions, euphoria, extrapyramidal reactions, headache, insomnia, lethargy, neuroleptic malignant syndrome (NMS), pseudoparkinsonian signs and symptoms, restlessness, seizure, tardive dyskinesia, tardive dystonia, vertigo

Dermatologic: Alopecia, contact dermatitis, hyperpigmentation, photosensitivity (rare), pruritus, rash

Endocrine & metabolic: Amenorrhea, breast engorgement, galactorrhea, gynecomastia, hyper-/hypoglycemia, hyponatremia, lactation, mastalgia, menstrual irregularities, sexual dysfunction

Gastrointestinal: Anorexia, constipation, diarrhea, dyspepsia, hypersalivation, nausea, vomiting, xerostomia

Genitourinary: Priapism, urinary retention

Hematologic: Cholestatic jaundice, obstructive jaundice

Ocular: Blurred vision

Respiratory: Bronchospasm, laryngospasm

Miscellaneous: Diaphoresis, heat stroke

Drug Interactions

Metabolism/Transport Effects Substrate of CYP1A2 (minor), 2D6 (major), 3A4 (major); **Inhibits** CYP2D6 (moderate), 3A4 (moderate)

◀ **Avoid Concomitant Use**

Avoid concomitant use of Haloperidol with any of the following: Artemether; Dronedarone; Everolimus; Lumefantrine; Nilotinib; Pimozide; QuiNINE; Tetrabenazine; Thioridazine; Tolvaptan; Ziprasidone

Increased Effect/Toxicity

Haloperidol may increase the levels/effects of: Alcohol (Ethyl); Anticholinergics; ChlorproMAZINE; CNS Depressants; Colchicine; CYP2D6 Substrates; CYP3A4 Substrates; Dronedarone; Eplerenone; Everolimus; FentaNYL; Fesoterodine; Nebivolol; Pimecrolimus; Pimozide; QTc-Prolonging Agents; QuiNINE; Salmeterol; Saxagliptin; Tamoxifen; Tetrabenazine; Thioridazine; Tolvaptan; Ziprasidone

The levels/effects of Haloperidol may be increased by: Acetylcholinesterase Inhibitors (Central); Alfuzosin; Artemether; Chloroquine; ChlorproMAZINE; Ciprofloxacin; CYP2D6 Inhibitors (Moderate); CYP2D6 Inhibitors (Strong); CYP3A4 Inhibitors (Moderate); CYP3A4 Inhibitors (Strong); Darunavir; Gadobutrol; Lithium formulations; Lumefantrine; Nilotinib; Pramlintide; QuiNIDine; QuiNINE; Selective Serotonin Reuptake Inhibitors; Tetrabenazine

Decreased Effect

Haloperidol may decrease the levels/effects of: Amphetamines; Anti-Parkinson's Agents (Dopamine Agonist); Codeine; TraMADol

The levels/effects of Haloperidol may be decreased by: CarBAMazepine; CYP3A4 Inducers (Strong); Deferasirox; Herbs (CYP3A4 Inducers); Lithium formulations; Peginterferon Alfa-2b

Ethanol/Nutrition/Herb Interactions

Ethanol: Avoid ethanol (may increase CNS depression).

Herb/Nutraceutical: Avoid valerian, St John's wort, kava kava, gotu kola (may increase CNS depression).

Dosage Forms Excipient information presented when available (limited, particularly for generics); consult specific product labeling. [DSC] = Discontinued product

Note: Strength expressed as base.

Injection, oil, as decanoate: 50 mg/mL (1 mL, 5 mL); 100 mg/mL (1 mL, 5 mL)

Haldol® Decanoate: 50 mg/mL (1 mL; 5 mL [DSC]); 100 mg/mL (1 mL; 5 mL [DSC]) [contains benzyl alcohol, sesame oil]

Injection, solution, as lactate: 5 mg/mL (1 mL, 10 mL)

Haldol®: 5 mg/mL (1 mL)

Solution, oral concentrate, as lactate: 2 mg/mL (15 mL, 120 mL)

Tablet: 0.5 mg, 1 mg, 2 mg, 5 mg, 10 mg, 20 mg

References

Barton MD, Libonati M, and Cohen PJ, "The Use of Haloperidol for Treatment of Postoperative Nausea and Vomiting - A Double-Blind Placebo-Controlled Trial," *Anesthesiology*, 1975, 42 (4):508-12.

Jacobi J, Fraser GL, Coursin DB, et al, "Clinical Practice Guidelines for the Sustained Use of Sedatives and Analgesics in the Critically Ill Adult," *Crit Care Med*, 2002, 30(1):119-41. Available at: http://www.sccm.org/pdf/sedatives.pdf.

Riker RR, Fraser GL, and Cox PM, "Continuous Infusion of Haloperidol Controls Agitation in Critically Ill Patients," *Crit Care Med*, 1994, 22(3):433-40.

Sharma ND, Rosman HS, Padhi ID, et al, "Torsades de Pointes Associated With Intravenous Haloperidol in Critically Ill Patients," *Am J Cardiol*, 1998, 81(2):238-40.

Wilt JL, Minnema AM, Johnson RF, et al, "Torsade de Pointes Associated With the Use of Intravenous Haloperidol," *Ann Intern Med*, 1993, 119(5):391-4.

◆ **Haloperidol Decanoate** *see* Haloperidol *on page 672*

◆ **Haloperidol Injection, USP (Can)** *see* Haloperidol *on page 672*

◆ **Haloperidol-LA (Can)** *see* Haloperidol *on page 672*

◆ **Haloperidol Lactate** *see* Haloperidol *on page 672*

◆ **Haloperidol-LA Omega (Can)** *see* Haloperidol *on page 672*

◆ **Haloperidol Long Acting (Can)** *see* Haloperidol *on page 672*

◆ **Harkoseride** *see* Lacosamide *on page 795*

◆ **Havrix® and Engerix-B®** *see* Hepatitis A Inactivated and Hepatitis B (Recombinant) Vaccine *on page 684*

◆ **HBIG** *see* Hepatitis B Immune Globulin *on page 685*

- ◆ **hBNP** *see* Nesiritide *on page 999*

- ◆ **HCTZ (error-prone abbreviation)** *see* Hydrochlorothiazide *on page 696*

- ◆ **HDCV** *see* Rabies Virus Vaccine *on page 1225*

- ◆ **Helixate® FS** *see* Antihemophilic Factor (Recombinant) *on page 124*

- ◆ **Hemorrhoidal HC** *see* Hydrocortisone *on page 699*

- ◆ **Hemril®-30** *see* Hydrocortisone *on page 699*

- ◆ **HepaGam B™** *see* Hepatitis B Immune Globulin *on page 685*

- ◆ **HepA-HepB** *see* Hepatitis A Inactivated and Hepatitis B (Recombinant) Vaccine *on page 684*

- ◆ **Hepalean® (Can)** *see* Heparin *on page 677*

- ◆ **Hepalean® Leo (Can)** *see* Heparin *on page 677*

- ◆ **Hepalean®-LOK (Can)** *see* Heparin *on page 677*

Heparin (HEP a rin)

Medication Safety Issues

Sound-alike/look-alike issues:
Heparin may be confused with Hespan®

High alert medication: The Institute for Safe Medication Practices (ISMP) includes this medication among its list of drugs which have a heightened risk of causing significant patient harm when used in error.

Heparin sodium injection 10,000 units/mL and Hep-Lock U/P 10 units/mL have been confused with each other. Fatal medication errors have occurred between the two whose labels are both blue. **Never rely on color as a sole indicator to differentiate product identity.**

Heparin lock flush solution is intended only to maintain patency of I.V. devices and is **not** to be used for anticoagulant therapy.

Note: The 100 unit/mL concentration should not be used in neonates or infants <10 kg. The 10 unit/mL concentration may cause systemic anticoagulation in infants <1 kg who receive frequent flushes.

2009 National Patient Safety Goals: The Joint Commission on Accreditation of Healthcare Organizations requires healthcare organizations that provide anticoagulant therapy to have a process in place to reduce the risk of anticoagulant-associated patient harm. Patients receiving anticoagulants should receive individualized care through a defined process that includes standardized ordering, dispensing, administration, monitoring and education. This does not apply to routine short-term use of anticoagulants for prevention of venous thromboembolism when the expectation is that the patient's laboratory values will remain within or close to normal values (NPSG.03.05.01).

Related Information

Anesthesia Considerations for Neurosurgery *on page 1514*
Anesthesia for Geriatric Patients *on page 1523*
Continuous Renal Replacement Therapy *on page 1557*
Dosing Considerations for the Critically-Ill Patient With Morbid Obesity *on page 1561*
Management of Postoperative Arrhythmias *on page 1571*
Perioperative / Periprocedural Management of Anticoagulant and Antiplatelet Therapy *on page 1607*
Regional Anesthesia in Patients Receiving Anticoagulant and Antiplatelet Therapy *on page 1642*

U.S. Brand Names Hep-Lock U/P; Hep-Lock®; HepFlush®-10
Canadian Brand Names Hepalean®; Hepalean® Leo; Hepalean®-LOK
Index Terms Heparin Calcium; Heparin Lock Flush; Heparin Sodium
Pharmacologic Category Anticoagulant
Generic Available Yes
Use Prophylaxis and treatment of thromboembolic disorders; as an anticoagulant for extracorporeal and dialysis procedures

◄ **Note:** Heparin lock flush solution is intended only to maintain patency of I.V. devices and is **not** to be used for anticoagulant therapy.

Unlabeled/Investigational Use ST-elevation myocardial infarction (STEMI) - combination regimen of heparin (unlabeled dose), tenecteplase (half dose), and abciximab (full dose)

Mechanism of Action Potentiates the action of antithrombin III and thereby inactivates thrombin (as well as activated coagulation factors IX, X, XI, XII, and plasmin) and prevents the conversion of fibrinogen to fibrin; heparin also stimulates release of lipoprotein lipase (lipoprotein lipase hydrolyzes triglycerides to glycerol and free fatty acids)

Pharmacodynamics/Kinetics

Onset of action: Anticoagulation: I.V.: Immediate; SubQ: ~20-30 minutes

Absorption: Oral, rectal: Erratic at best from these routes of administration; SubQ absorption is also erratic, but considered acceptable for prophylactic use

Distribution: Does not cross placenta; does not enter breast milk

Metabolism: Hepatic; may be partially metabolized in the reticuloendothelial system

Half-life elimination: Mean: 1.5 hours; Range: 1-2 hours; affected by obesity, renal function, hepatic function, malignancy, presence of pulmonary embolism, and infections

Excretion: Urine (small amounts as unchanged drug)

Dosage Note: Many concentrations of heparin are available ranging from 1 unit/mL to 20,000 units/mL. Carefully examine each prefilled syringe or vial prior to use ensuring that the correct concentration is chosen. Heparin lock flush solution is intended only to maintain patency of I.V. devices and is not to be used for anticoagulant therapy.

Children >1 year:

Prophylaxis for cardiac catheterization (arterial approach): I.V.: Bolus: 100-150 units/kg (Monagle, 2008)

Systemic heparinization:

Intermittent I.V.: Initial: 50-100 units/kg, then 50-100 units/kg every 4 hours (**Note:** Continuous I.V. infusion is preferred)

I.V. infusion: Initial loading dose: 75 units/kg given over 10 minutes, then initial maintenance dose: 20 units/kg/hour; adjust dose to maintain aPTT of 60-85 seconds (assuming this reflects an antifactor Xa level of 0.35-0.7 units/mL); see table.

Pediatric Protocol For Systemic Heparin Adjustment

To be used after initial loading dose and maintenance I.V. infusion dose (see usual dosage) to maintain aPTT of 60-85 seconds (assuming this reflects antifactor Xa level of 0.35-0.7 units/mL).

Obtain blood for aPTT 4 hours after heparin loading dose and 4 hours after every infusion rate change.

Obtain daily CBC and aPTT after aPTT is therapeutic.

aPTT (seconds)	Dosage Adjustment	Time to Repeat aPTT
<50	Give 50 units/kg bolus and increase infusion rate by 10%	4 h after rate change
50-59	Increase infusion rate by 10%	4 h after rate change
60-85	Keep rate the same	Next day
86-95	Decrease infusion rate by 10%	4 h after rate change
96-120	Hold infusion for 30 minutes and decrease infusion rate by 10%	4 h after rate change
>120	Hold infusion for 60 minutes and decrease infusion rate by 15%	4 h after rate change

Modified from Monagle P, Chalmers E, Chan A, et al, "Antithrombotic Therapy in Neonates and Children," *Chest*, 2008, 133(6 Suppl):887-968.

Adults:

Thromboprophylaxis (low-dose heparin): SubQ: 5000 units every 8-12 hours

Intermittent I.V.: Initial: 10,000 units, then 50-70 units/kg (5000-10,000 units) every 4-6 hours

I.V. infusion (weight-based dosing per institutional nomogram recommended):

Acute coronary syndromes:

STEMI: Fibrinolytic therapy:

Full-dose alteplase, reteplase, or tenecteplase with dosing as follows: Concurrent bolus of 60 units/kg (maximum: 4000 units), then 12 units/kg/ hour (maximum: 1000 units/hour) as continuous infusion. Check aPTT every 4-6 hours; adjust to target of 1.5-2 times the upper limit of control (50-70 seconds in clinical trials); usual range 10-30 units/kg/hour. Duration of heparin therapy depends on concurrent therapy and the specific patient risks for systemic or venous thromboembolism.

Combination regimen (unlabeled): Half-dose tenecteplase (15-25 mg based on weight) and abciximab 0.25 mg/kg bolus then 0.125 mcg/kg/minute (maximum 10 mcg/minute) for 12 hours with heparin dosing as follows: Concurrent bolus of 40 units/kg (maximum 3000 units), then 7 units/kg/ hour (maximum: 800 units/hour) as continuous infusion. Adjust to aPTT target of 50-70 seconds.

Percutaneous coronary intervention:

If no concurrent GPIIb/IIIa inhibitor: Initial bolus of 60-100 units/kg (target ACT 250-350 seconds)

or

If receiving GPIIb/IIIa inhibitor: Initial bolus of 50-70 units/kg (target ACT 200-250 seconds)

Treatment of unstable angina/non-ST-elevation myocardial infarction (NSTEMI): Initial bolus of 60 units/kg (maximum: 4000 units), followed by an initial infusion of 12 units/kg/hour (maximum: 1000 units/hour). The American College of Chest Physicians consensus conference has recommended dosage adjustments to correspond to a therapeutic range equivalent to heparin levels of 0.3-0.7 units/mL by antifactor Xa determinations.

Treatment of venous thromboembolism:

DVT/PE: I.V.: 80 units/kg (or 5000 units) I.V. push followed by continuous infusion of 18 units/kg/hour (or 1300 units/hour). The American College of Chest Physicians consensus conference has recommended dosage adjustments to correspond to a therapeutic range equivalent to heparin levels of 0.3-0.7 units/mL by antifactor Xa determinations.

DVT/PE: SubQ:

Monitored dosing regimen: Initial: 17,500 units or 250 units/kg then 250 units/kg every 12 hours. The American College of Chest Physicians consensus conference has recommended dosage adjustments to correspond to a therapeutic range equivalent to heparin levels of 0.3-0.7 units/mL by antifactor Xa determinations.

Unmonitored dosing regimen: Initial: 333 units/kg then 250 units/kg every 12 hours

Line flushing: When using daily flushes of heparin to maintain patency of single and double lumen central catheters, 10 units/mL is commonly used for younger infants (eg, <10 kg) while 100 units/mL is used for older infants, children, and adults. Capped PVC catheters and peripheral heparin locks require flushing more frequently (eg, every 6-8 hours). Volume of heparin flush is usually similar to volume of catheter (or slightly greater). Additional flushes should be given when stagnant blood is observed in catheter, after catheter is used for drug or blood administration, and after blood withdrawal from catheter.

Addition of heparin (0.5-3 unit/mL) to peripheral and central parenteral nutrition has not been shown to decrease catheter-related thrombosis. The final concentration of heparin used for TPN solutions may need to be decreased to 0.5 units/mL in small infants receiving larger amounts of volume in order to avoid approaching therapeutic amounts. Arterial lines are heparinized with a final concentration of 1 unit/mL.

Dosing adjustments in the elderly: Patients >60 years of age may have higher serum levels and clinical response (longer aPTTs) as compared to younger patients receiving similar dosages; lower dosages may be required

◀ **Stability**

Heparin solutions are colorless to slightly yellow; minor color variations do not affect therapeutic efficacy.

Heparin should be stored at controlled room temperature. Protect from freezing and temperatures >40°C.

Stability at room temperature and refrigeration:

Prepared bag: 24 hours.

Premixed bag: After seal is broken, 4 days.

Out of overwrap stability: 30 days.

Standard concentration/diluent: 25,000 units/500 mL D_5W (premixed). If preparing solution, mix thoroughly prior to administration.

Minimum volume: 250 mL D_5W.

Administration SubQ: Inject in subcutaneous tissue only (not muscle tissue). Injection sites should be rotated (usually left and right portions of the abdomen, above iliac crest).

Do not administer I.M. due to pain, irritation, and hematoma formation; central venous catheters must be flushed with heparin solution when newly inserted, daily (at the time of tubing change), after blood withdrawal or transfusion, and after an intermittent infusion through an injectable cap. A volume of at least 10 mL of blood should be removed and discarded from a heparinized line before blood samples are sent for coagulation testing.

Monitoring Parameters Hemoglobin, hematocrit, signs of bleeding; fecal occult blood test; aPTT (or antifactor Xa activity levels) or ACT depending upon indication

Platelet counts should be routinely monitored when the risk of HIT is >0.1% (eg, receiving therapeutic dose heparin, postoperative antithrombotic prophylaxis), if the patient has received heparin or low molecular weight heparin (eg, enoxaparin) within the past 100 days, if preexposure history is uncertain, or if anaphylactoid reaction to heparin occurs. When the risk of HIT is <0.1% (eg, medical/obstetrical patients receiving heparin flushes), routine platelet count monitoring is not recommended (Hirsh, 2008).

For intermittent I.V. injections, aPTT is measured 3.5-4 hours after I.V. injection.

For SubQ injections, when used for treatment (eg, monitored dosing regimen), aPTT is measured 6 hours after injection.

Note: Continuous I.V. infusion is preferred over I.V. intermittent injections. For full-dose heparin (ie, nonlow-dose), the dose should be titrated according to aPTT results. For anticoagulation, an aPTT 1.5-2.5 times normal is usually desired. Because of variation among hospitals in the control aPTT values, nomograms should be established at each institution, designed to achieve aPTT values in the target range (eg, for a control aPTT of 30 seconds, the target range [1.5-2.5 times control] would be 45-75 seconds). Measurements should be made prior to heparin therapy, 6 hours (pediatric: 4 hours) after initiation, and 6 hours (pediatric: 4 hours) after any dosage change, and should be used to adjust the heparin infusion until the aPTT exhibits a therapeutic level. When two consecutive aPTT values are therapeutic, subsequent measurements may be made every 24 hours, and if necessary, dose adjustment carried out. In addition, a significant change in the patient's clinical condition (eg, recurrent ischemia, bleeding, hypotension) should prompt an immediate aPTT determination, followed by dose adjustment if necessary. In general, may increase or decrease infusion by 2-4 units/kg/hour dependent upon aPTT.

Heparin infusion dose adjustment: A number of dose-adjustment nomograms have been developed which target an aPTT range of 1.5-2.5 times control (Cruickshank, 1991; Flaker, 1994; Hull, 1992; Raschke, 1993). However, institution-specific and indication-specific nomograms should be consulted for dose adjustment. **Note:** aPTT values vary throughout the day with maximum values occurring during the night (Decousus, 1985).

Reference Range Heparin: 0.3-0.7 unit/mL (by anti-Xa chromogenic assay) or 0.2-0.4 unit/mL (by protamine titration); aPTT: 1.5-2.5 times **the patient's baseline**

Anesthesia and Critical Care Concerns/Other Considerations
Evidence-Based Information:

Management of Intracerebral Hemorrhage (ICH) Due to Unfractionated Heparin (UFH): Overall management of ICH is similar regardless of cause; however, iatrogenic spontaneous ICH may have specific treatments. According to the 2007 ACC/ASA Guidelines for the Management of Spontaneous Intracerebral Hemorrhage, UFH-related ICH should be treated with I.V. protamine given by slow I.V. injection (not to exceed 5 mg/minute) with a maximum dose of 50 mg (Class I recommendation). Faster infusions of protamine can result in cardiovascular collapse. The use of protamine for reversal of low molecular weight heparins (eg, enoxaparin) is significantly less effective.

Thrombocytopenia: Heparin-associated thrombocytopenia (HAT) commonly occurs within 48-72 hours of initiation. Platelet counts usually fall below 100,000 cells/mm^3 and return to normal within 4 days with continued heparin therapy. Heparin-induced thrombocytopenia (HIT) is a serious, immunoglobulin-mediated reaction with a high risk for thromboembolic events. In HIT, thrombocytopenia usually begins 5-10 days following heparin initiation; HIT can begin within ~10 hours in patients who have received heparin within the previous 100 days (Warkentin, 2001). It can also occur up to several weeks after heparin has been discontinued. Thrombocytopenia can be severe; heparin of all forms must be stopped including flushes and heparin-coated indwelling catheters.

Pregnancy Risk Factor C

Contraindications Hypersensitivity to heparin or any component of the formulation (unless a life-threatening situation necessitates use and use of an alternative anticoagulant is not possible); severe thrombocytopenia; uncontrolled active bleeding except when due to disseminated intravascular coagulation (DIC); suspected intracranial hemorrhage; not for I.M. use; not for use when appropriate blood coagulation tests cannot be obtained at appropriate intervals (applies to full-dose heparin only)

Warnings/Precautions Hypersensitivity reactions can occur. Only in life-threatening situations when use of an alternative anticoagulant is not possible should heparin be cautiously used in patients with a documented hypersensitivity reaction. Hemorrhage is the most common complication. Monitor for signs and symptoms of bleeding. Certain patients are at increased risk of bleeding. Risk factors for bleeding include bacterial endocarditis; congenital or acquired bleeding disorders; active ulcerative or angiodysplastic GI diseases; continuous GI tube drainage; severe uncontrolled hypertension; history of hemorrhagic stroke; or use shortly after brain, spinal, or ophthalmology surgery; patient treated concomitantly with platelet inhibitors; conditions associated with increased bleeding tendencies (hemophilia, vascular purpura); recent GI bleeding; thrombocytopenia or platelet defects; severe liver disease; hypertensive or diabetic retinopathy; or in patients undergoing invasive procedures including spinal tap or spinal anesthesia. Many concentrations of heparin are available ranging from 1 unit/mL to 20,000 units/mL. Clinicians **must** carefully examine each prefilled syringe or vial prior to use ensuring that the correct concentration is chosen; fatal hemorrhages have occurred related to heparin overdose especially in pediatric patients. A higher incidence of bleeding has been reported in patients >60 years of age, particularly women. They are also more sensitive to the dose. Discontinue heparin if hemorrhage occurs; severe hemorrhage or overdosage may require protamine.

May cause thrombocytopenia; monitor platelet count closely. Patients who develop HIT may be at risk of developing a new thrombus (heparin-induced thrombocytopenia and thrombosis [HITT]). Discontinue therapy and consider alternatives if platelets are <100,000/mm^3 and/or thrombosis develops. HIT or HITT may be delayed and can occur up to several weeks after discontinuation of heparin. Osteoporosis may occur with prolonged use (>6 months) due to a reduction in bone mineral density. Monitor for hyperkalemia; can cause hyperkalemia by suppressing aldosterone production. Patients >60 years of age may require lower doses of heparin.

Some preparations contain benzyl alcohol as a preservative. In neonates, large amounts of benzyl alcohol (>100 mg/kg/day) have been associated with fatal toxicity (gasping syndrome). The use of preservative-free heparin is, therefore, recommended in neonates. Some preparations contain sulfite which may cause allergic reactions.

Heparin resistance may occur in patients with antithrombin deficiency, increased heparin clearance, elevations in heparin-binding proteins, elevations in factor VIII and/or fibrinogen; frequently encountered in patients with fever, thrombosis, thrombophlebitis, infections with thrombosing tendencies, MI, cancer, and in postsurgical patients; measurement of anticoagulant effects using antifactor Xa levels may be of benefit.

Adverse Reactions Frequency not defined.

Cardiovascular: Allergic vasospastic reaction (possibly related to thrombosis), chest pain, hemorrhagic shock, shock, thrombosis

Central nervous system: Chills, fever, headache

Dermatologic: Alopecia (delayed, transient), bruising (unexplained), cutaneous necrosis, dysesthesia pedis, erythematous plaques (case reports), eczema, urticaria, purpura,

Endocrine & metabolic: Adrenal hemorrhage, hyperkalemia (suppression of aldosterone synthesis), ovarian hemorrhage, rebound hyperlipidemia on discontinuation

Gastrointestinal: Constipation, hematemesis, nausea, tarry stools, vomiting

Genitourinary: Frequent or persistent erection

Hematologic: Bleeding from gums, epistaxis, hemorrhage, ovarian hemorrhage, retroperitoneal hemorrhage, thrombocytopenia (see **"Note"**)

Hepatic: Liver enzymes increased

Local: Irritation, erythema, pain, hematoma, and ulceration have been rarely reported with deep SubQ injections; I.M. injection (not recommended) is associated with a high incidence of these effects

Neuromuscular & skeletal: Peripheral neuropathy, osteoporosis (chronic therapy effect)

Ocular: Conjunctivitis (allergic reaction), lacrimation

Renal: Hematuria

Respiratory: Asthma, bronchospasm (case reports), hemoptysis, pulmonary hemorrhage, rhinitis

Miscellaneous: Allergic reactions, anaphylactoid reactions, heparin resistance, hypersensitivity (including chills, fever, and urticaria)

Note: Thrombocytopenia has been reported to occur at an incidence between 0% and 30%. It is often of no clinical significance. However, immunologically mediated heparin-induced thrombocytopenia (HIT) has been estimated to occur in 1% to 2% of patients, and is marked by a progressive fall in platelet counts and, in some cases, thromboembolic complications (skin necrosis, pulmonary embolism, gangrene of the extremities, stroke or MI). For recommendations regarding platelet monitoring during heparin therapy, see Monitoring Parameters.

Drug Interactions

Avoid Concomitant Use

Avoid concomitant use of Heparin with any of the following: Corticorelin

Increased Effect/Toxicity

Heparin may increase the levels/effects of: Anticoagulants; Corticorelin; Drotrecogin Alfa; Ibritumomab; Tositumomab and Iodine I 131 Tositumomab

The levels/effects of Heparin may be increased by: 5-ASA Derivatives; Antiplatelet Agents; Aspirin; Dasatinib; Herbs (Anticoagulant/Antiplatelet Properties); Nonsteroidal Anti-Inflammatory Agents; Pentosan Polysulfate Sodium; Pentoxifylline; Prostacyclin Analogues; Salicylates; Thrombolytic Agents

Decreased Effect

The levels/effects of Heparin may be decreased by: Nitroglycerin

Ethanol/Nutrition/Herb Interactions Herb/Nutraceutical: Avoid cat's claw, dong quai, evening primrose, feverfew, red clover, horse chestnut, garlic, green tea, ginseng, ginkgo (all have additional antiplatelet activity).

Test Interactions Increased thyroxine (competitive protein binding methods); increased PT

Aprotinin significantly increases aPTT and celite Activated Clotting Time (ACT) which may not reflect the actual degree of anticoagulation by heparin. Kaolin-based ACTs are not affected by aprotinin to the same degree as celite ACTs.

While institutional protocols may vary, a minimal celite ACT of 750 seconds or kaolin-ACT of 480 seconds is recommended in the presence of aprotinin. Consult the manufacturer's information on specific ACT test interpretation in the presence of aprotinin.

Dosage Forms Excipient information presented when available (limited, particularly for generics); consult specific product labeling.

Infusion, as sodium [premixed in NaCl 0.45%; porcine intestinal mucosa source]: 12,500 units (250 mL); 25,000 units (250 mL, 500 mL)

Infusion, as sodium [preservative free; premixed in D_5W; porcine intestinal mucosa source]: 10,000 units (100 mL) [contains sodium metabisulfite]; 12,500 units (250 mL) [contains sodium metabisulfite]; 20,000 units (500 mL) [contains sodium metabisulfite]; 25,000 units (250 mL, 500 mL) [contains sodium metabisulfite]

Infusion, as sodium [preservative free; premixed in NaCl 0.9%; porcine intestinal mucosa source]: 1000 units (500 mL); 2000 units (1000 mL)

Injection, solution, as sodium [lock flush preparation; porcine intestinal mucosa source; multidose vial]: 10 units/mL (1 mL, 10 mL, 30 mL) [contains parabens]; 100 units/mL (1 mL, 5 mL) [contains parabens]

Injection, solution, as sodium [lock flush preparation; porcine intestinal mucosa source; multidose vial]: 10 units/mL (10 mL, 30 mL); 100 units/mL (10 mL, 30 mL) [contains benzyl alcohol]

Hep-Lock®: 10 units/mL (1 mL, 2 mL, 10 mL, 30 mL); 100 units/mL (1 mL, 2 mL, 10 mL, 30 mL) [contains benzyl alcohol]

Injection, solution, as sodium [lock flush preparation; porcine intestinal mucosa source; prefilled syringe]: 10 units/mL (1 mL, 2 mL, 3 mL, 5 mL); 100 units/mL (1 mL, 2 mL, 3 mL, 5 mL) [contains benzyl alcohol]

Injection, solution, as sodium [preservative free; lock flush preparation; porcine intestinal mucosa source; prefilled syringe]: 1 unit/mL (2 mL, 3 mL, 5 mL); 2 units/mL (3 mL); 10 units/mL (2.5 mL, 3 mL, 5 mL, 10 mL); 100 units/mL (3 mL, 5 mL, 10 mL)

Injection, solution, as sodium [preservative free; lock flush preparation; porcine intestinal mucosa source; vial]:

HepFlush®-10: 10 units/mL (10 mL)

Hep-Lock U/P: 10 units/mL (1 mL); 100 units/mL (1 mL)

Injection, solution, as sodium [porcine intestinal mucosa source; multidose vial]: 1000 units/mL (1 mL, 10 mL, 30 mL) [contains benzyl alcohol]; 1000 units/mL (1 mL, 10 mL, 30 mL) [contains methylparabens]; 5000 units/mL (1 mL, 10 mL) [contains benzyl alcohol]; 5000 units/mL (1 mL) [contains methylparabens]; 10,000 units/mL (1 mL, 4 mL) [contains benzyl alcohol]; 10,000 units/mL (1 mL, 5 mL) [contains methylparabens]; 20,000 units/mL (1 mL) [contains methylparabens]

Injection, solution, as sodium [porcine intestinal mucosa source; prefilled syringe]: 5000 units/mL (1 mL) [contains benzyl alcohol]

Injection, solution, as sodium [preservative free; porcine intestinal mucosa source; prefilled syringe]: 10,000 units/mL (0.5 mL)

Injection, solution, as sodium [preservative free; porcine intestinal mucosa source; vial]: 1000 units/mL (2 mL); 2000 units/mL (5 mL); 2500 units/mL (10 mL)

References

Anderson JL, Adams CD, Antman EM, et al, "ACC/AHA 2007 Guidelines for the Management of Patients With Unstable Angina/Non-ST-Elevation Myocardial Infarction: A Report of the American College of Cardiology/American Heart Association Task Force on Practice Guidelines (Writing Committee to Revise the 2002 Guidelines for the Management of Patients With Unstable Angina/Non-ST-Elevation Myocardial Infarction) Developed in Collaboration With the American College of Emergency Physicians, the Society for Cardiovascular Angiography and Interventions, and the Society of Thoracic Surgeons endorsed by the American Association of Cardiovascular and Pulmonary Rehabilitation and the Society for Academic Emergency Medicine" *J Am Coll Cardiol*, 2007, 50(7):e1-e157.

Antman EM, Anbe DT, Armstrong PW, et al, "ACC/AHA Guidelines for the Management of Patients With ST-Elevation Myocardial Infarction: A Report of the American College of Cardiology/American Heart Association Task Force on Practice Guidelines (Committee to Revise the 1999 Guidelines for the Management of Patients with Acute Myocardial Infarction)," *Circulation*, 2004, 110(9):e82-292.

Broderick J, Connolly S, Feldmann E, et al, "Guidelines for the Management of Spontaneous Intracerebral Hemorrhage in Adults: 2007 Update: A Guideline From the American Heart Association/American Stroke Association Stroke Council, High Blood Pressure Research Council, and the Quality of Care and Outcomes in Research Interdisciplinary Working Group," *Stroke*, 2007, 38(6):2001-23. Available at http://stroke.ahajournals.org/cgi/content/short/STROKEAHA.107.183689.

Dager WE and White RH, "Pharmacotherapy of Heparin-Induced Thrombocytopenia," *Expert Opin Pharmacother*, 2003, 4(6):919-40.

Klerk CP, Smorenburg SM, and Buller HR, "Thrombosis Prophylaxis in Patient Populations With a Central Venous Catheter: A Systematic Review," *Arch Intern Med*, 2003, 163(16):1913-21.

Selleng K, Warkentin TE, and Greinacher A, "Heparin-Induced Thrombocytopenia in Intensive Care Patients," *Crit Care Med*, 2007, 35(4):1165-76.

Verma AK, Levine M, Shalansky SJ, et al, "Frequency of Heparin-Induced Thrombocytopenia in Critical Care Patients," *Pharmacotherapy*, 2003, 23(6):745-53.

Warkentin TE and Kelton JG, "Temporal Aspects of Heparin-Induced Thrombocytopenia," *N Engl J Med*, 2001, 344(17):1286-92.

Warkentin TE, Greinacher A, Koster A, et al, "Treatment and Prevention of Heparin-induced Thrombocytopenia: American College of Chest Physicians Evidence-Based Clinical Practice Guidelines (8th Edition)," *Chest*, 2008, 133(6 Suppl):340-80.

Warkentin TE, Levine MN, Hirsch J, et al, "Heparin-Induced Thrombocytopenia in Patients Treated With Low-Molecular Weight Heparin or Unfractionated Heparin," *N Engl J Med*, 1995, 332 (20):1330-5.

◆ **Heparin Calcium** *see* Heparin *on page* 677

◆ **Heparin Cofactor I** *see* Antithrombin III *on page* 127

◆ **Heparin Lock Flush** *see* Heparin *on page* 677

◆ **Heparin Sodium** *see* Heparin *on page* 677

◆ **HepatAmine®** *see* Amino Acid Injection *on page* 81

◆ **Hepatasol®** *see* Amino Acid Injection *on page* 81

Hepatitis A Inactivated and Hepatitis B (Recombinant) Vaccine (hep a TYE tis aye & hep a TYE tis bee ree KOM be nant vak SEEN)

U.S. Brand Names Twinrix®

Canadian Brand Names Twinrix®

Index Terms Engerix-B® and Havrix®; Havrix® and Engerix-B®; HepA-HepB; Hepatitis B and Hepatitis A Vaccine

Pharmacologic Category Vaccine, Inactivated (Viral)

Use Active immunization against disease caused by hepatitis A virus and hepatitis B virus (all known subtypes) in populations desiring protection against or at high risk of exposure to these viruses.

Populations include travelers or people living in or relocating to areas of intermediate/high endemicity for **both** HAV and HBV and are at increased risk of HBV infection due to behavioral or occupational factors; patients with chronic liver disease; laboratory workers who handle live HAV and HBV; healthcare workers, police, and other personnel who render first-aid or medical assistance; workers who come in contact with sewage; employees of day care centers and correctional facilities; patients/staff of hemodialysis units; male homosexuals; patients frequently receiving blood products; military personnel; users of injectable illicit drugs; close household contacts of patients with hepatitis A and hepatitis B infection; residents of drug and alcohol treatment centers

Pharmacodynamics/Kinetics

Onset of action: Seroconversion for antibodies against HAV and HBV were detected 1 month after completion of the 3-dose series.

Duration: Patients remained seropositive for at least 4 years during clinical studies.

Dosage I.M.: Adults: Primary immunization: Three doses (1 mL each) given on a 0-, 1-, and 6-month schedule

Alternative regimen: Accelerated regimen: Four doses (1 mL each) on day 0, 7, and 21-30, followed by a booster at 12 months

Additional Information Complete prescribing information for this medication should be consulted for additional detail.

Dosage Forms Excipient information presented when available (limited, particularly for generics); consult specific product labeling. [DSC] = Discontinued product

Injection, suspension [preservative free]:

Twinrix®: Hepatitis A virus antigen 720 ELISA units and hepatitis B surface antigen 20 mcg per mL (1 mL) [contains aluminum, yeast protein, and trace amounts of neomycin; prefilled syringe contains natural rubber/natural latex]

◆ **Hepatitis B and Hepatitis A Vaccine** *see* Hepatitis A Inactivated and Hepatitis B (Recombinant) Vaccine *on page 684*

Hepatitis B Immune Globulin
(hep a TYE tis bee i MYUN GLOB yoo lin YU man)

U.S. Brand Names HepaGam B™; HyperHEP B™ S/D; Nabi-HB®
Canadian Brand Names HepaGam B™; HyperHep B®
Index Terms HBIG
Pharmacologic Category Immune Globulin
Use

Passive prophylactic immunity to hepatitis B following: Acute exposure to blood containing hepatitis B surface antigen (HBsAg); perinatal exposure of infants born to HBsAg-positive mothers; sexual exposure to HBsAg-positive persons; household exposure to persons with acute HBV infection

Prevention of hepatitis B virus recurrence after liver transplantation in HBsAg-positive transplant patients

Note: Hepatitis B immune globulin is not indicated for treatment of active hepatitis B infection and is ineffective in the treatment of chronic active hepatitis B infection.

Pharmacodynamics/Kinetics

Duration: Postexposure prophylaxis: 3-6 months
Absorption: I.M.: Slow
Half-life: 17-25 days
Distribution: V_d: 7-15 L
Time to peak, serum: I.M.: 2-10 days

Dosage

I.M.:

Newborns: Perinatal exposure of infants born to HBsAg-positive mothers: 0.5 mL as soon after birth as possible (within 12 hours); active vaccination with hepatitis B vaccine may begin at the same time in a different site (if not contraindicated). If first dose of hepatitis B vaccine is delayed for as long as 3 months, dose may be repeated. If hepatitis B vaccine is refused, dose may be repeated at 3 and 6 months.

Infants <12 months: Household exposure prophylaxis: 0.5 mL (to be administered if mother or primary caregiver has acute HBV infection)

Children ≥12 months and Adults: Postexposure prophylaxis: 0.06 mL/kg as soon as possible after exposure (ie, within 24 hours of needlestick, ocular, or mucosal exposure or within 14 days of sexual exposure); usual dose: 3-5 mL; repeat at 28-30 days after exposure in nonresponders to hepatitis B vaccine or in patients who refuse vaccination

Note: HBIG may be administered at the same time (but at a different site) or up to 1 month preceding hepatitis B vaccination without impairing the active immune response

I.V.: Adults: Prevention of hepatitis B virus recurrence after liver transplantation (HepaGam B™): 20,000 int. units/dose according to the following schedule:
Anhepatic phase (Initial dose): One dose given with the liver transplant
Week 1 postop: One dose daily for 7 days (days 1-7)
Weeks 2-12 postop: One dose every 2 weeks starting day 14
Month 4 onward: One dose monthly starting on month 4
Dose adjustment: Adjust dose to reach anti-HBs levels of 500 int. units/L within the first week after transplantation. In patients with surgical bleeding, abdominal fluid drainage >500 mL or those undergoing plasmapheresis, administer 10,000 int. units/dose every 6 hours until target anti-HBs levels are reached.

Anesthesia and Critical Care Concerns/Other Considerations Hepatitis B immune globulin has been administered intravenously in hepatitis B-positive liver transplant patients.

Additional Information Complete prescribing information for this medication should be consulted for additional detail.

Dosage Forms Excipient information presented when available (limited, particularly for generics); consult specific product labeling.

◄ **Note:** Potency expressed in international units (as compared to the WHO standard) is noted by individual lot on the vial label.

Injection, solution [preservative free]:

HyperHEP B™ S/D: Anti-HBs ≥220 int. units/mL (0.5 mL, 1 mL, 5 mL)

Nabi-HB®: Anti-HBs >312 int. units/mL (1 mL, 5 mL) [contains polysorbate 80]

HepaGam B™: Anti-HBs 312 int. units/mL (1 mL, 5 mL) [contains maltose and polysorbate 80]

◆ **Hepatitis B Inactivated Virus Vaccine (recombinant DNA)** *see* Hepatitis B Vaccine *on page 686*

Hepatitis B Vaccine (hep a TYE tis bee vak SEEN ree KOM be nant)

U.S. Brand Names Engerix-B®; Recombivax HB®

Canadian Brand Names Engerix-B®; Recombivax HB®

Index Terms Hepatitis B Inactivated Virus Vaccine (recombinant DNA); HepB

Pharmacologic Category Vaccine, Inactivated (Viral)

Use Immunization against infection caused by all known subtypes of hepatitis B virus (HBV), in individuals seeking protection from HBV infection and/or in the following individuals considered at high risk of potential exposure to hepatitis B virus or HBsAg-positive materials:

Workplace Exposure:
- Healthcare workers[1] (including students, custodial staff, lab personnel, etc)
- Police and fire personnel
- Military personnel
- Morticians and embalmers
- Clients/staff of institutions for the developmentally disabled

Lifestyle Factors:
- Homosexual men
- Heterosexually-active persons with multiple partners in a 6-month period or those with recently acquired sexually-transmitted disease
- Intravenous drug users

Specific Patient Groups:
- Those on hemodialysis[2], receiving transfusions[3], or in hematology/oncology units
- Adolescents
- Infants born of HBsAG-positive mothers
- Individuals with chronic liver disease
- Individual with HIV infection

Others:
- Prison inmates and staff of correctional facilities
- Household and sexual contacts of HBV carriers
- Residents, immigrants, adoptees, and refugees from areas with endemic HBV infection (eg, Alaskan Eskimos, Pacific Islanders, Indochinese, and Haitian descent)
- International travelers to areas of endemic HBV
- Children born after 11/21/1991

[1]The risk of hepatitis B virus (HBV) infection for healthcare workers varies both between hospitals and within hospitals. Hepatitis B vaccination is recommended for all healthcare workers with blood exposure.

[2]Hemodialysis patients often respond poorly to hepatitis B vaccination; higher vaccine doses or increased number of doses are required. A special formulation of one vaccine is now available for such persons (Recombivax HB®, 40 mcg/mL). The anti-HB$_s$ (antibody to hepatitis B surface antigen) response of such persons should be tested after they are vaccinated, and those who have not responded should be revaccinated with 1-3 additional doses. Patients with chronic renal disease should be vaccinated as early as possible, ideally before they require hemodialysis. In addition, their anti-HB$_s$ levels should be monitored at 6- to 12-month intervals to assess the need for revaccination.

[3]Patients with hemophilia should be immunized subcutaneously, not intramuscularly.

In addition, the Advisory Committee on Immunization Practices (ACIP) recommends vaccination for any persons who are wounded in bombings or similar mass casualty events who have penetrating injuries or nonintact skin exposure, or who have contact with mucous membranes (exception - superficial contact with intact skin), and who cannot confirm receipt of a hepatitis B vaccination.

Pharmacodynamics/Kinetics Duration: Following a 3-dose series in children, up to 50% of patients will have low or undetectable anti-HB antibody 5-15 years postvaccination. However, anamnestic increases in anti-HB have been shown up to 23 years later suggesting a lifelong immune memory response.

Dosage I.M.:

Immunization regimen: Regimen consists of 3 doses (0, 1, and 6 months): First dose given on the elected date, second dose given 1 month later, third dose given 6 months after the first dose; see table.

When used for immediate prophylactic intervention (eg, administration to persons who are wounded in bombings or similar mass casualty events), vaccination should begin within 24 hours and no later than 7 days following the event.

Note: Infants born to mothers whose HBsAg status is unknown should follow the regimen for HBsAg-positive mothers, omitting the dose of HBIG.

Note: Preterm infants <2000 g and born to HBsAg-negative mothers should have the first dose delayed until 1 month after birth or hospital discharge due to decreased immune response in underweight infants.

Routine Immunization Regimen of Three I.M. Hepatitis B Vaccine Doses

Age	Initial		1 mo		2 mo	6 mo[1]	
	Recombivax HB® (mL)	Engerix-B® (mL)	Recombivax HB® (mL)	Engerix-B® (mL)	Engerix-B® (mL)	Recombivax HB® (mL)	Engerix-B® (mL)
Birth[2] to 19 y	0.5[3]	0.5[4]	0.5[3]	0.5[4]	–	0.5[3]	0.5[4]
≥20 y[5]	1[6]	1[7]	1[6]	1[7]	–	1[6]	1[7]
Dialysis or immunocompromised patients[8]	1[9]	2[10]	1[9]	2[10]	2[10]	1[9]	2[10]

[1] Final dose in series should not be administered before age of 24 weeks.

[2] Infants born of HBsAg **negative** mothers.

[3] 5 mcg/0.5 mL pediatric/adolescent formulation.

[4] 10 mcg/0.5 mL formulation.

[5] Alternately, doses may be administered at 0, 1, and 4 months **or** at 0, 2, and 4 months.

[6] 10 mcg/mL adult formulation.

[7] 20 mcg/mL formulation.

[8] Revaccinate if anti-HB$_s$ <10 mIU/mL ≥1-2 months after third dose.

[9] 40 mcg/mL dialysis formulation.

[10] Two 1 mL doses given at different sites using the 20 mcg/mL formulation.

Alternative dosing schedule for **Recombivax HB®**:

Children 11-15 years (10 mcg/mL adult formulation): First dose of 1 mL given on the elected date, second dose given 4-6 months later

Adults ≥20 years: Doses may be administered at 0, 1, and 4 months **or** at 0, 2, and 4 months

Alternative dosing schedules for **Engerix-B®**:

Children ≤10 years (10 mcg/0.5 mL formulation): High-risk children: 0.5 mL at 0, 1, 2, and 12 months; lower-risk children ages 5-10 who are candidates for an extended administration schedule may receive an alternative regimen of 0.5 mL at 0, 12, and 24 months. If booster dose is needed, revaccinate with 0.5 mL.

Adolescents 11-19 years (20 mcg/mL formulation): 1 mL at 0, 1, and 6 months. High-risk adolescents: 1 mL at 0, 1, 2, and 12 months; lower-risk adolescents 11-16 years who are candidates for an extended administration schedule may receive an alternative regimen of 0.5 mL (using the 10 mcg/0.5 mL) formulation at 0, 12, and 24 months. If booster dose is needed, revaccinate with 20 mcg.

◄ Adults ≥20 years:
Doses may be administered at 0, 1, and 4 months **or** at 0, 2, and 4 months
High-risk adults (20 mcg/mL formulation): 1 mL at 0, 1, 2, and 12 months. If booster dose is needed, revaccinate with 1 mL.

Postexposure prophylaxis: **Note:** High-risk individuals may include children born of hepatitis B-infected mothers, those who have been or might be exposed or those who have traveled to high-risk areas. See table.

**Postexposure Prophylaxis Recommended Dosage
for Infants Born to HBsAg-Positive Mothers**

Treatment	Birth ≤12 h	1 mo	6 mo
Engerix-B® (pediatric formulation 10 mcg/0.5 mL)[1]	0.5 mL[2]	0.5 mL	0.5 mL
Recombivax HB® (pediatric/adolescent formulation 5 mcg/0.5 mL)	0.5 mL[2]	0.5 mL	0.5 mL
Hepatitis B immune globulin	0.5 mL[2]	—	—

[1]An alternate regimen is administration of the vaccine at birth, and 1, 2, and 12 months later.

[2]The first dose of vaccine may be given at birth at the same time as HBIG, but give in the opposite anterolateral thigh. This may better ensure vaccine absorption. HBIG should be given immediately if mother is determined to be HBsAg-positive within 7 days of birth.

Additional Information Complete prescribing information for this medication should be consulted for additional detail.

Dosage Forms Excipient information presented when available (limited, particularly for generics); consult specific product labeling.
Injection, suspension [adult; preservative free]:
Engerix-B®: Hepatitis B surface antigen 20 mcg/mL (1 mL) [contains aluminum, trace amounts of thimerosal; prefilled syringes contain natural rubber/natural latex]
Recombivax HB®: Hepatitis B surface antigen 10 mcg/mL (1 mL, 3 mL) [contains aluminum and yeast protein]
Injection, suspension [pediatric/adolescent; preservative free]:
Engerix-B®: Hepatitis B surface antigen 10 mcg/0.5 mL (0.5 mL) [contains aluminum, trace amounts of thimerosal; prefilled syringes contain natural rubber/natural latex]
Recombivax HB®: Hepatitis B surface antigen 5 mcg/0.5 mL (0.5 mL) [contains aluminum and yeast protein]
Injection, suspension [dialysis formulation; preservative free]:
Recombivax HB®: Hepatitis B surface antigen 40 mcg/mL (1 mL) [contains aluminum and yeast protein]

◆ **HepB** *see* Hepatitis B Vaccine *on page 686*
◆ **HepFlush®-10** *see* Heparin *on page 677*
◆ **Hep-Lock®** *see* Heparin *on page 677*
◆ **Hep-Lock U/P** *see* Heparin *on page 677*
◆ **Heptovir® (Can)** *see* LamiVUDine *on page 797*
◆ **HES** *see* Hetastarch *on page 688*
◆ **Hespan®** *see* Hetastarch *on page 688*

Hetastarch (HET a starch)

Medication Safety Issues
Sound-alike/look-alike issues:
Hespan® may be confused with heparin
U.S. Brand Names Hespan®; Hextend®; Voluven®
Canadian Brand Names Hextend®; Voluven®
Index Terms HES; Hydroxyethyl Starch
Pharmacologic Category Plasma Volume Expander, Colloid
Generic Available Yes: Sodium chloride infusion

Use Blood volume expander used in treatment of hypovolemia; prevention of hypovolemia (Voluven®); adjunct in leukapheresis to improve harvesting and increase the yield of granulocytes by centrifugation (Hespan®)

Unlabeled/Investigational Use Hextend®: Priming fluid in pump oxygenators during cardiopulmonary bypass; plasma volume expansion during cardiopulmonary bypass

Mechanism of Action Produces plasma volume expansion by virtue of its highly colloidal starch structure, similar to albumin

Pharmacodynamics/Kinetics

Onset of action: Volume expansion: I.V.: ~30 minutes

Duration: 6-36 hours

Distribution: Voluven®: 5.9 L

Metabolism: Molecules >50,000 daltons require enzymatic degradation by the reticuloendothelial system or amylases in the blood

Half-life elimination: Voluven®: 12 hours

Excretion: Urine (33% to 40% within 24 hours; ~62% within 72 hours); smaller molecular weight molecules readily excreted

Dosage I.V. infusion (requires an infusion pump):

Plasma volume expansion:

Children:

<2 years: Voluven®: Average dose: 7-25 mL/kg; titrate to individual colloid needs, hemodynamic and hydration status

2-12 years: Not studied

>12 years: Voluven®: Up to 50 mL/kg/day

Adults: 500-1000 mL (up to 1500 mL/day) or 20 mL/kg/day (up to 1500 mL/day); larger volumes (15,000 mL/24 hours) have been used safely in small numbers of patients

Voluven®: Up to 50 mL/kg/day

Leukapheresis (Hextend®): 250-700 mL; **Note:** Citrate anticoagulant is added before use.

Dosing adjustment in renal impairment: Cl_{cr} <10 mL/minute: Initial dose is the same but subsequent doses should be reduced by 20% to 50% of normal

Stability Store at room temperature; do not freeze. Do not use if crystalline precipitate forms or is turbid deep brown. Do not use if crystalline precipitate forms or is turbid deep brown. In leukapheresis, admixtures of 500-560 mL of Hespan® with citrate concentrations up to 2.5% are compatible for 24 hours.

Administration Administer I.V. only; infusion pump is required. May administer up to 1.2 g/kg/hour (20 mL/kg/hour). Change I.V. tubing or flush copiously with normal saline before administering blood through the same line. Change I.V. tubing at least every 24 hours. Do not administer Hextend® with blood through the same administration set. Anaphylactoid reactions can occur, have epinephrine and resuscitative equipment available.

Leukapheresis: Mix Hespan® and citrate well. Administer to the input line of the centrifuge apparatus at a ration of 1:8 to 1:13 to venous whole blood.

Monitoring Parameters

Volume expansion: Blood pressure, heart rate, capillary refill time, CVP, RAP, MAP, urine output; if pulmonary artery catheter in place, monitor PCWP, SVR, and PVR; hemoglobin, hematocrit, serum electrolytes, renal function, acid-base balance, coagulation parameters, cardiac index

Leukapheresis: CBC, total leukocyte and platelet counts, leukocyte differential count, hemoglobin, hematocrit, PT, PTT

Anesthesia and Critical Care Concerns/Other Considerations

Clinical Pearls/Comments: Hetastarch is a synthetic polymer derived from a waxy starch composed of amylopectin.

Hespan®: 6% hetastarch in 0.9% sodium chloride

Molecular weight: 600,000

Sodium: 154 mEq/L

Chloride: 154 mEq/L

Osmolarity: ~309 mOsm/L

◄ Hextend®: 6% hetastarch in lactated electrolyte injection
  Molecular weight: ~670,000
  Sodium: 143 mEq/L
  Chloride: 124 mEq/L
  Calcium: 5 mEq/L
  Potassium: 3 mEq/L
  Magnesium: 0.9 mEq/L
  Lactate: 28 mEq/L
  Dextrose: 0.99 g/L
  Osmolarity: ~307 mOsm/L

Voluven®: 6% hetastarch (130/0.4) in 0.9% sodium chloride
  Molecular weight: ~130,000
  Sodium: 154 mEq/L
  Chloride: 154 mEq/L
  Osmolarity: 308 mOsm/L

Hextend®, Hespan®, and Voluven® will expand the intravascular volume the same as an equal volume of 5% albumin. Hetastarch will increase the intravascular volume up to 6-36 hours depending on the formulation. Hetastarch does not have oxygen-carrying capacity and is not a substitute for blood or plasma. Large volumes of Hespan®, Hextend®, or Voluven® may interfere with platelet function, prolong PT and PTT times, and cause hemodilution; however, clinically Hextend® has not been associated with coagulation abnormalities in doses >20 mL/kg up to a total of 5000 mL. Voluven®, because of its low molecular weight and reduced molar substitution, also has a low potential for affecting coagulation.

Hextend®: Formulated with near physiologic levels of sodium, chloride, calcium, potassium, magnesium; may be associated with less electrolyte abnormalities than Hespan®; not to be used for the treatment of lactic acidosis; should not be administered through the same line as blood products; use with caution in patients with heart failure.

Hespan®: Intraoperative use in patients undergoing cardiac surgery with cardiopulmonary bypass may increase bleeding; each 500 mL provides 77 mEq sodium chloride and may cause hyperchloremic metabolic acidosis in large volumes; critically-ill patients receiving hetastarch infusions (goal: PCWP 12-18 mm Hg) had an increase in cardiac index, oxygen delivery, and consumption.

Voluven®: Up to 50 mL/kg/day (or 3500 mL/day in a 70 kg patient) may be used without significant effects on coagulation parameters. Eliminated more rapidly resulting in a shorter duration of action (4-6 hours) compared to other HES products. Because of minimal accumulation, tissue storage is reduced and may result in a lower rate of delayed-onset pruritus seen with other HES products.

Hextend®, Hespan®, and Voluven®: May increase serum amylase temporarily without an association with pancreatitis; not eliminated by hemodialysis.

Pregnancy Risk Factor C

Contraindications Hypersensitivity to hydroxyethyl starch or any component of the formulation; renal failure with oliguria or anuria (not related to hypovolemia); any fluid overload condition (eg, pulmonary edema, congestive heart failure)

Hespan ® is also contraindicated in patients with pre-existing coagulation or bleeding disorders

Hextend® is also contraindicated with bleeding disorders; in the treatment of lactic acidosis and in leukapheresis

Voluven® is also contraindicated in patients receiving dialysis; severe hypernatremia; severe hyperchloremia; patients with intracranial bleeding

Warnings/Precautions Anaphylactoid reactions have occurred; use caution in patients allergic to corn (may have cross allergy to hetastarch); use with caution in patients with thrombocytopenia (may interfere with platelet function); large volume may cause drops in hemoglobin concentrations; use with caution in patients at risk from overexpansion of blood volume, including the very young or aged patients, those with HF; volumes >1500 mL may interfere with platelet function and prolong PT and PTT times; use with caution in patients with severe liver disease (may result in further reduction of coagulation factors, increasing the risk of bleeding). Note electrolyte content of Hextend® including calcium, lactate, and potassium; use caution in situations where electrolyte and/or acid-base disturbances may be exacerbated (renal impairment, respiratory alkalosis). The risk of adverse reactions may be increased in patients with renal impairment; monitor fluid status, urine output and infusion rate. Larger hetastarch molecules may leak into urine in patients with glomerular damage; may elevate urine specific gravity.

Adverse Reactions Frequency not defined.

Cardiovascular: Bradycardia, circulatory overload, heart failure, peripheral edema, tachycardia

Central nervous system: Chills, fever, headache, intracranial bleeding

Dermatologic: Itching, pruritus (dose dependant; may be delayed), rash

Endocrine & metabolic: Metabolic acidosis, parotid gland enlargement

Gastrointestinal: Amylase levels increased, vomiting

Hematologic: Anemia, bleeding, bleeding time prolonged, clotting time prolonged, dilutional coagulopathy, disseminated intravascular coagulopathy (rare), factor VIII:C plasma levels decreased, hemolysis (rare), plasma aggregation decreased, PT prolonged, PTT prolonged, thrombocytopenia, von Willebrand factor decreased, wound hemorrhage

Hepatic: Bilirubin increased (indirect)

Neuromuscular & skeletal: Myalgia

Respiratory: Bronchospasm, pulmonary edema (noncardiac)

Miscellaneous: Anaphylactoid reactions, flu-like syndrome (mild), hypersensitivity

Postmarketing and/or case reports: Hypotension, urticaria

Drug Interactions

Avoid Concomitant Use There are no known interactions where it is recommended to avoid concomitant use.

Increased Effect/Toxicity There are no known significant interactions involving an increase in effect.

Decreased Effect There are no known significant interactions involving a decrease in effect.

Test Interactions

Serum amylase levels may be temporarily elevated following administration; could interfere with the diagnosis of pancreatitis.

Large hetastarch volumes may result in decreased coagulation factors, plasma proteins, and /or hematocrit due to dilutional effect.

Dosage Forms Excipient information presented when available (limited, particularly for generics); consult specific product labeling.

Infusion [premixed in lactated electrolyte injection]:

Hextend®: 6% (500 mL)

Infusion, solution [premixed in NaCl 0.9%]: 6% (500 mL)

Hespan®, Voluven®: 6% (500 mL)

References

Abbott Laboratories, Hextend® Product Labeling, Revised January, 1999.

Bick RL, "Evaluation of a New Hydroxyethyl Starch Preparation (Hextend®) on Selected Coagulation Parameters," *Clin Appl Thrombosis/Hemostasis*, 1995, 1(3):215-29.

Boldt J, Heesen M, Müller M, et al, "The Effects of Albumin Versus Hydroxyethyl Starch Solution on Cardiorespiratory and Circulatory Variables in Critically Ill Patients," *Anesth Analg*, 1996, 83 (2):254-61.

Brutocao D, Bratton SL, Thomas JR, et al, "Comparison of Hetastarch With Albumin for Postoperative Volume Expansion in Children After Cardiopulmonary Bypass," *J Cardiothoracic Vasc Anesth*, 1996, 10(3):348-51.

Gan TJ, Bennett-Guerrero E, Phillips-Bute B, et al "Hextend®, a Physiologically Balanced Plasma Expander for Large Volume Use in Major Surgery: A Randomized Phase III Clinical Trial," *Anesth Analg*, 1999, 88(5):992-8.

Gan TJ, Wright D, Robertson C, et al, "Randomized Comparison of the Coagulation Profile When Hextend® or 5% Albumin is Used for Intraoperative Fluid Resuscitation," *Anesthesiology*, 2001, 95: A193.

Knutson JE, Deering JA, Hall FW, et al, "Does Intraoperative Hetastarch Administration Increase Blood Loss and Transfusion Requirements After Cardiac Surgery?" *Anesth Analg*, 2000, 90 (4):801-7.

Wilkes NJ, Woolf RL, Powanda MC, et al, "Hydroxyethyl Starch in Balanced Electrolyte Solution (Hextend®) - Pharmacokinetic and Pharmacodynamic Profiles in Healthy Volunteers," *Anesth Analg*, 2002, 94(3):538-44.

◆ **Hextend®** see Hetastarch on page 688

◆ **hGH** see Somatropin on page 1318

◆ **Hibiclens® [OTC]** see Chlorhexidine Gluconate on page 291

◆ **Hibidil® 1:2000 (Can)** see Chlorhexidine Gluconate on page 291

- **Hibistat® [OTC]** *see* Chlorhexidine Gluconate *on page 291*
- **Hirulog** *see* Bivalirudin *on page 193*
- **Histantil (Can)** *see* Promethazine *on page 1186*
- **Histaprin [OTC]** *see* DiphenhydrAMINE *on page 430*
- **HMR 3647** *see* Telithromycin *on page 1353*
- **Humalog®** *see* Insulin Lispro *on page 747*
- **Humalog® Mix 25 (Can)** *see* Insulin Lispro Protamine and Insulin Lispro *on page 748*
- **Humalog® Mix 50/50™** *see* Insulin Lispro Protamine and Insulin Lispro *on page 748*
- **Humalog® Mix 75/25™** *see* Insulin Lispro Protamine and Insulin Lispro *on page 748*
- **Human Albumin Grifols®** *see* Albumin *on page 46*
- **Human C1 Inhibitor** *see* C1 Inhibitor (Human) *on page 223*
- **Human Diploid Cell Cultures Rabies Vaccine** *see* Rabies Virus Vaccine *on page 1225*
- **Human Growth Hormone** *see* Somatropin *on page 1318*
- **Humatrope®** *see* Somatropin *on page 1318*
- **Humist® [OTC]** *see* Sodium Chloride *on page 1304*
- **Humist® for Kids [OTC]** *see* Sodium Chloride *on page 1304*
- **Humulin® 20/80 (Can)** *see* Insulin NPH and Insulin Regular *on page 749*
- **Humulin® 50/50 [DSC]** *see* Insulin NPH and Insulin Regular *on page 749*
- **Humulin® 70/30** *see* Insulin NPH and Insulin Regular *on page 749*
- **Humulin® N** *see* Insulin NPH and Insulin Regular *on page 749*
- **Humulin® R** *see* Insulin Regular *on page 750*
- **Humulin® R U-500** *see* Insulin Regular *on page 750*

Hyaluronidase (hye al yoor ON i dase)

Medication Safety Issues
Sound-alike/look-alike issues:
Wydase may be confused with Lidex®, Wyamine®
U.S. Brand Names Amphadase™; Hydase™; Hylenex™; Vitrase®
Pharmacologic Category Enzyme
Generic Available No
Use Increase the dispersion and absorption of other injected drugs; increase rate of absorption of parenteral fluids given by subcutaneous administration (hypodermoclysis)
Unlabeled/Investigational Use Management of drug extravasations; local anesthetic adjuvant in bupivacaine-lidocaine mixture for retrobulbar/peribulbar block
Mechanism of Action Modifies the permeability of connective tissue through hydrolysis of hyaluronic acid, one of the chief components of tissue cement which offers resistance to diffusion of liquids through tissues; hyaluronidase increases both the distribution and absorption of locally injected substances.
Pharmacodynamics/Kinetics
Onset of action: SubQ: Immediate
Duration: 24-48 hours
Dosage Note: A preliminary skin test for hypersensitivity can be performed.
Skin test: Intradermal: 0.02 mL (3 units) of a 150 units/mL solution. Positive reaction consists of a wheal with pseudopods appearing within 5 minutes and persisting for 20-30 minutes with localized itching.
Hypodermoclysis: SubQ: Infants and Children: 150 units followed by subcutaneous isotonic fluid administration at a rate appropriate for age, weight, and clinical condition of the patient; 150 units facilitates absorption of >1000 mL of solution **or** add 15 units to each 100 mL of I.V. fluid to be administered subcutaneously

Premature Infants and Neonates: Volume of a single clysis should not exceed 25 mL/kg and the rate of administration should not exceed 2 mL/minute

Children <3 years (Amphadase™, Hydase™, Vitrase®): Volume of a single clysis should not exceed 200 mL

Children ≥3 years and Adults: Rate and volume of a single clysis should not exceed those used for infusion of I.V. fluids

Extravasation (unlabeled use): Adults: SubQ: Inject 1 mL of a 150 unit/mL solution (as 5-10 injections of 0.1-0.2 mL) into affected area; doses of 15-250 units have been reported. **Note:** Do not use for extravasation of pressor agents (eg, dopamine, norepinephrine).

Elderly: See adult dosing. Adjust dose carefully to individual patient.

Stability

Amphadase™, Hydase™, Hylenex™: Store in refrigerator at 2°C to 8°C (35°F to 46°F); do not freeze.

Vitrase®: Store unopened vial in refrigerator at 2°C to 8°C (35°F to 46°F). Add 6.2 mL of NaCl to vial (1000 units/mL). Further dilute with NaCl before administration. After reconstitution, store at 20°C to 25°C (68°F to 77°F) and use within 6 hours.

For 50 units/mL, draw up 0.05 mL of hyaluronidase reconstituted solution (1000 units/mL) and add 0.95 mL of NaCl.

For 75 units/mL, draw up 0.075 mL of hyaluronidase reconstituted solution and add 0.925 mL of NaCl.

For 150 units/mL, draw up 0.15 mL of hyaluronidase reconstituted solution and add 0.85 mL of NaCl.

For 300 units/mL, draw up 0.3 mL of hyaluronidase reconstituted solution and add 0.7 mL of NaCl.

Administration Do **not** administer I.V.

Pregnancy Risk Factor C

Contraindications Hypersensitivity to hyaluronidase or any component of the formulation

Warnings/Precautions Do not inject in or around infected or inflamed areas; may spread localized infection. Should not be used for extravasation management of dopamine or alpha agonists, or to reduce swelling of bites or stings. Do not administer intravenously. Do not apply directly to the cornea. Discontinue if sensitization occurs.

Adverse Reactions

Frequency not defined:

Cardiovascular: Edema

Local: Injection site reactions

<1%: Allergic reactions, anaphylactic-like reactions (retrobulbar block or I.V. injections), angioedema, urticaria

Drug Interactions

Avoid Concomitant Use There are no known interactions where it is recommended to avoid concomitant use.

Increased Effect/Toxicity There are no known significant interactions involving an increase in effect.

Decreased Effect There are no known significant interactions involving a decrease in effect.

Dosage Forms Excipient information presented when available (limited, particularly for generics); consult specific product labeling.

Injection, powder for reconstitution:

Vitrase®: 6200 units [ovine derived; contains lactose]

Injection, solution:

Amphadase™: 150 units/mL (1 mL) [bovine derived; contains edetate disodium 1 mg, thimerosal ≤0.1 mg]

Injection, solution [preservative free]:

Hydase™: 150 units/mL (1 mL) [bovine derived; contains edetate disodium 1 mg]

Hylenex™: 150 units/mL (1 mL, 2 mL) [recombinant; contains human albumin and edetate disodium]

Vitrase®: 200 units/mL (2 mL) [ovine derived; contains lactose]

References

Kallio H, Paloheimo M, and Maunuksela EL, "Hyaluronidase as an Adjuvant in Bupivacaine-Lidocaine Mixture for Retrobulbar/Peribulbar Block," *Anesth Analg*, 2000, 91(4):934-7.

- ◆ **hycet™** *see* Hydrocodone and Acetaminophen *on page 697*
- ◆ **Hycort™ (Can)** *see* Hydrocortisone *on page 699*
- ◆ **Hydase™** *see* Hyaluronidase *on page 692*
- ◆ **Hydeltra T.B.A.® (Can)** *see* PrednisoLONE *on page 1164*
- ◆ **Hyderm (Can)** *see* Hydrocortisone *on page 699*

HydrALAZINE (hye DRAL a zeen)

Medication Safety Issues
Sound-alike/look-alike issues:
HydrALAZINE may be confused with hydrOXYzine
Related Information
Anesthesia Considerations for Neurosurgery *on page 1514*
Anesthetic Considerations in the Substance-Abusing Patient *on page 1613*
Heart Failure (Systolic) *on page 1739*
Hypertension *on page 1754*
Postoperative Hypertension *on page 1589*
Canadian Brand Names Apo-Hydralazine®; Apresoline®; Novo-Hylazin; Nu-Hydral
Index Terms Apresoline [DSC]; Hydralazine Hydrochloride
Pharmacologic Category Vasodilator
Generic Available Yes
Use Management of moderate-to-severe hypertension
Unlabeled/Investigational Use Heart failure; hypertension secondary to pre-eclampsia/eclampsia
Mechanism of Action Direct vasodilation of arterioles (with little effect on veins) with decreased systemic resistance
Pharmacodynamics/Kinetics
Onset of action: Oral: 20-30 minutes; I.V.: 5-20 minutes
Duration: Oral: Up to 8 hours; I.V.: 1-4 hours; **Note:** May vary depending on acetylator status of patient
Distribution: Crosses placenta; enters breast milk
Protein binding: 85% to 90%
Metabolism: Hepatically acetylated; extensive first-pass effect (oral)
Bioavailability: 30% to 50%; increased with food
Half-life elimination: Normal renal function: 2-8 hours; End-stage renal disease: 7-16 hours
Excretion: Urine (14% as unchanged drug)
Dosage
Children:
Oral: Initial: 0.75-1 mg/kg/day in 2-4 divided doses; increase over 3-4 weeks to maximum of 7.5 mg/kg/day in 2-4 divided doses; maximum daily dose: 200 mg/day
I.M., I.V.: 0.1-0.2 mg/kg/dose (not to exceed 20 mg) every 4-6 hours as needed, up to 1.7-3.5 mg/kg/day in 4-6 divided doses
Adults:
Oral:
Hypertension:
Initial dose: 10 mg 4 times/day for first 2-4 days; increase to 25 mg 4 times/day for the balance of the first week
Increase by 10-25 mg/dose gradually to 50 mg 4 times/day (maximum: 300 mg/day); usual dose range (JNC 7): 25-100 mg/day in 2 divided doses
Congestive heart failure:
Initial dose: 10-25 mg 3-4 times/day
Adjustment: Dosage must be adjusted based on individual response
Target dose: 225-300 mg/day in divided doses; use in combination with isosorbide dinitrate
I.M., I.V.:
Hypertension: Initial: 10-20 mg/dose every 4-6 hours as needed, may increase to 40 mg/dose; change to oral therapy as soon as possible.
Pre-eclampsia/eclampsia: 5 mg/dose then 5-10 mg every 20-30 minutes as needed.

Elderly: Oral: Initial: 10 mg 2-3 times/day; increase by 10-25 mg/day every 2-5 days.

Dosing interval in renal impairment:

Cl_{cr} 10-50 mL/minute: Administer every 8 hours.

Cl_{cr} <10 mL/minute: Administer every 8-16 hours in fast acetylators and every 12-24 hours in slow acetylators.

Hemodialysis: Supplemental dose is not necessary.

Peritoneal dialysis: Supplemental dose is not necessary.

Stability Intact ampuls/vials of hydralazine should not be stored under refrigeration because of possible precipitation or crystallization. Hydralazine should be diluted in NS for IVPB administration due to decreased stability in D_5W. Stability of IVPB solution in NS is 4 days at room temperature.

Administration Solution for injection: Administer as a slow I.V. push; maximum rate: 5 mg/minute

Monitoring Parameters Blood pressure (monitor closely with I.V. use), standing and sitting/supine, heart rate, ANA titer

Anesthesia and Critical Care Concerns/Other Considerations

Clinical Pearls/Comments: A common adverse event of intravenous hydralazine is unpredictable hypotension. Hypotension due to hydralazine may last longer (up to 12 hours) even though the circulating half-life is only ~3 hours. For this reason, intravenous hydralazine is not recommended for the treatment of hypertensive crisis (Marik, 2007). In patients with significant obstructive coronary disease, the use of intravenous hydralazine may be detrimental due to the production of reflex tachycardia; use with caution. Hydralazine is considered to be safe for the management of blood pressure during pregnancy (eg, pre-eclampsia); however, other agents may be considered.

Evidence-Based Information: May be combined with isosorbide dinitrate for the treatment of heart failure (HF) with ACE inhibitors, beta-blockers (eg, bisoprolol, carvedilol, metoprolol XL) and diuretics in patients who are self-identified as African-Americans. Hydralazine/isosorbide dinitrate combination may also be used in HF patients with reduced LVEF who are already on an ACE inhibitor and a beta-blocker for symptomatic heart failure and who have persistent symptoms or those unable to tolerate ACE inhibition or angiotensin II receptor blockade (Hunt, 2009).

Pregnancy Risk Factor C

Contraindications Hypersensitivity to hydralazine or any component of the formulation; mitral valve rheumatic heart disease

Warnings/Precautions May cause a drug-induced lupus-like syndrome (more likely on larger doses, longer duration). Discontinue hydralazine in patients who develop SLE-like syndrome or positive ANA. Use with caution in patients with severe renal disease or cerebral vascular accidents or with known or suspected coronary artery disease; monitor blood pressure closely with I.V. use. Slow acetylators, patients with decreased renal function, and patients receiving >200 mg/day (chronically) are at higher risk for SLE. Titrate dosage cautiously to patient's response. Hypotension effect after I.V. administration may be delayed and unpredictable in some patients. Usually administered with diuretic and a beta-blocker to counteract side effects of sodium and water retention and reflex tachycardia.

Adjust dose in severe renal dysfunction. Use with caution in CAD (increase in tachycardia may increase myocardial oxygen demand). Use with caution in pulmonary hypertension (may cause hypotension). Patients may be poorly compliant because of frequent dosing. Hydralazine-induced fluid and sodium retention may require addition or increased dosage of a diuretic.

Adverse Reactions Frequency not defined.

Cardiovascular: Tachycardia, angina pectoris, orthostatic hypotension (rare), dizziness (rare), paradoxical hypertension, peripheral edema, vascular collapse (rare), flushing

Central nervous system: Increased intracranial pressure (I.V., in patient with pre-existing increased intracranial pressure), fever (rare), chills (rare), anxiety*, disorientation*, depression*, coma*

Dermatologic: Rash (rare), urticaria (rare), pruritus (rare)

◀ Gastrointestinal: Anorexia, nausea, vomiting, diarrhea, constipation, adynamic ileus

Genitourinary: Difficulty in micturition, impotence

Hematologic: Hemolytic anemia (rare), eosinophilia (rare), decreased hemoglobin concentration (rare), reduced erythrocyte count (rare), leukopenia (rare), agranulocytosis (rare), thrombocytopenia (rare)

Neuromuscular & skeletal: Rheumatoid arthritis, muscle cramps, weakness, tremor, peripheral neuritis (rare)

Ocular: Lacrimation, conjunctivitis

Respiratory: Nasal congestion, dyspnea

Miscellaneous: Drug-induced lupus-like syndrome (dose related; fever, arthralgia, splenomegaly, lymphadenopathy, asthenia, myalgia, malaise, pleuritic chest pain, edema, positive ANA, positive LE cells, maculopapular facial rash, positive direct Coombs' test, pericarditis, pericardial tamponade), diaphoresis

*Seen in uremic patients and severe hypertension where rapidly escalating doses may have caused hypotension leading to these effects.

Drug Interactions

Metabolism/Transport Effects Inhibits CYP3A4 (weak)

Avoid Concomitant Use There are no known interactions where it is recommended to avoid concomitant use.

Increased Effect/Toxicity

HydrALAZINE may increase the levels/effects of: Amifostine; Antihypertensives; Hypotensive Agents; RiTUXimab

The levels/effects of HydrALAZINE may be increased by: Diazoxide; Herbs (Hypotensive Properties); MAO Inhibitors; Pentoxifylline; Phosphodiesterase 5 Inhibitors; Prostacyclin Analogues

Decreased Effect

The levels/effects of HydrALAZINE may be decreased by: Herbs (Hypertensive Properties); Methylphenidate; Nonsteroidal Anti-Inflammatory Agents; Yohimbine

Ethanol/Nutrition/Herb Interactions

Ethanol: Avoid ethanol (may increase CNS depression).

Food: Food enhances bioavailability of hydralazine.

Herb/Nutraceutical: Avoid dong quai if using for hypertension (has estrogenic activity). Avoid ephedra, yohimbe, ginseng (may worsen hypertension). Avoid garlic (may have increased antihypertensive effect).

Dietary Considerations Administer tablet with meals.

Dosage Forms Excipient information presented when available (limited, particularly for generics); consult specific product labeling.

Injection, solution, as hydrochloride: 20 mg/mL (1 mL)

Tablet, as hydrochloride: 10 mg, 25 mg, 50 mg, 100 mg

References

Erstad BL and Barletta JF, "Treatment of Hypertension in the Perioperative Patient," *Ann Pharmacother*, 2000, 34(1):66-79.

Hunt SA, Abraham WT, Chin MH, et al, "2009 Focused Update Incorporated into the ACC/AHA 2005 Guidelines for the Diagnosis and Management of Heart Failure in Adults: A Report of the American College of Cardiology Foundation/American Heart Association Task Force on Practice Guidelines Developed in Collaboration With the International Society for Heart and Lung Transplantation," *J Am Coll Cardiol*, 2009, 53(15):e1-e90.

Marik PE and Varon J, "Hypertensive Crises: Challenges and Management," *Chest*, 2007, 131(6):1949-62.

◆ **Hydralazine Hydrochloride** *see* HydrALAZINE *on page 694*

◆ **Hydramine [OTC]** *see* DiphenhydrAMINE *on page 430*

◆ **Hydrated Chloral** *see* Chloral Hydrate *on page 285*

◆ **Hydrea®** *see* Hydroxyurea *on page 712*

Hydrochlorothiazide (hye droe klor oh THYE a zide)

Related Information

Heart Failure (Systolic) *on page 1739*

U.S. Brand Names Microzide®

Canadian Brand Names Apo-Hydro®; Novo-Hydrazide; PMS-Hydrochlorothiazide

Index Terms HCTZ (error-prone abbreviation); Hydrodiuril

Pharmacologic Category Diuretic, Thiazide

Use Management of mild-to-moderate hypertension; treatment of edema in heart failure and nephrotic syndrome

Unlabeled/Investigational Use Treatment of lithium-induced diabetes insipidus

Pharmacodynamics/Kinetics
Onset of action: Diuresis: ~2 hours
  Peak effect: 4-6 hours
Duration: 6-12 hours
Absorption: ~50% to 80%
Distribution: 3.6-7.8 L/kg
Protein binding: 68%
Metabolism: Not metabolized
Bioavailability: 50% to 80%
Half-life elimination: 5.6-14.8 hours
Time to peak: 1-2.5 hours
Excretion: Urine (as unchanged drug)

Dosage Oral (effect of drug may be decreased when used every day):
Children (in pediatric patients, chlorothiazide may be preferred over hydrochlorothiazide as there are more dosage formulations [eg, suspension] available): Edema, hypertension:
<6 months: 1-3 mg/kg/day in 2 divided doses
>6 months to 2 years: 1-3 mg/kg/day in 2 divided doses; maximum: 37.5 mg/day
>2-17 years: Initial: 1 mg/kg/day; maximum: 3 mg/kg/day (50 mg/day)
Adults:
Edema: 25-100 mg/day in 1-2 doses; maximum: 200 mg/day
Hypertension: 12.5-50 mg/day; minimal increase in response and more electrolyte disturbances are seen with doses >50 mg/day
Elderly: 12.5-25 mg once daily

Dosing adjustment/comments in renal impairment: Cl_{cr} <10 mL/minute: Avoid use. Usually ineffective with GFR <30 mL/minute. Effective at lower GFR in combination with a loop diuretic.
  Note: ACC/AHA 2009 Heart Failure guidelines suggest that thiazides lose their efficacy when Cl_{cr} <40 mL/minute.

Anesthesia and Critical Care Concerns/Other Considerations If given the morning of surgery it may render the patient volume depleted and blood pressure may be labile during general anesthesia.

Thiazide diuretics are effective first-line therapeutic agents in the management of hypertension and have proven to be of benefit in terms of cardiovascular outcome. They may act synergistically to lower blood pressure when combined with an ACE inhibitor or beta-blocker.

Additional Information Complete prescribing information for this medication should be consulted for additional detail.

Dosage Forms Excipient information presented when available (limited, particularly for generics); consult specific product labeling.
Capsule: 12.5 mg
  Microzide®: 12.5 mg
Tablet: 25 mg, 50 mg

Hydrocodone and Acetaminophen
(hye droe KOE done & a seet a MIN oh fen)

Related Information
Acute Postoperative Pain *on page 1502*
Chronic Pain Management *on page 1546*

U.S. Brand Names Co-Gesic® [DSC]; hycet™; Lorcet® 10/650; Lorcet® Plus; Lortab®; Margesic® H; Maxidone®; Norco®; Stagesic™; Vicodin®; Vicodin® ES; Vicodin® HP; Xodol® 10/300; Xodol® 5/300; Xodol® 7.5/300; Zamicet™; Zydone®

Index Terms Acetaminophen and Hydrocodone

▶

◀ **Pharmacologic Category** Analgesic Combination (Opioid)
Restrictions C-III
Use Relief of moderate-to-severe pain
Pharmacodynamics/Kinetics
  Acetaminophen: See Acetaminophen monograph.
  Hydrocodone:
    Onset of action: Narcotic analgesic: 10-20 minutes
    Duration: 4-8 hours
    Distribution: Crosses placenta
    Metabolism: Hepatic; O-demethylation; N-demethylation and 6-ketosteroid reduction
    Half-life elimination: 3.3-4.4 hours
    Excretion: Urine
Dosage Oral (doses should be titrated to appropriate analgesic effect): Analgesic:
  Children 2-13 years or <50 kg: Hydrocodone 0.1-0.2 mg/kg/dose every 4-6 hours; do not exceed 6 doses/day or the maximum recommended dose of acetaminophen
  Children and Adults ≥50 kg: Average starting dose in opioid naive patients: Hydrocodone 5-10 mg 4 times/day; the dosage of acetaminophen should be limited to ≤4 g/day (and possibly less in patients with hepatic impairment or ethanol use).
    Dosage ranges (based on specific product labeling): Hydrocodone 2.5-10 mg every 4-6 hours; maximum: 60 mg hydrocodone/day (maximum dose of hydrocodone may be limited by the acetaminophen content of specific product)
  Elderly: Doses should be titrated to appropriate analgesic effect; 2.5-5 mg of the hydrocodone component every 4-6 hours. Do not exceed 4 g/day of acetaminophen.
  Dosage adjustment in hepatic impairment: Use with caution. Limited, low-dose therapy usually well tolerated in hepatic disease/cirrhosis; however, cases of hepatotoxicity at daily acetaminophen dosages <4 g/day have been reported. Avoid chronic use in hepatic impairment.
Anesthesia and Critical Care Concerns/Other Considerations Doses of agent must be individualized according to degree of pain; commonly used in place of Tylenol® with Codeine; patients on this drug chronically should have liver function monitored secondary to acetaminophen in the product. Keep acetaminophen dose ≤4 g/day. Patients with chronic alcoholism, liver disease, or those who are fasting can develop severe hepatic disease even at therapeutic doses.
Additional Information Complete prescribing information for this medication should be consulted for additional detail.
Dosage Forms Excipient information presented when available (limited, particularly for generics); consult specific product labeling. [DSC] = Discontinued product
  Capsule:
    Margesic® H, Stagesic™: Hydrocodone bitartrate 5 mg and acetaminophen 500 mg
  Elixir: Hydrocodone bitartrate 7.5 mg and acetaminophen 500 mg per 15 mL (480 mL)
    Lortab®: Hydrocodone bitartrate 7.5 mg and acetaminophen 500 mg per 15 mL (480 mL) [contains ethanol 7%, propylene glycol; tropical fruit punch flavor]
  Solution, oral: Hydrocodone bitartrate 7.5 mg and acetaminophen 500 mg per 15 mL (5 mL, 10 mL, 15 mL, 118 mL, 473 mL)
    hycet™: Hydrocodone bitartrate 7.5 mg and acetaminophen 325 mg per 15 mL (473 mL) [contains ethanol 6.7%, propylene glycol; fruit flavor]
    Zamicet™: Hydrocodone bitartrate 10 mg and acetaminophen 325 mg per 15 mL (473 mL) [contains ethanol 6.7%, propylene glycol; fruit flavor]
  Tablet:
    Hydrocodone bitartrate 2.5 mg and acetaminophen 500 mg
    Hydrocodone bitartrate 5 mg and acetaminophen 325 mg
    Hydrocodone bitartrate 5 mg and acetaminophen 500 mg
    Hydrocodone bitartrate 7.5 mg and acetaminophen 325 mg
    Hydrocodone bitartrate 7.5 mg and acetaminophen 500 mg
    Hydrocodone bitartrate 7.5 mg and acetaminophen 650 mg

Hydrocodone bitartrate 7.5 mg and acetaminophen 750 mg
Hydrocodone bitartrate 10 mg and acetaminophen 325 mg
Hydrocodone bitartrate 10 mg and acetaminophen 500 mg
Hydrocodone bitartrate 10 mg and acetaminophen 650 mg
Hydrocodone bitartrate 10 mg and acetaminophen 660 mg
Hydrocodone bitartrate 10 mg and acetaminophen 750 mg
Co-Gesic® 5/500: Hydrocodone bitartrate 5 mg and acetaminophen 500 mg [DSC]
Lorcet® 10/650: Hydrocodone bitartrate 10 mg and acetaminophen 650 mg
Lorcet® Plus: Hydrocodone bitartrate 7.5 mg and acetaminophen 650 mg
Lortab®:
  5/500: Hydrocodone bitartrate 5 mg and acetaminophen 500 mg
  7.5/500: Hydrocodone bitartrate 7.5 mg and acetaminophen 500 mg
  10/500: Hydrocodone bitartrate 10 mg and acetaminophen 500 mg
Maxidone®: Hydrocodone bitartrate 10 mg and acetaminophen 750 mg
Norco®:
  Hydrocodone bitartrate 5 mg and acetaminophen 325 mg
  Hydrocodone bitartrate 7.5 mg and acetaminophen 325 mg
  Hydrocodone bitartrate 10 mg and acetaminophen 325 mg
Vicodin®: Hydrocodone bitartrate 5 mg and acetaminophen 500 mg
Vicodin® ES: Hydrocodone bitartrate 7.5 mg and acetaminophen 750 mg
Vicodin® HP: Hydrocodone bitartrate 10 mg and acetaminophen 660 mg
Xodol®:
  5/300: Hydrocodone bitartrate 5 mg and acetaminophen 300 mg
  7.5/300: Hydrocodone bitartrate 7.5 mg and acetaminophen 300 mg
  10/300: Hydrocodone bitartrate 10 mg and acetaminophen 300 mg
Zydone®:
  Hydrocodone bitartrate 5 mg and acetaminophen 400 mg
  Hydrocodone bitartrate 7.5 mg and acetaminophen 400 mg
  Hydrocodone bitartrate 10 mg and acetaminophen 400 mg

References

"Principles of Analgesic Use in the Treatment of Acute Pain and Cancer Pain," 6th ed, Glenview, IL: American Pain Society, 2008.

Hydrocortisone (hye droe KOR ti sone)

Medication Safety Issues

Sound-alike/look-alike issues:
Hydrocortisone may be confused with hydrocodone, hydroxychloroquine, hydrochlorothiazide
Anusol® may be confused with Anusol-HC®, Aplisol®, Aquasol®
Anusol-HC® may be confused with Anusol®
Cortef® may be confused with Coreg®, Lortab®
Cortizone® may be confused with cortisone
HCT (occasional abbreviation for hydrocortisone) is an error-prone abbreviation (mistaken as hydrochlorothiazide)
Hytone® may be confused with Vytone®
Proctocort® may be confused with ProctoCream®
ProctoCream® may be confused with Proctocort®
Solu-Cortef® may be confused with Solu-Medrol®

International issues:
Hytone® may be confused with Hysone® [Australia]
Nutracort® may be confused with Nitrocor® which is a brand name of nitroglycerin in Chile and Italy

Related Information

Allergic Reactions *on page 1508*
Corticosteroids *on page 1676*
Desensitization Protocols *on page 1692*
Latex Allergy *on page 1511*
Skin Tests *on page 1707*
Stress Replacement of Corticosteroids *on page 1611*

◀ **U.S. Brand Names** Anucort-HC®; Anusol-HC®; Anusol® HC-1 [OTC]; Aquanil™ HC [OTC]; Beta-HC®; Caldecort® [OTC]; Cetacort® [DSC]; Colocort®; Cortaid® Intensive Therapy [OTC]; Cortaid® Maximum Strength [OTC]; Cortaid® Sensitive Skin [OTC]; Cortef®; Cortenema®; Corticool® [OTC]; Cortifoam®; Cortizone-10® Maximum Strength Cooling Relief [OTC]; Cortizone-10® Maximum Strength Easy Relief [OTC]; Cortizone-10® Maximum Strength Intensive Healing Formula [OTC]; Cortizone-10® Maximum Strength [OTC]; Cortizone-10® Plus Maximum Strength [OTC]; Cortizone-10® Quick Shot [OTC] [DSC]; Dermarest® Dricort® [OTC]; Dermtex® HC [OTC]; Encort™; Hemril®-30; Hydro-Rx; HydroZone Plus [OTC]; Hytone® [DSC]; IvySoothe® [OTC]; Locoid Lipocream®; Locoid®; Nupercainal® Hydrocortisone Cream [OTC]; Nutracort®; Pandel®; Post Peel Healing Balm [OTC]; Preparation H® Hydrocortisone [OTC]; Procto-Kit™; Procto-Pak™; Proctocort®; ProctoCream® HC; Proctosert; Proctosol-HC®; Proctozone-HC™; Sarnol®-HC [OTC]; Solu-Cortef®; Summer's Eve® SpecialCare™ Medicated Anti-Itch Cream [OTC] [DSC]; Texacort®; Tucks® Anti-Itch [OTC]; Westcort®

Canadian Brand Names Aquacort®; Cortamed®; Cortef®; Cortenema®; Cortifoam™; Emo-Cort®; Hycort™; Hyderm; HydroVal®; Locoid®; Prevex® HC; Sarna® HC; Solu-Cortef®; Westcort®

Index Terms A-hydroCort; Compound F; Cortisol; Hemorrhoidal HC; Hydrocortisone Acetate; Hydrocortisone Butyrate; Hydrocortisone Probutate; Hydrocortisone Sodium Succinate; Hydrocortisone Valerate

Pharmacologic Category Corticosteroid, Rectal; Corticosteroid, Systemic; Corticosteroid, Topical

Generic Available Yes: Excludes acetate foam, butyrate cream and ointment, gel as base, otic drops as base, probutate cream, sodium succinate injection

Use Management of adrenocortical insufficiency; relief of inflammation of corticosteroid-responsive dermatoses (low and medium potency topical corticosteroid); adjunctive treatment of ulcerative colitis

Unlabeled/Investigational Use Management of septic shock when blood pressure is poorly responsive to fluid resuscitation and vasopressor therapy

Mechanism of Action Decreases inflammation by suppression of migration of polymorphonuclear leukocytes and reversal of increased capillary permeability

Pharmacodynamics/Kinetics

Onset of action:

Hydrocortisone acetate: Slow

Hydrocortisone sodium succinate (water soluble): Rapid

Duration: Hydrocortisone acetate: Long

Absorption: Rapid by all routes, except rectally

Metabolism: Hepatic

Half-life elimination: Biologic: 8-12 hours

Excretion: Urine (primarily as 17-hydroxysteroids and 17-ketosteroids)

Dosage Dose should be based on severity of disease and patient response

Adrenal hyperplasia (congenital): Children: Oral: Initial: 10-20 mg/m^2/day in 3 divided doses; a variety of dosing schedules have been used. **Note:** Inconsistencies have occurred with liquid formulations; tablets may provide more reliable levels. Doses must be individualized by monitoring growth, bone age, and hormonal levels. Mineralocorticoid and sodium supplementation may be required based upon electrolyte regulation and plasma renin activity.

Adrenal insufficiency (acute): I.M., I.V.:

Infants and young Children: Succinate: 1-2 mg/kg/dose bolus, then 25-150 mg/day in divided doses every 6-8 hours

Older Children: Succinate: 1-2 mg/kg bolus then 150-250 mg/day in divided doses every 6-8 hours

Adults: Succinate: 100 mg I.V. bolus, then 300 mg/day in divided doses every 8 hours or as a continuous infusion for 48 hours; once patient is stable change to oral, 50 mg every 8 hours for 6 doses, then taper to 30-50 mg/day in divided doses

Adrenal insufficiency (chronic): Adults: Oral: 20-30 mg/day

Anti-inflammatory or immunosuppressive:
Infants and Children:
Oral: 2.5-10 mg/kg/day **or** 75-300 mg/m^2/day every 6-8 hours
I.M., I.V.: Succinate: 1-5 mg/kg/day **or** 30-150 mg/m^2/day divided every 12-24 hours
Adolescents and Adults: Oral, I.M., I.V.: Succinate: 15-240 mg every 12 hours
Physiologic replacement: Children:
Oral: 0.5-0.75 mg/kg/day **or** 20-25 mg/m^2/day every 8 hours
I.M.: Succinate: 0.25-0.35 mg/kg/day **or** 12-15 mg/m^2/day once daily
Rheumatic diseases: Adults:
Intralesional, intra-articular, soft tissue injection: Acetate:
Large joints: 25 mg (up to 37.5 mg)
Small joints: 10-25 mg
Tendon sheaths: 5-12.5 mg
Soft tissue infiltration: 25-50 mg (up to 75 mg)
Bursae: 25-37.5 mg
Ganglia: 12.5-25 mg
Septic shock (unlabeled use): I.V.: 50 mg every 6 hours (Annane, 2002; Marik, 2008). Taper slowly (for total of 11 days) and do not stop abruptly. **Note:** Fludrocortisone is optional with use of hydrocortisone.
Shock: I.M., I.V.: Succinate:
Children: Initial: 50 mg/kg, then repeated in 4 hours and/or every 24 hours as needed
Adolescents and Adults: 500 mg to 2 g every 2-6 hours
Status asthmaticus: Children and Adults: I.V.: Succinate: 1-2 mg/kg/dose every 6 hours for 24 hours, then maintenance of 0.5-1 mg/kg every 6 hours
Stress dosing (surgery) in patients known to be adrenally-suppressed or on chronic systemic steroids: I.V.: Adults:
Minor stress (ie, inguinal herniorrhaphy): 25 mg/day for 1 day
Moderate stress (ie, joint replacement, cholecystectomy): 50-75 mg/day (25 mg every 8-12 hours) for 1-2 days
Major stress (pancreatoduodenectomy, esophagogastrectomy, cardiac surgery): 100-150 mg/day (50 mg every 8-12 hours) for 2-3 days
Dermatosis: Children >2 years and Adults: Topical: Apply to affected area 2-4 times/day (Buteprate: Apply once or twice daily). Therapy should be discontinued when control is achieved; if no improvement is seen, reassessment of diagnosis may be necessary.
Ulcerative colitis: Adults: Rectal: 10-100 mg 1-2 times/day for 2-3 weeks

Stability Store at controlled room temperature 20°C to 25°C (68°F to 77°F). Protect from light. Hydrocortisone sodium phosphate and hydrocortisone sodium succinate are clear, light yellow solutions which are heat labile.

Sodium succinate: Reconstitute 100 mg vials with bacteriostatic water (not >2 mL). Act-O-Vial (self-contained powder for injection plus diluent) may be reconstituted by pressing the activator to force diluent into the powder compartment. Following gentle agitation, solution may be withdrawn via syringe through a needle inserted into the center of the stopper. May be administered (I.V. or I.M.) without further dilution. After initial reconstitution, hydrocortisone sodium succinate solutions are stable for 3 days at room temperature or under refrigeration when protected from light. Stability of parenteral admixture (Solu-Cortef®) at room temperature (25°C) and at refrigeration temperature (4°C) is concentration-dependent:
Stability of concentration 1 mg/mL: 24 hours.
Stability of concentration 2 mg/mL to 60 mg/mL: At least 4 hours.
Solutions for I.V. infusion: Reconstituted solutions may be added to an appropriate volume of compatible solution for infusion. Concentration should generally not exceed 1 mg/mL. However, in cases where administration of a small volume of fluid is desirable, 100-3000 mg may be added to 50 mL of D$_5$W or NS (stability limited to 4 hours).

Administration
Oral: Administer with food or milk to decrease GI upset
Parenteral: Hydrocortisone sodium succinate may be administered by I.M. or I.V. routes

◄   I.V. bolus: Dilute to 50 mg/mL and administer over 30 seconds or over 10 minutes for doses ≥500 mg

I.V. intermittent infusion: Dilute to 1 mg/mL and administer over 20-30 minutes

Topical: Apply a thin film to clean, dry skin and rub in gently

Monitoring Parameters Blood pressure, weight, serum glucose, and electrolytes

Reference Range Therapeutic: AM: 5-25 mcg/dL (SI: 138-690 nmol/L), PM: 2-9 mcg/dL (SI: 55-248 nmol/L) depending on test, assay

Anesthesia and Critical Care Concerns/Other Considerations

Clinical Pearls/Comments: Hydrocortisone is a long-acting corticosteroid with minimal sodium-retaining potential.

Evidence-Based Information:

Neuromuscular Effects: ICU-acquired paresis was recently studied in 5 ICUs (3 medical and 2 surgical ICUs) at 4 French hospitals. All ICU patients without pre-existing neuromuscular disease admitted from March 1999 through June 2000 were evaluated (De Jonghe, 2002). Each patient had to be mechanically ventilated for ≥7 days and was screened daily for awakening. The first day the patient was considered awake was Study Day 1. Patients with severe muscle weakness on Study Day 7 were considered to have ICU-acquired paresis. Among the 95 patients who were evaluated, about 25% developed ICU-acquired paresis. Independent predictors included: female gender, the number of days with ≥2 organ dysfunction, and administration of corticosteroids. Further studies may be required to verify and characterize the association between the development of ICU-acquired paresis and use of corticosteroids. Concurrent use of a corticosteroid and muscle relaxant appears to increase the risk of certain ICU myopathies; avoid or administer the corticosteroid at the lowest dose possible.

Adrenal Insufficiency: Patients will often have steroid-induced adverse effects on glucose tolerance and lipid profiles. When discontinuing steroid therapy in patients on long-term steroid supplementation, it is important that the steroid therapy be discontinued gradually. Abrupt withdrawal may result in adrenal insufficiency with hypotension and hyperkalemia. Patients on long-term steroid supplementation will require higher corticosteroid doses when subject to stress (eg, trauma, surgery, severe infection). Guidelines for glucocorticoid replacement during various surgical procedures have been published (Coursin, 2002; Salem, 1994).

Septic Shock: Annane, et al (2002) randomized 300 septic shock patients to either hydrocortisone (50 mg I.V. push every 6 hours) and fludrocortisone (50 mcg tablet daily via nasogastric tube) or matching placebos for 7 days. The mean Simplified Acute Physiology Score II (SAPS II) was 57 ± 19 in the placebo group and 60 ± 19 in the active treatment group. The Logistic Organ Dysfunction score was 9 ± 3 in the placebo group and 9 ± 3 in the active treatment group. In patients who did not appropriately respond to corticotropin (nonresponders), there were significantly fewer deaths in the active treatment group. Vasopressor therapy was withdrawn more frequently in this subset of the active treatment group. Adverse events were similar in both groups.

In the CORTICUS trial (Sprung, 2008), 484 septic shock patients were randomized within 72 hours of onset to receive either hydrocortisone (50 mg I.V. push every 6 hours) or placebo for 5 days followed by a 6-day taper. The primary endpoint was 28 day mortality in patients who did not respond to corticotropin. The SAPS II score in the treatment group was 49.5 ± 17.8 and 48.6 ± 16.7 in the placebo group. The Sequential Organ Failure Assessment scores were 10.6 ± 3.4 in the treatment group and 10.6 ± 3.2 in the placebo group. Different than the Annane study, in the patients who did not respond to corticotropin, there was no mortality difference at 28 days; 39.2% (95% CI: 30.5-47.9) mortality in the hydrocortisone group and 36.1 % (95% CI: 26.9-45.3, P=0.69) mortality in the placebo group. A trend towards increased incidence of superinfection was noted in hydrocortisone patients. New septic shock episodes, hyperglycemia, and hypernatremia were more frequent in the hydrocortisone group. Hydrocortisone did not improve survival in this population of septic shock patients regardless of corticotropin response.

The 2008 Surviving Sepsis Campaign Guidelines suggest the following: Intravenous hydrocortisone be given only to adult septic shock patients after blood pressure is identified to be poorly responsive to fluid resuscitation and vasopressor therapy (Grade 2C); ACTH stimulation test not be used to identify the subset of adults with septic shock who should receive hydrocortisone (Grade 2B); patients with septic shock should not receive dexamethasone if hydrocortisone is available (Grade 2B); the addition of fludrocortisone if hydrocortisone is not available and the steroid that is substituted does not have significant mineralocorticoid activity (Grade 2C); doses of corticosteroids comparable to >300 mg hydrocortisone daily not be used in severe sepsis or septic shock for the purpose of treating septic shock (Grade 1A). They also recommend corticosteroids not be administered for the treatment of sepsis in the absence of shock. There is, however, no contraindication to continuing maintenance steroid therapy or to using stress dose steroids if the patient's endocrine or corticosteroid administration history warrants (Grade 1D).

The 2008 Recommendations for the diagnosis and management of corticosteroid insufficiency in critically ill adult patients suggest a diagnosis of critical illness related corticosteroid insufficiency can be made by a delta cortisol level (after 250 mcg cosyntropin) of <9 mcg/dL or a random cortisol <10 mcg/dL (Grade 2B). However, they recommend **against** the use of ACTH stimulation test to determine if septic shock or ARDS patients should receive steroid therapy (Grade 2B). They recommend to consider using hydrocortisone in septic shock patients who have responded poorly to resuscitation and vasopressors (Grade 2B) and glucocorticoid treatment should be tapered slowly and not stopped abruptly (Grade 2B). Dexamethasone is **not** recommended for the treatment of septic shock or ARDS (Grade 1B). Fludrocortisone therapy is considered optional (Grade 2B).

Pregnancy Risk Factor C

Contraindications Hypersensitivity to hydrocortisone or any component of the formulation; serious infections, except septic shock or tuberculous meningitis; viral, fungal, or tubercular skin lesions; I.M. administration contraindicated in idiopathic thrombocytopenia purpura

Rectal suspension: Systemic fungal infections; ileocolostomy during the immediate or early postoperative period

Warnings/Precautions Use with caution in patients with thyroid disease, hepatic impairment, renal impairment, heart failure, hypertension, diabetes, glaucoma, cataracts, myasthenia gravis, patients at risk for osteoporosis, patients at risk for seizures, or GI diseases (diverticulitis, peptic ulcer, ulcerative colitis) due to perforation risk. Use caution following acute MI (corticosteroids have been associated with myocardial rupture). Because of the risk of adverse effects, systemic corticosteroids should be used cautiously in the elderly in the smallest possible effective dose for the shortest duration. May affect growth velocity; growth should be routinely monitored in pediatric patients. Withdraw therapy with gradual tapering of dose.

May cause hypercorticism or suppression of hypothalamic-pituitary-adrenal (HPA) axis, particularly in younger children or in patients receiving high doses for prolonged periods. HPA axis suppression may lead to adrenal crisis. Withdrawal and discontinuation of a corticosteroid should be done slowly and carefully. Particular care is required when patients are transferred from systemic corticosteroids to inhaled products due to possible adrenal insufficiency or withdrawal from steroids, including an increase in allergic symptoms. Patients receiving >20 mg per day of prednisone (or equivalent) may be most susceptible. Fatalities have occurred due to adrenal insufficiency in asthmatic patients during and after transfer from systemic corticosteroids to aerosol steroids; aerosol steroids do not provide the systemic steroid needed to treat patients having trauma, surgery, or infections. Avoid use of topical preparations with occlusive dressings or on weeping or exudative lesions. Some dosage forms may contain benzyl alcohol which has been associated with "gasping syndrome" in neonates.

Acute myopathy has been reported with high dose corticosteroids, usually in patients with neuromuscular transmission disorders; may involve ocular and/or respiratory muscles; monitor creatine kinase; recovery may be delayed. Corticosteroid use may cause psychiatric disturbances, including depression, euphoria, insomnia, mood swings, and personality changes. Pre-existing

◀ psychiatric conditions may be exacerbated by corticosteroid use. Prolonged use of corticosteroids may also increase the incidence of secondary infection, mask acute infection (including fungal infections), prolong or exacerbate viral infections, or limit response to vaccines. Exposure to chickenpox should be avoided; corticosteroids should not be used to treat ocular herpes simplex. Corticosteroids should not be used for cerebral malaria or viral hepatitis. Close observation is required in patients with latent tuberculosis and/or TB reactivity; restrict use in active TB (only in conjunction with antituberculosis treatment). Prolonged treatment with corticosteroids has been associated with the development of Kaposi's sarcoma (case reports); if noted, discontinuation of therapy should be considered. High-dose corticosteroids should not be used to manage acute head injury.

Adverse Reactions

Systemic: Frequency not defined:

Cardiovascular: Edema, hypertension

Central nervous system: Delirium, euphoria, hallucinations, headache, insomnia, nervousness, pseudotumor cerebri, psychoses, seizure, vertigo

Dermatologic: Bruising, hyperpigmentation, skin atrophy

Endocrine & metabolic: Adrenal suppression, alkalosis, amenorrhea, Cushing's syndrome, diabetes mellitus, glucose intolerance, growth suppression, hyperglycemia, hyperlipidemia, hypokalemia, pituitary-adrenal axis suppression, sodium and water retention

Gastrointestinal: Abdominal distention, appetite increased, indigestion, nausea, pancreatitis, peptic ulcer, ulcerative esophagitis, vomiting

Hematologic: Leukocytosis (transient)

Neuromuscular & skeletal: Arthralgia, fractures, muscle weakness, osteoporosis

Ocular: Cataracts, glaucoma

Miscellaneous: Avascular necrosis, hypersensitivity reactions, infection, secondary malignancy

Topical:

>10%: Dermatologic: Eczema (12.5%)

1% to 10%: Dermatologic: Pruritus (6%), stinging (2%), dry skin (2%)

<1% (Limited to important or life-threatening): Allergic contact dermatitis, burning, dermal atrophy, folliculitis, HPA axis suppression, hypopigmentation; metabolic effects (hyperglycemia, hypokalemia); striae

Drug Interactions

Metabolism/Transport Effects Substrate of CYP3A4 (minor); **Induces** CYP3A4 (weak)

Avoid Concomitant Use

Avoid concomitant use of Hydrocortisone with any of the following: Natalizumab; Vaccines (Live)

Increased Effect/Toxicity

Hydrocortisone may increase the levels/effects of: Acetylcholinesterase Inhibitors; Amphotericin B; CycloSPORINE; Leflunomide; Loop Diuretics; Natalizumab; NSAID (COX-2 Inhibitor); NSAID (Nonselective); Thiazide Diuretics; Vaccines (Live); Warfarin

The levels/effects of Hydrocortisone may be increased by: Antifungal Agents (Azole Derivatives, Systemic); Aprepitant; Calcium Channel Blockers (Nondihydropyridine); CycloSPORINE; Estrogen Derivatives; Fluconazole; Fosaprepitant; Macrolide Antibiotics; Neuromuscular-Blocking Agents (Nondepolarizing); P-Glycoprotein Inhibitors; Quinolone Antibiotics; Salicylates; Trastuzumab

Decreased Effect

Hydrocortisone may decrease the levels/effects of: Antidiabetic Agents; Calcitriol; Corticorelin; Isoniazid; Salicylates; Vaccines (Inactivated); Vaccines (Live)

The levels/effects of Hydrocortisone may be decreased by: Aminoglutethimide; Antacids; Barbiturates; Bile Acid Sequestrants; Echinacea; Mitotane; P-Glycoprotein Inducers; Primidone; Rifamycin Derivatives

Ethanol/Nutrition/Herb Interactions

Ethanol: Avoid ethanol (may enhance gastric mucosal irritation).

Food: Hydrocortisone interferes with calcium absorption.

Herb/Nutraceutical: St John's wort may decrease hydrocortisone levels. Avoid cat's claw, echinacea (have immunostimulant properties).

Dietary Considerations Systemic use of corticosteroids may require a diet with increased potassium, vitamins A, B$_6$, C, D, folate, calcium, zinc, phosphorus, and decreased sodium. Sodium content of 1 g (sodium succinate injection): 47.5 mg (2.07 mEq)

Dosage Forms Excipient information presented when available (limited, particularly for generics); consult specific product labeling. [DSC] = Discontinued product

Aerosol, rectal, as acetate:

Cortifoam®: 10% (15 g) [90 mg/applicator]

Cream, rectal, as acetate:

Nupercainal® Hydrocortisone Cream: 1% (30 g) [strength expressed as base]

Cream, topical, as acetate: 0.5% (9 g, 30 g, 60 g) [available with aloe]; 1% (30 g, 454 g) [available with aloe]

Cream, topical, as base: 0.5% (30 g); 1% (1.5 g, 30 g, 114 g, 454 g); 2.5% (20 g, 30 g, 454 g)

Anusol-HC®: 2.5% (30 g) [contains benzyl alcohol]

Caldecort®: 1% (30 g) [contains aloe vera gel]

Cortaid® Intensive Therapy: 1% (60 g)

Cortaid® Maximum Strength: 1% (15 g, 30 g, 40 g, 60 g) [contains aloe vera gel and benzyl alcohol]

Cortaid® Sensitive Skin: 0.5% (15 g) [contains aloe vera gel]

Cortizone-10® Maximum Strength: 1% (15 g, 30 g, 60 g) [contains aloe]

Cortizone-10® Maximum Strength Intensive Healing Formula: 1% (28 g, 56 g) [contains aloe, benzyl alcohol]

Cortizone-10® Plus Maximum Strength: 1% (30 g, 60 g) [contains vitamins A, D, E and aloe]

Dermarest® Dricort®: 1% (15 g, 30 g)

HydroZone Plus, Proctocort®, Procto-Pak™: 1% (30 g)

Hytone®: 1% (30 g), 2.5% (30 g, 60 g) [DSC]

IvySoothe®: 1% (30 g) [contains aloe]

Post Peel Healing Balm: 1% (23 g)

Preparation H® Hydrocortisone: 1% (27 g) [contains sodium benzoate]

ProctoCream® HC: 2.5% (30 g) [contains benzyl alcohol]

Procto-Kit™: 1% (30 g) [packaged with applicator tips and finger cots]; 2.5% (30 g) [packaged with applicator tips and finger cots]

Proctosol-HC®, Proctozone-HC™: 2.5% (30 g)

Summer's Eve® SpecialCare™ Medicated Anti-Itch Cream: 1% (30 g) [DSC]

Cream, topical, as butyrate:

Locoid®: 0.1% (15 g, 45 g)

Locoid Lipocream®: 0.1% (15 g, 45 g)

Cream, topical, as probutate:

Pandel®: 0.1% (15 g, 45 g, 80 g)

Cream, topical, as valerate: 0.2% (15 g, 45 g, 60 g)

Westcort®: 0.2% (15 g, 45 g, 60 g)

Gel, topical, as base:

Corticool®: 1% (45 g)

Cortizone-10® Maximum Strength Cooling Relief: 1% (28 g) [contains aloe, ethanol 15%]

Injection, powder for reconstitution, as sodium succinate:

A-Hydrocort®: 100 mg [contains monobasic sodium phosphate 0.8 mg, anhydrous dibasic sodium phosphate 8.73 mg; strength expressed as base]

Solu-Cortef®: 100 mg, 250 mg, 500 mg, 1 g [diluent contains benzyl alcohol; strength expressed as base]

Lotion, topical, as base [spray]:

Cortizone-10® Maximum Strength Easy Relief: 1% (36 mL) [contains aloe, ethanol 45%]

Lotion, topical, as base: 1% (120 mL); 2.5% (60 mL)

Aquanil™ HC: 1% (120 mL)

Beta-HC®

Cetacort® [DSC]

HydroZone Plus: 1% (120 mL)

Hytone®: 2.5% (60 mL) [DSC]

◀ Nutracort®: 1% (60 mL, 120 mL); 2.5% (60 mL, 120 mL)
Sarnol®-HC: 1% (60 mL)
Lotion, topical, as butyrate:
  Locoid®: 0.1% (60 mL)
Ointment, topical, as acetate: 1% (30 g) [strength expressed as base; available with aloe]
  Anusol® HC-1: 1% (21 g) [strength expressed as base]
  Cortaid® Maximum Strength: 1% (15 g, 30 g) [strength expressed as base]
Ointment, topical, as base: 0.5% (30 g); 1% (30 g, 454 g); 2.5% (20 g, 30 g, 454 g)
  Cortizone-10® Maximum Strength: 1% (30 g, 60 g)
  Hytone®: 2.5% (30 g) [DSC]
Ointment, topical, as butyrate:
  Locoid®: 0.1% (15 g, 45 g)
Ointment, topical, as valerate: 0.2% (15 g, 45 g, 60 g)
  Westcort®: 0.2% (15 g, 45 g, 60 g)
Powder, for prescription compounding [micronized]:
  Hydro-Rx: USP (10 g, 25 g, 50 g, 100 g)
Powder, for prescription compounding, as acetate [micronized]: USP (10 g, 25 g, 50 g)
Solution, topical, as base: 2.5% (30 mL)
  Texacort®: 2.5% (30 mL) [contains ethanol 48%]
Solution, topical, as butyrate: 0.1% (20 mL, 60 mL)
  Locoid®: 0.1% (20 mL, 60 mL) [contains alcohol 50%]
Solution, topical, as base [spray]:
  Cortaid® Intensive Therapy: 1% (60 mL) [contains alcohol]
  Cortizone-10® Quick Shot: 1% (44 mL) [contains benzyl alcohol] [DSC]
  Dermtex® HC: 1% (52 mL) [contains menthol 1%]
Suppository, rectal, as acetate: 25 mg (12s [DSC]; 24s, 100s)
  Anucort-HC®, Tucks® Anti-Itch: 25 mg (12s, 24s, 100s) [strength expressed as base; Anucort-HC® renamed Tucks® Anti-Itch]
  Anusol-HC®, Proctosol-HC®: 25 mg (12s, 24s)
  Encort™, Proctocort®: 30 mg (12s)
  Hemril®-30, Proctosert: 30 mg (12s, 24s)
Suspension, rectal, as base: 100 mg/60 mL (1s, 7s)
  Colocort®, Cortenema®: 100 mg/60 mL (1s, 7s)
Tablet, as base: 20 mg
  Cortef®: 5 mg, 10 mg, 20 mg

References

Abraham E and Evans T, "Corticosteroids and Septic Shock (editorial)," *JAMA*, 2002, 288(7):886-7.

Annane D, Sebille V, Charpentier C, et al, "Effect of Treatment With Low Doses of Hydrocortisone and Fludrocortisone on Mortality in Patients With Septic Shock," *JAMA*, 2002, 288(7):862-71.

Cooper MS and Stewart PM, "Corticosteroid Insufficiency in Acutely Ill Patients," *N Engl J Med*, 2003, 348(8):727-34.

Coursin DB and Wood KE, "Corticosteroid Supplementation for Adrenal Insufficiency," *JAMA*, 2002, 287(2):236-40.

de Jonghe B, Sharshar T, Lefaucheur JP, et al, "Paresis Acquired in the Intensive Care Unit. A Prospective Multicenter Study," *JAMA*, 2002, 288(22):2859-67.

Dellinger RP, Levy MM, Carlet JM, et al, "Surviving Sepsis Campaign: International Guidelines for Management of Severe Sepsis and Septic Shock: 2008," *Intensive Care Med*, 2008, 34(1): 17-60. Available at http://www.survivingsepsis.org/system/files/images/2008_20International_20SSC_20-Guidelines_1_.pdf

Hotchkiss RS and Karl IE, "The Pathophysiology and Treatment of Sepsis," *N Engl J Med*, 2003, 348 (2):138-50.

Marik PE, Pastores SM, Annane D, et al, "Recommendations for the Diagnosis and Management of Corticosteroid Insufficiency in Critically Ill Adult Patients: Consensus Statements From an International Task Force by the American College of Critical Care Medicine," *Crit Care Med*, 2008, 36(6):1937-49.

Salem M, Tainsh RE, Jr, Bromberg J, et al, "Perioperative Glucocorticoid Coverage: A Reassessment 42 Years After Emergence of a Problem," *Ann Surg*, 1994, 219(4):416-25.

Sprung CL, Annane D, Keh D, et al, "Hydrocortisone Therapy for Patients With Septic Shock," *N Engl J Med*, 2008, 358(2):111-24.

◆ **Hydrocortisone Acetate** *see* Hydrocortisone *on page 699*
◆ **Hydrocortisone Butyrate** *see* Hydrocortisone *on page 699*
◆ **Hydrocortisone Probutate** *see* Hydrocortisone *on page 699*
◆ **Hydrocortisone Sodium Succinate** *see* Hydrocortisone *on page 699*
◆ **Hydrocortisone Valerate** *see* Hydrocortisone *on page 699*

◆ **Hydrodiuril** *see* Hydrochlorothiazide *on page 696*

◆ **Hydromorph Contin® (Can)** *see* HYDROmorphone *on page 707*

◆ **Hydromorph-IR® (Can)** *see* HYDROmorphone *on page 707*

HYDROmorphone (hye droe MOR fone)

Medication Safety Issues
Sound-alike/look-alike issues:

Dilaudid® may be confused with Demerol®, Dilantin®

HYDROmorphone may be confused with morphine; significant overdoses have occurred when hydromorphone products have been inadvertently administered instead of morphine sulfate. Commercially available prefilled syringes of both products looks similar and are often stored in close proximity to each other. **Note:** Hydromorphone 1 mg oral is approximately equal to morphine 4 mg oral; hydromorphone 1 mg I.V. is approximately equal to morphine 5 mg I.V.

High alert medication: The Institute for Safe Medication Practices (ISMP) includes this medication among its list of drug classes which have a heightened risk of causing significant patient harm when used in error.

Dilaudid®, Dilaudid-HP®: Extreme caution should be taken to avoid confusing the highly-concentrated (Dilaudid-HP®) injection with the less-concentrated (Dilaudid®) injectable product.

Significant differences exist between oral and I.V. dosing. Use caution when converting from one route of administration to another.

Related Information
Acute Postoperative Pain *on page 1502*
Anesthesia Considerations for Neurosurgery *on page 1514*
Anesthesia for Patients With Liver Disease *on page 1537*
Chronic Pain Management *on page 1546*
Opioid Analgesics *on page 1688*
Opioids *on page 1641*

U.S. Brand Names Dilaudid-HP®; Dilaudid®

Canadian Brand Names Dilaudid-HP-Plus®; Dilaudid-HP®; Dilaudid-XP®; Dilaudid®; Dilaudid® Sterile Powder; Hydromorph Contin®; Hydromorph-IR®; Hydromorphone HP; Hydromorphone HP® 10; Hydromorphone HP® 20; Hydromorphone HP® 50; Hydromorphone HP® Forte; Hydromorphone Hydrochloride Injection, USP; PMS-Hydromorphone

Index Terms Dihydromorphinone; Hydromorphone Hydrochloride

Pharmacologic Category Analgesic, Opioid

Restrictions C-II

Generic Available Yes: Excludes capsule, liquid, powder for injection

Use Management of moderate-to-severe pain

Unlabeled/Investigational Use Antitussive

Mechanism of Action Binds to opiate receptors in the CNS, causing inhibition of ascending pain pathways, altering the perception of and response to pain; causes cough supression by direct central action in the medulla; produces generalized CNS depression

Pharmacodynamics/Kinetics
Onset of action: Analgesic: Immediate release formulations:
Oral: 15-30 minutes; Peak effect: 30-60 minutes
I.V.: 5 minutes; Peak effect: 10-20 minutes
Duration: Immediate release formulations: Oral, I.V.: 4-5 hours
Absorption: I.M.: Variable and delayed
Distribution: V_d: 4 L/kg
Protein binding: ~8% to 19%
Metabolism: Hepatic via glucuronidation; to inactive metabolites
Bioavailability: 62%
Half-life elimination: Immediate release formulations: 1-3 hours
Excretion: Urine (primarily as glucuronide conjugates)

◄ **Dosage**

Acute pain (moderate-to-severe): **Note:** These are guidelines and do not represent the maximum doses that may be required in all patients. Doses should be titrated to pain relief/prevention.

Children ≥6 months and <50 kg:

Oral: 0.03-0.08 mg/kg/dose every 3-4 hours as needed. **Note:** The American Pain Society recommends an initial dose of 0.06 mg/kg for severe pain in children.

I.V.: 0.015 mg/kg/dose every 3-6 hours as needed

Patient-controlled analgesia (PCA) (American Pain Society, 2008): **Note:** Opiate-naive: Consider lower end of dosing range:

Usual concentration: 0.2 mg/mL

Demand dose: Usual: 0.003-0.004 mg/kg/dose; range: 0.003-0.005 mg/kg/dose

Lockout interval: 6-10 minutes

Usual basal rate: 0-0.004 mg/kg/hour

Children >50 kg and Adults:

Oral: Initial: Opiate-naive: 2-4 mg every 3-6 hours as needed; elderly/debilitated patients may require lower doses; patients with prior opiate exposure may require higher initial doses; usual dosage range: 2-8 mg every 3-4 hours as needed. **Note:** The American Pain Society recommends an initial dose of 4-8 mg for severe pain in adults.

I.V.: Initial: Opiate-naive: 0.2-0.6 mg every 2-3 hours as needed; patients with prior opiate exposure may tolerate higher initial doses

Critically-ill patients (unlabeled dose): 0.7-2 mg (based on 70 kg patient) every 1-2 hours as needed. **Note:** More frequent dosing may be needed (eg, mechanically-ventilated patients).

Continuous infusion: Usual dosage range: 0.5-1 mg/hour (based on 70 kg patient) or 7-15 mcg/kg/hour

Patient-controlled analgesia (PCA): **Note:** Opiate-naive: Consider lower end of dosing range:

Usual concentration: 0.2 mg/mL

Demand dose: Usual: 0.1-0.2 mg; range: 0.05-0.4 mg

Lockout interval: 5-10 minutes

Epidural:

Bolus dose: 1-1.5 mg

Infusion concentration: 0.05-0.075 mg/mL

Infusion rate: 0.04-0.4 mg/hour

Demand dose: 0.15 mg

Lockout interval: 30 minutes

I.M., SubQ: **Note:** I.M. use may result in variable absorption and a lag time to peak effect.

Initial: Opiate-naive: 0.8-1 mg every 4-6 hours as needed; patients with prior opiate exposure may require higher initial doses; usual dosage range: 1-2 mg every 3-6 hours as needed

Rectal: 3 mg every 4-8 hours as needed

Chronic pain: Adults: Oral: **Note:** Patients taking opioids chronically may become tolerant and require doses higher than the usual dosage range to maintain the desired effect. Tolerance can be managed by appropriate dose titration. There is no optimal or maximal dose for hydromorphone in chronic pain. The appropriate dose is one that relieves pain throughout its dosing interval without causing unmanageable side effects.

Controlled release formulation (Hydromorph Contin®, not available in U.S.): 3-30 mg every 12 hours. **Note:** A patient's hydromorphone requirement should be established using prompt release formulations; conversion to long acting products may be considered when chronic, continuous treatment is required. Higher dosages should be reserved for use only in opioid-tolerant patients.

Antitussive (unlabeled use): Oral:

Children 6-12 years: 0.5 mg every 3-4 hours as needed

Children >12 years and Adults: 1 mg every 3-4 hours as needed

Dosing adjustment in hepatic impairment: Should be considered

Stability Store injection and oral dosage forms at 15°C to 30°C (59°F to 86°F). Protect tablets from light. A slightly yellowish discoloration has not been associated with a loss of potency.

Administration

Parenteral: May be given SubQ or I.M.; vial stopper contains latex

I.V.: For IVP, must be given slowly over 2-3 minutes (rapid IVP has been associated with an increase in side effects, especially respiratory depression and hypotension)

Oral: Hydromorph Contin®: Capsule should be swallowed whole; do not crush or chew; contents may be sprinkled on soft food and swallowed

Monitoring Parameters Pain relief, respiratory and mental status, blood pressure

Anesthesia and Critical Care Concerns/Other Considerations

Clinical Pearls/Comments: Hydromorphone does not have any active metabolites, has less protein binding than other opoids, and does not cause histamine release. If the patient has required high-dose analgesia or has used for a prolonged period (~7 days), taper dose to prevent withdrawal.

Evidence-Based Information: The 2002 ACCM/SCCM guidelines for analgesia (critically-ill adult) recommend fentanyl or hydromorphone in patients who are hypotensive or have renal dysfunction. Morphine or hydromorphone is recommended for intermittent, scheduled therapy. Both have a longer duration of action requiring less frequent administration.

Pregnancy Risk Factor C/D (prolonged use or high doses at term)

Contraindications Hypersensitivity to hydromorphone, any component of the formulation; acute or severe asthma, severe respiratory depression (in absence of resuscitative equipment or ventilatory support); severe CNS depression; pregnancy (prolonged use or high doses at term); obstetrical analgesia

Warnings/Precautions Use with caution in patients with hypersensitivity reactions to other phenanthrene derivative opioid agonists (codeine, hydrocodone, levorphanol, oxycodone, oxymorphone). Hydromorphone shares toxic potential of opiate agonists, including CNS depression and respiratory depression. Precautions associated with opiate agonist therapy should be observed. May cause CNS depression, which may impair physical or mental abilities; patients must be cautioned about performing tasks which require mental alertness (eg, operating machinery or driving). Myoclonus and seizures have been reported with high doses. Critical respiratory depression may occur, even at therapeutic dosages, particularly in elderly or debilitated patients or in patients with pre-existing respiratory compromise (hypoxia and/or hypercapnia). Use caution in COPD or other obstructive pulmonary disease. Use with caution in patients with hypersensitivity to other phenanthrene opiates, kyphoscoliosis, biliary tract disease, acute pancreatitis, morbid obesity, adrenocortical insufficiency, hypothyroidism, acute alcoholism, toxic psychoses, prostatic hyperplasia and/or urinary stricture, or severe liver or renal failure. Use extreme caution in patients with head injury, intracranial lesions, or elevated intracranial pressure; exaggerated elevation of ICP may occur (in addition, hydromorphone may complicate neurologic evaluation due to pupillary dilation and CNS depressant effects). Use with caution in patients with depleted blood volume or drugs which may exaggerate hypotensive effects (including phenothiazines or general anesthetics). May obscure diagnosis or clinical course of patients with acute abdominal conditions.

[U.S. Boxed Warning]: Hydromorphone has a high potential for abuse. Those at risk for opioid abuse include patients with a history of substance abuse or mental illness. Tolerance or drug dependence may result from extended use; however, concerns for abuse should not prevent effective management of pain. In general, abrupt discontinuation of therapy in dependent patients should be avoided.

An opioid-containing analgesic regimen should be tailored to each patient's needs and based upon the type of pain being treated (acute versus chronic), the route of administration, degree of tolerance for opioids (naive versus chronic user), age, weight, and medical condition. The optimal analgesic dose varies widely among patients. Doses should be titrated to pain relief/prevention. I.M. use may result in variable absorption and a lag time to peak effect.

Dosage form specific warnings:

[U.S. Boxed Warning]: Dilaudid-HP®: Extreme caution should be taken to avoid confusing the highly-concentrated (Dilaudid-HP®) injection with the less-concentrated (Dilaudid®) injectable product. Dilaudid-HP® should only be used in patients who are opioid-tolerant.

Controlled release: Capsules should only be used when continuous analgesia is required over an extended period of time. Controlled release products are not to be used on an "as needed" (PRN) basis.

Some dosage forms contain trace amounts of sodium metabisulfite which may cause allergic reactions in susceptible individuals.

Adverse Reactions Frequency not defined.

Cardiovascular: Bradycardia, flushing of face, hyper-/hypotension, palpitation, peripheral vasodilation, syncope, tachycardia

Central nervous system: Agitation, chills, CNS depression, dizziness, drowsiness, dysphoria, euphoria, fatigue, hallucinations, headache, increased intracranial pressure, insomnia, lightheadedness, mental depression, nervousness, restlessness, sedation, seizure

Dermatologic: Pruritus, rash, urticaria

Endocrine & metabolic: Antidiuretic hormone release

Gastrointestinal: Anorexia, biliary tract spasm, constipation, diarrhea, nausea, paralytic ileus, stomach cramps, taste perversion, vomiting, xerostomia

Genitourinary: Ureteral spasm, urinary retention, urinary tract spasm, urination decreased

Hepatic: LFTs increased

Local: Pain at injection site (I.M.), wheal/flare over vein (I.V.)

Neuromuscular & skeletal: Myoclonus, paresthesia, trembling, tremor, weakness

Ocular: Blurred vision, diplopia, miosis, nystagmus

Respiratory: Apnea, bronchospasm, dyspnea, laryngospasm, respiratory depression

Miscellaneous: Diaphoresis, histamine release, physical and psychological dependence

Drug Interactions

Avoid Concomitant Use There are no known interactions where it is recommended to avoid concomitant use.

Increased Effect/Toxicity

HYDROmorphone may increase the levels/effects of: Alcohol (Ethyl); Alvimopan; CNS Depressants; Desmopressin; Selective Serotonin Reuptake Inhibitors; Thiazide Diuretics

The levels/effects of HYDROmorphone may be increased by: Amphetamines; Antipsychotic Agents (Phenothiazines); Succinylcholine

Decreased Effect

HYDROmorphone may decrease the levels/effects of: Pegvisomant

The levels/effects of HYDROmorphone may be decreased by: Ammonium Chloride

Ethanol/Nutrition/Herb Interactions

Ethanol: Avoid ethanol (may increase CNS depression).

Herb/Nutraceutical: Avoid valerian, St John's wort, kava kava, gotu kola (may increase CNS depression).

Test Interactions Some quinolones may produce a false-positive urine screening result for opiates using commercially-available immunoassay kits. This has been demonstrated most consistently for levofloxacin and ofloxacin, but other quinolones have shown cross-reactivity in certain assay kits. Confirmation of positive opiate screens by more specific methods should be considered.

Dosage Forms Excipient information presented when available (limited, particularly for generics); consult specific product labeling. [DSC] = Discontinued product; [CAN] = Canadian brand name

Capsule, controlled release:

Hydromorph Contin® [CAN]: 3 mg, 6 mg, 12 mg, 18 mg, 24 mg, 30 mg [not available in U.S.]

Injection, powder for reconstitution, as hydrochloride:

Dilaudid-HP®: 250 mg [contains sodium metabisulfite]

Injection, solution, as hydrochloride: 1 mg/mL (1 mL); 2 mg/mL (1 mL, 20 mL); 4 mg/mL (1 mL)

Dilaudid®: 1 mg/mL (1 mL); 2 mg/mL (1 mL; 20 mL [DSC]) [20 mL size contains edetate sodium; natural rubber/natural latex in packaging]; 4 mg/mL (1 mL) [contains sodium metabisulfite]

Dilaudid-HP®: 10 mg/mL (1 mL, 5 mL) [contains sodium metabisulfite]

Dilaudid-HP®: 10 mg/mL (50 mL) [contains sodium metabisulfite; natural rubber/natural latex in packaging]

Injection, solution, as hydrochloride [preservative free]: 10 mg/mL (1 mL, 5 mL, 50 mL)

Liquid, oral, as hydrochloride:

Dilaudid®: 1 mg/mL (480 mL) [contains sodium metabisulfite (may have trace amounts)]

Powder, for prescription compounding: 100% (15 grain)

Suppository, rectal, as hydrochloride: 3 mg

Dilaudid®: 3 mg (6s) [DSC]

Tablet, as hydrochloride: 2 mg, 4 mg, 8 mg

Dilaudid®: 2 mg, 4 mg, 8 mg [contains sodium metabisulfite (may have trace amounts)]

References

Agency for Health Care Policy and Research, "Acute Pain Management in Infants, Children and Adolescents: Operative and Medical Procedures," *Am Fam Physician*, 1992, 46(2):469-79.

"Clinical Practice Guidelines for the Sustained Use of Sedatives and Analgesics in the Critically Ill Adult. Task Force of the American College of Critical Care Medicine (ACCM) of the Society of Critical Care Medicine (SCCM), American Society of Health-System Pharmacists (ASHP), American College of Chest Physicians," *Am J Health Syst Pharm*, 2002, 59(2):150-78.

Jacobi J, Fraser GL, Coursin DB, et al, "Clinical Practice Guidelines for the Sustained Use of Sedatives and Analgesics in the Critically Ill Adult," *Crit Care Med*, 2002, 30(1):119-41. Available at: http://www.sccm.org/pdf/sedatives.pdf.

Levy MH, "Pharmacologic Treatment of Cancer Pain," *N Engl J Med*, 1996, 335(15):1124-32.

Mokhlesi B, Leikin JB, Murray P, et al, "Adult Toxicology in Critical Care. Part II: Specific Poisonings," *Chest*, 2003, 123(3):897-922.

Nasraway SA, "Use of Sedative Medications in the Intensive Care Unit," *Sem Resp Crit Care Med*, 2001, 22(2):165-74.

"Principles of Analgesic Use in the Treatment of Acute Pain and Cancer Pain," 6th ed, Glenview, IL: American Pain Society, 2008.

◆ **Hydromorphone HP (Can)** *see* HYDROmorphone *on page* 707

◆ **Hydromorphone HP® 10 (Can)** *see* HYDROmorphone *on page* 707

◆ **Hydromorphone HP® 20 (Can)** *see* HYDROmorphone *on page* 707

◆ **Hydromorphone HP® 50 (Can)** *see* HYDROmorphone *on page* 707

◆ **Hydromorphone HP® Forte (Can)** *see* HYDROmorphone *on page* 707

◆ **Hydromorphone Hydrochloride** *see* HYDROmorphone *on page* 707

◆ **Hydromorphone Hydrochloride Injection, USP (Can)** *see* HYDROmorphone *on page* 707

◆ **Hydro-Rx** *see* Hydrocortisone *on page* 699

◆ **HydroVal® (Can)** *see* Hydrocortisone *on page* 699

Hydroxocobalamin (hye droks oh koe BAL a min)

U.S. Brand Names Cyanokit®

Index Terms Vitamin B$_{12a}$

Pharmacologic Category Antidote; Vitamin, Water Soluble

Use Treatment of pernicious anemia, vitamin B$_{12}$ deficiency due to dietary deficiencies or malabsorption diseases, inadequate secretion of intrinsic factor, and inadequate utilization of B$_{12}$ (eg, during neoplastic treatment); diagnostic agent for Schilling test

Cyanokit®: Treatment of cyanide poisoning (known or suspected)

Unlabeled/Investigational Use Neuropathies

Pharmacodynamics/Kinetics Following I.V. administration of Cyanokit®:

Protein binding: Significant; forms various cobalamin-(III) complexes

Half-life elimination: 26-31 hours

Excretion: Urine (50% to 60% within initial 72 hours)

◀ **Dosage**
Vitamin B$_{12}$ deficiency: I.M.:
Children: 100 mcg once daily for 2 or more weeks (total dose: 1-5 mg); maintenance: 30-50 mcg/month
Adults: 30 mcg/day for 5-10 days, followed by 100-200 mcg/month
Note: Larger doses may be required in critically-ill patients or if patient has neurologic disease, an infectious disease, or hyperthyroidism.
Schilling test: I.M.: Adults: 1000 mcg
Cyanide toxicity (Cyanokit®): I.V.: Adults: Initial: 5 g as single infusion; may repeat a second 5 g dose depending on severity of poisoning and clinical response. Maximum cumulative dose: 10 g. **Note:** If suspected, antidotal therapy must be given immediately.

Additional Information Complete prescribing information for this medication should be consulted for additional detail.

Dosage Forms Excipient information presented when available (limited, particularly for generics); consult specific product labeling.
Injection, solution: 1000 mcg/mL (30 mL)
Injection, powder for reconstitution:
Cyanokit®: 2.5 g (2 vials) [provided in a kit which also contains one I.V. infusion set]

References
Curry SC, Connor DA, and Raschke RA, "Effect of the Cyanide Antidote Hydroxocobalamin on Commonly Ordered Serum Chemistry Studies," *Ann Emerg Med*, 1994, 24(1):65-7.
Holland MA and Kozlowski LM, "Clinical Features and Management of Cyanide Poisoning," *Clin Pharm*, 1986, 5(9):737-41.
Huermer M, Simma B, Fowler B, et al, "Prenatal and Postnatal Treatment in Cobalamin C Defect," *J Pediatr*, 2005, 147(4):469-72.
Kayser SR and Kurisu S, "Hydroxocobalamin in Nitroprusside Induced Cyanide Toxicity," *Drug Intell Clin Pharm*, 1986, 20:365-6.
Lindenbaum J, Healton EB, Savage DG, et al, "Neuropsychiatric Disorders Caused by Cobalamin Deficiency in the Absence of Anemia or Macrocytosis," *N Engl J Med*, 1988, 318(26):1720-8.
Olszewski AJ, Szostak WB, Bialkowska M, et al, "Reduction of Plasma Lipid and Homocysteine Levels by Pyridoxine, Folate, Cobalamin, Choline, Riboflavin, and Troxerutin in Atherosclerosis," *Atherosclerosis*, 1989, 75(1):1-6.
Regland B, Gottfries CG, and Lindstedt G, "Dementia Patients With Low Serum Cobalamin Concentration: Relationship to Atrophic Gastritis," *Aging (Milano)*, 1992, 4(1):35-41.
Sauer SW and Keim ME, "Hydroxocobalamin: Improved Public Health Readiness for Cyanide Disasters," *Ann Emerg Med*, 2001, 37(6):635-41.

◆ **Hydroxycarbamide** see Hydroxyurea *on page 712*

◆ **Hydroxyethyl Starch** see Hetastarch *on page 688*

Hydroxyurea (hye droks ee yoor EE a)

Medication Safety Issues
Sound-alike/look-alike issues:
Hydroxyurea may be confused with hydrOXYzine

High alert medication: The Institute for Safe Medication Practices (ISMP) includes this medication among its list of drugs which have a heightened risk of causing significant patient harm when used in error.

International issues:
Hydrea® may be confused with Hydra® which is a brand name for isoniazid in Japan

U.S. Brand Names Droxia®; Hydrea®; Mylocel™

Canadian Brand Names Apo-Hydroxyurea®; Gen-Hydroxyurea; Hydrea®; Mylan-Hydroxyurea

Index Terms Hydroxycarbamide

Pharmacologic Category Antineoplastic Agent, Antimetabolite

Generic Available Yes: Capsule

Use Treatment of melanoma, refractory chronic myelocytic leukemia (CML), relapsed and refractory metastatic ovarian cancer; radiosensitizing agent in the treatment of squamous cell head and neck cancer (excluding lip cancer); adjunct in the management of sickle cell patients who have had at least three painful crises in the previous 12 months (to reduce frequency of these crises and the need for blood transfusions)

Unlabeled/Investigational Use Treatment of HIV; treatment of psoriasis, treatment of hematologic conditions such as essential thrombocythemia, polycythemia vera, hypereosinophilia, and hyperleukocytosis due to acute leukemia; treatment of uterine, cervix and nonsmall cell lung cancers; radio-sensitizing agent in the treatment of primary brain tumors

Mechanism of Action Thought to interfere (unsubstantiated hypothesis) with synthesis of DNA, during the S phase of cell division, without interfering with RNA synthesis; inhibits ribonucleoside diphosphate reductase, preventing conversion of ribonucleotides to deoxyribonucleotides; cell-cycle specific for the S phase and may hold other cells in the G_1 phase of the cell cycle. In sickle cell anemia, hydroxyurea increases red blood cell (RBC) hemoglobin F levels, RBC water content, deformability of sickled cells, and alters adhesion of RBCs to endothelium.

Pharmacodynamics/Kinetics

Absorption: Readily (≥80%)

Distribution: Readily crosses blood-brain barrier; distributes into intestine, brain, lung, kidney tissues, effusions and ascites

Metabolism: 60% via hepatic and GI tract

Half-life elimination: 3-4 hours

Time to peak: 1-4 hours

Excretion: Urine (80%, 50% as unchanged drug, 30% as urea); exhaled gases (as CO_2)

Dosage Oral (refer to individual protocols): All doses should be based on ideal or actual body weight, whichever is less:

Children (unlabeled use):

No FDA-approved dosage regimens have been established; dosages of 1500-3000 mg/m² as a single dose in combination with other agents every 4-6 weeks have been used in the treatment of pediatric astrocytoma, medulloblastoma, and primitive neuroectodermal tumors

CML: Initial: 10-20 mg/kg/day once daily; adjust dose according to hematologic response

Adults: Dose should always be titrated to patient response and WBC counts; usual oral doses range from 10-30 mg/kg/day or 500-3000 mg/day; if WBC count falls to <2500 cells/mm³, or the platelet count to <100,000/mm³, therapy should be stopped for at least 3 days and resumed when values rise toward normal

Solid tumors:

Intermittent therapy: 80 mg/kg as a single dose every third day

Continuous therapy: 20-30 mg/kg/day given as a single dose/day

Concomitant therapy with irradiation: 80 mg/kg as a single dose every third day starting at least 7 days before initiation of irradiation

Resistant chronic myelocytic leukemia: Continuous therapy: 20-30 mg/kg once daily

HIV (unlabeled use; in combination with antiretroviral agents): 1000-1500 mg daily in a single dose or divided doses

Psoriasis (unlabeled use): 1000-1500 mg/day in a single dose or divided doses

Sickle cell anemia (moderate/severe disease): Initial: 15 mg/kg/day, increased by 5 mg/kg every 12 weeks if blood counts are in an acceptable range until the maximum tolerated dose of 35 mg/kg/day is achieved or the dose that does not produce toxic effects

Acceptable range:

Neutrophils ≥2500 cells/mm³

Platelets ≥95,000/mm³

Hemoglobin >5.3 g/dL, and

Reticulocytes ≥95,000/mm³ if the hemoglobin concentration is <9 g/dL

Toxic range:

Neutrophils <2000 cells/mm³

Platelets <80,000/mm³

Hemoglobin <4.5 g/dL

Reticulocytes <80,000/mm³ if the hemoglobin concentration is <9 g/dL

Monitor for toxicity every 2 weeks; if toxicity occurs, stop treatment until the bone marrow recovers; restart at 2.5 mg/kg/day less than the dose at which toxicity occurs; if no toxicity occurs over the next 12 weeks, then the subsequent dose should be increased by 2.5 mg/kg/day; reduced dosage of hydroxyurea alternating with erythropoietin may decrease myelotoxicity and increase levels of fetal hemoglobin in patients who have not been helped by hydroxyurea alone

Dosing adjustment in renal impairment:
The FDA-approved labeling recommends the following adjustment:

Sickle cell anemia: Cl_{cr} <60 mL/minute or ESRD: Reduce initial dose to 7.5 mg/kg; titrate to response/avoidance of toxicity (refer to usual dosing).

Other indications: It is recommended to reduce the initial dose; however, no specific guidelines are available.

The following guidelines have been used by some clinicians:

Aronoff, 2007: Adults:
Cl_{cr} 10-50 mL/minute: Administer 50% of dose
Cl_{cr} <10 mL/minute: Administer 20% of dose

Hemodialysis: Administer dose after dialysis on dialysis days; supplemental dose is not necessary. Hydroxyurea is a low molecular weight compound with high aqueous solubility that may be freely dialyzable, however, clinical studies confirming this hypothesis have not been performed.

Continuous renal replacement therapy (CRRT): Administer 50% of dose

Kintzel, 1995:
Cl_{cr} 46-60 mL/minute: Administer 85% of dose
Cl_{cr} 31-45 mL/minute: Administer 80% of dose
Cl_{cr} <30 mL/minute: Administer 75% of dose

Dosing adjustment in hepatic impairment: Specific guidelines are not available for dosage adjustment in hepatic impairment. The FDA-approved labeling recommends closely monitoring for bone marrow toxicity in patients with hepatic impairment.

Stability Store at room temperature between 15°C and 30°C (59°F and 86°F).

Administration Capsules may be opened and emptied into water (will not dissolve completely); observe proper handling procedures

Monitoring Parameters CBC with differential and platelets, renal function and liver function tests, serum uric acid

Sickle cell disease: Monitor for toxicity every 2 weeks. If toxicity occurs, stop treatment until the bone marrow recovers; restart at 2.5 mg/kg/day less than the dose at which toxicity occurs. If no toxicity occurs over the next 12 weeks, then the subsequent dose should be increased by 2.5 mg/kg/day. Reduced dosage of hydroxyurea alternating with erythropoietin may decrease myelotoxicity and increase levels of fetal hemoglobin in patients who have not been helped by hydroxyurea alone.

Acceptable range: Neutrophils ≥2500 cells/mm^3, platelets ≥95,000/mm^3, hemoglobin >5.3 g/dL, and reticulocytes ≥95,000/mm^3 if the hemoglobin concentration is <9 g/dL

Toxic range: Neutrophils <2000 cells/mm^3, platelets <80,000/mm^3, hemoglobin <4.5 g/dL, and reticulocytes <80,000/mm^3 if the hemoglobin concentration is <9 g/dL

Pregnancy Risk Factor D

Contraindications Hypersensitivity to hydroxyurea or any component of the formulation; severe anemia; severe bone marrow suppression; WBC <2500/mm^3 or platelet count <100,000/mm^3 (neutrophils <2000/mm^3, platelets <80,000/mm^3, and hemoglobin <4.5 g/dL for sickle cell anemia); pregnancy

Warnings/Precautions Hazardous agent - use appropriate precautions for handling and disposal. Patients with a history of prior cytotoxic chemotherapy and radiation therapy are more likely to experience bone marrow depression. Patients with a history of radiation therapy are also at risk for exacerbation of post irradiation erythema. Megaloblastic erythropoiesis may be seen early in hydroxyurea treatment; plasma iron clearance may be delayed and the rate of utilization of iron by erythrocytes may be delayed. HIV-infected patients treated with hydroxyurea and antiretroviral agents (including didanosine) are at higher risk for potentially fatal pancreatitis, hepatotoxicity, hepatic failure, and severe peripheral neuropathy. **[U.S. Boxed Warning]: Hydroxyurea is mutagenic and clastogenic. Treatment of myeloproliferative disorders (polycythemia vera and thrombocythemia) with long-term hydroxyurea is associated with secondary leukemia; it is unknown if this is drug-related or disease-related.** Cutaneous vasculitic toxicities (vasculitic ulceration and gangrene) have been reported with hydroxyurea treatment, most often in patients with a history of or receiving concurrent interferon therapy; discontinue hydroxyurea and consider alternate cytoreductive therapy if cutaneous vasculitic toxicity develops. Use caution with renal dysfunction; may require dose reductions. **[U.S. Boxed Warning]: Should be administered under the supervision of a physician experienced in cancer chemotherapy or in the treatment of sickle cell anemia.**

Adverse Reactions Frequency not defined.

Cardiovascular: Edema

Central nervous system: Chills, disorientation, dizziness, drowsiness (dose-related), fever, hallucinations, headache, malaise, seizure

Dermatologic: Alopecia (rare), cutaneous vasculitic toxicities, dermatomyositis-like skin changes, dry skin, facial erythema, gangrene, hyperpigmentation, maculopapular rash, nail atrophy, nail pigmentation, peripheral erythema, scaling, skin atrophy, skin cancer, skin ulcer, vasculitis ulcerations, violet papules

Endocrine & metabolic: Hyperuricemia

Gastrointestinal: Anorexia, constipation, diarrhea, gastrointestinal irritation and mucositis, (potentiated with radiation therapy), nausea, pancreatitis, stomatitis, vomiting

Genitourinary: Dysuria (rare)

Hematologic: Myelosuppression (primarily leukopenia; onset: 24-48 hours; nadir: 10 days; recovery: 7 days after stopping drug; reversal of WBC count occurs rapidly but the platelet count may take 7-10 days to recover); thrombocytopenia and anemia, megaloblastic erythropoiesis, macrocytosis, hemolysis, serum iron decreased, persistent cytopenias, secondary leukemias (long-term use)

Hepatic: Hepatic enzymes increased, hepatotoxicity

Neuromuscular & skeletal: Peripheral neuropathy, weakness

Renal: BUN increased, creatinine increased

Respiratory: Acute diffuse pulmonary infiltrates (rare), dyspnea, pulmonary fibrosis (rare)

Drug Interactions

Avoid Concomitant Use

Avoid concomitant use of Hydroxyurea with any of the following: Natalizumab; Vaccines (Live)

Increased Effect/Toxicity

Hydroxyurea may increase the levels/effects of: Leflunomide; Natalizumab; Vaccines (Live)

The levels/effects of Hydroxyurea may be increased by: Didanosine; Trastuzumab

Decreased Effect

Hydroxyurea may decrease the levels/effects of: Vaccines (Inactivated); Vaccines (Live)

The levels/effects of Hydroxyurea may be decreased by: Echinacea

Dietary Considerations In sickle cell patients, supplemental administration of folic acid is recommended; hydroxyurea may mask development of folic acid deficiency.

Dosage Forms Excipient information presented when available (limited, particularly for generics); consult specific product labeling.

Capsule: 500 mg

Droxia®: 200 mg, 300 mg, 400 mg

Hydrea®: 500 mg

Tablet:

Mylocel™: 1000 mg

◆ **HydroZone Plus [OTC]** *see* Hydrocortisone *on page 699*

◆ **Hylenex™** *see* Hyaluronidase *on page 692*

◆ **Hyoscine Butylbromide** *see* Scopolamine Derivatives *on page 1278*

◆ **Hyoscine Hydrobromide** *see* Scopolamine Derivatives *on page 1278*

◆ **Hyperal** *see* Total Parenteral Nutrition *on page 1411*

◆ **Hyperalimentation** *see* Total Parenteral Nutrition *on page 1411*

◆ **HyperHep B® (Can)** *see* Hepatitis B Immune Globulin *on page 685*

◆ **HyperHEP B™ S/D** *see* Hepatitis B Immune Globulin *on page 685*

◆ **HyperRAB™ S/D** *see* Rabies Immune Globulin (Human) *on page 1224*

◆ **Hyper-Sal™** *see* Sodium Chloride *on page 1304*

◆ **HyperTET™ S/D** *see* Tetanus Immune Globulin (Human) *on page 1364*

◆ **Hytone® [DSC]** *see* Hydrocortisone *on page 699*

Ibandronate (eye BAN droh nate)

U.S. Brand Names Boniva®
Canadian Brand Names Bondronat®
Index Terms Ibandronate Sodium; Ibandronic Acid
Pharmacologic Category Bisphosphonate Derivative
Use Treatment and prevention of osteoporosis in postmenopausal females
Unlabeled/Investigational Use Hypercalcemia of malignancy; corticosteroid-induced osteoporosis; Paget's disease; reduce bone pain and skeletal complications from metastatic bone disease

Pharmacodynamics/Kinetics
Distribution: Terminal V_d: 90 L; 40% to 50% of circulating ibandronate binds to bone
Protein binding: 85.7% to 99.5%
Metabolism: Not metabolized
Bioavailability: Oral: Reduced by 90% following standard breakfast
Half-life elimination:
Oral: 150 mg dose: Terminal: 37-157 hours
I.V.: Terminal: ~5-25 hours
Time to peak, plasma: Oral: 0.5-2 hours
Excretion: Urine (50% to 60% of absorbed dose, excreted as unchanged drug); feces (unabsorbed drug)

Dosage
Oral:
Treatment of postmenopausal osteoporosis: 2.5 mg once daily **or** 150 mg once a month
Prevention of postmenopausal osteoporosis: 2.5 once daily **or** 150 mg once a month
Metastatic bone disease (unlabeled use): 50 mg once daily
I.V.:
Treatment of postmenopausal osteoporosis: 3 mg every 3 months
Hypercalcemia of malignancy (unlabeled use): 2-4 mg over 2 hours
Metastatic bone disease (unlabeled use): 6 mg over 1 hour every 3-4 weeks

Dosage adjustment in renal impairment:
Mild or moderate impairment: Dosing adjustment not needed
Severe impairment (Cl_{cr} <30 mL/minute): Use not recommended
Dose adjustment in renal impairment for oncologic uses (unlabeled): Severe impairment (Cl_{cr} <30 mL/minute):
Oral: 50 mg once weekly
I.V.: 2 mg over 1 hour every 3-4 weeks
Dosage adjustment in hepatic impairment: Dosing adjustment not needed
Additional Information Complete prescribing information for this medication should be consulted for additional detail.
Dosage Forms Excipient information presented when available (limited, particularly for generics); consult specific product labeling.
Injection, solution: 1 mg/mL (3 mL) [prefilled syringe]
Tablet: 2.5 mg [once-daily formulation]; 150 mg [once-monthly formulation]

References
Author Unknown, "Safety Update: Bone-Building Drugs: Risks Explained," *Consum Rep Health*, 2006, 18(5):3.
Barrett J, Worth E, Bauss F, et al, "Ibandronate: A Clinical Pharmacological and Pharmacokinetic Update," *J Clin Pharmacol*, 2004, 44(9):951-65.
Marx RE, Sawatari Y, Fortin M, et al, "Bisphosphonate-Induced Exposed Bone (Osteonecrosis/Osteopetrosis) of the Jaws: Risk Factors, Recognition, Prevention, and Treatment," *J Oral Maxillofac Surg*, 2005, 63(11):1567-75.

McCormack PL and Plosker GL, "Ibandronic Acid: A Review of its Use in the Treatment of Bone Metastases of Breast Cancer," *Drugs*, 2006, 66(5):711-28.

Tripathy D, Body JJ, and Bergstrom B, "Review of Ibandronate in the Treatment of Metastatic Bone Disease: Experience From Phase III Trials," *Clin Ther*, 2004, 26(12):1947-59.

Von Moos R, "Bisphosphonate Treatment Recommendations for Oncologists," *Oncologist*, 2005, 10 (Suppl 1):19-24.

◆ **Ibandronate Sodium** *see* Ibandronate *on page 716*

◆ **Ibandronic Acid** *see* Ibandronate *on page 716*

◆ **Ibidomide Hydrochloride** *see* Labetalol *on page 791*

◆ **Ibu®** *see* Ibuprofen *on page 717*

◆ **Ibu-200 [OTC]** *see* Ibuprofen *on page 717*

Ibuprofen (eye byoo PROE fen)

Medication Safety Issues
Sound-alike/look-alike issues:
  Haltran® may be confused with Halfprin®
  Motrin® may be confused with Neurontin®

Injectable formulations: Both ibuprofen and ibuprofen lysine are available for parenteral use. Ibuprofen lysine is **only** indicated for closure of a clinically-significant patent ductus arteriosus.

Medication Guide An FDA-approved patient medication guide, which is available with the product information and at http://www.fda.gov/downloads/Drugs/DrugSafety/ucm088647.pdf, must be dispensed with this medication for each new outpatient prescription and refill for oral administration.

Related Information
Acetaminophen and NSAIDS, Dosing in the Management of Pain *on page 1651*
Acute Postoperative Pain *on page 1502*
Chronic Pain Management *on page 1546*
Desensitization Protocols *on page 1692*
Nonsteroidal Anti-Inflammatory Agents *on page 1687*

U.S. Brand Names Addaprin [OTC]; Advil® Children's [OTC]; Advil® Infants' [OTC]; Advil® Migraine [OTC]; Advil® [OTC]; Caldolor™; Genpril® [OTC] [DSC]; I-Prin [OTC]; Ibu-200 [OTC]; Ibu®; Midol® Cramp and Body Aches [OTC]; Motrin® Children's [OTC]; Motrin® IB [OTC]; Motrin® Infants' [OTC]; Motrin® Junior [OTC]; NeoProfen®; Proprinal [OTC]; Ultraprin [OTC]

Canadian Brand Names Advil®; Apo-Ibuprofen®; Motrin® (Children's); Motrin® IB; Novo-Profen; Nu-Ibuprofen

Index Terms *p*-Isobutylhydratropic Acid; Ibuprofen Lysine

Pharmacologic Category Nonsteroidal Anti-inflammatory Drug (NSAID), Oral; Nonsteroidal Anti-inflammatory Drug (NSAID), Parenteral

Generic Available Yes: Caplet, suspension, tablet

Use
Oral: Inflammatory diseases and rheumatoid disorders including juvenile rheumatoid arthritis, mild-to-moderate pain, fever, dysmenorrhea, osteoarthritis

Ibuprofen injection (Caldolor™): Management of mild-to-moderate pain; management moderate-to-severe pain when used concurrently with an opioid analgesic; reduction of fever

Ibuprofen lysine injection (NeoProfen®): To induce closure of a clinically-significant patent ductus arteriosus (PDA) in premature infants weighing between 500-1500 g and who are ≤32 weeks gestational age (GA) when usual treatments are ineffective

Unlabeled/Investigational Use Cystic fibrosis, gout, ankylosing spondylitis, acute migraine headache

Mechanism of Action Reversibly inhibits cyclooxygenase-1 and 2 (COX-1 and 2) enzymes, which results in decreased formation of prostaglandin precursors; has antipyretic, analgesic, and anti-inflammatory properties

Other proposed mechanisms not fully elucidated (and possibly contributing to the anti-inflammatory effect to varying degrees), include inhibiting chemotaxis, altering lymphocyte activity, inhibiting neutrophil aggregation/activation, and decreasing proinflammatory cytokine levels.

Pharmacodynamics/Kinetics

Onset of action: Oral: Analgesic: 30-60 minutes; Anti-inflammatory: ≤7 days
  Peak effect: Oral: 1-2 weeks
Duration: Oral: 4-6 hours
Absorption: Oral: Rapid (85%)
Distribution: V_d: 6.35 L; premature infants with ductal closure (highly variable between studies):
  Day 3: 145-349 mL/kg
  Day 5: 72-222 mL/kg
Protein binding: 90% to 99%
Metabolism: Hepatic via oxidation
Half-life elimination:
  Premature infants (highly variable between studies):
    Day 3: 35-51 hours
    Day 5: 20-33 hours
  Children 3 months to 10 years: 1.6 ± 0.7 hours
  Adults: 2-4 hours; End-stage renal disease: Unchanged
Time to peak: Oral: ~1-2 hours
Excretion: Urine (primarily as metabolites; 1% as unchanged drug); some feces

Dosage

I.V.:
  Neonates: Ibuprofen lysine (NeoProfen®): Infants between 500-1500 g and ≤32 weeks GA: Patent ductus arteriosus: Initial dose: Ibuprofen 10 mg/kg, followed by two doses of 5 mg/kg at 24 and 48 hours. Dose should be based on birth weight.
  Adults (Caldolor™): **Note**: Patients should be well hydrated prior to administration
    Analgesic: 400-800 mg every 6 hours as needed (maximum: 3.2 g/day)
    Antipyretic: Initial: 400 mg, then every 4-6 hours or 100-200 mg every 4 hours as needed (maximum: 3.2 g/day)

Oral:
  Children:
  Antipyretic: 6 months to 12 years: Temperature <102.5°F (39°C): 5 mg/kg/dose; temperature >102.5°F: 10 mg/kg/dose given every 6-8 hours (maximum daily dose: 40 mg/kg/day)
  Juvenile rheumatoid arthritis: 30-50 mg/kg/24 hours divided every 8 hours; start at lower end of dosing range and titrate upward (maximum: 2.4 g/day)
  Analgesic: 4-10 mg/kg/dose every 6-8 hours
  Cystic fibrosis (unlabeled use): Chronic (>4 years) twice daily dosing adjusted to maintain serum concentration of 50-100 mcg/mL has been associated with slowing of disease progression in younger patients with mild lung disease
  OTC labeling (analgesic, antipyretic): **Note**: Treatment for >10 days is not recommended unless directed by healthcare provider.
    Children 6 months to 11 years: See table; use of weight to select dose is preferred; doses may be repeated every 6-8 hours (maximum: 4 doses/day)
    Children ≥12 years: 200 mg every 4-6 hours as needed (maximum: 1200 mg/24 hours)

Ibuprofen Dosing

Weight (lb)	Age	Dosage (mg)
12-17	6-11 mo	50
18-23	12-23 mo	75
24-35	2-3 y	100
36-47	4-5 y	150
48-59	6-8 y	200
60-71	9-10 y	250
72-95	11 y	300

Adults:

Inflammatory disease: 400-800 mg/dose 3-4 times/day (maximum dose: 3.2 g/day)

Analgesia/pain/fever/dysmenorrhea: 200-400 mg/dose every 4-6 hours (maximum daily dose: 1.2 g, unless directed by physician; under physician supervision daily doses ≤2.4 g may be used)

OTC labeling (analgesic, antipyretic): 200 mg every 4-6 hours as needed (maximum: 1200 mg/24 hours); treatment for >10 days is not recommended unless directed by healthcare provider.

Migraine: 2 capsules at onset of symptoms (maximum: 400 mg/24 hours unless directed by healthcare provider)

Dosing adjustment/comments in renal impairment: If anuria or oliguria evident, hold dose until renal function returns to normal

Dosing adjustment/comments in severe hepatic impairment: Avoid use

Stability

Ibuprofen injection (Caldolor™): Store intact vials at room temperature of 20°C to 25°C (68°F to 77°F). Must be diluted prior to use. Dilute with D_5W, NS or LR to a final concentration ≤4 mg/mL. Diluted solutions stable for 24 hours at room temperature.

Ibuprofen lysine injection (NeoProfen®): Store at room temperature of 20°C to 25°C (68°F to 77°F). Protect from light. Dilute with dextrose or saline to an appropriate volume. Following dilution, administer within 30 minutes of preparation.

Suspension, tablet: Store at room temperature of 20°C to 25°C (68°F to 77°F).

Administration

Oral: Administer with food

I.V.:

Caldolor™: For I.V. administration only; must be diluted to a final concentration of ≤4 mg/mL prior to administration; infuse over at least 30 minutes

NeoProfen® (ibuprofen lysine): For I.V. administration only; administration via umbilical arterial line has not been evaluated. Infuse over 15 minutes through port closest to insertion site. Avoid extravasation. Do not administer simultaneously via same line with TPN. If needed, interrupt TPN for 15 minutes prior to and after ibuprofen administration, keeping line open with dextrose or saline.

Monitoring Parameters CBC, chemistry profile, occult blood loss and periodic liver function tests; monitor response (pain, range of motion, grip strength, mobility, ADL function), inflammation; observe for weight gain, edema; monitor renal function (urine output, serum BUN and creatinine); observe for bleeding, bruising; evaluate gastrointestinal effects (abdominal pain, bleeding, dyspepsia); mental confusion, disorientation; with long-term therapy, periodic ophthalmic exams; signs of infection (ibuprofen lysine)

Reference Range Plasma concentrations >200 mcg/mL may be associated with severe toxicity

PDA: Minimum effective concentration: 10-12 mg/L

Anesthesia and Critical Care Concerns/Other Considerations The 2002 ACCM/SCCM guidelines for analgesia (critically-ill adult) suggest that NSAIDs may be used in combination with opioids in select patients for pain management. Concern about adverse events (increased risk of renal dysfunction, altered platelet function and gastrointestinal irritation) limits its use in patients who have other underlying risks for these events.

In short-term use, NSAIDs vary considerably in their effect on blood pressure. When NSAIDs are used in patients with hypertension, monitor blood pressure response, and duration of therapy, when possible, should be kept short. The use of NSAIDs in the treatment of patients with heart failure may be associated with an increased risk for fluid accumulation and edema; may precipitate renal failure in dehydrated patients by inhibition of prostaglandin-mediated autoregulation. Use extreme caution or avoid concurrent use with nephrotoxic agents.

Pregnancy Risk Factor C/D ≥30 weeks gestation

Contraindications Hypersensitivity to ibuprofen; history of asthma, urticaria, or allergic-type reaction to aspirin or other NSAIDs; aspirin triad (eg, bronchial asthma, aspirin intolerance, rhinitis); perioperative pain in the setting of coronary artery bypass graft (CABG) surgery

◀ Ibuprofen lysine (NeoProfen®): Preterm infants with untreated proven or suspected infection; congenital heart disease where patency of the PDA is necessary for pulmonary or systemic blood flow; bleeding (especially with active intracranial hemorrhage or GI bleed); thrombocytopenia; coagulation defects; proven or suspected necrotizing enterocolitis (NEC); significant renal dysfunction

Warnings/Precautions [U.S. Boxed Warning]: NSAIDs are associated with an increased risk of adverse cardiovascular thrombotic events, including fatal MI and stroke. Risk may be increased with duration of use or pre-existing cardiovascular risk factors or disease. Carefully evaluate individual cardiovascular risk profiles prior to prescribing. May cause new-onset hypertension or worsening of existing hypertension. Response to ACE inhibitors, thiazides, or loop diuretics may be impaired with concurrent use of NSAIDs. Use caution with fluid retention. Avoid use in heart failure. Concurrent administration of ibuprofen, and potentially other nonselective NSAIDs, may interfere with aspirin's cardioprotective effect. **[U.S. Boxed Warning]: Use is contraindicated for treatment of perioperative pain in the setting of coronary artery bypass graft (CABG) surgery.** Risk of MI and stroke may be increased with use following CABG surgery.

May increase the risk of aseptic meningitis, especially in patients with systemic lupus erythematosus (SLE) and mixed connective tissue disorders. Platelet adhesion and aggregation may be decreased; may prolong bleeding time; patients with coagulation disorders or who are receiving anticoagulants should be monitored closely. Anemia may occur; patients on long-term NSAID therapy should be monitored for anemia. Rarely, NSAID use may cause severe blood dyscrasias (eg, agranulocytosis, aplastic anemia, thrombocytopenia).

NSAID use may compromise existing renal function; dose-dependent decreases in prostaglandin synthesis may result from NSAID use, reducing renal blood flow which may cause renal decompensation. NSAID use may increase the risk for hyperkalemia. Patients with impaired renal function, dehydration, heart failure, liver dysfunction, those taking diuretics, and ACE inhibitors, and the elderly are at greater risk of renal toxicity and hyperkalemia. Rehydrate patient before starting therapy; monitor renal function closely. Not recommended for use in patients with advanced renal disease. Long-term NSAID use may result in renal papillary necrosis.

NSAIDs may increase risk of gastrointestinal irritation, inflammation, ulceration, bleeding, and perforation. These events can be fatal and may occur at any time during therapy and without warning. Use caution with a history of GI disease (bleeding or ulcers), concurrent therapy with aspirin, anticoagulants and/or corticosteroids, smoking, use of ethanol, the elderly or debilitated patients. When used concomitantly with ≤325 mg of aspirin, a substantial increase in the risk of gastrointestinal complications (eg, ulcer) occurs; concomitant gastro-protective therapy (eg, proton pump inhibitors) is recommended (Bhatt, 2008).

Use the lowest effective dose for the shortest duration of time, consistent with individual patient goals, to reduce risk of cardiovascular or GI adverse events. Alternate therapies should be considered for patients at high risk.

NSAIDs may cause serious skin adverse events including exfoliative dermatitis, Stevens-Johnson Syndrome (SJS) and toxic epidermal necrolysis (TEN); discontinue use at first sign of skin rash or hypersensitivity. Anaphylactoid reactions may occur, even without prior exposure; patients with "aspirin triad" (bronchial asthma, aspirin intolerance, rhinitis) may be at increased risk. Do not use in patients who experience bronchospasm, asthma, rhinitis, or urticaria with NSAID or aspirin therapy. Use caution in other forms of asthma.

NSAIDS may cause drowsiness, dizziness, blurred vision and other neurologic effects which may impair physical or mental abilities; patients must be cautioned about performing tasks which require mental alertness (eg, operating machinery or driving). Monitor vision with long-term therapy. Blurred/diminished vision, scotomata, and changes in color vision have been reported. Discontinue use with altered vision and perform ophthalmologic exam.

Use with caution in patients with decreased hepatic function. Closely monitor patients with any abnormal LFT. Severe hepatic reactions (eg, fulminant hepatitis, liver failure) have occurred with NSAID use, rarely; discontinue if signs or symptoms of liver disease develop, or if systemic manifestations occur.

The elderly are at increased risk for adverse effects (especially serious gastrointestinal events, CNS effects, renal toxicity) from NSAIDs even at low doses.

Withhold for at least 4-6 half-lives prior to surgical or dental procedures. Some products may contain phenylalanine. Ibuprofen injection (Caldolor™) must be diluted prior to administration; hemolysis can occur if not diluted.

Ibuprofen lysine injection (NeoProfen®): Hold second or third doses if urinary output is <0.6 mL/kg/hour. May alter signs of infection. May inhibit platelet aggregation; monitor for signs of bleeding. May displace bilirubin; use caution when total bilirubin is elevated. Long-term evaluations of neurodevelopment, growth, or diseases associated with prematurity following treatment have not been conducted. A second course of treatment, alternative pharmacologic therapy or surgery may be needed if the ductus arteriosus fails to close or reopens following the initial course of therapy.

Self medication (OTC use): Prior to self-medication, patients should contact healthcare provider if they have had recurring stomach pain or upset, ulcers, bleeding problems, high blood pressure, heart or kidney disease, other serious medical problems, are currently taking a diuretic, aspirin, anticoagulant, or are ≥60 years of age. If patients are using for migraines, they should also contact healthcare provider if they have not had a migraine diagnosis by healthcare provider, a headache that is different from usual migraine, worst headache of life, fever and neck stiffness, headache from head injury or coughing, first headache at ≥50 years of age, daily headache, or migraine requiring bed rest. Recommended dosages should not be exceeded, due to an increased risk of GI bleeding. Stop use and consult a healthcare provider if symptoms get worse, newly appear, fever lasts for >3 days or pain lasts >3 days (children) and >10 days (adults). Do not give for >10 days unless instructed by healthcare provider. Consuming ≥3 alcoholic beverages/day or taking longer than recommended may increase the risk of GI bleeding.

Adverse Reactions
Oral:
1% to 10%:
Cardiovascular: Edema (1% to 3%)
Central nervous system: Dizziness (3% to 9%), headache (1% to 3%), nervousness (1% to 3%)
Dermatologic: Rash (3% to 9%), itching (1% to 3%)
Endocrine & metabolic: Fluid retention (1% to 3%)
Gastrointestinal: Epigastric pain (3% to 9%), heartburn (3% to 9%), nausea (3% to 9%), abdominal pain/cramps/distress (1% to 3%), appetite decreased (1% to 3%), constipation (1% to 3%), diarrhea (1% to 3%), dyspepsia (1% to 3%), flatulence (1% to 3%), vomiting (1% to 3%)
Otic: Tinnitus (3% to 9%)
<1% (Limited to important or life-threatening): Acute renal failure, agranulocytosis, anaphylaxis, aplastic anemia, azotemia, blurred vision, bone marrow suppression, confusion, creatinine clearance decreased, duodenal ulcer, edema, eosinophilia, epistaxis, erythema multiforme, gastric ulcer, GI bleed, GI hemorrhage, GI ulceration, hallucinations, hearing decreased, hematuria, hematocrit decreased, hemoglobin decreased, hemolytic anemia, hepatitis, hypertension, inhibition of platelet aggregation, jaundice, liver function tests abnormal, leukopenia, melena, neutropenia, pancreatitis, photosensitivity, Stevens-Johnson syndrome, thrombocytopenia, toxic amblyopia, toxic epidermal necrolysis, urticaria, vesiculobullous eruptions, vision changes

Injection: Ibuprofen (Caldolor™): Abdominal pain, anemia, BUN increased, cough, dizziness, dyspepsia, edema, flatulence, headache, hemorrhage, hypokalemia, hypernatremia, hypertension, nausea, neutropenia, pruritus, urinary retention, vomiting

Injection: Ibuprofen lysine (NeoProfen®):
>10%:
Cardiovascular: Intraventricular hemorrhage (29%; grade 3/4: 15%)

Dermatologic: Skin irritation (16%)
Endocrine & metabolic: Hypocalcemia (12%), hypoglycemia (12%)
Gastrointestinal: GI disorders, non NEC (22%)
Hematologic: Anemia (32%)
Respiratory: Apnea (28%), respiratory infection (19%)
Miscellaneous: Sepsis (43%)

1% to 10%:
Cardiovascular: Edema (4%)
Endocrine & metabolic: Adrenal insufficiency (7%), hypernatremia (7%)
Genitourinary: Urinary tract infection (9%)
Renal: Urea increased (7%), renal impairment (6%), creatinine increased (3%), urine output decreased (3%; small decrease reported on days 2-6 with compensatory increase in output on day 9), renal failure (1%)
Respiratory: Respiratory failure (10%), atelectasis (4%)

Frequency not defined: Abdominal distension, cholestasis, feeding problems, gastritis, GI reflux, heart failure, hyperglycemia, hypotension, ileus, infection, inguinal hernia, injection site reaction, jaundice, neutropenia, seizure, tachycardia, thrombocytopenia

Postmarketing and/or case reports: GI perforation, necrotizing enterocolitis

Drug Interactions

Metabolism/Transport Effects Substrate (minor) of CYP2C9, 2C19; **Inhibits** CYP2C9 (strong)

Avoid Concomitant Use

Avoid concomitant use of Ibuprofen with any of the following: Ketorolac

Increased Effect/Toxicity

Ibuprofen may increase the levels/effects of: Aminoglycosides; Anticoagulants; Antiplatelet Agents; Bisphosphonate Derivatives; Carvedilol; CycloSPORINE; CYP2C9 Substrates (High risk); Desmopressin; Drotrecogin Alfa; Eplerenone; Ibritumomab; Lithium; Methotrexate; Nonsteroidal Anti-Inflammatory Agents; Pemetrexed; Potassium-Sparing Diuretics; Pralatrexate; Quinolone Antibiotics; Salicylates; Thrombolytic Agents; Tositumomab and Iodine I 131 Tositumomab; Vancomycin; Vitamin K Antagonists

The levels/effects of Ibuprofen may be increased by: Antidepressants (Tricyclic, Tertiary Amine); Corticosteroids (Systemic); Dasatinib; Herbs (Anticoagulant/ Antiplatelet Properties); Ketorolac; Nonsteroidal Anti-Inflammatory Agents; Omega-3-Acid Ethyl Esters; Pentosan Polysulfate Sodium; Pentoxifylline; Probenecid; Prostacyclin Analogues; Selective Serotonin Reuptake Inhibitors; Serotonin/Norepinephrine Reuptake Inhibitors; Treprostinil

Decreased Effect

Ibuprofen may decrease the levels/effects of: ACE Inhibitors; Angiotensin II Receptor Blockers; Antiplatelet Agents; Beta-Blockers; Eplerenone; HydrALA-ZINE; Loop Diuretics; Potassium-Sparing Diuretics; Salicylates; Thiazide Diuretics

The levels/effects of Ibuprofen may be decreased by: Bile Acid Sequestrants; Nonsteroidal Anti-Inflammatory Agents; Salicylates

Ethanol/Nutrition/Herb Interactions

Ethanol: Avoid ethanol (may enhance gastric mucosal irritation).
Food: Ibuprofen peak serum levels may be decreased if taken with food.
Herb/Nutraceutical: Avoid alfalfa, anise, bilberry, bladderwrack, bromelain, cat's claw, celery, chamomile, coleus, cordyceps, dong quai, evening primrose, fenugreek, feverfew, garlic, ginger, ginkgo biloba, ginseng (American, Panax, Siberian), grapeseed, green tea, guggul, horse chestnut seed, horseradish, licorice, prickly ash, red clover, reishi, SAMe (S-adenosylmethionine), sweet clover, turmeric, white willow (all have additional antiplatelet activity).

Dietary Considerations Should be taken with food. Chewable tablets may contain phenylalanine.

Dosage Forms Excipient information presented when available (limited, particularly for generics); consult specific product labeling. [DSC] = Discontinued product

Caplet: 200 mg [OTC]
Advil®: 200 mg [contains sodium benzoate]
Ibu-200: 200 mg

Motrin® IB: 200 mg
Motrin® Junior: 100 mg [scored]
Capsule, liquid-filled:
Advil®: 200 mg [solubilized ibuprofen; contains potassium 20 mg]
Advil® Migraine: 200 mg [solubilized ibuprofen; contains potassium 20 mg]
Gelcap:
Advil®: 200 mg [contains coconut oil]
Injection, solution:
Caldolor™: 100 mg/mL (4 mL, 8 mL)
Injection, solution, as lysine [preservative free]:
NeoProfen®: 17.1 mg/mL (2 mL) [equivalent to ibuprofen 10 mg/mL]
Suspension, oral: 100 mg/5 mL (5 mL, 10 mL, 120 mL, 240 mL, 480 mL)
Advil® Children's: 100 mg/5 mL (120 mL) [contains sodium benzoate, sodium, propylene glycol; blue raspberry, fruit, and grape flavors]
Motrin® Children's: 100 mg/5 mL (60 mL, 120 mL) [contains sodium benzoate; berry, dye free berry, bubble gum, and grape flavors]
Suspension, oral [concentrate, drops]: 40 mg/mL (15 mL)
Advil® Infants': 40 mg/mL (15 mL) [contains sodium benzoate; fruit, grape, and white grape flavors]
Motrin® Infants': 40 mg/mL (15 mL) [contains sodium benzoate; ethanol free; berry and dye-free berry flavors]
Tablet: 200 mg [OTC], 400 mg, 600 mg, 800 mg
Addaprin: 200 mg
Advil®: 200 mg [contains sodium benzoate]
Genpril®: 200 mg [DSC]
Ibu®: 400 mg, 600 mg, 800 mg
Ibu-200: 200 mg
I-Prin: 200 mg
Midol® Cramp and Body Aches: 200 mg
Motrin® IB: 200 mg
Proprinal: 200 mg [contains sodium benzoate]
Ultraprin: 200 mg [sugar free]
Tablet, chewable:
Advil® Children's: 50 mg [contains phenylalanine 2.1 mg; grape flavors]
Advil® Junior: 100 mg [contains phenylalanine 4.2 mg; grape flavors] [DSC]
Motrin® Junior: 100 mg [contains phenylalanine 2.1 mg; grape and orange flavors]

◆ **Ibuprofen Lysine** *see* Ibuprofen *on page* 717

Ibutilide (i BYOO ti lide)

Medication Safety Issues
High alert medication: The Institute for Safe Medication Practices (ISMP) includes this medication among its list of drugs which have a heightened risk of causing significant patient harm when used in error.

Related Information
Antiarrhythmic Drugs *on page* 1656
Management of Postoperative Arrhythmias *on page* 1571

U.S. Brand Names Corvert®
Index Terms Ibutilide Fumarate
Pharmacologic Category Antiarrhythmic Agent, Class III
Generic Available No

Use Acute termination of atrial fibrillation or flutter of recent onset; the effectiveness of ibutilide has not been determined in patients with arrhythmias >90 days in duration

Mechanism of Action Exact mechanism of action is unknown; prolongs the action potential in cardiac tissue

Pharmacodynamics/Kinetics
Onset of action: ~90 minutes after start of infusion ($\frac{1}{2}$ of conversions to sinus rhythm occur during infusion)
Distribution: V_d: 11 L/kg
Protein binding: 40%

Metabolism: Extensively hepatic; oxidation

Half-life elimination: 2-12 hours (average: 6 hours)

Excretion: Urine (82%; 7% as unchanged drug and metabolites); feces (19%)

Dosage I.V.: Initial:

Adults:

<60 kg: 0.01 mg/kg over 10 minutes

≥60 kg: 1 mg over 10 minutes

If the arrhythmia does not terminate within 10 minutes after the end of the initial infusion, a second infusion of equal strength may be infused over a 10-minute period

Elderly: Dose selection should be cautious, usually starting at the lower end of the dosing range.

Stability Admixtures are chemically and physically stable for 24 hours at room temperature and for 48 hours at refrigerated temperatures. May be administered undiluted or diluted in 50 mL diluent (0.9% NS or D_5W).

Administration May be administered undiluted or diluted in 50 mL diluent (0.9% NS or D_5W); infuse over 10 minutes

Monitoring Parameters Observe patient with continuous ECG monitoring for at least 4 hours following infusion or until QT_c has returned to baseline; skilled personnel and proper equipment should be available during administration of ibutilide and subsequent monitoring of the patient

Anesthesia and Critical Care Concerns/Other Considerations

Clinical Pearls/Comments: Ibutilide may lower the energy requirement for direct current cardioversion in atrial fibrillation; effective for termination of postsurgical atrial fibrillation or atrial flutter, but at the risk of precipitating ventricular arrhythmias (eg, torsade de pointes). Patients who receive ibutilide should be evaluated for risk of development of QT prolongation and subsequent torsade de pointes (TdP). A major risk factor for development of TdP is reduced left ventricular function, and therefore ibutilide should be avoided in these patients (Blomström-Lundqvist, 2003). Patients should be observed with continuous ECG monitoring during infusion and for at least 4 hours following infusion or until QT_c has returned to baseline.

The use of intravenous magnesium (2 g) immediately prior to and after ibutilide administration has been shown to be helpful in reducing QT interval prolongation due to ibutilide (Caron, 2003) and may enhance the efficacy of ibutilide (Kalus, 2003). Whether or not prophylactic magnesium reduces the incidence of TdP has yet to be determined; however, it is thought that this measure will reduce the incidence of TdP (Coleman, 2004).

Pregnancy Risk Factor C

Contraindications Hypersensitivity to ibutilide or any component of the formulation; QT_c >440 msec

Warnings/Precautions [U.S. Boxed Warning]: Potentially fatal arrhythmias (eg, polymorphic ventricular tachycardia) can occur with ibutilide, usually in association with torsade de pointes (QT prolongation). Studies indicate a 1.7% incidence of arrhythmias in treated patients. The drug should be given in a setting of continuous ECG monitoring and by personnel trained in treating arrhythmias particularly polymorphic ventricular tachycardia. **[U.S. Boxed Warning]: Patients with chronic atrial fibrillation may not be the best candidates for ibutilide since they often revert after conversion and the risks of treatment may not be justified when compared to alternative management.** Dosing adjustments are not required in patients with renal or hepatic dysfunction. Safety and efficacy in children have not been established. Use caution in elderly patients. Avoid concurrent use of any drug that can prolong QT interval. Correct hyperkalemia and hypomagnesemia before using. Monitor for heart block.

Adverse Reactions

1% to 10%:

Cardiovascular: Ventricular extrasystoles (5.1%), nonsustained monomorphic ventricular tachycardia (4.9%), nonsustained polymorphic ventricular tachycardia (2.7%), tachycardia/supraventricular tachycardia (2.7%), hypotension (2%), bundle branch block (1.9%), sustained polymorphic ventricular tachycardia (eg, torsade de pointes) (1.7%, often requiring cardioversion),

AV block (1.5%), bradycardia (1.2%), QT segment prolongation, hypertension (1.2%), palpitation (1%)

Central nervous system: Headache (4%)

Gastrointestinal: Nausea (>1%)

<1% (Limited to important or life-threatening): CHF, erythematous bullous lesions, idioventricular rhythm, nodal arrhythmia, renal failure, supraventricular extrasystoles, sustained monomorphic ventricular tachycardia, syncope (0.3%, not > placebo)

Drug Interactions

Avoid Concomitant Use

Avoid concomitant use of Ibutilide with any of the following: Artemether; Dronedarone; Lumefantrine; Nilotinib; Pimozide; QuiNINE; Tetrabenazine; Thioridazine; Ziprasidone

Increased Effect/Toxicity

Ibutilide may increase the levels/effects of: Dronedarone; Pimozide; QTc-Prolonging Agents; QuiNINE; Tetrabenazine; Thioridazine; Ziprasidone

The levels/effects of Ibutilide may be increased by: Alfuzosin; Artemether; Chloroquine; Ciprofloxacin; Gadobutrol; Lumefantrine; Nilotinib; QuiNINE

Decreased Effect There are no known significant interactions involving a decrease in effect.

Dosage Forms Excipient information presented when available (limited, particularly for generics); consult specific product labeling.

Injection, solution, as fumarate: 0.1 mg/mL (10 mL)

References

Blomström-Lundqvist C, Scheinman MM, Aliot EM, et al, "ACC/AHA/ESC Guidelines for the Management of Patients With Supraventricular Arrhythmias–Executive Summary. A Report of the American College of Cardiology/American Heart Association Task Force on Practice Guidelines and the European Society of Cardiology Committee for Practice Guidelines (Writing Committee to Develop Guidelines for the Management of Patients With Supraventricular Arrhythmias) Developed in Collaboration With NASPE-Heart Rhythm Society," *J Am Coll Cardiol*, 2003, 42(8):1493-531.

Caron MF, Kluger J, Tsikouris JP, et al, "Effects of Intravenous Magnesium Sulfate on the QT Interval in Patients Receiving Ibutilide," *Pharmacotherapy*, 2003, 23(3):296-300.

Coleman CI, Kalus JS, Caron MF, et al, "Model of Effect of Magnesium Prophylaxis on Frequency of Torsades de Pointes in Ibutilide-Treated Patients," *Am J Health Syst Pharm*, 2004, 61(7):685-8.

Kalus JS, Spencer AP, Tsikouris JP, et al, "Impact of Prophylactic I.V. Magnesium on the Efficacy of Ibutilide for Conversion of Atrial Fibrillation or Flutter," *Am J Health Syst Pharm*, 2003, 60 (22):2308-12.

◆ **Ibutilide Fumarate** *see* Ibutilide *on page 723*

◆ **ICI-D1033** *see* Anastrozole *on page 122*

◆ **IgG4-Kappa Monoclonal Antibody** *see* Natalizumab *on page 989*

◆ **IGIV** *see* Immune Globulin (Intravenous) *on page 732*

◆ **IGIVnex® (Can)** *see* Immune Globulin (Intravenous) *on page 732*

Iloperidone (eye loe PER i done)

U.S. Brand Names Fanapt™

Pharmacologic Category Antipsychotic Agent, Atypical

Use Acute treatment of schizophrenia

Additional Information Complete prescribing information for this medication should be consulted for additional detail.

Product Availability Fanapt™: FDA approved May 2009; availability expected by early 2010; consult prescribing information for additional information

Iloprost (EYE loe prost)

U.S. Brand Names Ventavis®

Index Terms Iloprost Tromethamine; Prostacyclin PGI$_2$

Pharmacologic Category Prostacyclin; Prostaglandin; Vasodilator

Generic Available No

Use Treatment of idiopathic pulmonary arterial hypertension in patients with NYHA Class III or IV symptoms

◀ **Mechanism of Action** Acutely, iloprost dilates systemic and pulmonary arterial vascular beds. With longer-term use, alters pulmonary vascular resistance and suppresses vascular smooth muscle proliferation. In addition, it is a mild endogenous inhibitor of platelet aggregation when aerosolized (Beghetti, 2002).

Pharmacodynamics/Kinetics

Duration: 30-60 minutes

Distribution: V_d: 0.7-0.8 L/kg

Protein binding: ~60%, primarily to albumin

Metabolism: Hepatic via beta oxidation of the carboxyl side chain; main metabolite, tetranor-iloprost (inactive in animal studies)

Half-life elimination: 20-30 minutes (effect), 7-9 minutes (elimination)

Time to peak, serum: Within 5 minutes after inhalation

Excretion: Urine (68% as metabolite); feces (12%)

Dosage Inhalation: Adults: Initial: 2.5 mcg/dose; if tolerated, increase to 5 mcg/dose; administer 6-9 times daily (dosing at intervals ≥2 hours while awake according to individual need and tolerability); maintenance dose: 2.5-5 mcg/dose; maximum daily dose: 45 mcg

Dosage adjustment in renal impairment: Adjustments are not necessary. Use caution in dialysis patients; may be more susceptible to hypotension.

Dosage adjustment in hepatic impairment: Use caution

Stability Store at controlled room temperature of 20°C to 25°C (68°F to 77°F).

Administration Do not mix with other medications. For inhalation only via the I-neb™ AAD® System or Prodose® AAD® System. Transfer entire contents of ampul into the medication chamber. Only use 1 mL ampul with I-neb™ AAD® System. After use, discard remainder of the medicine; not for reuse.

Monitoring Parameters Heart rate, blood pressure, and respiratory rate at baseline, with initiation and dosage adjustments. Monitor for improvements in pulmonary function, improved exercise tolerance, NYHA Class improvement; side effects

Pregnancy Risk Factor C

Contraindications There are no contraindications listed within the FDA-approved labeling.

Warnings/Precautions Intended for inhalation administration using only the I-neb™ AAD® System or Prodose® AAD® System. Solution should not come in contact with skin or eyes. Monitor vital signs during initiation. Avoid use in patients with hypotension (systolic BP <85 mm Hg). Use caution with concurrent conditions or medications that may increase risk of syncope. Dosage or therapy adjustment may be required if exertional syncope occurs. If pulmonary edema occurs during administration, discontinue therapy immediately. Use caution in patients with active bleeding or at increased risk of bleeding; mild inhibitor of platelet aggregation. Use caution in dialysis patients and in those with Child-Pugh classes B and C hepatic dysfunction. Safety and efficacy have not been established in patients with other concurrent pulmonary diseases (eg, COPD, severe asthma, or acute pulmonary infections); may induce bronchospasm in patients with hyper-reactive airways. Not FDA labeled for use in children.

Adverse Reactions

>10%:

Cardiovascular: Flushing (27%), hypotension (11%)

Central nervous system: Headache (30%)

Gastrointestinal: Nausea (13%)

Neuromuscular & skeletal: Trismus (12%), jaw pain (12%)

Respiratory: Cough increased (39%)

Miscellaneous: Flu-like syndrome (14%)

1% to 10%:

Cardiovascular: Syncope (8%), palpitation (7%)

Central nervous system: Insomnia (8%)

Gastrointestinal: Vomiting (7%)

Hepatic: Alkaline phosphatase increased (6%), GGT increased (6%)

Neuromuscular & skeletal: Back pain (7%), muscle cramps (6%)

Respiratory: Hemoptysis (5%), pneumonia (4%)

<1% (Limited to important or life-threatening): Bronchospasm, chest pain, CHF, diarrhea, dizziness, dyspnea, epistaxis, gingival bleeding, kidney failure,

paradoxical reaction (increased PVR), peripheral edema, supraventricular tachycardia, wheezing

Drug Interactions

Avoid Concomitant Use There are no known interactions where it is recommended to avoid concomitant use.

Increased Effect/Toxicity

Iloprost may increase the levels/effects of: Anticoagulants; Antihypertensives; Antiplatelet Agents

Decreased Effect There are no known significant interactions involving a decrease in effect.

Dosage Forms Excipient information presented when available (limited, particularly for generics); consult specific product labeling.

Solution for oral inhalation [preservative-free]:

Ventavis®: 10 mcg/mL (1 mL, 2 mL) [ampul]

References

Badesch DB, Abman SH, Ahearn GS, et al, "Medical Therapy for Pulmonary Arterial Hypertension: ACCP Evidence-Based Clinical Practice Guidelines," *Chest*, 2004, 126(1 Suppl):35-62.

Emmel M, Keuth B, and Schickendantz S, "Paradoxical Increase of Pulmonary Vascular Resistance During Testing of Inhaled Iloprost," *Heart*, 2004, 90(1):e2.

Humbert M, Sitbon O, and Simmoneau G, "Treatment of Pulmonary Arterial hypertension," *N Engl J Med*, 2004, 351(14):1425-36.

Olschewski H, Simonneau G, Galie N, et al, "Inhaled Iloprost for Severe Pulmonary Hypertension," *N Engl J Med*, 2002, 347(5):322-9.

◆ **Iloprost Tromethamine** *see* Iloprost *on page 725*

◆ **Imdur®** *see* Isosorbide Mononitrate *on page 774*

◆ **Imipemide** *see* Imipenem and Cilastatin *on page 727*

Imipenem and Cilastatin (i mi PEN em & sye la STAT in)

Medication Safety Issues

Sound-alike/look-alike issues:

Imipenem may be confused with ertapenem, meropenem

Primaxin® may be confused with Premarin®, Primacor®

U.S. Brand Names Primaxin®

Canadian Brand Names Primaxin®; Primaxin® I.V.

Index Terms Imipemide

Pharmacologic Category Antibiotic, Carbapenem

Generic Available No

Use Treatment of lower respiratory tract, urinary tract, intra-abdominal, gynecologic, bone and joint, skin and skin structure, and polymicrobic infections as well as bacterial septicemia and endocarditis. Antibacterial activity includes resistant gram-negative bacilli (*Pseudomonas aeruginosa* and *Enterobacter* sp), gram-positive bacteria (methicillin-sensitive *Staphylococcus aureus* and *Streptococcus* sp) and anaerobes.

Unlabeled/Investigational Use Hepatic abscess; neutropenic fever; melioidosis

Mechanism of Action Inhibits bacterial cell wall synthesis by binding to one or more of the penicillin binding proteins (PBPs); which in turn inhibits the final transpeptidation step of peptidoglycan synthesis in bacterial cell walls, thus inhibiting cell wall biosynthesis. Bacteria eventually lyse due to ongoing activity of cell wall autolytic enzymes (autolysins and murein hydrolases) while cell wall assembly is arrested. Cilastatin prevents renal metabolism of imipenem by competitive inhibition of dehydropeptidase along the brush border of the renal tubules.

Pharmacodynamics/Kinetics

Absorption: I.M.: Imipenem: 60% to 75%; cilastatin: 95% to 100%

Distribution: Rapidly and widely to most tissues and fluids including sputum, pleural fluid, peritoneal fluid, interstitial fluid, bile, aqueous humor, and bone; highest concentrations in pleural fluid, interstitial fluid, and peritoneal fluid; low concentrations in CSF

Protein binding: Imipenem: 20%; cilastatin: 40%

Metabolism: Imipenem is metabolized in the kidney by dehydropeptidase I; cilastatin prevents imipenem metabolism by this enzyme; cilastatin is partially metabolized renally

Half-life elimination: I.V.: Both drugs: 60 minutes; prolonged with renal impairment; I.M.: Imipenem: 2-3 hours

Time to peak: I.M.: 3.5 hours

Excretion: Both drugs: Urine (~70% as unchanged drug)

Dosage

Usual dosage ranges: Note: Dosage based on **imipenem** content:

Neonates ≤3 months and weight ≥1500 g: Non-CNS infections: I.V.:

<1 week: 25 mg/kg every 12 hours

1-4 weeks: 25 mg/kg every 8 hours

4 weeks to 3 months: 25 mg/kg every 6 hours

Children >3 months: Non-CNS infections: I.V.: 15-25 mg/kg every 6 hours; maximum dosage: Susceptible infections: 2 g/day; moderately-susceptible organisms: 4 g/day

Adults:

I.M.: 500-750 mg every 12 hours; maximum: 1500 mg/day

I.V.: Weight ≥70 kg: 250-1000 mg every 6-8 hours; maximum: 4 g/day. **Note:** For adults weighing <70 kg, refer to Dosing Adjustment in Renal Impairment:

Indication-specific dosing: Note: Doses based on imipenem content. I.M. administration is not intended for severe or life-threatening infections (eg, septicemia, endocarditis, shock), UTI, bone/joint or polymicrobic infections:

Children: I.V.:

Burkholderia mallei (melioidosis) (unlabeled use): 20 mg/kg every 8 hours for 10 days

Cystic fibrosis: Doses up to 90 mg/kg/day have been used

Adults:

Burkholderia mallei (melioidosis) (unlabeled use): I.V.: 20 mg/kg (up to 1 g) every 6-8 hours for 10 days

Intra-abdominal infections:

I.V.: Mild infection: 250-500 mg every 6 hours; severe: 500 mg every 6 hours

I.M.: Mild-to-moderate infection: 750 mg every 12 hours

Liver abscess (unlabeled use): I.V.: 500 mg every 6 hours for 2-3 weeks, then appropriate oral therapy for a total of 4-6 weeks

Lower respiratory tract, skin/skin structure, gynecologic infections: I.M.: Mild/moderate: 500-750 mg every 12 hours

Mild infection: Note: Rarely a suitable option in mild infections; normally reserved for moderate-severe cases:

I.M.: 500 mg every 12 hours

I.V.:

Fully-susceptible organisms: 250 mg every 6 hours

Moderately-susceptible organisms: 500 mg every 6 hours

Moderate infection:

I.M.: 750 mg every 12 hours

I.V.:

Fully-susceptible organisms: 500 mg every 6-8 hours

Moderately-susceptible organisms: 500 mg every 6 hours or 1 g every 8 hours

Neutropenic fever (unlabeled use): I.V.: 500 mg every 6 hours

Pseudomonas **infections:** I.V.: 500 mg every 6 hours; **Note:** Higher doses may be required based on organism sensitivity.

Severe infection: I.V.:

Fully-susceptible organisms: 500 mg every 6 hours

Moderately-susceptible organisms: 1 g every 6-8 hours

Maximum daily dose should not exceed 50 mg/kg or 4 g/day, whichever is lower

Urinary tract infection: I.V.:

Uncomplicated: 250 mg every 6 hours

Complicated: 500 mg every 6 hours

Dosage adjustment in renal impairment: I.V.: **Note:** Adjustments have not been established for I.M. dosing:

Patients with a Cl_{cr} ≤5 mL/minute/1.73 m^2 should not receive imipenem/cilastatin unless hemodialysis is instituted within 48 hours.

Patients weighing <30 kg with impaired renal function should not receive imipenem/cilastatin.

Hemodialysis: Use the dosing recommendation for patients with a Cl_{cr} 6-20 mL/ minute; administer dose after dialysis session and every 12 hours thereafter

Peritoneal dialysis: Dose as for Cl_{cr} 6-20 mL/minute

Continuous renal replacement therapy (CRRT): Drug clearance is highly dependent on the method of renal replacement, filter type, and flow rate. Appropriate dosing requires close monitoring of pharmacologic response, signs of adverse reactions due to drug accumulation, as well as drug levels in relation to target trough (if appropriate). The following are general recommendations only (based on dialysate flow/ultrafiltration rates of 1 L/ hour) and should not supersede clinical judgment:

CVVH: 250 mg every 6 hours or 500 mg every 8 hours

CVVHD/CVVHDF: 250 mg every 6 hours or 500 mg every 6-8 hours

Note: Data suggest that 500 mg every 12 hours may provide sufficient T>MIC to cover organisms with MIC values ≤2 mg/L; however, a higher dose of 500 mg every 6 hours is recommended for resistant organisms (particularly *Pseudomonas*) with MIC ≥4 mg/L (Fish, 2005).

Dosage adjustment in hepatic impairment: Hepatic dysfunction may further impair cilastatin clearance; consider decreasing the dosing frequency.

See table.

Imipenem and Cilastatin Dosage in Renal Impairment

Reduced I.V. Dosage Regimen Based on Creatinine Clearance (mL/minute/1.73 m^2) and/or Body Weight <70 kg				
Body Weight (kg)				
≥70	60	50	40	30
Total daily dose for normal renal function: 1 g/day				
Cl_{cr} ≥71	250 mg q6h	250 mg q8h	125 mg q6h	125 mg q6h	125 mg q8h
Cl_{cr} 41-70	250 mg q8h	125 mg q6h	125 mg q6h	125 mg q8h	125 mg q8h
Cl_{cr} 21-40	250 mg q12h	250 mg q12h	125 mg q8h	125 mg q12h	125 mg q12h
Cl_{cr} 6-20	250 mg q12h	125 mg q12h	125 mg q12h	125 mg q12h	125 mg q12h
Total daily dose for normal renal function: 1.5 g/day				
Cl_{cr} ≥71	500 mg q8h	250 mg q6h	250 mg q6h	250 mg q8h	125 mg q6h
Cl_{cr} 41-70	250 mg q6h	250 mg q8h	250 mg q8h	125 mg q6h	125 mg q8h
Cl_{cr} 21-40	250 mg q8h	250 mg q8h	250 mg q12h	125 mg q8h	125 mg q8h
Cl_{cr} 6-20	250 mg q12h	250 mg q12h	250 mg q12h	125 mg q12h	125 mg q12h
Total daily dose for normal renal function: 2 g/day				
Cl_{cr} ≥71	500 mg q6h	500 mg q8h	250 mg q6h	250 mg q6h	250 mg q8h
Cl_{cr} 41-70	500 mg q8h	250 mg q6h	250 mg q6h	250 mg q8h	250 mg q6h
Cl_{cr} 21-40	250 mg q6h	250 mg q8h	250 mg q8h	250 mg q12h	125 mg q6h
Cl_{cr} 6-20	250 mg q12h	250 mg q12h	250 mg q12h	250 mg q12h	125 mg q12h
Total daily dose for normal renal function: 3 g/day				
Cl_{cr} ≥71	1000 mg q8h	750 mg q8h	500 mg q6h	500 mg q8h	250 mg q6h
Cl_{cr} 41-70	500 mg q6h	500 mg q8h	500 mg q8h	250 mg q6h	250 mg q8h
Cl_{cr} 21-40	500 mg q8h	500 mg q8h	250 mg q6h	250 mg q8h	250 mg q8h
Cl_{cr} 6-20	500 mg q12h	500 mg q12h	250 mg q12h	250 mg q12h	250 mg q12h
Total daily dose for normal renal function: 4 g/day				
Cl_{cr} ≥71	1000 mg q8h	1000 mg q8h	750 mg q8h	500 mg q6h	500 mg q8h
Cl_{cr} 41-70	750 mg q8h	750 mg q8h	500 mg q6h	500 mg q8h	250 mg q6h
Cl_{cr} 21-40	500 mg q6h	500 mg q8h	500 mg q8h	250 mg q6h	250 mg q8h
Cl_{cr} 6-20	500 mg q12h	500 mg q12h	500 mg q12h	250 mg q12h	250 mg q12h

◀ **Stability** Imipenem/cilastatin powder for injection should be stored at <25°C (77°F).

I.M.: Prepare 500 mg vial with 2 mL 1% lidocaine (do not use lidocaine with epinephrine). The I.V. formulation does not form a stable suspension in lidocaine and cannot be used to prepare an I.M dose. The I.M. suspension should be used within 1 hour of reconstitution.

I.V.: Prior to use, dilute dose into 100-250 mL of an appropriate solution. Imipenem is inactivated at acidic or alkaline pH. Final concentration should not exceed 5 mg/mL. The I.M. formulation is not buffered and cannot be used to prepare I.V. solutions. Reconstituted I.V. solutions are stable for 4 hours at room temperature and 24 hours when refrigerated. Do not freeze.

Administration

I.M.: **Note:** I.M. administration is not intended for severe or life-threatening infections (eg, septicemia, endocarditis, shock). Administer by deep injection into a large muscle (gluteal or lateral thigh). **Only the I.M. formulation can be used for I.M. administration.**

I.V.: Do not administer I.V. push. Infuse doses ≤500 mg over 20-30 minutes; infuse doses ≥750 mg over 40-60 minutes. **Only the I.V. formulation can be used for I.V. administration.**

Monitoring Parameters Periodic renal, hepatic, and hematologic function tests; monitor for signs of anaphylaxis during first dose

Pregnancy Risk Factor C

Contraindications Hypersensitivity to imipenem/cilastatin or any component of the formulation

I.M. formulation (due to lidocaine diluent) additional contraindications: Hypersensitivity to amide-type anesthetics; severe shock or heart block

Warnings/Precautions Dosage adjustment required in patients with impaired renal function; elderly patients often require lower doses (adjust carefully to renal function). Prolonged use may result in fungal or bacterial superinfection, including *C. difficile*-associated diarrhea (CDAD) and pseudomembranous colitis; CDAD has been observed >2 months postantibiotic treatment. Has been associated with CNS adverse effects, including confusional states and seizures (myoclonic); use with caution in patients with a history of seizures or hypersensitivity to beta-lactams (including penicillins and cephalosporins); patients with impaired renal function are at increased risk of seizures if not properly dose adjusted. Not recommended in pediatric CNS infections due to seizure potential. Serious hypersensitivity reactions, including anaphylaxis, have been reported (some without a history of previous allergic reactions to beta-lactams). Doses for I.M. administration are mixed with lidocaine; consult information on lidocaine for associated warnings/precautions. Two different imipenem/cilastatin products are available; due to differences in formulation, the I.V. and I.M. preparations **cannot** be interchanged. Safety and efficacy of I.M. administration in children <12 years of age have not been established.

Adverse Reactions Adverse reactions reported with use for both I.V. and I.M. formulations in adults, except where noted.

1% to 10%:

Cardiovascular: Tachycardia (infants 2%; adults <1%)

Central nervous system: Seizure (infants 6%; adults <1%)

Dermatologic: Rash (≤1%, children 2%)

Gastrointestinal: Nausea (1% to 2%), diarrhea (children 3% to 4%; adults 1% to 2%), vomiting (≤2%)

Genitourinary: Oliguria/anuria (infants 2%; adults <1%)

Local: Phlebitis/thrombophlebitis (3%), pain at I.M. injection site (1.2%)

<1% (Limited to important or life-threatening): Abdominal pain, abnormal urinalysis, acute renal failure, alkaline phosphatase increased, anaphylaxis, anemia, angioneurotic edema, asthenia, bilirubin increased, bone marrow depression, BUN/creatinine increased, candidiasis, confusion, cyanosis, dizziness, drug fever, dyspnea, encephalopathy, eosinophilia, erythema multiforme, fever, flushing, gastroenteritis, glossitis, hallucinations, headache, hearing loss, hematocrit decreased, hemoglobin decreased, hemolytic anemia, hemorrhagic colitis, hepatitis (including fulminant onset), hepatic failure, hyperchloremia, hyperhidrosis, hyperkalemia, hypersensitivity, hyperventilation, hyponatremia, hypotension, injection site erythema, jaundice, lactate dehydrogenase increased, leukocytosis, leukopenia, myoclonus, neutropenia (including

agranulocytosis), palpitation, pancytopenia, paresthesia, pharyngeal pain, polyarthralgia, polyuria, positive Coombs' test, prothrombin time increased, pruritus, pruritus vulvae, pseudomembranous colitis, psychic disturbances, rash, resistant *P. aeruginosa*, salivation increased, somnolence, staining of teeth, Stevens-Johnson syndrome, taste perversion, thoracic spine pain, thrombocythemia, thrombocytopenia, tinnitus, tongue/tooth discoloration, tongue papillar hypertrophy, toxic epidermal necrolysis, transaminases increased, tremor, urine discoloration, urticaria, vertigo

Drug Interactions

Avoid Concomitant Use

Avoid concomitant use of Imipenem and Cilastatin with any of the following: Ganciclovir

Increased Effect/Toxicity

The levels/effects of Imipenem and Cilastatin may be increased by: Ganciclovir; Uricosuric Agents

Decreased Effect

Imipenem and Cilastatin may decrease the levels/effects of: Typhoid Vaccine; Valproic Acid

Test Interactions Interferes with urinary glucose determination using Clinitest®

Dietary Considerations Sodium content of 500 mg injection:

I.M.: 32 mg (1.4 mEq)

I.V.: 37.5 mg (1.6 mEq)

Dosage Forms Excipient information presented when available (limited, particularly for generics); consult specific product labeling.

Injection, powder for reconstitution [I.M.]:

Primaxin®: Imipenem 500 mg and cilastatin 500 mg [contains sodium 32 mg (1.4 mEq)]

Injection, powder for reconstitution [I.V.]:

Primaxin®: Imipenem 250 mg and cilastatin 250 mg [contains sodium 18.8 mg (0.8 mEq)]; imipenem 500 mg and cilastatin 500 mg [contains sodium 37.5 mg (1.6 mEq)]

References

American Thoracic Society and Infectious Diseases Society of America, "Guidelines for the Management of Adults With Hospital-Acquired, Ventilator-Associated, and Healthcare-Associated Pneumonia," *Am J Respir Crit Care Med*, 2005, 171(4):388-416.

Tegeder I, Bremer F, Oelkers R, et al, "Pharmacokinetics of Imipenem-Cilastatin in Critically Ill Patients Undergoing continuous Veno-Venous Hemofiltration," *Antimicrob Agents Chemother*, 1997, 41(12):2640-5.

Imipramine (im IP ra meen)

Related Information

Antidepressant Agents *on page 1660*

Chronic Pain Management *on page 1546*

U.S. Brand Names Tofranil-PM®; Tofranil®

Canadian Brand Names Apo-Imipramine®; Novo-Pramine; Tofranil®

Index Terms Imipramine Hydrochloride; Imipramine Pamoate

Pharmacologic Category Antidepressant, Tricyclic (Tertiary Amine)

Use Treatment of depression; treatment of nocturnal enuresis in children

Unlabeled/Investigational Use Analgesic for certain chronic and neuropathic pain; panic disorder; attention-deficit/hyperactivity disorder (ADHD); post-traumatic stress disorder (PTSD)

Pharmacodynamics/Kinetics

Onset of action: Peak antidepressant effect: Usually after ≥2 weeks

Absorption: Well absorbed

Distribution: Crosses placenta

Metabolism: Hepatic, primarily via CYP2D6 to desipramine (active) and other metabolites; significant first-pass effect

Half-life elimination: 6-18 hours

Excretion: Urine (as metabolites)

Dosage Oral:
Children:
Depression (unlabeled use): 1.5 mg/kg/day with dosage increments of 1 mg/kg every 3-4 days to a maximum dose of 5 mg/kg/day in 1-4 divided doses; monitor carefully especially with doses ≥3.5 mg/kg/day
Enuresis: ≥6 years: Initial: 25 mg at bedtime, if inadequate response still seen after 1 week of therapy, increase by 25 mg/day; dose should not exceed 2.5 mg/kg/day or 50 mg at bedtime if 6-12 years of age or 75 mg at bedtime if ≥12 years of age
Adjunct in the treatment of cancer pain (unlabeled use): Initial: 0.2-0.4 mg/kg at bedtime; dose may be increased by 50% every 2-3 days up to 1-3 mg/kg/dose at bedtime
Adolescents: Depression: Initial: 25-50 mg/day; increase gradually; maximum: 100 mg/day in single or divided doses
Adults:
Depression:
Outpatients: Initial: 75 mg/day; may increase gradually to 150 mg/day. May be given in divided doses or as a single bedtime dose; maximum: 200 mg/day
Inpatients: Initial: 100-150 mg/day; may increase gradually to 200 mg/day; if no response after 2 weeks, may further increase to 250-300 mg/day. May be given in divided doses or as a single bedtime dose; maximum: 300 mg/day.
Post-traumatic stress disorder (PTSD) (unlabeled use): 75-200 mg/day
Elderly: Depression: Initial: 25-50 mg at bedtime; may increase every 3 days for inpatients and weekly for outpatients if tolerated to a recommended maximum of 100 mg/day.
Additional Information Complete prescribing information for this medication should be consulted for additional detail.
Dosage Forms Excipient information presented when available (limited, particularly for generics); consult specific product labeling.
Capsule, as pamoate: 75 mg, 100 mg, 125 mg, 150 mg
Tofranil-PM®: 75 mg, 100 mg, 125 mg, 150 mg
Tablet, as hydrochloride: 10 mg, 25 mg, 50 mg
Tofranil®): 10 mg, 25 mg, 50 mg

◆ **Imipramine Hydrochloride** *see* Imipramine *on page 731*
◆ **Imipramine Pamoate** *see* Imipramine *on page 731*
◆ **Imitrex®** *see* SUMAtriptan *on page 1336*
◆ **Imitrex® DF (Can)** *see* SUMAtriptan *on page 1336*
◆ **Imitrex® Nasal Spray (Can)** *see* SUMAtriptan *on page 1336*

Immune Globulin (Intravenous) (i MYUN GLOB yoo lin, IN tra VEE nus)

Medication Safety Issues
Sound-alike/look-alike issues:
Gamimune® N may be confused with CytoGam®
Immune globulin (intravenous) may be confused with hepatitis B immune globulin
U.S. Brand Names Carimune® NF; Flebogamma®; Gammagard Liquid; Gammagard S/D; Gamunex®; Octagam®; Privigen™
Canadian Brand Names Gamimune® N; Gammagard Liquid; Gammagard S/D; Gamunex®; IGIVnex®; Privigen™
Index Terms IGIV; IV Immune Globulin; IVIG; Panglobulin
Pharmacologic Category Blood Product Derivative; Immune Globulin
Generic Available No
Use
Treatment of primary immunodeficiency syndromes (congenital agammaglobulinemia, severe combined immunodeficiency syndromes [SCIDS], common variable immunodeficiency, X-linked immunodeficiency, Wiskott-Aldrich syndrome) (Carimune® NF, Flebogamma®, Gammagard Liquid, Gammagard S/D, Gamunex®, Octagam®, Privigen™)
Treatment of immune (idiopathic) thrombocytopenic purpura (ITP) (Carimune® NF, Gammagard S/D, Gamunex®, Privigen™)

Treatment of chronic inflammatory demyelinating polyneuropathy (CIDP) (Gamunex®)

Prevention of coronary artery aneurysms associated with Kawasaki disease (in combination with aspirin) (Gammagard S/D)

Prevention of bacterial infection in B-cell chronic lymphocytic leukemia (CLL) (Gammagard S/D)

Unlabeled/Investigational Use Prevention of serious bacterial infections among HIV-infected children with hypogammaglobulinemia (IgG <400 mg/dL) (CDC guidelines); hematopoietic stem cell transplantation (HSCT), to prevent bacterial infections among allogeneic recipients with severe hypogammaglobulinemia (IgG <400 mg/dL) at <100 days post transplant (CDC guidelines); fetal-neonatal alloimmune thrombocytopenia; Guillain-Barré syndrome; pregnancy-associated ITP; prevention of gastroenteritis in children; multiple sclerosis (relapsing, remitting when other therapies cannot be used); hemolytic disease of the newborn; HIV-associated thrombocytopenia; acquired hypogammaglobulinemia secondary to malignancy; myasthenia gravis; refractory dermatomyositis/polymyositis

Mechanism of Action Replacement therapy for primary and secondary immunodeficiencies; interference with F_c receptors on the cells of the reticuloendothelial system for autoimmune cytopenias and ITP; possible role of contained antiviral-type antibodies

Pharmacodynamics/Kinetics

Onset of action: I.V.: Provides immediate antibody levels

Duration: Immune effect: 3-4 weeks (variable)

Distribution: V_d: 0.09-0.13 L/kg

Intravascular portion (primarily): Healthy subjects: 41% to 57%; Patients with congenital humoral immunodeficiencies: ~70%

Half-life elimination: IgG (variable among patients): Healthy subjects: 14-24 days; Patients with congenital humoral immunodeficiencies: 26-40 days; hypermetabolism associated with fever and infection have coincided with a shortened half-life

Dosage Approved doses and regimens may vary between brands; check manufacturer guidelines. **Note:** Some clinicians dose IVIG on ideal body weight or an adjusted ideal body weight in morbidly-obese patients.

Children: I.V.: Pediatric HIV, prevention of infection (CDC guidelines): 400 mg/kg every 2-4 weeks

Children and Adults: I.V.:

Primary immunodeficiency disorders: **Note:** Adjust dose/frequency based desired IgG levels and clinical response:

General dosing range: 200-800 mg/kg per month

Carimune® NF: 200 mg/kg every 4 weeks. May increase dose to 300 mg/kg every 4 weeks or may increase frequency based on patient response.

Flebogamma®, Gammagard Liquid, Gammagard S/D, Gamunex®, Octagam®: 300-600 mg/kg every 3-4 weeks; adjusted based on dosage and interval in conjunction with monitored serum IgG concentrations

Privigen™: 200-800 mg/kg every 3-4 weeks; adjusted based on dosage and interval in conjunction with monitored serum IgG concentrations

B-cell chronic lymphocytic leukemia (CLL) (Gammagard S/D): 400 mg/kg/dose every 3-4 weeks

Immune (idiopathic) thrombocytopenic purpura (ITP):

Carimune® NF:

Acute: 400 mg/kg/day for 2-5 days

Chronic: 400 mg/kg as needed to maintain platelet count ≥30,000/mm³ or to control significant bleeding; may increase dose if needed (range: 800-1000 mg/kg)

Gammagard S/D: 1000 mg/kg; adjust additional doses based on patient response or platelet count. Up to 3 separate doses may be administered on alternate days if required.

Gamunex®: 1000 mg/kg/day for 1-2 days, **or** 400 mg/kg/day for 5 days

Privigen™: 1000 mg/kg/day for 2 consecutive days

Chronic inflammatory demyelinating polyneuropathy (CIDP): Gamunex®: Loading dose: 2000 mg/kg divided over 2-4 consecutive days; Maintenance: 1000 mg/kg/day for 1 day every 3 weeks **or** 500 mg/kg/day for 2 consecutive days every 3 weeks

▶

◄   Kawasaki disease: Initiate IVIG therapy within 10 days of disease onset: Must be used in combination with aspirin: 80-100 mg/kg/day in 4 divided doses for 14 days; when fever subsides, dose aspirin at 3-5 mg/kg once daily for ≥6-8 weeks

AHA guidelines: 2000 mg/kg as a single dose

Gammagard S/D: 1000 mg/kg as a single dose administered over 10 hours, **or** 400 mg/kg/day for 4 days. Begin within 7 days of onset of fever.

Unlabeled uses:

Acquired hypogammaglobulinemia secondary to malignancy (unlabeled use): Adults: 400 mg/kg/dose every 3 weeks; reevaluate every 4-6 months

Guillain-Barré syndrome (unlabeled use): Children and Adults: Various regimens have been used, including:

400 mg/kg/day for 5 days

or

2000 mg/kg in divided doses administered over 2 days

Hematopoietic stem cell transplantation with hypogammaglobulinemia (CDC guidelines):

Children: 400 mg/kg per month; increase dose or frequency to maintain IgG levels >400 mg/dL

Adolescents and Adults: 500 mg/kg/week

HIV-associated thrombocytopenia (unlabeled use): Adults: 1000 mg/kg/day for 2 days

Multiple sclerosis (relapsing-remitting, when other therapies cannot be used) (unlabeled use): Adults: 1000 mg/kg per month, with or without an induction of 400 mg/kg/day for 5 days

Myasthenia gravis (severe exacerbation) (unlabeled use): Adults: Total dose of 2000 mg/kg over 2-5 days

Refractory dermatomyositis (unlabeled use): Adults: 2000 mg/kg per month administered over 2-5 days

Refractory polymyositis (unlabeled use): Adults: 2000 mg/kg per course administered over 2-5 days

Dosing adjustment/comments in renal impairment: Cl_{cr} <10 mL/minute: Avoid use; in patients at risk of renal dysfunction, consider infusion at a rate less than maximum.

Stability Stability is dependent upon the manufacturer and brand. Do not freeze. Dilution is dependent upon the manufacturer and brand. Gently swirl; do not shake; avoid foaming. Do not mix products from different manufacturers together. Discard unused portion of vials.

Carimune® NF: Prior to reconstitution, store at or below 30°C (86°F). Reconstitute with NS, D_5W, or SWFI. Following reconstitution, store under refrigeration. Begin infusion within 24 hours.

Flebogamma®: Store at 2°C to 25°C (36°F to 77°F). Dilution is not recommended.

Gammagard Liquid: May dilute in D_5W only. Prior to use, store at 2°C to 8°C (36°F to 46°F) for up to 36 months; do not freeze. May store at room temperature of 25°C (77°F) within the first 24 months of manufacturing. Storage time at room temperature varies with length of time previously refrigerated; refer to product labeling for details.

Gammagard S/D: Store at ≤25°C (≤77°F). Reconstitute with SWFI; may store diluted solution under refrigeration for up to 24 hours.

Gamunex®: May be stored for up to 36 months at 2°C to 8°C (36°F to 46°F); may be stored at ≤25°C (≤77°F) for up to 6 months. Dilute in D_5W only.

Octagam®: Store at 2°C to 25°C (36°F to 77°F).

Privigen™: Store at ≤25°C (≤77°F); do not freeze (do not use if previously frozen). Protect from light. If necessary to further dilute, D_5W may be used.

Administration I.V. infusion over 2-24 hours; for initial treatment, a lower concentration and/or a slower rate of infusion should be used. Initial rate of administration and titration is specific to each IVIG product. Consult specific product prescribing information for detailed recommendations.Administer in separate infusion line from other medications; if using primary line, flush with saline prior administration. Refrigerated product should be warmed to room temperature prior to infusion. Some products require filtration; refer to individual product labeling. Antecubital veins should be used, especially with concentrations

≥10% to prevent injection site discomfort. Decrease dose, rate and/or concentration of infusion in patients who may be at risk of renal failure. Decreasing the rate or stopping the infusion may help relieve some adverse effects (flushing, changes in pulse rate, changes in blood pressure). Epinephrine should be available during administration.

Monitoring Parameters Renal function, urine output, hemoglobin and hematocrit, platelets (in patients with ITP); infusion-related adverse reactions, anaphylaxis, signs and symptoms of hemolysis; blood viscosity (in patients at risk for hyperviscosity); presence of antineutrophil antibodies (if TRALI is suspected)

Pregnancy Risk Factor C

Contraindications Hypersensitivity to immune globulin or any component of the formulation; selective IgA deficiency; hyperprolinemia (Privigen™)

Warnings/Precautions [U.S. Boxed Warning]: Acute renal dysfunction (increased serum creatinine, oliguria, acute renal failure, osmotic nephrosis) can rarely occur; usually within 7 days of use (more likely with products stabilized with sucrose). Use with caution in the elderly, patients with renal disease, diabetes mellitus, volume depletion, sepsis, paraproteinemia, and nephrotoxic medications due to risk of renal dysfunction. In patients at risk of renal dysfunction, the rate of infusion and concentration of solution should be minimized. discontinue if renal function deteriorates. High-dose regimens (1000 mg/kg for 1-2 days) are not recommended for individuals with fluid overload or where fluid volume may be of concern. Hypersensitivity and anaphylactic reactions can occur; immediate treatment (including epinephrine 1:1000) should be available; product of human plasma; may potentially contain infectious agents which could transmit disease. Screening of donors, as well as testing and/or inactivation or removal of certain viruses, reduces the risk. Infections thought to be transmitted by this product should be reported to the manufacturer. Aseptic meningitis may occur with high doses (≥2 g/kg); syndrome usually appears within several hours to 2 days following treatment; usually resolves within several days after IVIG is discontinued; patients with a migraine history may be at higher risk for AMS.

Intravenous immune globulin has been associated with antiglobulin hemolysis; monitor for signs of hemolytic anemia. Patients should be adequately hydrated prior to initiation of therapy. Hyperproteinemia, increased serum viscosity and hyponatremia may occur; distinguish hyponatremia from pseudohyponatremia to prevent volume depletion and further increase in serum viscosity. Use caution in patients with a history of thrombotic events or a history of atherosclerosis or cardiovascular disease or patients with known/suspected hyperviscosity; there is clinical evidence of a possible association between thrombotic events and administration of intravenous immune globulin. Consider a baseline assessment of blood viscosity in patients at risk for hyperviscosity. For intravenous administration only. Patients should be monitored for adverse events during and after the infusion. Stop administration with signs of infusion reaction (fever, chills, nausea, vomiting, and rarely shock). Risk may be increased with initial treatment, when switching brands of immune globulin, and with treatment interruptions of >8 weeks. Monitor for transfusion-related acute lung injury (TRALI); noncardiogenic pulmonary edema has been reported with intravenous immune globulin use. TRALI is characterized by severe respiratory distress, pulmonary edema, hypoxemia, and fever (in the presence of normal left ventricular function) and usually occurs within 1-6 hours after infusion. Response to live vaccinations may be impaired. Some products may contain maltose, which may result in falsely-elevated blood glucose readings. Some products may contain sucrose. Some products may contain sorbitol; do not use in patients with fructose intolerance. Privigen™ contains the stabilizer L-proline and is contraindicated in patients with hyperprolinemia. Packaging of some products may contain natural latex/natural rubber.

Adverse Reactions Frequency not defined.

Cardiovascular: Chest tightness, edema, flushing of the face, hyper-/hypotension, palpitation, tachycardia

Central nervous system: Anxiety, aseptic meningitis syndrome, chills, dizziness, drowsiness, fatigue, fever, headache, irritability, lethargy, lightheadedness, malaise, migraine, pain

Dermatologic: Bruising, petechiae, pruritus, purpura, rash, urticaria

◄ Gastrointestinal: Abdominal cramps, abdominal pain, diarrhea, discomfort, dyspepsia, nausea, sore throat, vomiting

Hematologic: Anemia, autoimmune hemolytic anemia, hematocrit decreased, hemolysis (mild), hemorrhage, thrombocytopenia

Hepatic: Bilirubin increased, LDH increased, liver function test increased

Local: Pain or irritation at the infusion site

Neuromuscular & skeletal: Arthralgia, back or hip pain, leg cramps, muscle cramps, myalgia, neck pain, weakness

Otic: Ear pain

Renal: Acute renal failure, acute tubular necrosis, anuria, BUN increased, creatinine increased, oliguria, proximal tubular nephropathy, osmotic nephrosis

Respiratory: Asthma aggravated, bronchitis, cough, dyspnea, epistaxis, nasal congestion, pharyngeal pain, pharyngitis, rhinitis, rhinorrhea, sinus headache, sinusitis, upper respiratory infection, wheezing

Miscellaneous: Anaphylaxis, diaphoresis, flu-like syndrome, hypersensitivity reactions, infusion reaction

Postmarketing and/or case reports: Apnea, ARDS, autoimmune pure red cell aplasia (PRCA) exacerbation, bronchopneumonia, bronchospasm, bullous dermatitis, cardiac arrest, chest pain, coma, Coombs' test positive, cyanosis, epidermolysis, erythema multiforme, hepatic dysfunction, hypoxemia, leukopenia, loss of consciousness, pancytopenia, papular rash, pulmonary edema, pulmonary embolism, rigors, seizure, Stevens-Johnson syndrome, thromboembolism, transfusion-related acute lung injury (TRALI), tremor, vascular collapse

Drug Interactions

Avoid Concomitant Use There are no known interactions where it is recommended to avoid concomitant use.

Increased Effect/Toxicity There are no known significant interactions involving an increase in effect.

Decreased Effect

Immune Globulin (Intravenous) may decrease the levels/effects of: Vaccines (Live)

Test Interactions Octagam® contains maltose. Falsely-elevated blood glucose levels may occur when glucose monitoring devices and test strips utilizing the glucose dehydrogenase pyrroloquinolinequinone (GDH-PQQ) based methods are used. Glucose monitoring devices and test strips which utilize the glucose-specific method are recommended. Passively-transferred antibodies may yield false-positive serologic testing results; may yield false-positive direct and indirect Coombs' test.

Dietary Considerations Some products may contain sodium.

Dosage Forms Excipient information presented when available (limited, particularly for generics); consult specific product labeling.

Injection, powder for reconstitution [preservative free, nanofiltered]:

Carimune® NF: 3 g, 6 g, 12 g [contains sucrose]

Injection, powder for reconstitution [preservative free, solvent detergent-treated]:

Gammagard S/D: 2.5 g, 5 g, 10 g [stabilized with human albumin, glycine, glucose, and polyethylene glycol; packaging may contain natural latex/natural rubber]

Injection, solution [preservative free; solvent detergent-treated]:

Gammagard Liquid: 10% (10 mL, 25 mL, 50 mL, 100 mL, 200 mL) [latex free, sucrose free; stabilized with glycine]

Octagam®: 5% (20 mL, 50 mL, 100 mL, 200 mL) [sucrose free; contains sodium 30 mmol/L and maltose]

Injection, solution [preservative free]

Flebogamma®: 5% (10 mL, 50 mL, 100 mL, 200 mL) [contains polyethylene glycol and sorbitol]

Gamunex®: 10% (10 mL, 25 mL, 50 mL, 100 mL, 200 mL) [caprylate/chromatography purified]

Privigen™: 10% (50 mL, 100 mL, 200 mL) [sucrose free]

◆ **Immunine® VH (Can)** *see* Factor IX *on page 570*

◆ **Imogam® Rabies-HT** *see* Rabies Immune Globulin (Human) *on page 1224*

◆ **Imogam® Rabies Pasteurized (Can)** *see* Rabies Immune Globulin (Human) *on page 1224*

◆ **Imovax® Rabies** *see* Rabies Virus Vaccine *on page 1225*

◆ **Imuran®** *see* AzaTHIOprine *on page 167*

Inamrinone (eye NAM ri none)

Medication Safety Issues
Sound-alike/look-alike issues:
Amrinone may be confused with aMILoride, amiodarone

High alert medication: The Institute for Safe Medication Practices (ISMP) includes this medication among its list of drug classes which have a heightened risk of causing significant patient harm when used in error.

Related Information
Heart Failure (Systolic) *on page 1739*

Index Terms Amrinone Lactate

Pharmacologic Category Phosphodiesterase Enzyme Inhibitor

Generic Available Yes

Use Short-term therapy in patients with intractable heart failure

Mechanism of Action Inhibits myocardial cyclic adenosine monophosphate (cAMP) phosphodiesterase activity and increases cellular levels of cAMP resulting in a positive inotropic effect and increased cardiac output; also possesses systemic and pulmonary vasodilator effects resulting in pre- and afterload reduction; slightly increases atrioventricular conduction

Pharmacodynamics/Kinetics
Onset of action: I.V.: 2-5 minutes
Peak effect: ~10 minutes
Duration (dose dependent): Low dose: ~30 minutes; Higher doses: ~2 hours
Half-life elimination, serum: Adults: Healthy volunteers: 3.6 hours, Congestive heart failure: 5.8 hours
Excretion: Urine (10% to 40% as parent drug)

Dosage Dosage is based on clinical response (**Note:** Dose should not exceed 10 mg/kg/24 hours).
Infants (unlabeled population), Children (unlabeled population), and Adults: 0.75 mg/kg I.V. bolus over 2-3 minutes followed by maintenance infusion of 5-10 mcg/kg/minute; I.V. bolus may need to be repeated in 30 minutes.

Dosing adjustment in renal failure:
Infants and Children:
Cl_{cr} 30-50 mL/minute: Administer 100% of dose
Cl_{cr} 10-29 mL/minute: Administer 50% of dose
Cl_{cr} <10 mL/minute: Administer 25% of dose
Intermittent hemodialysis or peritoneal dialysis: Administer 25% of dose
Adults:
Cl_{cr} ≥10 mL/minute: Administer 100% of dose
Cl_{cr} <10 mL/minute: Administer 50% to 75% of dose

Stability Store at 15°C to 30°C (59°F to 86°F). Protect from light. Store in carton until ready for use. For continuous infusion, dilute with 0.45% or 0.9% sodium chloride to final concentration of 1-3 mg/mL. Use within 24 hours. Do not directly dilute with dextrose-containing solutions; chemical interaction occurs. May be administered I.V. into running dextrose infusions.

Administration May be administered undiluted for I.V. bolus doses. Dilute for use as continuous infusion.

Monitoring Parameters Platelet count, CBC, electrolytes (especially potassium and magnesium), liver function and renal function tests; ECG, CVP, SBP, DBP, heart rate; infusion rate

If pulmonary artery catheter is in place, monitor cardiac index, stroke volume, systemic vascular resistance, pulmonary capillary wedge pressure and pulmonary vascular resistance.

Pregnancy Risk Factor C

Contraindications Hypersensitivity to inamrinone, any component of the formulation, or bisulfites (contains sodium metabisulfite); patients with severe aortic or pulmonic valvular disease

Warnings/Precautions Due to a slight effect on AV conduction, may increase ventricular response rate in atrial fibrillation/atrial flutter; prior treatment with digoxin is recommended. Monitor liver function. Discontinue therapy if alteration in LFTs and clinical symptoms of hepatotoxicity occur. Observe for arrhythmias in this very high-risk patient population. Not recommended in acute MI treatment. Monitor fluid status closely; patients may require adjustment of diuretic and electrolyte replacement therapy. Can cause thrombocytopenia (dose dependent). Correct hypokalemia before initiating therapy. Increase risk of hospitalization and death with long-term therapy.

Adverse Reactions
1% to 10%:
Cardiovascular: Arrhythmias (3%; especially in high-risk patients), hypotension (1% to 2%; dose related)
Gastrointestinal: Nausea (1% to 2%), vomiting (1%)
Hematologic: Thrombocytopenia (~2%; dose related)
<1% (Limited to important or life-threatening): Abdominal pain, anorexia, chest pain, fever, hepatotoxicity, hyperbilirubinemia, hypersensitivity, injection site reactions, jaundice, liver enzymes increased

Drug Interactions
Avoid Concomitant Use There are no known interactions where it is recommended to avoid concomitant use.
Increased Effect/Toxicity There are no known significant interactions involving an increase in effect.
Decreased Effect There are no known significant interactions involving a decrease in effect.

Dosage Forms Excipient information presented when available (limited, particularly for generics); consult specific product labeling.
Injection, solution, as lactate: 5 mg/mL (20 mL) [contains sodium metabisulfite]

◆ **Inapsine® [DSC]** *see* Droperidol *on page 463*

◆ **Inderal® [DSC]** *see* Propranolol *on page 1198*

◆ **Inderal® (Can)** *see* Propranolol *on page 1198*

◆ **Inderal® LA** *see* Propranolol *on page 1198*

◆ **Indocid® P.D.A. (Can)** *see* Indomethacin *on page 738*

◆ **Indocin®** *see* Indomethacin *on page 738*

◆ **Indocin® I.V.** *see* Indomethacin *on page 738*

◆ **Indo-Lemmon (Can)** *see* Indomethacin *on page 738*

◆ **Indometacin** *see* Indomethacin *on page 738*

Indomethacin (in doe METH a sin)

Related Information
Chronic Pain Management *on page 1546*
Nonsteroidal Anti-Inflammatory Agents *on page 1687*
U.S. Brand Names Indocin®; Indocin® I.V.
Canadian Brand Names Apo-Indomethacin®; Indo-Lemmon; Indocid® P.D.A.; Indocin®; Indotec; Novo-Methacin; Nu-Indo; Rhodacine®
Index Terms Indometacin; Indomethacin Sodium Trihydrate
Pharmacologic Category Nonsteroidal Anti-inflammatory Drug (NSAID), Oral; Nonsteroidal Anti-inflammatory Drug (NSAID), Parenteral
Use Acute gouty arthritis, acute bursitis/tendonitis, moderate-to-severe osteo-arthritis, rheumatoid arthritis, ankylosing spondylitis; I.V. form used as alternative to surgery for closure of patent ductus arteriosus in neonates
Unlabeled/Investigational Use Management of preterm labor
Pharmacodynamics/Kinetics
Onset of action: ~30 minutes
Duration: 4-6 hours
Absorption: Oral: Immediate release: Prompt and extensive; Extended release: 90% over 12 hours
Distribution: V_d: 0.34-1.57 L/kg; crosses blood brain barrier
Protein binding: 99%

Metabolism: Hepatic; significant enterohepatic recirculation

Bioavailability: 100%

Half-life elimination: 4.5 hours; prolonged in neonates

Time to peak: Oral: Immediate release: 2 hours

Excretion: Urine (60%, primarily as glucuronide conjugates); feces (33%, primarily as metabolites)

Dosage

Patent ductus arteriosus:

Neonates: I.V.: Initial: 0.2 mg/kg, followed by 2 doses depending on postnatal age (PNA):

PNA **at time of first dose** <48 hours: 0.1 mg/kg at 12- to 24-hour intervals

PNA **at time of first dose** 2-7 days: 0.2 mg/kg at 12- to 24-hour intervals

PNA **at time of first dose** >7 days: 0.25 mg/kg at 12- to 24-hour intervals

In general, may use 12-hour dosing interval if urine output >1 mL/kg/hour after prior dose; use 24-hour dosing interval if urine output is <1 mL/kg/hour but >0.6 mL/kg/hour; doses should be withheld if patient has oliguria (urine output <0.6 mL/kg/hour) or anuria

Inflammatory/rheumatoid disorders: Oral: Use lowest effective dose.

Children ≥2 years: 1-2 mg/kg/day in 2-4 divided doses; maximum dose: 4 mg/kg/day; not to exceed 150-200 mg/day

Adults: 25-50 mg/dose 2-3 times/day; maximum dose: 200 mg/day; extended release capsule should be given on a 1-2 times/day schedule (maximum dose for extended release: 150 mg/day). In patients with arthritis and persistent night pain and/or morning stiffness may give the larger portion (up to 100 mg) of the total daily dose at bedtime.

Bursitis/tendonitis: Oral: Adults: Initial dose: 75-150 mg/day in 3-4 divided doses **or** 1-2 divided doses for extended release; usual treatment is 7-14 days

Acute gouty arthritis: Oral: Adults: 50 mg 3 times daily until pain is tolerable then reduce dose; usual treatment <3-5 days

Elderly: Refer to adult dosing. Use lowest recommended dose and frequency in elderly to initiate therapy for indications listed in adult dosing.

Dosage adjustment in renal impairment: Not recommended in patients with advanced renal disease

Anesthesia and Critical Care Concerns/Other Considerations The 2002 ACCM/SCCM guidelines for analgesia (critically-ill adult) suggest that NSAIDs may be used in combination with opioids in select patients for pain management. Concern about adverse events (increased risk of renal dysfunction, altered platelet function and gastrointestinal irritation) limits its use in patients who have other underlying risks for these events.

In short-term use, NSAIDs vary considerably in their effect on blood pressure. When NSAIDs are used in patients with hypertension, appropriate monitoring of blood pressure responses should be completed and the duration of therapy, when possible, kept short. The use of NSAIDs in the treatment of patients with congestive heart failure may be associated with an increased risk for fluid accumulation and edema; may precipitate renal failure in dehydrated patients.

Additional Information Complete prescribing information for this medication should be consulted for additional detail.

Dosage Forms Excipient information presented when available (limited, particularly for generics); consult specific product labeling.

Capsule: 25 mg, 50 mg

Capsule, extended release, oral: 75 mg

Injection, powder for reconstitution:

Indocin® I.V: 1 mg

Suppository, rectal: 50 mg (30s)

Suspension, oral:

Indocin®: 25 mg/5 mL (237 mL) [contains alcohol 1%; pineapple-coconut-mint flavor]

◆ **Indomethacin Sodium Trihydrate** *see* Indomethacin *on page* 738

◆ **Indotec (Can)** *see* Indomethacin *on page* 738

◆ **Infantaire [OTC]** *see* Acetaminophen *on page* 25

◆ **Infasurf®** *see* Calfactant *on page* 235

◆ **Inflamase® Mild (Can)** *see* PrednisoLONE *on page 1164*

InFLIXimab (in FLIKS e mab)

U.S. Brand Names Remicade®
Canadian Brand Names Remicade®
Index Terms Avakine; Infliximab, Recombinant
Pharmacologic Category Antirheumatic, Disease Modifying; Gastrointestinal Agent, Miscellaneous; Immunosuppressant Agent; Monoclonal Antibody; Tumor Necrosis Factor (TNF) Blocking Agent

Use
Treatment of moderately- to severely-active rheumatoid arthritis (with methotrexate)
Treatment of moderately- to severely-active Crohn's disease with inadequate response to conventional therapy (to reduce signs/symptoms and induce and maintain clinical remission) or to reduce the number of draining enterocutaneous and rectovaginal fistulas and maintain fistula closure
Treatment of psoriatic arthritis (to reduce signs/symptoms of active arthritis and inhibit progression of structural damage and improve physical function)
Treatment of chronic severe plaque psoriasis
Treatment of active ankylosing spondylitis (reduce signs/symptoms)
Treatment of moderately- to severely-active ulcerative colitis with inadequate response to conventional therapy (reduce signs/symptoms and induce and maintain clinical remission, mucosal healing and eliminate corticosteroid use)

Unlabeled/Investigational Use Acute graft-versus-host disease (GVHD)

Pharmacodynamics/Kinetics
Onset of action: Crohn's disease: ~2 weeks
Distribution: V_d: 3-6 L
Half-life elimination: 7-12 days

Dosage I.V.: **Note:** Premedication with antihistamines (H_1-antagonist and/or H_2-antagonist), acetaminophen and/or corticosteroids may be considered to prevent and/or manage infusion-related reactions:
Children: U.S. labeling ≥6 years, Canadian labeling ≥9 years: Crohn's disease: 5 mg/kg at 0, 2, and 6 weeks, followed by a maintenance dose of 5 mg/kg every 8 weeks; if no response by week 14, consider discontinuing therapy
Adults:
Crohn's disease: Induction regimen: 5 mg/kg at 0, 2, and 6 weeks, followed by 5 mg/kg every 8 weeks thereafter; dose may be increased to 10 mg/kg in patients who respond but then lose their response. If no response by week 14, consider discontinuing therapy.
Psoriatic arthritis (with or without methotrexate): 5 mg/kg at 0, 2, and 6 weeks, then every 8 weeks
Rheumatoid arthritis (in combination with methotrexate therapy): 3 mg/kg at 0, 2, and 6 weeks, then every 8 weeks thereafter; doses have ranged from 3-10 mg/kg intravenous infusion repeated at 4- to 8-week intervals
Ankylosing spondylitis: 5 mg/kg at 0, 2, and 6 weeks, followed by 5 mg/kg every 6 weeks thereafter
Plaque psoriasis: 5 mg/kg at 0, 2, and 6 weeks, then every 8 weeks thereafter
Ulcerative colitis: 5 mg/kg at 0, 2, and 6 weeks, followed by 5 mg/kg every 8 weeks thereafter
Acute GVHD (unlabeled use): 10 mg/kg weekly for up to 8 weeks (median 4 weeks of treatment)

Dosage adjustment with CHF: Weigh risk versus benefits for individual patient: NYHA Class III or IV: ≤5 mg/kg
Dosage adjustment in renal impairment: No specific adjustment is recommended
Dosage adjustment in hepatic impairment: No specific adjustment is recommended
Additional Information Complete prescribing information for this medication should be consulted for additional detail.
Dosage Forms Excipient information presented when available (limited, particularly for generics); consult specific product labeling.

Injection, powder for reconstitution [preservative free]:
Remicade®: 100 mg [contains sucrose 500 mg and polysorbate 80]

♦ **Infliximab, Recombinant** *see* InFLIXimab *on page 740*
♦ **Infumorph® 200** *see* Morphine Sulfate *on page 953*
♦ **Infumorph® 500** *see* Morphine Sulfate *on page 953*
♦ **INH** *see* Isoniazid *on page 767*
♦ **Inhibace® (Can)** *see* Cilazapril *on page 301*
♦ **Innohep®** *see* Tinzaparin *on page 1392*
♦ **InnoPran XL®** *see* Propranolol *on page 1198*
♦ **INOmax®** *see* Nitric Oxide *on page 1012*
♦ **Inspra™** *see* Eplerenone *on page 499*
♦ **Insta-Glucose® [OTC]** *see* Dextrose *on page 406*

Insulin Aspart (IN soo lin AS part)

Medication Safety Issues
Sound-alike/look-alike issues:
NovoLog® may be confused with Humalog®, Humulin® R, Novolin® N, Novolin® R, NovoLog® Mix 70/30

High alert medication: The Institute for Safe Medication Practices (ISMP) includes this medication among its list of drugs which have a heightened risk of causing significant patient harm when used in error. *Due to the number of insulin preparations, it is essential to identify/clarify the type of insulin to be used.*

Cross-contamination may occur if insulin pens are shared among multiple patients. Steps should be taken to prohibit sharing of insulin pens.

Related Information
Insulin Regular *on page 750*

U.S. Brand Names NovoLog®

Canadian Brand Names NovoRapid®

Index Terms Aspart Insulin

Pharmacologic Category Antidiabetic Agent, Insulin

Generic Available No

Use Treatment of type 1 diabetes mellitus (insulin dependent, IDDM) and type 2 diabetes mellitus (noninsulin dependent, NIDDM) to improve glycemic control

Unlabeled/Investigational Use Gestational diabetes mellitus (GDM); mild-to-moderate diabetic ketoacidosis (DKA); mild-to-moderate hyperosmolar hyperglycemic state (HHS)

Mechanism of Action Refer to Insulin Regular *on page 750*. Insulin aspart is a rapid-acting insulin analog.

Pharmacodynamics/Kinetics Note: Rate of absorption, onset, and duration of activity may be affected by site of injection, exercise, presence of lipodystrophy, local blood supply, and/or temperature.
Onset of action: 0.2-0.3 hours
Peak effect: 1-3 hours
Duration: 3-5 hours
Protein binding: <10%
Half-life elimination: SubQ: 81 minutes
Time to peak, plasma: 40-50 minutes
Excretion: Urine

Dosage Refer to Insulin Regular *on page 750*. Insulin aspart is a rapid-acting insulin analog which is normally administered as a premeal component of the insulin regimen. It is normally used along with a long-acting (basal) form of insulin.
Dosing adjustment in renal impairment: Insulin requirements are reduced due to changes in insulin clearance or metabolism.

Stability Unopened vials, cartridges, and prefilled pens may be stored under refrigeration between 2°C and 8°C (36°F to 46°F) until the expiration date or at room temperature <30°C (<86°F) for 28 days; do not freeze; keep away from heat and sunlight. Once punctured (in use), vials may be stored under refrigeration or ▶

◄ at room temperature <30°C (<86°F); use within 28 days. Cartridges and prefilled pens that have been punctured (in use) should be stored at temperatures <30°C (<86°F) and used within 28 days; do not freeze or refrigerate. When used for CSII, insulin aspart contained within an external insulin pump reservoir should be replaced at least every 6 days; discard if exposed to temperatures >37°C (>98.6°F).

For SubQ administration: *NovoLog® vials:* May be diluted with Insulin Diluting Medium for NovoLog® to a concentration of 10 units/mL (U-10) or 50 units/mL (U-50). According to the manufacturer, diluted insulin should be stored at temperatures <30°C (<86°F) and used within 28 days; do not dilute insulin contained in a cartridge, prefilled pen, or external insulin pump.

For I.V. infusion: May be diluted in NS, D_5W, or $D_{10}W$ to concentrations of 0.05-1 unit/mL. Stable for 24 hours at room temperature.

Administration

SubQ administration: Do not use if solution is viscous or cloudy; use only if clear and colorless. Insulin aspart should be administered immediately (within 5-10 minutes) before a meal. Cold injections should be avoided. SubQ administration is usually made into the thighs, arms, buttocks, or abdomen; rotate injection sites. When mixing insulin aspart with other preparations of insulin (eg, insulin NPH), insulin aspart should be drawn into syringe first. Do not dilute or mix other insulin formulations with insulin aspart contained in a cartridge or prefilled pen.

CSII administration: Do not use if solution is viscous or cloudy; use only if clear and colorless. Patients should be trained in the proper use of their external insulin pump and in intensive insulin therapy. Infusion sets and infusion set insertion sites should be changed at least every 3 days; rotate infusion sites. Do not dilute or mix other insulin formulations with insulin aspart that is to be used in an external insulin pump.

I.V. administration: Do not use if solution is viscous or cloudy; use only if clear and colorless. May be administered I.V. with close monitoring of blood glucose and serum potassium; appropriate medical supervision is required. **Do not administer insulin mixtures intravenously.**

I.V. infusions: To minimize adsorption to I.V. solution bag: **Note:** Refer to institution-specific protocols where appropriate.

*If new tubing is **not** needed:* Wait a minimum of 30 minutes between the preparation of the solution and the initiation of the infusion

If new tubing is needed: After receiving the insulin drip solution, the administration set should be attached to the I.V. container and the entire line should be flushed with a priming infusion of 20-50 mL of the insulin solution (Goldberg, 2006; Hirsch, 2006). Wait 30 minutes, and then flush the line again with the insulin solution prior to initiating the infusion.

Because of adsorption, the actual amount of insulin being administered via I.V. infusion could be substantially less than the apparent amount. Therefore, adjustment of the I.V. infusion rate should be based on effect and not solely on the apparent insulin dose. The apparent dose may be used as a starting point for determining the subsequent SubQ dosing regimen (Moghissi, 2009); however, the transition to SubQ administration requires continuous medical supervision, frequent monitoring of blood glucose, and careful adjustment of therapy. In addition, SubQ insulin should be given 1-4 hours prior to the discontinuation of I.V. insulin to prevent hyperglycemia (Moghissi, 2009).

Monitoring Parameters

Diabetes mellitus: Plasma glucose, electrolytes, Hb A_{1c}

I.V. administration: Close monitoring of blood glucose and serum potassium

Reference Range Refer to Insulin Regular on page 750.

Pregnancy Risk Factor B

Contraindications Hypersensitivity to insulin aspart or any component of the formulation; during episodes of hypoglycemia

Warnings/Precautions Refer to Insulin Regular on page 750.

In type 1 diabetes mellitus (insulin dependent, IDDM), insulin lispro (Humalog®) and insulin glulisine (Apidra™) should be used in combination with a long-acting insulin. However, in type 2 diabetes mellitus (noninsulin dependent, NIDDM), insulin lispro (Humalog®) may be used without a long-acting insulin when used in combination with a sulfonylurea.

Adverse Reactions Refer to Insulin Regular on page 750.

Drug Interactions

Metabolism/Transport Effects Refer to Insulin Regular on page 750.

Avoid Concomitant Use There are no known interactions where it is recommended to avoid concomitant use.

Increased Effect/Toxicity

Insulin Aspart may increase the levels/effects of: Antidiabetic Agents (Thiazolidinedione); Hypoglycemic Agents; Quinolone Antibiotics

The levels/effects of Insulin Aspart may be increased by: Beta-Blockers; Edetate CALCIUM Disodium; Edetate Disodium; Herbs (Hypoglycemic Properties); Pegvisomant

Decreased Effect

The levels/effects of Insulin Aspart may be decreased by: Corticosteroids (Orally Inhaled); Corticosteroids (Systemic); Luteinizing Hormone-Releasing Hormone Analogs; Somatropin; Thiazide Diuretics

Ethanol/Nutrition/Herb Interactions Refer to Insulin Regular on page 750.

Dietary Considerations Individualized medical nutrition therapy (MNT) based on ADA recommendations is an integral part of therapy.

Dosage Forms Excipient information presented when available (limited, particularly for generics); consult specific product labeling.

Injection, solution:

NovoLog®: 100 units/mL (3 mL) [FlexPen® prefilled syringe or PenFill® prefilled cartridge]; (10 mL) [vial]

References

American Diabetes Association, "Standards of Medical Care in Diabetes," *Diabetes Care*, 2007, 30 (Suppl 1):4-41.

◆ **Insulin Aspart and Insulin Aspart Protamine** *see* Insulin Aspart Protamine and Insulin Aspart *on page 743*

Insulin Aspart Protamine and Insulin Aspart

(IN soo lin AS part PROE ta meen & IN soo lin AS part)

Related Information

Insulin Regular *on page 750*

U.S. Brand Names NovoLog® Mix 70/30

Canadian Brand Names NovoMix® 30

Index Terms Insulin Aspart and Insulin Aspart Protamine; NovoLog 70/30

Pharmacologic Category Antidiabetic Agent, Insulin

Use Treatment of type 1 diabetes mellitus (insulin dependent, IDDM) and type 2 diabetes mellitus (noninsulin dependent, NIDDM) to improve glycemic control

Pharmacodynamics/Kinetics Note: Rate of absorption, onset, and duration of activity may be affected by site of injection, exercise, presence of lipodystrophy, local blood supply, and/or temperature.

Onset of action: 0.1-0.2 hours

Peak effect: 1-4 hours

Duration: 18-24 hours

Half-life elimination: ~8-9 hours

Time to peak, plasma: 1-1.5 hours

Excretion: Urine

Dosage Refer to Insulin Regular on page 750. Fixed ratio insulins (such as insulin aspart protamine and insulin aspart combination) are normally administered in 2 daily doses.

Dosing adjustment in renal impairment: Insulin requirements are reduced due to changes in insulin clearance or metabolism.

Additional Information Complete prescribing information for this medication should be consulted for additional detail.

Dosage Forms Excipient information presented when available (limited, particularly for generics); consult specific product labeling.

Injection, suspension:

NovoLog® Mix 70/30: Insulin aspart protamine suspension 70% [intermediate acting] and insulin aspart solution 30% [rapid acting]: 100 units/mL (3 mL) [FlexPen® prefilled syringe]; (10 mL) [vial]

References
American Diabetes Association, "Standards of Medical Care in Diabetes," *Diabetes Care*, 2007, 30 (Suppl 1):4-41.

Insulin Detemir (IN soo lin DE te mir)

Related Information
 Insulin Regular *on page 750*
U.S. Brand Names Levemir®
Canadian Brand Names Levemir®
Index Terms Detemir Insulin
Pharmacologic Category Antidiabetic Agent, Insulin
Use Treatment of type 1 diabetes mellitus (insulin dependent, IDDM) and type 2 diabetes mellitus (noninsulin dependent, NIDDM) to improve glycemic control
Pharmacodynamics/Kinetics Note: Rate of absorption, onset, and duration of activity may be affected by site of injection, exercise, presence of lipodystrophy, local blood supply, and/or temperature.
 Onset of action: 3-4 hours
  Peak effect: 3-9 hours (Plank, 2005)
 Duration: Dose dependent: 6-23 hours; **Note:** Duration is dose-dependent. At lower dosages (0.1-0.2 units/kg), mean duration is variable (5.7-12.1 hours). At 0.4 units/kg, the mean duration was 19.9 hours. At high dosages (≥0.8 units/kg) the duration is longer and less variable (mean of 22-23 hours) (Plank, 2005).
 Bioavailability: 60%
 Half-life elimination: 5-7 hours (dose-dependent)
 Protein binding: >98% (albumin)
 Distribution: V_d: 0.1 L/kg
 Time to peak, plasma: 6-8 hours
 Excretion: Urine
Dosage Also refer to Insulin Regular on page 750.

 Notes: Duration is dose-dependent. Dosage must be carefully titrated (adjustment of dose and timing. Adjustment of concomitant antidiabetic treatment (short-acting insulins or oral antidiabetic agents) may be required. In Canada, insulin detemir is not approved for use in children.

 SubQ: Children ≥6 years and Adults: Type 1 or type 2 diabetes:
  Basal insulin or basal-bolus: May be substituted on a unit-per-unit basis. Adjust dose to achieve glycemic targets.
  Insulin-naive patients (type 2 diabetes only): 0.1-0.2 units/kg once daily in the evening or 10 units once or twice daily. Adjust dose to achieve glycemic targets. Note: Canadian labeling recommends 10 units once daily (twice daily dosing is not included).
 Dosage adjustment in renal impairment: Insulin requirements are reduced due to changes in insulin clearance or metabolism.
Additional Information Complete prescribing information for this medication should be consulted for additional detail.
Dosage Forms Excipient information presented when available (limited, particularly for generics); consult specific product labeling.
 Injection, solution:
  Levemir®: 100 units/mL (3 mL) [FlexPen® prefilled syringe]; (10 mL) [vial]

References
American Diabetes Association, "Standards of Medical Care in Diabetes," *Diabetes Care*, 2007, 30 (Suppl 1):4-41.
Plank J, Bodenlenz M, Sinner F, et al, "A Double-Blind, Randomized, Dose-Response Study Investigating the Pharmacodynamic and Pharmacokinetic Properties of the Long-Acting Insulin Analog Detemir," *Diabetes Care*, 2005, 28(5):1107-12.

Insulin Glargine (IN soo lin GLAR jeen)

Related Information
 Insulin Regular *on page 750*
U.S. Brand Names Lantus®
Canadian Brand Names Lantus®; Lantus® OptiSet®

Index Terms Glargine Insulin

Pharmacologic Category Antidiabetic Agent, Insulin

Use Treatment of type 1 diabetes mellitus (insulin dependent, IDDM) and type 2 diabetes mellitus (noninsulin dependent, NIDDM) to improve glycemic control

Pharmacodynamics/Kinetics Note: Rate of absorption, onset, and duration of activity may be affected by site of injection, exercise, presence of lipodystrophy, local blood supply, and/or temperature.

Onset of action: 3-4 hours

Peak effect: No pronounced peak

Duration: Generally 24 hours or longer; reported range: 10.8 to >24 hours (up to 32 hours documented in some studies)

Absorption: Slow; upon injection into the subcutaneous tissue, microprecipitates form which allow small amounts of insulin glargine to release over time

Metabolism: Partially metabolized in the skin to form two active metabolites

Time to peak, plasma: No pronounced peak

Excretion: Urine

Dosage SubQ: Adults:

Type 1 diabetes: Refer to Insulin Regular on page 750.

Type 2 diabetes:

Patient not already on insulin: 10 units once daily, adjusted according to patient response (range in clinical study: 2-100 units/day)

Patient already receiving insulin: In clinical studies, when changing to insulin glargine from once-daily NPH or Ultralente® insulin, the initial dose was not changed; when changing from twice-daily NPH to once-daily insulin glargine, the total daily dose was reduced by 20% and adjusted according to patient response

Dosage adjustment in renal impairment: Insulin requirements are reduced due to changes in insulin clearance or metabolism.

Additional Information Complete prescribing information for this medication should be consulted for additional detail.

Dosage Forms Excipient information presented when available (limited, particularly for generics); consult specific product labeling.

Injection, solution:

Lantus®: 100 units/mL (3 mL) [OptiClik® prefilled cartridge or SoloStar® disposable insulin device]; (10 mL) [vial]

References

American Diabetes Association, "Standards of Medical Care in Diabetes," *Diabetes Care*, 2007, 30 (Suppl 1):4-41.

Insulin Glulisine (IN soo lin gloo LIS een)

Medication Safety Issues

Sound-alike/look-alike issues:

Insulin glulisine may be confused with insulin glargine

High alert medication: The Institute for Safe Medication Practices (ISMP) includes this medication among its list of drugs which have a heightened risk of causing significant patient harm when used in error. ***Due to the number of insulin preparations, it is essential to identify/clarify the type of insulin to be used.***

Cross-contamination may occur if insulin pens are shared among multiple patients. Steps should be taken to prohibit sharing of insulin pens.

Related Information

Insulin Regular *on page 750*

U.S. Brand Names Apidra®

Canadian Brand Names Apidra®

Index Terms Glulisine Insulin

Pharmacologic Category Antidiabetic Agent, Insulin

Generic Available No

Use Treatment of type 1 diabetes mellitus (insulin dependent, IDDM) and type 2 diabetes mellitus (noninsulin dependent, NIDDM) to improve glycemic control

Mechanism of Action Refer to Insulin Regular on page 750. Insulin glulisine is a rapid-acting insulin analog.

Pharmacodynamics/Kinetics Note: Rate of absorption, onset, and duration of activity may be affected by site of injection, exercise, presence of lipodystrophy, local blood supply, and/or temperature.

Onset of action: 0.2-0.5 hours

Peak effect: 1.6-2.8 hours

Duration: 3-4 hours

Distribution: I.V.: 13 L

Bioavailability: SubQ: ~70%

Half-life elimination:

I.V.: 13 minutes

SubQ: 42 minutes

Time to peak, plasma: 0.6-2 hours

Excretion: Urine

Dosage Refer to Insulin Regular on page 750.

Dosing adjustment in renal impairment: Insulin requirements are reduced due to changes in insulin clearance or metabolism.

Stability Unopened vials, cartridges, and prefilled pens may be stored under refrigeration between 2°C and 8°C (36°F to 46°F) until the expiration date or at room temperature for 28 days; do not freeze; keep away from heat and sunlight. Once punctured (in use), vials may be stored under refrigeration or at room temperature ≤25°C (≤77°F); use within 28 days. Cartridges and prefilled pens that have been punctured (in use) should be stored at temperatures ≤25°C (≤77°F) and used within 28 days; do not freeze or refrigerate. When used for CSII, insulin glulisine contained within an external insulin pump reservoir should be replaced every 48 hours; discard if exposed to temperatures >37°C (>98.6°F).

For I.V. infusion: May be diluted in NS to concentrations of 0.05-1 unit/mL. Stable for 48 hours at room temperature.

Administration

SubQ administration: Do not use if solution is viscous or cloudy; use only if clear and colorless. Insulin glulisine should be administered within 15 minutes before or within 20 minutes after starting a meal. Cold injections should be avoided. SubQ administration is usually made into the thighs, arms, buttocks, or abdomen; rotate injection sites. When mixing insulin glulisine with other preparations of insulin (eg, insulin NPH), insulin glulisine should be drawn into syringe first. Do not mix other insulin formulations with insulin glulisine contained in a cartridge or prefilled pen.

CSII administration: Do not use if solution is viscous or cloudy; use only if clear and colorless. Patients should be trained in the proper use of their external insulin pump and in intensive insulin therapy. Infusion sets, reservoirs, and infusion set insertion sites should be changed every 48 hours; rotate infusion sites. Do not dilute or mix other insulin formulations with insulin glulisine that is to be used in an external insulin pump.

I.V. administration: Do not use if solution is viscous or cloudy; use only if clear and colorless. May be administered I.V. with close monitoring of blood glucose and serum potassium; appropriate medical supervision is required. **Do not administer insulin mixtures intravenously.**

I.V. infusions: To minimize adsorption to I.V. solution bag: **Note:** Refer to institution-specific protocols where appropriate.

If new tubing is not needed: Wait a minimum of 30 minutes between the preparation of the solution and the initiation of the infusion.

If new tubing is needed: After receiving the insulin drip solution, the administration set should be attached to the I.V. container and the entire line should be flushed with a priming infusion of 20-50 mL of the insulin solution (Goldberg, 2006; Hirsch, 2006). Wait 30 minutes, and then flush the line again with the insulin solution prior to initiating the infusion.

Because of adsorption, the actual amount of insulin being administered via I.V. infusion could be substantially less than the apparent amount. Therefore, adjustment of the I.V. infusion rate should be based on effect and not solely on the apparent insulin dose. The apparent dose may be used as a starting point for determining the subsequent SubQ dosing regimen (Moghissi, 2009); however, the transition to SubQ administration requires continuous medical supervision, frequent monitoring of blood glucose, and careful adjustment of therapy. In addition, SubQ insulin should be given 1-4 hours prior to the discontinuation of I.V. insulin to prevent hyperglycemia (Moghissi, 2009).

Monitoring Parameters
Diabetes mellitus: Plasma glucose, electrolytes, Hb A$_{1c}$
I.V. administration: Close monitoring of blood glucose and serum potassium

Reference Range Refer to Insulin Regular on page 750.

Pregnancy Risk Factor C

Contraindications Hypersensitivity to insulin glulisine or any component of the formulation; during episodes of hypoglycemia

Warnings/Precautions Refer to Insulin Regular on page 750.
In type 1 diabetes mellitus (insulin dependent, IDDM), insulin lispro (Humalog®) and insulin glulisine (Apidra®) should be used in combination with a long-acting insulin. However, in type 2 diabetes mellitus (noninsulin dependent, NIDDM), insulin lispro (Humalog®) may be used without a long-acting insulin when used in combination with a sulfonylurea.

Adverse Reactions Refer to Insulin Regular on page 750.

Drug Interactions
Metabolism/Transport Effects Refer to Insulin Regular on page 750.

Avoid Concomitant Use There are no known interactions where it is recommended to avoid concomitant use.

Increased Effect/Toxicity
Insulin Glulisine may increase the levels/effects of: Antidiabetic Agents (Thiazolidinedione); Hypoglycemic Agents; Quinolone Antibiotics

The levels/effects of Insulin Glulisine may be increased by: Beta-Blockers; Edetate CALCIUM Disodium; Edetate Disodium; Herbs (Hypoglycemic Properties); Pegvisomant

Decreased Effect
The levels/effects of Insulin Glulisine may be decreased by: Corticosteroids (Orally Inhaled); Corticosteroids (Systemic); Luteinizing Hormone-Releasing Hormone Analogs; Somatropin; Thiazide Diuretics

Ethanol/Nutrition/Herb Interactions Refer to Insulin Regular on page 750.

Dietary Considerations Individualized medical nutrition therapy (MNT) based on ADA recommendations is an integral part of therapy.

Dosage Forms Excipient information presented when available (limited, particularly for generics); consult specific product labeling.
Injection, solution:
Apidra®: 100 units/mL (3 mL [cartridge], 3 mL [SoloStar® prefilled pen], 10 mL [vial])

References
American Diabetes Association, "Standards of Medical Care in Diabetes," *Diabetes Care,* 2007, 30 (Suppl 1):4-41.

Insulin Lispro (IN soo lin LYE sproe)

Related Information
Insulin Regular *on page 750*

U.S. Brand Names Humalog®

Canadian Brand Names Humalog®

Index Terms Lispro Insulin

Pharmacologic Category Antidiabetic Agent, Insulin

Use Treatment of type 1 diabetes mellitus (insulin dependent, IDDM) and type 2 diabetes mellitus (noninsulin dependent, NIDDM) to improve glycemic control

Unlabeled/Investigational Use Gestational diabetes mellitus (GDM); mild-to-moderate diabetic ketoacidosis (DKA); mild-to-moderate hyperosmolar hyperglycemic state (HHS)

Pharmacodynamics/Kinetics Note: Rate of absorption, onset, and duration of activity may be affected by site of injection, exercise, presence of lipodystrophy, local blood supply, and/or temperature.
Onset of action: 0.25-0.5 hours
Peak effect: 0.5-2.5 hours
Duration: ≤5 hours
Distribution: V$_d$: 0.26-0.36 L/kg

Bioavailability: 55% to 77%

Half-life elimination:

I.V.: ~0.5-1 hour (dose-dependent)

SubQ: 1 hour

Time to peak, plasma: 0.5-1.5 hours

Excretion: Urine

Dosage Refer to Insulin Regular on page 750. Insulin lispro is equipotent to insulin regular, but has a more rapid onset.

Dosing adjustment in renal impairment: Insulin requirements are reduced due to changes in insulin clearance or metabolism.

Additional Information Complete prescribing information for this medication should be consulted for additional detail.

Dosage Forms Excipient information presented when available (limited, particularly for generics); consult specific product labeling.

Injection, solution:

Humalog®: 100 units/mL (3 mL) [prefilled cartridge or prefilled disposable pen]; (10 mL) [vial]

References

American Diabetes Association, "Standards of Medical Care in Diabetes," *Diabetes Care*, 2007, 30 (Suppl 1):4-41.

◆ **Insulin Lispro and Insulin Lispro Protamine** *see* Insulin Lispro Protamine and Insulin Lispro *on page 748*

Insulin Lispro Protamine and Insulin Lispro
(IN soo lin LYE sproe PROE ta meen & IN soo lin LYE sproe)

Related Information

Insulin Regular *on page 750*

U.S. Brand Names Humalog® Mix 50/50™; Humalog® Mix 75/25™

Canadian Brand Names Humalog® Mix 25

Index Terms Insulin Lispro and Insulin Lispro Protamine

Pharmacologic Category Antidiabetic Agent, Insulin

Use Treatment of type 1 diabetes mellitus (insulin dependent, IDDM) and type 2 diabetes mellitus (noninsulin dependent, NIDDM) to improve glycemic control

Pharmacodynamics/Kinetics Note: Rate of absorption, onset, and duration of activity may be affected by site of injection, exercise, presence of lipodystrophy, local blood supply, and/or temperature.

Onset of action: 0.25-0.5 hours

Peak effect:

Humalog® Mix 50/50™: 0.8-4.8 hours

Humalog® Mix 75/25™: 1-6.5 hours

Duration: 14-24 hours

Time to peak, plasma:

Humalog® Mix 50/50™: 0.75-13.5 hours

Humalog® Mix 75/25™: 0.5-4 hours

Excretion: Urine

Dosage Refer to Insulin Regular on page 750. Fixed ratio insulins (such as insulin lispro protamine and insulin lispro) are normally administered in 2 daily doses.

Dosage adjustment in renal impairment: Insulin requirements are reduced due to changes in insulin clearance or metabolism.

Additional Information Complete prescribing information for this medication should be consulted for additional detail.

Dosage Forms Excipient information presented when available (limited, particularly for generics); consult specific product labeling.

Injection, suspension:

Humalog® Mix 50/50™: Insulin lispro protamine suspension 50% [intermediate acting] and insulin lispro solution 50% [rapid acting]: 100 units/mL (3 mL) [disposable pen]; (10 mL) [vial]

Humalog® Mix 75/25™: Insulin lispro protamine suspension 75% [intermediate acting] and insulin lispro solution 25% [rapid acting]: 100 units/mL (3 mL) [disposable pen]; (10 mL) [vial]

References

American Diabetes Association, "Standards of Medical Care in Diabetes," *Diabetes Care*, 2007, 30 (Suppl 1):4-41.

Insulin NPH (IN soo lin N P H)

Related Information

Insulin Regular *on page 750*

U.S. Brand Names Humulin® N; Novolin® N

Canadian Brand Names Humulin® N; Novolin® ge NPH

Index Terms Isophane Insulin; NPH Insulin

Pharmacologic Category Antidiabetic Agent, Insulin

Use Treatment of type 1 diabetes mellitus (insulin dependent, IDDM) and type 2 diabetes mellitus (noninsulin dependent, NIDDM) to improve glycemic control

Unlabeled/Investigational Use Gestational diabetes mellitus (GDM)

Pharmacodynamics/Kinetics Note: Rate of absorption, onset, and duration of activity may be affected by site of injection, exercise, presence of lipodystrophy, local blood supply, and/or temperature.

Onset of action: 1-2 hours

Peak effect: 4-12 hours

Duration: 14-24 hours

Time to peak, plasma: 6-10 hours

Excretion: Urine

Dosage Refer to Insulin Regular on page 750. Insulin NPH is usually administered 1-2 times daily.

Dosing adjustment in renal impairment: Insulin requirements are reduced due to changes in insulin clearance or metabolism.

Additional Information Complete prescribing information for this medication should be consulted for additional detail.

Dosage Forms Excipient information presented when available (limited, particularly for generics); consult specific product labeling. [CAN] = Canadian brand name

Injection, suspension:

Humulin® N: 100 units/mL (3 mL) [disposable pen]; (10 mL) [vial]

Novolin® ge NPH [CAN]: 100 units/mL (3 mL) [NovolinSet® prefilled syringe or PenFill® prefilled cartridge]; 10 mL [vial]

Novolin® N: 100 units/mL (3 mL) [InnoLet® prefilled syringe or PenFill® prefilled cartridge]; (10 mL) [vial]

References

American Diabetes Association, "Standards of Medical Care in Diabetes," *Diabetes Care*, 2007, 30 (Suppl 1):4-41.

Insulin NPH and Insulin Regular
(IN soo lin N P H & IN soo lin REG yoo ler)

Related Information

Insulin Regular *on page 750*

U.S. Brand Names Humulin® 50/50 [DSC]; Humulin® 70/30; Novolin® 70/30

Canadian Brand Names Humulin® 20/80; Humulin® 70/30; Novolin® ge 30/70; Novolin® ge 40/60; Novolin® ge 50/50

Index Terms Insulin Regular and Insulin NPH; Isophane Insulin and Regular Insulin; NPH Insulin and Regular Insulin

Pharmacologic Category Antidiabetic Agent, Insulin

Use Treatment of type 1 diabetes mellitus (insulin dependent, IDDM) and type 2 diabetes mellitus (noninsulin dependent, NIDDM) to improve glycemic control

Unlabeled/Investigational Use Gestational diabetes mellitus (GDM)

Pharmacodynamics/Kinetics Note: Rate of absorption, onset, and duration of activity may be affected by site of injection, exercise, presence of lipodystrophy, local blood supply, and/or temperature.

Onset of action: 0.5 hours

Peak effect: 2-12 hours

Duration: 18-24 hours

◀ Time to peak, plasma: Based on individual components:

Insulin regular: 0.8-2 hours

Insulin NPH: 6-10 hours

Excretion: Urine

Dosage Refer to Insulin Regular on page 750. Fixed ratio insulins are normally administered in 1-2 daily doses.

Additional Information Complete prescribing information for this medication should be consulted for additional detail.

Dosage Forms Excipient information presented when available (limited, particularly for generics); consult specific product labeling. [DSC] = Discontinued product

Injection, suspension:

Humulin® 50/50: Insulin NPH suspension 50% [intermediate acting] and insulin regular solution 50% [short acting]: 100 units/mL (10 mL) [vial] [DSC]

Humulin® 70/30: Insulin NPH suspension 70% [intermediate acting] and insulin regular solution 30% [short acting]: 100 units/mL (3 mL) [disposable pen]; (10 mL) [vial]

Novolin® 70/30: Insulin NPH suspension 70% [intermediate acting] and insulin regular solution 30% [short acting]: 100 units/mL (3 mL) [InnoLet® prefilled syringe or PenFill® prefilled cartridge]; (10 mL) [vial]

Additional formulations available in Canada: Injection, suspension:

Humulin® 20/80: Insulin regular solution 20% [short acting] and insulin NPH suspension 80% [intermediate acting]: 100 units/mL (3 mL) [PenFill® prefilled cartridge]

Novolin® ge 30/70: Insulin regular solution 30% [short acting] and insulin NPH suspension 70% [intermediate acting]: 100 units/mL (3 mL) [prefilled syringe or PenFill® prefilled cartridge]; (10 mL) [vial]

Novolin® ge 40/60: Insulin regular solution 40% [short acting] and insulin NPH suspension 60% [intermediate acting]: 100 units/mL (3 mL) [PenFill® prefilled cartridge]

Novolin® ge 50/50: Insulin regular solution 50% [short acting] and insulin NPH suspension 50% [intermediate acting]: 100 units/mL (3 mL) [PenFill® prefilled cartridge]

References

American Diabetes Association, "Standards of Medical Care in Diabetes," *Diabetes Care*, 2007, 30 (Suppl 1):4-41.

Insulin Regular (IN soo lin REG yoo ler)

Medication Safety Issues

Sound-alike/look-alike issues:

Humulin® R may be confused with Humalog®, Humira®, Humulin® 70/30, Humulin® N, Novolin® 70/30, Novolin® R, NovoLog®

Novolin® R may be confused with Humulin® R, Novolin® 70/30, Novolin® N, NovoLog®

High alert medication: The Institute for Safe Medication Practices (ISMP) includes this medication among its list of drugs which have a heightened risk of causing significant patient harm when used in error. *Due to the number of insulin preparations, it is essential to identify/clarify the type of insulin to be used.*

Concentrated solutions (eg, U-500) should not be available in patient care areas. U-500 regular insulin should be stored, dispensed, and administered separately from U-100 regular insulin. For patients who receive U-500 insulin in the hospital setting, highlighting the strength prominently on the patient's medical chart and medication record may help to reduce dispensing errors.

Cross-contamination may occur if insulin pens are shared among multiple patients. Steps should be taken to prohibit sharing of insulin pens.

Related Information

Insulin Aspart *on page 741*
Insulin Aspart Protamine and Insulin Aspart *on page 743*
Insulin Detemir *on page 744*
Insulin Glargine *on page 744*
Insulin Glulisine *on page 745*
Insulin Lispro *on page 747*
Insulin Lispro Protamine and Insulin Lispro *on page 748*
Insulin NPH *on page 749*
Insulin NPH and Insulin Regular *on page 749*

U.S. Brand Names Humulin® R; Humulin® R U-500; Novolin® R

Canadian Brand Names Humulin® R; Novolin® ge Toronto

Index Terms Regular Insulin

Pharmacologic Category Antidiabetic Agent, Insulin

Generic Available No

Use Treatment of type 1 diabetes mellitus (insulin dependent, IDDM) and type 2 diabetes mellitus (noninsulin dependent, NIDDM) to improve glycemic control

Unlabeled/Investigational Use Hyperkalemia; gestational diabetes mellitus (GDM), diabetic ketoacidosis (DKA); hyperosmolar hyperglycemic state (HHS); adjunct of parenteral nutrition

Mechanism of Action Insulin acts via specific membrane-bound receptors on target tissues to regulate metabolism of carbohydrate, protein, and fats. Target organs for insulin include the liver, skeletal muscle, and adipose tissue.

Within the liver, insulin stimulates hepatic glycogen synthesis. Insulin promotes hepatic synthesis of fatty acids, which are released into the circulation as lipoproteins. Skeletal muscle effects of insulin include increased protein synthesis and increased glycogen synthesis. Within adipose tissue, insulin stimulates the processing of circulating lipoproteins to provide free fatty acids, facilitating triglyceride synthesis and storage by adipocytes; also directly inhibits the hydrolysis of triglycerides. In addition, insulin stimulates the cellular uptake of amino acids and increases cellular permeability to several ions, including potassium, magnesium, and phosphate. By activating sodium-potassium ATPases, insulin promotes the intracellular movement of potassium.

Normally secreted by the pancreas, insulin products are manufactured for pharmacologic use through recombinant DNA technology using either *E. coli* or *Saccharomyces cerevisiae*. Insulins are categorized based on the onset, peak, and duration of effect (eg, rapid-, short-, intermediate- and long-acting insulin).

Pharmacodynamics/Kinetics Note: Rate of absorption, onset, and duration of activity may be affected by site of injection, exercise, presence of lipodystrophy, local blood supply, and/or temperature.

Onset of action: SubQ: 0.5 hours
  Peak effect: SubQ: 2.5-5 hours
Duration: SubQ:
  U-100: 4-12 hours (may increase with dose)
  U-500: Up to 24 hours
Distribution: V_d: 0.26-0.36 L/kg
Bioavailability: SubQ: 55% to 77%
Half-life elimination: I.V.: ~0.5-1 hour (dose-dependent); SubQ: 1 hour
Time to peak, plasma: SubQ: 0.8-2 hours
Excretion: Urine

Dosage

Diabetes mellitus: SubQ: **Note:** Insulin requirements vary dramatically between patients and therapy requires dosage adjustments with careful medical supervision. Specific formulations may require distinct administration procedures; please see individual agents.

Type 1: Children and Adults: **Note:** Multiple daily injections (MDI) guided by blood glucose monitoring or the use of continuous subcutaneous insulin infusions (CSII) is the standard of care for patients with type 1 diabetes. Combinations of insulin formulations are commonly used.

Initial dose: 0.5-1.0 units/kg/day in divided doses. Conservative initial doses of 0.2-0.4 units/kg/day may be recommended to avoid the potential for hypoglycemia.

◀ *Division of daily insulin requirement:* Generally, 50% to 75% of the total daily dose (TDD) is given as an intermediate- or long-acting form of insulin (in 1-2 daily injections). The remaining portion of the TDD is then divided and administered before or at mealtimes (depending on the formulation) as a rapid-acting or short-acting form of insulin. Premixed combinations are available that deliver the rapid- or short-acting component at the same time as the intermediate- or long-acting component. Some patients may benefit from the use of CSII which delivers rapid-acting insulin as a continuous infusion throughout the day and as boluses at mealtimes via an external pump device.

Adjustment of dose: Dosage must be titrated to achieve glucose control and avoid hypoglycemia. Adjust dose to maintain preprandial plasma glucose between 70-130 mg/dL for most patients. Since treatment regimens often consist of multiple formulations, dosage adjustments must address the specific phase of insulin release that is primarily contributing to the patient's impaired glycemic control. Treatment and monitoring regimens must be individualized.

Usual maintenance range: 0.5-1.2 units/kg/day in divided doses. Insulin requirements are patient-specific and may vary based on age, body weight, and/or activity factors:

Adolescents: May require as much as 1.5 units/kg/day during puberty (Silverstein, 2005)

Prepuberty: 0.7-1 unit/kg/day

Type 2: Children and Adults: The goal of therapy is to achieve an Hb A_{1c} <7% as quickly as possible using the safe titration of medications. According to a consensus statement by the ADA and European Association for the Study of Diabetes (EASD), basal insulin therapy (eg, intermediate- or long-acting insulin) should be considered in patients with type 2 diabetes who fail to achieve glycemic goals with lifestyle interventions and metformin ± a sulfonylurea. Pioglitazone or a GLP-1 agonist may also be considered prior to initiation of basal insulin therapy. In patients who continue to fail to achieve glycemic goals despite the addition of basal insulin, intensification of insulin therapy should be considered; this generally consists of multiple daily injections with a combination of insulin formulations (Nathan, 2009).

Initial basal insulin dose: 0.2 units/kg or 10 units/day (Nathan, 2009). **Note:** Current guidelines recommend that insulin therapy begin with intermediate- or long-acting insulin given at bedtime or long-acting insulin given in the morning (Nathan, 2009).

Adjustment of basal insulin dose: Increase dose by 2 units/day every 3 days until fasting glucose levels are consistently within target range (70-130 mg/dL); may increase dose in larger increments (eg, 4 units/day) if fasting glucose levels are >180 mg/dL (Nathan, 2009)

Note: If the patient experiences hypoglycemia following adjustment, reduce dose by 4 units/day or 10% of total daily dose, whichever is greater (Nathan, 2009). Additional algorithms, such as the "1-1-100", "2-4-6-8", "3-0-3", and "3-2-1" algorithms, exist to aid in the titration of basal insulin (Davies, 2005; Gerstein, 2006; Meneghini, 2007; Riddle, 2003); therapy should be individualized and based on patient-specific details.

Intensification of therapy: Add a second injection of a short-, rapid-, or intermediate-acting insulin as needed based on blood glucose monitoring; the timing of administration and type of insulin added for intensification of therapy depends on the blood glucose level that is consistently out of the target range (eg, preprandial glucose levels before lunch or dinner, postprandial glucose levels, and/or bedtime glucose levels). Additional injections and subsequent dosage adjustments must address the specific phase of insulin release that is primarily contributing to the patient's impaired glycemic control. Intensification of therapy can usually begin with a second injection of ~4 units/day followed by adjustments of ~2 units/day every 3 days until the targeted blood glucose is within range (Nathan, 2009).

In the setting of glucose toxicity (loss of beta-cell sensitivity to glucose concentrations), insulin therapy may be used for short-term management to restore sensitivity of beta-cells; in these cases, the dose may need to be rapidly reduced/withdrawn when sensitivity is re-established.

Diabetic ketoacidosis (DKA) (unlabeled use): Only I.V. regular insulin should be used for severe DKA; use of SubQ rapid-acting insulin analogs (eg, aspart, lispro) may be appropriate for mild-moderate DKA (Kitabchi, 2009). Treatment should continue until reversal of acid-base derangement/ketonemia. Serum glucose is not a direct indicator of these abnormalities, and may decrease more rapidly than correction of the metabolic abnormalities. Also, refer to institution-specific protocols where appropriate.

Children and Adults <20 years (Kitabchi, 2004):

I.V.:

Infusion: 0.1 units/kg/hour

Adjustment: If serum glucose does not fall by 50 mg/dL in the first hour, check hydration status; if acceptable, double insulin dose hourly until glucose levels fall at rate of 50-75 mg/dL per hour. Once serum glucose reaches 250 mg/dL, decrease dose to 0.05-0.1 units/kg/hour; dextrose-containing I.V. fluids should be administered to maintain serum glucose between 150-250 mg/dL until the acidosis clears. After resolution of DKA, supplement I.V. insulin with SubQ insulin as needed until the patient is able to eat and transition fully to a SubQ insulin regimen. An overlap of ~1-2 hours between discontinuation of I.V. insulin and administration of SubQ insulin is recommended to ensure adequate plasma insulin levels.

SubQ, I.M. (**Note:** Only use the SubQ and I.M route if I.V. infusion access is unavailable): 0.1-0.3 units/kg SubQ bolus, followed by 0.1 units/kg given every hour SubQ or I.M. or 0.15-0.2 units/kg every 2 hours SubQ; continue until acidosis clears, then decrease to 0.05 units/kg given every hour until SubQ replacement dosing can be initiated (Kitabchi, 2004; Wolfsdorf, 2007)

Adults ≥20 years (Kitabchi, 2009):

I.V.:

Bolus: 0.1 units/kg (optional)

Infusion: 0.1-0.14 units/kg/hour. **Note:** If no I.V. bolus was administered, patients should receive a continuous infusion of 0.14 units/kg/hour; lower doses may not achieve adequate insulin concentrations to suppress hepatic ketone body production.

Adjustment: If serum glucose does not fall by at least 10% in the first hour, give an I.V. bolus of 0.14 units/kg and continue previous regimen. In addition, if serum glucose does not fall by 50-70 mg/dL in the first hour, the insulin infusion dose should be increased hourly until a steady glucose decline is achieved Once serum glucose reaches 200 mg/dL, decrease infusion dose to 0.02-0.05 units/kg/hour or switch to SubQ rapid-acting insulin (eg, aspart, lispro) at 0.1 units/kg every 2 hours; dextrose-containing I.V. fluids should be administered to maintain serum glucose between 150-250 mg/dL until the acidosis clears. After resolution of DKA, supplement I.V. insulin with SubQ insulin as needed until the patient is able to eat and transition fully to a SubQ insulin regimen. An overlap of ~1-2 hours between discontinuation of I.V. insulin and administration of SubQ insulin is recommended to ensure adequate plasma insulin levels.

SubQ, I.M.: According to the 2009 ADA consensus statement on hyperglycemic crises, a rapid-acting insulin analog (eg, aspart, lispro) given every 1-2 hours via the SubQ route may be appropriate for mild-moderate DKA; however, specific dosing recommendations are not provided (Kitabchi, 2009). If using the I.V. route for severe DKA, consider switching to SubQ rapid-acting insulin once serum glucose reaches 200 mg/dL (Kitabchi, 2009). The following dosing regimen from the 2004 ADA position statement recommends regular insulin (Kitabchi, 2004):

Bolus: 0.4 units/kg; **Note:** Give half of the dose (0.2 units/kg) as an I.V. bolus and half of the dose (0.2 units/kg) as SubQ or I.M.

Intermittent: 0.1 units/kg given every hour SubQ or I.M.

Adjustment: If serum glucose does not fall by 50-70 mg/dL in the first hour, administer 10 units hourly by I.V. bolus until glucose levels fall at a rate of 50-70 mg/dL per hour. Once serum glucose reaches 250 mg/dL, decrease dose to 5-10 units SubQ every 2 hours; dextrose-containing I.V. fluids should be administered to maintain serum glucose between 150-250 mg/dL until the acidosis clears.

Gestational diabetes mellitus (unlabeled use): Insulin therapy should be considered when medical nutrition therapy has not achieved GDM glycemic goals (fasting plasma glucose: <95 mg/dL; 1-hour postprandial levels: <130-140 mg/dL; 2-hour postprandial levels: <120 mg/dL); dose and timing of administration should be based on frequent monitoring of plasma glucose levels (ACOG, 2001; ADA, 2004). Human insulin may be preferred (ADA, 2004); however, rapid-acting insulin analogues may also be considered (ACOG, 2001).

Hyperkalemia, moderate-to-severe (unlabeled use): I.V.:

Children: 0.1 units/kg regular insulin with dextrose 400 mg/kg infused over 15-30 minutes; ratio of ~1 unit of insulin to every 4 g of dextrose (Hegenbarth, 2008). **Note:** Dextrose monotherapy may be sufficient to correct hyperkalemia.

Adults: 10 units regular insulin mixed with 25 g dextrose (50 mL D_{50}W) given over 15-30 minutes (ACLS, 2005); alternatively, 50 mL D_{50}W over 5 minutes followed by 10 units regular insulin I.V. push over seconds may be administered in the setting of imminent cardiac arrest. In patients with ongoing cardiac arrest (eg, PEA with presumed hyperkalemia), administration of D_{50}W over <5 minutes is routine. Effects on potassium are temporary. As appropriate, consider methods of enhancing potassium removal/excretion.

Hyperosmolar hyperglycemic state (HHS) (unlabeled use): Only regular insulin should be used. Infusion should continue until reversal of mental status changes and hyperosmolality. Serum glucose is not a direct indicator of these abnormalities, and may decrease more rapidly than correction of the metabolic abnormalities. Also, refer to institution-specific protocols where appropriate.

Children and Adults <20 years (Kitabchi, 2004):

I.V.:

Infusion: 0.1 units/kg/hour

Adjustment: If serum glucose does not fall by 50 mg/dL in the first hour, check hydration status; if acceptable, double insulin dose hourly until glucose levels fall at rate of 50-75 mg/dL per hour. Once serum glucose reaches 300 mg/dL, decrease dose to 0.05-0.1 units/kg/hour; dextrose-containing I.V. fluids should be administered to maintain serum glucose between 250-300 mg/dL until hyperosmolality clears and mental status returns to normal. After resolution of HHS, supplement I.V. insulin with SubQ insulin as needed until the patient is able to eat and transition fully to a SubQ insulin regimen. An overlap of ~1-2 hours between discontinuation of I.V. insulin and administration of SubQ insulin is recommended to ensure adequate plasma insulin levels.

SubQ, I.M. (**Note:** Only use the SubQ and I.M route if I.V. infusion access is unavailable): 0.1-0.3 units/kg SubQ bolus, followed by 0.1 units/kg given every hour SubQ or I.M. or 0.15-0.2 units/kg every 2 hours SubQ; continue until resolution of hyperosmolality, then decrease to 0.05 units/kg given every hour until SubQ replacement dosing can be initiated (Kitabchi, 2004; Wolfsdorf, 2007)

Adults ≥20 years (Kitabchi, 2009):

I.V.:

Bolus: 0.1 units/kg bolus (optional)

Infusion: 0.1-0.14 units/kg/hour. **Note:** If no I.V. bolus was administered, patients should receive a continuous infusion of 0.14 units/kg/hour.

Adjustment: If serum glucose does not fall by at least 10% in the first hour, give an I.V. bolus of 0.14 units/kg and continue previous regimen. In addition, if serum glucose does not fall by 50-70 mg/dL in the first hour, the insulin infusion dose should be increased hourly until a steady glucose decline is achieved. Once serum glucose reaches 300 mg/dL, decrease dose to 0.02-0.05 units/kg/hour; dextrose-containing I.V. fluids should be administered to maintain serum glucose between 200-300 mg/dL until the patient is mentally alert. After resolution of HHS, supplement I.V. insulin with SubQ insulin as needed until the patient is able to eat and transition fully to a SubQ insulin regimen. An overlap of ~1-2 hours between discontinuation of I.V. insulin and administration of SubQ insulin is recommended to ensure adequate plasma insulin levels.

Dosing adjustment in renal impairment: Insulin requirements are reduced due to changes in insulin clearance or metabolism. Close monitoring of blood glucose and adjustment of therapy is required in renal impairment.

Cl_{cr} 10-50 mL/minute: Administer at 75% of normal dose and monitor glucose closely

Cl_{cr} <10 mL/minute: Administer at 25% to 50% of normal dose and monitor glucose closely

Hemodialysis: Because of a large molecular weight (6000 daltons), insulin is not significantly removed by hemodialysis; supplemental dose is not necessary

Peritoneal dialysis: Because of a large molecular weight (6000 daltons), insulin is not significantly removed by peritoneal dialysis; supplemental dose is not necessary

Continuous renal replacement therapy: Administer 75% of normal dose and monitor glucose closely; supplemental dose is not necessary

Dosing adjustment in hepatic impairment: Insulin requirements may be reduced. Close monitoring of blood glucose and adjustment of therapy is required in hepatic impairment.

Stability Store unopened vials, cartridges, and prefilled pens in refrigerator between 2°C and 8°C (36°F to 46°F); do not freeze; keep away from heat and sunlight. Once punctured (in use), vials may be stored under refrigeration or at room temperature. Cartridges and prefilled pens that have been punctured (in use) should be stored at temperatures <30°C (<86°F) and used within 28 days; do not freeze; refrigeration not required.

For SubQ administration:

Humulin® R vials: May be diluted with the universal diluent, Sterile Diluent for Humalog®, Humulin® N, Humulin® R, Humulin® 70/30, and Humulin® R U-500, to a concentration of 10 units/mL (U-10) or 50 units/mL (U-50). According to the manufacturer, diluted insulin should be stored at 30°C (86°F) and used within 14 days **or** at 5°C (41°F) and used within 28 days. Do not dilute insulin contained in a cartridge or prefilled pen.

Novolin® R: Insulin Diluting Medium for NovoLog® is **not** intended for use with Novolin® R or any insulin product other than insulin aspart.

For I.V. infusion:

Humulin® R: May be diluted in NS or D_5W to concentrations of 0.1-1 unit/mL. Stable for 48 hours at room temperature, 96 hours under refrigeration, or for 48 hours under refrigeration followed by 48 hours at room temperature.

Novolin® R: May be diluted in NS, D_5W, or $D_{10}W$ with 40 mEq/L potassium chloride at concentrations of 0.05-1 unit/mL. Stable for 24 hours at room temperature

Administration

SubQ administration: Do not use if solution is viscous or cloudy; use only if clear and colorless. Regular insulin should be administered within 30-60 minutes before a meal. Cold injections should be avoided. SubQ administration is usually made into the thighs, arms, buttocks, or abdomen; rotate injection sites. When mixing regular insulin with other preparations of insulin, regular insulin should be drawn into syringe first. Regular insulin is not recommended for use in external SubQ insulin infusion pump.

I.M. administration: Do not use if solution is viscous or cloudy; use only if clear and colorless. May be administered I.M. in selected clinical situations; close monitoring of blood glucose and serum potassium as well as medical supervision is required.

I.V. administration: Do not use if solution is viscous or cloudy; use only if clear and colorless. May be administered I.V. with close monitoring of blood glucose and serum potassium; appropriate medical supervision is required. If possible, avoid I.V. bolus administration in pediatric patients with DKA; may increase risk of cerebral edema. **Do not administer mixtures of insulin formulations intravenously.** I.V. administration of U-500 regular insulin is not recommended.

I.V. infusions: To minimize adsorption to I.V. solution bag (**Note:** Refer to institution-specific protocols where appropriate):

*If new tubing is **not** needed:* Wait a minimum of 30 minutes between the preparation of the solution and the initiation of the infusion.

If new tubing is needed: After receiving the insulin drip solution, the administration set should be attached to the I.V. container and the entire line should be flushed with a priming infusion of 20-50 mL of the insulin solution (Goldberg, 2006; Hirsch, 2006). Wait 30 minutes, then flush the line again with the insulin solution prior to initiating the infusion.

If insulin is required prior to the availability of the insulin drip, regular insulin should be administered by I.V. push injection.

Because of adsorption, the actual amount of insulin being administered via I.V. infusion could be substantially less than the apparent amount. Therefore, adjustment of the I.V. infusion rate should be based on effect and not solely on the apparent insulin dose. The apparent dose may be used as a starting point for determining the subsequent SubQ dosing regimen (Moghissi, 2009); however, the transition to SubQ administration requires continuous medical supervision, frequent monitoring of blood glucose, and careful adjustment of therapy. In addition, SubQ insulin should be given 1-4 hours prior to the discontinuation of I.V. insulin to prevent hyperglycemia (Moghissi, 2009).

Monitoring Parameters

Diabetes mellitus: Plasma glucose, electrolytes, Hb A_{1c}

DKA/HHS: Serum electrolytes, glucose, BUN, creatinine, osmolality, venous pH (repeat arterial blood gases are generally unnecessary), anion gap, urine output, urinalysis, mental status

Hyperkalemia: Serum potassium and glucose must be closely monitored to avoid hypokalemia, rebound hyperkalemia, and hypoglycemia.

Reference Range

Therapeutic, serum insulin (fasting): 5-20 µIU/mL (SI: 35-145 pmol/L)

Glucose, fasting:

Newborns: 60-110 mg/dL

Adults: 60-110 mg/dL

Elderly: 100-180 mg/dL

Recommendations for glycemic control in adults with diabetes mellitus (ADA, 2009):

Hb A_{1c}: <7%

Preprandial capillary plasma glucose: 70-130 mg/dL

Peak postprandial capillary plasma glucose: <180 mg/dL

Anesthesia and Critical Care Concerns/Other Considerations

Evidence-Based Information: *Intensive Insulin Therapy in the Critically-Ill:*

Surgical Patients: Van den Berghe and colleagues (2001) performed a single-center, prospective, randomized, controlled study in 1548 surgical intensive care patients (~63% cardiac surgery patients). Authors compared conventional control of blood glucose (180-200 mg/dL) versus intensive control of blood glucose (80-110 mg/dL). Primary outcome was ICU mortality. The authors showed an absolute ICU mortality reduction of 3.4% (8.0% vs 4.6%; p<0.04) in the intensive insulin therapy arm. Intensive insulin therapy also reduced bloodstream infections (7.8% vs 4.2%; p=0.003), acute renal failure requiring hemodialysis (8.2 vs 4.8%; p=0.007), and critical-illness polyneuropathy (51.9% vs 28.7%; p<0.001). Greatest ICU mortality reduction appeared in patients with an ICU stay >5 days, reducing mortality by 9.6% (20.2% vs 10.6%; p=0.005).

Medical Patients: A similar study (Van den Berghe, 2006) was done in adults admitted to the medical intensive care unit who were assumed to require ≥3 days of ICU care. The goal blood glucose was the same as the previous Van den Berghe study. The primary outcome was hospital mortality. Important secondary outcomes were mortality in the ICU, 90-day mortality, days to wean from mechanical ventilation, days in ICU and hospital, and new kidney injury. A subgroup analysis was planned for patients staying in the ICU for >3 days. Twelve hundred patients were randomized to conventional versus intensive blood glucose control. Intensive insulin therapy did not significantly reduce in-hospital mortality (40% conventional group vs 37.3% intensive group, p=0.33). Morbidity was significantly reduced in the intensive group by the prevention of newly-acquired kidney injury, accelerated weaning from mechanical ventilation and shortened stay in the ICU/hospital. For patients who stayed in the ICU for <3 days, mortality was greater in those receiving intensive insulin therapy. A subset of patients who remained in the ICU for ≥3 days was evaluated and in-hospital mortality was significantly reduced (52.5% vs 43%; p=0.009) in those who received intensive insulin therapy.

Sepsis: An additional study evaluated intensive insulin therapy in 537 medical ICU patients with severe sepsis. In this multicenter, two-by-two factorial design study, patients were randomized to intensive insulin therapy to maintain euglycemia (80-110 mg/dL) or conventional insulin therapy to maintain blood glucose levels between 180-200 mg/dL. For fluid resuscitation, patients were also randomized to 10% pentastarch, a low-molecular weight hydroxyethyl starch (HES), or Ringer's lactate. The coprimary endpoints of the trial were mortality at 28 days and morbidity as measured by the Sequential Organ Failure Assessment (SOFA) score. Of note, previous studies evaluated mortality as a single primary endpoint. Some of the secondary endpoints included rate of acute renal failure, mean SOFA subscores, mechanical ventilation duration, ICU length of stay, and 90-day mortality. Severe hypoglycemia was defined as a serum glucose ≤40 mg/dL. The trial was stopped early due to an increased number of hypoglycemic events with intensive insulin therapy compared to conventional insulin therapy (17% vs 4.1%, respectively; p<0.001). In addition, there was no significant difference in the rates of mortality or mean SOFA scores. Patients receiving conventional insulin therapy were continued on the randomized resuscitation fluid (HES or Ringer's lactate). Patients who received HES had a higher rate of renal failure and trended toward a higher rate of mortality at 90 days (Brunkhorst, 2008).

Medical and Surgical Patients: The largest study to date evaluating intensive insulin therapy in the critically-ill patient is the NICE-SUGAR study (2009). In this international open-label trial, 6104 medical (n=3796, 62%) and surgical (n=2233, 37%) patients expected to require treatment in the ICU on ≥3 consecutive days were randomized to either intensive glucose control (81-108 mg/dL) or conventional glucose control (144-180 mg/dL). The primary endpoint was death within 90 days of randomization. Secondary endpoints included survival time during the first 90 days, durations of mechanical ventilation, renal-replacement therapy, and ICU and hospital stays. Control of blood glucose was maintained using a continuous infusion of regular insulin (see algorithm at https://studies.thegeorgeinstitute.org/nice/docs/ALGORITHM.pdf). Severe hypoglycemia was defined as a serum glucose ≤40 mg/dL. Based on intention-to-treat analysis, 90-day mortality was significantly higher in the intensive glucose control group compared to the conventional control group (27.5% vs 24.9%; p=0.02) and was not different between medical and surgical patients. The number of patients who experienced severe hypoglycemia was higher in the intensive control group compared to the conventional control group (6.8% vs 0.5%; p<0.001). Study treatment was discontinued prematurely mostly due to reasons unrelated to adverse effects in 10% of patients in the intensive control group versus 7.4% of patients in the conventional control group which may have affected the results.

Guidelines: The 2008 Surviving Sepsis Campaign guidelines (Dellinger, 2008) have suggested targeting blood glucose levels <150 mg/dL by using a validated protocol for insulin adjustments (Grade 2C) and that all patients receiving I.V. insulin should receive a glucose calorie source. Concurrently blood glucose values should be monitored every 1-2 hours until glucose values and insulin infusion rates are stable, then monitored every 4 hours thereafter (Grade 1C).

More recently, as a result of a meta-analysis (Wiener, 2008) and the NICE-SUGAR study (2009), the American College of Endocrinology and the American Diabetes Association (Moghissi, 2009) recommended initiation of a continuous I.V. insulin infusion for the critically ill patient with persistent hyperglycemia (≥180 mg/dL) to maintain serum glucose levels between 140-180 mg/dL. Target serum glucose levels ≤110 mg/dL are no longer recommended. Frequent blood glucose monitoring (ie, every 0.5-2 hours) is necessary to reduce the incidence of hypoglycemia and achieve optimal glycemic control.

Contraindications Hypersensitivity to regular insulin or any component of the formulation; during episodes of hypoglycemia

Warnings/Precautions Hypoglycemia is the most common adverse effect of insulin. The timing of hypoglycemia differs among various insulin formulations. Hypoglycemia may result from increased work or exercise without eating; use of long-acting insulin preparations (eg, insulin detemir, insulin glargine) may delay recovery from hypoglycemia. Profound and prolonged episodes of hypoglycemia may result in convulsions, unconsciousness, temporary or permanent brain damage or even death. Insulin requirements may be altered during illness, emotional disturbances or other stressors. Insulin may produce hypokalemia which, if left untreated, may result in respiratory paralysis, ventricular arrhythmia and even death. Use with caution in patients at risk for hypokalemia (eg, I.V. insulin use). Use with caution in renal or hepatic impairment.

Human insulin differs from animal-source insulin. Any change of insulin should be made cautiously; changing manufacturers, type, and/or method of manufacture may result in the need for a change of dosage. U-500 regular insulin is a concentrated insulin formulation which contains 500 units of insulin per mL; for SubQ administration only using a U-100 insulin syringe or tuberculin syringe; **not for I.V. administration**. To avoid dosing errors when using a U-100 insulin syringe, the prescribed dose should be written in actual insulin units and as unit markings on the U-100 insulin syringe (eg, 50 units [10 units on a U-100 insulin syringe]). To avoid dosing errors when using a tuberculin syringe, the prescribed dose should be written in actual insulin units and as a volume (eg, 50 units [0.1 mL]). Mixing U-500 regular insulin with other insulin formulations is not recommended.

Regular insulin may be administered I.V. or I.M. in selected clinical situations; close monitoring of blood glucose and serum potassium, as well as medical supervision, is required.

The general objective of exogenous insulin therapy is to approximate the physiologic pattern of insulin secretion which is characterized by two distinct phases. Phase 1 insulin secretion suppresses hepatic glucose production and phase 2 insulin secretion occurs in response to carbohydrate ingestion; therefore, exogenous insulin therapy may consist of basal insulin (eg, intermediate- or long-acting insulin or via continuous subcutaneous insulin infusion [CSII]) and/or prandial insulin (eg, short- or rapid-acting insulin) (see Insulin Products in Appendix). Patients with type 1 diabetes do not produce endogenous insulin; therefore, these patients require both basal and preprandial insulin administration. Patients with type 2 diabetes retain some beta-cell function in the early stages of their disease; however, as the disease progresses, phase 1 insulin secretion may become completely impaired and phase 2 insulin secretion becomes delayed and/or inadequate in response to meals. Therefore, patients with type 2 diabetes may be treated with oral antidiabetic agents, basal insulin, and/or preprandial insulin depending on the stage of disease and current glycemic control. Since treatment regimens often consist of multiple agents, dosage adjustments must address the specific phase of insulin release that is primarily contributing to the patient's impaired glycemic control. Diabetes self-management education (DSME) is essential to maximize the effectiveness of therapy. Treatment and monitoring regimens must be individualized.

Adverse Reactions Frequency not defined.

Cardiovascular: Palpitation, pallor, peripheral edema, tachycardia

Central nervous system: Fatigue, headache, hypothermia, loss of consciousness, mental confusion

Dermatologic: Pruritus, rash, redness, urticaria

Endocrine & metabolic: Hypoglycemia, hypokalemia

Gastrointestinal: Hunger, nausea, numbness of mouth, weight gain

Local: Injection site reaction (including edema, itching, pain or warmth, stinging), lipoatrophy, lipodystrophy

Neuromuscular & skeletal: Muscle weakness, paresthesia, tremor

Ocular: Transient presbyopia or blurred vision

Miscellaneous: Anaphylaxis, antibodies to insulin (no change in efficacy), diaphoresis, local allergy, systemic allergic symptoms

Drug Interactions

Metabolism/Transport Effects Induces CYP1A2 (weak)

Avoid Concomitant Use There are no known interactions where it is recommended to avoid concomitant use.

Increased Effect/Toxicity

Insulin Regular may increase the levels/effects of: Antidiabetic Agents (Thiazolidinedione); Hypoglycemic Agents; Quinolone Antibiotics

The levels/effects of Insulin Regular may be increased by: Beta-Blockers; Edetate CALCIUM Disodium; Edetate Disodium; Herbs (Hypoglycemic Properties); Pegvisomant

Decreased Effect

The levels/effects of Insulin Regular may be decreased by: Corticosteroids (Orally Inhaled); Corticosteroids (Systemic); Luteinizing Hormone-Releasing Hormone Analogs; Somatropin; Thiazide Diuretics

Ethanol/Nutrition/Herb Interactions

Ethanol: Use caution with ethanol; may increase risk of hypoglycemia.

Herb/Nutraceutical: Use caution with alfalfa, aloe, bilberry, bitter melon, burdock, celery, damiana, fenugreek, garcinia, garlic, ginger, ginseng (American), gymnema, marshmallow, stinging nettle; may increase risk of hypoglycemia.

Dietary Considerations Individualized medical nutrition therapy (MNT) based on ADA recommendations is an integral part of therapy.

Dosage Forms Excipient information presented when available (limited, particularly for generics); consult specific product labeling.

Injection, solution:

Humulin® R: 100 units/mL (10 mL)

Novolin® R: 100 units/mL (3 mL) [InnoLet® prefilled syringe or PenFill® prefilled cartridge]; (10 mL) [vial]

Injection, solution [concentrate]:

Humulin® R U-500: 500 units/mL (20 mL vial)

References

American Diabetes Association, "Standards of Medical Care in Diabetes," *Diabetes Care*, 2007, 30 (Suppl 1):4-41.

Antman EM, Anbe SC, Alpert JS, et al, "ACC/AHA Guidelines for the Management of Patients With ST-Elevation Myocardial Infarction - Executive Summary: A Report of the American College of Cardiology/American Heart Association Task Force on Practice Guidelines (Writing Committee to Revise the 1999 Guidelines for the Management of Patients With Acute Myocardial Infarction)," *Circulation*, 2004, 110:588-636. Available at: http://www.circulationaha.org/cgi/content/full/110/5/588. Last accessed October 26, 2004.

Brown G and Dodek P, "Intravenous Insulin Nomogram Improves Blood Glucose Control in the Critically Ill," *Crit Care Med*, 2001, 29(9):1714-9.

Brunkhorst FM, Engel C, Bloos F, et al, "Intensive Insulin Therapy and Pentastarch Resuscitation in Severe Sepsis," *N Engl J Med*, 2008, 358(2):125-39.

Deedwania P, Kosiborod M, Barrett E, et al, "Hyperglycemia and Acute Coronary Syndrome: A Scientific Statement From the American Heart Association Diabetes Committee of the Council on Nutrition, Physical Activity, and Metabolism," *Circulation*, 2008, 117(12):1610-9.

Dellinger RP, Levy MM, Carlet JM, et al, "Surviving Sepsis Campaign: International Guidelines for Management of Severe Sepsis and Septic Shock: 2008," *Intensive Care Med*, 2008, 34(1): 17-60. Available at http://www.survivingsepsis.org/system/files/images/2008_20International_20SSC_20-Guidelines_1_.pdf

Holman RR and Turner RC, "Insulin Therapy in Type II Diabetes," *Diabetes Res Clin Pract*, 1995, (28 Suppl):179-84.

Joint Commission on Accreditation of Healthcare Organizations, "2005 National Patient Safety Goals," available at http://www.jcaho.org/accredited+organizations/patient+safety/05_npsg_guidelines.

Levine DF and Bulstrode C, "Managing Suicidal Insulin Overdose," *Br Med J (Clin Res Ed)*, 1982, 285 (6346):974-5.

Malhotra A, "Intensive Insulin in Intensive Care," *N Engl J Med*, 2006, 354(5):516-8.

Malmberg K, "Prospective Randomised Study of Intensive Insulin Treatment on Long Term Survival After Acute Myocardial Infarction in Patients With Diabetes Mellitus. DIGAMI (Diabetes Mellitus, Insulin Glucose Infusion in Acute Myocardial Infarction) Study Group," *BMJ*, 1997, 314 (7093):1512-5.

Moghissi ES, Korytkowski MT, DiNardo M, et al, "American Association of Clinical Endocrinologists and American Diabetes Association Consensus Statement on Inpatient Glycemic Control," *Endocrine Practice*, 2009, 15(4):1-17.

Mokhlesi B, Leikin JB, Murray P, et al, "Adult Toxicology in Critical Care: Part II: Specific Poisonings," *Chest*, 2003, 123(3):897-922.

Mueller-Schoop J, "Accidental Intravenous Self-Injection With Insulin Pen," *Lancet*, 1993, 341 (8849):894.

NICE-SUGAR Study Investigators, Finfer S, Chittock DR, et al, "Intensive Versus Conventional Glucose Control in Critically Ill Patients," *N Engl J Med*, 2009, 360(13):1283-97.

"Proceedings of the American College of Endocrinology Task Force on Inpatient Diabetes and Metabolic Control Consensus Conference, Washington, DC, USA, December 2003," *Endocr Pract*, 2004, (10 Suppl 2):3-108.

Roberge RJ, Martin TG, and Delbridge TR, "Intentional Massive Insulin Overdose: Recognition and Management," *Ann Emerg Med*, 1993, 22(2):228-34.

Silverstein J, Klingensmith G, Copeland K, et al, "Care of Children and Adolescents With Type 1 Diabetes: A Statement of the American Diabetes Association," *Diabetes Care*, 2005, 28 (1):186-212.

Simeon PS, Geffner ME, Levin SR, et al, "Continuous Insulin Infusions in Neonates: Pharmacologic Availability of Insulin in Intravenous Solutions," *J Pediatr*, 1994, 124(5 Pt 1):818-20.

Van den Berghe G, Wilmer A, Hermans G, et al, "Intensive Insulin Therapy in the Medical ICU," *N Engl J Med*, 2006, 354(5):449-6.

Van den Berghe G, Wouters P, Weekers F, et al, "Intensive Insulin Therapy in the Critically Ill Patients," *N Engl J Med*, 2001, 345(19):1359-67.

Wiener RS, Wiener DC, and Larson RJ, "Benefits and Risks of Tight Glucose Control in Critically Ill Adults: A Meta-Analysis," *JAMA*, 2008, 300(8):933-44.

- **Insulin Regular and Insulin NPH** *see* Insulin NPH and Insulin Regular *on page 749*
- **Integrilin®** *see* Eptifibatide *on page 511*
- **Intelence™** *see* Etravirine *on page 565*
- **Intralipid®** *see* Fat Emulsion *on page 578*
- **Intrapleural Talc** *see* Talc (Sterile) *on page 1349*
- **Intravenous Fat Emulsion** *see* Fat Emulsion *on page 578*
- **Intrifiban** *see* Eptifibatide *on page 511*
- **Intropin** *see* DOPamine *on page 448*
- **Invanz®** *see* Ertapenem *on page 513*

Ipratropium (i pra TROE pee um)

Medication Safety Issues
Sound-alike/look-alike issues:
Atrovent® may be confused with Alupent®, Serevent®
Ipratropium may be confused with tiotropium

U.S. Brand Names Atrovent®; Atrovent® HFA

Canadian Brand Names Alti-Ipratropium; Apo-Ipravent®; Atrovent®; Atrovent® HFA; Gen-Ipratropium; Mylan-Ipratropium Solution; Mylan-Ipratropium Sterinebs; Novo-Ipramide; Nu-Ipratropium; PMS-Ipratropium

Index Terms Ipratropium Bromide

Pharmacologic Category Anticholinergic Agent

Generic Available Yes: Solution for nebulization

Use
Oral inhalation: Anticholinergic bronchodilator used in bronchospasm associated with COPD, bronchitis, and emphysema

Nasal spray: Symptomatic relief of rhinorrhea associated with the common cold and allergic and nonallergic rhinitis

Unlabeled/Investigational Use Oral inhalation: Adjunct to short-acting beta-adrenergic agonists therapy in moderate-to-severe exacerbations of acute asthma

Mechanism of Action Blocks the action of acetylcholine at parasympathetic sites in bronchial smooth muscle causing bronchodilation; local application to nasal mucosa inhibits serous and seromucous gland secretions.

Pharmacodynamics/Kinetics
Onset of action: Bronchodilation: Within 15 minutes
Peak effect: 1-2 hours
Duration: 2-5 hours
Absorption: Negligible
Distribution: Inhalation: 15% of dose reaches lower airways
Protein Binding: ≤9%
Half-life elimination: 2 hours
Excretion: Urine

Dosage
Nebulization:
Children ≤12 years: Asthma exacerbation, acute (*NIH Asthma Guidelines, 2007*): 250-500 mcg every 20 minutes for 3 doses, then as needed. **Note:** Should be given in combination with a short-acting beta-adrenergic agonist.

Children >12 years and Adults:
Bronchodilator for COPD: 500 mcg (one unit-dose vial) 3-4 times/day with doses 6-8 hours apart
Asthma exacerbation, acute (*NIH Asthma Guidelines, 2007*): 500 mcg every 20 minutes for 3 doses, then as needed. **Note:** Should be given in combination with a short-acting beta-adrenergic agonist.

Oral inhalation: MDI:
  Children ≤12 years: Asthma exacerbation, acute (*NIH Asthma Guidelines, 2007*): 4-8 inhalations every 20 minutes as needed for up to 3 hours. **Note:** Should be given in combination with a short-acting beta-adrenergic agonist.
  Children >12 years and Adults:
    Bronchodilator for COPD: 2 inhalations 4 times/day, up to 12 inhalations/24 hours
    Asthma exacerbation, acute (*NIH Asthma Guidelines, 2007*): 8 inhalations every 20 minutes as needed for up to 3 hours. **Note:** Should be given in combination with a short-acting beta-adrenergic agonist.

Intranasal: Nasal spray:
  Symptomatic relief of rhinorrhea associated with the common cold (safety and efficacy of use beyond 4 days in patients with the common cold have not been established):
    Children 5-11 years: 0.06%: 2 sprays in each nostril 3 times/day
    Children ≥12 years and Adults: 0.06%: 2 sprays in each nostril 3-4 times/day
  Symptomatic relief of rhinorrhea associated with allergic/nonallergic rhinitis: Children ≥6 years and Adults: 0.03%: 2 sprays in each nostril 2-3 times/day
  Symptomatic relief of rhinorrhea associated with seasonal allergic rhinitis (safety and efficacy of use beyond 3 weeks in patients with seasonal allergic rhinitis has not been established): Children ≥5 years and Adults: 0.06%: 2 sprays in each nostril 4 times/day

Stability
Oral inhalation aerosol and nasal spray: Store at controlled room temperature of 25°C (77°F). Do not store near heat or open flame.
Oral inhalation solution: Store at 15°C to 30°C (59°F to 86°F). Protect from light.
Administration Avoid spraying into the eyes.
Atrovent® HFA: Prior to initial use, prime inhaler by releasing 2 test sprays into the air. If the inhaler has not been used for >3 days, reprime.
Nasal spray: Prior to initial use, prime inhaler by releasing 7 test sprays into the air. If the inhaler has not been used for >24 hours, reprime by releasing 2 test sprays into the air.

Pregnancy Risk Factor B

Contraindications Hypersensitivity to ipratropium, atropine (and its derivatives), or any component of the formulation

Warnings/Precautions Immediate hypersensitivity reactions (urticaria, angioedema, rash, bronchospasm) have been reported. Rarely, paradoxical bronchospasm may occur with use of inhaled bronchodilating agents; this should be distinguished from inadequate response. Not indicated for the initial treatment of acute episodes of bronchospasm where rescue therapy is required for rapid response. Should only be used in acute exacerbations of asthma in conjunction with short-acting beta-adrenergic agonists for acute episodes. Use with caution in patients with myasthenia gravis, narrow-angle glaucoma, benign prostatic hyperplasia (BPH), or bladder neck obstruction

Adverse Reactions
Inhalation aerosol and inhalation solution:
>10%: Respiratory: Upper respiratory tract infection (9% to 34%), bronchitis (10% to 23%), sinusitis (1% to 11%)
1% to 10%:
  Cardiovascular: Chest pain (3%), palpitation
  Central nervous system: Headache (6% to 7%), dizziness (2% to 3%)
  Gastrointestinal: Dyspepsia (1% to 5%), nausea (4%), xerostomia (2% to 4%)
  Genitourinary: Urinary tract infection (2% to 10%)
  Neuromuscular & skeletal: Back pain (2% to 7%)
  Respiratory: Dyspnea (7% to 10%), rhinitis (2% to 6%), cough (3% to 5%), pharyngitis (4%), bronchospasm (2%), sputum increased (1%)
  Miscellaneous: Flu-like syndrome (4% to 8%)
<1% (Limited to important or life-threatening): Anaphylactic reaction, angioedema, arthritis, atrial fibrillation, bitter taste, constipation, diarrhea, eye pain (acute), glaucoma, hypersensitivity reactions, hypotension, insomnia, laryngospasm, mydriasis, nervousness, pruritus, rash, tachycardia (including supraventricular), tremor, urinary retention, urticaria

Nasal spray:
1% to 10%:
   Central nervous system: Headache (4% to 10%)
   Gastrointestinal: Taste perversion (≤4%), xerostomia (1% to 4%), diarrhea (2%), nausea (2%)
   Respiratory: Upper respiratory tract infection (5% to 10%), epistaxis (6% to 9%), pharyngitis (≤8%), nasal dryness (<1% to 5%), nasal irritation (2%), nasal congestion (1%)
<2% (Limited to important or life-threatening): Anaphylactic reaction, angioedema, blurred vision, conjunctivitis, cough, dizziness, hoarseness, laryngospasm, nasal burning, ocular irritation, palpitation, rash, tachycardia, thirst, tinnitus, urticaria, xerostomia

Drug Interactions
   Avoid Concomitant Use There are no known interactions where it is recommended to avoid concomitant use.
   Increased Effect/Toxicity
     Ipratropium may increase the levels/effects of: Anticholinergics; Cannabinoids; Potassium Chloride

     The levels/effects of Ipratropium may be increased by: Pramlintide
   Decreased Effect
     Ipratropium may decrease the levels/effects of: Acetylcholinesterase Inhibitors (Central); Secretin

     The levels/effects of Ipratropium may be decreased by: Acetylcholinesterase Inhibitors (Central)

Dosage Forms Excipient information presented when available (limited, particularly for generics); consult specific product labeling.
   Aerosol for oral inhalation, as bromide:
     Atrovent® HFA: 17 mcg/actuation (12.9 g)
   Solution for nebulization, as bromide: 0.02% (2.5 mL)
   Solution, intranasal, as bromide [spray]:
     Atrovent®: 0.03% (30 mL); 0.06% (15 mL)

Ipratropium and Albuterol (i pra TROE pee um & al BYOO ter ole)

Related Information
   Albuterol *on page 49*
   Ipratropium *on page 760*
U.S. Brand Names Combivent®; DuoNeb®
Canadian Brand Names CO Ipra-Sal; Combivent UDV; Gen-Combo Sterinebs; ratio-Ipra Sal UDV
Index Terms Albuterol and Ipratropium; Salbutamol and Ipratropium
Pharmacologic Category Anticholinergic Agent; Beta$_2$-Adrenergic Agonist
Use Treatment of COPD in those patients who are currently on a regular bronchodilator who continue to have bronchospasms and require a second bronchodilator
Pharmacodynamics/Kinetics See individual agents.
Dosage Adults:
   Aerosol for inhalation: 2 inhalations 4 times/day (maximum: 12 inhalations/24 hours)
   Solution for nebulization: Initial: 3 mL every 6 hours (maximum: 3 mL every 4 hours)
Additional Information Complete prescribing information for this medication should be consulted for additional detail.
Dosage Forms Excipient information presented when available (limited, particularly for generics); consult specific product labeling.
   Aerosol for oral inhalation:
     Combivent®: Ipratropium bromide 18 mcg and albuterol sulfate 103 mcg per actuation (14.7 g) [contains chlorofluorocarbon, soya lecithin; 200 metered actuations]
   Solution for nebulization: Ipratropium bromide 0.5 mg and albuterol base 2.5 mg per 3 mL (30s, 60s)

DuoNeb®: Ipratropium bromide 0.5 mg and albuterol base 2.5 mg per 3 mL (30s, 60s)

♦ **Ipratropium Bromide** *see* Ipratropium *on page 760*
♦ **I-Prin [OTC]** *see* Ibuprofen *on page 717*
♦ **Iproveratril Hydrochloride** *see* Verapamil *on page 1468*
♦ **Iquix®** *see* Levofloxacin *on page 823*

Irbesartan (ir be SAR tan)

Related Information
Angiotensin Agents *on page 1652*
Heart Failure (Systolic) *on page 1739*

U.S. Brand Names Avapro®

Canadian Brand Names Avapro®

Pharmacologic Category Angiotensin II Receptor Blocker

Use Treatment of hypertension alone or in combination with other antihypertensives; treatment of diabetic nephropathy in patients with type 2 diabetes mellitus (noninsulin dependent, NIDDM) and hypertension

Unlabeled/Investigational Use To slow the rate of progression of aortic-root dilation in pediatric patients with Marfan's syndrome

Pharmacodynamics/Kinetics
Onset of action: Peak effect: 1-2 hours
Duration: >24 hours
Distribution: V_d: 53-93 L
Protein binding, plasma: 90%
Metabolism: Hepatic, primarily CYP2C9
Bioavailability: 60% to 80%
Half-life elimination: Terminal: 11-15 hours
Time to peak, serum: 1.5-2 hours
Excretion: Feces (80%); urine (20%)

Dosage Oral:
Hypertension:
Children:
<6 years: Safety and efficacy have not been established.
≥6-12 years: Initial: 75 mg once daily; may be titrated to a maximum of 150 mg once daily
Children ≥13 years and Adults: 150 mg once daily; patients may be titrated to 300 mg once daily
Note: Starting dose in volume-depleted patients should be 75 mg
Aortic-root dilation with Marfan's syndrome (unlabeled use): Children 14 months to 16 years: Initial: 1.4 mg/kg/day; can be increased to a maximum of 2 mg/kg/day (not to exceed adult maximum of 300 mg/day)
Nephropathy in patients with type 2 diabetes and hypertension: Adults: Target dose: 300 mg once daily

Dosage adjustment in renal impairment: No dosage adjustment necessary with mild to severe impairment unless the patient is also volume depleted.

Anesthesia and Critical Care Concerns/Other Considerations
Clinical Pearls/Comments: In patients on chronic angiotensin receptor blocker (ARB) therapy, intraoperative hypotension may occur with induction and maintenance of general anesthesia; however, discontinuation of therapy prior to surgery is controversial. If continued preoperatively, avoidance of hypotensive agents during surgery is prudent. Episodes of intraoperative hypotension may be managed by fluid administration and/or modest doses of alpha-adrenergic agents. Severe hypotension may occur in patients who are sodium- and/or volume-depleted; initiate lower doses and monitor closely when starting therapy in these patients. ARB therapy may elicit an increase in potassium and creatinine, especially when used in patients with bilateral renal artery stenosis. Concomitant NSAID therapy may attenuate blood pressure control; use of NSAIDs should be avoided or limited, with monitoring of blood pressure control. In the setting of heart failure, NSAID use may be associated with an increased risk for fluid accumulation and edema and therefore should be avoided.

Evidence-Based Information: The angiotensin II receptor antagonists have similar indications as ACE inhibitors. In heart failure, the angiotensin II receptor antagonists are especially useful in providing an alternative therapy in those patients who have intractable cough due to ACE inhibitor therapy. Candesartan has been studied as an alternative therapy in chronic heart failure patients who cannot tolerate an ACE-I (CHARM-Alternative) and as an added therapy in heart failure patients who are maintained on an ACE-I (CHARM-Added). In both studies, the combined endpoint of cardiovascular death or heart failure hospitalizations was significantly improved over the placebo-treated group.

Additional Information Complete prescribing information for this medication should be consulted for additional detail.

Dosage Forms Excipient information presented when available (limited, particularly for generics); consult specific product labeling.
Tablet: 75 mg, 150 mg, 300 mg

References

Brooke BS, Habashi JP, Judge DP, et al, "Angiotensin II Blockade and Aortic-Root Dilation in Marfan's Syndrome," *N Engl J Med*, 2008, 358(26):2787-95.

Chobanian AV, Bakris GL, Black HR, et al, "The Seventh Report of the Joint National Committee on Prevention, Detection, Evaluation, and Treatment of High Blood Pressure: The JNC 7 Report," *JAMA*, 2003, 289(19):2560-71.

Cohn JN and Tognoni G, "Valsartan Heart Failure Trial Investigators. A Randomized Trial of the Angiotensin-Receptor Blocker Valsartan in Chronic Heart Failure," *N Engl J Med*, 2001, 345 (23):1667-75.

Conlin P, Moore T, Swartz S, et al, "Effect of Indomethacin on Blood Pressure Lowering by Captopril and Losartan in Hypertensive Patients," *Hypertension*, 2000, 36(3):461-5.

"Consensus Recommendations for the Management of Chronic Heart Failure. On Behalf of the Membership of the Advisory Council to Improve Outcomes Nationwide in Heart Failure," *Am J Cardiol*, 1999, 83(2A):1A-38A.

Dahlof B, Devereux RB, Kjeldsen SE, et al, "Cardiovascular Morbidity and Mortality in the Losartan Intervention For Endpoint Reduction in Hypertension Study (LIFE): A Randomised Trial Against Atenolol," *Lancet*, 2002, 359(9311):995-1003.

Dickstein K, Kjeksnus J, et al, "Effects of Losartan and Captopril on Mortality and Morbidity in High-Risk Patients After Acute Myocardial Infarction: The OPTIMAAL Randomised Trial. Optimal Trial in Myocardial Infarction with Angiotensin II Antagonist Losartan," *Lancet* , 2002, 360(9335):752-60.

Epstein BJ and Gums JG, "Angiotensin Receptor Blockers Versus ACE Inhibitors: Prevention of Death and Myocardial Infarction in High-Risk Populations," *Ann Pharmacother*, 2005, 39(3):470-80.

Granger CB, McMurray JJ, Yusuf S, et al, "Effects of Candesartan in Patients With Chronic Heart Failure and Reduced Left-Ventricular Systolic Function Intolerant to Angiotensin-Converting-Enzyme Inhibitors: The CHARM-Alternative Trial," *Lancet*, 2003, 362(9386):772-6.

Hunt SA, Baker DW, Chin MH, et al, "ACC/AHA Guidelines for the Evaluation and Management of Chronic Heart Failure in the Adult: Executive Summary. A Report of the American College of Cardiology/American Heart Association Task Force on Practice Guidelines (Committee to Revise the 1995 Guidelines for the Evaluation and Management of Heart Failure)," *J Am Coll Cardiol*, 2001, 38(7):2101-13.

"K/DOQI Clinical Practice Guidelines for Chronic Kidney Disease: Evaluation, Classification, and Stratification. Kidney Disease Outcome Quality Initiative," *Am J Kidney Dis*, 2002, 39(2 Suppl 2):1-246. Available at: http://www.kidney.org/professionals/doqi/kdoqi/toc.htm. Accessed August 1, 2003.

McMurray JJ, Ostergren J, Swedberg K, et al, "Effects of Candesartan in Patients With Chronic Heart Failure and Reduced Left-Ventricular Systolic Function Taking Angiotensin-Converting-Enzyme Inhibitors: The CHARM-Added Trial," *Lancet*, 2003, 362(9386):767-71.

National High Blood Pressure Education Program Working Group on High Blood Pressure in Children and Adolescents, "The Fourth Report on the Diagnosis, Evaluation, and Treatment of High Blood Pressure in Children and Adolescents," *Pediatrics*, 2004, 114 (2 Suppl):555-76.

Pfeffer MA, McMurray JJ, Velazquez EJ, et al, "Valsartan, Captopril, or Both in Myocardial Infarction Complicated by Heart Failure, Left Ventricular Dysfunction, or Both," *N Engl J Med*, 2004, 350 (2):203.

Pitt B, Poole-Wilson PA, Segal R, et al, "Effect of Losartan Compared With Captopril on Mortality in Patients With Symptomatic Heart Failure: Randomised Trial - The Losartan Heart Failure Survival Study ELITE II," *Lancet*, 2000, 355(9215):1582-7.

Isocarboxazid (eye soe kar BOKS a zid)

Related Information
Antidepressant Agents *on page 1660*
U.S. Brand Names Marplan®
Pharmacologic Category Antidepressant, Monoamine Oxidase Inhibitor
Use Treatment of depression
Dosage Oral: Adults: Initial: 10 mg 2-4 times/day; may increase by 10 mg/day every 2-4 days to 40 mg/day by the end of the first week (divided into 2-4 doses). After first week, may increase by up to 20 mg/week to a maximum of 60 mg/day. May take 3-6 weeks to see effects. Dose should be reduced once maximum clinical effect is seen. If no response obtained within 6 weeks, additional titration is unlikely to be beneficial. **Note:** Use caution in patients on >40 mg/day; experience is limited.

Anesthesia and Critical Care Concerns/Other Considerations
Clinical Pearls/Comments: Patients receiving MAO inhibitors who undergo surgery may be at risk of developing significant hypertension when used with direct-acting adrenergic agents (eg, norepinephrine) and of lethal hypertension when administered with indirect-acting adrenergic agents (eg, ephedrine). The use of meperidine in these patients may also precipitate serotonin syndrome and is contraindicated. Years ago, it was advised that patients receiving MAO inhibitors have this drug discontinued for at least 10 days before elective surgery. However, the decision to continue or withhold MAO inhibitors must be done in collaboration with the patient's psychiatrist. Currently, an MAO-safe anesthetic technique which excludes the use of meperidine and indirect-acting adrenergic agonists is recommended for patients requiring continuing MAO therapy (Huyse, 2006).

Additional Information Complete prescribing information for this medication should be consulted for additional detail.

Dosage Forms Excipient information presented when available (limited, particularly for generics); consult specific product labeling.
Tablet: 10 mg

References

Huyse FJ, Touw DJ, van Schijndel RS, et al, "Psychotropic Drugs and the Perioperative Period: A Proposal for a Guideline in Elective Surgery," *Psychosomatics*, 2006, 47(1):8-22.

Pass SE and Simpson RW, "Discontinuation and Reinstitution of Medications During the Perioperative Period," *Am J Health Syst Pharm*, 2004, 61(9):899-912.

Shulman KI and Walker SE, "A Reevaluation of Dietary Restrictions for Irreversible Monoamine Oxidase Inhibitors," *Psychiatr Ann*, 2001, 31(6):378-84.

Shulman KI and Walker SE, "Refining the MAOI Diet: Tyramine Content of Pizzas and Soy Products," *J Clin Psychiatry*, 1999, 60(3):191-3.

Walker SE, Shulman KI, Tailor SA, et al, "Tyramine Content of Previously Restricted Foods in Monoamine Oxidase Inhibitor Diets," *J Clin Psychopharmacol*, 1996, 16(5):383-8.

◆ **Isochron™** *see* Isosorbide Dinitrate *on page 772*

Isoflurane (eye soe FLURE ane)

Medication Safety Issues
Sound-alike/look-alike issues:
Isoflurane may be confused with enflurane, isoflurophate

High alert medication: The Institute for Safe Medication Practices (ISMP) includes this medication among its list of drug classes which have a heightened risk of causing significant patient harm when used in error.

Related Information
Anesthesia Considerations for Neurosurgery *on page 1514*
Anesthesia for Geriatric Patients *on page 1523*
Anesthesia for Obstetric Patients in Nonobstetric Surgery *on page 1532*
Anesthetic Considerations in the Substance-Abusing Patient *on page 1613*
Inhalational Anesthetics *on page 1632*
U.S. Brand Names Forane®; Terrell™
Canadian Brand Names Forane®
Pharmacologic Category General Anesthetic, Inhalation

◀ **Generic Available** Yes

Use Induction and maintenance of general anesthesia

> **Note:** Use of isoflurane for induction of general anesthesia is not recommended due to its irritant properties and unpleasant odor, which causes breath-holding or coughing.

Unlabeled/Investigational Use Intraoperative cardio- and neuro-protection (ischemic preconditioning)

Pharmacodynamics/Kinetics

Onset of action: 7-10 minutes (pungent odor limits inhalation rate)

Duration: Emergence time: Depends on blood concentration when discontinued

Metabolism: Hepatic (0.2%)

Excretion: Exhaled gases

Dosage Inhalation: Adults:

Anesthesia: Minimum alveolar concentration (MAC), the concentration at which 50% of patients do not respond to surgical incision, is 1.15% (44 years of age) for isoflurane.

Induction: 1.5% to 3%

Maintenance: In nitrous oxide: 1% to 2.5%; in oxygen: 1.5% to 3.5%

Elderly: MAC is reduced

Stability Store at 15°C to 30°C (59°F to 86°F).

Administration Via isoflurane-specific calibrated vaporizer

Monitoring Parameters Blood pressure, heart rate and rhythm, serum potassium, oxygen saturation, end-tidal CO_2 and isoflurane concentrations should be monitored prior to and throughout anesthesia

Anesthesia and Critical Care Concerns/Other Considerations

> **Evidence-Based Information:** In animal studies, isoflurane and other inhaled anesthetics have shown a protective effect (ischemic preconditioning) of the heart and brain. A human randomized controlled clinical trial has also been conducted and has supported this effect (Lee, 2006).

Pregnancy Risk Factor C

Contraindications Hypersensitivity to isoflurane or any component of the formulation; known or suspected history of malignant hyperthermia

Warnings/Precautions Decrease in blood pressure is dose dependent due to peripheral vasodilation primarily in skin and muscle; cardiac output is maintained. Isoflurane may produce cardiac steal (due to coronary vasodilation) in patients with hypertension under certain conditions (eg, unusual coronary artery anatomy). Isoflurane may produce reflex tachycardia, but has less potential to alter atrioventricular conduction or sensitize the myocardium to epinephrine-induced arrhythmias compared to other inhaled anesthetics (eg. halothane, enflurane). Respiration is depressed as is the normal hyperventilatory response to hypoxia. Hypoxic pulmonary vasoconstriction is depressed which may lead to pulmonary shunt. Hypoxemia-induced increase in ventilation is abolished at low isoflurane concentration. Isoflurane can produce elevated carbon monoxide levels in the presence of a dry carbon dioxide absorbent within the circle breathing system of an anesthetic machine. Isoflurane dilates the cerebral vasculature and may, in certain conditions, increase intracranial pressure. Renal, splenic, and hepatic blood flow are reduced. May trigger malignant hyperthermia; avoid use in patients susceptible to malignant hyperthermia. Postoperative hepatic dysfunction and hepatitis have rarely been reported. Postmarketing reports of hepatic failure and necrosis have also been rarely associated with isoflurane. Use of other inhaled anesthetics has been associated with rare cases of perioperative hyperkalemia; concomitant use of succinylcholine was associated with many of the reported cases, but not all. Risk of hyperkalemia is increased in pediatric patients with underlying neuromuscular disease (eg, Duchenne muscular dystrophy). Other abnormalities may include elevation in CPK and myoglobinuria. Monitor closely for arrhythmias. Aggressively identify and treat hyperkalemia.

Adverse Reactions Potential safety issues exist for occupational exposure to inhaled anesthetic gases (primarily nitrous oxide). Although there are no documented adverse effects of chronic occupational exposure to halogenated anesthetic vapors, like isoflurane, some epidemiological studies suggest a link between these anesthetics and increased health problems (particularly spontaneous abortion). No conclusive relationship has been determined, but the National Institute for Occupational Safety and Health Administration (NIOSH) recommends no worker be exposed to >2 ppm (ceiling concentrations) over a period of 1 hour. Precautions (eg, adequate ventilation, scavenging-systems, minimizing leaks/spills) can help to lessen any potential risk.

Frequency not defined.

Cardiovascular: Arrhythmia, hypotension, myocardial depression, tachycardia (transient)

Central nervous system: Mood changes (may persist for ≤6 days after administration), cognitive function decreased (may persist for ≤3 days after administration)

Endocrine & metabolic: Cholesterol decreased, hyperglycemia, hyperkalemia (pediatric patients, perioperative)

Gastrointestinal: Ileus, nausea, vomiting

Hepatic: Hepatic dysfunction (mild to severe; rare), hepatitis (rare), alkaline phosphatase decreased

Renal: BUN decreased, creatinine increased

Respiratory: Respiratory depression/arrest; respiratory irritation (coughing, laryngospasms-related to induction)

Miscellaneous: Malignant hyperthermia, shivering

Postmarketing and/or case reports: Hepatic failure (rare), hepatic necrosis (rare)

Drug Interactions

Metabolism/Transport Effects Substrate of CYP2E1 (major); **Inhibits** CYP2B6 (weak)

Avoid Concomitant Use

Avoid concomitant use of Isoflurane with any of the following: Methylphenidate

Increased Effect/Toxicity

Isoflurane may increase the levels/effects of: EPINEPHrine; Neuromuscular-Blocking Agents (Nondepolarizing)

The levels/effects of Isoflurane may be increased by: CYP2E1 Inhibitors (Moderate); CYP2E1 Inhibitors (Strong); Methylphenidate

Decreased Effect There are no known significant interactions involving a decrease in effect.

Dosage Forms Excipient information presented when available (limited, particularly for generics); consult specific product labeling.

Liquid, for inhalation: >99.9% (100 mL, 250 mL)

Forane®: >99.9% (100 mL, 250 mL) [amber-colored bottle]

Forane®: >99.9% (100 mL, 250 mL) [aluminum bottle]

Terrell™: >99.9% (100 mL, 250 mL) [amber-colored bottle]

References

Campagna JA, Miller KW, and Forman SA, "Mechanisms of Action of Inhaled Anesthetics," *N Engl J Med*, 2003, 348(21):2110-23.

De Hert SG, Turani F, Mathur S, et al, "Cardioprotection With Volatile Anesthetics: Mechanisms and Clinical Implications," *Anesth Analg*, 2005, 100(6):1584-93.

Ebert TJ and Muzi M, "Sympathetic Hyperactivity During Desflurane Anesthesia in Healthy Volunteers. A Comparison With Isoflurane," *Anesthesiology*, 1993, 79(3):444-53.

Eger EI 2nd, "Isoflurane: A Review," *Anesthesiology*, 1981, 55(5):559-76.

Fee JP and Thompson GH, "Comparative Tolerability Profiles of the Inhaled Anaesthetics," *Drug Saf*, 1997, 16(3):157-70.

Lee MC, Chen CH, Kuo MC, et al, "Isoflurane Preconditioning-Induced Cardio-Protection in Patients Undergoing Coronary Artery Bypass Grafting," *Eur J Anaesthesiol*, 2006, 23(10):841-7.

Park KW, "Cardiovascular Effects of Inhalational Anesthetics," *Int Anesthesiol Clin*, 2002, 40(1):1-14.

Stachnik J, "Inhaled Anesthetic Agents," *Am J Health-Syst Pharm*, 2006, 63(7):623-34.

Wang L, Traystman RJ, and Murphy SJ, "Inhalational Anesthetics as Preconditioning Agents in Ischemic Brain," *Curr Opin Pharmacol*, 2008, 8(1):104-10.

Yasuda N, Lockhart SH, Eger EI 2nd, et al, "Comparison of Kinetics of Sevoflurane and Isoflurane in Humans," *Anesth Analg*, 1991, 72(3):316-24.

Yasuda N, Lockhart SH, Eger EI 2nd, et al, "Kinetics of Desflurane, Isoflurane, and Halothane in Humans," *Anesthesiology*, 1991, 74(3):489-98.

Isoniazid (eye soe NYE a zid)

Medication Safety Issues

International issues:

Hydra® [Japan] may be confused with Hydrea®

Canadian Brand Names Isotamine®; PMS-Isoniazid

Index Terms INH; Isonicotinic Acid Hydrazide

◄ **Pharmacologic Category** Antitubercular Agent

Generic Available Yes

Use Treatment of susceptible tuberculosis infections; treatment of latent tuberculosis infection (LTBI)

Mechanism of Action Unknown, but may include the inhibition of mycolic acid synthesis resulting in disruption of the bacterial cell wall

Pharmacodynamics/Kinetics

Absorption: Rapid and complete; rate can be slowed with food

Distribution: All body tissues and fluids including CSF; crosses placenta; enters breast milk

Protein binding: 10% to 15%

Metabolism: Hepatic with decay rate determined genetically by acetylation phenotype

Half-life elimination: Fast acetylators: 30-100 minutes; Slow acetylators: 2-5 hours; may be prolonged with hepatic or severe renal impairment

Time to peak, serum: 1-2 hours

Excretion: Urine (75% to 95%); feces; saliva

Dosage

Usual dosage ranges: Oral, I.M.:

Infants and Children: 10-15 mg/kg/day in 1-2 divided doses (maximum: 300 mg/day) or 20-40 mg/kg given 2-3 times per week (maximum: 900 mg/dose)

Adults: 5 mg/kg/day (usual: 300 mg/day) as a single daily dose or 15 mg/kg (maximum: 900 mg/dose) given 2-3 times per week

Indication-specific dosing: Oral, I.M.: Recommendations often change due to resistant strains and newly-developed information; consult *MMWR* for current CDC recommendations. Intramuscular injection is available for patients who are unable to either take or absorb oral therapy.

Infants and Children:

Tuberculosis, active:

Daily therapy: 10-15 mg/kg/day in 1-2 divided doses (maximum: 300 mg/day)

Twice weekly or 3 times/week directly observed therapy (DOT): 20-40 mg/kg (maximum: 900 mg)

Tuberculosis, latent infection (LTBI): 10 mg/kg/day as a single dose (maximum: 300 mg/day) **or** 20-30 mg/kg (maximum: 900 mg/dose) twice weekly for 9 months

Adults: **Note:** Concomitant administration of 10-50 mg/day pyridoxine is recommended in malnourished patients or those prone to neuropathy (eg, alcoholics, patients with diabetes).

Nontuberculous mycobacterium *(M. kansasii)* **(unlabeled use):** 5 mg/kg/day (maximum: 300 mg/day) for duration to include 12 months of culture-negative sputum; typically used in combination with ethambutol and rifampin

Tuberculosis, active:

Daily therapy: 5 mg/kg/day given daily (usual dose: 300 mg/day)

Twice weekly or 3 times/week directly observed therapy (DOT): 15 mg/kg (maximum: 900 mg). **Note:** CDC guidelines state that once-weekly therapy (15 mg/kg/dose) may be considered, but only after the first 2 months of initial therapy in HIV-negative patients, and only in combination with rifapentine.

Note: Treatment may be defined by the number of doses administered (eg, "six-month" therapy involves 182 doses of INH and rifampin, and 56 doses of pyrazinamide). Six months is the shortest interval of time over which these doses may be administered, assuming no interruption of therapy.

Tuberculosis, latent infection (LTBI): 300 mg/day or 900 mg twice weekly for 6-9 months in patients who do not have HIV infection (9 months is optimal, 6 months may be considered to reduce costs of therapy) and 9 months in patients who have HIV infection. Extend to 12 months of therapy if interruptions in treatment occur.

Dosing adjustment in renal impairment: No adjustment necessary

Hemodialysis: Dialyzable (50% to 100%); administer dose post dialysis

Dosing adjustment in hepatic impairment: No adjustment required, however, use with caution; may accumulate and additional liver damage may occur in patients with pre-existing liver disease. For ALT or AST >3 times the ULN: discontinue or temporarily withhold treatment. Treatment with isoniazid for latent tuberculosis infection should be deferred in patients with acute hepatic diseases.

Stability
Tablet: Store at 20°C to 25°C (68°F to 77°F). Protect from light.
Oral solution: Store at 15°C to 30°C (59°F to 86°F). Protect from light.

Administration Should be administered 1 hour before or 2 hours after meals on an empty stomach.

Monitoring Parameters Baseline and periodic (more frequently in patients with higher risk for hepatitis) liver function tests (ALT and AST); sputum cultures monthly (until 2 consecutive negative cultures reported); monitoring for prodromal signs of hepatitis

Reference Range Therapeutic: 1-7 mcg/mL (SI: 7-51 µmol/L); Toxic: 20-710 mcg/mL (SI: 146-5176 µmol/L)

Pregnancy Risk Factor C

Contraindications Hypersensitivity to isoniazid or any component of the formulation; acute liver disease; previous history of hepatic damage during isoniazid therapy; previous severe adverse reaction (drug fever, chills, arthritis) to isoniazid

Warnings/Precautions Use with caution in patients with severe renal impairment and liver disease. **[U.S. Boxed Warning]: Severe and sometimes fatal hepatitis may occur; usually occurs within the first 3 months of treatment, although may develop even after many months of treatment.** The risk of developing hepatitis is age-related; daily ethanol consumption may also increase the risk. Patients must report any prodromal symptoms of hepatitis, such as fatigue, weakness, malaise, anorexia, nausea, or vomiting. Treatment with isoniazid for latent tuberculosis infection should be deferred in patients with acute hepatic diseases. Periodic ophthalmic examinations are recommended even when usual symptoms do not occur. Pyridoxine (10-50 mg/day) is recommended in individuals at risk for development of peripheral neuropathies (eg, HIV infection, nutritional deficiency, diabetes, pregnancy). Children with low milk and low meat intake should receive concomitant pyridoxine therapy. Multidrug regimens should be utilized for the treatment of active tuberculosis to prevent the emergence of drug resistance.

Adverse Reactions Frequency not defined.
Cardiovascular: Hypertension, palpitation, tachycardia, vasculitis
Central nervous system: Depression, dizziness, encephalopathy, fever, lethargy, memory impairment, psychosis, seizure, slurred speech
Dermatologic: Flushing, rash (morbilliform, maculopapular, pruritic, or exfoliative)
Endocrine & metabolic: Gynecomastia, hyperglycemia, metabolic acidosis, pellagra, pyridoxine deficiency
Gastrointestinal: Anorexia, nausea, vomiting, stomach pain
Hematologic: Agranulocytosis, anemia (sideroblastic, hemolytic, or aplastic), eosinophilia, thrombocytopenia
Hepatic: LFTs mildly increased (10% to 20%); hyperbilirubinemia, bilirubinuria, jaundice, hepatitis (may involve progressive liver damage; risk increases with age; 2.3% in patients >50 years), hepatic dysfunction
Neuromuscular & skeletal: Arthralgia, hyper-reflexia, peripheral neuropathy (dose-related incidence, 10% to 20% incidence with 10 mg/kg/day), weakness
Ocular: Blurred vision, loss of vision, optic neuritis and atrophy
Miscellaneous: Lupus-like syndrome, lymphadenopathy, rheumatic syndrome

Drug Interactions
Metabolism/Transport Effects **Substrate** of CYP2E1 (major); **Inhibits** CYP1A2 (weak), 2A6 (moderate), 2C9 (weak), 2C19 (strong), 2D6 (moderate), 2E1 (moderate), 3A4 (strong); **Induces** CYP2E1 (after discontinuation) (weak)

Avoid Concomitant Use
Avoid concomitant use of Isoniazid with any of the following: Alfuzosin; Clopidogrel; Dronedarone; Eplerenone; Everolimus; Halofantrine; Nilotinib; Nisoldipine; Ranolazine; Rivaroxaban; Salmeterol; Silodosin; Thioridazine; Tolvaptan

◄ **Increased Effect/Toxicity**

Isoniazid may increase the levels/effects of: Acetaminophen; Alfuzosin; Almotriptan; Alosetron; Benzodiazepines (metabolized by oxidation); CarBAMazepine; Chlorzoxazone; Ciclesonide; Colchicine; CYP2A6 Substrates; CYP2C19 Substrates; CYP2D6 Substrates; CYP2E1 Substrates; CYP3A4 Substrates; Dronedarone; Dutasteride; Eplerenone; Everolimus; FentaNYL; Fesoterodine; Halofantrine; Ixabepilone; Maraviroc; Nebivolol; Nilotinib; Nisoldipine; Paricalcitol; Phenytoin; Pimecrolimus; Ranolazine; Rivaroxaban; Salmeterol; Saxagliptin; Silodosin; Sorafenib; Tadalafil; Tamoxifen; Theophylline Derivatives; Thioridazine; Tolvaptan

The levels/effects of Isoniazid may be increased by: CycloSERINE; Rifamycin Derivatives

Decreased Effect

Isoniazid may decrease the levels/effects of: Clopidogrel; Codeine; Prasugrel; TraMADol

The levels/effects of Isoniazid may be decreased by: Antacids; Corticosteroids (Systemic)

Ethanol/Nutrition/Herb Interactions

Ethanol: Avoid ethanol (increases the risk of hepatitis).

Food: Isoniazid should not be taken with food; serum levels may be decreased if taken with food. Has some ability to inhibit tyramine metabolism; several case reports of mild reactions (flushing, palpitations) after ingestion of cheese (with or without wine). Reactions resembling allergic symptoms following ingestion of fish rich in histamine content have been reported. Isoniazid decreases folic acid absorption. Isoniazid alters pyridoxine metabolism.

Test Interactions False-positive urinary glucose with Clinitest®

Dietary Considerations Should be taken 1 hour before or 2 hours after meals on an empty stomach; increase dietary intake of folate, niacin, magnesium. Avoid tyramine-containing foods; some examples include aged or matured cheese, air-dried or cured meats (including sausages and salamis), fava or broad bean pods, tap/draft beers, Marmite concentrate, sauerkraut, soy sauce and other soybean condiments. Avoid histamine-containing foods.

Dosage Forms Excipient information presented when available (limited, particularly for generics); consult specific product labeling.

Injection, solution: 100 mg/mL (10 mL)

Oral solution: 50 mg/5 mL (473 mL) [orange flavor]

Tablet: 100 mg, 300 mg

◆ **Isonicotinic Acid Hydrazide** *see* Isoniazid *on page 767*

◆ **Isonipecaine Hydrochloride** *see* Meperidine *on page 875*

◆ **Isophane Insulin** *see* Insulin NPH *on page 749*

◆ **Isophane Insulin and Regular Insulin** *see* Insulin NPH and Insulin Regular *on page 749*

Isoproterenol (eye soe proe TER e nole)

Medication Safety Issues

Sound-alike/look-alike issues:

Isuprel® may be confused with Disophrol®, Ismelin®, Isordil®

Related Information

Management of Postoperative Arrhythmias *on page 1571*

U.S. Brand Names Isuprel®

Index Terms Isoproterenol Hydrochloride

Pharmacologic Category Beta$_1$- & Beta$_2$-Adrenergic Agonist Agent

Generic Available No

Use Manufacturer's labeled indications (see **"Note"**): Mild or transient episodes of heart block that do not require electric shock or pacemaker therapy; serious episodes of heart block and Adams-Stokes attacks (except when caused by ventricular tachycardia or fibrillation); cardiac arrest until electric shock or pacemaker therapy is available; bronchospasm during anesthesia; adjunct to fluid and electrolyte replacement therapy and other drugs and procedures in the treatment of hypovolemic or septic shock and low cardiac output states (eg, decompensated heart failure, cardiogenic shock)

Note: The use of isoproterenol in advanced cardiac life support (ACLS) has largely been supplanted by the use of other adrenergic agents (eg, epinephrine and dopamine). The use of isoproterenol for bronchospasm during anesthesia and cardiogenic, hypovolemic, or septic shock is no longer recommended. See Unlabeled/Investigational Use field for more appropriate, yet unlabeled, uses

Unlabeled/Investigational Use Pharmacologic overdrive pacing for refractory torsade de pointes; pharmacologic provocation during tilt table testing for syncope; temporary control of bradycardia in denervated heart transplant patients unresponsive to atropine; ventricular arrhythmias due to AV nodal block; beta-blocker overdose

Mechanism of Action Stimulates beta$_1$- and beta$_2$-receptors resulting in relaxation of bronchial, GI, and uterine smooth muscle, increased heart rate and contractility, vasodilation of peripheral vasculature

Pharmacodynamics/Kinetics

Onset of action: I.V.: Immediate

Duration: I.V.: 10-15 minutes

Metabolism: Via conjugation in many tissues including hepatic and pulmonary

Half-life elimination: 2.5-5 minutes

Excretion: Urine (primarily as sulfate conjugates)

Dosage Continuous I.V. infusion:

Bradyarrhythmias, AV nodal block, or refractory torsade de pointes:

Children: 0.05-2 mcg/kg/minute; titrate to patient response

Adults: 2-10 mcg/minute; titrate to patient response

Tilt table testing for syncope (Benditt, 1996; Brignole, 2004): Adults: Initial: 1 mcg/minute; increase as necessary based on response to a maximum dose of 5 mcg/minute. **Note:** Timing of initiation and dose adjustment during test may be institution specific.

Stability Store undiluted solution at 20°C to 25°C (68°F to 77°F). Solution should not be used if a color or precipitate is present. Exposure to air, light, or increased temperature may cause a pink to brownish pink color to develop. Stability of parenteral admixture at room temperature (25°C) or at refrigeration (4°C) is 24 hours.

Standard admixture concentration: 1 mg/500 mL D_5W

Maximum admixture concentration: 1 mg/100 mL D_5W

Administration I.V. infusion administration requires the use of an infusion pump.

Monitoring Parameters ECG, heart rate, respiratory rate, arterial blood gas, arterial blood pressure, CVP; serum glucose, serum potassium, serum magnesium

Anesthesia and Critical Care Concerns/Other Considerations

Clinical Pearls/Comments: Isoproterenol can be effective in terminating torsade de pointes associated with bradycardia and drug-induced prolonged QT (adult case series; Keren, 1981).

Pregnancy Risk Factor C

Contraindications Angina, pre-existing ventricular arrhythmias, tachyarrhythmias; cardiac glycoside intoxication

Warnings/Precautions Use with extreme caution; not currently a treatment of choice; use with caution in elderly patients, patients with diabetes, cardiovascular disease, or hyperthyroidism; excessive or prolonged use may result in decreased effectiveness. Contains sulfites; may cause allergic reaction in susceptible individuals.

Adverse Reactions Frequency not defined.

Cardiovascular: Angina, flushing, hyper-/hypotension, pallor, palpitation, paradoxical bradycardia (with tilt table testing), premature ventricular beats, Stokes-Adams attacks, tachyarrhythmia, ventricular arrhythmia

Central nervous system: Dizziness, headache, nervousness, restlessness, Stokes-Adams seizure

Endocrine & metabolic: Hypokalemia, serum glucose increased

Gastrointestinal: Nausea, vomiting

Neuromuscular & skeletal: Tremor, weakness

Ocular: Blurred vision
Respiratory: Dyspnea, pulmonary edema
Miscellaneous: Diaphoresis

Drug Interactions

Avoid Concomitant Use There are no known interactions where it is recommended to avoid concomitant use.

Increased Effect/Toxicity
The levels/effects of Isoproterenol may be increased by: COMT Inhibitors

Decreased Effect There are no known significant interactions involving a decrease in effect.

Ethanol/Nutrition/Herb Interactions Herb/Nutraceutical: Avoid ephedra, yohimbe (may cause CNS stimulation).

Dosage Forms Excipient information presented when available (limited, particularly for generics); consult specific product labeling.

Injection, solution, as hydrochloride:

Isuprel®: 0.2 mg/mL (1:5000) (1 mL, 5 mL) [contains sodium metabisulfite]

References

"2005 American Heart Association Guidelines for Cardiopulmonary Resuscitation and Emergency Cardiovascular Care," *Circulation*, 2005, 112(24 Suppl):130.

Almquist A, Goldenberg IF, Milstein S, et al, "Provocation of Bradycardia and Hypotension by Isoproterenol and Upright Posture in Patients With Unexplained Syncope," *N Engl J Med*, 1989, 320 (6):346-51.

Hemstreet MP, Miles MV, and Rutland RO, "Effect of Intravenous Isoproterenol on Theophylline Kinetics," *J Allergy Clin Immunol*, 1982, 69(4):360-4.

Illi A, Sundberg S, Ojala-Karlsson P, et al, "The Effect of Entacapone on the Disposition and Hemodynamic Effects of Intravenous Isoproterenol and Epinephrine," *Clin Pharmacol Ther*, 1995, 58(2):221-7.

Keren A, Tzivoni D, Gavish D, et al, "Etiology, Warning Signs and Therapy of Torsade de Pointes. A Study of 10 Patients," *Circulation*, 1981, 64(6):1167-74.

Lang CC, Stein CM, Brown RM, et al, "Attenuation of Isoproterenol-Mediated Vasodilatation in Blacks," *N Engl J Med*, 1995, 333(3):155-60.

Rachelefsky GS and Siegel SC, "Asthma in Infants and Children - Treatment of Childhood Asthma: Part II," *J Allergy Clin Immunol*, 1985, 76(3):409-25.

Isosorbide Dinitrate (eye soe SOR bide dye NYE trate)

Related Information
Heart Failure (Systolic) *on page 1739*
Nitrates *on page 1686*

U.S. Brand Names Dilatrate®-SR; Isochron™; Isordil®

Canadian Brand Names Apo-ISDN®; Cedocard®-SR; Coronex®; Novo-Sorbide; PMS-Isosorbide

Index Terms ISD; ISDN

Pharmacologic Category Vasodilator

Use Prevention and treatment of angina pectoris; for congestive heart failure; to relieve pain, dysphagia, and spasm in esophageal spasm with GE reflux

Unlabeled/Investigational Use Esophageal spastic disorders

Pharmacodynamics/Kinetics

Onset of action: Sublingual tablet: 2-10 minutes; Chewable tablet: 3 minutes; Oral tablet: 45-60 minutes

Duration: Sublingual tablet: 1-2 hours; Chewable tablet: 0.5-2 hours; Oral tablet: 4-6 hours

Metabolism: Extensively hepatic to conjugated metabolites, including isosorbide 5-mononitrate (active) and 2-mononitrate (active)

Half-life elimination: Parent drug: 1-4 hours; Metabolite (5-mononitrate): 4 hours

Excretion: Urine and feces

Dosage Adults (elderly should be given lowest recommended daily doses initially and titrate upward): Oral:

Angina: 5-40 mg 4 times/day or 40 mg every 8-12 hours in sustained-release dosage form

Sublingual: 2.5-5 mg every 5-10 minutes for maximum of 3 doses in 15-30 minutes; may also use prophylactically 15 minutes prior to activities which may provoke an attack

Congestive heart failure:

Initial dose: 20 mg 3-4 times per day

Target dose: 120-160 mg/day in divided doses; use in combination with hydralazine

Esophageal spastic disorders (unlabeled use):

Oral: 5-10 mg before meals

Sublingual: 2.5 mg after meals

Tolerance to nitrate effects develops with chronic exposure: Dose escalation does not overcome this effect. Tolerance can only be overcome by short periods of nitrate absence from the body. Short periods (10-12 hours) of nitrate withdrawal help minimize tolerance. General recommendations are to take the last dose of short-acting agents no later than 7 PM; administer 2-3 times/day rather than 4 times/day. Sustained release preparations could be administered at times to allow a 15- to 17-hour interval between first and last daily dose. Example: Administer sustained release at 8 AM and 2 PM for a twice daily regimen.

Hemodialysis: During hemodialysis, administer dose postdialysis or administer supplemental 10-20 mg dose

Peritoneal dialysis: Supplemental dose is not necessary

Anesthesia and Critical Care Concerns/Other Considerations Nitrates used in right ventricular infarction may induce acute hypotension. Nitrate use in severe pericardial effusion may reduce cardiac filling pressure and precipitate cardiac tamponade. In the management of heart failure, the combination of isosorbide dinitrate and hydralazine confers beneficial effects on disease progression and cardiac outcomes.

Additional Information Complete prescribing information for this medication should be consulted for additional detail.

Dosage Forms Excipient information presented when available (limited, particularly for generics); consult specific product labeling. [DSC] = Discontinued product

Capsule, sustained release (Dilatrate®-SR): 40 mg

Tablet: 5 mg, 10 mg, 20 mg, 30 mg

Isordil®: 5 mg, 10 mg [DSC], 20 mg [DSC], 30 mg [DSC], 40 mg

Tablet, extended release (Isochron™): 40 mg

Tablet, sublingual: 2.5 mg, 5 mg

Isordil®: 2.5 mg, 5 mg, 10 mg [DSC]

References

Cheitlin MD, Hutter AM Jr, Brindis RG, et al, "ACC/AHA Expert Consensus Document. Use of Sildenafil (Viagra) in Patients With Cardiovascular Disease. American College of Cardiology/American Heart Association," *J Am Coll Cardiol*, 1999, 33(1):273-82.

Cohn JN, Archibald DG, Ziesche S, et al, "Effect of Vasodilator Therapy on Mortality in Chronic Congestive Heart Failure. Results of a Veterans Administration Cooperative Study," *N Engl J Med*, 1986, 314(24):1547-52.

Cohn JN, Johnson G, Ziesche S, et al, "A Comparison of Enalapril With Hydralazine-Isosorbide Dinitrate in the Treatment of Chronic Congestive Heart Failure," *N Engl J Med*, 1991, 325(5):303-10.

Gibbons RJ, Abrams J, Chatterjee K, et al, "ACC/AHA 2002 Guideline Update for the Management of Patients With Chronic Stable Angina - Summary Article: A Report of the American College of Cardiology/American Heart Association Task Force on Practice Guidelines (Committee on the Management of Patients With Chronic Stable Angina)," *J Am Coll Cardiol*, 2003, 41(1):159-68. Available at: http://http://www.acc.org/clinical/guidelines/stable/stable_clean.pdf. Accessed May 5, 2004.

Hunt SA, Abraham WT, Chin MH, et al, "2009 Focused Update Incorporated into the ACC/AHA 2005 Guidelines for the Diagnosis and Management of Heart Failure in Adults: A Report of the American College of Cardiology Foundation/American Heart Association Task Force on Practice Guidelines Developed in Collaboration With the International Society for Heart and Lung Transplantation," *J Am Coll Cardiol*, 2009, 53(15):e1-e90.

Parker JO, Fanell B, Lahey KA, et al, "Effect of Intervals Between Doses on the Development to Tolerance to Isosorbide Dinitrate," *N Engl J Med*, 1987, 316(23):1440-4.

Taylor AL, Ziesche S, Yancy C, et al, "Combination of Isosorbide Dinitrate and Hydralazine in Blacks With Heart Failure," *N Engl J Med*, 2004, 351(20):2049-57.

Isosorbide Mononitrate (eye soe SOR bide mon oh NYE trate)

Related Information
Heart Failure (Systolic) *on page 1739*
Nitrates *on page 1686*
U.S. Brand Names Imdur®; Ismo®; Monoket®
Canadian Brand Names Apo-ISMN®; Imdur®; PMS-ISMN; Pro-ISMN
Index Terms ISMN
Pharmacologic Category Vasodilator
Use Long-acting metabolite of the vasodilator isosorbide dinitrate used for the prophylactic treatment of angina pectoris
Pharmacodynamics/Kinetics
Onset of action: 30-60 minutes
Absorption: Nearly complete and low intersubject variability in its pharmacokinetic parameters and plasma concentrations
Metabolism: Hepatic
Half-life elimination: Mononitrate: ~4 hours
Excretion: Urine and feces
Dosage Adults and Geriatrics (start with lowest recommended dose): Oral:
Regular tablet: 5-20 mg twice daily with the two doses given 7 hours apart (eg, 8 AM and 3 PM) to decrease tolerance development; then titrate to 10 mg twice daily in first 2-3 days.
Extended release tablet: Initial: 30-60 mg given in morning as a single dose; titrate upward as needed, giving at least 3 days between increases; maximum daily single dose: 240 mg
Dosing adjustment in renal impairment: Not necessary for elderly or patients with altered renal or hepatic function.
Tolerance to nitrate effects develops with chronic exposure. Dose escalation does not overcome this effect. Tolerance can only be overcome by short periods of nitrate absence from the body. Short periods (10-12 hours) of nitrate withdrawal help minimize tolerance. Recommended dosage regimens incorporate this interval. General recommendations are to take the last dose of short-acting agents no later than 7 PM; administer 2 times/day rather than 4 times/day. Administer sustained release tablet once daily in the morning.

Anesthesia and Critical Care Concerns/Other Considerations Nitrates used in right ventricular infarction may induce acute hypotension. Nitrate use in severe pericardial effusion may reduce cardiac filling pressure and precipitate cardiac tamponade.

Additional Information Complete prescribing information for this medication should be consulted for additional detail.

Dosage Forms Excipient information presented when available (limited, particularly for generics); consult specific product labeling.
Tablet: 10 mg, 20 mg
Ismo®: 20 mg
Monoket®: 10 mg, 20 mg
Tablet, extended release: 30 mg, 60 mg, 120 mg
Imdur®: 30 mg, 60 mg, 120 mg

References

Cheitlin MD, Hutter AM Jr, Brindis RG, et al, "ACC/AHA Expert Consensus Document. Use of Sildenafil (Viagra) in Patients With Cardiovascular Disease. American College of Cardiology/American Heart Association," *J Am Coll Cardiol*, 1999, 33(1):273-82.

Flaherty JT, "Hemodynamic Attenuation and the Nitrate Dose-Free Interval: Alternative Dosing Strategies for Transdermal Nitroglycerin," *Am J Cardiol*, 1985, 56(17):321-71.

Gibbons RJ, Abrams J, Chatterjee K, et al, "ACC/AHA 2002 Guideline Update for the Management of Patients With Chronic Stable Angina - Summary Article: A Report of the American College of Cardiology/American Heart Association Task Force on Practice Guidelines (Committee on the Management of Patients With Chronic Stable Angina)," *J Am Coll Cardiol*, 2003, 41(1):159-68. Available at: http://http://www.acc.org/clinical/guidelines/stable/stable_clean.pdf. Accessed May 5, 2004.

Hunt SA, Baker DW, Chin MH, et al, "ACC/AHA Guidelines for the Evaluation and Management of Chronic Heart Failure in the Adult: Executive Summary. A Report of the American College of Cardiology/American Heart Association Task Force on Practice Guidelines (Committee to Revise the 1995 Guidelines for the Evaluation and Management of Heart Failure)," *J Am Coll Cardiol*, 2001, 38(7):2101-13.

Parker JO, "Eccentric Dosing With Isosorbide-5-Mononitrate in Angina Pectoris," *Am J Cardiol*, 1993, 72(12):871-6.

Parker JO, Fanell B, Lahey KA, et al, "Effect of Intervals Between Doses on the Development to Tolerance to Isosorbide Dinitrate," *N Engl J Med*, 1987, 316(23):1440-4.

Villaneuva C, Minana J, Ortiz J, et al, "Endoscopic Litigation Compared With Combined Treatment With Nadolol and Isosorbide Mononitrate to Prevent Recurrent Variceal Bleeding," *N Engl J Med*, 2001, 345(9):647-55.

Kanamycin (kan a MYE sin)

Medication Safety Issues
Sound-alike/look-alike issues:
Kanamycin may be confused with Garamycin®, gentamicin
U.S. Brand Names Kantrex®
Canadian Brand Names Kantrex®
Index Terms Kanamycin Sulfate
Pharmacologic Category Antibiotic, Aminoglycoside
Generic Available No
Use Treatment of serious infections caused by susceptible strains of *E. coli*, *Proteus* species, *Enterobacter aerogenes*, *Klebsiella pneumoniae*, *Serratia marcescens*, and *Acinetobacter* species; second-line treatment of *Mycobacterium tuberculosis*
Mechanism of Action Interferes with protein synthesis in bacterial cell by binding to ribosomal subunit
Pharmacodynamics/Kinetics
Absorption:
I.M.: Rapid
Oral: Minimal
Distribution:
Relative diffusion from blood into CSF: Good only with inflammation (exceeds usual MICs)
CSF:blood level ratio: Normal meninges: Nil; Inflamed meninges: 43%
Protein binding: 0%
Half-life elimination: 2-4 hours; Anuria: 80 hours; End-stage renal disease: 40-96 hours
Time to peak, serum: I.M.: 1-2 hours (decreased in burn patients)
Excretion: Urine (as unchanged drug)
Dosage Note: Dosing should be based on ideal body weight
Children: Infections: I.M., I.V.: 15 mg/kg/day in divided doses every 8-12 hours
Adults:
Infections: I.M., I.V.: 5-7.5 mg/kg/dose in divided doses every 8-12 hours (<15 mg/kg/day)
Intraperitoneal: After contamination in surgery: 500 mg
Irrigating solution: 0.25%; maximum 1.5 g/day (via all administration routes)
Aerosol: 250 mg 2-4 times/day

Dosing adjustment/interval in renal impairment:
Cl_{cr} 50-80 mL/minute: Administer 60% to 90% of dose or administer every 8-12 hours
Cl_{cr} 10-50 mL/minute: Administer 30% to 70% of dose or administer every 12 hours
Cl_{cr} <10 mL/minute: Administer 20% to 30% of dose or administer every 24-48 hours

Stability Store vial at controlled room temperature. Darkening of vials does not indicate loss of potency.
I.V.: Must be further diluted prior to I.V. infusion. For adults, dilute 500 mg in 100-200 mL of appropriate solution or 1 g in 200-400 mL. For pediatric patients, use sufficient amount to infuse solution over 30-60 minutes.
Intraperitoneal: Dilute dose in 20 mL sterile distilled water.
Aerosol: Dilute 250 mg in 3 mL normal saline.

Administration
I.M.: Administer deeply in upper outer quadrant of the gluteal muscle.
I.V.: Infuse over 30-60 minutes.

Some penicillins (eg, carbenicillin, ticarcillin and piperacillin) have been shown to inactivate aminoglycosides *in vitro*. This has been observed to a greater extent with tobramycin and gentamicin, while amikacin has shown greater stability against inactivation. Concurrent use of these agents may pose a risk of reduced antibacterial efficacy *in vivo*, particularly in the setting of profound renal impairment. However, definitive clinical evidence is lacking. If combination penicillin/aminoglycoside therapy is desired in a patient with renal dysfunction, separation of doses (if feasible), and routine monitoring of aminoglycoside levels, CBC, and clinical response should be considered.

Monitoring Parameters Serum creatinine and BUN every 2-3 days; peak and trough concentrations; hearing

Some penicillin derivatives may accelerate the degradation of aminoglycosides *in vitro*. This may be clinically-significant for certain penicillin (ticarcillin, piperacillin, carbenicillin) and aminoglycoside (gentamicin, tobramycin) combination therapy in patients with significant renal impairment. Close monitoring of aminoglycoside levels is warranted.

Reference Range Therapeutic: Peak: 15-30 mcg/mL; Trough: 5-10 mcg/mL; Toxic: Peak: >35 mcg/mL; Trough: >10 mcg/mL

Pregnancy Risk Factor D

Contraindications Hypersensitivity to kanamycin, any component of the formulation, or other aminoglycosides; pregnancy

Warnings/Precautions [U.S. Boxed Warning]: Aminoglycosides may cause neurotoxicity and/or nephrotoxicity; usual risk factors include pre-existing renal impairment, concomitant neuro-/nephrotoxic medications, advanced age, and dehydration. Ototoxicity may be directly proportional to the amount of drug given and the duration of treatment. Tinnitus or vertigo are indications of vestibular injury and impending hearing loss. Renal damage is usually reversible. May cause neuromuscular blockade and respiratory paralysis; especially when given soon after anesthesia or muscle relaxants.

Not intended for long-term therapy due to toxic hazards associated with extended administration. Use caution in pre-existing renal insufficiency, vestibular or cochlear impairment, myasthenia gravis, hypocalcemia, and conditions which depress neuromuscular transmission. Dosage modification required in patients with impaired renal function. Prolonged use may result in fungal or bacterial superinfection, including *C. difficile*-associated diarrhea (CDAD) and pseudomembranous colitis; CDAD has been observed >2 months postantibiotic treatment.

Adverse Reactions Frequency not defined.
Cardiovascular: Edema
Central nervous system: Neurotoxicity, drowsiness, headache, pseudomotor cerebri
Dermatologic: Skin itching, redness, rash, photosensitivity, erythema
Gastrointestinal: Nausea, vomiting, diarrhea, malabsorption syndrome (with prolonged and high-dose therapy of hepatic coma), anorexia, weight loss, salivation increased, enterocolitis

Hematologic: Granulocytopenia, agranulocytosis, thrombocytopenia
Local: Burning, stinging
Neuromuscular & skeletal: Weakness, tremor, muscle cramps
Otic: Ototoxicity (auditory), ototoxicity (vestibular)
Renal: Nephrotoxicity
Respiratory: Dyspnea

Drug Interactions

Avoid Concomitant Use

Avoid concomitant use of Kanamycin with any of the following: Gallium Nitrate

Increased Effect/Toxicity

Kanamycin may increase the levels/effects of: AbobotulinumtoxinA; Bisphosphonate Derivatives; CARBOplatin; Colistimethate; CycloSPORINE; Gallium Nitrate; Neuromuscular-Blocking Agents; OnabotulinumtoxinA; RimabotulinumtoxinB

The levels/effects of Kanamycin may be increased by: Amphotericin B; Capreomycin; CISplatin; Loop Diuretics; Nonsteroidal Anti-Inflammatory Agents; Vancomycin

Decreased Effect

Kanamycin may decrease the levels/effects of: Cardiac Glycosides; Typhoid Vaccine

The levels/effects of Kanamycin may be decreased by: Penicillins

Test Interactions Some penicillin derivatives may accelerate the degradation of aminoglycosides *in vitro*, leading to a potential underestimation of aminoglycoside serum concentration.

Dosage Forms Excipient information presented when available (limited, particularly for generics); consult specific product labeling.

Injection, solution, as sulfate: 1 g/3 mL (3 mL) [contains sodium bisulfate]

Ketamine (KEET a meen)

Medication Safety Issues

Sound-alike/look-alike issues:

Ketalar® may be confused with Kenalog®, ketorolac

High alert medication: The Institute for Safe Medication Practices (ISMP) includes this medication among its list of drugs which have a heightened risk of causing significant patient harm when used in error.

◀ **Related Information**
    Acute Postoperative Pain *on page 1502*
    Anesthesia Considerations for Neurosurgery *on page 1514*
    Anesthetic Considerations in the Substance-Abusing Patient *on page 1613*
    Chronic Renal Failure *on page 1552*
    Dosing Considerations for the Critically-Ill Patient With Morbid Obesity *on page 1561*
    Inhalational Anesthetics *on page 1632*
    Intravenous Anesthetic Agents *on page 1635*
U.S. Brand Names Ketalar®
Canadian Brand Names Ketalar®; Ketamine Hydrochloride Injection, USP
Index Terms Ketamine Hydrochloride
Pharmacologic Category General Anesthetic
Restrictions C-III
Generic Available Yes
Use Induction and maintenance of general anesthesia
Unlabeled/Investigational Use Analgesia, sedation
Mechanism of Action Produces a cataleptic-like state in which the patient is dissociated from the surrounding environment by direct action on the cortex and limbic system. Releases endogenous catecholamines (epinephrine, norepinephrine) which maintain blood pressure and heart rate. Reduces polysynaptic spinal reflexes.

Pharmacodynamics/Kinetics
  Onset of action:
    I.V.: Anesthetic effect: 30 seconds
    I.M.: Anesthetic effect: 3-4 minutes
  Duration: Anesthetic effect: I.V.: 5-10 minutes; I.M.: 12-25 minutes
  Metabolism: Hepatic via hydroxylation and N-demethylation; the metabolite norketamine is 33% as potent as parent compound
  Half-life elimination: Alpha: 10-15 minutes; Beta: 2.5 hours
  Excretion: Primarily urine
Dosage May be used in combination with anticholinergic agents to decrease hypersalivation.
  Children: **Note:** Titrate dose for desired effect.
    Oral: Sedation (unlabeled use/route): 6-10 mg/kg for 1 dose (mixed in 0.2-0.3 mL/kg of cola or other beverage) given 30 minutes before the procedure
    I.M.: Sedation/analgesia (unlabeled use): 4-5 mg/kg/dose; doses up to 13 mg/kg have been reported
    I.V.: Sedation/analgesia (unlabeled use): 1-2 mg/kg/dose; titrate repeat doses for desired effect
    Continuous I.V. infusion: Sedation (unlabeled use): 5-20 mcg/kg/minute; titrate to reach desired level of sedation
  Children ≥16 years and Adults:
    Induction of anesthesia:
      I.M.: 6.5-13 mg/kg; usual dose to produce 12-25 minutes of anesthesia: 10 mg/kg
      I.V.: 1-4.5 mg/kg; usual dose to produce 5-10 minutes of anesthesia: 2 mg/kg
      I.V. infusion: 1-2 mg/kg infuse over 0.5 mg/kg/minute; may administer with diazepam to prevent emergence reactions
    Maintenance of anesthesia: Supplemental doses of 1/2 to the full induction dose; may also be maintained with a continuous infusion of 0.1-5 mg/minute
Stability Store at 20°C to 25°C (68°F to 77°F). Protect from light. The 50 mg/mL and 100 mg/mL vials may be further diluted in D_5W or NS to a final concentration of 1 mg/mL (or 2 mg/mL in patients with fluid restrictions). The 10 mg/mL vials are not recommended to be further diluted. Do not mix with barbiturates or diazepam (precipitation may occur).
Administration
  Oral: Use 100 mg/mL I.V. solution and mix the appropriate dose in 0.2-0.3 mL/kg of cola or other beverage.
  Parenteral: I.V.: Do not exceed 0.5 mg/kg/minute or administer faster than 60 seconds. Solutions for infusion should not exceed final concentration of 2 mg/mL.

Monitoring Parameters Heart rate, blood pressure, respiratory rate, transcutaneous O_2 saturation, emergence reactions; cardiac function should be continuously monitored in patients with increased blood pressure or cardiac decompensation

Anesthesia and Critical Care Concerns/Other Considerations

Clinical Pearls/Comments: Can produce emergence psychosis, including auditory and visual hallucinations, restlessness, disorientation, vivid dreams, and irrational behavior in 5% to 30% of patients; risk factors include age >15 years, female gender, dose >2 mg/kg I.V., and a history of personality problems/ frequent dreams (White, 1982). Pretreatment with a benzodiazepine reduces incidence of psychosis by >50%. Spontaneous involuntary movements, nystagmus, hypertonus, and vocalizations are also commonly seen.

Bronchodilation is beneficial in asthmatic or COPD patients. Laryngeal reflexes may remain intact or may be obtunded. The direct myocardial depressant action of ketamine can be seen in stressed, catecholamine-deficient patients. Ketamine increases myocardial oxygen demand secondary to catecholamine release. Ketamine increases cerebral metabolism and cerebral blood flow while producing a noncompetitive block of the neuronal postsynaptic NMDA receptor. It lowers seizure threshold and stimulates salivary secretions. Recent laboratory/clinical studies support the use of low-dose ketamine to improve postoperative analgesia/ outcome (Adam, 2005; Menigaux, 2000).

Contraindications Hypersensitivity to ketamine or any component of the formulation; conditions in which an increase in blood pressure would be hazardous

Warnings/Precautions Use with caution in patients with coronary artery disease, catecholamine depletion, hypertension, and tachycardia. Cardiac function should be continuously monitored in patients with increased blood pressure or cardiac decompensation. Postanesthetic emergence reactions which can manifest as vivid dreams, hallucinations, and/or frank delirium occur; these reactions are less common in patients >65 years of age and when given intramuscularly. Emergence reactions, confusion, or irrational behavior may occur up to 24 hours postoperatively and may be reduced by pretreatment with a benzodiazepine and the use of ketamine at the lower end of the dosing range. Rapid I.V. administration or overdose may cause respiratory depression, apnea, and enhanced pressor response. Resuscitative equipment should be available during use. Use with caution in patients with CSF pressure elevation, the chronic alcoholic or acutely alcohol-intoxicated. May cause dependence (withdrawal symptoms on discontinuation) and tolerance with prolonged use. May cause CNS depression, which may impair physical or mental abilities; patients must be cautioned about performing tasks which require mental alertness (eg, operating machinery or driving). When used on an outpatient basis, patient should be accompanied by a responsible adult. Should be administered under the supervision of a physician experienced in administering general anesthetics.

Adverse Reactions Frequency not always defined.

Cardiovascular: Arrhythmia, bradycardia, hyper-/hypotension, pulse rate increased

Central nervous system: CSF pressure increased

Dermatologic: Erythema (transient), morbilliform rash (transient)

Gastrointestinal: Anorexia, nausea, vomiting

Local: Pain at the injection site, exanthema at the injection site

Neuromuscular & skeletal: Skeletal muscle tone enhanced (tonic-clonic movements)

Ocular: Diplopia, intraocular pressure increased, nystagmus

Respiratory: Airway obstruction, apnea, respiratory depression or stimulation, laryngospasm

Miscellaneous: Anaphylaxis, dependence with prolonged use, emergence reactions (~12%; includes confusion, delirium, dreamlike state, excitement, hallucinations, irrational behavior, vivid imagery)

Drug Interactions

Metabolism/Transport Effects Substrate (major) of CYP2B6, 2C9, 3A4

Avoid Concomitant Use There are no known interactions where it is recommended to avoid concomitant use.

▶

◀ **Increased Effect/Toxicity**

The levels/effects of Ketamine may be increased by: CYP2B6 Inhibitors (Moderate); CYP2B6 Inhibitors (Strong); CYP2C9 Inhibitors (Moderate); CYP2C9 Inhibitors (Strong); CYP3A4 Inhibitors (Moderate); CYP3A4 Inhibitors (Strong); Dasatinib

Decreased Effect

The levels/effects of Ketamine may be decreased by: CYP2C9 Inducers (Highly Effective); Peginterferon Alfa-2b

Dosage Forms Excipient information presented when available (limited, particularly for generics); consult specific product labeling.

Injection, solution: 10 mg/mL (20 mL); 50 mg/mL (10 mL); 100 mg/mL (5 mL)

Ketalar®: 10 mg/mL (20 mL); 50 mg/mL (10 mL); 100 mg/mL (5 mL)

References

Adam F, Chauvin M, Du Manoir B, et al, "Small-Dose Ketamine Infusion Improves Postoperative Analgesia and Rehabilitation After Total Knee Arthroplasty," *Anesth Analg*, 2005, 100(2):475-80.

Clements JA and Nimmo WS, "Pharmacokinetics and Analgesic Effect of Ketamine in Man," *Br J Anaesth*, 1981, 53(1):27-30.

Kohrs R and Durieux ME, "Ketamine: Teaching an Old Drug New Tricks," *Anesth Analg*, 1998, 87 (5):1186-93.

Menigaux C, Fletcher D, Dupont X, et al, "The Benefits of Intraoperative Small-Dose Ketamine on Postoperative Pain After Anterior Cruciate Ligament Repair," *Anesth Analg*, 2000, 90(1):129-35.

White PF, Way WL, and Trevor AJ, "Ketamine – Its Pharmacology and Therapeutic Uses," *Anesthesiology*, 1982, 56(2):119-36.

◆ **Ketamine Hydrochloride** *see* Ketamine *on page 777*

◆ **Ketamine Hydrochloride Injection, USP (Can)** *see* Ketamine *on page 777*

◆ **Ketek®** *see* Telithromycin *on page 1353*

Ketoconazole (kee toe KOE na zole)

Medication Safety Issues

Sound-alike/look-alike issues:

Kuric™ may be confused with Carac®

Nizoral® may be confused with Nasarel®, Neoral®, Nitrol®

Related Information

Antifungal Agents *on page 1664*

U.S. Brand Names Extina®; Kuric™; Nizoral®; Nizoral® A-D [OTC]; Xolegel®

Canadian Brand Names Apo-Ketoconazole®; Ketoderm®; Novo-Ketoconazole; Xolegel®

Pharmacologic Category Antifungal Agent, Oral; Antifungal Agent, Topical

Generic Available Yes: Cream, shampoo, tablet

Use

Systemic: Treatment of susceptible fungal infections, including candidiasis, oral thrush, blastomycosis, histoplasmosis, paracoccidioidomycosis, coccidioidomycosis, chromomycosis, candiduria, chronic mucocutaneous candidiasis, as well as certain recalcitrant cutaneous dermatophytoses

Topical:

Cream: Treatment of tinea corporis, tinea cruris, tinea versicolor, cutaneous candidiasis, seborrheic dermatitis

Foam, gel: Treatment of seborrheic dermatitis

Shampoo: Treatment of dandruff, seborrheic dermatitis, tinea versicolor

Unlabeled/Investigational Use Tablet: Treatment of prostate cancer (androgen synthesis inhibitor)

Mechanism of Action Alters the permeability of the cell wall by blocking fungal cytochrome P450; inhibits biosynthesis of triglycerides and phospholipids by fungi; inhibits several fungal enzymes that results in a build-up of toxic concentrations of hydrogen peroxide; also inhibits androgen synthesis

Pharmacodynamics/Kinetics

Absorption: Oral: Rapid (~75%); Shampoo: None; Gel: Minimal

Distribution: Well into inflamed joint fluid, saliva, bile, urine, breast milk, sebum, cerumen, feces, tendons, skin and soft tissue, and testes; crosses blood-brain barrier poorly; only negligible amounts reach CSF

Protein binding: 93% to 96%

Metabolism: Partially hepatic via CYP3A4 to inactive compounds

Bioavailability: Decreases as gastric pH increases
Half-life elimination: Biphasic: Initial: 2 hours; Terminal: 8 hours
Time to peak, serum: 1-2 hours
Excretion: Feces (57%); urine (13%)

Dosage

Oral:

Fungal infections:

Children ≥2 years: 3.3-6.6 mg/kg/day as a single dose for 1-2 weeks for candidiasis, for at least 4 weeks in recalcitrant dermatophyte infections, and for up to 6 months for other systemic mycoses

Adults: 200-400 mg/day as a single daily dose for durations as stated above

Prostate cancer (unlabeled use): Adults: 400 mg 3 times/day

Shampoo:

Seborrheic dermatitis (ketoconazole 1%): Children ≥12 years and Adults: Apply twice weekly for up to 8 weeks with at least 3 days between each shampoo

Tinea versicolor (ketoconazole 2%): Adults: Apply to damp skin, lather, leave on 5 minutes, and rinse (one application should be sufficient)

Topical:

Tinea infections: Adults: Cream: Rub gently into the affected area once daily. Duration of treatment: Tinea corporis, cruris: 2 weeks; tinea pedis: 6 weeks

Seborrheic dermatitis: Children ≥12 years and Adults:

Cream: Rub gently into the affected area twice daily for 4 weeks or until clinical response is noted

Foam: Apply to affected area twice daily for 4 weeks

Gel: Rub gently into the affected area once daily for 2 weeks

Dosing adjustment in renal impairment: Hemodialysis: Not dialyzable (0% to 5%)

Dosing adjustment in hepatic impairment: Dose reductions should be considered in patients with severe liver disease

Stability

Cream: Store at <25°C (<77°F).

Foam: Store at 20°C to 25°C (68°F to 77°F). Do not refrigerate. Do not store in direct sunlight. Contents are flammable.

Gel: Store at 15°C to 30°C (59°F to 86°F).

Shampoo:

Nizoral®: Store at ≤25°C (≤77°F). Protect from light.

Nizoral® A-D:Store between 2°C to 30°C (35°F to 86°F); protect from freezing. Protect from light.

Tablet: Store at 15°C to 25°C (59°F to 77°F).

Administration

Oral: Administer oral tablets 2 hours prior to antacids to prevent decreased absorption due to the high pH of gastric contents.

Cream, foam, gel, and shampoo are for external use only. Avoid exposure to flame or smoking immediately following application of gel or foam; do not apply directly to hands.

Monitoring Parameters Liver function tests

Pregnancy Risk Factor C

Contraindications Hypersensitivity to ketoconazole or any component of the formulation; CNS fungal infections (due to poor CNS penetration); coadministration with ergot derivatives, cisapride, or triazolam is contraindicated due to risk of potentially fatal cardiac arrhythmias

Warnings/Precautions [U.S. Boxed Warning]: Ketoconazole has been associated with hepatotoxicity, including some fatalities; use with caution in patients with impaired hepatic function and perform periodic liver function tests. **[U.S. Boxed Warning]: Concomitant use with cisapride is contraindicated due to the occurrence of ventricular arrhythmias.** High doses of ketoconazole may depress adrenocortical function. Cases of hypersensitivity reactions (including rare cases of anaphylaxis) have been reported.

Topical: Formulations may contain sulfites. Avoid exposure of gel to open flames during or immediately after application. Use of shampoo may remove curl from permanently wavy hair, cause hair discoloration, and changes in hair texture; avoid contact with eyes. Foam formulation contains alcohol and propane/butane;

◀ do not expose to open flame or smoking during or immediately after application; do not puncture or incinerate container.

Adverse Reactions

Oral:

1% to 10%:

Dermatologic: Pruritus (2%)

Gastrointestinal: Nausea/vomiting (3% to 10%), abdominal pain (1%)

<1% (Limited to important or life-threatening): Bulging fontanelles, chills, depression, diarrhea, dizziness, fever, gynecomastia, headache, hemolytic anemia, hepatotoxicity, impotence, leukopenia, photophobia, somnolence, thrombocytopenia

Topical cream/gel: Allergic reaction, contact dermatitis (possibly related to sulfites or propylene glycol), facial swelling, headache, impetigo, local burning, ocular irritation, paresthesia, pruritus, severe irritation, stinging (~5%)

Topical foam: Application site burning (10%), application site reaction (6%), contact sensitization, dryness, erythema, pruritus, rash

Shampoo: Abnormal hair texture, alopecia, application site reaction, burning sensation, contact dermatitis, hair discoloration, hair loss increased (<1%), hypersensitivity, irritation (<1%), itching, mild dryness of skin, oiliness/dryness of hair, pruritus, rash, scalp pustules, urticaria

Drug Interactions

Metabolism/Transport Effects Substrate of CYP3A4 (major); **Inhibits** CYP1A2 (strong), 2A6 (moderate), 2B6 (weak), 2C8 (weak), 2C9 (strong), 2C19 (moderate), 2D6 (moderate), 3A4 (strong)

Avoid Concomitant Use

Avoid concomitant use of Ketoconazole with any of the following: Alfuzosin; Cisapride; Clopidogrel; Conivaptan; Dabigatran Etexilate; Dofetilide; Dronedarone; Eplerenone; Everolimus; Halofantrine; Nilotinib; Nisoldipine; Pimozide; QuiNIDine; Ranolazine; Rivaroxaban; Salmeterol; Silodosin; Thioridazine; Tolvaptan; Topotecan

Increased Effect/Toxicity

Ketoconazole may increase the levels/effects of: Alfentanil; Alfuzosin; Aliskiren; Almotriptan; Alosetron; Aprepitant; Bendamustine; Benzodiazepines (metabolized by oxidation); Bosentan; BusPIRone; Busulfan; Calcium Channel Blockers; CarBAMazepine; Cardiac Glycosides; Carvedilol; Ciclesonide; Cilostazol; Cinacalcet; Cisapride; Colchicine; Conivaptan; Corticosteroids (Orally Inhaled); Corticosteroids (Systemic); CycloSPORINE; CYP1A2 Substrates; CYP2A6 Substrates; CYP2C19 Substrates; CYP2C9 Substrates (High risk); CYP2D6 Substrates; CYP3A4 Substrates; Dabigatran Etexilate; Docetaxel; Dofetilide; Dronedarone; Dutasteride; Eletriptan; Eplerenone; Erlotinib; Eszopiclone; Everolimus; FentaNYL; Fesoterodine; Fexofenadine; Fosaprepitant; Gefitinib; Halofantrine; HMG-CoA Reductase Inhibitors; Imatinib; Irinotecan; Ixabepilone; Losartan; Macrolide Antibiotics; Maraviroc; Methadone; Nebivolol; Nilotinib; Nisoldipine; Paricalcitol; P-Glycoprotein Substrates; Phenytoin; Phosphodiesterase 5 Inhibitors; Pimecrolimus; Pimozide; Praziquantel; Protease Inhibitors; Proton Pump Inhibitors; QuiNIDine; Ramelteon; Ranolazine; Repaglinide; Rifamycin Derivatives; Rivaroxaban; Salmeterol; Saxagliptin; Silodosin; Sirolimus; Solifenacin; Sorafenib; Sunitinib; Tacrolimus; Tadalafil; Tamoxifen; Temsirolimus; Thioridazine; Tolterodine; Tolvaptan; Topotecan; Trimetrexate; Vitamin K Antagonists; Ziprasidone; Zolpidem

The levels/effects of Ketoconazole may be increased by: Grapefruit Juice; Macrolide Antibiotics; Protease Inhibitors

Decreased Effect

Ketoconazole may decrease the levels/effects of: Amphotericin B; Clopidogrel; Codeine; Prasugrel; Saccharomyces boulardii; TraMADol

The levels/effects of Ketoconazole may be decreased by: Antacids; CYP3A4 Inducers (Strong); Deferasirox; Didanosine; H2-Antagonists; Herbs (CYP3A4 Inducers); Phenytoin; Proton Pump Inhibitors; Rifamycin Derivatives; Sucralfate

Ethanol/Nutrition/Herb Interactions

Food: Ketoconazole peak serum levels may be prolonged if taken with food.

Herb/Nutraceutical: St John's wort may decrease ketoconazole levels.

Dietary Considerations Tablet: May be taken with food or milk to decrease GI adverse effects.

Dosage Forms Excipient information presented when available (limited, particularly for generics); consult specific product labeling.

Aerosol, topical [foam]:

Extina®: 2% (50 g, 100 g)

Cream, topical: 2% (15 g, 30 g, 60 g)

Kuric™: 2%: (75 g)

Gel, topical:

Xolegel®: 2% (15 g, 45 g) [contains dehydrated alcohol 34%]

Shampoo, topical: 1% (120 mL), 2% (120 mL)

Nizoral®: 2% (120 mL)

Nizoral® A-D: 1% (120 mL, 210 mL)

Tablet: 200 mg

◆ **Ketoderm® (Can)** *see* Ketoconazole *on page 780*

Ketoprofen (kee toe PROE fen)

Related Information
Acetaminophen and NSAIDS, Dosing in the Management of Pain *on page 1651*
Chronic Pain Management *on page 1546*
Nonsteroidal Anti-Inflammatory Agents *on page 1687*

Canadian Brand Names Apo-Keto SR®; Apo-Keto-E®; Apo-Keto®; Novo-Keto; Novo-Keto-EC; Nu-Ketoprofen; Nu-Ketoprofen-E; Oruvail®; Rhodis SR™; Rhodis-EC™; Rhodis™

Pharmacologic Category Nonsteroidal Anti-inflammatory Drug (NSAID), Oral

Use Acute and long-term treatment of rheumatoid arthritis and osteoarthritis; primary dysmenorrhea; mild-to-moderate pain

Pharmacodynamics/Kinetics
Onset of action: Regular release: <30 minutes

Duration: Regular release: Up to 6 hours

Absorption: Almost complete

Protein binding: >99%, primarily to albumin; Hepatic impairment: Unbound fraction is approximately doubled

Metabolism: Hepatic via glucuronidation; metabolite can be converted back to parent compound; may have enterohepatic recirculation

Bioavailability: ~90%

Half-life elimination:

Regular release: 2-4 hours; Renal impairment: Mild: 3 hours; moderate-to-severe: 5-9 hours

Extended release: ~3-7.5 hours

Time to peak, serum:

Regular release: 0.5-2 hours

Extended release: 6-7 hours

Excretion: Urine (~80%, primarily as glucuronide conjugates)

Dosage Note: The extended release formulation is not recommended for the treatment of acute pain. Oral:

Adults:

Rheumatoid arthritis, osteoarthritis (lower doses may be used in small patients or in the elderly, or debilitated):

Regular release: 50 mg 4 times/day **or** 75 mg 3 times/day; up to a maximum of 300 mg/day

Extended release: 200 mg once daily

Dysmenorrhea, mild-to-moderate pain: Regular release: 25-50 mg every 6-8 hours up to a maximum of 300 mg/day

Elderly: Initial dose should be decreased in patients >75 years; use caution when dosage changes are made

◀ **Dosage adjustment in renal impairment:** In general, NSAIDs are not recommended for use in patients with advanced renal disease, but the manufacturer of ketoprofen does provide some guidelines for adjustment in renal dysfunction:

Mild impairment: Maximum dose: 150 mg/day

Severe impairment: Cl_{cr} <25 mL/minute: Maximum dose: 100 mg/day

Dosage adjustment in hepatic impairment and serum albumin <3.5 g/dL: Maximum dose: 100 mg/day

Anesthesia and Critical Care Concerns/Other Considerations The 2002 ACCM/SCCM guidelines for analgesia (critically-ill adult) suggest that NSAIDs may be used in combination with opioids in select patients for pain management. Concern about adverse events (increased risk of renal dysfunction, altered platelet function, and gastrointestinal irritation) limits its use in patients who have other underlying risks for these events.

In short-term use, NSAIDs vary considerably in their effect on blood pressure. When NSAIDs are used in patients with hypertension, appropriate monitoring of blood pressure responses should be completed and the duration of therapy, when possible, kept short. The use of NSAIDs in the treatment of patients with congestive heart failure may be associated with an increased risk for fluid accumulation and edema; may precipitate renal failure in dehydrated patients.

Additional Information Complete prescribing information for this medication should be consulted for additional detail.

Dosage Forms Excipient information presented when available (limited, particularly for generics); consult specific product labeling.

Capsule, regular release: 50 mg, 75 mg

Capsule, extended release: 200 mg

Ketorolac (KEE toe role ak)

Medication Safety Issues

Sound-alike/look-alike issues:

Acular® may be confused with Acthar®, Ocular®

Ketorolac may be confused with Ketalar®

Toradol® may be confused with Foradil®, Inderal®, Tegretol®, Torecan®, traMADol, tromethamine

International issues:

Toradol® may be confused with Theradol® which is a brand name for tramadol in the Netherlands

Medication Guide An FDA-approved patient medication guide, which is available with the product information and at http://www.fda.gov/downloads/Drugs/DrugSafety/ucm089165.pdf, must be dispensed with this medication for each new outpatient prescription and refill.

Related Information

Acetaminophen and NSAIDS, Dosing in the Management of Pain *on page 1651*
Acute Postoperative Pain *on page 1502*
Nonsteroidal Anti-Inflammatory Agents *on page 1687*

U.S. Brand Names Acular LS®; Acular®; Acular® PF [DSC]

Canadian Brand Names Acular LS®; Acular®; Apo-Ketorolac Injectable®; Apo-Ketorolac®; Ketorolac Tromethamine Injection, USP; Novo-Ketorolac; ratio-Ketorolac; Toradol®; Toradol® IM

Index Terms Ketorolac Tromethamine

Pharmacologic Category Nonsteroidal Anti-inflammatory Drug (NSAID), Ophthalmic; Nonsteroidal Anti-inflammatory Drug (NSAID), Oral; Nonsteroidal Anti-inflammatory Drug (NSAID), Parenteral

Generic Available Yes: Injection, tablet

Use

Oral, injection: Short-term (≤5 days) management of moderate-to-severe acute pain requiring analgesia at the opioid level

Ophthalmic: Temporary relief of ocular itching due to seasonal allergic conjunctivitis; postoperative inflammation following cataract extraction; reduction of ocular pain and photophobia following incisional refractive surgery; reduction of ocular pain, burning, and stinging following corneal refractive surgery

Mechanism of Action Reversibly inhibits cyclooxygenase-1 and 2 (COX-1 and 2) enzymes, which results in decreased formation of prostaglandin precursors; has antipyretic, analgesic, and anti-inflammatory properties

Other proposed mechanisms not fully elucidated (and possibly contributing to the anti-inflammatory effect to varying degrees), include inhibiting chemotaxis, altering lymphocyte activity, inhibiting neutrophil aggregation/activation, and decreasing proinflammatory cytokine levels.

Pharmacodynamics/Kinetics

Onset of action: Analgesic: I.M.: ~10 minutes
  Peak effect: Analgesic: 2-3 hours
Duration: Analgesic: 6-8 hours
Absorption: Oral: Well absorbed (100%)
Distribution: ~13 L; poor penetration into CSF; crosses placenta
Protein binding: 99%
Metabolism: Hepatic
Half-life elimination: 2-6 hours; prolonged 30% to 50% in elderly; up to 19 hours in renal impairment
Time to peak, serum: I.M.: 30-60 minutes
Excretion: Urine (92%, ~60% as unchanged drug); feces ~6%

Dosage

Children 2-16 years (unlabeled use): Limited pediatric studies. The maximum combined duration of treatment (for parenteral and oral) is 5 days. **Do not exceed adult doses. Note:** The manufacturer warns that oral ketorolac is not indicated for children.

  I.V.: Initial dose: 0.5 mg/kg, followed by 0.25-1 mg/kg every 6 hours for up to 48 hours (maximum daily dose: 90 mg)

  Oral: 0.25 mg/kg every 6 hours

Children ≥16 years and Adults (pain relief usually begins within 10 minutes with parenteral forms): **Note:** The maximum combined duration of treatment (for parenteral and oral) is 5 days; do not increase dose or frequency; supplement with low-dose opioids if needed for breakthrough pain. For patients <50 kg and/or ≥65 years, see Elderly dosing.

  I.M.: 60 mg as a single dose or 30 mg every 6 hours (maximum daily dose: 120 mg)

  I.V.: 30 mg as a single dose or 30 mg every 6 hours (maximum daily dose: 120 mg)

Children ≥17 years and Adults: Oral: 20 mg, followed by 10 mg every 4-6 hours; do not exceed 40 mg/day; oral dosing is intended to be a continuation of I.M. or I.V. therapy only

  Note: The maximum combined duration of treatment (for parenteral and oral) is 5 days; do not increase dose or frequency; supplement with low-dose opioids if needed for breakthrough pain. Therapy should not be initiated with oral formulation. For patients <50 kg and/or ≥65 years, see Elderly dosing.

Dosage adjustments in elderly (≥65 years), renal insufficiency, or low body weight (<50 kg): Note: These groups have an increased incidence of GI bleeding, ulceration, and perforation. The maximum combined duration of treatment (for parenteral and oral) is 5 days.

  I.M.: 30 mg as a single dose or 15 mg every 6 hours (maximum daily dose: 60 mg)

  I.V.: 15 mg as a single dose or 15 mg every 6 hours (maximum daily dose: 60 mg)

  Oral: 10 mg, followed by 10 mg every 4-6 hours; do not exceed 40 mg/day; oral dosing is intended to be a continuation of I.M. or I.V. therapy only

Ophthalmic: Children ≥3 years and Adults:

  Allergic conjunctivitis (relief of ocular itching) (Acular®): Instill 1 drop (0.25 mg) 4 times/day

  Inflammation following cataract extraction (Acular®): Instill 1 drop (0.25 mg) to affected eye(s) 4 times/day beginning 24 hours after surgery; continue for 2 weeks

  Pain and photophobia following incisional refractive surgery (Acular® PF): Instill 1 drop (0.25 mg) 4 times/day to affected eye for up to 3 days

◀   Pain following corneal refractive surgery (Acular LS®): Instill 1 drop 4 times/day as needed to affected eye for up to 4 days

Dosage adjustment in renal impairment: Contraindicated in patients with advanced renal impairment. Patients with moderately-elevated serum creatinine should use half the recommended dose, not to exceed 60 mg/day I.M./I.V.

Dosage adjustment in hepatic impairment: Use with caution, may cause elevation of liver enzymes; discontinue if clinical signs and symptoms of liver disease develop

Stability

Injection: Store at room temperature of 15°C to 30°C (59°F to 86°F). Protect from light. Injection is clear and has a slight yellow color. Precipitation may occur at relatively low pH values.

Ophthalmic solution: Store at room temperature 15°C to 25°C (59°F to 77°F). Protect from light.

Tablet: Store at room temperature of 15°C to 30°C (59°F to 86°F).

Administration

Oral: May take with food to reduce GI upset.

I.M.: Administer slowly and deeply into the muscle. Analgesia begins in 30 minutes and maximum effect within 2 hours.

I.V.: Administer I.V. bolus over a minimum of 15 seconds; onset within 30 minutes; peak analgesia within 2 hours.

Ophthalmic solution: Contact lenses should be removed before instillation. Acular® and Acular LS® have been safely administered with other ophthalmic medications including antibiotics, beta-blockers, carbonic anhydrase inhibitors, cycloplegics, and mydriatics.

Monitoring Parameters Monitor response (pain, range of motion, grip strength, mobility, ADL function), inflammation; observe for weight gain, edema; monitor renal function (serum creatinine, BUN, urine output); observe for bleeding, bruising; evaluate gastrointestinal effects (abdominal pain, bleeding, dyspepsia); mental confusion, disorientation, CBC and platelets, liver function tests

Reference Range Serum concentration: Therapeutic: 0.3-5 mcg/mL; Toxic: >5 mcg/mL

Anesthesia and Critical Care Concerns/Other Considerations

Evidence-Based Information: The 2002 ACCM/SCCM guidelines for analgesia (critically-ill adult) recommend that ketorolac therapy be limited to a maximum of 5 days. The risk of developing renal dysfunction or gastrointestinal bleeding further increases as treatment extends beyond 5 days.

In short-term use, NSAIDs vary considerably in their effect on blood pressure. When NSAIDs are used in patients with hypertension, blood pressure needs to be monitored and the duration of therapy kept short. The use of NSAIDs in patients with heart failure may be associated with an increased risk for fluid accumulation and edema; may precipitate renal failure in dehydrated patients by inhibition of prostaglandin-mediated autoregulation. Use extreme caution or avoid concurrent use with nephrotoxic agents.

Ketorolac is contraindicated during labor and delivery (may inhibit uterine contractions and adversely affect fetal circulation); avoid use of ketorolac ophthalmic solution during late pregnancy.

Using animal models of fracture healing, ketorolac has been shown to delay bone healing by inhibiting production of prostaglandin (Gerstenfeld, 2003). Further human clinical studies are required to determine the clinical implications of this finding. Of note, use of ketorolac (limited to 48 hours) following spinal fusion surgery did not significantly affect ultimate fusion rates (Pradhan, 2008).

Ketorolac produces reversible inhibition of platelet aggregation and prolongs bleeding time; has been reported to increase postoperative bleeding after tonsillectomy (Marret, 2003).

Pregnancy Risk Factor C/D (3rd trimester)

Contraindications

Oral, injection: Hypersensitivity to ketorolac, aspirin, other NSAIDs, or any component of the formulation; active or history of peptic ulcer disease; recent or history of GI bleeding or perforation; patients with advanced renal disease or risk of renal failure (due to volume depletion); prophylaxis before major surgery;

suspected or confirmed cerebrovascular bleeding; hemorrhagic diathesis, incomplete hemostasis, or high risk of bleeding; concurrent ASA or other NSAIDs; concomitant probenecid or pentoxifylline; epidural or intrathecal administration; perioperative pain in the setting of coronary artery bypass graft (CABG) surgery; labor and delivery; breast-feeding

Ophthalmic: Hypersensitivity to ketorolac or any component of the formulation

Warnings/Precautions [U.S. Boxed Warning]: May inhibit platelet function; contraindicated in patients with cerebrovascular bleeding (suspected or confirmed), hemorrhagic diathesis, incomplete hemostasis and patients at high risk for bleeding. Effects on platelet adhesion and aggregation may prolong bleeding time. Anemia may occur; patients on long-term NSAID therapy should be monitored for anemia. Rarely, NSAID use has been associated with potentially severe blood dyscrasias (eg, agranulocytosis, thrombocytopenia, aplastic anemia).

[U.S. Boxed Warning]: NSAIDs are associated with an increased risk of adverse cardiovascular thrombotic events, including MI and stroke. Risk may be increased with duration of use or pre-existing cardiovascular risk factors or disease. Carefully evaluate individual cardiovascular risk profiles prior to prescribing. May cause new-onset hypertension or worsening of existing hypertension. Use caution with fluid retention. Avoid use in heart failure. Concurrent administration of ibuprofen, and potentially other nonselective NSAIDs, may interfere with aspirin's cardioprotective effect. **[U.S. Boxed Warning]: Use is contraindicated as prophylactic analgesic before any major surgery and is contraindicated for treatment of perioperative pain in the setting of coronary artery bypass graft (CABG) surgery.** Risk of MI and stroke may be increased with use following CABG surgery. Wound bleeding and postoperative hematomas have been associated with ketorolac use in the perioperative setting. Withhold for at least 4-6 half-lives prior to surgical or dental procedures.

[U.S. Boxed Warning]: Ketorolac is contraindicated in patients with advanced renal impairment and in patients at risk for renal failure due to volume depletion. NSAID use may compromise existing renal function; dose-dependent decreases in prostaglandin synthesis may result from NSAID use, reducing renal blood flow which may cause renal decompensation. NSAID use may increase the risk for hyperkalemia. Patients with impaired renal function, dehydration, heart failure, liver dysfunction, those taking diuretics and ACE inhibitors, and the elderly are at greater risk of renal toxicity and hyperkalemia. Use with caution in patients with impaired renal function or history of kidney disease; dosage adjustment is required in patients with moderate elevation in serum creatinine. Monitor renal function closely. Acute renal failure, interstitial nephritis, and nephrotic syndrome have been reported with ketorolac use; papillary necrosis and renal injury have been reported with the use of NSAIDs. Use of NSAIDs can compromise existing renal function. Rehydrate patient before starting therapy.

[U.S. Boxed Warning]: NSAIDs may increase risk of gastrointestinal irritation, inflammation, ulceration, bleeding, and perforation. These events may occur at any time during therapy and without warning. Use caution with a history of GI disease (bleeding, ulcers, inflammatory bowel disease), concurrent therapy with aspirin, anticoagulants and/or corticosteroids, smoking, use of alcohol, the elderly, or debilitated patients. When used concomitantly with ≤325 mg of aspirin, a substantial increase in the risk of gastrointestinal complications (eg, ulcer) occurs; concomitant gastroprotective therapy (eg, proton pump inhibitors) is recommended (Bhatt, 2008).

NSAIDs may cause serious skin adverse events including exfoliative dermatitis, Stevens-Johnson syndrome (SJS), and toxic epidermal necrolysis (TEN); discontinue use at first sign of skin rash or hypersensitivity. Hypersensitivity or anaphylactoid reactions may occur, even without prior exposure; patients with "aspirin triad" (bronchial asthma, aspirin intolerance, rhinitis) may be at increased risk. Do not use in patients who experience bronchospasm, asthma, rhinitis, or urticaria with NSAID or aspirin therapy. **[U.S. Boxed Warning]: Ketorolac injection is contraindicated in patients with prior hypersensitivity reaction to aspirin or NSAIDs.** Use caution in other forms of asthma.

◀ Use with caution in patients with hepatic impairment or a history of liver disease. Closely monitor patients with any abnormal LFT. Rarely, severe hepatic reactions (eg, fulminant hepatitis, hepatic necrosis, liver failure) have occurred with NSAID use; discontinue if signs or symptoms of liver disease develop, or if systemic manifestations occur.

[U.S. Boxed Warning]: Dosage adjustment is required for patients ≥65 years of age. The elderly are at increased risk for adverse effects (especially peptic ulceration, CNS effects, renal toxicity) from NSAIDs, even at low doses. **[U.S. Boxed Warning]: Dosage adjustment is required for patients weighing <50 kg (<110 pounds). [U.S. Boxed Warning]: May inhibit uterine contractions and affect fetal circulation; inhibits prostaglandin synthesis in neonates; use is contraindicated in labor and delivery and breast-feeding women.** Avoid use in late pregnancy. **[U.S. Boxed Warning]: Concurrent use of ketorolac with aspirin or other NSAIDs is contraindicated due to the increased risk of adverse reactions.**

[U.S. Boxed Warning]: Contraindicated for epidural or intrathecal administration. [U.S. Boxed Warning]: Systemic ketorolac is indicated for short term (≤5 days) use in adults for treatment of moderately severe acute pain requiring opioid-level analgesia. Low doses of narcotics may be needed for breakthrough pain. **[U.S. Boxed Warning]: Oral therapy is only indicated for use as continuation treatment, following parenteral ketorolac and is not indicated for minor or chronic painful conditions. The maximum daily oral dose is 40 mg (adults); doses above 40 mg/day do not improve efficacy but may increase the risk of serious adverse effects.** The combined therapy duration (oral and parenteral) should not exceed 5 days. Use the lowest effective dose for the shortest duration of time, consistent with individual patient goals, to reduce risk of cardiovascular or GI adverse events. Alternate therapies should be considered for patients at high risk. **[U.S. Boxed Warning]: Oral ketorolac is not indicated for use in children.**

NSAIDS may cause drowsiness, dizziness, blurred vision and other neurologic effects which may impair physical or mental abilities; patients must be cautioned about performing tasks which require mental alertness (eg, operating machinery or driving). Discontinue use with blurred or diminished vision and perform ophthalmologic exam. Monitor vision with long-term therapy.

Ophthalmic: May increase bleeding time associated with ocular surgery. Use with caution in patients with known bleeding tendencies or those receiving anticoagulants. Healing time may be slowed or delayed. Corneal thinning, erosion, or ulceration have been reported with topical NSAIDs; discontinue if corneal epithelial breakdown occurs. Use caution with complicated ocular surgery, corneal denervation, corneal epithelial defects, diabetes, rheumatoid arthritis, ocular surface disease, or ocular surgeries repeated within short periods of time; risk of corneal epithelial breakdown (leading to possible loss of vision) may be increased. Use for >24 hours prior to or for >14 days following surgery also increases risk of corneal adverse effects. Do not administer while wearing soft contact lenses. Safety and efficacy in pediatric patients <3 years of age have not been established. Use with caution in patients with sensitivity to acetylsalicylic acid, phenylacetic acid derivatives, or other nonsteroidal anti-inflammatory agents. The safety and efficacy of Acular LS® have not been established in postcataract surgery patients.

Adverse Reactions

Systemic (frequencies noted for parenteral administration):

>10%:

Central nervous system: Headache (17%)

Gastrointestinal: Gastrointestinal pain (13%), dyspepsia (12%), nausea (12%)

>1% to 10%:

Cardiovascular: Edema (4%), hypertension

Central nervous system: Dizziness (7%), drowsiness (6%)

Dermatologic: Pruritus, purpura, rash

Gastrointestinal: Diarrhea (7%), constipation, flatulence, GI bleeding, GI fullness, GI perforation, GI ulcer, heartburn, stomatitis, vomiting

Hematologic: Anemia, bleeding time increased

Hepatic: Liver enzymes increased

Local: Injection site pain (2%)
Otic: Tinnitus
Renal: Renal function abnormal
Miscellaneous: Diaphoresis

<1% (Limited to important or life-threatening): Abnormal thinking, acute pancreatitis, acute renal failure, agranulocytosis, alopecia, anaphylactoid reaction, anaphylaxis, angioedema, anxiety, aplastic anemia, arrhythmia, aseptic meningitis, asthma, azotemia, blurred vision, bradycardia, bronchospasm, bruising, chest pain, CHF, cholestatic jaundice, coma, confusion, conjunctivitis, cough, cystitis, depression, dyspnea, dysuria, eosinophilia, epistaxis, eructation, erythema multiforme, esophagitis, euphoria, excessive thirst, exfoliative dermatitis, extrapyramidal symptoms, fever, flank pain, flushing, gastritis, GI hemorrhage, glossitis, hallucinations, hearing loss, hematemesis, hematuria, hemolytic anemia, hemolytic uremic syndrome, hepatitis, hyperglycemia, hyperkalemia, hyperkinesis, hypersensitivity reactions, hyponatremia, hypotension, inability to concentrate, infection, infertility, inflammatory bowel disease exacerbation, insomnia, interstitial nephritis, jaundice, laryngeal edema, leukopenia, liver failure, Lyell's syndrome, lymphadenopathy, maculopapular rash, melena, MI, nephritis, nervousness, oliguria, pallor, palpitation, pancytopenia, paresthesia, photosensitivity, pneumonia, polyuria, proteinuria, psychosis, pulmonary edema, rectal bleeding, renal failure, respiratory depression, rhinitis, seizure, sepsis, somnolence, Stevens-Johnson syndrome, stomatitis (ulcerative), stupor, syncope, tachycardia, thrombocytopenia, tongue edema, toxic epidermal necrolysis, tremor, urinary frequency increased, urinary retention, urticaria, vasculitis, vertigo, weakness, weight gain, wound hemorrhage (postoperative), xerostomia

Ophthalmic solution:
>10%: Ocular: Transient burning/stinging (Acular®: 40%; Acular® PF: 20%)
>1% to 10%:
Central nervous system: Headache
Ocular: Conjunctival hyperemia, corneal infiltrates, iritis, ocular edema, ocular inflammation, ocular irritation, ocular pain, superficial keratitis, superficial ocular infection
Miscellaneous: Allergic reactions
≤1% (Limited to important or life-threatening): Blurred vision, corneal ulcer, corneal erosion, corneal perforation, corneal thinning, dry eyes, epithelial breakdown

Drug Interactions

Avoid Concomitant Use

Avoid concomitant use of Ketorolac with any of the following: Aspirin; Nonsteroidal Anti-Inflammatory Agents; Pentoxifylline; Probenecid

Increased Effect/Toxicity

Ketorolac may increase the levels/effects of: Aminoglycosides; Anticoagulants; Antiplatelet Agents; Aspirin; Bisphosphonate Derivatives; CycloSPORINE; Desmopressin; Drotrecogin Alfa; Eplerenone; Ibritumomab; Lithium; Methotrexate; Neuromuscular-Blocking Agents (Nondepolarizing); Nonsteroidal Anti-Inflammatory Agents; Pemetrexed; Pentoxifylline; Potassium-Sparing Diuretics; Pralatrexate; Quinolone Antibiotics; Salicylates; Thrombolytic Agents; Tositumomab and Iodine I 131 Tositumomab; Vancomycin; Vitamin K Antagonists

The levels/effects of Ketorolac may be increased by: Antidepressants (Tricyclic, Tertiary Amine); Corticosteroids (Systemic); Dasatinib; Herbs (Anticoagulant/Antiplatelet Properties); Omega-3-Acid Ethyl Esters; Pentosan Polysulfate Sodium; Probenecid; Prostacyclin Analogues; Selective Serotonin Reuptake Inhibitors; Serotonin/Norepinephrine Reuptake Inhibitors; Treprostinil

Decreased Effect

Ketorolac may decrease the levels/effects of: ACE Inhibitors; Angiotensin II Receptor Blockers; Anticonvulsants; Antiplatelet Agents; Beta-Blockers; Eplerenone; HydrALAZINE; Latanoprost; Loop Diuretics; Potassium-Sparing Diuretics; Salicylates; Thiazide Diuretics

The levels/effects of Ketorolac may be decreased by: Bile Acid Sequestrants; Salicylates

◀ **Ethanol/Nutrition/Herb Interactions**
Ethanol: Avoid ethanol (may enhance gastric mucosal irritation).
Food: Oral: High-fat meals may delay time to peak (by ~1 hour) and decrease peak concentrations.
Herb/Nutraceutical: Avoid alfalfa, anise, bilberry, bladderwrack, bromelain, cat's claw, celery, chamomile, coleus, cordyceps, dong quai, evening primrose, fenugreek, feverfew, garlic, ginger, ginkgo biloba, ginseng (American, Panax, Siberian), grapeseed, green tea, guggul, horse chestnut seed, horseradish, licorice, prickly ash, red clover, reishi, SAMe (S-adenosylmethionine), sweet clover, turmeric, and white willow (all have additional antiplatelet activity).

Dietary Considerations Administer tablet with food or milk to decrease gastrointestinal distress.

Dosage Forms Excipient information presented when available (limited, particularly for generics); consult specific product labeling. [DSC] = Discontinued product
Injection, solution, as tromethamine: 15 mg/mL (1 mL); 30 mg/mL (1 mL, 2 mL, 10 mL) [contains ethanol]
Solution, ophthalmic, as tromethamine:
Acular®: 0.5% (3 mL, 5 mL, 10 mL) [contains benzalkonium chloride]
Acular LS®: 0.4% (5 mL) [contains benzalkonium chloride]
Solution, ophthalmic, as tromethamine [preservative free]:
Acular® PF: 0.5% (0.4 mL) [DSC]
Tablet, as tromethamine: 10 mg

References
Gerstenfeld LC, Thiede M, Seibert K, et al, "Differential Inhibition of Fracture Healing by Non-Selective and Cyclooxygenase-2 Selective Non-Steroidal Anti-Inflammatory Drugs," *J Orthop Res*, 2003, 21(4):670-5.
Jacobi J, Fraser GL, Coursin DB, et al, "Clinical Practice Guidelines for the Sustained Use of Sedatives and Analgesics in the Critically Ill Adult," *Crit Care Med*, 2002, 30(1):119-41. Available at: http://www.sccm.org/pdf/sedatives.pdf. Accessed August 2, 2003.
Marret E, Flahault A, Samama CM, et al, "Effects of Postoperative, Nonsteroidal, Antiinflammatory Drugs on Bleeding Risk After Tonsillectomy: Meta-Analysis of Randomized, Controlled Trials," *Anesthesiology*, 2003, 98(6):1497-502.
Pradhan BB, Tatsumi RL, Gallina J, et al, "Ketorolac and Spinal Fusion: Does the Perioperative Use of Ketorolac Really Inhibit Spinal Fusion?," *Spine*, 2008, 33(19):2079-82.

◆ **Ketorolac Tromethamine** *see* Ketorolac *on page 784*

◆ **Ketorolac Tromethamine Injection, USP (Can)** *see* Ketorolac *on page 784*

◆ **Kinlytic™** *see* Urokinase *on page 1438*

◆ **Kionex®** *see* Sodium Polystyrene Sulfonate *on page 1313*

◆ **Klonopin®** *see* ClonazePAM *on page 328*

◆ **Klonopin® Wafers [DSC]** *see* ClonazePAM *on page 328*

◆ **K-Lor®** *see* Potassium Chloride *on page 1151*

◆ **Klor-Con®** *see* Potassium Chloride *on page 1151*

◆ **Klor-Con® 8** *see* Potassium Chloride *on page 1151*

◆ **Klor-Con® 10** *see* Potassium Chloride *on page 1151*

◆ **Klor-Con®/25** *see* Potassium Chloride *on page 1151*

◆ **Klor-Con® M** *see* Potassium Chloride *on page 1151*

◆ **K-Lyte®/Cl (Can)** *see* Potassium Chloride *on page 1151*

◆ **KMD 3213** *see* Silodosin *on page 1290*

◆ **Kogenate® (Can)** *see* Antihemophilic Factor (Recombinant) *on page 124*

◆ **Kogenate® FS** *see* Antihemophilic Factor (Recombinant) *on page 124*

◆ **Konakion (Can)** *see* Phytonadione *on page 1128*

◆ **Kristalose®** *see* Lactulose *on page 796*

◆ **K-Tab®** *see* Potassium Chloride *on page 1151*

◆ **Kuric™** *see* Ketoconazole *on page 780*

◆ **Kuvan™** *see* Sapropterin *on page 1277*

◆ **Kytril®** *see* Granisetron *on page 669*

◆ **L-749,345** *see* Ertapenem *on page 513*

◆ **L-M-X™ 4 [OTC]** *see* Lidocaine *on page 836*

Labetalol (la BET a lole)

Medication Safety Issues
Sound-alike/look-alike issues:

Labetalol may be confused with betaxolol, Hexadrol®, lamoTRIgine, Lipitor®
Normodyne® may be confused with Norpramin®
Trandate® may be confused with traMADol, Trendar®, Trental®, Tridrate®

High alert medication: The Institute for Safe Medication Practices (ISMP) includes this medication among its list of drugs which have a heightened risk of causing significant patient harm when used in error.

Significant differences exist between oral and I.V. dosing. Use caution when converting from one route of administration to another.

Related Information
Anesthesia Considerations for Neurosurgery *on page 1514*
Anesthesia for Patients With Liver Disease *on page 1537*
Anesthetic Considerations in the Substance-Abusing Patient *on page 1613*
Beta-Blockers *on page 1669*
Chronic Renal Failure *on page 1552*
Dosing Considerations for the Critically-Ill Patient With Morbid Obesity *on page 1561*
Hypertension *on page 1754*
Postoperative Hypertension *on page 1589*
Preoperative Evaluation of the Cardiac Patient for Noncardiac Surgery *on page 1598*

U.S. Brand Names Trandate®

Canadian Brand Names Apo-Labetalol®; Labetalol Hydrochloride Injection, USP; Normodyne®; Trandate®

Index Terms Ibidomide Hydrochloride; Labetalol Hydrochloride

Pharmacologic Category Beta Blocker With Alpha-Blocking Activity

Generic Available Yes

Use Treatment of mild-to-severe hypertension; I.V. for severe hypertension (eg, hypertensive emergencies)

Unlabeled/Investigational Use Pediatric hypertension

Mechanism of Action Blocks alpha-, $beta_1$-, and $beta_2$-adrenergic receptor sites; elevated renins are reduced. The ratios of alpha- to beta-blockade differ depending on the route of administration: 1:3 (oral) and 1:7 (I.V.).

Pharmacodynamics/Kinetics
Onset of action: Oral: 20 minutes to 2 hours; I.V.: 2-5 minutes
Peak effect: Oral: 1-4 hours; I.V.: 5-15 minutes
Duration: Blood pressure response:
Oral: 8-12 hours (dose dependent)
I.V.: 2-18 hours (dose dependent; based on single and multiple sequential doses of 0.25-0.5 mg/kg with cumulative dosing up to 3.25 mg/kg)
Absorption: Complete
Distribution: V_d: Adults: 3-16 L/kg; mean: <9.4 L/kg; moderately lipid soluble, therefore, can enter CNS
Protein binding: 50%
Metabolism: Hepatic, primarily via glucuronide conjugation; extensive first-pass effect
Bioavailability: Oral: 25%; increased with liver disease, elderly, and concurrent cimetidine
Half-life elimination: Oral: 6-8 hours; I.V.: ~5.5 hours
Time to peak, plasma: Oral: 1-2 hours
Excretion: Urine (55% to 60% as glucuronide conjugates, <5% as unchanged drug)
Clearance: Possibly decreased in neonates/infants

Dosage

Children: Due to limited documentation of its use, labetalol should be initiated cautiously in pediatric patients with careful dosage adjustment and blood pressure monitoring.

Oral: Hypertension (unlabeled use): Initial: 1-3 mg/kg/day, in 2 divided doses; maximum: 10-12 mg/kg/day, up to 1200 mg/day

I.V., intermittent bolus doses of 0.3-1 mg/kg/dose have been reported.

For treatment of pediatric hypertensive emergencies, initial continuous infusions of 0.4-1 mg/kg/hour with a maximum of 3 mg/kg/hour have been used. Administration requires the use of an infusion pump.

Adults:

Oral: Initial: 100 mg twice daily, may increase as needed every 2-3 days by 100 mg twice daily (titration increments not to exceed 200 mg twice daily) until desired response is obtained; usual dose: 200-400 mg twice daily; may require up to 2.4 g/day.

Usual dose range (JNC 7): 200-800 mg/day in 2 divided doses

I.V.: 20 mg (0.25 mg/kg for an 80 kg patient) I.V. push over 2 minutes; may administer 40-80 mg at 10-minute intervals, up to 300 mg total dose.

I.V. infusion (acute loading): Initial: 2 mg/minute; titrate to response up to 300 mg total dose, if needed. Administration requires the use of an infusion pump.

I.V. infusion (500 mg/250 mL D_5W) rates:

1 mg/minute: 30 mL/hour

2 mg/minute: 60 mL/hour

3 mg/minute: 90 mL/hour

4 mg/minute: 120 mL/hour

5 mg/minute: 150 mL/hour

6 mg/minute: 180 mL/hour

Note: Although loading infusions are well described in the product labeling, the labeling is silent in specific clinical situations, such as in the patient who has an initial response to labetalol infusions but cannot be converted to an oral route for subsequent dosing. There is limited documentation of prolonged continuous infusions. In rare clinical situations, higher continuous infusion dosages (up to 6 mg/minute) have been used in the critical care setting (eg, aortic dissection). At the other extreme, continuous infusions at relatively low doses (0.03-0.1 mg/minute) have been used in some settings (following loading infusion in patients who are unable to be converted to oral regimens or in some cases as a continuation of outpatient oral regimens). These prolonged infusions should not be confused with loading infusions. Because of wide variation in the use of infusions, an awareness of institutional policies and practices is extremely important. Careful clarification of orders and specific infusion rates/units is required to avoid confusion. Due to the prolonged duration of action, careful monitoring should be extended for the duration of the infusion and for several hours after the infusion. Excessive administration may result in prolonged hypotension and/or bradycardia.

Elderly: Initial dose: Refer to adult dosing. Usual maintenance: 100-200 mg twice daily

Dosage adjustment in renal impairment: Dialysis: Not removed by hemo- or peritoneal dialysis; supplemental dose is not necessary.

Dosage adjustment in hepatic impairment: Dosage reduction may be necessary.

Stability

Tablets: Store tablets at 2°C to 30°C (36°F to 86°F). Protect from light and excessive moisture.

Vials: Store unopened injectable vials at 20°C to 25°C (68°F to 77°F); do not freeze. Protect from light. The solution is clear to slightly yellow.

Parenteral admixture: Stability of parenteral admixture at room temperature (25°C) and refrigeration temperature (4°C): 3 days.

Standard concentration: 500 mg/250 mL D_5W.

Minimum volume: 250 mL D_5W.

Administration Bolus dose may be administered I.V. push at a rate of 10 mg/minute; may follow with continuous I.V. infusion

Monitoring Parameters Blood pressure, standing and sitting/supine, pulse, cardiac monitor and blood pressure monitor required for I.V. administration

Anesthesia and Critical Care Concerns/Other Considerations

Clinical Pearls/Comments: Due to alterations in the beta-adrenergic autonomic nervous system, beta-adrenergic blockade may result in less hemodynamic response in the elderly than seen in younger adults. Despite decreased sensitivity to the chronotropic effects of beta-blockade with age, there appears to be an increased myocardial sensitivity to the negative inotropic effect during stress (eg, exercise).

Blood Pressure Management of Intracerebral Hemorrhage (ICH): In addition to standard management of ICH, blood pressure (BP) management in patients who are hypertensive is also of paramount importance when treating ICH. The primary rationale for lowering BP is to prevent further progression of the bleed. This can be accomplished using a number of different pharmacologic treatments (eg, nicardipine, labetalol, nitroprusside). Nitroprusside may increase ICP due to the pronounced vasodilatory actions and as a result may be less preferable. Specific BP targets are not supported by available evidence. The 2007 AHA/ASA Guidelines recommend initiating antihypertensive therapy if the SBP >180 mm Hg or if MAP >130 mm Hg (Broderick, 2007).

Pregnancy Risk Factor C (manufacturer); D (2nd and 3rd trimesters - expert analysis)

Contraindications Hypersensitivity to labetalol or any component of the formulation; severe bradycardia; heart block greater than first degree (except in patients with a functioning artificial pacemaker); cardiogenic shock; bronchial asthma; uncompensated cardiac failure; conditions associated with severe and prolonged hypotension

Warnings/Precautions Consider pre-existing conditions such as sick sinus syndrome before initiating. Symptomatic hypotension with or without syncope may occur with labetalol; close monitoring of patient is required especially with initial dosing and dosing increases; blood pressure must be lowered at a rate appropriate for the patient's clinical condition. Initiation with a low dose and gradual up-titration may help to decrease the occurrence of hypotension or syncope. Patients should be advised to avoid driving or other hazardous tasks during initiation of therapy due to the risk of syncope. Orthostatic hypotension may occur with I.V. administration; patient should remain supine during and for up to 3 hours after I.V. administration. Use with caution in impaired hepatic function; bioavailability is increased due to decreased first-pass metabolism. Severe hepatic injury including some fatalities have also been rarely reported with use: periodically monitor LFTs with prolonged use. Use with caution in patients with diabetes mellitus; may potentiate hypoglycemia and/or mask signs and symptoms. May also reduce release of insulin in response to hyperglycemia; dosage of antidiabetic agents may need to be adjusted. Elimination of labetalol is reduced in elderly patients; lower maintenance doses may be required.

Use only with extreme caution in compensated heart failure and monitor for a worsening of the condition. Beta-blocker therapy should not be withdrawn abruptly (particularly in patients with CAD), but gradually tapered to avoid acute tachycardia, hypertension, and/or ischemia. Use caution with concurrent use of beta-blockers and either verapamil or diltiazem; bradycardia or heart block can occur. Patients with bronchospastic disease should not receive beta-blockers; if used at all, should be used cautiously with close monitoring. Use with caution in patients with myasthenia gravis, psychiatric disease (may cause or exacerbate CNS depression), or peripheral vascular disease. If possible, obtain diagnostic tests for pheochromocytoma prior to use. May induce or exacerbate psoriasis. Labetalol has been shown to be effective in lowering blood pressure and relieving symptoms in patients with pheochromocytoma. However, some patients have experienced paradoxical hypertensive responses; use with caution in patients with pheochromocytoma. Additional alpha-blockade may be required during use of labetalol. Use caution with history of severe anaphylaxis to allergens; patients taking beta-blockers may become more sensitive to repeated challenges. Treatment of anaphylaxis (eg, epinephrine) in patients taking beta-blockers may be ineffective or promote undesirable effects. Use with caution in patients receiving anesthetic agents which decrease myocardial function.

Adverse Reactions

>10%:

Cardiovascular: Postural hypotension (I.V. use; ≤58%)

Central nervous system: Dizziness (1% to 20%), fatigue (1% to 11%)
Gastrointestinal: Nausea (≤19%)
1% to 10%:
Cardiovascular: Hypotension (1% to 5%), edema (≤2%), flushing (1%), ventricular arrhythmia (I.V. use; 1%)
Central nervous system: Somnolence (3%), headache (2%), vertigo (1% to 2%)
Dermatologic: Scalp tingling (≤7%), pruritus (1%), rash (1%)
Gastrointestinal: Dyspepsia (≤4%), vomiting (≤3%), taste disturbance (1%)
Genitourinary: Ejaculatory failure (≤5%), impotence (1% to 4%)
Hepatic: Transaminases increased (4%)
Neuromuscular & skeletal: Paresthesia (≤5%), weakness (1%)
Ocular: Vision abnormal (1%)
Renal: BUN increased (≤8%)
Respiratory: Nasal congestion (1% to 6%), dyspnea (2%)
Miscellaneous: Diaphoresis (≤4%)
<1% (Limited to important or life-threatening): Alopecia (reversible), anaphylactoid reaction, ANA positive, angioedema, bradycardia, bronchospasm, cholestatic jaundice, CHF, diabetes insipidus, heart block, hepatic necrosis, hepatitis, hypersensitivity, Peyronie's disease, Raynaud's syndrome, syncope, systemic lupus erythematosus, toxic myopathy, urinary retention, urticaria
Other adverse reactions noted with beta-adrenergic blocking agents include mental depression, catatonia, disorientation, short-term memory loss, emotional lability, clouded sensorium, intensification of pre-existing AV block, laryngospasm, respiratory distress, agranulocytosis, thrombocytopenic purpura, nonthrombocytopenic purpura, mesenteric artery thrombosis, and ischemic colitis.

Drug Interactions

Avoid Concomitant Use

Avoid concomitant use of Labelalol with any of the following: Methacholine

Increased Effect/Toxicity

Labelalol may increase the levels/effects of: Alpha-/Beta-Agonists (Direct-Acting); Alpha1-Blockers; Alpha2-Agonists; Amifostine; Antihypertensives; Antipsychotic Agents (Phenothiazines); Cardiac Glycosides; Hypotensive Agents; Insulin; Lidocaine; Methacholine; Midodrine; RiTUXimab; Sulfonylureas

The levels/effects of Labelalol may be increased by: Acetylcholinesterase Inhibitors; Aminoquinolines (Antimalarial); Amiodarone; Anilidopiperidine Opioids; Antipsychotic Agents (Phenothiazines); Calcium Channel Blockers (Nondihydropyridine); Diazoxide; Dipyridamole; Disopyramide; Dronedarone; Herbs (Hypotensive Properties); MAO Inhibitors; Pentoxifylline; Phosphodiesterase 5 Inhibitors; Propafenone; Propoxyphene; Prostacyclin Analogues; QuiNIDine; Reserpine; Selective Serotonin Reuptake Inhibitors

Decreased Effect

Labelalol may decrease the levels/effects of: Beta2-Agonists; Theophylline Derivatives

The levels/effects of Labelalol may be decreased by: Barbiturates; Herbs (Hypertensive Properties); Methylphenidate; Nonsteroidal Anti-Inflammatory Agents; Rifamycin Derivatives; Yohimbine

Ethanol/Nutrition/Herb Interactions

Food: Labelalol serum concentrations may be increased if taken with food.
Herb/Nutraceutical: Avoid dong quai if using for hypertension (has estrogenic activity). Avoid ephedra, yohimbe, ginseng (may worsen hypertension). Avoid natural licorice (causes sodium and water retention and increases potassium loss). Avoid garlic (may have increased antihypertensive effect).

Test Interactions False-positive urine catecholamines, vanillylmandelic acid (VMA) if measured by fluorometric or photometric methods; use HPLC or specific catecholamine radioenzymatic technique; false-positive amphetamine if measured by thin-layer chromatography or radioenzymatic assay (gas chromatographic-mass spectrometer technique should be used)

Dosage Forms Excipient information presented when available (limited, particularly for generics); consult specific product labeling.
Injection, solution, as hydrochloride: 5 mg/mL (4 mL, 8 mL, 20 mL, 40 mL)
Trandate®: 5 mg/mL (20 mL, 40 mL) [contains edetate disodium]

Tablet, as hydrochloride: 100 mg, 200 mg, 300 mg
  Trandate®: 100 mg, 200 mg [contains sodium benzoate], 300 mg

References
Erstad BL and Barletta JF, "Treatment of Hypertension in the Perioperative Patient," *Ann Pharmacother*, 2000, 34(1):66-79.
Mokhlesi B, Leikin JB, Murray P, et al, "Adult Toxicology in Critical Care. Part 11: Specific Poisonings," *Chest*, 2003, 123(3):897-922.

◆ **Labetalol Hydrochloride** *see* Labetalol *on page 791*

◆ **Labetalol Hydrochloride Injection, USP (Can)** *see* Labetalol *on page 791*

Lacosamide (la KOE sa mide)

U.S. Brand Names Vimpat®
Index Terms ADD 234037; Harkoseride; LCM; SPM 927
Pharmacologic Category Anticonvulsant, Miscellaneous
Restrictions
  C-V
Use Adjunctive therapy in the treatment of partial-onset seizures
Pharmacodynamics/Kinetics
  Absorption: Oral: Completely
  Distribution: V_d: ~0.6 L/kg
  Protein binding: <15%
  Metabolism: Hepatic; forms metabolite, O-desmethyl-lacosamide (inactive)
  Bioavailability: ~100%
  Half-life elimination: 13 hours
  Time to peak, plasma: Oral: 1-4 hours postdose
  Excretion: Urine (95%; 40% as unchanged drug, 30% as inactive metabolite, 20% as uncharacterized metabolite); feces (<0.5%)
Dosage Oral, I.V.: Adolescents ≥17 years and Adults: Partial onset seizure:
  Initial: 50 mg twice daily; may be increased at weekly intervals by 100 mg/day
  Maintenance dose: 200-400 mg/day
  Note: When switching from oral to I.V. formulations, the total daily dose and frequency should be the same; I.V. therapy should only be used temporarily.

  Dosing adjustment in renal impairment:
    Mild-to-moderate renal impairment: No dose adjustment necessary
    Severe renal impairment (Cl_{cr} ≤30 mL/minute): Maximum dose: 300 mg/day
    Hemodialysis: Removed by hemodialysis; after 4-hour HD treatment, a supplemental dose of up to 50% should be considered.
  Dosing adjustment in hepatic impairment:
    Mild-to-moderate hepatic impairment: Maximum dose: 300 mg/day
    Severe hepatic impairment: Use is not recommended
Additional Information Complete prescribing information for this medication should be consulted for additional detail.
Dosage Forms Excipient information presented when available (limited, particularly for generics); consult specific product labeling.
  Injection, solution:
    Vimpat®: 10 mg/mL (20 mL)
  Tablet:
    Vimpat®: 50 mg, 100 mg, 150 mg, 200 mg
References
Ben-Menachem E, Biton V, Jatuzis D, et al, "Efficacy and Safety of Oral Lacosamide as Adjunctive Therapy in Adults With Partial-Onset Seizures," *Epilepsia*, 2007, 48(7):1308-17.
Beyreuther BK, Freitag J, Heers C, et al, "Lacosamide: A Review of Preclinical Properties," *CNS Drug Rev*, 2007, 13(1):21-42.
Biton V, Rosenfeld WE, Whitesides J, et al, "Intravenous Lacosamide as Replacement for Oral Lacosamide in Patients With Partial-Onset Seizures," *Epilepsia*, 2008, 49(3):418-24.
Doty P, Rudd GD, Stoehr T, et al, "Lacosamide," *Neurotherapeutics*, 2007, 4(1):145-8.

◆ **LaCrosse Complete [OTC]** *see* Sodium Phosphates *on page 1309*

Lactulose (LAK tyoo lose)

Medication Safety Issues
Sound-alike/look-alike issues:
Lactulose may be confused with lactose

Related Information
Laxatives, Classification and Properties *on page 1683*

U.S. Brand Names Constulose; Enulose; Generlac; Kristalose®

Canadian Brand Names Acilac; Apo-Lactulose®; Laxilose; PMS-Lactulose

Pharmacologic Category Ammonium Detoxicant; Laxative, Osmotic

Generic Available Yes

Use Adjunct in the prevention and treatment of portal-systemic encephalopathy; treatment of chronic constipation

Mechanism of Action The bacterial degradation of lactulose resulting in an acidic pH inhibits the diffusion of NH_3 into the blood by causing the conversion of NH_3 to NH_4+; also enhances the diffusion of NH_3 from the blood into the gut where conversion to NH_4+ occurs; produces an osmotic effect in the colon with resultant distention promoting peristalsis

Pharmacodynamics/Kinetics
Absorption: Not appreciable

Metabolism: Via colonic flora to lactic acid and acetic acid; requires colonic flora for drug activation

Excretion: Primarily feces and urine (~3%)

Dosage Diarrhea may indicate overdosage and responds to dose reduction
Prevention of portal systemic encephalopathy (PSE): Oral:
Infants: 2.5-10 mL/day divided 3-4 times/day; adjust dosage to produce 2-3 stools/day
Older Children: Daily dose of 40-90 mL divided 3-4 times/day; if initial dose causes diarrhea, then reduce it immediately; adjust dosage to produce 2-3 stools/day

Constipation: Oral:
Children: 5 g/day (7.5 mL) after breakfast
Adults: 15-30 mL/day increased to 60 mL/day in 1-2 divided doses if necessary
Acute PSE: Adults:
Oral: 20-30 g (30-45 mL) every 1-2 hours to induce rapid laxation; adjust dosage daily to produce 2-3 soft stools; doses of 30-45 mL may be given hourly to cause rapid laxation, then reduce to recommended dose; usual daily dose: 60-100 g (90-150 mL) daily
Rectal administration: 200 g (300 mL) diluted with 700 mL of H_2O or NS; administer rectally via rectal balloon catheter and retain 30-60 minutes every 4-6 hours

Stability Keep solution at room temperature to reduce viscosity. Discard solution if cloudy or very dark.

Administration Dilute lactulose in water, usually 60-120 mL, prior to administering through a gastric or feeding tube. Syrup formulation has been used in preparation of rectal solution.

Monitoring Parameters Blood pressure, standing/supine; serum potassium, bowel movement patterns, fluid status, serum ammonia

Pregnancy Risk Factor B

Contraindications Hypersensitivity to lactulose or any component of the formulation; galactosemia (or patients requiring a low galactose diet)

Warnings/Precautions Use with caution in patients with diabetes mellitus; solution contains galactose and lactose; monitor periodically for electrolyte imbalance when lactulose is used >6 months or in patients predisposed to electrolyte abnormalities (eg, elderly); patients receiving lactulose and an oral anti-infective agent should be monitored for possible inadequate response to lactulose

Adverse Reactions Frequency not defined: Gastrointestinal: Abdominal discomfort, cramping, diarrhea (excessive dose), flatulence, nausea, vomiting

Drug Interactions
Avoid Concomitant Use There are no known interactions where it is recommended to avoid concomitant use.

Increased Effect/Toxicity There are no known significant interactions involving an increase in effect.

Decreased Effect There are no known significant interactions involving a decrease in effect.

Dietary Considerations Contraindicated in patients on galactose-restricted diet; may be mixed with fruit juice, milk, water, or citrus-flavored carbonated beverages.

Dosage Forms Excipient information presented when available (limited, particularly for generics); consult specific product labeling.

Crystals for solution, oral:

Kristalose®: 10 g/packet (30s), 20 g/packet (30s)

Solution, oral: 10 g/15 mL (15 mL, 30 mL, 237 mL, 473 mL, 946 mL, 1890 mL)

Constulose: 10 g/15 mL (240 mL, 960 mL)

Enulose: 10 g/15 mL (480 mL)

Generlac: 10 g/15 mL (480 mL, 1920 mL)

Solution, oral/rectal: 10 g/15 mL (237 mL, 473 mL, 946 mL)

◆ **L-AmB** see Amphotericin B (Liposomal) on page 110

◆ **Lamictal®** see LamoTRIgine on page 800

◆ **Lamictal® ODT™** see LamoTRIgine on page 800

◆ **Lamictal® XR™** see LamoTRIgine on page 800

LamiVUDine (la MI vyoo deen)

Medication Safety Issues

Sound-alike/look-alike issues:

LamiVUDine may be confused with lamoTRIgine

Epivir® may be confused with Combivir®

U.S. Brand Names Epivir-HBV®; Epivir®

Canadian Brand Names 3TC®; Heptovir®

Index Terms 3TC

Pharmacologic Category Antiretroviral Agent, Reverse Transcriptase Inhibitor (Nucleoside)

Generic Available No

Use

Epivir®: Treatment of HIV infection when antiretroviral therapy is warranted; should always be used as part of a multidrug regimen (at least three antiretroviral agents)

Epivir-HBV®: Treatment of chronic hepatitis B associated with evidence of hepatitis B viral replication and active liver inflammation

Unlabeled/Investigational Use Postexposure prophylaxis for HIV exposure as part of a multidrug regimen

Mechanism of Action Lamivudine is a cytosine analog. After lamivudine is triphosphorylated, the principle mode of action is inhibition of HIV reverse transcription via viral DNA chain termination; inhibits RNA- and DNA-dependent DNA polymerase activities of reverse transcriptase. The monophosphate form of lamivudine is incorporated into the viral DNA by hepatitis B virus polymerase, resulting in DNA chain termination.

Pharmacodynamics/Kinetics

Absorption: Rapid

Distribution: V_d: 1.3 L/kg

Protein binding, plasma: <36%

Metabolism: 4.2% to trans-sulfoxide metabolite

Bioavailability: Absolute; Cp_{max} decreased with food although AUC not significantly affected

Children: 66%

Adults: 86% to 87%

Half-life elimination: Children: 2 hours; Adults: 5-7 hours

Time to peak, plasma: Fed: 3.2 hours; Fasted: 0.9 hours

Excretion: Primarily urine (as unchanged drug)

Dosage Oral: **Note:** The formulation and dosage of Epivir-HBV® are not appropriate for patients infected with both HBV and HIV. Use with at least two other antiretroviral agents when treating HIV.

HIV:

Neonates <30 days (AIDS*info* guidelines): 2 mg/kg/dose twice daily

Infants 1-3 months (AIDS*info* guidelines): 4 mg/kg/dose twice daily

Infants and Children 3 months to 16 years: 4 mg/kg/dose twice daily (maximum: 150 mg/dose twice daily)

Alternate weight-based dosing using scored 150 mg tablets (AIDSinfo guidelines):

14-21 kg: 75 mg/dose twice daily (150 mg/day)

22-29 kg: 75 mg in the morning, 150 mg in the evening (225 mg/day)

≥30 kg: 150 mg/dose twice daily (300 mg/day)

Adults: 150 mg twice daily or 300 mg once daily

<50 kg (AIDS*info* guidelines): 4 mg/kg/dose twice daily (maximum: 150 mg/dose twice daily)

Treatment of hepatitis B (Epivir-HBV®): Note: Usual treatment duration is at least 1 year and varies with HBeAg status, consult current guidelines and literature.

Children 2-17 years: 3 mg/kg/dose once daily (maximum: 100 mg/day)

Adults: 100 mg/day

Postexposure prophylaxis for HIV exposure (unlabeled use): Adolescents and Adults: 150 mg twice daily (with zidovudine with or without a protease inhibitor, depending on risk)

Prevention of maternal-fetal HIV transmission (AIDSinfo guidelines): Note: Lamivudine may be used in combination with zidovudine and nevirapine in select situations (eg, infants born to mothers with suboptimal viral suppression at delivery, infants born to mothers with only intrapartum therapy or no therapy, or infants born to mothers with known antiretroviral drug-resistant virus). Lamivudine is used in this situation to reduce the development of nevirapine resistant virus:

Mother: 150 mg twice daily starting at onset of labor and continuing through 1 week postpartum

Neonate: 2 mg/kg/dose twice daily given at birth through 1 week of age

Dosing adjustment in renal impairment: HIV:

Patients ≤16 years: Insufficient data; however, dose reduction should be considered.

Patients >16 years:

Cl_{cr} 30-49 mL/minute: Administer 150 mg once daily

Cl_{cr} 15-29 mL/minute: Administer 150 mg first dose, then 100 mg once daily

Cl_{cr} 5-14 mL/minute: Administer 150 mg first dose, then 50 mg once daily

Cl_{cr} <5 mL/minute: Administer 50 mg first dose, then 25 mg once daily

Dosing adjustment in renal impairment: Hepatitis B: Adults:

Cl_{cr} 30-49: Administer 100 mg first dose then 50 mg once daily

Cl_{cr} 15-29: Administer 100 mg first dose then 25 mg once daily

Cl_{cr} 5-14: Administer 35 mg first dose then 15 mg once daily

Cl_{cr} <5: Administer 35 mg first dose then 10 mg once daily

Dialysis: Negligible amounts are removed by 4-hour hemodialysis or peritoneal dialysis. Supplemental dosing is not required.

Stability

Oral solution:

Epivir®: Store at 25°C (77°F) tightly closed.

Epivir-HBV®: Store at 20°C to 25°C (68°F to 77°F) tightly closed.

Tablet: Store at 25°C (77°F); excursions permitted to 15°C to 30°C (59°F to 86°F).

Administration May be administered without regard to meals. Adjust dosage in renal failure.

Monitoring Parameters Amylase, bilirubin, liver enzymes, hematologic parameters, viral load, and CD4 count; signs and symptoms of pancreatitis

Pregnancy Risk Factor C

Contraindications Hypersensitivity to lamivudine or any component of the formulation

Warnings/Precautions Use caution with renal impairment; dosage reduction recommended. Use with extreme caution in children with history of pancreatitis or risk factors for development of pancreatitis. Pancreatitis has been reported, particularly in HIV-infected children with a history of nucleoside use. Do not use as monotherapy in treatment of HIV. Treatment of HBV in patients with unrecognized/untreated HIV may lead to rapid HIV resistance. In addition, treatment of HIV in patients with unrecognized/untreated HBV may lead to rapid HBV resistance. Use with caution in combination with interferon alfa with or without ribavirin in HIV/HBV coinfected patients; monitor closely for hepatic decompensation, anemia, or neutropenia; dose reduction or discontinuation of interferon and/or ribavirin may be required if toxicity evident. **[U.S. Boxed Warning]: Do not use Epivir-HBV® tablets or Epivir-HBV® oral solution for the treatment of HIV.**

[U.S. Boxed Warning]: Lactic acidosis and severe hepatomegaly with steatosis have been reported, including fatal cases. Use caution in hepatic impairment. Pregnancy, obesity, and/or prolonged therapy may increase the risk of lactic acidosis and liver damage.

Immune reconstitution syndrome may develop resulting in the occurrence of an inflammatory response to an indolent or residual opportunistic infection. May be associated with fat redistribution.

[U.S. Boxed Warning]: Monitor patients closely for several months following discontinuation of therapy for chronic hepatitis B; clinical exacerbations may occur.

Adverse Reactions Reported for treatment of HIV or HBV in adults. Incidence data includes patients on combination therapy with other antiretroviral agents.
>10%:
   Central nervous system: Headache (21% to 35%), fatigue (24% to 27%), insomnia (11%)
   Gastrointestinal: Nausea (15% to 33%), diarrhea (14% to 18%), pancreatitis (range: 0.3% to 18%; higher percentage in pediatric patients), abdominal pain (9% to 16%), vomiting (13% to 15%)
   Hematologic: Neutropenia (7% to 15%)
   Hepatic: Transaminases increased (2% to 11%)
   Neuromuscular & skeletal: Myalgia (8% to 14%), neuropathy (12%), musculoskeletal pain (12%)
   Respiratory: Nasal signs and symptoms (20%), cough (18%), sore throat (13%)
   Miscellaneous: Infections (25%; includes ear, nose, and throat)
1% to 10%:
   Central nervous system: Dizziness (10%), depression (9%), fever (7% to 10%), chills (7% to 10%)
   Dermatologic: Rash (5% to 9%)
   Gastrointestinal: Anorexia (10%), lipase increased (10%), abdominal cramps (6%), dyspepsia (5%), amylase increased (<1% to 4%), heartburn
   Hematologic: Thrombocytopenia (1% to 4%), hemoglobinemia (2% to 3%)
   Neuromuscular & skeletal: Creatine phosphokinase increased (9%), arthralgia (5% to 7%)
<1% (Limited to important or life-threatening): Alopecia, anaphylaxis, anemia, body fat redistribution, hepatitis B exacerbation, hepatomegaly, hyperbilirubinemia, hyperglycemia, immune reconstitution syndrome, lactic acidosis, lymphadenopathy, muscle weakness, paresthesia, peripheral neuropathy, pruritus, red cell aplasia, rhabdomyolysis, splenomegaly, steatosis, stomatitis, urticaria, weakness, wheezing

Drug Interactions
Avoid Concomitant Use
   Avoid concomitant use of LamiVUDine with any of the following: Emtricitabine
Increased Effect/Toxicity
   LamiVUDine may increase the levels/effects of: Emtricitabine

   The levels/effects of LamiVUDine may be increased by: Ganciclovir-Valganciclovir; Ribavirin; Trimethoprim
Decreased Effect
   LamiVUDine may decrease the levels/effects of: Zalcitabine

◄ **Ethanol/Nutrition/Herb Interactions** Food: Food decreases the rate of absorption and C_{max}; however, there is no change in the systemic AUC. Therefore, may be taken with or without food.

Dietary Considerations May be taken without regard to meals. Some products may contain sucrose.

Dosage Forms Excipient information presented when available (limited, particularly for generics); consult specific product labeling.

Solution, oral:

Epivir®: 10 mg/mL (240 mL) [strawberry-banana flavor]

Epivir-HBV®: 5 mg/mL (240 mL) [strawberry-banana flavor]

Tablet:

Epivir®: 150 mg [scored], 300 mg

Epivir-HBV®: 100 mg

References

CDC and the National Foundation for Infectious Disease, "Update: Provisional Public Health Service Recommendations for Chemoprophylaxis After Occupational Exposure to HIV," *MMWR*, 1996, 45 (22):468-80.

Huang L, Quartin A, Jones D, et al, "Intensive Care of Patients With HIV Infection," *N Engl J Med*, 2006, 355(2):173-81.

LamoTRIgine (la MOE tri jeen)

Related Information

Chronic Pain Management *on page 1546*

Perioperative Management of Patients on Antiseizure Medication *on page 1577*

U.S. Brand Names Lamictal®; Lamictal® ODT™; Lamictal® XR™

Canadian Brand Names Apo-Lamotrigine®; Lamictal®; Mylan-Lamotrigine; Novo-Lamotrigine; PMS-Lamotrigine; ratio-Lamotrigine

Index Terms BW-430C; LTG

Pharmacologic Category Anticonvulsant, Miscellaneous

Use Adjunctive therapy in the treatment of generalized seizures of Lennox-Gastaut syndrome, primary generalized tonic-clonic seizures, and partial seizures in adults and children ≥2 years of age; conversion to monotherapy in adults (≥16 years of age) with partial seizures who are receiving treatment with valproic acid or a single enzyme-inducing antiepileptic drug (specifically carbamazepine, phenytoin, phenobarbital or primidone); maintenance treatment of bipolar I disorder in adults

Pharmacodynamics/Kinetics

Absorption: Immediate release: Rapid and complete

Distribution: V_d: 0.9-1.3 L/kg

Protein binding: ~55%

Metabolism: Hepatic and renal; metabolized primarily by glucuronic acid conjugation to inactive metabolites

Bioavailability: Immediate release: 98%; Extended release: ~77%

Half-life elimination: Immediate release: Adults: 25-33 hours, Elderly: 25-43 hours; Extended release: Similar to immediate release

Concomitant valproic acid therapy: 48-70 hours

Concomitant phenytoin, phenobarbital, primidone, or carbamazepine therapy: 13-14 hours

Chronic renal failure: 43 hours

Hemodialysis: 13 hours during dialysis; 57 hours between dialysis (~20% of a dose is eliminated in a 4-hour dialysis session)

Hepatic impairment:

Mild: 26-66 hours

Moderate: 28-116 hours

Severe without ascites: 56-78 hours

Severe with ascites: 52-148 hours

Time to peak, plasma: Immediate release: 1-1.5 hours; Extended release: 4-11 hours (dependent on adjunct therapy)

Excretion: Urine (94%, ~90% as glucuronide conjugates and ~10% unchanged); feces (2%)

Dosage Note: Only whole tablets should be used for dosing, round calculated dose down to the nearest whole tablet. Extended release formulation not approved for children ≤12 years of age. Enzyme-inducing regimens specifically refer to those containing carbamazepine, phenytoin, phenobarbital, or primidone. Oral:

Children 2-12 years: Lennox-Gastaut (adjunctive), primary generalized tonic-clonic seizures (adjunctive), or partial seizures (adjunctive): **Note:** Children <30 kg will likely require maintenance doses to be increased as much as 50% based on clinical response regardless of regimen below:

Immediate release formulations: Initial: 0.3 mg/kg/day in 1-2 divided doses for weeks 1 and 2, then increase to 0.6 mg/kg/day in 2 divided doses for weeks 3 and 4. Maintenance: Titrate dose to effect; after week 4, increase daily dose every 1-2 weeks by 0.6 mg/kg/day; usual maintenance: 4.5-7.5 mg/kg/day in 2 divided doses; maximum: 300 mg/day in 2 divided doses

Adjustment for AED regimens **containing** valproic acid (see **"Note"** below): Immediate release formulations: Initial: 0.15 mg/kg/day in 1-2 divided doses for weeks 1 and 2, then increase to 0.3 mg/kg/day in 1-2 divided doses for weeks 3 and 4. Maintenance: Titrate dose to effect; after week 4, increase daily dose every 1-2 weeks by 0.3 mg/kg/day; usual maintenance: 1-5 mg/kg/day in 2 divided doses; maximum: 200 mg/day in 1-2 divided doses

Note: For patients >6.7 kg and <14 kg, initial dosing should be 2 mg every other day for first 2 weeks, then increased to 2 mg daily for weeks 3-4. For patients taking lamotrigine with valproic acid alone, the usual maintenance dose is 1-3 mg/kg/day in 2 divided doses

Adjustment for **enzyme-inducing** AED regimens **without** valproic acid: Immediate release formulations: Initial: 0.6 mg/kg/day in 2 divided doses for weeks 1 and 2, then increase to 1.2 mg/kg/day in 2 divided doses for weeks 3 and 4. Maintenance: Titrate dose to effect; after week 4, increase daily dose every 1-2 weeks by 1.2 mg/kg/day; usual maintenance: 5-15 mg/kg/day in 2 divided doses; maximum: 400 mg/day in 2 divided doses

Children >12 years: Lennox-Gastaut (adjunctive), primary generalized tonic-clonic seizures (adjunctive), or partial seizures (adjunctive): Refer to adult dosing.

Children ≥16 years: Conversion from adjunctive therapy with valproic acid or a single enzyme-inducing AED regimen to monotherapy with lamotrigine: Refer to adult dosing.

Adults:

Lennox-Gastaut (adjunctive), primary generalized tonic-clonic seizures (adjunctive) or partial seizures (adjunctive): Immediate release formulations: Initial: 25 mg/day for weeks 1 and 2, then increase to 50 mg/day for weeks 3 and 4. Maintenance: Titrate dose to effect; after week 4 increase daily dose every 1-2 weeks by 50 mg/day; usual maintenance: 225-375 mg/day in 2 divided doses

Adjustment for AED regimens **containing** valproic acid (see **"Note"** below): Initial: 25 mg every other day for weeks 1 and 2, then increase to 25 mg every day for weeks 3 and 4. Maintenance: Titrate dose to effect; after week 4 increase daily dose every 1-2 weeks by 25-50 mg/day; usual maintenance: 100-400 mg/day in 1 or 2 divided doses

Note: For patients taking lamotrigine with valproic acid alone, the usual maintenance dose is 100-200 mg/day

Adjustment for **enzyme-inducing** AED regimens **without** valproic acid: Initial: 50 mg/day for weeks 1 and 2, then increase to 100 mg/day in 2 divided doses for weeks 3 and 4. Maintenance: titrate dose to effect; after week 4 increase daily dose every 1-2 weeks by 100 mg/day; usual maintenance: 300-500 mg/day in 2 divided doses. Doses as high as 700 mg/day have been used, though additional benefit has not been established.

Conversion to monotherapy with lamotrigine:

Conversion from adjunctive therapy with valproic acid: Initiate and titrate as per recommendations to a lamotrigine dose of 200 mg/day. Then taper valproic acid dose in decrements of not >500 mg/day at intervals of 1 week (or longer) to a valproic acid dosage of 500 mg/day; this dosage should be maintained for 1 week. The lamotrigine dosage should then be increased to 300 mg/day while valproic acid is decreased to 250 mg/day; this dosage should be maintained for 1 week. Valproic acid may then be discontinued, ▶

while the lamotrigine dose is increased by 100 mg/day at weekly intervals to achieve a lamotrigine maintenance dose of 500 mg/day.

Conversion from adjunctive therapy with carbamazepine, phenytoin, phenobarbital, or primidone: Initiate and titrate as per recommendations to a lamotrigine dose of 500 mg/day. Concomitant enzyme-inducing AED should then be withdrawn by 20% decrements each week over a 4-week period. Patients should be monitored for rash.

Conversion from adjunctive therapy with AED other than carbamazepine, phenytoin, phenobarbital, primidone or valproic acid: No specific guidelines available

Partial seizures (adjunctive): Extended release formulation: **Note:** Dose increases after week 8 should not exceed 100 mg/day at weekly intervals

Regimens **containing** valproic acid: Initial: Week 1 and 2: 25 mg every other day; Week 3 and 4: 25 mg once daily; Week 5: 50 mg once daily; Week 6: 100 mg once daily; Week 7: 150 mg once daily; Maintenance: 200-250 mg once daily

Regimens **containing** carbamazepine, phenytoin, phenobarbital, or primidone and **without** valproic acid: Initial: Week 1 and 2: 50 mg once daily; Week 3 and 4: 100 mg once daily; Week 5: 200 mg once daily; Week 6: 300 mg once daily; Week 7: 400 mg once daily; Maintenance: 400-600 mg once daily

Regimens **not containing** carbamazepine, phenytoin, phenobarbital, primidone, or valproic acid: Initial: Week 1 and 2: 25 mg once daily; Week 3 and 4: 50 mg once daily; Week 5: 100 mg once daily; Week 6: 150 mg once daily; Week 7: 200 mg once daily; Maintenance: 300-400 mg once daily

Bipolar disorder:

Initial: 25 mg/day for weeks 1 and 2, then increase to 50 mg/day for weeks 3 and 4, then increase to 100 mg/day for week 5; maintenance: increase dose to 200 mg/day beginning week 6

Adjustment for regimens **containing** valproic acid: Initial: 25 mg every other day for weeks 1 and 2, then increase to 25 mg every day for weeks 3 and 4, then increase to 50 mg/day for week 5; maintenance: 100 mg/day beginning week 6

Adjustment for **enzyme-inducing** regimens **without** valproic acid: Initial: 50 mg/day for weeks 1 and 2, then increase to 100 mg/day in divided doses for weeks 3 and 4, then increase to 200 mg/day in divided doses for week 5, then increase to 300 mg/day in divided dose for week 6; maintenance: 400 mg/day in divided doses beginning week 7

Adjustment following discontinuation of psychotropic medication:

Discontinuing valproic acid with current dose of lamotrigine 100 mg/day: 150 mg/day for week 1, then increase to 200 mg/day beginning week 2

Discontinuing carbamazepine, phenytoin, phenobarbital, primidone, or rifampin with current dose of lamotrigine 400 mg/day: 400 mg/day for week 1, then decrease to 300 mg/day for week 2, then decrease to 200 mg/day beginning week 3

Conversion from immediate release to extended release (Lamictal® XR™): Initial dose of the extended release tablet should match the total daily dose of the immediate-release formulation; monitor for seizure control, especially in patients on AED agents. Adjust dose as needed within the recommended dosing guidelines.

Discontinuing therapy: Children and Adults: Decrease dose by ~50% per week, over at least 2 weeks unless safety concerns require a more rapid withdrawal. Discontinuing carbamazepine, phenytoin, phenobarbital, or primidone should prolong the half-life of lamotrigine; discontinuing valproic acid should shorten the half-life of lamotrigine

Restarting therapy after discontinuation: If lamotrigine has been withheld for >5 half-lives, consider restarting according to initial dosing recommendations.

Dosage adjustment with estrogen-containing hormonal contraceptives: Follow initial lamotrigine dosing guidelines, maintenance dose should be adjusted as follows:

Patients taking concomitant carbamazepine, phenytoin, phenobarbital, primidone or rifampin: No dosing adjustment required

Patients **not** taking concomitant carbamazepine, phenytoin, phenobarbital, primidone or rifampin: Lamotrigine maintenance dose may need increased by twofold over target dose. If already taking a stable dose of lamotrigine and starting contraceptive, maintenance dose may need increased by twofold. Dose increases should start when contraceptive is started and titrated to clinical response increasing no more rapidly than 50-100 mg/day every week. Gradual increases of lamotrigine plasma levels may occur during the inactive "pill-free" week and will be greater when dose increases are made the week before. If increased adverse events consistently occur during "pill-free" week, overall maintenance dose adjustments may be required. When discontinuing estrogen-containing hormonal contraceptive, dose of lamotrigine may need decreased by as much as 50%; do not decrease by more than 25% of total daily dose over a 2-week period unless clinical response or plasma levels indicate otherwise. Dose adjustments during "pill-free" week are not recommended.

Dosage adjustment in renal impairment: Decreased maintenance dosage may be effective in patients with significant renal impairment; has not been adequately studied; use with caution

Dosage adjustment in hepatic impairment:
Mild impairment: No adjustment required
Moderate-to-severe impairment without ascites: Decrease initial, escalation, and maintenance doses by ~25%; adjust as clinically indicated
Moderate-to-severe impairment with ascites: Decrease initial, escalation, and maintenance doses by ~50%; adjust according to clinical response

Additional Information Complete prescribing information for this medication should be consulted for additional detail.

Dosage Forms Excipient information presented when available (limited, particularly for generics); consult specific product labeling.
Tablet, oral: 25 mg, 100 mg, 150 mg, 200 mg
Lamictal®: 25 mg, 100 mg, 150 mg, 200 mg
Tablet, oral [combination package; each unit-dose starter kit contains]:
Lamictal® [blue kit; for patients taking valproic acid]:
25 mg (35s)
Lamictal® [green kit; for patients taking carbamazepine, phenytoin, phenobarbital, primidone, or rifampin and **not** taking valproic acid]:
25 mg (84s)
100 mg (14s)
Lamictal® [orange kit; for patients **not** taking carbamazepine, phenytoin, phenobarbital, primidone, rifampin, or valproic acid]:
25 mg (42s)
100 mg (7s)
Tablet, dispersible/chewable, oral: 5 mg, 25 mg
Lamictal®: 2 mg, 25 mg [black currant flavor]
Lamictal®: 5 mg [scored; black currant flavor]
Tablet, extended release, oral:
Lamictal® XR™: 25 mg, 50 mg, 100 mg, 200 mg
Tablet, extended release, oral [combination package; each patient titration kit contains]:
Lamictal® XR™ [blue XR kit; for patients taking valproic acid]:
25 mg (21s)
50 mg (7s)
Lamictal® XR™ [green XR kit; for patients taking carbamazepine, phenytoin, phenobarbital, or primidone and **not** taking valproic acid]:
50 mg (14s)
100 mg (14s)
200 mg (7s)
Lamictal® XR™ [orange XR kit; for patients **not** taking carbamazepine, phenytoin, phenobarbital, primidone, or valproic acid]:
25 mg (14s)
50 mg (14s)
100 mg (7s)
Tablet, orally disintegrating, oral:
Lamictal® ODT™: 25 mg, 50 mg, 100 mg, 200 mg [cherry flavor]

◀ Tablet, orally disintegrating, oral [combination package; each patient titration kit contains]:

Lamictal® ODT™ [blue ODT kit; for patients taking valproic acid; cherry flavor]:

25 mg (21s)

50 mg (7s)

Lamictal® ODT™ [green ODT kit; for patients taking carbamazepine, phenytoin, phenobarbital, primidone, or rifampin and **not** taking valproic acid; cherry flavor]:

50 mg (42s)

100 mg (14s)

Lamictal® ODT™ [orange ODT kit; for patients **not** taking carbamazepine, phenytoin, phenobarbital, primidone, rifampin, or valproic acid; cherry flavor]:

25 mg (14s)

50 mg (14s)

100 mg (7s)

◆ **Lanoxicaps® [DSC]** *see* Digoxin *on page 417*

◆ **Lanoxicaps® (Can)** *see* Digoxin *on page 417*

◆ **Lanoxin®** *see* Digoxin *on page 417*

Lanreotide (lan REE oh tide)

U.S. Brand Names Somatuline® Depot

Canadian Brand Names Somatuline® Autogel®

Index Terms Lanreotide Acetate

Pharmacologic Category Somatostatin Analog

Use Long-term treatment of acromegaly in patients who are not candidates for or are unresponsive to surgery and/or radiotherapy

Canadian labeling: Also approved in Canada for relief of symptoms of acromegaly

Pharmacodynamics/Kinetics

Distribution: V_{ss}: ~0.2 L/kg

Protein binding: 79% to 83%

Metabolism: Extensively within GI tract after biliary excretion

Bioavailability: 69% to 83%

Half-life, elimination: 23-36 days

Time to peak, plasma: Mean: 7-12 hours

Excretion: Urine (<1% to 5% as unchanged drug); feces (<0.5% as unchanged drug)

Dosage SubQ: **Note: Differences in U.S. and Canadian labeled dosing:**

U.S. labeling: Adults: Acromegaly: 90 mg once every 4 weeks for 3 months; after initial 90 days of therapy, adjust dose based on clinical response of patient, growth hormone (GH) levels, and/or insulin-like growth factor 1 (IGF-1) levels as follows:

GH ≤1 ng/mL, IGF-1 normal, symptoms stable:60 mg once every 4 weeks

GH >1-2.5 ng/mL, IGF-1 normal, symptoms stable: 90 mg once every 4 weeks

GH >2.5 ng/mL, IGF-1 elevated and/or uncontrolled symptoms: 120 mg once every 4 weeks

Canadian labeling: Children ≥16 years and Adults: Acromegaly: 90 mg once every 4 weeks for 3 months; after initial 90 days of therapy, adjust dose based on clinical response of patient, growth hormone (GH) levels, and/or insulin-like growth factor 1 (IGF-1) levels as follows:

GH = 1 ng/mL, IGF-1 normal, symptoms stable: 60 mg once every 4 weeks

GH >1-2.5 ng/mL, IGF-1 normal, symptoms stable: 90 mg once every 4 weeks

GH >2.5 ng/mL, IGF-1 elevated and/or uncontrolled symptoms: 120 mg once every 4 weeks

Dosing adjustment in renal impairment:

U.S. labeling: Moderate-to-severe impairment: Recommended starting dose: 60 mg

Canadian labeling: No adjustment is necessary

Dosing adjustment in hepatic impairment:
  U.S. labeling: Moderate-to-severe impairment: Recommended starting dose: 60 mg
  Canadian labeling: No adjustment is necessary
Additional Information Complete prescribing information for this medication should be consulted for additional detail.
Dosage Forms Excipient information presented when available (limited, particularly for generics); consult specific product labeling. [CAN] = Canadian brand name
Injection, solution:
  Somatuline® Autogel® [CAN]: 60 mg/ 0.3 mL (0.3 mL); 90 mg/ 0.3 mL (0.3 mL); 120 mg/0.5 mL (0.5 mL) [packaging contains natural rubber/natural latex]
  Somatuline® Depot: 60 mg/~0.4 mL (~0.4 mL); 90 mg/~0.4 mL (~0.4 mL); 120 mg/~0.5 mL (~0.5 mL) [packaging contains natural rubber/natural latex]

References
Caron P, Beckers A, Cullen DR, et al, "Efficacy of the New Long-Acting Formulation of Lanreotide (Lanreotide Autogel) in the Management of Acromegaly," *J Clin Endocrinol Metab*, 2002, 87 (1):99-104.

Rasmussen E, Eriksson B, Oberg K, et al, "Selective Effects of Somatostatin Analogs on Human Drug-Metabolizing Enzymes," *Clin Pharmacol Ther*, 1998, 64(2):150-9.

Reubi JC, Waser B, Schaer JC, et al, "Somatostatin Receptor sst1-sst5 Expression in Normal and Neoplastic Human Tissues Using Receptor Autoradiography With Subtype-Selective Ligands," *Eur J Nucl Med*, 2001, 28(7):836-46.

◆ **Lanreotide Acetate** *see* Lanreotide *on page 804*

Lansoprazole (lan SOE pra zole)

Medication Safety Issues
  Sound-alike/look-alike issues:
    Lansoprazole may be confused with aripiprazole, dexlansoprazole
    Prevacid® may be confused with Pravachol®, Prevpac®, Prilosec®, Prinivil®
Related Information
  Helicobacter pylori Treatment *on page 1746*
U.S. Brand Names Prevacid®; Prevacid® SoluTab™
Canadian Brand Names Apo-Lansoprazole®; Prevacid®
Pharmacologic Category Proton Pump Inhibitor; Substituted Benzimidazole
Generic Available No
Use Short-term treatment of active duodenal ulcers; maintenance treatment of healed duodenal ulcers; as part of a multidrug regimen for *H. pylori* eradication to reduce the risk of duodenal ulcer recurrence; short-term treatment of active benign gastric ulcer; treatment of NSAID-associated gastric ulcer; to reduce the risk of NSAID-associated gastric ulcer in patients with a history of gastric ulcer who require an NSAID; short-term treatment of symptomatic GERD; short-term treatment for all grades of erosive esophagitis; to maintain healing of erosive esophagitis; long-term treatment of pathological hypersecretory conditions, including Zollinger-Ellison syndrome
Mechanism of Action Decreases acid secretion in gastric parietal cells through inhibition of (H+, K+)-ATPase enzyme system, blocking the final step in gastric acid production.
Pharmacodynamics/Kinetics
  Duration: >1 day
  Absorption: Rapid
  Distribution: V_d: 14-18 L
  Protein binding: 97%
  Metabolism: Hepatic via CYP2C19 and 3A4, and in parietal cells to two active metabolites that are not present in systemic circulation
  Bioavailability: 80%; decreased 50% to 70% if given 30 minutes after food
  Half-life elimination: 1-2 hours; Elderly: 2-3 hours; Hepatic impairment: ≤7 hours
  Time to peak, plasma: 1.7 hours
  Excretion: Feces (67%); urine (33%)
Dosage Oral:
  Children 1-11 years: GERD, erosive esophagitis:
    ≤30 kg: 15 mg once daily
    >30 kg: 30 mg once daily

Note: Doses were increased in some pediatric patients if still symptomatic after 2 or more weeks of treatment (maximum dose: 30 mg twice daily)

Children 12-17 years:

Nonerosive GERD: 15 mg once daily for up to 8 weeks

Erosive esophagitis: 30 mg once daily for up to 8 weeks

Adults:

Duodenal ulcer: Short-term treatment: 15 mg once daily for 4 weeks; maintenance therapy: 15 mg once daily

Gastric ulcer: Short-term treatment: 30 mg once daily for up to 8 weeks

NSAID-associated gastric ulcer (healing): 30 mg once daily for 8 weeks; controlled studies did not extend past 8 weeks of therapy

NSAID-associated gastric ulcer (to reduce risk): 15 mg once daily for up to 12 weeks; controlled studies did not extend past 12 weeks of therapy

Symptomatic GERD: Short-term treatment: 15 mg once daily for up to 8 weeks

Erosive esophagitis: Short-term treatment: 30 mg once daily for up to 8 weeks; continued treatment for an additional 8 weeks may be considered for recurrence or for patients who do not heal after the first 8 weeks of therapy; maintenance therapy: 15 mg once daily

Hypersecretory conditions: Initial: 60 mg once daily; adjust dose based upon patient response and to reduce acid secretion to <10 mEq/hour (5 mEq/hour in patients with prior gastric surgery); doses of 90 mg twice daily have been used; administer doses >120 mg/day in divided doses

Helicobacter pylori eradication:

Manufacturer labeling: 30 mg 3 times/day administered with amoxicillin 1000 mg 3 times/day for 14 days **or** 30 mg twice daily administered with amoxicillin 1000 mg *and* clarithromycin 500 mg twice daily for 10-14 days

American College of Gastroenterology guidelines (Chey, 2007):

Nonpenicillin allergy: 30 mg twice daily administered with amoxicillin 1000 mg *and* clarithromycin 500 mg twice daily for 10-14 days

Penicillin allergy: 30 mg twice daily administered with clarithromycin 500 mg *and* metronidazole 500 mg twice daily for 10-14 days **or** 30 mg once or twice daily administered with bismuth subsalicylate 525 mg *and* metronidazole 250 mg *plus* tetracycline 500 mg 4 times/day for 10-14 days

Elderly: No dosage adjustment is needed in elderly patients with normal hepatic function

Dosage adjustment in renal impairment: No dosage adjustment is needed

Dosing adjustment in hepatic impairment: Dose reduction is necessary for severe hepatic impairment

Stability Store at 25°C (77°F); excursions permitted to 15°C to 30°C (59°F to 86°F).

Administration

Oral: Administer before food; best if taken before breakfast. The intact granules should not be chewed or crushed; however, several options are available for those patients unable to swallow capsules:

Capsules may be opened and the intact granules sprinkled on 1 tablespoon of applesauce, Ensure® pudding, cottage cheese, yogurt, or strained pears. The granules should then be swallowed immediately.

Capsules may be opened and emptied into ~60 mL orange juice, apple juice, or tomato juice; mix and swallow immediately. Rinse the glass with additional juice and swallow to assure complete delivery of the dose.

Orally-disintegrating tablets: Should not be swallowed whole or chewed. Place tablet on tongue; allow to dissolve (with or without water) until particles can be swallowed. Orally-disintegrating tablets may also be administered via an oral syringe: Place the 15 mg tablet in an oral syringe and draw up ~4 mL water, or place the 30 mg tablet in an oral syringe and draw up ~10 mL water. After tablet has dispersed, administer within 15 minutes. Refill the syringe with water (2 mL for the 15 mg tablet; 4 mL for the 30 mg tablet), shake gently, then administer any remaining contents.

Nasogastric tube administration:

Capsule: Capsule can be opened, the granules mixed (not crushed) with 40 mL of apple juice and then injected through the NG tube into the stomach, then flush tube with additional apple juice. Do not mix with other liquids.

Orally-disintegrating tablet: Nasogastric tube ≥8 French: Place a 15 mg tablet in a syringe and draw up ~4 mL water, or place the 30 mg tablet in a syringe and draw up ~10 mL water. After tablet has dispersed, administer within 15 minutes. Refill the syringe with ~5 mL water, shake gently, and then flush the nasogastric tube.

Monitoring Parameters Patients with Zollinger-Ellison syndrome should be monitored for gastric acid output, which should be maintained at ≤10 mEq/hour during the last hour before the next lansoprazole dose; lab monitoring should include CBC, liver function, renal function, and serum gastrin levels

Anesthesia and Critical Care Concerns/Other Considerations
Evidence-Based Information:

Stress ulcer prophylaxis: The 2008 Surviving Sepsis Campaign guidelines recommend that stress ulcer prophylaxis using an H_2 blocker (Grade 1A) or proton pump inhibitor (Grade 1B) be given to patients with severe sepsis to prevent upper GI bleed. Benefit of prevention of upper GI bleed must be weighed against potential effect of increased stomach pH on development of ventilator-associated pneumonia.

Pregnancy Risk Factor B

Contraindications Hypersensitivity to lansoprazole, substituted benzimidazoles (ie, esomeprazole, omeprazole, pantoprazole, rabeprazole), or any component of the formulation

Warnings/Precautions Use of proton pump inhibitors may increase the risk of gastrointestinal infections (eg, *Salmonella, Campylobacter*). Relief of symptoms does not preclude the presence of a gastric malignancy. Atrophic gastritis (by biopsy) has been noted with long-term omeprazole therapy; this may also occur with lansoprazole. No reports of enterochromaffin-like (ECL) cell carcinoids, dysplasia, or neoplasia have occurred. Severe liver dysfunction may require dosage reductions. Decreased *H. pylori* eradication rates have been observed with short-term (≤7 days) combination therapy. The American College of Gastroenterology recommends 10-14 days of therapy (triple or quadruple) for eradication of *H. pylori* (Chey, 2007). Safety and efficacy have not been established in children <1 year of age.

Adverse Reactions
1% to 10%:
Central nervous system: Headache (children 1-11 years 3%, 12-17 years 7%)
Gastrointestinal: Abdominal pain (children 12-17 years 5%; adults 2%), constipation (children 1-11 years 5%; adults 1%), diarrhea (60 mg/day; adults 7%), nausea (children 12-17 years 3%; adults 1%)
<1% (Limited to important or life-threatening): Abnormal vision, agitation, allergic reaction, ALT increased, anaphylactoid reaction, anemia, angina, anxiety, aplastic anemia, arrhythmia, AST increased, chest pain, convulsion, depression, dizziness, dry eyes, dry mouth, erythema multiforme, esophagitis, gastrin levels increased, glucocorticoids increased, globulins increased, hemolysis, hemolytic anemia, hepatotoxicity, hyperglycemia, interstitial nephritis, LDH increased, maculopapular rash, myositis, pancreatitis, photophobia, rash, RBC abnormal, taste perversion, Stevens-Johnson syndrome, thrombocytopenia, tinnitus, toxic epidermal necrolysis, tremor, vertigo, visual field defect, vomiting, WBC abnormal

Drug Interactions
Metabolism/Transport Effects Substrate of CYP2C9 (minor), 2C19 (major), 3A4 (major); **Inhibits** CYP2C9 (weak), 2C19 (moderate), 2D6 (weak), 3A4 (weak); **Induces** CYP1A2 (weak)

Avoid Concomitant Use
Avoid concomitant use of Lansoprazole with any of the following: Delavirdine; Erlotinib; Nelfinavir; Posaconazole

Increased Effect/Toxicity
Lansoprazole may increase the levels/effects of: CYP2C19 Substrates; Imatinib; Methotrexate; Raltegravir; Saquinavir; Tacrolimus; Vitamin K Antagonists; Voriconazole

The levels/effects of Lansoprazole may be increased by: Fluconazole; Ketoconazole

◀ **Decreased Effect**

Lansoprazole may decrease the levels/effects of: Atazanavir; Clopidogrel; Dabigatran Etexilate; Dasatinib; Delavirdine; Erlotinib; Indinavir; Iron Salts; Itraconazole; Ketoconazole; Mesalamine; Mycophenolate; Nelfinavir; Posaconazole

The levels/effects of Lansoprazole may be decreased by: CYP2C19 Inducers (Strong); CYP3A4 Inducers (Strong); Deferasirox; Herbs (CYP3A4 Inducers); Tipranavir

Ethanol/Nutrition/Herb Interactions

Ethanol: Avoid ethanol (may cause gastric mucosal irritation).

Food: Lansoprazole serum concentrations may be decreased if taken with food.

Herb/Nutraceutical: Avoid St John's wort (may decrease the levels/effect of lansoprazole).

Dietary Considerations Should be taken before eating; best if taken before breakfast. Some products may contain phenylalanine.

Dosage Forms Excipient information presented when available (limited, particularly for generics); consult specific product labeling. [DSC] = Discontinued product

Capsule, delayed release:

Prevacid®: 15 mg, 30 mg

Tablet, delayed release, orally disintegrating:

Prevacid® SoluTab™: 15 mg [contains phenylalanine 2.5 mg; strawberry flavor]; 30 mg [contains phenylalanine 5.1 mg; strawberry flavor]

References

Allen ME, Kopp BJ, and Erstad BL, "Stress Ulcer Prophylaxis in the Postoperative Period," *Am J Health Syst Pharm*, 2004, 61(6):588-96.

Dellinger RP, Levy MM, Carlet JM, et al, "Surviving Sepsis Campaign: International Guidelines for Management of Severe Sepsis and Septic Shock: 2008," *Intensive Care Med*, 2008, 34(1): 17-60. Available at http://www.survivingsepsis.org/system/files/images/2008_20International_20SSC_20-Guidelines_1_.pdf

Jung R and MacLaren R, "Proton-Pump Inhibitors for Stress Ulcer Prophylaxis in Critically Ill Patients," *Ann Pharmacother*, 2002, 36(12):1929-37.

◆ **Lantus®** *see* Insulin Glargine *on page* 744

◆ **Lantus® OptiSet® (Can)** *see* Insulin Glargine *on page* 744

◆ **Largactil® (Can)** *see* ChlorproMAZINE *on page* 298

◆ **Lasix®** *see* Furosemide *on page* 645

◆ **Lasix® Special (Can)** *see* Furosemide *on page* 645

◆ **Lavacol® [OTC]** *see* Alcohol (Ethyl) *on page* 53

◆ **Laxilose (Can)** *see* Lactulose *on page* 796

◆ **LCM** *see* Lacosamide *on page* 795

◆ **L-Deprenyl** *see* Selegiline *on page* 1282

◆ **Leena™** *see* Ethinyl Estradiol and Norethindrone *on page* 554

Lepirudin (leh puh ROO din)

Medication Safety Issues

High alert medication: The Institute for Safe Medication Practices (ISMP) includes this medication among its list of drugs which have a heightened risk of causing significant patient harm when used in error.

Related Information

Continuous Renal Replacement Therapy *on page 1557*

U.S. Brand Names Refludan®

Canadian Brand Names Refludan®

Index Terms Lepirudin (rDNA); Recombinant Hirudin

Pharmacologic Category Anticoagulant, Thrombin Inhibitor

Generic Available No

Use Indicated for anticoagulation in patients with heparin-induced thrombocytopenia (HIT) and associated thromboembolic disease in order to prevent further thromboembolic complications

Unlabeled/Investigational Use Investigational: Prevention or reduction of ischemic complications associated with unstable angina

Mechanism of Action Lepirudin is a highly specific direct inhibitor of thrombin; lepirudin is a recombinant hirudin derived from yeast cells

Pharmacodynamics/Kinetics

Distribution: Two-compartment model; confined to extracellular fluids.

Metabolism: Via release of amino acids via catabolic hydrolysis of parent drug

Half-life elimination: Initial: ~10 minutes; Terminal: Healthy volunteers: 1.3 hours; Marked renal impairment (Cl_{cr} <15 mL/minute and on hemodialysis): ≤2 days

Excretion: Urine (~48%, 35% as unchanged drug and unchanged drug fragments of parent drug); systemic clearance is proportional to glomerular filtration rate or creatinine clearance

Dosage Note: Maximum infusion dose: Do not exceed 0.21 mg/kg/hour unless an evaluation of coagulation abnormalities limiting response has been completed.

Heparin-induced thrombocytopenia: Bolus dose: 0.4 mg/kg IVP (over 15-20 seconds), followed by continuous infusion at 0.15 mg/kg/hour (maximum initial bolus dose: 44 mg; maximum initial infusion dose: 16.5 mg/hour); bolus and infusion must be reduced in renal insufficiency

or

Alternate dosing regimen (unlabeled dose; Selleng, 2007; Warkentin, 2008): Bolus dose: 0.2 mg/kg (use only if life- or limb-threatening thrombosis present) followed by continuous infusion of 0.05-0.1 mg/kg/hour. Further dosage reduction may be required in patients with renal dysfunction. This alternate dosing regimen has been recommended due to higher rates of bleeding associated with the FDA-approved dosing regimen.

Concomitant use with thrombolytic therapy: Bolus dose: 0.2 mg/kg IVP (over 15-20 seconds), followed by continuous infusion at 0.1 mg/kg/hour

Dosing adjustments during infusions: Monitor first aPTT 4 hours after the start of the infusion. Subsequent determinations of aPTT should be obtained at least once daily during treatment. More frequent monitoring is recommended in renally- or hepatically-impaired patients. Any aPTT ratio measurement out of range (1.5-2.5) should be confirmed prior to adjusting dose, unless a clinical need for immediate reaction exists. If the aPTT is below target range, increase infusion by 20%. If the aPTT is in excess of the target range, stop infusion for 2 hours and when restarted the infusion rate should be decreased by 50%. A repeat aPTT should be obtained 4 hours after any dosing change.

Use in patients scheduled for switch to oral anticoagulants: Once platelets normalize, reduce lepirudin dose gradually to reach aPTT ratio just above 1.5 before starting warfarin therapy. Monitor PT/INR closely until results stabilize in therapeutic range. When lepirudin is discontinued, there may be a small reduction in INR.

Dosing adjustment in renal impairment: All patients with a creatinine clearance of <60 mL/minute or a serum creatinine of >1.5 mg/dL require dosage reduction; there is only limited information on the therapeutic use of lepirudin in patients with HIT and significant renal impairment; the following dosage recommendations are mainly based on single-dose studies in a small number of patients with renal impairment. An alternate dosing regimen has also been recommended for patients with serum creatinine >1 mg/dL (Warkentin, 2008).

Initial: Bolus dose: 0.2 mg/kg IVP (over 15-20 seconds), followed by adjusted infusion based on renal function; refer to the following infusion rate adjustments based on creatinine clearance (mL/minute) and serum creatinine (mg/dL):

Note: Acute renal failure or hemodialysis: Infusion is to be avoided or stopped. Following the bolus dose, additional bolus doses of 0.1 mg/kg may be administered every other day only if aPTT falls below lower therapeutic limit (1.5-times patient baseline [or mean laboratory] aPTT).

Lepirudin infusion rates in patients with renal impairment: See tables on next page. ▶

Lepirudin Infusion Rates in Patients With Renal Impairment

Creatinine Clearance (mL/min)	Serum Creatinine (mg/dL)	Adjusted Infusion Rate	
		% of Standard Initial Infusion Rate	mg/kg/h
45-60	1.6-2.0	50%	0.075
30-44	2.1-3.0	30%	0.045
15-29	3.1-6.0	15%	0.0225
<15	>6.0	Avoid or STOP infusion	

Alternate Dosing Regimen for Renal Impairment
(based on *Chest* 2008 guidelines[1])

Serum Creatinine (mg/dL)	Adjusted Infusion Rate	
	% of Standard Initial Infusion Rate[2]	mg/kg/h
1.0-1.6	50%	0.05
1.7-4.5	10%	0.01
>4.5-6.0	5%	0.005
>6.0	Avoid or STOP infusion[3]	

[1]Recommendation based on low or very low-quality evidence.

[2]Recommended standard initial infusion rate: 0.1 mg/kg/hour

[3]Recommendation based on manufacturer's labeling.

Note: The initial bolus should either be omitted, or in the case of perceived life- or limb-threatening thrombosis, be given at a reduced dose of 0.2 mg/kg.

Stability

Intact vials should be stored at 2°C to 25°C (36°F to 77°F).

Intravenous bolus: Use a solution with a concentration of 5 mg/mL.

Preparation of a lepirudin solution with a concentration of 5 mg/mL: Reconstitute one vial (50 mg) of lepirudin with 1 mL of sterile water for injection or 0.9% sodium chloride injection. The final concentration of 5 mg/mL is obtained by transferring the contents of the vial into a sterile, single-use syringe (of at least 10 mL capacity) and diluting the solution to a total volume of 10 mL using sterile water for injection, 0.9% sodium chloride, or 5% dextrose in water.

Intravenous infusion: For continuous intravenous infusion, solutions with concentrations of 0.2 or 0.4 mg/mL may be used.

Preparation of a lepirudin solution with a concentration of 0.2 mg/mL or 0.4 mg/mL: Reconstitute 2 vials (50 mg each) of lepirudin with 1 mL each using either sterile water for injection or 0.9% sodium chloride injection. The final concentration of 0.2 mg/mL or 0.4 mg/mL is obtained by transferring the contents of both vials into an infusion bag containing 500 mL or 250 mL of 0.9% sodium chloride injection or 5% dextrose injection.

Reconstituted solutions of lepirudin are stable for 24 hours at room temperature. Manufacturer recommends using reconstituted solution immediately after preparation.

Administration Administer **only** intravenously; administer I.V. bolus over 15-20 seconds

Monitoring Parameters Monitor aPTT levels; obtain baseline aPTT, then monitor first aPTT 4 hours after the start of the infusion and every 4 hours until steady state is reached (2 consecutive aPTTs in the same range) (Warkentin, 2008). Subsequent determinations of aPTT should be obtained at least once daily during treatment. More frequent monitoring is recommended in renally- or hepatically-impaired patients. Any aPTT ratio measurement out of range (1.5-2.5) should be confirmed prior to adjusting dose, unless a clinical need for immediate reaction exists

Reference Range aPTT 1.5 to 2.5 times the control value

Anesthesia and Critical Care Concerns/Other Considerations

Evidence-Based Information:

Heparin-Induced Thrombocytopenia (HIT): In a case series of 9 patients with HIT, the combination of lepirudin and a GP IIb/IIIa inhibitor was safe and effective during PCI (Pinto, 2003). Another case report describes use in patients with HIT during cardiopulmonary bypass (Liu, 2002). During prolonged treatment (>5 days) in HIT patients, anticoagulant activity should be monitored daily (Eichler, 2000). Antihirudin antibodies develop frequently and may enhance lepirudin's activity. In this trial, about half of the patients who developed antihirudin antibodies required a 45% (range: 17% to 90%) decrease in dose.

The American College of Chest Physicians Evidence Based Clinical Practice Guidelines (8th Edition, 2008) recommend reducing the initial lepirudin dose based on serum creatinine concentrations (Cr) for the treatment of heparin-induced thrombocytopenia (see Dosing: Renal Impairment).

Pregnancy Risk Factor B

Contraindications Hypersensitivity to hirudins or any component of the formulation

Warnings/Precautions Hemorrhagic events: Intracranial bleeding following concomitant thrombolytic therapy with rt-PA or streptokinase may be life threatening. For patients with an increased risk of bleeding, a careful assessment weighing the risk of lepirudin administration versus its anticipated benefit has to be made by the treating physician. In particular, this includes the following conditions: Recent puncture of large vessels or organ biopsy; anomaly of vessels or organs; recent cerebrovascular accident, stroke, intracerebral surgery, or other neuroaxial procedures; severe uncontrolled hypertension; bacterial endocarditis; advanced renal impairment; hemorrhagic diathesis; recent major surgery; and recent major bleeding (eg, intracranial, gastrointestinal, intraocular, or pulmonary bleeding). With renal impairment, relative overdose might occur even with standard dosage regimen. The bolus dose and rate of infusion must be reduced in patients with known or suspected renal insufficiency.

Formation of antihirudin antibodies may increase the anticoagulant effect of lepirudin possibly due to delayed renal elimination of active lepirudin-antihirudin complexes. Therefore, strict monitoring of aPTT is necessary also during prolonged therapy. No evidence of neutralization of lepirudin or of allergic reactions associated with positive antibody test results was found. Allergic and hypersensitivity reactions, including anaphylaxis have been reported and may occur frequently in patients treated concomitantly with streptokinase; caution is warranted during re-exposure (anaphylaxis has been reported).

Serious liver injury (eg, liver cirrhosis) may enhance the anticoagulant effect of lepirudin due to coagulation defects secondary to reduced generation of vitamin K-dependent clotting factors.

Clinical trials have provided limited information to support any recommendations for re-exposure to lepirudin (anaphylaxis has been reported). Safety and efficacy have not been established in children.

Adverse Reactions As with all anticoagulants, bleeding is the most common adverse event associated with lepirudin. Hemorrhage may occur at virtually any site. Risk is dependent on multiple variables.

HIT patients:

>10%: Hematologic: Anemia (12%), bleeding from puncture sites (11%), hematoma (11%)

1% to 10%:

Cardiovascular: Heart failure (3%), pericardial effusion (1%), ventricular fibrillation (1%)

Central nervous system: Fever (7%)

Dermatologic: Maculopapular rash (4%), eczema (3%)

Gastrointestinal: GI bleeding/rectal bleeding (5%)

Genitourinary: Vaginal bleeding (2%)

◀

Hepatic: Transaminases increased (6%)
Renal: Hematuria (4%)
Respiratory: Epistaxis (4%)

<1% (Limited to important or life-threatening): Allergic reactions, anaphylaxis, hemoperitoneum, hemoptysis, injection site reactions, intracranial bleeding, liver bleeding, mouth bleeding, pruritus, pulmonary bleeding, retroperitoneal bleeding, thrombocytopenia, urticaria

Non-HIT populations (including those receiving thrombolytics and/or contrast media):

1% to 10%: Respiratory: Bronchospasm/stridor/dyspnea/cough

<1% (Limited to important or life-threatening): Allergic reactions (unspecified), anaphylactoid reactions, anaphylaxis, angioedema, intracranial bleeding (0.6%), laryngeal edema, thrombocytopenia, tongue edema

Drug Interactions

Avoid Concomitant Use There are no known interactions where it is recommended to avoid concomitant use.

Increased Effect/Toxicity

Lepirudin may increase the levels/effects of: Anticoagulants; Ibritumomab; Tositumomab and Iodine I 131 Tositumomab

The levels/effects of Lepirudin may be increased by: Antiplatelet Agents; Dasatinib; Herbs (Anticoagulant/Antiplatelet Properties); Nonsteroidal Anti-Inflammatory Agents; Pentosan Polysulfate Sodium; Prostacyclin Analogues; Salicylates; Thrombolytic Agents

Decreased Effect There are no known significant interactions involving a decrease in effect.

Ethanol/Nutrition/Herb Interactions Herb/Nutraceutical: Avoid cat's claw, dong quai, evening primrose, feverfew, garlic, ginger, ginkgo, red clover, horse chestnut, green tea, ginseng (all have additional antiplatelet activity)

Test Interactions PT/INR levels may become elevated in the absence of warfarin. If warfarin is initiated, initial PT/INR goals while on lepirudin may require modification.

Dosage Forms Excipient information presented when available (limited, particularly for generics); consult specific product labeling.

Injection, powder for reconstitution: 50 mg

References

Eichler P, Friesen HJ, Lubenow N, et al, "Antihirudin Antibodies in Patients With Heparin-Induced Thrombocytopenia Treated With Lepirudin: Incidence, Effects on aPTT, and Clinical Relevance," *Blood*, 2000, 96(7):2373-8.

Liu H, Fleming NW, and Moore PG, "Anticoagulation for Patients With Heparin-Induced Thrombocytopenia Using Recombinant Hirudin During Cardiopulmonary Bypass," *J Clin Anesth*, 2002, 14(6):452-5.

Lubenow N, Eichler P, Lietz T, et al, "Lepirudin in Patients With Heparin-Induced Thrombocytopenia-Results of the Third Prospective Study (HAT-3) and a Combined Analysis of HAT-1. HAT-2, and HAT-3," *J Thromb Haemost*, 2005, 3(11):2428-36.

Pinto DS, Sperling RT, Tu TM, et al, "Combination Platelet Glycoprotein IIb/IIIa Receptor and Lepirudin Administration During Percutaneous Coronary Intervention in Patients With Heparin-Induced Thrombocytopenia," *Cathet Cardiovasc Intervent*, 2003, 58(1):65-8.

◆ **Lepirudin (rDNA)** *see* Lepirudin *on page 808*

◆ **Lescol®** *see* Fluvastatin *on page 623*

◆ **Lescol® XL** *see* Fluvastatin *on page 623*

◆ **Lessina™** *see* Ethinyl Estradiol and Levonorgestrel *on page 549*

Leucovorin Calcium (loo koe VOR in KAL see um)

Index Terms 5-Formyl Tetrahydrofolate; Calcium Leucovorin; Citrovorum Factor; Folinic Acid (error prone synonym)

Pharmacologic Category Antidote; Chemotherapy Modulating Agent; Rescue Agent (Chemotherapy); Vitamin, Water Soluble

Use Antidote for folic acid antagonists (methotrexate, trimethoprim, pyrimethamine) and rescue therapy following high-dose methotrexate; in combination with fluorouracil in the treatment of colon cancer; treatment of megaloblastic anemias when folate is deficient as in infancy, sprue, pregnancy, and nutritional deficiency when oral folate therapy is not possible

Pharmacodynamics/Kinetics
Absorption: Oral, I.M.: Well absorbed
Metabolism: Intestinal mucosa and hepatically to 5-methyl-tetrahydrofolate (5MTHF; active)
Bioavailability: Saturable at oral doses >25 mg; 25 mg (97%), 50 mg (75%), 100 mg (37%)
Half-life elimination: ~4-8 hours
Time to peak: Oral: ~2 hours; I.V.: Total folates: 10 minutes; 5MTHF: ~1 hour
Excretion: Urine (primarily); feces

Dosage
Children and Adults:
Treatment of folic acid antagonist overdosage: Oral: 5-15 mg/day
Folate-deficient megaloblastic anemia: I.M.: ≤1 mg/day
High-dose methotrexate-rescue dose: Initial: Oral, I.M., I.V.: 15 mg (~10 mg/m^2); start 24 hours after beginning methotrexate infusion; continue every 6 hours for 10 doses, until methotrexate level is <0.05 micromole/L. Adjust dose as follows:
Normal methotrexate elimination: Oral, I.M., I.V.: 15 mg every 6 hours
Delayed early methotrexate elimination: I.V.: 150 mg every 3 hours until methotrexate level is <1 micromole/L, then 15 mg every 3 hours until methotrexate level is <0.05 micromole/L
Adults:
Colorectal cancer (also refer to Combination Regimens):
I.V.: 200 mg/m^2 over at least 3 minutes (used in combination with fluorouracil 370 mg/m^2)
or
I.V.: 20 mg/m^2 (used in combination with fluorouracil 425 mg/m^2)
Pemetrexed toxicity (unlabeled use): I.V.: 100 mg/m^2 once, followed by 50 mg/m^2 every 6 hours for 8 days was used in clinical trial for CTC grade 4 leukopenia ≥3 days; CTC grade 4 neutropenia ≥3 days; immediately for CTC grade 4 thrombocytopenia, bleeding associated with grade 3 thrombocytopenia, or grade 3 or 4 mucositis

Additional Information Complete prescribing information for this medication should be consulted for additional detail.

Dosage Forms Excipient information presented when available (limited, particularly for generics); consult specific product labeling. **Note:** Strength expressed as base
Injection, powder for reconstitution: 50 mg, 100 mg, 200 mg, 350 mg
Injection, solution [preservative free]: 10 mg/mL (50 mL)
Tablet: 5 mg, 10 mg, 15 mg, 25 mg

Levalbuterol (leve al BYOO ter ole)

Medication Safety Issues
Sound-alike/look-alike issues:
Xopenex® may be confused with Xanax®
U.S. Brand Names Xopenex HFA™; Xopenex®
Canadian Brand Names Xopenex®
Index Terms Levalbuterol Hydrochloride; Levalbuterol Tartrate; R-albuterol
Pharmacologic Category Beta$_2$-Adrenergic Agonist
Generic Available Yes: Excludes aerosol
Use Treatment or prevention of bronchospasm in children and adults with reversible obstructive airway disease
Mechanism of Action Relaxes bronchial smooth muscle by action on beta$_2$-receptors with little effect on heart rate
Pharmacodynamics/Kinetics
Onset of action (as measured by a 15% increase in FEV$_1$):
Aerosol: 5.5-10.2 minutes
Peak effect: ~77 minutes
Nebulization: 10-17 minutes
Peak effect: 1.5 hours

Duration (as measured by a 15% increase in FEV_1):
  Aerosol: 3-4 hours (up to 6 hours in some patients)
  Nebulization: 5-6 hours (up to 8 hours in some patients)
Absorption: A portion of inhaled dose is absorbed to systemic circulation
Half-life elimination: 3.3-4 hours
Time to peak, serum:
  Aerosol: Children: 0.8 hours, Adults: 0.5 hours
  Nebulization: Children: 0.3-0.6 hours, Adults: 0.2 hours

Dosage

Metered-dose inhaler (45 mcg/puff):
  Children 5-11 years:
    Bronchospasm, quick relief: 1-2 puffs every 4-6 hours as needed
    Exacerbation of asthma (acute, severe) (NIH Guidelines, 2007): 4-8 puffs every 20 minutes for 3 doses, then every 1-4 hours as needed
  Children ≥12 years and Adults:
    Bronchospasm, quick relief: 1-2 puffs every 4-6 hours
    Exacerbation of asthma (acute, severe) (NIH Guidelines, 2007): 4-8 puffs every 20 minutes for up to 4 hours, then every 1-4 hours as needed
Solution for nebulization:
  Children: ≤4 years:
    Bronchospasm, quick relief (NIH Guidelines, 2007): 0.31-1.25 mg every 4-6 hours as needed
    Exacerbation of asthma (acute, severe) (NIH Guidelines, 2007): 0.075 mg/kg (minimum: 1.25 mg) every 20 minutes for 3 doses, then 0.075-0.15 mg/kg (maximum: 5 mg) every 1-4 hours as needed
  Children 5-11 years:
    Bronchospasm, quick relief: 0.31-0.63 mg every 8 hours as needed
    Exacerbation of asthma (acute severe) (NIH Guidelines, 2007): 0.075 mg/kg (minimum: 1.25 mg) every 20 minutes for 3 doses, then 0.075-0.15 mg/kg (maximum: 5 mg) every 1-4 hours as needed
  Children ≥12 years and Adults:
    Bronchospasm, quick relief: 0.63-1.25 mg every 8 hours as needed
    Exacerbation of asthma (acute, severe) (NIH Guidelines, 2007): 1.25-2.5 mg every 20 minutes for 3 doses, then 1.25-5 mg every 1-4 hours as needed
Elderly: Only a small number of patients have been studied. Although greater sensitivity of some elderly patients cannot be ruled out, no overall differences in safety or effectiveness were observed. An initial dose of 0.63 mg should be used in all patients >65 years of age.

Stability

Aerosol: Store at room temperature of 20°C to 25°C (68°F to 77°F); protect from freezing and direct sunlight. Store with mouthpiece down. Discard after 200 actuations.

Solution for nebulization: Store in protective foil pouch at room temperature of 20°C to 25°C (68°F to 77°F). Protect from light and excessive heat. Vials should be used within 2 weeks after opening protective pouch. Use within 1 week and protect from light if removed from pouch. Vials of concentrated solution should be used immediately after removing from protective pouch. Concentrated solution should be diluted with 2.5 mL NS prior to use.

Administration

Inhalation:
Metered-dose inhaler: Shake well before use; prime with 4 test sprays prior to first use or if inhaler has not been use of more than 3 days. Clean actuator (mouthpiece) weekly. A spacer device or valved holding chamber is recommended when using a metered-dose inhaler.

Solution for nebulization: Safety and efficacy were established when administered with the following nebulizers: PARI LC Jet™, PARI LC Plus™, as well as the following compressors: PARI Master®, Dura-Neb® 2000, and Dura-Neb® 3000. Concentrated solution should be diluted prior to use. Blow-by administration is not recommended, use a mask device if patient unable to hold mouthpiece in mouth for administration.

Monitoring Parameters Asthma symptoms; FEV_1, peak flow, and/or other pulmonary function tests; heart rate, blood pressure, CNS stimulation; arterial blood gases (if condition warrants); serum potassium, serum glucose (in selected patients)

Pregnancy Risk Factor C

Contraindications Hypersensitivity to levalbuterol, albuterol, or any component of the formulation

Warnings/Precautions Optimize anti-inflammatory treatment before initiating maintenance treatment with levalbuterol. Do not use as a component of chronic therapy without an anti-inflammatory agent. Only the mildest form of asthma (Step 1 and/or exercise-induced) would not require concurrent use based upon asthma guidelines. Patient must be instructed to seek medical attention in cases where acute symptoms are not relieved or a previous level of response is diminished. The need to increase frequency of use may indicate deterioration of asthma, and treatment must not be delayed. A spacer device or valved holding chamber is recommended when using a metered-dose inhaler.

Use caution in patients with cardiovascular disease (arrhythmia or hypertension or HF), convulsive disorders, diabetes, glaucoma, hyperthyroidism, or hypokalemia. Beta-agonists may cause elevation in blood pressure, heart rate, and result in CNS stimulation/excitation. Beta$_2$-agonists may increase risk of arrhythmia, increase serum glucose, or decrease serum potassium.

Immediate hypersensitivity reactions (urticaria, angioedema, rash, broncho-spasm) have been reported. Do not exceed recommended dose; serious adverse events including fatalities, have been associated with excessive use of inhaled sympathomimetics. Rarely, paradoxical bronchospasm may occur with use of inhaled bronchodilating agents; this should be distinguished from inadequate response. Use with caution during labor and delivery. Safety and efficacy have not been established in patients <4 years of age.

Adverse Reactions
>10%:

Endocrine & metabolic: Serum glucose increased, serum potassium decreased
Neuromuscular & skeletal: Tremor (≤7%)
Respiratory: Rhinitis (3% to 11%)
Miscellaneous: Viral infection (7% to 12%)

>2% to 10%:

Central nervous system: Headache (8% to 12%), nervousness (3% to 10%), dizziness (1% to 3%), anxiety (≤3%), migraine (≤3%), weakness (3%)
Cardiovascular: Tachycardia (~3%)
Dermatologic: Rash (≤8%)
Gastrointestinal: Diarrhea (2% to 6%), dyspepsia (1% to 3%)
Neuromuscular & skeletal: Leg cramps (≤3%)
Respiratory: Asthma (9%), pharyngitis (3% to 10%), cough (1% to 4%), sinusitis (1% to 4%), nasal edema (1% to 3%)
Miscellaneous: Flu-like syndrome (1% to 4%), accidental injury (≤3%)

<2% (Limited to important or life-threatening): Abnormal ECG, acne, anaphylaxis, angina, angioedema, arrhythmia, atrial fibrillation, chest pain, chills, constipation, conjunctivitis, cough, diaphoresis, dysmenorrhea, dyspnea, epistaxis, extra-systole, gastroenteritis, hematuria, hyper-/hypotension, hypoesthesia (hand), hypokalemia, insomnia, itching eyes, lymphadenopathy, myalgia, nausea, oropharyngeal dryness, paresthesia, supraventricular arrhythmia, syncope, vaginal moniliasis, vertigo, vomiting, wheezing, xerostomia

Note: Immediate hypersensitivity reactions have occurred (including angioedema, oropharyngeal edema, urticaria, and anaphylaxis).

Drug Interactions
Avoid Concomitant Use
Avoid concomitant use of Levalbuterol with any of the following: Iobenguane I 123

Increased Effect/Toxicity
Levalbuterol may increase the levels/effects of: Sympathomimetics

The levels/effects of Levalbuterol may be increased by: Atomoxetine; Cannabinoids; MAO Inhibitors; Tricyclic Antidepressants

Decreased Effect
Levalbuterol may decrease the levels/effects of: Iobenguane I 123

The levels/effects of Levalbuterol may be decreased by: Alpha-/Beta-Blockers; Beta-Blockers (Beta1 Selective); Beta-Blockers (Nonselective); Betahistine

◀ **Dosage Forms** Excipient information presented when available (limited, particularly for generics); consult specific product labeling.

Note: Strength expressed as base.

Aerosol, for oral inhalation, as tartrate:

Xopenex HFA™: 45 mcg/actuation (15 g) [200 actuations; chlorofluorocarbon free]

Solution for nebulization, as hydrochloride [preservative free]:

Xopenex®: 0.31 mg/3 mL (24s); 0.63 mg/3 mL (24s); 1.25 mg/3 mL (24s)

Solution for nebulization, as hydrochloride [concentrate; preservative free]: 1.25 mg/0.5 mL (30s)

Xopenex®: 1.25 mg/0.5 mL (30s)

References

Expert Panel Report 3, "Guidelines for the Diagnosis and Management of Asthma," *Clinical Practice Guidelines*, National Institutes of Health, National Heart, Lung, and Blood Institute, NIH Publication No. 08-4051, prepublication 2007. Available at http://www.nhlbi.nih.gov/guidelines/asthma/asthgdln.htm

◆ **Levalbuterol Hydrochloride** *see* Levalbuterol *on page 813*

◆ **Levalbuterol Tartrate** *see* Levalbuterol *on page 813*

◆ **Levaquin®** *see* Levofloxacin *on page 823*

◆ **Levarterenol Bitartrate** *see* Norepinephrine *on page 1024*

◆ **Levate® (Can)** *see* Amitriptyline *on page 89*

◆ **Levatol®** *see* Penbutolol *on page 1094*

◆ **Levemir®** *see* Insulin Detemir *on page 744*

Levetiracetam (lee va tye RA se tam)

Medication Safety Issues

Sound-alike/look-alike issues:

Keppra® may be confused with Keflex®, Keppra XR™

Levetiracetam may be confused with levofloxacin

Potential for dispensing errors between Keppra® and Kaletra® (lopinavir/ritonavir)

Medication Guide An FDA-approved patient medication guide, which is available with the product information and at http://www.fda.gov/downloads/Drugs/DrugSafety/UCM152832.pdf, must be dispensed with this medication for each new outpatient prescription and refill.

Related Information

Chronic Pain Management *on page 1546*

Perioperative Management of Patients on Antiseizure Medication *on page 1577*

U.S. Brand Names Keppra XR™; Keppra®

Canadian Brand Names Apo-Levetiracetam; CO Levetiracetam; DOM-Levetiracetam; Keppra®; PHL-Levetiracetam; PMS-Levetiracetam

Pharmacologic Category Anticonvulsant, Miscellaneous

Generic Available Yes: Oral solution, tablet

Use Adjunctive therapy in the treatment of partial onset, myoclonic, and/or primary generalized tonic-clonic seizures

Unlabeled/Investigational Use Bipolar disorder

Mechanism of Action The precise mechanism by which levetiracetam exerts its antiepileptic effect is unknown. However, several studies have suggested the mechanism may involve one or more of the following central pharmacologic effects: inhibition of voltage-dependent N-type calcium channels; facilitation of GABA-ergic inhibitory transmission through displacement of negative modulators; reduction of delayed rectifier potassium current; and/or binding to synaptic proteins which modulate neurotransmitter release.

Pharmacodynamics/Kinetics

Absorption: Oral: Rapid and almost complete

Distribution: V_d: Similar to total body water

Protein binding: <10%

Metabolism: Not extensive; primarily by enzymatic hydrolysis; forms metabolites (inactive)

Bioavailability: 100%

Half-life elimination: ~6-8 hours; extended release tablet: ~7 hours; half-life increased in renal dysfunction

Time to peak, plasma: Oral: Immediate release: ~1 hour; Extended release: ~4 hours

Excretion: Urine (66% as unchanged drug)

Dosage

Oral:

Children 4-15 years: Partial onset seizures: Immediate release: 10 mg/kg/dose given twice daily; may increase every 2 weeks by 10 mg/kg/dose to a maximum of 30 mg/kg/dose twice daily

Children 6-15 years: Tonic-clonic seizures: Immediate release: Initial: 10 mg/kg dose given twice daily; may increase every 2 weeks by 10 mg/kg/dose to the recommended dose of 30 mg/kg twice daily. Efficacy of doses >60 mg/kg/day has not been established.

Children ≥12 years and Adults: Myoclonic seizures: Immediate release: Initial: 500 mg twice daily; may increase every 2 weeks by 500 mg/dose to the recommended dose of 1500 mg twice daily. Efficacy of doses >3000 mg/day has not been established.

Children ≥16 years and Adults:

Partial onset seizure:

Immediate release: Initial: 500 mg twice daily; may increase every 2 weeks by 500 mg/dose to a maximum of 1500 mg twice daily. Doses >3000 mg/day have been used in trials; however, there is no evidence of increased benefit.

Extended release: Initial: 1000 mg once daily; may increase every 2 weeks by 1000 mg/day to a maximum of 3000 mg once daily.

Tonic-clonic seizures: Immediate release: Initial: 500 mg twice daily; may increase every 2 weeks by 500 mg/dose to the recommended dose of 1500 mg twice daily. Efficacy of doses >3000 mg/day has not been established.

Bipolar disorder (unlabeled use): Immediate release: Initial: 500 mg twice daily; if tolerated, increase by 500 mg twice daily; dose may be increased every 3 days until target dose of 3000 mg/day is reached; maximum: 4000 mg/day

Adults: Loading dose (unlabeled): Immediate release: Initial doses of 1500-2000 mg have been well-tolerated (Betts, 2000; Koubeissi, 2008), although the necessity of a loading dose has not been established

I.V.: Children ≥16 years and Adults: Partial onset seizure: Initial: 500 mg twice daily; may increase every 2 weeks by 500 mg/dose to a maximum of 1500 mg twice daily. Doses >3000 mg/day have been used in trials; however, there is no evidence of increased benefit.

Note: When switching from oral to I.V. formulations, the total daily dose should be the same.

Dosing adjustment in renal impairment: Adults:

Immediate release and I.V. formulations:

Cl_{cr} >80 mL/minute: 500-1500 mg every 12 hours

Cl_{cr} 50-80 mL/minute: 500-1000 mg every 12 hours

Cl_{cr} 30-50 mL/minute: 250-750 mg every 12 hours

Cl_{cr} <30 mL/minute: 250-500 mg every 12 hours

End-stage renal disease patients using dialysis: 500-1000 mg every 24 hours; a supplemental dose of 250-500 mg following dialysis is recommended

Extended release tablets:

Cl_{cr} >80 mL/minute: 1000-3000 mg every 24 hours

Cl_{cr} 50-80 mL/minute: 1000-2000 mg every 24 hours

Cl_{cr} 30-50 mL/minute: 500-1500 mg every 24 hours

Cl_{cr} <30 mL/minute: 500-1000 mg every 24 hours

Dosing adjustment in hepatic impairment: No adjustment required

Stability

Oral solution, tablets: Store at 25°C (77°F); excursions permitted to 15°C to 30°C (59°F to 86°F).

Injection solution: Store at 25°C (77°F); excursions permitted to 15°C to 30°C (59°F to 86°F). Must dilute dose in 100 mL of NS, LR, or D_5W. Admixed solution is stable for 24 hours in PVC bags kept at room temperature.

◀ **Administration**

I.V.: Infuse over 15 minutes

Oral: May be administered without regard to meals.

Oral solution: Should be administered with a calibrated measuring device (not a household teaspoon or tablespoon)

Tablet (immediate release and extended release): Only administer as whole tablet; do not crush, break or chew.

Monitoring Parameters Suicidality (eg, suicidal thoughts, depression, behavioral changes)

Pregnancy Risk Factor C

Contraindications Hypersensitivity to levetiracetam or any component of the formulation

Warnings/Precautions Antiepileptics are associated with an increased risk of suicidal behavior/thoughts with use (regardless of indication); patients should be monitored for signs/symptoms of depression, suicidal tendencies, and other unusual behavior changes during therapy and instructed to inform their healthcare provider immediately if symptoms occur.

Psychotic symptoms (psychosis, hallucinations) and behavioral symptoms (including aggression, anger, anxiety, depersonalization, depression, personality disorder) may occur; incidence may be increased in children. Dose reduction may be required. Levetiracetam should be withdrawn gradually to minimize the potential of increased seizure frequency. Use caution with renal impairment; dosage adjustment may be necessary. Weakness, dizziness, and somnolence occur mostly during the first month of therapy. Although rare, decreases in red blood cell counts, hemoglobin, hematocrit, white blood cell counts and neutrophils have been observed. Safety and efficacy in children <4 years of age (oral formulation) or <16 years (I.V. formulation and extended release tablets) have not been established.

Adverse Reactions

>10%:

Central nervous system: Behavioral symptoms (agitation, aggression, anger, anxiety, apathy, depersonalization, depression, emotional lability, hostility, hyperkinesias, irritability, nervousness, neurosis and personality disorder: adults 5% to 13%; children 5% to 38%), somnolence (8% to 23%), headache (14%), hostility (2% to 12%)

Gastrointestinal: Vomiting (15%), anorexia (3% to 13%)

Neuromuscular & skeletal: Weakness (9% to 15%)

Respiratory: Pharyngitis (6% to 14%), rhinitis (4% to 13%), cough (2% to 11%)

Miscellaneous: Accidental injury (17%), infection (2% to 13%)

1% to 10%:

Cardiovascular: Facial edema (2%)

Central nervous system: Fatigue (10%), nervousness (4% to 10%), dizziness (5% to 9%), personality disorder (8%), pain (6% to 7%), agitation (6%), irritability (6% to 7%), emotional lability (2% to 6%), mood swings (5%), depression (3% to 5%), vertigo (3% to 5%), ataxia (3%), amnesia (2%), anxiety (2%), confusion (2%)

Dermatologic: Bruising (4%), pruritus (2%), rash (2%), skin discoloration (2%)

Endocrine & metabolic: Dehydration (2%)

Gastrointestinal: Diarrhea (8%), nausea (5%), gastroenteritis (4%), constipation (3%)

Genitourinary: Urine abnormality (2%)

Hematologic: Leukocytes decreased (2% to 3%)

Neuromuscular & skeletal: Neck pain (2% to 8%), paresthesia (2%), reflexes increased (2%)

Ocular: Conjunctivitis (3%), diplopia (2%), amblyopia (2%)

Otic: Ear pain (2%)

Renal: Albuminuria (4%)

Respiratory: Influenza (5%), asthma (2%), sinusitis (2%)

Miscellaneous: Flu-like syndrome (3% to 8%), viral infection (2%)

<1% (Limited to important or life-threatening): Alopecia, anemia, catatonia, hematocrit decreased, hemoglobin decreased, hepatic failure, hepatitis, leukopenia, LFTs abnormal, neutropenia, pancreatitis, pancytopenia (with bone

marrow suppression), psychotic symptoms, red blood cells decreased, suicide attempt, suicide behavior, suicide ideation, thrombocytopenia, weight loss

Drug Interactions

Avoid Concomitant Use There are no known interactions where it is recommended to avoid concomitant use.

Increased Effect/Toxicity

Levetiracetam may increase the levels/effects of: Alcohol (Ethyl); CNS Depressants; Methotrimeprazine

The levels/effects of Levetiracetam may be increased by: Methotrimeprazine

Decreased Effect

The levels/effects of Levetiracetam may be decreased by: Ketorolac; Mefloquine

Ethanol/Nutrition/Herb Interactions

Ethanol: Avoid ethanol (may increase CNS depression).

Food: Food may delay, but does not affect the extent of absorption.

Dietary Considerations May be taken without regard to meals.

Dosage Forms Excipient information presented when available (limited, particularly for generics); consult specific product labeling.

Injection, solution:

Keppra®: 100 mg/mL (5 mL)

Solution, oral: 100 mg/mL (500 mL)

Keppra®: 100 mg/mL (480 mL) [dye free; grape flavor]

Tablet: 250 mg, 500 mg, 750 mg, 1000 mg

Keppra®: 250 mg, 500 mg, 750 mg, 1000 mg

Tablet, extended release:

Keppra XR™: 500 mg, 750 mg

◆ **Levlen®** *see* Ethinyl Estradiol and Levonorgestrel *on page 549*

◆ **Levlite™** *see* Ethinyl Estradiol and Levonorgestrel *on page 549*

Levobupivacaine (LEE voe byoo PIV a kane)

Medication Safety Issues

High alert medication: The Institute for Safe Medication Practices (ISMP) includes this medication (epidural administration) among its list of drug classes which have a heightened risk of causing significant patient harm when used in error.

U.S. Brand Names Chirocaine® [DSC]

Canadian Brand Names Chirocaine®

Pharmacologic Category Local Anesthetic

Generic Available No

Use Local or regional anesthesia for surgery and obstetrics, and for postoperative pain management

Mechanism of Action Levobupivacaine is the S-enantiomer of bupivacaine. It blocks both the initiation and transmission of nerve impulses by decreasing the neuronal membrane's permeability to sodium ions, which results in inhibition of depolarization with resultant blockade of conduction. Local anesthetics reversibly prevent generation and conduction of electrical impulses in neurons by decreasing the transient increase in permeability to sodium. The differential sensitivity generally depends on the size of the fiber; small fibers are more sensitive than larger fibers and require a longer period for recovery. Sensory pain fibers are usually blocked first, followed by fibers that transmit sensations of temperature, touch, and deep pressure. High concentrations block sympathetic somatic sensory and somatic motor fibers. The spread of anesthesia depends upon the distribution of the solution. This is primarily dependent on the site of administration and volume of drug injected.

Pharmacodynamics/Kinetics

Onset of action: Epidural: 10-14 minutes

Duration (dose dependent): 1-8 hours

Absorption: Dependent on route of administration and dose

Distribution: 67 L

Protein binding, plasma: >97%

Metabolism: Extensively hepatic via CYP3A4 and CYP1A2

◀ Half-life elimination: 1.3 hours
Time to peak: Epidural: 30 minutes
Excretion: Urine (71%) and feces (24%) as metabolites

Dosage Adults: **Note:** Rapid injection of a large volume of local anesthetic solution should be avoided. Fractional (incremental) doses are recommended.

Guidelines (individual response varies): See table.

	Concentration	Volume	Dose	Motor Block
Surgical Anesthesia				
Epidural for surgery	0.5%-0.75%	10-20 mL	50-150 mg	Moderate to complete
Epidural for C-section	0.5%	20-30 mL	100-150 mg	Moderate to complete
Peripheral nerve	0.25%-0.5%	0.4 mL/kg (30 mL)	1-2 mg/kg (75-150 mg)	Moderate to complete
Ophthalmic	0.75%	5-15 mL	37.5-112.5 mg	Moderate to complete
Local infiltration	0.25%	60 mL	150 mg	Not applicable
Pain Management				
Levobupivacaine can be used epidurally with fentanyl or clonidine; dilutions for epidural administration should be made with preservative free 0.9% saline according to standard hospital procedures for sterility				
Labor analgesia (epidural bolus)	0.25%	10-20 mL	25-50 mg	Minimal to moderate
Postoperative pain (epidural infusion)	0.125%[1]-0.25%	4-10 mL/h	5-25 mg/h	Minimal to moderate

[1]0.125%: Adjunct therapy with fentanyl or clonidine.

Maximum dosage: Epidural doses up to 375 mg have been administered incrementally to patients during a surgical procedure.

Intraoperative block and postoperative pain: 695 mg in 24 hours

Postoperative epidural infusion over 24 hours: 570 mg

Single-fractionated injection for brachial plexus block: 300 mg

Stability Store at room temperature (20°C to 25°C/68°F to 77°F). Disinfectants containing heavy metals should not be used for mucous membrane disinfection since they have been related to incidents of swelling and edema. Isopropyl or ethyl alcohol is recommended. Stability of solution in vial has been demonstrated following an autoclave cycle at 121°C for 15 minutes.

Administration Isopropyl or ethyl alcohol are recommended to disinfect the surface of the vial. Disinfectants containing heavy metals should not be used for mucous membrane disinfection since they have been related to incidents of swelling and edema. Prior to administration, it is essential that aspiration for blood or cerebrospinal fluid (where applicable) be performed prior to injecting any local anesthetic, both before the original dosage and at all subsequent doses (to avoid intravascular or intrathecal injection). A negative aspiration does not ensure against intrathecal or intravascular injection. Rapid injection of a large volume of local anesthetic solution should be avoided. Fractional (incremental) doses are recommended. Monitor patient during and after injection for symptoms of CNS or cardiac toxicity.

Monitoring Parameters Monitor the patient during and after injection for symptoms of CNS or cardiac toxicity

Anesthesia and Critical Care Concerns/Other Considerations

Local anesthetic toxicity: Cardiac arrest: Lipid infusion has been used in animal studies and several human cases (Bupivacaine: Rosenblatt, 2006; Levobupivacaine: Foxall, 2007; Ropivacaine: Litz, 2006) where cardiovascular toxicity, unresponsive to conventional resuscitation, resulted. Additional information is available at http://www.lipidrescue.org. The protocol from the website is: 20% Fat Emulsion: 1.5 mL/kg administered over 1 minute, followed immediately by an infusion of 0.25 mL/kg/minute. Continue chest compressions (lipid must circulate). Repeat bolus every 3-5 minutes up to 3 mL/kg total dose until circulation restored. Continue infusion until hemodynamic stability is restored. Increase the infusion rate to 0.5 mL/kg/minute if BP declines. A maximum total dose of 8 mL/kg is recommended.

Pregnancy Risk Factor B

Contraindications Hypersensitivity to levobupivacaine, any component of the formulation, bupivacaine, or any local anesthetic of the amide type

Warnings/Precautions Careful and constant monitoring of the patient's state of consciousness should be done following each local anesthetic injection; at such times, restlessness, anxiety, tinnitus, dizziness, blurred vision, tremors, depression, or drowsiness may be early warning signs of CNS toxicity. Treatment is primarily symptomatic and supportive. Intravascular injections should be avoided. Local anesthetics have been associated with rare occurrences of sudden respiratory arrest, seizures, and cardiac arrest. Local anesthetics should be administered only by clinicians familiar with the use of local anesthetic agents, procedures, and management of drug-related toxicity and other acute emergencies. Resuscitative equipment and medications should be readily available. Not for intravenous injection (cardiac arrest may occur) or obstetrical paracervical block. Risk of cardiac toxicity increases with higher concentration solutions. Avoid use of 0.75% solution with obstetrical patients. Use with caution in patients with hypotension, hypovolemia, heart block, hepatic impairment, cardiac impairment, or those receiving other local anesthetics or structurally-related agents. Safety and efficacy have not been established in children.

Adverse Reactions

>10%:
    Cardiovascular: Hypotension (20% to 31%)
    Central nervous system: Pain (postoperative) (7% to 18%), fever (7% to 17%)
    Gastrointestinal: Nausea (12% to 21%), vomiting (8% to 14%)
    Hematologic: Anemia (10% to 12%)

1% to 10%:
    Central nervous system: Pain (4% to 8%), headache (5% to 7%), dizziness (5% to 6%), hypoesthesia (3%), somnolence (1%), anxiety (1%), hypothermia (2%)
    Cardiovascular: Abnormal ECG (3%), bradycardia (2%), tachycardia (2%), hypertension (1%)
    Dermatologic: Pruritus (4% to 9%), purpura (1%)
    Endocrine & metabolic: Breast pain - female (1%)
    Gastrointestinal: Constipation (3% to 7%), enlarged abdomen (3%), flatulence (2%), abdominal pain (2%), dyspepsia (2%), diarrhea (1%)
    Genitourinary: Urinary incontinence (1%), urine flow decreased (1%), urinary tract infection (1%)
    Hematologic: Leukocytosis (1%)
    Local: Anesthesia (1%)
    Neuromuscular & skeletal: Back pain (6%), rigors (3%), paresthesia (2%)
    Ocular: Diplopia (3%)
    Renal: Albuminuria (3%), hematuria (2%)
    Respiratory: Cough (1%)
    Miscellaneous: Fetal distress (5% to 10%), delayed delivery (6%), hemorrhage in pregnancy (2%), uterine abnormality (2%), increased wound drainage (1%)

<1% (Limited to important or life-threatening): Apnea, arrhythmia, atrial fibrillation, bronchospasm, cardiac arrest, confusion, dyspnea, generalized spasm, ileus, involuntary muscle contraction, pulmonary edema, skin discoloration, syncope

Drug Interactions

Metabolism/Transport Effects Substrate (minor) of CYP1A2, 3A4

Avoid Concomitant Use There are no known interactions where it is recommended to avoid concomitant use.

Increased Effect/Toxicity There are no known significant interactions involving an increase in effect.

Decreased Effect There are no known significant interactions involving a decrease in effect.

Ethanol/Nutrition/Herb Interactions Herb/Nutraceutical: St John's wort may decrease levobupivacaine levels.

Dosage Forms Excipient information presented when available (limited, particularly for generics); consult specific product labeling. [DSC] = Discontinued product

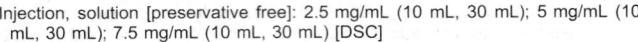

Injection, solution [preservative free]: 2.5 mg/mL (10 mL, 30 mL); 5 mg/mL (10 mL, 30 mL); 7.5 mg/mL (10 mL, 30 mL) [DSC]

References

Corcoran W, Butterworth J, Weller RS, et al, "Local Anesthetic-Induced Cardiac Toxicity: A Survey of Contemporary Practice Strategies Among Academic Anesthesiology Departments," *Anesth Analg*, 2006, 103(5):1322-6.

Foxall G, McCahon R, Lamb J, et al, "Levobupivacaine-Induced Seizures and Cardiovascular Collapse Treated With Intralipid," *Anaesthesia*, 2007, 62(5):516-8.

Litz RJ, Popp M, Stehr SN, et al, "Successful Resuscitation of a Patient With Ropivacaine-Induced Asystole After Axillary Plexus Block Using lipid infusion," *Anaesthesia*, 2006, 61(8):800-1.

Rosenblatt MA, Abel M, Fischer GW, et al, "Successful Use of a 20% Lipid Emulsion to Resuscitate a Patient After a Presumed Bupivacaine-Related Cardiac Arrest," *Anesthesiology*, 2006, 105 (1):217-8.

Levodopa and Carbidopa (kar bi DOE pa & lee voe DOE pa)

U.S. Brand Names Parcopa™; Sinemet®; Sinemet® CR

Canadian Brand Names Apo-Levocarb®; Apo-Levocarb® CR; Endo®-Levodopa/Carbidopa; Novo-Levocarbidopa; Nu-Levocarb; Pro-Levocarb; Sinemet®; Sinemet® CR

Index Terms Levodopa and Carbidopa

Pharmacologic Category Anti-Parkinson's Agent, Dopamine Agonist

Use Idiopathic Parkinson's disease; postencephalitic parkinsonism; symptomatic parkinsonism

Unlabeled/Investigational Use Restless leg syndrome

Pharmacodynamics/Kinetics

Duration: Variable, 6-12 hours; longer with sustained release forms

Dosage Oral: Adults:

Parkinson's disease:

Immediate release tablet:

Initial: Carbidopa 25 mg/levodopa 100 mg 3 times/day

Dosage adjustment: Alternate tablet strengths may be substituted according to individual carbidopa/levodopa requirements. Increase by 1 tablet every other day as necessary, except when using the carbidopa 25 mg/levodopa 250 mg tablets where increases should be made using 1/2-1 tablet every 1-2 days. Use of more than 1 dosage strength or dosing 4 times/day may be required (maximum: 8 tablets of any strength/day or 200 mg of carbidopa and 2000 mg of levodopa)

Sustained release tablet:

Initial: Carbidopa 50 mg/levodopa 200 mg 2 times/day, at intervals not <6 hours

Dosage adjustment: May adjust every 3 days; intervals should be between 4-8 hours during the waking day (maximum: 8 tablets/day)

Restless leg syndrome (unlabeled use): Carbidopa 25 mg/levodopa 100 mg given 30-60 minutes before bedtime; may repeat dose once

Elderly: Initial: Carbidopa 25 mg/levodopa 100 mg twice daily, increase as necessary

Anesthesia and Critical Care Concerns/Other Considerations

Clinical Pearls/Comments: Consider use of alternative therapies before attempting to use levodopa containing products. 50-100 mg/day of carbidopa is needed to block the peripheral conversion of levodopa to dopamine. "On-off" (a clinical syndrome characterized by sudden periods of drug activity/inactivity), can be managed by giving smaller, more frequent doses of Sinemet® or adding a dopamine agonist or selegiline; when adding a new agent, doses of Sinemet® can usually be decreased. Protein in the diet should be distributed throughout the day to avoid fluctuations in levodopa absorption. Levodopa is the drug of choice when rigidity is the predominant presenting symptom.

Additional Information Complete prescribing information for this medication should be consulted for additional detail.

Dosage Forms Excipient information presented when available (limited, particularly for generics); consult specific product labeling.

Tablet: 10/100: Carbidopa 10 mg and levodopa 100 mg; 25/100: Carbidopa 25 mg and levodopa 100 mg; 25/250: Carbidopa 25 mg and levodopa 250 mg

Sinemet®:
  10/100: Carbidopa 10 mg and levodopa 100 mg
  25/100: Carbidopa 25 mg and levodopa 100 mg
  25/250: Carbidopa 25 mg and levodopa 250 mg
Tablet, extended release: 25/100: Carbidopa 25 mg and levodopa 100 mg; 50/200: Carbidopa 50 mg and levodopa 200 mg
Tablet, orally disintegrating: 10/100: Carbidopa 10 mg and levodopa 100 mg; 25/100: Carbidopa 25 mg and levodopa 100 mg; 25/250: Carbidopa 25 mg and levodopa 250 mg
  Parcopa™:
    10/100: Carbidopa 10 mg and levodopa 100 mg [contains phenylalanine 3.4 mg/tablet; mint flavor]
    25/100: Carbidopa 25 mg and levodopa 100 mg [contains phenylalanine 3.4 mg/tablet; mint flavor]
    25/250: Carbidopa 25 mg and levodopa 250 mg [contains phenylalanine 8.4 mg/tablet; mint flavor]
Tablet, sustained release: 25/100: Carbidopa 25 mg and levodopa 100 mg; 50/200: Carbidopa 50 mg and levodopa 200 mg
  Sinemet® CR:
    25/100: Carbidopa 25 mg and levodopa 100 mg
    50/200: Carbidopa 50 mg and levodopa 200 mg

◆ **Levodopa and Carbidopa** see Levodopa and Carbidopa on page 822
◆ **Levo-Dromoran®** see Levorphanol on page 829

Levofloxacin (lee voe FLOKS a sin)

Medication Safety Issues
Sound-alike/look-alike issues:
  Levaquin® may be confused with Levoxyl®, Levsin/SL®, Lovenox®
  Levofloxacin may be confused with levetiracetam, levodopa, levothyroxine
Medication Guide An FDA-approved patient medication guide, which is available with the product information and at http://www.fda.gov/downloads/Drugs/DrugSafety/ucm088619.pdf, must be dispensed with this medication for each new outpatient prescription and refill.
Related Information
  Prevention of Wound Infection and Sepsis in Surgical Patients on page 1721
U.S. Brand Names Iquix®; Levaquin®; Quixin®
Canadian Brand Names Apo-Levofloxacin®; CO Levofloxacin; Levaquin®; Mylan-Levofloxacin; Novo-Levofloxacin; PMS-Levofloxacin; Sandoz-Levofloxacin
Pharmacologic Category Antibiotic, Quinolone; Respiratory Fluoroquinolone
Generic Available No
Use
Systemic: Treatment of community-acquired pneumonia, including multidrug resistant strains of *S. pneumoniae* (MDRSP); nosocomial pneumonia; chronic bronchitis (acute bacterial exacerbation); acute bacterial sinusitis; prostatitis; urinary tract infection (uncomplicated or complicated); acute pyelonephritis; skin or skin structure infections (uncomplicated or complicated); reduce incidence or disease progression of inhalational anthrax (postexposure)
Ophthalmic: Treatment of bacterial conjunctivitis caused by susceptible organisms (Quixin® 0.5% ophthalmic solution); treatment of corneal ulcer caused by susceptible organisms (Iquix® 1.5% ophthalmic solution)
Unlabeled/Investigational Use Diverticulitis, enterocolitis (*Shigella* spp.), epididymitis (nongonococcal), gonococcal infections, Legionnaires' disease, peritonitis, PID
Note: As of April 2007, the CDC no longer recommends the use of fluoroquinolones for the treatment of gonococcal disease.
Mechanism of Action As the S (-) enantiomer of the fluoroquinolone, ofloxacin, levofloxacin, inhibits DNA-gyrase in susceptible organisms thereby inhibits relaxation of supercoiled DNA and promotes breakage of DNA strands. DNA gyrase (topoisomerase II), is an essential bacterial enzyme that maintains the superhelical structure of DNA and is required for DNA replication and transcription, DNA repair, recombination, and transposition.

Pharmacodynamics/Kinetics

Absorption: Rapid and complete

Distribution: V_d: 74-112 L; CSF concentrations ~15% of serum levels; high concentrations are achieved in prostate, lung, and gynecological tissues, sinus, saliva

Protein binding: ~24% to 38%; primarily to albumin

Metabolism: Minimally hepatic

Bioavailability: ~99%

Half-life elimination: ~6-8 hours

Time to peak, serum: Oral: 1-2 hours

Excretion: Urine (~87% as unchanged drug, <5% as metabolites); feces (<4%)

Dosage Note: Sequential therapy (intravenous to oral) may be instituted based on prescriber's discretion.

Usual dosage range:

Children ≥1 year: Ophthalmic: 1-2 drops every 2-6 hours

Adults:

Ophthalmic: 1-2 drops every 2-6 hours

Oral, I.V.: 250-500 mg every 24 hours; severe or complicated infections: 750 mg every 24 hours

Indication-specific dosing:

Children ≥1 year and Adults: Ophthalmic:

Conjunctivitis (0.5% ophthalmic solution):

Treatment day 1 and day 2: Instill 1-2 drops into affected eye(s) every 2 hours while awake, up to 8 times/day

Treatment day 3 through day 7: Instill 1-2 drops into affected eye(s) every 4 hours while awake, up to 4 times/day

Children ≥6 years and Adults: Ophthalmic:

Corneal ulceration (1.5% ophthalmic solution):

Treatment day 1 through day 3: Instill 1-2 drops into affected eye(s) every 30 minutes to 2 hours while awake and 4-6 hours after retiring

Treatment day 4 through completion: Instill 1-2 drops into affected eye(s) every 1-4 hours while awake

Children ≥6 months and Adults: Oral, I.V.:

Anthrax (inhalational, postexposure):

≤50 kg: 8 mg/kg every 12 hours for 60 days (do not exceed 250 mg/dose), beginning as soon as possible after exposure

>50 kg and Adults: 500 mg every 24 hours for 60 days, beginning as soon as possible after exposure

Adults: Oral, I.V.:

Chronic bronchitis (acute bacterial exacerbation): 500 mg every 24 hours for at least 7 days

Diverticulitis, peritonitis (unlabeled use): 750 mg every 24 hours for 7-10 days; use adjunctive metronidazole therapy

Dysenteric enterocolitis, _Shigella_ spp. (unlabeled use): 500 mg every 24 hours for 3-5 days

Epididymitis, nongonococcal (unlabeled use): 500 mg once daily for 10 days

Gonococcal infection (unlabeled use):

Cervicitis, urethritis: 250 mg for one dose with azithromycin or doxycycline; **Note:** As of April 2007, the CDC no longer recommends the use of fluoroquinolones for the treatment of uncomplicated gonococcal disease.

Disseminated infection: 250 mg I.V. once daily; 24 hours after symptoms improve may change to 500 mg orally every 24 hours to complete total therapy of 7 days; **Note:** As of April 2007, the CDC no longer recommends the use of fluoroquinolones for the treatment of more serious gonococcal disease, unless no other options exist and susceptibility can be confirmed via culture.

Pelvic inflammatory disease (unlabeled use): 500 mg once daily for 14 days with or without adjunctive metronidazole; **Note:** The CDC recommends use only if standard cephalosporin therapy is not feasible and community prevalence of quinolone-resistant gonococcal organisms is low. Culture sensitivity must be confirmed.

Pneumonia:
  Community-acquired: 500 mg every 24 hours for 7-14 days or 750 mg every 24 hours for 5 days (efficacy of 5-day regimen for MDRSP not established)
  Nosocomial: 750 mg every 24 hours for 7-14 days
Prostatitis (chronic bacterial): 500 mg every 24 hours for 28 days
Sinusitis (acute bacterial): 500 mg every 24 hours for 10-14 days or 750 mg every 24 hours for 5 days
Skin and skin structure infections:
  Uncomplicated: 500 mg every 24 hours for 7-10 days
  Complicated: 750 mg every 24 hours for 7-14 days
Traveler's diarrhea (unlabeled use): 500 mg for one dose
Urinary tract infections:
  Uncomplicated: 250 mg once daily for 3 days
  Complicated, including pyelonephritis: 250 mg once daily for 10 days **or** 750 mg once daily for 5 days

Dosing adjustment in renal impairment:
  Normal renal function dosing of 750 mg/day:
    Cl_{cr} 20-49 mL/minute: Administer 750 mg every 48 hours
    Cl_{cr} 10-19 mL/minute: Administer 750 mg initial dose, followed by 500 mg every 48 hours
    Hemodialysis/CAPD: Administer 750 mg initial dose, followed by 500 mg every 48 hours
  Normal renal function dosing of 500 mg/day:
    Cl_{cr} 20-49 mL/minute: Administer 500 mg initial dose, followed by 250 mg every 24 hours
    Cl_{cr} 10-19 mL/minute: Administer 500 mg initial dose, followed by 250 mg every 48 hours
    Hemodialysis/CAPD: Administer 500 mg initial dose, followed by 250 mg every 48 hours
  Normal renal function dosing of 250 mg/day:
    Cl_{cr} 20-49 mL/minute: No dosage adjustment required
    Cl_{cr} 10-19 mL/minute: Administer 250 mg every 48 hours (except in uncomplicated UTI, where no dosage adjustment is required)
    Hemodialysis/CAPD: No information available
  CRRT: **Note:** Clearance dependent on filter type, flow rates, and other variables.
  CVVH/CVVHD/CVVHDF: Alternative recommendations exist:
    500 mg every 48 hours **or**
    250 mg every 24 hours (**Note:** This regimen has been shown to be equivalent to 500 mg/day in normal renal function. Appropriateness of this regimen for target dosing equal to 750 mg/day is not known.)

Stability

Solution for injection:
  Vial: Store at room temperature. Protect from light. When diluted to 5 mg/mL in a compatible I.V. fluid, solution is stable for 72 hours when stored at room temperature; stable for 14 days when stored under refrigeration. When frozen, stable for 6 months; do not refreeze. Do not thaw in microwave or by bath immersion.
  Premixed: Store at ≤25°C (77°F); do not freeze. Brief exposure to 40°C (104°F) does not affect product. Protect from light.
  Tablet, oral solution: Store at 25°C (77°F); excursions permitted to 15°C to 30°C (59°F to 86°F).
  Ophthalmic solution: Store at 15°C to 25°C (59°F to 77°F).

Administration

Oral: Tablets may be administered without regard to meals. Oral solution should be administered 1 hour before or 2 hours after meals. Maintain adequate hydration of patient to prevent crystalluria.
I.V.: Infuse 250-500 mg I.V. solution over 60 minutes; infuse 750 mg I.V. solution over 90 minutes. Too rapid of infusion can lead to hypotension. Avoid administration through an intravenous line with a solution containing multivalent cations (eg, magnesium, calcium). Maintain adequate hydration of patient to prevent crystalluria.

◄ **Monitoring Parameters** Evaluation of organ system functions (renal, hepatic, ophthalmologic, and hematopoietic) is recommended periodically during therapy; the possibility of crystalluria should be assessed; WBC and signs of infection

Pregnancy Risk Factor C

Contraindications Hypersensitivity to levofloxacin, any component of the formulation, or other quinolones

Warnings/Precautions

Systemic: [U.S. Boxed Warning]: There have been reports of tendon inflammation and/or rupture with quinolone antibiotics; risk may be increased with concurrent corticosteroids, organ transplant recipients, and in patients >60 years of age. Rupture of the Achilles tendon sometimes requiring surgical repair has been reported most frequently; but other tendon sites (eg, rotator cuff, biceps) have also been reported. Strenuous physical activity, rheumatoid arthritis, and renal impairment may be an independent risk factor for tendonitis. Discontinue at first sign of tendon inflammation or pain. May occur even after discontinuation of therapy. Use with caution in patients with rheumatoid arthritis; may increase risk of tendon rupture. Systemic use is only recommended in children <18 years of age for the prevention of inhalational anthrax (postexposure); increased incidence of musculoskeletal disorders (eg, arthralgia, tendon rupture) has been observed in children; CNS stimulation may occur (tremor, restlessness, confusion, and very rarely hallucinations or seizures). Potential for seizures, although very rare, may be increased with concomitant NSAID therapy. Use with caution in individuals at risk of seizures, with known or suspected CNS disorders or renal dysfunction. Avoid excessive sunlight and take precautions to limit exposure (eg, loose fitting clothing, sunscreen); may cause moderate-to-severe phototoxicity reactions. Discontinue use if photosensitivity occurs.

Rare cases of torsade de pointes have been reported in patients receiving levofloxacin. Use caution in patients with known prolongation of QT interval, bradycardia, hypokalemia, hypomagnesemia, or in those receiving concurrent therapy with Class Ia or Class III antiarrhythmics.

Severe hypersensitivity reactions, including anaphylaxis, have occurred with quinolone therapy. Reactions may present as typical allergic symptoms after a single dose, or may manifest as severe idiosyncratic dermatologic, vascular, pulmonary, renal, hepatic, and/or hematologic events, usually after multiple doses. Prompt discontinuation of drug should occur if skin rash or other symptoms arise. Prolonged use may result in fungal or bacterial superinfection, including *C. difficile*-associated diarrhea (CDAD) and pseudomembranous colitis; CDAD has been observed >2 months postantibiotic treatment. Peripheral neuropathies have been linked to levofloxacin use; discontinue if numbness, tingling, or weakness develops. Quinolones may exacerbate myasthenia gravis. Unrelated to hypersensitivity, severe hepatotoxicity (including acute hepatitis and fatalities) has been reported. Elderly patients may be at greater risk. Discontinue therapy immediately if signs and symptoms of hepatitis occur. Hemolytic reactions may (rarely) occur with quinolone use in patients with latent or actual G6PD deficiency.

Fluoroquinolones have been associated with the development of serious, and sometimes fatal, hypoglycemia, most often in elderly diabetics, but also in patients without diabetes. This occurred most frequently with gatifloxacin (no longer available systemically) but may occur at a lower frequency with other quinolones.

Ophthalmic solution: For topical use only. Do not inject subconjunctivally or introduce into anterior chamber of the eye. Contact lenses should not be worn during treatment for bacterial conjunctivitis. Safety and efficacy in children <1 year of age (Quixin®) or <6 years of age (Iquix®) have not been established. **Note:** Indications for ophthalmic solutions are product concentration-specific and should not be used interchangeably.

Adverse Reactions

1% to 10%:

Cardiovascular: Chest pain (1%), edema (1%)

Central nervous system: Headache (6%), insomnia (4%), dizziness (3%), fatigue (1%), pain (1%)

Dermatologic: Rash (2%), pruritus (1%)

Gastrointestinal: Taste disturbance (8% to 10% [ophthalmic]), nausea (7%), diarrhea (5%), constipation (3%), abdominal pain (2%), dyspepsia (2%), vomiting (2%)

Genitourinary: Vaginitis (1%)

Local: Injection site reaction (1%)

Ocular (with ophthalmic solution use): Decreased vision (transient), foreign body sensation, transient ocular burning, ocular pain or discomfort, photophobia

Respiratory: Pharyngitis (4%), dyspnea (1%)

Miscellaneous: Moniliasis (1%)

<1% (Limited to important or life-threatening):

Systemic: Acute renal failure, agitation, agranulocytosis; allergic reaction (including anaphylaxis, angioedema, pneumonitis rash, pneumonitis, and serum sickness); anaphylactoid reaction, arrhythmia (including atrial/ventricular tachycardia/fibrillation and torsade de pointes), aplastic anemia, arthralgia, ascites, bradycardia, bronchospasm, carcinoma, cardiac failure, cholecystitis, cholelithiasis, confusion, depression, EEG abnormalities, encephalopathy, eosinophilia, erythema multiforme, GI hemorrhage, granulocytopenia, hallucination, heart block, hemolytic anemia, hemoptysis, hepatic failure (some fatal), hepatitis, hyper-/hypoglycemia, hyperkalemia, hyperkinesias, hyper-/hypotension, infection, INR increased, intestinal obstruction, intracranial hypertension, involuntary muscle contractions, jaundice, leukocytosis, leukopenia, leukorrhea, lymphadenopathy, MI, migraine, multiple organ failure, myalgia, nephritis (interstitial), palpitation, pancreatitis, pancytopenia, paralysis, paresthesia, peripheral neuropathy, photosensitivity (<0.1%), pleural effusion, pneumonitis, postural hypotension, prothrombin time increased/decreased, pseudomembraneous colitis, psychosis, pulmonary edema, pulmonary embolism, purpura, QT_c prolongation, respiratory depression, rhabdomyolysis, seizure, skin disorder, somnolence, speech disorder, Stevens-Johnson syndrome, stupor, suicide attempt/ideation, syncope, tendonitis, tendon rupture, tongue edema, toxic epidermal necrolysis, transaminases increased, thrombocythemia, thrombocytopenia, tremor, urticaria, WBC abnormality

Ophthalmic solution: Allergic reaction, lid edema, ocular dryness, ocular itching

Drug Interactions

Avoid Concomitant Use

Avoid concomitant use of Levofloxacin with any of the following: Artemether; Dronedarone; Lumefantrine; Nilotinib; Pimozide; QuiNINE; Tetrabenazine; Thioridazine; Ziprasidone

Increased Effect/Toxicity

Levofloxacin may increase the levels/effects of: Corticosteroids (Systemic); Dronedarone; Pimozide; QTc-Prolonging Agents; QuiNINE; Sulfonylureas; Tetrabenazine; Thioridazine; Vitamin K Antagonists; Ziprasidone

The levels/effects of Levofloxacin may be increased by: Alfuzosin; Artemether; Chloroquine; Ciprofloxacin; Gadobutrol; Insulin; Lumefantrine; Nilotinib; Nonsteroidal Anti-Inflammatory Agents; Probenecid; QuiNINE

Decreased Effect

Levofloxacin may decrease the levels/effects of: Mycophenolate; Sulfonylureas; Typhoid Vaccine

The levels/effects of Levofloxacin may be decreased by: Antacids; Calcium Salts; Didanosine; Iron Salts; Magnesium Salts; Quinapril; Sevelamer; Sucralfate; Zinc Salts

Test Interactions Some quinolones may produce a false-positive urine screening result for opiates using commercially-available immunoassay kits. This has been demonstrated most consistently for levofloxacin and ofloxacin, but other quinolones have shown cross-reactivity in certain assay kits. Confirmation of positive opiate screens by more specific methods should be considered.

Dietary Considerations Tablets may be taken without regard to meals. Oral solution should be administered on an empty stomach (1 hour before or 2 hours after a meal). Take 2 hours before or 2 hours after multiple vitamins, antacids, or other products containing magnesium, aluminum, iron, or zinc.

Dosage Forms Excipient information presented when available (limited, particularly for generics); consult specific product labeling. [DSC] = Discontinued product

Infusion, premixed in D_5W [preservative free]:
Levaquin®: 250 mg (50 mL); 500 mg (100 mL); 750 mg (150 mL)
Injection, solution [preservative free]
Levaquin®: 25 mg/mL (20 mL, 30 mL)
Solution, ophthalmic [drops]:
Iquix®: 1.5% (5 mL)
Quixin®: 0.5% (5 mL) [contains benzalkonium chloride]
Solution, oral:
Levaquin®: 25 mg/mL (480 mL) [contains benzyl alcohol, propylene glycol]
Tablet, oral:
Levaquin®: 250 mg, 500 mg, 750 mg [DSC]
Levaquin® Leva-Pak: 750 mg (5s) [DSC]

References
American Thoracic Society and Infectious Diseases Society of America, "Guidelines for the Management of Adults With Hospital-Acquired, Ventilator-Associated, and Healthcare-Associated Pneumonia," *Am J Respir Crit Care Med*, 2005, 171(4):388-416.

Trotman RL, Williamson JC, Shoemaker DM, et al, "Antibiotic Dosing in Critically Ill Adult Patients Receiving Continuous Renal Replacement Therapy," *Clin Infect Dis*, 2005, 41(8):1159-66.

◆ **Levo-folinic Acid** *see* LEVOleucovorin *on page 828*

LEVOleucovorin (lee voe loo koe VOR in)

U.S. Brand Names Fusilev™
Index Terms 6S-leucovorin; Calcium Levoleucovorin; L-leucovorin; Levo-folinic Acid; Levo-leucovorin; Levoleucovorin Calcium Pentahydrate; S-leucovorin
Pharmacologic Category Antidote; Rescue Agent (Chemotherapy)
Use Rescue agent after high-dose methotrexate therapy in osteosarcoma; antidote for impaired methotrexate elimination and for inadvertent overdosage of folic acid antagonists
Unlabeled/Investigational Use Treatment of colorectal cancer (in combination with fluorouracil)
Pharmacodynamics/Kinetics
Metabolism: Converted to the active reduced form of folate, 5-methyl-tetrahydrofolate (5-methyl-THF; active)
Half-life elimination: 15 mg: 5-7 hours; 300 mg: elimination half life: 16-30 hours
Time to peak, serum: I.V.: 0.9 hours
Dosage Note: Levoleucovorin is dosed at **one-half** the usual dose of the racemic form (leucovorin calcium):
High-dose methotrexate rescue: Children and Adults: I.V.: Usual dose: 7.5 mg ($\sim$5 mg/m^2) every 6 hours for 10 doses, beginning 24 hours after the start of the methotrexate infusion (based on a methotrexate dose of 12 g/m^2 I.V. over 4 hours). Levoleucovorin (and hydration and urinary alkalinization) should be continued and/or adjusted until the methotrexate level is <0.05 micromolar (5 x 10^{-8} M) as follows:
Normal methotrexate elimination (serum methotrexate levels $\sim$10 micromolar at 24 hours post administration, 1 micromolar at 48 hours and <0.2 micromolar at 72 hours post infusion): 7.5 mg I.V. every 6 hours for 10 doses
Delayed late methotrexate elimination (serum methotrexate levels >0.2 micromolar at 72 hours and >0.05 micromolar at 96 hours post methotrexate infusion): Continue 7.5 mg I.V. every 6 hours until methotrexate level is <0.05 micromolar
Delayed early methotrexate elimination and/or evidence of acute renal injury (serum methotrexate level $\geq$50 micromolar at 24 hours, $\geq$5 micromolar at 48 hours or a doubling or more of the serum creatinine level at 24 hours post methotrexate infusion): 75 mg I.V. every 3 hours until methotrexate level is <1 micromolar, followed by 7.5 mg I.V. every 3 hours until methotrexate level is <0.05 micromolar
Significant clinical toxicity in the presence of less severe abnormalities in methotrexate elimination or renal function (as described above): Extend levoleucovorin treatment for an additional 24 hours (total of 14 doses) in subsequent treatment cycles.

Delayed methotrexate elimination due to third space fluid accumulation, renal insufficiency, or inadequate hydration: May require higher levoleucovorin doses or prolonged administration.

Methotrexate overdose (inadvertent): Children and Adults: I.V.: 7.5 mg (~5 mg/m^2) every 6 hours; continue until the methotrexate level is <0.01 micromolar (10^{-8} M). Initiate treatment as soon as possible after methotrexate overdose. Increase the levoleucovorin dose to 50 mg/m^2 I.V. every 3 hours if the 24 hour serum creatinine has increased 50% over baseline, or if the 24-hour methotrexate level is >5 micromolar (5 x 10^{-6} M), or if the 48-hour methotrexate level is >0.9 micromolar (9 x 10^{-7} M); continue levoleucovorin until the methotrexate level is <0.01 micromolar (10^{-8} M). Hydration (3 L/day) and urinary alkalinization (with sodium bicarbonate) should also be maintained.

Treatment of colorectal cancer (in combination with fluorouracil; unlabeled use): Adults: I.V.: Levoleucovorin is dosed at **one-half** the usual dose of the racemic form (leucovorin)

Additional Information Complete prescribing information for this medication should be consulted for additional detail.

Dosage Forms Excipient information presented when available (limited, particularly for generics); consult specific product labeling.

Note: Strength expressed as base.

Injection, powder for reconstitution:

Fusilev™: 50 mg

References

Comella P, De Vita F, Mancarella S, et al, "Biweekly Irinotecan or Raltitrexed Plus 6S-Leucovorin and Bolus 5-Fluorouracil in Advanced Colorectal Carcinoma: A Southern Italy Cooperative Oncology Group Phase II-III Randomized Trial," *Ann Oncol,* 2000, 11(10):1323-33.

Goorin A, Strother D, Poplack D, et al, "Safety and Efficacy of l-leucovorin Rescue Following High-Dose Methotrexate for Osteosarcoma," *Med Pediatr Oncol,* 1995, 24(6):362-7.

Hempel G, Lingg R, and Boos J, "Interactions of Carboxypeptidase G2 With 6S-Leucovorin and 6R-Leucovorin *in vitro*: Implications for the Application in Case of Methotrexate Intoxications," *Cancer Chemother Pharmacol,* 2005, 55(4):347-53.

Jaffe N, Jorgensen K, Robertson R, et al, "Substitution of l-leucovorin for d,l-leucovorin in the Rescue from High-Dose Methotrexate Treatment in Patients With Osteosarcoma," *Anticancer Drugs,* 1993, 4(5):559-64.

Labianca R, Cascinu S, Frontini L, et al, "High-Versus Low-Dose Levo-Leucovorin as a Modulator of 5-Fluorouracil in Advanced Colorectal Cancer: A 'GISCAD' Phase III Study," *Ann Oncol,* 1997, 8 (2):169-74.

Mader RM, Steger GG, Rizovsky B, et al, "Pharmacokinetics of Rac-Leucovorin vs [S]-Leucovorin in Patients With Advanced Gastrointestinal Cancer," *Br J Clin Pharmacol,* 1994, 37(3):243-8.

Scheithauer W, Kornek G, Marczell A, et al, "Fluorouracil Plus Racemic Leucovorin Versus Fluorouracil Combined With the Pure L-Isomer of Leucovorin for the Treatment of Advanced Colorectal Cancer: A Randomized Phase III Study," *J Clin Oncol,* 1997, 15(3):908-14.

Tournigand C, Cervantes A, Figer A, et al, "OPTIMOX1: A Randomized Study of FOLFOX4 or FOLFOX7 With Oxaliplatin in a Stop-and-Go Fashion in Advanced Colorectal Cancer–A GERCOR Study," *J Clin Oncol,* 2006, 24(3):394-400.

♦ **Levo-leucovorin** *see* LEVOleucovorin *on page 828*

♦ **Levoleucovorin Calcium Pentahydrate** *see* LEVOleucovorin *on page 828*

♦ **Levonorgestrel and Ethinyl Estradiol** *see* Ethinyl Estradiol and Levonorgestrel *on page 549*

♦ **Levophed®** *see* Norepinephrine *on page 1024*

♦ **Levora®** *see* Ethinyl Estradiol and Levonorgestrel *on page 549*

Levorphanol (lee VOR fa nole)

Medication Safety Issues

High alert medication: The Institute for Safe Medication Practices (ISMP) includes this medication among its list of drug classes which have a heightened risk of causing significant patient harm when used in error.

Related Information

Opioid Analgesics *on page 1688*

U.S. Brand Names Levo-Dromoran®

Index Terms Levorphan Tartrate; Levorphanol Tartrate

Pharmacologic Category Analgesic, Opioid

Restrictions C-II

Generic Available Yes: Tablet

◀ **Use** Relief of moderate-to-severe pain; preoperative sedation/analgesia; management of chronic pain (eg, cancer) requiring opoid therapy

Mechanism of Action Levorphanol tartrate is a synthetic opioid agonist that is
classified as a morphinan derivative. Opioids interact with stereospecific opioid
receptors in various parts of the central nervous system and other tissues.
Analgesic potency parallels the affinity for these binding sites. These drugs do not
alter the threshold or responsiveness to pain, but the perception of pain.

Pharmacodynamics/Kinetics

Onset of action: Oral: 10-60 minutes

Duration: 4-8 hours

Metabolism: Hepatic

Half-life elimination: 11-16 hours

Excretion: Urine (as inactive metabolite)

Dosage Adults: **Note:** These are guidelines and do not represent the maximum
doses that may be required in all patients. Doses should be titrated to pain relief/
prevention.

Acute pain (moderate-to-severe):

Oral: Initial: Opiate-naive: 2 mg every 6-8 hours as needed; patients with prior
opiate exposure may require higher initial doses; usual dosage range: 2-4 mg
every 6-8 hours as needed

Note: The American Pain Society recommends an initial dose of 2-4 mg for
severe pain in adults.

I.M., SubQ: Initial: Opiate-naive: 1 mg every 6-8 hours as needed; patients with
prior opiate exposure may require higher initial doses; usual dosage range:
1-2 mg every 6-8 hours as needed

Slow I.V.: Initial: Opiate-naive: Up to 1 mg/dose every 3-6 hours as needed;
patients with prior opiate exposure may require higher initial doses

Chronic pain: Patients taking opioids chronically may become tolerant and require
doses higher than the usual dosage range to maintain the desired effect.
Tolerance can be managed by appropriate dose titration. **There is no optimal or
maximal dose for levorphanol in chronic pain. The appropriate dose is one
that relieves pain throughout its dosing interval without causing
unmanageable side effects.**

Premedication: I.M., SubQ: 1-2 mg/dose 60-90 minutes prior to surgery; older or
debilitated patients usually require less drug

Dosing adjustment in hepatic disease: Reduction is necessary in patients with
liver disease

Stability Store at room temperature; do not freeze.

Administration I.V.: Inject 3 mg over 4-5 minutes

Monitoring Parameters Pain relief, respiratory and mental status, blood
pressure

Pregnancy Risk Factor B/D (prolonged use or high doses at term)

Contraindications Hypersensitivity to levorphanol or any component of the
formulation; pregnancy (prolonged use or high doses at term)

Warnings/Precautions An opioid-containing analgesic regimen should be
tailored to each patient's needs and based upon the type of pain being treated
(acute versus chronic), the route of administration, degree of tolerance for opioids
(naive versus chronic user), age, weight, and medical condition. The optimal
analgesic dose varies widely among patients. Doses should be titrated to pain
relief/prevention.

May cause CNS depression, which may impair physical or mental abilities;
patients must be cautioned about performing tasks which require mental alertness
(eg, operating machinery or driving). Effects may be potentiated when used with
other sedative drugs or ethanol. Use with caution in patients with hypersensitivity
reactions to other phenanthrene derivative opioid agonists (morphine, hydrocodone, hydromorphone, oxycodone, oxymorphone); respiratory diseases
including asthma, emphysema, COPD, hypothyroidism, head trauma, morbid
obesity, adrenal insufficiency, prostatic hyperplasia/urinary stricture, or severe
liver or renal insufficiency. Use with caution in patients with biliary tract
dysfunction; acute pancreatitis may cause constriction of sphincter of Oddi.
Some preparations contain sulfites which may cause allergic reactions. May be
habit-forming. May cause hypotension; use with caution in patients with depleted
blood volume or drugs which may exaggerate hypotensive effects (including

phenothiazines or general anesthetics). May obscure diagnosis or clinical course of patients with acute abdominal conditions. Concurrent use of agonist/antagonist analgesics may precipitate withdrawal symptoms and/or reduced analgesic efficacy in patients following prolonged therapy with mu opioid agonists. Abrupt discontinuation following prolonged use may also lead to withdrawal symptoms. Elderly and debilitated patients may be particularly susceptible to the adverse effects of narcotics. Safety and efficacy have not been established in children.

Adverse Reactions Frequency not defined.

Cardiovascular: Palpitation, hypotension, bradycardia, peripheral vasodilation, cardiac arrest, shock, tachycardia

Central nervous system: CNS depression, fatigue, drowsiness, dizziness, nervousness, headache, restlessness, anorexia, malaise, confusion, coma, convulsion, insomnia, amnesia, mental depression, hallucinations, paradoxical CNS stimulation, intracranial pressure increased

Dermatologic: Pruritus, urticaria, rash

Endocrine & metabolic: Antidiuretic hormone release

Gastrointestinal: Nausea, vomiting, dyspepsia, stomach cramps, xerostomia, constipation, abdominal pain, dry mouth, biliary tract spasm, paralytic ileus

Genitourinary: Decreased urination, urinary tract spasm, urinary retention

Local: Pain at injection site

Neuromuscular & skeletal: Weakness

Ocular: Miosis, diplopia

Respiratory: Respiratory depression, apnea, hypoventilation, cyanosis

Miscellaneous: Histamine release, physical and psychological dependence

Drug Interactions

Avoid Concomitant Use There are no known interactions where it is recommended to avoid concomitant use.

Increased Effect/Toxicity

Levorphanol may increase the levels/effects of: Alcohol (Ethyl); Alvimopan; CNS Depressants; Desmopressin; Selective Serotonin Reuptake Inhibitors; Thiazide Diuretics

The levels/effects of Levorphanol may be increased by: Amphetamines; Antipsychotic Agents (Phenothiazines); Succinylcholine

Decreased Effect

Levorphanol may decrease the levels/effects of: Pegvisomant

The levels/effects of Levorphanol may be decreased by: Ammonium Chloride

Ethanol/Nutrition/Herb Interactions

Ethanol: Avoid or limit ethanol (may increase CNS depression). Watch for sedation.

Herb/Nutraceutical: Avoid valerian, St John's wort, kava kava, gotu kola (may increase CNS depression).

Dosage Forms Excipient information presented when available (limited, particularly for generics); consult specific product labeling.

Injection, solution, as tartrate:
Levo-Dromoran®: 2 mg/mL (1 mL, 10 mL)
Tablet, as tartrate: 2 mg

References

Mokhlesi B, Leikin JB, Murray P, et al, "Adult Toxicology in Critical Care: Part II: Specific Poisonings," *Chest*, 2003, 123(3):897-922.

◆ **Levorphanol Tartrate** *see* Levorphanol *on page 829*

◆ **Levorphan Tartrate** *see* Levorphanol *on page 829*

◆ **Levothroid®** *see* Levothyroxine *on page 831*

Levothyroxine (lee voe thye ROKS een)

Medication Safety Issues

Sound-alike/look-alike issues:

Levothyroxine may be confused with lamoTRIgine, Lanoxin®, levofloxacin, liothyronine

Levoxyl® may be confused with Lanoxin®, Levaquin®, Luvox®

Synthroid® may be confused with Symmetrel®

◄ To avoid errors due to misinterpretation of a decimal point, always express dosage in mcg (**not** mg).

Significant differences exist between oral and I.V. dosing. Use caution when converting from one route of administration to another.

U.S. Brand Names Levothroid®; Levoxyl®; Synthroid®; Unithroid®

Canadian Brand Names Eltroxin®; Euthyrox; Levothyroxine Sodium; Synthroid®

Index Terms *L*-Thyroxine Sodium; Levothyroxine Sodium; T_4

Pharmacologic Category Thyroid Product

Generic Available Yes

Use Replacement or supplemental therapy in hypothyroidism; pituitary TSH suppression

Unlabeled/Investigational Use Management of hemodynamically unstable potential organ donors increasing the quantity of organs available for transplantation

Mechanism of Action Levothyroxine (T_4) is a synthetic form of thyroxine, an endogenous hormone secreted by the thyroid gland. T_4 is converted to its active metabolite, L-triiodothyronine (T_3). Thyroid hormones (T_4 and T_3) then bind to thyroid receptor proteins in the cell nucleus and exert metabolic effects through control of DNA transcription and protein synthesis; involved in normal metabolism, growth, and development; promotes gluconeogenesis, increases utilization and mobilization of glycogen stores, and stimulates protein synthesis, increases basal metabolic rate

Pharmacodynamics/Kinetics

Onset of action: Therapeutic: Oral: 3-5 days; I.V. 6-8 hours
Peak effect: I.V.: 24 hours

Absorption: Oral: Erratic (40% to 80%); may be decreased by age and specific foods and drugs

Protein binding: >99% bound to plasma proteins including thyroxine-binding globulin, thyroxine-binding prealbumin, and albumin

Metabolism: Hepatic to triiodothyronine (active); T_4 deiodination in kidney and periphery; glucuronidation/conjugation also occurs; undergoes enterohepatic recirculation

Time to peak, serum: 2-4 hours

Half-life elimination: Euthyroid: 6-7 days; Hypothyroid: 9-10 days; Hyperthyroid: 3-4 days

Excretion: Urine (major route of elimination; decreases with age); feces (~20%)

Dosage Doses should be adjusted based on clinical response and laboratory parameters.

Oral:

Neonates, Infants, and Children: Hypothyroidism: Daily dosage based on body weight and age as listed below:

0-3 months: 10-15 mcg/kg/day; if the infant is at risk for development of cardiac failure, use a lower starting dose of 25 mcg/day; if the initial serum T_4 is very low (<5 mcg/dL) begin treatment at a higher dosage of 50 mcg/day

3-6 months: 8-10 mcg/kg/day **or** 25-50 mcg/day

6-12 months: 6-8 mcg/kg/day **or** 50-75 mcg/day

1-5 years: 5-6 mcg/kg/day **or** 75-100 mcg/day

6-12 years: 4-5 mcg/kg/day **or** 100-125 mcg/day

>12 years: 2-3 mcg/kg/day **or** ≥150 mcg/day

Growth and puberty complete: 1.7 mcg/kg/day; refer to Adult dosing.

Dosing modifications:

Hyperactivity in older children may be minimized by starting at 1/4 of the recommended dose and increasing each week by that amount until the full dose is achieved (4 weeks).

Children with severe or chronic hypothyroidism should be started at 25 mcg/day; adjust dose by 25 mcg every 2-4 weeks.

Adults (including children in whom growth and puberty are complete, healthy adults <50 years of age, and older adults who have been recently treated for hyperthyroidism or who have been hypothyroid for only a few months):

Hypothyroidism: ~1.7 mcg/kg/day; usual doses are ≤200 mcg/day (range: 100-125 mcg/day [70 kg adult]); doses ≥300 mcg/day are rare (consider poor compliance, malabsorption, and/or drug interactions). Titrate dose every 6 weeks.

Patients >50 years or patients with cardiac disease: Refer to Elderly dosing.

Severe hypothyroidism: Initial: 12.5-25 mcg/day; adjust dose by 25 mcg/day every 2-4 weeks as appropriate

Myxedema: Oral agents are not recommended for myxedema: Refer to I.V. dosing.

Subclinical hypothyroidism (if treated): 1 mcg/kg/day

TSH suppression:

Well-differentiated thyroid cancer: Highly individualized; Doses >2 mcg/kg/day may be needed to suppress TSH to <0.1 mIU/mL. High-risk tumors may need a target level of <0.01 mIU/mL for TSH suppression.

Benign nodules and nontoxic multinodular goiter: Routine use of T_4 for TSH suppression is not recommended in patients with benign thyroid nodules. In patients deemed appropriate candidates, treatment should never be fully suppressive (TSH <0.1 mIU/mL) (Gharib, 2006; Cooper, 2006). **Note:** Avoid use if TSH is already suppressed.

Elderly: Hypothyroidism (elderly patients may require <1 mcg/kg/day):

>50 years without cardiac disease **or** <50 years with cardiac disease: Initial: 25-50 mcg/day; adjust dose by 12.5-25 mcg increments at 6- to 8-week intervals as needed

>50 years with cardiac disease: Initial: 12.5-25 mcg/day; adjust dose by 12.5-25 mcg increments at 4- to 6-week intervals (many clinicians prefer to adjust at 6- to 8-week intervals)

Note: Patients with combined hypothyroidism and cardiac disease should be monitored carefully for changes in stability.

I.M., I.V.: Children, Adults, Elderly: Hypothyroidism: 50% of the oral dose

I.V.:

Adults: Myxedema coma or stupor: 200-500 mcg, then 100-300 mcg the next day if necessary; smaller doses should be considered in patients with cardiovascular disease

Elderly: Myxedema coma: Refer to adult dosing; lower doses may be needed

Stability

Tablet: Store at room temperature of 15°C to 30°C (59°F to 86°F). Protect from light and moisture.

Injection: Store at room temperature of 15°C to 30°C (59°F to 86°F). Dilute vials for injection with 5 mL normal saline. Reconstituted concentrations for the 200 mcg and 500 mcg vials are 40 mcg/mL and 100 mcg/mL, respectively. Shake well and use immediately after reconstitution (manufacturer recommendation); discard any unused portions.

Additional stability data: Stability in polypropylene syringes (100 mcg/mL in NS) at 5°C ± 1°C is 7 days (Gupta, 2000).

Administration

Oral: Administer in the morning on an empty stomach, at least 30 minutes before food. Tablets may be crushed and suspended in 1-2 teaspoonfuls of water; suspension should be used immediately. Levoxyl® should be administered with a full glass of water to prevent gagging (due to tablet swelling).

Parenteral: Dilute vial with 5 mL normal saline; use immediately after reconstitution; should not be admixed with other solutions

Monitoring Parameters Thyroid function test (serum thyroxine, thyrotropin concentrations), resin triiodothyronine uptake (rT_3U), free thyroxine index (FTI), T_4, TSH, heart rate, blood pressure, clinical signs of hypo- and hyperthyroidism; TSH is the most reliable guide for evaluating adequacy of thyroid replacement dosage. TSH may be elevated during the first few months of thyroid replacement despite patients being clinically euthyroid. In cases where T_4 remains low and TSH is within normal limits, an evaluation of "free" (unbound) T_4 is needed to evaluate further increase in dosage

Infants: Monitor closely for cardiac overload, arrhythmias, and aspiration from avid suckling

Infants/children: Monitor closely for under/overtreatment. Undertreatment may decrease intellectual development and linear growth, and lead to poor school performance due to impaired concentration and slowed mentation. Overtreatment may adversely affect brain maturation, accelerate bone age (leading to premature ▶

closure of the epiphyses and reduced adult height); craniosynostosis has been reported in infants. Treated children may experience a period of catch-up growth. Monitor TSH and total or free T_4 at 2 and 4 weeks after starting treatment; every 1-2 months for first year of life; every 2-3 months during years 1-3; every 3-12 months until growth completed. Perform routine clinical examinations at regular intervals (to assess mental and physical growth and development).

Adults: Monitor TSH every 6-8 weeks until normalized; 8-12 weeks after dosage changes; every 6-12 months throughout therapy

Reference Range Pediatrics: Cord T_4 and values in the first few weeks are much higher, falling over the first months and years. ≥10 years: ~5.8-11 mcg/dL (SI: 75-142 nmol/L). Borderline low: ≤4.5-5.7 mcg/dL (SI: 58-73 nmol/L); low: ≤4.4 mcg/dL (SI: 57 nmol/L); results <2.5 mcg/dL (SI: <32 nmol/L) are strong evidence for hypothyroidism.

Approximate adult normal range: 4-12 mcg/dL (SI: 51-154 nmol/L). Borderline high: 11.1-13 mcg/dL (SI: 143-167 nmol/L); high: ≥13.1 mcg/dL (SI: 169 nmol/L). Normal range is increased in women on birth control pills (5.5-12 mcg/dL); normal range in pregnancy: ~5.5-16 mcg/dL (SI: ~71-206 nmol/L). TSH: 0.4-10 (for those ≥80 years) mIU/L; T_4: 4-12 mcg/dL (SI: 51-154 nmol/L); T_3 (RIA) (total T_3): 80-230 ng/dL (SI: 1.2-3.5 nmol/L); T_4 free (free T_4): 0.7-1.8 ng/dL (SI: 9-23 pmol/L).

Anesthesia and Critical Care Concerns/Other Considerations

Clinical Pearls/Comments: Equivalent doses: The following statement on relative potency of thyroid products is included in a joint statement by American Thyroid Association (ATA), American Association of Clinical Endocrinologists (AACE), and The Endocrine Society (TES): For purposes of conversion, levothyroxine sodium (T_4) 100 mcg is usually considered equivalent to desiccated thyroid 60 mg, thyroglobulin 60 mg, or liothyronine sodium (T_3) 25 mcg. However, these are rough guidelines only and do not obviate the careful re-evaluation of a patient when switching thyroid hormone preparations, including a change from one brand of levothyroxine to another. Joint position statement is available at http://www.thyroid.org/professionals/advocacy/04_12_08_thyroxine.html.

Note: Several medications have effects on thyroid production or conversion. The impact in thyroid replacement has not been specifically evaluated, but patient response should be monitored:
   Antithyroid agents: Methimazole decreases thyroid hormone secretion, while propylthiouracil decreases thyroid hormone secretion and conversion of T_4 to T_3.
   Beta-adrenergic antagonists: Decrease conversion of T_4 to T_3 (dose related, propranolol ≥160 mg/day); patients may be clinically euthyroid.
   Iodide, iodine-containing radiographic contrast agents may decrease thyroid hormone secretion; may also increase thyroid hormone secretion, especially in patients with Graves' disease.

Other agents reported to impact on thyroid production/conversion include aminoglutethimide, amiodarone, chloral hydrate, diazepam, ethionamide, interferon-alpha, interleukin-2, lithium, lovastatin (case report), glucocorticoids (dose-related), mercaptopurine, sulfonamides, thiazide diuretics, and tolbutamide.

In addition, a number of medications have been noted to cause transient depression in TSH secretion, which may complicate interpretation of monitoring tests for levothyroxine, including corticosteroids, octreotide, and dopamine. Metoclopramide may increase TSH secretion.

Soy protein may interfere with absorption of levothyroxine sodium. An enteral formula without soy protein should be selected and thyroid function monitored during tube feeding.

Evidence-Based Information: Cadaveric organ donation: Hemodynamically unstable donors: Hormonal resuscitation: Intravenous levothyroxine (20 mcg bolus followed by 10 mcg/hour) given concomitantly with an ampule of 50% dextrose, 2 grams of methylprednisolone sodium succinate, and 20 units of regular insulin has been successfully used in hemodynamically unstable brain-dead donors to increase the quantity and quality of organs available for transplantation (Salim, 2007). Another protocol using liothyronine (T_3) has been used with success (Rosendale, 2003; Rosengard, 2002). Of note, stability of further diluted injectable levothyroxine (after reconstitution) and liothyronine solutions has not been adequately studied.

Pregnancy Risk Factor A

Contraindications Hypersensitivity to levothyroxine sodium or any component of the formulation; acute MI; thyrotoxicosis of any etiology; uncorrected adrenal insufficiency

Warnings/Precautions [U.S. Boxed Warning]: Thyroid supplements are ineffective and potentially toxic when used for the treatment of obesity or for weight reduction, especially in euthyroid patients. High doses may produce serious or even life-threatening toxic effects particularly when used with some anorectic drugs (eg, sympathomimetic amines). Routine use of T_4 for TSH suppression is not recommended in patients with benign thyroid nodules. In patients deemed appropriate candidates, treatment should never be fully suppressive (TSH <0.1 mIU/mL). Use with caution and reduce dosage in patients with angina pectoris or other cardiovascular disease; decrease initial dose. Use cautiously in the elderly since they may be more likely to have compromised cardiovascular functions. Patients with adrenal insufficiency, myxedema, diabetes mellitus and insipidus may have symptoms exaggerated or aggravated. Chronic hypothyroidism predisposes patients to coronary artery disease. Long-term therapy can decrease bone mineral density. Levoxyl® may rapidly swell and disintegrate causing choking or gagging (should be administered with a full glass of water); use caution in patients with dysphagia or other swallowing disorders.

Adverse Reactions Frequency not defined.

Cardiovascular: Angina, arrhythmia, cardiac arrest, flushing, heart failure, hypertension, MI, palpitation, pulse increased, tachycardia

Central nervous system: Anxiety, emotional lability, fatigue, fever, headache, hyperactivity, insomnia, irritability, nervousness, pseudotumor cerebri (children), seizure (rare)

Dermatologic: Alopecia

Endocrine & metabolic: Fertility impaired, menstrual irregularities

Gastrointestinal: Abdominal cramps, appetite increased, diarrhea, vomiting, weight loss

Hepatic: Liver function tests increased

Neuromuscular & skeletal: Bone mineral density decreased, muscle weakness, tremor, slipped capital femoral epiphysis (children)

Respiratory: Dyspnea

Miscellaneous: Diaphoresis, heat intolerance, hypersensitivity (to inactive ingredients, symptoms include urticaria, pruritus, rash, flushing, angioedema, GI symptoms, fever, arthralgia, serum sickness, wheezing)

Levoxyl®: Choking, dysphagia, gagging

Drug Interactions

Avoid Concomitant Use

Avoid concomitant use of Levothyroxine with any of the following: Sodium Iodide I131

Increased Effect/Toxicity

Levothyroxine may increase the levels/effects of: Vitamin K Antagonists

Decreased Effect

Levothyroxine may decrease the levels/effects of: Sodium Iodide I131; Theophylline Derivatives

The levels/effects of Levothyroxine may be decreased by: Bile Acid Sequestrants; Calcium Salts; CarBAMazepine; Estrogen Derivatives; Iron Salts; Orlistat; Phenytoin; Raloxifene; Rifampin; Sevelamer; Sucralfate

Ethanol/Nutrition/Herb Interactions Food: Taking levothyroxine with enteral nutrition may cause reduced bioavailability and may lower serum thyroxine levels leading to signs or symptoms of hypothyroidism. Soybean flour (infant formula), cottonseed meal, walnuts, and dietary fiber may decrease absorption of levothyroxine from the GI tract.

Test Interactions Many drugs may have effects on thyroid function tests. Pregnancy, infectious hepatitis, and acute intermittent porphyria may increase TBG concentrations; nephrosis, severe hypoproteinemia, severe liver disease, and acromegaly may decrease TBG concentrations.

Dietary Considerations Should be taken on an empty stomach, at least 30 minutes before food.

◄ **Dosage Forms** Excipient information presented when available (limited, particularly for generics); consult specific product labeling.

Injection, powder for reconstitution, as sodium: 0.2 mg, 0.5 mg

Tablet, as sodium: 25 mcg, 50 mcg, 75 mcg, 88 mcg, 100 mcg, 112 mcg, 125 mcg, 137 mcg, 150 mcg, 175 mcg, 200 mcg, 300 mcg

Levothroid®: 25 mcg, 75 mcg, 88 mcg, 100 mcg, 112 mcg, 125 mcg, 137 mcg, 150 mcg, 175 mcg, 200 mcg, 300 mcg [scored]

Levothroid®: 50 mcg [scored; dye free]

Levoxyl®: 25 mcg, 75 mcg, 88 mcg, 100 mcg, 112 mcg, 125 mcg, 137 mcg, 150 mcg, 175 mcg, 200 mcg [scored]

Levoxyl®: 50 mcg [scored; dye free]

Synthroid®: 25 mcg, 75 mcg, 88 mcg, 100 mcg, 112 mcg, 125 mcg, 137 mcg, 150 mcg, 175 mcg, 200 mcg, 300 mcg [scored]

Synthroid®: 50 mcg [scored; dye free]

Unithroid®: 25 mcg, 75 mcg, 88 mcg, 100 mcg, 112 mcg, 125 mcg, 150 mcg, 175 mcg, 200 mcg, 300 mcg [scored]

Unithroid®: 50 mcg [scored; dye free]

References
Gupta VD, "Stability of Levothyroxine Sodium Injection in Polypropylene Syringes," *Int J Pharm Compound*, 2000, 4(6):482-3.

Rosendale JD, Kauffman HM, McBride MA, et al, "Aggressive Pharmacologic Donor Management Results in More Transplanted Organs," *Transplantation*, 2003, 75(4):482-7.

Rosengard BR, Feng S, Alfrey EJ, et al, "Report of the Crystal City Meeting to Maximize the Use of Organs Recovered From the Cadaver Donor," *Am J Transplant*, 2002, 2(8):701-11.

Salim A, Martin M, Brown C, et al, "Using Thyroid Hormone in Brain-Dead Donors to Maximize the Number of Organs Available for Transplantation," *Clin Transplant*, 2007, 21(3):405-9.

♦ **Levothyroxine Sodium** see Levothyroxine on page 831

♦ **Levoxyl®** see Levothyroxine on page 831

♦ **Lexapro®** see Escitalopram on page 521

♦ **Lialda™** see Mesalamine on page 884

♦ **Librium®** see ChlordiazePOXIDE on page 290

♦ **LidaMantle®** see Lidocaine on page 836

Lidocaine (LYE doe kane)

Medication Safety Issues

High alert medication: The Institute for Safe Medication Practices (ISMP) includes this medication (epidural administration; I.V. formulation) among its list of drugs which have a heightened risk of causing significant patient harm when used in error.

Transdermal patch may contain conducting metal (eg, aluminum); remove patch prior to MRI.

International issues:

Lidpen® may be confused with Linoten® which is a brand name for pamidronate in Spain

Related Information

Acute Postoperative Pain on page 1502

Anesthesia Considerations for Neurosurgery on page 1514

Anesthesia for Obstetric Patients in Nonobstetric Surgery on page 1532

Anesthesia for Patients With Liver Disease on page 1537

Antiarrhythmic Drugs on page 1656

Chronic Pain Management on page 1546

Dosing Considerations for the Critically-Ill Patient With Morbid Obesity on page 1561

Local Anesthetics on page 1636

Management of Postoperative Arrhythmias on page 1571

U.S. Brand Names Akten™; Anestacon®; Anestafoam™ [OTC]; Band-Aid® Hurt-Free™ Antiseptic Wash [OTC]; Burn Jel® [OTC]; Burn-O-Jel® [OTC]; BurnaMycin [OTC]; L-M-X™ 4 [OTC]; L-M-X™ 5 [OTC]; LidaMantle®; Lidoderm®; LTA® 360; Premjact® [OTC]; Solarcaine® Aloe Extra Burn Relief [OTC]; Topicaine® [OTC]; Unburn®; Xylocaine®; Xylocaine® Dental; Xylocaine® MPF; Xylocaine® Viscous; Zilactin-L® [OTC]; Zingo™ [DSC]

Canadian Brand Names Betacaine®; Lidodan™; Lidoderm®; Xylocaine®; Xylocard®; Zilactin®

Index Terms Lidocaine Hydrochloride; Lignocaine Hydrochloride

Pharmacologic Category Analgesic, Topical; Antiarrhythmic Agent, Class Ib; Local Anesthetic; Local Anesthetic, Ophthalmic

Generic Available Yes: Cream, infusion, injection, jelly, lotion, ointment, solution

Use Local and regional anesthesia by infiltration, nerve block, epidural, or spinal techniques; acute treatment of ventricular arrhythmias from myocardial infarction or cardiac manipulation

Ophthalmic: To provide local anesthesia to ocular surface during ophthalmologic procedures

Rectal: Temporary relief of pain and itching due to anorectal disorders

Topical: Local anesthetic for oral muscous membrane; use in laser/cosmetic surgeries; minor burns, cuts, and abrasions of the skin

Lidoderm® Patch: Relief of allodynia (painful hypersensitivity) and chronic pain in postherpetic neuralgia

Unlabeled/Investigational Use ACLS guidelines (not considered drug of choice): Stable monomorphic VT (preserved ventricular function), polymorphic VT (preserved ventricular function), drug-induced monomorphic VT; I.V. infusion for chronic pain syndrome

Mechanism of Action Class Ib antiarrhythmic; suppresses automaticity of conduction tissue, by increasing electrical stimulation threshold of ventricle, His-Purkinje system, and spontaneous depolarization of the ventricles during diastole by a direct action on the tissues; blocks both the initiation and conduction of nerve impulses by decreasing the neuronal membrane's permeability to sodium ions, which results in inhibition of depolarization with resultant blockade of conduction

Pharmacodynamics/Kinetics

Onset of action: Single bolus dose: 45-90 seconds; Ophthalmic: 20 seconds to 5 minutes (median: 40 seconds)

Duration: 10-20 minutes; Ophthalmic: 5-30 minutes (median: 15 minutes)

Distribution: V_d: 1.1-2.1 L/kg; alterable by many patient factors; decreased in CHF and liver disease; crosses blood-brain barrier

Protein binding: 60% to 80% to alpha$_1$ acid glycoprotein

Metabolism: 90% hepatic; active metabolites monoethylglycinexylidide (MEGX) and glycinexylidide (GX) can accumulate and may cause CNS toxicity

Half-life elimination: Biphasic: Prolonged with congestive heart failure, liver disease, shock, severe renal disease; Initial: 7-30 minutes; Terminal: Infants, premature: 3.2 hours, Adults: 1.5-2 hours

Excretion: Urine (<10% as unchanged drug, ~90% as metabolites)

Dosage

Antiarrhythmic:

Children:

I.V., I.O.: **Note:** For use in pulseless VT or VF, give after defibrillation, CPR, and epinephrine:

Loading dose: 1 mg/kg (maximum 100 mg); follow with continuous infusion; may administer second bolus of 0.5-1 mg/kg if delay between bolus and start of infusion is >15 minutes

Continuous infusion: 20-50 mcg/kg/minute. Use 20 mcg/kg/minute in patients with shock, hepatic disease, cardiac arrest, mild CHF; moderate-to-severe CHF may require 1/2 loading dose and lower infusion rates to avoid toxicity.

E.T.: 2-3 mg/kg; flush with 5 mL of NS and follow with 5 assisted manual ventilations

Adults:

Ventricular fibrillation or pulseless ventricular tachycardia (after defibrillation, CPR, and vasopressor administration): I.V.: Initial: 1-1.5 mg/kg. Refractory ventricular tachycardia or ventricular fibrillation, a repeat 0.5-0.75 mg/kg bolus may be given every 5-10 minutes after initial dose for a maximum of 3 doses. Total dose should not exceed 3 mg/kg. Follow with continuous infusion (1-4 mg/minute) after return of perfusion. Reappearance of arrhythmia during constant infusion: 0.5 mg/kg bolus and reassessment of infusion.

E.T. (loading dose only): 2-2.5 times the recommended I.V. dose; dilute in 10 mL NS or distilled water. **Note:** Absorption is greater with distilled water, but causes more adverse effects on PaO_2.

◄ Hemodynamically stable VT: 0.5-0.75 mg/kg followed by synchronized cardioversion

Note: Decrease dose in patients with CHF, shock, or hepatic disease.

Anesthetic, local injectable: Children and Adults: Varies with procedure, degree of anesthesia needed, vascularity of tissue, duration of anesthesia required, and physical condition of patient; maximum: 4.5 mg/kg/dose; do not repeat within 2 hours.

Anesthesia, ocular: Children and Adults: Apply 2 drops to ocular surface in area where procedure will occur; may reapply to maintain effect.

Anesthesia, topical: Unless otherwise noted, the following traditional pediatric guideline for topical lidocaine dosage may be observed: Apply to affected area as needed; maximum dose: 3 mg/kg/dose; do not repeat within 2 hours (Benitz, 1988)

Cream:

LidaMantle®: Skin irritation: Children and Adults: Apply to affected area 2-3 times/day as needed

L-M-X™ 4: Children ≥2 years and Adults: Apply 1/4 inch thick layer to intact skin. Leave on until adequate anesthetic effect is obtained. Remove cream and cleanse area before beginning procedure.

L-M-X™ 5: Relief of anorectal pain and itching: Children ≥12 years and Adults: Rectal: Apply topically to clean, dry area **or** using applicator, insert rectally, up to 6 times/day

Gel, ointment, solution: Adults: Apply to affected area ≤3 times/day as needed (maximum dose: 4.5 mg/kg, not to exceed 300 mg)

Jelly:

Children ≥10 years: Dose varies with age and weight (maximum dose: 4.5 mg/kg)

Adults (maximum dose: 30 mL [600 mg] in any 12-hour period):

Anesthesia of male urethra: 5-30 mL

Anesthesia of female urethra: 3-5 mL

Lubrication of endotracheal tube: Apply a moderate amount to external surface only

Liquid: Cold sores and fever blisters: Children ≥5 years and Adults: Apply to affected area every 6 hours as needed

Patch: Postherpetic neuralgia: Adults: Apply patch to most painful area. Up to 3 patches may be applied in a single application. Patch may remain in place for up to 12 hours in any 24-hour period.

Dosage adjustment in renal impairment: Not dialyzable (0% to 5%) by hemo- or peritoneal dialysis; supplemental dose is not necessary.

Dosage adjustment in hepatic impairment: Reduce dose in acute hepatitis and decompensated cirrhosis by 50%.

Stability

Injection: Stable at room temperature. Stability of parenteral admixture at room temperature (25°C) is the expiration date on premixed bag; out of overwrap stability is 30 days.

Standard concentration/diluent: 2 g/250 mL D_5W.

Ophthalmic: Store at 15°C to 25°C (59°F to 77°F). Protect from light. Discard after use.

Administration

Endotracheal: Dilute in NS or distilled water. Absorption is greater with distilled water, but causes more adverse effects on PaO_2. Pass catheter beyond tip of tracheal tube, stop compressions, spray drug quickly down tube. Follow immediately with several quick insufflations and continue chest compressions.

I.V.: Use microdrip (60 gtt/mL) or infusion pump to administer an accurate dose

Infusion rates: 2 g/250 mL D_5W (infusion pump should be used):

1 mg/minute: 7.5 mL/hour

2 mg/minute: 15 mL/hour

3 mg/minute: 22.5 mL/hour

4 mg/minute: 30 mL/hour

Buffered lidocaine for injectable local anesthetic: Add 2 mL of sodium bicarbonate 8.4% to 18 mL of lidocaine 1%

Topical:
Gel (Topicaine®): Avoid mucous membranes; remove prior to laser treatment.
Transdermal: Apply to painful area of skin immediately after removal from protective envelope. May be cut to appropriate size. After removal from skin, fold used transdermal systems so the adhesive side sticks to itself. Remove immediately if burning sensation occurs. Wash hands after application.

Reference Range
Therapeutic: 1.5-5.0 mcg/mL (SI: 6-21 μmol/L)
Potentially toxic: >6 mcg/mL (SI: >26 μmol/L)
Toxic: >9 mcg/mL (SI: >38 μmol/L)

Anesthesia and Critical Care Concerns/Other Considerations
Cardiac Arrest: In out-of-hospital cardiac arrest victims, lidocaine is not as effective as amiodarone for improving intermediate outcomes, but neither has improved survival to hospital discharge among patients with shock-resistant VF cardiac arrest (Dorian, 2002).

Monitoring: Toxic effects of lidocaine may appear earlier in the elderly and in patients with heart failure, shock, or hepatic disease. The half-life of lidocaine increases after 24-48 hours as the drug inhibits its own hepatic metabolism. The dose should be reduced after 24 hours or blood levels should be monitored. Lidocaine toxicity may elicit seizures, respiratory arrest, and cardiac toxicity (eg, sinus arrest, AV block, asystole, and hypotension).

Local anesthetic toxicity: Cardiac arrest: Lipid infusion has been used in animal studies and several human cases (*Bupivacaine:* Rosenblatt, 2006; *Levobupivacaine:* Foxall, 2007; *Ropivacaine:* Litz, 2006) where cardiovascular toxicity, unresponsive to conventional resuscitation, resulted. Additional information is available at http://www.lipidrescue.org. The protocol from the website is: 20% Fat Emulsion: 1.5 mL/kg administered over 1 minute, followed immediately by an infusion of 0.25 mL/kg/minute. Continue chest compressions (lipid must circulate). Repeat bolus every 3-5 minutes up to 3 mL/kg total dose until circulation restored. Continue infusion until hemodynamic stability is restored. Increase the infusion rate to 0.5 mL/kg/minute if BP declines. A maximum total dose of 8 mL/kg is recommended.

Administration issue: The On-Q® infusion pump is used to slowly administer local anesthetics (eg, bupivacaine, lidocaine, ropivacaine) to or around surgical wound sites and/or in close proximity to nerves for pre- or postoperative regional anesthesia. When infused directly into the shoulder joint instead of the tissue around the shoulder, destruction of articular artilage (chondrolysis) has occurred. On-Q® pumps should never be placed directly into any joint (see https://www.ismp.org/Newsletters/acutecare/archives/May09.asp).

Pregnancy Risk Factor B

Contraindications Hypersensitivity to lidocaine or any component of the formulation; hypersensitivity to another local anesthetic of the amide type; Adam-Stokes syndrome; severe degrees of SA, AV, or intraventricular heart block (except in patients with a functioning artificial pacemaker); premixed injection may contain corn-derived dextrose and its use is contraindicated in patients with allergy to corn-related products

Warnings/Precautions Use caution in patients with severe hepatic dysfunction or pseudocholinesterase deficiency; may have increased risk of lidocaine toxicity.

Intravenous: Constant ECG monitoring is necessary during I.V. administration. Use cautiously in hepatic impairment, any degree of heart block, Wolff-Parkinson-White syndrome, HF, marked hypoxia, severe respiratory depression, hypovolemia, history of malignant hyperthermia, or shock. Increased ventricular rate may be seen when administered to a patient with atrial fibrillation. Correct electrolyte disturbances, especially hypokalemia or hypomagnesemia, prior to use and throughout therapy. Correct any underlying causes of ventricular arrhythmias. Monitor closely for signs and symptoms of CNS toxicity. The elderly may be prone to increased CNS and cardiovascular side effects. Reduce dose in hepatic dysfunction and CHF.

Injectable anesthetic: Follow appropriate administration techniques so as not to administer any intravascularly. Solutions containing antimicrobial preservatives should not be used for epidural or spinal anesthesia. Some solutions contain a bisulfite; avoid in patients who are allergic to bisulfite. Resuscitative equipment, medicine and oxygen should be available in case of emergency. Use products containing epinephrine cautiously in patients with significant vascular disease, compromised blood flow, or during or following general anesthesia (increased risk of arrhythmias). Adjust the dose for the elderly, pediatric, acutely ill, and debilitated patients.

Ophthalmic: For ophthalmic use only; not for injection. Prolonged use may cause permanent corneal ulceration and/or opacification with loss of vision.

Topical: Do not leave on large body areas for >2 hours. Potentially life threatening side effects (eg, irregular heart beat, seizures, coma, respiratory depression, death) have occurred when used prior to cosmetic procedures. Observe young children closely to prevent accidental ingestion. Not for ophthalmic use. Some products are not recommended for use on mucous membranes; consult specific product labeling.

Transdermal patch: Safety and efficacy have not been established in children.

Adverse Reactions Effects vary with route of administration. Many effects are dose related.

Frequency not defined.

Cardiovascular: Arrhythmia, bradycardia, arterial spasms, cardiovascular collapse, defibrillator threshold increased, edema, flushing, heart block, hypotension, sinus node supression, vascular insufficiency (periarticular injections)

Central nervous system: Agitation, anxiety, apprehension, coma, confusion, disorientation, dizziness, drowsiness, euphoria, hallucinations, headache, hyperesthesia, hypoesthesia, lethargy, lightheadedness, nervousness, psychosis, seizure, slurred speech, somnolence, unconsciousness

Dermatologic: Angioedema, bruising (transdermal system), contact dermatitis, depigmentation (transdermal system), edema of the skin, itching, petechia (transdermal system), pruritus, rash, urticaria

Gastrointestinal: Metallic taste, nausea, vomiting

Local: Burning (ophthalmic), irritation (transdermal system), thrombophlebitis

Neuromuscular & skeletal: Pain exacerbation (transdermal system), paresthesia, transient radicular pain (subarachnoid administration; up to 1.9%), tremor, twitching, weakness

Ocular: Conjunctival hyperemia (ophthalmic), corneal epithelial changes (ophthalmic), diplopia, visual changes

Otic: Tinnitus

Respiratory: Bronchospasm, dyspnea, respiratory depression or arrest

Miscellaneous: Allergic reactions, anaphylactoid reaction, sensitivity to temperature extremes

Following spinal anesthesia: Positional headache (3%), shivering (2%) nausea, peripheral nerve symptoms, respiratory inadequacy and double vision (<1%), hypotension, cauda equina syndrome

Postmarketing and/or case reports: ARDS (inhalation), asystole, disorientation, methemoglobinemia, skin reaction

Drug Interactions

Metabolism/Transport Effects Substrate of CYP1A2 (minor), 2A6 (minor), 2B6 (minor), 2C9 (minor), 2D6 (major), 3A4 (major); **Inhibits** CYP1A2 (strong), 2D6 (moderate), 3A4 (moderate)

Avoid Concomitant Use

Avoid concomitant use of Lidocaine with any of the following: Everolimus; Thioridazine; Tolvaptan

Increased Effect/Toxicity

Lidocaine may increase the levels/effects of: Bendamustine; Colchicine; CYP1A2 Substrates; CYP2D6 Substrates; CYP3A4 Substrates; Eplerenone; Everolimus; Fesoterodine; Halofantrine; Pimecrolimus; Ranolazine; Salmeterol; Saxagliptin; Tamoxifen; Thioridazine; Tolvaptan

The levels/effects of Lidocaine may be increased by: Amiodarone; Beta-Blockers; CYP2D6 Inhibitors (Moderate); CYP2D6 Inhibitors (Strong); CYP3A4 Inhibitors (Moderate); CYP3A4 Inhibitors (Strong); Darunavir; Dasatinib; Disopyramide; P-Glycoprotein Inhibitors

Decreased Effect

Lidocaine may decrease the levels/effects of: TraMADol

The levels/effects of Lidocaine may be decreased by: CYP3A4 Inducers (Strong); Deferasirox; Herbs (CYP3A4 Inducers); Peginterferon Alfa-2b; P-Glycoprotein Inducers

Ethanol/Nutrition/Herb Interactions Herb/Nutraceutical: St John's wort may decrease lidocaine levels; avoid concurrent use.

Dietary Considerations Premixed injection may contain corn-derived dextrose and its use is contraindicated in patients with allergy to corn-related products.

Product Availability Zingo™: FDA approved August 2007; the product is not available following a non-safety recall and market withdrawal by the manufacturer, Anesiva, in November 2008

Dosage Forms Excipient information presented when available (limited, particularly for generics); consult specific product labeling. [DSC] = Discontinued product

Aerosol, topical [foam]:
  Anestafoam™: 4% (30 g) [contains benzalkonium chloride and benzyl alcohol]
Cream, rectal: 5% (15 g)
  L-M-X™ 5: 5% (15 g) [contains benzyl alcohol; packaged with applicator]; (30 g) [contains benzyl alcohol]
Cream, topical: 4% (5 g, 15, g, 30 g)
  L-M-X™ 4: 4% (5 g) [contains benzyl alcohol; packaged with Tegaderm™ dressing]; (15 g, 30 g) [contains benzyl alcohol]
Cream, topical, as hydrochloride: 3% (30 g)
  LidaMantle®: 3% (30 g, 85 g)
Gel, ophthalmic, as hydrochloride [preservative free]:
  Akten™: 3.5% (5 mL)
Gel, topical:
  Burn-O-Jel: 0.5% (90 g)
  Topicaine®: 4% (10 g, 30 g, 113 g) [contains alcohol 35%, benzyl alcohol, aloe vera, and jojoba]
Gel, topical, as hydrochloride:
  Burn Jel®: 2% (3.5 g, 60 mL, 120 mL)
  Solarcaine® Aloe Extra Burn Relief: 0.5% (113 g, 226 g) [contains aloe vera gel and tartrazine]
  Unburn®: 2.5% (3.5 g, 59 mL, 118 mL) [contains vitamin E]
Infusion, as hydrochloride [premixed in D_5W]: 0.4% [4 mg/mL] (250 mL, 500 mL); 0.8% [8 mg/mL] (250 mL, 500 mL)
Injection, solution, as hydrochloride: 0.5% [5 mg/mL] (50 mL); 1% [10 mg/mL] (2 mL, 10 mL, 20 mL, 30 mL, 50 mL); 2% [20 mg/mL] (2 mL, 5 mL, 20 mL, 50 mL)
  Xylocaine®: 0.5% [5 mg/mL] (50 mL); 1% [10 mg/mL] (10 mL, 20 mL, 50 mL); 2% [20 mg/mL] (10 mL, 20 mL, 50 mL)
Injection, solution, as hydrochloride [for dental use]:
  Xylocaine® Dental: 2% (1.8 mL)
Injection, solution, as hydrochloride [premixed in $D_{7.5}W$, preservative free]: 5% [50 mg/mL] (2 mL)
Injection, solution, as hydrochloride [preservative free]: 0.5% [5 mg/mL] (50 mL); 1% [10 mg/mL] (2 mL, 5 mL, 30 mL); 1.5% [15 mg/mL] (20 mL); 2% [20 mg/mL] (2 mL, 5 mL, 10 mL); 4% [40 mg/mL] (5 mL)
  Xylocaine®: 10% [100 mg/mL] (5 mL) [for ventricular arrhythmias]
  Xylocaine® MPF: 0.5% [5 mg/mL] (50 mL); 1% [10 mg/mL] (2 mL, 5 mL, 10 mL, 30 mL); 1.5% [15 mg/mL] (10 mL, 20 mL); 2% [20 mg/mL] (2 mL, 5 mL, 10 mL); 4% [40 mg/mL] (5 mL)
Jelly, topical, as hydrochloride: 2% (5 mL, 30 mL)
  Anestacon®: 2% (15 mL) [contains benzalkonium chloride]
  Xylocaine®: 2% (5 mL, 30 mL)
Liquid, topical:
  Zilactin®-L: 2.5% (7.5 mL)
Lotion, topical, as hydrochloride: 3% (177 mL)
  LidaMantle®: 3% (177 mL)
Ointment, topical: 5% (30 g, 37 g, 50 g)
Powder, intradermal, as hydrochloride:
  Zingo™: 0.5 mg [DSC]

▶

◀ Solution, topical, as hydrochloride: 4% [40 mg/mL] (50 mL)
　Band-Aid® Hurt-Free™ Antiseptic Wash: 2% (180 mL)
　LTA® 360: 4% [40 mg/mL] (4 mL) [packaged with cannula for laryngotracheal administration]
　Xylocaine®: 4% [40 mg/mL] (50 mL)
Solution, topical [spray]:
　BurnaMycin: 0.5% (60 mL) [contains aloe vera gel and menthol]
　Premjact®: 9.6% (13 mL)
　Solarcaine® Aloe Extra Burn Relief: 0.5% (127 g) [contains aloe vera]
Solution, viscous, oral, as hydrochloride: 2% [20 mg/mL] (20 mL, 100 mL)
　Xylocaine® Viscous: 2% [20 mg/mL] (100 mL, 450 mL)
Transdermal system, topical:
　Lidoderm®: 5% (30s)

References

"2005 American Heart Association Guidelines for Cardiopulmonary Resuscitation and Emergency Cardiovascular Care," *Circulation*, 2005, 112(24 Suppl):IV1-203.

American Pain Society, "Principles of Analgesic Use in the Treatment of Acute Pain and Cancer Pain," 6th ed, Glenview, IL: American Pain Society, 2008.

Corcoran W, Butterworth J, Weller RS, et al, "Local Anesthetic-Induced Cardiac Toxicity: A Survey of Contemporary Practice Strategies Among Academic Anesthesiology Departments," *Anesth Analg*, 2006, 103(5):1322-6.

Dorian P, Cass D, Schwartz B, et al, "Amiodarone as Compared With Lidocaine for Shock-Resistant Ventricular Fibrillation," *N Engl J Med*, 2002, 346(12):884-90.

Foxall G, McCahon R, Lamb J, et al, "Levobupivacaine-Induced Seizures and Cardiovascular Collapse Treated With Intralipid," *Anaesthesia*, 2007, 62(5):516-8.

Litz RJ, Popp M, Stehr SN, et al, "Successful Resuscitation of a Patient With Ropivacaine-Induced Asystole After Axillary Plexus Block Using lipid Infusion," *Anaesthesia*, 2006, 61(8):800-1.

Marchettini P, Lacerenza M, Marangoni C, et al, "Lidocaine Test in Neuralgia," *Pain*, 1992, 48 (3):377-82.

Rosenblatt MA, Abel M, Fischer GW, et al, "Successful Use of a 20% Lipid Emulsion to Resuscitate a Patient After a Presumed Bupivacaine-Related Cardiac Arrest," *Anesthesiology*, 2006, 105 (1):217-8.

Schnider TW, Gaeta R, Brose W, et al, "Derivation and Cross-Validation of Pharmacokinetic Parameters for Computer-Controlled Infusion of Lidocaine in Pain Therapy," *Anesthesiology*, 1996, 84(5):1043-50.

Linezolid (li NE zoh lid)

Medication Safety Issues
Sound-alike/look-alike issues:
　Zyvox® may be confused with Ziox™, Zosyn®, Zovirax®

Related Information
Dosing Considerations for the Critically-Ill Patient With Morbid Obesity *on page 1561*

U.S. Brand Names Zyvox®

Canadian Brand Names Zyvoxam®

Pharmacologic Category Antibiotic, Oxazolidinone

Generic Available No

Use Treatment of vancomycin-resistant *Enterococcus faecium* (VRE) infections, nosocomial pneumonia caused by *Staphylococcus aureus* including MRSA or *Streptococcus pneumoniae* (including multidrug-resistant strains [MDRSP]), complicated and uncomplicated skin and skin structure infections (including diabetic foot infections without concomitant osteomyelitis), and community-acquired pneumonia caused by susceptible gram-positive organisms

Mechanism of Action Inhibits bacterial protein synthesis by binding to bacterial 23S ribosomal RNA of the 50S subunit. This prevents the formation of a functional 70S initiation complex that is essential for the bacterial translation process. Linezolid is bacteriostatic against enterococci and staphylococci and bactericidal against most strains of streptococci.

Pharmacodynamics/Kinetics

Absorption: Rapid and extensive

Distribution: V_{dss}: Adults: 40-50 L

Protein binding: Adults: 31%

Metabolism: Hepatic via oxidation of the morpholine ring, resulting in two inactive metabolites (aminoethoxyacetic acid, hydroxyethyl glycine); does not involve CYP

Bioavailability: Oral: ~100%

Half-life elimination: Children ≥1 week (full-term) to 11 years: 1.5-3 hours; Adults: 4-5 hours

Time to peak: Adults: Oral: 1-2 hours

Excretion: Urine (30% as parent drug, 50% as metabolites); feces (9% as metabolites)

Nonrenal clearance: ~65%; increased in children ≥1 week to 11 years

Dosage

Oral, I.V.:

VRE infections including concurrent bacteremia:

Preterm neonates (<34 weeks gestational age): 10 mg/kg every 12 hours; neonates with a suboptimal clinical response can be advanced to 10 mg/kg every 8 hours. By day 7 of life, all neonates should receive 10 mg/kg every 8 hours.

Infants (excluding preterm neonates <1 week) and Children ≤11 years: 10 mg/kg every 8 hours for 14-28 days

Children ≥12 years and Adults: 600 mg every 12 hours for 14-28 days

MRSA: Adults: 600 mg every 12 hours

Nosocomial pneumonia, complicated skin and skin structure infections, community acquired pneumonia including concurrent bacteremia: Oral, I.V.:

Preterm neonates (<34 weeks gestational age): 10 mg/kg every 12 hours; neonates with a suboptimal clinical response can be advanced to 10 mg/kg every 8 hours. By day 7 of life, all neonates should receive 10 mg/kg every 8 hours.

Infants (excluding preterm neonates <1 week) and Children ≤11 years: 10 mg/kg every 8 hours for 10-14 days

Children ≥12 years and Adults: 600 mg every 12 hours for 10-14 days

Uncomplicated skin and skin structure infections: Oral:

Preterm neonates (<34 weeks gestational age): 10 mg/kg every 12 hours; neonates with a suboptimal clinical response can be advanced to 10 mg/kg every 8 hours. By day 7 of life, all neonates should receive 10 mg/kg every 8 hours.

Infants (excluding preterm neonates <1 week) and Children <5 years: 10 mg/kg every 8 hours for 10-14 days

Children 5-11 years: 10 mg/kg every 12 hours for 10-14 days

Children ≥12-18 years: 600 mg every 12 hours for 10-14 days

Adults: 400 mg every 12 hours for 10-14 days

Note: 400 mg dose is recommended in the product labeling; however, 600 mg dose is commonly employed clinically

Elderly: No dosage adjustment required

Dosage adjustment in renal impairment: No adjustment is recommended. The two primary metabolites may accumulate in patients with renal impairment but the clinical significance is unknown. Weigh the risk of accumulation of metabolites versus the benefit of therapy. Monitor for hematopoietic (eg, anemia, leukopenia, thrombocytopenia) and neuropathic (eg, peripheral neuropathy) adverse events when administering for extended periods. Both linezolid and the two metabolites are eliminated by dialysis. Linezolid should be given after hemodialysis.

Continuous renal replacement therapy (CRRT): No adjustment needed.

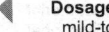

Dosage adjustment in hepatic impairment: No dosage adjustment required for mild-to-moderate hepatic insufficiency (Child-Pugh Class A or B). Use in severe hepatic insufficiency has not been adequately evaluated.

Stability
Infusion: Store at 25°C (77°F). Protect from light. Keep infusion bags in overwrap until ready for use. Protect infusion bags from freezing.

Oral suspension: Reconstitute with 123 mL of distilled water (in 2 portions); shake vigorously. Concentration is 100 mg/5 mL. Prior to administration mix gently by inverting bottle; do not shake. Following reconstitution, store at 25°C (77°F). Use reconstituted suspension within 21 days. Protect from light.

Tablet: Store at 25°C (77°F). Protect from light; protect from moisture.

Administration
I.V.: Administer intravenous infusion over 30-120 minutes. Do not mix or infuse with other medications. When the same intravenous line is used for sequential infusion of other medications, flush line with D_5W, NS, or LR before and after infusing linezolid. The yellow color of the injection may intensify over time without affecting potency.

Oral suspension: Invert gently to mix prior to administration, do not shake. Administer without regard to meals.

Monitoring Parameters
Weekly CBC and platelet counts, particularly in patients at increased risk of bleeding, with pre-existing myelosuppression, on concomitant medications that cause bone marrow suppression, in those who require >2 weeks of therapy, or in those with chronic infection who have received previous or concomitant antibiotic therapy; visual function with extended therapy (≥3 months) or in patients with new onset visual symptoms, regardless of therapy length

Anesthesia and Critical Care Concerns/Other Considerations
Clinical Pearls/Comments: Linezolid has mild MAO inhibitor properties and should be used with caution in patients with cardiovascular disease, particularly those with hypertension. Avoid use with sympathomimetic and dopaminergic agents (serotonin reuptake inhibitors, tricyclic antidepressants, serotonin 5-HT$_1$ receptor agonists, meperidine, or buspirone).

Linezolid has time-dependent kill characteristics; time for which the serum concentration remains above the MIC for a dosing period is the best predictor of efficacy. With prolonged exposure (>2 weeks), monitor closely for anemia, leukopenia, and thrombocytopenia.

Evidence-Based Information:

Trial Showing Increased Rate of Death in Catheter-Related Bloodstream Infections - March, 2007: The U.S. Food and Drug Administration (FDA) has issued an alert to healthcare professionals regarding an increased rate of death among patients treated with linezolid (Zyvox®) for catheter-related bacteremia and catheter-site infections. Healthcare professionals are reminded that linezolid is not approved for the treatment of catheter-related bloodstream, catheter-site, or gram-negative infections. Additional information is available at http://www.fda.gov/Safety/MedWatch/SafetyInformation/SafetyAlertsforHumanMedicalProducts/ucm152993.htm

Pregnancy Risk Factor C

Contraindications Hypersensitivity to linezolid or any other component of the formulation; concurrent use or within 2 weeks of MAO inhibitors; patients with uncontrolled hypertension, pheochromocytoma, thyrotoxicosis, and/or taking sympathomimetics (eg, pseudoephedrine), vasopressive agents (eg, epinephrine, norepinephrine), or dopaminergic agents (eg, dopamine, dobutamine) unless closely monitored for increased blood pressure; patients with carcinoid syndrome and/or taking SSRIs, tricyclic antidepressants, serotonin 5-HT$_{1B,1D}$ receptor agonists, meperidine, or buspirone unless closely monitored for sign/symptoms of serotonin syndrome

Warnings/Precautions Myelosuppression has been reported and may be dependent on duration of therapy (generally >2 weeks of treatment); use with caution in patients with pre-existing myelosuppression, in patients receiving other drugs which may cause bone marrow suppression, or in chronic infection (previous or concurrent antibiotic therapy). Weekly CBC monitoring is recommended. Discontinue linezolid in patients developing myelosuppression (or in whom myelosuppression worsens during treatment).

Lactic acidosis has been reported with use. Linezolid exhibits mild MAO inhibitor properties and has the potential to have the same interactions as other MAO inhibitors; use with caution and monitor closely in patients with uncontrolled hypertension, pheochromocytoma, carcinoid syndrome, or untreated hyperthyroidism; use is contraindicated in the absence of close monitoring. Symptoms of agitation, confusion, hallucinations, hyper-reflexia, myoclonus, shivering, and tachycardia may occur with concomitant proserotonergic drugs (eg, SSRIs/SNRIs or triptans) or agents which reduce linezolid's metabolism; concurrent use with these medications is contraindicated unless patient is closely monitored for signs/symptoms of serotonin syndrome. Unnecessary use may lead to the development of resistance to linezolid; consider alternatives before initiating outpatient treatment.

Peripheral and optic neuropathy (with vision loss) has been reported and may occur primarily with extended courses of therapy >28 days; any symptoms of visual change or impairment warrant immediate ophthalmic evaluation and possible discontinuation of therapy. Seizures have been reported; use with caution in patients with a history of seizures. Prolonged use may result in fungal or bacterial superinfection, including *C. difficile*-associated diarrhea (CDAD) and pseudomembranous colitis; CDAD has been observed >2 months postantibiotic treatment.

Due to inconsistent concentrations in the CSF, empiric use in pediatric patients with CNS infections is not recommended by the manufacturer; however, there are multiple case reports describing successful treatment of documented VRE and *Staphylococcus aureus* CNS and shunt infections in the literature. Oral suspension contains phenylalanine.

Adverse Reactions Percentages as reported in adults; frequency similar in pediatric patients

>10%:

Central nervous system: Headache (<1% to 11%)

Gastrointestinal: Diarrhea (3% to 11%)

1% to 10%:

Central nervous system: Insomnia (3%), dizziness (≤2%), fever (2%)

Dermatologic: Rash (2%)

Gastrointestinal: Nausea (3% to 10%), vomiting (1% to 4%), pancreatic enzymes increased (≤4%), constipation (2%), taste alteration (1% to 2%), tongue discoloration (≤1%), oral moniliasis (≤1%), pancreatitis

Genitourinary: Vaginal moniliasis (1% to 2%)

Hematologic: Hemoglobin decreased (1% to 7%), thrombocytopenia (≤3%), anemia, leukopenia, neutropenia; **Note:** Myelosuppression (including anemia, leukopenia, pancytopenia, and thrombocytopenia; may be more common in patients receiving linezolid for >2 weeks)

Hepatic: Abnormal LFTs (≤10%), bilirubin increased (≤1%)

Renal: BUN increased (≤2%)

Miscellaneous: Fungal infection (0.1% to 2%), lactate dehydrogenase increased (<1% to 2%)

<1% or frequency not defined (limited to important or life-threatening): Anaphylaxis, angioedema, bullous skin disorders, *C. difficile*-related complications, dyspepsia, increased creatinine, hypertension, localized abdominal pain, pruritus, lactic acidosis, peripheral neuropathy, optic neuropathy, seizures, serotonin syndrome (with concurrent use of other serotonergic agents), Stevens-Johnson syndrome, vision loss

Drug Interactions

Avoid Concomitant Use

Avoid concomitant use of Linezolid with any of the following: Alpha-/Beta-Agonists (Indirect-Acting); Alpha1-Agonists; Alpha2-Agonists (Ophthalmic); Amphetamines; Anilidopiperidine Opioids; Atomoxetine; BuPROPion; BusPIRone; CarBAMazepine; Cyclobenzaprine; Dexmethylphenidate; Dextromethorphan; MAO Inhibitors; Maprotiline; Meperidine; Methyldopa; Methylphenidate; Mirtazapine; Propoxyphene; Selective Serotonin Reuptake Inhibitors; Serotonin 5-HT1D Receptor Agonists; Serotonin/Norepinephrine Reuptake Inhibitors; Sibutramine; Tapentadol; Tetrabenazine; Tricyclic Antidepressants

◀ **Increased Effect/Toxicity**

Linezolid may increase the levels/effects of: Alpha-/Beta-Agonists (Direct-Acting); Alpha-/Beta-Agonists (Indirect-Acting); Alpha1-Agonists; Alpha2-Agonists (Ophthalmic); Amphetamines; Antihypertensives; Atomoxetine; Beta2-Agonists; BuPROPion; Dexmethylphenidate; Dextromethorphan; Lithium; Meperidine; Methyldopa; Methylphenidate; Mirtazapine; Orthostasis Producing Agents; Rauwolfia Alkaloids; Selective Serotonin Reuptake Inhibitors; Serotonin 5-HT1D Receptor Agonists; Serotonin Modulators; Serotonin/Norepinephrine Reuptake Inhibitors; Tricyclic Antidepressants

The levels/effects of Linezolid may be increased by: Altretamine; Anilidopiperidine Opioids; BusPIRone; CarBAMazepine; COMT Inhibitors; Cyclobenzaprine; Levodopa; MAO Inhibitors; Maprotiline; Propoxyphene; Sibutramine; Tapentadol; Tetrabenazine; TraMADol

Decreased Effect There are no known significant interactions involving a decrease in effect.

Ethanol/Nutrition/Herb Interactions

Ethanol: Avoid ethanol (based on CNS depressant effects and potential tyramine content)

Food: Concurrent ingestion of foods rich in tyramine may cause sudden and severe high blood pressure (hypertensive crisis). Avoid tyramine-containing foods with MAO-Is. Food's freshness is also an important concern; improperly stored or spoiled food can create an environment where tyramine concentrations may increase.

Herb/Nutraceutical: Avoid supplements containing caffeine, tyrosine, tryptophan or phenylalanine. Ingestion of large quantities may increase the risk of severe side effects (eg, hypertensive reactions, serotonin syndrome).

Dietary Considerations Take without regard to meals. Avoid consuming large amounts of tyramine-containing foods/beverages. Some examples include aged or matured cheese, air-dried or cured meats (including sausages and salamis), fava or broad bean pods, tap/draft beers, Marmite concentrate, sauerkraut, soy sauce and other soybean condiments.

Some products may contain phenylalanine.

Dosage Forms Excipient information presented when available (limited, particularly for generics); consult specific product labeling.

Infusion [premixed]:

Zyvox®: 200 mg (100 mL) [contains sodium 1.7 mEq]; 600 mg (300 mL) [contains sodium 5 mEq]

Powder for oral suspension:

Zyvox®: 20 mg/mL (150 mL) [contains phenylalanine 20 mg/5 mL, sodium benzoate, and sodium 0.4 mEq/5 mL; orange flavor]

Tablet:

Zyvox®: 600 mg [contains sodium 0.1 mEq/tablet]

References

American Thoracic Society and Infectious Diseases Society of America, "Guidelines for the Management of Adults With Hospital-Acquired, Ventilator-Associated, and Healthcare-Associated Pneumonia," *Am J Respir Crit Care Med*, 2005, 171(4):388-416.

Mandell LA, Wunderink RG, Anzueto A, et al, "Infectious Diseases Society of America/American Thoracic Society Consensus Guidelines on the Management of Community-Acquired Pneumonia in Adults," *Clin Infect Dis*, 2007, 44 Suppl 2:S27-72.

Roberts JA and Lipman J, "Antibacterial Dosing in Intensive Care: Pharmacokinetics, Degree of Disease and Pharmacodynamics of Sepsis," *Clin Pharmacokinet*, 2006, 45(8):755-73.

Trotman RL, Williamson JC, Shoemaker DM, et al, "Antibiotic Dosing in Critically Ill Adult Patients Receiving Continuous Renal Replacement Therapy," *Clin Infect Dis*, 2005, 41(8):1159-66.

◆ **Lin-Sotalol (Can)** *see* Sotalol *on page 1321*

◆ **Lioresal®** *see* Baclofen *on page 178*

◆ **Liotec (Can)** *see* Baclofen *on page 178*

Liothyronine (lye oh THYE roe neen)

Medication Safety Issues

Sound-alike/look-alike issues:

Liothyronine may be confused with levothyroxine

T3 is an error-prone abbreviation (mistaken as acetaminophen and codeine [ie, Tylenol® #3])

U.S. Brand Names Cytomel®; Triostat®

Canadian Brand Names Cytomel®

Index Terms Liothyronine Sodium; Sodium L-Triiodothyronine; T_3 Sodium (error-prone abbreviation)

Pharmacologic Category Thyroid Product

Generic Available Yes

Use

Oral: Replacement or supplemental therapy in hypothyroidism; management of nontoxic goiter; a diagnostic aid

I.V.: Treatment of myxedema coma/precoma

Unlabeled/Investigational Use Management of hemodynamically unstable potential organ donors increasing the quantity of organs available for transplantation

Mechanism of Action Exact mechanism of action is unknown; however, it is believed the thyroid hormone exerts its many metabolic effects through control of DNA transcription and protein synthesis; involved in normal metabolism, growth, and development; promotes gluconeogenesis, increases utilization and mobilization of glycogen stores, and stimulates protein synthesis, increases basal metabolic rate

Pharmacodynamics/Kinetics

Onset of action: 2-4 hours

Peak response: 2-3 days

Absorption: Oral: Well absorbed (95% in 4 hours)

Half-life elimination: 2.5 days

Excretion: Urine

Dosage Doses should be adjusted based on clinical response and laboratory parameters.

Children: Congenital hypothyroidism: Oral: 5 mcg/day increase by 5 mcg every 3-4 days until the desired response is achieved. Usual maintenance dose: 20 mcg/day for infants, 50 mcg/day for children 1-3 years of age, and adult dose for children >3 years.

Adults:

Hypothyroidism: Oral: 25 mcg/day increase by increments of 12.5-25 mcg/day every 1-2 weeks to a maximum of 100 mcg/day; usual maintenance dose: 25-75 mcg/day.

Patients with cardiovascular disease: Refer to Elderly dosing.

T_3 suppression test: Oral: 75-100 mcg/day for 7 days; use lowest dose for elderly

Myxedema: Oral: Initial: 5 mcg/day; increase in increments of 5-10 mcg/day every 1-2 weeks. When 25 mcg/day is reached, dosage may be increased at intervals of 5-25 mcg/day every 1-2 weeks. Usual maintenance dose: 50-100 mcg/day.

Myxedema coma: I.V.: 25-50 mcg

Patients with known or suspected cardiovascular disease: 10-20 mcg

Note: Normally, at least 4 hours should be allowed between doses to adequately assess therapeutic response and no more than 12 hours should elapse between doses to avoid fluctuations in hormone levels. Oral therapy should be resumed as soon as the clinical situation has been stabilized and the patient is able to take oral medication. If levothyroxine rather than liothyronine sodium is used in initiating oral therapy, the physician should bear in mind that there is a delay of several days in the onset of levothyroxine activity and that I.V. therapy should be discontinued gradually.

Simple (nontoxic) goiter: Oral: Initial: 5 mcg/day; increase by 5-10 mcg every 1-2 weeks; after 25 mcg/day is reached, may increase dose by 12.5-25 mcg. Usual maintenance dose: 75 mcg/day

Elderly: Oral: 5 mcg/day; increase by 5 mcg/day every 2 weeks

Stability Vials must be stored under refrigeration at 2°C to 8°C (36°F to 46°F). Store tablets at 15°C to 30°C (59°F to 86°F).

Administration I.V.: For I.V. use only; **do not administer I.M. or SubQ**

Administer doses at least 4 hours, and no more than 12 hours, apart

◄ Resume oral therapy as soon as the clinical situation has been stabilized and the patient is able to take oral medication

When switching to tablets, discontinue the injectable, initiate oral therapy at a low dosage and increase gradually according to response

If **levothyroxine** is used for oral therapy, there is a delay of several days in the onset of activity; therefore, discontinue I.V. therapy gradually.

Monitoring Parameters T_3, TSH, heart rate, blood pressure, renal function, clinical signs of hypo- and hyperthyroidism; TSH is the most reliable guide for evaluating adequacy of thyroid replacement dosage. TSH may be elevated during the first few months of thyroid replacement despite patients being clinically euthyroid. In cases where T_4 remains low and TSH is within normal limits, an evaluation of "free" (unbound) T_4 is needed to evaluate further increase in dosage.

Reference Range Free T_3, serum: 250-390 pg/dL; TSH: 0.4 and up to 10 ($\geq$80 years) mIU/L; remains normal in pregnancy

Anesthesia and Critical Care Concerns/Other Considerations

Clinical Pearls/Comments: Equivalent doses: The following statement on relative potency of thyroid products is included in a joint statement by American Thyroid Association (ATA), American Association of Clinical Endocrinologists (AACE) and The Endocrine Society (TES): For purposes of conversion, levothyroxine sodium (T_4) 100 mcg is usually considered equivalent to desiccated thyroid 60 mg, thyroglobulin 60 mg, or liothyronine sodium (T_3) 25 mcg. However, these are rough guidelines only and do not obviate the careful re-evaluation of a patient when switching thyroid hormone preparations, including a change from one brand of levothyroxine to another. Joint position statement is available at http://www.thyroid.org/professionals/advocacy/04_12_08_thyroxine.html.

Evidence-Based Information: Cadaveric organ donation: Hemodynamically unstable donors: Hormonal resuscitation: Intravenous liothyronine (4 mcg bolus followed by 3 mcg/hour) given concomitantly with a continuous infusion of insulin (1 unit/hour minimum; titrated to BG 120-180 mg/dL), 15 mg/kg of methylprednisolone, and vasopressin (1 unit bolus followed by 0.5-4 units/hour; titrate to SVR 800-1200 dyne·s/cm^5) has been successfully used in hemodynamically unstable brain-dead donors to increase the quantity and quality of organs available for transplantation (Rosendale, 2003; Rosengard, 2002). Of note, stability of further diluted injectable levothyroxine (after reconstitution) and liothyronine solutions has not been adequately studied.

Pregnancy Risk Factor A

Contraindications Hypersensitivity to liothyronine sodium or any component of the formulation; undocumented or uncorrected adrenal insufficiency; recent myocardial infarction or thyrotoxicosis; artificial rewarming (injection)

Warnings/Precautions [U.S. Boxed Warning]: Ineffective and potentially toxic for weight reduction. High doses may produce serious or even life-threatening toxic effects particularly when used with some anorectic drugs. Use with extreme caution in patients with angina pectoris or other cardiovascular disease (including hypertension) or coronary artery disease. Use with caution in elderly patients since they may be more likely to have compromised cardiovascular function. Patients with adrenal insufficiency, myxedema, diabetes mellitus and insipidus may have symptoms exaggerated or aggravated. Thyroid replacement requires periodic assessment of thyroid status. Chronic hypothyroidism predisposes patients to coronary artery disease.

Adverse Reactions

1% to 10%: Cardiovascular: Arrhythmia (6%), tachycardia (3%), cardiopulmonary arrest (2%), hypotension (2%), MI (2%)

<1% (Limited to important or life-threatening): Allergic skin reactions, angina, CHF, fever, hypertension, phlebitis, twitching

Drug Interactions

Avoid Concomitant Use

Avoid concomitant use of Liothyronine with any of the following: Sodium Iodide I131

Increased Effect/Toxicity

Liothyronine may increase the levels/effects of: Vitamin K Antagonists

Decreased Effect

Liothyronine may decrease the levels/effects of: Sodium Iodide I131; Theophylline Derivatives

The levels/effects of Liothyronine may be decreased by: Bile Acid Sequestrants; Calcium Salts; CarBAMazepine; Estrogen Derivatives; Phenytoin; Rifampin

Dosage Forms Excipient information presented when available (limited, particularly for generics); consult specific product labeling.

Injection, solution: 10 mcg/mL (1 mL)

Triostat®: 10 mcg/mL (1 mL) [contains ethanol 6.8%]

Tablet, oral: 5 mcg, 25 mcg, 50 mcg

Cytomel®: 5 mcg, 25 mcg, 50 mcg

References

Rosendale JD, Kauffman HM, McBride MA, et al, "Aggressive Pharmacologic Donor Management Results in More Transplanted Organs," *Transplantation*, 2003, 75(4):482-7.

Rosengard BR, Feng S, Alfrey EJ, et al, "Report of the Crystal City Meeting to Maximize the Use of Organs Recovered From the Cadaver Donor," *Am J Transplant*, 2002, 2(8):701-11.

Salim A, Martin M, Brown C, et al, "Using Thyroid Hormone in Brain-Dead Donors to Maximize the Number of Organs Available for Transplantation," *Clin Transplant*, 2007, 21(3):405-9.

◆ **Liothyronine Sodium** *see* Liothyronine *on page 846*

◆ **Lipidil EZ® (Can)** *see* Fenofibrate *on page 582*

◆ **Lipidil Micro® (Can)** *see* Fenofibrate *on page 582*

◆ **Lipidil Supra® (Can)** *see* Fenofibrate *on page 582*

◆ **Lipitor®** *see* Atorvastatin *on page 158*

◆ **Lipofen®** *see* Fenofibrate *on page 582*

◆ **Liposyn® II** *see* Fat Emulsion *on page 578*

◆ **Liposyn® III** *see* Fat Emulsion *on page 578*

◆ **Liquid Antidote** *see* Charcoal *on page 283*

Lisinopril (lyse IN oh pril)

Related Information

Angiotensin Agents *on page 1652*

Heart Failure (Systolic) *on page 1739*

U.S. Brand Names Prinivil®; Zestril®

Canadian Brand Names Apo-Lisinopril®; CO Lisinopril; Gen-Lisinopril; Mylan-Lisinopril; Novo-Lisinopril; PMS-Lisinopril; Prinivil®; Pro-Lisinopril; Ran-Lisinopril; ratio-Lisinopril; Riva-Lisinopril; Zestril®

Pharmacologic Category Angiotensin-Converting Enzyme (ACE) Inhibitor

Use Treatment of hypertension, either alone or in combination with other antihypertensive agents; adjunctive therapy in treatment of heart failure (afterload reduction); treatment of acute myocardial infarction within 24 hours in hemodynamically-stable patients to improve survival; treatment of left ventricular dysfunction after myocardial infarction

Pharmacodynamics/Kinetics

Onset of action: 1 hour

Peak effect: Hypotensive: Oral: ~6 hours

Duration: 24 hours

Absorption: Well absorbed; unaffected by food

Protein binding: 25%

Metabolism: Not metabolized

Bioavailability: Decreased with NYHA Class II-IV heart failure

Half-life elimination: 11-12 hours

Time to peak: ~7 hours

Excretion: Primarily urine (as unchanged drug)

Dosage Oral:

Heart failure: Adults: Initial: 2.5-5 mg once daily; then increase by no more than 10 mg increments at intervals no less than 2 weeks to a maximum daily dose of 40 mg. Usual maintenance: 5-40 mg/day as a single dose. Target dose: 20-40 mg once daily (ACC/AHA 2009 Heart Failure Guidelines)

◀ **Note:** If patient has hyponatremia (serum sodium <130 meq/L) or renal impairment (Cl$_{cr}$ <30 mL/minute or creatinine >3 mg/dL), then initial dose should be 2.5 mg/day

Hypertension:

Children ≥6 years: Initial: 0.07 mg/kg once daily (up to 5 mg); increase dose at 1- to 2-week intervals; doses >0.61 mg/kg or >40 mg have not been evaluated.

Adults: Usual dosage range (JNC 7): 10-40 mg/day

Not maintained on diuretic: Initial: 10 mg/day

Maintained on diuretic: Initial: 5 mg/day

Note: Antihypertensive effect may diminish toward the end of the dosing interval especially with doses of 10 mg/day. An increased dose may aid in extending the duration of antihypertensive effect. Doses up to 80 mg/day have been used, but do not appear to give greater effect.

Elderly: Initial: 2.5-5 mg/day; increase doses 2.5-5 mg/day at 1- to 2-week intervals; maximum daily dose: 40 mg

Patients taking diuretics should have them discontinued 2-3 days prior to initiating lisinopril if possible. Restart diuretic after blood pressure is stable if needed. If diuretic cannot be discontinued prior to therapy, begin with 5 mg with close supervision until stable blood pressure. In patients with hyponatremia (<130 mEq/L), start dose at 2.5 mg/day

Acute myocardial infarction (within 24 hours in hemodynamically stable patients): Oral: 5 mg immediately, then 5 mg at 24 hours, 10 mg at 48 hours, and 10 mg every day thereafter for 6 weeks. Patients should continue to receive standard treatments such as thrombolytics, aspirin, and beta-blockers.

Dosing adjustment in renal impairment:

Heart failure: Adults: Cl$_{cr}$ <30 mL/minute or creatinine >3 mg/dL: Initial: 2.5 mg/day

Hypertension:

Adults: Initial doses should be modified and upward titration should be cautious, based on response (maximum: 40 mg/day)

Cl$_{cr}$ >30 mL/minute: Initial: 10 mg/day

Cl$_{cr}$ 10-30 mL/minute: Initial: 5 mg/day

Hemodialysis: Initial: 2.5 mg/day; dialyzable (50%)

Children: Use in not recommended in pediatric patients with GFR <30 mL/minute/1.73 m^2

Anesthesia and Critical Care Concerns/Other Considerations

Clinical Pearls/Comments: In patients on chronic ACE inhibitor therapy, intraoperative hypotension may occur with induction and maintenance of general anesthesia; however, discontinuation of therapy prior to surgery is controversial. If continued preoperatively, avoidance of hypotensive agents during surgery is prudent. Episodes of intraoperative hypotension may be managed by fluid administration and/or modest doses of alpha-adrenergic agents. Severe hypotension may occur in patients who are sodium- and/or volume-depleted, initiate lower doses and monitor closely when starting therapy in these patients. ACE inhibitor therapy may elicit an increase in potassium and creatinine, especially when used in patients with bilateral renal artery stenosis. In those patients experiencing cough on an ACE inhibitor, the ACE inhibitor may be discontinued and, if necessary, angiotensin-receptor blocker therapy instituted. Concomitant NSAID therapy may attenuate blood pressure control; use of NSAIDs should be avoided or limited, with monitoring of blood pressure control. In the setting of heart failure, NSAID use may be associated with an increased risk for fluid accumulation and edema. Because of the potent teratogenic effects of ACE inhibitors, these drugs should be avoided, if possible, when treating women of childbearing potential not on effective birth control measures. Aging patients with a decrease in glomerular filtration (also creatinine clearance), severe heart failure, and renal failure may experience an exaggerated response with administration of ACE inhibitors. Diabetic proteinuria is reduced and insulin sensitivity is enhanced.

Evidence-Based Information: ACE inhibitors decrease morbidity and mortality in patients with asymptomatic and symptomatic left ventricular dysfunction. In this situation, they decrease hospitalizations for, and retard progression to, decompensated heart failure. ACE inhibitors are also indicated in patients postmyocardial infarction in whom left ventricular ejection fraction is <40%. When used in patients with heart failure, the target dose or maximum tolerated dose should be achieved, if possible. Lower daily doses of ACE inhibitors have not demonstrated the same cardioprotective effects. ACE inhibitors have renal protective effects in patients with diabetic proteinuria. The HOPE trial examined the use of ramipril at a dose of between 2.5-10 mg daily in patients without heart failure at high risk for cardiovascular events and documented a significant improvement in cardiovascular outcome compared to placebo.

Additional Information Complete prescribing information for this medication should be consulted for additional detail.

Dosage Forms Excipient information presented when available (limited, particularly for generics); consult specific product labeling.
Tablet: 2.5 mg, 5 mg, 10 mg, 20 mg, 30 mg, 40 mg
  Prinivil®: 5 mg, 10 mg, 20 mg
  Zestril®: 2.5 mg, 5 mg, 10 mg, 20 mg, 30 mg, 40 mg

◆ **Lispro Insulin** see Insulin Lispro on page 747
◆ **Lithane™ (Can)** see Lithium on page 851

Lithium (LITH ee um)

Related Information
  Inhalational Anesthetics on page 1632
U.S. Brand Names Lithobid®
Canadian Brand Names Apo-Lithium® Carbonate; Apo-Lithium® Carbonate SR; Carbolith™; Duralith®; Euro-Lithium; Lithane™; PMS-Lithium Carbonate; PMS-Lithium Citrate
Index Terms Eskalith; Lithium Carbonate; Lithium Citrate
Pharmacologic Category Antimanic Agent
Use Management of bipolar disorders; treatment of mania in individuals with bipolar disorder (maintenance treatment prevents or diminishes intensity of subsequent episodes)
Unlabeled/Investigational Use Potential augmenting agent for antidepressants; aggression, post-traumatic stress disorder, conduct disorder in children
Pharmacodynamics/Kinetics
Absorption: Rapid and complete
Distribution: V_d: Initial: 0.3-0.4 L/kg; V_{dss}: 0.7-1 L/kg; crosses placenta; enters breast milk at 35% to 50% the concentrations in serum; distribution is complete in 6-10 hours
  CSF, liver concentrations: $1/3$ to $1/2$ of serum concentration
  Erythrocyte concentration: ~$1/2$ of serum concentration
  Heart, lung, kidney, muscle concentrations: Equivalent to serum concentration
  Saliva concentration: 2-3 times serum concentration
  Thyroid, bone, brain tissue concentrations: Increase 50% over serum concentrations
Protein binding: Not protein bound
Metabolism: Not metabolized
Bioavailability: Not affected by food; Capsule, immediate release tablet: 95% to 100%; Extended release tablet: 60% to 90%; Syrup: 100%
Half-life elimination: 18-24 hours; can increase to more than 36 hours in elderly or with renal impairment
Time to peak, serum: Nonsustained: ~0.5-2 hours; slow release: 4-12 hours; syrup: 15-60 minutes
Excretion: Urine (90% to 98% as unchanged drug); sweat (4% to 5%); feces (1%)
  Clearance: 80% of filtered lithium is reabsorbed in the proximal convoluted tubules; therefore, clearance approximates 20% of GFR or 20-40 mL/minute
Dosage Oral: Monitor serum concentrations and clinical response (efficacy and toxicity) to determine proper dose

Children 6-12 years:
  Bipolar disorder (unlabeled use): 15-60 mg/kg/day in 3-4 divided doses; dose not to exceed usual adult dosage
  Conduct disorder (unlabeled use): 15-30 mg/kg/day in 3-4 divided doses; dose not to exceed usual adult dosage

◀ Adults: Bipolar disorder: 900-2400 mg/day in 3-4 divided doses or 900-1800 mg/day (sustained release) in 2 divided doses

Elderly: Bipolar disorder: Initial dose: 300 mg once or twice daily; increase weekly in increments of 300 mg/day, monitoring levels; rarely need >900-1200 mg/day

Dosing adjustment in renal impairment:

Cl_{cr} 10-50 mL/minute: Administer 50% to 75% of normal dose

Cl_{cr} <10 mL/minute: Administer 25% to 50% of normal dose

Hemodialysis: Dialyzable (50% to 100%); 4-7 times more efficient than peritoneal dialysis

Additional Information Complete prescribing information for this medication should be consulted for additional detail.

Dosage Forms Excipient information presented when available (limited, particularly for generics); consult specific product labeling.

Capsule, as carbonate: 150 mg, 300 mg, 600 mg

Solution, as citrate: 300 mg/5 mL (5 mL, 500 mL) [equivalent to amount of lithium in lithium carbonate]

Syrup, as citrate: 300 mg/5 mL (480 mL) [equivalent to amount of lithium in lithium carbonate]

Tablet, as carbonate: 300 mg

Tablet, controlled release, as carbonate: 450 mg

Tablet, slow release, as carbonate: 300 mg

Lithobid®: 300 mg

References

Mokhlesi B, Leikin JB, Murray P, et al, "Adult Toxicology in Critical Care. Part 11: Specific Poisonings," *Chest*, 2003, 123(3):897-922.

Szerlip HM, Heeger P, and Feldman GM, "Comparison Between Acetate and Bicarbonate Dialysis for the Treatment of Lithium Intoxication," *Am J Nephrol*, 1992, 12(1-2):116-20.

◆ **Lithium Carbonate** see Lithium on page 851

◆ **Lithium Citrate** see Lithium on page 851

◆ **Lithobid®** see Lithium on page 851

◆ **Little Fevers™ [OTC]** see Acetaminophen on page 25

◆ **Little Noses® Decongestant [OTC]** see Phenylephrine on page 1114

◆ **Little Noses® Saline [OTC]** see Sodium Chloride on page 1304

◆ **Little Noses® Stuffy Nose Kit [OTC]** see Sodium Chloride on page 1304

◆ **Livalo®** see Pitavastatin on page 1140

◆ **L-leucovorin** see LEVOleucovorin on page 828

◆ **LMD®** see Dextran on page 402

◆ **L-methylfolate** see Methylfolate on page 906

◆ **Locoid®** see Hydrocortisone on page 699

◆ **Locoid Lipocream®** see Hydrocortisone on page 699

◆ **Lodine** see Etodolac on page 562

◆ **Loestrin®** see Ethinyl Estradiol and Norethindrone on page 554

◆ **Loestrin™ 1.5/30 (Can)** see Ethinyl Estradiol and Norethindrone on page 554

◆ **Loestrin® 24 Fe** see Ethinyl Estradiol and Norethindrone on page 554

◆ **Loestrin® Fe** see Ethinyl Estradiol and Norethindrone on page 554

◆ **Lofibra®** see Fenofibrate on page 582

◆ **Loniten® (Can)** see Minoxidil on page 943

◆ **Lo/Ovral®-28** see Ethinyl Estradiol and Norgestrel on page 560

◆ **Lopressor®** see Metoprolol on page 922

LORazepam (lor A ze pam)

Medication Safety Issues

Sound-alike/look-alike issues:

LORazepam may be confused with ALPRAZolam, clonazePAM, diazepam, Lovaza®, temazepam, zolpidem

Ativan® may be confused with Ambien®, Atarax®, Atgam®, Avitene®

Injection dosage form contains propylene glycol. Monitor for toxicity when administering continuous lorazepam infusions.

Related Information

Anesthesia Considerations for Neurosurgery *on page 1514*
Anesthesia for Patients With Liver Disease *on page 1537*
Benzodiazepines *on page 1666*
Dosing Considerations for the Critically-Ill Patient With Morbid Obesity *on page 1561*
Intravenous Anesthetic Agents *on page 1635*
Moderate Sedation *on page 1566*
Perioperative Management of Patients on Antiseizure Medication *on page 1577*
Sedative Agents in the Intensive Care Unit *on page 1690*
Status Epilepticus *on page 1737*

U.S. Brand Names Ativan®; Lorazepam Intensol™

Canadian Brand Names Apo-Lorazepam®; Ativan®; Lorazepam Injection, USP; Novo-Lorazepam; Nu-Loraz; PHL-Lorazepam; PMS-Lorazepam; Riva-Lorazepam

Pharmacologic Category Benzodiazepine

Restrictions C-IV

Generic Available Yes

Use

Oral: Management of anxiety disorders or short-term (≤4 months) relief of the symptoms of anxiety or anxiety associated with depressive symptoms
I.V.: Status epilepticus, amnesia, sedation

Unlabeled/Investigational Use Ethanol detoxification; insomnia; psychogenic catatonia; partial complex seizures; agitation (I.V.); antiemetic adjunct

Mechanism of Action Binds to stereospecific benzodiazepine receptors on the postsynaptic GABA neuron at several sites within the central nervous system, including the limbic system, reticular formation. Enhancement of the inhibitory effect of GABA on neuronal excitability results by increased neuronal membrane permeability to chloride ions. This shift in chloride ions results in hyperpolarization (a less excitable state) and stabilization.

Pharmacodynamics/Kinetics

Onset of action:
  Hypnosis: I.M.: 20-30 minutes
  Sedation: I.V.: 5-20 minutes
  Anticonvulsant: I.V.: 5 minutes, oral: 30-60 minutes
Duration: 6-8 hours
Absorption: Oral, I.M.: Prompt
Distribution:
  V_d: Neonates: 0.76 L/kg, Adults: 1.3 L/kg; crosses placenta; enters breast milk
Protein binding: 85%; free fraction may be significantly higher in elderly
Metabolism: Hepatic to inactive compounds
Bioavailability: Oral: 90%
Half-life elimination: Neonates: 40.2 hours; Older children: 10.5 hours; Adults: 12.9 hours; Elderly: 15.9 hours; End-stage renal disease: 32-70 hours
Time to peak: Oral: 2 hours
Excretion: Urine; feces (minimal)

Dosage

Antiemetic (unlabeled use):
  Children 2-15 years: I.V.: 0.05 mg/kg (up to 2 mg/dose) prior to chemotherapy
  Adults: Oral, I.V. (**Note:** May be administered sublingually; not a labeled route): 0.5-2 mg every 4-6 hours as needed

Anxiety and sedation (unlabeled in children except for oral use in children >12 years):
  Infants and Children: Oral, I.M., I.V.: Usual: 0.05 mg/kg/dose (range: 0.02-0.09 mg/kg) every 4-8 hours
    I.V.: May use smaller doses (eg, 0.01-0.03 mg/kg) and repeat every 20 minutes, as needed to titrate to effect
  Adults: Oral: 1-10 mg/day in 2-3 divided doses; usual dose: 2-6 mg/day in divided doses
  Elderly: 0.5-4 mg/day; initial dose not to exceed 2 mg

Insomnia: Adults: Oral: 2-4 mg at bedtime

◀ Preoperative: Adults:
  I.M.: 0.05 mg/kg administered 2 hours before surgery (maximum: 4 mg/dose)
  I.V.: 0.044 mg/kg 15-20 minutes before surgery (usual maximum: 2 mg/dose)
Preprocedural anxiety (dental use): Adults: Oral: 1-2 mg 1 hour before procedure
Operative amnesia: Adults: I.V.: Up to 0.05 mg/kg (maximum: 4 mg/dose)
Sedation (preprocedure): Infants and Children (unlabeled):
  Oral, I.M., I.V.: Usual: 0.05 mg/kg (range: 0.02-0.09 mg/kg)
    I.V.: May use smaller doses (eg, 0.01-0.03 mg/kg) and repeat every 20 minutes, as needed to titrate to effect
Status epilepticus: I.V.:
  Infants and Children (unlabeled): 0.05-0.1 mg/kg (maximum: 4 mg/dose) slow I.V. (maximum rate: 2 mg/minute); may repeat every 10-15 minutes as needed (Hegenbarth, 2008; Sabo-Graham, 1998)
  Adults: 4 mg/dose slow I.V. (maximum rate: 2 mg/minute); may repeat in 10-15 minutes; usual maximum dose: 8 mg
Rapid tranquilization of agitated patient (administer every 30-60 minutes): Adults:
  Oral: 1-2 mg
  I.M.: 0.5-1 mg
  Average total dose for tranquilization: Oral, I.M.: 4-8 mg
Agitation in the ICU patient (unlabeled): Adults:
  I.V.: 0.02-0.06 mg/kg every 2-6 hours
  I.V. infusion: 0.01-0.1 mg/kg/hour
  Concurrent use of probenecid or valproic acid: Reduce lorazepam dose by 50%

Dosage adjustment in renal impairment: I.V.: Risk of propylene glycol toxicity. Monitor closely if using for prolonged periods of time or at high doses.
Dosage adjustment in hepatic impairment: Use cautiously.
Stability
  I.V.: Intact vials should be refrigerated. Protect from light. Do not use discolored or precipitate-containing solutions. May be stored at room temperature for up to 60 days. Parenteral admixture is stable at room temperature (25°C) for 24 hours. Dilute I.V. dose with equal volume of compatible diluent (D_5W, NS, SWI).
    Infusion: Use 2 mg/mL injectable vial to prepare; there may be deceased stability when using 4 mg/mL vial. Dilute ≤1 mg/mL and mix in glass bottle. Precipitation may develop. Can also be administered undiluted via infusion.
  Tablet: Store at room temperature.
Administration
  I.M.: Should be administered deep into the muscle mass
  I.V.: Do not exceed 2 mg/minute or 0.05 mg/kg over 2-5 minutes; dilute I.V. dose with equal volume of compatible diluent (D_5W, NS, SWI). Avoid intra-arterial administration. Monitor I.V. site for extravasation.
Monitoring Parameters Respiratory and cardiovascular status, blood pressure, heart rate, symptoms of anxiety
  Clinical signs of propylene glycol toxicity (for continuous high-dose and/or long duration intravenous use): Serum creatinine, BUN, serum lactate, osmol gap
Reference Range Therapeutic: 50-240 ng/mL (SI: 156-746 nmol/L)
Anesthesia and Critical Care Concerns/Other Considerations Lorazepam 2 mg/mL and 4 mg/mL each contain propylene glycol 830 mg/mL (80% v/v). In addition, lorazepam 2 mg/mL oral solution (Intensol™) contains propylene glycol.

Agitation in the ICU Patient: Lorazepam has a slower onset of action than midazolam or diazepam, making it less useful for treatment of acute agitation. The polyethylene glycol and propylene glycol solvents in lorazepam injection can accumulate and lead to reversible acute tubular necrosis, lactic acidosis, and hyperosmolar states with prolonged, high-dose infusions.

A prospective, observational study was performed in a medical intensive care unit evaluating patients receiving high-dose lorazepam (≥10 mg/hour) infusions (Arroliga, 2004). The primary objective was to evaluate the relationship between high-dose lorazepam and serum propylene glycol concentrations. Nine patients met the criteria for entry. Baseline creatinine clearances were 50-100 mL/minute. Propylene glycol accumulation was observed in these patients receiving high-dose lorazepam infusions for ≥48 hours. A significant correlation between high-dose lorazepam infusion rate and serum propylene glycol concentrations was observed. However, osmol gap was the strongest predictor ($R^2 = 0.80$) of serum propylene glycol concentrations. Study findings suggest that in critically ill adults with normal renal function, serum propylene glycol concentrations may be predicted by the osmol gap. Based on these findings, propylene glycol accumulation may occur as early as 48 hours when using high-dose lorazepam infusions.

To calculate osmolarity: [2 x sodium (mEq/L)] + [glucose (mg/dL)/18] + [BUN (mg/dL)/2.8]

To calculate osmol gap (normal range: 0-5): (measured osmolality minus calculated osmolarity)

However, Nelsen et al (2008) conducted a prospective evaluation of 50 adult critically-ill patients (median APACHE II = 20) receiving lorazepam continuous infusion for ≥48 hours in the surgical, medical or burn/trauma ICU. Eight patients exhibited PG accumulation (>25 mg/dL) associated with a median lorazepam infusion rate of 6.4 mg/hour, despite lack of correlation with osmolal gap or serum lactate levels. Of note, reduced clearance of PG correlated with increasing APACHE II scores.

Lorazepam is recommended for the sedation of most patients. Use a defined endpoint in titration of the dose. Use a system to minimize prolonged sedative effects. If patient has received high-dose or >7 days of continuous therapy, consider tapering infusion to prevent withdrawal symptoms.

In the MENDS trial, compared to dexmedetomidine the use of lorazepam for ICU sedation of mechanically-ventilated patients increased the number of days alive with delirium or coma. A nonsignificant increase in 28-day mortality was noted in the lorazepam group when compared to dexmedetomidine (27% vs 17%, respectively; p=0.18) (Pandharipande, 2007).

Pregnancy Risk Factor D

Contraindications Hypersensitivity to lorazepam or any component of the formulation (cross-sensitivity with other benzodiazepines may exist); acute narrow-angle glaucoma; sleep apnea (parenteral); intra-arterial injection of parenteral formulation; severe respiratory insufficiency (except during mechanical ventilation)

Warnings/Precautions Use with caution in elderly or debilitated patients, patients with hepatic disease (including alcoholics) or renal impairment. Use with caution in patients with respiratory disease (COPD or sleep apnea) or limited pulmonary reserve, or impaired gag reflex. Initial doses in elderly or debilitated patients should be at the lower end of the dosing range. May worsen hepatic encephalopathy.

Causes CNS depression (dose-related) resulting in sedation, dizziness, confusion, or ataxia which may impair physical and mental capabilities. Patients must be cautioned about performing tasks which require mental alertness (eg, operating machinery or driving). Use with caution in patients receiving other CNS depressants or psychoactive agents. Effects with other sedative drugs or ethanol may be potentiated. Benzodiazepines have been associated with falls and traumatic injury and should be used with extreme caution in patients who are at risk of these events (especially the elderly).

Lorazepam may cause anterograde amnesia. Paradoxical reactions, including hyperactive or aggressive behavior have been reported with benzodiazepines, particularly in adolescent/pediatric or psychiatric patients. Does not have analgesic, antidepressant, or antipsychotic properties.

Use caution in patients with depression, particularly if suicidal risk may be present. Pre-existing depression may worsen or emerge during therapy. Not recommended for use in primary depressive or psychotic disorders. Use with caution in patients with a history of drug dependence, alcoholism, or significant personality disorders. Benzodiazepines have been associated with dependence and acute withdrawal symptoms on discontinuation or reduction in dose. Acute withdrawal, including seizures, may be precipitated after administration of flumazenil to patients receiving long-term benzodiazepine therapy.

As a hypnotic agent, should be used only after evaluation of potential causes of sleep disturbance. Failure of sleep disturbance to resolve after 7-10 days may ▶

◀ indicate psychiatric or medical illness. A worsening of insomnia or the emergence of new abnormalities of thought or behavior may represent unrecognized psychiatric or medical illness and requires immediate and careful evaluation.

Parenteral formulation of lorazepam contains polyethylene glycol which has resulted in toxicity during high-dose and/or longer-term infusions. Parenteral formulation also contains propylene glycol (PG); may be associated with dose-related toxicity and can occur ≥48 hours after initiation of lorazepam. Limited data suggest increased risk of PG accumulation at doses of ≥6 mg/hour for 48 hours or more (Nelson, 2008). Consider monitoring for signs of toxicity which may include acute renal failure, lactic acidosis, and/or osmol gap. In high-risk patients requiring higher doses/extended treatment durations, use of enteral delivery of lorazepam tablets may be beneficial (Jacobi, 2002). Also contains benzyl alcohol; avoid in neonates.

Safety and efficacy have not been established in children <12 years of age.

Adverse Reactions

>10%:

Central nervous system: Sedation

Respiratory: Respiratory depression

1% to 10%:

Cardiovascular: Hypotension

Central nervous system: Akathisia, amnesia, ataxia, confusion, depression, disorientation, dizziness, headache

Dermatologic: Dermatitis, rash

Gastrointestinal: Changes in appetite, nausea, weight gain/loss

Neuromuscular & skeletal: Weakness

Ocular: Visual disturbances

Respiratory: Apnea, hyperventilation, nasal congestion

<1% or frequency not defined (Limited to important or life-threatening): Asthenia, blood dyscrasias, disinhibition, euphoria, fatigue, increased salivation, menstrual irregularities, physical and psychological dependence (with prolonged use), reflex slowing, polyethylene glycol or propylene glycol poisoning (prolonged I.V. infusion), suicidal ideation, seizure, vertigo

Drug Interactions

Avoid Concomitant Use There are no known interactions where it is recommended to avoid concomitant use.

Increased Effect/Toxicity

LORazepam may increase the levels/effects of: Alcohol (Ethyl); Clozapine; CNS Depressants; Methotrimeprazine; Phenytoin

The levels/effects of LORazepam may be increased by: Loxapine; Methotrimeprazine; Probenecid; Valproic Acid

Decreased Effect

The levels/effects of LORazepam may be decreased by: Theophylline Derivatives; Yohimbine

Ethanol/Nutrition/Herb Interactions

Ethanol: Avoid or limit ethanol (may increase CNS depression).

Herb/Nutraceutical: Avoid valerian, St John's wort, kava kava, gotu kola (may increase CNS depression).

Dosage Forms Excipient information presented when available (limited, particularly for generics); consult specific product labeling. [DSC] = Discontinued product

Injection, solution: 2 mg/mL (1 mL, 10 mL); 4 mg/mL (1 mL, 10 mL)

Ativan®: 2 mg/mL (1 mL; 10 mL [DSC]); 4 mg/mL (1 mL, 10 mL) [contains benzyl alcohol, polyethylene glycol 400, and propylene glycol]

Injection, solution [preservative free]: 2 mg/mL (1 mL); 4 mg/mL (1 mL)

Solution, oral [concentrate]: 2 mg/mL (30 mL)

Lorazepam Intensol™: 2 mg/mL (30 mL) [ethanol free, sugar free, dye free; contains propylene glycol]

Tablet: 0.5 mg, 1 mg, 2 mg

Ativan®: 0.5 mg

Ativan®: 1 mg, 2 mg [scored]

References

Alldredge BK, Gelb AM, Isaacs SM, et al, "A Comparison of Lorazepam, Diazepam, and Placebo for the Treatment of Out-of-Hospital Status Epilepticus," *N Engl J Med*, 2001, 345(9):631-7.

Arroliga AC, Shehab N, McCarthy K, et al, "Relationship of Continuous Infusion Lorazepam to Serum Propylene Glycol Concentration in Critically Ill Adults," *Crit Care Med*, 2004, 32(8):1709-14.

Barnes BJ, Gerst C, Smith JR, et al, "Osmol Gap as a Surrogate Marker for Serum Propylene Glycol Concentrations in Patients Receiving Lorazepam for Sedation," *Pharmacotherapy*, 2006, 26 (1):23-33.

Bleck TP, "Seizures, Stroke, and Other Neurologic Emergencies," *Multidisciplinary Critical Care Review*, Zimmerman JL and Roberts PR, eds, Des Plaines, IL: Society of Critical Care Medicine, 2003, 325-34.

Crawford TO, Mitchell WG, and Snodgrass SR, "Lorazepam in Childhood Status Epilepticus and Serial Seizures: Effectiveness and Tachyphylaxis," *Neurology*, 1987, 37(2):190-5.

Hayman M, Seidl EC, Ali M, et al, "Acute Tubular Necrosis Associated With Propylene Glycol From Concomitant Administration of Intravenous Lorazepam and Trimethoprim-Sulfamethoxazole," *Pharmacotherapy*, 2003, 23(9):1190-4.

Jacobi J, Fraser GL, Coursin DB, et al, "Clinical Practice Guidelines for the Sustained Use of Sedatives and Analgesics in the Critically Ill Adult," *Crit Care Med*, 2002, 30(1):119-41. Available at: http://www.sccm.org/pdf/sedatives.pdf.

Manno EM, "New Management Strategies in the Treatment of Status Epilepticus," *Mayo Clin Proc*, 2003, 78(4):508-18.

Mokhlesi B, Leikin JB, Murray P, et al, "Adult Toxicology in Critical Care. Part II: Specific Poisonings," *Chest*, 2003, 123(3):897-922.

Nelsen JL, Haas CE, Habtemariam B, et al, "A Prospective Evaluation of Propylene Glycol Clearance and Accumulation During Continuous-Infusion Lorazepam in Critically Ill Patients," *J Intensive Care Med*, 2008, 23(3):184-94.

"New Treatment Strategies in the Treatment of Status Epilepticus," *Mayo Clin Proc*, 2003, 78 (4):508-18.

Pandharipande PP, Pun BT, Herr DL, et al, "Effect of Sedation With Dexmedetomidine Vs Lorazepam on Acute Brain Dysfunction in Mechanically Ventilated Patients: The MENDS Randomized Controlled Trial," *JAMA*, 2007, 298(22):2644-53.

"Treatment of Convulsive Status Epilepticus. Recommendations of the Epilepsy Foundation of America's Working Group on Status Epilepticus," *JAMA*, 1993, 270(7):854-9.

Treiman DM, Meyers PD, Walton NY, et al, "A Comparison of Four Treatments for Generalized Convulsive Status Epilepticus. Veterans Affairs Status Epilepticus Cooperative Study Group," *N Engl J Med*, 1998, 339(12):792-8.

Yaucher NE, Fish JT, Smith HW, et al, "Propylene Glycol-Associated Renal Toxicity From Lorazepam Infusion," *Pharmacotherapy*, 2003, 23(9):1094-9.

◆ **Lorazepam Injection, USP (Can)** *see* LORazepam *on page 852*

◆ **Lorazepam Intensol™** *see* LORazepam *on page 852*

◆ **Lorcet® 10/650** *see* Hydrocodone and Acetaminophen *on page 697*

◆ **Lorcet® Plus** *see* Hydrocodone and Acetaminophen *on page 697*

◆ **Lortab®** *see* Hydrocodone and Acetaminophen *on page 697*

Losartan (loe SAR tan)

Related Information
Angiotensin Agents *on page 1652*
Heart Failure (Systolic) *on page 1739*
Preoperative Evaluation of the Cardiac Patient for Noncardiac Surgery *on page 1598*

U.S. Brand Names Cozaar®

Canadian Brand Names Cozaar®

Index Terms DuP 753; Losartan Potassium; MK594

Pharmacologic Category Angiotensin II Receptor Blocker

Use Treatment of hypertension (HTN); treatment of diabetic nephropathy in patients with type 2 diabetes mellitus (noninsulin dependent, NIDDM) and a history of hypertension; stroke risk reduction in patients with HTN and left ventricular hypertrophy (LVH)

Unlabeled/Investigational Use To slow the rate of progression of aortic-root dilation in pediatric patients with Marfan's syndrome

Pharmacodynamics/Kinetics
Onset of action: 6 hours

Distribution: V_d: Losartan: 34 L; E-3174: 12 L; does not cross blood brain barrier

Protein binding, plasma: High

Metabolism: Hepatic (14%) via CYP2C9 and 3A4 to active metabolite, E-3174 (40 times more potent than losartan); extensive first-pass effect

◄ Bioavailability: 25% to 33%; AUC of E-3174 is four times greater than that of losartan

Half-life elimination: Losartan: 1.5-2 hours; E-3174: 6-9 hours

Time to peak, serum: Losartan: 1 hour; E-3174: 3-4 hours

Excretion: Urine (4% as unchanged drug, 6% as active metabolite)

Clearance: Plasma: Losartan: 600 mL/minute; Active metabolite: 50 mL/minute

Dosage Oral:

Hypertension:

Children 6-16 years:

U.S. labeling: 0.7 mg/kg once daily (maximum: 50 mg/day); doses >1.4 mg/kg (maximum: 100 mg) have not been studied

Canadian labeling:

≥20 kg to <50 kg: 25 mg once daily (maximum: 50 mg once daily)

≥50 kg: 50 mg once daily (maximum: 100 mg once daily)

Adults: Usual starting dose: 50 mg once daily; can be administered once or twice daily with total daily doses ranging from 25-100 mg

Patients receiving diuretics or with intravascular volume depletion: Usual initial dose: 25 mg once daily

Aortic-root dilation with Marfan's syndrome (unlabeled use): Children 14 months to 16 years: Initial: 0.6 mg/kg/day; can be increased to a maximum of 1.4 mg/kg/day (not to exceed adult maximum of 100 mg/day)

Nephropathy in patients with type 2 diabetes and hypertension: Adults: Initial: 50 mg once daily; can be increased to 100 mg once daily based on blood pressure response

Stroke reduction (HTN with LVH): Adults: 50 mg once daily (maximum daily dose: 100 mg); may be used in combination with a thiazide diuretic

Dosing adjustment in renal impairment:

Children: Use is not recommended if GFR <30 mL/minute/1.73 m^2

Adults: No adjustment necessary.

Dosing adjustment in hepatic impairment:

Children 6-16 years:

U.S. labeling: No specific dosing recommendations are provided in the approved labeling, however it may be advisable to initiate therapy at a reduced dosage.

Canadian labeling: Use is not recommended.

Adults: Reduce the initial dose to 25 mg/day

Anesthesia and Critical Care Concerns/Other Considerations

Clinical Pearls/Comments: In patients on chronic angiotensin receptor blocker (ARB) therapy, intraoperative hypotension may occur with induction and maintenance of general anesthesia; however, discontinuation of therapy prior to surgery is controversial. If continued preoperatively, avoidance of hypotensive agents during surgery is prudent. Episodes of intraoperative hypotension may be managed by fluid administration and/or modest doses of alpha-adrenergic agents. Severe hypotension may occur in patients who are sodium- and/or volume-depleted; initiate lower doses and monitor closely when starting therapy in these patients. ARB therapy may elicit an increase in potassium and creatinine, especially when used in patients with bilateral renal artery stenosis. Concomitant NSAID therapy may attenuate blood pressure control; use of NSAIDs should be avoided or limited, with monitoring of blood pressure control. In the setting of heart failure, NSAID use may be associated with an increased risk for fluid accumulation and edema and therefore should be avoided.

Evidence-Based Information: The angiotensin II receptor antagonists have similar indications as ACE inhibitors. In heart failure, the angiotensin II receptor antagonists are especially useful in providing an alternative therapy in those patients who have intractable cough due to ACE inhibitor therapy. Candesartan has been studied as an alternative therapy in chronic heart failure patients who cannot tolerate an ACE-I (CHARM-Alternative) and as an added therapy in heart failure patients who are maintained on an ACE-I (CHARM-Added). In both studies, the combined endpoint of cardiovascular death or heart failure hospitalizations was significantly improved over the placebo-treated group.

Additional Information Complete prescribing information for this medication should be consulted for additional detail.

Dosage Forms Excipient information presented when available (limited, particularly for generics); consult specific product labeling.
Tablet, oral, as potassium:
  Cozaar®: 25 mg [contains potassium 2.12 mg (0.054 mEq)]
  Cozaar®: 50 mg [contains potassium 4.24 mg (0.108 mEq)]
  Cozaar®: 100 mg [contains potassium 8.48 mg (0.216 mEq)]

♦ **Losartan Potassium** *see Losartan on page 857*
♦ **LoSeasonique™** *see Ethinyl Estradiol and Levonorgestrel on page 549*
♦ **Losec® (Can)** *see Omeprazole on page 1048*
♦ **Losec MUPS® (Can)** *see Omeprazole on page 1048*
♦ **Lotemax®** *see Loteprednol on page 859*
♦ **Lotensin®** *see Benazepril on page 182*

Loteprednol (loe te PRED nol)

U.S. Brand Names Alrex®; Lotemax®
Canadian Brand Names Alrex®; Lotemax®
Index Terms Loteprednol Etabonate
Pharmacologic Category Corticosteroid, Ophthalmic
Use
  Suspension, 0.2% (Alrex®): Temporary relief of signs and symptoms of seasonal allergic conjunctivitis
  Suspension, 0.5% (Lotemax®): Inflammatory conditions (treatment of steroid-responsive inflammatory conditions of the palpebral and bulbar conjunctiva, cornea, and anterior segment of the globe such as allergic conjunctivitis, acne rosacea, superficial punctate keratitis, herpes zoster keratitis, iritis, cyclitis, selected infective conjunctivitis, when the inherent hazard of steroid use is accepted to obtain an advisable diminution in edema and inflammation) and treatment of postoperative inflammation following ocular surgery
Pharmacodynamics/Kinetics Absorption: None
Dosage Adults: Ophthalmic:
  Suspension, 0.2% (Alrex®): Instill 1 drop into affected eye(s) 4 times/day
  Suspension, 0.5% (Lotemax®):
    Inflammatory conditions: Apply 1-2 drops into the conjunctival sac of the affected eye(s) 4 times/day. During the initial treatment within the first week, the dosing may be increased up to 1 drop every hour. Advise patients not to discontinue therapy prematurely. If signs and symptoms fail to improve after 2 days, re-evaluate the patient.
    Postoperative inflammation: Apply 1-2 drops into the conjunctival sac of the operated eye(s) 4 times/day beginning 24 hours after surgery and continuing throughout the first 2 weeks of the postoperative period
Additional Information Complete prescribing information for this medication should be consulted for additional detail.
Dosage Forms Excipient information presented when available (limited, particularly for generics); consult specific product labeling.
Suspension, ophthalmic, as etabonate:
  Alrex®: 0.2% (5 mL, 10 mL) [contains benzalkonium chloride]
  Lotemax®: 0.5% (2.5 mL, 5 mL, 10 mL, 15 mL) [contains benzalkonium chloride]

♦ **Loteprednol Etabonate** *see Loteprednol on page 859*

Lovastatin (LOE va sta tin)

Related Information
  Hyperlipidemia Management *on page 1747*
  Preoperative Evaluation of the Cardiac Patient for Noncardiac Surgery *on page 1598*
U.S. Brand Names Altoprev®; Mevacor®
Canadian Brand Names Apo-Lovastatin®; CO Lovastatin; DOM-Lovastatin; Gen-Lovastatin; Mevacor®; Mylan-Lovastatin; Novo-Lovastatin; Nu-Lovastatin;

◀ PHL-Lovastatin; PMS-Lovastatin; PRO-Lovastatin; RAN™-Lovastatin; ratio-Lovastatin; Riva-Lovastatin; Sandoz-Lovastatin

Index Terms Mevinolin; Monacolin K

Pharmacologic Category Antilipemic Agent, HMG-CoA Reductase Inhibitor

Use

Adjunct to dietary therapy to decrease elevated serum total and LDL-cholesterol concentrations in primary hypercholesterolemia

Primary prevention of coronary artery disease (patients without symptomatic disease with average or moderately elevated total and LDL-cholesterol and below average HDL-cholesterol); slow progression of coronary atherosclerosis in patients with coronary heart disease

Adjunct to dietary therapy in adolescent patients (10-17 years of age, females >1 year postmenarche) with heterozygous familial hypercholesterolemia having LDL >189 mg/dL, **or** LDL >160 mg/dL with positive family history of premature cardiovascular disease (CVD), **or** LDL >160 mg/dL with the presence of at least two other CVD risk factors

Pharmacodynamics/Kinetics

Onset of action: LDL-cholesterol reductions: 3 days

Absorption: 30%; increased with extended release tablets when taken in the fasting state

Protein binding: 95%

Metabolism: Hepatic; extensive first-pass effect; hydrolyzed to B-hydroxy acid (active)

Bioavailability: Increased with extended release tablets

Half-life elimination: 1.1-1.7 hours

Time to peak, serum: 2-4 hours

Excretion: Feces (~80% to 85%); urine (10%)

Dosage Oral:

Adolescents 10-17 years: Immediate release tablet:

LDL reduction <20%: Initial: 10 mg/day with evening meal

LDL reduction ≥20%: Initial: 20 mg/day with evening meal

Usual range: 10-40 mg with evening meal, then adjust dose at 4-week intervals

Adults: Initial: 20 mg with evening meal, then adjust at 4-week intervals; maximum dose: 80 mg/day immediate release tablet **or** 60 mg/day extended release tablet

Dosage modification/limits based on concurrent therapy:

Cyclosporine and other immunosuppressant drugs: Initial dose: 10 mg/day with a maximum recommended dose of 20 mg/day

Concurrent therapy with fibrates, danazol, and/or lipid-lowering doses of niacin (>1 g/day): Maximum recommended dose: 20 mg/day. Concurrent use with fibrates should be avoided unless risk to benefit favors use.

Concurrent therapy with amiodarone or verapamil: Maximum recommended dose: 40 mg/day of regular release or 20 mg/day with extended release.

Dosage adjustment in renal impairment: Cl_{cr} <30 mL/minute: Use doses >20 mg/day with caution.

Anesthesia and Critical Care Concerns/Other Considerations

Clinical Pearls/Comments: Myopathy: Currently-marketed HMG-CoA reductase inhibitors appear to have a similar potential for causing myopathy. Incidence of severe myopathy is about 0.08% to 0.09%. The factors that increase risk include advanced age (especially >80 years), gender (occurs in women more frequently than men), small body frame, frailty, multisystem disease (eg, chronic renal insufficiency especially due to diabetes), multiple medications, and drug interactions (use with caution or avoid).

Based on current research and clinical guidelines (Fleisher, 2007), HMG-CoA reductase inhibitors should be continued in the perioperative period. Postoperative discontinuation of statin therapy is associated with an increased risk of cardiac morbidity and mortality.

Additional Information Complete prescribing information for this medication should be consulted for additional detail.

Dosage Forms Excipient information presented when available (limited, particularly for generics); consult specific product labeling.

Tablet: 10 mg, 20 mg, 40 mg

Mevacor®: 20 mg, 40 mg

Tablet, extended release:
Altoprev®: 20 mg, 40 mg, 60 mg
References
Pasternak RC, Smith SC Jr, Bairey-Merz CN, et al, "ACC/AHA/NHLBI Clinical Advisory on the Use and Safety of Statins," *Stroke,* 2002, 33(9):2337-41. Available at: http://www.acc.org/clinical/alerts/statins_june02.htm. accessed June 18, 2003.

◆ **Lovenox®** *see* Enoxaparin *on page 485*

◆ **Lovenox® HP (Can)** *see* Enoxaparin *on page 485*

◆ **Low-Ogestrel®** *see* Ethinyl Estradiol and Norgestrel *on page 560*

◆ **LTA® 360** *see* Lidocaine *on page 836*

◆ **LTG** *see* LamoTRIgine *on page 800*

◆ ***L*-Thyroxine Sodium** *see* Levothyroxine *on page 831*

◆ **Lu-26-054** *see* Escitalopram *on page 521*

◆ **Luminal® Sodium** *see* PHENobarbital *on page 1109*

◆ **Lunesta®** *see* Eszopiclone *on page 540*

◆ **Lusedra™** *see* Fospropofol *on page 642*

◆ **LuSonal™** *see* Phenylephrine *on page 1114*

◆ **Lutera™** *see* Ethinyl Estradiol and Levonorgestrel *on page 549*

◆ **Luxiq®** *see* Betamethasone *on page 186*

◆ **LY139603** *see* Atomoxetine *on page 157*

◆ **LY146032** *see* DAPTOmycin *on page 372*

◆ **LY170053** *see* OLANZapine *on page 1043*

◆ **LY246736** *see* Alvimopan *on page 75*

◆ **LY248686** *see* DULoxetine *on page 469*

◆ **LY303366** *see* Anidulafungin *on page 123*

◆ **LY-640315** *see* Prasugrel *on page 1160*

◆ **LY2148568** *see* Exenatide *on page 566*

◆ **Lybrel™** *see* Ethinyl Estradiol and Levonorgestrel *on page 549*

◆ **Lyrica®** *see* Pregabalin *on page 1171*

Mafenide (MA fe nide)

U.S. Brand Names Sulfamylon®
Index Terms Mafenide Acetate
Pharmacologic Category Antibiotic, Topical
Generic Available No
Use
Cream: Adjunctive antibacterial agent in the treatment of second- and third-degree burns
Solution: Adjunctive antibacterial agent for use under moist dressings over meshed autografts on excised burn wounds
Mechanism of Action As a sulfonamide, mafenide interferes with bacterial folic acid synthesis through competitive inhibition of para-aminobenzoic acid. Spectrum of activity encompasses both gram positive and negative organisms, including *Pseudomonas* and some anaerobes.
Pharmacodynamics/Kinetics
Absorption: Diffuses through devascularized areas and is rapidly absorbed from burned surface
Metabolism: To para-carboxybenzene sulfonamide; mafenide and metabolite are carbonic anhydrase inhibitors
Time to peak, serum: Cream 11%: 2-4 hours
Burn tissue: Cream 11%: 2 hours, Solution 5%: 4 hours
Excretion: Urine (as metabolites)
Dosage Children and Adults: Topical:
Cream: Apply once or twice daily with a sterile-gloved hand; apply to a thickness of approximately 1/16 inch; the burned area should be covered with cream at all times

Solution: Cover graft area with 1 layer of fine mesh gauze. Wet an 8-ply burn dressing with mafenide solution and cover graft area. Keep dressing wet using syringe or irrigation tubing every 4 hours (or as necessary), or by moistening dressing every 6-8 hours (or as necessary). Irrigation dressing should be secured with bolster dressing and wrapped as appropriate. May leave dressings in place for up to 5 days.

Dosage adjustment for acidosis: Discontinuing treatment for 24-48 hours may aid in restoring acid-base balance

Stability

Cream: Avoid exposure to excessive heat, >40°C (>104°F).

Powder: Prior to reconstitution, store powder at room temperature of 15°C to 30°C (59°F to 86°F). To prepare a 5% topical solution, add mafenide 50 g to 1000 mL of NS for irrigation or sterile water for irrigation. Mix until dissolved. Store prepared solution at 20°C to 25°C (68°F to 77°F); may store at room temperature for limited periods. Solution may be stored in unopened containers for up to 28 days; once container is open, discard unused portion within 48 hours.

Administration Cream: Keep burn area covered with cream at all times; use thinner layer if dressings are used. Apply to clean debrided area with a sterile gloved hand

Monitoring Parameters Acid base balance; signs of infection; signs of healing

Pregnancy Risk Factor C

Contraindications Hypersensitivity to mafenide or any component of the formulation

Warnings/Precautions Use with caution in patients with renal impairment; accumulation of parent drug and metabolite may enhance carbonic anhydrase inhibition and increase risk of metabolic acidosis. Use caution in patients with G6PD deficiency; may increase risk of DIC or hemolytic anemia. Use caution in patients with hypersensitivity to sulfonamides (cross sensitivity not known). Prolonged use may result in fungal or bacterial superinfection, including *C. difficile*-associated diarrhea (CDAD) and pseudomembranous colitis; CDAD has been observed >2 months postantibiotic treatment. Some dosage forms contain sulfites which may cause allergic reactions in certain individuals.

Adverse Reactions Frequency not defined.

Cardiovascular: Edema, facial edema

Dermatologic: Erythema, maceration, pruritus, rash, urticaria

Endocrine & metabolic: Hyperchloremia, metabolic acidosis

Gastrointestinal: Diarrhea (following accidental ingestion)

Hematologic: Bleeding, bone marrow suppression, DIC, eosinophilia, hemolytic anemia, porphyria

Local: Blisters, burning sensation, excoriation, pain

Respiratory: Dyspnea, hyperventilation, pCO_2 decreased, tachypnea

Miscellaneous: Hypersensitivity

Drug Interactions

Avoid Concomitant Use There are no known interactions where it is recommended to avoid concomitant use.

Increased Effect/Toxicity There are no known significant interactions involving an increase in effect.

Decreased Effect There are no known significant interactions involving a decrease in effect.

Dosage Forms Excipient information presented when available (limited, particularly for generics); consult specific product labeling.

Cream, topical:

Sulfamylon®: 85 mg/g (60 g, 120 g, 454 g) [contains sodium metabisulfite]

Powder, for topical solution, as acetate:

Sulfamylon®: 50 g/packet (5s)

◆ **Mafenide Acetate** *see* Mafenide *on page 861*

◆ **Magnacet™** *see* Oxycodone and Acetaminophen *on page 1072*

Magnesium Sulfate (mag NEE zhum SUL fate)

Medication Safety Issues
Sound-alike/look-alike issues:

Magnesium sulfate may be confused with manganese sulfate, morphine sulfate

$MgSO_4$ is an error-prone abbreviation (mistaken as morphine sulfate)

High alert medication: The Institute for Safe Medication Practices (ISMP) includes this medication (I.V. formulation) among its list of drugs which have a heightened risk of causing significant patient harm when used in error.

Index Terms Epsom Salts; $MgSO_4$ (error-prone abbreviation)

Pharmacologic Category Anticonvulsant, Miscellaneous; Electrolyte Supplement, Parenteral; Magnesium Salt

Generic Available Yes

Use Treatment and prevention of hypomagnesemia; prevention and treatment of seizures in severe pre-eclampsia or eclampsia, pediatric acute nephritis; torsade de pointes; treatment of cardiac arrhythmias (VT/VF) caused by hypomagnesemia; soaking aid

Unlabeled/Investigational Use Asthma exacerbation (life-threatening)

Mechanism of Action When taken orally, magnesium promotes bowel evacuation by causing osmotic retention of fluid which distends the colon with increased peristaltic activity; parenterally, magnesium decreases acetylcholine in motor nerve terminals and acts on myocardium by slowing rate of S-A node impulse formation and prolonging conduction time. Magnesium is necessary for the movement of calcium, sodium, and potassium in and out of cells, as well as stabilizing excitable membranes.

Pharmacodynamics/Kinetics
Onset of action: Anticonvulsant: I.M.: 1 hour; I.V.: Immediate
Duration of anticonvulsant activity: I.M.: 3-4 hours; I.V.: 30 minutes
Distribution: Bone (50% to 60%); extracellular fluid (1% to 2%)
Protein binding: 30%, to albumin
Excretion: Urine (as magnesium)

Dosage Dose represented as magnesium sulfate unless stated otherwise. **Note:** Serum magnesium is poor reflection of repletional status as the majority of magnesium is intracellular; serum levels may be transiently normal for a few hours after a dose is given, therefore, aim for consistently high normal serum levels in patients with normal renal function for most efficient repletion.

Note: 1 g of magnesium sulfate = 98.6 mg elemental magnesium = 8.12 mEq elemental magnesium

Hypomagnesemia: Note: Treatment depends on severity and clinical status:
Children: I.V., I.O.: 25-50 mg/kg/dose over 10-20 minutes (faster in cardiac arrest); maximum single dose: 2000 mg
Adults:
Mild deficiency: I.M.: 1 g every 6 hours for 4 doses, or as indicated by serum magnesium levels
Severe deficiency:
I.M.: Up to 250 mg/kg within a 4-hour period
I.V.: Severe, nonlife-threatening: 1-2 g/hour for 3-6 hours then 0.5-1 g/hour as needed to correct deficiency
Symptomatic deficiency: I.V.: 1-2 g over 5-60 minutes; maintenance infusion may be required to correct deficiency (0.5-1 g/hour).
Arrhythmia (ACLS guidelines, 2005), hypomagnesemia-induced (life-threatening): 1-2 g over 5-20 minutes (torsades with cardiac arrest) or over 5-60 minutes (symptomatic arrhythmias without cardiac arrest)
Seizures, hypomagnesemia-induced: I.V.: 2 g over 10 minutes; calcium administration may also be appropriate as many patients are also hypocalcemic.

Asthma (life-threatening or severe exacerbation after 1 hour of intensive conventional therapy; unlabeled use): I.V.:
Children: 25-75 mg/kg (maximum: 2 g)
Adults: 2 g

◄ **Eclampsia:** Adults:
I.V.: 4-5 g infusion; followed by a 1-2 g/hour continous infusion; or may follow with I.M. doses of 4-5 g in each buttock every 4 hours. **Note:** Initial infusion may be given over 3-4 minutes if eclampsia is severe; maximum: 40 g/24 hours
ACOG Practice Bulletin 2002: 4-6 g over 15-20 minutes followed by 2 g/hour continuous infusion

Pre-eclampsia (severe): Adults: I.V. 4-5 g infusion; followed by a 1-2 g/hour continous infusion; or may follow with I.M. doses of 4-5 g in each buttock every 4 hours; maximum: 40 g/24 hour

Torsade de pointes: Adults: I.V.:
Pulseless: 1-2 g over 5-20 minutes
With pulse: 1-2 g over 5-60 minutes. **Note:** Slower administration preferable for stable patients.

Parenteral nutrition supplementation: I.V.:
Children:
<50 kg: 0.3-0.5 mEq elemental magnesium/kg/day
>50 kg: 10-30 mEq elemental magnesium/day
Adults: 8-24 mEq elemental magnesium/day

Soaking aid: Topical: Adults: Dissolve 2 cupfuls of powder per gallon of warm water

RDA:
Children:
1-3 years: 80 mg elemental magnesium/day
4-8 years: 130 mg elemental magnesium/day
9-13 years: 240 mg elemental magnesium/day
14-18 years:
Female: 360 mg elemental magnesium/day
Pregnant female: 400 mg elemental magnesium/day
Male: 410 mg elemental magnesium/day
Adults:
19-30 years:
Female: 310 mg elemental magnesium/day
Pregnant female: 350 mg elemental magnesium/day
Male: 400 mg elemental magnesium/day
≥31 years:
Female: 320 mg elemental magnesium/day
Pregnant female: 360 mg elemental magnesium/day
Male: 420 mg elemental magnesium/day

Dosage adjustment in renal impairment: Cl_{cr} <30 mL/minute: Use with caution; monitor for hypermagnesemia; do not exceed 20 g/48 hours as per manufacturer. Close monitoring is required.

Stability Prior to use, store at room temperature of 20°C to 25°C (68°F to 77°F). Refrigeration of solution may result in precipitation or crystallization.

Administration
Injection: May be administered I.M. or I.V.
I.M.: A 25% or 50% concentration may be used for adults and dilution to a ≤20% solution is recommended for children
I.V.: Magnesium should be diluted to a ≤20% solution for I.V. infusion and may be administered IVP, IVPB or I.V.; when giving I.V. push, must dilute first and should not be given any faster than 150 mg/minute. Hypotension and asystole may occur with rapid administration.
Maximal rate of infusion: 2 g/hour to avoid hypotension; doses of 4 g/hour have been given in emergencies (eclampsia, seizures); optimally, should add magnesium to I.V. fluids, but bolus doses are also effective
Topical: Dissolve 2 cups of powder per gallon of warm water to use as a soaking aid. To make a compress, dissolve 2 cups of powder per 2 cups of hot water and use a towel to apply as a wet dressing.

Monitoring Parameters
I.V.: Rapid administration: ECG monitoring, vital signs, deep tendon reflexes; magnesium, calcium, and potassium levels; renal function during administration

Obstetrics: Patient status including vital signs, oxygen saturation, deep tendon reflexes, level of consciousness, fetal heart rate, maternal uterine activity.

Reference Range Serum magnesium: 1.5-2.5 mg/dL; slightly different ranges are reported by different laboratories

Anesthesia and Critical Care Concerns/Other Considerations

Clinical Pearls/Comments: Hypomagnesemia can hinder the replenishment of intracellular potassium and should be corrected in order to correct hypokalemia.

Pregnancy Risk Factor A/C (manufacturer dependent)

Contraindications Hypersensitivity to any component of the formulation; heart block; myocardial damage

Warnings/Precautions Use magnesium with caution in patients with impaired renal function (accumulation of magnesium may lead to magnesium intoxication). Use with extreme caution in patients with myasthenia gravis or other neuro-muscular disease. Magnesium toxicity can lead to fatal cardiovascular arrest and/or respiratory paralysis; close monitoring of serum magnesium, respiratory rate, and presence of deep tendon reflex necessary during parenteral administration, particularly with repeated dosing. Vigilant monitoring and safe administration techniques (ISMP Medication Safety Alert, 2005) recommended to avoid potential for errors resulting in toxicity when used in obstetrics; monitor patient and fetal status, and serum magnesium levels closely. Solution for injection may contain aluminum; toxic levels may occur following prolonged administration in premature neonates or patients with renal dysfunction. Concurrent hypokalemia or hypocalcemia can accompany a magnesium deficit.

Adverse Reactions Adverse effects on neuromuscular function may occur at lower levels in patients with neuromuscular disease (eg, myasthenia gravis). Frequency not defined:

Cardiovascular: Flushing (I.V.; dose related), hypotension (I.V.; rate related), vasodilation (I.V.; rate related)

Gastrointestinal: Diarrhea

Drug Interactions

Avoid Concomitant Use There are no known interactions where it is recommended to avoid concomitant use.

Increased Effect/Toxicity

Magnesium Sulfate may increase the levels/effects of: Alcohol (Ethyl); Calcium Channel Blockers; CNS Depressants; Methotrimeprazine; Neuromuscular-Blocking Agents

The levels/effects of Magnesium Sulfate may be increased by: Calcitriol; Calcium Channel Blockers; Methotrimeprazine

Decreased Effect

Magnesium Sulfate may decrease the levels/effects of: Bisphosphonate Derivatives; Eltrombopag; Mycophenolate; Phosphate Supplements; Quinolone Antibiotics; Tetracycline Derivatives; Trientine

The levels/effects of Magnesium Sulfate may be decreased by: Ketorolac; Mefloquine; Trientine

Ethanol/Nutrition/Herb Interactions Ethanol: Magnesium may enhance the CNS depressant effect of alcohol (ethyl).

Dietary Considerations Whole grains, legumes and dark-green leafy vegetables are dietary sources of magnesium.

Dosage Forms Excipient information presented when available (limited, particularly for generics); consult specific product labeling.

Infusion [premixed in D_5W]: 10 mg/mL (100 mL); 20 mg/mL (500 mL)

Infusion [premixed in water for injection]: 40 mg/mL (100 mL, 500 mL, 1000 mL); 80 mg/mL (50 mL)

Injection, solution: 500 mg/mL (2 mL, 10 mL, 20 mL, 50 mL)

Powder, oral/topical: Magnesium sulfate USP (227 g, 454 g, 480 g, 1810 g, 1920 g, 2720 g)

References

"2005 American Heart Association Guidelines for Cardiopulmonary Resuscitation and Emergency Cardiovascular Care," *Circulation*, 2005, 112(24 Suppl):1-211.

"ACOG Practice Bulletin. Diagnosis and Management of Preeclampsia and Eclampsia. Number 33, January 2002," *Obstet Gynecol*, 2002, 99(1):159-67.

Dubé L and Granry JC, "The Therapeutic Use of Magnesium in Anesthesiology, Intensive Care and Emergency Medicine: A Review," *Can J Anaesth*, 2003, 50(7):732-46.

◀

Mirtallo J, Canada T, Johnson D, et al, "Safe Practices for Parenteral Nutrition," *JPEN J Parenter Enteral Nutr*, 2004, 28(6):39-70.

National Asthma Education and Prevention Program Coordinating Committee, "Expert Panel Report 3 (EPR 3): Guidelines for the Diagnosis and Management of Asthma," 2007. Available online at: http://www.nhlbi.nih.gov/guidelines/asthma/asthgdln.htm. Last accessed October 8, 2007

Mannitol (MAN i tole)

Medication Safety Issues
Sound-alike/look-alike issues:
Osmitrol® may be confused with esmolol

Related Information
Anesthesia Considerations for Neurosurgery *on page 1514*
Malignant Hyperthermia *on page 1638*

U.S. Brand Names Osmitrol®; Resectisol®

Canadian Brand Names Osmitrol®

Index Terms *D*-Mannitol

Pharmacologic Category Diuretic, Osmotic; Genitourinary Irrigant

Generic Available Yes

Use Reduction of increased intracranial pressure associated with cerebral edema; promotion of diuresis in the prevention and/or treatment of oliguria or anuria due to acute renal failure; reduction of increased intraocular pressure; promoting urinary excretion of toxic substances; genitourinary irrigant in transurethral prostatic resection or other transurethral surgical procedures

Mechanism of Action Increases the osmotic pressure of glomerular filtrate, which inhibits tubular reabsorption of water and electrolytes and increases urinary output

Pharmacodynamics/Kinetics
Onset of action: Diuresis: Injection: 1-3 hours; Reduction in intracranial pressure: ~15-30 minutes

Duration: Reduction in intracranial pressure: 1.5-6 hours

Distribution: Remains confined to extracellular space (except in extreme concentrations); does not penetrate the blood-brain barrier (generally, penetration is low)

Metabolism: Minimally hepatic to glycogen

Half-life elimination: 1.1-1.6 hours

Excretion: Primarily urine (as unchanged drug)

Dosage
Children: I.V.:
Test dose (to assess adequate renal function): 200 mg/kg over 3-5 minutes to produce a urine flow of at least 1 mL/kg for 1-3 hours
Initial: 0.25-1 g/kg
Maintenance: 0.25-0.5 g/kg given every 4-6 hours

Adults:
I.V.:
Test dose (to assess adequate renal function): 12.5 g (200 mg/kg) over 3-5 minutes to produce a urine flow of at least 30-50 mL of urine per hour. If urine flow does not increase, a second test dose may be given. If test dose does not produce an acceptable urine output, then need to reassess management.
Initial: 0.5-1 g/kg
Maintenance: 0.25-0.5 g/kg every 4-6 hours; usual daily dose: 20-200 g/24 hours
Intracranial pressure: Cerebral edema: 0.25-1.5 g/kg/dose I.V. as a 15% to 20% solution over ≥30 minutes; maintain serum osmolality 310 to <320 mOsm/kg
Prevention of acute renal failure (oliguria): 50-100 g dose
Treatment of oliguria: 100 g dose
Preoperative for neurosurgery: 1.5-2 g/kg administered 1-1.5 hours prior to surgery
Reduction of intraocular pressure: 1.5-2 g/kg as a 15% to 20% solution; administer over 30 minutes

Topical: Transurethral irrigation: Use urogenital solution as required for irrigation

Elderly: Consider initiation at lower end of dosing range

Dosage adjustment in renal impairment: Contraindicated in severe renal impairment. If test dose does not produce adequate urine output reassess options. Use caution in patients with underlying renal disease.

Dosage adjustment in hepatic impairment: No adjustment required.

Stability Should be stored at room temperature (15°C to 30°C); do not freeze. Crystallization may occur at low temperatures; do not use solutions that contain crystals. Heating in a hot water bath and vigorous shaking may be utilized for resolubilization. Cool solutions to body temperature before using.

Administration Inspect for crystals prior to administration. If crystals present redissolve by warming solution. Use filter-type administration set; in-line 5-micron filter set should always be used for mannitol infusion with concentrations ≥20%; administer test dose (for oliguria) I.V. push over 3-5 minutes; avoid extravasation; for cerebral edema or elevated ICP, administer over 20-30 minutes; crenation and agglutination of red blood cells may occur if administered with whole blood.

Monitoring Parameters Renal function, daily fluid I & O, serum electrolytes, serum and urine osmolality; for treatment of elevated intracranial pressure, maintain serum osmolality 310 to <320 mOsm/kg.

Anesthesia and Critical Care Concerns/Other Considerations

Clinical Pearls/Comments: Other information:

May autoclave or heat mannitol solution to redissolve crystals.

Mannitol 20% has an approximate osmolarity of 1100 mOsm/L.

Mannitol 25% has an approximate osmolarity of 1375 mOsm/L.

Evidence-Based Information:

Management of Intracerebral Hemorrhage (ICH): The 2007 AHA/ASA Guidelines for the Management of Spontaneous Intracerebral Hemorrhage in Adults recommends mannitol as a treatment option to decrease intracranial pressure (ICP) (Class IIa recommendation).

Pregnancy Risk Factor C

Contraindications Hypersensitivity to mannitol or any component or the formulation; severe renal disease (anuria); severe dehydration; active intracranial bleeding except during craniotomy; progressive heart failure, pulmonary congestion, or renal dysfunction after mannitol administration; severe pulmonary edema or congestion

Warnings/Precautions Should not be administered until adequacy of renal function and urine flow is established; use 1-2 test doses to assess renal response. Excess amounts can lead to profound diuresis with fluid and electrolyte loss; close medical supervision and dose evaluation are required. Watch for and correct electrolyte disturbances; adjust dose to avoid dehydration. May cause renal dysfunction especially with high doses; use caution in patients taking other nephrotoxic agents, with sepsis or pre-existing renal disease. To minimize adverse renal effects, adjust to keep serum osmolality less than 320 mOsm/L. Discontinue if evidence of acute tubular necrosis.

In patients being treated for cerebral edema, mannitol may accumulate in the brain (causing rebound increases in intracranial pressure) if circulating for long periods of time as with continuous infusion; intermittent boluses preferred. Cardiovascular status should also be evaluated; do not administer electrolyte-free mannitol solutions with blood. If hypotension occurs monitor cerebral perfusion pressure to insure adequate.

Adverse Reactions Frequency not defined.

Cardiovascular: Chest pain, CHF, circulatory overload, hyper-/hypotension, tachycardia

Central nervous system: Chills, convulsions, dizziness, headache

Dermatologic: Rash, urticaria

Endocrine & metabolic: Fluid and electrolyte imbalance, dehydration and hypovolemia secondary to rapid diuresis, hyperglycemia, hypernatremia, hyponatremia (dilutional), hyperosmolality-induced hyperkalemia, metabolic acidosis (dilutional), osmolar gap increased, water intoxication

Gastrointestinal: Nausea, vomiting, xerostomia

Genitourinary: Dysuria, polyuria

Local: Pain, thrombophlebitis, tissue necrosis

Ocular: Blurred vision

◄ Renal: Acute renal failure, acute tubular necrosis (>200 g/day; serum osmolality >320 mOsm/L)

Respiratory: Pulmonary edema, rhinitis

Miscellaneous: Allergic reactions

Drug Interactions

Avoid Concomitant Use There are no known interactions where it is recommended to avoid concomitant use.

Increased Effect/Toxicity

Mannitol may increase the levels/effects of: Amifostine; Antihypertensives; Hypotensive Agents; RiTUXimab

The levels/effects of Mannitol may be increased by: Diazoxide; Herbs (Hypotensive Properties); MAO Inhibitors; Pentoxifylline; Phosphodiesterase 5 Inhibitors; Prostacyclin Analogues

Decreased Effect

The levels/effects of Mannitol may be decreased by: Herbs (Hypertensive Properties); Methylphenidate; Yohimbine

Dosage Forms Excipient information presented when available (limited, particularly for generics); consult specific product labeling.

Injection, solution: 5% [50 mg/mL] (1000 mL); 10% [100 mg/mL] (500 mL, 1000 mL); 15% [150 mg/mL] (500 mL); 20% [200 mg/mL] (150 mL, 250 mL, 500 mL); 25% [250 mg/mL] (50 mL)

Osmitrol®: 5% [50 mg/mL] (1000 mL); 10% [100 mg/mL] (500 mL, 1000 mL); 15% [150 mg/mL] (500 mL); 20% [200 mg/mL] (250 mL, 500 mL)

Solution, urogenital (Resectisol®): 5% [50 mg/mL] (2000 mL, 4000 mL)

References

Adelson PD, Bratton SL, Carney NA, et al, "Guidelines for the Acute Medical Management of Severe Traumatic Brain Injury in Infants, Children, and Adolescents," *Pediatr Crit Care Med*, 2003, 4(3 Suppl):40-4.

Broderick J, Connolly S, Feldmann E, et al, "Guidelines for the Management of Spontaneous Intracerebral Hemorrhage in Adults: 2007 Update: A Guideline From the American Heart Association/American Stroke Association Stroke Council, High Blood Pressure Research Council, and the Quality of Care and Outcomes in Research Interdisciplinary Working Group," *Stroke*, 2007, 38(6):2001-23. Available at http://stroke.ahajournals.org/cgi/content/short/STROKEAHA.107.183689.

Procaccio F, Stocchetti N, Citerio G, et al, "Guidelines for the Treatment of Adults With Severe Head Trauma (Part II). Criteria for Medical Treatment," *J Neurosurg Sci*, 2000, 44(1):11-8.

◆ **Mapap [OTC]** *see* Acetaminophen *on page 25*

◆ **Mapap Children's [OTC]** *see* Acetaminophen *on page 25*

◆ **Mapap Extra Strength [OTC]** *see* Acetaminophen *on page 25*

◆ **Mapap Infants [OTC]** *see* Acetaminophen *on page 25*

◆ **Mapap Jr. Strength [OTC]** *see* Acetaminophen *on page 25*

◆ **Mapezine® (Can)** *see* CarBAMazepine *on page 241*

◆ **Marcaine®** *see* Bupivacaine *on page 211*

◆ **Marcaine® Spinal** *see* Bupivacaine *on page 211*

◆ **Margesic® H** *see* Hydrocodone and Acetaminophen *on page 697*

◆ **Marinol®** *see* Dronabinol *on page 460*

◆ **Marplan®** *see* Isocarboxazid *on page 765*

◆ **Marvelon® (Can)** *see* Ethinyl Estradiol and Desogestrel *on page 544*

◆ **3M™ Avagard™ [OTC]** *see* Chlorhexidine Gluconate *on page 291*

◆ **Mavik®** *see* Trandolapril *on page 1419*

◆ **Mavik™ (Can)** *see* Trandolapril *on page 1419*

◆ **Maxalt®** *see* Rizatriptan *on page 1258*

◆ **Maxalt™ (Can)** *see* Rizatriptan *on page 1258*

◆ **Maxalt-MLT®** *see* Rizatriptan *on page 1258*

◆ **Maxalt RPD™ (Can)** *see* Rizatriptan *on page 1258*

◆ **Maxidex®** *see* Dexamethasone *on page 391*

◆ **Maxidone®** *see* Hydrocodone and Acetaminophen *on page 697*

◆ **Maxipime®** *see* Cefepime *on page 253*

◆ **MDL 73,147EF** *see* Dolasetron *on page 444*

Meclofenamate (me kloe fen AM ate)

Related Information
Acetaminophen and NSAIDS, Dosing in the Management of Pain *on page 1651*
Chronic Pain Management *on page 1546*
Nonsteroidal Anti-Inflammatory Agents *on page 1687*

Canadian Brand Names Meclomen®
Index Terms Meclofenamate Sodium
Pharmacologic Category Nonsteroidal Anti-inflammatory Drug (NSAID), Oral
Use Treatment of inflammatory disorders, arthritis, mild-to-moderate pain, dysmenorrhea

Pharmacodynamics/Kinetics
Duration: 2-4 hours
Distribution: Crosses placenta
Protein binding: 99%
Half-life elimination: 2-3.3 hours
Time to peak, serum: 0.5-1.5 hours
Excretion: Primarily urine and feces (as metabolites)

Dosage Children >14 years and Adults: Oral:
Mild-to-moderate pain: 50 mg every 4-6 hours; increases to 100 mg may be required; maximum dose: 400 mg
Rheumatoid arthritis and osteoarthritis: 50 mg every 4-6 hours; increase, over weeks, to 200-400 mg/day in 3-4 divided doses; do not exceed 400 mg/day; maximal benefit for any dose may not be seen for 2-3 weeks

Anesthesia and Critical Care Concerns/Other Considerations The 2002 ACCM/SCCM guidelines for analgesia (critically-ill adult) suggest that NSAIDs may be used in combination with opioids in select patients for pain management. Concern about adverse events (increased risk of renal dysfunction, altered platelet function and gastrointestinal irritation) limits its use in patients who have other underlying risks for these events.

In short-term use, NSAIDs vary considerably in their effect on blood pressure. When NSAIDs are used in patients with hypertension, appropriate monitoring of blood pressure responses should be completed and the duration of therapy, when possible, kept short. The use of NSAIDs in the treatment of patients with congestive heart failure may be associated with an increased risk for fluid accumulation and edema; may precipitate renal failure in dehydrated patients.

Additional Information Complete prescribing information for this medication should be consulted for additional detail.

Dosage Forms Excipient information presented when available (limited, particularly for generics); consult specific product labeling.
Capsule, as sodium: 50 mg, 100 mg

◆ **Meclofenamate Sodium** *see* Meclofenamate *on page 869*
◆ **Meclomen® (Can)** *see* Meclofenamate *on page 869*
◆ **Med-Diltiazem (Can)** *see* Diltiazem *on page 425*
◆ **Medicinal Carbon** *see* Charcoal *on page 283*
◆ **Medicinal Charcoal** *see* Charcoal *on page 283*
◆ **Medicone® Suppositories [OTC]** *see* Phenylephrine *on page 1114*
◆ **Medi-Phenyl [OTC]** *see* Phenylephrine *on page 1114*
◆ **Mediproxen [OTC]** *see* Naproxen *on page 987*
◆ **MED-Metformin (Can)** *see* MetFORMIN *on page 886*
◆ **Medrol®** *see* MethylPREDNISolone *on page 911*
◆ **Medrol Dose Pack** *see* MethylPREDNISolone *on page 911*
◆ **Medroxyprogesterone and Estrogens (Conjugated)** *see* Estrogens (Conjugated/Equine) and Medroxyprogesterone *on page 539*
◆ **MED-Sotalol (Can)** *see* Sotalol *on page 1321*
◆ **Med-Verapamil (Can)** *see* Verapamil *on page 1468*

◆ **Mefenamic-250 (Can)** *see* Mefenamic Acid *on page 870*

Mefenamic Acid (me fe NAM ik AS id)

Related Information
Acetaminophen and NSAIDS, Dosing in the Management of Pain *on page 1651*
Chronic Pain Management *on page 1546*
Nonsteroidal Anti-Inflammatory Agents *on page 1687*

U.S. Brand Names Ponstel®

Canadian Brand Names Apo-Mefenamic®; Dom-Mefenamic Acid; Mefenamic-250; Nu-Mefenamic; PMS-Mefenamic Acid; Ponstan®

Pharmacologic Category Nonsteroidal Anti-inflammatory Drug (NSAID), Oral

Use Short-term relief of mild-to-moderate pain including primary dysmenorrhea

Pharmacodynamics/Kinetics
Onset of action: Peak effect: 2-4 hours

Duration: ≤6 hours

Protein binding: High

Metabolism: Conjugated hepatically

Half-life elimination: 3.5 hours

Excretion: Urine (50%) and feces as unchanged drug and metabolites

Dosage Children >14 years and Adults: Oral: 500 mg to start then 250 mg every 4 hours as needed; maximum therapy: 1 week

Dosing adjustment/comments in renal impairment: Not recommended for use

Anesthesia and Critical Care Concerns/Other Considerations The 2002 ACCM/SCCM guidelines for analgesia (critically-ill adult) suggest that NSAIDs may be used in combination with opioids in select patients for pain management. Concern about adverse events (increased risk of renal dysfunction, altered platelet function and gastrointestinal irritation) limits its use in patients who have other underlying risks for these events.

In short-term use, NSAIDs vary considerably in their effect on blood pressure. When NSAIDs are used in patients with hypertension, appropriate monitoring of blood pressure responses should be completed and the duration of therapy, when possible, kept short. The use of NSAIDs in the treatment of patients with congestive heart failure may be associated with an increased risk for fluid accumulation and edema; may precipitate renal failure in dehydrated patients.

Additional Information Complete prescribing information for this medication should be consulted for additional detail.

Dosage Forms Excipient information presented when available (limited, particularly for generics); consult specific product labeling.
Capsule:
Ponstel®: 250 mg

Meloxicam (mel OKS i kam)

Medication Guide An FDA-approved patient medication guide, which is available with the product information and at http://www.fda.gov/downloads/Drugs/DrugSafety/ucm088646.pdf, must be dispensed with this medication for each new outpatient prescription and refill.

Related Information
Nonsteroidal Anti-Inflammatory Agents *on page 1687*

U.S. Brand Names Mobic®

Canadian Brand Names Apo-Meloxicam®; CO Meloxicam; Gen-Meloxicam; Mobicox®; Mobic®; Mylan-Meloxicam; Novo-Meloxicam; PMS-Meloxicam

Pharmacologic Category Nonsteroidal Anti-inflammatory Drug (NSAID), Oral

Generic Available Yes: Tablet

Use Relief of signs and symptoms of osteoarthritis, rheumatoid arthritis, and juvenile rheumatoid arthritis (JRA)

Mechanism of Action Reversibly inhibits cyclooxygenase-1 and 2 (COX-1 and 2) enzymes, which results in decreased formation of prostaglandin precursors; has antipyretic, analgesic, and anti-inflammatory properties

Other proposed mechanisms not fully elucidated (and possibly contributing to the anti-inflammatory effect to varying degrees), include inhibiting chemotaxis, altering lymphocyte activity, inhibiting neutrophil aggregation/activation, and decreasing proinflammatory cytokine levels.

Pharmacodynamics/Kinetics

Distribution: 10 L

Protein binding: ~99%, primarily to albumin

Metabolism: Hepatic via CYP2C9 and CYP3A4 (minor); forms 4 metabolites (inactive)

Bioavailability: 89%

Half-life elimination: Adults: 15-20 hours

Time to peak: Initial: 4-5 hours; Secondary: 12-14 hours

Excretion: Urine and feces (as inactive metabolites)

Dosage Oral:

Children ≥2 years: JRA: 0.125 mg/kg/day; maximum dose: 7.5 mg/day

Adults: Osteoarthritis, rheumatoid arthritis: Initial: 7.5 mg once daily; some patients may receive additional benefit from increasing dose to 15 mg once daily; maximum dose: 15 mg/day

Elderly: Increased concentrations may occur in elderly patients (particularly in females); however, no specific dosage adjustment is recommended

Dosage adjustment in renal impairment:

Mild-to-moderate impairment: No specific dosage recommendations

Significant impairment (Cl_{cr} ≤15 mL/minute): Patients with severe renal impairment have not been adequately studied; use not recommended.

Hemodialysis: Supplemental dose after dialysis not necessary.

Dosage adjustment in hepatic impairment:

Mild (Child-Pugh class A) to moderate (Child-Pugh class B) hepatic dysfunction: No dosage adjustment is necessary

Severe hepatic impairment: Patients with severe hepatic impairment have not been adequately studied

Stability Store at 25°C (77°F). Protect tablets from moisture.

Administration Administer with food or milk to minimize gastrointestinal irritation.

Monitoring Parameters Periodic CBC, serum chemistries, liver function, renal function (serum BUN, and creatinine) with long-term use; signs and symptoms of bleeding

Anesthesia and Critical Care Concerns/Other Considerations

Clinical Pearls/Comments: The 2002 ACCM/SCCM guidelines for analgesia (critically-ill adult) suggest that NSAIDs may be used in combination with opioids in select patients for pain management. Concern about adverse events (increased risk of renal dysfunction, altered platelet function and gastrointestinal irritation) limits its use in patients who have other underlying risks for these events.

In short-term use, NSAIDs vary considerably in their effect on blood pressure. When NSAIDs are used in patients with hypertension, blood pressure needs to be monitored and the duration of therapy kept short. The use of NSAIDs in patients with heart failure may be associated with an increased risk for fluid accumulation and edema; may precipitate renal failure in dehydrated patients by inhibition of prostaglandin-mediated autoregulation. Use extreme caution or avoid concurrent use with nephrotoxic agents.

Pregnancy Risk Factor C/D (3rd trimester)

Contraindications Hypersensitivity (eg, asthma, urticaria, allergic-type reactions) to meloxicam, aspirin, other NSAIDs, or any component of the formulation; perioperative pain in the setting of coronary artery bypass graft (CABG) surgery

Warnings/Precautions [U.S. Boxed Warning]: NSAIDs are associated with an increased risk of adverse cardiovascular thrombotic events, including MI and stroke. Risk may be increased with duration of use or pre-existing cardiovascular risk factors or disease. Carefully evaluate individual cardiovascular risk profiles prior to prescribing. May cause new-onset hypertension or worsening of existing hypertension. Use caution with fluid retention. Avoid use in heart failure. Concurrent administration of ibuprofen, and potentially other nonselective ▶

NSAIDs, may interfere with aspirin's cardioprotective effect. **[U.S. Boxed Warning]: Use is contraindicated for treatment of perioperative pain in the setting of coronary artery bypass graft (CABG) surgery.** Risk of MI and stroke may be increased with use following CABG surgery.

Platelet adhesion and aggregation may be decreased; may prolong bleeding time; patients with coagulation disorders or who are receiving anticoagulants should be monitored closely. Anemia may occur; patients on long-term NSAID therapy should be monitored for anemia. Rarely, NSAID use may cause severe blood dyscrasias (eg, agranulocytosis, aplastic anemia, thrombocytopenia).

NSAID use may compromise existing renal function; dose-dependent decreases in prostaglandin synthesis may result from NSAID use, reducing renal blood flow which may cause renal decompensation. NSAID use may increase the risk for hyperkalemia. Patients with impaired renal function, dehydration, heart failure, liver dysfunction, those taking diuretics, and ACE inhibitors, and the elderly are at greater risk of renal toxicity and hyperkalemia. Rehydrate patient before starting therapy; monitor renal function closely. Not recommended for use in patients with advanced renal disease. Long-term NSAID use may result in renal papillary necrosis.

[U.S. Boxed Warning]: NSAIDs may increase risk of gastrointestinal irritation, inflammation, ulceration, bleeding, and perforation. These events may occur at any time during therapy and without warning. Use caution with a history of GI disease (bleeding or ulcers), concurrent therapy with aspirin, anticoagulants and/or corticosteroids, smoking, use of alcohol, the elderly or debilitated patients. When used concomitantly with ≤325 mg of aspirin, a substantial increase in the risk of gastrointestinal complications (eg, ulcer) occurs; concomitant gastroprotective therapy (eg, proton pump inhibitors) is recommended (Bhatt, 2008).

Use the lowest effective dose for the shortest duration of time, consistent with individual patient goals, to reduce risk of cardiovascular or GI adverse events. Alternate therapies should be considered for patients at high risk.

NSAIDs may cause serious skin adverse events including exfoliative dermatitis, Stevens-Johnson syndrome (SJS) and toxic epidermal necrolysis (TEN); discontinue use at first sign of skin rash or hypersensitivity. Anaphylactoid reactions may occur, even without prior exposure; patients with "aspirin triad" (bronchial asthma, aspirin intolerance, rhinitis) may be at increased risk. Do not use in patients who experience bronchospasm, asthma, rhinitis, or urticaria with NSAID or aspirin therapy. Use caution in other forms of asthma.

Use with caution in patients with decreased hepatic function. Closely monitor patients with any abnormal LFT. Severe hepatic reactions (eg, fulminant hepatitis, liver failure) have occurred with NSAID use, rarely; discontinue if signs or symptoms of liver disease develop, or if systemic manifestations occur.

NSAIDS may cause drowsiness, dizziness, blurred vision and other neurologic effects which may impair physical or mental abilities; patients must be cautioned about performing tasks which require mental alertness (eg, operating machinery or driving). Discontinue use with blurred or diminished vision and perform ophthalmologic exam. Monitor vision with long-term therapy.

The elderly are at increased risk for adverse effects (especially peptic ulceration, CNS effects, renal toxicity) from NSAIDs even at low doses.

Withhold for at least 4-6 half-lives prior to surgical or dental procedures. Safety and efficacy have not been established in pediatric patients <2 years of age.

Adverse Reactions Percentages reported in adult patients; abdominal pain, diarrhea, fever, headache, pyrexia, and vomiting were reported more commonly in pediatric patients

2% to 10%:

Cardiovascular: Edema (≤5%)

Central nervous system: Headache (2% to 8%), pain (1% to 5%), dizziness (≤4%), insomnia (≤4%)

Dermatologic: Pruritus (≤2%), rash (≤3%)

Gastrointestinal: Dyspepsia (4% to 10%), diarrhea (2% to 8%), nausea (2% to 7%), abdominal pain (2% to 5%), constipation (≤3%), flatulence (≤3%), vomiting (≤3%)

Genitourinary: Urinary tract infection (≤7%), micturition (≤2%)

Hematologic: Anemia (≤4%)

Neuromuscular & skeletal: Arthralgia (≤5%), back pain (≤3%)

Respiratory: Upper respiratory infection (≤8%), cough (≤2%), pharyngitis (≤3%)

Miscellaneous: Flu-like syndrome (2% to 6%), falls (≤3%)

<2% (Limited to important or life-threatening): Abnormal dreams, abnormal vision, agranulocytosis, albuminuria, allergic reaction, alopecia, anaphylactoid reactions, angina, angioedema, anxiety, appetite increased, arrhythmia, asthma, bilirubinemia, bronchospasm, bullous eruption, BUN increased, cardiac failure, colitis, confusion, conjunctivitis, creatinine increased, dehydration, depression, diaphoresis, duodenal perforation, duodenal ulcer, dyspnea, edema (facial), eructation, erythema multiforme, esophagitis, exfoliative dermatitis, fatigue, fever, gastric perforation, gastric ulcer, gastritis, gastroesophageal reflux, gastrointestinal hemorrhage, GGT increased, hematemesis, hematuria, hepatic failure, hepatitis, hot flushes, hyper-/hypotension, interstitial nephritis, intestinal perforation, jaundice, leukopenia, malaise, melena, MI, mood alterations, nervousness, palpitation, pancreatitis, paresthesia, photosensitivity reaction, pruritus, purpura, renal failure, seizure, shock, somnolence, Stevens-Johnson syndrome, syncope, tachycardia, taste perversion, thrombocytopenia, tinnitus, toxic epidermal necrolysis, transaminases increased, tremor, ulcerative stomatitis, urinary retention (acute), urticaria, vasculitis, vertigo, xerostomia, weight gain/loss

Drug Interactions

Metabolism/Transport Effects Substrate (minor) of CYP2C9, 3A4; **Inhibits** CYP2C9 (weak)

Avoid Concomitant Use

Avoid concomitant use of Meloxicam with any of the following: Ketorolac

Increased Effect/Toxicity

Meloxicam may increase the levels/effects of: Aminoglycosides; Anticoagulants; Antiplatelet Agents; Bisphosphonate Derivatives; CycloSPORINE; Desmopressin; Drotrecogin Alfa; Eplerenone; Ibritumomab; Lithium; Methotrexate; Nonsteroidal Anti-Inflammatory Agents; Pemetrexed; Potassium-Sparing Diuretics; Pralatrexate; Quinolone Antibiotics; Salicylates; Thrombolytic Agents; Tositumomab and Iodine I 131 Tositumomab; Vancomycin; Vitamin K Antagonists

The levels/effects of Meloxicam may be increased by: Antidepressants (Tricyclic, Tertiary Amine); Corticosteroids (Systemic); Dasatinib; Herbs (Anticoagulant/Antiplatelet Properties); Ketorolac; Nonsteroidal Anti-Inflammatory Agents; Omega-3-Acid Ethyl Esters; Pentosan Polysulfate Sodium; Pentoxifylline; Probenecid; Prostacyclin Analogues; Selective Serotonin Reuptake Inhibitors; Serotonin/Norepinephrine Reuptake Inhibitors; Treprostinil

Decreased Effect

Meloxicam may decrease the levels/effects of: ACE Inhibitors; Angiotensin II Receptor Blockers; Antiplatelet Agents; Beta-Blockers; Eplerenone; HydrALAZINE; Loop Diuretics; Potassium-Sparing Diuretics; Salicylates; Thiazide Diuretics

The levels/effects of Meloxicam may be decreased by: Bile Acid Sequestrants; Nonsteroidal Anti-Inflammatory Agents; Salicylates

Ethanol/Nutrition/Herb Interactions

Ethanol: Avoid ethanol (may enhance gastric mucosal irritation).

Herb/Nutraceutical: Avoid alfalfa, anise, bilberry, bladderwrack, bromelain, cat's claw, celery, chamomile, coleus, cordyceps, dong quai, evening primrose, fenugreek, feverfew, garlic, ginger, ginkgo biloba, ginseng (American, Panax, Siberian), grapeseed, green tea, guggul, horse chestnut seed, horseradish, licorice, prickly ash, red clover, reishi, SAMe (S-adenosylmethionine), sweet clover, turmeric, white willow (all have additional antiplatelet activity).

Dietary Considerations Should be taken with food or milk to minimize gastrointestinal irritation.

◀ **Dosage Forms** Excipient information presented when available (limited, particularly for generics); consult specific product labeling. [DSC] = Discontinued product

Suspension: 7.5 mg/5 mL (100 mL) [DSC]

Mobic®: 7.5 mg/5 mL (100 mL) [contains sodium benzoate; raspberry flavor]

Tablet: 7.5 mg, 15 mg

Mobic®: 7.5 mg, 15 mg

References

Jacobi J, Fraser GL, Coursin DB, et al, "Clinical Practice Guidelines for the Sustained Use of Sedatives and Analgesics in the Critically Ill Adult," *Crit Care Med*, 2002, 30(1):119-41. Available at: http://www.sccm.org/pdf/sedatives.pdf.

Memantine (me MAN teen)

U.S. Brand Names Namenda™

Canadian Brand Names Ebixa®

Index Terms Memantine Hydrochloride

Pharmacologic Category N-Methyl-D-Aspartate Receptor Antagonist

Use Treatment of moderate-to-severe dementia of the Alzheimer's type

Unlabeled/Investigational Use Treatment of mild-to-moderate vascular dementia; mild cognitive impairment

Pharmacodynamics/Kinetics

Distribution: 9-11 L/kg

Protein binding: 45%

Metabolism: Forms 3 metabolites (minimal activity)

Half-life elimination: Terminal: 60-80 hours; severe renal impairment (Cl_{cr} 5-29 mL/minute): 117-156 hours

Time to peak, serum: 3-7 hours

Excretion: Urine (57% to 82% unchanged); excretion reduced by alkaline urine pH

Dosage Oral: Adults:

Alzheimer's disease: Initial: 5 mg/day; increase dose by 5 mg/day to a target dose of 20 mg/day; wait at least 1 week between dosage changes. Doses >5 mg/day should be given in 2 divided doses.

Suggested titration: 5 mg/day for ≥1 week; 5 mg twice daily for ≥1 week; 15 mg/day given in 5 mg and 10 mg separated doses for ≥1 week; then 10 mg twice daily

Mild-to-moderate vascular dementia (unlabeled use): 10 mg twice daily

Dosage adjustment in renal impairment:

Mild-to-moderate impairment: No adjustment required

Severe impairment: Cl_{cr} 5-29 mL/minute): 5 mg twice daily

Additional Information Complete prescribing information for this medication should be consulted for additional detail.

Dosage Forms Excipient information presented when available (limited, particularly for generics); consult specific product labeling.

Solution, oral: 2 mg/mL (360 mL) [alcohol free, dye free, sugar free; peppermint flavor]

Tablet, as hydrochloride: 5 mg, 10 mg

Combination package [titration pack contains two separate tablet formulations]: Memantine hydrochloride 5 mg (28s) and memantine hydrochloride 10 mg (21s)

References

Lipton, SA, "Failures and Successes of NMDA Receptor Antagonists: Molecular Basis for the Use of Open-Channel Blockers like Memantine in the Treatment of Acute and Chronic Neurologic Insults," *NeuroRx*, 2004, 1:101-10.

Orgogozo JM, Rigaud AS, Stoffler A et al, "Efficacy and Safety of Memantine in Patients with Mild to Moderate Vascular Dementia: A Randomized, Placebo-Controlled Trial (MMM 300)," *Stroke*, 2002, 33:1834-39.

Reisberg B, Doody R, Stoffler A, et al, "Memantine in Moderate-to-Severe Alzheimer's Disease," *N Engl J Med*, 2003, 348(14):1333-41.

Tariot PN, Farlow MR, Grossberg GT, et al, "Memantine Treatment in Patients With Moderate to Severe Alzheimer Disease Already Receiving Donepezil: A Randomized Controlled Trial. The Memantine Study Group," *JAMA*, 2004, 291(3):317-24.

Wilcock G, Mobius HJ, Stoffler A et al, "A Double-Blind, Placebo-Controlled Multicentre Study of Memantine in Mild to Moderate Vascular Dementia (MMM 500)," *Int Clin Psychopharmacol*, 2002, 17(6):297-305.

◆ **Memantine Hydrochloride** see Memantine on page 874

◆ **Menostar®** *see* Estradiol *on page 531*

Meperidine (me PER i deen)

Medication Safety Issues

Avoid the use of meperidine for pain control, especially in elderly and renally-compromised patients because of the risk of neurotoxicity (Institute for Safe Medication Practices [ISMP], 2007; American Pain Society, 2008)

Sound-alike/look-alike issues:

Meperidine may be confused with meprobamate

Demerol® may be confused with Demulen®, Desyrel®, dicumarol, Dilaudid®, Dymelor®, Pamelor®

High alert medication: The Institute for Safe Medication Practices (ISMP) includes this medication among its list of drug classes which have a heightened risk of causing significant patient harm when used in error.

Related Information

Acute Postoperative Pain *on page 1502*
Anesthetic Considerations in the Substance-Abusing Patient *on page 1613*
Chronic Pain Management *on page 1546*
Chronic Renal Failure *on page 1552*
Moderate Sedation *on page 1566*
Opioid Analgesics *on page 1688*
Perioperative Management of Patients on Antiseizure Medication *on page 1577*

U.S. Brand Names Demerol®

Canadian Brand Names Demerol®

Index Terms Isonipecaine Hydrochloride; Meperidine Hydrochloride; Pethidine Hydrochloride

Pharmacologic Category Analgesic, Opioid

Restrictions C-II

Generic Available Yes

Use Management of moderate-to-severe pain; adjunct to anesthesia and preoperative sedation

Unlabeled/Investigational Use Reduce postoperative shivering; reduce rigors from amphotericin B (conventional)

Mechanism of Action Binds to opiate receptors in the CNS, causing inhibition of ascending pain pathways, altering the perception of and response to pain; produces generalized CNS depression

Pharmacodynamics/Kinetics

Onset of action: Analgesic: Oral, SubQ: 10-15 minutes; I.V.: ~5 minutes
  Peak effect: SubQ.: ~1 hour; Oral: 2 hours
Duration: Oral, SubQ.: 2-4 hours
Absorption: I.M.: Erratic and highly variable
Distribution: Crosses placenta; enters breast milk
Protein binding: 65% to 75%
Metabolism: Hepatic; hydrolyzed to meperidinic acid (inactive) or undergoes N-demethylation to normeperidine (active; has $1/2$ the analgesic effect and 2-3 times the CNS effects of meperidine)
Bioavailability: ~50% to 60%; increased with liver disease
Half-life elimination:
  Parent drug: Terminal phase: Adults: 2.5-4 hours, Liver disease: 7-11 hours
  Normeperidine (active metabolite): 15-30 hours; can accumulate with high doses (>600 mg/day) or with decreased renal function
Excretion: Urine (as metabolites)

Dosage Note: The American Pain Society (2008) and ISMP (2007) do not recommend meperidine's use as an analgesic.

Children: Pain: Oral, I.M., I.V., SubQ: 1-1.5 mg/kg/dose every 3-4 hours as needed; 1-2 mg/kg as a single dose preoperative medication may be used; maximum 100 mg/dose (**Note:** Oral route is not recommended for acute pain.) ▶

◀ Adults: Pain:

Oral: Initial: Opiate-naive: 50 mg every 3-4 hours as needed; usual dosage range: 50-150 mg every 2-4 hours as needed (manufacturers recommendation; oral route is not recommended for acute pain)

I.M., SubQ: Initial: Opiate-naive: 50-75 mg every 3-4 hours as needed; patients with prior opiate exposure may require higher initial doses

Slow I.V.: Initial: 5-10 mg every 5 minutes as needed

Preoperatively: 50-100 mg given 30-90 minutes before the beginning of anesthesia

Note: If use in acute pain (in patients without renal or CNS disease) cannot be avoided, treatment should be limited to ≤48 hours and doses should not exceed 600 mg/24 hours.

Elderly:

Oral: 50 mg every 4 hours

I.M.: 25 mg every 4 hours

Dosing adjustment in renal impairment: Avoid use in renal impairment

Dosing adjustment/comments in hepatic disease: Increased narcotic effect in cirrhosis; reduction in dose more important for oral than I.V. route

Stability Meperidine injection should be stored at room temperature; do not freeze. Protect from light. Protect oral dosage forms from light.

Administration

Solution for injection: Meperidine may be administered I.M., SubQ, or I.V.; I.V. push should be administered slowly, use of a 10 mg/mL concentration has been recommended. For continuous I.V. infusions, a more dilute solution (eg, 1 mg/mL) should be used.

Oral solution: Administer solution in 1/2 glass of water; undiluted solution may exert topical anesthetic effect on mucous membranes

Monitoring Parameters Pain relief, respiratory and mental status, blood pressure; observe patient for excessive sedation, CNS depression, seizures, respiratory depression

Reference Range Therapeutic: 70-500 ng/mL (SI: 283-2020 nmol/L); Toxic: >1000 ng/mL (SI: >4043 nmol/L)

Anesthesia and Critical Care Concerns/Other Considerations

Clinical Pearls/Comments: Accumulation of normeperidine can cause anxiety, tremors, or seizures. Meperidine inhibits serotonin reuptake; potential for serotonin syndrome when administered with other serotonergic agents (eg, SSRI, MAO inhibitor). Combination of meperidine and an MAO inhibitor is an absolute contraindication. Euphoria is more common with meperidine than with other opioids.

Evidence-Based Information: The 2002 ACCM/SCCM guidelines for analgesia (critically-ill adult) recommend against using meperidine repetitively.

Pregnancy Risk Factor C/D (prolonged use or high doses at term)

Contraindications Hypersensitivity to meperidine or any component of the formulation; use with or within 14 days of MAO inhibitors; pregnancy (prolonged use or high doses near term)

Warnings/Precautions Oral meperidine is not recommended for acute/chronic pain management. Meperidine should not be used for acute/cancer pain because of the risk of neurotoxicity. Normeperidine (an active metabolite and CNS stimulant) may accumulate and precipitate anxiety, tremors, or seizures; risk increases with CNS or renal dysfunction, prolonged use (>48 hours), and cumulative dose (>600 mg/24 hours). The Institute for Safe Medication Practice recommends avoiding the use of meperidine for pain control, especially in the elderly and renally-impaired (ISMP, 2007).

May cause CNS depression, which may impair physical or mental abilities; patients must be cautioned about performing tasks which require mental alertness (eg, operating machinery or driving). Effects may be potentiated when used with other sedative drugs or ethanol. Use only with extreme caution (if at all) in patients with head injury or increased intracranial pressure (ICP). Use caution with pulmonary, hepatic, or renal disorders, supraventricular tachycardias, acute abdominal conditions, hypothyroidism, toxic psychosis, kyphoscoliosis, morbid obesity, Addison's disease, BPH, or urethral stricture. Use with caution in patients with biliary tract dysfunction; acute pancreatitis may cause constriction of sphincter of Oddi. May cause hypotension; use with caution in patients with depleted blood volume or drugs which may exaggerate hypotensive effects (including phenothiazines or general anesthetics).

An opioid-containing analgesic regimen should be tailored to each patient's needs and based upon the type of pain being treated (acute versus chronic), the route of administration, degree of tolerance for opioids (naive versus chronic user), age, weight, and medical condition. The optimal analgesic dose varies widely among patients. Some preparations contain sulfites which may cause allergic reaction. Tolerance or drug dependence may result from extended use. Healthcare provider should be alert to problems of abuse, misuse, and diversion. Concurrent use of agonist/antagonist analgesics may precipitate withdrawal symptoms and/or reduced analgesic efficacy in patients following prolonged therapy with mu opioid agonists. Abrupt discontinuation following prolonged use may also lead to withdrawal symptoms. Avoid use in the elderly.

Adverse Reactions Frequency not defined.

Cardiovascular: Hypotension

Central nervous system: Fatigue, drowsiness, dizziness, nervousness, headache, restlessness, malaise, confusion, mental depression, hallucinations, paradoxical CNS stimulation, increased intracranial pressure, seizure (associated with metabolite accumulation), serotonin syndrome

Dermatologic: Rash, urticaria

Gastrointestinal: Nausea, vomiting, constipation, anorexia, stomach cramps, xerostomia, biliary spasm, paralytic ileus, sphincter of Oddi spasm

Genitourinary: Ureteral spasms, decreased urination

Local: Pain at injection site

Neuromuscular & skeletal: Weakness

Respiratory: Dyspnea

Miscellaneous: Anaphylaxis, histamine release, hypersensitivity reactions, physical and psychological dependence

Drug Interactions

Metabolism/Transport Effects Substrate (minor) of CYP2B6, 2C19, 3A4

Avoid Concomitant Use

Avoid concomitant use of Meperidine with any of the following: MAO Inhibitors; Sibutramine

Increased Effect/Toxicity

Meperidine may increase the levels/effects of: Alcohol (Ethyl); Alvimopan; CNS Depressants; Desmopressin; Selective Serotonin Reuptake Inhibitors; Serotonin Modulators; Thiazide Diuretics

The levels/effects of Meperidine may be increased by: Amphetamines; Antipsychotic Agents (Phenothiazines); Barbiturates; MAO Inhibitors; Protease Inhibitors; Sibutramine; Succinylcholine

Decreased Effect

Meperidine may decrease the levels/effects of: Pegvisomant

The levels/effects of Meperidine may be decreased by: Ammonium Chloride; Phenytoin; Protease Inhibitors

Ethanol/Nutrition/Herb Interactions

Ethanol: Avoid or limit ethanol (may increase CNS depression). Watch for sedation.

Herb/Nutraceutical: Avoid valerian, St John's wort, kava kava, gotu kola (may increase CNS depression).

Test Interactions Increased amylase (S), increased BSP retention, increased CPK (I.M. injections)

Dosage Forms Excipient information presented when available (limited, particularly for generics); consult specific product labeling. [DSC] = Discontinued product

Injection, solution, as hydrochloride [ampul]: 25 mg/0.5 mL (0.5 mL); 25 mg/mL (1 mL); 50 mg/mL (1 mL, 1.5 mL, 2 mL); 75 mg/mL (1 mL); 100 mg/mL (1 mL)

Injection, solution, as hydrochloride [prefilled syringe]: 25 mg/mL (1 mL); 50 mg/mL (1 mL); 75 mg/mL (1 mL); 100 mg/mL (1 mL)

Injection, solution, as hydrochloride [for PCA pump]: 10 mg/mL (30 mL, 50 mL [DSC], 60 mL)

Injection, solution, as hydrochloride [vial]: 25 mg/mL (1 mL); 50 mg/mL (1 mL, 30 mL); 75 mg/mL (1 mL); 100 mg/mL (1 mL, 20 mL) [may contain sodium metabisulfite]

Solution, oral, as hydrochloride: 50 mg/5 mL (500 mL)

Tablet, as hydrochloride: 50 mg, 100 mg

Demerol®: 50 mg, 100 mg

References

American Academy of Pediatrics Committee on Drugs, "The Transfer of Drugs and Other Chemicals Into Human Milk," *Pediatrics*, 2001, 108(3):776-89.

American Academy of Pediatrics Committee on Drugs, "Reappraisal of Lytic Cocktail/Demerol®, Phenergan®, and Thorazine® (DPT) for the Sedation of Children," *Pediatrics*, 1995, 95(4):598-602.

Armstrong PJ and Bersten A, "Normeperidine Toxicity," *Anesth Analg*, 1986, 65(5):536-8.

Buchanan JF and Brown CR, "Designer Drugs: A Problem in Clinical Toxicology," *Med Toxicol Adverse Drug Exp*, 1988, 3(1):1-17.

Clark RF, Wei EM, and Anderson PO, "Meperidine: Therapeutic Use and Toxicity," *J Emerg Med*, 1995,13(6):797-802.

Cole TB, Sprinkle RH, Smith SJ, et al, "Intravenous Narcotic Therapy for Children With Severe Sickle Cell Pain Crisis," *Am J Dis Child*, 1986, 140(12):1255-9.

Ferrell BA, "Pain Management in Elderly People," *J Am Geriatr Soc*, 1991, 39(1):64-73.

Golembiewski J, "Safety Concerns With Meperidine," *J Perianesth Nurs*, 2002, 17(2):123-5.

Institute for Safe Medication Practice, "High Alert Medication Feature: Reducing Patient Harm From Opiates," *ISMP Medication Safety Alert*, 2007, 12 (4):1-3.

Jacobi J, Fraser GL, Coursin DB, et al, "Clinical Practice Guidelines for the Sustained Use of Sedatives and Analgesics in the Critically Ill Adult," *Crit Care Med*, 2002, 30(1):119-41. Available at: http://www.sccm.org/pdf/sedatives.pdf.

Kyff JV and Rice TL, "Meperidine-Associated Seizures in a Child," *Clin Pharm*, 1990, 9(5):337-8.

Latta KS, Ginsberg B, and Barkin RL, "Meperidine: A Critical Review," *Am J Ther*, 2002, 9(1):53-68.

Miller RR and Jick H, "Clinical Effects of Meperidine in Hospitalized Medical Patients," *J Clin Pharmacol*, 1978, 18(4):180-9.

Mokhlesi B, Leikin JB, Murray P, et al, "Adult Toxicology in Critical Care. Part II: Specific Poisonings," *Chest*, 2003, 123(3):897-922.

Olkkola KT, Hamunen K, and Maunuksela EL, "Clinical Pharmacokinetics and Pharmacodynamics of Opioid Analgesics in Infants and Children," *Clin Pharmacokinet*, 1995, 28(5):385-404.

Pokela ML, Olkkola KT, Koivisto ME, et al, "Pharmacokinetics and Pharmacodynamics of Intravenous Meperidine in Neonates and Infants," *Clin Pharmacol Ther*, 1992, 52(4):342-9.

"Principles of Analgesic Use in the Treatment of Acute Pain and Cancer Pain," 6th ed, Glenview, IL: American Pain Society, 2008.

Stone PA, Macintyre PE, and Jarvis DA, "Norpethidine Toxicity and Patient Controlled Analgesia," *Br J Anaesth*, 1993, 71(5):738-40.

◆ **Meperidine Hydrochloride** *see* Meperidine *on page 875*

◆ **Mephyton®** *see* Phytonadione *on page 1128*

Mepivacaine (me PIV a kane)

Medication Safety Issues

Sound-alike/look-alike issues:

Mepivacaine may be confused with bupivacaine

Polocaine® may be confused with prilocaine

High alert medication: The Institute for Safe Medication Practices (ISMP) includes this medication (epidural administration) among its list of drug classes which have a heightened risk of causing significant patient harm when used in error.

Related Information

Acute Postoperative Pain *on page 1502*

Local Anesthetics *on page 1636*

U.S. Brand Names Carbocaine®; Polocaine®; Polocaine® Dental; Polocaine® MPF; Scandonest® 3% Plain

Canadian Brand Names Carbocaine®; Polocaine®

Index Terms Mepivacaine Hydrochloride

Pharmacologic Category Local Anesthetic

Generic Available No

Use Local or regional analgesia; anesthesia by local infiltration, peripheral and central neural techniques (epidural and caudal); **not** for use in spinal anesthesia

Mechanism of Action Mepivacaine is an amide local anesthetic similar to lidocaine; like all local anesthetics, mepivacaine acts by preventing the generation and conduction of nerve impulses

Pharmacodynamics/Kinetics

Onset of action (route and dose dependent): Range: 3-20 minutes
Duration (route and dose dependent): 2-2.5 hours
Protein binding: ~75%
Metabolism: Primarily hepatic via N-demethylation, hydroxylation, and glucuronidation
Half-life elimination: Neonates: 8.7-9 hours; Adults: 1.9-3 hours
Excretion: Urine (95% as metabolites)

Dosage

Injectable local anesthetic: Dose varies with procedure, degree of anesthesia needed, vascularity of tissue, duration of anesthesia required, and physical condition of patient. The smallest dose and concentration required to produce the desired effect should be used.

Children: Maximum dose: 5-6 mg/kg; only concentrations <2% should be used in children <3 years or <14 kg (30 lbs)

Adults: Maximum dose: 400 mg; do not exceed 1000 mg/24 hours

Cervical, brachial, intercostal, pudenal nerve block: 5-40 mL of a 1% solution (maximum: 400 mg) **or** 5-20 mL of a 2% solution (maximum: 400 mg). For pudenal block, inject 1/2 the total dose each side.

Transvaginal block (paracervical plus pudenal): Up to 30 mL (both sides) of a 1% solution (maximum: 300 mg). Inject 1/2 the total dose each side.

Paracervical block: Up to 20 mL (both sides) of a 1% solution (maximum: 200 mg). Inject 1/2 the total dose to each side. This is the maximum recommended dose per 90-minute procedure; inject slowly with 5 minutes between sides.

Caudal and epidural block (preservative free solutions only): 15-30 mL of a 1% solution (maximum: 300 mg) **or** 10-25 mL of a 1.5% solution (maximum: 375 mg) **or** 10-20 mL of a 2% solution (maximum: 400 mg)

Infiltration: Up to 40 mL of a 1% solution (maximum: 400 mg)

Therapeutic block (pain management): 1-5 mL of a 1% solution (maximum: 50 mg) **or** 1-5 mL of a 2% solution (maximum: 100 mg)

Dental anesthesia: Adults:

Single site in upper or lower jaw: 54 mg (1.8 mL) as a 3% solution

Infiltration and nerve block of entire oral cavity: 270 mg (9 mL) as a 3% solution. Manufacturer's maximum recommended dose is not more than 400 mg to normal healthy adults.

Stability Store at controlled room temperature of 15°C to 30°C (59°F to 86°F). Brief exposure up to 40°C (104°F) does not adversely affect the product. Solutions may be sterilized. Dental solutions should be protected from light.

Administration Before injecting, withdraw syringe plunger to ensure injection is not into vein or artery

Monitoring Parameters Vital signs, state of consciousness; signs of CNS toxicity

Anesthesia and Critical Care Concerns/Other Considerations

Clinical Pearls/Comments:

Local anesthetic toxicity: Cardiac arrest: Lipid infusion has been used in animal studies and several human cases (*Bupivacaine:* Rosenblatt, 2006; *Levobupivacaine:* Foxall, 2007; *Ropivacaine:* Litz, 2006) where cardiovascular toxicity, unresponsive to conventional resuscitation, resulted. Additional information is available at http://www.lipidrescue.org. The protocol from the website is: 20% Fat Emulsion: 1.5 mL/kg administered over 1 minute, followed immediately by an infusion of 0.25 mL/kg/minute. Continue chest compressions (lipid must circulate). Repeat bolus every 3-5 minutes up to 3 mL/kg total dose until circulation restored. Continue infusion until hemodynamic stability is restored. Increase the infusion rate to 0.5 mL/kg/minute if BP declines. A maximum total dose of 8 mL/kg is recommended.

Pregnancy Risk Factor C

Contraindications Hypersensitivity to mepivacaine, other amide-type local anesthetics, or any component of the formulation

Warnings/Precautions Careful and constant monitoring of the patient's state of consciousness should be done following each local anesthetic injection; at such times, restlessness, anxiety, tinnitus, dizziness, blurred vision, tremors, depression, or drowsiness may be early warning signs of CNS toxicity. Treatment is primarily symptomatic and supportive. Use with caution in patients with cardiac disease, hepatic or renal disease, or hyperthyroidism. Local anesthetics have been associated with rare occurrences of sudden respiratory arrest; convulsions due to systemic toxicity leading to cardiac arrest have been reported presumably due to intravascular injection. A test dose is recommended prior to epidural administration and all reinforcing doses with continuous catheter technique. Do not use solutions containing preservatives for caudal or epidural block. Use caution in debilitated, elderly, or acutely-ill patients; dose reduction may be required. Resuscitative equipment, oxygen, and other resuscitative drugs should be available for immediate use.

Adverse Reactions Degree of adverse effects in the CNS and cardiovascular system is directly related to the blood levels of mepivacaine, route of administration, and physical status of the patient. The effects below are more likely to occur after systemic administration rather than infiltration.

Cardiovascular: Bradycardia, cardiac arrest, cardiac output decreased, heart block, hyper-/hypotension, myocardial depression, syncope, tachycardia, ventricular arrhythmias

Central nervous system: Anxiety, chills, convulsions, depression, dizziness, excitation, restlessness, tremors

Dermatologic: Angioneurotic edema, diaphoresis, erythema, pruritus, urticaria

Gastrointestinal: Fecal incontinence, nausea, vomiting

Genitourinary: Incontinence, urinary retention

Neuromuscular & skeletal: Paralysis

Ocular: Blurred vision, pupil constriction

Otic: Tinnitus

Respiratory: Apnea, hypoventilation, sneezing

Miscellaneous: Allergic reaction, anaphylactoid reaction

Drug Interactions

Avoid Concomitant Use There are no known interactions where it is recommended to avoid concomitant use.

Increased Effect/Toxicity There are no known significant interactions involving an increase in effect.

Decreased Effect There are no known significant interactions involving a decrease in effect.

Dosage Forms Excipient information presented when available (limited, particularly for generics); consult specific product labeling. [DSC] = Discontinued product

Injection, solution, as hydrochloride:
Carbocaine®: 1% (50 mL); 2% (50 mL) [contains methylparaben]
Polocaine®: 1% (50 mL); 2% (50 mL) [contains methylparaben]

Injection, solution, as hydrochloride [for dental use]: 3% (1.8 mL)
Carbocaine®: 3% (1.7 mL)
Polocaine® Dental: 3% (1.7 mL, 1.8 mL [DSC])
Scandonest® 3% Plain: 3% (1.7 mL)

Injection, solution, as hydrochloride [preservative free]:
Carbocaine®: 1% (30 mL); 1.5% (30 mL); 2% (20 mL)
Polocaine® MPF: 1% (30 mL); 1.5% (30 mL); 2% (20 mL)

References

Corcoran W, Butterworth J, Weller RS, et al, "Local Anesthetic-Induced Cardiac Toxicity: A Survey of Contemporary Practice Strategies Among Academic Anesthesiology Departments," *Anesth Analg*, 2006, 103(5):1322-6.

Foxall G, McCahon R, Lamb J, et al, "Levobupivacaine-Induced Seizures and Cardiovascular Collapse Treated With Intralipid," *Anaesthesia*, 2007, 62(5):516-8.

Litz RJ, Popp M, Stehr SN, et al, "Successful Resuscitation of a Patient With Ropivacaine-Induced Asystole After Axillary Plexus Block Using lipid Infusion," *Anaesthesia*, 2006, 61(8):800-1.

Rosenblatt MA, Abel M, Fischer GW, et al, "Successful Use of a 20% Lipid Emulsion to Resuscitate a Patient After a Presumed Bupivacaine-Related Cardiac Arrest," *Anesthesiology*, 2006, 105 (1):217-8.

◆ **Mepivacaine Hydrochloride** *see* Mepivacaine *on page 878*

◆ **Mercapturic Acid** *see* Acetylcysteine *on page 35*

Meropenem (mer oh PEN em)

Medication Safety Issues
Sound-alike/look-alike issues:
Meropenem may be confused with ertapenem, imipenem, metronidazole.

Related Information
Dosing Considerations for the Critically-Ill Patient With Morbid Obesity *on page 1561*

U.S. Brand Names Merrem® I.V.

Canadian Brand Names Merrem®

Pharmacologic Category Antibiotic, Carbapenem

Generic Available No

Use Treatment of intra-abdominal infections (complicated appendicitis and peritonitis); treatment of bacterial meningitis in pediatric patients ≥3 months of age caused by *S. pneumoniae*, *H. influenzae*, and *N. meningitidis*; treatment of complicated skin and skin structure infections caused by susceptible organisms

Unlabeled/Investigational Use *Burkholderia pseudomallei* (melioidosis), febrile neutropenia, liver abscess, meningitis (adults), otitis externa, pneumonia, urinary tract infections

Mechanism of Action Inhibits bacterial cell wall synthesis by binding to several of the penicillin-binding proteins, which in turn inhibit the final transpeptidation step of peptidoglycan synthesis in bacterial cell walls, thus inhibiting cell wall biosynthesis; bacteria eventually lyse due to ongoing activity of cell wall autolytic enzymes (autolysins and murein hydrolases) while cell wall assembly is arrested

Pharmacodynamics/Kinetics
Distribution: V_d: Adults: ~0.3 L/kg, Children: 0.4-0.5 L/kg; penetrates well into most body fluids and tissues; CSF concentrations approximate those of the plasma

Protein binding: ~2%

Metabolism: Hepatic; metabolized to open beta-lactam form (inactive)

Half-life elimination:
Normal renal function: 1-1.5 hours
Cl_{cr} 30-80 mL/minute: 1.9-3.3 hours
Cl_{cr} 2-30 mL/minute: 3.82-5.7 hours

Time to peak, tissue: 1 hour following infusion

Excretion: Urine (~25% as inactive metabolites)

Dosage
Usual dosage ranges:
Neonates: I.V.:
Postnatal age 0-7 days: 20 mg/kg/dose every 12 hours
Postnatal age >7 days:
Weight 1200-2000 g: 20 mg/kg/dose every 12 hours
Weight >2000 g: 20 mg/kg/dose every 8 hours
Children ≥3 months: I.V.: 30-120 mg/kg/day divided every 8 hours (maximum dose: 6 g/day)
Adults: I.V.: 1.5-6 g/day divided every 8 hours

Indication-specific dosing:
Children ≥3 months (<50 kg): I.V.:
Febrile neutropenia (unlabeled use): 20 mg/kg every 8 hours (maximum dose: 1 g every 8 hours)
Intra-abdominal infections: 20 mg/kg every 8 hours (maximum dose: 1 g every 8 hours)
Meningitis: 40 mg/kg every 8 hours (maximum dose: 2 g every 8 hours)
Skin and skin structure infections (complicated): 10 mg/kg every 8 hours (maximum dose: 500 mg every 8 hours)
Children >50 kg and Adults: I.V.:
***Burkholderia pseudomallei* (melioidosis) (unlabeled use), *Pseudomonas*:** 1 g every 8 hours
Cholangitis, intra-abdominal infections: 1 g every 8 hours
Febrile neutropenia, otitis externa, pneumonia (unlabeled uses): 1 g every 8 hours

Liver abscess (unlabeled use): 1 g every 8 hours for 2-3 weeks, then oral therapy for duration of 4-6 weeks

Meningitis (unlabeled use): 2 g every 8 hours

Mild-to-moderate infection, other severe infections (unlabeled use): 1.5-3 g/day divided every 8 hours

Skin and skin structure infections (complicated): 500 mg every 8 hours; diabetic foot: 1 g every 8 hours

Urinary tract infections, complicated (unlabeled use): 500 mg to 1 g every 8 hours

Dosing adjustment in renal impairment: Adults:

Cl_{cr} 26-50 mL/minute: Administer recommended dose based on indication every 12 hours

Cl_{cr} 10-25 mL/minute: Administer one-half recommended dose based on indication every 12 hours

Cl_{cr} <10 mL/minute: Administer one-half recommended dose based on indication every 24 hours

Dialysis: Meropenem and its metabolites are readily dialyzable; administer dose after dialysis

Continuous renal replacement therapy (CRRT): Drug clearance is highly dependent on the method of renal replacement, filter type, and flow rate. Appropriate dosing requires close monitoring of pharmacologic response, signs of adverse reactions due to drug accumulation, as well as drug levels in relation to target trough (if appropriate). The following are general recommendations only (based on dialysate flow/ultrafiltration rates of 1 L/hour) and should not supersede clinical judgment:

CVVH or CVVHD/CVVHDF: 1 g every 12 hours to achieve target trough of ~4 mg/L; 500 mg every 12 hours may be considered for highly sensitive organisms. **Note:** Substantial variability exists in various published recommendations, ranging from 1-3 g/day given in 2-3 divided doses.

Stability Dry powder should be stored at controlled room temperature 20°C to 25°C (68°F to 77°F). Meropenem infusion vials may be reconstituted with SWFI or a compatible diluent (eg, NS). The 500 mg vials should be reconstituted with 10 mL, and 1 g vials with 20 mL. May be further diluted with compatible solutions for infusion. Consult detailed reference/product labeling for compatibility.

Injection reconstitution: Stability in vial when constituted (up to 50 mg/mL) with:

SWFI: Stable for up to 2 hours at controlled room temperature of 15°C to 25°C (59°F to 77°F) or for up to 12 hours under refrigeration.

Sodium chloride: Stable for up to 2 hours at controlled room temperature of 15°C to 25°C (59°F to 77°F) or for up to 18 hours under refrigeration.

Dextrose 5% injection: Stable for 1 hour at controlled room temperature of 15°C to 25°C (59°F to 77°F) or for 8 hours under refrigeration.

Infusion admixture (1-20 mg/mL): Solution stability when diluted in NS is 4 hours at controlled room temperature of 15°C to 25°C (59°F to 77°F) or 24 hours under refrigeration. Stability in D_5W is 1 hour at controlled room temperature of 15°C to 25°C (59°F to 77°F) or 4 hours under refrigeration.

Administration Administer I.V. infusion over 15-30 minutes; I.V. bolus injection over 3-5 minutes

Monitoring Parameters Perform culture and sensitivity testing prior to initiating therapy. Monitor for signs of anaphylaxis during first dose. During prolonged therapy, monitor renal function, liver function, CBC.

Pregnancy Risk Factor B

Contraindications Hypersensitivity to meropenem, any component of the formulation, or other carbapenems (eg, imipenem); patients who have experienced anaphylactic reactions to other beta-lactams

Warnings/Precautions Serious hypersensitivity reactions, including anaphylaxis, have been reported (some without a history of previous allergic reactions to beta-lactams). Has been associated with CNS adverse effects, including confusional states and seizures; use caution with CNS disorders (eg, brain lesions, history of seizures, or renal impairment). Prolonged use may result in fungal or bacterial superinfection, including *C. difficile*-associated diarrhea (CDAD) and pseudomembranous colitis; CDAD has been observed >2 months postantibiotic treatment. Use with caution in patients with renal impairment; dosage adjustment required in patients with moderate-to-severe renal dysfunction. Thrombocytopenia has been reported in patients with renal dysfunction. Lower doses (based upon renal function) are often required in the elderly.

Adverse Reactions

1% to 10%:

Cardiovascular: Peripheral vascular disorder

Central nervous system: Headache (2% to 8%), pain (≤5%)

Dermatologic: Rash (2% to 3%, includes diaper-area moniliasis in pediatrics), pruritus (1%)

Endocrine & metabolic: Hypoglycemia

Gastrointestinal: Diarrhea (4% to 7%), nausea/vomiting (1% to 8%), constipation (1% to 7%), oral moniliasis (up to 2% in pediatric patients), glossitis (1%)

Hematologic: Anemia (≤6%)

Local: Inflammation at the injection site (2%), phlebitis/thrombophlebitis (1%), injection site reaction (1%)

Respiratory: Apnea (1%), pharyngitis, pneumonia

Miscellaneous: Sepsis (2%), shock (1%)

<1% (Limited to important or life-threatening): Abdominal enlargement, abdominal pain, agitation/delirium, agranulocytosis, alkaline phosphatase increased, ALT increased, AST increased, anemia (hypochromic), angioedema, anorexia, anxiety, asthma, back pain, bilirubin increased, bradycardia, BUN increased, chest pain, chills, cholestatic jaundice/jaundice, confusion, cough, creatinine increased, depression, diaphoresis, dizziness, dyspepsia, dyspnea, dysuria, eosinophilia, epistaxis (0.2%), erythema multiforme, fever, flatulence, gastrointestinal hemorrhage (0.5%), hallucinations, heart failure, hemoglobin/hematocrit decreased, hemolytic anemia, hemoperitoneum (0.2%), hepatic failure, hyper-/hypotension, hypervolemia, hypokalemia, hypoxia, ileus, insomnia, intestinal obstruction, LDH increased, leukocytosis, leukopenia, melena (0.3%), MI, nervousness, neutropenia, paresthesia, pelvic pain, peripheral edema, platelets decreased/increased, pleural effusion, prothrombin time decreased, pulmonary edema, positive Coombs test, pulmonary embolism, renal failure, respiratory disorder, seizure, skin ulcer, somnolence, Stevens-Johnson syndrome, syncope, tachycardia, toxic epidermal necrolysis, urinary incontinence, urticaria, vaginal moniliasis, weakness, WBC decreased, whole body pain

Drug Interactions

Avoid Concomitant Use There are no known interactions where it is recommended to avoid concomitant use.

Increased Effect/Toxicity

The levels/effects of Meropenem may be increased by: Uricosuric Agents

Decreased Effect

Meropenem may decrease the levels/effects of: Typhoid Vaccine; Valproic Acid

Dietary Considerations Some products may contain sodium.

Dosage Forms Excipient information presented when available (limited, particularly for generics); consult specific product labeling.

Injection, powder for reconstitution:

Merrem® I.V: 500 mg [contains sodium 45.1 mg as sodium carbonate (1.96 mEq)]; 1 g [contains sodium 90.2 mg as sodium carbonate (3.92 mEq)]

References

American Thoracic Society and Infectious Diseases Society of America, "Guidelines for the Management of Adults With Hospital-Acquired, Ventilator-Associated, and Healthcare-Associated Pneumonia," *Am J Respir Crit Care Med*, 2005, 171(4):388-416.

Krueger WA, Schroeder TH, Hutchison M, et al, "Pharmacokinetics of Meropenem in Critically Ill Patients With Acute Renal Failure Treated by Continuous Hemodiafiltration," *Antimicrob Agents Chemother*, 1998, 42(9):2421-4.

Tunkel AR, Hartman BJ, Kaplan SL, et al, "Practice Guidelines for the Management of Bacterial Meningitis," *Clin Infect Dis*, 2004, 39(9):1267-84.

Ververs TF, van Dijk A, Vinks SA, et al, "Pharmacokinetics and Dosing Regimen of Meropenem in Critically Ill Patients Receiving Continuous Venovenous Hemofiltration," *Crit Care Med*, 2000, 28 (10):3412-6.

◆ **Merrem® (Can)** *see* Meropenem *on page 881*

◆ **Merrem® I.V.** *see* Meropenem *on page 881*

Mesalamine (me SAL a meen)

U.S. Brand Names Apriso™; Asacol®; Asacol® HD; Canasa®; Lialda™; Pentasa®; Rowasa®

Canadian Brand Names Asacol®; Asacol® 800; Mesasal®; Mezavant®; Novo-5 ASA; Pentasa®; Salofalk®

Index Terms 5-Aminosalicylic Acid; 5-ASA; Fisalamine; Mesalazine

Pharmacologic Category 5-Aminosalicylic Acid Derivative

Use

Oral: Treatment and maintenance of remission of mildly- to moderately-active ulcerative colitis

Asacol® HD: Treatment of moderately-active ulcerative colitis

Rectal: Treatment of active mild-to-moderate distal ulcerative colitis, proctosigmoiditis, or proctitis

Pharmacodynamics/Kinetics

Absorption: Rectal: Variable and dependent upon retention time, underlying GI disease, and colonic pH; Oral: Tablet: ~20% to 28%, Capsule: ~20% to 40%

Distribution: ~18 L

Protein binding: 43%

Metabolism: Hepatic and via GI tract to N-acetyl-5-aminosalicylic acid

Half-life elimination: 5-ASA: 0.5-10 hours; N-acetyl-5-ASA: 2-15 hours

Time to peak, serum:

Capsule: Apriso™: ~4 hours; Pentasa®: 3 hours

Rectal: 4-7 hours

Tablet: Asacol®: 4-12 hours; Asacol® HD: 10-16 hours; Lialda™: 9-12 hours; Mezavant®: 8 hours

Excretion: Urine (primarily as metabolites, <8% as unchanged drug); feces (<2%)

Dosage Adults:

Oral:

Treatment of ulcerative colitis (usual course of therapy is 3-8 weeks):

Capsule: 1 g 4 times/day

Tablet: Initial:

Asacol®: 800 mg 3 times/day for 6 weeks

Asacol® HD: 1.6 g 3 times/day for 6 weeks

Lialda™, Mezavant®: 2.4-4.8 g once daily for up to 8 weeks

Maintenance of remission of ulcerative colitis:

Capsule:

Apriso™: 1.5 g once daily in the morning

Pentasa®: 1 g 4 times/day

Tablet (Asacol®): 1.6 g/day in divided doses; **Note:** Asacol® HD, Lialda™, and Mezavant® tablets are approved for treatment only.

Rectal:

Retention enema: 60 mL (4 g) at bedtime, retained overnight, approximately 8 hours

Rectal suppository (Canasa®): Insert one 1000 mg suppository in rectum daily at bedtime

Note: Suppositories should be retained for at least 1-3 hours to achieve maximum benefit.

Note: Some patients may require rectal and oral therapy concurrently.

Elderly: See adult dosing; use with caution

Additional Information Complete prescribing information for this medication should be consulted for additional detail.

Dosage Forms Excipient information presented when available (limited, particularly for generics); consult specific product labeling. [CAN] = Canadian brand name

Capsule, controlled release:

Pentasa®: 250 mg, 500 mg

Capsule, delayed and extended release:

Apriso™: 0.375 g [contains phenylalanine 0.56 mg/capsule]

Suppository, rectal:

Canasa®: 1000 mg [contains saturated vegetable fatty acid esters]

Suspension, rectal: 4 g/60 mL (7s, 28s) [contains potassium metabisulfite and sodium benzoate]

Rowasa®: 4 g/60 mL (7s, 28s) [contains potassium metabisulfite and sodium benzoate]

Tablet, delayed release [enteric coated]:

Asacol®: 400 mg

Asacol® HD: 800 mg

Lialda™: 1.2 g

Tablet, delayed and extended release:

Mezavant® [CAN]: 1.2 g [not available in U.S.]

References

Grand RJ, Ramakrishna J, and Calenda KA, "Inflammatory Bowel Disease in the Pediatric Patient," *Gastroenterol Clin North Am*, 1995, 24(3):613-32.

♦ **Mesalazine** *see* Mesalamine *on page 884*

♦ **Mesasal® (Can)** *see* Mesalamine *on page 884*

♦ **M-Eslon® (Can)** *see* Morphine Sulfate *on page 953*

♦ **Mestinon®** *see* Pyridostigmine *on page 1210*

♦ **Mestinon®-SR (Can)** *see* Pyridostigmine *on page 1210*

♦ **Mestinon® Timespan®** *see* Pyridostigmine *on page 1210*

♦ **Metacortandralone** *see* PrednisoLONE *on page 1164*

♦ **Metadate CD®** *see* Methylphenidate *on page 908*

♦ **Metadate® ER** *see* Methylphenidate *on page 908*

♦ **Metadol™ (Can)** *see* Methadone *on page 888*

♦ **Metadol-D™ (Can)** *see* Methadone *on page 888*

Metaproterenol (met a proe TER e nol)

U.S. Brand Names Alupent® [DSC]

Canadian Brand Names Apo-Orciprenaline®; ratio-Orciprenaline®; Tanta-Orciprenaline®

Index Terms Metaproterenol Sulfate; Orciprenaline Sulfate

Pharmacologic Category Beta$_2$-Adrenergic Agonist

Use Bronchodilator in reversible airway obstruction due to asthma or COPD

Pharmacodynamics/Kinetics

Onset of action: Bronchodilation: Oral: ~30 minutes; Inhalation (nebulization): 5-30 minutes

Peak effect: Oral: ~1 hour

Duration: ~2-6 hours

Dosage

Oral:

Children:

<2 years: 0.4 mg/kg/dose given 3-4 times/day; in infants, the dose can be given every 8-12 hours

2-6 years: 1-2.6 mg/kg/day divided every 6 hours

6-9 years: 10 mg/dose 3-4 times/day

Children >9 years and Adults: 20 mg 3-4 times/day

Elderly: Initial: 10 mg 3-4 times/day, increasing as necessary up to 20 mg 3-4 times/day

Inhalation: Children >12 years and Adults: 2-3 inhalations every 3-4 hours, up to 12 inhalations in 24 hours

Nebulizer:

Infants and Children: 0.01-0.02 mL/kg of 5% solution; minimum dose: 0.1 mL; maximum dose: 0.3 mL diluted in 2-3 mL normal saline every 4-6 hours (may be given more frequently according to need)

Adolescents and Adults: 5-20 breaths of full strength 5% metaproterenol **or** 0.2 to 0.3 mL 5% metaproterenol in 2.5-3 mL normal saline until nebulized every 4-6 hours (can be given more frequently according to need)

Anesthesia and Critical Care Concerns/Other Considerations Hypertension and tachycardia are increased with exogenous sympathomimetics. Beta$_2$-specific agent is more appropriate for use.

◀ **Additional Information** Complete prescribing information for this medication should be consulted for additional detail.

Dosage Forms Excipient information presented when available (limited, particularly for generics); consult specific product labeling. [DSC] = Discontinued product

Aerosol for oral inhalation, as sulfate:
   Alupent®: 0.65 mg/inhalation (14 g) [contains chlorofluorocarbon; 200 doses] [DSC]
Solution for nebulization, as sulfate [preservative free]: 0.4% [4 mg/mL] (2.5 mL); 0.6% [6 mg/mL] (2.5 mL)
Syrup, as sulfate: 10 mg/5 mL (480 mL)
Tablet, as sulfate: 10 mg, 20 mg

◆ **Metaproterenol Sulfate** *see* Metaproterenol *on page 885*

Metaxalone (me TAKS a lone)

U.S. Brand Names Skelaxin®
Canadian Brand Names Skelaxin®
Pharmacologic Category Skeletal Muscle Relaxant
Use Relief of discomfort associated with acute, painful musculoskeletal conditions
Pharmacodynamics/Kinetics
   Onset of action: ~1 hour
   Duration: ~4-6 hours
   Distribution: V_d: ~800 L
   Metabolism: Hepatic via CYP1A2, CYP2D6, CYP2E1, CYP3A4 and to lesser extent CYP2C8, CPY2C9, and CYP2C19
   Bioavailability: Not established; food may increase
   Half-life elimination: 4-14 hours
   Time to peak: T_{max}: ~3 hours
   Excretion: Urine (as metabolites)
Dosage Oral: Children >12 years and Adults: Muscle discomfort: 800 mg 3-4 times/day
   Dosage adjustment in renal impairment: Use caution in patients with mild-to-moderate renal impairment; contraindicated with significant impairment. No specific recommendation are provided in approved labeling.
   Dosage adjustment in hepatic impairment: Use caution in patients with mild-to-moderate hepatic impairment; contraindicated with significant impairment. No specific recommendation are provided in approved labeling.
Additional Information Complete prescribing information for this medication should be consulted for additional detail.
Dosage Forms Excipient information presented when available (limited, particularly for generics); consult specific product labeling. [DSC] = Discontinued product
   Tablet: 400 mg [DSC], 800 mg
References
   Toth PP and Urtis J, "Commonly Used Muscle Relaxant Therapies for Acute Low Back Pain: A Review of Carisoprodol, Cyclobenzaprine Hydrochloride, and Metaxalone," *Clin Ther*, 2004, 26 (9):1355-67.

MetFORMIN (met FOR min)

Related Information
   Heart Failure (Systolic) *on page 1739*
   Perioperative Management of the Diabetic Patient *on page 1584*
U.S. Brand Names Fortamet®; Glucophage®; Glucophage® XR; Glumetza™; Riomet®
Canadian Brand Names Apo-Metformin®; CO Metformin; Dom-Metformin; Gen-Metformin; Glucophage®; Glumetza™; Glycon; MED-Metformin; Mylan-Metformin; Novo-Metformin; Nu-Metformin; PHL-Metformin; PMS-Metformin; Pro-Metformin; RAN™-Metformin; ratio-Metformin; Rhoxal-metformin; Riva-Metformin; Sandoz-Metformin FC; ZYM-Metformin
Index Terms Metformin Hydrochloride

Pharmacologic Category Antidiabetic Agent, Biguanide

Use Management of type 2 diabetes mellitus (noninsulin dependent, NIDDM) as monotherapy when hyperglycemia cannot be managed with diet and exercise alone. In adults, may be used concomitantly with a sulfonylurea or insulin to improve glycemic control.

Unlabeled/Investigational Use Gestational diabetes mellitus (GDM); polycystic ovary syndrome (PCOS)

Pharmacodynamics/Kinetics
Onset of action: Within days; maximum effects up to 2 weeks
Distribution: V_d: 654 ± 358 L; partitions into erythrocytes
Protein binding: Negligible
Metabolism: Not metabolized by the liver
Bioavailability: Absolute: Fasting: 50% to 60%
Half-life elimination: Plasma: 4-9 hours
Time to peak, serum: Immediate release: 2-3 hours; Extended release: 7 hours (range: 4-8 hours)
Excretion: Urine (90% as unchanged drug; active secretion)

Dosage Type 2 diabetes management: **Note:** Allow 1-2 weeks between dose titrations. Generally, clinically significant responses are not seen at doses <1500 mg daily; however, a lower recommended starting dose and gradual increased dosage is recommended to minimize gastrointestinal symptoms.

Immediate release tablet or solution: Oral:
Children 10-16 years: Initial: 500 mg twice daily; increases in daily dosage should be made in increments of 500 mg at weekly intervals, given in divided doses, up to a maximum of 2000 mg/day
Chidlren ≥17 years and Adults: Initial: 500 mg twice daily **or** 850 mg once daily; increase dosage incrementally.
Incremental dosing recommendations based on dosage form:
500 mg tablet: One tablet/day at weekly intervals
850 mg tablet: One tablet/day every other week
Oral solution: 500 mg twice daily every other week
Doses of up to 2000 mg/day may be given twice daily. If a dose >2000 mg/day is required, it may be better tolerated in three divided doses. Maximum recommended dose 2550 mg/day.

Extended release tablet: Oral: **Note:** If glycemic control is not achieved at maximum dose, may divide dose and administer twice daily.
Children ≥17 years and Adults:
Fortamet®: Initial: 1000 mg once daily; dosage may be increased by 500 mg weekly; maximum dose: 2500 mg once daily
Glucophage® XR: Initial: 500 mg once daily; dosage may be increased by 500 mg weekly; maximum dose: 2000 mg once daily
Adults: Glumetza™: Initial: 1000 mg once daily; dosage may be increased by 500 mg weekly; maximum dose: 2000 mg once daily

Elderly: The initial and maintenance dosing should be conservative, due to the potential for decreased renal function. Generally, elderly patients should not be titrated to the maximum dose of metformin. Do not use in patients ≥80 years of age unless normal renal function has been established.

Transfer from other antidiabetic agents: No transition period is generally necessary except when transferring from chlorpropamide. When transferring from chlorpropamide, care should be exercised during the first 2 weeks because of the prolonged retention of chlorpropamide in the body, leading to overlapping drug effects and possible hypoglycemia.

Concomitant metformin and oral sulfonylurea therapy: If patients have not responded to 4 weeks of the maximum dose of metformin monotherapy, consider a gradual addition of an oral sulfonylurea, even if prior primary or secondary failure to a sulfonylurea has occurred. Continue metformin at the maximum dose. If adequate response has not occurred following 3 months of metformin and sulfonylurea combination therapy, consider switching to insulin with or without metformin.

Failed sulfonylurea therapy: Patients with prior failure on glyburide may be treated by gradual addition of metformin. Initiate with glyburide 20 mg and metformin 500 mg daily. Metformin dosage may be increased by 500 mg/day at

◄ weekly intervals, up to a maximum metformin dose (dosage of glyburide maintained at 20 mg/day).

Concomitant metformin and insulin therapy: Initial: 500 mg metformin once daily, continue current insulin dose; increase by 500 mg metformin weekly until adequate glycemic control is achieved

Maximum daily dose: Immediate release and solution: 2550 mg metformin; Extended release: 2000-2500 mg (varies by product)

Decrease insulin dose 10% to 25% when FPG <120 mg/dL; monitor and make further adjustments as needed

Dosing adjustment/comments in renal impairment: The plasma and blood half-life of metformin is prolonged and the renal clearance is decreased in proportion to the decrease in creatinine clearance. Per the manufacturer, metformin is contraindicated in the presence of renal dysfunction defined as a serum creatinine ≥1.5 mg/dL in males, or ≥1.4 mg/dL in females and in patients with abnormal clearance. Clinically, it has been recommended that metformin be avoided in patients with Cl_{cr} <60-70 mL/minute (DeFronzo, 1999).

Dosing adjustment in hepatic impairment: Avoid metformin; liver disease is a risk factor for the development of lactic acidosis during metformin therapy.

Anesthesia and Critical Care Concerns/Other Considerations

Clinical Pearls/Comments: While megaloblastic anemia has been rarely seen with metformin, if suspected, vitamin B_{12} deficiency should be excluded. Metformin has a large volume of distribution in liver, kidney, and GI tract where concentration is much larger than in the plasma.

Lactic acidosis is an uncommon side effect in patients without renal or respiratory insufficiency, hepatic failure, or conditions that predispose to hypoxemia.

Additional Information Complete prescribing information for this medication should be consulted for additional detail.

Dosage Forms Excipient information presented when available (limited, particularly for generics); consult specific product labeling.

Solution, oral, as hydrochloride:
Riomet®: 100 mg/mL (118 mL, 473 mL) [contains saccharin; cherry flavor]
Tablet, as hydrochloride: 500 mg, 850 mg, 1000 mg
Glucophage®: 500 mg, 850 mg, 1000 mg
Tablet, extended release, as hydrochloride: 500 mg, 750 mg
Fortamet®: 500 mg, 1000 mg
Glucophage® XR: 500 mg
Glumetza™: 500 mg, 1000 mg

References
"Standards of Medical Care for Patients With Diabetes Mellitus. American Diabetes Association," *Diabetes Care*, 2007, 30(Suppl 1):4-41.

◆ **Metformin Hydrochloride** *see* MetFORMIN *on page 886*

Methadone (METH a done)

Medication Safety Issues

Sound-alike/look-alike issues:
Methadone may be confused with dexmethylphenidate, Mephyton®, methyl-phenidate, Metadate® CD, and Metadate® ER

High alert medication: The Institute for Safe Medication Practices (ISMP) includes this medication among its list of drug classes which have a heightened risk of causing significant patient harm when used in error.

Related Information

Anesthesia for Patients With Liver Disease *on page 1537*
Anesthetic Considerations in the Substance-Abusing Patient *on page 1613*
Chronic Pain Management *on page 1546*
Opioid Analgesics *on page 1688*

U.S. Brand Names Dolophine®; Methadone Diskets®; Methadone Intensol™; Methadose®

Canadian Brand Names Metadol-D™; Metadol™

Index Terms Methadone Hydrochloride

Pharmacologic Category Analgesic, Opioid

Restrictions C-II

When used for treatment of opioid addiction: May only be dispensed in accordance to guidelines established by the Substance Abuse and Mental Health Services Administration's (SAMHSA) Center for Substance Abuse Treatment (CSAT). Regulations regarding methadone use may vary by state and/or country. Obtain advice from appropriate regulatory agencies and/or consult with pain management/palliative care specialists.

Note: Regulatory Exceptions to the General Requirement to Provide Opioid Agonist Treatment (per manufacturer's labeling):
1. During inpatient care, when the patient was admitted for any condition other than concurrent opioid addiction, to facilitate the treatment of the primary admitting diagnosis.
2. During an emergency period of no longer than 3 days while definitive care for the addiction is being sought in an appropriately licensed facility.

Generic Available Yes

Use Management of moderate-to-severe pain; detoxification and maintenance treatment of opioid addiction as part of an FDA-approved program

Mechanism of Action Binds to opiate receptors in the CNS, causing inhibition of ascending pain pathways, altering the perception of and response to pain; produces generalized CNS depression

Pharmacodynamics/Kinetics

Onset of action: Oral: Analgesic: 0.5-1 hour; Parenteral: 10-20 minutes
  Peak effect: Parenteral: 1-2 hours; Oral: continuous dosing: 3-5 days
Duration of analgesia: Oral: 4-8 hours, increases to 22-48 hours with repeated doses
Distribution: V_{dss}: 1-8 L/kg
Protein binding: 85% to 90%
Metabolism: Hepatic; N-demethylation primarily via CYP3A4, CYP2B6, and CYP2C19 to inactive metabolites
Bioavailability: Oral: 36% to 100%
Half-life elimination: 8-59 hours; may be prolonged with alkaline pH, decreased during pregnancy
Time to peak, plasma: 1-7.5 hours
Excretion: Urine (<10% as unchanged drug); increased with urine pH <6

Dosage Regulations regarding methadone use may vary by state and/or country. Obtain advice from appropriate regulatory agencies and/or consult with pain management/palliative care specialists. **Note:** These are guidelines and do not represent the maximum doses that may be required in all patients. Methadone accumulates with repeated doses and dosage may need reduction after 3-5 days to prevent CNS depressant effects. Some patients may benefit from every 8-12 hour dosing interval for chronic pain management. Doses should be titrated to appropriate effects.

Children (unlabeled use):
  Pain (analgesia):
    Oral: Initial: 0.1-0.2 mg/kg 4-8 hours initially for 2-3 doses, then every 6-12 hours as needed. Dosing interval may range from 4-12 hours during initial therapy; decrease in dose or frequency may be required (~days 2-5) due to accumulation with repeated doses (maximum dose: 5-10 mg)
    I.V.: 0.1 mg/kg every 4-8 hours initially for 2-3 doses, then every 6-12 hours as needed. Dosing interval may range from 4-12 hours during initial therapy; decrease in dose or frequency may be required (~days 2-5) due to accumulation with repeated doses (maximum dose: 5-8 mg)
  Iatrogenic narcotic dependency: Oral: General guidelines: Initial: 0.05-0.1 mg/kg/dose every 6 hours; increase by 0.05 mg/kg/dose until withdrawal symptoms are controlled; after 24-48 hours, the dosing interval can be lengthened to every 12-24 hours; to taper dose, wean by 0.05 mg/kg/day; if withdrawal symptoms recur, taper at a slower rate
Adults:
  Acute pain (moderate-to-severe):
    Oral: Opioid-naive: Initial: 2.5-10 mg every 8-12 hours; more frequent administration may be required during initiation to maintain adequate analgesia. Dosage interval may range from 4-12 hours, since duration of

analgesia is relatively short during the first days of therapy, but increases substantially with continued administration.

Chronic pain (opioid-tolerant): **Conversion from oral morphine to oral methadone: Note:** 1) There is not a linear relationship when converting to methadone from oral morphine. The higher the daily morphine equivalent dose the more potent methadone is, and 2) conversion to methadone is more of a process than a calculation. Patient response to methadone needs to be monitored closely throughout the process of the conversion.

Daily oral morphine dose <100 mg: Estimated daily oral methadone dose: 20% to 30% of total daily morphine dose

Daily oral morphine dose 100-300 mg: Estimated daily oral methadone dose: 10% to 20% of total daily morphine dose

Daily oral morphine dose 300-600 mg: Estimated daily oral methadone dose: 8% to 12% of total daily morphine dose

Daily oral morphine dose 600-1000 mg: Estimated daily oral methadone dose: 5% to 10% of total daily morphine dose.

Daily oral morphine dose >1000 mg: Estimated daily oral methadone dose: <5% of total daily morphine dose.

Note: The total daily methadone dose should then be divided to reflect the intended dosing schedule.

Or, per American Pain Society:

Daily oral morphine or equivalent dose per day <90 mg: Estimated daily oral methadone dose: 25% of total daily morphine dose

Daily oral morphine or equivalent dose per day 90-300 mg: Estimated daily oral methadone dose: 12% of total daily morphine dose

Daily oral morphine or equivalent dose per day >300 mg: Estimated daily oral methadone dose: 8% of total daily morphine dose

Note: The estimated total daily methadone dose should then be divided by 3 and administered every 8 hours.

I.V.: Manufacturers labeling: Initial: 2.5-10 mg every 8-12 hours in opioid-naive patients; titrate slowly to effect; may also be administered by SubQ or I.M. injection

Conversion from oral methadone to parenteral methadone dose: Initial dose: Parenteral:Oral ratio: 1:2 (eg, 5 mg parenteral methadone equals 10 mg oral methadone)

Detoxification: Oral:

Initial: A single dose of 20-30 mg is generally sufficient to suppress symptoms. Should not exceed 30 mg; lower doses should be considered in patients with low tolerance at initiation (eg, absence of opioids ≥5 days); an additional 5-10 mg of methadone may be provided if withdrawal symptoms have not been suppressed or if symptoms reappear after 2-4 hours; total daily dose on the first day should not exceed 40 mg, unless the program physician documents in the patient's record that 40 mg did not control opiate abstinence symptoms.

Maintenance: Titrate to a dosage which attenuates craving, blocks euphoric effects of other opiates, and tolerance to sedative effect of methadone. Usual range: 80-120 mg/day (titration should occur cautiously)

Withdrawal: Dose reductions should be <10% of the maintenance dose, every 10-14 days

Detoxification (short-term): Oral:

Initial: Titrate to ~40 mg/day in divided doses to achieve stabilization, may continue 40 mg dose for 2-3 days

Maintenance: Titrate to a dosage which prevents/attenuates euphoric effects of self-administered opioids, reduces drug craving, and withdrawal symptoms are prevented for 24 hours.

Withdrawal: Requires individualization. Decrease daily or every other day, keeping withdrawal symptoms tolerable; hospitalized patients may tolerate a 20% reduction/day; ambulatory patients may require a slower reduction

Dosage adjustment during pregnancy: Methadone dose may need to be increased, or the dosing interval decreased; use should be reserved for cases where the benefits clearly outweigh the risks

Dosage adjustment for toxicity:

QT_c >450-499 msecs: Monitor QT_c more frequently

QT_c ≥500 msecs: Consider discontinuation or reducing methadone dose

Dosage adjustment in renal impairment: Cl_{cr} <10 mL/minute: Administer 50% to 75% of normal dose

Dosage adjustment in hepatic impairment: Avoid in severe liver disease

Stability

Injection: Store at controlled room temperature of 15°C to 30°C (59°F to 86°F). Protect from light.

Oral concentrate, oral solution, tablet: Store at controlled room temperature of 15°C to 30°C (59°F to 86°F).

Administration Oral dose for detoxification and maintenance may be administered in fruit juice or water. Dispersible tablet should not be chewed or swallowed; add to liquid and allow to dissolve before administering. May rinse if residual remains.

Monitoring Parameters Obtain baseline ECG (evaluate QT_c interval), within 30 days of initiation, and then annually for all patients receiving methadone. Increase ECG monitoring if patient receiving >100 mg/day or if unexplained syncope or seizure occurs while on methadone (Krantz, 2008).

If before or at anytime during therapy:

QT_c >450-499 msecs: Discuss potential risks and benefits; monitor QT_c more frequently

QT_c ≥500 msecs: Consider discontinuation or reducing methadone dose **or** eliminate factors promoting QT_c prolongation (eg, potassium-wasting drugs) **or** use alternative therapy (eg, buprenorphine)

Pain relief, respiratory and mental status, blood pressure

Reference Range Prevention of opiate withdrawal: Therapeutic: 100-400 ng/mL (SI: 0.32-1.29 µmol/L); Toxic: >2 mcg/mL (SI: >6.46 µmol/L)

Pregnancy Risk Factor C/D (prolonged use or high doses at term)

Contraindications Hypersensitivity to methadone or any component of the formulation; respiratory depression (in the absence of resuscitative equipment or in an unmonitored setting); acute bronchial asthma or hypercarbia; paralytic ileus; concurrent use of selegiline

Warnings/Precautions An opioid-containing analgesic regimen should be tailored to each patient's needs and based upon the type of pain being treated (acute versus chronic), the route of administration, degree of tolerance for opioids (naive versus chronic user), age, weight, and medical condition. The optimal analgesic dose varies widely among patients. Doses should be titrated to pain relief/prevention. Patients maintained on stable doses of methadone may need higher and/or more frequent doses in case of acute pain (eg, postoperative pain, physical trauma). Methadone is ineffective for the relief of anxiety.

[U.S. Boxed Warning]: May prolong the QT_c interval and increase risk for torsade de pointes. Patients should be informed of the potential arrhythmia risk, evaluated for any history of structural heart disease, arrhythmia, syncope, and for existence of potential drug interactions including drugs that possess QT_c interval-prolonging properties, promote hypokalemia, hypomagnesemia, or hypocalcemia, or reduce elimination of methadone (eg, CYP3A4 inhibitors). Obtain baseline ECG for all patients and risk stratify according to QT_c interval (see Monitoring Parameters). Use with caution in patients at risk for QT_c prolongation, with medications known to prolong the QT_c interval, promote electrolyte depletion, or inhibit CYP3A4, or history of conduction abnormalities. QT_c interval prolongation and torsade de pointes may be associated with doses >100 mg/day, but have also been observed with lower doses. May cause severe hypotension; use caution with severe volume depletion or other conditions which may compromise maintenance of normal blood pressure. Use caution with cardiovascular disease or patients predisposed to dysrhythmias.

[U.S. Boxed Warning]: May cause respiratory depression. Use caution in patients with respiratory disease or pre-existing respiratory conditions (eg, severe obesity, asthma, COPD, sleep apnea, CNS depression). Because the respiratory effects last longer than the analgesic effects, slow titration is required. Use extreme caution during treatment initiation, dose titration and conversion from other opioid agonists. Incomplete cross tolerance may occur; patients tolerant to other mu opioid agonists may not be tolerant to methadone. Abrupt cessation may precipitate withdrawal symptoms.

May cause CNS depression, which may impair physical or mental abilities. Patients must be cautioned about performing tasks which require mental alertness (eg, operating machinery or driving). Effects with other sedative drugs or ethanol may be potentiated. Use with caution in patients with depression or suicidal tendencies, or in patients with a history of drug abuse. Tolerance or psychological and physical dependence may occur with prolonged use.

Use with caution in patients with head injury or increased intracranial pressure. May obscure diagnosis or clinical course of patients with acute abdominal conditions. Elderly may be more susceptible to adverse effects (eg, CNS, respiratory, gastrointestinal). Decrease initial dose and use caution in the elderly or debilitated; with hyper/hypothyroidism, morbid obesity, adrenal insufficiency, prostatic hyperplasia, or urethral stricture; or with severe renal or hepatic failure. Use with caution in patients with biliary tract dysfunction; acute pancreatitis may cause constriction of sphincter of Oddi. Safety and efficacy have not been established in children. **[U.S. Boxed Warning]: For oral administration only; excipients to deter use by injection are contained in tablets.**

[U.S. Boxed Warning]: When used for treatment of narcotic addiction: May only be dispensed by opioid treatment programs certified by the Substance Abuse and Mental Health Services Administration (SAMHSA) and certified by the designated state authority. Exceptions include inpatient treatment of other conditions and emergency period (not >3 days) while definitive substance abuse treatment is being sought.

Adverse Reactions Frequency not defined. During prolonged administration, adverse effects may decrease over several weeks; however, constipation and sweating may persist.

Cardiovascular: Arrhythmia, bigeminal rhythms, bradycardia, cardiac arrest, cardiomyopathy, ECG changes, edema, extrasystoles, faintness, flushing, heart failure, hypotension, palpitation, peripheral vasodilation, phlebitis, orthostatic hypotension, QT interval prolonged, shock, syncope, tachycardia, torsade de pointes, T-wave inversion, ventricular fibrillation, ventricular tachycardia,

Central nervous system: Agitation, confusion, disorientation, dizziness, drowsiness, dysphoria, euphoria, hallucination, headache, insomnia, lightheadedness, sedation, seizure

Dermatologic: Hemorrhagic urticaria, pruritus, rash, urticaria

Endocrine & metabolic: Antidiuretic effect, amenorrhea, hypokalemia, hypomagnesemia, libido decreased

Gastrointestinal: Abdominal pain, anorexia, biliary tract spasm, constipation, glossitis, nausea, stomach cramps, vomiting, weight gain, xerostomia

Genitourinary: Impotence, urinary retention or hesitancy

Hematologic: Thrombocytopenia (reversible, reported in patients with chronic hepatitis)

Neuromuscular & skeletal: Weakness

Local: I.M./SubQ injection: Erythema, pain, swelling; I.V. injection: Hemorrhagic urticaria (rare), pruritus, urticaria, rash

Ocular: Miosis, visual disturbances

Respiratory: Pulmonary edema, respiratory depression, respiratory arrest

Miscellaneous: Death, diaphoresis, physical and psychological dependence

Drug Interactions

Metabolism/Transport Effects Substrate of CYP2C9 (minor), 2C19 (minor), 2D6 (minor), 3A4 (major); **Inhibits** CYP2D6 (moderate), 3A4 (weak)

Avoid Concomitant Use

Avoid concomitant use of Methadone with any of the following: Artemether; Dronedarone; Lumefantrine; Nilotinib; Pimozide; QuiNINE; Tetrabenazine; Thioridazine; Ziprasidone

Increased Effect/Toxicity

Methadone may increase the levels/effects of: Alcohol (Ethyl); Alvimopan; CNS Depressants; CYP2D6 Substrates; Desmopressin; Dronedarone; Fesoterodine; Nebivolol; Pimozide; QTc-Prolonging Agents; QuiNINE; Selective Serotonin Reuptake Inhibitors; Tamoxifen; Tetrabenazine; Thiazide Diuretics; Thioridazine; Zidovudine; Ziprasidone

The levels/effects of Methadone may be increased by: Alfuzosin; Amphetamines; Antifungal Agents (Azole Derivatives, Systemic); Antipsychotic Agents

(Phenothiazines); Artemether; Chloroquine; Ciprofloxacin; CYP2B6 Inhibitors (Moderate); CYP2B6 Inhibitors (Strong); CYP3A4 Inhibitors (Moderate); CYP3A4 Inhibitors (Strong); Gadobutrol; Lumefantrine; Nilotinib; QuiNINE; Selective Serotonin Reuptake Inhibitors; Succinylcholine

Decreased Effect

Methadone may decrease the levels/effects of: Codeine; Didanosine; Pegvisomant; TraMADol

The levels/effects of Methadone may be decreased by: Ammonium Chloride; Barbiturates; CarBAMazepine; CYP2B6 Inducers (Strong); CYP3A4 Inducers (Strong); Deferasirox; Etravirine; Herbs (CYP3A4 Inducers); Phenytoin; Protease Inhibitors; Reverse Transcriptase Inhibitors (Non-Nucleoside); Rifamycin Derivatives

Ethanol/Nutrition/Herb Interactions

Ethanol: Avoid ethanol (may increase CNS effects). Watch for sedation.

Herb/Nutraceutical: Avoid St John's wort (may decrease methadone levels; may increase CNS depression). Avoid valerian, kava kava, gotu kola (may increase CNS depression). Methadone is metabolized by CYP3A4 in the intestines; avoid concurrent use of grapefruit juice.

Test Interactions Some quinolones may produce a false-positive urine screening result for opiates using commercially-available immunoassay kits. This has been demonstrated most consistently for levofloxacin and ofloxacin, but other quinolones have shown cross-reactivity in certain assay kits. Confirmation of positive opiate screens by more specific methods should be considered.

Dosage Forms Excipient information presented when available (limited, particularly for generics); consult specific product labeling. [DSC] = Discontinued product

Injection, solution, as hydrochloride: 10 mg/mL (20 mL)

Solution, oral, as hydrochloride: 5 mg/5 mL (500 mL); 10 mg/5 mL (500 mL) [contains alcohol 8%; citrus flavor]

Solution, oral, as hydrochloride [concentrate]: 10 mg/mL (946 mL)

Methadone Intensol™: 10 mg/mL (30 mL) [dye free, sugar free; contains sodium benzoate; unflavored]

Methadose®: 10 mg/mL (1000 mL) [contains propylene glycol; cherry flavor]

Methadose®: 10 mg/mL (1000 mL) [dye free, sugar free; contains sodium benzoate; unflavored]

Tablet, as hydrochloride: 5 mg, 10 mg

Dolophine®: 5 mg, 10 mg

Methadose®: 5 mg, 10 mg [DSC]

Tablet, dispersible, as hydrochloride: 40 mg

Methadose®: 40 mg

Methadone Diskets®: 40 mg [orange-pineapple flavor]

References

Mercadante S, Casuccio A, Fulfaro F, et al, "Switching From Morphine to Methadone to Improve Analgesia and Tolerability in Cancer Patients: A Prospective Study," *J Clin Oncol*, 2001, 19 (11):2898-904.

"Principles of Analgesic Use in the Treatment of Acute Pain and Cancer Pain," 6th ed, Glenview, IL: American Pain Society, 2008.

Weschules DJ and Bain KT, "A Systematic Review of Opioid Conversion Ratios Used With Methadone for the Treatment of Pain," *Pain Med*, 2008, 9(5):595-612.

♦ **Methadone Diskets®** *see* Methadone *on page 888*

♦ **Methadone Hydrochloride** *see* Methadone *on page 888*

♦ **Methadone Intensol™** *see* Methadone *on page 888*

♦ **Methadose®** *see* Methadone *on page 888*

♦ **Methaminodiazepoxide Hydrochloride** *see* ChlordiazePOXIDE *on page 290*

♦ **Methergine®** *see* Methylergonovine *on page 904*

Methimazole (meth IM a zole)

Medication Safety Issues

Sound-alike/look-alike issues:

Methimazole may be confused with metolazone

U.S. Brand Names Northyx™; Tapazole®

◀ **Canadian Brand Names** Dom-Methimazole; PHL-Methimazole; Tapazole®
Index Terms Thiamazole
Pharmacologic Category Antithyroid Agent; Thioamide
Generic Available Yes
Use Palliative treatment of hyperthyroidism, return the hyperthyroid patient to a normal metabolic state prior to thyroidectomy, and to control thyrotoxic crisis that may accompany thyroidectomy
Mechanism of Action Inhibits the synthesis of thyroid hormones by blocking the oxidation of iodine in the thyroid gland, blocking iodine's ability to combine with tyrosine to form thyroxine and triiodothyronine (T_3), does not inactivate circulating T_4 and T_3

Pharmacodynamics/Kinetics
  Onset of action: Antithyroid: Oral: 12-18 hours
  Duration: 36-72 hours
  Distribution: Concentrated in thyroid gland; crosses placenta; enters breast milk (1:1)
  Protein binding, plasma: None
  Metabolism: Hepatic
  Bioavailability: 80% to 95%
  Half-life elimination: 4-13 hours
  Excretion: Urine (80%)

Dosage Oral: Administer in 3 equally divided doses at approximately 8-hour intervals
  Children: Initial: 0.4 mg/kg/day in 3 divided doses; maintenance: 0.2 mg/kg/day in 3 divided doses up to 30 mg/24 hours maximum
    Alternatively: Initial: 0.5-0.7 mg/kg/day **or** 15-20 mg/m^2/day in 3 divided doses
    Maintenance: $1/3$ to $2/3$ of the initial dose beginning when the patient is euthyroid
    Maximum: 30 mg/24 hours
  Adults: Initial: 15 mg/day in 3 divided doses (approximately every 8 hours) for mild hyperthyroidism; 30-40 mg/day in moderately-severe hyperthyroidism; 60 mg/day in severe hyperthyroidism; maintenance: 5-15 mg/day (may be given as a single daily dose in many cases)
    Adjust dosage as required to achieve and maintain serum T_3, T_4, and TSH levels in the normal range. An elevated T_3 may be the sole indicator of inadequate treatment. An elevated TSH indicates excessive antithyroid treatment.
    Thyrotoxic crisis (recommendations vary widely and have not been evaluated in comparative trials): Dosages of 20-30 mg every 6-12 hours have been recommended for short-term initial therapy, followed by gradual reduction to a maintenance dosage (5-15 mg/day). Rectal administration has been described (Nabil, 1982).

  Dosing adjustment in renal impairment: Adjustment is not necessary
Stability Protect from light.
Administration In thyroid storm, rectal administration has been attempted (Nabil, 1982).
Monitoring Parameters Monitor for signs of hypothyroidism, hyperthyroidism, T_4, T_3; CBC with differential, liver function (baseline and as needed), serum thyroxine, free thyroxine index

Anesthesia and Critical Care Concerns/Other Considerations
  Clinical Pearls/Comments: Agranulocytosis, when it occurs, is usually seen during the first several months of therapy and with maintenance doses >40 mg/day.

Pregnancy Risk Factor D
Contraindications Hypersensitivity to methimazole or any component of the formulation; breast-feeding (per manufacturer; however, expert analysis and the AAP state this drug may be used in nursing mothers)
Warnings/Precautions Antithyroid agents have been associated (rarely) with significant bone marrow depression. The most severe manifestation is agranulocytosis. Aplastic anemia, thrombocytopenia, and leukopenia may also occur. Use with extreme caution in patients receiving other drugs known to cause myelosuppression particularly agranulocytosis, patients >40 years of age; avoid doses >40 mg/day (increased myelosuppression). Discontinue if significant bone marrow suppression occurs, particularly agranulocytosis or aplastic anemia.

Rare, severe hepatic reactions (hepatic necrosis, hepatitis) may occur. Symptoms suggestive of hepatic dysfunction should prompt evaluation. Discontinue in the presence of hepatitis (transaminase >3 times upper limit of normal). In addition, other rare hypersensitivity reactions to antithyroid agents have been reported, including the development of ANCA-positive vasculitis, drug fever, interstitial pneumonitis, exfoliative dermatitis, glomerulonephritis, leukocytoclastic vasculitis, and a lupus-like syndrome; prompt discontinuation is warranted in patients who develop symptoms consistent with a form of autoimmunity or other hyper-sensitivity during therapy. Minor dermatologic reactions may not require discontinuation, depending on severity.

May cause hypoprothrombinemia and bleeding; use with particular caution in patients >40 years of age.

Adverse Reactions Frequency not defined.

Cardiovascular: ANCA-positive vasculitis, edema, leukocytoclastic vasculitis, periarteritis

Central nervous system: CNS stimulation, depression, drowsiness, fever, headache, vertigo

Dermatologic: Alopecia, erythema nodosum, exfoliative dermatitis, pruritus, skin pigmentation, skin rash, urticaria

Endocrine & metabolic: Goiter

Gastrointestinal: Nausea, vomiting, stomach pain, abnormal taste, constipation, weight gain, salivary gland swelling

Hematologic: Agranulocytosis, aplastic anemia, granulocytopenia, hypoprothrom-binemia, leukopenia, thrombocytopenia

Hepatic: Cholestatic jaundice, hepatitis, jaundice

Neuromuscular & skeletal: Arthralgia, paresthesia

Renal: Nephritis, nephrotic syndrome

Miscellaneous: SLE-like syndrome

Drug Interactions

Metabolism/Transport Effects Inhibits CYP1A2 (weak), 2A6 (weak), 2B6 (weak), 2C9 (weak), 2C19 (weak), 2D6 (moderate), 2E1 (weak), 3A4 (weak)

Avoid Concomitant Use

Avoid concomitant use of Methimazole with any of the following: Sodium Iodide I131

Increased Effect/Toxicity There are no known significant interactions involving an increase in effect.

Decreased Effect

Methimazole may decrease the levels/effects of: Sodium Iodide I131; Vitamin K Antagonists

Dietary Considerations Should be taken consistently in relation to meals every day.

Dosage Forms Excipient information presented when available (limited, particularly for generics); consult specific product labeling.

Tablet: 5 mg, 10 mg, 20 mg

Northyx™: 5 mg, 10 mg, 15 mg, 20 mg

Tapazole®: 5 mg, 10 mg

Methohexital (meth oh HEKS i tal)

Medication Safety Issues

Sound-alike/look-alike issues:

Brevital® may be confused with Brevibloc®

High alert medication: The Institute for Safe Medication Practices (ISMP) includes this medication among its list of drugs which have a heightened risk of causing significant patient harm when used in error.

◀ **Related Information**

Anesthesia Considerations for Neurosurgery *on page 1514*
Anesthesia for Geriatric Patients *on page 1523*
Anesthesia for Patients With Liver Disease *on page 1537*
Intravenous Anesthetic Agents *on page 1635*
Moderate Sedation *on page 1566*
Perioperative Management of Patients on Antiseizure Medication *on page 1577*

U.S. Brand Names Brevital® Sodium

Canadian Brand Names Brevital®

Index Terms Methohexital Sodium

Pharmacologic Category Barbiturate; General Anesthetic

Restrictions C-IV

Generic Available No

Use For induction of anesthesia prior to the use of other general anesthetic agents; as an adjunct to subpotent inhalational anesthetic agents for short surgical procedures; for short surgical, diagnostic, or therapeutic procedures associated with minimal painful stimuli

Additional indications for adults: For use with other parenteral agents, usually narcotic analgesics, to supplement subpotent inhalational anesthetic agents for longer surgical procedures; as an agent to induce a hypnotic state

Unlabeled/Investigational Use Wada test

Mechanism of Action Ultra short-acting I.V. barbiturate anesthetic

Pharmacodynamics/Kinetics

Onset of action: I.V.: Immediate; I.M. (pediatrics): 2-10 minutes; Rectal (pediatrics): 5-15 minutes
Duration: Single dose: I.V.: 10-20 minutes; Rectal: 45 minutes
Metabolism: Hepatic via demethylation and oxidation
Excretion: Urine

Dosage Doses must be titrated to effect.

Infants <1 month: Safety and efficacy not established

Infants ≥1 month and Children:

Anesthesia induction:

I.M.: 6.6-10 mg/kg of a 5% solution
Rectal: Usual: 25 mg/kg of a 1% solution
I.V. (unlabeled dose): 1-2 mg/kg/dose of a 1% solution

Procedural sedation (unlabeled dose):

I.V.: Initial: 0.5 mg/kg given immediately prior to procedure; if sedation not adequate, repeat 0.5 mg/kg to a maximum total dose of 2 mg/kg
Rectal: 25 mg/kg of a 10% (100 mg/mL) solution given 5-15 minutes prior to procedure; maximum dose 500 mg

Adults: I.V.:

Induction: 1-1.5 mg/kg; maintenance: 50-120 mcg/kg/minute (or 20-40 mg every 4-7 minutes)
Wada test (unlabeled): 2-4 mg

Dosing adjustment/comments in hepatic impairment: Lower dosage and monitor closely

Stability Do not dilute with solutions containing bacteriostatic agents. Solutions should be freshly prepared and used promptly. Store at 20°C to 25°C (68°F to 77°F). Reconstituted solutions are chemically stable at room temperature for 24 hours; 0.2% (2 mg/mL) solutions in D_5W or NS are stable at room temperature for 24 hours.

Reconstitution:

For a 1% (10 mg/mL) solution:

500 mg vial: Dilute with 50 mL with SWFI (preferred), D_5W, or NS
2.5 g vial: Dilute with 15 mL of SWFI (preferred), D_5W, or NS, then add to 235 mL for a total volume of 250 mL

For a 5% (50 mg/mL) solution:

500 mg vial: Dilute with 10 mL of SWFI (preferred), D_5W, or NS
2.5 g vial: Dilute with 50 mL of SWFI (preferred), D_5W, or NS

For a 10% (100 mg/mL) solution:

500 mg vial: Dilute with 5 mL of SWFI (Pomeranz, 2000)
2.5 g vial: Dilute with 25 mL of SWFI (Pomeranz, 2000)

For continuous I.V. anesthesia: Prepare a 0.2% (2 mg/mL) solution by adding 500 mg to 250 mL of D_5W or NS. Do not dilute with SWFI (use of SWFI to make the 0.2% solution will result in extreme hypotonicity).

Administration
I.V.: Dilute to a maximum concentration of 1% for I.V. use

Induction and maintenance of anesthesia: 1% (10 mg/mL) solution is administered I.V. at a rate of ~1 mL/5 seconds or ~2 mg/second

Wada testing: Dilution of 0.1% (1 mg/mL) has been used; administer I.V. at a rate of 1 mg/second

Continuous I.V. infusion: Use 0.2% (2 mg/mL) solution

I.M. administration: Use 5% (50 mg/mL) solution

Rectal administration: Use 1% (10 mg/mL) solution; 10% (100 mg/mL) solution has also been used (Pomeranz, 2000)

Monitoring Parameters Respiratory status (for conscious sedation, includes pulse oximetry), cardiovascular status, CNS status (when used for procedures monitor sedation score); cardiac monitor and blood pressure monitor required

Anesthesia and Critical Care Concerns/Other Considerations Methohexital does not possess analgesic properties.

Pregnancy Risk Factor B

Contraindications Hypersensitivity to barbiturates, methohexital, or any component of the formulation; porphyria (latent or manifest); patients in whom general anesthesia is contraindicated

Warnings/Precautions Use with caution in patients with liver impairment, renal impairment, cardiovascular disease (including heart failure), severe anemia, extreme obesity, or seizure disorder, the elderly and children. May cause hypotension; use with caution in hemodynamically unstable patients (hypotension or shock) or severe hypertension. May cause respiratory depression; use with caution in patients with pulmonary disease. Use with caution in patients with asthma and chronic obstructive pulmonary disease. Use with extreme caution in patients with ongoing status asthmaticus; hiccups, coughing, laryngospasm, and muscle twitching have occurred impairing ventilation.

Postmarketing studies have indicated that the use of hypnotic/sedative agents for sleep has been associated with hypersensitivity reactions including anaphylaxis as well as angioedema. Effects with other sedative drugs or ethanol may be potentiated. Repeated dosing or continuous infusions may cause cumulative effects. Ensure patient has intravenous access; extravasation or intra-arterial injection causes necrosis. **[U.S. Boxed Warning]: Should only be administered in hospitals or ambulatory care settings with continuous monitoring of respiratory function; resuscitative drugs, age- and size-appropriate and intubation equipment and trained personnel experienced in handling their use should be readily available. For deeply sedated patients, a healthcare provider other than the individual performing the procedure should be present to continuously monitor the patient.**

Adverse Reactions Frequency not defined.
Cardiovascular: Cardiorespiratory arrest, circulatory depression, hypotension, peripheral vascular collapse, tachycardia

Central nervous system: Anxiety, emergence delirium, headache, restlessness, seizure

Dermatologic: Erythema, pruritus, urticaria

Gastrointestinal: Abdominal pain, nausea, salivation, vomiting

Hepatic: Transaminases increased

Local: Injection site pain, nerve injury adjacent to injection site, thrombophlebitis

Neuromuscular & skeletal: Involuntary muscle movement, radial nerve palsy, rigidity, tremor, twitching

Respiratory: Apnea, bronchospasm, cough, dyspnea, hiccups, laryngospasm, respiratory depression, rhinitis

Miscellaneous: Anaphylaxis (rare)

Drug Interactions
Avoid Concomitant Use There are no known interactions where it is recommended to avoid concomitant use.

Increased Effect/Toxicity
Methohexital may increase the levels/effects of: Alcohol (Ethyl); CNS Depressants; Meperidine; Thiazide Diuretics

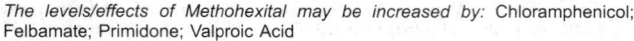

The levels/effects of Methohexital may be increased by: Chloramphenicol; Felbamate; Primidone; Valproic Acid

Decreased Effect

Methohexital may decrease the levels/effects of: Acetaminophen; Beta-Blockers; Calcium Channel Blockers; Chloramphenicol; Contraceptive (Progestins); Corticosteroids (Systemic); CycloSPORINE; Disopyramide; Doxycycline; Etoposide; Etoposide Phosphate; LamoTRIgine; Methadone; Oral Contraceptive (Estrogens); Propafenone; QuiNIDine; Teniposide; Theophylline Derivatives; Tricyclic Antidepressants; Valproic Acid; Vitamin K Antagonists

The levels/effects of Methohexital may be decreased by: Pyridoxine; Rifamycin Derivatives

Dosage Forms Excipient information presented when available (limited, particularly for generics); consult specific product labeling.

Injection, powder for reconstitution, as sodium:
Brevital® Sodium: 500 mg, 2.5 g

◆ **Methohexital Sodium** *see* Methohexital *on page 895*

Methotrexate (meth oh TREKS ate)

U.S. Brand Names Rheumatrex®; Trexall™

Canadian Brand Names Apo-Methotrexate®; ratio-Methotrexate

Index Terms Amethopterin; Methotrexate Sodium; Methotrexatum; MTX (error-prone abbreviation)

Pharmacologic Category Antineoplastic Agent, Antimetabolite (Antifolate); Antirheumatic, Disease Modifying

Use

Oncology-related uses: Treatment of trophoblastic neoplasms (gestational choriocarcinoma, chorioadenoma destruens and hydatidiform mole), acute lymphocytic leukemia (ALL), meningeal leukemia, breast cancer, head and neck cancer (epidermoid), cutaneous T-Cell lymphoma (advanced mycosis fungoides), lung cancer (squamous cell and small cell), advanced non-Hodgkin's lymphomas (NHL), osteosarcoma

Nononcology uses: Treatment of psoriasis (severe, recalcitrant, disabling) and severe rheumatoid arthritis (RA), including polyarticular-course juvenile rheumatoid arthritis (JRA)

Unlabeled/Investigational Use Treatment and maintenance of remission in Crohn's disease; ectopic pregnancy; dermatomyositis; bladder cancer, central nervous system tumors (including nonleukemic meningeal cancers), acute promyelocytic leukemia (maintenance treatment), soft tissue sarcoma (desmoid tumors)

Pharmacodynamics/Kinetics

Onset of action: Antirheumatic: 3-6 weeks; additional improvement may continue longer than 12 weeks

Absorption: Oral: Rapid; well absorbed at low doses (<30 mg/m^2), incomplete after large doses; I.M.: Complete

Distribution: Penetrates slowly into 3rd space fluids (eg, pleural effusions, ascites), exits slowly from these compartments (slower than from plasma); crosses placenta; small amounts enter breast milk; sustained concentrations retained in kidney and liver

Protein binding: 50%

Metabolism: <10%; degraded by intestinal flora to DAMPA by carboxypeptidase; hepatic aldehyde oxidase converts methotrexate to 7-OH methotrexate; polyglutamates are produced intracellularly and are just as potent as methotrexate; their production is dose- and duration-dependent and they are slowly eliminated by the cell once formed

Half-life elimination: Low dose: 3-10 hours; High dose: 8-12 hours

Time to peak, serum: Oral: 1-2 hours; I.M.: 30-60 minutes

Excretion: Urine (44% to 100%); feces (small amounts)

Dosage Details concerning dosing in combination regimens should also be consulted.

Note: Doses between 100-500 mg/m^2 **may require** leucovorin rescue. Doses >500 mg/m^2 **require** leucovorin rescue: Oral, I.M., I.V.: Leucovorin 10-15 mg/m^2 every 6 hours for 8 or 10 doses, starting 24 hours after the start of methotrexate infusion. Continue until the methotrexate level is ≤0.1 micromolar (10^{-7} M). Some clinicians continue leucovorin until the methotrexate level is <0.05 micromolar (5 x 10^{-8} M) or 0.01 micromolar (10^{-8} M).

If the 48-hour methotrexate level is >1 micromolar (10^{-6} M) or the 72-hour methotrexate level is >0.2 micromolar (2 x 10^{-7} M): I.V., I.M, Oral: Leucovorin 100 mg/m^2 every 6 hours until the methotrexate level is ≤0.1 micromolar (10^{-7}M). Some clinicians continue leucovorin until the methotrexate level is <0.05 micromolar (5 x 10^{-8} M) or 0.01 micromolar (10^{-8} M).

Children:

Dermatomyositis (unlabeled use): Oral: 15-20 mg/m^2/week as a single dose once weekly **or** 0.3-1 mg/kg/dose once weekly

Juvenile rheumatoid arthritis: Oral, I.M.: 10 mg/m^2 once weekly, then 5-15 mg/m^2/week as a single dose **or** as 3 divided doses given 12 hours apart

Antineoplastic dosage range:

Oral, I.M.: 7.5-30 mg/m^2/week **or** every 2 weeks

I.V.: 10-18,000 mg/m^2 bolus dosing **or** continuous infusion over 6-42 hours

Pediatric solid tumors (high-dose): I.V.:

<12 years: 12-25 g/m^2

≥12 years: 8 g/m^2

Acute lymphocytic leukemia (intermediate-dose): I.V.: Loading: 100 mg/m^2 bolus dose, followed by 900 mg/m^2/day infusion over 23-41 hours.

Meningeal leukemia: I.T.: 6-12 mg/dose based on age:

<1 year: 6 mg/dose

1 year: 8 mg/dose

2 years: 10 mg/dose

≥3 years: 12 mg/dose

Adults: I.V.: Range is wide from 30-40 mg/m^2/week to 100-12,000 mg/m^2 with leucovorin rescue

Trophoblastic neoplasms:

Oral, I.M.: 15-30 mg/day for 5 days; repeat in 7 days for 3-5 courses

I.V.: 11 mg/m^2 days 1 through 5 every 3 weeks

Head and neck cancer: Oral, I.M., I.V.: 25-50 mg/m^2 once weekly

Mycosis fungoides (cutaneous T-cell lymphoma): Oral, I.M.: Initial (early stages):

5-50 mg once weekly **or**

15-37.5 mg twice weekly

Breast cancer: I.V.: 30-60 mg/m^2 days 1 and 8 every 3-4 weeks

Lymphoma, non-Hodgkin's: I.V.:

30 mg/m^2 days 3 and 10 every 3 weeks **or**

120 mg/m^2 day 8 and 15 every 3-4 weeks **or**

200 mg/m^2 day 8 and 15 every 3 weeks **or**

400 mg/m^2 every 4 weeks for 3 cycles **or**

1 g/m^2 every 3 weeks **or**

1.5 g/m^2 every 4 weeks

Meningeal leukemia: I.T.: Usual dose: 12 mg/dose

Osteosarcoma: I.V.: 8-12 g/m^2 weekly for 2-4 weeks

Rheumatoid arthritis: **Note:** Some experts recommend concomitant folic acid at a dose of at least 5 mg/week (except the day of methotrexate) to reduce hematologic, gastrointestinal, and hepatic adverse events related to methotrexate.

Oral (manufacturer labeling): 7.5 mg once weekly or 2.5 mg every 12 hours for 3 doses/week (dosage exceeding 20 mg/week may cause a higher incidence and severity of adverse events); *alternatively,* 10-15 mg once weekly, increased by 5 mg every 2-4 weeks to a maximum of 20-30 mg once weekly has been recommended by some experts (Visser, 2009)

I.M., SubQ (unlabeled route): 15 mg once weekly (dosage varies, similar to oral) (Braun, 2008)

◀ Psoriasis: **Note:** Some experts recommend concomitant folic acid 1-5 mg/day (except the day of methotrexate) to reduce hematologic, gastrointestinal, and hepatic adverse events related to methotrexate.

Oral: 2.5-5 mg/dose every 12 hours for 3 doses given weekly **or**

Oral, I.M., SubQ: 10-25 mg/dose given once weekly; titrate to lowest effective dose

Note: An initial test dose of 2.5-5 mg is recommended in patients with risk factors for hematologic toxicity or renal impairment. (Kalb, 2009)

Bladder cancer (unlabeled use): I.V.:

30 mg/m^2 day 1 and 8 every 3 weeks **or**

30 mg/m^2 day 1, 15, and 22 every 4 weeks

Ectopic pregnancy (unlabeled use): I.M.:

Single-dose regimen: Methotrexate 50 mg/m^2 on day 1; Measure serum hCG levels on days 4 and 7; if needed, repeat dose on day 7 (Barnhart 2009)

Two-dose regimen: Methotrexate 50 mg/m^2 on day 1; Measure serum hCG levels on day 4 and administer a second dose of methotrexate 50 mg/m^2; Measure serum hCG levels on day 7 and if needed, administer a third dose of 50 mg/m^2 (Barnhart 2009)

Multidose regimen: Methotrexate 1 mg/kg on day 1; leucovorin 0.1 mg/kg I.M. on day 2; measure serum hCG on day 2; methotrexate 1mg/kg on day 3; leucovorin 0.1 mg/kg on day 4; measure serum hCG on day 4; continue up to a total of 4 courses based on hCG concentrations (Barnhart 2009)

Active Crohn's disease (unlabeled use): Induction of remission: I.M., SubQ: 15-25 mg once weekly; remission maintenance: 15 mg once weekly

Note: Oral dosing has been reported as effective but oral absorption is highly variable. If patient relapses after a switch to oral, may consider returning to injectable.

Nonleukemic meningeal cancer (unlabeled uses): I.T.: 10-12 mg/dose twice weekly for 4 weeks, then weekly for 4 weeks, then monthly (NCCN CNS cancer guidelines v.2.2009) **or** 12 mg/dose twice weekly for 4 weeks, then weekly for 4 doses, then monthly for 4 doses (Glantz, 1998) **or** 10 mg twice weekly for 4 weeks, then weekly for 1 month, then every 2 weeks for 2 months (Glantz, 1999)

Elderly: Rheumatoid arthritis/psoriasis: Oral: Initial: 5-7.5 mg/week, not to exceed 20 mg/week

Dosing adjustment in renal impairment: The FDA-approved labeling does not contain dosage adjustment guidelines. The following guidelines have been used by some clinicians:

Cl$_{cr}$ 61-80 mL/minute: Administer 75% of dose

Cl$_{cr}$ 51-60 mL/minute: Administer 70% of dose

Cl$_{cr}$ 10-50 mL/minute: Administer 30% to 50% of dose

Cl$_{cr}$ <10 mL/minute: Avoid use

Hemodialysis: Not dialyzable (0% to 5%); supplemental dose is not necessary

Peritoneal dialysis effects: Supplemental dose is not necessary

CAVH effects: Unknown

Aronoff, 2007:

Children:

Cl$_{cr}$ 10-50 mL/minute: Administer 50% of dose

Cl$_{cr}$ <10 mL/minute: Administer 30% of dose

Hemodialysis: Administer 30% of dose

Continuous ambulatory peritoneal dialysis (CAPD): Administer 30% of dose

Continuous renal replacement therapy (CRRT): Administer 50% of dose

Adults:

Cl$_{cr}$ 10-50 mL/minute: Administer 50% of dose

Cl$_{cr}$ <10 mL/minute: Avoid use

Hemodialysis: Administer 50% of dose

Continuous renal replacement therapy (CRRT): Administer 50% of dose

Kintzel, 1995:

Cl$_{cr}$ 46-60 mL/minute: Administer 65% of normal dose

Cl$_{cr}$ 31-45 mL/minute: Administer 50% of normal dose

Cl$_{cr}$ <30 mL/minute: Avoid use

Dosage adjustment in hepatic impairment: The FDA-approved labeling does not contain dosage adjustment guidelines. The following guidelines have been used by some clinicians (Floyd, 2006):

Bilirubin 3.1-5 mg/dL **or** transaminases >3 times ULN: Administer 75% of dose

Bilirubin >5 mg/dL: Avoid use

Additional Information Complete prescribing information for this medication should be consulted for additional detail.

Dosage Forms Excipient information presented when available (limited, particularly for generics); consult specific product labeling.

Injection, powder for reconstitution: 1 g

Injection, solution: 25 mg/mL (2 mL, 10 mL) [contains benzyl alcohol]

Injection, solution [preservative free]: 25 mg/mL (2 mL, 4 mL, 8 mL, 10 mL, 40 mL)

Tablet: 2.5 mg

Trexall™: 5 mg, 7.5 mg, 10 mg, 15 mg

Tablet [dose pack]: 2.5 mg (4 cards with 2, 3, 4, 5, or 6 tablets each)

Rheumatrex®: 2.5 mg (4 cards with 2, 3, 4, 5, or 6 tablets each)

◆ **Methotrexate Sodium** *see* Methotrexate *on page* 898

◆ **Methotrexatum** *see* Methotrexate *on page* 898

Methyldopa (meth il DOE pa)

Medication Safety Issues

Sound-alike/look-alike issues:

Methyldopa may be confused with L-dopa, levodopa

Related Information

Allergic Reactions *on page* 1508

Hypertension *on page* 1754

Canadian Brand Names Apo-Methyldopa®; Nu-Medopa

Index Terms Aldomet; Methyldopate Hydrochloride

Pharmacologic Category Alpha-Adrenergic Inhibitor; Alpha$_2$-Adrenergic Agonist

Generic Available Yes

Use Management of moderate-to-severe hypertension

Mechanism of Action Stimulation of central alpha-adrenergic receptors by a false transmitter that results in a decreased sympathetic outflow to the heart, kidneys, and peripheral vasculature

Pharmacodynamics/Kinetics

Onset of action: Peak effect: Hypotensive: Oral/parenteral: 3-6 hours

Duration: 12-24 hours

Distribution: Crosses placenta; enters breast milk

Protein binding: <15%

Metabolism: Intestinal and hepatic

Half-life elimination: 75-80 minutes; End-stage renal disease: 6-16 hours

Excretion: Urine (85% as metabolites) within 24 hours

Dosage

Children:

Oral: Initial: 10 mg/kg/day in 2-4 divided doses; increase every 2 days as needed to maximum dose of 65 mg/kg/day; do not exceed 3 g/day.

I.V.: 5-10 mg/kg/dose every 6-8 hours up to a total dose of 65 mg/kg/24 hours or 3 g/24 hours

Adults:

Oral: Initial: 250 mg 2-3 times/day; increase every 2 days as needed (maximum dose: 3 g/day): usual dose range (JNC 7): 250-1000 mg/day in 2 divided doses

I.V.: 250-500 mg every 6-8 hours; maximum dose: 1 g every 6 hours

Dosing interval in renal impairment:

Cl$_{cr}$ >50 mL/minute: Administer every 8 hours.

Cl$_{cr}$ 10-50 mL/minute: Administer every 8-12 hours.

Cl$_{cr}$ <10 mL/minute: Administer every 12-24 hours.

Hemodialysis: Slightly dialyzable (5% to 20%)

Stability Injectable dosage form is most stable at acid to neutral pH. Stability of parenteral admixture at room temperature (25°C) is 24 hours. Stability of parenteral admixture at refrigeration temperature (4°C) is 4 days.
Standard diluent: 250-500 mg/100 mL D_5W.

Administration When methyldopa is administered with antihypertensives other than thiazides, limit initial doses to 500 mg/day.

Monitoring Parameters Blood pressure, standing and sitting/lying down, CBC, liver enzymes, Coombs' test (direct); blood pressure monitor required during I.V. administration

Anesthesia and Critical Care Concerns/Other Considerations Most effective if used with diuretic. Titrate dose to optimal blood pressure control with minimal side effects. Patients on methyldopa may need less anesthetic agents. Hypotension readily responds to vasopressors because the adrenergic receptors remain sensitive.

It is used in the management of pregnancy-associated hypertension. Although the drug crosses the placenta and may cause hypotension, there is a large body of experience using this drug in the treatment of pregnancy-associated hypertension. Overall, the medication appears to be safe during pregnancy and lactation.

Pregnancy Risk Factor B

Contraindications Hypersensitivity to methyldopa or any component of the formulation; active hepatic disease; liver disorders previously associated with use of methyldopa; on MAO inhibitors; bisulfite allergy if using oral suspension or injectable

Warnings/Precautions May rarely produce hemolytic anemia and liver disorders; positive Coombs' test occurs in 10% to 20% of patients (perform periodic CBCs); sedation usually transient may occur during initial therapy or whenever the dose is increased. Use with caution in patients with previous liver disease or dysfunction, the active metabolites of methyldopa accumulate in uremia. Patients with impaired renal function may respond to smaller doses. Tolerance may occur usually between the second and third month of therapy. Adding a diuretic or increasing the dosage of methyldopa frequently restores blood pressure control. Elderly patients may experience syncope (avoid by giving smaller doses). Because of its CNS effects, methyldopa is not considered a drug of first choice in the elderly. Often considered the drug of choice for treatment of hypertension in pregnancy. Do not use injectable if bisulfite allergy.

Adverse Reactions
>10%: Cardiovascular: Peripheral edema
1% to 10%:
    Central nervous system: Drug fever, mental depression, anxiety, nightmares, drowsiness, headache
    Gastrointestinal: Dry mouth
<1% (Limited to important or life-threatening): Bradycardia (sinus), cholestasis or hepatitis and heptocellular injury, cirrhosis, dyspnea, gynecomastia, hemolytic anemia, hyperprolactinemia, increased liver enzymes, jaundice, leukopenia, orthostatic hypotension, positive Coombs' test, sexual dysfunction, SLE-like syndrome, sodium retention, thrombocytopenia, transient leukopenia or granulocytopenia

Drug Interactions

Avoid Concomitant Use
Avoid concomitant use of Methyldopa with any of the following: Iobenguane I 123; MAO Inhibitors

Increased Effect/Toxicity
Methyldopa may increase the levels/effects of: Lithium

The levels/effects of Methyldopa may be increased by: COMT Inhibitors; MAO Inhibitors

Decreased Effect
Methyldopa may decrease the levels/effects of: Iobenguane I 123

The levels/effects of Methyldopa may be decreased by: Iron Salts

Ethanol/Nutrition/Herb Interactions Herb/Nutraceutical: Avoid dong quai if using for hypertension (has estrogenic activity). Avoid ephedra, yohimbe, ginseng (may worsen hypertension). Avoid valerian, St John's wort, kava kava, gotu kola (may increase CNS depression). Avoid natural licorice (causes sodium and water retention and increases potassium loss). Avoid garlic (may have increased antihypertensive effect).

Test Interactions Methyldopa interferes with the following laboratory tests: urinary uric acid, serum creatinine (alkaline picrate method), AST (colorimetric method), and urinary catecholamines (falsely high levels)

Dietary Considerations Dietary requirements for vitamin B_{12} and folate may be increased with high doses of methyldopa.

Dosage Forms Excipient information presented when available (limited, particularly for generics); consult specific product labeling.

Injection, solution, as methyldopa hydrochloride: 50 mg/mL (5 mL) [contains sodium bisulfite]

Tablet: 250 mg, 500 mg

◆ **Methyldopate Hydrochloride** *see* Methyldopa *on page 901*

Methylene Blue (METH i leen bloo)

Medication Safety Issues Due to potential toxicity (hemolytic anemia), do not use methylene blue to color enteral feedings to detect aspiration.

Pharmacologic Category Antidote

Generic Available Yes

Use Antidote for cyanide poisoning and drug-induced methemoglobinemia, indicator dye

Unlabeled/Investigational Use Treatment/prevention of ifosfamide-induced encephalopathy; topically, in conjunction with polychromatic light to photo-inactivate viruses such as herpes simplex; alone or in combination with vitamin C for the management of chronic urolithiasis

Mechanism of Action Weak germicide in low concentrations, hastens the conversion of methemoglobin to hemoglobin; has opposite effect at high concentrations by converting ferrous ion of reduced hemoglobin to ferric ion to form methemoglobin; in cyanide toxicity, it combines with cyanide to form cyanmethemoglobin preventing the interference of cyanide with the cytochrome system

Pharmacodynamics/Kinetics

Onset of action: Reduction of methemoglobin: I.V.: 30-60 minutes

Absorption: Oral: 53% to 97%

Excretion: Urine and feces

Dosage

Children and Adults: Methemoglobinemia: I.V.: 1-2 mg/kg or 25-50 mg/m^2 over several minutes; may be repeated in 1 hour if necessary

Adults: Ifosfamide-induced encephalopathy (unlabeled use): **Note:** Treatment may not be necessary; encephalopathy may improve spontaneously: I.V.:

Prevention: 50 mg every 6-8 hours

Treatment: 50 mg as a single dose or every 4-8 hours until symptoms resolve

Administration I.V.: Administer undiluted by direct I.V. injection over several minutes. For the treatment of ifosfamide-induced encephalopathy, methylene blue may be administered either undiluted as a slow I.V. push over at least 5 minutes or diluted in 50 mL NS or D_5W and infused over at least 5 minutes. Consider concomitant dextrose administration, especially in patients who are hypoglycemic, to ensure efficacy of methylene blue.

Monitoring Parameters Arterial blood gases; cardiac monitoring (patients with pre-existing pulmonary and/or cardiac disease); CBC; methemoglobin levels (co-oximetry yields a direct and accurate measure of methemoglobin levels); pulse oximeter (will not provide accurate measurement of oxygenation when methemoglobin levels are >35%); renal function; signs and symptoms of methemoglobinemia such as pallor, cyanosis, nausea, muscle weakness, dizziness, confusion, agitation, dyspnea and tachycardia; transcutaneous O_2 saturation

Reference Range Methemoglobin levels: **Note:** The level of methemoglobin is expressed as a percent of total hemoglobin affected.

10% to 25%: Cyanosis

35% to 40%: Fatigue, dizziness, dyspnea, headache, tachycardia

60%: Lethargy, stupor
>70%: Death (adults)

Pregnancy Risk Factor C

Contraindications Hypersensitivity to methylene blue or any component of the formulation; intraspinal injection; renal insufficiency

Warnings/Precautions Do not inject SubQ or intrathecally; use with caution in young patients and in patients with G6PD deficiency; continued use can cause profound anemia. At high doses or in patients with G6PD-deficiency and infants, methylene blue may catalyze the oxidation of ferrous iron in hemoglobin to ferric iron causing paradoxical methemoglobinemia; monitor methemoglobin concentrations regularly during administration. Methylene blue should not be added to enteral feeding products (Durfee, 2006; Wessel, 2005); safety and efficacy have not been established.

Adverse Reactions Frequency not defined.
Cardiovascular: Hypertension, precordial pain
Central nervous system: Dizziness, mental confusion, headache, fever
Dermatologic: Staining of skin
Gastrointestinal: Fecal discoloration (blue-green), nausea, vomiting, abdominal pain
Genitourinary: Discoloration of urine (blue-green), bladder irritation
Hematologic: Anemia
Miscellaneous: Diaphoresis

Drug Interactions

Avoid Concomitant Use There are no known interactions where it is recommended to avoid concomitant use.

Increased Effect/Toxicity There are no known significant interactions involving an increase in effect.

Decreased Effect There are no known significant interactions involving a decrease in effect.

Dosage Forms Excipient information presented when available (limited, particularly for generics); consult specific product labeling.
Injection, solution: 10 mg/mL (1 mL, 10 mL)

♦ **Methylergometrine Maleate** see Methylergonovine on page 904

Methylergonovine (meth il er goe NOE veen)

Medication Safety Issues
Sound-alike/look-alike issues:
Methergine® may be confused with Brethine
Methylergonovine and terbutaline parenteral dosage forms look similar. Due to their contrasting indications, use care when administering these agents.

U.S. Brand Names Methergine®

Canadian Brand Names Methergine®

Index Terms Methylergometrine Maleate; Methylergonovine Maleate

Pharmacologic Category Ergot Derivative

Generic Available No

Use Prevention and treatment of postpartum and postabortion hemorrhage caused by uterine atony or subinvolution

Mechanism of Action Similar smooth muscle actions as seen with ergotamine; however, it affects primarily uterine smooth muscles producing sustained contractions and thereby shortens the third stage of labor and reduces blood loss.

Pharmacodynamics/Kinetics
Onset of action: Oxytocic: Oral: 5-10 minutes; I.M.: 2-5 minutes; I.V.: Immediately
Duration: Oral: ~3 hours; I.M.: ~3 hours; I.V.: 45 minutes
Absorption: Rapid
Distribution: V_d: 39-73 L
Rapid; primarily to plasma and extracellular fluid following I.V. administration; tissues
Metabolism: Hepatic
Bioavailability: Oral: 60%; I.M.: 78%

Half-life elimination: Biphasic: Initial: 1-5 minutes; Terminal: 0.5-2 hours
Time to peak, serum: Oral: 0.3-2 hours; I.M.: 0.2-0.6 hours
Excretion: Urine and feces

Dosage Adults:

Oral: 0.2 mg 3-4 times/day in the puerperium for 2-7 days

I.M., I.V.: 0.2 mg after delivery of anterior shoulder, after delivery of placenta, or during puerperium; may be repeated as required at intervals of 2-4 hours

Stability

Ampul: Store under refrigeration at 2°C to 8°C (36°F to 46°F). Protect from light.
Tablet: Store below 25°C (77°F).

Administration Administer over ≥60 seconds. Should not be routinely administered I.V. because of possibility of inducing sudden hypertension and cerebrovascular accident.

Anesthesia and Critical Care Concerns/Other Considerations

Clinical Pearls/Comments: This drug should be used with extreme caution because of potent vasoconstrictor action; I.V. use may induce sudden hypertension and cerebrovascular accidents and therefore should be administered by this route as a last resort. If administered I.V., must be given slowly over several minutes and blood pressure monitored closely.

Pregnancy Risk Factor C

Contraindications Hypersensitivity to methylergonovine or any component of the formulation; ergot alkaloids are contraindicated with potent inhibitors of CYP3A4 (includes protease inhibitors, azole antifungals, and some macrolide antibiotics); hypertension; toxemia; pregnancy

Warnings/Precautions Use caution in patients with sepsis, obliterative vascular disease, cardiovascular disease, hepatic or renal involvement, or second stage of labor; administer with extreme caution if using intravenously. Pleural and peritoneal fibrosis have been reported with prolonged daily use of other ergot alkaloids. Cardiac valvular fibrosis has also been associated with ergot alkaloids. Ergot alkaloid use may result in ergotism (intense vasoconstriction) resulting in peripheral vascular ischemia and possible gangrene. Concomitant use with potent inhibitors of CYP3A4 (includes protease inhibitors, azole antifungals, and some macrolide antibiotics) and ergot alkaloids has been associated with acute ergot toxicity (ergotism); concurrent use of certain ergot alkaloids (eg, ergotamine and dihydroergotamine) are not recommended by the manufacturer. Use with caution in the elderly. Safety and efficacy have not been established in children.

Adverse Reactions Frequency not defined.

Cardiovascular: Acute MI, arterial spasm, bradycardia, hyper-/hypotension, palpitation, tachycardia, temporary chest pain

Central nervous system: Dizziness, hallucinations, headache, seizure

Dermatologic: Rash

Endocrine & metabolic: Water intoxication

Gastrointestinal: Diarrhea, foul taste, nausea, vomiting

Local: Thrombophlebitis

Neuromuscular & skeletal: Leg cramps

Otic: Tinnitus

Renal: Hematuria

Respiratory: Dyspnea, nasal congestion

Miscellaneous: Anaphylaxis, diaphoresis

Drug Interactions

Metabolism/Transport Effects Substrate of CYP3A4 (major)

Avoid Concomitant Use

Avoid concomitant use of Methylergonovine with any of the following: Efavirenz; Itraconazole; Posaconazole; Protease Inhibitors; Serotonin 5-HT1D Receptor Agonists; Sibutramine; Voriconazole

Increased Effect/Toxicity

Methylergonovine may increase the levels/effects of: Serotonin 5-HT1D Receptor Agonists; Serotonin Modulators

The levels/effects of Methylergonovine may be increased by: CYP3A4 Inhibitors (Moderate); CYP3A4 Inhibitors (Strong); Dasatinib; Efavirenz; Itraconazole; Macrolide Antibiotics; Posaconazole; Protease Inhibitors; Serotonin 5-HT1D Receptor Agonists; Sibutramine; Voriconazole

◀ **Decreased Effect** There are no known significant interactions involving a decrease in effect.

Dosage Forms Excipient information presented when available (limited, particularly for generics); consult specific product labeling.

Injection, solution, as maleate: 0.2 mg/mL (1 mL)

Methergine®: 0.2 mg/mL (1 mL)

Tablet, as maleate:

Methergine®: 0.2 mg

◆ **Methylergonovine Maleate** *see* Methylergonovine *on page 904*

Methylfolate (meth il FO late)

U.S. Brand Names Deplin™

Index Terms 6(S)-5-methyltetrahydrofolate; 6(S)-5-MTHF; L-methylfolate

Pharmacologic Category Dietary Supplement

Use Medicinal food for management of patients with low plasma and/or low red blood cell folate

Dosage Oral: Adults: One tablet (7.5 mg) daily

Additional Information Information in this monograph is currently limited to the fields presented. Consult product labeling for additional details.

The manufacturer of Deplin™ indicates a use of methylfolate in individuals who have a major depressive disorder that has not fully responded or may not fully respond to antidepressant therapy. Limited data exists of the investigational use of folate supplementation as an adjunct to the treatment of major depressive disorder. Adjunctive use in major depressive disorders requires further studies, but some studies (using various forms of folic acid) suggest a possible benefit of supplementation by augmentation of response to antidepressants, particularly in patients with low serum folate levels prior to supplementation.

Dosage Forms Excipient information presented when available (limited, particularly for generics); consult specific product labeling.

Tablet:

Deplin™: L-methylfolate 7.5 mg [gluten free, lactose free, sugar free, yeast free]

References

Alpert JE, Mischoulon D, Rubenstein GE, et al, "Folinic Acid (Leucovorin) as an Adjunctive Treatment for SSRI-Refractory Depression," *Ann Clin Psychiatry*, 2002, 14(1):33-8.

Coppen A and Bailey J, "Enhancement of the Antidepressant Action of Fluoxetine by Folic Acid: A Randomised, Placebo Controlled Trial," *J Affect Disord*, 2000, 60(2):121-30.

Papakostas GI, Petersen T, Mischoulon D, et al, "Serum Folate, Vitamin B_{12}, and Homocysteine in Major Depressive Disorder, Part 1: Predictors of Clinical Response in Fluoxetine-Resistant Depression," *J Clin Psychiatry*, 2004, 65(8):1090-5.

Papakostas GI, Petersen T, Mischoulon D, et al, "Serum Folate, Vitamin B_{12}, and Homocysteine in Major Depressive Disorder, Part 1: Predictors of Clinical Response in Fluoxetine-Resistant Depression," *J Clin Psychiatry*, 2004, 65(8):1096-8.

◆ **Methylin®** *see* Methylphenidate *on page 908*

◆ **Methylin® ER** *see* Methylphenidate *on page 908*

◆ **Methylmorphine** *see* Codeine *on page 340*

Methylnaltrexone (meth il nal TREKS one)

Medication Safety Issues

Sound-alike/look-alike issues:

Methylnaltrexone may be confused with naltrexone

U.S. Brand Names Relistor™

Canadian Brand Names Relistor™

Index Terms Methylnaltrexone Bromide; N-methylnaltrexone Bromide

Pharmacologic Category Gastrointestinal Agent, Miscellaneous; Opioid Antagonist, Peripherally-Acting

Generic Available No

Use Treatment of opioid-induced constipation in patients with advanced illness receiving palliative care with inadequate response to conventional laxative regimens

Mechanism of Action An opioid receptor antagonist which blocks opioid binding at the mu receptor, methylnaltrexone is a quaternary derivative of naltrexone with ability to cross the blood-brain barrier restricted. It therefore functions as a peripheral acting opioid antagonist, including actions on the gastrointestinal tract to inhibit opioid-induced decreased gastrointestinal motility and delay in gastrointestinal transit time, decreasing opioid-induced constipation. Does not affect opioid analgesic effects or induce opioid withdrawal symptoms.

Pharmacodynamics/Kinetics

Onset of action: Usually within 30-60 minutes (in responding patients)

Absorption: SubQ: Rapid

Distribution: V_{ss}: 1.1 L/kg

Protein binding: 11% to 15%

Metabolism: Metabolized to methyl-6-naltrexol isomers, methylnaltrexone sulfate. and other minor metabolites

Half-life elimination: Terminal: ~8 hours

Time to peak, plasma: SubQ: 30 minutes

Excretion: Urine (~50%, primarily as unchanged drug); feces (<50%, primarily as unchanged drug)

Dosage SubQ: Adults: Opioid-induced constipation: Dosing is according to body weight: Administer 1 dose every other day as needed; maximum: 1 dose/24 hours

<38 kg: 0.15 mg/kg (round dose up to nearest 0.1 mL of volume)

38 to <62 kg: 8 mg

62-114 kg: 12 mg

>114 kg: 0.15 mg/kg (round dose up to nearest 0.1 mL of volume)

Dosage adjustment in renal impairment:

Mild-to-moderate renal impairment: No adjustment required

Severe renal impairment (Cl_{cr} <30 mL/minute): Administer 50% of normal dose

End-stage renal impairment (dialysis-dependent): Has not been studied

Dosage adjustment in hepatic impairment:

Mild-to-moderate hepatic impairment (Child-Pugh class A and B): No adjustment required

Severe hepatic impairment: Has not been studied

Stability Store intact vials at room temperature of 20°C to 25°C (68°F to 77°F); excursions permitted to 15°C to 30°C (59°F to 86°F); do not freeze. Protect from light. Solution for injection is stable in a syringe for 24 hours at room temperature (protection from light during this 24 hours is not necessary).

Administration SubQ: Administer subcutaneously into upper arm, abdomen, or thigh. Rotate injection site. Do not use tender, bruised, red, or hard areas.

Pregnancy Risk Factor B

Contraindications Known or suspected mechanical bowel obstruction

Warnings/Precautions Discontinue treatment for severe or persistent diarrhea. Use with caution in patients with renal impairment; dosage adjustment recommended for severe renal impairment (Cl_{cr} <30 mL/minute). Has not been studied in patients with end-stage renal impairment requiring dialysis. Discontinue methylnaltrexone if opioids are discontinued. Use has not been studied in patients with peritoneal catheters. Use beyond 4 months has not been studied. Safety and efficacy have not been established in children.

Adverse Reactions

>10%: Gastrointestinal: Abdominal pain (29%), flatulence (13%), nausea (12%)

1% to 10%:

Central nervous system: Dizziness (7%)

Gastrointestinal: Diarrhea (6%)

<1% (Limited to important or life-threatening): Abdominal cramps, body temperature increased, muscle spasm, syncope

Drug Interactions

Metabolism/Transport Effects Inhibits CYP2D6 (weak)

Avoid Concomitant Use There are no known interactions where it is recommended to avoid concomitant use.

Increased Effect/Toxicity There are no known significant interactions involving an increase in effect.

◄ **Decreased Effect**
The levels/effects of Methylnaltrexone may be decreased by: Peginterferon Alfa-2b

Dosage Forms Excipient information presented when available (limited, particularly for generics); consult specific product labeling.

Injection, solution:

Relistor™: 12 mg/0.6 mL (0.6 mL) [contains edetate calcium disodium]

References

Portenoy RK, Thomas J, Moehl Boatwright ML, et al, "Subcutaneous Methylnaltrexone for the Treatment of Opioid-Induced Constipation in Patients With Advanced Illness: A Double-Blind Randomized, Parallel Group, Dose-Ranging Study," *J Pain Symptom Manage*, 2008, 35(5):458-68.

Thomas H, "Opioid-Induced Bowel Dysfunction," *J Pain Symptom Manage*, 2008, 35(1):103-13.

Yuan CS, "Methylnaltrexone Mechanisms of Action and Effects on Opioid Bowel Dysfunction and Other Opioid Adverse Effects," *Ann Pharmacother*, 2007, 41(6):984-93.

◆ **Methylnaltrexone Bromide** *see* Methylnaltrexone *on page 906*

Methylphenidate (meth il FEN i date)

U.S. Brand Names Concerta®; Daytrana™; Metadate CD®; Metadate® ER; Methylin®; Methylin® ER; Ritalin LA®; Ritalin-SR®; Ritalin®

Canadian Brand Names Apo-Methylphenidate®; Apo-Methylphenidate® SR; Biphentin®; Concerta®; PHL-Methylphenidate; PMS-Methylphenidate; ratio-Methylphenidate; Ritalin®; Ritalin® SR; Sandoz® Methylphenidate SR

Index Terms Methylphenidate Hydrochloride

Pharmacologic Category Central Nervous System Stimulant

Restrictions C-II

Use Treatment of attention-deficit/hyperactivity disorder (ADHD); symptomatic management of narcolepsy

Unlabeled/Investigational Use Depression (especially elderly or medically ill)

Pharmacodynamics/Kinetics

Onset of action: Peak effect:

Immediate release tablet: Cerebral stimulation: ~2 hours

Extended release capsule (Metadate CD®): Biphasic; initial peak similar to immediate release product, followed by second rising portion (corresponding to extended release portion)

Sustained release tablet: 4-7 hours

Osmotic release tablet (Concerta®): Initial: 1-2 hours

Transdermal: ~2 hours; may be expedited by the application of external heat

Duration: Immediate release tablet: 3-6 hours; Sustained release tablet: 8 hours; Extended release tablet: Methylin® ER, Metadate® ER: 8 hours, Concerta®: 12 hours

Absorption:

Oral: Readily absorbed

Transdermal: Absorption increased when applied to inflamed skin or exposed to heat. Absorption is continuous for 9 hours after application.

Metabolism: Hepatic via de-esterification to minimally active metabolite

Half-life elimination: *d*-methylphenidate: 3-4 hours; *l*-methylphenidate: 1-3 hours

Time to peak: Concerta®: C_{max}: 6-8 hours; Daytrana™: 7.5-10.5 hours

Excretion: Urine (90% as metabolites and unchanged drug)

Dosage

ADHD:

Oral:

Immediate release products Children ≥6 years and Adults: Initial: 5 mg/dose (~0.3 mg/kg/dose) given twice daily before breakfast and lunch; increase by 5-10 mg/day (0.2 mg/kg/day) at weekly intervals; maximum dose: 60 mg/day (2 mg/kg/day). **Note:** Discontinue periodically to re-evaluate or if no improvement occurs within 1 month.

Extended release products

Children ≥6 years and Adults:

Metadate® ER, Methylin® ER, Ritalin® SR: May be given in place of immediate release products, once the daily dose is titrated and the titrated 8-hour dosage corresponds to sustained or extended release tablet size; maximum: 60 mg/day

Metadate CD®, Ritalin LA®: Initial: 20 mg once daily; may be adjusted in 10-20 mg increments at weekly intervals; maximum: 60 mg/day

Children 6-12 years and Adolescents 13-17 years: *Concerta®:*

Patients not currently taking methylphenidate: Initial dose: 18 mg once daily in the morning

Patients currently taking methylphenidate: **Note:** Initial dose: Dosing based on current regimen and clinical judgment; suggested dosing listed below:
- Patients taking methylphenidate 5 mg 2-3 times/day: 18 mg once every morning
- Patients taking methylphenidate 10 mg 2-3 times/day: 36 mg once every morning
- Patients taking methylphenidate 15 mg 2-3 times/day: 54 mg once every morning

Dose adjustment: May increase dose in increments of 18 mg; dose may be adjusted at weekly intervals. A dosage strength of 27 mg is available for situations in which a dosage between 18-36 mg is desired. Maximum dose should not exceed 2 mg/kg/day **or** 54 mg/day in children 6-12 years or 72 mg/day in children 13-17 years.

Adults: *Concerta®:*

Patients not currently taking methylphenidate: Initial dose: 18-36 mg once daily in the morning

Patients currently taking methylphenidate: **Note:** Initial dose: Dosing based on current regimen and clinical judgment; suggested dosing listed below:
- Patients taking methylphenidate 5 mg 2-3 times/day: 18 mg once every morning
- Patients taking methylphenidate 10 mg 2-3 times/day: 36 mg once every morning
- Patients taking methylphenidate 15 mg 2-3 times/day: 54 mg once every morning
- Patients taking methylphenidate 20 mg 2-3 times/day: 72 mg once every morning

Dose adjustment: May increase dose in increments of 18 mg; dose may be adjusted at weekly intervals. A dosage strength of 27 mg is available for situations in which a dosage between 18-36 mg is desired. Maximum dose should not exceed 72 mg/day.

Transdermal (Daytrana™): Children ≥6 years: Initial: 10 mg patch once daily; remove up to 9 hours after application. Titrate based on response and tolerability; may increase to next transdermal dose no more frequently than every week. **Note:** Application should occur 2 hours prior to desired effect. Drug absorption may continue for a period of time after patch removal; patients converting from another formulation of methylphenidate should be initiated at 10 mg regardless of their previous dose and titrated as needed due to the differences in bioavailability of the transdermal formulation.

Narcolepsy: Oral: Adults: 10 mg 2-3 times/day, up to 60 mg/day

Depression (unlabeled use): Oral: Adults: Initial: 2.5 mg every morning before 9 AM; dosage may be increased by 2.5-5 mg every 2-3 days as tolerated to a maximum of 20 mg/day; may be divided (ie, 7 AM and 12 noon), but should not be given after noon; do not use sustained release product

Additional Information Complete prescribing information for this medication should be consulted for additional detail.

Dosage Forms Excipient information presented when available (limited, particularly for generics); consult specific product labeling. [DSC] = Discontinued product

Capsule, extended release, oral, as hydrochloride [bi-modal release]:

Metadate CD®: 10 mg [contains sucrose; 3 mg immediate release, 7 mg extended release]

Metadate CD®: 20 mg [contains sucrose; 6 mg immediate release, 14 mg extended release]

Metadate CD®: 30 mg [contains sucrose; 9 mg immediate release, 21 mg extended release]

Metadate CD®: 40 mg [contains sucrose; 12 mg immediate release, 28 mg extended release]

Metadate CD®: 50 mg [contains sucrose; 15 mg immediate release, 35 mg extended release]

Metadate CD®: 60 mg [contains sucrose; 18 mg immediate release, 42 mg extended release]

Ritalin LA®: 10 mg [5 mg immediate release, 5 mg extended release]

Ritalin LA®: 20 mg [10 mg immediate release, 10 mg extended release]

Ritalin LA®: 30 mg [15 mg immediate release, 15 mg extended release]

Ritalin LA®: 40 mg [20 mg immediate release, 20 mg extended release]

Solution, oral, as hydrochloride:

Methylin®: 5 mg/5 mL (500 mL) [grape flavor]; 10 mg/5 mL (500 mL) [grape flavor]

Tablet, as hydrochloride: 5 mg, 10 mg, 20 mg

Methylin®, Ritalin®: 5 mg, 10 mg, 20 mg

Tablet, chewable, as hydrochloride:

Methylin®: 2.5 mg [contains phenylalanine 0.42 mg/tablet; grape flavor]; 5 mg [contains phenylalanine 0.84 mg/tablet; grape flavor]; 10 mg [scored; contains phenylalanine 1.68 mg/tablet; grape flavor]

Tablet, extended release, as hydrochloride: 20 mg [DSC]

Metadate® ER: 10 mg [contains lactose] [DSC]; 20 mg [contains lactose]

Methylin® ER: 10 mg, 20 mg

Tablet, extended release, as hydrochloride [bi-modal release]:

Concerta®: 18 mg [4 mg immediate release, 14 mg extended release]

Concerta®: 27 mg [6 mg immediate release, 21 mg extended release]

Concerta®: 36 mg [8 mg immediate release, 28 mg extended release]

Concerta®: 54 mg [12 mg immediate release, 42 mg extended release]

Tablet, sustained release, as hydrochloride: 20 mg

Ritalin-SR®: 20 mg [dye free]

Transdermal system [once-daily patch]:

Daytrana™: 10 mg/9 hours (10s [DSC], 30s) [12.5 cm^2, total methylphenidate 27.5 mg]

Daytrana™: 15 mg/9 hours (10s [DSC], 30s) [18.75 cm^2, total methylphenidate 41.3 mg]

Daytrana™: 20 mg/9 hours (10s [DSC], 30s) [25 cm^2, total methylphenidate 55 mg]

Daytrana™: 30 mg/9 hours (10s [DSC], 30s) [37.5 cm^2, total methylphenidate 82.5 mg]

References

Berkovitch M, Pope E, Phillips J, et al, "Pemoline-Associated Fulminant Liver Failure: Testing the Evidence for Causation," *Clin Pharmacol Ther*, 1995, 57(6):696-8.

Bond WS, "Recognition and Treatment of Attention Deficit Disorder," *Clin Pharm*, 1987, 6(8):617-24.

Emptage RE and Semla TP, "Depression in the Medically Ill Elderly: A Focus on Methylphenidate," *Ann Pharmacother*, 1996, 30(2):151-7.

Friberg TR, Gragoudas ES, and Regan CD, "Talc Emboli and Macular Ischemia in Intravenous Drug Abuse," *Arch Ophthalmol*, 1979, 97(6):1089-91.

Greenhill LL, "Pharmacologic Treatment of Attention Deficit Hyperactivity Disorder," *Psychiatr Clin North Am*, 1992, 15(1):1-27.

Gurian B and Rosowsky E, "Low-Dose Methylphenidate in the Very Old," *J Geriatr Psychiatry Neurol*, 1990, 3(3):152-4.

Hackett LP, Kristensen JH, Hale TW, et al, "Methylphenidate and Breast-Feeding," *Ann Pharmacother*, 2006, 40(10):1890-1.

Katon W and Raskind M, "Treatment of Depression in the Medically Ill Elderly With Methylphenidate," *Am J Psychiatry*, 1980, 137:963-5.

Kelly DP and Aylward GP, "Attention Deficits in School-Aged Children and Adolescents," *Pediatr Clin North Am*, 1992, 39(3):487-512.

Lazarus LW, Moberg PJ, Langsley PR, et al, "Methylphenidate and Nortriptyline in the Treatment of Poststroke Depression: A Retrospective Comparison," *Arch Phys Med Rehabil*, 1994, 75(4):403-6.

Modi NB, Lindemulder B, and Gupta SK, " Single- and Multiple-Dose Pharmacokinetics of an Oral Once-a-day Osmotic Controlled-release OROS (Methylphenidate HCl) Formulation," *J Clin Pharmacol*, 2000, 40(4):379-88.

Nissen SE, "ADHD and Cardiovascular Risk," *N Engl J Med*, 2006, 354:1445-8.

Parran TV Jr and Jasinski DR, "Intravenous Methylphenidate Abuse: Prototype for Prescription Drug Abuse," *Arch Intern Med*, 1991, 151(4):781-3.

Pleak RR, "Adverse Effects of Chewing Methylphenidate," *Am J Psychiatry*, 1995, 152(5):811.

Shaywitz SE and Shaywitz BA, "Diagnosis and Management of Attention Deficit Disorder: A Pediatric Perspective," *Pediatr Clin North Am*, 1984, 31(2):429-57.

Stecyk O, Loludice TA, Demeter S, et al, "Multiple Organ Failure Resulting From Intravenous Abuse of Methylphenidate Hydrochloride," *Ann Emerg Med*, 1985, 14(6):597-9.

Wallace AE, Kofoed LL and West AN, "Double-Blind, Placebo-Controlled Trial of Methylphenidate in Older, Depressed, Medically Ill Patients," *Am J Psychiatry*, 1995, 152(6):929-31.

Warden C and Winger J, "Choreoathetoid Reaction Associated With a Methylphenidate Ingestion in a Toddler," *Clin Toxicol*, 1995, 33(5):522.

Weiss MD and Weiss JR, "A Guide to the Treatment of Adults With ADHD," *J Clin Psychiatry*, 2004, 65(Suppl 3):27-37.

Wilens TE and Biederman J, "The Stimulants," *Psychiatr Clin North Am*, 1992, 15(1):191-222.

◆ **Methylphenidate Hydrochloride** *see* Methylphenidate *on page 908*

◆ **Methylphenoxy-Benzene Propanamine** *see* Atomoxetine *on page 157*

◆ **Methylphytyl Napthoquinone** *see* Phytonadione *on page 1128*

MethylPREDNISolone (meth il pred NIS oh lone)

Medication Safety Issues
Sound-alike/look-alike issues:

MethylPREDNISolone may be confused with medroxyPROGESTERone, methotrexate, predniSONE

Depo-Medrol® may be confused with Solu-Medrol®

Medrol® may be confused with Mebaral®

Solu-Medrol® may be confused with Depo-Medrol®, salmeterol, Solu-Cortef®

International issues:

Medor® may be confused with Medral® which is a brand name for omeprazole in Mexico

Related Information
Allergic Reactions *on page 1508*

Contrast Media Reactions, Premedication for Prophylaxis *on page 1735*

Corticosteroids *on page 1676*

Desensitization Protocols *on page 1692*

Stress Replacement of Corticosteroids *on page 1611*

U.S. Brand Names A-Methapred®; Depo-Medrol®; Medrol®; Solu-Medrol®

Canadian Brand Names Depo-Medrol®; Medrol®; Methylprednisolone Acetate; Solu-Medrol®

Index Terms 6-α-Methylprednisolone; A-Methapred; Medrol Dose Pack; Methylprednisolone Acetate; Methylprednisolone Sodium Succinate; Solumedrol

Pharmacologic Category Corticosteroid, Systemic

Generic Available Yes

Use Primarily as an anti-inflammatory or immunosuppressant agent in the treatment of a variety of diseases including those of hematologic, allergic, inflammatory, neoplastic, and autoimmune origin. Prevention and treatment of graft-versus-host disease following allogeneic bone marrow transplantation.

Mechanism of Action In a tissue-specific manner, corticosteroids regulate gene expression subsequent to binding specific intracellular receptors and translocation into the nucleus. Corticosteroids exert a wide array of physiologic effects including modulation of carbohydrate, protein, and lipid metabolism and maintenance of fluid and electrolyte homeostasis. Moreover cardiovascular, immunologic, musculoskeletal, endocrine, and neurologic physiology are influenced by corticosteroids. Decreases inflammation by suppression of migration of polymorphonuclear leukocytes and reversal of increased capillary permeability.

Pharmacodynamics/Kinetics
Onset of action: Peak effect (route dependent): Oral: 1-2 hours; I.M.: 4-8 days; Intra-articular: 1 week; methylprednisolone sodium succinate is highly soluble and has a rapid effect by I.M. and I.V. routes

Duration (route dependent): Oral: 30-36 hours; I.M.: 1-4 weeks; Intra-articular: 1-5 weeks; methylprednisolone acetate has a low solubility and has a sustained I.M. effect

Distribution: V_d: 0.7-1.5 L/kg

Half-life elimination: 3-3.5 hours; reduced in obese

Excretion: Clearance: Reduced in obese

Dosage Dosing should be based on the lesser of ideal body weight or actual body weight

Only sodium succinate may be given I.V.; methylprednisolone sodium succinate is highly soluble and has a rapid effect by I.M. and I.V. routes. Methylprednisolone acetate has a low solubility and has a sustained I.M. effect.

◀ Children:

Acute spinal cord injury: I.V. (sodium succinate): 30 mg/kg over 15 minutes, followed in 45 minutes by a continuous infusion of 5.4 mg/kg/hour for 23 hours

Anti-inflammatory or immunosuppressive: Oral, I.M., I.V. (sodium succinate): 0.5-1.7 mg/kg/day **or** 5-25 mg/m^2/day in divided doses every 6-12 hours; "Pulse" therapy: 15-30 mg/kg/dose over ≥30 minutes given once daily for 3 days

Asthma exacerbations, including status asthmaticus (emergency medical care or hospital doses) (NIH Asthma Guidelines, NAEPP, 2007): Children <12 years: Oral, I.V.: 1-2 mg/kg/day in 2 divided doses (maximum: 60 mg/day) until peak expiratory flow is 70% of predicted or personal best

Lupus nephritis: I.V. (sodium succinate): 30 mg/kg over ≥30 minutes every other day for 6 doses

Status asthmaticus: I.V. (sodium succinate): Previous NAEPP guidelines still encountered in clinical practice: Loading dose: 2 mg/kg/dose, then 0.5-1 mg/kg/dose every 6 hours for up to 5 days; **Note:** See new dosing guidelines for asthma exacerbations.

Adults: **Only sodium succinate may be given I.V.;** methylprednisolone sodium succinate is highly soluble and has a rapid effect by I.M. and I.V. routes. Methylprednisolone acetate has a low solubility and has a sustained I.M. effect.

Acute spinal cord injury: I.V. (sodium succinate): 30 mg/kg over 15 minutes, followed in 45 minutes by a continuous infusion of 5.4 mg/kg/hour for 23 hours

Allergic conditions: Oral: Tapered-dosage schedule:

Day 1: 24 mg on day 1 administered as 8 mg before breakfast, 4 mg after lunch, 4 mg after supper, and 8 mg at bedtime **OR** 24 mg as a single dose or divided into 2 or 3 doses upon initiation (regardless of time of day)

Day 2: 20 mg on day 2 administered as 4 mg before breakfast, 4 mg after lunch, 4 mg after supper, and 8 mg at bedtime

Day 3: 16 mg on day 3 administered as 4 mg before breakfast, 4 mg after lunch, 4 mg after supper, and 4 mg at bedtime

Day 4: 12 mg on day 4 administered as 4 mg before breakfast, 4 mg after lunch, and 4 mg at bedtime

Day 5: 8 mg on day 5 administered as 4 mg before breakfast and 4 mg at bedtime

Day 6: 4 mg on day 6 administered as 4 mg before breakfast

Anti-inflammatory or immunosuppressive:

Oral: 2-60 mg/day in 1-4 divided doses to start, followed by gradual reduction in dosage to the lowest possible level consistent with maintaining an adequate clinical response.

I.M. (sodium succinate): 10-80 mg/day once daily

I.M. (acetate): 10-80 mg every 1-2 weeks

I.V. (sodium succinate): 10-40 mg over a period of several minutes and repeated I.V. or I.M. at intervals depending on clinical response; when high dosages are needed, give 30 mg/kg over a period ≥30 minutes and may be repeated every 4-6 hours for 48 hours.

Dermatitis, acute severe: I.M. (acetate): 80-120 mg as a single dose

Dermatitis, chronic: I.M. (acetate): 40-120 mg every 5-10 days

Status asthmaticus: I.V. (sodium succinate): Loading dose: 2 mg/kg/dose, then 0.5-1 mg/kg/dose every 6 hours for up to 5 days

Lupus nephritis: High-dose "pulse" therapy: I.V. (sodium succinate): 1 g/day for 3 days

Aplastic anemia: I.V. (sodium succinate): 1 mg/kg/day or 40 mg/day (whichever dose is higher), for 4 days. After 4 days, change to oral and continue until day 10 or until symptoms of serum sickness resolve, then rapidly reduce over approximately 2 weeks.

Pneumocystis pneumonia in AIDS patients: I.V.: 30 mg twice daily for 5 days, then 30 mg once daily for 5 days, then 15 mg once daily for 11 days

Intra-articular (acetate): Administer every 1-5 weeks.

Large joints: 20-80 mg

Small joints: 4-10 mg

Intralesional (acetate): 20-60 mg every 1-5 weeks

Stability

Intact vials of methylprednisolone sodium succinate should be stored at controlled room temperature of 20°C to 25°C (68°F to 77°F). Protect from light.

Reconstituted solutions of methylprednisolone sodium succinate should be stored at room temperature of 20°C to 25°C (68°F to 77°F), and used within 48 hours.

Stability of parenteral admixture at room temperature (25°C) and at refrigeration temperature (4°C) is 48 hours.

Standard diluent (Solu-Medrol®): 40 mg/50 mL D_5W; 125 mg/50 mL D_5W.

Minimum volume (Solu-Medrol®): 50 mL D_5W.

Administration

Administer with meals to decrease GI upset.

Parenteral: Methylprednisolone sodium succinate may be administered I.M. or I.V.; I.V. administration may be IVP over one to several minutes or IVPB or continuous I.V. infusion. **Acetate salt should not be given I.V.**

I.V.: Succinate:

Low dose: ≤1.8 mg/kg or ≤125 mg/dose: I.V. push over 3-15 minutes

Moderate dose: ≥2 mg/kg or 250 mg/dose: I.V. over 15-30 minutes

High dose: 15 mg/kg or ≥500 mg/dose: I.V. over ≥30 minutes

Doses >15 mg/kg or ≥1 g: Administer over 1 hour

Do **not** administer high-dose I.V. push; hypotension, cardiac arrhythmia, and sudden death have been reported in patients given high-dose methylprednisolone I.V. push (>0.5 g over <10 minutes); intermittent infusion over 15-60 minutes; maximum concentration: I.V. push 125 mg/mL

I.M.: Acetate: Avoid injection into the deltoid muscle due to a high incidence of subcutaneous atrophy. Do not inject into areas that have evidence of acute local infection.

Monitoring Parameters Blood pressure, blood glucose, electrolytes

Anesthesia and Critical Care Concerns/Other Considerations

Evidence-Based Information:

Neuromuscular Effects: ICU-acquired paresis was recently studied in five ICUs (three medical and two surgical ICUs) at four French hospitals. All ICU patients without pre-existing neuromuscular disease admitted from March 1999 through June 2000 were evaluated (de Jonghe, 2002). Each patient had to be mechanically-ventilated for ≥7 days and was screened daily for awakening. The first day the patient was considered awake was Study Day 1. Patients with severe muscle weakness on Study Day 7 were considered to have ICU-acquired paresis. Among the 95 patients who were evaluated, about 25% developed ICU-acquired paresis. Independent predictors included female gender, the number of days with ≥2 organ dysfunction, and administration of corticosteroids. Further studies may be required to verify and characterize the association between the development of ICU-acquired paresis and use of corticosteroids. Concurrent use of a corticosteroid and muscle relaxant appears to increase the risk of certain ICU myopathies; avoid or administer the corticosteroid at the lowest dose possible.

Adrenal Insufficiency: Patients will often have steroid-induced adverse effects on glucose tolerance and lipid profiles. When discontinuing steroid therapy in patients on long-term steroid supplementation, it is important that the steroid therapy be discontinued gradually. Abrupt withdrawal may result in adrenal insufficiency with hypotension and hyperkalemia. Patients on long-term steroid supplementation will require higher corticosteroid doses when subject to stress (eg, trauma, surgery, severe infection). Guidelines for glucocorticoid replacement during various surgical procedures have been published (Coursin, 2002; Salem, 1994).

Septic Shock: Annane, et al (2002) randomized 300 septic shock patients to either hydrocortisone (50 mg I.V. push every 6 hours) and fludrocortisone (50 mcg tablet daily via nasogastric tube) or matching placebos for 7 days. The mean Simplified Acute Physiology Score II (SAPS II) was 57 ± 19 in the placebo group and 60 ± 19 in the active treatment group. The Logistic Organ Dysfunction score was 9 ± 3 in the placebo group and 9 ± 3 in the active treatment group. In patients who did not appropriately respond to corticotropin (nonresponders), there were significantly fewer deaths in the active treatment group. Vasopressor therapy was withdrawn more frequently in this subset of the active treatment group. Adverse events were similar in both groups.

In the CORTICUS trial (Sprung, 2008), 484 septic shock patients were randomized within 72 hours of onset to receive either hydrocortisone (50 mg I.V. push every 6 hours) or placebo for 5 days followed by a 6-day taper. The primary endpoint was 28 day mortality in patients who did not respond to corticotropin. The SAPS II score in the treatment group was 49.5 ± 17.8 and 48.6 ± 16.7 in the placebo group. The Sequential Organ Failure Assessment scores were 10.6 ± 3.4 in the treatment group and 10.6 ± 3.2 in the placebo group. Different than the Annane study, in the patients who did not respond to corticotropin, there was no mortality difference at 28 days; 39.2% (95% CI: 30.5-47.9) mortality in the hydrocortisone group and 36.1% (95% CI: 26.9-45.3, P=0.69) mortality in the placebo group. A trend towards increased incidence of superinfection was noted in hydrocortisone patients. New septic shock episodes, hyperglycemia, and hypernatremia were more frequent in the hydrocortisone group. Hydrocortisone did not improve survival in this population of septic shock patients regardless of corticotropin response.

The 2008 Surviving Sepsis Campaign Guidelines suggest the following: Intravenous hydrocortisone be given only to adult septic shock patients after blood pressure is identified to be poorly responsive to fluid resuscitation and vasopressor therapy (Grade 2C); ACTH stimulation test not be used to identify the subset of adults with septic shock who should receive hydrocortisone (Grade 2B); patients with septic shock should not receive dexamethasone if hydrocortisone is available (Grade 2B); the addition of fludrocortisone if hydrocortisone is not available and the steroid that is substituted does not have significant mineralocorticoid activity (Grade 2C); doses of corticosteroids comparable to >300 mg hydrocortisone daily **not** be used in severe sepsis or septic shock for the purpose of treating septic shock (Grade 1A). They also recommend corticosteroids **not** be administered for the treatment of sepsis in the absence of shock. There is, however, no contraindication to continuing maintenance steroid therapy or to using stress dose steroids if the patient's endocrine or corticosteroid administration history warrants (Grade 1D).

The 2008 Recommendations for the diagnosis and management of corticosteroid insufficiency in critically ill adult patients recommend a diagnosis of critical illness related corticosteroid insufficiency can be made by a delta cortisol level (after 250 mcg cosyntropin) of <9 mcg/dL or a random cortisol <10 mcg/dL (Grade 2B). However, they recommend **against** the use of ACTH stimulation test to determine if septic shock or ARDS patients should receive steroid therapy (Grade 2B). They recommend to consider using hydrocortisone in septic shock patients who have responded poorly to resuscitation and vasopressors (Grade 2B) and glucocorticoid treatment should be tapered slowly and not stopped abruptly (Grade 2B). Dexamethasone is **not** recommended for the treatment of septic shock or ARDS (Grade 1B). Fludrocortisone therapy is considered optional (Grade 2B).

Contraindications Hypersensitivity to methylprednisolone or any component of the formulation; systemic fungal infection (except intra-articular injection in localized joint conditions); administration of live virus vaccines. methylprednisolone formulations containing benzyl alcohol preservative are contraindicated in infants; I.M. administration in idiopathic thrombocytopenia purpura; intrathecal administration of methylprednisolone acetate suspension

Warnings/Precautions Use with caution in patients with thyroid disease, hepatic impairment, renal impairment, cardiovascular disease, diabetes, glaucoma, cataracts, myasthenia gravis, patients at risk for osteoporosis, patients at risk for seizures, or GI diseases (diverticulitis, peptic ulcer, ulcerative colitis) due to perforation risk. Not recommended for the treatment of optic neuritis; may increase frequency of new episodes. Use caution following acute MI (corticosteroids have been associated with myocardial rupture). Cardiomegaly and congestive heart failure have been reported following concurrent use of amphotericin B and hydrocortisone for the management of fungal infections.

Because of the risk of adverse effects, systemic corticosteroids should be used cautiously in the elderly in the smallest possible effective dose for the shortest duration. May affect growth velocity; growth should be routinely monitored in pediatric patients. Withdraw therapy with gradual tapering of dose.

May cause hypercorticism or suppression of hypothalamic-pituitary-adrenal (HPA) axis, particularly in younger children or in patients receiving high doses for prolonged periods. HPA axis suppression may lead to adrenal crisis. Withdrawal and discontinuation of a corticosteroid should be done slowly and carefully. Particular care is required when patients are transferred from systemic corticosteroids to inhaled products due to possible adrenal insufficiency or withdrawal from steroids, including an increase in allergic symptoms. Patients receiving >20 mg per day of prednisone (or equivalent) may be most susceptible. Fatalities have occurred due to adrenal insufficiency in asthmatic patients during and after transfer from systemic corticosteroids to aerosol steroids; aerosol steroids do not provide the systemic steroid needed to treat patients having trauma, surgery, or infections.

Acute myopathy has been reported with high dose corticosteroids, usually in patients with neuromuscular transmission disorders; may involve ocular and/or respiratory muscles; monitor creatine kinase; recovery may be delayed. Corticosteroid use may cause psychiatric disturbances, including depression, euphoria, insomnia, mood swings, and personality changes. Pre-existing psychiatric conditions may be exacerbated by corticosteroid use. Prolonged use of corticosteroids may also increase the incidence of secondary infection, cause activation of latent infections, mask acute infection (including fungal infections), prolong or exacerbate viral or parasitic infections, or limit response to vaccines. Exposure to chickenpox or measles should be avoided; corticosteroids should not be used to treat ocular herpes simplex. Corticosteroids should not be used for cerebral malaria or viral hepatitis. Close observation is required in patients with latent tuberculosis and/or TB reactivity; restrict use in active TB (only in conjunction with antituberculosis treatment). Amebiasis should be ruled out in any patient with recent travel to tropic climates or unexplained diarrhea prior to initiation of corticosteroids. Prolonged treatment with corticosteroids has been associated with the development of Kaposi's sarcoma (case reports); discontinuation may result in clinical improvement.

High-dose corticosteroids should not be used to manage acute head injury. Rare cases of anaphylactoid reactions have been observed in patients receiving corticosteroids. Dermal and/or subdermal skin depression may occur at the site of methylprednisolone acetate injection. Avoid injection or leakage into the dermis. Some dosage forms contain benzyl alcohol which has been associated with "gasping syndrome" in neonates.

Adverse Reactions Frequency not defined.

Cardiovascular: Arrhythmias, bradycardia, cardiac arrest, cardiomegaly, circulatory collapse, congestive heart failure, edema, fat embolism, hypertension, hypertrophic cardiomyopathy in premature infants, myocardial rupture (post MI), syncope, tachycardia, thromboembolism, vasculitis

Central nervous system: Delirium, depression, emotional instability, euphoria, hallucinations, headache, intracranial pressure increased, insomnia, malaise, mood swings, nervousness, neuritis, personality changes, psychic disorders, pseudotumor cerebri (usually following discontinuation), seizure, vertigo

Dermatologic: Acne, allergic dermatitis, alopecia, dry scaly skin, ecchymoses, edema, erythema, hirsutism, hyper-/hypopigmentation, hypertrichosis, impaired wound healing, petechiae, rash, skin atrophy, sterile abscess, skin test reaction impaired, striae, urticaria

Endocrine & metabolic: Adrenal suppression, amenorrhea, carbohydrate intolerance increased, Cushing's syndrome, diabetes mellitus, fluid retention, glucose intolerance, growth suppression (children), hyperglycemia, hyperlipidemia, hypokalemia, hypokalemic alkalosis, menstrual irregularities, negative nitrogen balance, pituitary-adrenal axis suppression, protein catabolism, sodium and water retention

Gastrointestinal: Abdominal distention, appetite increased, bowel/bladder dysfunction (after intrathecal administration), gastrointestinal hemorrhage, gastrointestinal perforation, nausea, pancreatitis, peptic ulcer, perforation of the small and large intestine, ulcerative esophagitis, vomiting, weight gain

Hematologic: Leukocytosis (transient)

Hepatic: Hepatomegaly, transaminases increased

Local: Postinjection flare (intra-articular use), thrombophlebitis

Neuromuscular & skeletal: Arthralgia, arthropathy, aseptic necrosis (femoral and humoral heads), fractures, muscle mass loss, muscle weakness, myopathy (particularly in conjunction with neuromuscular disease or neuromuscular-blocking agents), neuropathy, osteoporosis, parasthesia, tendon rupture, vertebral compression fractures, weakness

Ocular: Cataracts, exophthalmoses, glaucoma, intraocular pressure increased

Renal: Glycosuria

Respiratory: Pulmonary edema

Miscellaneous: Abnormal fat disposition, anaphylactoid reaction, anaphylaxis, angioedema, avascular necrosis, diaphoresis, hiccups, hypersensitivity reactions, infections, secondary malignancy

Drug Interactions

Metabolism/Transport Effects Substrate of CYP3A4 (major); **Inhibits** CYP2C8 (weak), 3A4 (weak)

Avoid Concomitant Use

Avoid concomitant use of MethylPREDNISolone with any of the following: Natalizumab; Vaccines (Live)

Increased Effect/Toxicity

MethylPREDNISolone may increase the levels/effects of: Acetylcholinesterase Inhibitors; Amphotericin B; CycloSPORINE; Leflunomide; Loop Diuretics; Natalizumab; NSAID (COX-2 Inhibitor); NSAID (Nonselective); Thiazide Diuretics; Vaccines (Live); Warfarin

The levels/effects of MethylPREDNISolone may be increased by: Antifungal Agents (Azole Derivatives, Systemic); Aprepitant; Calcium Channel Blockers (Nondihydropyridine); CycloSPORINE; Estrogen Derivatives; Fluconazole; Fosaprepitant; Macrolide Antibiotics; Neuromuscular-Blocking Agents (Non-depolarizing); Quinolone Antibiotics; Salicylates; Trastuzumab

Decreased Effect

MethylPREDNISolone may decrease the levels/effects of: Antidiabetic Agents; Calcitriol; Corticorelin; Isoniazid; Salicylates; Vaccines (Inactivated); Vaccines (Live)

The levels/effects of MethylPREDNISolone may be decreased by: Aminoglutethimide; Antacids; Barbiturates; Bile Acid Sequestrants; Echinacea; Mitotane; Primidone; Rifamycin Derivatives

Ethanol/Nutrition/Herb Interactions

Ethanol: Avoid ethanol (may increase gastric mucosal irritation).

Food: Methylprednisolone interferes with calcium absorption. Limit caffeine.

Herb/Nutraceutical: St John's wort may decrease methylprednisolone levels. Avoid cat's claw, echinacea (have immunostimulant properties).

Test Interactions Interferes with skin tests

Dietary Considerations Take with meals to decrease GI upset.; need diet rich in pyridoxine, vitamin C, vitamin D, folate, calcium, phosphorus, and protein.

Dosage Forms Excipient information presented when available (limited, particularly for generics); consult specific product labeling.

Injection, powder for reconstitution, as sodium succinate: 40 mg, 125 mg, 500 mg, 1 g [strength expressed as base]

A-Methapred®: 40 mg, 125 mg [strength expressed as base]

Solu-Medrol®: 40 mg, 125 mg, 500 mg, 1 g, 2 g [contains benzyl alcohol (in diluent); strength expressed as base]

Solu-Medrol®: 500 mg, 1 g [strength expressed as base]

Injection, suspension, as acetate: 40 mg/mL (1 mL, 5 mL, 10 mL); 80 mg/mL (1 mL, 5 mL)

Depo-Medrol®: 20 mg/mL (5 mL); 40 mg/mL (5 mL, 10 mL); 80 mg/mL (5 mL) [contains benzyl alcohol, polysorbate 80]

Depo-Medrol®: 40 mg/mL (1 mL); 80 mg/mL (1 mL)

Tablet, oral: 4 mg

Medrol®: 2 mg, 4 mg, 8 mg, 16 mg, 32 mg

Tablet, oral [dose-pack]: 4 mg (21s) [scored]

Medrol® Dosepak™: 4 mg (21s) [scored]

References

Abraham E and Evans T, "Corticosteroids and Septic Shock (editorial)," *JAMA*, 2002, 288(7):886-7.

Annane D, Sebille V, Charpentier C, et al, "Effect of Treatment With Low Doses of Hydrocortisone and Fludrocortisone on Mortality in Patients With Septic Shock," *JAMA*, 2002, 288(7):862-71.

Bracken MB, Shepard MJ, Collins WF, et al, "A Randomized, Controlled Trial of Methylprednisolone or Naloxone in the Treatment of Acute Spinal-Cord Injury. Results of the Second National Acute Spinal Cord Injury Study," *N Engl J Med*, 1990, 322(20):1405-11.

Cooper MS and Stewart PM, "Corticosteroid Insufficiency in Acutely Ill Patients," *N Engl J Med*, 2003, 348(8):727-34.

Coursin DB and Wood KE, "Corticosteroid Supplementation for Adrenal Insufficiency," *JAMA*, 2002, 287(2):236-40.

de Jonghe B, Sharshar T, Lefaucheur JP, et al, "Paresis Acquired in the Intensive Care Unit. A Prospective Multicenter Study," *JAMA*, 2002, 288(22):2859-67.

Dellinger RP, Levy MM, Carlet JM, et al, "Surviving Sepsis Campaign: International Guidelines for Management of Severe Sepsis and Septic Shock: 2008," *Intensive Care Med*, 2008, 34(1): 17-60. Available at http://www.survivingsepsis.org/system/files/images/2008_20International_20SSC_20-Guidelines_1_.pdf

Expert Panel Report 3, "Guidelines for the Diagnosis and Management of Asthma," *Clinical Practice Guidelines*, National Institutes of Health, National Heart, Lung, and Blood Institute, NIH Publication No. 08-4051, prepublication 2007. Available at http://www.nhlbi.nih.gov/guidelines/asthma/asthgdln.htm

Hotchkiss RS and Karl IE, "The Pathophysiology and Treatment of Sepsis," *N Engl J Med*, 2003, 348 (2):138-50.

Marik PE, Pastores SM, Annane D, et al, "Recommendations for the Diagnosis and Management of Corticosteroid Insufficiency in Critically Ill Adult Patients: Consensus Statements From an International Task Force by the American College of Critical Care Medicine," *Crit Care Med*, 2008, 36(6):1937-49.

Salem M, Tainsh RE Jr, Bromberg J, et al, "Perioperative Glucocorticoid Coverage: A Reassessment 42 Years After Emergence of a Problem," *Ann Surg*, 1994, 219(4):416-25.

Sprung CL, Annane D, Keh D, et al, "Hydrocortisone Therapy for Patients With Septic Shock," *N Engl J Med*, 2008, 358(2):111-24.

Steinberg KP, Hudson LD, Goodman RB, et al, "Efficacy and Safety of Corticosteroids for Persistent Acute Respiratory Distress Syndrome. National Heart, Lung and Blood Institute Acute Respiratory Distress Syndrome (ARDS) Clinical Trials Network," *N Engl J Med*, 2006, 354(16):1671-84.

◆ **6-α-Methylprednisolone** see MethylPREDNISolone *on page 911*

◆ **Methylprednisolone Acetate** see MethylPREDNISolone *on page 911*

◆ **Methylprednisolone Sodium Succinate** see MethylPREDNISolone *on page 911*

◆ **4-Methylpyrazole** see Fomepizole *on page 625*

Metoclopramide (met oh KLOE pra mide)

Medication Safety Issues
Sound-alike/look-alike issues:
Metoclopramide may be confused with metolazone, metoprolol, metroNIDAZOLE
Reglan® may be confused with Megace®, Regonol®, Renagel®

Medication Guide An FDA-approved patient medication guide, which is available with the product information and as follows, must be dispensed with this medication for each new outpatient prescription and refill for oral administration.
Metozolv™ ODT: http://www.accessdata.fda.gov/drugsatfda_docs/label/2009/022246s000lbl.pdf
Reglan® injection: http://www.fda.gov/downloads/Drugs/DrugSafety/UCM176362.pdf
Reglan® tablet: http://www.alavenpharm.com/downloads/ReglanTab-lets_MedicationGuide.pdf

Related Information
Anesthesia for Obstetric Patients in Nonobstetric Surgery *on page 1532*
Perioperative Management of Patients on Antiseizure Medication *on page 1577*
Postoperative Nausea and Vomiting *on page 1593*

U.S. Brand Names Metozolv™ ODT; Reglan®

Canadian Brand Names Apo-Metoclop®; Metoclopramide Hydrochloride Injection; Metoclopramide Omega; Nu-Metoclopramide; PMS-Metoclopramide

Pharmacologic Category Antiemetic; Gastrointestinal Agent, Prokinetic

Generic Available Yes: Excludes oral-disintegrating tablet

Use
Oral: Symptomatic treatment of diabetic gastroparesis; gastroesophageal reflux

I.V., I.M.: Symptomatic treatment of diabetic gastroparesis; postpyloric placement of enteral feeding tubes; prevention and/or treatment of nausea and vomiting associated with chemotherapy, or postsurgery; to stimulate gastric emptying and intestinal transit of barium during radiological examination of the stomach/small intestine

Mechanism of Action Blocks dopamine receptors and (when given in higher doses) also blocks serotonin receptors in chemoreceptor trigger zone of the CNS; enhances the response to acetylcholine of tissue in upper GI tract causing enhanced motility and accelerated gastric emptying without stimulating gastric, biliary, or pancreatic secretions; increases lower esophageal sphincter tone

Pharmacodynamics/Kinetics

Onset of action: Oral: 30-60 minutes; I.V.: 1-3 minutes; I.M.: 10-15 minutes
Duration: Therapeutic: 1-2 hours, regardless of route
Absorption: Oral: Rapid
Distribution: V_d: ~3.5 L/kg
Protein binding: ~30%
Bioavailability: Oral: Range: 65% to 95%
Half-life elimination: Normal renal function: Children: ~4 hours; Adults: 5-6 hours (may be dose dependent)
Time to peak, serum: Oral: 1-2 hours
Excretion: Urine (~85%)

Dosage

Children:
Gastroesophageal reflux (unlabeled use): Oral: 0.1-0.2 mg/kg/dose 4 times/day
Antiemetic (chemotherapy-induced emesis) (unlabeled): I.V.: 1-2 mg/kg 30 minutes before chemotherapy and every 2-4 hours (maximum: 5 doses/day); pretreatment with diphenhydramine will decrease risk of extrapyramidal reactions to this dosage
Postpyloric feeding tube placement: I.V.:
<6 years: 0.1 mg/kg as a single dose
6-14 years: 2.5-5 mg as a single dose
>14 years: Refer to adult dosing.

Adults:
Gastroesophageal reflux: Oral: 10-15 mg/dose up to 4 times/day 30 minutes before meals or food and at bedtime; single doses of 20 mg are occasionally needed prior to provoking situations. Treatment >12 weeks is not recommended.
Diabetic gastroparesis:
Oral: 10 mg/dose up to 4 times/day 30 minutes before meals or food and at bedtime for 2-8 weeks
I.M., I.V. (for severe symptoms): 10 mg over 1-2 minutes; 10 days of I.V. therapy may be necessary before symptoms are controlled to allow transition to oral administration
Chemotherapy-induced emesis prophylaxis: I.V.: 1-2 mg/kg 30 minutes before chemotherapy and repeated every 2 hours for 2 doses, then every 3 hours for 3 doses (manufacturer labeling); pretreatment with diphenhydramine will decrease risk of extrapyramidal reactions
Alternate dosing: **Note:** Metoclopramide is considered an antiemetic with a low therapeutic index; use is generally reserved for agents with low emetogenic potential or in patients intolerant/refractory to first-line antiemetics.
Low-risk chemotherapy (unlabeled): I.V., Oral: 10-40 mg prior to dose, then every 4-6 hours as needed (NCCN Antiemesis guidelines, v.4.2009)
Breakthrough treatment (unlabeled): I.V., Oral: 10-40 mg every 4-6 hours (NCCN Antiemesis guidelines, v.4.2009)
Delayed-emesis prophylaxis (unlabeled): Oral: 20-40 mg/dose (or 0.5 mg/kg/dose) 2-4 times/day for 3-4 days (in combination with dexamethasone [ASCO guidelines, 2006])
Refractory or intolerant to antiemetics with a higher therapeutic index (unlabeled; Hesketh, 2008):
I.V.: 1-2 mg/kg/dose before chemotherapy and repeat 2 hours after chemotherapy
Oral: 0.5 mg/kg every 6 hours on days 2-4
Postoperative nausea and vomiting prophylaxis: I.M.: 10-20 mg near end of surgery
Postpyloric feeding tube placement, radiological exam: I.V.: 10 mg as a single dose
Elderly: Initial: Dose at the lower end of the recommended range. Refer to adult dosing.

Dosing adjustment in renal impairment: Cl_{cr} <40 mL/minute: Administer at 50% of normal dose

Hemodialysis: Not dialyzable (0% to 5%); supplemental dose is not necessary

Stability

Injection: Store intact vial at controlled room temperature. Injection is photosensitive and should be protected from light during storage. Parenteral admixtures in D_5W or NS are stable for at least 24 hours and do not require light protection if used within 24 hours.

Tablet: Store at controlled room temperature of 20°C to 25°C (68°F to 77°F).

Administration

Injection solution: May be given I.M., direct I.V. push, short infusion (15-30 minutes), or continuous infusion; lower doses (≤10 mg) of metoclopramide can be given I.V. push undiluted over 1-2 minutes; higher doses (>10 mg) to be diluted in 50 mL of compatible solution (preferably NS) and given IVPB over at least 15 minutes; continuous SubQ infusion and rectal administration have been reported. **Note:** Rapid I.V. administration may be associated with a transient (but intense) feeling of anxiety and restlessness, followed by drowsiness.

Orally-disintegrating tablets: Administer on an empty stomach at least 30 minutes prior to food. Do not remove from packaging until time of administration. If tablet breaks or crumbles while handling, discard and remove new tablet. Using dry hands, place tablet on tongue and allow to dissolve. Swallow with saliva.

Monitoring Parameters Dystonic reactions; signs of hypoglycemia in patients using insulin and those being treated for gastroparesis; agitation, and confusion

Anesthesia and Critical Care Concerns/Other Considerations

Evidence-Based Information: The consensus guidelines for postoperative nausea and vomiting (Gan, 2003) does not recommend the use of metoclopramide.

Pregnancy Risk Factor B

Contraindications Hypersensitivity to metoclopramide or any component of the formulation; GI obstruction, perforation or hemorrhage; pheochromocytoma; history of seizures or concomitant use of other agents likely to increase extrapyramidal reactions

Warnings/Precautions [U.S. Boxed Warning]: May cause tardive dyskinesia, which is often irreversible; duration of treatment and total cumulative dose are associated with an increased risk. Therapy durations >12 weeks should be avoided (except in rare cases following risk:benefit assessment). Risk appears to be increased in the elderly, women, and diabetics; however, it is not possible to predict which patients will develop tardive dyskinesia. Therapy should be discontinued in any patient if signs/symptoms of tardive dyskinesia appear.

May cause extrapyramidal symptoms, generally manifested as acute dystonic reactions within the initial 24-48 hours of use. Risk of these reactions is increased at higher doses, and in pediatric patients, and adults <30 years of age. Pseudoparkinsonism (eg, bradykinesia, tremor, rigidity) may also occur (usually within first 6 months of therapy) and is generally reversible following discontinuation. Use with caution or avoid in patients with Parkinson's disease. Use caution in the elderly; may have increased risk of tardive dyskinesia, particularly older women. Neuroleptic malignant syndrome (NMS) has been reported (rarely) with metoclopramide.

May cause transient increase in serum aldosterone; use caution in patients who are at risk of fluid overload (HF, cirrhosis). Use caution in patients with hypertension or following surgical anastomosis/closure. Use caution with a history of mental illness; has been associated with depression. Abrupt discontinuation may (rarely) result in withdrawal symptoms (dizziness, headache, nervousness). Use caution and adjust dose in renal impairment. Patients with NADH-cytochrome b5 reductase deficiency are at increased risk of methemoglobinemia and/or sulfhemoglobinemia. Neonates may have an increased risk of methemoglobinemia due to decreased levels of NADH-cytochrome b5 reductase deficiency and prolonged clearance of metoclopramide.

Adverse Reactions Frequency not always defined.

Cardiovascular: AV block, bradycardia, HF, fluid retention, flushing (following high I.V. doses), hyper-/hypotension, supraventricular tachycardia

◀ Central nervous system: Drowsiness (~10% to 70%; dose related), acute dystonic reactions (<1% to 25%; dose and age related), fatigue (2% to 10%), lassitude (~10%), restlessness (~10%), headache (4% to 5%), dizziness (1% to 4%), somnolence (2% to 3%), akathisia, confusion, depression, hallucinations (rare), insomnia, neuroleptic malignant syndrome (rare), Parkinsonian-like symptoms, suicidal ideation, seizure, tardive dyskinesia

Dermatologic: Angioneurotic edema (rare), rash, urticaria

Endocrine & metabolic: Amenorrhea, galactorrhea, gynecomastia, hyperprolacti-nemia, impotence

Gastrointestinal: Nausea (4% to 6%), vomiting (1% to 2%), diarrhea

Genitourinary: Incontinence, urinary frequency

Hematologic: Agranulocytosis, leukopenia, neutropenia, porphyria

Hepatic: Hepatotoxicity (rare)

Ocular: Visual disturbance

Respiratory: Bronchospasm, laryngeal edema (rare), laryngospasm (rare)

Miscellaneous: Allergic reactions, methemoglobinemia, sulfhemoglobinemia

Drug Interactions

Metabolism/Transport Effects Substrate (minor) of CYP1A2, 2D6; **Inhibits** CYP2D6 (weak)

Avoid Concomitant Use There are no known interactions where it is recommended to avoid concomitant use.

Increased Effect/Toxicity
Metoclopramide may increase the levels/effects of: CycloSPORINE; Sertraline; Venlafaxine

Decreased Effect
Metoclopramide may decrease the levels/effects of: Anti-Parkinson's Agents (Dopamine Agonist); Posaconazole

The levels/effects of Metoclopramide may be decreased by: Peginterferon Alfa-2b

Ethanol/Nutrition/Herb Interactions Ethanol: Avoid ethanol (may increase CNS depression).

Test Interactions Increased aminotransferase [ALT/AST] (S), increased amylase (S)

Dosage Forms Excipient information presented when available (limited, particularly for generics); consult specific product labeling.

Injection, solution [preservative free]: 5 mg/mL (2 mL)
  Reglan®: 5 mg/mL (2 mL, 10 mL, 30 mL)
Solution, oral: 5 mg/5 mL (10 mL, 480 mL)
Tablet: 5 mg, 10 mg
  Reglan®: 5 mg, 10 mg
Tablet, orally disintegrating:
  Metozolv™ ODT: 5 mg, 10 mg [mint flavor]

References

Gan TJ, Meyer T, Apfel CC, et al, "Consensus Guidelines for Managing Postoperative Nausea and Vomiting," *Anesth Analg*, 2003, 97(1):62-71.

◆ **Metoclopramide Hydrochloride Injection (Can)** *see* Metoclopramide *on page 917*

◆ **Metoclopramide Omega (Can)** *see* Metoclopramide *on page 917*

Metolazone (me TOLE a zone)

Medication Safety Issues
Sound-alike/look-alike issues:
  Metolazone may be confused with metaxalone, methazolamide, methimazole, methotrexate, metoclopramide, metoprolol, minoxidil
  Zaroxolyn® may be confused with Zarontin®

Related Information
  Heart Failure (Systolic) *on page 1739*

U.S. Brand Names Zaroxolyn®

Canadian Brand Names Zaroxolyn®

Pharmacologic Category Diuretic, Thiazide-Related

Generic Available Yes

Use Management of mild-to-moderate hypertension; treatment of edema in heart failure and nephrotic syndrome, impaired renal function

Mechanism of Action Inhibits sodium reabsorption in the distal tubules causing increased excretion of sodium and water, as well as, potassium and hydrogen ions

Pharmacodynamics/Kinetics

Onset of action: Diuresis: ~60 minutes

Duration: ≥24 hours

Absorption: Incomplete

Distribution: Crosses placenta; enters breast milk

Protein binding: 95%

Half-life elimination: 20 hours

Excretion: Urine (80%); bile (10%)

Dosage Oral:

Adults:

Edema: Initial: 2.5-10 mg once daily; may increase as necessary to 20 mg once daily (ACC/AHA 2009 Heart Failure Guidelines)

Hypertension: 2.5-5 mg/dose every 24 hours

Elderly: Initial: 2.5 mg/day or every other day

Dosage adjustment in renal impairment: Dialysis: Not dialyzable (0% to 5%) via hemo- or peritoneal dialysis; supplemental dose is not necessary

Administration May be taken with food or milk. Take early in day to avoid nocturia. Take the last dose of multiple doses no later than 6 PM unless instructed otherwise.

Monitoring Parameters Serum electrolytes (potassium, sodium, chloride, bicarbonate), renal function, blood pressure (standing, sitting/supine)

Anesthesia and Critical Care Concerns/Other Considerations

Clinical Pearls/Comments: Metolazone 5 mg is approximately equivalent to hydrochlorothiazide 50 mg. When taken the day of surgery, it may cause hypovolemia and the hypertensive patient undergoing general anesthesia to have labile blood pressure; use with caution prior to surgery or perioperatively

Metolazone is a potent diuretic with a duration of action exceeding 24 hours and is often used in patients refractory to thiazide or loop diuretics. It is important that the patient be closely monitored to avoid profound volume depletion and electrolyte disturbances (eg, hyponatremia, hypochloremia, and hypomagnesemia).

Pregnancy Risk Factor B (manufacturer); D (expert analysis)

Contraindications Hypersensitivity to metolazone, any component of the formulation, other thiazides, and sulfonamide derivatives; anuria; hepatic coma; pregnancy (expert analysis)

Warnings/Precautions Electrolyte disturbances (hypokalemia, hypochloremic alkalosis, hyponatremia) can occur. Large or prolonged fluid and electrolyte losses may occur with concomitant furosemide administration. Use with caution in severe hepatic dysfunction; hepatic encephalopathy can be caused by electrolyte disturbances. Gout can be precipitate in certain patients with a history of gout, a familial predisposition to gout, or chronic renal failure. Cautious use in patients with prediabetes or diabetes; may see a change in glucose control. Can cause SLE exacerbation or activation. Use caution in severe renal impairment. Use with caution in patients with moderate or high cholesterol concentrations. Photo-sensitization may occur.

Chemical similarities are present among sulfonamides, sulfonylureas, carbonic anhydrase inhibitors, thiazides, and loop diuretics (except ethacrynic acid). Use in patients with thiazide or sulfonamide allergy is specifically contraindicated in product labeling, however, a risk of cross-reaction exists in patients with allergy to any of these compounds; avoid use when previous reaction has been severe. Discontinue if signs of hypersensitivity are noted.

Adverse Reactions Frequency not defined.

Cardiovascular: Chest pain/discomfort, necrotizing angiitis, orthostatic hypotension, palpitation, syncope, venous thrombosis, vertigo, volume depletion

Central nervous system: Chills, depression, dizziness, drowsiness, fatigue, headache, lightheadedness, restlessness

Dermatologic: Petechiae, photosensitivity, pruritus, purpura, rash, skin necrosis, Stevens-Johnson syndrome, toxic epidermal necrolysis, urticaria

Endocrine & metabolic: Gout attacks, hypercalcemia, hyperglycemia, hyperuricemia, hypochloremia, hypochloremic alkalosis, hypokalemia, hypomagnesemia, hyponatremia, hypophosphatemia

Gastrointestinal: Abdominal bloating, abdominal pain, anorexia, constipation, diarrhea, epigastric distress, nausea, pancreatitis, vomiting, xerostomia

Genitourinary: Impotence

Hematologic: Agranulocytosis, aplastic/hypoplastic anemia, hemoconcentration, leukopenia, thrombocytopenia

Hepatic: Cholestatic jaundice, hepatitis

Neuromuscular & skeletal: Joint pain, muscle cramps/spasm, neuropathy, paresthesia, weakness

Ocular: Blurred vision (transient)

Renal: BUN increased, glucosuria

Drug Interactions

Avoid Concomitant Use

Avoid concomitant use of Metolazone with any of the following: Dofetilide

Increased Effect/Toxicity

Metolazone may increase the levels/effects of: ACE Inhibitors; Allopurinol; Amifostine; Antihypertensives; Calcitriol; Calcium Salts; Dofetilide; Hypotensive Agents; Lithium; RiTUXimab

The levels/effects of Metolazone may be increased by: Alcohol (Ethyl); Analgesics (Opioid); Barbiturates; Corticosteroids (Orally Inhaled); Corticosteroids (Systemic); Herbs (Hypotensive Properties); MAO Inhibitors; Pentoxifylline; Phosphodiesterase 5 Inhibitors; Prostacyclin Analogues

Decreased Effect

Metolazone may decrease the levels/effects of: Antidiabetic Agents

The levels/effects of Metolazone may be decreased by: Bile Acid Sequestrants; Herbs (Hypertensive Properties); Methylphenidate; Nonsteroidal Anti-Inflammatory Agents; Yohimbine

Ethanol/Nutrition/Herb Interactions

Ethanol: May potentiate hypotensive effect of metazolone.

Herb/Nutraceutical: Avoid herbs with *hypertensive* properties (bayberry, blue cohosh, cayenne, ephedra, ginger, ginseng [American], kola, licorice); may diminish the antihypertensive effect of metolazone. Avoid herbs with *hypotensive* properties (black cohosh, California poppy, coleus, golden seal, hawthorn, mistletoe, periwinkle, quinine, shepherd's purse); may enhance the hypotensive effect of metolazone.

Dietary Considerations Should be taken after breakfast; may require potassium supplementation

Dosage Forms Excipient information presented when available (limited, particularly for generics); consult specific product labeling. [DSC] = Discontinued product

Tablet: 2.5 mg, 5 mg, 10 mg

Zaroxolyn®: 2.5 mg, 5 mg; 10 mg [DSC]

Metoprolol (me toe PROE lole)

Medication Safety Issues

Sound-alike/look-alike issues:

Lopressor® may be confused with Lyrica®

Metoprolol may be confused with metaproterenol, metoclopramide, metolazone, misoprostol

Toprol-XL® may be confused with Tegretol®, Tegretol®-XL, Topamax®

High alert medication: The Institute for Safe Medication Practices (ISMP) includes this medication among its list of drugs which have a heightened risk of causing significant patient harm when used in error.

Significant differences exist between oral and I.V. dosing. Use caution when converting from one route of administration to another.

Related Information

U.S. Brand Names Lopressor®; Toprol-XL®

Canadian Brand Names Apo-Metoprolol®; Betaloc®; Betaloc® Durules®; Dom-Metoprolol; Gen-Metoprolol; Lopressor®; Metoprolol Tartrate Injection, USP; Metoprolol-25; Mylan-Metoprolol (Type L); Novo-Metoprolol; Nu-Metop; PHL-Metoprolol; PMS-Metoprolol; Riva-Metoprolol; Sandoz-Metoprolol; Toprol-XL®

Index Terms Metoprolol Succinate; Metoprolol Tartrate

Pharmacologic Category Beta Blocker, Beta$_1$ Selective

Generic Available Yes

Use Treatment of angina pectoris, hypertension, or hemodynamically-stable acute myocardial infarction

Extended release: Treatment of angina pectoris or hypertension; to reduce mortality/hospitalization in patients with heart failure (stable NYHA Class II or III) already receiving ACE inhibitors, diuretics, and/or digoxin

Unlabeled/Investigational Use Treatment of ventricular arrhythmias, atrial ectopy; migraine prophylaxis, essential tremor, aggressive behavior (not recommended for dementia-associated aggression); prevention of reinfarction and sudden death after myocardial infarction; prevention and treatment of atrial fibrillation and atrial flutter; multifocal atrial tachycardia; symptomatic treatment of hypertrophic obstructive cardiomyopathy

Mechanism of Action Selective inhibitor of beta$_1$-adrenergic receptors; competitively blocks beta$_1$-receptors, with little or no effect on beta$_2$-receptors at doses <100 mg; does not exhibit any membrane stabilizing or intrinsic sympathomimetic activity

Pharmacodynamics/Kinetics

Onset of action: Peak effect: Oral: 1.5-4 hours; I.V.: 20 minutes (when infused over 10 minutes)

Duration: Oral: Immediate release: 10-20 hours, Extended release: ~24 hours; I.V.: 5-8 hours

Absorption: 95%, rapid and complete

Distribution: V_d: 5.5 L/kg

Protein binding: 12% to albumin

Metabolism: Extensively hepatic via CYP2D6; significant first-pass effect (~50%)

Bioavailability: Oral: ~50%

Half-life elimination: 3-8 hours (dependent on rate of CYP2D6 metabolism)

Excretion: Urine (<5% to 10% as unchanged drug)

Dosage

Children: Hypertension: Oral:

1-17 years: Immediate release tablet: (National High Blood Pressure Education Program Working Group on High Blood Pressure in Children and Adolescents, 2004): Initial: 1-2 mg/kg/day; maximum 6 mg/kg/day (≤200 mg/day); administer in 2 divided doses

≥6 years: Extended release tablet: Initial: 1 mg/kg once daily (maximum initial dose: 50 mg/day). Adjust dose based on patient response (maximum: 2 mg/kg/day or 200 mg/day)

Adults:

Angina: Oral:

Immediate release: Initial: 50 mg twice daily; usual dosage range: 50-200 mg twice daily; maximum: 400 mg/day; increase dose at weekly intervals to desired effect

Extended release: Initial: 100 mg/day (maximum: 400 mg/day)

Atrial fibrillation (ventricular rate control), supraventricular tachycardia (SVT) (acute treatment; unlabeled use; Antman, 2004; Fuster, 2006): I.V.: 2.5-5 mg every 2-5 minutes (maximum total dose: 15 mg over a 10-15 minute period). **Note:** Initiate cautiously in patients with concomitant heart failure

Maintenance: Oral (immediate release): 25-100 mg twice daily

Heart failure: Oral (extended release): Initial: 25 mg once daily (reduce to 12.5 mg once daily in NYHA class higher than class II); may double dosage every 2 weeks as tolerated (maximum: 200 mg/day)

Hypertension: Oral:

Immediate release: Initial: 50 mg twice daily; effective dosage range: 100-450 mg/day in 2-3 divided doses; increase dose at weekly intervals to desired effect; maximum: 450 mg/day; usual dosage range (JNC 7): 50-100 mg/day

Extended release: Initial: 25-100 mg once daily; increase doses at weekly (or longer) intervals to desired effect; maximum: 400 mg/day; usual dosage range (JNC 7): 50-100 mg/day

Hypertension/ventricular rate control: I.V. (in patients having nonfunctioning GI tract): Initial: 1.25-5 mg every 6-12 hours; titrate initial dose to response. Initially, low doses may be appropriate to establish response; however, up to 15 mg every 3-6 hours has been employed.

Myocardial infarction:

Acute: I.V.: 5 mg every 2 minutes for 3 doses in early treatment of myocardial infarction; thereafter, give 50 mg orally every 6 hours beginning 15 minutes after last I.V. dose and continue for 48 hours; then administer a maintenance dose of 100 mg twice daily. **Note:** If initial I.V. dosing is not tolerated, may give 25-50 mg orally (depending on degree of intolerance) every 6 hours beginning 15 minutes after the last I.V. dose or as soon as clinical condition permits.

Secondary prevention (unlabeled use; Olsson, 1992): Oral: Immediate release: 25-100 mg twice daily; optimize dose based on heart rate and blood pressure; continue indefinitely.

Elderly: Initiate at the lower end of the dosage range

Note: Switching dosage forms:

When switching from immediate release metoprolol to extended release, the same total daily dose of metoprolol should be used.

When switching between oral and intravenous dosage forms, equivalent beta-blocking effect is achieved when doses in a 2.5:1 (Oral:I.V.) ratio is used. For example, if the patient is receiving an oral dose of 25 mg twice daily (50 mg/day), this would translate to 5 mg I.V. every 6 hours; consider reducing initial I.V. dose to evaluate patient response.

Dosing adjustment in renal impairment: No adjustment required.

Dosing adjustment in hepatic impairment: Reduced dose may be necessary

Stability

Injection: Store at controlled room temperature of 25°C (77°F). Protect from light.

Tablet: Store at controlled room temperature of 25°C (77°F). Protect from moisture.

Administration

Oral: Extended release tablets may be divided in half; do not crush or chew.

I.V.: I.V. dose is much smaller than oral dose. When administered acutely for cardiac treatment, monitor ECG and blood pressure; may administer by rapid infusion (I.V. push) over 1 minute. May also be administered by slow infusion (ie, 5-10 mg of metoprolol in 50 mL of fluid) over ~30-60 minutes during less urgent situations (eg, substitution for oral metoprolol).

Monitoring Parameters Acute cardiac treatment: Monitor ECG and blood pressure with I.V. administration; heart rate and blood pressure with oral administration. Necessary monitoring for surgical patients who are unable to take oral beta-blockers (prolonged ileus) has not been defined. Some institutions require monitoring of baseline and postinfusion heart rate and blood pressure when a patient's response to beta-blockade has not been characterized (ie, the patient's initial dose or following a change in dose). Consult individual institutional policies and procedures.

Anesthesia and Critical Care Concerns/Other Considerations

Clinical Pearls/Comments:Surgery: Based on available evidence, beta-blockers should be started days to weeks before elective surgery in selected patients when possible and titrated to a heart rate <65 beats per minute. Additional data suggest that long acting beta-blockers may be superior to short acting ones (Redelmeier, 2005). The ACC/AHA 2007 guidelines on perioperative cardiovascular evaluation and care for noncardiac surgery recommend beta-blockers be continued in patients undergoing surgery who are receiving beta-blockers to treat angina, symptomatic arrhythmias, hypertension, or other ACC/AHA Class I guideline indications (Class I recommendation). The guidelines also recommend that beta-blockers be given to patients undergoing vascular surgery who have myocardial ischemia demonstrated during preoperative testing (Class I recommendation).

The guidelines also state that beta-blockers are probably recommended in patients undergoing intermediate risk (eg, carotid endarterectomy, prostate surgery) or vascular surgery in whom preoperative assessment identifies coronary heart disease or high cardiac risk (Class IIa recommendation). High cardiac risk is defined as having >1 of the following clinical risk factors: History of ischemic heart disease, compensated or prior heart failure, cerebrovascular disease, diabetes mellitus, or renal insufficiency. The use of beta-blockers is uncertain in patients undergoing intermediate risk or vascular surgery with ≤1 clinical risk factor (Class IIb recommendation).

The majority of published trials suggest a benefit of perioperative beta-blocker use during noncardiac surgery; however, more recent clinical trials have not shown a benefit to perioperative beta-blockade for noncardiac surgery (Juul, 2006; POISE Study Group, 2008; Yang, 2006). One such clinical trial randomized 8351 patients with, or at risk of, atherosclerotic disease who underwent noncardiac surgery to either extended release metoprolol succinate or placebo. To receive study drug, first dose (metoprolol extended release 100 mg or matching placebo) administered 2-4 hours prior to surgery, patients were to have a heart rate ≥50 bpm or systolic blood pressure (SBP) ≥100 mm Hg. If during the first 6 hours after surgery heart rate was ≥80 bpm and SBP ≥100 mm Hg, the first postoperative dose (metoprolol extended release 100 mg or matching placebo) was administered. If not given during the first 6 hours, metoprolol extended release 100 mg (or matching placebo) was administered at 6 hours after surgery. Twelve hours after administration of the first postoperative dose, metoprolol extended release 200 mg (or matching placebo) was administered once daily for 30 days. Therefore, patients may have received up to 400 mg during the first 24 hours; an initial dose not recommended for any indication. Study drug was withheld when heart rate was consistently <45 bpm or systolic blood pressure was <100 mm Hg. The primary outcome of the trial was a composite of cardiovascular death, nonfatal MI, and nonfatal cardiac arrest at 30 days after randomization. Compared to those who received placebo, fewer patients receiving metoprolol experienced the primary outcome (244 [5.8%] vs 290 [6.9%], p=0.0399) or developed MI (176 [4.2%] vs 239 [5.7%], p=0.0017). However, more deaths occurred in the metoprolol group compared to placebo (129 [3.1%] vs 97 [2.3%], p=0.0317). In addition, more strokes occurred in the metoprolol group compared to placebo (41 [1%] vs 19 [0.5%], p=0.0053). Death was associated with a number of risk factors (eg, clinically significant hypotension, MI, significant bleeding). Stroke was associated with history of stroke or TIA, postoperative hypotension, new-onset atrial fibrillation, and significant bleeding (POISE Study Group, 2008). The negative results of this trial are thought to be due to the aggressive administration of metoprolol leading to an excessive amount of clinically significant hypotension which then contributed to the incidence of stroke and mortality. Therefore, when administering beta-blockers to eligible patients undergoing elective surgery, patients should be titrated days to weeks in advance when possible and careful monitoring of heart rate (goal <65 bpm) and blood pressure is necessary.

Extemporaneously Prepared: To prepare a metoprolol 10 mg/mL liquid, crush 12 metoprolol tartrate 100 mg tablets into a fine powder. Add ~20 mL of either Ora-Sweet® and Ora-Plus® (1:1 preparation), or Ora-Sweet® SF and Ora-Plus® (1:1 preparation), or cherry syrup. Mix to a uniform paste. Continue to add the vehicle to bring the final volume to 120 mL. The preparation is stable for 60 days; shake well before using and protect from light.

Pregnancy Risk Factor C (manufacturer); D (2nd and 3rd trimesters - expert analysis)

Contraindications

Hypersensitivity to metoprolol, any component of the formulation, or other beta-blockers

Note: Additional contraindications are formulation and/or indication specific.

Immediate release tablets/injectable formulation:

Hypertension and angina: Sinus bradycardia; second- and third-degree heart block; cardiogenic shock; overt heart failure; sick sinus syndrome (except in patients with a functioning artificial pacemaker); severe peripheral arterial disease; pheochromocytoma (without alpha blockade)

Myocardial infarction: Severe sinus bradycardia (heart rate <45 beats/minute); significant first-degree heart block (P-R interval ≥0.24 seconds); second- and third-degree heart block; systolic blood pressure <100 mm Hg; moderate-to-severe cardiac failure

Extended release tablet: Severe bradycardia, second- and third degree heart block; cardiogenic shock; decompensated heart failure; sick sinus syndrome (except in patients with a functioning artificial pacemaker)

Warnings/Precautions [U.S. Boxed Warning]: Beta-blocker therapy should not be withdrawn abruptly (particularly in patients with CAD), but gradually tapered over 1-2 weeks to avoid acute tachycardia, hypertension, and/or ischemia. Consider pre-existing conditions such as sick sinus syndrome before initiating. Metoprolol commonly produces mild first-degree heart block (P-R interval >0.2-0.24 sec). May also produce severe first- (P-R interval ≥0.26 sec), second-, or third-degree heart block. Patients with acute MI (especially right ventricular MI) have a high risk of developing heart block of varying degrees. If severe heart block occurs, metoprolol should be discontinued and measures to increase heart rate should be employed. Symptomatic hypotension may occur with use. Use caution in patients with PVD (can aggravate arterial insufficiency). Use caution with concurrent use of beta-blockers and either verapamil or diltiazem; bradycardia or heart block can occur; avoid concurrent I.V. use of both agents.

In general, beta-blockers should be avoided in patients with bronchospastic disease. Metoprolol, with B_1 selectivity, should be used cautiously in bronchospastic disease with close monitoring. Use cautiously in patients with diabetes because it can mask prominent hypoglycemic symptoms. Use caution in hyperthyroidism since beta-blockade may mask signs of thyrotoxicosis. Use caution with hepatic dysfunction. Use with caution in patients with myasthenia gravis or psychiatric disease (may cause CNS depression). Use caution with inhalation anesthetic agents which may decrease myocardial function. Use of beta-blockers may unmask cardiac failure in patients without a history of dysfunction. Adequate alpha-blockade is required prior to use of any beta-blocker for patients with untreated pheochromocytoma. May induce or exacerbate psoriasis. Use caution with history of severe anaphylaxis to allergens; patients taking beta-blockers may become more sensitive to repeated allergen challenges. Treatment of anaphylaxis (eg, epinephrine) in patients taking beta-blockers may be ineffective or promote undesirable effects. Safety and efficacy have not been established in children <1 year of age.

Extended release: Use with caution in patients with compensated heart failure; monitor for a worsening of heart failure.

Adverse Reactions Frequency may not be defined.

Cardiovascular: Hypotension (1% to 27%), bradycardia (2% to 16%), first-degree heart block (P-R interval ≥0.26 sec; 5%), arterial insufficiency (usually Raynaud type; 1%), chest pain (1%), CHF (1%), edema (peripheral; 1%), palpitation (1%), syncope (1%)

Central nervous system: Dizziness (2% to 10%), fatigue (1% to 10%), depression (5%), confusion, hallucinations, headache, insomnia, memory loss (short-term), nightmares, sleep disturbances, somnolence, vertigo

Dermatology: Pruritus (5%), rash (5%), photosensitivity, psoriasis exacerbated

Endocrine & metabolic: Libido decreased, Peyronie's disease (<1%), diabetes exacerbated

Gastrointestinal: Diarrhea (5%), constipation (1%), flatulence (1%), gastro-intestinal pain (1%), heartburn (1%), nausea (1%), xerostomia (1%), vomiting

Hematologic: Claudication

Neuromuscular & skeletal: Musculoskeletal pain

Ocular: Blurred vision, visual disturbances

Otic: Tinnitus

Respiratory: Dyspnea (1% to 3%), bronchospasm (1%), wheezing (1%), rhinitis

Miscellaneous: Cold extremities (1%)

Postmarketing and/or case reports: Agranulocytosis, alkaline phosphatase increased, alopecia (reversible), arthralgia, arthritis, anxiety, cardiogenic shock, diaphoresis increased, dry eyes, gangrene, hepatitis, HDL decreased, impotence, jaundice, lactate dehydrogenase increased, nervousness, pares-thesia, retroperitoneal fibrosis, second-degree heart block, taste disturbance, third-degree heart block, thrombocytopenia, transaminases increased, triglycer-ides increased, urticaria, vomiting, weight gain

Other events reported with beta-blockers: Catatonia, emotional lability, fever, hypersensitivity reactions, laryngospasm, nonthrombocytopenic purpura, respi-ratory distress, thrombocytopenic purpura

Drug Interactions

Metabolism/Transport Effects Substrate of CYP2C19 (minor), 2D6 (major); **Inhibits** CYP2D6 (weak)

Avoid Concomitant Use

Avoid concomitant use of Metoprolol with any of the following: Methacholine

Increased Effect/Toxicity

Metoprolol may increase the levels/effects of: Alpha-/Beta-Agonists (Direct-Acting); Alpha1-Blockers; Alpha2-Agonists; Amifostine; Antihypertensives; Antipsychotic Agents (Phenothiazines); Cardiac Glycosides; Hypotensive Agents; Insulin; Lidocaine; Methacholine; Midodrine; RiTUXimab; Sulfonylureas

The levels/effects of Metoprolol may be increased by: Acetylcholinesterase Inhibitors; Aminoquinolines (Antimalarial); Amiodarone; Anilidopiperidine Opioids; Antipsychotic Agents (Phenothiazines); Calcium Channel Blockers (Nondihydropyridine); CYP2D6 Inhibitors (Moderate); CYP2D6 Inhibitors (Strong); Darunavir; Diazoxide; Dipyridamole; Disopyramide; Dronedarone; Herbs (Hypotensive Properties); MAO Inhibitors; Pentoxifylline; Phosphodiester-ase 5 Inhibitors; Propafenone; Propoxyphene; Prostacyclin Analogues; QuiNIDine; Reserpine; Selective Serotonin Reuptake Inhibitors

Decreased Effect

Metoprolol may decrease the levels/effects of: Beta2-Agonists; Theophylline Derivatives

The levels/effects of Metoprolol may be decreased by: Barbiturates; Herbs (Hypertensive Properties); Methylphenidate; Nonsteroidal Anti-Inflammatory Agents; Peginterferon Alfa-2b; Rifamycin Derivatives; Yohimbine

Ethanol/Nutrition/Herb Interactions

Food: Food increases absorption. Metoprolol serum levels may be increased if taken with food.

Herb/Nutraceutical: Avoid bayberry, blue cohosh, cayenne, ephedra, ginger, ginseng (American), gotu kola, licorice, (may worsen hypertension). Avoid black cohosh, California poppy, coleus, golden seal, hawthorn, mistletoe, periwinkle, quinine, shepherd's purse (may have increased antihypertensive effect).

Dietary Considerations Regular tablets should be taken with food. Extended release tablets may be taken without regard to meals.

Dosage Forms Excipient information presented when available (limited, particularly for generics); consult specific product labeling.

Injection, solution, as tartrate: 1 mg/mL (5 mL)

Lopressor®: 1 mg/mL (5 mL)

Tablet, as tartrate: 25 mg, 50 mg, 100 mg

Lopressor®: 50 mg, 100 mg

Tablet, extended release, as succinate: 25 mg, 50 mg, 100 mg, 200 mg [expressed as mg equivalent to tartrate]

Toprol-XL®: 25 mg, 50 mg, 100 mg, 200 mg [expressed as mg equivalent to tartrate]

◀ **References**

Allen LV Jr and Erickson III MA, "Stability of Labetalol Hydrochloride, Metoprolol Tartrate, Verapamil Hydrochloride, and Spironolactone With Hydrochlorothiazide in Extemporaneously Compounded Oral Liquids," *Am J Health Syst Pharm*, 1996, 53(19):2304-9.

Fleisher LA, Beckman JA, Brown KA, et al, "ACC/AHA 2006 Guideline Update on Perioperative Cardiovascular Evaluation for Noncardiac Surgery: Focused Update on Perioperative Beta-Blocker Therapy: A Report of the American College of Cardiology/American Heart Association Task Force on Practice Guidelines (Writing Committee to Update the 2002 Guidelines on Perioperative Cardiovascular Evaluation for Noncardiac Surgery) Developed in Collaboration With the American Society of Echocardiography, American Society of Nuclear Cardiology, Heart Rhythm Society, Society of Cardiovascular Anesthesiologists, Society for Cardiovascular Angiography and Interventions, and Society for Vascular Medicine and Biology," *J Am Coll Cardiol*, 2006, 47 (11):2343-55.

Juul AB, Wetterslev J, Gluud C, et al, "Effect of Perioperative Beta-Blockade in Patients With Diabetes Undergoing Major Noncardiac Surgery: Randomized Placebo Controlled, Blinded Multicentre Trial," *BMJ*, 2006, 332(7556):1482.

Lindenauer PK, Pekow P, Wang K, et al, "Perioperative Beta-Blocker Therapy and Mortality After Major Noncardiac Surgery," *N Engl J Med*, 2005, 353(4):349-61.

Mokhlesi B, Leikin JB, Murray P, et al, "Adult Toxicology in Critical Care: Part II: Specific Poisonings," *Chest*, 2003, 123(3):897-922.

Radack K and Deck C, "Beta-Adrenergic Blocker Therapy Does Not Worsen Intermittent Claudication in Subjects With Peripheral Arterial Disease. A Meta-Analysis of Randomized Controlled Trials," *Arch Intern Med*, 1991, 151(9):1769-76.

Yang H, Raymer K, Butler R, et al, "The Effects of Perioperative Beta-Blockade: Results of the Metoprolol After Vascular Surgery (MaVS) Study, A Randomized Controlled Trial," *Am Heart J*, 2006, 152(5):983-90.

◆ **Metoprolol-25 (Can)** *see* Metoprolol *on page 922*

◆ **Metoprolol Succinate** *see* Metoprolol *on page 922*

◆ **Metoprolol Tartrate** *see* Metoprolol *on page 922*

◆ **Metoprolol Tartrate Injection, USP (Can)** *see* Metoprolol *on page 922*

◆ **Metozolv™ ODT** *see* Metoclopramide *on page 917*

◆ **MetroCream®** *see* MetroNIDAZOLE *on page 928*

◆ **MetroGel®** *see* MetroNIDAZOLE *on page 928*

◆ **Metrogel® (Can)** *see* MetroNIDAZOLE *on page 928*

◆ **MetroGel-Vaginal®** *see* MetroNIDAZOLE *on page 928*

◆ **MetroLotion®** *see* MetroNIDAZOLE *on page 928*

MetroNIDAZOLE (met roe NYE da zole)

Medication Safety Issues
Sound-alike/look-alike issues:
MetroNIDAZOLE may be confused with mebendazole, meropenem, metFOR-MIN, methotrexate, metoclopramide, miconazole

Related Information
Helicobacter pylori Treatment *on page 1746*
Prevention of Wound Infection and Sepsis in Surgical Patients *on page 1721*

U.S. Brand Names Flagyl®; Flagyl® 375; Flagyl® ER; MetroCream®; MetroGel-Vaginal®; MetroGel®; MetroLotion®; Noritate®; Vandazole®

Canadian Brand Names Apo-Metronidazole®; Flagyl®; Florazole® ER; MetroCream®; Metrogel®; Nidagel™; Noritate®; Trikacide

Index Terms Metronidazole Hydrochloride

Pharmacologic Category Amebicide; Antibiotic, Miscellaneous; Antibiotic, Topical; Antiprotozoal, Nitroimidazole

Generic Available Yes: Capsule, cream, gel, infusion, lotion, tablet

Use Treatment of susceptible anaerobic bacterial and protozoal infections in the following conditions: Amebiasis, symptomatic and asymptomatic trichomoniasis; skin and skin structure infections, bone and joint infections, CNS infections, endocarditis, gynecologic infections, intra-abdominal infections (as part of combination regimen), respiratory tract infections (lower), systemic anaerobic infections; treatment of antibiotic-associated pseudomembranous colitis (AAPC); as part of a multidrug regimen for *H. pylori* eradication to reduce the risk of duodenal ulcer recurrence; surgical prophylaxis (colorectal)
Topical: Treatment of inflammatory lesions and erythema of rosacea
Vaginal gel: Bacterial vaginosis

Unlabeled/Investigational Use Crohn's disease

Mechanism of Action After diffusing into the organism, interacts with DNA to cause a loss of helical DNA structure and strand breakage resulting in inhibition of protein synthesis and cell death in susceptible organisms

Pharmacodynamics/Kinetics

Absorption: Oral: Well absorbed; Topical: Concentrations achieved systemically after application of 1 g topically are 10 times less than those obtained after a 250 mg oral dose

Distribution: To saliva, bile, seminal fluid, bone, liver, and liver abscesses, lung and vaginal secretions; crosses blood-brain barrier

CSF:blood level ratio: Normal meninges: 16% to 43%; Inflamed meninges: 100%

Protein binding: <20%

Metabolism: Hepatic (30% to 60%)

Half-life elimination: Neonates: 25-75 hours; Others: 6-8 hours, prolonged with hepatic impairment; End-stage renal disease: 21 hours

Time to peak, serum: Oral: Immediate release: 1-2 hours

Excretion: Urine (60% to 80% as unchanged drug); feces (6% to 15%)

Dosage

Infants and Children:

Amebiasis: Oral: 35-50 mg/kg/day in divided doses every 8 hours for 10 days

Trichomoniasis: Oral: 15-30 mg/kg/day in divided doses every 8 hours for 7 days

Anaerobic infections:

Oral: 15-35 mg/kg/day in divided doses every 8 hours

I.V.: 30 mg/kg/day in divided doses every 6 hours

Clostridium difficile (antibiotic-associated colitis): Oral: 20 mg/kg/day divided every 6 hours

Maximum dose: 2 g/day

Adults:

Anaerobic infections (diverticulitis, intra-abdominal, peritonitis, cholangitis, or abscess): Oral, I.V.: 500 mg every 6-8 hours, not to exceed 4 g/day; **Note:** Initial: 1 g I.V. loading dose may be administered

Acne rosacea: Topical:

0.75%: Apply and rub a thin film twice daily, morning and evening, to entire affected areas after washing. Significant therapeutic results should be noticed within 3 weeks. Clinical studies have demonstrated continuing improvement through 9 weeks of therapy.

1%: Apply thin film to affected area once daily

Amebiasis: Oral: 500-750 mg every 8 hours for 5-10 days

Antibiotic-associated pseudomembranous colitis: Oral: 250-500 mg 3-4 times/day for 10-14 days

Note: Due to the emergence of a new strain of *C. difficile*, some clinicians recommend converting to oral vancomycin therapy if the patient does not show a clear clinical response after 2 days of metronidazole therapy.

Giardiasis: 500 mg twice daily for 5-7 days

Helicobacter pylori eradication: Oral: 250-500 mg with meals and at bedtime for 14 days; requires combination therapy with at least one other antibiotic and an acid-suppressing agent (proton pump inhibitor or H_2 blocker)

Bacterial vaginosis or vaginitis due to *Gardnerella*, *Mobiluncus*:

Oral: 500 mg twice daily (regular release) or 750 mg once daily (extended release tablet) for 7 days

Vaginal: 1 applicatorful (~37.5 mg metronidazole) intravaginally once or twice daily for 5 days; apply once in morning and evening if using twice daily, if daily, use at bedtime

Trichomoniasis: Oral: 250 mg every 8 hours for 7 days **or** 375 mg twice daily for 7 days **or** 2 g as a single dose **or** 1 g twice daily for 2 doses (on same day)

Surgical prophylaxis (colorectal): I.V. 15 mg/kg 1 hour prior to surgery; followed by 7.5 mg/kg 6 and 12 hours after initial dose

Elderly: Use lower end of dosing recommendations for adults, do not administer as a single dose

◄ **Dosing adjustment in renal impairment:** Cl_{cr} <10 mL/minute, but not on dialysis: Recommendations vary: To reduce possible accumulation in patients receiving multiple doses, consider reduction to 50% of dose or every 12 hours; **Note:** Dosage reduction is unnecessary in short courses of therapy. Clinical recommendations and practice vary. Some references do not recommend reduction at any level of renal impairment (Lamp, 1999).

Hemodialysis: Extensively removed by hemodialysis and peritoneal dialysis (50% to 100%); dosage reduction not recommended; administer full dose posthemodialysis

Peritoneal dialysis: Dose as for Cl_{cr} <10 mL/minute

Continuous arteriovenous or venovenous hemofiltration: Administer usual dose

Dosing adjustment/comments in hepatic disease: Unchanged in mild liver disease; reduce dosage in severe liver disease

Stability

Injection: Store at controlled room temperature of 15°C to 30°C (59°C to 86°C). Protect from light. Keep in overwrap until ready to use. Product may be refrigerated but crystals may form. Crystals redissolve on warming to room temperature. Prolonged exposure to light will cause a darkening of the product. However, short-term exposure to normal room light does not adversely affect metronidazole stability. Direct sunlight should be avoided. Stability of parenteral admixture at room temperature (25°C); Out of overwrap stability: 30 days. Standard diluent: 500 mg/100 mL NS.

Tablets: Store at room temperature. Protect from light and moisture.

Topical cream, gel, lotion: Store at controlled room temperature of 20°C to 25°C (68°C to 77°C).

Vaginal gel: Store at controlled room temperature of 15°C to 30°C (59°C to 86°C); do not freeze.

Administration

I.V.: Infuse intravenously over 30-60 minutes. Avoid contact of drug solution with equipment containing aluminum.

Oral: May be taken with food to minimize stomach upset. Extended release tablets should be taken on an empty stomach (1 hour before or 2 hours after meals).

Topical: No disulfiram-like reactions have been reported after **topical** application, although metronidazole can be detected in the blood. Apply to clean, dry skin. Cosmetics may be used after application (wait at least 5 minutes after using lotion).

Pregnancy Risk Factor B (may be contraindicated in 1st trimester)

Contraindications Hypersensitivity to metronidazole, nitroimidazole derivatives, or any component of the formulation; pregnancy (first trimester)

Warnings/Precautions Use with caution in patients with severe liver impairment due to potential accumulation, blood dyscrasias; history of seizures, CHF or other sodium-retaining states; reduce dosage in patients with severe liver impairment, CNS disease, and consider dosage reduction in longer-term therapy with severe renal failure (Cl_{cr} <10 mL/minute); if *H. pylori* is not eradicated in patients being treated with metronidazole in a regimen, it should be assumed that metronidazole-resistance has occurred and it should not again be used; aseptic meningitis, encephalopathy, seizures, and neuropathies have been reported especially with increased doses and chronic treatment; monitor and consider discontinuation of therapy if symptoms occur. **[U.S. Boxed Warning]: Possibly carcinogenic based on animal data.** Prolonged use may result in fungal or bacterial superinfection, including *C. difficile*-associated diarrhea (CDAD) and pseudo-membranous colitis; CDAD has been observed >2 months postantibiotic treatment. Candidiasis infection (known or unknown) maybe more prominent during metronidazole treatment, antifungal treatment required.

Adverse Reactions

Systemic: Frequency not defined:

Cardiovascular: Flattening of the T-wave, flushing, syncope

Central nervous system: Aseptic meningitis, ataxia, confusion, coordination impaired, depression, dizziness, encephalopathy, fever, headache, insomnia, irritability, seizure, vertigo

Dermatologic: Erythematous rash, pruritus, Stevens-Johnson syndrome, urticaria

Endocrine & metabolic: Disulfiram-like reaction, dysmenorrhea

Gastrointestinal: Nausea (~12%), anorexia, abdominal cramping, constipation, diarrhea, epigastric distress, furry tongue, glossitis, pancreatitis (rare), proctitis, stomatitis, unusual/metallic taste, vomiting, xerostomia

Genitourinary: Cystitis, darkened urine (rare), dyspareunia, dysuria, incontinence, libido decreased, pelvic pressure, polyuria, vaginal dryness, vaginitis

Hematologic: Neutropenia (reversible), thrombocytopenia (reversible, rare)

Local: Thrombophlebitis

Neuromuscular & skeletal: Dysarthria, peripheral neuropathy, weakness

Ocular: Optic neuropathy

Respiratory: Nasal congestion, pharyngitis, rhinitis, sinusitis, pharyngitis

Miscellaneous: Flu-like syndrome, joint pains resembling serum sickness, moniliasis

Topical: Frequency not defined:

Cardiovascular: Hypertension

Central nervous system: Headache

Dermatologic: Burning, contact dermatitis, dryness, erythema, irritation, pruritus, rash

Gastrointestinal: Constipation, nausea, unusual/metallic taste

Genitourinary: Urinary tract infection

Local: Local allergic reaction

Neuromuscular & skeletal: Tingling/numbness of extremities

Ocular: Eye irritation

Miscellaneous: Flu-like syndrome

Vaginal:

>10%:

Genitourinary: Vaginal discharge (12%)

Miscellaneous: Fungal infection (9% to 12%)

1% to 10%:

Central nervous system: Headache (5% to 7%), dizziness (2%)

Dermatological: Rash (1%)

Endocrine & metabolic: Dysmenorrhea (3%), breast pain (1%), metrorrhagia (1%)

Gastrointestinal: Gastrointestinal discomfort (7%), abdominal pain (5%), nausea and/or vomiting (3% to 4%), unusual/metallic taste (2%), diarrhea (1%)

Genitourinary: Vaginitis (10%), vulva/vaginal irritation (9%), pelvic discomfort (3%)

Hematologic: WBC increased (2%)

Respiratory: Pharyngitis (2%)

<1% (Limited to important or life-threatening): Abdominal bloating, abdominal gas, darkened urine, depression, fatigue, itching, rash, thirst, xerostomia

Drug Interactions

Metabolism/Transport Effects Inhibits CYP2C9 (weak), 3A4 (moderate)

Avoid Concomitant Use

Avoid concomitant use of MetroNIDAZOLE with any of the following: Amprenavir; Everolimus; Tolvaptan

Increased Effect/Toxicity

MetroNIDAZOLE may increase the levels/effects of: Alcohol (Ethyl); Amprenavir; Busulfan; Calcineurin Inhibitors; Colchicine; CYP3A4 Substrates; Eplerenone; Everolimus; FentaNYL; Halofantrine; Pimecrolimus; Ranolazine; Salmeterol; Saxagliptin; Tipranavir; Tolvaptan; Vitamin K Antagonists

The levels/effects of MetroNIDAZOLE may be increased by: Disulfiram; Mebendazole

Decreased Effect

MetroNIDAZOLE may decrease the levels/effects of: Mycophenolate; Typhoid Vaccine

Ethanol/Nutrition/Herb Interactions

Ethanol: The manufacturer recommends to avoid all ethanol or any ethanol-containing drugs (may cause disulfiram-like reaction characterized by flushing, headache, nausea, vomiting, sweating, or tachycardia).

Food: Peak antibiotic serum concentration lowered and delayed, but total drug absorbed not affected.

◀ **Test Interactions** May interfere with AST, ALT, triglycerides, glucose, and LDH testing

Dietary Considerations Take on an empty stomach. Drug may cause GI upset; if GI upset occurs, take with food. Extended release tablets should be taken on an empty stomach (1 hour before or 2 hours after meals). Some products may contain sodium. The manufacturer recommends that ethanol be avoided during treatment and for 3 days after therapy is complete.

Dosage Forms Excipient information presented when available (limited, particularly for generics); consult specific product labeling.

Capsule, oral: 375 mg
  Flagyl® 375: 375 mg
Cream, topical: 0.75% (45 g)
  MetroCream®: 0.75% (45 g) [contains benzyl alcohol]
  Noritate®: 1% (60 g)
Gel, topical: 1% (45 g)
  MetroGel®: 1% (60 g) [60 g tube also packaged in a kit with Cetaphil® skin cleanser]
Gel, vaginal: 0.75% (70 g)
  MetroGel-Vaginal®, Vandazole®: 0.75% (70 g)
Infusion [premixed iso-osmotic sodium chloride solution]: 500 mg (100 mL)
Lotion, topical: 0.75% (60 mL)
  MetroLotion®: 0.75% (60 mL) [contains benzyl alcohol]
Tablet, oral: 250 mg, 500 mg
  Flagyl®: 250 mg, 500 mg
Tablet, extended release, oral:
  Flagyl® ER: 750 mg

References
"Antimicrobial Prophylaxis for Surgery," *Treat Guidel Med Lett*, 2004, 2(20):27-32.

◆ **Metronidazole Hydrochloride** *see* MetroNIDAZOLE *on page 928*

◆ **Mevacor®** *see* Lovastatin *on page 859*

◆ **Mevinolin** *see* Lovastatin *on page 859*

Mexiletine (meks IL e teen)

Related Information
  Antiarrhythmic Drugs *on page 1656*
Canadian Brand Names Novo-Mexiletine
Pharmacologic Category Antiarrhythmic Agent, Class Ib
Use Management of serious ventricular arrhythmias; suppression of PVCs
Unlabeled/Investigational Use Diabetic neuropathy
Pharmacodynamics/Kinetics
  Absorption: Well absorbed; elderly have a slightly slower rate, but extent of absorption is the same as young adults
  Distribution: V_d: 5-7 L/kg
  Protein binding: 50% to 60%
  Metabolism: Hepatic; low first-pass effect
  Bioavailability: 80% to 95%
  Half-life elimination: Adults: 10-14 hours (average: elderly: 14.4 hours, younger adults: 12 hours); prolonged with hepatic impairment or heart failure
  Time to peak, serum: 2-3 hours
  Excretion: Urine (10% to 15% as unchanged drug); urinary acidification increases excretion, alkalinization decreases excretion
Dosage Adults: Oral: Initial: 200 mg every 8 hours (may load with 400 mg if necessary); adjust dose every 2-3 days; usual dose: 200-300 mg every 8 hours; maximum dose: 1.2 g/day (some patients respond to every 12-hour dosing). When switching from another antiarrhythmic, initiate a 200 mg dose 6-12 hours after stopping former agents, 3-6 hours after stopping procainamide.
  Dosage adjustment in hepatic impairment: Reduce dose to 25% to 30% of usual dose
Anesthesia and Critical Care Concerns/Other Considerations As with other antiarrhythmic agents, mexiletine is also proarrhythmic, particularly in patients with underlying cardiovascular disease and electrolyte abnormalities.

Additional Information Complete prescribing information for this medication should be consulted for additional detail.

Dosage Forms Excipient information presented when available (limited, particularly for generics); consult specific product labeling.

Capsule, as hydrochloride: 150 mg, 200 mg, 250 mg

◆ **Mezavant® (Can)** *see* Mesalamine *on page 884*

◆ **MgSO₄ (error-prone abbreviation)** *see* Magnesium Sulfate *on page 863*

◆ **Miacalcin®** *see* Calcitonin *on page 226*

◆ **Miacalcin® NS (Can)** *see* Calcitonin *on page 226*

Micafungin (mi ka FUN gin)

Related Information
Antifungal Agents *on page 1664*
U.S. Brand Names Mycamine®
Canadian Brand Names Mycamine®
Index Terms Micafungin Sodium
Pharmacologic Category Antifungal Agent, Parenteral; Echinocandin
Generic Available No
Use Treatment of esophageal candidiasis; *Candida* prophylaxis in patients undergoing hematopoietic stem cell transplant (HSCT); treatment of candidemia, acute disseminated candidiasis, and other *Candida* infections (peritonitis and abscesses)
Unlabeled/Investigational Use Treatment of infections due to *Aspergillus* spp; prophylaxis of HIV-related esophageal candidiasis
Mechanism of Action Concentration-dependent inhibition of 1,3-beta-D-glucan synthase resulting in reduced formation of 1,3-beta-D-glucan, an essential polysaccharide comprising 30% to 60% of *Candida* cell walls (absent in mammalian cells); decreased glucan content leads to osmotic instability and cellular lysis
Pharmacodynamics/Kinetics
Distribution: 0.28-0.5 L/kg
Protein binding: >99%; primarily to albumin
Metabolism: Hepatic; forms M-1 (catechol) and M-2 (methoxy) metabolites (activity unknown)
Half-life elimination: 11-21 hours
Excretion: Primarily feces (71%); urine (<15%)
Dosage I.V.: Adults:
Candidemia, acute disseminated candidiasis, and *Candida* peritonitis and abscesses: 100 mg daily; mean duration of therapy (from clinical trials) was 15 days (range: 10-47 days)
Esophageal candidiasis: 150 mg daily; mean duration of therapy (from clinical trials) was 15 days (range: 10-30 days)
Prophylaxis of *Candida* infection in hematopoietic stem cell transplantation: 50 mg daily

Dosing adjustment in renal impairment: No adjustment required
Dosing adjustment in hepatic impairment: No dosage adjustment required for moderate hepatic impairment (Child-Pugh score 7-9). Patients with severe hepatic dysfunction have not been studied.
Stability Store at controlled room temperature of 25°C (77°F). Reconstituted and diluted solutions are stable for 24 hours at room temperature. Protect from light. Aseptically add 5 mL of NS (preservative-free) to each 50 or 100 mg vial. Swirl to dissolve; do not shake. Further dilute 50-150 mg in 100 mL NS. Protect from light. Alternatively, D₅W may be used for reconstitution and dilution.
Administration For intravenous use only; infuse over 1 hour. Flush line with NS prior to administration.
Monitoring Parameters Liver function tests
Pregnancy Risk Factor C
Contraindications Hypersensitivity to micafungin, other echinocandins, or any component of the formulation

Warnings/Precautions Anaphylactic reactions, including shock, have been reported. New onset or worsening hepatic failure has been reported; use caution in pre-existing mild-moderate hepatic impairment; safety in severe liver failure has not been evaluated. Hemolytic anemia and hemoglobinuria have been reported. Increased BUN, serum creatinine, renal dysfunction, and/or acute renal failure has been reported; use caution in patients with pre-existing renal impairment and monitor closely. Safety and efficacy in pediatric patients have not been established.

Adverse Reactions Percentages reflect incidence across all approved indications (prophylaxis and treatment); however, in general, a higher frequency of adverse reactions was observed in studies with HSCT patients.

>10%:
Central nervous system: Fever (20%), headache (16%)
Endocrine & metabolic: Hypokalemia (18%), hypomagnesemia (13%)
Gastrointestinal: Diarrhea (23%), nausea (22%), vomiting (22%), mucosal inflammation (14%), constipation (11%)
Hematologic: Thrombocytopenia (15%), neutropenia (14%)

1% to 10%:
Cardiovascular: Hypotension (9%), tachycardia (8%), hypertension (7%), peripheral edema (7%), phlebitis (6%), edema (5%)
Central nervous system: Insomnia (10%), anxiety (6%), fatigue (6%)
Dermatologic: Rash (9%), pruritus (6%)
Endocrine & metabolic: Hypocalcemia (7%), hyperglycemia (6%)
Gastrointestinal: Abdominal pain (10%), anorexia (6%), dyspepsia (6%)
Hematologic: Anemia (10%), febrile neutropenia (6%)
Hepatic: AST increased (6%), ALT increased (5%), serum alkaline phosphatase increased (5%)
Neuromuscular & skeletal: Rigors (9%), back pain (5%)
Respiratory: Cough (8%), dyspnea (6%), epistaxis (6%)
Miscellaneous: Bacteremia (6%), sepsis (5%)

<1% (Limited to important or life-threatening) or frequency not defined: Acidosis, acute renal failure, anuria, apnea, arrhythmia, arthralgia, atrial fibrillation, BUN increased, cardiac arrest, coagulopathy, creatinine increased, cyanosis, deep vein thrombosis, delirium, hypoxia, encephalopathy, erythema multiforme, facial edema, hemoglobinuria, hemolysis, hemolytic anemia, hepatic dysfunction, hepatic failure, hepatocellular damage, hepatomegaly, hiccups, hyperbilirubinemia, hyponatremia, hypoxia, infection, injection site necrosis, injection site thrombosis, intracranial hemorrhage, jaundice, MI, mucosal inflammation, oliguria, pancytopenia, pneumonia, pulmonary embolism, renal impairment, renal tubular necrosis, seizure, shock, skin necrosis, thrombotic thrombocytopenia purpura, thrombophlebitis, urticaria, vasodilatation, WBC decreased

Drug Interactions

Metabolism/Transport Effects Substrate of CYP3A4 (minor); **Inhibits** CYP3A4 (weak)

Avoid Concomitant Use There are no known interactions where it is recommended to avoid concomitant use.

Increased Effect/Toxicity There are no known significant interactions involving an increase in effect.

Decreased Effect
Micafungin may decrease the levels/effects of: Saccharomyces boulardii

Dosage Forms Excipient information presented when available (limited, particularly for generics); consult specific product labeling.
Injection, powder for reconstitution, as sodium [preservative-free]:
Mycamine®: 50 mg, 100 mg [contains lactose]

♦ **Micafungin Sodium** *see* Micafungin *on page 933*

♦ **Micardis®** *see* Telmisartan *on page 1356*

♦ **Microgestin™** *see* Ethinyl Estradiol and Norethindrone *on page 554*

♦ **Microgestin™ Fe** *see* Ethinyl Estradiol and Norethindrone *on page 554*

♦ **microK®** *see* Potassium Chloride *on page 1151*

♦ **microK® 10** *see* Potassium Chloride *on page 1151*

♦ **Micro-K Extencaps® (Can)** *see* Potassium Chloride *on page 1151*

◆ **Micronase® [DSC]** *see* GlyBURIDE *on page* 666
◆ **Microzide®** *see* Hydrochlorothiazide *on page* 696

Midazolam (MID aye zoe lam)

Medication Safety Issues
Sound-alike/look-alike issues:
Versed may be confused with VePesid®, Vistaril®

High alert medication: The Institute for Safe Medication Practices (ISMP) includes this medication among its list of drugs which have a heightened risk of causing significant patient harm when used in error.

Related Information
Anesthesia Considerations for Neurosurgery *on page* 1514
Anesthesia for Geriatric Patients *on page* 1523
Anesthesia for Patients With Liver Disease *on page* 1537
Benzodiazepines *on page* 1666
Chronic Renal Failure *on page* 1552
Intravenous Anesthetic Agents *on page* 1635
Moderate Sedation *on page* 1566
Perioperative Management of Patients on Antiseizure Medication *on page* 1577
Sedative Agents in the Intensive Care Unit *on page* 1690
Status Epilepticus *on page* 1737

Canadian Brand Names Apo-Midazolam®; Midazolam Injection
Index Terms Midazolam Hydrochloride; Versed
Pharmacologic Category Benzodiazepine
Restrictions C-IV
Generic Available Yes

Use Preoperative sedation; moderate sedation prior to diagnostic or radiographic procedures; ICU sedation (continuous infusion); induction and maintenance of general anesthesia

Unlabeled/Investigational Use Anxiety, status epilepticus

Mechanism of Action Binds to stereospecific benzodiazepine receptors on the postsynaptic GABA neuron at several sites within the central nervous system, including the limbic system, reticular formation. Enhancement of the inhibitory effect of GABA on neuronal excitability results by increased neuronal membrane permeability to chloride ions. This shift in chloride ions results in hyperpolarization (a less excitable state) and stabilization.

Pharmacodynamics/Kinetics
Onset of action: I.M.: Sedation: ~15 minutes; I.V.: 1-5 minutes
Peak effect: I.M.: 0.5-1 hour
Duration: I.M.: Up to 6 hours; Mean: 2 hours
Absorption: Oral: Rapid
Distribution: V_d: 0.8-2.5 L/kg; increased with congestive heart failure (CHF) and chronic renal failure
Protein binding: 95%
Metabolism: Extensively hepatic via CYP3A4
Bioavailability: Mean: 45%
Half-life elimination: 1-4 hours; prolonged with cirrhosis, congestive heart failure, obesity, and elderly
Excretion: Urine (as glucuronide conjugated metabolites); feces (~2% to 10%)

Dosage The dose of midazolam needs to be individualized based on the patient's age, underlying diseases, and concurrent medications. Decrease dose (by ~30%) if narcotics or other CNS depressants are administered concomitantly. **Personnel and equipment needed for standard respiratory resuscitation should be immediately available during midazolam administration.**

Children <6 years may require higher doses and closer monitoring than older children; calculate dose on ideal body weight
Conscious sedation for procedures or preoperative sedation:
Oral: 0.25-0.5 mg/kg as a single dose preprocedure, up to a maximum of 20 mg; administer 30-45 minutes prior to procedure. Children <6 years or less cooperative patients may require as much as 1 mg/kg as a single dose; 0.25 mg/kg may suffice for children 6-16 years of age.

◀ Intranasal (not an approved route): 0.2 mg/kg (up to 0.4 mg/kg in some studies), to a maximum of 15 mg; may be administered 30-45 minutes prior to procedure

I.M.: 0.1-0.15 mg/kg 30-60 minutes before surgery or procedure; range 0.05-0.15 mg/kg; doses up to 0.5 mg/kg have been used in more anxious patients; maximum total dose: 10 mg

I.V.:

Infants <6 months: Limited information is available in nonintubated infants; dosing recommendations not clear; infants <6 months are at higher risk for airway obstruction and hypoventilation; titrate dose in small increments to desired effect; monitor carefully

Infants 6 months to Children 5 years: Initial: 0.05-0.1 mg/kg; titrate dose carefully; total dose of 0.6 mg/kg may be required; usual maximum total dose: 6 mg

Children 6-12 years: Initial: 0.025-0.05 mg/kg; titrate dose carefully; total doses of 0.4 mg/kg may be required; usual maximum total dose: 10 mg

Children 12-16 years: Dose as adults; usual maximum total dose: 10 mg

Conscious sedation during mechanical ventilation: Children: Loading dose: 0.05-0.2 mg/kg, followed by initial continuous infusion: 0.06-0.12 mg/kg/hour (1-2 mcg/kg/minute); titrate to the desired effect; usual range: 0.4-6 mcg/kg/minute

Status epilepticus refractory to standard therapy (unlabeled use): Infants >2 months and Children: Loading dose: 0.15 mg/kg followed by a continuous infusion of 0.06 mg/kg/hour (1 mcg/kg/min); titrate dose upward every 5 minutes until clinical seizure activity is controlled; mean infusion rate required in 24 children was 0.14 mg/kg/hour (2.3 mcg/kg/minute) with a range of 0.06-1.1 mg/kg/hour (Rivera, 1993)

Adults:

Preoperative sedation:

I.M.: 0.07-0.08 mg/kg 30-60 minutes prior to surgery/procedure; usual dose: 5 mg; **Note:** Reduce dose in patients with COPD, high-risk patients, patients ≥60 years of age, and patients receiving other narcotics or CNS depressants

I.V.: 0.02-0.04 mg/kg; repeat every 5 minutes as needed to desired effect or up to 0.1-0.2 mg/kg

Intranasal (not an approved route): 0.2 mg/kg (up to 0.4 mg/kg in some studies); administer 30-45 minutes prior to surgery/procedure

Conscious sedation: I.V.: Initial: 0.5-2 mg slow I.V. over at least 2 minutes; slowly titrate to effect by repeating doses every 2-3 minutes if needed; usual total dose: 2.5-5 mg; use decreased doses in elderly

Healthy Adults <60 years: Some patients respond to doses as low as 1 mg; no more than 2.5 mg should be administered over a period of 2 minutes. Additional doses of midazolam may be administered after a 2-minute waiting period and evaluation of sedation after each dose increment. A total dose >5 mg is generally not needed. If narcotics or other CNS depressants are administered concomitantly, the midazolam dose should be reduced by 30%.

Anesthesia: I.V.:

Induction:

Unpremedicated patients: 0.3-0.35 mg/kg (up to 0.6 mg/kg in resistant cases)

Premedicated patients: 0.15-0.35 mg/kg

Maintenance: 0.05-0.3 mg/kg as needed, or continuous infusion 0.25-1.5 mcg/kg/minute

Sedation in mechanically-ventilated patients: I.V. continuous infusion: 100 mg in 250 mL D₅W or NS (if patient is fluid-restricted, may concentrate up to a maximum of 0.5 mg/mL); initial dose: 0.02-0.08 mg/kg (~1 mg to 5 mg in 70 kg adult) initially and repeated at 5- to 15-minute intervals until adequate sedation is achieved; may use continuous infusion to maintain sedation; usual dosage range for continuous infusion: 0.04-0.2 mg/kg/hour (Jacobi, 2002). Titrate to reach desired level of sedation.

Refractory status epilepticus (unlabeled use): I.V.: 0.15-0.3 mg/kg (usual dose: 5-15 mg); may repeat every 10-15 minutes as needed **or** continuous infusion of 0.05-0.6 mg/kg/hour

Elderly: I.V.: Conscious sedation: Initial: 0.5 mg slow I.V.; give no more than 1.5 mg in a 2-minute period; if additional titration is needed, give no more than

1 mg over 2 minutes, waiting another 2 or more minutes to evaluate sedative effect; a total dose of >3.5 mg is rarely necessary

Dosage adjustment in renal impairment:
Hemodialysis: Supplemental dose is not necessary
Peritoneal dialysis: Significant drug removal is unlikely based on physiochemical characteristics

Stability The manufacturer states that midazolam, at a final concentration of 0.5 mg/mL, is stable for up to 24 hours when diluted with D_5W or NS. A final concentration of 1 mg/mL in NS has been documented to be stable for up to 10 days (McMullen, 1995). Admixtures do not require protection from light for short-term storage.

Administration

Intranasal: Administer using a 1 mL needleless syringe into the nostrils over 15 seconds; use the 5 mg/mL injection; 1/2 of the dose may be administered to each nostril

Oral: Do not mix with any liquid (such as grapefruit juice) prior to administration
Parenteral:
I.M.: Administer deep I.M. into large muscle.
I.V.: Administer by slow I.V. injection over at least 2-5 minutes at a concentration of 1-5 mg/mL or by I.V. infusion. Continuous infusions should be administered via an infusion pump.

Monitoring Parameters Respiratory and cardiovascular status, blood pressure, blood pressure monitor required during I.V. administration

Anesthesia and Critical Care Concerns/Other Considerations

Clinical Pearls/Comments: Midazolam may accumulate in patients who are obese or in patients with hypoalbuminemia or renal failure. Concurrent use of CYP3A4 inhibitors may inhibit metabolism of midazolam and prolong its sedative effects.

In healthy volunteers, the combination of midazolam (0.05 mg/kg) with fentanyl (2 mcg/kg) produces synergistic respiratory depression (92% incidence of hypoxemia (SaO_2 <90%) and 50% incidence of apnea (Bailey, 1990).

Evidence-Based Information: Agitation in the ICU Patient: Diazepam or midazolam is recommended for rapid sedation of the acutely-agitated patient. The 2002 ACCM/SCCM task force does not recommend midazolam use for ongoing sedation in the critically-ill adult. Midazolam is 3-4 times as potent as diazepam. Paradoxical reactions associated with midazolam use in children (eg, agitation, restlessness, combativeness) have been successfully treated with flumazenil.

Pregnancy Risk Factor D

Contraindications Hypersensitivity to midazolam or any component of the formulation, including benzyl alcohol (cross-sensitivity with other benzodiazepines may exist); parenteral form is not for intrathecal or epidural injection; narrow-angle glaucoma; concurrent use of potent inhibitors of CYP3A4 (amprenavir, atazanavir, or ritonavir); pregnancy

Warnings/Precautions [U.S. Boxed Warning]: May cause severe respiratory depression, respiratory arrest, or apnea. Use with extreme caution, particularly in noncritical care settings. Appropriate resuscitative equipment and qualified personnel must be available for administration and monitoring. Initial dosing must be cautiously titrated and individualized, particularly in elderly or debilitated patients, patients with hepatic impairment (including alcoholics), or in renal impairment, particularly if other CNS depressants (including opiates) are used concurrently. **[U.S. Boxed Warning]: Initial doses in elderly or debilitated patients should be conservative; as little as 1 mg, but not to exceed 2.5 mg.** Use with caution in patients with respiratory disease or impaired gag reflex. Use during upper airway procedures may increase risk of hypoventilation. Prolonged responses have been noted following extended administration by continuous infusion (possibly due to metabolite accumulation) or in the presence of drugs which inhibit midazolam metabolism.

Causes CNS depression (dose-related) resulting in sedation, dizziness, confusion, or ataxia which may impair physical and mental capabilities. Patients must be cautioned about performing tasks which require mental alertness (eg, operating machinery or driving). A minimum of 1 day should elapse after

◄ midazolam administration before attempting these tasks. Use with caution in patients receiving other CNS depressants or psychoactive agents. Effects with other sedative drugs or ethanol may be potentiated. Benzodiazepines have been associated with falls and traumatic injury and should be used with extreme caution in patients who are at risk of these events (especially the elderly).

May cause hypotension - hemodynamic events are more common in pediatric patients or patients with hemodynamic instability. Hypotension and/or respiratory depression may occur more frequently in patients who have received opioid analgesics. Use with caution in obese patients, chronic renal failure, and HF. Does not protect against increases in heart rate or blood pressure during intubation. Should not be used in shock, coma, or acute alcohol intoxication. **[U.S. Boxed Warning]: Parenteral form contains benzyl alcohol; avoid rapid injection in neonates or prolonged infusions.** Avoid intra-arterial administration or extravasation of parenteral formulation.

Midazolam causes anterograde amnesia. Paradoxical reactions, including hyperactive or aggressive behavior have been reported with benzodiazepines, particularly in adolescent/pediatric or psychiatric patients. Does not have analgesic, antidepressant, or antipsychotic properties.

Benzodiazepines have been associated with dependence and acute withdrawal symptoms on discontinuation or reduction in dose. Acute withdrawal, including seizures, may be precipitated after administration of flumazenil to patients receiving long-term benzodiazepine therapy.

Adverse Reactions As reported in adults unless otherwise noted:

>10%: Respiratory: Decreased tidal volume and/or respiratory rate decrease, apnea (3% children)

1% to 10%:

Cardiovascular: Hypotension (3% children)

Central nervous system: Drowsiness (1%), oversedation, headache (1%), seizure-like activity (1% children)

Gastrointestinal: Nausea (3%), vomiting (3%)

Local: Pain and local reactions at injection site (4% I.M., 5% I.V.; severity less than diazepam)

Ocular: Nystagmus (1% children)

Respiratory: Cough (1%)

Miscellaneous: Physical and psychological dependence with prolonged use, hiccups (4%, 1% children), paradoxical reaction (2% children)

<1% (Limited to important or life-threatening): Agitation, amnesia, bigeminy, bronchospasm, emergence delirium, euphoria, hallucinations, laryngospasm, rash

Drug Interactions

Metabolism/Transport Effects Substrate of CYP2B6 (minor), 3A4 (major); **Inhibits** CYP2C8 (weak), 2C9 (weak), 3A4 (weak)

Avoid Concomitant Use

Avoid concomitant use of Midazolam with any of the following: Atazanavir; Efavirenz; Fosamprenavir

Increased Effect/Toxicity

Midazolam may increase the levels/effects of: Alcohol (Ethyl); Clozapine; CNS Depressants; Methotrimeprazine; Phenytoin

The levels/effects of Midazolam may be increased by: Antifungal Agents (Azole Derivatives, Systemic); Aprepitant; Atazanavir; Atorvastatin; Calcium Channel Blockers (Nondihydropyridine); Cimetidine; CYP3A4 Inhibitors (Moderate); CYP3A4 Inhibitors (Strong); Dasatinib; Disulfiram; Efavirenz; Fluconazole; Fosamprenavir; Fosaprepitant; Grapefruit Juice; Isoniazid; Macrolide Antibiotics; Methotrimeprazine; Nefazodone; Oral Contraceptive (Estrogens); Oral Contraceptive (Progestins); Protease Inhibitors; Proton Pump Inhibitors; Selective Serotonin Reuptake Inhibitors

Decreased Effect

The levels/effects of Midazolam may be decreased by: CarBAMazepine; CYP3A4 Inducers (Strong); Deferasirox; Ginkgo Biloba; Rifamycin Derivatives; St Johns Wort; Theophylline Derivatives; Yohimbine

Ethanol/Nutrition/Herb Interactions

Ethanol: Avoid ethanol (may increase CNS depression).

Food: Grapefruit juice may increase serum concentrations of midazolam; avoid concurrent use with oral form.

Herb/Nutraceutical: Avoid concurrent use with St John's wort (may decrease midazolam levels, may increase CNS depression). Avoid concurrent use with valerian, kava kava, gotu kola (may increase CNS depression).

Dietary Considerations Avoid grapefruit juice with oral syrup.

Dosage Forms Excipient information presented when available (limited, particularly for generics); consult specific product labeling.

Injection, solution: 1 mg/mL (2 mL, 5 mL, 10 mL); 5 mg/mL (1 mL, 2 mL, 5 mL, 10 mL) [contains benzyl alcohol 1%]

Injection, solution [preservative free]: 1 mg/mL (2 mL, 5 mL); 5 mg/mL (1 mL, 2 mL)

Syrup: 2 mg/mL (118 mL) [contains sodium benzoate; cherry flavor]

References

Bailey PL, Pace NL, Ashburn MA, et al, "Frequent Hypoxemia and Apnea After Sedation With Midazolam and Fentanyl," *Anesthesiology*, 1990, 73(5):826-30.

Hughes J, Gill A, Leach HJ, et al, "A Prospective Study of the Adverse Effects of Midazolam on Withdrawal in Critically Ill Children," *Acta Paediatr*, 1994, 83(11):1194-9.

Jacobi J, Fraser GL, Coursin DB, et al, "Clinical Practice Guidelines for the Sustained Use of Sedatives and Analgesics in the Critically Ill Adult," *Crit Care Med*, 2002, 30(1):119-41. Available at: http://www.sccm.org/pdf/sedatives.pdf.

Mokhlesi B, Leikin JB, Murray P, et al, "Adult Toxicology in Critical Care. Part II: Specific Poisonings," *Chest*, 2003, 123(3):897-922.

Rivera R, Segnini M, Baltodano A, et al, "Midazolam in the Treatment of Status Epilepticus in Children," *Crit Care Med*, 1993, 21(7):991-4.

◆ **Midazolam Hydrochloride** *see* Midazolam *on page* 935

◆ **Midazolam Injection (Can)** *see* Midazolam *on page* 935

Midodrine (MI doe dreen)

Medication Safety Issues

Sound-alike/look-alike issues:

Midodrine may be confused with Midrin®, minoxidil

ProAmatine® may be confused with protamine

U.S. Brand Names ProAmatine®

Canadian Brand Names Amatine®; Apo-Midodrine®

Index Terms Midodrine Hydrochloride

Pharmacologic Category Alpha$_1$ Agonist

Generic Available Yes

Use Orphan drug: Treatment of symptomatic orthostatic hypotension

Unlabeled/Investigational Use Management of urinary incontinence; vasovagal syncope; prevention of dialysis-induced hypotension

Mechanism of Action Midodrine forms an active metabolite, desglymidodrine, which is an alpha$_1$-agonist. This agent increases arteriolar and venous tone resulting in a rise in standing, sitting, and supine systolic and diastolic blood pressure in patients with orthostatic hypotension.

Pharmacodynamics/Kinetics

Onset of action: ~1 hour

Duration: 2-3 hours

Absorption: Rapid

Distribution: V_d (desglymidodrine): <1.6 L/kg; poorly across membrane (eg, blood brain barrier)

Protein binding: Minimal

Metabolism: Hepatic and many other tissues; midodrine is a prodrug which undergoes rapid deglycination to desglymidodrine (active metabolite)

Bioavailability: Desglymidodrine: 93%

Half-life elimination: Desglymidodrine: ~3-4 hours; Midodrine: 25 minutes

Time to peak, serum: Desglymidodrine: 1-2 hours; Midodrine: 30 minutes

Excretion: Urine (Midodrine: Insignificant; Desglymidodrine: 80% by active renal secretion)

◀ **Dosage** Adults: Oral:

Orthostatic hypotension: 10 mg 3 times/day during daytime hours (every 3-4 hours) when patient is upright (maximum: 40 mg/day)

Prevention of hemodialysis-induced hypotension (unlabeled use): 2.5-10 mg given 15-30 minutes prior to dialysis session (Cruz, 1998; Prakash, 2004; KDOQI, 2005)

Vasovagal syncope (unlabeled use): Initial: 5 mg 3 times/day during daytime hours (every 6 hours) increased up to 15 mg/dose if necessary (Ward, 1998; Perez-Lugones, 2001)

Dosing adjustment in renal impairment: Orthostatic hypotension: 2.5 mg 3 times/day, gradually increasing as tolerated

Hemodialysis: Dialyzable; dose after hemodialysis unless used for prevention of hemodialysis-induced hypotension.

Administration Doses may be given in approximately 3- to 4-hour intervals (eg, shortly before or upon rising in the morning, at midday, in the late afternoon not later than 6 PM). Avoid dosing after the evening meal or within 4 hours of bedtime. Continue therapy only in patients who appear to attain symptomatic improvement during initial treatment. Standing systolic blood pressure may be elevated 15-30 mm Hg at 1 hour after a 10 mg dose. Some effect may persist for 2-3 hours.

Monitoring Parameters Blood pressure, renal and hepatic function

Pregnancy Risk Factor C

Contraindications Hypersensitivity to midodrine or any component of the formulation; severe organic heart disease; acute renal failure; urinary retention; pheochromocytoma; thyrotoxicosis; persistent and significant supine hypertension

Warnings/Precautions [U.S. Boxed Warning]: Indicated for patients for whom orthostatic hypotension significantly impairs their daily life despite standard clinical care. May cause hypertension. Use is not recommended with supine hypertension. May slow heart rate primarily due to vagal reflex. Use caution when administered concurrently with negative chronotropes (eg, digoxin, beta blockers). Use is not recommended with supine hypertension. Use cautiously in patients with renal impairment and initiate with a reduced dose; contraindicated in patients with acute renal failure. Caution should be exercised in patients with diabetes, visual problems (especially if receiving fludrocortisone), urinary retention (reduce initial dose), or hepatic dysfunction; monitor renal and hepatic function prior to and periodically during therapy; safety and efficacy have not been established in children.

Adverse Reactions

>10%:

Cardiovascular: Supine hypertension (7% to 13%)

Dermatologic: Piloerection (13%), pruritus (12%)

Genitourinary: Urinary urgency, retention, or polyuria, dysuria (up to 13%)

Neuromuscular & skeletal: Paresthesia (18%)

1% to 10%:

Central nervous system: Chills (5%), pain (5%)

Dermatologic: Rash (2%)

Gastrointestinal: Abdominal pain

<1% (Limited to important or life-threatening): Anxiety, backache, canker sore, confusion, dizziness, dry skin, erythema multiforme, facial flushing, flatulence, flushing, GI distress, headache, heartburn, hyperesthesia, insomnia, ICP increased, leg cramps, nausea, somnolence, visual field defect, weakness, xerostomia

Drug Interactions

Avoid Concomitant Use

Avoid concomitant use of Midodrine with any of the following: Iobenguane I 123; MAO Inhibitors

Increased Effect/Toxicity

Midodrine may increase the levels/effects of: Sympathomimetics

The levels/effects of Midodrine may be increased by: Atomoxetine; Beta-Blockers; Calcium Channel Blockers (Nondihydropyridine); Cannabinoids; Cardiac Glycosides; MAO Inhibitors; Tricyclic Antidepressants

Decreased Effect

Midodrine may decrease the levels/effects of: Iobenguane I 123

Dosage Forms Excipient information presented when available (limited, particularly for generics); consult specific product labeling.

Tablet, as hydrochloride: 2.5 mg, 5 mg, 10 mg

ProAmatine®: 2.5 mg, 5 mg, 10 mg [scored]

♦ **Midodrine Hydrochloride** *see* Midodrine *on page 939*

♦ **Midol® Cramp and Body Aches [OTC]** *see* Ibuprofen *on page 717*

♦ **Midol® Extended Relief [OTC]** *see* Naproxen *on page 987*

♦ **Millipred™** *see* PrednisoLONE *on page 1164*

Milrinone (MIL ri none)

Medication Safety Issues

Sound-alike/look-alike issues:

Primacor® may be confused with Primaxin®

High alert medication: The Institute for Safe Medication Practices (ISMP) includes this medication among its list of drugs which have a heightened risk of causing significant patient harm when used in error.

Related Information

Heart Failure (Systolic) *on page 1739*

Hemodynamic Support, Intravenous *on page 1681*

U.S. Brand Names Primacor® [DSC]

Canadian Brand Names Milrinone Lactate Injection; Primacor®

Index Terms Milrinone Lactate

Pharmacologic Category Phosphodiesterase Enzyme Inhibitor

Generic Available Yes

Use Short-term I.V. therapy of acutely-decompensated heart failure

Unlabeled/Investigational Use Inotropic therapy for patients unresponsive to other acute heart failure therapies (eg, dobutamine); outpatient inotropic therapy for heart transplant candidates; palliation of symptoms in end-stage heart failure patients who cannot otherwise be discharged from the hospital and are not transplant candidates

Mechanism of Action A selective phosphodiesterase inhibitor in cardiac and vascular tissue, resulting in vasodilation and inotropic effects with little chronotropic activity.

Pharmacodynamics/Kinetics

Onset of action: I.V.: 5-15 minutes

Distribution: V_{dss}: 0.32-0.45 L/kg

Protein binding, plasma: ~70%

Metabolism: Hepatic (12%)

Half-life elimination: Normal renal function: ~2.5 hours; CVVH: 20.1 hours (Taniguchi, 2000)

Excretion: Urine (85% as unchanged drug) within 24 hours; active tubular secretion is a major elimination pathway for milrinone

Dosage Adults: I.V.: Loading dose (optional): 50 mcg/kg administered over 10 minutes followed by a maintenance dose titrated according to the hemodynamic and clinical response; Maintenance dose: I.V. infusion: 0.375-0.75 mcg/kg/minute.

Dosing adjustment in renal impairment:

Cl_{cr} 50 mL/minute: Administer 0.43 mcg/kg/minute

Cl_{cr} 40 mL/minute: Administer 0.38 mcg/kg/minute

Cl_{cr} 30 mL/minute: Administer 0.33 mcg/kg/minute

Cl_{cr} 20 mL/minute: Administer 0.28 mcg/kg/minute

Cl_{cr} 10 mL/minute: Administer 0.23 mcg/kg/minute

Cl_{cr} 5 mL/minute: Administer 0.2 mcg/kg/minute

Stability Store at 15°C to 30°C (59°F to 86°F); avoid freezing. Stable at 0.2 mg/mL in 1/2NS, NS, or D_5W for 72 hours at room temperature in normal light.

Standard dilution: For a final concentration of 0.2 mg/mL: Dilute Primacor® 1 mg/mL (20 mL) with 80 mL diluent (final volume: 100 mL). May also dilute 1 mg/mL (10 mL) with 40 mL diluent (final volume: 50 mL).

◄ **Administration** Infuse via infusion pump

Monitoring Parameters Platelet count, CBC, electrolytes (especially potassium and magnesium), liver function and renal function tests; ECG, CVP, SBP, DBP, heart rate; infusion site

If pulmonary artery catheter is in place, monitor cardiac index, stroke volume, systemic vascular resistance, pulmonary capillary wedge pressure and pulmonary vascular resistance.

Anesthesia and Critical Care Concerns/Other Considerations

Clinical Pearls/Comments: If hypotension is a problem, loading doses may be omitted and maintenance infusions initiated. There is some delay in hemodynamic effects, but it is minimal (1-3 hours). Lower initial maintenance infusions have also been used (0.18-0.25 mcg/kg/minute).

Evidence-Based Information: Milrinone is ~85% renally eliminated and therefore requires dosage adjustment in patients with renal impairment. In patients with decompensated heart failure receiving CVVH, it has been demonstrated that milrinone continuous infusions (0.25 mcg/kg/minute) resulted in steady-state concentrations >4 times the concentrations obtained in patients with normal renal function. In addition, the half-life is prolonged (~20.1 hours vs 2.5 hours) (Taniguchi, 2000).

Pregnancy Risk Factor C

Contraindications Hypersensitivity to milrinone, inamrinone, or any component of the formulation; concurrent use of inamrinone

Warnings/Precautions Monitor closely for hypotension. Avoid in severe obstructive aortic or pulmonic valvular disease. Milrinone may aggravate outflow tract obstruction in hypertrophic subaortic stenosis. Supraventricular and ventricular arrhythmias have developed in high-risk patients. Ensure that ventricular rate controlled in atrial fibrillation/flutter prior to initiating milrinone. Not recommended for use in acute MI patients. Monitor and correct fluid and electrolyte problems. Adjust dose in renal dysfunction. Discontinue therapy if dose-related elevations in LFTs and clinical symptoms of hepatotoxicity occur.

Adverse Reactions

>10%: Cardiovascular: Ventricular arrhythmia (ectopy 9%, NSVT 3%, sustained ventricular tachycardia 1%, ventricular fibrillation <1%)

1% to 10%:

Cardiovascular: Supraventricular arrhythmia (4%), hypotension (3%), angina/chest pain (1%)

Central nervous system: Headache (3%)

<1% (Limited to important or life-threatening): Anaphylaxis, atrial fibrillation, bronchospasm, hypokalemia, injection site reaction, liver function abnormalities, MI, rash, thrombocytopenia, torsade de pointes, tremor, ventricular fibrillation

Drug Interactions

Avoid Concomitant Use There are no known interactions where it is recommended to avoid concomitant use.

Increased Effect/Toxicity There are no known significant interactions involving an increase in effect.

Decreased Effect There are no known significant interactions involving a decrease in effect.

Dosage Forms Excipient information presented when available (limited, particularly for generics); consult specific product labeling. [DSC] = Discontinued product

Infusion [premixed in D_5W]: 200 mcg/mL (100 mL, 200 mL)

Primacor®: 200 mcg/mL (200 mL) [DSC]

Injection, solution: 1 mg/mL (10 mL, 20 mL, 50 mL)

References

Cuffe MS, Califf RM, Adams KF Jr, et al, "Short-Term Intravenous Milrinone for Acute Exacerbation of Chronic Heart Failure: A Randomized Controlled Trial," *JAMA*, 2002, 287(12):1541-7.

Hunt SA, Abraham WT, Chin MH, et al, "ACC/AHA 2005 Guideline Update for the Diagnosis and Management of Chronic Heart Failure in the Adult: A Report of the American College of Cardiology/American Heart Association Task Force on Practice Guidelines (Writing Committee to Update the 2001 Guidelines for the Evaluation and Management of Heart Failure)." Available at http://www.acc.org/qualityandscience/clinical/guidelines/failure/index.pdf.

Pamboukian SV, Carere RG, Webb JG, et al, "The Use of Milrinone in Pretransplant Assessment of Patients With Congestive Heart Failure and Pulmonary Hypertension," *J Heart Lung Transplant*, 1999, 18(4):367-71.

Taniguchi T, Shibata K, Saito S, et al, "Pharmacokinetics of Milrinone in Patients With Congestive Heart Failure During Continuous Venovenous Hemofiltration," *Intensive Care Med*, 2000, 26 (8):1089-93.

- ◆ **Milrinone Lactate** *see* Milrinone *on page 941*
- ◆ **Milrinone Lactate Injection (Can)** *see* Milrinone *on page 941*
- ◆ **Minestrin™ 1/20 (Can)** *see* Ethinyl Estradiol and Norethindrone *on page 554*
- ◆ **Minirin® (Can)** *see* Desmopressin *on page 386*
- ◆ **Minitran™** *see* Nitroglycerin *on page 1014*
- ◆ **Min-Ovral® (Can)** *see* Ethinyl Estradiol and Levonorgestrel *on page 549*
- ◆ **Minox (Can)** *see* Minoxidil *on page 943*

Minoxidil (mi NOKS i dil)

Medication Safety Issues
Sound-alike/look-alike issues:
Loniten® may be confused with Lipitor®
Minoxidil may be confused with metolazone, midodrine, Minipress®, Minocin®, Monopril®, Noxafil®

International issues:
Noxidil® [Thailand] may be confused with Noxafil® which is a brand name for posaconazole in the U.S.

Related Information
Hypertension *on page 1754*

U.S. Brand Names Rogaine® Extra Strength for Men [OTC]; Rogaine® for Men [OTC]; Rogaine® for Women [OTC]

Canadian Brand Names Apo-Gain®; Loniten®; Minox; Rogaine®

Pharmacologic Category Topical Skin Product; Vasodilator, Direct-Acting

Generic Available Yes: Excludes aerosol, topical solution

Use Management of severe hypertension (usually in combination with a diuretic and beta-blocker); treatment (topical formulation) of alopecia androgenetica in males and females

Mechanism of Action Produces vasodilation by directly relaxing arteriolar smooth muscle, with little effect on veins; effects may be mediated by cyclic AMP; stimulation of hair growth is secondary to vasodilation, increased cutaneous blood flow and stimulation of resting hair follicles

Pharmacodynamics/Kinetics
Onset of action: Hypotensive: Oral: ~30 minutes
 Peak effect: 2-8 hours
Duration: 2-5 days
Protein binding: None
Metabolism: 88%, primarily via glucuronidation
Bioavailability: Oral: 90%
Half-life elimination: Adults: 3.5-4.2 hours
Excretion: Urine (12% as unchanged drug)

Dosage
Children <12 years: Hypertension: Oral: Initial: 0.1-0.2 mg/kg once daily; maximum: 5 mg/day; increase gradually every 3 days; usual dosage range: 0.25-1 mg/kg/day in 1-2 divided doses; maximum: 50 mg/day
Children ≥12 years and Adults: Hypertension: Oral: Initial: 5 mg once daily, increase gradually every 3 days (maximum: 100 mg/day); usual dosage range (JNC 7): 2.5-80 mg/day in 1-2 divided doses
 Note: Dosage adjustment is needed when added to concomitant therapy.
Adults: Alopecia: Topical: Apply twice daily; 4 months of therapy may be necessary for hair growth.
Elderly: Hypertension: Oral: Initial: 2.5 mg once daily; increase gradually.

Dosing adjustment in renal impairment: Patient with renal failure and/or receiving dialysis may require dosage reduction.
Supplemental dose is not necessary after hemo- or peritoneal dialysis.

▶

◀ **Stability**
Tablet: Store at controlled room temperature of 15°C to 30°C (59°F to 86°F).
Topical: Store at controlled room temperature of 20°C to 25°C (68°F to 77°F).

Monitoring Parameters Blood pressure, standing and sitting/supine; fluid and electrolyte balance and body weight should be monitored. Any tests that are abnormal at the time of initiation (including, renal function tests, ECG, echocardiogram, chest x-ray) should be repeated initially every 1-3 months then every 6-12 months once stable.

Pregnancy Risk Factor C

Contraindications Hypersensitivity to minoxidil or any component of the formulation; pheochromocytoma

Warnings/Precautions **[U.S. Boxed Warning]: Minoxidil may cause pericarditis and pericardial effusion that may progress to tamponade;** patients with renal impairment not on dialysis may be at higher risk. Observe patients closely. **[U.S. Boxed Warning]: May increase oxygen demand and exacerbate angina pectoris;** concomitant use with a beta-blocker (if no contraindication exists may help reduce the effect. Use with caution in patients with pulmonary hypertension, significant renal failure, or HF; use with caution in patients with coronary artery disease or recent myocardial infarction; renal failure or dialysis patients may require smaller doses; usually used with a beta-blocker (to treat minoxidil-induced tachycardia) and a diuretic (for treatment of water retention/edema. Compared to placebo minoxidil increased the frequency of clinical events, including increased need for diuretics, angina, ventricular arrhythmias, worsening heart failure and death (Franciosa, 1984). Use with caution in the elderly; initiate at the low end of the dosage range and monitor closely.

[U.S. Boxed Warning]: Maximum therapeutic doses of a diuretic and two antihypertensives should be used before this drug is ever added. Should be given with a diuretic to minimize fluid gain and a beta-blocker (if no contraindications) to prevent tachycardia. Anyone with malignant hypertension should be hospitalized with close medical supervision to ensure blood pressure is reducing and to prevent too rapid of a reduction in blood pressure. Inform patients of excessive hair growth before initiating therapy; may take 1-6 months for hypertrichosis to reverse itself after discontinuation of the drug.

Adverse Reactions

Oral: Incidence of reactions not always reported.
Cardiovascular: ECG changes (T-wave changes 60%), peripheral edema (7%), pericardial effusion with tamponade (3%), pericardial effusion without tamponade (3%), angina pectoris, heart failure, pericarditis, rebound hypertension (in children after a gradual withdrawal), sodium and water retention, tachycardia
Dermatologic: Hypertrichosis (common; 80%), bullous eruption (rare), rash, Stevens-Johnson syndrome (rare)
Endocrine & metabolic: Breast tenderness (rare; <1%)
Gastrointestinal: Nausea, vomiting, weight gain
Hematologic: Leukopenia (rare), thrombocytopenia (rare), transient decreased erythrocyte count (hemodilution), transient decreased hematocrit/hemoglobin (hemodilution)
Hepatic: Increased alkaline phosphatase
Renal: Transient increase in serum BUN and creatinine
Respiratory: Pulmonary edema
Topical: Incidence of adverse events is not always reported.
Cardiovascular: Blood pressure increased/decreased, cardiac output increased, chest pain (transient), edema, left ventricular mass increased, left ventricular end-diastolic volume increased, palpitation, tachycardia
Central nervous system: Anxiety (rare), dizziness, faintness, headache, mental depression (rare), taste alterations
Dermatologic: Allergic contact dermatitis (7.4%), alopecia, dryness, eczema, exacerbation of hair loss, flushing, folliculitis; hair growth increased outside the area of application (face, beard, eyebrows, ear, arm); hypertrichosis, local erythema, papular rash, pruritus, scaling/flaking, seborrhea
Endocrine & metabolic: Menstrual changes

Gastrointestinal: Diarrhea, nausea

Genitourinary: Urinary tract infection (rare), renal calculi (rare), urethritis (rare), prostatitis (rare), epididymitis (rare), impotence (rare)

Hematologic: Lymphadenopathy, thrombocytopenia

Neuromuscular & skeletal: Fractures, back pain, retrosternal chest pain of muscular origin, tendonitis (2.6%), weakness

Ocular: Conjunctivitis, visual disturbances, decreased visual acuity

Respiratory: Bronchitis, upper respiratory infection

Drug Interactions

Avoid Concomitant Use There are no known interactions where it is recommended to avoid concomitant use.

Increased Effect/Toxicity

Minoxidil may increase the levels/effects of: Amifostine; Antihypertensives; Hypotensive Agents; RiTUXimab

The levels/effects of Minoxidil may be increased by: CycloSPORINE; Diazoxide; Herbs (Hypotensive Properties); MAO Inhibitors; Pentoxifylline; Phosphodiesterase 5 Inhibitors; Prostacyclin Analogues

Decreased Effect

The levels/effects of Minoxidil may be decreased by: Herbs (Hypertensive Properties); Methylphenidate; Yohimbine

Ethanol/Nutrition/Herb Interactions Herb/Nutraceutical: Bayberry, blue cohosh, cayenne, ephedra, ginger, ginseng (American), kola, licorice may diminish the antihypertensive effects of minoxidil. Black cohosh, California poppy, coleus, golden seal, hawthorn, mistletoe, periwinkle, quinine, shepherd's purse may enhance the hypotensive effects of minoxidil.

Dosage Forms Excipient information presented when available (limited, particularly for generics); consult specific product labeling. [DSC] = Discontinued product

Aerosol, topical [foam]:
  Rogaine for Men®: 5% (60 g)
Solution, topical: 2% (60 mL); 5% (60 mL)
  Rogaine® for Men: 2% (60 mL) [DSC] [supplied with dropper applicator]
  Rogaine® for Women: 2% (60 mL) [supplied with dropper applicator]
  Rogaine® Extra Strength for Men: 5% (60 mL) [supplied with dropper applicator]
Tablet: 2.5 mg, 10 mg

References

Allon M, Hall D, and Macon EJ, "Prolonged Hypotension After Initial Minoxidil Dose," *Arch Intern Med*, 1986, 146(10):2075-6.

Chobanian AV, Bakris GL, Black HR, et al, "The Seventh Report of the Joint National Committee on Prevention, Detection, Evaluation, and Treatment of High Blood Pressure: The JNC 7 Report," *JAMA*, 2003, 289 (19):2560-71.

Franciosa JA, Jordan RA, Wilen MM, et al, "Minoxidil in Patients With Chronic Left Heart Failure: Contrasting Hemodynamic and Clinical Effects in a Controlled Trial," *Circulation*, 1984, 70(1):63-8.

National High Blood Pressure Education Program Working Group on High Blood Pressure in Children and Adolescents "Fourth Report on High Blood Pressure in Children and Adolescents," *Pediatrics*, 2004, 114(2 Suppl): 555-76.

◆ **Mint-Ciprofloxacin (Can)** *see* Ciprofloxacin *on page 306*

◆ **MINT-Ondansetron (Can)** *see* Ondansetron *on page 1057*

◆ **Mint-Topiramate (Can)** *see* Topiramate *on page 1408*

◆ **Miochol®-E** *see* Acetylcholine *on page 34*

◆ **Miostat®** *see* Carbachol *on page 241*

◆ **Mirapex®** *see* Pramipexole *on page 1159*

◆ **Mircette®** *see* Ethinyl Estradiol and Desogestrel *on page 544*

Misoprostol (mye soe PROST ole)

Medication Safety Issues

Sound-alike/look-alike issues:
  Cytotec® may be confused with Cytoxan®, Sytobex®
  Misoprostol may be confused with metoprolol, mifepristone

U.S. Brand Names Cytotec®

Canadian Brand Names Apo-Misoprostol®; Novo-Misoprostol

◀ **Pharmacologic Category** Prostaglandin

Generic Available Yes

Use Prevention of NSAID-induced gastric ulcers; medical termination of pregnancy of ≤49 days (in conjunction with mifepristone)

Unlabeled/Investigational Use Cervical ripening and labor induction; NSAID-induced nephropathy; fat malabsorption in cystic fibrosis

Mechanism of Action Misoprostol is a synthetic prostaglandin E_1 analog that replaces the protective prostaglandins consumed with prostaglandin-inhibiting therapies (eg, NSAIDs); has been shown to induce uterine contractions

Pharmacodynamics/Kinetics

Absorption: Rapid

Metabolism: Hepatic; rapidly de-esterified to misoprostol acid (active)

Half-life elimination: Metabolite: 20-40 minutes

Time to peak, serum: Active metabolite: Fasting: 15-30 minutes

Excretion: Urine (64% to 73%) and feces (15%) within 24 hours

Dosage

Oral:

Children 8-16 years: Fat absorption in cystic fibrosis (unlabeled use): 100 mcg 4 times/day

Adults: Prevention of NSAID-induced gastric ulcers: 200 mcg 4 times/day with food; if not tolerated, may decrease dose to 100 mcg 4 times/day with food or 200 mcg twice daily with food; last dose of the day should be taken at bedtime

Intravaginal: Adults: Labor induction or cervical ripening (unlabeled uses): 25 mcg (1/4 of 100 mcg tablet); may repeat at intervals no more frequent than every 3-6 hours. Do not use in patients with previous cesarean delivery or prior major uterine surgery.

Stability Store at or below 25°C (77°F).

Administration Incidence of diarrhea may be lessened by having patient take dose right after meals. Therapy is usually begun on the second or third day of the next normal menstrual period.

Pregnancy Risk Factor X

Contraindications Hypersensitivity to misoprostol, prostaglandins, or any component of the formulation; pregnancy (when used to reduce NSAID-induced ulcers)

Warnings/Precautions Safety and efficacy have not been established in children <18 years of age; use with caution in patients with renal impairment, cardiovascular disease and the elderly. **[U.S. Boxed Warning]: Not to be used in pregnant women or women of childbearing potential unless woman is capable of complying with effective contraceptive measures;** therapy is normally begun on the second or third day of next normal menstrual period. Uterine perforation and/or rupture have been reported in association with intravaginal use to induce labor or with combined oral/intravaginal use to induce abortion. Should not be used as a cervical-ripening agent for induction of labor. However, The American College of Obstetricians and Gynecologists (ACOG) continues to support this off-label use.

Adverse Reactions

>10%: Gastrointestinal: Diarrhea, abdominal pain

1% to 10%:

Central nervous system: Headache

Gastrointestinal: Constipation, flatulence, nausea, dyspepsia, vomiting

<1% (Limited to important or life-threatening): Anaphylaxis, anxiety, appetite changes, arrhythmia, arterial thrombosis, bronchospasm, confusion, cramps, depression, drowsiness, edema, fetal or infant death (when used during pregnancy), fever, GI bleeding, GI inflammation, gingivitis, gout, hyper-/hypotension, impotence, loss of libido, MI, neuropathy, neurosis, pulmonary embolism, purpura, rash, reflux, rigors, thrombocytopenia, uterine rupture, weakness, weight changes

Drug Interactions

Avoid Concomitant Use There are no known interactions where it is recommended to avoid concomitant use.

Increased Effect/Toxicity

Misoprostol may increase the levels/effects of: Oxytocin

Decreased Effect There are no known significant interactions involving a decrease in effect.

Ethanol/Nutrition/Herb Interactions Food: Misoprostol peak serum concentrations may be decreased if taken with food (not clinically significant).

Dietary Considerations Should be taken with food; incidence of diarrhea may be lessened by having patient take dose right after meals.

Dosage Forms Excipient information presented when available (limited, particularly for generics); consult specific product labeling.
Tablet: 100 mcg, 200 mcg

- ◆ **MK-217** *see* Alendronate *on page 57*
- ◆ **MK383** *see* Tirofiban *on page 1397*
- ◆ **MK-0431** *see* SitaGLIPtin *on page 1300*
- ◆ **MK462** *see* Rizatriptan *on page 1258*
- ◆ **MK-0518** *see* Raltegravir *on page 1229*
- ◆ **MK594** *see* Losartan *on page 857*
- ◆ **MK0826** *see* Ertapenem *on page 513*
- ◆ **MK 869** *see* Aprepitant *on page 132*
- ◆ **MMF** *see* Mycophenolate *on page 966*
- ◆ **Mobic®** *see* Meloxicam *on page 870*
- ◆ **Mobicox® (Can)** *see* Meloxicam *on page 870*

Modafinil (moe DAF i nil)

U.S. Brand Names Provigil®
Canadian Brand Names Alertec®; APO-Modafinil
Pharmacologic Category Stimulant
Restrictions C-IV
Use Improve wakefulness in patients with excessive daytime sleepiness associated with narcolepsy and shift work sleep disorder (SWSD); adjunctive therapy for obstructive sleep apnea/hypopnea syndrome (OSAHS)
Unlabeled/Investigational Use Attention-deficit/hyperactivity disorder (ADHD); treatment of fatigue in MS and other disorders
Pharmacodynamics/Kinetics Modafinil is a racemic compound (10% *d*-isomer and 90% *l*-isomer at steady state) whose enantiomers have different pharmacokinetics

Distribution: V_d: 0.9 L/kg
Protein binding: 60%, primarily to albumin
Metabolism: Hepatic; multiple pathways including CYP3A4
Half-life elimination: Effective half-life: 15 hours; Steady-state: 2-4 days
Time to peak, serum: 2-4 hours
Excretion: Urine (as metabolites, <10% as unchanged drug)
Dosage Oral:
Children: ADHD (unlabeled use): 50-100 mg once daily
Adults:
ADHD (unlabeled use): 100-300 mg once daily
Narcolepsy, obstructive sleep apnea/hypopnea syndrome (OSAHS): Initial: 200 mg as a single daily dose in the morning
Shift work sleep disorder (SWSD): Initial: 200 mg as a single dose taken ~1 hour prior to start of work shift
Note: Doses of 400 mg/day, given as a single dose, have been well tolerated, but there is no consistent evidence that this dose confers additional benefit.
Elderly: Elimination of modafinil and its metabolites may be reduced as a consequence of aging and as a result, consider initiating dose at 100 mg once daily.
Dosing adjustment in renal impairment: Safety and efficacy have not been established in severe renal impairment.
Dosing adjustment in hepatic impairment: Dose should be reduced to one-half of that recommended for patients with normal liver function.

◄ **Additional Information** Complete prescribing information for this medication should be consulted for additional detail.

Dosage Forms Excipient information presented when available (limited, particularly for generics); consult specific product labeling.

Tablet:

Provigil®: 100 mg, 200 mg

References

Broughton, RJ, "Randomized, Double-Blind, Placebo-Controlled Crossover Trial of Modafinil in the Treatment of Excessive Daytime Sleepiness in Narcolepsy," *Neurology*, 1997, 49(2):444-451.

Grozinger M, "Interaction of Modafinil and Clomipramine as Comedication in a Narcoleptic Patient," *Clin Neuropharmacol*, 1998, 21(2):127-129.

Rugino TA and Copley TC, "Effects of Modafinil in Children With Attention-Deficit/Hyperactivity Disorder: An Open-Label Study," *J Am Acad Child Adolesc Psychiatry*, 2001, 40(2):230-5.

Taylor FB and Russo J, "Efficacy of Modafinil Compared to Dextroamphetamine for the Treatment of Attention Deficit Hyperactivity Disorder in Adults," *J Child Adolesc Psychopharmacol*, 2000, 10 (4):311-20.

U.S. Modafinil in Narcolepsy Multicenter Study Group, "Randomized Trial of Modafinil for the Treatment of Pathological Somnolence in Narcolepsy," *Ann Neurol*, 1998, 43(1):88-97.

Wong, YN, "Single-Dose Pharmacokinetics of Modafinil and Methylphenidate Given Alone or in Combination in Healthy Male Volunteers," *J Clin Pharmacol*, 1998, 38(3):276-282.

◆ **Modicon®** *see* Ethinyl Estradiol and Norethindrone *on page 554*

Moexipril (mo EKS i pril)

Related Information

Angiotensin Agents *on page 1652*

Preoperative Evaluation of the Cardiac Patient for Noncardiac Surgery *on page 1598*

U.S. Brand Names Univasc®

Index Terms Moexipril Hydrochloride

Pharmacologic Category Angiotensin-Converting Enzyme (ACE) Inhibitor

Use Treatment of hypertension, alone or in combination with thiazide diuretics

Pharmacodynamics/Kinetics

Absorption: Incomplete

Onset of action: Peak effect: 1-2 hours

Duration: >24 hours

Distribution: V_d (moexiprilat): 180 L

Protein binding, plasma: Moexipril: 90%; Moexiprilat: 50% to 70%

Metabolism: Parent drug: Hepatic and via GI tract to moexiprilat, 1000 times more potent than parent

Bioavailability: Moexiprilat: 13%; reduced with food (AUC decreased by ~40%)

Half-life elimination: Moexipril: 1 hour; Moexiprilat: 2-9 hours

Time to peak: 1.5 hours

Excretion: Feces (50%)

Dosage Adults: Oral: Initial: 7.5 mg once daily (in patients **not** receiving diuretics), 1 hour prior to a meal **or** 3.75 mg once daily (when combined with thiazide diuretics); maintenance dose: 7.5-30 mg/day in 1 or 2 divided doses 1 hour before meals

Dosing adjustment in renal impairment: Cl_{cr} ≤40 mL/minute: Patients may be cautiously placed on 3.75 mg once daily, then upwardly titrated to a maximum of 15 mg/day.

Anesthesia and Critical Care Concerns/Other Considerations

Clinical Pearls/Comments: In patients on chronic ACE inhibitor therapy, intraoperative hypotension may occur with induction and maintenance of general anesthesia; however, discontinuation of therapy prior to surgery is controversial. If continued preoperatively, avoidance of hypotensive agents during surgery is prudent. Episodes of intraoperative hypotension may be managed by fluid administration and/or modest doses of alpha-adrenergic agents. Severe hypotension may occur in patients who are sodium- and/or volume-depleted, initiate lower doses and monitor closely when starting therapy in these patients. ACE inhibitor therapy may elicit an increase in potassium and creatinine, especially when used in patients with bilateral renal artery stenosis. In those patients experiencing cough on an ACE inhibitor, the ACE inhibitor may be discontinued and, if necessary, angiotensin-receptor blocker therapy instituted.

Concomitant NSAID therapy may attenuate blood pressure control; use of NSAIDs should be avoided or limited, with monitoring of blood pressure control. In the setting of heart failure, NSAID use may be associated with an increased risk for fluid accumulation and edema. Because of the potent teratogenic effects of ACE inhibitors, these drugs should be avoided, if possible, when treating women of childbearing potential not on effective birth control measures. Aging patients with a decrease in glomerular filtration (also creatinine clearance), severe heart failure, and renal failure may experience an exaggerated response with administration of ACE inhibitors. Diabetic proteinuria is reduced and insulin sensitivity is enhanced.

Evidence-Based Information: ACE inhibitors decrease morbidity and mortality in patients with asymptomatic and symptomatic left ventricular dysfunction. In this situation, they decrease hospitalizations for, and retard progression to, decompensated heart failure. ACE inhibitors are also indicated in patients postmyocardial infarction in whom left ventricular ejection fraction is <40%. When used in patients with heart failure, the target dose or maximum tolerated dose should be achieved, if possible. Lower daily doses of ACE inhibitors have not demonstrated the same cardioprotective effects. ACE inhibitors have renal protective effects in patients with diabetic proteinuria. The HOPE trial examined the use of ramipril at a dose of between 2.5-10 mg daily in patients without heart failure at high risk for cardiovascular events and documented a significant improvement in cardiovascular outcome compared to placebo.

Additional Information Complete prescribing information for this medication should be consulted for additional detail.

Dosage Forms Excipient information presented when available (limited, particularly for generics); consult specific product labeling.
Tablet, as hydrochloride [scored]: 7.5 mg, 15 mg
  Univasc®: 7.5 mg, 15 mg

- ◆ **Moexipril Hydrochloride** *see* Moexipril *on page 948*
- ◆ **Monacolin K** *see* Lovastatin *on page 859*
- ◆ **Monitan® (Can)** *see* Acebutolol *on page 24*
- ◆ **Monocor® (Can)** *see* Bisoprolol *on page 192*
- ◆ **Monodox®** *see* Doxycycline *on page 456*
- ◆ **Monoethanolamine** *see* Ethanolamine Oleate *on page 543*
- ◆ **Monoket®** *see* Isosorbide Mononitrate *on page 774*
- ◆ **MonoNessa®** *see* Ethinyl Estradiol and Norgestimate *on page 558*
- ◆ **Mononine®** *see* Factor IX *on page 570*
- ◆ **Monopril®** *see* Fosinopril *on page 636*
- ◆ **Morning After Pill** *see* Ethinyl Estradiol and Norgestrel *on page 560*

Morphine and Naltrexone (MOR feen & nal TREKS one)

Medication Safety Issues
Sound-alike/look-alike issues:
  Morphine may be confused with HYDROmorphone
  Morphine sulfate may be confused with magnesium sulfate
  Naltrexone may be confused with methylnaltrexone, naloxone
MSO_4 and MS are error-prone abbreviations (mistaken as magnesium sulfate)

Medication Guide An FDA-approved patient medication guide, which is available with the product information and at http://www.fda.gov/downloads/Drugs/DrugSafety/UCM179172.pdf, must be dispensed with this medication for each new outpatient prescription and refill.

U.S. Brand Names Embeda™

Index Terms Morphine Sulfate and Naltrexone Hydrochloride; MS (error-prone abbreviation and should not be used); MSO_4 (error-prone abbreviation and should not be used); Naltrexone and Morphine

Pharmacologic Category Analgesic, Opioid; Opioid Antagonist

Restrictions C-II

Generic Available No

Use Relief of moderate-to-severe pain when continual, around-the-clock therapy is needed for an extended period of time

Mechanism of Action

Morphine binds to opiate receptors in the CNS, causing inhibition of ascending pain pathways, altering the perception of and response to pain; produces generalized CNS depression.

Naltrexone (a pure opioid antagonist) is a cyclopropyl derivative of oxymorphone similar in structure to naloxone and nalorphine (a morphine derivative); it acts as a competitive antagonist at opioid receptor sites, showing the highest affinity for mu receptors. Naltrexone is not an active component unless tablet is chewed, crushed, or dissolved.

Pharmacodynamics/Kinetics

Onset (patient dependent; dosing must be individualized): ~ 8 hours

Absorption: Rate and extent of morphine decreased by high-fat meal; total bioavailability not affected

Distribution: V_d: Morphine: ~3-4 L/kg

Protein binding: Morphine: 30% to 35%

Metabolism:

Morphine: Hepatic via conjugation with glucuronic acid primarily to morphine-6-glucoronide (active analgesic) morphine-3-glucuronide (inactive as analgesic); minor metabolites include morphine-3-6-diglucuronide; other minor metabolites include normorphine (active) and morphine 3-ethereal sulfate

Naltrexone: Noncytochrome-mediated dehydrogenase conversion to 6-beta-naltrexol and related minor metabolites

Half-life elimination: Terminal: ~29 hours

Time to peak, plasma: 7.5 hours

Excretion: Urine (55% to 65%, as morphine-6- glucuronide and morphine-3-glucuronide, ~10 as unchanged); feces (~7% to 10%). It has been suggested that accumulation of morphine-6-glucuronide might cause toxicity with renal insufficiency. All of the metabolites (ie, morphine-3-glucuronide, morphine-6-glucuronide, and normorphine) have been suggested as possible causes of neurotoxicity (eg, myoclonus).

Dosage Oral: Moderate-to-severe pain: **Note:** These are guidelines and do not represent the doses that may be required in all patients. Treatment should be individualized based on patient's prior analgesic treatment experience/tolerance and pain relief. Not intended for use as a prn medication.

Adults: Opiate-naive: Initial: 20 mg/0.8 mg once or twice daily; 100 mg/4 mg strength for use in opioid-tolerant patients only

Titration: Do not increase dose more frequently than every other day. May supplement dose with a short-acting analgesic (<20% of total daily dose) for breakthrough pain. If once-daily dosing is inadequate may switch to twice daily dosing.

Conversion from other oral morphine products to Embeda™: Administer one-half of the patient's total daily oral morphine dose as Embeda™ every 12 hours or all of the patient's total daily oral morphine dose as Embeda™ once daily.

Conversion from other oral/parenteral opioids or parenteral morphine to Embeda™: Must first convert to oral morphine equivalent.

Conversion from parenteral to oral morphine: It may take 2-6 mg of oral morphine to provide pain relief equivalent to 1 mg of parenteral morphine. An oral dose 3 times the daily parenteral dose may be sufficient in chronic pain settings.

Conversion from other oral/parenteral opioids to oral morphine: Specific recommendations are not available; refer to published relative potency data realizing that such ratios are only approximations. It is generally safest to give half the estimated daily morphine requirement as the initial dose and manage inadequate relief with immediate release morphine.

Note: When converting from other opioid analgesics it is better to underestimate the patient's 24-hour oral requirement and provide breakthrough treatment than to overestimate and manage an adverse event.

Elderly or debilitated patients: Use with caution; may require dose reduction

Dosing adjustment in renal impairment: Use with caution in patients with severe impairment; no specific dosing recommendations are provided by the manufacturer.

Dosing adjustment/comments in hepatic disease: Use with caution in patients with severe impairment; no specific dosing recommendations are provided by the manufacturer.

Stability Store at 25°C (77°F); excursions permitted to 15°C to 30°C (59°F to 86°F). Protect from light.

Administration Capsule should be swallowed whole. Contents of the capsule may be sprinkled on applesauce (do not divide in separate doses) and swallowed immediately. Rinse mouth to ensure all contents have been swallowed. Do not crush, chew, or dissolve pellets in the capsule prior to swallowing. Not for nasogastric/gastric tube administration. First dose may be taken at the same time as the last dose of immediate release opioid medication.

Monitoring Parameters Pain relief, respiratory and mental status, blood pressure

Pregnancy Risk Factor C

Contraindications Hypersensitivity to morphine, naltrexone, or any component of the formulation; patients with significant respiratory depression, acute/severe bronchial asthma, or hypercapnia in unmonitored settings or in the absence of resuscitative equipment; patients with or suspected of having paralytic ileus; any situation where opioids are contraindicated

Warnings/Precautions An opioid-containing analgesic regimen should be tailored to each patient's needs and based upon the type of pain being treated (acute versus chronic), the route of administration, degree of tolerance for opioids (naive versus chronic user), age, weight, and medical condition. The optimal analgesic dose varies widely among patients. Doses should be titrated to pain relief/prevention. **[U.S. Boxed Warnings]: Morphine and naltrexone is not intended for use as a prn analgesic; indicated for management of moderate-to-severe pain when a continuous, around-the-clock opioid analgesic is needed for an extended period of time. High potential for abuse; healthcare provider should be alert to problems of abuse, misuse, and diversion.**

May cause respiratory depression; use with caution in patients (particularly elderly or debilitated) with impaired respiratory function, adrenal insufficiency, prostatic hyperplasia, urinary stricture, severe renal impairment, or severe hepatic dysfunction and in patients with hypersensitivity reactions to other phenanthrene derivative opioid agonists (codeine, hydrocodone, hydromorphone, levorphanol, oxycodone, oxymorphone). Use with caution in patients with biliary tract dysfunction; acute pancreatitis may cause constriction of sphincter of Oddi.

May cause CNS depression, which may impair physical or mental abilities; patients must be cautioned about performing tasks which require mental alertness (eg, operating machinery or driving). Effects may be potentiated when used with other sedative drugs or ethanol. **[U.S. Boxed Warning]: Patients should not consume alcoholic beverages or medication containing ethanol while taking morphine and naltrexone; ethanol may increase morphine plasma levels resulting in a potentially fatal overdose.** Use caution in patients with acute alcoholism or delirium tremors. May cause hypotension in patients with acute myocardial infarction, volume depletion, or concurrent drug therapy which may exaggerate vasodilation. Use with extreme caution in patients with head injury, intracranial lesions, or elevated intracranial pressure; exaggerated elevation of ICP may occur. May cause seizures if high doses are used; use with caution in patients with seizure disorders. Tolerance or drug dependence may result from extended use. May obscure diagnosis or clinical course of patients with acute abdominal conditions. **[U.S. Boxed Warnings]: Capsules and pellets within the capsule are to be swallowed whole; do not chew, crush, or dissolve. Chewing, crushing, or dissolving capsule will result in the release of naltrexone which may precipitate withdrawal in opioid-tolerant patients.** Symptoms of withdrawal (eg, confusion, somnolence, visual hallucination, vomiting, diarrhea) usually appear within 5 minutes of naltrexone ingestion and may last for up to 48 hours. Abrupt discontinuation following prolonged use may also lead to withdrawal symptoms. Stop therapy and use parenteral short-acting opioids 24 hours prior to cordotomy. Do not use concurrently in patient taking MAO inhibitors; discontinue MAO inhibitor 14 days prior to starting morphine and naltrexone. Elderly and debilitated patients may be particularly susceptible to adverse effects of narcotics.

◀ **[U.S. Boxed Warning:] Embeda™ 100 mg/4 mg capsules are for use in opioid-tolerant patients only; may cause fatal respiratory depression in patients not already tolerant to high doses of opioids.**

Adverse Reactions Frequency not always defined.

>10%:
Central nervous system: Somnolence (1% to 14%)
Gastrointestinal: Constipation (7% to 31%), nausea (11% to 22%)

1% to 10%:
Cardiovascular: Flushing (≤2%), peripheral edema
Central nervous system: Dizziness (1% to 8%), headache (2% to 7%), fatigue (1% to 4%), insomnia (1% to 3%), anxiety (2%), chills, depression, irritability, lethargy, restlessness, sedation
Dermatologic: Pruritus (≤6%), hyperhidrosis (3%)
Endocrine & metabolic: Hot flashes
Gastrointestinal: Vomiting (4% to 8%), xerostomia (2% to 6%), diarrhea (≤2%), abdominal pain/discomfort, anorexia, appetite decreased, dyspepsia, flatulence
Neuromuscular & skeletal: Arthralgia, muscle spasms, tremor

<1% (Limited to important or life-threatening): Abdominal distention, abdominal tenderness, abnormal dreams/thinking, ALT increased, AST increased, blurred vision, cholecystitis, cold sweats, confusion, coordination abnormal, CNS depression, disorientation, dyspnea, dysuria, erectile dysfunction, euphoria, hallucination, hypotension, hypotension (orthostatic), jittery, malaise, memory impairment, mental impairment, mental status change, mood swings, myalgia, nervousness, night sweats, pancreatitis, paresthesia, physical and psychological dependence, piloerection, rash, rhinorrhea, stupor, urinary retention, weakness, withdrawal syndrome

Drug Interactions

Avoid Concomitant Use There are no known interactions where it is recommended to avoid concomitant use.

Increased Effect/Toxicity There are no known significant interactions involving an increase in effect.

Decreased Effect There are no known significant interactions involving a decrease in effect.

Ethanol/Nutrition/Herb Interactions

Ethanol: Alcoholic beverages or ethanol-containing products may disrupt extended-release formulation resulting in rapid release of entire morphine dose. Concurrent use may also increase/potentiate CNS depressant effects.

Herb/Nutraceutical: Avoid valerian, St John's wort, kava kava, gotu kola (may increase CNS depression).

Test Interactions Some quinolones may produce a false-positive urine screening result for opioids using commercially-available immunoassay kits. This has been demonstrated most consistently for levofloxacin and ofloxacin, but other quinolones have shown cross-reactivity in certain assay kits. Confirmation of positive opioids screens by more specific methods should be considered.

Dietary Considerations Morphine may cause GI upset; take with food if GI upset occurs. Be consistent when taking morphine with or without meals.

Dosage Forms Excipient information presented when available (limited, particularly for generics); consult specific product labeling.
Capsule, extended release, oral:
Embeda™ 20/0.8: Morphine sulfate 20 mg and naltrexone hydrochloride 0.8 mg
Embeda™ 30/1.2: Morphine sulfate 30 mg and naltrexone hydrochloride 1.2 mg
Embeda™ 50/2: Morphine sulfate 50 mg and naltrexone hydrochloride 2 mg
Embeda™ 60/2.4: Morphine sulfate 60 mg and naltrexone hydrochloride 2.4 mg
Embeda™ 80/3.2: Morphine sulfate 80 mg and naltrexone hydrochloride 3.2 mg
Embeda™ 100/4: Morphine sulfate 100 mg and naltrexone hydrochloride 4 mg

◆ **Morphine HP® (Can)** see Morphine Sulfate on page 953

◆ **Morphine LP® Epidural (Can)** see Morphine Sulfate on page 953

Morphine Sulfate (MOR feen SUL fate)

Medication Safety Issues
Sound-alike/look-alike issues:
Morphine may be confused with HYDROmorphone
Morphine sulfate may be confused with magnesium sulfate
MS Contin® may be confused with Oxycontin®
MSO$_4$ and MS are error-prone abbreviations (mistaken as magnesium sulfate)
Avinza® may be confused with Evista®, Invanz®
Roxanol™ may be confused with OxyFast®, Roxicet™, Roxicodone®

High alert medication: The Institute for Safe Medication Practices (ISMP) includes this medication (I.V. formulation) among its list of drug classes which have a heightened risk of causing significant patient harm when used in error.

Use care when prescribing and/or administering morphine solutions. These products are available in different concentrations. Always prescribe dosage in mg; **not** by volume (mL).

Use caution when selecting a morphine formulation for use in neurologic infusion pumps (eg, Medtronic delivery systems). The product should be appropriately labeled as "preservative-free" and suitable for intraspinal use via continuous infusion. In addition, the product should be formulated in a pH range that is compatible with the device operation specifications.

Significant differences exist between oral and I.V. dosing. Use caution when converting from one route of administration to another.

Related Information
Acute Postoperative Pain *on page 1502*
Anesthesia Considerations for Neurosurgery *on page 1514*
Anesthesia for Patients With Liver Disease *on page 1537*
Anesthetic Considerations in the Substance-Abusing Patient *on page 1613*
Chronic Pain Management *on page 1546*
Chronic Renal Failure *on page 1552*
Dosing Considerations for the Critically-Ill Patient With Morbid Obesity *on page 1561*
Moderate Sedation *on page 1566*
Opioid Analgesics *on page 1688*
Opioids *on page 1641*
Skin Tests *on page 1707*

U.S. Brand Names Astramorph/PF™; Avinza®; DepoDur®; Duramorph®; Infumorph® 200; Infumorph® 500; Kadian®; MS Contin®; Oramorph® SR; Roxanol™

Canadian Brand Names Doloral; Kadian®; M-Eslon®; M.O.S.-SR®; M.O.S.-Sulfate®; M.O.S.® 10; M.O.S.® 20; M.O.S.® 30; Morphine HP®; Morphine LP® Epidural; MS Contin®; MS-IR®; Novo-Morphine SR; PMS-Morphine Sulfate SR; ratio-Morphine; ratio-Morphine SR; Statex®; Zomorph®

Index Terms MS (error-prone abbreviation and should not be used); MSO$_4$ (error-prone abbreviation and should not be used)

Pharmacologic Category Analgesic, Opioid

Restrictions C-II

Generic Available Yes: Excludes capsule, controlled release tablet, sustained release tablet, extended release liposomal suspension for injection

Use Relief of moderate-to-severe acute and chronic pain; relief of pain of myocardial infarction; relief of dyspnea of acute left ventricular failure and pulmonary edema; preanesthetic medication

DepoDur®: Epidural (lumbar) single-dose management of surgical pain

Infumorph®: Used in continuous microinfusion devices for intrathecal or epidural administration in treatment of intractable chronic pain

Controlled, extended, or sustained release products: Only intended/indicated for use when repeated doses for an extended period of time are required. The 100 mg and 200 mg tablets or capsules of Kadian®, MS Contin®, and morphine sulfate controlled-release tablets and the 60 mg, 90 mg, and 120 mg capsules of Avinza® should only be used in opioid-tolerant patients.

▶

◀ **Mechanism of Action** Binds to opiate receptors in the CNS, causing inhibition of ascending pain pathways, altering the perception of and response to pain; produces generalized CNS depression

Pharmacodynamics/Kinetics

Onset of action (patient dependent; dosing must be individualized): Oral (immediate release): ~30 minutes; I.V.: 5-10 minutes

Duration (patient dependent; dosing must be individualized): Pain relief:
Immediate release formulations: 4 hours
Extended release capsule and tablet: 8-24 hours (formulation dependent)
Extended release epidural injection (DepoDur®): >48 hours

Absorption: Variable

Distribution: V_d: 3-4 L/kg; binds to opioid receptors in the CNS and periphery (eg, GI tract)

Protein binding: 30% to 35%

Metabolism: Hepatic via conjugation with glucuronic acid primarily to morphine-6-glucoronide (active analgesic) morphine-3-glucuronide (inactive as analgesic); minor metabolites include morphine-3-6-diglucuronide; other minor metabolites include normorphine (active) and morphine 3-ethereal sulfate

Bioavailability: Oral: 17% to 33% (first-pass effect limits oral bioavailability; oral: parenteral effectiveness reportedly varies from 1:6 in opioid naive patients to 1:3 with chronic use)

Half-life elimination: Adults: 2-4 hours (immediate release forms)

Time to peak, plasma: Avinza®: 30 minutes (maintained for 24 hours); Kadian®: ~10 hours; Oramorph® SR: ~4 hours

Excretion: Urine (primarily as morphine-3-glucuronide, ~2% to 12% excreted unchanged); feces (~7% to 10%). It has been suggested that accumulation of morphine-6-glucuronide might cause toxicity with renal insufficiency. All of the metabolites (ie, morphine-3-glucuronide, morphine-6-glucuronide, and normorphine) have been suggested as possible causes of neurotoxicity (eg, myoclonus).

Dosage Note: These are guidelines and do not represent the doses that may be required in all patients. Doses and dosage intervals should be titrated to pain relief/prevention.

Children >6 months and <50 kg: Acute pain (moderate-to-severe):

Oral (immediate release formulations): 0.15-0.3 mg/kg every 3-4 hours as needed. **Note:** The American Pain Society recommends an initial dose of 0.3 mg/kg for children with severe pain.

I.M., I.V.: 0.1-0.2 mg/kg every 3-4 hours as needed

I.V. infusion: Range: 10-60 mcg/kg/hour

Patient-controlled analgesia (PCA) (American Pain Society, 2008): **Note:** Opiate-naive: Consider lower end of dosing range:
Usual concentration: 1 mg/mL
Demand dose: Usual: 0.02 mg/kg/dose; range: 0.01-0.03 mg/kg/dose
Lockout interval: 6-8 minutes
Usual basal rate: 0-0.03 mg/kg/hour

Adults:

Acute pain (moderate-to-severe):

Oral (immediate release formulations): Opiate-naive: Initial: 10 mg every 4 hours as needed; patients with prior opiate exposure may require higher initial doses: usual dosage range: 10-30 mg every 4 hours as needed

I.M., SubQ: **Note:** Repeated SubQ administration causes local tissue irritation, pain, and induration.
Initial: Opiate-naive: 5-10 mg every 4 hours as needed; patients with prior opiate exposure may require higher initial doses; usual dosage range: 5-20 mg every 4 hours as needed

Rectal: 10-20 mg every 3-4 hours

I.V.: Initial: Opiate-naive: 2.5-5 mg every 3-4 hours; patients with prior opiate exposure may require higher initial doses. **Note:** Repeated doses (up to every 5 minutes if needed) in small increments (eg, 1-4 mg) may be preferred to larger and less frequent doses.
Acute myocardial infarction, analgesia (ACC/AHA 2004 guidelines): Initial management: 2-4 mg, give 2-8 mg every 5-15 minutes as needed.

Critically-ill patients (unlabeled dose): 0.7-10 mg (based on 70 kg patient) **or** 0.01-0.15 mg/kg every 1-2 hours as needed. **Note:** More frequent dosing may be needed (eg, mechanically-ventilated patients).

I.V., SubQ continuous infusion: 0.8-10 mg/hour; usual range: Up to 80 mg/hour
Continuous infusion: Usual dosage range: 5-35 mg/hour (based on 70 kg patient) **or** 0.07-0.5 mg/kg/hour
Patient-controlled analgesia (PCA): **Note:** Opiate-naive: Consider lower end of dosing range:
Usual concentration: 1 mg/mL
Demand dose: Usual: 1 mg; range: 0.5-2.5 mg
Lockout interval: 5-10 minutes

Intrathecal (I.T.): **Note: Must be preservative-free.** Administer with extreme caution and in reduced dosage to geriatric or debilitated patients. I.T. dose is usually ¹/₁₀ that of epidural dosage.
Opioid-naive: 0.2-1 mg/dose (may provide adequate relief for up to 24 hours); repeat doses are **not** recommended. **Note:** The American Pain Society recommends 0.1-0.3 mg/dose; adjust dose for age, injection site, and patient's medical condition and degree of opioid tolerance.
Continuous microinfusion (Infumorph®): Initial: 0.2-1 mg/day
Opioid-tolerant: 1-10 mg/day
Continuous microinfusion (Infumorph®): Initial: 1-10 mg/day, titrate to effect; usual maximum is ~20 mg/day

Epidural: Pain management: **Note: Must be preservative-free.** Administer with extreme caution and in reduced dosage to geriatric or debilitated patients. Vigilant monitoring is particularly important in these patients.
Single-dose (Astromorph/PF™, Duramorph®): Initial: 5 mg, if pain relief not achieved in 1 hour, careful administration of 1-2 mg at intervals sufficient to assess effectiveness may be given; maximum: 10 mg/24 hours (single doses may provide adequate relief for up to 24 hours)
Infusion: Bolus dose: 1-6 mg; infusion rate: 0.1-0.2 mg/hour; maximum dose: 10 mg/24 hours.
Note: The American Pain Society recommends 1-6 mg/dose as a single dose or an infusion of 0.1-1 mg/hour; adjust dose for age, injection site, and patient's medical condition and degree of opioid tolerance.
Continuous microinfusion (Infumorph®):
Opioid-naive: Initial: 0.2-1 mg/day
Opioid-tolerant: Initial: 1-10 mg/day, titrate to effect; usual maximum is ~20 mg/day

Surgical anesthesia: Epidural: Single-dose (extended release, DepoDur®): Lumbar epidural only; not recommended in patients <18 years of age:
Cesarean section: 10 mg (after clamping umbilical cord)
Lower abdominal/pelvic surgery: 10-15 mg
Major orthopedic surgery of lower extremity: 15 mg
For DepoDur®: To minimize the pharmacokinetic interaction resulting in higher peak serum concentrations of morphine, administer the test dose of the local anesthetic at least 15 minutes prior to DepoDur® administration. Use of DepoDur® with epidural local anesthetics has not been studied. Other medications should not be administered into the epidural space for at least 48 hours after administration of DepoDur®.
Note: Some patients may benefit from a 20 mg dose; however, the incidence of adverse effects may be increased.

Chronic pain: Note: Patients taking opioids chronically may become tolerant and require doses higher than the usual dosage range to maintain the desired effect. Tolerance can be managed by appropriate dose titration. There is no optimal or maximal dose for morphine in chronic pain. The appropriate dose is one that relieves pain throughout its dosing interval without causing unmanageable side effects.
Oral: Controlled-, extended-, or sustained-release formulations: A patient's morphine requirement should be established using prompt-release formulations. Conversion to long-acting products may be considered when chronic, continuous treatment is required. Higher dosages should be reserved for use only in opioid-tolerant patients.
Capsules, extended release (Avinza®): Daily dose administered once daily (for best results, administer at same time each day)

Capsules, sustained release (Kadian®): Daily dose administered once daily or in 2 divided doses daily (every 12 hours)

Tablets, controlled release (MS Contin®), sustained release (Oramorph SR®), or extended release: Daily dose divided and administered every 8 or every 12 hours

Elderly or debilitated patients: Use with caution; may require dose reduction

Dosing adjustment in renal impairment:

Cl_{cr} 10-50 mL/minute: Children and Adults: Administer at 75% of normal dose

Cl_{cr} <10 mL/minute: Children and Adults: Administer at 50% of normal dose

Intermittent HD:

Children: Administer 50% of normal dose

Adults: No dosage adjustment necessary

Peritoneal dialysis: Children: Administer 50% of normal dose

CRRT: Children and Adults: Administer 75% of normal dose, titrate

Dosing adjustment/comments in hepatic disease: Unchanged in mild liver disease; substantial extrahepatic metabolism may occur; excessive sedation may occur in cirrhosis

Stability

Capsule, sustained release (Avinza®, Kadian®): Store at 25°C (77°F); excursions permitted to 15°C to 30°C (59°F to 86°F). Protect from light and moisture.

Injection: Store at controlled room temperature of 20°C to 25°C (68°F to 77°F); do not freeze. Protect from light. Degradation depends on pH and presence of oxygen; relatively stable in pH ≤4; darkening of solutions indicate degradation. Usual concentration for continuous I.V. infusion: 0.1-1 mg/mL in D_5W.

DepoDur®: Store under refrigeration at 2°C to 8°C (36°F to 46°F); keep vials in carton during refrigeration; do not freeze. Check freeze indicator before administration; do not administer if bulb is pink or purple. May store at room temperature for up to 30 days in sealed, unopened vials. DepoDur® may be diluted in preservative-free NS to a volume of 5 mL. Gently invert to suspend particles prior to removal from vial. Once vial is opened, use within 4 hours.

Oral solution: Store at controlled room temperature of 25°C (68°F to 77°F); do not freeze.

Suppositories: Store at controlled room temperature 25°C (77°F). Protect from light.

Tablet, extended release: Store at controlled room temperature of 25°C (77°F).

Tablet, immediate release: Store at controlled room temperature of 25°C (77°F). Protect from moisture.

Administration

Oral: Do not crush controlled release drug product, swallow whole. Kadian® and Avinza® can be opened and sprinkled on applesauce; do not crush or chew the beads. Contents of Kadian® capsules may be opened and sprinkled over 10 mL water and flushed through prewetted 16F gastrostomy tube; do not administer Kadian® through nasogastric tube.

I.V.: When giving morphine I.V. push, it is best to first dilute with sterile water or NS for a final concentration of 1-2 mg/mL and then administer slowly.

Epidural: Use preservative-free solutions

Epidural, extended release liposomal suspension (DepoDur®): Intended for lumbar administration only. Thoracic administration has not been studied. May be administered undiluted or diluted up to 5 mL total volume in preservative-free NS. Do not use an in-line filter during administration. Not for I.V., I.M., or intrathecal administration.

Resedation may occur following epidural administration; this may be delayed ≥48 hours in patients receiving extended-release (DepoDur®) injections.

Administration of an epidural test dose (lidocaine 1.5% and epinephrine 1:200,000) may affect the release of morphine from the liposomal preparation. Delaying the dose for an interval of at least 15 minutes following the test dose minimizes this pharmacokinetic interaction. Except for a test dose, other epidural local anesthetics or medications should not be administered epidurally before or after this product for a minimum of 48 hours.

Intrathecal: Use preservative-free solutions

Monitoring Parameters Pain relief, respiratory and mental status, blood pressure

Astromorph/PF™, Duramorph®, Infumorph®: Patients should be observed in a fully-equipped and staffed environment for at least 24 hours following initiation, and as appropriate for the first several days after catheter implantation.

DepoDur®: Patient should be monitored for at least 48 hours following administration.

Reference Range Therapeutic: Surgical anesthesia: 65-80 ng/mL (SI: 227-280 nmol/L); Toxic: 200-5000 ng/mL (SI: 700-17,500 nmol/L)

Anesthesia and Critical Care Concerns/Other Considerations

Clinical Pearls/Comments: Synergistic respiratory depression occurs when combined with a benzodiazepine.

Evidence-Based Information: The 2002 ACCM/SCCM guidelines for analgesia (critically-ill adult) recommend morphine or hydromorphone for intermittent, scheduled therapy. Both have a longer duration of action requiring less frequent administration. If the patient has required high-dose analgesia or has used for a prolonged period (~7 days), taper dose to prevent withdrawal. Use only preservative-free injections for epidural or intrathecal administration.

Pregnancy Risk Factor C/D (prolonged use or high doses at term)

Contraindications Note: Some contraindications are product specific. For details, please see detailed product prescribing information.

Hypersensitivity to morphine sulfate or any component of the formulation; severe respiratory depression (without resuscitative equipment); acute or severe asthma; known or suspected paralytic ileus; sustained release products are not recommended with gastrointestinal obstruction or in acute/postoperative pain; pregnancy (prolonged use or high doses at term). Oral solutions contraindicated in patients with heart failure due to chronic lung disease, cardiac arrhythmias, head injuries, brain tumors, acute alcoholism, deliriums tremens, seizure disorders, Injectable solution contraindicated during labor when a premature birth is anticipated. Some products contraindicated in patients with head injuries or increased intracranial pressure. DepoDur® contraindicated in circulatory shock and upper airway obstruction. MS Contin® and Kadian® contraindicated in patients with hypercarbia. Some immediate release formulations (tablets and solution) contraindicated in post biliary tract surgery, suspected surgical abdomen, surgical anastomosis, MAO inhibitor use (concurrent or within 14 days), general CNS depression.

Warnings/Precautions An opioid-containing analgesic regimen should be tailored to each patient's needs and based upon the type of pain being treated (acute versus chronic), the route of administration, degree of tolerance for opioids (naive versus chronic user), age, weight, and medical condition. The optimal analgesic dose varies widely among patients. Doses should be titrated to pain relief/prevention. When used as an epidural injection, monitor for delayed sedation. **[U.S. Boxed Warning]: Healthcare provider should be alert to problems of abuse, misuse, and diversion.**

May cause respiratory depression; use with caution in patients (particularly elderly or debilitated) with impaired respiratory function, morbid obesity, adrenal insufficiency, prostatic hyperplasia, urinary stricture, renal impairment, or severe hepatic dysfunction and in patients with hypersensitivity reactions to other phenanthrene derivative opioid agonists (codeine, hydrocodone, hydromorphone, levorphanol, oxycodone, oxymorphone). Use with caution in patients with biliary tract dysfunction; acute pancreatitis may cause constriction of sphincter of Oddi. Some preparations contain sulfites which may cause allergic reactions; infants <3 months of age are more susceptible to respiratory depression, use with caution and generally in reduced doses in this age group.

May cause CNS depression, which may impair physical or mental abilities; patients must be cautioned about performing tasks which require mental alertness (eg, operating machinery or driving). Effects may be potentiated when used with other sedative drugs or ethanol. May cause hypotension in patients with acute myocardial infarction, volume depletion, or concurrent drug therapy which may exaggerate vasodilation. Use with extreme caution in patients with head injury, intracranial lesions, or elevated intracranial pressure; exaggerated elevation of ICP may occur. May cause seizures if high doses are used; use with caution in patients with seizure disorders. Tolerance or drug dependence may result from extended use. Concurrent use of agonist/antagonist analgesics may precipitate ▶

withdrawal symptoms and/or reduced analgesic efficacy in patients following prolonged therapy with mu opioid agonists. Abrupt discontinuation following prolonged use may also lead to withdrawal symptoms. Elderly may be particularly susceptible to adverse effects of narcotics. May obscure diagnosis or clinical course of patients with acute abdominal conditions.

Extended or sustained-release formulations:

[U.S. Boxed Warning]: Extended or sustained release dosage forms should not be crushed or chewed. Controlled-, extended-, or sustained-release products are not intended for "as needed (PRN)" use. **MS Contin® 100 or 200 mg tablets and Kadian® 100 mg or 200 mg capsules are for use only in opioid-tolerant patients.** Avinza®, Kadian®, MS Contin®: **[U.S. Boxed Warning]: Indicated for the management of moderate-to-severe pain when around the clock pain control is needed for an extended time period.**

[U.S. Boxed Warning]: Avinza®: Do not administer with alcoholic beverages or ethanol-containing products, which may disrupt extended-release characteristic of product.

Injections: Note: Products are designed for administration by specific routes (I.V., intrathecal, epidural). Use caution when prescribing, dispensing, or administering to use formulations only by intended route(s).

[U.S. Boxed Warning]: Duramorph®: Due to the risk of severe and/or sustained cardiopulmonary depressant effects of Duramorph® must be administered in a fully equipped and staffed environment. Naloxone injection should be immediately available. Patient should remain in this environment for at least 24 hours following the initial dose.

[U.S. Boxed Warning]: Intrathecal dosage is usually $1/10$ that of epidural dosage.

Infumorph® solutions are **for use in microinfusion devices only**; not for I.V., I.M., or SubQ administration, or for single-dose administration.

When used as an epidural injection, monitor for delayed sedation.

DepoDur®: **For lumbar administration only.** Intrathecal administration has resulted in prolonged respiratory depression. Freezing may adversely affect modified-release mechanism of drug; check freeze indicator within carton prior to administration.

Adverse Reactions Note: Individual patient differences are unpredictable, and percentage may differ in acute pain (surgical) treatment. Reactions may be dose, formulation, and/or route dependent.

Frequency not defined:
  Cardiovascular: Circulatory depression, flushing, shock
  Central nervous system: Physical and psychological dependence, sedation
  Endocrine & metabolic: Antidiuretic hormone release
>10%:
  Cardiovascular: Bradycardia, hypotension
  Central nervous system: Drowsiness (9% to 48%; tolerance usually develops to drowsiness with regular dosing for 1-2 weeks), dizziness (6% to 20%), fever (<3% to >10%), confusion, headache (following epidural or intrathecal use)
  Dermatologic: Pruritus (may be dose related)
  Gastrointestinal: Xerostomia (78%), constipation (9% to 40%; tolerance develops very slowly if at all), nausea (7% to 28%; tolerance usually develops to nausea and vomiting with chronic use), vomiting
  Genitourinary: Urinary retention (16%; may be prolonged, up to 20 hours, following epidural or intrathecal use)
  Hematologic: Anemia (following intrathecal use)
  Local: Pain at injection site
  Neuromuscular & skeletal: Weakness
  Respiratory: Oxygen saturation decreased
  Miscellaneous: Histamine release
1% to 10%:
  Cardiovascular: Atrial fibrillation (<3%), chest pain (<3%), edema, hypertension, palpitation, peripheral edema, syncope, tachycardia, vasodilation

Central nervous system: Amnesia, agitation, anxiety, apathy, ataxia, chills, coma, delirium, depression, dream abnormalities, euphoria, false sense of well being, hallucination, hypoesthesia, insomnia, lethargy, malaise, nervousness, restlessness, seizure, slurred speech, somnolence, vertigo

Dermatologic: Dry skin, rash, urticaria

Endocrine & metabolic: Gynecomastia (<3%), hypokalemia, hyponatremia, libido decreased

Gastrointestinal: Abdominal distension, abdominal pain, anorexia, biliary colic, diarrhea, dyspepsia, dysphagia, flatulence, gastroenteritis, GERD, GI irritation, paralytic ileus, rectal disorder, taste perversion, weight loss

Genitourinary: Bladder spasm, dysuria, ejaculation abnormal, impotence, urination decreased

Hematologic: Leukopenia (<3%), thrombocytopenia (<3%), hematocrit decreased

Hepatic: Liver function tests increased

Neuromuscular & skeletal: Arthralgia, back pain, bone pain, foot drop, gait abnormalities, paresthesia, rigors, skeletal muscle rigidity, tremor

Ocular: Amblyopia, conjunctivitis, eye pain, vision problems/disturbance

Renal: Oliguria

Respiratory: Asthma, atelectasis, dyspnea, hiccups, hypercapnia, hypoxia, pulmonary edema (noncardiogenic), respiratory depression, rhinitis

Miscellaneous: Diaphoresis, flu-like syndrome, infection, thirst, voice alteration, withdrawal syndrome

<1% (Limited to important or life-threatening): Amenorrhea, anaphylaxis, apnea, biliary tract spasm, blurred vision, bronchospasm, cardiac arrest, cough reflex decreased, dehydration, diplopia, disorientation, hemorrhagic urticaria, intestinal obstruction, intracranial pressure increased, laryngospasm, menstrual irregularities, miosis, myoclonus, nystagmus, paradoxical CNS stimulation, respiratory arrest, sepsis, urinary tract spasm, thermal dysregulation, toxic psychoses

Drug Interactions

Metabolism/Transport Effects Substrate of CYP2D6 (minor)

Avoid Concomitant Use There are no known interactions where it is recommended to avoid concomitant use.

Increased Effect/Toxicity

Morphine Sulfate may increase the levels/effects of: Alcohol (Ethyl); Alvimopan; CNS Depressants; Desmopressin; Selective Serotonin Reuptake Inhibitors; Thiazide Diuretics

The levels/effects of Morphine Sulfate may be increased by: Amphetamines; Antipsychotic Agents (Phenothiazines); Succinylcholine

Decreased Effect

Morphine Sulfate may decrease the levels/effects of: Pegvisomant; Trovafloxacin

The levels/effects of Morphine Sulfate may be decreased by: Ammonium Chloride; Peginterferon Alfa-2b; Rifamycin Derivatives

Ethanol/Nutrition/Herb Interactions

Ethanol: Avoid ethanol, including alcoholic beverages or ethanol-containing products (may increase CNS depression).

Avinza®: Alcoholic beverages or ethanol-containing products may disrupt extended-release formulation resulting in rapid release of entire morphine dose.

Food: Administration of oral morphine solution with food may increase bioavailability (ie, a report of 34% increase in morphine AUC when morphine oral solution followed a high-fat meal). The bioavailability of Avinza®, Oramorph SR®, or Kadian® does not appear to be affected by food.

Herb/Nutraceutical: Avoid valerian, St John's wort, kava kava, gotu kola (may increase CNS depression).

Test Interactions Some quinolones may produce a false-positive urine screening result for opiates using commercially-available immunoassay kits. This has been demonstrated most consistently for levofloxacin and ofloxacin, but other quinolones have shown cross-reactivity in certain assay kits. Confirmation of positive opiate screens by more specific methods should be considered. ▶

◀ **Dietary Considerations** Morphine may cause GI upset; take with food if GI upset occurs. Be consistent when taking morphine with or without meals.

Dosage Forms Excipient information presented when available (limited, particularly for generics); consult specific product labeling. [DSC] = Discontinued product; [CAN] Canadian brand name

Capsule, extended release, oral:
  Avinza®: 30 mg, 45 mg, 60 mg, 75 mg, 90 mg, 120 mg
  Kadian®: 10 mg, 20 mg, 30 mg, 50 mg, 60 mg, 80 mg, 100 mg, 200 mg
Infusion [premixed in D$_5$W]: 1 mg/mL (100 mL, 250 mL)
Injection, extended release liposomal suspension [lumbar epidural injection, preservative free]:
  DepoDur®: 10 mg/mL (1 mL, 1.5 mL)
Injection, solution: 1 mg/mL (10 mL); 2 mg/mL (1 mL); 4 mg/mL (1 mL); 5 mg/mL (1 mL); 8 mg/mL (1 mL); 10 mg/0.7 mL (0.7 mL); 10 mg/mL (1 mL, 10 mL); 15 mg/mL (1 mL, 20 mL); 25 mg/mL (4 mL, 10 mL, 20 mL, 40 mL, 50 mL, 100 mL, 250 mL); 50 mg/mL (20 mL, 40 mL, 50 mL) [some preparations contain sodium metabisulfite]
Injection, solution [epidural, intrathecal, or I.V. infusion; preservative free]:
  Astramorph/PF™: 0.5 mg/mL (2 mL, 10 mL); 1 mg/mL (2 mL, 10 mL)
  Duramorph®: 0.5 mg/mL (10 mL); 1 mg/mL (10 mL)
Injection, solution [epidural or intrathecal infusion via microinfusion device; preservative free]:
  Infumorph® 200: 10 mg/mL (20 mL)
  Infumorph® 500: 25 mg/mL (20 mL)
Injection, solution [for PCA pump]: 1 mg/mL (30 mL; 50 mL [DSC]); 5 mg/mL (30 mL; 50 mL [DSC])
Injection, solution [for PCP pump, preservative free]: 1 mg/mL (30 mL)
Injection, solution [preservative free]: 0.5 mg/mL (10 mL); 1 mg/mL (10 mL); 25 mg/mL (10 mL)
Solution, oral: 10 mg/5 mL (5 mL, 100 mL, 500 mL)
  Doloral [CAN]: 1 mg/mL (10 mL, 250 mL, 500 mL); 5 mg/mL (10 mL, 250 mL, 500 mL) [not available in U.S.]
Solution, oral [concentrate]: 5 mg/0.25 mL (0.25 mL) [DSC]; 10 mg/0.5 mL (0.5 mL) [DSC]; 20 mg/mL (1 mL [DSC], 15 ml, 30 mL, 120 mL, 240 mL)
  Roxanol™: 20 mg/mL (30 mL, 120 mL); 100 mg/5 mL (240 mL)
Suppository, rectal: 5 mg (12s), 10 mg (12s), 20 mg (12s), 30 mg (12s)
Tablet, oral: 10 mg [DSC], 15 mg, 30 mg
Tablet, controlled release, oral: 15 mg, 30 mg, 60 mg, 100 mg, 200 mg
  MS Contin®: 15 mg, 30 mg, 60 mg, 100 mg, 200 mg
Tablet, extended release, oral: 15 mg, 30 mg, 60 mg, 100 mg, 200 mg
Tablet, sustained release, oral:
  Oramorph® SR: 15 mg, 30 mg, 60 mg, 100 mg

References

Braunwald E, Antman EM, Beasley JW, et al, "ACC/AHA Guidelines for the Management of Patients With Unstable Angina and Non-ST-Segment Elevation Myocardial Infarction. A Report of the American College of Cardiology/American Heart Association Task Force on Practice Guidelines (Committee on the Management of Patients With Unstable Angina)," *J Am Coll Cardiol*, 2000, 36 (3):970-1062.

Golianu B, Krane EJ, Galloway KS, et al, "Pediatric Acute Pain Management," *Pediatr Clin North Am*, 2000, 47(3):559-87.

Jacobi J, Fraser GL, Coursin DB, et al, "Clinical Practice Guidelines for the Sustained Use of Sedatives and Analgesics in the Critically Ill Adult," *Crit Care Med*, 2002, 30(1):119-41. Available at: http://www.sccm.org/pdf/sedatives.pdf.

Mokhlesi B, Leikin JB, Murray P, et al, "Adult Toxicology in Critical Care. Part 11: Specific Poisonings," *Chest*, 2003, 123(3):897-922.

"Principles of Analgesic Use in the Treatment of Acute Pain and Cancer Pain," 6th ed, Glenview, IL: American Pain Society, 2008.

◆ **Morphine Sulfate and Naltrexone Hydrochloride** *see* Morphine and Naltrexone *on page 949*

◆ **M.O.S.® 10 (Can)** *see* Morphine Sulfate *on page 953*

◆ **M.O.S.® 20 (Can)** *see* Morphine Sulfate *on page 953*

◆ **M.O.S.® 30 (Can)** *see* Morphine Sulfate *on page 953*

◆ **M.O.S.-SR® (Can)** *see* Morphine Sulfate *on page 953*

◆ **M.O.S.-Sulfate® (Can)** *see* Morphine Sulfate *on page 953*

◆ **Motrin® Children's [OTC]** *see* Ibuprofen *on page 717*

◆ **Motrin® (Children's) (Can)** *see* Ibuprofen *on page 717*

◆ **Motrin® IB [OTC]** *see* Ibuprofen *on page 717*

◆ **Motrin® IB (Can)** *see* Ibuprofen *on page 717*

◆ **Motrin® Infants' [OTC]** *see* Ibuprofen *on page 717*

◆ **Motrin® Junior [OTC]** *see* Ibuprofen *on page 717*

◆ **Moxatag™** *see* Amoxicillin *on page 95*

Moxifloxacin (moxs i FLOKS a sin)

Medication Safety Issues
Sound-alike/look-alike issues:
Avelox® may be confused with Avonex®

International issues:
Vigamox® may be confused with Fisamox® which is a brand name for amoxicillin in Australia

Medication Guide An FDA-approved patient medication guide, which is available with the product information and at http://www.accessdata.fda.gov/drugsatfda_docs/label/2009/021085s042,021277s036lbl.pdf, must be dispensed with this medication for each new outpatient prescription and refill.

Related Information
Prevention of Wound Infection and Sepsis in Surgical Patients *on page 1721*

U.S. Brand Names Avelox®; Avelox® I.V.; Vigamox®

Canadian Brand Names Avelox®; Avelox® I.V.; Vigamox®

Index Terms Moxifloxacin Hydrochloride

Pharmacologic Category Antibiotic, Ophthalmic; Antibiotic, Quinolone; Respiratory Fluoroquinolone

Generic Available No

Use Treatment of mild-to-moderate community-acquired pneumonia, including multidrug-resistant *Streptococcus pneumoniae* (MDRSP); acute bacterial exacerbation of chronic bronchitis; acute bacterial sinusitis; complicated and uncomplicated skin and skin structure infections; complicated intra-abdominal infections; bacterial conjunctivitis (ophthalmic formulation)

Unlabeled/Investigational Use *Legionella*

Mechanism of Action Moxifloxacin is a DNA gyrase inhibitor, and also inhibits topoisomerase IV. DNA gyrase (topoisomerase II) is an essential bacterial enzyme that maintains the superhelical structure of DNA. DNA gyrase is required for DNA replication and transcription, DNA repair, recombination, and transposition; inhibition is bactericidal.

Pharmacodynamics/Kinetics
Absorption: Well absorbed; not affected by high-fat meal or yogurt

Distribution: V_d: 1.7 to 2.7 L/kg; tissue concentrations often exceed plasma concentrations in respiratory tissues, alveolar macrophages, abdominal tissues/fluids, and sinus tissues

Protein binding: ~30% to 50%

Metabolism: Hepatic (~52% of dose) via glucuronide (~14%) and sulfate (~38%) conjugation

Bioavailability: ~90%

Half-life elimination: Single dose: Oral: 12-16 hours; I.V.: 8-15 hours

Excretion: Urine (as unchanged drug [20%] and glucuronide conjugates); feces (as unchanged drug [25%] and sulfate conjugates)

Dosage
Usual dosage range:
Children ≥1 year and Adults: Ophthalmic: Instill 1 drop into affected eye(s) 3 times/day for 7 days

Adults: Oral, I.V.: 400 mg every 24 hours

Indication-specific dosing:
Children ≥1 year and Adults: Ophthalmic:
Bacterial conjunctivitis: Instill 1 drop into affected eye(s) 3 times/day for 7 days

Adults: Oral, I.V.:

Acute bacterial sinusitis: 400 mg every 24 hours for 10 days

Chronic bronchitis, acute bacterial exacerbation: 400 mg every 24 hours for 5 days

Intra-abdominal infections (complicated): 400 mg every 24 hours for 5-14 days (initiate with I.V.)

Pneumonia, community-acquired (including MDRSP): 400 mg every 24 hours for 7-14 days

Skin and skin structure infections:

Complicated: 400 mg every 24 hours for 7-21 days

Uncomplicated: 400 mg every 24 hours for 7 days

Elderly: No dosage adjustments are required based on age

Dosage adjustment in renal impairment: No dosage adjustment is required, including patients on hemodialysis, CRRT, or CAPD.

Dosage adjustment in hepatic impairment: No dosage adjustment is required in mild, moderate, or severe hepatic insufficiency (Child-Pugh class A, B, or C); however, use with caution in this patient population secondary to the risk of QT prolongation.

Stability Store at controlled room temperature of 25°C (77°F). Do not refrigerate infusion solution.

Administration Administer without regard to meals.

I.V.: Infuse over 60 minutes; do not infuse by rapid or bolus intravenous infusion

Monitoring Parameters WBC, signs of infection

Anesthesia and Critical Care Concerns/Other Considerations

Clinical Pearls/Comments: Moxifloxacin causes a dose-dependent QT prolongation. Coadministration of moxifloxacin with other drugs that also prolong the QT interval or induce bradycardia (eg, beta-blockers, amiodarone) should be avoided. Careful consideration should be given in the use of moxifloxacin in patients with cardiovascular disease, in those with conduction abnormalities.

Pregnancy Risk Factor C

Contraindications Hypersensitivity to moxifloxacin, other quinolone antibiotics, or any component of the formulation

Warnings/Precautions [U.S. Boxed Warning]: There have been reports of tendon inflammation and/or rupture with quinolone antibiotics; risk may be increased with concurrent corticosteroids, organ transplant recipients, and in patients >60 years of age. Rupture of the Achilles tendon sometimes requiring surgical repair has been reported most frequently; but other tendon sites (eg, rotator cuff, biceps) have also been reported. Strenuous physical activity, rheumatoid arthritis, and renal impairment may be an independent risk factor for tendonitis. Discontinue at first sign of tendon inflammation or pain. Tendon rupture may occur even after discontinuation of therapy. Use with caution in patients with rheumatoid arthritis or renal impairment; may increase risk of tendon rupture.

Use with caution in patients with significant bradycardia or acute myocardial ischemia. Moxifloxacin causes a concentration-dependent QT prolongation. Do not exceed recommended dose or infusion rate. Avoid use with uncorrected hypokalemia, with other drugs that prolong the QT interval or induce bradycardia, or with class Ia or III antiarrhythmic agents. Use with caution in individuals at risk of seizures (CNS disorders or concurrent therapy with medications which may lower seizure threshold). Potential for seizures, although very rare, may be increased with concomitant NSAID therapy. Discontinue in patients who experience significant CNS adverse effects (dizziness, hallucinations, suicidal ideation or actions). Use with caution in patients with mild, moderate, or severe hepatic impairment or liver cirrhosis; may increase the risk of QT prolongation. Use with caution in diabetes; glucose regulation may be altered.

Fluoroquinolones have been associated with the development of serious, and sometimes fatal, hypoglycemia, most often in elderly diabetics, but also in patients without diabetes. This occurred most frequently with gatifloxacin (no longer available systemically) but may occur at a lower frequency with other quinolones.

Severe hypersensitivity reactions, including anaphylaxis, have occurred with quinolone therapy. Reactions may present as typical allergic symptoms after a single dose, or may manifest as severe idiosyncratic dermatologic, vascular, pulmonary, renal, hepatic, and/or hematologic events, usually after multiple doses. Prompt discontinuation of drug should occur if skin rash or other symptoms arise. Avoid excessive sunlight and take precautions to limit exposure (eg, loose fitting clothing, sunscreen); may cause moderate-to-severe phototoxicity reactions. Discontinue use if photosensitivity occurs. Prolonged use may result in fungal or bacterial superinfection, including *C. difficile*-associated diarrhea (CDAD) and pseudomembranous colitis; CDAD has been observed >2 months postantibiotic treatment. Quinolones may exacerbate myasthenia gravis. Peripheral neuropathy may rarely occur. Hemolytic reactions may (rarely) occur with quinolone use in patients with latent or actual G6PD deficiency. Adverse effects (eg, tendon rupture, QT changes) may be increased in the elderly. Some quinolones may exacerbate myasthenia gravis, use with caution (rare, potentially life-threatening weakness of respiratory muscles may occur). Safety and efficacy of systemically administered moxifloxacin (oral, intravenous) in patients <18 years of age have not been established.

Ophthalmic: Eye drops should not be injected subconjunctivally or introduced directly into the anterior chamber of the eye. Contact lenses should not be worn during therapy.

Adverse Reactions

Systemic:

2% to 10%:

Central nervous system: Dizziness (2%)

Endocrine & metabolic: Serum chloride increased (≥2%), serum ionized calcium increased (≥2%), serum glucose decreased (≥2%)

Gastrointestinal: Nausea (6%), diarrhea (5%), amylase decreased (≥2%)

Hematologic: Decreased serum levels of the following (≥2%): Basophils, eosinophils, hemoglobin, RBC, neutrophils; increased serum levels of the following (≥2%): MCH, neutrophils, WBC

Hepatic: Bilirubin decreased/increased (≥2%)

Renal: Serum albumin increased (≥2%)

Respiratory: PO_2 decreased (≥2%)

0.1% to <2%:

Cardiovascular: Cardiac arrhythmias, palpitation, QT_c prolongation, tachycardia, vasodilation

Central nervous system: Anxiety, headache, insomnia, malaise, nervousness, pain, somnolence, vertigo

Dermatologic: Pruritus, rash (maculopapular, purpuric, pustular), urticaria

Gastrointestinal: Abdominal pain, amylase increased, anorexia, constipation, dyspepsia, flatulence, glossitis, lactic dehydrogenase increased, stomatitis, taste perversion, vomiting, xerostomia

Genitourinary: Vaginal moniliasis, vaginitis

Hematologic: Eosinophilia, leukopenia, prothrombin time prolonged, increased INR, thrombocythemia

Hepatic: GGTP increased, liver function test abnormal

Local: Injection site reaction

Neuromuscular & skeletal: Arthralgia, myalgia, tremor, weakness

Respiratory: Pharyngitis, pneumonia, rhinitis, sinusitis

Miscellaneous: Allergic reaction, infection, diaphoresis, oral moniliasis

<0.1% (Limited to important or life-threatening): Abnormal dreams, abnormal gait, agitation, amblyopia, amnesia, anaphylactic reaction, anaphylactic shock, anemia, angioedema, aphasia, arthritis, asthma, atrial fibrillation, back pain, *C. difficile*-positive diarrhea, chest pain, cholestasis, confusion, depersonalization, depression, dysphagia, dyspnea, ECG abnormalities, emotional lability, face edema, gastritis, hallucinations, hepatic failure, hepatitis, hyperglycemia, hyperlipidemia, hyper-/hypotension, hypertonia, hyperuricemia, hypoesthesia, incoordination, INR decreased, jaundice (cholestatic), laryngeal edema, leg pain, nightmares, paresthesia, parosmia, pelvic pain, peripheral edema, peripheral neuropathy, photosensitivity/toxicity, prothrombin time decreased, pseudomembranous colitis, psychotic reaction, renal dysfunction, renal failure, seizure, sleep disorder, speech disorder, Stevens-Johnson syndrome, supraventricular tachycardia, syncope, taste loss, tendonitis, tendon rupture, thinking abnormal, thrombocytopenia, thromboplastin decreased, tinnitus, tongue discoloration, toxic epidermal necrolysis, ventricular tachyarrhythmias (including

◀ torsade de pointes and cardiac arrest [usually in patients with concurrent, severe proarrhythmic conditions]), vision abnormalities

Additional reactions with **ophthalmic** preparation: 1% to 6%: Conjunctivitis, dry eye, ocular discomfort, ocular hyperemia, ocular pain, ocular pruritus, subconjunctival hemorrhage, tearing, visual acuity decreased

Drug Interactions

Avoid Concomitant Use

Avoid concomitant use of Moxifloxacin with any of the following: Artemether; Dronedarone; Lumefantrine; Nilotinib; Pimozide; QuiNINE; Tetrabenazine; Thioridazine; Ziprasidone

Increased Effect/Toxicity

Moxifloxacin may increase the levels/effects of: Corticosteroids (Systemic); Dronedarone; Pimozide; QTc-Prolonging Agents; QuiNINE; Sulfonylureas; Tetrabenazine; Thioridazine; Vitamin K Antagonists; Ziprasidone

The levels/effects of Moxifloxacin may be increased by: Alfuzosin; Artemether; Chloroquine; Ciprofloxacin; Gadobutrol; Insulin; Lumefantrine; Nilotinib; Non-steroidal Anti-Inflammatory Agents; Probenecid; QuiNINE

Decreased Effect

Moxifloxacin may decrease the levels/effects of: Mycophenolate; Sulfonylureas; Typhoid Vaccine

The levels/effects of Moxifloxacin may be decreased by: Antacids; Didanosine; Iron Salts; Magnesium Salts; Quinapril; Sevelamer; Sucralfate; Zinc Salts

Ethanol/Nutrition/Herb Interactions Food: Absorption is not affected by administration with a high-fat meal or yogurt.

Test Interactions Some quinolones may produce a false-positive urine screening result for opiates using commercially-available immunoassay kits. This has been demonstrated most consistently for levofloxacin and ofloxacin, but other quinolones have shown cross-reactivity in certain assay kits. Confirmation of positive opiate screens by more specific methods should be considered.

Dietary Considerations May be taken without regard to meals. Take 4 hours before or 8 hours after multiple vitamins, antacids, or other products containing magnesium, aluminum, iron, or zinc.

Avelox® I.V. infusion (premixed in sodium chloride 0.8%) contains sodium 34.2 mEq (~787 mg)/250 mL.

Dosage Forms Excipient information presented when available (limited, particularly for generics); consult specific product labeling.

Infusion, premixed in sodium chloride 0.8% [preservative free]:

Avelox® I.V.: 400 mg (250 mL) [contains sodium ~787 mg (34.2 mEq)/250 mL]

Solution, ophthalmic:

Vigamox®: 0.5% (3 mL)

Tablet:

Avelox®: 400 mg

Avelox® ABC Pack: 400 mg (5s)

References

Graumlich JF, Habis S, Avelino RR, et al, "Hypoglycemia in Inpatients After Gatifloxacin or Levofloxacin Therapy: Nested Case-Control Study," *Pharmacotherapy*, 2005, 25(10):1296-302.

Malone RS, Fish DN, Abraham E, et al, "Pharmacokinetics of Levofloxacin and Ciprofloxacin During Continuous Renal Replacement Therapy in Critically Ill Patients," *Antimicrob Agents Chemother*, 2001, 45(10):2949-54.

Trotman RL, Williamson JC, Shoemaker DM, et al, "Antibiotic Dosing in Critically Ill Adult Patients Receiving Continuous Renal Replacement Therapy," *Clin Infect Dis*, 2005, 41(8):1159-66.

◆ **Moxifloxacin Hydrochloride** *see* Moxifloxacin *on page 961*

◆ **4-MP** *see* Fomepizole *on page 625*

◆ **MPA** *see* Mycophenolate *on page 966*

◆ **MPA and Estrogens (Conjugated)** *see* Estrogens (Conjugated/Equine) and Medroxyprogesterone *on page 539*

◆ **MS Contin®** *see* Morphine Sulfate *on page 953*

◆ **MS (error-prone abbreviation and should not be used)** *see* Morphine and Naltrexone *on page 949*

◆ **MS (error-prone abbreviation and should not be used)** *see* Morphine Sulfate *on page 953*

- **MS-IR® (Can)** *see* Morphine Sulfate *on page 953*
- **MSO₄ (error-prone abbreviation and should not be used)** *see* Morphine and Naltrexone *on page 949*
- **MSO₄ (error-prone abbreviation and should not be used)** *see* Morphine Sulfate *on page 953*
- **MTX (error-prone abbreviation)** *see* Methotrexate *on page 898*
- **Mucomyst** *see* Acetylcysteine *on page 35*
- **Mucomyst® (Can)** *see* Acetylcysteine *on page 35*
- **Multaq®** *see* Dronedarone *on page 461*

Mupirocin (myoo PEER oh sin)

Medication Safety Issues
Sound-alike/look-alike issues:
Bactroban® may be confused with bacitracin, baclofen, Bactrim™
U.S. Brand Names Bactroban Cream®; Bactroban Nasal®; Bactroban®
Canadian Brand Names Bactroban®
Index Terms Mupirocin Calcium; Pseudomonic Acid A
Pharmacologic Category Antibiotic, Topical
Generic Available Yes: Topical ointment
Use
Intranasal: Eradication of nasal colonization with MRSA in adult patients and healthcare workers
Topical: Treatment of impetigo or secondary infected traumatic skin lesions due to *S. aureus* and *S. pyogenes*
Unlabeled/Investigational Use Intranasal: Surgical prophylaxis to prevent wound infections
Mechanism of Action Binds to bacterial isoleucyl transfer-RNA synthetase resulting in the inhibition of protein synthesis
Pharmacodynamics/Kinetics
Absorption: Topical: Penetrates outer layers of skin; systemic absorption minimal through intact skin
Metabolism: Skin: 3% to monic acid (inactive)
Excretion: Urine
Dosage
Intranasal: Children ≥12 years and Adults: Eradication of nasal MRSA: Approximately one-half of the ointment from the single-use tube should be applied into one nostril and the other half into the other nostril twice daily for 5 days
Topical:
Children ≥2 months and Adults: Impetigo: Ointment: Apply to affected area 3 times/day; re-evaluate after 3-5 days if no clinical response
Children ≥3 months and Adults: Secondary skin infections: Cream: Apply to affected area 3 times/day for 10 days; re-evaluate after 3-5 days if no clinical response
Administration
Intranasal ointment: After application into nostrils, press sides of nose together and gently massage to spread ointment throughout the insides of the nostrils; discard tube after use
Topical cream, ointment: For external use only; area may be covered with gauze if desired
Pregnancy Risk Factor B
Contraindications Hypersensitivity to mupirocin or any component of the formulation
Warnings/Precautions Potentially toxic amounts of polyethylene glycol contained in some topical products may be absorbed percutaneously in patients with extensive burns or open wounds; use caution with renal impairment. Prolonged use may result in over growth of nonsusceptible organisms. For external use only; avoid contact with eyes. Not for treatment of pressure sores. If skin irritation occurs, discontinue use. Safety and efficacy of the nasal product have not been established in children <12 years of age.

◄ **Adverse Reactions** Frequency not defined.

Central nervous system: Dizziness, headache

Dermatologic: Cellulitis, dermatitis, dry skin, erythema, hives, pruritus, rash

Gastrointestinal: Abdominal pain, diarrhea, nausea, taste perversion, ulcerative stomatitis, xerostomia

Local: Burning, edema, pain, stinging, tenderness

Ocular: Blepharitis

Otic: Ear pain

Respiratory: Cough, pharyngitis, rhinitis, upper respiratory tract congestion

Miscellaneous: Secondary wound infection

Drug Interactions

Avoid Concomitant Use There are no known interactions where it is recommended to avoid concomitant use.

Increased Effect/Toxicity There are no known significant interactions involving an increase in effect.

Decreased Effect

Mupirocin may decrease the levels/effects of: Typhoid Vaccine

Dosage Forms Excipient information presented when available (limited, particularly for generics); consult specific product labeling.

Note: Strength expressed as base

Cream, topical, as calcium:

Bactroban Cream®: 2% (15 g, 30 g) [contains benzyl alcohol]

Ointment, intranasal, as calcium:

Bactroban Nasal®: 2% (1 g) [single-use tube]

Ointment, topical: 2% (0.9 g, 22 g)

Bactroban®: 2% (22 g) [contains polyethylene glycol]

References

Perl TM, Cullen JJ, Wenzel RP, et al, "Intranasal Mupirocin to Prevent Postoperative *Staphylococcus aureus* Infections," *N Engl J Med*, 2002, 346(24):1871-7.

◆ **Mupirocin Calcium** *see* Mupirocin *on page 965*

◆ **Muro 128® [OTC]** *see* Sodium Chloride *on page 1304*

◆ **Muse®** *see* Alprostadil *on page 66*

◆ **Muse® Pellet (Can)** *see* Alprostadil *on page 66*

◆ **Mycamine®** *see* Micafungin *on page 933*

◆ **Mycinaire™ [OTC] [DSC]** *see* Sodium Chloride *on page 1304*

Mycophenolate (mye koe FEN oh late)

Medication Guide An FDA-approved medication guide must be distributed when dispensing an outpatient prescription (new or refill) if this medication is to be used without direct supervision of a healthcare provider. Medication guides are available:

Myfortic®: http://www.accessdata.fda.gov/drugsatfda_docs/label/2008/050791s004lbl.pdf

CellCept®: http://www.fda.gov/downloads/Drugs/DrugSafety/UCM170919.pdf

U.S. Brand Names CellCept®; Myfortic®

Canadian Brand Names CellCept®; Myfortic®

Index Terms MMF; MPA; Mycophenolate Mofetil; Mycophenolate Sodium; Mycophenolic Acid

Pharmacologic Category Immunosuppressant Agent

Generic Available Yes: Capsule, tablet

Use Prophylaxis of organ rejection concomitantly with cyclosporine and corticosteroids in patients receiving allogeneic renal (CellCept®, Myfortic®), cardiac (CellCept®), or hepatic (CellCept®) transplants

Unlabeled/Investigational Use Treatment of rejection in liver transplant patients unable to tolerate tacrolimus or cyclosporine due to neurotoxicity; mild rejection in heart transplant patients; treatment of moderate-severe psoriasis; treatment of proliferative lupus nephritis; treatment of myasthenia gravis; prevention and treatment of graft-versus-host disease (GVHD)

Mechanism of Action MPA exhibits a cytostatic effect on T and B lymphocytes. It is an inhibitor of inosine monophosphate dehydrogenase (IMPDH) which inhibits *de novo* guanosine nucleotide synthesis. T and B lymphocytes are dependent on this pathway for proliferation.

Pharmacodynamics/Kinetics

Onset of action: Peak effect: Correlation of toxicity or efficacy is still being developed, however, one study indicated that 12-hour AUCs >40 mcg/mL/hour were correlated with efficacy and decreased episodes of rejection

T_{max}: Oral: MPA:
  CellCept®: 1-1.5 hours
  Myfortic®: 1.5-2.75 hours

Absorption: AUC values for MPA are lower in the early post-transplant period versus later (>3 months) post-transplant period. The extent of absorption in pediatrics is similar to that seen in adults, although there was wide variability reported.
  Oral: Myfortic®: 93%

Distribution:
  CellCept®: MPA: Oral: 4 L/kg; I.V.: 3.6 L/kg
  Myfortic®: MPA: Oral: 54 L (at steady state); 112 L (elimination phase)
Protein binding: MPA: >98%, MPAG 82%

Metabolism: Hepatic and via GI tract; CellCept® is completely hydrolyzed in the liver to mycophenolic acid (MPA; active metabolite); enterohepatic recirculation of MPA may occur; MPA is glucuronidated to MPAG (inactive metabolite)

Bioavailability: Oral: CellCept®: 94%; Myfortic®: 72%

Half-life elimination:
  CellCept®: MPA: Oral: 18 hours; I.V.: 17 hours
  Myfortic®: MPA: Oral: 8-16 hours; MPAG: 13-17 hours

Excretion:
  CellCept®: MPA: Urine (<1%), feces (6%); MPAG: Urine (87%)
  Myfortic®: MPA: Urine (3%), feces; MPAG: Urine (>60%)

Dosage

Children: Renal transplant: Oral:
  CellCept® suspension: 600 mg/m²/dose twice daily; maximum dose: 1 g twice daily
    Alternatively, may use solid dosage forms according to BSA as follows:
    BSA 1.25-1.5 m²: 750 mg capsule twice daily
    BSA >1.5 m²: 1 g capsule or tablet twice daily
  Myfortic®: 400 mg/m²/dose twice daily; maximum dose: 720 mg twice daily
    BSA <1.19 m²: Use of this formulation is not recommended
    BSA 1.19-1.58 m²: 540 mg twice daily (maximum: 1080 mg/day)
    BSA >1.58 m²: 720 mg twice daily (maximum: 1440 mg/day)

Adults: **Note:** May be used I.V. for up to 14 days; transition to oral therapy as soon as tolerated.
  Renal transplant:
    CellCept®:
      Oral: 1 g twice daily. Doses >2 g/day are not recommended.
      I.V.: 1 g twice daily
    Myfortic®: Oral: 720 mg twice daily (1440 mg/day)
  Cardiac transplantation:
    Oral (CellCept®): 1.5 g twice daily
    I.V. (CellCept®): 1.5 g twice daily
  Hepatic transplantation:
    Oral (CellCept®): 1.5 g twice daily
    I.V. (CellCept®): 1 g twice daily
  Myasthenia gravis (unlabeled use): Oral (CellCept®): 1 g twice daily (range 1-3 g/day)

Elderly: Dosage is the same as younger patients, however, dosing should be cautious due to possibility of increased hepatic, renal or cardiac dysfunction; elderly patients may be at an increased risk of certain infections, gastrointestinal hemorrhage, and pulmonary edema, as compared to younger patients

Dosing adjustment for toxicity (neutropenia): Neutropenia (ANC <1.3 x 10³/µL): Dosing should be interrupted or the dose reduced, appropriate diagnostic tests performed and patients managed appropriately

Dosing adjustment in renal impairment:
Renal transplant: GFR <25 mL/minute/1.73 m^2 in patients outside the immediate post-transplant period:
CellCept®: Doses of >1 g administered twice daily should be avoided; patients should also be carefully observed; no dose adjustments are needed in renal transplant patients experiencing delayed graft function postoperatively
Myfortic®: No dose adjustments are needed in renal transplant patients experiencing delayed graft function postoperatively; however, monitor carefully for potential concentration dependent adverse events
Cardiac or liver transplant: No data available; mycophenolate may be used in cardiac or hepatic transplant patients with severe chronic renal impairment if the potential benefit outweighs the potential risk
Hemodialysis: Not removed; supplemental dose is not necessary
Peritoneal dialysis: Supplemental dose is not necessary
Dosage adjustment in hepatic impairment: No dosage adjustment is recommended for renal patients with severe hepatic parenchymal disease; however, it is not currently known whether dosage adjustments are necessary for hepatic disease with other etiologies

Stability
Capsules: Store at room temperature of 15°C to 30°C (59°F to 86°F).
Tablets: Store at room temperature of 15°C to 30°C (59°F to 86°F). Protect from moisture and light.
Oral suspension: Store powder for oral suspension at room temperature of 15°C to 30°C (59°F to 86°F). Should be constituted prior to dispensing to the patient and **not** mixed with any other medication. Add 47 mL of water to the bottle and shake well for ~1 minute. Add another 47 mL of water to the bottle and shake well for an additional minute. Final concentration is 200 mg/mL of mycophenolate mofetil. Once reconstituted, the oral solution may be stored at room temperature or under refrigeration. Do not freeze. The mixed suspension is stable for 60 days.
I.V.: Store intact vials at room temperature 15°C to 30°C (59°F to 86°F). Reconstitute the contents of each vial with 14 mL of 5% dextrose injection; dilute the contents of a vial with 5% dextrose in water to a final concentration of 6 mg mycophenolate mofetil per mL. Begin infusion within 4 hours of reconstitution. **Note:** Vial is vacuum-sealed; if a lack of vacuum is noted during preparation, the vial should not be used. Store solutions at 15°C to 30°C (59°F to 86°F).

Administration
Oral dosage formulations (tablet, capsule, suspension) should be administered on an empty stomach to avoid variability in MPA absorption. The oral solution may be administered via a nasogastric tube (minimum 8 French, 1.7 mm interior diameter); oral suspension should not be mixed with other medications. Delayed release tablets should not be crushed, cut, or chewed.
Intravenous solutions should be administered over at least 2 hours (either peripheral or central vein); do **not** administer intravenous solution by rapid or bolus injection.
Monitoring Parameters Complete blood count (weekly for first month, twice monthly during months 2 and 3, then monthly thereafter through the first year); renal and liver function; signs and symptoms of infection; pregnancy test (prior to initiation in females of childbearing potential)

Anesthesia and Critical Care Concerns/Other Considerations

Clinical Pearls/Comments: Hypertension may accompany the use of mycophenolate in patients post-transplantation. Furthermore, this drug may also increase cholesterol, impair glucose tolerance, deplete phosphate, and have variable effects on potassium hemeostasis.

Pregnancy Risk Factor D
Contraindications Hypersensitivity to mycophenolate mofetil, mycophenolic acid, mycophenolate sodium, or any component of the formulation; intravenous formulation is contraindicated in patients who are allergic to polysorbate 80

Warnings/Precautions Hazardous agent - use appropriate precautions for handling and disposal. **[U.S. Boxed Warning]: Risk for infection and development of lymphoma and skin malignancy is increased.** Opportunistic infections, sepsis, and/or fatal infections may occur with immunosuppressive therapy. Patients should be monitored appropriately. Instruct patients to limit exposure to sunlight/UV light and give supportive treatment should these conditions occur. Pure red cell aplasia (PRCA) or progressive multifocal leukoencephalopathy (PML) may occur rarely, particularly in immunosuppressed patients or those receiving immunosuppressant therapy; monitor for signs of PRCA (anemia, fatigue, lethargy, pallor, dyspnea) or PML (neurologic impairment, apathy, ataxia, cognitive deficiencies, confusion, and hemiparesis); may require dosage reduction or discontinuation of therapy. Neutropenia (including severe neutropenia) may occur, requiring dose reduction or interruption of treatment (risk greater from day 31-180 post-transplant). Use caution with active peptic ulcer disease; may be associated with gastric or duodenal ulcers, GI bleeding and/or perforation. Use caution in renal impairment as toxicity may be increased; may require dosage adjustment in severe impairment.

[U.S. Boxed Warning]: Mycophenolate is associated with an increased risk of congenital malformations and spontaneous abortions when used during pregnancy. Females of childbearing potential should have a negative pregnancy test within 1 week prior to beginning therapy. Two reliable forms of contraception should be used beginning 4 weeks prior to, during, and for 6 weeks after therapy. Because mycophenolate mofetil has demonstrated teratogenic effects in rats and rabbits, tablets should not be crushed, and capsules should not be opened or crushed. Avoid inhalation or direct contact with skin or mucous membranes of the powder contained in the capsules and the powder for oral suspension. Caution should be exercised in the handling and preparation of solutions of intravenous mycophenolate. Avoid skin contact with the intravenous solution and reconstituted suspension. If such contact occurs, wash thoroughly with soap and water, rinse eyes with plain water.

Theoretically, use should be avoided in patients with the rare hereditary deficiency of hypoxanthine-guanine phosphoribosyltransferase (such as Lesch-Nyhan or Kelley-Seegmiller syndrome). Intravenous solutions should be given over at least 2 hours; never administer intravenous solution by rapid or bolus injection. **[U.S. Boxed Warning]: Should be administered under the supervision of a physician experienced in immunosuppressive therapy.**

Note: CellCept® and Myfortic® dosage forms should not be used interchangeably due to differences in absorption. Some dosage forms may contain phenylalanine.

Adverse Reactions As reported in adults following oral dosing of CellCept® alone in renal, cardiac, and hepatic allograft rejection studies. In general, lower doses used in renal rejection patients had less adverse effects than higher doses. Rates of adverse effects were similar for each indication, except for those unique to the specific organ involved. The type of adverse effects observed in pediatric patients was similar to those seen in adults; abdominal pain, anemia, diarrhea, fever, hypertension, infection, pharyngitis, respiratory tract infection, sepsis, and vomiting were seen in higher proportion; lymphoproliferative disorder was the only type of malignancy observed. Percentages of adverse reactions were similar in studies comparing CellCept® to Myfortic® in patients following renal transplant.

>20%:
Cardiovascular: Hypertension (28% to 77%), hypotension (up to 33%), peripheral edema (27% to 64%), edema (27% to 28%), chest pain (26%), tachycardia (20% to 22%)

Central nervous system: Pain (31% to 76%), headache (16% to 54%), insomnia (41% to 52%), fever (21% to 52%), dizziness (up to 29%), anxiety (28%)

Dermatologic: Rash (up to 22%)

Endocrine & metabolic: Hyperglycemia (44% to 47%), hypercholesterolemia (41%), hypomagnesemia (up to 39%), hypokalemia (32% to 37%), hypocalcemia (up to 30%), hyperkalemia (up to 22%)

Gastrointestinal: Abdominal pain (25% to 63%), nausea (20% to 55%), diarrhea (31% to 51%), constipation (19% to 41%), vomiting (33% to 34%), anorexia (up to 25%), dyspepsia (22%)

Genitourinary: Urinary tract infection (37%)

Hematologic: Leukopenia (23% to 46%), anemia (26% to 43%; hypochromic 25%), leukocytosis (22% to 40%), thrombocytopenia (24% to 38%)

Hepatic: Liver function tests abnormal (up to 25%), ascites (24%)

Neuromuscular & skeletal: Back pain (35% to 47%), weakness (35% to 43%), tremor (24% to 34%), paresthesia (21%)

Renal: Creatinine increased (up to 39%), BUN increased (up to 35%)

Respiratory: Dyspnea (31% to 37%), respiratory tract infection (22% to 37%), pleural effusion (34%), cough (31%), lung disorder (22% to 30%), sinusitis (26%)

Miscellaneous: Infection (18% to 27%), *Candida* (17% to 22%), herpes simplex (10% to 21%)

3% to <20%:

Cardiovascular: Angina, arrhythmia, arterial thrombosis, atrial fibrillation, atrial flutter, bradycardia, cardiac arrest, cardiac failure, CHF, extrasystole, facial edema, hypervolemia, pallor, palpitation, pericardial effusion, peripheral vascular disorder, postural hypotension, supraventricular extrasystoles, supraventricular tachycardia, syncope, thrombosis, vasodilation, vasospasm, venous pressure increased, ventricular extrasystole, ventricular tachycardia

Central nervous system: Agitation, chills with fever, confusion, convulsion, delirium, depression, emotional lability, hallucinations, hypoesthesia, malaise, nervousness, psychosis, somnolence, thinking abnormal, vertigo

Dermatologic: Acne, alopecia, bruising, cellulitis, hirsutism, petechia, pruritus, skin carcinoma, skin hypertrophy, skin ulcer, vesiculobullous rash

Endocrine & metabolic: Acidosis, Cushing's syndrome, dehydration, diabetes mellitus, gout, hypercalcemia, hyperlipemia, hyperphosphatemia, hyperuricemia, hypochloremia, hypoglycemia, hyponatremia, hypoproteinemia, hypothyroidism, parathyroid disorder, weight gain/loss

Gastrointestinal: Abdomen enlarged, dry mouth, dysphagia, esophagitis, flatulence, gastritis, gastroenteritis, gastrointestinal hemorrhage, gastrointestinal moniliasis, gingivitis, gum hyperplasia, ileus, melena, mouth ulceration, oral moniliasis, stomach disorder, stomatitis

Genitourinary: Impotence, nocturia, pelvic pain, prostatic disorder, scrotal edema, urinary frequency, urinary incontinence, urinary retention, urinary tract disorder

Hematologic: Coagulation disorder, hemorrhage, neutropenia, pancytopenia, polycythemia, prothrombin time increased, thromboplastin increased

Hepatic: Alkaline phosphatase increased, alkalosis, bilirubinemia, cholangitis, cholestatic jaundice, GGT increased, hepatitis, jaundice, liver damage, transaminases increased

Local: Abscess

Neuromuscular & skeletal: Arthralgia, hypertonia, joint disorder, leg cramps, myalgia, myasthenia, neck pain, neuropathy, osteoporosis

Ocular: Amblyopia, cataract, conjunctivitis, eye hemorrhage, lacrimation disorder, vision abnormal

Otic: Deafness, ear disorder, ear pain, tinnitus

Renal: Albuminuria, creatinine increased, dysuria, hematuria, hydronephrosis, kidney failure, kidney tubular necrosis, oliguria

Respiratory: Apnea, asthma, atelectasis, bronchitis, epistaxis, hemoptysis, hiccup, hyperventilation, hypoxia, respiratory acidosis, lung edema, pharyngitis, pneumonia, pneumothorax, pulmonary hypertension, respiratory moniliasis, rhinitis, sputum increased, voice alteration

Miscellaneous: *Candida* (mucocutaneous 16% to 18%), CMV viremia/syndrome (12% to 14%), CMV tissue invasive disease (6% to 11%), herpes zoster cutaneous disease (4% to 10%), cyst, diaphoresis, flu-like syndrome, fungal dermatitis, healing abnormal, hernia, ileus infection, lactic dehydrogenase increased, peritonitis, pyelonephritis, sepsis, thirst

Postmarketing and/or case reports: Atypical mycobacterial infection, colitis, gastrointestinal perforation, gastrointestinal ulcers, infectious endocarditis, interstitial lung disorder, intestinal villous atrophy, meningitis, pancreatitis, progressive multifocal leukoencephalopathy, pulmonary fibrosis (fatal), pure red cell aplasia, tuberculosis

Drug Interactions

Avoid Concomitant Use

Avoid concomitant use of Mycophenolate with any of the following: Cholestyramine Resin; Natalizumab; Rifamycin Derivatives; Vaccines (Live)

Increased Effect/Toxicity

Mycophenolate may increase the levels/effects of: Acyclovir-Valacyclovir; Ganciclovir-Valganciclovir; Leflunomide; Natalizumab; Vaccines (Live)

The levels/effects of Mycophenolate may be increased by: Acyclovir-Valacyclovir; Ganciclovir-Valganciclovir; Probenecid; Trastuzumab

Decreased Effect

Mycophenolate may decrease the levels/effects of: Oral Contraceptive (Estrogens); Oral Contraceptive (Progestins); Vaccines (Inactivated); Vaccines (Live)

The levels/effects of Mycophenolate may be decreased by: Antacids; Cholestyramine Resin; CycloSPORINE; Echinacea; Magnesium Salts; MetroNIDAZOLE; Penicillins; Proton Pump Inhibitors; Quinolone Antibiotics; Rifamycin Derivatives; Sevelamer

Ethanol/Nutrition/Herb Interactions

Food: Decreases C_{max} of MPA by 40% following CellCept® administration and 33% following Myfortic® use; the extent of absorption is not changed

Herb/Nutraceutical: Avoid cat's claw, echinacea (have immunostimulant properties)

Dietary Considerations Oral dosage formulations should be taken on an empty stomach to avoid variability in MPA absorption. However, in stable renal transplant patients, may be administered with food if necessary. Oral suspension contains phenylalanine; use caution if administered to patients with phenylketonuria.

Dosage Forms Excipient information presented when available (limited, particularly for generics); consult specific product labeling.

Capsule, oral, as mofetil: 250 mg
  CellCept®: 250 mg
Injection, powder for reconstitution, as mofetil hydrochloride:
  CellCept®: 500 mg [contains polysorbate 80]
Powder for suspension, oral, as mofetil:
  CellCept®: 200 mg/mL (175 mL) [contains phenylalanine 0.56 mg/mL; mixed fruit flavor]
Tablet, oral, as mofetil: 500 mg
  CellCept®: 500 mg [may contain ethyl alcohol]
Tablet, delayed release, as mycophenolic acid:
  Myfortic®: 180 mg, 360 mg [formulated as a sodium salt]

- **Mylan-Captopril (Can)** *see* Captopril *on page* 239
- **Mylan-Carbamazepine CR (Can)** *see* CarBAMazepine *on page* 241
- **Mylan-Cilazapril (Can)** *see* Cilazapril *on page* 301
- **Mylan-Cimetidine (Can)** *see* Cimetidine *on page* 305
- **Mylan-Ciprofloxacin (Can)** *see* Ciprofloxacin *on page* 306
- **Mylan-Clarithromycin (Can)** *see* Clarithromycin *on page* 317
- **Mylan-Clindamycin (Can)** *see* Clindamycin *on page* 324
- **Mylan-Clonazepam (Can)** *see* ClonazePAM *on page* 328
- **Mylan-Divalproex (Can)** *see* Valproic Acid and Derivatives *on page* 1445
- **Mylan-Enalapril (Can)** *see* Enalapril *on page* 478
- **Mylan-Famotidine (Can)** *see* Famotidine *on page* 575
- **Mylan-Fenofibrate Micro (Can)** *see* Fenofibrate *on page* 582
- **Mylan-Fluconazole (Can)** *see* Fluconazole *on page* 607
- **Mylan-Fluoxetine (Can)** *see* FLUoxetine *on page* 616
- **Mylan-Fosinopril (Can)** *see* Fosinopril *on page* 636
- **Mylan-Gabapentin (Can)** *see* Gabapentin *on page* 650
- **Mylan-Glybe (Can)** *see* GlyBURIDE *on page* 666
- **Mylan-Hydroxyurea (Can)** *see* Hydroxyurea *on page* 712
- **Mylan-Ipratropium Solution (Can)** *see* Ipratropium *on page* 760
- **Mylan-Ipratropium Sterinebs (Can)** *see* Ipratropium *on page* 760
- **Mylan-Lamotrigine (Can)** *see* LamoTRIgine *on page* 800
- **Mylan-Levofloxacin (Can)** *see* Levofloxacin *on page* 823
- **Mylan-Lisinopril (Can)** *see* Lisinopril *on page* 849
- **Mylan-Lovastatin (Can)** *see* Lovastatin *on page* 859
- **Mylan-Meloxicam (Can)** *see* Meloxicam *on page* 870
- **Mylan-Metformin (Can)** *see* MetFORMIN *on page* 886
- **Mylan-Metoprolol (Type L) (Can)** *see* Metoprolol *on page* 922
- **Mylan-Nabumetone (Can)** *see* Nabumetone *on page* 973
- **Mylan-Naproxen EC (Can)** *see* Naproxen *on page* 987
- **Mylan-Nifedipine Extended Release (Can)** *see* NIFEdipine *on page* 1006
- **Mylan-Nitro Sublingual Spray (Can)** *see* Nitroglycerin *on page* 1014
- **Mylan-Omeprazole (Can)** *see* Omeprazole *on page* 1048
- **Mylan-Ondansetron (Can)** *see* Ondansetron *on page* 1057
- **Mylan-Oxybutynin (Can)** *see* Oxybutynin *on page* 1068
- **Mylan-Pantoprazole (Can)** *see* Pantoprazole *on page* 1084
- **Mylan-Paroxetine (Can)** *see* PARoxetine *on page* 1089
- **Mylan-Pioglitazone (Can)** *see* Pioglitazone *on page* 1132
- **Mylan-Pravastatin (Can)** *see* Pravastatin *on page* 1162
- **Mylan-Propafenone (Can)** *see* Propafenone *on page* 1189
- **Mylan-Quetiapine (Can)** *see* QUEtiapine *on page* 1212
- **Mylan-Ramipril (Can)** *see* Ramipril *on page* 1229
- **Mylan-Ranitidine (Can)** *see* Ranitidine *on page* 1231
- **Mylan-Salbutamol Respirator Solution (Can)** *see* Albuterol *on page* 49
- **Mylan-Salbutamol Sterinebs P.F. (Can)** *see* Albuterol *on page* 49
- **Mylan-Selegiline (Can)** *see* Selegiline *on page* 1282
- **Mylan-Simvastatin (Can)** *see* Simvastatin *on page* 1293
- **Mylan-Sotalol (Can)** *see* Sotalol *on page* 1321
- **Mylan-Sumatriptan (Can)** *see* SUMAtriptan *on page* 1336
- **Mylan-Ticlopidine (Can)** *see* Ticlopidine *on page* 1385
- **Mylan-Timolol (Can)** *see* Timolol *on page* 1390

- ◆ **Mylan-Topiramate (Can)** *see* Topiramate *on page 1408*
- ◆ **Mylan-Trazodone (Can)** *see* TraZODone *on page 1423*
- ◆ **Mylan-Triazolam (Can)** *see* Triazolam *on page 1434*
- ◆ **Mylan-Valproic (Can)** *see* Valproic Acid and Derivatives *on page 1445*
- ◆ **Mylan-Venlafaxine XR (Can)** *see* Venlafaxine *on page 1466*
- ◆ **Mylan-Verapamil (Can)** *see* Verapamil *on page 1468*
- ◆ **Mylan-Verapamil SR (Can)** *see* Verapamil *on page 1468*
- ◆ **Mylan-Warfarin (Can)** *see* Warfarin *on page 1479*
- ◆ **Mylocel™** *see* Hydroxyurea *on page 712*
- ◆ **Nabi-HB®** *see* Hepatitis B Immune Globulin *on page 685*

Nabumetone (na BYOO me tone)

Related Information
  Chronic Pain Management *on page 1546*
  Nonsteroidal Anti-Inflammatory Agents *on page 1687*
Canadian Brand Names Apo-Nabumetone®; Gen-Nabumetone; Mylan-Nabumetone; Novo-Nabumetone; Relafen®; Rhoxal-nabumetone; Sandoz-Nabumetone
Index Terms Relafen
Pharmacologic Category Nonsteroidal Anti-inflammatory Drug (NSAID), Oral
Use Management of osteoarthritis and rheumatoid arthritis
Unlabeled/Investigational Use Moderate pain
Pharmacodynamics/Kinetics
  Onset of action: Several days
  Distribution: Diffusion occurs readily into synovial fluid
    V_d: 6MNA: 29-82 L
  Protein binding: 6MNA: >99%
  Metabolism: Prodrug, rapidly metabolized in the liver to an active metabolite [6-methoxy-2-naphthylacetic acid (6MNA)] and inactive metabolites; extensive first-pass effect
  Half-life elimination: 6MNA: ~24 hours
  Time to peak, serum: 6MNA: Oral: 2.5-4 hours; Synovial fluid: 4-12 hours
  Excretion: 6MNA: Urine (80%) and feces (9%)
Dosage Adults: Oral: 1000 mg/day; an additional 500-1000 mg may be needed in some patients to obtain more symptomatic relief; may be administered once or twice daily (maximum dose: 2000 mg/day)
  Note: Patients <50 kg are less likely to require doses >1000 mg/day.

  Dosage adjustment in renal impairment: In general, NSAIDs are not recommended for use in patients with advanced renal disease, but the manufacturer of nabumetone does provide some guidelines for adjustment in renal dysfunction:
    Moderate impairment (Cl_{cr} 30-49 mL/minute): Initial dose: 750 mg/day; maximum dose: 1500 mg/day
    Severe impairment (Cl_{cr} <30 mL/minute): Initial dose: 500 mg/day; maximum dose: 1000 mg/day
Anesthesia and Critical Care Concerns/Other Considerations The 2002 ACCM/SCCM guidelines for analgesia (critically-ill adult) suggest that NSAIDs may be used in combination with opioids in select patients for pain management. Concern about adverse events (increased risk of renal dysfunction, altered platelet function and gastrointestinal irritation) limits its use in patients who have other underlying risks for these events.

In short-term use, NSAIDs vary considerably in their effect on blood pressure. When NSAIDs are used in patients with hypertension, appropriate monitoring of blood pressure responses should be completed and the duration of therapy, when possible, kept short. The use of NSAIDs in the treatment of patients with congestive heart failure may be associated with an increased risk for fluid accumulation and edema; may precipitate renal failure in dehydrated patients.
Additional Information Complete prescribing information for this medication should be consulted for additional detail.

◀ **Dosage Forms** Excipient information presented when available (limited, particularly for generics); consult specific product labeling.
Tablet: 500 mg, 750 mg

◆ **NAC** *see Acetylcysteine on page 35*

◆ *N*-**Acetyl-L-cysteine** *see Acetylcysteine on page 35*

◆ *N*-**Acetylcysteine** *see Acetylcysteine on page 35*

◆ **N-Acetyl-P-Aminophenol** *see Acetaminophen on page 25*

◆ **NaCl** *see Sodium Chloride on page 1304*

Nadolol (NAY doe lol)

Related Information
Antiarrhythmic Drugs *on page 1656*
Beta-Blockers *on page 1669*
Preoperative Evaluation of the Cardiac Patient for Noncardiac Surgery *on page 1598*

U.S. Brand Names Corgard®

Canadian Brand Names Alti-Nadolol; Apo-Nadol®; Corgard®; Novo-Nadolol

Pharmacologic Category Beta-Adrenergic Blocker, Nonselective

Use Treatment of hypertension and angina pectoris; prophylaxis of migraine headaches

Unlabeled/Investigational Use Primary and secondary prophylaxis of variceal hemorrhage

Pharmacodynamics/Kinetics
Duration: 17-24 hours
Absorption: 30% to 40%
Distribution: V_d: 1.9 L/kg
Protein binding: 30%
Metabolism: Not metabolized
Half-life elimination: Adults: 10-24 hours; prolonged with renal impairment; End-stage renal disease: 45 hours
Time to peak, serum: 2-4 hours
Excretion: Urine (as unchanged drug)

Dosage Oral:
Adults: Initial: 40 mg/day, increase dosage gradually by 40-80 mg increments at 3- to 7-day intervals until optimum clinical response is obtained with profound slowing of heart rate; doses up to 160-240 mg/day in angina and 240-320 mg/day in hypertension may be necessary.
Hypertension: Usual dosage range (JNC 7): 40-120 mg once daily
Variceal hemorrhage prophylaxis (unlabeled use; Garcia-Tsao, 2007):
Primary prophylaxis: Initial: 40 mg once daily; adjust to maximal tolerated dose. **Note:** Risk factors for hemorrhage include Child-Pugh class B/C or variceal red wale markings on endoscopy.
Secondary prophylaxis: Initial: 40 mg once daily; adjust to maximal tolerated dose
Elderly: Initial: 20 mg/day; increase doses by 20 mg increments at 3- to 7-day intervals; usual dosage range: 20-240 mg/day.
Dosing adjustment in renal impairment:
Cl_{cr} 31-40 mL/minute: Administer every 24-36 hours or administer 50% of normal dose.
Cl_{cr} 10-30 mL/minute: Administer every 24-48 hours or administer 50% of normal dose.
Cl_{cr} <10 mL/minute: Administer every 40-60 hours or administer 25% of normal dose.
Hemodialysis: Moderately dialyzable (20% to 50%); administer dose postdialysis or administer 40 mg supplemental dose.
Peritoneal dialysis: Supplemental dose is not necessary.
Dosing adjustment/comments in hepatic disease: Reduced dose probably necessary.

Anesthesia and Critical Care Concerns/Other Considerations Surgery: Based on available evidence, beta-blockers should be started days to weeks before elective surgery in selected patients when possible and titrated to a heart rate <65 beats per minute. Additional data suggest that long acting beta-blockers may be superior to short acting ones (Redelmeier, 2005). The ACC/AHA 2007 guidelines on perioperative cardiovascular evaluation and care for noncardiac surgery recommend beta-blockers be continued in patients undergoing surgery who are receiving beta-blockers to treat angina, symptomatic arrhythmias, hypertension, or other ACC/AHA Class I guideline indications (Class I recommendation). The guidelines also recommend that beta-blockers be given to patients undergoing vascular surgery who have myocardial ischemia demonstrated during preoperative testing (Class I recommendation).

The guidelines also state that beta-blockers are probably recommended in patients undergoing intermediate risk (eg, carotid endarterectomy, prostate surgery) or vascular surgery in whom preoperative assessment identifies coronary heart disease or high cardiac risk (Class IIa recommendation). High cardiac risk is defined as having >1 of the following clinical risk factors: History of ischemic heart disease, compensated or prior heart failure, cerebrovascular disease, diabetes mellitus, or renal insufficiency. The use of beta-blockers is uncertain in patients undergoing intermediate risk or vascular surgery with ≤1 clinical risk factor (Class IIb recommendation).

The majority of published trials suggest a benefit of perioperative beta-blocker use during noncardiac surgery especially in high-risk patients; however, more recent clinical trials have not shown a benefit to perioperative beta-blockade for noncardiac surgery (Jul, 2006; Yang, 2006).

Additional Information Complete prescribing information for this medication should be consulted for additional detail.

Dosage Forms Excipient information presented when available (limited, particularly for generics); consult specific product labeling. [DSC] = Discontinued product

Tablet: 20 mg, 40 mg, 80 mg

Corgard®: 20 mg, 40 mg, 80 mg, 120 mg [DSC], 160 mg [DSC]

References

Fleisher LA, Beckman JA, Brown KA, et al, "ACC/AHA 2006 Guideline Update on Perioperative Cardiovascular Evaluation for Noncardiac Surgery: Focused Update on Perioperative Beta-Blocker Therapy: A Report of the American College of Cardiology/American Heart Association Task Force on Practice Guidelines (Writing Committee to Update the 2002 Guidelines on Perioperative Cardiovascular Evaluation for Noncardiac Surgery) Developed in Collaboration With the American Society of Echocardiography, American Society of Nuclear Cardiology, Heart Rhythm Society, Society of Cardiovascular Anesthesiologists, Society for Cardiovascular Angiography and Interventions, and Society for Vascular Medicine and Biology," *J Am Coll Cardiol*, 2006, 47 (11):2343-55.

Juul AB, Wetterslev J, Gluud C, et al, "Effect of Perioperative Beta-Blockade in Patients With Diabetes Undergoing Major Noncardiac Surgery: Randomized Placebo Controlled, Blinded Multicentre Trial," *BMJ*, 2006, 332(7556):1482.

Yang H, Raymer K, Butler R, et al, "The Effects of Perioperative Beta-Blockade: Results of the Metoprolol After Vascular Surgery (MaVS) Study, A Randomized Controlled Trial," *Am Heart J* 2006, 152(5):983-90.

Nafcillin (naf SIL in)

Related Information

Anesthesia for Patients With Liver Disease *on page 1537*
Extravasation Treatment of Drugs *on page 1789*
Skin Tests *on page 1707*

Canadian Brand Names Nallpen®; Unipen®

Index Terms Ethoxynaphthamido Penicillin Sodium; Nafcillin Sodium; Nallpen; Sodium Nafcillin

Pharmacologic Category Antibiotic, Penicillin

Generic Available Yes

Use Treatment of infections such as osteomyelitis, septicemia, endocarditis, and CNS infections caused by susceptible strains of staphylococci species

◄ **Mechanism of Action** Interferes with bacterial cell wall synthesis during active multiplication, causing cell wall death and resultant bactericidal activity against susceptible bacteria

Pharmacodynamics/Kinetics

Distribution: Widely distributed; CSF penetration is poor but enhanced by meningeal inflammation

Protein binding: ~90%; primarily to albumin

Metabolism: Primarily hepatic; undergoes enterohepatic recirculation

Half-life elimination:

Neonates: <3 weeks: 2.2-5.5 hours; 4-9 weeks: 1.2-2.3 hours

Children 3 months to 14 years: 0.75-1.9 hours

Adults: Normal renal/hepatic function: 30-60 minutes

Time to peak, serum: I.M.: 30-60 minutes

Excretion: Primarily feces; urine (10% to 30% as unchanged drug)

Dosage

Usual dosage range:

Neonates: I.M., I.V.:

1200-2000 g, <7 days: 50 mg/kg/day divided every 12 hours

>2000 g, <7 days: 75 mg/kg/day divided every 8 hours

1200-2000 g, ≥7 days: 75 mg/kg/day divided every 8 hours

>2000 g, ≥7 days: 100-140 mg/kg/day divided every 6 hours

Children:

I.M.: 25 mg/kg twice daily

I.V.: 50-200 mg/kg/day in divided doses every 4-6 hours (maximum: 12 g/day)

Adults:

I.M.: 500 mg every 4-6 hours

I.V.: 500-2000 mg every 4-6 hours

Indication-specific dosing:

Children:

Mild-to-moderate infections: I.M., I.V.: 50-100 mg/kg/day in divided doses every 6 hours

Severe infections: I.M., I.V.: 100-200 mg/kg/day in divided doses every 4-6 hours (maximum dose: 12 g/day)

Staphylococcal endocarditis: I.V.:

Native valve: 200 mg/kg/day in divided doses every 4-6 hours for 6 weeks

Prosthetic valve: 200 mg/kg/day in divided doses every 4-6 hours for ≥6 weeks (use with rifampin and gentamicin)

Adults: I.V.:

Endocarditis: MSSA:

Native valve: 12 g/24 hours in 4-6 divided doses for 6 weeks

Prosthetic valve: 12 g/24 hours in 6 divided doses for ≥6 weeks (use with rifampin and gentamicin)

Joint:

Bursitis, septic: 2 g every 4 hours

Prosthetic: 2 g every 4-6 hours with rifampin for 6 weeks

***Staphylococcus aureus*, methicillin-susceptible infections, including brain abscess, empyema, erysipelas, mastitis, myositis, orbital cellulitis, osteomyelitis, pneumonia, splenic abscess, toxic shock, urinary tract (perinephric abscess):** 2 g every 4 hours

Dosing adjustment in renal impairment: Not necessary unless renal impairment is in the setting of concomitant hepatic impairment

Dialysis: Not dialyzable (0% to 5%) via hemodialysis; supplemental dosage not necessary with hemo- or peritoneal dialysis or continuous arteriovenous or venovenous hemofiltration

Dosing adjustment in hepatic impairment: In patients with both hepatic and renal impairment, modification of dosage may be necessary; no data available.

Stability

Premixed infusions: Store in a freezer at -20°C (4°F). Thaw at room temperature or under refrigeration only. Thawed bags are stable for 21 days under refrigeration or 72 hours at room temperature. Do not refreeze.

Vials: Reconstituted parenteral solution is stable for 3 days at room temperature and 7 days when refrigerated or 12 weeks when frozen. For I.V. infusion in NS or

D$_5$W, solution is stable for 24 hours at room temperature and 96 hours when refrigerated.

Administration

I.M.: Rotate injection sites

I.V.: Vesicant. Administer around-the-clock to promote less variation in peak and trough serum levels; infuse over 30-60 minutes

Extravasation management: Use cold packs. Hyaluronidase: Add 1 mL NS to 150 unit vial to make 150 units/mL of concentration; mix 0.1 mL of above with 0.9 mL NS in 1 mL syringe to make final concentration = 15 units/mL.

Monitoring Parameters Baseline and periodic CBC with differential; periodic urinalysis, BUN, serum creatinine, AST and ALT; observe for signs and symptoms of anaphylaxis during first dose

Pregnancy Risk Factor B

Contraindications Hypersensitivity to nafcillin, or any component of the formulation, or penicillins; premixed injection may contain corn-derived dextrose and its use is contraindicated in patients with allergy to corn-related products

Warnings/Precautions Serious and occasionally severe or fatal hypersensitivity (anaphylactoid) reactions have been reported in patients on penicillin therapy, especially with a history of beta-lactam hypersensitivity, history of sensitivity to multiple allergens, or previous IgE-mediated reactions (eg, anaphylaxis, angioedema, urticaria). Use with caution in asthmatic patients. Extravasation of I.V. infusions should be avoided. Modification of dosage is necessary in patients with both severe renal and hepatic impairment. Elimination rate will be slow in neonates. Prolonged use may result in fungal or bacterial superinfection, including *C. difficile*-associated diarrhea (CDAD) and pseudomembranous colitis; CDAD has been observed >2 months postantibiotic treatment.

Adverse Reactions Frequency not defined.

Central nervous system: Neurotoxicity (high doses)

Gastrointestinal: Pseudomembranous colitis

Hematologic: Agranulocytosis, bone marrow depression, neutropenia

Local: Inflammation, pain, phlebitis, skin sloughing, swelling, and thrombophlebitis at the injection site; oxacillin (less likely to cause phlebitis) is often preferred in pediatric patients; tissue necrosis with sloughing (SubQ extravasation)

Renal: Interstitial nephritis (rare), renal tubular damage (rare)

Miscellaneous: Anaphylaxis, hypersensitivity reactions (immediate and delayed; general incidence of 1% to 10% for penicillins), serum sickness

Drug Interactions

Metabolism/Transport Effects Induces CYP3A4 (strong)

Avoid Concomitant Use

Avoid concomitant use of Nafcillin with any of the following: Dronedarone; Everolimus; Nilotinib; Ranolazine; Tolvaptan

Increased Effect/Toxicity

Nafcillin may increase the levels/effects of: Methotrexate

The levels/effects of Nafcillin may be increased by: Uricosuric Agents

Decreased Effect

Nafcillin may decrease the levels/effects of: Calcium Channel Blockers; CycloSPORINE; CYP3A4 Substrates; Dronedarone; Everolimus; Maraviroc; Mycophenolate; Nilotinib; Oral Contraceptive (Estrogens); Ranolazine; Saxagliptin; Sorafenib; Tadalafil; Tolvaptan; Typhoid Vaccine; Vitamin K Antagonists

The levels/effects of Nafcillin may be decreased by: Fusidic Acid; Tetracycline Derivatives

Test Interactions Positive Coombs' test (direct), false-positive urinary and serum proteins; may inactivate aminoglycosides *in vitro*

Dietary Considerations Premixed injection may contain corn-derived dextrose and its use is contraindicated in patients with allergy to corn-related products. Sodium content of 1 g: 76.6 mg (3.33 mEq).

Dosage Forms Excipient information presented when available (limited, particularly for generics); consult specific product labeling.

Infusion [premixed iso-osmotic dextrose solution]: 1 g (50 mL); 2 g (100 mL)

Injection, powder for reconstitution, as sodium: 1 g, 2 g, 10 g

References

Baddour LM, Wilson WR, Bayer AS, et al, "Infective Endocarditis. Diagnosis, Antimicrobial Therapy, and Management of Complications. A Statement for Healthcare Professionals From the Committee on Rheumatic Fever, Endocarditis, and Kawasaki Disease, Council on Cardiovascular Disease in the Young, and the Councils on Clinical Cardiology, Stroke, and Cardiovascular Surgery and Anesthesia, American Heart Association," *Circulation*, 2005, 111(23):e394-434.

◆ **Nafcillin Sodium** *see* Nafcillin *on page 975*

◆ **NaHCO₃** *see* Sodium Bicarbonate *on page 1301*

Nalbuphine (NAL byoo feen)

Medication Safety Issues

Sound-alike/look-alike issues:

Nubain® may be confused with Navane®, Nebcin®

High alert medication: The Institute for Safe Medication Practices (ISMP) includes this medication among its list of drug classes which have a heightened risk of causing significant patient harm when used in error.

Related Information

Opioid Analgesics *on page 1688*

Opioids *on page 1641*

U.S. Brand Names Nubain®

Index Terms Nalbuphine Hydrochloride

Pharmacologic Category Analgesic, Opioid

Generic Available Yes

Use Relief of moderate-to-severe pain; preoperative analgesia, postoperative and surgical anesthesia, and obstetrical analgesia during labor and delivery

Unlabeled/Investigational Use Opioid-induced pruritus

Mechanism of Action Agonist of kappa opiate receptors and partial antagonist of mu opiate receptors in the CNS, causing inhibition of ascending pain pathways, altering the perception of and response to pain; produces generalized CNS depression

Pharmacodynamics/Kinetics

Onset of action: Peak effect: SubQ, I.M.: <15 minutes; I.V.: 2-3 minutes

Metabolism: Hepatic

Half-life elimination: 5 hours

Excretion: Feces; urine (~7% as metabolites)

Dosage

Children ≥1 year (unlabeled use): Pain management: I.M., I.V., SubQ: 0.1-0.2 mg/kg every 3-4 hours as needed; maximum: 20 mg/dose and/or 160 mg/day

Adults:

Pain management: I.M., I.V., SubQ: 10 mg/70 kg every 3-6 hours; maximum single dose in nonopioid-tolerant patients: 20 mg; maximum daily dose: 160 mg

Surgical anesthesia supplement: I.V.: Induction: 0.3-3 mg/kg over 10-15 minutes; maintenance doses of 0.25-0.5 mg/kg may be given as required

Opioid-induced pruritus (unlabeled use): I.V. 2.5-5 mg; may repeat dose

Dosing adjustment in renal impairment: Use with caution and reduce dose; monitor.

Dosing adjustment in hepatic impairment: Use with caution and reduce dose.

Stability Store at room temperature of 15°C to 30°C (59°F to 86°F). Protect from light.

Administration Administer I.M., SubQ, or I.V.

Monitoring Parameters Relief of pain, respiratory and mental status, blood pressure

Anesthesia and Critical Care Concerns/Other Considerations

Clinical Pearls/Comments: Abrupt discontinuation after sustained use (generally >10 days) may cause withdrawal symptoms.

Mixed agonist-antagonist: Incidence of psychomimetic effect is lower than with pentazocine.

Pregnancy Risk Factor B/D (prolonged use or high doses at term)

Contraindications Hypersensitivity to nalbuphine or any component of the formulation

Warnings/Precautions Use caution in CNS depression. Sedation and psychomotor impairment are likely, and are additive with other CNS depressants or ethanol. May cause respiratory depression. Ambulatory patients must be cautioned about performing tasks which require mental alertness (eg, operating machinery or driving). Effects may be potentiated when used with other sedative drugs or ethanol. Use with caution in patients with recent myocardial infarction, biliary tract impairment, morbid obesity, thyroid dysfunction, head trauma, or increased intracranial pressure. Use caution in patients with prostatic hyperplasia and/or urinary stricture, adrenal insufficiency, decreased hepatic or renal function. Use with caution in patients with pre-existing respiratory compromise (hypoxia and/or hypercapnia), COPD or other obstructive pulmonary disease; critical respiratory depression may occur, even at therapeutic dosages. May cause hypotension; use with caution in patients with hypovolemia, cardiovascular disease (including acute MI), or drugs which may exaggerate hypotensive effects (including phenothiazines or general anesthetics). May obscure diagnosis or clinical course of patients with acute abdominal conditions. May result in tolerance and/or drug dependence with chronic use; use with caution in patients with a history of drug dependence. Abrupt discontinuation following prolonged use may lead to withdrawal symptoms. May precipitate withdrawal symptoms in patients following prolonged therapy with mu opioid agonists. Use with caution in pregnancy (close neonatal monitoring required when used in labor and delivery). Use with caution in the elderly and debilitated patients; may be more sensitive to adverse effects. Safety and efficacy in children have not been established.

Adverse Reactions

>10%: Central nervous system: Sedation (36%)

1% to 10%:

Central nervous system: Dizziness (5%), headache (3%)

Gastrointestinal: Nausea/vomiting (6%), xerostomia (4%)

Miscellaneous: Clamminess (9%)

<1% (Limited to important or life-threatening): Abdominal pain, agitation, allergic reaction, anaphylaxis, anaphylactoid reaction, anxiety, asthma, bitter taste, blurred vision, bradycardia, cardiac arrest, confusion, crying, delusion, depersonalization, depression, diaphoresis, dreams (abnormal), dyspepsia, dysphoria, dyspnea, euphoria, faintness, fever, floating sensation, flushing, gastrointestinal cramps, hallucinations, hostility, hypertension, hypotension, injection site reactions (pain, swelling, redness, burning); laryngeal edema, loss of consciousness, nervousness, numbness, pruritus, pulmonary edema, rash, respiratory depression, respiratory distress, restlessness, seizure, sensation of warmth/burning, somnolence, speech disorder, stridor, tachycardia, tingling, tremor, unreality, urinary urgency, urticaria

Drug Interactions

Avoid Concomitant Use There are no known interactions where it is recommended to avoid concomitant use.

Increased Effect/Toxicity

Nalbuphine may increase the levels/effects of: Alcohol (Ethyl); Alvimopan; CNS Depressants; Desmopressin; Selective Serotonin Reuptake Inhibitors; Thiazide Diuretics

The levels/effects of Nalbuphine may be increased by: Amphetamines; Antipsychotic Agents (Phenothiazines); Succinylcholine

Decreased Effect

Nalbuphine may decrease the levels/effects of: Pegvisomant

The levels/effects of Nalbuphine may be decreased by: Ammonium Chloride

Ethanol/Nutrition/Herb Interactions

Ethanol: Avoid ethanol (may increase CNS depression).

Herb/Nutraceutical: Avoid valerian, St John's wort, kava kava, gotu kola (may increase CNS depression).

◀ **Dosage Forms** Excipient information presented when available (limited, particularly for generics); consult specific product labeling. [DSC] = Discontinued product

Injection, solution, as hydrochloride: 10 mg/mL (10 mL); 20 mg/mL (10 mL)
  Nubain®: 10 mg/mL (10 mL) [DSC]; 20 mg/mL (10 mL)
Injection, solution, as hydrochloride [preservative free]: 10 mg/mL (1 mL); 20 mg/mL (1 mL)
  Nubain®: 10 mg/mL (1 mL); 20 mg/mL (1 mL)

References

Mokhlesi B, Leikin JB, Murray P, et al, "Adult Toxicology in Critical Care: Part II: Specific Poisonings," Chest, 2003, 123(3):897-922.

♦ **Nalbuphine Hydrochloride** see Nalbuphine on page 978

♦ **Nalfon®** see Fenoprofen on page 586

♦ **Nallpen** see Nafcillin on page 975

♦ **Nallpen® (Can)** see Nafcillin on page 975

♦ **N-allylnoroxymorphine Hydrochloride** see Naloxone on page 982

Nalmefene (NAL me feen)

Medication Safety Issues
Sound-alike/look-alike issues:
  Revex® may be confused with Nimbex®, ReVia®

Color-coded ampuls denote indication-specific concentrations:
  Blue-labeled ampul (for postoperative use) contains 1 mL (100 mcg/mL)
  Green-labeled ampul (for overdose management) contains 2 mL (1 mg/mL)

International issues:
  Revex® may be confused with Brivex® which is a brand name for brivudine in Switzerland
  Revex® may be confused with Rubex® which is a brand name for ascorbic acid in Ireland

U.S. Brand Names Revex® [DSC]

Index Terms Nalmefene Hydrochloride

Pharmacologic Category Antidote; Opioid Antagonist

Generic Available No

Use Complete or partial reversal of opioid drug effects, including respiratory depression; management of known or suspected opioid overdose

Mechanism of Action As a 6-methylene analog of naltrexone, nalmefene acts as a competitive antagonist at opioid receptor sites, preventing or reversing the respiratory depression, sedation, and hypotension induced by opiates; no pharmacologic activity of its own (eg, opioid agonist activity) has been demonstrated

Pharmacodynamics/Kinetics
Onset of action: I.M., SubQ: 5-15 minutes
Distribution: V_d: 8.6 L/kg; rapid
Protein binding: 45%
Metabolism: Hepatic via glucuronide conjugation to metabolites with little or no activity
Bioavailability: I.M., SubQ: 100%
Half-life elimination: 10.8 hours
Time to peak, serum: Serum: I.M.: 2.3 hours; I.V.: <2 minutes; SubQ: 1.5 hours
Excretion: Feces (17%); urine (<5% as unchanged drug)
  Clearance: 0.8 L/hour/kg

Dosage I.M., I.V., SubQ:
Reversal of postoperative opioid depression: Blue-labeled product (100 mcg/mL): Titrate to reverse the undesired effects of opioids; initial dose for nonopioid dependent patients: 0.25 mcg/kg followed by 0.25 mcg/kg incremental doses at 2- to 5-minute intervals; after a total dose >1 mcg/kg, further therapeutic response is unlikely
  Note: In patients with increased cardiovascular risks, dilute 1:1 in NS or SWFI, and initiate/titrate with 0.1 mcg/kg doses.

Management of known/suspected opioid overdose: **Note:** I.V. route is preferred. Green-labeled product (1 mg/mL): Adults:

Nonopioid-dependent patients: 0.5 mg/70 kg; may repeat with 1 mg/70 kg in 2-5 minutes; further increase beyond a total dose of 1.5 mg/70 kg will not likely result in improved response and may result in cardiovascular stress and precipitated withdrawal syndrome

Opioid-dependent patients: Administer a challenge dose of 0.1 mg/70 kg; if no withdrawal symptoms are observed in 2 minutes, give 0.5 mg/70 kg; may repeat with 1 mg/70 kg in 2-5 minutes; further increase beyond a total dose of 1.5 mg/70 kg will not likely result in improved response and may result in cardiovascular stress and precipitated withdrawal syndrome

Note: If recurrence of respiratory depression is noted, dose may again be titrated to clinical effect using incremental doses.

Note: If I.V. access is lost or not readily obtainable, a single SubQ or I.M. dose of 1 mg may be effective in 5-15 minutes.

Dosing adjustment in renal impairment: Not necessary with single use, however, slow administration (over 60 seconds) of incremental doses is recommended to minimize hypertension and dizziness

Dosing adjustment in hepatic impairment: No adjustment necessary with single use.

Stability Store at controlled room temperature.

Administration Check dosage strength carefully before use to avoid error. Slow administration (over 60 seconds) of incremental doses is recommended to minimize hypertension and dizziness in renal patients. Dilute drug (1:1) with diluent and use smaller doses in patients known to be at increased cardiovascular risk. May be administered via I.M. or SubQ routes if I.V. access is not feasible. A single SubQ or I.M. dose of 1 mg may be effective in 5-15 minutes.

Monitoring Parameters Symptoms of withdrawal; neurological status, oxygenation, pain, vital signs

Anesthesia and Critical Care Concerns/Other Considerations

Clinical Pearls/Comments: The goal of treatment in the postoperative setting is to achieve reversal of excessive opioid effects without inducing a complete reversal and acute pain. If opioid dependence is suspected, nalmefene should only be used in opioid overdose if the likelihood of overdose is high, based on history or the clinical presentation of respiratory depression with concurrent pupillary constriction present.

Pregnancy Risk Factor B

Contraindications Hypersensitivity to nalmefene or any component of the formulation

Warnings/Precautions May induce symptoms of acute withdrawal in opioid-dependent patients; recurrence of respiratory depression is possible if the opioid involved is long-acting; observe patients until there is no reasonable risk of recurrent respiratory depression. Nalmefene is structurally similar to both naltrexone and naloxone; patients with hypersensitivity to these agents may also react to nalmefene. Concurrent use of flumazenil and nalmefene may increase the risk of seizures. Safety and efficacy have not been established in children. Avoid abrupt reversal of opioid effects in patients of high cardiovascular risk or who have received potentially cardiotoxic drugs. Pulmonary edema and cardiovascular instability have been reported in association with abrupt reversal with other narcotic antagonists. Animal studies indicate nalmefene may not completely reverse buprenorphine-induced respiratory depression. Use caution with renal impairment. Excessive dosages should be avoided after use of opiates in surgery. Abrupt postoperative reversal may result in nausea, vomiting, sweating, tachycardia, hypertension, seizures, and other cardiovascular events (including pulmonary edema and arrhythmias). Discharged patients who are opioid-dependent may attempt to override the narcotic-blocking effect of nalmefene. Patients are at a greater risk of overdose when nalmefene wears off if megadosing of opiates has occurred. Adequate duration of monitoring should be provided.

Two products are available at different concentrations. A blue-labeled ampul contains a 100 mcg/mL solution of nalmefene and is intended for postoperative use. A green-labeled ampul contains a 1 mg/mL (**10** times as concentrated; **20** times as much drug) and is intended to be used for the management of an overdose.

Adverse Reactions

>10%: Gastrointestinal: Nausea (18%)

1% to 10%:

Cardiovascular: Tachycardia (5%), hypertension (5%), hypotension (1%), vasodilation (1%)

Central nervous system: Fever (3%), dizziness (3%), headache (1%), chills (1%)

Gastrointestinal: Vomiting (9%)

Miscellaneous: Postoperative pain (4%)

<1% (Limited to important or life-threatening): Agitation, arrhythmia, AST increased, bradycardia, confusion, depression, diarrhea, myoclonus, nervousness, pharyngitis, pruritus, pulmonary edema, somnolence, tremor, urinary retention, withdrawal syndrome, xerostomia

Postmarketing and/or case reports:

Drug Interactions

Avoid Concomitant Use There are no known interactions where it is recommended to avoid concomitant use.

Increased Effect/Toxicity There are no known significant interactions involving an increase in effect.

Decreased Effect There are no known significant interactions involving a decrease in effect.

Dosage Forms Excipient information presented when available (limited, particularly for generics); consult specific product labeling.

Injection, solution:

Revex®: 100 mcg/mL (1 mL) [blue label]; 1 mg/mL (2 mL) [green label] [DSC]

References

Mokhlesi B, Leikin JB, Murray P, et al, "Adult Toxicology in Critical Care: Part II: Specific Poisonings," *Chest*, 2003, 123(3):897-922.

◆ **Nalmefene Hydrochloride** *see* Nalmefene *on page 980*

Naloxone (nal OKS one)

Medication Safety Issues

Sound-alike/look-alike issues:

Naloxone may be confused with Lanoxin®, naltrexone

Narcan® may be confused with Marcaine®, Norcuron®

International issues:

Narcan® may be confused with Marcen® which is a brand name for ketazolam in Spain

Related Information

Moderate Sedation *on page 1566*

Canadian Brand Names Naloxone Hydrochloride Injection®

Index Terms *N*-allylnoroxymorphine Hydrochloride; Naloxone Hydrochloride; Narcan

Pharmacologic Category Antidote; Opioid Antagonist

Generic Available Yes

Use Complete or partial reversal of opioid drug effects, including respiratory depression; management of known or suspected opioid overdose; diagnosis of suspected opioid dependence or acute opioid overdose

Unlabeled/Investigational Use Opioid-induced pruritus

Mechanism of Action Pure opioid antagonist that competes and displaces narcotics at opioid receptor sites

Pharmacodynamics/Kinetics

Onset of action: Endotracheal, I.M., SubQ: 2-5 minutes; I.V.: ~2 minutes

Duration: ~30-120 minutes depending on route of administration; I.V. has a shorter duration of action than I.M. administration; since naloxone's action is shorter than that of most opioids, repeated doses are usually needed

Distribution: Crosses placenta

Metabolism: Primarily hepatic via glucuronidation

Half-life elimination: Neonates: 3-4 hours; Adults: 0.5-1.5 hours

Excretion: Urine (as metabolites)

Dosage Note: I.M., I.V. (preferred), and SubQ routes are available. Endotracheal administration is the least desirable and is supported by only anecdotal evidence (case report) (ACLS guidelines, 2005):

Infants and Children: Postoperative reversal: 0.01 mg/kg; may repeat every 2-3 minutes as needed based on response (adequate ventilation without significant pain)

Children:

Opioid intoxication: Respiratory depression:

I.V.:

Birth (including premature infants) to 5 years or <20 kg: Initial: 0.1 mg/kg (maximum dose: 2 mg); repeat every 2-3 minutes if needed (*Drugs for Pediatric Emergencies*, 1998)

>5 years or ≥20 kg: 2 mg/dose; if no response, repeat every 2-3 minutes (*Drugs for Pediatric Emergencies*, 1998)

Continuous infusion: I.V.: If continuous infusion is required, calculate dosage/hour based on effective intermittent dose used and duration of adequate response seen **or** use $2/3$ of the initial effective naloxone bolus on an hourly basis; titrate dose (typically 0.04-0.16 mg/kg/hour for 2-5 days in children); $1/2$ of the initial bolus dose should be readministered 15 minutes after initiation of the continuous infusion to prevent a drop in naloxone levels; increase infusion rate as needed to assure adequate ventilation and prevent withdrawal symptoms

Adults:

Opioid intoxication: Respiratory depression: I.V.: 0.4-2 mg; may need to repeat doses every 2-3 minutes; after reversal, may need to readminister dose(s) at a later interval (ie, 20-60 minutes) depending on type/duration of opioid. If no response is observed after 10 mg, consider other causes of respiratory depression. **Note:** Opioid-dependent patients may require lower doses (0.1 mg) titrated incrementally to avoid precipitating acute withdrawal.

Continuous infusion: I.V.: Calculate dosage/hour based on effective intermittent dose used and duration of adequate response seen **or** use $2/3$ of the initial effective naloxone bolus on an hourly basis (typically 0.25-6.25 mg/hour); $1/2$ of the initial bolus dose should be readministered 15 minutes after initiation of the continuous infusion to prevent a drop in naloxone levels; adjust infusion rate as needed to assure adequate ventilation and prevent withdrawal symptoms

Opioid-dependent patients being treated for cancer pain (unlabeled; NCCN guidelines, 2008): I.V.: 0.04-0.08 mg (40-80 mcg) slow I.V. push; administer every 30-60 seconds until improvement in symptoms, if no response is observed after total naloxone dose 1 mg, consider other causes of respiratory depression. **Note:** May dilute 0.4 mg/mL (1 mL) ampule into 9 mL of normal saline for a total volume of 10 mL to achieve a 0.04 mg/mL (40 mcg/mL) concentration.

Postoperative reversal: I.V.: 0.1-0.2 mg every 2-3 minutes until desired response (adequate ventilation and alertness without significant pain). **Note:** Repeat doses may be needed within 1-2 hour intervals depending on type, dose, and timing of the last dose of opioid administered.

Opioid-induced pruritus (unlabeled use): I.V. infusion: 0.25 mcg/kg/hour; **Note:** Monitor pain control; verify that the naloxone is not reversing analgesia.

Stability Store at 25°C (77°F). Protect from light. Stable in 0.9% sodium chloride and D_5W at 4 mcg/mL for 24 hours.

Administration

Endotracheal: There is only anecdotal support for this route of administration. May require a slightly higher dose than used in other routes. Dilute to 1-2 mL with normal saline; flush with 5 cc of saline and then administer 5 ventilations

Intratracheal: Dilute to 1-2 mL with normal saline

I.V. push: Administer over 30 seconds as undiluted preparation **or** (unlabeled) administer as diluted preparation slow I.V. push by diluting 0.4 mg (1 mL) ampul with 9 mL of normal saline for a total volume of 10 mL to achieve a concentration of 0.04 mg/mL

I.V. continuous infusion: Dilute to 4 mcg/mL in D_5W or normal saline

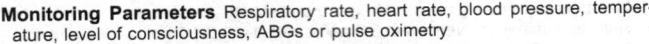

Monitoring Parameters Respiratory rate, heart rate, blood pressure, temperature, level of consciousness, ABGs or pulse oximetry

Anesthesia and Critical Care Concerns/Other Considerations

Clinical Pearls/Comments: Naloxone may contain methyl and propylparabens. The goal of treatment in the postoperative setting is to achieve reversal of excessive opioid effects without inducing a complete reversal and acute pain.

Pregnancy Risk Factor C

Contraindications Hypersensitivity to naloxone or any component of the formulation

Warnings/Precautions Due to an association between naloxone and acute pulmonary edema, use with caution in patients with cardiovascular disease or in patients receiving medications with potential adverse cardiovascular effects (eg, hypotension, pulmonary edema, or arrhythmias). Administration of naloxone causes the release of catecholamines; may precipitate acute withdrawal or unmask pain in those who regularly take opioids. Excessive dosages should be avoided after use of opiates in surgery. Abrupt postoperative reversal may result in nausea, vomiting, sweating, tachycardia, hypertension, seizures, and other cardiovascular events (including pulmonary edema and arrhythmias). May precipitate withdrawal symptoms in patients addicted to opiates, including pain, hypertension, sweating, agitation, irritability; in neonates: shrill cry, failure to feed; carefully titrate dose to reverse hypoventilation; do not fully awaken patient or reverse analgesic effect (postoperative patient). Use caution in patients with history of seizures; avoid use in treatment of meperidine-induced seizures. Recurrence of respiratory depression is possible if the opioid involved is long-acting; observe patients until there is no reasonable risk of recurrent respiratory depression.

Adverse Reactions Adverse reactions are related to reversing dependency and precipitating withdrawal. Withdrawal symptoms are the result of sympathetic excess. Adverse events occur secondarily to reversal (withdrawal) of narcotic analgesia and sedation.

Central nervous system: Narcotic withdrawal

Drug Interactions

Avoid Concomitant Use There are no known interactions where it is recommended to avoid concomitant use.

Increased Effect/Toxicity There are no known significant interactions involving an increase in effect.

Decreased Effect There are no known significant interactions involving a decrease in effect.

Dosage Forms Excipient information presented when available (limited, particularly for generics); consult specific product labeling.

Injection, solution, as hydrochloride: 0.4 mg/mL (1 mL, 10 mL)

Injection, solution, as hydrochloride [preservative free]: 0.4 mg/mL (1 mL); 1 mg/mL (2 mL)

References

Boeuf B, Gauvin F, Guerguerian AM, et al, "Therapy of Shock With Naloxone: A Meta-Analysis," *Crit Care Med*, 1998, 26(11):1910-6.

Goldfrank L, Weisman RS, Errick JK, et al, "A Dosing Nomogram for Continuous Infusion Intravenous Naloxone," *Ann Emerg Med*, 1986, 15(5):566-70.

Mokhlesi B, Leikin JB, Murray P, et al, "Adult Toxicology in Critical Care. Part 11: Specific Poisonings," *Chest*, 2003, 123(3):897-922.

Tandberg D and Abercrombie D, "Treatment of Heroin Overdose With Endotracheal Naloxone," *Ann Emerg Med*, 1982, 11(8):443-5.

Trujillo MH, Guerrero J, Fragachan C, et al, "Pharmacologic Antidotes in Critical Care Medicine: A Practical Guide for Drug Administration," *Crit Care Med*, 1998, 26(2):377-91.

◆ **Naloxone Hydrochloride** *see* Naloxone *on page* 982

◆ **Naloxone Hydrochloride Injection® (Can)** *see* Naloxone *on page* 982

Naltrexone (nal TREKS one)

Medication Safety Issues

Sound-alike/look-alike issues:

Naltrexone may be confused with methylnaltrexone, naloxone

ReVia® may be confused with Revatio®, Revex®

Administration issues: Vivitrol™: For intramuscular (I.M.) gluteal injection only

U.S. Brand Names Depade®; ReVia®; Vivitrol™

Canadian Brand Names ReVia®

Index Terms Naltrexone Hydrochloride

Pharmacologic Category Antidote; Opioid Antagonist

Generic Available Yes: Tablet

Use Treatment of ethanol dependence; blockade of the effects of exogenously administered opioids

Mechanism of Action Naltrexone (a pure opioid antagonist) is a cyclopropyl derivative of oxymorphone similar in structure to naloxone and nalorphine (a morphine derivative); it acts as a competitive antagonist at opioid receptor sites, showing the highest affinity for mu receptors.

Pharmacodynamics/Kinetics

Duration: Oral: 50 mg: 24 hours; 100 mg: 48 hours; 150 mg: 72 hours; I.M.: 4 weeks

Absorption: Oral: Almost complete

Distribution: V_d: 19 L/kg; widely throughout the body but considerable interindividual variation exists

Protein binding: 21%

Metabolism: Noncytochrome-mediated dehydrogenase conversion to 6-beta-naltrexol and related minor metabolites; Oral: Extensive first-pass effect

Half-life elimination: Oral: 4 hours; 6-beta-naltrexol: 13 hours; I.M.: naltrexone and 6-beta-naltrexol: 5-10 days

Time to peak, serum: Oral: ~60 minutes; I.M.: Biphasic: 2 hours (first peak), 2-3 days (second peak)

Excretion: Primarily urine (as metabolites and unchanged drug)

Dosage Adults: Do not give until patient is opioid-free for 7-10 days as determined by urinalysis

Oral: Alcohol dependence, opioid antidote: 25 mg; if no withdrawal signs within 1 hour give another 25 mg; maintenance regimen is flexible, variable and individualized (50 mg/day to 100-150 mg 3 times/week for 12 weeks); up to 800 mg/day has been tolerated in a small number of healthy adults without an adverse effect

I.M.: Alcohol dependence: 380 mg once every 4 weeks

Dosage adjustment in renal impairment: Use caution. No adjustment needed in mild impairment. Not adequately studied in moderate-to-severe renal impairment.

Dosage adjustment in hepatic impairment: Use caution. An increase in naltrexone AUC of approximately five- and 10-fold in patients with compensated or decompensated liver cirrhosis respectively, compared with normal liver function has been reported No adjustment required with mild-to-moderate hepatic impairment. Not adequately studied in severe hepatic impairment.

Stability

Injection: Store unopened kit at 2°C to 8°C (36°F to 46°F). Kit may be kept at room temperature of ≤25°C (77°F) for ≤7 days prior to use; do not freeze.

Tablet: Store at 20°C to 25°C (68°F to 77°F).

Administration If there is any question of occult opioid dependence, perform a naloxone challenge test; do not attempt treatment until naloxone challenge is negative.

Oral: To minimize adverse gastrointestinal effects, administer with food or antacids or after meals; advise patient not to self-administer opiates while receiving naltrexone therapy.

I.M.: Vivitrol™: Administer I.M. into the upper outer quadrant of the gluteal area; use provided 1.5 inch 20-gauge needle for administration. Avoid inadvertent injection into a blood vessel; do not administer I.V., SubQ, or into fatty tissue (the risk of serious injection site reaction is increased if given SubQ or into fatty tissue. Injection should alternate between the two buttocks. Do not substitute any components of the dose-pack.

Monitoring Parameters For narcotic withdrawal; liver function tests; injection site reactions

Pregnancy Risk Factor C

Contraindications Hypersensitivity to naltrexone or any component of the formulation; narcotic dependence or current use of opioid analgesics; acute opioid withdrawal; failure to pass Narcan® challenge or positive urine screen for opioids; acute hepatitis; liver failure

Warnings/Precautions

[U.S. Boxed Warning]: Dose-related hepatocellular injury is possible; the margin of separation between the apparent safe and hepatotoxic doses appears to be ≤ fivefold.

May precipitate withdrawal symptoms in patients addicted to opiates; patients should be opioid-free for a minimum of 7-10 days; use naloxone challenge test to confirm. Use with caution in patients with hepatic or renal impairment. Patients may respond to lower opioid doses than previously used. This could result in potentially life-threatening opioid intoxication. Use of naltrexone does not eliminate or diminish withdrawal symptoms. Warn patients that attempts to overcome opioid blockade could lead to fatal overdose. Suicidal thoughts and depression have been reported; monitor closely. Cases of eosinophilic pneumonia have been reported; monitor for hypoxia and dyspnea. Use with caution in patients with a history of bleeding disorders (including thrombocytopenia) and/or patients on anticoagulant therapy; bleeding/hematoma may occur from I.M. administration. Serious injection site reactions (eg, cellulitis, induration, hematoma, abscess, necrosis) have been reported with use. Patients should report injection site pain, swelling, bruising, pruritus, or redness that does not improve (or worsens) within 2 weeks; consider surgical consult for worsening reactions. For I.M. use only; do not administer I.V., SubQ, or into fatty tissue; may increase the risk of injection site reactions. Vehicle used in injectable (polylactide-co-glycolide microspheres) has rarely been associated with retinal artery occlusion in patients with abnormal arteriovenous anastomosis. Safety and efficacy in children have not been established.

Adverse Reactions Combined reporting of adverse events from oral and injectable formulations:

>10%:

Cardiovascular: Syncope (13%)

Central nervous system: Headache (25%), insomnia (14%), dizziness (13%), anxiety (12%), somnolence (4%), nervousness, fatigue

Gastrointestinal: Nausea (33%), vomiting (14%), appetite decreased (14%), diarrhea (13%), abdominal pain (11%), abdominal cramping

Local: Injection site reaction (69%; includes bruising, induration, nodules, pain, pruritus, swelling, tenderness)

Neuromuscular & skeletal: Arthralgia (12%), CPK increased (11%)

Respiratory: Upper respiratory tract infection (13%), pharyngitis (11%)

1% to 10%:

Central nervous system: Depression (8%), suicidal thoughts (1%), energy increased, feeling down

Dermatologic: Rash (6%)

Endocrine & metabolic: Polydipsia

Gastrointestinal: Dry mouth (5%)

Genitourinary: Delayed ejaculation, impotency

Hepatic: AST increased (2%)

Neuromuscular & skeletal: Muscle cramps (8%), back pain (6%)

<1% (Limited to important or life-threatening): ALT increased, angina, atrial fibrillation, blood pressure increased, cerebral aneurysm, chest pain, chest tightness, CHF, cholecystitis, cholelithiasis, colitis, COPD, dehydration, delirium, disorientation, DVT, dyspnea, eosinophilic pneumonia, euphoria, GI hemorrhage, hallucinations, hypercholesterolemia, hypersensitivity reaction (includes angioedema and urticaria), hypertension, influenza, ischemic stroke, leukocytosis, lymphadenopathy, MI, narcotic withdrawal, palpitation, paralytic ileus,

paranoia, PE, perirectal abscess, pneumonia, pyrexia, rigors, seizure, suicide attempts, tachycardia, thrombocytopenia, tooth abscess, UTI

Drug Interactions

Avoid Concomitant Use There are no known interactions where it is recommended to avoid concomitant use.

Increased Effect/Toxicity There are no known significant interactions involving an increase in effect.

Decreased Effect There are no known significant interactions involving a decrease in effect.

Test Interactions May cause cross-reactivity with some opioid immunoassay methods.

Dosage Forms Excipient information presented when available (limited, particularly for generics); consult specific product labeling.

Injection, microspheres for suspension, extended release:
Vivitrol™: 380 mg [contains polylactide-co-glycolide; packaged with diluent, syringe, needles, and safety device]

Tablet, as hydrochloride: 50 mg
Depade®: 25 mg, 50 mg, 100 mg
ReVia®: 50 mg

References

Mokhlesi B, Leikin JB, Murray P, et al, "Adult Toxicology in Critical Care. Part 11: Specific Poisonings," Chest, 2003, 123(3):897-922.

O'Connor PG and Kosten TR, "Rapid and Ultrarapid Opioid Detoxification Techniques," JAMA, 1998, 279(3):229-34.

◆ **Naltrexone and Morphine** see Morphine and Naltrexone on page 949

◆ **Naltrexone Hydrochloride** see Naltrexone on page 985

◆ **Namenda™** see Memantine on page 874

◆ **Naprelan®** see Naproxen on page 987

◆ **Naprosyn®** see Naproxen on page 987

Naproxen (na PROKS en)

Related Information

Acetaminophen and NSAIDS, Dosing in the Management of Pain on page 1651
Acute Postoperative Pain on page 1502
Chronic Pain Management on page 1546
Nonsteroidal Anti-Inflammatory Agents on page 1687

U.S. Brand Names Aleve® [OTC]; Anaprox®; Anaprox® DS; EC-Naprosyn®; Mediproxen [OTC]; Midol® Extended Relief [OTC]; Naprelan®; Naprosyn®; Pamprin® Maximum Strength All Day Relief [OTC]

Canadian Brand Names Anaprox®; Anaprox® DS; Apo-Napro-Na DS®; Apo-Napro-Na®; Apo-Naproxen EC®; Apo-Naproxen SR®; Apo-Naproxen®; Gen-Naproxen EC; Mylan-Naproxen EC; Naprosyn®; Naxen®; Naxen® EC; Novo-Naproc EC; Novo-Naprox; Novo-Naprox Sodium; Novo-Naprox Sodium DS; Novo-Naprox SR; Nu-Naprox; PMS-Naproxen EC; Pro-Naproxen EC; Riva-Naproxen; Sab-Naproxen

Index Terms Naproxen Sodium

Pharmacologic Category Nonsteroidal Anti-inflammatory Drug (NSAID), Oral

Use Management of ankylosing spondylitis, osteoarthritis, and rheumatoid disorders (including juvenile rheumatoid arthritis); acute gout; mild-to-moderate pain; tendonitis, bursitis; dysmenorrhea; fever

Pharmacodynamics/Kinetics

Onset of action: Analgesic: 1 hour; Anti-inflammatory: ~2 weeks
Peak effect: Anti-inflammatory: 2-4 weeks
Duration: Analgesic: ≤7 hours; Anti-inflammatory: ≤12 hours
Absorption: Almost 100%
Distribution: 0.16 L/kg
Protein binding: >99% to albumin; increased free fraction in elderly
Metabolism: Hepatic to metabolites
Bioavailability: 95%
Half-life elimination: Normal renal function: 12-17 hours; End-stage renal disease: No change

Time to peak, serum: 1-4 hours

Excretion: Urine (95%; primarily as metabolites); feces (≤3%)

Dosage Note: Dosage expressed as naproxen base; 200 mg naproxen base is equivalent to 220 mg naproxen sodium.

Oral:

Children >2 years: Juvenile arthritis: 10 mg/kg/day in 2 divided doses

Adults:

Gout, acute: Initial: 750 mg, followed by 250 mg every 8 hours until attack subsides. **Note:** EC-Naprosyn® is not recommended.

Migraine, acute (unlabeled use): Initial: 500-750 mg; an additional 250-500 mg may be given if needed (maximum: 1250 mg in 24 hours). **Note:** EC-Naprosyn® is not recommended.

Pain (mild-to-moderate), dysmenorrhea, acute tendonitis, bursitis: Initial: 500 mg, then 250 mg every 6-8 hours; maximum: 1250 mg/day naproxen base

Rheumatoid arthritis, osteoarthritis, and ankylosing spondylitis: 500-1000 mg/day in 2 divided doses; may increase to 1.5 g/day of naproxen base for limited time period

OTC labeling: Pain/fever:

Children ≥12 years and Adults ≤65 years: 200 mg naproxen base every 8-12 hours; if needed, may take 400 mg naproxen base for the initial dose; maximum: 600 mg naproxen base/24 hours

Adults >65 years: 200 mg naproxen base every 12 hours

Dosing adjustment in renal impairment: Cl_{cr} <30 mL/minute: use is not recommended

Anesthesia and Critical Care Concerns/Other Considerations The 2002 ACCM/SCCM guidelines for analgesia (critically-ill adult) suggest that NSAIDs may be used in combination with opioids in select patients for pain management. Concern about adverse events (increased risk of renal dysfunction, altered platelet function and gastrointestinal irritation) limits its use in patients who have other underlying risks for these events.

In short-term use, NSAIDs vary considerably in their effect on blood pressure. When NSAIDs are used in patients with hypertension, appropriate monitoring of blood pressure responses should be completed and the duration of therapy, when possible, kept short. The use of NSAIDs in the treatment of patients with congestive heart failure may be associated with an increased risk for fluid accumulation and edema; may precipitate renal failure in dehydrated patients. Should not be used to treat perioperative pain after coronary bypass surgery (CABG).

Additional Information Complete prescribing information for this medication should be consulted for additional detail.

Dosage Forms Excipient information presented when available (limited, particularly for generics); consult specific product labeling. [DSC] = Discontinued product

Caplet, as sodium: 220 mg [equivalent to naproxen 200 mg and sodium 20 mg]

Aleve®, Midol® Extended Relief, Pamprin® Maximum Strength All Day Relief: 220 mg [equivalent to naproxen 200 mg and sodium 20 mg]

Capsule, liquid gel, as sodium:

Aleve®: 220 mg [equivalent to naproxen 200 mg and sodium 20 mg]

Gelcap, as sodium:

Aleve®: 220 mg [equivalent to naproxen 200 mg and sodium 20 mg]

Suspension, oral: 125 mg/5 mL (500 mL)

Naprosyn®: 125 mg/5 mL (473 mL) [contains sodium 39 mg (1.5 mEq)/5 mL; orange-pineapple flavor]

Tablet: 250 mg, 375 mg, 500 mg

Naprosyn®: 250 mg, 375 mg, 500 mg

Tablet, as sodium: 220 mg [equivalent to naproxen 200 mg and sodium 20 mg]; 275 mg [equivalent to naproxen 250 mg and sodium 25 mg]; 550 mg [equivalent to naproxen 500 mg and sodium 50 mg]

Aleve®: 220 mg [equivalent to naproxen 200 mg and sodium 20 mg]

Anaprox®: 275 mg [equivalent to naproxen 250 mg and sodium 25 mg]

Anaprox® DS: 550 mg [equivalent to naproxen 500 mg and sodium 50 mg]

Mediproxen: 220 mg [equivalent to naproxen 200 mg and sodium 20 mg]

Tablet, controlled release, as sodium:
Naprelan®: 412.5 mg [equivalent to naproxen 375 mg and sodium 37.5 mg]
Naprelan®: 550 mg [equivalent to naproxen 500 mg and sodium 50 mg]
Naprelan®: 825 mg [equivalent to naproxen 750 mg and sodium 75 mg]
Tablet, delayed release, enteric coated: 375 mg, 500 mg
EC-Naprosyn®: 375 mg, 500 mg
Tablet, extended release, as sodium: 550 mg [equivalent to naproxen 500 mg and sodium 50 mg] [DSC]

◆ **Naproxen Sodium** see Naproxen on page 987

Naratriptan (NAR a trip tan)

U.S. Brand Names Amerge®
Canadian Brand Names Amerge®
Index Terms Naratriptan Hydrochloride
Pharmacologic Category Antimigraine Agent; Serotonin 5-HT$_{1B, 1D}$ Receptor Agonist
Use Treatment of acute migraine headache with or without aura
Pharmacodynamics/Kinetics
Onset of action: 30 minutes
Absorption: Well absorbed
Protein binding, plasma: 28% to 31%
Metabolism: Hepatic via CYP
Bioavailability: 70%
Time to peak: 2-3 hours
Excretion: Urine
Dosage
Adults: Oral: 1-2.5 mg at the onset of headache; it is recommended to use the lowest possible dose to minimize adverse effects. If headache returns or does not fully resolve, the dose may be repeated after 4 hours; do not exceed 5 mg in 24 hours.
Elderly: Not recommended for use in the elderly
Dosing in renal impairment:
Cl$_{cr}$ 18-39 mL/minute: Initial: 1 mg; do not exceed 2.5 mg in 24 hours
Cl$_{cr}$ <15 mL/minute: Do not use
Dosing in hepatic impairment: Contraindicated in patients with severe liver failure; maximum dose: 2.5 mg in 24 hours for patients with mild or moderate liver failure; recommended starting dose: 1 mg
Anesthesia and Critical Care Concerns/Other Considerations Naratriptan should not be used in patients with a history of vasospastic disease, Prinzmetal's angina, or any critical vascular disease.
Additional Information Complete prescribing information for this medication should be consulted for additional detail.
Dosage Forms Excipient information presented when available (limited, particularly for generics); consult specific product labeling.
Tablet: 1 mg, 2.5 mg

◆ **Naratriptan Hydrochloride** see Naratriptan on page 989
◆ **Narcan** see Naloxone on page 982
◆ **Nardil®** see Phenelzine on page 1108
◆ **Naropin®** see Ropivacaine on page 1266
◆ **Nasacort® AQ** see Triamcinolone on page 1429
◆ **Nasal Moist® Saline [OTC]** see Sodium Chloride on page 1304
◆ **Nasal Spray [OTC]** see Sodium Chloride on page 1304
◆ **Nasop12™ [DSC]** see Phenylephrine on page 1114

Natalizumab (na ta LIZ u mab)

Medication Guide An FDA-approved patient medication guide, which is available with the product information and at http://www.fda.gov/downloads/Drugs/DrugSafety/ucm089809.pdf, must be dispensed with this medication for each new outpatient prescription and refill.

◀ **U.S. Brand Names** Tysabri®

Canadian Brand Names Tysabri®

Index Terms AN100226; Anti-4 Alpha Integrin; IgG4-Kappa Monoclonal Antibody

Pharmacologic Category Gastrointestinal Agent, Miscellaneous; Monoclonal Antibody, Selective Adhesion-Molecule Inhibitor

Restrictions Patients must be enrolled in the Tysabri® Outreach Unified Commitment to Health (TOUCH™) Prescribing Program (800-456-2255) to receive natalizumab (MS-TOUCH™ for multiple sclerosis or CD-TOUCH™ for Crohn's disease). Healthcare providers must also register with the program in order to prescribe, dispense or administer natalizumab. Treatment must be reauthorized every 6 months. Natalizumab is available only through infusion centers registered with the TOUCH™ program; infusion center information is available at 1-800-456-2255.

Generic Available No

Use

U.S. labeling: Monotherapy for the treatment of relapsing forms of multiple sclerosis; treatment of moderately- to severely-active Crohn's disease

Canada labeling: Treatment of relapsing forms of multiple sclerosis

Mechanism of Action Natalizumab is a monoclonal antibody against the alpha-4 subunit of integrin molecules. These molecules are important to adhesion and migration of cells from the vasculature into inflamed tissue. Natalizumab blocks integrin association with vascular receptors, limiting adhesion and transmigration of leukocytes. Efficacy in specific disorders may be related to reduction in specific inflammatory cell populations in target tissues. In multiple sclerosis, efficacy may be related to blockade of T-lymphocyte migration into the central nervous system; treatment results in a decreased frequency of relapse. In Crohn's disease, natalizumab decreases inflammation by binding to alpha-4 integrin, blocking adhesion and migration of leukocytes in the gut.

Pharmacodynamics/Kinetics

Distribution: Crohn's disease: 2.4-8 L; Multiple sclerosis: 3.8-7.6 L

Half-life elimination: Crohn's disease: 3-17 days; Multiple sclerosis: 7-15 days

Dosage I.V.: Adults:

Multiple sclerosis: 300 mg infused over 1 hour every 4 weeks

Crohn's disease: 300 mg infused over 1 hour every 4 weeks; discontinue if therapeutic benefit is not observed within initial 12 weeks of therapy

Concomitant use with corticosteroids: For patients who begin treatment while on chronic oral corticosteroids, begin tapering oral steroids when the onset of natalizumab therapeutic benefit is observed; discontinue use if patient cannot be tapered off of oral corticosteroids within 6 months of therapy initiation. If additional concomitant corticosteroids are required and exceed 3 months/year (in addition to initial corticosteroid taper), consider discontinuing therapy.

Dosage adjustment in renal impairment: Not studied

Dosage adjustment in hepatic impairment: Not studied. Discontinue use with jaundice or signs/symptoms of hepatic injury.

Stability Store concentrated solution under refrigeration between 2°C to 8°C (36°F to 46°F); do not freeze. Protect from light. Do not shake. Dilute natalizumab 300 mg in NS 100 mL to a final concentration of 2.6 mg/mL. Gently invert to mix; do not shake. Following dilution, may store refrigerated for use within up to 8 hours.

Administration Solution may be warmed to room temperature prior to administration. Diluted solution should be infused over 1 hour; do not administer by I.V. bolus or push. Patients should be closely monitored for signs and symptoms of hypersensitivity during the infusion and for at least 1 hour after the infusion is complete. The infusion should be discontinued if a reaction occurs, and treatment of the reaction should be instituted. Following infusion, flush line with NS.

Monitoring Parameters Monitor for symptoms of hepatotoxicity (eg, elevated serum transaminases, bilirubin); hypersensitivity reactions during, and for 1 hour after, infusion; symptoms of persistent antibody-positivity (eg, anxiety, dizziness, dyspnea, feeling cold, flushing, headache, hypertension, myalgia, nausea, pruritus, pyrexia, rigors, tachycardia, tremor, urticaria or, vomiting). Antibody testing is recommended if persistent antibodies are suspected and repeated in

3 months in all patients with documented positivity on initial test. Consider antibody testing in patients that resume therapy following a period of dosage interruption.

Baseline brain MRI scan; if PML is suspected, obtain gadolinium-enhanced brain MRI scan and CSF analysis for JC viral DNA. Evaluate for signs or symptoms of progressive multifocal leukoencephalopathy (focal neurologic deficits, which may present as hemiparesis, visual field deficits, cognitive impairment, aphasia, ataxia, and/or cranial nerve deficits) at 3 and 6 months after first infusion; every 6 months thereafter. **Note:** Transient and reversible leukocytosis (excluding neutrophils) and mildly reduced hemoglobin may occur with treatment and may require ~4 months for return to baseline values after the last dose.

Pregnancy Risk Factor C

Contraindications Hypersensitivity to natalizumab, murine proteins, or any component of the formulation; current or history of progressive multifocal leukoencephalopathy (PML)

Canada labeling: Additional contraindications (not in U.S. labeling): Immunocompromised patients as a result of immunosuppressant or antineoplastic therapy, or immunodeficiencies (eg, HIV, leukemia, lymphoma)

Warnings/Precautions [U.S. Boxed Warning]: Increased risk of developing fatal or disabling progressive multifocal leukoencephalopathy (PML), an opportunistic infection caused by the JC virus; patients must be routinely monitored for signs of PML with baseline and periodic MRI evaluations; access to and provision of therapy requires registration of patients and healthcare providers; with the TOUCH™ prescribing program; concurrent immunomodulator therapy or immunosuppression may be risk factors for the development of PML, however, PML has also been reported with natalizumab monotherapy. Use may be associated with an increased risk of infections, including opportunistic infections and serious herpes infections (rare, postmarketing reports; concurrent use of antineoplastic, immunosuppressant [including short-course corticosteroids], or immunomodulating agents may increase this risk). In the presence of a serious herpes infection, discontinue therapy until successful resolution of the infection. A brain MRI scan (baseline) should be obtained prior to initiating therapy in MS patients and should be considered in Crohn's patients. Use should be restricted to patients with inadequate response to or intolerant to other therapies for Crohn's disease or multiple sclerosis.

During clinical studies, up to 24% of patients experienced an infusion-related reaction; serious systemic hypersensitivity reactions occurred in ≤1% of patients. Severe reactions, including anaphylaxis, occur rarely. Patients treated with brief initial courses of therapy (≤3 infusions) followed by an extended interruption in therapy (≥3 months) may be at an increased risk for hypersensitivity reactions following reinitiation of therapy. Retreatment is not recommended in patients developing hypersensitivity reactions. Infusion-related reactions may occur more frequently in patients with antibodies to natalizumab. Antibody formation (which occurs in about 10% of patients) is associated with a decrease in natalizumab levels and a decrease in the efficacy of natalizumab. Antibody testing should be performed in any patient when there is a suspicion of persistent antibodies and should be considered in patients that resume therapy following a period of dosage interruption.

Natalizumab should not be used in combination with immunosuppressants or tumor necrosis factor (TNF) inhibitors in patients with Crohn's disease; aminosalicylates may be used concurrently with natalizumab. For patients who begin treatment while on chronic oral corticosteroids, begin tapering oral steroids when the onset of natalizumab therapeutic benefit is observed; discontinue use if patient cannot be tapered off of oral corticosteroids within 6 months of therapy initiation. If additional concomitant corticosteroids are required and exceed 3 months/year (in addition to initial corticosteroid taper), consider discontinuing therapy.

Hepatotoxicity, including transaminase and bilirubin elevation, has been reported with use; may occur as early as 6 days after the first dose; may recur with treatment rechallenge; discontinue with jaundice or signs/symptoms of hepatic injury. Use caution in patients with a history of depression; closely monitor. Safety and efficacy have not been established in chronic progressive multiple sclerosis, for therapy >2 years, or in children (<18 years of age).

Adverse Reactions

>10%:

Central nervous system: Headache (32% to 38%), fatigue (10% to 27%), depression (≤19%)

Dermatologic: Rash (6% to 12%)

Gastrointestinal: Nausea (≤17%), gastroenteritis (≤11%), abdominal discomfort (≤11%)

Genitourinary: Urinary tract infection (3% to 21%)

Neuromuscular & skeletal: Arthralgia (8% to 19%), extremity pain (16%), back pain (≤12%)

Respiratory: Upper respiratory infection (≤22%), lower respiratory infection (≤17%)

Miscellaneous: Infusion-related reaction (11% to 24%), influenza (≤12%), flu-like syndrome (≤11%)

1% to 10%:

Cardiovascular: Peripheral edema (5% to 6%), chest discomfort (≤5%)

Central nervous system: Vertigo (≤6%), dysesthesia (3%), syncope (≤2%), somnolence (≤2%)

Dermatologic: Dermatitis (≤7%), pruritus (≤4%), urticaria (≤2%), dry skin (≤1%)

Endocrine & metabolic: Dysmenorrhea (2% to 6%), menstrual irregularities (≤5%), amenorrhea (≤2%), ovarian cyst (≤2%)

Gastrointestinal: Diarrhea (10%), dyspepsia (≤5%), abdominal pain (≤4%), constipation (≤4%), flatulence (≤3%), aphthous stomatitis (≤2%), weight changes (≤2%), cholelithiasis (≤1%), gingival infection (1%)

Genitourinary: Vaginitis/vaginal infections (4% to 10%), urinary frequency (≤9%), urinary incontinence (≤4%)

Hematologic: Hematoma (1%)

Hepatic: Transaminase increased (≤5%)

Local: Bleeding at injection site (≤3%)

Neuromuscular & skeletal: Muscle cramp (≤5%), tremor (1% to 3%), rigors (≤3%), joint swelling (≤2%)

Respiratory: Sinusitis (≤8%), cough (≤7%), tonsillitis (≤7%), pharyngolaryngeal pain (≤6%), epistaxis (2%)

Miscellaneous: Antibody formation (9% to 10%), tooth infection (≤9%), herpes infection (≤8%), viral infection (≤7%), hypersensitivity reactions (acute: 2% to 4%; serious acute: ≤1%; delayed: ≤5%), toothache (≤4%), serious infection (2% to 3%), night sweats (≤1%)

<1% (Limited to important or life-threatening): Acne, agitation, anaphylaxis/anaphylactoid reactions, anemia, angina, appendicitis, bilirubin increased, bronchopulmonary aspergillosis, Burkholderia cepacia, Crohn's disease exacerbation, cryptosporidial gastroenteritis, cytomegalovirus hepatitis, dizziness, dyspnea, erythema, fever, flushing, hemoglobin decreased (mild, transient), hepatotoxicity, herpes encephalitis, herpes meningitis, hypotension, joint stiffness, lethargy, leukocytosis, nasopharyngitis, opportunistic infections (including progressive multifocal leukoencephalopathy [PML], meningitis, and bronchopulmonary infections), muscle spasms, muscle weakness, onychorrhexis, paresis, petechiae, pharyngitis, Pneumocystis jiroveci pneumonia, pneumonia, psychomotor hyperactivity, pulmonary Mycobacterium avium intracellulare, suicidal ideation, tachycardia, thrombocytopenia, thrombophlebitis, varicella pneumonia, vasodilatation

Drug Interactions

Avoid Concomitant Use

Avoid concomitant use of Natalizumab with any of the following: Immunosuppressants; Vaccines (Live)

Increased Effect/Toxicity

Natalizumab may increase the levels/effects of: Leflunomide; Vaccines (Live)

The levels/effects of Natalizumab may be increased by: Immunosuppressants; Trastuzumab

Decreased Effect

Natalizumab may decrease the levels/effects of: Vaccines (Inactivated); Vaccines (Live)

The levels/effects of Natalizumab may be decreased by: Echinacea

Dosage Forms Excipient information presented when available (limited, particularly for generics); consult specific product labeling.

Injection, solution [preservative free]:

Tysabri®: 300 mg/15 mL (15 mL) [contains polysorbate-80]

References

Ghosh S, Goldin E, Gordon FH, et al, "Natalizumab for Active Crohn's Disease," *N Engl J Med*, 2003, 348(1):24-32.

♦ **Natrecor®** *see* Nesiritide *on page 999*

♦ **Natriuretic Peptide** *see* Nesiritide *on page 999*

♦ **Natural Lung Surfactant** *see* Beractant *on page 185*

♦ **Nature-Throid™** *see* Thyroid, Desiccated *on page 1379*

♦ **Naxen® (Can)** *see* Naproxen *on page 987*

♦ **Naxen® EC (Can)** *see* Naproxen *on page 987*

♦ **Na-Zone® [OTC]** *see* Sodium Chloride *on page 1304*

Nebivolol (ne BIV oh lole)

Related Information

Beta-Blockers *on page 1669*

Preoperative Evaluation of the Cardiac Patient for Noncardiac Surgery *on page 1598*

U.S. Brand Names Bystolic™

Index Terms Nebivolol Hydrochloride

Pharmacologic Category Beta Blocker, Beta$_1$ Selective

Use Treatment of hypertension, alone or in combination with other agents

Unlabeled/Investigational Use Heart failure

Pharmacodynamics/Kinetics

Absorption: Rapid

Distribution: V_d: 8-12 L/kg

Protein binding: ~98%, primarily to albumin

Metabolism: Hepatic; via glucuronidation and CYP2D6; extensive first-pass metabolism to multiple active metabolites with variable activity

Bioavailability: ~12% (extensive metabolizers); 96% (poor metabolizers)

Half-life elimination: Terminal: 10-12 hours (extensive metabolizers); 19-32 hours in poor metabolizers

Time to peak, plasma: 0.5-4 hours

Excretion: Urine (38%; 67% in poor metabolizers; <0.5% of unchanged drug); feces (44%; 13% in poor metabolizers; <0.5% of unchanged drug)

Dosage Oral:

Adults:

Hypertension: Initial: 5 mg once daily; if initial response is inadequate, may be increased at 2-week intervals to a maximum dose of 40 mg once daily

Heart failure (unlabeled use): Adults ≥70 years: Initial: 1.25 mg once daily; if tolerated, may increase by 2.5 mg at 1- to 2-week intervals to a maximum dose of 10 mg once daily

Elderly: Refer to adult dosing.

Dosing adjustment in renal impairment: Severe impairment (Cl$_{cr}$ <30 mL/minute): Initial: 2.5 mg/day; increase cautiously

Dosage adjustment in hepatic impairment: Moderate impairment (Child-Pugh class B): Initial: 2.5 mg/day; increase cautiously

Anesthesia and Critical Care Concerns/Other Considerations

Surgery: Based on available evidence, beta-blockers should be started days to weeks before elective surgery in selected patients when possible and titrated to a heart rate <65 beats per minute. Additional data suggest that long acting beta-blockers may be superior to short acting ones (Redelmeier, 2005). The ACC/AHA 2007 guidelines on perioperative cardiovascular evaluation and care for ▶

◄ noncardiac surgery recommend beta-blockers be continued in patients under-going surgery who are receiving beta-blockers to treat angina, symptomatic arrhythmias, hypertension, or other ACC/AHA Class I guideline indications (Class I recommendation). The guidelines also recommend that beta-blockers be given to patients undergoing vascular surgery who have myocardial ischemia demonstrated during preoperative testing (Class I recommendation).

The guidelines also state that beta-blockers are probably recommended in patients undergoing intermediate risk (eg, carotid endarterectomy, prostate surgery) or vascular surgery in whom preoperative assessment identifies coronary heart disease or high cardiac risk (Class IIa recommendation). High cardiac risk is defined as having >1 of the following clinical risk factors: History of ischemic heart disease, compensated or prior heart failure, cerebrovascular disease, diabetes mellitus, or renal insufficiency. The use of beta-blockers is uncertain in patients undergoing intermediate risk or vascular surgery with ≤1 clinical risk factor (Class IIb recommendation).

The majority of published trials suggest a benefit of perioperative beta-blocker use during noncardiac surgery especially in high-risk patients; however, more recent clinical trials have not shown a benefit to perioperative beta-blockade for noncardiac surgery (Juul. 2006; Yang, 2006).

Additional Information Complete prescribing information for this medication should be consulted for additional detail.

Dosage Forms Excipient information presented when available (limited, particularly for generics); consult specific product labeling.

Tablet:

Bystolic™: 2.5 mg, 5 mg, 10 mg

References

Brixius K, Bundkirchen A, Bolck B, et al, "Nebivolol, Bucindolol, Metoprolol and Carvedilol are Devoid of Intrinsic Sympathomimetic Activity in Human Myocardium," *Br J Pharmacol*, 2001, 133 (8):1330-8.

Cazzola M, Noschese P, D'Amato M, Det al, "Comparison of the Effects of Single Oral Doses of Nebivolol and Celiprolol on Airways in Patients With Mild Asthma," *Chest*, 2000, 118(5):1322-6.

Cheymol G, Woestenborghs R, Snoeck E, et al. "Pharmacokinetic Study and Cardiovascular Monitoring of Nebivolol in Normal and Obese Subjects," *Eur J Clin Pharmacol*, 1997, 51(6):493-8.

Chobanian AV, Bakris GL, Black HR, et al, "The Seventh Report of the Joint National Committee on Prevention, Detection, Evaluation, and Treatment of High Blood Pressure: The JNC 7 Report," *JAMA*, 2003, 289(19):2560-71.

Flather MD, Shibata MC, Coats AJ, et al, "Randomized Trial to Determine the Effect of Nebivolol on Mortality and Cardiovascular Hospital Admission in Elderly Patients With Heart Failure (SENIORS)," *Eur Heart J*, 2005, 26(3):215-25.

Fleisher LA, Beckman JA, Brown KA, et al, "ACC/AHA 2007 Guidelines on Perioperative Cardiovascular Evaluation for Noncardiac Surgery: A Report of the American College of Cardiology/American Heart Association Task Force on Practice Guidelines (Writing Committee to Revise the 2002 Guidelines on Perioperative Cardiovascular Evaluation for Noncardiac Surgery) Developed in Collaboration With the American Society of Echocardiography, American Society of Nuclear Cardiology, Heart Rhythm Society, Society of Cardiovascular Anesthesiologists, Society for Cardiovascular Angiography and Interventions, Society for Vascular Medicine and Biology, and Society for Vascular Surgery," *J Am Coll Cardiol*, 2007, 50(17):e159-241.

Fogari R, Zoppi A, Lazzari P, et al, "Comparative Effects of Nebivolol and Atenolol on Blood Pressure and Insulin Sensitivity in Hypertensive Subjects With Type II Diabetes," *J Hum Hypertens*, 1997, 11 (11):753-7.

Heart Failure Society of America, "HFSA 2006 Comprehensive Heart Failure Practice Guideline," *J Card Fail*, 2006, 12(1):e1-119.

Juul AB, Wetterslev J, Gluud C, et al, "Effect of Perioperative Beta Blockade in Patients With Diabetes Undergoing Major Non-Cardiac Surgery: Randomized Placebo Controlled, Blinded Multicentre Trial. DIPOM Trial Group," *BMJ*, 2006, 332(7556):1482.

Kamali F, Howes A, Thomas SHL, et al, "A Pharmacokinetic and Pharmacodynamic Interaction Study Between Nebivolol and the H2-Receptor Antagonists Cimetidine and Ranitidine," *Br J Clin Pharmacol*, 1997, 43(2):201-4.

Lang DM, "Anaphylactoid and Anaphylactic Reactions. Hazards of Beta-Blockers," *Drug Saf*, 1995, 12(5):299-304.

Lindenauer PK, Pekow P, Wang K, et al, "Perioperative Beta-Blocker Therapy and Mortality After Major Noncardiac Surgery," *N Engl J Med*, 2005, 353(4):349-61.

Mokhlesi B, Leikin JB, Murray P, et al, "Adult Toxicology in Critical Care: Part II: Specific Poisonings," *Chest*, 2003, 123(3):897-922.

Nuttall SL, Routledge HC, and Kendall MJ, "A Comparison of the Beta1-Selectivity of Three Beta1-Selective Beta-Blockers," *J Clin Pharm Ther*, 2003, 28(3):179-86.

Patrianakos AP, Parthenakis FI, Mavrakis HE, et al, "Comparative Efficacy of Nebivolol versus Carvedilol on Left Ventricular Function and Exercise Capacity in Patients With Non-Ischemic Cardiomyopathy. A 12-Month Study," *Am Heart J*, 2005, 150(5):985.

Prisant LM, "Nebivolol: Pharmacologic Profile of an Ultraselective, Vasodilatory [Beta]1–Blocker," *J Clin Pharm*, 2007 [epub ahead of print].

UK Prospective Diabetes Study Group, "Efficacy of Atenolol and Captopril in Reducing Risk of Macrovascular and Microvascular Complications in Type 2 Diabetes: UKPDS 39," *BMJ*, 1998, 317 (7160):713-20.

Yang H, Raymer K, Butler R, et al, "The Effects of Perioperative Beta-Blockade: Results of the Metoprolol After Vascular Surgery (MaVS) Study, a Randomized Controlled Trial," *Am Hear J*, 2006, 152(5):983-90.

- ◆ **Nebivolol Hydrochloride** *see* Nebivolol *on page* 993
- ◆ **NebuPent®** *see* Pentamidine *on page* 1097
- ◆ **Necon® 0.5/35** *see* Ethinyl Estradiol and Norethindrone *on page* 554
- ◆ **Necon® 1/35** *see* Ethinyl Estradiol and Norethindrone *on page* 554
- ◆ **Necon® 7/7/7** *see* Ethinyl Estradiol and Norethindrone *on page* 554
- ◆ **Necon® 10/11** *see* Ethinyl Estradiol and Norethindrone *on page* 554
- ◆ **Nembutal®** *see* PENTobarbital *on page* 1101
- ◆ **Nembutal® Sodium (Can)** *see* PENTobarbital *on page* 1101
- ◆ **Neo-Fradin™** *see* Neomycin *on page* 995
- ◆ **Neofrin™** *see* Phenylephrine *on page* 1114

Neomycin (nee oh MYE sin)

Related Information
Prevention of Wound Infection and Sepsis in Surgical Patients *on page* 1721

U.S. Brand Names Neo-Fradin™; Neo-Rx

Index Terms Neomycin Sulfate

Pharmacologic Category Ammonium Detoxicant; Antibiotic, Aminoglycoside; Antibiotic, Topical

Generic Available Yes

Use Orally to prepare GI tract for surgery; topically to treat minor skin infections; treatment of diarrhea caused by *E. coli*; adjunct in the treatment of hepatic encephalopathy; bladder irrigation; ocular infections

Mechanism of Action Interferes with bacterial protein synthesis by binding to 30S ribosomal subunits

Pharmacodynamics/Kinetics
Absorption: Oral, percutaneous: Poor (3%)

Distribution: 97% of an orally administered dose remains in the GI tract. Absorbed neomycin distributes to tissues and concentrates in the renal cortex. With repeated doses, accumulation also occurs in the inner ear.

V_d: 0.36 L/kg

Protein binding: 0% to 30%

Metabolism: Slightly hepatic

Half-life elimination (age and renal function dependent): 3 hours

Time to peak, serum: Oral: 1-4 hours

Excretion: Feces (97% of oral dose as unchanged drug); urine (30% to 50% of absorbed drug as unchanged drug)

Dosage
Children: Oral:

Preoperative intestinal antisepsis: 90 mg/kg/day divided every 4 hours for 2 days; or 25 mg/kg at 1 PM, 2 PM, and 11 PM on the day preceding surgery as an adjunct to mechanical cleansing of the intestine and in combination with erythromycin base

Hepatic encephalopathy: 50-100 mg/kg/day in divided doses every 6-8 hours or 2.5-7 g/m^2/day divided every 4-6 hours for 5-6 days not to exceed 12 g/day

Children and Adults: Topical: Topical solutions containing 0.1% to 1% neomycin have been used for irrigation

Adults: Oral:

Preoperative intestinal antisepsis: 1 g each hour for 4 doses then 1 g every 4 hours for 5 doses; or 1 g at 1 PM, 2 PM, and 11 PM on day preceding surgery as an adjunct to mechanical cleansing of the bowel and oral erythromycin; or 6 g/day divided every 4 hours for 2-3 days

Hepatic encephalopathy: 500-2000 mg every 6-8 hours or 4-12 g/day divided every 4-6 hours for 5-6 days

Chronic hepatic insufficiency: 4 g/day for an indefinite period

Monitoring Parameters Renal function tests, audiometry in symptomatic patients

Pregnancy Risk Factor D

Contraindications Hypersensitivity to neomycin or any component of the formulation, or other aminoglycosides; intestinal obstruction

Warnings/Precautions [U.S. Boxed Warning]: May cause neurotoxicity, nephrotoxicity, and/or neuromuscular blockade and respiratory paralysis; usual risk factors include pre-existing renal impairment, concomitant neuro-/nephrotoxic medications, advanced age and dehydration. The drug's neurotoxicity can result in respiratory paralysis from neuromuscular blockade, especially when the drug is given soon after anesthesia or muscle relaxants. Use with caution in patients with renal impairment, pre-existing hearing impairment, neuromuscular disorders; neomycin is more toxic than other aminoglycosides when given parenterally; **do not administer parenterally;** topical neomycin is a contact sensitizer with sensitivity occurring in 5% to 15% of patients treated with the drug; symptoms include itching, reddening, edema, and failure to heal; **do not use as peritoneal lavage** due to significant systemic adsorption of the drug. Prolonged use may result in fungal or bacterial superinfection, including *C. difficile*-associated diarrhea (CDAD) and pseudomembranous colitis; CDAD has been observed >2 months postantibiotic treatment.

Adverse Reactions

Oral:

>10%: Gastrointestinal: Nausea, diarrhea, vomiting, irritation or soreness of the mouth or rectal area

<1% (Limited to important or life-threatening): Dyspnea, eosinophilia, nephrotoxicity, neurotoxicity, ototoxicity (auditory), ototoxicity (vestibular)

Topical: >10%: Dermatologic: Contact dermatitis

Drug Interactions

Avoid Concomitant Use

Avoid concomitant use of Neomycin with any of the following: Gallium Nitrate

Increased Effect/Toxicity

Neomycin may increase the levels/effects of: AbobotulinumtoxinA; Bisphosphonate Derivatives; CARBOplatin; Colistimethate; CycloSPORINE; Gallium Nitrate; Neuromuscular-Blocking Agents; OnabotulinumtoxinA; RimabotulinumtoxinB

The levels/effects of Neomycin may be increased by: Amphotericin B; Capreomycin; CISplatin; Loop Diuretics; Nonsteroidal Anti-Inflammatory Agents; Vancomycin

Decreased Effect

Neomycin may decrease the levels/effects of: Cardiac Glycosides

The levels/effects of Neomycin may be decreased by: Penicillins

Dosage Forms Excipient information presented when available (limited, particularly for generics); consult specific product labeling.

Powder, micronized, as sulfate [for prescription compounding] (Neo-Rx): (10 g, 100 g)

Solution, oral, as sulfate (Neo-Fradin™): 125 mg/5 mL (60 mL, 480 mL) [contains benzoic acid; cherry flavor]

Tablet, as sulfate: 500 mg

References

"Antimicrobial Prophylaxis for Surgery," *Treat Guidel Med Lett*, 2004, 2(20):27-32.

Neostigmine (nee oh STIG meen)

Medication Safety Issues
Sound-alike/look-alike issues:
Prostigmin® may be confused with physostigmine

Related Information
Anesthesia for Obstetric Patients in Nonobstetric Surgery *on page 1532*
Chronic Renal Failure *on page 1552*
Postoperative Nausea and Vomiting *on page 1593*

U.S. Brand Names Prostigmin®

Canadian Brand Names Prostigmin®

Index Terms Neostigmine Bromide; Neostigmine Methylsulfate

Pharmacologic Category Acetylcholinesterase Inhibitor

Generic Available Yes: Injection

Use Reversal of the effects of nondepolarizing neuromuscular-blocking agents; treatment of myasthenia gravis; prevention and treatment of postoperative bladder distention and urinary retention

Mechanism of Action Inhibits destruction of acetylcholine by acetylcholinesterase which facilitates transmission of impulses across myoneural junction

Pharmacodynamics/Kinetics
Onset of action: I.M.: 20-30 minutes; I.V.: 1-20 minutes
Duration: I.M.: 2.5-4 hours; I.V.: 1-2 hours
Absorption: Oral: Poor, <2%
Metabolism: Hepatic
Half-life elimination: Normal renal function: 0.5-2.1 hours; End-stage renal disease: Prolonged
Excretion: Urine (50% as unchanged drug)

Dosage
Myasthenia gravis: Diagnosis: I.M.:
Children: 0.04 mg/kg as a single dose
Adults: 0.02 mg/kg as a single dose
Myasthenia gravis: Treatment:
Children:
Oral: 2 mg/kg/day divided every 3-4 hours
I.M., I.V., SubQ: 0.01-0.04 mg/kg every 2-4 hours
Adults:
Oral: 15 mg/dose every 3-4 hours up to 375 mg/day maximum; interval between doses must be individualized to maximal response
I.M., I.V., SubQ: 0.5-2.5 mg every 1-3 hours up to 10 mg/24 hours maximum
Reversal of nondepolarizing neuromuscular blockade after surgery in conjunction with atropine (must administer atropine several minutes prior to neostigmine): I.V.:
Infants: 0.025-0.1 mg/kg/dose
Children: 0.025-0.08 mg/kg/dose
Adults: 0.5-2.5 mg; total dose not to exceed 5 mg
Bladder atony: Adults: I.M., SubQ:
Prevention: 0.25 mg every 4-6 hours for 2-3 days
Treatment: 0.5-1 mg every 3 hours for 5 doses after bladder has emptied
Dosing adjustment in renal impairment:
Cl_{cr} 10-50 mL/minute: Administer 50% of normal dose
Cl_{cr} <10 mL/minute: Administer 25% of normal dose

Administration May be administered undiluted by slow I.V. injection over several minutes

Anesthesia and Critical Care Concerns/Other Considerations
Clinical Pearls/Comments: Neostigmine has occasionally been used to improve gastrointestinal motility (Ponec, 1999; van der Spoel, 2001). Atropine may be needed to treat symptomatic bradycardia.

Evidence-based Information: Atropine or glycopyrrolate should be administered along with edrophonium when reversing the effects of nondepolarizing agents to antagonize the cholinergic effects at the muscarinic receptors.

Pregnancy Risk Factor C

Contraindications Hypersensitivity to neostigmine, bromides, or any component of the formulation; GI or GU obstruction

Warnings/Precautions Does **not** antagonize and may prolong the Phase I block of depolarizing muscle relaxants (eg, succinylcholine). Use with caution in patients with epilepsy, asthma, bradycardia, hyperthyroidism, cardiac arrhythmias, or peptic ulcer; not generally recommended for use in patients with vagotonia. Adequate facilities should be available for cardiopulmonary resuscitation when testing and adjusting dose for myasthenia gravis. Have atropine and epinephrine ready to treat hypersensitivity reactions. Overdosage may result in cholinergic crisis, this must be distinguished from myasthenic crisis. Anticholinesterase insensitivity can develop for brief or prolonged periods.

Adverse Reactions Frequency not defined.

Cardiovascular: Arrhythmias (especially bradycardia), hypotension, tachycardia, AV block, nodal rhythm, nonspecific ECG changes, cardiac arrest, syncope, flushing

Central nervous system: Convulsions, dysarthria, dysphonia, dizziness, loss of consciousness, drowsiness, headache

Dermatologic: Skin rash, thrombophlebitis (I.V.), urticaria

Gastrointestinal: Hyperperistalsis, nausea, vomiting, salivation, diarrhea, stomach cramps, dysphagia, flatulence

Genitourinary: Urinary urgency

Neuromuscular & skeletal: Weakness, fasciculations, muscle cramps, spasms, arthralgia

Ocular: Small pupils, lacrimation

Respiratory: Increased bronchial secretions, laryngospasm, bronchiolar constriction, respiratory muscle paralysis, dyspnea, respiratory depression, respiratory arrest, bronchospasm

Miscellaneous: Diaphoresis increased, anaphylaxis, allergic reactions

Drug Interactions

Avoid Concomitant Use There are no known interactions where it is recommended to avoid concomitant use.

Increased Effect/Toxicity

Neostigmine may increase the levels/effects of: Beta-Blockers; Cholinergic Agonists; Succinylcholine

The levels/effects of Neostigmine may be increased by: Corticosteroids (Systemic); Ginkgo Biloba

Decreased Effect

Neostigmine may decrease the levels/effects of: Neuromuscular-Blocking Agents (Nondepolarizing)

Dosage Forms Excipient information presented when available (limited, particularly for generics); consult specific product labeling.

Injection, solution, as methylsulfate: 0.5 mg/mL (1 mL, 10 mL); 1 mg/mL (10 mL)

Tablet, as bromide: 15 mg

References

Ponec RJ, Saunders MD, and Kimmey MB, "Neostigmine for the Treatment of Acute Colonic Pseudo-Obstruction," *N Engl J Med*, 1999, 341(3):137-41.

van der Spoel JI, Oudemans-van Straaten HM, Stoutenbeek CP, et al, "Neostigmine Resolves Critical Illness-Related Colonic Ileus in Intensive Care Patients With Multiple Organ Failure–A Prospective, Double-Blind, Placebo-Controlled Trial," *Intensive Care Med*, 2001, 27(5):822-7.

◆ **Neostigmine Bromide** *see* Neostigmine *on page 997*

◆ **Neostigmine Methylsulfate** *see* Neostigmine *on page 997*

◆ **Neo-Synephrine® (Can)** *see* Phenylephrine *on page 1114*

◆ **Neo-Synephrine® Extra Strength [OTC]** *see* Phenylephrine *on page 1114*

◆ **Neo-Synephrine® Injection** *see* Phenylephrine *on page 1114*

◆ **Neo-Synephrine® Mild [OTC]** *see* Phenylephrine *on page 1114*

◆ **Neo-Synephrine® Regular Strength [OTC]** *see* Phenylephrine *on page 1114*

◆ **NephrAmine®** *see* Amino Acid Injection *on page 81*

◆ **Nesacaine®** *see* Chloroprocaine *on page 293*

◆ **Nesacaine®-CE (Can)** *see* Chloroprocaine *on page 293*

◆ **Nesacaine®-MPF** *see* Chloroprocaine *on page 293*

Nesiritide (ni SIR i tide)

Medication Safety Issues

High alert medication: The Institute for Safe Medication Practices (ISMP) includes this medication among its list of drugs which have a heightened risk of causing significant patient harm when used in error.

International issues:
Natrecor® may be confused with Nitrocor® which is a brand name for nitroglycerin in Chile and Italy

Related Information
Hemodynamic Support, Intravenous *on page 1681*

U.S. Brand Names Natrecor®

Canadian Brand Names Natrecor®

Index Terms B-type Natriuretic Peptide (Human); hBNP; Natriuretic Peptide

Pharmacologic Category Natriuretic Peptide, B-Type, Human; Vasodilator

Generic Available No

Use Treatment of acutely decompensated heart failure (HF) with dyspnea at rest or with minimal activity

Mechanism of Action Binds to guanylate cyclase receptor on vascular smooth muscle and endothelial cells, increasing intracellular cyclic GMP, resulting in smooth muscle cell relaxation. Has been shown to produce dose-dependent reductions in pulmonary capillary wedge pressure (PCWP) and systemic arterial pressure.

Pharmacodynamics/Kinetics

Onset of action: 15 minutes (60% of 3-hour effect achieved)

Duration: >60 minutes (up to several hours) for systolic blood pressure; hemodynamic effects persist longer than serum half-life would predict

Distribution: V_{ss}: 0.19 L/kg

Metabolism: Proteolytic cleavage by vascular endopeptidases and proteolysis following binding to the membrane bound natriuretic peptide (NPR-C) and cellular internalization

Half-life elimination: Initial (distribution) 2 minutes; Terminal: 18 minutes

Time to peak: 1 hour

Excretion: Primarily eliminated by metabolism; also excreted in the urine

Dosage Adults: I.V.: Initial: 2 mcg/kg (bolus); followed by continuous infusion at 0.01 mcg/kg/minute. **Note:** Should not be initiated at a dosage higher than initial recommended dose. There is limited experience with increasing the dose >0.01 mcg/kg/minute; in one trial, a limited number of patients received higher doses that were increased no faster than every 3 hours by 0.005 mcg/kg/minute (preceded by a bolus of 1 mcg/kg), up to a maximum of 0.03 mcg/kg/minute. Increases beyond the initial infusion rate should be limited to selected patients and accompanied by close hemodynamic and renal function monitoring.

Patients experiencing hypotension during the infusion: Infusion dose should be reduced or discontinued. Other measures to support blood pressure should be initiated (eg, I.V. fluids, Trendelenburg position). May attempt to restart at a lower dose (reduce previous infusion dose by 30% and omit bolus).

Dosage adjustment in renal impairment: No adjustment required, but use cautiously in patients with renal impairment or those patients who rely on the renin-angiotensin-aldosterone system for renal perfusion. Monitor renal function closely.

Dosage adjustment in hepatic impairment: No dosage adjustment recommended.

Stability Vials may be stored below 25°C (77°F); do not freeze. Protect from light. Following reconstitution, vials are stable at 2°C to 25°C (36°F to 77°F) for up to 24 hours. Use reconstituted solution within 24 hours.

Reconstitute 1.5 mg vial with 5 mL of diluent removed from a prefilled 250 mL plastic I.V. bag (compatible with D_5W, $D_5^{1/2}NS$, $D_5^{1/4}NS$, NS). Do not shake vial to dissolve (roll gently). Withdraw entire contents of vial and add to 250 mL I.V. bag. Invert several times to mix. Resultant concentration of solution is ~6 mcg/mL.

Administration Do not administer through a heparin-coated catheter (concurrent administration of heparin via a separate catheter is acceptable, per manufacturer).

◄ Prime I.V. tubing with 5 mL of infusion prior to connection with vascular access port and prior to administering bolus or starting the infusion. Withdraw bolus from the prepared infusion bag and administer over 60 seconds. Begin infusion immediately following administration of the bolus.

Monitoring Parameters Blood pressure, hemodynamic responses (PCWP, RAP, CI), BUN, creatinine; urine output

Pregnancy Risk Factor C

Contraindications Hypersensitivity to natriuretic peptide or any component of the formulation; cardiogenic shock (when used as primary therapy); hypotension (systolic blood pressure <90 mm Hg)

Warnings/Precautions May cause hypotension; administer in clinical situations when blood pressure may be closely monitored. Use caution in patients systolic blood pressure <100 mm Hg (contraindicated if <90 mm Hg); more likely to experience hypotension. Effects may be additive with other agents capable of causing hypotension. Hypotensive effects may last for several hours.

Should not be used in patients with low cardiac filling pressures, or in patients with conditions which depend on venous return including significant valvular stenosis, restrictive or obstructive cardiomyopathy, constrictive pericarditis, and pericardial tamponade. May be associated with development of azotemia; use caution in patients with renal impairment or in patients where renal perfusion is dependent on renin-angiotensin-aldosterone system; avoid initiation at doses higher than recommended.

Monitor for allergic or anaphylactic reactions. Use caution with prolonged infusions; limited experience with infusions >48 hours. Safety and efficacy in pediatric patients have not been established.

Adverse Reactions Note: Frequencies cited below were recorded in VMAC trial at dosages similar to approved labeling. Higher frequencies have been observed in trials using higher dosages of nesiritide. The percentages marked with an asterisk (*) indicate frequency less than or equal to placebo or other standard therapy.

>10%:
  Cardiovascular: Hypotension (total: 11%; symptomatic: 4% at recommended dose, up to 17% at higher doses)
  Renal: Increased serum creatinine (28% with >0.5 mg/dL increase over baseline)
1% to 10%:
  Cardiovascular: Ventricular tachycardia (3%)*, ventricular extrasystoles (3%)*, angina (2%)*, bradycardia (1%), tachycardia, atrial fibrillation, AV node conduction abnormalities
  Central nervous system: Headache (8%)*, dizziness (3%), insomnia (2%)*, anxiety (3%), confusion, fever, paresthesia, somnolence, tremor
  Dermatologic: Pruritus, rash
  Gastrointestinal: Nausea (4%)*, abdominal pain (1%)*, vomiting (1%)*
  Hematologic: Anemia
  Local: Injection site reaction, catheter pain
  Neuromuscular & skeletal: Back pain (4%), leg cramps
  Ocular: Amblyopia
  Respiratory: Apnea, cough increased, hemoptysis
  Miscellaneous: Diaphoresis
Postmarketing and/or case reports: Hypersensitivity reactions (rare)

Drug Interactions

Avoid Concomitant Use There are no known interactions where it is recommended to avoid concomitant use.

Increased Effect/Toxicity
  Nesiritide may increase the levels/effects of: Hypotensive Agents

Decreased Effect There are no known significant interactions involving a decrease in effect.

Ethanol/Nutrition/Herb Interactions Herb/Nutraceutical: Avoid bayberry, blue cohosh, cayenne, ephedra, ginger, ginseng (American), kola, and licorice (may increase blood pressure). Avoid black cohosh, California poppy, coleus, golden seal, hawthorn, mistletoe, periwinkle, quinine, and shepherd's purse (may enhance decreased blood pressure).

Dosage Forms Excipient information presented when available (limited, particularly for generics); consult specific product labeling.
Injection, powder for reconstitution:
  Natrecor®: 1.5 mg

References
Sackner-Bernstein JD, Skopicki HA, and Aaronson KD, "Risk of Worsening Renal Function With Nesiritide in Patients With Acutely Decompensated Heart Failure," *Circulation*, 2005, 111 (12):1487-9.

◆ **Neupogen®** *see* Filgrastim *on page 601*

◆ **Neurontin®** *see* Gabapentin *on page 650*

◆ **Neut®** *see* Sodium Bicarbonate *on page 1301*

◆ **Neutra-Phos®-K [OTC] [DSC]** *see* Potassium Phosphate *on page 1154*

◆ **Nexium®** *see* Esomeprazole *on page 526*

Niacin (NYE a sin)

Related Information
  Hyperlipidemia Management *on page 1747*
U.S. Brand Names Niacin-Time®; Niacor®; Niaspan®; Slo-Niacin® [OTC]
Canadian Brand Names Niaspan®
Index Terms Nicotinic Acid; Vitamin B_3
Pharmacologic Category Antilipemic Agent, Miscellaneous; Vitamin, Water Soluble
Use Adjunctive treatment of dyslipidemias (types IIa and IIb or primary hypercholesterolemia) to lower the risk of recurrent MI and/or slow progression of coronary artery disease, including combination therapy with other antidyslipidemic agents when additional triglyceride-lowering or HDL-increasing effects are desired; treatment of hypertriglyceridemia in patients at risk of pancreatitis; treatment of peripheral vascular disease and circulatory disorders; treatment of pellagra; dietary supplement
Pharmacodynamics/Kinetics
  Absorption: Rapid and extensive (60% to 76%)
  Distribution: Mainly to hepatic, renal, and adipose tissue
  Metabolism: Extensive first-pass effects; converted to nicotinamide adenine dinucleotide, nicotinuric acid, and other metabolites
  Half-life elimination: 20-45 minutes
  Time to peak, serum: Immediate release formulation: 30-60 minutes; extended release formulation: 4-5 hours
  Excretion: Urine 60% to 88% (unchanged drug and metabolites)
Dosage Note: Formulations of niacin (regular release versus extended release) are not interchangeable.
  Children: Oral:
    Pellagra: 50-100 mg/dose 3 times/day
    Recommended daily allowances:
      0-0.5 years: 5 mg/day
      0.5-1 year: 6 mg/day
      1-3 years: 9 mg/day
      4-6 years: 12 mg/day
      7-10 years: 13 mg/day
  Children and Adolescents: Recommended daily allowances:
    Male:
      11-14 years: 17 mg/day
      15-18 years: 20 mg/day
      19-24 years: 19 mg/day
    Female: 11-24 years: 15 mg/day
  Adults: Oral:
    Recommended daily allowances:
      Male: 25-50 years: 19 mg/day; >51 years: 15 mg/day
      Female: 25-50 years: 15 mg/day; >51 years: 13 mg/day
    Hyperlipidemia: Usual target dose: Regular release: 1.5-6 g/day in 3 divided doses with or after meals using a dosage titration schedule. Extended release: 500 mg to 2 g once daily at bedtime.

◄ Regular release formulation (Niacor®): Initial: 250 mg once daily (with evening meal); increase frequency and/or dose every 4-7 days to desired response or first-level therapeutic dose (1.5-2 g/day in 2-3 divided doses); after 2 months, may increase at 2- to 4-week intervals to 3 g/day in 3 divided doses (maximum dose: 6 g/day in 3 divided doses)

Extended release formulation (Niaspan®): Initial: 500 mg at bedtime for 4 weeks, then 1 g at bedtime for 4 weeks; adjust dose to response and tolerance; can increase to a maximum of 2 g/day, but only at 500 mg/day at 4-week intervals

With lovastatin: Recommended initial dose: 20 mg/day; Maximum lovastatin dose: 40 mg/day

Pellagra: 50-100 mg 3-4 times/day, maximum: 500 mg/day

Niacin deficiency: 10-20 mg/day, maximum: 100 mg/day

Dosage adjustment in renal impairment: Use with caution

Dosage adjustment in hepatic impairment: Contraindicated in patients with significant or unexplained hepatic dysfunction, active liver disease or unexplained transaminase elevations.

Dosage adjustment for hepatic toxicity: Transaminases rise ≥3 times ULN, either persistent or if symptoms of nausea, fever, and/or malaise occur: Discontinue therapy.

Additional Information Complete prescribing information for this medication should be consulted for additional detail.

Dosage Forms Excipient information presented when available (limited, particularly for generics); consult specific product labeling. [DSC] = Discontinued product

Caplet, timed release, oral: 500 mg

Capsule, oral: 50 mg, 250 mg

Capsule, extended release, oral: 250 mg; 400 mg [DSC]; 500 mg

Capsule, timed release, oral: 250 mg, 400 mg, 500 mg

Tablet, oral: 50 mg, 100 mg, 250 mg, 500 mg

Niacor®: 500 mg [scored]

Tablet, controlled release, oral:

Slo-Niacin®: 250 mg, 500 mg, 750 mg [scored]

Tablet, extended release, oral:

Niaspan®: 500 mg, 750 mg, 1000 mg

Tablet, timed release, oral: 250 mg, 500 mg, 750 mg, 1000 mg

Niacin-Time®: 500 mg

References

Carlson LA and Rosenhamer G, "Reduction of Mortality in the Stockholm Ischaemic Heart Disease Secondary Prevention Study by Combined Treatment With Clofibrate and Nicotinic Acid," *Acta Med Scand*, 1988, 223(5):405-18.

"Clofibrate and Niacin in Coronary Heart Disease," *JAMA*, 1975, 231(4):360-81.

"Executive Summary of The Third Report of The National Cholesterol Education Program (NCEP) Expert Panel on Detection, Evaluation, and Treatment of High Blood Cholesterol in Adults (Adult Treatment Panel III)," *JAMA*, 2001, 285(19):2486-97.

Knopp RH, Ginsberg J, Albers JJ, et al, "Contrasting Effects of Unmodified and Time-Release Forms of Niacin on Lipoproteins in Hyperlipidemic Subjects: Clues to Mechanism of Action of Niacin," *Metabolism*, 1985, 34(7):642-50.

Mahley RW and Bersot TP, "Drug Therapy for Hypercholesterolemia and Dyslipidemia," *Goodman and Gilman's The Pharmacological Basis of Therapeutics*, 10th ed, Hardman JE and Limbird LE, eds, New York, NY: McGraw-Hill, 2001, 993-5.

McKenney JM, Proctor JD, Harris S, et al, "A Comparison of the Efficacy and Toxic Effects of Sustained- vs Immediate-Release Niacin in Hypercholesterolemic Patients," *JAMA*, 1994, 271 (9):672-7.

◆ **Niacin-Time®** *see* Niacin *on page 1001*

◆ **Niacor®** *see* Niacin *on page 1001*

◆ **Niaspan®** *see* Niacin *on page 1001*

◆ **Niastase® (Can)** *see* Factor VIIa (Recombinant) *on page 567*

NiCARdipine (nye KAR de peen)

Medication Safety Issues

Sound-alike/look-alike issues:

NiCARdipine may be confused with niacinamide, NIFEdipine, niMODipine

Cardene® may be confused with Cardizem®, Cardura®, codeine

International issues:

Cardene® may be confused with Cardem® which is a brand name for celiprolol in Spain

Cardene® may be confused with Cardin® which is a brand name for methyldopa in Brazil and a brand name for simvastatin in Poland

Significant differences exist between oral and I.V. dosing. Use caution when converting from one route of administration to another.

Related Information

Anesthesia Considerations for Neurosurgery *on page 1514*
Calcium Channel Blockers *on page 1672*
Chronic Renal Failure *on page 1552*
Hypertension *on page 1754*
Postoperative Hypertension *on page 1589*

U.S. Brand Names Cardene®; Cardene® I.V.; Cardene® SR

Index Terms Nicardipine Hydrochloride

Pharmacologic Category Calcium Channel Blocker; Calcium Channel Blocker, Dihydropyridine

Generic Available Yes: Capsule, injection

Use Chronic stable angina (immediate-release product only); management of hypertension (immediate and sustained release products); parenteral only for short-term use when oral treatment is not feasible

Unlabeled/Investigational Use Congestive heart failure, control of blood pressure in acute ischemic stroke and spontaneous intracranial hemorrhage, postoperative hypertension associated with carotid endarterectomy, perioperative hypertension, prevention of migraine headaches, subarachnoid hemorrhage associated cerebral vasospasm

Mechanism of Action Inhibits calcium ion from entering the "slow channels" or select voltage-sensitive areas of vascular smooth muscle and myocardium during depolarization, producing a relaxation of coronary vascular smooth muscle and coronary vasodilation; increases myocardial oxygen delivery in patients with vasospastic angina

Pharmacodynamics/Kinetics

Onset of action: Oral: 0.5-2 hours; I.V.: 10 minutes; Hypotension: ~20 minutes

Duration:

I.V.: ≤8 hours

Oral: Immediate release capsules: ≤8 hours; Sustained release capsules: 8-12 hours

Absorption: Oral: ~100%

Protein binding: >95%

Metabolism: Hepatic; CYP3A4 substrate (major); extensive first-pass effect (saturable)

Bioavailability: 35%

Half-life elimination: 2-4 hours

Time to peak, serum: Oral: Immediate release: 30-120 minutes; Sustained release: 60-240 minutes

Excretion: Urine (49% to 60% as metabolites); feces (43% as metabolites)

Dosage

Adults:

Oral:

Immediate release: Initial: 20 mg 3 times/day; usual: 20-40 mg 3 times/day (allow 3 days between dose increases)

Sustained release: Initial: 30 mg twice daily, titrate up to 60 mg twice daily

Note: The total daily dose of immediate-release product may not automatically be equivalent to the daily sustained-release dose; use caution in converting.

I.V.:

Acute hypertension: Initial: 5 mg/hour increased by 2.5 mg/hour every 15 minutes to a maximum of 15 mg/hour; consider reduction to 3 mg/hour after response is achieved. Monitor and titrate to lowest dose necessary to maintain stable blood pressure.

Substitution for oral therapy (approximate equivalents):

20 mg every 8 hours oral, equivalent to 0.5 mg/hour I.V. infusion

30 mg every 8 hours oral, equivalent to 1.2 mg/hour I.V. infusion

40 mg every 8 hours oral, equivalent to 2.2 mg/hour I.V. infusion

Elderly: Initiate at the low end of the dosage range. Specific guidelines for adjustment of nicardipine are not available, but careful monitoring is warranted and adjustment may be necessary.

Dosing adjustment in renal impairment: Titrate dose beginning with 20 mg 3 times/day (immediate release capsule) or 30 mg twice daily (sustained release capsule). Specific guidelines for adjustment of nicardipine are not available, but careful monitoring is warranted and adjustment may be necessary.

Dosing adjustment in hepatic impairment: Starting dose: 20 mg twice daily (immediate release) with titration. Specific guidelines for adjustment of nicardipine are not available, but careful monitoring is warranted and adjustment may be necessary.

Stability

I.V.:

Premixed bags: Store at controlled room temperature of 20°C to 25°C (68°F to 77°F). Protect from light and excessive heat. Do not freeze.

Vials: Store at controlled room temperature of 20°C to 25°C (68°F to 77°F). Protect from light. Dilute 25 mg ampul with 240 mL of compatible solution to provide a 250 mL total volume solution and a final concentration of 0.1 mg/mL. Diluted solution (0.1 mg/mL) is stable at room temperature for 24 hours in glass or PVC containers. Stability has also been demonstrated at room temperature at concentrations up to 0.5 mg/mL in PVC containers for 24 hours or in glass containers for up to 7 days (Baaske, 1996).

Oral (Cardene®, Cardene SR®): Store at 15°C to 30°C (59°F to 86°F). Protect from light. Freezing does not affect stability.

Administration

Oral: The total daily dose of immediate-release product may not automatically be equivalent to the daily sustained-release dose; use caution in converting. Do not chew or crush the sustained release formulation, swallow whole. Do not open or cut capsules.

I.V.:

Ampuls must be diluted before use. Administer as a slow continuous infusion at a concentration of 0.1 mg/mL. Concentrations of 0.5 mg/mL may be administered via a central line only.

Premixed bags: No further dilution needed. For single use only, discard any unused portion. Use only if solution is clear; the manufacturer recommends not to admix or run in the same line as other medications.

Anesthesia and Critical Care Concerns/Other Considerations

Clincial Pearls/Comments: As a dihydropyridine calcium channel antagonist, the primary mechanism of action of nicardipine is potent peripheral vasodilation, which can result in reflex tachycardia. Nicardipine has minimal direct effects on inotropy; however, decreases in systemic vascular resistance may increase cardiac index without increasing work of the heart. Because nicardipine does not slow cardiac conduction, it has no antiarrhythmic effect.

Pregnancy Risk Factor C

Contraindications Hypersensitivity to nicardipine or any component of the formulation; advanced aortic stenosis

Warnings/Precautions Symptomatic hypotension with or without syncope can rarely occur; blood pressure must be lowered at a rate appropriate for the patient's clinical condition. Reflex tachycardia may occur resulting in angina and/or MI in patients with obstructive coronary disease especially in the absence of concurrent beta blockade. The most common side effect is peripheral edema (dose-dependent); occurs within 2-3 weeks of starting therapy. Use with caution in CAD (can cause increase in angina), HF (can worsen heart failure symptoms), aortic stenosis (may reduce coronary perfusion resulting in ischemia; use is contra-indicated in patients with advanced aortic stenosis), and hypertrophic cardiomyopathy with outflow tract obstruction. To minimize infusion site reactions, peripheral infusion sites (for I.V. therapy) should be changed every 12 hours; use of small peripheral veins should be avoided. Titrate I.V. dose cautiously in patients with HF, renal or hepatic dysfunction. Use the I.V. form cautiously in patients with portal hypertension (can cause increase in hepatic pressure gradient). Initiate at the low end of the dosage range in the elderly. Concurrent use of fentanyl anesthesia may result in hypotension. Abrupt withdrawal may cause rebound angina in patients with CAD. Safety and efficacy have not been established in pediatric patients.

Adverse Reactions

1% to 10%:

Cardiovascular: Cardiovascular: Flushing (6% to 10%), peripheral edema (dose related; 6% to 8%), hypotension (I.V. 6%), increased angina (dose related; 6%), palpitation (3% to 4%), tachycardia (1% to 4%), vasodilation (1% to 5%), chest pain (I.V. 1%), ECG abnormal (I.V. 1%), extrasystoles (I.V. 1%), hemopericardium (I.V. 1%), hypertension (I.V. 1%), orthostasis (1%), supraventricular tachycardia (I.V. 1%), syncope (1%), ventricular extrasystoles (I.V. 1%), ventricular tachycardia (I.V. 1%)

Central nervous system: Headache (6% to 15%), dizziness (1% to 7%), hypoesthesia (1%), intracranial hemorrhage (1%) pain (1%), somnolence (1%)

Dermatologic: Rash (1%)

Endocrine & metabolic: Hypokalemia (I.V. 1%)

Gastrointestinal: Nausea (2% to 5%), vomiting (I.V. 5%), dyspepsia (oral 2%), abdominal pain (I.V. 1%), dry mouth (1%)

Genitourinary: Polyuria (1%)

Local: Injection site pain (I.V. 1%), injection site reaction (I.V. 1%)

Neuromuscular & skeletal: Weakness (1% to 6%), myalgia (1%), paresthesia (1%)

Renal: Hematuria (1%)

Respiratory: Dyspnea (1%)

Miscellaneous: Diaphoresis (1%)

<1% (Limited to important or life-threatening): Allergic reaction, confusion, constipation, deep vein thrombophlebitis; ECG effects (AV block, inverted T wave, ST segment depression); gingival hyperplasia, hypertonia, hypophosphatemia, insomnia, malaise, nervousness, nocturia, parotitis, thrombocytopenia, tinnitus, tremor

Drug Interactions

Metabolism/Transport Effects Substrate of CYP1A2 (minor), 2C9 (minor), 2D6 (minor), 2E1 (minor), 3A4 (major); **Inhibits** CYP2C9 (strong), 2C19 (moderate), 2D6 (moderate), 3A4 (strong)

Avoid Concomitant Use

Avoid concomitant use of NiCARdipine with any of the following: Alfuzosin; Dabigatran Etexilate; Dronedarone; Eplerenone; Everolimus; Halofantrine; Nilotinib; Nisoldipine; Ranolazine; Rivaroxaban; Salmeterol; Silodosin; Thioridazine; Tolvaptan; Topotecan

Increased Effect/Toxicity

NiCARdipine may increase the levels/effects of: Alfuzosin; Almotriptan; Alosetron; Amifostine; Antihypertensives; Ciclesonide; Colchicine; CYP2C19 Substrates; CYP2C9 Substrates (High risk); CYP2D6 Substrates; CYP3A4 Substrates; Dabigatran Etexilate; Dronedarone; Dutasteride; Eplerenone; Everolimus; FentaNYL; Fesoterodine; Halofantrine; Hypotensive Agents; Ixabepilone; Magnesium Salts; Maraviroc; Neuromuscular-Blocking Agents (Nondepolarizing); Nilotinib; Nisoldipine; Nitroprusside; Paricalcitol; P-Glycoprotein Substrates; Phenytoin; Pimecrolimus; Ranolazine; RiTUXimab; Rivaroxaban; Salmeterol; Saxagliptin; Silodosin; Sorafenib; Tacrolimus; Tadalafil; Tamoxifen; Thioridazine; Tolvaptan; Topotecan

The levels/effects of NiCARdipine may be increased by: Alpha1-Blockers; Antifungal Agents (Azole Derivatives, Systemic); Calcium Channel Blockers (Nondihydropyridine); CycloSPORINE; CYP3A4 Inhibitors (Moderate); CYP3A4 Inhibitors (Strong); Dasatinib; Diazoxide; Fluconazole; Grapefruit Juice; Herbs (Hypotensive Properties); Macrolide Antibiotics; Magnesium Salts; MAO Inhibitors; Pentoxifylline; P-Glycoprotein Inhibitors; Phosphodiesterase 5 Inhibitors; Prostacyclin Analogues; Protease Inhibitors; Quinupristin

Decreased Effect

NiCARdipine may decrease the levels/effects of: Clopidogrel; Codeine; Prasugrel; QuiNIDine; TraMADol

The levels/effects of NiCARdipine may be decreased by: Barbiturates; Calcium Salts; CarBAMazepine; CYP3A4 Inducers (Strong); Deferasirox; Herbs (CYP3A4 Inducers); Herbs (Hypertensive Properties); Methylphenidate; Nafcillin; Peginterferon Alfa-2b; P-Glycoprotein Inducers; Rifamycin Derivatives; Yohimbine

◄ **Ethanol/Nutrition/Herb Interactions**
Ethanol: Avoid ethanol (may increase CNS depression).
Food: Nicardipine average peak concentrations may be decreased if taken with food. Serum concentrations/toxicity of nicardipine may be increased by grapefruit juice; avoid concurrent use.
Herb/Nutraceutical: St John's wort may decrease levels. Avoid bayberry, blue cohosh, cayenne, ephedra, ginger, ginseng (American), kola, licorice (may worsen hypertension). Avoid black cohosh, California poppy, coleus, golden seal, hawthorn, mistletoe, periwinkle, quinine, shepherd's purse (may have increased antihypertensive effect).

Dosage Forms Excipient information presented when available (limited, particularly for generics); consult specific product labeling.
Capsule, oral, as hydrochloride: 20 mg, 30 mg
Cardene®: 20 mg, 30 mg
Capsule, sustained release, oral, as hydrochloride:
Cardene® SR: 30 mg, 45 mg, 60 mg
Infusion, premixed in iso-osmotic dextrose, as hydrochloride:
Cardene® I.V.: 20 mg (200 mL); 40 mg (200 mL)
Infusion, premixed in iso-osmotic sodium chloride, as hydrochloride:
Cardene® I.V.: 20 mg (200 mL); 40 mg (200 mL)
Injection, solution, as hydrochloride: 2.5 mg/mL (10 mL)
Cardene® I.V.: 2.5 mg/mL (10 mL)

References

Broderick J, Connolly S, Feldmann E, et al, "Guidelines for the Management of Spontaneous Intracerebral Hemorrhage in Adults: 2007 Update: A Guideline From the American Heart Association/American Stroke Association Stroke Council, High Blood Pressure Research Council, and the Quality of Care and Outcomes in Research Interdisciplinary Working Group," *Stroke*, 2007, 38(6):2001-23. Available at http://stroke.ahajournals.org/cgi/content/short/STROKEAHA.107.183689.
Erstad BL and Barletta JF, "Treatment of Hypertension in the Perioperative Patient," *Ann Pharmacother*, 2000, 34(1):66-79.

◆ **Nicardipine Hydrochloride** *see* NiCARdipine *on page* 1002

◆ **Nicotinic Acid** *see* Niacin *on page* 1001

◆ **Nidagel™ (Can)** *see* MetroNIDAZOLE *on page* 928

◆ **Nifediac CC®** *see* NIFEdipine *on page* 1006

◆ **Nifedical XL®** *see* NIFEdipine *on page* 1006

NIFEdipine (nye FED i peen)

Medication Safety Issues
Sound-alike/look-alike issues:
NIFEdipine may be confused with niCARdipine, niMODipine, nisoldipine
Procardia XL® may be confused with Cartia XT®

International issues:
Nipin® [Italy and Singapore] may be confused with Nipent® which is a brand name for pentostatin in the U.S.

Related Information
Calcium Channel Blockers *on page* 1672
Hypertension *on page* 1754

U.S. Brand Names Adalat® CC; Afeditab® CR; Nifediac CC®; Nifedical XL®; Procardia XL®; Procardia®

Canadian Brand Names Adalat® XL®; Apo-Nifed PA®; Apo-Nifed®; GEN-Nifedipine XL; Mylan-Nifedipine Extended Release; Nifedipine PA; Nu-Nifed; Nu-Nifedipine-PA; PMS-Nifedipine

Pharmacologic Category Calcium Channel Blocker; Calcium Channel Blocker, Dihydropyridine

Generic Available Yes

Use Management of chronic stable or vasospastic angina; treatment of hypertension (sustained release products only)

Unlabeled/Investigational Use Management of pulmonary hypertension, preterm labor, Raynaud's phenomenon

Mechanism of Action Inhibits calcium ion from entering the "slow ci.
select voltage-sensitive areas of vascular smooth muscle and myocardiu.
depolarization, producing a relaxation of coronary vascular smooth musc
coronary vasodilation; increases myocardial oxygen delivery in patients
vasospastic angina; also reduces peripheral vascular resistance, producing
reduction in arterial blood pressure.

Pharmacodynamics/Kinetics
Onset of action: Immediate release: ~20 minutes

Protein binding (concentration dependent): 92% to 98%

Metabolism: Hepatic via CYP3A4 to inactive metabolites

Bioavailability: Capsule: 40% to 77%; Sustained release: 65% to 89% relative to
immediate release capsules; bioavailability increased with significant hepatic
disease

Half-life elimination: Adults: Healthy: 2-5 hours; Cirrhosis: 7 hours; Elderly: 7
hours (extended release tablet)

Excretion: Urine (60% to 80% as inactive metabolites); feces

Dosage Oral:
Children 1-17 years: Hypertension: Extended release tablet: Initial: 0.25-0.5 mg/
kg/day once daily or in 2 divided doses; maximum: 3 mg/kg/day up to 120 mg/
day

Adults: **Note:** Dosage adjustments should occur at 7- to 14-day intervals, to allow
for adequate assessment of new dose; when switching from immediate release
to sustained release formulations, use same total daily dose.

Chronic stable or vasospastic angina:
Immediate release: Initial: 10 mg 3 times/day; usual dose: 10-20 mg 3 times/
day; maximum: 180 mg/day; **Note:** Do not use for acute anginal episodes; may
precipitate myocardial infarction

Extended release: Initial: 30 or 60 mg once daily; maximum: 120-180 mg/day
Hypertension: Extended release: Initial: 30 or 60 mg once daily; maximum:
90-120 mg/day

Pulmonary hypertension (unlabeled use; Galie, 2004): Extended release:
Dosage range: 60-240 mg once daily

Raynaud's phenomenon (unlabeled use; Wigley, 2002): Extended release:
Dosage range: 30-120 mg once daily

Hemodialysis: Supplemental dose is not necessary

Peritoneal dialysis effects: Supplemental dose is not necessary

Dosing adjustment in hepatic impairment: Reduce dose by 50% to 60% in
patients with cirrhosis

Administration
Immediate release: In general, may be administered with or without food.

Extended release: Tablets should be swallowed whole; do not crush or chew.
Adalat® CC, Afeditab® CR, Nifediac CC®: Administer on an empty stomach
(per manufacturer). Other extended release products may not have this
recommendation; consult product labeling.

Monitoring Parameters Heart rate, blood pressure, signs and symptoms of
CHF, peripheral edema

Anesthesia and Critical Care Concerns/Other Considerations
Evidence-Based Information: Considerable attention has been directed to
potential increases in mortality and morbidity when short-acting nifedipine is used
in treating hypertension. The rapid reduction in blood pressure may precipitate
adverse cardiovascular events.

Short-acting nifedipine should not be used for acute anginal episodes since this
may precipitate myocardial infarction. Extended-release formulations are
preferred for the management of chronic or vasospastic angina (Poole-Wilson,
2004).

Pregnancy Risk Factor C

Contraindications Hypersensitivity to nifedipine or any component of the
formulation; immediate release preparation for treatment of urgent or emergent
hypertension; acute MI

Warnings/Precautions Symptomatic hypotension with or without syncope can
rarely occur; blood pressure must be lowered at a rate appropriate for the patient's
clinical condition. **The use of immediate release nifedipine (sublingually or** ▸

orally) in hypertensive emergencies and urgencies is neither safe nor effective. Serious adverse events (eg, death, cerebrovascular ischemia, syncope, stroke, acute myocardial infarction, and fetal distress) have been reported. **Immediate release nifedipine should not be used for acute blood pressure reduction.**

Blood pressure lowering should be done at a rate appropriate for the patient's condition. Rapid drops in blood pressure can lead to arterial insufficiency. Increased angina and/or MI have occurred with initiation or dosage titration of dihydropyridine calcium channel blockers; use with caution in patients with obstructive coronary disease especially in the absence of concurrent beta-blockade. Use with caution before major surgery. Cardiopulmonary bypass, intraoperative blood loss or vasodilating anesthesia may result in severe hypotension and/or increased fluid requirements. Consider withdrawing nifedipine (>36 hours) before surgery if possible.

The most common side effect is peripheral edema; occurs within 2-3 weeks of starting therapy. Reflex tachycardia may occur with use. Use with caution in HF or severe aortic stenosis (especially with concomitant beta-adrenergic blocker), severe left ventricular dysfunction, renal impairment, hypertrophic cardiomyopathy (especially obstructive), concomitant therapy with beta-blockers or digoxin, and edema. Use caution in patients with severe hepatic impairment (may need dosage adjustment). Mild and transient elevations in liver function enzymes may be apparent within 8 weeks of therapy initiation. Abrupt withdrawal may cause rebound angina in patients with CAD. The elderly may be more susceptible to adverse effects. Immediate release formulations should not be used to manage essential hypertension, adequate studies to evaluate outcomes have not been conducted. Avoid use of extended release tablets (Procardia XL®) in patients with known stricture/narrowing of the GI tract.

Adverse Reactions
>10%:
  Cardiovascular: Flushing (10% to 25%; extended release products 3% to 4%), peripheral edema (dose related 7% to 30%)
  Central nervous system: Dizziness/lightheadedness/giddiness (10% to 27%), headache (10% to 23%)
  Gastrointestinal: Nausea/heartburn (10% to 11%)
≥1% to 10%:
  Cardiovascular: Palpitation (≤2% to 7%), transient hypotension (dose related 5%), CHF (2%)
  Central nervous system: Nervousness/mood changes (≤2% to 7%), fatigue (6%), shakiness (≤2%), jitteriness (≤2%), sleep disturbances (≤2%), difficulties in balance (≤2%), fever (≤2%), chills (≤2%)
  Dermatologic: Dermatitis (≤2%), pruritus (≤2%), urticaria (≤2%)
  Endocrine & metabolic: Sexual difficulties (≤2%)
  Gastrointestinal: Diarrhea (≤2%), constipation (≤2%), cramps (≤2%), flatulence (≤2%), gingival hyperplasia (≤10%)
  Neuromuscular & skeletal: Muscle cramps/tremor (≤2% to 8%), weakness (<3%), inflammation (≤2%), joint stiffness (≤2%)
  Ocular: Blurred vision (≤2%)
  Respiratory: Cough/wheezing (6%), nasal congestion/sore throat (≤2% to 6%), chest congestion (≤2%), dyspnea (≤2%)
  Miscellaneous: Diaphoresis (≤2%)
<1% (Limited to important or life-threatening): Agranulocytosis, allergic hepatitis, alopecia, anemia, aplastic anemia, angina, angioedema, arrhythmia, arthritis with positive ANA, bezoars (sustained-release preparations), cerebral ischemia, depression, EPS, dysosmia, erythema multiforme, erythromelalgia, epistaxis, exfoliative dermatitis, facial edema, gastroesophageal reflux, gynecomastia, hematuria, ischemia, leukopenia, memory dysfunction, migraine, myalgia, myoclonus, nocturia, paranoid syndrome, parotitis, periorbital edema, photosensitivity, polyuria, purpura, Stevens-Johnson syndrome, syncope, tachycardia, taste perversion, thrombocytopenia, tinnitus, transient blindness, ventricular arrhythmia
Reported with use of sublingual short-acting nifedipine: Acute MI, cerebrovascular ischemia, ECG changes, fetal distress, heart block, severe hypotension, sinus arrest, stroke, syncope

Drug Interactions

Metabolism/Transport Effects Substrate of CYP2D6 (minor), 3A4 (major); Inhibits CYP1A2 (moderate), 2C9 (weak), 2D6 (weak), 3A4 (weak)

Avoid Concomitant Use

Avoid concomitant use of NIFEdipine with any of the following: Grapefruit Juice

Increased Effect/Toxicity

NIFEdipine may increase the levels/effects of: Amifostine; Antihypertensives; CYP1A2 Substrates; Hypotensive Agents; Magnesium Salts; Neuromuscular-Blocking Agents (Nondepolarizing); Nitroprusside; Phenytoin; RiTUXimab; Tacrolimus; VinCRIStine

The levels/effects of NIFEdipine may be increased by: Alcohol (Ethyl); Alpha1-Blockers; Antifungal Agents (Azole Derivatives, Systemic); Calcium Channel Blockers (Nondihydropyridine); Cimetidine; Cisapride; CycloSPORINE; CYP3A4 Inhibitors (Moderate); CYP3A4 Inhibitors (Strong); Dasatinib; Diazoxide; Fluconazole; Grapefruit Juice; Herbs (Hypotensive Properties); Macrolide Antibiotics; Magnesium Salts; MAO Inhibitors; Pentoxifylline; Phosphodiesterase 5 Inhibitors; Prostacyclin Analogues; Protease Inhibitors; Quinupristin

Decreased Effect

NIFEdipine may decrease the levels/effects of: Clopidogrel; QuiNIDine

The levels/effects of NIFEdipine may be decreased by: Barbiturates; Calcium Salts; CarBAMazepine; CYP3A4 Inducers (Strong); Deferasirox; Herbs (CYP3A4 Inducers); Herbs (Hypertensive Properties); Methylphenidate; Nafcillin; Peginterferon Alfa-2b; Rifamycin Derivatives; Yohimbine

Ethanol/Nutrition/Herb Interactions

Ethanol: Avoid ethanol (may increase CNS depression and may increase the effects of nifedipine). Monitor.

Food: Nifedipine serum levels may be decreased if taken with food. Food may decrease the rate but not the extent of absorption of Procardia XL®. Increased therapeutic and vasodilator side effects, including severe hypotension and myocardial ischemia, may occur if nifedipine is taken by patients ingesting grapefruit.

Herb/Nutraceutical: St John's wort may decrease nifedipine levels. Avoid bayberry, blue cohosh, cayenne, ephedra, ginger, ginseng (American), kola, licorice (may worsen hypertension). Avoid black cohosh, California poppy, coleus, golden seal, hawthorn, mistletoe, periwinkle, quinine, shepherd's purse (may have increased antihypertensive effect).

Dietary Considerations Avoid grapefruit juice with all products.

Immediate release: Capsule is rapidly absorbed orally if it is administered without food, but may result in vasodilator side effects; if flushing is problematic, administration with low-fat meals may decrease. In general, can take with or without food.

Extended release: Adalat® CC, Afeditab® CR, Nifediac CC®: Take on an empty stomach (manufacturer recommendation). Other extended release products may not have this recommendation; consult product labeling.

Dosage Forms Excipient information presented when available (limited, particularly for generics); consult specific product labeling.

Capsule, softgel: 10 mg, 20 mg
    Procardia®: 10 mg
Tablet, extended release: 30 mg, 60 mg, 90 mg
    Adalat® CC, Procardia XL®: 30 mg, 60 mg, 90 mg
    Afeditab® CR, Nifedical XL®: 30 mg, 60 mg
    Nifediac CC®: 30 mg, 60 mg, 90 mg [90 mg tablet contains tartrazine]

◆ **Nifedipine PA (Can)** *see* NIFEdipine *on page 1006*

◆ **Nilstat (Can)** *see* Nystatin *on page 1032*

◆ **Nimbex®** *see* Cisatracurium *on page 314*

NiMODipine (nye MOE di peen)

Medication Safety Issues

Sound-alike/look-alike issues:

NiMODipine may be confused with niCARdipine, NIFEdipine, nisoldipine

Administration issues: **For oral administration only.** For patients unable to swallow a capsule, the drug should be dispensed in an oral syringe labeled **"for oral use only."** Nimodipine has inadvertently been administered I.V. when withdrawn from capsules into a syringe for subsequent nasogastric administration. Severe cardiovascular adverse events, including fatalities, have resulted. Employ precautions against such an event.

Related Information

Calcium Channel Blockers *on page 1672*

U.S. Brand Names Nimotop® [DSC]

Canadian Brand Names Nimotop®

Pharmacologic Category Calcium Channel Blocker; Calcium Channel Blocker, Dihydropyridine

Generic Available Yes

Use Vasospasm following subarachnoid hemorrhage from ruptured intracranial aneurysms

Unlabeled/Investigational Use Prevention of migraines (inconsistent data)

Mechanism of Action Nimodipine shares the pharmacology of other calcium channel blockers; animal studies indicate that nimodipine has a greater effect on cerebral arterials than other arterials; this increased specificity may be due to the drug's increased lipophilicity and cerebral distribution as compared to nifedipine; inhibits calcium ion from entering the "slow channels" or select voltage sensitive areas of vascular smooth muscle and myocardium during depolarization

Pharmacodynamics/Kinetics

Protein binding: >95%

Metabolism: Extensively hepatic

Bioavailability: 13%

Half-life elimination: 1-2 hours; prolonged with renal impairment

Time to peak, serum: ~1 hour

Excretion: Urine (50%) and feces (32%) within 4 days

Dosage Note: Capsules and contents are for oral administration **ONLY.**

Adults: Oral: 60 mg every 4 hours for 21 days, start therapy within 96 hours after subarachnoid hemorrhage.

Dialysis: Not removed by hemo- or peritoneal dialysis; supplemental dose is not necessary.

Dosing adjustment in hepatic impairment: Reduce dosage to 30 mg every 4 hours in patients with liver failure.

Administration For oral administration **ONLY.** If the capsules cannot be swallowed, the liquid may be removed by making a hole in each end of the capsule with an 18-gauge needle and extracting the contents into a syringe. If administered via NG tube, follow with a flush of 30 mL NS.

Anesthesia and Critical Care Concerns/Other Considerations

Clinical Pearls/Comments: Studies suggest nimodipine has preferential action on cerebral arterioles, possibly due to its lipophilicity which may increase cerebral distribution.

Pregnancy Risk Factor C

Contraindications Hypersensitivity to nimodipine or any component of the formulation

Warnings/Precautions Increased angina and/or MI has occurred with initiation or dosage titration of calcium channel blockers. The most common side effect is peripheral edema; occurs within 2-3 weeks of starting therapy. Reflex tachycardia may occur with use. Symptomatic hypotension with or without syncope can rarely occur; blood pressure must be lowered at a rate appropriate for the patient's clinical condition. Use caution in hepatic impairment. Intestinal pseudo-obstruction and ileus have been reported during the use of nimodipine. Use caution in patients with decreased GI motility of a history of bowel obstruction. Use caution when treating patients with hypertrophic cardiomyopathy. Safety and efficacy have not been established in children.

[U.S. Boxed Warning]: Nimodipine has inadvertently been administered I.V. when withdrawn from capsules into a syringe for subsequent nasogastric administration. Severe cardiovascular adverse events, including fatalities, have resulted; precautions should be employed against such an event.

Adverse Reactions
1% to 10%:
Cardiovascular: Reductions in systemic blood pressure (1% to 8%)
Central nervous system: Headache (1% to 4%)
Dermatologic: Rash (1% to 2%)
Gastrointestinal: Diarrhea (2% to 4%), abdominal discomfort (2%)
<1% (Limited to important or life-threatening): Anemia, CHF, deep vein thrombosis, depression, disseminated intravascular coagulation, dyspnea, ECG abnormalities, GI hemorrhage, hemorrhage, hepatitis, jaundice, neurological deterioration, rebound vasospasm, thrombocytopenia, vomiting

Drug Interactions
Metabolism/Transport Effects Substrate of CYP3A4 (major)
Avoid Concomitant Use
Avoid concomitant use of NiMODipine with any of the following: Grapefruit Juice
Increased Effect/Toxicity
NiMODipine may increase the levels/effects of: Amifostine; Antihypertensives; Hypotensive Agents; Magnesium Salts; Neuromuscular-Blocking Agents (Non-depolarizing); Nitroprusside; Phenytoin; RiTUXimab; Tacrolimus

The levels/effects of NiMODipine may be increased by: Alpha1-Blockers; Antifungal Agents (Azole Derivatives, Systemic); Calcium Channel Blockers (Nondihydropyridine); Cimetidine; CycloSPORINE; CYP3A4 Inhibitors (Moderate); CYP3A4 Inhibitors (Strong); Dasatinib; Diazoxide; Fluconazole; Grapefruit Juice; Herbs (Hypotensive Properties); Macrolide Antibiotics; Magnesium Salts; MAO Inhibitors; Pentoxifylline; Phosphodiesterase 5 Inhibitors; Prostacyclin Analogues; Protease Inhibitors; Quinupristin

Decreased Effect
NiMODipine may decrease the levels/effects of: Clopidogrel; QuiNIDine

The levels/effects of NiMODipine may be decreased by: Barbiturates; Calcium Salts; CarBAMazepine; CYP3A4 Inducers (Strong); Deferasirox; Herbs (CYP3A4 Inducers); Herbs (Hypertensive Properties); Methylphenidate; Nafcillin; Rifamycin Derivatives; Yohimbine

Ethanol/Nutrition/Herb Interactions
Food: Nimodipine has shown a 1.5-fold increase in bioavailability when taken with grapefruit juice; avoid concurrent use.
Herb/Nutraceutical: St John's wort may decrease levels. Avoid dong quai if using for hypertension (has estrogenic activity). Avoid ephedra, yohimbe, ginseng (may worsen hypertension). Avoid garlic (may have increased antihypertensive effect).

Dosage Forms Excipient information presented when available (limited, particularly for generics); consult specific product labeling. [DSC] = Discontinued product
Capsule, liquid filled: 30 mg
Nimotop®: 30 mg [DSC]

◆ **Nimotop® [DSC]** *see* NiMODipine *on page 1009*

◆ **Nimotop® (Can)** *see* NiMODipine *on page 1009*

◆ **Niravam™** *see* ALPRAZolam *on page 64*

Nisoldipine (nye SOL di peen)

Related Information
Calcium Channel Blockers *on page 1672*
U.S. Brand Names Sular®
Pharmacologic Category Calcium Channel Blocker; Calcium Channel Blocker, Dihydropyridine
Use Management of hypertension, alone or in combination with other antihypertensive agents
Pharmacodynamics/Kinetics
Duration: >24 hours
Absorption: Well absorbed. Peak concentrations significantly increased with high-lipid meals; however, AUC is reduced.
Protein binding: >99%

Metabolism: Extensively hepatic; 1 active metabolite (10% of activity of parent); first-pass effect

Bioavailability: ~5%

Half-life elimination: 9-18 hours

Time to peak: 4-14 hours

Excretion: Urine (60% to 80% as inactive metabolites); feces

Dosage Oral:

Sular® (Geomatrix® delivery system):

Adults: Initial: 17 mg once daily, then increase by 8.5 mg/week (or longer intervals) to attain adequate control of blood pressure

Usual dose range: 17-34 mg once daily; doses >34 mg once daily are not recommended

Elderly: Initial dose: 8.5 mg once daily, increase by 8.5 mg/week (or longer intervals) to attain adequate blood pressure control

Nisoldipine extended-release tablet (original formulation):

Adults: Oral: Initial: 20 mg once daily, then increase by 10 mg/week (or longer intervals) to attain adequate control of blood pressure

Usual dose range (JNC 7): 10-40 mg once daily; doses >60 mg once daily are not recommended

Elderly: Initial dose: 10 mg once daily, increase by 10 mg/week (or longer intervals) to attain adequate blood pressure control

Conversion from nisoldipine extended-release (original formulation) to Sular® Geomatrix® delivery system:

Nisoldipine Extended Release Dosing Equivalency

Original Extended Release Formulation	Sular® Extended Release (Geomatrix® delivery system)
10 mg	8.5 mg
20 mg	17 mg
30 mg	25.5 mg
40 mg	34 mg

Dosage adjustment in hepatic impairment:

Sular® (Geomatrix® delivery system): An initial dose exceeding 8.5 mg once daily is not recommended for patients with hepatic impairment.

Nisoldipine extended-release (original formulation): An initial dose exceeding 10 mg once daily is not recommended for patients with hepatic impairment.

Additional Information Complete prescribing information for this medication should be consulted for additional detail.

Dosage Forms Excipient information presented when available (limited, particularly for generics); consult specific product labeling.

Tablet, extended release [original formulation]: 20 mg, 30 mg, 40 mg

Sular®: 10 mg, 20 mg, 30 mg 40 mg [DSC]

Tablet, extended release [Geomatrix® delivery system]:

Sular®: 8.5 mg; 17 mg [contains tartrazine]; 25.5 mg, 34 mg

References

Braunwald E, Antman EM, Beasley JW, et al, "ACC/AHA Guidelines for the Management of Patients With Unstable Angina and Non-ST-Segment Elevation Myocardial Infarction. A Report of the American College of Cardiology/American Heart Association Task Force on Practice Guidelines (Committee on the Management of Patients With Unstable Angina)," *J Am Coll Cardiol*, 2000, 36 (3):970-1062.

Chobanian AV, Bakris GL, Black HR, et al, "The Seventh Report of the Joint National Committee on Prevention, Detection, Evaluation, and Treatment of High Blood Pressure: The JNC 7 Report," *JAMA*, 2003, 289(19):2560-71.

Estacio RO, Jeffers BW, Hiatt WR, et al, "The Effect of Nisoldipine as Compared With Enalapril on Cardiovascular Outcomes in Patients With Noninsulin-Dependent Diabetes and Hypertension," *N Engl J Med*, 1998, 338(10):645-52.

Nitric Oxide (NYE trik OKS ide)

Related Information

Anesthesia for Geriatric Patients *on page 1523*

Postoperative Hypertension *on page 1589*

U.S. Brand Names INOmax®

Canadian Brand Names INOmax®
Pharmacologic Category Vasodilator, Pulmonary
Generic Available No

Use Treatment of term and near-term (>34 weeks) neonates with hypoxic respiratory failure associated with pulmonary hypertension; used concurrently with ventilatory support and other agents

Unlabeled/Investigational Use Treatment of adult respiratory distress syndrome (ARDS); acute vasodilator testing in pulmonary artery hypertension (PAH)

Mechanism of Action In neonates with persistent pulmonary hypertension, nitric oxide improves oxygenation. Nitric oxide relaxes vascular smooth muscle by binding to the heme moiety of cytosolic guanylate cyclase, activating guanylate cyclase and increasing intracellular levels of cyclic guanosine 3',5'-monophosphate, which leads to vasodilation. When inhaled, pulmonary vasodilation occurs and an increase in the partial pressure of arterial oxygen results. Dilation of pulmonary vessels in well ventilated lung areas redistributes blood flow away from lung areas where ventilation/perfusion ratios are poor.

Pharmacodynamics/Kinetics

Absorption: Systemic after inhalation

Metabolism: Nitric oxide combines with hemoglobin that is 60% to 100% oxygenated. Nitric oxide combines with oxyhemoglobin to produce methemoglobin and nitrate. Within the pulmonary system, nitric oxide can combine with oxygen and water to produce nitrogen dioxide and nitrite respectively, which interact with oxyhemoglobin to then produce methemoglobin and nitrate. At 80 ppm the methemoglobin percent is ~5% after 8 hours of administration. Methemoglobin levels >7% were attained only in patients receiving 80 ppm.

Excretion: Urine (as nitrate)

Clearance: Nitrate: At a rate approaching the glomerular filtration rate

Dosage Inhalation:

Neonates (up to 14 days old): Hypoxic respiratory failure associated with pulmonary hypertension: 20 ppm. Treatment should be maintained up to 14 days or until the underlying oxygen desaturation has resolved and the neonate is ready to be weaned from therapy. In the CINRGI trial, patients whose oxygenation improved had their dose reduced to 5 ppm at the end of 4 hours of treatment. Doses above 20 ppm should not be used because of the risk of methemoglobinemia and elevated NO_2.

Adults: Acute vasodilator testing in pulmonary artery hypertension (unlabeled use; McLaughlin, 2009): 10-80 ppm for 5 minutes; commonly used doses: 20-40 ppm. **Note:** Measure hemodynamics while on nitric oxide.

Stability Store at 25°C (77°F).

Administration In the ventilated neonate, precise monitoring of inspired nitric oxide and NO_2 should be instituted using a calibrated analysis device with alarms. Sample gas for analysis should be drawn before the Y-piece, proximal to the patient. In addition, oxygen levels should be measured. A backup delivery system should be available in the event of power failure. Do not discontinue abruptly.

Monitoring Parameters Respiratory status including arterial blood gases with close attention to PaO_2, methemoglobin, NO_2, vital signs, blood sugar, signs and symptoms of infection.

Pregnancy Risk Factor C

Contraindications Hypersensitivity to nitric oxide or any component of the formulation; neonates dependent on right-to-left shunting of blood

Warnings/Precautions Use in patients with left ventricular dysfunction may increase pulmonary capillary wedge pressure and cause pulmonary edema. Abrupt discontinuation may lead to worsening hypotension, oxygenation, and increasing pulmonary artery pressure (PAP). Worsening oxygenation and increasing PAP may occur in patients who do not respond. Doses above 20 ppm should not be used because of the increased risk of methemoglobinemia and elevated nitrogen dioxide (NO_2) levels. Methemoglobin levels and NO_2 should be monitored.

Pulmonary artery hypertension (PAH): Acute vasodilator testing (not an approved use): Use with extreme caution in patients with concomitant heart failure (LV systolic dysfunction with significantly elevated left heart filling pressures) or pulmonary veno-occlusive disease/pulmonary capillary hemangiomatosis; significant decompensation has occurred resulting in acute pulmonary edema.

Adverse Reactions

>10%:

Cardiovascular: Hypotension (13%)

Miscellaneous: Withdrawal syndrome (12%)

1% to 10%:

Dermatologic: Cellulitis (5%)

Endocrine & metabolic: Hyperglycemia (8%)

Genitourinary: Hematuria (8%)

Respiratory: Atelectasis (9% - same as placebo), stridor (5%)

Miscellaneous: Sepsis (7%), infection (6%)

Postmarketing and/or case reports: Headache (environmental exposure, eg, hospital staff); hypoxemia; pulmonary edema

Drug Interactions

Avoid Concomitant Use There are no known interactions where it is recommended to avoid concomitant use.

Increased Effect/Toxicity There are no known significant interactions involving an increase in effect.

Decreased Effect There are no known significant interactions involving a decrease in effect.

Dosage Forms Excipient information presented when available (limited, particularly for generics); consult specific product labeling.

Gas, for inhalation:

100 ppm [nitric oxide 0.01% and nitrogen 99.99%] (353 L) [delivers 344 L], (1963 L) [delivers 1918 L]

800 ppm [nitric oxide 0.08% and nitrogen 99.92%] (353 L) [delivers 344 L], (1963 L) [delivers 1918 L]

References

Davidson D, Barefield ES, Kattwinkel J, et al, "Inhaled Nitric Oxide for the Early Treatment of Persistent Pulmonary Hypertension of the Term Newborn: A Randomized, Double-Masked, Placebo-Controlled, Dose-Response, Multicenter Study: I-NO/PPHN Study Group," *Pediatrics*, 1998, 101(3 Pt 1):325-34.

"Inhaled Nitric Oxide in Full-Term and Nearly Full-Term Infants With Hypoxic Respiratory Failure, The Neonatal Inhaled Nitric Oxide Study Group," *N Engl J Med*, 1997, 336(9):597-604.

◆ **Nitro-Bid®** *see* Nitroglycerin *on page* 1014

◆ **Nitro-Dur®** *see* Nitroglycerin *on page* 1014

Nitroglycerin (nye troe GLI ser in)

Medication Safety Issues

Sound-alike/look-alike issues:

Nitroglycerin may be confused with nitrofurantoin, nitroprusside

Nitro-Bid® may be confused with Macrobid®, Nicobid®

Nitroderm may be confused with NicoDerm®

Nitrol® may be confused with Nizoral®

Nitrostat® may be confused with Nilstat®, nystatin

Nitroglycerin transdermal patches should be removed prior to defibrillation or MRI study.

International issues:

Nitrocor® [Chile and Italy] may be confused with Natrecor® which is a brand name for nesiritide in the U.S.

Nitrocor® [Chile and Italy] may be confused with Nutracort® which is a brand name for hydrocortisone in the U.S.

Nitro-Dur® may be confused with Nitrocor® [Chile and Italy]

Related Information

U.S. Brand Names Minitran™; Nitro-Bid®; Nitro-Dur®; Nitro-Time®; Nitrolingual®; NitroQuick® [DSC]; Nitrostat®

Canadian Brand Names Gen-Nitro; Minitran™; Mylan-Nitro Sublingual Spray; Nitro-Dur®; Nitroglycerin Injection, USP; Nitrol®; Nitrostat™; Rho®-Nitro; Transderm-Nitro®; Trinipatch® 0.2; Trinipatch® 0.4; Trinipatch® 0.6

Index Terms Glyceryl Trinitrate; Nitroglycerol; NTG; Tridil

Pharmacologic Category Vasodilator

Generic Available Yes: Capsule, injection, patch, tablet

Use Treatment of angina pectoris; I.V. for congestive heart failure (especially when associated with acute myocardial infarction); pulmonary hypertension; perioperative hypertension (especially during cardiovascular surgery); induction of intraoperative hypotension

Unlabeled/Investigational Use Esophageal spastic disorders (sublingual)

Mechanism of Action Works by relaxation of smooth muscle, producing a vasodilator effect on the peripheral veins and arteries with more prominent effects on the veins. Primarily reduces cardiac oxygen demand by decreasing preload (left ventricular end-diastolic pressure); may modestly reduce afterload; dilates coronary arteries and improves collateral flow to ischemic regions

Pharmacodynamics/Kinetics

Onset of action: Sublingual tablet: 1-3 minutes; Translingual spray: 2 minutes; Sustained release: 20-45 minutes; Topical: 15-60 minutes; Transdermal: 40-60 minutes; I.V. drip: Immediate

Peak effect: Sublingual tablet: 4-8 minutes; Translingual spray: 4-10 minutes; Sustained release: 45-120 minutes; Topical: 30-120 minutes; Transdermal: 60-180 minutes; I.V. drip: Immediate

Duration: Sublingual tablet: 30-60 minutes; Translingual spray: 30-60 minutes; Sustained release: 4-8 hours; Topical: 2-12 hours; Transdermal: 18-24 hours; I.V. drip: 3-5 minutes

Protein binding: 60%

Metabolism: Extensive first-pass effect

Half-life elimination: 1-4 minutes

Excretion: Urine (as inactive metabolites)

Dosage Note: Hemodynamic and antianginal tolerance often develop within 24-48 hours of continuous nitrate administration. Nitrate-free interval (10-12 hours/day) is recommended to avoid tolerance development; gradually decrease dose in patients receiving NTG for prolonged period to avoid withdrawal reaction.

Children: Pulmonary hypertension: Continuous infusion: Start 0.25-0.5 mcg/kg/minute and titrate by 1 mcg/kg/minute at 20- to 60-minute intervals to desired effect; usual dose: 1-3 mcg/kg/minute; maximum: 5 mcg/kg/minute

Adults:

Oral: 2.5-9 mg 2-4 times/day (up to 26 mg 4 times/day)

I.V.: 5 mcg/minute, increase by 5 mcg/minute every 3-5 minutes to 20 mcg/minute; if no response at 20 mcg/minute increase by 10 mcg/minute every 3-5 minutes, up to 200 mcg/minute

Ointment: 1/2" upon rising and 1/2" 6 hours later; the dose may be doubled and even doubled again as needed

Patch, transdermal: Initial: 0.2-0.4 mg/hour, titrate to doses of 0.4-0.8 mg/hour; tolerance is minimized by using a patch-on period of 12-14 hours and patch-off period of 10-12 hours

Sublingual: 0.2-0.6 mg every 5 minutes for maximum of 3 doses in 15 minutes; may also use prophylactically 5-10 minutes prior to activities which may provoke an attack

Esophageal spastic disorders (unlabeled use): 0.3-0.4 mg 5 minutes before meals

Translingual: 1-2 sprays into mouth under tongue every 3-5 minutes for maximum of 3 doses in 15 minutes, may also be used 5-10 minutes prior to activities which may provoke an attack prophylactically

Hemodialysis: Supplemental dose is not necessary

Peritoneal dialysis: Supplemental dose is not necessary

Elderly: In general, dose selection should be cautious, usually starting at the low end of the dosing range

Stability Doses should be made in glass bottles, Excell® or PAB® containers. Adsorption occurs to soft plastic (ie, PVC).

Nitroglycerin diluted in D_5W or NS in glass containers is physically and chemically stable for 48 hours at room temperature and 7 days under refrigeration. In D_5W or NS in Excell®/PAB® containers it is physically and chemically stable for 24 hours at room temperature and 14 days under refrigeration.

Premixed bottles are stable according to the manufacturer's expiration dating.

Standard diluent: 50 mg/250 mL D_5W; 50 mg/500 mL D_5W.

Minimum volume: 100 mg/250 mL D_5W; concentration should not exceed 400 mcg/mL.

Store sublingual tablets and ointment in tightly closed containers at 15°C to 30°C. Store spray and transdermal patch at 25°C; excursions permitted to 15°C to 30°C (59°F to 86°F).

Administration

I.V.: I.V. must be prepared in glass bottles; use special sets intended for nitroglycerin. Glass I.V. bottles and administration sets provided by manufacturer.

Sublingual: Do not crush sublingual product (tablet). Place under tongue and allow to dissolve.

Translingual spray: Do not shake container. Release spray onto or under tongue. Do not rinse the mouth for at least 5-10 minutes. Priming sprays should be directed away from patient and others. The end of the pump should be covered by the fluid in the bottle.

Nitrolingual®: Prime prior to first use (5 sprays into the air). If unused for 6 weeks, a single priming spray should be completed.

Monitoring Parameters Blood pressure, heart rate

Anesthesia and Critical Care Concerns/Other Considerations

Clinical Pearls/Comments: In the treatment of unstable angina/non-ST-segment elevation MI, nitroglycerin (sublingual tablet or spray), followed by intravenous administration, is recommended for immediate relief of ischemia and associated symptoms. Note that nitrate use may result in significant hypotension in individuals who are volume depleted.

Nitrate use in right ventricular infarction may induce acute hypotension. Nitrate use in severe pericardial effusion may reduce cardiac filling pressure and precipitate cardiac tamponade.

Pregnancy Risk Factor C

Contraindications Hypersensitivity to organic nitrates; hypersensitivity to isosorbide, nitroglycerin, or any component of the formulation; concurrent use with phosphodiesterase-5 (PDE-5) inhibitors (sildenafil, tadalafil, or vardenafil); angle-closure glaucoma (intraocular pressure may be increased); head trauma or cerebral hemorrhage (increase intracranial pressure); severe anemia; allergy to adhesive (transdermal product)

Additional contraindications for I.V. product: Hypotension; uncorrected hypovolemia; inadequate cerebral circulation; constrictive pericarditis; pericardial tamponade

Warnings/Precautions Severe hypotension can occur. Use with caution in volume depletion, hypotension, and right ventricular infarctions. Paradoxical bradycardia and increased angina pectoris can accompany hypotension. Orthostatic hypotension can also occur. Ethanol can accentuate this. Tolerance does develop to nitrates and appropriate dosing is needed to minimize this (drug-free interval). Avoid use of long-acting agents in acute MI or HF; cannot easily reverse. Nitrate may aggravate angina caused by hypertrophic cardiomyopathy. Nitroglycerin transdermal patches should be removed prior to defibrillation or MRI study. Avoid concurrent use with PDE-5 inhibitors. Safety and efficacy have not been established in children.

Adverse Reactions

Frequency not always defined:

Cardiovascular: Hypotension (4%), crescendo angina (2%), flushing, peripheral edema, postural hypotension, tachycardia

Central nervous system: Headache (most common; 50% to 63%), lightheaded-ness (6%), syncope (4%), dizziness

Gastrointestinal: Bowel incontinence, nausea, vomiting, xerostomia

Genitourinary: Urinary incontinence

Ocular: Blurred vision

Miscellaneous: Diaphoresis

<1% (Limited to important or life-threatening): Allergic reactions, application site irritation (patch), cardiovascular collapse, exfoliative dermatitis, methemoglobi-nemia (rare; overdose), pallor, palpitation, rash, rebound hypertension, rest-lessness, shock, vertigo, weakness

Drug Interactions

Avoid Concomitant Use

Avoid concomitant use of Nitroglycerin with any of the following: Phosphodies-terase 5 Inhibitors

Increased Effect/Toxicity

Nitroglycerin may increase the levels/effects of: Hypotensive Agents; Rosiglitazone

The levels/effects of Nitroglycerin may be increased by: Phosphodiesterase 5 Inhibitors

Decreased Effect

Nitroglycerin may decrease the levels/effects of: Alteplase; Heparin

Ethanol/Nutrition/Herb Interactions

Ethanol: Avoid ethanol (may increase the hypotensive effects of nitroglycerin). Monitor.

Herb/Nutraceutical: Avoid bayberry, blue cohosh, cayenne, ephedra, ginger, ginseng (american), kola, licorice (may worsen hypertension). Avoid black cohosh, California poppy, coleus, golden seal, hawthorn, mistletoe, periwinkle, quinine, shepherd's purse (may cause hypotension).

Dosage Forms Excipient information presented when available (limited, particularly for generics); consult specific product labeling. [DSC] = Discontinued product

Capsule, extended release: 2.5 mg, 6.5 mg, 9 mg

Nitro-Time®: 2.5 mg, 6.5 mg, 9 mg

Infusion [premixed in D_5W]: 25 mg (250 mL) [0.1 mg/mL]; 50 mg (250 mL) [0.2 mg/mL]; 50 mg (500 mL) [0.1 mg/mL]; 100 mg (250 mL) [0.4 mg/mL]; 200 mg (500 mL) [0.4 mg/mL]

Injection, solution: 5 mg/mL (5 mL, 10 mL) [contains ethanol and propylene glycol]

Ointment, topical:

Nitro-Bid®: 2% [20 mg/g] (1 g, 30 g, 60 g)

Solution, translingual [spray]:

Nitrolingual®: 0.4 mg/metered spray (4.9 g) [contains ethanol 20%; 60 metered sprays]; (12 g) [contains ethanol 20%; 200 metered sprays]; (16.9 g) [contains ethanol 20%; 260 metered sprays]

Tablet, sublingual: 0.3 mg, 0.4 mg, 0.6 mg

NitroQuick® [DSC], Nitrostat®: 0.3 mg, 0.4 mg, 0.6 mg

Transdermal system [once-daily patch]: 0.1 mg/hour (30s); 0.2 mg/hour (30s); 0.4 mg/hour (30s); 0.6 mg/hour (30s)

Minitran™: 0.1 mg/hour (30s); 0.2 mg/hour (30s); 0.4 mg/hour (30s); 0.6 mg/hour (30s)

Nitro-Dur®: 0.1 mg/hour (30s); 0.2 mg/hour (30s); 0.3 mg/hour (30s); 0.4 mg/hour (30s); 0.6 mg/hour (30s); 0.8 mg/hour (30s)

References

Antman EM, Anbe SC, Alpert JS, et al, "ACC/AHA Guidelines for the Management of Patients With ST-Elevation Myocardial Infarction - Executive Summary: A Report of the American College of Cardiology/American Heart Association Task Force on Practice Guidelines (Writing Committee to Revise the 1999 Guidelines for the Management of Patients With Acute Myocardial Infarction)," *Circulation*, 2004, 110(5):588-636. Available at: http://www.circulationaha.org/cgi/content/full/110/5/588. Last accessed October 26, 2004.

◀ Erstad BL and Barletta JF, "Treatment of Hypertension in the Perioperative Patient," *Ann. Pharmacother*, 2000, 34(1):66-79.

♦ **Nitroglycerin Injection, USP (Can)** *see* Nitroglycerin *on page 1014*

♦ **Nitroglycerol** *see* Nitroglycerin *on page 1014*

♦ **Nitrol® (Can)** *see* Nitroglycerin *on page 1014*

♦ **Nitrolingual®** *see* Nitroglycerin *on page 1014*

♦ **Nitropress®** *see* Nitroprusside *on page 1018*

Nitroprusside (nye troe PRUS ide)

Medication Safety Issues
Sound-alike/look-alike issues:
  Nitroprusside may be confused with nitroglycerin

High alert medication: The Institute for Safe Medication Practices (ISMP) includes this medication among its list of drugs which have a heightened risk of causing significant patient harm when used in error.

Related Information
Anesthesia Considerations for Neurosurgery *on page 1514*
Chronic Renal Failure *on page 1552*
Hemodynamic Support, Intravenous *on page 1681*
Hypertension *on page 1754*
Postoperative Hypertension *on page 1589*

U.S. Brand Names Nitropress®

Index Terms Nitroprusside Sodium; Sodium Nitroferricyanide; Sodium Nitroprusside

Pharmacologic Category Vasodilator

Generic Available Yes

Use Management of hypertensive crises; acute decompensated heart failure (HF); used for controlled hypotension to reduce bleeding during surgery

Mechanism of Action Causes peripheral vasodilation by direct action on venous and arteriolar smooth muscle, thus reducing peripheral resistance; will increase cardiac output by decreasing afterload; reduces aortal and left ventricular impedance

Pharmacodynamics/Kinetics
Onset of action: BP reduction <2 minutes
Duration: 1-10 minutes
Metabolism: Nitroprusside is converted to cyanide ions in the bloodstream; decomposes to prussic acid which in the presence of sulfur donor is converted to thiocyanate (hepatic and renal rhodanase systems)
Half-life elimination: Parent drug: <10 minutes; Thiocyanate: 2.7-7 days
Excretion: Urine (as thiocyanate)

Dosage Administration requires the use of an infusion pump. Average dose: 5 mcg/kg/minute.

Children: Pulmonary hypertension: I.V.: Initial: 1 mcg/kg/minute by continuous I.V. infusion; increase in increments of 1 mcg/kg/minute at intervals of 20-60 minutes; titrating to the desired response; usual dose: 3 mcg/kg/minute, rarely need >4 mcg/kg/minute; maximum: 5 mcg/kg/minute.

Adults: I.V. Initial: 0.3-0.5 mcg/kg/minute; increase in increments of 0.5 mcg/kg/minute, titrating to the desired hemodynamic effect or the appearance of headache or nausea; usual dose: 3 mcg/kg/minute; rarely need >4 mcg/kg/minute; maximum: 10 mcg/kg/minute. When administered by prolonged infusion faster than 2 mcg/kg/minute, cyanide is generated faster than an unaided patient can handle.

Stability
Nitroprusside sodium should be reconstituted freshly by diluting 50 mg in 250-1000 mL of D_5W.

Use only clear solutions; solutions of nitroprusside exhibit a color described as brownish, brown, brownish-pink, light orange, and straw. Solutions are highly sensitive to light. Exposure to light causes decomposition, resulting in a highly colored solution of orange, dark brown or blue. **A blue color indicates almost complete degradation and breakdown to cyanide.**

Solutions should be wrapped with aluminum foil or other opaque material to protect from light (do as soon as possible).

Stability of parenteral admixture at room temperature (25°C) and at refrigeration temperature (4°C) is 24 hours.

Administration I.V. infusion only, not for direct injection

Monitoring Parameters Blood pressure, heart rate; monitor for cyanide and thiocyanate toxicity; monitor acid-base status as acidosis can be the earliest sign of cyanide toxicity; monitor thiocyanate levels if requiring prolonged infusion (>3 days) or dose ≥4 mcg/kg/minute or patient has renal dysfunction; monitor cyanide blood levels in patients with decreased hepatic function; cardiac monitor and blood pressure monitor required

Reference Range Serum thiocyanate levels are not helpful in detecting toxicity. A level may be confirmatory if a patient is exhibiting signs and symptoms of thiocyanate toxicity. Initial signs of toxicity (eg, tinnitus) may be observed at levels >35 mcg/mL (manufacturer suggests 60 mcg/mL), but serious toxicity typically may not occur with levels <100 mcg/mL.

Anesthesia and Critical Care Concerns/Other Considerations

Clinical Pearls/Comments: Elderly patients may have an increased sensitivity to nitroprusside possibly due to a decreased baroreceptor reflex, altered sensitivity to vasodilating effects or a resistance of cardiac adrenergic receptors to stimulation by catecholamines.

Thiocyanate levels should be monitored if high doses are used for more than 24 hours. Nitroprusside may also be useful for afterload reduction in patients with severe heart failure. Nitroprusside should be avoided in patients with aortic stenosis or coarctation. Nitroprusside should also be used cautiously in patients with acute myocardial infarction, because of hemodynamic effects and possible coronary steal.

Blood Pressure Management of Intracerebral Hemorrhage (ICH): In addition to standard management of ICH, blood pressure (BP) management while maintaining cerebral perfusion pressure in patients who are hypertensive is also of paramount importance when treating ICH. The primary rationale for lowering BP is to prevent further progression of the bleed. This can be accomplished using a number of different pharmacologic treatments (eg, nicardipine, labetalol, nitroprusside). Nitroprusside may increase ICP due to the pronounced vasodilatory actions and therefore may be less preferable. Specific BP targets are not supported by available evidence. The 2007 AHA/ASA guidelines for the management of spontaneous intracerebral hemorrhage in adults recommend initiating antihypertensive therapy if the SBP >180 mm Hg or if MAP >130 mm Hg (Broderick, 2007).

Pregnancy Risk Factor C

Contraindications Hypersensitivity to nitroprusside or any component of the formulation; treatment of compensatory hypertension (aortic coarctation, arteriovenous shunting); high output failure; congenital optic atrophy or tobacco amblyopia

Warnings/Precautions **[U.S. Boxed Warning]: Continuous blood pressure monitoring is needed. Except when used briefly or at low (<2 mcg/kg/minute) infusion rates, nitroprusside gives rise to large cyanide quantities. Do not use the maximum dose for more than 10 minutes; if blood pressure not controlled then discontinue infusion. Monitor for cyanide toxicity via acid-base balance and venous oxygen concentration.** Use with extreme caution in patients with elevated intracranial pressure (head trauma, cerebral hemorrhage), severe renal impairment, hepatic failure, hypothyroidism. Use the lowest end of the dosage range with renal impairment. Cyanide toxicity may occur in patients with decreased liver function. Thiocyanate toxicity occurs in patients with renal impairment or those on prolonged infusions. **[U.S. Boxed Warning]: Should not be administered by direct injection; must be further diluted with 5% dextrose in water.**

Adverse Reactions Frequency not defined.

Cardiovascular: Excessive hypotensive response, palpitation, substernal distress

Central nervous system: Disorientation, psychosis, headache, restlessness

Endocrine & metabolic: Thyroid suppression (due to thiocyanate)

Gastrointestinal: Nausea, vomiting

◀ Neuromuscular & skeletal: Hyperreflexia (thiocyanate toxicity), muscle spasm, weakness
Ocular: Miosis (thiocyanate toxicity)
Otic: Tinnitus (thiocyanate toxicity)
Respiratory: Hypoxia
Miscellaneous: Diaphoresis

Drug Interactions

Avoid Concomitant Use There are no known interactions where it is recommended to avoid concomitant use.

Increased Effect/Toxicity

Nitroprusside may increase the levels/effects of: Amifostine; Antihypertensives; Hypotensive Agents; RiTUXimab

The levels/effects of Nitroprusside may be increased by: Calcium Channel Blockers; Diazoxide; Herbs (Hypotensive Properties); MAO Inhibitors; Pentoxifylline; Phosphodiesterase 5 Inhibitors; Prostacyclin Analogues

Decreased Effect

The levels/effects of Nitroprusside may be decreased by: Herbs (Hypertensive Properties); Methylphenidate; Yohimbine

Dosage Forms Excipient information presented when available (limited, particularly for generics); consult specific product labeling.
Injection, solution, as sodium: 25 mg/mL (2 mL)

References

Broderick J, Connolly S, Feldmann E, et al, "Guidelines for the Management of Spontaneous Intracerebral Hemorrhage in Adults: 2007 Update: A Guideline From the American Heart Association/American Stroke Association Stroke Council, High Blood Pressure Research Council, and the Quality of Care and Outcomes in Research Interdisciplinary Working Group," *Stroke*, 2007, 38(6):2001-23. Available at http://stroke.ahajournals.org/cgi/content/short/STROKEAHA.107.183689.

Erstad BL and Barletta JF, "Treatment of Hypertension in the Perioperative Patient," *Ann Pharmacother*, 2000, 34(1):66-79.

Hunt SA, Abraham WT, Chin MH, et al, "ACC/AHA 2005 Guideline Update for the Diagnosis and Management of Chronic Heart Failure in the Adult: A Report of the American College of Cardiology/American Heart Association Task Force on Practice Guidelines (Writing Committee to Update the 2001 Guidelines for the Evaluation and Management of Heart Failure)," available at http://www.acc.org/qualityandscience/clinical/guidelines/failure/update/index.pdf.

♦ **Nitroprusside Sodium** *see* Nitroprusside *on page 1018*

♦ **NitroQuick® [DSC]** *see* Nitroglycerin *on page 1014*

♦ **Nitrostat®** *see* Nitroglycerin *on page 1014*

♦ **Nitrostat™ (Can)** *see* Nitroglycerin *on page 1014*

♦ **Nitro-Time®** *see* Nitroglycerin *on page 1014*

Nitrous Oxide (NYE trus OKS ide)

Medication Safety Issues

High alert medication: The Institute for Safe Medication Practices (ISMP) includes this medication among its list of drug classes which have a heightened risk of causing significant patient harm when used in error.

Related Information

Anesthesia Considerations for Neurosurgery *on page 1514*
Anesthesia for Obstetric Patients in Nonobstetric Surgery *on page 1532*
Inhalational Anesthetics *on page 1632*
Moderate Sedation *on page 1566*
Postoperative Nausea and Vomiting *on page 1593*

Pharmacologic Category Dental Gases; General Anesthetic

Generic Available Yes

Use Sedation, analgesia, and amnesia; principal adjunct to inhalation and intravenous general anesthesia

Mechanism of Action General CNS depressant action; may act similarly as inhalant general anesthetics by stabilizing axonal membranes to partially inhibit action potentials leading to sedation; may partially act on opiate receptor systems to cause mild analgesia; central sympathetic stimulating action supports blood pressure, systemic vascular resistance, and cardiac output; it does not depress carbon dioxide drive to breath. Nitrous oxide increases cerebral blood flow and intracranial pressure while decreasing hepatic and renal blood flow; has analgesic action similar to morphine.

Pharmacodynamics/Kinetics

Onset of action: Inhalation: 2-5 minutes

Absorption: Rapid via lungs; blood/gas partition coefficient is 0.47

Metabolism: Body: <0.004%

Excretion: Primarily exhaled gases; skin (minimal amounts)

Dosage Children and Adults:

Surgical: For sedation and analgesia: Concentrations of 25% to 50% nitrous oxide with oxygen. For general anesthesia, concentrations of 40% to 70% via mask or endotracheal tube. Minimal alveolar concentration (MAC), which can be considered the ED_{50} of inhalational anesthetics, is 105%; therefore delivery in a hyperbaric chamber is necessary to use as a complete anesthetic. When administered at 70%, reduces the MAC of other anesthetics by half.

Dental: For sedation and analgesia: Concentrations of 25% to 50% nitrous oxide with oxygen

Anesthesia and Critical Care Concerns/Other Considerations

Evidence-Based Information: Nitrous oxide's central sympathetic stimulating action supports blood pressure, systemic vascular resistance, and cardiac output. It does not depress carbon dioxide drive to breathe. It increases cerebral blood flow and intracranial pressure while decreasing hepatic and renal blood flow. Nitrous oxide has analgesic action similar to morphine. It causes minimal skeletal muscle relaxation. Because of nitrous oxide's capacity to diffuse into air-containing spaces (based on concentration and blood flow), there is a relative contraindication to its use in pneumothorax, pneumocephalus, middle ear surgery, or bowel obstruction.

Pregnancy Risk Factor No data reported

Contraindications Hypersensitivity to nitrous oxide or any component of the formulation; nitrous oxide should not be administered without oxygen

Warnings/Precautions Nausea and vomiting occurs postoperatively in ~15% of patients. Prolonged use may produce bone marrow suppression and/or neurologic dysfunction. Oxygen should be briefly administered during emergence from prolonged anesthesia with nitrous oxide to prevent diffusion hypoxia. Patients with vitamin B_{12} deficiency (pernicious anemia) and those with other nutritional deficiencies (alcoholics) are at increased risk of developing neurologic disease and bone marrow suppression with exposure to nitrous oxide. May be associated with abuse and/or addiction.

Adverse Reactions Frequency not defined.

Cardiovascular: Hypotension

Central nervous system: Headache, dizziness, confusion, CNS excitation

Gastrointestinal: Possibly nausea and vomiting

Respiratory: Apnea

Miscellaneous: Personnel exposed to unscavenged nitrous oxide have an increased risk of renal and hepatic diseases and peripheral neuropathy similar to that of vitamin B_{12} deficiency. Female dental personnel who were exposed to unscavenged nitrous oxide for more than 5 hours/week were significantly less fertile than women who were not exposed, or who were exposed to lower levels of scavenged or unscavenged nitrous oxide.

Drug Interactions

Avoid Concomitant Use There are no known interactions where it is recommended to avoid concomitant use.

Increased Effect/Toxicity There are no known significant interactions involving an increase in effect.

Decreased Effect There are no known significant interactions involving a decrease in effect.

Dosage Forms Excipient information presented when available (limited, particularly for generics); consult specific product labeling.

Supplied in blue cylinders

Nizatidine (ni ZA ti deen)

Medication Safety Issues

Sound-alike/look-alike issues:

Axid® may be confused with Ansaid®

International issues:

Tazac® [Australia] may be confused with Tiazac® which is a brand name for diltiazem in the U.S.

U.S. Brand Names Axid®; Axid® AR [OTC]

Canadian Brand Names Apo-Nizatidine®; Axid®; Gen-Nizatidine; Novo-Nizatidine; Nu-Nizatidine; PMS-Nizatidine

Pharmacologic Category Histamine H_2 Antagonist

Generic Available Yes: Capsule

Use Treatment and maintenance of duodenal ulcer; treatment of benign gastric ulcer; treatment of gastroesophageal reflux disease (GERD); OTC tablet used for the prevention of meal-induced heartburn, acid indigestion, and sour stomach

Unlabeled/Investigational Use Part of a multidrug regimen for *H. pylori* eradication to reduce the risk of duodenal ulcer recurrence

Mechanism of Action Competitive inhibition of histamine at H_2-receptors of the gastric parietal cells resulting in reduced gastric acid secretion, gastric volume and hydrogen ion concentration reduced. In healthy volunteers, nizatidine suppresses gastric acid secretion induced by pentagastrin infusion or food.

Pharmacodynamics/Kinetics

Distribution: V_d: 0.8-1.5 L/kg

Protein binding: 35% to α_1-acid glycoprotein

Metabolism: Partially hepatic; forms metabolites

Bioavailability: >70%

Half-life elimination: 1-2 hours; prolonged with renal impairment

Time to peak, plasma: 0.5-3.0 hours

Excretion: Urine (90%; ~60% as unchanged drug); feces (<6%)

Dosage Oral:

Children:

<12 years: GERD (unlabeled use): 10 mg/kg/day in divided doses given twice daily; may not be as effective in children <12 years

≥12 years:

GERD: Refer to adult dosing

Meal-induced heartburn, acid indigestion and sour stomach: Refer to adult dosing

Adults:

Duodenal ulcer:

Treatment of active ulcer: 300 mg at bedtime or 150 mg twice daily

Maintenance of healed ulcer: 150 mg/day at bedtime

Gastric ulcer: 150 mg twice daily or 300 mg at bedtime

GERD: 150 mg twice daily

Meal-induced heartburn, acid indigestion, and sour stomach: 75 mg tablet [OTC] twice daily, 30 to 60 minutes prior to consuming food or beverages

Helicobacter pylori eradication (unlabeled use): 150 mg twice daily; requires combination therapy

Dosing adjustment in renal impairment:

Active treatment:

Cl_{cr} 20-50 mL/minute: 150 mg/day

Cl_{cr} <20 mL/minute: 150 mg every other day

Maintenance treatment:

Cl_{cr} 20-50 mL/minute: 150 mg every other day

Cl_{cr} <20 mL/minute: 150 mg every 3 days

Pregnancy Risk Factor B

Contraindications Hypersensitivity to nizatidine or any component of the formulation; hypersensitivity to other H_2 antagonists (cross-sensitivity has been observed)

Warnings/Precautions Relief of symptoms does not preclude the presence of a gastric malignancy. Use with caution in children <12 years of age. Use with caution in patients with liver and renal impairment. Dosage modification required in patients with renal impairment

Adverse Reactions
>10%: Central nervous system: Headache (16%)
1% to 10%:
Central nervous system: Anxiety, dizziness, fever (reported in children), insomnia, irritability (reported in children), somnolence, nervousness
Dermatologic: Pruritus, rash
Gastrointestinal: Abdominal pain, anorexia, constipation, diarrhea, dry mouth, flatulence, heartburn, nausea, vomiting
Respiratory: Reported in children: Cough, nasal congestion, nasopharyngitis
<1% (Limited to important or life-threatening): Alkaline phosphatase increased, ALT increased, anaphylaxis, anemia, AST increased, bronchospasm, confusion, eosinophilia, exfoliative dermatitis, gynecomastia, hepatitis, jaundice, laryngeal edema, serum-sickness like reactions, thrombocytopenia, thrombocytopenic purpura, vasculitis, ventricular tachycardia

Drug Interactions
Metabolism/Transport Effects Inhibits 3A4 (weak)
Avoid Concomitant Use
Avoid concomitant use of Nizatidine with any of the following: Delavirdine; Erlotinib
Increased Effect/Toxicity
Nizatidine may increase the levels/effects of: Saquinavir
Decreased Effect
Nizatidine may decrease the levels/effects of: Antifungal Agents (Azole Derivatives, Systemic); Atazanavir; Cefpodoxime; Cefuroxime; Dasatinib; Delavirdine; Erlotinib; Fosamprenavir; Indinavir; Iron Salts; Mesalamine; Nelfinavir

Ethanol/Nutrition/Herb Interactions
Ethanol: Avoid ethanol (may cause gastric mucosal irritation).
Food: Administration with apple juice may decrease absorption.

Test Interactions False-positive urine protein using Multistix®, gastric acid secretion test, skin tests allergen extracts, serum creatinine and serum transaminase concentrations, urine protein test

Dosage Forms Excipient information presented when available (limited, particularly for generics); consult specific product labeling.
Capsule:
Axid®: 150 mg, 300 mg [DSC]
Solution, oral:
Axid®: 15 mg/mL (120 mL, 480 mL) [bubble gum flavor]
Tablet:
Axid® AR: 75 mg

◆ **Nizoral®** *see* Ketoconazole *on page 780*

◆ **Nizoral® A-D [OTC]** *see* Ketoconazole *on page 780*

◆ **N-methylnaltrexone Bromide** *see* Methylnaltrexone *on page 906*

◆ **No Doz® Maximum Strength [OTC]** *see* Caffeine *on page 225*

◆ **Noradrenaline** *see* Norepinephrine *on page 1024*

◆ **Noradrenaline Acid Tartrate** *see* Norepinephrine *on page 1024*

◆ **Norco®** *see* Hydrocodone and Acetaminophen *on page 697*

◆ **Norcuron** *see* Vecuronium *on page 1463*

◆ **Norcuron® (Can)** *see* Vecuronium *on page 1463*

◆ **Nordeoxyguanosine** *see* Ganciclovir *on page 654*

◆ **Nordette®** *see* Ethinyl Estradiol and Levonorgestrel *on page 549*

◆ **Norditropin®** *see* Somatropin *on page 1318*

◆ **Norditropin® NordiFlex®** *see* Somatropin *on page 1318*

◆ **Norelgestromin and Ethinyl Estradiol** *see* Ethinyl Estradiol and Norelgestromin *on page 552*

Norepinephrine (nor ep i NEF rin)

Medication Safety Issues
High alert medication: The Institute for Safe Medication Practices (ISMP) includes this medication among its list of drugs which have a heightened risk of causing significant patient harm when used in error.

Related Information
Allergic Reactions *on page 1508*
Anesthesia Considerations for Neurosurgery *on page 1514*
Chronic Pain Management *on page 1546*
Extravasation Treatment of Drugs *on page 1789*
Hemodynamic Support, Intravenous *on page 1681*
Latex Allergy *on page 1511*

U.S. Brand Names Levophed®

Canadian Brand Names Levophed®

Index Terms Levarterenol Bitartrate; Noradrenaline; Noradrenaline Acid Tartrate; Norepinephrine Bitartrate

Pharmacologic Category Alpha/Beta Agonist

Generic Available Yes

Use Treatment of shock which persists after adequate fluid volume replacement

Mechanism of Action Stimulates $beta_1$-adrenergic receptors and alpha-adrenergic receptors causing increased contractility and heart rate as well as vasoconstriction, thereby increasing systemic blood pressure and coronary blood flow; clinically alpha effects (vasoconstriction) are greater than beta effects (inotropic and chronotropic effects)

Pharmacodynamics/Kinetics
Onset of action: I.V.: Very rapid-acting
Duration: vasopressor: 1-2 minutes
Metabolism: Via catechol-o-methyltransferase (COMT) and monoamine oxidase (MAO)
Excretion: Urine (84% to 96% as inactive metabolites)

Dosage Administration requires the use of an infusion pump!
Note: Norepinephrine dosage is stated in terms of norepinephrine base.
Continuous I.V. infusion:
Children: Initial: 0.05-0.1 mcg/kg/minute; titrate to desired effect; maximum dose: 2 mcg/kg/minute
Adults: Initial: 0.5-1 mcg/minute and titrate to desired response; 8-30 mcg/minute is usual range
ACLS dosing range: 0.5-30 mcg/minute
Alternative weight-based dosing (Hollenberg, 2004): 0.01-3 mcg/kg/minute

Stability Readily oxidized. Protect from light. Do not use if brown coloration. Dilute with D_5W, D_5NS, or NS; dilution in NS is not recommended by the manufacturer; however, stability in NS has been demonstrated (Tremblay, 2008). Stability of parenteral admixture at room temperature (25°C) is 24 hours.

Administration Administer into large vein to avoid the potential for extravasation; potent drug, must be diluted prior to use; do not administer $NaHCO_3$ through an I.V. line containing norepinephrine.

Anesthesia and Critical Care Concerns/Other Considerations
Clinical Pearls/Comments: Norepinephrine is effective at increasing arterial blood pressure through vasoconstriction with little change in heart rate or cardiac output. Adequate fluid resuscitation is essential to the success of norepinephrine in raising blood pressure; may successfully increase blood pressure without causing a deterioration in cardiac index or organ function in patients with septic shock. It should be used early and not withheld as a last resort. The 2008 Surviving Sepsis Campaign guidelines recommend that either norepinephrine or dopamine is the first-choice vasopressor agent in adult patients (Grade 1C). Norepinephrine is more potent than dopamine and may be more effective at reversing hypotension in septic shock.

Extravasation Management: Antidote for peripheral ischemia caused by norepinephrine extravasation: To prevent sloughing and necrosis in ischemic areas, the area should be infiltrated as soon as possible with 5-10 mg of Regitine® (phentolamine), an adrenergic blocking agent, diluted in 10-15 mL of saline. A syringe with a fine hypodermic needle should be used and the solution liberally infiltrated throughout the ischemic area. Sympathetic blockade with phentolamine causes immediate and conspicuous local hyperemic changes if the area is infiltrated within 12 hours. Therefore, phentolamine should be given as soon as possible after the extravasation is noted, as phentolamine may be ineffective if given >12 hours after extravasation.

Evidence-Based Information: The 2008 Surviving Sepsis Campaign guidelines recommend that either norepinephrine or dopamine is the first-choice vasopressor agent in adult patients (Grade 1C). Norepinephrine is more potent than dopamine and may be more effective at reversing hypotension in septic shock.

Pregnancy Risk Factor C

Contraindications Hypersensitivity to norepinephrine, bisulfites (contains metabisulfite), or any component of the formulation; hypotension from hypovolemia except as an emergency measure to maintain coronary and cerebral perfusion until volume could be replaced; mesenteric or peripheral vascular thrombosis unless it is a lifesaving procedure; during anesthesia with cyclopropane or halothane anesthesia (risk of ventricular arrhythmias)

Warnings/Precautions Assure adequate circulatory volume to minimize need for vasoconstrictors. Avoid hypertension; monitor blood pressure closely and adjust infusion rate. Use with extreme caution in patients taking MAO-Inhibitors. Avoid extravasation; infuse into a large vein if possible. Avoid infusion into leg veins. Watch I.V. site closely. **[U.S. Boxed Warning]: If extravasation occurs, infiltrate the area with diluted phentolamine (5-10 mg in 10-15 mL of saline) with a fine hypodermic needle. Phentolamine should be administered as soon as possible after extravasation is noted.** Product may contain sodium metasulfite.

Adverse Reactions Frequency not defined.

Cardiovascular: Arrhythmias, bradycardia, peripheral (digital) ischemia

Central nervous system: Anxiety, headache (transient)

Local: Skin necrosis (with extravasation)

Respiratory: Dyspnea, respiratory difficulty

Drug Interactions

Avoid Concomitant Use

Avoid concomitant use of Norepinephrine with any of the following: Iobenguane I 123

Increased Effect/Toxicity

Norepinephrine may increase the levels/effects of: Bromocriptine; Sympathomimetics

The levels/effects of Norepinephrine may be increased by: Antacids; Atomoxetine; Beta-Blockers; Cannabinoids; Carbonic Anhydrase Inhibitors; COMT Inhibitors; MAO Inhibitors; Serotonin/Norepinephrine Reuptake Inhibitors; Tricyclic Antidepressants

Decreased Effect

Norepinephrine may decrease the levels/effects of: Iobenguane I 123

The levels/effects of Norepinephrine may be decreased by: Spironolactone

Dosage Forms Excipient information presented when available (limited, particularly for generics); consult specific product labeling. Strength expressed as base:

Injection, solution: 1 mg/mL (4 mL) [contains sodium metabisulfite]

References

Dellinger RP, Levy MM, Carlet JM, et al, "Surviving Sepsis Campaign: International Guidelines for Management of Severe Sepsis and Septic Shock: 2008," *Intensive Care Med*, 2008, 34(1): 17-60. Available at http://www.survivingsepsis.org/system/files/images/2008_20International_20SSC_20-Guidelines_1_.pdf

Martin C, Papazian L, Perrin G, et al, "Norepinephrine or Dopamine for the Treatment of Hyperdynamic Septic Shock?" *Chest*, 1993, 103(6):1826-31.

◆ **Norepinephrine Bitartrate** *see* Norepinephrine *on page 1024*

◆ **Norethindrone Acetate and Ethinyl Estradiol** *see* Ethinyl Estradiol and Norethindrone *on page 554*

◆ **Norgestimate and Ethinyl Estradiol** *see* Ethinyl Estradiol and Norgestimate *on page 558*

Nortriptyline (nor TRIP ti leen)

Related Information
Antidepressant Agents *on page 1660*
Chronic Pain Management *on page 1546*

U.S. Brand Names Pamelor®

Canadian Brand Names Alti-Nortriptyline; Apo-Nortriptyline®; Aventyl®; Gen-Nortriptyline; Norventyl; Novo-Nortriptyline; Nu-Nortriptyline; PMS-Nortriptyline

Index Terms Nortriptyline Hydrochloride

Pharmacologic Category Antidepressant, Tricyclic (Secondary Amine)

Use Treatment of symptoms of depression

Unlabeled/Investigational Use Chronic pain (including neuropathic pain), anxiety disorders, enuresis, attention-deficit/hyperactivity disorder (ADHD); adjunctive therapy for smoking cessation

Pharmacodynamics/Kinetics
Onset of action: Therapeutic: 1-3 weeks
Distribution: V_d: 21 L/kg
Protein binding: 93% to 95%
Metabolism: Primarily hepatic; extensive first-pass effect
Half-life elimination: 28-31 hours
Time to peak, serum: 7-8.5 hours
Excretion: Urine (as metabolites and small amounts of unchanged drug); feces (small amounts)

Dosage Oral:
Nocturnal enuresis: Children (unlabeled use): 10-20 mg/day; titrate to a maximum of 40 mg/day
Depression: Children (unlabeled use): 1-3 mg/kg/day
Depression:
Adults: 25 mg 3-4 times/day up to 150 mg/day; doses may be given once daily
Elderly: Initial: 30-50 mg/day, given as a single daily dose or in divided doses
Note: Nortriptyline is one of the best tolerated TCAs in the elderly)
Myofascial pain, neuralgia, burning mouth syndrome (dental use): Adults: Initial: 10-25 mg at bedtime; dosage may be increased by 25 mg/day weekly, if tolerated; usual maintenance dose: 75 mg as a single bedtime dose or 2 divided doses
Chronic urticaria, angioedema, nocturnal pruritus (unlabeled use): Adults: Oral: 75 mg/day
Smoking cessation (unlabeled use; Fiore, 2008): Adults: Initial: 25 mg/day; titrate dose to 75-100 mg/day 10-28 days prior to selected "quit" date; continue therapy for ≥12 weeks after "quit" day

Dosing adjustment in hepatic impairment: Lower doses and slower titration dependent on individualization of dosage is recommended

Additional Information Complete prescribing information for this medication should be consulted for additional detail.

Dosage Forms Excipient information presented when available (limited, particularly for generics); consult specific product labeling.
Capsule: 10 mg, 25 mg, 50 mg, 75 mg
  Pamelor®: 10 mg, 25 mg, 50 mg, 75 mg [may contain benzyl alcohol; 50 mg may also contain sodium bisulfite]
Solution:
  Pamelor®: 10 mg/5 mL (473 mL) [contains ethanol 4% and benzoic acid]

◆ **Nortriptyline Hydrochloride** see Nortriptyline on page 1026
◆ **Norvasc®** see AmLODIPine on page 93
◆ **Norventyl (Can)** see Nortriptyline on page 1026
◆ **Norvir®** see Ritonavir on page 1251
◆ **Norvir® SEC (Can)** see Ritonavir on page 1251
◆ **Novamoxin® (Can)** see Amoxicillin on page 95
◆ **Novasen (Can)** see Aspirin on page 147
◆ **Novo-5 ASA (Can)** see Mesalamine on page 884
◆ **Novo-Acebutolol (Can)** see Acebutolol on page 24
◆ **Novo-Acyclovir (Can)** see Acyclovir on page 40
◆ **Novo-Alendronate (Can)** see Alendronate on page 57
◆ **Novo-Alprazol (Can)** see ALPRAZolam on page 64
◆ **Novo-Amiodarone (Can)** see Amiodarone on page 86
◆ **Novo-Amlodipine (Can)** see AmLODIPine on page 93
◆ **Novo-Ampicillin (Can)** see Ampicillin on page 115
◆ **Novo-Atenol (Can)** see Atenolol on page 155
◆ **Novo-Azathioprine (Can)** see AzaTHIOprine on page 167
◆ **Novo-Azithromycin (Can)** see Azithromycin on page 169
◆ **Novo-Benzydamine (Can)** see Benzydamine on page 184
◆ **Novo-Bisoprolol (Can)** see Bisoprolol on page 192
◆ **Novo-Bupropion SR (Can)** see BuPROPion on page 217
◆ **Novo-Buspirone (Can)** see BusPIRone on page 219
◆ **Novo-Captopril (Can)** see Captopril on page 239
◆ **Novo-Carbamaz (Can)** see CarBAMazepine on page 241
◆ **Novo-Carvedilol (Can)** see Carvedilol on page 244
◆ **Novo-Chlorpromazine (Can)** see ChlorproMAZINE on page 298
◆ **Novo-Cilazapril (Can)** see Cilazapril on page 301
◆ **Novo-Cimetidine (Can)** see Cimetidine on page 305
◆ **Novo-Ciprofloxacin (Can)** see Ciprofloxacin on page 306
◆ **Novo-Clavamoxin (Can)** see Amoxicillin and Clavulanate Potassium on page 98
◆ **Novo-Clindamycin (Can)** see Clindamycin on page 324
◆ **Novo-Clonazepam (Can)** see ClonazePAM on page 328
◆ **Novo-Clonidine (Can)** see CloNIDine on page 329
◆ **Novo-Clopate (Can)** see Clorazepate on page 337
◆ **Novo-Desmopressin (Can)** see Desmopressin on page 386
◆ **Novo-Difenac ECT (Can)** see Diclofenac on page 414
◆ **Novo-Difenac K (Can)** see Diclofenac on page 414
◆ **Novo-Difenac-SR (Can)** see Diclofenac on page 414
◆ **Novo-Difenac Suppositories (Can)** see Diclofenac on page 414
◆ **Novo-Diflunisal (Can)** see Diflunisal on page 416
◆ **Novo-Digoxin (Can)** see Digoxin on page 417
◆ **Novo-Diltazem (Can)** see Diltiazem on page 425
◆ **Novo-Diltazem-CD (Can)** see Diltiazem on page 425
◆ **Novo-Diltazem HCl ER (Can)** see Diltiazem on page 425

- ◆ **Novo-Naproc EC (Can)** *see* Naproxen *on page 987*
- ◆ **Novo-Naprox (Can)** *see* Naproxen *on page 987*
- ◆ **Novo-Naprox Sodium (Can)** *see* Naproxen *on page 987*
- ◆ **Novo-Naprox Sodium DS (Can)** *see* Naproxen *on page 987*
- ◆ **Novo-Naprox SR (Can)** *see* Naproxen *on page 987*
- ◆ **Novo-Nizatidine (Can)** *see* Nizatidine *on page 1022*
- ◆ **Novo-Nortriptyline (Can)** *see* Nortriptyline *on page 1026*
- ◆ **Novo-Ofloxacin (Can)** *see* Ofloxacin *on page 1038*
- ◆ **Novo-Olanzapine (Can)** *see* OLANZapine *on page 1043*
- ◆ **Novo-Ondansetron (Can)** *see* Ondansetron *on page 1057*
- ◆ **Novo-Oxybutynin (Can)** *see* Oxybutynin *on page 1068*
- ◆ **Novo-Oxycodone Acet (Can)** *see* Oxycodone and Acetaminophen *on page 1072*
- ◆ **Novo-Pantoprazole (Can)** *see* Pantoprazole *on page 1084*
- ◆ **Novo-Paroxetine (Can)** *see* PARoxetine *on page 1089*
- ◆ **Novo-Peridol (Can)** *see* Haloperidol *on page 672*
- ◆ **Novo-Pindol (Can)** *see* Pindolol *on page 1130*
- ◆ **Novo-Pioglitazone (Can)** *see* Pioglitazone *on page 1132*
- ◆ **Novo-Pirocam (Can)** *see* Piroxicam *on page 1139*
- ◆ **Novo-Pramine (Can)** *see* Imipramine *on page 731*
- ◆ **Novo-Pramipexole (Can)** *see* Pramipexole *on page 1159*
- ◆ **Novo-Pranol (Can)** *see* Propranolol *on page 1198*
- ◆ **Novo-Pravastatin (Can)** *see* Pravastatin *on page 1162*
- ◆ **Novo-Prednisolone (Can)** *see* PrednisoLONE *on page 1164*
- ◆ **Novo-Prednisone (Can)** *see* PredniSONE *on page 1166*
- ◆ **Novo-Profen (Can)** *see* Ibuprofen *on page 717*
- ◆ **Novo-Purol (Can)** *see* Allopurinol *on page 62*
- ◆ **Novo-Quetiapine (Can)** *see* QUEtiapine *on page 1212*
- ◆ **Novo-Quinidin (Can)** *see* QuiNIDine *on page 1216*
- ◆ **Novo-Rabeprazole EC (Can)** *see* Rabeprazole *on page 1221*
- ◆ **Novo-Raloxifene (Can)** *see* Raloxifene *on page 1228*
- ◆ **Novo-Ramipril (Can)** *see* Ramipril *on page 1229*
- ◆ **Novo-Ranidine (Can)** *see* Ranitidine *on page 1231*
- ◆ **NovoRapid® (Can)** *see* Insulin Aspart *on page 741*
- ◆ **Novo-Rythro Estolate (Can)** *see* Erythromycin *on page 516*
- ◆ **Novo-Rythro Ethylsuccinate (Can)** *see* Erythromycin *on page 516*
- ◆ **Novo-Selegiline (Can)** *see* Selegiline *on page 1282*
- ◆ **Novo-Semide (Can)** *see* Furosemide *on page 645*
- ◆ **NovoSeven [DSC]** *see* Factor VIIa (Recombinant) *on page 567*
- ◆ **NovoSeven® RT** *see* Factor VIIa (Recombinant) *on page 567*
- ◆ **Novo-Simvastatin (Can)** *see* Simvastatin *on page 1293*
- ◆ **Novo-Sorbide (Can)** *see* Isosorbide Dinitrate *on page 772*
- ◆ **Novo-Sotalol (Can)** *see* Sotalol *on page 1321*
- ◆ **Novo-Sucralate (Can)** *see* Sucralfate *on page 1329*
- ◆ **Novo-Sumatriptan (Can)** *see* SUMAtriptan *on page 1336*
- ◆ **Novo-Sundac (Can)** *see* Sulindac *on page 1335*
- ◆ **Novo-Temazepam (Can)** *see* Temazepam *on page 1357*
- ◆ **Novo-Theophyl SR (Can)** *see* Theophylline *on page 1373*
- ◆ **Novo-Ticlopidine (Can)** *see* Ticlopidine *on page 1385*
- ◆ **Novo-Topiramate (Can)** *see* Topiramate *on page 1408*
- ◆ **Novo-Trazodone (Can)** *see* TraZODone *on page 1423*

- **Novo-Trimel (Can)** *see* Sulfamethoxazole and Trimethoprim *on page 1333*
- **Novo-Trimel D.S. (Can)** *see* Sulfamethoxazole and Trimethoprim *on page 1333*
- **Novo-Triptyn (Can)** *see* Amitriptyline *on page 89*
- **Novo-Venlafaxine XR (Can)** *see* Venlafaxine *on page 1466*
- **Novo-Veramil (Can)** *see* Verapamil *on page 1468*
- **Novo-Veramil SR (Can)** *see* Verapamil *on page 1468*
- **Novo-Warfarin (Can)** *see* Warfarin *on page 1479*
- **Noxafil®** *see* Posaconazole *on page 1148*
- **NPH Insulin** *see* Insulin NPH *on page 749*
- **NPH Insulin and Regular Insulin** *see* Insulin NPH and Insulin Regular *on page 749*
- **Nplate™** *see* Romiplostim *on page 1263*
- **NSC-15200** *see* Gallium Nitrate *on page 654*
- **NSC-125066** *see* Bleomycin *on page 197*
- **NSC-614629** *see* Filgrastim *on page 601*
- **NSC-671663** *see* Octreotide *on page 1033*
- **NSC-714371** *see* Dalteparin *on page 366*
- **NSC-724223** *see* Epoetin Alfa *on page 500*
- **NSC-729969** *see* Darbepoetin Alfa *on page 375*
- **NTG** *see* Nitroglycerin *on page 1014*
- **Nu-Acebutolol (Can)** *see* Acebutolol *on page 24*
- **Nu-Acyclovir (Can)** *see* Acyclovir *on page 40*
- **Nu-Alprax (Can)** *see* ALPRAZolam *on page 64*
- **Nu-Amoxi (Can)** *see* Amoxicillin *on page 95*
- **Nu-Ampi (Can)** *see* Ampicillin *on page 115*
- **Nu-Atenol (Can)** *see* Atenolol *on page 155*
- **Nu-Baclo (Can)** *see* Baclofen *on page 178*
- **Nubain®** *see* Nalbuphine *on page 978*
- **Nu-Buspirone (Can)** *see* BusPIRone *on page 219*
- **Nu-Capto (Can)** *see* Captopril *on page 239*
- **Nu-Carbamazepine (Can)** *see* CarBAMazepine *on page 241*
- **Nu-Cimet (Can)** *see* Cimetidine *on page 305*
- **Nu-Clonazepam (Can)** *see* ClonazePAM *on page 328*
- **Nu-Clonidine (Can)** *see* CloNIDine *on page 329*
- **Nu-Cotrimox (Can)** *see* Sulfamethoxazole and Trimethoprim *on page 1333*
- **Nucynta™** *see* Tapentadol *on page 1350*
- **Nu-Desipramine (Can)** *see* Desipramine *on page 384*
- **Nu-Diclo (Can)** *see* Diclofenac *on page 414*
- **Nu-Diclo-SR (Can)** *see* Diclofenac *on page 414*
- **Nu-Diflunisal (Can)** *see* Diflunisal *on page 416*
- **Nu-Diltiaz (Can)** *see* Diltiazem *on page 425*
- **Nu-Diltiaz-CD (Can)** *see* Diltiazem *on page 425*
- **Nu-Divalproex (Can)** *see* Valproic Acid and Derivatives *on page 1445*
- **Nu-Doxycycline (Can)** *see* Doxycycline *on page 456*
- **Nu-Erythromycin-S (Can)** *see* Erythromycin *on page 516*
- **Nu-Famotidine (Can)** *see* Famotidine *on page 575*
- **Nu-Fenofibrate (Can)** *see* Fenofibrate *on page 582*
- **Nu-Fluoxetine (Can)** *see* FLUoxetine *on page 616*
- **Nu-Flurprofen (Can)** *see* Flurbiprofen *on page 619*
- **Nu-Furosemide (Can)** *see* Furosemide *on page 645*
- **Nu-Glyburide (Can)** *see* GlyBURIDE *on page 666*

- ◆ **Nu-Hydral (Can)** *see* HydrALAZINE *on page 694*
- ◆ **Nu-Ibuprofen (Can)** *see* Ibuprofen *on page 717*
- ◆ **Nu-Indo (Can)** *see* Indomethacin *on page 738*
- ◆ **Nu-Ipratropium (Can)** *see* Ipratropium *on page 760*
- ◆ **Nu-Ketoprofen (Can)** *see* Ketoprofen *on page 783*
- ◆ **Nu-Ketoprofen-E (Can)** *see* Ketoprofen *on page 783*
- ◆ **Nu-Levocarb (Can)** *see* Levodopa and Carbidopa *on page 822*
- ◆ **Nu-Loraz (Can)** *see* LORazepam *on page 852*
- ◆ **Nu-Lovastatin (Can)** *see* Lovastatin *on page 859*
- ◆ **Nu-Medopa (Can)** *see* Methyldopa *on page 901*
- ◆ **Nu-Mefenamic (Can)** *see* Mefenamic Acid *on page 870*
- ◆ **Nu-Metformin (Can)** *see* MetFORMIN *on page 886*
- ◆ **Nu-Metoclopramide (Can)** *see* Metoclopramide *on page 917*
- ◆ **Nu-Metop (Can)** *see* Metoprolol *on page 922*
- ◆ **Nu-Naprox (Can)** *see* Naproxen *on page 987*
- ◆ **Nu-Nifed (Can)** *see* NIFEdipine *on page 1006*
- ◆ **Nu-Nifedipine-PA (Can)** *see* NIFEdipine *on page 1006*
- ◆ **Nu-Nizatidine (Can)** *see* Nizatidine *on page 1022*
- ◆ **Nu-Nortriptyline (Can)** *see* Nortriptyline *on page 1026*
- ◆ **Nu-Oxybutyn (Can)** *see* Oxybutynin *on page 1068*
- ◆ **Nupercainal® Hydrocortisone Cream [OTC]** *see* Hydrocortisone *on page 699*
- ◆ **Nu-Pindol (Can)** *see* Pindolol *on page 1130*
- ◆ **Nu-Pirox (Can)** *see* Piroxicam *on page 1139*
- ◆ **NU-Pravastatin (Can)** *see* Pravastatin *on page 1162*
- ◆ **Nu-Prochlor (Can)** *see* Prochlorperazine *on page 1180*
- ◆ **Nu-Propranolol (Can)** *see* Propranolol *on page 1198*
- ◆ **Nu-Ranit (Can)** *see* Ranitidine *on page 1231*
- ◆ **Nu-Selegiline (Can)** *see* Selegiline *on page 1282*
- ◆ **Nu-Simvastatin (Can)** *see* Simvastatin *on page 1293*
- ◆ **Nu-Sotalol (Can)** *see* Sotalol *on page 1321*
- ◆ **Nu-Sucralate (Can)** *see* Sucralfate *on page 1329*
- ◆ **Nu-Sundac (Can)** *see* Sulindac *on page 1335*
- ◆ **Nu-Temazepam (Can)** *see* Temazepam *on page 1357*
- ◆ **Nu-Ticlopidine (Can)** *see* Ticlopidine *on page 1385*
- ◆ **Nu-Timolol (Can)** *see* Timolol *on page 1390*
- ◆ **Nutracort®** *see* Hydrocortisone *on page 699*
- ◆ **Nu-Trazodone (Can)** *see* TraZODone *on page 1423*
- ◆ **Nutropin®** *see* Somatropin *on page 1318*
- ◆ **Nutropin AQ®** *see* Somatropin *on page 1318*
- ◆ **Nutropin® AQ (Can)** *see* Somatropin *on page 1318*
- ◆ **NuvaRing®** *see* Ethinyl Estradiol and Etonogestrel *on page 547*
- ◆ **Nu-Verap (Can)** *see* Verapamil *on page 1468*
- ◆ **Nu-Verap SR (Can)** *see* Verapamil *on page 1468*
- ◆ **Nuvigil™** *see* Armodafinil *on page 146*
- ◆ **Nyaderm (Can)** *see* Nystatin *on page 1032*
- ◆ **Nyamyc™** *see* Nystatin *on page 1032*

Nystatin (nye STAT in)

Medication Safety Issues
Sound-alike/look-alike issues:

Nystatin may be confused with HMG-CoA reductase inhibitors (also known as "statins"; eg, atorvastatin, fluvastatin, lovastatin, pitavastatin, pravastatin, rosuvastatin, simvastatin), Nilstat®, Nitrostat®

Nilstat may be confused with Nitrostat®, nystatin

Related Information
Antifungal Agents *on page 1664*

U.S. Brand Names Bio-Statin®; Mycostatin®; Nyamyc™; Nystat-Rx®; Nystop®; Paddock Nystatin™; Pedi-Dri®

Canadian Brand Names Candistatin®; Nilstat; Nyaderm; PMS-Nystatin

Pharmacologic Category Antifungal Agent, Oral Nonabsorbed; Antifungal Agent, Topical; Antifungal Agent, Vaginal

Generic Available Yes: Cream, ointment, powder, suspension, tablet

Use Treatment of susceptible cutaneous, mucocutaneous, and oral cavity fungal infections normally caused by the *Candida* species

Mechanism of Action Binds to sterols in fungal cell membrane, changing the cell wall permeability allowing for leakage of cellular contents

Pharmacodynamics/Kinetics
Onset of action: Symptomatic relief from candidiasis: 24-72 hours

Absorption: Topical: None through mucous membranes or intact skin; Oral: Poorly absorbed

Excretion: Feces (as unchanged drug)

Dosage
Oral candidiasis:

Suspension (swish and swallow orally):

Premature infants: 100,000 units 4 times/day

Infants: 200,000 units 4 times/day or 100,000 units to each side of mouth 4 times/day

Children and Adults: 400,000-600,000 units 4 times/day

Powder for compounding: Children and Adults: 1/8 teaspoon (500,000 units) to equal approximately 1/2 cup of water; give 4 times/day

Mucocutaneous infections: Children and Adults: Topical: Apply 2-3 times/day to affected areas; very moist topical lesions are treated best with powder

Intestinal infections: Adults: Oral: 500,000-1,000,000 units every 8 hours

Vaginal infections: Adults: Vaginal tablets: Insert 1 tablet/day at bedtime for 2 weeks

Stability
Vaginal insert: Store in refrigerator. Protect from temperature extremes, moisture, and light.

Oral tablet, ointment, topical powder, and oral suspension: Store at controlled room temperature of 15°C to 25°C (59°F to 77°F).

Administration Suspension: Shake well before using. Should be swished about the mouth and retained in the mouth for as long as possible (several minutes) before swallowing.

Pregnancy Risk Factor B/C (oral)

Contraindications Hypersensitivity to nystatin or any component of the formulation

Adverse Reactions
Frequency not defined: Dermatologic: Contact dermatitis, Stevens-Johnson syndrome

1% to 10%: Gastrointestinal: Diarrhea, nausea, stomach pain, vomiting

<1% (Limited to important or life-threatening): Hypersensitivity reactions

Drug Interactions
Avoid Concomitant Use There are no known interactions where it is recommended to avoid concomitant use.

Increased Effect/Toxicity There are no known significant interactions involving an increase in effect.

Decreased Effect

Nystatin may decrease the levels/effects of: Saccharomyces boulardii

Dosage Forms Excipient information presented when available (limited, particularly for generics); consult specific product labeling. [DSC] = Discontinued product
Capsule:
  Bio-Statin®: 500,000 units, 1 million units
Cream: 100,000 units/g (15 g, 30 g)
  Mycostatin®: 100,000 units/g (30 g)
Ointment, topical: 100,000 units/g (15 g, 30 g)
Powder, for prescription compounding: 50 million units (10 g); 150 million units (30 g); 500 million units (100 g); 2 billion units (400 g)
  Nystat-Rx®: 50 million units (10 g); 150 million units (30 g); 500 million units (100 g); 1 billion units (190 g); 2 billion units (350 g)
Powder, for prescription compounding: 50 million units (10 g); 150 million units (30 g); 500 million units (100 g); 1 billion units (190 g); 2 billion units (350 g)
  Bio-Statin®: 2 billion units (30 g)
Powder for suspension, oral [preservative free]:
  Paddock Nystatin™: 50 million units (10 g); 150 million units (30 g); 500 million units (100 g); 2 billion units (400 g) [sugar free]
Powder, topical:
  Mycostatin®: 100,000 units/g (15 g) [contains talc] [DSC]
  Nyamyc™: 100,000 units/g (15 g, 30 g) [contains talc]
  Nystop®: 100,000 units/g (15 g, 30 g, 60 g) [contains talc]
  Pedi-Dri®: 100,000 units/g (56.7 g) [contains talc]
Suspension, oral: 100,000 units/mL (5 mL, 60 mL, 480 mL)
Tablet: 500,000 units
Tablet, vaginal: 100,000 units (15s) [packaged with applicator]

◆ **Nystat-Rx®** see Nystatin on page 1032
◆ **Nystop®** see Nystatin on page 1032
◆ **Nytol® (Can)** see DiphenhydrAMINE on page 430
◆ **Nytol® Extra Strength (Can)** see DiphenhydrAMINE on page 430
◆ **Nytol® Quick Caps [OTC]** see DiphenhydrAMINE on page 430
◆ **Nytol® Quick Gels [OTC]** see DiphenhydrAMINE on page 430
◆ **NāSal™ [OTC]** see Sodium Chloride on page 1304
◆ **NāSop™ [DSC]** see Phenylephrine on page 1114
◆ **OCBZ** see OXcarbazepine on page 1066
◆ **Ocean® [OTC]** see Sodium Chloride on page 1304
◆ **Ocean® for Kids [OTC]** see Sodium Chloride on page 1304
◆ **Ocella™** see Ethinyl Estradiol and Drospirenone on page 546
◆ **Octagam®** see Immune Globulin (Intravenous) on page 732
◆ **Octostim® (Can)** see Desmopressin on page 386

Octreotide (ok TREE oh tide)

Medication Safety Issues
Sound-alike/look-alike issues:
  Sandostatin® may be confused with Sandimmune®, Sandostatin LAR®, sargramostim, simvastatin
U.S. Brand Names Sandostatin LAR®; Sandostatin®
Canadian Brand Names Octreotide Acetate Injection; Octreotide Acetate Omega; Sandostatin LAR®; Sandostatin®
Index Terms NSC-671663; Octreotide Acetate
Pharmacologic Category Antidiarrheal; Antidote; Somatostatin Analog
Generic Available Yes: Injection solution (excludes depot formulation)
Use Control of symptoms in patients with metastatic carcinoid and vasoactive intestinal peptide-secreting tumors (VIPomas); treatment of acromegaly
Unlabeled/Investigational Use Secretory diarrhea (AIDS-associated [including *Cryptosporidiosis*], chemotherapy-induced, graft-versus-host disease (GVHD) induced, and postgastrectomy dumping syndrome); control of bleeding of esophageal varices; second-line treatment for thymic malignancies; Cushing's

syndrome (ectopic); insulinomas; small bowel fistulas; pancreatic tumors; gastrinoma; Zollinger-Ellison syndrome; congenital hyperinsulinism; hypothalamic obesity; treatment of hypoglycemia secondary to sulfonylurea poisoning

Mechanism of Action Mimics natural somatostatin by inhibiting serotonin release, and the secretion of gastrin, VIP, insulin, glucagon, secretin, motilin, and pancreatic polypeptide. Decreases growth hormone and IGF-1 in acromegaly. Octreotide provides more potent inhibition of growth hormone, glucagon, and insulin as compared to endogenous somatostatin. Also suppresses LH response to GnRH, secretion of thyroid-stimulating hormone and decreases splanchnic blood flow.

Pharmacodynamics/Kinetics

Duration: SubQ: 6-12 hours

Absorption: SubQ: Rapid and complete; I.M. (depot formulation): Released slowly (via microsphere degradation in the muscle)

Distribution: V_d: 14 L (13-30 L in acromegaly)

Protein binding: 65%, mainly to lipoprotein (41% in acromegaly)

Metabolism: Extensively hepatic

Bioavailability: SubQ: 100%; I.M. 60% to 63% of SubQ dose

Half-life elimination: 1.7-1.9 hours; Increased in elderly patients; Cirrhosis: Up to 3.7 hours; Fatty liver disease: Up to 3.4 hours; Renal impairment: Up to 3.1 hours

Time to peak, plasma: SubQ: 0.4 hours (0.7 hours acromegaly); I.M.: 1 hour

Excretion: Urine (32% as unchanged drug)

Dosage

Acromegaly: Adults:

SubQ, I.V.: Initial: 50 mcg 3 times/day; titrate to achieve growth hormone levels <5 ng/mL or IGF-I (somatomedin C) levels <1.9 units/mL in males and <2.2 units/mL in females. Usual effective dose 100-200 mcg 3 times/day; range 300-1500 mcg/day. **Note:** Should be withdrawn yearly for a 4-week interval (8 weeks for depot injection) in patients who have received irradiation. Resume if levels increase and signs/symptoms recur.

I.M. depot injection: Patients must be stabilized on subcutaneous octreotide for at least 2 weeks before switching to the long-acting depot. Upon switch: 20 mg I.M. intragluteally every 4 weeks for 3 months, then the dose may be modified based upon response.

Dosage adjustment for acromegaly: After 3 months of depot injections, the dosage may be continued or modified as follows:

GH ≤1 ng/mL, IGF-1 normal, and symptoms controlled: Reduce octreotide LAR® to 10 mg I.M. every 4 weeks

GH ≤2.5 ng/mL, IGF-1 normal, and symptoms controlled: Maintain octreotide LAR® at 20 mg I.M. every 4 weeks

GH >2.5 ng/mL, IGF-1 elevated, and/or symptoms uncontrolled: Increase octreotide LAR® to 30 mg I.M. every 4 weeks

Note: Patients not adequately controlled at a dose of 30 mg may increase dose to 40 mg every 4 weeks. Dosages >40 mg are not recommended.

Carcinoid tumors: Adults:

SubQ, I.V.: Initial 2 weeks: 100-600 mcg/day in 2-4 divided doses; usual range: 50-750 mcg/day (some patients may require up to 1500 mcg/day)

I.M. depot injection: Patients must be stabilized on subcutaneous octreotide for at least 2 weeks before switching to the long-acting depot. Upon switch: 20 mg I.M. intragluteally every 4 weeks for 2 months, then the dose may be modified based upon response.

Note: Patients should continue to receive their SubQ injections for the first 2 weeks at the same dose in order to maintain therapeutic levels (some patients may require 3-4 weeks of continued SubQ injections). Patients who experience periodic exacerbations of symptoms may require temporary SubQ injections in addition to depot injections (at their previous SubQ dosing regimen) until symptoms have resolved.

Dosage adjustment: See dosing adjustment for VIPomas.

VIPomas: Adults:

SubQ, I.V.: Initial 2 weeks: 200-300 mcg/day in 2-4 divided doses; titrate dose based on response/tolerance. Range: 150-750 mcg/day (doses >450 mcg/day are rarely required)

I.M. depot injection: Patients must be stabilized on subcutaneous octreotide for at least 2 weeks before switching to the long-acting depot. Upon switch: 20 mg I.M. intragluteally every 4 weeks for 2 months, then the dose may be modified based upon response.

Note: Patients receiving depot injection should continue to receive their SubQ injections for the first 2 weeks at the same dose in order to maintain therapeutic levels (some patients may require 3-4 weeks of continued SubQ injections). Patients who experience periodic exacerbations of symptoms may require temporary SubQ injections in addition to depot injections (at their previous SubQ dosing regimen) until symptoms have resolved.

Dosage adjustment for carcinoid tumors and VIPomas: After 2 months of depot injections, the dosage may be continued or modified as follows:

Increase to 30 mg I.M. every 4 weeks if symptoms are inadequately controlled

Decrease to 10 mg I.M. every 4 weeks, for a trial period, if initially responsive to 20 mg dose

Dosage >30 mg is not recommended

Congenital hyperinsulinism (unlabeled use): Infants and Children: SubQ: Doses of 3-40 mcg/kg/day have been used

Diarrhea (unlabeled use):

Infants and Children: I.V., SubQ: Doses of 1-10 mcg/kg every 12 hours have been used in children beginning at the low end of the range and increasing by 0.3 mcg/kg/dose at 3-day intervals. Suppression of growth hormone (animal data) is of concern when used as long-term therapy.

Adults: I.V.: Initial: 50-100 mcg every 8 hours; increase by 100 mcg/dose at 48-hour intervals; maximum dose: 500 mcg every 8 hours

Esophageal varices bleeding (unlabeled use): Adults: I.V. bolus: 25-50 mcg followed by continuous I.V. infusion of 25-50 mcg/hour

Hypoglycemia in sulfonylurea poisoning (unlabeled use): Note: SubQ is the preferred route of administration; repeat dosing, dose escalation, or initiation of a continuous infusion may be required in patients who experience recurrent hypoglycemia. Duration of treatment may exceed 24 hours. Optimal care decisions should be made based upon patient-specific details:

Children: SubQ: 1-1.5 mcg/kg; repeat in 6-12 hours as needed based upon blood glucose concentrations

Adults:

SubQ: 50-100 mcg; repeat in 6-12 hours as needed based upon blood glucose concentrations

I.V.: Doses up to 100-125 mcg/hour have been used successfully

Elderly: Elimination half-life is increased by 46% and clearance is decreased by 26%; dose adjustment may be required. Dosing should generally begin at the lower end of dosing range.

Dosage adjustment in renal impairment:

Nondialysis-dependent renal impairment: No dosage adjustment required

Dialysis-dependent renal impairment: Depot injection: Initial dose: 10 mg I.M. every 4 weeks; titrate based upon response (clearance is reduced by ~50%)

Dosage adjustment in hepatic impairment: Patients with established cirrhosis of the liver: Depot injection: Initial dose: 10 mg I.M. every 4 weeks; titrate based upon response

Stability

Solution: Octreotide is a clear solution and should be stored at refrigerated temperatures between 2°C and 8°C (36°F and 46°F). Protect from light. May be stored at room temperature of 20°C to 30°C (70°F and 86°F) for up to 14 days when protected from light. Stability of parenteral admixture is stable in NS for 96 hours at room temperature (25°C) and in D_5W for 24 hours. Discard multidose vials within 14 days after initial entry.

Suspension: Prior to dilution, store at refrigerated temperatures between 2°C and 8°C (36°F and 46°F) and protect from light. Depot drug product kit may be at room temperature for 30-60 minutes prior to use. Use suspension immediately after preparation.

◀ **Administration**

Regular injection formulation (do not use if solution contains particles or is discolored): Administer SubQ or I.V.; I.V. administration may be IVP, IVPB, or continuous I.V. infusion (unlabeled route):

IVP should be administered undiluted over 3 minutes

IVPB should be administered over 15-30 minutes

Continuous I.V. infusion rates have ranged from 25-50 mcg/hour for the treatment of esophageal variceal bleeding (unlabeled route/use); continuous I.V. infusion rates of 100-125 mcg/hour have been used for the treatment of sulfonylurea-induced hypoglycemia (unlabeled use).

SubQ: Use the concentration with smallest volume to deliver dose to reduce injection site pain. Rotate injection site; may bring to room temperature prior to injection.

Depot formulation: Administer I.M. intragluteal (avoid deltoid administration); alternate gluteal injection sites to avoid irritation. Do not administer Sandostatin LAR® intravenously or subcutaneously; must be administered immediately after mixing.

Monitoring Parameters

Acromegaly: Growth hormone, somatomedin C (IGF-1)

Carcinoid: 5-HIAA, plasma serotonin and plasma substance P

VIPomas: Vasoactive intestinal peptide

Chronic therapy: Thyroid function (baseline and periodic), vitamin B_{12} level, blood glucose, cardiac function (heart rate, ECG), zinc level (patients with excessive fluid loss maintained on TPN)

Reference Range Vasoactive intestinal peptide: <75 ng/L; levels vary considerably between laboratories

Pregnancy Risk Factor B

Contraindications Hypersensitivity to octreotide or any component of the formulation

Warnings/Precautions May impair gallbladder function; monitor patients for cholelithiasis. Use with caution in patients with renal and/or hepatic impairment; dosage adjustment is required in patients receiving dialysis and in patients with established cirrhosis. Somatostatin analogs may affect glucose regulation. In type I diabetes, severe hypoglycemia may occur; in type II diabetes or patients without diabetes, hyperglycemia may occur. Insulin and other hypoglycemic medication requirements may change. Do not use depot formulation for the treatment of sulfonylurea-induced hypoglycemia. Bradycardia, conduction abnormalities, and arrhythmia have been observed in acromegalic and carcinoid syndrome patients; use caution with CHF or concomitant medications that alter heart rate or rhythm. Cardiovascular medication requirements may change. Octreotide may enhance the adverse/toxic effects of other QT_c-prolonging agents. May alter absorption of dietary fats; monitor for pancreatitis. May reduce excessive fluid loss in patients with conditions that cause such loss; monitor for elevations in zinc levels in such patients that are maintained on total parenteral nutrition (TPN). Chronic treatment has been associated with abnormal Schillings test; monitor vitamin B_{12} levels. Suppresses secretion of TSH; monitor for hypothyroidism. Therapy may restore fertility; females of childbearing potential should use adequate contraception. Dosage adjustment may be necessary in the elderly; significant increases in elimination half-life have been observed in older adults. Vehicle used in depot injection (polylactide-co-glycolide microspheres) has rarely been associated with retinal artery occlusion in patients with abnormal arteriovenous anastomosis.

Adverse Reactions Adverse reactions vary by route of administration and dosage form. Frequency of cardiac, endocrine, and gastrointestinal adverse reactions was generally higher in acromegalics.

>16%:

Cardiovascular: Sinus bradycardia (19% to 25%), chest pain (≤20%; non-depot formulations)

Central nervous system: Fatigue (1% to 32%), headache (6% to 30%), malaise (16% to 20%), fever (16% to 20%), dizziness (5% to 20%)

Dermatologic: Pruritus (≤18%)

Endocrine & metabolic: Hyperglycemia (2% to 27%)

Gastrointestinal: Abdominal pain (5% to 61%), loose stools (5% to 61%), nausea (5% to 61%), diarrhea (34% to 58%), flatulence (≤38%), cholelithiasis (13% to 38%; length of therapy dependent), biliary sludge (24%; length of therapy dependent), constipation (9% to 21%), vomiting (4% to 21%), biliary duct dilatation (12%)

Local: Injection site pain (2% to 50%; dose and formulation related)

Neuromuscular & skeletal: Back pain (1% to 27%), arthropathy (8% to 19%), myalgia (≤18%)

Respiratory: Upper respiratory infection (10% to 23%), dyspnea (≤20%; non-depot formulations)

Miscellaneous: Antibodies to octreotide (up to 25%; no efficacy change), flu symptoms (1% to 20%)

5% to 15%:

Cardiovascular: Hypertension (≤13%), conduction abnormalities (9% to 10%), arrhythmia (3% to 9%), palpitation, peripheral edema

Central nervous system: Pain (4% to 15%), anxiety, confusion, hypoesthesia, insomnia

Dermatologic: Rash (15%; depot formulation), alopecia (≤13%)

Endocrine & metabolic: Hypothyroidism (≤12%; non-depot formulations), goiter (≤8%; non-depot formulations)

Gastrointestinal: Anorexia, cramping, tenesmus (4% to 6%), dyspepsia (4% to 6%), steatorrhea (4% to 6%), feces discoloration (4% to 6%)

Hematologic: Anemia (≤15%; non-depot formulations: <1%)

Neuromuscular & skeletal: Arthralgia, myalgia, paresthesia, rigors, weakness

Otic: Earache

Renal: Renal calculus

Respiratory: Cough, pharyngitis, sinusitis, rhinitis

Miscellaneous: Allergy, diaphoresis

1% to 4%:

Cardiovascular: Angina, cardiac failure, edema, flushing, hematoma, phlebitis

Central nervous system: Abnormal gait, amnesia, depression, dysphonia, hallucinations, nervousness, neuralgia, somnolence, vertigo

Dermatologic: Acne, bruising, cellulitis

Endocrine & metabolic: Hypoglycemia (2% to 4%), hypokalemia, hypoproteinemia, gout, cachexia, breast pain, impotence

Gastrointestinal: Colitis, diverticulitis, dysphagia, fat malabsorption, gastritis, gastroenteritis, gingivitis, glossitis, melena, stomatitis, taste perversion, xerostomia

Genitourinary: Incontinence, pollakuria (non-depot formulations), urinary tract infection

Local: Injection site hematoma

Neuromuscular & skeletal: Hyperkinesia, hypertonia, joint pain, neuropathy, tremor

Ocular: Blurred vision, visual disturbance

Otic: Tinnitus

Renal: Albuminuria, renal abscess

Respiratory: Bronchitis, epistaxis

Miscellaneous: Bacterial infection, cold symptoms, moniliasis

<1% (Limited to important or life-threatening): Anaphylactic shock, anaphylactoid reaction, aneurysm, aphasia, appendicitis, arthritis, ascending cholangitis, ascites, atrial fibrillation, basal cell carcinoma, Bell's palsy, biliary obstruction, breast carcinoma, cardiac arrest, cerebral vascular disorder, CHF, cholestatic hepatitis, CK increased, creatinine increased, deafness, diabetes insipidus, diabetes mellitus, facial edema, fatty liver, galactorrhea, gallbladder polyp, GI bleeding, GI hemorrhage, GI ulcer, glaucoma, gynecomastia, hearing loss, hematuria, hemiparesis, hemorrhoids, hepatitis, hyperesthesia, hypertensive reaction, hypoadrenalism, intestinal obstruction, intracranial hemorrhage, intraocular pressure increased, ischemia, jaundice, joint effusion, lactation, LFTs increased, libido decreased, malignant hyperpyrexia, menstrual irregularities, MI, migraine, nephrolithiasis, neuritis, orthostatic hypotension, pancreatitis, pancytopenia, paresis, petechiae, pituitary apoplexy, pleural effusion, pneumonia, pneumothorax, pulmonary embolism, pulmonary hypertension, pulmonary nodule, Raynaud's syndrome, rectal bleeding, renal failure, renal insufficiency, retinal vein thrombosis, scotoma, seizure, status asthmaticus, suicide attempt, syncope, tachycardia, thrombocytopenia, thrombophlebitis, thrombosis, urticaria, visual field defect, weight loss, wheal/erythema

◀ **Drug Interactions**
Avoid Concomitant Use
Avoid concomitant use of Octreotide with any of the following: Artemether; Dronedarone; Lumefantrine; Nilotinib; Pimozide; QuiNINE; Tetrabenazine; Thioridazine; Ziprasidone

Increased Effect/Toxicity
Octreotide may increase the levels/effects of: Codeine; Dronedarone; Hypoglycemic Agents; Pegvisomant; Pimozide; QTc-Prolonging Agents; QuiNINE; Tetrabenazine; Thioridazine; Ziprasidone

The levels/effects of Octreotide may be increased by: Alfuzosin; Artemether; Chloroquine; Ciprofloxacin; Gadobutrol; Herbs (Hypoglycemic Properties); Lumefantrine; Nilotinib; QuiNINE

Decreased Effect
Octreotide may decrease the levels/effects of: CycloSPORINE

Ethanol/Nutrition/Herb Interactions
Herb/Nutraceutical: Avoid hypoglycemic herbs, including alfalfa, aloe, bilberry, bitter melon, burdock, celery, damiana, fenugreek, garcinia, garlic, ginger, ginseng (American), gymnema, marshmallow, and stinging nettle (may enhance the hypoglycemic effect of octreotide).

Dietary Considerations Schedule injections between meals to decrease GI effects. May alter absorption of dietary fats.

Dosage Forms Excipient information presented when available (limited, particularly for generics); consult specific product labeling.
Injection, microspheres for suspension, as acetate [depot formulation]:
Sandostatin LAR®: 10 mg, 20 mg, 30 mg [contains polylactide-co-glycolide; packaged with diluent and syringe]
Injection, solution, as acetate: 0.2 mg/mL (5 mL); 1 mg/mL (5 mL)
Sandostatin®: 0.2 mg/mL (5 mL); 1 mg/mL (5 mL)
Injection, solution, as acetate [preservative free]: 0.05 mg/mL (1 mL); 0.1 mg/mL (1 mL); 0.5 mg/mL (1 mL)
Sandostatin®: 0.05 mg/mL (1 mL); 0.1 mg/mL (1 mL); 0.5 mg/mL (1 mL)

References
Braatvedt GD, "Octreotide for the Treatment of Sulphonylurea Induced Hypoglycaemia in Type 2 Diabetes," *N Z Med J*, 1997, 110(1044):189-90.
Corley DA, Cello JP, Adkisson W, et al, "Octreotide for Acute Esophageal Variceal Bleeding: A Meta-Analysis," *Gastroentology*, 2001, 120(4):946-54.
Erstad BL, "Octreotide For Acute Variceal Bleeding," *Ann Pharmacother*, 2001, 35(5):618-26.

◆ **Octreotide Acetate** *see* Octreotide *on page 1033*

◆ **Octreotide Acetate Injection (Can)** *see* Octreotide *on page 1033*

◆ **Octreotide Acetate Omega (Can)** *see* Octreotide *on page 1033*

◆ **Ocufen®** *see* Flurbiprofen *on page 619*

◆ **Ocuflox®** *see* Ofloxacin *on page 1038*

◆ **OcuNefrin™ [OTC]** *see* Phenylephrine *on page 1114*

◆ **O-desmethylvenlafaxine** *see* Desvenlafaxine *on page 390*

◆ **ODV** *see* Desvenlafaxine *on page 390*

◆ **Oesclim® (Can)** *see* Estradiol *on page 531*

Ofloxacin (oh FLOKS a sin)

Medication Safety Issues
Sound-alike/look-alike issues:
Floxin® may be confused with Flexeril®
Ocuflox® may be confused with Occlusal®-HP, Ocufen®

International issues:
Floxin® may be confused with Flogen® which is a brand name for naproxen in Mexico
Floxin® may be confused with Fluoxin® which is a brand name for fluoxetine in the Czech Republic and Romania
Floxin® may be confused with Flexin® which is a brand name for orphenadrine in Israel and indomethacin in Great Britain

Medication Guide An FDA-approved patient medication guide, which is available with the product information and at http://www.fda.gov/downloads/Drugs/DrugSafety/ucm088599.pdf, must be dispensed with this medication for each new outpatient prescription and refill.

Related Information

Prevention of Wound Infection and Sepsis in Surgical Patients *on page 1721*

U.S. Brand Names Floxin®; Ocuflox®

Canadian Brand Names Apo-Ofloxacin®; Apo-Oflox®; Floxin®; Novo-Ofloxacin; Ocuflox®; PMS-Ofloxacin

Index Terms Floxin Otic Singles

Pharmacologic Category Antibiotic, Quinolone

Generic Available Yes

Use

Quinolone antibiotic for the treatment of acute exacerbations of chronic bronchitis, community-acquired pneumonia, skin and skin structure infections (uncomplicated), urethral and cervical gonorrhea (acute, uncomplicated), urethritis and cervicitis (nongonococcal), mixed infections of the urethra and cervix, pelvic inflammatory disease (acute), cystitis (uncomplicated), urinary tract infections (complicated), prostatitis

Note: As of April 2007, the CDC no longer recommends the use of fluoroquinolones for the treatment of gonococcal disease.

Ophthalmic: Treatment of superficial ocular infections involving the conjunctiva or cornea due to strains of susceptible organisms

Otic: Otitis externa, chronic suppurative otitis media, acute otitis media

Unlabeled/Investigational Use Epididymitis (nongonococcal), leprosy, Traveler's diarrhea

Mechanism of Action Ofloxacin is a DNA gyrase inhibitor. DNA gyrase is an essential bacterial enzyme that maintains the superhelical structure of DNA. DNA gyrase is required for DNA replication and transcription, DNA repair, recombination, and transposition; bactericidal

Pharmacodynamics/Kinetics

Absorption: Well absorbed; food causes only minor alterations

Distribution: V_d: 2.4-3.5 L/kg

Protein binding: 32%

Bioavailability: Oral: 98%

Half-life elimination: Biphasic: 4-5 hours and 20-25 hours (accounts for <5%); prolonged with renal impairment

Excretion: Primarily urine (as unchanged drug)

Dosage

Usual dosage range:

Children ≥6 months: Otic: 5 drops daily

Children >1 year: Ophthalmic: 1-2 drops every 30 minutes to 4 hours initially, decreasing to every 4-6 hours

Children >12 years: Otic: 10 drops once or twice daily

Adults:

Ophthalmic: 1-2 drops every 30 minutes to 4 hours initially, decreasing to every 4-6 hours

Oral: 200-400 mg every 12 hours

Otic: 10 drops once or twice daily

Indication-specific dosing:

Children 6 months to 13 years: Otic:

Otitis externa: Instill 5 drops (or the contents of 1 single-dose container) into affected ear(s) once daily for 7 days

Children 1-12 years: Otic:

Acute otitis media with tympanostomy tubes: Instill 5 drops (or the contents of 1 single-dose container) into affected ear(s) twice daily for 10 days

Children >1 year and Adults: Ophthalmic:

Conjunctivitis: Instill 1-2 drops in affected eye(s) every 2-4 hours for the first 2 days, then use 4 times/day for an additional 5 days

Corneal ulcer: Instill 1-2 drops every 30 minutes while awake and every 4-6 hours after retiring for the first 2 days; beginning on day 3, instill 1-2 drops every hour while awake for 4-6 additional days; thereafter, 1-2 drops 4 times/day until clinical cure.

Children >12 years and Adults: Otic:
Otitis media, chronic suppurative with perforated tympanic membranes: Instill 10 drops (or the contents of 2 single-dose containers) into affected ear twice daily for 14 days
Children ≥13 years and Adults: Otic:
Otitis externa: Instill 10 drops (or the contents of 2 single-dose containers) into affected ear(s) once daily for 7 days
Adults: Oral:
Cervicitis/urethritis:
Nongonococcal: 300 mg every 12 hours for 7 days
Gonococcal (acute, uncomplicated): 400 mg as a single dose; **Note:** As of April 2007, the CDC no longer recommends the use of fluoroquinolones for the treatment of uncomplicated gonococcal disease.
Chronic bronchitis (acute exacerbation), community-acquired pneumonia, skin and skin structure infections (uncomplicated): 400 mg every 12 hours for 10 days
Epididymitis, nongonococcal (unlabeled use): 300 mg twice daily for 10 days
Leprosy (unlabeled use): 400 mg once daily
Pelvic inflammatory disease (acute): 400 mg every 12 hours for 10-14 days with or without metronidazole; **Note:** The CDC recommends use only if standard cephalosporin therapy is not feasible and community prevalence of quinolone-resistant gonococcal organisms is low. Culture sensitivity must be confirmed.
Prostatitis:
Acute: 400 mg for 1 dose, then 300 mg twice daily for 10 days
Chronic: 200 mg every 12 hours for 6 weeks
Traveler's diarrhea (unlabeled use): 300 mg twice daily for 3 days
UTI:
Uncomplicated: 200 mg every 12 hours for 3-7 days
Complicated: 200 mg every 12 hours for 10 days

Dosing adjustment/interval in renal impairment: Adults: Oral: After a normal initial dose, adjust as follows:
Cl_{cr} 20-50 mL/minute: Administer usual dose every 24 hours
Cl_{cr} <20 mL/minute: Administer half the usual dose every 24 hours
Continuous arteriovenous or venovenous hemodiafiltration effects: Administer 300 mg every 24 hours
Dosing adjustment in hepatic impairment: Severe impairment: Maximum dose: 400 mg/day

Stability
Ophthalmic and otic solution: Store at 15°C to 25°C (59°F to 77°F).
Otic Singles™: Store at 15°C to 30°C (59°F to 86°F). Store in pouch to protect from light.
Tablet: Store below 30°C (86°F).

Administration
Ophthalmic: For ophthalmic use only; avoid touching tip of applicator to eye or other surfaces.
Oral: Do not take within 2 hours of food or any antacids which contain zinc, magnesium, or aluminum.
Otic: Prior to use, warm solution by holding container in hands for 1-2 minutes. Patient should lie down with affected ear upward and medication instilled. Pump tragus 4 times to ensure penetration of medication. Patient should remain in this position for 5 minutes.

Pregnancy Risk Factor C

Contraindications Hypersensitivity to ofloxacin or other members of the quinolone group, such as nalidixic acid, oxolinic acid, cinoxacin, norfloxacin, and ciprofloxacin; hypersensitivity to any component of the formulation

Warnings/Precautions [U.S. Boxed Warning]: There have been reports of tendon inflammation and/or rupture with quinolone antibiotics; risk may be increased with concurrent corticosteroids, organ transplant recipients, and in patients >60 years of age. Rupture of the Achilles tendon sometimes requiring surgical repair has been reported most frequently; but other tendon sites (eg, rotator cuff, biceps) have also been reported. Strenuous physical activity, rheumatoid arthritis, and renal impairment may be an independent risk factor for tendonitis. Discontinue at first sign of tendon inflammation or pain. May occur even after discontinuation of therapy. Use with caution in patients with rheumatoid arthritis; may increase risk of tendon rupture. Use with caution in patients with epilepsy or other CNS diseases which could predispose seizures; potential for seizures, although very rare, may be increased with concomitant NSAID therapy. Tremor, restlessness, confusion, and very rarely hallucinations or seizures may occur; use with caution in patients with known or suspected CNS disorder. Discontinue in patients who experience significant CNS adverse effects (eg, dizziness, hallucinations, suicidal ideations or actions). Use with caution in patients with renal or hepatic impairment. Peripheral neuropathies have been linked to ofloxacin use; discontinue if numbness, tingling, or weakness develops.

Fluoroquinolones have been associated with the development of serious, and sometimes fatal, hypoglycemia, most often in elderly diabetics, but also in patients without diabetes. This occurred most frequently with gatifloxacin (no longer available systemically) but may occur at a lower frequency with other quinolones.

Rare cases of torsade de pointes have been reported in patients receiving ofloxacin and other quinolones. Risk may be minimized by avoiding use in patients with known prolongation of the QT interval, bradycardia, hypokalemia, hypomagnesemia, cardiomyopathy, or in those receiving concurrent therapy with Class Ia or Class III antiarrhythmics.

Severe hypersensitivity reactions, including anaphylaxis, have occurred with quinolone therapy. Reactions may present as typical allergic symptoms after a single dose, or may manifest as severe idiosyncratic dermatologic, vascular, pulmonary, renal, hepatic, and/or hematologic events, usually after multiple doses. Prompt discontinuation of drug should occur if skin rash or other symptoms arise. Prolonged use may result in fungal or bacterial superinfection, including *C. difficile*-associated diarrhea (CDAD) and pseudomembranous colitis; CDAD has been observed >2 months postantibiotic treatment. Quinolones may exacerbate myasthenia gravis. Avoid excessive sunlight and take precautions to limit exposure (eg, loose fitting clothing, sunscreen); may cause moderate-to-severe phototoxicity reactions. Discontinue use if photosensitivity occurs. Since ofloxacin is ineffective in the treatment of syphilis and may mask symptoms, all patients should be tested for syphilis at the time of gonorrheal diagnosis and 3 months later. Hemolytic reactions may (rarely) occur with quinolone use in patients with latent or actual G6PD deficiency. Safety and efficacy have not been established in children.

Adverse Reactions
Systemic:
1% to 10%:

Cardiovascular: Chest pain (1% to 3%)

Central nervous system: Headache (1% to 9%), insomnia (3% to 7%), dizziness (1% to 5%), fatigue (1% to 3%), somnolence (1% to 3%), sleep disorders (1% to 3%), nervousness (1% to 3%), pyrexia (1% to 3%)

Dermatologic: Rash/pruritus (1% to 3%)

Gastrointestinal: Diarrhea (1% to 4%), vomiting (1% to 4%), GI distress (1% to 3%), abdominal cramps (1% to 3%), flatulence (1% to 3%), abnormal taste (1% to 3%), xerostomia (1% to 3%), appetite decreased (1% to 3%), nausea (3% to 10%), constipation (1% to 3%)

Genitourinary: Vaginitis (1% to 5%), external genital pruritus in women (1% to 3%)

Ocular: Visual disturbances (1% to 3%)

Respiratory: Pharyngitis (1% to 3%)

Miscellaneous: Trunk pain

<1%, postmarketing, and/or case reports (limited to important or life-threatening): Anaphylaxis reactions, anxiety, blurred vision, chills, cognitive change, cough, depression, dream abnormality, ecchymosis, edema, erythema nodosum, euphoria, extremity pain, hallucinations, hearing acuity decreased, hepatic dysfunction, hepatic failure (some fatal), hepatitis, hyper-/hypoglycemia, hypertension, interstitial nephritis, lightheadedness, malaise, myasthenia gravis exacerbation, palpitation, paresthesia, peripheral neuropathy, photophobia, photosensitivity, pneumonitis, psychotic reactions, rhabdomyolysis, seizure,

Stevens-Johnson syndrome, syncope, tendonitis and tendon rupture, thirst, tinnitus, torsade de pointes, Tourette's syndrome, toxic epidermal necrolysis, vasculitis, vasodilation, vertigo, weakness, weight loss

Ophthalmic: Frequency not defined:
Central nervous system: Dizziness
Gastrointestinal: Nausea
Ocular: Blurred vision, burning, chemical conjunctivitis/keratitis, discomfort, dryness, edema, eye pain, foreign body sensation, itching, photophobia, redness, stinging, tearing

Otic:
>10%: Local: Application site reaction (<1% to 17%)
1% to 10%:
Central nervous system: Dizziness (≤1%), vertigo (≤1%)
Dermatologic: Pruritus (1% to 4%), rash (1%)
Gastrointestinal: Taste perversion (7%)
Neuromuscular & skeletal: Paresthesia (1%)
<1% (Limited to important or life-threatening): Diarrhea, fever, headache, hearing loss (transient), hypertension, nausea, otorrhagia, tinnitus, transient neuropsychiatric disturbances, tremor, vomiting, xerostomia

Drug Interactions
Metabolism/Transport Effects Inhibits CYP1A2 (strong)
Avoid Concomitant Use There are no known interactions where it is recommended to avoid concomitant use.

Increased Effect/Toxicity
Ofloxacin may increase the levels/effects of: Bendamustine; Corticosteroids (Systemic); CYP1A2 Substrates; Sulfonylureas; Theophylline Derivatives; Vitamin K Antagonists

The levels/effects of Ofloxacin may be increased by: Insulin; Nonsteroidal Anti-Inflammatory Agents; Probenecid

Decreased Effect
Ofloxacin may decrease the levels/effects of: Mycophenolate; Sulfonylureas; Typhoid Vaccine

The levels/effects of Ofloxacin may be decreased by: Antacids; Calcium Salts; Didanosine; Iron Salts; Magnesium Salts; Quinapril; Sevelamer; Sucralfate; Zinc Salts

Ethanol/Nutrition/Herb Interactions
Food: Ofloxacin average peak serum concentrations may be decreased by 20% if taken with food.
Herb/Nutraceutical: Avoid dong quai, St John's wort (may also cause photosensitization).

Test Interactions Some quinolones may produce a false-positive urine screening result for opiates using commercially-available immunoassay kits. This has been demonstrated most consistently for levofloxacin and ofloxacin, but other quinolones have shown cross-reactivity in certain assay kits. Confirmation of positive opiate screens by more specific methods should be considered.

Dosage Forms Excipient information presented when available (limited, particularly for generics); consult specific product labeling. [DSC] = Discontinued product

Solution, ophthalmic [drops]: 0.3% (5 mL, 10 mL)
Ocuflox®: 0.3% (5 mL) [contains benzalkonium chloride]
Solution, otic [drops]: 0.3% (5 mL, 10 mL)
Floxin®: 0.3% (5 mL, 10 mL) [contains benzalkonium chloride]
Floxin® Otic Singles™: 0.3% (0.25 mL) [contains benzalkonium chloride; packaged as 2 single-dose containers per pouch, 10 pouches per carton, total net volume 5 mL] [DSC]
Tablet: 200 mg, 300 mg, 400 mg

References
Graumlich JF, Habis S, Avelino RR, et al, "Hypoglycemia in Inpatients After Gatifloxacin or Levofloxacin Therapy: Nested Case-Control Study," *Pharmacotherapy*, 2005, 25(10):1296-302.
Malone RS, Fish DN, Abraham E, et al, "Pharmacokinetics of Levofloxacin and Ciprofloxacin During Continuous Renal Replacement Therapy in Critically Ill Patients," *Antimicrob Agents Chemother*, 2001, 45(10):2949-54.

Trotman RL, Williamson JC, Shoemaker DM, et al, "Antibiotic Dosing in Critically Ill Adult Patients Receiving Continuous Renal Replacement Therapy," *Clin Infect Dis*, 2005, 41(8):1159-66.

♦ **Ogestrel®** *see* Ethinyl Estradiol and Norgestrel *on page 560*

OLANZapine (oh LAN za peen)

U.S. Brand Names Zyprexa®; Zyprexa® IntraMuscular; Zyprexa® Zydis®
Canadian Brand Names Novo-Olanzapine; PMS-Olanzapine; Zyprexa®; Zyprexa® Zydis®
Index Terms LY170053; Zyprexa Zydis
Pharmacologic Category Antimanic Agent; Antipsychotic Agent, Atypical
Use Treatment of the manifestations of schizophrenia; treatment of acute or mixed mania episodes associated with bipolar I disorder (as monotherapy or in combination with lithium or valproate); maintenance treatment of bipolar disorder; acute agitation (patients with schizophrenia or bipolar mania); in combination with fluoxetine for treatment-resistant or bipolar I depression
Unlabeled/Investigational Use Treatment of psychosis/schizophrenia in children or adolescents; chronic pain; prevention of chemotherapy-associated delayed nausea or vomiting; psychosis/agitation related to Alzheimer's dementia
Pharmacodynamics/Kinetics
Absorption:
  I.M.: Rapidly absorbed
  Oral: Well absorbed; not affected by food; tablets and orally-disintegrating tablets are bioequivalent
Distribution: V_d: Extensive, 1000 L
Protein binding, plasma: 93% bound to albumin and alpha$_1$-glycoprotein
Metabolism: Highly metabolized via direct glucuronidation and cytochrome P450 mediated oxidation (CYP1A2, CYP2D6); 40% removed via first pass metabolism
Bioavailability: >57%
Half-life elimination: 21-54 hours; ~1.5 times greater in elderly
Time to peak, plasma: Maximum plasma concentrations after I.M. administration are 5 times higher than maximum plasma concentrations produced by an oral dose.
  I.M.: 15-45 minutes
  Oral: ~6 hours
Excretion: Urine (57%, 7% as unchanged drug); feces (30%)
  Clearance: 40% increase in olanzapine clearance in smokers; 30% decrease in females

Dosage
Children: Schizophrenia/bipolar disorder (unlabeled use): Oral: Initial: 2.5 mg/day; titrate as necessary to 20 mg/day (0.12-0.29 mg/kg/day)
Adults:
  Agitation (acute, associated with bipolar I mania or schizophrenia): I.M.: Initial dose: 5-10 mg (a lower dose of 2.5 mg may be considered when clinical factors warrant); additional doses (2.5-10 mg) may be considered; however, 2-4 hours should be allowed between doses to evaluate response (maximum total daily dose: 30 mg, per manufacturer's recommendation)
  Bipolar I acute mixed or manic episodes: Oral:
    Monotherapy: Initial: 10-15 mg once daily; increase by 5 mg/day at intervals of not less than 24 hours. Maintenance: 5-20 mg/day; recommended maximum dose: 20 mg/day.
    Combination therapy (with lithium or valproate): Initial: 10 mg once daily; dosing range: 5-20 mg/day; recommended maximum dose: 20 mg/day.
  Depression associated with bipolar disorder (in combination with fluoxetine): Oral: Initial: 5 mg in the evening; adjust as tolerated to usual range of 5-12.5 mg/day. See **"Note."**
  Schizophrenia: Oral: Initial: 5-10 mg once daily (increase to 10 mg once daily within 5-7 days); thereafter, adjust by 5 mg/day at 1-week intervals, up to a recommended maximum of 20 mg/day. Maintenance: 10-20 mg once daily. Doses of 30-50 mg/day have been used; however, doses >10 mg/day have not demonstrated better efficacy, and safety and efficacy of doses >20 mg/day have not been evaluated.

Treatment-resistant depression (in combination with fluoxetine): Oral: Initial: 5 mg in the evening; adjust as tolerated to usual range of 5-12.5 mg/day. See **"Note."**

Note: When using individual components of fluoxetine with olanzapine rather than fixed dose combination product (Symbyax®), approximate dosage correspondence is as follows:

Olanzapine 2.5 mg + fluoxetine 20 mg = Symbyax® 3/25

Olanzapine 5 mg + fluoxetine 20 mg = Symbyax® 6/25

Olanzapine 12.5 mg + fluoxetine 20 mg = Symbyax® 12/25

Olanzapine 5 mg + fluoxetine 50 mg = Symbyax® 6/50

Olanzapine 12.5 mg + fluoxetine 50 mg = Symbyax® 12/50

Prevention of chemotherapy-associated delayed nausea or vomiting (unlabeled use; in combination with a corticosteroid and serotonin [5HT$_3$] antagonist): Oral: 10 mg once daily for 3-5 days, beginning on day 1 of chemotherapy **or** 5 mg once daily for 2 days before chemotherapy, followed by 10 mg once daily (beginning on the day of chemotherapy) for 3-8 days

Elderly: Oral, I.M.: Consider lower starting dose of 2.5-5 mg/day for elderly or debilitated patients; may increase as clinically indicated and tolerated with close monitoring of orthostatic blood pressure

Psychosis/agitation related to Alzheimer's dementia (unlabeled use): Initial: 1.25-5 mg/day; if necessary, gradually increase as tolerated not to exceed 10 mg/day

Dosage adjustment in renal impairment: No adjustment required. Not removed by dialysis.

Dosage adjustment in hepatic impairment: Dosage adjustment may be necessary, however, there are no specific recommendations. Monitor closely.

Additional Information Complete prescribing information for this medication should be consulted for additional detail.

Dosage Forms Excipient information presented when available (limited, particularly for generics); consult specific product labeling.

Injection, powder for reconstitution:

Zyprexa® IntraMuscular: 10 mg [contains lactose 50 mg]

Tablet, oral:

Zyprexa®: 2.5 mg, 5 mg, 7.5 mg, 10 mg, 15 mg, 20 mg

Tablet, orally disintegrating:

Zyprexa® Zydis®:

5 mg [contains phenylalanine 0.34 mg/tablet]

10 mg [contains phenylalanine 0.45 mg/tablet]

15 mg [contains phenylalanine 0.67 mg/tablet]

20 mg [contains phenylalanine 0.9 mg/tablet]

References

American Diabetes Association; American Psychiatric Association; American Association of Clinical Endocrinologists; North American Association for the Study of Obesity, "Consensus Development Conference on Antipsychotic Drugs and Obesity and Diabetes," *Diabetes Care*, 2004, 27 (2):596-601.

Baldwin DS and Montgomery SA, "First Clinical Experience With Olanzapine (LY 170053): Results of an Open-Label Safety and Dose-Ranging Study in Patients With Schizophrenia," *Int Clin Psychopharmacol*, 1995, 10(4):239-44.

Carrillo JA, Herraiz AG, Ramos SI, et al, "Role of the Smoking-Induced Cytochrome P450 (CYP)1A2 and Polymorphic CYP2D6 in Steady-State Concentration of Olanzapine," *J Clin Psychopharmacol*, 23(2):119-27.

Davis JM, Chen N, and Glick ID, "A Meta-analysis of the Efficacy of Second-Generation Antipsychotics," *Arch Gen Psychiatry*, 2003, 60(6):553-64.

Duggal HS, Gates C, and Pathak PC, "Olanzapine-Induced Neutropenia: Mechanism and Treatment," *J Clin Psychopharmacol*, 2004, 24(2):234-5.

Farwell WR, Stump TE, Wang J, et al, "Weight Gain and New Onset Diabetes Associated With Olanzapine and Risperidone," *J Gen Intern Med*, 2004, 19(12):1200-5.

Goldberg RJ, "Managing Psychosis-Related Behavioral Problems in the Elderly," *Consult Pharm*, 1997, 12(Suppl C):4-10.

Gorski ED and Willis KC, "Report of Three Cases Studied With Olanzapine for Chronic Pain," *J Pain*, 2003, 4:166-8.

Khojainova N, Santiago-Palma J, Kornick C, et al, "Olanzapine in the Management of Cancer Pain," *J Pain Symptom Manage*, 2002, 23(4):346-50.

Kiser RS, Cohen HM, Freedenfeld RN, et al, "Olanzapine for the Treatment of Fibromyalgia Symptoms," *J Pain Symptom Manage*, 2001, 22(2):704-8.

Krishnamoorthy J and King BH, "Open-Label Olanzapine Treatment in Five Preadolescent Children," *J Child Adolesc Psychopharmacol*, 1998, 8(2):107-13.

Kumra S, Jacobsen LK, Lenane M et al, "Childhood-Onset Schizophrenia: An Open-Label Study of Olanzapine in Adolescents," *J Am Acad Child Adolesc Psychiatry*, 1998, 37(4):377-385.

Rozen TD, "New Treatments in Cluster Headache," *Curr Neurol Neurosci Rep*, 2002, 2(2):114-21.

Schneider LS, Tariot PN, Dagerman KS, et al, "Effectiveness of Atypical Antipsychotic Drugs in Patients With Alzheimer's Disease," *N Engl J Med*, 2006, 355(15):1525-38.

Shaw P, Sporn A, Gogtay N et al, "Childhood-Onset Schizophrenia: A Double-Blind, Randomized Clozapine-Olanzapine Comparison," *Arch Gen Psychiatry*, 2006, 63(7):721-30.

Sorsaburu S, Hornbuckle K, Blake D, et al, "The First 21 Months of Safety Experience With Postmarketing Use of Olanzapine's Intramuscular Formulation," College of Psychiatric and Neurologic Pharmacists, April, 2006, Baltimore, MD.

Soutullo CA, Sorter MT, Foster KD, et al, "Olanzapine in the Treatment of Adolescent Acute Mania: A Report of Seven Cases," *J Affect Disord*, 1999, 53(3):279-83.

Thangadurai P, Jyothi KS, Gopalakrishman R, et al, "Reversible Neutropenia With Olanzapine Following Clozapine-Induced Neutropenia," *Am J Psychiatry*, 2006, 163(7):1298.

Thinn SS, Liew E, May AL, et al, "Reversible Delayed Onset Olanzapine-Associated Leukopenia and Neutropenia in a Clozapine-Naive Patient on Concomitant Depot Antipsychotic," *J Clin Psychopharmacol*, 2007, 27(4):394-5.

Olmesartan (ole me SAR tan)

Related Information

Angiotensin Agents *on page 1652*

Heart Failure (Systolic) *on page 1739*

Preoperative Evaluation of the Cardiac Patient for Noncardiac Surgery *on page 1598*

U.S. Brand Names Benicar®

Canadian Brand Names Olmetec®

Index Terms Olmesartan Medoxomil

Pharmacologic Category Angiotensin II Receptor Blocker

Use Treatment of hypertension with or without concurrent use of other antihypertensive agents

Pharmacodynamics/Kinetics

Distribution: 17 L; does not cross the blood-brain barrier (animal studies)

Protein binding: 99%

Metabolism: Olmesartan medoxomil is hydrolyzed in the GI tract to active olmesartan. No further metabolism occurs.

Bioavailability: 26%

Half-life elimination: Terminal: 13 hours

Time to peak: 1-2 hours

Excretion: All as unchanged drug: Feces (50% to 65%); urine (35% to 50%)

Dosage Oral:

Adults: Initial: Usual starting dose is 20 mg once daily; if initial response is inadequate, may be increased to 40 mg once daily after 2 weeks. May administer with other antihypertensive agents if blood pressure inadequately controlled with olmesartan. Consider lower starting dose in patients with possible depletion of intravascular volume (eg, patients receiving diuretics).

Elderly: No dosage adjustment necessary

Dosage adjustment in renal impairment: No specific guidelines for dosage adjustment; patients undergoing hemodialysis have not been studied.

Dosage adjustment in hepatic impairment: No adjustment necessary.

Anesthesia and Critical Care Concerns/Other Considerations

Clinical Pearls/Comments: In patients on chronic angiotensin receptor blocker (ARB) therapy, intraoperative hypotension may occur with induction and maintenance of general anesthesia; however, discontinuation of therapy prior to surgery is controversial. If continued preoperatively, avoidance of hypotensive agents during surgery is prudent. Episodes of intraoperative hypotension may be managed by fluid administration and/or modest doses of alpha-adrenergic agents. Severe hypotension may occur in patients who are sodium- and/or volume-depleted; initiate lower doses and monitor closely when starting therapy in these patients. ARB therapy may elicit an increase in potassium and creatinine, especially when used in patients with bilateral renal artery stenosis. Concomitant NSAID therapy may attenuate blood pressure control; use of NSAIDs should be avoided or limited, with monitoring of blood pressure control. In the setting of heart failure, NSAID use may be associated with an increased risk for fluid accumulation and edema and therefore should be avoided.

◄ **Evidence-Based Information:** The angiotensin II receptor antagonists have similar indications as ACE inhibitors. In heart failure, the angiotensin II receptor antagonists are especially useful in providing an alternative therapy in those patients who have intractable cough due to ACE inhibitor therapy. Candesartan has been studied as an alternative therapy in chronic heart failure patients who cannot tolerate an ACE-I (CHARM-Alternative) and as an added therapy in heart failure patients who are maintained on an ACE-I (CHARM-Added). In both studies, the combined endpoint of cardiovascular death or heart failure hospitalizations was significantly improved over the placebo-treated group.

Additional Information Complete prescribing information for this medication should be consulted for additional detail.

Dosage Forms Excipient information presented when available (limited, particularly for generics); consult specific product labeling.
Tablet, as medoxomil:
Benicar®: 5 mg, 20 mg, 40 mg

◆ **Olmesartan and Amlodipine** *see* Amlodipine and Olmesartan *on page 94*

◆ **Olmesartan Medoxomil** *see* Olmesartan *on page 1045*

◆ **Olmetec® (Can)** *see* Olmesartan *on page 1045*

Omalizumab (oh mah lye ZOO mab)

Medication Safety Issues
Sound-alike/look-alike issues:
Omalizumab may be confused with ofatumumab

Medication Guide An FDA-approved patient medication guide, which is available with the product information and at http://www.fda.gov/downloads/Drugs/DrugSafety/ucm089829.pdf, must be dispensed with this medication for each new outpatient prescription and refill.

Related Information
Asthma *on page 1728*

U.S. Brand Names Xolair®

Canadian Brand Names Xolair®

Index Terms rhuMAb-E25

Pharmacologic Category Monoclonal Antibody, Anti-Asthmatic

Generic Available No

Use Treatment of moderate-to-severe, persistent allergic asthma not adequately controlled with inhaled corticosteroids

Mechanism of Action Omalizumab is an IgG monoclonal antibody (recombinant DNA derived) which inhibits IgE binding to the high-affinity IgE receptor on mast cells and basophils. By decreasing bound IgE, the activation and release of mediators in the allergic response (early and late phase) is limited. Serum-free IgE levels and the number of high-affinity IgE receptors are decreased. Long-term treatment in patients with allergic asthma showed a decrease in asthma exacerbations and corticosteroid usage.

Pharmacodynamics/Kinetics
Absorption: Slow following SubQ injection

Distribution: V_d: 78 ± 32 mL/kg

Metabolism: Hepatic; IgG degradation by reticuloendothelial system and endothelial cells

Bioavailability: 62%

Half-life elimination: 26 days

Time to peak: 7-8 days

Excretion: Primarily via hepatic degradation; intact IgG may be secreted in bile

Dosage SubQ: Children ≥12 years and Adults: Asthma: Dose is based on pretreatment IgE serum levels and body weight. Dosing should not be adjusted based on IgE levels taken during treatment or <1 year following discontinuation of therapy; doses should be adjusted during treatment for significant changes in body weight.
IgE ≥30-100 int. units/mL:
30-90 kg: 150 mg every 4 weeks
>90-150 kg: 300 mg every 4 weeks

IgE >100-200 int. units/mL:
  30-90 kg: 300 mg every 4 weeks
  >90-150 kg: 225 mg every 2 weeks
IgE >200-300 int. units/mL:
  30-60 kg: 300 mg every 4 weeks
  >60-90 kg: 225 mg every 2 weeks
  >90-150 kg: 300 mg every 2 weeks
IgE >300-400 int. units/mL:
  30-70 kg: 225 mg every 2 weeks
  >70-90 kg: 300 mg every 2 weeks
  >90 kg: Do not administer dose
IgE >400-500 int. units/mL:
  30-70 kg: 300 mg every 2 weeks
  >70-90 kg: 375 mg every 2 weeks
  >90 kg: Do not administer dose
IgE >500-600 int. units/mL:
  30-60 kg: 300 mg every 2 weeks
  >60-70 kg: 375 mg every 2 weeks
  >70 kg: Do not administer dose
IgE >600-700 int. units/mL:
  30-60 kg: 375 mg every 2 weeks
  >60 kg: Do not administer dose

Stability Prior to reconstitution, store under refrigeration at 2°C to 8°C (36°F to 46°F); product may be shipped at room temperature. Prepare using SWFI, USP only; add SWFI 1.4 mL to upright vial and swirl gently for 5-10 seconds every 5 minutes until dissolved; may take >20 minutes to dissolve completely. Resulting solution is 150 mg/1.2 mL. Do not use if powder takes >40 minutes to dissolve. Following reconstitution, protect from direct sunlight. May be stored for up to 8 hours if refrigerated or 4 hours if stored at room temperature.

Administration For SubQ injection only; doses >150 mg should divided over more than one site. Injections may take 5-10 seconds to administer. Administer only under direct medical supervision and observe patient for a minimum of 2 hours following administration of any dose given.

Monitoring Parameters Anaphylactic/hypersensitivity reactions, baseline IgE; FEV_1, peak flow, and/or other pulmonary function tests; monitor for signs of infection

Pregnancy Risk Factor B

Contraindications Hypersensitivity to omalizumab or any component of the formulation; acute bronchospasm, status asthmaticus

Warnings/Precautions [U.S. Boxed Warning]: Anaphylaxis, including delayed-onset anaphylaxis, has been reported following administration; reactions usually occur within 2 hours of administration, but may occur up to 24 hours and in some cases >1 year after initiation of regular treatment. Patients should receive treatment only under direct medical supervision and be observed for a minimum of 2 hours following administration; appropriate medications for the treatment of anaphylactic reactions should be available. Hypersensitivity reactions may occur following any dose, even during chronic therapy; discontinue therapy following any severe reaction.

For use in patients with a documented reactivity to a perennial aeroallergen and with symptoms uncontrolled using inhaled corticosteroids; not used to control acute asthma symptoms. Dosing is based on pretreatment IgE serum levels and body weight. IgE levels remain elevated up to 1 year following treatment, therefore, levels taken during treatment cannot be used as a dosage guide. Corticosteroid therapy should be tapered gradually, do not discontinue abruptly. Malignant neoplasms have been reported with use in short-term studies; impact of long-term use is not known. Use caution with and monitor patients at risk for parasitic (helminth) infections (risk of infection may be increased). Safety and efficacy in children <12 years of age have not been established.

Adverse Reactions
>10%:
  Central nervous system: Headache (15%)

Local: Injection site reaction (45%; placebo 43%; severe 12%). Most reactions occurred within 1 hour, lasted <8 days, and decreased in frequency with additional dosing.

Respiratory: Upper respiratory tract infection (20%), sinusitis (16%), pharyngitis (11%)

Miscellaneous: Viral infection (23%)

1% to 10%:

Central nervous system: Pain (7%), fatigue (3%), dizziness (3%)

Dermatologic: Dermatitis (2%), pruritus (2%)

Neuromuscular & skeletal: Arthralgia (8%), leg pain (4%), arm pain (2%), fracture (2%)

Otic: Earache (2%)

<1% (Limited to important or life-threatening): Alopecia; anaphylaxis (angioedema of the throat or tongue, bronchospasm, chest tightness, cough, cutaneous angioedema, dyspnea, hypotension, generalized pruritus, syncope, and urticaria); antibody formation to omalizumab, hot flushes, malignancy (0.5%; placebo 0.2%), throat edema, thrombocytopenia, tongue edema, urticaria, wheezing

Drug Interactions

Avoid Concomitant Use

Avoid concomitant use of Omalizumab with any of the following: Natalizumab; Vaccines (Live)

Increased Effect/Toxicity

Omalizumab may increase the levels/effects of: Leflunomide; Natalizumab; Vaccines (Live)

The levels/effects of Omalizumab may be increased by: Trastuzumab

Decreased Effect

Omalizumab may decrease the levels/effects of: Vaccines (Inactivated); Vaccines (Live)

The levels/effects of Omalizumab may be decreased by: Echinacea

Test Interactions Total IgE levels are elevated for up to 1 year following treatment. Total serum IgE may be retested after interruption of therapy for 1 year or more.

Dosage Forms Excipient information presented when available (limited, particularly for generics); consult specific product labeling.

Injection, powder for reconstitution [preservative free]:

Xolair®: 150 mg [contains sucrose 145.5 g]

References

Expert Panel Report 3, "Guidelines for the Diagnosis and Management of Asthma," *Clinical Practice Guidelines*, National Institutes of Health, National Heart, Lung, and Blood Institute, NIH Publication No. 08-4051, prepublication 2007. Available at http://www.nhlbi.nih.gov/guidelines/asthma/asthgdln.htm

---

Omeprazole (oh MEP ra zole)

Medication Safety Issues

Sound-alike/look-alike issues:

Omeprazole may be confused with aripiprazole, fomepizole

Prilosec® may be confused with Plendil®, Prevacid®, predniSONE, prilocaine, Prinivil®, Proventil®, Prozac®

International issues:

Norpramin®: Brand name for desipramine in the U.S.

Related Information

Helicobacter pylori Treatment *on page 1746*

U.S. Brand Names Prilosec OTC™ [OTC]; Prilosec®

Canadian Brand Names Apo-Omeprazole®; Losec MUPS®; Losec®; Mylan-Omeprazole; PMS-Omeprazole; PMS-Omeprazole DR; ratio-Omeprazole; Sandoz Omeprazole

Index Terms Omeprazole Magnesium

Pharmacologic Category Proton Pump Inhibitor; Substituted Benzimidazole

Generic Available Yes: Excludes granules for suspension

Use Short-term (4-8 weeks) treatment of active duodenal ulcer disease or active benign gastric ulcer; treatment of heartburn and other symptoms associated with gastroesophageal reflux disease (GERD); short-term (4-8 weeks) treatment of endoscopically-diagnosed erosive esophagitis; maintenance healing of erosive esophagitis; long-term treatment of pathological hypersecretory conditions; as part of a multidrug regimen for *H. pylori* eradication to reduce the risk of duodenal ulcer recurrence

OTC labeling: Short-term treatment of frequent, uncomplicated heartburn occurring ≥2 days/week

Unlabeled/Investigational Use Healing NSAID-induced ulcers; prevention of NSAID-induced ulcer; stress-ulcer prophylaxis in the critically-ill

Mechanism of Action Proton pump inhibitor; suppresses gastric basal and stimulated acid secretion by inhibiting the parietal cell H+/K+ ATP pump

Pharmacodynamics/Kinetics
Onset of action: Antisecretory: ~1 hour
  Peak effect: Within 2 hours
Duration: Up to 72 hours; 50% of maximum effect at 24 hours; after stopping treatment, secretory activity gradually returns over 3-5 days
Absorption: Rapid
Protein binding: ~95%
Metabolism: Extensively hepatic by cytochrome P450 system to inactive metabolites; saturable first-pass effect
Bioavailability: Oral: ~30% to 40%; increased in Asian patients, elderly patients, and patients with hepatic dysfunction
Half-life elimination: 0.5-1 hour; hepatic impairment: ~3 hours
Time to peak, plasma: 0.5-3.5 hours
Excretion: Urine (~77% as metabolites, very small amount as unchanged drug); feces

Dosage Oral:
Children 1-16 years: GERD or other acid-related disorders:
  5 kg to <10 kg: 5 mg once daily
  10 kg to <20 kg: 10 mg once daily
  ≥20 kg: 20 mg once daily
Adults:
  Active duodenal ulcer: 20 mg/day for 4-8 weeks
  Gastric ulcers: 40 mg/day for 4-8 weeks
  Symptomatic GERD (without esophageal lesions): 20 mg/day for up to 4 weeks
  Erosive esophagitis: 20 mg/day for 4-8 weeks; maintenance of healing: 20 mg/day for up to 12 months total therapy (including treatment period of 4-8 weeks)
  Helicobacter pylori eradication: Dose varies with regimen:
    Manufacturer labeling: 40 mg once daily administered with clarithromycin 500 mg 3 times/day for 14 days **or** 20 mg twice daily administered with amoxicillin 1000 mg *and* clarithromycin 500 mg twice daily for 10 days. **Note:** Presence of ulcer at time of therapy initiation may necessitate an additional 14-18 days of omeprazole 20 mg/day (monotherapy) after completion of combination therapy.
    American College of Gastroenterology guidelines (Chey, 2007):
      Nonpenicillin allergy: 20 mg twice daily administered with amoxicillin 1000 mg *and* clarithromycin 500 mg twice daily for 10-14 days
      Penicillin allergy: 20 mg twice daily administered with clarithromycin 500 mg *and* metronidazole 500 mg twice daily for 10-14 days **or** 20 mg once or twice daily administered with bismuth subsalicylate 525 mg *and* metronidazole 250 mg *plus* tetracycline 500 mg 4 times/day for 10-14 days
  Pathological hypersecretory conditions: Initial: 60 mg once daily; doses up to 120 mg 3 times/day have been administered; administer daily doses >80 mg in divided doses
  Stress-ulcer prophylaxis (ICU patients; unlabeled use): 40 mg once daily; periodically evaluate patient for continued need.
  Frequent heartburn (OTC labeling): 20 mg/day for 14 days; treatment may be repeated after 4 months if needed

Dosage adjustment in hepatic impairment: Bioavailability is increased with chronic liver disease. Consider dosage adjustment, especially for maintenance of erosive esophagitis. Specific guidelines are not available.

◄ **Stability**
Capsules, tablets: Store at 15°C to 30°C (59°F to 86°F). Protect from light and moisture.

Granules for oral suspension: Store at 25°C (77°F); excursions permitted to 15°C to 30°C (59°F to 86°F). For oral administration, empty the contents of the 2.5 mg packet into 5 mL of water (10 mg packet into 15 mL of water); stir. For NG administration, add 5 mL of water into a catheter-tipped syringe, and then add the contents of a 2.5 mg packet (15 mL water for the 10 mg packet); shake. **Note:** Regardless of the route of administration, the suspension should be left to thicken for 2-3 minutes prior to administration.

Administration
Oral: Best if administered before breakfast.

Capsule: Should be swallowed whole; do not chew or crush. Delayed release capsule may be opened and contents added to 1 tablespoon of applesauce (use immediately after adding to applesauce).

Oral suspension: Following reconstitution, the suspension should be left to thicken for 2-3 minutes and administered within 30 minutes. If any material remains after administration, add more water, stir, and administer immediately.

Tablet: Should be swallowed whole; do not crush or chew.

Nasogastric tube administration:

Capsule: When using capsules to extemporaneously prepare a solution for NG administration, the manufacturers of Prilosec® recommend the use of an acidic juice for preparation and administration

Oral suspension: Following reconstitution in a catheter-tipped syringe, shake the suspension well and leave to thicken for 2-3 minutes. Administer within 30 minutes of reconstitution. Use an NG tube or gastric tube that is a French size 6 or larger; flush the syringe and tube with water.

Anesthesia and Critical Care Concerns/Other Considerations
Clinical Pearls/Comments: A 2 mg/mL oral omeprazole solution (Simplified Omeprazole Solution) can be prepared with five omeprazole 20 mg delayed release capsules and 50 mL 8.4% sodium bicarbonate. Empty capsules into beaker. Add sodium bicarbonate solution. Gently stir (about 15 minutes) until a white suspension is formed. Transfer to amber-colored syringe or bottle. Stable for 14 days at room temperature or for 30 days under refrigeration.

DiGiancinto JL, Olsen KM, Bergman KL, et al, "Stability of Suspension Formulations of Lansoprazole and Omeprazole Stored in Amber-Colored Plastic Oral Syringes," *Ann Pharmacother*, 2000, 34:600-5.

Quercia R, Fan C, Liu X, et al, "Stability of Omeprazole in an Extemporaneously Prepared Oral Liquid," *Am J Health Syst Pharm*, 1997, 54:1833-6.

Sharma V, "Comparison of 24-Hour Intragastric pH Using Four Liquid Formulations of Lansoprazole and Omeprazole," *Am J Health Syst Pharm*, 1999, 56(Suppl 4):S18-21.

Evidence-Based Information: The 2008 Surviving Sepsis Campaign guidelines recommend that stress ulcer prophylaxis using an H_2 blocker (Grade 1A) or proton pump inhibitor (Grade 1B) be given to patients with severe sepsis to prevent upper GI bleed. Benefit of prevention of upper GI bleed must be weighed against potential effect of increased stomach pH on development of ventilator-associated pneumonia.

Pregnancy Risk Factor C
Contraindications Hypersensitivity to omeprazole or any component of the formulation

Warnings/Precautions Use of proton pump inhibitors may increase the risk of gastrointestinal infections (eg, *Salmonella, Campylobacter*). Relief of symptoms does not preclude the presence of a gastric malignancy. Atrophic gastritis (by biopsy) has been noted with long-term omeprazole therapy. In long-term (2-year) studies in rats, omeprazole produced a dose-related increase in gastric carcinoid tumors. While available endoscopic evaluations and histologic examinations of biopsy specimens from human stomachs have not detected a risk from short-term exposure to omeprazole, further human data on the effect of sustained hypochlorhydria and hypergastrinemia are needed to rule out the possibility of an increased risk for the development of tumors in humans receiving long-term therapy.

Decreased *H. pylori* eradication rates have been observed with short-term (≤7 days) combination therapy. The American College of Gastroenterology recommends 10-14 days of therapy (triple or quadruple) for eradication of *H. pylori* (Chey, 2007). Bioavailability may be increased in Asian populations and with hepatic dysfunction; consider dosage reductions, especially for maintenance healing of erosive esophagitis. Bioavailability may be increased in the elderly. Safety and efficacy have not been established in children <1 year of age. When used for self-medication (OTC), do not use for >14 days. Treatment should not be repeated more often than every 4 months. OTC use is not approved for children <18 years of age.

Adverse Reactions

1% to 10%:

Central nervous system: Headache (3% to 7%), dizziness (2%)

Dermatologic: Rash (2%)

Gastrointestinal: Abdominal pain (2% to 5%), diarrhea (3% to 4%), nausea (2% to 4%), vomiting (2% to 3%), flatulence (≤3%), acid regurgitation (2%), constipation (1% to 2%), taste perversion

Neuromuscular & skeletal: Back pain (1%), weakness (1%)

Respiratory: Upper respiratory infection (2%), cough (1%)

1% (Limited to important or life-threatening; adverse event occurrence may vary based on formulation): Abdominal swelling, abnormal dreams, aggression, agitation, agranulocytosis, alkaline phosphatase increased, allergic reactions, alopecia, ALT increased, AST increased, anaphylaxis, anemia, angina, angioedema, anorexia, anxiety, apathy, atrophic gastritis, benign gastric polyps, bilirubin increased, blurred vision, bradycardia, bronchospasm, chest pain, cholestatic hepatitis, confusion, creatinine increased, depression, diaphoresis, double vision, dry skin, epistaxis, erythema multiforme, esophageal candidiasis, fatigue, fecal discoloration, fever, gastroduodenal carcinoids, GGT increased, glycosuria, gynecomastia, hallucinations, hematuria, hemifacial dysesthesia, hemolytic anemia, hepatic encephalopathy, hepatic failure, hepatic necrosis, hepatitis, hepatocellular hepatitis, hyperhidrosis, hypersensitivity, hypertension, hypoglycemia, hyponatremia, insomnia, interstitial nephritis, irritable colon, jaundice, joint pain, leg pain, leukocytosis, leukopenia, liver disease (hepatocellular, cholestatic, mixed), malaise, microscopic pyuria, mucosal atrophy (tongue), muscle cramps, muscle weakness, myalgia, nervousness, neutropenia, ocular irritation, optic atrophy, optic neuritis, optic neuropathy (anterior ischemic), pain, palpitation, pancreatitis, pancytopenia, paresthesia, peripheral edema, petechiae, pharyngeal pain, photosensitivity, pneumothorax, proteinuria, pruritus, psychiatric disturbance, purpura, skin inflammation, sleep disturbance, somnolence, Stevens-Johnson syndrome, stomatitis, tachycardia, testicular pain, thrombocytopenia, tinnitus, toxic epidermal necrolysis, tremor, urinary frequency, urinary tract infection, urticaria, vertigo, weight gain, xerophthalmia, xerostomia

Drug Interactions

Metabolism/Transport Effects Substrate of CYP2A6 (minor), 2C9 (minor), 2C19 (major), 2D6 (minor), 3A4 (major); **Inhibits** CYP1A2 (weak), 2C9 (moderate), 2C19 (strong), 2D6 (weak), 3A4 (weak); **Induces** CYP1A2 (weak)

Avoid Concomitant Use

Avoid concomitant use of Omeprazole with any of the following: Delavirdine; Erlotinib; Nelfinavir; Posaconazole

Increased Effect/Toxicity

Omeprazole may increase the levels/effects of: Benzodiazepines (metabolized by oxidation); Carvedilol; Cilostazol; Clozapine; CycloSPORINE; CYP2C19 Substrates; CYP2C9 Substrates (High risk); Methotrexate; Phenytoin; Raltegravir; Saquinavir; Tacrolimus; Vitamin K Antagonists; Voriconazole

The levels/effects of Omeprazole may be increased by: Fluconazole; Ketoconazole

Decreased Effect

Omeprazole may decrease the levels/effects of: Atazanavir; Clopidogrel; Clozapine; Dabigatran Etexilate; Dasatinib; Delavirdine; Erlotinib; Indinavir; Iron Salts; Itraconazole; Ketoconazole; Mesalamine; Mycophenolate; Nelfinavir; Posaconazole ▶

◄ *The levels/effects of Omeprazole may be decreased by:* CYP2C19 Inducers (Strong); Peginterferon Alfa-2b; Tipranavir

Ethanol/Nutrition/Herb Interactions
Ethanol: Avoid ethanol (may cause gastric mucosal irritation).
Food: Food delays absorption.

Dietary Considerations Should be taken on an empty stomach; best if taken before breakfast.

Dosage Forms Excipient information presented when available (limited, particularly for generics); consult specific product labeling.
Capsule, delayed release: 10 mg, 20 mg, 40 mg
  Prilosec®: 10 mg, 20 mg, 40 mg
Granules for suspension, delayed release, enteric coated, oral:
  Prilosec®: 2.5 mg/packet (30s); 10 mg/packet (30s)
Tablet, delayed release: 20 mg
  Prilosec OTC™: 20 mg

References

Allen ME, Kopp BJ, and Erstad BL, "Stress Ulcer Prophylaxis in the Postoperative Period," *Am J Health Syst Pharm*, 2004, 61(6):588-96.

Dellinger RP, Levy MM, Carlet JM, et al, "Surviving Sepsis Campaign: International Guidelines for Management of Severe Sepsis and Septic Shock: 2008," *Intensive Care Med*, 2008, 34(1): 17-60. Available at http://www.survivingsepsis.org/system/files/images/2008_20International_20SSC_20-Guidelines_1_.pdf

Jung R and MacLaren R, "Proton-Pump Inhibitors for Stress Ulcer Prophylaxis in Critically Ill Patients," *Ann Pharmacother*, 2002, 36(12):1929-37.

Lau JY, Sung JJ, Lee KK, et al, "Effect of Intravenous Omeprazole on Recurrent Bleeding After Endoscopic Treatment of Bleeding Peptic Ulcers," *N Engl J Med*, 2000, 343(5):310-6.

Lin HJ, Lo WC, Lee FY, et al, "A Prospective Randomized Comparative Trial Showing That Omeprazole Prevents Rebleeding in Patients With Bleeding Peptic Ulcer After Successful Endoscopic Therapy," *Arch Intern Med*, 1998, 158(1):54-8.

Omeprazole and Sodium Bicarbonate
(oh MEP ra zole & SOW dee um bye KAR bun ate)

U.S. Brand Names Zegerid®

Index Terms Sodium Bicarbonate and Omeprazole

Pharmacologic Category Proton Pump Inhibitor; Substituted Benzimidazole

Use Short-term (4-8 weeks) treatment of active duodenal ulcer disease or active benign gastric ulcer; treatment of heartburn and other symptoms associated with gastroesophageal reflux disease (GERD); short-term (4-8 weeks) treatment of endoscopically-diagnosed erosive esophagitis; maintenance healing of erosive esophagitis; reduction of risk of upper gastrointestinal bleeding in critically-ill patients

Pharmacodynamics/Kinetics
Onset of action: Antisecretory: ~1 hour
  Peak effect: 2 hours
Duration: 72 hours
Protein binding: 95%
Metabolism: Extensively hepatic to inactive metabolites
Bioavailability: Oral: 30% to 40%; increased in Asian patients and patients with hepatic dysfunction
Half-life elimination: 0.4-3.2 hours
Excretion: Urine (77% as metabolites, very small amount as unchanged drug); feces

Dosage Oral: Adults:
Active duodenal ulcer: 20 mg/day for 4-8 weeks
Gastric ulcers: 40 mg/day for 4-8 weeks
Symptomatic GERD: 20 mg/day for up to 4 weeks
Erosive esophagitis: 20 mg/day for 4-8 weeks; maintenance of healing: 20 mg/day for up to 12 months total therapy (including treatment period of 4-8 weeks)
Risk reduction of upper GI bleeding in critically-ill patients (Zegerid® powder for oral suspension):
  Loading dose: Day 1: 40 mg every 6-8 hours for two doses
  Maintenance dose: 40 mg/day for up to 14 days; therapy >14 days has not been evaluated

Dosage adjustment in renal impairment: No adjustment necessary

Dosage adjustment in hepatic impairment: Specific guidelines are not available; bioavailability is increased with chronic liver disease

Additional Information Complete prescribing information for this medication should be consulted for additional detail.

Dosage Forms Excipient information presented when available (limited, particularly for generics); consult specific product labeling.

Capsule, immediate release:

Zegerid®: 20 mg, 40 mg [both strengths contain sodium bicarbonate 1100 mg, equivalent to sodium 300 mg (13 mEq) per capsule]

Powder for oral suspension:

Zegerid®: 20 mg/packet (30s), 40 mg/packet (30s) [both strengths contain sodium bicarbonate 1680 mg, equivalent to sodium 460 mg per packet]

References

Lau JY, Sung JJ, Lee KK, et al, "Effect of Intravenous Omeprazole on Recurrent Bleeding After Endoscopic Treatment of Bleeding Peptic Ulcers," *N Engl J Med*, 2000, 343(5):310-6.

◆ **Omeprazole Magnesium** *see* Omeprazole *on page 1048*

◆ **Omnicef®** *see* Cefdinir *on page 252*

◆ **Omnipred™** *see* PrednisoLONE *on page 1164*

◆ **Omnitrope®** *see* Somatropin *on page 1318*

OnabotulinumtoxinA (oh nuh BOT yoo lin num TOKS in aye)

Medication Safety Issues

Botulinum products are not interchangeable; potency differences may exist between the products.

Medication Guide An FDA-approved patient medication guide, which is available with the product information and at http://www.fda.gov/downloads/Drugs/DrugSafety/UCM176360.pdf, must be dispensed with this medication for each new outpatient prescription and refill.

U.S. Brand Names Botox®; Botox® Cosmetic

Canadian Brand Names Botox®; Botox® Cosmetic

Index Terms Botulinum Toxin Type A; BTX-A

Pharmacologic Category Neuromuscular Blocker Agent, Toxin; Ophthalmic Agent, Toxin

Generic Available No

Use Treatment of strabismus and blepharospasm associated with dystonia (including benign essential blepharospasm or VII nerve disorders) in patients ≥12 years of age; cervical dystonia (spasmodic torticollis) in patients ≥16 years of age; temporary improvement in the appearance of lines/wrinkles of the face (moderate-to-severe glabellar lines associated with corrugator and/or procerus muscle activity) in adult patients ≤65 years of age; treatment of severe primary axillary hyperhidrosis in adults not adequately controlled with topical treatments

Canadian labeling: Additional use (not in U.S. labeling): Focal spasticity, including treatment of stroke related upper limb spasticity; dynamic equines foot deformity in pediatric cerebral palsy patients

Unlabeled/Investigational Use Treatment of oromandibular dystonia, spasmodic dysphonia (laryngeal dystonia) and other dystonias (ie, writer's cramp, focal task-specific dystonias); migraine treatment and prophylaxis; treatment of dynamic muscle contracture in pediatric cerebral palsy patients

Mechanism of Action OnabotulinumtoxinA (previously known as botulinum toxin type A) is a neurotoxin produced by *Clostridium botulinum*, spore-forming anaerobic bacillus, which appears to affect only the presynaptic membrane of the neuromuscular junction in humans, where it prevents calcium-dependent release of acetylcholine and produces a state of denervation. Muscle inactivation persists until new fibrils grow from the nerve and form junction plates on new areas of the muscle-cell walls. Intradermal injection results in temporary sweat gland denervation, reducing local sweating.

Pharmacodynamics/Kinetics

Onset of action (improvement):

Blepharospasm: ~3 days

Cervical dystonia: ~2 weeks

Reduction of glabellar lines (Botox® Cosmetic): 1-2 days, increasing in intensity during first week

Spasticity (focal and cerebral palsy related): <2 weeks

Strabismus: ~1-2 days

Duration:

Blepharospasm: ~3 months

Cervical dystonia: <3 months

Primary axillary hyperhidrosis: 201 days (mean)

Reduction of glabellar lines (Botox® Cosmetic): ~3-4 months

Spasticity (cerebral palsy related): ~3-3.5 months

Strabismus: ~2-6 weeks

Absorption: Not expected to be present in peripheral blood at recommended doses following intramuscular (I.M.) injection

Time to peak:

Blepharospasm: 1-2 weeks

Cervical dystonia: ~6 weeks

Spasticity (focal): 4-6 weeks

Strabismus: Within first week

Dosage

Cervical dystonia: Children ≥16 years and Adults: I.M.: For dosing guidance, the mean dose is 236 units (25th to 75th percentile range 198-300 units) divided among the affected muscles in patients previously treated with botulinum toxin. Initial dose in previously untreated patients should be lower. Sequential dosing should be based on the patient's head and neck position, localization of pain, muscle hypertrophy, patient response, and previous adverse reactions. The total dose injected into the sternocleidomastoid muscles should be ≤100 units to decrease the occurrence of dysphagia.

Canadian labeling (not in U.S. labeling): Effective range of 200-360 units has been used in clinical practice; maximum dose: 6 units/kg every 2 months

Blepharospasm: Children ≥12 years and Adults: I.M.: Initial dose: 1.25-2.5 units injected into the medial and lateral pretarsal orbicularis oculi of the upper lid and lateral pretarsal orbicularis oculi of lower lid; dose may be increased up to twice the previous dose if the response from the initial dose lasted ≤2 months; maximum dose per site: 5 units. Tolerance may occur if treatments are given more often than every 3 months, but the effect is not usually permanent. Cumulative dose:

U.S. labeling: ≤200 units in 30-day period

Canadian labeling (not in U.S. labeling): ≤200 units in 60-day period

Strabismus: Children ≥12 years and Adults: I.M.: **Note:** Several minutes prior to injection, administration of local anesthetic and ocular decongestant drops are recommended.

Initial dose:

Vertical muscles and for horizontal strabismus <20 prism diopters: 1.25-2.5 units in any one muscle

Horizontal strabismus of 20-50 prism diopters: 2.5-5 units in any one muscle

Persistent VI nerve palsy ≥1 month: 1.25-2.5 units in the medial rectus muscle

Re-examine patients 7-14 days after each injection to assess the effect of that dose. Subsequent doses for patients experiencing incomplete paralysis of the target may be increased up to twice the previous administered dose. The maximum recommended dose as a single injection for any one muscle is 25 units. Do not administer subsequent injections until the effects of the previous dose are gone.

Primary axillary hyperhidrosis: Adults ≥18 years: Intradermal: 50 units/axilla. Injection area should be defined by standard staining techniques. Injections should be evenly distributed into multiple sites (10-15), administered in 0.1-0.2 mL aliquots, ~1-2 cm apart. May repeat when clinical effect diminishes.

Reduction of glabellar lines: Adults ≤65 years: I.M.: An effective dose is determined by gross observation of the patient's ability to activate the superficial muscles injected. The location, size and use of muscles may vary markedly among individuals. Inject 0.1 mL (4 units) dose into each of five sites, two in each corrugator muscle and one in the procerus muscle for a total dose 0.5 mL (20 units) administered no more frequently than every 3-4 months.

Spasticity (cerebral palsy related; Canadian labeling [not approved in U.S. labeling]): Children ≥2 years: I.M.: 4 units/kg (total dose) divided into two injections into medial and lateral heads of the gastrocnemius of affected limb; if clinically indicated, may repeat every 2 months (maximum dose: 200 units)

Spasticity (focal; Canadian labeling [not approved in U.S. labeling]): Adults ≥18 years: I.M.: Individualize dose based on patient size, extent, and location of muscle involvement, degree of spasticity, local muscle weakness, and response to prior treatment. In clinical trials total doses up to 360 units were administered as separate injections typically divided among flexor muscles of the elbow, wrist, and fingers; may repeat therapy at 3-4 months with appropriate dosage based upon the clinical condition of patient at time of retreatment.

Suggested guidelines for the treatment of stroke-related upper limb spasticity: **Note:** Dose listed is total dose administered as individual or separate intramuscular injection(s):

Biceps brachii: 100-200 units (up to 4 sites)

Flexor digitorum profundus: 15-50 units (1-2 sites)

Flexor digitorum sublimes: 15-50 units (1-2 sites)

Flexor carpi radialis: 15-60 units (1-2 sites)

Flexor carpi ulnaris: 10-50 units (1-2 sites)

Adductor pollicis: 20 units (1-2 sites)

Flexor pollicis longus: 20 units (1-2 sites)

Elderly: No specific adjustment recommended

Dosage adjustment in renal impairment: No specific adjustment recommended

Dosage adjustment in hepatic impairment: No specific adjustment recommended

Stability Store undiluted vials under refrigeration at 2°C to 8°C for up to 24 months (Botox® Cosmetic) or up to 36 months (Botox®). Reconstitute with sterile, preservative free 0.9% sodium chloride. Mix gently. After reconstitution, store in refrigerator (2°C to 8°C) and use within 4 hours (does not contain preservative).

Botox®: Reconstitute vials with 1 mL of diluent to obtain concentration of 10 units per 0.1 mL; 2 mL of diluent to obtain concentration of 5 units per 0.1 mL; 4 mL of diluent to obtain concentration of 2.5 units per 0.1 mL; 8 mL of diluent to obtain concentration of 1.25 units per 0.1 mL.

Botox® Cosmetic: Reconstitute vials with 2.5 mL of diluent to obtain concentration of 4 units per 0.1 mL (20 units per 0.5 mL).

Administration

Cervical dystonia: Use 25-, 27-, or 30-gauge needle for superficial muscles and a longer 22-gauge needle for deeper musculature; electromyography may help localize the involved muscles.

Blepharospasm: Use a 27- or 30-gauge needle without electromyography guidance. Avoid injecting near the levator palpebrae superioris (may decrease ptosis); avoid medial lower lid injections (may decrease diplopia). Apply pressure at the injection site to prevent ecchymosis in the soft eyelid tissues.

Spasticity (cerebral palsy related; Canadian labeling [not in U.S. labeling]): Use a 23- to 26-gauge needle for administration into the medial and lateral heads of the gastrocnemius muscle of the affected limb.

Spasticity (focal; Canadian labeling [not in U.S. labeling]): Use a 25-, 27-, or 30-gauge needle for superficial muscles and a longer 22-gauge needle for deeper musculature; electromyography or nerve stimulation may help localize the involved muscles.

Strabismus injections: Must use surgical exposure or electromyographic guidance; use the electrical activity recorded from the tip of the injections needle as a guide to placement within the target muscle. Local anesthetic and ocular decongestant should be given before injection. The volume of injection should be 0.05-0.15 mL per muscle. Many patients will require additional doses because of inadequate response to initial dose.

Primary axillary hyperhidrosis: Inject each dose intradermally to a depth of ~2 mm and at a 45° angle. Do not inject directly into areas marked in ink (to avoid permanent tattoo effect). Prior to administration, injection area should be defined by standard staining techniques such as Minor's Iodine-Starch Test.

Instructions for Minor's Iodine-Starch Test: Patient should shave underarms and refrain from using deodorants or antiperspirants for 24 hours prior to test. At 30 minutes prior to test, patient should be at rest, no exercise, and not consume hot beverages. Underarm area should be dried and immediately painted with iodine solution. After area dries, lightly sprinkle with starch powder. Gently blow off excess powder. A deep blue-black color will develop over the hyperhidrotic area in ~10 minutes.

Reduction of glabellar lines (Botox® Cosmetic): Use a 30-gauge needle. Ensure injected volume/dose is accurate and where feasible keep to a minimum. Avoid injection near the levator palpebrae superioris. Medial corrugator injections should be at least 1 cm above the bony supraorbital ridge. Do not inject toxin closer than 1 cm above the central eyebrow.

Pregnancy Risk Factor C

Contraindications Hypersensitivity to albumin, botulinum toxin, or any component of the formulation; infection at the proposed injection site(s)

Canadian labeling: Additional contraindications (not in U.S. labeling): Myasthenia gravis or Eaton-Lambert syndrome

Warnings/Precautions Systemic toxicity, including difficulty breathing and swallowing, aspiration pneumonia, respiratory depression, muscular weakness, facial and eyelid drooping, double vision, speech disorder, and constipation have been reported when the toxin spreads beyond the site of local injection. Higher doses or more frequent administration may result in neutralizing antibody formation and loss of efficacy. Product contains albumin and may carry a remote risk of virus transmission. Use caution if there is excessive weakness or atrophy at the proposed injection site(s); use is contraindicated if infection is present at injection site. Have appropriate support in case of anaphylactic reaction. Use with caution in patients with neuromuscular diseases (such as myasthenia gravis), neuropathic disorders (such as amyotrophic lateral sclerosis), patients taking aminoglycosides, neuromuscular-blocking agents, or other drugs that interfere with neuromuscular transmission and patients with pre-existing cardiovascular disease (rare reports of arrhythmia and MI). Long-term effects of chronic therapy unknown.

Cervical dystonia: Dysphagia is common. It may be severe requiring alternative feeding methods and may persist anywhere from 2 weeks up to 5 months after administration. Risk of upper respiratory infection may be increased. Risk factors include smaller neck muscle mass, bilateral injections into the sternocleidomastoid muscle, or injections into the levator scapulae.

Ocular disease: Blepharospasm: Reduced blinking from injection of the orbicularis muscle can lead to corneal exposure and ulceration. Strabismus: Retrobulbar hemorrhages may occur from needle penetration into orbit. Spatial disorientation, double vision, or past pointing may occur if one or more extraocular muscles are paralyzed. Covering the affected eye may help. Careful testing of corneal sensation, avoidance of lower lid injections, and treatment of epithelial defects are necessary. Use with caution in angle closure glaucoma.

Primary axillary hyperhidrosis: Evaluate for secondary causes prior to treatment (eg, hyperthyroidism). Safety and efficacy for treatment of hyperhidrosis in other areas of the body have not been established.

Temporary reduction in glabellar lines: Do not use more frequently than every 3 months. Patients with marked facial asymmetry, ptosis, excessive dermatochalasis, deep dermal scarring, thick sebaceous skin, or the inability to substantially lessen glabellar lines by physically spreading them apart were excluded from clinical trials. Reduced blinking from injection of the orbicularis muscle can lead to corneal exposure and ulceration. Spatial disorientation, double vision, or past pointing may occur if one or more extraocular muscles are paralyzed.

Adverse Reactions Adverse effects usually occur in 1 week and may last up to several months

>10%:
Cervical dystonia:
Central nervous system: Pain (32%), headache (up to 11%)
Gastrointestinal: Dysphagia (19%)
Neuromuscular & skeletal: Focal weakness (17%), neck pain (11%)
Respiratory: Upper respiratory infection (12%)
Other indications (blepharospasm, primary axillary hyperhidrosis, strabismus):
Neuromuscular & skeletal: Primary axillary hyperhidrosis (3% to 10%)
Ocular: Ptosis (blepharospasm 21%; strabismus 1% to 38%), vertical deviation (strabismus 17%)

2% to 10%:
Cervical dystonia:
  Central nervous system: Dizziness, drowsiness, fever, malaise, speech disorder
  Gastrointestinal: Nausea, xerostomia
  Local: Injection site reaction: Soreness
  Neuromuscular & skeletal: Back pain, hypertonia, weakness, stiffness
  Respiratory: Cough, rhinitis
  Miscellaneous: Flu-like syndrome
Cerebral palsy spasticity:
  Central nervous system: Pain (1% to 2%), fever (1%), lethargy (1%)
  Neuromuscular & skeletal: Falling, weakness
Focal spasticity:
  Central nervous system: Arm pain (1% to 3%)
  Dermatologic: Bruising (1% to 3%)
  Local: Injection site reactions: burning, pain (1% to 3%)
  Neuromuscular & skeletal: Hypertonia (1% to 3%), weakness (1% to 3%)
Other indications (blepharospasm, primary axillary hyperhidrosis, reduction of glabellar lines, strabismus):
  Central nervous system: Anxiety, dizziness
  Dermatologic: Pruritus
  Gastrointestinal: Nausea
  Local: Injection site reaction: Soreness
  Neuromuscular & skeletal: Back pain, facial pain, weakness
  Ocular: Irritation/tearing (includes dry eye, lagophthalmos, photophobia); ptosis, superficial punctate keratitis
  Respiratory: Pharyngitis
  Miscellaneous: Flu-like syndrome, infection, nonaxillary sweating

<2% (Limited to important or life-threatening): *Any indication:* Abdominal pain, acute angle closure glaucoma, allergic reactions, anaphylaxis, ankle pain, anterior segment eye ischemia, appetite decreased, arrhythmia, arthralgia, aspiration pneumonia, blurred vision, brachial plexopathy, bruising, ciliary ganglion damage, corneal perforation, dermatitis, diaphoresis, diarrhea, diplopia, dyspepsia, dysphonia, dyspnea, ectropion, entropion, erythema multiforme, eyelid edema, facial weakness, focal facial paralysis, glaucoma, hearing loss, hypoesthesia, hypertension, knee pain, leg cramps, lethargy, malaise, MI, myalgia, myasthenia gravis exacerbation, neutralizing antibody formation, numbness, pneumonia, pruritus, psoriasiform eruption, ptosis, rash, reduced blinking leading to corneal ulceration, retinal vein occlusion, retrobulbar hemorrhage, seizure, skin tightness, syncope, tooth disorder, urticaria, vertigo with nystagmus, vitreous hemorrhage, vomiting

Drug Interactions
  Avoid Concomitant Use There are no known interactions where it is recommended to avoid concomitant use.
  Increased Effect/Toxicity
    OnabotulinumtoxinA may increase the levels/effects of: AbobotulinumtoxinA; RimabotulinumtoxinB

    The levels/effects of OnabotulinumtoxinA may be increased by: Aminoglycosides; Neuromuscular-Blocking Agents
  Decreased Effect There are no known significant interactions involving a decrease in effect.
  Dosage Forms Excipient information presented when available (limited, particularly for generics); consult specific product labeling.
    Injection, powder for reconstitution [preservative free]:
      Botox®, Botox® Cosmetic: OnabotulinumtoxinA 100 units [contains human albumin]

Ondansetron (on DAN se tron)

Medication Safety Issues
  Sound-alike/look-alike issues:
    Ondansetron may be confused with dolasetron, granisetron, palonosetron
    Zofran® may be confused with Zantac®, Zosyn®

Related Information
Postoperative Nausea and Vomiting *on page 1593*

U.S. Brand Names Zofran®; Zofran® ODT

Canadian Brand Names Apo-Ondansetron®; DOM-Ondansetron; Gen-Ondansetron; JAMP-Ondansetron; MINT-Ondansetron; Mylan-Ondansetron; Novo-Ondansetron; Ondansetron Injection; Ondansetron-Omega; PHL-Ondansetron; PMS-Ondansetron; RAN-Ondansetron; ratio-Ondansetron; Sandoz-Ondansetron; Zofran®; Zofran® ODT

Index Terms GR38032R; Ondansetron Hydrochloride

Pharmacologic Category Antiemetic; Selective 5-HT$_3$ Receptor Antagonist

Generic Available Yes

Use Prevention of nausea and vomiting associated with moderately- to highly-emetogenic cancer chemotherapy; radiotherapy; prevention of postoperative nausea and vomiting (PONV); treatment of PONV if no prophylactic dose of ondansetron received

Unlabeled/Investigational Use Hyperemesis gravidarum; breakthrough treatment of nausea and vomiting associated with chemotherapy

Mechanism of Action Selective 5-HT$_3$-receptor antagonist, blocking serotonin, both peripherally on vagal nerve terminals and centrally in the chemoreceptor trigger zone

Pharmacodynamics/Kinetics
Onset of action: ~30 minutes

Distribution: V_d: Children: 1.7-3.7 L/kg; Adults: 2.2-2.5 L/kg

Protein binding, plasma: 70% to 76%

Metabolism: Extensively hepatic via hydroxylation, followed by glucuronide or sulfate conjugation; CYP1A2, CYP2D6, and CYP3A4 substrate; some demethylation occurs

Bioavailability: Oral: 56% to 71%; Rectal: 58% to 74%

Half-life elimination: Children <15 years: 2-7 hours; Adults: 3-6 hours
Mild-to-moderate hepatic impairment: Adults: 12 hours
Severe hepatic impairment (Child-Pugh C): Adults: 20 hours

Time to peak: Oral: ~2 hours

Excretion: Urine (44% to 60% as metabolites, 5% to 10% as unchanged drug); feces (~25%)

Dosage Note: Studies in adults have shown a single daily dose of 8-12 mg I.V. or 8-24 mg orally to be as effective as mg/kg dosing, and should be considered for **all** patients whose mg/kg dose exceeds 8-12 mg I.V.; oral solution and ODT formulations are bioequivalent to corresponding doses of tablet formulation
Children:
I.V.:
Prevention of chemotherapy-induced emesis: 6 months to 18 years: 0.15 mg/kg/dose administered 30 minutes prior to chemotherapy, 4 and 8 hours after the first dose **or** 0.45 mg/kg/day as a single dose
Prevention of postoperative nausea and vomiting: 1 month to 12 years:
≤40 kg: 0.1 mg/kg as a single dose
>40 kg: 4 mg as a single dose
Oral: Prevention of chemotherapy-induced emesis:
4-11 years: 4 mg 30 minutes before chemotherapy; repeat 4 and 8 hours after initial dose, then 4 mg every 8 hours for 1-2 days after chemotherapy completed
≥12 years: Refer to adult dosing.

Adults:
I.V.:
Prevention of chemotherapy-induced emesis:
0.15 mg/kg 3 times/day beginning 30 minutes prior to chemotherapy **or**
0.45 mg/kg once daily **or**
8-10 mg 1-2 times/day **or**
24 mg or 32 mg once daily
Treatment of hyperemesis gravidum (unlabeled use): 8 mg administered over 15 minutes every 12 hours **or** 1 mg/hour infused continuously for up to 24 hours

I.M., I.V.: Postoperative nausea and vomiting (PONV): 4 mg as a single dose approximately 30 minutes before the end of anesthesia (see **"Note"**) or as treatment if vomiting occurs after surgery (Gan, 2007).

Note: The manufacturer recommends administration immediately before induction of anesthesia; however, this has been shown not to be as effective as administration at the end of surgery (Sun, 1997). Repeat doses given in response to inadequate control of nausea/vomiting from preoperative doses are generally ineffective.

Oral:

Chemotherapy-induced emesis:

Highly-emetogenic agents/single-day therapy: 24 mg given 30 minutes prior to the start of therapy

Moderately-emetogenic agents: 8 mg every 12 hours beginning 30 minutes before chemotherapy, continuously for 1-2 days after chemotherapy completed

Total body irradiation: 8 mg 1-2 hours before daily each fraction of radiotherapy

Single high-dose fraction radiotherapy to abdomen: 8 mg 1-2 hours before irradiation, then 8 mg every 8 hours after first dose for 1-2 days after completion of radiotherapy

Daily fractionated radiotherapy to abdomen: 8 mg 1-2 hours before irradiation, then 8 mg 8 hours after first dose for each day of radiotherapy

Postoperative nausea and vomiting: 16 mg given 1 hour prior to induction of anesthesia

Treatment of hyperemesis gravidum (unlabeled use): 8 mg every 12 hours

Elderly: No dosing adjustment required

Dosage adjustment in renal impairment: No dosing adjustment required
Dosage adjustment in hepatic impairment: Severe liver disease (Child-Pugh C): Maximum daily dose: 8 mg

Stability

Oral solution: Store between 15°C and 30°C (59°F and 86°F). Protect from light.
Premixed bag: Store between 2°C and 30°C (36°F and 86°F). Protect from light.
Tablet: Store between 2°C and 30°C (36°F and 86°F).
Vial: Store between 2°C and 30°C (36°F and 86°F). Protect from light. Prior to I.V. infusion, dilute in 50 mL D_5W or NS. Solution is stable for 48 hours at room temperature.

Administration

Oral: Oral dosage forms should be administered 30 minutes prior to chemotherapy; 1-2 hours before radiotherapy; 1 hour prior to the induction of anesthesia.

Orally-disintegrating tablets: Do not remove from blister until needed. Peel backing off the blister, do not push tablet through. Using dry hands, place tablet on tongue and allow to dissolve. Swallow with saliva.

I.M.: Should be administered undiluted.

I.V.:

IVPB: Dilute in 50 mL D_5W or NS. Infuse over 15-30 minutes; 24-hour continuous infusions have been reported, but are rarely used.

Chemotherapy-induced nausea and vomiting: Give first dose 30 minutes prior to beginning chemotherapy.

I.V. push: Prevention of postoperative nausea and vomiting: Single doses may be administered I.V. injection over 2-5 minutes as undiluted solution.

Monitoring Parameters Closely monitor patients <4 months of age
Pregnancy Risk Factor B
Contraindications Hypersensitivity to ondansetron, other selective 5-HT$_3$ antagonists, or any component of the formulation
Warnings/Precautions Ondansetron should be used on a scheduled basis, not on an "as needed" (PRN) basis, since data support the use of this drug only in the prevention of nausea and vomiting (due to antineoplastic therapy) and not in the rescue of nausea and vomiting. Ondansetron should only be used in the first 24-48 hours of chemotherapy. Data do not support any increased efficacy of ondansetron in delayed nausea and vomiting. Does not stimulate gastric or intestinal peristalsis; may mask progressive ileus and/or gastric distension. Use with caution in patients allergic to other 5-HT$_3$ receptor antagonists; cross-reactivity has been reported.

◀ Use with caution in patients with congenital long QT syndrome or other risk factors for QT prolongation (eg, medications known to prolong QT interval, electrolyte abnormalities, and cumulative high-dose anthracycline therapy). 5-HT$_3$ antagonists have been associated with a number of dose-dependent increases in ECG intervals (eg, PR, QRS duration, QT/QT$_c$, JT), usually occurring 1-2 hours after I.V. administration. In general, these changes are not clinically relevant, however, when used in conjunction with other agents that prolong these intervals, arrhythmia may occur. When used with agents that prolong the QT interval (eg, Class I and III antiarrhythmics), clinically relevant QT interval prolongation may occur resulting in torsade de pointes. I.V. formulations of 5-HT$_3$ antagonists have more association with ECG interval changes, compared to oral formulations.

Orally-disintegrating tablets contain phenylalanine. Safety and efficacy for children <1 month of age have not been established.

Adverse Reactions Note: Percentages reported in adult patients.

>10%:

Central nervous system: Headache (9% to 27%), malaise/fatigue (9% to 13%)

Gastrointestinal: Constipation (6% to 11%)

1% to 10%:

Central nervous system: Drowsiness (8%), fever (2% to 8%), dizziness (4% to 7%), anxiety (6%), cold sensation (2%)

Dermatologic: Pruritus (2% to 5%), rash (1%)

Gastrointestinal: Diarrhea (2% to 7%)

Genitourinary: Gynecological disorder (7%), urinary retention (5%)

Hepatic: ALT increased (1% to 5%), AST increased (1% to 5%)

Local: Injection site reaction (4%; pain, redness, burning)

Neuromuscular & skeletal: Paresthesia (2%)

Respiratory: Hypoxia (9%)

<1% (Limited to important or life-threatening): Anaphylactoid reactions, anaphylaxis, angina, angioedema, arrhythmia, blindness (transient/following infusion; lasting ≤48 hours), blurred vision (transient/following infusion), bradycardia, bronchospasm, cardiopulmonary arrest, dyspnea, dystonic reaction, ECG changes, electrocardiographic alterations (second-degree heart block and ST-segment depression), extrapyramidal symptoms, flushing, grand mal seizure, hiccups, hypersensitivity reaction, hypokalemia, hypotension, laryngeal edema, laryngospasm, oculogyric crisis, palpitation, premature ventricular contractions (PVC), QT interval increased, shock, stridor, supraventricular tachycardia, syncope, tachycardia, urticaria, vascular occlusive events, ventricular arrhythmia

Drug Interactions

Metabolism/Transport Effects Substrate of CYP1A2 (minor), 2C9 (minor), 2D6 (minor), 2E1 (minor), 3A4 (major); **Inhibits** CYP1A2 (weak), 2C9 (weak), 2D6 (weak)

Avoid Concomitant Use

Avoid concomitant use of Ondansetron with any of the following: Apomorphine

Increased Effect/Toxicity

Ondansetron may increase the levels/effects of: Apomorphine

The levels/effects of Ondansetron may be increased by: P-Glycoprotein Inhibitors

Decreased Effect

The levels/effects of Ondansetron may be decreased by: CYP3A4 Inducers (Strong); Deferasirox; Herbs (CYP3A4 Inducers); Peginterferon Alfa-2b; P-Glycoprotein Inducers; Rifamycin Derivatives

Ethanol/Nutrition/Herb Interactions

Food: Food increases the extent of absorption. The C_{max} and T_{max} do not change much.

Herb/Nutraceutical: St John's wort may decrease ondansetron levels.

Dietary Considerations Take without regard to meals.

Orally-disintegrating tablet contains <0.03 mg phenylalanine

Dosage Forms Excipient information presented when available (limited, particularly for generics); consult specific product labeling. [DSC] = Discontinued product

Infusion, premixed in D_5 [preservative free]: 32 mg (50 mL)
  Zofran®: 32 mg (50 mL) [DSC]
Infusion, premixed in sodium chloride [preservative free]: 32 mg (50 mL)
Injection, solution: 2 mg/mL (2 mL, 20 mL)
  Zofran®: 2 mg/mL (2 mL, 20 mL)
Injection, solution [preservative free]: 2 mg/mL (2 mL)
Solution, oral: 4 mg/5 mL (50 mL)
  Zofran®: 4 mg/5 mL (50 mL) [contains sodium benzoate; strawberry flavor]
Tablet: 4 mg; 8 mg
  Zofran®: 4 mg; 8 mg
Tablet, orally disintegrating: 4 mg; 8 mg
  Zofran® ODT: 4 mg, 8 mg [each strength contains phenylalanine <0.03 mg/tablet; strawberry flavor]

References

Gan TJ, Meyer TA, Apfel CC, et al, "Society for Ambulatory Anesthesia Guidelines for the Management of Postoperative Nausea and Vomiting," *Anesth Analg*, 2007, 105(6):1615-28.

Sun R, Klein KW, and White PF, "The Effect of Timing of Ondansetron Administration in Outpatients Undergoing Otolaryngologic Surgery," *Anesth Analg*, 1997, 84(2):331-6.

Tramer MR, Moore RA, Reynolds DJ, et al, "A Quantitative Systematic Review of Ondansetron in Treatment of Established Postoperative Nausea and Vomiting," *BMJ*, 1997, 314(7087):1088-92.

♦ **Ondansetron Hydrochloride** *see* Ondansetron *on page 1057*

♦ **Ondansetron Injection (Can)** *see* Ondansetron *on page 1057*

♦ **Ondansetron-Omega (Can)** *see* Ondansetron *on page 1057*

♦ **Onsolis™** *see* FentaNYL *on page 587*

♦ **Opana®** *see* Oxymorphone *on page 1074*

♦ **Opana® ER** *see* Oxymorphone *on page 1074*

♦ **OPC-13013** *see* Cilostazol *on page 303*

♦ **OPC-14597** *see* Aripiprazole *on page 143*

♦ **OPC-41061** *see* Tolvaptan *on page 1406*

♦ **Operand® Chlorhexidine Gluconate [OTC]** *see* Chlorhexidine Gluconate *on page 291*

♦ **Ophtho-Tate® (Can)** *see* PrednisoLONE *on page 1164*

♦ **Optivar®** *see* Azelastine *on page 168*

♦ **Optive™ [OTC]** *see* Carboxymethylcellulose *on page 243*

♦ **Oracea™** *see* Doxycycline *on page 456*

♦ **Oracort (Can)** *see* Triamcinolone *on page 1429*

♦ **Oramorph® SR** *see* Morphine Sulfate *on page 953*

♦ **Orapred®** *see* PrednisoLONE *on page 1164*

♦ **Orapred ODT®** *see* PrednisoLONE *on page 1164*

♦ **OraVerse™** *see* Phentolamine *on page 1112*

♦ **Oraxyl™** *see* Doxycycline *on page 456*

♦ **Orciprenaline Sulfate** *see* Metaproterenol *on page 885*

♦ **ORG 946** *see* Rocuronium *on page 1259*

♦ **ORG NC 45** *see* Vecuronium *on page 1463*

♦ **ORO-Clense (Can)** *see* Chlorhexidine Gluconate *on page 291*

♦ **Ortho® 0.5/35 (Can)** *see* Ethinyl Estradiol and Norethindrone *on page 554*

♦ **Ortho® 1/35 (Can)** *see* Ethinyl Estradiol and Norethindrone *on page 554*

♦ **Ortho® 7/7/7 (Can)** *see* Ethinyl Estradiol and Norethindrone *on page 554*

♦ **Ortho Cept** *see* Ethinyl Estradiol and Desogestrel *on page 544*

♦ **Ortho-Cept®** *see* Ethinyl Estradiol and Desogestrel *on page 544*

♦ **Ortho Cyclen** *see* Ethinyl Estradiol and Norgestimate *on page 558*

♦ **Ortho-Cyclen®** *see* Ethinyl Estradiol and Norgestimate *on page 558*

♦ **Ortho-Evra** *see* Ethinyl Estradiol and Norelgestromin *on page 552*

♦ **Ortho Evra®** *see* Ethinyl Estradiol and Norelgestromin *on page 552*

♦ **Ortho Novum** *see* Ethinyl Estradiol and Norethindrone *on page 554*

◆ **Ortho-Novum®** *see* Ethinyl Estradiol and Norethindrone *on page 554*

◆ **Ortho-Novum® 7/7/7** *see* Ethinyl Estradiol and Norethindrone *on page 554*

◆ **Ortho Tri Cyclen** *see* Ethinyl Estradiol and Norgestimate *on page 558*

◆ **Ortho Tri-Cyclen®** *see* Ethinyl Estradiol and Norgestimate *on page 558*

◆ **Ortho Tri-Cyclen® Lo** *see* Ethinyl Estradiol and Norgestimate *on page 558*

◆ **Oruvail® (Can)** *see* Ketoprofen *on page 783*

Oseltamivir (oh sel TAM i vir)

Medication Safety Issues

Sound-alike/look-alike issues:

Tamiflu® may be confused with Thera-Flu®

Tamiflu® may be confused with Tambocor™

Dispensing issues:

Oseltamivir (Tamiflu®) oral suspension is packaged with an oral syringe. Healthcare providers dispensing this medication should be aware that the syringe is calibrated in 30 mg, 45 mg, and 60 mg graduations. **When the oral syringe is dispensed, instructions to the patient should be provided based on these units of measure (not mL or teaspoon). When dispensing the oral suspension for children <1 year of age, the oral syringe provided from the manufacturer should be removed and NOT provided to the caregiver.** Pharmacists and healthcare providers should instead supply an oral syringe capable of measuring mL doses. Patients should always be provided with a measuring device calibrated the same way as their labeled instructions.

Oseltamivir (Tamiflu®) 75 mg capsules can be compounded into a suspension when oseltamivir oral suspension is not commercially available. The commercially-available oral suspension concentration is 12 mg/mL; however, the extemporaneously prepared suspension concentration is 15 mg/mL. Prescriptions written in mL or teaspoons should specify the oral suspension concentration to be dispensed.

U.S. Brand Names Tamiflu®

Canadian Brand Names Tamiflu®

Pharmacologic Category Antiviral Agent; Neuraminidase Inhibitor

Generic Available No

Use Treatment of uncomplicated acute illness due to influenza (A or B) infection in children ≥1 year of age and adults who have been symptomatic for no more than 2 days; prophylaxis against influenza (A or B) infection in children ≥1 year of age and adults

The Advisory Committee on Immunization Practices (ACIP) recommends that **treatment** be considered for the following:

• Persons hospitalized with laboratory confirmed influenza (may also have benefit if started >48 hours after onset of illness).

• Persons with laboratory confirmed influenza pneumonia.

• Persons with laboratory confirmed influenza and bacterial infections.

• Persons with laboratory confirmed influenza and who are at higher risk for influenza complications.

• Persons presenting for care within 48 hours of laboratory confirmed influenza onset and who want to decrease duration and/or severity of their symptoms or decrease the risk of transmission to those at high risk for complications.

The ACIP recommends that **prophylaxis** be considered for the following:

• Persons at high risk for influenza infection during the first 2 weeks following vaccination (eg, children <9 years and not previously vaccinated) if the virus is circulating in the community.

• Persons at high risk for influenza infection, but the vaccination is contraindicated.

• Unvaccinated family members or healthcare providers with prolonged exposure to or close contact with high-risk persons, unvaccinated persons, or infants <6 months of age.

- Persons at high risk for influenza infection, their family members and close contacts, and healthcare workers when the circulating strain of influenza is not matched with the vaccine.
- Persons with immune deficiency or those who may not respond to vaccination.
- Unvaccinated staff and persons during response to an outbreak in a closed institutional setting that has patients at high risk for infection (eg, extended care facilities).

Unlabeled/Investigational Use Treatment and chemoprophylaxis of novel influenza A (H1N1) virus

Mechanism of Action Oseltamivir, a prodrug, is hydrolyzed to the active form, oseltamivir carboxylate (OC). OC inhibits influenza virus neuraminidase, an enzyme known to cleave the budding viral progeny from its cellular envelope attachment point (neuraminic acid) just prior to release.

Pharmacodynamics/Kinetics

Absorption: Well absorbed

Distribution: V_d: 23-26 L (oseltamivir carboxylate)

Protein binding, plasma: Oseltamivir carboxylate: 3%; Oseltamivir: 42%

Metabolism: Hepatic (90%) to oseltamivir carboxylate; neither the parent drug nor active metabolite has any effect on the cytochrome P450 system

Bioavailability: 75% as oseltamivir carboxylate

Half-life elimination: Oseltamivir: 1-3 hours; Oseltamivir carboxylate: 6-10 hours

Excretion: Urine (>90% as oseltamivir carboxylate); feces

Dosage Oral:

Treatment of seasonal influenza and uncomplicated 2009 H1N1 influenza: Initiate treatment within 2 days of onset of symptoms; duration of treatment: 5 days unless severely ill and hospitalized:

Children <1 year (interim recommendations for treatment of 2009 H1N1 influenza [CDC, 2009]):

<3 months: 12 mg twice daily

3-5 months: 20 mg twice daily

6-11 months: 25 mg twice daily

Alternate dosing based on weight:

<9 months: 3 mg/kg/dose twice daily

≥9 months: 3.5 mg/kg/dose twice daily

Children: 1-12 years:

≤15 kg: 30 mg twice daily

>15 kg to ≤23 kg: 45 mg twice daily

>23 kg to ≤40 kg: 60 mg twice daily

>40 kg: 75 mg twice daily

Adolescents ≥13 years and Adults: 75 mg twice daily

Treatment of 2009 H1N1 influenza infection: Severely-ill hospitalized patients [interim recommendations (CDC, 2009)]: **Note:** Initiate as early as possible in any hospitalized patient with suspected/confirmed influenza; may be administered via naso- or orogastric tube in mechanically-ventilated patients (Taylor, 2008)

Children: Use twice the standard treatment dose according to the age and weight of the patient and extend the treatment duration (minimum of a 10-day course)

Adults: 150 mg twice daily and extend treatment duration (minimum of a 10-day course)

Prophylaxis: Initiate treatment within 2 days of contact with an infected individual; duration of treatment: 10 days

Children <1 year (interim recommendations for chemoprophylaxis of 2009 H1N1 influenza [CDC, 2009]):

<3 months: Not recommended unless clinically critical

3-5 months: 20 mg once daily

6-11 months: 25 mg once daily

Alternate dosing based on weight:

<9 months: 3 mg/kg/dose once daily

≥9 months: 3.5 mg/kg/dose once daily

◀ Children: 1-12 years:

   ≤15 kg: 30 mg once daily

   >15 kg to ≤23 kg: 45 mg once daily

   >23 kg to ≤40 kg: 60 mg once daily

   >40 kg: 75 mg once daily

Adolescents ≥13 years and Adults: 75 mg once daily. During community outbreaks, dosing is 75 mg once daily. May be used for up to 6 weeks; duration of protection lasts for length of dosing period

Dosage adjustment in renal impairment: Adults:

Cl_{cr} 10-30 mL/minute:

   Treatment: Reduce dose to 75 mg once daily for 5 days

      High-dose treatment (unlabeled [eg, severely-ill hospitalized patients with 2009 H1N1 influenza]): Currently no data are available; consider 150 mg once daily

   Prophylaxis: 75 mg every other day or 30 mg once daily

   CAPD (unlabeled dose): 30 mg once weekly (Robson, 2006)

   Hemodialysis (unlabeled dose): 30 mg after every other session (Robson, 2006)

Dosage adjustment in hepatic impairment:

   Mild-to-moderate impairment: No adjustment necessary

   Severe impairment: Pharmacokinetics and safety have not been evaluated

Stability

Capsules: Store at 25°C (77°F).

Oral suspension: Store powder for suspension at 25°C (77°F). Reconstitute with 23 mL of water (to make 25 mL total suspension). Once reconstituted, store suspension under refrigeration at 2°C to 8°C (36°F to 46°F); do not freeze. Use within 10 days of preparation.

Administration

Capsules may be opened and mixed with sweetened liquid (eg, chocolate syrup).

Mechanically-ventilated critically-ill patients: May administer via naso- or orogastric (NG/OG) tube. For a 150 mg dose, dissolve powder from 150 mg capsule in 20 mL of sterile water and inject down the NG/OG tube; follow with a 10 mL sterile water flush (Taylor, 2008).

Monitoring Parameters Signs or symptoms of unusual behavior, including attempts at self-injury, confusion, and/or delirium

Critically-ill patients: Repeat rRT-PCR or viral culture may help to determine on-going viral replication

Anesthesia and Critical Care Concerns/Other Considerations

2009 H1N1 influenza: Clinical characteristics of 272 hospitalized patients who tested positive for the 2009 H1N1 influenza virus have been described (Jain, 2009). Of these patients, 67 (25%) were admitted to the ICU with 45 (67%) having an underlying medical condition (asthma/COPD: 28%; immunosuppression: 18%; pregnancy: 9%). Forty-two patients required mechanical ventilation, 24 had acute respiratory distress syndrome (ARDS), and 21 developed sepsis. There was no description of specific antiviral therapy for patients admitted to the ICU; however, of the total group, 188 received oseltamivir, 19 zanamivir, 13 amantadine/oseltamivir, and 14 rimantadine/oseltamivir. Of the ICU patients who received antiviral drugs (56/65, 86%; data not available in 2 patients), the median time to initiation was 6 days (range, 0 to 24 days); only 23% received antiviral drugs within 48 hours after onset of illness. Of the patients who expired (19/272, 7%), all were admitted to the ICU and required mechanical ventilation. These patients were less likely to have been vaccinated for seasonal influenza during the 2008-9 season and had a longer time between onset of illness and antiviral therapy initiation compared to non-ICU patients. In a multivariable analysis, the only variable associated with a positive outcome was initiation of antiviral therapy within 2 days after onset of illness. Also see http://www.cdc.gov/h1n1flu/EUA/peramivir_recommendations.htm

Pregnancy Risk Factor C

Contraindications Hypersensitivity to oseltamivir or any component of the formulation

Warnings/Precautions Oseltamivir is not a substitute for the influenza virus vaccine. Use caution with renal impairment; dosage adjustment is required for creatinine clearance <30 mL/minute. Also consider primary or concomitant bacterial infections. Safety and efficacy for use in severe hepatic impairment or for treatment or prophylaxis in immunocompromised patients have not been established. Efficacy has not been established if treatment begins >40 hours after the onset of symptoms or in the treatment of patients with chronic cardiac and/or respiratory disease. Rare but severe hypersensitivity reactions (anaphylaxis, severe dermatologic reactions) have been associated with use. Rare occurrences of neuropsychiatric events (including confusion, delirium, hallucinations, and/or self-injury) have been reported from postmarketing surveillance (primarily in pediatric patients); direct causation is difficult to establish (influenza infection may also be associated with behavioral and neurologic changes). Monitor closely for signs of any unusual behavior. Safety and efficacy in children (<1 year of age) have not been established.

Adverse Reactions
>10%: Gastrointestinal: Vomiting (2% to 15%)
1% to 10%: Gastrointestinal: Nausea (3% to 10%), abdominal pain (2% to 5%)
<1% (Limited to important or life-threatening): Allergy, anaphylactic/anaphylactoid reaction, arrhythmia, confusion, dermatitis, diabetes aggravation, eczema, erythema multiforme, hepatitis, liver function tests abnormal, neuropsychiatric events (self-injury, confusion, delirium), rash, seizure, Stevens-Johnson syndrome, swelling of face or tongue, toxic epidermal necrolysis, urticaria

Drug Interactions
Avoid Concomitant Use There are no known interactions where it is recommended to avoid concomitant use.
Increased Effect/Toxicity There are no known significant interactions involving an increase in effect.
Decreased Effect
Oseltamivir may decrease the levels/effects of: Influenza Virus Vaccine

Dietary Considerations Take with or without food; take with food to improve tolerance.

Dosage Forms Excipient information presented when available (limited, particularly for generics); consult specific product labeling.
Capsule, as phosphate:
Tamiflu®: 30 mg, 45 mg, 75 mg
Powder for oral suspension:
Tamiflu®: 12 mg/mL (25 mL) [contains sodium benzoate; tutti-frutti flavor]

References
Centers for Disease Control, "Prevention and Control of Influenza. Recommendations of the Advisory Committee on Immunization Practices (ACIP)," *MMWR Recomm Rep*, 2007, 56 (early release):1-54. Available at http://www.cdc.gov/mmwr/preview/mmwrhtml/rr56e629a1.htm

◆ **Osmitrol®** *see* Mannitol *on page 866*

◆ **OsmoPrep®** *see* Sodium Phosphates *on page 1309*

◆ **OTFC (Oral Transmucosal Fentanyl Citrate)** *see* FentaNYL *on page 587*

◆ **Ovcon®** *see* Ethinyl Estradiol and Norethindrone *on page 554*

◆ **Ovral® (Can)** *see* Ethinyl Estradiol and Norgestrel *on page 560*

Oxaprozin (oks a PROE zin)

Related Information
Nonsteroidal Anti-Inflammatory Agents *on page 1687*
U.S. Brand Names Daypro®
Canadian Brand Names Apo-Oxaprozin®; Daypro®
Pharmacologic Category Nonsteroidal Anti-inflammatory Drug (NSAID), Oral
Use Acute and long-term use in the management of signs and symptoms of osteoarthritis and rheumatoid arthritis; juvenile rheumatoid arthritis

Pharmacodynamics/Kinetics
Absorption: Almost complete
Protein binding: >99%
Metabolism: Hepatic via oxidation and glucuronidation; no active metabolites
Half-life elimination: 40-50 hours
Time to peak: 2-4 hours
Excretion: Urine (5% unchanged, 65% as metabolites); feces (35% as metabolites)

◄ **Dosage** Oral (individualize dosage to lowest effective dose to minimize adverse effects):

Children 6-16 years: Juvenile rheumatoid arthritis:
  22-31 kg: 600 mg once daily
  32-54 kg: 900 mg once daily
  ≥55 kg: 1200 mg once daily

Adults:
  Osteoarthritis: 600-1200 mg once daily; patients should be titrated to lowest dose possible; patients with low body weight should start with 600 mg daily
  Rheumatoid arthritis: 1200 mg once daily; a one-time loading dose of up to 1800 mg/day or 26 mg/kg (whichever is lower) may be given
  Maximum doses:
    Patient <50 kg: Maximum: 1200 mg/day
    Patient >50 kg with normal renal/hepatic function and low risk of peptic ulcer: Maximum: 1800 mg or 26 mg/kg (whichever is lower) in divided doses

Dosing adjustment in renal impairment: In general, NSAIDs are not recommended for use in patients with advanced renal disease but the manufacturer of oxaprozin does provide some guidelines for adjustment in renal dysfunction.

Severe renal impairment or on dialysis: 600 mg once daily; may increase cautiously to 1200 mg/day with close monitoring

Dosing adjustment in hepatic impairment: Use caution in patients with severe dysfunction

Anesthesia and Critical Care Concerns/Other Considerations The 2002 ACCM/SCCM guidelines for analgesia (critically-ill adult) suggest that NSAIDs may be used in combination with opioids in select patients for pain management. Concern about adverse events (increased risk of renal dysfunction, altered platelet function and gastrointestinal irritation) limits its use in patients who have other underlying risks for these events.

In short-term use, NSAIDs vary considerably in their effect on blood pressure. When NSAIDs are used in patients with hypertension, appropriate monitoring of blood pressure responses should be completed and the duration of therapy, when possible, kept short. The use of NSAIDs in the treatment of patients with congestive heart failure may be associated with an increased risk for fluid accumulation and edema; may precipitate renal failure in dehydrated patients.

Additional Information Complete prescribing information for this medication should be consulted for additional detail.

Dosage Forms Excipient information presented when available (limited, particularly for generics); consult specific product labeling.
Tablet: 600 mg

OXcarbazepine (ox car BAZ e peen)

Related Information
  Perioperative Management of Patients on Antiseizure Medication *on page 1577*
U.S. Brand Names Trileptal®
Canadian Brand Names Trileptal®
Index Terms GP 47680; OCBZ
Pharmacologic Category Anticonvulsant, Miscellaneous
Use Monotherapy or adjunctive therapy in the treatment of partial seizures in adults and children ≥4 years of age with epilepsy; adjunctive therapy in the treatment of partial seizures in children ≥2 years of age with epilepsy
Unlabeled/Investigational Use Bipolar disorder; treatment of neuropathic pain
Pharmacodynamics/Kinetics
  Absorption: Complete; food has no affect on rate or extent
  Distribution: MHD: V_d: 49 L
  Protein binding, serum: MHD: 40%
  Metabolism: Hepatic to 10-monohydroxy metabolite (MHD; active); MHD is further glucuronidated or oxidized to a 10,11-dihydroxy metabolite (DHD; inactive)
  Bioavailability: Decreased in children <8 years; increased in elderly >60 years
  Half-life elimination: Parent drug: 2 hours; MHD: 9 hours; renal impairment (Cl_{cr} 30 mL/minute): MHD: 19 hours

Clearance of MHD is increased in younger children (~80% in children 2-4 years of age) and approaches that of adults by ~13 years of age

Time to peak, serum (median): Tablets: 4.5 hours; oral suspension: 6 hours

Excretion: Urine (95%, <1% as unchanged oxcarbazepine, 27% as unchanged MHD, 49% as MHD glucuronides); feces (<4%)

Dosage Oral:

Children 2-3 years:

Adjunctive therapy: 8-10 mg/kg/day, not to exceed 600 mg/day, given in 2 divided daily doses. Maintenance dose should be achieved over 2 weeks, and is dependent upon patient weight.

<20 kg: Consider initiating dose at 16-20 mg/kg/day; maximum maintenance dose should be achieved over 2-4 weeks and should not exceed 60 mg/kg/day

Children 4-16 years:

Adjunctive therapy: 8-10 mg/kg/day, not to exceed 600 mg/day, given in 2 divided daily doses. Maintenance dose should be achieved over 2 weeks, and is dependent upon patient weight, according to the following:

20-29 kg: 900 mg/day in 2 divided doses

29.1-39 kg: 1200 mg/day in 2 divided doses

>39 kg: 1800 mg/day in 2 divided doses

Children 4-16 years:

Conversion to monotherapy: Oxcarbazepine 8-10 mg/kg/day in twice daily divided doses, while simultaneously initiating the reduction of the dose of the concomitant antiepileptic drug; the concomitant drug should be withdrawn over 3-6 weeks. Oxcarbazepine dose may be increased by a maximum of 10 mg/kg/day at weekly intervals. See below for recommended total daily dose by weight.

Initiation of monotherapy: Oxcarbazepine should be initiated at 8-10 mg/kg/day in twice daily divided doses; doses may be titrated by 5 mg/kg/day every third day. See below for recommended total daily dose by weight.

Range of maintenance doses by weight during monotherapy:

20 kg: 600-900 mg/day

25-30 kg: 900-1200 mg/day

35-40 kg: 900-1500 mg/day

45 kg: 1200-1500 mg/day

50-55 kg: 1200-1800 mg/day

60-65 kg: 1200-2100 mg/day

70 kg: 1500-2100 mg/day

Adults:

Adjunctive therapy: Initial: 300 mg twice daily; dose may be increased by as much as 600 mg/day at weekly intervals; recommended daily dose: 1200 mg/day in 2 divided doses. Although daily doses >1200 mg/day were somewhat more efficacious, most patients were unable to tolerate 2400 mg/day (due to CNS effects).

Conversion to monotherapy: Oxcarbazepine 600 mg/day in twice daily divided doses while simultaneously initiating the reduction of the dose of the concomitant antiepileptic drug. The concomitant dosage should be withdrawn over 3-6 weeks, while the maximum dose of oxcarbazepine should be reached in about 2-4 weeks. Recommended daily dose: 2400 mg/day.

Initiation of monotherapy: Oxcarbazepine should be initiated at a dose of 600 mg/day in twice daily divided doses; doses may be titrated upward by 300 mg/day every third day to a final dose of 1200 mg/day given in 2 daily divided doses

Dosing adjustment in renal impairment: Cl$_{cr}$ <30 mL/minute: Therapy should be initiated at one-half the usual starting dose (300 mg/day in adults) and increased slowly to achieve the desired clinical response

Dosing adjustment in hepatic impairment: Adjustment not needed for mild-to-moderate impairment. No data in patients with severe impairment.

Additional Information Complete prescribing information for this medication should be consulted for additional detail.

Dosage Forms Excipient information presented when available (limited, particularly for generics); consult specific product labeling.

Suspension, oral:
Trileptal® 300 mg/5 mL (250 mL) [contains ethanol; packaged with oral syringe]
Tablet: 150 mg, 300 mg, 600 mg
Trileptal® 150 mg, 300 mg, 600 mg

References

American Academy of Pediatrics Committee on Drugs, "The Transfer of Drugs and Other Chemicals Into Human Milk," *Pediatrics*, 2001, 108(3):776-89.

Carrazana E and Mikoshiba I, "Rationale and Evidence for the Use of Oxcarbazepine in Neuropathic Pain," *J Pain Symptom Manage*, 2003, 25(5 Suppl):31-5.

Irving GA, "Contemporary Assessment and Management of Neuropathic Pain," *Neurology*, 2005, 28;64(12 Suppl 3):21-7.

Myllynen P, Pienimaki P, Jouppila P, et al, "Transplacental Passage of Oxcarbazepine and its Metabolites *in vivo*," *Epilepsia*, 2001, 42(11):1482-5.

Rey E, Bulteau C, Motte J, et al, "Oxcarbazepine Pharmacokinetics and Tolerability in Children With Inadequately Controlled Epilepsy," *J Clin Pharmacol*, 2004, 44(11):1290-300.

◆ **Oxeze® Turbuhaler® (Can)** *see* Formoterol *on page 631*

◆ **Oxidized Regenerated Cellulose** *see* Cellulose (Oxidized Regenerated) *on page 280*

◆ **Oxybutyn (Can)** *see* Oxybutynin *on page 1068*

Oxybutynin (oks i BYOO ti nin)

U.S. Brand Names Ditropan XL®; Ditropan®; Gelnique™; Oxytrol®
Canadian Brand Names Apo-Oxybutynin®; Ditropan XL®; Ditropan®; Dom-Oxybutynin; Mylan-Oxybutynin; Novo-Oxybutynin; Nu-Oxybutyn; Oxybutyn; Oxytrol®; PHL-Oxybutynin; PMS-Oxybutynin; Riva-Oxybutynin; Uromax®
Index Terms Oxybutynin Chloride
Pharmacologic Category Antispasmodic Agent, Urinary
Use Antispasmodic for neurogenic bladder (urgency, frequency, leakage, urge incontinence, dysuria); extended release formulation also indicated for treatment of symptoms associated with detrusor overactivity due to a neurological condition (eg, spina bifida)

Pharmacodynamics/Kinetics

Onset of action: Oral: 30-60 minutes
Peak effect: 3-6 hours
Duration: 6-10 hours (up to 24 hours for extended release oral formulation)
Absorption: Oral: Rapid and well absorbed; Transdermal: High
Distribution: I.V.: V_d: 193 L
Metabolism: Hepatic via CYP3A4; Oral: High first-pass metabolism; forms active and inactive metabolites
Bioavailability: Oral: ~6%
Half-life elimination: I.V.: ~2 hours (parent drug), 7-8 hours (metabolites); Oral: ~2-3 hours
Time to peak, serum: Oral: Immediate release: ~60 minutes; Extended release: 4-6 hours; Transdermal: 24-48 hours
Excretion: Urine, as metabolites and unchanged drug (<0.1%)

Dosage

Oral:
Children:
1-5 years (unlabeled use): 0.2 mg/kg/dose 2-4 times/day
>5 years: 5 mg twice daily, up to 5 mg 3 times/day maximum
>6 years: Extended release: 5 mg once daily; adjust dose in 5 mg increments; maximum dose: 20 mg/day
Adults: 5 mg 2-3 times/day up to 5 mg 4 times/day maximum
Extended release: Initial: 5-10 mg once daily, adjust dose in 5 mg increments at weekly intervals; maximum: 30 mg daily
Elderly: Regular release: Initial dose: 2.5 mg 2-3 times/day; increase as needed to 5 mg 2-3 times/day
Topical gel: Adults: Apply contents of 1 sachet (100 mg/g) once daily
Transdermal: Adults: Apply one 3.9 mg/day patch twice weekly (every 3-4 days)

Note: Should be discontinued periodically to determine whether the patient can manage without the drug and to minimize resistance to the drug

Additional Information Complete prescribing information for this medication should be consulted for additional detail.

Dosage Forms Excipient information presented when available (limited, particularly for generics); consult specific product labeling.

Gel, topical, as chloride:
Gelnique™: 10% (1 g) [contains ethanol]
Syrup, as chloride: 5 mg/5 mL (473 mL)
Tablet, as chloride: 5 mg
Ditropan®: 5 mg
Tablet, extended release, as chloride: 5 mg, 10 mg, 15 mg
Ditropan XL®: 5 mg, 10 mg, 15 mg
Transdermal system:
Oxytrol®: 3.9 mg/day (8s) [39 cm^2; total oxybutynin 36 mg]

♦ **Oxybutynin Chloride** *see* Oxybutynin *on page 1068*

♦ **Oxycocet® (Can)** *see* Oxycodone and Acetaminophen *on page 1072*

OxyCODONE (oks i KOE done)

Medication Safety Issues
Sound-alike/look-alike issues:
OxyCODONE may be confused with HYDROcodone, OxyContin®, oxymorphone
OxyContin® may be confused with MS Contin®, oxybutynin, oxycodone
OxyFast® may be confused with Roxanol™
Roxicodone® may be confused with Roxanol™

High alert medication: The Institute for Safe Medication Practices (ISMP) includes this medication among its list of drug classes which have a heightened risk of causing significant patient harm when used in error.

Related Information
Acute Postoperative Pain *on page 1502*
Anesthetic Considerations in the Substance-Abusing Patient *on page 1613*
Chronic Pain Management *on page 1546*
Opioid Analgesics *on page 1688*

U.S. Brand Names ETH-Oxydose™ [DSC]; OxyContin®; OxyIR®; Roxicodone®
Canadian Brand Names Oxy.IR®; OxyContin®; PMS-Oxycodone; Supeudol®
Index Terms Dihydrohydroxycodeinone; Oxycodone Hydrochloride
Pharmacologic Category Analgesic, Opioid
Restrictions C-II
Generic Available Yes
Use Management of moderate-to-severe pain, normally used in combination with nonopioid analgesics

OxyContin® is indicated for around-the-clock management of moderate-to-severe pain when an analgesic is needed for an extended period of time.

Mechanism of Action Binds to opiate receptors in the CNS, causing inhibition of ascending pain pathways, altering the perception of and response to pain; produces generalized CNS depression

Pharmacodynamics/Kinetics
Onset of action: Pain relief: 10-15 minutes
Peak effect: 0.5-1 hour
Duration: Immediate release: 3-6 hours; Controlled release: ≤12 hours
Distribution: V_d: 2.6 L/kg; distributed to skeletal muscle, liver, intestinal tract, lungs, spleen, brain, and breast milk
Protein binding: ~45%
Metabolism: Hepatically via CYP3A4 to noroxycodone (has weak analgesic), noroxymorphone, and alpha- and beta-noroxycodol. CYP2D6 mediated metabolism produces oxymorphone (has analgesic activity; low plasma concentrations), alpha- and beta-oxymorphol.
Bioavailability: Controlled release, immediate release: 60% to 87%
Half-life elimination: Immediate release: 2-3 hours; controlled release: ~5 hours
Excretion: Urine (~19% as parent; >64% as metabolites)

◀ **Dosage** Oral:

Children: Immediate release: 6-18 years: Initial: 0.1-0.2 mg/kg/dose every 6 hours as needed (maximum initial dose: 5 mg for moderate pain; 10 mg for severe pain)

Note: The American Pain Society recommends an initial dose of 0.1-0.2 mg/kg for moderate pain and 0.2 mg/kg for severe pain in children.

Adults:

Immediate release: Initial: 5-10 mg every 4-6 hours as needed; dosing range: 2.5-15 mg/dose. For severe chronic pain, administer on a regularly scheduled basis, every 4-6 hours, at the lowest dose that will achieve adequate analgesia.

Controlled release:

Opioid naive: 10 mg every 12 hours

Concurrent CNS depressants: Reduce usual dose by $1/3$ to $1/2$

Conversion from transdermal fentanyl: For each 25 mcg/hour transdermal dose, substitute 10 mg controlled release oxycodone every 12 hours; should be initiated 18 hours after the removal of the transdermal fentanyl patch

Currently on opioids: Use standard conversion chart to convert daily dose to oxycodone equivalent. Divide daily dose in 2 (for twice-daily dosing, usually every 12 hours) and round down to nearest dosage form.

Note: 60 mg, 80 mg, or 160 mg tablets are for use **only** in opioid-tolerant patients. Special safety considerations must be addressed when converting to OxyContin® doses ≥160 mg every 12 hours. Dietary caution must be taken when patients are initially titrated to 160 mg tablets. Using different strengths to obtain the same daily dose is equivalent (eg, four 40 mg tablets, two 80 mg tablets, one 160 mg tablet); all produce similar blood levels.

Multiplication factors for converting the daily dose of current oral opioid to the daily dose of oral oxycodone:

Current opioid mg/day dose x factor = Oxycodone mg/day dose

Codeine mg/day oral dose **x** 0.15 = Oxycodone mg/day dose

Hydrocodone mg/day oral dose **x** 0.9 = Oxycodone mg/day dose

Hydromorphone mg/day oral dose **x** 4 = Oxycodone mg/day dose

Levorphanol mg/day oral dose **x** 7.5 = Oxycodone mg/day dose

Meperidine mg/day oral dose **x** 0.1 = Oxycodone mg/day dose

Methadone mg/day oral dose **x** 1.5 = Oxycodone mg/day dose

Morphine mg/day oral dose **x** 0.5 = Oxycodone mg/day dose

Note: Divide the oxycodone mg/day dose into the appropriate dosing interval for the specific form being used.

Dosing adjustment in hepatic impairment: Reduce dosage in patients with severe liver disease

Stability Store at 15°C to 30°C (59°F to 86°F). Protect from light.

Administration Do not crush, break, or chew controlled-release tablets; 60 mg, 80 mg, and 160 mg tablets are for use **only** in opioid-tolerant patients. Do not administer OxyContin® 160 mg tablet with a high-fat meal. Controlled release tablets are not indicated for rectal administration; increased risk of adverse events due to better rectal absorption.

Monitoring Parameters Pain relief, respiratory and mental status, blood pressure

Reference Range Blood level of 5 mg/L associated with fatality

Pregnancy Risk Factor B/D (prolonged use or high doses at term)

Contraindications Hypersensitivity to oxycodone or any component of the formulation; significant respiratory depression; hypercarbia; acute or severe bronchial asthma; OxyContin® is also contraindicated in paralytic ileus (known or suspected); pregnancy (prolonged use or high doses at term)

Warnings/Precautions May cause CNS depression, which may impair physical or mental abilities; patients must be cautioned about performing tasks which require mental alertness (eg, operating machinery or driving). Effects may be potentiated when used with other sedative drugs or ethanol. Use with caution in patients with hypersensitivity reactions to other phenanthrene derivative opioid agonists (morphine, hydrocodone, hydromorphone, levorphanol, oxymorphone), respiratory diseases including asthma, emphysema, or COPD. Use with caution in pancreatitis or biliary tract disease, acute alcoholism (including delirium tremens), morbid obesity, adrenocortical insufficiency, history of seizure disorders, CNS depression/coma, kyphoscoliosis (or other skeletal disorder which may alter respiratory function), hypothyroidism (including myxedema), prostatic hyper-plasia, urethral stricture, and toxic psychosis. May obscure diagnosis or clinical course of patients with acute abdominal conditions.

Use with caution in the elderly, debilitated, severe hepatic or renal function. Hemodynamic effects (hypotension, orthostasis) may be exaggerated in patients with hypovolemia, concurrent vasodilating drugs, or in patients with head injury. Respiratory depressant effects and capacity to elevate CSF pressure may be exaggerated in presence of head injury, other intracranial lesion, or pre-existing intracranial pressure.

Use the oral concentrate formulation with caution in patients with latex sensitivity; dropper dispenser contains dry, natural rubber. Concurrent use of agonist/antagonist analgesics may precipitate withdrawal symptoms and/or reduced analgesic efficacy in patients following prolonged therapy with mu opioid agonists. Abrupt discontinuation following prolonged use may also lead to withdrawal symptoms.

[U.S. Boxed Warning]: Healthcare provider should be alert to problems of abuse, misuse, and diversion. Tolerance or drug dependence may result from extended use.

Controlled-release formulations:

[U.S. Boxed Warning]: OxyContin® is not intended for use as an "as needed" analgesic or for immediately-postoperative pain management (should be used postoperatively only if the patient has received it prior to surgery or if severe, persistent pain is anticipated). **[U.S. Boxed Warning]: Do NOT crush, break, or chew controlled-release tablets;** 60 mg, 80 mg, and 160 mg strengths are for use only in opioid-tolerant patients.

Adverse Reactions

>10%:
Central nervous system: Somnolence (23% to 24%), dizziness (13% to 16%)
Dermatologic: Pruritus (12% to 13%)
Gastrointestinal: Nausea (23% to 27%), constipation (23% to 26%), vomiting (12% to 14%)

1% to 10%:
Cardiovascular: Postural hypotension (1% to 5%)
Central nervous system: Headache (7% to 8%), abnormal dreams (1% to 5%), anxiety (1% to 5%), chills (1% to 5%), confusion (1% to 5%), euphoria (1% to 5%), fever (1% to 5%), insomnia (1% to 5%), nervousness (1% to 5%), thought abnormalities (1% to 5%)
Dermatologic: Rash (1% to 5%)
Gastrointestinal: Xerostomia (6% to 7%), abdominal pain (1% to 5%), anorexia (1% to 5%), diarrhea (1% to 5%), dyspepsia (1% to 5%), gastritis (1% to 5%)
Neuromuscular & skeletal: Weakness (6% to 7%), twitching (1% to 5%)
Respiratory: Dyspnea (1% to 5%), hiccups (1% to 5%)
Miscellaneous: Diaphoresis (5% to 6%)
<1% (Limited to important or life-threatening): Agitation, amenorrhea, amnesia, anaphylaxis, anaphylactoid reaction, appetite increased, chest pain, cough, dehydration, depression, dysphagia, dysuria, edema, emotional lability, eructation, exfoliative dermatitis, facial edema, hallucinations, hematuria, histamine release, hyperkinesia, hypoesthesia, hyponatremia, hypotonia, ileus, impotence, intracranial pressure increased, libido decreased, malaise, migraine, paradoxical CNS stimulation, paralytic ileus, paresthesia, pharyngitis, physical dependence, polyuria, psychological dependence, seizure, SIADH, speech disorder, ST segment depression, stomatitis, stupor, syncope, tablet in stool (OxyContin®), taste perversion, thirst, tinnitus, tremor, urinary retention, urticaria, vasodilation, vertigo, vision change, voice alteration, withdrawal syndrome

Drug Interactions

Metabolism/Transport Effects Substrate (minor) of CYP2D6, 3A

Avoid Concomitant Use There are no known interactions where it is recommended to avoid concomitant use.

◄ **Increased Effect/Toxicity**
OxyCODONE may increase the levels/effects of: Alcohol (Ethyl); Alvimopan; CNS Depressants; Desmopressin; Selective Serotonin Reuptake Inhibitors; Thiazide Diuretics

The levels/effects of OxyCODONE may be increased by: Amphetamines; Antipsychotic Agents (Phenothiazines); Succinylcholine

Decreased Effect
OxyCODONE may decrease the levels/effects of: Pegvisomant

The levels/effects of OxyCODONE may be decreased by: Ammonium Chloride

Ethanol/Nutrition/Herb Interactions
Ethanol: Avoid ethanol (may increase CNS depression).
Food: When taken with a high-fat meal, peak concentration is 25% greater following a single OxyContin® 160 mg tablet as compared to two 80 mg tablets.
Herb/Nutraceutical: Avoid valerian, St John's wort, kava kava, gotu kola (may increase CNS depression).

Test Interactions Some quinolones may produce a false-positive urine screening result for opiates using commercially-available immunoassay kits. This has been demonstrated most consistently for levofloxacin and ofloxacin, but other quinolones have shown cross-reactivity in certain assay kits. Confirmation of positive opiate screens by more specific methods should be considered.

Dietary Considerations Instruct patient to avoid high-fat meals when taking OxyContin® 160 mg tablets.

Dosage Forms Excipient information presented when available (limited, particularly for generics); consult specific product labeling. [DSC] = Discontinued product
Capsule, immediate release, as hydrochloride: 5 mg
OxyIR®: 5 mg
Liquid, oral, as hydrochloride [concentrate]:
Roxicodone®: 20 mg/mL (30 mL) [contains sodium benzoate]
Solution, oral, as hydrochloride: 5 mg/5 mL (100 mL, 500 mL)
Roxicodone®: 5 mg/5 mL (5 mL, 500 mL) [contains ethanol]
Solution, oral, as hydrochloride [concentrate]: 20 mg/mL (30 mL)
ETH-Oxydose™: 20 mg/mL (1 mL, 30 mL) [contains sodium benzoate; berry flavor] [DSC]
Tablet, as hydrochloride: 5 mg, 10 mg, 15 mg, 20 mg, 30 mg
Roxicodone®: 5 mg, 15 mg, 30 mg
Tablet, controlled release, as hydrochloride:
OxyContin®: 10 mg, 15 mg, 20 mg, 30 mg, 40 mg, 60 mg, 80 mg
Tablet, extended release, as hydrochloride: 10 mg, 20 mg, 40 mg, 80 mg [DSC]

References
Mokhlesi B, Leikin JB, Murray P, et al, "Adult Toxicology in Critical Care: Part II: Specific Poisonings," *Chest*, 2003, 123(3):897-922.

Oxycodone and Acetaminophen (oks i KOE done & a seet a MIN oh fen)

U.S. Brand Names Endocet®; Magnacet™; Percocet®; Primalev™; Roxicet™; Roxicet™ 5/500; Tylox®
Canadian Brand Names Endocet®; Novo-Oxycodone Acet; Oxycocet®; Percocet®; Percocet®-Demi; PMS-Oxycodone-Acetaminophen
Index Terms Acetaminophen and Oxycodone
Pharmacologic Category Analgesic, Opioid
Restrictions C-II
Use Management of moderate-to-severe pain
Pharmacodynamics/Kinetics See individual agents.
Dosage Oral: Doses should be given every 4-6 hours as needed and titrated to appropriate analgesic effects. **Note:** Initial dose is based on the **oxycodone** content; however, the maximum daily dose is based on the **acetaminophen** content.

Children: Maximum acetaminophen dose: Children <45 kg: 90 mg/kg/day; children >45 kg: 4 g/day

Mild-to-moderate pain: Initial dose, **based on oxycodone content:** 0.05-0.1 mg/kg/dose

Severe pain: Initial dose, **based on oxycodone content:** 0.3 mg/kg/dose

Adults:

Mild-to-moderate pain: Initial dose, **based on oxycodone content:** 2.5-5 mg

Severe pain: Initial dose, **based on oxycodone content:** 10-30 mg. Do not exceed acetaminophen 4 g/day.

Elderly: Doses should be titrated to appropriate analgesic effects: Initial dose, **based on oxycodone content:** 2.5-5 mg every 6 hours. Do not exceed acetaminophen 4 g/day.

Dosage adjustment in hepatic impairment: Dose should be reduced in patients with severe liver disease.

Additional Information Complete prescribing information for this medication should be consulted for additional detail.

Dosage Forms Excipient information presented when available (limited, particularly for generics); consult specific product labeling.

Caplet:

Roxicet™ 5/500: Oxycodone hydrochloride 5 mg and acetaminophen 500 mg

Capsule: 5/500: Oxycodone hydrochloride 5 mg and acetaminophen 500 mg

Tylox®: 5/500: Oxycodone hydrochloride 5 mg and acetaminophen 500 mg [contains sodium benzoate and sodium metabisulfite]

Solution, oral:

Roxicet™: Oxycodone hydrochloride 5 mg and acetaminophen 325 mg per 5 mL (5 mL, 500 mL) [contains ethanol <0.5%; mint flavor]

Tablet: 2.5/325: Oxycodone hydrochloride 2.5 mg and acetaminophen 325 mg; 5/325: Oxycodone hydrochloride 5 mg and acetaminophen 325 mg; 7.5/325: Oxycodone hydrochloride 7.5 mg and acetaminophen 325 mg; 7.5/500: Oxycodone hydrochloride 7.5 mg and acetaminophen 500 mg; 10/325: Oxycodone hydrochloride 10 mg and acetaminophen 325 mg; 10/650: Oxycodone hydrochloride 10 mg and acetaminophen 650 mg

Endocet® 5/325 [scored]: Oxycodone hydrochloride 5 mg and acetaminophen 325 mg

Endocet® 7.5/325: Oxycodone hydrochloride 7.5 mg and acetaminophen 325 mg

Endocet® 7.5/500: Oxycodone hydrochloride 7.5 mg and acetaminophen 500 mg

Endocet® 10/325: Oxycodone hydrochloride 10 mg and acetaminophen 325 mg

Endocet® 10/650: Oxycodone hydrochloride 10 mg and acetaminophen 650 mg

Magnacet™ 2.5/400: Oxycodone hydrochloride 2.5 mg and acetaminophen 400 mg

Magnacet™ 5/400: Oxycodone hydrochloride 5 mg and acetaminophen 400 mg

Magnacet™ 7.5/400: Oxycodone hydrochloride 7.5 mg and acetaminophen 400 mg

Magnacet™ 10/400: Oxycodone hydrochloride 10 mg and acetaminophen 400 mg

Percocet® 2.5/325: Oxycodone hydrochloride 2.5 mg and acetaminophen 325 mg

Percocet® 5/325 [scored]: Oxycodone hydrochloride 5 mg and acetaminophen 325 mg

Percocet® 7.5/325: Oxycodone hydrochloride 7.5 mg and acetaminophen 325 mg

Percocet® 7.5/500: Oxycodone hydrochloride 7.5 mg and acetaminophen 500 mg

Percocet® 10/325: Oxycodone hydrochloride 10 mg and acetaminophen 325 mg

Percocet® 10/650: Oxycodone hydrochloride 10 mg and acetaminophen 650 mg

Primalev™ 2.5/300: Oxycodone hydrochloride 2.5 mg and acetaminophen 300 mg

Primalev™ 5/300: Oxycodone hydrochloride 5 mg and acetaminophen 300 mg

Primalev™ 7.5/300: Oxycodone hydrochloride 7.5 mg and acetaminophen 300 mg

Primalev™ 10/300: Oxycodone hydrochloride 10 mg and acetaminophen 300 mg

Roxicet™ [scored]: Oxycodone hydrochloride 5 mg and acetaminophen 325 mg

References

Mokhlesi B, Leikin JB, Murray P, et al, "Adult Toxicology in Critical Care: Part II: Specific Poisonings," *Chest*, 2003, 123(3):897-922.

◆ **Oxycodone Hydrochloride** *see* OxyCODONE *on page 1069*

◆ **OxyContin®** *see* OxyCODONE *on page 1069*

◆ **OxyIR®** *see* OxyCODONE *on page 1069*

◆ **Oxy.IR® (Can)** *see* OxyCODONE *on page 1069*

Oxymorphone (oks i MOR fone)

Medication Safety Issues

Sound-alike/look-alike issues:

Oxymorphone may be confused with oxycodone, oxymetholone

High alert medication: The Institute for Safe Medication Practices (ISMP) includes this medication among its list of drug classes which have a heightened risk of causing significant patient harm when used in error.

Related Information

Chronic Pain Management *on page 1546*

Opioid Analgesics *on page 1688*

U.S. Brand Names Opana®; Opana® ER

Index Terms Oxymorphone Hydrochloride

Pharmacologic Category Analgesic, Opioid

Restrictions C-II

Generic Available No

Use

Parenteral: Management of moderate-to-severe pain

Oral, regular release: Management of moderate-to-severe pain

Oral, extended release: Management of moderate-to-severe pain in patients requiring around-the-clock opioid treatment for an extended period of time

Mechanism of Action Oxymorphone hydrochloride (Numorphan®) is a potent narcotic analgesic with uses similar to those of morphine. The drug is a semisynthetic derivative of morphine (phenanthrene derivative) and is closely related to hydromorphone chemically (Dilaudid®).

Pharmacodynamics/Kinetics

Onset of action: Parenteral: 5-10 minutes

Duration: Analgesic: Parenteral: 3-6 hours

Distribution: V_d: I.V.: 1.94-4.22 L/kg

Protein binding: 10% to 12%

Metabolism: Hepatic via glucuronidation to active and inactive metabolites

Bioavailability: Oral: 10%

Half-life elimination: Oral: Immediate release: 7-9 hours; Extended release: 9-11 hours

Excretion: Urine (<1% as unchanged drug); feces

Dosage Adults: **Note:** Dosage must be individualized.

I.M., SubQ: Initial: 1-1.5 mg; may repeat every 4-6 hours as needed

Labor analgesia: I.M.: 0.5-1 mg

I.V.: Initial: 0.5 mg

Oral:

Immediate release:

Opioid-naive: 10-20 mg every 4-6 hours as needed. Initial dosages as low as 5 mg may be considered in selected patients and/or patients with renal impairment. Dosage adjustment should be based on level of analgesia, side effects, and pain intensity. Initiation of therapy with initial dose >20 mg is **not** recommended.

Note: The American Pain Society recommends an initial dose of 5-10 mg for adult patients with severe pain.

Currently on stable dose of parenteral oxymorphone: ~10 times the daily parenteral requirement. The calculated amount should be divided and given in 4-6 equal doses.

Currently on other opioids: Use standard conversion chart to convert daily dose to oxymorphone equivalent. Generally start with $1/2$ the calculated daily oxymorphone dosage and administered in divided doses every 4-6 hours.

Extended release (Opana® ER):

Opioid-naive: Initial: 5 mg every 12 hours. Supplemental doses of immediate-release oxymorphone may be used as "rescue" medication as dosage is titrated.

Note: Continued requirement for supplemental dosing may be used to titrate the dose of extended-release continuous therapy. Adjust therapy incrementally, by 5-10 mg every 12 hours at intervals of every 3-7 days. Ideally, basal dosage may be titrated to generally mild pain or no pain with the regular use of fewer than 2 supplemental doses per 24 hours.

Currently on stable dose of parenteral oxymorphone: Approximately 10 times the daily parenteral requirement. The calculated amount should be given in 2 divided doses (every 12 hours).

Currently on opioids: Use conversion chart (see **"Note"**) to convert daily dose to oxymorphone equivalent. Generally start with $1/2$ the calculated daily oxymorphone dosage. Divide daily dose in 2 (for every 12-hour dosing) and round down to nearest dosage form. **Note:** Per manufacturer, the following approximate oral dosages are equivalent to oxymorphone 10 mg:

Hydrocodone 20 mg

Oxycodone 20 mg

Methadone 20 mg

Morphine 30 mg

Conversion of stable dose of immediate-release oxymorphone to extended-release oxymorphone: Administer $1/2$ of the daily dose of immediate-release oxymorphone (Opana®) as the extended-release formulation (Opana® ER) every 12 hours

Elderly: Initiate dosing at the lower end of the dosage range

Dosing adjustment in renal impairment: Cl_{cr} <50 mL/minute: Reduce initial dosage of oral formulations (bioavailability increased 57% to 65%). Begin therapy at lowest dose and titrate carefully.

Dosing adjustment in hepatic impairment: Generally, contraindicated for use in patients with moderate-to-severe liver disease. Initiate with lowest possible dose and titrate slowly in mild impairment.

Stability Injection solution, tablet: Store at 15°C to 30°C (59°F to 86°F).

Administration Administer immediate release and extended release tablets 1 hour before or 2 hours after eating. Opana® ER tablet should be swallowed; do not break, crush, or chew.

Monitoring Parameters Respiratory rate, heart rate, blood pressure, CNS activity

Pregnancy Risk Factor C/D (prolonged use or high doses at term)

Contraindications Hypersensitivity to oxymorphone, other morphine analogs (phenanthrene derivatives), or any component of the formulation; paralytic ileus (known or suspected); increased intracranial pressure; moderate-to-severe hepatic impairment; severe respiratory depression (unless in monitored setting with resuscitative equipment); acute/severe bronchial asthma; hypercarbia; pregnancy (prolonged use or high doses at term).

Note: Injection formulation is also contraindicated in the treatment of upper airway obstruction and pulmonary edema due to a chemical respiratory irritant.

Warnings/Precautions An opioid-containing analgesic regimen should be tailored to each patient's needs and based upon the type of pain being treated (acute versus chronic), the route of administration, degree of tolerance for opioids (naive versus chronic user), age, weight, and medical condition. The optimal analgesic dose varies widely among patients. Doses should be titrated to pain relief/prevention.

May cause CNS depression, which may impair physical or mental abilities; patients must be cautioned about performing tasks which require mental alertness (eg, operating machinery or driving). Effects may be potentiated when used with other sedative drugs or ethanol. Use with caution in patients with hypersensitivity reactions to other phenanthrene-derivative opioid agonists (codeine, hydro-codone, hydromorphone, levorphanol, oxycodone). May cause respiratory depression. Use extreme caution in patients with COPD or other chronic respiratory conditions characterized by hypoxia, hypercapnia, or diminished respiratory reserve (myxedema, cor pulmonale, kyphoscoliosis, obstructive sleep apnea, severe obesity). Use with caution in patients (particularly elderly or debilitated) with impaired respiratory function, adrenal disease, morbid obesity, thyroid dysfunction, prostatic hyperplasia, or renal impairment. Use caution in mild hepatic dysfunction; use is contraindicated in moderate-to-severe hepatic impairment. Use only with extreme caution (if at all) in patients with head injury or increased intracranial pressure (ICP); potential to elevate ICP and/or blunt papillary response may be greatly exaggerated in these patients. Use with caution in biliary tract disease or acute pancreatitis (may cause constriction of sphincter of Oddi). May obscure diagnosis or clinical course of patients with acute abdominal conditions.

Oxymorphone shares the toxic potential of opiate agonists and usual precautions of opiate agonist therapy should be observed; may cause hypotension in patients with acute myocardial infarction, volume depletion, or concurrent drug therapy which may exaggerate vasodilation. The elderly may be particularly susceptible to adverse effects of narcotics. Safety and efficacy have not been established in children <18 years of age.

[U.S. Boxed Warning]: Healthcare provider should be alert to problems of abuse, misuse, and diversion. Tolerance or drug dependence may result from extended use. Use caution in patients with a history of drug dependence or abuse. Abrupt discontinuation may precipitate withdrawal syndrome.

Extended release formulation:

[U.S. Boxed Warnings]: Opana® ER is an extended release oral formulation of oxymorphone and is not suitable for use as an "as needed" analgesic. Tablets should not be broken, chewed, dissolved, or crushed; tablets should be swallowed whole. Opana® ER is intended for use in long-term, continuous management of moderate-to-severe chronic pain. It is not indicated for use in the immediate postoperative period (12-24 hours). **[U.S. Boxed Warning]: The coingestion of ethanol or ethanol-containing medications with Opana® ER may result in accelerated release of drug from the dosage form, abruptly increasing plasma levels, which may have fatal consequences.**

Adverse Reactions Frequency not defined.

Cardiovascular: Bradycardia, cardiac shock, flushing, hypotension, orthostatic hypotension, palpitation, peripheral vasodilation, shock, tachycardia

Central nervous system: Agitation, amnesia, anorexia, anxiety, CNS depression, coma, confusion, convulsion, dizziness, drowsiness, dysphoria, euphoria, fatigue, fever, hallucinations, headache, insomnia, intracranial pressure increased, malaise, mental depression, mental impairment, nervousness, restlessness, paradoxical CNS stimulation

Dermatologic: Pruritus, urticaria, rash

Endocrine & metabolic: Antidiuretic hormone release, weight loss

Gastrointestinal: Abdominal pain, appetite depression, biliary tract spasm, constipation, dehydration, dry mouth, dyspepsia, flatulence, nausea, paralytic ileus, stomach cramps, vomiting, xerostomia

Genitourinary: Urination decreased, urinary retention, urinary tract spasm

Local: Pain/reaction at injection site

Neuromuscular & skeletal: Weakness

Ocular: Blurred vision, diplopia, miosis

Renal: Oliguria

Respiratory: Apnea, bronchospasm, cyanosis, dyspnea, hypoventilation, laryngeal edema, laryngeal spasm, respiratory depression

Miscellaneous: Diaphoresis, histamine release, physical and psychological dependence

Drug Interactions

Avoid Concomitant Use There are no known interactions where it is recommended to avoid concomitant use.

Increased Effect/Toxicity

Oxymorphone may increase the levels/effects of: Alcohol (Ethyl); Alvimopan; CNS Depressants; Desmopressin; Selective Serotonin Reuptake Inhibitors; Thiazide Diuretics

The levels/effects of Oxymorphone may be increased by: Amphetamines; Antipsychotic Agents (Phenothiazines); Succinylcholine

Decreased Effect

Oxymorphone may decrease the levels/effects of: Pegvisomant

The levels/effects of Oxymorphone may be decreased by: Ammonium Chloride

Ethanol/Nutrition/Herb Interactions

Ethanol: Avoid ethanol (may increase CNS depression). Ethanol ingestion with extended-release tablets is specifically contraindicated due to possible accelerated release and potentially fatal overdose.

Food: When taken orally with a high-fat meal, peak concentration is 38% to 50% greater. Both immediate-release and extended-release tablets should be taken 1 hour before or 2 hours after eating.

Herb/Nutraceutical: Avoid valerian, St John's wort, kava kava, gotu kola (may increase CNS depression).

Test Interactions Some quinolones may produce a false-positive urine screening result for opiates using commercially-available immunoassay kits. This has been demonstrated most consistently for levofloxacin and ofloxacin, but other quinolones have shown cross-reactivity in certain assay kits. Confirmation of positive opiate screens by more specific methods should be considered. May cause elevation in amylase (due to constriction of the sphincter of Oddi).

Dietary Considerations Immediate release and extended release tablets should be taken 1 hour before or 2 hours after eating.

Dosage Forms Excipient information presented when available (limited, particularly for generics); consult specific product labeling.

Injection, solution, as hydrochloride:

Opana®: 1 mg/mL (1 mL)

Tablet, as hydrochloride:

Opana®: 5 mg, 10 mg

Tablet, extended release, as hydrochloride:

Opana®: ER: 5 mg, 7.5 mg, 10 mg, 15 mg, 20 mg, 30 mg, 40 mg

References

"Drugs for Pain," *Treat Guidel Med Lett*, 2004, 2(23):47-54.

"Principles of Analgesic Use in the Treatment of Acute Pain and Cancer Pain," 6th ed, Glenview, IL: American Pain Society, 2008.

♦ **Oxymorphone Hydrochloride** *see* Oxymorphone *on page 1074*

Oxytocin (oks i TOE sin)

Medication Safety Issues

High alert medication: The Institute for Safe Medication Practices (ISMP) includes this medication among its list of drugs which have a heightened risk of causing significant patient harm when used in error.

U.S. Brand Names Pitocin®

Canadian Brand Names Pitocin®; Syntocinon®

Index Terms Pit

Pharmacologic Category Oxytocic Agent

Generic Available Yes

Use Induction of labor at term; control of postpartum bleeding; adjunctive therapy in management of abortion

Mechanism of Action Produces the rhythmic uterine contractions characteristic to delivery

Pharmacodynamics/Kinetics

Onset of action: Uterine contractions: I.M.: 3-5 minutes; I.V.: ~1 minute

Duration: I.M.: 2-3 hour; I.V.: 1 hour

Metabolism: Rapidly hepatic and via plasma (by oxytocinase) and to a smaller degree the mammary gland

Half-life elimination: 1-5 minutes

Excretion: Urine

Dosage I.V. administration requires the use of an infusion pump. Adults:

Induction of labor: I.V.: 0.5-1 milliunits/minute; gradually increase dose in increments of 1-2 milliunits/minute until desired contraction pattern is established; dose may be decreased after desired frequency of contractions is reached and labor has progressed to 5-6 cm dilation. Infusion rates of 6 milliunits/minute provide oxytocin levels similar to those in spontaneous labor; rates >9-10 milliunits/minute are rarely required.

Postpartum bleeding:

I.M.: Total dose of 10 units after delivery

I.V.: 10-40 units by I.V. infusion in 1000 mL of intravenous fluid at a rate sufficient to control uterine atony

Adjunctive treatment of abortion: I.V.: 10-20 milliunits/minute; maximum total dose: 30 units/12 hours

Stability Store oxytocin at 2°C to 8°C (36°F to 46°F); do not freeze. Pitocin® may also be stored at 15°C to 25°C (59°F to 77°F) for up to 30 days. Reconstitution: I.V.:

Induction or stimulation of labor: Add oxytocin 10 units to NS or LR 1000 mL to yield a solution containing oxytocin 10 milliunits/mL. Rotate solution to mix.

Postpartum uterine bleeding: Add oxytocin 10-40 units to running I.V. infusion; maximum: 40 units/1000 mL.

Adjunctive management of abortion: Add oxytocin 10 units to 500 mL of a physiologic saline solution or D_5W.

Administration I.V.: Refer to Stability (reconstitution) for dilution information; an infusion pump is required for administration

Monitoring Parameters Fluid intake and output during administration; fetal monitoring

Pregnancy Risk Factor X

Contraindications Hypersensitivity to oxytocin or any component of the formulation; significant cephalopelvic disproportion; unfavorable fetal positions; fetal distress; hypertonic or hyperactive uterus; contraindicated vaginal delivery (invasive cervical cancer, active genital herpes, prolapse of the cord, cord presentation, total placenta previa, or vasa previa)

Warnings/Precautions [U.S. Boxed Warning]: To be used for medical rather than elective induction of labor. May produce antidiuretic effect (ie, water intoxication and excess uterine contractions). High doses or hypersensitivity to oxytocin may cause uterine hypertonicity, spasm, tetanic contraction, or rupture of the uterus. Severe water intoxication with convulsions, coma, and death is associated with a slow oxytocin infusion over 24 hours.

Adverse Reactions Frequency not defined.

Fetus or neonate:

Cardiovascular: Arrhythmias (including premature ventricular contractions), bradycardia

Central nervous system: Brain or CNS damage (permanent), neonatal seizure

Hepatic: Neonatal jaundice

Ocular: Neonatal retinal hemorrhage

Miscellaneous: Fetal death, low Apgar score (5 minute)

Mother:

Cardiovascular: Arrhythmias, hypertensive episodes, premature ventricular contractions

Gastrointestinal: Nausea, vomiting

Genitourinary: Pelvic hematoma, postpartum hemorrhage, uterine hypertonicity, tetanic contraction of the uterus, uterine rupture, uterine spasm

Hematologic: Afibrinogenemia (fatal)

Miscellaneous: Anaphylactic reaction, subarachnoid hemorrhage

Drug Interactions

Avoid Concomitant Use There are no known interactions where it is recommended to avoid concomitant use.

Increased Effect/Toxicity

The levels/effects of Oxytocin may be increased by: Dinoprostone; Misoprostol

Decreased Effect There are no known significant interactions involving a decrease in effect.

Dosage Forms Excipient information presented when available (limited, particularly for generics); consult specific product labeling.

Injection, solution: 10 units/mL (1 mL, 10 mL, 30 mL)

Pitocin®: 10 units/mL (1 mL, 10 mL)

♦ **Oxytrol®** *see* Oxybutynin *on page 1068*

♦ **P-071** *see* Cetirizine *on page 282*

♦ **Pacerone®** *see* Amiodarone *on page 86*

♦ **Paddock Nystatin™** *see* Nystatin *on page 1032*

♦ **Pain Eze [OTC]** *see* Acetaminophen *on page 25*

Palonosetron (pal oh NOE se tron)

Medication Safety Issues
Sound-alike/look-alike issues:
Aloxi® may be confused with Eloxatin®, oxaliplatin
Palonosetron may be confused with dolasetron, granisetron, ondansetron

U.S. Brand Names Aloxi®

Index Terms Palonosetron Hydrochloride; RS-25259; RS-25259-197

Pharmacologic Category Antiemetic; Selective 5-HT$_3$ Receptor Antagonist

Generic Available No

Use
I.V.: Prevention of chemotherapy-associated nausea and vomiting; indicated for prevention of acute (highly-emetogenic therapy) as well as acute and delayed (moderately-emetogenic therapy) nausea and vomiting; prevention of post-operative nausea and vomiting (PONV)

Oral: Prevention of chemotherapy-associated nausea and vomiting (moderately-emetogenic therapy)

Mechanism of Action Selective 5-HT$_3$ receptor antagonist, blocking serotonin, both on vagal nerve terminals in the periphery and centrally in the chemoreceptor trigger zone

Pharmacodynamics/Kinetics
Absorption: Oral: Well absorbed

Distribution: V_d: 8.3 ± 2.5 L/kg

Protein binding: ~62%

Metabolism: ~50% metabolized via CYP enzymes (and likely other pathways) to relatively inactive metabolites (N-oxide-palonosetron and 6-S-hydroxy-palono-setron); CYP1A2, 2D6, and 3A4 contribute to its metabolism

Bioavailability: Oral: 97%

Half-life elimination: I.V.: Terminal: ~40 hours; Oral: 29-45 hours (healthy patients), 38-62 hours (cancer patients)

Time to peak, plasma: Oral: 3-7 hours (healthy patients); ~5 hours (cancer patients)

Excretion: Urine (80% to 93%, 40% as unchanged drug); feces (5% to 8%)

Dosage Adults:
Chemotherapy-associated nausea and vomiting:
I.V.: 0.25 mg 30 minutes prior to the start of chemotherapy administration
Oral: 0.5 mg 1 hour prior to the start of chemotherapy
Breakthrough: Palonosetron has not been shown to be effective in terminating nausea or vomiting once it occurs and should not be used for this purpose.
PONV: I.V.: 0.075 mg immediately prior to anesthesia induction
Elderly: No dosage adjustment necessary

Dosage adjustment in renal/hepatic impairment: No dosage adjustment necessary

Stability
Capsule: Store at room temperature of 25°C (77°F); excursions permitted to 15°C to 30°C (59°F to 86°F). Protect from light.

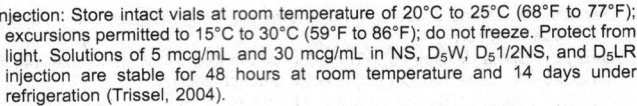

Injection: Store intact vials at room temperature of 20°C to 25°C (68°F to 77°F); excursions permitted to 15°C to 30°C (59°F to 86°F); do not freeze. Protect from light. Solutions of 5 mcg/mL and 30 mcg/mL in NS, D_5W, $D_51/2NS$, and D_5LR injection are stable for 48 hours at room temperature and 14 days under refrigeration (Trissel, 2004).

Administration
I.V.: Flush I.V. line with NS prior to and following administration.
Chemotherapy-associated nausea and vomiting: Infuse over 30 seconds, 30 minutes prior to the start of chemotherapy
PONV: Infuse over 10 seconds immediately prior to anesthesia induction
Oral: May administer with or without meals.

Pregnancy Risk Factor B

Contraindications Hypersensitivity to palonosetron or any component of the formulation

Warnings/Precautions Hypersensitivity has been observed rarely with I.V. palonosetron. Use caution in patients allergic to other $5-HT_3$ receptor antagonists; cross-reactivity is possible. Some selective $5-HT_3$ receptor antagonists have been associated with dose-dependent increases in ECG intervals (eg, PR, QRS duration, QT/QT_c, JT), usually occurring 1-2 hours after I.V. administration. In general, these changes are not clinically relevant, however, when these agents are used in conjunction with other agents that prolong these intervals, arrhythmia may occur. When used with agents that prolong the QT interval (eg, Class I and III antiarrhythmics), clinically relevant QT interval prolongation could result in torsade de pointes. A number of trials have shown that $5-HT_3$ antagonists produce QT interval prolongation to variable degrees. Use with caution in patients at risk of QT prolongation and/or ventricular arrhythmia. Reduction in heart rate may also occur with the $5-HT_3$ antagonists. Use with caution in patients with congenital long QT syndrome or other risk factors for QT prolongation (eg, medications known to prolong QT interval, electrolyte abnormalities, and cumulative high dose anthracycline therapy).

Not intended for treatment of nausea and vomiting or for chronic continuous therapy. **For chemotherapy, should be used on a scheduled basis, not on an "as needed" (PRN) basis,** since data support the use of this drug only in the prevention of nausea and vomiting (due to antineoplastic therapy) and not in the rescue of nausea and vomiting. For PONV, may use for low expectation of PONV if it is essential to avoid nausea and vomiting in the postoperative period; use is not recommended if there is little expectation of nausea and vomiting. Safety and efficacy in children have not been established.

Adverse Reactions Adverse events may vary according to indication. In general, adverse reactions similar between I.V. and oral dosage forms.
1% to 10%:
Cardiovascular: QT prolongation (chemotherapy-associated <1%; PONV 1% to 5%), bradycardia (chemotherapy-associated 1%; PONV 4%), hypotension (≤1%), sinus bradycardia (≤1%), tachycardia (nonsustained) (≤1%)
Central nervous system: Headache (chemotherapy-associated 4% to 9%; PONV 3%), anxiety (1%), dizziness (≤1%), fatigue (≤1%)
Dermatologic: Pruritus (≤1%)
Endocrine & metabolic: Hyperkalemia (1%)
Gastrointestinal: Constipation (1% to 5%), diarrhea (≤1%), flatulence (≤1%)
Genitourinary: Urinary retention (≤1%)
Hepatic: ALT increased (≤1%; transient), AST increased (≤1%; transient)
Neuromuscular & skeletal: Weakness (1%)
<1% (Limited to important or life-threatening): Abdominal pain, abnormal taste, allergic dermatitis, alopecia, amblyopia, anemia, anorexia, appetite decreased, arrhythmia, arthralgia, atrioventricular block (first and second degree), bilirubin increased (transient), chills, dyspepsia, dyspnea, edema (generalized), electrolyte fluctuations, epistaxis, erythema, euphoric mood, extrasystoles, eye irritation/edema, fever, flu-like syndrome, gastritis, glycosuria, hiccups, hot flash, hyperglycemia, hypersensitivity (rare), hypersomnia, hypertension, hypokalemia, hypoventilation, injection site reactions (burning/discomfort/induration/pain; rare), insomnia, intestinal hypomotility, joint stiffness, laryngospasm, metabolic acidosis, motion sickness, myalgia, myocardial ischemia, pain in extremities, paresthesia, platelets decreased, rash, salivation increased, sinus arrhythmia,

sinus tachycardia, sinusitis, somnolence, supraventricular extrasystoles, tinnitus, T-wave amplitude decreased, vein discoloration, vein distention, ventricular extrasystoles, xerostomia

Drug Interactions

Metabolism/Transport Effects Substrate (minor) of CYP1A2, 2D6, 3A4

Avoid Concomitant Use

Avoid concomitant use of Palonosetron with any of the following: Apomorphine

Increased Effect/Toxicity

Palonosetron may increase the levels/effects of: Apomorphine

Decreased Effect

The levels/effects of Palonosetron may be decreased by: Peginterferon Alfa-2b

Dietary Considerations Capsule: May be taken with or without meals.

Product Availability Aloxi® capsules: FDA approved August 2008; anticipated availability currently undetermined

Dosage Forms Excipient information presented when available (limited, particularly for generics); consult specific product labeling.

Capsule:

Aloxi®: 0.5 mg

Injection, solution:

Aloxi®: 0.05 mg/mL (1.5 mL, 5 mL) [contains edetate disodium]

References

Trissel LA, Trusley C, Ben M, et al, "Physical and Chemical Stability of Palonosetron Hydrochloride With Five Opiate Agonists During Simulated Y-Site Administration," *Am J Health-Syst Pharm*, 2007, 64 (11):1209-13.

◆ **Palonosetron Hydrochloride** *see* Palonosetron *on page 1079*

◆ **2-PAM** *see* Pralidoxime *on page 1157*

◆ **Pamelor®** *see* Nortriptyline *on page 1026*

◆ **Pamprin® Maximum Strength All Day Relief [OTC]** *see* Naproxen *on page 987*

Pancuronium (pan kyoo ROE nee um)

Medication Safety Issues

Sound-alike/look-alike issues:

Pancuronium may be confused with pipecuronium

High alert medication: The Institute for Safe Medication Practices (ISMP) includes this medication among its list of drugs which have a heightened risk of causing significant patient harm when used in error.

United States Pharmacopeia (USP) 2006: The Interdisciplinary Safe Medication Use Expert Committee of the USP has recommended the following:
- Hospitals, clinics, and other practice sites should institute special safeguards in the storage, labeling, and use of these agents and should include these safeguards in staff orientation and competency training.
- Healthcare professionals should be on high alert (especially vigilant) whenever a neuromuscular-blocking agent (NMBA) is stocked, ordered, prepared, or administered.

Related Information

Allergic Reactions *on page 1508*

Anesthesia Considerations for Neurosurgery *on page 1514*

Anesthetic Considerations in the Substance-Abusing Patient *on page 1613*

Chronic Renal Failure *on page 1552*

Neuromuscular-Blocking Agents *on page 1684*

Canadian Brand Names Pancuronium Bromide®

Index Terms Pancuronium Bromide; Pavulon [DSC]

Pharmacologic Category Neuromuscular Blocker Agent, Nondepolarizing

Generic Available Yes

Use Facilitation of endotracheal intubation and relaxation of skeletal muscles during surgery; facilitation of mechanical ventilation in ICU patients; does not relieve pain or produce sedation

Mechanism of Action Blocks neural transmission at the myoneural junction by binding with cholinergic receptor sites

Pharmacodynamics/Kinetics
Onset of effect: Peak effect: I.V.: 2-3 minutes
Duration (dose dependent): 60-100 minutes
Metabolism: Hepatic (30% to 45%); active metabolite 3-hydroxypancuronium ($\frac{1}{3}$ to $\frac{1}{2}$ the activity of parent drug)
Half-life elimination: 110 minutes
Excretion: Urine (55% to 70% as unchanged drug)

Dosage Administer I.V.; dose to effect; doses will vary due to interpatient variability; use ideal body weight for obese patients
Surgery:
Neonates <1 month:
Test dose: 0.02 mg/kg to measure responsiveness
Initial: 0.03 mg/kg/dose repeated twice at 5- to 10-minute intervals as needed; maintenance: 0.03-0.09 mg/kg/dose every 30 minutes to 4 hours as needed
Infants >1 month, Children, and Adults: Initial: 0.06-0.1 mg/kg or 0.05 mg/kg after initial dose of succinylcholine for intubation; maintenance dose: 0.01 mg/kg 60-100 minutes after initial dose and then 0.01 mg/kg every 25-60 minutes
Pretreatment/priming: 10% of intubating dose given 3-5 minutes before initial dose
ICU: 0.05-0.1 mg/kg bolus followed by 0.8-1.7 mcg/kg/minute once initial recovery from bolus observed or 0.1-0.2 mg/kg every 1-3 hours

Dosing adjustment in renal impairment: Elimination half-life is doubled, plasma clearance is reduced and rate of recovery is sometimes much slower
Cl_{cr} 10-50 mL/minute: Administer 50% of normal dose
Cl_{cr} <10 mL/minute: Do not use

Dosing adjustment/comments in hepatic/biliary tract disease: Elimination half-life is doubled, plasma clearance is reduced, recovery time is prolonged, volume of distribution is increased (50%) and results in a slower onset, higher total initial dosage and prolongation of neuromuscular blockade

Stability Refrigerate; however, stable for up to 6 months at room temperature.

Administration May be administered undiluted by rapid I.V. injection

Monitoring Parameters Heart rate, blood pressure, assisted ventilation status; cardiac monitor, blood pressure monitor, and ventilator required

Anesthesia and Critical Care Concerns/Other Considerations
Evidence-Based Information: Classified as a long-duration, neuromuscular-blocking agent; neuromuscular blockade will be prolonged in patients with decreased renal function; may produce cumulative effect on duration of blockade; produces tachycardia secondary to vagolytic activity and sympathetic stimulation; synergistic effect when combined with benzylisoquinoline nondepolarizing neuromuscular muscle relaxants (Meretoja, 1994)

Critically-Ill Adult Patients:
The 2008 Surviving Sepsis Campaign guidelines recommend avoiding use of neuromuscular blockers if at all possible in the septic patient due to the risk of prolonged neuromuscular blockade following discontinuation. If one is required, monitor the depth of blockade (Grade 1B).
The 2002 ACCM/SCCM/ASHP clinical practice guidelines for sustained neuromuscular blockade in the adult critically-ill patient recommend:
Optimize sedatives and analgesics prior to initiation and monitor and adjust accordingly during course. Neuromuscular blockers do not relieve pain or produce sedation.
Protect patient's eyes from development of keratitis and corneal abrasion by administering ophthalmic ointment and taping eyelids closed or using eye patches. Reposition patient routinely to protect pressure points from breakdown. Address DVT prophylaxis.
Concurrent use of a neuromuscular blocker and corticosteroids appear to increase the risk of ICU myopathies; avoid or administer the corticosteroid at the lowest dose possible. Reassess need for neuromuscular blocker daily.
Using daily drug holidays (stopping neuromuscular-blocking agent until patient requires it again) may decrease the incidence of acute quadriplegic myopathy syndrome.
Tachyphylaxis can develop. Monitor patients clinically and via "Train of Four" (TOF) testing with a goal of adjusting the degree of blockade to 1-2 twitches.

Pregnancy Risk Factor C

Contraindications Hypersensitivity to pancuronium, bromide, or any component of the formulation

Warnings/Precautions Ventilation must be supported during neuromuscular blockade; use with caution in patients with renal and/or hepatic impairment (adjust dose appropriately); certain clinical conditions may result in potentiation or antagonism of neuromuscular blockade:

Potentiation: Electrolyte abnormalities, severe hyponatremia, severe hypocalcemia, severe hypokalemia, hypermagnesemia, neuromuscular diseases, acidosis, acute intermittent porphyria, renal failure, hepatic failure

Antagonism: Alkalosis, hypercalcemia, demyelinating lesions, peripheral neuropathies, diabetes mellitus

Increased sensitivity in patients with myasthenia gravis, Eaton-Lambert syndrome; resistance in burn patients (>30% of body) for period of 5-70 days postinjury; resistance in patients with muscle trauma, denervation, immobilization, infection. Cross-sensitivity with other neuromuscular-blocking agents may occur; use extreme caution in patients with previous anaphylactic reactions. Use caution in the elderly. **[U.S. Boxed Warning]: Should be administered by adequately trained individuals familiar with its use.** Some dosage forms may contain benzyl alcohol which has been associated with "gasping syndrome" in neonates.

Adverse Reactions Frequency not defined.

Cardiovascular: Elevation in pulse rate, elevated blood pressure and cardiac output, tachycardia, edema, skin flushing, circulatory collapse

Dermatologic: Rash, itching, erythema, burning sensation along the vein

Gastrointestinal: Excessive salivation

Neuromuscular & skeletal: Profound muscle weakness

Respiratory: Wheezing, bronchospasm

Miscellaneous: Hypersensitivity reaction

Postmarketing and/or case reports: Acute quadriplegic myopathy syndrome (prolonged use), myositis ossificans (prolonged use)

Drug Interactions

Avoid Concomitant Use

Avoid concomitant use of Pancuronium with any of the following: QuiNINE

Increased Effect/Toxicity

Pancuronium may increase the levels/effects of: Cardiac Glycosides; Corticosteroids (Systemic); OnabotulinumtoxinA; RimabotulinumtoxinB

The levels/effects of Pancuronium may be increased by: AbobotulinumtoxinA; Aminoglycosides; Calcium Channel Blockers; Capreomycin; Colistimethate; Inhalational Anesthetics; Ketorolac; Lincosamide Antibiotics; Lithium; Loop Diuretics; Magnesium Salts; Polymyxin B; Procainamide; QuiNIDine; QuiNINE; Spironolactone; Tetracycline Derivatives; Vancomycin

Decreased Effect

The levels/effects of Pancuronium may be decreased by: Acetylcholinesterase Inhibitors; Loop Diuretics

Dosage Forms Excipient information presented when available (limited, particularly for generics); consult specific product labeling.

Injection, solution, as bromide: 1 mg/mL (10 mL); 2 mg/mL (2 mL, 5 mL) [may contain benzyl alcohol]

References

Dellinger RP, Levy MM, Carlet JM, et al, "Surviving Sepsis Campaign: International Guidelines for Management of Severe Sepsis and Septic Shock: 2008," *Intensive Care Med*, 2008, 34(1): 17-60. Available at http://www.survivingsepsis.org/system/files/images/2008_20International_20SSC_20-Guidelines_1_.pdf

Meretoja OA, Taivainen T, Jalkanen L, et al, "Synergism Between Atracurium and Vecuronium in Infants and Children During Nitrous Oxide-Oxygen-Alfentanil Anaesthesia," *Br J Anaesth*, 1994, 73 (5):605-7.

Murray MJ, Cowen J, DeBlock H, et al, "Clinical Practice Guidelines for Sustained Neuromuscular Blockade in the Adult Critically Ill Patient. Task Force of the American College of Critical Care Medicine (ACCM) of the Society of Critical Care Medicine (SCCM), American Society of Health-System Pharmacists, American College of Chest Physicians," *Crit Care Med*, 2002, 30(1):142-56; viewable at http://www.sccm.org/pdf/NeuromuscularBlockade.pdf.

◆ **Pancuronium Bromide** see Pancuronium on page 1081

◆ **Pancuronium Bromide® (Can)** see Pancuronium on page 1081

◆ **Pandel®** see Hydrocortisone on page 699

- ◆ **Panglobulin** *see* Immune Globulin (Intravenous) *on page 732*
- ◆ **Panto™ I.V. (Can)** *see* Pantoprazole *on page 1084*
- ◆ **Pantoloc® (Can)** *see* Pantoprazole *on page 1084*

Pantoprazole (pan TOE pra zole)

Medication Safety Issues
Sound-alike/look-alike issues:
  Pantoprazole may be confused with aripiprazole
  Protonix® may be confused with Lotronex®, Lovenox®, protamine

Vials containing Protonix® I.V. for injection are not recommended for use with spiked I.V. system adaptors. Nurses and pharmacists have reported breakage of the glass vials during attempts to connect spiked I.V. system adaptors, which may potentially result in injury to healthcare professionals.

International issues:
  Protonix® may be confused with Pretanix® which is a brand name for indapamide in Hungary

U.S. Brand Names Protonix®

Canadian Brand Names Apo-Pantoprazole®; CO Pantoprazole; Gen-Pantoprazole; Mylan-Pantoprazole; Novo-Pantoprazole; Pantoloc®; Panto™ I.V.; PMS-Pantoprazole; Protonix®; Ran-Pantoprazole; ratio-Pantoprazole; Riva-Pantoprazole; Sandoz-Pantoprazole; Tecta™; ZYM-Pantoprazole

Pharmacologic Category Proton Pump Inhibitor; Substituted Benzimidazole

Generic Available Yes: Delayed release tablet

Use
Oral: Treatment and maintenance of healing of erosive esophagitis associated with GERD; reduction in relapse rates of daytime and nighttime heartburn symptoms in GERD; hypersecretory disorders associated with Zollinger-Ellison syndrome or other GI hypersecretory disorders

I.V.: Short-term treatment (7-10 days) of patients with gastroesophageal reflux disease (GERD) and a history of erosive esophagitis; hypersecretory disorders associated with Zollinger-Ellison syndrome or other neoplastic disorders

Unlabeled/Investigational Use Peptic ulcer disease, active ulcer bleeding (parenteral formulation); adjunct treatment with antibiotics for *Helicobacter pylori* eradication; stress-ulcer prophylaxis in the critically-ill

Mechanism of Action Suppresses gastric acid secretion by inhibiting the parietal cell H^+/K^+ ATP pump

Pharmacodynamics/Kinetics
Absorption: Rapid, well absorbed
Distribution: V_d: 11-24 L
Protein binding: 98%, primarily to albumin
Metabolism: Extensively hepatic; CYP2C19 (demethylation), CYP3A4; no evidence that metabolites have pharmacologic activity
Bioavailability: 77%
Half-life elimination: 1 hour; increased to 3.5-10 hours with CYP2C19 deficiency
Time to peak: Oral: 2.5 hours
Excretion: Urine (71%); feces (18%)

Dosage
Oral:
  Children ≥5 years (unlabeled use): GERD, erosive esophagitis associated with GERD: 20-40 mg once daily
  Adults:
    Erosive esophagitis associated with GERD:
      Treatment: 40 mg once daily for up to 8 weeks; an additional 8 weeks may be used in patients who have not healed after an 8-week course
      Maintenance of healing: 40 mg once daily
      Note: Lower doses (20 mg once daily) have been used successfully in mild GERD treatment and maintenance of healing
    Hypersecretory disorders (including Zollinger-Ellison): Initial: 40 mg twice daily; adjust dose based on patient needs; doses up to 240 mg/day have been administered

Helicobacter pylori eradication (unlabeled use): American College of Gastroenterology guidelines (Chey, 2007):

Nonpenicillin allergy: 40 mg twice daily administered with amoxicillin 1000 mg *and* clarithromycin 500 mg twice daily for 10-14 days

Penicillin allergy: 40 mg twice daily administered with clarithromycin 500 mg *and* metronidazole 500 mg twice daily for 10-14 days **or** 40 mg once or twice daily administered with bismuth subsalicylate 525 mg *and* metronidazole 250 mg *plus* tetracycline 500 mg 4 times/day for 10-14 days

I.V.:

Erosive esophagitis associated with GERD: 40 mg once daily for 7-10 days

Hypersecretory disorders: 80 mg twice daily; adjust dose based on acid output measurements; 160-240 mg/day in divided doses has been used for a limited period (up to 7 days)

Prevention of rebleeding in peptic ulcer bleed (unlabeled use): 80 mg, followed by 8 mg/hour infusion for 72 hours. **Note:** A daily infusion of 40 mg does not raise gastric pH sufficiently to enhance coagulation in active GI bleeds.

Elderly: Dosage adjustment not required

Dosage adjustment in renal impairment: Not required; pantoprazole is not removed by hemodialysis

Dosage adjustment in hepatic impairment: Not required

Stability

Oral: Store tablet and oral suspension at controlled room temperature of 20°C to 25°C (68°F to 77°F).

I.V.: Prior to reconstitution, store at controlled room temperature of 20°C to 25°C (68°F to 77°F). Protect from light. Reconstitute with 10 mL NS (final concentration 4 mg/mL). Reconstituted solution may be given intravenously (over 2 minutes) or may be added to 100 mL D_5W, NS, or LR (for 15-minute infusion). When reconstituted, solution is stable up to 96 hours at room temperature (Johnson, 2005). The preparation should be stored at 3°C to 5°C (37°F to 41°F) if it is stored beyond 48 hours to minimize discoloration. If further diluting in 100 mL of D_5W, LR, or NS, dilute within 6 hours of reconstitution. Diluted solution is stable at room temperature for up to 24 hours from the time of initial reconstitution; protection from light is not required.

Administration

I.V.: Flush I.V. line before and after administration. In-line filter not required.

2-minute infusion: The volume of reconstituted solution (4 mg/mL) to be injected may be administered intravenously over at least 2 minutes.

15-minute infusion: Infuse over 15 minutes at a rate not to exceed 7 mL/minute (3 mg/minute).

Oral:

Tablet: Should be swallowed whole, do not crush or chew. Best if taken before breakfast.

Delayed-release oral suspension: Should only be administered in apple juice or applesauce and taken ~30 minutes before a meal. Do not administer with any other liquid (eg, water) or foods.

Oral administration in **applesauce**: Sprinkle intact granules on 1 tablespoon of applesauce and swallow within 10 minutes of preparation.

Oral administration in **apple juice**: Empty intact granules into 5 mL of apple juice (~1 teaspoonful), stir for 5 seconds, and swallow immediately after preparation. Rinse container once or twice with apple juice and swallow immediately.

Nasogastric tube administration: Separate the plunger from the barrel of a 60 mL catheter tip syringe and connect to a ≥16 French nasogastric tube. Holding the syringe attached to the tubing as high as possible, empty the contents of the packet into barrel of the syringe, add 10 mL of apple juice and gently tap/shake the barrel of the syringe to help empty the syringe. Add an additional 10 mL of apple juice and gently tap/shake the barrel to help rinse. Repeat rinse with at least 2-10 mL aliquots of apple juice. No granules should remain in the syringe.

Monitoring Parameters Hypersecretory disorders: Acid output measurements, target level <10 mEq/hour (<5 mEq/hour if prior gastric acid-reducing surgery)

◀ **Anesthesia and Critical Care Concerns/Other Considerations**
Evidence-Based Information:

Acute ulcer: Pre-endoscopy therapy: Lau and associates (2007) evaluated the effects of preemptive infusion of omeprazole before endoscopy in upper gastrointestinal bleeding. Consecutive patients (n=638) were stabilized and then randomly assigned to intravenous omeprazole (80 mg bolus followed by a continuous infusion of 8 mg/hour) or placebo infusion before endoscopy the next morning. The primary endpoint was the need for endoscopic therapy (eg, epinephrine, thermocoagulation). Seven patients were excluded from the analysis. The need for endoscopic treatment was significantly lower in the omeprazole group (60/314 patients; 19%) than in the placebo group (90/317; 28%). The active treatment group had a significantly shorter hospital stay. Duration of infusion before endoscopy was similar in both groups (~8-21 hours).

Acute ulcer: Postendoscopy therapy: Intravenous omeprazole has been studied in prevention of rebleeding in ulcer patients who are at high risk for rebleeding (endoscopic findings of active bleeding or nonbleeding visible vessel) after successful hemostasis (Lin, 1998; Lau, 2000). Lin and his group treated 100 ulcer patients (actively bleeding ulcers or ulcers with nonbleeding visible vessels) endoscopically and then randomized them to cimetidine (300 mg bolus followed by 50 mg/hour infusion) or omeprazole (40 mg bolus, ~7 mg/hour infusion) for 72 hours. Patients were discharged on the oral form of the drug arm they were assigned to. The omeprazole group maintained an intragastric pH >6 for about 84% of the infusion duration, while the cimetidine group maintained their pH >6 only about 50% of the time. Rebleeding occurred significantly more often in the cimetidine group.

Lau and his colleagues treated patients with actively bleeding ulcers or ulcers with nonbleeding visible vessels with an epinephrine infusion followed by thermocoagulation. They were then randomized to omeprazole (80 mg bolus followed by a continuous infusion of 8 mg/hour for 72 hours) or placebo. All patients were discharged on oral omeprazole (20 mg/day) for 8 weeks and received *H. pylori* treatment if indicated. The primary goal was to evaluate the rate of rebleeding during the first 30 days after endoscopy. Two hundred and forty patients were enrolled with randomization of 120 into each group. Bleeding recurred in significantly more patients receiving placebo than omeprazole infusion. The authors concluded that after endoscopic therapy, omeprazole reduces the risk of rebleeding in patients with actively bleeding ulcers or ulcers with nonbleeding visible vessels.

Stress ulcer prophylaxis: The 2008 Surviving Sepsis Campaign guidelines recommend that stress ulcer prophylaxis using an H_2 blocker (Grade 1A) or proton pump inhibitor (Grade 1B) be given to patients with severe sepsis to prevent upper GI bleed. Benefit of prevention of upper GI bleed must be weighed against potential effect of increased stomach pH on development of ventilator-associated pneumonia.

Pregnancy Risk Factor B

Contraindications Hypersensitivity to pantoprazole, substituted benzamidazoles (eg, esomeprazole, lansoprazole, omeprazole, rabeprazole), or any component of the formulation

Canadian labeling: Additional contraindication (not in U.S. labeling): Concomitant use with atazanavir

Warnings/Precautions Use of proton pump inhibitors may increase the risk of gastrointestinal infections (eg, *Salmonella, Campylobacter*). Relief of symptoms does not preclude the presence of a gastric malignancy. Long-term pantoprazole therapy (especially in patients who were *H. pylori* positive) has caused biopsy-proven atrophic gastritis. No reports of enterochromaffin-like (ECL) cell carcinoids, dysplasia, or neoplasia such as those seen in rodent studies have occurred in humans. Not indicated for maintenance therapy; safety and efficacy for use beyond 16 weeks have not been established. Prolonged treatment (typically >3 years) may lead to vitamin B_{12} malabsorption and subsequent deficiency. Intravenous preparation contains edetate sodium (EDTA); use caution in patients who are at risk for zinc deficiency if other EDTA-containing solutions are coadministered. Decreased *H. pylori* eradication rates have been observed with short-term (≤7 days) combination therapy. The American College of

Gastroenterology recommends 10-14 days of therapy (triple or quadruple) for eradication of *H. pylori* (Chey, 2007).

Adverse Reactions

≥1%:

Cardiovascular: Chest pain

Central nervous system: Headache (2% to 9%), insomnia (≤1%), anxiety, dizziness, migraine, pain

Dermatologic: Rash (≤2%)

Endocrine & metabolic: Hyperglycemia (≤1%), hyperlipidemia

Gastrointestinal: Diarrhea (2% to 6%), flatulence (2% to 4%), abdominal pain (1% to 4%), nausea (≤2%), vomiting (≤2%), eructation (≤1%), constipation, dyspepsia, gastroenteritis, rectal disorder

Genitourinary: Urinary frequency, UTI

Hepatic: Liver function tests abnormal (≤2%)

Local: Injection site reaction (includes thrombophlebitis and abscess)

Neuromuscular & skeletal: Arthralgia, back pain, hypertonia, neck pain, weakness

Respiratory: Bronchitis, cough, dyspnea, pharyngitis, rhinitis, sinusitis, upper respiratory tract infection

Miscellaneous: Flu syndrome, infection

<1% (Limited to important or life-threatening): Abnormal dreams, acne, albuminuria, alkaline phosphatase increased, allergic reaction, alopecia, anaphylaxis, anemia, angioedema, angina pectoris, anorexia, aphthous stomatitis, appetite increased, arrhythmia, asthma exacerbation, atrial fibrillation/flutter, atrophic gastritis, balanitis, biliary pain, blurred vision, bone pain, breast pain, bursitis, cataract, CHF, chills, cholecystitis, cholelithiasis, CPK increased, colitis, confusion, contact dermatitis, creatinine increased, cystitis, deafness, decreased reflexes, dehydration, depression, diabetes mellitus, diaphoresis, diplopia, duodenitis, dysarthria, dysmenorrhea, dysphagia, dysuria, ecchymosis, ECG abnormality, eczema, eosinophilia, epididymitis, epistaxis, erythema multiforme, esophagitis, extraocular palsy, facial edema, fever, fungal dermatitis, gastrointestinal carcinoma, gastrointestinal hemorrhage, gastrointestinal moniliasis, generalized edema, GGT increased, gingivitis, glaucoma, glossitis, glycosuria, goiter, gout, halitosis, hallucinations, heat stroke, hematemesis, hematuria, hemorrhage, hepatic failure, hepatitis, hernia, herpes simplex, herpes zoster, hiccup, hyperbilirubinemia, hyperesthesia, hyper-/hypotension, hyperkinesia, hyperuricemia, hypokinesia, impaired urination, impotence, interstitial nephritis, jaundice, kidney calculus, kidney pain, laryngitis, leg cramps, leukocytosis, leukopenia, libido decreased, lichenoid dermatitis, maculopapular rash, malaise, melena, mouth ulceration, myalgia, myocardial infarction, myocardial ischemia, neoplasm, nervousness, neuralgia, neuritis, nocturia, optic neuropathy (including anterior ischemic), otitis externa, palpitation, pancreatitis, pancytopenia, paresthesia, periodontal abscess, periodontitis, photosensitivity, pneumonia, pruritus, pyelonephritis, rectal hemorrhage, retinal vascular disorder, rhabdomyolysis, salivation increased, scrotal edema, seizure, skin ulcer, somnolence, Stevens-Johnson syndrome, stomach ulcer, stomatitis, syncope, tachycardia, taste perversion, tenosynovitis, thrombocytopenia, thrombosis, tinnitus, tongue discoloration, toxic epidermal necrolysis, tremor, urethral pain, urethritis, urticaria, vaginitis, vasodilation, vertigo, vision abnormal, weight changes, xerostomia

Drug Interactions

Metabolism/Transport Effects Substrate of CYP2C19 (major), 2C9 (minor), 2D6 (minor), 3A4 (minor); **Inhibits** 2C9 (weak); **Induces** CYP1A2 (weak), 3A4 (weak)

Avoid Concomitant Use

Avoid concomitant use of Pantoprazole with any of the following: Delavirdine; Erlotinib; Nelfinavir; Posaconazole

Increased Effect/Toxicity

Pantoprazole may increase the levels/effects of: Methotrexate; Raltegravir; Saquinavir; Topotecan; Voriconazole

The levels/effects of Pantoprazole may be increased by: Fluconazole; Ketoconazole

◀ **Decreased Effect**
Pantoprazole may decrease the levels/effects of: Atazanavir; Clopidogrel; Dabigatran Etexilate; Dasatinib; Delavirdine; Erlotinib; Indinavir; Iron Salts; Itraconazole; Ketoconazole; Mesalamine; Mycophenolate; Nelfinavir; Posaconazole

The levels/effects of Pantoprazole may be decreased by: CYP2C19 Inducers (Strong); Peginterferon Alfa-2b; Tipranavir

Ethanol/Nutrition/Herb Interactions
Ethanol: Avoid ethanol (may cause gastric mucosal irritation).
Herb/Nutraceutical: Prolonged treatment (typically >3 years) may lead to vitamin B_{12} malabsorption and subsequent deficiency.

Test Interactions False-positive urine screening tests for tetrahydrocannabinol (THC) have been noted in patients receiving proton pump inhibitors, including pantoprazole.

Dietary Considerations
Oral: May be taken with or without food; best if taken before breakfast.
I.V.: Due to EDTA in preparation, zinc supplementation may be needed in patients prone to zinc deficiency.

Dosage Forms Excipient information presented when available (limited, particularly for generics); consult specific product labeling. [CAN] = Canadian brand name
Note: Strength expressed as base
Granules for suspension, delayed release, enteric coated, as sodium, oral:
  Protonix®: 40 mg/packet (30s)
Injection, powder for reconstitution, as sodium:
  Protonix®: 40 mg [contains edetate sodium 1 mg]
Tablet, delayed release, as sodium: 20 mg, 40 mg
  Protonix®: 20 mg, 40 mg
Tablet, enteric coated, as magnesium:
  Pantoloc® M [CAN]: 40 mg [not available in the U.S.]

References
Allen ME, Kopp BJ, and Erstad BL, "Stress Ulcer Prophylaxis in the Postoperative Period," *Am J Health Syst Pharm*, 2004, 61(6):588-96.
Bardhan KD, Dillon J, Axon AT, et al, "Triple Therapy for *Helicobacter pylori* Eradication: A Comparison of Pantoprazole Once Versus Twice Daily," *Aliment Pharmacol Ther*, 2000, 14 (1):59-67.
Brunner G, Luna P, Hartmann M, et al, "Optimizing the Intragastric pH as a Supportive Therapy in Upper Gastrointestinal Bleeding," *Yale J Biol Med*, 1996, 69(3):225-31.
Dellinger RP, Levy MM, Carlet JM, et al, "Surviving Sepsis Campaign: International Guidelines for Management of Severe Sepsis and Septic Shock: 2008," *Intensive Care Med*, 2008, 34(1): 17-60. Available at http://www.survivingsepsis.org/system/files/images/2008_20International_20SSC_20-Guidelines_1_.pdf
Jung R and MacLaren R, "Proton-Pump Inhibitors for Stress Ulcer Prophylaxis in Critically Ill Patients," *Ann Pharmacother*, 2002, 36(12):1929-37.
Lau JY, Leung WK, Wu JC, et al, "Omeprazole Before Endoscopy in Patients With Gastrointestinal Bleeding," *N Engl J Med*, 2007, 356(16):1631-40.
Lau JY, Sung JJ, Lee KK, et al, "Effect of Intravenous Omeprazole on Recurrent Bleeding After Endoscopic Treatment of Bleeding Peptic Ulcers," *N Engl J Med*, 2000, 343(5):310-6.
Lew EA, Pisegna JR, Starr JA, et al, "Intravenous Pantoprazole Rapidly Controls Gastric Acid Hypersecretion in Patients With Zollinger-Ellison Syndrome," *Gastroenterology*, 2000, 118 (4):696-704.
Lin HJ, Lo WC, Lee FY, et al, "A Prospective Randomized Comparative Trial Showing That Omeprazole Prevents Rebleeding in Patients With Bleeding Peptic Ulcer After Successful Endoscopic Therapy," *Arch Intern Med*, 1998, 158(1):54-8.
Morgan D, "Intravenous Proton-Pump Inhibitors in the Critical Care Setting," *Crit Care Med*, 2002, 30 (Suppl):369-72.

PARoxetine (pa ROKS e teen)

Related Information
 Antidepressant Agents *on page 1660*

U.S. Brand Names Paxil CR®; Paxil®; Pexeva®

Canadian Brand Names Apo-Paroxetine®; CO Paroxetine; Mylan-Paroxetine; Novo-Paroxetine; Paxil CR®; Paxil®; PHL-Paroxetine; PMS-Paroxetine; ratio-Paroxetine; Riva-paroxetine; Sandoz-Paroxetine; ZYM-Paroxetine

Index Terms Paroxetine Hydrochloride; Paroxetine Mesylate

Pharmacologic Category Antidepressant, Selective Serotonin Reuptake Inhibitor

Use Treatment of major depressive disorder (MDD); treatment of panic disorder with or without agoraphobia; obsessive-compulsive disorder (OCD); social anxiety disorder (social phobia); generalized anxiety disorder (GAD); post-traumatic stress disorder (PTSD); premenstrual dysphoric disorder (PMDD)

Unlabeled/Investigational Use May be useful in eating disorders, impulse control disorders, self-injurious behavior; vasomotor symptoms of menopause; treatment of depression and obsessive-compulsive disorder (OCD) in children; treatment of mild dementia-associated agitation in nonpsychotic patients

Pharmacodynamics/Kinetics

Onset of action: Depression: The onset of action is within a week; however, individual response varies greatly and full response may not be seen until 8-12 weeks after initiation of treatment.

Absorption: Completely absorbed following oral administration

Distribution: V_d: 8.7 L/kg (3-28 L/kg)

Protein binding: 93% to 95%

Metabolism: Extensively hepatic via CYP2D6 enzymes; primary metabolites are formed via oxidation and methylation of parent drug, with subsequent glucuronide/sulfate conjugation; nonlinear pharmacokinetics (via 2D6 saturation) may be seen with higher doses and longer duration of therapy. Metabolites exhibit ~2% potency of parent compound. C_{min} concentrations are 70% to 80% greater in the elderly compared to nonelderly patients; clearance is also decreased.

Half-life elimination: 21 hours (3-65 hours)

Time to peak: Immediate release: 5.2 hours; controlled release: 6-10 hours

Excretion: Urine (64%, 2% as unchanged drug); feces (36% primarily via bile, <1% as unchanged drug)

Dosage Oral:

Children:

Depression (unlabeled use; not recommended by FDA): Initial: 10 mg/day and adjusted upward on an individual basis to 20 mg/day

Obsessive-compulsive disorder (unlabeled use): Initial: 10 mg/day and titrate up as necessary to 60 mg/day

Self-injurious behavior (unlabeled use): 20 mg/day

Social anxiety disorder (unlabeled use): 2.5-15 mg/day

Adults:

Major depressive disorder:

Paxil®, Pexeva®: Initial: 20 mg once daily, preferably in the morning; increase if needed by 10 mg/day increments at intervals of at least 1 week; maximum dose: 50 mg/day

Paxil CR®: Initial: 25 mg once daily; increase if needed by 12.5 mg/day increments at intervals of at least 1 week; maximum dose: 62.5 mg/day

Generalized anxiety disorder (Paxil®, Pexeva®): Initial: 20 mg once daily, preferably in the morning (if dose is increased, adjust in increments of 10 mg/day at 1-week intervals); doses of 20-50 mg/day were used in clinical trials, however, no greater benefit was seen with doses >20 mg.

Obsessive-compulsive disorder (Paxil®, Pexeva™): Initial: 20 mg once daily, preferably in the morning; increase if needed by 10 mg/day increments at intervals of at least 1 week; recommended dose: 40 mg/day; range: 20-60 mg/day; maximum dose: 60 mg/day

Panic disorder:

Paxil®, Pexeva®: Initial: 10 mg once daily, preferably in the morning; increase if needed by 10 mg/day increments at intervals of at least 1 week; recommended dose: 40 mg/day; range: 10-60 mg/day; maximum dose: 60 mg/day

Paxil CR®: Initial: 12.5 mg once daily; increase if needed by 12.5 mg/day at intervals of at least 1 week; maximum dose: 75 mg/day

Premenstrual dysphoric disorder (Paxil CR®): Initial: 12.5 mg once daily in the morning; may be increased to 25 mg/day; dosing changes should occur at intervals of at least 1 week. May be given daily throughout the menstrual cycle or limited to the luteal phase.

Post-traumatic stress disorder (PTSD) (Paxil®): Initial: 20 mg once daily, preferably in the morning; increase if needed by 10 mg/day increments at intervals of at least 1 week; range: 20-50 mg. Limited data suggest doses of 40 mg/day were not more efficacious than 20 mg/day.

Social anxiety disorder:

Paxil®: Initial: 20 mg once daily, preferably in the morning; recommended dose: 20 mg/day; range: 20-60 mg/day; doses >20 mg may not have additional benefit

Paxil CR®: Initial: 12.5 mg once daily, preferably in the morning; may be increased by 12.5 mg/day at intervals of at least 1 week; maximum dose: 37.5 mg/day

Vasomotor symptoms of menopause (unlabeled use, Paxil CR®): 12.5-25 mg/day

Elderly:

Paxil®, Pexeva®: Initial: 10 mg/day; increase if needed by 10 mg/day increments at intervals of at least 1 week; maximum dose: 40 mg/day

Paxil CR®: Initial: 12.5 mg/day; increase if needed by 12.5 mg/day increments at intervals of at least 1 week; maximum dose: 50 mg/day

Note: Upon discontinuation of paroxetine therapy, gradually taper dose:

Paxil®, Pexeva®: 10 mg/day at weekly intervals; when 20 mg/day dose is reached, continue for 1 week before treatment is discontinued. Some patients may need to be titrated to 10 mg/day for 1 week before discontinuation.

Paxil CR®: Patients receiving 37.5 mg/day in clinical trials had their dose decreased by 12.5 mg/day to a dose of 25 mg/day and remained at a dose of 25 mg/day for 1 week before treatment was discontinued.

Dosage adjustment in renal impairment: Adults:

Cl_{cr} <30 mL/minute: Mean plasma concentration is ~4 times that seen in normal function.

Cl_{cr} 30-60 mL/minute: Plasma concentration is 2 times that seen in normal function.

Paxil®, Pexeva®: Initial: 10 mg/day; increase if needed by 10 mg/day increments at intervals of at least 1 week; maximum dose: 40 mg/day

Paxil CR®: Initial: 12.5 mg/day; increase if needed by 12.5 mg/day increments at intervals of at least 1 week; maximum dose: 50 mg/day

Dosage adjustment in severe hepatic impairment: Adults: In hepatic dysfunction, plasma concentration is 2 times that seen in normal function.

Paxil®, Pexeva®: Initial: 10 mg/day; increase if needed by 10 mg/day increments at intervals of at least 1 week; maximum dose: 40 mg/day

Paxil CR®: Initial: 12.5 mg/day; increase if needed by 12.5 mg/day increments at intervals of at least 1 week; maximum dose: 50 mg/day

Additional Information Complete prescribing information for this medication should be consulted for additional detail.

Dosage Forms Excipient information presented when available (limited, particularly for generics); consult specific product labeling.

Note: Strength expressed as base:

Suspension, oral, as hydrochloride: 10 mg/5 mL (250 mL)

Paxil®: 10 mg/5 mL (250 mL) [contains propylene glycol; orange flavor]

Tablet, as hydrochloride: 10 mg, 20 mg, 30 mg, 40 mg

Paxil®: 10 mg, 20 mg, 30 mg, 40 mg

Tablet, as mesylate:

Pexeva®: 10 mg, 20 mg, 30 mg, 40 mg

Tablet, controlled release, enteric coated, as hydrochloride: 37.5 mg
  Paxil CR®: 12.5 mg, 25 mg, 37.5 mg
Tablet, extended release, enteric coated, as hydrochloride: 12.5 mg, 25 mg

Peginterferon Alfa-2a and Ribavirin
(peg in ter FEER on AL fa too aye & rye ba VYE rin)

Canadian Brand Names Pegasys® RBV
Index Terms Ribavirin and Peginterferon Alfa-2a
Pharmacologic Category Antiviral Agent; Interferon
Restrictions Not available in U.S.
Use Combination therapy for the treatment of chronic hepatitis C (HCV) in patients without cirrhosis and patients with compensated cirrhosis; includes patients coinfected with stable HIV disease
Pharmacodynamics/Kinetics
Dosage Adults: Canadian Consensus Guidelines recommend peginterferon plus ribavirin as treatment of choice for chronic hepatitis C (Sherman, 2007).
  Chronic hepatitis C (HCV) monoinfection:
    Genotypes 1,4:
      <75 kg: Peginterferon alfa-2a (SubQ): 180 mcg/once weekly **and** ribavirin (oral) 1000 mg/day (divided into 2 doses)
      ≥75 kg: Peginterferon alfa-2a (SubQ): 180 mcg/once weekly **and** ribavirin (oral) 1200 mg/day (divided into 2 doses)
    Genotypes 2,3: Peginterferon alfa-2a (SubQ): 180 mcg/once weekly **and** ribavirin (oral) 800 mg/day (divided into 2 doses)
  HIV-HCV coinfection: HCV genotypes 1,2,3,4: Peginterferon alfa-2a (SubQ): 180 mcg/once weekly **and** ribavirin (oral) 800 mg/day (divided into 2 doses)
  Treatment duration (Canadian Consensus Guidelines [Sherman, 2007]):
    HCV genotype 1: Treatment recommended for 48 weeks or may consider extended therapy up to 72 weeks in slow responders; may reduce treatment to 24 weeks in patients achieving RVR at 4 weeks **AND** without poor response predictors (eg, high viral load, advanced fibrosis, elderly); discontinue therapy in patients failing to achieve EVR at 12 weeks or with detectable HCV RNA at 24 weeks; retreatment for 48 weeks is required in patients who relapse after discontinuing abbreviated therapy (24 weeks)
    HCV genotypes 2,3: Treatment recommended for 24 weeks; may consider abbreviated therapy (12 or 16 weeks) in patients with weight-based ribavirin dosing and RVR; if relapse occurs following abbreviated therapy, retreat for 24 weeks
    HCV genotype 4,5, and 6: Treatment recommended for 48 weeks; discontinue therapy in patients failing to achieve EVR at 12 weeks or with detectable HCV RNA at 24 weeks

◄ *HCV-HIV coinfection:* Treatment recommended for 48 weeks; discontinue therapy in patients failing to achieve EVR at 12 weeks

Relapsing or nonresponding patients (regardless of genotype): Peginterferon/ribavirin therapy may be considered in patients that have relapsed or were nonresponsive to prior interferon monotherapy or interferon/ribavirin combination therapy; discontinue therapy if EVR not achieved after 12 weeks.

Dosing adjustment for toxicity: Note: Recommendations (per manufacturer labeling - also refer to dosing in renal and hepatic impairment):

Adverse events/toxicity: For moderate-to-severe adverse reactions (clinical and/or laboratory): Reduce peginterferon alfa-2a dose to 135 mcg/once weekly; may need decreased to 90 mcg/once weekly in some cases

Depression:

Mild depression: No dosage adjustment required; monitor closely

Moderate depression: Decrease peginterferon alfa-2a dose to 90-135 mcg/once weekly; monitor closely

Severe depression: Discontinue combination therapy; obtain immediate psychiatric consultation

Hemoglobin (patients without cardiac disease):

Hemoglobin <10 g/dL: Decrease ribavirin dose to 600 mg/day

Hemoglobin <8.5 g/dL: Discontinue ribavirin; upon resolution of decreased hemoglobin, may reinitiate ribavirin therapy at 600 mg/day with subsequent increase to 800 mg/day as tolerated; higher doses are not recommended

Hemoglobin (patients with stable cardiac disease):

Hemoglobin decrease >2 g/dL in any 4-week period: Permanently decrease ribavirin dose to 600 mg/day

Hemoglobin <12 g/dL after ribavirin dose is decreased for 4 weeks: Discontinue ribavirin; upon resolution of decreased hemoglobin, may reinitiate ribavirin therapy at 600 mg/day with subsequent increase to 800 mg/day as tolerated; higher doses are not recommended

Neutrophils:

Neutrophils <0.75 x 10^9/L: Decrease peginterferon alfa-2a dose to 135 mcg/week

Neutrophils <0.5 x 10^9/L: Interrupt peginterferon alfa-2a therapy; may reinitiate therapy at 90 mcg/week when ANC >1 x 10^9/L

Platelets:

Platelet count <50 x 10^9/L: Decrease peginterferon alfa-2a dose to 90 mcg/week

Platelet count <25 x 10^9/L: Permanently discontinue peginterferon alfa-2a and ribavirin

Dosing adjustment in renal impairment:

Peginterferon alfa-2a: SubQ:

Cl_{cr} >20 mL/minute: No dosage adjustment required. Monitor closely as dose reduction may be warranted with onset of adverse events.

End-stage renal disease requiring hemodialysis: Reduce initial dosage to 135 mcg/once weekly

Ribavirin: Oral: Cl_{cr} <50 mL/minuteUse is not recommended

Dosing adjustment in hepatic impairment: Avoid use in decompensated hepatic disease (eg, Child-Pugh class B or C). Use is contraindicated in HCV-HIV coinfected patients with cirrhosis and baseline Child-Pugh score ≥6.

Peginterferon alfa-2a: SubQ: Reduce dose to 90 mcg/once weekly in the presence of progressive ALT increases greater than baseline. Therapy discontinuation may be necessary for persistently marked ALT elevations despite dose reduction and/or with accompanying elevated bilirubin or with evidence of hepatic decompensation.

Ribavirin: Oral: Dosage adjustments are not required in patients with compensated hepatic impairment

Additional Information Complete prescribing information for this medication should be consulted for additional detail.

Dosage Forms Excipient information presented when available (limited, particularly for generics); consult specific product labeling. [CAN] = Canadian product; not available in the U.S.

Combination package:
Pegasys RBV® [CAN; 1-week package]:
Tablet, oral: Ribavirin 200 mg (28s)
Injection, solution: Peginterferon alfa-2a: 180 mcg/0.5 mL (0.5 mL) (1s)
[contains polysorbate 80, benzyl alcohol; prefilled syringe]

Tablet, oral: Ribavirin 200 mg (35s)
Injection, solution: Peginterferon alfa-2a: 180 mcg/0.5 mL (0.5 mL) (1s)
[contains polysorbate 80, benzyl alcohol; prefilled syringe]

Tablet, oral: Ribavirin 200 mg (42s)
Injection, solution: Peginterferon alfa-2a: 180 mcg/0.5 mL (0.5 mL) (1s)
[contains polysorbate 80, benzyl alcohol; prefilled syringe]

Pegasys RBV® [CAN; 1-week package]:
Tablet, oral: Ribavirin 200 mg (28s)
Injection, solution: Peginterferon alfa-2a: 180 mcg/mL (1 mL) (1s) [contains
polysorbate 80, benzyl alcohol; single-use vial]

Tablet, oral: Ribavirin 200 mg (35s)
Injection, solution: Peginterferon alfa-2a: 180 mcg/mL (1 mL) (1s) [contains
polysorbate 80, benzyl alcohol; single-use vial]

Tablet, oral: Ribavirin 200 mg (42s)
Injection, solution: Peginterferon alfa-2a: 180 mcg/mL (1 mL) (1s) [contains
polysorbate 80, benzyl alcohol; single-use vial]

Pegasys RBV® [CAN; 4-week package]:
Tablet, oral: Ribavirin 200 mg (112s)
Injection, solution: Peginterferon alfa-2a: 180 mcg/0.5 mL (0.5 mL) (4s)
[contains polysorbate 80, benzyl alcohol; prefilled syringe]

Tablet, oral: Ribavirin 200 mg (140s)
Injection, solution: Peginterferon alfa-2a: 180 mcg/0.5 mL (0.5 mL) (4s)
[contains polysorbate 80, benzyl alcohol; prefilled syringe]

Tablet, oral: Ribavirin 200 mg (168s)
Injection, solution: Peginterferon alfa-2a: 180 mcg/0.5 mL (0.5 mL) (4s)
[contains polysorbate 80, benzyl alcohol; prefilled syringe]

Tablet, oral: Ribavirin 200 mg (168s + 28s)
Injection, solution: Peginterferon alfa-2a: 180 mcg/0.5 mL (0.5 mL) (4s)
[contains polysorbate 80, benzyl alcohol; prefilled syringe]

Pegasys RBV® [CAN; 4-week package]:
Tablet, oral: Ribavirin 200 mg (112s)
Injection, solution: Peginterferon alfa-2a: 180 mcg/mL (1 mL) (4s) [contains
polysorbate 80, benzyl alcohol; single-use vial]

Tablet, oral: Ribavirin 200 mg (140s)
Injection, solution: Peginterferon alfa-2a: 180 mcg/mL (1 mL) (4s) [contains
polysorbate 80, benzyl alcohol; single-use vial]

Tablet, oral: Ribavirin 200 mg (168s)
Injection, solution: Peginterferon alfa-2a: 180 mcg/mL (1 mL) (4s) [contains
polysorbate 80, benzyl alcohol; single-use vial]

References

Berg T, Von Wagner M, Nasser S, et al, "Extended Treatment Duration for Hepatitis C Virus Type 1: Comparing 48 Versus 72 Weeks of Peginterferon-Alfa-2a Plus Ribavirin," *Gastroenterology*, 2006, 130(4):1086-97.

Dienstag JL and McHutchinson JG, "American Gastroenterological Association Medical Position Statement on the Management of Hepatitis C," *Gastroenterology*, 2006, 130(1):225-30.

Ghany MG, Strader DB, Thomas DL, et al, "Diagnosis, Management and Treatment of Hepatitis C: An Update," *Hepatology*, 2009, 49(4):1335-74.

Hoofnagle JH and Seeff LB,"Peginterferon and Ribavirin for Chronic Hepatitis C," *N Engl J Med*, 2006, 355(23):2444-51.

Pearlman BL, Ehleben C, and Saifee S, "Treatment Extension to 72 Weeks of Peginterferon and Ribavirin in Hepatitis C Genotype 1-Infected Slow Responders," *Hepatology*, 2007, 46(6):1688-94.

Sherman M, Shafran S, Burak K, et al, "Management of Chronic Hepatitis C: Consensus Guidelines," *Can J Gastroenterology*, 2007, 21(Suppl C):25-34.

Penbutolol (pen BYOO toe lole)

Related Information
Beta-Blockers *on page 1669*
Preoperative Evaluation of the Cardiac Patient for Noncardiac Surgery *on page 1598*

U.S. Brand Names Levatol®
Canadian Brand Names Levatol®
Index Terms Penbutolol Sulfate
Pharmacologic Category Beta Blocker With Intrinsic Sympathomimetic Activity
Use Treatment of mild-to-moderate arterial hypertension

Pharmacodynamics/Kinetics
Onset of action: Peak effect: 1.3-3 hours
Duration: >20 hours
Absorption: ~100%
Protein binding: 80% to 98%
Metabolism: Extensively hepatic (oxidation and conjugation)
Bioavailability: ~100%
Half-life elimination: Penbutolol: 5 hours; Conjugated metabolite: ~20 hours with normal renal function, 100 hours with end-stage renal disease
Time to peak, plasma: 2-3 hours
Excretion: Urine

Dosage Adults: Oral: Initial: 20 mg once daily, full effect of a 20 or 40 mg dose is seen by the end of a 2-week period, doses of 40-80 mg have been tolerated but have shown little additional antihypertensive effects; usual dose range (JNC 7): 10-40 mg once daily

Anesthesia and Critical Care Concerns/Other Considerations Penbutolol possesses intrinsic sympathomimetic activity. While beta-blockers with intrinsic sympathomimetic activity induce fewer side effects, the cardiovascular benefits are less clear.

Additional Information Complete prescribing information for this medication should be consulted for additional detail.

Dosage Forms Excipient information presented when available (limited, particularly for generics); consult specific product labeling.
Tablet, as sulfate: 20 mg

References
Braunwald E, Antman EM, Beasley JW, et al, "ACC/AHA 2002 Guideline Update for the Management of Patients With Unstable Angina and Non-ST-Segment Elevation Myocardial Infarction - Summary Article: A Report of the American College of Cardiology/American Heart Association Task Force on Practice Guidelines (Committee on the Management of Patients With Unstable Angina)," *J Am Coll Cardiol*, 2002, 40(7):1366-74. Available at: http://www.acc.org/clinical/guidelines/unstable/incorporated/index.htm. Accessed May 20, 2003.

Chobanian AV, Bakris GL, Black HR, et al, "The Seventh Report of the Joint National Committee on Prevention, Detection, Evaluation, and Treatment of High Blood Pressure: The JNC 7 Report," *JAMA*, 2003, 289(19):2560-71.

"Consensus Recommendations for the Management of Chronic Heart Failure. On Behalf of the Membership of the Advisory Council to Improve Outcomes Nationwide in Heart Failure," *Am J Cardiol*, 1999, 83(2A):1A-38A.

Gibbons RJ, Abrams J, Chatterjee K, et al, "ACC/AHA 2002 Guideline Update for the Management of Patients With Chronic Stable Angina - Summary Article: A Report of the American College of Cardiology/American Heart Association Task Force on Practice Guidelines (Committee on the Management of Patients With Chronic Stable Angina)," *J Am Coll Cardiol*, 2003, 41(1):159-68.

Lang DM, "Anaphylactoid and Anaphylactic Reactions. Hazards of Beta-Blockers," *Drug Saf*, 1995, 12(5):299-304.

Mokhlesi B, Leikin JB, Murray P, et al, "Adult Toxicology in Critical Care: Part II: Specific Poisonings," *Chest*, 2003, 123(3):897-922.

◆ **Penbutolol Sulfate** *see* Penbutolol *on page 1094*

Penicillin G (Parenteral/Aqueous)
(pen i SIL in jee, pa REN ter al, AYE kwee us)

Medication Safety Issues
Sound-alike/look-alike issues:
Penicillin may be confused with penicillamine

Related Information
Prevention of Wound Infection and Sepsis in Surgical Patients *on page 1721*
U.S. Brand Names Pfizerpen®
Canadian Brand Names Crystapen®
Index Terms Benzylpenicillin Potassium; Benzylpenicillin Sodium; Crystalline Penicillin; Penicillin G Potassium; Penicillin G Sodium
Pharmacologic Category Antibiotic, Penicillin
Generic Available Yes

Use Treatment of infections (including sepsis, pneumonia, pericarditis, endocarditis, meningitis, anthrax) caused by susceptible organisms; active against some gram-positive organisms, generally not *Staphylococcus aureus*; some gram-negative organisms such as *Neisseria gonorrhoeae*, and some anaerobes and spirochetes

Mechanism of Action Interferes with bacterial cell wall synthesis during active multiplication, causing cell wall death and resultant bactericidal activity against susceptible bacteria

Pharmacodynamics/Kinetics
Distribution: Poor penetration across blood-brain barrier, despite inflamed meninges
Relative diffusion from blood into CSF: Poor unless meninges inflamed (exceeds usual MICs)
CSF:blood level ratio: Normal meninges: <1%; Inflamed meninges: 2% to 6%
Protein binding: 65%
Metabolism: Hepatic (30%) to penicilloic acid
Half-life elimination:
Neonates: <6 days old: 3.2-3.4 hours; 7-13 days old: 1.2-2.2 hours; >14 days old: 0.9-1.9 hours
Children and Adults: Normal renal function: 30-50 minutes
End-stage renal disease: 3.3-5.1 hours
Time to peak, serum: I.M.: ~30 minutes; I.V.: ~1 hour
Excretion: Urine (58% to 85% as unchanged drug)

Dosage
Usual dosage range:
Infants >1 month and Children: I.M., I.V.: 100,000-400,000 units/kg/day in divided doses every 4-6 hours (maximum dose: 24 million units/day)
Adults: I.M., I.V.: 2-30 million units/day in divided doses every 4-6 hours depending on sensitivity of the organism and severity of the infection
Indication-specific dosing:
Infants >1 month and Children:
Meningitis **(gonococcal):** I.V.: 250,000 units/kg/day in 4 divided doses
Moderate infections: I.M., I.V.: 100,000-250,000 units/kg/day in 4 divided doses
Severe infections: I.M., I.V.: 250,000-400,000 units/kg/day in divided doses every 4-6 hours (maximum dose: 24 million units/day)
Syphilis (congenital): Infants: I.V.: 50,000 units/kg every 4-6 hours for 10 days
Adults:
Actinomyces **species:** I.V.: 10-20 million units/day in divided doses every 4-6 hours for 4-6 weeks
Clostridium perfringens: I.V.: 24 million units/day in divided doses every 4-6 hours with clindamycin
Corynebacterium diphtheriae: I.V.: 2-3 million units/day in divided doses every 4-6 hours for 10-12 days
Erysipelas: I.V.: 1-2 million units every 4-6 hours
Erysipelothrix: I.V.: 2-4 million units every 4 hours
Fascial space infections: I.V.: 2-4 million units every 4-6 hours with metronidazole
Leptospirosis: I.V.: 1.5 million units every 6 hours for 7 days
Listeria: I.V.: 15-20 million units/day in divided doses every 4-6 hours for 2 weeks (meningitis) or 4 weeks (endocarditis)
Lyme disease (meningitis): I.V.: 20 million units/day in divided doses
Neurosyphilis: I.V.: 18-24 million units/day in divided doses every 4 hours (or by continuous infusion) for 10-14 days

◄

Streptococcus:
Brain abscess: I.V.: 18-24 million units/day in divided doses every 4 hours with metronidazole
Endocarditis or osteomyelitis: I.V.: 3-4 million units every 4 hours for at least 4 weeks
Pregnancy (prophylaxis GBS): I.V.: 5 million units x 1 dose, then 2.5 million units every 4 hours until delivery (AGOG, 2002; CDC, 2002)
Skin and soft tissue: I.V.: 3-4 million units every 4 hours for 10 days
Toxic shock: I.V.: 24 million units/day in divided doses with clindamycin
Streptococcal pneumonia: I.V.: 2-3 million units every 4 hours
Whipple's disease: I.V.: 2 million units every 4 hours for 2 weeks, followed by oral trimethoprim/sulfamethoxazole or doxycycline for 1 year
Relapse or CNS involvement: 4 million units every 4 hours for 4 weeks

Dosing interval in renal impairment:
Uremic patients with Cl_{cr} >10 mL/minute/1.73 m^2: Administer full loading dose followed by $1/2$ of the loading dose given every 4-5 hours
Cl_{cr} <10 mL/minute/1.73 m^2: Administer full loading dose followed by $1/2$ of the loading dose given every 8-10 hours

Stability
Penicillin G potassium powder for injection should be stored below 86°F (30°C). Following reconstitution, solution may be stored for up to 7 days under refrigeration. Premixed bags for infusion should be stored in the freezer (-20°C to -4°F); frozen bags may be thawed at room temperature or in refrigerator. Once thawed, solution is stable for 14 days if stored in refrigerator or for 24 hours when stored at room temperature. Do not refreeze once thawed.
Penicillin G sodium powder for injection should be stored at controlled room temperature. Reconstituted solution may be stored under refrigeration for up to 3 days.

Administration Administer I.M. by deep injection in the upper outer quadrant of the buttock

Monitoring Parameters Periodic electrolyte, hepatic, renal, cardiac and hematologic function tests during prolonged/high-dose therapy; observe for signs and symptoms of anaphylaxis during first dose

Anesthesia and Critical Care Concerns/Other Considerations
Clinical Pearls/Comments: One million units is approximately equal to 625 mg.

Pregnancy Risk Factor B

Contraindications Hypersensitivity to penicillin or any component of the formulation

Warnings/Precautions Avoid intra-arterial administration or injection into or near major peripheral nerves or blood vessels since such injections may cause severe and/or permanent neurovascular damage; use with caution in patients with renal impairment (dosage reduction required), concomitant renal and hepatic impairment (further dosage adjustment may be required), pre-existing seizure disorders, or with a history of hypersensitivity to cephalosporins. Prolonged use may result in fungal or bacterial superinfection, including *C. difficile*-associated diarrhea (CDAD) and pseudomembranous colitis; CDAD has been observed >2 months postantibiotic treatment. Serious and occasionally severe or fatal hypersensitivity (anaphylactoid) reactions have been reported in patients on penicillin therapy, especially with a history of beta-lactam hypersensitivity, history of sensitivity to multiple allergens, or previous IgE-mediated reactions (eg, anaphylaxis, angioedema, urticaria). Use with caution in asthmatic patients. Extended duration of therapy or use associated with high serum concentrations may be associated with an increased risk for some adverse reactions. Neonates may have decreased renal clearance of penicillin and require frequent dosage adjustments depending on age. Product contains sodium and potassium; high doses of I.V. therapy may alter serum levels.

Adverse Reactions Frequency not defined.
Central nervous system: Coma (high doses), hyperreflexia (high doses), seizures (high doses)
Dermatologic: Contact dermatitis, rash
Endocrine & metabolic: Electrolyte imbalance (high doses)
Gastrointestinal: Pseudomembranous colitis
Hematologic: Neutropenia, positive Coombs' hemolytic anemia (rare, high doses)

Local: Injection site reaction, phlebitis, thrombophlebitis

Neuromuscular & skeletal: Myoclonus (high doses)

Renal: Acute interstitial nephritis (high doses), renal tubular damage (high doses)

Miscellaneous: Anaphylaxis, hypersensitivity reactions (immediate and delayed), Jarisch-Herxheimer reaction, serum sickness

Drug Interactions

Avoid Concomitant Use There are no known interactions where it is recommended to avoid concomitant use.

Increased Effect/Toxicity

Penicillin G (Parenteral/Aqueous) may increase the levels/effects of: Methotrexate

The levels/effects of Penicillin G (Parenteral/Aqueous) may be increased by: Uricosuric Agents

Decreased Effect

Penicillin G (Parenteral/Aqueous) may decrease the levels/effects of: Mycophenolate; Typhoid Vaccine

The levels/effects of Penicillin G (Parenteral/Aqueous) may be decreased by: Fusidic Acid; Tetracycline Derivatives .

Test Interactions False-positive or negative urinary glucose determination using Clinitest®; positive Coombs' [direct]; false-positive urinary and/or serum proteins

Dietary Considerations

Injection powder for reconstitution as potassium contains sodium 6.8 mg (0.3 mEq) and potassium 65.6 mg (1.68 mEq) per 1 million units

Injection solution (premixed) as a potassium contains sodium 23.5 mg (1.02 mEq) and potassium 66.5 mg (1.7 mEq) per 1 million units

Dosage Forms Excipient information presented when available (limited, particularly for generics); consult specific product labeling.

Infusion, as potassium [premixed iso-osmotic dextrose solution, frozen]: 1 million units (50 mL), 2 million units (50 mL), 3 million units (50 mL) [contains sodium 1.02 mEq and potassium 1.7 mEq per 1 million units]

Injection, powder for reconstitution, as potassium (Pfizerpen®): 5 million units, 20 million units [contains sodium 6.8 mg (0.3 mEq) and potassium 65.6 mg (1.68 mEq) per 1 million units]

Injection, powder for reconstitution, as sodium: 5 million units [contains sodium 1.68 mEq per 1 million units]

References

Gilbert DN, Moellering RC, Eliopoulos GM, et al, eds, *The Sanford Guide To Antimicrobial Therapy*, 2006, 36th ed, Hyde Park, VT: Antimicrobial Therapy, Inc, 2006, 6-7.

Tunkel AR, Hartman BJ, Kaplan SL, et al, "Practice Guidelines for the Management of Bacterial Meningitis," *Clin Infect Dis*, 2004, 39(9):1267-84.

◆ **Penicillin G Potassium** *see* Penicillin G (Parenteral/Aqueous) *on page 1094*

◆ **Penicillin G Sodium** *see* Penicillin G (Parenteral/Aqueous) *on page 1094*

◆ **Pennsaid® (Can)** *see* Diclofenac *on page 414*

◆ **Pentahydrate** *see* Sodium Thiosulfate *on page 1316*

◆ **Pentam®-300** *see* Pentamidine *on page 1097*

Pentamidine (pen TAM i deen)

U.S. Brand Names NebuPent®; Pentam®-300

Index Terms Pentamidine Isethionate

Pharmacologic Category Antibiotic, Miscellaneous; Antiprotozoal

Generic Available No

Use Treatment and prevention of pneumonia caused by *Pneumocystis jiroveci* pneumonia (PCP)

Unlabeled/Investigational Use Treatment of African trypanosomiasis, cutaneous leishmaniasis, and amebic meningoencephalitis

Mechanism of Action Interferes with RNA/DNA, phospholipids and protein synthesis, through inhibition of oxidative phosphorylation and/or interference with incorporation of nucleotides and nucleic acids into RNA and DNA, in protozoa

◄ **Pharmacodynamics/Kinetics**
Absorption: I.M.: Well absorbed; Inhalation: Limited systemic absorption
Distribution: V_{dss}: I.V.: 286-1356 L; I.M.: 1658-3790 L
Half-life elimination: I.V.: 5-8 hours; I.M.: 7-11 hours; may be prolonged with severe renal impairment
Excretion: Urine (I.V.: ≤12% as unchanged drug)

Dosage
Children:
PCP:
FDA-approved labeling: Children >4 months: Treatment: I.M., I.V.: 4 mg/kg once daily for 14-21 days
CDC recommendation:
Prevention (children ≥5 years): Inhalation: 300 mg/dose monthly via Respirgard® II nebulizer
Treatment: I.V.: 3-4 mg/kg once daily for 21 days
AIDS*info* guidelines (2009):
Prevention: Children ≥5 years: Inhalation: 300 mg/dose monthly via Respirgard® II nebulizer
Treatment: I.V.: 4 mg/kg once daily, if clinical improvement may change to atovaquone after 7-10 days
PCP prevention in pediatric oncology patients (age <5 years, intolerant to trimethoprim-sulfamethoxazole; unlabeled use): 4 mg/kg I.V. once monthly (Kim, 2008; Prasad, 2007)
Cutaneous leishmaniasis (unlabeled use; CDC recommendation): I.M., I.V.: 2-3 mg/kg once daily or every second day for 4-7 doses
Trypanosomiasis (unlabeled use; CDC recommendation): I.M.: 4 mg/kg once daily for 7 days
Adults:
PCP:
FDA-approved labeling:
Prevention: Inhalation: 300 mg every 4 weeks via Respirgard® II nebulizer
Treatment: I.M., I.V.: 4 mg/kg once daily for 14-21 days
CDC recommendation:
Prevention: Inhalation: 300 mg monthly via Respirgard® II nebulizer
Treatment: I.V.: 3-4 mg/kg once daily for 21 days
AIDS*info* guidelines (2009):
Prevention: Inhalation: 300 mg/dose monthly via Respirgard® II nebulizer
Treatment: I.V.: 4 mg/kg once daily, 3 mg/kg may be used by some clinicians
Cutaneous leishmaniasis (unlabeled use; CDC recommendation): I.M., I.V.: 2-3 mg/kg once daily or every second day for 4-7 doses
Trypanosomiasis (unlabeled use; CDC recommendation): I.M.: 4 mg/kg once daily for 7 days

Dosing adjustment in renal impairment: I.V.: The FDA-approved labeling recommends that caution should be used in patients with renal impairment; however, no specific dosage adjustment guidelines are available. The following guidelines have been used by some clinicians (Aronoff, 2007):
Children:
Cl_{cr} >30 mL/minute: No adjustment required
Cl_{cr} 10-30 mL/minute: Administer 4 mg/kg every 36 hours
Cl_{cr} <10 mL/minute and peritoneal dialysis: Administer 4 mg/kg every 48 hours
Hemodialysis: Administer 4 mg/kg every 48 hours, after dialysis on dialysis days
Adults:
Cl_{cr} ≥10 mL/minute: No adjustment required
Cl_{cr} <10 mL/minute: Administer 4 mg/kg every 24-36 hours

Stability Store intact vials at 20°C to 25°C (68°F to 77°F); protect from light. Do not use sodium chloride for initial reconstitution (sodium chloride will cause precipitation).
Aerosol: Reconstitute with 6 mL SWFI. The manufacturer recommends the use of freshly prepared solutions for inhalation; however, may be stored for up to 48 hours in the vial at room temperature if protected from light. Do not mix with other nebulizer solutions.

Injection: I.M.: Reconstitute with 3 mL SWFI; I.V.: Reconstitute with 3-5 mL SWFI or D_5W; the manufacturer recommends further dilution in 50-250 mL D_5W; however, stability with further dilution in NS has also been documented. Store at room temperature to avoid crystallization. Reconstituted solution is stable for 48 hours in the vial at room temperature and protected from light. Solutions for injection (1-2.5 mg/mL) in D_5W are stable for at least 24 hours at room temperature.

Administration Do not use NS to reconstitute.

Inhalation: Deliver via Respirgard® II nebulizer until nebulizer is emptied (30-45 minutes). Use appropriate precautions to minimize exposure to healthcare personnel; refer to individual institutional policy.

I.V.: Infuse slowly over 60-120 minutes. Avoid extravasation; assess catheter position before and during infusion.

I.M.: Administer deep I.M.

Monitoring Parameters Liver function tests, renal function tests, blood glucose, serum potassium and calcium, CBC and platelets; ECG, blood pressure

Pregnancy Risk Factor C

Contraindications Hypersensitivity to pentamidine isethionate or any component of the formulation

Warnings/Precautions Severe hypotension (some fatalities) has been observed (even after a single dose); may occur with either I.V. or I.M administration, although more common with rapid I.V. administration; monitor blood pressure during (and after) infusion. Use with caution in patients with pre-existing cardiovascular disease; hyper-/hypotension and arrhythmia, including ventricular tachycardia have been reported.

Use with caution in patients with diabetes mellitus or hypocalcemia; hyper-/ hypoglycemia and pancreatic islet cell necrosis with hyperinsulinemia has been reported. Symptoms may occur months after therapy; monitor blood glucose daily on therapy and periodically thereafter. Use with caution in patients with a history of pancreatic disease or elevated amylase/lipase levels; acute pancreatitis (with fatality) has been reported. Concurrent use with other bone marrow suppressants may increase the risk for myelotoxicity; use with caution in patients with current evidence and/or prior history of hematologic disorders; anemia, leukopenia and/or thrombocytopenia have been reported. Use with caution in patients with hepatic or renal disease. Concurrent use with other nephrotoxic drugs may increase the risk for nephrotoxicity. Stevens-Johnson syndrome has been reported with use. Avoid extravasation; may cause tissue ulceration, necrosis, and/or sloughing; if extravasation occurs, treat symptomatically. Assess catheter position before and during infusion.

Aerosolized pentamidine may induce bronchospasm or cough, especially in patients with a smoking or asthma history (an inhaled bronchodilator prior to pentamidine may ameliorate symptoms). Use appropriate precautions to minimize exposure to healthcare personnel; refer to individual institutional policy. Acute PCP may develop despite aerosolized pentamidine prophylaxis. Although rare, extrapulmonary PCP disease may occur and has been associated with aerosolized pentamidine.

Adverse Reactions

Aerosol:

>10%:

Central nervous system: Fatigue (66%), fever (51%), dizziness/lightheadedness (45%)

Gastrointestinal: Appetite decreased (50%)

Respiratory: Cough (1% to 63%), dyspnea (48%), wheezing (32%)

Miscellaneous: Infection (15%)

1% to 10%:

Central nervous system: Headache

Gastrointestinal: Diarrhea, nausea, oral candida, taste alteration

Hematologic: Anemia

Respiratory: Bronchitis, chest pain, pharyngitis, sinusitis, upper respiratory tract infection

Miscellaneous: Herpes infection, influenza, night sweats

Injection:
>10%:
  Local: Local reactions at I.M. injection site (11%; includes sterile abscess, necrosis, pain, induration)
  Renal: Renal function impaired (29%), creatinine increased (24%)
1% to 10%:
  Cardiovascular: Hypotension (5%)
  Central nervous system: Confusion/hallucinations (2%)
  Dermatologic: Rash (3%)
  Endocrine & metabolic: Hypoglycemia (6%)
  Gastrointestinal: Nausea/anorexia (6%), taste alteration (2%)
  Hematologic: Leukopenia (10%), thrombocytopenia (3%), anemia (1%)
  Hepatic: Liver function tests increased (9%)
  Renal: Azotemia (9%), BUN increased (7%)

Aerosol or injection: <1% (Limited to important or life-threatening): Abdominal pain, allergic reaction, anaphylaxis, anxiety, arthralgia, asthma, blepharitis, blurred vision, bronchitis, bronchospasm, cardiac arrhythmia, central venous line related sepsis, cerebrovascular accident, chest tightness, chills, clotting time prolonged, CMV infection, colitis, confusion, congestion (chest, nasal), conjunctivitis, cough, cryptococcal meningitis, cyanosis, defibrination, depression, dermatitis, desquamation, diabetes mellitus, diabetic ketoacidosis, diarrhea, dizziness, drowsiness, dyspepsia, dyspnea, emotional lability, eosinophilia, erythema, esophagitis, extrapulmonary pneumocystosis, extravasation (tissue ulceration, necrosis, and/or sloughing), facial edema, flank pain, gait unsteady, gagging, gingivitis, headache, hearing loss, hematochezia, hematuria, hemoptysis, hepatic dysfunction, hepatitis, hepatomegaly, histoplasmosis, hyperglycemia, hyperkalemia, hypersalivation, hypertension, hyperventilation, hypesthesia, hypocalcemia, hypomagnesemia, incontinence, insomnia, laryngitis, laryngospasm, leg edema, melena, memory loss, nephritis, nervousness, neuralgia, neuropathy, neutropenia, night sweats, palpitation, pancreatitis, pancytopenia, paranoia, paresthesia, peripheral neuropathy, phlebitis, pleuritis, pneumonitis (eosinophilic or interstitial), pneumothorax, pruritus, rales, renal dysfunction, renal failure, rhinitis, seizure, splenomegaly, Stevens-Johnson syndrome, ST segment abnormal, syncope, syndrome of inappropriate antidiuretic hormone (SIADH), tachycardia, tachypnea, temperature abnormal, torsade de pointes, tremor, vasodilation, vasculitis, ventricular tachycardia, vertigo, vomiting, urticaria, xerostomia

Drug Interactions

Metabolism/Transport Effects Substrate of CYP2C19 (major); **Inhibits** CYP2C8/9 (weak), 2C19 (weak), 2D6 (weak), 3A4 (weak)

Avoid Concomitant Use
  Avoid concomitant use of Pentamidine with any of the following: Artemether; Dronedarone; Lumefantrine; Nilotinib; Pimozide; QuiNINE; Tetrabenazine; Thioridazine; Ziprasidone

Increased Effect/Toxicity
  Pentamidine may increase the levels/effects of: Dronedarone; Pimozide; QTc-Prolonging Agents; QuiNINE; Tetrabenazine; Thioridazine; Ziprasidone

  The levels/effects of Pentamidine may be increased by: Alfuzosin; Artemether; Chloroquine; Ciprofloxacin; CYP2C19 Inhibitors (Moderate); CYP2C19 Inhibitors (Strong); Gadobutrol; Lumefantrine; Nilotinib; QuiNINE

Decreased Effect
  Pentamidine may decrease the levels/effects of: Typhoid Vaccine

  The levels/effects of Pentamidine may be decreased by: CYP2C19 Inducers (Strong)

Ethanol/Nutrition/Herb Interactions Ethanol: Avoid ethanol (may increase CNS depression or aggravate hypoglycemia).

Dosage Forms Excipient information presented when available (limited, particularly for generics); consult specific product labeling.
Injection, powder for reconstitution, as isethionate [preservative free]:
  Pentam®-300: 300 mg
Powder for solution, for nebulization, as isethionate [preservative free]:
  NebuPent®: 300 mg

◆ **Pentamidine Isethionate** *see* Pentamidine *on page 1097*
◆ **Pentamycetin® (Can)** *see* Chloramphenicol *on page 287*
◆ **Pentasa®** *see* Mesalamine *on page 884*
◆ **Pentasodium Colistin Methanesulfonate** *see* Colistimethate *on page 346*
◆ **Pentaspan®** *see* Pentastarch *on page 1101*

Pentastarch (PEN ta starch)

U.S. Brand Names Pentaspan®
Canadian Brand Names Pentaspan®
Pharmacologic Category Blood Modifiers
Generic Available No
Use Orphan drug: Adjunct in leukapheresis to improve harvesting and increase yield of leukocytes by centrifugal means
Dosage 250-700 mL to which citrate anticoagulant has been added is administered by adding to the input line of the centrifugation apparatus at a ratio of 1:8-1:13 to venous whole blood
Drug Interactions
  Avoid Concomitant Use There are no known interactions where it is recommended to avoid concomitant use.
  Increased Effect/Toxicity There are no known significant interactions involving an increase in effect.
  Decreased Effect There are no known significant interactions involving a decrease in effect.
Dosage Forms Excipient information presented when available (limited, particularly for generics); consult specific product labeling.
  Infusion [premixed in NS]: 10% (500 mL)

PENTobarbital (pen toe BAR bi tal)

Medication Safety Issues
  Sound-alike/look-alike issues:
  PENTobarbital may be confused with PHENobarbital
  Nembutal® may be confused with Myambutol®
Related Information
  Anesthesia Considerations for Neurosurgery *on page 1514*
  Status Epilepticus *on page 1737*
U.S. Brand Names Nembutal®
Canadian Brand Names Nembutal® Sodium
Index Terms Pentobarbital Sodium
Pharmacologic Category Anticonvulsant, Barbiturate; Barbiturate
Restrictions C-II
Generic Available No
Use Sedative/hypnotic; refractory status epilepticus
Unlabeled/Investigational Use Barbiturate coma in patients with severe brain injury (eg, hemorrhagic stroke, traumatic brain injury) and increased intracranial pressure
Mechanism of Action Short-acting barbiturate with sedative, hypnotic, and anticonvulsant properties. Barbiturates depress the sensory cortex, decrease motor activity, alter cerebellar function, and produce drowsiness, sedation, and hypnosis. In high doses, barbiturates exhibit anticonvulsant activity; barbiturates produce dose-dependent respiratory depression.
Pharmacodynamics/Kinetics
  Onset of action: I.M.: 10-15 minutes; I.V.: ~1 minute
  Duration: I.V.: 15 minutes
  Distribution: V_d: Children: 0.8 L/kg; Adults: 1 L/kg
  Protein binding: 35% to 55%
  Metabolism: Extensively hepatic via hydroxylation and oxidation pathways
  Half-life elimination: Terminal: Children: 25 hours; Adults: Healthy: 22 hours (range: 15-50 hours)
  Excretion: Urine (<1% as unchanged drug)

◀ **Dosage**
Children:
Hypnotic: I.M.: 2-6 mg/kg; maximum: 100 mg/dose
Preoperative/preprocedure sedation: ≥6 months:
Note: Limited information is available for infants <6 months of age.
I.M.: 2-6 mg/kg; maximum: 100 mg/dose
I.V.: 1-3 mg/kg to a maximum of 100 mg until asleep
Conscious sedation prior to a procedure: Children 5-12 years: I.V.: 2 mg/kg 5-10 minutes before procedures, may repeat one time
Adolescents: Conscious sedation: I.V.: 100 mg prior to a procedure
Children and Adults: Barbiturate coma in head injury patients (unlabeled use): I.V.: Loading dose: 5-10 mg/kg given slowly over 1-2 hours; monitor blood pressure and respiratory rate; maintenance infusion: Initial: 1 mg/kg/hour; may increase to 2-3 mg/kg/hour; maintain burst suppression on EEG
Status epilepticus: I.V.: **Note:** Intubation required; monitor hemodynamics
Children: Loading dose: 5-15 mg/kg given slowly over 1-2 hours; maintenance infusion: 0.5-5 mg/kg/hour
Adults: Loading dose: 10-20 mg/kg given slowly over 1-2 hours; maintenance infusion: 0.5-3 mg/kg/hour
Adults:
Hypnotic:
I.M.: 150-200 mg
I.V.: Initial: 100 mg, may repeat every 1-3 minutes up to 200-500 mg total dose
Preoperative sedation: I.M.: 150-200 mg
Barbiturate coma in severe brain injury patients (unlabeled use; Bratton, 2007): I.V.: Loading dose: 10 mg/kg given over 30 minutes (or ≤25 mg/minute), followed by 5 mg/kg every hour for 3 doses; monitor blood pressure and respiratory rate. Maintenance infusion: Initial: 1 mg/kg/hour; may increase to 2-4 mg/kg/hour; maintain burst suppression on EEG.
Refractory status epilepticus: I.V.: Loading dose: 10-20 mg/kg given slowly over 1-2 hours; maintenance infusion: 0.5-3 mg/kg/hour. **Note:** Intubation required; monitor hemodynamics.
Dosing adjustment in hepatic impairment: Reduce dosage in patients with severe liver dysfunction.
Stability Protect from freezing. Aqueous solutions are not stable; a commercially available vehicle (containing propylene glycol) is more stable. When mixed with an acidic solution, precipitate may form. Use only clear solution.
Administration Pentobarbital may be administered by deep I.M. or slow I.V. injection.
I.M.: No more than 5 mL (250 mg) should be injected at any one site because of possible tissue irritation.
I.V.: I.V. push doses can be given undiluted, but should be administered no faster than 50 mg/minute; parenteral solutions are highly alkaline; avoid extravasation; avoid rapid I.V. administration >50 mg/minute; avoid intra-arterial injection
Monitoring Parameters Respiratory status (for conscious sedation, includes pulse oximetry), cardiovascular status, CNS status; cardiac monitor and blood pressure monitor required; temperature with high doses (eg, barbiturate coma)
Reference Range
Therapeutic:
Hypnotic: 1-5 mcg/mL (SI: 4-22 µmol/L)
Coma: 10-50 mcg/mL (SI: 88-221 µmol/L)
Toxic: >10 mcg/mL (SI: >44 µmol/L)
Anesthesia and Critical Care Concerns/Other Considerations
Clinical Pearls/Comments: For refractory status epilepticus, patients may require arterial and central venous monitoring to guide fluid and vasoactive therapy for maintenance of blood pressure. High-dose pentobarbital generally produces poikilothermia. High doses of barbiturates are potentially immunosuppressive.
Pregnancy Risk Factor D
Contraindications Hypersensitivity to barbiturates or any component of the formulation; marked hepatic impairment; dyspnea or airway obstruction; porphyria; pregnancy

Warnings/Precautions Tolerance to hypnotic effect can occur; do not use for >2 weeks to treat insomnia. Potential for drug dependency exists, abrupt cessation may precipitate withdrawal, including status epilepticus in epileptic patients. Do not administer to patients in acute pain. Use caution in elderly, debilitated, renally impaired, hepatic dysfunction, or pediatric patients. May cause paradoxical responses, including agitation and hyperactivity, particularly in acute pain and pediatric patients. Use with caution in patients with depression or suicidal tendencies, or in patients with a history of drug abuse. Tolerance, psychological and physical dependence may occur with prolonged use.

May cause CNS depression, which may impair physical or mental abilities. Patients must be cautioned about performing tasks which require mental alertness (eg, operating machinery or driving). Effects with other sedative drugs or ethanol may be potentiated. Use of this agent as a hypnotic in the elderly is not recommended due to its long half-life and potential for physical and psychological dependence.

May cause respiratory depression or hypotension, particularly when administered intravenously. Use with caution in hemodynamically unstable patients or patients with respiratory disease. High doses (loading doses of 15-35 mg/kg given over 1-2 hours) have been utilized to induce pentobarbital coma, but these higher doses often cause hypotension requiring vasopressor therapy.

Adverse Reactions Frequency not defined.
Cardiovascular: Bradycardia, hypotension, syncope
Central nervous system: Drowsiness, lethargy, CNS excitation or depression, impaired judgment, "hangover" effect, confusion, somnolence, agitation, hyperkinesia, ataxia, nervousness, headache, insomnia, nightmares, hallucinations, anxiety, dizziness
Dermatologic: Rash, exfoliative dermatitis, Stevens-Johnson syndrome
Gastrointestinal: Nausea, vomiting, constipation
Hematologic: Agranulocytosis, thrombocytopenia, megaloblastic anemia
Local: Pain at injection site, thrombophlebitis with I.V. use
Renal: Oliguria
Respiratory: Laryngospasm, respiratory depression, apnea (especially with rapid I.V. use), hypoventilation
Miscellaneous: Gangrene with inadvertent intra-arterial injection

Drug Interactions
Metabolism/Transport Effects Induces CYP2A6 (strong), 3A4 (strong)
Avoid Concomitant Use
Avoid concomitant use of PENTobarbital with any of the following: Dronedarone; Everolimus; Nilotinib; Ranolazine; Tolvaptan
Increased Effect/Toxicity
PENTobarbital may increase the levels/effects of: Alcohol (Ethyl); CNS Depressants; Meperidine; Thiazide Diuretics

The levels/effects of PENTobarbital may be increased by: Carbonic Anhydrase Inhibitors; Chloramphenicol; Felbamate; Primidone; Valproic Acid
Decreased Effect
PENTobarbital may decrease the levels/effects of: Acetaminophen; Beta-Blockers; Calcium Channel Blockers; Chloramphenicol; Contraceptive (Progestins); Corticosteroids (Systemic); CycloSPORINE; CYP2A6 Substrates; CYP3A4 Substrates; Disopyramide; Doxycycline; Dronedarone; Etoposide; Etoposide Phosphate; Everolimus; Griseofulvin; LamoTRIgine; Maraviroc; Methadone; Nilotinib; Oral Contraceptive (Estrogens); Propafenone; QuiNIDine; Ranolazine; Saxagliptin; Sorafenib; Tadalafil; Teniposide; Theophylline Derivatives; Tolvaptan; Tricyclic Antidepressants; Valproic Acid; Vitamin K Antagonists

The levels/effects of PENTobarbital may be decreased by: Ketorolac; Mefloquine; Pyridoxine; Rifamycin Derivatives
Ethanol/Nutrition/Herb Interactions Ethanol: Avoid ethanol (may increase CNS depression).
Dosage Forms Excipient information presented when available (limited, particularly for generics); consult specific product labeling.
Injection, solution, as sodium: 50 mg/mL (20 mL, 50 mL) [contains alcohol 10% and propylene glycol 40%]

References

Brain Trauma Foundation; American Association of Neurological Surgeons; Congress of Neurological Surgeons, et al, "Guidelines for the Management of Severe Traumatic Brain Injury. XI. Anesthetics, Analgesics, and Sedatives," *J Neurotrauma*, 2007, (24 Suppl)1:S71-6.

Chapman MG, Smith M, and Hirsch NP, "Status Epilepticus," *Anaesthesia*, 2001, 56(7):648-59.

Eisenberg HM, Frankowski RF, Contant CF, et al, "High-Dose Barbiturate Control of Elevated Intracranial Pressure in Patients With Severe Head Injury," *J Neurosurg*, 1988, 69(1):15-23.

Fischer JH and Raineri DL, "Pentobarbital Anesthesia for Status Epilepticus," *Clin Pharm*, 1987, 6 (8):601-2.

Hubbard AM, Markowitz RI, Kimmel B, et al, "Sedation for Pediatric Patients Undergoing CT and MRI," *J Comput Assist Tomogr*, 1992, 16(1):3-6.

Manno EM, "New Management Strategies in the Treatment of Status Epilepticus," *Mayo Clin Proc*, 2003, 78(4):508-18.

"The Brain Trauma Foundation. The American Association of Neurological Surgeons. The Joint Section on Neurotrauma and Critical Care, "Use of Barbiturates in the Control of Intracranial Hypertension," *J Neurotrauma*, 2000, 17(6-7):527-30.

◆ **Pentobarbital Sodium** *see* PENTobarbital *on page 1101*

◆ **Pentothal®** *see* Thiopental *on page 1377*

◆ **Pepcid®** *see* Famotidine *on page 575*

◆ **Pepcid® AC [OTC]** *see* Famotidine *on page 575*

◆ **Pepcid® AC (Can)** *see* Famotidine *on page 575*

◆ **Pepcid® AC Maximum Strength [OTC]** *see* Famotidine *on page 575*

◆ **Pepcid® I.V. (Can)** *see* Famotidine *on page 575*

Peramivir (pe RA mi veer)

Index Terms BCX-1812; RWJ-270201

Pharmacologic Category Antiviral Agent; Neuraminidase Inhibitor

Restrictions Investigational agent (not FDA approved) – only available in the U.S. under an Emergency Use Authorization (EUA). For information on eligibility or to request the emergency use, refer to http://www.cdc.gov/h1n1flu/eua/.

Peramivir is **not** for the treatment of seasonal influenza A or B virus infections, for outpatients with acute uncomplicated 2009 H1N1 virus infection, or for pre- or postexposure chemoprophylaxis (prevention) of influenza.

Under the terms of the EUA, reporting of all medication errors and selected adverse events occurring during treatment is mandatory (within 7 days from event onset) using the FDA MedWatch Form 3500 (available online at http://www.fda.gov/medwatch/safety/FDA-3500_fillable.pdf). The patient's healthcare provider is also required to provide any follow-up request by the FDA or CDC. Adverse events which require reporting to the FDA include death, neuropsychiatric events, renal events, serious skin reactions (eg, Stevens-Johnson syndrome, toxic epidermal necrolysis), hypersensitivity reactions (eg, anaphylaxis, urticaria, angioedema), severe I.V. administration adverse events (eg, infiltrated I.V.), and other serious events (eg, congenital anomaly, birth defect, permanent disability).

Unlabeled/Investigational Use Emergency Use Authorization (EUA): Treatment of certain *hospitalized* patients with suspected or laboratory-confirmed 2009 H1N1 infection or infection due to nonsubtypable influenza A virus suspected to be 2009 H1N1. Eligible patients include:
- Adult or pediatric patients not responding to appropriate oral or inhaled antiviral therapy
- Adult or pediatric patients for whom drug delivery by a route other than I.V. (eg, enteral oseltamivir or inhaled zanamivir) is not feasible or not expected to be dependable
- Adult patients that the clinician judges I.V. therapy is appropriate due to other circumstances

Mechanism of Action Peramivir, a cyclopentane analogue, selectively inhibits the neuraminidase enzyme, thus preventing the release of particles from infected cells.

Pharmacodynamics/Kinetics

Bioavailability: Oral: ≤3% (agent investigated only as a parenteral formulation due to low oral bioavailability)

Half-life elimination: Range: 8-21 hours (normal renal function)

Excretion: Urine (primarily unchanged)

Dosage I.V.: Influenza treatment of 2009 H1N1 infection (patients meeting criteria of EUA):

Children (age/weight-based dosing): Calculated mg/kg dose (maximum dose: 600 mg) over 60 minutes once daily for 5-10 days:

≤30 days of age: 6 mg/kg

31-90 days: 8 mg/kg

91-180 days: 10 mg/kg

181 days to 5 years: 12 mg/kg

6-17 years: 10 mg/kg

Adults: 600 mg over 30 minutes once daily for 5-10 days; **Note:** Treatment duration >10 days may be permitted in certain situations such as critical illness (eg, respiratory failure or intensive care unit admission), continued viral shedding, or unresolved clinical influenza illness.

Dosing adjustment in renal impairment: Dosage must be adjusted in patients with a Cl_{cr} <50 mL/minute. **Note:** Cl_{cr} may be estimated in pediatrics using the Schwartz formula at http://www-users.med.cornell.edu/~spon/picu/calc/crclschw.htm and in adults using the Cockroft and Gault equation.

Cl_{cr} 50-80 mL/minute:

≤30 days of age: 6 mg/kg once daily

31-90 days: 8 mg/kg once daily

91-180 days: 10 mg/kg once daily

181 days to 5 years: 12 mg/kg once daily

6-17 years: 10 mg/kg once daily

Adults: 600 mg once daily

Cl_{cr} 31-49 mL/minute:

≤30 days of age: 1.5 mg/kg once daily

31-90 days: 2 mg/kg once daily

91-180 days: 2.5 mg/kg once daily

181 days to 5 year: 3 mg/kg once daily

6-17 years: 2.5 mg/kg once daily

Adults: 150 mg once daily

Cl_{cr} 10-30 mL/minute:

≤30 days of age: 1 mg/kg once daily

31-90 days: 1.3 mg/kg once daily

91-180 days: 1.6 mg/kg once daily

181 days to 5 years: 1.9 mg/kg once daily

6-17 years: 1.6 mg/kg once daily

Adults: 100 mg once daily

Cl_{cr} <10 mL/minute (or hemodialysis):

≤30 days of age: 0.15 mg/kg once daily

31-90 days: 0.2 mg/kg once daily

91-180 days: 0.25 mg/kg once daily

181 days to 5 years: 0.3 mg/kg once daily

6-17 years: 0.25 mg/kg once daily

Adults: 15 mg once daily

Hemodialysis: Adjust dose according to Cl_{cr} <10 mL/minute and administer peramivir after hemodialysis is completed

Peritoneal dialysis: No information available

Continuous veno-venous hemofiltration (CVVH) dialysis: No information available

Dosing adjustment in hepatic impairment: No dosage adjustment necessary; not significantly metabolized hepatically

Stability Store undiluted vials at 15°C to 30°C (59°F to 86°F). Once diluted, use immediately or refrigerate. If refrigerated, use within 24 hours following preparation. Any unused portion of the single use vial must be discarded following dilution. Maintain adequate records of all vials of peramivir showing receipt, use, and disposition of product, including unused, intact vials.

Further dilute prior to infusion; add calculated dose to an empty sterile I.V. container and dilute with either 0.9% NS or 0.45% NS. Do not dilute using solutions containing electrolytes or dextrose.

Pediatrics (≤17 years): Dilute calculated dose to make a final concentration ≤6 mg/mL

Adults: Dilute 600 mg (60 mL) to make a total volume of 100 mL. Maximum concentration: 6 mg/mL

Administration Administer diluted dose intravenously over 30 minutes (adults) or 60 minutes (pediatrics). Do not exceed an infusion rate of 40 mg/minute. Alternatively, in pediatrics, may administer an undiluted dose using an infusion device (eg, piggy back system, timed syringe system or pump) to allow infusion into an open I.V. line with NS.

Monitoring Parameters CBC with differential and BMP (initiation, day 3, and end of therapy); liver function tests including AST, ALT, alkaline phosphatase, total and direct bilirubin (initiation, end of therapy, and as needed); urinalysis (initiation, end of therapy, and as needed); renal function (prior to initiation and during therapy); vital signs (daily at minimum); development of diarrhea; signs or symptoms of unusual behavior (including attempts at self-injury, confusion, and/or delirium)

Contraindications Hypersensitivity to peramivir, other neuraminidase inhibitors, or any component of the formulation

Warnings/Precautions Diarrhea, nausea, and vomiting have commonly occurred during clinical trials. Neutropenia has occurred; monitor during therapy. Rare occurrences of neuropsychiatric events (including confusion, delirium, hallucinations, and/or self-injury) have been reported with the use of other neuraminidase inhibitors from postmarketing surveillance; direct causation is difficult to establish (influenza infection may also be associated with behavioral and neurologic changes). Elimination is primarily renal; dosage adjustment is required in renal impairment. Recommended pediatric doses are based on modeling from adult use; peramivir has not been administered to pediatric patients in clinical trials. Prior to use, patients must be informed and understand peramivir is an investigational agent and safety and efficacy have not been established. Peramivir should not be used in the setting of highly suspected or documented oseltamivir resistance.

Adverse Reactions Frequency unknown (investigational agent).

Cardiovascular: Blood pressure increased, ECG abnormalities (prolonged QT_c interval)

Central nervous system: Dizziness, headache, nervousness, neuropsychiatric events (including anxiety, confusion, delirium, depression, insomnia, nightmares, restlessness, and mood alterations), somnolence

Endocrine & metabolic: Hyperglycemia

Gastrointestinal: Anorexia, diarrhea, nausea, vomiting

Genitourinary: Cystitis, hematuria, proteinuria

Hematologic: Neutropenia

Hepatic: Hyperbilirubinemia

Dosage Forms Excipient information presented when available (limited, particularly for generics); consult specific product labeling.

Injection, solution: 10 mg/mL (20 mL)

References

Hayden F, "Developing New Antiviral Agents for Influenza Treatment: What Does the Future Hold?" *Clin Infect Dis*, 2009, 48 Suppl 1:3-13.

Kohono S, MY Yen, HJ Cheong, et al, "Single-Intravenous Peramivir vs Oral Oseltamivir to Treat Acute, Uncomplicated Influenza in the Outpatient Setting: A Phase III Randomized, Double-Blind Trial," ICAAC 2009, Abstract V-537a.

Ong AK and Hayden FG, "John F. Enders Lecture 2006: Antivirals for Influenza," *J Infect Dis*, 2007, 196(2):181-90.

◆ **Percocet®** *see* Oxycodone and Acetaminophen *on page 1072*

◆ **Percocet®-Demi (Can)** *see* Oxycodone and Acetaminophen *on page 1072*

◆ **Perforomist™** *see* Formoterol *on page 631*

◆ **Peridex®** *see* Chlorhexidine Gluconate *on page 291*

◆ **Peridex® Oral Rinse (Can)** *see* Chlorhexidine Gluconate *on page 291*

◆ **Peridol (Can)** *see* Haloperidol *on page 672*

Perindopril Erbumine (per IN doe pril er BYOO meen)

Related Information
Angiotensin Agents *on page 1652*
Heart Failure (Systolic) *on page 1739*

U.S. Brand Names Aceon®

Canadian Brand Names Apo-Perindopril®; Coversyl®

Pharmacologic Category Angiotensin-Converting Enzyme (ACE) Inhibitor

Use Treatment of hypertension; reduction of cardiovascular mortality or nonfatal myocardial infarction in patients with stable coronary artery disease

Unlabeled/Investigational Use Treatment of heart failure; to delay the progression of nephropathy and reduce risks of cardiovascular events in hypertensive patients with type 1 or 2 diabetes mellitus

Pharmacodynamics/Kinetics
Onset of action: Peak effect: 1-2 hours

Protein binding: Perindopril: 60%; Perindoprilat: 10% to 20%

Metabolism: Hepatically hydrolyzed to active metabolite, perindoprilat (~17% to 20% of a dose) and other inactive metabolites

Bioavailability: Perindopril: 75%; Perindoprilat ~25% (~16% with food)

Half-life elimination: Parent drug: 1.5-3 hours; Metabolite: Effective: 3-10 hours, Terminal: 30-120 hours

Time to peak: Chronic therapy: Perindopril: 1 hour; Perindoprilat: 3-7 hours (maximum perindoprilat serum levels are 2-3 times higher and T_{max} is shorter following chronic therapy); CHF: Perindoprilat: 6 hours

Excretion: Urine (75%, 4% to 12% as unchanged drug)

Dosage Oral:
Adults:

Heart failure (unlabeled use): Initial: 2 mg once daily; increase at 1- to 2-week intervals; target dose: 8-16 mg once daily (ACC/AHA 2009 Heart Failure Guidelines)

Hypertension: Initial: 4 mg/day but may be titrated to response; usual range: 4-8 mg/day (may be given in 2 divided doses); increase at 1- to 2-week intervals (maximum: 16 mg/day)

Concomitant therapy with diuretics: To reduce the risk of hypotension, discontinue diuretic, if possible, 2-3 days prior to initiating perindopril. If unable to stop diuretic, initiate perindopril at 2-4 mg/day and monitor blood pressure closely for the first 2 weeks of therapy, and after any dose adjustment of perindopril or diuretic.

Stable coronary artery disease: Initial: 4 mg once daily for 2 weeks; increase as tolerated to 8 mg once daily.

Elderly:

Hypertension: >65 years of age: Initial: 4 mg/day; maintenance: 8 mg/day; experience with doses >8 mg/day is limited

Stable coronary artery disease: >70 years of age: Initial: 2 mg/day for 1 week; increase as tolerated to 4 mg/day for 1 week; then increase as tolerated to 8 mg/day; experience with doses >8 mg/day is limited

Dosing adjustment in renal impairment:
Cl_{cr} >30 mL/minute: Initial: 2 mg/day; maintenance dosing not to exceed 8 mg/day

Cl_{cr} <30 mL/minute: Safety and efficacy not established.

Hemodialysis: Perindopril and its metabolites are dialyzable

Dosing adjustment in hepatic impairment: No adjustment necessary

Anesthesia and Critical Care Concerns/Other Considerations
Clinical Pearls/Comments: In patients on chronic ACE inhibitor therapy, intraoperative hypotension may occur with induction and maintenance of general anesthesia; however, discontinuation of therapy prior to surgery is controversial. If continued preoperatively, avoidance of hypotensive agents during surgery is prudent. Episodes of intraoperative hypotension may be managed by fluid administration and/or modest doses of alpha-adrenergic agents. Severe hypotension may occur in patients who are sodium- and/or volume-depleted, initiate lower doses and monitor closely when starting therapy in these patients. ACE inhibitor therapy may elicit an increase in potassium and creatinine,

especially when used in patients with bilateral renal artery stenosis. In those patients experiencing cough on an ACE inhibitor, the ACE inhibitor may be discontinued and, if necessary, angiotensin-receptor blocker therapy instituted. Concomitant NSAID therapy may attenuate blood pressure control; use of NSAIDs should be avoided or limited, with monitoring of blood pressure control. In the setting of heart failure, NSAID use may be associated with an increased risk for fluid accumulation and edema. Because of the potent teratogenic effects of ACE inhibitors, these drugs should be avoided, if possible, when treating women of childbearing potential not on effective birth control measures. Aging patients with a decrease in glomerular filtration (also creatinine clearance), severe heart failure, and renal failure may experience an exaggerated response with administration of ACE inhibitors. Diabetic proteinuria is reduced and insulin sensitivity is enhanced.

Evidence-Based Information: ACE inhibitors decrease morbidity and mortality in patients with asymptomatic and symptomatic left ventricular dysfunction. In this situation, they decrease hospitalizations for, and retard progression to, decompensated heart failure. ACE inhibitors are also indicated in patients postmyocardial infarction in whom left ventricular ejection fraction is <40%. When used in patients with heart failure, the target dose or maximum tolerated dose should be achieved, if possible. Lower daily doses of ACE inhibitors have not demonstrated the same cardioprotective effects. ACE inhibitors have renal protective effects in patients with diabetic proteinuria. The HOPE trial examined the use of ramipril at a dose of between 2.5-10 mg daily in patients without heart failure at high risk for cardiovascular events and documented a significant improvement in cardiovascular outcome compared to placebo.

Additional Information Complete prescribing information for this medication should be consulted for additional detail.

Dosage Forms Excipient information presented when available (limited, particularly for generics); consult specific product labeling.
Tablet: 2 mg, 4 mg, 8 mg

- ◆ **PerioChip®** *see* Chlorhexidine Gluconate *on page 291*
- ◆ **PerioGard®** *see* Chlorhexidine Gluconate *on page 291*
- ◆ **Periostat®** *see* Doxycycline *on page 456*
- ◆ **Persantine®** *see* Dipyridamole *on page 435*
- ◆ **Pethidine Hydrochloride** *see* Meperidine *on page 875*
- ◆ **Pexeva®** *see* PARoxetine *on page 1089*
- ◆ **PFA** *see* Foscarnet *on page 632*
- ◆ **Pfizerpen®** *see* Penicillin G (Parenteral/Aqueous) *on page 1094*
- ◆ **PGE₁** *see* Alprostadil *on page 66*
- ◆ **PGI₂** *see* Epoprostenol *on page 506*
- ◆ **PGX** *see* Epoprostenol *on page 506*
- ◆ **Phenadoz™** *see* Promethazine *on page 1186*

Phenelzine (FEN el zeen)

Related Information
Antidepressant Agents *on page 1660*
U.S. Brand Names Nardil®
Canadian Brand Names Nardil®
Index Terms Phenelzine Sulfate
Pharmacologic Category Antidepressant, Monoamine Oxidase Inhibitor
Use Symptomatic treatment of atypical, nonendogenous, or neurotic depression
Unlabeled/Investigational Use Selective mutism
Pharmacodynamics/Kinetics
Onset of action: Therapeutic: 2-4 weeks; geriatric patients receiving an average of 55 mg/day developed a mean platelet MAO activity inhibition of about 85%.
Duration: May continue to have a therapeutic effect and interactions 2 weeks after discontinuing therapy
Absorption: Well absorbed

Metabolism: Oxidized via monoamine oxidase (primary pathway) and acetylation (minor pathway)

Half-life elimination: 11 hours

Excretion: Urine (primarily as metabolites and unchanged drug)

Dosage Oral:

Children: Selective mutism (unlabeled use): 30-60 mg/day

Adults: Depression: 15 mg 3 times/day; may increase to 60-90 mg/day during early phase of treatment, then reduce dose for maintenance therapy slowly after maximum benefit is obtained; takes 2-4 weeks for a significant response to occur

Elderly: Depression: Initial: 7.5 mg/day; increase by 7.5-15 mg/day every 3-4 days as tolerated; usual therapeutic dose: 15-60 mg/day in 3-4 divided doses

Anesthesia and Critical Care Concerns/Other Considerations

Clinical Pearls/Comments: Patients receiving MAO inhibitors who undergo surgery may be at risk of developing significant hypertension when used with direct-acting adrenergic agents (eg, norepinephrine) and of lethal hypertension when administered with indirect-acting adrenergic agents (eg, ephedrine). The use of meperidine in these patients may also precipitate serotonin syndrome and is contraindicated. Years ago, it was advised that patients receiving MAO inhibitors have this drug discontinued for at least 10 days before elective surgery. However, the decision to continue or withhold MAO inhibitors must be done in collaboration with the patient's psychiatrist. Currently, an MAO-safe anesthetic technique which excludes the use of meperidine and indirect-acting adrenergic agonists is recommended for patients requiring continuing MAO therapy (Huyse, 2006).

Additional Information Complete prescribing information for this medication should be consulted for additional detail.

Dosage Forms Excipient information presented when available (limited, particularly for generics); consult specific product labeling.

Tablet: 15 mg

References

Huyse FJ, Touw DJ, van Schijndel RS, et al, "Psychotropic Drugs and the Perioperative Period: A Proposal for a Guideline in Elective Surgery," *Psychosomatics*, 2006, 47(1):8-22.

♦ **Phenelzine Sulfate** *see* Phenelzine *on page 1108*

♦ **Phenergan®** *see* Promethazine *on page 1186*

PHENobarbital (fee noe BAR bi tal)

Medication Safety Issues

Sound-alike/look-alike issues:

PHENobarbital may be confused with PENTobarbital, Phenergan®, phenytoin
Luminal® may be confused with Tuinal®

Related Information

Anesthesia Considerations for Neurosurgery *on page 1514*
Anesthesia for Patients With Liver Disease *on page 1537*
Perioperative Management of Patients on Antiseizure Medication *on page 1577*
Status Epilepticus *on page 1737*

U.S. Brand Names Luminal® Sodium

Canadian Brand Names PMS-Phenobarbital

Index Terms Phenobarbital Sodium; Phenobarbitone; Phenylethylmalonylurea

Pharmacologic Category Anticonvulsant, Barbiturate; Barbiturate

Restrictions C-IV

Generic Available Yes

Use Management of generalized tonic-clonic (grand mal), status epilepticus, and partial seizures; sedative/hypnotic

Unlabeled/Investigational Use Prevention and treatment of neonatal hyperbilirubinemia and lowering of bilirubin in chronic cholestasis; neonatal seizures

Mechanism of Action Long-acting barbiturate with sedative, hypnotic, and anticonvulsant properties. Barbiturates depress the sensory cortex, decrease motor activity, alter cerebellar function, and produce drowsiness, sedation, and hypnosis. In high doses, barbiturates exhibit anticonvulsant activity; barbiturates produce dose-dependent respiratory depression.

◄ **Pharmacodynamics/Kinetics**
　Onset of action: Oral: Hypnosis: 20-60 minutes; I.V.: ~5 minutes
　　Peak effect: I.V.: ~30 minutes
　Duration: Oral: 6-10 hours; I.V.: 4-10 hours
　Absorption: Oral: 70% to 90%
　Protein binding: 20% to 45%; decreased in neonates
　Metabolism: Hepatic via hydroxylation and glucuronide conjugation
　Half-life elimination: Neonates: 45-500 hours; Infants: 20-133 hours; Children: 37-73 hours; Adults: 53-140 hours
　Time to peak, serum: Oral: 1-6 hours
　Excretion: Urine (20% to 50% as unchanged drug)

Dosage
　Children:
　　Sedation: Oral: 2 mg/kg 3 times/day
　　Hypnotic: I.M., I.V.: 3-5 mg/kg at bedtime
　　Preoperative sedation: Oral, I.M., I.V.: 1-3 mg/kg 1-1.5 hours before procedure
　Adults:
　　Sedation: Oral, I.M.: 30-120 mg/day in 2-3 divided doses
　　Hypnotic: Oral, I.M., I.V.: 100-320 mg at bedtime
　　Preoperative sedation: I.M.: 100-200 mg 1-1.5 hours before procedure

　Anticonvulsant: Status epilepticus **Loading dose:** I.V.:
　　Infants and Children: 15-20 mg/kg (maximum: 1000 mg/dose, maximum rate ≤30 mg/minute in children <60 kg); may repeat dose after 15 minutes as needed (maximum total dose: 40 mg/kg)
　　Adults: 10-20 mg/kg (maximum rate ≤60 mg/minute in patients ≥60 kg); may repeat dose in 20-minute intervals as needed (maximum total dose: 30 mg/kg)
　Anticonvulsant maintenance dose: Oral, I.V.:
　　Infants: 5-8 mg/kg/day in 1-2 divided doses
　　Children:
　　　1-5 years: 6-8 mg/kg/day in 1-2 divided doses
　　　5-12 years: 4-6 mg/kg/day in 1-2 divided doses
　　Children >12 years and Adults: 1-3 mg/kg/day in divided doses or 50-100 mg 2-3 times/day
　Sedative/hypnotic withdrawal (unlabeled use): Initial daily requirement is determined by substituting phenobarbital 30 mg for every 100 mg pentobarbital used during tolerance testing; then daily requirement is decreased by 10% of initial dose

Dosing interval in renal impairment: Cl_{cr} <10 mL/minute: Administer every 12-16 hours
Hemodialysis: Moderately dialyzable (20% to 50%)
Dosing adjustment/comments in hepatic disease: Increased side effects may occur in severe liver disease; monitor plasma levels and adjust dose accordingly
Stability Protect elixir from light. Not stable in aqueous solutions; use only clear solutions. Do not add to acidic solutions; precipitation may occur.
Administration May be administered I.V., I.M. or orally. Avoid rapid I.V. administration >60 mg/minute in adults and >30 mg/minute in children; intra-arterial injection is contraindicated; avoid subcutaneous administration; parenteral solutions are highly alkaline; avoid extravasation. For I.M. administration, inject deep into muscle. Do not exceed 5 mL per injection site due to potential for tissue irritation
Monitoring Parameters Phenobarbital serum concentrations, mental status, CBC, LFTs, seizure activity
Reference Range
　Therapeutic:
　　Infants and children: 15-30 mcg/mL (SI: 65-129 μmol/L)
　　Adults: 20-40 mcg/mL (SI: 86-172 μmol/L)
　Toxic: >40 mcg/mL (SI: >172 μmol/L)
　Toxic concentration: Slowness, ataxia, nystagmus: 35-80 mcg/mL (SI: 150-344 μmol/L)
　Coma with reflexes: 65-117 mcg/mL (SI: 279-502 μmol/L)
　Coma without reflexes: >100 mcg/mL (SI: >430 μmol/L)
Pregnancy Risk Factor D

Contraindications Hypersensitivity to barbiturates or any component of the formulation; marked hepatic impairment; dyspnea or airway obstruction; porphyria (manifest and latent); intra-arterial administration, subcutaneous administration (not recommended); use in patients with a history of sedative/hypnotic addiction is not recommended; nephritic patients (large doses)

Warnings/Precautions Potential for drug dependency exists, abrupt cessation may precipitate withdrawal, including status epilepticus in epileptic patients. Do not administer to patients in acute pain. Use caution in elderly, debilitated, renal or hepatic dysfunction, and pediatric patients. May cause paradoxical responses, including agitation and hyperactivity, particularly in acute pain and pediatric patients. Use with caution in patients with depression or suicidal tendencies, or in patients with a history of drug abuse. Tolerance, psychological and physical dependence may occur with prolonged use. May cause CNS depression, which may impair physical or mental abilities. Effects with other sedative drugs or ethanol may be potentiated. May cause respiratory depression or hypotension, particularly when administered intravenously. Use with caution in hemodynamically unstable patients (hypovolemic shock, CHF) or patients with respiratory disease. Due to its long half-life and risk of dependence, phenobarbital is not recommended as a sedative in the elderly. Use has been associated with cognitive deficits in children. Use with caution in patients with hypoadrenalism. Intra-arterial administration may cause reactions ranging from transient pain to gangrene and is contraindicated. Subcutaneous administration may cause tissue irritation (eg, redness, tenderness, necrosis) and is not recommended.

Adverse Reactions Frequency not defined.

Cardiovascular: Bradycardia, hypotension, syncope

Central nervous system: Drowsiness, lethargy, CNS excitation or depression, impaired judgment, "hangover" effect, confusion, somnolence, agitation, hyperkinesia, ataxia, nervousness, headache, insomnia, nightmares, hallucinations, anxiety, dizziness

Dermatologic: Rash, exfoliative dermatitis, Stevens-Johnson syndrome

Gastrointestinal: Nausea, vomiting, constipation

Hematologic: Agranulocytosis, thrombocytopenia, megaloblastic anemia

Local: Pain at injection site, thrombophlebitis with I.V. use

Renal: Oliguria

Respiratory: Laryngospasm, respiratory depression, apnea (especially with rapid I.V. use), hypoventilation

Miscellaneous: Gangrene with inadvertent intra-arterial injection

Drug Interactions

Metabolism/Transport Effects Substrate of CYP2C9 (minor), 2C19 (major), 2E1 (minor); **Induces** CYP1A2 (strong), 2A6 (strong), 2B6 (strong), 2C8 (strong), 2C9 (strong), 3A4 (strong)

Avoid Concomitant Use

Avoid concomitant use of PHENobarbital with any of the following: Darunavir; Dronedarone; Etravirine; Everolimus; Nilotinib; Ranolazine; Tolvaptan; Voriconazole

Increased Effect/Toxicity

PHENobarbital may increase the levels/effects of: Alcohol (Ethyl); CNS Depressants; Meperidine; Thiazide Diuretics

The levels/effects of PHENobarbital may be increased by: Carbonic Anhydrase Inhibitors; Chloramphenicol; CYP2C19 Inhibitors (Moderate); CYP2C19 Inhibitors (Strong); Felbamate; Primidone; Rufinamide; Valproic Acid

Decreased Effect

PHENobarbital may decrease the levels/effects of: Acetaminophen; Aminocamptothecin; Bendamustine; Beta-Blockers; Calcium Channel Blockers; Chloramphenicol; Contraceptive (Progestins); Corticosteroids (Systemic); CycloSPORINE; CYP1A2 Substrates; CYP2A6 Substrates; CYP2B6 Substrates; CYP2C8 Substrates (High risk); CYP2C9 Substrates (High risk); CYP3A4 Substrates; Darunavir; Deferasirox; Disopyramide; Doxycycline; Dronedarone; Etoposide; Etoposide Phosphate; Etravirine; Everolimus; Griseofulvin; Irinotecan; Lacosamide; LamoTRIgine; Maraviroc; Methadone; Nilotinib; Oral Contraceptive (Estrogens); OXcarbazepine; Propafenone; QuiNIDine; Ranolazine; Rufinamide; Saxagliptin; Sorafenib; Tadalafil; Teniposide; Theophylline Derivatives; Tipranavir; Tolvaptan; Treprostinil; Tricyclic Antidepressants; Valproic Acid; Vitamin K Antagonists; Voriconazole; Zonisamide

▶

The levels/effects of PHENobarbital may be decreased by: Amphetamines; Cholestyramine Resin; CYP2C19 Inducers (Strong); Folic Acid; Ketorolac; Leucovorin-Levoleucovorin; Mefloquine; Methylfolate; Pyridoxine; Rifamycin Derivatives; Tipranavir

Ethanol/Nutrition/Herb Interactions

Ethanol: Avoid ethanol (may increase CNS depression).

Food: May cause decrease in vitamin D and calcium.

Herb/Nutraceutical: Avoid evening primrose (seizure threshold decreased). Avoid valerian, St John's wort, kava kava, gotu kola (may increase CNS depression).

Test Interactions Assay interference of LDH

Dietary Considerations Vitamin D: Loss in vitamin D due to malabsorption; increase intake of foods rich in vitamin D. Supplementation of vitamin D and/or calcium may be necessary. Sodium content of injection (65 mg, 1 mL): 6 mg (0.3 mEq).

Dosage Forms Excipient information presented when available (limited, particularly for generics); consult specific product labeling.

Elixir: 20 mg/5 mL (5 mL, 7.5 mL, 15 mL, 480 mL) [contains ethanol]

Injection, solution, as sodium: 65 mg/mL (1 mL); 130 mg/mL (1 mL) [contains ethanol and propylene glycol]

Luminal® Sodium: 60 mg/mL (1 mL); 130 mg/mL (1 mL) [contains ethanol 10% and propylene glycol 67.8%]

Tablet: 15 mg, 30 mg, 60 mg, 100 mg

References

Treiman DM, Meyers PD, Walton NY, et al, "A Comparison of Four Treatments for Generalized Convulsive Status Epilepticus. Veterans Affairs Status Epilepticus Cooperative Study Group," *N Engl J Med*, 1998, 339(12):792-8.

◆ **Phenobarbital Sodium** *see* PHENobarbital *on page* 1109

◆ **Phenobarbitone** *see* PHENobarbital *on page* 1109

◆ **Phenoptin** *see* Sapropterin *on page* 1277

Phentolamine (fen TOLE a meen)

Medication Safety Issues

Sound-alike/look-alike issues:

Phentolamine may be confused with phentermine, Ventolin®

Related Information

Extravasation Treatment of Drugs *on page* 1789

Hypertension *on page* 1754

U.S. Brand Names OraVerse™

Canadian Brand Names Regitine®; Rogitine®

Index Terms Phentolamine Mesylate; Regitine [DSC]

Pharmacologic Category Alpha$_1$ Blocker

Generic Available Yes

Use Diagnosis of pheochromocytoma and treatment of hypertension associated with pheochromocytoma or other forms of hypertension caused by excess sympathomimetic amines; treatment of dermal necrosis after extravasation of drugs with alpha-adrenergic effects (ie, dopamine, epinephrine, norepinephrine, phenylephrine)

OraVerse™: Reversal of soft tissue anesthesia and the associated functional deficits resulting from a local dental anesthetic containing a vasoconstrictor

Unlabeled/Investigational Use Treatment of pralidoxime-induced hypertension

Mechanism of Action Competitively blocks alpha-adrenergic receptors to produce brief antagonism of circulating epinephrine and norepinephrine to reduce hypertension caused by alpha effects of these catecholamines; also has a positive inotropic and chronotropic effect on the heart

OraVerse™: Causes vasodilation and increased blood flow in injection area via alpha-adrenergic blockade to accelerate reversal of soft tissue anesthetic

Pharmacodynamics/Kinetics

Onset of action: I.M.: 15-20 minutes; I.V.: Immediate

Peak effect: OraVerse™: 10-20 minutes

Duration: I.M.: 30-45 minutes; I.V.: 15-30 minutes
Metabolism: Hepatic
Half-life elimination: 19 minutes
Excretion: Urine (10% as unchanged drug)

Dosage

Treatment of alpha-adrenergic agonist drug extravasation: SubQ:

Children: Infiltrate area with a small amount (eg, 1 mL given in 0.2 mL aliquots) of a 0.5-1 mg/mL solution (made by diluting 5-10 mg in 10 mL of NS) within 12 hours of extravasation; in general, do not exceed 0.1-0.2 mg/kg or 5 mg total

Adults: Infiltrate area with small amount of solution made by diluting 5-10 mg in 10 mL 0.9% sodium chloride within 12 hours of extravasation; in general, do not exceed 0.1-0.2 mg/kg (5 mg total); typically doses of ≤5 mg are effective; a case using 50 mg for a large extravasation has been reported (Cooper, 1989). If dose is effective, normal skin color should return to the blanched area within 1 hour

Diagnosis of pheochromocytoma: I.M., I.V.:

Children: 0.05-0.1 mg/kg/dose, maximum single dose: 5 mg

Adults: 5 mg

Surgery for pheochromocytoma: Hypertension: I.M., I.V.:

Children: 0.05-0.1 mg/kg/dose given 1-2 hours before procedure; repeat as needed every 2-4 hours until hypertension is controlled; maximum single dose: 5 mg

Adults: 5 mg given 1-2 hours before procedure and repeated as needed every 2-4 hours

Hypertensive crisis: Adults: 5-20 mg

Treatment of pralidoxime-induced hypertension (unlabeled use): I.V.:

Children: 1 mg

Adults and Elderly: 5 mg

Reversal of soft tissue (lip, tongue) anesthesia (OraVerse™): Infiltration or block technique: Submucosal oral injection:

Children: 15-30 kg: 0.2 mg maximum dose

Children >30 kg and <12 years: 0.4 mg maximum dose

Adults: **Note:** Dose is based upon the number of cartridges of local anesthetic administered. Infiltration or block injection:

0.2 mg if one-half cartridge of anesthesia was administered

0.4 mg if 1 cartridge of anesthesia was administered

0.8 mg if 2 cartridges of anesthesia were administered

Stability Reconstituted solution is stable for 48 hours at room temperature and 1 week when refrigerated.

OraVerse™: Store at 20°C to 25°C (68°F to 77°F); excursions permitted between 15°C to 30°C (59°F to 86°F).

Administration

Vasoconstrictor (alpha-adrenergic agonist) extravasation: Infiltrate the area of extravasation with multiple small injections using only 27- or 30-gauge needles and changing the needle between each skin entry. Be careful not to cause so much swelling of the extremity or digit that a compartment syndrome occurs. If infiltration is severe, may also need to consult vascular surgeon.

Pheochromocytoma: Inject each 5 mg over 1 minute.

Monitoring Parameters Blood pressure, heart rate; area of infiltration; monitor patient for orthostasis; assist with ambulation

Pregnancy Risk Factor C

Contraindications Hypersensitivity to phentolamine or any component of the formulation; renal impairment; coronary or cerebral arteriosclerosis; concurrent use with phosphodiesterase-5 (PDE-5) inhibitors including sildenafil (>25 mg), tadalafil, or vardenafil

OraVerse™: There are no contraindications listed in the manufacturer's labeling.

Warnings/Precautions Myocardial infarction, cerebrovascular spasm, and cerebrovascular occlusion have occurred following administration; use with caution in patients with gastritis or peptic ulcer, tachycardia, or a history of cardiac arrhythmias. Discontinue if symptoms of angina occur or worsen. OraVerse™: Efficacy has not been established in children <6 years of age or <15 kg (33 pounds).

◀ **Adverse Reactions** Frequency not always defined.

Cardiovascular: Arrhythmia, flushing, hypertension (OraVerse™), hypotension, orthostatic hypotension, tachycardia (OraVerse™ ≤6%), bradycardia (OraVerse™ ≤4%)

Central nervous system: Dizziness, headache (OraVerse™ ≤6%)

Dermatologic: Pruritus (OraVerse™)

Gastrointestinal: Nausea, vomiting, diarrhea

Local: Injection site pain (OraVerse™ 4% to 6%)

Neuromuscular & skeletal: Paresthesia (OraVerse™), weakness

Respiratory: Nasal congestion

Postmarketing and/or case reports: Pulmonary hypertension

Drug Interactions

Avoid Concomitant Use

Avoid concomitant use of Phentolamine with any of the following: Alfuzosin; Silodosin; Tamsulosin

Increased Effect/Toxicity

Phentolamine may increase the levels/effects of: Alfuzosin; Amifostine; Antihypertensives; Calcium Channel Blockers; RiTUXimab; Silodosin; Tamsulosin

The levels/effects of Phentolamine may be increased by: Alfuzosin; Beta-Blockers; Diazoxide; Herbs (Hypotensive Properties); MAO Inhibitors; Pentoxifylline; Phosphodiesterase 5 Inhibitors; Prostacyclin Analogues; Silodosin; Tamsulosin

Decreased Effect

The levels/effects of Phentolamine may be decreased by: Herbs (Hypertensive Properties); Methylphenidate; Yohimbine

Test Interactions Increased LFTs rarely

Dosage Forms Excipient information presented when available (limited, particularly for generics); consult specific product labeling.

Injection, powder for reconstitution, as mesylate: 5 mg

Injection, solution, as mesylate [preservative free]:

OraVerse™: 0.4 mg/1.7 mL (1.7 mL) [contains edetate disodium; dental cartridge]

◆ **Phentolamine Mesylate** *see* Phentolamine *on page 1112*

Phenylephrine (fen il EF rin)

Medication Safety Issues

Sound-alike/look-alike issues:

Mydfrin® may be confused with Midrin®

Neo-Synephrine® (phenylephrine) may be confused with Neo-Synephrine® (oxymetazoline)

Sudafed PE™ may be confused with Sudafed®

High alert medication: The Institute for Safe Medication Practices (ISMP) includes this medication among its list of drugs which have a heightened risk of causing significant patient harm when used in error.

Related Information

Anesthesia Considerations for Neurosurgery *on page 1514*

Anesthetic Considerations in the Substance-Abusing Patient *on page 1613*

Extravasation Treatment of Drugs *on page 1789*

Hemodynamic Support, Intravenous *on page 1681*

U.S. Brand Names 4 Way® Fast Acting [OTC]; 4 Way® Menthol [OTC]; 4 Way® No Drip [OTC]; AK-Dilate®; Altafrin; Anu-Med [OTC]; Dimetapp® Toddler's [OTC]; Formulation R™ [OTC]; Little Noses® Decongestant [OTC]; LuSonal™; Medi-Phenyl [OTC]; Medicone® Suppositories [OTC]; Mydfrin®; Nasop12™ [DSC]; Neo-Synephrine® Extra Strength [OTC]; Neo-Synephrine® Injection; Neo-Synephrine® Mild [OTC]; Neo-Synephrine® Regular Strength [OTC]; Neofrin™; NãSop™ [DSC]; OcuNefrin™ [OTC]; Preparation H® [OTC]; Rectacaine [OTC]; Relief® [OTC] [DSC]; Rhinall [OTC]; Sudafed PE™ [OTC]; Triaminic® Infant Thin Strips® Decongestant [OTC] [DSC]; Triaminic® Thin Strips® Cold [OTC];

Tronolane® Suppository [OTC]; Vicks® Sinex® Nasal Spray [OTC]; Vicks® Sinex® UltraFine Mist [OTC]

Canadian Brand Names Dionephrine®; Mydfrin®; Neo-Synephrine®

Index Terms Phenylephrine Hydrochloride; Phenylephrine Tannate

Pharmacologic Category Alpha/Beta Agonist; Ophthalmic Agent, Antiglaucoma; Ophthalmic Agent, Mydriatic

Generic Available Yes: Excludes chewable tablet, cream, filmstrip, liquid, suspension

Use Treatment of hypotension, vascular failure in shock; as a vasoconstrictor in regional analgesia; as a mydriatic in ophthalmic procedures and treatment of wide-angle glaucoma; supraventricular tachycardia

For OTC use as symptomatic relief of nasal and nasopharyngeal mucosal congestion, treatment of hemorrhoids, relief of redness of the eye due to irritation

Mechanism of Action Potent, direct-acting alpha-adrenergic stimulator with weak beta-adrenergic activity; causes vasoconstriction of the arterioles of the nasal mucosa and conjunctiva; activates the dilator muscle of the pupil to cause contraction; produces vasoconstriction of arterioles in the body; produces systemic arterial vasoconstriction

Pharmacodynamics/Kinetics

Onset of action: I.M., SubQ: 10-15 minutes; I.V.: Immediate; Ophthalmic: 10-15 minutes

Duration: I.M.: 0.5-2 hours; I.V.: 15-30 minutes; SubQ: 1 hour; Ophthalmic: Maximal mydriasis: 1 hour, recover time: 3-6 hours

Metabolism: Hepatic, via intestinal monoamine oxidase to phenolic conjugates

Excretion: Urine (90%)

Dosage

Hemorrhoids: Children ≥12 years and Adults: Rectal:

Cream/ointment: Apply to clean dry area, up to 4 times/day; may be used externally or inserted rectally using applicator.

Suppository: Insert 1 suppository rectally, up to 4 times/day

Hypotension/shock:

Children:

I.V. bolus: 5-20 mcg/kg/dose every 10-15 minutes as needed

I.V. infusion: 0.1-0.5 mcg/kg/minute

Adults:

I.V. bolus: 0.1-0.5 mg/dose every 10-15 minutes as needed (initial dose should not exceed 0.5 mg)

I.V. infusion: Initial dose: 100-180 mcg/minute, **or alternatively**, 0.5 mcg/kg/minute; titrate to desired response. Dosing ranges between 0.4-9.1 mcg/kg/minute have been reported (Gregory, 1991).

Nasal decongestant:

Children:

2-6 years:

Intranasal: Instill 1 drop every 2-4 hours of 0.125% solution as needed. (**Note:** Therapy should not exceed 3 continuous days.)

Oral: Tannate salt (NāSop™ suspension): 1.87-3.75 mg every 12 hours

6-12 years:

Intranasal: Instill 1-2 sprays or instill 1-2 drops every 4 hours of 0.25% solution as needed. (**Note:** Therapy should not exceed 3 continuous days.)

Oral:

Hydrochloride salt: 10 mg every 4 hours

Tannate salt:

NāSop™ suspension: 3.75-7.5 mg every 12 hours

Nasop12™ chewable tablet: 1/2 to 1 tablet (5-10 mg) every 12 hours

Children >12 years and Adults:

Intranasal: Instill 1-2 sprays or instill 1-2 drops every 4 hours of 0.25% to 0.5% solution as needed; 1% solution may be used in adult in cases of extreme nasal congestion; do not use nasal solutions more than 3 days

Oral:

Hydrochloride salt: 10-20 mg every 4 hours

Tannate salt:

NāSop™ suspension: 7.5-15 mg every 12 hours

Nasop12™ chewable tablet: 1-2 tablets (10-20 mg) every 12 hours

Ocular procedures:
   Infants <1 year: Instill 1 drop of 2.5% 15-30 minutes before procedures
   Children and Adults: Instill 1 drop of 2.5% or 10% solution, may repeat in 10-60 minutes as needed
Ophthalmic irritation (OTC formulation for relief of eye redness): Adults: Instill 1-2 drops 0.12% solution into affected eye, up to 4 times/day; do not use for >72 hours
Paroxysmal supraventricular tachycardia: I.V.:
   Children: 5-10 mcg/kg/dose over 20-30 seconds
   Adults: 0.25-0.5 mg/dose over 20-30 seconds

Stability

Solution for injection: Store vials at controlled room temperature of 15°C to 30°C (59°F to 86°F). Protect from light. Do not use solution if brown or contains a precipitate.
   I.V. infusion: May dilute 10 mg in 500 mL NS or D_5W.
   I.V. injection: Dilute with SWFI to a concentration of 1 mg/mL.
Ophthalmic solution:
   0.12%: Store at controlled room temperature. Protect from light and excessive heat.
   2.5% and 10%: Refer to product labeling. Some products are labeled to store at room temperature, others should be stored under refrigeration at 2°C to 8°C (36°F to 46°F). Do not use solution if brown or contains a precipitate.
Tablet, chewable: Store at controlled room temperature of 15°C to 30°C (59°F to 86°F). Protect from light.

Administration

I.V.: May cause necrosis or sloughing tissue if extravasation occurs during I.V. administration or SubQ administration.
Extravasation management: Use phentolamine as antidote; mix 5 mg with 9 mL of NS. Inject a small amount of this dilution subcutaneously into extravasated area. Blanching should reverse immediately. Monitor site. If blanching should recur, additional injections of phentolamine may be needed.

Oral: Chewable tablet: Chew or crush well. May mix crushed tablet with food. Do not swallow whole.

Monitoring Parameters Blood pressure, pulse; excitability, irritability, anxiety

Anesthesia and Critical Care Concerns/Other Considerations

Clinical Pearls/Comments: Phenylephrine allows for close titration of blood pressure and may be used in patients with hypotension or shock due to peripheral vasodilation; can increase blood pressure in fluid-resuscitated septic shock patients; does not impair cardiac or renal function in patients without structural heart disease at baseline (eg, heart failure) or those with hyperdynamic sepsis. In patients with heart failure, the use of phenylephrine without inotropic support (eg, dobutamine) may result in a dose-dependent reduction in stroke volume and cardiac output due to the increase in systemic vascular resistance (Yamazaki, 1982; Goertz, 1993). Therefore, phenylephrine is not recommended in the treatment of hypotension with comorbid left ventricular dysfunction. Phenylephrine may be a good choice when tachyarrhythmias limit use of other vasopressors. Experience in patients with septic shock is limited. An increase in oxygen delivery and consumption may occur in >15% of patients according to one study (Flancbaum, 1997).

Evidence Based Information:
Septic Shock: The 2008 Surviving Sepsis Campaign Guidelines (Dellinger, 2008) state that phenylephrine should not be administered as the initial vasopressor in septic shock (Grade 2C). Either norepinephrine or dopamine is recommended as the first choice for septic shock (Grade 1C).

Extravasation Management: Antidote for peripheral ischemia caused by phenylephrine extravasation: To prevent sloughing and necrosis in ischemic areas, the area should be infiltrated as soon as possible with 5-10 mg of Regitine® (phentolamine), an adrenergic blocking agent, diluted in 10-15 mL of saline. A syringe with a fine hypodermic needle should be used, and the solution liberally infiltrated throughout the ischemic area. Sympathetic blockade with phentolamine causes immediate and conspicuous local hyperemic changes if the area is infiltrated within 12 hours. Therefore, phentolamine should be given as soon as possible after the extravasation is noted, as phentolamine may be ineffective if given >12 hours after extravasation.

Pregnancy Risk Factor C

Contraindications Hypersensitivity to phenylephrine or any component of the formulation; hypertension; ventricular tachycardia

Oral: Use with or within 14 days of MAO inhibitor therapy

Nasop12™: Additional contraindications: Use in newborns; breast-feeding

Ophthalmic: Narrow-angle glaucoma

Warnings/Precautions Some products contain sulfites which may cause allergic reactions in susceptible individuals. Use with extreme caution in patients taking MAO inhibitors.

Intravenous: Use with caution in the elderly, patients with hyperthyroidism, bradycardia, partial heart block, myocardial disease, or severe CAD. Assure adequate circulatory volume to minimize need for vasoconstrictors. Avoid hypertension; monitor blood pressure closely and adjust infusion rate. Avoid extravasation; infuse into a large vein if possible. Avoid infusion into leg veins. Watch I.V. site closely. If extravasation occurs, infiltrate the area subcutaneously with diluted phentolamine (5-10 mg in 10-15 mL of saline) with a fine hypodermic needle. Phentolamine should be administered as soon as possible after extravasation is noted. **[U.S. Boxed Warning]: Should be administered by adequately trained individuals familiar with its use.**

Nasal, oral, rectal: Use caution with asthma, bowel obstruction/narrowing, hyperthyroidism, diabetes mellitus, cardiovascular disease, ischemic heart disease, increased intraocular pressure, prostatic hyperplasia or in the elderly. Rebound congestion may occur when nasal products are discontinued after chronic use. When used for self-medication (OTC), notify healthcare provider if symptoms do not improve within 7 days (oral, rectal) or 3 days (nasal), are accompanied by fever (oral), or if bleeding occurs (rectal). Not for OTC use in children <2 years of age.

Ophthalmic: When used for self-medication (OTC), notify healthcare provider in case of vision changes, continued redness, or if symptoms worsen or do not improve within 3 days.

Adverse Reactions Frequency not defined.

Cardiovascular: Arrhythmia (rare), decreased cardiac output, hypertension, pallor, precordial pain or discomfort, reflex bradycardia, severe peripheral and visceral vasoconstriction

Central nervous system: Anxiety, dizziness, excitability, giddiness, headache, insomnia, nervousness, restlessness

Endocrine & metabolic: Metabolic acidosis

Gastrointestinal: Gastric irritation, nausea

Local: I.V.: Extravasation which may lead to necrosis and sloughing of surrounding tissue, blanching of skin

Neuromuscular & skeletal: Paresthesia, pilomotor response, tremor, weakness

Renal: Decreased renal perfusion, reduced urine output

Respiratory: Respiratory distress

Miscellaneous: Hypersensitivity reactions (including rash, urticaria, leukopenia, agranulocytosis, thrombocytopenia)

Drug Interactions

Avoid Concomitant Use

Avoid concomitant use of Phenylephrine with any of the following: Iobenguane I 123; MAO Inhibitors

Increased Effect/Toxicity

Phenylephrine may increase the levels/effects of: Sympathomimetics

The levels/effects of Phenylephrine may be increased by: Atomoxetine; Cannabinoids; MAO Inhibitors; Tricyclic Antidepressants

Decreased Effect

Phenylephrine may decrease the levels/effects of: Iobenguane I 123

Ethanol/Nutrition/Herb Interactions Herb/Nutraceutical: Avoid ephedra, yohimbe (may cause CNS stimulation).

Dietary Considerations NãSop™ contains phenylalanine 4 mg/tablet. LuSonal™ contains phenylalanine. Sudafed PE™ contains phenylalanine 1 mg/strip.

◀ **Dosage Forms** Excipient information presented when available (limited, particularly for generics); consult specific product labeling. [DSC] = Discontinued product

Cream, rectal, as hydrochloride:
Formulation R™: 0.25% (54 g) [contains sodium benzoate]

Filmstrip, orally disintegrating, as hydrochloride:
Sudafed PE™: 10 mg (5s, 10s) [contains phenylalanine 1 mg/strip; cherry menthol flavor]
Triaminic® Infant Thin Strips® Decongestant: 1.25 mg [mixed berry flavor] [DSC]
Triaminic® Thin Strips® Cold: 2.5 mg [raspberry flavor]

Injection, solution, as hydrochloride: 1% [10 mg/mL] (1 mL, 5 mL, 10 mL) [may contain sodium metabisulfite]
Neo-Synephrine®: 1% (1 mL) [contains sodium metabisulfite]

Liquid, oral, as hydrochloride:
LuSonal™: 7.5 mg/5 mL (480 mL) [contains phenylalanine; strawberry flavor]

Liquid, oral, as hydrochloride [drops]:
Dimetapp® Toddler's: 1.25 mg/0.8 mL (15 mL) [alcohol free; contains sodium benzoate; grape flavor]

Ointment, rectal, as hydrochloride:
Formulation R™, Preparation H®: 0.25% (30 g, 60 g) [contains benzoic acid]
Rectacaine: 0.25% (30 g)

Solution, intranasal, as hydrochloride [drops]:
Little Noses® Decongestant: 0.125% (15 mL) [contains benzalkonium chloride]
Neo-Synephrine® Extra Strength: 1% (15 mL) [contains benzalkonium chloride]
Neo-Synephrine® Regular Strength: 0.5% (15 mL) [contains benzalkonium chloride]
Rhinall: 0.25% (30 mL) [contains benzalkonium chloride and sodium bisulfite]

Solution, intranasal, as hydrochloride [spray]:
4 Way® Fast Acting: 1% (15 mL, 30 mL) [contains benzalkonium chloride]
4 Way® Menthol: 1% (15 mL) [contains benzalkonium chloride and menthol]
4 Way® No Drip: 1% (15 mL) [contains benzalkonium chloride]
Neo-Synephrine® Extra Strength: 1% (15 mL) [contains benzalkonium chloride]
Neo-Synephrine® Mild: 0.25% (15 mL) [contains benzalkonium chloride]
Neo-Synephrine® Regular Strength: 0.5% (15 mL) [contains benzalkonium chloride]
Rhinall: 0.25% (40 mL) [contains benzalkonium chloride and sodium bisulfite]
Vicks® Sinex®, Vicks® Sinex® UltraFine Mist: 0.5% (15 mL) [contains benzalkonium chloride]

Solution, ophthalmic, as hydrochloride: 2.5% (2 mL, 3 mL, 5 mL, 15 mL) [may contain sodium bisulfite]
AK-Dilate®: 2.5% (2 mL, 15 mL); 10% (5 mL) [contains benzyl alcohol]
Altrafrin: 0.12% (15 mL) [OTC]; 2.5% (15 mL) [RX; contains benzalkonium chloride]; 10% (5 mL) [RX; contains benzalkonium chloride]
Mydfrin®: 2.5% (3 mL, 5 mL) [contains sodium bisulfite]
Neofrin™: 2.5% (15 mL); 10% (15 mL)
OcuNefrin™: 0.12% (15 mL)
Relief®: 0.12% (15 mL) [contains benzalkonium chloride] [DSC]

Suppository, rectal, as hydrochloride: 0.25% (12s)
Anu-Med: 0.25% (12s)
Formulation R™, Preparation H®: 0.25% (12s, 24s, 48s)
Medicone®, Tronolane®: 0.25% (12s, 24s)
Rectacaine: 0.25% (12s)

Suspension, oral, as tannate:
NāSop™: 7.5 mg/5 mL (120 mL) [orange flavor] [DSC]

Tablet, chewable, as tannate:
Nasop12™: 10 mg [grape flavor] [DSC]

Tablet, as hydrochloride: 10 mg
Medi-Phenyl: 5 mg
Sudafed PE™: 10 mg

Tablet, orally dissolving, as hydrochloride:
NāSop™: 10 mg [contains phenylalanine 4 mg/tablet; bubble gum flavor] [DSC]

References

Beale RJ, Hollenberg SM, Vincent JL, et al, "Vasopressor and Inotropic Support in Septic Shock: An Evidence Based Review," *Crit Care Med*, 2004, 32(11 Suppl):455-65.

Bonfiglio MF, Dasta JF, Gregory JS, et al, "High-Dose Phenylephrine Infusion in the Hemodynamic Support of Septic Shock," *DICP*, 1990, 24(10):936-9.

Dellinger RP, Levy MM, Carlet JM, et al, "Surviving Sepsis Campaign: International Guidelines for Management of Severe Sepsis and Septic Shock: 2008," *Intensive Care Med*, 2008, 34(1): 17-60. Available at http://www.survivingsepsis.org/system/files/images/2008_20International_20SSC_20-Guidelines_1_.pdf

Flancbaum L, Dick M, Dasta J, et al, "A Dose-Response Study of Phenylephrine in Critically Ill, Septic Surgical Patients," *Eur J Clin Pharmacol*, 1997, 51(6):461-5.

Goertz AW, Lindner KH, Seefelder C, et al, "Effect of Phenylephrine Bolus Administration on Global Left Ventricular Function in Patients With Coronary Artery Disease and Patients With Valvular Aortic Stenosis," *Anesthesiology*, 1993, 78(5):834-41.

Gregory JS, Bonfiglio MF, Dasta JF, et al, "Experience With Phenylephrine as a Component of the Pharmacologic Support of Septic Shock," *Crit Care Med*, 1991, 19(11):1395-400.

Hollenberg SM, Ahrens TS, Annane D, et al, "Practice Parameters for Hemodynamic Support of Sepsis in Adult Patients: 2004 Update," *Crit Care Med*, 2004, 32(9):1928-48.

"Task Force of the American College of Critical Care Medicine and Society of Critical Care Medicine. Practice Parameters for Hemodynamic Support of Sepsis in Adult Patients," *Crit Care Med*, 1999, 27(3):639-60. Available at: http://www.sccm.org/pdf/Hemodynamic%20Support.pdf.

Yamazaki T, Shimada Y, Taenaka N, et al, "Circulatory Responses to Afterloading with Phenylephrine in Hyperdynamic Sepsis," *Crit Care Med*, 1992, 10(7):432-35.

◆ **Phenylephrine Hydrochloride** *see* Phenylephrine *on page 1114*

◆ **Phenylephrine Tannate** *see* Phenylephrine *on page 1114*

◆ **Phenylethylmalonylurea** *see* PHENobarbital *on page 1109*

◆ **Phenytek®** *see* Phenytoin *on page 1119*

Phenytoin (FEN i toyn)

Medication Safety Issues

Sound-alike/look-alike issues:

Phenytoin may be confused with phenelzine, phentermine, PHENobarbital

Dilantin® may be confused with Dilaudid®, diltiazem, Dipentum®

High alert medication: The Institute for Safe Medication Practices (ISMP) includes this medication (I.V. formulation) among its list of drug classes which have a heightened risk of causing significant patient harm when used in error.

International issues:

Dilantin® may be confused with Dolantine® which is a brand name for pethidine in Belgium and Switzerland

Related Information

Anesthesia for Patients With Liver Disease *on page 1537*

Chronic Pain Management *on page 1546*

Chronic Renal Failure *on page 1552*

Dosing Considerations for the Critically-Ill Patient With Morbid Obesity *on page 1561*

Extravasation Treatment of Drugs *on page 1789*

Perioperative Management of Patients on Antiseizure Medication *on page 1577*

Status Epilepticus *on page 1737*

Stress Replacement of Corticosteroids *on page 1611*

U.S. Brand Names Dilantin®; Phenytek®

Canadian Brand Names Dilantin®

Index Terms Diphenylhydantoin; DPH; Phenytoin Sodium; Phenytoin Sodium, Extended; Phenytoin Sodium, Prompt

Pharmacologic Category Antiarrhythmic Agent, Class Ib; Anticonvulsant, Hydantoin

Generic Available Yes: Excludes chewable tablet

Use Management of generalized tonic-clonic (grand mal), complex partial seizures; prevention of seizures following head trauma/neurosurgery

Mechanism of Action Stabilizes neuronal membranes and decreases seizure activity by increasing efflux or decreasing influx of sodium ions across cell membranes in the motor cortex during generation of nerve impulses; prolongs effective refractory period and suppresses ventricular pacemaker automaticity, shortens action potential in the heart

▶

◀ **Pharmacodynamics/Kinetics**
Onset of action: I.V.: ~0.5-1 hour
Absorption: Oral: Slow
Distribution: V_d:
  Neonates: Premature: 1-1.2 L/kg; Full-term: 0.8-0.9 L/kg
  Infants: 0.7-0.8 L/kg
  Children: 0.7 L/kg
  Adults: 0.6-0.7 L/kg
Protein binding:
  Neonates: ≥80% (≤20% free)
  Infants: ≥85% (≤15% free)
  Adults: 90% to 95%
  Others: Decreased protein binding
    Disease states resulting in a decrease in serum albumin concentration:
    Burns, hepatic cirrhosis, nephrotic syndrome, pregnancy, cystic fibrosis
    **Disease states resulting in an apparent decrease in affinity of phenytoin
    for serum albumin**: Renal failure, jaundice (severe), other drugs
    (displacers), hyperbilirubinemia (total bilirubin >15 mg/dL), Cl_{cr} <25 mL/
    minute (unbound fraction is increased two- to threefold in uremia)
Metabolism: Follows dose-dependent capacity-limited (Michaelis-Menten) phar-
macokinetics with increased V_{max} in infants >6 months of age and children
versus adults; major metabolite (via oxidation), HPPA, undergoes enterohepatic
recirculation
Bioavailability: Form dependent
Half-life elimination: Oral: 22 hours (range: 7-42 hours)
Time to peak, serum (form dependent): Oral: Extended-release capsule: 4-12
hours; Immediate release preparation: 2-3 hours
Excretion: Urine (<5% as unchanged drug); as glucuronides
  Clearance: Highly variable, dependent upon intrinsic hepatic function and dose
  administered; increased clearance and decreased serum concentrations with
  febrile illness

Dosage
Status epilepticus: I.V.:
  Infants and Children: Loading dose: 15-20 mg/kg in a single or divided dose;
  maintenance dose: Initial: 5 mg/kg/day in 2 divided doses; usual doses:
    6 months to 3 years: 8-10 mg/kg/day
    4-6 years: 7.5-9 mg/kg/day
    7-9 years: 7-8 mg/kg/day
    10-16 years: 6-7 mg/kg/day, some patients may require every 8 hours dosing
  Adults: Loading dose: Manufacturer recommends 10-15 mg/kg, however,
  15-20 mg/kg is generally recommended; maximum rate: 50 mg/minute
Anticonvulsant: Children and Adults: Oral:
  Loading dose: 15-20 mg/kg; based on phenytoin serum concentrations and
  recent dosing history; administer oral loading dose in 3 divided doses given
  every 2-4 hours to decrease GI adverse effects and to ensure complete oral
  absorption; maintenance dose: same as I.V.
  Neurosurgery (prophylactic): 100-200 mg at approximately 4-hour intervals
  during surgery and during the immediate postoperative period
Dosage adjustment in obesity: Adults: Loading dose: Use adjusted body weight
  (ABW) correction based on a pharmacokinetic study of phenytoin loading doses
  in obese patients (Abernethy, 1985). The larger correction factor (ie, 1.33) is due
  to a doubling of V_d estimated in these obese patients.
  ABW = [(Actual body weight – IBW) x 1.33] + IBW
  Maximum loading dose: 2000 mg (Erstad, 2004)
  Maintenance doses should be based on ideal body weight, conventional daily
  doses with adjustments based upon therapeutic drug monitoring and clinical
  effectiveness. (Abernethy, 1985; Erstad, 2002; Erstad, 2004)

Dosing adjustment/comments in renal impairment or hepatic disease: Safe
in usual doses in mild liver disease; clearance may be substantially reduced in
cirrhosis and plasma level monitoring with dose adjustment advisable. Free
phenytoin levels should be monitored closely.
Stability
Capsule, tablet: Store below 30°C (86°F). Protect from light and moisture.

Oral suspension: Store at room temperature of 20°C to 25°C (68°F to 77°F); do not freeze. Protect from light.

Solution for injection: Store at room temperature of 15°C to 30°C (59°F to 86°F). Use only clear solutions free of precipitate and haziness; slightly yellow solutions may be used. Precipitation may occur if solution is refrigerated and may dissolve at room temperature.

Further dilution of the solution for I.V. infusion is controversial and no consensus exists as to the optimal concentration and length of stability. Stability is concentration and pH dependent. Based on limited clinical consensus, NS or LR are recommended diluents. Dilutions of 1-10 mg/mL have been used and should be administered as soon as possible after preparation (some recommend to discard if not used within 4 hours). Do not refrigerate.

Administration

Oral: Suspension: Shake well prior to use. Absorption is impaired when phenytoin suspension is given concurrently to patients who are receiving continuous nasogastric feedings. A method to resolve this interaction is to divide the daily dose of phenytoin and withhold the administration of nutritional supplements for 1-2 hours before and after each phenytoin dose.

I.M.: Although approved for I.M. use, I.M. administration is not recommended due to erratic absorption and pain on injection. Fosphenytoin may be considered.

I.V.: Vesicant. Fosphenytoin may be considered for loading in patients who are in status epilepticus, hemodynamically unstable, or develop hypotension/brady-cardia with I.V. administration of phenytoin. Phenytoin may be administered by IVP or IVPB administration. The maximum rate of I.V. administration is 50 mg/ minute. Highly sensitive patients (eg, elderly, patients with pre-existing cardiovascular conditions) should receive phenytoin more slowly (eg, 20 mg/ minute). An in-line 0.22-5 micron filter is recommended for IVPB solutions due to the high potential for precipitation of the solution. Avoid extravasation. Following I.V. administration, NS should be injected through the same needle or I.V. catheter to prevent irritation.

pH: 10.0-12.3

SubQ: SubQ administration is not recommended because of the possibility of local tissue damage (due to high pH).

Monitoring Parameters Blood pressure, vital signs (with I.V. use); plasma phenytoin level, CBC, liver function. **Note:** If available, free phenytoin concentrations should be obtained in patients with renal impairment and/or hypoalbuminemia. If free phenytoin levels are unavailable, the adjusted total level is based upon equations in adult patients. Monitor for suicidality (eg, suicidal thoughts, depression, behavioral changes).

Reference Range Timing of serum samples: Because it is slowly absorbed, peak blood levels may occur 4-8 hours after ingestion of an oral dose. The serum half-life varies with the dosage and the drug follows Michaelis-Menten kinetics. The average adult half-life is about 24 hours. Steady-state concentrations are reached in 5-10 days.

Children and Adults: Toxicity is measured clinically, and some patients require levels outside the suggested therapeutic range

Therapeutic range:

Total phenytoin: 10-20 mcg/mL (children and adults), 8-15 mcg/mL (neonates)

Concentrations of 5-10 mcg/mL may be therapeutic for some patients but concentrations <5 mcg/mL are not likely to be effective

50% of patients show decreased frequency of seizures at concentrations >10 mcg/mL

86% of patients show decreased frequency of seizures at concentrations >15 mcg/mL

Add another anticonvulsant if satisfactory therapeutic response is not achieved with a phenytoin concentration of 20 mcg/mL

Free phenytoin: 1-2.5 mcg/mL

Total phenytoin:

Toxic: >30 mcg/mL (SI: <120-200 µmol/L)

Lethal: >100 mcg/mL (SI: >400 µmol/L)

When to draw levels: This is dependent on the disease state being treated and the clinical condition of the patient

◀ **Key points:**

Slow absorption of extended capsules and prolonged half-life minimize fluctuations between peak and trough concentrations, timing of sampling not crucial

Trough concentrations are generally recommended for routine monitoring. Daily levels are not necessary and may result in incorrect dosage adjustments. If it is determined essential to monitor free phenytoin concentrations, concomitant monitoring of total phenytoin concentrations is not necessary and expensive.

After a loading dose: If rapid therapeutic levels are needed, initial levels may be drawn after 1 hour (I.V. loading dose) or within 24 hours (oral loading dose) to aid in determining maintenance dose or need to reload.

Rapid achievement: Draw within 2-3 days of therapy initiation to ensure that the patient's metabolism is not remarkably different from that which would be predicted by average literature-derived pharmacokinetic parameters; early levels should be used cautiously in design of new dosing regimens

Second concentration: Draw within 6-7 days with subsequent doses of phenytoin adjusted accordingly

If plasma concentrations have not changed over a 3- to 5-day period, monitoring interval may be increased to once weekly in the acute clinical setting

In stable patients requiring long-term therapy, generally monitor levels at 3- to 12-month intervals

Adjustment of serum concentration: See tables.

Note: Although it is ideal to obtain free phenytoin concentrations to assess serum concentrations in patients with hypoalbuminemia or renal failure (Cl_{cr} ≤10 mL/minute), it may not always be possible. If free phenytoin concentrations are unavailable, the following equations may be utilized in adult patients.

Adjustment of Serum Concentration in Adults With Low Serum Albumin

Measured Total Phenytoin Concentration (mcg/mL)	Patient's Serum Albumin (g/dL)			
	3.5	3	2.5	2
	Adjusted Total Phenytoin Concentration (mcg/mL)[1]			
5	6	7	8	10
10	13	14	17	20
15	19	21	25	30

[1]Adjusted concentration = measured total concentration divided by [(0.2 x albumin) + 0.1].

Adjustment of Serum Concentration in Adults With Renal Failure (Cl_{cr} ≤10 mL/min)

Measured Total Phenytoin Concentration (mcg/mL)	Patient's Serum Albumin (g/dL)				
	4	3.5	3	2.5	2
	Adjusted Total Phenytoin Concentration (mcg/mL)[1]				
5	10	11	13	14	17
10	20	22	25	29	33
15	30	33	38	43	50

[1]Adjusted concentration = measured total concentration divided by [(0.1 x albumin) + 0.1].

Anesthesia and Critical Care Concerns/Other Considerations

Clinical Pearls/Comments: Because phenytoin induces the metabolism of many drugs, it may alter their effective blood concentration.

The vehicle, which contains propylene glycol and ethanol, may cause hypotension, bradycardia, arrhythmias (refractory to defibrillation), or asystole. Phenytoin 50 mg/mL contains propylene glycol 414.4 mg/mL (40% v/v). Rapid intravenous administration may cause hypotension. Infuse at a rate not exceeding 50 mg/minute in adults or 25 mg/minute in the elderly.

Patients on chronic phenytoin therapy (>7 days) require larger and more frequent doses of nondepolarizing neuromuscular blocking agents (NMBAs) to attain the same degree of muscle relaxation. The most likely reason for this reduced sensitivity is increased clearance of the NMBA due to hepatic enzyme induction (Hans, 1997; Richard, 2005; Wright, 2004).

Status Epilepticus: A randomized, double-blind trial (Treiman, 1998) evaluated the efficacy of four treatments in overt status epilepticus. Treatment arms were designed based upon accepted practices of North American neurologists. The treatments were: 1) lorazepam 0.1 mg/kg, 2) diazepam 0.15 mg/kg followed by phenytoin 18 mg/kg, 3) phenytoin 18 mg/kg alone, and 4) phenobarbital 15 mg/kg. Treatment was considered successful if the seizures were terminated (clinically and by EEG) within 20 minutes of start of therapy without seizure recurrence within 60 minutes from the start of therapy. Patients who failed the first treatment received a second and a third, if necessary. Patients did not receive randomized treatments after the first one but the treating physician remained blinded. Treatment success: Lorazepam 64.9%, phenobarbital 58.2%, diazepam/phenytoin 55.8%, and phenytoin alone 43.6%. Using an intention to treat analysis, there was no statistical difference between the groups. Results of subsequent treatments in patients who failed the first therapy indicated that response rate significantly dropped regardless of treatment. Aggregate response rate to the second treatment was 7% and third treatment 2.3%.

Pregnancy Risk Factor D

Contraindications Hypersensitivity to phenytoin, other hydantoins, or any component of the formulation; pregnancy

Warnings/Precautions Antiepileptics are associated with an increased risk of suicidal behavior/thoughts with use (regardless of indication); patients should be monitored for signs/symptoms of depression, suicidal tendencies, and other unusual behavior changes during therapy and instructed to inform their healthcare provider immediately if symptoms occur.

May increase frequency of petit mal seizures; I.V. form may cause hypotension, skin necrosis at I.V. site; avoid I.V. administration in small veins; use with caution in patients with porphyria; discontinue if rash or lymphadenopathy occurs; a spectrum of hematologic effects have been reported with use (eg, neutropenia, leukopenia, thrombocytopenia, pancytopenia, and anemias); use with caution in patients with hepatic dysfunction, sinus bradycardia, S-A block, or AV block; use with caution in elderly or debilitated patients, or in any condition associated with low serum albumin levels, which will increase the free fraction of phenytoin in the serum and, therefore, the pharmacologic response. Sedation, confusional states, or cerebellar dysfunction (loss of motor coordination) may occur at higher total serum concentrations, or at lower total serum concentrations when the free fraction of phenytoin is increased. Effects with other sedative drugs or ethanol may be potentiated. Abrupt withdrawal may precipitate status epilepticus. Severe reactions, including toxic epidermal necrolysis and Stevens-Johnson syndromes, although rarely reported, have resulted in fatalities; drug should be discontinued if there are any signs of rash. Patients of Asian descent with the variant *HLA-B*1502* may be at an increased risk of developing Stevens-Johnson syndrome and/or toxic epidermal necrolysis.

Adverse Reactions I.V. effects: Hypotension, bradycardia, cardiac arrhythmia, cardiovascular collapse (especially with rapid I.V. use), venous irritation and pain, thrombophlebitis

Effects not related to plasma phenytoin concentrations: Hypertrichosis, gingival hypertrophy, thickening of facial features, carbohydrate intolerance, folic acid deficiency, peripheral neuropathy, vitamin D deficiency, osteomalacia, systemic lupus erythematosus

Concentration-related effects: Nystagmus, blurred vision, diplopia, ataxia, slurred speech, dizziness, drowsiness, lethargy, coma, rash, fever, nausea, vomiting, gum tenderness, confusion, mood changes, folic acid depletion, osteomalacia, hyperglycemia

Related to elevated concentrations:
>20 mcg/mL: Far lateral nystagmus
>30 mcg/mL: 45° lateral gaze nystagmus and ataxia
>40 mcg/mL: Decreased mentation
>100 mcg/mL: Death

Cardiovascular: Hypotension, bradycardia, cardiac arrhythmia, cardiovascular collapse

Central nervous system: Psychiatric changes, slurred speech, dizziness, drowsiness, headache, insomnia

Dermatologic: Rash

Gastrointestinal: Constipation, nausea, vomiting, gingival hyperplasia, enlargement of lips

Hematologic: Leukopenia, thrombocytopenia, agranulocytosis

Hepatic: Hepatitis

Local: Thrombophlebitis

Neuromuscular & skeletal: Tremor, peripheral neuropathy, paresthesia

Ocular: Diplopia, nystagmus, blurred vision

Rarely seen effects: Blood dyscrasias, coarsening of facial features, dyskinesias, hepatitis, hypertrichosis, lymphadenopathy, lymphoma, pseudolymphoma, SLE-like syndrome, Stevens-Johnson syndrome, toxic epidermal necrolysis, venous irritation and pain

Drug Interactions

Metabolism/Transport Effects Substrate of CYP2C9 (major), 2C19 (major), 3A4 (minor); **Induces** CYP2B6 (strong), 2C8 (strong), 2C9 (strong), 2C19 (strong), 3A4 (strong)

Avoid Concomitant Use

Avoid concomitant use of Phenytoin with any of the following: Darunavir; Dronedarone; Etravirine; Everolimus; Nilotinib; Ranolazine; Tolvaptan

Increased Effect/Toxicity

Phenytoin may increase the levels/effects of: Alcohol (Ethyl); Amprenavir; CNS Depressants; Fosamprenavir; Lithium; Methotrimeprazine; Vitamin K Antagonists

The levels/effects of Phenytoin may be increased by: Amiodarone; Antifungal Agents (Azole Derivatives, Systemic); Benzodiazepines; Calcium Channel Blockers; Capecitabine; CarBAMazepine; Carbonic Anhydrase Inhibitors; Chloramphenicol; Cimetidine; CYP2C19 Inhibitors (Moderate); CYP2C19 Inhibitors (Strong); CYP2C9 Inhibitors (Moderate); CYP2C9 Inhibitors (Strong); Dexmethylphenidate; Disulfiram; Efavirenz; Felbamate; Floxuridine; Fluconazole; Fluorouracil; Isoniazid; Methotrimeprazine; Methylphenidate; OXcarbazepine; Proton Pump Inhibitors; Rufinamide; Selective Serotonin Reuptake Inhibitors; Sulfonamide Derivatives; Tacrolimus; Ticlopidine; Topiramate; Trimethoprim; Vitamin K Antagonists

Decreased Effect

Phenytoin may decrease the levels/effects of: Acetaminophen; Aminocamptothecin; Amiodarone; Antifungal Agents (Azole Derivatives, Systemic); CarBAMazepine; Caspofungin; Chloramphenicol; Clozapine; Contraceptive (Progestins); CycloSPORINE; CYP2B6 Substrates; CYP2C19 Substrates; CYP2C8 Substrates (High risk); CYP2C9 Substrates (High risk); CYP3A4 Substrates; Darunavir; Deferasirox; Disopyramide; Doxycycline; Dronedarone; Efavirenz; Etoposide; Etoposide Phosphate; Etravirine; Everolimus; Felbamate; Flunarizine; HMG-CoA Reductase Inhibitors; Irinotecan; Lacosamide; LamoTRIgine; Levodopa; Loop Diuretics; Lopinavir; Maraviroc; Mebendazole; Meperidine; Methadone; Metyrapone; Mexiletine; Nilotinib; Oral Contraceptive (Estrogens); OXcarbazepine; Primidone; QUEtiapine; QuiNIDine; Ranolazine; Ritonavir; Rufinamide; Saxagliptin; Sirolimus; Sorafenib; Tacrolimus; Tadalafil; Temsirolimus; Teniposide; Theophylline Derivatives; Thyroid Products; Tipranavir; Tolvaptan; Topiramate; Treprostinil; Valproic Acid; Vecuronium; Zonisamide

The levels/effects of Phenytoin may be decreased by: Amphetamines; Amprenavir; Antacids; CarBAMazepine; Ciprofloxacin; Colesevelam; CYP2C19 Inducers (Strong); CYP2C9 Inducers (Highly Effective); Diazoxide; Folic Acid; Fosamprenavir; Ketorolac; Leucovorin-Levoleucovorin; Lopinavir; Mefloquine; Methylfolate; Peginterferon Alfa-2b; Pyridoxine; Rifamycin Derivatives; Ritonavir; Theophylline Derivatives; Tipranavir; Valproic Acid; Vigabatrin

Ethanol/Nutrition/Herb Interactions

Ethanol:

Acute use: Avoid or limit ethanol (inhibits metabolism of phenytoin). Watch for sedation.

Chronic use: Avoid or limit ethanol (stimulates metabolism of phenytoin).

Food: Phenytoin serum concentrations may be altered if taken with food. If taken with enteral nutrition, phenytoin serum concentrations may be decreased. Tube feedings decrease bioavailability; hold tube feedings 1-2 hours before and 1-2 hours after phenytoin administration. May decrease calcium, folic acid, and vitamin D levels.

Herb/Nutraceutical: Avoid evening primrose (seizure threshold decreased). Avoid valerian, St John's wort, kava kava, gotu kola (may increase CNS depression).

Dietary Considerations

Folic acid: Phenytoin may decrease mucosal uptake of folic acid; to avoid folic acid deficiency and megaloblastic anemia, some clinicians recommend giving patients on anticonvulsants prophylactic doses of folic acid and cyanocobalamin. However, folate supplementation may increase seizures in some patients (dose dependent). Discuss with healthcare provider prior to using any supplements.

Calcium: Hypocalcemia has been reported in patients taking prolonged high-dose therapy with an anticonvulsant. Some clinicians have given an additional 4000 units/week of vitamin D (especially in those receiving poor nutrition and getting no sun exposure) to prevent hypocalcemia.

Vitamin D: Phenytoin interferes with vitamin D metabolism and osteomalacia may result; may need to supplement with vitamin D

Tube feedings: Tube feedings decrease phenytoin absorption. To avoid decreased serum levels with continuous NG feeds, hold feedings for 1-2 hours prior to and 1-2 hours after phenytoin administration, if possible. There is a variety of opinions on how to administer phenytoin with enteral feedings. Be **consistent** throughout therapy.

Sodium content of 1 g injection: 88 mg (3.8 mEq)

Dosage Forms Excipient information presented when available (limited, particularly for generics); consult specific product labeling.

Capsule, extended release, as sodium: 100 mg

Dilantin®: 30 mg [contains sodium benzoate], 100 mg

Phenytek®: 200 mg, 300 mg

Capsule, prompt release, as sodium: 100 mg

Injection, solution, as sodium: 50 mg/mL (2 mL, 5 mL) [contains alcohol and propylene glycol]

Suspension, oral: 100 mg/4 mL (4 mL); 125 mg/5 mL (240 mL)

Dilantin®: 125 mg/5 mL (240 mL) [contains alcohol <0.6%, sodium benzoate; orange vanilla flavor]

Tablet, chewable:

Dilantin®: 50 mg

References

Bleck TP, "Seizures, Stroke, and Other Neurologic Emergencies," *Multidisciplinary Critical Care Review*, Zimmerman JL and Roberts PR, eds, Des Plaines, IL: Society of Critical Care Medicine, 2003, 325-34.

Chapman MG, Smith M, and Hirsch NP, "Status Epilepticus," *Anaesthesia*, 2001, 56(7):648-59.

Hans P, Brichant JF, Pieron F, et al, "Elevated Plasma Alpha 1-Acid Glycoprotein Levels: Lack of Connection to Resistance to Vecuronium Blockade Induced by Anticonvulsant Therapy," *J Neurosurg Anesthesiol*, 1997, 9(1):3-7.

Manno EM, "New Management Strategies in the Treatment of Status Epilepticus," *Mayo Clin Proc*, 2003, 78(4):508-18.

Richard A, Girard F, Girard DC, et al, "Cisatracurium-Induced Neuromuscular Blockade is Affected by Chronic Phenytoin or Carbamazepine Treatment in Neurosurgical Patients," *Anesth Analg*, 2005, 100(2):538-44.

Soriano SG, Sullivan LJ, Venkatakrishnan K, et al, "Pharmacokinetics and Pharmacodynamics of Vecuronium in Children Receiving Phenytoin or Carbamazepine for Chronic Anticonvulsant Therapy," *Br J Anaesth*, 2001, 86(2):223-9.

"Treatment of Convulsive Status Epilepticus. Recommendations of the Epilepsy Foundation of America's Working Group on Status Epilepticus." *JAMA*, 1993, 270(7):854-9.

Treiman DM, Meyers PD, Walton NY, et al, "A Comparison of Four Treatments for Generalized Convulsive Status Epilepticus. Veterans Affairs Status Epilepticus Cooperative Study Group," *N Engl J Med*, 1998, 339(12):792-8.

Wright PM, McCarthy G, Szenohradszky J, et al, "Influence of Chronic Phenytoin Administration on the Pharmacokinetics and Pharmacodynamics of Vecuronium," *Anesthesiology*, 2004, 100 (3):626-33.

- **Phenytoin Sodium** *see* Phenytoin *on page 1119*
- **Phenytoin Sodium, Extended** *see* Phenytoin *on page 1119*
- **Phenytoin Sodium, Prompt** *see* Phenytoin *on page 1119*
- **PHL-Alendronate (Can)** *see* Alendronate *on page 57*
- **PHL-Alendronate-FC (Can)** *see* Alendronate *on page 57*
- **PHL-Amiodarone (Can)** *see* Amiodarone *on page 86*
- **PHL-Amlodipine (Can)** *see* AmLODIPine *on page 93*
- **PHL-Amoxicillin (Can)** *see* Amoxicillin *on page 95*
- **PHL-Azithromycin (Can)** *see* Azithromycin *on page 169*
- **PHL-Carbamazepine (Can)** *see* CarBAMazepine *on page 241*
- **PHL-Carvedilol (Can)** *see* Carvedilol *on page 244*
- **PHL-Cilazapril (Can)** *see* Cilazapril *on page 301*
- **PHL-Ciprofloxacin (Can)** *see* Ciprofloxacin *on page 306*
- **PHL-Divalproex (Can)** *see* Valproic Acid and Derivatives *on page 1445*
- **PHL-Fenofibrate Supra (Can)** *see* Fenofibrate *on page 582*
- **PHL-Fluconazole (Can)** *see* Fluconazole *on page 607*
- **PHL-Fluoxetine (Can)** *see* FLUoxetine *on page 616*
- **PHL-Gabapentin (Can)** *see* Gabapentin *on page 650*
- **PHL-Levetiracetam (Can)** *see* Levetiracetam *on page 816*
- **PHL-Lorazepam (Can)** *see* LORazepam *on page 852*
- **PHL-Lovastatin (Can)** *see* Lovastatin *on page 859*
- **PHL-Metformin (Can)** *see* MetFORMIN *on page 886*
- **PHL-Methimazole (Can)** *see* Methimazole *on page 893*
- **PHL-Methylphenidate (Can)** *see* Methylphenidate *on page 908*
- **PHL-Metoprolol (Can)** *see* Metoprolol *on page 922*
- **PHL-Ondansetron (Can)** *see* Ondansetron *on page 1057*
- **PHL-Oxybutynin (Can)** *see* Oxybutynin *on page 1068*
- **PHL-Paroxetine (Can)** *see* PARoxetine *on page 1089*
- **PHL-Pioglitazone (Can)** *see* Pioglitazone *on page 1132*
- **PHL-Pravastatin (Can)** *see* Pravastatin *on page 1162*
- **PHL-Simvastatin (Can)** *see* Simvastatin *on page 1293*
- **PHL-Sotalol (Can)** *see* Sotalol *on page 1321*
- **PHL-Sumatriptan (Can)** *see* SUMAtriptan *on page 1336*
- **PHL-Temazepam (Can)** *see* Temazepam *on page 1357*
- **PHL-Topiramate (Can)** *see* Topiramate *on page 1408*
- **PHL-Trazodone (Can)** *see* TraZODone *on page 1423*
- **PHL-Valproic Acid (Can)** *see* Valproic Acid and Derivatives *on page 1445*
- **PHL-Valproic Acid E.C. (Can)** *see* Valproic Acid and Derivatives *on page 1445*
- **PHL-Verapamil (Can)** *see* Verapamil *on page 1468*
- **PhosLo®** *see* Calcium Acetate *on page 227*
- **Phosphate, Potassium** *see* Potassium Phosphate *on page 1154*
- **Phosphates, Sodium** *see* Sodium Phosphates *on page 1309*
- **Phosphonoformate** *see* Foscarnet *on page 632*
- **Phosphonoformic Acid** *see* Foscarnet *on page 632*
- **Phoxal-timolol (Can)** *see* Timolol *on page 1390*
- ***p*-Hydroxyampicillin** *see* Amoxicillin *on page 95*
- **Phylloquinone** *see* Phytonadione *on page 1128*

Physostigmine (fye zoe STIG meen)

Medication Safety Issues
  Sound-alike/look-alike issues:
    Physostigmine may be confused with Prostigmin®, pyridostigmine
Canadian Brand Names Eserine®; Isopto® Eserine
Index Terms Eserine Salicylate; Physostigmine Salicylate; Physostigmine Sulfate
Pharmacologic Category Acetylcholinesterase Inhibitor
Generic Available Yes
Use Reverse toxic, life-threatening delirium caused by atropine, diphenhydramine, dimenhydrinate, *Atropa belladonna* (deadly nightshade), or jimson weed (*Datura* spp)
Mechanism of Action Inhibits destruction of acetylcholine by acetylcholinesterase which facilitates transmission of impulses across myoneural junction and prolongs the central and peripheral effects of acetylcholine
Pharmacodynamics/Kinetics
  Onset of action: ~5 minutes
  Duration: 1-2 hours
  Absorption: I.M.: Readily absorbed
  Distribution: Crosses blood-brain barrier readily and reverses both central and peripheral anticholinergic effects
  Metabolism: Hepatic and via hydrolysis by cholinesterases
  Half-life elimination: 15-40 minutes
Dosage Reversal of toxic anticholinergic effects: **Note:** Administer slowly over 5 minutes to prevent respiratory distress and seizures. Continuous infusions of physostigmine should never be used.
  Children: **Note:** Reserve for life-threatening situations only: I.V.: 0.01-0.03 mg/kg/dose; may repeat after 5-10 minutes to a maximum total dose of 2 mg or until response occurs or adverse cholinergic effects occur
  Adults: I.M., I.V.: 0.5-2 mg to start, repeat every 20 minutes until response occurs or adverse effect occurs; repeat 1-4 mg every 30-60 minutes as life-threatening symptoms recur
Stability Do not use solution if cloudy or dark brown.
Administration Injection: Infuse slowly I.V. over 5 minutes. Too rapid administration can cause bradycardia and hypersalivation leading to respiratory distress and seizures.
Monitoring Parameters ECG, vital signs
Anesthesia and Critical Care Concerns/Other Considerations
  Clinical Pearls/Comments: Cholinergic effects of physostigmine include bradycardia and bradydysrhythmias.
Pregnancy Risk Factor C
Contraindications Hypersensitivity to physostigmine or any component of the formulation; GI or GU obstruction; asthma; gangrene; diabetes; cardiovascular disease; any vagotonic state; coadministration of choline esters and depolarizing neuromuscular-blocking agents
Warnings/Precautions Patient must have a normal QRS interval, as measured by ECG, in order to receive; use caution in poisoning with agents known to prolong intraventricular conduction. Concomitant administration of choline esters or depolarizing neuromuscular-blocking agents (ie, succinylcholine) are contra-indicated. Use with caution in patients with epilepsy, asthma, diabetes, gangrene, cardiovascular disease, bradycardia. Discontinue if excessive salivation or emesis, frequent urination or diarrhea occur. Reduce dosage if excessive sweating or nausea occurs. Administer slowly over 5 minutes to prevent respiratory distress and seizures. Continuous infusions should never be used. Due to the possibility of hypersensitivity or overdose/cholinergic crisis, atropine should be readily available; not intended as a first-line agent for anticholinergic toxicity or Parkinson's disease. Asystole and seizures have been reported when physostigmine was administered to TCA poisoned patients. Physostigmine is not recommended in patients with known or suspected TCA intoxication. Products may contain benzyl alcohol. Products may contain sodium bisulfate.
Adverse Reactions Frequency not defined.
  Cardiovascular: Asystole, bradycardia, palpitation

◀ Central nervous system: Hallucinations, nervousness, restlessness, seizure
Gastrointestinal: Diarrhea, nausea, salivation, stomach pain
Genitourinary: Urinary frequency
Neuromuscular & skeletal: Twitching
Ocular: Lacrimation, miosis
Respiratory: Bronchospasm, dyspnea, pulmonary edema, respiratory paralysis
Miscellaneous: Diaphoresis

Drug Interactions

Avoid Concomitant Use There are no known interactions where it is recommended to avoid concomitant use.

Increased Effect/Toxicity

Physostigmine may increase the levels/effects of: Beta-Blockers; Cholinergic Agonists; Succinylcholine

The levels/effects of Physostigmine may be increased by: Corticosteroids (Systemic); Ginkgo Biloba

Decreased Effect

Physostigmine may decrease the levels/effects of: Neuromuscular-Blocking Agents (Nondepolarizing)

Ethanol/Nutrition/Herb Interactions Herb/Nutraceutical: Ginkgo biloba may enhance the adverse/toxic effect of physostigmine; monitor.

Test Interactions Increased aminotransferase [ALT/AST] (S), increased amylase (S)

Dosage Forms Excipient information presented when available (limited, particularly for generics); consult specific product labeling.

Injection, solution, as salicylate: 1 mg/mL (2 mL) [contains benzyl alcohol and sodium metabisulfite]

◆ **Physostigmine Salicylate** *see* Physostigmine *on page 1127*

◆ **Physostigmine Sulfate** *see* Physostigmine *on page 1127*

◆ **Phytomenadione** *see* Phytonadione *on page 1128*

Phytonadione (fye toe na DYE one)

Medication Safety Issues
Sound-alike/look-alike issues:
Mephyton® may be confused with melphalan, methadone

U.S. Brand Names Mephyton®

Canadian Brand Names AquaMEPHYTON®; Konakion; Mephyton®

Index Terms Methylphytyl Napthoquinone; Phylloquinone; Phytomenadione; Vitamin K_1

Pharmacologic Category Vitamin, Fat Soluble

Generic Available Yes

Use Prevention and treatment of hypoprothrombinemia caused by coumarin derivative-induced or other drug-induced vitamin K deficiency, hypoprothrombinemia caused by malabsorption or inability to synthesize vitamin K; hemorrhagic disease of the newborn

Unlabeled/Investigational Use Treatment of hypoprothrombinemia caused by anticoagulant rodenticides

Mechanism of Action Promotes liver synthesis of clotting factors (II, VII, IX, X); however, the exact mechanism as to this stimulation is unknown. Menadiol is a water soluble form of vitamin K; phytonadione has a more rapid and prolonged effect than menadione; menadiol sodium diphosphate (K_4) is half as potent as menadione (K_3).

Pharmacodynamics/Kinetics
Onset of action: Increased coagulation factors: Oral: 6-10 hours; I.V.: 1-2 hours
Peak effect: INR values return to normal: Oral: 24-48 hours; I.V.: 12-14 hours
Absorption: Oral: From intestines in presence of bile; SubQ: Variable
Metabolism: Rapidly hepatic
Excretion: Urine and feces

Dosage Note: According to the manufacturer, SubQ is the preferred parenteral route; I.M. route should be avoided due to the risk of hematoma formation; I.V. route should be restricted for emergency use only. The American College of Chest

Physicians recommends the I.V. route in patients with serious or life-threatening bleeding secondary to use of vitamin K antagonists.

Adequate intake:

Children:

1-3 years: 30 mcg/day

4-8 years: 55 mcg/day

9-13 years: 60 mcg/day

14-18 years: 75 mcg/day

Adults: Males: 120 mcg/day; Females: 90 mcg/day

Hemorrhagic disease of the newborn:

Prophylaxis: I.M.: 0.5-1 mg within 1 hour of birth

Treatment: I.M., SubQ: 1 mg/dose/day; higher doses may be necessary if mother has been receiving oral anticoagulants

Hypoprothrombinemia due to drugs (other than coumarin derivatives) or factors limiting absorption or synthesis: Adults: Oral, SubQ, I.M., I.V.: Initial: 2.5-25 mg (rarely up to 50 mg)

Vitamin K deficiency (supratherapeutic INR) secondary to coumarin derivative (Ansell, 2008): Adults:

If INR above therapeutic range to <5 (no significant bleeding and rapid reversal unnecessary): Lower or hold next dose and monitor frequently; when INR approaches desired range, resume dosing with a lower dose.

If INR ≥5 and <9 (no significant bleeding): If no risk factors for bleeding exist, omit next 1 or 2 doses, monitor INR more frequently, and resume with an appropriately adjusted dose when INR in desired range.

Alternatively, if other risk factors for bleeding exist, omit next dose and administer vitamin K orally 1-2.5 mg; resume with an appropriately adjusted dose when INR in desired range.

If INR ≥5 and <9 (no significant bleeding and rapid reversal required for surgery): Administer vitamin K orally ≤5 mg and hold warfarin. Expect INR to be reduced within 24 hours; if INR still elevated, another 1-2 mg of vitamin K orally may be given.

If INR ≥9 (no significant bleeding): Hold warfarin, administer vitamin K orally 2.5-5 mg, expect INR to be reduced within 24-48 hours, monitor INR more frequently and give additional vitamin K at an appropriate dose if necessary. Resume warfarin at an appropriately adjusted dose when INR is in desired range.

If serious bleeding at any INR elevation: Hold warfarin, administer vitamin K 10 mg by slow I.V. infusion and supplement with FFP, PCC, or rFVIIa depending on the urgency of the situation; I.V. Vitamin K may be repeated every 12 hours.

If life-threatening bleeding: Hold warfarin, give FFP, PCC, or rFVIIa supplemented with vitamin K 10 mg slow I.V. infusion; repeat if necessary, depending on INR.

Notes:

If mild-moderate INR elevation without major bleeding occurs, administer vitamin K orally instead of subcutaneously.

Use of high doses of vitamin K (eg, 10-15 mg) may cause warfarin resistance for ≥1 week. During this period of resistance, heparin or low molecular weight heparin may be given until INR responds.

FFP=fresh frozen plasma; PCC=prothrombin complex concentrate; rFVIIa=recombinant factor VIIa

Stability

Injection: Store at 15°C to 30°C (59°F to 86°F). Dilute in preservative-free NS, D_5W, or D_5NS.

Note: Store Hospira product at 20°C to 25°C (68°F to 77°F).

Oral: Store tablets at 15°C to 30°C (59°F to 86°F). Protect from light.

Administration

I.V. administration: Infuse slowly; rate of infusion should not exceed 1 mg/minute (3 mg/m^2/minute in children and infants). The injectable route should be used only if the oral route is not feasible or there is a greater urgency to reverse anticoagulation.

Oral: The parenteral preparation has been administered orally to neonates.

Monitoring Parameters PT, INR

Pregnancy Risk Factor C

◀ **Contraindications** Hypersensitivity to phytonadione or any component of the formulation

Warnings/Precautions [U.S. Boxed Warning]: Severe reactions resembling hypersensitivity (eg, anaphylaxis) reactions have occurred rarely during or immediately after I.V. administration. Allergic reactions have also occurred with I.M. and SubQ injections; oral administration is the safest. In obstructive jaundice or with biliary fistulas concurrent administration of bile salts is necessary. Manufacturers recommend the SubQ route over other parenteral routes. SubQ is less predictable when compared to the oral route. The American College of Chest Physicians recommends the I.V. route in patients with serious or life-threatening bleeding secondary to warfarin. The I.V. route should be restricted to emergency situations where oral phytonadione cannot be used. Efficacy is delayed regardless of route of administration; patient management may require other treatments in the interim. Administer a dose that will quickly lower the INR into a safe range without causing resistance to warfarin. High phytonadione doses may lead to warfarin resistance for at least one week. Use caution in newborns especially premature infants; hemolysis, jaundice and hyperbilirubinemia have been reported with larger than recommended doses. Some dosage forms contain benzyl alcohol which has been associated with "gasping syndrome" in premature infants. In liver disease, if initial doses do not reverse coagulopathy then higher doses are unlikely to have any effect. Ineffective in hereditary hypoprothrombinemia. Use caution with renal dysfunction (including premature infants). Injectable products may contain aluminum; may result in toxic levels following prolonged administration. Product may contain polysorbate 80.

Adverse Reactions Parenteral administration: Frequency not defined.

Cardiovascular: Cyanosis, flushing, hypotension

Central nervous system: Dizziness

Dermatologic: Scleroderma-like lesions

Endocrine & metabolic: Hyperbilirubinemia (newborn; greater than recommended doses)

Gastrointestinal: Abnormal taste

Local: Injection site reactions

Respiratory: Dyspnea

Miscellaneous: Anaphylactoid reactions, diaphoresis, hypersensitivity reactions

Drug Interactions

Avoid Concomitant Use There are no known interactions where it is recommended to avoid concomitant use.

Increased Effect/Toxicity There are no known significant interactions involving an increase in effect.

Decreased Effect

Phytonadione may decrease the levels/effects of: Vitamin K Antagonists

The levels/effects of Phytonadione may be decreased by: Mineral Oil; Orlistat

Dosage Forms Excipient information presented when available (limited, particularly for generics); consult specific product labeling.

Injection, aqueous colloidal: 2 mg/mL (0.5 mL); 10 mg/mL (1 mL) [contains benzyl alcohol]

Injection, aqueous colloidal [preservative free]: 2 mg/mL (0.5 mL) [contains polysorbate 80, propylene glycol 10.4 mg/0.5 mL]

Tablet: 100 mcg [OTC]

Mephyton®: 5 mg

References

Ansell J, Hirsh J, Poller L, et al, "The Pharmacology and Management of the Vitamin K Antagonists: The Seventh ACCP Conference on Antithrombotic and Thrombolytic Therapy," *Chest*, 2004, 126(3 Suppl):204-33.

Pindolol (PIN doe lole)

Related Information

Beta-Blockers *on page 1669*

Preoperative Evaluation of the Cardiac Patient for Noncardiac Surgery *on page 1598*

Canadian Brand Names Apo-Pindol®; Gen-Pindolol; Novo-Pindol; Nu-Pindol; PMS-Pindolol; Visken®

Pharmacologic Category Beta Blocker With Intrinsic Sympathomimetic Activity
Use Treatment of hypertension, alone or in combination with other agents
Unlabeled/Investigational Use Potential augmenting agent for antidepressants; ventricular arrhythmias/tachycardia, antipsychotic-induced akathisia, situational anxiety; aggressive behavior associated with dementia
Pharmacodynamics/Kinetics
Absorption: Rapid, 50% to 95%
Distribution: V_d: ~2 L/kg
Protein binding: 40%
Metabolism: Hepatic (60% to 65%) to conjugates
Half-life elimination: 3-4 hours; prolonged with advanced age, and cirrhosis (range: 2.5-30 hours)
Time to peak, serum: ~1 hour
Excretion: Urine (35% to 40% as unchanged drug); feces (6% to 9%)
Dosage Oral:
Adults:
Hypertension: Initial: 5 mg twice daily, increase as necessary by 10 mg/day every 3-4 weeks (maximum daily dose: 60 mg); usual dose range (JNC 7): 10-40 mg twice daily
Antidepressant augmentation (unlabeled use): 2.5 mg 3 times/day
Elderly: Initial: 5 mg once daily, increase as necessary by 5 mg/day every 3-4 weeks

Dosing adjustment in renal impairment: Use with caution. Clearance significantly decreased in uremic patients. Dosage reduction may be necessary.
Dosage adjustment in hepatic impairment: Use with caution. Elimination half-life in cirrhotic patients may be 10 times as long compared to normal patients. Dosage reduction is necessary in severely impaired.
Anesthesia and Critical Care Concerns/Other Considerations Pindolol possesses intrinsic sympathomimetic activity. While beta-blockers with intrinsic sympathomimetic activity induce fewer side effects, the cardiovascular benefits are less clear than for beta-blockers without intrinsic sympathomimetic activity.

Withdrawal: Beta-blocker therapy should not be withdrawn abruptly, but gradually tapered over 1-2 weeks to avoid acute tachycardia and hypertension.
Additional Information Complete prescribing information for this medication should be consulted for additional detail.
Dosage Forms Excipient information presented when available (limited, particularly for generics); consult specific product labeling.
Tablet: 5 mg, 10 mg
References
Artigas F, Romero L, de Montigny C, et al, "Acceleration of the effect of Selected Antidepressant Drugs in Major Depression by 5-HT1A Antagonists," *Trends Neurosci*, 1996, 19(9):378–83

Chobanian AV, Bakris GL, Black HR, et al, "The Seventh Report of the Joint National Committee on Prevention, Detection, Evaluation, and Treatment of High Blood Pressure: The JNC 7 Report," *JAMA*, 2003, 289(19):2560-71.

"Consensus Recommendations for the Management of Chronic Heart Failure. On Behalf of the Membership of the Advisory Council to Improve Outcomes Nationwide in Heart Failure," *Am J Cardiol*, 1999, 83(2A):1-38.

Ekbom T, Dahlof B, Hansson L, et al, "Antihypertensive Efficacy and Side Effects of Three Beta-blockers and a Diuretic in Elderly Hypertensives: a report from the STOP-Hypertension Study," *J Hypertens*, 1992, 10(12):1525-30.

Erstad BL and Barletta JF, "Treatment of Hypertension in the Perioperative Patient," *Ann Pharmacother*, 2000, 34(1):66-79.

Fraker TD, Fihn SD, Gibbons RJ, et al, "2007 Chronic Angina Focused Update of the ACC/AHA 2002 Guidelines for the Management of Patients With Chronic Stable Angina: A Report of the American College of Cardiology/American Heart Association Task Force on Practice Guidelines Writing Group to Develop the Focused Update of the 2002 Guidelines for the Management of Patients With Chronic Stable Angina," *Circulation*, 2007, 116(23):2762-72.

Fuster V, Ryden LE, Cannom DS, et al, "ACC/AHA/ESC 2006 Guidelines for the Management of Patients With Atrial Fibrillation-Executrive Summary. A Report of the American College of Cardiology/American Heart Association Task Force on Practice Guidelines and the European Society of Cardiology Committee for Practice Guidelines (Writing Committee to Revise the 2001 Guidelines for the Management of Patients With Atrial Fibrillation). Developed in Collaboration With the European Heart Rhythm Association and the Heart Rhythm Society," *J Am Coll Cardiol*, 2006, 48(4):854-906.

Geretsegger C, Bitterlich W, Stelzig R, et al, "Paroxetine With Pindolol Augmentation: A Double-blind, Randomized, Placebo-Controlled Study in Depressed In-Patients," *Eur Neuropsychopharmacol*, 2008, 18(2):141-6.

Gibbons RJ, Abrams J, Chatterjee K, et al, "ACC/AHA 2002 Guideline Update for the Management of Patients With Chronic Stable Angina - Summary Article: A Report of the American College of Cardiology/American Heart Association Task Force on Practice Guidelines (Committee on the Management of Patients With Chronic Stable Angina)," *J Am Coll Cardiol*, 2003, 41(1):159-68.

Lang DM, "Anaphylactoid and Anaphylactic Reactions. Hazards of Beta-Blockers," *Drug Saf*, 1995, 12(5):299-304.

Mokhlesi B, Leikin JB, Murray P, et al, "Adult Toxicology in Critical Care: Part II: Specific Poisonings," *Chest*, 2003, 123(3):897-922.

Ohnhaus EE, Heidemann H, Meier J, et al, "Metabolism of Pindolol in Patients with Renal Failure," *Eur J Clin Pharmacol*, 1982, 22(5):423-8.

UK Prospective Diabetes Study Group, "Efficacy of Atenolol and Captopril in Reducing Risk of Macrovascular and Microvascular Complications in Type 2 Diabetes: UKPDS 39," *BMJ*, 1998, 317 (7160):713-20.

Pioglitazone (pye oh GLI ta zone)

U.S. Brand Names Actos®

Canadian Brand Names Actos®; Apo-Pioglitazone; CO Pioglitazone; Gen-Pioglitazone; Mylan-Pioglitazone; Novo-Pioglitazone; PHL-Pioglitazone; PMS-Pioglitazone; ratio-Pioglitazone; Sandoz-Pioglitazone; SPEF-Pioglitazone

Pharmacologic Category Antidiabetic Agent, Thiazolidinedione

Use

Type 2 diabetes mellitus (noninsulin dependent, NIDDM), monotherapy: Adjunct to diet and exercise, to improve glycemic control

Type 2 diabetes mellitus (noninsulin dependent, NIDDM), combination therapy with sulfonylurea, metformin, or insulin: When diet, exercise, and a single agent alone does not result in adequate glycemic control

Unlabeled/Investigational Use Polycystic ovary syndrome (PCOS)

Pharmacodynamics/Kinetics

Onset of action: Delayed

Peak effect: Glucose control: Several weeks

Distribution: V_{ss} (apparent): 0.63 L/kg

Protein binding: 99.8%; primarily to albumin

Metabolism: Hepatic (99%) via CYP2C8 and 3A4 to both active and inactive metabolites

Half-life elimination: Parent drug: 3-7 hours; Total: 16-24 hours

Time to peak: ~2 hours; delayed with food

Excretion: Urine (15% to 30%) and feces as metabolites

Dosage Oral:

Adults:

Monotherapy: Initial: 15-30 mg once daily; if response is inadequate, the dosage may be increased in increments up to 45 mg once daily; maximum recommended dose: 45 mg once daily

Combination therapy: Maximum recommended dose: 45 mg/day

With sulfonylureas: Initial: 15-30 mg once daily; dose of sulfonylurea should be reduced if the patient reports hypoglycemia

With metformin: Initial: 15-30 mg once daily; it is unlikely that the dose of metformin will need to be reduced due to hypoglycemia

With insulin: Initial: 15-30 mg once daily; dose of insulin should be reduced by 10% to 25% if the patient reports hypoglycemia or if the plasma glucose falls to <100 mg/dL.

Dosage adjustment in patients with CHF (NYHA Class II) in mono- or combination therapy: Initial: 15 mg once daily; may be increased after several months of treatment, with close attention to heart failure symptoms

Elderly: No dosage adjustment is recommended in elderly patients.

Dosage adjustment in renal impairment: No dosage adjustment is required.

Dosage adjustment in hepatic impairment: Clearance is significantly lower in hepatic impairment (Child-Pugh Grade B/C). Therapy should not be initiated if the patient exhibits active liver disease or increased transaminases (>2.5 times ULN) at baseline. During treatment if ALT levels elevate >3 times ULN, the test should be repeated as soon as possible. If ALT levels remain >3 times ULN or if the patient is jaundiced, therapy should be discontinued.

Additional Information Complete prescribing information for this medication should be consulted for additional detail.

Dosage Forms Excipient information presented when available (limited, particularly for generics); consult specific product labeling.
Tablet:
Actos®: 15 mg, 30 mg, 45 mg

References

Dormandy JA, Charbonnel B, Eckland DJ, et al, "Secondary Prevention of Macrovascular Events in Patients With Type 2 Diabetes in the PROactive Study (PROspective PioglitAzone Clinical Trial In MacroVascular Events): A Randomised Controlled Trial," *Lancet*, 2005, 366(9493):1279-89.

Glueck CJ, Moreira A, Goldenberg N, et al, "Pioglitazone and Metformin in Obese Women With Polycystic Ovary Syndrome Not Optimally Responsive to Metformin," *Hum Reprod*, 2003, 18 (8):1618-25

Romualdi D, Guido M, Ciampelli M, et al, "Selective Effects of Pioglitazone on Insulin and Androgen Abnormalities in Normo- and Hyperinsulinaemic Obese Patients With Polycystic Ovary Syndrome," *Hum Reprod*, 2003, 18(6):1210-8.

Ryden L, Thrainsdottir I, and Swedberg K, "Adjudication of Serious Heart Failure in Patients From PROactive," *Lancet*, 2007, 369(9557):189-90.

Piperacillin (pi PER a sil in)

Related Information
Prevention of Infective Endocarditis *on page 1718*
Canadian Brand Names Piperacillin for Injection, USP
Index Terms Piperacillin Sodium
Pharmacologic Category Antibiotic, Penicillin
Generic Available Yes
Use Treatment of susceptible infections such as septicemia, acute and chronic respiratory tract infections, skin and soft tissue infections, and urinary tract infections due to susceptible strains of *Pseudomonas*, *Proteus*, and *Escherichia coli* and *Enterobacter*; active against some streptococci and some anaerobic bacteria; febrile neutropenia (as part of combination regimen)
Mechanism of Action Inhibits bacterial cell wall synthesis by binding to one or more of the penicillin binding proteins (PBPs); which in turn inhibits the final transpeptidation step of peptidoglycan synthesis in bacterial cell walls, thus inhibiting cell wall biosynthesis. Bacteria eventually lyse due to ongoing activity of cell wall autolytic enzymes (autolysins and murein hydrolases) while cell wall assembly is arrested.
Pharmacodynamics/Kinetics
Absorption: I.M.: 70% to 80%
Protein binding: ~16%
Bioavailability: Not well absorbed when given orally
Half-life elimination (dose dependent; prolonged with moderately severe renal or hepatic impairment):
Neonates: 1-5 days old: 3.6 hours; >6 days old: 2.1-2.7 hours
Children: 1-6 months: 0.79 hour; 6 months to 12 years: 0.39-0.5 hour
Adults: 36-80 minutes
Time to peak, serum: I.M.: 30-50 minutes
Excretion: Primarily urine; partially feces
Dosage
Usual dosage range:
Neonates: I.M., I.V.: 100 mg/kg every 12 hours
Infants and Children: I.M., I.V.: 200-300 mg/kg/day in divided doses every 4-6 hours
Adults: I.M., I.V.: 2-4 g/dose every 4-6 hours (maximum: 24 g/day)
Indication-specific dosing:
Children: I.M., I.V.:
Cystic fibrosis: 350-500 mg/kg/day in divided doses every 4-6 hours
Adults:
Burn wound sepsis: I.V.: 4 g every 4 hours with vancomycin and amikacin
Cholangitis, acute: I.V.: 4 g every 6 hours
Keratitis *(Pseudomonas)*: Ophthalmic: 6-12 mg/mL every 15-60 minutes around the clock for 24-72 hours, then slow reduction
Malignant otitis externa: I.V.: 4-6 g every 4-6 hours with tobramycin
Moderate infections: I.M., I.V.: 2-3 g/dose every 6-12 hours (maximum: 2 g I.M./site)
Prosthetic joint *(Pseudomonas)*: I.V.: 3 g every 6 hours with aminoglycoside

◄ **Pseudomonas infections:** I.V.: 4 g every 4 hours
Severe infections: I.M., I.V.: 3-4 g/dose every 4-6 hours (maximum: 24 g/24 hours)
Urinary tract infections: I.V.: 2-3 g/dose every 6-12 hours
Uncomplicated gonorrhea: I.M.: 2 g in a single dose accompanied by 1 g probenecid 30 minutes prior to injection

Dosing adjustment in renal impairment: Adults: I.V.:
Cl_{cr} 20-40 mL/minute: Administer 3-4 g every 8 hours
Cl_{cr} <20 mL/minute: Administer 3-4 g every 12 hours
Moderately dialyzable (20% to 50%)
Continuous arteriovenous or venovenous hemodiafiltration effects: Dose as for Cl_{cr} 10-50 mL/minute

Stability Reconstituted solution is stable (I.V. infusion) in NS or D_5W for 24 hours at room temperature, 7 days when refrigerated, or 4 weeks when frozen. After freezing, thawed solution is stable for 24 hours at room temperature or 48 hours when refrigerated. 40 g bulk vial should **not** be frozen after reconstitution.

Administration Administer around-the-clock to promote less variation in peak and trough serum levels. Give at least 1 hour apart from aminoglycosides. Rapid administration can lead to seizures. Administer direct I.V. over 3-5 minutes. Intermittently infusion over 30 minutes. Do not administer more than 2 g per I.M. injection site.

Some penicillins (eg, carbenicillin, ticarcillin and piperacillin) have been shown to inactivate aminoglycosides *in vitro*. This has been observed to a greater extent with tobramycin and gentamicin, while amikacin has shown greater stability against inactivation. Concurrent use of these agents may pose a risk of reduced antibacterial efficacy *in vivo*, particularly in the setting of profound renal impairment. However, definitive clinical evidence is lacking. If combination penicillin/aminoglycoside therapy is desired in a patient with renal dysfunction, separation of doses (if feasible), and routine monitoring of aminoglycoside levels, CBC, and clinical response should be considered.

Monitoring Parameters Observe for signs and symptoms of anaphylaxis during first dose

Pregnancy Risk Factor B

Contraindications Hypersensitivity to piperacillin, other beta-lactam antibiotics (penicillins or cephalosporins), or any component of the formulation

Warnings/Precautions Serious and occasionally severe or fatal hypersensitivity (anaphylactoid) reactions have been reported in patients on penicillin therapy, especially with a history of beta-lactam hypersensitivity, history of sensitivity to multiple allergens, or previous IgE-mediated reactions (eg, anaphylaxis, angioedema, urticaria). Use with caution in asthmatic patients. Bleeding disorders have been observed, particularly in patients with renal impairment; discontinue if thrombocytopenia or bleeding occurs. Due to sodium load and adverse effects (anemia, neuropsychological changes), use with caution and modify dosage in patients with renal impairment. Use caution in patients with history of seizure activity. Leukopenia and neutropenia have been reported (during prolonged therapy). An increased frequency of fever and rash has been reported in patients with cystic fibrosis. Prolonged use may result in fungal or bacterial superinfection, including *C. difficile*-associated diarrhea (CDAD) and pseudomembranous colitis; CDAD has been observed >2 months postantibiotic treatment.

Adverse Reactions Frequency not defined.
Central nervous system: Confusion, convulsions, drowsiness, fever, Jarisch-Herxheimer reaction
Dermatologic: Rash, toxic epidermal necrolysis, urticaria
Endocrine & metabolic: Electrolyte imbalance, hypokalemia
Hematologic: Abnormal platelet aggregation and prolonged PT (high doses), agranulocytosis, Coombs' reaction (positive), hemolytic anemia, pancytopenia
Local: Thrombophlebitis
Neuromuscular & skeletal: Myoclonus
Renal: Acute interstitial nephritis, acute renal failure
Miscellaneous: Anaphylaxis, hypersensitivity reactions

Drug Interactions
Avoid Concomitant Use There are no known interactions where it is recommended to avoid concomitant use.

Increased Effect/Toxicity
Piperacillin may increase the levels/effects of: Methotrexate

The levels/effects of Piperacillin may be increased by: Uricosuric Agents
Decreased Effect
Piperacillin may decrease the levels/effects of: Aminoglycosides; Mycophenolate; Typhoid Vaccine

The levels/effects of Piperacillin may be decreased by: Fusidic Acid; Tetracycline Derivatives

Test Interactions May interfere with urinary glucose tests using cupric sulfate (Benedict's solution, Clinitest®); false-positive urinary and serum proteins, positive Coombs' test [direct]. False-positive Platelia® *Aspergillus* EIA test (Bio-Rad Laboratories) has been reported.

Some penicillin derivatives may accelerate the degradation of aminoglycosides *in vitro*, leading to a potential underestimation of aminoglycoside serum concentration.

Dietary Considerations Sodium content of 1 g: 1.85 mEq

Dosage Forms Excipient information presented when available (limited, particularly for generics); consult specific product labeling.

Injection, powder for reconstitution: 2 g, 3 g, 4 g, 40 g

References
Capellier G, Cornette C, Boillot A, et al, "Removal of Piperacillin in Critically Ill Patients Undergoing Continuous Veno-Venous Hemofiltration," *Crit Care Med*, 1998, 26(1):88-91.

Chow MS, Quintiliani, and Nightingale CH, "*In Vivo* Inactivation of Tobramycin by Ticarcillin. A Case Report," *JAMA*, 1982, 247(5):658-9.

Daly JS, Dodge RA, Glew RH, et al, "Effect of Time and Temperature on Inactivation of Aminoglycosides by Ampicillin at Neonatal Dosages," *J Perinatol*, 1997, 17(1):42-5.

Donowitz GR and Mandell GL, "Beta-Lactam Antibiotics," *N Engl J Med*, 1988, 318(7):419-26 and 318(8):490-500.

Dowell JA, Korth-Bradley J, Milisci M, et al, "Evaluating Possible Pharmacokinetic Interactions Between Tobramycin, Piperacillin, and a Combination of Piperacillin and Tazobactam in Patients With Various Degrees of Renal Impairment," *J Clin Pharmacol*, 2001, 41:979-86.

Farchione LA, "Inactivation of Aminoglycosides by Penicillins," *J Antimicrob Chemother*, 1982, 8 (Suppl A):27-36.

Fuchs PC, Stickel S, Anderson PH, et al, "*In Vitro* Inactivation of Aminoglycosides by Sulbactam, Other Beta-Lactams, and Sulbactam-Beta-Lactam Combinations," *Antimicrob Agents Chemother*, 1991, 35(1):182-4.

Halstenson CE, Wong MO, Herman CS, et al, "Effect of Concomitant Administration of Piperacillin on the Dispositions on Isepamicin and Gentamicin in Patients With End-Stage Renal Disease," *Antimicrob Agents Chemother*, 1992, 36(9):1832-36.

Hitt CM, Patel KB, Nicolau DP, et al, "Influence of Piperacillin-Tazobactam on Pharmacokinetics of Gentamicin Given Once Daily," *Am J Health Syst Pharm*, 1997, 54(23):2704-8.

Keller E, Bohler J, Busse-Grawitz A, et al, "Single Dose Kinetics of Piperacillin During Continuous Arteriovenous Hemodialysis in Intensive Care Patients," *Clin Nephrol*, 1995, 43(Suppl 1):20-3.

Konishi H, Goto M, Nakamoto Y, et al, "Tobramycin Inactivation by Carbenicillin, Ticarcillin, and Piperacillin," *Antimicrob Agents Chemother*, 1983, 23(5):653-57.

Lau A, Lee M, Flascha S, et al, "Effect of Piperacillin on Tobramycin Pharmacokinetics in Patients with Normal Renal Function," *Antimicrob Agents Chemother*, 1983, 24(4):533-37.

Placzek M, Whitelaw A, Want S, et al, "Piperacillin in Early Neonatal Infection," *Arch Dis Child*, 1983, 58(12):1006-9.

Prince AS and Neu HC, "Use of Piperacillin, A Semisynthetic Penicillin, in the Therapy of Acute Exacerbations of Pulmonary Disease in Patients With Cystic Fibrosis," *J Pediatr*, 1980, 97 (1):148-51.

Russoe ME and Atkins-Thor E, "Gentamicin and Ticarcillin in Subjects With End-Stage Renal Disease. Comparison of Two Assay Methods and Evaluation of Inactivation Rate," *Clin Nephrol*, 1981, 15(4):175-80.

Tan JS and File TM Jr, "Antipseudomonal Penicillins," *Med Clin North Am*, 1995, 79(4):679-93.

Thirumoorthi MC, Asmar BI, Buckley JA, et al, "Pharmacokinetics of Intravenously Administered Piperacillin in Preadolescent Children," *J Pediatr*, 1983, 102(6):941-6.

Thompson MIB, Russo ME, Saxon BJ, et al, "Gentamicin Inactivation by Piperacillin or Carbenicillin in Patients With End-Stage Renal Disease," *Antimicrob Agents Chemother*, 1982, 21(2):268-73.

Viollier AF, Standiford HC, Drusano GL, et al, "Comparative Pharmacokinetics and Serum Bactericidal Activity of Mezlocillin, Ticarcillin and Piperacillin, With and Without Gentamicin," *J Antimicrob Chemother*, 1985, 15(5):597-606.

Walterspiel JN, Feldman S, Van R, et al, "Comparative Inactivation of Isepamicin, Amikacin, and Gentamicin by Nine Beta-Lactams and Two Beta-Lactamase Inhibitors, Cilastatin and Heparin," *Antimicrob Agents Chemother*, 1991, 35(9):1875-8.

Wright AJ, "The Penicillins," *Mayo Clin Proc*, 1999, 74(3):290-307.

Yoshikawa TT, "Antimicrobial Therapy for the Elderly Patient," *J Am Geriatr Soc*, 1990, 38 (12):1353-72.

Piperacillin and Tazobactam Sodium
(pi PER a sil in & ta zoe BAK tam SOW dee um)

Medication Safety Issues
Sound-alike/look-alike issues:
Zosyn® may be confused with Zofran®, Zyvox®

U.S. Brand Names Zosyn®

Canadian Brand Names Tazocin®

Index Terms Piperacillin Sodium and Tazobactam Sodium; Tazobactam and Piperacillin

Pharmacologic Category Antibiotic, Penicillin

Generic Available No

Use Treatment of moderate-to-severe infections caused by susceptible organisms, including infections of the lower respiratory tract (community-acquired pneumonia, nosocomial pneumonia); urinary tract; uncomplicated and complicated skin and skin structures; gynecologic (endometritis, pelvic inflammatory disease); bone and joint infections; intra-abdominal infections (appendicitis with rupture/abscess, peritonitis); and septicemia. Tazobactam expands activity of piperacillin to include beta-lactamase producing strains of *S. aureus*, *H. influenzae*, *Bacteroides*, and other gram-negative bacteria.

Mechanism of Action Inhibits bacterial cell wall synthesis by binding to one or more of the penicillin binding proteins (PBPs); which in turn inhibits the final transpeptidation step of peptidoglycan synthesis in bacterial cell walls, thus inhibiting cell wall biosynthesis. Bacteria eventually lyse due to ongoing activity of cell wall autolytic enzymes (autolysins and murein hydrolases) while cell wall assembly is arrested. Tazobactam inhibits many beta-lactamases, including staphylococcal penicillinase and Richmond and Sykes types II, III, IV, and V, including extended spectrum enzymes; it has only limited activity against class I beta-lactamases other than class Ic types.

Pharmacodynamics/Kinetics Both AUC and peak concentrations are dose proportional; hepatic impairment does not affect kinetics

Distribution: Well into lungs, intestinal mucosa, skin, muscle, uterus, ovary, prostate, gallbladder, and bile; penetration into CSF is low in subject with noninflamed meninges

Protein binding: Piperacillin and tazobactam: ~30%

Metabolism:
Piperacillin: 6% to 9% to desethyl metabolite (weak activity)
Tazobactam: ~26% to inactive metabolite

Bioavailability:
Piperacillin: I.M.: 71%
Tazobactam: I.M.: 84%

Half-life elimination: Piperacillin and tazobactam: 0.7-1.2 hours

Time to peak, plasma: Immediately following infusion of 30 minutes

Excretion: Clearance of both piperacillin and tazobactam are directly proportional to renal function
Piperacillin: Urine (68% as unchanged drug); feces (10% to 20%)
Tazobactam: Urine (80% as unchanged drug; remainder as inactive metabolite)

Dosage
Usual dosage range:
Children: I.V.:
2-8 months: 80 mg of piperacillin component/kg every 8 hours
≥9 months and ≤40 kg: 100 mg of piperacillin component/kg every 8 hours
Adults: I.V.: 3.375 g every 6 hours **or** 4.5 g every 6-8 hours; maximum: 18 g/day
Indication-specific dosing: I.V.:
Children: **Note:** Dosing based on piperacillin component:
Appendicitis, peritonitis:
2-8 months: 80 mg/kg every 8 hours
≥9 months and ≤40 kg: 100 mg/kg every 8 hours
>40 kg: refer to Adult dosing
Cystic fibrosis, pseudomonal infections (unlabeled use): 350-450 mg/kg/day in divided doses

Adults:

Diverticulitis, intra-abdominal abscess, peritonitis: I.V.: 3.375 g every 6 hours; **Note:** Some clinicians use 4.5 g every 8 hours for empiric coverage since the %time>MIC is similar between the regimens for most pathogens; however, this regimen is NOT recommended for nosocomial pneumonia or *Pseudomonas* coverage.

Pneumonia (nosocomial): I.V.: 4.5 g every 6 hours for 7-14 days (when used empirically, combination with an aminoglycoside or antipseudomonal fluoroquinolone is recommended; consider discontinuation of additional agent if *P. aeruginosa* is not isolated)

Severe infections: I.V.: 3.375 g every 6 hours for 7-10 days; **Note:** Some clinicians use 4.5 g every 8 hours for empiric coverage since the %time>MIC is similar between the regimens for most pathogens; however, this regimen is NOT recommended for nosocomial pneumonia or *Pseudomonas* coverage.

Dosing interval in renal impairment:

Cl_{cr} 20-40 mL/minute: Administer 2.25 g every 6 hours (3.375 g every 6 hours for nosocomial pneumonia)

Cl_{cr} <20 mL/minute: Administer 2.25 g every 8 hours (2.25 g every 6 hours for nosocomial pneumonia)

Hemodialysis/CAPD: Administer 2.25 g every 12 hours (2.25 g every 8 hours for nosocomial pneumonia) with an additional dose of 0.75 g after each hemodialysis session

Continuous renal replacement therapy (CRRT): Drug clearance is highly dependent on the method of renal replacement, filter type, and flow rate. Appropriate dosing requires close monitoring of pharmacologic response, signs of adverse reactions due to drug accumulation, as well as drug levels in relation to target trough (if appropriate). The following are general recommendations only (based on dialysate flow/ultrafiltration rates of 1 L/hour) and should not supersede clinical judgment:

CVVH: 2.25 g every 6 hours

CVVHD/CVVHDF: 2.25-3.375 g every 6 hours

Note: Higher dose of 3.375 g should be considered when treating resistant pathogens (especially *Pseudomonas*); alternative recommendations suggest dosing of 4.5 g every 8 hours; regardless of regimen, there is some concern of tazobactam (TAZ) accumulation, given its lower clearance relative to piperacillin (PIP). Some clinicians advocate dosing with PIP to alternate with PIP/TAZ, particularly in CVVH-dependent patients, to lessen this concern.

Stability

Vials: Store at controlled room temperature of 20°C to 25°C (68°F to 77°F). Use single-dose vials immediately after reconstitution (discard unused portions after 24 hours at room temperature and 48 hours if refrigerated). Reconstitute with 5 mL of diluent per 1 g of piperacillin and then further dilute. After reconstitution, vials or solution are stable in NS or D_5W for 24 hours at room temperature and 48 hours (vials) or 7 days (solution) when refrigerated.

Premixed solution: Store frozen at -20°C (-4°F). Thawed solution is stable for 24 hours at room temperature or 14 days under refrigeration; do not refreeze.

Administration Administer by I.V. infusion over 30 minutes

Some penicillins (eg, carbenicillin, ticarcillin and piperacillin) have been shown to inactivate aminoglycosides *in vitro*. This has been observed to a greater extent with tobramycin and gentamicin, while amikacin has shown greater stability against inactivation. Concurrent use of these agents may pose a risk of reduced antibacterial efficacy *in vivo*, particularly in the setting of profound renal impairment. However, definitive clinical evidence is lacking. If combination penicillin/aminoglycoside therapy is desired in a patient with renal dysfunction, separation of doses (if feasible), and routine monitoring of aminoglycoside levels, CBC, and clinical response should be considered. **Note:** Reformulated Zosyn® containing EDTA has been shown to be compatible *in vitro* for Y-site infusion with amikacin and gentamicin, but not compatible with tobramycin.

Monitoring Parameters Creatinine, BUN, CBC with differential, PT, PTT; signs of bleeding; monitor for signs of anaphylaxis during first dose

Pregnancy Risk Factor B

Contraindications Hypersensitivity to penicillins, beta-lactamase inhibitors, or any component of the formulation

◀ **Warnings/Precautions** Bleeding disorders have been observed, particularly in patients with renal impairment; discontinue if thrombocytopenia or bleeding occurs. Due to sodium load and to the adverse effects of high serum concentrations of penicillins, dosage modification is required in patients with impaired or underdeveloped renal function; use with caution in patients with seizures or in patients with history of beta-lactam allergy; associated with an increased incidence of rash and fever in cystic fibrosis patients. Prolonged use may result in fungal or bacterial superinfection, including *C. difficile*-associated diarrhea (CDAD) and pseudomembranous colitis; CDAD has been observed >2 months postantibiotic treatment. Safety and efficacy have not been established in children <2 months of age.

Adverse Reactions

>10%: Gastrointestinal: Diarrhea (7% to 11%)

>1% to 10%:

Cardiovascular: Hypertension (2%)

Central nervous system: Insomnia (7%), headache (8%), fever (2% to 5%), agitation (2%), pain (2%)

Dermatologic: Rash (4%), pruritus (3%)

Gastrointestinal: Constipation (1% to 8%), nausea (7%), vomiting (3% to 4%), dyspepsia (3%), stool changes (2%), abdominal pain (1% to 2%)

Hepatic: Transaminases increased

Local: Local reaction (3%), abscess (2%)

Respiratory: Pharyngitis (2%)

Miscellaneous: Moniliasis (2%), sepsis (2%), infection (2%)

≤1% (Limited to important and life-threatening): Agranulocytosis, anaphylaxis/anaphylactoid reaction, anemia, anxiety, arrhythmia, arthralgia, atrial fibrillation, back pain, bradycardia, bronchospasm, candidiasis, cardiac arrest, cardiac failure, circulatory failure, chest pain, cholestatic jaundice, confusion, convulsions, coughing, depression, diaphoresis, dizziness, dyspnea, dysuria, edema, epistaxis, erythema multiforme, flatulence, flushing, gastritis, genital pruritus, hallucination, hematuria, hemolytic anemia, hemorrhage, hepatitis, hiccough, hypoglycemia, hypotension, ileus, incontinence, inflammation, injection site reaction, interstitial nephritis, leukorrhea, malaise, mesenteric embolism, myalgia, myocardial infarction, oliguria, pancytopenia, phlebitis, photophobia, pseudomembranous colitis, pulmonary edema, pulmonary embolism, purpura, renal failure, rhinitis, rigors, Stevens-Johnson syndrome, syncope, tachycardia (supraventricular and ventricular), taste perversion, thirst, thrombocytopenia, thrombocytosis, thrombophlebitis, tinnitus, toxic epidermal necrolysis, tremor, ulcerative stomatitis, urinary retention, vaginitis, ventricular fibrillation, vertigo

Drug Interactions

Avoid Concomitant Use There are no known interactions where it is recommended to avoid concomitant use.

Increased Effect/Toxicity

Piperacillin and Tazobactam Sodium may increase the levels/effects of: Methotrexate

The levels/effects of Piperacillin and Tazobactam Sodium may be increased by: Uricosuric Agents

Decreased Effect

Piperacillin and Tazobactam Sodium may decrease the levels/effects of: Aminoglycosides; Mycophenolate; Typhoid Vaccine

The levels/effects of Piperacillin and Tazobactam Sodium may be decreased by: Fusidic Acid; Tetracycline Derivatives

Test Interactions Positive Coombs' [direct] test; false positive reaction for urine glucose using copper-reduction method (Clinitest®); may result in false positive results with the Platelia® *Aspergillus* enzyme immunoassay (EIA)

Some penicillin derivatives may accelerate the degradation of aminoglycosides *in vitro*, leading to a potential underestimation of aminoglycoside serum concentration. **Note:** Reformulated Zosyn® containing EDTA has been shown to be compatible *in vitro* for Y-site infusion with amikacin and gentamicin, but not compatible with tobramycin.

Dietary Considerations

Infusion, premixed: 2.25 g contains sodium 5.58 mEq (128 mg); 3.375 g contains sodium 8.38 mEq (192 mg); 4.5 g contains sodium 11.17 mEq (256 mg)

Injection, powder for reconstitution: 2.25 g contains sodium 5.58 mEq (128 mg); 3.375 g contains sodium 8.38 mEq (192 mg); 4.5 g contains sodium 11.17 mEq (256 mg); 40.5 g contains sodium 100.4 mEq (2304 mg, bulk pharmacy vial)

Dosage Forms Excipient information presented when available (limited, particularly for generics); consult specific product labeling.

Note: 8:1 ratio of piperacillin sodium/tazobactam sodium

Infusion [premixed iso-osmotic solution, frozen]:

2.25 g: Piperacillin 2 g and tazobactam 0.25 g (50 mL) [contains sodium 5.58 mEq (128 mg) and EDTA]

3.375 g: Piperacillin 3 g and tazobactam 0.375 g (50 mL) [contains sodium 8.38 mEq (192 mg) and EDTA]

4.5 g: Piperacillin 4 g and tazobactam 0.5 g (50 mL) [contains sodium 11.17 mEq (256 mg) and EDTA]

Injection, powder for reconstitution:

2.25 g: Piperacillin 2 g and tazobactam 0.25 g [contains sodium 5.58 mEq (128 mg) and EDTA]

3.375 g: Piperacillin 3 g and tazobactam 0.375 g [contains sodium 8.38 mEq (192 mg) and EDTA]

4.5 g: Piperacillin 4 g and tazobactam 0.5 g [contains sodium 11.17 mEq (256 mg) and EDTA]

40.5 g: Piperacillin 36 g and tazobactam 4.5 g [contains sodium 100.4 mEq (2304 mg) and EDTA; bulk pharmacy vial]

References

American Thoracic Society and Infectious Diseases Society of America, "Guidelines for the Management of Adults With Hospital-Acquired, Ventilator-Associated, and Healthcare-Associated Pneumonia," *Am J Respir Crit Care Med*, 2005, 171(4):388-416.

◆ **Piperacillin for Injection, USP (Can)** *see* Piperacillin *on page 1133*

◆ **Piperacillin Sodium** *see* Piperacillin *on page 1133*

◆ **Piperacillin Sodium and Tazobactam Sodium** *see* Piperacillin and Tazobactam Sodium *on page 1136*

Piroxicam (peer OKS i kam)

Related Information

Chronic Pain Management *on page 1546*

Nonsteroidal Anti-Inflammatory Agents *on page 1687*

U.S. Brand Names Feldene®

Canadian Brand Names Apo-Piroxicam®; Dom-Piroxicam; Gen-Piroxicam; Novo-Pirocam; Nu-Pirox; PMS-Piroxicam; Pro-Piroxicam

Pharmacologic Category Nonsteroidal Anti-inflammatory Drug (NSAID), Oral

Use Symptomatic treatment of acute and chronic rheumatoid arthritis and osteoarthritis

Unlabeled/Investigational Use Ankylosing spondylitis

Pharmacodynamics/Kinetics

Onset of action: Analgesic: ~1 hour

Distribution: V_d: 0.14 L/kg

Protein binding: 99%

Metabolism: Hepatic

Half-life elimination: 50 hours

Time to peak: 3-5 hours

Excretion: Primarily urine and feces (small amounts) as unchanged drug (5%) and metabolites

Dosage Oral:

Children (unlabeled use): 0.2-0.3 mg/kg/day once daily; maximum dose: 15 mg/day

Adults: 10-20 mg/day once daily; although associated with increase in GI adverse effects, doses >20 mg/day have been used (ie, 30-40 mg/day)

◀ **Dosing adjustment in renal impairment:** Not recommended in patients with advanced renal disease

Dosing adjustment in hepatic impairment: Reduction of dosage is necessary

Anesthesia and Critical Care Concerns/Other Considerations The 2002 ACCM/SCCM guidelines for analgesia (critically-ill adult) suggest that NSAIDs may be used in combination with opioids in select patients for pain management. Concern about adverse events (increased risk of renal dysfunction, altered platelet function and gastrointestinal irritation) limits its use in patients who have other underlying risks for these events.

In short-term use, NSAIDs vary considerably in their effect on blood pressure. When NSAIDs are used in patients with hypertension, appropriate monitoring of blood pressure responses should be completed and the duration of therapy, when possible, kept short. The use of NSAIDs in the treatment of patients with congestive heart failure may be associated with an increased risk for fluid accumulation and edema; may precipitate renal failure in dehydrated patients.

Additional Information Complete prescribing information for this medication should be consulted for additional detail.

Dosage Forms Excipient information presented when available (limited, particularly for generics); consult specific product labeling.
Capsule: 10 mg, 20 mg

◆ *p*-Isobutylhydratropic Acid *see* Ibuprofen *on page 717*
◆ **Pit** *see* Oxytocin *on page 1077*

Pitavastatin (pi TA va sta tin)

Related Information
    Hyperlipidemia Management *on page 1747*
    Preoperative Evaluation of the Cardiac Patient for Noncardiac Surgery *on page 1598*

U.S. Brand Names Livalo®

Index Terms Pitavastatin Calcium

Pharmacologic Category Antilipemic Agent, HMG-CoA Reductase Inhibitor

Use Adjunct to dietary therapy to reduce elevations in total cholesterol (TC), LDL-C, apolipoprotein B (Apo B), and triglycerides (TG), and to increase low HDL-C in patients with primary hyperlipidemia and mixed dyslipidemia

Pharmacodynamics/Kinetics
    Distribution: V_d: ~148 L
    Protein binding: >99%
    Metabolism: Hepatic, via UGT1A3 and UGT 2B7; minimal metabolism via CYP2C9 and CYP2C8
    Bioavailability: 51%
    Half-life elimination: ~12 hours
    Time to peak, plasma: ~1 hour
    Excretion: Feces (79%); urine (15%)

Dosage Oral: **Note:** Doses should be individualized according to the baseline LDL-cholesterol levels, the recommended goal of therapy, and patient response; adjustments should be made at intervals of 4 weeks.
    Adults: Primary hyperlipidemia and mixed dyslipidemia: Initial: 2 mg once daily; may be increased to maximum 4 mg once daily
    Dosage adjustment with concomitant medications:
    Erythromycin: Pitavastatin dose should not exceed 1 mg once daily
    Rifampin: Pitavastatin dose should not exceed 2 mg once daily

Dosing adjustment in renal impairment:
    Moderate renal impairment (Cl_{cr} 30-60 mL/minute/1.73 m^2) or end-stage renal disease receiving hemodialysis: Initial: 1 mg once daily; do not exceed 2 mg once daily
    Severe renal impairment (Cl_{cr} <30 mL/minute/1.73 m^2) not receiving hemodialysis: Not recommended

Dosing adjustment in hepatic impairment: Contraindicated in active liver disease or in patients with unexplained persistent elevations of serum transaminases

Anesthesia and Critical Care Concerns/Other Considerations
Evidence-Based Information:

Myopathy: Currently-marketed HMG-CoA reductase inhibitors appear to have a similar potential for causing myopathy. Incidence of severe myopathy is about 0.08% to 0.09%. The factors that increase risk include advanced age (especially >80 years), gender (occurs in women more frequently than men), small body frame, frailty, multisystem disease (eg, chronic renal insufficiency especially due to diabetes), multiple medications, and drug interactions (use with caution or avoid).

Perioperative use: Based on current research and clinical guidelines (Fleisher, 2007), HMG-CoA reductase inhibitors should be continued in the perioperative period. Postoperative discontinuation of statin therapy is associated with an increased risk of cardiac morbidity and mortality.

Additional Information Complete prescribing information for this medication should be consulted for additional detail.

Product Availability Livalo®: FDA approved in August 2009; availability anticipated first quarter 2010

Dosage Forms Excipient information presented when available (limited, particularly for generics); consult specific product labeling.
Tablet:
Livalo®: 1 mg, 2 mg, 4 mg

References

American Diabetes Association, "Standards of Medical Care in Diabetes Mellitus – 2009," *Diabetes Care*, 2009, 32(Suppl 1):13-61.

Cannon CP, Braunwald E, McCabe CH, et al, "Intensive Versus Moderate Lipid Lowering With Statins After Acute Coronary Syndromes. Pravastatin or Atorvastatin Evaluation and Infection Therapy-Thrombolysis in Myocardial Infarction 22 Investigators," *N Engl J Med*, 2004, 350(15):1495-504.

de Denus S and Spinler SA, "Early Statin Therapy for Acute Coronary Syndromes," *Ann Pharmacother*, 2002, 36(11):1749-58.

"Executive Summary of The Third Report of The National Cholesterol Education Program (NCEP) Expert Panel on Detection, Evaluation, and Treatment of High Blood Cholesterol in Adults (Adult Treatment Panel III)," *JAMA*, 2001, 285(19):2486-97.

Fleisher LA, Beckman JA, Brown KA, et al, "ACC/AHA 2007 Guidelines on Perioperative Cardiovascular Evaluation and Care for Noncardiac Surgery: A Report of the American College of Cardiology/American Heart Association Task Force on Practice Guidelines (Writing Committee to Revise the 2002 Guidelines on Perioperative Cardiovascular Evaluation for Noncardiac Surgery) Developed in Collaboration With the American Society of Echocardiography, American Society of Nuclear Cardiology, Heart Rhythm Society, Society of Cardiovascular Anesthesiologists, Society for Cardiovascular Angiography and Interventions, Society for Vascular Medicine and Biology, and Society for Vascular Surgery," *J Am Coll Cardiol*, 2007, 50(17):e159-241.

Grundy SM, Cleeman JI, Merz CN, et al, "Implications of Recent Clinical Trials for the National Cholesterol Education Program Adult Treatment Panel III Guidelines," *J Am Coll Cardiol*, 2004, 44 (3):720-32.

Heeschen C, Hamm CW, Laufs U, et al, "Withdrawal of Statins Increases Event Rates in Patients With Acute Coronary Syndromes," *Circulation*, 2002, 105(12):1446-52.

LaRosa JC, Grundy SM, Waters DD, et al, "Intensive Lipid Lowering With Atorvastatin in Patients With Stable Coronary Disease," *N Engl J Med*, 2005, 352(14):1425-35.

LeManach Y, Godet G, Coriat P, et al, "The Impact of Postoperative Discontinuation or Continuation of Chronic Statin Therapy on Cardiac Outcome After Major Vascular Surgery," *Anesth Analg*, 2007, 104(6):1326-33.

"MRC/BHF Heart Protection Study of Cholesterol Lowering With Simvastatin in 20,536 High-Risk Individuals: A Randomised Placebo-Controlled Trial. Heart Protection Study Collaborative Group," *Lancet*, 2002, 360(9326):7-22.

Neuvonen PJ, Niemi M, and Backman JT, "Drug Interactions with Lipid-lowering Drugs: Mechanisms and Clinical Relevance," *Clin Pharmacol Ther*, 2006, 80(6):565-81.

Pasternak RC, Smith SC Jr, Bairey-Merz CN, et al, "ACC/AHA/NHLBI Clinical Advisory on the Use and Safety of Statins," *Stroke*, 2002, 33(9):2337-41. Available at: http://www.acc.org/clinical/alerts/statins_june02.htm. Accessed June 18, 2003.

Poldermans D, Bax JJ, Kertai MD, et al, "Statins Are Associated With a Reduced Incidence of Perioperative Mortality in Patients Undergoing Major Noncardiac Vascular Surgery," *Circulation*, 2003, 107(14):1848-51.

Ridker PM, Danielson E, Fonseca FAH, et al, "Rosuvastatin to Prevent Vascular Events in Men and Women With Elevated C-Reactive Protein," *N Engl J Med*, 2008, 359(21):2195-207.

Sever PS, Dahlof B, Poulter NR, et al, "Prevention of Coronary and Stroke Events With Atorvastatin in Hypertensive Patients Who Have Average or Lower-Than-Average Cholesterol Concentrations, in the Anglo-Scandinavian Cardiac Outcomes Trial - Lipid-Lowering Arm (ASCOT-LLA): A Multicentre Randomised Controlled Trial," *Lancet*, 2003, 361(9364):1149-58.

Shepherd J, Cobbe SM, Ford I, et al, "Prevention of Coronary Heart Disease With Pravastatin in Men With Hypercholesterolemia. West of Scotland Coronary Prevention Study Group," *N Engl J Med*, 1995, 333(20):1301-7.

◀ Smith SC Jr, Allen J, Blair SN, et al, "AHA/ACC Guidelines for Secondary Prevention for Patients With Coronary and Other Atherosclerotic Vascular Disease: 2006 Update: Endorsed by the National Heart, Lung, and Blood Institute," *J Am Coll Cardiol*, 2006, 47(10):2130-9.

- **Pitavastatin Calcium** *see* Pitavastatin *on page 1140*
- **Pitocin®** *see* Oxytocin *on page 1077*
- **Pitressin®** *see* Vasopressin *on page 1458*
- **Plasbumin®** *see* Albumin *on page 46*
- **Plasbumin®-5 (Can)** *see* Albumin *on page 46*
- **Plasbumin®-25 (Can)** *see* Albumin *on page 46*
- **Plavix®** *see* Clopidogrel *on page 333*
- **Pletal®** *see* Cilostazol *on page 303*
- **PMS-Alendronate (Can)** *see* Alendronate *on page 57*
- **PMS-Alendronate-FC (Can)** *see* Alendronate *on page 57*
- **PMS-Amantadine (Can)** *see* Amantadine *on page 77*
- **PMS-Amiodarone (Can)** *see* Amiodarone *on page 86*
- **PMS-Amitriptyline (Can)** *see* Amitriptyline *on page 89*
- **PMS-Amlodipine (Can)** *see* AmLODIPine *on page 93*
- **PMS-Amoxicillin (Can)** *see* Amoxicillin *on page 95*
- **PMS-Atenolol (Can)** *see* Atenolol *on page 155*
- **PMS-Azithromycin (Can)** *see* Azithromycin *on page 169*
- **PMS-Baclofen (Can)** *see* Baclofen *on page 178*
- **PMS-Benzydamine (Can)** *see* Benzydamine *on page 184*
- **PMS-Bisoprolol (Can)** *see* Bisoprolol *on page 192*
- **PMS-Bromocriptine (Can)** *see* Bromocriptine *on page 203*
- **PMS-Bupropion SR (Can)** *see* BuPROPion *on page 217*
- **PMS-Buspirone (Can)** *see* BusPIRone *on page 219*
- **PMS-Butorphanol (Can)** *see* Butorphanol *on page 220*
- **PMS-Captopril (Can)** *see* Captopril *on page 239*
- **PMS-Carbamazepine (Can)** *see* CarBAMazepine *on page 241*
- **PMS-Carvedilol (Can)** *see* Carvedilol *on page 244*
- **PMS-Cetirizine (Can)** *see* Cetirizine *on page 282*
- **PMS-Chloral Hydrate (Can)** *see* Chloral Hydrate *on page 285*
- **PMS-Cilazapril (Can)** *see* Cilazapril *on page 301*
- **PMS-Cimetidine (Can)** *see* Cimetidine *on page 305*
- **PMS-Ciprofloxacin (Can)** *see* Ciprofloxacin *on page 306*
- **PMS-Clarithromycin (Can)** *see* Clarithromycin *on page 317*
- **PMS-Clindamycin (Can)** *see* Clindamycin *on page 324*
- **PMS-Clonazepam (Can)** *see* ClonazePAM *on page 328*
- **PMS-Desipramine (Can)** *see* Desipramine *on page 384*
- **PMS-Desmopressin (Can)** *see* Desmopressin *on page 386*
- **PMS-Dexamethasone (Can)** *see* Dexamethasone *on page 391*
- **PMS-Diclofenac (Can)** *see* Diclofenac *on page 414*
- **PMS-Diclofenac-K (Can)** *see* Diclofenac *on page 414*
- **PMS-Diclofenac SR (Can)** *see* Diclofenac *on page 414*
- **PMS-Diphenhydramine (Can)** *see* DiphenhydrAMINE *on page 430*
- **PMS-Enalapril (Can)** *see* Enalapril *on page 478*
- **PMS-Erythromycin (Can)** *see* Erythromycin *on page 516*
- **PMS-Fenofibrate Micro (Can)** *see* Fenofibrate *on page 582*
- **PMS-Fluconazole (Can)** *see* Fluconazole *on page 607*
- **PMS-Fluoxetine (Can)** *see* FLUoxetine *on page 616*
- **PMS-Fosinopril (Can)** *see* Fosinopril *on page 636*

Polymyxin B (pol i MIKS in bee)

Medication Safety Issues
High alert medication: The Institute for Safe Medication Practices (ISMP) includes this medication (intrathecal administration) among its list of drug classes which have a heightened risk of causing significant patient harm when used in error.

U.S. Brand Names Poly-Rx

Index Terms Polymyxin B Sulfate

Pharmacologic Category Antibiotic, Irrigation; Antibiotic, Miscellaneous

Generic Available Yes

Use Treatment of acute infections caused by susceptible strains of *Pseudomonas aeruginosa*; used occasionally for gut decontamination; parenteral use of polymyxin B has mainly been replaced by less toxic antibiotics, reserved for life-threatening infections caused by organisms resistant to the preferred drugs (eg, pseudomonal meningitis - intrathecal administration)

Mechanism of Action Binds to phospholipids, alters permeability, and damages the bacterial cytoplasmic membrane permitting leakage of intracellular constituents

Pharmacodynamics/Kinetics
Absorption: Well absorbed from peritoneum; minimal from GI tract (except in neonates) from mucous membranes or intact skin. Clinically insignificant amounts are absorbed following irrigation of an intact urinary bladder; systemic absorption may occur from a denuded bladder. Small amounts are systemically absorbed following ophthalmic installation.

Distribution: Minimal into CSF; V_d: 71-194 mL/kg

Protein binding: 79% to 92% (critically ill patients)

Half-life elimination: 6 hours; 2-3 days with anuria

Time to peak, serum: I.M.: ~2 hours

Excretion: Urine (<1% as unchanged drug)

Dosage

Otic (in combination with other drugs): 1-2 drops, 3-4 times/day; should be used sparingly to avoid accumulation of excess debris

Infants <2 years:

I.M.: Up to 40,000 units/kg/day divided every 6 hours (not routinely recommended due to pain at injection sites)

I.V.: Up to 40,000 units/kg/day divided every 12 hours

Intrathecal: 20,000 units/day for 3-4 days, then 25,000 units every other day for at least 2 weeks after CSF cultures are negative and CSF (glucose) has returned to within normal limits

Children ≥2 years and Adults:

I.M.: 25,000-30,000 units/kg/day divided every 4-6 hours (not routinely recommended due to pain at injection sites)

I.V.: 15,000-25,000 units/kg/day divided every 12 hours

Intrathecal: 50,000 units/day for 3-4 days, then every other day for at least 2 weeks after CSF cultures are negative and CSF (glucose) has returned to within normal limits

Total daily dose should not exceed 2,000,000 units/day

Bladder irrigation: Continuous irrigant or rinse in the urinary bladder for up to 10 days using 20 mg (equal to 200,000 units) added to 1 L of normal saline; usually no more than 1 L of irrigant is used per day unless urine flow rate is high; administration rate is adjusted to patient's urine output

Topical irrigation or topical solution: 500,000 units/L of normal saline; topical irrigation should not exceed 2 million units/day in adults

Gut sterilization: Oral: 15,000-25,000 units/kg/day in divided doses every 6 hours

Clostridium difficile enteritis: Oral: 25,000 units every 6 hours for 10 days

Ophthalmic: A concentration of 0.1% to 0.25% is administered as 1-3 drops every hour, then increasing the interval as response indicates to 1-2 drops 4-6 times/day

Dosing adjustment/interval in renal impairment:

Cl_{cr} 20-50 mL/minute: Administer 75% to 100% of the normal daily dose given in divided doses every 12 hours

Cl_{cr} 5-20 mL/minute: Administer 50% of normal daily dose given in divided doses every 12 hours

Cl_{cr} <5 mL/minute: Administer 15% of normal daily dose given in divided doses every 12 hours

Stability Prior to reconstitution, store at room temperature of 15°C to 30°C (59°F to 86°F). Protect from light. After reconstitution, store under refrigeration at 2°C to 8°C (36°F to 46°F). Discard any unused solution after 72 hours.

Administration Dissolve 500,000 units in 300-500 mL D_5W for continuous I.V. drip; dissolve 500,000 units in 2 mL water for injection, saline, or 1% procaine solution for I.M. injection; dissolve 500,000 units in 10 mL physiologic solution for intrathecal administration

Extravasation management: Monitor I.V. site closely; extravasation may cause serious injury with possible necrosis and tissue sloughing. Rotate infusion site frequently.

Monitoring Parameters Neurologic symptoms and signs of superinfection; renal function (decreasing urine output and increasing BUN may require discontinuance of therapy)

Reference Range Serum concentrations >5 mcg/mL are toxic in adults

Pregnancy Risk Factor B

Contraindications Hypersensitivity to polymyxin B or any component of the formulation; concurrent use of neuromuscular blockers

Warnings/Precautions [U.S. Boxed Warning]: May cause neurotoxicity, nephrotoxicity, and/or neuromuscular blockade and respiratory paralysis; usual risk factors include pre-existing renal impairment, concomitant neuro-/nephrotoxic medications, advanced age and dehydration. Use with caution in patients with impaired renal function (modify dosage); polymyxin B-induced nephrotoxicity may be manifested by albuminuria, cellular casts, and azotemia.

◄ Discontinue therapy with decreasing urinary output and increasing BUN; neurotoxic reactions are usually associated with high serum levels, often in patients with renal dysfunction. Avoid concurrent or sequential use of other nephrotoxic and neurotoxic drugs (eg, aminoglycosides). The drug's neurotoxicity can result in respiratory paralysis from neuromuscular blockade, especially when the drug is given soon after anesthesia or muscle relaxants. Polymyxin B sulfate is most toxic when given parenterally; avoid parenteral use whenever possible. Prolonged use may result in fungal or bacterial superinfection, including *C. difficile*-associated diarrhea (CDAD) and pseudomembranous colitis; CDAD has been observed >2 months postantibiotic treatment. **[U.S. Boxed Warnings]: Safety in pregnant women not established; intramuscular/intrathecal administration only to hospitalized patients.**

Adverse Reactions Frequency not defined (limited to important or life-threatening):

Central nervous system: Neurotoxicity (irritability, drowsiness, ataxia, perioral paresthesia, numbness of the extremities, and blurred vision); dizziness

Neuromuscular & skeletal: Neuromuscular blockade

Renal: Nephrotoxicity

Respiratory: Respiratory arrest

Drug Interactions

Avoid Concomitant Use There are no known interactions where it is recommended to avoid concomitant use.

Increased Effect/Toxicity

Polymyxin B may increase the levels/effects of: Colistimethate; Neuromuscular-Blocking Agents

The levels/effects of Polymyxin B may be increased by: Capreomycin

Decreased Effect There are no known significant interactions involving a decrease in effect.

Dosage Forms Excipient information presented when available (limited, particularly for generics); consult specific product labeling.

Injection, powder for reconstitution: 500,000 units

Powder [for prescription compounding]:

Poly-Rx: 100 million units (13 g)

◆ **Polymyxin B Sulfate** *see* Polymyxin B *on page 1144*

◆ **Poly-Rx** *see* Polymyxin B *on page 1144*

◆ **Ponstan® (Can)** *see* Mefenamic Acid *on page 870*

◆ **Ponstel®** *see* Mefenamic Acid *on page 870*

◆ **Pontocaine®** *see* Tetracaine *on page 1367*

◆ **Pontocaine® Niphanoid®** *see* Tetracaine *on page 1367*

Poractant Alfa (por AKT ant AL fa)

U.S. Brand Names Curosurf®

Canadian Brand Names Curosurf®

Pharmacologic Category Lung Surfactant

Generic Available No

Use Treatment of respiratory distress syndrome (RDS) in premature infants

Mechanism of Action Endogenous pulmonary surfactant reduces surface tension at the air-liquid interface of the alveoli during ventilation and stabilizes the alveoli against collapse at resting transpulmonary pressures. A deficiency of pulmonary surfactant in preterm infants results in respiratory distress syndrome characterized by poor lung expansion, inadequate gas exchange, and atelectasis. Poractant alpha compensates for the surfactant deficiency and restores surface activity to the infant's lungs. It reduces mortality and pneumothoraces associated with RDS.

Pharmacodynamics/Kinetics Information limited to animal models. No human pharmacokinetic information is available.

Dosage Intratracheal use **only**: Premature infant with RDS: Initial dose is 2.5 mL/kg of birth weight. Up to 2 subsequent doses of 1.25 mL/kg birth weight can be administered at 12-hour intervals if needed in infants who continue to require mechanical ventilation and supplemental oxygen. Maximum total dose: 5 mL/kg (sum of the initial dose and 2 repeat doses)

Stability Store under refrigeration at defined temperature of 2°C to 8°C (36°F to 46°F). Unopened, unused vials that have been warmed to room temperature can be returned to refrigerator storage within 24 hours for future use. Do not warm and then refrigerate more than once. Vials are for single use only. Protect from light. Do not shake.

Administration Take from refrigerator and warm to room temperature. Inspect for discoloration. The color should be white to creamy white. Gently turn the vial upside down to get a uniform suspension. Do not shake. Slowly withdraw the entire contents into a 3 mL or 5 mL plastic syringe through a large gauge needle (at least 20 gauge). Attach the catheter to the syringe. Fill the catheter with poractant alfa. Discard the excess through the catheter so that only the total dose to be given remains in the syringe.

Before administering, assure proper placement and patency of the endotracheal tube. The endotracheal tube may be suctioned before administering the poractant alpha. The drug is administered intratracheally through a 5-French end-hole catheter cut to a standard length of 8 cm **or** through a secondary lumen of a dual-lumen endotracheal tube (without interrupting mechanical ventilation). Up to 2 repeated doses may be administered, using the same technique at 12-hour intervals.

Administration using a 5-French end-hole catheter: The infant should be stable before proceeding with dosing. The infant's ventilator settings should be changed to a rate of 40-60 breaths/minute, inspiratory time 0.5 seconds, and supplemental oxygen to maintain SaO_2 >92%. Keep the head and body of the infant in alignment without inclination. Briefly disconnect the endotracheal tube from the ventilator, insert the 5-French catheter. This catheter is inserted into the infant's endotracheal tube with the tip positioned distally in the endotracheal tube. The catheter tip should not extend beyond the distal tip of the endotracheal tube. Each dose should be administered in two aliquots with each aliquot administered into one of the two main bronchi by positioning the infant with either the right or left side dependent.

Insert the first aliquot (1.25 mL/kg birth weight) and position the infant so that either the right or left side is dependent for the aliquot. Remove the catheter and manually ventilate the infant with 100% oxygen at a rate of 40-60 breaths/minute for 1 minute. When the infant is stable, reposition the infant such that the other side is dependent and administer the remaining aliquot using the same technique. Remove the catheter without flushing. Do not suction the airways for 1 hour after instillation unless signs of significant airway obstruction occur. Resume ventilator management and clinical care.

Administration using the secondary lumen of a dual-lumen endotracheal tube: Slowly withdraw the entire vial content into a 3 mL or 5 mL plastic syringe through a large gauge needle (at least 20 gauge). Keep infant in neutral position and administer poractant through the proximal end of the secondary lumen of the endotracheal tube as a single dose over 1 minute (without interrupting mechanical ventilation); transient increases in F_1O_2, ventilatory rate, or peak inspiratory pressure (PIP) may be required.

pH: 6.2 (5.5-6.5; adjusted as required with sodium bicarbonate)

Monitoring Parameters Arterial blood gases, ventilator measurement assessment

Contraindications No known contraindications

Warnings/Precautions For intratracheal administration only. Correct acidosis, hypotension, anemia, hypoglycemia, and hypothermia before use. Rapidly affects oxygenation and lung compliance; restrict use to a highly-supervised clinical setting with immediate availability of clinicians experienced in intubation and ventilatory management of premature infants. Transient episodes of bradycardia, decreased oxygen saturation, hypotension, or endotracheal tube blockage may occur. Discontinue dosing procedure and initiate measures to alleviate the condition; may reinstitute after the patient is stable. Pulmonary hemorrhage is a known complication of premature birth and very low birth-weight; has been reported in both clinical trials and postmarketing reports in infants who have received poractant. Produces rapid improvements in lung oxygenation and compliance; may require frequent adjustments to oxygen delivery and ventilator settings.

Adverse Reactions Frequency not defined.

Cardiovascular: Bradycardia, hypotension

Respiratory: Endotracheal tube blockage, oxygen desaturation

Postmarketing and/or case reports: Pulmonary hemorrhage

Drug Interactions

Avoid Concomitant Use There are no known interactions where it is recommended to avoid concomitant use.

Increased Effect/Toxicity There are no known significant interactions involving an increase in effect.

Decreased Effect There are no known significant interactions involving a decrease in effect.

Dosage Forms Excipient information presented when available (limited, particularly for generics); consult specific product labeling.

Suspension, intratracheal [preservative free; porcine derived]:

Curosurf®: 80 mg/mL (1.5 mL, 3 mL)

◆ **Portia™** see Ethinyl Estradiol and Levonorgestrel on page 549

Posaconazole (poe sa KON a zole)

Medication Safety Issues

Sound-alike/look-alike issues:

Noxafil® may be confused with minoxidil

International issues:

Noxafil® may be confused with Noxidil® which is a brand name for minoxidil in Thailand

Related Information

Antifungal Agents on page 1664

U.S. Brand Names Noxafil®

Canadian Brand Names Posanol™

Index Terms SCH 56592

Pharmacologic Category Antifungal Agent, Oral

Generic Available No

Use Prophylaxis of invasive *Aspergillus* and *Candida* infections in severely-immunocompromised patients [eg, hematopoietic stem cell transplant (HSCT) recipients with graft-versus-host disease (GVHD) or those with prolonged neutropenia secondary to chemotherapy for hematologic malignancies]; treatment of oropharyngeal candidiasis (including patients refractory to itraconazole and/or fluconazole)

Unlabeled/Investigational Use Salvage therapy of refractory invasive fungal infections; mucormycosis

Mechanism of Action Interferes with fungal cytochrome P450 (latosterol-14α-demethylase) activity, decreasing ergosterol synthesis (principal sterol in fungal cell membrane) and inhibiting fungal cell membrane formation.

Pharmacodynamics/Kinetics

Absorption: Coadministration with food, liquid nutritional supplements, and/or acidic carbonated beverages (eg, ginger ale) increases absorption; fasting states do not provide sufficient absorption to ensure adequate plasma concentrations.

Distribution: V_d: 465-1774 L

Protein binding: >98%; predominantly bound to albumin

Metabolism: Not significantly metabolized; ~15% to 17% undergoes non-CYP-mediated metabolism, primarily via hepatic glucuronidation into metabolites

Half-life elimination: 35 hours (range: 20-66 hours)

Time to peak, plasma: ~3-5 hours

Excretion: Feces 71% to 77% (~66% of the total dose as unchanged drug); urine 13% to 14% (<0.2% of the total dose as unchanged drug)

Dosage Oral:

Children ≥13 years and Adults:

Aspergillosis, invasive:

Prophylaxis: 200 mg 3 times/day

Salvage treatment of refractory infection (unlabeled use): 200 mg 4 times/day initially; after disease stabilization may decrease frequency to 400 mg twice daily (Walsh, 2007). **Note:** Duration of therapy should be a minimum of 6-12 weeks or throughout period of immunosuppression.

Candidal infections:

Prophylaxis: 200 mg 3 times/day

Treatment of oropharyngeal infection: Initial: 100 mg twice daily for 1 day; maintenance: 100 mg once daily for 13 days

Treatment of refractory oropharyngeal infection: 400 mg twice daily

Adults: **Mucormycosis (unlabeled use):** 800 mg/day in 2 or 4 divided doses (Greenburg, 2006)

Dosage adjustment in renal impairment:

Mild-to-moderate renal insufficiency (Cl_{cr} 20-80 mL/minute): No adjustment necessary

Severe renal insufficiency (Cl_{cr} <20 mL/minute): No adjustment necessary; however, monitor for breakthrough fungal infections due to variability in posaconazole exposure.

Dosage adjustment in hepatic impairment:

Mild-to-severe hepatic insufficiency (Child-Pugh classes A, B, and C): No adjustment necessary

Clinical signs and symptoms of liver disease due to posaconazole: Consider discontinuing therapy

Stability Store at 25°C (77°F); excursions permitted to 15°C to 30°C (59°F to 86°C). Do not freeze.

Administration Oral: Shake well before use. Must be administered during or within 20 minutes following a full meal or an oral liquid nutritional supplement; alternatively, posaconazole may be administered with an acidic carbonated beverage (eg, ginger ale). In patients able to swallow, administer oral suspension using dosing spoon provided by the manufacturer; spoon should be rinsed clean with water after each use and before storage.

Monitoring Parameters Hepatic function (eg, AST/ALT, alkaline phosphatase and bilirubin) prior to initiation and during treatment; renal function; electrolyte disturbances (eg, calcium, magnesium, potassium); CBC

Pregnancy Risk Factor C

Contraindications Hypersensitivity to posaconazole or any component of the formulation; coadministration of cisapride, ergot alkaloids, pimozide, quinidine, or sirolimus

Warnings/Precautions Hepatic dysfunction has occurred, ranging from reversible mild/moderate increases of ALT, AST, alkaline phosphatase, total bilirubin, and/or clinical hepatitis to severe reactions (cholestasis, hepatic failure including death). Consider discontinuation of therapy in patients who develop clinical evidence of liver disease that may be secondary to posaconazole. Use caution in patients with an increased risk of arrhythmia (long QT syndrome, concurrent QT_c-prolonging drugs, hypokalemia). Correct electrolyte abnormalities (eg, potassium, magnesium, and calcium) before initiating therapy. Concurrent use may significantly increase cyclosporine levels and may result in rare serious adverse events (eg, nephrotoxicity, leukoencephalopathy, and death); dose reduction and close monitoring are recommended with initiation of posaconazole therapy.

Use caution in hypersensitivity with other azole antifungal agents; cross-reaction may occur, but has not been established. Consider alternative therapy or closely monitor for breakthrough fungal infections in patients receiving drugs that decrease absorption or increase the metabolism of posaconazole or in any patient unable to eat or tolerate an oral liquid nutritional supplement. Use caution in severe renal impairment or GI disturbances; monitor for breakthrough fungal infections. Safety and efficacy have not been established in children <13 years of age.

Adverse Reactions Note: A higher frequency of adverse reactions was observed in studies with refractory oropharyngeal candidiasis patients and percentages are included below.

>10%: Gastrointestinal: Diarrhea (3% to 11%)

1% to 10%:

Cardiovascular: QT_c prolongation (≤4%), hypertension (≤1%)

Central nervous system: Headache (1% to 8%), dizziness (1% to 3%), fatigue (1% to 3%), insomnia (1% to 3%), fever (≤3%), somnolence (≤1%)

Dermatologic: Rash (1% to 4%), pruritus (1% to 2%)

Endocrine & metabolic: Hypokalemia (≤3%)

Gastrointestinal: Nausea (5% to 8%), vomiting (4% to 7%), abdominal pain (1% to 5%), flatulence (1% to 5%), anorexia (1% to 3%), mucositis (≤2%), dyspepsia (1% to 2%), xerostomia (1% to 2%), constipation (≤1%), taste perversion (≤1%)

Hematologic: Neutropenia (2% to 8%), anemia (≤3%), thrombocytopenia (≤2%)

Hepatic: ALT increased (2% to 17%), AST increased (2% to 17%), alkaline phosphatase increased (1% to 13%), bilirubin increased (2% to 9%), GGT increased (2% to 3%), hepatocellular damage (≤1%)

Neuromuscular & skeletal: Weakness (1% to 3%), myalgia (≤2%), tremor (≤1%)

Ocular: Blurred vision (≤1%)

Renal: Serum creatinine increased (≤2%)

<1% (Limited to important or life-threatening): Adrenal insufficiency, allergic/hypersensitivity reactions, atrial fibrillation, cholestasis, ejection fraction decreased, hemolytic uremic syndrome, hepatic failure, hepatitis, jaundice, pulmonary embolus, syncope, thrombotic thrombocytopenic purpura, torsade de pointes

Drug Interactions

Metabolism/Transport Effects Inhibits CYP3A4 (strong)

Avoid Concomitant Use

Avoid concomitant use of Posaconazole with any of the following: Alfuzosin; Cisapride; Conivaptan; Dofetilide; Dronedarone; Efavirenz; Eplerenone; Ergot Derivatives; Everolimus; Halofantrine; Nilotinib; Nisoldipine; Pimozide; Proton Pump Inhibitors; QuiNIDine; Ranolazine; Rivaroxaban; Salmeterol; Silodosin; Sirolimus; Tolvaptan

Increased Effect/Toxicity

Posaconazole may increase the levels/effects of: Alfentanil; Alfuzosin; Almotriptan; Alosetron; Antineoplastic Agents (Vinca Alkaloids); Aprepitant; Benzodiazepines (metabolized by oxidation); Bosentan; BusPIRone; Busulfan; Calcium Channel Blockers; CarBAMazepine; Cardiac Glycosides; Ciclesonide; Cilostazol; Cinacalcet; Cisapride; Colchicine; Conivaptan; Corticosteroids (Orally Inhaled); Corticosteroids (Systemic); CycloSPORINE; CYP3A4 Substrates; Docetaxel; Dofetilide; Dronedarone; Dutasteride; Eletriptan; Eplerenone; Ergot Derivatives; Erlotinib; Eszopiclone; Everolimus; FentaNYL; Fesoterodine; Fosaprepitant; Gefitinib; Halofantrine; HMG-CoA Reductase Inhibitors; Imatinib; Irinotecan; Ixabepilone; Losartan; Macrolide Antibiotics; Maraviroc; Methadone; Nilotinib; Nisoldipine; Paricalcitol; Phenytoin; Phosphodiesterase 5 Inhibitors; Pimecrolimus; Pimozide; Protease Inhibitors; QuiNIDine; Ramelteon; Ranolazine; Repaglinide; Rifamycin Derivatives; Rivaroxaban; Salmeterol; Saxagliptin; Silodosin; Sirolimus; Solifenacin; Sorafenib; Sunitinib; Tacrolimus; Tadalafil; Temsirolimus; Tolterodine; Tolvaptan; Trimetrexate; Vitamin K Antagonists; Ziprasidone; Zolpidem

The levels/effects of Posaconazole may be increased by: Grapefruit Juice; Macrolide Antibiotics; Protease Inhibitors

Decreased Effect

Posaconazole may decrease the levels/effects of: Amphotericin B; Prasugrel; Saccharomyces boulardii

The levels/effects of Posaconazole may be decreased by: Antacids; Didanosine; Efavirenz; H2-Antagonists; Metoclopramide; Phenytoin; Proton Pump Inhibitors; Rifamycin Derivatives; Sucralfate

Ethanol/Nutrition/Herb Interactions Food: Bioavailability increased ~3 times when posaconazole is administered with a nonfat meal or an oral liquid nutritional supplement; increased ~4 times when administered with a high-fat meal.

Grapefruit juice may decrease the levels/effects of posaconazole; concurrent use should be avoided.

Dietary Considerations Give during or within 20 minutes following a full meal or liquid nutritional supplement; alternatively, posaconazole may be administered with an acidic carbonated beverage (eg, ginger ale). Consider alternative antifungal therapy in patients with inadequate oral intake or severe diarrhea/ vomiting; if alternative therapy is not an option, closely monitoring for breakthrough fungal infections. Adequate posaconazole absorption from GI tract and subsequent plasma concentrations are dependent on food for efficacy. Lower average plasma concentrations have been associated with an increased risk of treatment failure.

Dosage Forms Excipient information presented when available (limited, particularly for generics); consult specific product labeling.

Suspension, oral:

Noxafil®: 40 mg/mL (123 mL) [contains sodium benzoate; delivers 105 mL of suspension; cherry flavor; packaged with calibrated dosing spoon]

References

Herbrecht R, "Posaconazole: A Potent, Extended-Spectrum Triazole Anti-Fungal for the Treatment of Serious Fungal Infections," *Int J Clin Pract*, 2004, 58(6): 612-24.

Keating G, "Posaconazole," *Drugs*, 2005, 65(11):1553-67.

Raad II, Graybill JR, Bustamante AB, "Safety of Long-Term Oral Posaconazole Use in the Treatment of Refractory Invasive Fungal Infections," *Clin Infect Dis*, 2006, 42(12):1726-34.

♦ **Posanol™ (Can)** *see* Posaconazole *on page 1148*

♦ **Post Peel Healing Balm [OTC]** *see* Hydrocortisone *on page 699*

Potassium Chloride (poe TASS ee um KLOR ide)

Medication Safety Issues

Sound-alike/look-alike issues:

Kaon-Cl-10® may be confused with kaolin

KCl may be confused with HCl

K-Lor® may be confused with Klor-Con®

Klor-Con® may be confused with Klaron®, K-Lor®

microK® may be confused with Macrobid®, Micronase®

High alert medication: The Institute for Safe Medication Practices (ISMP) includes this medication (I.V. formulation) among its list of drugs which have a heightened risk of causing significant patient harm when used in error.

Per JCAHO recommendations, concentrated electrolyte solutions should not be available in patient care areas.

Consider special storage requirements for intravenous potassium salts; I.V. potassium salts have been administered IVP in error, leading to fatal outcomes.

U.S. Brand Names K-Lor®; K-Tab®; Kaon-Cl-10®; Kay Ciel® [DSC]; Klor-Con®; Klor-Con® 10; Klor-Con® 8; Klor-Con® M; Klor-Con®/25; microK®; microK® 10

Canadian Brand Names Apo-K®; K-10®; K-Dur®; K-Lor®; K-Lyte®/Cl; Micro-K Extencaps®; Roychlor®; Slo-Pot; Slow-K®

Index Terms KCl; Kdur

Pharmacologic Category Electrolyte Supplement, Oral; Electrolyte Supplement, Parenteral

Generic Available Yes

Use Treatment or prevention of hypokalemia

Mechanism of Action Potassium is the major cation of intracellular fluid and is essential for the conduction of nerve impulses in heart, brain, and skeletal muscle; contraction of cardiac, skeletal and smooth muscles; maintenance of normal renal function, acid-base balance, carbohydrate metabolism, and gastric secretion

Pharmacodynamics/Kinetics

Absorption: Well absorbed from upper GI tract

Distribution: Enters cells via active transport from extracellular fluid

Excretion: Primarily urine; skin and feces (small amounts); most intestinal potassium reabsorbed

◀ **Dosage** I.V. doses should be incorporated into the patient's maintenance I.V. fluids; intermittent I.V. potassium administration should be reserved for severe depletion situations in patients undergoing ECG monitoring. Doses expressed as mEq of potassium.

Normal daily requirements: Oral, I.V.:
  Children: 1-2 mEq/kg/day
  Adults: 40-80 mEq/day
Prevention of hypokalemia: Oral:
  Children: 1-2 mEq/kg/day in 1-2 divided doses
  Adults: 20-40 mEq/day in 1-2 divided doses
Treatment of hypokalemia: Children:
  Oral: 1-2 mEq/kg initially, then as needed based on frequently obtained lab values. If deficits are severe or ongoing losses are great, I.V. route should be considered.
  I.V. intermittent infusion: 0.5-1 mEq/kg/dose (maximum dose: 40 mEq). If infusion exceeds 0.5 mEq/kg/hour, physician should be at bedside and patient should have continuous ECG monitoring; repeat as needed based on frequently obtained lab values.
Treatment of hypokalemia: Adults:
  Oral:
    Asymptomatic, mild hypokalemia: Usual dosage range: 40-100 mEq/day divided in 2-5 doses; generally recommended to limit doses to 20-25 mEq/dose to avoid GI discomfort.
    Mild-to-moderate hypokalemia: Some clinicians may administer up to 120-240 mEq/day divided in 3-4 doses; limit doses to 40-60 mEq/dose. If deficits are severe or ongoing losses are great, I.V. route should be considered.
  I.V. intermittent infusion: Peripheral or central line: ≤10 mEq/hour; repeat as needed based on frequently obtained lab values; central line infusion and continuous ECG monitoring highly recommended for infusions >10 mEq/hour.
    Potassium dosage/rate of infusion general guidelines (per product labeling):
    Note: High variability exists in dosing/infusion rate recommendations; therapy guided by patient condition and specific institutional guidelines.
    Serum potassium >2.5 mEq/L: Maximum infusion rate: 10 mEq/hour; maximum concentration: 40 mEq/L; maximum 24-hour dose: 200 mEq
    Serum potassium <2 mEq/L and symptomatic (excluding emergency treatment of cardiac arrest): Maximum infusion rate (central line only): 40 mEq/hour in presence of continuous ECG monitoring and frequent lab monitoring; In selected situations, patients may require up to 400 mEq/24 hours.

Stability
Capsule: MicroK®: Store between 20°C to 25°C (68°F to 77°F).
Powder for oral solution: Klor-Con®: Store at room temperature of 15°C to 30°C (59°F to 86°F).
Solution for injection: Store at room temperature; do not freeze. Use only clear solutions. Use admixtures within 24 hours.
Tablet: K-Tab®: Store below 30°C (86°F).

Administration
Parenteral: Potassium must be diluted prior to parenteral administration. Do not administer I.V. push. In general, the dose, concentration of infusion and rate of administration may be dependant on patient condition and specific institution policy. Some clinicians recommend that the maximum concentration for peripheral infusion is 10 mEq/100 mL and maximum rate of administration for peripheral infusion is 10 mEq/hour. ECG monitoring is recommended for peripheral or central infusions >10 mEq/hour in adults. Concentrations and rates of infusion may be greater with central line administration. Some clinicians recommend that the maximum concentration for central infusion is 20-40 mEq/100 mL and maximum rate of administration for central infusion is 40 mEq/hour.
Oral: Oral dosage forms should be taken with meals and a full glass of water or other liquid.
  Capsule: MicroK®: Swallow whole, do not chew. Capsules may also be opened and contents sprinkled on a spoonful of applesauce or pudding and should be swallowed immediately without chewing. No more than 20 mEq should be given as a single dose.

Powder: Klor-Con®: Dissolve in 4-5 ounces of water or other beverage prior to administration.

Tablet: K-Tab®, Kaon-Cl®, Klor-Con®: Swallow tablets whole; do not crush, chew or suck on tablet. No more than 20 mEq should be given as a single dose.

Klor-Con® M: Tablet may also be broken in half and each half swallowed separately; the whole tablet may be dissolved in ~4 ounces of water (allow ~2 minutes to dissolve, stir well and drink immediately)

Monitoring Parameters Serum potassium, glucose, chloride, pH, urine output (if indicated), cardiac monitor (if intermittent infusion or potassium infusion rates 0.5 mEq/kg/hour in children or >10 mEq/hour in adults)

Pregnancy Risk Factor C

Contraindications Hypersensitivity to any component of the formulation; hyperkalemia. In addition, solid oral dosage forms are contraindicated in patients in whom there is a structural, pathological, and/or pharmacologic cause for delay or arrest in passage through the GI tract.

Warnings/Precautions Close monitoring of serum potassium concentrations is needed to avoid hyperkalemia. Use with caution in patients with renal impairment, cardiac disease, acid/base disorders, or potassium-altering conditions/disorders. Use with caution in digitalized patients or patients receiving concomitant medications or therapies that increase potassium (eg, ACEI, potassium-sparing diuretics, potassium containing salt substitutes). Do **NOT** administer undiluted or I.V. push; inappropriate parenteral administration may be fatal. Always administer potassium further diluted; refer to appropriate dilution and administration rate recommendations. Pain and phlebitis may occur during parenteral infusion requiring a decrease in infusion rate or potassium concentration. Avoid administering potassium diluted in dextrose solutions during initial therapy; potential for transient decreases in serum potassium due to intracellular shift of potassium from dextrose-stimulated insulin release. May cause GI upset (eg, nausea, vomiting, diarrhea, abdominal pain, discomfort) and lead to GI ulceration, bleeding, perforation and/or obstruction. Oral liquid preparations (not solid) should be used in patients with esophageal compression or delayed gastric emptying.

Adverse Reactions Frequency not defined.

Dermatologic: Rash

Endocrine & metabolic: Hyperkalemia

Gastrointestinal: Abdominal pain/discomfort, diarrhea, flatulence, GI bleeding (oral), GI obstruction (oral), GI perforation (oral), nausea, vomiting

Drug Interactions

Avoid Concomitant Use There are no known interactions where it is recommended to avoid concomitant use.

Increased Effect/Toxicity

Potassium Chloride may increase the levels/effects of: ACE Inhibitors; Angiotensin II Receptor Blockers; Potassium-Sparing Diuretics

The levels/effects of Potassium Chloride may be increased by: Anticholinergic Agents; Eplerenone

Decreased Effect There are no known significant interactions involving a decrease in effect.

Dietary Considerations Administer with plenty of fluid to decrease stomach irritation and discomfort. Some dietary sources of potassium include leafy green vegetables (eg, spinach, cabbage), tomatoes, cucumbers, zucchini, fruits (eg, apples, oranges, and bananas), root vegetables (eg, carrots, radishes), beans, and peas.

Dosage Forms Excipient information presented when available (limited, particularly for generics); consult specific product labeling. [DSC] = Discontinued product

Capsule, extended release, microencapsulated: 8 mEq [600 mg]; 10 mEq [750 mg]

microK®: 8 mEq [600 mg]

microK® 10: 10 mEq [750 mg]

Infusion [premixed in D_5W]: 20 mEq (1000 mL); 30 mEq (1000 mL); 40 mEq (1000 mL)

Infusion [premixed in D_5W and LR]: 20 mEq (1000 mL); 30 mEq (1000 mL); 40 mEq (1000 mL)

◀ Infusion [premixed in D_5W and sodium chloride 0.2%]: 5 mEq (250 mL); 10 mEq (500 mL, 1000 mL); 20 mEq (1000 mL); 30 mEq (1000 mL); 40 mEq (1000 mL)

Infusion [premixed in D_5W and sodium chloride 0.225%]: 10 mEq (500 mL, 1000 mL); 20 mEq (1000 mL); 30 mEq (1000 mL); 40 mEq (1000 mL)

Infusion [premixed in D_5W and sodium chloride 0.3%]: 10 mEq (500 mL); 20 mEq (1000 mL)

Infusion [premixed in D_5W and sodium chloride 0.33%]: 10 mEq (500 mL); 20 mEq (1000 mL)

Infusion [premixed in D_5W and sodium chloride 0.45%]: 10 mEq (500 mL, 1000 mL); 20 mEq (1000 mL); 30 mEq (1000 mL); 40 mEq (1000 mL)

Infusion [premixed in D_5W and NS]: 20 mEq (1000 mL); 40 mEq (1000 mL)

Infusion [premixed in $D_{10}W$ and sodium chloride 0.2%]: 5 mEq (250 mL)

Infusion [premixed in sodium chloride 0.45%]: 20 mEq (1000 mL); 40 mEq (1000 mL)

Infusion [premixed in NS]: 20 mEq (1000 mL); 40 mEq (1000 mL)

Infusion [premixed in SWFI; highly concentrated]: 10 mEq (50 mL, 100 mL); 20 mEq (50 mL, 100 mL); 30 mEq (100 mL); 40 mEq (100 mL)

Injection, solution [concentrate]: 2 mEq/mL (5 mL, 10 mL, 15 mL, 20 mL, 30 mL, 250 mL, 500 mL)

Powder, for oral solution: 20 mEq/packet (30s, 100s, 1000s)

K-Lor®: 20 mEq/packet (30s, 100s) [fruit flavor]

Kay Ciel® 10%: 20 mEq/packet (30s, 100s) [sugar free] [DSC]

Klor-Con®: 20 mEq/packet (30s, 100s) [sugar free; fruit flavor]

Klor-Con®/25: 25 mEq/packet (30s, 100s) [sugar free; fruit flavor]

Solution, oral: 20 mEq/15 mL (15 mL, 30 mL, 480 mL, 3840 mL); 40 mEq/15 mL (15 mL, 480 mL)

Tablet, extended release: 8 mEq [600 mg]; 10 mEq [750 mg]; 20 mEq [1500 mg]

K-Tab®: 10 mEq [750 mg]

Kaon-Cl® 10: 10 mEq [750 mg]

Tablet, extended release, microencapsulated: 10 mEq, 20 mEq

Klor-Con® M10: 10 mEq [750 mg]

Klor-Con® M15: 15 mEq [1125 mg; scored]

Klor-Con® M20: 20 mEq [1500 mg; scored]

Tablet, extended release, wax matrix: 8 mEq, 10 mEq

Klor-Con® 8: 8 mEq [600 mg]

Clor-Con® 10: 10 mEq [750 mg]

References

Alfonzo AV, Isles C, Geddes C, et al, "Potassium Disorders - Clinical Spectrum and Emergency Management," *Resuscitation*, 2006, 70(1):10-25.

ASPEN Board of Directors and the Clinical Guidelines Task Force, "Guidelines for the Use of Parenteral and Enteral Nutrition in Adult and Pediatric Patients," *JPEN J Parenter Enteral Nutr*, 2002, 26(1 Suppl):22-4.

ASPEN Board of Directors and the Clinical Guidelines Task Force, "Guidelines for the Use of Parenteral and Enteral Nutrition in Adult and Pediatric Patients," *JPEN J Parenter Enteral Nutr*, 2002, 26(1 Suppl):25-32.

"Dietary Reference Intakes for Water, Potassium, Sodium, Chloride, and Sulfate. Standing Committee on the Scientific Evaluation of Dietary Reference Intakes, Food and Nutrition Board, Institute of Medicine," National Academy of Sciences, Washington, DC: National Academy Press, 2004. Available at http://www.nap.edu.

Hamill RJ, Robinson LM, Wexler HR, et al, "Efficacy and Safety of Potassium Infusion Therapy in Hypokalemic Critically Ill Patients," *Crit Care Med*, 1991, 19(5):694-9.

Khilnani P, "Electrolyte Abnormalities in Critically Ill Children," *Crit Care Med*, 1992, 20(2):241-50.

Joint Commission on Accreditation of Healthcare Organizations, "2005 National Patient Safety Goals," available at http://www.jcaho.org/accredited+organizations/patient+safety/05_npsg_guidelines Last accessed October 15, 2004.

Weiss-Guillet EM, Takala J, and Jakob SM, "Diagnosis and Management of Electrolyte Emergencies," *Best Pract Res Clin Endocrinol Metab*, 2003, 17(4):623-51.

Potassium Phosphate (poe TASS ee um FOS fate)

Medication Safety Issues

Sound-alike/look-alike issues:

Neutra-Phos®-K may be confused with K-Phos Neutral®

High alert medication: The Institute for Safe Medication Practices (ISMP) includes this medication (I.V. formulation) among its list of drugs which have a heightened risk of causing significant patient harm when used in error.

Per JCAHO recommendations, concentrated electrolyte solutions should not be available in patient care areas.

Consider special storage requirements for intravenous potassium salts; I.V. potassium salts have been administered IVP in error, leading to fatal outcomes.

Safe Prescribing: Because inorganic phosphate exists as monobasic and dibasic anions, with the mixture of valences dependent on pH, ordering by mEq amounts is unreliable and may lead to large dosing errors. In addition, I.V. phosphate is available in the sodium and potassium salt; therefore, the content of these cations must be considered when ordering phosphate. The most reliable method of ordering I.V. phosphate is by millimoles, then specifying the potassium or sodium salt. For example, an order for 15 mmol of phosphate as potassium phosphate in one liter of normal saline.

U.S. Brand Names Neutra-Phos®-K [OTC] [DSC]

Index Terms Phosphate, Potassium

Pharmacologic Category Electrolyte Supplement, Oral; Electrolyte Supplement, Parenteral

Generic Available Yes: Injection

Use Treatment and prevention of hypophosphatemia; **Note:** The concomitant amount of potassium must be calculated into the total electrolyte content. For each 1 mmol of phosphate, ~1.5 mEq of potassium will be administered. Therefore, if ordering 30 mmol of potassium phosphate, the patient will receive ~45 mEq of potassium.

Dosage

Oral:

Normal Requirements Elemental Phosphorus:

0-6 months: 100 mg

7-12 months: 275 mg

1-3 years: 460 mg

4-8 years: 500 mg

9-18 years: 1250 mg

Adults: 700 mg

Oral maintenance:

Children <4 years: 250 mg phosphorus/8 mmol 4 times/day; dilute as instructed

Children >4 years and Adults: 250-500 mg phosphorus/8-16 mmol 4 times/day; dilute as instructed

I.V.: **Caution: The concomitant amount of potassium must be calculated into the total electrolyte content. For each 1 mmol of phosphate, ~1.5 mEq of potassium will be administered. Therefore, if ordering 30 mmol of potassium phosphate, the patient will receive ~45 mEq of potassium. With orders for I.V. phosphate, there is considerable confusion associated with the use of millimoles (mmol) versus milliequivalents (mEq) to express the phosphate requirement.** The most reliable method of ordering I.V. phosphate is by millimoles, then specifying the potassium or sodium salt. Doses listed as mmol of phosphate.

Acute treatment of hypophosphatemia: It is recommended that repletion of severe hypophosphatemia be done I.V. because large doses of oral phosphate may cause diarrhea and intestinal absorption may be unreliable. Intermittent I.V. infusion should be reserved for severe depletion situations; requires continuous cardiac monitoring. Guidelines differ based on degree of illness, need/use of TPN, and severity of hypophosphatemia. If potassium >4.0 mEq/L consider phosphate replacement strategy without potassium (eg, sodium phosphates). Obese patients and/or severe renal impairment were excluded from phosphate supplement trials. **Note:** 1 mmol phosphate = 31 mg phosphorus; 1 mg phosphorus = 0.032 mmol phosphate.

Children and Adults: **Note:** There are no prospective studies of parenteral phosphate replacement in children. The following weight-based guidelines for adult dosing may be cautiously employed in pediatric patients.

◀ **General replacement guidelines** (Lentz, 1978):

Low dose: 0.08 mmol/kg over 6 hours; use if losses are recent and uncomplicated

Intermediate dose: 0.16-0.24 mmol/kg over 4-6 hours; use if serum phosphorus level 0.5-1 mg/dL (0.16-0.32 mmol/L)

Note: The initial dose may be increased by 25% to 50% if the patient is symptomatic secondary to hypophosphatemia and lowered by 25% to 50% if the patient is hypercalcemic.

Critically-ill adult trauma patients receiving concurrent TPN (Brown, 2006):

Low dose: 0.32 mmol/kg over 4-6 hours; use if serum phosphorus level 2.3-3 mg/dL (0.73-0.96 mmol/L)

Intermediate dose: 0.64 mmol/kg over 4-6 hours; use if serum phosphorus level 1.6-2.2 mg/dL (0.51-0.72 mmol/L)

High dose: 1 mmol/kg over 8-12 hours; use if serum phosphorus <1.5 mg/dL (<0.5 mmol/L)

Parenteral nutrition: Adults: 10-15 mmol/1000 kcal (Hicks, 2001) **or** 20-40 mmol/24 hours (Mirtallo, 2004 [ASPEN guidelines])

Stability Store at room temperature; do not freeze. Use only clear solutions. Up to 10-15 mEq of calcium may be added per liter before precipitate may occur.

Stability of parenteral admixture at room temperature (25°C) is 24 hours.

Phosphate salts may precipitate when mixed with calcium salts. Solubility is improved in amino acid parenteral nutrition solutions. Check with a pharmacist to determine compatibility.

Administration Injection must be diluted in appropriate I.V. solution and volume prior to administration and administered over a minimum of 4 hours

Monitoring Parameters Serum potassium, calcium, phosphate, magnesium; cardiac monitor (when intermittent infusion or high-dose I.V. replacement needed); after I.V. phosphate repletion, repeat serum phosphate level should be checked 2-4 hours later

Pregnancy Risk Factor C

Contraindications Hyperphosphatemia, hyperkalemia, hypocalcemia, hypomagnesemia, renal failure (oral product)

Warnings/Precautions Close monitoring of serum potassium concentrations is needed to avoid hyperkalemia. Use with caution in patients with renal insufficiency, cardiac disease, metabolic alkalosis. Use with caution in digitalized patients and patients receiving concomitant potassium-altering therapies. Oral formulations may cause GI upset. Admixture of phosphate and calcium in I.V. fluids can result in calcium phosphate precipitation. Use extreme caution when administering potassium phosphate parenterally. Parenteral potassium may cause pain and phlebitis, requiring a decrease in infusion rate or potassium concentration. Solutions for injection may contain aluminum; toxic levels may occur following prolonged administration in premature neonates or patients with renal impairment.

Adverse Reactions Frequency not defined.

Cardiovascular: Arrhythmia, bradycardia, chest pain, ECG changes, edema, heart block, hypotension

Central nervous system: Listlessness, mental confusion, tetany (with large doses of phosphate)

Endocrine & metabolic: Hyperkalemia

Gastrointestinal: Diarrhea, flatulence, nausea, stomach pain, vomiting

Genitourinary: Urine output decreased

Local: Phlebitis

Neuromuscular & skeletal: Paralysis, paresthesia, weakness

Renal: Acute renal failure

Respiratory: Dyspnea

Drug Interactions

Avoid Concomitant Use There are no known interactions where it is recommended to avoid concomitant use.

Increased Effect/Toxicity

Potassium Phosphate may increase the levels/effects of: ACE Inhibitors; Angiotensin II Receptor Blockers; Potassium-Sparing Diuretics

The levels/effects of Potassium Phosphate may be increased by: Bisphosphonate Derivatives; Eplerenone

Decreased Effect

The levels/effects of Potassium Phosphate may be decreased by: Antacids; Calcium Salts; Iron Salts; Magnesium Salts; Sucralfate

Ethanol/Nutrition/Herb Interactions Food: Avoid administering with oxalate (berries, nuts, chocolate, beans, celery, tomato) or phytate-containing foods (bran, whole wheat).

Dosage Forms Excipient information presented when available (limited, particularly for generics); consult specific product labeling. [DSC] = Discontinued product

Injection, solution: Potassium 4.4 mEq and phosphorus 3 mmol per mL (5 mL, 15 mL, 50 mL) [equivalent to potassium 170 mg and elemental phosphorus 93 mg per mL]

Powder for oral solution:

Neutra-Phos®-K: Monobasic potassium phosphate and dibasic potassium phosphate per packet (100s) [equivalent to elemental potassium 556 mg (14.25 mEq) and phosphorus 250 mg (14.25 mEq) per packet; sodium and sugar free; fruit flavor] [DSC]

References

Brown KA, Dickerson RN, Morgan LM, et al, "A New Graduated Dosing Regimen for Phosphorus Replacement in Patients Receiving Nutrition Support," *JPEN J Parenter Enteral Nutr*, 2006, 30 (3):209-14.

Charron T, Bernard F, Skrobik Y, et al, "Intravenous Phosphate in the Intensive Care Unit: More Aggressive Repletion Regimens for Moderate and Severe Hypophosphatemia," *Intensive Care Med*, 2003, 29(8):1273-8.

Clark CL, Sacks GS, Dickerson RN, et al, "Treatment of Hypophosphatemia in Patients Receiving Specialized Nutrition Support Using a Graduated Dosing Scheme: Results From a Prospective Clinical Trial," *Crit Care Med*, 1995, 23(9):1504-1.

Joint Commission on Accreditation of Healthcare Organizations, "2005 National Patient Safety Goals," available at http://www.jcaho.org/accredited+organizations/patient+safety/05_npsg_guidelines Last accessed October 15, 2004.

Lentz RD, Brown DM, and Kjellstrand CM, "Treatment of Severe Hypophosphatemia," *Ann Intern Med*, 1978, 89(6):941-4.

Perreault MM, Ostrop NJ, and Tierney MG, "Efficacy and Safety of Intravenous Phosphate Replacement in Critically Ill Patients," *Ann Pharmacother*, 1997, 31(6):683-8.

Rosen GH, Boullata JI, O'Rangers EA, et al, "Intravenous Phosphate Repletion Regimen for Critically Ill Patients With Moderate Hypophosphatemia," *Crit Care Med*, 1995, 23(7):1204-10.

Vannatta JB, Whang R, and Papper S, "Efficacy of Intravenous Phosphorus Therapy in the Severely Hypophosphatemic Patient," *Arch Intern Med*, 1981, 141(7):885-7.

Pralidoxime (pra li DOKS eem)

Medication Safety Issues

Sound-alike/look-alike issues:

Pralidoxime may be confused with pramoxine, pyridoxine

Protopam® may be confused with protamine, Protropin®

U.S. Brand Names Protopam®

Canadian Brand Names Protopam®

Index Terms 2-PAM; 2-Pyridine Aldoxime Methochloride; Pralidoxime Chloride

Pharmacologic Category Antidote

Generic Available No

Use Reverse muscle paralysis caused by toxic exposure to organophosphate acetylcholinesterase-inhibiting pesticides and chemicals; control of overdose of acetylcholinesterase medications used to treat myasthenia gravis (ambenonium, neostigmine, pyridostigmine)

Unlabeled/Investigational Use Treatment of nerve agent toxicity (chemical warfare) in combination with atropine

Mechanism of Action Reactivates cholinesterase that had been inactivated by phosphorylation due to exposure to organophosphate pesticides by displacing the enzyme from its receptor sites; removes the phosphoryl group from the active site of the inactivated enzyme

Pharmacodynamics/Kinetics

Protein binding: None

Metabolism: Hepatic

Half-life elimination: 74-77 minutes

◀ Time to peak, serum: I.V.: 5-15 minutes

Excretion: Urine (80% to 90% as metabolites and unchanged drug)

Dosage

Organic phosphorus poisoning (use in conjunction with atropine; atropine effects should be established before pralidoxime is administered): I.V. (may be given I.M. or SubQ if I.V. is not feasible):

Children: 20-50 mg/kg/dose; repeat in 1-2 hours if muscle weakness has not been relieved, then at 8- to 12-hour intervals if cholinergic signs recur

Adults: Initial: 30 mg/kg over 20 minutes, maintenance: I.V. infusion: 4-8 mg/kg/hour

Treatment of acetylcholinesterase inhibitor toxicity: Adults: I.V.: Initial: 1-2 g followed by increments of 250 mg every 5 minutes until response is observed

Nerve agent toxicity management (unlabeled use): **Note:** Atropine is a component of the management of nerve agent toxicity; consult atropine monograph for specific route and dose. To be effective, pralidoxime must be administered within minutes to a few hours following exposure (depending on the nerve agent).

Infants and Children:

Prehospital ("in the field"): Mild-to-moderate symptoms: I.M.: 15 mg/kg; severe symptoms: 25 mg/kg

Hospital/emergency department: Mild-to-severe symptoms: I.V.: 15 mg/kg (up to 1 g)

Adults:

Prehospital ("in the field"): Mild-to-moderate symptoms: I.M.: 600 mg; severe symptoms: 1800 mg

Hospital/emergency department: Mild-to-severe symptoms: I.V.: 15 mg/kg (up to 1 g)

Frail patients, elderly:

Prehospital ("in the field"): Mild-to-moderate symptoms: I.M.: 10 mg/kg; severe symptoms: 25 mg/kg

Hospital/emergency department: Mild-to-severe symptoms: I.V.: 5-10 mg/kg

Elderly: Refer to adult dosing; dosing should be cautious, considering possibility of decreased hepatic, renal, or cardiac function

Dosing adjustment in renal impairment: Dose should be reduced

Stability Store at controlled room temperature of 20°C to 25°C (68°F to 77°F). For I.V. administration, dilute 1 g with 20 mL SWI. Solution should be further diluted and administered as 1-2 g in 100 mL NS. If not practical or in cases of fluid overload, may prepare as a 5% solution.

Administration I.V.: Infuse over 15-30 minutes at a rate not to exceed 200 mg/minute; may administer I.M. or SubQ if I.V. is not accessible. If a more concentrated 5% solution is used, infuse over at least 5 minutes.

Monitoring Parameters Heart rate, respiratory rate, blood pressure, continuous ECG; cardiac monitor and blood pressure monitor required for I.V. administration

Reference Range Minimum therapeutic concentration: 4 mcg/mL

Anesthesia and Critical Care Concerns/Other Considerations

Clinical Pearls/Comments: Use I.V. phentolamine for treatment of pralidoxime-induced hypertension (children: 1 mg; adults: 5 mg).

Pregnancy Risk Factor C

Contraindications Hypersensitivity to pralidoxime or any component of the formulation; poisonings due to phosphorus, inorganic phosphates, or organic phosphates without anticholinesterase activity; poisonings due to pesticides of carbamate class (may increase toxicity of carbaryl)

Warnings/Precautions Use with caution in patients with myasthenia gravis; dosage modification required in patients with impaired renal function. Clinical symptoms consistent with highly-suspected organophosphorous poisoning should be treated with antidote immediately; administration should not be delayed for confirmatory laboratory tests. Treatment should always include proper evacuation and decontamination procedures; medical personnel should protect themselves from inadvertent contamination. Antidotal administration is intended only for initial management; definitive and more extensive medical care is required following administration. Individuals should not rely solely on antidote for treatment, as other supportive measures (eg, artificial respiration) may still be required.

Adverse Reactions Frequency not defined.
Cardiovascular: Hypertension, tachycardia
Central nervous system: Dizziness, drowsiness, headache
Dermatologic: Rash
Gastrointestinal: Nausea
Hepatic: ALT increased (transient), AST increased (transient)
Local: Pain at injection site after I.M. administration
Neuromuscular & skeletal: Muscle rigidity, weakness
Ocular: Accommodation impaired, blurred vision, diplopia
Renal: Renal function decreased
Respiratory: Hyperventilation, laryngospasm

Drug Interactions

Avoid Concomitant Use There are no known interactions where it is recommended to avoid concomitant use.

Increased Effect/Toxicity There are no known significant interactions involving an increase in effect.

Decreased Effect There are no known significant interactions involving a decrease in effect.

Dosage Forms Excipient information presented when available (limited, particularly for generics); consult specific product labeling.
Injection, powder for reconstitution, as chloride:
Protopam®: 1 g
Injection, solution: 300 mg/mL (2 mL) [contains benzyl alcohol; prefilled auto injector]

References

"Medical Management Guidelines (MMGs) for Nerve Agents: Tabun (GA); Sarin (GB); Soman (GD); and VX," available at www.atsdr.cdc.gov/MHMI/mmg166.html.
Mokhlesi B, Leikin JB, Murray P, et al, "Adult Toxicology in Critical Care: Part II: Specific Poisonings," *Chest*, 2003, 123(3):897-922.

◆ **Pralidoxime Chloride** *see* Pralidoxime *on page 1157*

Pramipexole (pra mi PEKS ole)

U.S. Brand Names Mirapex®
Canadian Brand Names Apo-Pramipexole; CO Pramipexole; Mirapex®; Novo-Pramipexole; PMS-Pramipexole; SANDOZ-Pramipexole
Pharmacologic Category Anti-Parkinson's Agent, Dopamine Agonist
Use Treatment of the signs and symptoms of idiopathic Parkinson's disease; treatment of moderate-to-severe primary Restless Legs Syndrome (RLS)
Unlabeled/Investigational Use Treatment of depression; treatment of fibromyalgia

Pharmacodynamics/Kinetics
Absorption: Rapid
Distribution: V_d: 500 L
Protein binding: 15%
Bioavailability: >90%
Half-life elimination: ~8 hours; Elderly: 12-14 hours
Time to peak, serum: ~2 hours
Excretion: Urine (90% as unchanged drug)

Dosage Oral: Adults:
Parkinson's disease: Initial: 0.375 mg/day given in 3 divided doses, increase gradually by 0.125 mg/dose every 5-7 days; range: 1.5-4.5 mg/day
Restless legs syndrome: Initial: 0.125 mg once daily 2-3 hours before bedtime. Dose may be doubled every 4-7 days up to 0.5 mg/day. Maximum dose: 0.5 mg/day (manufacturer's recommendation).
Note: Most patients require <0.5 mg/day, but higher doses have been used (2 mg/day). If augmentation occurs, dose earlier in the day.
Depression (unlabeled use): Initial: 0.25-0.375 mg/day given in 2-3 divided doses with a gradual titration; mean dose: 1.6-1.7 mg/day
Fibromyalgia (unlabeled use): Initial: 0.25 mg once daily at bedtime; may be increased weekly by 0.25 mg/day increments up to 4.5 mg/day (Holman, 2005)

Dosage adjustment in renal impairment: Use caution; renally-eliminated

Parkinson's disease:

Cl_{cr} 35-59 mL/minute: Initial: 0.125 mg twice daily (maximum dose: 1.5 mg twice daily)

Cl_{cr} 15-34 mL/minute: Initial: 0.125 mg once daily (maximum dose: 1.5 mg once daily)

Cl_{cr} <15 mL/minute (or hemodialysis patients): Not adequately studied

Restless legs syndrome:

Cl_{cr} 20-60 mL/minute: Duration between titration should be increased to 14 days

Cl_{cr} <20 mL/minute: Not adequately studied

Additional Information Complete prescribing information for this medication should be consulted for additional detail.

Dosage Forms Excipient information presented when available (limited, particularly for generics); consult specific product labeling. [CAN] = Canadian product

Tablet, as dihydrochloride monohydrate: 0.25 mg [CAN; generic not available in U.S.], 0.5 mg [CAN; generic not available in U.S.], 1 mg [CAN; generic not available in U.S.], 1.5 mg [CAN; generic not available in U.S.]

Mirapex®: 0.125 mg, 0.25 mg, 0.5 mg, 0.75 mg, 1 mg, 1.5 mg

References

Guttman M, "Double-Blind Comparison of Pramipexole and Bromocriptine Treatment With Placebo in Advanced Parkinson's Disease," International Pramipexole-Bromocriptine Study Group, *Neurology*, 1997, 49(4):1060-5.

Lieberman A, Ranhosky A, and Korts D, "Clinical Evaluation of Pramipexole in Advanced Parkinson's Disease: Results of a Double-Blind, Placebo-Controlled, Parallel-Group Study," *Neurology*, 1997, 49(1):162-8.

Molho ES, Factor SA, Weiner WJ, et al, "The Use of Pramipexole, a Novel Dopamine (DA) Agonist, in Advanced Parkinson's Disease," *J Neural Trans*, 195, 45(Suppl):225-30.

Piercey MF, Hoffman WE, Smith MW, et al, "Inhibition of Dopamine Neuron Firing by Pramipexole, a Dopamine D(3) Receptor-Preferring Agonist: Comparison to Other Dopamine Receptor Agonists," *Eur J Pharmacol*, 1996, 312(1):35-44.

"RLS Medical Bulletin," Restless Legs Syndrome Foundation, 2005, 1-34. Available at www.rls.org. Last accessed December 13, 2006.

"Safety and Efficacy of Pramipexole in Early Parkinson Disease. Parkinson Study Group," *JAMA*, 1997, 278(2):125-30.

Shannon KM, Bennet JP Jr, and Friedman JH, "Efficacy of Pramipexole, A Novel Dopamine Agonist, as Monotherapy in Mild to Moderate Parkinson's Disease," The Pramipexole Study Group, *Neurology*, 1997, 49(3):724-8.

Silber MH, Girish M, and Izurieta R, "Pramipexole in the Management of Resless Legs Syndrome: An Extended Study," *Sleep*, 2003, 26(7):819-21.

Stern MB, "Contemporary Approaches to the Pharmacotherapeutic Management of Parkinson's Disease: An Overview," *Neurology*, 1997, 49(1 Suppl 1):2-9.

Szegedi A, Wetzel H, Hillert A, et al, "Pramipexole, A Novel Selective Dopamine Agonist, in Major Depression," *Mov Disord*, 1996, 11(Suppl):266.

Ting RM and Force RW, "Pramipexole for Parkinson's Disease," *J Fam Pract*, 1998, 46(1):19-20.

Watts RL, "The Role of Dopamine Agonists in Early Parkinson's Disease," *Neurology*, 1997, 49(1 Suppl 1):34-48.

Winkelman JW and Johnston L, "Augmentation and Tolerance With Long-Term Pramipexole Treatment of Restless Legs Syndrome (RLS)," *Sleep Med*, 2004, 5(1):9-14.

Prasugrel (PRA soo grel)

Medication Guide An FDA-approved patient medication guide, which is available with the product information and at http://pi.lilly.com/us/effient-ppi.pdf, must be dispensed with this medication for each new outpatient prescription and refill.

Related Information

Perioperative / Periprocedural Management of Anticoagulant and Antiplatelet Therapy *on page 1607*

Preoperative Evaluation of the Cardiac Patient for Noncardiac Surgery *on page 1598*

Regional Anesthesia in Patients Receiving Anticoagulant and Antiplatelet Therapy *on page 1642*

U.S. Brand Names Effient™

Index Terms CS-747; LY-640315; Prasugrel Hydrochloride

Pharmacologic Category Antiplatelet Agent; Antiplatelet Agent, Thienopyridine

Generic Available No

Use Reduces rate of thrombotic cardiovascular (eg, stent thrombosis) events in patients with unstable angina, non-ST-segment elevation MI, or ST-elevation MI (STEMI) managed with percutaneous coronary intervention (PCI)

Mechanism of Action Prasugrel is a prodrug that is metabolized to both active (R-138727) and inactive metabolites. The active metabolite irreversibly blocks the $P2Y_{12}$ component of ADP receptors on the platelet, which prevents activation of the GPIIb/IIIa receptor complex, thereby reducing platelet activation and aggregation. Platelet aggregation returns to baseline within 5-9 days of discontinuation.

Pharmacodynamics/Kinetics

Onset of action: Inhibition of platelet aggregation (IPA): Dose dependent: 60 mg loading dose: <30 minutes; median time to reach 20% IPA: 30 minutes (Brandt, 2007)

Peak effect: Time to maximal IPA: Dose-dependent: **Note:** Degree of IPA based on adenosine diphosphate (ADP) concentration used during light aggregometry: 60 mg loading dose: Occurs 4 hours post administration; mean IPA (ADP 5 μmol/L): 78.8%: mean IPA (ADP 20 μmol/L): 84.1%

Duration of effect: >3 days; platelet aggregation gradually returns to baseline values over 5-9 days after discontinuation; reflective of new platelet production

Absorption: Rapid; ≥79%

Distribution: V_d: 44-68 L

Protein binding: Active metabolite: ~98%

Metabolism: Rapid intestinal and serum metabolism via esterase-mediated hydrolysis to a thiolactone (inactive), which is then converted, via CYP450-mediated (primarily CYP3A4 and CYP2B6) oxidation, to an active metabolite (R-138727)

Half-life elimination: Active metabolite: ~7 hours (range 2-15 hours)

Time to peak, plasma: Active metabolite: ~30 minutes (peak plasma levels begin to decrease at ~24 hours); with high-fat/high-calorie meal: 1.5 hours

Excretion: Urine (~68% inactive metabolites); feces (27% inactive metabolites)

Dosage Oral:

Adults: ≥60 kg: Loading dose: 60 mg; Maintenance dose: 10 mg once daily (in combination with aspirin 75-325 mg/day)

Note: In patients weighing <60 kg, consider decreasing maintenance dose to 5 mg once daily.

Elderly: Refer to adult dosing. Patients ≥75 years: Use not recommended; may be considered in high-risk situations (eg, patients with diabetes or history of MI)

Dosing adjustment in renal impairment: No dosage adjustment necessary

Dosing adjustment in hepatic impairment: No dosage adjustment necessary for mild-to-moderate hepatic impairment; use in severe hepatic impairment has not been evaluated

Stability Store at 25°C (77°F); excursions permitted to 15°C to 30°C (59°F to 86°F).

Administration Administer without regard to meals.

Monitoring Parameters Hemoglobin and hematocrit periodically

Pregnancy Risk Factor B

Contraindications Active pathological bleeding such as peptic ulcer disease (PUD) or intracranial hemorrhage; history of transient ischemic attack (TIA) or stroke

Warnings/Precautions [U.S. Boxed Warning]: May cause significant or fatal bleeding. Use is contraindicated in patients with active pathological bleeding or history of TIA or stroke. Use with caution in patients who may be at risk of increased bleeding, including patients with active PUD, recent or recurrent GI bleeding, severe hepatic impairment, trauma, or surgery. Additional risk factors include body weight <60 kg, CABG or other surgical procedure, concomitant use of medications that increase risk of bleeding.

[U.S. Boxed Warning]: In patients ≥75 years of age, use is not recommended due to increased risk of fatal and intracranial bleeding and uncertain benefit; use may be considered in high-risk situations (eg, patients with diabetes or history of MI). **[U.S. Boxed Warning]: Discontinue ≥7 days before CABG;** increased risk of bleeding; do not initiate therapy in patients likely to undergo CABG.

◀ If necessary, temporarily discontinue therapy for active bleeding, elective surgery, stroke, or TIA; reinitiate therapy as soon as possible. If possible, manage bleeding without discontinuing prasugrel. Use caution in concurrent treatment with oral anticoagulants (eg, warfarin), NSAIDs, or fibrinolytic agents; bleeding risk is increased. Use with caution in patients with severe liver impairment or end-stage renal disease (experience is limited). Cases of thrombotic thrombocytopenic purpura (usually occurring within the first 2 weeks of therapy), resulting in some fatalities, have been reported with other thienopyridines; urgent plasmapheresis is required. In patients <60 kg, consider lower maintenance dose. Safety and efficacy have not been established in pediatric patients.

Adverse Reactions As with all drugs which may affect hemostasis, bleeding is associated with prasugrel. Hemorrhage may occur at virtually any site. Risk is dependent on multiple variables, including patient susceptibility and concurrent use of multiple agents which alter hemostasis.

2% to 10%:

Cardiovascular: Hypertension (8%), hypotension (4%), atrial fibrillation (3%), bradycardia (3%), noncardiac chest pain (3%), peripheral edema (3%)

Central nervous system: Headache (6%), dizziness (4%), fatigue (4%), fever (3%), extremity pain (3%)

Dermatologic: Rash (3%)

Endocrine & metabolic: Hypercholesterolemia/hyperlipidemia (7%)

Gastrointestinal: Nausea (5%), diarrhea (2%), gastrointestinal hemorrhage (2%)

Hematologic: Leukopenia (3%), anemia (2%)

Neuromuscular & skeletal: Back pain (5%)

Respiratory: Epistaxis (6%), dyspnea (5%), cough (4%)

<2% (Limited to important or life-threatening): Allergic reaction, angioedema, hematoma, hemoptysis, hemorrhage (postprocedural, retinal, retroperitoneal), liver function (abnormal), thrombocytopenia

Drug Interactions

Avoid Concomitant Use There are no known interactions where it is recommended to avoid concomitant use.

Increased Effect/Toxicity

Prasugrel may increase the levels/effects of: Anticoagulants; Antiplatelet Agents; Drotrecogin Alfa; Ibritumomab; Salicylates; Thrombolytic Agents; Tositumomab and Iodine I 131 Tositumomab

The levels/effects of Prasugrel may be increased by: Dasatinib; Herbs (Anticoagulant/Antiplatelet Properties); Nonsteroidal Anti-Inflammatory Agents; Omega-3-Acid Ethyl Esters; Pentosan Polysulfate Sodium; Pentoxifylline; Prostacyclin Analogues

Decreased Effect

The levels/effects of Prasugrel may be decreased by: CYP3A4 Inhibitors (Strong); Nonsteroidal Anti-Inflammatory Agents; Ranitidine; Rifampin

Dietary Considerations May be taken without regard to meals.

Dosage Forms Excipient information presented when available (limited, particularly for generics); consult specific product labeling.

Tablet:

Effient™: 5 mg, 10 mg

References
Brandt JT, Payne CD, Wiviott SD, et al, "A Comparison of Prasugrel and Clopidogrel Loading Doses on Platelet Function: Magnitude of Platelet Inhibition is Related to Active Metabolite Formation," *Am Heart J*, 2007, 153(1):66.e9-16.

◆ **Prasugrel Hydrochloride** *see* Prasugrel *on page 1160*

◆ **Pravachol®** *see* Pravastatin *on page 1162*

Pravastatin (prav a STAT in)

Related Information

Hyperlipidemia Management *on page 1747*

Preoperative Evaluation of the Cardiac Patient for Noncardiac Surgery *on page 1598*

U.S. Brand Names Pravachol®

Canadian Brand Names Apo-Pravastatin®; CO Pravastatin; DOM-Pravastatin; GEN-Pravastatin; Mylan-Pravastatin; Novo-Pravastatin; NU-Pravastatin; PHL-Pravastatin; PMS-Pravastatin; Pravachol®; RAN-Pravastatin; ratio-Pravastatin; Riva-Pravastatin; Sandoz-Pravastatin

Index Terms Pravastatin Sodium

Pharmacologic Category Antilipemic Agent, HMG-CoA Reductase Inhibitor

Use Use with dietary therapy for the following:

Primary prevention of coronary events: In hypercholesterolemic patients without established coronary heart disease to reduce cardiovascular morbidity (myocardial infarction, coronary revascularization procedures) and mortality.

Secondary prevention of cardiovascular events in patients with established coronary heart disease: To slow the progression of coronary atherosclerosis; to reduce cardiovascular morbidity (myocardial infarction, coronary vascular procedures) and to reduce mortality; to reduce the risk of stroke and transient ischemic attacks

Hyperlipidemias: Reduce elevations in total cholesterol, LDL-C, apolipoprotein B, and triglycerides (elevations of 1 or more components are present in Fredrickson type IIa, IIb, III, and IV hyperlipidemias)

Heterozygous familial hypercholesterolemia (HeFH): In pediatric patients, 8-18 years of age, with HeFH having LDL-C ≥190 mg/dL **or** LDL ≥160 mg/dL with positive family history of premature cardiovascular disease (CVD) or 2 or more CVD risk factors in the pediatric patient

Pharmacodynamics/Kinetics

Onset of action: Several days

Peak effect: 4 weeks

Absorption: Rapidly absorbed; average absorption 34%

Protein binding: 50%

Metabolism: Hepatic to at least two metabolites

Bioavailability: 17%

Half-life elimination: ~2-3 hours

Time to peak, serum: 1-1.5 hours

Excretion: Feces (70%); urine (≤20%, 8% as unchanged drug)

Dosage Oral: **Note:** Doses should be individualized according to the baseline LDL-cholesterol levels, the recommended goal of therapy, and patient response; adjustments should be made at intervals of 4 weeks or more; doses may need adjusted based on concomitant medications

Children: HeFH:

8-13 years: 20 mg/day

14-18 years: 40 mg/day

Dosage adjustment for pravastatin based on concomitant cyclosporine: Refer to adult dosing section

Adults: Hyperlipidemias, primary prevention of coronary events, secondary prevention of cardiovascular events: Initial: 40 mg once daily; titrate dosage to response; usual range: 10-80 mg; (maximum dose: 80 mg once daily)

Dosage adjustment for pravastatin based on concomitant cyclosporine: Initial: 10 mg/day, titrate with caution (maximum dose: 20 mg/day)

Elderly: No specific dosage recommendations. Clearance is reduced in the elderly, resulting in an increase in AUC between 25% to 50%. However, substantial accumulation is not expected.

Dosing adjustment in renal impairment: Initial: 10 mg/day

Dosing adjustment in hepatic impairment: Initial: 10 mg/day

Anesthesia and Critical Care Concerns/Other Considerations

Clinical Pearls/Comments: Myopathy: Currently-marketed HMG-CoA reductase inhibitors appear to have a similar potential for causing myopathy. Incidence of severe myopathy is about 0.08% to 0.09%. The factors that increase risk include advanced age (especially >80 years), gender (occurs in women more frequently than men), small body frame, frailty, multisystem disease (eg, chronic renal insufficiency especially due to diabetes), multiple medications, and drug interactions (use with caution or avoid).

Based on current research and clinical guidelines (Fleisher, 2007), HMG-CoA reductase inhibitors should be continued in the perioperative period. Post-operative discontinuation of statin therapy is associated with an increased risk of cardiac morbidity and mortality.

◄ **Additional Information** Complete prescribing information for this medication should be consulted for additional detail.

Dosage Forms Excipient information presented when available (limited, particularly for generics); consult specific product labeling.

Tablet, as sodium: 10 mg, 20 mg, 40 mg, 80 mg

Pravachol®: 10 mg, 20 mg, 40 mg, 80 mg

References

Pasternak RC, Smith SC Jr, Bairey-Merz CN, et al, "ACC/AHA/NHLBI Clinical Advisory on the Use and Safety of Statins," *Stroke*, 2002, 33(9):2337-41. Available at: http://www.acc.org/clinical/alerts/statins_june02.htm. Accessed June 18, 2003.

◆ **Pravastatin Sodium** *see* Pravastatin *on page 1162*

◆ **Praxis ASA EC 81 Mg Daily Dose (Can)** *see* Aspirin *on page 147*

◆ **Precedex®** *see* Dexmedetomidine *on page 397*

◆ **Pred Forte®** *see* PrednisoLONE *on page 1164*

◆ **Pred Mild®** *see* PrednisoLONE *on page 1164*

PrednisoLONE (pred NISS oh lone)

Related Information

Corticosteroids *on page 1676*

Stress Replacement of Corticosteroids *on page 1611*

U.S. Brand Names Econopred® Plus [DSC]; Millipred™; Omnipred™; Orapred ODT®; Orapred®; Pediapred®; Pred Forte®; Pred Mild®; Prelone®; Veripred™ 20

Canadian Brand Names Diopred®; Hydeltra T.B.A.®; Inflamase® Mild; Novo-Prednisolone; Ophtho-Tate®; Pediapred®; Pred Forte®; Pred Mild®; Sab-Prenase

Index Terms Deltahydrocortisone; Metacortandralone; Prednisolone Acetate; Prednisolone Acetate, Ophthalmic; Prednisolone Sodium Phosphate; Prednisolone Sodium Phosphate, Ophthalmic

Pharmacologic Category Corticosteroid, Ophthalmic; Corticosteroid, Systemic

Use Treatment of palpebral and bulbar conjunctivitis; corneal injury from chemical, radiation, thermal burns, or foreign body penetration; endocrine disorders, rheumatic disorders, collagen diseases, dermatologic diseases, allergic states, ophthalmic diseases, respiratory diseases, hematologic disorders, neoplastic diseases, edematous states, and gastrointestinal diseases; resolution of acute exacerbations of multiple sclerosis; management of fulminating or disseminated tuberculosis and trichinosis; acute or chronic solid organ rejection

Pharmacodynamics/Kinetics

Duration: 18-36 hours

Protein binding (concentration dependent): 65% to 91%; decreased in elderly

Metabolism: Primarily hepatic, but also metabolized in most tissues, to inactive compounds

Half-life elimination: 3.6 hours; End-stage renal disease: 3-5 hours

Excretion: Primarily urine (as glucuronides, sulfates, and unconjugated metabolites)

Dosage Dose depends upon condition being treated and response of patient; dosage for infants and children should be based on severity of the disease and response of the patient rather than on strict adherence to dosage indicated by age, weight, or body surface area. Oral dosage expressed in terms of prednisolone base. Consider alternate day therapy for long-term therapy. Discontinuation of long-term therapy requires gradual withdrawal by tapering the dose. Patients undergoing unusual stress while receiving corticosteroids, should receive increased doses prior to, during, and after the stressful situation.

Children: Oral:

Acute asthma: 1-2 mg/kg/day in divided doses 1-2 times/day for 3-5 days

Anti-inflammatory or immunosuppressive dose: 0.1-2 mg/kg/day in divided doses 1-4 times/day

Nephrotic syndrome:
  Initial (first 3 episodes): 2 mg/kg/day **or** 60 mg/m^2/day (maximum: 80 mg/day) in divided doses 3-4 times/day until urine is protein free for 3 consecutive days (maximum: 28 days); followed by 1-1.5 mg/kg/dose **or** 40 mg/m^2/dose given every other day for 4 weeks
  Maintenance (long-term maintenance dose for frequent relapses): 0.5-1 mg/kg/dose given every other day for 3-6 months
Adults: Oral:
  Usual range: 5-60 mg/day
  Multiple sclerosis: 200 mg/day for 1 week followed by 80 mg every other day for 1 month
  Rheumatoid arthritis: Initial: 5-7.5 mg/day; adjust dose as necessary

Ophthalmic suspension/solution: Conjunctivitis, corneal injury: Children and Adults: Instill 1-2 drops into conjunctival sac every hour during day, every 2 hours at night until favorable response is obtained, then use 1 drop every 4 hours.
Elderly: Use lowest effective dose
Dosing adjustment in hyperthyroidism: Prednisolone dose may need to be increased to achieve adequate therapeutic effects
Hemodialysis: Slightly dialyzable (5% to 20%); administer dose posthemodialysis
Peritoneal dialysis: Supplemental dose is not necessary

Anesthesia and Critical Care Concerns/Other Considerations

Evidence-Based Information:

Neuromuscular Effects: ICU-acquired paresis was recently studied in five ICUs (three medical and two surgical ICUs) at four French hospitals. All ICU patients without pre-existing neuromuscular disease admitted from March 1999 through June 2000 were evaluated (de Jonghe, 2002). Each patient had to be mechanically-ventilated for ≥7 days and was screened daily for awakening. The first day the patient was considered awake was Study Day 1. Patients with severe muscle weakness on Study Day 7 were considered to have ICU-acquired paresis. Among the 95 patients who were evaluated, about 25% developed ICU-acquired paresis. Independent predictors included female gender, the number of days with ≥2 organ dysfunction, and administration of corticosteroids. Further studies may be required to verify and characterize the association between the development of ICU-acquired paresis and use of corticosteroids. Concurrent use of a corticosteroid and muscle relaxant appears to increase the risk of certain ICU myopathies; avoid or administer the corticosteroid at the lowest dose possible.

Adrenal Insufficiency: Patients will often have steroid-induced adverse effects on glucose tolerance and lipid profiles. When discontinuing steroid therapy in patients on long-term steroid supplementation, it is important that the steroid therapy be discontinued gradually. Abrupt withdrawal may result in adrenal insufficiency with hypotension and hyperkalemia. Patients on long-term steroid supplementation will require higher corticosteroid doses when subject to stress (eg, trauma, surgery, severe infection). Guidelines for glucocorticoid replacement during various surgical procedures have been published (Coursin, 2002; Salem, 1994).

Additional Information Complete prescribing information for this medication should be consulted for additional detail.

Dosage Forms Excipient information presented when available (limited, particularly for generics); consult specific product labeling. [DSC] = Discontinued product

Solution, ophthalmic, as sodium phosphate: 1% (5 mL, 10 mL, 15 mL) [contains benzalkonium chloride]

Solution, oral, as base: 15 mg/5 mL (240 mL, 480 mL)

Solution, oral, as sodium phosphate: Prednisolone base 5 mg/5 mL (120 mL, 240 mL); prednisolone base 15 mg/5 mL (240 mL)

  Millipred™: Prednisolone base 10 mg/5 mL (237 mL) [dye free; grape flavor]

  Orapred®: Prednisolone base 15 mg/5 mL (20 mL, 240 mL) [dye free; contains ethanol 2%, sodium benzoate; grape flavor]

  Pediapred®: Prednisolone base 5 mg/5 mL (120 mL) [dye free; raspberry flavor]

  Veripred™ 20: Prednisolone base 20 mg/5 mL (237 mL) [dye free, ethanol free; grape flavor]

◀ Suspension, ophthalmic, as acetate: 1% (5 mL, 10 mL, 15 mL)
  Econopred® Plus [DSC], Omnipred™: 1% (5 mL, 10 mL) [contains benzalkonium chloride]
  Pred Forte®: 1% (1 mL, 5 mL, 10 mL, 15 mL) [contains benzalkonium chloride and sodium bisulfite]
  Pred Mild®: 0.12% (5 mL, 10 mL) [contains benzalkonium chloride and sodium bisulfite]
Syrup, as base: 5 mg/5 mL (120 mL); 15 mg/5 mL (5 mL [DSC], 240 mL, 480 mL)
  Prelone®: 15 mg/5 mL (240 mL, 480 mL) [contains ethanol 5%, benzoic acid, propylene glycol; wild cherry flavor]
Tablet, as base: 5 mg
Tablet, orally disintegrating, as sodium phosphate [strength expressed as base]:
  Orapred ODT®: 10 mg, 15 mg, 30 mg [grape flavor]

References

Abraham E and Evans T, "Corticosteroids and Septic Shock [editorial]," *JAMA*, 2002, 288(7):886-7.

Annane D, Sebille V, Charpentier C, et al, "Effect of Treatment With Low Doses of Hydrocortisone and Fludrocortisone on Mortality in Patients With Septic Shock," *JAMA*, 2002, 288(7):862-71.

Beitins IZ, Bayard F, Ances IG, et al, "The Transplacental Passage of Prednisone and Prednisolone in Pregnancy Near Term," *J Pediatr*, 1972, 81(5):936-45.

Cooper MS and Stewart PM, "Corticosteroid Insufficiency in Acutely Ill Patients," *N Engl J Med*, 2003, 348(8):727-34.

Coursin DB and Wood KE, "Corticosteroid Supplementation for Adrenal Insufficiency," *JAMA*, 2002, 287(2):236-40.

de Jonghe B, Sharshar T, Lefaucheur JP, et al, "Paresis Acquired in the Intensive Care Unit. A Prospective Multicenter Study," *JAMA*, 2002, 288(22):2859-67.

Frey BM and Frey FJ, "Clinical Pharmacokinetics of Prednisone and Prednisolone," *Clin Pharmacokinet*, 1990, 19(2):126-46.

Frey FJ, "Kinetics and Dynamics of Prednisolone," *Endocr Rev*, 1987, 8(4):453-73.

Gambertoglio JG, Amend WJ Jr and Benet LZ, "Pharmacokinetics and Bioavailability of Prednisone and Prednisolone in Healthy Volunteers and Patients: A Review," *J Pharmacokinet Biopharm*, 1980, 8(1):1-52.

Gamsu HR, Mullinger BM, Donnai P, et al, "Antenatal Administration of Betamethasone to Prevent Respiratory Distress Syndrome in Preterm Infants: Report of a UK Multicentre Trial," *Br J Obstet Gynaecol*, 1989, 96(4):401-10.

Goedert JJ, Vitale F, Lauria C, et al, "Risk Factors for Classical Kaposi's Sarcoma," *J Natl Cancer Inst*, 2002, 94(22):1712-8.

Hotchkiss RS and Karl IE, "The Pathophysiology and Treatment of Sepsis," *N Engl J Med*, 2003, 348 (2):138-50.

Lawrence RA, "Corticosteroid Effect on Lactation," *JAMA*, 1991, 265(18):2409.

Liggins GC and Howie RN, "A Controlled Trial of Antepartum Glucocorticoid Treatment of Respiratory Distress Syndrome in Premature Infants," *Pediatrics*, 1972, 50:515-25.

McGee S and Hirschmann J, "Use of Corticosteroids in Treating Infectious Diseases," *Arch Intern Med*, 2008, 168(10):1034-46.

Ost L, Wettrell G, Björkhem I, et al, "Prednisolone Excretion in Human Milk," *J Pediatr*, 1985, 106 (6):1008-11.

Ostensen M, "Optimisation of Antirheumatic Drug Treatment in Pregnancy," *Clin Pharmacokinet*, 1994, 27(6):486-503.

Pradat P, Robert-Gnansia E, Di Tanna GL, et al, "First Trimester Exposure to Corticosteroids and Oral Clefts," *Birth Defects Res A Clin Mol Teratol*, 2003, 67(12):968-70.

Report of a Workshop by the British Association for Paediatric Nephrology and Research Unit, Royal College of Physicians, "Consensus Statement on Management and Audit Potential for Steroid Responsive Nephrotic Syndrome," *Arch Dis Child*, 1994, 70(2):151-7.

Salem M, Tainsh RE Jr, Bromberg J, et al, "Perioperative Glucocorticoid Coverage. A Reassessment 42 Years After Emergence of a Problem," *Ann Surg*, 1994, 219(4):416-25.

van Runnard Heimel PJ, Schobben AF, Huisjes AJ, et al, "The Transplacental Passage of Prednisolone in Pregnancies Complicated by Early-Onset HELLP Syndrome," *Placenta*, 2005, 26 (10):842-5.

◆ **Prednisolone Acetate** *see* PrednisoLONE *on page 1164*

◆ **Prednisolone Acetate, Ophthalmic** *see* PrednisoLONE *on page 1164*

◆ **Prednisolone Sodium Phosphate** *see* PrednisoLONE *on page 1164*

◆ **Prednisolone Sodium Phosphate, Ophthalmic** *see* PrednisoLONE *on page 1164*

PredniSONE (PRED ni sone)

Medication Safety Issues

Sound-alike/look-alike issues:
  PredniSONE may be confused with methylPREDNISolone, Pramosone®, prazosin, prednisoLONE, Prilosec®, primidone, promethazine

Related Information

Chronic Pain Management *on page 1546*
Contrast Media Reactions, Premedication for Prophylaxis *on page 1735*
Corticosteroids *on page 1676*
Desensitization Protocols *on page 1692*
Latex Allergy *on page 1511*
Stress Replacement of Corticosteroids *on page 1611*

U.S. Brand Names PredniSONE Intensol™; Sterapred®; Sterapred® DS [DSC]
Canadian Brand Names Apo-Prednisone®; Novo-Prednisone; Winpred™
Index Terms Deltacortisone; Deltadehydrocortisone
Pharmacologic Category Corticosteroid, Systemic
Generic Available Yes
Use Treatment of a variety of diseases, including:

Allergic states (including adjunctive treatment of anaphylaxis)
Autoimmune disorders (including systemic lupus erythematosus [SLE])
Collagen diseases
Dermatologic conditions/diseases
Edematous states (including nephrotic syndrome)
Endocrine disorders
Gastrointestinal diseases
Hematologic disorders (including idiopathic thrombocytopenia purpura [ITP])
Multiple sclerosis exacerbations
Neoplastic diseases
Ophthalmic diseases
Respiratory diseases (including acute asthma exacerbation)
Rheumatic disorders (including rheumatoid arthritis)
Trichinosis with neurologic or myocardial involvement
Tuberculous meningitis

Unlabeled/Investigational Use Adjunctive therapy for *Pneumocystis jiroveci* (formerly *carinii*) pneumonia (PCP); autoimmune hepatitis; adjunctive therapy for pain management in immunocompetent patients with herpes zoster; tuberculosis (severe, paradoxical reactions)

Mechanism of Action Decreases inflammation by suppression of migration of polymorphonuclear leukocytes and reversal of increased capillary permeability; suppresses the immune system by reducing activity and volume of the lymphatic system; suppresses adrenal function at high doses. Antitumor effects may be related to inhibition of glucose transport, phosphorylation, or induction of cell death in immature lymphocytes. Antiemetic effects are thought to occur due to blockade of cerebral innervation of the emetic center via inhibition of prostaglandin synthesis.

Pharmacodynamics/Kinetics

Absorption: 50% to 90% (may be altered in IBS or hyperthyroidism)
Protein binding (concentration dependent): 65% to 91%
Metabolism: Hepatically converted from prednisone (inactive) to prednisolone (active); may be impaired with hepatic dysfunction
Half-life elimination: Normal renal function: ~3.5 hours
Excretion: Urine (small portion)

Dosage Oral:

General dosing range: Children and Adults: Initial: 5-60 mg/day: **Note:** Dose depends upon condition being treated and response of patient; dosage for infants and children should be based on severity of the disease and response of the patient rather than on strict adherence to dosage indicated by age, weight, or body surface area. Consider alternate day therapy for long-term therapy. Discontinuation of long-term therapy requires gradual withdrawal by tapering the dose.

Prednisone taper (other regimens also available):
Day 1: 30 mg divided as 10 mg before breakfast, 5 mg at lunch, 5 mg at dinner, 10 mg at bedtime
Day 2: 5 mg at breakfast, 5 mg at lunch, 5 mg at dinner, 10 mg at bedtime
Day 3: 5 mg 4 times/day (with meals and at bedtime)
Day 4: 5 mg 3 times/day (breakfast, lunch, bedtime)
Day 5: 5 mg 2 times/day (breakfast, bedtime)
Day 6: 5 mg before breakfast

◄ **Indication-specific dosing:**
Children:

Acute asthma (NIH guidelines, 2007):
0-11 years 1-2 mg/kg/day for 3-10 days (maximum: 60 mg/day)
≥12 years: Refer to Adult dosing

Autoimmune hepatitis (unlabeled use; Czaja 2002): Initial treatment: 2 mg/kg/day for 2 weeks (maximum: 60 mg/day), followed by a taper over 6-8 weeks to a dose of 0.1-0.2 mg/kg/day or 5 mg/day

Nephrotic syndrome (Pediatric Nephrology Panel recommendations [Hogg, 2000]): Initial: 2 mg/kg/day or 60 mg/m^2/day given every day in 1-3 divided doses (maximum: 80 mg/day) until urine is protein free or for 4-6 weeks; followed by maintenance dose: 2 mg/kg/dose or 40 mg/m^2/dose given every other day in the morning; gradually taper and discontinue after 4-6 weeks. **Note:** No definitive treatment guidelines exist. Dosing is dependant on institution protocols and individual response.

PCP pneumonia (AIDSinfo guidelines, 2008): 1 mg/kg twice daily for 5 days, *followed by* 0.5-1 mg/kg twice daily for 5 days, *followed by* 0.5 mg/kg once daily for 11-21 days

Adolescents and Adults:

PCP pneumonia (AIDSinfo guidelines, 2008): Note: Begin within 72 hours of PCP therapy: 40 mg twice daily for 5 days, *followed by* 40 mg once daily for 5 days, *followed by* 20 mg once daily for 11 days or until antimicrobial regimen is completed

Adults:

Acute asthma (NIH guidelines, 2007): 40-60 mg per day for 3-10 days; administer as single or 2 divided doses

Anaphylaxis, adjunctive treatment (Lieberman 2005): 0.5 mg/kg

Antineoplastic: Usual range: 10 mg/day to 100 mg/m^2/day (depending on indication). **Note:** Details concerning dosing in combination regimens should also be consulted.

Autoimmune hepatitis (unlabeled use; Czaja 2002): Initial treatment: 60 mg/day for 1 week, *followed by* 40 mg/day for 1 week, *then* 30 mg/day for 2 weeks, *then* 20 mg/day. Half this dose should be given when used in combination with azathioprine

Herpes zoster (unlabeled use; Dworkin 2007): 60 mg/day for 7 days, *followed by* 30 mg/day for 7 days, *then* 15 mg/day for 7 days

Idiopathic thrombocytopenia purpura (American Society of Hematology 1997): 1-2 mg/kg/day

Rheumatoid arthritis (American College of Rheumatology 2002): ≤10 mg/day

Systemic lupus erythematosus (American College of Rheumatology 1999):
Mild SLE: ≤10 mg/day
Refractory or severe organ-threatening disease: 20-60 mg/day

Thyrotoxicosis (type II amiodarone induced; unlabeled use): 30-40 mg/day for 7-14 days, gradually taper over 3 months

Tuberculosis, severe, paradoxical reactions (unlabeled use, AIDSinfo guidelines 2008): 1 mg/kg/day, gradually reduce after 1-2 weeks

Elderly: Use the lowest effective dose

Dosing adjustment in hepatic impairment: Prednisone is inactive and must be metabolized by the liver to prednisolone. This conversion may be impaired in patients with liver disease, however, prednisolone levels are observed to be higher in patients with severe liver failure than in normal patients. Therefore, compensation for the inadequate conversion of prednisone to prednisolone occurs.

Dosing adjustment in hyperthyroidism: Prednisone dose may need to be increased to achieve adequate therapeutic effects

Hemodialysis: Supplemental dose is not necessary

Peritoneal dialysis: Supplemental dose is not necessary

Administration Administer with food to decrease gastrointestinal upset

Monitoring Parameters Blood pressure, blood glucose, electrolytes

Following prolonged use: Bone mass density, growth in children, signs and symptoms of infection, cataract formation

Anesthesia and Critical Care Concerns/Other Considerations
Evidence-Based Information:

Neuromuscular Effects: ICU-acquired paresis was recently studied in 5 ICUs (3 medical and 2 surgical ICUs) at 4 French hospitals. All ICU patients without pre-existing neuromuscular disease admitted from March 1999 through June 2000 were evaluated (De Jonghe, 2002). Each patient had to be mechanically ventilated for ≥7 days and was screened daily for awakening. The first day the patient was considered awake was Study Day 1. Patients with severe muscle weakness on Study Day 7 were considered to have ICU-acquired paresis. Among the 95 patients who were evaluated, about 25% developed ICU-acquired paresis. Independent predictors included female gender, the number of days with ≥2 organ dysfunction, and administration of corticosteroids. Further studies may be required to verify and characterize the association between the development of ICU-acquired paresis and use of corticosteroids. Concurrent use of a corticosteroid and muscle relaxant appears to increase the risk of certain ICU myopathies; avoid or administer the corticosteroid at the lowest dose possible.

Adrenal Insufficiency: Patients will often have steroid-induced adverse effects on glucose tolerance and lipid profiles. When discontinuing steroid therapy in patients on long-term steroid supplementation, it is important that the steroid therapy be discontinued gradually. Abrupt withdrawal may result in adrenal insufficiency with hypotension and hyperkalemia. Patients on long-term steroid supplementation will require higher corticosteroid doses when subject to stress (ie, trauma, surgery, severe infection). Guidelines for glucocorticoid replacement during various surgical procedures have been published (Coursin, 2002; Salem, 1994).

Contraindications Hypersensitivity to any component of the formulation; systemic fungal infections; administration of live or live attenuated vaccines with immunosuppressive doses of prednisone

Warnings/Precautions May cause hypercorticism or suppression of hypothalamic-pituitary-adrenal (HPA) axis, particularly in younger children or in patients receiving high doses for prolonged periods. HPA axis suppression may lead to adrenal crisis. Withdrawal and discontinuation of a corticosteroid should be done slowly and carefully. Particular care is required when patients are transferred from systemic corticosteroids to inhaled products due to possible adrenal insufficiency or withdrawal from steroids, including an increase in allergic symptoms. Patients receiving >20 mg per day of prednisone (or equivalent) may be most susceptible. Fatalities have occurred due to adrenal insufficiency in asthmatic patients during and after transfer from systemic corticosteroids to aerosol steroids; aerosol steroids do **not** provide the systemic steroid needed to treat patients having trauma, surgery, or infections.

Acute myopathy has been reported with high dose corticosteroids, usually in patients with neuromuscular transmission disorders; may involve ocular and/or respiratory muscles; monitor creatine kinase; recovery may be delayed. Prolonged use of corticosteroids may increase the incidence of secondary infection, mask acute infection (including fungal infections), prolong or exacerbate viral infections, or limit response to vaccines. Exposure to chickenpox should be avoided. Corticosteroids should not be used to treat ocular herpes simplex or cerebral malaria. Close observation is required in patients with latent tuberculosis and/or TB reactivity; restrict use in active TB (only in conjunction with antituberculosis treatment). Prolonged treatment with corticosteroids has been associated with the development of Kaposi's sarcoma (case reports); if noted, discontinuation of therapy should be considered. Prolonged use may cause posterior subcapsular cataracts, glaucoma (with possible nerve damage) and may increase the risk for ocular infections. Corticosteroid use may cause psychiatric disturbances, including depression, euphoria, insomnia, mood swings, and personality changes. Pre-existing psychiatric conditions may be exacerbated by corticosteroid use.

Use with caution in patients with HF, diabetes, GI diseases (diverticulitis, peptic ulcer, ulcerative colitis; due to risk of perforation), hepatic impairment, myasthenia gravis, MI, patients with or who are at risk for osteoporosis, seizure disorders or thyroid disease. May affect growth velocity; growth should be routinely monitored in pediatric patients.

◄ Prior to use, the dose and duration of treatment should be based on the risk versus benefit for each individual patient. In general, use the smallest effective dose for the shortest duration of time to minimize adverse events. A gradual tapering of dose may be required prior to discontinuing therapy.

Adverse Reactions Frequency not defined.

Cardiovascular: Congestive heart failure (in susceptible patients), hypertension

Central nervous system: Emotional instability, headache, intracranial pressure increased (with papilledema), psychic derangements (including euphoria, insomnia, mood swings, personality changes, severe depression), seizure, vertigo

Dermatologic: Bruising, facial erythema, petechiae, thin fragile skin, urticaria, wound healing impaired

Endocrine & metabolic: Adrenocortical and pituitary unresponsiveness (in times of stress), carbohydrate intolerance, Cushing's syndrome, diabetes mellitus, fluid retention, growth suppression (in children), hypokalemic alkalosis, hypo-thyroidism enhanced, menstrual irregularities, negative nitrogen balance due to protein catabolism, potassium loss, sodium retention

Gastrointestinal: Abdominal distension, pancreatitis, peptic ulcer (with possible perforation and hemorrhage), ulcerative esophagitis

Hepatic: ALT increased, AST increased, alkaline phosphatase increased

Neuromuscular & skeletal: Aseptic necrosis of femoral and humeral heads, muscle mass loss, muscle weakness, osteoporosis, pathologic fracture of long bones, steroid myopathy, tendon rupture (particularly Achilles tendon), vertebral compression fractures

Ocular: Exophthalmos, glaucoma, intraocular pressure increased, posterior subcapsular cataracts

Miscellaneous: Allergic reactions, anaphylactic reactions, diaphoresis, hyper-sensitivity reactions, infections, Kaposi's sarcoma

Drug Interactions

Metabolism/Transport Effects **Substrate** of CYP3A4 (minor); **Induces** CYP2C19 (weak), 3A4 (weak)

Avoid Concomitant Use

Avoid concomitant use of PredniSONE with any of the following: Natalizumab; Vaccines (Live)

Increased Effect/Toxicity

PredniSONE may increase the levels/effects of: Acetylcholinesterase Inhibitors; Amphotericin B; CycloSPORINE; Leflunomide; Loop Diuretics; Natalizumab; NSAID (COX-2 Inhibitor); NSAID (Nonselective); Thiazide Diuretics; Vaccines (Live); Warfarin

The levels/effects of PredniSONE may be increased by: Antifungal Agents (Azole Derivatives, Systemic); Aprepitant; Calcium Channel Blockers (Non-dihydropyridine); CycloSPORINE; Estrogen Derivatives; Fluconazole; Fosapre-pitant; Macrolide Antibiotics; Neuromuscular-Blocking Agents (Nondepolarizing); Quinolone Antibiotics; Salicylates; Trastuzumab

Decreased Effect

PredniSONE may decrease the levels/effects of: Antidiabetic Agents; Calcitriol; Corticorelin; Isoniazid; Salicylates; Vaccines (Inactivated); Vaccines (Live)

The levels/effects of PredniSONE may be decreased by: Aminoglutethimide; Antacids; Barbiturates; Bile Acid Sequestrants; Echinacea; Mitotane; Primidone; Rifamycin Derivatives; Somatropin

Ethanol/Nutrition/Herb Interactions

Ethanol: Avoid ethanol (may increase gastric mucosal irritation)

Food: Prednisone interferes with calcium absorption. Limit caffeine.

Herb/Nutraceutical: St John's wort may decrease prednisone levels. Avoid cat's claw, echinacea (have immunostimulant properties).

Test Interactions Decreased response to skin tests

Dietary Considerations Should be taken after meals or with food or milk; may require increased dietary intake of pyridoxine, vitamin C, vitamin D, folate, calcium, and phosphorus; may require decreased dietary intake of sodium

Dosage Forms Excipient information presented when available (limited, particularly for generics); consult specific product labeling. [DSC] = Discontinued product

Solution, oral: 1 mg/mL (5 mL, 120 mL, 500 mL) [contains ethanol 5%, sodium benzoate; peppermint vanilla flavor]

Solution, oral [concentrate]:

PredniSONE Intensol™: 5 mg/mL (30 mL) [dye free, sugar free; contains ethanol 30%, propylene glycol]

Tablet: 1 mg, 2.5 mg, 5 mg, 10 mg, 20 mg, 50 mg

Sterapred®: 5 mg [scored; supplied as 21 tablet 6-day unit-dose package or 48 tablet 12-day unit-dose package]

Sterapred® DS: 10 mg [supplied as 21 tablet 6-day unit-dose package or 48 tablet 12-day unit-dose package] [DSC]

References

Abraham E and Evans T, "Corticosteroids and Septic Shock (editorial)," *JAMA*, 2002, 288(7):886-7.

Annane D, Sebille V, Charpentier C, et al, "Effect of Treatment With Low Doses of Hydrocortisone and Fludrocortisone on Mortality in Patients With Septic Shock," *JAMA*, 2002, 288(7):862-71.

Cooper MS and Stewart PM, "Corticosteroid Insufficiency in Acutely Ill Patients," *N Engl J Med*, 2003, 348(8):727-34.

Coursin DB and Wood KE, "Corticosteroid Supplementation for Adrenal Insufficiency," *JAMA*, 2002, 287(2):236-40.

de Jonghe B, Sharshar T, Lefaucheur JP, et al, "Paresis Acquired in the Intensive Care Unit. A Prospective Multicenter Study," *JAMA*, 2002, 288(22):2859-67.

Dellinger RP, Levy MM, Carlet JM, et al, "Surviving Sepsis Campaign: International Guidelines for Management of Severe Sepsis and Septic Shock: 2008," *Intensive Care Med*, 2008, 34(1): 17-60. Available at http://www.survivingsepsis.org/system/files/images/2008_20International_20SSC_20-Guidelines_1_.pdf

Expert Panel Report 3, "Guidelines for the Diagnosis and Management of Asthma," *Clinical Practice Guidelines*, National Institutes of Health, National Heart, Lung, and Blood Institute, NIH Publication No. 08-4051, prepublication 2007. Available at http://www.nhlbi.nih.gov/guidelines/asthma/asthgdln.htm

Hotchkiss RS and Karl IE, "The Pathophysiology and Treatment of Sepsis," *N Engl J Med*, 2003, 348 (2):138-50.

Salem M, Tainsh RE, Jr, Bromberg J, et al, "Perioperative Glucocorticoid Coverage: A Reassessment 42 Years After Emergence of a Problem," *Ann Surg*, 1994, 219(4):416-25.

◆ **PredniSONE Intensol™** *see* PredniSONE *on page 1166*

Pregabalin (pre GAB a lin)

Medication Safety Issues

Sound-alike/look-alike issues:

Lyrica® may be confused with Lopressor®

Medication Guide An FDA-approved patient medication guide, which is available with the product information and at http://www.fda.gov/downloads/Drugs/DrugSafety/UCM152825.pdf, must be dispensed with this medication for each new outpatient prescription and refill.

Related Information

Acute Postoperative Pain *on page 1502*

Chronic Pain Management *on page 1546*

Perioperative Management of Patients on Antiseizure Medication *on page 1577*

U.S. Brand Names Lyrica®

Canadian Brand Names Lyrica®

Index Terms CI-1008; S-(+)-3-isobutylgaba

Pharmacologic Category Analgesic, Miscellaneous; Anticonvulsant, Miscellaneous

Restrictions C-V

Generic Available No

Use Management of pain associated with diabetic peripheral neuropathy; management of postherpetic neuralgia; adjunctive therapy for partial-onset seizure disorder in adults; management of fibromyalgia

Mechanism of Action Binds to alpha$_2$-delta subunit of voltage-gated calcium channels within the CNS, inhibiting excitatory neurotransmitter release. Although structurally related to GABA, it does not bind to GABA or benzodiazepine receptors. Exerts antinociceptive and anticonvulsant activity. Decreases symptoms of painful peripheral neuropathies and, as adjunctive therapy in partial seizures, decreases the frequency of seizures.

Pharmacodynamics/Kinetics

Onset of action: Pain management: Effects may be noted as early as the first week of therapy.

◄ Distribution: V_d: 0.5 L/kg
Protein binding: 0%
Metabolism: Negligible
Bioavailability: >90%
Half-life elimination: 6.3 hours
Time to peak, plasma: 1.5 hours (3 hours with food)
Excretion: Urine (90% as unchanged drug; minor metabolites)

Dosage Oral: Adults:

Fibromyalgia: Initial: 150 mg/day in divided doses (75 mg 2 times/day); may be increased to 300 mg/day (150 mg 2 times/day) within 1 week based on tolerability and effect; may be further increased to 450 mg/day (225 mg 2 times/day). Maximum dose: 450 mg/day (dosages up to 600 mg/day were evaluated with no significant additional benefit and an increase in adverse effects)

Neuropathic pain (diabetes-associated): Initial: 150 mg/day in divided doses (50 mg 3 times/day); may be increased within 1 week based on tolerability and effect; maximum dose: 300 mg/day (dosages up to 600 mg/day were evaluated with no significant additional benefit and an increase in adverse effects)

Postherpetic neuralgia: Initial: 150 mg/day in divided doses (75 mg 2 times/day or 50 mg 3 times/day); may be increased to 300 mg/day within 1 week based on tolerability and effect; further titration (to 600 mg/day) after 2-4 weeks may be considered in patients who do not experience sufficient relief of pain provided they are able to tolerate pregabalin. Maximum dose: 600 mg/day

Partial-onset seizures (adjunctive therapy): Initial: 150 mg per day in divided doses (75 mg 2 times/day or 50 mg 3 times/day); may be increased based on tolerability and effect (optimal titration schedule has not been defined). Maximum dose: 600 mg/day

Discontinuing therapy: Pregabalin should not be abruptly discontinued; taper dosage over at least 1 week

Dosage adjustment in renal impairment: In renally-impaired patients, dosage adjustment depends on renal function and daily dosage.

Pregabalin Renal Impairment Dosing

Cl_{cr} (mL/minute)	Total Pregabalin Daily Dose (mg/day)				Dosing Frequency
≥60	150	300	450	600	2-3 divided doses
30-60	75	150	225	300	2-3 divided doses
15-30	25-50	75	100-150	150	1-2 divided doses
<15	25	25-50	50-75	75	Single daily dose

Posthemodialysis supplementary dosage (as a single additional dose):
25 mg/day schedule: Single supplementary dose of 25 mg **or** 50 mg
25-50 mg/day schedule: Single supplementary dose of 50 mg **or** 75 mg
50-75 mg/day schedule: Single supplementary dose of 75 mg **or** 100 mg
75 mg/day schedule: Single supplementary dose of 100 mg **or** 150 mg

Stability Store at 15°C to 30°C (59°F to 86°F).

Administration May be administered with or without food.

Monitoring Parameters Measures of efficacy (pain intensity/seizure frequency); degree of sedation; symptoms of myopathy or ocular disturbance; weight gain/edema; CPK; skin integrity (in patients with diabetes); suicidality (eg, suicidal thoughts, depression, behavioral changes)

Pregnancy Risk Factor C

Contraindications Hypersensitivity to pregabalin or any component of the formulation

Warnings/Precautions Antiepileptics are associated with an increased risk of suicidal behavior/thoughts with use (regardless of indication); patients should be monitored for signs/symptoms of depression, suicidal tendencies, and other unusual behavior changes during therapy and instructed to inform their healthcare provider immediately if symptoms occur.

Angioedema has been reported; may be life threatening; use with caution in patients with a history of angioedema episodes. Concurrent use with other drugs known to cause angioedema (eg, ACE inhibitors) may increase risk. Hypersensitivity reactions, including skin redness, blistering, hives, rash, dyspnea and wheezing have been reported; discontinue treatment of hypersensitivity occurs. May cause CNS depression and/or dizziness, which may impair physical or mental abilities. Patients must be cautioned about performing tasks which require mental alertness (eg, operating machinery or driving). Effects with other sedative drugs or ethanol may be potentiated. Visual disturbances (blurred vision, decreased acuity and visual field changes) have been associated with pregabalin therapy; patients should be instructed to notify their physician if these effects are noted.

Pregabalin has been associated with increases in CPK and rare cases of rhabdomyolysis. Patients should be instructed to notify their prescriber if unexplained muscle pain, tenderness, or weakness, particularly if fever and/or malaise are associated with these symptoms. Use may be associated with weight gain and peripheral edema; use caution in patients with congestive heart failure, hypertension, or diabetes. Effect on weight gain/edema may be additive to thiazolidinedione antidiabetic agent; particularly in patients with prior cardiovascular disease. May decrease platelet count or prolong PR interval.

Has been noted to be tumorigenic (increased incidence of hemangiosarcoma) in animal studies; significance of these findings in humans is unknown. Pregabalin has been associated with discontinuation symptoms following abrupt cessation, and increases in seizure frequency (when used as an antiepileptic) may occur. Should not be discontinued abruptly; dosage tapering over at least 1 week is recommended. Use caution in renal impairment; dosage adjustment required. Safety and efficacy have not been established in pediatric patients.

Adverse Reactions Note: Frequency of adverse effects may be influenced by dose or concurrent therapy. In add-on trials in epilepsy, frequency of CNS and adverse effects were higher than those reported in pain management trials. Range noted below is inclusive of all trials.

>10%:
Cardiovascular: Peripheral edema (up to 16%)
Central nervous system: Dizziness (8% to 45%), somnolence (4% to 28%), ataxia (up to 20%), headache (up to 14%)
Gastrointestinal: Weight gain (up to 16%), xerostomia (1% to 15%)
Neuromuscular & skeletal: Tremor (up to 11%)
Ocular: Blurred vision (1% to 12%), diplopia (up to 12%)
Miscellaneous: Infection (up to 14%), accidental injury (2% to 11%)

1% to 10%:
Cardiovascular: Chest pain (up to 4%), edema (up to 6%)
Central nervous system: Neuropathy (up to 9%), thinking abnormal (up to 9%), fatigue (up to 8%), confusion (up to 7%), euphoria (up to 7%), speech disorder (up to 7%), attention disturbance (up to 6%), incoordination (up to 6%), amnesia (up to 6%), pain (up to 5%), memory impaired (up to 4%), vertigo (up to 4%), feeling abnormal (up to 3%), hypoesthesia (up to 3%), anxiety (up to 2%), depression (up to 2%), disorientation (up to 2%), lethargy (up to 2%), fever (≥1%), depersonalization (≥1%), hypertonia (≥1%), stupor (≥1%), nervousness (up to 1%)
Dermatologic: Facial edema (up to 3%), bruising (≥1%), pruritus (≥1%)
Endocrine & metabolic: Fluid retention (up to 3%), hypoglycemia (up to 3%), libido decreased (≥1%)
Gastrointestinal: Constipation (up to 10%), appetite increased (up to 7%), flatulence (up to 3%), vomiting (up to 3%), abdominal distension (up to 2%), abdominal pain (≥1%), gastroenteritis (≥1%)
Genitourinary: Incontinence (up to 2%), anorgasmia (≥1%), impotence (≥1%), urinary frequency (≥1%)
Hematologic: Thrombocytopenia (3%)
Neuromuscular & skeletal: Balance disorder (up to 9%), abnormal gait (up to 8%), weakness (up to 7%), arthralgia (up to 6%), twitching (up to 5%), back pain (up to 4%), muscle spasm (up to 4%), myoclonus (up to 4%), paresthesia (>2%), CPK increased (2%), leg cramps (≥1%), myalgia (≥1%), myasthenia (up to 1%)

Ocular: Visual abnormalities (up to 5%), visual field defect (≥2%), eye disorder (up to 2%), nystagmus (>2%), conjunctivitis (≥1%)

Otic: Otitis media (≥1%), tinnitus (≥1%)

Respiratory: Sinusitis (up to 7%), dyspnea (up to 3%), bronchitis (up to 3%), pharyngolaryngeal pain (up to 3%)

Miscellaneous: Flu-like syndrome (up to 2%), allergic reaction (≥1%)

<1% (Limited to important or life-threatening): Abscess, acute renal failure, addiction (rare), agitation, albuminuria, anaphylactoid reaction, anemia, angioedema, aphasia, aphthous stomatitis, apnea, ascites, atelectasis, blepharitis, blindness, bronchiolitis, cellulitis, cerebellar syndrome, cervicitis, chills, cholecystitis, cholelithiasis, chondrodystrophy, circumoral paresthesia, cogwheel rigidity, colitis, coma, corneal ulcer, crystalluria (urate), delirium, delusions, diarrhea, dysarthria, dysautonomia, dyskinesia, dysphagia, dystonia, dysuria, encephalopathy, eosinophilia, esophageal ulcer, esophagitis, exfoliative dermatitis, extraocular palsy, extrapyramidal syndrome, gastritis, GI hemorrhage, glomerulitis, glucose tolerance decreased, granuloma, Guillain-Barré syndrome, hallucinations, heart failure, hematuria, hostility, hyper-/hypokinesia; hypersensitivity (including skin redness, blistering, hives, rash, dyspnea, and wheezing); hypotension, hypotonia, intracranial hypertension, laryngismus, leukopenia, leukorrhea, leukocytosis, lymphadenopathy, manic reaction, melena, myelofibrosis, nausea, nephritis, neuralgia, ocular hemorrhage, oliguria, optic atrophy, pancreatitis, papilledema, paranoid reaction, pelvic pain, periodontal abscess, peripheral neuritis, polycythemia, postural hypotension, prothrombin decreased, psychotic depression, ptosis, pulmonary edema, pulmonary fibrosis, purpura, pyelonephritis, rectal hemorrhage, renal calculus, retinal edema, retinal vascular disorder, retroperitoneal fibrosis, rhabdomyolysis, schizophrenic reaction, shock, skin necrosis, skin ulcer, spasm (generalized), ST depression, Stevens-Johnson syndrome, subcutaneous nodule, suicide, suicide attempt, syncope, thrombocythemia, thrombophlebitis, tongue edema, torticollis, trismus, uveitis, ventricular fibrillation

Drug Interactions

Avoid Concomitant Use There are no known interactions where it is recommended to avoid concomitant use.

Increased Effect/Toxicity

Pregabalin may increase the levels/effects of: Alcohol (Ethyl); Antidiabetic Agents (Thiazolidinedione); CNS Depressants; Methotrimeprazine

The levels/effects of Pregabalin may be increased by: Methotrimeprazine

Decreased Effect

The levels/effects of Pregabalin may be decreased by: Ketorolac; Mefloquine

Ethanol/Nutrition/Herb Interactions

Ethanol: Avoid ethanol (may increase CNS depression).

Herb/Nutraceutical: Avoid valerian, St John's wort, kava kava, gotu kola (may increase CNS depression).

Dietary Considerations May be taken with or without food.

Dosage Forms Excipient information presented when available (limited, particularly for generics); consult specific product labeling.

Capsule:

Lyrica®: 25 mg, 50 mg, 75 mg, 100 mg, 150 mg, 200 mg, 225 mg, 300 mg

References

Hill CM, Balkenohl M, Thomas DW, et al, "Pregabalin in Patients With Postoperative Dental Pain," *Eur J Pain*, 2001, 5(2):119-24.

- ◆ **Prempro™** *see* Estrogens (Conjugated/Equine) and Medroxyprogesterone *on page 539*
- ◆ **Preparation H® [OTC]** *see* Phenylephrine *on page 1114*
- ◆ **Preparation H® Hydrocortisone [OTC]** *see* Hydrocortisone *on page 699*
- ◆ **Pressyn® (Can)** *see* Vasopressin *on page 1458*
- ◆ **Pressyn® AR (Can)** *see* Vasopressin *on page 1458*
- ◆ **Pretz® [OTC]** *see* Sodium Chloride *on page 1304*
- ◆ **Prevacare® [OTC]** *see* Alcohol (Ethyl) *on page 53*
- ◆ **Prevacid®** *see* Lansoprazole *on page 805*
- ◆ **Prevacid® SoluTab™** *see* Lansoprazole *on page 805*
- ◆ **Prevex® B (Can)** *see* Betamethasone *on page 186*
- ◆ **Prevex® HC (Can)** *see* Hydrocortisone *on page 699*
- ◆ **Previfem®** *see* Ethinyl Estradiol and Norgestimate *on page 558*
- ◆ **Prilosec®** *see* Omeprazole *on page 1048*
- ◆ **Prilosec OTC™ [OTC]** *see* Omeprazole *on page 1048*
- ◆ **Primacor® [DSC]** *see* Milrinone *on page 941*
- ◆ **Primacor® (Can)** *see* Milrinone *on page 941*
- ◆ **Primalev™** *see* Oxycodone and Acetaminophen *on page 1072*
- ◆ **Primatene® Mist [OTC]** *see* EPINEPHrine *on page 492*
- ◆ **Primaxin®** *see* Imipenem and Cilastatin *on page 727*
- ◆ **Primaxin® I.V. (Can)** *see* Imipenem and Cilastatin *on page 727*
- ◆ **Primene® (Can)** *see* Amino Acid Injection *on page 81*
- ◆ **Prinivil®** *see* Lisinopril *on page 849*
- ◆ **Pristinamycin** *see* Quinupristin and Dalfopristin *on page 1219*
- ◆ **Pristiq®** *see* Desvenlafaxine *on page 390*
- ◆ **Privigen™** *see* Immune Globulin (Intravenous) *on page 732*
- ◆ **ProAir® HFA** *see* Albuterol *on page 49*
- ◆ **ProAmatine®** *see* Midodrine *on page 939*
- ◆ **PRO-Amiodarone (Can)** *see* Amiodarone *on page 86*
- ◆ **PRO-Azithromycin (Can)** *see* Azithromycin *on page 169*

Probenecid (proe BEN e sid)

Canadian Brand Names Benuryl™
Index Terms Benemid [DSC]
Pharmacologic Category Uricosuric Agent
Use Prevention of hyperuricemia associated with gout or gouty arthritis; prolongation and elevation of beta-lactam plasma levels
Pharmacodynamics/Kinetics
Onset of action: Effect on penicillin levels: 2 hours
Absorption: Rapid and complete
Metabolism: Hepatic
Half-life elimination (dose dependent): Normal renal function: 6-12 hours
Time to peak, serum: 2-4 hours
Excretion: Urine
Dosage Oral:
Children:
<2 years: Contraindicated
2-14 years: Prolong penicillin serum levels: Initial: 25 mg/kg, then 40 mg/kg/day given 4 times/day (maximum: 500 mg/dose)
Gonorrhea: >45 kg: Refer to adult guidelines
Adults:
Hyperuricemia with gout: 250 mg twice daily for one week; increase to 250-500 mg/day; may increase by 500 mg/month, if needed, to maximum of 2-3 g/day (dosages may be increased by 500 mg every 6 months if serum urate concentrations are controlled)

Prolong penicillin serum levels: 500 mg 4 times/day

Gonorrhea: CDC guidelines (alternative regimen): Probenecid 1 g orally with cefoxitin 2 g I.M.

Pelvic inflammatory disease: CDC guidelines: Cefoxitin 2 g I.M. plus probenecid 1 g orally as a single dose

Neurosyphilis: CDC guidelines (alternative regimen): Procaine penicillin 2.4 million units/day I.M. plus probenecid 500 mg 4 times/day; both administered for 10-14 days

Dosing adjustment in renal impairment: Cl_{cr} <30 mL/minute: Avoid use

Additional Information Complete prescribing information for this medication should be consulted for additional detail.

Dosage Forms Excipient information presented when available (limited, particularly for generics); consult specific product labeling.
Tablet: 500 mg

♦ **PRO-Bisoprolol (Can)** *see* Bisoprolol *on page 192*

Procainamide (pro KANE a mide)

Medication Safety Issues
Sound-alike/look-alike issues:
Procanbid may be confused with probenecid, Procan SR®
Procan SR® may be confused with procanbid
Pronestyl may be confused with Ponstel®

High alert medication: The Institute for Safe Medication Practices (ISMP) includes this medication among its list of drugs which have a heightened risk of causing significant patient harm when used in error.

Procainamide hydrochloride is available in 10 mL vials of 100 mg/mL and in 2 mL vials with 500 mg/mL. Note that **BOTH** vials contain 1 gram of drug; confusing the strengths can lead to massive overdoses or underdoses.

PCA is an error-prone abbreviation (mistaken as patient controlled analgesia)

Related Information
Antiarrhythmic Drugs *on page 1656*
Chronic Renal Failure *on page 1552*
Dosing Considerations for the Critically-Ill Patient With Morbid Obesity *on page 1561*
Management of Postoperative Arrhythmias *on page 1571*

Canadian Brand Names Apo-Procainamide®; Procainamide Hydrochloride Injection, USP ; Procan SR®

Index Terms PCA (error-prone abbreviation); Procainamide Hydrochloride; Procaine Amide Hydrochloride; Procanbid; Pronestyl

Pharmacologic Category Antiarrhythmic Agent, Class Ia

Generic Available Yes

Use
Intravenous: Treatment of ventricular arrhythmias (eg, sustained ventricular tachycardia [VT]); **Note:** Due to proarrhythmic effects, use should be reserved for life-threatening arrhythmias

Oral (Canadian labeling; not available in U.S.): Treatment of supraventricular arrhythmias. **Note:** In the treatment of atrial fibrillation, use only when preferred treatment is ineffective or cannot be used. Use in paroxysmal atrial tachycardia when reflex stimulation or other measures are ineffective.

Unlabeled/Investigational Use
Paroxysmal supraventricular tachycardia (PSVT); prevent recurrence of ventricular tachycardia; symptomatic premature ventricular contractions

ACLS guidelines: I.V.: Treatment of the following arrhythmias in patients with preserved left ventricular function: Stable monomorphic VT; atrial fibrillation or atrial flutter, including pre-excitation syndrome; AV re-entrant narrow complex tachycardias (eg, re-entrant SVT), uncontrolled by adenosine and vagal maneuvers; and stable wide complex regular tachycardia (likely VT)

PALS guidelines: I.V.: Tachycardia with pulses and poor perfusion (probable SVT [unresponsive to vagal maneuvers and adenosine or synchronized cardioversion]; probable VT [unresponsive to synchronized cardioversion or adenosine])

Mechanism of Action Decreases myocardial excitability and conduction velocity and may depress myocardial contractility, by increasing the electrical stimulation threshold of ventricle, His-Purkinje system and through direct cardiac effects

Pharmacodynamics/Kinetics

Onset of action: I.M. 10-30 minutes

Distribution: V_d: Children: 2.2 L/kg; Adults: 2 L/kg; decreased with congestive heart failure or shock

Protein binding: 15% to 20%

Metabolism: Hepatic via acetylation to produce N-acetyl procainamide (NAPA) (active metabolite)

Half-life elimination:

Procainamide (hepatic acetylator, phenotype, cardiac and renal function dependent):

Children: 1.7 hours; Adults: 2.5-4.7 hours; Anephric: 11 hours

NAPA (dependent upon renal function):

Children: 6 hours; Adults: 6-8 hours; Anephric: 42 hours

Time to peak, serum: I.M.: 15-60 minutes

Excretion: Urine (30% to 60% unchanged procainamide; 6% to 52% as NAPA); feces (<5% unchanged procainamide. **Note:** >80% of formed NAPA is renally eliminated in contrast to procainamide which is ~50% renally eliminated (Gibson, 1977).

Dosage Must be titrated to patient's response

Children:

I.M.: 20-30 mg/kg/day divided every 4-6 hours; maximum: 4 g/day

I.V.:

Load: 3-6 mg/kg/dose over 5 minutes not to exceed 100 mg/dose; may repeat every 5-10 minutes to maximum of 15 mg/kg/load

Maintenance as continuous I.V. infusion: 20-80 mcg/kg/minute; maximum: 2 g/ 24 hours

Possible VT (pulses and poor perfusion) [PALS 2005 Guidelines]: I.V.; I.O.: 15 mg/kg over 30-60 minutes

Adults:

I.M.: 50 mg/kg/day divided every 3-6 hours **or** 0.5-1 g every 4-8 hours (Koch-Weser, 1971)

I.V.:

Loading dose: 15-18 mg/kg administered as slow infusion over 25-30 minutes **or** 100 mg/dose at a rate not to exceed 50 mg/minute repeated every 5 minutes as needed to a total dose of 1 g.

ACLS guidelines: Loading dose: Infuse 20 mg/minute (up to 50 mg/minute for more urgent situations) until arrhythmia is controlled, hypotension occurs, QRS complex widens by 50% of its original width, or total of 17 mg/kg is given; followed by continuous infusion of 1-4 mg/minute. **Note:** Not recommended for use in ongoing ventricular fibrillation (VF) or pulseless ventricular tachycardia (VT) due to prolonged administration time and uncertain efficacy.

Maintenance dose: 1-4 mg/minute by continuous infusion. Maintenance infusions should be reduced by one-third in patients with moderate renal or cardiac impairment and by two-thirds in patients with severe renal or cardiac impairment.

Oral (not available in the U.S.; Canadian labeling): Sustained release formulation (Procan SR®): Maintenance: 50 mg/kg/24 hours given in divided doses every 6 hours

Suggested Procan SR® maintenance dose:

<55 kg: 500 mg every 6 hours

55-91 kg: 750 mg every 6 hours

>91 kg: 1000 mg every 6 hours

Elderly: Initiate doses at lower end of dosage range.

Dosing interval in renal impairment:

Oral:

Cl_{cr} 10-50 mL/minute: Administer every 6-12 hours.

Cl_{cr} <10 mL/minute: Administer every 8-24 hours.

I.V.:

Loading dose: Reduce dose to 12 mg/kg in severe renal impairment.

Maintenance infusion: Reduce dose by one-third in patients with mild renal impairment. Reduce dose by two-thirds in patients with severe renal impairment.

Dialysis:

Procainamide: Moderately hemodialyzable (20% to 50%): Monitor procainamide/N-acetylprocainamide (NAPA) levels; supplementation may be necessary.

NAPA: Not dialyzable (0% to 5%)

Procainamide/NAPA: Not peritoneal dialyzable (0% to 5%)

Procainamide/NAPA: Replace by blood level during continuous arteriovenous or venovenous hemofiltration

Dosing adjustment in hepatic impairment: Reduce dose by 50%.

Stability Store undiluted vials at room temperature of 15°C to 30°C (59°F to 86°F). The solution is initially colorless but may turn slightly yellow on standing. Injection of air into the vial causes solution to darken. Discard solutions darker than light amber. Color formation may occur upon refrigeration.

Maximum concentration (loading dose only): 20 mg/mL

Maximum admixture concentration: 8 mg/mL

Usual admixture concentration: 1 g/250 mL NS/D_5W or 1 g/500 mL NS/D_5W

When admixed in NS or D_5W to a final concentration of 2-4 mg/mL, solution is stable at room temperature for 24 hours and for 7 days under refrigeration.

Some information indicates that procainamide may be subject to greater decomposition in D_5W unless the admixture is refrigerated or the pH is adjusted. Procainamide is believed to form an association complex with dextrose - the bioavailability of procainamide in this complex is not known and the complex formation is reversible (Raymond, 1988).

Administration

Oral: Do **not** crush or chew sustained release drug products (not available in the U.S.).

I.V.: Must dilute prior to I.V. administration. Loading dose: Maximum rate: 50 mg/minute

Monitoring Parameters ECG, blood pressure, renal function; with prolonged use monitor CBC with differential, platelet count; procainamide and NAPA blood levels in patients with hepatic impairment, renal impairment, or receiving constant infusion >3 mg/minute for longer than 24 hours; ANA titers

Reference Range

Timing of serum samples: Draw 6-12 hours after I.V. infusion has started; half-life is 2.5-5 hours

Therapeutic levels: Procainamide: 4-10 mcg/mL; NAPA 15-25 mcg/mL; Combined: 10-30 mcg/mL

Toxic concentration: Procainamide: >10-12 mcg/mL

Anesthesia and Critical Care Concerns/Other Considerations

Clinical Pearls/Comments: In patients with pre-existing cardiovascular disease, the incidence of proarrhythmia and mortality may be increased with Class Ia antiarrhythmic agents.

Procainamide may be used to pharmacologically convert atrial fibrillation to normal sinus rhythm. In this setting, it is important that AV nodal conduction be controlled (eg, digoxin, beta-blocker, calcium channel blocker) prior to cardioversion to inhibit procainamide-induced increases in ventricular response. Patients should be monitored (ECG and BP) in a controlled setting when initiating therapy.

Pregnancy Risk Factor C

Contraindications Hypersensitivity to procainamide, procaine, other ester-type local anesthetics, or any component of the formulation; complete heart block; second-degree AV block or various types of hemiblock (without a functional artificial pacemaker); SLE; torsade de pointes

Warnings/Precautions Monitor and adjust dose to prevent QT_c prolongation. Watch for proarrhythmic effects. May precipitate or exacerbate HF due to negative inotropic actions. Correct electrolyte disturbances, especially hypokalemia or hypomagnesemia, prior to use and throughout therapy. Reduce dosage in renal impairment. May increase ventricular response rate in patients with atrial fibrillation or flutter; control AV conduction before initiating. Correct hypokalemia before initiating therapy; hypokalemia may worsen toxicity. Reduce dose if first-degree heart block occurs. Use caution with concurrent use of other antiarrhythmics; may exacerbate or increase the risk of conduction disturbances. Avoid use in myasthenia gravis (may worsen condition). Use caution and dose cautiously; renal clearance of procainamide/NAPA declines in patients ≥50 years of age (independent of creatinine clearance reductions) and in the presence of concomitant renal impairment. This product contains sodium metabisulfite which may cause allergic-type reactions, including anaphylactic symptoms and life-threatening asthmatic episodes in susceptible people; this is seen more frequently in asthmatics.

[U.S. Boxed Warning]: Potentially fatal blood dyscrasias (eg, agranulocytosis) have occurred with therapeutic doses; weekly monitoring is recommended during the first 3 months of therapy and periodically thereafter. Discontinue procainamide if this occurs.

[U.S. Boxed Warning]: Long-term administration leads to the development of a positive antinuclear antibody (ANA) test in 50% of patients which may result in a drug-induced lupus erythematosus-like syndrome (in 20% to 30% of patients); discontinue procainamide with rising ANA titers or with SLE symptoms and choose an alternative agent.

[U.S. Boxed Warning] In the Cardiac Arrhythmia Suppression Trial (CAST), recent (>6 days but <2 years ago) myocardial infarction patients with asymptomatic, non-life-threatening ventricular arrhythmias did not benefit and may have been harmed by attempts to suppress the arrhythmia with flecainide or encainide. An increased mortality or nonfatal cardiac arrest rate (7.7%) was seen in the active treatment group compared with patients in the placebo group (3%). The applicability of the CAST results to other populations is unknown. Procainamide should be reserved for patients with life-threatening ventricular arrhythmias.

Adverse Reactions

>1%:

Cardiovascular: Hypotension (I.V. up to 5%)

Dermatologic: Rash

Gastrointestinal: Diarrhea (oral: 3% to 4%), nausea (oral: 3% to 4%), taste disorder (oral: 3% to 4%), vomiting (oral: 3% to 4%)

Miscellaneous: Positive ANA (≤50%), SLE-like syndrome (≤30%, increased incidence with long-term therapy or slow acetylators; syndrome may include abdominal pain, arthralgia, arthritis, chills, fever, hepatomegaly, myalgia, pericarditis, pleural effusion, pulmonary infiltrates, rash)

<1% (Limited to important or life-threatening): Agranulocytosis, alkaline phosphatase increased, angioedema, anorexia, aplastic anemia, arrhythmia exacerbated, arthralgia, asystole, bone marrow suppression, cerebellar ataxia, confusion, demyelinating polyradiculoneuropathy, disorientation, dizziness, drug fever, fever, first degree heart block, flushing, granulomatous hepatitis, hallucinations, hemolytic anemia, hepatic failure, hyperbilirubinemia, hypoplastic anemia, intrahepatic cholestasis, leukopenia, lightheadedness, maculopapular rash, mania, mental depression, myasthenia gravis worsened, myocardial contractility depressed, myocarditis, myopathy, neuromuscular blockade, neutropenia, pancreatitis, pancytopenia, paradoxical increase in ventricular rate in atrial fibrillation/flutter, peripheral/polyneuropathy, pleural effusion, positive Coombs' test, proarrhythmia, pseudo-obstruction, psychosis, pulmonary embolism, QT_c-interval prolongation, pruritus, rash, respiratory failure due to myopathy, second-degree heart block, tachycardia, thrombocytopenia, torsade de pointes, transaminases increased, urticaria, vasculitis, ventricular fibrillation, weakness

Drug Interactions

Metabolism/Transport Effects Substrate of CYP2D6 (major)

Avoid Concomitant Use

Avoid concomitant use of Procainamide with any of the following: Artemether; Dronedarone; Lumefantrine; Nilotinib; Pimozide; QuiNINE; Tetrabenazine; Thioridazine; Ziprasidone

◀ **Increased Effect/Toxicity**

Procainamide may increase the levels/effects of: Amiodarone; Dronedarone; Neuromuscular-Blocking Agents; Pimozide; QTc-Prolonging Agents; QuiNINE; Tetrabenazine; Thioridazine; Ziprasidone

The levels/effects of Procainamide may be increased by: Alfuzosin; Artemether; Chloroquine; Cimetidine; Ciprofloxacin; CYP2D6 Inhibitors (Moderate); CYP2D6 Inhibitors (Strong); Darunavir; Gadobutrol; Lumefantrine; Nilotinib; QuiNINE; Ranitidine; Trimethoprim

Decreased Effect

The levels/effects of Procainamide may be decreased by: Amiodarone; Peginterferon Alfa-2b

Ethanol/Nutrition/Herb Interactions

Ethanol: Avoid ethanol (acute ethanol administration reduces procainamide serum concentrations).

Herb/Nutraceutical: Avoid ephedra (may worsen arrhythmia).

Test Interactions In the presence of propranolol or suprapharmacologic concentrations of lidocaine or meprobamate, tests which depend on fluorescence to measure procainamide/NAPA concentrations may be affected.

Dosage Forms Excipient information presented when available (limited, particularly for generics); consult specific product labeling. [CAN] = Canadian brand name

Injection, solution, as hydrochloride: 100 mg/mL (10 mL); 500 mg/mL (2 mL) [contains sodium metabisulfite]

Tablet, sustained release, oral, as hydrochloride:

Procan SR® [CAN]: 250 mg, 500 mg, 750 mg [not available in U.S.]

References

"2005 American Heart Association Guidelines for Cardiopulmonary Resuscitation and Emergency Cardiovascular Care," *Circulation*, 2005, 112(24 Suppl): 1-211.

◆ **Procainamide Hydrochloride** *see* Procainamide *on page 1176*

◆ **Procainamide Hydrochloride Injection, USP (Can)** *see* Procainamide *on page 1176*

◆ **Procaine Amide Hydrochloride** *see* Procainamide *on page 1176*

◆ **Pro-Calcitonin (Can)** *see* Calcitonin *on page 226*

◆ **Procanbid** *see* Procainamide *on page 1176*

◆ **Procan SR® (Can)** *see* Procainamide *on page 1176*

◆ **Procardia®** *see* NIFEdipine *on page 1006*

◆ **Procardia XL®** *see* NIFEdipine *on page 1006*

◆ **Pro-Cefuroxime (Can)** *see* Cefuroxime *on page 272*

◆ **Procetofene** *see* Fenofibrate *on page 582*

◆ **Prochieve®** *see* Progesterone *on page 1184*

Prochlorperazine (proe klor PER a zeen)

Medication Safety Issues

Sound-alike/look-alike issues:

Prochlorperazine may be confused with chlorproMAZINE

Compazine® may be confused with Copaxone®, Coumadin®

CPZ (occasional abbreviation for Compazine®) is an error-prone abbreviation (mistaken as chlorpromazine)

Related Information

Postoperative Nausea and Vomiting *on page 1593*

U.S. Brand Names Compro™

Canadian Brand Names Apo-Prochlorperazine®; Nu-Prochlor; Stemetil®

Index Terms Chlormeprazine; Compazine; Prochlorperazine Edisylate; Prochlorperazine Maleate

Pharmacologic Category Antiemetic; Antipsychotic Agent, Typical, Phenothiazine

Generic Available Yes: Injection, tablet, suppository

Use Management of nausea and vomiting; psychotic disorders, including schizophrenia and anxiety

Unlabeled/Investigational Use Behavioral syndromes in dementia; psychosis/agitation related to Alzheimer's dementia

Mechanism of Action Prochlorperazine is a piperazine phenothiazine antipsychotic which blocks postsynaptic mesolimbic dopaminergic D_1 and D_2 receptors in the brain, including the chemoreceptor trigger zone; exhibits a strong alpha-adrenergic and anticholinergic blocking effect and depresses the release of hypothalamic and hypophyseal hormones; believed to depress the reticular activating system, thus affecting basal metabolism, body temperature, wakefulness, vasomotor tone and emesis

Pharmacodynamics/Kinetics

Onset of action: Oral: 30-40 minutes; I.M.: 10-20 minutes; Rectal: ~60 minutes
Peak antiemetic effect: I.V.: 30-60 minutes

Duration: Rectal: 12 hours; Oral: 3-4 hours; I.M., I.V.: Adults: 4-6 hours; I.M.: Children: 12 hours

Distribution: V_d: 1400-1548 L; crosses placenta; enters breast milk

Metabolism: Primarily hepatic; N-desmethyl prochlorperazine (major active metabolite)

Bioavailability: Oral: 12.5%

Half-life elimination: Oral: 6-10 hours (single dose), 14-22 hours (repeated dosing); I.V.: 6-10 hours

Dosage

Antiemetic: Children (therapy >1 day usually not required): **Note:** Not recommended for use in children <9 kg or <2 years:
Oral, rectal: >9 kg: 0.4 mg/kg/24 hours in 3-4 divided doses; **or**
9-13 kg: 2.5 mg every 12-24 hours as needed; maximum: 7.5 mg/day
13.1-17 kg: 2.5 mg every 8-12 hours as needed; maximum: 10 mg/day
17.1-37 kg: 2.5 mg every 8 hours or 5 mg every 12 hours as needed; maximum: 15 mg/day
I.M.: 0.13 mg/kg/dose; change to oral as soon as possible

Antiemetic: Adults:
Oral (tablet): 5-10 mg 3-4 times/day; usual maximum: 40 mg/day; larger doses may rarely be required
I.M. (deep): 5-10 mg every 3-4 hours; usual maximum: 40 mg/day
I.V.: 2.5-10 mg; maximum 10 mg/dose or 40 mg/day; may repeat dose every 3-4 hours as needed
Rectal: 25 mg twice daily

Surgical nausea/vomiting: Adults: **Note:** Should not exceed 40 mg/day
I.M.: 5-10 mg 1-2 hours before induction or to control symptoms during or after surgery; may repeat once if necessary
I.V. (administer slow IVP <5 mg/minute): 5-10 mg 15-30 minutes before induction or to control symptoms during or after surgery; may repeat once if necessary
Rectal (unlabeled use): 25 mg

Antipsychotic:
Children 2-12 years (not recommended in children <9 kg or <2 years):
Oral, rectal: 2.5 mg 2-3 times/day; do not give more than 10 mg the first day; increase dosage as needed to maximum daily dose of 20 mg for 2-5 years and 25 mg for 6-12 years
I.M.: 0.13 mg/kg/dose; change to oral as soon as possible
Adults:
Oral: 5-10 mg 3-4 times/day; titrate dose slowly every 2-3 days; doses up to 150 mg/day may be required in some patients for treatment of severe disturbances
I.M.: Initial: 10-20 mg; if necessary repeat initial dose every 1-4 hours to gain control; more than 3-4 doses are rarely needed. If parenteral administration is still required; give 10-20 mg every 4-6 hours; change to oral as soon as possible.

Nonpsychotic anxiety: Oral (tablet): Adults: Usual dose: 15-20 mg/day in divided doses; do not give doses >20 mg/day or for longer than 12 weeks

Elderly: Behavioral symptoms associated with dementia (unlabeled use): Initial: 2.5-5 mg 1-2 times/day; increase dose at 4- to 7-day intervals by 2.5-5 mg/day; increase dosing intervals (twice daily, 3 times/day, etc) as necessary to control response or side effects; maximum daily dose should probably not exceed 75 mg in elderly; gradual increases (titration) may prevent some side effects or decrease their severity

Stability

Injection: Store at <30°C (<86°F); do not freeze. Protect from light. Clear or slightly yellow solutions may be used.

I.V. infusion: Injection may be diluted in 50-100 mL NS or D_5W.

Suppository, tablet: Store at 15°C to 30°C (59°F to 86°F). Protect from light.

Administration May be administered orally, I.M., or I.V.

I.M.: Inject by deep IM into outer quadrant of buttocks.

I.V.: Doses should be given as a short (~30 minute) infusion to avoid orthostatic hypotension; administer at ≤5 mg/minute

Monitoring Parameters Vital signs; lipid profile, fasting blood glucose/Hgb A_{1c}; BMI; mental status, abnormal involuntary movement scale (AIMS); periodic ophthalmic exams (if chronically used); extrapyramidal symptoms (EPS)

Anesthesia and Critical Care Concerns/Other Considerations

Clinical Pearls/Comments: When compared with ondansetron (4 mg I.V.), prochlorperazine (10 mg I.M.) administered at the end of surgery more effectively reduced postoperative nausea and the need for rescue antiemetics in patients undergoing total hip or knee replacement. In patients undergoing tympanoplasty, prophylactic prochlorperazine (0.02 mg/kg I.M.) administered at the end of surgery was as effective as ondansetron (0.06 mg/kg I.V.) for reducing PONV.

Evidence-Based Information: Prochlorperazine has a faster onset of action and causes less sedation than promethazine.

Contraindications Hypersensitivity to prochlorperazine or any component of the formulation (cross-reactivity between phenothiazines may occur); severe CNS depression; coma; pediatric surgery; Reye's syndrome; should not be used in children <2 years of age or <9 kg

Warnings/Precautions [U.S. Boxed Warning]: Elderly patients with dementia-related psychosis treated with antipsychotics are at an increased risk of death compared to placebo. Most deaths appeared to be either cardiovascular (eg, heart failure, sudden death) or infectious (eg, pneumonia) in nature. Prochlorperazine is not approved for the treatment of dementia-related psychosis.

Leukopenia, neutropenia, and agranulocytosis (sometimes fatal) have been reported in clinical trials and postmarketing reports with antipsychotic use; presence of risk factors (eg, pre-existing low WBC or history of drug-induced leuko-/neutropenia) should prompt periodic blood count assessment. Discontinue therapy at first signs of blood dyscrasias or if absolute neutrophil count <1000/ mm^3.

May be sedating; use with caution in disorders where CNS depression is a feature. May obscure intestinal obstruction or brain tumor. May impair physical or mental abilities. Effects with other sedative drugs or ethanol may be potentiated. Use with caution in Parkinson's disease; hemodynamic instability; predisposition to seizures; subcortical brain damage; and in severe cardiac, hepatic, or renal disease. May alter temperature regulation or mask toxicity of other drugs. Use caution with exposure to heat. May alter cardiac conduction. May cause orthostatic hypotension. Hypotension may occur following administration, particularly when parenteral form is used or in high dosages. Antipsychotic use has been associated with esophageal dysmotility and aspiration; use with caution in patients at risk of pneumonia (ie, Alzheimer's disease).

May cause pigmentary retinopathy, and lenticular and corneal deposits, particularly with prolonged therapy. Use associated with increased prolactin levels; clinical significance of hyperprolactinemia in patients with breast cancer or other prolactin-dependent tumors is unknown.

Phenothiazines may cause anticholinergic effects; therefore, they should be used with caution in patients with decreased gastrointestinal motility, urinary retention, BPH, xerostomia, or visual problems. Conditions which also may be exacerbated by cholinergic blockade include narrow-angle glaucoma and worsening of myasthenia gravis. May cause extrapyramidal symptoms (EPS), including pseudoparkinsonism, acute dystonic reactions, akathisia, and tardive dyskinesia (risk of these reactions is high relative to other neuroleptics). Risk of dystonia (and possibly other EPS) may be greater with increased doses, use of conventional antipsychotics, males, and younger patients. Use caution in the elderly. Children with acute illness or dehydration are more susceptible to neuromuscular reactions; use cautiously. May be associated with neuroleptic malignant syndrome (NMS). Injection contains benzyl alcohol which has been associated with "gasping syndrome" in neonates.

Adverse Reactions Reported with prochlorperazine or other phenothiazines. Frequency not defined.

Cardiovascular: Cardiac arrest, hypotension, peripheral edema, Q-wave distortions, T-wave distortions

Central nervous system: Agitation, catatonia, cerebral edema, cough reflex suppressed, dizziness, drowsiness, fever (mild - I.M.), headache, hyperactivity, hyperpyrexia, impairment of temperature regulation, insomnia, neuroleptic malignant syndrome (NMS), paradoxical excitement, restlessness, seizure

Dermatologic: Angioedema, contact dermatitis, discoloration of skin (blue-gray), epithelial keratopathy, erythema, eczema, exfoliative dermatitis (injectable), itching, photosensitivity, rash, skin pigmentation, urticaria

Endocrine & metabolic: Amenorrhea, breast enlargement, galactorrhea, gynecomastia, glucosuria, hyperglycemia, hypoglycemia, lactation, libido (changes in), menstrual irregularity, SIADH

Gastrointestinal: Appetite increased, atonic colon, constipation, ileus, nausea, weight gain, xerostomia

Genitourinary: Ejaculating dysfunction, ejaculatory disturbances, impotence, incontinence, polyuria, priapism, urinary retention, urination difficulty

Hematologic: Agranulocytosis, aplastic anemia, eosinophilia, hemolytic anemia, leukopenia, pancytopenia, thrombocytopenic purpura

Hepatic: Biliary stasis, cholestatic jaundice, hepatotoxicity

Neuromuscular & skeletal: Dystonias (torticollis, opisthotonos, carpopedal spasm, trismus, oculogyric crisis, protusion of tongue); extrapyramidal symptoms (pseudoparkinsonism, akathisia, dystonias, tardive dyskinesia); SLE-like syndrome, tremor

Ocular: blurred vision, cornea and lens changes, lenticular/corneal deposits, miosis, mydriasis, pigmentary retinopathy

Respiratory: Asthma, laryngeal edema, nasal congestion

Miscellaneous: Allergic reactions, diaphoresis

Drug Interactions

Avoid Concomitant Use

Avoid concomitant use of Prochlorperazine with any of the following: Dofetilide

Increased Effect/Toxicity

Prochlorperazine may increase the levels/effects of: Alcohol (Ethyl); Analgesics (Opioid); Anticholinergics; Beta-Blockers; CNS Depressants; Dofetilide; Methotrimeprazine

The levels/effects of Prochlorperazine may be increased by: Acetylcholinesterase Inhibitors (Central); Antimalarial Agents; Beta-Blockers; Lithium formulations; Methotrimeprazine; Pramlintide; Tetrabenazine

Decreased Effect

Prochlorperazine may decrease the levels/effects of: Amphetamines; Anti-Parkinson's Agents (Dopamine Agonist)

The levels/effects of Prochlorperazine may be decreased by: Antacids; Lithium formulations

Ethanol/Nutrition/Herb Interactions

Ethanol: Avoid ethanol (may increase CNS depression).

Food: Limit caffeine.

Herb/Nutraceutical: Avoid dong quai, St John's wort (may also cause photosensitization). Avoid kava kava, gotu kola, valerian, St John's wort (may increase CNS depression).

Test Interactions False-positives for phenylketonuria, pregnancy, urinary amylase, uroporphyrins, urobilinogen

Dietary Considerations Increase dietary intake of riboflavin; should be administered with food or water. Rectal suppositories may contain coconut and palm oil.

◀ **Dosage Forms** Excipient information presented when available (limited, particularly for generics); consult specific product labeling.
Injection, solution, as edisylate: 5 mg/mL (2 mL, 10 mL) [contains benzyl alcohol]
Suppository, rectal: 25 mg (12s) [may contain coconut and palm oil]
  Compro™: 25 mg (12s) [contains coconut and palm oils]
Tablet, as maleate: 5 mg, 10 mg [strength expressed as base]

References

Gan TJ, Meyer TA, Apfel CC, et al, "Society for Ambulatory Anesthesia Guidelines for the Management of Postoperative Nausea and Vomiting," *Anesth Analg*, 2007, 105(6):1615-28.
Golembiewski J, Chernin E, and Chopra T, "Prevention and Treatment of Postoperative Nausea and Vomiting," *Am J Health-Syst Pharm*, 2005, 62:1247-60.

◆ **Prochlorperazine Edisylate** *see* Prochlorperazine *on page 1180*
◆ **Prochlorperazine Maleate** *see* Prochlorperazine *on page 1180*
◆ **PRO-Ciprofloxacin (Can)** *see* Ciprofloxacin *on page 306*
◆ **Pro-Clonazepam (Can)** *see* ClonazePAM *on page 328*
◆ **Procrit®** *see* Epoetin Alfa *on page 500*
◆ **Proctocort®** *see* Hydrocortisone *on page 699*
◆ **ProctoCream® HC** *see* Hydrocortisone *on page 699*
◆ **Proctofene** *see* Fenofibrate *on page 582*
◆ **Procto-Kit™** *see* Hydrocortisone *on page 699*
◆ **Procto-Pak™** *see* Hydrocortisone *on page 699*
◆ **Proctosert** *see* Hydrocortisone *on page 699*
◆ **Proctosol-HC®** *see* Hydrocortisone *on page 699*
◆ **Proctozone-HC™** *see* Hydrocortisone *on page 699*
◆ **Procytox® (Can)** *see* Cyclophosphamide *on page 354*
◆ **Pro-Diclo-Rapide (Can)** *see* Diclofenac *on page 414*
◆ **Pro-Enalapril (Can)** *see* Enalapril *on page 478*
◆ **Pro-Feno-Super (Can)** *see* Fenofibrate *on page 582*
◆ **Profilnine® SD** *see* Factor IX Complex (Human) *on page 573*
◆ **Pro-Fluconazole (Can)** *see* Fluconazole *on page 607*
◆ **PRO-Fluoxetine (Can)** *see* FLUoxetine *on page 616*
◆ **PRO-Gabapentin (Can)** *see* Gabapentin *on page 650*

Progesterone (proe JES ter one)

U.S. Brand Names Crinone®; Endometrin®; First™-Progesterone VGS; Prochieve®; Prometrium®
Canadian Brand Names Crinone®; Prometrium®
Index Terms Pregnenedione; Progestin
Pharmacologic Category Progestin
Use
  Oral: Prevention of endometrial hyperplasia in nonhysterectomized, postmenopausal women who are receiving conjugated estrogen tablets; secondary amenorrhea
  I.M.: Amenorrhea; abnormal uterine bleeding due to hormonal imbalance
  Intravaginal gel: Part of assisted reproductive technology (ART) for infertile women with progesterone deficiency; secondary amenorrhea
  Vaginal tablet: Part of ART for infertile women with progesterone deficiency
Pharmacodynamics/Kinetics
  Absorption: Vaginal gel: Prolonged
    Absorption half-life: 25-50 hours
  Protein binding: Albumin (50% to 54%) and cortisol-binding protein (43% to 48%)
  Metabolism: Hepatic to metabolites
  Half-life elimination: Vaginal gel: 5-20 minutes
  Time to peak: Oral: Within 3 hours; I.M.: ~8 hours; Vaginal tablet: ~17-24 hours
  Excretion: Urine, bile, feces

Dosage Adults:

I.M.: Females:

Amenorrhea: 5-10 mg/day for 6-8 consecutive days

Functional uterine bleeding: 5-10 mg/day for 6 doses

Oral: Females:

Prevention of endometrial hyperplasia (in postmenopausal women with a uterus who are receiving daily conjugated estrogen tablets): 200 mg as a single daily dose every evening for 12 days sequentially per 28-day cycle

Amenorrhea: 400 mg every evening for 10 days

Intravaginal gel: Females:

ART in women who require progesterone supplementation: 90 mg (8% gel) once daily; if pregnancy occurs, may continue treatment for up to 10-12 weeks

ART in women with partial or complete ovarian failure: 90 mg (8% gel) intravaginally twice daily; if pregnancy occurs, may continue up to 10-12 weeks

Secondary amenorrhea: 45 mg (4% gel) intravaginally every other day for up to 6 doses; women who fail to respond may be increased to 90 mg (8% gel) every other day for up to 6 doses

Intravaginal tablet: Females: ART: 100 mg 2-3 times daily starting at oocyte retrieval and continuing for up to 10 weeks.

Additional Information Complete prescribing information for this medication should be consulted for additional detail.

Dosage Forms Excipient information presented when available (limited, particularly for generics); consult specific product labeling.

Capsule:

Prometrium®: 100 mg, 200 mg [contains peanut oil]

Gel, vaginal:

Crinone®: 8% (1.45 g) [90 mg/dose; contains palm oil; 6 or 18 prefilled applicators]

Prochieve®: 4% (1.45 g) [45 mg/dose; contains palm oil; 6 prefilled applicators]; 8% (1.45 g) [90 mg/dose; contains palm oil; 6 or 18 prefilled applicators]

Injection, oil: 50 mg/mL (10 mL) [contains benzyl alcohol 10%, sesame oil]

Powder, for prescription compounding [micronized]: Progesterone USP (10 g, 25 g, 100 g, 1000 g)

Powder, for prescription compounding [wettable]: Progesterone USP (10 g, 25 g, 100 g, 1000 g)

First™-Progesterone VGS 25: Progesterone USP (0.75 g) [makes 30 progesterone 25 mg vaginal suppositories; kit contains fatty acid base, suppository mold, stirrer, filling tool, guide plate, mold cover with dispensing tool]

First™-Progesterone VGS 50: Progesterone USP (1.5 g) [makes 30 progesterone 50 mg vaginal suppositories; kit contains fatty acid base, suppository mold, stirrer, filling tool, guide plate, mold cover with dispensing tool]

First™-Progesterone VGS 100: Progesterone USP (3 g) [makes 30 progesterone 100 mg vaginal suppositories; kit contains fatty acid base, suppository mold, stirrer, filling tool, guide plate, mold cover with dispensing tool]

First™-Progesterone VGS 200: Progesterone USP (6 g) [makes 30 progesterone 200 mg vaginal suppositories; kit contains fatty acid base, suppository mold, stirrer, filling tool, guide plate, mold cover with dispensing tool]

First™-Progesterone VGS 400: Progesterone USP (12 g) [makes 30 progesterone 400 mg vaginal suppositories; kit contains fatty acid base, suppository mold, stirrer, filling tool, guide plate, mold cover with dispensing tool]

Tablet, vaginal:

Endometrin®: 100 mg (21s) [packaged with applicators]

References

"American Academy of Pediatrics Committee on Drugs. The Transfer of Drugs and Other Chemicals Into Human Milk," *Pediatrics*, 2001, 108(3):776-89.

American College of Obstetricians and Gynecologists, "ACOG Committee Opinion. Use of Progesterone to Reduce Preterm Birth," *Obstet Gynecol*, 2003, 102(5 Pt 1):1115-6.

Doody K, Shamma N, Paulson R, et al. "Endometrin® for Luteal Phase Support in a Randomized, Controlled, Open-Label, Prospective IVF Clinical Trial Using a Combination of Menopur® and Bravelle®," *Fertil Steril*, 2007, 87(4 Suppl 2):24 [abstract].

◀ Ng EH, Chan CC, Tang OS, et al, "A Randomized Comparison of Side Effects and Patient Convenience Between Cyclogest® Suppositories and Endometrin® Tablets Used for Luteal Phase Support in IVF Treatment," *Eur J Obstet Gynecol Reprod Biol*, 2007, 131(2):182-8.

◆ **Progestin** *see* Progesterone *on page 1184*
◆ **PRO-Glyburide (Can)** *see* GlyBURIDE *on page 666*
◆ **Prograf®** *see* Tacrolimus *on page 1338*
◆ **Pro-ISMN (Can)** *see* Isosorbide Mononitrate *on page 774*
◆ **Pro-Levocarb (Can)** *see* Levodopa and Carbidopa *on page 822*
◆ **Pro-Lisinopril (Can)** *see* Lisinopril *on page 849*
◆ **PRO-Lovastatin (Can)** *see* Lovastatin *on page 859*
◆ **Promacta®** *see* Eltrombopag *on page 477*
◆ **Pro-Metformin (Can)** *see* MetFORMIN *on page 886*

Promethazine (proe METH a zeen)

Medication Safety Issues
Sound-alike/look-alike issues:
Promethazine may be confused with chlorproMAZINE, predniSONE, promazine
Phenergan® may be confused with Phenaphen®, PHENobarbital, Phrenilin®, Theragran®

High alert medication: The Institute for Safe Medication Practices (ISMP) includes this medication (I.V. formulation) among its list of drugs which have a heightened risk of causing significant patient harm when used in error.

Administration issues:
To prevent or minimize tissue damage during I.V. administration, the Institute for Safe Medication Practices (ISMP) has the following recommendations:
Limit concentration available to the 25 mg/mL product
Consider limiting initial doses to 6.25-12.5 mg
Further dilute the 25 mg/mL strength into 10-20 mL NS
Administer through a large bore vein (not hand or wrist)
Administer via running I.V. line at port farthest from patient's vein
Consider administering over 10-15 minutes
Instruct patients to report immediately signs of pain or burning

Related Information
Postoperative Nausea and Vomiting *on page 1593*

U.S. Brand Names Phenadoz™; Phenergan®; Promethegan™

Canadian Brand Names Bioniche Promethazine; Histantil; Phenergan®; PMS-Promethazine

Index Terms Promethazine Hydrochloride

Pharmacologic Category Antiemetic; Histamine H_1 Antagonist; Histamine H_1 Antagonist, First Generation

Generic Available Yes

Use Symptomatic treatment of various allergic conditions; antiemetic; motion sickness; sedative

Mechanism of Action Blocks postsynaptic mesolimbic dopaminergic receptors in the brain; exhibits a strong alpha-adrenergic blocking effect and depresses the release of hypothalamic and hypophyseal hormones; competes with histamine for the H_1-receptor; muscarinic-blocking effect may be responsible for antiemetic activity; reduces stimuli to the brainstem reticular system

Pharmacodynamics/Kinetics
Onset of action: Oral, I.M.: ~20 minutes; I.V.: 3-5 minutes
Peak effect: C_{max}: 9.04 ng/mL (suppository); 19.3 ng/mL (syrup)
Duration: Usually 4-6 hours (up to 12 hours)
Absorption:
I.M.: Bioavailability may be greater than with oral or rectal administration
Oral: Rapid and complete; large first pass effect limits systemic bioavailability
Distribution: V_d: 171 L
Protein binding: 93%
Metabolism: Hepatic; primarily oxidation; forms metabolites
Half-life elimination: 9-16 hours

Time to maximum serum concentration: 4.4 hours (syrup); 6.7-8.6 hours (suppositories)

Excretion: Primarily urine and feces (as inactive metabolites)

Dosage

Children ≥2 years:

Allergic conditions: Oral, rectal: 0.1 mg/kg/dose (maximum: 12.5 mg) every 6 hours during the day and 0.5 mg/kg/dose (maximum: 25 mg) at bedtime as needed

Antiemetic: Oral, I.M., I.V., rectal: 0.25-1 mg/kg 4-6 times/day as needed (maximum: 25 mg/dose)

Motion sickness: Oral, rectal: 0.5 mg/kg/dose 30 minutes to 1 hour before departure, then every 12 hours as needed (maximum dose: 25 mg twice daily)

Sedation: Oral, I.M., I.V., rectal: 0.5-1 mg/kg/dose every 6 hours as needed (maximum: 50 mg/dose)

Adults:

Allergic conditions (including allergic reactions to blood or plasma):

Oral, rectal: 25 mg at bedtime **or** 12.5 mg before meals and at bedtime (range: 6.25-12.5 mg 3 times/day)

I.M., I.V.: 25 mg, may repeat in 2 hours when necessary; switch to oral route as soon as feasible

Antiemetic: Oral, I.M., I.V., rectal: 12.5-25 mg every 4-6 hours as needed

Motion sickness: Oral, rectal: 25 mg 30-60 minutes before departure, then every 12 hours as needed

Sedation: Oral, I.M., I.V., rectal: 12.5-50 mg/dose

Stability

Injection: Prior to dilution, store at room temperature. Protect from light. Solutions in NS or D_5W are stable for 24 hours at room temperature.

Suppositories: Store refrigerated at 2°C to 8°C (36°F to 46°F).

Tablets, oral solution: Store at room temperature. Protect from light.

Administration Formulations available for oral, rectal, I.M./I.V.; not for SubQ or intra-arterial administration. Administer I.M. into deep muscle (preferred route of administration). I.V. administration is **not** the preferred route; severe tissue damage may occur. Solution for injection should be administered in a maximum concentration of 25 mg/mL (more dilute solutions are recommended). Administer via running I.V. line at port farthest from patient's vein, or through a large bore vein (not hand or wrist). Consider administering over 10-15 minutes (maximum: 25 mg/minute). Discontinue immediately if burning or pain occurs with administration.

Monitoring Parameters Relief of symptoms, mental status

Pregnancy Risk Factor C

Contraindications Hypersensitivity to promethazine or any component of the formulation (cross-reactivity between phenothiazines may occur); coma; treatment of lower respiratory tract symptoms, including asthma; children <2 years of age

Warnings/Precautions [U.S. Boxed Warning]: Respiratory fatalities have been reported in children <2 years of age. Contraindicated in children <2 years of age. In children ≥2 years, use the lowest possible dose; other drugs with respiratory depressant effects should be avoided. Not for SubQ or intra-arterial administration. Injection may contain sodium metabisulfite. I.M. is the preferred route of parenteral administration. I.V. use has been associated with severe tissue damage; follow specific administration techniques to minimize risk; discontinue immediately if burning or pain occurs with administration. May be sedating; use with caution in disorders where CNS depression is a feature. May impair physical or mental abilities; patients must be cautioned about performing tasks which require mental alertness. Use with caution in Parkinson's disease; hemodynamic instability; bone marrow suppression; subcortical brain damage; and in severe cardiac, hepatic or respiratory disease. Avoid use in Reye's syndrome. May lower seizure threshold; use caution in persons with seizure disorders or in persons using narcotics or local anesthetics which may also affect seizure threshold. May alter temperature regulation or mask toxicity of other drugs due to antiemetic effects. May alter cardiac conduction (life-threatening arrhythmias have occurred with therapeutic doses of phenothiazines). May cause orthostatic hypotension; use with caution in patients at risk of hypotension or where transient hypotensive episodes would be poorly tolerated (cardiovascular disease or cerebrovascular disease).

◀ Phenothiazines may cause anticholinergic effects; therefore, they should be used with caution in patients with decreased gastrointestinal motility, GI or GU obstruction, urinary retention, BPH, xerostomia, or visual problems. Conditions which also may be exacerbated by cholinergic blockade include narrow-angle glaucoma (screening is recommended) and worsening of myasthenia gravis. May cause extrapyramidal symptoms, including pseudoparkinsonism, acute dystonic reactions, akathisia, and tardive dyskinesia. May be associated with neuroleptic malignant syndrome (NMS). Use cautiously in the elderly.

Adverse Reactions

Cardiovascular: Bradycardia, hypertension, nonspecific QT changes, postural hypotension, tachycardia

Central nervous system: Akathisia, catatonic states, confusion, delirium, disorientation, dizziness, drowsiness, dystonias, euphoria, excitation, extrapyramidal symptoms, fatigue, hallucinations, hysteria, insomnia, lassitude, nervousness, neuroleptic malignant syndrome, nightmares, pseudoparkinsonism, sedation, seizure, somnolence, tardive dyskinesia

Dermatologic: Angioneurotic edema, dermatitis, photosensitivity, skin pigmentation (slate gray), urticaria

Endocrine & metabolic: Amenorrhea, breast engorgement, gynecomastia, hyperglycemia, lactation

Gastrointestinal: Constipation, nausea, vomiting, xerostomia

Genitourinary: Ejaculatory disorder, impotence, urinary retention

Hematologic: Agranulocytosis, aplastic anemia, eosinophilia, hemolytic anemia, leukopenia, thrombocytopenia, thrombocytopenic purpura

Hepatic: Jaundice

Local: Venous thrombosis; injection site reactions (burning, erythema, pain, edema)

Neuromuscular & skeletal: Incoordination, tremor

Ocular: Blurred vision, corneal and lenticular changes, diplopia, epithelial keratopathy, pigmentary retinopathy

Otic: Tinnitus

Respiratory: Apnea, asthma, nasal congestion, respiratory depression

Drug Interactions

Metabolism/Transport Effects Substrate (major) of CYP2B6, 2D6; **Inhibits** CYP2D6 (weak)

Avoid Concomitant Use

Avoid concomitant use of Promethazine with any of the following: Sibutramine

Increased Effect/Toxicity

Promethazine may increase the levels/effects of: Anticholinergics; Serotonin Modulators

The levels/effects of Promethazine may be increased by: CYP2B6 Inhibitors (Moderate); CYP2B6 Inhibitors (Strong); CYP2D6 Inhibitors (Moderate); CYP2D6 Inhibitors (Strong); Darunavir; MAO Inhibitors; Pramlintide; Sibutramine

Decreased Effect

Promethazine may decrease the levels/effects of: Acetylcholinesterase Inhibitors (Central)

The levels/effects of Promethazine may be decreased by: Acetylcholinesterase Inhibitors (Central); CYP2B6 Inducers (Strong); Peginterferon Alfa-2b

Ethanol/Nutrition/Herb Interactions

Ethanol: Avoid ethanol (may increase CNS depression).

Herb/Nutraceutical: Avoid valerian, St John's wort, kava kava, gotu kola (may increase CNS depression).

Test Interactions Alters the flare response in intradermal allergen tests; hCG-based pregnancy tests may result in false-negatives or false-positives

Dietary Considerations Increase dietary intake of riboflavin.

Dosage Forms Excipient information presented when available (limited, particularly for generics); consult specific product labeling.

Injection, solution, as hydrochloride: 25 mg/mL (1 mL); 50 mg/mL (1 mL)

Phenergan®: 25 mg/mL (1 mL); 50 mg/mL (1 mL) [contains edetate disodium, sodium metabisulfite]

Suppository, rectal, as hydrochloride: 12.5 mg (12s); 25 mg (12s)
  Phenadoz™: 12.5 mg (12s); 25 mg (12s)
  Promethegan™: 12.5 mg (12s); 25 mg (12s); 50 mg (12s)
Syrup, as hydrochloride: 6.25 mg/5 mL (120 mL, 480 mL)
Tablet, as hydrochloride: 12.5 mg, 25 mg, 50 mg

♦ **Promethazine Hydrochloride** *see* Promethazine *on page 1186*
♦ **Promethegan™** *see* Promethazine *on page 1186*
♦ **Prometrium®** *see* Progesterone *on page 1184*
♦ **Pro-Naproxen EC (Can)** *see* Naproxen *on page 987*
♦ **Pronestyl** *see* Procainamide *on page 1176*

Propafenone (pro PAF en one)

Related Information
  Antiarrhythmic Drugs *on page 1656*
U.S. Brand Names Rythmol®; Rythmol® SR
Canadian Brand Names Apo-Propafenone®; Mylan-Propafenone; PMS-Propafenone; Rythmol® Gen-Propafenone
Index Terms Propafenone Hydrochloride
Pharmacologic Category Antiarrhythmic Agent, Class Ic
Use Treatment of life-threatening ventricular arrhythmias
  Rythmol® SR: Maintenance of normal sinus rhythm in patients with symptomatic atrial fibrillation
Unlabeled/Investigational Use Supraventricular tachycardias, including those patients with Wolff-Parkinson-White syndrome
Pharmacodynamics/Kinetics
  Absorption: Well absorbed
  Distribution: V_d: Adults: 2-5 L/kg
  Protein binding: 85% to 95%
  Metabolism: Hepatic; two genetically determined metabolism groups exist (extensive and poor metabolizers); 10% of Caucasians are poor metabolizers. Exhibits nonlinear pharmacokinetics; when dose is increased from 300-900 mg/day, serum concentrations increase tenfold; this nonlinearity is thought to be due to saturable first-pass effect.
  Bioavailability: 150 mg: 3.4%; 300 mg: 10.6%
  Half-life elimination: Extensive metabolizers: 2-10 hours; Poor metabolizers: 10-32 hours
  Time to peak, serum: 3.5 hours
Dosage Oral: Adults: **Note:** Patients who exhibit significant widening of QRS complex or second- or third-degree AV block may need dose reduction.
  Ventricular arrhythmias:
    Immediate release tablet: Initial: 150 mg every 8 hours, increase at 3- to 4-day intervals up to 300 mg every 8 hours.
    Extended release capsule: Initial: 225 mg every 12 hours; dosage increase may be made at a minimum of 5-day intervals; may increase to 325 mg every 12 hours; if further increase is necessary, may increase to 425 mg every 12 hours
  Paroxysmal atrial fibrillation (unlabeled dose): Immediate release tablet: Outpatient: "Pill-in-the-pocket" dose: 450 mg (weight <70 kg); 600 mg (weight ≥70 kg). May not repeat in ≤24 hours. **Note:** An initial inpatient conversion trial should have been successful before sending patient home on this approach. Patient must be taking an AV nodal-blocking agent (eg, beta-blocker, nondihydropyridine calcium channel blocker) prior to initiation of antiarrhythmic.

Dosing adjustment in hepatic impairment: Reduction is necessary; however, specific guidelines are not available.
Anesthesia and Critical Care Concerns/Other Considerations As with other class 1c agents, avoid use in patients with cardiovascular disease.
Additional Information Complete prescribing information for this medication should be consulted for additional detail.
Dosage Forms Excipient information presented when available (limited, particularly for generics); consult specific product labeling.

◀ Capsule, extended release, as hydrochloride (Rythmol® SR): 225 mg, 325 mg, 425 mg [contains soy lecithin]

Tablet, as hydrochloride (Rythmol®): 150 mg, 225 mg, 300 mg

◆ **Propafenone Hydrochloride** see Propafenone on page 1189

◆ **Propecia®** see Finasteride on page 604

◆ **Pro-Piroxicam (Can)** see Piroxicam on page 1139

Propofol (PROE po fole)

Medication Safety Issues

Sound-alike/look-alike issues:

Diprivan® may be confused with Diflucan®, Ditropan®

Propofol may be confused with fospropofol

High alert medication: The Institute for Safe Medication Practices (ISMP) includes this medication among its list of drugs which have a heightened risk of causing significant patient harm when used in error.

Related Information

Allergic Reactions on page 1508
Anesthesia Considerations for Neurosurgery on page 1514
Anesthesia for Geriatric Patients on page 1523
Anesthesia for Patients With Liver Disease on page 1537
Anesthetic Considerations in the Substance-Abusing Patient on page 1613
Dosing Considerations for the Critically-Ill Patient With Morbid Obesity on page 1561
Inhalational Anesthetics on page 1632
Intravenous Anesthetic Agents on page 1635
Moderate Sedation on page 1566
Postoperative Nausea and Vomiting on page 1593
Sedative Agents in the Intensive Care Unit on page 1690
Status Epilepticus on page 1737

U.S. Brand Names Diprivan®

Canadian Brand Names Diprivan®

Pharmacologic Category General Anesthetic

Generic Available Yes

Use Induction of anesthesia in patients ≥3 years of age; maintenance of anesthesia in patients >2 months of age; in adults, for monitored anesthesia care sedation during procedures; sedation in intubated, mechanically-ventilated ICU patients

Unlabeled/Investigational Use Postoperative antiemetic; refractory delirium tremens (case reports)

Mechanism of Action Propofol is a sterically hindered, alkyl-phenolic compound with intravenous general anesthetic properties. The drug is unrelated to any of the currently used barbiturate, opioid, benzodiazepine, arylcyclohexylamine, or imidazole intravenous anesthetic agents.

Pharmacodynamics/Kinetics

Onset of action: Anesthetic: Bolus infusion (dose dependent): 9-51 seconds (average 30 seconds)

Duration (dose and rate dependent): 3-10 minutes

Distribution: V_d: 2-10 L/kg; after a 10-day infusion, V_d approaches 60 L/kg; decreased in the elderly

Protein binding: 97% to 99%

Metabolism: Hepatic to water-soluble sulfate and glucuronide conjugates (~50%)

Half-life elimination: Biphasic: Initial: 40 minutes; Terminal: 4-7 hours (after 10-day infusion, may be up to 1-3 days)

Excretion: Urine (~88% as metabolites, 40% as glucuronide metabolite); feces (<2%)

Dosage Dosage must be individualized based on total body weight and titrated to the desired clinical effect; wait at least 3-5 minutes between dosage adjustments to clinically assess drug effects; smaller doses are required when used with narcotics; the following are general dosing guidelines:

General anesthesia:

Induction: I.V.:

Children (healthy) 3-16 years, ASA-PS 1 or 2: 2.5-3.5 mg/kg over 20-30 seconds; use a lower dose for children ASA-PS 3 or 4

Adults (healthy), ASA-PS 1 or 2, <55 years: 2-2.5 mg/kg (~40 mg every 10 seconds until onset of induction)

Elderly, debilitated, or ASA-PS 3 or 4: 1-1.5 mg/kg (~20 mg every 10 seconds until onset of induction); **do not use rapid bolus dose (single or repeated)**

Maintenance: I.V. infusion:

Children (healthy) 2 months to 16 years, ASA-PS 1 or 2: Initial: 200-300 mcg/kg/minute; after 30 minutes, if clinical signs of light anesthesia are absent, decrease the infusion rate; usual infusion rate: 125-150 mcg/kg/minute (range: 125-300 mcg/kg/minute); children ≤5 years may require larger infusion rates compared to older children

Adults (healthy), ASA-PS 1 or 2, <55 years: Initial: 100-200 mcg/kg/minute for 10-15 minutes; decrease by 30% to 50% during first 30 minutes of maintenance; usual infusion rate: 50-100 mcg/kg/minute to optimize recovery time

Elderly, debilitated, ASA-PS 3 or 4: 50-100 mcg/kg/minute

Maintenance: I.V. intermittent bolus: Adults (healthy), ASA-PS 1 or 2, <55 years: 25-50 mg increments as needed

Monitored anesthesia care sedation:

Initiation:

Adults (healthy), ASA-PS 1 or 2, <55 years: Slow I.V. infusion: 100-150 mcg/kg/minute for 3-5 minutes **or** slow injection: 0.5 mg/kg over 3-5 minutes

Elderly, debilitated, or ASA-PS 3 or 4 patients: Use 80% of healthy adult dose; **do not use rapid bolus doses (single or repeated)**

Maintenance:

Adults (healthy), ASA-PS 1 or 2, <55 years: I.V. infusion using variable rates (preferred over intermittent boluses): 25-75 mcg/kg/minute **or** incremental bolus doses: 10 mg or 20 mg

Elderly, debilitated, or ASA-PS 3 or 4 patients: Use 80% of healthy adult dose; **do not use rapid bolus doses (single or repeated)**

ICU sedation in intubated mechanically-ventilated patients: Avoid rapid bolus injection; individualize dose and titrate to response. Continuous infusion: Initial: 5 mcg/kg/minute; increase by 5-10 mcg/kg/minute every 5-10 minutes until desired sedation level is achieved (Jacobi, 2002); usual maintenance (Jacobi, 2002): 5-80 mcg/kg/minute; use 80% of healthy adult dose in elderly, debilitated, and ASA-PS 3 or 4 patients; reduce dose after adequate sedation established and adjust to response (eg, evaluate frequently to use minimum dose for sedation). Daily interruption with retitration is recommended to minimize prolonged sedative effects (Jacobi, 2002).

Postoperative nausea and vomiting (PONV), rescue therapy (unlabeled use; Gan, 2007; Unlugenc, 2004): Adults: I.V.: 20 mg, may be repeated

Refractory status epilepticus (unlabeled use): Adults: 1-2 mg/kg bolus, then 1.5-10 mg/kg/hour (intubation required)

Stability Store between 4°C to 22°C (40°F to 72°F); refrigeration is not required. Do not freeze. Protect from light. If transferred to a syringe or other container prior to administration, use within 6 hours. If used directly from vial/prefilled syringe, use within 12 hours. Shake well before use. Do not use if there is evidence of separation of phases of emulsion.

Does not need to be diluted; however, propofol may be further diluted in 5% dextrose in water to a concentration of ≥2 mg/mL and is stable for 8 hours at room temperature.

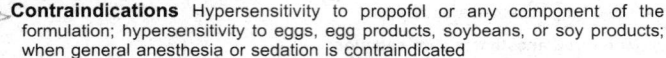

Administration Strict aseptic technique must be maintained in handling although a preservative has been added. Do not use if contamination is suspected. Do not administer through the same I.V. catheter with blood or plasma. Tubing and any unused portions of propofol vials should be discarded after 12 hours.

To reduce pain associated with injection, use larger veins of forearm or antecubital fossa; lidocaine I.V. (1 mL of a 1% solution) may also be used prior to administration or it may be added to propofol immediately before administration in a quantity not to exceed 20 mg lidocaine per 200 mg propofol. Do not use filter <5 micron for administration.

Monitoring Parameters Cardiac monitor, blood pressure, oxygen saturation (during monitored anesthesia care sedation), arterial blood gas (with prolonged infusions). With prolonged infusions (eg, ICU sedation), monitor for metabolic acidosis, hyperkalemia, rhabdomyolysis or elevated CPK, hepatomegaly, and progression of cardiac and renal failure.

ICU sedation: Assess and adjust sedation according to scoring system; assess CNS function daily. Serum triglyceride levels should be obtained prior to initiation of therapy and every 3-7 days thereafter, especially if receiving for >48 hours with doses exceeding 50 mcg/kg/minute (Devlin, 2005); use intravenous port opposite propofol infusion or temporarily suspend infusion and flush port prior to blood draw.

Diprivan®: Monitor zinc levels in patients predisposed to deficiency (burns, diarrhea, major sepsis) or after 5 days of treatment.

Pregnancy Risk Factor B

Contraindications Hypersensitivity to propofol or any component of the formulation; hypersensitivity to eggs, egg products, soybeans, or soy products; when general anesthesia or sedation is contraindicated

Warnings/Precautions May rarely cause hypersensitivity, anaphylaxis, anaphylactoid reactions, angioedema, bronchospasm, and erythema; medications for the treatment of hypersensitivity reactions should be available for immediate use. The major cardiovascular effect of propofol is hypotension especially if patient is hypovolemic or if bolus dosing is used; use with caution in patients who are hemodynamically unstable, hypovolemic, or have abnormally low vascular tone (eg, sepsis). Use requires careful patient monitoring, should only be used by experienced personnel who are not actively engaged in the procedure or surgery. If used in a nonintubated and/or nonmechanically-ventilated patient, qualified personnel and appropriate equipment for rapid institution of respiratory and/or cardiovascular support must be immediately available. Use to induce moderate (conscious) sedation in patients warrants monitoring equivalent to that seen with deep anesthesia.

Use a lower induction dose, a slower maintenance rate of administration, and avoid rapidly administered boluses in the elderly, debilitated, or ASA-PS (American Society of Anesthesiologists - Physical Status) 3/4 patients to reduce the incidence of unwanted cardiorespiratory depressive events. Use caution in patients with severe cardiac disease (ejection fraction <50%) or respiratory disease; may have more profound adverse cardiovascular responses to propofol. Use caution in patients with a history of epilepsy or seizures; seizure may occur during recovery phase. Use caution in patients with increased intracranial pressure or impaired cerebral circulation; substantial decreases in mean arterial pressure and subsequent decreases in cerebral perfusion pressure may occur; consider continuous infusion or administer as a slow bolus.

Propofol-related infusion syndrome is a serious side effect with a high mortality rate characterized by dysrhythmia (eg, bradycardia or tachycardia), heart failure, hyperkalemia, lipemia, metabolic acidosis, and/or rhabdomyolysis or myoglobinuria with subsequent renal failure. Risk factors include poor oxygen delivery, sepsis, serious cerebral injury, and the administration of high doses of propofol (usually doses >83 mcg/kg/minute or >5 mg/kg/hour for >48 hours), but has also been reported following large dose, short term infusions during surgical anesthesia. The onset of the syndrome is rapid, occurring within 4 days of initiation. Alternate sedative therapy should be considered for patients with escalating doses of vasopressors or inotropes, when cardiac failure occurs during high-dose propofol infusion, when metabolic acidosis is observed, or in whom lengthy and/or high-dose sedation is needed.

Because propofol is formulated within a 10% fat emulsion, hypertriglyceridemia is an expected side effect. Patients who develop hypertriglyceridemia (eg, >500 mg/dL) are at risk of developing pancreatitis. An alternative sedative agent should be employed if significant hypertriglyceridemia occurs. Use with caution in patients with preexisting pancreatitis; use of propofol may exacerbate this condition. Use caution in patients with preexisting hyperlipidemia as evidenced by increased serum triglyceride levels or serum turbidity. Transient local pain may occur during I.V. injection; perioperative myoclonia has occurred. Propofol should only be used in pregnancy if clearly needed. Not recommended for use in obstetrics, including cesarean section deliveries. Safety and efficacy in pediatric intensive care unit patients have not been established. Concurrent use of fentanyl and propofol in pediatric patients may result in bradycardia.

Concomitant use may lead to increased sedative or anesthetic effects of propofol, more pronounced decreases in systolic, diastolic, and mean arterial pressures and cardiac output. Lower doses of propofol may be needed. In addition, fentanyl may cause serious bradycardia when used with propofol in pediatric patients. Alfentanil use with propofol has precipitated seizure activity in patients without any history of epilepsy. Discontinue opioids and paralytic agents prior to weaning. Avoid abrupt discontinuation prior to weaning or daily wake up assessments. Abrupt discontinuation can result in rapid awakening, anxiety, agitation, and resistance to mechanical ventilation; wean the infusion rate so the patient awakens slowly. Propofol lacks analgesic properties; pain management requires specific use of analgesic agents, at effective dosages, propofol must be titrated separately from the analgesic agent.

Propofol vials and prefilled syringes have the potential to support the growth of various microorganisms despite product additives intended to suppress microbial growth. To limit the potential for contamination, recommendations in product labeling for handling and administering propofol should be strictly adhered to. Some formulations may contain edetate disodium which may lead to decreased zinc levels in patients with prolonged therapy (>5 days) or a predisposition to zinc deficiency (eg, burns, diarrhea, or sepsis). A holiday from propofol infusion should take place after 5 days of therapy to allow for evaluation and necessary replacement of zinc. Some formulations may contain sulfites. Some products may contain benzyl alcohol; benzyl alcohol has been associated with the "gasping syndrome" in neonates and low-birth-weight infants.

Adverse Reactions

>10%:
  Cardiovascular: Hypotension (children 17%; adults 3% to 26%)
  Central nervous system: Movement (children 17%; adults 3% to 10%)
  Local: Injection site burning, stinging, or pain (children 10%; adults 18%)
  Respiratory: Apnea lasting 30-60 seconds (children 10%; adults 24%), apnea lasting >60 seconds (children 5%; adults 12%)

1% to 10%:
  Cardiovascular: Hypertension (children 8%), arrhythmia (1% to 3%), bradycardia (1% to 3%), cardiac output decreased (1% to 3%; concurrent opioid use increases incidence), tachycardia (1% to 3%)
  Dermatologic: Pruritus (1% to 3%), rash (children 5%; adults 1% to 3%)
  Endocrine & metabolic: Hypertriglyceridemia (3% to 10%)
  Respiratory: Respiratory acidosis during weaning (3% to 10%)

<1% (Limited to important or life-threatening): Agitation, amblyopia, anaphylaxis, anaphylactoid reaction, anticholinergic syndrome, asystole, atrial arrhythmia, bigeminy, cardiac arrest, chills, cough, dizziness, delirium, discoloration (green [urine, hair, or nailbeds]), extremity pain, fever, flushing, hemorrhage, hyper-salivation, hypertonia, hypomagnesemia, hypoxia, infusion site reactions (including pain, swelling, blisters and/or tissue necrosis following accidental extravasation); laryngospasm, leukocytosis, lung function decreased, myalgia, myoclonia (rarely including convulsions and opisthotonos), nausea, pancreatitis, paresthesia, phlebitis, postoperative unconsciousness with or without increase in muscle tone, premature atrial contractions, premature ventricular contractions,

pulmonary edema, propofol-related infusion syndrome, rhabdomyolysis, somnolence, syncope, thrombosis, urine cloudy, vision abnormality, wheezing

Drug Interactions

Metabolism/Transport Effects Substrate of CYP1A2 (minor), 2A6 (minor), 2B6 (major), 2C9 (major), 2C19 (minor), 2D6 (minor), 2E1 (minor), 3A4 (minor); **Inhibits** CYP1A2 (moderate), 2C9 (weak), 2C19 (moderate), 2D6 (weak), 2E1 (weak), 3A4 (strong)

Avoid Concomitant Use There are no known interactions where it is recommended to avoid concomitant use.

Increased Effect/Toxicity

Propofol may increase the levels/effects of: Ropivacaine

The levels/effects of Propofol may be increased by: Alfentanil; CYP2B6 Inhibitors (Moderate); CYP2B6 Inhibitors (Strong)

Decreased Effect

The levels/effects of Propofol may be decreased by: Peginterferon Alfa-2b

Ethanol/Nutrition/Herb Interactions Food: Edetate disodium, an ingredient of propofol emulsion, may lead to decreased zinc levels in patients on prolonged therapy (>5 days) or those predisposed to deficiency (burns, diarrhea, and/or major sepsis).

Dietary Considerations Propofol is formulated in an oil-in-water emulsion. If on parenteral nutrition, may need to adjust the amount of lipid infused. Propofol emulsion contains 1.1 kcal/mL. Soybean fat emulsion is used as a vehicle for propofol. Formulations also contain egg phosphatide and glycerol.

Dosage Forms Excipient information presented when available (limited, particularly for generics); consult specific product labeling.

Injection, emulsion: 10 mg/mL (20 mL, 50 mL, 100 mL) [products may contain egg lecithin, and soybean oil; may contain benzyl alcohol, sodium benzoate, or sodium metabisulfite]

Diprivan®: 10 mg/mL (20 mL, 50 mL, 100 mL) [contains egg lecithin, soybean oil, and disodium edetate]

References

Burow BK, Johnson ME, and Packer DL, "Metabolic Acidosis Associated With Propofol in the Absence of Other Causative Factors," *Anesthesiology*, 2004, 101(1):239-41.

Cawley MJ, Guse TM, Laroia A, et al, "Propofol Withdrawal Syndrome in an Adult Patient With Thermal Injury," *Pharmacotherapy*, 2003, 23(7):933-9.

Corbett SM, Moore J, Rebuck JA, et al, "Survival of Propofol Infusion Syndrome in a Head-Injured Patient," *Crit Care Med*, 2006, 34(9):2479-83.

Ernest D and French C, "Propofol Infusion Syndrome - Report of an Adult Fatality," *Anaesth Intensive Care*, 2003, 31(3):316-9.

Funston JS and Prough DS, "Two Reports of Propofol Anesthesia Associated With Metabolic Acidosis in Adults," *Anesthesiology*, 2004, 101(1):6-8.

Gan TJ, Meyer TA, Apfel CC, et al, "Society for Ambulatory Anesthesia Guidelines for the Management of Postoperative Nausea and Vomiting," *Anesth Analg*, 2007, 105(6):1615-28.

Jacobi J, Fraser GL, Coursin DB, et al, "Clinical Practice Guidelines for the Sustained Use of Sedatives and Analgesics in the Critically Ill Adult," *Crit Care Med*, 2002, 30(1):119-41. Available at: http://www.sccm.org/pdf/sedatives.pdf.

Kang TM, "Propofol Infusion Syndrome in Critically Ill Patients," *Ann Pharmacother*, 2002, 36 (9):1453-6.

Kress JP, Pohlman AS, O'Connor MF, et al, "Daily Interruption of Sedative Infusions in Critically Ill Patients Undergoing Mechanical Ventilation," *N Engl J Med*, 2000, 342(20):1471-7.

McCowan C and Marik P, "Refractory Delirium Tremens Treated With Propofol: A Case Series," *Crit Care Med*, 2000, 28(6):1781-4.

Salengros JC, Velghe-Lenelle CE, Bollens R, et al, "Lactic Acidosis During Propofol-Remifentanil Anesthesia in an Adult," *Anesthesiology*, 2004, 101(1):241-3.

Short TG and Young Y, "Toxicity of Intravenous Anaesthetics," *Best Pract Res Clin Anaesthesiol*, 2003, 17(1):77-89.

Unlugenc H, Guler T, Gunes Y, et al, "Comparative Study of the Antiemetic Efficacy of Ondansetron, Propofol and Midazolam in the Early Postoperative Period," *Eur J Anaesthesiol*, 2004, 21(1):60-5.

Propoxyphene (proe POKS i feen)

Medication Safety Issues

Sound-alike/look-alike issues:

Propoxyphene may be confused with proparacaine

Darvon® may be confused with Devrom®, Diovan®

Darvon-N® may be confused with Darvocet-N®

High alert medication: The Institute for Safe Medication Practices (ISMP) includes this medication among its list of drug classes which have a heightened risk of causing significant patient harm when used in error.

Related Information
Acute Postoperative Pain *on page 1502*
Anesthetic Considerations in the Substance-Abusing Patient *on page 1613*
Chronic Pain Management *on page 1546*
Opioid Analgesics *on page 1688*

U.S. Brand Names Darvon-N®; Darvon®

Canadian Brand Names 642® Tablet; Darvon-N®

Index Terms Dextropropoxyphene; Propoxyphene Hydrochloride; Propoxyphene Napsylate

Pharmacologic Category Analgesic, Opioid

Restrictions C-IV

Generic Available Yes: Capsule

Use Management of mild-to-moderate pain

Mechanism of Action Propoxyphene is a weak narcotic analgesic which acts through binding to opiate receptors to inhibit ascending pain pathways. Propoxyphene, as with other narcotic (opiate) analgesics, blocks pain perception in the cerebral cortex by binding to specific receptor molecules (opiate receptors) within the neuronal membranes of synapses. This binding results in a decreased synaptic chemical transmission throughout the CNS thus inhibiting the flow of pain sensations into the higher centers. Mu and kappa are the two subtypes of the opiate receptor which propoxyphene binds to cause analgesia.

Pharmacodynamics/Kinetics
Onset of action: 0.5-1 hour
Duration: 4-6 hours
Metabolism: Hepatic to active metabolite (norpropoxyphene) and inactive metabolites; first-pass effect
Half-life elimination: Adults: Parent drug: 6-12 hours; Norpropoxyphene: 30-36 hours
Excretion: Urine (primarily as metabolites)

Dosage Oral:
Children: Doses for children are not well established; doses of the hydrochloride of 2-3 mg/kg/d divided every 6 hours have been used
Adults:
Hydrochloride: 65 mg every 3-4 hours as needed for pain; maximum: 390 mg/day
Napsylate: 100 mg every 4 hours as needed for pain; maximum: 600 mg/day
Elderly:
Hydrochloride: 65 mg every 4-6 hours as needed for pain
Napsylate: 100 mg every 4-6 hours as needed for pain

Dosing adjustment in renal impairment: Serum concentrations of propoxyphene may be increased or elimination may be delayed. Avoid use in Cl_{cr} <10 mL/minute. Specific dosing recommendations not available for less severe impairment.
Not dialyzable (0% to 5%)

Dosing adjustment in hepatic impairment: Serum concentrations of propoxyphene may be increased or elimination may be delayed; specific dosing recommendations not available.

Stability Store at controlled room temperature of 15°C to 30°C (59°F to 86°F).

Administration Should be administered with glass of water on an empty stomach. Food may decrease rate of absorption, but may slightly increase bioavailability.

Monitoring Parameters Pain relief, respiratory and mental status, blood pressure

Reference Range
Therapeutic: Ranges published vary between laboratories and may not correlate with clinical effect
Therapeutic concentration: 0.1-0.4 mcg/mL (SI: 0.3-1.2 µmol/L)
Toxic: >0.5 mcg/mL (SI: >1.5 µmol/L)

◄ **Anesthesia and Critical Care Concerns/Other Considerations**

Clinical Pearls/Comments: Equivalent dosing: 100 mg of propoxyphene napsylate = 65 mg of propoxyphene hydrochloride

Pregnancy Risk Factor C/D (prolonged use)

Contraindications Hypersensitivity to propoxyphene or any component of the formulation

Warnings/Precautions [U.S. Boxed Warning]: When given in excessive doses, either alone or in combination with other CNS depressants (including alcohol), propoxyphene is a major cause of drug-related deaths; recommended dosage must not be exceeded and alcohol intake should be limited. Avoid use in severely depressed or suicidal patients. Should not be prescribed in patients who are addiction prone or suicidal. Use caution in patients taking CNS depressant medications or antidepressants, and in patients who use alcohol in excess. Use with caution in patients with CNS depression coma, head trauma, thyroid dysfunction, adrenal insufficiency, morbid obesity, and prostatic hyperplasia/urinary stricture. Use with caution in patients with biliary tract dysfunction; acute pancreatitis may cause constriction of sphincter of Oddi. May cause hypotension; use with caution in patients with hypovolemia, cardiovascular disease (including acute MI), or drugs which may exaggerate hypotensive effects (including phenothiazines or general anesthetics). May obscure diagnosis or clinical course of patients with acute abdominal conditions.

May cause CNS depression, which may impair physical or mental abilities; patients must be cautioned about performing tasks which require mental alertness (eg, operating machinery or driving). Effects may be potentiated when used with other sedative drugs or ethanol. Use caution in patients dependent on opiates, substitution may result in acute opiate withdrawal symptoms. Tolerance or drug dependence may result from extended use. Propoxyphene should be used with caution in patients with renal or hepatic dysfunction, debilitated patients or in the elderly; consider dosing adjustment.

An opioid-containing analgesic regimen should be tailored to each patient's needs and based upon the type of pain being treated (acute versus chronic), the route of administration, degree of tolerance for opioids (naive versus chronic user), age, weight, and medical condition. The optimal analgesic dose varies widely among patients; doses should be titrated to pain relief/prevention. Safety and efficacy have not been established in children.

Adverse Reactions Frequency not defined.

Cardiovascular: Bundle branch block, hypotension

Central nervous system: Confusion, dizziness, dysphoria, drowsiness, fatigue, hallucinations, headache, increased intracranial pressure, lightheadedness, malaise, mental depression, nervousness, paradoxical CNS stimulation, paradoxical excitement and insomnia, restlessness, sedation, vertigo

Dermatologic: Rash, urticaria

Endocrine & metabolic: Hypoglycemia, urinary 17-OHCS decreased

Gastrointestinal: Abdominal pain, anorexia, biliary spasm, constipation, nausea, paralytic ileus, stomach cramps, vomiting, xerostomia

Genitourinary: Ureteral spasms, urination decreased

Hepatic: Jaundice, LFTs increased

Neuromuscular & skeletal: Weakness

Ocular: Visual disturbances

Respiratory: Dyspnea

Miscellaneous: Histamine release, hypersensitivity reaction psychologic and physical dependence with prolonged use

Drug Interactions

Metabolism/Transport Effects Inhibits CYP2C9 (weak), 2D6 (weak), 3A4 (weak)

Avoid Concomitant Use

Avoid concomitant use of Propoxyphene with any of the following: MAO Inhibitors

Increased Effect/Toxicity

Propoxyphene may increase the levels/effects of: Alcohol (Ethyl); Alvimopan; Beta-Blockers; CarBAMazepine; CNS Depressants; Desmopressin; MAO Inhibitors; Selective Serotonin Reuptake Inhibitors; Thiazide Diuretics; Tricyclic Antidepressants; Vitamin K Antagonists

The levels/effects of Propoxyphene may be increased by: Amphetamines; Antipsychotic Agents (Phenothiazines); Succinylcholine

Decreased Effect

Propoxyphene may decrease the levels/effects of: Pegvisomant

The levels/effects of Propoxyphene may be decreased by: Ammonium Chloride

Ethanol/Nutrition/Herb Interactions

Ethanol: Avoid or limit ethanol (may increase CNS depression). Watch for sedation.

Food: May decrease rate of absorption, but may slightly increase bioavailability.

Test Interactions False-positive methadone test

Dietary Considerations May administer with food if gastrointestinal distress occurs.

Dosage Forms Excipient information presented when available (limited, particularly for generics); consult specific product labeling.

Capsule, as hydrochloride: 65 mg
  Darvon®: 65 mg
Tablet, as napsylate:
  Darvon-N®: 100 mg

References

Mokhlesi B, Leikin JB, Murray P, et al, "Adult Toxicology in Critical Care: Part II: Specific Poisonings," *Chest*, 2003, 123(3):897-922.

Propoxyphene and Acetaminophen

(proe POKS i feen & a seet a MIN oh fen)

U.S. Brand Names Balacet 325™; Darvocet A500®; Darvocet-N® 100; Darvocet-N® 50

Canadian Brand Names Darvocet-N® 100; Darvocet-N® 50

Index Terms Acetaminophen and Propoxyphene; Propoxyphene Hydrochloride and Acetaminophen; Propoxyphene Napsylate and Acetaminophen

Pharmacologic Category Analgesic Combination (Opioid)

Restrictions C-IV

Use Management of mild-to-moderate pain

Pharmacodynamics/Kinetics See individual agents.

Dosage Oral: Adults:

Darvocet A500®, Darvocet-N® 100: 1 tablet every 4 hours as needed; maximum: 600 mg propoxyphene napsylate/day

Darvocet-N® 50: 1-2 tablets every 4 hours as needed; maximum: 600 mg propoxyphene napsylate/day

Propoxyphene hydrochloride 65 mg and acetaminophen 650 mg: 1 tablet every 4 hours as needed; maximum: 390 mg/day propoxyphene hydrochloride, 4 g/day acetaminophen)

Note: Formulations contain significant amounts of acetaminophen; intake should be limited to <4 g acetaminophen/day (less in patients with hepatic impairment/ethanol abuse)

Elderly: Refer to adult dosing

Dosing adjustment in renal/hepatic impairment: Serum concentrations of propoxyphene may be increased or elimination may be delayed; specific dosing recommendations not available.

Anesthesia and Critical Care Concerns/Other Considerations

Clinical Pearls/Comments: Equivalent dosing: 100 mg of propoxyphene napsylate = 65 mg of propoxyphene hydrochloride

Additional Information Complete prescribing information for this medication should be consulted for additional detail.

Dosage Forms Excipient information presented when available (limited, particularly for generics); consult specific product labeling.

Tablet, 50/325:
   Darvocet-N® 50: Propoxyphene napsylate 50 mg and acetaminophen 325 mg
Tablet, 65/650: Propoxyphene hydrochloride 65 mg and acetaminophen 650 mg
Tablet, 100/325: Propoxyphene napsylate 100 mg and acetaminophen 325 mg
   Balacet 325™: Propoxyphene napsylate 100 mg and acetaminophen 325 mg
Tablet, 100/500: Propoxyphene hydrochloride 100 mg and acetaminophen 500 mg
   Darvocet A500®: Propoxyphene napsylate 100 mg and acetaminophen 500 mg
Tablet, 100/650: Propoxyphene napsylate 100 mg and acetaminophen 650 mg
   Darvocet-N® 100: Propoxyphene napsylate 100 mg and acetaminophen 650 mg

References
Mokhlesi B, Leikin JB, Murray P, et al, "Adult Toxicology in Critical Care: Part II: Specific Poisonings," *Chest*, 2003, 123(3):897-922.

◆ **Propoxyphene Hydrochloride** *see* Propoxyphene *on page 1194*

◆ **Propoxyphene Hydrochloride and Acetaminophen** *see* Propoxyphene and Acetaminophen *on page 1197*

◆ **Propoxyphene Napsylate** *see* Propoxyphene *on page 1194*

◆ **Propoxyphene Napsylate and Acetaminophen** *see* Propoxyphene and Acetaminophen *on page 1197*

Propranolol (proe PRAN oh lole)

Medication Safety Issues
Sound-alike/look-alike issues:
   Propranolol may be confused with Pravachol®, Propulsid®
   Inderal® may be confused with Adderall®, Enduron®, Enduronyl®, Imdur®, Imuran®, Inderide®, Isordil®, Toradol®
   Inderal® 40 may be confused with Enduronyl® Forte

High alert medication: The Institute for Safe Medication Practices (ISMP) includes this medication among its list of drugs which have a heightened risk of causing significant patient harm when used in error.

Significant differences exist between oral and I.V. dosing. Use caution when converting from one route of administration to another.

International issues:
   Inderal® may be confused with Indiaral® which is a brand name for loperamide in France

Related Information
Anesthesia for Patients With Liver Disease *on page 1537*
Anesthetic Considerations in the Substance-Abusing Patient *on page 1613*
Antiarrhythmic Drugs *on page 1656*
Beta-Blockers *on page 1669*
Desensitization Protocols *on page 1692*
Preoperative Evaluation of the Cardiac Patient for Noncardiac Surgery *on page 1598*

U.S. Brand Names Inderal® [DSC]; Inderal® LA; InnoPran XL®

Canadian Brand Names Apo-Propranolol®; Dom-Propranolol; Inderal®; Inderal® LA; Novo-Pranol; Nu-Propranolol; PMS-Propranolol; Propranolol Hydrochloride Injection, USP

Index Terms Propranolol Hydrochloride

Pharmacologic Category Antiarrhythmic Agent, Class II; Beta-Adrenergic Blocker, Nonselective

Generic Available Yes

Use Management of hypertension; angina pectoris; pheochromocytoma; essential tremor; supraventricular arrhythmias (such as atrial fibrillation and flutter, AV nodal re-entrant tachycardias), ventricular tachycardias (catecholamine-induced arrhythmias, digoxin toxicity); prevention of myocardial infarction; migraine headache prophylaxis; symptomatic treatment of hypertrophic subaortic stenosis (hypertrophic obstructive cardiomyopathy)

Unlabeled/Investigational Use Tremor due to Parkinson's disease; ethanol withdrawal; aggressive behavior (not recommended for dementia-associated aggression), anxiety, schizophrenia; antipsychotic-induced akathisia; primary and secondary prophylaxis of variceal hemorrhage; acute panic; thyrotoxicosis; tetralogy of Fallot (TOF) hypercyanotic spells

Mechanism of Action Nonselective beta-adrenergic blocker (class II antiarrhythmic); competitively blocks response to beta$_1$- and beta$_2$-adrenergic stimulation which results in decreases in heart rate, myocardial contractility, blood pressure, and myocardial oxygen demand. Nonselective beta-adrenergic blockers (propranolol, nadolol) reduce portal pressure by producing splanchnic vasoconstriction (beta$_2$ effect) thereby reducing portal blood flow.

Pharmacodynamics/Kinetics

Onset of action: Beta-blockade: Oral: 1-2 hours

Duration: Immediate release: 6-12 hours; Extended-release formulations: ~24-27 hours

Absorption: Oral: Rapid and complete

Distribution: V_d: 4 L/kg in adults

Protein binding: Newborns: 68%; Adults: ~90% (S-isomer primarily to alpha$_1$-acid glycoprotein; R-isomer primarily to albumin)

Metabolism: Hepatic via CYP2D6, and CYP1A2 to 4-hydroxypropranolol (active) and inactive compounds; extensive first-pass effect

Bioavailability: ~25% reaches systemic circulation due to high first-pass metabolism; protein-rich foods increase bioavailability by ~50%

Half-life elimination: Neonates and Infants: Possible increased half-life; Children: 3.9-6.4 hours; Adults: Immediate release formulation: 3-6 hours; Extended-release formulations: 8-10 hours

Time to peak: Immediate release: 1-4 hours; Extended-release formulations: ~6-14 hours

Excretion: Metabolites are excreted primarily in urine (96% to 99%); <1% excreted in urine as unchanged drug

Dosage

Akathisia (unlabeled use): Oral: Adults: 30-120 mg/day in 2-3 divided doses

Essential tremor: Oral: Adults: 40 mg twice daily initially; maintenance doses: Usually 120-320 mg/day

Hypertension:

Oral:

Children (unlabeled use): Initial: 0.5-1 mg/kg/day in divided doses every 6-12 hours; increase gradually every 5-7 days; maximum: 16 mg/kg/24 hours

Adults: Initial: 40 mg twice daily; increase dosage every 3-7 days; usual dose: 120-240 mg divided in 2-3 doses/day; maximum daily dose: 640 mg; usual dosage range (JNC 7): 40-160 mg/day in 2 divided doses

Extended release formulations:

Inderal® LA: Initial: 80 mg once daily; usual maintenance: 120-160 mg once daily; maximum daily dose: 640 mg; usual dosage range (JNC 7): 60-180 mg/day once daily

InnoPran XL®: Initial: 80 mg once daily at bedtime; if initial response is inadequate, may be increased at 2-3 week intervals to a maximum dose of 120 mg

Hypertrophic subaortic stenosis: Oral: Adults: 20-40 mg 3-4 times/day

Inderal® LA: 80-160 mg once daily

Migraine headache prophylaxis: Oral:

Children (unlabeled use): Initial: 2-4 mg/kg/day **or**

≤35 kg: 10-20 mg 3 times/day

>35 kg: 20-40 mg 3 times/day

Adults: Initial: 80 mg/day divided every 6-8 hours; increase by 20-40 mg/dose every 3-4 weeks to a maximum of 160-240 mg/day given in divided doses every 6-8 hours; if satisfactory response not achieved within 6 weeks of starting therapy, drug should be withdrawn gradually over several weeks

Inderal® LA: Initial: 80 mg once daily; effective dose range: 160-240 mg once daily

Post-MI mortality reduction: Oral: Adults: Initial: 40 mg 3 times/day; usual dosage range: 180-240 mg/day in 3-4 divided doses

Pheochromocytoma: Oral: Adults: 30-60 mg/day in divided doses

◄ Stable angina: Oral: Adults: 80-320 mg/day in doses divided 2-4 times/day
Inderal® LA: Initial: 80 mg once daily; maximum dose: 320 mg once daily
Tachyarrhythmias:
Oral:
Children (unlabeled use): Initial: 0.5-1 mg/kg/day in divided doses every 6-8 hours; titrate dosage upward every 3-7 days; usual dose: 2-6 mg/kg/day; higher doses may be needed; do not exceed 16 mg/kg/day or 60 mg/day
Adults: 10-30 mg/dose every 6-8 hours
Elderly: Initial: 10 mg twice daily; increase dosage every 3-7 days; usual dosage range: 10-320 mg given in 2 divided doses
I.V.:
Children (unlabeled use): 0.01-0.1 mg/kg/dose slow IVP over 10 minutes; maximum dose: 1 mg for infants; 3 mg for children
Adults: 1-3 mg/dose slow IVP; repeat every 2-5 minutes up to a total of 5 mg; titrate initial dose to desired response
or
0.1 mg/kg divided into 3 equal doses given at 2-3 minute intervals. May repeat total dose in 2 minutes if necessary (ACLS guidelines, 2005)
Note: Once response achieved or maximum dose administered, additional doses should not be given for at least 4 hours.
Elderly: Use caution; initiate at lower end of the dosing range.
Hypercyanotic spells (TOF) (unlabeled use): Children:
Oral: Palliation: Initial: 1 mg/kg/day every 6 hours; if ineffective, may increase dose after 1 week by 1 mg/kg/day to a maximum of 5 mg/kg/day; if patient becomes refractory, may increase slowly to a maximum of 10-15 mg/kg/day. Allow 24 hours between dosing changes.
I.V.: 0.01-0.2 mg/kg/dose infused over 10 minutes; maximum dose: 5 mg
Thyrotoxicosis (unlabeled use):
Oral:
Children: 2 mg/kg/day, divided every 6-8 hours, titrate to effective dose
Adolescents and Adults: Oral: 10-40 mg/dose every 6 hours
I.V.: Adults: 1-3 mg/dose slow IVP as a single dose
Variceal hemorrhage prophylaxis (unlabeled use; Garcia-Tsao, 2007): Oral: Adults:
Primary prophylaxis: Initial: 20 mg twice daily; adjust to maximal tolerated dose.
Note: Risk factors for hemorrhage include Child-Pugh class B/C or variceal red wale markings on endoscopy.
Secondary prophylaxis: Initial: 20 mg twice daily; adjust to maximal tolerated dose

Dosing adjustment in renal impairment:
Not dialyzable (0% to 5%); supplemental dose is not necessary.
Peritoneal dialysis effects: Supplemental dose is not necessary.

Dosing adjustment in hepatic disease: Marked slowing of heart rate may occur in chronic liver disease with conventional doses; low initial dose and regular heart rate monitoring

Stability
Injection: Store at 20°C to 25°C (68°F to 77°F); protect from freezing or excessive heat. Once diluted, propranolol is stable for 24 hours at room temperature in D_5W or NS. Protect from light. Solution has a maximum stability at pH of 3 and decomposes rapidly in alkaline pH.
Capsule, tablet: Store at 20°C to 25°C (68°F to 77°F); protect from freezing or excessive heat. Protect from light and moisture.

Administration I.V. dose is much smaller than oral dose. When administered acutely for cardiac treatment, monitor ECG and blood pressure. May administer by rapid infusion (I.V. push) at a rate of 1 mg/minute or by slow infusion over ~30 minutes. Necessary monitoring for surgical patients who are unable to take oral beta-blockers (prolonged ileus) has not been defined. Some institutions require monitoring of baseline and postinfusion heart rate and blood pressure when a patient's response to beta-blockade has not been characterized (ie, the patient's initial dose or following a change in dose). Consult individual institutional policies and procedures. Do not crush long-acting oral forms.

Monitoring Parameters Acute cardiac treatment: Monitor ECG, heart rate, and blood pressure with I.V. administration; heart rate and blood pressure with oral administration

Reference Range Therapeutic: 50-100 ng/mL (SI: 190-390 nmol/L) at end of dose interval

Anesthesia and Critical Care Concerns/Other Considerations
Clinical Pearls/Comments:

Surgery: Based on available evidence, beta-blockers should be started days to weeks before elective surgery in selected patients when possible and titrated to a heart rate <65 beats per minute. Additional data suggest that long acting beta-blockers may be superior to short acting ones (Redelmeier, 2005). The ACC/AHA 2007 guidelines on perioperative cardiovascular evaluation and care for noncardiac surgery recommend beta-blockers be continued in patients under-going surgery who are receiving beta-blockers to treat angina, symptomatic arrhythmias, hypertension, or other ACC/AHA Class I guideline indications (Class I recommendation). The guidelines also recommend that beta-blockers be given to patients undergoing vascular surgery who have myocardial ischemia demonstrated during preoperative testing (Class I recommendation).

The guidelines also state that beta-blockers are probably recommended in patients undergoing intermediate risk (eg, carotid endarterectomy, prostate surgery) or vascular surgery in whom preoperative assessment identifies coronary heart disease or high cardiac risk (Class IIa recommendation). High cardiac risk is defined as having >1 of the following clinical risk factors: History of ischemic heart disease, compensated or prior heart failure, cerebrovascular disease, diabetes mellitus, or renal insufficiency. The use of beta-blockers is uncertain in patients undergoing intermediate risk or vascular surgery with ≤1 clinical risk factor (Class IIb recommendation).

The majority of published trials suggest a benefit of perioperative beta-blocker use during noncardiac surgery especially in high-risk patients; however, more recent clinical trials have not shown a benefit to perioperative beta-blockade for noncardiac surgery (Juul, 2006; Yang, 2006).

Pregnancy Risk Factor C (manufacturer); D (2nd and 3rd trimesters - expert analysis)

Contraindications Hypersensitivity to propranolol, beta-blockers, or any component of the formulation; uncompensated congestive heart failure (unless the failure is due to tachyarrhythmias being treated with propranolol), cardiogenic shock, severe sinus bradycardia or heart block (2nd or 3rd degree), severe hyperactive airway disease (asthma or COPD)

Warnings/Precautions Consider pre-existing conditions such as sick sinus syndrome before initiating. Administer cautiously in compensated heart failure and monitor for a worsening of the condition (efficacy of propranolol in HF has not been demonstrated). **[U.S. Boxed Warning]: Beta-blocker therapy should not be withdrawn abruptly (particularly in patients with CAD), but gradually tapered to avoid acute tachycardia, hypertension, and/or ischemia.** Use caution in patient with peripheral vascular disease (PVD). Use caution with concurrent use of beta-blockers and either verapamil or diltiazem; bradycardia or heart block can occur. Avoid concurrent I.V. use of both agents.

Use cautiously in patients with diabetes because it can mask prominent hypoglycemic symptoms. Use caution in hyperthyroidism since beta-blockade may mask signs of thyrotoxicosis. May alter thyroid-function tests. Use with caution in myasthenia gravis or psychiatric disease (may cause CNS depression). Use cautiously in renal and hepatic dysfunction; dosage adjustment required in hepatic impairment. Use care with anesthetic agents which decrease myocardial function. In general, patients with bronchospastic disease should not receive beta-blockers; if used at all, should be used cautiously with close monitoring. Adequate alpha-blockade is required prior to use of any beta-blocker for patients with untreated pheochromocytoma. May induce or exacerbate psoriasis. Use caution with history of severe anaphylaxis to allergens; patients taking beta-blockers may become more sensitive to repeated challenges. Treatment of anaphylaxis (eg, epinephrine) in patients taking beta-blockers may be ineffective or promote undesirable effects. Safety and efficacy in children have not been established.

◀ **Adverse Reactions** Frequency not defined.

Cardiovascular: Angina, arterial insufficiency, AV conduction disturbance increased, bradycardia, cardiogenic shock, CHF, hypotension, impaired myocardial contractility, mesenteric arterial thrombosis (rare), Raynaud's syndrome, syncope

Central nervous system: Amnesia, catatonia, cognitive dysfunction, confusion, depression, dizziness, emotional lability, fatigue, hallucinations, hypersomnolence, insomnia, lethargy, lightheadedness, psychosis, vertigo, vivid dreams

Dermatologic: Alopecia, contact dermatitis, cutaneous ulcers, eczematous eruptions, erythema multiforme, exfoliative dermatitis, hyperkeratosis, nail changes, oculomucocutaneous reactions, pruritus, psoriasiform eruptions, rash, Stevens-Johnson syndrome, toxic epidermal necrolysis, ulcers, ulcerative lichenoid, urticaria

Endocrine & metabolic: Hyper-/hypoglycemia, hyperkalemia, hyperlipidemia

Gastrointestinal: Anorexia, cramping, constipation, diarrhea, ischemic colitis, nausea, stomach discomfort, vomiting

Genitourinary: Impotence, interstitial nephritis (rare), oliguria (rare), Peyronie's disease, proteinuria (rare)

Hematologic: Agranulocytosis, nonthrombocytopenic purpura, thrombocytopenia, thrombocytopenic purpura

Hepatic: Alkaline phosphatase increased, transaminases increased

Neuromuscular & skeletal: Arthropathy, carpal tunnel syndrome (rare), myotonus, paresthesia, polyarthritis, weakness

Ocular: Hyperemia of the conjunctiva, mydriasis, visual acuity decreased, visual disturbances, xerophthalmia

Renal: BUN increased

Respiratory: Bronchospasm, dyspnea, laryngospasm, pharyngitis, pulmonary edema, respiratory distress, wheezing

Miscellaneous: Anaphylactic/anaphylactoid allergic reaction, cold extremities, lupus-like syndrome (rare)

Drug Interactions

Metabolism/Transport Effects Substrate of CYP1A2 (major), 2C19 (minor), 2D6 (major), 3A4 (minor); **Inhibits** CYP1A2 (weak), 2D6 (weak)

Avoid Concomitant Use

Avoid concomitant use of Propranolol with any of the following: Dabigatran Etexilate; Methacholine; Topotecan

Increased Effect/Toxicity

Propranolol may increase the levels/effects of: Alpha-/Beta-Agonists (Direct-Acting); Alpha1-Blockers; Alpha2-Agonists; Amifostine; Antihypertensives; Antipsychotic Agents (Phenothiazines); Cardiac Glycosides; Colchicine; Dabigatran Etexilate; Hypotensive Agents; Insulin; Lidocaine; Methacholine; Midodrine; P-Glycoprotein Substrates; RiTUXimab; Rivaroxaban; Rizatriptan; Sulfonylureas; Topotecan; Zolmitriptan

The levels/effects of Propranolol may be increased by: Acetylcholinesterase Inhibitors; Alcohol (Ethyl); Aminoquinolines (Antimalarial); Amiodarone; Anilidopiperidine Opioids; Antipsychotic Agents (Phenothiazines); Calcium Channel Blockers (Nondihydropyridine); CYP1A2 Inhibitors (Moderate); CYP1A2 Inhibitors (Strong); CYP2D6 Inhibitors (Moderate); CYP2D6 Inhibitors (Strong); Darunavir; Diazoxide; Dipyridamole; Disopyramide; Dronedarone; Fluvoxamine; Herbs (Hypotensive Properties); MAO Inhibitors; Pentoxifylline; Phosphodiesterase 5 Inhibitors; Propafenone; Propoxyphene; Prostacyclin Analogues; QuiNIDine; Reserpine; Selective Serotonin Reuptake Inhibitors; Zileuton

Decreased Effect

Propranolol may decrease the levels/effects of: Beta2-Agonists; Theophylline Derivatives

The levels/effects of Propranolol may be decreased by: Alcohol (Ethyl); Barbiturates; Bile Acid Sequestrants; CYP1A2 Inducers (Strong); Herbs (Hypertensive Properties); Methylphenidate; Nonsteroidal Anti-Inflammatory Agents; Peginterferon Alfa-2b; Rifamycin Derivatives; Yohimbine

Ethanol/Nutrition/Herb Interactions

Ethanol: Ethanol may increase or decrease plasma levels of propranolol. Reports are variable and have shown both enhanced as well as inhibited hepatic metabolism (of propranolol). Caution advised with consumption of alcohol and monitor for heart rate and/or blood pressure changes.

Food: Propranolol serum levels may be increased if taken with food. Protein-rich foods may increase bioavailability; a change in diet from high carbohydrate/low protein to low carbohydrate/high protein may result in increased oral clearance.

Cigarette: Smoking may decrease plasma levels of propranolol by increasing metabolism.

Herb/Nutraceutical: Avoid dong quai if using for hypertension (has estrogenic activity). Avoid bayberry, blue cohosh, cayenne, ephedra, ginger, ginseng (american), gotu kola, licorice, yohimbe (may worsen hypertension). Avoid black cohosh, california poppy, coleus, garlic, golden seal, hawthorn, mistletoe, periwinkle, quinine, shepherd's purse (have antihypertensive activity, may cause hypotension).

Dietary Considerations Tablets (immediate release) should be taken on an empty stomach; capsules (extended release) may be taken with or without food, but should always be taken consistently (with food or on an empty stomach)

Dosage Forms Excipient information presented when available (limited, particularly for generics); consult specific product labeling. [DSC] = Discontinued product

Capsule, extended release, as hydrochloride: 60 mg, 80 mg, 120 mg, 160 mg
  InnoPran XL®: 80 mg, 120 mg

Capsule, sustained release, as hydrochloride:
  Inderal® LA: 60 mg, 80 mg, 120 mg, 160 mg

Injection, solution, as hydrochloride: 1 mg/mL (1 mL)
  Inderal®: 1 mg/mL (1 mL) [DSC]

Solution, oral, as hydrochloride: 4 mg/mL (500 mL); 8 mg/mL (500 mL)

Tablet, as hydrochloride: 10 mg, 20 mg, 40 mg, 60 mg, 80 mg

References

Fleisher LA, Beckman JA, Brown KA, et al, "ACC/AHA 2006 Guideline Update on Perioperative Cardiovascular Evaluation for Noncardiac Surgery: Focused Update on Perioperative Beta-Blocker Therapy: A Report of the American College of Cardiology/American Heart Association Task Force on Practice Guidelines (Writing Committee to Update the 2002 Guidelines on Perioperative Cardiovascular Evaluation for Noncardiac Surgery) Developed in Collaboration With the American Society of Echocardiography, American Society of Nuclear Cardiology, Heart Rhythm Society, Society of Cardiovascular Anesthesiologists, Society for Cardiovascular Angiography and Interventions, and Society for Vascular Medicine and Biology," *J Am Coll Cardiol*, 2006, 47 (11):2343-55.

Juul AB, Wetterslev J, Gluud C, et al, "Effect of Perioperative Beta-Blockade in Patients With Diabetes Undergoing Major Noncardiac Surgery: Randomized Placebo Controlled, Blinded Multicentre Trial," *BMJ*, 2006, 332(7556):1482.

Lindenauer PK, Pekow P, Wang K, et al, "Perioperative Beta-Blocker Therapy and Mortality After Major Noncardiac Surgery," *N Engl J Med*, 2005, 353(4):349-61.

Mokhlesi B, Leikin JB, Murray P, et al, "Adult Toxicology in Critical Care: Part II: Specific Poisonings," *Chest*, 2003, 123(3):897-922.

Radack K and Deck C, "Beta-Adrenergic Blocker Therapy Does Not Worsen Intermittent Claudication in Subjects With Peripheral Arterial Disease. A Meta-Analysis of Randomized Controlled Trials," *Arch Intern Med*, 1991, 151(9):1769-76.

Yang H, Raymer K, Butler R, et al, "The Effects of Perioperative Beta-Blockade: Results of the Metoprolol After Vascular Surgery (MaVS) Study, A Randomized Controlled Trial," *Am Heart J*, 2006, 152(5):983-90.

◆ **Propranolol Hydrochloride** see Propranolol on page 1198

◆ **Propranolol Hydrochloride Injection, USP (Can)** see Propranolol on page 1198

◆ **Proprinal [OTC]** see Ibuprofen on page 717

◆ **2-Propylpentanoic Acid** see Valproic Acid and Derivatives on page 1445

Propylthiouracil (proe pil thye oh YOOR a sil)

Medication Safety Issues
Sound-alike/look-alike issues:
  Propylthiouracil may be confused with Purinethol®
  PTU is an error-prone abbreviation (mistaken as mercaptopurine [Purinethol®; 6-MP])

Canadian Brand Names Propyl-Thyracil®

Index Terms PTU (error-prone abbreviation)

Pharmacologic Category Antithyroid Agent; Thioamide

Generic Available Yes

Use Palliative treatment of hyperthyroidism as an adjunct to ameliorate hyperthyroidism in preparation for surgical treatment or radioactive iodine therapy; management of thyrotoxic crisis

Mechanism of Action Inhibits the synthesis of thyroid hormones by blocking the oxidation of iodine in the thyroid gland; blocks synthesis of thyroxine and triiodothyronine

Pharmacodynamics/Kinetics
Onset of action: Therapeutic: 24-36 hours
 Peak effect: Remission: 4 months of continued therapy
Duration: 2-3 hours
Distribution: Concentrated in the thyroid gland
Protein binding: 75% to 80%
Metabolism: Hepatic
Bioavailability: 80% to 95%
Half-life elimination: 1.5-5 hours; End-stage renal disease: 8.5 hours
Time to peak, serum: ~1 hour
Excretion: Urine (35%)

Dosage Oral: Administer in 3 equally divided doses at approximately 8-hour intervals. Adjust dosage to maintain T_3, T_4, and TSH levels in normal range; elevated T_3 may be sole indicator of inadequate treatment. Elevated TSH indicates excessive antithyroid treatment.

Children: Initial: 5-7 mg/kg/day **or** 150-200 mg/m^2/day in divided doses every 8 hours
 or
 6-10 years: 50-150 mg/day
 >10 years: 150-300 mg/day
 Maintenance: Determined by patient response **or** $1/3$ to $2/3$ of the initial dose in divided doses every 8-12 hours. This usually begins after 2 months on an effective initial dose.
Adults: Initial: 300-400 mg/day in divided doses every 6-8 hours. In patients with severe hyperthyroidism, very large goiters, or both, the initial dosage is usually 400 mg/day; an occasional patient will require 600-900 mg/day; maintenance: 100-150 mg/day in divided doses every 8-12 hours
 Thyrotoxic crisis (recommendations vary widely and have not been evaluated in comparative trials): Dosages of 200-300 mg every 4-6 hours have been recommended for short-term initial therapy (until initial response), followed by gradual reduction to a maintenance dosage (100-150 mg/day in divided doses).

Elderly: Use lower dose recommendations; Initial: 150-300 mg/day
Withdrawal of therapy: Therapy should be withdrawn gradually with evaluation of the patient every 4-6 weeks for the first 3 months then every 3 months for the first year after discontinuation of therapy to detect any reoccurrence of a hyperthyroid state.

Dosing adjustment in renal impairment: Adjustment is not necessary

Monitoring Parameters CBC with differential, prothrombin time, liver function tests, thyroid function tests (TSH, T_3, T_4); periodic blood counts are recommended chronic therapy

Reference Range Normal laboratory values:
Total T_4: 5-12 mcg/dL
Serum T_3: 90-185 ng/dL
Free thyroxine index (FT_4 I): 6-10.5
TSH: 0.5-4.0 microunits/mL

Anesthesia and Critical Care Concerns/Other Considerations
Clinical Pearls/Comments: Agranulocytosis, when it occurs, is usually seen during the first several months of therapy.

The use of antithyroid thioamides is as effective in elderly as in younger adults; however, the expense, potential adverse effects, and inconvenience (compliance, monitoring) make them undesirable. The use of radioiodine, due to ease of administration and less concern for long-term side effects and reproduction problems, makes it a more appropriate therapy.

Pregnancy Risk Factor D

Contraindications Hypersensitivity to propylthiouracil or any component of the formulation; breast-feeding (per manufacturer; however, expert analysis and the AAP state this drug may be used in nursing mothers)

Warnings/Precautions Has been associated (rarely) with significant bone marrow depression. The most severe manifestation is agranulocytosis. Aplastic anemia, thrombocytopenia, and leukopenia may also occur. Use with caution in patients receiving other drugs known to cause myelosuppression particularly agranulocytosis. Discontinue if significant bone marrow suppression occurs, particularly agranulocytosis or aplastic anemia.

Rare, severe hepatic reactions (hepatic necrosis, hepatitis) may occur. Symptoms suggestive of hepatic dysfunction should prompt evaluation. Discontinue in the presence of hepatitis (transaminase >3x upper limit of normal). In addition, other rare hypersensitivity reactions have been reported, including the development of ANCA-positive vasculitis, drug fever, interstitial pneumonitis, exfoliative dermatitis, glomerulonephritis, leukocytoclastic vasculitis, and a lupus-like syndrome; prompt discontinuation is warranted in patients who develop symptoms consistent with a form of autoimmunity or other hypersensitivity during therapy.

May cause hypoprothrombinemia and bleeding; use with particular caution in patients >40 years of age. Thyroid hyperplasia or carcinoma may occur with prolonged usage (>1 year). Safety and efficacy have not been established in children <6 years of age.

Adverse Reactions Frequency not defined.

Cardiovascular: ANCA-positive vasculitis, cutaneous vasculitis, edema, leukocytoclastic vasculitis

Central nervous system: Dizziness, drowsiness, drug fever, fever, headache, neuritis, vertigo

Dermatologic: Alopecia, erythema nodosum, exfoliative dermatitis, pruritus, skin rash, urticaria

Endocrine & metabolic: Goiter, swollen salivary glands, weight gain

Gastrointestinal: Constipation, loss of taste perception, nausea, stomach pain, vomiting

Hematologic: Agranulocytosis, aplastic anemia, bleeding, leukopenia, thrombocytopenia

Hepatic: Cholestatic jaundice, hepatitis

Neuromuscular & skeletal: Arthralgia, paresthesia

Renal: Acute renal failure, glomerulonephritis, nephritis

Respiratory: Alveolar hemorrhage, interstitial pneumonitis

Miscellaneous: SLE-like syndrome

Drug Interactions

Avoid Concomitant Use

Avoid concomitant use of Propylthiouracil with any of the following: Sodium Iodide I131

Increased Effect/Toxicity There are no known significant interactions involving an increase in effect.

Decreased Effect

Propylthiouracil may decrease the levels/effects of: Sodium Iodide I131; Vitamin K Antagonists

Ethanol/Nutrition/Herb Interactions Food: Propylthiouracil serum levels may be altered if taken with food.

Dietary Considerations Administer at the same time in relation to meals each day, either always with meals or always between meals.

Dosage Forms Excipient information presented when available (limited, particularly for generics); consult specific product labeling.

Tablet: 50 mg

- ◆ **Prosol** *see* Amino Acid Injection *on page* 81
- ◆ **PRO-Sotalol (Can)** *see* Sotalol *on page* 1321
- ◆ **Prostacyclin** *see* Epoprostenol *on page* 506
- ◆ **Prostacyclin PGI$_2$** *see* Iloprost *on page* 725
- ◆ **Prostaglandin E$_1$** *see* Alprostadil *on page* 66
- ◆ **Prostigmin®** *see* Neostigmine *on page* 997
- ◆ **Prostin® VR (Can)** *see* Alprostadil *on page* 66
- ◆ **Prostin VR Pediatric®** *see* Alprostadil *on page* 66

Protamine Sulfate (PROE ta meen SUL fate)

Medication Safety Issues
Sound-alike/look-alike issues:
Protamine may be confused with ProAmatine®, Protonix®, Protopam®, Protropin®

Pharmacologic Category Antidote

Generic Available Yes

Use Treatment of heparin overdosage; neutralize heparin during surgery or dialysis procedures

Unlabeled/Investigational Use Treatment of low molecular weight heparin (LMWH) overdose

Mechanism of Action Combines with strongly acidic heparin to form a stable complex (salt) neutralizing the anticoagulant activity of both drugs

Pharmacodynamics/Kinetics Onset of action: I.V.: Heparin neutralization: ~5 minutes

Dosage
Heparin neutralization: I.V.: Protamine dosage is determined by the dosage of heparin; 1 mg of protamine neutralizes 90 USP units of heparin (lung) and 115 USP units of heparin (intestinal); maximum dose: 50 mg

Heparin overdosage, following intravenous administration: I.V.: Since blood heparin concentrations decrease rapidly **after** administration, adjust the protamine dosage depending upon the duration of time since heparin administration as follows: See table.

Time Elapsed	Dose of Protamine (mg) to Neutralize 100 units of Heparin
Immediate	1-1.5
30-60 min	0.5-0.75
>2 h	0.25-0.375

Heparin overdosage, following SubQ injection: I.V.: 1-1.5 mg protamine per 100 units heparin; this may be done by a portion of the dose (eg, 25-50 mg) given slowly I.V. followed by the remaining portion as a continuous infusion over 8-16 hours (the expected absorption time of the SubQ heparin dose)

LMWH overdose (unlabeled use): **Note:** Antifactor Xa activity never completely neutralized (maximum: ~60% to 75%)

Enoxaparin: 1 mg protamine for each mg of enoxaparin; if PTT prolonged 2-4 hours after first dose, consider additional dose of 0.5 mg for each mg of enoxaparin.

Dalteparin or tinzaparin: 1 mg protamine for each 100 anti-Xa int. units of dalteparin or tinzaparin; if PTT prolonged 2-4 hours after first dose, consider additional dose of 0.5 mg for each 100 anti-Xa int. units of dalteparin or tinzaparin.

Note: Excessive protamine doses may worsen bleeding potential.

Stability Refrigerate; do not freeze. Stable for at least 2 weeks at room temperature. Preservative-free formulation does not require refrigeration. Reconstitute vial with 5 mL sterile water. If using protamine in neonates, reconstitute with preservative-free sterile water for injection; resulting solution equals 10 mg/mL.

Administration For I.V. use only; **incompatible** with cephalosporins and penicillins; administer slow IVP (50 mg over 10 minutes); rapid I.V. infusion causes hypotension; resulting solution equals 10 mg/mL; inject without further dilution over 1-3 minutes; maximum of 50 mg in any 10-minute period

Monitoring Parameters Coagulation test, aPTT or ACT, cardiac monitor and blood pressure monitor required during administration

Anesthesia and Critical Care Concerns/Other Considerations

Clinical Pearls/Comments: Monitor vital signs closely during protamine therapy because of possible hypotension during administration.

Anaphylaxis or hypersensitivity responses with acute hypotension to protamine may present with its use, especially in patients with allergies to fish, previous exposure to protamine (through previous use of protamine or protamine-containing insulin), infertile or vasectomized males.

Evidence-Based Information:
Management of Intracerebral Hemorrhage (ICH) Due to Unfractionated Heparin (UFH): Overall management of ICH is similar regardless of cause; however, iatrogenic spontaneous ICH may have specific treatments. According to the 2007 ACC/ASA Guidelines for the Management of Spontaneous Intracerebral Hemorrhage, UFH-related ICH should be treated with I.V. protamine given by slow I.V. injection (not to exceed 5 mg/minute) with a maximum dose of 50 mg (Class I recommendation). Faster infusions of protamine can result in cardiovascular collapse.

Protamine's reversal of LMWHs is not as complete or predictable as with heparin. Protamine neutralizes the antithrombin activity of LMWHs, but the cationic protein neutralizes the antifactor Xa activity incompletely. A recent case illustrates a failure to reverse enoxaparin (Makris, 2000). Protamine will not reverse the effects of thrombin inhibitors such as lepirudin, bivalirudin, or argatroban.

Pregnancy Risk Factor C

Contraindications Hypersensitivity to protamine or any component of the formulation

Warnings/Precautions May not be totally effective in some patients following cardiac surgery despite adequate doses. May cause hypersensitivity reaction in patients (have epinephrine 1:1000 and resuscitation equipment available). **[U.S. Boxed Warning]: Hypotension, cardiovascular collapse, noncardiogenic pulmonary edema, pulmonary vasoconstriction, and pulmonary hypertension may occur. Risk factors for such events include: use of high doses or overdose, repeated doses, previous protamine administration (including protamine-containing drugs), fish allergy, vasectomy, severe left ventricular dysfunction, abnormal preoperative pulmonary hemodynamics.** Too rapid administration can cause severe hypotension and anaphylactoid-like reactions. Heparin rebound associated with anticoagulation and bleeding has been reported to occur occasionally; symptoms typically occur 8-9 hours after protamine administration, but may occur as long as 18 hours later.

Adverse Reactions Frequency not defined.
Cardiovascular: Sudden fall in blood pressure, bradycardia, flushing, hypotension
Central nervous system: Lassitude
Gastrointestinal: Nausea, vomiting
Hematologic: Hemorrhage
Respiratory: Dyspnea, pulmonary hypertension
Miscellaneous: Hypersensitivity reactions

Drug Interactions

Avoid Concomitant Use There are no known interactions where it is recommended to avoid concomitant use.

Increased Effect/Toxicity There are no known significant interactions involving an increase in effect.

Decreased Effect There are no known significant interactions involving a decrease in effect.

Dosage Forms Excipient information presented when available (limited, particularly for generics); consult specific product labeling.
Injection, solution, as sulfate [preservative free]: 10 mg/mL (5 mL, 25 mL)

◀ **References**
Aren C, "Heparin and Protamine Therapy," *Semin Thorac Cardiovasc Surg*, 1990, 2(4):364-72.

Broderick J, Connolly S, Feldmann E, et al, "Guidelines for the Management of Spontaneous Intracerebral Hemorrhage in Adults: 2007 Update: A Guideline From the American Heart Association/American Stroke Association Stroke Council, High Blood Pressure Research Council, and the Quality of Care and Outcomes in Research Interdisciplinary Working Group," *Stroke*, 2007, 38(6):2001-23. Available at http://stroke.ahajournals.org/cgi/content/short/STROKEAHA.107.183689.

Kondo NI, Maddi R, Ewenstein BM, et al, "Anticoagulation and Hemostasis in Cardiac Surgical Patients," *J Card Surg*, 1994, 9(4):443-61.

Makris M, Hough RE, and Kitchen S, et al, "Poor Reversal of Low Molecular Weight Heparin by Protamine," *Br J Haematol*, 2000, 108(4): 884-5.

Michelson AD, Bovill E, Monagle P, et al, "Antithrombic Therapy in Children," *Chest*, 1998, 114(5 Suppl):748-69.

Mokhlesi B, Leikin JB, Murray P, et al, "Adult Toxicology in Critical Care. Part 11: Specific Poisonings," *Chest*, 2003, 123(3):897-922.

Wakefield TW and Stanley JC, "Intraoperative Heparin Anticoagulation and Its Reversal," *Semin Vasc Surg*, 1996, 9(4):296-302.

◆ **Protection Plus® [OTC]** *see* Alcohol (Ethyl) *on page 53*

◆ **Protein C** *see* Protein C Concentrate (Human) *on page 1208*

◆ **Protein C (Activated), Human, Recombinant** *see* Drotrecogin Alfa *on page 466*

Protein C Concentrate (Human)
(PROE teen cee KON suhn trate HYU man)

Medication Safety Issues
Sound-alike/look-alike issues:
Ceprotin may be confused with aprotinin, Cipro®
Protein C concentrate (human) may be confused with activated protein C (human, recombinant) which refers to drotrecogin alfa

U.S. Brand Names Ceprotin

Index Terms Protein C

Pharmacologic Category Anticoagulant

Generic Available No

Use Replacement therapy for severe congenital protein C deficiency for the prevention and/or treatment of venous thromboembolism and purpura fulminans

Mechanism of Action Converted to activated protein C (APC). APC is a serine protease which inactivates factors Va and VIIIa, limiting thrombotic formation. *In vitro* data also suggest inhibition of plasminogen activator inhibitor-1 (PAF-1) resulting in profibrinolytic activity, inhibition of macrophage production of tumor necrosis factor, blocking of leukocyte adhesion, and limitation of thrombin-induced inflammatory responses.

Pharmacodynamics/Kinetics
Distribution: V_d: 0.074L/kg
Metabolism: Activated protein C (APC) inactivated by plasma protease inhibitors
Half-life elimination: Median: 9.8 hours; range 4.9-14.7 hours
Time to peak, plasma: T_{max}: 0.5 hours

Dosage Patient variables (including age, clinical condition, and plasma levels of protein C) will influence dosing and duration of therapy. Individualize dosing based on protein C activity and patient pharmacokinetic profile. Dosing is dependent on the severity of protein C deficiency, age of patient, clinical condition, and patient's level of protein C. The frequency, duration, and dose should be individualized.

I.V.: Children and Adults: Severe congenital protein C deficiency:
Acute episode/short-term prophylaxis: Initial dose: 100-120 int. units/kg (for determination of recovery and half-life)
Subsequent 3 doses: 60-80 int. units/kg every 6 hours (adjust to maintain peak protein C activity of 100%)
Maintenance dose: 45-60 int. units/kg every 6 or 12 hours (adjust to maintain recommended maintenance trough protein C activity levels >25%)
Long-term prophylaxis: Maintenance dose: 45-60 int. units/kg every 12 hours (recommended maintenance trough protein C activity levels >25%)

Note: Maintain target peak protein C activity of 100% during acute episodes and short-term prophylaxis. Maintain trough levels of protein C activity >25%. Higher peak levels of protein C may be necessary in prophylactic therapy of patients at increased risk for thrombosis (eg, infection, trauma, surgical intervention).

Stability Store under refrigeration at 2°C to 8°C (36°F to 46°F); do not freeze. Protect from light. Allow Ceprotin and sterile water vial to warm to room temperature. Reconstitute 500 int. units vial with 5 mL and 1000 int. units vial with 10 mL sterile water for injection (resultant concentration ~100 int. units/mL). Gently swirl vial after adding the diluent until powder is completely dissolved. Use provided filter needle to withdraw solution from vial; remove filter needle prior to administration. The resulting solution (which is preservative free) should be administered within 3 hours and any unused portion should be discarded.

Administration Administer by intravenous injection at a rate not to exceed 2 mL/minute. In children <10 kg, administration should not exceed a rate of 0.2 mL/kg/minute. Administration must be completed within 3 hours of solution preparation.

Monitoring Parameters Protein C activity (chromogenic assay) prior to and during therapy; signs and symptoms of bleeding; hemoglobin/hematocrit; PT/INR, platelet count

Reference Range Maintain target peak protein C activity of 100% during acute episodes and short-term prophylaxis. Maintain trough levels of protein C activity >25%. Higher peak levels of protein C may be necessary in prophylactic therapy of patients at increased risk for thrombosis (eg, infection, trauma, surgical intervention).

Pregnancy Risk Factor C

Contraindications Hypersensitivity to protein C or any component of the formulation

Warnings/Precautions Formulation may contain small amounts of mouse protein and/or heparin. Hypersensitivity reactions may occur. Discontinue use in the presence of allergy related symptoms. Use of products derived from human plasma carries the potential risk for the transmission of infectious agents including viruses. Consideration should be given for patients to receive appropriate vaccinations during therapy. Concomitant use with other anticoagulants may increase risk of bleeding. Small amounts of heparin within formulation may induce thrombocytopenia. Use with caution in patients with renal impairment or in whom sodium overload is a concern.

Adverse Reactions As with all drugs which may affect hemostasis, bleeding may be associated with protein C administration. Hemorrhage may occur at virtually any site. Risk is dependent on multiple variables, including the concurrent use of multiple agents that alter hemostasis and patient susceptibility. Frequency not defined.

Central nervous system: Lightheadedness

Hematologic: Bleeding

Miscellaneous: Hypersensitivity reactions (itching and rash)

Postmarketing and/or case reports: Fever, hemothorax, hypotension, hyperhidrosis, restlessness

Drug Interactions

Avoid Concomitant Use There are no known interactions where it is recommended to avoid concomitant use.

Increased Effect/Toxicity

Protein C Concentrate (Human) may increase the levels/effects of: Anticoagulants; Ibritumomab; Tositumomab and Iodine I 131 Tositumomab

The levels/effects of Protein C Concentrate (Human) may be increased by: Antiplatelet Agents; Dasatinib; Herbs (Anticoagulant/Antiplatelet Properties); Nonsteroidal Anti-Inflammatory Agents; Pentosan Polysulfate Sodium; Prostacyclin Analogues; Salicylates; Thrombolytic Agents

Decreased Effect There are no known significant interactions involving a decrease in effect.

Ethanol/Nutrition/Herb Interactions Herb/Nutraceutical: Recent use/intake of herbs with anticoagulant or antiplatelet activity (including cat's claw, feverfew, garlic, ginkgo, ginseng, and horse chestnut seed) may increase the risk of bleeding.

Dietary Considerations At maximum daily doses, product formulation contains sodium >200 mg.

◀ **Dosage Forms**

Injection, powder for reconstitution:

Ceprotin: ~500 int. units [actual potency printed on vial label; contains human albumin and sodium; may contain trace amounts of mouse protein or heparin; packaged with diluent]; ~1000 int. units [actual potency printed on vial label; contains human albumin and sodium; may contain trace amounts of mouse protein or heparin; packaged with diluent]

◆ **Prothrombin Complex Concentrate** *see* Factor IX Complex (Human) *on page 573*

◆ **Protonix®** *see* Pantoprazole *on page 1084*

◆ **Protopam®** *see* Pralidoxime *on page 1157*

◆ **Protopic®** *see* Tacrolimus *on page 1338*

◆ **PRO-Topiramate (Can)** *see* Topiramate *on page 1408*

◆ **Pro-Valacyclovir (Can)** *see* Valacyclovir *on page 1441*

◆ **Proventil® HFA** *see* Albuterol *on page 49*

◆ **PRO-Verapamil SR (Can)** *see* Verapamil *on page 1468*

◆ **Provigil®** *see* Modafinil *on page 947*

◆ **Prozac®** *see* FLUoxetine *on page 616*

◆ **Prozac® Weekly™** *see* FLUoxetine *on page 616*

◆ **Prudoxin™** *see* Doxepin *on page 455*

◆ **Pseudomonic Acid A** *see* Mupirocin *on page 965*

◆ **PTU (error-prone abbreviation)** *see* Propylthiouracil *on page 1203*

◆ **Pulmicort® (Can)** *see* Budesonide *on page 206*

◆ **Pulmicort Flexhaler™** *see* Budesonide *on page 206*

◆ **Pulmicort Respules®** *see* Budesonide *on page 206*

◆ **Pulmophylline (Can)** *see* Theophylline *on page 1373*

◆ **Purell® [OTC]** *see* Alcohol (Ethyl) *on page 53*

◆ **Purell® 2 in 1 [OTC]** *see* Alcohol (Ethyl) *on page 53*

◆ **Purell® Lasting Care [OTC]** *see* Alcohol (Ethyl) *on page 53*

◆ **Purell® Moisture Therapy [OTC]** *see* Alcohol (Ethyl) *on page 53*

◆ **Purell® with Aloe [OTC]** *see* Alcohol (Ethyl) *on page 53*

◆ **Purified Chick Embryo Cell** *see* Rabies Virus Vaccine *on page 1225*

◆ **2-Pyridine Aldoxime Methochloride** *see* Pralidoxime *on page 1157*

Pyridostigmine (peer id oh STIG meen)

Medication Safety Issues

Sound-alike/look-alike issues:

Pyridostigmine may be confused with physostigmine

Mestinon® may be confused with Metatensin®

Regonol® may be confused with Reglan®, Renagel®

Related Information

Chronic Renal Failure *on page 1552*

U.S. Brand Names Mestinon®; Mestinon® Timespan®; Regonol®

Canadian Brand Names Mestinon®; Mestinon®-SR

Index Terms Pyridostigmine Bromide

Pharmacologic Category Acetylcholinesterase Inhibitor

Generic Available Yes: Tablet

Use Symptomatic treatment of myasthenia gravis; antagonism of nondepolarizing neuromuscular blockers

Military use: Pretreatment for Soman nerve gas exposure

Mechanism of Action Inhibits destruction of acetylcholine by acetylcholinesterase which facilitates transmission of impulses across myoneural junction

Pharmacodynamics/Kinetics

Onset of action: Oral, I.M.: 15-30 minutes; I.V. injection: 2-5 minutes

Duration: Oral: Up to 6-8 hours (due to slow absorption); I.V.: 2-3 hours

Absorption: Oral: Very poor
Distribution: 19 ± 12 L
Metabolism: Hepatic
Bioavailability: 10% to 20%
Half-life elimination: 1-2 hours; Renal failure: ≤6 hours
Excretion: Urine (80% to 90% as unchanged drug)

Dosage

Myasthenia gravis:

Oral:

Children: 7 mg/kg/24 hours divided into 5-6 doses

Adults: Highly individualized dosing ranges: 60-1500 mg/day, usually 600 mg/day divided into 5-6 doses, spaced to provide maximum relief

Sustained release formulation: Highly individualized dosing ranges: 180-540 mg once or twice daily (doses separated by at least 6 hours); **Note:** Most clinicians reserve sustained release dosage form for bedtime dose only.

I.M., slow I.V. push:

Children: 0.05-0.15 mg/kg/dose

Adults: To supplement oral dosage pre- and postoperatively during labor and postpartum, during myasthenic crisis, or when oral therapy is impractical: ~1/30th of oral dose; observe patient closely for cholinergic reactions

or

I.V. infusion: Initial: 2 mg/hour with gradual titration in increments of 0.5-1 mg/hour, up to a maximum rate of 4 mg/hour

Reversal of nondepolarizing muscle relaxants: **Note:** Atropine sulfate (0.6-1.2 mg) I.V. immediately prior to pyridostigmine to minimize side effects: I.V.:

Children: Dosing range: 0.1-0.25 mg/kg/dose*

Adults: 0.1-0.25 mg/kg/dose; 10-20 mg is usually sufficient*

*Full recovery usually occurs ≤15 minutes, but ≥30 minutes may be required

Pretreatment for Soman nerve gas exposure (military use): Oral: Adults: 30 mg every 8 hours beginning several hours prior to exposure; discontinue at first sign of nerve agent exposure, then begin atropine and pralidoxime

Dosage adjustment in renal dysfunction: Lower dosages may be required due to prolonged elimination; no specific recommendations have been published

Stability

Injection: Protect from light.

Tablet:

30 mg: Store under refrigeration at 2°C to 8°C (36°F to 46°F). Protect from light. Stable at room temperature for up to 3 months.

Mestinon®: Store at 25°C (77°F). Protect from moisture.

Administration Do **not** crush sustained release tablet.

Monitoring Parameters Observe for cholinergic reactions, particularly when administered I.V.

Anesthesia and Critical Care Concerns/Other Considerations

Clinical Pearls/Comments: For reversal of neuromuscular blockade, atropine or glycopyrrolate must be administered with pyridostigmine to minimize its cholinergic effects. For patients with myasthenia gravis, extended release products may be preferred at bedtime for patients who are very weak upon rising in the morning.

Pregnancy Risk Factor B

Contraindications Hypersensitivity to pyridostigmine, bromides, or any component of the formulation; GI or GU obstruction

Warnings/Precautions Use with caution in patients with epilepsy, bradycardia, hyperthyroidism, cardiac arrhythmias, or peptic ulcer; use with extreme caution in patients with asthma or bronchospastic disease; adequate facilities should be available for cardiopulmonary resuscitation when testing and adjusting dose for myasthenia gravis; have atropine and epinephrine ready to treat hypersensitivity reactions; overdosage may result in cholinergic crisis, this must be distinguished from myasthenic crisis; anticholinesterase insensitivity can develop for brief or prolonged periods. Regonol® injection contains 1% benzyl alcohol as the preservative (not intended for use in newborns). **[U.S. Boxed Warning]: Regonol® injection must be administered by trained personnel.**

◀ **Adverse Reactions** Frequency not defined.

Cardiovascular: Arrhythmias (especially bradycardia), AV block, cardiac arrest, decreased carbon monoxide, flushing, hypotension, nodal rhythm, nonspecific ECG changes, syncope, tachycardia

Central nervous system: Convulsions, dizziness, drowsiness, dysphonia, headache, loss of consciousness

Dermatologic: Skin rash, thrombophlebitis (I.V.), urticaria

Gastrointestinal: Abdominal pain, diarrhea, dysphagia, flatulence, hyperperistalsis, nausea, salivation, stomach cramps, vomiting

Genitourinary: Urinary urgency

Neuromuscular & skeletal: Arthralgia, dysarthria, fasciculations, muscle cramps, myalgia, spasms, weakness

Ocular: Amblyopia, lacrimation, small pupils

Respiratory: Bronchial secretions increased, bronchiolar constriction, bronchospasm, dyspnea, laryngospasm, respiratory arrest, respiratory depression, respiratory muscle paralysis

Miscellaneous: Allergic reactions, anaphylaxis, diaphoresis increased

Drug Interactions

Avoid Concomitant Use There are no known interactions where it is recommended to avoid concomitant use.

Increased Effect/Toxicity

Pyridostigmine may increase the levels/effects of: Beta-Blockers; Cholinergic Agonists; Succinylcholine

The levels/effects of Pyridostigmine may be increased by: Corticosteroids (Systemic); Ginkgo Biloba

Decreased Effect

Pyridostigmine may decrease the levels/effects of: Neuromuscular-Blocking Agents (Nondepolarizing)

The levels/effects of Pyridostigmine may be decreased by: Methocarbamol

Test Interactions Increased aminotransferase [ALT/AST] (S), increased amylase (S)

Dosage Forms Excipient information presented when available (limited, particularly for generics); consult specific product labeling.

Injection, solution, as bromide:
Regonol®: 5 mg/mL (2 mL) [contains benzyl alcohol]

Syrup, as bromide:
Mestinon®: 60 mg/5 mL (480 mL) [raspberry flavor; contains alcohol 5%, sodium benzoate]

Tablet, as bromide: 60 mg
Mestinon®: 60 mg

Tablet, sustained release, as bromide:
Mestinon® Timespan®: 180 mg

◆ **Pyridostigmine Bromide** see Pyridostigmine on page *1210*

◆ **Quasense™** see Ethinyl Estradiol and Levonorgestrel on page *549*

◆ **Quelicin®** see Succinylcholine on page *1326*

QUEtiapine (kwe TYE a peen)

U.S. Brand Names Seroquel XR®; Seroquel®

Canadian Brand Names Apo-Quetiapine®; CO Quetiapine; Gen-Quetiapine; Mylan-Quetiapine; Novo-Quetiapine; PMS-Quetiapine; PRO-Quetiapine; ratio-Quetiapine; Riva-Quetiapine; Sandoz-Quetiapine; Seroquel XR®; Seroquel®; ZYM-Quetiapine

Index Terms Quetiapine Fumarate

Pharmacologic Category Antipsychotic Agent, Atypical

Use Treatment of schizophrenia; treatment of acute manic episodes associated with bipolar I disorder (as monotherapy or in combination with lithium or divalproex); maintenance treatment of bipolar I disorder (in combination with lithium or divalproex); treatment of depressive episodes associated with bipolar disorder

Unlabeled/Investigational Use Autism, psychosis (children); psychosis/agitation related to Alzheimer's dementia

Pharmacodynamics/Kinetics

Absorption: Rapidly absorbed following oral administration

Distribution: V_d: 6-14 L/kg; V_{dss}: ~2 days

Protein binding, plasma: 83%

Metabolism: Primarily hepatic; via CYP3A4; forms the metabolite N-desalkyl quetiapine (active) and two inactive metabolites

Bioavailability: 9% ± 4%; tablet is 100% bioavailable relative to solution

Half-life elimination:

Mean: Terminal: Quetiapine: ~6 hours; Extended release: ~7 hours

Metabolite: N-desalkyl quetiapine: 9-12 hours

Time to peak, plasma: Immediate release: 1.5 hours; Extended release: 6 hours

Excretion: Urine (73% as metabolites, <1% as unchanged drug); feces (20%)

Dosage Oral:

Children and Adolescents:

Autism (unlabeled use): 100-350 mg/day (1.6-5.2 mg/kg/day)

Psychosis and mania (unlabeled use): Initial: 25 mg twice daily; titrate as necessary to 450 mg/day

Adults:

Bipolar disorder:

Depression:

Immediate release tablet: Initial: 50 mg/day the first day; increase to 100 mg/day on day 2, further increasing by 100 mg/day each day until a target dose of 300 mg/day is reached by day 4. Further increases up to 600 mg/day by day 8 have been evaluated in clinical trials, but no additional antidepressant efficacy was noted.

Extended release tablet: Initial: 50 mg/day the first day; increase to 100 mg on day 2, further increasing by 100 mg/day each day until a target dose of 300 mg/day is reached by day 4.

Mania:

Immediate release tablet: Initial: 50 mg twice daily on day 1, increase dose in increments of 100 mg/day to 200 mg twice daily on day 4; may increase to a target dose of 800 mg/day by day 6 at increments ≤200 mg/day. Usual dosage range: 400-800 mg/day.

Extended release tablet: Initial: 300 mg on day 1; increase to 600 mg on day 2 and adjust dose to 400-800 mg once daily on day 3, depending on response and tolerance.

Maintenance therapy: Immediate release tablet: 200-400 mg twice daily with lithium or divalproex; **Note:** Average time of stabilization was 15 weeks in clinical trials.

Schizophrenia/psychoses:

Immediate release tablet: Initial: 25 mg twice daily; increase in increments of 25-50 mg 2-3 times/day on the second and third day, if tolerated, to a target dose of 300-400 mg/day in 2-3 divided doses by day 4. Make further adjustments as needed at intervals of at least 2 days in adjustments of 25-50 mg twice daily. Usual maintenance range: 300-800 mg/day.

Extended release tablet: Initial: 300 mg once daily; increase in increments of up to 300 mg/day (in intervals of ≥1 day). Usual maintenance range: 400-800 mg/day.

Note: Dose reductions should be attempted periodically to establish lowest effective dose in patients with psychosis. Patients being restarted after 1 week of no drug need to be titrated as above.

Elderly: 40% lower mean oral clearance of quetiapine in adults >65 years of age; higher plasma levels expected and, therefore, dosage adjustment may be needed; elderly patients usually require 50-200 mg/day of immediate release tablets or 50 mg/day of extended release tablets with a slower titration schedule. Increase immediate release dose by 25-50 mg/day or extended release dose by 50 mg/day to effective dose, based on clinical response and tolerability. If initiated with immediate release tablets, patient may transition to extended release formulation (at equivalent total daily dose) when effective dose has been reached. See **"Note"** in adult dosing.

◀ Psychosis/agitation related to Alzheimer's dementia (unlabeled use): Initial: 12.5-50 mg/day; if necessary, gradually increase as tolerated not to exceed 200-300 mg/day

Dosing comments in renal insufficiency: 25% lower mean oral clearance of quetiapine than normal subjects; however, plasma concentrations similar to normal subjects receiving the same dose; no dosage adjustment required

Dosing comments in hepatic insufficiency: 30% lower mean oral clearance of quetiapine than normal subjects; higher plasma levels expected in hepatically impaired subjects; dosage adjustment may be needed

Immediate release tablet: Initial: 25 mg/day, increase dose by 25-50 mg/day to effective dose, based on clinical response and tolerability to patient. If initiated with immediate-release formulation, patient may transition to extended-release formulation (at equivalent total daily dose) when effective dose has been reached.

Extended release tablet: Initial: 50 mg/day; increase dose by 50 mg/day to effective dose, based on clinical response and tolerability to patient.

Anesthesia and Critical Care Concerns/Other Considerations Quetiapine has a very low incidence of extrapyramidal symptoms such as restlessness and abnormal movement, and is at least as effective as conventional antipsychotics. For patients who have been off quetiapine for more than 1 week, dose titration is necessary when restarting the medication.

Additional Information Complete prescribing information for this medication should be consulted for additional detail.

Dosage Forms Excipient information presented when available (limited, particularly for generics); consult specific product labeling.

Tablet:

Seroquel®: 25 mg, 50 mg, 100 mg, 200 mg, 300 mg, 400 mg

Tablet, extended release:

Seroquel XR®: 50 mg, 150 mg, 200 mg, 300 mg, 400 mg

References

American Diabetes Association; American Psychiatric Association; American Association of Clinical Endocrinologists; North American Association for the Study of Obesity, "Consensus Development Conference on Antipsychotic Drugs and Obesity and Diabetes," *Diabetes Care*, 2004, 27 (2):596-601.

Davis JM, Chen N, and Glick ID, "A Meta-analysis of the Efficacy of Second-Generation Antipsychotics," *Arch Gen Psychiatry*, 2003, 60(6):553-64.

DelBello MP, Schwiers ML, Rosenberg HL, et al, "Quetiapine as Adjunctive Treatment for Adolescent Mania," Poster presented at Fourth International Conference on Bipolar Disorder, Pittsburgh, PA: Jun 14.

Goldberg RJ, "Managing Psychosis-Related Behavioral Problems in the Elderly," *Consult Pharm*, 1997, 12(Suppl C):4-10.

Martin A, Koenig K, Scahill L, et al, "Open-Label Quetiapine in the Treatment of Children and Adolescents With Autistic Disorder," *J Child Adolesc Psychopharmacol*, 1999, 9(2):99-107.

McConville BJ, Arvanitis LA, Thyrum PT, et al, "Pharmacokinetics, Tolerability, and Clinical Effectiveness of Quetiapine Fumarate: An Open-Label Trial in Adolescents With Psychotic Disorders," *J Clin Psychiatry*, 2000, 61(4):252-60.

Schneider LS, Tariot PN, Dagerman KS, et al, "Effectiveness of Atypical Antipsychotic Drugs in Patients With Alzheimer's Disease," *N Engl J Med*, 2006, 355(15):1525-38.

Shaw JA, Lewis JE, Pascal S, et al, "An Open Trial of Quetiapine in Adolescents With a Diagnosis of a Psychotic Disorder," Poster presented at NCDEU 41st Annual Meeting, Phoenix, AZ: May 28.

◆ **Quetiapine Fumarate** *see* QUEtiapine *on page 1212*

Quinapril (KWIN a pril)

Related Information

Angiotensin Agents *on page 1652*

Heart Failure (Systolic) *on page 1739*

Preoperative Evaluation of the Cardiac Patient for Noncardiac Surgery *on page 1598*

U.S. Brand Names Accupril®

Canadian Brand Names Accupril®; GD-Quinapril

Index Terms Quinapril Hydrochloride

Pharmacologic Category Angiotensin-Converting Enzyme (ACE) Inhibitor

Use Treatment of hypertension; treatment of heart failure

Unlabeled/Investigational Use Treatment of left ventricular dysfunction after myocardial infarction; pediatric hypertension; to delay the progression of nephropathy and reduce risks of cardiovascular events in hypertensive patients with type 1 or 2 diabetes mellitus

Pharmacodynamics/Kinetics
Onset of action: 1 hour
Duration: 24 hours
Absorption: Quinapril: ≥60%
Protein binding: Quinapril: 97%; Quinaprilat: 97%
Metabolism: Rapidly hydrolyzed to quinaprilat, the active metabolite
Half-life elimination: Quinapril: 0.8 hours; Quinaprilat: 3 hours; increases as Cl_{cr} decreases
Time to peak, serum: Quinapril: 1 hour; Quinaprilat: ~2 hours
Excretion: Urine (50% to 60% primarily as quinaprilat)

Dosage Oral:
Children (unlabeled use): Hypertension: Initial 5-10 mg once daily; maximum: 80 mg/day
Adults:
Heart failure: Initial: 5 mg once or twice daily, titrated at weekly intervals to 20-40 mg daily in 2 divided doses; target dose (heart failure): 20 mg twice daily (ACC/AHA 2009 Heart Failure Guidelines)
Hypertension: Initial: 10-20 mg once daily, adjust according to blood pressure response at peak and trough blood levels; initial dose may be reduced to 5 mg in patients receiving diuretic therapy if the diuretic is continued; usual dose range (JNC 7): 10-40 mg once daily
Elderly: Initial: 2.5-5 mg/day; increase dosage at increments of 2.5-5 mg at 1- to 2-week intervals.

Dosing adjustment in renal impairment: Lower initial doses should be used; after initial dose (if tolerated), administer initial dose twice daily; may be increased at weekly intervals to optimal response:
Heart failure: Initial:
Cl_{cr} >30 mL/minute: Administer 5 mg/day
Cl_{cr} 10-30 mL/minute: Administer 2.5 mg/day
Hypertension: Initial:
Cl_{cr} >60 mL/minute: Administer 10 mg/day
Cl_{cr} 30-60 mL/minute: Administer 5 mg/day
Cl_{cr} 10-30 mL/minute: Administer 2.5 mg/day

Dosing comments in hepatic impairment: In patients with alcoholic cirrhosis, hydrolysis of quinapril to quinaprilat is impaired; however, the subsequent elimination of quinaprilat is unaltered.

Anesthesia and Critical Care Concerns/Other Considerations

Clinical Pearls/Comments: In patients on chronic ACE inhibitor therapy, intraoperative hypotension may occur with induction and maintenance of general anesthesia; however, discontinuation of therapy prior to surgery is controversial. If continued preoperatively, avoidance of hypotensive agents during surgery is prudent. Episodes of intraoperative hypotension may be managed by fluid administration and/or modest doses of alpha-adrenergic agents. Severe hypotension may occur in patients who are sodium- and/or volume-depleted; initiate lower doses and monitor closely when starting therapy in these patients. ACE inhibitor therapy may elicit an increase in potassium and creatinine, especially when used in patients with bilateral renal artery stenosis. In those patients experiencing cough on an ACE inhibitor, the ACE inhibitor may be discontinued and, if necessary, angiotensin-receptor blocker therapy instituted. Concomitant NSAID therapy may attenuate blood pressure control; use of NSAIDs should be avoided or limited, with monitoring of blood pressure control. In the setting of heart failure, NSAID use may be associated with an increased risk for fluid accumulation and edema. Because of the potent teratogenic effects of ACE inhibitors, these drugs should be avoided, if possible, when treating women of childbearing potential not on effective birth control measures. Aging patients with a decrease in glomerular filtration (also creatinine clearance), severe heart failure, and renal failure may experience an exaggerated response with administration of ACE inhibitors. Diabetic proteinuria is reduced and insulin sensitivity is enhanced.

Evidence-Based Information: ACE inhibitors decrease morbidity and mortality in patients with asymptomatic and symptomatic left ventricular dysfunction. In this situation, they decrease hospitalizations for, and retard progression to, decompensated heart failure. ACE inhibitors are also indicated in patients postmyocardial infarction in whom left ventricular ejection fraction is <40%. When used in patients with heart failure, the target dose or maximum tolerated dose should be achieved, if possible. Lower daily doses of ACE inhibitors have not demonstrated the same cardioprotective effects. ACE inhibitors have renal protective effects in patients with diabetic proteinuria. The HOPE trial examined the use of ramipril at a dose of between 2.5-10 mg daily in patients without heart failure at high risk for cardiovascular events and documented a significant improvement in cardiovascular outcome compared to placebo.

Additional Information Complete prescribing information for this medication should be consulted for additional detail.

Dosage Forms Excipient information presented when available (limited, particularly for generics); consult specific product labeling.
Tablet: 5 mg, 10 mg, 20 mg, 40 mg
Accupril®: 5 mg, 10 mg, 20 mg, 40 mg

◆ **Quinapril Hydrochloride** see Quinapril on page 1214
◆ **Quinate® (Can)** see QuiNIDine on page 1216

QuiNIDine (KWIN i deen)

Medication Safety Issues
Sound-alike/look-alike issues:
QuiNIDine may be confused with cloNIDine, quiNINE, Quinora®

High alert medication: The Institute for Safe Medication Practices (ISMP) includes this medication (I.V. formulation) among its list of drug classes which have a heightened risk of causing significant patient harm when used in error.

Related Information
Allergic Reactions on page 1508
Antiarrhythmic Drugs on page 1656

Canadian Brand Names Apo-Quinidine®; BioQuin® Durules™; Novo-Quinidin; Quinate®

Index Terms Quinidine Gluconate; Quinidine Polygalacturonate; Quinidine Sulfate

Pharmacologic Category Antiarrhythmic Agent, Class Ia

Generic Available Yes

Use
Quinidine gluconate and sulfate salts: Conversion and prevention of relapse into atrial fibrillation and/or flutter; suppression of ventricular arrhythmias. **Note:** Due to proarrhythmic effects, use should be reserved for life-threatening arrhythmias. Moreover, the use of quinidine has largely been replaced by more effective/safer antiarrhythmic agents and/or nonpharmacologic therapies (eg, radiofrequency ablation).

Quinidine gluconate (I.V. formulation): Conversion of atrial fibrillation/flutter and ventricular tachycardia. **Note:** The use of I.V. quinidine gluconate for these indications has been replaced by more effective/safer antiarrhythmic agents (eg, amiodarone and procainamide).

Quinidine gluconate (I.V. formulation) and quinidine sulfate: Treatment of malaria (*Plasmodium falciparum*)

Unlabeled/Investigational Use Paroxysmal supraventricular tachycardia, paroxysmal AV junctional rhythm, and symptomatic atrial or ventricular premature contractions

Mechanism of Action Class Ia antiarrhythmic agent; depresses phase O of the action potential; decreases myocardial excitability and conduction velocity, and myocardial contractility by decreasing sodium influx during depolarization and potassium efflux in repolarization; also reduces calcium transport across cell membrane

Pharmacodynamics/Kinetics
Distribution: V_d: Adults: 2-3 L/kg, decreased with congestive heart failure, malaria; increased with cirrhosis; crosses placenta; enters breast milk

Protein binding:
  Newborns: 50% to 70%; decreased protein binding with cyanotic congenital heart disease, cirrhosis, or acute myocardial infarction
  Adults: 80% to 90%
Metabolism: Extensively hepatic (50% to 90%) to inactive compounds
Bioavailability: Sulfate: 80%; Gluconate: 70%
Half-life elimination, plasma: Children: 2.5-6.7 hours; Adults: 6-8 hours; prolonged with elderly, cirrhosis, and congestive heart failure
Time to peak, serum: Sulfate: 2 hours; Gluconate: 3-5 hours
Excretion: Urine (15% to 25% as unchanged drug)

Dosage Dosage expressed in terms of the salt: 267 mg of quinidine gluconate = 200 mg of quinidine sulfate.

Children: Test dose for idiosyncratic reaction (sulfate, oral or gluconate, I.M.): 2 mg/kg or 60 mg/m^2
  Oral (quinidine sulfate): 15-60 mg/kg/day in 4-5 divided doses or 6 mg/kg every 4-6 hours; usual 30 mg/kg/day or 900 mg/m^2/day given in 5 daily doses
  I.V. **not** recommended (quinidine gluconate): 2-10 mg/kg/dose given at a rate ≤10 mg/minute every 3-6 hours as needed
Adults: Test dose: Oral, I.M.: 200 mg administered several hours before full dosage (to determine possibility of idiosyncratic reaction)
  Oral (for malaria):
    Sulfate: 100-600 mg/dose every 4-6 hours; begin at 200 mg/dose and titrate to desired effect (maximum daily dose: 3-4 g)
    Gluconate: 324-972 mg every 8-12 hours
  I.M.: 400 mg/dose every 2-6 hours; initial dose: 600 mg (gluconate)
  I.V.: 200-400 mg/dose diluted and given at a rate ≤10 mg/minute; may require as much as 500-750 mg

Dosing adjustment in renal impairment: Cl$_{cr}$ <10 mL/minute: Administer 75% of normal dose.
Hemodialysis: Slightly hemodialyzable (5% to 20%); 200 mg supplemental dose posthemodialysis is recommended.
Peritoneal dialysis: Not dialyzable (0% to 5%)

Dosing adjustment/comments in hepatic impairment: Larger loading dose may be indicated; reduce maintenance doses by 50% and monitor serum levels closely.

Stability Do not use discolored parenteral solution.

Administration Administer around-the-clock to promote less variation in peak and trough serum levels
Oral: Do not crush, chew, or break sustained release dosage forms.
Parenteral: When injecting I.M., aspirate carefully to avoid injection into a vessel; maximum I.V. infusion rate: 10 mg/minute.

Monitoring Parameters Cardiac monitor required during I.V. administration; CBC, liver and renal function tests, should be routinely performed during long-term administration

Reference Range Therapeutic: 2-5 mcg/mL (SI: 6.2-15.4 µmol/L). Patient-dependent therapeutic response occurs at levels of 3-6 mcg/mL (SI: 9.2-18.5 µmol/L). Optimal therapeutic level is method dependent; >6 mcg/mL (SI: >18 µmol/L).

Pregnancy Risk Factor C

Contraindications Hypersensitivity to quinidine or any component of the formulation; thrombocytopenia; thrombocytopenic purpura; myasthenia gravis; heart block greater than first degree; idioventricular conduction delays (except in patients with a functioning artificial pacemaker); those adversely affected by anticholinergic activity; concurrent use of quinolone antibiotics which prolong QT interval, cisapride, amprenavir, or ritonavir

Warnings/Precautions Monitor and adjust dose to prevent QT$_c$ prolongation. Watch for proarrhythmic effects. Correct hypokalemia before initiating therapy. Hypokalemia may worsen toxicity. **[U.S. Boxed Warning]: Antiarrhythmic drugs have not been shown to enhance survival in non-life-threatening ventricular arrhythmias and may increase mortality; the risk is greatest with structural heart disease. Quinidine may increase mortality in treatment of atrial fibrillation/flutter.** May precipitate or exacerbate HF. Reduce dosage in hepatic impairment. Use may cause digoxin-induced toxicity (adjust digoxin's dose). Use

◀ caution with concurrent use of other antiarrhythmics. Hypersensitivity reactions can occur. Can unmask sick sinus syndrome (causes bradycardia); use with caution in patients with heart block. Has been associated with severe hepatotoxic reactions, including granulomatous hepatitis. Hemolysis may occur in patients with G6PD (glucose-6-phosphate dehydrogenase) deficiency. Different salt products are not interchangeable.

Adverse Reactions

Frequency not defined: Hypotension, syncope

>10%:

Cardiovascular: QT_c prolongation (modest prolongation is common, however, excessive prolongation is rare and indicates toxicity)

Central nervous system: Lightheadedness (15%)

Gastrointestinal: Diarrhea (35%), upper GI distress, bitter taste, diarrhea, anorexia, nausea, vomiting, stomach cramping (22%)

1% to 10%:

Cardiovascular: Angina (6%), palpitation (7%), new or worsened arrhythmia (proarrhythmic effect)

Central nervous system: Syncope (1% to 8%), headache (7%), fatigue (7%), sleep disturbance (3%), tremor (2%), nervousness (2%), incoordination (1%)

Dermatologic: Rash (5%)

Neuromuscular & skeletal: Weakness (5%)

Ocular: Blurred vision

Otic: Tinnitus

Respiratory: Wheezing

<1% (Limited to important or life-threatening): Abnormal pigmentation, acute psychotic reactions, agranulocytosis, angioedema, arthralgia, bronchospasm, cerebral hypoperfusion (possibly resulting in ataxia, apprehension, and seizure), cholestasis, confusion, delirium, depression, drug-induced lupus-like syndrome, eczematous dermatitis, esophagitis, exacerbated bradycardia (in sick sinus syndrome), exfoliative rash, fever, flushing, granulomatous hepatitis, hallucinations, heart block, hemolytic anemia, hepatotoxic reaction (rare), hearing impaired, CPK increased, lichen planus, livedo reticularis, lymphadenopathy, melanin pigmentation of the hard palate, myalgia, mydriasis, nephropathy, optic neuritis, pancytopenia, paradoxical increase in ventricular rate during atrial fibrillation/flutter, photosensitivity, pneumonitis, pruritus, psoriaform rash, QT_c prolongation (excessive), respiratory depression, sicca syndrome, tachycardia, thrombocytopenia, thrombocytopenic purpura, torsade de pointes, urticaria, uveitis, vascular collapse, vasculitis, ventricular fibrillation, ventricular tachycardia, vertigo, visual field loss

Note: Cinchonism, a syndrome which may include tinnitus, high-frequency hearing loss, deafness, vertigo, blurred vision, diplopia, photophobia, headache, confusion, and delirium has been associated with quinidine use. Usually associated with chronic toxicity, this syndrome has also been described after brief exposure to a moderate dose in sensitive patients. Vomiting and diarrhea may also occur as isolated reactions to therapeutic quinidine levels.

Drug Interactions

Metabolism/Transport Effects Substrate of CYP2C9 (minor), 2E1 (minor), 3A4 (major); **Inhibits** CYP2C9 (weak), 2D6 (strong), 3A4 (strong)

Avoid Concomitant Use

Avoid concomitant use of QuiNIDine with any of the following: Alfuzosin; Antifungal Agents (Azole Derivatives, Systemic); Artemether; Dabigatran Etexilate; Dronedarone; Eplerenone; Everolimus; Halofantrine; Lumefantrine; Mefloquine; Nilotinib; Nisoldipine; Pimozide; Protease Inhibitors; QuiNINE; Ranolazine; Rivaroxaban; Salmeterol; Silodosin; Tamoxifen; Tetrabenazine; Thioridazine; Tolvaptan; Topotecan; Ziprasidone

Increased Effect/Toxicity

QuiNIDine may increase the levels/effects of: Alfuzosin; Almotriptan; Alosetron; Amiodarone; Atomoxetine; Beta-Blockers; Cardiac Glycosides; Ciclesonide; Colchicine; CYP2D6 Substrates; CYP3A4 Substrates; Dabigatran Etexilate; Dextromethorphan; Dronedarone; Dutasteride; Eplerenone; Everolimus; FentaNYL; Fesoterodine; Halofantrine; Haloperidol; Ixabepilone; Maraviroc; Mefloquine; Neuromuscular-Blocking Agents; Nilotinib; Nisoldipine; Paricalcitol; P-Glycoprotein Substrates; Pimecrolimus; Pimozide; QTc-Prolonging Agents;

QuiNINE; Ranolazine; Rivaroxaban; Salmeterol; Saxagliptin; Silodosin; Sorafenib; Tadalafil; Tamoxifen; Tetrabenazine; Thioridazine; Tolvaptan; Topotecan; Tricyclic Antidepressants; Vitamin K Antagonists; Ziprasidone

The levels/effects of QuiNIDine may be increased by: Alfuzosin; Antacids; Antifungal Agents (Azole Derivatives, Systemic); Artemether; Calcium Channel Blockers (Nondihydropyridine); Carbonic Anhydrase Inhibitors; Chloroquine; Cimetidine; Ciprofloxacin; CYP3A4 Inhibitors (Moderate); CYP3A4 Inhibitors (Strong); Fluconazole; Gadobutrol; Lumefantrine; Macrolide Antibiotics; Nilotinib; P-Glycoprotein Inhibitors; Protease Inhibitors; QuiNINE; Selective Serotonin Reuptake Inhibitors; Tricyclic Antidepressants

Decreased Effect

QuiNIDine may decrease the levels/effects of: Codeine; Dihydrocodeine; Hydrocodone; Prasugrel; TraMADol

The levels/effects of QuiNIDine may be decreased by: Amiodarone; Barbiturates; Calcium Channel Blockers (Dihydropyridine); CYP3A4 Inducers (Strong); Deferasirox; Herbs (CYP3A4 Inducers); Kaolin; P-Glycoprotein Inducers; Phenytoin; Potassium-Sparing Diuretics; Primidone; Rifamycin Derivatives; Sucralfate

Ethanol/Nutrition/Herb Interactions

Food: Dietary salt intake may alter the rate and extent of quinidine absorption. A decrease in dietary salt may lead to an increase in quinidine serum concentrations. Avoid changes in dietary salt intake. Quinidine serum levels may be increased if taken with food. Food has a variable effect on absorption of sustained release formulation. The rate of absorption of quinidine may be decreased following the ingestion of grapefruit juice. In addition, CYP3A4 metabolism of quinidine may be reduced by grapefruit juice. Grapefruit juice should be avoided. Excessive intake of fruit juices or vitamin C may decrease urine pH and result in increased clearance of quinidine with decreased serum concentration. Alkaline foods may result in increased quinidine serum concentrations.

Herb/Nutraceutical: St John's wort may decrease quinidine levels. Avoid ephedra (may worsen arrhythmia).

Dietary Considerations Administer with food or milk to decrease gastrointestinal irritation. Avoid changes in dietary salt intake.

Dosage Forms Excipient information presented when available (limited, particularly for generics); consult specific product labeling.

Injection, solution, as gluconate: 80 mg/mL (10 mL) [equivalent to quinidine base 50 mg/mL]

Tablet, as sulfate: 200 mg, 300 mg

Tablet, extended release, as gluconate: 324 mg [equivalent to quinidine base 202 mg]

Tablet, extended release, as sulfate: 300 mg [equivalent to quinidine base 249 mg]

◆ **Quinidine Gluconate** *see* QuiNIDine *on page 1216*

◆ **Quinidine Polygalacturonate** *see* QuiNIDine *on page 1216*

◆ **Quinidine Sulfate** *see* QuiNIDine *on page 1216*

Quinupristin and Dalfopristin (kwi NYOO pris tin & dal FOE pris tin)

U.S. Brand Names Synercid®

Canadian Brand Names Synercid®

Index Terms Dalfopristin and Quinupristin; Pristinamycin; RP-59500

Pharmacologic Category Antibiotic, Streptogramin

Generic Available No

Use Treatment of serious or life-threatening infections associated with vancomycin-resistant *Enterococcus faecium* bacteremia; treatment of complicated skin and skin structure infections caused by methcillin-susceptible *Staphylococcus aureus* or *Streptococcus pyogenes*

Has been studied in the treatment of a variety of infections caused by *Enterococcus faecium* (not *E. fecalis*) including vancomycin-resistant strains. ▶

May also be effective in the treatment of serious infections caused by *Staphylococcus* species including those resistant to methicillin.

Mechanism of Action Quinupristin/dalfopristin inhibits bacterial protein synthesis by binding to different sites on the 50S bacterial ribosomal subunit thereby inhibiting protein synthesis

Pharmacodynamics/Kinetics

Distribution: Quinupristin: 0.45 L/kg; Dalfopristin: 0.24 L/kg

Protein binding: Moderate

Metabolism: To active metabolites via nonenzymatic reactions

Half-life elimination: Quinupristin: 0.85 hour; Dalfopristin: 0.7 hour (mean elimination half-lives, including metabolites: 3 and 1 hours, respectively)

Excretion: Feces (75% to 77% as unchanged drug and metabolites); urine (15% to 19%)

Dosage I.V.:

Children (limited information): Dosages similar to adult dosing have been used in the treatment of complicated skin/soft tissue infections and infections caused by vancomycin-resistant *Enterococcus faecium*

CNS shunt infection due to vancomycin-resistant *Enterococcus faecium*: 7.5 mg/kg/dose every 8 hours; concurrent intrathecal doses of 1-2 mg/day have been administered for up to 68 days

Adults:

Vancomycin-resistant *Enterococcus faecium*: 7.5 mg/kg every 8 hours

Complicated skin and skin structure infection: 7.5 mg/kg every 12 hours

Dosage adjustment in renal impairment: No adjustment required in renal failure, hemodialysis, or peritoneal dialysis

Dosage adjustment in hepatic impairment: Pharmacokinetic data suggest dosage adjustment may be necessary; however, specific recommendations have not been proposed

Elderly: No dosage adjustment is required

Stability Store unopened vials under refrigeration at 2°C to 8°C (36°F to 46°F). Reconstitute single dose vial with 5 mL of 5% dextrose in water or sterile water for injection. Swirl gently to dissolve; do not shake (to limit foam formation). The reconstituted solution should be diluted within 30 minutes. Stability of the diluted solution prior to the infusion is established as 5 hours at room temperature or 54 hours if refrigerated at 2°C to 8°C (36°F to 46°F). Reconstituted solution should be added to at least 250 mL of 5% dextrose in water for peripheral administration (increase to 500 mL or 750 mL if necessary to limit venous irritation). An infusion volume of 100 mL may be used for central line infusions. Do not freeze solution.

Administration Line should be flushed with 5% dextrose in water prior to and following administration. Infusion should be completed over 60 minutes (toxicity may be increased with shorter infusion). If severe venous irritation occurs following peripheral administration of quinupristin/dalfopristin diluted in 250 mL 5% dextrose in water, consideration should be given to increasing the infusion volume to 500 mL or 750 mL, changing the infusion site, or infusing by a peripherally-inserted central catheter (PICC) or a central venous catheter.

Pregnancy Risk Factor B

Contraindications Hypersensitivity to quinupristin, dalfopristin, pristinamycin, or virginiamycin, or any component of the formulation

Warnings/Precautions [U.S. Boxed Warning]: For the treatment of serious or life-threatening vancomycin-resistant *Enterococcus faecium* infections (VREF). Use with caution in patients with hepatic or renal dysfunction. May cause pain and phlebitis when infused through a peripheral line (not relieved by hydrocortisone or diphenhydramine). Prolonged use may result in fungal or bacterial superinfection, including *C. difficile*-associated diarrhea (CDAD) and pseudomembranous colitis; CDAD has been observed >2 months postantibiotic treatment. May cause arthralgias, myalgias, and hyperbilirubinemia. May inhibit the metabolism of many drugs metabolized by CYP3A4. Concurrent therapy with cisapride (which may prolong QT_c interval and lead to arrhythmias) should be avoided. Safety and efficacy have not been established in children <16 years of age.

Adverse Reactions

>10%:

Hepatic: Hyperbilirubinemia (3% to 35%)

Local: Local pain (40% to 44%), inflammation at infusion site (38% to 42%), local edema (17% to 18%), infusion site reaction (12% to 13%)

Neuromuscular & skeletal: Arthralgia (up to 47%), myalgia (up to 47%)

1% to 10%:

Central nervous system: Pain (2% to 3%), headache (2%)

Dermatologic: Rash (3%), pruritus (2%)

Endocrine & metabolic: Hyperglycemia (1%)

Gastrointestinal: Nausea (3% to 5%), vomiting (3% to 4%), diarrhea (3%)

Hematologic: Anemia (3%)

Hepatic: GGT increased (2%), LDH increased (3%)

Local: Thrombophlebitis (2%)

Neuromuscular & skeletal: CPK increased (2%)

<1% (Limited to important or life-threatening): Allergic reaction, anaphylactoid reaction, angina, apnea, arrhythmia, cardiac arrest, coagulation disorder, dysautonomia, dyspnea, encephalopathy, gout, hematuria, hemolytic anemia, hepatitis, hyperkalemia, hypotension, maculopapular rash, mesenteric artery occlusion, myasthenia, neuropathy, pancreatitis, pancytopenia, paraplegia, paresthesia, pericarditis, pleural effusion, pseudomembranous colitis, respiratory distress, seizure, shock, stomatitis, syncope, thrombocytopenia, urticaria

Drug Interactions

Metabolism/Transport Effects Quinupristin: **Inhibits** CYP3A4 (weak)

Avoid Concomitant Use There are no known interactions where it is recommended to avoid concomitant use.

Increased Effect/Toxicity

Quinupristin and Dalfopristin may increase the levels/effects of: Calcium Channel Blockers; CycloSPORINE

Decreased Effect There are no known significant interactions involving a decrease in effect.

Dosage Forms Excipient information presented when available (limited, particularly for generics); consult specific product labeling.

Injection, powder for reconstitution:

Synercid®: 500 mg: Quinupristin 150 mg and dalfopristin 350 mg

♦ **Quixin®** *see* Levofloxacin *on page 823*

♦ **RabAvert®** *see* Rabies Virus Vaccine *on page 1225*

Rabeprazole (ra BEP ra zole)

Medication Safety Issues

Sound-alike/look-alike issues:

AcipHex® may be confused with Acephen®, Accupril®, Aricept®, pHisoHex®

Rabeprazole may be confused with aripiprazole, donepezil, lansoprazole, omeprazole, raloxifene

Related Information

Helicobacter pylori Treatment *on page 1746*

U.S. Brand Names AcipHex®

Canadian Brand Names AcipHex®; Novo-Rabeprazole EC; Pariet®; PMS-Rabeprazole; Pro-Rabeprazole; Ran-Rabeprazole; Riva-Rabeprazole EC; Sandoz-Rabeprazole; Zym-Rabeprazole

Index Terms Pariprazole

Pharmacologic Category Proton Pump Inhibitor; Substituted Benzimidazole

Generic Available No

Use Short-term (4-8 weeks) treatment and maintenance of erosive or ulcerative gastroesophageal reflux disease (GERD); symptomatic GERD; short-term (up to 4 weeks) treatment of duodenal ulcers; long-term treatment of pathological hypersecretory conditions, including Zollinger-Ellison syndrome; *H. pylori* eradication (in combination therapy)

Canadian labeling: Additional uses (not in U.S. labeling): Treatment of nonerosive reflux disease (NERD); treatment of gastric ulcers

Unlabeled/Investigational Use Maintenance of duodenal ulcer

Mechanism of Action Potent proton pump inhibitor; suppresses gastric acid secretion by inhibiting the parietal cell H+/K+ ATP pump

◀ **Pharmacodynamics/Kinetics**
  Onset of action: Within 1 hour
  Duration: 24 hours
  Absorption: Oral: Well absorbed within 1 hour
  Protein binding, serum: ~96%
  Metabolism: Hepatic via CYP3A and 2C19 to inactive metabolites
  Bioavailability: Oral: ~52%
  Half-life elimination (dose dependent): 1-2 hours
  Time to peak, plasma: 2-5 hours
  Excretion: Urine (90% primarily as thioether carboxylic acid metabolites); remainder in feces

Dosage Oral:
  Children ≥12 years: *U.S. labeling:* Short-term treatment of GERD: 20 mg once daily for ≤8 weeks
  Adults >18 years and Elderly:
  Erosive/ulcerative GERD: Treatment: 20 mg once daily for 4-8 weeks; if inadequate response, may repeat up to an additional 8 weeks; maintenance: 20 mg once daily
    Canadian labeling: 20 mg once daily for 4 weeks; if inadequate response, may repeat for an additional 4 weeks (lack of symptom control after 4 weeks warrants further evaluation); maintenance: 10 mg once daily (maximum: 20 mg once daily)
  Symptomatic GERD: Treatment: 20 mg once daily for 4 weeks; if inadequate response, may repeat for an additional 4 weeks
    Canadian labeling: 10 mg once daily (maximum: 20 mg once daily) for 4 weeks; lack of symptom control after 4 weeks warrants further evaluation
  Duodenal ulcer: 20 mg/day before breakfast for 4 weeks; additional therapy may be required for some patients
  Gastric ulcers (*Canadian labeling*): 20 mg once daily up to 6 weeks; additional therapy may be required for some patients
  Helicobacter pylori eradication:
    Manufacturer labeling: 20 mg twice daily administered with amoxicillin 1000 mg *and* clarithromycin 500 mg twice daily for 7 days
    American College of Gastroenterology guidelines (Chey, 2007):
      Nonpenicillin allergy: 20 mg twice daily administered with amoxicillin 1000 mg *and* clarithromycin 500 mg twice daily for 10-14 days
      Penicillin allergy: 20 mg twice daily administered with clarithromycin 500 mg *and* metronidazole 500 mg twice daily for 10-14 days **or** 20 mg once or twice daily administered with bismuth subsalicylate 525 mg *and* metronidazole 250 mg *plus* tetracycline 500 mg 4 times/day for 10-14 days
  Hypersecretory conditions: 60 mg once daily; dose may need to be adjusted as necessary. Doses as high as 100 mg once daily and 60 mg twice daily have been used, and continued as long as necessary (up to 1 year in some patients).
  NERD (*Canadian labeling*): Treatment: 10 mg (maximum: 20 mg once daily) for 4 weeks; lack of symptom control after 4 weeks warrants further evaluation

  Dosage adjustment in renal impairment: No dosage adjustment required
  Dosage adjustment in hepatic impairment:
    Mild-to-moderate: Elimination decreased; no dosage adjustment required
    Severe: Use caution

Stability Store at 25°C (77°F). Protect from moisture.

Administration May be administered with or without food; best if taken before breakfast. Do not crush, split, or chew tablet. May be administered with an antacid.

Pregnancy Risk Factor B

Contraindications Hypersensitivity to rabeprazole, substituted benzimidazoles (ie, esomeprazole, lansoprazole, omeprazole, pantoprazole), or any component of the formulation

Warnings/Precautions Use of proton pump inhibitors may increase the risk of gastrointestinal infections (eg, *Salmonella, Campylobacter*). Use caution in severe hepatic impairment. Relief of symptoms with rabeprazole does not preclude the presence of a gastric malignancy. Decreased *H. pylori* eradication rates have been observed with short-term (≤7 days) combination therapy. The American College of Gastroenterology recommends 10-14 days of therapy (triple or quadruple) for eradication of *H. pylori* (Chey, 2007). Safety and efficacy have not been established in patients <12 years of age.

Adverse Reactions

1% to 10%:

Central nervous system: Pain (3%), headache (2% to 5%)

Gastrointestinal: Diarrhea (3%), flatulence (3%), constipation (2%), nausea (2%)

Respiratory: Pharyngitis (3%)

Miscellaneous: Infection (2%)

<1% (Limited to important or life-threatening): Abdomen enlarged, abdominal pain, abnormal stools, abnormal vision, agitation, agranulocytosis, albuminuria, allergic reaction, alopecia, amblyopia, anaphylaxis, anemia, angina pectoris, angioedema, anorexia, apnea, arrhythmia, arthralgia, arthritis, ascites, asthma, bloody diarrhea, bone pain, bradycardia, breast enlargement, bullous and other drug eruptions of skin, bundle branch block, bursitis, cataract, cellulitis, cerebral hemorrhage, chest pain substernal, cholangitis, cholecystitis, cholelithiasis, colitis, coma, constipation, contact dermatitis, convulsions, corneal opacity, CPK increased, cystitis, deafness, delirium, depression, diaphoresis, diabetes mellitus, diplopia, disorientation, dizziness, duodenitis, dysmenorrhea, dyspepsia, dysphagia, dyspnea, dysuria, edema, electrocardiogram abnormal, embolus, epistaxis, erythema multiforme, esophageal stenosis, esophagitis, extrapyramidal syndrome, eye hemorrhage, facial edema, fever, flatulence, fungal dermatitis, gastritis, gastroenteritis, gastrointestinal hemorrhage, gingivitis, glaucoma, glossitis, gout, gynecomastia, hematuria, hemolytic anemia, hepatic encephalopathy, hepatic cirrhosis, hepatic enzymes increased, hepatitis, hepatoma, hernia, hyperammonemia, hypercholesteremia, hyperglycemia, hyperkinesia, hyperlipemia, hypertension, hyper-/hypothyroidism, hypertonia, hypokalemia, hyponatremia, hypoxia, impotence, injection site hemorrhage/pain/reaction, insomnia, interstitial nephritis, interstitial pneumonia, jaundice, kidney calculus, leukocytosis, leukopenia, leukorrhea, liver fatty deposit, lymphadenopathy, malaise, melena, menorrhagia, metrorrhagia, MI, migraine, myalgia, nausea, neck rigidity, nervousness, neuralgia, neuropathy, neutropenia, orchitis, palpitation, pancreatitis, pancytopenia, paresthesia, peripheral edema, photosensitivity, polycystic kidney, polyuria, proctitis, pruritus, PSA increased, psoriasis, pulmonary embolus, QT_c prolongation, rash, rectal hemorrhage, retinal degeneration, rhabdomyolysis, salivary gland enlargement, sinus bradycardia, skin discoloration, somnolence, Stevens-Johnson syndrome, stomatitis, strabismus, sudden death, supraventricular tachycardia, syncope, tachycardia, taste abnormal, thrombocytopenia, thrombophlebitis, thrombosis, thirst (rare) tinnitus, toxic epidermal necrolysis, tremor, TSH increased, ulcerative colitis, urinary incontinence, urticaria, vasodilation, ventricular arrhythmias, vertigo, vomiting, weakness, weight gain/loss, xerostomia

Drug Interactions

Metabolism/Transport Effects Substrate (major) of CYP2C19, 3A4; **Inhibits** CYP2C8 (moderate), 2C19 (moderate), 2DC (weak), 3A4 (weak)

Avoid Concomitant Use

Avoid concomitant use of Rabeprazole with any of the following: Delavirdine; Erlotinib; Nelfinavir; Posaconazole

Increased Effect/Toxicity

Rabeprazole may increase the levels/effects of: CYP2C19 Substrates; CYP2C8 Substrates (High risk); Methotrexate; Raltegravir; Saquinavir; Tacrolimus; Voriconazole

The levels/effects of Rabeprazole may be increased by: Fluconazole; Ketoconazole

Decreased Effect

Rabeprazole may decrease the levels/effects of: Atazanavir; Clopidogrel; Dabigatran Etexilate; Dasatinib; Delavirdine; Erlotinib; Indinavir; Iron Salts; Itraconazole; Ketoconazole; Mesalamine; Mycophenolate; Nelfinavir; Posaconazole

The levels/effects of Rabeprazole may be decreased by: CYP2C19 Inducers (Strong); CYP3A4 Inducers (Strong); Deferasirox; Herbs (CYP3A4 Inducers); Tipranavir

◀ **Ethanol/Nutrition/Herb Interactions**
Ethanol: Avoid ethanol (may cause gastric mucosal irritation).
Food: High-fat meals may delay absorption, but C_{max} and AUC are not altered.
Herb/Nutraceutical: St John's wort may increase the metabolism and thus decrease the levels/effects of rabeprazole.

Dietary Considerations May be taken with or without food; best if taken before breakfast.

Dosage Forms Excipient information presented when available (limited, particularly for generics); consult specific product labeling. [CAN] = Canadian brand name
Tablet, delayed release, enteric coated, as sodium:
  AcipHex®: 20 mg
  Pariet® [CAN]: 10 mg, 20 mg

Rabies Immune Globulin (Human)
(RAY beez i MYUN GLOB yoo lin, HYU man)

U.S. Brand Names HyperRAB™ S/D; Imogam® Rabies-HT
Canadian Brand Names HyperRAB™ S/D; Imogam® Rabies Pasteurized
Index Terms RIG
Pharmacologic Category Blood Product Derivative; Immune Globulin
Generic Available No

Use Part of postexposure prophylaxis of persons with rabies exposure who lack a history of pre-exposure or postexposure prophylaxis with rabies vaccine or a recently documented neutralizing antibody response to previous rabies vaccination

Mechanism of Action Rabies immune globulin is a solution of globulins dried from the plasma or serum of selected adult human donors who have been immunized with rabies vaccine and have developed high titers of rabies antibody. It generally contains 10% to 18% of protein of which not less than 80% is monomeric immunoglobulin G.

Dosage Children and Adults: Postexposure prophylaxis: Local wound infiltration: 20 units/kg in a single dose, RIG should always be administered as part of rabies vaccine regimen. If anatomically feasible, the full rabies immune globulin dose should be infiltrated around and into the wound(s); remaining volume should be administered I.M. at a site distant from the vaccine administration site. If rabies vaccine was initiated without rabies immune globulin, rabies immune globulin may be administered through the seventh day after the administration of the first dose of the vaccine. Administration of RIG is not recommended after the seventh day post vaccine since an antibody response to the vaccine is expected during this time period.

Note: Persons known to have an adequate titer or who have previously received postexposure prophylaxis with rabies vaccine should not receive RIG.

Stability Store between 2°C to 8°C (36°F to 46°F); do not freeze. Discard product exposed to freezing.

Administration Do not administer I.V.
Postexposure wound infiltration: If anatomically feasible, the full rabies immune globulin dose should be infiltrated around and into the wound(s); remaining volume should be administered I.M. in the deltoid muscle of the upper arm or lateral thigh muscle. The gluteal area should be avoided to reduce the risk of sciatic nerve damage. Do not administer rabies vaccine in the same syringe or at the same administration site as RIG.

Pregnancy Risk Factor C

Contraindications There are no contraindications listed within the FDA-approved manufacturer's labeling.

Warnings/Precautions Hypersensitivity and anaphylactic reactions can occur; immediate treatment (including epinephrine 1:1000) should be available. Use with caution in patients with isolated immunoglobulin A deficiency or a history of systemic hypersensitivity to human immunoglobulins. Use with caution in patients with thrombocytopenia or coagulation disorders; I.M. injections may be contra-indicated. Product of human plasma; may potentially contain infectious agents which could transmit disease. Screening of donors, as well as testing and/or inactivation or removal of certain viruses, reduces the risk. Infections thought to be transmitted by this product should be reported to the manufacturer. Not for intravenous administration.

Adverse Reactions Frequency not defined.

Central nervous system: Fever (mild), headache, malaise

Dermatologic: Angioedema, rash, urticaria

Local: Soreness at injection site, tenderness, stiffness

Renal: Nephrotic syndrome

Miscellaneous: Anaphylaxis

Drug Interactions

Avoid Concomitant Use There are no known interactions where it is recommended to avoid concomitant use.

Increased Effect/Toxicity There are no known significant interactions involving an increase in effect.

Decreased Effect

Rabies Immune Globulin (Human) may decrease the levels/effects of: Vaccines (Live)

Dosage Forms Excipient information presented when available (limited, particularly for generics); consult specific product labeling.

Injection, solution [preservative free]:

HyperRAB™ S/D: 150 int. units/mL (2 mL, 10 mL) [solvent/detergent treated]

Imogam® Rabies-HT: 150 int. units/mL (2 mL, 10 mL) [heat treated]

Rabies Virus Vaccine (RAY beez vak SEEN)

U.S. Brand Names Imovax® Rabies; RabAvert®

Canadian Brand Names Imovax® Rabies; RabAvert®

Index Terms HDCV; Human Diploid Cell Cultures Rabies Vaccine; PCEC; Purified Chick Embryo Cell

Pharmacologic Category Vaccine, Inactivated (Viral)

Generic Available No

Use Pre-exposure and postexposure vaccination against rabies

The Advisory Committee on Immunization Practices (ACIP) recommends a primary course of prophylactic immunization (pre-exposure vaccination) for the following:

• Persons with continuous risk of infection including rabies research laboratory and biologics production workers

• Persons with frequent risk of infection in areas where rabies is enzootic, including rabies diagnostic laboratory workers, cavers, veterinarians and their staff, animal control and wildlife workers; persons who frequently handle bats

• Persons with infrequent risk of infection, including veterinarians and animal control staff with terrestrial animals in areas where rabies infection is rare, veterinary students, travelers visiting areas where rabies is enzootic and immediate access to medical care and biologicals is limited

The ACIP recommends the use of postexposure vaccination for a particular person be assessed by the severity and likelihood versus the actual risk of acquiring rabies. Consideration should include the type of exposure, epidemiology of rabies in the area, species of the animal, circumstances of the incident, and the availability of the exposing animal for observation or rabies testing. Postexposure vaccination is used in both previously vaccinated and previously unvaccinated individuals.

Mechanism of Action Rabies vaccine is an inactivated virus vaccine which promotes immunity by inducing an active immune response. The production of specific antibodies requires about 7-10 days to develop. Rabies immune globulin or antirabies serum, equine (ARS) is given in conjunction with rabies vaccine to provide immune protection until an antibody response can occur.

Pharmacodynamics/Kinetics

Onset of action: I.M.: Rabies antibody: ~7-10 days

Peak effect: ~30-60 days

Duration: ≥1 year

◀ **Dosage**

Pre-exposure vaccination: 1 mL I.M. on days 0, 7, and 21 to 28. **Note:** Prolonging the interval between doses does not interfere with immunity achieved after the concluding dose of the basic series.

Postexposure vaccination: All postexposure treatment should begin with immediate cleansing of the wound with soap and water

Persons not previously immunized as above: I.M.: 5 doses (1 mL each) on days 0, 3, 7, 14, 28. In addition, patients should also receive rabies immune globulin with the first dose (day 0). **Note:** A regimen of 4 doses (1 mL each) on days 0, 3, 7, 14 may be used in persons who are not immununosuppressed (ACIP Provisional Recommendations, 2009).

Persons who have previously received postexposure prophylaxis with rabies vaccine, received a recommended I.M. pre-exposure series of rabies vaccine or have a previously documented rabies antibody titer considered adequate: I.M.: Two doses (1 mL each) on days 0 and 3; do not administer rabies immune globulin

Booster (for persons with continuous or frequent risk of infection): 1 mL I.M. based on antibody titers

Stability Prior to reconstitution, store under refrigeration at 2°C to 8°C (36°F to 46°F); do not freeze. Protect from light. Reconstitute with provided diluent; gently swirl to dissolve. Use immediately after reconstitution.

Imovax®: Suspension will appear pink to red

RabAvert®: Suspension will appear clear to slightly opaque

Administration For I.M. administration only; this rabies vaccine product must not be administered intradermally; in adults and children, administer I.M. injections in the deltoid muscle, not the gluteal; for younger children, use the outer aspect of the thigh.

For patients at risk of hemorrhage following intramuscular injection, the ACIP recommends "it should be administered intramuscularly if, in the opinion of the physician familiar with the patients bleeding risk, the vaccine can be administered with reasonable safety by this route. If the patient receives antihemophilia or other similar therapy, intramuscular vaccination can be scheduled shortly after such therapy is administered. A fine needle (23 gauge or smaller) can be used for the vaccination and firm pressure applied to the site (without rubbing) for at least 2 minutes. The patient should be instructed concerning the risk of hematoma from the injection."

Administration with other vaccines:

Rabies vaccine with other inactivated vaccines: May be given simultaneously or at any interval between doses.

Rabies vaccine with live vaccines: May be given simultaneously or at any interval between doses.

Vaccine administration with antibody-containing products: Rabies vaccine may be given simultaneously at different sites or at any interval between doses. Examples of antibody containing products include I.M. and I.V. immune globulin, hepatitis B immune globulin, tetanus immune globulin, varicella zoster immune globulin, rabies immune globulin, whole blood, packed red cells, plasma, and platelet products.

Monitoring Parameters Monitor for syncope for ≥15 minutes following vaccination.

Antibody response to vaccination is not recommended for otherwise healthy persons who complete the pre-exposure or Postexposure regimen. Serologic testing to determine if the antibody titer is at an acceptable level is required for the following persons (booster vaccination recommended if titer is below the acceptable level):

Persons with continuous risk of infection: Serologic testing every 6 months

Persons with frequent risk of infection: Serologic testing every 2 years

Monitoring of antibody response to vaccination is not recommended for otherwise healthy persons who complete the pre-exposure or Postexposure regimen.

Reference Range Adequate adaptive immune response: antibody titers of 0.5 int. units/mL [WHO] or complete virus neutralization at a 1:5 serum dilution by the rapid fluorescent focus inhibition test (RFFIT) [ACIP]

Pregnancy Risk Factor C

Contraindications

Pre-exposure prophylaxis: Hypersensitivity to rabies vaccine or any component of the formulation

Postexposure prophylaxis: There are no contraindications listed within the FDA-approved manufacturer's labeling.

Warnings/Precautions Rabies vaccine should not be used in persons with a confirmed diagnosis of rabies; use after the onset of symptoms may be detrimental. Postexposure vaccination may begin regardless of the length of time from documented or likely exposure, as long as clinical signs of rabies are not present. Immediate treatment (including epinephrine 1:1000) for anaphylactoid and/or hypersensitivity reactions should be available during vaccine use. Once postexposure prophylaxis has begun, administration should generally not be interrupted or discontinued due to local or mild adverse events. Continuation of vaccination following severe systemic reactions should consider the persons risk of developing rabies. Report serious reactions to the State Health Department or the manufacturer/distributor. An immune complex reaction is possible 2-21 days following booster doses of HDCV. Symptoms may include arthralgia, arthritis, angioedema, fever, generalized urticaria, malaise, nausea, and vomiting Immune response may be decreased in immunosuppressed patients. Imovax® Rabies contains albumin and neomycin. RabAvert® contains amphotericin B, bovine gelatin, chicken protein, chlortetracycline, and neomycin. For I. M. administration only.

Adverse Reactions All serious adverse reactions must be reported to the U.S. Department of Health and Human Services (DHHS) Vaccine Adverse Event Reporting System (VAERS) 1-800-822-7967.

>10%:
Central nervous system: Dizziness, headache, malaise
Gastrointestinal: Abdominal pain, nausea
Local: Erythema, itching, pain, swelling
Neuromuscular & skeletal: Myalgia
Miscellaneous: Lymphadenopathy

Uncommon, frequency not defined, postmarketing, and/or case reports:
Cardiovascular: Circulatory reactions, edema, palpitation
Central nervous system: Chills, fatigue, fever >38°C (100°F), Guillain-Barré syndrome, encephalitis, meningitis, multiple sclerosis, myelitis, neuroparalysis, vertigo
Dermatologic: Pruritus, urticaria, urticaria pigmentosa
Endocrine & metabolic: Hot flashes
Local: Limb swelling (extensive)
Neuromuscular & skeletal: Limb pain, monoarthritis, paralysis (transient), paresthesias (transient)
Otic: Retrobulbar neuritis, visual disturbances
Respiratory: Bronchospasm
Miscellaneous: Allergic reactions, anaphylaxis, hypersensitivity reactions, swollen lymph nodes

Drug Interactions

Avoid Concomitant Use There are no known interactions where it is recommended to avoid concomitant use.

Increased Effect/Toxicity There are no known significant interactions involving an increase in effect.

Decreased Effect

The levels/effects of Rabies Vaccine may be decreased by: Chloroquine; Immunosuppressants

Dosage Forms Injection, powder for reconstitution [preservative free]:

Imovax® Rabies: ≥2.5 int. units [HDCV; grown in human diploid cell culture; contains albumin (human), neomycin (may have trace amounts)]

RabAvert®: ≥2.5 int. units [contains albumin (human), amphotericin B (may have trace amounts), bovine gelatin, chicken egg protein, chlortetracycline (may have trace amounts), neomycin (may have trace amounts); PCEC; grown in chicken fibroblast culture]

◆ **Racemic Epinephrine** *see* EPINEPHrine *on page 492*

◆ **Racepinephrine** *see* EPINEPHrine *on page 492*

- ◆ **rAHF** *see* Antihemophilic Factor (Recombinant) *on page 124*
- ◆ **R-albuterol** *see* Levalbuterol *on page 813*
- ◆ **Ralivia™ ER (Can)** *see* TraMADol *on page 1415*

Raloxifene (ral OKS i feen)

U.S. Brand Names Evista®

Canadian Brand Names Apo-Raloxifene; Evista®; Novo-Raloxifene

Index Terms Keoxifene Hydrochloride; Raloxifene Hydrochloride

Pharmacologic Category Selective Estrogen Receptor Modulator (SERM)

Use Prevention and treatment of osteoporosis in postmenopausal women; risk reduction for invasive breast cancer in postmenopausal women with osteoporosis and in postmenopausal women with high risk for invasive breast cancer

Pharmacodynamics/Kinetics

Onset of action: 8 weeks

Absorption: Rapid; ~60%

Distribution: 2348 L/kg

Protein binding: >95% to albumin and α-glycoprotein; does not bind to sex-hormone-binding globulin

Metabolism: Hepatic, extensive first-pass effect; metabolized to glucuronide conjugates

Bioavailability: ~2%

Half-life elimination: 28-33 hours

Excretion: Primarily feces; urine (<0.2% as unchanged drug; <6% as glucuronide conjugates)

Dosage Adults: Females: Oral:

Osteoporosis: 60 mg once daily

Invasive breast cancer risk reduction: 60 mg once daily for 5 years per ASCO guidelines (Visvanathan, 2009)

Dosage adjustment in renal impairment: Moderate-to-severe impairment: Use caution; safety and efficacy have not been established.

Dosage adjustment in hepatic impairment: Mild impairment (Child-Pugh class A): Plasma concentrations were higher and correlated with total bilirubin. Safety and efficacy in hepatic insufficiency have not been established.

Additional Information Complete prescribing information for this medication should be consulted for additional detail.

Dosage Forms Excipient information presented when available (limited, particularly for generics); consult specific product labeling.

Tablet, as hydrochloride:

Evista®: 60 mg

References

Barrett-Connor E, Mosca L, Collins P, et al, "Raloxifene Use for The Heart (RUTH) Trial Investigators. Effects of Raloxifene on Cardiovascular Events and Breast Cancer in Postmenopausal Women," *N Engl J Med*, 2006, 355(2):125-37.

Chlebowski RT, Col N, Winer EP, et al, "American Society of Clinical Oncology Technology Assessment of Pharmacologic Interventions for Breast Cancer Risk Reduction Including Tamoxifen, Raloxifene, and Aromatase Inhibition," *J Clin Oncol* , 2002, 20(15):3328-43.

Cummings SR, Eckert S, Krueger KA, et al, "The Effect of Raloxifene on Risk of Breast Cancer in Postmenopausal Women: Results from the MORE Randomized Trial," *JAMA*, 1999, 281(23) 2189-97.

Delmas PD, Bjarnason NH, Mitlak BH, et al, "Effects of Raloxifene on Bone Mineral Density, Serum Cholesterol Concentrations, and Uterine Endometrium in Postmenopausal Women," *N Engl J Med*, 1997, 337(23):1641-7.

Draper MW, Flowers DE, Huster WJ, et al, "A Controlled Trial of Raloxifene (LY139481) HCl: Impact on Bone Turnover and Serum Lipid Profile in Healthy Postmenopausal Women," *J Bone Miner Res*, 1996, 11(6):835-42.

Heaney RP and Draper MW, "Raloxifene and Estrogen: Comparative Bone-Remodeling Kinetics," *J Clin Endocrinol Metab*, 1997, 2(10):3425-9.

Martino S, Cauley JA, Barrett-Connor E, et al, "Continuing Outcomes Relevant to Evista: Breast Cancer Incident in Postmenopausal Women in a Randomized Trial of Raloxifene," *J Natl Cancer Inst*, 2004, 96(23):1751-61.

- ◆ **Raloxifene Hydrochloride** *see* Raloxifene *on page 1228*

Raltegravir (ral TEG ra vir)

U.S. Brand Names Isentress®
Canadian Brand Names Isentress®
Index Terms MK-0518
Pharmacologic Category Antiretroviral Agent, Integrase Inhibitor
Use Treatment of HIV-1 infection in combination with other antiretroviral agents
Pharmacodynamics/Kinetics
  Absorption: AUC increased ~19% with high-fat meal
  Protein binding: ~83%
  Metabolism: Primarily hepatic glucuronidation mediated by UGT1A1
  Half-life elimination: ~9 hours
  Time to peak, plasma: ~3 hours
  Excretion: Feces (~51%, as unchanged drug); urine (~32%; 9% as unchanged drug)
Dosage Oral: Adolescents ≥16 years and Adults: 400 mg twice daily
  Dosage adjustment for rifampin coadministration: 800 mg twice daily
  Dosage adjustment in renal impairment: Severe renal impairment: No dosage adjustment required
  Dosage adjustment in hepatic impairment:
    Mild-to-moderate hepatic impairment: No dosage adjustment required
    Severe impairment: No data available
Additional Information Complete prescribing information for this medication should be consulted for additional detail.
Dosage Forms Excipient information presented when available (limited, particularly for generics); consult specific product labeling.
  Tablet:
    Isentress®: 400 mg
References

  Grinsztejn B, Nguyen BY, Katlama C, et al, "Safety and Efficacy of the HIV-1 Integrase inhibitor Raltegravir (MK-0518) in Treatment-Experienced Patients with Multidrug-Resistant Virus: A Phase II Randomised Controlled Trial," *Lancet*, 2007, 369(9569):1261-9.
  Kassahun K, McIntosh I, Cui D, et al, "Metabolism and Disposition in Humans of Raltegravir (MK-0518), an Anti-AIDS Drug Targeting the Human Immunodeficiency Virus 1 Integrase Enzyme," *Drug Metab Dispos*, 2007, 35(9):1657-63.
  Nair V and Chi G, "HIV Integrase Inhibitors as Therapeutic Agents in AIDS," *Rev Med Virol*, 2007, 17 (4):277-95.

Ramipril (RA mi pril)

Related Information
  Angiotensin Agents *on page 1652*
  Heart Failure (Systolic) *on page 1739*
  Preoperative Evaluation of the Cardiac Patient for Noncardiac Surgery *on page 1598*
U.S. Brand Names Altace®
Canadian Brand Names Altace®; Apo-Ramipril®; CO Ramipril; Mylan-Ramipril; Novo-Ramipril; PMS-Ramipril; RAN-Ramipril; ratio-Ramipril; Sandoz-Ramipril
Pharmacologic Category Angiotensin-Converting Enzyme (ACE) Inhibitor
Use Treatment of hypertension, alone or in combination with thiazide diuretics; treatment of left ventricular dysfunction after MI; to reduce risk of MI, stroke, and death in patients at increased risk for these events
Unlabeled/Investigational Use Treatment of heart failure; to delay the progression of nephropathy and reduce risks of cardiovascular events in hypertensive patients with type 1 or 2 diabetes mellitus
Pharmacodynamics/Kinetics
  Onset of action: 1-2 hours
  Duration: 24 hours
  Absorption: Well absorbed (50% to 60%)
  Distribution: Plasma levels decline in a triphasic fashion; rapid decline is a distribution phase to peripheral compartment, plasma protein and tissue ACE (half-life: 2-4 hours); second phase is an apparent elimination phase representing the clearance of free ramiprilat (half-life: 9-18 hours); and final

phase is the terminal elimination phase representing the equilibrium phase between tissue binding and dissociation

Protein binding:
   Ramipril: 73%
   Ramiprilat: 56%
Metabolism: Hepatic to the active form, ramiprilat
Bioavailability:
   Ramipril: 28%
   Ramiprilat: 44%
Half-life elimination: Ramiprilat: Effective: 13-17 hours; Terminal: >50 hours
Time to peak, serum:
   Ramipril: ~1 hour
   Ramiprilat: 2-4 hours
Excretion: Urine (60%) and feces (40%) as parent drug and metabolites

Dosage Adults: Oral:
   Heart failure (unlabeled use): Initial: 1.25-2.5 mg once daily; target dose: 10 mg once daily (ACC/AHA 2009 Heart Failure Guidelines)
   Hypertension: 2.5-5 mg once daily, maximum: 20 mg/day
   LV dysfunction postmyocardial infarction: Initial: 2.5 mg twice daily titrated upward, if possible, to 5 mg twice daily
   Reduction in risk of MI, stroke, and death from cardiovascular causes: Initial: 2.5 mg once daily for 1 week, then 5 mg once daily for the next 3 weeks, then increase as tolerated to 10 mg once daily (may be given as divided dose)
   Note: The dose of any concomitant diuretic should be reduced. If the diuretic cannot be discontinued, initiate therapy with 1.25 mg. After the initial dose, the patient should be monitored carefully until blood pressure has stabilized.

Dosing adjustment in renal impairment:
   Cl_{cr} <40 mL/minute: Administer 25% of normal dose.
   Renal failure and heart failure: Administer 1.25 mg once daily, increasing to 1.25 mg twice daily up to 2.5 mg twice daily as tolerated.
   Renal failure and hypertension: Administer 1.25 mg once daily, titrated upward as possible; maximum daily dose 5 mg

Anesthesia and Critical Care Concerns/Other Considerations

Clinical Pearls/Comments: In patients on chronic ACE inhibitor therapy, intraoperative hypotension may occur with induction and maintenance of general anesthesia; however, discontinuation of therapy prior to surgery is controversial. If continued preoperatively, avoidance of hypotensive agents during surgery is prudent. Episodes of intraoperative hypotension may be managed by fluid administration and/or modest doses of alpha-adrenergic agents. Severe hypotension may occur in patients who are sodium- and/or volume-depleted, initiate lower doses and monitor closely when starting therapy in these patients. ACE inhibitor therapy may elicit an increase in potassium and creatinine, especially when used in patients with bilateral renal artery stenosis. In those patients experiencing cough on an ACE inhibitor, the ACE inhibitor may be discontinued and, if necessary, angiotensin-receptor blocker therapy instituted. Concomitant NSAID therapy may attenuate blood pressure control; use of NSAIDs should be avoided or limited, with monitoring of blood pressure control. In the setting of heart failure, NSAID use may be associated with an increased risk for fluid accumulation and edema. Because of the potent teratogenic effects of ACE inhibitors, these drugs should be avoided, if possible, when treating women of childbearing potential not on effective birth control measures. Aging patients with a decrease in glomerular filtration (also creatinine clearance), severe heart failure, and renal failure may experience an exaggerated response with administration of ACE inhibitors. Diabetic proteinuria is reduced and insulin sensitivity is enhanced.

Evidence-Based Information: ACE inhibitors decrease morbidity and mortality in patients with asymptomatic and symptomatic left ventricular dysfunction. In this situation, they decrease hospitalizations for, and retard progression to, decompensated heart failure. ACE inhibitors are also indicated in patients postmyocardial infarction in whom left ventricular ejection fraction is <40%. When used in patients with heart failure, the target dose or maximum tolerated dose should be achieved, if possible. Lower daily doses of ACE inhibitors have not demonstrated the same cardioprotective effects. ACE inhibitors have renal protective effects in patients with diabetic proteinuria. The HOPE trial examined the use of ramipril at a dose of between 2.5-10 mg daily in patients without heart failure at high risk for cardiovascular events and documented a significant improvement in cardiovascular outcome compared to placebo.

Additional Information Complete prescribing information for this medication should be consulted for additional detail.

Dosage Forms Excipient information presented when available (limited, particularly for generics); consult specific product labeling.

Capsule: 1.25 mg, 2.5 mg, 5 mg, 10 mg
  Altace®: 1.25 mg, 2.5 mg, 5 mg, 10 mg
Tablet:
  Altace®: 1.25 mg, 2.5 mg, 5 mg, 10 mg

♦ **Ran-Amlodipine (Can)** *see* AmLODIPine *on page* 93

♦ **RAN™-Atenolol (Can)** *see* Atenolol *on page* 155

♦ **RAN™-Carvedilol (Can)** *see* Carvedilol *on page* 244

♦ **RAN-Ciprofloxacin (Can)** *see* Ciprofloxacin *on page* 306

♦ **Ranexa®** *see* Ranolazine *on page* 1235

♦ **RAN™-Fentanyl Transdermal System (Can)** *see* FentaNYL *on page* 587

♦ **RAN-Fosinopril (Can)** *see* Fosinopril *on page* 636

♦ **Ran-Gabapentin (Can)** *see* Gabapentin *on page* 650

Ranitidine (ra NI ti deen)

Medication Safety Issues

Sound-alike/look-alike issues:
  Ranitidine may be confused with amantadine, rimantadine
  Zantac® may be confused with Xanax®, Zarontin®, Zofran®, Zyrtec®

International issues:
  Antagon®: Brand name for astemizole in Mexico; brand name for ganirelix in the U.S.

Related Information

Allergic Reactions *on page* 1508
Anesthesia for Obstetric Patients in Nonobstetric Surgery *on page* 1532
Desensitization Protocols *on page* 1692
Latex Allergy *on page* 1511

U.S. Brand Names Zantac 150® [OTC]; Zantac 75® [OTC]; Zantac®; Zantac® EFFERdose®

Canadian Brand Names Acid Reducer; Acid Reducer Maximum Strength Non Prescription; Apo-Ranitidine®; CO Ranitidine; Dom-Ranitidine; Gen-Ranidine; Mylan-Ranitidine; Novo-Ranidine; Nu-Ranit; PMS-Ranitidine; Ranitidine Injection, USP; ratio-Ranitidine; Riva-Ranitidine; Sandoz-Ranitidine; ScheinPharm Ranitidine; Zantac 75®; Zantac Maximum Strength Non-Prescription; Zantac®

Index Terms Ranitidine Hydrochloride

Pharmacologic Category Histamine H_2 Antagonist

Generic Available Yes: Excludes effervescent tablet

Use

Zantac®: Short-term and maintenance therapy of duodenal ulcer, gastric ulcer, gastroesophageal reflux disease (GERD), active benign ulcer, erosive esophagitis, and pathological hypersecretory conditions; as part of a multidrug regimen for *H. pylori* eradication to reduce the risk of duodenal ulcer recurrence

Zantac 75® [OTC]: Relief of heartburn, acid indigestion, and sour stomach

Unlabeled/Investigational Use Recurrent postoperative ulcer, upper GI bleeding, prevention of acid-aspiration pneumonitis during surgery, and prevention of stress-induced ulcers

Mechanism of Action Competitive inhibition of histamine at H_2-receptors of the gastric parietal cells, which inhibits gastric acid secretion, gastric volume, and hydrogen ion concentration are reduced. Does not affect pepsin secretion, pentagastrin-stimulated intrinsic factor secretion, or serum gastrin.

Pharmacodynamics/Kinetics

Absorption: Oral: 50%

◄ Distribution: Normal renal function: V_d: ~1.4 L/kg; Cl_{cr} 25-35 mL/minute: 1.76 L/kg minimally penetrates the blood-brain barrier; enters breast milk

Protein binding: 15%

Metabolism: Hepatic to N-oxide, S-oxide, and N-desmethyl metabolites

Bioavailability: Oral: 48% to 50%; I.M.: 90% to 100%

Half-life elimination:

Oral: Normal renal function: 2.5-3 hours; Cl_{cr} 25-35 mL/minute: 4.8 hours

I.V.: Normal renal function: 2-2.5 hours

Time to peak, serum: Oral: 2-3 hours; I.M.: ≤15 minutes

Excretion: Urine: Oral: 30%, I.V.: 70% (as unchanged drug); feces (as metabolites)

Dosage

Children 1 month to 16 years:

Duodenal and gastric ulcer:

Oral:

Treatment: 4-8 mg/kg/day divided twice daily; maximum: 300 mg/day

Maintenance: 2-4 mg/kg/day once daily; maximum: 150 mg/day

I.V.: 2-4 mg/kg/day divided every 6-8 hours; maximum: 200 mg/day

GERD and erosive esophagitis:

Oral: 5-10 mg/kg/day divided twice daily; maximum: GERD: 300 mg/day, erosive esophagitis: 600 mg/day

I.V. (unlabeled): 2-4 mg/kg/day divided every 6-8 hours; maximum: 200 mg/day **or as an alternative**

Continuous infusion: Initial: 1 mg/kg/dose for one dose followed by infusion of 0.08-0.17 mg/kg/hour or 2-4 mg/kg/day

Children ≥12 years: Prevention of heartburn: Oral: Zantac 75® [OTC]: 75 mg 30-60 minutes before eating food or drinking beverages which cause heartburn; maximum: 150 mg/24 hours; do not use for more than 14 days

Adults:

Duodenal ulcer: Oral: Treatment: 150 mg twice daily, or 300 mg once daily after the evening meal or at bedtime; maintenance: 150 mg once daily at bedtime

Helicobacter pylori eradication: 150 mg twice daily; requires combination therapy

Pathological hypersecretory conditions:

Oral: 150 mg twice daily; adjust dose or frequency as clinically indicated; doses of up to 6 g/day have been used

I.V.: Continuous infusion for Zollinger-Ellison: Initial: 1 mg/kg/hour; measure gastric acid output at 4 hours, if >10 mEq or if patient is symptomatic, increase dose in increments of 0.5 mg/kg/hour; doses of up to 2.5 mg/kg/hour (or 220 mg/hour) have been used

Gastric ulcer, benign: Oral: 150 mg twice daily; maintenance: 150 mg once daily at bedtime

GERD: Oral: 150 mg twice daily

Erosive esophagitis: Oral: Treatment: 150 mg 4 times/day; maintenance: 150 mg twice daily

Prevention of heartburn: Oral: Zantac 75® [OTC]: 75 mg 30-60 minutes before eating food or drinking beverages which cause heartburn; maximum: 150 mg in 24 hours; do not use for more than 14 days

Patients not able to take oral medication:

I.M.: 50 mg every 6-8 hours

I.V.: Intermittent bolus or infusion: 50 mg every 6-8 hours

Continuous I.V. infusion: 6.25 mg/hour

Elderly: Ulcer healing rates and incidence of adverse effects are similar in the elderly, when compared to younger patients; dosing adjustments not necessary based on age alone

Dosing adjustment in renal impairment: Adults: Cl_{cr} <50 mL/minute:

Oral: 150 mg every 24 hours; adjust dose cautiously if needed

I.V.: 50 mg every 18-24 hours; adjust dose cautiously if needed

Hemodialysis: Adjust dosing schedule so that dose coincides with the end of hemodialysis

Dosing adjustment/comments in hepatic disease: Patients with hepatic impairment may have minor changes in ranitidine half-life, distribution, clearance, and bioavailability; dosing adjustments not necessary, monitor

Stability

Injection: Vials: Store between 4°C to 25°C (39°F to 77°F); excursion permitted to 30°C (86°F). Protect from light. Solution is a clear, colorless to yellow solution; slight darkening does not affect potency.

Premixed bag: Store between 2°C to 25°C (36°F to 77°F). Protect from light.

EFFERdose® formulations: Store between 2°C to 30°C (36°F to 86°F).

Syrup: Store between 4°C to 25°C (39°F to 77°F). Protect from light.

Tablet: Store in dry place, between 15°C to 30°C (59°F to 86°F). Protect from light.

Vials can be mixed with NS or D_5W; solutions are stable for 48 hours at room temperature.

Intermittent bolus injection, continuous infusion: Dilute to maximum of 2.5 mg/mL.

Intermittent infusion: Dilute to maximum of 0.5 mg/mL.

Administration

Ranitidine injection may be administered I.M. or I.V.:

I.M.: Injection is administered undiluted

I.V.: Must be diluted; may be administered I.V. push, intermittent I.V. infusion, or continuous I.V. infusion

I.V. push: Ranitidine (usually 50 mg) should be diluted to a total of 20 mL (or a concentration not exceeding 2.5 mg/mL) with NS or D_5W and administered over at least 5 minutes or a maximum rate of 10 mg/minute

Intermittent I.V. infusion: Dilute to a maximum concentration of 0.5 mg/mL; administer over 15-20 minutes

Continuous I.V. infusion: Dilute to a maximum concentration of 2.5 mg/mL. Titrate dosage based on gastric pH.

EFFERdose®: Should not be chewed, swallowed whole, or dissolved on tongue: 25 mg tablet: Dissolve in at least 5 mL (1 teaspoonful) of water; wait until completely dissolved before administering

Monitoring Parameters AST, ALT, serum creatinine; when used to prevent stress-related GI bleeding, measure the intragastric pH and try to maintain pH >4; signs and symptoms of peptic ulcer disease, occult blood with GI bleeding, monitor renal function to correct dose

Anesthesia and Critical Care Concerns/Other Considerations

Clinical Pearls/Comments: Ranitidine causes fewer CNS adverse reactions and drug interactions compared to cimetidine.

Evidence-Based Information: The 2008 Surviving Sepsis Campaign guidelines recommend that stress ulcer prophylaxis using an H_2 blocker (Grade 1A) or proton pump inhibitor (Grade 1B) be given to patients with severe sepsis to prevent upper GI bleed. Benefit of prevention of upper GI bleed must be weighed against potential effect of increased stomach pH on development of ventilator-associated pneumonia.

Pregnancy Risk Factor B

Contraindications Hypersensitivity to ranitidine or any component of the formulation

Warnings/Precautions Ranitidine has been associated with confusional states (rare). Use with caution in patients with hepatic impairment; use with caution in renal impairment, dosage modification required. Avoid use in patients with history of acute porphyria (may precipitate attacks); long-term therapy may be associated with vitamin B_{12} deficiency. Symptoms of GI distress may be associated with a variety of conditions; symptomatic response to H_2 antagonists does not rule out the potential for significant pathology (eg, malignancy). EFFERdose® formulation contains phenylalanine. Safety and efficacy of ranitidine have not been established for pediatric patients <1 month of age

Adverse Reactions Frequency not defined.

Cardiovascular: Asystole, atrioventricular block, bradycardia (with rapid I.V. administration), premature ventricular beats, tachycardia, vasculitis

Central nervous system: Agitation, dizziness, depression, hallucinations, headache, insomnia, malaise, mental confusion, somnolence, vertigo

Dermatologic: Alopecia, erythema multiforme, rash

Endocrine & metabolic: Prolactin levels increased

◄ Gastrointestinal: Abdominal discomfort/pain, constipation, diarrhea, nausea, pancreatitis, vomiting

Hematologic: Acquired immune hemolytic anemia, acute porphyritic attack, agranulocytosis, aplastic anemia, granulocytopenia, leukopenia, pancytopenia, thrombocytopenia

Hepatic: Cholestatic hepatitis, hepatic failure, hepatitis, jaundice

Local: Transient pain, burning or itching at the injection site

Neuromuscular & skeletal: Arthralgia, involuntary motor disturbance, myalgia

Ocular: Blurred vision

Renal: Acute interstitial nephritis, serum creatinine increased

Respiratory: Pneumonia (causal relationship not established)

Miscellaneous: Anaphylaxis, angioneurotic edema, hypersensitivity reactions (eg, bronchospasm, fever, eosinophilia)

Drug Interactions

Metabolism/Transport Effects Substrate (minor) of CYP1A2, 2C19, 2D6; **Inhibits** CYP1A2 (weak), 2D6 (weak)

Avoid Concomitant Use

Avoid concomitant use of Ranitidine with any of the following: Delavirdine; Erlotinib

Increased Effect/Toxicity

Ranitidine may increase the levels/effects of: Procainamide; Saquinavir; Sulfonylureas; Warfarin

The levels/effects of Ranitidine may be increased by: P-Glycoprotein Inhibitors

Decreased Effect

Ranitidine may decrease the levels/effects of: Antifungal Agents (Azole Derivatives, Systemic); Atazanavir; Cefpodoxime; Cefuroxime; Dasatinib; Delavirdine; Erlotinib; Fosamprenavir; Gefitinib; Indinavir; Iron Salts; Mesalamine; Nelfinavir; Prasugrel

The levels/effects of Ranitidine may be decreased by: Peginterferon Alfa-2b; P-Glycoprotein Inducers

Ethanol/Nutrition/Herb Interactions

Ethanol: Avoid ethanol (may cause gastric mucosal irritation).

Food: Does not interfere with absorption of ranitidine.

Test Interactions False-positive urine protein using Multistix®; gastric acid secretion test; skin test allergen extracts

Dietary Considerations Oral dosage forms may be taken with or without food.

Zantac® EFFERdose®: Effervescent tablet 25 mg contains sodium 1.33 mEq/tablet and phenylalanine 2.81 mg/tablet

Dosage Forms Excipient information presented when available (limited, particularly for generics); consult specific product labeling.

Capsule 150 mg, 300 mg

Infusion, premixed in 1/2NS [preservative free]:

Zantac®: 50 mg (50 mL)

Injection, solution: 25 mg/mL (2 mL, 6 mL, 40 mL)

Zantac®: 25 mg/mL (2 mL, 6 mL, 40 mL) [contains phenol 0.5% as preservative]

Syrup: 15 mg/mL (5 mL, 10 mL, 473 mL)

Zantac®: 15 mg/mL (473 mL) [contains ethanol 7.5%; peppermint flavor]

Tablet: 75 mg [OTC], 150 mg, 300 mg

Zantac®: 150 mg, 300 mg

Zantac 75®: 75 mg

Zantac 150®: 150 mg

Tablet, for solution, oral [effervescent]:

Zantac® EFFERdose®: 25 mg [contains phenylalanine 2.81 mg/tablet, sodium 1.33 mEq/tablet, sodium benzoate]

References

Allen ME, Kopp BJ, and Erstad BL, "Stress Ulcer Prophylaxis in the Postoperative Period," *Am J Health Syst Pharm*, 2004, 61(6):588-96.

"ASHP Therapeutic Guidelines on Stress Ulcer Prophylaxis. ASHP Commission on Therapeutics and Approved by the ASHP Board of Directors on November 14, 1998," *Am J Health Syst Pharm*, 1999, 56(4):347-79.

Cook D, Guyatt G, Marshall J, et al, "A Comparison of Sucralfate and Ranitidine for the Prevention of Upper Gastrointestinal Bleeding in Patients Requiring Mechanical Ventilation. Canadian Critical Care Trials Group," *N Engl J Med*, 1998, 338(12):791-7.

Dellinger RP, Levy MM, Carlet JM, et al, "Surviving Sepsis Campaign: International Guidelines for Management of Severe Sepsis and Septic Shock: 2008," *Intensive Care Med*, 2008, 34(1): 17-60. Available at http://www.survivingsepsis.org/system/files/images/2008_20International_20SSC_20-Guidelines_1_.pdf

◆ **Ranitidine Hydrochloride** *see* Ranitidine *on page 1231*

◆ **Ranitidine Injection, USP (Can)** *see* Ranitidine *on page 1231*

◆ **Ran-Lisinopril (Can)** *see* Lisinopril *on page 849*

◆ **RAN™-Lovastatin (Can)** *see* Lovastatin *on page 859*

◆ **RAN™-Metformin (Can)** *see* MetFORMIN *on page 886*

Ranolazine (ra NOE la zeen)

U.S. Brand Names Ranexa®
Pharmacologic Category Cardiovascular Agent, Miscellaneous
Use Treatment of chronic angina
Pharmacodynamics/Kinetics
 Absorption: Highly variable; ranolazine is a substrate of P-glycoprotein; concurrent use of P-glycoprotein inhibitors may increase absorption
 Protein binding: ~62%
 Metabolism: Hepatic via CYP3A (major) and 2D6 (minor); gut
 Bioavailability: 35% to 55%
 Half-life elimination: Terminal: 7 hours
 Time to peak, plasma: 2-5 hours
 Excretion: Primarily urine (75% mostly as metabolites); feces (25% mostly as metabolites); in feces and urine, <5% to 7% excreted unchanged
Dosage Oral: Chronic angina:
 Adults: Initial: 500 mg twice daily; maximum recommended dose: 1000 mg twice daily
 Elderly: Select dose cautiously, starting at the lower end of the dosing range

 Dosage adjustment for ranolazine with concomitant medications:
  Diltiazem, verapamil, and other moderate CYP3A inhibitors: Dose should not exceed 500 mg twice daily
  P-glycoprotein inhibitors (eg, cyclosporine): Down-titrate ranolazine based on clinical response

 Dosage adjustment in renal impairment: Dosage adjustment recommendations have not been established. However, plasma ranolazine levels increased ~50% in patients with varying degrees of renal dysfunction. Patients with severe renal dysfunction had an increase in mean diastolic blood pressure of 10-15 mm Hg. Monitor blood pressure closely in these patients. Ranolazine has not been evaluated in patients requiring dialysis.
 Dosage adjustment in hepatic impairment: Use with caution in patients with mild (Child-Pugh class A) and moderate (Child-Pugh class B) hepatic impairment. Use is contraindicated with clinically significant hepatic impairment.
Additional Information Complete prescribing information for this medication should be consulted for additional detail.
Dosage Forms Excipient information presented when available (limited, particularly for generics); consult specific product labeling.
 Tablet, extended release:
  Ranexa®: 500 mg, 1000 mg
References
Abdallah H and Jerling M, "Effect of Hepatic Impairment on the Multiple-Dose Pharmacokinetics of Ranolazine Sustained Release Tablets," *J Clin Pharmacol*, 2005, 45(7):802-9.
Chaitman BR, Pepine CJ, Parker JO, et al, "Effects of Ranolazine With Atenolol, Amlodipine, or Diltiazem on Exercise Tolerance and Angina Frequency in Patients With Severe Chronic Angina. A Randomized Controlled Trial," *JAMA*, 2004, 291(3):309-16.
Jerling M and Abdallah H, "Effect of Renal Impairment on Multiple-Dose Pharmacokinetics of Extended Release Ranolazine," *Clin Pharmacol Ther*, 2005, 78(3):288-97.
Morrow DA, Scirica BM, Karwatowska-Prokopczuk E, et al, "Effects of Ranolazine on Recurrent Cardiovascular Events in Patients With Non-ST-Elevation Acute Coronary Syndromes. The MERLIN-TIMI 36 Randomized Trial," *JAMA*, 2007, 297(16):1775-83.

◆ **RAN-Ondansetron (Can)** *see* Ondansetron *on page 1057*

◆ **Ran-Pantoprazole (Can)** *see* Pantoprazole *on page 1084*

Rasagiline (ra SA ji leen)

U.S. Brand Names Azilect®
Index Terms AGN 1135; Rasagiline Mesylate; TVP-1012
Pharmacologic Category Anti-Parkinson's Agent, MAO Type B Inhibitor
Use Initial monotherapy or as adjunct to levodopa in the treatment of idiopathic Parkinson's disease
Pharmacodynamics/Kinetics
Onset of action: Therapeutic: Within 1 hour
Duration: ~1 week (irreversible inhibition); may require ~14-40 days for complete restoration of (brain) MAO-B activity
Absorption: Rapid
Protein binding: 88% to 94%
Metabolism: Hepatic N-dealkylation and/or hydroxylation via CYP1A2 to multiple inactive metabolites (nonamphetamine derivatives)
Distribution: V_{dss}: 87 L
Bioavailability: 36%
Half-life elimination: ~1.3-3 hours (no correlation with biologic effect due to irreversible inhibition)
Time to peak, plasma: 30 minutes to 1 hour
Excretion: Urine (62%, >99% as metabolites); feces (7%)
Dosage Oral: Adults: Parkinson's disease:
Monotherapy: 1 mg once daily
Adjunctive therapy with levodopa: Initial: 0.5 mg once daily; may increase to 1 mg once daily based on response and tolerability
Note: When added to existing levodopa therapy, a dose reduction of levodopa may be required to avoid exacerbation of dyskinesias; typical dose reductions of ~9% to 13% were employed in clinical trials

Dose reduction with concomitant ciprofloxacin or other CYP1A2 inhibitors: 0.5 mg once daily

Dosage adjustment in renal impairment:
Mild impairment: No adjustment necessary
Moderate-to-severe impairment: No data available
Dosage adjustment in hepatic impairment:
Mild impairment (Child-Pugh ≤6): 0.5 mg once daily
Moderate-to-severe impairment: Not recommended
Anesthesia and Critical Care Concerns/Other Considerations
Clinical Pearls/Comments: Patients receiving MAO inhibitors who undergo surgery may be at risk of developing significant hypertension when used with direct-acting adrenergic agents (eg, norepinephrine) and of lethal hypertension when administered with indirect-acting adrenergic agents (eg, ephedrine). The use of meperidine in these patients may also precipitate serotonin syndrome and is contraindicated. Years ago, it was advised that patients receiving MAO inhibitors have this drug discontinued for at least 10 days before elective surgery. However, the decision to continue or withhold MAO inhibitors must be done in collaboration with the patient's psychiatrist. Currently, an MAO-safe anesthetic technique which excludes the use of meperidine and indirect-acting adrenergic agonists is recommended for patients requiring continuing MAO therapy (Huyse, 2006).
Additional Information When adding rasagiline to levodopa/carbidopa, the dose of the latter can usually be decreased. Studies are investigating the use of

rasagiline in early Parkinson's disease to slow the progression of the disease. Complete prescribing information for this medication should be consulted for additional detail.

Dosage Forms Excipient information presented when available (limited, particularly for generics); consult specific product labeling.

Tablet:

Azilect®: 0.5 mg, 1 mg

References

Chen JJ and Ly A-V, "Rasagiline: A Second-Generation Monoamine Oxidase Type-B Inhibitor for the Treatment of Parkinson's Disease," *Am J Health-Syst Pharm*, 2006, 63(10):915-28.

Chen JJ and Swope DM, "Clinical Pharmacology of Rasagiline: A Novel, Second-Generation Propargylamine for the Treatment of Parkinson Disease," *J Clin Pharmacol*, 2005, 45(8):878-94.

Freedman NM, Mishani E, Krausz Y, et al, "In Vivo Measurement of Brain Monoamine Oxidase B Occupancy by Rasagiline, Using L-[11C]deprenyl and PET," *J Nucl Med*, 2005, 46(10):1618-24.

Hubalek F, Binda C, Li M et al, "Inactivation of Purified Human Recombinant Monoamine Oxidases A and B by Rasagiline and its Analogues," *J Med Chem*, 2004, 47(7):1760-66.

Huyse FJ, Touw DJ, van Schijndel RS, et al, "Psychotropic Drugs and the Perioperative Period: A Proposal for a Guideline in Elective Surgery," *Psychosomatics*, 2006, 47(1):8-22.

Parkinson Study Group, "A Randomized Placebo-Controlled Trial of Rasagiline in Levodopa-Treated Patients with Parkinson Disease and Motor Fluctuations. The PRESTO Study," *Arch Neurol*, 2005 62(2):241-8.

Parkinson Study Group, "A Controlled, Randomized, Delayed-Start Study of Rasagiline in Early Parkinson Disease," *Arch Neurol*, 2004, 6(4):561-66.

Parkinson Study Group, "A Controlled Trial of Rasagiline in Early Parkinson Disease: the TEMPO Study," *Arch Neurol*, 2002, 59(12):1937-43.

Rascol O, Brooks DJ, Melamed E et al, "Rasagiline as an Adjunct to Levodopa in Patients with Parkinson's Disease and Motor Fluctuations (LARGO, Lasting effect in Adjunct therapy With Rasagiline Given Once Daily, Study): A Randomized, Double-Blind, Parallel-Group Trial," *Lancet*, 2005, 365(9463):947-54.

Shulman KI and Walker SE, "A Reevaluation of Dietary Restrictions for Irreversible Monoamine Oxidase Inhibitors," *Psychiatr Ann*, 2001, 31(6):378-84.

Shulman KI and Walker SE, "Refining the MAOI Diet: Tyramine Content of Pizzas and Soy Products," *J Clin Psychiatry*, 1999, 60(3):191-3.

Walker SE, Shulman KI, Tailor SA, et al, "Tyramine Content of Previously Restricted Foods in Monoamine Oxidase Inhibitor Diets," *J Clin Psychopharmacol*, 1996, 16(5):383-8.

- ◆ **ratio-Glyburide (Can)** *see* GlyBURIDE *on page 666*
- ◆ **ratio-Inspra-Sal (Can)** *see* Albuterol *on page 49*
- ◆ **ratio-Ipra Sal UDV (Can)** *see* Ipratropium and Albuterol *on page 762*
- ◆ **ratio-Ketorolac (Can)** *see* Ketorolac *on page 784*
- ◆ **ratio-Lamotrigine (Can)** *see* LamoTRIgine *on page 800*
- ◆ **ratio-Lenoltec (Can)** *see* Acetaminophen and Codeine *on page 29*
- ◆ **ratio-Lisinopril (Can)** *see* Lisinopril *on page 849*
- ◆ **ratio-Lovastatin (Can)** *see* Lovastatin *on page 859*
- ◆ **ratio-Metformin (Can)** *see* MetFORMIN *on page 886*
- ◆ **ratio-Methotrexate (Can)** *see* Methotrexate *on page 898*
- ◆ **ratio-Methylphenidate (Can)** *see* Methylphenidate *on page 908*
- ◆ **ratio-Morphine (Can)** *see* Morphine Sulfate *on page 953*
- ◆ **ratio-Morphine SR (Can)** *see* Morphine Sulfate *on page 953*
- ◆ **ratio-Omeprazole (Can)** *see* Omeprazole *on page 1048*
- ◆ **ratio-Ondansetron (Can)** *see* Ondansetron *on page 1057*
- ◆ **ratio-Orciprenaline® (Can)** *see* Metaproterenol *on page 885*
- ◆ **ratio-Pantoprazole (Can)** *see* Pantoprazole *on page 1084*
- ◆ **ratio-Paroxetine (Can)** *see* PARoxetine *on page 1089*
- ◆ **ratio-Pioglitazone (Can)** *see* Pioglitazone *on page 1132*
- ◆ **ratio-Pravastatin (Can)** *see* Pravastatin *on page 1162*
- ◆ **ratio-Quetiapine (Can)** *see* QUEtiapine *on page 1212*
- ◆ **ratio-Ramipril (Can)** *see* Ramipril *on page 1229*
- ◆ **ratio-Ranitidine (Can)** *see* Ranitidine *on page 1231*
- ◆ **ratio-Salbutamol (Can)** *see* Albuterol *on page 49*
- ◆ **ratio-Simvastatin (Can)** *see* Simvastatin *on page 1293*
- ◆ **ratio-Sotalol (Can)** *see* Sotalol *on page 1321*
- ◆ **ratio-Sumatriptan (Can)** *see* SUMAtriptan *on page 1336*
- ◆ **ratio-Temazepam (Can)** *see* Temazepam *on page 1357*
- ◆ **ratio-Theo-Bronc (Can)** *see* Theophylline *on page 1373*
- ◆ **ratio-Topiramate (Can)** *see* Topiramate *on page 1408*
- ◆ **ratio-Trazodone (Can)** *see* TraZODone *on page 1423*
- ◆ **ratio-Valproic (Can)** *see* Valproic Acid and Derivatives *on page 1445*
- ◆ **ratio-Valproic ECC (Can)** *see* Valproic Acid and Derivatives *on page 1445*
- ◆ **ratio-Venlafaxine XR (Can)** *see* Venlafaxine *on page 1466*
- ◆ **6R-BH4** *see* Sapropterin *on page 1277*
- ◆ **Reactine™ (Can)** *see* Cetirizine *on page 282*
- ◆ **Reclipsen™** *see* Ethinyl Estradiol and Desogestrel *on page 544*
- ◆ **Recombinant Hirudin** *see* Lepirudin *on page 808*
- ◆ **Recombinant Human Platelet-Derived Growth Factor B** *see* Becaplermin *on page 180*
- ◆ **Recombinant Plasminogen Activator** *see* Reteplase *on page 1242*
- ◆ **Recombinate** *see* Antihemophilic Factor (Recombinant) *on page 124*
- ◆ **Recombivax HB®** *see* Hepatitis B Vaccine *on page 686*
- ◆ **Rectacaine [OTC]** *see* Phenylephrine *on page 1114*
- ◆ **ReFacto® [DSC]** *see* Antihemophilic Factor (Recombinant) *on page 124*
- ◆ **ReFacto® (Can)** *see* Antihemophilic Factor (Recombinant) *on page 124*
- ◆ **Refludan®** *see* Lepirudin *on page 808*
- ◆ **Refresh Liquigel® [OTC]** *see* Carboxymethylcellulose *on page 243*
- ◆ **Refresh Plus® [OTC]** *see* Carboxymethylcellulose *on page 243*
- ◆ **Refresh Plus® (Can)** *see* Carboxymethylcellulose *on page 243*
- ◆ **Refresh Tears® [OTC]** *see* Carboxymethylcellulose *on page 243*

- **Refresh Tears® (Can)** *see* Carboxymethylcellulose *on page* 243
- **Regitine [DSC]** *see* Phentolamine *on page* 1112
- **Regitine® (Can)** *see* Phentolamine *on page* 1112
- **Reglan®** *see* Metoclopramide *on page* 917
- **Regonol®** *see* Pyridostigmine *on page* 1210
- **Regranex®** *see* Becaplermin *on page* 180
- **Regular Insulin** *see* Insulin Regular *on page* 750
- **Relafen** *see* Nabumetone *on page* 973
- **Relafen® (Can)** *see* Nabumetone *on page* 973
- **Relenza®** *see* Zanamivir *on page* 1486
- **Relief® [OTC] [DSC]** *see* Phenylephrine *on page* 1114
- **Relistor™** *see* Methylnaltrexone *on page* 906
- **Relpax®** *see* Eletriptan *on page* 477
- **Remicade®** *see* InFLIXimab *on page* 740

Remifentanil (rem i FEN ta nil)

Medication Safety Issues
Sound-alike/look-alike issues:
  Remifentanil may be confused with alfentanil

High alert medication: The Institute for Safe Medication Practices (ISMP) includes this medication among its list of drug classes which have a heightened risk of causing significant patient harm when used in error.

Related Information
Anesthesia Considerations for Neurosurgery *on page* 1514
Anesthesia for Geriatric Patients *on page* 1523
Anesthesia for Patients With Liver Disease *on page* 1537
Chronic Renal Failure *on page* 1552
Dosing Considerations for the Critically-Ill Patient With Morbid Obesity *on page* 1561

U.S. Brand Names Ultiva®
Canadian Brand Names Ultiva®
Index Terms GI87084B
Pharmacologic Category Analgesic, Opioid; Anilidopiperidine Opioid
Restrictions C-II
Generic Available No
Use Analgesic for use during the induction and maintenance of general anesthesia; for continued analgesia into the immediate postoperative period; analgesic component of monitored anesthesia
Unlabeled/Investigational Use Management of pain in mechanically-ventilated patients
Mechanism of Action Binds with stereospecific mu-opioid receptors at many sites within the CNS, increases pain threshold, alters pain reception, inhibits ascending pain pathways

Pharmacodynamics/Kinetics
Onset of action: I.V.: 1-3 minutes
Distribution: V_d: 100 mL/kg; increased in children
Protein binding: ~70% (primarily alpha$_1$ acid glycoprotein)
Metabolism: Rapid via blood and tissue esterases
Half-life elimination (dose dependent): Terminal: 10-20 minutes; effective: 3-10 minutes
Excretion: Urine

Dosage I.V. continuous infusion: Dose should be based on ideal body weight (IBW) in obese patients (>30% over IBW).
Children Birth to 2 months: Maintenance of anesthesia with nitrous oxide (70%): 0.4 mcg/kg/minute (range: 0.4-1 mcg/kg/minute); supplemental bolus dose of 1 mcg/kg may be administered, smaller bolus dose may be required with potent inhalation agents, potent neuraxial anesthesia, significant comorbidities,

significant fluid shifts, or without atropine pretreatment. Clearance in neonates is highly variable; dose should be carefully titrated.

Children 1-12 years: Maintenance of anesthesia with halothane, sevoflurane, or isoflurane: 0.25 mcg/kg/minute (range: 0.05-1.3 mcg/kg/minute); supplemental bolus dose of 1 mcg/kg may be administered every 2-5 minutes. Consider increasing concomitant anesthetics with infusion rate >1 mcg/kg/minute. Infusion rate can be titrated upward in increments up to 50% or titrated downward in decrements of 25% to 50%. May titrate every 2-5 minutes.

Adults:

Induction of anesthesia: 0.5-1 mcg/kg/minute; if endotracheal intubation is to occur in <8 minutes, an initial dose of 1 mcg/kg may be given over 30-60 seconds

Coronary bypass surgery: 1 mcg/kg/minute

Maintenance of anesthesia: **Note:** Supplemental bolus dose of 1 mcg/kg may be administered every 2-5 minutes. Consider increasing concomitant anesthetics with infusion rate >1 mcg/kg/minute. Infusion rate can be titrated upward in increments of 25% to 100% or downward in decrements of 25% to 50%. May titrate every 2-5 minutes.

With nitrous oxide (66%): 0.4 mcg/kg/minute (range: 0.1-2 mcg/kg/minute)

With isoflurane: 0.25 mcg/kg/minute (range: 0.05-2 mcg/kg/minute)

With propofol: 0.25 mcg/kg/minute (range: 0.05-2 mcg/kg/minute)

Coronary bypass surgery: 1 mcg/kg/minute (range: 0.125-4 mcg/kg/minute); supplemental dose: 0.5-1 mcg/kg

Continuation as an analgesic in immediate postoperative period: 0.1 mcg/kg/minute (range: 0.025-0.2 mcg/kg/minute). Infusion rate may be adjusted every 5 minutes in increments of 0.025 mcg/kg/minute. Bolus doses are not recommended. Infusion rates >0.2 mcg/kg/minute are associated with respiratory depression.

Coronary bypass surgery, continuation as an analgesic into the ICU: 1 mcg/kg/minute (range: 0.05-1 mcg/kg/minute)

Analgesic component of monitored anesthesia care: **Note:** Supplemental oxygen is recommended:

Single I.V. dose given 90 seconds prior to local anesthetic:

Remifentanil alone: 1 mcg/kg over 30-60 seconds

With midazolam: 0.5 mcg/kg over 30-60 seconds

Continuous infusion beginning 5 minutes prior to local anesthetic:

Remifentanil alone: 0.1 mcg/kg minute

With midazolam: 0.05 mcg/kg/minute

Continuous infusion given after local anesthetic:

Remifentanil alone: 0.05 mcg/kg/minute (range: 0.025-0.2 mcg/kg/minute)

With midazolam: 0.025 mcg/kg/minute (range: 0.025-0.2 mcg/kg/minute)

Note: Following local or anesthetic block, infusion rate should be decreased to 0.05 mcg/kg/minute; rate adjustments of 0.025 mcg/kg/minute may be done at 5-minute intervals

Critically-ill patients (unlabeled dose): Continuous infusion: 42-1050 mcg/hour (based on 70 kg patient) **or** 0.6-15 mcg/kg/hour

Elderly: Elderly patients have an increased sensitivity to effect of remifentanil; doses should be decreased by 50% and titrated.

Stability Prior to reconstitution, store at 2°C to 25°C (36°F to 77°F). Prepare solution by adding 1 mL of diluent per 1 mg of remifentanil. Shake well. Further dilute to a final concentration of 20, 25, 50, or 250 mcg/mL. Stable for 24 hours at room temperature after reconstitution and further dilution to concentrations of 20-250 mcg/mL (4 hours if diluted with LR).

Administration An infusion device should be used to administer continuous infusions. During the maintenance of general anesthesia, I.V. boluses may be administered over 30-60 seconds. Injections should be given into I.V. tubing close to the venous cannula; tubing should be cleared after treatment to prevent residual effects when other fluids are administered through the same I.V. line.

Monitoring Parameters Respiratory and cardiovascular status, blood pressure, heart rate

Anesthesia and Critical Care Concerns/Other Considerations

Clinical Pearls/Comments: Remifentanil should be used in combination with other induction agents; bolus doses are not recommended for sedation cases and in treatment of postoperative pain due to risk of respiratory depression and muscle rigidity; due to remifentanil's short duration of action, when postoperative pain is anticipated, discontinuation of an infusion of remifentanil should be preceded by an adequate postoperative analgesic (ie, fentanyl, morphine). Remifentanil demonstrates synergistic respiratory depression when combined with benzodiazepines.

No metabolic interactions occur with other esterase-hydrolyzed drugs (eg, succinylcholine, esmolol, atracurium).

Elderly patients have an increased sensitivity to the effect of remifentanil; doses should be decreased by 50% and titrated.

Evidence-Based Information: Ultra short-acting opioid that is unique compared to other short-acting opioids because it does not accumulate during infusion and its rapid metabolism.

Pregnancy Risk Factor C

Contraindications Not for intrathecal or epidural administration, due to the presence of glycine in the formulation; hypersensitivity to remifentanil, fentanyl, or fentanyl analogs, or any component of the formulation

Warnings/Precautions Remifentanil is not recommended as the sole agent in general anesthesia, because the loss of consciousness cannot be assured and due to the high incidence of apnea, hypotension, tachycardia and muscle rigidity; it should be administered by individuals specifically trained in the use of anesthetic agents and should not be used in diagnostic or therapeutic procedures outside the monitored anesthesia setting; resuscitative and intubation equipment should be readily available. May cause hypotension; use with caution in patients with hypovolemia, cardiovascular disease (including acute MI), or drugs which may exaggerate hypotensive effects (including phenothiazines or general anesthetics). Shares the toxic potentials of opiate agonists, and precautions of opiate agonist therapy should be observed. In patients <55 years of age, intraoperative awareness has been reported when used with propofol rates of ≤75 mcg/kg/minute.

Use with caution when administering to patients with bradycardia. Inject slowly over 3-5 minutes; rapid I.V. infusion may result in skeletal muscle and chest wall rigidity, impaired ventilation, or respiratory distress/arrest; nondepolarizing skeletal muscle relaxant may be required. Interruption of an infusion will result in offset of effects within 5-10 minutes; the discontinuation of remifentanil infusion should be preceded by the establishment of adequate postoperative analgesia orders, especially for patients in whom postoperative pain is anticipated. Use caution in the morbidly obese. Safety and efficacy for postoperative analgesic or monitored anesthesia care have not been established in children.

Adverse Reactions

>10%: Gastrointestinal: Nausea, vomiting

1% to 10%:

Cardiovascular: Bradycardia (dose dependent), hypertension, hypotension (dose dependent), tachycardia

Central nervous system: Agitation, dizziness, fever, headache

Dermatologic: Pruritus

Neuromuscular & skeletal: Muscle rigidity (dose dependent)

Ocular: Visual disturbances

Respiratory: Apnea, hypoxia, respiratory depression

Miscellaneous: Postoperative pain, shivering

<1% (Limited to important or life-threatening): Anaphylactic/anaphylactoid reactions, anemia, anxiety, arrhythmia, asystole, bronchospasm, confusion, constipation, CPK-MB increased, diarrhea, dysphagia, electrolyte disorders, hallucinations, heart block, pleural effusion, prolonged emergence from anesthesia, pulmonary edema, syncope, thrombocytopenia, xerostomia

Drug Interactions

Avoid Concomitant Use

Avoid concomitant use of Remifentanil with any of the following: MAO Inhibitors ▶

Increased Effect/Toxicity

Remifentanil may increase the levels/effects of: Alcohol (Ethyl); Alvimopan; Beta-Blockers; Calcium Channel Blockers (Nondihydropyridine); CNS Depressants; Desmopressin; MAO Inhibitors; Selective Serotonin Reuptake Inhibitors; Thiazide Diuretics

The levels/effects of Remifentanil may be increased by: Amphetamines; Antipsychotic Agents (Phenothiazines); Succinylcholine

Decreased Effect

Remifentanil may decrease the levels/effects of: Pegvisomant

The levels/effects of Remifentanil may be decreased by: Ammonium Chloride

Dosage Forms Excipient information presented when available (limited, particularly for generics); consult specific product labeling.

Injection, powder for reconstitution: 1 mg, 2 mg, 5 mg [contains glycine 15 mg]

References

"Clinical Practice Guidelines for the Sustained Use of Sedatives and Analgesics in the Critically Ill Adult. Task Force of the American College of Critical Care Medicine (ACCM) of the Society of Critical Care Medicine (SCCM), American Society of Health-System Pharmacists (ASHP), American College of Chest Physicians," *Am J Health Syst Pharm*, 2002, 59(2):150-78.

Hogue CW, Bowdle TA, O'Leary C, et al, "A Multicenter Evaluation of Total Intravenous Anesthesia With Remifentanil and Propofol for Elective Inpatient Surgery," *Anesth Analg*, 1996, 83(2):279-85.

Jacobi J, Fraser GL, Coursin DB, et al, "Clinical Practice Guidelines for the Sustained Use of Sedatives and Analgesics in the Critically Ill Adult," *Crit Care Med*, 2002, 30(1):119-41. Available at: http://www.sccm.org/pdf/sedatives.pdf.

Mokhlesi B, Leikin JB, Murray P, et al, "Adult Toxicology in Critical Care. Part II: Specific Poisonings," *Chest*, 2003, 123(3):897-922.

"Principles of Analgesic Use in the Treatment of Acute Pain and Chronic Cancer Pain," 5th ed, Glenview, IL: American Pain Society, 2003.

Warner DS, Hindman BJ, Todd MM, et al, "Intracranial Pressure and Hemodynamic Effects of Remifentanil Versus Alfentanil in Patients Undergoing Supratentorial Craniotomy," *Anesth Analg*, 1996, 83(2):348-53.

Westmoreland CL, Hoke JF, Sebel PS, et al, "Pharmacokinetics of Remifentanil (GI87084B) and Its Major Metabolite (GI90291) in Patients Undergoing Elective Inpatient Surgery," *Anesthesiology*, 1993, 79(5):893-903.

Reteplase (RE ta plase)

Medication Safety Issues

High alert medication: The Institute for Safe Medication Practices (ISMP) includes this medication (I.V.) among its list of drugs which have a heightened risk of causing significant patient harm when used in error.

U.S. Brand Names Retavase®

Canadian Brand Names Retavase®

Index Terms r-PA; Recombinant Plasminogen Activator

Pharmacologic Category Thrombolytic Agent

Generic Available No

Use Management of ST-elevation myocardial infarction (STEMI); improvement of ventricular function; reduction of the incidence of CHF and the reduction of mortality following AMI

Recommended criteria for treatment: STEMI: Chest pain ≥20 minutes duration, onset of chest pain within 12 hours of treatment (or within prior 12-24 hours in patients with continuing ischemic symptoms), and ST-segment elevation >0.1 mV in at least two contiguous precordial leads or two adjacent limb leads on ECG or new or presumably new left bundle branch block (LBBB)

Mechanism of Action Reteplase is a nonglycosylated form of tPA produced by recombinant DNA technology using *E. coli*; it initiates local fibrinolysis by binding to fibrin in a thrombus (clot) and converts entrapped plasminogen to plasmin

Pharmacodynamics/Kinetics

Onset of action: Thrombolysis: 30-90 minutes

Half-life elimination: 13-16 minutes

Excretion: Feces and urine

Clearance: Plasma: 250-450 mL/minute

Dosage

Children: Not recommended

Adults: 10 units I.V. over 2 minutes, followed by a second dose 30 minutes later of 10 units I.V. over 2 minutes; withhold second dose if serious bleeding or anaphylaxis occurs

Note: All patients should receive 162-325 mg of chewable nonenteric coated aspirin as soon as possible and then daily. Administer concurrently with heparin 60 units/kg bolus (maximum: 4000 units) followed by continuous infusion of 12 units/kg/hour (maximum: 1000 units/hour) and adjust to aPTT target of 50-70 seconds (or 1.5-2 times the upper limit of control).

Stability Dosage kits should be stored at 2°C to 25°C (36°F to 77°F) and remain sealed until use in order to protect from light. Reteplase should be reconstituted using the diluent, syringe, needle, and dispensing pin provided with each kit.

Administration Reteplase should be reconstituted using the diluent, syringe, needle and dispensing pin provided with each kit and the each reconstituted dose should be administered I.V. over 2 minutes; no other medication should be added to the injection solution

Monitoring Parameters Monitor for signs of bleeding (hematuria, GI bleeding, gingival bleeding)

Anesthesia and Critical Care Concerns/Other Considerations

Evidence-Based Information:

Management of Intracerebral Hemorrhage (ICH) Due to Thrombolysis: Overall management of ICH is similar regardless of cause; however, iatrogenic spontaneous ICH may have specific treatments. According to the 2007 ACC/ASA Guidelines for the Management of Spontaneous Intracerebral Hemorrhage, fibrinolytic-related ICH should be treated with infusion of platelets (6-8 units) and cryoprecipitate which contains factor VIII (Class IIb recommendation).

Pregnancy Risk Factor C

Contraindications Hypersensitivity to reteplase or any component of the formulation; active internal bleeding; history of cerebrovascular accident; recent intracranial or intraspinal surgery or trauma; intracranial neoplasm, arteriovenous malformations, or aneurysm; known bleeding diathesis; severe uncontrolled hypertension

Warnings/Precautions Concurrent heparin anticoagulation can contribute to bleeding; careful attention to all potential bleeding sites. I.M. injections and nonessential handling of the patient should be avoided. Venipunctures should be performed carefully and only when necessary. If arterial puncture is necessary, use an upper extremity vessel that can be manually compressed. If serious bleeding occurs then the infusion of anistreplase and heparin should be stopped.

For the following conditions the risk of bleeding is higher with use of reteplase and should be weighed against the benefits of therapy: recent major surgery (eg, CABG, obstetrical delivery, organ biopsy, previous puncture of noncompressible vessels), cerebrovascular disease, recent gastrointestinal or genitourinary bleeding, recent trauma including CPR, hypertension (systolic BP >180 mm Hg and/or diastolic BP >110 mm Hg), high likelihood of left heart thrombus (eg, mitral stenosis with atrial fibrillation), acute pericarditis, subacute bacterial endocarditis, hemostatic defects including ones caused by severe renal or hepatic dysfunction, significant hepatic dysfunction, pregnancy, diabetic hemorrhagic retinopathy or other hemorrhagic ophthalmic conditions, septic thrombophlebitis or occluded AV

◄ cannula at seriously infected site, advanced age (eg, >75 years), patients receiving oral anticoagulants, any other condition in which bleeding constitutes a significant hazard or would be particularly difficult to manage because of location.

Coronary thrombolysis may result in reperfusion arrhythmias. Follow standard MI management. Rare anaphylactic reactions can occur. Safety and efficacy in pediatric patients have not been established.

Adverse Reactions Bleeding is the most frequent adverse effect associated with reteplase. Heparin and aspirin have been administered concurrently with reteplase in clinical trials. The incidence of adverse events is a reflection of these combined therapies, and are comparable with comparison thrombolytics.

>10%: Local: Injection site bleeding (4.6% to 48.6%)

1% to 10%:

Gastrointestinal: Bleeding (1.8% to 9.0%)

Genitourinary: Bleeding (0.9% to 9.5%)

Hematologic: Anemia (0.9% to 2.6%)

<1% (Limited to important or life-threatening): Allergic/anaphylactoid reactions, cholesterol embolization, intracranial hemorrhage (0.8%)

Other adverse effects noted are frequently associated with MI (and therefore may or may not be attributable to Retavase®) and include arrhythmia, arrest, cardiac reinfarction, cardiogenic shock, embolism, hypotension, pericarditis, pulmonary edema, tamponade, thrombosis

Drug Interactions

Avoid Concomitant Use There are no known interactions where it is recommended to avoid concomitant use.

Increased Effect/Toxicity

Reteplase may increase the levels/effects of: Anticoagulants; Drotrecogin Alfa

The levels/effects of Reteplase may be increased by: Antiplatelet Agents; Herbs (Anticoagulant/Antiplatelet Properties); Nonsteroidal Anti-Inflammatory Agents; Salicylates

Decreased Effect

The levels/effects of Reteplase may be decreased by: Aprotinin

Dosage Forms Excipient information presented when available (limited, particularly for generics); consult specific product labeling.

Injection, powder for reconstitution [preservative free]:

Retavase®: 10.4 units [equivalent to reteplase 18.1 mg; contains sucrose and polysorbate 80; packaged with sterile water for injection]

References

Antman EM, Anbe SC, Alpert JS, et al, "ACC/AHA Guidelines for the Management of Patients With ST-Elevation Myocardial Infarction - Executive Summary: A Report of the American College of Cardiology/American Heart Association Task Force on Practice Guidelines (Writing Committee to Revise the 1999 Guidelines for the Management of Patients With Acute Myocardial Infarction)," *Circulation*, 2004, 110:588-636. Available at: http://www.circulationaha.org/cgi/content/full/110/5/588.

Broderick J, Connolly S, Feldmann E, et al, "Guidelines for the Management of Spontaneous Intracerebral Hemorrhage in Adults: 2007 Update: A Guideline From the American Heart Association/American Stroke Association Stroke Council, High Blood Pressure Research Council, and the Quality of Care and Outcomes in Research Interdisciplinary Working Group," *Stroke*, 2007, 38(6):2001-23. Available at http://stroke.ahajournals.org/cgi/content/short/STROKEAHA.107.183689.

- **Rho®-Clonazepam (Can)** *see* ClonazePAM *on page* 328
- **Rhodacine® (Can)** *see* Indomethacin *on page* 738
- **Rhodis™ (Can)** *see* Ketoprofen *on page* 783
- **Rhodis-EC™ (Can)** *see* Ketoprofen *on page* 783
- **Rhodis SR™ (Can)** *see* Ketoprofen *on page* 783
- **Rho®-Nitro (Can)** *see* Nitroglycerin *on page* 1014
- **Rhotral (Can)** *see* Acebutolol *on page* 24
- **Rhoxal-acebutolol (Can)** *see* Acebutolol *on page* 24
- **Rhoxal-atenolol (Can)** *see* Atenolol *on page* 155
- **Rhoxal-cyclosporine (Can)** *see* CycloSPORINE *on page* 357
- **Rhoxal-metformin (Can)** *see* MetFORMIN *on page* 886
- **Rhoxal-nabumetone (Can)** *see* Nabumetone *on page* 973
- **Rhoxal-salbutamol (Can)** *see* Albuterol *on page* 49
- **Rhoxal-sotalol (Can)** *see* Sotalol *on page* 1321
- **Rhoxal-sumatriptan (Can)** *see* SUMAtriptan *on page* 1336
- **Rhoxal-ticlopidine (Can)** *see* Ticlopidine *on page* 1385
- **Rhoxal-valproic (Can)** *see* Valproic Acid and Derivatives *on page* 1445
- **rHuEPO-α** *see* Epoetin Alfa *on page* 500
- **rhuMAb-E25** *see* Omalizumab *on page* 1046
- **RiaSTAP™** *see* Fibrinogen Concentrate (Human) *on page* 600
- **Ribavirin and Peginterferon Alfa-2a** *see* Peginterferon Alfa-2a and Ribavirin *on page* 1091
- **Rifadin®** *see* Rifampin *on page* 1245
- **Rifampicin** *see* Rifampin *on page* 1245

Rifampin (rif AM pin)

Medication Safety Issues
Sound-alike/look-alike issues:
Rifadin® may be confused with Rifater®, Ritalin®
Rifampin may be confused with ribavirin, rifabutin, Rifamate®, rifapentine, rifaximin

Related Information
Desensitization Protocols *on page* 1692
Stress Replacement of Corticosteroids *on page* 1611

U.S. Brand Names Rifadin®

Canadian Brand Names Rifadin®; Rofact™

Index Terms Rifampicin

Pharmacologic Category Antibiotic, Miscellaneous; Antitubercular Agent

Generic Available Yes

Use Management of active tuberculosis in combination with other agents; elimination of meningococci from the nasopharynx in asymptomatic carriers

Unlabeled/Investigational Use Prophylaxis of *Haemophilus influenzae* type b infection; *Legionella* pneumonia; used in combination with other anti-infectives in the treatment of staphylococcal infections; treatment of *M. leprae* infections

Mechanism of Action Inhibits bacterial RNA synthesis by binding to the beta subunit of DNA-dependent RNA polymerase, blocking RNA transcription

Pharmacodynamics/Kinetics
Duration: ≤24 hours
Absorption: Oral: Well absorbed; food may delay or slightly reduce peak
Distribution: Highly lipophilic; crosses blood-brain barrier well
Relative diffusion from blood into CSF: Adequate with or without inflammation (exceeds usual MICs)
CSF:blood level ratio: Inflamed meninges: 25%
Protein binding: 80%
Metabolism: Hepatic; undergoes enterohepatic recirculation

◄ Half-life elimination: 3-4 hours; prolonged with hepatic impairment; End-stage renal disease: 1.8-11 hours

Time to peak, serum: Oral: 2-4 hours

Excretion: Feces (60% to 65%) and urine (~30%) as unchanged drug

Dosage

Usual dosage ranges: Oral, I.V.:

Infants and Children: 10-20 mg/kg/day as a single dose or in 2 divided doses; maximum: 600 mg/day

Adults: 600 mg once or twice daily

Indication-specific dosing: Oral, I.V.:

H. influenzae prophylaxis (unlabeled use):

Infants and Children: 20 mg/kg/day every 24 hours for 4 days, not to exceed 600 mg/dose

Adults: 600 mg every 24 hours for 4 days

Leprosy (unlabeled use): Adults:

Multibacillary: 600 mg once monthly for 24 months in combination with ofloxacin and minocycline

Paucibacillary: 600 mg once monthly for 6 months in combination with dapsone

Single lesion: 600 mg as a single dose in combination with ofloxacin 400 mg and minocycline 100 mg

Meningitis *(Pneumococcus* or *Staphylococcus)* (unlabeled use): Recommended only for organisms known to be rifampin-susceptible and highly penicillin- or cephalosporin-resistant. May be used in place of or in addition to vancomycin when dexamethasone therapy employed.

Infants and Children: 20 mg/kg/day as a single dose or in 2 divided doses; maximum: 600 mg/day

Adults: 600 mg once daily

Meningococcal meningitis prophylaxis (unlabeled use):

Infants <1 month: 10 mg/kg/day in divided doses every 12 hours for 2 days

Infants ≥1 month and Children: 20 mg/kg/day in divided doses every 12 hours for 2 days (maximum: 600 mg/dose)

Adults: 600 mg every 12 hours for 2 days

Nasal carriers of *Staphylococcus aureus* (unlabeled use):

Children: 15 mg/kg/day divided every 12 hours for 5-10 days in combination with other antibiotics

Adults: 600 mg/day for 5-10 days in combination with other antibiotics

Nontuberculous mycobacterium *(M. kansasii)* (unlabeled use): Adults: 10 mg/kg/day (maximum: 600 mg/day) for duration to include 12 months of culture-negative sputum; typically used in combination with ethambutol and isoniazid

Synergy for *Staphylococcus aureus* infections (unlabeled use): Adults: 300-600 mg twice daily with other antibiotics

Tuberculosis, active: Note: A four-drug regimen (isoniazid, rifampin, pyrazinamide, and ethambutol) is preferred for the initial, empiric treatment of TB. When the drug susceptibility results are available, the regimen should be altered as appropriate.

Infants and Children <12 years:

Daily therapy: 10-20 mg/kg/day usually as a single dose (maximum: 600 mg/day)

Twice weekly directly observed therapy (DOT): 10-20 mg/kg (maximum: 600 mg)

Adults:

Daily therapy: 10 mg/kg/day (maximum: 600 mg/day)

Twice weekly directly observed therapy (DOT): 10 mg/kg (maximum: 600 mg); 3 times/week: 10 mg/kg (maximum: 600 mg)

Tuberculosis, latent infection (LTBI): As an alternative to isoniazid:

Children: 10-20 mg/kg/day (maximum: 600 mg/day) for 6 months

Adults: 10 mg/kg/day (maximum: 600 mg/day) for 4 months. **Note:** Combination with pyrazinamide should not generally be offered (*MMWR*, Aug 8, 2003).

Dosing adjustment in hepatic impairment: Dose reductions may be necessary to reduce hepatotoxicity

Hemodialysis or peritoneal dialysis: Plasma rifampin concentrations are not significantly affected by hemodialysis or peritoneal dialysis.

Stability Rifampin powder is reddish brown. Intact vials should be stored at room temperature and protected from excessive heat and light. Reconstitute powder for injection with SWFI. Prior to injection, dilute in appropriate volume of compatible diluent (eg, 100 mL D_5W). Reconstituted vials are stable for 24 hours at room temperature.

Stability of parenteral admixture at room temperature (25°C) is 4 hours for D_5W and 24 hours for NS.

Administration

I.V.: Administer I.V. preparation once daily by slow I.V. infusion over 30 minutes to 3 hours at a final concentration not to exceed 6 mg/mL.

Oral: Administer on an empty stomach (ie, 1 hour prior to, or 2 hours after meals or antacids) to increase total absorption. The compounded oral suspension must be shaken well before using. May mix contents of capsule with applesauce or jelly.

Monitoring Parameters Periodic (baseline and every 2-4 weeks during therapy) monitoring of liver function (AST, ALT, bilirubin), CBC; hepatic status and mental status, sputum culture, chest x-ray 2-3 months into treatment

Anesthesia and Critical Care Concerns/Other Considerations

Clinical Pearls/Comments: Rifampin causes body secretions to turn orange and may stain contact lenses.

Pregnancy Risk Factor C

Contraindications Hypersensitivity to rifampin, any rifamycins, or any component of the formulation; concurrent use of amprenavir, saquinavir/ritonavir (possibly other protease inhibitors)

Warnings/Precautions Use with caution and modify dosage in patients with liver impairment; observe for hyperbilirubinemia; discontinue therapy if this in conjunction with clinical symptoms or any signs of significant hepatocellular damage develop. Use with caution in patients receiving concurrent medications associated with hepatotoxicity. Use with caution in patients with a history of alcoholism (even if ethanol consumption is discontinued during therapy). Since rifampin since rifampin has enzyme-inducing properties, porphyria exacerbation is possible; use with caution in patients with porphyria; do not use for meningococcal disease, only for short-term treatment of asymptomatic carrier states

Regimens of >600 mg once or twice weekly have been associated with a high incidence of adverse reactions including a flu-like syndrome, hypersensitivity, thrombocytopenia, leukopenia, and anemia. Urine, feces, saliva, sweat, tears, and CSF may be discolored to red/orange; remove soft contact lenses during therapy since permanent staining may occur. Do not administer I.V. form via I.M. or SubQ routes; restart infusion at another site if extravasation occurs. Prolonged use may result in fungal or bacterial superinfection, including *C. difficile*-associated diarrhea (CDAD) and pseudomembranous colitis; CDAD has been observed >2 months postantibiotic treatment. Monitor for compliance in patients on intermittent therapy.

Adverse Reactions

Frequency not defined:

Cardiovascular: Edema, flushing

Central nervous system: Ataxia, behavioral changes, concentration impaired, confusion, dizziness, drowsiness, fatigue, fever, headache, numbness, psychosis

Dermatologic: Pemphigoid reaction, pruritus, urticaria

Endocrine & metabolic: Adrenal insufficiency, menstrual disorders

Hematologic: Agranulocytosis (rare), DIC, eosinophilia, hemoglobin decreased, hemolysis, hemolytic anemia, leukopenia, thrombocytopenia (especially with high-dose therapy)

Hepatic: Hepatitis (rare), jaundice

Neuromuscular & skeletal: Myalgia, osteomalacia, weakness

Ocular: Exudative conjunctivitis, visual changes

Renal: Acute renal failure, BUN increased, hemoglobinuria, hematuria, interstitial nephritis, uric acid increased

Miscellaneous: Flu-like syndrome

◀ 1% to 10%:
Dermatologic: Rash (1% to 5%)
Gastrointestinal (1% to 2%): Anorexia, cramps, diarrhea, epigastric distress, flatulence, heartburn, nausea, pseudomembranous colitis, pancreatitis vomiting
Hepatic: LFTs increased (up to 14%)

Drug Interactions

Metabolism/Transport Effects Induces CYP1A2 (strong), 2A6 (strong), 2B6 (strong), 2C8 (strong), 2C9 (strong), 2C19 (strong), 3A4 (strong)

Avoid Concomitant Use

Avoid concomitant use of Rifampin with any of the following: Atazanavir; Dronedarone; Etravirine; Everolimus; Mycophenolate; Nilotinib; Praziquantel; QuiNINE; Ranolazine; Tolvaptan; Voriconazole

Increased Effect/Toxicity

Rifampin may increase the levels/effects of: Clopidogrel; Gadoxetate; HMG-CoA Reductase Inhibitors; Isoniazid; Leflunomide

The levels/effects of Rifampin may be increased by: Antifungal Agents (Azole Derivatives, Systemic); Delavirdine; Eltrombopag; Fluconazole; Macrolide Antibiotics; P-Glycoprotein Inhibitors; Protease Inhibitors; Pyrazinamide; Voriconazole

Decreased Effect

Rifampin may decrease the levels/effects of: Alfentanil; Amiodarone; Angiotensin II Receptor Blockers; Antidiabetic Agents (Thiazolidinedione); Antiemetics (5HT3 Antagonists); Antifungal Agents (Azole Derivatives, Systemic); Aprepitant; Atazanavir; Atovaquone; Barbiturates; Bendamustine; Benzodiazepines (metabolized by oxidation); Beta-Blockers; BusPIRone; Calcium Channel Blockers; Caspofungin; Chloramphenicol; Contraceptive (Progestins); Corticosteroids (Systemic); CycloSPORINE; CYP1A2 Substrates; CYP2A6 Substrates; CYP2B6 Substrates; CYP2C19 Substrates; CYP2C8 Substrates (High risk); CYP2C9 Substrates (High risk); CYP3A4 Substrates; Dabigatran Etexilate; Dapsone; Deferasirox; Delavirdine; Disopyramide; Dronedarone; Efavirenz; Erlotinib; Etravirine; Everolimus; Exemestane; FentaNYL; Fexofenadine; Fluconazole; Fosaprepitant; Gefitinib; HMG-CoA Reductase Inhibitors; Imatinib; LamoTRIgine; Maraviroc; Methadone; Morphine Sulfate; Mycophenolate; Nevirapine; Nilotinib; Oral Contraceptive (Estrogens); P-Glycoprotein Substrates; Phenytoin; Prasugrel; Praziquantel; Propafenone; Protease Inhibitors; QuiNIDine; QuiNINE; Raltegravir; Ramelteon; Ranolazine; Repaglinide; Saxagliptin; Sirolimus; Sorafenib; Sulfonylureas; Sunitinib; Tacrolimus; Tadalafil; Tamoxifen; Temsirolimus; Terbinafine; Thyroid Products; Tocainide; Tolvaptan; Treprostinil; Typhoid Vaccine; Valproic Acid; Vitamin K Antagonists; Voriconazole; Zaleplon; Zidovudine; Zolpidem

The levels/effects of Rifampin may be decreased by: P-Glycoprotein Inducers

Ethanol/Nutrition/Herb Interactions

Ethanol: Avoid ethanol (may increase risk of hepatotoxicity).
Food: Food decreases the extent of absorption; rifampin concentrations may be decreased if taken with food.
Herb/Nutraceutical: St John's wort may decrease rifampin levels.

Test Interactions Positive Coombs' reaction [direct], rifampin inhibits standard assay's ability to measure serum folate and B_{12}; transient increase in LFTs and decreased biliary excretion of contrast media

Dietary Considerations Rifampin should be taken on an empty stomach.

Dosage Forms Excipient information presented when available (limited, particularly for generics); consult specific product labeling.
Capsule: 150 mg, 300 mg
Injection, powder for reconstitution: 600 mg

References

Tunkel AR, Hartman BJ, Kaplan SL, et al, "Practice Guidelines for the Management of Bacterial Meningitis," *Clin Infect Dis*, 2004, 39(9):1267-84.

◆ **RIG** *see* Rabies Immune Globulin (Human) *on page 1224*

Rimantadine (ri MAN ta deen)

Medication Safety Issues
Sound-alike/look-alike issues:
Rimantadine may be confused with amantadine, ranitidine, Rimactane®
Flumadine® may be confused with fludarabine, flunisolide, flutamide
U.S. Brand Names Flumadine®
Canadian Brand Names Flumadine®
Index Terms Rimantadine Hydrochloride
Pharmacologic Category Antiviral Agent; Antiviral Agent, Adamantane
Generic Available Yes: Tablet

Use Prophylaxis (adults and children >1 year of age) and treatment (adults) of influenza A viral infection (per manufacturer labeling; also refer to current ACIP guidelines for recommendations during current flu season)

Note: In certain circumstances, the ACIP recommends use of rimantadine in combination with oseltamivir for the treatment or prophylaxis of influenza A infection when resistance to oseltamivir is suspected.

Mechanism of Action Exerts its inhibitory effect on three antigenic subtypes of influenza A virus (H1N1, H2N2, H3N2) early in the viral replicative cycle, possibly inhibiting the uncoating process; it has no activity against influenza B virus and is two- to eightfold more active than amantadine

Pharmacodynamics/Kinetics
Onset of action: Antiviral activity: No data exist establishing a correlation between plasma concentration and antiviral effect
Absorption: Tablet and syrup formulations are equally absorbed
Metabolism: Extensively hepatic
Half-life elimination: 25.4 hours; prolonged in elderly
Time to peak: 6 hours
Excretion: Urine (<25% as unchanged drug)
Clearance: Hemodialysis does not contribute to clearance

Dosage Oral:
Prophylaxis:
Children 1-10 years: CDC recommendation: 5 mg/kg/day in 2 divided doses; maximum: 150 mg/day
Children >10 years and Adults: 100 mg twice daily
Elderly: 100 mg/day in nursing home patients or all elderly patients who may experience adverse effects using the adult dose
Treatment:
Adults: 100 mg twice daily
Elderly: 100 mg once daily in patients ≥65 years
Dosage adjustment in renal impairment:
Cl_{cr} >10 mL/minute: Dose adjustment not required
Cl_{cr} ≤10 mL/minute: 100 mg/day
Dosage adjustment in hepatic impairment: Severe dysfunction: 100 mg/day

Stability Store at 15°C to 30°C (59°F to 86°F).

Administration Initiation of rimantadine within 48 hours of the onset of influenza A illness halves the duration of illness and significantly reduces the duration of viral shedding and increased peripheral airways resistance; continue therapy for 5-7 days after symptoms begin

Monitoring Parameters Monitor for CNS or GI effects in elderly or patients with renal or hepatic impairment

Pregnancy Risk Factor C

Contraindications Hypersensitivity to drugs of the adamantine class, including rimantadine and amantadine, or any component of the formulation

Warnings/Precautions Use with caution in patients with renal and hepatic dysfunction; avoid use, if possible, in patients with recurrent and eczematoid dermatitis, uncontrolled psychosis, or severe psychoneurosis. An increase in seizure incidence may occur in patients with seizure disorders; discontinue drug if seizures occur; resistance may develop during treatment; viruses exhibit cross-resistance between amantadine and rimantadine. Due to increased resistance, the ACIP has recommended that rimantadine and amantadine no longer be used for the treatment or prophylaxis of influenza A in the United States until susceptibility has been re-established; consult current guidelines.

◀ **Adverse Reactions**
1% to 10%:
Central nervous system: Insomnia (2% to 3%), concentration impaired (2%), dizziness (1% to 2%), nervousness (1% to 2%), anxiety (1%), fatigue (1%), headache (1%)
Gastrointestinal: Nausea (3%), anorexia (2%), vomiting (2%), xerostomia (2%), abdominal pain (1%)
Neuromuscular & skeletal: Weakness (1%)
<1% (Limited to important or life-threatening): Agitation, ataxia, bronchospasm, cardiac failure, confusion, convulsions, cough, depression, diarrhea, dyspepsia, dyspnea, euphoria, gait abnormality, hallucinations, heart block, hyperkinesias, hypertension, lactation, palpitation, pallor, parosmia, pedal edema, rash, somnolence, syncope, tachycardia, taste alteration, tinnitus, tremor

Drug Interactions
Avoid Concomitant Use There are no known interactions where it is recommended to avoid concomitant use.
Increased Effect/Toxicity
The levels/effects of Rimantadine may be increased by: MAO Inhibitors
Decreased Effect
Rimantadine may decrease the levels/effects of: Influenza Virus Vaccine

Ethanol/Nutrition/Herb Interactions Food: Food does not affect rate or extent of absorption

Dosage Forms Excipient information presented when available (limited, particularly for generics); consult specific product labeling. [DSC] = Discontinued product
Syrup, as hydrochloride:
Flumadine®: 50 mg/5 mL (240 mL) [raspberry flavor] [DSC]
Tablet, as hydrochloride: 100 mg
Flumadine®: 100 mg

References
Bentley DW, Karki SD, and Betts RF, "Rimantadine and Seizures," *Ann Intern Med*, 1989, 110 (4):323-4.
Centers for Disease Control, "Prevention and Control of Influenza. Recommendations of the Advisory Committee on Immunization Practices (ACIP)," *MMWR Recomm Rep*, 2008, 56 (early release):1-60. Available at http://www.cdc.gov/mmwr/preview/mmwrhtml/rr57e717a1.htm
Dolin R, Reichman RC, Madore HP, et al, "A Controlled Trial of Amantadine and Rimantadine in the Prophylaxis of Influenza A Infection," *N Engl J Med*, 1982, 307(10):580-4.
Douglas RG Jr, "Prophylaxis and Treatment of Influenza," *N Engl J Med*, 1990, 322(7):443-50.
"Drugs for Non-HIV Viral Infections," *Med Lett Drugs Ther*, 1994, 36(919):27.
Guay DR, "Amantadine and Rimantadine Prophylaxis of Influenza A in Nursing Homes," *Drugs Aging*, 1994, 5(1):8-19.
Keating MR, "Antiviral Agents," *Mayo Clin Proc*, 1992, 67(2):160-78.
Patriarca PA, Kater NA, Kendal AP, et al, "Safety of Prolonged Administration of Rimantadine Hydrochloride in the Prophylaxis of Influenza A Virus Infections in Nursing Homes," *Antimicrob Agents Chemother*, 1984, 26(1):101-3.
Wintermeyer SM and Nahata MC, "Rimantadine: A Clinical Perspective," *Ann Pharmacother*, 1995, 29(3):299-310.

◆ **Rimantadine Hydrochloride** *see* Rimantadine *on page 1249*

◆ **Riomet®** *see* MetFORMIN *on page 886*

Risedronate (ris ED roe nate)

U.S. Brand Names Actonel®
Canadian Brand Names Actonel®
Index Terms Risedronate Sodium
Pharmacologic Category Bisphosphonate Derivative
Use Treatment of Paget's disease of the bone; treatment and prevention of glucocorticoid-induced osteoporosis; treatment and prevention of osteoporosis in postmenopausal women; treatment of osteoporosis in men
Pharmacodynamics/Kinetics
Onset of action: May require weeks
Absorption: Rapid
Distribution: V_d: 13.8 L/kg
Protein binding: ~24%

Metabolism: None
Bioavailability: Poor, ~0.54% to 0.75%
Half-life elimination: Initial: 1.5 hours; Terminal: 480-561 hours
Time to peak, serum: 1 hour
Excretion: Urine (up to 85%); feces (as unabsorbed drug)

Dosage Oral: Adults:

Paget's disease of bone: 30 mg once daily for 2 months
Retreatment may be considered (following post-treatment observation of at least 2 months) if relapse occurs, or if treatment fails to normalize serum alkaline phosphatase. For retreatment, the dose and duration of therapy are the same as for initial treatment. No data are available on more than one course of retreatment.

Osteoporosis (postmenopausal) prevention and treatment: 5 mg once daily **or** 35 mg once weekly **or** one 75 mg tablet taken on 2 consecutive days once a month (total of 2 tablets/month) **or** 150 mg once a month

Osteoporosis (male) treatment: 35 mg once weekly

Osteoporosis (glucocorticoid-induced) prevention and treatment: 5 mg once daily

Dosage adjustment in renal impairment:
Cl_{cr} ≥30 mL/minute: No adjustment required
Cl_{cr} <30 mL/minute: **Not** recommended for use

Additional Information Complete prescribing information for this medication should be consulted for additional detail.

Dosage Forms Excipient information presented when available (limited, particularly for generics); consult specific product labeling. [DSC] = Discontinued product

Tablet, as sodium:
Actonel®: 5 mg, 30 mg, 35 mg, 75 mg [DSC], 150 mg

References

Author Unknown, "Safety Update: Bone-Building Drugs: Risks Explained," *Consum Rep Health*, 2006, 18(5):3.
French AE, Kaplan N, Lishner M, et al, "Taking Bisphosphonates During Pregnancy," *Can Fam Physician*, 2003, 49:1281-2.
Marx RE, Sawatari Y, Fortin M, et al, "Bisphosphonate-Induced Exposed Bone (Osteonecrosis/ Osteopetrosis) of the Jaws: Risk Factors, Recognition, Prevention, and Treatment," *J Oral Maxillofac Surg*, 2005, 63(11):1567-75.

◆ **Risedronate Sodium** *see* Risedronate *on page 1250*

◆ **Ritalin®** *see* Methylphenidate *on page 908*

◆ **Ritalin LA®** *see* Methylphenidate *on page 908*

◆ **Ritalin-SR®** *see* Methylphenidate *on page 908*

◆ **Ritalin® SR (Can)** *see* Methylphenidate *on page 908*

Ritonavir (ri TOE na veer)

Medication Safety Issues
Sound-alike/look-alike issues:
Ritonavir may be confused with Retrovir®
Norvir® may be confused with Norvasc®

U.S. Brand Names Norvir®

Canadian Brand Names Norvir®; Norvir® SEC

Pharmacologic Category Antiretroviral Agent, Protease Inhibitor

Generic Available No

Use Treatment of HIV infection; should always be used as part of a multidrug regimen (at least three antiretroviral agents); may be used as a pharmacokinetic "booster" for other protease inhibitors

Mechanism of Action Binds to the site of HIV-1 protease activity and inhibits cleavage of viral Gag-Pol polyprotein precursors into individual functional proteins required for infectious HIV. This results in the formation of immature, noninfectious viral particles.

Pharmacodynamics/Kinetics
Absorption: Variable; increased with food
Distribution: High concentrations in serum and lymph nodes; V_d: 0.16-0.66 L/kg
Protein binding: 98% to 99%

◀ Metabolism: Hepatic via CYP3A4 and 2D6; five metabolites, low concentration of an active metabolite (M-2) achieved in plasma (oxidative)

Half-life elimination: 3-5 hours

Time to peak, plasma: Oral solution: 2 hours (fasted); 4 hours (nonfasted)

Excretion: Urine (~11%; ~4% as unchanged drug); feces (~86%; ~34% as unchanged drug)

Dosage Treatment of HIV infection: Oral:

Children >1 month: 350-400 mg/m^2 twice daily (maximum dose: 600 mg twice daily). Initiate dose at 250 mg/m^2 twice daily; titrate dose upward every 2-3 days by 50 mg/m^2 twice daily.

Adults: 600 mg twice daily; dose escalation tends to avoid nausea that many patients experience upon initiation of full dosing. Escalate the dose as follows: 300 mg twice daily for 1 day, 400 mg twice daily for 2 days, 500 mg twice daily for 1 day, then 600 mg twice daily. Ritonavir may be better tolerated when used in combination with other antiretrovirals by initiating the drug alone and subsequently adding the second agent within 2 weeks.

Pharmacokinetic "booster" in combination with other protease inhibitors: 100-400 mg/day

Refer to individual monographs; specific dosage recommendations often require adjustment of both agents.

Note: Dosage adjustments for ritonavir when administered in combination therapy:

Amprenavir: Adjustments necessary for each agent:

Amprenavir 1200 mg with ritonavir 200 mg once daily **or**

Amprenavir 600 mg with ritonavir 100 mg twice daily

Amprenavir plus efavirenz (3-drug regimen): Amprenavir 1200 mg twice daily plus ritonavir 200 mg twice daily plus efavirenz at standard dose

Indinavir: Adjustments necessary for both agents:

Indinavir 800 mg twice daily plus ritonavir 100-200 mg twice daily **or**

Indinavir 400 mg twice daily plus ritonavir 400 mg twice daily

Nelfinavir: Ritonavir 400 mg twice daily

Rifabutin: Decrease rifabutin dose to 150 mg every other day

Saquinavir: Ritonavir 400 mg twice daily

Dosing adjustment in renal impairment: None necessary

Dosing adjustment in hepatic impairment: No adjustment required in mild or moderate impairment; however, careful monitoring is required in moderate hepatic impairment (levels may be decreased); caution advised with severe impairment (no data available)

Stability

Capsule: Store under refrigeration at 2°C to 8°C (36°F to 46°F); may be left out at room temperature of <25°C (<77°F) if used within 30 days. Protect from light. Avoid exposure to excessive heat.

Solution: Store at room temperature at 20°C to 25°C (68°F to 77°F); do not refrigerate. Avoid exposure to excessive heat.

Administration Administer with food. Liquid formulations usually have an unpleasant taste. Consider mixing it with chocolate milk or a liquid nutritional supplement. Whenever possible, administer oral solution with calibrated dosing syringe. Shake liquid well before use.

Monitoring Parameters Triglycerides, cholesterol, CBC, LFTs, CPK, uric acid, basic HIV monitoring, viral load, CD4 count, glucose, serum amylase and lipase

Pregnancy Risk Factor B

Contraindications Hypersensitivity to ritonavir or any component of the formulation; concurrent alfuzosin, amiodarone, cisapride, dihydroergotamine, ergonovine, ergotamine, flecainide, methylergonovine, midazolam, pimozide, propafenone, quinidine, triazolam, and voriconazole (when ritonavir ≥800 mg/day)

Warnings/Precautions [U.S. Boxed Warning]: Ritonavir may interact with many medications, resulting in potentially serious and/or life-threatening adverse events. Use with caution in patients taking strong CYP3A4 inhibitors, moderate or strong CYP3A4 inducers and major CYP3A4 substrates (see Drug Interactions); consider alternative agents that avoid or lessen the potential for CYP-mediated interactions. Not recommended for use with alfuzosin, amiodarone, cisapride, ergot derivatives, flecainide, lovastatin, midazolam, pimozide, propafenone quinidine, simvastatin, St John's wort, triazolam, or voriconazole. Pancreatitis has been observed; use with caution in patients with increased triglycerides; monitor serum lipase and amylase and for gastrointestinal symptoms. Increases in total cholesterol and triglycerides have been reported; screening should be done prior to therapy and periodically throughout treatment.

Protease inhibitors have been associated with a variety of hypersensitivity events (some severe), including rash, anaphylaxis (rare), angioedema, bronchospasm, erythema multiforme, and/or Stevens-Johnson syndrome (rare). It is generally recommended to discontinue treatment if severe rash or moderate symptoms accompanied by other systemic symptoms occur. Use with caution in patients with cardiomyopathy, ischemic heart disease, pre-existing conduction abnormalities, or structural heart disease; may be at increased risk of conduction abnormalities (eg, second- or third-degree AV block). Ritonavir has been associated with AV block due to prolongation of PR interval; use caution with drugs that prolong the PR interval. Use with caution in patients with hemophilia A or B; increased bleeding during protease inhibitor therapy has been reported. Changes in glucose tolerance, hyperglycemia, exacerbation of diabetes, DKA, and new-onset diabetes mellitus have been reported in patients receiving protease inhibitors. May be associated with fat redistribution (buffalo hump, increased abdominal girth, breast engorgement, facial atrophy, and dyslipidemia). Immune reconstitution syndrome may develop resulting in the occurrence of an inflammatory response to an indolent or residual opportunistic infection; further evaluation and treatment may be required. May cause hepatitis or exacerbate pre-existing hepatic dysfunction; use with caution in patients with hepatitis B or C and in hepatic disease. Safety and efficacy have not been established in children <1 month of age.

Adverse Reactions Percentages as reported for combined experiences in both treatment-naive and experienced adults:

>10%:

  Endocrine & metabolic: Hypercholesterolemia (>240 mg/dL: 37% to 45%), triglycerides increased (>800 mg/dL: 17% to 34%; >1500 mg/dL: 1% to 13%)

  Gastrointestinal: Nausea (26% to 30%), diarrhea (15% to 23%), vomiting (14% to 17%), taste perversion (7% to 11%)

  Hepatic: GGT increased (5% to 20%)

  Neuromuscular & skeletal: Weakness (10% to 15%), creatine phosphokinase increased (9% to 12%)

2% to 10%:

  Cardiovascular: Vasodilation (2%)

  Central nervous system: Fever (1% to 5%), dizziness (3% to 4%), insomnia (2% to 3%), somnolence (2% to 3%), depression (2%), anxiety (up to 2%)

  Dermatologic: Rash (up to 4%)

  Endocrine & metabolic: Uric acid increased (up to 4%)

  Gastrointestinal: Abdominal pain (6% to 8%), anorexia (2% to 8%), dyspepsia (up to 6%), local throat irritation (2% to 3%)

  Hepatic: Transaminases increased (6% to 10%)

  Neuromuscular & skeletal: Paresthesia (3% to 7%), arthralgia (up to 2%), myalgia (2%)

  Respiratory: Pharyngitis (≤1% to 3%)

  Miscellaneous: Diaphoresis (2% to 3%)

<2% (Limited to important or life-threatening): Abnormal vision. acute myeloblastic leukemia, adrenal cortex insufficiency, adrenal suppression, anaphylaxis, allergic reaction, amnesia, anemia, angioedema, aphasia, asthma, atrioventricular block (first, second, or third degree), bleeding increased (in patients with hemophilia A or B), bronchospasm, cachexia, cerebral ischemia, cerebral venous thrombosis, chest pain, cholestatic jaundice, coma, Cushing's syndrome, dehydration, dementia, depersonalization, diabetes mellitus, dyspnea, edema, esophageal ulcer, gastroenteritis, gastrointestinal hemorrhage, hallucinations, hepatic coma, hepatitis, hepatomegaly, hepatosplenomegaly, hyper-/hypotension, hypercholesteremia, hypothermia, hypoventilation, ileus, interstitial pneumonia, kidney failure, larynx edema, leukopenia, lymphadenopathy, lymphocytosis, manic reaction, MI, myeloproliferative disorder, neuropathy, orthostatic hypotension, palpitation, pancreatitis, paralysis, postural hypotension, pseudomembranous colitis, rectal hemorrhage, redistribution of body fat, right bundle branch block, seizure, skin melanoma, Stevens-Johnson syndrome,

subdural hematoma, syncope, tachycardia, thrombocytopenia, tongue edema, ulcerative colitis, urticaria, vasospasm

Drug Interactions

Metabolism/Transport Effects Substrate of CYP1A2 (minor), 2B6 (minor), 2D6 (major), 3A4 (major); **Inhibits** CYP2C8 (strong), 2C9 (weak), 2C19 (weak), 2D6 (strong), 2E1 (weak), 3A4 (strong); **Induces** CYP1A2 (weak), 2C8 (weak), 2C9 (weak), 3A4 (weak)

Avoid Concomitant Use

Avoid concomitant use of Ritonavir with any of the following: Alfuzosin; Amiodarone; Cisapride; Dabigatran Etexilate; Disulfiram; Dronedarone; Eplerenone; Ergot Derivatives; Etravirine; Everolimus; Flecainide; Halofantrine; Nilotinib; Nisoldipine; Pimozide; Pitavastatin; Propafenone; QuiNIDine; Ranolazine; Rivaroxaban; Salmeterol; Silodosin; St Johns Wort; Tamoxifen; Thioridazine; Tolvaptan; Topotecan; Voriconazole

Increased Effect/Toxicity

Ritonavir may increase the levels/effects of: Alfuzosin; Almotriptan; Alosetron; Amiodarone; Antifungal Agents (Azole Derivatives, Systemic); Atomoxetine; Benzodiazepines (metabolized by oxidation); Bosentan; Calcium Channel Blockers (Dihydropyridine); Calcium Channel Blockers (Nondihydropyridine); CarBAMazepine; Ciclesonide; Cisapride; Clarithromycin; Colchicine; Corticosteroids (Orally Inhaled); CycloSPORINE; CYP2C8 Substrates (High risk); CYP2D6 Substrates; CYP3A4 Substrates; Dabigatran Etexilate; Digoxin; Dronabinol; Dronedarone; Dutasteride; Enfuvirtide; Eplerenone; Ergot Derivatives; Everolimus; FentaNYL; Fesoterodine; Flecainide; Fusidic Acid; Halofantrine; HMG-CoA Reductase Inhibitors; Ixabepilone; Maraviroc; Meperidine; Nebivolol; Nefazodone; Nilotinib; Nisoldipine; Paricalcitol; P-Glycoprotein Substrates; Pimecrolimus; Pimozide; Pitavastatin; Propafenone; Protease Inhibitors; QuiNIDine; Ranolazine; Rifamycin Derivatives; Rivaroxaban; Salmeterol; Saxagliptin; Sildenafil; Silodosin; Sirolimus; Sorafenib; Tacrolimus; Tadalafil; Tamoxifen; Temsirolimus; Tenofovir; Tetrabenazine; Thioridazine; Tolvaptan; Topotecan; TraZODone; Treprostinil; Tricyclic Antidepressants; Vardenafil; VinBLAStine; VinCRIStine

The levels/effects of Ritonavir may be increased by: Antifungal Agents (Azole Derivatives, Systemic); Clarithromycin; CycloSPORINE; Delavirdine; Disulfiram; Efavirenz; Enfuvirtide; Fusidic Acid; P-Glycoprotein Inhibitors

Decreased Effect

Ritonavir may decrease the levels/effects of: Abacavir; Atovaquone; BuPROPion; Clarithromycin; Codeine; Deferasirox; Delavirdine; Etravirine; LamoTRIgine; Meperidine; Methadone; Oral Contraceptive (Estrogens); Phenytoin; Prasugrel; Theophylline Derivatives; TraMADol; Valproic Acid; Voriconazole; Warfarin; Zidovudine

The levels/effects of Ritonavir may be decreased by: Antacids; CarBAMazepine; CYP3A4 Inducers (Strong); Efavirenz; Garlic; Nevirapine; Oral Contraceptive (Estrogens); Peginterferon Alfa-2b; P-Glycoprotein Inducers; Phenytoin; Rifamycin Derivatives; St Johns Wort; Tenofovir

Ethanol/Nutrition/Herb Interactions

Food: Food enhances absorption.

Herb/Nutraceutical: St John's wort may decrease ritonavir serum levels. Avoid use.

Dietary Considerations Should be taken with food. Oral solution contains 43% ethanol by volume.

Dosage Forms Excipient information presented when available (limited, particularly for generics); consult specific product labeling.

Capsule, soft gelatin:

Norvir®: 100 mg [contains ethanol and polyoxyl 35 castor oil]

Solution:

Norvir®: 80 mg/mL (240 mL) [contains ethanol, polyoxyl 35 castor oil, and propylene glycol; peppermint and caramel flavor]

References

Huang L, Quartin A, Jones D, et al, "Intensive Care of Patients With HIV Infection," *N Engl J Med*, 2006, 355(2):173-81.

◆ **Riva-Alendronate (Can)** *see* Alendronate *on page 57*

- **Riva-Amiodarone (Can)** *see* Amiodarone *on page* 86
- **Riva-Amlodipine (Can)** *see* AmLODIPine *on page* 93
- **Riva-Atenolol (Can)** *see* Atenolol *on page* 155
- **Riva-Azithromycin (Can)** *see* Azithromycin *on page* 169
- **Riva-Buspirone (Can)** *see* BusPIRone *on page* 219
- **Riva-Ciprofloxacin (Can)** *see* Ciprofloxacin *on page* 306
- **Riva-Clindamycin (Can)** *see* Clindamycin *on page* 324
- **Riva-Enalapril (Can)** *see* Enalapril *on page* 478
- **Riva-Famotidine (Can)** *see* Famotidine *on page* 575
- **Riva-Fenofibrate Micro (Can)** *see* Fenofibrate *on page* 582
- **Riva-Fluconazole (Can)** *see* Fluconazole *on page* 607
- **Riva-Fluoxetine (Can)** *see* FLUoxetine *on page* 616
- **Riva-Fosinopril (Can)** *see* Fosinopril *on page* 636
- **Riva-Gabapentin (Can)** *see* Gabapentin *on page* 650
- **Riva-Lisinopril (Can)** *see* Lisinopril *on page* 849
- **Riva-Lorazepam (Can)** *see* LORazepam *on page* 852
- **Riva-Lovastatin (Can)** *see* Lovastatin *on page* 859
- **Riva-Metformin (Can)** *see* MetFORMIN *on page* 886
- **Riva-Metoprolol (Can)** *see* Metoprolol *on page* 922
- **Riva-Naproxen (Can)** *see* Naproxen *on page* 987
- **Riva-Oxybutynin (Can)** *see* Oxybutynin *on page* 1068
- **Riva-Pantoprazole (Can)** *see* Pantoprazole *on page* 1084
- **Riva-paroxetine (Can)** *see* PARoxetine *on page* 1089
- **Riva-Pravastatin (Can)** *see* Pravastatin *on page* 1162
- **Riva-Quetiapine (Can)** *see* QUEtiapine *on page* 1212
- **Riva-Rabeprazole EC (Can)** *see* Rabeprazole *on page* 1221
- **Riva-Ranitidine (Can)** *see* Ranitidine *on page* 1231

Rivaroxaban (riv a ROX a ban)

Canadian Brand Names Xarelto®
Index Terms BAY 59-7939
Pharmacologic Category Factor Xa Inhibitor
Restrictions Not available in U.S.
Generic Available No
Use Postoperative thromboprophylaxis in patients who have undergone elective total hip or knee replacement procedures
Mechanism of Action Inhibits platelet activation and fibrin clot formation via direct, selective and reversible inhibition of factor Xa (FXa) in both the intrinsic and extrinsic coagulation pathways. FXa, as part of the prothrombinase complex consisting also of factor Va, calcium ions, factor II and phospholipid, catalyzes the conversion of prothrombin to thrombin. Thrombin both activates platelets and catalyzes the conversion of fibrinogen to fibrin.

Pharmacodynamics/Kinetics
Absorption: Rapid
Distribution: V_{dss}: ~50 L
Protein binding: 92% to 95% (primarily to albumin)
Metabolism: Hepatic via CYP3A4, CYP3A5, and CYP2J2
Bioavailability: Absolute bioavailability: ~100%
Half-life elimination: Young individual: 5-9 hours; Elderly: 11-13 hours
Time to peak, plasma: 2-4 hours
Excretion: Urine (33% as unchanged drug; 33% as inactive metabolites); feces (33% as inactive metabolites)

◀ **Dosage** Oral: **Note:** Therapy should not be initiated until hemostasis has been established.

Adults: Postoperative thromboprophylaxis:

Knee replacement: 10 mg once daily; initial dose should be administered within 6-10 hours after completion of surgery and establishment of hemostasis (total duration of therapy: 14 days)

Hip replacement: 10 mg once daily; initial dose should be administered within 6-10 hours after completion of surgery and establishment of hemostasis (total duration of therapy: 35 days)

Elderly: Refer to adult dosing.

Dosing adjustment in renal impairment:

Moderate renal impairment (Cl_{cr} 30-49 mL/minute): Use with caution; no specific dosage adjustments are specified in approved labeling

Severe renal impairment (Cl_{cr} <30 mL/minute): Use not recommended

Dosing adjustment in hepatic impairment:

Mild hepatic impairment: Manufacturer provides no specific dosing recommendations in approved labeling. Limited data indicates pharmacokinetics and pharmacodynamic response were similar to healthy subjects.

Significant hepatic impairment (including Child-Pugh classes B and C): Use is contraindicated

Stability Store at 15°C to 30°C (59°F to 86°F).

Administration May be administered without regard to meals.

Monitoring Parameters Prothrombin time (PT), CBC with differential, renal function, hepatic function; **Note:** In major clinical trials, monitoring of aPTT, PT/INR, or antifactor Xa levels did not occur. However, certain patient populations (eg, renal insufficiency, hepatic impairment, low body weight, extreme obesity) may require monitoring of the PT time which correlates well with rivaroxaban concentrations (Kubitza, 2005; Abrams, 2009).

Contraindications Hypersensitivity to rivaroxaban or any component of the formulation; hepatic disease (including Child-Pugh classes B and C) associated with coagulopathy and clinically relevant bleeding risk; clinically significant active bleeding, including hemorrhagic manifestations and bleeding diathesis; lesions at increased risk of clinically significant bleeding (eg, hemorrhagic or ischemic cerebral infarction) within previous 6 months; spontaneous hemostasis impairment; concomitant systemic treatment with strong CYP3A4 and P-glycoprotein (P-gp) inhibitors; pregnancy; lactation

Warnings/Precautions Most common complication is bleeding. Certain patients are at increased risk of bleeding; risk factors include bacterial endocarditis, congenital or acquired bleeding disorders, thrombocytopenia, recent puncture of large vessels or organ biopsy, stroke, intracerebral surgery, or other neuraxial procedure, severe uncontrolled hypertension, renal impairment, recent major surgery, recent major bleeding (intracranial, GI, intraocular, or pulmonary). Monitor for signs and symptoms of bleeding. Prompt clinical evaluation is warranted with any unexplained decrease in hemoglobin or blood pressure. Avoid use with direct thrombin inhibitors (eg, bivalirudin), unfractionated heparin or heparin derivatives, low molecular weight heparins (eg, enoxaparin), aspirin, coumarin derivatives, and sulfinpyrazone. NSAIDs and other platelet aggregation inhibitors (eg, clopidogrel) should be used cautiously.

Avoid use in patients undergoing anesthesia with postoperative indwelling epidural catheters. Hematomas (spinal or epidural) resulting in extended or permanent paralysis may occur. Avoid removal of epidural catheter for at least 18 hours following last rivaroxaban dose. Avoid rivaroxaban administration for at least 6 hours following epidural catheter removal. Monitor for signs of neurologic impairment (eg, numbness/weakness of legs, bowel/bladder dysfunction); prompt diagnosis and treatment are necessary.

Use in significant hepatic dysfunction was not evaluated during clinical trials. Use is contraindicated in hepatic dysfunction (including Child-Pugh classes B and C) associated with coagulopathy and clinically significant risk of bleeding. Limited data in patients with mild hepatic dysfunction without coagulopathy suggests use may be appropriate. Use caution in patients with moderate renal impairment (Cl_{cr} 30-49 mL/minute) including patients receiving concomitant drug therapy that may increase rivaroxaban systemic exposure and those with deteriorating renal function. Use in severe renal impairment (Cl_{cr} <30 mL/minute) has not been studied and is not recommended. Discontinue use with onset of acute renal failure.

Use caution if used concomitantly with strong CYP3A4 inducers. Concomitant use of strong CYP3A4/P-gp inhibitors is contraindicated. Use with caution in patients <50 kg. Safety and efficacy have not been established in patients <18 years of age. Formulation contains lactose; use is not recommended in patients with lactose or galactose intolerance (eg, Lapp lactase deficiency, glucose-galactose malabsorption).

Adverse Reactions

1% to 10%:

Gastrointestinal: Nausea (1%)

Hematologic: Bleeding: Major: (<1% to 2%, includes surgical site bleeding events with decreased hemoglobin or transfusion); Nonmajor: (4% to 7%), anemia (1%)

Hepatic: Transaminases increased (2%; ALT >3 X upper limit of normal [ULN] 2% to 6%), GGT increased (1%)

<1% (Limited to important or life-threatening): Abdominal pain, alkaline phosphatase increased, allergic dermatitis, amylase increased, bilirubin increased, BUN increased, constipation, creatinine increased, diarrhea, dizziness, dyspepsia, ecchymosis, fatigue, fever, headache, hematuria, hypersensitivity, hypotension, jaundice, LDH increased, lipase increased, pain, peripheral edema, pruritus, rash, syncope, tachycardia, thrombocythemia, urticaria, vomiting, weakness, xerostomia

Drug Interactions

Avoid Concomitant Use

Avoid concomitant use of Rivaroxaban with any of the following: CYP3A4 Inhibitors (Strong)

Increased Effect/Toxicity

Rivaroxaban may increase the levels/effects of: Anticoagulants; Ibritumomab; Tositumomab and Iodine I 131 Tositumomab

The levels/effects of Rivaroxaban may be increased by: Antiplatelet Agents; CYP3A4 Inhibitors (Strong); Dasatinib; Erythromycin; Herbs (Anticoagulant/ Antiplatelet Properties); Nonsteroidal Anti-Inflammatory Agents; Pentosan Polysulfate Sodium; P-Glycoprotein Inhibitors; Prostacyclin Analogues; Salicylates; Thrombolytic Agents

Decreased Effect

The levels/effects of Rivaroxaban may be decreased by: CYP3A4 Inducers (Strong); Deferasirox; Herbs (CYP3A4 Inducers); P-Glycoprotein Inducers

Ethanol/Nutrition/Herb Interactions

Food: Grapefruit juice may increase levels/effects of rivaroxaban; use caution.

Herb/Nutraceutical: Avoid St John's wort (may decrease levels/effects of rivaroxaban; avoid concomitant use if possible; use with caution if concomitant use can not be avoided).

Test Interactions Prolongs activated partial thromboplastin time (aPTT), HepTest®, and Russell viper venom time

Dietary Considerations May be taken without regard to meals.

Dosage Forms Excipient information presented when available (limited, particularly for generics); consult specific product labeling. [CAN] = Canadian brand name

Tablet:

Xarelto® [CAN]: 10 mg [contains lactose] [not available in U.S.]

References

Eriksson BI, Borris LC, Friedman RJ, et al, "Rivaroxaban Versus Enoxaparin for Thromboprophylaxis After Hip Arthroplasty," *N Engl J Med*, 2008, 358(26): 2765-75.

Gulseth MP, Michaud J, Nutescu EA, "Rivaroxaban: An Oral Direct Inhibitor of Factor Xa," *Am J Health Syst Pharm*, 2008, 65(16): 1520-9.

Kubitza D, Becka M, Voith B, et al, "Safety, Pharmacodynamics, and Pharmacokinetics of Single Doses of BAY 59-7939, an Oral, Direct Factor Xa Inhibitor," *Clin Pharmacol Ther*, 2005, 78 (4):412-21.

Lassen MR, Ageno W, Borris LC, et al, "Rivaroxaban Versus Enoxaparin for Thromboprophylaxis After Total Knee Arthroplasty," *N Engl J Med*, 2008, 358(26):2776-86.

Turpie AG, "New Oral Anticoagulants in Atrial Fibrillation," *Eur Heart J*, 2007, 29(2):155-65.

◆ **Riva-Simvastatin (Can)** *see* Simvastatin *on page 1293*

◆ **Riva-Sotalol (Can)** *see* Sotalol *on page 1321*

◆ **Riva-Sumatriptan (Can)** *see* SUMAtriptan *on page 1336*

◆ **Riva-Valacyclovir (Can)** *see* Valacyclovir *on page 1441*

◆ **Riva-Venlafaxine XR (Can)** *see* Venlafaxine *on page 1466*

◆ **Riva-Verapamil SR (Can)** *see* Verapamil *on page 1468*

◆ **Rivotril® (Can)** *see* ClonazePAM *on page 328*

Rizatriptan (rye za TRIP tan)

U.S. Brand Names Maxalt-MLT®; Maxalt®
Canadian Brand Names Maxalt RPD™; Maxalt™
Index Terms MK462
Pharmacologic Category Antimigraine Agent; Serotonin 5-HT$_{1B, 1D}$ Receptor Agonist
Use Acute treatment of migraine with or without aura
Pharmacodynamics/Kinetics
Onset of action: ~30 minutes
Duration: 14-16 hours
Protein binding: 14%
Metabolism: Via monoamine oxidase-A; first-pass effect
Bioavailability: 40% to 50%
Half-life elimination: 2-3 hours
Time to peak: 1-1.5 hours
Excretion: Urine (82%, 8% to 16% as unchanged drug); feces (12%)
Dosage Note: In patients with risk factors for coronary artery disease, following adequate evaluation to establish the absence of coronary artery disease, the initial dose should be administered in a setting where response may be evaluated (physician's office or similarly staffed setting). ECG monitoring may be considered.
Oral: 5-10 mg, repeat after 2 hours if significant relief is not attained; maximum: 30 mg in a 24-hour period (use 5 mg dose in patients receiving propranolol with a maximum of 15 mg in 24 hours)
Note: For orally-disintegrating tablets (Maxalt-MLT®): Patient should be instructed to place tablet on tongue and allow to dissolve. Dissolved tablet will be swallowed with saliva.
Anesthesia and Critical Care Concerns/Other Considerations Clinical Pearls/Comments: Rizatriptan should not be used in patients with a history of vasospastic disease, Prinzmetal's angina, or any critical vascular disease.
Additional Information Complete prescribing information for this medication should be consulted for additional detail.
Dosage Forms Excipient information presented when available (limited, particularly for generics); consult specific product labeling.
Tablet:
Maxalt®: 5 mg, 10 mg
Tablet, orally disintegrating:
Maxalt-MLT®: 5 mg [contains phenylalanine 1.05 mg/tablet; peppermint flavor]; 10 mg [contains phenylalanine 2.1 mg/tablet; peppermint flavor]
References
Boyer EW and Shannon M, "The Serotonin Syndrome," *N Engl J Med*, 2005, 352:1112-20.

◆ **R-modafinil** *see* Armodafinil *on page 146*

◆ **Robinul®** *see* Glycopyrrolate *on page 667*

◆ **Robinul® Forte** *see* Glycopyrrolate *on page 667*

◆ **Rocephin®** *see* CefTRIAXone *on page 267*

Rocuronium (roe kyoor OH nee um)

Medication Safety Issues

Sound-alike/look-alike issues:

Zemuron® may be confused with Remeron®

High alert medication: The Institute for Safe Medication Practices (ISMP) includes this medication among its list of drugs which have a heightened risk of causing significant patient harm when used in error.

United States Pharmacopeia (USP) 2006: The Interdisciplinary Safe Medication Use Expert Committee of the USP has recommended the following:

- Hospitals, clinics, and other practice sites should institute special safeguards in the storage, labeling, and use of these agents and should include these safeguards in staff orientation and competency training.
- Healthcare professionals should be on high alert (especially vigilant) whenever a neuromuscular-blocking agent (NMBA) is stocked, ordered, prepared, or administered.

Related Information

Allergic Reactions *on page 1508*
Anesthesia Considerations for Neurosurgery *on page 1514*
Anesthesia for Patients With Liver Disease *on page 1537*
Chronic Renal Failure *on page 1552*
Dosing Considerations for the Critically-Ill Patient With Morbid Obesity *on page 1561*
Neuromuscular-Blocking Agents *on page 1684*
Perioperative Management of Patients on Antiseizure Medication *on page 1577*

U.S. Brand Names Zemuron®

Canadian Brand Names Zemuron®

Index Terms ORG 946; Rocuronium Bromide

Pharmacologic Category Neuromuscular Blocker Agent, Nondepolarizing

Generic Available Yes

Use Facilitate both rapid sequence and routine endotracheal intubation and to relax skeletal muscles during surgery; to facilitate mechanical ventilation in ICU patients

Mechanism of Action Blocks acetylcholine from binding to receptors on motor endplate inhibiting depolarization

Pharmacodynamics/Kinetics

Onset of action: Good intubation conditions within 1-2 minutes (depending on dose administered); maximum neuromuscular blockade within 4 minutes

Duration: ~30 minutes (with standard doses, increases with higher doses and inhalational anesthetic agents; patient age dependent)

Distribution: V_d: ~0.25 L/kg

Protein binding: ~30%

Metabolism: Minimally hepatic; 17-desacetylrocuronium (5% to 10% activity of parent drug)

Half-life elimination: 60-70 minutes

Excretion: Feces (50%); urine (30%)

Dosage Administer I.V.; dose to effect; doses will vary due to interpatient variability. Dosing also dependent on anesthetic technique and age of patient.

Neonates <28 days, Infants 28 days to 3 months, and Children ≥3 months: **Note:** In general, onset is shortened and duration is prolonged as dose increases. Duration is shortest in children >2 to ≤11 years and longest in neonates and infants.

Suggested Pediatric Dosing Based on Indication

Indication	Dose
Rapid sequence intubation (unlabeled use)[1]	0.9 mg/kg
	1.2 mg/kg
Tracheal intubation	0.45 mg/kg
	0.6 mg/kg
Maintenance for continued surgical relaxation	0.15 mg/kg[2]
	7-10 mcg/kg/min as a continuous infusion[3]

[1]Not recommended, per the manufacturer, for rapid sequence intubation in pediatric patients; however, it has been used successfully in clinical trials for this indication in children >1 year of age (Cheng, 2002; Fuchs-Buder, 1996; Mazurek, 1998; Naguib, 1997). An alternative dose of 1 mg/kg may also be used.

[2]Redosing interval is guided by monitoring with a peripheral nerve stimulator.

[3]Use lower end of the continuous infusion dosing range for neonates and infants up to age 28 days and the upper end for children >2 to ≤11 years of age.

Adults:

Rapid sequence intubation: I.V.: 0.6-1.2 mg/kg in appropriately premedicated and anesthetized patients

Tracheal intubation: I.V.: **Note:** May use ideal body weight (IBW) for morbidly obese (BMI >40 kg/m^2) adult patients (Leykin, 2004); onset time may be slightly delayed using IBW. The manufacturer recommends dosing based on actual body weight in all obese patients; however, this may prolong the duration of action to 25% return of twitch tension.

Initial: 0.45-0.6 mg/kg; administration of 0.3 mg/kg may also provide optimal conditions for tracheal intubation (Barclay, 1997)

Maintenance for continued surgical relaxation: 0.1-0.2 mg/kg administered at 25% recovery of control T_1 or a continuous infusion of 8-12 mcg/kg/minute only after early evidence of spontaneous recovery of neuromuscular function is evident; infusion rates have ranged from 4-16 mcg/kg/minute

Note: Inhaled anesthetic agents prolong the duration of action of rocuronium. Use lower end of the dosing range when anesthesia is maintained with an inhaled anesthetic agent, with the redosing interval guided by monitoring with a peripheral nerve stimulator.

ICU paralysis (eg, facilitate mechanical ventilation) in selected adequately sedated patients (Murray, 2002; Rudis, 1996; Sparr, 1997): Initial bolus dose: 0.6-1 mg/kg, then a continuous I.V. infusion of 8-12 mcg/kg/minute; monitor depth of blockade every 2-3 hours initially until stable dose, then every 8-12 hours; adjust rate of administration by 10% increments according to peripheral nerve stimulation response (eg, train-of-four [TOF] count) or desired clinical response as long as TOF count >1/4 is present.

Note: When possible, minimize depth and duration of paralysis. Stopping the infusion for some time until forced to restart based on patient condition is recommended to reduce post-paralytic complications (eg, acute quadriplegic myopathy syndrome [AQMS]) (Murray, 2002).

Intermittent dosing has also been described with an initial loading dose of 50 mg followed by 25 mg given when TOF count >1/4 (TOF monitored every 15 minutes). After the initial loading dose, the frequency of intermittent dosing reduced over the first 6-9 hours and remained constant thereafter (Sparr, 1997).

Dosing adjustment in renal impairment: No adjustments required; duration of neuromuscular blockade may vary in patients with renal impairment.

Dosing adjustment in hepatic impairment: Reductions may be necessary in patients with liver disease; duration of neuromuscular blockade may be prolonged. When rapid sequence intubation is required in adult patients with ascites, a dose on the higher end of the dosage range may be necessary to achieve adequate neuromuscular blockade.

Stability Store unopened/undiluted vials under refrigeration at 2°C to 8°C (36°F to 46°F); do not freeze. When stored at room temperature, it is stable for 60 days; once opened, use within 30 days. Dilutions up to 5 mg/mL in 0.9% sodium chloride, dextrose 5% in water, 5% dextrose in sodium chloride 0.9%, or lactated Ringer's are stable for up to 24 hours at room temperature.

Administration Administer I.V. only; may be administered undiluted as a bolus injection or via a continuous infusion using an infusion pump

Monitoring Parameters Peripheral nerve stimulator measuring twitch response, heart rate, blood pressure, assisted ventilation status

Anesthesia and Critical Care Concerns/Other Considerations

Clinical Pearls/Comments: Classified as an intermediate-duration, neuro-muscular-blocking agent; do not mix in same syringe with barbiturates; synergistic effect when combined with benzylisoquinoline nondepolarizing neuromuscular muscle relaxants (Meretoja, 1994).

Critically-Ill Adult Patients:

The 2008 Surviving Sepsis Campaign guidelines recommend avoiding use of neuromuscular blockers if at all possible in the septic patient due to the risk of prolonged neuromuscular blockade following discontinuation. If one is required, monitor the depth of blockade (Grade 1B).

The 2002 ACCM/SCCM/ASHP clinical practice guidelines for sustained neuro-muscular blockade in the adult critically-ill patient recommend:

Optimize sedatives and analgesics prior to initiation and monitor and adjust accordingly during course. Neuromuscular blockers do not relieve pain or produce sedation.

Protect patient's eyes from development of keratitis and corneal abrasion by administering ophthalmic ointment and taping eyelids closed or using eye patches. Reposition patient routinely to protect pressure points from breakdown. Address DVT prophylaxis.

Concurrent use of a neuromuscular blocker and corticosteroids appear to increase the risk of certain ICU myopathies; avoid or administer the corticosteroid at the lowest dose possible. Reassess need for neuromuscular blocker daily.

Using daily drug holidays (stopping neuromuscular-blocking agent until patient requires it again) may decrease the incidence of acute quadriplegic myopathy syndrome.

Tachyphylaxis can develop.

Monitor patients clinically and via "Train of Four" (TOF) testing with a goal of adjusting the degree of blockade to 1-2 twitches.

Issues Related to Pregnancy: Rocuronium crosses the placenta; umbilical venous plasma levels are ~18% of the maternal concentration. The manufacturer does not recommend use for rapid sequence induction during cesarean section.

Pregnancy Risk Factor C

Contraindications Hypersensitivity to rocuronium, other neuromuscular-blocking agents, or any component of the formulation

Warnings/Precautions Use with caution in patients with cardiovascular disease and pulmonary disease; ventilation must be supported during neuromuscular blockade; certain clinical conditions may result in potentiation or antagonism of neuromuscular blockade:

Potentiation: Electrolyte abnormalities, severe hyponatremia, severe hypocalce-mia, severe hypokalemia, hypermagnesemia, cachexia, neuromuscular diseases, metabolic acidosis, metabolic alkalosis, Eaton-Lambert syndrome, and myasthenia gravis

Antagonism: Respiratory alkalosis, hypercalcemia, demyelinating lesions, peripheral neuropathies, denervation, infection, and muscle trauma

Use with caution in patients with hepatic impairment; clinical duration may be prolonged. Resistance may occur in burn patients (>30% of body) for period of 5-70 days postinjury or in immobilized patients. Cross-sensitivity with other neuromuscular-blocking agents may occur; use caution in patients with previous anaphylactic reactions to other neuromuscular blockers. Use with caution in patients with pulmonary hypertension or valvular heart disease. Use caution in the elderly. Should be administered by adequately trained individuals familiar with its use. Use appropriate anesthesia, pain control, and sedation. In patients requiring long-term administration in the ICU, use of a peripheral nerve stimulator to monitor drug effects is strongly recommended. Additional doses of rocuronium or any other neuromuscular-blocking agent should be avoided unless definite excessive response to nerve stimulation is present.

Some patients may experience prolonged recovery of neuromuscular function after administration (especially after prolonged use). Patients should be adequately recovered prior to extubation. Other factors associated with prolonged recovery should be considered (eg, corticosteroid use, patient condition). In addition to prolonging recovery from neuromuscular blockade, concomitant use with corticosteroids has been associated with development of acute quadriplegic myopathy syndrome (AQMS). Current guidelines recommend neuromuscular blockers be discontinued as soon as possible in patients receiving corticosteroids or interrupted daily until necessary to restart based on clinical condition (Murray, 2002). Numerous drugs either *antagonize* (eg, acetylcholinesterase inhibitors) or *potentiate* (eg, calcium channel blockers, certain antimicrobials, inhalation anesthetics) the effects of neuromuscular blockade; use with caution in patients receiving these agents. Immediate treatment (including epinephrine 1:1000) for anaphylactoid and/or hypersensitivity reactions should be available during use. Not recommended by the manufacturer for rapid sequence intubation in pediatric patients; however, it has been used successfully in clinical trials for this indication.

Adverse Reactions
>1%: Cardiovascular: Hypertension (≤2%), hypotension (transient; ≤2%)
<1% (Limited to important or life-threatening): Abnormal ECG, anaphylactoid reaction, anaphylaxis, arrhythmia, bronchospasm, injection site edema, hiccups, pruritus, nausea, pulmonary vascular resistance (increased), rash, rhonchi, shock, tachycardia, vomiting, wheezing

Drug Interactions

Avoid Concomitant Use
Avoid concomitant use of Rocuronium with any of the following: QuiNINE

Increased Effect/Toxicity
Rocuronium may increase the levels/effects of: Cardiac Glycosides; Corticosteroids (Systemic); OnabotulinumtoxinA; RimabotulinumtoxinB

The levels/effects of Rocuronium may be increased by: AbobotulinumtoxinA; Aminoglycosides; Calcium Channel Blockers; Capreomycin; Colistimethate; Inhalational Anesthetics; Ketorolac; Lincosamide Antibiotics; Lithium; Loop Diuretics; Magnesium Salts; Polymyxin B; Procainamide; QuiNIDine; QuiNINE; Spironolactone; Tetracycline Derivatives; Vancomycin

Decreased Effect
The levels/effects of Rocuronium may be decreased by: Acetylcholinesterase Inhibitors; Loop Diuretics

Dosage Forms Excipient information presented when available (limited, particularly for generics); consult specific product labeling.
Injection, solution, as bromide: 10 mg/mL (5 mL, 10 mL)
Zemuron®: 10 mg/mL (5 mL, 10 mL)

References
Bartkowski RR, Witkowski TA, Azad S, et al, "Rocuronium Onset of Action: A Comparison With Atracurium and Vecuronium," *Anesth Analg*, 1993, 77(3):574-8.

Dellinger RP, Levy MM, Carlet JM, et al, "Surviving Sepsis Campaign: International Guidelines for Management of Severe Sepsis and Septic Shock: 2008," *Intensive Care Med*, 2008, 34(1): 17-60. Available at http://www.survivingsepsis.org/system/files/images/2008_20International_20SSC_20-Guidelines_1_.pdf

Khuenl-Brady KS, Sparr H, Puhringer F, et al, "Rocuronium Bromide in the ICU: Dose Finding and Pharmacokinetics," *Eur J Anaesthesiol Suppl*, 1995, 11:79-80.

Meretoja OA, Taivainen T, Jalkanen L, et al, "Synergism Between Atracurium and Vecuronium in Infants and Children During Nitrous Oxide-Oxygen-Alfentanil Anaesthesia," *Br J Anaesth*, 1994, 73 (5):605-7.

Murray MJ, Cowen J, DeBlock H, et al, "Clinical Practice Guidelines for Sustained Neuromuscular Blockade in the Adult Critically Ill Patient. Task Force of the American College of Critical Care Medicine (ACCM) of the Society of Critical Care Medicine (SCCM), American Society of Health-System Pharmacists, American College of Chest Physicians," *Crit Care Med*, 2002, 30(1):142-56. Available at: http://www.sccm.org/pdf/NeuromuscularBlockade.pdf. Accessed August 6, 2003.

Puhringer FK, Khuenl-Brady KS, and Mitterschiffthaler G, "Rocuronium Bromide: Time-Course of Action in Underweight, Normal Weight, Overweight and Obese Patients," *Eur J Anaesthesiol Suppl*, 1995, 11:107-10.

- ◆ **Rocuronium Bromide** *see* Rocuronium *on page 1259*
- ◆ **Rofact™ (Can)** *see* Rifampin *on page 1245*
- ◆ **Rogaine® (Can)** *see* Minoxidil *on page 943*
- ◆ **Rogaine® Extra Strength for Men [OTC]** *see* Minoxidil *on page 943*
- ◆ **Rogaine® for Men [OTC]** *see* Minoxidil *on page 943*
- ◆ **Rogaine® for Women [OTC]** *see* Minoxidil *on page 943*
- ◆ **Rogitine® (Can)** *see* Phentolamine *on page 1112*
- ◆ **Romazicon®** *see* Flumazenil *on page 613*

Romiplostim (roe mi PLOE stim)

Medication Guide An FDA-approved patient medication guide, which is available with the product information and at http://www.fda.gov/downloads/Drugs/DrugSafety/ucm088667.pdf, must be dispensed with this medication for each new outpatient prescription and refill.

U.S. Brand Names Nplate™

Canadian Brand Names Nplate™

Index Terms AMG 531

Pharmacologic Category Colony Stimulating Factor; Thrombopoietic Agent

Restrictions Approved for use only under a risk management and restricted distribution program, Nplate™ NEXUS (Network of Experts Understanding and Supporting Nplate™ and Patients) program (1-877-675-2831 or www.nplate.com). Prescribers and patients must be registered with the program.

Generic Available No

Use Treatment of thrombocytopenia in patients with chronic immune (idiopathic) thrombocytopenia purpura (ITP) who have had insufficient response to corticosteroids, immune globulin, or splenectomy

Mechanism of Action Thrombopoietin (TPO) peptide mimetic which increases platelet counts in ITP by binding to and activating the human TPO receptor.

Pharmacodynamics/Kinetics

Onset of action: Platelet count increase: SubQ: 4-9 days; Peak platelet count increase: Days 12-16

Duration: Platelet counts return to baseline by day 28

Absorption: SubQ: Slow

Half-life elimination: Median: 3.5 days (range: 1-34 days)

Time to peak, plasma: SubQ: Median: 14 hours (range: 7-50 hours)

Dosage Note: Initial dose is based on actual body weight. Discontinue if platelet count does not respond to a level that avoids clinically important bleeding after 4 weeks at the maximum recommended dose.

SubQ: Adults: ITP: Initial: 1 mcg/kg once weekly; adjust dose by 1 mcg/kg/week to achieve platelet count ≥50,000/mm^3 and to reduce the risk of bleeding; Maximum: 10 mcg/kg (median dose needed to achieve response in clinical trials: 2 mcg/kg)

Dosage adjustment recommendations:

Platelet count <50,000/mm^3: Increase dose by 1 mcg/kg

Platelet count >200,000/mm^3 for 2 consecutive weeks: Reduce dose by 1 mcg/kg

Platelet count >400,000/mm^3: Withhold dose; assess platelet count weekly; when platelet count <200,000/mm^3, resume with the dose reduced by 1 mcg/kg

Stability Store intact vials refrigerated at 2°C to 8°C (36°F to 46°F); do not freeze. Protect from light. Reconstitute with preservative free SWFI to a final concentration of 500 mcg/mL. Gently invert vial and swirl; do not shake. Reconstituted solution may be stored at room temperature of 25°C (77°F) or refrigerated at 2°C to 8°C (36°F to 46°F) for up to 24 hours. Protect reconstituted solution from light.

Administration Administer SubQ. Administration volume may be small; use appropriate syringe (with graduations to 0.01 mL) for administration.

Monitoring Parameters CBC with differential and platelets (baseline, during treatment [weekly until platelet response stable for 4 weeks then monthly] and weekly for at least 2 weeks following completion of treatment)

Evaluate for neutralizing antibodies in patients with inadequate response (blood samples may be submitted to Amgen for assay [1-800-772-6436]).

Reference Range Target platelet count of 50,000-200,000/mm^3; platelet life span: 8-11 days

Pregnancy Risk Factor C

Contraindications There are no contraindications listed within the manufacturer's labeling.

Warnings/Precautions May increase the risk for bone marrow reticulin formation or progression. Collagen fibrosis with cytopenias was not observed in clinical trials, although patients receiving romiplostim may be at risk for marrow fibrosis with cytopenias. Onset of new or worsening cellular abnormalities or cytopenias may warrant therapy discontinuation and subsequent bone marrow biopsy. Thromboembolism may occur with treatment; use with caution in patients with a history of cerebrovascular disease. Stimulation of cell surface thrombopoietin (TPO) receptors may increase the risk for hematologic malignancies; may increase the risk for progression of underlying myelodysplastic syndrome (MDS).

Inadequate platelet response may be due to neutralizing antibodies (to romiplostim or TPO) or bone marrow fibrosis. Indicated only when the degree of thrombocytopenia and clinical conditions increase the risk for bleeding; use the lowest dose necessary to achieve and maintain platelet count platelet count ≥50,000/mm^3. Do not use to normalize platelet counts. Discontinue if platelet count does not respond to a level to avoid clinically important bleeding after 4 weeks at the maximum recommended dose. May be used in combination with other therapies for ITP, including corticosteroids, danazol, azathioprine, immune globulin, or Rho(D) immune globulin. Reduce dose of or discontinue ITP medications when platelet count ≥50,000/mm^3.

Upon discontinuation of therapy, thrombocytopenia may worsen. Severity may be greater than pretreatment level. Risk of bleeding is increased, particularly in patients receiving anticoagulants or antiplatelet agents; monitor closely. Rebound thrombocytopenia generally resolves within 14 days.

Use with caution in patients with hepatic and renal impairment (has not been studied). Safety and efficacy have not been established in children.

Adverse Reactions

>10%:

Central nervous system: Headache (35%), fatigue (33%), dizziness (17%), insomnia (16%)

Gastrointestinal: Diarrhea (17%), nausea (13%), abdominal pain (11%)

Neuromuscular & skeletal: Arthralgia (26%), myalgia (14%), back pain (13%), limb pain (13%)

Respiratory: Epistaxis (32%), upper respiratory tract infection (17%)

1% to 10%:

Gastrointestinal: Dyspepsia (7%)

Hematologic: Rebound thrombocytopenia (7%), bone marrow reticulin formation/deposition (4%)

Neuromuscular & skeletal: Shoulder pain (8%), paresthesia (6%)

Miscellaneous: Antibody formation (romiplostim 10%; TPO 5%)

<1% (Limited to important or life-threatening): Thromboembolism

Drug Interactions

Avoid Concomitant Use There are no known interactions where it is recommended to avoid concomitant use.

Increased Effect/Toxicity There are no known significant interactions involving an increase in effect.

Decreased Effect There are no known significant interactions involving a decrease in effect.

Dietary Considerations Nplate™ 250 mcg vial contains sucrose 15 mg and 500 mcg vial contains sucrose 25 mg.

Dosage Forms Excipient information presented when available (limited, particularly for generics); consult specific product labeling.

Injection, powder for reconstitution:

Nplate™: 250 mcg [contains sucrose 15 mg/vial]; 500 mcg [contains sucrose 25 mg/vial]

References

Bussel JB, Kuter DJ, George JN, et al, "AMG 531, a Thrombopoiesis-Stimulating Protein, for Chronic ITP," *N Engl J Med*, 2006, 355(16):1672-81.

Kuter DJ, "New Thrombopoietic Growth Factors," *Blood*, 2007, 109(11):4607-16.

Kuter DJ, Bussel JB, Lyons RM, et al, "Efficacy of Romiplostim in Patients With Chronic Immune Thrombocytopenic Purpura: A Double-Blind Randomised Controlled Trial," *Lancet*, 2008, 371 (9610):395-403.

Wang B, Nichol JL, and Sullivan JT, "Pharmacodynamics and Pharmacokinetics of AMG 531, a Novel Thrombopoietin Receptor Ligand," *Clin Pharmacol Ther*, 2004, 76(6):628-38.

♦ **Romycin®** *see* Erythromycin *on page 516*

Ropinirole (roe PIN i role)

U.S. Brand Names Requip®; Requip® XL™

Canadian Brand Names CO Ropinirole; PMS-Ropinirole; RAN-Ropinirole; Requip®

Index Terms Ropinirole Hydrochloride

Pharmacologic Category Anti-Parkinson's Agent, Dopamine Agonist

Use Treatment of idiopathic Parkinson's disease; in patients with early Parkinson's disease who were not receiving concomitant levodopa therapy as well as in patients with advanced disease on concomitant levodopa; treatment of moderate-to-severe primary Restless Legs Syndrome (RLS)

Pharmacodynamics/Kinetics

Absorption: Not affected by food

Distribution: V_d: 525 L

Protein binding: 40%

Metabolism: Extensively hepatic via CYP1A2 to inactive metabolites; first-pass effect

Bioavailability: Absolute: 45% to 55%

Half-life elimination: ~6 hours

Time to peak: Immediate release: ~1-2 hours; Extended release: 6-10 hours; T_{max} increased by 2.5-3 hours when drug taken with food

Excretion: Urine (<10% as unchanged drug, 60% as metabolites)

Clearance: Reduced by 15% to 30% in patients >65 years of age

Dosage Oral: Adults:

Parkinson's disease:

Immediate release tablet: The dosage should be increased to achieve a maximum therapeutic effect, balanced against the principal side effects of nausea, dizziness, somnolence and dyskinesia. Recommended starting dose is 0.25 mg 3 times/day; based on individual patient response, the dosage should be titrated with weekly increments as described below:

• Week 1: 0.25 mg 3 times/day; total daily dose: 0.75 mg

• Week 2: 0.5 mg 3 times/day; total daily dose: 1.5 mg

• Week 3: 0.75 mg 3 times/day; total daily dose: 2.25 mg

• Week 4: 1 mg 3 times/day; total daily dose: 3 mg

Note: After week 4, if necessary, daily dosage may be increased by 1.5 mg/day on a weekly basis up to a dose of 9 mg/day, and then by up to 3 mg/day weekly to a total of 24 mg/day

Parkinson's disease discontinuation taper: Ropinirole should be gradually tapered over 7 days as follows: reduce frequency of administration from 3 times daily to twice daily for 4 days, then reduce to once daily for remaining 3 days.

Extended release tablet: Initial: 2 mg once daily for 1-2 weeks, followed by increases of 2 mg/day at weekly or longer intervals based on therapeutic response and tolerability (maximum: 24 mg/day); **Note:** When discontinuing gradually taper over 7 days.

Restless legs syndrome: Immediate release tablets: Initial: 0.25 mg once daily 1-3 hours before bedtime. Dose may be increased after 2 days to 0.5 mg daily, and after 7 days to 1 mg daily. Dose may be further titrated upward in 0.5 mg increments every week until reaching a daily dose of 3 mg during week 6. If symptoms persist or reappear, the daily dose may be increased to a maximum of 4 mg beginning week 7.

Note: Doses up to 4 mg per day may be discontinued without tapering.

◄ **Converting from ropinirole immediate release tablets to ropinirole extended-release tablets:** Choose a once daily extended-release dose that most closely matches current immediate-release daily dose.

Dosage adjustment in renal impairment: No adjustment needed in patients with moderate renal impairment (Cl_{cr} 30-50 mL/minute); has not been studied in patients with severe impairment.

Removal by hemodialysis is unlikely.

Dosage adjustment in hepatic impairment: Titrate with caution; has not been studied.

Anesthesia and Critical Care Concerns/Other Considerations If therapy with a drug known to be a potent inhibitor of CYP1A2 is stopped or started during treatment with ropinirole, adjustment of ropinirole dose may be required.

Additional Information Complete prescribing information for this medication should be consulted for additional detail.

Dosage Forms Excipient information presented when available (limited, particularly for generics); consult specific product labeling. [DSC] = Discontinued product

Combination package:

Requip® [starter kit; contents per each administration card]: Tablet: 0.25 mg (2s), 0.5 mg (5s), 1 mg (7s) [DSC]

Tablet: 0.25 mg, 0.5 mg, 1 mg, 2 mg, 3 mg, 4 mg, 5 mg

Requip®: 0.25 mg, 0.5 mg, 1 mg, 2 mg, 3 mg, 4 mg, 5 mg

Tablet, extended-release:

Requip® XL™: 2 mg, 4 mg, 6 mg, 8 mg, 12 mg

References

Olanow CW, Watts RL, and Koller WC, "An Algorithm (Decision Tree) for the Management of Parkinson's Disease (2001): Treatment Guidelines," *Neurology*, 2001, 56(11 Suppl 5):1-88.

Stern MB, "Contemporary Approaches to the Pharmacotherapeutic Management of Parkinson's Disease: An Overview," *Neurology*, 1997, 49(1 Suppl 1):2-9.

Watts RL, "The Role of Dopamine Agonists in Early Parkinson's Disease," *Neurology*, 1997, 49(1 Suppl 1):34-48.

♦ **Ropinirole Hydrochloride** *see* Ropinirole *on page 1265*

Ropivacaine (roe PIV a kane)

Medication Safety Issues

Sound-alike/look-alike issues:

Ropivacaine may be confused with bupivacaine, ropinirole

High alert medication: The Institute for Safe Medication Practices (ISMP) includes this medication (epidural administration) among its list of drug classes which have a heightened risk of causing significant patient harm when used in error.

Related Information

Acute Postoperative Pain *on page 1502*

Local Anesthetics *on page 1636*

U.S. Brand Names Naropin®

Canadian Brand Names Naropin®

Index Terms Ropivacaine Hydrochloride

Pharmacologic Category Local Anesthetic

Generic Available No

Use Local anesthetic for use in surgery, postoperative pain management, and obstetrical procedures when local or regional anesthesia is needed

Mechanism of Action Blocks both the initiation and conduction of nerve impulses by decreasing the neuronal membrane's permeability to sodium ions, which results in inhibition of depolarization with resultant blockade of conduction

Pharmacodynamics/Kinetics

Onset of action: Anesthesia (route dependent): 3-15 minutes

Duration (dose and route dependent): 3-15 hours

Metabolism: Hepatic, via CYP1A2 to metabolites

Half-life elimination: Epidural: 5-7 hours

Excretion: Urine (86% as metabolites)

Dosage Dose varies with procedure, onset and depth of anesthesia desired, vascularity of tissues, duration of anesthesia, and condition of patient: Adults:

Surgical anesthesia:
  Lumbar epidural: 15-30 mL of 0.5% to 1% solution
  Lumbar epidural block for cesarean section:
    20-30 mL dose of 0.5% solution
    15-20 mL dose of 0.75% solution
  Thoracic epidural block: 5-15 mL dose of 0.5% to 0.75% solution
  Major nerve block:
    35-50 mL dose of 0.5% solution (175-250 mg)
    10-40 mL dose of 0.75% solution (75-300 mg)
  Field block: 1-40 mL dose of 0.5% solution (5-200 mg)
  Labor pain management: Lumbar epidural: Initial: 10-20 mL 0.2% solution; continuous infusion dose: 6-14 mL/hour of 0.2% solution with incremental injections of 10-15 mL/hour of 0.2% solution
  Postoperative pain management:
    Lumbar or thoracic epidural: Continuous infusion dose: 6-14 mL/hour of 0.2% solution
  Infiltration/minor nerve block:
    1-100 mL dose of 0.2% solution
    1-40 mL dose of 0.5% solution

Stability Store at 20°C to 25°C (68°F to 77°F). Infusions should be discarded after 24 hours.

Administration Administered via local infiltration, epidural block and epidural infusion, or intermittent bolus

Monitoring Parameters Heart rate, blood pressure, ECG monitoring (if used with antiarrhythmics)

Anesthesia and Critical Care Concerns/Other Considerations

Local anesthetic toxicity: Cardiac arrest: Lipid infusion has been used in animal studies and several human cases (*Bupivacaine:* Rosenblatt, 2006; *Levobupivacaine:* Foxall, 2007; *Ropivacaine:* Litz, 2006) where cardiovascular toxicity, unresponsive to conventional resuscitation, resulted. Additional information is available at http://www.lipidrescue.org. The protocol from the website is: 20% Fat Emulsion: 1.5 mL/kg administered over 1 minute, followed immediately by an infusion of 0.25 mL/kg/minute. Continue chest compressions (lipid must circulate). Repeat bolus every 3-5 minutes up to 3 mL/kg total dose until circulation restored. Continue infusion until hemodynamic stability is restored. Increase the infusion rate to 0.5 mL/kg/minute if BP declines. A maximum total dose of 8 mL/kg is recommended.

Administration issue: The On-Q® infusion pump is used to slowly administer local anesthetics (eg, bupivacaine, lidocaine, ropivacaine) to or around surgical wound sites and/or in close proximity to nerves for pre- and postoperative regional anesthesia. When infused directly into the shoulder joint instead of the tissue around the shoulder, destruction of articular cartilage (chondrolysis) has occurred. On-Q® pumps should never be placed directly into any joint (see https://www.ismp.org/Newsletters/acutecare/archives/May09.asp).

Pregnancy Risk Factor B

Contraindications Hypersensitivity to ropivacaine, amide-type local anesthetics (eg, bupivacaine, mepivacaine, lidocaine), or any component of the formulation

Warnings/Precautions Careful and constant monitoring of the patient's state of consciousness should be done following each local anesthetic injection; at such times, restlessness, anxiety, tinnitus, dizziness, blurred vision, tremors, depression, or drowsiness may be early warning signs of CNS toxicity. Treatment is primarily symptomatic and supportive. Intravascular injections should be avoided. Local anesthetics have been associated with rare occurrences of sudden respiratory arrest, seizures, and cardiac arrest. When administering this agent, have ready access to drugs and equipment for resuscitation. Use with caution in patients with liver disease, cardiovascular disease, neurological or psychiatric disorders, and in the elderly or debilitated; these patients may be at greater risk for toxicity. Cardiovascular adverse events (bradycardia, hypotension) may be age-related (more common in patients >61 years of age). Use caution in patients on type III antiarrhythmics (eg, amiodarone); consider ECG monitoring since cardiac effects may be additive. Use cautiously in hypotension, hypovolemia, or heart block. Ropivacaine is not recommended for use in emergency situations where rapid administration is necessary. Safety and efficacy have not been established in pediatric patients.

Adverse Reactions

>10%:

Cardiovascular: Hypotension (dose-related and age-related: 32% to 69%), bradycardia (6% to 20%)

Gastrointestinal: Nausea (11% to 29%), vomiting (7% to 14%)

Neuromuscular & skeletal: Back pain (7% to 16%)

1% to 10%:

Cardiovascular: Hypertension, tachycardia, chest pain (1% to 5%)

Central nervous system: Fever (3% to 9%), headache (5% to 8%), dizziness (3%), chills (2% to 3%), anxiety (1%), lightheadedness

Dermatologic: Pruritus (1% to 5%)

Endocrine & metabolic: Hypokalemia

Genitourinary: Urinary retention (1% to 5%), urinary tract infection (1% to 5%)

Hematologic: Anemia (6%)

Neuromuscular & skeletal: Paresthesia (2% to 6%), hypoesthesia, rigors, circumoral paresthesia

Renal: Oliguria

Respiratory: Dyspnea

Miscellaneous: Shivering

<1% (Limited to important or life-threatening): Accidental I.V. injection (0.2%), angioedema, allergic reaction, apnea (usually associated with epidural block in head/neck region), bronchospasm, cardiac arrest, cardiovascular collapse, dyskinesia, hallucination, hyperthermia, laryngeal edema, myocardial depression, MI, rash, seizure, syncope, tinnitus, urticaria, ventricular arrhythmia

Drug Interactions

Metabolism/Transport Effects Substrate of CYP1A2 (major), 2B6 (minor), 2D6 (minor), 3A4 (minor; may be major in cases of 1A2 inhibition/deficiency)

Avoid Concomitant Use There are no known interactions where it is recommended to avoid concomitant use.

Increased Effect/Toxicity

The levels/effects of Ropivacaine may be increased by: Ciprofloxacin; CYP1A2 Inhibitors (Moderate); CYP1A2 Inhibitors (Strong); Fluvoxamine; Fospropofol; Propofol

Decreased Effect

The levels/effects of Ropivacaine may be decreased by: Peginterferon Alfa-2b

Dosage Forms Excipient information presented when available (limited, particularly for generics); consult specific product labeling.

Infusion, as hydrochloride:

Naropin®: 2 mg/mL (100 mL, 200 mL)

Injection, solution, as hydrochloride [preservative free]:

Naropin®: 2 mg/mL (10 mL, 20 mL); 5 mg/mL (20 mL, 30 mL); 7.5 mg/mL (20 mL); 10 mg/mL (10 mL, 20 mL)

References

Alahuhta S, Rasanen J, Jouppila P, et al, "The Effects of Epidural Ropivacaine and Bupivacaine for Cesarean Section on Uteroplacental and Fetal Circulation," *Anesthesiology*, 1995, 83(1):23-32.

Corcoran W, Butterworth J, Weller RS, et al, "Local Anesthetic-Induced Cardiac Toxicity: A Survey of Contemporary Practice Strategies Among Academic Anesthesiology Departments," *Anesth Analg*, 2006, 103(5):1322-6.

Datta S, Camann W, Bader A, et al, "Clinical Effects and Maternal and Fetal Plasma Concentrations of Epidural Ropivacaine Versus Bupivacaine for Cesarean Section," *Anesthesiology*, 1995, 82 (6):1346-52.

Foxall G, McCahon R, Lamb J, et al, "Levobupivacaine-Induced Seizures and Cardiovascular Collapse Treated With Intralipid," *Anaesthesia*, 2007, 62(5):516-8.

Litz RJ, Popp M, Stehr SN, et al, "Successful Resuscitation of a Patient With Ropivacaine-Induced Asystole After Axillary Plexus Block Using Lipid Infusion," *Anaesthesia*, 2006, 61(8):800-1.

McClure JH, "Ropivacaine," *Br J Anaesth*, 1996, 76(2):300-7.

Rosenblatt MA, Abel M, Fischer GW, et al, "Successful Use of a 20% Lipid Emulsion to Resuscitate a Patient After a Presumed Bupivacaine-Related Cardiac Arrest," *Anesthesiology*, 2006, 105 (1):217-8.

Scott DB, Lee A, Fagan D, et al, "Acute Toxicity of Ropivacaine Compared With That of Bupivacaine," *Anesth Analg*, 1989, 69(5):563-9.

Wood MB and Rubin AP, "A Comparison of Epidural 1% Ropivacaine and 0.75% Bupivacaine for Lower Abdominal Gynecologic Surgery," *Anesth Analg*, 1993, 76(6):1274-8.

Zaric D, Axelsson K, Nydahl P, et al, "Sensory and Motor Blockade During Epidural Analgesia With 1%, 0.75%, and 0.5% Ropivacaine - A Double-Blind Study," *Anesth Analg*, 1991, 72(4):509-15.

◆ **Ropivacaine Hydrochloride** *see* Ropivacaine *on page 1266*

Rosiglitazone (roh si GLI ta zone)

U.S. Brand Names Avandia®
Canadian Brand Names Avandia®
Pharmacologic Category Antidiabetic Agent, Thiazolidinedione
Use Type 2 diabetes mellitus (noninsulin dependent, NIDDM):
  Monotherapy: Improve glycemic control as an adjunct to diet and exercise
    Note: Canadian labeling approves use as monotherapy only when metformin is contraindicated or not tolerated.
  Combination therapy: **Note:** Use when diet, exercise, and a single agent do not result in adequate glycemic control.
    U.S. labeling: In combination with a sulfonylurea, metformin, or sulfonylurea plus metformin
    Canadian labeling: In combination with metformin; in combination with a sulfonylurea only when metformin use is contraindicated or not tolerated
Unlabeled/Investigational Use Polycystic ovary syndrome (PCOS)
Pharmacodynamics/Kinetics
  Onset of action: Delayed; Maximum effect: Up to 12 weeks
  Distribution: V_{dss} (apparent): 17.6 L
  Protein binding: 99.8%; primarily albumin
  Metabolism: Hepatic (99%) via CYP2C8; minor metabolism via CYP2C9
  Bioavailability: 99%
  Half-life elimination: 3-4 hours
  Time to peak, plasma: 1 hour; delayed with food
  Excretion: Urine (64%) and feces (23%) as metabolites
Dosage Oral:
  Adults: **Note:** All patients should be initiated at the lowest recommended dose.
    Monotherapy: Initial: 4 mg daily as a single daily dose or in divided doses twice daily. If response is inadequate after 8-12 weeks of treatment, the dosage may be increased to 8 mg daily as a single daily dose or in divided doses twice daily. In clinical trials, the 4 mg twice-daily regimen resulted in the greatest reduction in fasting plasma glucose and Hb A_{1c}.
    Combination therapy: When adding rosiglitazone to existing therapy, continue current dose(s) of previous agents:
      U.S. labeling: With sulfonylureas or metformin (or sulfonylurea plus metformin): Initial: 4 mg daily as a single daily dose or in divided doses twice daily. If response is inadequate after 8-12 weeks of treatment, the dosage may be increased to 8 mg daily as a single daily dose or in divided doses twice daily. Reduce dose of sulfonylurea if hypoglycemia occurs. It is unlikely that the dose of metformin will need to be reduced due to hypoglycemia.
      Canadian labeling:
        With metformin: Initial: 4 mg daily as a single daily dose or in divided doses twice daily. If response is inadequate after 8-12 weeks of treatment, the dosage may be increased to 8 mg daily as a single daily dose or in divided doses twice daily.
        With a sulfonylurea: 4 mg daily as a single daily dose or in divided doses twice daily. Dose should not exceed 4 mg daily when using in combination with a sulfonylurea. Reduce dose of sulfonylurea if hypoglycemia occurs.
    Elderly: No dosage adjustment is recommended .

  Dosage adjustment in renal impairment: No dosage adjustment is required
  Dosage comment in hepatic impairment: Clearance is significantly lower in hepatic impairment. Therapy should not be initiated if the patient exhibits active liver disease or increased transaminases (ALT >2.5 times the upper limit of normal) at baseline.
Additional Information Complete prescribing information for this medication should be consulted for additional detail.
Dosage Forms Excipient information presented when available (limited, particularly for generics); consult specific product labeling. ▶

Tablet:
Avandia®: 2 mg, 4 mg, 8 mg

References

Al-Salman J, Arjomand H, Kemp DG, et al, "Hepatocellular Injury in a Patient Receiving Rosiglitazone. A Case Report," *Ann Intern Med*, 2000, 132(2):121-4.

Belli SH, Graffigna MN, Oneto A, et al, "Effect of Rosiglitazone on Insulin Resistance, Growth Factors, and Reproductive Disturbances in Women With Polycystic Ovary Syndrome," *Fertil Steril*, 2004, 81 (3):624-9.

Cataldo NA, Abbasi F, McLaughlin TL, et al, "Metabolic and Ovarian Effects of Rosiglitazone Treatment for 12 Weeks in Insulin-Resistant Women With Polycystic Ovary Syndrome," *Hum Reprod*, 2006, 21(1):109-20.

Dormandy JA, Charbonnel B, Eckland DJ, et al, "Secondary Prevention of Macrovascular Events in Patients With Type 2 Diabetes in the PROactive Study (PROspective PioglitAzone Clinical Trial In MacroVascular Events): A Randomised Controlled Trial," *Lancet*, 2005, 366(9493):1279-89.

Freid J, Everitt D, and Boscia J, "Rosiglitazone and Hepatic Failure," *Ann Intern Med*, 2000, 132 (2):164-6.

Gerstein HC, Yusuf S, Bosch J, et al, "Effect Of Rosiglitazone On The Frequency Of Diabetes In Patients With Impaired Glucose Tolerance or Impaired Fasting Glucose: A Randomized Controlled Trial. DREAM (Diabetes REduction Assessment with ramipril and rosiglitazone Medication)Trial Investigators," *Lancet*, 2006,368(9541):2096-105.

Gutschi LM, Malcolm JC, Favreau CM, et al, "Paradoxically Decreased HDL-Cholesterol Levels Associated With Rosiglitazone Therapy," *Ann Pharmacother*, 2006, 40(9):1672-6.

Kahn SE, Haffner SM, Heise MA, et al, "Glycemic Durability of Rosiglitazone, Metformin, or Glyburide Monotherapy," *N Engl J Med*, 2006:355(23):2427-43.

Liu S, Huang T, Sahud MA, "Rosiglitazone-Induced Immune Thrombocytopenia," *Platelets*, 2006, 17 (3):143-8.

Nissen SE, Wolski K, "Effects Of Rosiglitazone On The Risk of Myocardial Infarction and Death From Cardiovascular Causes," *N Engl J Med*, 2007. Available online at http://content.nejm.org/cgi/content/full/NEJMoa072761 May 21, 2007.

Rosuvastatin (roe soo va STAT in)

Related Information

Hyperlipidemia Management *on page 1747*
Preoperative Evaluation of the Cardiac Patient for Noncardiac Surgery *on page 1598*

U.S. Brand Names Crestor®

Canadian Brand Names Crestor®

Index Terms Rosuvastatin Calcium

Pharmacologic Category Antilipemic Agent, HMG-CoA Reductase Inhibitor

Use Used with dietary therapy for hyperlipidemias to reduce elevations in total cholesterol (TC), LDL-C, apolipoprotein B, nonHDL-C, and triglycerides (TG) in patients with primary hypercholesterolemia (elevations of 1 or more components are present in Fredrickson type IIa, IIb, and IV hyperlipidemias); treatment of primary dysbetalipoproteinemia (Fredrickson type III hyperlipidemia); treatment of homozygous familial hypercholesterolemia (FH); to slow progression of atherosclerosis as an adjunct to diet to lower TC and LDL-C

Pharmacodynamics/Kinetics

Onset of action: Within 1 week; maximal at 4 weeks

Distribution: V_d: 134 L

Protein binding: 88%

Metabolism: Hepatic (10%), via CYP2C9 (1 active metabolite identified)

Bioavailability: 20% (high first-pass extraction by liver)

Asian patients have been noted to have increased bioavailability.

Half-life elimination: 19 hours

Time to peak, plasma: 3-5 hours

Excretion: Feces (90%), primarily as unchanged drug

Dosage Adults: Oral:

Hyperlipidemia, mixed dyslipidemia, hypertriglyceridemia, primary dysbetalipoproteinemia, slowing progression of atherosclerosis:

Initial dose:

General dosing: 10 mg once daily; 20 mg once daily may be used in patients with severe hyperlipidemia (LDL >190 mg/dL) and aggressive lipid targets

Conservative dosing: Patients requiring less aggressive treatment or predisposed to myopathy (including patients of Asian descent): 5 mg once daily

Titration: After 2 weeks, may be increased by 5-10 mg once daily; dosing range: 5-40 mg/day (maximum dose: 40 mg once daily)

Note: The 40 mg dose should be reserved for patients who have not achieved goal cholesterol levels on a dose of 20 mg/day, including patients switched from another HMG-CoA reductase inhibitor.

Homozygous familial hypercholesterolemia (FH): Initial: 20 mg once daily (maximum dose: 40 mg/day)

Dosage adjustment with concomitant medications:
Cyclosporine: Rosuvastatin dose should not exceed 5 mg/day
Gemfibrozil or lopinavir/ritonavir: Rosuvastatin dose should not exceed 10 mg/day

Dosage adjustment for hematuria and/or persistent, unexplained proteinuria while on 40 mg/day: Reduce dose and evaluate causes

Dosage adjustment in renal impairment:
Mild-to-moderate impairment: No dosage adjustment required.
Cl_{cr} <30 mL/minute/1.73 m^2: Initial: 5 mg/day; do not exceed 10 mg once daily

Anesthesia and Critical Care Concerns/Other Considerations
Clinical Pearls/Comments: Based on the atorvastatin component: **Myopathy:** Currently-marketed HMG-CoA reductase inhibitors appear to have a similar potential for causing myopathy. Incidence of severe myopathy is about 0.08% to 0.09%. The factors that increase risk include advanced age (especially >80 years), gender (occurs in women more frequently than men), small body frame, frailty, multisystem disease (eg, chronic renal insufficiency especially due to diabetes), multiple medications, and drug interactions (use with caution or avoid).

Based on current research and clinical guidelines (Fleisher, 2007), HMG-CoA reductase inhibitors should be continued in the perioperative period. Postoperative discontinuation of statin therapy is associated with an increased risk of cardiac morbidity and mortality.

Additional Information Complete prescribing information for this medication should be consulted for additional detail.

Dosage Forms Excipient information presented when available (limited, particularly for generics); consult specific product labeling.
Tablet:
Crestor®: 5 mg, 10 mg, 20 mg, 40 mg

References
Pasternak RC, Smith SC Jr, Bairey-Merz CN, et al, "ACC/AHA/NHLBI Clinical Advisory on the Use and Safety of Statins," *J Am Coll Cardiol*, 2002, 40(3):567-72. Available at: http://www.nhlbi.nih.gov/guidelines/cholesterol/statins.pdf. Accessed March 14, 2003.

◆ **Rosuvastatin Calcium** *see* Rosuvastatin *on page 1270*

◆ **Rowasa®** *see* Mesalamine *on page 884*

◆ **Roxanol™** *see* Morphine Sulfate *on page 953*

◆ **Roxicet™** *see* Oxycodone and Acetaminophen *on page 1072*

◆ **Roxicet™ 5/500** *see* Oxycodone and Acetaminophen *on page 1072*

◆ **Roxicodone®** *see* OxyCODONE *on page 1069*

◆ **Roychlor® (Can)** *see* Potassium Chloride *on page 1151*

◆ **RP-59500** *see* Quinupristin and Dalfopristin *on page 1219*

◆ **r-PA** *see* Reteplase *on page 1242*

◆ **rPDGF-BB** *see* Becaplermin *on page 180*

◆ **(R,R)-Formoterol L-Tartrate** *see* Arformoterol *on page 137*

◆ **RS-25259** *see* Palonosetron *on page 1079*

◆ **RS-25259-197** *see* Palonosetron *on page 1079*

◆ **RUF 331** *see* Rufinamide *on page 1271*

Rufinamide (roo FIN a mide)

U.S. Brand Names Banzel™
Index Terms CGP 33101; E 2080; RUF 331; Xilep
Pharmacologic Category Anticonvulsant, Triazole Derivative

◀ **Use** Adjunctive therapy in the treatment of generalized seizures of Lennox-Gastaut syndrome

Pharmacodynamics/Kinetics

Absorption: Slow; extensive ≥85%; increased with food

Distribution: V_d: ~50 L

Protein binding: 34%, primarily to albumin

Metabolism: Extensively via carboxylesterase-mediated hydrolysis of the carboxylamide group to CGP 47292 (inactive metabolite); weak inhibitor of CYP2E1 and weak inducer of CYP3A4

Bioavailability: Extent decreased with increased dose

Half-life elimination: ~6-10 hours

Time to peak, plasma: 4-6 hours

Excretion: Urine (85%, ~66% as CGP 47292, <2% as unchanged drug)

Dosage Oral: Lennox-Gastaut (adjunctive):

Children ≥4 years: Initial: 10 mg/kg/day in 2 equally divided doses; increase dose by ~10 mg/kg/day every other day to a target dose of 45 mg/kg/day or 3200 mg/day (whichever is lower) in 2 equally divided doses

Adults: Initial: 400-800 mg/day in 2 equally divided doses; increase dose by 400-800 mg/day every 2 days until maximum daily dose: 3200 mg/day in 2 equally divided doses

Dosage adjustment in renal impairment: Cl_{cr} <30 mL/minute: No dosage adjustment needed

Hemodialysis: No specific guidelines available; consider dosage adjustment for loss of drug

Dosage adjustment in hepatic impairment:

Mild-to-moderate impairment: Use caution

Severe impairment: Use in severe impairment has not been studied and is not recommended

Additional Information Complete prescribing information for this medication should be consulted for additional detail.

Dosage Forms Excipient information presented when available (limited, particularly for generics); consult specific product labeling.

Tablet:

Banzel™: 200 mg, 400 mg

References

Deeks ED and Scott LJ, "Rufinamide," *CNS Drugs*, 2006, 20(9):751-60.

Glauser T, Kluger G, Sachdeo R, et al, "Rufinamide for Generalized Seizures Associated With Lennox-Gastaut Syndrome," *Neurology*, 2008, 70(21):1950-8.

Perucca E, Cloyd J, Critchley D, et al, "Rufinamide: Clinical Pharmacokinetics and Concentration-Response Relationships in Patients With Epilepsy," *Epilepsia*, 2008, 49(7):1123-41.

- ◆ **Salbu-2 (Can)** *see* Albuterol *on page* 49
- ◆ **Salbu-4 (Can)** *see* Albuterol *on page* 49
- ◆ **Salbutamol** *see* Albuterol *on page* 49
- ◆ **Salbutamol and Ipratropium** *see* Ipratropium and Albuterol *on page* 762
- ◆ **Salbutamol Sulphate** *see* Albuterol *on page* 49
- ◆ **Salflex® (Can)** *see* Salsalate *on page* 1275
- ◆ **Salicylsalicylic Acid** *see* Salsalate *on page* 1275
- ◆ **Saline Mist [OTC]** *see* Sodium Chloride *on page* 1304
- ◆ **SalineX® [OTC] [DSC]** *see* Sodium Chloride *on page* 1304

Salmeterol (sal ME te role)

Medication Safety Issues
Sound-alike/look-alike issues:
Salmeterol may be confused with Salbutamol, Solu-Medrol®
Serevent® may be confused with Atrovent®, Combivent®, Serentil®, sertraline, Sinemet®, Spiriva®, Zoloft®

Medication Guide An FDA-approved patient medication guide, which is available with the product information and at http://www.fda.gov/downloads/Drugs/DrugSafety/ucm089125.pdf, must be dispensed with this medication for each new outpatient prescription and refill.

U.S. Brand Names Serevent® Diskus®

Canadian Brand Names Serevent® Diskhaler® Disk; Serevent® Diskus®

Index Terms Salmeterol Xinafoate

Pharmacologic Category Beta$_2$-Adrenergic Agonist; Beta$_2$-Adrenergic Agonist, Long-Acting

Generic Available No

Use Maintenance treatment of asthma; prevention of bronchospasm with reversible obstructive airway disease, including patients with symptoms of nocturnal asthma; prevention of exercise-induced bronchospasm; maintenance treatment of bronchospasm associated with COPD

Mechanism of Action Relaxes bronchial smooth muscle by selective action on beta$_2$-receptors with little effect on heart rate; salmeterol acts locally in the lung.

Pharmacodynamics/Kinetics
Onset of action: Asthma: 30-48 minutes, COPD: 2 hours
Peak effect: Asthma: 3 hours, COPD: 2-5 hours
Duration: 12 hours
Absorption: Systemic: Inhalation: Undetectable to poor
Protein binding: 96%
Metabolism: Hepatic; hydroxylated via CYP3A4
Half-life elimination: 5.5 hours
Time to peak, serum: ~20 minutes
Excretion: Feces (60%), urine (25%)

Dosage Inhalation, powder (50 mcg/inhalation):
Asthma, maintenance and prevention: Children ≥4 years and Adults: One inhalation twice daily (~12 hours apart); maximum: 1 inhalation twice daily. **Note:** For long-term asthma control, long acting beta$_2$-agonists (LABAs) should be used in combination with inhaled corticosteroids and not as monotherapy.

Exercise-induced asthma, prevention: Children ≥4 years and Adults: One inhalation at least 30 minutes prior to exercise; additional doses should not be used for 12 hours; should not be used in individuals already receiving salmeterol twice daily. **Note:** Because LABAs may disguise poorly controlled persistent asthma, frequent or chronic use of LABAs for exercise-induced bronchospasm is discouraged by the NIH Asthma Guidelines (NIH, 2007).

COPD maintenance: Adults: One inhalation twice daily (~12 hours apart); maximum: 1 inhalation twice daily

Dosage adjustment in hepatic impairment: No dosage adjustment required; manufacturer suggests close monitoring of patients with hepatic impairment.

Stability Inhalation powder: Store at controlled room temperature 20°C to 25°C (68°F to 77°F) in a dry place away from direct heat or sunlight. Stable for 6 weeks after removal from foil pouch.

◄ **Administration** Inhalation: **Not** to be used for the relief of acute attacks. Not for use with a spacer device. Administer with Diskus® in a level, horizontal position. Do not wash mouthpiece; Diskus® should be kept dry.

Monitoring Parameters FEV_1, peak flow, and/or other pulmonary function tests; blood pressure, heart rate; CNS stimulation. Monitor for increased use of short-acting beta$_2$-agonist inhalers; may be marker of a deteriorating asthma condition.

Pregnancy Risk Factor C

Contraindications Hypersensitivity to salmeterol or any component of the formulation

Warnings/Precautions

Asthma treatment: [U.S. Boxed Warning]: Long-acting beta$_2$-agonists (LABAs) may increase the risk of asthma-related deaths. Salmeterol should only be used as adjuvant therapy in patients not adequately controlled on inhaled corticosteroids or whose disease requires two maintenance therapies. In a large, randomized clinical trial (SMART, 2006), salmeterol was associated with a small, but statistically significant increase in asthma-related deaths (when added to usual asthma therapy); risk may be greater in African-American patients versus Caucasians. Do **not** use for acute asthmatic symptoms. Short-acting beta$_2$-agonist (eg, albuterol) should be used for acute symptoms and symptoms occurring between treatments. Do **not** initiate in patients with significantly worsening or acutely deteriorating asthma; reports of severe (sometimes fatal) respiratory events have been reported when salmeterol has been initiated in this situation. Salmeterol is not a substitute for inhaled or oral corticosteroids; should not be used as monotherapy for the treatment of asthma. Corticosteroids should not be stopped or reduced when salmeterol is initiated. During the initiation of salmeterol watch for signs of worsening asthma. Patients must be instructed to use short-acting beta$_2$-agonists (eg, albuterol) for acute asthmatic or COPD symptoms and to seek medical attention in cases where acute symptoms are not relieved or a previous level of response is diminished. The need to increase frequency of use of short-acting beta$_2$-agonist may indicate deterioration of asthma, and treatment must not be delayed. Because LABAs may disguise poorly controlled persistent asthma, frequent or chronic use of LABAs for exercise-induced bronchospasm is discouraged by the NIH Asthma Guidelines (NIH, 2007). Salmeterol should not be used more than twice daily; do not use with other long-acting beta$_2$-agonists.

Concurrent diseases: Use caution in patients with cardiovascular disease (eg, arrhythmia, hypertension, or HF), seizure disorders, diabetes, glaucoma, hyperthyroidism, hepatic impairment, or hypokalemia. Beta-agonists may cause elevation in blood pressure, heart rate, CNS stimulation/excitation, increased risk of arrhythmia, increase serum glucose, or decrease serum potassium.

Adverse events: Immediate hypersensitivity reactions (urticaria, angioedema, rash, bronchospasm) have been reported. There have been reports of laryngeal spasm, irritation, swelling (stridor, choking) with use. Salmeterol should not be used more than twice daily; do not exceed recommended dose; do not use with other long-acting beta$_2$-agonists; serious adverse events have been associated with excessive use of inhaled sympathomimetics. Rarely, paradoxical broncho-spasm may occur with use of inhaled bronchodilating agents; this should be distinguished from inadequate response. Powder for oral inhalation contains lactose; very rare anaphylactic reactions have been reported in patients with severe milk protein allergy.

Safety and efficacy have not been established in children <4 years of age.

Adverse Reactions

>10%:
  Central nervous system: Headache (13% to 17%)
  Neuromuscular & skeletal: Pain (1% to 12%)

1% to 10%:
  Cardiovascular: Hypertension (4%), edema (1% to 3%), pallor
  Central nervous system: Dizziness (4%), sleep disturbance (1% to 3%), fever (1% to 3%), anxiety (1% to 3%), migraine (1% to 3%)
  Dermatologic: Rash (1% to 4%), contact dermatitis (1% to 3%), eczema (1% to 3%), urticaria (3%), photodermatitis (1% to 2%)
  Endocrine & metabolic: Hyperglycemia (1% to 3%)

Gastrointestinal: Throat irritation (7%), nausea (1% to 3%), dyspepsia (1% to 3%), dental pain (1% to 3%), gastrointestinal infection (1% to 3%), oropharyngeal candidiasis (1% to 3%), xerostomia (1% to 3%)

Neuromuscular & skeletal: Muscular cramps/spasm (3%), articular rheumatism (1% to 3%), arthralgia (1% to 3%), joint pain (1% to 3%), muscular stiffness (1% to 3%), paresthesia (1% to 3%), rigidity (1% to 3%)

Ocular: Keratitis/conjunctivitis (1% to 3%)

Respiratory: Nasal congestion (4% to 9%), tracheitis/bronchitis (7%), pharyngitis (≤6%), cough (5%), influenza (5%), viral respiratory tract infection (5%), sinusitis (4% to 5%), rhinitis (4% to 5%), asthma (3% to 4%)

<1% (Limited to important or life-threatening): Abdominal pain, agitation, aggression, anaphylactic reaction (Diskus®: severe milk allergy), angioedema, aphonia, arrhythmia, atrial fibrillation, bronchospasm and immediate broncho-spasm, cataracts, chest congestion, chest tightness, choking, contusions, Cushing syndrome, Cushingoid features, depression, dysmenorrhea, dyspnea, earache, ecchymoses, edema (facial, oropharyngeal), eosinophilic conditions, glaucoma, growth velocity reduction in children/adolescents, hypercorticism, hypersensitivity reaction (immediate and delayed), hypokalemia, hypothyroid-ism, intraocular pressure increased, laryngeal spasm/irritation, irregular menstruation, myositis, osteoporosis, pallor, paradoxical tracheitis, paranasal sinus pain, PID, restlessness, stridor, supraventricular tachycardia, syncope, tremor, vaginal candidiasis, vaginitis, vulvovaginitis, rare cases of vasculitis (Churg-Strauss syndrome), ventricular tachycardia, weight gain

Drug Interactions

Metabolism/Transport Effects Substrate of CYP3A4 (major)

Avoid Concomitant Use

Avoid concomitant use of Salmeterol with any of the following: CYP3A4 Inhibitors (Strong); Iobenguane I 123

Increased Effect/Toxicity

Salmeterol may increase the levels/effects of: Sympathomimetics

The levels/effects of Salmeterol may be increased by: Atomoxetine; Cannabinoids; CYP3A4 Inhibitors (Moderate); CYP3A4 Inhibitors (Strong); MAO Inhibitors; Tricyclic Antidepressants

Decreased Effect

Salmeterol may decrease the levels/effects of: Iobenguane I 123

The levels/effects of Salmeterol may be decreased by: Alpha-/Beta-Blockers; Beta-Blockers (Beta1 Selective); Beta-Blockers (Nonselective); Betahistine

Dietary Considerations Powder for oral inhalation contains lactose; very rare anaphylactic reactions have been reported in patients with severe milk protein allergy.

Dosage Forms Excipient information presented when available (limited, particularly for generics); consult specific product labeling. [CAN] = Canadian brand name

Powder for oral inhalation:

Serevent® Diskus®: Salmeterol xinafoate 50 mcg (28s, 60s) [delivers 50 mcg/inhalation; contains lactose]

Serevent® Diskhaler® Disk [CAN]: Salmeterol xinafoate 50 mcg (60s) [delivers 50 mcg/inhalation; contains lactose] [not available in U.S]

References

Expert Panel Report 3, "Guidelines for the Diagnosis and Management of Asthma," *Clinical Practice Guidelines*, National Institutes of Health, National Heart, Lung, and Blood Institute, NIH Publication No. 08-4051, prepublication 2007. Available at http://www.nhlbi.nih.gov/guidelines/asthma/asthgdln.htm

◆ **Salmeterol Xinafoate** see Salmeterol on page 1273

◆ **Salofalk® (Can)** see Mesalamine on page 884

Salsalate (SAL sa late)

Related Information

Nonsteroidal Anti-Inflammatory Agents on page 1687

U.S. Brand Names Amigesic® [DSC]

Canadian Brand Names Amigesic®; Salflex®

◀ **Index Terms** Disalicylic Acid; Salicylsalicylic Acid
Pharmacologic Category Salicylate
Use Treatment of minor pain or fever; arthritis
Pharmacodynamics/Kinetics
Onset of action: Therapeutic: 3-4 days of continuous dosing
Absorption: Complete from small intestine
Metabolism: Hepatically hydrolyzed to two moles of salicylic acid (active)
Half-life elimination: 7-8 hours
Excretion: Primarily urine
Dosage Adults: Oral: 3 g/day in 2-3 divided doses
Dosing comments in renal impairment: In patients with end-stage renal disease undergoing hemodialysis: 750 mg twice daily with an additional 500 mg after dialysis
Anesthesia and Critical Care Concerns/Other Considerations Salsalate does not appear to inhibit platelet aggregation.
Additional Information Complete prescribing information for this medication should be consulted for additional detail.
Dosage Forms Excipient information presented when available (limited, particularly for generics); consult specific product labeling. [DSC] = Discontinued product
Tablet: 500 mg, 750 mg
Amigesic®: 500 mg [DSC], 750 mg [DSC]

- **Sandoz Fenofibrate S (Can)** *see* Fenofibrate *on page 582*
- **Sandoz-Fluoxetine (Can)** *see* FLUoxetine *on page 616*
- **Sandoz-Glyburide (Can)** *see* GlyBURIDE *on page 666*
- **Sandoz-Levofloxacin (Can)** *see* Levofloxacin *on page 823*
- **Sandoz-Lovastatin (Can)** *see* Lovastatin *on page 859*
- **Sandoz-Metformin FC (Can)** *see* MetFORMIN *on page 886*
- **Sandoz® Methylphenidate SR (Can)** *see* Methylphenidate *on page 908*
- **Sandoz-Metoprolol (Can)** *see* Metoprolol *on page 922*
- **Sandoz-Nabumetone (Can)** *see* Nabumetone *on page 973*
- **Sandoz Omeprazole (Can)** *see* Omeprazole *on page 1048*
- **Sandoz-Ondansetron (Can)** *see* Ondansetron *on page 1057*
- **Sandoz-Pantoprazole (Can)** *see* Pantoprazole *on page 1084*
- **Sandoz-Paroxetine (Can)** *see* PARoxetine *on page 1089*
- **Sandoz-Pioglitazone (Can)** *see* Pioglitazone *on page 1132*
- **SANDOZ-Pramipexole (Can)** *see* Pramipexole *on page 1159*
- **Sandoz-Pravastatin (Can)** *see* Pravastatin *on page 1162*
- **Sandoz-Quetiapine (Can)** *see* QUEtiapine *on page 1212*
- **Sandoz-Rabeprazole (Can)** *see* Rabeprazole *on page 1221*
- **Sandoz-Ramipril (Can)** *see* Ramipril *on page 1229*
- **Sandoz-Ranitidine (Can)** *see* Ranitidine *on page 1231*
- **Sandoz-Simvastatin (Can)** *see* Simvastatin *on page 1293*
- **Sandoz-Sotalol (Can)** *see* Sotalol *on page 1321*
- **Sandoz-Sumatriptan (Can)** *see* SUMAtriptan *on page 1336*
- **Sandoz-Ticlopidine (Can)** *see* Ticlopidine *on page 1385*
- **Sandoz-Timolol (Can)** *see* Timolol *on page 1390*
- **Sandoz-Tobramycin (Can)** *see* Tobramycin *on page 1400*
- **Sandoz-Topiramate (Can)** *see* Topiramate *on page 1408*
- **Sandoz-Valproic (Can)** *see* Valproic Acid and Derivatives *on page 1445*
- **Sandoz-Venlafaxine XR (Can)** *see* Venlafaxine *on page 1466*
- **Sans Acne® (Can)** *see* Erythromycin *on page 516*

Sapropterin (sap roe TER in)

U.S. Brand Names Kuvan™
Index Terms 6R-BH4; Phenoptin; Sapropterin Dihydrochloride
Pharmacologic Category Enzyme Cofactor
Use Adjunct to dietary management in the treatment of tetrahydrobioterin (BH4) responsive phenylketonuria (PKU)
Pharmacodynamics/Kinetics
Onset of action: Within 24 hours; maximum effect: 1-2 months
Duration: 24 hours
Absorption: Absorption is enhanced when administered with food (high fat/high calorie)
Half-life elimination: ~7 hours (range: 4-17 hours)
Dosage Oral: PKU: Children ≥4 years and Adults: Initial: 10 mg/kg once daily; adjust after 1 month based on blood phenylalanine levels (if phenylalanine levels do not decrease from baseline, increase dose to 20 mg/kg once daily); discontinue if phenylalanine levels do not decrease after 1 month of treatment at 20 mg/kg/day (nonresponder). Maintenance range: 5-20 mg/kg once daily
Additional Information Complete prescribing information for this medication should be consulted for additional detail.
Dosage Forms Excipient information presented when available (limited, particularly for generics); consult specific product labeling.
Tablet, as dihydrochloride:
Kuvan™: 100 mg

References

Burton BK, Grange DK, Milanowski A, et al, "The Response of Patients With Phenylketonuria and Elevated Serum Phenylalanine to Treatment With Oral Sapropterin Dihydrochloride (6R-Tetrahydrobiopterin): A Phase II, Multicentre, Open-Label, Screening Study," *J Inherit Metab Dis*, 2007, 30(5):700-7.

Koch R, Hanley W, Levy H, et al, "The Maternal Phenylketonuria International Study: 1984-2002," *Pediatrics*, 2003, 112(6 Pt 2):1523-9.

Levy H, Burton B, Cederbaum S, et al, "Recommendations for Evaluation of Responsiveness to Tetrahydrobiopterin (BH4) in Phenylketonuria and its Use in Treatment," *Mol Genet Metab*, 2007, 92 (4):287-291.

Levy HL, Milanowski A, Chakrapani A, et al, "Efficacy of Sapropterin Dihydrochloride (Tetrahydrobiopterin, 6R-BH4) for Reduction of Phenylalanine Concentration in Patients With Phenylketonuria: A Phase III Randomised Placebo-Controlled Study," *Lancet*, 2007, 370 (9586):504-10.

Maillot F, Cook P, Lilburn M, et al, "A Practical Approach to Maternal Phenylketonuria Management," *J Inherit Metab Dis*, 2007, 30(2):198-201.

◆ **Sapropterin Dihydrochloride** *see* Sapropterin *on page 1277*

◆ **Sarafem®** *see* FLUoxetine *on page 616*

◆ **Sarna® HC (Can)** *see* Hydrocortisone *on page 699*

◆ **Sarnol®-HC [OTC]** *see* Hydrocortisone *on page 699*

◆ **SB-497115** *see* Eltrombopag *on page 477*

◆ **SB-497115-GR** *see* Eltrombopag *on page 477*

◆ **Scandonest® 3% Plain** *see* Mepivacaine *on page 878*

◆ **SCH 56592** *see* Posaconazole *on page 1148*

◆ **ScheinPharm Ranitidine (Can)** *see* Ranitidine *on page 1231*

◆ **S-Citalopram** *see* Escitalopram *on page 521*

◆ **Sclerosol®** *see* Talc (Sterile) *on page 1349*

◆ **Scopace™** *see* Scopolamine Derivatives *on page 1278*

◆ **Scopolamine Base** *see* Scopolamine Derivatives *on page 1278*

◆ **Scopolamine Butylbromide** *see* Scopolamine Derivatives *on page 1278*

Scopolamine Derivatives (skoe POL a meen dah RIV ah tives)

Medication Safety Issues
Transdermal patch may contain conducting metal (eg, aluminum); remove patch prior to MRI.

Related Information
Cycloplegic Mydriatics *on page 1679*
Postoperative Nausea and Vomiting *on page 1593*

U.S. Brand Names Isopto® Hyoscine; Scopace™; Transderm Scōp®

Canadian Brand Names Buscopan®; Transderm-V®

Index Terms Hyoscine Butylbromide; Hyoscine Hydrobromide; Scopolamine Base; Scopolamine Butylbromide; Scopolamine Hydrobromide

Pharmacologic Category Anticholinergic Agent

Generic Available Yes: Injection

Use

Scopolamine base:

Transdermal: Prevention of nausea/vomiting associated with motion sickness and recovery from anesthesia and surgery

Scopolamine hydrobromide:

Injection: Preoperative medication to produce amnesia, sedation, tranquilization, antiemetic effects, and decrease salivary and respiratory secretions

Ophthalmic: Produce cycloplegia and mydriasis; treatment of iridocyclitis

Oral: Symptomatic treatment of postencephalitic parkinsonism and paralysis agitans; in spastic states; inhibits excessive motility and hypertonus of the gastrointestinal tract in such conditions as the irritable colon syndrome, mild dysentery, diverticulitis, pylorospasm, and cardiospasm

Scopolamine butylbromide [not available in the U.S.]:
Oral/injection: Treatment of smooth muscle spasm of the genitourinary or gastrointestinal tract; injection may also be used to prior to radiological/diagnostic procedures to prevent spasm

Mechanism of Action Blocks the action of acetylcholine at parasympathetic sites in smooth muscle, secretory glands and the CNS; increases cardiac output, dries secretions, antagonizes histamine and serotonin; dilates pupils

Pharmacodynamics/Kinetics
Onset of action: Oral, I.M.: 0.5-1 hour; I.V.: 10 minutes
  Peak effect: 20-60 minutes; may take 3-7 days for full recovery; transdermal: 24 hours
Duration: Oral, I.M.: 4-6 hours; I.V.: 2 hours
Absorption: Tertiary salts (hydrobromide) are well absorbed; quaternary salts (butylbromide) are poorly absorbed (local concentrations in the GI tract following oral dosing may be high)
Metabolism: Hepatic
Half-life elimination: Hyoscine-N-butylbromide: 4.8 hours; Scopolamine: 9.5 hours
Excretion: Urine (<10%, as parent drug and metabolites)

Dosage Note: Scopolamine (hyoscine) hydrobromide should not be interchanged with scopolamine butylbromide formulations. Dosages are not equivalent.

Scopolamine base: Transdermal patch: Adults:
  Preoperative: Apply 1 patch to hairless area behind ear the night before surgery or 1 hour prior to cesarean section (apply no sooner than 1 hour before surgery to minimize newborn exposure); remove 24 hours after surgery
  Motion sickness: Apply 1 patch behind the ear at least 4 hours prior to exposure and every 3 days as needed; effective if applied as soon as 2-3 hours before anticipated need, best if 12 hours before

Scopolamine hydrobromide:
Antiemetic: SubQ:
  Children: 0.006 mg/kg
  Adults: 0.6-1 mg
Preoperative: I.M., I.V., SubQ:
  Children 6 months to 3 years: 0.1-0.15 mg
  Children 3-6 years: 0.2-0.3 mg
  Adults: 0.3-0.65 mg
Sedation, tranquilization: I.M., I.V., SubQ: Adults: 0.6 mg 3-4 times/day
Refraction: Ophthalmic:
  Children: Instill 1 drop of 0.25% to eye(s) twice daily for 2 days before procedure
  Adults: Instill 1-2 drops of 0.25% to eye(s) 1 hour before procedure
Iridocyclitis: Ophthalmic:
  Children: Instill 1 drop of 0.25% to eye(s) up to 3 times/day
  Adults: Instill 1-2 drops of 0.25% to eye(s) up to 4 times/day
Parkinsonism, spasticity, motion sickness: Adults: Oral: 0.4-0.8 mg. May repeat every 8-12 hours as needed; the dosage may be cautiously increased in parkinsonism and spastic states. For motion sickness, administration at least 1 hour before exposure is recommended.

Scopolamine butylbromide:
Gastrointestinal/genitourinary spasm (Buscopan® [CAN]; not available in the U.S.): Adults:
Oral: 10-20 mg daily (1-2 tablets); maximum: 6 tablets/day
I.M., I.V., SubQ: 10-20 mg; maximum: 100 mg/day. Intramuscular injections should be administered 10-15 minutes prior to radiological/diagnostic procedures

Stability
Injection: Store at room temperature of 15°C to 30°C (58°F to 86°F). Protect from light.
  Hydrobromide injection: Avoid acid solutions, hydrolysis occurs at pH <3.
  Butylbromide injection: Stable in D_5W, NS, $D_{10}W$, and LR for up to 8 hours.
Ophthalmic solution: Store at 8°C to 27°C (46°F to 80°F). Protect from light.
Tablet: Store at room temperature of 15°C to 30°C (58°F to 86°F).
Transdermal system: Store at 20°C to 25°C (68°F to 77°F).

◀ **Administration**

I.V.:

Hydrobromide: Dilute with an equal volume of sterile water and administer by direct I.V.; inject over 2-3 minutes

Butylbromide: No dilution is necessary prior to injection; inject at a rate of 1 mL/minute

Ophthalmic: Remove contact lenses prior to administration; wait 15 minutes before reinserting if using products containing benzalkonium chloride. Wash hands following administration.

Transdermal: Topical patch is programmed to deliver 1 mg over 3 days. Once applied, do not remove the patch for 3 full days. Apply to hairless area of skin behind the ear. Wash hands before and after applying the disc to avoid drug contact with eyes.

Monitoring Parameters Body temperature, heart rate, urinary output, intraocular pressure

Anesthesia and Critical Care Concerns/Other Considerations

Clinical Pearls/Comments: In administering scopolamine, it is important to recognize that lower doses (0.1 mg) may have vagal mimetic effects (ie, increase vagal tone causing paradoxical bradycardia). It is likely that the vagotonic effects of scopolamine are mediated by blockade of muscarinic receptors at the level of the brain. Transdermal patch is programmed to deliver *in vivo* 1 mg over 3 days.

Pregnancy Risk Factor C

Contraindications Hypersensitivity to scopolamine, other belladonna alkaloids, or any component of the formulation; narrow-angle glaucoma; acute hemorrhage; paralytic ileus; tachycardia secondary to cardiac insufficiency; myasthenia gravis

Tablet formulations are contraindicated in patients with prostatic hyperplasia, pyloric obstruction, or patients with an idiosyncrasy to anticholinergic drugs.

Injectable formulations are contraindicated in patients with chronic lung disease (repeated administration).

Warnings/Precautions Use with caution in patients with coronary artery disease, tachyarrhythmias, heart failure, or hypertension; evaluate tachycardia prior to administration. Use with caution with hepatic or renal impairment; adverse CNS effects occur more often in these patients. Use with caution in infants and children since they may be more susceptible to adverse effects of scopolamine. Use injectable, ophthalmic, and transdermal products with caution in patients with prostatic hyperplasia (nonobstructive) or urinary retention; oral products are contraindicated. Discontinue if patient reports unusual visual disturbances or pain within the eye. Use caution in hiatal hernia, reflux esophagitis, and ulcerative colitis. Use with caution in patients with a history of seizure or psychosis; may exacerbate these conditions. Patients with idiosyncratic reaction to anticholinergics, including scopolamine, may experience disorientation, delirium and/or marked somnolence; may be accompanied by dilated pupils, rapid pulse and xerostomia. May cause CNS depression, which may impair physical or mental abilities; patients must be cautioned about performing tasks which require mental alertness (eg, operating machinery or driving).

Transdermal patch may contain conducting metal (eg, aluminum); remove patch prior to MRI. Ophthalmic products may contain benzalkonium chloride which may be absorbed by contact lenses; remove contacts prior to administration and wait 15 minutes before reinserting. Scopolamine (hyoscine) hydrobromide should not be interchanged with scopolamine butylbromide formulations; dosages are not equivalent. Safety and efficacy have not been established for the use of transdermal and oral scopolamine in children.

Adverse Reactions Frequency not defined.

Ophthalmic: Note: Systemic adverse effects have been reported following ophthalmic administration.

Central nervous system: Drowsiness, somnolence, visual hallucination

Dermatologic: Eczematoid dermatitis

Ocular: Blurred vision, edema, exudate, follicular conjunctivitis, increased intraocular pressure, local irritation, photophobia, vascular congestion

Respiratory: Congestion

Systemic:

Cardiovascular: Flushing, orthostatic hypotension, palpitation, tachycardia, ventricular fibrillation

Central nervous system: Acute toxic psychosis (rare), agitation (rare), ataxia, confusion, delusion (rare), disorientation, dizziness, drowsiness, fatigue, hallucination (rare), headache, loss of memory, paranoid behavior (rare), restlessness

Dermatologic: Dry skin, erythema, increased sensitivity to light, rash

Endocrine & metabolic: Decreased flow of breast milk, thirst

Gastrointestinal: Bloated feeling, constipation, dry throat, dysphagia, nausea, vomiting, xerostomia

Genitourinary: Dysuria, urinary retention

Local: Irritation at injection site

Neuromuscular & skeletal: Tremor, weakness

Ocular: Accommodation impaired, blurred vision, cycloplegia, dryness, glaucoma (narrow-angle), increased intraocular pain, itching, photophobia, pupil dilation

Respiratory: Dry nose

Miscellaneous: Diaphoresis decreased, heat intolerance

Drug Interactions

Avoid Concomitant Use There are no known interactions where it is recommended to avoid concomitant use.

Increased Effect/Toxicity

Scopolamine Derivatives may increase the levels/effects of: Alcohol (Ethyl); Anticholinergics; Cannabinoids; CNS Depressants; Methotrimeprazine; Potassium Chloride

The levels/effects of Scopolamine Derivatives may be increased by: Methotrimeprazine; Pramlintide

Decreased Effect

Scopolamine Derivatives may decrease the levels/effects of: Acetylcholinesterase Inhibitors (Central); Secretin

The levels/effects of Scopolamine Derivatives may be decreased by: Acetylcholinesterase Inhibitors (Central)

Ethanol/Nutrition/Herb Interactions Ethanol: Avoid ethanol (may increase CNS depression).

Test Interactions Interferes with gastric secretion test

Dosage Forms Excipient information presented when available (limited, particularly for generics); consult specific product labeling. [CAN] = Canadian brand name

Injection, solution, as hydrobromide: 0.4 mg/mL (1 mL)

Injection, solution, as hyoscine-N-butylbromide:

Buscopan® [CAN]: 20 mg/mL [not available in U.S.]

Solution, ophthalmic, as hydrobromide:

Isopto® Hyoscine: 0.25% (5 mL) [contains benzalkonium chloride]

Tablet, as hyoscine-N-butylbromide:

Buscopan® [CAN]: 10 mg [not available in U.S.]

Tablet, soluble, as hydrobromide:

Scopace™: 0.4 mg

Transdermal system:

Transderm Scōp®: 1.5 mg (4s, 10s, 24s) [releases ~1 mg over 72 hours]

References

Hamilton R, Perrone J, Meggs WJ, et al, "Epidemic Anticholinergic Poisoning From Scopolamine Tainted Heroin," *Clin Toxicol*, 1995, 33(5):502-3.

Hooper RG, Conner CS, and Rumack BH, "Acute Poisoning From Over-The-Counter Sleep Preparations," *JACEP*, 1979, 8(3):98-100.

◆ **Scopolamine Hydrobromide** *see* Scopolamine Derivatives *on page 1278*

◆ **Seasonale®** *see* Ethinyl Estradiol and Levonorgestrel *on page 549*

◆ **Seasonique™** *see* Ethinyl Estradiol and Levonorgestrel *on page 549*

◆ **Sectral®** *see* Acebutolol *on page 24*

◆ **Select™ 1/35 (Can)** *see* Ethinyl Estradiol and Norethindrone *on page 554*

Selegiline (se LE ji leen)

Related Information
Antidepressant Agents *on page 1660*

U.S. Brand Names Eldepryl®; Emsam®; Zelapar™

Canadian Brand Names Apo-Selegiline®; Gen-Selegiline; Mylan-Selegiline; Novo-Selegiline; Nu-Selegiline

Index Terms Deprenyl; L-Deprenyl; Selegiline Hydrochloride

Pharmacologic Category Anti-Parkinson's Agent, MAO Type B Inhibitor; Antidepressant, Monoamine Oxidase Inhibitor

Use Adjunct in the management of parkinsonian patients in which levodopa/carbidopa therapy is deteriorating (oral products); treatment of major depressive disorder (transdermal product)

Unlabeled/Investigational Use Early Parkinson's disease; attention-deficit/hyperactivity disorder (ADHD); negative symptoms of schizophrenia; extrapyramidal symptoms

Pharmacodynamics/Kinetics
Onset of action: Therapeutic: Oral: Within 1 hour

Duration: Oral: 24-72 hours

Absorption:
  Orally disintegrating tablet: Rapid; greater bioavailability than capsule/tablet
  Transdermal: 25% to 30% (of total selegiline content) over 24 hours

Protein binding: ~90%

Metabolism: Hepatic, primarily via CYP2B6 to active (N-desmethylselegiline, amphetamine, methamphetamine) and inactive metabolites

Half-life elimination: Oral: 10 hours; Transdermal: 18-25 hours

Excretion: Urine (primarily metabolites); feces

Dosage
Capsule/tablet:
  Children and Adolescents: ADHD (unlabeled use): 5-15 mg/day
  Adults: Parkinson's disease: 5 mg twice daily with breakfast and lunch or 10 mg in the morning
  Elderly: Parkinson's disease: Initial: 5 mg in the morning, may increase to a total of 10 mg/day

Orally disintegrating tablet (Zelapar™): Adults: Parkinson's disease: Initial 1.25 mg daily for at least 6 weeks; may increase to 2.5 mg daily based on clinical response (maximum: 2.5 mg daily)

Transdermal (Emsam®): Depression:
  Adults: Initial: 6 mg/24 hours once daily; may titrate based on clinical response in increments of 3 mg/day every 2 weeks up to a maximum of 12 mg/24 hours
  Elderly: 6 mg/24 hours

Dosage adjustment in renal impairment: No adjustment necessary.

Dosage adjustment in hepatic impairment: No adjustment necessary in mild-moderate hepatic impairment.

Anesthesia and Critical Care Concerns/Other Considerations
Clinical Pearls/Comments: Patients receiving MAO inhibitors who undergo surgery may be at risk of developing significant hypertension when used with direct-acting adrenergic agents (eg, norepinephrine) and of lethal hypertension when administered with indirect-acting adrenergic agents (eg, ephedrine). The use of meperidine in these patients may also precipitate serotonin syndrome and is contraindicated. Years ago, it was advised that patients receiving MAO inhibitors have this drug discontinued for at least 10 days before elective surgery. However, the decision to continue or withhold MAO inhibitors must be done in collaboration with the patient's psychiatrist. Currently, an MAO-safe anesthetic technique which excludes the use of meperidine and indirect-acting adrenergic agonists is recommended for patients requiring continuing MAO therapy (Huyse, 2006).

Additional Information When adding selegiline to levodopa/carbidopa, the dose of the latter can usually be decreased. Complete prescribing information for this medication should be consulted for additional detail.

Dosage Forms Excipient information presented when available (limited, particularly for generics); consult specific product labeling.

Capsule, oral, as hydrochloride: 5 mg
  Eldepryl®: 5 mg
Tablet, oral, as hydrochloride: 5 mg
Tablet, orally-disintegrating:
  Zelapar™: 1.25 mg [contains phenylalanine 1.25 mg/tablet]
Transdermal system, topical [once-daily patch]:
  Emsam®: 6 mg/24 hours (30s) [20 cm^2, total selegiline 20 mg]; 9 mg/24 hours (30s) [30 cm^2, total selegiline 30 mg]; 12 mg/24 hours (30s) [40 cm^2, total selegiline 40 mg]

References

Burke WJ, Roccaforte WH, Wengel SP, et al, "L-Deprenyl in the Treatment of Mild Dementia of the Alzheimer Type: Results of a 15-Month Trial," *J Am Geriatr Soc*, 1993, 41(11):1219-25.

Collier DS, Berg MJ, and Fincham RW, "Parkinsonism Treatment: Part III - Update," *Ann Pharmacother*, 1992, 26(2):227-33.

Huyse FJ, Touw DJ, van Schijndel RS, et al, "Psychotropic Drugs and the Perioperative Period: A Proposal for a Guideline in Elective Surgery," *Psychosomatics*, 2006, 47(1):8-22.

Jankovic J, "Deprenyl in Attention Deficit Associated With Tourette's Syndrome," *Arch Neurol*, 1993, 50(3):286-8.

Koller WC, Silver DE, and Lieberman A, "An Algorithm for the Management of Parkinson's Disease," *Neurology*, 1994, 44(12 Suppl 10):1-52.

Lawlor BA, Aisen PS, and Green C, "Selegiline in the Treatment of Behavioural Disturbances in Alzheimer's Disease," *Int J Geriatr Psychiatry*, 1997, 12(3):319-22.

Sano M, Ernesto C, Thomas RG, et al, "A Controlled Trial of Selegiline, Alpha-Tocopherol, or Both as Treatment for Alzheimer's Disease," *N Engl J Med*, 1997, 336(17):1216-22.

Schneider LS, Pollock VE, Zemansky MF, et al, "A Pilot Study of Low-Dose L-Deprenyl in Alzheimer's Disease," *J Geriatr Psychiatry Neurol*, 1991, 4(3):143-8.

Shulman KI and Walker SE, "A Reevaluation of Dietary Restrictions for Irreversible Monoamine Oxidase Inhibitors," *Psychiatr Ann*, 2001, 31(6):378-84.

Shulman KI and Walker SE, "Refining the MAOI Diet: Tyramine Content of Pizzas and Soy Products," *J Clin Psychiatry*, 1999, 60(3):191-3.

Stern MB, "Contemporary Approaches to the Pharmacotherapeutic Management of Parkinson's Disease: An Overview," *Neurology*, 1997, 49(1 Suppl 1):2-9.

The Parkinson Study Group, "Effect of Deprenyl on the Progression of Disability in Early Parkinson's Disease," *N Engl J Med*, 1989, 321(20):1364-71.

The Parkinson Study Group, "Effects of Tocopherol and Deprenyl on the Progression of Disability in Early Parkinson's Disease," *N Engl J Med*, 1993, 328(3):176-83.

Walker SE, Shulman KI, Tailor SA, et al, "Tyramine Content of Previously Restricted Foods in Monoamine Oxidase Inhibitor Diets," *J Clin Psychopharmacol*, 1996, 16(5):383-8.

♦ **Selegiline Hydrochloride** *see* Selegiline *on page 1282*

♦ **Selfemra™** *see* FLUoxetine *on page 616*

♦ **Sensorcaine®** *see* Bupivacaine *on page 211*

♦ **Sensorcaine®-MPF** *see* Bupivacaine *on page 211*

♦ **Sensorcaine®-MPF Spinal** *see* Bupivacaine *on page 211*

♦ **Septra®** *see* Sulfamethoxazole and Trimethoprim *on page 1333*

♦ **Septra® DS** *see* Sulfamethoxazole and Trimethoprim *on page 1333*

♦ **Septra® Injection (Can)** *see* Sulfamethoxazole and Trimethoprim *on page 1333*

♦ **Serevent® Diskhaler® Disk (Can)** *see* Salmeterol *on page 1273*

♦ **Serevent® Diskus®** *see* Salmeterol *on page 1273*

♦ **Seroquel®** *see* QUEtiapine *on page 1212*

♦ **Seroquel XR®** *see* QUEtiapine *on page 1212*

♦ **Serostim®** *see* Somatropin *on page 1318*

Sevoflurane (see voe FLOO rane)

Medication Safety Issues

Sound-alike/look-alike issues:
  Ultane® may be confused with Ultram®

High alert medication: The Institute for Safe Medication Practices (ISMP) includes this medication among its list of drug classes which have a heightened risk of causing significant patient harm when used in error.

◀ **Related Information**

Anesthesia Considerations for Neurosurgery *on page 1514*
Anesthesia Considerations for Geriatric Patients *on page 1523*
Anesthetic Considerations in the Substance-Abusing Patient *on page 1613*
Chronic Renal Failure *on page 1552*
Inhalational Anesthetics *on page 1632*
Perioperative Management of Patients on Antiseizure Medication *on page 1577*

U.S. Brand Names Sojourn™; Ultane®

Canadian Brand Names Sevorane® AF

Pharmacologic Category General Anesthetic, Inhalation

Generic Available Yes

Use Induction and maintenance of general anesthesia

Unlabeled/Investigational Use Intraoperative cardio-, hepatic-, and neuro-protection (ischemic preconditioning)

Mechanism of Action Inhaled anesthetics alter activity of neuronal ion channels particularly the fast synaptic neurotransmitter receptors (nicotinic acetylcholine, GABA, and glutamate receptors). Limited effects on sympathetic stimulation including cardiovascular system. Seroflurane does not cause respiratory irritation or circulatory stimulation. May depress myocardial contractility, decrease blood pressure through a decrease in systemic vascular resistance and decrease sympathetic nervous activity.

Pharmacodynamics/Kinetics Sevoflurane has a low blood/gas partition coefficient and therefore is associated with a rapid onset of anesthesia and recovery

Onset of action: Time to induction: Within 2 minutes

Duration: Emergence time: Depends on blood concentration when sevoflurane is discontinued. The rate of change of anesthetic concentration in the lung is rapid with sevoflurane because of its low blood gas solubility (0.63). The 90% decrement time (time required for anesthetic concentration in vessel-rich tissues to decrease by 90%) for sevoflurane is short when the duration of anesthesia is <2 hours but increases dramatically as the duration of administration is lengthened.

Metabolism: 3% to 5% hepatic via CYP2E1

Excretion: Exhaled gases

Dosage Minimum alveolar concentration (MAC), the concentration that abolishes movement in response to a noxious stimulus (surgical incision) in 50% of patients, is 2.6% (25 years of age) for sevoflurane. Surgical levels of anesthesia are generally achieved with concentrations from 0.5% to 3%; the concentration at which amnesia and loss of awareness occur is 0.6%.

Minimum alveolar concentrations (MAC) values for surgical levels of anesthesia:

0 to 1 month old full-term neonates: Sevoflurane in oxygen: 3.3%

1 to <6 months: Sevoflurane in oxygen: 3%

6 months to <3 years:
  Sevoflurane in oxygen: 2.8%
  Sevoflurane in 60% N_2O/40% oxygen: 2%

3-12 years: Sevoflurane in oxygen: 2.5%

25 years:
  Sevoflurane in oxygen: 2.6%
  Sevoflurane in 65% N_2O/35% oxygen: 1.4%

40 years:
  Sevoflurane in oxygen: 2.1%
  Sevoflurane in 65% N_2O/35% oxygen: 1.1%

60 years:
  Sevoflurane in oxygen: 1.7%
  Sevoflurane in 65% N_2O/35% oxygen: 0.9%

80 years:
  Sevoflurane in oxygen: 1.4%
  Sevoflurane in 65% N_2O/35% oxygen: 0.7%

Dosage adjustment in renal impairment: Use with caution in renal insufficiency.

Dosage adjustment in hepatic impairment: Use with caution in patients with underlying hepatic conditions.

Stability Store at 15°C to 30°C (59°F to 86°F).

Administration Via sevoflurane-specific calibrated vaporizers; use cautiously in low-flow or closed-circuit systems since sevoflurane is unstable and potentially toxic breakdown products have been liberated.

Monitoring Parameters Blood pressure, temperature, heart rate and rhythm, oxygen saturation, end-tidal CO_2 and end-tidal sevoflurane concentrations should be monitored prior to and throughout anesthesia; temperature of CO_2 absorbent canister

Anesthesia and Critical Care Concerns/Other Considerations

Evidence-Based Information: In animal studies, sevoflurane and other inhaled anesthetics have shown a protective effect (ischemic preconditioning) of the heart and brain. A human randomized controlled clinical trial has also been conducted supporting this effect (Bein, 2008). In patients undergoing liver surgery with inflow occlusion, sevoflurane has demonstrated a protective effect of preconditioning (Beck-Schimmer, 2008).

Pregnancy Risk Factor B

Contraindications Previous hypersensitivity to sevoflurane, other halogenated anesthetics, or any component of the formulation; known or suspected susceptibility to malignant hyperthermia

Warnings/Precautions Reaction of sevoflurane with CO_2 absorbents that become desiccated within circle breathing equipment can lead to formation of formaldehyde (causing respiratory irritation) and carbon monoxide; maintain fresh absorbent as per manufacturer guidelines regardless of state of colorimetric indicator. Exothermic reaction of sevoflurane with desiccated CO_2 absorbents has been reported to generate extreme heat, smoke and/or fire within breathing circuit. This reaction also leads to formation of a fluorinated byproduct, compound A, which has been reported to cause nephrotoxicity (eg, proteinuria, glycosuria) in animal studies. Compound A-induced renal toxicity is dose- and exposure time-dependent; minimize exposure risk by not exceeding 2 MAC hours and fresh flow rates <2 L/minute (low fresh gas flow rates maximize rebreathing of the anesthetic). Steps that might reduce the risk of these events include: Replace CO_2 absorbent if it has not been used for an extended period of time, shut off anesthesia machine at the end of clinical use or after any case when a subsequent extended period of nonuse is expected, turn off all vaporizers when not in use, verify the integrity of new CO_2 absorbents prior to use, monitor the temperature of the CO_2 absorbent canisters, and monitor the correlation between sevoflurane vaporizer setting and the inspired concentration.

Causes dose-dependent respiratory depression and blunted ventilatory response to hypoxia and hypercapnia. Hypoxic pulmonary vasoconstriction is blunted which may lead to increased pulmonary shunt. May dilate the cerebral vasculature and increase intracranial pressure. Use cautiously in patients with risk of elevation in intracranial pressure. May trigger malignant hyperthermia; avoid use in patients susceptible to malignant hyperthermia. Use of other inhaled anesthetics has been associated with rare cases of perioperative hyperkalemia; concomitant use of succinylcholine was associated with many of the reported cases, but not all. Risk of hyperkalemia is increased in pediatric patients with underlying neuromuscular disease (eg, Duchenne muscular dystrophy). Other abnormalities may include elevation in CPK and myoglobinuria. Monitor closely for arrhythmias. Aggressively identify and treat hyperkalemia. Use cautiously in patients with renal dysfunction. Use with caution in patients at risk for seizures; seizures have been reported in children and young adults. Monitor for emergence agitation or delirium. Postoperative hepatitis or hepatic dysfunction with or without jaundice has rarely been reported. Safety in patients with severe renal dysfunction or severe hepatic dysfunction has not been determined.

Adverse Reactions
>10%:
  Cardiovascular: Hypotension (4% to 11% dose dependent)
  Central nervous system: Agitation (7% to 15%)
  Gastrointestinal: Nausea (25%), vomiting (18%)
  Respiratory: Cough increased (5% to 11%)
1% to 10%:
  Cardiovascular: Bradycardia (5%), tachycardia (2% to 6%), hypertension (2%)
  Central nervous system: Somnolence (8%), dizziness (4%), hypothermia (1%), headache (1%), fever (1%), emergence delirium

◀ Gastrointestinal: Salivation (2% to 4%)

Respiratory: Airway obstruction (8%), laryngospasm (2% to 8%), breath-holding (2% to 5%), apnea (2%)

Miscellaneous: Shivering (6%)

<1% (Limited to important or life-threatening): Acidosis, albuminuria, alkaline phosphatase increased, allergic reactions, ALT increased, amblyopia, anaphylactic/anaphylactoid reaction, arrhythmia, asthenia, AST increased, atrial arrhythmia, atrial fibrillation, bigeminy, bilirubinemia, bronchospasm, BUN increased, complete AV block, confusion, conjunctivitis, creatinine increased, creatine phosphokinase increased, crying, dry mouth, dyspnea, fluorosis, glycosuria, hemorrhage, hepatic dysfunction, hepatic failure, hepatic necrosis, hepatitis, hiccup, hyperglycemia, hyperkalemia (pediatric patients, postoperative), hypertonia, hyper-/hypoventilation, hypophosphatemia, hypoxia, insomnia, inverted T wave, jaundice, leukocytosis, LDH increased, liver enzymes increased, malignant hyperthermia, myoglobinuria, nervousness, oliguria, pain, pharyngitis, pruritus, rash, second-degree AV block, seizure, sputum, ST depression, stridor, supraventricular extrasystoles, syncope, taste perversion, thrombocytopenia, urinary retention, ventricular extrasystoles, wheezing

Drug Interactions

Metabolism/Transport Effects Substrate of CYP2A6 (minor), 2B6 (minor), 2E1 (major), 3A4 (minor)

Avoid Concomitant Use

Avoid concomitant use of Sevoflurane with any of the following: Methylphenidate

Increased Effect/Toxicity

Sevoflurane may increase the levels/effects of: EPINEPHrine; Neuromuscular-Blocking Agents (Nondepolarizing)

The levels/effects of Sevoflurane may be increased by: CYP2E1 Inhibitors (Moderate); CYP2E1 Inhibitors (Strong); Methylphenidate

Decreased Effect There are no known significant interactions involving a decrease in effect.

Dosage Forms Excipient information presented when available (limited, particularly for generics); consult specific product labeling.

Liquid for inhalation: 100% (250 mL)

Sojourn™, Ultane®: 100% (250 mL)

References

Beck-Schimmer B, Breitenstein S, Urech S, et al, "A randomized Controlled Trial on Pharmacological Preconditioning in Liver Surgery Using a Volatile Anesthetic," *Ann Surg*, 2008, 248(6):909-18.

Bein B, Renner J, Caliebe D, et al, "The Effects of Interrupted or Continuous Administration of Sevoflurane on Preconditioning Before Cardio-Pulmonary Bypass in Coronary Artery Surgery: Comparison With Continuous Propofol," *Anaesthesia*, 2008, 63(10):1046-55.

Campagna JA, Miller KW, and Forman SA, "Mechanisms of Action of Inhaled Anesthetics," *N Engl J Med*, 2003, 348(21):2110-24.

De Hert SG, Turani F, Mathur S, et al, "Cardioprotection With Volatile Anesthetics: Mechanisms and Clinical Implications," *Anesth Analg*, 2005, 100(6):1584-93.

Doi M and Ikeda K, "Airway Irritation Produced by Volatile Anaesthetics During Brief Inhalation: Comparison of Halothane, Enflurane, Isoflurane and Sevoflurane," *Can J Anaesth*, 1993, 40 (2):122-6.

Eger EI 2nd, "Characteristics of Anesthetic Agents Used for Induction and Maintenance of General Anesthesia," *Am J Health Syst Pharm*, 2004, 61(Suppl 4):3-10.

FDA/CDER resources page, Food and Drug Administration Website, available at: http://www.fda.gov/medwatch/SAFETY/2003/Ultane_deardoc.pdf.

Frink EJ Jr, Ghantous H, Malan TP, et al, "Plasma Inorganic Fluoride With Sevoflurane Anesthesia: Correlation With Indices of Hepatic and Renal Function," *Anesth Analg*, 1992, 74(2):231-5.

Golembiewski J, "Considerations in Selecting an Inhaled Anesthetic Agent: Case Studies," *Am J Health Syst Pharm*, 2004, 61 (Suppl 4):10-17.

Jones RM, "Desflurane and Sevoflurane: Inhalation Anaesthetics for This Decade?" *Br J Anaesth*, 1990, 65(4):527-36.

Katoh T, Suguro Y, Nakajima R, et al, "Blood Concentrations of Sevoflurane and Isoflurane on Recovery From Anaesthesia," *Br J Anaesth*, 1992, 69(3):259-62.

Smith I, Ding Y, and White PF, "Comparison of Induction, Maintenance, and Recovery Characteristics of Sevoflurane-N20 and Propofol-Sevoflurane-N(2)O With Propofol-Isoflurane-N(2)O Anesthesia," *Anesth Analg*, 1992, 74(2):253-9.

Strum DP and Eger EI 2d, "Partition Coefficients for Sevoflurane in Human Blood, Saline, and Olive Oil," *Anesth Analg*, 1987, 66(7):654-6.

Wang L, Traystman RJ, and Murphy SJ, "Inhalational Anesthetics as Preconditioning Agents in Ischemic Brain," *Curr Opin Pharmacol*, 2008, 8(1):104-10.

Yasuda N, Lockhart SH, Eger EI 2nd, et al, "Comparison of Kinetics of Sevoflurane and Isoflurane in Humans," *Anesth Analg*, 1991, 72(3):316-24.

◆ **Sevorane® AF (Can)** *see* Sevoflurane *on page 1283*

◆ **Siladryl Allergy [OTC]** *see* DiphenhydrAMINE *on page 430*

◆ **Silapap Children's [OTC]** *see* Acetaminophen *on page 25*

◆ **Silapap Infant's [OTC]** *see* Acetaminophen *on page 25*

Sildenafil (sil DEN a fil)

Medication Safety Issues
Sound-alike/look-alike issues:
Revatio® may be confused with ReVia®
Sildenafil may be confused with silodosin, tadalafil, vardenafil
Viagra® may be confused with Allegra®, Vaniqa™

U.S. Brand Names Revatio®; Viagra®
Canadian Brand Names Viagra®
Index Terms UK92480
Pharmacologic Category Phosphodiesterase-5 Enzyme Inhibitor
Generic Available No
Use
Revatio®: Treatment of pulmonary arterial hypertension (WHO Group I) to improve exercise ability and delay clinical worsening
Viagra®: Treatment of erectile dysfunction (ED)

Unlabeled/Investigational Use Pulmonary arterial hypertension in children

Mechanism of Action
Erectile dysfunction: Does not directly cause penile erections, but affects the response to sexual stimulation. The physiologic mechanism of erection of the penis involves release of nitric oxide (NO) in the corpus cavernosum during sexual stimulation. NO then activates the enzyme guanylate cyclase, which results in increased levels of cyclic guanosine monophosphate (cGMP), producing smooth muscle relaxation and inflow of blood to the corpus cavernosum. Sildenafil enhances the effect of NO by inhibiting phosphodiesterase type 5 (PDE-5), which is responsible for degradation of cGMP in the corpus cavernosum; when sexual stimulation causes local release of NO, inhibition of PDE-5 by sildenafil causes increased levels of cGMP in the corpus cavernosum, resulting in smooth muscle relaxation and inflow of blood to the corpus cavernosum; at recommended doses, it has no effect in the absence of sexual stimulation.

Pulmonary arterial hypertension (PAH): Inhibits phosphodiesterase type 5 (PDE-5) in smooth muscle of pulmonary vasculature where PDE-5 is responsible for the degradation of cyclic guanosine monophosphate (cGMP). Increased cGMP concentration results in pulmonary vasculature relaxation; vasodilation in the pulmonary bed and the systemic circulation (to a lesser degree) may occur.

Pharmacodynamics/Kinetics
Onset of action: ~60 minutes
Duration: 2-4 hours
Absorption: Rapid; slower with a high-fat meal
Distribution: V_{dss}: 105 L
Protein binding, plasma: ~96%
Metabolism: Hepatic via CYP3A4 (major) and CYP2C9 (minor route); forms N-desmethyl metabolite (active)
Bioavailability: 40% (25% to 63%)
Half-life elimination: 4 hours; the elderly and those with severe renal impairment have reduced clearance of sildenafil and its active N-desmethyl metabolite
Time to peak: 30-120 minutes; delayed by 60 minutes with a high-fat meal
Excretion: Feces (80%); urine (13%)

Dosage Oral:
Children ≥1 month: Pulmonary arterial hypertension (unlabeled use): 0.25-2 mg/kg/dose every 4-6 hours. Most reports used 0.5 mg/kg/dose and titrated up to 2 mg/kg/dose

◀ Adults:

Erectile dysfunction (Viagra®): Usual dose: 50 mg once daily 1 hour (range: 30 minutes to 4 hours) before sexual activity; dosing range: 25-100 mg once daily

Pulmonary arterial hypertension (Revatio®): Pulmonary arterial hypertension (Revatio®): 20 mg 3 times/day, taken 4-6 hours apart

Note: A delay in clinical worsening was observed in a short-term trial in which most patients achieved a target dose of 80 mg 3 times daily (unlabeled dose). The patients had an incremental dosage escalation while on a stable epoprostenol regimen (Simonneau, 2008).

Elderly >65 years: Use with caution

Revatio®: Refer to adult dosing.

Viagra®: Starting dose of 25 mg should be considered.

Dosage considerations for patients stable on alpha-blockers: Viagra®: Initial 25 mg

Dosage adjustment for concomitant use of potent CYP34A inhibitors:

Revatio®:

Erythromycin, saquinavir: No dosage adjustment

Itraconazole, ketoconazole, ritonavir: Not recommended

Viagra®:

Erythromycin, itraconazole, ketoconazole, saquinavir: Starting dose of 25 mg should be considered

Ritonavir: Maximum: 25 mg every 48 hours

Dosage adjustment in renal impairment:

Revatio®: Dose adjustment not necessary

Viagra®: Cl_{cr} <30 mL/minute: Starting dose of 25 mg should be considered

Dosage adjustment in hepatic impairment:

Revatio®: Child-Pugh class A and B: Dose adjustment not necessary

Viagra®: Child-Pugh class A and B: Starting dose of 25 mg should be considered; not studied in severe impairment (Child-Pugh class C)

Stability Store tablets at controlled room temperature of 25°C (77°F); excursions permitted to 15°C to 30°C (59°F to 86°F).

Administration

Revatio®: Administer tablets at least 4-6 hours apart

Viagra®: Administer orally 30 minutes to 4 hours before sexual activity

Anesthesia and Critical Care Concerns/Other Considerations

Clinical Pearls/Comments:

Cardiovascular effects of sildenafil may be potentially hazardous in patients with:
- active coronary ischemia (not on nitrates)
- heart failure and with low blood pressure and low volume status
- complicated, multidrug antihypertensive regimens
- potential for drug-drug interactions that may prolong sildenafil half-life (eg, drugs that predominantly inhibit CYP3A4, such as certain HMG-CoA reductase inhibitors, protease inhibitors, certain macrolide antibiotics, imidazole antibiotics)

Use of sildenafil is contraindicated in patients currently taking nitrate preparations. When nitrate administration becomes medically necessary in patients who received sildenafil, the ACC/AHA 2004 guidelines on treatment of ST-segment elevation MI and the ACC/AHA 2007 guidelines on treatment of unstable angina/non-ST-segment elevation MI support administration of nitrates only if 24 hours have elapsed after use of sildenafil.

Pregnancy Risk Factor B

Contraindications Hypersensitivity to sildenafil or any component of the formulation; concurrent use (regularly/intermittently) of organic nitrates in any form (eg, nitroglycerin, isosorbide dinitrate)

Warnings/Precautions Decreases in blood pressure may occur due to vasodilator effects; use with caution in patients with left ventricular outflow obstruction (aortic stenosis or hypertrophic obstructive cardiomyopathy); may be more sensitive to hypotensive actions. Concurrent use with alpha-adrenergic antagonist therapy or substantial ethanol consumption may cause symptomatic hypotension; patients should be hemodynamically stable prior to initiating therapy at the lowest possible dose. Use with caution in patients with hypotension (<90/50 mm Hg); uncontrolled hypertension (>170/110 mm Hg); life-threatening arrhythmias, stroke or MI within the last 6 months; cardiac failure or coronary artery disease causing unstable angina; safety and efficacy have not been studied in these patients. There is a degree of cardiac risk associated with sexual activity; therefore, physicians should consider the cardiovascular status of their patients prior to initiating any treatment for erectile dysfunction.

Sildenafil should be used with caution in patients with anatomical deformation of the penis (angulation, cavernosal fibrosis, or Peyronie's disease) and in patients who have conditions which may predispose them to priapism (sickle cell anemia, multiple myeloma, leukemia). All patients should be instructed to seek medical attention if erection persists >4 hours.

Vision loss may occur rarely and be a sign of nonarteritic anterior ischemic optic neuropathy (NAION). Risk may be increased with history of vision loss. Other risk factors for NAION include low cup-to-disc ratio ("crowded disc"), coronary artery disease, diabetes, hypertension, hyperlipidemia, smoking, and age >50 years. May cause dose-related impairment of color discrimination. Use caution in patients with retinitis pigmentosa; a minority have genetic disorders of retinal phosphodiesterases (no safety information available). Sudden decrease or loss of hearing has been reported rarely; hearing changes may be accompanied by tinnitus and dizziness. A direct relationship between therapy and vision or hearing loss has not been determined.

The potential underlying causes of erectile dysfunction should be evaluated prior to treatment. The safety and efficacy of sildenafil with other treatments for erectile dysfunction have not been established; use is not recommended. Efficacy with concurrent bosentan therapy has not been evaluated; use with caution. Use with caution in patients taking strong CYP3A4 inhibitors or alpha-blockers. Concomitant use with all forms of nitrates is contraindicated. If nitrate administration is medically necessary, it is not known when nitrates can be safely administered following the use of sildenafil (per manufacturer); the ACC/AHA 2007 guidelines supports administration of nitrates only if 24 hours have elapsed.

Avoid abrupt discontinuation, especially if used as monotherapy in PAH as exacerbation may occur. Use caution in patients with bleeding disorders or with active peptic ulcer disease; safety and efficacy have not been established. Use with caution in the elderly, or patients with renal or hepatic dysfunction; dose adjustment may be needed.

Adverse Reactions Based upon normal doses for either indication. (Adverse effects such as flushing, diarrhea, myalgia, and visual disturbances may be increased with doses >100 mg/24 hours.)

>10%:
  Central nervous system: Headache (16% to 46%)
  Gastrointestinal: Dyspepsia (7% to 17%; dose related)
2% to 10%:
  Cardiovascular: Flushing (10%)
  Central nervous system: Insomnia ($\leq$7%), pyrexia (6%), dizziness (2%)
  Dermatologic: Erythema (6%), rash (2%)
  Gastrointestinal: Diarrhea (3% to 9%), gastritis ($\leq$3%)
  Genitourinary: Urinary tract infection (3%)
  Hepatic: LFTs increased
  Neuromuscular & skeletal: Myalgia ($\leq$7%), paresthesia ($\leq$3%)
  Ocular: Abnormal vision (color changes, blurred vision, or increased sensitivity to light 3% to 11%; dose related)
  Respiratory: Epistaxis (9% to 13%), dyspnea exacerbated ($\leq$7%), nasal congestion (4%), rhinitis (4%), sinusitis (3%)
<2% (Limited to important or life-threatening): Allergic reaction, amnesia (transient global), anemia, angina pectoris, anorgasmia, asthma, AV block, cardiac arrest, cardiomyopathy, cataract, cerebral thrombosis, cerebrovascular hemorrhage, colitis, cystitis, depression, dysphagia, edema, exfoliative dermatitis, eye hemorrhage, gout, hearing decreased, hearing loss, heart failure, hematuria, hemorrhage, hyper-/hypoglycemia, hypernatremia, hyper-/hypotension, hyper-uricemia, intracerebral hemorrhage, intraocular pressure increased, leukopenia, migraine, myocardial ischemia, MI, myasthenia, mydriasis, neuralgia, non-arteritic ischemic optic neuropathy (NAION), palpitation, postural hypotension, priapism, pulmonary hemorrhage, rectal hemorrhage, retinal vascular disease or bleeding, seizure, shock, stomatitis, subarachnoid hemorrhage, syncope,

◄ tachycardia, tendon rupture, TIA, urinary incontinence, ventricular arrhythmia, vertigo, visual field loss, vitreous detachment/traction, vomiting

Drug Interactions

Metabolism/Transport Effects Substrate of CYP2C9 (minor), 3A4 (major); **Inhibits** CYP1A2 (weak), 2C9 (weak), 2C19 (weak), 2D6 (weak), 2E1 (weak), 3A4 (weak)

Avoid Concomitant Use

Avoid concomitant use of Sildenafil with any of the following: Phosphodiesterase 5 Inhibitors; Vasodilators (Organic Nitrates)

Increased Effect/Toxicity

Sildenafil may increase the levels/effects of: Alpha1-Blockers; Antihypertensives; Bosentan; HMG-CoA Reductase Inhibitors; Phosphodiesterase 5 Inhibitors; Vasodilators (Organic Nitrates)

The levels/effects of Sildenafil may be increased by: Antifungal Agents (Azole Derivatives, Systemic); CYP3A4 Inhibitors (Moderate); CYP3A4 Inhibitors (Strong); Dasatinib; Macrolide Antibiotics; Protease Inhibitors; Sapropterin

Decreased Effect

The levels/effects of Sildenafil may be decreased by: Bosentan; CYP3A4 Inducers (Strong); Deferasirox; Etravirine; Herbs (CYP3A4 Inducers); Peginterferon Alfa-2b

Ethanol/Nutrition/Herb Interactions

Food: Amount and rate of absorption of sildenafil is reduced when taken with a high-fat meal. Serum concentrations/toxicity may be increased with grapefruit juice; avoid concurrent use.

Herb/Nutraceutical: St John's wort may decrease sildenafil levels.

Dosage Forms Excipient information presented when available (limited, particularly for generics); consult specific product labeling.

Tablet:

Revatio®: 20 mg

Viagra®: 25 mg, 50 mg, 100 mg

References

Badesch DB, Abman SH, Ahearn GS, et al, "Medical Therapy for Pulmonary Arterial Hypertension: ACCP Evidence-Based Clinical Practice Guidelines," *Chest*, 2004, 126(1 Suppl):35-62.

Galie N, Ghofrani HA, Torbicki A, et al, "Sildenafil Citrate Therapy for Pulmonary Arterial Hypertension," *N Engl J Med*, 2005, 353(20):2148-57.

Humbert M, Sitbon O, and Simmoneau G, "Treatment of Pulmonary Arterial Hypertension," *N Engl J Med*, 2004, 351(14):1425-36.

Jackson G and Chambers J, "Sildenafil for Primary Pulmonary Hypertension: Short and Long-Term Symptomatic Benefit," *Int J Clin Pract*, 2002 56(5):397-8.

Prasad S, Wilkinson J, and Gatzoulis MA, "Sildenafil in Primary Pulmonary Hypertension," *N Engl J Med*, 2000, 343(18):1342.

Watanabe H, Ohashi K, Takeuchi K, et al, "Sildenafil for Primary and Secondary Pulmonary Hypertension," *Clin Pharmacol Ther*, 2002, 71(5):398-402.

Silodosin (SI lo doe sin)

U.S. Brand Names Rapaflo™

Index Terms KMD 3213

Pharmacologic Category Alpha$_1$ Blocker

Use Treatment of signs and symptoms of benign prostatic hyperplasia (BPH)

Pharmacodynamics/Kinetics

Distribution: V_d: 49.5 L

Protein binding: ~97%

Metabolism: Extensive, via CYP3A4, glucuronidation, and alcohol and aldehyde dehydrogenase pathways; KMD-3213G (active *in vitro*) and KMD-3293 (not significant) metabolites formed

Bioavailability: ~32%

Half-life elimination: Healthy volunteers: Silodosin: 5-21 hours; KMD-3213G: ~24 hours

Time to peak, plasma: ~3 hours

Excretion: Feces (55%); urine (34%)

Dosage Oral: Adults: BPH: 8 mg once daily with a meal

Dosage adjustment in renal impairment:

Cl_{cr} >50 mL/minute: No adjustment needed

Cl_{cr} 30-50 mL/minute: 4 mg once daily

Cl_{cr} <30 mL/minute: Use is contraindicated

Dosage adjustment in hepatic impairment:

Mild-to-moderate impairment (Child-Pugh classes A and B): No adjustment needed

Severe impairment (Child-Pugh class C): Use is contraindicated

Additional Information Complete prescribing information for this medication should be consulted for additional detail.

Dosage Forms Excipient information presented when available (limited, particularly for generics); consult specific product labeling.

Capsule:

Rapaflo™: 4 mg, 8 mg

References

Chang DF and Campbell JR, "Intraoperative Floppy Iris Syndrome Associated With Tamsulosin," *J Cataract Refract Surg*, 2005, 31(4):664-73.

◆ **Silphen Cough [OTC]** *see* DiphenhydrAMINE *on page 430*

◆ **Silvadene®** *see* Silver Sulfadiazine *on page 1292*

Silver Nitrate (SIL ver NYE trate)

Index Terms $AgNO_3$

Pharmacologic Category Antibiotic, Topical; Cauterizing Agent, Topical; Topical Skin Product, Antibacterial

Generic Available Yes

Use Cauterization of wounds and sluggish ulcers, removal of granulation tissue and warts; aseptic prophylaxis of burns

Mechanism of Action Free silver ions precipitate bacterial proteins by combining with chloride in tissue forming silver chloride; coagulates cellular protein to form an eschar; silver ions or salts or colloidal silver preparations can inhibit the growth of both gram-positive and gram-negative bacteria. This germicidal action is attributed to the precipitation of bacterial proteins by liberated silver ions. Silver nitrate coagulates cellular protein to form an eschar, and this mode of action is the postulated mechanism for control of benign hematuria, rhinitis, and recurrent pneumothorax.

Pharmacodynamics/Kinetics

Absorption: Because silver ions readily combine with protein, there is minimal GI and cutaneous absorption of the 0.5% and 1% preparations

Excretion: Highest amounts of silver noted on autopsy have been in kidneys, excretion in urine is minimal

Dosage Children and Adults:

Sticks: Apply to mucous membranes and other moist skin surfaces only on area to be treated 2-3 times/week for 2-3 weeks

Topical solution: Apply a cotton applicator dipped in solution on the affected area 2-3 times/week for 2-3 weeks

Stability Must be stored in a dry place. Store in a tight, light-resistant container. Exposure to light causes silver to oxidize and turn brown. Dipping in water causes oxidized film to readily dissolve.

Administration Applicators are **not** for ophthalmic use.

Monitoring Parameters With prolonged use, monitor methemoglobin levels

Pregnancy Risk Factor C

Contraindications Hypersensitivity to silver nitrate or any component of the formulation; not for use on broken skin, cuts, or wounds

Warnings/Precautions Do not use applicator sticks on the eyes. Prolonged use may result in skin discoloration.

Adverse Reactions Frequency not defined.

Dermatologic: Burning and skin irritation, staining of the skin

Endocrine & metabolic: Hyponatremia

Hematologic: Methemoglobinemia

Drug Interactions

Avoid Concomitant Use There are no known interactions where it is recommended to avoid concomitant use.

◀ **Increased Effect/Toxicity** There are no known significant interactions involving an increase in effect.

Decreased Effect There are no known significant interactions involving a decrease in effect.

Dosage Forms Excipient information presented when available (limited, particularly for generics); consult specific product labeling.

Applicator sticks, topical: Silver nitrate 75% and potassium nitrate 25% (6", 12", 18")

Solution, topical: 0.5% (960 mL); 10% (30 mL); 25% (30 mL); 50% (30 mL)

Silver Sulfadiazine (SIL ver sul fa DYE a zeen)

U.S. Brand Names Silvadene®; SSD®; SSD® AF; Thermazene®
Canadian Brand Names Flamazine®
Pharmacologic Category Antibiotic, Topical
Generic Available Yes
Use Prevention and treatment of infection in second and third degree burns
Mechanism of Action Acts upon the bacterial cell wall and cell membrane. Bactericidal for many gram-negative and gram-positive bacteria and is effective against yeast. Active against *Pseudomonas aeruginosa*, *Pseudomonas maltophilia*, *Enterobacter* species, *Klebsiella* species, *Serratia* species, *Escherichia coli*, *Proteus mirabilis*, *Morganella morganii*, *Providencia rettgeri*, *Proteus vulgaris*, *Providencia* species, *Citrobacter* species, *Acinetobacter calcoaceticus*, *Staphylococcus aureus*, *Staphylococcus epidermidis*, *Enterococcus* species, *Candida albicans*, *Corynebacterium diphtheriae*, and *Clostridium perfringens*

Pharmacodynamics/Kinetics
Absorption: Significant percutaneous absorption of silver sulfadiazine can occur especially when applied to extensive burns
Half-life elimination: 10 hours; prolonged with renal impairment
Time to peak, serum: 3-11 days of continuous therapy
Excretion: Urine (~50% as unchanged drug)

Dosage Children and Adults: Topical: Apply once or twice daily with a sterile-gloved hand; apply to a thickness of 1/16"; burned area should be covered with cream at all times

Stability Silvadene® cream will occasionally darken either in the jar or after application to the skin. This color change results from a light catalyzed reaction which is a common characteristic of all silver salts. A similar analogy is the oxidation of silverware. The product of this color change reaction is silver oxide which ranges in color from gray to black. Silver oxide has rarely been associated with permanent skin discoloration. Additionally, the antimicrobial activity of the product is not substantially diminished because the color change reaction involves such a small amount of the active drug and is largely a surface phenomenon.

Administration Apply with a sterile-gloved hand. Apply to a thickness 1/16". Burned area should be covered with cream at all times.

Monitoring Parameters Serum electrolytes, urinalysis, renal function tests, CBC in patients with extensive burns on long-term treatment

Pregnancy Risk Factor B

Contraindications Hypersensitivity to silver sulfadiazine or any component of the formulation; premature infants or neonates <2 months of age (sulfonamides may displace bilirubin and cause kernicterus); pregnancy (approaching or at term)

Warnings/Precautions Use with caution in patients with G6PD deficiency, renal impairment, or history of allergy to other sulfonamides; sulfadiazine may accumulate in patients with impaired hepatic or renal function. Prolonged use may result in fungal or bacterial superinfection, including *C. difficile*-associated diarrhea (CDAD) and pseudomembranous colitis; CDAD has been observed >2 months postantibiotic treatment. Use of analgesic might be needed before application; systemic absorption may be significant and adverse reactions may occur

Adverse Reactions Frequency not defined.
Dermatologic: Discoloration of skin, erythema multiforme, itching, photosensitivity, rash
Hematologic: Agranulocytosis, aplastic anemia, hemolytic anemia, leukopenia

Hepatic: Hepatitis

Renal: Interstitial nephritis

Miscellaneous: Allergic reactions may be related to sulfa component

Drug Interactions

Avoid Concomitant Use There are no known interactions where it is recommended to avoid concomitant use.

Increased Effect/Toxicity There are no known significant interactions involving an increase in effect.

Decreased Effect There are no known significant interactions involving a decrease in effect.

Dosage Forms Excipient information presented when available (limited, particularly for generics); consult specific product labeling.

Cream, topical: 1% (25 g, 50 g, 85 g, 400 g)

Silvadene®, Thermazene®: 1% (20 g, 50 g, 85 g, 400 g, 1000 g)

SSD®: 1% (25 g, 50 g, 85 g, 400 g)

SSD® AF: 1% (50 g, 400 g)

◆ **Similac® Glucose** *see* Dextrose *on page* 406

◆ **Simply Saline® [OTC]** *see* Sodium Chloride *on page* 1304

◆ **Simply Saline® Baby [OTC]** *see* Sodium Chloride *on page* 1304

◆ **Simply Saline® Nasal Moist® [OTC]** *see* Sodium Chloride *on page* 1304

◆ **Simply Sleep™ [OTC]** *see* DiphenhydrAMINE *on page* 430

◆ **Simply Sleep® (Can)** *see* DiphenhydrAMINE *on page* 430

◆ **Simulect®** *see* Basiliximab *on page* 179

Simvastatin (sim va STAT in)

Related Information

Hyperlipidemia Management *on page* 1747

Preoperative Evaluation of the Cardiac Patient for Noncardiac Surgery *on page* 1598

U.S. Brand Names Zocor®

Canadian Brand Names Apo-Simvastatin®; CO Simvastatin; Dom-Simvastatin; Gen-Simvastatin; Mylan-Simvastatin; Novo-Simvastatin; Nu-Simvastatin; PHL-Simvastatin; PMS-Simvastatin; Ran-Simvastatin; ratio-Simvastatin; Riva-Simvastatin; Sandoz-Simvastatin; Taro-Simvastatin; Zocor®; ZYM-Simvastatin

Pharmacologic Category Antilipemic Agent, HMG-CoA Reductase Inhibitor

Use Used with dietary therapy for the following:

Secondary prevention of cardiovascular events in hypercholesterolemic patients with established coronary heart disease (CHD) or at high risk for CHD: To reduce cardiovascular morbidity (myocardial infarction, coronary revascularization procedures) and mortality; to reduce the risk of stroke and transient ischemic attacks

Hyperlipidemias: To reduce elevations in total cholesterol, LDL-C, apolipoprotein B, and triglycerides, and increase HDL-C in patients with primary hypercholesterolemia (elevations of 1 or more components are present in Fredrickson type IIa, IIb, III, and IV hyperlipidemias); treatment of homozygous familial hypercholesterolemia

Heterozygous familial hypercholesterolemia (HeFH): In adolescent patients (10-17 years of age, females >1 year postmenarche) with HeFH having LDL-C ≥190 mg/dL **or** LDL ≥160 mg/dL with positive family history of premature cardiovascular disease (CVD), or 2 or more CVD risk factors in the adolescent patient

Pharmacodynamics/Kinetics

Onset of action: >3 days

Peak effect: 2 weeks

Absorption: 85%

Protein binding: ~95%

Metabolism: Hepatic via CYP3A4; extensive first-pass effect

Bioavailability: <5%

◀ Half-life elimination: Unknown

Time to peak: 1.3-2.4 hours

Excretion: Feces (60%); urine (13%)

Dosage Oral: **Note:** Doses should be individualized according to the baseline LDL-cholesterol levels, the recommended goal of therapy, and the patient's response; adjustments should be made at intervals of 4 weeks or more; doses may need adjusted based on concomitant medications

Children 10-17 years (females >1 year postmenarche): HeFH: 10 mg once daily in the evening; range: 10-40 mg/day (maximum: 40 mg/day)

Dosage adjustment for simvastatin with concomitant amiodarone, cyclosporine, danazol, gemfibrozil, or verapamil: Refer to drug-specific dosing in adult dosing section

Adults:

Homozygous familial hypercholesterolemia: 40 mg once daily in the evening **or** 80 mg/day (given as 20 mg, 20 mg, and 40 mg evening dose)

Prevention of cardiovascular events, hyperlipidemias: 20-40 mg once daily in the evening; range: 5-80 mg/day

Patients requiring only moderate reduction of LDL-cholesterol may be started at 10 mg once daily

Patients requiring reduction of >45% in low-density lipoprotein (LDL) cholesterol may be started at 40 mg once daily in the evening

Patients with CHD or at high risk for CHD: Dosing should be started at 40 mg once daily in the evening; simvastatin should be started simultaneously with diet therapy.

Dosage adjustment with concomitant medications:

Cyclosporine or danazol: Initial: 5 mg simvastatin, should **not** exceed 10 mg/day

Gemfibrozil: Simvastatin dose should **not** exceed 10 mg/day

Amiodarone or verapamil: Simvastatin dose should **not** exceed 20 mg/day

Dosing adjustment/comments in renal impairment: Because simvastatin does not undergo significant renal excretion, modification of dose should not be necessary in patients with mild-to-moderate renal insufficiency.

Severe renal impairment: Cl_{cr} <10 mL/minute: Initial: 5 mg/day with close monitoring.

Anesthesia and Critical Care Concerns/Other Considerations

Clinical Pearls/Comments: Myopathy: Currently-marketed HMG-CoA reductase inhibitors appear to have a similar potential for causing myopathy. Incidence of severe myopathy is about 0.08% to 0.09%. The factors that increase risk include advanced age (especially >80 years), gender (occurs in women more frequently than men), small body frame, frailty, multisystem disease (eg, chronic renal insufficiency especially due to diabetes), multiple medications, and drug interactions (use with caution or avoid).

Based on current research and clinical guidelines (Fleisher, 2007), HMG-CoA reductase inhibitors should be continued in the perioperative period. Postoperative discontinuation of statin therapy is associated with an increased risk of cardiac morbidity and mortality.

Additional Information Complete prescribing information for this medication should be consulted for additional detail.

Dosage Forms Excipient information presented when available (limited, particularly for generics); consult specific product labeling.

Tablet: 5 mg, 10 mg, 20 mg, 40 mg, 80 mg

Zocor®: 5 mg, 10 mg, 20 mg, 40 mg, 80 mg

References

Pasternak RC, Smith SC Jr, Bairey-Merz CN, et al, "ACC/AHA/NHLBI Clinical Advisory on the Use and Safety of Statins," *Stroke*, 2002, 33(9):2337-41. Available at: http://www.acc.org/clinical/alerts/statins_june02.htm. Accessed June 18, 2003.

◆ **Sinemet®** *see* Levodopa and Carbidopa *on page 822*

◆ **Sinemet® CR** *see* Levodopa and Carbidopa *on page 822*

◆ **Sinequan® [DSC]** *see* Doxepin *on page 455*

◆ **Sinequan® (Can)** *see* Doxepin *on page 455*

Sirolimus (sir OH li mus)

Medication Safety Issues
Sound-alike/look-alike issues:
Rapamune® may be confused with Rapaflo™
Sirolimus may be confused with everolimus, tacrolimus, temsirolimus

Related Information
Perioperative / Periprocedural Management of Anticoagulant and Antiplatelet Therapy *on page 1607*

U.S. Brand Names Rapamune®

Canadian Brand Names Rapamune®

Pharmacologic Category Immunosuppressant Agent; mTOR Kinase Inhibitor

Generic Available No

Use Prophylaxis of organ rejection in patients receiving renal transplants

Unlabeled/Investigational Use Prophylaxis of organ rejection in heart transplant recipients; immunosuppression in peripheral stem cell/bone marrow transplantation

Mechanism of Action Sirolimus inhibits T-lymphocyte activation and proliferation in response to antigenic and cytokine stimulation and inhibits antibody production. Its mechanism differs from other immunosuppressants. Sirolimus binds to FKBP-12, an intracellular protein, to form an immunosuppressive complex which inhibits the regulatory kinase, mTOR (mammalian target of rapamycin). This inhibition suppresses cytokine mediated T-cell proliferation, halting progression from the G1 to the S phase of the cell cycle. It inhibits acute rejection of allografts and prolongs graft survival.

Pharmacodynamics/Kinetics
Absorption: Rapid

Distribution: 12 L/kg (range: 4-20 L/kg)

Protein binding: ~92%, primarily to albumin

Metabolism: Extensive; in intestinal wall via P-gp and hepatic via CYP3A4; to 7 major metabolites

Bioavailability: Oral solution: 14%; Oral tablet: 18%

Half-life elimination: Mean: 62 hours (range: 46-78 hours); extended in hepatic impairment (Child-Pugh class A or B) to 113 hours

Time to peak: Oral solution: 1-3 hours; Tablet: 1-6 hours

Excretion: Feces (91% due to P-glycoprotein-mediated efflux into gut lumen); urine (2%)

Dosage Oral:
Combination therapy with cyclosporine: Doses should be taken 4 hours after cyclosporine, and should be taken consistently either with or without food.

Low-to-moderate immunologic risk renal transplant patients: Children ≥13 years and Adults: Dosing by body weight:
<40 kg: Loading dose: 3 mg/m^2 on day 1, followed by maintenance dosing of 1 mg/m^2 once daily

≥40 kg: Loading dose: 6 mg on day 1; maintenance: 2 mg once daily

High immunologic risk renal transplant patients: Adults: Loading dose: Up to 15 mg on day 1; maintenance: 5 mg/day; obtain trough concentration between days 5-7 and adjust accordingly. Continue concurrent cyclosporine/sirolimus therapy for 1 year following transplantation. Further adjustment of the regimen must be based on clinical status.

Dosage adjustment: Sirolimus dosages should be adjusted to maintain trough concentrations within desired range based on risk and concomitant therapy. Maximum daily dose: 40 mg. Dosage should be adjusted at intervals of 7-14 days to account for the long half-life of sirolimus. In general, dose proportionality may be assumed. New sirolimus dose **equals** current dose **multiplied by** (target concentration/current concentration). **Note:** If large dose increase is required, consider loading dose calculated as:
Loading dose **equals** (new maintenance dose **minus** current maintenance dose) **multiplied by** 3

Maximum dose in 1 day: 40 mg; if required dose is >40 mg (due to loading dose), divide over 2 days. Serum concentrations should not be used as the ▶

sole basis for dosage adjustment (monitor clinical signs/symptoms, tissue biopsy, and laboratory parameters).

Maintenance therapy after withdrawal of cyclosporine: Cyclosporine withdrawal is not recommended in high immunological risk patients. Following 2-4 months of combined therapy, withdrawal of cyclosporine may be considered in low-to-moderate immunologic risk patients. Cyclosporine should be discontinued over 4-8 weeks, and a necessary increase in the dosage of sirolimus (up to fourfold) should be anticipated due to removal of metabolic inhibition by cyclosporine and to maintain adequate immunosuppressive effects. Dose-adjusted trough target concentrations are typically 16-24 ng/mL for the first year post-transplant and 12-20 ng/mL thereafter (measured by chromatographic methodology).

Dosage adjustment in renal impairment: No dosage adjustment (in loading or maintenance dose) is necessary in renal impairment. However, adjustment of regimen (including discontinuation of therapy) should be considered when used concurrently with cyclosporine and elevated or increasing serum creatinine is noted.

Dosage adjustment in hepatic impairment:

Loading dose: No adjustment required

Maintenance dose:

Mild-to-moderate hepatic impairment: reduce maintenance dose by ~33%

Severe hepatic impairment: reduce maintenance dose by ~50%

Stability

Oral solution: Store under refrigeration, 2°C to 8°C (36°F to 46°F). Protect from light. A slight haze may develop in refrigerated solutions, but the quality of the product is not affected. After opening, solution should be used in 1 month. If necessary, may be stored at temperatures up to 25°C (77°F) for ≤15 days after opening. Product may be stored in amber syringe for a maximum of 24 hours (at room temperature or refrigerated). Solution should be used immediately following dilution.

Tablet: Store at room temperature of 20°C to 25°C (68°F to 77°F). Protect from light.

Administration Initial dose should be administered as soon as possible after transplant. Sirolimus should be taken 4 hours after oral cyclosporine (Neoral® or Gengraf®).

Solution: Mix with at least 2 ounces of water or orange juice. No other liquids should be used for dilution. Patient should drink diluted solution immediately. The cup should then be refilled with an additional 4 ounces of water or orange juice, stirred vigorously, and the patient should drink the contents at once.

Tablet: Do not crush, split, or chew.

Monitoring Parameters Monitor LFTs and CBC during treatment. Monitor sirolimus levels in all patients (especially in pediatric patients, patients ≥13 years of age weighing <40 kg, patients with hepatic impairment, or on concurrent potent inhibitors or inducers of CYP3A4 or P-gp, and/or if cyclosporine dosing is markedly reduced or discontinued), and when changing dosage forms of sirolimus. Also monitor serum cholesterol and triglycerides, blood pressure, serum creatinine, and urinary protein. Serum drug concentrations should be determined 3-4 days after loading doses and 7-14 days after dosage adjustments; however, these concentrations should not be used as the sole basis for dosage adjustment, especially during withdrawal of cyclosporine (monitor clinical signs/symptoms, tissue biopsy, and laboratory parameters). **Note:** Specific ranges will vary with assay methodology (chromatographic or immunoassay) and are not interchangeable.

Reference Range Note: Differences in sensitivity and specificity exist between methods of detection (eg, immunoassay vs HPLC); on average, chromatographic methods yield values ~20% lower than (whole blood) immunoassay determinations. Target range may vary based on assay methodology.

Serum trough concentrations (based on HPLC methods):

Concomitant cyclosporine: 4-12 ng/mL

After cyclosporine withdrawal: 16-24 ng/mL for the first year after transplant; after 1 year: 12-20 ng/mL

Note: Trough concentrations vary based on clinical context and use of additional immunosuppressants. The following represents typical ranges.

When combined with tacrolimus and mycophenolate mofetil (MMF) without steroids: 6-8 ng/mL

As a substitute for tacrolimus (starting 4-8 weeks post-transplant), in combination with MMF and steroids: 8-12 ng/mL

Following conversion from tacrolimus to sirolimus >6 months post-transplant due to chronic allograft nephropathy: 4-6 ng/mL

Pregnancy Risk Factor C

Contraindications Hypersensitivity to sirolimus or any component of the formulation

Warnings/Precautions [U.S. Boxed Warning]: Immunosuppressive agents, including sirolimus, increase the risk of infection and may be associated with the development of lymphoma. Immune suppression may also increase the risk of opportunistic infections, fatal infections, and sepsis. Prophylactic treatment for *Pneumocystis jirovec* pneumonia (PCP) should be administered for 1 year post-transplant; prophylaxis for cytomegalovirus (CMV) should be taken for 3 months post-transplant in patients at risk for CMV.

[U.S. Boxed Warning]: Sirolimus is not recommended for *de novo* use in liver or lung transplant patients. Bronchial anastomotic dehiscence cases have been reported in lung transplant patients when sirolimus was used as part of an immunosuppressive regimen; most of these reactions were fatal. Studies indicate an association with an increase risk of hepatic artery thrombosis (HAT), graft failure, and increased mortality (with evidence of infection) in liver transplant patients when sirolimus is used in combination with cyclosporine and/or tacrolimus. Most cases of HAT occurred within 30 days of transplant.

In renal transplant patients, *de novo* use without cyclosporine has been associated with higher rates of acute rejection. Sirolimus should be used in combination with cyclosporine (and corticosteroids) initially. Cyclosporine may be withdrawn in low-to-moderate immunologic risk patients after 2-4 months, in conjunction with an increase in sirolimus dosage. In high immunologic risk patients, use in combination with cyclosporine and corticosteroids is recommended for the first year. Safety and efficacy of combination therapy with cyclosporine in high-risk patients has not been studied beyond 12 months of treatment; adjustment of immunosuppressive therapy beyond 12 months should be considered based on clinical judgement. Monitor renal function closely when combined with cyclosporine; consider dosage adjustment or discontinue in patients with increasing serum creatinine. Separate dosing; sirolimus should be administered 4 hours after oral cyclosporine dose.

May increase serum creatinine and decrease GFR. Use caution when used concurrently with medications which may alter renal function. May delay recovery of renal function in patients with delayed allograft function. Increased urinary protein excretion has been observed when converting renal transplant patients from calcineurin inhibitors to sirolimus during maintenance therapy. A higher level of proteinuria prior to sirolimus conversion correlates with a higher degree of proteinuria after conversion. In some patients, proteinuria may reach nephrotic levels; nephrotic syndrome (new onset) has been reported.

Use caution with hepatic impairment; a reduction in the maintenance dose is recommended. Has been associated with an increased risk of fluid accumulation and lymphocele; peripheral edema, lymphedema, and pleural and pericardial effusions (including significant effusions and tamponade) were reported; use with caution in patients in whom fluid accumulation may be poorly tolerated, such as in cardiovascular disease (heart failure or hypertension) and pulmonary disease. Cases of interstitial lung disease (eg, pneumonitis, bronchiolitis obliterans organizing pneumonia [BOOP], pulmonary fibrosis) have been observed; risk may be increased with higher trough levels. Avoid concurrent use of strong CYP3A4 and/or P-glycoprotein (P-gp) inhibitors (eg, clarithromycin, erythromycin, telithromycin, itraconazole, ketoconazole, voriconazole) and strong inducers of CYP3A4 and/or P-gp (eg, rifampin, rifabutin). Concurrent use with a calcineurin inhibitor (cyclosporine, tacrolimus) may increase the risk of calcineurin inhibitor- ▶

◄ induced hemolytic uremic syndrome/thrombotic thrombocytopenic purpura/ thrombotic microangiopathy (HUS/TTP/TMA).

Hypersensitivity reactions, including anaphylactic/anaphylactoid reactions, angioedema, exfoliative dermatitis, and hypersensitivity vasculitis have been reported. Concurrent use with other drugs known to cause angioedema (eg, ACE inhibitors) may increase risk. Immunosuppressant therapy is associated with an increased risk of skin cancer; limit sun and ultraviolet light exposure; use appropriate sun protection. May increase serum lipids (cholesterol and triglycerides); use with caution in patients with hyperlipidemia. May be associated with wound dehiscence and impaired healing; use caution in the perioperative period. Patients with a body mass index (BMI) >30 kg/m^2 are at increased risk for abnormal wound healing. Not labeled for use in children <13 years of age, or in adolescent patients <18 years of age considered at high immunological risk.

Adverse Reactions Incidence of many adverse effects is dose related.

>20%:

Cardiovascular: Peripheral edema (54% to 64%), hypertension (39% to 49%), edema (16% to 24%), chest pain (16% to 24%)

Central nervous system: Fever (23% to 34%), headache (23% to 34%), pain (24% to 33%), insomnia (13% to 22%)

Dermatologic: Acne (20% to 31%)

Endocrine & metabolic: Hypertriglyceridemia (38% to 57%), hypercholesterolemia (38% to 46%), hypophosphatemia (15% to 23%), hypokalemia (11% to 21%)

Gastrointestinal: Diarrhea (25% to 42%), constipation (28% to 38%), abdominal pain (28% to 36%), nausea (25% to 36%), vomiting (19% to 25%), dyspepsia (17% to 25%), weight gain (8% to 21%)

Genitourinary: Urinary tract infection (20% to 33%)

Hematologic: Anemia (23% to 37%), thrombocytopenia (13% to 30%)

Neuromuscular & skeletal: Weakness (22% to 40%), arthralgia (25% to 31%), tremor (21% to 31%), back pain (16% to 26%)

Renal: Serum creatinine increased (35% to 40%)

Respiratory: Dyspnea (22% to 30%), upper respiratory infection (20% to 26%), pharyngitis (16% to 21%)

3% to 20%:

Cardiovascular: Atrial fibrillation, CHF, DVT, facial edema, hypervolemia, hypotension, palpitation, peripheral vascular disorder, postural hypotension, syncope, tachycardia, thrombosis, vasodilation, venous thromboembolism

Central nervous system: Chills, malaise, anxiety, confusion, depression, dizziness, emotional lability, hypoesthesia, hypotonia, neuropathy, somnolence

Dermatologic: Rash (10% to 20%), dermatitis (fungal), hirsutism, pruritus, skin hypertrophy, dermal ulcer, ecchymosis, cellulitis, skin carcinoma (up to 3%; includes basal cell carcinoma, squamous cell carcinoma, melanoma), wound healing abnormal

Endocrine & metabolic: Hyperkalemia (12% to 17%), Cushing's syndrome, diabetes mellitus, glycosuria, acidosis, dehydration, hypercalcemia, hyperglycemia, hyperphosphatemia, hypocalcemia, hypoglycemia, hypomagnesemia, hyponatremia

Gastrointestinal: Enlarged abdomen, anorexia, dysphagia, eructation, esophagitis, flatulence, gastritis, gastroenteritis, gingivitis, gingival hyperplasia, ileus, mouth ulceration, oral moniliasis, stomatitis, weight loss

Genitourinary: Pelvic pain, scrotal edema, testis disorder, impotence

Hematologic: Leukopenia (9% to 15%), leukocytosis, polycythemia, TTP, hemolytic-uremic syndrome, hemorrhage

Hepatic: Abnormal liver function tests, alkaline phosphatase increased, ascites, LDH increased, transaminases increased

Local: Thrombophlebitis

Neuromuscular & skeletal: Arthrosis, bone necrosis, CPK increased, leg cramps, myalgia, osteoporosis, tetany, hypertonia, paresthesia

Ocular: Abnormal vision, cataract, conjunctivitis

Otic: Ear pain, otitis media, tinnitus

Renal: Albuminuria, bladder pain, BUN increased, dysuria, hematuria, hydronephrosis, kidney pain, tubular necrosis, nocturia, oliguria, pyelonephritis, pyuria, nephropathy (toxic), urinary frequency, urinary incontinence, urinary retention

Respiratory: Asthma, atelectasis, bronchitis, cough, epistaxis, hypoxia, lung edema, pleural effusion, pneumonia, pulmonary embolism, rhinitis, sinusitis

Miscellaneous: Abscess, diaphoresis, flu-like syndrome, herpesvirus infection, hernia, infection (including opportunistic), lymphadenopathy, lymphocele, lymphoproliferative disease/lymphoma (1% to 3%), peritonitis, sepsis

Infrequent, postmarketing, and/or case reports: Alveolar proteinosis, anaphylactoid reaction, anaphylaxis, anastomotic disruption, angioedema, azoospermia, cytomegalovirus, Epstein-Barr virus, exfoliative dermatitis, fascial dehiscence, focal segmental glomerulosclerosis, hepatic necrosis, hepatotoxicity, hypersensitivity reaction, hypersensitivity vasculitis; incisional hernia; interstitial lung disease (dose-related; includes pneumonitis, pulmonary fibrosis, and bronchiolitis obliterans organizing pneumonia [BOOP] with no identified infectious etiology); joint disorders, lymphedema, nephrotic syndrome, neutropenia, pancreatitis, pancytopenia, pericardial effusion, *Pneumocystis* pneumonia, proteinuria, pulmonary hemorrhage, tamponade, tuberculosis, wound dehiscence

Note: Hepatic artery thrombosis (HAT) and graft failure have been reported in liver transplant patients (not an approved use); bronchial anastomotic dehiscence has been reported in lung transplant patients (not an approved use); and calcineurin inhibitor-induced hemolytic uremic syndrome/thrombotic thrombocytopenic purpura/thrombotic microangiopathy (HUS/TTP/TMA) has been reported with concurrent cyclosporine and/or tacrolimus.

Drug Interactions

Metabolism/Transport Effects Substrate of CYP3A4 (major), P-glycoprotein; **Inhibits** CYP3A4 (weak)

Avoid Concomitant Use

Avoid concomitant use of Sirolimus with any of the following: Natalizumab; Posaconazole; Tacrolimus; Vaccines (Live); Voriconazole

Increased Effect/Toxicity

Sirolimus may increase the levels/effects of: ACE Inhibitors; CycloSPORINE; Hypoglycemic Agents; Leflunomide; Natalizumab; Tacrolimus; Vaccines (Live)

The levels/effects of Sirolimus may be increased by: CycloSPORINE; CYP3A4 Inhibitors (Moderate); CYP3A4 Inhibitors (Strong); Dasatinib; Fluconazole; Herbs (Hypoglycemic Properties); Itraconazole; Ketoconazole; Macrolide Antibiotics; Miconazole; P-Glycoprotein Inhibitors; Posaconazole; Protease Inhibitors; Tacrolimus; Trastuzumab; Voriconazole

Decreased Effect

Sirolimus may decrease the levels/effects of: Vaccines (Inactivated); Vaccines (Live)

The levels/effects of Sirolimus may be decreased by: CYP3A4 Inducers (Strong); Deferasirox; Echinacea; Herbs (CYP3A4 Inducers); P-Glycoprotein Inducers; Phenytoin; Rifampin

Ethanol/Nutrition/Herb Interactions

Food: Avoid grapefruit juice; may decrease clearance of sirolimus. Ingestion with high-fat meals decreases peak concentrations but increases AUC by 23% to 35%. Sirolimus should be taken consistently (either with or without food) to minimize variability.

Herb/Nutraceutical: St John's wort may decrease sirolimus levels; avoid concurrent use. Avoid cat's claw, echinacea (have immunostimulant properties); consider therapy modifications). Herbs with hypoglycemic properties may increase the risk of sirolimus-induced hypoglycemia; includes alfalfa, aloe, bilberry, bitter melon, burdock, celery, damiana, fenugreek, garcinia, garlic, ginger, ginseng (American), gymnema, marshmallow, stinging nettle.

Dietary Considerations Take consistently (with or without food) to minimize variability of absorption.

Dosage Forms Excipient information presented when available (limited, particularly for generics); consult specific product labeling.

Solution, oral:

Rapamune®: 1 mg/mL (60 mL) [contains ethanol 1.5% to 2.5%; packaged with oral syringes and a carrying case]

Tablet:
Rapamune®: 1 mg, 2 mg

SitaGLIPtin (sit a GLIP tin)

U.S. Brand Names Januvia™
Index Terms MK-0431; Sitagliptin Phosphate
Pharmacologic Category Antidiabetic Agent, Dipeptidyl Peptidase IV (DPP-IV) Inhibitor
Use
U.S. labeling: Management of type 2 diabetes mellitus (noninsulin dependent, NIDDM) as an adjunct to diet and exercise as monotherapy or in combination therapy with other antidiabetic agents
Canadian labeling: Management of NIDDM in combination with metformin therapy, diet, and exercise. **Note:** Use as monotherapy is not approved in Canadian labeling.
Pharmacodynamics/Kinetics
Absorption: Rapid
Distribution: ~198 L
Protein binding: 38%
Metabolism: Not extensively metabolized; minor metabolism via CYP3A4 and 2C8 to metabolites (inactive) suggested by *in vitro* studies
Bioavailability: ~87%
Half-life elimination: 12 hours
Time to peak, plasma: 1-4 hours
Excretion: Urine 87% (79% as unchanged drug, 16% as metabolites); feces 13%
Dosage Oral: Adults: Type 2 diabetes: 100 mg once daily
Concomitant use with sulfonylureas: Reduced dose of sulfonylurea may be needed
Dosage adjustment in renal impairment:
Cl_{cr} ≥50 mL/minute: No adjustment required
Cl_{cr} ≥30 to <50 mL/minute: 50 mg once daily
S_{cr}: Males: >1.7 to ≤3.0 mg/dL; Females: >1.5 to ≤2.5 mg/dL: 50 mg once daily
Cl_{cr}<30 mL/minute: 25 mg once daily
S_{cr}: Males: >3.0 mg/dL; Females: >2.5 mg/dL: 25 mg once daily
ESRD requiring hemodialysis or peritoneal dialysis: 25 mg once daily; administered without regard to timing of hemodialysis
Dosage adjustment in hepatic impairment:
Mild-to-moderate impairment (Child-Pugh score 7-9): No dosage adjustment required
Severe impairment (Child-Pugh score >9): Not studied
Additional Information Complete prescribing information for this medication should be consulted for additional detail.
Dosage Forms Excipient information presented when available (limited, particularly for generics); consult specific product labeling.
Tablet:
Januvia™: 25 mg, 50 mg, 100 mg

- ◆ **Sitagliptin Phosphate** *see* SitaGLIPtin *on page 1300*
- ◆ **Skelaxin®** *see* Metaxalone *on page 886*
- ◆ **Sleep-ettes D [OTC]** *see* DiphenhydrAMINE *on page 430*
- ◆ **Sleepinal® [OTC]** *see* DiphenhydrAMINE *on page 430*
- ◆ **Sleep-Tabs [OTC]** *see* DiphenhydrAMINE *on page 430*
- ◆ **S-leucovorin** *see* LEVOleucovorin *on page 828*
- ◆ **6S-leucovorin** *see* LEVOleucovorin *on page 828*
- ◆ **Slo-Niacin® [OTC]** *see* Niacin *on page 1001*
- ◆ **Slo-Pot (Can)** *see* Potassium Chloride *on page 1151*
- ◆ **Slow-K® (Can)** *see* Potassium Chloride *on page 1151*
- ◆ **SMZ-TMP** *see* Sulfamethoxazole and Trimethoprim *on page 1333*
- ◆ **(+)-(S)-N-Methyl-γ-(1-naphthyloxy)-2-thiophenepropylamine Hydrochloride** *see* DULoxetine *on page 469*

◆ **Sodium *L*-Triiodothyronine** *see* Liothyronine *on page 846*

Sodium Acetate (SOW dee um AS e tate)

Pharmacologic Category Electrolyte Supplement, Parenteral
Generic Available Yes
Use Sodium source in large volume I.V. fluids to prevent or correct hyponatremia in patients with restricted intake; used to counter acidosis through conversion to bicarbonate
Dosage Sodium acetate is metabolized to bicarbonate on an equimolar basis outside the liver; administer in large volume I.V. fluids as a sodium source. Refer to Sodium Bicarbonate monograph.
Maintenance electrolyte requirements of sodium in parenteral nutrition solutions:
Daily requirements: 3-4 mEq/kg/24 hours or 25-40 mEq/1000 kcal/24 hours
Maximum: 100-150 mEq/24 hours
Stability Protect from light, heat, and freezing.
Administration Must be diluted prior to I.V. administration; infusion hypertonic solutions (>154 mEq/L) via a central line; maximum rate of administration: 1 mEq/kg/hour
Pregnancy Risk Factor C
Contraindications Alkalosis, hypocalcemia, low sodium diets, edema, cirrhosis
Warnings/Precautions Avoid extravasation, use with caution in patients with edema, heart failure, severe hepatic failure or renal impairment. Use with caution in patients with acid/base alterations; contains acetate, monitor closely during acid/base correction. Close monitoring of serum sodium concentrations is needed to avoid hypernatremia. Solution for injection contains aluminum; use with caution in patients with impaired renal function and in premature infants.
Adverse Reactions 1% to 10%:
Cardiovascular: Thrombosis, hypervolemia
Dermatologic: Chemical cellulitis at injection site (extravasation)
Endocrine & metabolic: Hypernatremia, dilution of serum electrolytes, overhydration, hypokalemia, metabolic alkalosis, hypocalcemia
Gastrointestinal: Gastric distension, flatulence
Local: Phlebitis
Respiratory: Pulmonary edema
Miscellaneous: Congestive conditions
Drug Interactions
Avoid Concomitant Use There are no known interactions where it is recommended to avoid concomitant use.
Increased Effect/Toxicity There are no known significant interactions involving an increase in effect.
Decreased Effect There are no known significant interactions involving a decrease in effect.
Dietary Considerations Sodium acetate anhydrous (2 mEq/mL): 1 mL = 164 mg sodium acetate anhydrous = 2 mEq of sodium (46 mg) and acetate (118 mg)
Dosage Forms Excipient information presented when available (limited, particularly for generics); consult specific product labeling. [DSC] = Discontinued product
Injection, solution, as anhydrous [concentrate]: 2 mEq/mL (20 mL, 50 mL, 100 mL; 250 mL [DSC]); 4 mEq/mL (50 mL, 100 mL)

◆ **Sodium Acid Carbonate** *see* Sodium Bicarbonate *on page 1301*
◆ **Sodium Benzoate and Caffeine** *see* Caffeine *on page 225*

Sodium Bicarbonate (SOW dee um bye KAR bun ate)

Related Information
Allergic Reactions *on page 1508*
U.S. Brand Names Brioschi® [OTC]; Neut®
Index Terms Baking Soda; NaHCO$_3$; Sodium Acid Carbonate; Sodium Hydrogen Carbonate

◀ **Pharmacologic Category** Alkalinizing Agent; Antacid; Electrolyte Supplement, Oral; Electrolyte Supplement, Parenteral

Generic Available Yes: Excludes granules

Use Management of metabolic acidosis; gastric hyperacidity; as an alkalinization agent for the urine; treatment of hyperkalemia; management of overdose of certain drugs, including tricyclic antidepressants and aspirin

Unlabeled/Investigational Use Prevention of contrast-induced nephropathy (CIN)

Mechanism of Action Dissociates to provide bicarbonate ion which neutralizes hydrogen ion concentration and raises blood and urinary pH

Pharmacodynamics/Kinetics

Onset of action: Oral: Rapid; I.V.: 15 minutes

Duration: Oral: 8-10 minutes; I.V.: 1-2 hours

Absorption: Oral: Well absorbed

Excretion: Urine (<1%)

Dosage

Cardiac arrest: **Routine use of NaHCO₃ is not recommended.** May be considered in the setting of prolonged cardiac arrest only after adequate alveolar ventilation has been established and effective cardiac compressions. **Note:** In some cardiac arrest situations (eg, metabolic acidosis, hyperkalemia, or tricyclic antidepressant overdose), sodium bicarbonate may be beneficial.

Infants and Children: I.V.: 0.5-1 mEq/kg/dose repeated every 10 minutes or as indicated by arterial blood gases; rate of infusion should not exceed 10 mEq/minute; neonates and children <2 years of age should receive 4.2% (0.5 mEq/mL) solution

Adults: I.V.: Initial: 1 mEq/kg/dose one time; maintenance: 0.5 mEq/kg/dose every 10 minutes or as indicated by arterial blood gases

Metabolic acidosis: Infants, Children, and Adults: Dosage should be based on the following formula if blood gases and pH measurements are available:

HCO_3^- (mEq) = 0.3 x weight (kg) x base deficit (mEq/L)

Administer ¹/₂ dose initially, then remaining ¹/₂ dose over the next 24 hours; monitor pH, serum HCO_3^-, and clinical status

Note: If acid-base status is not available: Dose for older Children and Adults: 2-5 mEq/kg I.V. infusion over 4-8 hours; subsequent doses should be based on patient's acid-base status

Chronic renal failure: Oral: Initiate when plasma HCO_3^- <15 mEq/L

Children: 1-3 mEq/kg/day

Adults: Start with 20-36 mEq/day in divided doses, titrate to bicarbonate level of 18-20 mEq/L

Hyperkalemia: Adults: I.V.: 50 mEq over 5 minutes (as appropriate, consider methods of enhancing potassium removal/excretion)

Renal tubular acidosis: Oral:

Distal:

Children: 2-3 mEq/kg/day

Adults: 0.5-2 mEq/kg/day in 4-5 divided doses

Proximal: Children and Adults: Initial: 5-10 mEq/kg/day; maintenance: Increase as required to maintain serum bicarbonate in the normal range

Urine alkalinization: Oral:

Children: 1-10 mEq (84-840 mg)/kg/day in divided doses every 4-6 hours; dose should be titrated to desired urinary pH

Adults: Initial: 48 mEq (4 g), then 12-24 mEq (1-2 g) every 4 hours; dose should be titrated to desired urinary pH; doses up to 16 g/day (200 mEq) in patients <60 years and 8 g (100 mEq) in patients >60 years

Antacid: Adults: Oral: 325 mg to 2 g 1-4 times/day

Prevention of contrast-induced nephropathy (unlabeled use): Adults: I.V. infusion: 154 mEq/L sodium bicarbonate in D₅W solution: 3 mL/kg/hour for 1 hour immediately before contrast injection, then 1mL/kg/hour during contrast exposure and for 6 hours after procedure

To prepare solution, remove 154 mL from 1000 mL bag of D₅W; replace with 154 mL of 8.4% sodium bicarbonate; resultant concentration is 154 mEq/L (Merten, 2004); more practically, institutions may remove 150 mL from 1000 mL bag of D₅W and replace with 150 mL of 8.4% sodium bicarbonate; resultant concentration is 150 mEq/L

Stability Store injection at room temperature; do not freeze. Protect from heat. Use only clear solutions.

Prevention of contrast-induced nephropathy (unlabeled use): Remove 154 mL from 1000 mL bag of D_5W; replace with 154 mL of 8.4% sodium bicarbonate; resultant concentration is 154 mEq/L (Merten, 2004); more practically, institutions may remove 150 mL from 1000 mL bag of D_5W and replace with 150 mL of 8.4% sodium bicarbonate; resultant concentration is 150 mEq/L

Administration For I.V. administration to infants, use the 0.5 mEq/mL solution or dilute the 1 mEq/mL solution 1:1 with **sterile water**; for direct I.V. infusion in emergencies, administer slowly (maximum rate in infants: 10 mEq/minute); for infusion, dilute to a maximum concentration of 0.5 mEq/mL in dextrose solution and infuse over 2 hours (maximum rate of administration: 1 mEq/kg/hour)

Anesthesia and Critical Care Concerns/Other Considerations

Clinical Pearls/Comments: The use of bicarbonate for the treatment of lactic acidosis has not been proven useful. Increased pCO_2 after bicarbonate administration may result in an acute decrease in intracellular pH. Bicarbonate does not improve any hemodynamic parameters resulting in improved cardiovascular function. Many clinicians do not use bicarbonate in the treatment of lactic acidosis regardless of the patient's pH level.

Evidence-Based Information: The 2008 Surviving Sepsis Campaign guidelines recommend avoiding use of sodium bicarbonate therapy for the purpose of improving hemodynamics or reducing vasopressor requirements in patients with hypoperfusion-induced lactic academia with pH ≥7.15 (Grade 1B).

Pregnancy Risk Factor C

Contraindications Alkalosis, hypernatremia, severe pulmonary edema, hypocalcemia, unknown abdominal pain

Warnings/Precautions Rapid administration in neonates and children <2 years of age has led to hypernatremia, decreased CSF pressure and intracranial hemorrhage. **Use of I.V. NaHCO$_3$ should be reserved for documented metabolic acidosis and for hyperkalemia-induced cardiac arrest.** Routine use in cardiac arrest is not recommended. Avoid extravasation, tissue necrosis can occur due to the hypertonicity of NaHCO$_3$. May cause sodium retention especially if renal function is impaired; not to be used in treatment of peptic ulcer; use with caution in patients with HF, edema, cirrhosis, or renal failure. Not the antacid of choice for the elderly because of sodium content and potential for systemic alkalosis.

Adverse Reactions Frequency not defined.

Cardiovascular: Cerebral hemorrhage, CHF (aggravated), edema

Central nervous system: Tetany

Gastrointestinal: Belching, flatulence (with oral), gastric distension

Endocrine & metabolic: Hypernatremia, hyperosmolality, hypocalcemia, hypokalemia, increased affinity of hemoglobin for oxygen-reduced pH in myocardial tissue necrosis when extravasated, intracranial acidosis, metabolic alkalosis, milk-alkali syndrome (especially with renal dysfunction)

Respiratory: Pulmonary edema

Drug Interactions

Avoid Concomitant Use There are no known interactions where it is recommended to avoid concomitant use.

Increased Effect/Toxicity

Sodium Bicarbonate may increase the levels/effects of: Alpha-/Beta-Agonists; Amphetamines; Flecainide; Memantine; QuiNIDine; QuiNINE; Tocainide

Decreased Effect

Sodium Bicarbonate may decrease the levels/effects of: ACE Inhibitors; Anticonvulsants (Hydantoin); Antifungal Agents (Azole Derivatives, Systemic); Antipsychotic Agents (Phenothiazines); Atazanavir; Bisacodyl; Cefpodoxime; Cefuroxime; Chloroquine; Corticosteroids (Oral); CycloSPORINE; Dabigatran Etexilate; Dasatinib; Delavirdine; Erlotinib; Flecainide; Iron Salts; Isoniazid; Lithium; Mesalamine; Methenamine; Penicillamine; Phosphate Supplements; Protease Inhibitors; Tetracycline Derivatives; Trientine

Ethanol/Nutrition/Herb Interactions Herb/Nutraceutical: Concurrent doses with iron may decrease iron absorption.

Dietary Considerations Oral product should be administered 1-3 hours after meals.

◄ Sodium content:

Injection: 50 mL, 8.4% = 1150 mg = 50 mEq; each mL of 8.4% NaHCO$_3$ contains 23 mg sodium; 1 mEq NaHCO$_3$ = 84 mg

Granules: 2.69 g packet or capful = 770 mg sodium

Powder: 30 mEq sodium per 1/2 teaspoon

Dosage Forms Excipient information presented when available (limited, particularly for generics); consult specific product labeling.

Granules, for solution, oral [effervescent]:

Brioschi®: 2.69 g/packet (12s) [contains sodium 770 mg/packet; lemon flavor]; 2.69 g/capful (120 g, 240 g) [contains sodium 770 mg/capful; lemon flavor]

Infusion [premixed in water for injection]: 5% (500 mL) [5.95 mEq/10 mL]

Injection, solution:

4.2% (10 mL) [5 mEq/10 mL]

7.5% (50 mL) [8.92 mEq/10 mL]

8.4% (10 mL, 50 mL, 250 mL, 500 mL) [10 mEq/10 mL]

Neut® 4% (5 mL) [2.4 mEq/5 mL; contains edetate disodium]

Powder: Sodium bicarbonate USP (120 g, 480 g) [contains sodium 30 mEq per 1/2 teaspoon]

Tablet: 325 mg [3.8 mEq]; 650 mg [7.6 mEq]

References

Dellinger RP, Levy MM, Carlet JM, et al, "Surviving Sepsis Campaign: International Guidelines for Management of Severe Sepsis and Septic Shock: 2008," *Intensive Care Med*, 2008, 34(1): 17-60. Available at http://www.survivingsepsis.org/system/files/images/2008_20International_20SSC_20-Guidelines_1_.pdf

Forsythe SM and Schmidt GA, "Sodium Bicarbonate for the Treatment of Lactic Acidosis," *Chest*, 2000, 117(1):260-7.

Merten GJ, Burgess WP, Gray LV, et al, "Prevention of Contrast-Induced Nephropathy With Sodium Bicarbonate: A Randomized Controlled Trial," *JAMA*, 2004, 291(19):2328-34.

Mokhlesi B, Leikin JB, Murray P, et al, "Adult Toxicology in Critical Care: Part II: Specific Poisonings," *Chest*, 2003, 123(3):897-922.

◆ **Sodium Bicarbonate and Omeprazole** *see* Omeprazole and Sodium Bicarbonate *on page 1052*

Sodium Chloride (SOW dee um KLOR ide)

U.S. Brand Names 4-Way® Saline Moisturizing Mist [OTC]; Altachlore [OTC]; Altamist [OTC]; Ayr® Allergy Sinus [OTC]; Ayr® Baby Saline [OTC]; Ayr® Saline No-Drip [OTC]; Ayr® Saline [OTC]; Breathe Free® [OTC]; Deep Sea [OTC]; Entsol® [OTC]; Humist® for Kids [OTC]; Humist® [OTC]; Hyper-Sal™; Little Noses® Saline [OTC]; Little Noses® Stuffy Nose Kit [OTC] ; Muro 128® [OTC]; Mycinaire™ [OTC] [DSC]; Na-Zone® [OTC]; Nasal Moist® Saline [OTC]; Nasal Spray [OTC]; NāSal™ [OTC]; Ocean® for Kids [OTC]; Ocean® [OTC]; Pretz® [OTC]; Saline Mist [OTC]; SalineX® [OTC] [DSC]; Simply Saline® Baby [OTC]; Simply Saline® Nasal Moist® [OTC] ; Simply Saline® [OTC]; Syrex; Wound Wash Saline™ [OTC]

Index Terms NaCl; Normal Saline; Salt

Pharmacologic Category Electrolyte Supplement, Parenteral; Genitourinary Irrigant; Irrigant; Lubricant, Ocular; Sodium Salt

Use

Parenteral: Restores sodium ion in patients with restricted oral intake (especially hyponatremia states or low salt syndrome).

Concentrated sodium chloride: Additive for parenteral fluid therapy

Hypertonic sodium chloride: For severe hyponatremia and hypochloremia

Hypotonic sodium chloride: Hydrating solution

Normal saline: Restores water/sodium losses

Ophthalmic: Reduces corneal edema

Inhalation: Restores moisture to pulmonary system; loosens and thins congestion caused by colds or allergies; diluent for bronchodilator solutions that require dilution before inhalation

Intranasal: Restores moisture to nasal membranes

Irrigation: Wound cleansing, irrigation, and flushing

Unlabeled/Investigational Use Refractory elevated intracranial pressure (ICP) due to various etiologies (eg, subarachnoid hemorrhage, neoplasm); transtentorial herniation syndrome; traumatic brain injury with elevated ICP. **Note:** May be used in patients in whom mannitol may not be recommended (eg, renal failure).

Pharmacodynamics/Kinetics

Absorption: Oral, I.V.: Rapid

Distribution: Widely distributed

Excretion: Primarily urine; also sweat, tears, saliva

Dosage

Children: I.V.: Hypertonic solutions (>0.9%) should only be used for the initial treatment of acute serious symptomatic hyponatremia; maintenance: 3-4 mEq/kg/day; maximum: 100-150 mEq/day; dosage varies widely depending on clinical condition

Replacement: Determined by laboratory determinations mEq

Sodium deficiency (mEq/kg) = [% dehydration (L/kg)/100 x 70 (mEq/L)] + [0.6 (L/kg) x (140 - serum sodium) (mEq/L)]

Children ≥2 years and Adults:

Intranasal: 2-3 sprays in each nostril as needed

Irrigation: Spray affected area

Children and Adults: Inhalation: Bronchodilator diluent: 1-3 sprays (1-3 mL) to dilute bronchodilator solution in nebulizer prior to administration

Adults:

Refractory elevated ICP due to various etiologies (eg, subarachnoid hemorrhage, trauma, neoplasm), transtentorial herniation syndromes (unlabeled use): I.V.: Hypertonic saline: 23.4% (30-60 mL) given over 2-20 minutes administered via central venous access only (Suarez, 1998; Koenig, 2008; Ware, 2005)

Subarachnoid hemorrhage with hyponatremia (ie, ≤135 mEq/L) to enhance cerebral perfusion (unlabeled use): I.V.: Hypertonic saline: 3% sodium chloride/acetate (50:50 mixture) 100-200 mL/hour administered via central venous catheter; titrate to clinical response up to a maximum serum sodium between 150-160 mEq/L (achieved at a rate of 0.5-1 mEq/L/hour) (Suarez, 1999)

Traumatic brain injury with elevated ICP (unlabeled use): I.V.: Hypertonic saline: **Note:** Optimal dose has not been established; due to insufficient evidence, the Brain Trauma Foundation guidelines (Bratton, 2007) do not make specific recommendations on the use of hypertonic saline for the treatment of traumatic intracranial hypertension. Clinical trials are small; few are prospective. **Some concentrations may not be commercially available; administer via central venous catheter;** protocols include:

3%: 300 mL administered over 20 minutes when ICP values exceed 20 mm Hg (Huang, 2006)

7.2%: 1.5 mL/kg administered over 15 minutes when ICP values exceed 15 mm Hg (Munar, 2000)

7.5%: 2 mL/kg administered over 20 minutes when ICP values exceed 25 mm Hg (Vialet, 2003)

23.4%: 30 mL administered over 2 minutes (Ware, 2005) **or** over >30 minutes when ICP values exceed 20 mm Hg (Kerwin, 2009)

GU irrigant: 1-3 L/day by intermittent irrigation

Replacement I.V.: Determined by laboratory determinations mEq

Hyponatremia: Sodium deficiency (mEq/kg) = [% dehydration (L/kg)/100 x 70 (mEq/L)] + [0.6 (L/kg) x (140 - serum sodium) (mEq/L)]

To correct acute, serious hyponatremia: mEq sodium = [desired sodium (mEq/L) - actual sodium (mEq/L)] x [0.6 x wt (kg)]; for acute correction use 125 mEq/L as the desired serum sodium; acutely correct serum sodium in 5 mEq/L/dose increments; more gradual correction in increments of 10 mEq/L/day is indicated in the asymptomatic patient

Chloride maintenance electrolyte requirement in parenteral nutrition: 2-4 mEq/kg/24 hours or 25-40 mEq/1000 kcals/24 hours; maximum: 100-150 mEq/24 hours

Sodium maintenance electrolyte requirement in parenteral nutrition: 3-4 mEq/kg/24 hours or 25-40 mEq/1000 kcals/24 hours; maximum: 100-150 mEq/24 hours.

Approximate Deficits of Water and Electrolytes in Moderately Severe Dehydration[1]

Condition	Water (mL/kg)	Sodium (mEq/kg)
Fasting and thirsting	100-120	5-7
Diarrhea		
isonatremic	100-120	8-10
hypernatremic	100-120	2-4
hyponatremic	100-120	10-12
Pyloric stenosis	100-120	8-10
Diabetic acidosis	100-120	9-10

[1]A **negative** deficit indicates total body **excess** prior to treatment.

Adapted from Behrman RE, Kleigman RM, Nelson WE, et al, eds, *Nelson Textbook of Pediatrics*, 14th ed, WB Saunders Co, 1992.

Ophthalmic:

Ointment: Apply once daily or more often

Solution: Instill 1-2 drops into affected eye(s) every 3-4 hours

Anesthesia and Critical Care Concerns/Other Considerations An Australian/New Zealand group recently published results from their evaluation of resuscitation fluid (4% albumin versus normal saline) in a heterogeneous intensive care population (Finfer, 2004). They conducted this multicenter, randomized, double-blind trial to compare the effects of resuscitation fluid on mortality from any cause during the 28-day period after randomization. Patients were eligible for inclusion if the treating clinician judged that fluid resuscitation was required for intravascular fluid depletion as supported by one of the following criteria:

Heart rate >90 bpm

Systolic BP <100 mm Hg

Mean arterial BP <75 mm Hg

Decrease of 40 mm Hg in systolic or mean arterial BP (as compared with baseline)

CVP <10 mm Hg

PCWP <12 mm Hg

Respiratory variation in systolic or mean BP >5 mm Hg

Capillary refill time >1 second

Urine output <0.5 mL/kg for 1 hour

Patients were excluded for a variety of reasons, including ICU transfer following cardiac or liver transplantation surgery, or burn treatment. Almost 7000 patients were randomized; 3497 to albumin and 3500 to saline. Baseline characteristics were similar between the groups, except CVP pressure was slightly higher in the albumin group (9.0 in albumin versus 8.6 in saline). There was no significant mortality difference between groups (726 deaths in albumin group; 729 deaths in saline group). There were no significant differences in secondary endpoints (length of stay in the ICU or hospital, days of mechanical ventilation, and days of renal replacement therapy). Similar outcomes resulted from use of either fluid for resuscitation in this patient population.

The 2008 Surviving Sepsis Campaign guidelines suggest that during the first 6 hours of resuscitation, the goals of sepsis-induced hypoperfusion should include central venous pressure 8-12 mm Hg, mean arterial pressure ≥65 mm Hg, urine output >0.5 mL/kg/hour, central venous (superior vena cava) oxygen saturation ≥70% or mixed venous oxygen saturation ≥65% (Grade 2C).

Management of Elevated Intracranial Pressure (ICP): Hypertonic saline has been used to treat refractory elevated ICP. In a retrospective study, 23.4% NaCl (30 mL over 20 minutes) reduced refractory elevated ICP for at least 3 hours (Suarez, 1998). A prospective, randomized study demonstrated greater efficacy of 7.5% saline compared to 20% mannitol in decreasing ICP in traumatic brain injury patients. Unfortunately, the osmolar load in the two arms was substantially different (Vialet, 2003). Several studies have demonstrated that the use of hypertonic saline solutions enhance cerebral perfusion in patients with subarachnoid hemorrhage (Suarez, 1999; Tseng, 2003). In addition, a retrospective study of 23.4% NaCl demonstrated rapid reversal of transtentorial herniation and reduced ICP (Koenig, 2008).

Additional Information Complete prescribing information for this medication should be consulted for additional detail.

Dosage Forms Excipient information presented when available (limited, particularly for generics); consult specific product labeling. [DSC] = Discontinued product

Aerosol, intranasal [spray; preservative free]:
 Entsol®: 3% (100 mL) [chlorofluorocarbon free]

Gel, intranasal:
 Ayr® Saline: <0.5% (14 g) [contains soybean oil and aloe]
 Entsol®: 3% (20 g) [contains benzalkonium chloride; with aloe and vitamin E]
 Simply Saline® Nasal Moist®: 0.65% (30 g) [contains aloe]

Gel, intranasal [spray]:
 Ayr® Saline No-Drip: <0.5% (22 mL) [contains benzalkonium chloride, benzyl alcohol, and soybean oil]

Injection, solution: 0.45% (25 mL, 50 mL, 100 mL, 250 mL, 500 mL, 1000 mL); 0.9% (25 mL, 50 mL, 100 mL, 150 mL, 250 mL, 500 mL, 1000 mL, 1 g); 3% (500 mL); 5% (500 mL)

Injection, solution [preservative free]: 0.9% (2 mL, 3 mL, 5 mL, 10 mL, 20 mL, 50 mL, 100 mL)

Injection, solution [I.V. flush]: 0.9% (10 mL)

Injection, solution [I.V. flush; preservative free]: 0.9% (1 mL, 2 mL, 2.5 mL, 3 mL, 5 mL, 10 mL)
 Syrex: 0.9% (2.5 mL, 3 mL, 5 mL, 10 mL)

Injection, solution [bacteriostatic]: 0.9% (10 mL, 20 mL, 30 mL)

Injection, solution [concentrate]: 14.6% (40 mL); 23.4% (100 mL, 250 mL)

Injection, solution [concentrate; preservative free]: 14.6% (20 mL, 40 mL); 23.4% (30 mL, 100 mL, 200 mL)

Ointment, ophthalmic: 5% (3.5 g)
 Altachlore: 5% (3.5 g)

Ointment, ophthalmic [preservative free]:
 Muro 128®: 5% (3.5 g)

Powder for solution, intranasal [preservative free]:
 Entsol®: 3% (10.5 g)

Solution for blood processing [not for injection]: 0.9% (3000 mL)

Solution for inhalation [preservative free]: 0.9% (3 mL, 5 mL, 15 mL); 3% (15 mL)

Solution for inhalation [hypertonic; preservative free]: 10% (15 mL)

Solution for inhalation [hypotonic; preservative free]: 0.45% (5 mL)

Solution for injection [I.V. flush; preservative free]: 0.9% (2.5 mL, 5 mL, 10 mL)

Solution for irrigation: 0.45% (2000 mL); 0.9% (250 mL, 500 mL, 1000 mL, 1500 mL, 2000 mL, 3000 mL, 4000 mL, 5000 mL)

Solution for irrigation [preservative free]: 0.45% (1500 mL [DSC]; 2000 mL); 0.9% (250 mL, 500 mL, 1000 mL, 1500 mL, 2000 mL, 3000 mL)

Solution for irrigation [slush solution]: 0.9% (1000 mL)

Solution for nebulization [preservative free]:
 Hyper-Sal™: 7% (4 mL)

Solution, intranasal [preservative free]:
 Simply Saline®: 3% (44 mL)

Solution, intranasal [drops]:
 Ayr® Saline: 0.65% (50 mL) [alcohol free; contains benzalkonium chloride]
 NāSal™: 0.65% (15 mL) [alcohol free; contains benzalkonium chloride]
 SalineX®: 0.4% (15 mL) [contains benzalkonium chloride] [DSC]

Solution, intranasal [drops, mist, spray]
 Humist®: 0.65% (45 mL) [ethanol free]
 Humist® for Kids: 0.65% (30 mL) [ethanol free; bubblegum flavor]
 Ocean®: 0.65% (45 mL, 473 mL) [gluten free; contains benzalkonium chloride and benzyl alcohol]
 Ocean® for Kids: 0.65% (37.5 mL) [alcohol free; contains benzalkonium chloride]

Solution, intranasal [drops, spray]:
 Ayr® Baby Saline: 0.65% (30 mL) [ethanol free; contains benzalkonium chloride]
 Little Noses® Saline: 0.65% (30 mL) [contains benzalkonium chloride]
 Little Noses® Stuffy Nose Kit: 0.65% (15 mL) [contains benzalkonium chloride]
Solution, intranasal [drops, spray, stream]:
 Saline Mist: 0.65% (45 mL) [contains benzalkonium chloride] [DSC]
Solution, intranasal [irrigation]:
 Pretz®: 0.75% (237 mL, 960 mL) [contains benzalkonium chloride and sodium
  benzoate; with yerba santa]
Solution, intranasal [mist]:
 Ayr® Allergy Sinus: 2.65% (50 mL)
 Ayr® Saline: 0.65% (50 mL) [ethanol free; contains benzalkonium chloride]
 Entsol®: 3% (30 mL) [contains benzalkonium chloride]
 Mycinaire™: 0.65% (30 mL) [contains benzalkonium chloride] [DSC]
 Saline Mist: 0.65% (45 mL) [contains benzalkonium chloride]
 SalineX®: 0.4% (50 mL) [contains benzalkonium chloride] [DSC]
 4-Way® Moisturizing Mist: 0.74% (29.6 mL) [ethanol free; contains benzalko-
  nium chloride and menthol]
Solution, intranasal [mist, preservative free]:
 Simply Saline®: 0.9% (44 mL, 90 mL)
 Simply Saline® Baby: 0.9% (45 mL)
Solution, intranasal [nasal wash; preservative free]:
 Entsol®: 3% (240 mL)
Solution, intranasal [spray]:
 Altamist: 0.65% (60 mL) [contains benzalkonium chloride]
 Breathe Free®: 0.65% (44.3 mL) [contains benzalkonium chloride]
 Deep Sea: 0.65% (45 mL) [contains benzalkonium chloride and benzyl alcohol]
 Na-Zone®: 0.65% (60 mL) [contains benzalkonium chloride]
 Nasal Moist® Saline: 0.65% (45 mL)
 Nasal Spray: 0.65% (45 mL) [contains benzalkonium chloride and benzyl
  alcohol]
 NäSal™: 0.65% (30 mL) [ethanol free; contains benzalkonium chloride and
  thimerosal]
Solution, intranasal [spray, isotonic, buffered]:
 Pretz®: 0.75% (50 mL) [contains benzalkonium chloride and sodium benzoate;
  with yerba santa]
Solution, ophthalmic: 5% (15 mL)
Solution, ophthalmic [drops]: 5% (15 mL)
 Altachlore: 5% (15 mL, 30 mL)
 Muro 128®: 2% (15 mL); 5% (15 mL, 30 mL)
Solution, topical [preservative free]:
 Wound Wash Saline™: 0.9% (90 mL, 210 mL)
Swab, intranasal:
 Ayr® Saline: <0.5% (20) [contains aloe and soybean oil]
Tablet for solution, topical: 1000 mg

References

Bhardwaj A and Ulatowski JA, "Hypertonic Saline Solutions in Brain Injury," *Curr Opin Crit Care*,
 2004, 10(2):126-31.
Cooper DJ, Myles PS, McDermott FT, et al, "Prehospital Hypertonic Saline Resuscitation of Patients
 With Hypotension and Severe Traumatic Brain Injury: A Randomized Controlled Trial," *JAMA*, 2004,
 291(11):1350-7.
Dellinger RP, Levy MM, Carlet JM, et al, "Surviving Sepsis Campaign: International Guidelines for
 Management of Severe Sepsis and Septic Shock: 2008," *Intensive Care Med*, 2008, 34(1):17-60.
 Available at http://www.survivingsepsis.org/system/files/images/2008_20International_20SSC_20-
 Guidelines_1_.pdf
Doyle JA, Davis DP, and Hoyt DB, "The Use of Hypertonic Saline in the Treatment of Traumatic Brain
 Injury," *J Trauma*, 2001, 50(2):367-83.
Finfer S, Bellomo R, Boyce N, et al, "A Comparison of Albumin and Saline for Fluid Resuscitation in
 the Intensive Care Unit. SAFE Study Investigators," *N Engl J Med*, 2004, 350(22):2247-56.
Forsyth LL, Liu-DeRyke X, Parker D, et al, "Role of Hypertonic Saline for the Management of
 Intracranial Hypertension After Stroke and Traumatic Brain Injury," *Pharmacotherapy*, 2008, 28
 (4):469-84.
Huang SJ, Chang L, Han YY, et al, "Efficacy and Safety of Hypertonic Saline Solutions in the
 Treatment of Severe Head Injury," *Surg Neurol*, 2006, 65(6):539-46.
Kerwin AJ, Schinco MA, Tepas JJ 3rd, et al, "The Use of 23.4% Hypertonic Saline for the
 Management of Elevated Intracranial Pressure in Patients With Severe Traumatic Brain Injury: A
 Pilot Study," *J Trauma*, 2009, 67(2):277-82.

Koenig MA, Bryan M, Lewin JL 3rd, et al, "Reversal of Transtentorial Herniation With Hypertonic Saline," *Neurology*, 2008, 70(13):1023-9.

Munar F, Ferrer AM, de Nadal M, et al, "Cerebral Hemodynamic Effects of 7.2% Hypertonic Saline in Patients With Head Injury and Raised Intracranial Pressure," *J Neurotrauma*, 2000, 17(1):41-51.

SAFE Study Investigators, Australian and New Zealand Intensive Care Society Clinical Trials Group, Australian Red Cross Blood Service, et al, "Saline or Albumin for Fluid Resuscitation in Patients With Traumatic Brain Injury," *N Engl J Med*, 2007, 357(9):874-84

Suarez JI, Qureshi, AI, Bhardwaj A, et al, "Treatment of Refractory Intracranial Hypertension With 23.4% Saline," *Crit Care Med*, 1998, 26(6):1118-22.

Suarez JI, Qureshi AI, Parekh PD, et al, "Administration of Hypertonic (3%) Sodium Chloride/Acetate in Hyponatremic Patients With Symptomatic Vasospasm Following Subarachnoid Hemorrhage," *J Neurosurg Anesthesiol*, 1999, 11(3):178-84.

Tseng MY, Al-Rawi PG, Pickard JD, et al, "Effect of Hypertonic Saline on Cerebral Blood Flow in Poor-Grade Patients With Subarachnoid Hemorrhage," *Stroke*, 2003, 34(6):1389-96.

Vialet R, Albanese J, Thomachot L, et al, "Isovolume Hypertonic Solutes (Sodium Chloride or Mannitol) in the Treatment of Refractory Posttraumatic Intracranial Hypertension: 2 mL/kg 7.5% Saline is More Effective Than 2 mL/kg 20% Mannitol," *Crit Care Med*, 2003, 31(6):1683-7.

Ware ML, Nemani VM, Meeker M, et al, "Effects of 23.4% Sodium Chloride Solution in Reducing Intracranial Pressure in Patients With Traumatic Brain Injury: A Preliminary Study," *Neurosurgery*, 2005, 57(4):727-36.

◆ **Sodium Diuril®** *see* Chlorothiazide *on page 295*

◆ **Sodium Edecrin®** *see* Ethacrynic Acid *on page 541*

◆ **Sodium Fusidate** *see* Fusidic Acid *on page 649*

◆ **Sodium Hydrogen Carbonate** *see* Sodium Bicarbonate *on page 1301*

◆ **Sodium Hyposulfate** *see* Sodium Thiosulfate *on page 1316*

◆ **Sodium Nafcillin** *see* Nafcillin *on page 975*

◆ **Sodium Nitroferricyanide** *see* Nitroprusside *on page 1018*

◆ **Sodium Nitroprusside** *see* Nitroprusside *on page 1018*

Sodium Phosphates (SOW dee um FOS fates)

Medication Safety Issues

Sound-alike/look-alike issues:

Visicol® may be confused with Asacol®, VESIcare®

Enemas and oral solution are available in pediatric and adult sizes; prescribe by "volume" not by "bottle."

Safe Prescribing: Because inorganic phosphate exists as monobasic and dibasic anions, with the mixture of valences dependent on pH, ordering by mEq amounts is unreliable and may lead to large dosing errors. In addition, I.V. phosphate is available in the sodium and potassium salt; therefore, the content of these cations must be considered when ordering phosphate. The most reliable method of ordering I.V. phosphate is by millimoles, then specifying the potassium or sodium salt.

Medication Guide An FDA-approved patient medication guide, which is available with the product information and as follows, must be dispensed with each new outpatient prescription and refill.

OsmoPrep®:http://www.fda.gov/downloads/Drugs/DrugSafety/UCM135936.pdf
Visicol®:http://www.fda.gov/downloads/Drugs/DrugSafety/UCM134684.pdf

U.S. Brand Names Fleet® Enema Extra® [OTC]; Fleet® Enema [OTC]; Fleet® Pedia-Lax™ Enema [OTC]; Fleet® Phospho-soda® EZ-Prep™ [OTC] [DSC]; Fleet® Phospho-soda® [OTC] [DSC]; LaCrosse Complete [OTC]; OsmoPrep®; Visicol®

Canadian Brand Names Fleet Enema®

Index Terms Phosphates, Sodium

Pharmacologic Category Cathartic; Electrolyte Supplement, Parenteral; Laxative, Bowel Evacuant

Generic Available Yes: Enema, injection, oral solution

Use

Oral, rectal: Short-term treatment of constipation and to evacuate the colon for rectal and bowel exams

I.V.: Source of phosphate in large volume I.V. fluids and parenteral nutrition; treatment and prevention of hypophosphatemia

Mechanism of Action As a laxative, exerts osmotic effect in the small intestine by drawing water into the lumen of the gut, producing distention and promoting peristalsis and evacuation of the bowel; phosphorous participates in bone deposition, calcium metabolism, utilization of B complex vitamins, and as a buffer in acid-base equilibrium

Pharmacodynamics/Kinetics

Onset of action: Cathartic: 3-6 hours; Rectal: 2-5 minutes

Absorption: Oral: ~1% to 20%

Excretion: Urine

Dosage Caution: With orders for I.V. phosphate, there is considerable confusion associated with the use of millimoles (mmol) versus milliequivalents (mEq) to express the phosphate requirement. The most reliable method of ordering I.V. phosphate is by millimoles, then specifying the potassium or sodium salt. Intravenous doses listed as mmol of phosphate.

Acute treatment of hypophosphatemia: I.V.: It is difficult to provide concrete guidelines for the treatment of severe hypophosphatemia because the extent of total body deficits and response to therapy are difficult to predict. Aggressive doses of phosphate may result in a transient serum elevation followed by redistribution into intracellular compartments or bone tissue. It is recommended that repletion of severe hypophosphatemia be done I.V. because large doses of oral phosphate may cause diarrhea and intestinal absorption may be unreliable. Intermittent I.V. infusion should be reserved for severe depletion situations; requires continuous cardiac monitoring. Guidelines differ based on degree of illness, need/use of TPN, and severity of hypophosphatemia. If hypokalemia exists (some clinicians recommend threshold of <4 mmol/L), consider phosphate replacement strategy with potassium (eg, potassium phosphates). Obese patients and/or severe renal impairment were excluded from phosphate supplement trials.

Children and Adults: There are no prospective studies of parenteral phosphate replacement in children. The following weight-based guidelines for adult dosing may be cautiously employed in pediatric patients. **Note:** 1 mmol phosphate = 31 mg phosphorus; 1 mg phosphorus = 0.032 mmol phosphate

General replacement guidelines (Lentz, 1978):

Low dose: 0.08 mmol/kg over 6 hours; use if losses are recent and uncomplicated

Intermediate dose: 0.16-0.24 mmol/kg over 4-6 hours; use if serum phosphorus level 0.5-1 mg/dL (0.16-0.32 mmol/L)

Note: The initial dose may be increased by 25% to 50% if the patient is symptomatic secondary to hypophosphatemia and lowered by 25% to 50% if the patient is hypercalcemic.

Critically-ill adult trauma patients receiving concurrent TPN (Brown, 2006):

Low dose: 0.32 mmol/kg over 4-6 hours; use if serum phosphorus level 2.3-3 mg/dL (0.73-0.96 mmol/L)

Intermediate dose: 0.64 mmol/kg over 4-6 hours; use if serum phosphorus level 1.6-2.2 mg/dL (0.51-0.72 mmol/L)

High dose: 1 mmol/kg over 8-12 hours; use if serum phosphorus <1.5 mg/dL (<0.5 mmol/L)

Parenteral nutrition: I.V.:

Infants and Children: 0.5-2 mmol/kg/24 hours (Mirtallo, 2004 [ASPEN guidelines])

Children >50 kg and Adolescents: 10-40 mmol/24 hours (Mirtallo, 2004 [ASPEN guidelines])

Adults: 10-15 mmol/1000 kcal (Hicks, 2001) **or** 20-40 mmol/24 hours (Mirtallo, 2004 [ASPEN guidelines])

Laxative (Fleet®): Rectal:

Children 2-<5 years: One-half contents of one 2.25 oz pediatric enema

Children 5-12 years: Contents of one 2.25 oz pediatric enema, may repeat

Children ≥12 years and Adults: Contents of one 4.5 oz enema as a single dose, may repeat

Laxative (Fleet® Phospho-soda®): Oral: Take on an empty stomach; dilute dose with 8 ounces cool water, then follow dose with 8 ounces water; **do not repeat dose within 24 hours**

Children 5-9 years: 7.5 mL as a single dose; maximum daily dose: 7.5 mL
Children 10-12 years: 15 mL as a single dose; maximum daily dose: 15 mL
Children ≥12 years and Adults: 15 mL as a single dose; maximum daily dose: 45 mL

Bowel cleansing prior to colonoscopy: Adults: Oral: **Note:** Each dose should be taken with a minimum of 8 ounces of clear liquids. Do not repeat treatment within 7 days. Do not use additional agents, especially sodium phosphate products.

Fleet® Phospho-Soda® (as component of Fleet® Prep Kit 3): Prior to procedure (timing of doses determined by prescriber): Mix 15 mL with 240 mL clear liquid; drink, then follow with 240 mL clear liquid; repeat every 10 minutes for a total of 45 mL

Visicol®: A total of 40 tablets divided as follows:
Evening before colonoscopy: 3 tablets every 15 minutes for 6 doses, then 2 additional tablets in 15 minutes (total of 20 tablets)
3-5 hours prior to colonoscopy: 3 tablets every 15 minutes for 6 doses, then 2 additional tablets in 15 minutes (total of 20 tablets)

OsmoPrep®: A total of 32 tablets divided as follows:
Evening before colonoscopy: 4 tablets every 15 minutes for 5 doses (total of 20 tablets)
3-5 hours prior to colonoscopy: 4 tablets every 15 minutes for 3 doses (total of 12 tablets)

Elderly: Use with caution due to increased risk of renal impairment in the elderly

Dosage adjustment in renal impairment: Use with caution; ionized inorganic phosphate is excreted by the kidneys; oral solution is contraindicated in patients with kidney disease

Dosage adjustment in hepatic impairment: Not expected to be metabolized in the liver

Stability Store at 15°C to 30°C (59°F to 86°F).

Administration

Intermittent I.V. infusion: Dilute to a maximum concentration of 0.12 mmol/mL and infuse over 4-6 hours; maximum rate of infusion: 0.06 mmol/kg/hour

Bowel cleansing: Have patient drink ~8 ounces of water with each dose of sodium phosphate (total of 2 quarts/64 ounces); have patient rehydrate before and after colonoscopy

Monitoring Parameters

I.V.: Serum calcium, magnesium, and phosphate levels; renal function; after I.V. phosphate repletion, repeat serum phosphate level should be checked 2-4 hours later

Oral: Bowel cleansing: Baseline and postprocedure labs (electrolytes, calcium, phosphate, BUN, creatinine) in patients at risk for acute renal nephropathy, seizure, or who have a history of electrolyte abnormality; ECG in patients with risks for prolonged QT or arrhythmias. Ensure euvolemia before initiating bowel preparation.

Pregnancy Risk Factor C

Contraindications Hypersensitivity to sodium phosphate salts or any component of the formulation; additional contraindications vary by product:

Enema: Ascites, clinically significant renal impairment, heart failure, imperforate anus, known or suspected GI obstruction, megacolon (congenital or acquired)

Intravenous preparation: Diseases with hyperphosphatemia, hypocalcemia, or hypernatremia

Oral preparation: Acute phosphate nephropathy (biopsy proven), bowel obstruction, congenital megacolon, toxic megacolon

Warnings/Precautions [U.S. Boxed Warning]: Acute phosphate nephropathy has been reported (rarely) with use of oral products as a colon cleanser prior to colonoscopy. Some cases have resulted in permanent renal impairment (some requiring dialysis). Risk factors for acute phosphate nephropathy may include increased age (>55 years of age), pre-existing renal dysfunction, bowel obstruction, active colitis, or dehydration, and the use of medicines that affect renal perfusion or function (eg, ACE inhibitors, angiotensin receptor blockers, diuretics, and possibly NSAIDs), although some cases have been reported in patients without apparent risk factors. Other preventive measures may include avoid exceeding maximum recommended doses and concurrent use of other laxatives containing sodium phosphate; encourage patients to adequately hydrate before, during, and after use; obtain baseline and postprocedure labs in patients at risk; consider hospitalization and intravenous hydration during bowel cleansing for patients unable to hydrate themselves (eg, frail patients).

Use with caution in patients with impaired renal dysfunction, pre-existing electrolyte imbalances, risk of electrolyte disturbance (hypocalcemia, hyper-phosphatemia, hypernatremia), or dehydration. If using as a bowel evacuant, correct electrolyte abnormalities before administration. Use caution in patients with unstable angina, history of myocardial infarction arrhythmia, cardiomyopathy; use caution in patients with or at risk for arrhythmias (eg, cardiomyopathy, prolonged QT interval, history of uncontrolled arrhythmias, recent MI) or with concurrent use of other QT-prolonging medications; pre-/postdose ECGs should be considered in high-risk patients.

Use caution in inflammatory bowel disease; may induce colonic aphthous ulceration. Use caution in patients with any of the following: Bowel obstruction (including pseudo) or perforation, gastric retention or hypomotility, ileus, severe, chronic constipation, colitis, gastric bypass or bariatric surgery.

Use with caution in patients with a history of seizures and those at higher risk of seizures. Inadequate fluid intake may lead to dehydration. Use with caution in debilitated patients; consider each patient's ability to hydrate properly. Use with caution in geriatric patients. Laxatives and purgatives have the potential for abuse by bulimia nervosa patients. Other oral medications may not be well absorbed when given during bowel evacuation because of rapid intestinal peristalsis. Solutions for injection may contain aluminum; toxic levels may occur following prolonged administration in premature neonates or patients with renal impairment. Enemas and oral solution are available in pediatric and adult sizes; prescribe by "volume" not by "bottle." Safety and efficacy of tablets in children have not been established.

Visicol®: Use caution with history of swallowing difficulties or esophageal narrowing. Tablet particles may be seen in the stool.

Adverse Reactions Frequency not defined.

Cardiovascular: Edema, hypotension

Central nervous system: Dizziness, headache

Endocrine & metabolic: Calcium phosphate precipitation, hypernatremia, hyper-phosphatemia, hypocalcemia

Gastrointestinal: Abdominal bloating, abdominal pain, diarrhea, mucosal bleeding, nausea, superficial mucosal ulcerations, vomiting

Renal: Acute renal failure

Postmarketing and/or case reports: Acute phosphate nephropathy, anaphylaxis, arrhythmia, atrial fibrillation (following severe vomiting [tablet formulation]), BUN increased, creatinine increased, nephrocalcinosis (oral solution), pruritus, rash, renal tubular necrosis, swelling (face, lips, tongue), urticaria, seizure

Drug Interactions

Avoid Concomitant Use There are no known interactions where it is recommended to avoid concomitant use.

Increased Effect/Toxicity

The levels/effects of Sodium Phosphates may be increased by: Bisphosphonate Derivatives

Decreased Effect

The levels/effects of Sodium Phosphates may be decreased by: Antacids; Calcium Salts; Iron Salts; Magnesium Salts; Sucralfate

Dietary Considerations Should be taken on an empty stomach with water; a clear liquid diet should be used for 12 hours prior to tablet administration.

Oral solution contains 556 mg (24.17 mEq) sodium/ 5 mL; 20.6 mmol phosphate/5 mL

Oral tablet contains 312 mg (13.6 mEq) sodium/tablet; 336 mg (10.8 mmol phosphate) elemental phosphorus/tablet

Whole cow's milk: 0.03 mmol/mL phosphate; 0.025 mEq/mL sodium; 0.035 mEq/mL potassium

Dosage Forms Excipient information presented when available (limited, particularly for generics); consult specific product labeling. [DSC] = Discontinued product

Kit [packaged as a two-dose kit which contains]:

Fleet® Phospho-soda® EZ-Prep™ [DSC]:

Solution, oral: Monobasic sodium phosphate monohydrate 2.4 g and dibasic sodium phosphate heptahydrate 0.9 g per 5 mL (30 mL) [sugar-free; contains sodium 556 mg/5 mL and phosphate 62.25 mEq/5 mL; packaged with lemonade flavor packets which contain phenylalanine]

Solution, oral: Monobasic sodium phosphate monohydrate 2.4 g and dibasic sodium phosphate heptahydrate 0.9 g per 5 mL (45 mL) [sugar-free; contains sodium 556 mg/5 mL and phosphate 62.25 mEq/5 mL; packaged with lemonade flavor packets which contain phenylalanine]

Injection, solution [concentrate; preservative free]: Phosphorus 3 mmol and sodium 4 mEq per 1 mL (5 mL, 15 mL, 50 mL) [equivalent to phosphorus 93 mg and sodium 92 mg per 1 mL; source of electrolytes; monobasic and dibasic sodium phosphate]

Solution, oral: Monobasic sodium phosphate monohydrate 2.4 g and dibasic sodium phosphate heptahydrate 0.9 g per 5 mL (45 mL)

Fleet® Phospho-soda®: Monobasic sodium phosphate monohydrate 2.4 g and dibasic sodium phosphate heptahydrate 0.9 g per 5 mL (45 mL) [sugar free; contains sodium 556 mg/5 mL, sodium benzoate, and phosphate 62.25 mEq/5 mL; unflavored or ginger-lemon flavor] [DSC]

Solution, rectal [enema]: Monobasic sodium phosphate monohydrate 19 g and dibasic sodium phosphate heptahydrate 7 g per 118 mL delivered dose (133 mL)

Fleet® Enema: Monobasic sodium phosphate monohydrate 19 g and dibasic sodium phosphate heptahydrate 7 g per 118 mL delivered dose (133 mL) [contains sodium 4.4 g/118 mL]

Fleet® Enema Extra®: Monobasic sodium phosphate monohydrate 19 g and dibasic sodium phosphate heptahydrate 7 g per 197 mL delivered dose (230 mL) [contains sodium 4.4 g/197 mL]

Fleet® Pedia-Lax™ Enema: Monobasic sodium phosphate monohydrate 9.5 g and dibasic sodium phosphate heptahydrate 3.5 g per 59 mL delivered dose (66 mL) [contains sodium 2.2 g/59 mL]

LaCrosse Complete: Monobasic sodium phosphate monohydrate 19 g and dibasic sodium phosphate heptahydrate 7 g per 118 mL delivered dose (133 mL) [contains sodium 4.4 g/118 mL]

Tablet, oral [scored]:

OsmoPrep®, Visicol®: Monobasic sodium phosphate monohydrate 1.102 g and dibasic sodium phosphate anhydrous 0.398 g [sodium phosphate 1.5 g per tablet; gluten free]

References

Clark CL, Sacks GS, Dickerson RN, et al, "Treatment of Hypophosphatemia in Patients Receiving Specialized Nutrition Support Using a Graduated Dosing Scheme: Results From a Prospective Clinical Trial," *Crit Care Med*, 1995, 23(9):1504-11.

Dickerson R, "Treating Hypophosphatemia," *Hosp Pharm*, 1985, 20:920-24.

Lentz RD, Brown BM, and Kjellstrand CM, "Treatment of Severe Hypophosphatemia," *Ann Intern Med*, 1978, 89(6):941-4.

Lloyd CW and Johnson CE, "Management of Hypophosphatemia," *Clin Pharm*, 1988, 7(2):123-8.

Rosen GH, Boullata JI, O'Rangers EA, et al, "Intravenous Phosphate Repletion Regimen for Critically Ill Patients With Moderate Hypophosphatemia," *Crit Care Med*, 1995, 23(7):1204-10.

"Safe Practices for Parenteral Nutrition Formulations," National Advisory Group on Standards and Practice Guidelines for Parenteral Nutrition, *J Parenter Enteral Nutr*, 1998, 22(2):49-66.

Sodium Polystyrene Sulfonate

(SOW dee um pol ee STYE reen SUL fon ate)

Medication Safety Issues

Sound-alike/look-alike issues:

Kayexalate® may be confused with Kaopectate®

Always prescribe either one-time doses or as a specific number of doses (eg, 15 g q6h x 2 doses). Scheduled doses with no dosage limit could be given for days leading to dangerous hypokalemia.

▶

◀ International issues:
Kionex™ may be confused with Kinex® which is a brand name for biperiden in Mexico

U.S. Brand Names Kalexate; Kayexalate®; Kionex®; SPS®

Canadian Brand Names Kayexalate®; PMS-Sodium Polystyrene Sulfonate

Pharmacologic Category Antidote

Generic Available No

Use Treatment of hyperkalemia

Mechanism of Action Removes potassium by exchanging sodium ions for potassium ions in the intestine before the resin is passed from the body

Pharmacodynamics/Kinetics
Onset of action: 2-24 hours
Absorption: None
Excretion: Completely feces (primarily as potassium polystyrene sulfonate)

Dosage
Children:
Oral: 1 g/kg/dose every 6 hours
Rectal: 1 g/kg/dose every 2-6 hours (In small children and infants, employ lower doses by using the practical exchange ratio of 1 mEq K$^+$/g of resin as the basis for calculation)
Adults: Hyperkalemia:
Oral: 15 g 1-4 times/day
Rectal: 30-50 g every 6 hours

Stability Store prepared suspensions at 15°C to 30°C (59°F to 86°F). Store repackaged product in refrigerator and use within 14 days. Freshly prepared suspensions should be used within 24 hours. Do not heat resin suspension.

Administration
Oral: Administer orally (or NG) as a suspension using the commercially available suspension or the powder for suspension. **Do not mix in orange juice.** Chilling the oral mixture will increase palatability. Shake suspension well prior to administration.
Powder for suspension: For each 1 g of the powdered resin, add 3-4 mL of water or syrup (amount of fluid usually ranges from 20-100 mL)
Rectal: Enema route is less effective than oral administration. Administer cleansing enema first. Retain enema in colon for at least 30-60 minutes and for several hours, if possible. Enema should be followed by irrigation with normal saline to prevent necrosis.

Monitoring Parameters Exchange capacity is 1 mEq/g *in vivo*, and *in vitro* capacity is 3.1 mEq/g, therefore, a wide range of exchange capacity exists such that close monitoring of serum electrolytes (potassium, sodium, calcium, magnesium) is necessary; ECG

Reference Range Serum potassium: Adults: 3.5-5.2 mEq/L

Anesthesia and Critical Care Concerns/Other Considerations
Clinical Pearls/Comments: While sodium polystyrene sulfonate can be used in the treatment of hyperkalemia, if hyperkalemia is associated with ECG changes, more emergent therapy needs to be used (ie, glucose-insulin or calcium). Sodium polystyrene sulfonate should be used with caution in patients with severe heart failure, hypertension, or renal failure. While rectal administration of sodium polystyrene sulfonate achieves a more rapid action, oral administration results in a more sustained potassium reduction.

Colonic necrosis is a rare but deadly complication of sodium polystyrene sulfonate-sorbitol when used orally or as an enema in the critically ill patient with hyperkalemia. The clinician should be keenly aware of this devastating side effect and its management. After administration, patients should be closely monitored for abdominal pain, fever, and hypotension. If possible, critically ill patients should receive alternative therapies for potassium removal (eg, hemodialysis).

Pregnancy Risk Factor C

Contraindications Hypersensitivity to sodium polystyrene sulfonate or any component of the formulation; hypernatremia, hypokalemia, obstructive bowel disease

Warnings/Precautions Use with caution in patients with severe HF, hypertension, edema, or renal failure; avoid using the commercially available liquid product in neonates due to the preservative content; large oral doses may cause fecal impaction (especially in elderly); enema will reduce the serum potassium faster than oral administration, but the oral route will result in a greater reduction over several hours.

Adverse Reactions Frequency not defined.

Endocrine & metabolic: Hypernatremia, hypokalemia, hypocalcemia, hypomagnesemia

Gastrointestinal: Anorexia, colonic necrosis (rare), constipation, fecal impaction, intestinal obstruction (due to concretions in association with aluminum hydroxide), nausea, vomiting

Drug Interactions

Avoid Concomitant Use There are no known interactions where it is recommended to avoid concomitant use.

Increased Effect/Toxicity

Sodium Polystyrene Sulfonate may increase the levels/effects of: Antacids

Decreased Effect There are no known significant interactions involving a decrease in effect.

Dietary Considerations Do **not** mix in orange juice. Powder for suspension contains sodium 100 mg/g (4.1 mEq/g). SPS® suspension contains sodium 1500 mg/60 mL (65 mEq/60 mL).

Dosage Forms Excipient information presented when available (limited, particularly for generics); consult specific product labeling.

Powder for suspension, oral/rectal:

Kalexate: 15 g/4 level teaspoons (454 g) [contains sodium 100 mg (4.1 mEq)/g]

Kayexalate®: 15 g/4 level teaspoons (480 g) [contains sodium 100 mg (4.1 mEq)/g]

Kionex®: 15 g/4 level teaspoons (454 g) [contains sodium 100 mg (4.1 mEq)/g]

Suspension, oral/rectal:

SPS®: 15 g/60 mL (60 mL, 120 mL, 480 mL) [contains alcohol 0.3%, sodium 1500 mg (65 mEq)/60 mL, propylene glycol, and sorbitol; cherry flavor]

References

Mokhlesi B, Leikin JB, Murray P, et al, "Adult Toxicology in Critical Care: Part II: Specific Poisonings," *Chest*, 2003, 123(3):897-922.

Sodium Tetradecyl (SOW dee um tetra DEK il)

U.S. Brand Names Sotradecol®

Canadian Brand Names Trombovar®

Index Terms Sodium Tetradecyl Sulfate

Pharmacologic Category Sclerosing Agent

Generic Available No

Use Treatment of small, uncomplicated varicose veins of the lower extremities

Mechanism of Action Acts by irritation of the vein intimal endothelium and causes thrombosis formation leading to occlusion of the injected vein

Dosage I.V.: Test dose: 0.5 mL given several hours prior to administration of larger dose; 0.5-2 mL (preferred maximum: 1 mL) in each vein, maximum: 10 mL per treatment session; 3% solution reserved for large varices

Stability Store at controlled room temperature.

Administration Inject slowly.

Monitoring Parameters Monitor for DVT or PE (up to 4 weeks after injection)

Pregnancy Risk Factor C

Contraindications Hypersensitivity to sodium tetradecyl or any component of the formulation; arterial disease, acute thrombophlebitis; valvular or deep vein incompetence, phlebitis migrans, cellulitis, acute infections; bedridden patients; patients with uncontrolled systemic disease such as diabetes, toxic hyperthyroidism, tuberculosis, asthma, neoplasm, sepsis, blood dyscrasias, and acute respiratory or skin diseases; huge superficial veins with wide open communications to deeper veins; allergic conditions; varicosities caused by abdominal and pelvic tumors (unless tumor has been removed)

◀ **Warnings/Precautions** Use caution with thromboangiitis obliterans or peripheral arteriosclerosis. Avoid extravasation. Observe for hypersensitivity/anaphylactic reaction; emergency resuscitation equipment should be available. Deep vein thrombosis (DVT) and pulmonary embolism (PE) have occurred following treatment. Valvular and venous competency should be evaluated prior to use.

Adverse Reactions Frequency not defined.

Central nervous system: Headache

Dermatologic: Discoloration at site of injection, sloughing and tissue necrosis following extravasation

Gastrointestinal: Nausea, vomiting

Local: Pain, itching, or ulceration at injection site

Miscellaneous: Allergic reaction (including hives, asthma, hay fever); anaphylactic shock

Drug Interactions

Avoid Concomitant Use There are no known interactions where it is recommended to avoid concomitant use.

Increased Effect/Toxicity There are no known significant interactions involving an increase in effect.

Decreased Effect There are no known significant interactions involving a decrease in effect.

Dosage Forms Excipient information presented when available (limited, particularly for generics); consult specific product labeling.

Injection, as sulfate:

Sotradecol®: 1% (2 mL) [contains benzyl alcohol]; 3% (2 mL) [contains benzyl alcohol]

◆ **Sodium Tetradecyl Sulfate** *see* Sodium Tetradecyl *on page 1315*

Sodium Thiosulfate (SOW dee um thye oh SUL fate)

U.S. Brand Names Versiclear™

Index Terms Disodium Thiosulfate Pentahydrate; Pentahydrate; Sodium Hyposulfate; Sodium Thiosulphate; Thiosulfuric Acid Disodium Salt

Pharmacologic Category Antidote

Generic Available Yes: Injection

Use

Parenteral: Used alone or with sodium nitrite or amyl nitrite in cyanide poisoning; reduce the risk of nephrotoxicity associated with cisplatin therapy; treatment of cyanide poisoning due to nitroprusside

Topical: Treatment of tinea versicolor

Unlabeled/Investigational Use Management of I.V. extravasation

Mechanism of Action

Cyanide toxicity: Accelerates the clearance of cyanide via the rhodanase-catalyzed detoxification of cyanide to thiocyanate (much less toxic than cyanide). The accelerated action of rhodanase is a result of the exogenous sulfur provided by sodium thiosulfate.

Cisplatin toxicity: Complexes with cisplatin to form a compound that is nontoxic to either normal or cancerous cells

Pharmacodynamics/Kinetics

Absorption: Oral: Poor

Distribution: Extracellular fluid

Half-life elimination: 0.65 hour

Excretion: Urine (28.5% as unchanged drug)

Dosage

Cyanide poisoning: I.V.: **Note:** Death from cyanide poisoning may occur rapidly, do not delay antidote administration in the event of highly suspected or confirmed cyanide poisoning; usually given in conjunction with amyl nitrite and sodium nitrite

Children: 7 g/m^2 (maximum dose: 12.5 g) given over 10 minutes; may repeat at $1/2$ the original dose if symptoms return

Adults: 12.5 g given over 10 minutes; may repeat at $1/2$ the original dose if symptoms return

Cisplatin rescue should be given before or during cisplatin administration: I.V. infusion (in sterile water): 12 g/m^2 over 6 hours or 9 g/m^2 I.V. push followed by 1.2 g/m^2 continuous infusion for 6 hours

Tinea versicolor: Children and Adults: Topical: 20% to 25% solution: Apply a thin layer to affected areas twice daily

Drug extravasation (unlabeled use): Children and Adults: SubQ: 1/6 M (~4%) solution: Inject into the affected area; various volumes have also been suggested for direct injection into existing I.V. line; however, the optimal volume and efficacy of such practices have not been thoroughly evaluated. **Note:** Use only for large cisplatin infiltrates (>20 mL) and cisplatin concentrations >0.5 mg/mL.

Administration

I.V.: Inject slowly, over at least 10 minutes; rapid administration may cause hypotension.

Topical: Do not apply to or near eyes.

Monitoring Parameters Monitor for signs of thiocyanate toxicity; monitor for hypotension and hypersensitivity reactions

Pregnancy Risk Factor C

Contraindications Hypersensitivity to sodium thiosulfate or any component of the formulation

Warnings/Precautions Safety in pregnancy has not been established; discontinue topical use if irritation or sensitivity occurs; rapid I.V. infusion has caused transient hypotension and ECG changes in dogs; can increase risk of thiocyanate intoxication; use caution with renal impairment.

Fire victims may present with both cyanide and carbon monoxide poisoning. Collection of pretreatment blood cyanide concentrations does not preclude administration and should not delay administration in the emergency management of highly suspected or confirmed cyanide toxicity. Patients receiving treatment for acute cyanide toxicity must be monitored for return of symptoms for 24-48 hours.

Adverse Reactions Frequency not defined

Cardiovascular: Hypotension (infusion rate-dependent)

Dermatologic: Contact dermatitis, local irritation

Gastrointestinal: Nausea, vomiting

Miscellaneous: Hypersensitivity reactions

Drug Interactions

Avoid Concomitant Use There are no known interactions where it is recommended to avoid concomitant use.

Increased Effect/Toxicity There are no known significant interactions involving an increase in effect.

Decreased Effect There are no known significant interactions involving a decrease in effect.

Dosage Forms Excipient information presented when available (limited, particularly for generics); consult specific product labeling.

Injection, solution [preservative free]: 100 mg/mL (10 mL); 250 mg/mL (50 mL)

Lotion: Sodium thiosulfate 25% and salicylic acid 1% (120 mL) [contains isopropyl alcohol 10%]

References

Geller RJ, Barthold C, Saiers JA, et al, "Pediatric Cyanide Poisoning: Causes, Manifestations, Management, and Unmet Needs," *Pediatrics*, 2006, 118(5):2146-58.

Mokhlesi B, Leikin JB, Murray P, et al, "Adult Toxicology in Critical Care: Part II: Specific Poisonings," *Chest*, 2003, 123(3):897-922.

Somatropin (soe ma TROE pin)

U.S. Brand Names Genotropin Miniquick®; Genotropin®; Humatrope®; Norditropin®; Norditropin® NordiFlex®; Nutropin AQ®; Nutropin®; Omnitrope®; Saizen®; Serostim®; Tev-Tropin®; Zorbtive®

Canadian Brand Names Humatrope®; Nutropin®; Nutropin® AQ; Saizen®; Serostim®

Index Terms Growth Hormone, Human; hGH; Human Growth Hormone; Somatrem

Pharmacologic Category Growth Hormone

Use

Children:

Treatment of growth failure due to inadequate endogenous growth hormone secretion (Genotropin®, Humatrope®, Norditropin®, Nutropin®, Nutropin AQ®, Omnitrope®, Saizen®, Tev-Tropin®)

Treatment of short stature associated with Turner syndrome (Genotropin®, Humatrope®, Norditropin®, Nutropin®, Nutropin AQ®)

Treatment of Prader-Willi syndrome (Genotropin®)

Treatment of growth failure associated with chronic renal insufficiency (CRI) up until the time of renal transplantation (Nutropin®, Nutropin AQ®)

Treatment of growth failure in children born small for gestational age who fail to manifest catch-up growth by 2 years of age (Genotropin®) or by 2-4 years of age (Humatrope®, Norditropin®)

Treatment of idiopathic short stature (nongrowth hormone-deficient short stature) defined by height standard deviation score (SDS) ≤ -2.25 and growth rate not likely to attain normal adult height (Genotropin®, Humatrope®, Nutropin®, Nutropin AQ®)

Treatment of short stature or growth failure associated with short stature homeobox gene (SHOX) deficiency (Humatrope®)

Treatment of short stature associated with Noonan syndrome (Norditropin®)

Adults:

HIV patients with wasting or cachexia with concomitant antiviral therapy (Serostim®)

Replacement of endogenous growth hormone in patients with adult growth hormone deficiency who meet both of the following criteria (Genotropin®, Humatrope®, Norditropin®, Nutropin®, Nutropin AQ®, Omnitrope®, Saizen®):

Biochemical diagnosis of adult growth hormone deficiency by means of a subnormal response to a standard growth hormone stimulation test (peak growth hormone ≤5 mcg/L). Confirmatory testing may not be required in patients with congenital/genetic growth hormone deficiency or multiple pituitary hormone deficiencies due to organic diseases.

and

Adult-onset: Patients who have adult growth hormone deficiency whether alone or with multiple hormone deficiencies (hypopituitarism) as a result of pituitary disease, hypothalamic disease, surgery, radiation therapy, or trauma

or

Childhood-onset: Patients who were growth hormone deficient during child-hood, confirmed as an adult before replacement therapy is initiated

Treatment of short-bowel syndrome (Zorbtive®)

Unlabeled/Investigational Use Investigational: Pediatric HIV patients with wasting/cachexia (Serostim®); HIV-associated adipose redistribution syndrome (HARS) (Serostim®)

Pharmacodynamics/Kinetics

Duration: Maintains supraphysiologic levels for 18-20 hours

Absorption: I.M., SubQ: Well absorbed

Distribution: ~1 L/kg

Metabolism: Hepatic and renal (~90%)

Bioavailability: SubQ: ~70% to 90%; **Note:** Variable; product-dependent

Half-life elimination: Preparation and route of administration dependent; SubQ: ~2-4 hours

Excretion: Urine (small amount)

Dosage

Children (individualize dose):

Chronic renal insufficiency (CRI): Nutropin®, Nutropin® AQ: SubQ: Weekly dosage: 0.35 mg/kg divided into daily injections; continue until the time of renal transplantation

Dosage recommendations in patients treated for CRI who require dialysis:

Hemodialysis: Administer dose at night prior to bedtime or at least 3-4 hours after hemodialysis to prevent hematoma formation from heparin

CCPD: Administer dose in the morning following dialysis

CAPD: Administer dose in the evening at the time of overnight exchange

Growth hormone deficiency:

Genotropin®, Omnitrope®: SubQ: Weekly dosage: 0.16-0.24 mg/kg divided into equal doses 6-7 days per week

Humatrope®: SubQ: Weekly dosage: 0.18-0.3 mg/kg divided into equal doses 6-7 days per week

Norditropin®: SubQ: 0.024-0.034 mg/kg/day, 6-7 days per week

Nutropin®, Nutropin® AQ: SubQ: Weekly dosage: 0.3 mg/kg divided into equal daily doses; pubertal patients: ≤0.7 mg/kg divided into equal daily doses

Tev-Tropin®: SubQ: Up to 0.1 mg/kg administered 3 days per week

Saizen®: I.M., SubQ: Weekly dosage: 0.18 mg/kg divided into equal daily doses **or** as 0.06 mg/kg/dose administered 3 days per week **or** as 0.03 mg/kg/dose administered 6 days per week

Note: Therapy should be discontinued when patient has reached satisfactory adult height, when epiphyses have fused, or when the patient ceases to respond. Growth of 5 cm/year or more is expected, if growth rate does not exceed 2.5 cm in a 6-month period, double the dose for the next 6 months; if there is still no satisfactory response, discontinue therapy

HIV patients with wasting or cachexia (unlabeled use): Serostim®: SubQ: Limited data; doses of 0.04 mg/kg/day were reported in five children, 6-17 years of age; doses of 0.07 mg/kg/day were reported in six children, 8-14 years of age

Idiopathic short stature:

Genotropin®: SubQ: Weekly dosage: 0.47 mg/kg divided into equal doses 6-7 days per week

Humatrope®: SubQ: Weekly dosage: 0.37 mg/kg divided into equal doses 6-7 days per week

Nutropin®, Nutropin AQ®: SubQ: Weekly dosage: Up to 0.3 mg/kg divided into equal daily doses

Noonan syndrome: Norditropin®: SubQ: Up to 0.066 mg/kg/day

Prader-Willi syndrome: Genotropin®: SubQ: Weekly dosage: 0.24 mg/kg divided into equal doses 6-7 days per week

SHOX deficiency: Humatrope®: SubQ: Weekly dosage: 0.35 mg/kg divided into equal doses 6-7 days per week

Small for gestational age:

Genotropin®: SubQ: Weekly dosage: 0.48 mg/kg divided into equal doses 6-7 days per week

Humatrope®: SubQ: Weekly dosage: 0.47 mg/kg divided into equal doses 6-7 days per week

Norditropin®: SubQ: Up to 0.067 mg/kg/day

Alternate dosing (small for gestational age): In older/early pubertal children or children with very short stature, consider initiating therapy at higher doses (0.067 mg/kg/day) and then consider reducing the dose (0.033 mg/kg/day) if substantial catch-up growth observed. In younger children (<4 years) with less severe short stature, consider initiating therapy with lower doses (0.033 mg/kg/day) and then titrating the dose upwards as needed.

Turner syndrome:

Genotropin®: SubQ: Weekly dosage: 0.33 mg/kg divided into equal doses 6-7 days per week

Humatrope®: SubQ: Weekly dosage: 0.375 mg/kg divided into equal doses 6-7 days per week

Norditropin®: SubQ: Up to 0.067 mg/kg/day

Nutropin®, Nutropin® AQ: SubQ: Weekly dosage: ≤0.375 mg/kg divided into equal doses 3-7 days per week

◀ **Adults:**

Growth hormone deficiency: Adjust dose based on individual requirements: To minimize adverse events in older or overweight patients, reduced dosages may be necessary. During therapy, dosage should be decreased if required by the occurrence of side effects or excessive IGF-I levels.

Weight-based dosing:

Norditropin®: SubQ: Initial dose ≤0.004 mg/kg/day; after 6 weeks of therapy, may increase dose up to 0.016 mg/kg/day

Nutropin®, Nutropin® AQ: SubQ: ≤0.006 mg/kg/day; dose may be increased up to a maximum of 0.025 mg/kg/day in patients <35 years of age, or up to a maximum of 0.0125 mg/kg/day in patients ≥35 years of age

Humatrope®: SubQ: ≤0.006 mg/kg/day; dose may be increased up to a maximum of 0.0125 mg/kg/day

Genotropin®, Omnitrope®: SubQ: Weekly dosage: ≤0.04 mg/kg divided into equal doses 6-7 days per week; dose may be increased at 4- to 8-week intervals to a maximum of 0.08 mg/kg/week

Saizen®: SubQ: ≤0.005 mg/kg/day; dose may be increased to not more than 0.01 mg/kg/day after 4 weeks

Nonweight-based dosing: SubQ: Initial: 0.2 mg/day (range: 0.15-0.3 mg/day); may increase every 1-2 months by 0.1-0.2 mg/day based on response and/or serum IGF-I levels

Dosage adjustment with estrogen supplementation (growth hormone deficiency): Larger doses of somatropin may be needed for women taking oral estrogen replacement products; dosing not affected by topical products

HARS (unlabeled use): Serostim®: SubQ: Induction: 4 mg once daily at bedtime for 12 weeks; Maintenance: 2 mg or 4 mg every other day at bedtime for 12-24 weeks. **Note:** Every-other-day dosing during induction has also been studied. Although a greater response was seen with daily dosing, it was associated with an increased incidence of adverse events.

HIV patients with wasting or cachexia: Serostim®: SubQ: 0.1 mg/kg once daily at bedtime (maximum: 6 mg/day). Alternately, patients at risk for side effects may be started at 0.1 mg/kg every other day. Patients who continue to lose weight after 12 weeks should be re-evaluated for opportunistic infections or other clinical events; rotate injection sites to avoid lipodystrophy Adjust dose if needed to manage side effects.

Daily dose based on body weight:

<35 kg: 0.1 mg/kg

35-45 kg: 4 mg

45-55 kg: 5 mg

>55 kg: 6 mg

Short-bowel syndrome (Zorbtive®): SubQ: 0.1 mg/kg once daily for 4 weeks (maximum: 8 mg/day)

Fluid retention (moderate) or arthralgias: Treat symptomatically or reduce dose by 50%

Severe toxicity: Discontinue therapy for up to 5 days; when symptoms resolve, restart at 50% of dose. If severe toxicity recurs or does not disappear within 5 days after discontinuation, permanently discontinue treatment.

Elderly: Patients ≥65 years of age may be more sensitive to the action of growth hormone and more prone to adverse effects; in general, dosing should be cautious, beginning at low end of dosing range

Dosage adjustment in renal impairment Reports indicate patients with chronic renal failure tend to have decreased clearance; specific dosing suggestions not available

Dosage adjustment in hepatic impairment: Clearance may be reduced in patients with severe hepatic dysfunction; specific dosing suggestions not available

Additional Information Complete prescribing information for this medication should be consulted for additional detail.

Dosage Forms Excipient information presented when available (limited, particularly for generics); consult specific product labeling. [DSC] = Discontinued product

Injection, powder for reconstitution [rDNA origin]:
Genotropin®: 5.8 mg [~15 int. units/mL; delivers 5 mg/mL; contains m-cresol]; 13.8 mg [~36 int. units/mL; delivers 12 mg/mL; contains m-cresol]
Genotropin Miniquick® [preservative free]: 0.2 mg, 0.4 mg, 0.6 mg, 0.8 mg, 1 mg, 1.2 mg, 1.4 mg, 1.6 mg, 1.8 mg, 2 mg [each strength delivers 0.25 mL]
Humatrope®: 5 mg [15 int. units], 6 mg [18 int. units], 12 mg [36 int. units], 24 mg [72 int. units]
Nutropin®: 5 mg [~15 int. units; packaged with diluent containing benzyl alcohol]; 10 mg [~30 int. units; packaged with diluent containing benzyl alcohol]
Omnitrope®: 5.8 mg [~17.4 int. units; packaged with diluent containing benzyl alcohol]
Saizen®: 5 mg [~15 int. units; contains sucrose 34.2 mg; packaged with diluent containing benzyl alcohol]; 8.8 mg [~26.4 int. units; contains sucrose 60.2 mg; packaged with diluent containing benzyl alcohol]
Serostim®: 4 mg [~12 int. units; contains sucrose 27.3 mg; packaged with diluent containing benzyl alcohol; 5 mg [~15 int. units; contains sucrose 34.2 mg]; 6 mg [~18 int. units; contains sucrose 41 mg]; 8.8 mg [DSC] [~26.4 int. units; contains sucrose 60.19 mg; packaged with diluent containing benzyl alcohol]
Tev-Tropin®: 5 mg [15 int. units/mL; packaged with diluent containing benzyl alcohol]
Zorbtive®: 8.8 mg [~26.4 int. units; contains sucrose 60.19 mg; packaged with diluent containing benzyl alcohol]
Injection, solution [rDNA origin]:
Norditropin®: 5 mg/1.5 mL (1.5 mL); 15 mg/1.5 mL (1.5 mL)
Norditropin® NordiFlex®: 5 mg/1.5 mL (1.5 mL); 10 mg/1.5 mL (1.5 mL); 15 mg/ 1.5 mL (1.5 mL)
Nutropin AQ®: 5 mg/mL (2 mL) [~15 int. units/mL]
Omnitrope®: 5 mg/1.5 mL (1.5 mL); 10 mg/1.5 mL (1.5 mL)

◆ **Somatuline® Autogel® (Can)** *see* Lanreotide *on page* 804

◆ **Somatuline® Depot** *see* Lanreotide *on page* 804

◆ **Sominex® [OTC]** *see* DiphenhydrAMINE *on page* 430

◆ **Sominex® Maximum Strength [OTC]** *see* DiphenhydrAMINE *on page* 430

◆ **Somnote®** *see* Chloral Hydrate *on page* 285

◆ **Som Pam (Can)** *see* Flurazepam *on page* 618

◆ **Sorine®** *see* Sotalol *on page* 1321

Sotalol (SOE ta lole)

Medication Safety Issues
Sound-alike/look-alike issues:
Sotalol may be confused with Stadol®, Sudafed®
Betapace® may be confused with Betapace AF®
Betapace AF® may be confused with Betapace®

Related Information
Antiarrhythmic Drugs *on page* 1656
Beta-Blockers *on page* 1669
Management of Postoperative Arrhythmias *on page* 1571
Preoperative Evaluation of the Cardiac Patient for Noncardiac Surgery *on page* 1598

U.S. Brand Names Betapace AF®; Betapace®; Sorine®

Canadian Brand Names Apo-Sotalol®; Betapace AF®; CO Sotalol; DOM-Sotalol; Gen-Sotalol; Lin-Sotalol; MED-Sotalol; Mylan-Sotalol; Novo-Sotalol; Nu-Sotalol; PHL-Sotalol; PMS-Sotalol; PRO-Sotalol; ratio-Sotalol; Rhoxal-sotalol; Riva-Sotalol; Rylosol; Sandoz-Sotalol; ZYM-Sotalol

Index Terms Sotalol Hydrochloride

Pharmacologic Category Antiarrhythmic Agent, Class II; Antiarrhythmic Agent, Class III; Beta-Adrenergic Blocker, Nonselective

Generic Available Yes

Use Treatment of documented ventricular arrhythmias (ie, sustained ventricular tachycardia), that in the judgment of the physician are life-threatening;

◄ maintenance of normal sinus rhythm in patients with symptomatic atrial fibrillation and atrial flutter who are currently in sinus rhythm. Manufacturer states substitutions should not be made for Betapace AF® since Betapace AF® is distributed with a patient package insert specific for atrial fibrillation/flutter.

Mechanism of Action

Beta-blocker which contains both beta-adrenoreceptor-blocking (Vaughan Williams Class II) and cardiac action potential duration prolongation (Vaughan Williams Class III) properties

Class II effects: Increased sinus cycle length, slowed heart rate, decreased AV nodal conduction, and increased AV nodal refractoriness

Class III effects: Prolongation of the atrial and ventricular monophasic action potentials, and effective refractory prolongation of atrial muscle, ventricular muscle, and atrioventricular accessory pathways in both the antegrade and retrograde directions

Sotalol is a racemic mixture of d- and l-sotalol; both isomers have similar Class III antiarrhythmic effects while the l-isomer is responsible for virtually all of the beta-blocking activity

Sotalol has both beta$_1$- and beta$_2$-receptor blocking activity

The beta-blocking effect of sotalol is a noncardioselective [half maximal at about 80 mg/day and maximal at doses of 320-640 mg/day]. Significant beta-blockade occurs at oral doses as low as 25 mg/day.

The Class III effects are seen only at oral doses ≥160 mg/day

Pharmacodynamics/Kinetics

Onset of action: Rapid, 1-2 hours

Duration: 8-16 hours

Absorption: Decreased 20% to 30% by meals compared to fasting

Distribution: V_d: 1.2-2.4 L/kg

Protein binding: None

Metabolism: None

Bioavailability: 90% to 100%

Half-life elimination: 12 hours; Children: 9.5 hours; terminal half-life decreases with age <2 years (time to steady state may be ≥1 week in neonates); increases with renal dysfunction

Time to peak, serum: 2.5-4 hours

Excretion: Urine (as unchanged drug)

Dosage Sotalol should be initiated and doses increased in a hospital with facilities for cardiac rhythm monitoring and assessment. Proarrhythmic events can occur after initiation of therapy and with each upward dosage adjustment.

Children: Oral: The safety and efficacy of sotalol in children have not been established

Note: Dosing per manufacturer, based on pediatric pharmacokinetic data; wait at least 36 hours between dosage adjustments to allow monitoring of QT intervals

≤2 years: Dosage should be adjusted (decreased) by plotting of the child's age on a logarithmic scale; see graph on next page or refer to manufacturer's package labeling.

>2 years: Initial: 90 mg/m^2/day in 3 divided doses; may be incrementally increased to a maximum of 180 mg/m^2/day

Adults: Oral:

Ventricular arrhythmias (Betapace®, Sorine®):

Initial: 80 mg twice daily

Dose may be increased gradually to 240-320 mg/day; allow 3 days between dosing increments in order to attain steady-state plasma concentrations and to allow monitoring of QT intervals

Most patients respond to a total daily dose of 160-320 mg/day in 2-3 divided doses.

Some patients, with life-threatening refractory ventricular arrhythmias, may require doses as high as 480-640 mg/day; however, these doses should only be prescribed when the potential benefit outweighs the increased of adverse events.

Atrial fibrillation or atrial flutter (Betapace AF®): Initial: 80 mg twice daily

If the initial dose does not reduce the frequency of relapses of atrial fibrillation/flutter and is tolerated without excessive QT prolongation (not >520 msec)

after 3 days, the dose may be increased to 120 mg twice daily. This may be further increased to 160 mg twice daily if response is inadequate and QT prolongation is not excessive.

Sotalol Age Factor Nomogram for Patients ≤2 Years of Age

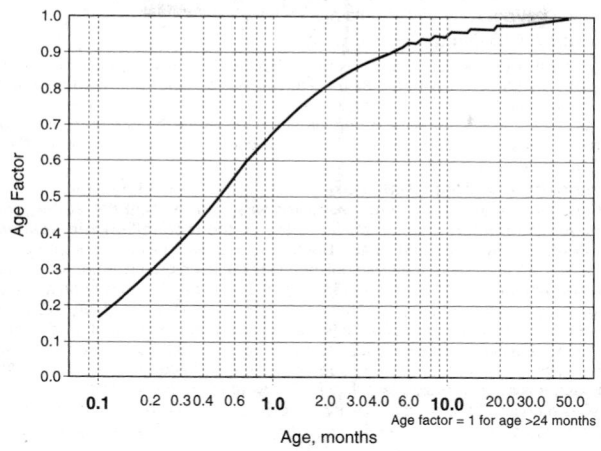

Age, months

Adapted from U.S. Food and Drug Administration.
http://www.fda.gov/cder/foi/label/2001/2115s3lbl.PDF

Elderly: Age does not significantly alter the pharmacokinetics of sotalol, but impaired renal function in elderly patients can increase the terminal half-life, resulting in increased drug accumulation

Dosage adjustment in renal impairment: Adults: Impaired renal function can increase the terminal half-life, resulting in increased drug accumulation. Sotalol (Betapace AF®) is contraindicated per the manufacturer for treatment of atrial fibrillation/flutter in patients with a Cl_{cr} <40 mL/minute.

Ventricular arrhythmias (Betapace®, Sorine®):

Cl_{cr} >60 mL/minute: Administer every 12 hours

Cl_{cr} 30-60 mL/minute: Administer every 24 hours

Cl_{cr} 10-30 mL/minute: Administer every 36-48 hours

Cl_{cr} <10 mL/minute: Individualize dose

Atrial fibrillation/flutter (Betapace AF®):

Cl_{cr} >60 mL/minute: Administer every 12 hours

Cl_{cr} 40-60 mL/minute: Administer every 24 hours

Cl_{cr} <40 mL/minute: Use is contraindicated

Dialysis: Hemodialysis would be expected to reduce sotalol plasma concentrations because sotalol is not bound to plasma proteins and does not undergo extensive metabolism; administer dose postdialysis or administer supplemental 80 mg dose; peritoneal dialysis does not remove sotalol; supplemental dose is not necessary

Stability Store at 25°C (77°F); excursions permitted to 15°C to 30°C (59°F to 86°F).

Administration Food may decrease absorption.

Monitoring Parameters Serum magnesium, potassium, ECG

Anesthesia and Critical Care Concerns/Other Considerations

Clinical Pearls/Comments: Monitor QT_c interval closely and adjust dose as appropriate, especially in patients with renal impairment. Risk of torsade de pointes with sotalol is highest in women, patients with baseline QT interval >450 msecs, renal impairment, significant bradycardia, or concomitant heart failure (see Contraindications). Avoid concomitant use of QT-prolonging agents.

Withdrawal: Beta-blocker therapy should not be withdrawn abruptly, but gradually tapered to avoid acute tachycardia and hypertension.

Pregnancy Risk Factor B

Contraindications Hypersensitivity to sotalol or any component of the formulation; bronchial asthma; sinus bradycardia; second- and third-degree AV block (unless a functioning pacemaker is present); congenital or acquired long QT syndromes; cardiogenic shock; uncontrolled congestive heart failure. Betapace AF® is contraindicated in patients with significantly reduced renal filtration (Cl_{cr} <40 mL/minute).

Warnings/Precautions [U.S. Boxed Warning] Manufacturer recommends initiation (or reinitiation) and doses increased in a hospital setting with continuous monitoring and staff familiar with the recognition and treatment of life-threatening arrhythmias. Some experts will initiate therapy on an outpatient basis in a patient without heart disease or bradycardia, who has a baseline uncorrected QT interval <450 msec, and normal serum potassium and magnesium levels; close ECG monitoring during this time is necessary. ACC/AHA guidelines for management of atrial fibrillation also recommend that for outpatient initiation the patient not have risk factors predisposing to drug-induced ventricular proarrhythmia (Fuster, 2001). Dosage should be adjusted gradually with 3 days between dosing increments to achieve steady-state concentrations, and to allow time to monitor QT intervals. Creatinine clearance must be calculated prior to dosing. Use cautiously in the renally-impaired (dosage adjustment required).

Watch for proarrhythmic effects; monitor and adjust dose to prevent QTc prolongation. Concurrent use with other QT_c-prolonging drugs (including Class I and Class III antiarrhythmics) is generally not recommended; withhold for 3 half-lives. Correct electrolyte imbalances before initiating (especially hypokalemia and hypomagnesemia). Consider pre-existing conditions such as sick sinus syndrome before initiating. Conduction abnormalities can occur particularly sinus bradycardia. Use cautiously within the first 2 weeks post-MI (experience limited). Administer cautiously in compensated heart failure and monitor for a worsening of the condition. Use caution in patients with PVD (can aggravate arterial insufficiency). Beta-blocker therapy should not be withdrawn abruptly (particularly in patients with CAD), but gradually tapered to avoid acute tachycardia, hypertension, and/or ischemia. Use caution with concurrent use of beta-blockers and either verapamil or diltiazem; bradycardia or heart block can occur. Use cautiously in diabetics because it can mask prominent hypoglycemic symptoms. Use with caution in patients with bronchospastic disease, myasthenia gravis, peripheral vascular disease, or psychiatric disease. Use care with anesthetic agents which decrease myocardial function. Adequate alpha-blockade is required prior to use of any beta-blocker for patients with untreated pheochromocytoma. Use caution with history of severe anaphylaxis to allergens; patients taking beta-blockers may become more sensitive to repeated challenges. Treatment of anaphylaxis (eg, epinephrine) in patients taking beta-blockers may be ineffective or promote undesirable effects.

[U.S. Boxed Warning]: Betapace® should not be substituted for Betapace® AF; Betapace® AF is distributed with an educational insert specifically for patients with atrial fibrillation/flutter.

Adverse Reactions

>10%:

Cardiovascular: Bradycardia (16%), chest pain (16%), palpitation (14%)

Central nervous system: Fatigue (20%), dizziness (20%), lightheadedness (12%)

Neuromuscular & skeletal: Weakness (13%)

Respiratory: Dyspnea (21%)

1% to 10%:

Cardiovascular: Edema (8%), abnormal ECG (7%), hypotension (6%), proarrhythmia (5%), syncope (5%), CHF (5%), peripheral vascular disorders (3%)

Central nervous system: Headache (8%), sleep problems (8%), mental confusion (6%), anxiety (4%), depression (4%)

Dermatologic: Itching/rash (5%)

Endocrine & metabolic: Sexual ability decreased (3%)

Gastrointestinal: Nausea/vomiting (10%), diarrhea (7%), stomach discomfort (3% to 6%), flatulence (2%)

Genitourinary: Impotence (2%)

Hematologic: Bleeding (2%)

Neuromuscular & skeletal: Extremity pain (7%), paresthesia (4%), back pain (3%)

Ocular: Visual problems (5%)

Respiratory: Upper respiratory problems (5% to 8%), asthma (2%)

<1% (Limited to important or life-threatening): Alopecia, bronchiolitis obliterans with organized pneumonia (BOOP), cold extremities, diaphoresis, eosinophilia, leukocytoclastic vasculitis, leukopenia, paralysis, phlebitis, photosensitivity reaction, pruritus, pulmonary edema, Raynaud's phenomenon, red crusted skin, retroperitoneal fibrosis, serum transaminases increased, skin necrosis after extravasation, thrombocytopenia, vertigo

Drug Interactions

Avoid Concomitant Use

Avoid concomitant use of Sotalol with any of the following: Artemether; Dronedarone; Lumefantrine; Methacholine; Nilotinib; Pimozide; QuiNINE; Tetrabenazine; Thioridazine; Ziprasidone

Increased Effect/Toxicity

Sotalol may increase the levels/effects of: Alpha-/Beta-Agonists (Direct-Acting); Alpha1-Blockers; Alpha2-Agonists; Amifostine; Antihypertensives; Antipsychotic Agents (Phenothiazines); Cardiac Glycosides; Dronedarone; Hypotensive Agents; Insulin; Lidocaine; Methacholine; Midodrine; Pimozide; QTc-Prolonging Agents; QuiNINE; RiTUXimab; Sulfonylureas; Tetrabenazine; Thioridazine; Ziprasidone

The levels/effects of Sotalol may be increased by: Acetylcholinesterase Inhibitors; Alfuzosin; Aminoquinolines (Antimalarial); Amiodarone; Anilidopiperidine Opioids; Antipsychotic Agents (Phenothiazines); Artemether; Calcium Channel Blockers (Nondihydropyridine); Chloroquine; Ciprofloxacin; Diazoxide; Dipyridamole; Disopyramide; Dronedarone; Gadobutrol; Herbs (Hypotensive Properties); Lumefantrine; MAO Inhibitors; Nilotinib; Pentoxifylline; Phosphodiesterase 5 Inhibitors; Propafenone; Propoxyphene; Prostacyclin Analogues; QuiNIDine; QuiNINE; Reserpine; Selective Serotonin Reuptake Inhibitors

Decreased Effect

Sotalol may decrease the levels/effects of: Beta2-Agonists; Theophylline Derivatives

The levels/effects of Sotalol may be decreased by: Barbiturates; Herbs (Hypertensive Properties); Methylphenidate; Nonsteroidal Anti-Inflammatory Agents; Rifamycin Derivatives; Yohimbine

Ethanol/Nutrition/Herb Interactions

Food: Sotalol peak serum concentrations may be decreased if taken with food.

Herb/Nutraceutical: Avoid ephedra (may worsen arrhythmia).

Dietary Considerations Take on an empty stomach. Food may decrease absorption.

Dosage Forms Excipient information presented when available (limited, particularly for generics); consult specific product labeling.

Tablet, as hydrochloride: 80 mg, 80 mg [atrial fibrillation], 120 mg, 120 mg [atrial fibrillation], 160 mg, 160 mg [atrial fibrillation], 240 mg

Betapace®: 80 mg, 120 mg, 160 mg, 240 mg

Betapace AF®: 80 mg, 120 mg, 160 mg [atrial fibrillation]

Sorine®: 80 mg, 120 mg, 160 mg, 240 mg

References

Fuster V, Ryden LE, Asinger RW, et al, "ACC/AHA/ESC Guidelines for the Mangement of Patients With Atrial Fibrillation. A Report of the American College of Cardiology/ American Heart Associateion Task Force on Practice Guidelines and the European Society of Cardiology Committee for Practice Guidelines and Policy Conferences (Committee to Develop Guidelines for the Management of Patients With Atrial Fibrillation)," *J Am Coll Cardiol*, 2001, 38(4):1231-66.

Mokhlesi B, Leikin JB, Murray P, et al, "Adult Toxicology in Critical Care: Part II: Specific Poisonings," *Chest*, 2003, 123(3):897-922.

- **Sotalol Hydrochloride** *see* Sotalol *on page 1321*
- **Sotradecol®** *see* Sodium Tetradecyl *on page 1315*
- **SPA** *see* Albumin *on page 46*
- **SPD417** *see* CarBAMazepine *on page 241*
- **SPEF-Pioglitazone (Can)** *see* Pioglitazone *on page 1132*
- **Spiriva® (Can)** *see* Tiotropium *on page 1395*
- **Spiriva® HandiHaler®** *see* Tiotropium *on page 1395*
- **SPM 927** *see* Lacosamide *on page 795*
- **SPP100** *see* Aliskiren *on page 61*
- **Sprintec®** *see* Ethinyl Estradiol and Norgestimate *on page 558*
- **SPS®** *see* Sodium Polystyrene Sulfonate *on page 1313*
- **SR33589** *see* Dronedarone *on page 461*
- **Sronyx™** *see* Ethinyl Estradiol and Levonorgestrel *on page 549*
- **SSD®** *see* Silver Sulfadiazine *on page 1292*
- **SSD® AF** *see* Silver Sulfadiazine *on page 1292*
- **Stadol** *see* Butorphanol *on page 220*
- **Stagesic™** *see* Hydrocodone and Acetaminophen *on page 697*
- **Statex® (Can)** *see* Morphine Sulfate *on page 953*
- **Stavzor™** *see* Valproic Acid and Derivatives *on page 1445*
- **Stemetil® (Can)** *see* Prochlorperazine *on page 1180*
- **Sterapred®** *see* PredniSONE *on page 1166*
- **Sterapred® DS [DSC]** *see* PredniSONE *on page 1166*
- **Sterile Talc** *see* Talc (Sterile) *on page 1349*
- **Sterile Talc Powder™** *see* Talc (Sterile) *on page 1349*
- **Stimate®** *see* Desmopressin *on page 386*
- **St. Joseph® Adult Aspirin [OTC]** *see* Aspirin *on page 147*
- **Strattera®** *see* Atomoxetine *on page 157*
- **Striant®** *see* Testosterone *on page 1362*
- **Sublimaze®** *see* FentaNYL *on page 587*
- **Subutex®** *see* Buprenorphine *on page 214*

Succinylcholine (suks in il KOE leen)

Medication Safety Issues

High alert medication: The Institute for Safe Medication Practices (ISMP) includes this medication among its list of drugs which have a heightened risk of causing significant patient harm when used in error.

United States Pharmacopeia (USP) 2006: The Interdisciplinary Safe Medication Use Expert Committee of the USP has recommended the following:
- Hospitals, clinics, and other practice sites should institute special safeguards in the storage, labeling, and use of these agents and should include these safeguards in staff orientation and competency training.
- Healthcare professionals should be on high alert (especially vigilant) whenever a neuromuscular-blocking agent (NMBA) is stocked, ordered, prepared, or administered.

Related Information

Allergic Reactions *on page 1508*
Anesthesia Considerations for Neurosurgery *on page 1514*
Anesthesia for Obstetric Patients in Nonobstetric Surgery *on page 1532*
Anesthetic Considerations in the Substance-Abusing Patient *on page 1613*
Chronic Renal Failure *on page 1552*
Dosing Considerations for the Critically-Ill Patient With Morbid Obesity *on page 1561*
Malignant Hyperthermia *on page 1638*
Management of Postoperative Arrhythmias *on page 1571*
Neuromuscular-Blocking Agents *on page 1684*

U.S. Brand Names Anectine®; Quelicin®

Canadian Brand Names Quelicin®

Index Terms Succinylcholine Chloride; Suxamethonium Chloride

Pharmacologic Category Neuromuscular Blocker Agent, Depolarizing

Generic Available No

Use To facilitate both rapid sequence and routine endotracheal intubation and to relax skeletal muscles during surgery; to reduce the intensity of muscle contractions of pharmacologically- or electrically-induced convulsions; does not relieve pain or produce sedation

Mechanism of Action Acts similar to acetylcholine, produces depolarization of the motor endplate at the myoneural junction which causes sustained flaccid skeletal muscle paralysis produced by state of accommodation that developes in adjacent excitable muscle membranes

Pharmacodynamics/Kinetics

Onset of action: I.M.: 2-3 minutes; I.V.: Complete muscular relaxation: 30-60 seconds

Duration: I.M.: 10-30 minutes; I.V.: 4-6 minutes with single administration

Metabolism: Rapidly hydrolyzed by plasma pseudocholinesterase

Excretion: Urine

Dosage I.M., I.V.: Dose to effect; doses will vary due to interpatient variability; use ideal body weight for obese patients

I.M.: Children and Adults: Up to 3-4 mg/kg, total dose should not exceed 150 mg

I.V.:

Children: **Note:** Because of the risk of malignant hyperthermia, use of continuous infusions is not recommended in infants and children

Smaller Children: Intermittent: Initial: 2 mg/kg/dose one time; maintenance: 0.3-0.6 mg/kg/ dose every 5-10 minutes as needed

Older Children and Adolescents: Intermittent: Initial: 1 mg/kg/dose one time; maintenance: 0.3-0.6 mg/kg every 5-10 minutes as needed

Adults: Initial:

Short surgical procedures: 0.6 mg/kg (range 0.3-1.1 mg/kg)

Long surgical procedures:

Continuous infusion: 2.5-4.3 mg/minute; adjust dose based on response

Intermittent: Initial: 0.3-1.1 mg/kg; maintenance: 0.04-0.07 mg/kg/dose as required

Note: Initial dose of succinylcholine must be increased when nondepolarizing agent pretreatment used because of the antagonism between succinylcholine and nondepolarizing neuromuscular-blocking agents.

Dose adjustment with reduced plasma cholinesterase activity: Administer a test dose of 5-10 mg to evaluate sensitivity, or cautiously administer 1 mg/mL by slow I.V. infusion to produce neuromuscular blockade

Dosing adjustment in hepatic impairment: Dose should be decreased in patients with severe liver disease

Stability Manufacturer recommends refrigeration at 2°C to 8°C (36°F to 46°F) and may be stored at room temperature for 14 days; however, additional testing has demonstrated stability for ≤6 months unrefrigerated (25°C) (Ross, 1988; Roy, 2008). May dilute to a final concentration of 1-2 mg/mL. Do not mix with alkaline solutions (pH >8.5). Stability in polypropylene syringes (20 mg/mL) at room temperature (25°C) is 45 days (Storms, 2003). Stability of parenteral admixture (1-2 mg/mL) at refrigeration temperature (4°C) is 24 hours in D_5W or NS.

◄ **Administration** May be administered by rapid I.V. injection without further dilution. I.M. injections should be made deeply, preferably high into deltoid muscle; use only when I.V. access is not available.

Monitoring Parameters Monitor cardiac, blood pressure, and oxygenation during administration; temperature, serum potassium and calcium, assisted ventilator status; neuromuscular function with a peripheral nerve stimulator

Pregnancy Risk Factor C

Contraindications Hypersensitivity to succinylcholine or any component of the formulation; personal or familial history of malignant hyperthermia; myopathies associated with elevated serum creatine phosphokinase (CPK) values; acute phase of injury following major burns, multiple trauma, extensive denervation of skeletal muscle or upper motor neuron injury

Warnings/Precautions [U.S. Boxed Warning]: Use caution in children and adolescents. Acute rhabdomyolysis with hyperkalemia, ventricular arrhythmias and cardiac arrest have been reported (rarely) in children with undiagnosed skeletal muscle myopathy. Use in children should be reserved for emergency intubation or where immediate airway control is necessary. Use with caution in patients with pre-existing hyperkalemia, extensive or severe burns; severe hyperkalemia may develop in patients with chronic abdominal infections, burn injuries, children with skeletal muscle myopathy, subarachnoid hemorrhage, or conditions which cause degeneration of the nervous system. Alkalosis, hypercalcemia, demyelinating lesions, peripheral neuropathies, denervation, infection, muscle trauma, and diabetes mellitus may result in antagonism of neuromuscular blockade. Electrolyte abnormalities, severe hyponatremia, severe hypocalcemia, severe hypokalemia, hypermagnesemia, neuromuscular diseases, acidosis, acute intermittent porphyria, Eaton-Lambert syndrome, myasthenia gravis, renal failure, and hepatic failure may result in potentiation of neuromuscular blockade. May increase vagal tone.

Succinylcholine is metabolized by plasma cholinesterase; use with caution (if at all) in patients suspected of being homozygous for the atypical plasma cholinesterase gene.

Use with caution in patients with extensive or severe burns; risk of hyperkalemia is increased following injury. May increase intraocular pressure; use caution with narrow angle glaucoma or penetrating eye injuries. Risk of bradycardia may be increased with second dose and may occur more in children. Use may be associated with acute onset of malignant hyperthermia; risk may be increased with concomitant administration of volatile anesthetics. Use with caution in the elderly; effects and duration are more variable.

Maintenance of an adequate airway and respiratory support is critical. Should be administered by adequately trained individuals familiar with its use.

Adverse Reactions
Frequency not defined.
Cardiovascular: Arrhythmias, bradycardia (higher with second dose, more frequent in children), cardiac arrest, hyper-/hypotension, tachycardia
Dermatologic: Rash
Endocrine & metabolic: Hyperkalemia
Gastrointestinal: Salivation (excessive)
Neuromuscular & skeletal: Jaw rigidity, muscle fasciculation, postoperative muscle pain, rhabdomyolysis (with possible myoglobinuric acute renal failure)
Ocular: Intraocular pressure increased
Renal: Acute renal failure (secondary to rhabdomyolysis)
Respiratory: Apnea, respiratory depression (prolonged)
Miscellaneous: Anaphylaxis, malignant hyperthermia
Postmarketing and/or case reports: Acute quadriplegic myopathy syndrome (prolonged use), myositis ossificans (prolonged use)

Drug Interactions

Avoid Concomitant Use
Avoid concomitant use of Succinylcholine with any of the following: QuiNINE

Increased Effect/Toxicity
Succinylcholine may increase the levels/effects of: Analgesics (Opioid); Cardiac Glycosides; OnabotulinumtoxinA; RimabotulinumtoxinB

The levels/effects of Succinylcholine may be increased by: AbobotulinumtoxinA; Acetylcholinesterase Inhibitors; Aminoglycosides; Capreomycin; Colistimethate; Cyclophosphamide; Echothiophate Iodide; Lincosamide Antibiotics; Lithium; Loop Diuretics; Magnesium Salts; Phenelzine; Polymyxin B; Procainamide; QuiNIDine; QuiNINE; Tetracycline Derivatives; Vancomycin

Decreased Effect

The levels/effects of Succinylcholine may be decreased by: Loop Diuretics

Dosage Forms Excipient information presented when available (limited, particularly for generics); consult specific product labeling.

Injection, solution, as chloride:
Anectine®: 20 mg/mL (10 mL):
Quelicin®: 20 mg/mL (10 mL)

Injection, solution, as chloride [preservative free]:
Quelicin®: 100 mg/mL (10 mL)

◆ **Succinylcholine Chloride** *see* Succinylcholine *on page 1326*

Sucralfate (soo KRAL fate)

Medication Safety Issues
Sound-alike/look-alike issues:
Sucralfate may be confused with salsalate
Carafate® may be confused with Cafergot®

U.S. Brand Names Carafate®

Canadian Brand Names Novo-Sucralate; Nu-Sucralate; PMS-Sucralate; Sulcrate®; Sulcrate® Suspension Plus

Index Terms Aluminum Sucrose Sulfate, Basic

Pharmacologic Category Gastrointestinal Agent, Miscellaneous

Generic Available Yes

Use Short-term (≤8 weeks) management of duodenal ulcers; maintenance therapy for duodenal ulcers

Unlabeled/Investigational Use Gastric ulcers; suspension may be used topically for treatment of stomatitis due to cancer chemotherapy and other causes of esophageal and gastric erosions; GERD, esophagitis; treatment of NSAID mucosal damage; prevention of stress ulcers; postsclerotherapy for esophageal variceal bleeding

Mechanism of Action Forms a complex by binding with positively charged proteins in exudates, forming a viscous paste-like, adhesive substance. This selectively forms a protective coating that acts locally to protect the gastric lining against peptic acid, pepsin, and bile salts.

Pharmacodynamics/Kinetics
Onset of action: Paste formation and ulcer adhesion: 1-2 hours
Duration: Up to 6 hours
Absorption: Oral: <5%
Distribution: Acts locally at ulcer sites; unbound in GI tract to aluminum and sucrose octasulfate
Metabolism: None
Excretion: Urine (small amounts as unchanged compounds)

Dosage Oral:
Children (unlabeled use): Doses of 40-80 mg/kg/day divided every 6 hours have been used
Stomatitis (unlabeled use): 5-10 mL (1 g/10 mL suspension), swish and spit or swish and swallow 4 times/day
Adults:
Stress ulcer (unlabeled use):
Prophylaxis: 1 g 4 times/day
Treatment: 1 g every 4 hours
Duodenal ulcer:
Treatment: 1 g 4 times/day on an empty stomach and at bedtime for 4-8 weeks, or alternatively 2 g twice daily; treatment is recommended for 4-8 weeks in adults
Maintenance: Prophylaxis: 1 g twice daily

Stomatitis (unlabeled use): 10 mL (1 g/10 mL suspension), swish and spit or swish and swallow 4 times/day

Dosage comment in renal impairment: Aluminum salt is minimally absorbed (<5%), however, may accumulate in renal failure

Stability Suspension: Shake well. Store at 20°C to 25°C (68°F to 77°F); do **not** freeze.

Administration Tablet may be broken or dissolved in water before ingestion. Administer with water on an empty stomach.

Pregnancy Risk Factor B

Contraindications Hypersensitivity to sucralfate or any component of the formulation

Warnings/Precautions Because sucralfate acts locally at the ulcer site, successful therapy with sucralfate should not be expected to alter the posthealing frequency of recurrence or the severity of duodenal ulceration. Use with caution in patients with chronic renal failure; sucralfate is an aluminum complex, small amounts of aluminum are absorbed following oral administration. Excretion of aluminum may be decreased in patients with chronic renal failure. Because of the potential for sucralfate to alter the absorption of some drugs, separate administration (take other medication 2 hours before sucralfate) should be considered when alterations in bioavailability are believed to be critical. Safety and efficacy have not been established in children.

Adverse Reactions

1% to 10%: Gastrointestinal: Constipation (2%)

<1% (Limited to important or life-threatening): Back pain, bezoar formation, diarrhea, dizziness, flatulence, headache, gastric discomfort; hypersensitivity (urticaria, angioedema, facial swelling, laryngospasm, respiratory difficulty, rhinitis); indigestion, insomnia, nausea, pruritus, rash, sleepiness, vertigo, vomiting, xerostomia

Drug Interactions

Avoid Concomitant Use There are no known interactions where it is recommended to avoid concomitant use.

Increased Effect/Toxicity There are no known significant interactions involving an increase in effect.

Decreased Effect

Sucralfate may decrease the levels/effects of: Antifungal Agents (Azole Derivatives, Systemic); Digoxin; Eltrombopag; Levothyroxine; Phosphate Supplements; QuiNIDine; Quinolone Antibiotics; Tetracycline Derivatives; Vitamin K Antagonists

Ethanol/Nutrition/Herb Interactions Food: Sucralfate may interfere with absorption of vitamin A, vitamin D, vitamin E, and vitamin K.

Dietary Considerations Take with water on an empty stomach.

Dosage Forms Excipient information presented when available (limited, particularly for generics); consult specific product labeling.

Suspension, oral: 1 g/10 mL (10 mL)

Carafate®: 1 g/10 mL (420 mL)

Tablet: 1 g

Carafate®: 1 g

References

Collard HR, Saint S, and Matthay MA, "Prevention of Ventilator-Associated Pneumonia: An Evidence-Based Systematic Review," *Ann Intern Med*, 2003, 138(6):494-501.

Cook D, Guyatt G, Marshall J, et al, "A Comparison of Sucralfate and Ranitidine for the Prevention of Upper Gastrointestinal Bleeding in Patients Requiring Mechanical Ventilation. Canadian Critical Care Trials Group," *N Engl J Med*, 1998, 338(12):791-7.

♦ **Sudafed PE™ [OTC]** *see* Phenylephrine *on page 1114*

♦ **Sufenta®** *see* SUFentanil *on page 1330*

SUFentanil (soo FEN ta nil)

Medication Safety Issues

Sound-alike/look-alike issues:

SUFentanil may be confused with alfentanil, fentaNYL

Sufenta® may be confused with Alfenta®, Sudafed®, Survanta®

High alert medication: The Institute for Safe Medication Practices (ISMP) includes this medication among its list of drugs which have a heightened risk of causing significant patient harm when used in error.

Related Information

Acute Postoperative Pain *on page 1502*

Anesthesia Considerations for Neurosurgery *on page 1514*

Anesthesia for Patients With Liver Disease *on page 1537*

Chronic Pain Management *on page 1546*

Chronic Renal Failure *on page 1552*

Dosing Considerations for the Critically-Ill Patient With Morbid Obesity *on page 1561*

Opioids *on page 1641*

U.S. Brand Names Sufenta®

Canadian Brand Names Sufentanil Citrate Injection, USP; Sufenta®

Index Terms Sufentanil Citrate

Pharmacologic Category Analgesic, Opioid; Anilidopiperidine Opioid; General Anesthetic

Restrictions C-II

Generic Available Yes

Use Analgesic supplement in maintenance of general anesthesia; epidural analgesic in conjunction with a local anesthetic

Mechanism of Action Binds to opioid receptors throughout the CNS. Once receptor binding occurs, effects are exerted by opening K+ channels and inhibiting Ca++ channels. These mechanisms increase pain threshold, alter pain perception, inhibit ascending pain pathways; short-acting narcotic; dose-related inhibition of catecholamine release (up to 30 mcg/kg) controls sympathetic response to surgical stress.

Pharmacodynamics/Kinetics

Onset of action: Analgesia: I.V.: 1-3 minutes; epidural: 10 minutes

Duration: Dose dependent; Epidural:10-15 mcg with bupivacaine: 1.7 hours

Protein binding: Neonates: 79%; Adults: 91% to 93%

Metabolism: Primarily hepatic and small intestine

Half-life elimination: Neonates: 5-10 hours; Infants & Children: 55-139 minutes; Adults: 164 minutes

Excretion: Primarily urine as metabolites (2% excreted as unchanged drug)

Dosage

I.V.:

Children 2-12 years: Induction: 10-25 mcg/kg (10-15 mcg/kg most common dose) with 100% O_2; Maintenance: Up to 1-2 mcg/kg total dose

Adults: Dose should be based on body weight. **Note:** In obese patients (eg, >20% above ideal body weight), use lean body weight to determine dosage.

Surgical analgesia (surgery 1-2 hours long): Total dose: 1-2 mcg/kg; ≥75% of dose administered prior to intubation; administered with N_2O/O_2; Maintenance: 5-20 mcg as needed. Total dose should not exceed 1 mcg/kg/hour of expected surgical time.

Epidural: Adults: Analgesia: Labor and delivery: 10-15 mcg with 10 mL bupivacaine 0.125% with/without epinephrine. May repeat at ≥1-hour interval for 2 additional doses.

Monitoring Parameters Pain relief, respiratory and mental status, blood pressure

Anesthesia and Critical Care Concerns/Other Considerations

Clinical Pearls/Comments: Sufentanil is 5-10 times more potent than fentanyl; it is packaged in the same concentration as fentanyl (50 mcg/mL); keep in mind the differences in potency to prevent overdose with sufentanil. Sufentanil may be diluted to decrease concentration; this will decrease the potential for administering excessive doses. Sufentanil demonstrates synergistic respiratory depression when combined with benzodiazepines.

Pregnancy Risk Factor C/D (prolonged use or high doses at term)

Contraindications Hypersensitivity to sufentanil or any component of the formulation

Warnings/Precautions Sufentanil shares the toxic potentials of opiate agonists, and precautions of opiate agonist therapy should be observed. Use with caution in ▶

◀ patients with bradycardia, head trauma (eg, head injury, intracranial lesions, elevated intracranial pressure), hepatic impairment, or renal impairment. Use with caution in patients with pre-existing respiratory compromise (hypoxia and/or hypercapnia), COPD or other obstructive pulmonary disease, and kyphoscoliosis or other skeletal disorder which may alter respiratory function; critical respiratory depression may occur, even at therapeutic dosages. Use caution in patients who are morbidly obese, debilitated, or elderly. Use caution in neonates as sufentanil clearance is slow much slower than adults; neonates with cardiovascular disease have an even slower clearance. Inject slowly over 3-5 minutes; rapid I.V. infusion may result in skeletal muscle and chest wall rigidity, impaired ventilation, or respiratory distress/arrest; nondepolarizing skeletal muscle relaxant may be required. Due to the high incidence of apnea, hypotension, tachycardia, and muscle rigidity, it should be administered by individuals specifically trained in the use of anesthetic agents and should not be used in diagnostic or therapeutic procedures outside the monitored anesthesia setting; resuscitative and intubation equipment should be readily available.

Adverse Reactions

>10%: Dermatologic: Pruritus (epidural: 25%)

1% to 10%:

Cardiovascular: Bradycardia (dose related; 3% to 9%), hyper-/hypotension (3% to 9%; more common with I.V. administration)

Central nervous system: Somnolence (3% to 9%), CNS depression, confusion

Gastrointestinal: Nausea (3% to 9%), vomiting (3% to 9%)

Neuromuscular & skeletal: Chest wall rigidity (dose related; 3% to 9%)

Ocular: Blurred vision

<1% (Limited to important or life-threatening): Anaphylaxis, apnea, arrhythmia, biliary spasm, bronchospasm, cardiac arrest, chills, circulatory depression; cold, clammy skin; dizziness, dysesthesia, erythema, itching, laryngospasm, mental depression, paradoxical CNS excitation or delirium, physical and psychological dependence with prolonged use, respiratory depression (dose related), seizure, skeletal muscle rigidity, skin rash, tachycardia, urinary retention, urinary tract spasm, urticaria

Drug Interactions

Metabolism/Transport Effects Substrate of CYP3A4 (major)

Avoid Concomitant Use

Avoid concomitant use of SUFentanil with any of the following: MAO Inhibitors

Increased Effect/Toxicity

SUFentanil may increase the levels/effects of: Alcohol (Ethyl); Alvimopan; Beta-Blockers; Calcium Channel Blockers (Nondihydropyridine); CNS Depressants; Desmopressin; MAO Inhibitors; Selective Serotonin Reuptake Inhibitors; Thiazide Diuretics

The levels/effects of SUFentanil may be increased by: Amphetamines; Antipsychotic Agents (Phenothiazines); CYP3A4 Inhibitors (Moderate); CYP3A4 Inhibitors (Strong); Dasatinib; Succinylcholine

Decreased Effect

SUFentanil may decrease the levels/effects of: Pegvisomant

The levels/effects of SUFentanil may be decreased by: Ammonium Chloride

Dosage Forms Excipient information presented when available (limited, particularly for generics); consult specific product labeling.

Injection, solution [preservative free]: 50 mcg/mL (1 mL, 2 mL, 5 mL)

Sufenta®: 50 mcg/mL (1 mL, 2 mL, 5 mL)

References

Bovill JG, Sebel PS, Blackburn CL, et al, "The Pharmacokinetics of Sufentanil in Surgical Patients," *Anesthesiology*, 1984, 61(5):502-6.

Bowdle TA, "Myoclonus Following Sufentanil Without EEG Seizure Activity," *Anesthesiology*, 1987, 67(4):593-5.

Guay J, Gaudreault P, Tang A, et al, "Pharmacokinetics of Sufentanil in Normal Children," *Can J Anaesth*, 1992, 39(1):14-20.

Gust R and Böhrer H, "Stiff-Man Syndrome Associated With Continuous Sufentanil Administration," *Anaesthesia*, 1995, 50(6):575.

Mokhlesi B, Leikin JB, Murray P, et al, "Adult Toxicology in Critical Care. Part 11: Specific Poisonings," *Chest*, 2003, 123(3):897-922.

Rosow CE, "Sufentanil Citrate: A New Opioid Analgesic for Use in Anaesthesia," *Pharmacotherapy*, 1984, 4(1):11-9.

Scholz J, Steinfath M, and Schulz M, "Clinical Pharmacokinetics of Alfentanil, Fentanyl, and Sufentanil. An Update," *Clin Pharmacokinet*, 1996, 31(4):275-92.

Seguin JH, Erenberg A, and Leff RD, "Safety and Efficacy of Sufentanil Therapy in the Ventilated Infant," *Neonatal Netw*, 1994, 13(4):37-40.

◆ **Sufentanil Citrate** *see* SUFentanil *on page 1330*

◆ **Sufentanil Citrate Injection, USP (Can)** *see* SUFentanil *on page 1330*

◆ **Sular®** *see* Nisoldipine *on page 1011*

◆ **Sulbactam and Ampicillin** *see* Ampicillin and Sulbactam *on page 118*

◆ **Sulcrate® (Can)** *see* Sucralfate *on page 1329*

◆ **Sulcrate® Suspension Plus (Can)** *see* Sucralfate *on page 1329*

Sulfamethoxazole and Trimethoprim
(sul fa meth OKS a zole & trye METH oh prim)

U.S. Brand Names Bactrim™; Bactrim™ DS; Septra®; Septra® DS; Sulfatrim®

Canadian Brand Names Apo-Sulfatrim®; Apo-Sulfatrim® DS; Apo-Sulfatrim® Pediatric; Novo-Trimel; Novo-Trimel D.S.; Nu-Cotrimox; Septra® Injection

Index Terms Co-Trimoxazole; SMZ-TMP; Sulfatrim; TMP-SMZ; Trimethoprim and Sulfamethoxazole

Pharmacologic Category Antibiotic, Miscellaneous; Antibiotic, Sulfonamide Derivative

Use

Oral treatment of urinary tract infections due to *E. coli*, *Klebsiella* and *Enterobacter* sp, *M. morganii*, *P. mirabilis* and *P. vulgaris*; acute otitis media in children; acute exacerbations of chronic bronchitis in adults due to susceptible strains of *H. influenzae* or *S. pneumoniae*; treatment and prophylaxis of *Pneumocystis jiroveci* pneumonitis (PCP); traveler's diarrhea due to enterotoxigenic *E. coli*; treatment of enteritis caused by *Shigella flexneri* or *Shigella sonnei*

I.V. treatment or severe or complicated infections when oral therapy is not feasible, for documented PCP, empiric treatment of PCP in immune compromised patients; treatment of documented or suspected shigellosis, typhoid fever, *Nocardia asteroides* infection, or other infections caused by susceptible bacteria

Unlabeled/Investigational Use Cholera and *Salmonella*-type infections and nocardiosis; chronic prostatitis; as prophylaxis in neutropenic patients with *P. jiroveci* infections, in leukemia patients, and in patients following renal transplantation, to decrease incidence of PCP; treatment of *Cyclospora* infection, typhoid fever, *Nocardia asteroides* infection; prophylaxis against urinary tract infection; skin/soft tissue infections due to community-acquired MRSA

Pharmacodynamics/Kinetics

Absorption: Oral: Almost completely, 90% to 100%

Protein binding: SMX: 68%, TMP: 45%

Metabolism: SMX: N-acetylated and glucuronidated; TMP: Metabolized to oxide and hydroxylated metabolites

Half-life elimination: SMX: 9 hours, TMP: 6-17 hours; both are prolonged in renal failure

Time to peak, serum: Within 1-4 hours

Excretion: Both are excreted in urine as metabolites and unchanged drug

Effects of aging on the pharmacokinetics of both agents has been variable; increase in half-life and decreases in clearance have been associated with reduced creatinine clearance

Dosage Dosage recommendations are based on the trimethoprim component. double strength tablets are equivalent to sulfamethoxazole 800 mg and trimethoprim 160 mg.

Usual dosage ranges:

Children >2 months:

Mild-to-moderate infections: Oral: 8-12 mg TMP/kg/day in divided doses every 12 hours

Serious infection:

Oral: 20 mg TMP/kg/day in divided doses every 6 hours

I.V.: 8-12 mg TMP/kg/day in divided doses every 6 hours

Adults:
Oral: One double strength tablet (sulfamethoxazole 800 mg; trimethoprim 160 mg) every 12-24 hours
I.V.: 8-20 mg TMP/kg/day divided every 6-12 hours

Indication-specific dosing:

Children >2 months:

Acute otitis media: Oral: 8 mg TMP/kg/day in divided doses every 12 hours for 10 days. **Note:** Recommended by the American Academy of Pediatrics as an alternative agent in penicillin-allergic patients at a dose of 6-10 mg TMP/kg/day (AOM guidelines, 2004).

Cyclospora **(unlabeled use):** Oral, I.V.: 5 mg TMP/kg twice daily for 7-10 days

Pneumocystis jiroveci:
Treatment: Oral, I.V.: 15-20 mg TMP/kg/day in divided doses every 6-8 hours
Prophylaxis: Oral, 150 mg TMP/m^2/day in divided doses every 12 hours for 3 days/week; dose should not exceed trimethoprim 320 mg and sulfamethoxazole 1600 mg daily
Alternative prophylaxis dosing schedules include:
150 mg TMP/m^2/day as a single daily dose 3 times/week on consecutive days
or
150 mg TMP/m^2/day in divided doses every 12 hours administered 7 days/week
or
150 mg TMP/m^2/day in divided doses every 12 hours administered 3 times/week on alternate days

Shigellosis:
Oral: 8 mg TMP/kg/day in divided doses every 12 hours for 5 days
I.V.: 8-10 mg TMP/kg/day in divided doses every 6, 8, or 12 hours for up to 5 days

Urinary tract infection:
Treatment:
Oral: 6-12 mg TMP/kg/day in divided doses every 12 hours
I.V.: 8-10 mg TMP/kg/day in divided doses every 6, 8, or 12 hours for up to 14 days with serious infections
Prophylaxis: Oral: 2 mg TMP/kg/dose daily or 5 mg TMP/kg/dose twice weekly

Adults:

Chronic bronchitis (acute): Oral: One double strength tablet every 12 hours for 10-14 days

Cyclospora (unlabeled use): Oral, I.V.: 160 mg TMP twice daily for 7-10 days. **Note:** AIDS patients: Oral: One double strength tablet 2-4 times/day for 10 days, then 1 double strength tablet 3 times/week for 10 weeks (Pape, 1994; Verdier, 2000).

Meningitis (bacterial): I.V.: 10-20 mg TMP/kg/day in divided doses every 6-12 hours

Nocardia (unlabeled use): Oral, I.V.:
Cutaneous infections: 5-10 mg TMP/kg/day in 2-4 divided doses
Severe infections (pulmonary/cerebral): 15 mg TMP/kg/day in 2-4 divided doses for 3-4 weeks, then 10 mg TMP/kg/day in 2-4 divided doses. Treatment duration is controversial; an average of 7 months has been reported.
Note: Therapy for severe infection may be initiated I.V. and converted to oral therapy (frequently converted to approximate dosages of oral solid dosage forms: 2 DS tablets every 8-12 hours). Although not widely available, sulfonamide levels should be considered in patients with questionable absorption, at risk for dose-related toxicity, or those with poor therapeutic response.

Pneumocystis jiroveci:
Prophylaxis: Oral: One double strength tablet daily or 3 times/week
Treatment: Oral, I.V.: 15-20 mg TMP/kg/day in 3-4 divided doses

Sepsis: I.V.: 20 TMP/kg/day divided every 6 hours

Shigellosis:
Oral: One double strength tablet every 12 hours for 5 days
I.V.: 8-10 mg TMP/kg/day in divided doses every 6, 8, or 12 hours for up to 5 days

Skin/soft tissue infection due to community-acquired MRSA (unlabeled use): Oral: 1-2 double strength tablets every 12 hours (Stevens, 2005)

Travelers' diarrhea: Oral: One double strength tablet every 12 hours for 5 days

Urinary tract infection:

Oral: One double strength tablet every 12 hours
Duration of therapy: Uncomplicated: 3-5 days; Complicated: 7-10 days
Pyelonephritis: 14 days
Prostatitis: Acute: 2 weeks; Chronic: 2-3 months
I.V.: 8-10 mg TMP/kg/day in divided doses every 6, 8, or 12 hours for up to 14 days with severe infections

Dosing adjustment in renal impairment: Oral, I.V.:
Cl_{cr} 15-30 mL/minute: Administer 50% of recommended dose
Cl_{cr} <15 mL/minute: Use is not recommended

Additional Information Complete prescribing information for this medication should be consulted for additional detail.

Dosage Forms Excipient information presented when available (limited, particularly for generics); consult specific product labeling. **Note:** The 5:1 ratio (SMX:TMP) remains constant in all dosage forms.

Injection, solution: Sulfamethoxazole 80 mg and trimethoprim 16 mg per mL (5 mL, 10 mL, 30 mL) [contains benzyl alcohol, ethanol 12.2%, propylene glycol 400 mg/mL, sodium metabisulfite]

Suspension, oral: Sulfamethoxazole 200 mg and trimethoprim 40 mg per 5 mL (480 mL)
Sulfatrim®: Sulfamethoxazole 200 mg and trimethoprim 40 mg per 5 mL (100 mL, 480 mL) [contains alcohol ≤0.5% propylene glycol; cherry flavor]

Tablet: Sulfamethoxazole 400 mg and trimethoprim 80 mg
Bactrim™: Sulfamethoxazole 400 mg and trimethoprim 80 mg
Septra®: Sulfamethoxazole 400 mg and trimethoprim 80 mg

Tablet, double strength: Sulfamethoxazole 800 mg and trimethoprim 160 mg
Bactrim™ DS: Sulfamethoxazole 800 mg and trimethoprim 160 mg
Septra® DS: Sulfamethoxazole 800 mg and trimethoprim 160 mg

References

Gilbert DN, Moellering RC, Eliopoulos GM, et al, eds, *The Sanford Guide To Antimicrobial Therapy,* 2006, 36th ed, Hyde Park, VT: Antimicrobial Therapy, Inc, 2006, 6-7.
Tunkel AR, Hartman BJ, Kaplan SL, et al, "Practice Guidelines for the Management of Bacterial Meningitis," *Clin Infect Dis,* 2004, 39(9):1267-84.

♦ **Sulfamylon®** *see* Mafenide *on page 861*

♦ **Sulfatrim** *see* Sulfamethoxazole and Trimethoprim *on page 1333*

♦ **Sulfatrim®** *see* Sulfamethoxazole and Trimethoprim *on page 1333*

Sulindac (SUL in dak)

Related Information

Acetaminophen and NSAIDS, Dosing in the Management of Pain *on page 1651*
Nonsteroidal Anti-Inflammatory Agents *on page 1687*

U.S. Brand Names Clinoril®

Canadian Brand Names Apo-Sulin®; Novo-Sundac; Nu-Sundac

Pharmacologic Category Nonsteroidal Anti-inflammatory Drug (NSAID), Oral

Use Management of inflammatory diseases including osteoarthritis, rheumatoid arthritis, acute gouty arthritis, ankylosing spondylitis, acute painful shoulder (bursitis/tendonitis)

Unlabeled/Investigational Use Management of preterm labor

Pharmacodynamics/Kinetics

Absorption: 90%

Distribution: Crosses blood-brain barrier (brain concentrations <4% of plasma concentrations)

Protein binding: Sulindac: 93%, sulfone metabolite: 95%, sulfide metabolite: 98%; primarily to albumin

Metabolism: Hepatic; prodrug metabolized to sulfide metabolite (active) for therapeutic effects and to sulfone metabolites (inactive); parent and inactive sulfone metabolite undergo extensive enterohepatic recirculation

Half-life elimination: Sulindac: ~8 hours; Sulfide metabolite: ~16 hours

◀ Time to peak: Sulindac: 3-4 hours; Sulfide and sulfone metabolites: 5-6 hours
Excretion: Urine (~50%, primarily as inactive metabolites, <1% as active metabolite); feces (~25%, primarily as metabolites)

Dosage Oral:

Children: Dose not established

Adults: **Note:** Maximum daily dose: 400 mg

Osteoarthritis, rheumatoid arthritis, ankylosing spondylitis: 150 mg twice daily

Acute painful shoulder (bursitis/tendonitis): 200 mg twice daily; usual treatment: 7-14 days

Acute gouty arthritis: 200 mg twice daily; usual treatment: 7 days

Dosing adjustment in renal impairment: Not recommended with advanced renal impairment; if required, decrease dose and monitor closely

Dosing adjustment in hepatic impairment: Dose reduction is necessary; discontinue if abnormal liver function tests occur

Anesthesia and Critical Care Concerns/Other Considerations The 2002 ACCM/SCCM guidelines for analgesia (critically-ill adult) suggest that NSAIDs may be used in combination with opioids in select patients for pain management. Concern about adverse events (increased risk of renal dysfunction, altered platelet function and gastrointestinal irritation) limits its use in patients who have other underlying risks for these events.

In short-term use, NSAIDs vary considerably in their effect on blood pressure. When NSAIDs are used in patients with hypertension, appropriate monitoring of blood pressure responses should be completed and the duration of therapy, when possible, kept short. The use of NSAIDs in the treatment of patients with congestive heart failure may be associated with an increased risk for fluid accumulation and edema; may precipitate renal failure in dehydrated patients.

Sulindac is associated with the highest incidence of upper GI bleeds among NSAIDs. It may be less likely to inhibit renal prostaglandin synthesis and adversely affect renal function than most other NSAIDs. Maximum therapeutic response may not be realized for up to 3 weeks.

Additional Information Complete prescribing information for this medication should be consulted for additional detail.

Dosage Forms Excipient information presented when available (limited, particularly for generics); consult specific product labeling.

Tablet: 150 mg, 200 mg

Clinoril®: 200 mg

SUMAtriptan (soo ma TRIP tan)

U.S. Brand Names Imitrex®

Canadian Brand Names Apo-Sumatriptan®; CO Sumatriptan; Dom-Sumatriptan; Gen-Sumatriptan; Imitrex®; Imitrex® DF; Imitrex® Nasal Spray; Mylan-Sumatriptan; Novo-Sumatriptan; PHL-Sumatriptan; PMS-Sumatriptan; ratio-Sumatriptan; Rhoxal-sumatriptan; Riva-Sumatriptan; Sandoz-Sumatriptan; Sumatryx

Index Terms Sumatriptan Succinate

Pharmacologic Category Antimigraine Agent; Serotonin 5-HT$_{1B, 1D}$ Receptor Agonist

Use

Oral, SubQ: Acute treatment of migraine with or without aura

SubQ: Acute treatment of cluster headache episodes

Pharmacodynamics/Kinetics

Onset of action: ~30 minutes

Distribution: V_d: 2.4 L/kg

Protein binding: 14% to 21%

Metabolism: Hepatic, primarily via MAO-A isoenzyme

Bioavailability: SubQ: 97% ± 16% of that following I.V. injection; Oral: 15%

Half-life elimination: Injection, tablet: 2.5 hours; Nasal spray: 2 hours

Time to peak, serum: 5-20 minutes

Excretion:

Injection: Urine (38% as indole acetic acid metabolite, 22% as unchanged drug)

Nasal spray: Urine (42% as indole acetic acid metabolite, 3% as unchanged drug)

Tablet: Urine (60% as indole acetic acid metabolite, 3% as unchanged drug); feces (40%)

Dosage Adults:

Oral: A single dose of 25 mg, 50 mg, or 100 mg (taken with fluids). If a satisfactory response has not been obtained at 2 hours, a second dose may be administered. Results from clinical trials show that initial doses of 50 mg and 100 mg are more effective than doses of 25 mg, and that 100 mg doses do not provide a greater effect than 50 mg and may have increased incidence of side effects. Although doses of up to 300 mg/day have been studied, the total daily dose should not exceed 200 mg. The safety of treating an average of >4 headaches in a 30-day period have not been established.

Intranasal: A single dose of 5 mg, 10 mg, or 20 mg administered in one nostril. A 10 mg dose may be achieved by administering a single 5 mg dose in each nostril. If headache returns, the dose may be repeated once after 2 hours, not to exceed a total daily dose of 40 mg. The safety of treating an average of >4 headaches in a 30-day period has not been established.

SubQ: Up to 6 mg; if side effects are dose-limiting, lower doses may be used. A second injection may be administered at least 1 hour after the initial dose, but not more than 2 injections in a 24-hour period.

Dosage adjustment in renal impairment: Dosage adjustment not necessary

Dosage adjustment in hepatic impairment: Bioavailability of oral sumatriptan is increased with liver disease. If treatment is needed, do not exceed single doses of 50 mg. The nasal spray has not been studied in patients with hepatic impairment, however, because the spray does not undergo first-pass metabolism, levels would not be expected to alter. Use of all dosage forms is contraindicated with severe hepatic impairment.

Anesthesia and Critical Care Concerns/Other Considerations

Clincal!Pearls/Comments: Sumatriptan should not be used in patients with a history of vasospastic disease, Prinzmetal's angina, or any critical vascular disease.

Additional Information Complete prescribing information for this medication should be consulted for additional detail.

Dosage Forms Excipient information presented when available (limited, particularly for generics); consult specific product labeling. **Note:** Strength expressed as sumatriptan base

Injection, solution, as succinate: 8 mg/mL (0.5 mL); 12 mg/mL (0.5 mL)

Imitrex®: 8 mg/mL (0.5 mL); 12 mg/mL (0.5 mL)

Solution, intranasal [spray]: 5 mg/0.1 mL (6s); 20 mg/0.1 mL (6s)

Imitrex®: 5 mg/0.1 mL (6s); 20 mg/0.1 mL (6s)

Tablet, as succinate: 25 mg, 50 mg, 100 mg

Imitrex®: 25 mg, 50 mg, 100 mg

- **Synphasic® (Can)** *see* Ethinyl Estradiol and Norethindrone *on page* *554*
- **Synthroid®** *see* Levothyroxine *on page* *831*
- **Syntocinon® (Can)** *see* Oxytocin *on page* *1077*
- **Syrex** *see* Sodium Chloride *on page* *1304*
- **T_3 Sodium (error-prone abbreviation)** *see* Liothyronine *on page* *846*
- **T_4** *see* Levothyroxine *on page* *831*
- **642® Tablet (Can)** *see* Propoxyphene *on page* *1194*

Tacrolimus (ta KROE li mus)

Medication Safety Issues

Sound-alike/look-alike issues:

Prograf® may be confused with Gengraf®, Prozac®

Tacrolimus may be confused with everolimus, pimecrolimus, sirolimus, temsirolimus

Medication Guide An FDA-approved patient medication guide, which is available with the product information and at http://www.fda.gov/downloads/Drugs/DrugSafety/ucm088996.pdf, must be dispensed with this medication for each new outpatient prescription and refill.

U.S. Brand Names Prograf®; Protopic®

Canadian Brand Names Advagraf™; Prograf®; Protopic®

Index Terms FK506

Pharmacologic Category Calcineurin Inhibitor; Immunosuppressant Agent; Topical Skin Product

Generic Available Yes: Capsule

Use

Oral/injection: Prevention of organ rejection in heart, kidney, or liver transplant recipients

Topical: Moderate-to-severe atopic dermatitis in patients not responsive to conventional therapy or when conventional therapy is not appropriate

Unlabeled/Investigational Use Prevention of organ rejection in lung, small bowel transplant recipients; prevention and treatment of graft-versus-host disease (GVHD) in allogenic hematopoietic stem cell transplantation

Mechanism of Action Suppresses cellular immunity (inhibits T-lymphocyte activation), by binding to an intracellular protein, FKBP-12 and complexes with calcineurin dependant proteins to inhibit calcineurin phosphatase activity

Pharmacodynamics/Kinetics

Absorption: Better in resected patients with a closed stoma; unlike cyclosporine, clamping of the T-tube in liver transplant patients does not alter trough concentrations or AUC

Oral: Incomplete and variable; the rate and extent of absorption is affected by food and may be most pronounced with a high-fat meal

Topical: Minimally absorbed; serum concentrations range from undetectable to 20 ng/mL (~2 ng/mL in majority of adult patients studied)

Distribution: V_d: Children: 0.5-4.7 L/kg; Adults: 0.55-2.47 L/kg

Protein binding: 99% primarily to albumin and alpha$_1$-acid glycoprotein glycoprotein

Metabolism: Extensively hepatic via CYP3A4 to eight possible metabolites (major metabolite, 31-demethyl tacrolimus, shows same activity as tacrolimus *in vitro*)

Bioavailability: Oral: Children: 7% to 55%, Adults: 7% to 32%; Topical: <0.5%; Absolute: Unknown

Half-life elimination: Variable, 23-46 hours in healthy volunteers; 2.1-36 hours in transplant patients

Time to peak: 0.5-6 hours

Excretion: Feces (~93%); urine (<2% as unchanged drug)

Dosage

Oral:

Prevention of organ rejection in transplant recipients: The initial dose of tacrolimus should begin no sooner than 6 hours post-transplant; adjunctive therapy with corticosteroids is recommended early post-transplant. I.V. route should only be used in patients not able to take oral medications and continued only until oral medication can be tolerated; anaphylaxis has been reported with I.V. administration. If switching from I.V. to oral, the oral dose should be started 8-12 hours after stopping the infusion.

Children: Patients without pre-existing renal or hepatic dysfunction have required (and tolerated) higher doses than adults to achieve similar blood concentrations. It is recommended that therapy be initiated at **high end** of the recommended adult I.V. and oral dosing ranges; dosage adjustments may be required.

Liver transplant: Initial dose: 0.15-0.20 mg/kg/day in 2 divided doses, given every 12 hours

Adults:

Heart transplant: Initial dose: 0.075 mg/kg/day in 2 divided doses, given every 12 hours. Use in combination with azathioprine or mycophenolate mofetil is recommended.

Kidney transplant: Initial dose: 0.2 mg/kg/day in combination with azathioprine **or** 0.1 mg/kg/day in combination with mycophenolate mofetil. Administer in 2 divided doses, given every 12 hours; initial dose may be given within 24 hours of transplant, but should be delayed until renal function has recovered; African-American patients may require larger doses to maintain trough concentration.

Liver transplant: Initial dose: 0.1-0.15 mg/kg/day in 2 divided doses, given every 12 hours

Prevention of graft-versus-host disease (unlabeled use): Children and Adults: Convert from I.V. to oral dose (1:4 ratio): Multiply total daily I.V. dose times 4 and administer in 2 divided oral doses per day, every 12 hours (Uberti, 1999; Yanik, 2000).

Treatment of graft-versus-host disease (unlabeled use): Adults: 0.06 mg/kg twice daily (Furlong, 2000; Przepiorka, 1999)

I.V.:

Prevention of organ rejection in transplant recipients: The initial dose of tacrolimus should begin no sooner than 6 hours post-transplant; adjunctive therapy with corticosteroids is recommended early post-transplant. I.V. route should only be used in patients not able to take oral medications and continued only until oral medication can be tolerated; anaphylaxis has been reported with I.V. administration. If switching from I.V. to oral, the oral dose should be started 8-12 hours after stopping the infusion.

Children: It is recommended that therapy be initiated at the **high end** of the dosing range.

Liver transplant: Initial dose: 0.03-0.05 mg/kg/day as a continuous infusion

Adults: It is recommended that therapy be initiated at the **lower end** of the dosing range.

Heart transplant: Initial dose: 0.01 mg/kg/day as a continuous infusion. Use in combination with azathioprine or mycophenolate mofetil is recommended.

Kidney transplant: Initial dose: 0.03-0.05 mg/kg/day as a continuous infusion. Use in combination with azathioprine or mycophenolate mofetil is recommended.

Liver transplant: Initial dose: 0.03-0.05 mg/kg/day as a continuous infusion.

Prevention of graft-versus-host disease (unlabeled use): Children and Adults: Initial: 0.03 mg/kg/day (based on lean body weight) as continuous infusion. Treatment should begin at least 24 hours prior to stem cell infusion and continued only until oral medication can be tolerated (Przepiorka, 1999; Yanik, 2000).

Treatment of graft-versus-host disease (unlabeled use): Adults: Initial: 0.03 mg/kg/day (based on lean body weight) as continuous infusion (Furlong, 2000; Przepiorka, 1999)

Topical:

Atopic dermatitis (moderate-to-severe):

Children ≥2 years: Apply minimum amount of 0.03% ointment to affected area twice daily; rub in gently and completely. Discontinue use when symptoms have cleared. If no improvement within 6 weeks, patients should be re-examined to confirm diagnosis.

Adults: Apply minimum amount of 0.03% or 0.1% ointment to affected area twice daily; rub in gently and completely. Discontinue use when symptoms have cleared. If no improvement within 6 weeks, patients should be re-examined to confirm diagnosis.

Dosing adjustment in renal impairment: Systemic therapy: Evidence suggests that lower doses should be used; patients should receive doses at the lowest value of the recommended I.V. and oral dosing ranges; further reductions in dose below these ranges may be required.

Tacrolimus therapy should usually be delayed up to 48 hours or longer in patients with postoperative oliguria.

Hemodialysis: Not removed by hemodialysis; supplemental dose is not necessary.

Peritoneal dialysis: Significant drug removal is unlikely based on physiochemical characteristics.

Dosing adjustment in hepatic impairment: Systemic therapy: Use of tacrolimus in liver transplant recipients experiencing post-transplant hepatic impairment may be associated with increased risk of developing renal insufficiency related to high whole blood levels of tacrolimus. The presence of moderate-to-severe hepatic dysfunction (serum bilirubin >2 mg/dL; Child-Pugh score ≥10) appears to affect the metabolism of tacrolimus. The half-life of the drug was prolonged and the clearance reduced after I.V. administration. The bioavailability of tacrolimus was also increased after oral administration. The higher plasma concentrations as determined by ELISA, in patients with severe hepatic dysfunction are probably due to the accumulation of metabolites of lower activity. These patients should be monitored closely and dosage adjustments should be considered. Some evidence indicates that lower doses could be used in these patients.

Stability

Injection: Prior to dilution, store at 5°C to 25°C (41°F to 77°F). Following dilution, stable for 24 hours in D_5W or NS in glass or polyethylene containers. Dilute with 5% dextrose injection or 0.9% sodium chloride injection to a final concentration between 0.004 mg/mL and 0.02 mg/mL.

Capsules and ointment: Store at room temperature of 25°C (77°F); excursions permitted to 15°C to 30°C (59°F to 86°F).

Administration

I.V.: If I.V. administration is necessary, administer by continuous infusion only. Do not use PVC tubing when administering diluted solutions. Tacrolimus is usually intended to be administered as a continuous infusion over 24 hours. Do not mix with solutions with a pH ≥9 (eg, acyclovir or ganciclovir) due to chemical degradation of tacrolimus (use different ports in multilumen lines). Do not alter dose with concurrent T-tube clamping. Adsorption of the drug to PVC tubing may become clinically significant with low concentrations.

Oral: Administer on an empty stomach; be consistent with timing and composition of meals if GI intolerance occurs and administration with food becomes necessary (per manufacturer). If dosed once daily (not common), administer in the morning. If dosed twice daily, doses should be 12 hours apart. If the morning and evening doses differ, the larger dose (differences are never >0.5-1 mg) should be given in the morning. If dosed 3 times/day, separate doses by 8 hours.

Topical: Do not use with occlusive dressings. Burning at the application site is most common in first few days; improves as atopic dermatitis improves. Limit application to involved areas. Continue as long as signs and symptoms persist; discontinue if resolution occurs; re-evaluate if symptoms persist >6 weeks.

Monitoring Parameters Renal function, hepatic function, serum electrolytes (especially potassium), glucose and blood pressure, measure 3 times/week for first few weeks, then gradually decrease frequency as patient stabilizes. Whole blood concentrations should be used for monitoring (trough for oral therapy). Signs/symptoms of anaphylactic reactions during infusion should also be monitored. Patients should be monitored during the first 30 minutes of the infusion, and frequently thereafter.

Reference Range

Heart: Typical whole blood trough concentrations:

Months 1-3: 10-20 ng/mL

Months ≥4: 5-15 ng/mL

Kidney transplant: Whole blood trough concentrations:
  In combination with azathioprine:
    Months 1-3: 7-20 ng/mL
    Months 4-12: 5-15 ng/mL
  In combination with mycophenolate mofetil/IL-2 receptor antagonist (eg, daclizumab): Months 1-2: 4-11 ng/mL
Liver transplant: Whole blood trough concentrations: Months 1-12: 5-20 ng/mL
Prevention of graft-versus-host disease (unlabeled use): 10-20 ng/mL (Uberti, 1999) although some institutions use a lower limit of 5 ng/mL and an upper limit of 15 ng/mL (Przepiorka, 1999; Yanik, 2000)

Anesthesia and Critical Care Concerns/Other Considerations

Clinical Pearls/Comments: Additional dosing considerations:
  Switch from I.V. to oral therapy: initiate oral therapy 8-12 hours after discontinuation of I.V.

Tacrolimus is associated with more neurotoxicity, nephrotoxicity, and glucose intolerance but less hypertension, dyslipidemia, gingival hyperplasia, or hirsutism than cyclosporine.

Pregnancy Risk Factor C

Contraindications Hypersensitivity to tacrolimus or any component of the formulation

Warnings/Precautions

Oral/injection: [U.S. Boxed Warning]: Increased susceptibility to infection and the possible development of lymphoma may result from immunosuppression with tacrolimus. The risk of developing other malignancies may also be increased. Insulin-dependent post-transplant diabetes mellitus (PTDM) has been reported including in patients without pretransplant history of diabetes mellitus; risk increases in African-American and Hispanic kidney transplant patients. Posterior reversible encephalopathy syndrome (PRES) may occur with therapy; symptoms are reversible with dose reduction or discontinuation of immunosuppressant therapy; stabilize blood pressure and reduce dose with suspected or confirmed diagnosis. Nephrotoxicity has has been reported, especially with higher doses; to avoid excess nephrotoxicity do not administer simultaneously with other nephrotoxic drugs (eg sirolimus, cyclosporine). Neurotoxicity may occur especially when used in high doses; tremor headache, coma and delirium have been reported and are associated with serum concentrations. Seizures may also occur. Monitoring of serum concentrations (trough for oral therapy) is essential to prevent organ rejection and reduce drug-related toxicity. Variable absorption is seen in bone marrow transplantation relative to total body radiation and/or methotrexate use. A period of ≥24 hours should elapse between discontinuation of cyclosporine and the initiation of tacrolimus. Delay initiation further with persistently elevated tacrolimus/cyclosporine levels. Use caution in renal or hepatic dysfunction, dosing adjustments may be required. Delay initiation if postoperative oliguria occurs. Use may be associated with the development of hypertension (common); hyperkalemia has been reported; avoid use of potassium-sparing diuretics. Myocardial hypertrophy has been reported (rare). Each mL of injection contains polyoxyl 60 hydrogenated castor oil (HCO-60) (200 mg) and dehydrated alcohol USP 80% v/v. Anaphylaxis has been reported with the injection, use should be reserved for those patients not able to take oral medications. **[U.S. Boxed Warning]: Should be administered under the supervision of a physician experienced in immunosuppressive therapy and organ transplantation in a facility appropriate for monitoring and managing therapy.**

Topical: [U.S. Boxed Warning]: Topical calcineurin inhibitors have been associated with rare cases of malignancy (including skin and lymphoma), therefore it should be limited to short-term and intermittent treatment using the minimum amount necessary for the control of symptoms and only on involved areas. Use in children <2 years of age is not recommended, children ages 2-15 should only use the 0.03% ointment. Avoid use on malignant or premalignant skin conditions (eg cutaneous T-cell lymphoma). Should not be used in immunocompromised patients. Do not apply to areas of active bacterial or viral infection; infections at the treatment site should be cleared prior to therapy. Topical calcineurin agents are considered second-line therapies in the treatment of atopic dermatitis/eczema, and should be limited to use in patients who have failed treatment with other therapies. Patients with atopic dermatitis are predisposed to skin infections, and tacrolimus therapy has been associated with risk of developing eczema herpeticum, varicella zoster, and herpes simplex. If atopic dermatitis is not improved in <6 weeks, re-evaluate to confirm diagnosis. May be associated with development of lymphadenopathy; possible infectious causes should be investigated. Discontinue use in patients with unknown cause of lymphadenopathy or acute infectious mononucleosis. Acute renal failure has been observed (rarely) with topical use. Not recommended for use in patients with skin disease which may increase systemic absorption (eg, Netherton's syndrome). Minimize sunlight exposure during treatment. Safety not established in patients with generalized erythroderma. Safety of intermittent use for >1 year has not been established, particularly since the effect on immune system development is unknown.

Adverse Reactions As reported for kidney, liver, and heart transplantation:

Oral, I.V.:

≥15%:

Cardiovascular: Hypertension (13% to 62%), edema (peripheral 11% to 36%), chest pain (19%), edema (18%), pericardial effusion (heart transplant 15%)

Central nervous system: Headache (25% to 64%), insomnia (30% to 64%), pain (24% to 63%), fever (19% to 48%), postprocedural pain (kidney transplant 29%), dizziness (19%)

Dermatologic: Pruritus (15% to 36%), rash (10% to 24%)

Endocrine & metabolic: Hypophosphatemia (28% to 49%), hypomagnesemia (16% to 48%), hyperglycemia (21% to 47%), hyperkalemia (8% to 45%), hyperlipemia (10% to 31%), hypokalemia (13% to 29%), diabetes mellitus (24% to 26%)

Gastrointestinal: Diarrhea (24% to 72%), abdominal pain (29% to 59%), nausea (32% to 46%), constipation (23% to 36%), anorexia (7% to 34%), vomiting (14% to 29%), dyspepsia (18% to 28%)

Genitourinary: Urinary tract infection (16% to 34%)

Hematologic: Anemia (5% to 50%), leukopenia (13% to 48%), leukocytosis (8% to 32%), thrombocytopenia (14% to 24%)

Hepatic: Liver function tests abnormal (6% to 36%), ascites (7% to 27%)

Local: Incision site complication (kidney transplant 28%)

Neuromuscular & skeletal: Tremor (34% to 56%; heart transplant 15%), weakness (11% to 52%), paresthesia (17% to 40%), back pain (17% to 30%), arthralgia (25%)

Renal: Abnormal kidney function (36% to 56%), creatinine increased (23% to 45%), BUN increased (12% to 30%), oliguria (18% to 19%)

Respiratory: Atelectasis (5% to 28%), pleural effusion (30% to 36%), dyspnea (5% to 29%), cough increased (18%), bronchitis (17%)

Miscellaneous: Infection (24% to 45%), CMV infection (32%), graft dysfunction (kidney transplant 24%)

<15%:

Cardiovascular: Abnormal ECG (QRS or ST segment abnormal), arrhythmia, atrial fibrillation, atrial flutter, bradycardia, cardiopulmonary failure, deep thrombophlebitis, heart failure, heart rate decreased, hemorrhage, hemorrhagic stroke, hypervolemia, hypotension, peripheral vascular disorder, phlebitis, postural hypotension, syncope, tachycardia, thrombosis, vasodilation, ventricular fibrillation

Central nervous system: Abnormal dreams, abnormal thinking, agitation, amnesia, anxiety, chills, confusion, depression, emotional lability, encephalopathy, flaccid paralysis, hallucinations, mood elevated, nervousness, psychosis, quadriparesis, seizure, somnolence

Dermatologic: Acne, alopecia, bruising, cellulitis, exfoliative dermatitis, fungal dermatitis, hirsutism, photosensitivity reaction, skin discoloration, skin disorder, skin neoplasm, skin ulcer, wound healing impaired

Endocrine & metabolic: Acidosis, alkalosis, bicarbonate decreased, Cushing's syndrome, dehydration, gout, hypercholesterolemia, hyper-/hypocalcemia, hyperphosphatemia, hyperuricemia, hypoproteinemia, serum iron decreased

Gastrointestinal: Appetite increased, cramps, duodenitis, dysphagia, enlarged abdomen, esophagitis (including ulcerative), flatulence, gastritis, gastroesophagitis, GI perforation/hemorrhage, ileus, oral moniliasis, pancreatic pseudocyst, rectal disorder, stomatitis, weight gain

Genitourinary: Bladder spasm, cystitis, dysuria, nocturia, urge incontinence, urinary frequency, urinary incontinence, urinary retention, vaginitis

Hematologic: Coagulation disorder, decreased prothrombin, hypochromic anemia, polycythemia

Hepatic: Alkaline phosphatase increased, bilirubinemia, cholangitis, cholestatic jaundice, GGT increased, hepatitis (including granulomatous), jaundice, LDH increased, liver damage

Local: Phlebitis

Neuromuscular & skeletal: Hypertonia, incoordination, joint disorder, leg cramps, myalgia, myasthenia, myoclonus, nerve compression, neuropathy, osteoporosis

Ocular: Abnormal vision, amblyopia

Otic: Ear pain, otitis media, tinnitus

Renal: Acute renal failure, albuminuria, BK nephropathy, hematuria, hydronephrosis, renal tubular necrosis, toxic nephropathy

Respiratory: Asthma, lung disorder, pharyngitis, pneumonia, pneumothorax, pulmonary edema, respiratory disorder, rhinitis, sinusitis, voice alteration

Miscellaneous: Abscess, abnormal healing, allergic reaction, crying, diaphoresis, flu-like syndrome, generalized spasm, hernia, herpes simplex, peritonitis, sepsis, writing impaired

Topical (as reported in children and adults, unless otherwise noted):
>10%:

Central nervous system: Headache (5% to 20%), fever (1% to 21%)

Dermatologic: Skin burning (43% to 58%; tends to improve as lesions resolve), pruritus (41% to 46%), erythema (12% to 28%)

Respiratory: Increased cough (children 18%)

Miscellaneous: Flu-like syndrome (23% to 31%), allergic reaction (4% to 12%)
1% to 10%:

Cardiovascular: Peripheral edema (adults 3% to 4%)

Central nervous system: Hyperesthesia (adults 3% to 7%), pain (1% to 2%)

Dermatologic: Skin tingling (2% to 8%), acne (adults 4% to 7%), localized flushing (following ethanol consumption; adults 3% to 7%), folliculitis (2% to 6%), urticaria (1% to 6%), rash (2% to 5%), pustular rash (2% to 4%), vesiculobullous rash (children 4%), contact dermatitis (3% to 4%), cyst (adults 1% to 3%), eczema herpeticum (1% to 2%), fungal dermatitis (adults 1% to 2%), sunburn (adults 1% to 2%), alopecia (adults 1%), dry skin (children 1%)

Endocrine & metabolic: Dysmenorrhea (adult females 4%)

Gastrointestinal: Diarrhea (3% to 5%), dyspepsia (adults 1% to 4%), abdominal pain (children 3%), vomiting (adults 1%), gastroenteritis (adults 2%), nausea (children 1%), tooth disorder (adults 1%)

Neuromuscular & skeletal: Paresthesia (adults 3%), myalgia (adults 2% to 3%), weakness (adults 2% to 3%), arthralgia (adults 1% to 3%), back pain (adults 2%)

Ocular: Conjunctivitis (2% adults)

Otic: Otitis media (12% children)

Respiratory: Rhinitis (6% children), sinusitis (2% to 4% adults), bronchitis (2% adults), pneumonia (1% adults)

Miscellaneous: Varicella/herpes zoster (1% to 5%), lymphadenopathy (3% children)

Oral, I.V., topical: Postmarketing and/or case reports (limited to important or life-threatening): Acute renal failure, anaphylaxis, anaphylactoid reaction, angioedema, ARDS, arrhythmia, atrial fibrillation, atrial flutter, basal cell carcinoma, bile duct stenosis, blindness, cardiac arrest, cerebral infarction, cerebrovascular accident, deafness, delirium, DIC, hemiparesis, hemolytic-uremic syndrome, hemorrhagic cystitis, hepatic necrosis, hepatotoxicity, interstitial lung disease, leukoencephalopathy, lymphoproliferative disorder (related to EBV), malignant melanoma, myocardial hypertrophy (associated with ventricular dysfunction; reversible upon discontinuation), MI, neutropenia, osteomyelitis, pancreatitis (hemorrhagic and necrotizing), pancytopenia, paresthesia, photosensitivity reaction (topical), posterior reversible encephalopathy syndrome (PRES), progressive multifocal leukoencephalopathy (PML), quadriplegia, QT_c prolongation, respiratory failure, seizure, septicemia, skin discoloration (topical), squamous cell carcinoma, Stevens-Johnson syndrome, syncope, toxic epidermal necrolysis, thrombocytopenic purpura, torsade de pointes, TTP, veno-occlusive hepatic disease, venous thrombosis, ventricular fibrillation

Note: Calcineurin inhibitor-induced hemolytic uremic syndrome/thrombotic thrombocytopenic purpura/thrombotic microangiopathy (HUS/TTP/TMA) have been reported (with concurrent sirolimus).

Drug Interactions

Metabolism/Transport Effects Substrate of CYP3A4 (major); **Inhibits** CYP3A4 (weak)

Avoid Concomitant Use

Avoid concomitant use of Tacrolimus with any of the following: Artemether; CycloSPORINE; Dabigatran Etexilate; Dronedarone; Grapefruit Juice; Lumefantrine; Natalizumab; Nilotinib; Pimozide; QuiNINE; Silodosin; Sirolimus; Tetrabenazine; Thioridazine; Topotecan; Vaccines (Live); Ziprasidone

Increased Effect/Toxicity

Tacrolimus may increase the levels/effects of: Alcohol (Ethyl); Colchicine; CycloSPORINE; Dabigatran Etexilate; Dronedarone; Leflunomide; Natalizumab; P-Glycoprotein Substrates; Phenytoin; Pimozide; QTc-Prolonging Agents; QuiNINE; Rivaroxaban; Silodosin; Sirolimus; Tetrabenazine; Thioridazine; Topotecan; Vaccines (Live); Ziprasidone

The levels/effects of Tacrolimus may be increased by: Alfuzosin; Antidepressants (Serotonin Reuptake Inhibitor/Antagonist); Antifungal Agents (Azole Derivatives, Systemic); Artemether; Calcium Channel Blockers (Dihydropyridine); Calcium Channel Blockers (Nondihydropyridine); Chloroquine; Ciprofloxacin; CycloSPORINE; CYP3A4 Inhibitors (Moderate); CYP3A4 Inhibitors (Strong); Fluconazole; Gadobutrol; Grapefruit Juice; Lumefantrine; Macrolide Antibiotics; MetroNIDAZOLE; Nilotinib; P-Glycoprotein Inhibitors; Protease Inhibitors; Proton Pump Inhibitors; QuiNINE; Sirolimus; Temsirolimus; Trastuzumab

Decreased Effect

Tacrolimus may decrease the levels/effects of: Vaccines (Inactivated); Vaccines (Live)

The levels/effects of Tacrolimus may be decreased by: Caspofungin; Cinacalcet; CYP3A4 Inducers (Strong); Deferasirox; Echinacea; P-Glycoprotein Inducers; Phenytoin; Rifamycin Derivatives; St Johns Wort

Ethanol/Nutrition/Herb Interactions

Ethanol: Localized flushing (redness, warm sensation) may occur at application site of topical tacrolimus following ethanol consumption.

Food: Decreases rate and extent of absorption. High-fat meals have most pronounced effect (37% decrease in AUC, 77% decrease in C_{max}). Grapefruit juice, CYP3A4 inhibitor, may increase serum level and/or toxicity of tacrolimus; avoid concurrent use.

Herb/Nutraceutical: St John's wort: May reduce tacrolimus serum concentrations (avoid concurrent use).

Dietary Considerations Capsule: Take on an empty stomach; be consistent with timing and composition of meals if GI intolerance occurs and administration with food becomes necessary (per manufacturer). Avoid grapefruit juice.

Dosage Forms Excipient information presented when available (limited, particularly for generics); consult specific product labeling.

Capsule: 0.5 mg, 1 mg, 5 mg

Prograf®: 0.5 mg, 1 mg, 5 mg

Injection, solution:

Prograf®: 5 mg/mL (1 mL) [contains dehydrated alcohol 80% and polyoxyl 60 hydrogenated castor oil]

Ointment, topical:

Protopic®: 0.03% (30 g, 60 g, 100 g); 0.1% (30 g, 60 g, 100 g)

References

Winkel E, DiSesa VJ, and Costanzo MR, "Advances in Heart Transplantation," *Dis Mon*, 1999, 45 (3):62-87.

Tadalafil (tah DA la fil)

Medication Safety Issues
Sound-alike/look-alike issues:
Tadalafil may be confused with sildenafil, vardenafil
Adcirca™ may be confused with Advair® Diskus®, Advair® HFA, Advicor®

U.S. Brand Names Adcirca™; Cialis®

Canadian Brand Names Cialis®

Index Terms GF196960

Pharmacologic Category Phosphodiesterase-5 Enzyme Inhibitor

Generic Available No

Use
Adcirca™: Treatment of pulmonary arterial hypertension (PAH) (WHO Group I) to improve exercise ability
Cialis®: Treatment of erectile dysfunction (ED)

Mechanism of Action
Erectile dysfunction: Does not directly cause penile erections, but affects the response to sexual stimulation. The physiologic mechanism of erection of the penis involves release of nitric oxide (NO) in the corpus cavernosum during sexual stimulation. NO then activates the enzyme guanylate cyclase, which results in increased levels of cyclic guanosine monophosphate (cGMP), producing smooth muscle relaxation and inflow of blood to the corpus cavernosum. Tadalafil enhances the effect of NO by inhibiting phosphodiesterase type 5 (PDE-5), which is responsible for degradation of cGMP in the corpus cavernosum; when sexual stimulation causes local release of NO, inhibition of PDE-5 by tadalafil causes increased levels of cGMP in the corpus cavernosum, resulting in smooth muscle relaxation and inflow of blood to the corpus cavernosum. At recommended doses, it has no effect in the absence of sexual stimulation.

PAH: Inhibits phosphodiesterase type 5 (PDE-5) in smooth muscle of pulmonary vasculature where PDE-5 is responsible for the degradation of cyclic guanosine monophosphate (cGMP). Increased cGMP concentration results in pulmonary vasculature relaxation; vasodilation in the pulmonary bed and the systemic circulation (to a lesser degree) may occur.

Pharmacodynamics/Kinetics
Onset of action: Within 1 hour
Peak effect (pulmonary artery vasodilation): 75-90 minutes (Ghofrani, 2004)
Duration: Erectile dysfunction: Up to 36 hours
Distribution: V_d: 63-77 L
Protein binding: 94%
Metabolism: Hepatic, via CYP3A4 to metabolites (inactive)
Half-life elimination: 15-17.5 hours; Pulmonary hypertension (not receiving bosentan): 35 hours
Time to peak, plasma: ~2-4 hours (range: 30 minutes to 8 hours)
Excretion: Feces (~61%, predominantly as metabolites); urine (~36%, predominantly as metabolites)

Dosage Oral: Adults:
Erectile dysfunction (Cialis®):
As-needed dosing: 10 mg at least 30 minutes prior to anticipated sexual activity (dosing range: 5-20 mg); to be given as one single dose and not given more than once daily. **Note:** Erectile function may be improved for up to 36 hours following a single dose; adjust dose.
Once-daily dosing: 2.5 mg once daily (dosing range: 2.5-5 mg/day) to be given at approximately the same time daily without regard to timing of sexual activity
Dosing adjustment with concomitant medications:
Alpha$_1$-blockers: If stabilized on either alpha-blockers or tadalafil therapy, initiate new therapy with the other agent at the lowest possible dose.
CYP3A4 inhibitors: Dose reduction of tadalafil is recommended with strong CYP3A4 inhibitors. When used on an as-needed basis, the dose of tadalafil should not exceed 10 mg, and tadalafil should not be taken more frequently than once every 72 hours. When used on a once-daily basis, the dose of tadalafil should not exceed 2.5 mg. Examples of such inhibitors include amprenavir, atazanavir, clarithromycin, conivaptan, delavirdine, diclofenac,

◄   fosamprenavir, imatinib, indinavir, isoniazid, itraconazole, ketoconazole, miconazole, nefazodone, nelfinavir, nicardipine, propofol, quinidine, ritonavir, and telithromycin.

Pulmonary arterial hypertension (Adcirca™): 40 mg once daily

Dosing adjustment with concomitant medications:

  Concomitant ritonavir:

    If patient receiving ritonavir for at least 1 week: Initiate tadalafil at 20 mg once daily; increase to 40 mg once daily based on individual tolerability.

    If patient receiving tadalafil when initiating ritonavir: Stop tadalafil at least 24 hours prior to starting ritonavir. After at least 1 week following the initiation of ritonavir, resume tadalafil at 20 mg once daily; increase to 40 mg once daily based on individual tolerability.

  Other potent CYP3A4 inhibitors: Avoid concurrent use when tadalafil used for PAH. Examples of such inhibitors include amprenavir, atazanavir, clarithromycin, conivaptan, delavirdine, diclofenac, fosamprenavir, imatinib, indinavir, isoniazid, itraconazole, ketoconazole, miconazole, nefazodone, nelfinavir, nicardipine, propofol, quinidine, and telithromycin.

  Potent CYP3A4 inducers (eg, rifampin): Avoid concurrent use when tadalafil used for PAH.

Elderly: No dose adjustment for patients >65 years of age in the absence of renal or hepatic impairment

Dosage adjustment in renal impairment:

  Erectile dysfunction (Cialis®):

  As-needed use:

    Cl_{cr} ≥51 mL/minute: Dosage adjustment not required

    Cl_{cr} 31-50 mL/minute: Initial: 5 mg once daily; maximum: 10 mg (not to be given more frequently than every 48 hours)

    Cl_{cr} <30 mL/minute and on hemodialysis: Maximum: 5 mg (not to be given more frequently than every 72 hours)

  Once-daily use:

    Cl_{cr} ≥31 mL/minute: Dose adjustment not required

    Cl_{cr} <30 mL/minute and on hemodialysis: Use not recommended

  Pulmonary arterial hypertension (Adcirca™):

    Cl_{cr} 31-80 mL/minute: Initial: 20 mg once daily; increase to 40 mg once daily based on individual tolerability

    Cl_{cr} <30 mL/minute and on hemodialysis: Avoid use due to increased tadalafil exposure, limited clinical experience, and lack of ability to influence clearance by dialysis.

Dosage adjustment in hepatic impairment:

  Erectile dysfunction (Cialis®):

  As-needed use:

    Mild-to-moderate hepatic impairment (Child-Pugh class A or B): Use with caution; dose should not exceed 10 mg once daily

    Severe hepatic impairment (Child-Pugh class C): Use is not recommended

  Once-daily use:

    Mild-to-moderate hepatic impairment (Child-Pugh class A or B): Use with caution

    Severe hepatic impairment (Child-Pugh class C): Use is not recommended

  Pulmonary arterial hypertension (Adcirca™):

    Mild-to-moderate hepatic impairment (Child-Pugh class A or B): Use with caution; consider initial dose of 20 mg once daily

    Severe hepatic impairment (Child-Pugh class C): Avoid use; has not been studied in patients with severe hepatic cirrhosis.

Stability Store at controlled room temperature of 25°C (77°F); excursions permitted to 15°C to 30°C (59°F to 86°F).

Administration May be administered with or without food.

  Adcirca™: Administer daily dose all at once; dividing doses throughout the day is not advised.

  Cialis®: When used on an as-needed basis, should be taken at least 30 minutes prior to sexual activity. When used on a once-daily basis, should be taken at the same time each day, without regard to timing of sexual activity.

Monitoring Parameters Blood pressure; response and adverse effects

Anesthesia and Critical Care Concerns/Other Considerations
Clinical Pearls/Comments:
Cardiovascular effects of PDE-5 inhibitors may be potentially hazardous in patients with:
- active coronary ischemia (not on nitrates)
- heart failure and with borderline low blood pressure and borderline low volume status
- complicated, multidrug antihypertensive regimens
- potential for drug-drug interactions that may prolong PDE-5 inhibitor half-life (eg, drugs that inhibit cytochrome P450 3A4)

Use of tadalafil is contraindicated in patients currently taking nitrate preparations. When nitrate administration becomes medically necessary in patients who received tadalafil, the ACC/AHA 2004 guidelines on treatment of ST-segment elevation MI and the ACC/AHA 2007 guidelines on treatment of unstable angina/ non ST-segment elevation MI support administration of nitrates only if 48 hours have elapsed after use of tadalafil.

Pregnancy Risk Factor B

Contraindications Known serious hypersensitivity to tadalafil; concurrent use (regularly/intermittently) of organic nitrates in any form (eg, nitroglycerin, isosorbide dinitrate)

Warnings/Precautions There is a degree of cardiac risk associated with sexual activity; therefore, physicians should consider the cardiovascular status of their patients prior to initiation. Use for erectile dysfunction is not recommended in patients with hypotension (<90/50 mm Hg), uncontrolled hypertension (>170/100 mm Hg), NYHA class II-IV heart failure within the last 6 months, uncontrolled arrhythmias, stroke within the last 6 months, MI within the last 3 months, unstable angina or angina during sexual intercourse; safety and efficacy have not been evaluated in these patients. Safety and efficacy in PAH have not been evaluated in patients with clinically significant aortic and/or mitral valve disease, life-threatening arrhythmias, hypotension (<90/50 mm Hg), uncontrolled hypertension, significant left ventricular dysfunction, pericardial constriction, restrictive or congestive cardiomyopathy, symptomatic coronary artery disease. Use caution in patients with left ventricular outflow obstruction (eg, aortic stenosis, hypertrophic obstructive cardiomyopathy); may be more sensitive to vasodilator effects.

Patients experiencing anginal chest pain after tadalafil administration should seek immediate medical attention. Concomitant use (regularly/intermittently) with all forms of nitrates is contraindicated. When used for either erectile dysfunction or PAH and nitrate administration is medically necessary following use, at least 48 hours should elapse after the tadalafil dose and nitrate administration. When used for PAH, per the manufacturer, nitrate may be administered within 48 hours of tadalafil. For both situations, administration of nitrates should only be done under close medical supervision with hemodynamic monitoring.

Concurrent use with alpha-adrenergic antagonist therapy or substantial alcohol consumption may cause symptomatic hypotension; patients should be hemodynamically stable prior to initiating tadalafil therapy at the lowest possible dose. When used for erectile dysfunction, use caution in patients receiving strong CYP3A4 inhibitors. When used for PAH, avoid use in patients taking strong CYP3A4 inducers/inhibitors. Use in patients receiving or about to receive ritonavir requires dosage adjustment or interruption of therapy, respectively. Pulmonary vasodilators may exacerbate the cardiovascular status in patients with pulmonary veno-occlusive disease (PVOD); use is not recommended. In patients with unrecognized PVOD, signs of pulmonary edema should prompt investigation into this diagnosis. Use with caution in patients with mild-to-moderate hepatic impairment; dosage adjustment/limitation is needed. Use is not recommended in patients with severe hepatic impairment or cirrhosis. Use with caution in patients with renal impairment; dosage adjustment/limitation is needed. Safety and efficacy with other tadalafil brands or other PDE-5 inhibitors (ie, sildenafil and vardenafil) have not been established. Patients should be informed not to take with other tadalafil brands or other PDE-5 inhibitors. Use caution in patients with bleeding disorders or peptic ulcer disease due to effect on platelets (bleeding).

When used to treat erectile dysfunction, potential underlying causes of erectile dysfunction should be evaluated prior to treatment. Use with caution in patients with anatomical deformation of the penis (angulation, cavernosal fibrosis, or Peyronie's disease), or who have conditions which may predispose them to priapism (sickle cell anemia, multiple myeloma, leukemia). Instruct patients to seek immediate medical attention if erection persists >4 hours. Safety and efficacy with other tadalafil brands or other PDE-5 inhibitors (ie, sildenafil and vardenafil) have not been established. Patients should be informed not to take with other tadalafil brands or other PDE-5 inhibitors. The safety and efficacy of tadalafil with other treatments for erectile dysfunction have not been studied and are, therefore, not recommended as combination therapy.

Rare cases of nonarteritic anterior ischemic optic neuropathy (NAION) have been reported; risk may be increased with history of vision loss or NAION in one eye. Other risk factors for NAION include heart disease, diabetes, hypertension, smoking, age >50 years, or history of certain eye problems. Sudden decrease or loss of hearing has been reported rarely; hearing changes may be accompanied by tinnitus and dizziness. A direct relationship between therapy and vision or hearing loss has not been determined.

Patients with genetic retinal disorders (eg, retinitis pigmentosa) were not evaluated in clinical trials; use is not recommended. Use with caution in the elderly. Safety and efficacy in children ≤18 years of age have not been established.

Adverse Reactions Based upon usual doses for either indication. For erectile dysfunction, similar adverse events are reported with once-daily versus intermittent dosing, but are generally lower than with doses used intermittently.
>10%:
Cardiovascular: Flushing (1% to 13%; dose related)
Central nervous system: Headache (3% to 42%; dose related)
Gastrointestinal: Dyspepsia (1% to 13%), nausea (10% to 11%)
Neuromuscular & skeletal: Myalgia (1% to 14%; dose related), back pain (2% to 12%), extremity pain (1% to 11%)
Respiratory: Respiratory tract infection (3% to 13%), nasopharyngitis (2% to 13%)
2% to 10%:
Cardiovascular: Hypertension (1% to 3%)
Genitourinary: Urinary tract infection (≤2%)
Respiratory: Nasal congestion (≤9%), cough (2% to 4%)
<2% (Limited to important or life-threatening): Abdominal pain (upper), amnesia (transient global), angina pectoris, arthralgia, blurred vision, chest pain, color perception change, color vision decreased, conjunctival hyperemia, conjunctivitis, diaphoresis, diarrhea, dizziness, dysphagia, dyspnea, epistaxis, esophagitis, exfoliative dermatitis, eye pain, eyelid swelling, facial edema, fatigue, gastritis, hearing decreased, hearing loss, hepatic enzymes increased, hypoesthesia, hypotension, GGTP increased, lacrimation, migraine, MI, neck pain, nonarteritic ischemic optic neuropathy (NAION), pain, palpitation, paresthesia, photophobia, postural hypotension, priapism, pruritus, rash, retinal artery occlusion, retinal vein occlusion, seizure, somnolence, Stevens-Johnson syndrome, stroke, sudden cardiac death, syncope, tachycardia, tinnitus, urticaria, vertigo, visual field loss, vomiting, weakness, xerostomia

Drug Interactions
Metabolism/Transport Effects Substrate of CYP3A4 (major)
Avoid Concomitant Use
Avoid concomitant use of Tadalafil with any of the following: Phosphodiesterase 5 Inhibitors; Vasodilators (Organic Nitrates)
Increased Effect/Toxicity
Tadalafil may increase the levels/effects of: Alpha1-Blockers; Antihypertensives; Bosentan; Phosphodiesterase 5 Inhibitors; Vasodilators (Organic Nitrates)

The levels/effects of Tadalafil may be increased by: Antifungal Agents (Azole Derivatives, Systemic); CYP3A4 Inhibitors (Moderate); CYP3A4 Inhibitors (Strong); Dasatinib; Macrolide Antibiotics; Ritonavir; Sapropterin
Decreased Effect
The levels/effects of Tadalafil may be decreased by: Bosentan; CYP3A4 Inducers (Strong); Etravirine

Ethanol/Nutrition/Herb Interactions

Ethanol: Substantial consumption of ethanol may increase the risk of hypotension and orthostasis. Lower ethanol consumption has not been associated with significant changes in blood pressure or increase in orthostatic symptoms.

Food: Rate and extent of absorption are not affected by food. Grapefruit juice may increase serum levels/toxicity of tadalafil. Use tadalafil with caution in patients who regularly consume grapefruit juice. In general, use of grapefruit juice should be limited or avoided; the manufacturer does not give specific recommendations.

Herb/Nutraceutical: St John's wort: Use caution with concomitant use.

Dietary Considerations May be taken with or without food.

Dosage Forms Excipient information presented when available (limited, particularly for generics); consult specific product labeling.

Tablet:

Adcirca™: 20 mg

Cialis®: 2.5 mg, 5 mg, 10 mg, 20 mg

- ◆ **Tagamet® HB (Can)** *see* Cimetidine *on page 305*
- ◆ **Tagamet® HB 200 [OTC]** *see* Cimetidine *on page 305*
- ◆ **Talc** *see* Talc (Sterile) *on page 1349*
- ◆ **Talc for Pleurodesis** *see* Talc (Sterile) *on page 1349*

Talc (Sterile) (talk STARE il)

U.S. Brand Names Sclerosol®; Sterile Talc Powder™

Index Terms Intrapleural Talc; Sterile Talc; Talc; Talc for Pleurodesis

Pharmacologic Category Sclerosing Agent

Use Prevention of recurrence of malignant pleural effusion in symptomatic patients

Mechanism of Action Induces an inflammatory reaction that promotes adherence of the visceral to the parietal pleura, therefore, preventing reaccumulation of pleural fluid.

Dosage Adults: Pleural effusion:

Intrapleural aerosol: 4-8 g (1-2 cans) as a single dose

Intrapleural instillation: 5 g

Stability

Sclerosol® Intrapleural Aerosol: Store at room temperature 15°C to 30°C (59°F to 86°F); do not freeze. Protect from heat and light.

Sterile Talc Powder™: Store at controlled room temperature of 18°C to 25°C (64°F to 77°F). Protect from light. Vent bottle with needle; slowly add 50 mL of NS to bottle using aseptic technique. For doses >5 g, use a second bottle. Swirl the bottle to disperse talc and avoid settling. Divide the contents of each bottle into two 60 mL irrigation syringes (25 mL of talc slurry in each). Add an additional 25 mL of NS to each syringe for a total of 50 mL (2.5 g/50 mL). If not used immediately, label "For IntraPleural Use Only." Use within 12 hours of slurry preparation.

Administration Administer after adequate drainage of the effusion.

Sclerosol® Intrapleural Aerosol: Shake well and attach delivery tube. Insert delivery tube through pleural trocar, manually press on actuator button of canister to release; point in several different directions to distribute to all pleural surfaces. Keep canister in an upright position. Rate of delivery is 0.4 g per second.

Sterile Talc Powder™: Administer as a slurry. Shake well before instillation. Empty contents of each syringe into chest cavity through the chest tube by gently applying pressure to syringe plunger. After administration, flush with 10-25 mL of NS. Clamp chest tube and have patient rotate from supine to alternating decubitus positions at 20-30 minute intervals for 2 hours. For intrapleural use only; **not for I.V. administration.**

Pregnancy Risk Factor B

Contraindications There are no contraindications listed within the manufacturer's labeling.

Warnings/Precautions Acute pneumonitis and acute respiratory distress syndrome (including one death) have rarely been reported with higher doses (10 g). Should not be used to treat malignancies; does not have antineoplastic ▶

activity. Clinicians should evaluate need for future diagnostic procedures before use; sclerosis of pleural space may preclude subsequent procedures (eg, pneumonectomy for transplantation). Sclerosol® contents under pressure and should be kept away from any heat source.

Adverse Reactions Frequency not defined.

Cardiovascular: Asystolic arrest, chest pain, hypotension (transient), hypovolemia, MI, tachycardia

Central nervous system: Fever (generally lasting <24 hours)

Local: Bleeding (localized), infection at administration site, pain

Respiratory: ARDS, bronchopleural fistula, dyspnea, empyema, hemoptysis, hypoxemia, pneumonia, pulmonary edema, pulmonary embolism, subcutaneous emphysema

Dosage Forms Excipient information presented when available (limited, particularly for generics); consult specific product labeling.

Aerosol, intrapleural [powder]:

Sclerosol®: 4 g [contains chlorofluorocarbon]

Powder, intrapleural:

Sterile Talc Powder™: Talc USP (5 g)

References

Dresler CM, Olak J, Herndon JE, et al, "Phase III Intergroup Study of Talc Poudrage vs Talc Slurry Sclerosis for Malignant Pleural Effusion," *Chest*, 2005, 127(3):909-15.

Kvale PA, Seleecky PA, and Prakash UB, "Palliative Care in Lung Cancer: ACCP Evidence-Based Clinical Practice Guidelines (2nd Edition)," *Chest*, 2007, 132(3 Suppl):368-403.

◆ **Tambocor™** *see* Flecainide *on page 605*

◆ **Tamiflu®** *see* Oseltamivir *on page 1062*

◆ **Tanta-Orciprenaline® (Can)** *see* Metaproterenol *on page 885*

◆ **Tantum® (Can)** *see* Benzydamine *on page 184*

◆ **Tapazole®** *see* Methimazole *on page 893*

Tapentadol (ta PEN ta dol)

Medication Safety Issues

Sound-alike/look-alike issues:

Tapentadol may be confused with traMADol

Medication Guide An FDA-approved patient medication guide, which is available with the product information and at http://img.medscape.com/pi/alert/tapentadol/NucyntaPI.pdf, must be dispensed with this medication for each new outpatient prescription and refill.

U.S. Brand Names Nucynta™

Index Terms CG5503; Tapentadol Hydrochloride

Pharmacologic Category Analgesic, Opioid

Restrictions C-II

Generic Available No

Use Relief of moderate-to-severe acute pain

Mechanism of Action Binds to µ-opiate receptors in the CNS causing inhibition of ascending pain pathways, altering the perception of and response to pain; also inhibits the reuptake of norepinephrine, which also modifies the ascending pain pathway

Pharmacodynamics/Kinetics

Absorption: Rapid and complete

Distribution: V_d: I.V.: 442-638 L

Protein binding: ~20%

Metabolism: Extensive metabolism, including first pass metabolism; metabolized primarily via phase 2 glucuronidation to glucuronides (major metabolite: tapentadol-O-glucuronide); minimal phase 1 oxidative metabolism; also metabolized to a lesser degree by CYP2C9, CYP2C19, and CYP2D6; all metabolites pharmacologically inactive

Bioavailability: ~32%

Half-life elimination: ~4 hours

Time to peak, plasma: 1.25 hours

Excretion: Urine (99%: 70% conjugated metabolites; 3% unchanged drug)

Dosage Oral: **Note:** Dose and dosage intervals should be individualized according to pain severity with respect to patient's previous experience with similar opioid analgesics.

Adults: Acute moderate-severe pain: Day 1: 50-100 mg every 4-6 hours as needed; may administer a second dose ≥1 hour after the initial dose (maximum dose on first day: 700 mg/day); Day 2 and subsequent dosing: 50-100 mg every 4-6 hours as needed (maximum: 600 mg/day)

Elderly: Initial: Consider initiating at lower range of dosing. Refer to adult dosing.

Dosage adjustment in renal impairment:
Mild-moderate renal impairment: No adjustment necessary
Severe renal impairment: Not recommended (not studied)

Dosage adjustment in hepatic impairment:
Mild hepatic impairment: No adjustment necessary
Moderate hepatic impairment: Initial: 50 mg every 8 hours or longer (maximum: 3 doses/24 hours). Further dose adjustments may be achieved by either shortening or lengthening the dosing interval.
Severe hepatic impairment: Not recommended (not studied)

Stability Store at room temperature up to 25°C (77°F); excursions permitted to 15°C to 30°C (59°F to 86°F). Protect from moisture.

Administration Administer orally with or without food.

Pregnancy Risk Factor C

Contraindications Impaired pulmonary function (severe respiratory depression, acute or severe asthma or hypercapnia) in unmonitored settings or in absence of resuscitative equipment or ventilatory support; paralytic ileus; use of MAO inhibitors within 14 days

Warnings/Precautions Use with caution in patients with respiratory disease or respiratory compromise (eg, asthma, chronic obstructive pulmonary disease [COPD], cor pulmonale, sleep apnea, severe obesity, kyphoscoliosis, hypoxia, hypercapnia); critical respiratory depression may occur, even at therapeutic dosages. May cause CNS depression, which may impair physical or mental abilities; patients must be cautioned about performing tasks which require mental alertness (eg, operating machinery or driving). Use with caution in patients with CNS depression or coma. Effects may be potentiated when used with other sedative drugs or ethanol.

Serotonin syndrome (SS) may occur with serotonin/norepinephrine reuptake inhibitors (SNRIs), including tapentadol. Signs of SS may include agitation, tachycardia, hyperthermia, nausea, and vomiting. Avoid use with serotonergic agents such as TCAs, triptans, venlafaxine, trazodone, lithium, sibutramine, meperidine, dextromethorphan, St John's wort, SNRIs and SSRIs; concomitant use has been associated with the development of serotonin syndrome. Contraindicated with MAO inhibitor use within 14 days.

Use caution in patients with biliary tract dysfunction or acute pancreatitis; opioids may cause spasm of the sphincter of Oddi. Opioid use may obscure diagnosis or clinical course of patients with acute abdominal conditions. Use with extreme caution in patients with head injury, intracranial lesions, or elevated intracranial pressure (ICP); exaggerated elevation of ICP may occur. Serum concentrations are increased in hepatic impairment; use with caution in patients with moderate hepatic impairment (dosage adjustment required). Not recommended for use in severe hepatic impairment (not studied). Use with caution in patients with mild-to-moderate renal impairment (no dosage adjustment recommended). Not recommended for use in severe renal impairment (not studied). Use caution in patients with a history of seizures or conditions predisposing patients to seizures; patients with a history of seizures were excluded in clinical trials of tapentadol. Tramadol, an analgesic with similar pharmacologic properties to tapentadol, has been associated with seizures, particularly in patients with predisposing factors.

Approved for acute pain (not approved for chronic use); prolonged use increases risk of abuse, addiction, and withdrawal symptoms. An opioid-containing regimen should be tailored to each patient's needs with respect to degree of tolerance for opioids (naïve versus chronic user), age, weight, and medical condition. Healthcare provider should be alert to problems of abuse, misuse, and diversion. Abrupt discontinuation may lead to withdrawal symptoms. Symptoms may be

◀ decreased by tapering prior to discontinuation. Use opioids with caution in elderly; consider decreasing initial dose. Use caution in debilitated patients; there is a greater potential for critical respiratory depression, even at therapeutic dosages. Safety and efficacy have not been established in children <18 years of age.

Adverse Reactions

>10%:

Central nervous system: Dizziness (24%), somnolence (15%)

Gastrointestinal: Nausea (30%), vomiting (18%)

1% to 10%:

Central nervous system: Fatigue (3%), insomnia (2%), anxiety (1%), confusion (1%), dreams abnormal (1%), lethargy (1%)

Dermatologic: Pruritus (3% to 5%), hyperhidrosis (3%), rash (1%)

Endocrine & metabolic: Hot flushes (1%)

Gastrointestinal: Constipation (8%), xerostomia (4%), appetite decreased (2%), dyspepsia (2%)

Genitourinary: Urinary tract infection (1%)

Neuromuscular & skeletal: Arthralgia (1%), tremor (1%)

Respiratory: Nasopharyngitis (1%), upper respiratory tract infection (1%)

<1% (Limited to important or life-threatening): Abdominal discomfort, agitation, ALT increased, AST increased, ataxia, attention disturbances, blood pressure decreased, bradycardia, consciousness decreased, coordination abnormal, cough, diarrhea, disorientation, drunk feeling, dysarthria, dyspnea, ear pain, edema, euphoria, gastric emptying impaired, GGT increased, headache, heart rate increased/decreased, heaviness sensation, hypersensitivity, hypertension, hypoesthesia, involuntary muscle contractions, irritability, memory impairment, nervousness, oxygen saturation decreased, paresthesia, pharyngolaryngeal pain, pollakiuria, presyncope, respiratory depression, restlessness, sedation, seizure, syncope, thinking abnormal, urticaria, urinary hesitation, visual disturbance, weakness, withdrawal syndrome

Drug Interactions

Avoid Concomitant Use

Avoid concomitant use of Tapentadol with any of the following: MAO Inhibitors; Sibutramine

Increased Effect/Toxicity

Tapentadol may increase the levels/effects of: Alcohol (Ethyl); Alvimopan; CNS Depressants; Desmopressin; MAO Inhibitors; Selective Serotonin Reuptake Inhibitors; Serotonin Modulators; Thiazide Diuretics

The levels/effects of Tapentadol may be increased by: Amphetamines; Antipsychotic Agents (Phenothiazines); Sibutramine; Succinylcholine

Decreased Effect

Tapentadol may decrease the levels/effects of: Pegvisomant

The levels/effects of Tapentadol may be decreased by: Ammonium Chloride; Peginterferon Alfa-2b

Ethanol/Nutrition/Herb Interactions

Food: When administered after a high fat/calorie meal, the AUC and C_{max} increased by 25% and 16%, respectively; may administer without regard to meals.

Herb/Nutraceutical: Avoid St John's wort (may increase CNS depression and risk of serotonin syndrome).

Dietary Considerations May be taken without regard to meals.

Dosage Forms

Excipient information presented when available (limited, particularly for generics); consult specific product labeling.

Tablet, oral, as hydrochloride:

Nucynta™: 50 mg, 75 mg, 100 mg

◆ **Tapentadol Hydrochloride** *see* Tapentadol *on page 1350*

◆ **Taro-Carbamazepine Chewable (Can)** *see* CarBAMazepine *on page 241*

◆ **Taro-Ciprofloxacin (Can)** *see* Ciprofloxacin *on page 306*

◆ **Taro-Clindamycin (Can)** *see* Clindamycin *on page 324*

◆ **Taro-Enalapril (Can)** *see* Enalapril *on page 478*

- **Taro-Fluconazole (Can)** *see* Fluconazole *on page 607*
- **Taro-Simvastatin (Can)** *see* Simvastatin *on page 1293*
- **Taro-Sone® (Can)** *see* Betamethasone *on page 186*
- **Taro-Warfarin (Can)** *see* Warfarin *on page 1479*
- **Tazicef®** *see* Ceftazidime *on page 263*
- **Tazobactam and Piperacillin** *see* Piperacillin and Tazobactam Sodium *on page 1136*
- **Tazocin® (Can)** *see* Piperacillin and Tazobactam Sodium *on page 1136*
- **Taztia XT®** *see* Diltiazem *on page 425*
- **3TC** *see* LamiVUDine *on page 797*
- **3TC® (Can)** *see* LamiVUDine *on page 797*
- **TD-6424** *see* Telavancin *on page 1353*
- **Tears Again® Gel Drops™ [OTC]** *see* Carboxymethylcellulose *on page 243*
- **Tears Again® Night and Day™ [OTC]** *see* Carboxymethylcellulose *on page 243*
- **Tecta™ (Can)** *see* Pantoprazole *on page 1084*
- **Tegretol®** *see* CarBAMazepine *on page 241*
- **Tegretol®-XR** *see* CarBAMazepine *on page 241*
- **Tekturna®** *see* Aliskiren *on page 61*

Telavancin (tel a VAN sin)

Medication Safety Issues
Sound-alike/look-alike issues:
Telavancin may be confused with telithromycin
Vibativ™ may be confused with Viactiv®, Vibra-Tabs®, Vibramycin®, vigabatrin

U.S. Brand Names Vibativ™

Index Terms TD-6424; Telavancin Hydrochloride

Pharmacologic Category Antibiotic, Miscellaneous

Use Treatment of complicated skin and skin structure infections caused by susceptible gram-positive organisms including methicillin-susceptible or -resistant *Staphylococcus aureus*, vancomycin-susceptible *Enterococcus faecalis*, and *Streptococcus pyogenes*, *Streptococcus agalactiae*, or *Streptococcus anginosus* group

Product Availability
Vibativ™: FDA-approved September 2009; availability expected by end of 2009; consult prescribing information for additional information

- **Telavancin Hydrochloride** *see* Telavancin *on page 1353*

Telithromycin (tel ith roe MYE sin)

Medication Safety Issues
Sound-alike/look-alike issues:
Telithromycin may be confused with telavancin

Medication Guide An FDA-approved patient medication guide, which is available with the product information and at http://www.fda.gov/downloads/Drugs/DrugSafety/ucm088615.pdf, must be dispensed with this medication for each new outpatient prescription and refill.

U.S. Brand Names Ketek®

Canadian Brand Names Ketek®

Index Terms HMR 3647

Pharmacologic Category Antibiotic, Ketolide

Generic Available No

Use Treatment of community-acquired pneumonia (mild-to-moderate) caused by susceptible strains of *Streptococcus pneumoniae* (including multidrug-resistant isolates), *Haemophilus influenzae*, *Chlamydophila pneumoniae*, *Moraxella catarrhalis*, and *Mycoplasma pneumoniae*

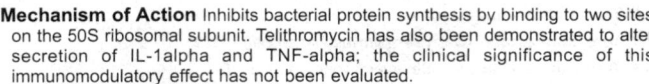

Mechanism of Action Inhibits bacterial protein synthesis by binding to two sites on the 50S ribosomal subunit. Telithromycin has also been demonstrated to alter secretion of IL-1alpha and TNF-alpha; the clinical significance of this immunomodulatory effect has not been evaluated.

Pharmacodynamics/Kinetics

Absorption: Rapid

Distribution: 2.9 L/kg

Protein binding: 60% to 70%; primarily to albumin

Metabolism: Hepatic, via CYP3A4 (50%) and non-CYP-mediated pathways

Bioavailability: 57% (significant first-pass metabolism)

Half-life elimination: 10 hours

Time to peak, plasma: 1 hour

Excretion: Urine (13% unchanged drug, remainder as metabolites); feces (7%)

Dosage Oral:

Children ≥13 years and Adults: Tonsillitis/pharyngitis (unlabeled use; Canadian indication): 800 mg once daily for 5 days

Adults:

Community-acquired pneumonia: 800 mg once daily for 7-10 days

Dosage adjustment in renal impairment:

U.S. product labeling: Cl_{cr} <30 mL/minute, including dialysis: 600 mg once daily; when renal impairment is accompanied by hepatic impairment, reduce dosage to 400 mg once daily

Canadian product labeling: Cl_{cr} <30 mL/minute: Reduce dose to 400 mg once daily

Hemodialysis: Administer following dialysis

Dosage adjustment in hepatic impairment: No adjustment recommended, unless concurrent severe renal impairment is present

Stability Store at 15°C to 30°C (59°F to 86°F).

Administration May be administered with or without food.

Monitoring Parameters Liver function tests; signs/symptoms of liver failure (eg, jaundice, fatigue, malaise, anorexia, nausea, bilirubinemia, acholic stools, liver tenderness, hepatomegaly); visual acuity

Pregnancy Risk Factor C

Contraindications Hypersensitivity to telithromycin, macrolide antibiotics, or any component of the formulation; myasthenia gravis; history of hepatitis and/or jaundice associated with telithromycin or other macrolide antibiotic use; concurrent use of cisapride or pimozide

Warnings/Precautions Acute hepatic failure and severe liver injury, including hepatitis and hepatic necrosis (leading to some fatalities) have been reported, in some cases after only a few doses; if signs/symptoms of hepatitis or liver damage occur, discontinue therapy and initiate liver function tests. **[U.S. Boxed Warning]: Life-threatening (including fatal) respiratory failure has occurred in patients with myasthenia gravis;** use in these patients is contraindicated. May prolong QT_c interval, leading to a risk of ventricular arrhythmias; closely-related antibiotics have been associated with malignant ventricular arrhythmias and torsade de pointes. Avoid in patients with prolongation of QTc interval due to congenital causes, history of long QT syndrome, uncorrected electrolyte disturbances (hypokalemia or hypomagnesemia), significant bradycardia (<50 bpm), or concurrent therapy with QT_c-prolonging drugs (eg, class Ia and class III antiarrhythmics). Avoid use in patients with a prior history of confirmed cardiogenic syncope or ventricular arrhythmias while receiving macrolide antibiotics or other QT_c-prolonging drugs. May cause severe visual disturbances (eg, changes in accommodation ability, diplopia, blurred vision). May cause loss of consciousness (possibly vagal-related); caution patients that these events may interfere with ability to operate machinery or drive, and to use caution until effects are known. Use caution in renal impairment; severe impairment (Cl_{cr} <30 mL/minute) requires dosage adjustment. Pseudomembranous colitis has been reported. Safety and efficacy not established in pediatric patients <13 years of age per Canadian approved labeling and <18 years of age per U.S. approved labeling.

Adverse Reactions

>10%: Gastrointestinal: Diarrhea (10% to 11%)

2% to 10%:

Central nervous system: Headache (2% to 6%), dizziness (3% to 4%)

Gastrointestinal: Nausea (7% to 8%), vomiting (2% to 3%), loose stools (2%), dysgeusia (2%)

≥0.2% to <2%:

Central nervous system: Fatigue, insomnia, somnolence, vertigo

Dermatologic: Rash

Gastrointestinal: Abdominal distension, abdominal pain, anorexia, constipation, dyspepsia, flatulence, gastritis, gastroenteritis, GI upset, glossitis, stomatitis, watery stools, xerostomia

Genitourinary: Vaginal candidiasis, vaginitis

Hematologic: Platelets increased

Hepatic: Transaminases increased

Ocular: Blurred vision, accommodation delayed, diplopia

Miscellaneous: Candidiasis, diaphoresis increased

<0.2% (Limited to important or life-threatening): Acute repiratory failure, alkaline phosphatase increased, allergic reaction, anaphylaxis, angioedema, anxiety, arrhythmia, bilirubin increased, bradycardia, edema (facial), eosinophilia, erythema multiforme, flushing, hepatitis, hepatitis, hepatocellular injury (including necrosis), hypotension, jaundice, liver failure, loss of consciousness (may be vagal-related), muscle cramps, myasthenia gravis exacerbation (rare), palpitation, pancreatitis, paresthesia, pruritus, pseudomembranous colitis, QT_c prolongation, syncope, torsade de pointes

Drug Interactions

Metabolism/Transport Effects Substrate of CYP1A2 (minor), 3A4 (major); **Inhibits** CYP2D6 (weak), 3A4 (strong)

Avoid Concomitant Use

Avoid concomitant use of Telithromycin with any of the following: Alfuzosin; Artemether; Cisapride; Disopyramide; Dronedarone; Eplerenone; Everolimus; Halofantrine; Lumefantrine; Nilotinib; Nisoldipine; Pimozide; QuiNINE; Ranolazine; Rivaroxaban; Salmeterol; Silodosin; Tetrabenazine; Thioridazine; Tolvaptan; Ziprasidone

Increased Effect/Toxicity

Telithromycin may increase the levels/effects of: Alfentanil; Alfuzosin; Almotriptan; Alosetron; Antifungal Agents (Azole Derivatives, Systemic); Antineoplastic Agents (Vinca Alkaloids); Benzodiazepines (metabolized by oxidation); BusPIRone; Calcium Channel Blockers; CarBAMazepine; Cardiac Glycosides; Ciclesonide; Cilostazol; Cisapride; Clozapine; Colchicine; Corticosteroids (Systemic); CycloSPORINE; CYP3A4 Substrates; Disopyramide; Dronedarone; Dutasteride; Eletriptan; Eplerenone; Ergot Derivatives; Everolimus; FentaNYL; Fesoterodine; Halofantrine; HMG-CoA Reductase Inhibitors; Ixabepilone; Maraviroc; Nilotinib; Nisoldipine; Paricalcitol; Phosphodiesterase 5 Inhibitors; Pimecrolimus; Pimozide; QTc-Prolonging Agents; QuiNIDine; QuiNINE; Ranolazine; Repaglinide; Rifamycin Derivatives; Rivaroxaban; Salmeterol; Saxagliptin; Selective Serotonin Reuptake Inhibitors; Silodosin; Sirolimus; Sorafenib; Tacrolimus; Tadalafil; Temsirolimus; Tetrabenazine; Thioridazine; Tolvaptan; Vitamin K Antagonists; Ziprasidone; Zopiclone

The levels/effects of Telithromycin may be increased by: Alfuzosin; Antifungal Agents (Azole Derivatives, Systemic); Artemether; Chloroquine; Ciprofloxacin; CYP3A4 Inhibitors (Moderate); CYP3A4 Inhibitors (Strong); Gadobutrol; Lumefantrine; Nilotinib; QuiNINE

Decreased Effect

Telithromycin may decrease the levels/effects of: Clopidogrel; Prasugrel; Typhoid Vaccine

The levels/effects of Telithromycin may be decreased by: CYP3A4 Inducers (Strong); Deferasirox; Etravirine; Herbs (CYP3A4 Inducers)

Ethanol/Nutrition/Herb Interactions Herb/nutraceutical: St John's wort: May decrease the levels/effects of telithromycin.

Dietary Considerations May be taken with or without food.

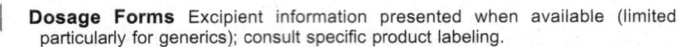

Dosage Forms Excipient information presented when available (limited, particularly for generics); consult specific product labeling.
Tablet:
Ketek®: 300 mg [not available in Canada], 400 mg

Telmisartan (tel mi SAR tan)

Related Information
Angiotensin Agents *on page 1652*
Heart Failure (Systolic) *on page 1739*
Preoperative Evaluation of the Cardiac Patient for Noncardiac Surgery *on page 1598*

U.S. Brand Names Micardis®

Canadian Brand Names Micardis®

Pharmacologic Category Angiotensin II Receptor Blocker

Use Treatment of hypertension; may be used alone or in combination with other antihypertensive agents

Pharmacodynamics/Kinetics Orally active, not a prodrug
Onset of action: 1-2 hours
Peak effect: 0.5-1 hours
Duration: Up to 24 hours
Protein binding: >99.5%
Metabolism: Hepatic via conjugation to inactive metabolites; not metabolized via CYP
Bioavailability (dose dependent): 42% to 58%
Half-life elimination: Terminal: 24 hours
Excretion: Feces (97%)
Clearance: Total body: 800 mL/minute

Dosage Adults: Oral: Initial: 40 mg once daily; usual maintenance dose range: 20-80 mg/day. Patients with volume depletion should be initiated on the lower dosage with close supervision.

Dosage adjustment in renal impairment: No adjustment required; hemodialysis patients are more susceptible to orthostatic hypotension

Dosage adjustment in hepatic impairment: Supervise patients closely.

Anesthesia and Critical Care Concerns/Other Considerations

Clinical Pearls/Comments: In patients on chronic angiotensin receptor blocker (ARB) therapy, intraoperative hypotension may occur with induction and maintenance of general anesthesia; however, discontinuation of therapy prior to surgery is controversial. If continued preoperatively, avoidance of hypotensive agents during surgery is prudent. Episodes of intraoperative hypotension may be managed by fluid administration and/or modest doses of alpha-adrenergic agents. Severe hypotension may occur in patients who are sodium- and/or volume-depleted; initiate lower doses and monitor closely when starting therapy in these patients. ARB therapy may elicit an increase in potassium and creatinine, especially when used in patients with bilateral renal artery stenosis. Concomitant NSAID therapy may attenuate blood pressure control; use of NSAIDs should be avoided or limited, with monitoring of blood pressure control. In the setting of heart failure, NSAID use may be associated with an increased risk for fluid accumulation and edema and therefore should be avoided.

Evidence-Based Information: The angiotensin II receptor antagonists have similar indications as ACE inhibitors. In heart failure, the angiotensin II antagonists are especially useful in providing an alternative therapy in those patients who have intractable cough due to ACE inhibitor therapy. Candesartan has been studied as an alternative therapy in chronic heart failure patients who cannot tolerate an ACE-I (CHARM-Alternative) and as an added therapy in heart failure patients who are maintained on an ACE-I (CHARM-Added). In both studies, the combined endpoint of cardiovascular death or heart failure hospitalizations was significantly improved over the placebo-treated group.

Additional Information Complete prescribing information for this medication should be consulted for additional detail.

Dosage Forms Excipient information presented when available (limited, particularly for generics); consult specific product labeling.
Tablet: 20 mg, 40 mg, 80 mg

Temazepam (te MAZ e pam)

Related Information
Benzodiazepines *on page 1666*
U.S. Brand Names Restoril™
Canadian Brand Names Apo-Temazepam®; CO Temazepam; Dom-Temazepam; Gen-Temazepam; Novo-Temazepam; Nu-Temazepam; PHL-Temazepam; PMS-Temazepam; ratio-Temazepam; Restoril™
Pharmacologic Category Hypnotic, Benzodiazepine
Restrictions C-IV
Use Short-term treatment of insomnia
Unlabeled/Investigational Use Treatment of anxiety; adjunct in the treatment of depression; management of panic attacks
Pharmacodynamics/Kinetics
Distribution: V_d: 1.4 L/kg
Protein binding: 96%
Metabolism: Hepatic
Half-life elimination: 9.5-12.4 hours
Time to peak, serum: 2-3 hours
Excretion: Urine (80% to 90% as inactive metabolites)
Dosage Oral:
Adults: 15-30 mg at bedtime
Elderly or debilitated patients: 15 mg
Anesthesia and Critical Care Concerns/Other Considerations Chronic use of this agent may increase perioperative benzodiazepine dose needed to achieve desired effect. Abrupt discontinuation after sustained use (generally >10 days) may cause withdrawal symptoms. Benzodiazepines, as a class, may depress respiration; may exacerbate sleep-disordered breathing.
Additional Information Complete prescribing information for this medication should be consulted for additional detail.
Dosage Forms Excipient information presented when available (limited, particularly for generics); consult specific product labeling.
Capsule: 7.5 mg, 15 mg, 22.5 mg, 30 mg
Restoril™: 7.5 mg, 15 mg, 22.5 mg, 30 mg

◆ **Tempra® (Can)** *see* Acetaminophen *on page 25*

Tenecteplase (ten EK te plase)

Medication Safety Issues
Sound-alike/look-alike issues:
TNKase® may be confused with Activase®, t-PA
TNK (occasional abbreviation for TNKase®) is an error-prone abbreviation (mistaken as TPA)

High alert medication: The Institute for Safe Medication Practices (ISMP) includes this medication (I.V.) among its list of drugs which have a heightened risk of causing significant patient harm when used in error.
U.S. Brand Names TNKase®
Canadian Brand Names TNKase®
Pharmacologic Category Thrombolytic Agent
Generic Available No
Use Thrombolytic agent used in the management of ST-elevation myocardial infarction (STEMI) for the lysis of thrombi in the coronary vasculature to restore perfusion and reduce mortality.

◄ Recommended criteria for treatment: STEMI: Chest pain ≥20 minutes duration, onset of chest pain within 12 hours of treatment (or within prior 12-24 hours in patients with continuing ischemic symptoms), and S-T segment elevation >0.1 mV in at least two contiguous precordial leads or two adjacent limb leads on ECG or new or presumably new left bundle branch block (LBBB)

Unlabeled/Investigational Use Acute MI - combination regimen of tenecteplase (unlabeled dose), abciximab, and heparin (unlabeled dose)

Mechanism of Action Initiates fibrinolysis by binding to fibrin and converting plasminogen to plasmin.

Pharmacodynamics/Kinetics

Distribution: V_d is weight related and approximates plasma volume

Metabolism: Primarily hepatic

Half-life elimination: 90-130 minutes

Excretion: Clearance: Plasma: 99-119 mL/minute

Dosage I.V.:

Adult: Recommended total dose should not exceed 50 mg and is based on patient's weight; administer as a bolus over 5 seconds

If patient's weight:

<60 kg, dose: 30 mg

≥60 to <70 kg, dose: 35 mg

≥70 to <80 kg, dose: 40 mg

≥80 to <90 kg, dose: 45 mg

≥90 kg, dose: 50 mg

Note: All patients should receive 162-325 mg of chewable nonenteric coated aspirin as soon as possible and then daily. Administer concurrently with heparin 60 units/kg bolus (maximum: 4000 units) followed by continuous infusion of 12 units/kg/hour (maximum: 1000 units/hour) and adjust to aPTT target of 50-70 seconds (or 1.5-2 times the upper limit of control).

Elderly: Although dosage adjustments are not recommended, the elderly have a higher incidence of morbidity and mortality with the use of tenecteplase. The 30-day mortality in the ASSENT-2 trial was 2.5% for patients <65 years, 8.5% for patients 65-74 years, and 16.2% for patients ≥75 years. The intracranial hemorrhage rate was 0.4% for patients <65, 1.6% for patients 65-74 years, and 1.7% for patients ≥75 years. The risks and benefits of use should be weighted carefully in the elderly.

Combination regimen (unlabeled): Half-dose tenecteplase (15-25 mg based on weight) and abciximab 0.25 mg/kg bolus then 0.125 mcg/kg/minute (maximum: 10 mcg/minute) for 12 hours with heparin dosing as follows: Concurrent bolus of 40 units/kg (maximum: 3000 units), then 7 units/kg/hour (maximum: 800 units/hour) as continuous infusion. Adjust to aPTT target of 50-70 seconds.

Note: The 2004 ACC/AHA guidelines for the management of patients with STEMI suggests that abciximab and half-dose reteplase or tenecteplase may be considered for prevention of reinfarction in patients with anterior MI, who are <75 years of age and have no risk factors for bleeding. However, more recently the American College of Chest Physicians recommends against the combination of half-dose reteplase or tenecteplase and standard-dose abciximab (with low dose unfractionated heparin) in any patient with STEMI due to the lack of mortality benefit and the risk of major bleeding (Goodman, 2008).

Dosage adjustment in renal impairment: No formal recommendations for renal impairment

Dosage adjustment in hepatic impairment: Severe hepatic failure is a relative contraindication. Recommendations were not made for mild-to-moderate hepatic impairment.

Stability Store at room temperature not to exceed 30°C (86°F) or under refrigeration 2°C to 8°C (36°F to 46°F). Tenecteplase should be reconstituted using the supplied 10 mL syringe with TwinPak™ Dual Cannula Device and 10 mL sterile water for injection. If reconstituted and not used immediately, store in refrigerator and use within 8 hours.

Administration Tenecteplase should be reconstituted using the supplied 10 mL syringe with TwinPak™ dual cannula device and 10 mL sterile water for injection. Do not shake when reconstituting. Slight foaming is normal and will dissipate if left standing for several minutes. The reconstituted solution is 5 mg/mL. Any unused solution should be discarded. Tenecteplase is **incompatible** with dextrose solutions. Dextrose-containing lines must be flushed with a saline solution before and after administration. Administer as a single I.V. bolus over 5 seconds. Avoid I.M. injections and nonessential handling of patient.

Monitoring Parameters CBC, aPTT, signs and symptoms of bleeding, ECG monitoring

Anesthesia and Critical Care Concerns/Other Considerations
Evidence-Based Information:

Management of Intracerebral Hemorrhage (ICH) Due to Thrombolysis: Overall management of ICH is similar regardless of cause; however, iatrogenic spontaneous ICH may have specific treatments. According to the 2007 ACC/ASA Guidelines for the Management of Spontaneous Intracerebral Hemorrhage, fibrinolytic-related ICH should be treated with infusion of platelets (6-8 units) and cryoprecipitate which contains factor VIII (Class IIb recommendation).

Pregnancy Risk Factor C

Contraindications Hypersensitivity to tenecteplase or any component of the formulation; active internal bleeding; history of stroke; intracranial/intraspinal surgery or trauma within 2 months; intracranial neoplasm; arteriovenous malformation or aneurysm; bleeding diathesis; severe uncontrolled hypertension

Warnings/Precautions Stop antiplatelet agents and heparin if serious bleeding occurs. Avoid I.M. injections and nonessential handling of the patient for a few hours after administration. Monitor for bleeding complications. Venipunctures should be performed carefully and only when necessary. If arterial puncture is necessary, then use an upper extremity that can be easily compressed manually. For the following conditions, the risk of bleeding is higher with use of tenecteplase and should be weighed against the benefits: Recent major surgery, cerebrovascular disease, recent GI or GU bleed, recent trauma, uncontrolled hypertension (systolic BP ≥180 mm Hg and/or diastolic BP ≥110 mm Hg), suspected left heart thrombus, acute pericarditis, subacute bacterial endocarditis, hemostatic defects, severe hepatic dysfunction, pregnancy, hemorrhagic diabetic retinopathy or other hemorrhagic ophthalmic conditions, septic thrombophlebitis or occluded arteriovenous cannula at seriously infected site, advanced age (see Dosage, Elderly), anticoagulants, recent administration of GP IIb/IIIa inhibitors. Coronary thrombolysis may result in reperfusion arrhythmias. Caution with readministration of tenecteplase. Safety and efficacy have not been established in pediatric patients. Cholesterol embolism has rarely been reported.

Adverse Reactions As with all drugs which may affect hemostasis, bleeding is the major adverse effect associated with tenecteplase. Hemorrhage may occur at virtually any site. Risk is dependent on multiple variables, including the dosage administered, concurrent use of multiple agents which alter hemostasis, and patient predisposition. Rapid lysis of coronary artery thrombi by thrombolytic agents may be associated with reperfusion-related arterial and/or ventricular arrhythmia.

>10%:
  Local: Hematoma (12% minor)
  Hematologic: Bleeding (22% minor; ASSENT-2 trial)
1% to 10%:
  Central nervous system: Stroke (2%)
  Gastrointestinal: GI hemorrhage (1% major, 2% minor), epistaxis (2% minor)
  Genitourinary: GU bleeding (4% minor)
  Hematologic: Bleeding (5% major; ASSENT-2 trial)
  Local: Bleeding at catheter puncture site (4% minor), hematoma (2% major)
  Respiratory: Pharyngeal (3% minor)
The incidence of stroke and bleeding increase with age above 65 years.
<1% (Limited to important or life-threatening): Anaphylaxis, angioedema, bleeding at catheter puncture site (<1% major), cholesterol embolism (clinical features may include livedo reticularis, "purple toe" syndrome, acute renal failure, gangrenous digits, hypertension, pancreatitis, MI, cerebral infarction, spinal cord infarction, retinal artery occlusion, bowel infarction, rhabdomyolysis), GU bleeding (<1% major), intracranial hemorrhage (0.9%), laryngeal edema, rash, respiratory tract bleeding, retroperitoneal bleeding, urticaria
Additional cardiovascular events associated with use in MI: Arrhythmias, AV block, cardiac arrest, cardiac tamponade, cardiogenic shock, electromechanical ▶

dissociation, embolism, fever, heart failure, hypotension, mitral regurgitation, myocardial reinfarction, myocardial rupture, nausea, pericardial effusion, pericarditis, pulmonary edema, recurrent myocardial ischemia, thrombosis, vomiting

Drug Interactions

Avoid Concomitant Use There are no known interactions where it is recommended to avoid concomitant use.

Increased Effect/Toxicity

Tenecteplase may increase the levels/effects of: Anticoagulants; Drotrecogin Alfa

The levels/effects of Tenecteplase may be increased by: Antiplatelet Agents; Herbs (Anticoagulant/Antiplatelet Properties); Nonsteroidal Anti-Inflammatory Agents; Salicylates

Decreased Effect

The levels/effects of Tenecteplase may be decreased by: Aprotinin

Dosage Forms Excipient information presented when available (limited, particularly for generics); consult specific product labeling.

Injection, powder for reconstitution [recombinant]:
TNKase®: 50 mg

References

Broderick J, Connolly S, Feldmann E, et al, "Guidelines for the Management of Spontaneous Intracerebral Hemorrhage in Adults: 2007 Update: A Guideline From the American Heart Association/American Stroke Association Stroke Council, High Blood Pressure Research Council, and the Quality of Care and Outcomes in Research Interdisciplinary Working Group," *Stroke*, 2007, 38(6):2001-23. Available at http://stroke.ahajournals.org/cgi/content/short/STROKEAHA.107.183689.

- ◆ **Tenolin (Can)** *see* Atenolol *on page 155*
- ◆ **Tenormin®** *see* Atenolol *on page 155*
- ◆ **Tensilon® (Can)** *see* Edrophonium *on page 474*

Terbutaline (ter BYOO ta leen)

Medication Safety Issues

Sound-alike/look-alike issues:

Brethine may be confused with Methergine®

Terbutaline may be confused with terbinafine, TOLBUTamide

Terbutaline and methylergonovine parenteral dosage forms look similar. Due to their contrasting indications, use care when administering these agents.

Canadian Brand Names Bricanyl®

Index Terms Brethaire [DSC]; Brethine; Bricanyl [DSC]

Pharmacologic Category Beta$_2$-Adrenergic Agonist

Generic Available Yes

Use Bronchodilator in reversible airway obstruction and bronchial asthma

Unlabeled/Investigational Use Tocolytic agent (management of preterm labor)

Mechanism of Action Relaxes bronchial smooth muscle by action on beta$_2$-receptors with less effect on heart rate

Pharmacodynamics/Kinetics

Onset of action: Oral: 30-45 minutes; SubQ: 6-15 minutes

Protein binding: 25%

Metabolism: Hepatic to inactive sulfate conjugates

Bioavailability: SubQ doses are more bioavailable than oral

Half-life elimination: 11-16 hours

Excretion: Urine

Dosage

Children <12 years: Bronchoconstriction:

Oral: Initial: 0.05 mg/kg/dose 3 times/day, increased gradually as required; maximum: 0.15 mg/kg/dose 3-4 times/day or a total of 5 mg/24 hours

SubQ: 0.005-0.01 mg/kg/dose to a maximum of 0.3 mg/dose; may repeat in 15-20 minutes

Children ≥6 years and Adults: Bronchospasm (acute): Inhalation (Bricanyl® [CAN] MDI: 500 mcg/puff, *not labeled for use in the U.S.*): One puff as needed; may repeat with 1 inhalation (after 5 minutes); more than 6 inhalations should not be necessary in any 24 hour period. **Note:** If a previously effective dosage regimen fails to provide the usual relief, or the effects of a dose last for >3 hours, medical advice should be sought immediately; this is a sign of seriously worsening asthma that requires reassessment of therapy.

Children >12 years and Adults: Bronchoconstriction:

Oral:

12-15 years: 2.5 mg every 6 hours 3 times/day; not to exceed 7.5 mg in 24 hours

>15 years: 5 mg/dose every 6 hours 3 times/day; if side effects occur, reduce dose to 2.5 mg every 6 hours; not to exceed 15 mg in 24 hours

SubQ: 0.25 mg/dose; may repeat in 15-30 minutes (maximum: 0.5 mg/4-hour period)

Adults: Premature labor (tocolysis; unlabeled use):

Acute: I.V. 2.5-10 mcg/minute; increased gradually every 10-20 minutes; effective maximum dosages from 17.5-30 mcg/minute have been used with caution. Duration of infusion is at least 12 hours.

Maintenance: Oral: 2.5-10 mg every 4-6 hours for as long as necessary to prolong pregnancy depending on patient tolerance

Dosing adjustment/comments in renal impairment:

Cl_{cr} 10-50 mL/minute: Administer at 50% of normal dose

Cl_{cr} <10 mL/minute: Avoid use

Stability Store injection at room temperature; do not freeze. Protect from heat and light. Use only clear solutions. Store powder for inhalation (Bricanyl® Turbuhaler [CAN]) at room temperature between 15°C and 30°C (58°F and 86°F).

Administration

I.V.: Use infusion pump.

Oral: Administer around-the-clock to promote less variation in peak and trough serum levels

Monitoring Parameters Serum potassium, glucose; heart rate, blood pressure, respiratory rate; monitor for signs and symptoms of pulmonary edema (when used as a tocolytic); monitor FEV_1, peak flow, and/or other pulmonary function tests (when used as bronchodilator)

Anesthesia and Critical Care Concerns/Other Considerations

Evidence-Based Information: Beta$_2$-selective agents lose much of their receptor selectivity when delivered parenterally or orally. Subcutaneous beta-agonist therapy has a deleterious therapeutic to toxicity ratio when compared with inhalation. There is no proven benefit of systemic therapy over aerosolized (Expert Report Panel 3, 2007).

Pregnancy Risk Factor B

Contraindications Hypersensitivity to terbutaline or any component of the formulation; cardiac arrhythmias associated with tachycardia; tachycardia caused by digitalis intoxication

Warnings/Precautions When used for tocolysis, there is some risk of maternal pulmonary edema, which has been associated with the following risk factors, excessive hydration, multiple gestation, occult sepsis and underlying cardiac disease. To reduce risk, limit fluid intake to 2.5-3 L/day, limit sodium intake, maintain maternal pulse to <130 beats/minute.

Use caution in patients with cardiovascular disease (arrhythmia or hypertension or HF), convulsive disorders, diabetes, glaucoma, hyperthyroidism, or hypokalemia. Beta-agonists may cause elevation in blood pressure, heart rate, and result in CNS stimulation/excitation. Beta$_2$-agonists may increase risk of arrhythmia, increase serum glucose, or decrease serum potassium.

When used as a bronchodilator, optimize anti-inflammatory treatment before initiating maintenance treatment with terbutaline. Do not use as a component of chronic therapy without an anti-inflammatory agent. Only the mildest form of asthma (Step 1 and/or exercise-induced) would not require concurrent use based upon asthma guidelines. Patient must be instructed to seek medical attention in cases where acute symptoms are not relieved or a previous level of response is diminished. The need to increase frequency of use may indicate deterioration of asthma, and treatment must not be delayed.

Immediate hypersensitivity reactions (urticaria, angioedema, rash, bronchospasm) have been reported. Do not exceed recommended dose; serious adverse

◀ events including fatalities, have been associated with excessive use of inhaled sympathomimetics. Rarely, paradoxical bronchospasm may occur with use of inhaled bronchodilating agents; this should be distinguished from inadequate response.

Adverse Reactions

>10%:

Central nervous system: Nervousness, restlessness

Endocrine & metabolic: Serum glucose increased, serum potassium decreased

Neuromuscular & skeletal: Trembling

1% to 10%:

Cardiovascular: Tachycardia, hypertension, pounding heartbeat

Central nervous system: Dizziness, lightheadedness, drowsiness, headache, insomnia

Gastrointestinal: Dry mouth, nausea, vomiting, bad taste in mouth

Neuromuscular & skeletal: Muscle cramps, weakness

Miscellaneous: Diaphoresis

<1% (Limited to important or life-threatening): Arrhythmia, chest pain, hypokalemia, paradoxical bronchospasm

Drug Interactions

Avoid Concomitant Use

Avoid concomitant use of Terbutaline with any of the following: Iobenguane I 123

Increased Effect/Toxicity

Terbutaline may increase the levels/effects of: Sympathomimetics

The levels/effects of Terbutaline may be increased by: Atomoxetine; Cannabinoids; MAO Inhibitors; Tricyclic Antidepressants

Decreased Effect

Terbutaline may decrease the levels/effects of: Iobenguane I 123

The levels/effects of Terbutaline may be decreased by: Alpha-/Beta-Blockers; Beta-Blockers (Beta1 Selective); Beta-Blockers (Nonselective); Betahistine

Ethanol/Nutrition/Herb Interactions Herb/Nutraceutical: Avoid ephedra, yohimbe (may cause CNS stimulation).

Dosage Forms Excipient information presented when available (limited, particularly for generics); consult specific product labeling. [CAN] = Canadian brand name

Injection, solution, as sulfate: 1 mg/mL (1 mL)

Powder for oral inhalation:

Bricanyl® Turbuhaler [CAN]: 500 mcg/actuation [50 or 200 metered actuations] [not available in U.S.]

Tablet, as sulfate: 2.5 mg, 5 mg

References

Expert Panel Report 3, "Guidelines for the Diagnosis and Management of Asthma," *Clinical Practice Guidelines*, National Institutes of Health, National Heart, Lung, and Blood Institute, NIH Publication No. 08-4051, prepublication 2007. Available at http://www.nhlbi.nih.gov/guidelines/asthma/asthgdln.htm

◆ **Terrell™** *see* Isoflurane *on page 765*

◆ **Testim®** *see* Testosterone *on page 1362*

◆ **Testopel®** *see* Testosterone *on page 1362*

Testosterone (tes TOS ter one)

U.S. Brand Names Androderm®; AndroGel®; Delatestryl®; Depo®-Testosterone; First®-Testosterone; First®-Testosterone MC; Striant®; Testim®; Testopel®

Canadian Brand Names Andriol®; Androderm®; AndroGel®; Andropository®; Delatestryl®; Depotest® 100; Everone® 200; PMS-Testosterone; Testim®

Index Terms Testosterone Cypionate; Testosterone Enanthate

Pharmacologic Category Androgen

Restrictions C-III

Use

Injection: Androgen replacement therapy in the treatment of delayed male puberty; male hypogonadism (primary or hypogonadotropic); inoperable metastatic female breast cancer (enanthate only)

Pellet: Androgen replacement therapy in the treatment of delayed male puberty; male hypogonadism (primary or hypogonadotropic)

Topical (buccal system, gel, transdermal system): Male hypogonadism (primary or hypogonadotropic)

Capsule (not available in U.S.): Androgen replacement therapy in the treatment of delayed male puberty; male hypogonadism (primary or hypogonadotropic); replacement therapy in impotence or for male climacteric symptoms due to androgen deficiency

Unlabeled/Investigational Use Androgen deficiency in men with AIDS wasting; postmenopausal women with decreased sexual desire (in combination with estrogen therapy)

Pharmacodynamics/Kinetics

Duration (route and ester dependent): I.M.: Cypionate and enanthate esters have longest duration, ≤2-4 weeks; gel: 24-48 hours

Absorption: Transdermal gel: ~10% of applied dose

Protein binding: 98%; bound to sex hormone-binding globulin (40%) and albumin

Metabolism: Hepatic; forms metabolites, including dihydrotestosterone (DHT) and estradiol (both active)

Half-life elimination: 10-100 minutes

Excretion: Urine (90%); feces (6%)

Dosage

Adolescents and Adults: Male:

I.M.:

Hypogonadism: Testosterone enanthate or testosterone cypionate: 50-400 mg every 2-4 weeks (FDA-approved dosing range); 75-100 mg/week or 150-200 mg every 2 weeks (per practice guidelines)

Delayed puberty: Testosterone enanthate: 50-200 mg every 2-4 weeks for a limited duration

Pellet (for subcutaneous implantation): Delayed male puberty, male hypogonadism: 150-450 mg every 3-6 months

Oral: Delayed puberty, hypogonadism, or hypogonadotropic hypogonadism: Capsule (Andriol®; not available in U.S.): Initial: 120-160 mg/day in 2 divided doses for 2-3 weeks; adjust according to individual response; usual maintenance dose: 40-120 mg/day (in divided doses)

Adults:

I.M.: Females: Inoperable metastatic breast cancer: Testosterone enanthate: 200-400 mg every 2-4 weeks

Topical: Primary male hypogonadism **or** hypogonadotropic hypogonadism:

Buccal: 30 mg twice daily (every 12 hours) applied to the gum region above the incisor tooth

Transdermal system: Androderm®: Initial: Apply 5 mg/day once nightly to clean, dry area on the back, abdomen, upper arms, or thighs (do **not** apply to scrotum); dosing range: 2.5-7.5 mg/day; in nonvirilized patients, dose may be initiated at 2.5 mg/day

Gel: AndroGel®, Testim®: 5 g (to deliver 50 mg of testosterone with 5 mg systemically absorbed) applied once daily (preferably in the morning) to clean, dry, intact skin of the shoulder and upper arms. AndroGel® may also be applied to the abdomen. Dosage may be increased to a maximum of 10 g (100 mg). **Do not apply testosterone gel to the genitals.**

Dose adjustment based on testosterone levels:

Less than normal range: Increase dose from 5 g to 7.5 g to 10 g

Greater than normal range: Decrease dose. Discontinue if consistently above normal at 5 g/day

Dosing adjustment/comments in hepatic disease: Reduce dose

Additional Information Complete prescribing information for this medication should be consulted for additional detail.

Dosage Forms Excipient information presented when available (limited, particularly for generics); consult specific product labeling. [CAN] = Canadian brand name

Capsule, gelatin, as undecanoate:

Andriol™ [CAN]: 40 mg (10s) [not available in U.S.]

◀ Gel, topical:

AndroGel®:

1.25 g/actuation (75 g) [1% metered-dose pump; delivers 5 g/4 actuations; provides sixty 1.25 g actuations; contains ethanol 67%; may be chemically synthesized from soy]

2.5 g (30s) [1% unit dose packets; contains ethanol 67%; may be chemically synthesized from soy]

5 g (30s) [1% unit dose packets; contains ethanol; may be chemically synthesized from soy]

Testim®: 5 g (30s) [1% unit-dose tube; contains ethanol 74%; may be chemically synthesized from soy]

Implant, subcutaneous:

Testopel®: 75 mg (10s, 100s)

Injection, in oil, as cypionate: 100 mg/mL (10 mL); 200 mg/mL (1 mL, 10 mL)

Depo®-Testosterone: 100 mg/mL (10 mL); 200 mg/mL (1 mL, 10 mL) [contains benzyl alcohol, benzyl benzoate, and cottonseed oil]

Injection, in oil, as enanthate: 200 mg/mL (5 mL)

Delatestryl®: 200 mg/mL (1 mL, 5 mL) [contains sesame oil]

Kit [for prescription compounding; testosterone 2%]:

First®-Testosterone:

Injection, in oil: Testosterone propionate 100 mg/mL (12 mL) [contains sesame oil and benzyl alcohol]

Ointment: White petrolatum (48 g)

First®-Testosterone MC:

Injection, in oil: Testosterone propionate 100 mg/mL (12 mL) [contains sesame oil and benzyl alcohol]

Cream: Moisturizing cream (48 g)

Mucoadhesive, for buccal application [buccal system]:

Striant®: 30 mg (10s) [may be chemically synthesized from soy]

Transdermal system, topical:

Androderm®: 2.5 mg/day (60s) [contains ethanol]; 5 mg/day (30s) [contains ethanol]

References

Bhasin S, Cunningham GR, Hayes FJ, et al, "Testosterone Therapy in Adult Men With Androgen Deficiency Syndromes: An Endocrine Society Clinical Practice Guideline," *J Clin Endocrinol Metab*, 2006, 91(6):1995-2010.

Borhan-Manesh F and Farnum JB, "Methyltestosterone-Induced Cholestasis. The Importance of Disproportionately Low Serum Alkaline Phosphatase Level," *Arch Intern Med*, 1989, 149(12):2127-9.

Cunningham GR, Cordero E, and Thornby JI, "Testosterone Replacement With Transdermal Therapeutic Systems. Physiological Serum Testosterone and Elevated Dihydrotestosterone Levels," *JAMA*, 1989, 261(17):2525-30.

Daigle RD, "Anabolic Steroids," *J Psychoactive Drugs*, 1990, 22(1):77-80.

Moller BB and Ekelund B, "Toxicity of Cyclosporine During Treatment With Androgens," *N Engl J Med*, 1985, 313(22):1416.

NAMS Board of Trustees, "The Role of Testosterone Therapy in Postmenopausal Women: Position Statement of The North American Menopause Society," *Menopause*, 2005, 12(5):497-511.

Ruch W and Jenny P, "Priapism Following Testosterone Administration for Delayed Male Puberty," *Am J Med*, 1989, 86(2):256.

◆ **Testosterone Cypionate** *see* Testosterone *on page 1362*

◆ **Testosterone Enanthate** *see* Testosterone *on page 1362*

Tetanus Immune Globulin (Human)

(TET a nus i MYUN GLOB yoo lin HYU man)

U.S. Brand Names HyperTET™ S/D

Canadian Brand Names HyperTET™ S/D

Index Terms TIG

Pharmacologic Category Immune Globulin

Generic Available No

Use Prophylaxis against tetanus following injury in patients where immunization status is not known or uncertain

The Advisory Committee on Immunization Practices (ACIP) recommends passive immunization with TIG for the following:

- Persons with a wound that is not clean or minor and in whom contraindications to a tetanus-toxoid containing vaccine exist and they have not completed a primary series of tetanus toxoid immunization.
- Persons who are wounded in bombings or similar mass casualty events who have penetrating injuries or nonintact skin exposure and who cannot confirm receipt of a tetanus booster within the previous 5 years. In case of shortage, use should be reserved for persons ≥60 years of age.

Mechanism of Action Passive immunity toward tetanus

Pharmacodynamics/Kinetics Absorption: Well absorbed

Dosage I.M.:

Prophylaxis of tetanus:

Children <7 years: 4 units/kg; some recommend administering 250 units to small children

Children ≥7 years and Adults: 250 units

Treatment of tetanus: Children and Adults: 500-6000 units. Infiltration of part of the dose around the wound is recommended.

Tetanus Prophylaxis in Wound Management

Number of Prior Tetanus Toxoid Doses	Clean, Minor Wounds		All Other Wounds	
	Td[1] or Tdap	TIG[2]	Td[1] or Tdap	TIG[2]
Unknown or <3	Yes	No	Yes	Yes
≥3[3]	No[4]	No	No[5]	No

[1]Adult tetanus and diphtheria toxoids; use pediatric preparations (DT or DTP) if the patient is <7 years old. **Note:** Tdap is preferred in adolescents ≥10 years and adults who have never received Tdap. Td is preferred to TT in adolescents ≥10 years and adults who received Tdap previously or when Tdap is not available. If TT and TIG are both used, tetanus toxoid (adsorbed) rather than tetanus toxoid (fluid) should be used.

[2]Tetanus immune globulin.

[3]If only three doses of fluid tetanus toxoid have been received, a fourth dose of toxoid, preferably an adsorbed toxoid, should be given.

[4]Yes, if ≥10 years since last dose.

[5]Yes, if ≥5 years since last dose.

Adapted from Centers for Disease Control publications *MMWR*, 1991, 40(RR-10); *MMWR*, 2009, 58(14):374-5; *MMWR*, 2006, 55(early release);1-34; *MMWR Recomm Rep*, 2006, 55(RR-17):1-37.

Stability Store at 2°C to 8°C (26°F to 46°F). Do not use if frozen.

Administration Do not administer I.V.; I.M. use only. Administer in the anterolateral aspects of the upper thigh or the deltoid muscle of the upper arm. Avoid gluteal region due to risk of injury to sciatic nerve; if gluteal region is used, administer only in the upper outer quadrant. If tetanus vaccine and tetanus immune globulin are administered simultaneously, separate sites should be used for each injection. When used for the treatment of tetanus, infiltration of part of the dose around the wound is recommended.

Vaccine administration with antibody-containing products*:

Antibody-containing products and inactivated vaccines: May be given simultaneously at different sites or at any interval between doses.

Antibody-containing products and live vaccines: Do not give simultaneously.

*Examples of antibody-containing products include I.M. and I.V. immune globulin, hepatitis B immune globulin, tetanus immune globulin, varicella zoster immune globulin, rabies immune globulin, whole blood, packed red cells, plasma, and platelet products.

Pregnancy Risk Factor C

Warnings/Precautions Hypersensitivity and anaphylactic reactions can occur; immediate treatment (including epinephrine 1:1000) should be available. Use caution in patients with isolated immunoglobulin A deficiency or a history of systemic hypersensitivity to human immunoglobulins. Use with caution in patients with thrombocytopenia or coagulation disorders; I.M. injections may be contra-indicated. Product of human plasma; may potentially contain infectious agents which could transmit disease. Screening of donors, as well as testing and/or

◀ inactivation or removal of certain viruses, reduces the risk. Infections thought to be transmitted by this product should be reported to the manufacturer. Skin testing should not be performed as local irritation can occur and be misinterpreted as a positive reaction. Not for intravenous administration.

Adverse Reactions Frequency not defined.

Central nervous system: Temperature increased

Dermatologic: Angioneurotic edema (rare)

Local: Injection site: pain, soreness, tenderness

Renal: Nephritic syndrome (rare)

Miscellaneous: Anaphylactic shock (rare)

Drug Interactions

Avoid Concomitant Use There are no known interactions where it is recommended to avoid concomitant use.

Increased Effect/Toxicity There are no known significant interactions involving an increase in effect.

Decreased Effect

Tetanus Immune Globulin (Human) may decrease the levels/effects of: Vaccines (Live)

Dosage Forms Excipient information presented when available (limited, particularly for generics); consult specific product labeling.

Injection, solution [preservative free]:

HyperTET™ S/D: 250 units/mL (1 mL) [prefilled syringe]

Tetanus Toxoid (Adsorbed) (TET a nus TOKS oyd, ad SORBED)

Medication Safety Issues

Sound-alike/look-alike issues:

Tetanus toxoid products may be confused with influenza virus vaccine and tuberculin products. Medication errors have occurred when tetanus toxoid products have been inadvertently administered instead of tuberculin skin tests (PPD) and influenza virus vaccine. These products are refrigerated and often stored in close proximity to each other.

Index Terms TT

Pharmacologic Category Vaccine, Inactivated (Bacterial)

Generic Available No

Use Active immunization against tetanus when combination antigen preparations are not indicated. **Note:** Tetanus and diphtheria toxoids for adult use (Td) is the preferred immunizing agent for most adults and for children after their seventh birthday. Young children should receive trivalent DTaP (diphtheria/tetanus/ acellular pertussis), as part of their childhood immunization program, unless pertussis is contraindicated, then DT is warranted.

Mechanism of Action Tetanus toxoid preparations contain the toxin produced by virulent tetanus bacilli (detoxified growth products of *Clostridium tetani*). The toxin has been modified by treatment with formaldehyde so that it has lost toxicity but still retains ability to act as antigen and produce active immunity; the aluminum salt, a mineral adjuvant, delays the rate of absorption and prolongs and enhances its properties; duration ~10 years.

Pharmacodynamics/Kinetics Duration: Primary immunization: ~10 years

Dosage Children ≥7 years and Adults: I.M.:

Primary immunization: 0.5 mL; repeat 0.5 mL at 4-8 weeks after first dose and at 6-12 months after second dose

Routine booster dose: Recommended every 10 years

Note: In most patients, Td is the recommended product for primary immunization, booster doses, and tetanus immunization in wound management

Stability Store at 2°C to 8°C (26°F to 46°F); do not freeze.

Administration Inject intramuscularly in the area of the vastus lateralis (midthigh laterally) or deltoid. Do not inject into gluteal area. Shake well prior to withdrawing dose; do not use if product does not form a suspension.

For patients at risk of hemorrhage following intramuscular injection, the ACIP recommends "it should be administered intramuscularly if, in the opinion of the physician familiar with the patients bleeding risk, the vaccine can be administered with reasonable safety by this route. If the patient receives antihemophilia or other similar therapy, intramuscular vaccination can be scheduled shortly after such therapy is administered. A fine needle (23 gauge or smaller) can be used for the vaccination and firm pressure applied to the site (without rubbing) for at least 2 minutes. The patient should be instructed concerning the risk of hematoma from the injection."

Administration with other vaccines:

Tetanus toxoid vaccine with other inactivated vaccines: May be given simultaneously or at any interval between doses.

Tetanus toxoid vaccine with live vaccines: May be given simultaneously or at any interval between doses

Vaccine administration with antibody-containing products: Tetanus toxoid vaccine may be be given simultaneously at different sites or at any interval between doses. Examples of antibody-containing products include I.M. and I.V. immune globulin, hepatitis B immune globulin, tetanus immune globulin, varicella zoster immune globulin, rabies immune globulin, whole blood, packed red cells, plasma, and platelet products.

Pregnancy Risk Factor C

Contraindications Hypersensitivity to tetanus toxoid or any component of the formulation

Warnings/Precautions Avoid injection into a blood vessel; allergic reactions may occur; epinephrine 1:1000 must be available. Patients who are immunocompromised may have reduced response; may be used in patients with HIV infection. May defer elective immunization during febrile illness or acute infection; defer elective immunization during outbreaks of poliomyelitis. In patients with a history of severe local reaction (Arthus-type) or temperature of >39.4°C (>103°F) following previous dose, do not give further routine or emergency doses of tetanus and diphtheria toxoids for 10 years. Use caution in patients on anticoagulants, with thrombocytopenia, or bleeding disorders (bleeding may occur following intramuscular injection). Use with caution if Guillain-Barré syndrome occurred within 6 weeks of prior tetanus toxoid. Contains thimerosal; vial stopper may contain natural latex rubber. This product is not indicated for use in children <7 years of age. In order to maximize vaccination rates, the ACIP recommends simultaneous administration of all age-appropriate vaccines (live or inactivated) for which a person is eligible at a single clinic visit, unless contraindications exist.

Adverse Reactions All serious adverse reactions must be reported to the U.S. Department of Health and Human Services (DHHS) Vaccine Adverse Event Reporting System (VAERS) 1-800-822-7967.
Frequency not defined.

Cardiovascular: Hypotension

Central nervous system: Brachial neuritis, fever, malaise, pain

Gastrointestinal: Nausea

Local: Edema, induration (with or without tenderness), rash, redness, urticaria, warmth

Neuromuscular: Arthralgia, Guillain-Barré syndrome

Miscellaneous: Anaphylactic reaction, Arthus-type hypersensitivity reaction

Drug Interactions

Avoid Concomitant Use There are no known interactions where it is recommended to avoid concomitant use.

Increased Effect/Toxicity There are no known significant interactions involving an increase in effect.

Decreased Effect

The levels/effects of Tetanus Toxoid (Adsorbed) may be decreased by: Immunosuppressants

Dosage Forms Excipient information presented when available (limited, particularly for generics); consult specific product labeling.

Injection, suspension: Tetanus 5 Lf units per 0.5 mL (0.5 mL) [contains trace amounts of thimerosal]

Tetracaine (TET ra kane)

Related Information

Local Anesthetics *on page 1636*

U.S. Brand Names Pontocaine®; Pontocaine® Niphanoid®

▶

◀ **Canadian Brand Names** Ametop™; Pontocaine®

Index Terms Amethocaine Hydrochloride; Tetracaine Hydrochloride

Pharmacologic Category Local Anesthetic

Generic Available Yes: Ophthalmic solution, solution for injection

Use Spinal anesthesia; local anesthesia in the eye for various diagnostic and examination purposes; topically applied to nose and throat for diagnostic procedures

Mechanism of Action Ester local anesthetic blocks both the initiation and conduction of nerve impulses by decreasing the neuronal membrane's permeability to sodium ions, which results in inhibition of depolarization with resultant blockade of conduction

Pharmacodynamics/Kinetics

Onset of action: Anesthetic: Rhinolaryngology: 5-10 minutes

Duration: Rhinolaryngology: ~30 minutes

Metabolism: Hepatic; detoxified by plasma esterases to aminobenzoic acid

Excretion: Urine

Dosage Adults:

Ophthalmic: Short-term anesthesia of the eye: 0.5% solution: Instill 1-2 drops; prolonged use (especially for at-home self-medication) is not recommended

Injection: Spinal anesthesia: **Note:** Dosage varies with the anesthetic procedure, the degree of anesthesia required, and the individual patient response; it is administered by subarachnoid injection for spinal anesthesia.

Perineal anesthesia: 5 mg

Perineal and lower extremities: 10 mg

Anesthesia extending up to costal margin: 15 mg; doses up to 20 mg may be given, but are reserved for exceptional cases

Low spinal anesthesia (saddle block): 2-5 mg

Topical mucous membranes (rhinolaryngology): Used as a 0.25% or 0.5% solution by direct application or nebulization; total dose should not exceed 20 mg

Stability

Solution for injection: Store solution under refrigeration. Protect from light.

Hyperbaric solution: May be made by mixing equal volumes of the 1% solution and $D_{10}W$.

Powder for injection: Following reconstitution, store solution under refrigeration. Protect from light.

Hyperbaric solution: Dissolve 10 mg of Pontocaine® Niphanoid® in 1 mL $D_{10}W$. Further dilute with equal volume of spinal fluid. Resulting solution is D_5W with tetracaine 5 mg/mL.

Hypobaric solution: Dissolve 1 mg of Pontocaine® Niphanoid® in 1 mL SWFI.

Ophthalmic and topical solutions: Store under refrigeration at 2°C to 8°C.

Administration Before injection, withdraw syringe plunger to make sure injection is not into vein or artery

Anesthesia and Critical Care Concerns/Other Considerations

Local anesthetic toxicity: Cardiac arrest: Lipid infusion has been used in animal studies and several human cases (*Bupivacaine:* Rosenblatt, 2006; *Levobupivacaine:* Foxall, 2007; *Ropivacaine:* Litz, 2006) where cardiovascular toxicity, unresponsive to conventional resuscitation, resulted. Additional information is available at http://www.lipidrescue.org. The protocol from the website is: 20% Fat Emulsion: 1.5 mL/kg administered over 1 minute, followed immediately by an infusion of 0.25 mL/kg/minute. Continue chest compressions (lipid must circulate). Repeat bolus every 3-5 minutes up to 3 mL/kg total dose until circulation restored. Continue infusion until hemodynamic stability is restored. Increase the infusion rate to 0.5 mL/kg/minute if BP declines. A maximum total dose of 8 mL/kg is recommended.

Pregnancy Risk Factor C

Contraindications Hypersensitivity to tetracaine, ester-type anesthetics, aminobenzoic acid, or any component of the formulation; injection should not be used when spinal anesthesia is contraindicated

Warnings/Precautions Use with caution in patients with cardiac disease, hyperthyroidism, abnormal or decreased levels of plasma esterases. Use of the lowest effective dose is recommended. Acutely ill, elderly, debilitated, obstetric patients, or patients with increased intra-abdominal pressure may require decreased doses. Products may contain sodium bisulfite which may cause allergic reactions in some individuals. Resuscitative equipment, oxygen, and other resuscitative drugs should be available for immediate use.

Ophthalmic: May delay wound healing. Prolonged use is not recommended. The anesthetized eye should be protected from irritation, foreign bodies, and rubbing to prevent inadvertent damage.

Adverse Reactions Frequency not defined.

Injection: Note: Adverse effects listed are those characteristics of local anesthetics.

Cardiovascular: Cardiac arrest, hypotension

Central nervous system: Chills, convulsions, dizziness, drowsiness, nervousness, unconsciousness

Gastrointestinal: Nausea, vomiting

Neuromuscular & skeletal: Tremors

Ocular: Blurred vision, pupil constriction

Otic: Tinnitus

Respiratory: Respiratory arrest

Miscellaneous: Allergic reaction

Ophthalmic: Ocular: Chemosis, lacrimation, photophobia, transient stinging

With chronic use: Corneal erosions, corneal healing retardation, corneal opacification (permanent), corneal scarring, keratitis (severe)

Drug Interactions

Avoid Concomitant Use There are no known interactions where it is recommended to avoid concomitant use.

Increased Effect/Toxicity There are no known significant interactions involving an increase in effect.

Decreased Effect There are no known significant interactions involving a decrease in effect.

Dosage Forms Excipient information presented when available (limited, particularly for generics); consult specific product labeling.

Injection, powder for reconstitution, as hydrochloride [preservative free]:
Pontocaine® Niphanoid®: 20 mg

Injection, solution, as hydrochloride [preservative free]: 1% [10 mg/mL] (2 mL)
Pontocaine®): 1% [10 mg/mL] (2 mL) [contains sodium bisulfite]

Solution, ophthalmic, as hydrochloride: 0.5% [5 mg/mL] (2 mL, 15 mL)

Solution, topical, as hydrochloride (Pontocaine®): 2% [20 mg/mL] (30 mL, 118 mL) [for rhinolaryngology]

References

Corcoran W, Butterworth J, Weller RS, et al, "Local Anesthetic-Induced Cardiac Toxicity: A Survey of Contemporary Practice Strategies Among Academic Anesthesiology Departments," *Anesth Analg*, 2006, 103(5):1322-6.

Foxall G, McCahon R, Lamb J, et al, "Levobupivacaine-Induced Seizures and Cardiovascular Collapse Treated With Intralipid," *Anaesthesia*, 2007, 62(5):516-8.

Litz RJ, Popp M, Stehr SN, et al, "Successful Resuscitation of a Patient With Ropivacaine-Induced Asystole After Axillary Plexus Block Using lipid Infusion," *Anaesthesia*, 2006, 61(8):800-1.

Rosenblatt MA, Abel M, Fischer GW, et al, "Successful Use of a 20% Lipid Emulsion to Resuscitate a Patient After a Presumed Bupivacaine-Related Cardiac Arrest," *Anesthesiology*, 2006, 105(1):217-8.

♦ **Tetracaine Hydrochloride** *see* Tetracaine *on page 1367*

♦ **Tetracosactide** *see* Cosyntropin *on page 352*

♦ **Tetrahydrocannabinol** *see* Dronabinol *on page 460*

♦ **Teveten®** *see* Eprosartan *on page 510*

♦ **Tev-Tropin®** *see* Somatropin *on page 1318*

♦ **Texacort®** *see* Hydrocortisone *on page 699*

Thalidomide (tha LI doe mide)

Medication Safety Issues

Sound-alike/look-alike issues:

Thalidomide may be confused with flutamide, lenalidomide

Thalomid® may be confused with thiamine

◄ **High alert medication:** The Institute for Safe Medication Practices (ISMP) includes this medication among its list of drugs which have a heightened risk of causing significant patient harm when used in error.

International issues:
Thalomid® may be confused with Thilomide® which is a brand name for Iodoxamide in Greece and Turkey

Related Information
Anesthesia for Obstetric Patients in Nonobstetric Surgery *on page 1532*

U.S. Brand Names Thalomid®

Canadian Brand Names Thalomid®

Pharmacologic Category Angiogenesis Inhibitor; Immunomodulator, Systemic; Tumor Necrosis Factor (TNF) Blocking Agent

Restrictions Thalidomide is approved for marketing only under a special distribution program. This program, called the "System for Thalidomide Education and Prescribing Safety" (STEPS® 1-888-423-5436), has been approved by the FDA. Prescribers and pharmacists must be registered with the program. No more than a 4-week supply should be dispensed. Blister packs should be dispensed intact (do not repackage capsules). Prescriptions must be filled within 7 days. Subsequent prescriptions may be filled only if fewer than 7 days of therapy remain on the previous prescription. A new prescription is required for further dispensing (a telephone prescription may not be accepted.)

Generic Available No

Use Treatment of multiple myeloma; treatment and maintenance of cutaneous manifestations of erythema nodosum leprosum (ENL)

Unlabeled/Investigational Use Treatment of Crohn's disease; graft-versus-host reactions after bone marrow transplantation; AIDS-related aphthous stomatitis; Behçet's syndrome; Waldenström's macroglobulinemia; Langerhans cell histiocytosis

Mechanism of Action Has immunomodulatory and antiangiogenic characteristics. Immunologic effects may vary based on conditions; may suppress excessive tumor necrosis factor-alpha production in patients with ENL, yet may increase plasma tumor necrosis factor-alpha levels in HIV-positive patients. In multiple myeloma, thalidomide is associated with an increase in natural killer cells and increased levels of interleukin-2 and interferon gamma. Other proposed mechanisms of action include suppression of angiogenesis, prevention of free-radical-mediated DNA damage, increased cell mediated cytotoxic effects, and altered expression of cellular adhesion molecules.

Pharmacodynamics/Kinetics
Distribution: V_d: 120 L
Protein binding: 55% to 66%
Metabolism: Nonenzymatic hydrolysis in plasma; forms multiple metabolites
Half-life elimination: 5-7 hours
Time to peak, plasma: 3-6 hours
Excretion: Urine (<1% as unchanged drug)

Dosage Oral:
Multiple myeloma: 200 mg once daily (with dexamethasone 40 mg daily on days 1-4, 9-12, and 17-20 of a 28-day treatment cycle)
Cutaneous ENL:
Initial: 100-300 mg/day taken once daily at bedtime with water (at least 1 hour after evening meal)
Patients weighing <50 kg: Initiate at lower end of the dosing range
Severe cutaneous reaction or patients previously requiring high dose may be initiated at 400 mg/day; doses may be divided, but taken 1 hour after meals
Maintenance: Dosing should continue until active reaction subsides (usually at least 2 weeks), then tapered in 50 mg decrements every 2-4 weeks
Patients who flare during tapering or with a history or requiring prolonged maintenance should be maintained on the minimum dosage necessary to control the reaction. Efforts to taper should be repeated every 3-6 months, in increments of 50 mg every 2-4 weeks.
Behçet's syndrome (unlabeled use): 100-400 mg/day
Graft-vs-host reactions (unlabeled use): 100-1600 mg/day; usual initial dose: 200 mg 4 times/day for use up to 700 days

AIDS-related aphthous stomatitis (unlabeled use): 200 mg twice daily for 5 days, then 200 mg/day for up to 8 weeks

Stability Store at 15°C to 30°C (50°F to 86°F). Protect from light. Keep in original package.

Administration Oral: Administer with water, preferably at bedtime once daily on an empty stomach, at least 1 hour after the evening meal. Doses >400 mg/day may be given in 2-3 divided doses. Avoid extensive handling of capsules; capsules should remain in blister pack until ingestion. If exposed to the powder content from broken capsules or body fluids from patients receiving thalidomide, the exposed area should be washed with soap and water.

Monitoring Parameters CBC with differential, platelets; signs of neuropathy monthly for the first 3 months, then periodically during treatment; consider monitoring of sensory nerve application potential amplitudes (at baseline and every 6 months) to detect asymptomatic neuropathy. In HIV-seropositive patients: viral load after 1 and 3 months, then every 3 months. Pregnancy testing (sensitivity of at least 50 mIU/mL) is required within 24 hours prior to initiation of therapy, weekly during the first 4 weeks, then every 4 weeks in women with regular menstrual cycles or every 2 weeks in women with irregular menstrual cycles.

Reference Range Therapeutic plasma thalidomide levels in graft-vs-host reactions are 5-8 mcg/mL, although it has been suggested that lower plasma levels (0.5-1.5 mcg/mL) may be therapeutic; peak serum thalidomide level after a 200 mg dose: 1.2 mcg/mL

Pregnancy Risk Factor X

Contraindications Hypersensitivity to thalidomide or any component of the formulation; neuropathy (peripheral); patient unable to comply with STEPS® program (including males); women of childbearing potential unless alternative therapies are inappropriate and adequate precautions are taken to avoid pregnancy; pregnancy

Warnings/Precautions Hazardous agent - use appropriate precautions for handling and disposal. **[U.S. Boxed Warning]: Thalidomide is a known teratogen; effective contraception must be used for at least 4 weeks before initiating therapy, during therapy, and for 4 weeks following discontinuation of thalidomide for women of childbearing potential.** Use caution with drugs which may decrease the efficacy of hormonal contraceptives.

[U.S. Boxed Warning]: Thrombotic events have been reported, generally in patients with other risk factors for thrombosis (neoplastic disease, inflammatory disease, or concurrent therapy with combination chemo-therapy. Use in combination with dexamethasone is associated with increased risk for deep vein thrombosis (DVT) and pulmonary embolism (PE), monitor for signs and symptoms of thromboembolism; patients at risk may benefit from prophylactic anticoagulation or aspirin.

May cause sedation; patients must be warned to use caution when performing tasks which require alertness. Use caution in patients with renal or hepatic impairment, neurological disorders, or constipation. Thalidomide has been associated with the development of peripheral neuropathy, which may be irreversible; use caution with other medications which may cause peripheral neuropathy. Consider immediate discontinuation (if clinically appropriate) in patients who develop neuropathy. May cause seizures; use caution in patients with a history of seizures, concurrent therapy with drugs which alter seizure threshold, or conditions which predispose to seizures. May cause neutropenia; discontinue therapy if absolute neutrophil count decreases to <750/mm^3. Use caution in patients with HIV infection; has been associated with increased viral loads. May cause orthostasis and/or bradycardia; use with caution in patients with cardiovascular disease or in patients who would not tolerate transient hypotensive episodes. Hypersensitivity, Stevens-Johnson syndrome (SJS) and toxic epi-dermal necrolysis (TEN) have been reported; withhold therapy and evaluate with skin rashes; permanently discontinue if rash is exfoliative, purpuric, bullous or if SJS or TEN is suspected. Safety and efficacy have not been established in children <12 years of age.

◀ **Adverse Reactions**

>10%:

Cardiovascular: Edema (57%), thrombosis/embolism (23%; grade 3: 13%, grade 4: 9%), hypotension (16%)

Central nervous system: Fatigue (79%; grade 3: 3%, grade 4: 1%), somnolence (36% to 38%), dizziness (4% to 20%), sensory neuropathy (54%), confusion (28%), anxiety/agitation (9% to 26%), fever (19% to 23%), motor neuropathy (22%), headache (13% to 19%)

Dermatologic: Rash (21% to 31%), rash/desquamation (30%; grade 3: 4%), dry skin (21%), maculopapular rash (4% to 19%), acne (3% to 11%)

Endocrine & metabolic: Hypocalcemia (72%)

Gastrointestinal: Constipation (3% to 55%), anorexia (3% to 28%), nausea (4% to 24%), weight loss (23%), weight gain (22%), diarrhea (4% to 19%), oral moniliasis (4% to 11%)

Hematologic: Leukopenia (17% to 35%), neutropenia (31%), anemia (6% to 13%), lymphadenopathy (6% to 13%)

Hepatic: AST increased (3% to 25%), bilirubin increased (14%)

Neuromuscular & skeletal: Muscle weakness (40%), tremor (4% to 26%), weakness (6% to 22%), myalgia (17%), paresthesia (6% to 16%), arthralgia (13%)

Renal: Hematuria (11%)

Respiratory: Dyspnea (42%)

Miscellaneous: Diaphoresis (13%)

1% to 10%:

Cardiovascular: Facial edema (4%), peripheral edema (3% to 8%)

Central nervous system: Insomnia (9%), nervousness (3% to 9%), malaise (8%), vertigo (8%), pain (3% to 8%)

Dermatologic: Dermatitis (fungal 4% to 9%), pruritus (3% to 8%), nail disorder (3% to 4%)

Endocrine & metabolic: Hyperlipemia (6% to 9%)

Gastrointestinal: Xerostomia (8% to 9%), flatulence (8%), tooth pain (4%)

Genitourinary: Impotence (3% to 8%)

Hepatic: LFTs abnormal (9%)

Neuromuscular & skeletal: Neuropathy (8%), back pain (4% to 6%), neck pain (4%), neck rigidity (4%)

Renal: Albuminuria (3% to 8%)

Respiratory: Pharyngitis (4% to 8%), rhinitis (4%), sinusitis (4% to 8%)

Miscellaneous: Infection (6% to 8%)

Postmarketing and/or case reports (limited to important or life-threatening): Acute renal failure, alkaline phosphatase increased, ALT increased, amenorrhea, aphthous stomatitis, arrhythmia, atrial fibrillation, bile duct obstruction, bradycardia, BUN increased, carpal tunnel, CML, creatinine clearance decreased, creatinine increased, deafness, depression, diplopia, dysesthesia, ECG abnormalities, electrolyte imbalances, enuresis, eosinophilia, epistaxis, erythema multiforme, erythema nodosum, erythroleukemia, exfoliative dermatitis, febrile neutropenia, foot drop, galactorrhea, granulocytopenia, gynecomastia, hepatomegaly, Hodgkin's disease, hypercalcemia, hyper-/hypokalemia, hypersensitivity, hypertension, hyper-/hypothyroidism, hyperuricemia, hypomagnesemia, hyponatremia, hypoproteinemia, intestinal obstruction, intestinal perforation, interstitial pneumonitis, LDH increased, lethargy, leukocytosis, lymphedema, lymphopenia, mental status changes, metrorrhagia, migraine, myxedema, nystagmus, oliguria, orthostatic hypotension, pancytopenia, paresthesia, petechiae, peripheral neuritis, photosensitivity, pleural effusion, prothrombin time changes, psychosis, pulmonary embolus, pulmonary hypertension, purpura, Raynaud's syndrome, seizure, status epilepticus, Stevens-Johnson syndrome, stomach ulcer, stupor, suicide attempt, syncope, tachycardia, thrombocytopenia, toxic epidermal necrolysis, tumor lysis syndrome

Drug Interactions

Avoid Concomitant Use

Avoid concomitant use of Thalidomide with any of the following: Abatacept; Anakinra; Canakinumab; Certolizumab Pegol; Natalizumab; Rilonacept; Vaccines (Live)

Increased Effect/Toxicity

Thalidomide may increase the levels/effects of: Abatacept; Alcohol (Ethyl); Anakinra; Canakinumab; Certolizumab Pegol; CNS Depressants; Leflunomide; Methotrimeprazine; Natalizumab; Pamidronate; Rilonacept; Vaccines (Live); Zoledronic Acid

The levels/effects of Thalidomide may be increased by: Dexamethasone; Methotrimeprazine; Trastuzumab

Decreased Effect

Thalidomide may decrease the levels/effects of: Vaccines (Inactivated); Vaccines (Live)

The levels/effects of Thalidomide may be decreased by: Echinacea

Ethanol/Nutrition/Herb Interactions

Ethanol: Avoid ethanol (may increase sedation).

Herb/Nutraceutical: Avoid cat's claw and echinacea (have immunostimulant properties; consider therapy modifications).

Dietary Considerations Should be taken at least 1 hour after the evening meal.

Dosage Forms Excipient information presented when available (limited, particularly for generics); consult specific product labeling.

Capsule:

Thalomid®: 50 mg, 100 mg, 150 mg, 200 mg

◆ **Thalomid®** *see* Thalidomide *on page 1369*

◆ **THC** *see* Dronabinol *on page 460*

◆ **Theo-24®** *see* Theophylline *on page 1373*

◆ **Theochron™** *see* Theophylline *on page 1373*

◆ **Theochron® SR (Can)** *see* Theophylline *on page 1373*

Theophylline (thee OFF i lin)

Related Information

Asthma *on page 1728*

U.S. Brand Names Elixophyllin®; Theo-24®; Theochron™; Uniphyl®

Canadian Brand Names Apo-Theo LA®; Novo-Theophyl SR; PMS-Theophylline; Pulmophylline; ratio-Theo-Bronc; Theochron® SR; Uniphyl® SRT

Index Terms Theophylline Anhydrous

Pharmacologic Category Theophylline Derivative

Generic Available Yes: Extended release tablet, infusion

Use Treatment of symptoms and reversible airway obstruction due to chronic asthma, or other chronic lung diseases; apnea of prematurity

Note: The National Heart, Lung, and Blood Institute Guidelines (2007) do not recommend oral theophylline as a long-term control medication for asthma in children ≤4 years of age; use may be considered as an alternative (but not preferred) agent in older children and adults. The guidelines do not recommend theophylline I.V. for the treatment of exacerbations of asthma.

Mechanism of Action Causes bronchodilatation, diuresis, CNS and cardiac stimulation, and gastric acid secretion by blocking phosphodiesterase which increases tissue concentrations of cyclic adenine monophosphate (cAMP) which in turn promotes catecholamine stimulation of lipolysis, glycogenolysis, and gluconeogenesis and induces release of epinephrine from adrenal medulla cells

Pharmacodynamics/Kinetics

Absorption: Oral: Dosage form dependent

Distribution: 0.45 L/kg (range: 0.3-0.7 L/kg) based on ideal body weight; distributes poorly into body fat; V_d may increase in premature neonates, patients with hepatic cirrhosis, acidemia (uncorrected), the elderly

Metabolism: Children >1 year and Adults: Hepatic; involves CYP1A2, 2E1 and 3A4; forms active metabolites (caffeine and 3-methylxanthine)

Protein binding: 40%, primarily to albumin

Half-life elimination: Highly variable and dependent upon age, liver function, cardiac function, lung disease, and smoking history

Premature infants, postnatal age 3-15 days: 30 hours (range: 17-43 hours)

Premature infants, postnatal age 25-57 days: 20 hours (range: 9.4-30.6 hours)
Children 6-17 years: 3.7 hours (range: 1.5-5.9 hours)
Adults 16-60 years with asthma, nonsmoking, otherwise healthy: 8.7 hours
  (range: 6.1-12.8 hours)
Time to peak, serum:
  Oral: Liquid: 1 hour; Tablet, enteric-coated: 5 hours; Tablet, uncoated: 2 hours
  I.V.: Within 30 minutes
Excretion: Urine
  Neonates: 50% as unchanged theophylline
  Children >3 months and Adults: ~10% as unchanged theophylline

Dosage Note: Doses should be individualized based on peak serum concentrations and should be based on ideal body weight.

Acute symptoms: Loading dose: Children and Adults: Oral, I.V.:

If no theophylline received within the previous 24 hours: 4.6 mg/kg loading dose (~5.8 mg/kg hydrous aminophylline) I.V. or 5 mg/kg orally. Loading dose intended to achieve a serum level of approximately 10 mcg/mL; loading doses should be given intravenously (preferred) or with a rapidly absorbed oral product (not an extended-release product). **Note:** On the average, for every 1 mg/kg theophylline given, blood levels will rise 2 mcg/mL.

If theophylline has been administered in the previous 24 hours: A loading dose is not recommended without obtaining a serum theophylline concentration. The loading dose should be calculated as follows:

Dose = (desired serum theophylline concentration - measured serum
  theophylline concentration) (V_d)

Acute symptoms: Maintenance dose: Children and Adults: I.V.: **Note:** To achieve a target concentration of 10 mcg/mL unless otherwise noted. Lower initial doses may be required in patients with reduced theophylline clearance. Dosage should be adjusted according to serum level measurements during the first 12- to 24-hour period.

Neonates ≤24 days: 1 mg/kg every 12 hours to achieve a target concentration of 7.5 mcg/mL for apnea of prematurity
Neonates >24 days: 1.5 mg/kg every 12 hours to achieve a target concentration of 7.5 mcg/mL for apnea of prematurity
Infants 6-52 weeks: mg/kg/hour = (0.008) (age in weeks) + 0.21
Children 1-9 years: 0.8 mg/kg/hour
Children 9-12 years: 0.7 mg/kg/hour
Adolescents 12-16 years (cigarette or marijuana smokers): 0.7 mg/kg/hour
Adolescents 12-16 years (nonsmokers): 0.5 mg/kg/hour; maximum 900 mg/day unless serum levels indicate need for larger dose
Adults 16-60 years (otherwise healthy, nonsmokers): 0.4 mg/kg/hour; maximum 900 mg/day unless serum levels indicate need for larger dose
Adults >60 years: 0.3 mg/kg/hour; maximum 400 mg/day unless serum levels indicate need for larger dose
Cardiac decompensation, cor pulmonale, hepatic dysfunction, sepsis with multiorgan failure, shock: 0.2 mg/kg/hour; maximum 400 mg/day unless serum levels indicate need for larger dose

Treatment of chronic conditions: Oral:

Infants <1 year: **Note:** Doses should be adjusted to maintain the peak steady state serum concentrations. The time to reach steady state will vary based on age and the presence of risk factors which may affect theophylline clearance. Theophylline serum levels obtained prior to reaching steady state should not be used to increase the maintenance dose even if the serum concentration is <10 mcg/mL. Peak steady state theophylline serum concentrations should be 5-10 mcg/mL in neonates and 10-15 mcg/mL in older infants.
Premature Neonates <24 days postnatal age: 1 mg/kg/dose every 12 hours
Premature Neonates ≥24 days postnatal age: 1.5 mg/kg/dose every 12 hours
Full-term Infants and Infants <26 weeks: Total daily dose (mg)= [(0.2 x age in weeks) +5] x (weight in kg); divide dose into 3 equal amounts and administer at 8-hour intervals
Full-term Infants and Infants ≥26 weeks and <52 weeks: Total daily dose (mg) = [(0.2 x age in weeks) +5] x (weight in kg); divide dose into 4 equal amounts and administer at 6-hour intervals

Children 1-15 years and <45 kg **without** risk factors for impaired theophylline clearance: 12-14 mg/kg/day in divided doses, every 4-6 hours for 3 days (maximum dose: 300 mg/day), then increase to 16 mg/kg/day in divided doses every 4-6 hours for 3 days (maximum dose: 400 mg/day); maintenance dose: 20 mg/kg/day in divided doses every 4-6 hours (maximum dose: 600 mg/day)

Increase dose only if tolerated. Consider lowering dose or using a slower titration if caffeine-like adverse events occur. Smaller doses given more frequently may be used in patients with a more rapid metabolism to prevent breakthrough symptoms which could occur due to low trough concentration prior to the next dose. Reliably absorbed slow release formulations can be used to decrease serum fluctuations and permit longer dosing intervals.

Adults 16-60 years **without** risk factors for impaired theophylline clearance: 300 mg/day in divided doses every 6-8 hours for 3 days, then increase to 400 mg/day in divided doses every 6-8 hours for 3 days; maintenance dose: 600 mg/day in divided doses every 6-8 hours

Increase dose only if tolerated. Consider lowering dose or using a slower titration if caffeine-like adverse events occur. Smaller doses given more frequently may be used in patients with a more rapid metabolism to prevent breakthrough symptoms which could occur due to low trough concentration prior to the next dose. Reliably absorbed slow release formulations can be used to decrease serum fluctuations and permit longer dosing intervals.

Dose adjustment in patients **with** risk factors for impaired theophylline clearance and patients in whom monitoring serum theophylline levels is not feasible:

Children 1-15 years: Do not exceed a dose of 16 mg/kg/day or 400 mg/day

Children ≥16 and Adults: Do not exceed a dose of 400 mg/day

Dose adjustment in the elderly (>60 years): Do not exceed a dose of 400 mg/day

Dosage adjustment after serum theophylline measurement:

Within normal limits: 10-19.9 mcg/mL: Maintain dosage if tolerated. Recheck serum theophylline concentration at 24-hour intervals (for acute I.V. dosing) or at 6- to 12-month intervals (for oral dosing). Finer adjustments in dosage may be needed for some patients. If levels ≥15 mcg/mL, consider 10% dose reduction to improve safety margin.

Too high:

20-24.9 mcg/mL: Decrease doses by about 25%. Recheck serum theophylline concentrations (see **"Note"**).

25-30 mcg/mL: Skip next dose (oral) or stop infusion for 12 hours (children) or 24 hours (adults) and decrease subsequent doses by about 25%. Recheck serum theophylline concentrations (see **"Note"**).

>30 mcg/mL: Stop dosing and treat overdose; if resumed, decrease subsequent doses by 50%. Recheck serum theophylline concentrations (see **"Note"**).

Too low: <9.9 mcg/mL: If tolerated, but symptoms remain, increase dose by about 25%. Recheck serum theophylline concentrations (see **"Note"**).

Note: Recheck serum theophylline levels after 3 days when using oral dosing, or after 12 hours (children) or 24 hours (adults) when dosing intravenously. Patients maintained with oral therapy may be reassessed at 6- to 12-month intervals.

Stability Elixir, tablet, premixed infusion: Store at controlled room temperature of 25°C (77°F).

Administration Oral: Long-acting preparations should be taken with a full glass of water, swallowed whole, or cut in half if scored. Do **not** crush. Extended release capsule forms may be opened and the contents sprinkled on soft foods; do **not** chew beads.

Monitoring Parameters Monitor heart rate, CNS effects (insomnia, irritability); respiratory rate (COPD patients often have resting controlled respiratory rates in low 20s); arterial or capillary blood gases (if applicable)

Theophylline levels: Serum theophylline levels should be monitored prior to making dose increases; in the presence of signs or symptoms of toxicity; or when a new illness, worsening of a present illness, or medication changes occur that may change theophylline clearance

I.V. loading dose: Measure serum concentrations 30 minutes after the end of an I.V. loading dose

◀ I.V. infusion: Measure serum concentrations one half-life after starting a continuous infusion, then every 12-24 hours

Reference Range Therapeutic levels:

Asthma: 5-15 mcg/mL (peak level)

Toxic concentration: >20 mcg/mL

Pregnancy Risk Factor C

Contraindications Hypersensitivity to theophylline or any component of the formulation; premixed injection may contain corn-derived dextrose and its use is contraindicated in patients with allergy to corn-related products

Warnings/Precautions If a patient develops signs and symptoms of theophylline toxicity (eg, persistent, repetitive vomiting), a serum theophylline level should be measured and subsequent doses held. Due to potential saturation of theophylline clearance at serum levels in or (in some patients) less than the therapeutic range, dosage adjustment should be made in small increments (maximum: 25%). Due to wider interpatient variability, theophylline serum level measurements must be used to optimize therapy and prevent serious toxicity. Use with caution in patients with peptic ulcer, hyperthyroidism, seizure disorders, and patients with tachyarrhythmias (eg, sinus tachycardia, atrial fibrillation); use may exacerbate these conditions. Theophylline clearance may be decreased in patients with acute pulmonary edema, congestive heart failure, cor-pulmonale, fever, hepatic disease, acute hepatitis, cirrhosis, hypothyroidism, sepsis with multiorgan failure, and shock; clearance may also be decreased in neonates, infants <3 months of age with decreased renal function, children <1 year of age, the elderly >60 years of age, and patients following cessation of smoking.

Adverse Reactions Frequency not defined. Adverse events observed at therapeutic serum levels:

Cardiovascular: Flutter, tachycardia

Central nervous system: Headache, hyperactivity (children), insomnia, restlessness, seizures

Endocrine & metabolic: Hypercalcemia (with concomitant hyperthyroid disease)

Gastrointestinal: Nausea, reflux or ulcer aggravation, vomiting

Genitourinary: Difficulty urinating (elderly males with prostatism)

Neuromuscular & skeletal: Tremor

Renal: Diuresis (transient)

Drug Interactions

Metabolism/Transport Effects Substrate of CYP1A2 (major), 2C9 (minor), 2D6 (minor), 2E1 (major), 3A4 (major); **Inhibits** CYP1A2 (weak)

Avoid Concomitant Use

Avoid concomitant use of Theophylline with any of the following: Febuxostat; Iobenguane I 123

Increased Effect/Toxicity

Theophylline may increase the levels/effects of: Sympathomimetics

The levels/effects of Theophylline may be increased by: Allopurinol; Atomoxetine; Cannabinoids; Cimetidine; CYP1A2 Inhibitors (Moderate); CYP1A2 Inhibitors (Strong); CYP3A4 Inhibitors (Moderate); CYP3A4 Inhibitors (Strong); Dasatinib; Disulfiram; Febuxostat; Fluvoxamine; Interferons; Isoniazid; Macrolide Antibiotics; Mexiletine; Pentoxifylline; QuiNINE; Quinolone Antibiotics; Tacrine; Thiabendazole; Ticlopidine; Zileuton

Decreased Effect

Theophylline may decrease the levels/effects of: Adenosine; Benzodiazepines; Iobenguane I 123; Lithium; Phenytoin; Regadenoson; Zafirlukast

The levels/effects of Theophylline may be decreased by: Aminoglutethimide; Barbiturates; Beta-Blockers (Beta1 Selective); Beta-Blockers (Nonselective); CarBAMazepine; CYP1A2 Inducers (Strong); CYP3A4 Inducers (Strong); Deferasirox; Herbs (CYP3A4 Inducers); Moricizine; Phenytoin; Protease Inhibitors; Thyroid Products

Ethanol/Nutrition/Herb Interactions Food: Food does not appreciably affect the absorption of liquid, fast-release products, and most sustained release products; however, food may induce a sudden release (dose-dumping) of once-daily sustained release products resulting in an increase in serum drug levels and potential toxicity. Avoid excessive amounts of caffeine. Avoid extremes of dietary protein and carbohydrate intake. Changes in diet may affect the elimination of theophylline; charbroiled foods may increase elimination, reducing half-life by 50%.

Test Interactions Plasma glucose, uric acid, free fatty acids, total cholesterol, HDL, HDL/LDL ratio, and urinary free cortisol excretion may be increased by theophylline. Theophylline may decrease triiodothyronine.

Dietary Considerations Should be taken with water 1 hour before or 2 hours after meals. Premixed injection may contain corn-derived dextrose and its use is contraindicated in patients with allergy to corn-related products.

Dosage Forms Excipient information presented when available (limited, particularly for generics); consult specific product labeling.

Capsule, extended release:
Theo-24®: 100 mg, 200 mg, 300 mg, 400 mg [24 hours]
Elixir:
Elixophyllin®: 80 mg/15 mL (473 mL) [contains alcohol 20%; mixed fruit flavor]
Infusion [premixed in D₅W]: 200 mg (50 mL, 100 mL); 400 mg (250 mL, 500 mL); 800 mg (250 mL, 500 mL, 1000 mL)
Tablet, controlled release:
Uniphyl®: 400 mg, 600 mg [24 hours]
Tablet, extended release: 100 mg, 200 mg, 300 mg, 400 mg, 450 mg, 600 mg
Theochron™: 100 mg, 200 mg, 300 mg, 450 mg [12-24 hours]

References

Expert Panel Report 3, "Guidelines for the Diagnosis and Management of Asthma," *Clinical Practice Guidelines*, National Institutes of Health, National Heart, Lung, and Blood Institute, NIH Publication No. 08-4051, prepublication 2007. Available at http://www.nhlbi.nih.gov/guidelines/asthma/asthgdln.htm

Mokhlesi B, Leikin JB, Murray P, et al, "Adult Toxicology in Critical Care: Part II: Specific Poisonings," *Chest*, 2003, 123(3):897-922.

♦ **Theophylline Anhydrous** *see* Theophylline *on page 1373*

♦ **Theraflu® Thin Strips® Multi Symptom [OTC]** *see* DiphenhydrAMINE *on page 430*

♦ **Theratears® [OTC]** *see* Carboxymethylcellulose *on page 243*

♦ **Thermazene®** *see* Silver Sulfadiazine *on page 1292*

♦ **Thiamazole** *see* Methimazole *on page 893*

Thiopental (thye oh PEN tal)

Medication Safety Issues
High alert medication: The Institute for Safe Medication Practices (ISMP) includes this medication among its list of drugs which have a heightened risk of causing significant patient harm when used in error.

Related Information
Anesthesia Considerations for Neurosurgery *on page 1514*
Anesthesia for Geriatric Patients *on page 1523*
Anesthesia for Obstetric Patients in Nonobstetric Surgery *on page 1532*
Anesthesia for Patients With Liver Disease *on page 1537*
Anesthetic Considerations in the Substance-Abusing Patient *on page 1613*
Chronic Renal Failure *on page 1552*
Dosing Considerations for the Critically-Ill Patient With Morbid Obesity *on page 1561*
Intravenous Anesthetic Agents *on page 1635*

U.S. Brand Names Pentothal®
Canadian Brand Names Pentothal®
Index Terms Thiopental Sodium
Pharmacologic Category Anticonvulsant, Barbiturate; Barbiturate; General Anesthetic
Restrictions C-III
Generic Available No
Use Induction of anesthesia; control of convulsive states; treatment of elevated intracranial pressure
Mechanism of Action Short-acting barbiturate with sedative, hypnotic, and anticonvulsant properties. Barbiturates depress the sensory cortex, decrease motor activity, alter cerebellar function, and produce drowsiness, sedation, and ▶

◀ hypnosis. In high doses, barbiturates exhibit anticonvulsant activity; barbiturates produce dose-dependent respiratory depression.

Pharmacodynamics/Kinetics
Onset of action: Anesthetic: I.V.: 30-60 seconds
Duration: 5-30 minutes
Distribution: V_d: ~1.6 L/kg
Protein binding: 72% to 86%
Metabolism: Hepatic, primarily to inactive metabolites but pentobarbital is also formed
Half-life elimination: 3-11.5 hours; decreased in children

Dosage I.V.:
Induction anesthesia:
Infants: 5-8 mg/kg
Children 1-12 years: 5-6 mg/kg
Adults: 3-5 mg/kg
Maintenance anesthesia:
Children: 1 mg/kg as needed
Adults: 25-100 mg as needed
Increased intracranial pressure: Children and Adults: 1.5-5 mg/kg/dose; repeat as needed to control intracranial pressure
Seizures:
Children: 2-3 mg/kg/dose; repeat as needed
Adults: 75-250 mg/dose; repeat as needed

Dosing adjustment in renal impairment: Cl_{cr} <10 mL/minute: Administer at 75% of normal dose

Note: Accumulation may occur with chronic dosing due to lipid solubility; prolonged recovery may result from redistribution of thiopental from fat stores

Stability Reconstituted solutions remain stable for 3 days at room temperature and 7 days when refrigerated.

Administration Administer slowly over 20-30 seconds. Rapid I.V. injection may cause hypotension or decreased cardiac output; avoid extravasation, necrosis may occur. Check I.V. catheter placement prior to administration. If inadvertent intra-arterial administration occurs, treat with a local anesthetic (eg, lidocaine 1%, 5 mL) and/or papaverine (20-40 mg), preferably through the catheter used for the thiopental injection.

Monitoring Parameters Respiratory rate, heart rate, blood pressure

Reference Range Therapeutic: Hypnotic: 1-5 mcg/mL (SI: 4.1-20.7 μmol/L); Coma: 30-100 mcg/mL (SI: 124-413 μmol/L); Anesthesia: 7-130 mcg/mL (SI: 29-536 μmol/L); Toxic: >10 mcg/mL (SI: >41 μmol/L)

Anesthesia and Critical Care Concerns/Other Considerations
Clinical Pearls/Comments: Thiopental switches from linear to nonlinear pharmacokinetics following prolonged continuous infusions. The initial CNS action is terminated by redistribution. Once the total volume of distribution is filled (after 2.5 hours of infusion or repeated large doses), termination of action by hepatic metabolism occurs. To avoid an overdose, calculate dose based on lean body mass. May precipitate in the I.V. when mixed with acidic drugs (eg, succinylcholine, vecuronium, rocuronium).

Pregnancy Risk Factor C

Contraindications Hypersensitivity to thiopental, barbiturates, or any component of the formulation; status asthmaticus; severe cardiovascular disease; porphyria (variegate or acute intermittent); should not be administered by intra-arterial injection

Warnings/Precautions Laryngospasm or bronchospasms may occur; use with extreme caution in patients with reactive airway diseases (asthma or COPD). Use with caution when the hypnotic may be prolonged or potentiated (excessive premedication, Addison's disease, hepatic or renal dysfunction, myxedema, increased blood urea, severe anemia, or myasthenia gravis). Potential for drug dependency exists, abrupt cessation may precipitate withdrawal, including status epilepticus in epileptic patients. Do not administer to patients in acute pain. Use caution in patients with unstable aneurysms, cardiovascular disease, renal impairment, or hepatic disease. Use caution in elderly, debilitated, or pediatric patients. May cause paradoxical responses, including agitation and hyperactivity, particularly in acute pain and pediatric patients. Effects with other sedative drugs or ethanol may be potentiated. May cause respiratory depression or hypotension. Use with caution in hemodynamically unstable patients (hypotension or shock) or patients with respiratory disease. Repeated dosing or continuous infusions may cause cumulative effects. Administer only by I.V. route.

Adverse Reactions Frequency not defined.

Cardiovascular: Bradycardia, hypotension, syncope

Central nervous system: Drowsiness, lethargy, CNS excitation or depression, impaired judgment, "hangover" effect, confusion, somnolence, agitation, hyperkinesia, ataxia, nervousness, headache, insomnia, nightmares, hallucinations, anxiety, dizziness, shivering

Dermatologic: Rash, exfoliative dermatitis, Stevens-Johnson syndrome

Gastrointestinal: Nausea, vomiting, constipation

Hematologic: Agranulocytosis, thrombocytopenia, megaloblastic anemia, immune hemolytic anemia (rare)

Local: Pain at injection site, thrombophlebitis with I.V. use

Renal: Oliguria

Respiratory: Laryngospasm, respiratory depression, apnea (especially with rapid I.V. use), hypoventilation, sneezing, cough, bronchospasm

Miscellaneous: Gangrene with inadvertent intra-arterial injection, anaphylaxis, anaphylactic reactions

Drug Interactions

Avoid Concomitant Use There are no known interactions where it is recommended to avoid concomitant use.

Increased Effect/Toxicity

Thiopental may increase the levels/effects of: Alcohol (Ethyl); CNS Depressants; Meperidine; Thiazide Diuretics

The levels/effects of Thiopental may be increased by: Carbonic Anhydrase Inhibitors; Chloramphenicol; Felbamate; Primidone; Valproic Acid

Decreased Effect

Thiopental may decrease the levels/effects of: Acetaminophen; Beta-Blockers; Calcium Channel Blockers; Chloramphenicol; Contraceptive (Progestins); Corticosteroids (Systemic); CycloSPORINE; Disopyramide; Doxycycline; Etoposide; Etoposide Phosphate; LamoTRIgine; Methadone; Oral Contraceptive (Estrogens); Propafenone; QuiNIDine; Teniposide; Theophylline Derivatives; Tricyclic Antidepressants; Valproic Acid; Vitamin K Antagonists

The levels/effects of Thiopental may be decreased by: Ketorolac; Mefloquine; Pyridoxine; Rifamycin Derivatives

Dietary Considerations Sodium content of 1 g (injection): 105 mg (4.5 mEq)

Dosage Forms Excipient information presented when available (limited, particularly for generics); consult specific product labeling.

Injection, powder for reconstitution, as sodium:

Pentothal®: 250 mg, 400 mg, 500 mg, 1 g [contains sodium 105 mg/g]

◆ **Thiopental Sodium** *see* Thiopental *on page 1377*

◆ **Thiosulfuric Acid Disodium Salt** *see* Sodium Thiosulfate *on page 1316*

◆ **Thorazine** *see* ChlorproMAZINE *on page 298*

◆ **Thrombate III®** *see* Antithrombin III *on page 127*

Thyroid, Desiccated (THYE roid DES i kay tid)

U.S. Brand Names Armour® Thyroid; Nature-Throid™; Westhroid™

Index Terms Desiccated Thyroid; Thyroid Extract; Thyroid USP

Pharmacologic Category Thyroid Product

Use Replacement or supplemental therapy in hypothyroidism; pituitary TSH suppressants (thyroid nodules, thyroiditis, multinodular goiter, thyroid cancer), thyrotoxicosis, diagnostic suppression tests

Pharmacodynamics/Kinetics

Absorption: T_4: 48% to 79%; T_3: 95%; desiccated thyroid contains thyroxine, liothyronine, and iodine (primarily bound)

Metabolism: Thyroxine: Largely converted to liothyronine

Half-life elimination, serum: Liothyronine: 1-2 days; Thyroxine: 6-7 days

Dosage Oral:

Children: See table.

Recommended Pediatric Dosage for Congenital Hypothyroidism

Age	Daily Dose (mg)	Daily Dose/kg (mg)
0-6 mo	15-30	4.8-6
6-12 mo	30-45	3.6-4.8
1-5 y	45-60	3-3.6
6-12 y	60-90	2.4-3
>12 y	>90	1.2-1.8

Adults: Initial: 15-30 mg; increase with 15 mg increments every 2-4 weeks; use 15 mg in patients with cardiovascular disease or myxedema. Maintenance dose: Usually 60-120 mg/day; monitor TSH and clinical symptoms.

Thyroid cancer: Requires larger amounts than replacement therapy

Anesthesia and Critical Care Concerns/Other Considerations Equivalent doses: The following statement on relative potency of thyroid products is included in a joint statement by American Thyroid Association (ATA), American Association of Clinical Endocrinologists (AACE) and The Endocrine Society (TES): For purposes of conversion, levothyroxine sodium (T_4) 100 mcg is usually considered equivalent to desiccated thyroid 60 mg, thyroglobulin 60 mg, or liothyronine sodium (T_3) 25 mcg. However, these are rough guidelines only and do not obviate the careful re-evaluation of a patient when switching thyroid hormone preparations, including a change from one brand of levothyroxine to another. Joint position statement is available at http://www.thyroid.org/professionals/advocacy/04_12_08_thyroxine.html.

Additional Information Complete prescribing information for this medication should be consulted for additional detail.

Dosage Forms Excipient information presented when available (limited, particularly for generics); consult specific product labeling. [DSC] = Discontinued product

Tablet: 30 mg [DSC], 32.5 mg [DSC], 60 mg, 65 mg [DSC], 120 mg, 130 mg [DSC], 180 mg [DSC]

Armour® Thyroid: 15 mg, 30 mg, 60 mg, 90 mg, 120 mg, 180 mg, 240 mg, 300 mg

Nature-Throid™: 16.25 mg, 32.5 mg, 65 mg, 130 mg, 195 mg

Westhroid™: 32.5 mg, 65 mg, 130 mg

References

Bhasin S, Wallace W, Lawrence JB, et al, "Sudden Death Associated With Thyroid Hormone Abuse," *Am J Med*, 1981, 71(5):887-90.

Helfand M and Crapo LM, "Monitoring Therapy in Patients Taking Levothyroxine," *Ann Intern Med*, 1990, 113(6):450-4.

Johnson DG and Campbell S, "Hormonal and Metabolic Agents," *Geriatric Pharmacology*, Bressler R and Katz MD, eds, New York, NY: McGraw-Hill, 1993, 427-50.

Sanders LR, "Pituitary, Thyroid, Adrenal and Parathyroid Diseases in the Elderly," *Geriatric Medicine*, 1990, 475-87.

Sawin CT, Geller A, Hershman JM, et al, "The Aging Thyroid. The Use of Thyroid Hormone in Older Persons," *JAMA*, 1989, 261(18):2653-5.

Tunget CL, Clark RF, Turchen SG, et al, "Raising the Decontamination Level for Thyroid Hormone Ingestions," *Am J Emerg Med*, 1995, 13(1):9-13.

Watts NB, "Use of a Sensitive Thyrotropin Assay for Monitoring Treatment With Levothyroxine," *Arch Intern Med*, 1989, 149(2):309-12.

◆ **Thyroid Extract** *see* Thyroid, Desiccated *on page 1379*

◆ **Thyroid USP** *see* Thyroid, Desiccated *on page 1379*

◆ *L*-**Thyroxine Sodium** *see* Levothyroxine *on page 831*

TiaGABine (tye AG a been)

Related Information
Chronic Pain Management *on page 1546*
Perioperative Management of Patients on Antiseizure Medication *on page 1577*

U.S. Brand Names Gabitril®
Canadian Brand Names Gabitril®
Index Terms Tiagabine Hydrochloride
Pharmacologic Category Anticonvulsant, Miscellaneous
Use Adjunctive therapy in adults and children ≥12 years of age in the treatment of partial seizures

Pharmacodynamics/Kinetics
Absorption: Rapid (45 minutes); prolonged with food
Protein binding: 96%, primarily to albumin and α_1-acid glycoprotein
Metabolism: Hepatic via CYP (primarily 3A4)
Bioavailability: Oral: Absolute: 90%
Half-life elimination: 2-5 hours when administered with enzyme inducers; 7-9 hours when administered without enzyme inducers
Time to peak, plasma: 45 minutes
Excretion: Feces (63%); urine (25%); 2% as unchanged drug; primarily as metabolites

Dosage Oral (administer with food):
Patients receiving enzyme-inducing AED regimens:
Children 12-18 years: 4 mg once daily for 1 week; may increase to 8 mg daily in 2 divided doses for 1 week; then may increase by 4-8 mg weekly to response or up to 32 mg daily in 2-4 divided doses
Adults: 4 mg once daily for 1 week; may increase by 4-8 mg weekly to response or up to 56 mg daily in 2-4 divided doses; usual maintenance: 32-56 mg/day
Patients **not** receiving enzyme-inducing AED regimens: The estimated plasma concentrations of tiagabine in patients not taking enzyme-inducing medications is twice that of patients receiving enzyme-inducing AEDs. Lower doses are required; slower titration may be necessary.

Additional Information Complete prescribing information for this medication should be consulted for additional detail.

Dosage Forms Excipient information presented when available (limited, particularly for generics); consult specific product labeling.
Tablet, as hydrochloride:
Gabitril®: 2 mg, 4 mg, 12 mg, 16 mg

◆ **Tiagabine Hydrochloride** *see* TiaGABine *on page 1381*

◆ **Tiazac®** *see* Diltiazem *on page 425*

◆ **Tiazac® XC (Can)** *see* Diltiazem *on page 425*

Ticarcillin and Clavulanate Potassium
(tye kar SIL in & klav yoo LAN ate poe TASS ee um)

U.S. Brand Names Timentin®
Canadian Brand Names Timentin®
Index Terms Ticarcillin and Clavulanic Acid
Pharmacologic Category Antibiotic, Penicillin
Generic Available No

Use Treatment of lower respiratory tract, urinary tract, skin and skin structures, bone and joint, gynecologic (endometritis) and intra-abdominal (peritonitis) infections, and septicemia caused by susceptible organisms. Clavulanate expands activity of ticarcillin to include beta-lactamase producing strains of *S. aureus, H. influenzae, Bacteroides* species, and some other gram-negative bacilli

Mechanism of Action Inhibits bacterial cell wall synthesis by binding to one or more of the penicillin binding proteins (PBPs); which in turn inhibits the final transpeptidation step of peptidoglycan synthesis in bacterial cell walls, thus inhibiting cell wall biosynthesis. Bacteria eventually lyse due to ongoing activity of cell wall autolytic enzymes (autolysins and murein hydrolases) while cell wall assembly is arrested.

◀ **Pharmacodynamics/Kinetics**
    Absorption: Ticarcillin: Not absorbed orally
    Protein binding: Ticarcillin: ~45%; Clavulanic acid: ~25%
    Metabolism: Clavulanic acid: Hepatic
    Half-life elimination: Ticarcillin: 1.1 hours;Clavulanic acid: 1.1 hours
    Excretion: Ticarcillin: Urine (60% to 70%); Clavulanic acid: Urine (35% to 45% as unchanged drug)
    Clearance: Clavulanic acid does not affect clearance of ticarcillin

Dosage Note: Timentin® (ticarcillin/clavulanate) is a combination product; each 3.1 g dosage form contains 3 g ticarcillin disodium and 0.1 g clavulanic acid.

Usual dosage range:
    Children and Adults <60 kg: I.V.: 200-300 mg of ticarcillin component/kg/day in divided doses every 4-6 hours
    Children ≥60 kg and Adults: I.V.: 3.1 g (ticarcillin 3 g plus clavulanic acid 0.1 g) every 4-6 hours (maximum: 24 g of ticarcillin component/day)

Indication-specific dosing:
    Children: I.V.:
        Bite wounds (animal): 200 mg of ticarcillin component/kg/day in divided doses
        Neutropenic fever: 75 mg of ticarcillin component/kg every 6 hours (maximum: 3.1 g/dose)
        Pneumonia (nosocomial): 300 mg of ticarcillin component/kg/day in 4 divided doses (maximum: 18-24 g of ticarcillin component/day)
    Children ≥60 kg and Adults: I.V.:
        Amnionitis, cholangitis, diverticulitis, endometritis, epididymo-orchitis, mastoiditis, orbital cellulitis, peritonitis, pneumonia (aspiration): 3.1 g every 6 hours
        Liver abscess, parafascial space infections, septic thrombophlebitis: 3.1 g every 4 hours
        ***Pseudomonas* infections:** 3.1 g every 4 hours
        Urinary tract infections: 3.1 g every 6-8 hours

Dosing adjustment in renal impairment: Loading dose: I.V.: 3.1 g one dose, followed by maintenance dose based on creatinine clearance:
    Cl_{cr} 30-60 mL/minute: Administer 2 g of ticarcillin component every 4 hours or 3.1 g every 8 hours
    Cl_{cr} 10-30 mL/minute: Administer 2 g of ticarcillin component every 8 hours or 3.1 g every 12 hours
    Cl_{cr} <10 mL/minute: Administer 2 g of ticarcillin component every 12 hours
    Cl_{cr} <10 mL/minute with concomitant hepatic dysfunction: 2 g of ticarcillin component every 24 hours
    Moderately dialyzable (20% to 50%)
    Continuous ambulatory peritoneal dialysis: 3.1 g every 12 hours
    Hemodialysis: 2 g of ticarcillin component every 12 hours; supplemented with 3.1 g after each dialysis
    Continuous renal replacement therapy (CRRT): Drug clearance is highly dependent on the method of renal replacement, filter type, and flow rate. Appropriate dosing requires close monitoring of pharmacologic response, signs of adverse reactions due to drug accumulation, as well as drug levels in relation to target trough (if appropriate). The following are general recommendations only (based on dialysate flow/ultrafiltration rates of 1 L/hour) and should not supersede clinical judgment:
    CVVH: 2 g every 6-8 hours
    CVVHD/CVVHDF: 3.1 g every 6 hours
    Note: Do not administer in intervals exceeding every 8 hours. Clavulanate component is hepatically eliminated; extending the dosing interval beyond 8 hours may result in loss of beta-lactamase inhibition.

Dosing adjustment in hepatic dysfunction: With concomitant renal dysfunction (Cl_{cr} <10 mL/minute): 2 g of ticarcillin component every 24 hours

Stability
    Vials: Store intact vials at <24°C (<75°F). Reconstituted solution is stable for 6 hours at room temperature and 72 hours when refrigerated. I.V. infusion in NS or LR is stable for 24 hours at room temperature, 7 days when refrigerated, or 30 days when frozen. I.V. infusion in D_5W solution is stable for 24 hours at room

temperature, 3 days when refrigerated, or 7 days when frozen. After freezing, thawed solution is stable for 8 hours at room temperature. Darkening of drug indicates loss of potency of clavulanate potassium.

Premixed solution: Store frozen at ≤-20°C (-4°F). Thawed solution is stable for 24 hours at room temperature or 7 days under refrigeration; do not refreeze.

Administration Infuse over 30 minutes.

Some penicillins (eg, carbenicillin, ticarcillin, and piperacillin) have been shown to inactivate aminoglycosides *in vitro*. This has been observed to a greater extent with tobramycin and gentamicin, while amikacin has shown greater stability against inactivation. Concurrent use of these agents may pose a risk of reduced antibacterial efficacy *in vivo*, particularly in the setting of profound renal impairment. However, definitive clinical evidence is lacking. If combination penicillin/aminoglycoside therapy is desired in a patient with renal dysfunction, separation of doses (if feasible), and routine monitoring of aminoglycoside levels, CBC, and clinical response should be considered.

Monitoring Parameters Observe for signs and symptoms of anaphylaxis during first dose.

Pregnancy Risk Factor B

Contraindications Hypersensitivity to ticarcillin, clavulanate, any penicillin, or any component of the formulation

Warnings/Precautions Use with caution and modify dosage in patients with renal impairment; serious and occasionally severe or fatal hypersensitivity (anaphylactoid) reactions have been reported in patients on penicillin therapy (especially with a history of beta-lactam hypersensitivity and/or a history of sensitivity to multiple allergens); use with caution in patients with seizures and in patients with HF due to high sodium load. Particularly in patients with renal impairment, bleeding disorders have been observed; discontinue if thrombocytopenia or bleeding occurs. Prolonged use may result in fungal or bacterial superinfection, including *C. difficile*-associated diarrhea (CDAD) and pseudomembranous colitis; CDAD has been observed >2 months postantibiotic treatment. Safety and efficacy have not been established in children <3 months of age.

Adverse Reactions Frequency not defined.

Central nervous system: Confusion, drowsiness, fever, headache, Jarisch-Herxheimer reaction, seizure

Dermatologic: Erythema multiforme, pruritus, rash, Stevens-Johnson syndrome, toxic epidermal necrolysis, urticaria

Endocrine & metabolic: Electrolyte imbalance

Gastrointestinal: *Clostridium difficile* colitis, diarrhea, nausea, vomiting

Hematologic: Bleeding, eosinophilia, hemolytic anemia, leukopenia, neutropenia, positive Coombs' reaction, prothrombin time prolonged, thrombocytopenia

Hepatic: Hepatotoxicity, jaundice

Local: Injection site reaction (pain, burning, induration); thrombophlebitis

Neuromuscular & skeletal: Myoclonus

Renal: BUN increased, interstitial nephritis (acute), serum creatinine increased

Miscellaneous: Anaphylaxis, hypersensitivity reactions

Drug Interactions

Avoid Concomitant Use There are no known interactions where it is recommended to avoid concomitant use.

Increased Effect/Toxicity

Ticarcillin and Clavulanate Potassium may increase the levels/effects of: Methotrexate

The levels/effects of Ticarcillin and Clavulanate Potassium may be increased by: Uricosuric Agents

Decreased Effect

Ticarcillin and Clavulanate Potassium may decrease the levels/effects of: Aminoglycosides; Mycophenolate; Typhoid Vaccine

The levels/effects of Ticarcillin and Clavulanate Potassium may be decreased by: Fusidic Acid; Tetracycline Derivatives

◀ **Test Interactions** Positive Coombs' test, false-positive urinary proteins

Some penicillin derivatives may accelerate the degradation of aminoglycosides *in vitro*, leading to a potential underestimation of aminoglycoside serum concentration.

Dietary Considerations Sodium content of 1 g: 4.51 mEq; potassium content of 1 g: 0.15 mEq

Dosage Forms Excipient information presented when available (limited, particularly for generics); consult specific product labeling.

Infusion [premixed, frozen]: Ticarcillin 3 g and clavulanic acid 0.1 g (100 mL) [contains sodium 4.51 mEq and potassium 0.15 mEq per g]

Injection, powder for reconstitution: Ticarcillin 3 g and clavulanic acid 0.1 g (3.1 g, 31 g) [contains sodium 4.51 mEq and potassium 0.15 mEq per g]

References

Begue P, Quiniou F, Quinet B, "Efficacy and Pharmacokinetics of Timentin® in Paediatric Infections," *J Antimicrob Chemother*, 1986, 17(Suppl C):81-91.

Chow MS, Quintiliani, and Nightingale CH, "*In Vivo* Inactivation of Tobramycin by Ticarcillin. A Case Report," *JAMA*, 1982, 247(5):658-9.

Daly JS, Dodge RA, Glew RH, et al, "Effect of Time and Temperature on Inactivation of Aminoglycosides by Ampicillin at Neonatal Dosages," *J Perinatol*, 1997, 17(1):42-5.

Donowitz GR and Mandell GL, "Beta-Lactam Antibiotics," *N Engl J Med*, 1988, 318(7):419-26 and 318(8):490-500.

Dowell JA, Korth-Bradley J, Milisci M, et al, "Evaluating Possible Pharmacokinetic Interactions Between Tobramycin, Piperacillin, and a Combination of Piperacillin and Tazobactam in Patients With Various Degrees of Renal Impairment," *J Clin Pharmacol*, 2001, 41:979-86.

Farchione LA, "Inactivation of Aminoglycosides by Penicillins," *J Antimicrob Chemother*, 1982, 8 (Suppl A):27-36.

Fuchs PC, Stickel S, Anderson PH, et al, "*In Vitro* Inactivation of Aminoglycosides by Sulbactam, Other Beta-Lactams, and Sulbactam-Beta-Lactam Combinations," *Antimicrob Agents Chemother*, 1991, 35(1):182-4.

Halstenson CE, Wong MO, Herman CS, et al, "Effect of Concomitant Administration of Piperacillin on the Dispositions on Isepamicin and Gentamicin in Patients With End-Stage Renal Disease," *Antimicrob Agents Chemother*, 1992, 36(9):1832-36.

Hitt CM, Patel KB, Nicolau DP, et al, "Influence of Piperacillin-Tazobactam on Pharmacokinetics of Gentamicin Given Once Daily," *Am J Health Syst Pharm*, 1997, 54(23):2704-8.

Itokazu GS and Danziger LH, "Ampicillin-Sulbactam and Ticarcillin-Clavulanic Acid: A Comparison of Their *In Vitro* Activity and Review of Their Clinical Efficacy," *Pharmacotherapy*, 1991, 11(5):382-414.

Konishi H, Goto M, Nakamoto Y, et al, "Tobramycin Inactivation by Carbenicillin, Ticarcillin, and Piperacillin," *Antimicrob Agents Chemother*, 1983, 23(5):653-57.

Lau A, Lee M, Flascha S, et al, "Effect of Piperacillin on Tobramycin Pharmacokinetics in Patients with Normal Renal Function," *Antimicrob Agents Chemother*, 1983, 24(4):533-37.

Reed MD, Yamashita TS, and Blumer JL, "Pharmacokinetic-Based Ticarcillin/Clavulanic Acid Dose Recommendations for Infants and Children," *J Clin Pharmacol*, 1995, 35(7):658-65.

Russoe ME and Atkins-Thor E, "Gentamicin and Ticarcillin in Subjects With End-Stage Renal Disease. Comparison of Two Assay Methods and Evaluation of Inactivation Rate," *Clin Nephrol*, 1981, 15(4):175-80.

Stutman HR and Marks MI, "Review of Pediatric Antimicrobial Therapies," *Semin Pediatr Infect Dis*, 1991, 2:3-17.

Thompson MIB, Russo ME, Saxon BJ, et al, "Gentamicin Inactivation by Piperacillin or Carbenicillin in Patients With End-Stage Renal Disease," *Antimicrob Agents Chemother*, 1982, 21(2):268-73.

Trotman RL, Williamson JC, Shoemaker DM, et al, "Antibiotic Dosing in Critically Ill Adult Patients Receiving Continuous Renal Replacement Therapy," *Clin Infect Dis*, 2005, 41(8):1159-66.

Viollier AF, Standiford HC, Drusano GL, et al, "Comparative Pharmacokinetics and Serum Bactericidal Activity of Mezlocillin, Ticarcillin and Piperacillin, With and Without Gentamicin," *J Antimicrob Chemother*, 1985, 15(5):597-606.

Walterspiel JN, Feldman S, Van R, et al, "Comparative Inactivation of Isepamicin, Amikacin, and Gentamicin by Nine Beta-Lactams and Two Beta-Lactamase Inhibitors, Cilastatin and Heparin," *Antimicrob Agents Chemother*, 1991, 35(9):1875-8.

Wright AJ, "The Penicillins," *Mayo Clin Proc*, 1999, 74(3):290-307.

◆ **Ticarcillin and Clavulanic Acid** *see* Ticarcillin and Clavulanate Potassium *on page 1381*

◆ **Ticlid® [DSC]** *see* Ticlopidine *on page 1385*

◆ **Ticlid® (Can)** *see* Ticlopidine *on page 1385*

Ticlopidine (tye KLOE pi deen)

Related Information

Perioperative / Periprocedural Management of Anticoagulant and Antiplatelet Therapy *on page 1607*

Preoperative Evaluation of the Cardiac Patient for Noncardiac Surgery *on page 1598*

Regional Anesthesia in Patients Receiving Anticoagulant and Antiplatelet Therapy *on page 1642*

U.S. Brand Names Ticlid® [DSC]

Canadian Brand Names Alti-Ticlopidine; Apo-Ticlopidine®; Gen-Ticlopidine; Mylan-Ticlopidine; Novo-Ticlopidine; Nu-Ticlopidine; Rhoxal-ticlopidine; Sandoz-Ticlopidine; Ticlid®

Index Terms Ticlopidine Hydrochloride

Pharmacologic Category Antiplatelet Agent; Antiplatelet Agent, Thienopyridine

Generic Available Yes

Use Platelet aggregation inhibitor that reduces the risk of thrombotic stroke in patients who have had a stroke or stroke precursors. **Note:** Due to its association with life-threatening hematologic disorders, ticlopidine should be reserved for patients who are intolerant to aspirin, or who have failed aspirin therapy. Adjunctive therapy (with aspirin) following successful coronary stent implantation to reduce the incidence of subacute stent thrombosis.

Unlabeled/Investigational Use Protection of aortocoronary bypass grafts, diabetic microangiopathy, ischemic heart disease, prevention of postoperative DVT, reduction of graft loss following renal transplant

Mechanism of Action Ticlopidine requires *in vivo* biotransformation to an unidentified active metabolite. This active metabolite irreversibly blocks the P2Y12 component of ADP receptors, which prevents activation of the GPIIb/IIIa receptor complex, thereby reducing platelet aggregation. Platelets blocked by ticlopidine are affected for the remainder of their lifespan.

Pharmacodynamics/Kinetics

Onset of action: ~6 hours

Peak effect: 3-5 days; serum levels do not correlate with clinical antiplatelet activity

Absorption: Well absorbed

Protein binding: Parent drug: 98%; <15% bound to alpha$_1$-acid glycoprotein

Metabolism: Extensively hepatic; has at least 1 active metabolite

Half-life elimination: 13 hours

Time to peak, serum: ~2 hours

Excretion: Urine (60%); feces (23%)

Dosage Oral: Adults:

Stroke prevention: 250 mg twice daily

Coronary artery stenting (initiate after successful implantation): 250 mg twice daily (in combination with antiplatelet doses of aspirin) for up to 30 days

Unstable angina, non-ST-segment elevation myocardial infarction (UA/NSTEMI) undergoing percutaneous coronary intervention (PCI) in patients unable to receive clopidogrel (unlabeled dosing): Initial: 500 mg loading dose given at least 6 hours prior to PCI, followed by 250 mg twice daily (in combination with aspirin 75-325 mg once daily). Duration of therapy dependent upon type of stent implanted during PCI.

Note: *Coronary artery stents:* Duration of ticlopidine (clopidogrel preferred) in combination with aspirin: According to the ACC/AHA/SCAI guidelines, ideally 12 months following drug-eluting stent (DES) placement in patients not at high risk for bleeding; at a minimum, 1, 3, and 6 months for bare metal (BMS), sirolimus-eluting, and paclitaxel-eluting stents, respectively, for uninterrupted therapy (Smith, 2005). The 2008 *Chest* guidelines recommend for patients who undergo PCI and receive a BMS (with ongoing ACS) or a DES (with or without ongoing ACS) that ticlopidine (clopidogrel preferred) be continued for at least 12 months. In patients receiving a BMS without ongoing ACS, ticlopidine (or clopidogrel) may be continued for at least 1 month. In patients receiving a DES, therapy with ticlopidine (or clopidogrel) beyond 12 months may be considered in patients without bleeding or tolerability issues (Becker, 2008). Premature ▶

interruption of therapy may result in stent thrombosis with subsequent fatal and nonfatal myocardial infarction.

Dosage adjument in renal impairment: No adjustment is necessary

Dosage adjustment in hepatic impairment: No specific guidelines for patients with hepatic impairment; use with caution. Use is contraindicated with severe renal impairment.

Administration Administer with food.

Monitoring Parameters Signs of bleeding; CBC with differential every 2 weeks starting the second week through the third month of treatment; more frequent monitoring is recommended for patients whose absolute neutrophil counts have been consistently declining or are 30% less than baseline values. The peak incidence of TTP occurs between 3-4 weeks, the peak incidence of neutropenia occurs at approximately 4-6 weeks, and the incidence of aplastic anemia peaks after 4-8 weeks of therapy. Few cases have been reported after 3 months of treatment. Liver function tests (alkaline phosphatase and transaminases) should be performed in the first 4 months of therapy if liver dysfunction is suspected.

Anesthesia and Critical Care Concerns/Other Considerations The adverse effect profile including neutropenia and thrombotic thrombocytopenia purpura (TTP), along with twice-daily dosing and GI upset, makes ticlopidine a less attractive option than clopidogrel. Neutropenia usually resolves within 1-3 weeks of discontinuation of therapy. TTP, although rare, is life-threatening and requires immediate plasma exchange.

Perioperative Management of Ticlopidine: In patients with coronary stents the risk of stent thrombosis becomes elevated depending on the type of stent deployed (bare metal vs drug-eluting stent) and the time from implantation. According to the American College of Chest Physicians (Becker, 2008), the recommended length of therapy for ticlopidine (clopidogrel preferred) is at least 12 months in patients with ACS who undergo PCI with a bare metal stent (BMS) or drug-eluting stent (DES). In patients receiving a BMS without ongoing ACS, ticlopidine (clopidogrel preferred) can be continued for at least 1 month. Early discontinuation of ticlopidine (or clopidogrel) may result in stent thrombosis leading to nonfatal and fatal myocardial infarction. The perioperative recommendations for clopidogrel are below (Douketis, 2008):

Patients undergoing noncardiac surgery (low risk of cardiac event without coronary stent): Ticlopidine and other antiplatelet agents should be temporarily discontinued 5-10 days prior to surgery and resumed ~24 hours (or the next morning) after the procedure when adequate hemostasis is achieved.

Patients without coronary stent undergoing cardiac surgery (eg, CABG) or noncardiac surgery (high risk of cardiac event): Discontinue ticlopidine at least 5 days and, preferably, 10 days prior to surgery while continuing aspirin up to and beyond the time of surgery. If aspirin is interrupted, it should be reinitiated 6-48 hours after surgery; may resume ticlopidine ~24 hours (or the next morning) after the procedure when adequate hemostasis is achieved.

Patients undergoing cardiac surgery (eg, CABG) or noncardiac surgery (with coronary stent): Based on the risk of stent thrombosis, patients with a BMS who require surgery within 6 weeks of implantation or with a DES who require surgery within 12 months of implantation should continue on both aspirin and ticlopidine (clopidogrel preferred) during the perioperative period.

The AHA/ACC/SCAI/ACS/ADA Science Advisory (2007) published recommendations (*Circulation*, February 13, 2007) to prevent premature discontinuation of dual antiplatelet therapy (clopidogrel and aspirin) in patients with coronary artery stents. The advisory panel agreed with the 2004 ACC/AHA guidelines stressing the importance of 12 months of dual antiplatelet therapy after placement of a drug-eluting stent (DES) in patients who are not at high risk of bleeding. The advisory panel included these recommendations. Minor surgery, teeth cleaning, and tooth extraction can usually be performed without increased bleeding on the dual antiplatelet regimen. If increased bleeding is anticipated, then the procedure should be delayed until the antiplatelet regimen is completed. Elective procedures with a significant risk of bleeding should be postponed until the antiplatelet regimen is completed. The advisory panel recommends healthcare providers who perform invasive or surgical procedures contact the patient's cardiologist before discontinuing antiplatelet therapy. For patients with drug-eluting stents who must undergo a procedure that requires discontinuation of thienopyridine therapy, aspirin should be continued if possible and the thienopyridine restarted as soon as possible after the procedure. "Bridging" stent patients with warfarin, other antithrombins, or glycoprotein IIb/IIIa agents is not supported by the Advisory Committee.

For the complete review and additional recommendations available at http://www.acc.org/qualityandscience/clinical/pdfs/Final_Dual_Antiplatelet_Statement_010507.pdf

Pregnancy Risk Factor B

Contraindications Hypersensitivity to ticlopidine or any component of the formulation; active pathological bleeding such as peptic ulcer disease (PUD) or intracranial hemorrhage; severe liver dysfunction; hematopoietic disorders (neutropenia, thrombocytopenia, a past history of TTP or aplastic anemia)

Warnings/Precautions Use with caution in patients who may be at risk of increased bleeding (eg, PUD, trauma, or surgery). Consider discontinuing 10-14 days before elective surgery (except in patients with cardiac stents that have not completed their full course of dual antiplatelet therapy; patient-specific situations need to be discussed with cardiologist; AHA/ACC/SCAI/ACS/ADA Science Advisory provides recommendations). Use caution in concurrent treatment with anticoagulants (eg, heparin, warfarin) or other antiplatelet drugs; bleeding risk is increased. Use with caution in patients with mild-to-moderate hepatic impairment; use is contraindicated with severe hepatic impairment. Use with caution in patients with moderate-to-severe renal impairment (experience is limited); bleeding times may be significantly prolonged and the risk of hematologic adverse effects (eg, neutropenia) may be increased. **[U.S. Boxed Warning]: May cause life-threatening hematologic reactions, including neutropenia, agranulocytosis, thrombotic thrombocytopenia purpura (TTP), and aplastic anemia.** Routine monitoring is required (see Monitoring Parameters). Monitor for signs and symptoms of neutropenia including WBC count. Discontinue if the absolute neutrophil count falls to <1200/mm^3 or if the platelet count falls to <80,000/mm^3. Safety and efficacy have not been established in children.

Adverse Reactions As with all drugs which may affect hemostasis, bleeding is associated with ticlopidine. Hemorrhage may occur at virtually any site. Risk is dependent on multiple variables, including the use of multiple agents which alter hemostasis and patient susceptibility.

>10%:

Endocrine & metabolic: Total cholesterol increased (increases of ~8% to 10% within 1 month of therapy), triglycerides increased

Gastrointestinal: Diarrhea (13%)

1% to 10%:

Central nervous system: Dizziness (1%)

Dermatologic: Rash (5%), purpura (2%), pruritus (1%)

Gastrointestinal: Nausea (7%), dyspepsia (7%), gastrointestinal pain (4%), vomiting (2%), flatulence (2%), anorexia (1%)

Hematologic: Neutropenia (2%)

Hepatic: Alkaline phosphatase increased (>2 x upper limit of normal; 8%), abnormal liver function test (1%)

<1% (Limited to important or life-threatening): Agranulocytosis, anaphylaxis, angioedema, aplastic anemia, arthropathy, bilirubin increased, bone marrow suppression, bronchiolitis obliterans-organized pneumonia, chronic diarrhea, conjunctival bleeding, eosinophilia, erythema multiforme, erythema nodosum, exfoliative dermatitis, gastrointestinal bleeding, hematuria, hemolytic anemia, hepatic necrosis, hepatitis, hyponatremia, intracranial bleeding (rare), jaundice, maculopapular rash, menorrhagia, myositis, nephrotic syndrome, pancytopenia, peptic ulcer, peripheral neuropathy, pneumonitis (allergic), positive ANA, renal failure, sepsis, serum creatinine increased, serum sickness, Stevens-Johnson syndrome, systemic lupus erythematosus, thrombocytopenia (immune), thrombocytosis, thrombotic thrombocytopenic purpura, urticaria, vasculitis

Drug Interactions

Metabolism/Transport Effects Substrate of CYP3A4 (major); **Inhibits** CYP1A2 (weak), 2C9 (weak), 2C19 (strong), 2D6 (moderate), 2E1 (weak), 3A4 (weak)

◀ **Avoid Concomitant Use**
Avoid concomitant use of Ticlopidine with any of the following: Clopidogrel; Thioridazine

Increased Effect/Toxicity
Ticlopidine may increase the levels/effects of: Anticoagulants; Antiplatelet Agents; CYP2B6 Substrates; CYP2C19 Substrates; CYP2D6 Substrates; Drotrecogin Alfa; Fesoterodine; Ibritumomab; Nebivolol; Phenytoin; Salicylates; Tamoxifen; Theophylline Derivatives; Thioridazine; Thrombolytic Agents; Tositumomab and Iodine I 131 Tositumomab

The levels/effects of Ticlopidine may be increased by: Dasatinib; Herbs (Anticoagulant/Antiplatelet Properties); Nonsteroidal Anti-Inflammatory Agents; Omega-3-Acid Ethyl Esters; Pentosan Polysulfate Sodium; Pentoxifylline; Prostacyclin Analogues

Decreased Effect
Ticlopidine may decrease the levels/effects of: Clopidogrel; Codeine; TraMADol

The levels/effects of Ticlopidine may be decreased by: CYP3A4 Inducers (Strong); Deferasirox; Herbs (CYP3A4 Inducers); Nonsteroidal Anti-Inflammatory Agents

Ethanol/Nutrition/Herb Interactions
Food: Ticlopidine bioavailability may be increased (20%) if taken with food. High-fat meals increase absorption, antacids decrease absorption.
Herb/Nutraceutical: Avoid alfalfa, anise, bilberry, bladderwrack, bromelain, cat's claw, chamomile, coleus, cordyceps, dong quai, evening primrose oil, fenugreek, feverfew, garlic, ginger, ginkgo biloba, ginseng (American), ginseng (Panax), ginseng (Siberian), grape seed, green tea, guggul, horse chestnut seed, horseradish, licorice, prickly ash, red clover, reishi, SAMe (S-adenosylmethionine), sweet clover, turmeric, white willow (all have additional antiplatelet activity).

Dietary Considerations Should be taken with food to reduce stomach upset.

Dosage Forms Excipient information presented when available (limited, particularly for generics); consult specific product labeling. [DSC] = Discontinued product
Tablet, as hydrochloride: 250 mg
Ticlid®: 250 mg [DSC]

◆ **Ticlopidine Hydrochloride** *see* Ticlopidine *on page 1385*
◆ **TIG** *see* Tetanus Immune Globulin (Human) *on page 1364*
◆ **Tigan®** *see* Trimethobenzamide *on page 1435*

Tigecycline (tye ge SYE kleen)

U.S. Brand Names Tygacil®
Index Terms GAR-936
Pharmacologic Category Antibiotic, Glycylcycline
Generic Available No
Use Treatment of complicated skin and skin structure infections caused by susceptible organisms, including methicillin-resistant *Staphylococcus aureus* and vancomycin-sensitive *Enterococcus faecalis*; complicated intra-abdominal infections; community-acquired pneumonia
Mechanism of Action A glycylcycline antibiotic that binds to the 30S ribosomal subunit of susceptible bacteria, thereby, inhibiting protein synthesis. Generally considered bacteriostatic; however, bactericidal activity has been demonstrated against isolates of *S. pneumoniae* and *L. pneumophila*. Tigecycline is a derivative of minocycline (9-t-butylglycylamido minocycline), and while not classified as a tetracycline, it may share some class-associated adverse effects. Tigecycline has demonstrated activity against a variety of gram-positive and -negative bacterial pathogens including methicillin-resistant staphylococci.
Pharmacodynamics/Kinetics **Note:** Systemic clearance is reduced by 55% and half-life increased by 43% in severe hepatic impairment.
Distribution: V_d: 7-9 L/kg; extensive tissue distribution
Protein binding: 71% to 89%

Metabolism: Hepatic, via glucuronidation, N-acetylation, and epimerization to several metabolites, each <10% of the dose

Half-life elimination: Single dose: 27 hours; following multiple doses: 42 hours

Excretion: Feces (59%, primarily as unchanged drug); urine (33%, with 22% of the total dose as unchanged drug)

Dosage I.V.: Adults: **Note:** Duration of therapy dependant on severity/site of infection and clinical status and response to therapy.

Community-acquired pneumonia: Initial: 100 mg as a single dose; Maintenance dose: 50 mg every 12 hours for 7-14 days

Complicated intra-abdominal infections: Initial: 100 mg as a single dose; Maintenance dose: 50 mg every 12 hours for 5-14 days

Complicated skin/skin structure infections: Initial: 100 mg as a single dose; Maintenance dose: 50 mg every 12 hours for 5-14 days

Dosage adjustment in renal impairment: No dosage adjustment required in renal impairment or in patients undergoing hemodialysis.

Dosage adjustment in hepatic impairment:

Mild-to-moderate hepatic impairment (Child-Pugh classes A and B): No dosage adjustment required

Severe hepatic impairment (Child-Pugh class C): Initial: 100 mg single dose; Maintenance: 25 mg every 12 hours

Stability Prior to reconstitution, store at 20°C to 25°C (68°F to 77°F); excursions permitted to 15°C to 30°C (59°F to 86°F). Add 5.3 mL NS, D_5W, or LR to each 50 mg vial. Swirl gently to dissolve. Resulting solution is 10 mg/mL. Reconstituted solution must be further diluted to allow I.V. administration. Transfer to 100 mL I.V. bag for infusion (final concentration should not exceed 1 mg/mL). Reconstituted solution may be stored at room temperature for up to 6 hours or up to 24 hours if further diluted in a compatible I.V. solution. Alternatively, may be stored refrigerated at 2°C to 8°C (36°F to 46°F) for up to 48 hours following immediate transfer of the reconstituted solution into NS or D_5W. Reconstituted solution should be yellow-orange; discard if not this color.

Administration Infuse over 30-60 minutes through dedicated line or via Y-site

Pregnancy Risk Factor D

Contraindications Hypersensitivity to tigecycline or any component of the formulation

Warnings/Precautions May cause life-threatening anaphylaxis/anaphylactoid reactions. Due to structural similarity with tetracyclines, use caution in patients with prior hypersensitivity and/or severe adverse reactions associated with tetracycline use. Due to structural similarities with tetracyclines, may be associated with photosensitivity, pseudotumor cerebri, pancreatitis, and anti-anabolic effects (including increased BUN, azotemia, acidosis, and hyperphosphatemia) observed with this class. May cause fetal harm if used during pregnancy; patients should be advised of potential risks associated with use. Permanent discoloration of the teeth may occur if used during tooth development (fetal stage through children up to 8 years of age).

Use caution in hepatic impairment; dosage adjustment recommended in severe hepatic impairment. Abnormal liver function tests (increased total bilirubin, prothrombin time, transaminases) have been reported. Isolated cases of significant hepatic dysfunction and hepatic failure have occurred. Closely monitor for worsening hepatic function in patients that develop abnormal liver function tests during therapy. Adverse hepatic effects may occur after drug discontinuation.

Prolonged use may result in fungal or bacterial superinfection, including *C. difficile*-associated diarrhea (CDAD) and pseudomembranous colitis; CDAD has been observed >2 months postantibiotic treatment. Use with caution if using as monotherapy for patients with intestinal perforation (in the small sample of available cases, septic shock occurred more frequently than patients treated with imipenem/cilastatin comparator). Inferior efficacy (versus comparator antibiotic), including lower cure rates and increased mortality, have been observed in patients treated with tigecycline for hospital-acquired pneumonia. Safety and efficacy in children <18 years of age have not been established.

Adverse Reactions Note: Frequencies relative to placebo are not available; some frequencies are lower than those experienced with comparator drugs.

◀ >10%: Gastrointestinal: Nausea (26%; severe: 1%), vomiting (18%; severe: 1%), diarrhea (12%)

2% to 10%:

Central nervous system: Headache (6%), dizziness (3%)

Dermatologic: Rash (3%)

Endocrine & metabolic: Hypoproteinemia (5%)

Gastrointestinal: Abdominal pain (6%), dyspepsia (2%)

Hematologic: Anemia (4%)

Hepatic: ALT increased (5%), AST increased (4%), alkaline phosphatase increased (4%), amylase increased (3%), bilirubin increased (2%)

Local: Phlebitis (3%)

Neuromuscular & skeletal: Weakness (3%)

Renal: BUN increased (2%)

Miscellaneous: Infection (8%), abnormal healing (4%), abscess (3%)

<2% (Limited to important or life-threatening): Abnormal stools, anaphylaxis/anaphylactoid reactions, anorexia, aPTT prolonged, chills, creatinine increased, eosinophilia, hepatic cholestasis, hypocalcemia, hypoglycemia, hyponatremia, injection site edema, injection site inflammation, injection site pain, injection site phlebitis, injection site reaction, jaundice, leukorrhea, pancreatitis (acute), pruritus, PT prolonged, septic shock, taste perversion, thrombocytopenia, thrombophlebitis, vaginal moniliasis, vaginitis

Drug Interactions

Avoid Concomitant Use There are no known interactions where it is recommended to avoid concomitant use.

Increased Effect/Toxicity

Tigecycline may increase the levels/effects of: Warfarin

Decreased Effect There are no known significant interactions involving a decrease in effect.

Dosage Forms Excipient information presented when available (limited, particularly for generics); consult specific product labeling.

Injection, powder for reconstitution:

Tygacil®: 50 mg [contains lactose 100 mg]

◆ **Tikosyn®** *see* Dofetilide *on page 441*

◆ **Tilia™ Fe** *see* Ethinyl Estradiol and Norethindrone *on page 554*

◆ **Tim-AK (Can)** *see* Timolol *on page 1390*

◆ **Timentin®** *see* Ticarcillin and Clavulanate Potassium *on page 1381*

Timolol (TIM oh lol)

Related Information

Antiarrhythmic Drugs *on page 1656*

Beta-Blockers *on page 1669*

Desensitization Protocols *on page 1692*

Preoperative Evaluation of the Cardiac Patient for Noncardiac Surgery *on page 1598*

U.S. Brand Names Betimol®; Istalol®; Timolol GFS; Timoptic-XE®; Timoptic®; Timoptic® in OcuDose®

Canadian Brand Names Alti-Timolol; Apo-Timol®; Apo-Timop®; Gen-Timolol; Mylan-Timolol; Nu-Timolol; Phoxal-timolol; PMS-Timolol; Sandoz-Timolol; Tim-AK; Timoptic-XE®; Timoptic®

Index Terms Blocadren; Timolol Hemihydrate; Timolol Maleate

Pharmacologic Category Beta-Adrenergic Blocker, Nonselective; Ophthalmic Agent, Antiglaucoma

Use

Ophthalmic: Treatment of elevated intraocular pressure such as glaucoma or ocular hypertension

Oral: Treatment of hypertension and angina; to reduce mortality following myocardial infarction; prophylaxis of migraine

Pharmacodynamics/Kinetics

Onset of action:

Hypotensive: Oral: 15-45 minutes

Peak effect: 0.5-2.5 hours

Intraocular pressure reduction: Ophthalmic: 30 minutes
  Peak effect: 1-2 hours
Duration: ~4 hours; Ophthalmic: Intraocular: 24 hours
Absorption: Oral: Rapid and complete (~90%); Timolol is measurable in the serum following ophthalmic use
Distribution: V_d: 1.7 L/kg
Protein binding: 60%
Metabolism: Extensively hepatic; extensive first-pass effect
Bioavailability: 50%
Half-life elimination: 2-2.7 hours; prolonged with renal impairment
Time to peak, plasma: Oral: 1-2 hours
Excretion: Urine (15% to 20% as unchanged drug)

Dosage

Ophthalmic:
  Children and Adults:
    Solution: Initial: Instill 1 drop (0.25% solution) into affected eye(s) twice daily; increase to 0.5% solution if response not adequate; decrease to 1 drop/day if controlled; do not exceed 1 drop twice daily of 0.5% solution
    Gel-forming solution (Timolol GFS, Timoptic-XE®): Instill 1 drop (either 0.25% or 0.5% solution) once daily
  Adults: Solution (Istalol®): Instill 1 drop (0.5% solution) once daily in the morning
Oral: Adults:
  Hypertension: Initial: 10 mg twice daily, increase gradually every 7 days, usual dosage: 20-40 mg/day in 2 divided doses; maximum: 60 mg/day
  Prevention of myocardial infarction: 10 mg twice daily initiated within 1-4 weeks after infarction
  Migraine headache: Initial: 10 mg twice daily, increase to maximum of 30 mg/day

Anesthesia and Critical Care Concerns/Other Considerations Surgery:

Based on available evidence, beta-blockers should be started days to weeks before elective surgery in selected patients when possible and titrated to a heart rate <65 beats per minute. Additional data suggest that long acting beta-blockers may be superior to short acting ones (Redelmeier, 2005). The ACC/AHA 2007 guidelines update on perioperative cardiovascular evaluation and care for noncardiac surgery recommend beta-blockers be continued in patients undergoing surgery who are receiving beta-blockers to treat angina, symptomatic arrhythmias, hypertension, or other ACC/AHA Class I guideline indications (Class I recommendation). The guidelines also recommend that beta-blockers be given to patients undergoing vascular surgery who have myocardial ischemia demonstrated during preoperative testing (Class I recommendation).

The guidelines also state that beta-blockers are probably recommended in patients undergoing intermediate risk (eg, carotid endarterectomy, prostate surgery) or vascular surgery in whom preoperative assessment identifies coronary heart disease or high cardiac risk (Class IIa recommendation). High cardiac risk is defined as having >1 of the following clinical risk factors: History of ischemic heart disease, compensated or prior heart failure, cerebrovascular disease, diabetes mellitus, or renal insufficiency. The use of beta-blockers is uncertain in patients undergoing intermediate risk or vascular surgery with ≤1 clinical risk factor (Class IIb recommendation).

The majority of published trials suggest a benefit of perioperative beta-blocker use during noncardiac surgery especially in high-risk patients; however, more recent clinical trials have not shown a benefit to perioperative beta-blockade for noncardiac surgery (Juul, 2006; Yang, 2006).

Additional Information Complete prescribing information for this medication should be consulted for additional detail.

Dosage Forms Excipient information presented when available (limited, particularly for generics); consult specific product labeling. [DSC] = Discontinued product

Note: Unless otherwise specified, strength expressed as base.

Gel-forming solution, ophthalmic, as maleate:
  Timolol GFS: 0.25% (2.5 mL [DSC], 5 mL); 0.5% (2.5 mL [DSC], 5 mL)
  Timoptic-XE®: 0.25% (5 mL); 0.5% (5 mL)

◀ Solution, ophthalmic, as hemihydrate:
  Betimol®: 0.25% (5 mL, 10 mL [DSC], 15 mL [DSC]); 0.5% (5 mL, 10 mL, 15 mL) [contains benzalkonium chloride]
Solution, ophthalmic, as maleate: 0.25% (5 mL, 10 mL, 15 mL); 0.5% (5 mL, 10 mL, 15 mL)
  Istalol®: 0.5% (10 mL) [contains benzalkonium chloride and potassium sorbate]
  Timoptic®: 0.25% (5 mL); 0.5% (5 mL, 10 mL) [contains benzalkonium chloride]
Solution, ophthalmic, as maleate [preservative free]:
  Timoptic® in OcuDose®: 0.25% (0.2 mL); 0.5% (0.2 mL)
Tablet, as maleate: 5 mg, 10 mg, 20 mg [strength expressed as salt]

References

Fleisher LA, Beckman JA, Brown KA, et al, "ACC/AHA 2006 Guideline Update on Perioperative Cardiovascular Evaluation for Noncardiac Surgery: Focused Update on Perioperative Beta-Blocker Therapy: A Report of the American College of Cardiology/American Heart Association Task Force on Practice Guidelines (Writing Committee to Update the 2002 Guidelines on Perioperative Cardiovascular Evaluation for Noncardiac Surgery) Developed in Collaboration With the American Society of Echocardiography, American Society of Nuclear Cardiology, Heart Rhythm Society, Society of Cardiovascular Anesthesiologists, Society for Cardiovascular Angiography and Interventions, and Society for Vascular Medicine and Biology," *J Am Coll Cardiol*, 2006, 47 (11):2343-55.

Juul AB, Wetterslev J, Gluud C, et al, "Effect of Perioperative Beta-Blockade in Patients With Diabetes Undergoing Major Noncardiac Surgery: Randomized Placebo Controlled, Blinded Multicentre Trial," *BMJ*, 2006, 332(7556):1482.

Yang H, Raymer K, Butler R, et al, "The Effects of Perioperative Beta-Blockade: Results of the Metoprolol After Vascular Surgery (MaVS) Study, A Randomized Controlled Trial," *Am Heart J* 2006, 152(5):983-90.

◆ **Timolol GFS** *see Timolol on page 1390*

◆ **Timolol Hemihydrate** *see Timolol on page 1390*

◆ **Timolol Maleate** *see Timolol on page 1390*

◆ **Timoptic®** *see Timolol on page 1390*

◆ **Timoptic® in OcuDose®** *see Timolol on page 1390*

◆ **Timoptic-XE®** *see Timolol on page 1390*

Tinzaparin (tin ZA pa rin)

Medication Safety Issues

High alert medication: The Institute for Safe Medication Practices (ISMP) includes this medication among its list of drug classes which have a heightened risk of causing significant patient harm when used in error.

2009 National Patient Safety Goals: The Joint Commission on Accreditation of Healthcare Organizations requires healthcare organizations that provide anticoagulant therapy to have a process in place to reduce the risk of anticoagulant-associated patient harm. Patients receiving anticoagulants should receive individualized care through a defined process that includes standardized ordering, dispensing, administration, monitoring and education. This does not apply to routine short-term use of anticoagulants for prevention of venous thromboembolism when the expectation is that the patient's laboratory values will remain within or close to normal values (NPSG.03.05.01).

U.S. Brand Names Innohep®
Canadian Brand Names Innohep®
Index Terms Tinzaparin Sodium
Pharmacologic Category Low Molecular Weight Heparin
Generic Available No
Use Treatment of acute symptomatic deep vein thrombosis, with or without pulmonary embolism, in conjunction with warfarin sodium
Mechanism of Action Standard heparin consists of components with molecular weights ranging from 4000-30,000 daltons with a mean of 16,000 daltons. Heparin acts as an anticoagulant by enhancing the inhibition rate of clotting proteases by antithrombin III, impairing normal hemostasis and inhibition of factor Xa. Low molecular weight heparins have a small effect on the activated partial thromboplastin time and strongly inhibit factor Xa. The primary inhibitory activity of tinzaparin is through antithrombin. Tinzaparin is derived from porcine heparin that undergoes controlled enzymatic depolymerization. The average molecular

weight of tinzaparin ranges between 5500 and 7500 daltons which is distributed as <2000 daltons (<10%), 2000-8000 daltons (60% to 72%), and >8000 daltons (22% to 36%). The anti-Xa activity is approximately 100 int. units/mg.

Pharmacodynamics/Kinetics
Onset of action: 2-3 hours
Distribution: 3-5 L
Half-life elimination: 3-4 hours
Metabolism: Partially metabolized by desulphation and depolymerization
Bioavailability: 87%
Time to peak: 4-5 hours
Excretion: Urine

Dosage SubQ:
Adults: DVT with or without pulmonary embolism (PE): 175 anti-Xa int. units/kg of body weight once daily. The 2008 *Chest* guidelines recommend starting warfarin on the first treatment day and continuing tinzaparin until INR is between 2 and 3 (usually 5-7 days). Administer tinzaparin for at least 5 days and until INR ≥2 for at least 24 hours (Hirsh, 2008).
  Note: To calculate the volume of solution to administer per dose: Volume to be administered (mL) = patient weight (kg) x 0.00875 mL/kg (may be rounded off to the nearest 0.05 mL)
Elderly: No significant differences in safety or response were seen when used in patients ≥65 years of age. However, increased sensitivity to tinzaparin in elderly patients may be possible due to a decline in renal function. Increased all-cause mortality noted in patients ≥70 years of age with Cl_{cr} ≤30 mL/minute or ≥75 years of age and Cl_{cr} ≤60 mL/minute; consider alternative treatments in these patients.
Dosing adjustment in obesity: Weight based dosing (175 anti-Xa int. units/kg of body weight once daily) provided in product labeling for patients up to 162 kg. Limited clinical experience in patients with a BMI >40 kg/m^2.
Dosage adjustment in renal impairment:
  Cl_{cr} ≤50 mL/minute: Use with caution; clearance is decreased
  Cl_{cr} <30 mL/minute: Per manufacturer's labeling, use with caution. The 2008 *Chest* guidelines recommend avoiding use (in patients requiring therapeutic anticoagulation); if used, consider monitoring anti-Xa levels (Hirsh, 2008).
Dosage adjustment in hepatic impairment: No specific dosage adjustment has been recommended.

Stability Store at 15°C to 30°C (59°F to 86°F).

Administration Patient should be lying down or sitting. Administer by deep SubQ injection, alternating between the left and right anterolateral and left and right posterolateral abdominal wall. Vary site daily. The entire needle should be introduced into the skin fold formed by the thumb and forefinger. Hold the skin fold until injection is complete. To minimize bruising, do not rub the injection site.

Monitoring Parameters CBC including platelet count and hematocrit or hemoglobin, and stool for occult blood; the monitoring of PT and/or aPTT is not of clinical value. Patients receiving both warfarin and tinzaparin should have their INR drawn just prior to the next scheduled dose of tinzaparin.

According to 2008 *Chest* guidelines, routine monitoring of anti-Xa levels is generally not recommended; however, anti-Xa levels may be beneficial in certain patients (eg, obese patients, patients with severe renal insufficiency receiving therapeutic doses, and possibly pregnant women receiving therapeutic doses; Hirsh, 2008)

Pregnancy Risk Factor B

Contraindications Hypersensitivity to tinzaparin sodium, heparin, or any component of the formulation; active major bleeding; heparin-induced thrombocytopenia (current or history of)

Warnings/Precautions [U.S. Boxed Warning]: Patients with recent or anticipated neuraxial anesthesia (epidural or spinal anesthesia) are at risk of spinal or epidural hematoma and subsequent paralysis. Consider risk versus benefit prior to neuraxial anesthesia; risk is increased by concomitant agents that may alter hemostasis, as well as traumatic or repeated epidural or spinal puncture, and indwelling epidural catheters. Patient should be observed closely for signs and symptoms of neurological impairment. Not to be used interchangeably (unit for unit) with heparin or any other low molecular weight heparins.

◄ Monitor patient closely for signs or symptoms of bleeding. Certain patients are at increased risk of bleeding. Risk factors include bacterial endocarditis; congenital or acquired bleeding disorders; active ulcerative or angiodysplastic GI diseases; severe uncontrolled hypertension; history of hemorrhagic stroke; use shortly after brain, spinal, or ophthalmologic surgery; patients treated concomitantly with platelet inhibitors; recent GI bleeding; thrombocytopenia or platelet defects; severe liver disease; hypertensive or diabetic retinopathy; or in patients undergoing invasive procedures. Monitor platelet count closely. Rare cases of thrombocytopenia have occurred. Manufacturer recommends discontinuation of therapy if platelets are <100,000/mm^3. Rare cases of thrombocytopenia with thrombosis have occurred.

Reduced tinzaparin clearance was observed in patients with moderate-to-severe renal impairment; use with caution or avoid use in patients with renal insufficiency. The 2008 *Chest* guidelines recommend that patients with Cl$_{cr}$ <30 mL/minute be treated with unfractionated heparin instead of LMWH (Hirsh, 2008). Use with caution in the elderly (delayed elimination may occur). Use in patients ≥70 years of age with renal insufficiency (Cl$_{cr}$ ≤30 mL/minute or ≥75 years of age and Cl$_{cr}$ ≤60 mL/minute) has been associated with an increased risk of death compared to use of unfractionated heparin; consider alternative treatments in these patients. Safety and efficacy in pediatric patients have not been established.

Heparin can cause hyperkalemia by suppressing aldosterone production; similar reactions could occur with LMWHs. Monitor for hyperkalemia which most commonly occurs in patients with risk factors for the development of hyperkalemia (eg, renal dysfunction, concomitant use of potassium-sparing diuretics or potassium supplements, hematoma in body tissues). For subcutaneous use only; do not administer intramuscularly or intravenously. Clinical experience is limited in patients with BMI >40 kg/m^2. Derived from porcine intestinal mucosa. Contains benzyl alcohol and sodium metabisulfite

Adverse Reactions As with all anticoagulants, bleeding is the major adverse effect of tinzaparin. Hemorrhage may occur at virtually any site. Risk is dependent on multiple variables.

>10%:
Hepatic: ALT increased (13%)
Local: Injection site hematoma (16%)
1% to 10%:
Cardiovascular: Angina pectoris, chest pain (2%), hyper-/hypotension, tachycardia
Central nervous system: Confusion, dizziness, fever (2%), headache (2%), insomnia, pain (2%)
Dermatologic: Bullous eruption, pruritus, rash (1%), skin disorder
Gastrointestinal: Constipation (1%), dyspepsia, flatulence, nausea (2%), nonspecified gastrointestinal disorder, vomiting (1%)
Genitourinary: Dysuria, urinary retention, urinary tract infection (4%)
Hematologic: Anemia, hematoma, hemorrhage (2%), thrombocytopenia (1%)
Hepatic: AST increased (9%)
Local: Thrombophlebitis (deep)
Neuromuscular & skeletal: Back pain (2%)
Renal: Hematuria (1%)
Respiratory: Dyspnea (1%), epistaxis (2%), pneumonia, pulmonary embolism (2%), respiratory disorder
Miscellaneous: Impaired healing, infection, unclassified reactions
<1% (Limited to important or life-threatening): Abscess, acute febrile reaction, agranulocytosis, allergic purpura, allergic reaction, angioedema, anaphylactoid reaction, anorectal bleeding, cardiac arrhythmia, cellulitis, cerebral hemorrhage, cholestatic hepatitis, coronary thrombosis, dependent edema, epidermal necrolysis, erythematous gastrointestinal hemorrhage, granulocytopenia, hemarthrosis, hematemesis, hemoptysis, injection site bleeding, intracranial hemorrhage, ischemic necrosis, melena, MI, necrosis, neoplasm, ocular hemorrhage, pancytopenia, peripheral ischemia, priapism, purpura, rash, retroperitoneal/intra-abdominal bleeding, severe thrombocytopenia, skin

necrosis, spinal epidural hematoma, Stevens-Johnson syndrome, thromboembolism, urticaria, vaginal hemorrhage, wound hematoma

Drug Interactions

Avoid Concomitant Use There are no known interactions where it is
recommended to avoid concomitant use.

Increased Effect/Toxicity
Tinzaparin may increase the levels/effects of: Anticoagulants; Drotrecogin Alfa;
Ibritumomab; Tositumomab and Iodine I 131 Tositumomab

The levels/effects of Tinzaparin may be increased by: 5-ASA Derivatives;
Antiplatelet Agents; Dasatinib; Herbs (Anticoagulant/Antiplatelet Properties);
Nonsteroidal Anti-Inflammatory Agents; Pentosan Polysulfate Sodium; Pentox-
ifylline; Prostacyclin Analogues; Salicylates; Thrombolytic Agents

Decreased Effect There are no known significant interactions involving a
decrease in effect.

Dosage Forms Excipient information presented when available (limited,
particularly for generics); consult specific product labeling.

Injection, solution, as sodium:
Innohep®: 20,000 anti-Xa int. units/mL (2 mL) [contains benzyl alcohol and
sodium metabisulfite]

◆ **Tinzaparin Sodium** *see* Tinzaparin *on page 1392*

Tiotropium (ty oh TRO pee um)

Medication Safety Issues
Sound-alike/look-alike issues:
Spiriva® may be confused with Inspra™, Serevent®
Tiotropium may be confused with ipratropium
Spiriva® capsules for inhalation are for administration via HandiHaler® device
and are **not** for oral use

U.S. Brand Names Spiriva® HandiHaler®

Canadian Brand Names Spiriva®

Index Terms Tiotropium Bromide Monohydrate

Pharmacologic Category Anticholinergic Agent

Generic Available No

Use Maintenance treatment of bronchospasm associated with COPD (including
bronchitis and emphysema)

Mechanism of Action Competitively and reversibly inhibits the action of
acetylcholine at type 3 muscarinic (M_3) receptors in bronchial smooth muscle
causing bronchodilation

Pharmacodynamics/Kinetics
Absorption: Poorly absorbed from GI tract, systemic absorption may occur from
lung
Distribution: V_d: 32 L/kg
Protein binding: 72%
Metabolism: Hepatic (minimal), via CYP2D6 and CYP3A4
Bioavailability: Following inhalation, 19.5%; oral solution: 2% to 3%
Half-life elimination: 5-6 days
Time to peak, plasma: 5 minutes (following inhalation)
Excretion: Urine (14% of an inhaled dose); feces (primarily nonabsorbed drug)

Dosage Oral inhalation: Adults: Contents of 1 capsule (18 mcg) inhaled once daily
using HandiHaler® device
Dosage adjustment in renal impairment: Plasma concentrations may increase
in renal impairment. Use caution in moderate-severe impairment (Cl_{cr} ≤50 mL/
minute); although no dosage adjustment is required, monitor closely.

Stability Store at 25°C (77°F); excursions permitted to 15°C to 30°C (59°F to
86°F). Avoid excessive temperatures and moisture. Do not store capsules in
HandiHaler® device. Capsules should be stored in the blister pack and only
removed immediately before use. Once protective foil is peeled back and/or
removed the capsule should be used immediately; if capsule is not used
immediately it should be discarded.

◀ **Administration** Administer once daily at the same time each day. Remove capsule from foil blister immediately before use. Capsule should not be swallowed. Place capsule in the capsule-chamber in the base of the HandiHaler® Inhaler. Must only use the HandiHaler® Inhaler. Close mouthpiece until a click is heard, leaving dustcap open. Exhale fully. Do not exhale into inhaler. Tilt head slightly back and inhale (rapidly, steadily and deeply); the capsule vibration may be heard within the device. Hold breath as long as possible. If any powder remains in capsule, exhale and inhale again. Repeat until capsule is empty. Throw away empty capsule; do not leave in inhaler. Do not use a spacer with the HandiHaler® Inhaler. Do not use HandiHaler® device for other medications. Always keep capsules and inhaler dry.

Delivery of dose: Instruct patient to place mouthpiece gently between teeth, closing lips around inhaler. Instruct patient to inhale deeply and hold breath held for 5-10 seconds. The amount of drug delivered is small, and the individual will not sense the medication as it is inhaled. Remove mouthpiece prior to exhalation. Patient should not breathe out through the mouthpiece.

Monitoring Parameters FEV_1, peak flow (or other pulmonary function studies)

Pregnancy Risk Factor C

Contraindications Hypersensitivity to tiotropium, atropine or its derivatives, including ipratropium, or any component of the formulation (contains lactose)

Warnings/Precautions Rarely, paradoxical bronchospasm may occur with use of inhaled bronchodilating agents; this should be distinguished from inadequate response. Not indicated for the initial (rescue) treatment of acute episodes of bronchospasm. Use with caution in patients with myasthenia gravis, narrow-angle glaucoma, prostatic hyperplasia, moderate-severe renal impairment (Cl_{cr} ≤50 mL/minute), or bladder neck obstruction; avoid inadvertent instillation of powder into the eyes. Immediate hypersensitivity reactions may occur; discontinue immediately if signs/symptoms occur. The contents of Spiriva® capsules are for inhalation only via the HandiHaler® device. There have been reports of incorrect administration (swallowing of the capsules). Safety and efficacy have not been established in pediatric patients.

Adverse Reactions

>10%:
  Gastrointestinal: Xerostomia (16%)
  Respiratory: Upper respiratory tract infection (41%), sinusitis (11%)

1% to 10%:
  Cardiovascular: Chest pain (1% to 7%), edema (dependent, 5%)
  Central nervous system: Depression (1% to 3%), dysphonia (1% to 3%)
  Dermatologic: Rash (4%)
  Endocrine & metabolic: Hypercholesterolemia (1% to 3%), hyperglycemia (1% to 3%)
  Gastrointestinal: Dyspepsia (6%), abdominal pain (5%), constipation (4%), vomiting (4%), gastroesophageal reflux (1% to 3%), stomatitis (including ulcerative; 1% to 3%)
  Genitourinary: Urinary tract infection (7%)
  Neuromuscular & skeletal: Myalgia (4%), arthritis (≥3%), leg pain (1% to 3%), paresthesia (1% to 3%), skeletal pain (1% to 3%)
  Ocular: Cataract (1% to 3%)
  Respiratory: Pharyngitis (9%), rhinitis (6%), epistaxis (4%), cough (≥3%), laryngitis (1% to 3%)
  Miscellaneous: Infection (4%), moniliasis (4%), flu-like syndrome (≥3%), allergic reaction (1% to 3%), herpes zoster (1% to 3%)

<1% (Limited to important or life-threatening): Angioedema; application site irritation (glossitis, mouth ulceration, pharyngolaryngeal pain); atrial fibrillation, blurred vision, candidiasis (oral), dizziness, dysphagia, glaucoma, hoarseness, hypersensitivity reactions, ileus (paralytic), intestinal obstruction, intraocular pressure increased, palpitation, paradoxical bronchospasm, pruritus, pupil dilation (if powder comes in contact with eyes), stroke, supraventricular tachycardia, tachycardia, throat irritation, urinary difficulty, urinary retention, urticaria

Drug Interactions

Metabolism/Transport Effects Substrate (minor) of CYP2D6, 3A4

Avoid Concomitant Use There are no known interactions where it is recommended to avoid concomitant use.

Increased Effect/Toxicity

Tiotropium may increase the levels/effects of: Anticholinergics; Cannabinoids; Potassium Chloride

The levels/effects of Tiotropium may be increased by: Pramlintide

Decreased Effect

Tiotropium may decrease the levels/effects of: Acetylcholinesterase Inhibitors (Central); Secretin

The levels/effects of Tiotropium may be decreased by: Acetylcholinesterase Inhibitors (Central); Peginterferon Alfa-2b

Dosage Forms Excipient information presented when available (limited, particularly for generics); consult specific product labeling.

Powder for oral inhalation [capsule]:

Spiriva® HandiHaler®: 18 mcg/capsule (5s, 30s, 90s) [contains lactose]

◆ **Tiotropium Bromide Monohydrate** *see* Tiotropium *on page 1395*

Tirofiban (tye roe FYE ban)

Medication Safety Issues

Sound-alike/look-alike issues:

Aggrastat® may be confused with Aggrenox®, argatroban

High alert medication: The Institute for Safe Medication Practices (ISMP) includes this medication among its list of drugs which have a heightened risk of causing significant patient harm when used in error.

Related Information

Regional Anesthesia in Patients Receiving Anticoagulant and Antiplatelet Therapy *on page 1642*

U.S. Brand Names Aggrastat®

Canadian Brand Names Aggrastat®

Index Terms MK383; Tirofiban Hydrochloride

Pharmacologic Category Antiplatelet Agent, Glycoprotein IIb/IIIa Inhibitor

Generic Available No

Use In combination with heparin, is indicated for the treatment of acute coronary syndrome, including patients who are to be managed medically and those undergoing PTCA or atherectomy. In this setting, it has been shown to decrease the rate of a combined endpoint of death, new myocardial infarction or refractory ischemia/repeat cardiac procedure.

Mechanism of Action A reversible antagonist of fibrinogen binding to the GP IIb/IIIa receptor, the major platelet surface receptor involved in platelet aggregation. When administered intravenously, it inhibits *ex vivo* platelet aggregation in a dose- and concentration-dependent manner. When given according to the recommended regimen, >90% inhibition is attained by the end of the 30-minute infusion. Platelet aggregation inhibition is reversible following cessation of the infusion.

Pharmacodynamics/Kinetics

Distribution: 35% unbound

Metabolism: Minimally hepatic

Half-life elimination: 2 hours

Excretion: Urine (65%) and feces (25%) primarily as unchanged drug

Clearance: Elderly: Reduced by 19% to 26%

Dosage Adults: I.V.: Initial rate of 0.4 mcg/kg/minute for 30 minutes and then continued at 0.1 mcg/kg/minute; dosing should be continued through angiography and for 12-24 hours after angioplasty or atherectomy. See table on next page.

Tirofiban Dosing (Using 50 mcg/mL Concentration)

Patient Weight (kg)	Patients With Normal Renal Function		Patients With Renal Dysfunction	
	30-Min Loading Infusion Rate (mL/h)	Maintenance Infusion Rate (mL/h)	30-Min Loading Infusion Rate (mL/h)	Maintenance Infusion Rate (mL/h)
30-37	16	4	8	2
38-45	20	5	10	3
46-54	24	6	12	3
55-62	28	7	14	4
63-70	32	8	16	4
71-79	36	9	18	5
80-87	40	10	20	5
88-95	44	11	22	6
96-104	48	12	24	6
105-112	52	13	26	7
113-120	56	14	28	7
121-128	60	15	30	8
128-137	64	16	32	8
138-145	68	17	34	9
146-153	72	18	36	9

Dosing adjustment in severe renal impairment: Cl_{cr} <30 mL/minute: Reduce dose to 50% of normal rate.

Stability Store at 25°C (77°F); do not freeze. Protect from light during storage.

Administration Intended for intravenous delivery using sterile equipment and technique. Do not add other drugs or remove solution directly from the bag with a syringe. Do not use plastic containers in series connections; such use can result in air embolism by drawing air from the first container if it is empty of solution. Discard unused solution 24 hours following the start of infusion. May be administered through the same catheter as heparin. Tirofiban injection must be diluted to a concentration of 50 mcg/mL (premixed solution does not require dilution). Infuse over 30 minutes.

Monitoring Parameters Platelet count. Hemoglobin and hematocrit should be monitored prior to treatment, within 6 hours following loading infusion, and at least daily thereafter during therapy. Platelet count may need to be monitored earlier in patients who received prior glycoprotein IIb/IIa antagonists. Persistent reductions of platelet counts <90,000/mm^3 may require interruption or discontinuation of infusion. Because tirofiban requires concurrent heparin therapy, aPTT levels should also be followed. Monitor vital signs and laboratory results prior to, during, and after therapy. Assess infusion insertion site during and after therapy (every 15 minutes or as institutional policy). Observe and teach patient bleeding precautions (avoid invasive procedures and activities that could result in injury). Monitor closely for signs of unusual or excessive bleeding (eg, CNS changes, blood in urine, stool, or vomitus, unusual bruising or bleeding). Breast-feeding is contraindicated.

Anesthesia and Critical Care Concerns/Other Considerations Clinical Pearls/Comments: Platelet Effects: As a reversible inhibitor of the platelet glycoprotein (GP) IIb/IIIa receptor, tirofiban has a short duration of action and hemostasis is restored within about 4 hours after discontinuation in patients with normal renal function.

Tirofiban-induced thrombocytopenia: Acute profound thrombocytopenia has been associated with tirofiban use and may occur within 24 hours of initiation (Demirkan, 2006).

Platelet count monitoring is recommended 2-4 hours after initiation, and at 24 hours or prior to discharge, whichever is first. Specific management guidelines for GP IIb/IIIa induced thrombocytopenia have been published (Huxtable, 2006; Llevadot, 2000). Platelet counts should recover rapidly (within 1-5 days) after discontinuation of tirofiban. Although sustained thrombocytopenia is less of a risk with tirofiban compared to abciximab, the presence of active bleeding at any time, emergent invasive procedure, or a platelet level of <20,000 cells/microL should prompt the consideration of platelet transfusion.

Pregnancy Risk Factor B

Contraindications Hypersensitivity to tirofiban or any component of the formulation; active internal bleeding or a history of bleeding diathesis within the previous 30 days; history of intracranial hemorrhage, intracranial neoplasm, arteriovenous malformation, or aneurysm; history of thrombocytopenia following prior exposure; history of CVA within 30 days or any history of hemorrhagic stroke; major surgical procedure or severe physical trauma within the previous month; history, symptoms, or findings suggestive of aortic dissection; severe hypertension (systolic BP >180 mm Hg and/or diastolic BP >110 mm Hg); concomitant use of another parenteral GP IIb/IIIa inhibitor; acute pericarditis

Warnings/Precautions Bleeding is the most common complication encountered during this therapy; most major bleeding occurs at the arterial access site for cardiac catheterization. Caution in patients with platelets <150,000/mm^3; patients with hemorrhagic retinopathy; chronic dialysis patients; when used in combination with other drugs impacting on coagulation. To minimize bleeding complications, care must be taken in sheath insertion/removal. Sheath hemostasis should be achieved at least 4 hours before hospital discharge. Other trauma and vascular punctures should be minimized. Avoid obtaining vascular access through a noncompressible site (eg, subclavian or jugular vein). Patients with severe renal insufficiency require dosage reduction. Safety and efficacy have not been established in children.

Adverse Reactions Bleeding is the major drug-related adverse effect. Patients received background treatment with aspirin and heparin. Major bleeding was reported in 1.4% to 2.2%; minor bleeding in 10.5% to 12%; transfusion was required in 4% to 4.3%.

>1% (nonbleeding adverse events):
  Cardiovascular: Coronary artery dissection (5%), bradycardia (4%), edema (2%)
  Central nervous system: Dizziness (3%), vasovagal reaction (2%), fever (>1%), headache (>1%)
  Gastrointestinal: Nausea (>1%)
  Genitourinary: Pelvic pain (6%)
  Hematologic: Thrombocytopenia: <90,000/mm^3 (1.5%), <50,000/mm^3 (0.3%)
  Neuromuscular & skeletal: Leg pain (3%)
  Miscellaneous: Diaphoresis (2%)
<1% (Limited to important or life-threatening): Acutely decreased platelets in association with fever, anaphylaxis, GI bleeding (0.1% to 0.2%), GU bleeding (up to 0.1%), hemopericardium, intracranial bleeding (up to 0.1%), pulmonary alveolar hemorrhage, rash, retroperitoneal bleeding (up to 0.6%), severe (<10,000/mm^3) thrombocytopenia (rare), spinal-epidural hematoma

Drug Interactions

Avoid Concomitant Use There are no known interactions where it is recommended to avoid concomitant use.

Increased Effect/Toxicity

Tirofiban may increase the levels/effects of: Anticoagulants; Antiplatelet Agents; Drotrecogin Alfa; Ibritumomab; Salicylates; Thrombolytic Agents; Tositumomab and Iodine I 131 Tositumomab

The levels/effects of Tirofiban may be increased by: Dasatinib; Herbs (Anticoagulant/Antiplatelet Properties); Nonsteroidal Anti-Inflammatory Agents; Omega-3-Acid Ethyl Esters; Pentosan Polysulfate Sodium; Pentoxifylline; Prostacyclin Analogues

Decreased Effect

The levels/effects of Tirofiban may be decreased by: Nonsteroidal Anti-Inflammatory Agents

◀ **Dosage Forms** Excipient information presented when available (limited, particularly for generics); consult specific product labeling. [DSC] = Discontinued product

Infusion [premixed in sodium chloride]:
  Aggrastat®: 50 mcg/mL (100 mL, 250 mL)
Injection, solution:
  Aggrastat®: 250 mcg/mL (50 mL) [DSC]

References

Demirkan B, Guray Y, Guray U, et al, "Differential Diagnosis and Management of Acute Profound Thrombocytopenia by Tirofiban: A Case Report," *J Thromb Thrombolysis*, 2006, 22(1):77-8.

Huxtable LM, Tafreshi MJ, and Rakkar AN, "Frequency and Management of Thrombocytopenia With the Glycoprotein IIb/IIIa Receptor Antagonists," *Am J Cardiol*, 2006, 97(3):426-9.

Llevadot J, Coulter SA, and Giugliano RP, "A Practical Approach to the Diagnosis and Management of Thrombocytopenia Associated With Glycoprotein IIb/IIIa Receptor Inhibitors," *J Thromb Thrombolysis*, 2000, 9(2):175-80.

♦ **Tirofiban Hydrochloride** *see* Tirofiban *on page 1397*

♦ **TMC125** *see* Etravirine *on page 565*

♦ **TMP-SMZ** *see* Sulfamethoxazole and Trimethoprim *on page 1333*

♦ **TNKase®** *see* Tenecteplase *on page 1357*

♦ **TOBI®** *see* Tobramycin *on page 1400*

Tobramycin (toe bra MYE sin)

Medication Safety Issues

Sound-alike/look-alike issues:

Tobramycin may be confused with Trobicin®, vancomycin
AKTob® may be confused with AK-Trol®
Nebcin® may be confused with Inapsine®, Naprosyn®, Nubain®
Tobrex® may be confused with TobraDex®

High alert medication: The Institute for Safe Medication Practices (ISMP) includes this medication (intrathecal administration) among its list of drug classes which have a heightened risk of causing significant patient harm when used in error.

Related Information

Prevention of Wound Infection and Sepsis in Surgical Patients *on page 1721*

U.S. Brand Names AKTob®; TOBI®; Tobrex®

Canadian Brand Names PMS-Tobramycin; Sandoz-Tobramycin; TOBI®; Tobramycin Injection, USP; Tobrex®

Index Terms Tobramycin Sulfate

Pharmacologic Category Antibiotic, Aminoglycoside; Antibiotic, Ophthalmic

Generic Available Yes: Excludes ophthalmic ointment, solution for nebulization

Use Treatment of documented or suspected infections caused by susceptible gram-negative bacilli including *Pseudomonas aeruginosa*; topically used to treat superficial ophthalmic infections caused by susceptible bacteria. Tobramycin solution for inhalation is indicated for the management of cystic fibrosis patients (>6 years of age) with *Pseudomonas aeruginosa*.

Mechanism of Action Interferes with bacterial protein synthesis by binding to 30S and 50S ribosomal subunits resulting in a defective bacterial cell membrane

Pharmacodynamics/Kinetics

Absorption:

Oral: Poorly absorbed
I.M.: Rapid and complete
Inhalation: Peak serum concentrations are ~1 mcg/mL following a 300 mg dose

Distribution: V_d: 0.2-0.3 L/kg; Pediatrics: 0.2-0.7 L/kg; to extracellular fluid including serum, abscesses, ascitic, pericardial, pleural, synovial, lymphatic, and peritoneal fluids; poor penetration into CSF, eye, bone, prostate

Inhalation: Tobramycin remains concentrated primarily in the airways

Protein binding: <30%

Half-life elimination:

Neonates: ≤1200 g: 11 hours; >1200 g: 2-9 hours
Adults: 2-3 hours; directly dependent upon glomerular filtration rate
Adults with impaired renal function: 5-70 hours

Time to peak, serum: I.M.: 30-60 minutes; I.V.: ~30 minutes

Excretion: Normal renal function: Urine (~90% to 95%) within 24 hours

Dosage Note: Dosage individualization is **critical** because of the low therapeutic index.

Use of ideal body weight (IBW) for determining the mg/kg/dose appears to be more accurate than dosing on the basis of total body weight (TBW). In morbid obesity, dosage requirement may best be estimated using a dosing weight of IBW + 0.4 (TBW - IBW).

Initial and periodic plasma drug levels (eg, peak and trough with conventional dosing) should be determined, particularly in critically-ill patients with serious infections or in disease states known to significantly alter aminoglycoside pharmacokinetics (eg, cystic fibrosis, burns, or major surgery).

Usual dosage range:

Infants and Children <5 years: I.M., I.V.: 2.5 mg/kg/dose every 8 hours

Children ≥5 years: I.M., I.V.: 2-2.5 mg/kg/dose every 8 hours

  Note: Higher individual doses and/or more frequent intervals (eg, every 6 hours) may be required in selected clinical situations (cystic fibrosis) or serum levels document the need.

Children and Adults:

Inhalation:

  Aerosolized tobramycin injection (unlabeled use): 80 mg 2 times/day. **Note:** Injectable formulation may contain preservatives, which may increase risk of bronchospasm.

  TOBI®: Children ≥6 years and Adults: 300 mg every 12 hours (do not administer doses <6 hours apart); administer in repeated cycles of 28 days on drug followed by 28 days off drug.

Intrathecal: 4-8 mg/day

Ophthalmic: Children ≥2 months and Adults:

  Ointment: Instill 1/2" (1.25 cm) 2-3 times/day every 3-4 hours

  Solution: Instill 1-2 drops every 2-4 hours, up to 2 drops every hour for severe infections

Topical: Apply 3-4 times/day to affected area

Adults: I.M., I.V.:

  Conventional: 1-2.5 mg/kg/dose every 8-12 hours; to ensure adequate peak concentrations early in therapy, higher initial dosage may be considered in selected patients when extracellular water is increased (edema, septic shock, postsurgical, and/or trauma)

  Once-daily: 4-7 mg/kg/dose once daily; some clinicians recommend this approach for all patients with normal renal function; this dose is at least as efficacious with similar, if not less, toxicity than conventional dosing.

Indication-specific dosing:

Neonates:

Meningitis: I.M., I.V.:

  0-7 days: <2000 g: 2.5 mg/kg every 18-24 hours; >2000 g: 2.5 mg/kg every 12 hours

  8-28 days: <2000 g: 2.5 mg/kg every 8-12 hours; >2000 g: 2.5 mg/kg every 8 hours

Children:

Cystic fibrosis:

  I.M., I.V.: 2.5-3.3 mg/kg every 6-8 hours; **Note:** Some patients may require larger or more frequent doses if serum levels document the need (eg, cystic fibrosis or febrile granulocytopenic patients).

  Inhalation: See adult dosing.

Adults:

I.M., I.V.:

Brucellosis: 240 mg (I.M.) daily or 5 mg/kg (I.V.) daily for 7 days; either regimen recommended in combination with doxycycline

Cholangitis: 4-6 mg/kg once daily with ampicillin

Diverticulitis, complicated: 1.5-2 mg/kg every 8 hours (with ampicillin and metronidazole)

Infective endocarditis or synergy (for gram-positive infections): I.M., I.V.: 1 mg/kg every 8 hours (with ampicillin)

◄ **Meningitis** *(Enterococcus or Pseudomonas aeruginosa):* I.V.: Loading dose: 2 mg/kg, then 1.7 mg/kg/dose every 8 hours (administered with another bacteriocidal drug)

Pelvic inflammatory disease: Loading dose: 2 mg/kg, then 1.5 mg/kg every 8 hours **or** 4.5 mg/kg once daily

Plague *(Yersinia pestis):* Treatment: 5 mg/kg/day, followed by postexposure prophylaxis with doxycycline

Pneumonia, hospital- or ventilator-associated: 7 mg/kg/day (with anti-pseudomonal beta-lactam or carbapenem)

Prophylaxis against endocarditis (dental, oral, upper respiratory procedures, GI/GU procedures): 1.5 mg/kg with ampicillin (50 mg/kg) 30 minutes prior to procedure. **Note:** AHA guidelines now recommend prophylaxis only in patients undergoing invasive procedures and in whom underlying cardiac conditions may predispose to a higher risk of adverse outcomes should infection occur. As of April 2007, routine prophylaxis no longer recommended by the AHA.

Tularemia: 5 mg/kg/day divided every 8 hours for 1-2 weeks

Urinary tract infection: 1.5 mg/kg/dose every 8 hours

Inhalation:

Cystic fibrosis:

Aerosolized tobramycin injection (unlabeled use): 80 mg 2 times/day; **Note:** Injectable formulation may contain preservatives, which may increase risk of bronchospasm.

TOBI®: 300 mg every 12 hours (do not administer doses <6 hours apart); administer in repeated cycles of 28 days on drug followed by 28 days off drug.

Dosing interval in renal impairment: I.M., I.V.:

Conventional dosing:

Cl_{cr} ≥60 mL/minute: Administer every 8 hours

Cl_{cr} 40-60 mL/minute: Administer every 12 hours

Cl_{cr} 20-40 mL/minute: Administer every 24 hours

Cl_{cr} 10-20 mL/minute: Administer every 48 hours

Cl_{cr} <10 mL/minute: Administer every 72 hours

High-dose therapy: Interval may be extended (eg, every 48 hours) in patients with moderate renal impairment (Cl_{cr} 30-59 mL/minute) and/or adjusted based on serum level determinations.

Hemodialysis: Dialyzable; 30% removal of aminoglycosides occurs during 4 hours of HD - administer dose after dialysis and follow levels

Continuous arteriovenous or venovenous hemofiltration: Dose as for Cl_{cr} of 10-40 mL/minute and follow levels

Administration in CAPD fluid:

Gram-negative infection: 4-8 mg/L (4-8 mcg/mL) of CAPD fluid

Gram-positive infection (ie, synergy): 3-4 mg/L (3-4 mcg/mL) of CAPD fluid

Administration IVPB/I.M.: Dose as for Cl_{cr} <10 mL/minute and follow levels

Dosing adjustment/comments in hepatic disease: Monitor plasma concentrations

Stability

Injection: Stable at room temperature both as the clear, colorless solution and as the dry powder. Reconstituted solutions remain stable for 24 hours at room temperature and 96 hours when refrigerated. Dilute in 50-100 mL NS, D_5W for I.V. infusion.

Separate administration of extended-spectrum penicillins (eg, carbenicillin, ticarcillin, piperacillin) from tobramycin in patients with severe renal impairment; tobramycin's efficacy may be reduced if given concurrently.

Ophthalmic solution: Store at 8°C to 27°C (46°F to 80°F).

Solution, for inhalation (TOBI®): Store under refrigeration at 2°C to 8°C (36°F to 46°F). May be stored in foil pouch at room temperature of 25°C (77°F) for up to 28 days. Avoid intense light. Solution may darken over time; however, do not use if cloudy or contains particles.

Administration

I.V.: Infuse over 30-60 minutes. Flush with saline before and after administration.

Inhalation (TOBI®): To be inhaled over ~15 minutes using a handheld nebulizer (PARI-LC PLUS™). If multiple different nebulizer treatments are required, administer bronchodilator first, followed by chest physiotherapy, any other nebulized medications, and then TOBI® last. Do not mix with other nebulizer medications.

Ophthalmic: Contact lenses should not be worn during treatment of ophthalmic infections.

Ointment: Do not touch tip of tube to eye. Instill ointment into pocket between eyeball and lower lid; patient should look downward before closing eye.

Solution: Allow 5 minutes between application of "multiple-drop" therapy.

Suspension: Shake well before using; tilt head back, instill suspension in conjunctival sac and close eye(s). Do not touch dropper to eye. Apply light finger pressure on lacrimal sac for 1 minute following instillation.

Some penicillins (eg, carbenicillin, ticarcillin and piperacillin) have been shown to inactivate aminoglycosides *in vitro*. This has been observed to a greater extent with tobramycin and gentamicin, while amikacin has shown greater stability against inactivation. Concurrent use of these agents may pose a risk of reduced antibacterial efficacy *in vivo*, particularly in the setting of profound renal impairment. However, definitive clinical evidence is lacking. If combination penicillin/aminoglycoside therapy is desired in a patient with renal dysfunction, separation of doses (if feasible), and routine monitoring of aminoglycoside levels, CBC, and clinical response should be considered.

Monitoring Parameters Urinalysis, urine output, BUN, serum creatinine, peak and trough plasma tobramycin levels; be alert to ototoxicity; hearing should be tested before and during treatment

Some penicillin derivatives may accelerate the degradation of aminoglycosides *in vitro*. This may be clinically-significant for certain penicillin (ticarcillin, piperacillin, carbenicillin) and aminoglycoside (gentamicin, tobramycin) combination therapy in patients with significant renal impairment. Close monitoring of aminoglycoside levels is warranted.

Reference Range

Timing of serum samples: Draw peak 30 minutes after 30-minute infusion has been completed or 1 hour following I.M. injection or beginning of infusion; draw trough immediately before next dose

Therapeutic levels:

Peak:

Serious infections: 6-8 mcg/mL (SI: 12-17 μmol/L)

Life-threatening infections: 8-10 mcg/mL (SI: 17-21 μmol/L)

Urinary tract infections: 4-6 mcg/mL (SI: 7-12 μmol/L)

Synergy against gram-positive organisms: 3-5 mcg/mL

Trough:

Serious infections: 0.5-1 mcg/mL

Life-threatening infections: 1-2 mcg/mL

The American Thoracic Society (ATS) recommends trough levels of <1 mcg/mL for patients with hospital-acquired pneumonia.

Monitor serum creatinine and urine output; obtain drug levels after the third dose unless otherwise directed

Inhalation: Serum levels are ~1 mcg/mL one hour following a 300 mg dose in patients with normal renal function.

Pregnancy Risk Factor D (injection, inhalation); B (ophthalmic)

Contraindications Hypersensitivity to tobramycin, other aminoglycosides, or any component of the formulation; pregnancy (injection/inhalation)

Warnings/Precautions [U.S. Boxed Warning]: Aminoglycosides may cause neurotoxicity and/or nephrotoxicity; usual risk factors include pre-existing renal impairment, concomitant neuro-/nephrotoxic medications, advanced age and dehydration. Ototoxicity may be directly proportional to the amount of drug given and the duration of treatment; tinnitus or vertigo are indications of vestibular injury and impending hearing loss; renal damage is usually reversible. May cause neuromuscular blockade and respiratory paralysis; especially when given soon after anesthesia or muscle relaxants.

Not intended for long-term therapy due to toxic hazards associated with extended administration; use caution in pre-existing renal insufficiency, vestibular or cochlear impairment, myasthenia gravis, hypocalcemia, conditions which depress neuromuscular transmission. Dosage modification required in patients with impaired renal function. Prolonged use may result in fungal or bacterial

◄ superinfection, including *C. difficile*-associated diarrhea (CDAD) and pseudo-membranous colitis; CDAD has been observed >2 months postantibiotic treatment. Solution may contain sodium metabisulfate; use caution in patients with sulfite allergy.

Adverse Reactions

Injection: Frequency not defined:

Central nervous system: Confusion, disorientation, dizziness, fever, headache, lethargy, vertigo

Dermatologic: Exfoliative dermatitis, itching, rash, urticaria

Endocrine & metabolic: Serum calcium, magnesium, potassium, and/or sodium decreased

Gastrointestinal: Diarrhea, nausea, vomiting

Hematologic: Anemia, eosinophilia, granulocytopenia, leukocytosis, leukopenia, thrombocytopenia

Hepatic: ALT increased, AST increased, bilirubin increased, LDH increased

Local: Pain at the injection site

Otic: Hearing loss, tinnitus, ototoxicity (auditory), ototoxicity (vestibular), roaring in the ears

Renal: BUN increased, cylindruria, serum creatinine increased, oliguria, proteinuria

Inhalation:

>10%:

Gastrointestinal: Sputum discoloration (21%)

Respiratory: Voice alteration (13%)

1% to 10%:

Central nervous system: Malaise (6%)

Otic: Tinnitus (3%)

Postmarketing and/or case reports: Hearing loss

Ophthalmic: <1% (Limited to important or life-threatening): Ocular: Conjunctival erythema, lid itching, lid swelling

Drug Interactions

Avoid Concomitant Use

Avoid concomitant use of Tobramycin with any of the following: Gallium Nitrate

Increased Effect/Toxicity

Tobramycin may increase the levels/effects of: AbobotulinumtoxinA; Bisphosphonate Derivatives; CARBOplatin; Colistimethate; CycloSPORINE; Gallium Nitrate; Neuromuscular-Blocking Agents; OnabotulinumtoxinA; RimabotulinumtoxinB

The levels/effects of Tobramycin may be increased by: Amphotericin B; Capreomycin; CISplatin; Loop Diuretics; Nonsteroidal Anti-Inflammatory Agents; Vancomycin

Decreased Effect

Tobramycin may decrease the levels/effects of: Typhoid Vaccine

The levels/effects of Tobramycin may be decreased by: Penicillins

Test Interactions Some penicillin derivatives may accelerate the degradation of aminoglycosides *in vitro*, leading to a potential underestimation of aminoglycoside serum concentration.

Dietary Considerations May require supplementation of calcium, magnesium, potassium.

Dosage Forms Excipient information presented when available (limited, particularly for generics); consult specific product labeling.

Infusion [premixed in NS]: 60 mg (50 mL); 80 mg (100 mL)

Injection, powder for reconstitution: 1.2 g

Injection, solution: 10 mg/mL (2 mL, 8 mL); 40 mg/mL (2 mL, 30 mL, 50 mL) [may contain sodium metabisulfite]

Ointment, ophthalmic (Tobrex®): 0.3% (3.5 g)

Solution for nebulization [preservative free] (TOBI®): 60 mg/mL (5 mL)

Solution, ophthalmic (AKTob®, Tobrex®): 0.3% (5 mL) [contains benzalkonium chloride]

References

American Thoracic Society and Infectious Diseases Society of America, "Guidelines for the Management of Adults With Hospital-Acquired, Ventilator-Associated, and Healthcare-Associated Pneumonia," *Am J Respir Crit Care Med*, 2005, 171(4):388-416.

Kahler DA, Schowengerdt KO, Fricker FJ, et al, "Toxic Serum Trough Concentrations After Administration of Nebulized Tobramycin," *Pharmacotherapy*, 2003, 23(4):543-5.

Ramsey BW, Burns J, Smith A, et al, "Safety and Efficacy of Tobramycin for Inhalation in Patients With Cystic Fibrosis: The Results of Two Phase III Placebo Controlled Clinical Trials," *Pediatr Pulmonol*, 1997, (Suppl 14):137-8, S10.3.

Ramsey BW, Dorkin HL, Eisenberg JD, et al, "Efficacy of Aerosolized Tobramycin in Patients With Cystic Fibrosis," *N Engl J Med*, 1993, 328(24):1740-6.

Shaw PK, Braun TL, Liebergen A, et al, "Aerosolized Tobramycin Pharmacokinetics in Cystic Fibrosis Patients," *J Pediatr Pharm Pract*, 1997, 2(1):23-6.

Tunkel AR, Hartman BJ, Kaplan SL, et al, "Practice Guidelines for the Management of Bacterial Meningitis," *Clin Infect Dis*, 2004, 39(9):1267-84.

Wilson W, Taubert KA, Gewitz M, et al, "Prevention of Infective Endocarditis. Guidelines From the American Heart Association. A Guideline From the American Heart Association Rheumatic Fever, Endocarditis, and Kawasaki Disease Committee, Council on Cardiovascular Disease in the Young, and the Council on Clinical Cardiology, Council on Cardiovascular Surgery and Anesthesia, and the Quality of Care and Outcomes Research Interdisciplinary Working Group," *Circulation*, 2007, 115. Available at http://circ.ahajournals.org/cgi/reprint/CIRCULATIONAHA.106.183095v1; last accessed July 26, 2007.

◆ **Tobramycin Injection, USP (Can)** *see* Tobramycin *on page 1400*

◆ **Tobramycin Sulfate** *see* Tobramycin *on page 1400*

◆ **Tobrex®** *see* Tobramycin *on page 1400*

◆ **Tofranil®** *see* Imipramine *on page 731*

◆ **Tofranil-PM®** *see* Imipramine *on page 731*

◆ **Tolectin** *see* Tolmetin *on page 1405*

Tolmetin (TOLE met in)

Related Information

Nonsteroidal Anti-Inflammatory Agents *on page 1687*

Index Terms Tolectin; Tolmetin Sodium

Pharmacologic Category Nonsteroidal Anti-inflammatory Drug (NSAID), Oral

Use Treatment of rheumatoid arthritis and osteoarthritis, juvenile rheumatoid arthritis

Pharmacodynamics/Kinetics

Onset of action: Analgesic: 1-2 hours; Anti-inflammatory: Days to weeks

Absorption: Well absorbed, rapid

Bioavailability: Reduced 16% with food or milk

Half-life elimination: Biphasic: Rapid: 1-2 hours; Slow: 5 hours

Time to peak, serum: 30-60 minutes

Excretion: Urine (as inactive metabolites or conjugates) within 24 hours

Dosage Oral:

Children ≥2 years:

JRA: Initial: 20 mg/kg/day in 3-4 divided doses, then 15-30 mg/kg/day in 3-4 divided doses (maximum dose: 30 mg/kg/day)

Analgesic (unlabeled use): 5-7 mg/kg/dose every 6-8 hours

Adults: RA, osteoarthritis: 400 mg 3 times/day; usual dose: 600 mg to 1.8 g/day; maximum: 1.8 g/day

Anesthesia and Critical Care Concerns/Other Considerations The 2002 ACCM/SCCM guidelines for analgesia (critically-ill adult) suggest that NSAIDs may be used in combination with opioids in select patients for pain management. Concern about adverse events (increased risk of renal dysfunction, altered platelet function and gastrointestinal irritation) limits its use in patients who have other underlying risks for these events.

In short-term use, NSAIDs vary considerably in their effect on blood pressure. When NSAIDs are used in patients with hypertension, appropriate monitoring of blood pressure responses should be completed and the duration of therapy, when possible, kept short. The use of NSAIDs in the treatment of patients with congestive heart failure may be associated with an increased risk for fluid accumulation and edema; may precipitate renal failure in dehydrated patients.

Additional Information Complete prescribing information for this medication should be consulted for additional detail.

Dosage Forms Excipient information presented when available (limited, particularly for generics); consult specific product labeling.
Capsule: 400 mg
Tablet: 200 mg, 600 mg

♦ **Tolmetin Sodium** *see* Tolmetin *on page 1405*

Tolvaptan (tol VAP tan)

U.S. Brand Names Samsca™
Index Terms OPC-41061
Pharmacologic Category Vasopressin Antagonist
Generic Available No
Use Treatment of clinically significant hypervolemic or euvolemic hyponatremia (associated with heart failure, cirrhosis or SIADH) with either a serum sodium <125 mEq/L or less marked hyponatremia that is symptomatic and resistant to fluid restriction
Mechanism of Action An arginine vasopressin (AVP) receptor antagonist with affinity for AVP receptor subtypes V_2 and V_{1a} in a ratio of 29:1. Antagonism of the V_2 receptor by tolvaptan promotes the excretion of free water (without loss of serum electrolytes) resulting in net fluid loss, increased urine output, decreased urine osmolality, and subsequent restoration of normal serum sodium levels.
Pharmacodynamics/Kinetics
Onset of action: 2-4 hours
Peak effect: 4-8 hours
Duration: 60% peak serum sodium elevation is retained at 24 hours; urinary excretion of free water is no longer elevated
Distribution: V_d: 3 L/kg
Protein binding: 99%
Metabolism: Hepatic via CYP3A4
Bioavailability: ~40%
Half-life elimination: 5-12 hours; dominant half-life <12 hours
Time to peak, plasma: 2-4 hours
Excretion: Feces
Dosage Oral: Adults: Hyponatremia: Initial: 15 mg once daily; after at least 24 hours, may increase to 30 mg once daily to a maximum of 60 mg once daily titrating at 24-hour intervals to desired serum sodium concentration
Stability Store at 25°C (77°F); excursions permitted between 15°C and 30°C (59°F and 86°F).
Administration Treatment should be initiated or reinitiated in a hospital. May be administered without regards to meals.
Monitoring Parameters Serum sodium concentration, rate of serum sodium increase, serum potassium concentration (if >5 mEq/L prior to administration or receiving medications known to elevate serum potassium); volume status
Pregnancy Risk Factor C
Contraindications Hypovolemic hyponatremia; urgent need to raise serum sodium acutely; use in patients unable to sense or appropriately respond to thirst; anuria; concurrent use with strong CYP3A inhibitors (eg, ketoconazole, itraconazole, ritonavir, indinavir, nelfinavir, saquinavir, nefazodone, telithromycin, clarithromycin)
Warnings/Precautions [U.S. Boxed Warning]: Tolvaptan should be initiated and reinitiated in patients only in a hospital where serum sodium can be closely monitored. Too rapid correction of hyponatremia (ie, >12 mEq/L/24 hours) can cause osmotic demyelination resulting in dysarthria, mutism, dysphagia, lethargy, affective changes, spastic quadriparesis, seizures, coma, and death. In susceptible patients (including those with severe malnutrition, alcoholism, or advanced liver disease), slower rates of correction may be advisable. Patients with SIADH or very low baseline serum sodium concentrations may be at greater risk of overly-rapid correction.

Interrupt or discontinue therapy in patients who develop medically significant signs or symptoms of hypovolemia. Patients should ingest fluids in response to thirst. Gastrointestinal bleeding can occur in patients with cirrhosis; use only if the need to treat outweighs the risk. Reductions in extracellular fluid volumes may cause hyperkalemia. Patients with a pretreatment serum potassium >5 mEq/L should be monitored after initiation of therapy.

Use in patients with creatinine clearance <10 mL/minute has not been studied. Do not use in anuric patients. Use with hypertonic saline is not recommended. Use contraindicated in patients taking strong CYP3A inhibitors; avoid use in patients taking moderate CYP3A4 inhibitors. If possible, avoid use with CYP3A4 inducers; if administered with CYP3A4 inducers, dose increases may be necessary. Dose reductions may be necessary if administered with P-gp inhibitors. Consider alternative agents that avoid or lessen the potential for CYP- or P-gp mediated interactions. Patients receiving medications known to increase potassium should be monitored for hyperkalemia. Safety and efficacy have not been established in children.

Monitor closely for rate of serum sodium increase and neurological status; rapid serum sodium correction (>12 mEq/L/24 hours) can lead to permanent neurological damage. Discontinue use if rate of serum sodium increase is undesirable; fluid restriction during the first 24 hours of sodium correction can increase the risk of overly-rapid correction and should generally be avoided; not intended for urgent correction of serum sodium to prevent or treat serious neurologic symptoms; it has not been demonstrated that raising serum sodium with tolvaptan provides a symptomatic benefit.

Adverse Reactions

>10%:

Gastrointestinal: Nausea (21%), xerostomia (7% to 13%)

Renal: Pollakiuria (4% to 11%), polyuria (4% to 11%)

Miscellaneous: Thirst (12% to 16%)

2% to 10%:

Central nervous system: Pyrexia (4%)

Endocrine & metabolic: Hyperglycemia (6%)

Gastrointestinal: Constipation (7%), anorexia (4%)

Neuromuscular & skeletal: Weakness (9%)

<2% (Limited to important or life-threatening): Cerebrovascular accident, deep vein thrombosis, diabetic ketoacidosis, disseminated intravascular coagulation, intracardiac thrombus, ischemic colitis, prothrombin time prolonged, pulmonary embolism, respiratory failure, rhabdomyolysis, urethral hemorrhage, vaginal hemorrhage, ventricular fibrillation

Drug Interactions

Avoid Concomitant Use

Avoid concomitant use of Tolvaptan with any of the following: CYP3A4 Inducers (Strong); CYP3A4 Inhibitors (Moderate); CYP3A4 Inhibitors (Strong); Sodium Chloride

Increased Effect/Toxicity

Tolvaptan may increase the levels/effects of: ACE Inhibitors; Angiotensin II Receptor Blockers; Potassium-Sparing Diuretics

The levels/effects of Tolvaptan may be increased by: CYP3A4 Inhibitors (Moderate); CYP3A4 Inhibitors (Strong); Dasatinib; P-Glycoprotein Inhibitors; Sodium Chloride

Decreased Effect

The levels/effects of Tolvaptan may be decreased by: CYP3A4 Inducers (Strong); Deferasirox; Herbs (CYP3A4 Inducers); P-Glycoprotein Inducers

Ethanol/Nutrition/Herb Interactions

Food: Tolvaptan exposure may be doubled when taken with grapefruit juice.

Herb/Nutraceutical: St John's wort may decrease tolvaptan serum concentrations.

Dietary Considerations May be taken without regards to meals. Avoid grapefruit juice.

Dosage Forms Excipient information presented when available (limited, particularly for generics); consult specific product labeling.

Tablet, oral:

Samsca™: 15 mg, 30 mg

◄ **References**

Ali F, Guglin M, Vaitkevicus P, et al, "Therapeutic Potential of Vasopressin Receptor Antagonists," *Drugs*, 2007, 67(6):847-58.

Decaux G, Soupart A, Vassart G, "Non-Peptide Arginine-Vasopressin Antagonists: The Vaptans," *Lancet*, 2008, 371(9624):1624-32.

Gheorghiade M, Konstam MA, Burnett JC Jr, "Short-term Clinical Effects of Tolvaptan, an Oral Vasopressin Antagonist, in Patients Hospitalized for Heart Failure," *JAMA*, 2007, 297(12):1332-43.

Konstam MA, Gheorghiade M, Burnett JC Jr, et al, "Effects of Oral Tolvaptan in Patients Hospitalized for Worsening Heart Failure: The EVEREST Outcome Trial," *JAMA*, 2007, 297(12):1319-31.

Oghlakian G and Klapholz M, "Vasopressin and Vasopressin Receptor Antagonists in Heart Failure," *Cardiol Rev*, 2009, 17(1):10-15.

Shoaf SE, Bramer SL, Bricmont P, et al, "Pharmacokinetic and Pharmacodynamic Interaction Between Tolvaptan, a Non-peptide AVP Antagonist, and Furosemide or Hydrochlorothiazide," *J Cardiovasc Pharmacol*, 2007, 50(2):213-22.

Shoaf SE, Elizari MV, Wang Z, et al, "Tolvaptan Administration Does Not Affect Steady State Amiodarone Concentrations in Patients With Cardiac Arrhythmias," *J Cardiovasc Pharmacol Ther*, 2005, 10(3):165-71.

◆ **Tomoxetine** *see* Atomoxetine *on page 157*

◆ **Topamax®** *see* Topiramate *on page 1408*

◆ **Topicaine® [OTC]** *see* Lidocaine *on page 836*

◆ **Topilene® (Can)** *see* Betamethasone *on page 186*

Topiramate (toe PYRE a mate)

Related Information
Chronic Pain Management *on page 1546*
Perioperative Management of Patients on Antiseizure Medication *on page 1577*

U.S. Brand Names Topamax®

Canadian Brand Names Apo-Topiramate®; CO Topiramate; Dom-Topiramate; Mint-Topiramate; Mylan-Topiramate; Novo-Topiramate; PHL-Topiramate; PMS-Topiramate; PRO-Topiramate; ratio-Topiramate; Sandoz-Topiramate; Topamax®; ZYM-Topiramate

Pharmacologic Category Anticonvulsant, Miscellaneous

Use Monotherapy or adjunctive therapy for partial onset seizures and primary generalized tonic-clonic seizures; adjunctive treatment of seizures associated with Lennox-Gastaut syndrome; prophylaxis of migraine headache

Unlabeled/Investigational Use Infantile spasms, neuropathic pain, cluster headache

Pharmacodynamics/Kinetics
Absorption: Good, rapid; unaffected by food
Protein binding: 15% to 41% (inversely related to plasma concentrations)
Metabolism: Hepatic via P450 enzymes
Bioavailability: 80%
Half-life elimination: Mean: Adults: Normal renal function: 21 hours; shorter in pediatric patients; clearance is 50% higher in pediatric patients; Elderly: ~24 hours
Time to peak, serum: ~1-4 hours
Excretion: Urine (~70% to 80% as unchanged drug)
Dialyzable: ~30%

Dosage Oral: **Note:** Do not abruptly discontinue therapy; taper dosage gradually to prevent rebound effects. (In clinical trials, adult doses were withdrawn by decreasing in weekly intervals of 50-100 mg/day gradually over 2-8 weeks for seizure treatment, and by decreasing in weekly intervals by 25-50 mg/day for migraine prophylaxis.)

Epilepsy, monotherapy: Children ≥10 years and Adults: Partial onset seizure and primary generalized tonic-clonic seizure: Initial: 25 mg twice daily; may increase weekly by 50 mg/day up to 100 mg twice daily (week 4 dose); thereafter, may further increase weekly by 100 mg/day up to the recommended maximum of 200 mg twice daily.

Epilepsy, adjunctive therapy:
Children 2-16 years:
Partial onset seizure or seizure associated with Lennox-Gastaut syndrome: Initial dose titration should begin at 25 mg (or less, based on a range of 1-3 mg/kg/day) nightly for the first week; dosage may be increased in

increments of 1-3 mg/kg/day (administered in 2 divided doses) at 1- or 2-week intervals to a total daily dose of 5-9 mg/kg/day

Primary generalized tonic-clonic seizure: Use initial dose listed above, but use slower initial titration rate; titrate to recommended maintenance dose by the end of 8 weeks

Adolescents ≥17 years and Adults:

Partial onset seizures: Initial: 25-50 mg/day (given in 2 divided doses) for 1 week; increase at weekly intervals by 25-50 mg/day until response; usual maintenance dose: 100-200 mg twice daily. Doses >1600 mg/day have not been studied.

Primary generalized tonic-clonic seizures: Use initial dose as listed above for partial onset seizures, but use slower initial titration rate; titrate upwards to recommended dose by the end of 8 weeks; usual maintenance dose: 200 mg twice daily. Doses >1600 mg/day have not been studied.

Adults:

Migraine prophylaxis: Initial: 25 mg/day (in the evening), titrated at weekly intervals in 25 mg increments, up to the recommended total daily dose of 100 mg/day given in 2 divided doses

Cluster headache (unlabeled use): Initial: 25 mg/day, titrated at weekly intervals in 25 mg increments, up to 200 mg/day

Neuropathic pain (unlabeled use): Initial: 25 mg/day, titrated at weekly intervals in 25-50 mg increments to target dose of 400 mg daily in 2 divided doses. Reported dosage range studied: 25-800 mg/day

Dosing adjustment in renal impairment: Cl_{cr} <70 mL/minute: Administer 50% dose and titrate more slowly

Hemodialysis: Supplemental dose may be needed during hemodialysis

Dosing adjustment in hepatic impairment: Clearance may be reduced

Additional Information Complete prescribing information for this medication should be consulted for additional detail.

Dosage Forms Excipient information presented when available (limited, particularly for generics); consult specific product labeling.

Capsule, sprinkle: 15 mg, 25 mg

Topamax®: 15 mg, 25 mg

Tablet: 25 mg, 50 mg, 100 mg, 200 mg

Topamax®: 25 mg, 50 mg, 100 mg, 200 mg

◆ **Topisone® (Can)** see Betamethasone on page 186

◆ **Toprol-XL®** see Metoprolol on page 922

◆ **Toradol® (Can)** see Ketorolac on page 784

◆ **Toradol® IM (Can)** see Ketorolac on page 784

Torsemide (TORE se mide)

Medication Safety Issues

Sound-alike/look-alike issues:

Torsemide may be confused with furosemide

Demadex® may be confused with Denorex®

Related Information

Diuretics, Loop on page 1680

Heart Failure (Systolic) on page 1739

U.S. Brand Names Demadex®

Pharmacologic Category Diuretic, Loop

Generic Available Yes: Tablet

Use Management of edema associated with heart failure and hepatic or renal disease; used alone or in combination with antihypertensives in treatment of hypertension; I.V. form is indicated when rapid onset is desired

Mechanism of Action Inhibits reabsorption of sodium and chloride in the ascending loop of Henle and distal renal tubule, interfering with the chloride-binding cotransport system, thus causing increased excretion of water, sodium, chloride, magnesium, and calcium; does not alter GFR, renal plasma flow, or acid-base balance

◀ **Pharmacodynamics/Kinetics**
Onset of action: Diuresis: 30-60 minutes
  Peak effect: 1-4 hours
Duration: ~6 hours
Absorption: Oral: Rapid
Protein binding, plasma: ~97% to 99%
Metabolism: Hepatic (80%) via CYP
Bioavailability: 80% to 90%
Half-life elimination: 2-4; Cirrhosis: 7-8 hours
Excretion: Urine (20% as unchanged drug)

Dosage Adults: Oral, I.V.:
Chronic renal failure: 20 mg once daily; increase as described above
Heart failure: Initial: 10-20 mg once daily; may increase gradually for chronic treatment by doubling dose until the diuretic response is apparent (for acute treatment, I.V. dose may be repeated every 2 hours with double the dose as needed). **Note:** ACC/AHA 2009 guidelines for heart failure recommend a maximum daily oral dose of 200 mg; maximum single I.V. dose of 100-200 mg
  Continuous I.V. infusion (Hunt, 2009): 20 mg I.V. load then 5-20 mg/hour
Hepatic cirrhosis: 5-10 mg once daily with an aldosterone antagonist or a potassium-sparing diuretic; increase as described above
Hypertension: 2.5-5 mg once daily; increase to 10 mg after 4-6 weeks if an adequate hypotensive response is not apparent; if still not effective, an additional antihypertensive agent may be added

Stability If torsemide is to be administered via continuous infusion, stability has been demonstrated through 24 hours at room temperature in plastic containers for the following fluids and concentrations:
200 mg torsemide (10 mg/mL) added to 250 mL D_5W, 250 mL NS or 500 mL 0.45% sodium chloride.
50 mg torsemide (10 mg/mL) added to 500 mL D_5W, 250 mL NS or 500 mL 0.45% sodium chloride.

Administration I.V. injections should be administered over ≥2 minutes; the oral form may be administered regardless of meal times; patients may be switched from the I.V. form to the oral and vice-versa with no change in dose; no dosage adjustment is needed in the elderly or patients with hepatic impairment
To administer as a continuous infusion: 50 mg or 200 mg torsemide should be diluted in 250 mL or 500 mL of compatible solution in plastic containers

Monitoring Parameters Renal function, electrolytes, and fluid status (weight and I & O), blood pressure

Anesthesia and Critical Care Concerns/Other Considerations
Clinical Pearls/Comments: If given the morning of surgery, it may render the patient volume depleted and blood pressure may be labile during general anesthesia. Torsemide may induce potent diuretic effects and, as with other potent diuretics, electrolytes and volume status needs to be closely monitored.

Dose equivalency (approximate): Bumetanide 1 mg = furosemide 40 mg = torsemide 10 mg

Pregnancy Risk Factor B
Contraindications Hypersensitivity to torsemide, any component of the formulation, or any sulfonylureas; anuria

Warnings/Precautions Loop diuretics are potent diuretics; excess amounts can lead to profound diuresis with fluid and electrolyte loss; close medical supervision and dose evaluation are required. Watch for and correct electrolyte disturbances; adjust dose to avoid dehydration. In cirrhosis, avoid electrolyte and acid/base imbalances that might lead to hepatic encephalopathy. Coadministration of antihypertensives may increase the risk of hypotension.

Monitor fluid status and renal function in an attempt to prevent oliguria, azotemia, and reversible increases in BUN and creatinine; close medical supervision of aggressive diuresis required. Rapid I.V. administration (associated with other loop diuretics), renal impairment, excessive doses, and concurrent use of other ototoxins is associated with ototoxicity; has been seen with oral torsemide.

Chemical similarities are present among sulfonamides, sulfonylureas, carbonic anhydrase inhibitors, thiazides, and loop diuretics (except ethacrynic acid). Use in patients with sulfonylurea allergy is specifically contraindicated in product labeling, however, a risk of cross-reaction exists in patients with allergy to any of these compounds; avoid use when previous reaction has been severe. Discontinue if signs of hypersensitivity are noted.

Adverse Reactions

1% to 10%:

Cardiovascular: ECG abnormality (2%), edema (1.1%), chest pain (1.2%)

Central nervous system: Headache (7.3%), dizziness (3.2%), insomnia (1.2%), nervousness (1%)

Endocrine & metabolic: Hyperglycemia, hyperuricemia, hypokalemia

Gastrointestinal: Diarrhea (2%), constipation (1.8%), nausea (1.8%), dyspepsia (1.6%), sore throat (1.6%)

Genitourinary: Excessive urination (6.7%)

Neuromuscular & skeletal: Weakness (2%), arthralgia (1.8%), myalgia (1.6%)

Respiratory: Rhinitis (2.8%), cough increase (2%)

<1% (Limited to important or life-threatening): Angioedema, atrial fibrillation, GI hemorrhage, hypernatremia hypotension, hypovolemia, rash, rectal bleeding, shunt thrombosis, syncope, ventricular tachycardia

Drug Interactions

Metabolism/Transport Effects Substrate of CYP2C8 (minor), 2C9 (major); **Inhibits** CYP2C19 (weak)

Avoid Concomitant Use There are no known interactions where it is recommended to avoid concomitant use.

Increased Effect/Toxicity

Torsemide may increase the levels/effects of: ACE Inhibitors; Allopurinol; Amifostine; Aminoglycosides; Antihypertensives; Dofetilide; Hypotensive Agents; Lithium; Neuromuscular-Blocking Agents; RiTUXimab; Salicylates; Warfarin

The levels/effects of Torsemide may be increased by: Corticosteroids (Orally Inhaled); Corticosteroids (Systemic); CYP2C9 Inhibitors (Moderate); CYP2C9 Inhibitors (Strong); Diazoxide; Eltrombopag; Herbs (Hypotensive Properties); MAO Inhibitors; Pentoxifylline; Phosphodiesterase 5 Inhibitors; Prostacyclin Analogues

Decreased Effect

Torsemide may decrease the levels/effects of: Lithium; Neuromuscular-Blocking Agents

The levels/effects of Torsemide may be decreased by: Bile Acid Sequestrants; CYP2C9 Inducers (Highly Effective); Herbs (Hypertensive Properties); Methylphenidate; Nonsteroidal Anti-Inflammatory Agents; Peginterferon Alfa-2b; Phenytoin; Salicylates; Yohimbine

Ethanol/Nutrition/Herb Interactions Herb/Nutraceutical: Avoid herbs with *hypertensive* properties (bayberry, blue cohosh, cayenne, ephedra, ginger, ginseng [American], kola, licorice); may diminish the antihypertensive effect of torsemide. Avoid herbs with *hypotensive* properties (black cohosh, California poppy, coleus, golden seal, hawthorn, mistletoe, periwinkle, quinine, shepherd's purse); may enhance the hypotensive effect of torsemide.

Dosage Forms Excipient information presented when available (limited, particularly for generics); consult specific product labeling. [DSC] = Discontinued product

Injection, solution:

Demadex®: 10 mg/mL (2 mL [DSC], 5 mL [DSC])

Tablet: 5 mg, 10 mg, 20 mg, 100 mg

Demadex®: 5 mg, 10 mg, 20 mg, 100 mg [scored]

Total Parenteral Nutrition (TOE tal par EN ter al noo TRISH un)

Medication Safety Issues

High alert medication: The Institute for Safe Medication Practices (ISMP) includes this medication among its list of drugs which have a heightened risk of causing significant patient harm when used in error.

Related Information

Fat Emulsion *on page 578*

Index Terms Hyperal; Hyperalimentation; Parenteral Nutrition; PN; TPN

◀ **Pharmacologic Category** Caloric Agent; Intravenous Nutritional Therapy

Use Infusion of nutrient solutions into the bloodstream to support nutritional needs during a time when patient is unable to absorb nutrients via the gastrointestinal tract, cannot take adequate nutrition orally or enterally, or have had (or are expected to have) inadequate oral intake for 7-14 days

Dosage PN is a highly-individualized therapy. The following general guidelines may be used in the estimation of needs. Electrolytes, vitamins, and trace minerals should be added to TPN mixtures based on patients individualized needs.

Neonates: I.V.: **Note:** When indicated for premature neonates, start on day 1 of life if possible.

Total calories:

Term: 85-105 kcal/kg/day

Preterm (stable): 90-120 kcal/kg/day

Fluid:

<1.5 kg: 130-150 mL/kg/day

1.5-2 kg: 110-130 mL/kg/day

2-10 kg: 100 mL/kg/day

Carbohydrate (dextrose): 40% to 50 % of caloric intake; advance as tolerated

Term: Initial: 6-8 mg/kg/minute; goal: 10-14 mg/kg/minute

Premature: Initial: 6 mg/kg/minute; goal: 10-13 mg/kg/minute

Protein (amino acids):

Term: Initial: 2.5 g/kg/day; goal: 3 g/kg/day

Extremely (<1000 g) and very (<1500 g) low-birth-weight (stable): Initial: 1-1.5 g/kg/day; goal: 3.5-3.85 g/kg/day to promote utero growth rates.

Sepsis, hypoxia: Initial: 1 g/kg/day; goal: 3-3.85 g/kg/day

Fat:

Term: Initial: 0.5-1 g/kg/day (maximum: 3 g/kg/day); administer over 24 hours

Preterm: Initial: 0.25-0.5 g/kg/day (maximum: 3 g/kg/day or 1 g/kg/day if on phototherapy); administer over 24 hours

Note: Monitor triglycerides while receiving intralipids. If triglycerides >200 mg/dL, stop infusion and restart at 0.5-1g/kg/day

Heparin: 1 unit/mL of parenteral nutrition fluids should be added to enhance clearance of lipid emulsions

Children: I.V.: **Note:** Give within 5-7 days if unable to meet needs orally or with enteral nutrition:

Total calories:

<6 months: 85-105 kcal/kg/day

6-12 months: 80-100 kcal/kg/day

1-7 years: 75-90 kcal/kg/day

7-12 years: 50-75 kcal/kg/day

12-18 years: 30-50 kcal/kg/day

Fluid:

2-10 kg: 100 mL/kg

>10-20 kg: 1000 mL for 10 kg plus 50 mL/kg for each kg >10

>20 kg: 1500 mL for 10 kg plus 20 mL/kg for each kg >20

Carbohydrate (dextrose): 40% to 50% of caloric intake

<1 year: Initial: 6-8 mg/kg/minute; goal: 10-14 mg/kg/minute

1-10 years: Initial: 10% to 12.5%; daily increase: 5% increments (maximum: 15 mg/kg/minute)

>10 years: Initial: 10% to 15%; daily increase: 5% increments (maximum: 8.5 mg/kg/minute)

Protein (amino acids):

1-12 months: Initial: 2-3 g/kg/day; daily increase: 1 g/kg/day (maximum: 3 g/kg/day)

1-10 years: Initial: 1-2 g/kg/day; daily increase: 1 g/kg/day (maximum: 2-2.5 g/kg/day)

>10 years: Initial: 0.8-1.5 g/kg/day; daily increase: 1 g/kg/day (maximum: 1.5-2 g/kg/day)

Fat: Initial: 1 g/kg/day; daily increase: 1 g/kg/day (maximum: 3 g/kg/day); **Note:** Monitor triglycerides while receiving intralipids.

Adults: I.V.:

Total calories: Calculate using Harris-Benedict equation or based on stress level as indicated below:

Harris-Benedict Equation (BEE):

Females: 655.1 + [(9.56 x W) + (1.85 x H) - (4.68 x A)]

Males: 66.47 + [(13.75 x W) + (5 x H) - (6.76 x A)]

Then multiply BEE x (activity factor) x (stress factor)

W = weight in kg; H = height in cm; A = age in years

Activity factor = 1.2 sedentary, 1.3 normal activity, 1.4 active, 1.5 very active

Stress factor = 1.5 for trauma, stressed, or surgical patients and underweight (to promote weight gain); 2.0 for severe burn patients

Stress level:

Normal/mild stress level: 20-25 kcal/kg/day

Moderate stress level: 25-30 kcal/kg/day

Severe stress level: 30-40 kcal/kg/day

Pregnant women in second or third trimester: Add an additional 300 kcal/day

Fluid: mL/day = 30-40 mL/kg

Carbohydrate (dextrose):

5 g/kg/day or 3.5 mg/kg/minute (maximum rate: 4-7 mg/kg/minute)

Minimum recommended amount: 400 calories/day or 100 g/day

Protein (amino acids):

Maintenance: 0.8-1 g/kg/day

Normal/mild stress level: 1-1.2 g/kg/day

Moderate stress level: 1.2-1.5 g/kg/day

Severe stress level: 1.5-2 g/kg/day

Burn patients (severe): Increase protein until significant wound healing achieved

Solid organ transplant: Perioperative: 1.5-2 g/kg/day

Renal failure:

Acute (severely malnourished or hypercatabolic): 1.5-1.8 g/kg/day

Chronic, with dialysis: 1.2-1.3 g/kg/day

Chronic, without dialysis: 0.6-0.8 g/kg/day

Continuous hemofiltration: ≥1 g/kg/day

Hepatic failure:

Acute management when other treatments have failed:

With encephalopathy: 0.6-1 g/kg/day

Without encephalopathy: 1-1.5 g/kg/day

Chronic encephalopathy: Use branch chain amino acid enriched diets only if unresponsive to pharmacotherapy

Pregnant women in second or third trimester: Add an additional 10-14 g/day

Fat:

Initial: 20% to 40 % of total calories (maximum: 60% of total calories or 2.5 g/kg/day); **Note:** Monitor triglycerides while receiving intralipids.

Safe for use in pregnancy

I.V. lipids are safe in adults with pancreatitis if triglyceride levels <400 mg/dL

Stability USP Chapter 797 Guidelines consider TPN a medium-risk preparation and state that (in the absence of passing a sterility test) storage period should not exceed 30 hours at room temperature, 7 days at cold temperature, and 45 days in a solid frozen state at -20°C or colder. For patients on home TPN, multiple vitamins should be added prior to TPN administration, due to limited stability of multiple vitamins.

Administration For I.V. administration only, usually via a central venous catheter; can be administered by continuous infusion over 24 hours or cyclic infusion over 12-14 hours. Cyclic infusion is used with a tapering-up period at the beginning and a tapering-down period at the end to avoid hyper-/hypoglycemia. For infants <2 years, taper over 1-2 hours. Change tubing after each infusion. Hang fat emulsion higher than other fluids (has low specific gravity and could run up into other lines). Infuse via pump using either peripheral or central venous line. Do not use in-line filter.

Monitoring Parameters

Electrolytes: Sodium, potassium, chloride, and bicarbonate should be monitored frequently upon initiation and until stable; phosphate should be monitored closely in patients with pulmonary disease.

Efficacy: Nutrition and outcome parameters should be measured serially.

◄ Glucose: In patients with diabetes or patients with glucose intolerance risk factors, monitor closely. Monitor frequently upon initiation of therapy and with any changes in insulin dose or renal function.

Line site: Monitor for signs and symptoms of infection.

Liver function tests: Monitor periodically.

Triglycerides: Before initiation of lipid therapy and at least weekly during therapy.

Refeeding syndrome: Patients at risk should have phosphorus, magnesium, potassium, and glucose levels monitored closely at initiation.

Bone densitometry: Perform upon initiation of long-term therapy.

Vitamin A status: Should be carefully monitored in patients with chronic renal failure.

Neonates: Sodium, calcium and phosphate should be monitored closely. Frequent (some advise daily) platelet counts should be performed in neonatal patients receiving parenteral lipids.

Contraindications Varies by composition:

Lipid-containing formulations are contraindicated in patients with hypersensitivity to fat emulsion or any component of the formulation; severe egg or legume (soybean) allergies; pathologic hyperlipidemia, lipoid nephrosis, pancreatitis with hyperlipemia

Dextrose is contraindicated in patients with hypersensitivity to corn or corn products; hypertonic solutions in patients with intracranial or intraspinal hemorrhage; glucose-galactose malabsorption syndrome

Amino acids are contraindicated in patients with hypersensitivity to one or more amino acids; severe liver disease or hepatic coma

Warnings/Precautions Monitor fluid and electrolyte status carefully. Use with caution in patients at risk for refeeding syndrome. Refeeding syndrome is a medical emergency; it can consist of electrolyte disturbances (eg, potassium, phosphorus), respiratory distress, and cardiac arrhythmias, resulting in cardiopulmonary arrest. It is usually seen in patients with long-standing or severe malnutrition; initiate cautiously; approach goals slowly. Do not overfeed patients; caloric replacement should match as closely as possible to intake. Use caution in patients with diabetes or insulin resistance. Use caution in patients who may be sensitive to volume overload (eg, HF, renal failure, hepatic failure). Use caution and limit protein in patients with hepatic disease. If TPN is discontinued abruptly, infuse 10% dextrose at same rate and monitor blood glucose for hypoglycemia.

Adverse Reactions Frequency not defined (unless noted).

Endocrine & metabolic: Fluid overload, hypercapnia, hyperglycemia, hyper-/hypokalemia, hyper-/hypophosphatemia, metabolic bone disease, nonanion gap metabolic acidosis, refeeding syndrome

Hepatic: Cholestasis, cirrhosis (<1%), gallstones, liver function tests increased, pancreatitis, steatosis, triglycerides increased

Renal: Azotemia, BUN increased

Miscellaneous: Bacteremia, catheter-induced infection, exit-site infections

Dosage Forms TPN is usually compounded from optimal combinations of macronutrients (water, protein, dextrose, and lipids) and micronutrients (electrolytes, trace elements, and vitamins) to meet the specific nutritional requirements of a patient. Individual hospitals may have designated standard TPN formulas. There are a few commercially-available amino acids with electrolytes solutions; however, these products may not meet an individual's specific nutrition requirements.

References

ASPEN Board of Directors and the Clinical Guidelines Task Force, "Guidelines for the Use of Parenteral and Enteral Nutrition in Adult and Pediatric Patients," *JPEN J Parenter Enteral Nutr*, 2002, 26(1 Suppl):1-138.

Dersch D and Schoen J, "Weight-Based Ordering: An Evaluation of Increased Guideline Use in Hospital Total Parenteral Nutrition Dosing," *Nutr Clin Pract*, 2002, 17(5):296-303.

Fulford A, Scolapio JS, and Aranda-Michel J, "Parenteral Nutrition-Associated Hepatotoxicity," *Nutr Clin Pract*, 2004, 19(3):274-83.

Mayhew SL and Gonzalez ER, "Neonatal Nutrition: A Focus on Parenteral Nutrition and Early Enteral Nutrition," *Nutr Clin Pract*, 2003, 18(5):406-13.

Mirtallo J, Canada T, Johnson D, et al, "Safe Practices for Parenteral Nutrition. Task Force for the Revision of Safe Practices for Parenteral Nutrition," *JPEN J Parenter Enteral Nutr*, 2004, 28(6): S39-70.

U.S. Pharmacopeia Convention, Inc, U.S. Pharmacopeia 27, Chapter <797> Pharmaceutical Compounding — Sterile Preparations. Rockville, MD: U.S. Pharmacopeial Convention, Inc, 2003, 2350-70.

♦ **Toviaz™** *see* Fesoterodine *on page 599*

♦ **tPA** *see* Alteplase *on page 67*

♦ **TPN** *see* Total Parenteral Nutrition *on page 1411*

♦ **Tracleer®** *see* Bosentan *on page 199*

TraMADol (TRA ma dole)

Medication Safety Issues
Sound-alike/look-alike issues:
TraMADol may be confused with tapentadol, Toradol®, Trandate®, traZODone, Voltaren®
Ultram® may be confused with Ultane®, Ultracet®, Voltaren®

International issues:
Theradol® [Netherlands] may be confused with Foradil® which is a brand name for formoterol in the U.S.
Theradol® [Netherlands] may be confused with Terazol® which is a brand name for terconazole in the U.S.
Theradol® [Netherlands] may be confused with Toradol® which is a brand name for ketorolac in the U.S.

Related Information
Acute Postoperative Pain *on page 1502*
Chronic Pain Management *on page 1546*

U.S. Brand Names Ryzolt™; Ultram®; Ultram® ER

Canadian Brand Names Ralivia™ ER; Tridural™; Zytram® XL

Index Terms Tramadol Hydrochloride

Pharmacologic Category Analgesic, Opioid

Generic Available Yes: Excludes extended release tablet

Use Relief of moderate to moderately-severe pain
Extended release formulations are indicated for patients requiring around-the-clock management of moderate to moderately-severe pain for an extended period of time

Mechanism of Action Tramadol and its active metabolite (M1) binds to μ-opiate receptors in the CNS causing inhibition of ascending pain pathways, altering the perception of and response to pain; also inhibits the reuptake of norepinephrine and serotonin, which also modifies the ascending pain pathway

Pharmacodynamics/Kinetics
Onset of action: Immediate release: ~1 hour
Duration: 9 hours
Absorption: Immediate release formulation: Rapid and complete; Extended release formulation: Delayed
Distribution: V_d: 2.5-3 L/kg
Protein binding, plasma: 20%
Metabolism: Extensively hepatic via demethylation (mediated by CYP3A4 and CYP2B6), glucuronidation, and sulfation; has pharmacologically active metabolite formed by CYP2D6 (M1; O-desmethyl tramadol)
Bioavailability: Immediate release: 75%; Extended release: Ultram® ER: 85% to 90% (as compared to immediate release), Zytram® XL, Tridural™: 70%, Ryzolt™: ~95% (as compared to immediate release)
Half-life elimination: Tramadol: ~6-8 hours; Active metabolite: 7-9 hours; prolonged in elderly, hepatic or renal impairment; Zytram® XL: ~16 hours; Ralivia™ ER, Ryzolt™, Tridural™: ~5-9 hours
Time to peak: Immediate release: ~2 hours; Extended release: Ultram® ER: ~12 hours, Ryzolt™, Tridural™: ~4 hours
Excretion: Urine (30% as unchanged drug; 60% as metabolites)

Dosage Oral: Moderate-to-severe pain:
Children 7-16 years (unlabeled use): 1-2 mg/kg/dose every 4-6 hours; maximum: 400 mg/day
Children ≥17 years and Adults: Immediate release formulation: 50-100 mg every 4-6 hours (not to exceed 400 mg/day)
For patients not requiring rapid onset of effect, tolerability may be improved by starting dose at 25 mg/day and titrating dose by 25 mg every 3 days, until reaching 25 mg 4 times/day. The total daily dose may then be increased by

◄ 50 mg every 3 days as tolerated, to reach dose of 50 mg 4 times/day. After titration, 50-100 mg may be given every 4-6 hours as needed up to a maximum 400 mg/day.

Adults: Extended release formulations:

Ultram® ER:

Patients not currently on immediate-release: 100 mg once daily; titrate every 5 days (maximum: 300 mg/day)

Patients currently on immediate-release: Calculate 24-hour immediate release total dose and initiate total extended release daily dose (round dose to the next lowest 100 mg increment); titrate (maximum: 300 mg/day)

Ralivia™ ER (Canadian labeling, not available in U.S.): 100 mg once daily; titrate every 5 days as needed based on clinical response and severity of pain (maximum: 300 mg/day)

Ryzolt™:

Patients not currently on immediate-release: 100 mg once daily; titrate every 2-3 days by 100 mg/day increments; usual daily dose: 200-300 mg/day (maximum: 300 mg/day)

Patients currently on immediate-release: Calculate 24 hour immediate release total dose and initiate total extended release daily dose (round dose to the next lowest 100 mg increment); titrate (maximum: 300 mg/day)

Tridural™ (Canadian labeling, not available in U.S.): 100 mg once daily; titrate by 100 mg/day every 2 days as needed based on clinical response and severity of pain (maximum: 300 mg/day)

Zytram® XL (Canadian labeling, not available in U.S.): 150 mg once daily; if pain relief is not achieved may titrate by increasing dosage incrementally, with sufficient time to evaluate effect of increased dosage; generally not more often than every 7 days (maximum: 400 mg/day)

Elderly >65 years: Use caution and initiate at the lower end of the dosing range

Immediate release: Elderly >75 years: Do not exceed 300 mg/day; see dosing adjustments for renal and hepatic impairment.

Extended release formulation: Elderly >75 years: Use with great caution. See adult, renal, and hepatic dosing.

Dosing adjustment in renal impairment:

Immediate release: Cl_{cr} <30 mL/minute: Administer 50-100 mg dose every 12 hours (maximum: 200 mg/day)

Extended release: Should not be used in patients with Cl_{cr} <30 mL/minute

Dosing adjustment in hepatic impairment:

Immediate release: Cirrhosis: Recommended dose: 50 mg every 12 hours

Extended release: Should not be used in patients with severe (Child-Pugh class C) hepatic dysfunction; Ryzolt™ should not be used in any degree of hepatic impairment

Stability Store at controlled room temperature of 25°C (77°F).

Administration Extended release tablet: Swallow whole; do not crush, chew, or split

Monitoring Parameters Pain relief, respiratory rate, blood pressure, and pulse; signs of tolerance or abuse

Reference Range 100-300 ng/mL; however, serum level monitoring is not required

Anesthesia and Critical Care Concerns/Other Considerations Tramadol 50 mg is comparable to codeine 60 mg; tramadol 100 mg is comparable to aspirin 650 mg/codeine 60 mg. Tramadol is 5-10 times less potent than morphine and reported to cause less respiratory depression.

Pregnancy Risk Factor C

Contraindications Hypersensitivity to tramadol, opioids, or any component of the formulation; opioid-dependent patients; acute intoxication with alcohol, hypnotics, centrally-acting analgesics, opioids, or psychotropic drugs

Additional contraindications for Ryzolt™: Severe/acute bronchial asthma, hypercapnia, or significant respiratory depression in the absence of appropriately monitored setting and/or resuscitative equipment

Note: Based on Canadian product labeling:

Tramadol is contraindicated during or within 14 days following MAO inhibitor therapy

Extended release formulations (Ralivia™ ER [CAN], Tridural™[CAN], and Zytram® XL [CAN]): Additional contraindications: Severe (Cl$_{cr}$ <30 mL/minute) renal dysfunction, severe (Child-Pugh class C) hepatic dysfunction

Warnings/Precautions Rare but serious anaphylactoid reactions (including fatalities) often following initial dosing have been reported. Pruritus, hives, bronchospasm, angioedema, toxic epidermal necrolysis (TEN) and Stevens-Johnson syndrome also have been reported with use. Previous anaphylactoid reactions to opioids may increase risks for similar reactions to tramadol. Caution patients to swallow extended release tablets whole. Rapid release and absorption of tramadol from extended release tablets that are broken, crushed, or chewed may lead to a potentially lethal overdose. May cause CNS depression, which may impair physical or mental abilities; patients must be cautioned about performing tasks which require mental alertness (eg, operating machinery or driving). May cause CNS depression and/or respiratory depression, particularly when combined with other CNS depressants. Use with caution and reduce dosage when administered to patients receiving other CNS depressants. An increased risk of seizures may occur in patients receiving serotonin reuptake inhibitors (SSRIs or anorectics), tricyclic antidepressants, other cyclic compounds (including cyclobenzaprine, promethazine), neuroleptics, or drugs which may lower seizure threshold. Patients with a history of seizures, or with a risk of seizures (head trauma, metabolic disorders, CNS infection, or malignancy, or during ethanol/drug withdrawal) are also at increased risk. Avoid use with serotonergic agents such as TCAs, MAO inhibitors (contraindicated in Canadian product labeling), triptans, venlafaxine, trazodone, lithium, sibutramine, meperidine, dextromethorphan, St John's wort, SNRIs and SSRIs; concomitant use has been associated with the development of serotonin syndrome.

Elderly (particularly >75 years of age), debilitated patients and patients with chronic respiratory disorders may be at greater risk of adverse events. Use with caution in patients with increased intracranial pressure or head injury. Avoid use in patients who are suicidal or addiction prone. Healthcare provider should be alert to problems of abuse, misuse, and diversion. Use caution in heavy alcohol users. Use caution in treatment of acute abdominal conditions; may mask pain. Use tramadol with caution and reduce dosage in patients with liver disease or renal dysfunction. Avoid using extended release tablets in severe hepatic impairment. Do not use Ryzolt™ in any degree of hepatic impairment. Tolerance or drug dependence may result from extended use (withdrawal symptoms have been reported); abrupt discontinuation should be avoided. Tapering of dose at the time of discontinuation limits the risk of withdrawal symptoms. Safety and efficacy in pediatric patients have not been established.

Adverse Reactions

>10%:

Cardiovascular: Flushing (8% to 16%)

Central nervous system: Dizziness (10% to 33%), headache (4% to 32%), somnolence (7% to 25%), insomnia (2% to 11%)

Dermatologic: Pruritus (5% to 12%)

Gastrointestinal: Constipation (10% to 46%), nausea (15% to 40%), vomiting (5% to 17%), dyspepsia (1% to 13%)

Neuromuscular & skeletal: Weakness (4% to 12%)

1% to 10%:

Cardiovascular: Postural hypotension (2% to 5%), chest pain (1% to <5%), vasodilation (1% to <5%)

Central nervous system: Anxiety (1% to <5%), confusion (1% to <5%), coordination impaired (1% to <5%), depression (1% to <5%), euphoria (1% to <5%), hypoesthesia (1% to <5%), lethargy (1% to <5%), nervousness (1% to <5%), pain (1% to <5%), pyrexia (1% to <5%), restlessness (1% to <5%), malaise (<1% to <5%), fatigue (2%), vertigo (2%)

Dermatologic: Dermatitis (1% to <5%), rash (1% to <5%)

Endocrine & metabolic: Hot flashes (2% to 9%), menopausal symptoms (1% to <5%)

Gastrointestinal: Diarrhea (5% to 10%), xerostomia (3% to 10%), anorexia (1% to <6%), abdominal pain (1% to <5%), appetite decreased (1% to <5%), weight loss (1% to <5%), flatulence (<1% to <5%)

Genitourinary: Urinary tract infection (1% to <5%), urinary frequency (<1% to <5%), urinary retention (<1% to <5%)

Neuromuscular & skeletal: Arthralgia (1% to <5%), back pain (1% to <5%), hypertonia (1% to <5%), rigors (1% to <5%), paresthesia (1% to <5%), tremor (1% to <5%), creatine phosphokinase increased (1% to <5%)

Ocular: Blurred vision (1% to <5%), miosis (1% to <5%)

Respiratory: Bronchitis (1% to <5%), congestion (nasal/sinus) (1% to <5%), cough (1% to <5%), dyspnea (1% to <5%), nasopharyngitis (1% to <5%), rhinorrhea (1% to <5%), sinusitis (1% to <5%), sneezing (1% to <5%), sore throat (1% to <5%), upper respiratory infection (1% to <5%)

Miscellaneous: Diaphoresis (2% to 9%), flu-like syndrome (1% to <5%), shivering (<1% to <5%)

<1% (Limited to important or life-threatening): Abnormal ECG, abnormal gait, agitation, allergic reaction, amnesia, anaphylactoid reactions, anaphylaxis, anemia, angioedema, appendicitis, ALT increased/decreased, AST increased/decreased, bradycardia, bronchospasm, cataracts, cellulitis, cholecystitis, cholelithiasis, clamminess, cognitive dysfunction, concentration difficulty, creatinine increased, deafness, disorientation, diverticulitis, dreams abnormal, dysphagia, dysuria, ear infection, edema, fecal impaction, gastroenteritis, gastrointestinal bleeding, hallucination, hematuria, hemoglobin decreased, hepatitis, hyperglycemia, hyper-/hypotension, hypersensitivity, irritability, joint stiffness, libido decreased, liver enzymes increased, liver failure, menstrual disorder, MI, migraine, muscle cramps, muscle spasms, muscle twitching, myalgia, myocardial ischemia, night sweats, orthostatic hypotension, palpitation, pancreatitis, peripheral edema, peripheral ischemia, pneumonia, proteinuria, pulmonary edema, pulmonary embolism, sedation, seizure, serotonin syndrome, sleep disorder, speech disorder, Stevens-Johnson syndrome, stomatitis, suicidal tendency, syncope, taste perversion, tachycardia, thrombocytopenia, tinnitus, toxic epidermal necrolysis, urticaria, vesicles, visual disturbance

A withdrawal syndrome may occur with abrupt discontinuation; includes anxiety, diarrhea, hallucinations (rare), nausea, pain, piloerection, rigors, sweating, and tremor. Uncommon discontinuation symptoms may include severe anxiety, panic attacks, or paresthesia.

Drug Interactions

Metabolism/Transport Effects Substrate of CYP2D6 (major), 3A4 (major)

Avoid Concomitant Use

Avoid concomitant use of TraMADol with any of the following: Sibutramine

Increased Effect/Toxicity

TraMADol may increase the levels/effects of: Alcohol (Ethyl); CNS Depressants; MAO Inhibitors; Methotrimeprazine; Selective Serotonin Reuptake Inhibitors; Serotonin Modulators

The levels/effects of TraMADol may be increased by: CYP3A4 Inhibitors (Moderate); CYP3A4 Inhibitors (Strong); Dasatinib; Methotrimeprazine; Selective Serotonin Reuptake Inhibitors; Sibutramine; Tricyclic Antidepressants

Decreased Effect

The levels/effects of TraMADol may be decreased by: CYP2D6 Inhibitors (Moderate); CYP2D6 Inhibitors (Strong); CYP3A4 Inducers (Strong); Deferasirox

Ethanol/Nutrition/Herb Interactions

Ethanol: Avoid ethanol (may increase CNS depression).

Food:

Immediate release: Does not affect the rate or extent of absorption.

Extended release: Reduced C_{max} and AUC and T_{max} occurred 3 hours earlier when taken with a high-fat meal.

Ryzolt™: Increased C_{max}; no effect on AUC.

Herb/Nutraceutical: Avoid valerian, St John's wort, kava kava, gotu kola (may increase CNS depression).

Dietary Considerations May be taken with or without food. Ultram® ER: Be consistent; always give with food or always give on an empty stomach.

Dosage Forms Excipient information presented when available (limited, particularly for generics); consult specific product labeling. [CAN] = Canadian brand name

Tablet, as hydrochloride: 50 mg
Ultram®: 50 mg
Tablet, extended release, as hydrochloride:
Ultram® ER: 100 mg, 200 mg, 300 mg
Ralivia™ ER [CAN]: 100 mg, 200 mg, 300 mg [not available in the U.S.]
Ryzolt™: 100 mg, 200 mg, 300 mg
Tridural™ [CAN]: 100 mg, 200 mg, 300 mg [not available in the U.S.]
Zytram® XL [CAN]: 150 mg, 200 mg, 300 mg, 400 mg [not available in the U.S.]

◆ **Tramadol Hydrochloride** *see* TraMADol *on page 1415*
◆ **Trandate®** *see* Labetalol *on page 791*

Trandolapril (tran DOE la pril)

Related Information
Angiotensin Agents *on page 1652*
Heart Failure (Systolic) *on page 1739*
U.S. Brand Names Mavik®
Canadian Brand Names Mavik™
Pharmacologic Category Angiotensin-Converting Enzyme (ACE) Inhibitor
Generic Available Yes
Use Treatment of hypertension alone or in combination with other antihypertensive agents; treatment of heart failure or left ventricular dysfunction after myocardial infarction
Unlabeled/Investigational Use To delay the progression of nephropathy and reduce risks of cardiovascular events in hypertensive patients with type 1 or 2 diabetes mellitus
Mechanism of Action Trandolapril is an ACE inhibitor which prevents the formation of angiotensin II from angiotensin I. Trandolapril must undergo enzymatic hydrolysis, mainly in liver, to its biologically active metabolite, trandolaprilat. A CNS mechanism may also be involved in the hypotensive effect as angiotensin II increases adrenergic outflow from the CNS. Vasoactive kallikrein's may be decreased in conversion to active hormones by ACE inhibitors, thus reducing blood pressure.

Pharmacodynamics/Kinetics
Onset of action: 1-2 hours
Peak effect: Reduction in blood pressure: 6 hours
Duration: Prolonged; 72 hours after single dose
Absorption: Rapid
Distribution:
Trandolapril: ~18L
Trandolaprilat (active metabolite) is very lipophilic in comparison to other ACE inhibitors
Protein binding: 80%
Metabolism: Hepatically hydrolyzed to active metabolite, trandolaprilat
Bioavailability:
Trandolapril: 10%
Trandolaprilat: 70%
Half-life elimination:
Trandolapril: 6 hours; Trandolaprilat: Effective: 10 hours, Terminal: 24 hours
Time to peak: Parent: 1 hour; Active metabolite trandolaprilat: 4-10 hours
Excretion: Urine (33%); feces (66%)
Clearance: Reduce dose in renal failure; creatinine clearances ≤30 mL/minute result in accumulation of active metabolite

Dosage Adults: Oral:
Heart failure postmyocardial infarction or left ventricular dysfunction postmyo-cardial infarction: Initial: 1 mg/day; titrate patients (as tolerated) towards the target dose of 4 mg/day. If a 4 mg dose is not tolerated, patients can continue therapy with the greatest tolerated dose.
Hypertension: Initial dose in patients not receiving a diuretic: 1 mg/day (2 mg/day in black patients). Adjust dosage according to the blood pressure response. Make dosage adjustments at intervals of ≥1 week. Most patients have required dosages of 2-4 mg/day. There is a little experience with doses >8 mg/day.

Patients inadequately treated with once daily dosing at 4 mg may be treated with twice daily dosing. If blood pressure is not adequately controlled with trandolapril monotherapy, a diuretic may be added.

Usual dose range (JNC 7): 1-4 mg once daily

Dosing adjustment in renal impairment: Cl_{cr} ≤30 mL/minute: Recommended starting dose: 0.5 mg/day.

Dosing adjustment in hepatic impairment: Cirrhosis: Recommended starting dose: 0.5 mg/day.

Monitoring Parameters Blood pressure; serum creatinine and potassium; if patient has collagen vascular disease and/or renal impairment, periodically monitor CBC with differential

Anesthesia and Critical Care Concerns/Other Considerations

Clinical Pearls/Comments: In patients on chronic ACE inhibitor therapy, intraoperative hypotension may occur with induction and maintenance of general anesthesia; however, discontinuation of therapy prior to surgery is controversial. If continued preoperatively, avoidance of hypotensive agents during surgery is prudent. Episodes of intraoperative hypotension may be managed by fluid administration and/or modest doses of alpha-adrenergic agents. Severe hypotension may occur in patients who are sodium- and/or volume-depleted, initiate lower doses and monitor closely when starting therapy in these patients. ACE inhibitor therapy may elicit an increase in potassium and creatinine, especially when used in patients with bilateral renal artery stenosis. In those patients experiencing cough on an ACE inhibitor, the ACE inhibitor may be discontinued and, if necessary, angiotensin-receptor blocker therapy instituted. Concomitant NSAID therapy may attenuate blood pressure control; use of NSAIDs should be avoided or limited, with monitoring of blood pressure control. In the setting of heart failure, NSAID use may be associated with an increased risk for fluid accumulation and edema. Because of the potent teratogenic effects of ACE inhibitors, these drugs should be avoided, if possible, when treating women of childbearing potential not on effective birth control measures. Aging patients with a decrease in glomerular filtration (also creatinine clearance), severe heart failure, and renal failure may experience an exaggerated response with administration of ACE inhibitors. Diabetic proteinuria is reduced and insulin sensitivity is enhanced.

Evidence-Based Information: ACE inhibitors decrease morbidity and mortality in patients with asymptomatic and symptomatic left ventricular dysfunction. In this situation, they decrease hospitalizations for, and retard progression to, decompensated heart failure. ACE inhibitors are also indicated in patients postmyocardial infarction in whom left ventricular ejection fraction is <40%. When used in patients with heart failure, the target dose or maximum tolerated dose should be achieved, if possible. Lower daily doses of ACE inhibitors have not demonstrated the same cardioprotective effects. ACE inhibitors have renal protective effects in patients with diabetic proteinuria. The HOPE trial examined the use of ramipril at a dose of between 2.5-10 mg daily in patients without heart failure at high risk for cardiovascular events and documented a significant improvement in cardiovascular outcome compared to placebo.

Pregnancy Risk Factor C (1st trimester); D (2nd and 3rd trimesters)

Contraindications Hypersensitivity to trandolapril or any component of the formulation; history of angioedema related to previous treatment with an ACE inhibitor

Warnings/Precautions Anaphylactic reactions may occur rarely with ACE inhibitors. At any time during treatment (especially following first dose) angioedema may occur rarely with ACE inhibitors; it may involve the head and neck (potentially compromising the airway) or the intestine (presenting with abdominal pain). African-Americans and patients with idiopathic or hereditary angioedema may be at an increased risk. Prolonged frequent monitoring may be required especially if tongue, glottis, or larynx are involved as they are associated with airway obstruction. Patients with a history of airway surgery may have a higher risk of airway obstruction. Aggressive early and appropriate management is critical. Use in patients with previous angioedema associated with ACE inhibitor therapy is contraindicated. Severe anaphylactoid reactions may be seen during hemodialysis (eg, CVVHD) with high-flux dialysis membranes (eg, AN69). Rare cases of anaphylactoid reactions have been reported in patients undergoing sensitization treatment with hymenoptera (bee, wasp) venom while receiving ACE inhibitors.

Symptomatic hypotension with or without syncope can occur with ACE inhibitors (usually with the first several doses); effects are most often observed in volume-depleted patients; correct volume depletion prior to initiation; close monitoring of patient is required especially with initial dosing and dosing increases; blood pressure must be lowered at a rate appropriate for the patient's clinical condition. Initiation of therapy in patients with ischemic heart disease or cerebrovascular disease warrants close observation due to the potential consequences posed by falling blood pressure (eg, MI, stroke). Use with caution in hypertrophic cardiomyopathy with outflow tract obstruction, severe aortic stenosis, or before, during, or immediately after major surgery. **[U.S. Boxed Warning]: Based on human data, ACEIs can cause injury and death to the developing fetus when used in the second and third trimesters. ACEIs should be discontinued as soon as possible once pregnancy is detected.**

Hyperkalemia may occur with ACE inhibitors; risk factors include renal dysfunction, diabetes mellitus, concomitant use of potassium-sparing diuretics, potassium supplements, and/or potassium-containing salts. Use cautiously, if at all, with these agents and monitor potassium closely. Cough may occur with ACE inhibitors. Other causes of cough should be considered (eg, pulmonary congestion in patients with heart failure) and excluded prior to discontinuation.

Dosage adjustment needed in severe renal dysfunction (Cl_{cr} <30 mL/minute) or hepatic cirrhosis. May be associated with deterioration of renal function and/or increases in serum creatinine, particularly in patients with low renal blood flow (eg, renal artery stenosis, heart failure) whose glomerular filtration rate (GFR) is dependent on efferent arteriolar vasoconstriction by angiotensin II; deterioration may result in oliguria, acute renal failure, and progressive azotemia. Small increases in serum creatinine may occur following initiation; consider discontinuation only in patients with progressive and/or significant deterioration in renal function. Use with caution in patients with unstented unilateral/bilateral renal artery stenosis. When unstented bilateral renal artery stenosis is present, use is generally avoided due to the elevated risk of deterioration in renal function unless possible benefits outweigh risks.

Rare toxicities associated with ACE inhibitors include cholestatic jaundice (which may progress to fulminant hepatic necrosis), agranulocytosis, neutropenia, or leukopenia with myeloid hypoplasia. Patients with collagen vascular diseases (especially with concomitant renal impairment) or renal impairment alone may be at increased risk for hematologic toxicity; periodically monitor CBC with differential in these patients. Safety and efficacy have not been established in children.

Adverse Reactions Note: Frequency ranges include data from hypertension and heart failure trials. Higher rates of adverse reactions have generally been noted in patients with CHF. However, the frequency of adverse effects associated with placebo is also increased in this population.

>1%:
  Cardiovascular: Hypotension (<1% to 11%), bradycardia (<1% to 4.7%), intermittent claudication (3.8%), stroke (3.3%), syncope (5.9%)

  Central nervous system: Dizziness (1.3% to 23%), asthenia (3.3%)

  Endocrine & metabolic: Elevated uric acid (15%), hyperkalemia (5.3%), hypocalcemia (4.7%)

  Gastrointestinal: Dyspepsia (6.4%), gastritis (4.2%)

  Neuromuscular & skeletal: Myalgia (4.7%)

  Renal: Elevated BUN (9%), elevated serum creatinine (1.1% to 4.7%)

  Respiratory: Cough (1.9% to 35%)

  <1% (Limited to important or life-threatening): Angina, angioedema, anxiety, AV block (first-degree), dyspnea, gout, impotence, increased ALT, increased serum creatinine, insomnia, laryngeal edema, muscle pain, neutropenia, pancreatitis, paresthesia, pruritus, rash, symptomatic hypotension, thrombocytopenia, vertigo. Worsening of renal function may occur in patients with bilateral renal artery stenosis or in hypovolemic patients. In addition, a syndrome which may include fever, myalgia, arthralgia, interstitial nephritis, vasculitis, rash,

◄ eosinophilia and positive ANA, and elevated ESR has been reported with ACE inhibitors.

Drug Interactions

Avoid Concomitant Use There are no known interactions where it is recommended to avoid concomitant use.

Increased Effect/Toxicity

Trandolapril may increase the levels/effects of: Allopurinol; Amifostine; Antihypertensives; AzaTHIOprine; CycloSPORINE; Ferric Gluconate; Gold Sodium Thiomalate; Hypotensive Agents; Iron Dextran Complex; Lithium; RiTUXimab

The levels/effects of Trandolapril may be increased by: Angiotensin II Receptor Blockers; Diazoxide; Eplerenone; Herbs (Hypotensive Properties); Loop Diuretics; MAO Inhibitors; Pentoxifylline; Phosphodiesterase 5 Inhibitors; Potassium Salts; Potassium-Sparing Diuretics; Prostacyclin Analogues; Sirolimus; Temsirolimus; Thiazide Diuretics; Tolvaptan; Trimethoprim

Decreased Effect

The levels/effects of Trandolapril may be decreased by: Antacids; Aprotinin; Herbs (Hypertensive Properties); Methylphenidate; Nonsteroidal Anti-Inflammatory Agents; Salicylates; Yohimbine

Ethanol/Nutrition/Herb Interactions Herb/Nutraceutical: Avoid bayberry, blue cohosh, cayenne, ephedra, ginger, ginseng (American), kola, licorice (may worsen hypertension). Avoid black cohosh, California poppy, coleus, golden seal, hawthorn, mistletoe, periwinkle, quinine, shepherd's purse (may have increased antihypertensive effect).

Dosage Forms Excipient information presented when available (limited, particularly for generics); consult specific product labeling.
Tablet: 1 mg, 2 mg, 4 mg
Mavik®: 1 mg, 2 mg, 4 mg

- ◆ **Transamine Sulphate** *see* Tranylcypromine *on page 1422*
- ◆ **Transderm-V® (Can)** *see* Scopolamine Derivatives *on page 1278*
- ◆ **Transderm-Nitro® (Can)** *see* Nitroglycerin *on page 1014*
- ◆ **Transderm Scōp®** *see* Scopolamine Derivatives *on page 1278*
- ◆ **Tranxene® SD™** *see* Clorazepate *on page 337*
- ◆ **Tranxene® SD™-Half Strength** *see* Clorazepate *on page 337*
- ◆ **Tranxene T-Tab®** *see* Clorazepate *on page 337*
- ◆ **Tranxene® T-Tab®** *see* Clorazepate *on page 337*

Tranylcypromine (tran il SIP roe meen)

Related Information

Antidepressant Agents *on page 1660*

U.S. Brand Names Parnate®

Canadian Brand Names Parnate®

Index Terms Transamine Sulphate; Tranylcypromine Sulfate

Pharmacologic Category Antidepressant, Monoamine Oxidase Inhibitor

Use Treatment of major depressive episode without melancholia

Unlabeled/Investigational Use Post-traumatic stress disorder

Pharmacodynamics/Kinetics

Onset of action: Therapeutic: 2 days to 3 weeks continued dosing
Half-life elimination: 90-190 minutes
Time to peak, serum: ~2 hours
Excretion: Urine

Dosage Adults: Oral: 10 mg twice daily, increase by 10 mg increments at 1- to 3-week intervals; maximum: 60 mg/day; usual effective dose: 30 mg/day

Anesthesia and Critical Care Concerns/Other Considerations

Clinical Pearls/Comments: Patients receiving MAO inhibitors who undergo surgery may be at risk of developing significant hypertension when used with direct-acting adrenergic agents (eg, norepinephrine) and of lethal hypertension when administered with indirect-acting adrenergic agents (eg, ephedrine). The use of meperidine in these patients may also precipitate serotonin syndrome and is contraindicated. Years ago, it was advised that patients receiving MAO inhibitors have this drug discontinued for at least 10 days before elective surgery. However, the decision to continue or withhold MAO inhibitors must be done in collaboration with the patient's psychiatrist. Currently, an MAO-safe anesthetic technique which excludes the use of meperidine and indirect-acting adrenergic agonists is recommended for patients requiring continuing MAO therapy (Huyse, 2006).

Additional Information Complete prescribing information for this medication should be consulted for additional detail.

Dosage Forms Excipient information presented when available (limited, particularly for generics); consult specific product labeling.

Tablet: 10 mg

References

Huyse FJ, Touw DJ, van Schijndel RS, et al, "Psychotropic Drugs and the Perioperative Period: A Proposal for a Guideline in Elective Surgery," *Psychosomatics*, 2006, 47(1):8-22.

♦ **Tranylcypromine Sulfate** *see* Tranylcypromine *on page 1422*

♦ **Trasylol®** *see* Aprotinin *on page 134*

♦ **Travasol®** *see* Amino Acid Injection *on page 81*

TraZODone (TRAZ oh done)

Medication Safety Issues

Sound-alike/look-alike issues:

Desyrel® may be confused with Demerol®, Delsym®, Zestril®

TraZODone may be confused with traMADol

International issues:

Desyrel® may be confused with Deseril® which is a brand name for methysergide in multiple international markets

Medication Guide An FDA-approved patient medication guide, which is available with the product information and at http://www.fda.gov/downloads/Drugs/DrugSafety/ucm089126.pdf, must be dispensed with this medication for each new outpatient prescription and refill.

Related Information

Antidepressant Agents *on page 1660*

Canadian Brand Names Apo-Trazodone D®; Apo-Trazodone®; Desyrel®; Dom-Trazodone; Mylan-Trazodone; Novo-Trazodone; Nu-Trazodone; PHL-Trazodone; PMS-Trazodone; ratio-Trazodone; Trazorel®; ZYM-Trazodone

Index Terms Trazodone Hydrochloride

Pharmacologic Category Antidepressant, Serotonin Reuptake Inhibitor/Antagonist

Generic Available Yes

Use Treatment of depression

Unlabeled/Investigational Use Potential augmenting agent for antidepressants, hypnotic

Mechanism of Action Inhibits reuptake of serotonin, causes adrenoreceptor subsensitivity, and induces significant changes in 5-HT presynaptic receptor adrenoreceptors. Trazodone also significantly blocks histamine (H_1) and alpha$_1$-adrenergic receptors.

Pharmacodynamics/Kinetics

Onset of action: Therapeutic (antidepressant): 1-3 weeks; sleep aid: 1-3 hours

Protein binding: 85% to 95%

Metabolism: Hepatic via CYP3A4 to an active metabolite (mCPP)

Half-life elimination: 7-8 hours, two compartment kinetics

Time to peak, serum: 30-100 minutes; delayed with food (up to 2.5 hours)

Excretion: Primarily urine; secondarily feces

Dosage Oral: Therapeutic effects may take up to 6 weeks to occur; therapy is normally maintained for 6-12 months after optimum response is reached to prevent recurrence of depression

Children 6-12 years: Depression (unlabeled use): Initial: 1.5-2 mg/kg/day in divided doses; increase gradually every 3-4 days as needed; maximum: 6 mg/kg/day in 3 divided doses

◄ Adolescents: Depression (unlabeled use): Initial: 25-50 mg/day; increase to 100-150 mg/day in divided doses

Adults:

Depression: Initial: 150 mg/day in 3 divided doses (may increase by 50 mg/day every 3-7 days); maximum: 600 mg/day

Sedation/hypnotic (unlabeled use): 25-50 mg at bedtime (often in combination with daytime SSRIs); may increase up to 200 mg at bedtime

Elderly: 25-50 mg at bedtime with 25-50 mg/day dose increase every 3 days for inpatients and weekly for outpatients, if tolerated; usual dose: 75-150 mg/day

Administration Dosing after meals may decrease lightheadedness and postural hypotension

Monitoring Parameters Suicidal ideation (especially at the beginning of therapy or when doses are increased or decreased)

Reference Range

Plasma levels do not always correlate with clinical effectiveness

Therapeutic: 0.5-2.5 mcg/mL

Potentially toxic: >2.5 mcg/mL

Toxic: >4 mcg/mL

Pregnancy Risk Factor C

Contraindications Hypersensitivity to trazodone or any component of the formulation

Warnings/Precautions [U.S. Boxed Warning]: Antidepressants increase the risk of suicidal thinking and behavior in children, adolescents, and young adults (18-24 years of age) with major depressive disorder (MDD) and other psychiatric disorders; consider risk prior to prescribing. Short-term studies did not show an increased risk in patients >24 years of age and showed a decreased risk in patients ≥65 years. Closely monitor for clinical worsening, suicidality, or unusual changes in behavior; the patient's family or caregiver should be instructed to closely observe the patient and communicate condition with healthcare provider. A medication guide should be dispensed with each prescription. **Trazodone is not FDA approved for use in children.**

The possibility of a suicide attempt is inherent in major depression and may persist until remission occurs. Monitor for worsening of depression or suicidality, especially during initiation of therapy (generally first 1-2 months) or with dose increases or decreases. Use caution in high-risk patients. Worsening depression and severe abrupt suicidality that are not part of the presenting symptoms may require discontinuation or modification of drug therapy. The patient's family or caregiver should be alerted to monitor patients for the emergence of suicidality and associated behaviors (such as agitation, irritability, hostility, impulsivity, and hypomania) and call healthcare provider.

May worsen psychosis in some patients or precipitate a shift to mania or hypomania in patients with bipolar disorder. Patients presenting with depressive symptoms should be screened for bipolar disorder. Monotherapy in patients with bipolar disorder should be avoided. **Trazodone is not FDA approved for the treatment of bipolar depression.**

Priapism, including cases resulting in permanent dysfunction, has occurred with the use of trazodone. Not recommended for use in a patient during the acute recovery phase of MI. Trazodone should be initiated with caution in patients who are receiving concurrent or recent therapy with a MAO inhibitor.

The risks of sedation and/or postural hypotension are high relative to other antidepressants. Trazodone frequently causes sedation, which may result in impaired performance of tasks requiring alertness (eg, operating machinery or driving). Sedative effects may be additive with other CNS depressants and ethanol. Use with caution in patients with a history of cardiovascular disease (including previous MI, stroke, tachycardia, or conduction abnormalities). The risk of conduction abnormalities with this agent is low relative to other antidepressants.

Consider discontinuing, when possible, prior to elective surgery. Therapy should not be abruptly discontinued in patients receiving high doses for prolonged periods. Use caution in patients with a previous seizure disorder or condition predisposing to seizures such as brain damage, alcoholism, or concurrent therapy with other drugs which lower the seizure threshold. Use with caution in patients with hepatic or renal dysfunction and in elderly patients.

Adverse Reactions

>10%:

Central nervous system: Dizziness, headache, sedation

Gastrointestinal: Nausea, xerostomia

Ocular: Blurred vision

1% to 10%:

Cardiovascular: Syncope, hyper-/hypotension, edema

Central nervous system: Concentration decreased, confusion, fatigue, incoordination

Gastrointestinal: Diarrhea, constipation, weight gain/loss

Neuromuscular & skeletal: Tremor, myalgia

Respiratory: Nasal congestion

<1% (Limited to important or life-threatening): Agitation, allergic reactions, alopecia, anxiety, bradycardia, extrapyramidal symptoms, hepatitis, priapism, rash, seizure, speech impairment, tachycardia, urinary retention

Drug Interactions

Metabolism/Transport Effects Substrate of CYP2D6 (minor), 3A4 (major); **Inhibits** CYP2D6 (moderate), 3A4 (weak)

Avoid Concomitant Use

Avoid concomitant use of TraZODone with any of the following: Sibutramine

Increased Effect/Toxicity

TraZODone may increase the levels/effects of: Alcohol (Ethyl); CNS Depressants; Serotonin Modulators

The levels/effects of TraZODone may be increased by: BusPIRone; CYP3A4 Inhibitors (Moderate); CYP3A4 Inhibitors (Strong); Dasatinib; MAO Inhibitors; Protease Inhibitors; Selective Serotonin Reuptake Inhibitors; Sibutramine; Venlafaxine

Decreased Effect

TraZODone may decrease the levels/effects of: Dabigatran Etexilate; P-Glycoprotein Substrates

The levels/effects of TraZODone may be decreased by: CYP3A4 Inducers (Strong); Deferasirox; Peginterferon Alfa-2b

Ethanol/Nutrition/Herb Interactions

Ethanol: Avoid ethanol (may increase CNS depression).

Food: Time to peak serum levels may be increased if trazodone is taken with food.

Herb/Nutraceutical: Avoid valerian, St John's wort, SAMe, kava kava (may increase risk of serotonin syndrome and/or excessive sedation).

Dosage Forms Excipient information presented when available (limited, particularly for generics); consult specific product labeling.

Tablet, as hydrochloride: 50 mg, 100 mg, 150 mg, 300 mg

References

Mokhlesi B, Leikin JB, Murray P, et al, "Adult Toxicology in Critical Care: Part II: Specific Poisonings," *Chest*, 2003, 123(3):897-922.

◆ **Trazodone Hydrochloride** *see* TraZODone *on page 1423*

◆ **Trazorel® (Can)** *see* TraZODone *on page 1423*

Treprostinil (tre PROST in il)

U.S. Brand Names Remodulin®; Tyvaso™

Canadian Brand Names Remodulin®

Index Terms Treprostinil Sodium

Pharmacologic Category Prostacyclin; Prostaglandin; Vasodilator

Generic Available No

◄ **Use**

Injection: Treatment of pulmonary arterial hypertension (PAH) in patients with NYHA Class II-IV symptoms to decrease exercise-associated symptoms; to diminish clinical deterioration when transitioning from epoprostenol (I.V.)

Inhalation: Treatment of pulmonary arterial hypertension (PAH) in patients with NYHA Class III symptoms to increase walk distance. **Note:** Nearly all controlled clinical trial experience has been with concomitant bosentan or sildenafil.

Mechanism of Action Treprostinil is a direct vasodilator of both pulmonary and systemic arterial vascular beds; also inhibits platelet aggregation.

Pharmacodynamics/Kinetics

Absorption: SubQ: Rapidly and completely

Distribution: 14 L/70 kg lean body weight

Protein binding: 91%

Metabolism: Hepatic (primarily by CYP2C8); forms 5 metabolites (HU1-HU5)

Bioavailability: Inhalation: 64% to 72% (dose-dependent); SubQ: 100%

Half-life elimination: Terminal: ~4 hours

Excretion: Urine (79%; 4% as unchanged drug, 64% as metabolites); feces (13%)

Dosage

Adults: PAH:

Inhalation: **Note:** Prior to initiation, patients should be carefully evaluated for ability to administer treprostinil and care for the inhalation system and accessories required for administration. Immediate access to a back-up inhalation device, accessories, and medication is essential to prevent treatment interruptions.

Initial: 18 mcg (or 3 inhalations) every 4 hours 4 times/day; if 3 inhalations are not tolerated, reduce to 1-2 inhalations, then increase to 3 inhalations as tolerated

Maintenance: If tolerated, increase dose by an additional 3 inhalations at approximately 1- to 2-week intervals; maximum dose: 54 mcg (or 9 inhalations) 4 times/day

SubQ (preferred) or I.V. infusion: **Note:** Prior to initiation, patients should be carefully evaluated for ability to administer treprostinil and care for the infusion system outside of inpatient setting. Immediate access to a back-up pump, infusion sets, and medication is essential to prevent treatment interruptions.

Initial: New to prostacyclin therapy: 1.25 ng/kg/minute continuous; if dose cannot be tolerated due to systemic effects, reduce to 0.625 ng/kg/minute. Increase at rate not >1.25 ng/kg/minute per week for first 4 weeks, and not >2.5 ng/kg/minute per week for remainder of therapy. Limited experience with doses >40 ng/kg/minute. **Note:** Dose must be carefully and individually titrated (symptom improvement with minimal adverse effects). Avoid abrupt withdrawal. If infusion is restarted within a few hours of discontinuation, the same dose rate may be used. Interruptions for longer periods may require retitration.

Transitioning from epoprostenol (see table on next page): SubQ (preferred) or I.V. infusion: **Note:** Transition should occur in a hospital setting to follow response (eg, walking distance, sign/symptoms of disease progression). May take 24-48 hours to transition. Transition is accomplished by initiating the infusion of treprostinil, and increasing it while simultaneously reducing the dose of intravenous epoprostenol. During transition, increases in PAH symptoms should be first treated with an increase in treprostinil dose. Occurrence of prostacyclin associated side effects should be treated by decreasing the dose of epoprostenol.

Transitioning From I.V. Epoprostenol to SubQ (Preferred) or I.V. Treprostinil

Step	Epoprostenol Dose	Treprostinil Dose
1	Maintain current dose	Initiate at 10% initial epoprostenol dose
2	Decrease to 80% initial dose	Increase to 30% initial epoprostenol dose
3	Decrease to 60% initial dose	Increase to 50% initial epoprostenol dose
4	Decrease to 40% initial dose	Increase to 70% initial epoprostenol dose
5	Decrease to 20% initial dose	Increase to 90% initial epoprostenol dose
6	Decrease to 5% initial dose	Increase to 110% initial epoprostenol dose
7	Discontinue epoprostenol	Maintain current dose plus additional 5% to 10% as needed

Elderly: Limited experience in patients ≥65 years; refer to adult dosing; use caution

Dosage adjustment in renal impairment:
  Inhalation: Titrate slowly in patients with renal impairment.
  I.V./SubQ: No specific dosage adjustment recommended; use with caution.

Dosage adjustment in hepatic impairment:
  Mild-to-moderate:
    Inhalation: Titrate slowly in patients with hepatic impairment.
    I.V./SubQ: Initial: 0.625 mg/kg/minute; increase with caution.
  Severe: Has not been studied in patients with severe hepatic impairment.

Stability Injection solution: Store vials at 15°C to 30°C (59°F to 86°F). Contents of a vial should not be used past 30 days after initial needle access into the vial. For SubQ infusion, **product should not be diluted prior to use**. Contents of a single-reservoir syringe of treprostinil can be administered up to 72 hours at 37°C. For I.V. infusion, dilute in SWFI, NS, or Flolan® sterile diluent to a final volume of either 50 mL or 100 mL (dependent on system reservoir and calculated dose). Stability for up to 48 hours has been shown for concentrations as low as 4000 ng/mL. Solutions diluted for infusion may be used for up to 48 hours at 37°C.

Solution for inhalation: Store ampules in foil packs at 25°C (77°F); excursions permitted to 15°C to 30°C (59°F to 89°F). Protect from light. Once foil pack is opened, ampules should be used within 7 days. Following transfer of solution to inhalation device, solution should remain in device for no more than 24 hours; discard unused portion.

Administration Regardless of administration route (inhalation, I.V., or SubQ), treatment interruptions or rapid large dosage reductions should be avoided. Immediate access to medication, a back-up inhalation device, or pump and infusion sets is essential to prevent treatment interruptions.

  Inhalation: Do not mix with other medications. For inhalation only via the Tyvaso™ Inhalation System; consists of the Optineb-ir Model ON-100/7 (an ultrasonic, pulsed-delivery device) and accessories. Prior to the first treatment session of each day, transfer the entire contents of one ampule into the medicine chamber; one ampule contains sufficient volume of medication for all 4 treatment sessions in a single day. Between each session, the device should be capped and stored upright with the remaining medication inside. At the end of each day, the medicine chamber and any remaining medication must be discarded. Avoid contact of solution with eyes or skin; wash hands after handling.

  I.V. infusion: I.V. use is recommended when SubQ infusion is not tolerated or when the benefit outweighs the potential risks of an indwelling central venous catheter. Solution must be diluted in SWFI or NS prior to use and administered by continuous infusion using a central indwelling catheter and infusion pump. Peripheral infusion may be used temporarily until central line is established.

◄ SubQ infusion (preferred): Administer undiluted via continuous SubQ infusion using an appropriately-designed infusion pump. Infusion site reactions may be helped by moving the infusion site every 3 days, local application of topical hot and cold packs, topical or oral analgesics. Injection site pain and erythema may improve after several months of therapy.

Monitoring Parameters BP, dyspnea, fatigue, activity tolerance, symptoms of excessive dose (eg, headache, nausea, vomiting)

Pregnancy Risk Factor B

Contraindications There are no contraindications listed in the FDA-approved labeling.

Warnings/Precautions May produce symptomatic hypotension; use with caution in patients with low systemic arterial blood pressure. Abrupt withdrawal/large dosage reductions may worsen symptoms of PAH. I.V./SubQ: If infusion is restarted within a few hours of discontinuation, the same dose rate may be used. Interruptions for longer periods may require retitration. Regardless of administration route (inhalation, I.V., or SubQ), treatment interruptions should be avoided. Immediate access to medication, back-up inhalation device, or pump and infusion sets is essential to prevent treatment interruptions. Chronic continuous I.V. infusion of treprostinil via a chronic indwelling central venous catheter has been associated with serious blood stream infections. This method of administration should be reserved for patients who are intolerant of the SubQ route or in whom the benefit outweighs the potential risks. Treprostinil should only be used by clinicians experienced in the treatment of PAH. Prior to initiation, patients should be carefully evaluated for ability to administer treprostinil, either as an I.V./SubQ infusion or inhalation, and care for the infusion system/inhalation device. Initiation of infusion must occur in a setting where adequate personnel and equipment necessary for hemodynamic monitoring and emergency treatment is available. Use with caution in patients with hepatic impairment; dose reduction is recommended for the initial dose (I.V./SubQ) in patients with mild-to-moderate hepatic insufficiency; titrate dose (inhalation) slowly in patients with hepatic insufficiency; has not been studied in severe hepatic impairment. Has not been studied in renal impairment; use with caution in renal impairment; titrate dose (inhalation) slowly in patients with renal insufficiency. Use with caution in patients ≥65 years of age. Inhalation: Safety and efficacy have not been established in patients with underlying pulmonary disease (eg, asthma, COPD). Patients with acute pulmonary infections should be monitored closely for exacerbation or reduced efficacy. Treprostinil inhibits platelet aggregation, increasing the risk of bleeding; use with caution in patients receiving concurrent anticoagulant/antiplatelet therapy. Safety and efficacy have not been established in children ≤16 years of age (I.V., SubQ) or <18 years of age (inhalation).

Adverse Reactions

>10%:

Cardiovascular: Flushing (inhalation: 15%), vasodilation (11%)

Central nervous system: Headache (27% to 41%)

Dermatologic: Rash (14%)

Gastrointestinal: Diarrhea (25%), nausea (19% to 22%)

Local: Infusion site pain (SubQ: 85%; may improve after several months of therapy); infusion site reaction (SubQ: 83%)

Neuromuscular & skeletal: Jaw pain (13%)

Respiratory: Cough (inhalation: 54%), throat irritation/pharyngolaryngeal pain (inhalation: 25%)

1% to 10%:

Cardiovascular: Edema (9%), syncope (inhalation: 6%), hypotension (4%), epistaxis (inhalation), wheezing (inhalation)

Central nervous system: Dizziness (9%)

Dermatologic: Pruritus (8%)

Respiratory: Pneumonia (inhalation: 4%), hemoptysis (inhalation: 2%)

<1% (Limited to important or life-threatening): Anxiety, arm swelling, bone pain, cellulitis, central venous catheter-related line infections, central venous catheter-related sepsis, hematoma, pain, paresthesia, restlessness, thrombocytopenia, thrombophlebitis

Drug Interactions

Avoid Concomitant Use There are no known interactions where it is recommended to avoid concomitant use.

Increased Effect/Toxicity

Treprostinil may increase the levels/effects of: Anticoagulants; Antihypertensives; Antiplatelet Agents; Nonsteroidal Anti-Inflammatory Agents; Salicylates

The levels/effects of Treprostinil may be increased by: CYP2C8 Inhibitors (Strong)

Decreased Effect

The levels/effects of Treprostinil may be decreased by: CYP2C8 Inducers (Highly Effective)

Dietary Considerations Sodium chloride content of solution for injection:

1 mg/mL, 2.5 mg/mL, and 5 mg/mL each contain sodium chloride 5.3 mg/mL

10 mg/mL contains sodium chloride 4 mg/mL

Dosage Forms Excipient information presented when available (limited, particularly for generics); consult specific product labeling.

Injection, solution:

Remodulin®: 1 mg/mL (20 mL) [contains sodium chloride 5.3 mg/mL]; 2.5 mg/mL (20 mL) [contains sodium chloride 5.3 mg/mL]; 5 mg/mL (20 mL) [contains sodium chloride 5.3 mg/mL]; 10 mg/mL (20 mL) [contains sodium chloride 4 mg/mL]

Solution for oral inhalation:

Tyvaso™: 0.6 mg/mL (2.9 mL) [delivers ~6 mcg/inhalation]

References

Badesch DB, Abman SH, Ahearn GS, et al, "Medical Therapy for Pulmonary Arterial Hypertension: ACCP Evidence-Based Clinical Practice Guidelines," *Chest*, 2004, 126(1 Suppl):35-62.

Gildea TR, Arroliga AC, and Minai OA, "Treatments and Strategies to Optimize the Comprehensive Management of Patients With Pulmonary Arterial Hypertension," *Cleve Clin J Med*, 2003, 70(Suppl 1):18-27.

Gomberg-Maitland M, Tapson VF, Benza RL, et al, "Transition from Intravenous Epoprostenol to Intravenous Treprostinil in Pulmonary Hypertension," *Am J Respir Crit Care Med*, 2005, 172 (12):1586-9.

Humbert M, Sitbon O, and Simmoneau G, "Treatment of Pulmonary Arterial hypertension," *N Engl J Med*, 2004, 351(14):1425-36.

McLaughlin VV, Gaine SP, Barst RJ, et al, "Efficacy and Safety of Treprostinil: An Epoprostenol Analog for Primary Pulmonary Hypertension," *J Cardiovasc Pharmacol*, 2003, 41(2):293-9.

Rubin LJ and American College of Chest Physicians, "Diagnosis and Management of Pulmonary Arterial Hypertension: ACCP Evidence-Based Clinical Practice Guidelines," *Chest*, 2004, 126(1 Suppl):4-6.

◆ **Treprostinil Sodium** *see* Treprostinil *on page 1425*

◆ **Trexall™** *see* Methotrexate *on page 898*

◆ **Triaderm (Can)** *see* Triamcinolone *on page 1429*

Triamcinolone (trye am SIN oh lone)

Related Information

Asthma *on page 1728*

Corticosteroids *on page 1676*

Stress Replacement of Corticosteroids *on page 1611*

U.S. Brand Names Aristospan®; Azmacort®; Kenalog-10®; Kenalog-40®; Kenalog®; Nasacort® AQ; Tri-Nasal® [DSC]; Triderm®; Triesence™; Trivaris™; Zytopic™

Canadian Brand Names Aristospan®; Kenalog®; Kenalog® in Orabase; Nasacort® AQ; Oracort; Triaderm; Trinasal®

Index Terms Triamcinolone Acetonide, Aerosol; Triamcinolone Acetonide, Parenteral; Triamcinolone Hexacetonide; Triamcinolone, Oral

Pharmacologic Category Corticosteroid, Inhalant (Oral); Corticosteroid, Nasal; Corticosteroid, Ophthalmic; Corticosteroid, Systemic; Corticosteroid, Topical

Use

Intra-articular (soft tissue): Acute gouty arthritis, acute/subacute bursitis, acute tenosynovitis, epicondylitis, rheumatoid arthritis, synovitis of osteoarthritis

◀ Intralesional: Alopecia areata, discoid lupus erythematosus, keloids, granuloma annulare lesions (localized hypertrophic, infiltrated, or inflammatory), lichen planus plaques, lichen simplex chronicus plaques, psoriatic plaques, necrobiosis lipoidica diabeticorum, cystic tumors of aponeurosis or tendon (ganglia)

Nasal inhalation: Management of seasonal and perennial allergic rhinitis

Ophthalmic: Intravitreal: treatment of sympathetic ophthalmia, temporal arteritis, uveitis, ocular inflammatory conditions unresponsive to topical corticosteroids

Triesence™: Visualization during vitrectomy

Oral inhalation: Control of bronchial asthma and related bronchospastic conditions

Oral topical: Adjunctive treatment and temporary relief of symptoms associated with oral inflammatory lesions and ulcerative lesions resulting from trauma

Systemic: Adrenocortical insufficiency, dermatologic diseases, endocrine disorders, gastrointestinal diseases, hematologic and neoplastic disorders, nervous system disorders, nephrotic syndrome, rheumatic disorders, allergic states, respiratory diseases, systemic lupus erythematosus (SLE), and other diseases requiring anti-inflammatory or immunosuppressive effects

Topical: Inflammatory dermatoses responsive to steroids

Pharmacodynamics/Kinetics

Duration: Oral: 8-12 hours

Absorption: Topical: Systemic

Distribution: V_d: 99.5 L

Protein binding: ~68%

Time to peak: I.M.: 8-10 hours

Half-life elimination: Biologic: 18-36 hours; Intravitreal: Nonvitrectomized patients: 13-24 days, Vitrectomized patients: ~3 days (based upon 1 patient)

Excretion: Urine (~40%); feces (~60%)

Dosage The lowest possible dose should be used to control the condition; when dose reduction is possible, the dose should be reduced gradually. Parenteral dose is usually 1/3 to 1/2 the oral dose given every 12 hours. In life-threatening situations, parenteral doses larger than the oral dose may be needed.

Injection:

Acetonide:

Intra-articular, intrabursal, tendon sheaths: Adults: Initial: Smaller joints: 2.5-5 mg, larger joints: 5-15 mg; may require up to 10 mg for small joints and up to 40 mg for large joints; maximum dose/treatment (several joints at one time): 20-80 mg

Intradermal: Adults: Initial: 1 mg

I.M.: Range: 2.5-100 mg/day

Children: Initial: 0.11-1.6 mg/kg/day in 3-4 divided doses

Children 6-12 years: Initial: 40 mg

Children >12 years and Adults: Initial: 60 mg

Hay fever/pollen asthma: 40-100 mg as a single injection/season

Multiple sclerosis (acute exacerbation): 160 mg daily for 1 week, followed by 64 mg every other day for 1 month

Hexacetonide: Adults:

Intralesional, sublesional: Up to 0.5 mg/square inch of affected skin; range: 2-48 mg

Intra-articular: Average dose: 2-20 mg; smaller joints: 2-6 mg; larger joints: 10-20 mg. Frequency of injection into a single joint is every 3-4 weeks as necessary; to avoid possible joint destruction use as infrequently as possible.

Triamcinolone Dosing

	Acetonide	Hexacetonide
Intrasynovial	5-40 mg	
Intralesional	1-30 mg (usually 1 mg per injection site); 10 mg/mL suspension usually used	Up to 0.5 mg/sq inch affected area
Sublesional	1-30 mg	
Systemic I.M.	2.5-60 mg/dose (usual adult dose: 60 mg; may repeat with 20-100 mg dose when symptoms recur)	
Intra-articular	2.5-40 mg	2-20 mg average
large joints	5-15 mg	10-20 mg
small joints	2.5-5 mg	2-6 mg
Tendon sheaths	2.5-10 mg	
Intradermal	1 mg/site	

Intranasal: Perennial allergic rhinitis, seasonal allergic rhinitis:
Nasal spray:
Children 2-5 years: 110 mcg/day as 1 spray in each nostril once daily (maximum: 110 mcg/day)
Children 6-11 years: 110 mcg/day as 1 spray in each nostril once daily; may increase to 220 mcg/day as 2 sprays in each nostril if response not adequate; once symptoms controlled may reduce to 110 mcg/day
Children ≥12 years and Adults: 220 mcg/day as 2 sprays in each nostril once daily; once symptoms controlled reduce to 110 mcg/day
Nasal inhaler:
Children 6-11 years: Initial: 220 mcg/day as 2 sprays in each nostril once daily
Children ≥12 years and Adults: Initial: 220 mcg/day as 2 sprays in each nostril once daily; may increase dose to 440 mcg/day (given once daily or divided and given 2 or 4 times/day)

Ophthalmic injection: Intravitreal: Children and Adults
Ocular disease: Initial: 4 mg as a single dose; additional doses may be given as needed over the course of treatment
Visualization during vitrectomy (Triesence™): 1-4 mg

Oral inhalation: Asthma:
Children 6-12 years: 75-150 mcg 3-4 times/day **or** 150-300 mcg twice daily; maximum dose: 900 mcg/day
Children >12 years and Adults: 150 mcg 3-4 times/day **or** 300 mcg twice daily; maximum dose: 1200 mcg/day
NIH Asthma Guidelines (NIH, 2007) (administer in divided doses twice daily):
Children: 5-11 years:
"Low" dose: 300-600 mcg/day
"Medium" dose: >600-900 mcg/day
"High" dose: >900 mcg/day
Children ≥12 years and Adults:
"Low" dose: 300-750 mcg/day
"Medium" dose: >750-1500 mcg/day
"High" dose: >1500 mcg/day

Oral topical: Oral inflammatory lesions/ulcers: Press a small dab (about ¼ inch) to the lesion until a thin film develops. A larger quantity may be required for coverage of some lesions. For optimal results use only enough to coat the lesion with a thin film; do not rub in.

Topical:
Cream, Ointment:
0.025%: Apply thin film to affected areas 2-4 times/day
0.1% or 0.5%: Apply thin film to affected areas 2-3 times/day
Spray: Apply to affected area 3-4 times/day

◀ **Anesthesia and Critical Care Concerns/Other Considerations**
Clinical Pearls/Comments: Triamcinolone is a long-acting corticosteroid with minimal sodium-retaining potential.

Evidence-Based Information:
Neuromuscular Effects: ICU-acquired paresis was recently studied in five ICUs (three medical and two surgical ICUs) at four French hospitals. All ICU patients without pre-existing neuromuscular disease admitted from March 1999 through June 2000 were evaluated (de Jonghe, 2002). Each patient had to be mechanically ventilated for ≥7 days and was screened daily for awakening. The first day the patient was considered awake was Study Day 1. Patients with severe muscle weakness on Study Day 7 were considered to have ICU-acquired paresis. Among the 95 patients who were evaluated, about 25% developed ICU-acquired paresis. Independent predictors included female gender, the number of days with ≥2 organ dysfunction, and administration of corticosteroids. Further studies may be required to verify and characterize the association between the development of ICU-acquired paresis and use of corticosteroids. Concurrent use of a corticosteroid and muscle relaxant appears to increase the risk of certain ICU myopathies; avoid or administer the corticosteroid at the lowest dose possible.

Adrenal Insufficiency: Patients will often have steroid-induced adverse effects on glucose tolerance and lipid profiles. When discontinuing steroid therapy in patients on long-term steroid supplementation, it is important that the steroid therapy be discontinued gradually. Abrupt withdrawal may result in adrenal insufficiency with hypotension and hyperkalemia. Patients on long-term steroid supplementation will require higher corticosteroid doses when subject to stress (eg, trauma, surgery, severe infection). Guidelines for glucocorticoid replacement during various surgical procedures have been published (Coursin, 2002; Salem, 1994).

Additional Information Complete prescribing information for this medication should be consulted for additional detail.

Product Availability Trivaris™: FDA approved June 2008; availability currently undetermined

Dosage Forms Excipient information presented when available (limited, particularly for generics); consult specific product labeling. [DSC] = Discontinued product

Aerosol for oral inhalation, as acetonide:
  Azmacort®: 75 mcg per actuation (20 g) [contains chlorofluorocarbon; 240 actuations]
Aerosol, topical, as acetonide:
  Kenalog®: 0.2 mg/2-second spray (63 g) [contains dehydrated ethanol 10.3%]
Cream, as acetonide: 0.025% (15 g, 80 g, 454 g); 0.1% (15 g, 80 g, 454 g, 2270 g); 0.5% (15 g)
  Triderm®: 0.1% (30 g, 85 g)
  Zytopic™: 0.1% (85 g)
Injection, suspension, as acetonide:
  Kenalog-10®: 10 mg/mL (5 mL) [contains benzyl alcohol, polysorbate 80; not for I.V. or I.M. use]
  Kenalog-40®: 40 mg/mL (1 mL, 5 mL, 10 mL) [contains benzyl alcohol, polysorbate 80; not for I.V. or intradermal use]
  Triesence™: 40 mg/mL (1 mL) [contains polysorbate 80; not for I.V. use]
  Trivaris™: 80 mg/mL (0.1 mL) [preservative free; not for I.V. use; (for intra-articular, intramuscular, intravitreal use)]
Injection, suspension, as hexacetonide:
  Aristospan®: 5 mg/mL (5 mL); 20 mg/mL (1 mL, 5 mL) [contains benzyl alcohol, polysorbate 80; not for I.V. use]
Lotion, as acetonide: 0.025% (60 mL); 0.1% (60 mL)
Ointment, topical, as acetonide: 0.025% (15 g, 80 g, 454 g); 0.05% (430 g); 0.1% (15 g, 80 g, 454 g); 0.5% (15 g)
Paste, oral, topical, as acetonide: 0.1% (5 g)
Powder, for prescription compounding, as acetonide [micronized]: Triamcinolone acetonide USP (5 g)
Solution, intranasal, as acetonide [spray]:
  Tri-Nasal®: 50 mcg/inhalation (15 mL) [120 actuations] [DSC]

Suspension, intranasal, as acetonide [spray]:
Nasacort® AQ: 55 mcg/inhalation (16.5 g) [120 actuations]

References

Abraham E and Evans T, "Corticosteroids and Septic Shock [editorial]," *JAMA*, 2002, 288(7):886-7.
American Academy of Pediatrics Committee on Drugs: "Transfer of Drugs and Other Chemicals Into Human Milk," *Pediatrics*, 2001, 108(3):776-89.
Annane D, Sebille V, Charpentier C, et al, "Effect of Treatment With Low Doses of Hydrocortisone and Fludrocortisone on Mortality in Patients With Septic Shock," *JAMA*, 2002, 288(7):862-71.
Boot AM, Nauta J, Hokken-Koelega AC, et al, "Renal Transplantation and Osteoporosis," *Arch Dis Child*, 1995, 72(6):502-6.
Bowman H and Lennard TW, "Immunosuppressive Drugs," *Br J Hosp Med*, 1992, 48(9):570-3.
Cooper MS and Stewart PM, "Corticosteroid Insufficiency in Acutely Ill Patients," *N Engl J Med*, 2003, 348(8):727-34.
Coursin DB and Wood KE, "Corticosteroid Supplementation for Adrenal Insufficiency," *JAMA*, 2002, 287(2):236-40.
de Jonghe B, Sharshar T, Lefaucheur JP, et al, "Paresis Acquired in the Intensive Care Unit. A Prospective Multicenter Study," *JAMA*, 2002, 288(22):2859-67.
Expert Panel Report 3, "Guidelines for the Diagnosis and Management of Asthma," *Clinical Practice Guidelines*, National Institutes of Health, National Heart, Lung, and Blood Institute, NIH Publication No. 08-4051, prepublication 2007. Available at http://www.nhlbi.nih.gov/guidelines/asthma/asthgdln.htm
Frey BM and Frey FJ, "Clinical Pharmacokinetics of Prednisone and Prednisolone," *Clin Pharmacokinet*, 1990, 19(2):126-46.
Gamsu HR, Mullinger BM, Donnai P, et al, "Antenatal Administration of Betamethasone to Prevent Respiratory Distress Syndrome in Preterm Infants: Report of a UK Multicentre Trial," *Br J Obstet Gynaecol*, 1989, 96(4):401-10.
Goedert JJ, Vitale F, Lauria C, et al, "Risk Factors for Classical Kaposi's Sarcoma," *J Natl Cancer Inst*, 2002, 94(22):1712-8.
Grotz WH, Mundinger FA, Gugel B, et al, "Bone Mineral Density After Kidney Transplantation: A Cross-Sectional Study in 190-Graft Recipients Up to 20 Years After Transplantation," *Transplantation*, 1995, 59(7):982-6.
Gutin PH, "Corticosteroid Therapy in Patients With Brain Tumors," *Natl Cancer Inst Monogr*, 1977, 46:151-6.
Hotchkiss RS and Karl IE, "The Pathophysiology and Treatment of Sepsis," *N Engl J Med*, 2003, 348(2):138-50.
Kimberly RP, "Glucocorticoids," *Curr Opin Rheumatol*, 1994, 6(3):273-80.
Liggins GC and Howie RN, "A Controlled Trial of Antepartum Glucocorticoid Treatment of Respiratory Distress Syndrome in Premature Infants," *Pediatrics*, 1972, 50:515-25.
Lowenthal RM and Jestrimski KW, "Corticosteroid Drugs: Their Role in Oncological Practice," *Med J Aust*, 1986, 144(2):81-5.
Murphy CM, Coonce SL, and Simon PA, "Treatment of Asthma in Children," *Clin Pharm*, 1991, 10(9):685-703.
Reed B, "Dermatologic Drugs, Pregnancy, and Lactation. A Conservative Guide," *Arch Dermatol*, 1997, 133:894-8.
Report of a Workshop by the British Association for Paediatric Nephrology and Research Unit, Royal College of Physicians, "Consensus Statement on Management and Audit Potential for Steroid Responsive Nephrotic Syndrome," *Arch Dis Child*, 1994, 70(2):151-7.
Salem M, Tainsh RE Jr, Bromberg J, et al, "Perioperative Glucocorticoid Coverage. A Reassessment 42 Years After Emergence of a Problem," *Ann Surg*, 1994, 219(4):416-25.
Todd GR, Acerini CL, Buck JJ, et al, "Acute Adrenal Crisis in Asthmatics Treated With High-Dose Fluticasone Propionate," *Eur Respir J*, 2002, 19(6):1207-9.
Todd GR, Acerini CL, Ross-Russell R, et al, "Survey of Adrenal Crisis Associated With Inhaled Corticosteroids in the United Kingdom," *Arch Dis Child*, 2002, 87(6):457-61.

◆ **Triamcinolone Acetonide, Aerosol** *see* Triamcinolone *on page 1429*

◆ **Triamcinolone Acetonide, Parenteral** *see* Triamcinolone *on page 1429*

◆ **Triamcinolone Hexacetonide** *see* Triamcinolone *on page 1429*

◆ **Triamcinolone, Oral** *see* Triamcinolone *on page 1429*

◆ **Triaminic® Infant Thin Strips® Decongestant [OTC] [DSC]** *see* Phenylephrine *on page 1114*

◆ **Triaminic Thin Strips® Children's Cough and Runny Nose [OTC]** *see* DiphenhydrAMINE *on page 430*

◆ **Triaminic® Thin Strips® Cold [OTC]** *see* Phenylephrine *on page 1114*

◆ **Triatec-8 (Can)** *see* Acetaminophen and Codeine *on page 29*

◆ **Triatec-8 Strong (Can)** *see* Acetaminophen and Codeine *on page 29*

◆ **Triatec-30 (Can)** *see* Acetaminophen and Codeine *on page 29*

Triazolam (trye AY zoe lam)

Related Information
　Antidepressant Agents *on page 1660*
　Benzodiazepines *on page 1666*
U.S. Brand Names Halcion®
Canadian Brand Names Apo-Triazo®; Gen-Triazolam; Halcion®; Mylan-Triazolam
Pharmacologic Category Hypnotic, Benzodiazepine
Restrictions C-IV
Use Short-term treatment of insomnia
Pharmacodynamics/Kinetics
　Onset of action: Hypnotic: 15-30 minutes
　Duration: 6-7 hours
　Distribution: V_d: 0.8-1.8 L/kg
　Protein binding: 89%
　Metabolism: Extensively hepatic
　Half-life elimination: 1.5-5.5 hours
　Excretion: Urine as unchanged drug and metabolites
Dosage Oral (onset of action is rapid, patient should be in bed when taking medication):
　Children <18 years: Dosage not established
　Adults:
　　Insomnia (short-term): 0.125-0.25 mg at bedtime (maximum dose: 0.5 mg/day)
　　Preprocedure sedation (dental): 0.25 mg taken the evening before oral surgery; or 0.25 mg 1 hour before procedure
　Elderly: Insomnia (short-term use): Initial: 0.125 mg at bedtime; maximum dose: 0.25 mg/day
　Dosing adjustment/comments in hepatic impairment: Reduce dose or avoid use in cirrhosis
Anesthesia and Critical Care Concerns/Other Considerations Chronic use of this agent may increase the perioperative benzodiazepine dose needed to achieve desired effect. Abrupt discontinuation after sustained use (generally >10 days) may cause withdrawal symptoms.
Additional Information Complete prescribing information for this medication should be consulted for additional detail.
Dosage Forms Excipient information presented when available (limited, particularly for generics); consult specific product labeling. [DSC] = Discontinued product
　Tablet: 0.125 mg, 0.25 mg
　　Halcion®: 0.125 mg [DSC], 0.25 mg

◆ **Trichloroacetaldehyde Monohydrate** *see* Chloral Hydrate *on page 285*

◆ **TriCor®** *see* Fenofibrate *on page 582*

◆ **Tricosal** *see* Choline Magnesium Trisalicylate *on page 299*

◆ **Tri-Cyclen® (Can)** *see* Ethinyl Estradiol and Norgestimate *on page 558*

◆ **Tri-Cyclen® Lo (Can)** *see* Ethinyl Estradiol and Norgestimate *on page 558*

◆ **Triderm®** *see* Triamcinolone *on page 1429*

◆ **Tridil** *see* Nitroglycerin *on page 1014*

◆ **Tridural™ (Can)** *see* TraMADol *on page 1415*

◆ **Triesence™** *see* Triamcinolone *on page 1429*

◆ **Triglide™** *see* Fenofibrate *on page 582*

◆ **Trikacide (Can)** *see* MetroNIDAZOLE *on page 928*

◆ **Tri-Legest™ Fe** *see* Ethinyl Estradiol and Norethindrone *on page 554*

◆ **Trileptal®** *see* OXcarbazepine *on page 1066*

◆ **TriLipix™** *see* Fenofibric Acid *on page 583*

◆ **Trilisate** *see* Choline Magnesium Trisalicylate *on page 299*

◆ **Tri-Lo-Sprintec™** *see* Ethinyl Estradiol and Norgestimate *on page 558*

Trimethobenzamide (trye meth oh BEN za mide)

Medication Safety Issues
Sound-alike/look-alike issues:
Tigan® may be confused with Tiazac®, Ticar®, Ticlid®
Trimethobenzamide may be confused with metoclopramide, trimethoprim

U.S. Brand Names Tigan®

Canadian Brand Names Tigan®

Index Terms Trimethobenzamide Hydrochloride

Pharmacologic Category Anticholinergic Agent; Antiemetic

Generic Available Yes

Use Treatment of postoperative nausea and vomiting; treatment of nausea associated with gastroenteritis

Mechanism of Action Acts centrally to inhibit the medullary chemoreceptor trigger zone by blocking emetic impulses to the vomiting center

Pharmacodynamics/Kinetics
Onset of action: Antiemetic: Oral: 10-40 minutes; I.M.: 15-35 minutes
Duration: 3-4 hours
Metabolism: Via oxidation, forms metabolite trimethobenzamide N-oxide
Bioavailability: Oral: 60% to 100%
Half-life elimination: 7-9 hours
Time to peak: Oral: ~45 minutes; I.M.: ~30 minutes
Excretion: Urine (30% to 50%, as unchanged drug)

Dosage
Children >40 kg: Oral: 300 mg 3-4 times/day
Adults:
Oral: 300 mg 3-4 times/day
I.M.: 200 mg 3-4 times/day
Postoperative nausea and vomiting (PONV): I.M.: 200 mg, followed 1 hour later by a second 200 mg dose
Elderly: Refer to adult dosing. Consider dosage reduction or increasing dosing interval in elderly patients with renal impairment (specific adjustment guidelines are not provided in the manufacturer's labeling).

Dosage adjustment in renal impairment: Cl_{cr} ≤70 mL/minute: Consider dosage reduction or increasing dosing interval (specific adjustment guidelines are not provided in the manufacturer's labeling)

Stability Store capsules and injection solution at room temperature of 25°C (77°F); excursions permitted to 15°C to 30°C (59°F to 86°F).

Administration
Injection: Administer I.M. only; not for I.V. administration. Inject deep into upper outer quadrant of gluteal muscle. Capsule: Administer capsule orally without regard to meals.

Monitoring Parameters Renal function (at baseline)

Contraindications Hypersensitivity to trimethobenzamide or any component of the formulation; injection contraindicated in children

Warnings/Precautions May mask emesis due to Reye's syndrome or mimic CNS effects of Reye's syndrome in patients with emesis of other etiologies. Antiemetic effects may mask toxicity of other drugs or conditions (eg, intestinal obstruction). May cause drowsiness; patient should avoid tasks requiring alertness (eg, driving, operating machinery). May cause extrapyramidal symptoms (EPS) which may be confused with CNS symptoms of primary disease responsible for emesis. Risk of CNS adverse effects (eg, coma, EPS, seizure) may be increased in patients with acute febrile illness, dehydration, electrolyte imbalance, encephalitis, or gastroenteritis; use caution. Allergic-type skin reactions have been reported with use; discontinue with signs of sensitization. Trimethobenzamide clearance is predominantly renal; dosage reductions may be recommended in patient with renal impairment. Use capsule formulation with caution in children; antiemetics are not recommended for uncomplicated vomiting in children, limit antiemetic use to prolonged vomiting of known etiology. Use of injection is contraindicated in children.

Adverse Reactions Frequency not defined.
Cardiovascular: Hypotension (I.V. administration)

Central nervous system: Coma, depression, disorientation, dizziness, drowsiness, EPS, headache, Parkinson-like symptoms, seizure

Dermatologic: Allergic-type skin reactions

Gastrointestinal: Diarrhea

Hematologic: Blood dyscrasias

Hepatic: Jaundice

Local: Injection site burning, pain, redness, stinging, or swelling

Neuromuscular & skeletal: Muscle cramps, opisthotonos

Ocular: Blurred vision

Miscellaneous: Hypersensitivity reactions

Drug Interactions

Avoid Concomitant Use There are no known interactions where it is recommended to avoid concomitant use.

Increased Effect/Toxicity

Trimethobenzamide may increase the levels/effects of: Anticholinergics; Cannabinoids; Potassium Chloride

The levels/effects of Trimethobenzamide may be increased by: Pramlintide

Decreased Effect

Trimethobenzamide may decrease the levels/effects of: Acetylcholinesterase Inhibitors (Central); Secretin

The levels/effects of Trimethobenzamide may be decreased by: Acetylcholinesterase Inhibitors (Central)

Ethanol/Nutrition/Herb Interactions Ethanol: Concomitant use should be avoided (sedative effects may be additive).

Dosage Forms Excipient information presented when available (limited, particularly for generics); consult specific product labeling.

Capsule, as hydrochloride: 300 mg

Tigan®: 300 mg

Injection, solution, as hydrochloride: 100 mg/mL (2 mL)

Tigan®: 100 mg/mL (20 mL)

Injection, solution, as hydrochloride [preservative free]:

Tigan®: 100 mg/mL (2 mL)

Tropicamide (troe PIK a mide)

Related Information
Cycloplegic Mydriatics *on page 1679*

U.S. Brand Names Mydral™; Mydriacyl®; Tropicacyl®

Canadian Brand Names Diotrope®; Mydriacyl®

Index Terms Bistropamide

Pharmacologic Category Ophthalmic Agent, Mydriatic

Use Short-acting mydriatic used in diagnostic procedures; as well as preoperatively and postoperatively; treatment of some cases of acute iritis, iridocyclitis, and keratitis

Pharmacodynamics/Kinetics
Onset of action: Mydriasis: ~20-40 minutes; Cycloplegia: ~30 minutes
Duration: Mydriasis: ~6-7 hours; Cycloplegia: <6 hours

Dosage Ophthalmic: Children and Adults (individuals with heavily pigmented eyes may require larger doses):
Cycloplegia: Instill 1-2 drops (1%); may repeat in 5 minutes
Exam must be performed within 30 minutes after the repeat dose; if the patient is not examined within 20-30 minutes, instill an additional drop
Mydriasis: Instill 1-2 drops (0.5%) 15-20 minutes before exam; may repeat every 30 minutes as needed

Additional Information Complete prescribing information for this medication should be consulted for additional detail.

Dosage Forms Excipient information presented when available (limited, particularly for generics); consult specific product labeling.
Solution, ophthalmic [drops]: 0.5% (15 mL); 1% (2 mL, 3 mL, 15 mL)
Mydriacyl®: 1% (3 mL, 15 mL) [contains benzalkonium chloride]
Mydral™, Tropicacyl®: 0.5% (15 mL); 1% (15 mL) [contains benzalkonium chloride]

- **TT** *see* Tetanus Toxoid (Adsorbed) *on page 1366*
- **Tucks® Anti-Itch [OTC]** *see* Hydrocortisone *on page 699*
- **TVP-1012** *see* Rasagiline *on page 1236*
- **Twilite® [OTC]** *see* DiphenhydrAMINE *on page 430*
- **Twinject®** *see* EPINEPHrine *on page 492*
- **Twinrix®** *see* Hepatitis A Inactivated and Hepatitis B (Recombinant) Vaccine *on page 684*
- **Tycolene [OTC] [DSC]** *see* Acetaminophen *on page 25*
- **Tycolene Maximum Strength [OTC]** *see* Acetaminophen *on page 25*
- **Tygacil®** *see* Tigecycline *on page 1388*
- **Tylenol® [OTC]** *see* Acetaminophen *on page 25*
- **Tylenol® (Can)** *see* Acetaminophen *on page 25*
- **Tylenol #3** *see* Acetaminophen and Codeine *on page 29*
- **Tylenol® 8 Hour [OTC]** *see* Acetaminophen *on page 25*
- **Tylenol® Arthritis Pain Extended Relief [OTC]** *see* Acetaminophen *on page 25*
- **Tylenol® Children's [OTC]** *see* Acetaminophen *on page 25*
- **Tylenol® Children's Meltaways [OTC]** *see* Acetaminophen *on page 25*
- **Tylenol Elixir with Codeine (Can)** *see* Acetaminophen and Codeine *on page 29*
- **Tylenol® Extra Strength [OTC]** *see* Acetaminophen *on page 25*
- **Tylenol® Infant's Concentrated [OTC]** *see* Acetaminophen *on page 25*
- **Tylenol® Jr. Meltaways [OTC]** *see* Acetaminophen *on page 25*
- **Tylenol No. 1 (Can)** *see* Acetaminophen and Codeine *on page 29*
- **Tylenol No. 1 Forte (Can)** *see* Acetaminophen and Codeine *on page 29*
- **Tylenol No. 2 with Codeine (Can)** *see* Acetaminophen and Codeine *on page 29*
- **Tylenol No. 3 with Codeine (Can)** *see* Acetaminophen and Codeine *on page 29*
- **Tylenol No. 4 with Codeine (Can)** *see* Acetaminophen and Codeine *on page 29*

- **Tylenol® with Codeine No. 3** *see* Acetaminophen and Codeine *on page* 29
- **Tylenol® with Codeine No. 4** *see* Acetaminophen and Codeine *on page* 29
- **Tylox®** *see* Oxycodone and Acetaminophen *on page* 1072
- **Tysabri®** *see* Natalizumab *on page* 989
- **Tyvaso™** *see* Treprostinil *on page* 1425
- **UCB-P071** *see* Cetirizine *on page* 282
- **UK** *see* Urokinase *on page* 1438
- **UK92480** *see* Sildenafil *on page* 1287
- **UK109496** *see* Voriconazole *on page* 1474
- **Ulcidine (Can)** *see* Famotidine *on page* 575
- **Ultane®** *see* Sevoflurane *on page* 1283
- **Ultiva®** *see* Remifentanil *on page* 1239
- **Ultram®** *see* TraMADol *on page* 1415
- **Ultram® ER** *see* TraMADol *on page* 1415
- **Ultraprin [OTC]** *see* Ibuprofen *on page* 717
- **Unasyn®** *see* Ampicillin and Sulbactam *on page* 118
- **Unburn®** *see* Lidocaine *on page* 836
- **Unipen® (Can)** *see* Nafcillin *on page* 975
- **Uniphyl®** *see* Theophylline *on page* 1373
- **Uniphyl® SRT (Can)** *see* Theophylline *on page* 1373
- **Unisom® SleepGels® Maximum Strength [OTC]** *see* DiphenhydrAMINE *on page* 430
- **Unisom® SleepMelts™ [OTC]** *see* DiphenhydrAMINE *on page* 430
- **Unithroid®** *see* Levothyroxine *on page* 831
- **Univasc®** *see* Moexipril *on page* 948

Urokinase (ur oh KYE nase)

Medication Safety Issues
High alert medication: The Institute for Safe Medication Practices (ISMP) includes this medication among its list of drugs which have a heightened risk of causing significant patient harm when used in error.

U.S. Brand Names Kinlytic™

Index Terms Abbokinase; UK

Pharmacologic Category Thrombolytic Agent

Generic Available No

Use Thrombolytic agent for the lysis of acute massive pulmonary emboli or pulmonary emboli with unstable hemodynamics

Unlabeled/Investigational Use Thrombolytic agent used in treatment of recent severe or massive deep vein thrombosis, and occluded I.V. or dialysis cannulas; peripheral arterial occlusive disease

Mechanism of Action Promotes thrombolysis by directly activating plasminogen to plasmin, which degrades fibrin, fibrinogen, and other procoagulant plasma proteins

Pharmacodynamics/Kinetics
Onset of action: I.V.: Fibrinolysis occurs rapidly

Duration: ≥4 hours

Distribution: 11.5 L

Half-life elimination: 6.4-18.8 minutes

Excretion: Urine and feces (small amounts)

Dosage
Children and Adults: Deep vein thrombosis (unlabeled use): I.V.: Loading: 4400 units/kg over 10 minutes, then 4400 units/kg/hour for 12 hours

Adults:

Acute pulmonary embolism: I.V.: Loading: 4400 int. units/kg over 10 minutes; maintenance: 4400 int. units/kg/hour for 12 hours. To prevent recurrent thrombosis, anticoagulation treatment is recommended after the completion of urokinase infusion; if heparin is used, do not administer heparin loading dose. Do not start anticoagulation until aPTT has decreased to less than twice the normal control value.

Acute peripheral arterial occlusion of leg (unlabeled use; Ouriel, 1998): I.V.: 4000 int. units/minute for 4 hours, followed by 2000 int. units/minute for up to a total duration of therapy of 48 hours. **Note:** Systemic heparinization should not be given concurrently.

Occluded I.V. catheters (unlabeled use):

5000 units in each lumen over 1-2 minutes, leave in lumen for 1-4 hours, then aspirate; may repeat with 10,000 units in each lumen if 5000 units fails to clear the catheter; **do not infuse into the patient**; volume to instill into catheter is equal to the volume of the catheter

I.V. infusion: 200 units/kg/hour in each lumen for 12-48 hours at a rate of at least 20 mL/hour

Dialysis patients: 5000 units is administered in each lumen over 1-2 minutes; leave urokinase in lumen for 1-2 days, then aspirate

Stability Prior to reconstitution, store in refrigerator at 2°C to 8°C (36°F to 46°F). Reconstitute vial with 5 mL preservative free sterile water for injection by gently rolling and tilting; do not shake. Contains no preservatives; should not be reconstituted until immediately before using. Discard unused portion. Solution will look pale and straw colored. May filter through ≤0.45 micron filter. Prior to infusion, solution should be further diluted in D_5W or NS; the manufacturer recommends a total infusion volume of 195 mL.

Administration Solution may be filtered with ≤0.45 micron filter during I.V. therapy. Administer using an infusion pump. When prepared to a total volume of 195 mL, the loading dose should be administered at 90 mL/hour over 10 minutes. The maintenance dose should be administered at 15 mL/hour over 12 hours. I.V. tubing should be flushed with NS or D_5W to ensure total dose is administered.

Monitoring Parameters Blood pressure (avoid using lower extremities for BP), pulse; CBC, platelet count, aPTT, urinalysis

Anesthesia and Critical Care Concerns/Other Considerations
Evidence-Based Information:

Acute Pulmonary Embolism (PE): The American College of Chest Physicians (Kearon, 2008) recommends the following:

All patients with acute PE: All patients with diagnosed PE should undergo rapid risk stratification based on risk of death from PE and bleeding. In general, the majority of patients with PE will not require treatment with thrombolytics; however, treatment with anticoagulation (eg, enoxaparin, heparin) will be necessary unless contraindicated.

Patients with acute PE without hemodynamic compromise: In general, patients without hemodynamic compromise should not receive thrombolytic therapy. However, patients without hemodynamic compromise but with poor prognostic indicators (elevated troponin, right ventricular dysfunction on echocardiogram, etc) are at high risk of an adverse outcome and may derive benefit from receiving systemic thrombolysis. Therefore, the most recent recommendation is to administer thrombolysis in these selected high-risk patients who have a low risk of bleeding. The use of regimens with short infusion times (eg, 2-hour infusion) is recommended over longer infusion times (eg, 12-hour infusions). The most widely used thrombolytic for this indication is alteplase which is administered as an infusion of 100 mg over 2 hours. Urokinase may also be used; however, the administration time for urokinase is 12 hours.

Patients with acute PE with hemodynamic compromise: Since thrombolytic therapy has been shown to accelerate thrombolysis resulting in more rapid resolution of perfusion scan abnormalities, decrement angiographic thrombus, reduction in elevated pulmonary artery pressures, and normalization of right ventricular dysfunction in patients with PE and hemodynamic compromise (usually defined as SBP <90 mm Hg requiring vasopressor therapy), the use of thrombolytic therapy via a peripheral vein is recommended unless major contraindications exist. The use of regimens with short infusion times (eg, 2-hour infusion) is recommended over longer infusion times (eg, 12-hour infusions). The most widely used thrombolytic for this indication is alteplase which is

◄ administered as an infusion of 100 mg over 2 hours. Urokinase may also be used; however, the administration time for urokinase is 12 hours.

Patients with PE experiencing cardiac arrest: According to the 2005 ACLS guidelines, when PE is responsible for cardiac arrest and the patient is unresponsive to cardiopulmonary resuscitation (CPR), it is reasonable to administer bolus thrombolytic therapy, specifically alteplase (Böttiger, 2001). However, routine use in cardiac arrest or undifferentiated pulseless electrical activity (PEA) is not recommended. Of note, ongoing CPR is not a contra-indication in this setting.

Pregnancy Risk Factor B

Contraindications Hypersensitivity to urokinase or any component of the formulation; active internal bleeding; recent (within 2 months) CVA, intracranial surgery or intraspinal surgery; recent trauma (including cardiopulmonary resuscitation); intracranial neoplasm, arteriovenous malformation, or aneurysm; known bleeding diathesis; severe uncontrolled arterial hypertension

Warnings/Precautions The risk of bleeding is increased with use; fatal hemorrhage has been reported. Concurrent heparin anticoagulation can contribute to bleeding; careful attention to all potential bleeding sites. I.M. injections and nonessential handling of the patient should be avoided. Venipunctures should be performed carefully and only when necessary. If arterial puncture is necessary, use an upper extremity vessel that can be manually compressed. If serious bleeding occurs, then the infusion of urokinase and heparin should be stopped.

For the following conditions, the risk of bleeding is higher with use of thrombolytics and should be weighed against the benefits of therapy: recent (within 10 days) major surgery, obstetrical delivery, organ biopsy, or previous puncture of noncompressible vessels; pregnancy, cerebrovascular disease, recent (within 10 days) gastrointestinal bleeding, high likelihood of left heart thrombus (in the setting of mitral stenosis with atrial fibrillation), subacute bacterial endocarditis, hemostatic defects including those caused by severe renal or hepatic dysfunction, diabetic hemorrhagic retinopathy, and/or any other condition in which bleeding constitutes a significant hazard or would be particularly difficult to manage because of location. Use is contraindicated in recent trauma, including CPR. Use with caution in patients receiving oral anticoagulants or platelet inhibitors; increased risk of bleeding. Cholesterol embolization has been reported rarely with the use of thrombolytics, usually associated with invasive vascular procedures and/or anticoagulant therapy. Hypersensitivity reactions, including fatal anaphylaxis (rare), bronchospasm, orolingual edema and urticaria have been reported. Infusion reactions (eg, chills, rigor, hypoxia, hyper-/hypotension, tachycardia) may also occur. Reactions usually occur within the first hour of infusion. Safety and efficacy in pediatric patients have not been established.

Adverse Reactions As with all drugs which may affect hemostasis, bleeding is the major adverse effect associated with urokinase. Hemorrhage may occur at virtually any site. Risk is dependent on multiple variables, including the dosage administered, concurrent use of multiple agents which alter hemostasis, and patient predisposition.

>10%: Local: Injection site: Bleeding (5% decrease in hematocrit reported in 37% patients; most bleeding occurring at external incisions or injection sites, but also reported in other areas)

<1% (Limited to important or life-threatening): Allergic reaction (includes anaphylaxis, bronchospasm, orolingual edema, urticaria, skin rash, pruritus), cardiac arrest, cerebral vascular accident, chest pain, cholesterol embolism, diaphoresis, hemiplegia, intracranial hemorrhage, retroperitoneal hemorrhage, MI, pulmonary edema, recurrent pulmonary embolism, reperfusion ventricular arrhythmia, stroke, substernal pain, thrombocytopenia, vascular embolization (cerebral and distal); infusion reactions (most occurring within 1 hour) including acidosis, back pain, chills, cyanosis, dyspnea, fever, hyper-/hypotension, hypoxia, nausea, rigors, tachycardia, vomiting

Drug Interactions

Avoid Concomitant Use There are no known interactions where it is recommended to avoid concomitant use.

Increased Effect/Toxicity

Urokinase may increase the levels/effects of: Anticoagulants; Drotrecogin Alfa

The levels/effects of Urokinase may be increased by: Antiplatelet Agents; Herbs (Anticoagulant/Antiplatelet Properties); Nonsteroidal Anti-Inflammatory Agents; Salicylates

Decreased Effect

The levels/effects of Urokinase may be decreased by: Aprotinin

Product Availability

Kinlytic™: ImaRx Therapeutics retired the trade name Abbokinase® for urokinase and had intended to market urokinase under the trade name Kinlytic™. As of September, 2009, Microbix Biosystems, Inc. has acquired all rights to Kinlytic™, but have not yet gained FDA approval so no product is available.

- ◆ **Uromax® (Can)** *see* Oxybutynin *on page 1068*
- ◆ **Utradol™ (Can)** *see* Etodolac *on page 562*
- ◆ **Vagifem®** *see* Estradiol *on page 531*

Valacyclovir (val ay SYE kloe veer)

U.S. Brand Names Valtrex®

Canadian Brand Names Apo-Valacyclovir®; PMS-Valacyclovir; Pro-Valacyclovir; Riva-Valacyclovir; Valtrex®

Index Terms Valacyclovir Hydrochloride

Pharmacologic Category Antiviral Agent; Antiviral Agent, Oral

Use Treatment of herpes zoster (shingles) in immunocompetent patients; treatment of first-episode and recurrent genital herpes; suppression of recurrent genital herpes and reduction of heterosexual transmission of genital herpes in immunocompetent patients; suppression of genital herpes in HIV-infected individuals; treatment of herpes labialis (cold sores); chickenpox in immunocompetent children

Unlabeled/Investigational Use Prophylaxis of cancer-related HSV, VZV, and CMV infections; treatment of cancer-related HSV, VZV infection

Pharmacodynamics/Kinetics

Absorption: Rapid

Distribution: Acyclovir is widely distributed throughout the body including brain, kidney, lungs, liver, spleen, muscle, uterus, vagina, and CSF

Protein binding: ~14% to 18%

Metabolism: Hepatic; valacyclovir is rapidly and nearly completely converted to acyclovir and L-valine by first-pass effect; acyclovir is hepatically metabolized to a very small extent by aldehyde oxidase and by alcohol and aldehyde dehydrogenase (inactive metabolites)

Bioavailability: ~55% once converted to acyclovir

Half-life elimination: Normal renal function: Adults: Acyclovir: 2.5-3.3 hours, Valacyclovir: ~30 minutes; End-stage renal disease: Acyclovir: 14-20 hours; During hemodialysis: 4 hours

Excretion: Urine, primarily as acyclovir (89%); **Note:** Following oral administration of radiolabeled valacyclovir, 46% of the label is eliminated in the feces (corresponding to nonabsorbed drug), while 47% of the radiolabel is eliminated in the urine.

Dosage Oral:

Children 2 to <18 years: Chickenpox: 20 mg/kg/dose 3 times/day for 5 days (maximum: 1 g 3 times/day)

Children ≥12 and Adults: Herpes labialis (cold sores): 2 g twice daily for 1 day (separate doses by ~12 hours)

Adults:

CMV prophylaxis in allogeneic HSCT recipients (unlabeled use): 2 g 4 times/day

Herpes zoster (shingles): 1 g 3 times/day for 7 days

HSV, VZV in cancer patients (unlabeled use): Prophylaxis: 500 mg 2-3 times/day; Treatment: 1 g 3 times/day

Genital herpes:

Initial episode: 1 g twice daily for 10 days

Recurrent episode: 500 mg twice daily for 3 days

◀ Reduction of transmission: 500 mg once daily (source partner)
Suppressive therapy:
Immunocompetent patients: 1000 mg once daily (500 mg once daily in patients with <9 recurrences per year)
HIV-infected patients (CD4 ≥100 cells/mm^3): 500 mg twice daily

Dosing adjustment in renal impairment:
Herpes zoster: Adults:
Cl_{cr} 30-49 mL/minute: 1 g every 12 hours
Cl_{cr} 10-29 mL/minute: 1 g every 24 hours
Cl_{cr} <10 mL/minute: 500 mg every 24 hours
Genital herpes: Adults:
Initial episode:
Cl_{cr} 10-29 mL/minute: 1 g every 24 hours
Cl_{cr} <10 mL/minute: 500 mg every 24 hours
Recurrent episode: Cl_{cr} <29 mL/minute: 500 mg every 24 hours
Suppressive therapy: Cl_{cr} <29 mL/minute:
For usual dose of 1 g every 24 hours, decrease dose to 500 mg every 24 hours
For usual dose of 500 mg every 24 hours, decrease dose to 500 mg every 48 hours
HIV-infected patients: 500 mg every 24 hours
Herpes labialis: Adolescents and Adults:
Cl_{cr} 30-49 mL/minute: 1 g every 12 hours for 2 doses
Cl_{cr} 10-29 mL/minute: 500 mg every 12 hours for 2 doses
Cl_{cr} <10 mL/minute: 500 mg as a single dose
Hemodialysis: Dialyzable (~33% removed during 4-hour session); administer dose postdialysis
Chronic ambulatory peritoneal dialysis/continuous arteriovenous hemofiltration dialysis: Pharmacokinetic parameters are similar to those in patients with ESRD; supplemental dose not needed following dialysis

Dosing adjustment in hepatic impairment: No adjustment required.

Additional Information Complete prescribing information for this medication should be consulted for additional detail.

Dosage Forms Excipient information presented when available (limited, particularly for generics); consult specific product labeling.
Caplet:
Valtrex®: 500 mg, 1000 mg

References
Acosta EP and Fletcher CV, "Valacyclovir," *Ann Pharmacother*, 1997, 31(2):185-91.

Alrabiah FA and Sacks SL, "New Antiherpesvirus Agents. Their Targets and Therapeutic Potential," *Drugs*, 1996, 52(1):17-32.

Beutner KR, Friedman DJ, Forszpaniak C, et al, "Valacyclovir Compared With Acyclovir for Improved Therapy for Herpes Zoster in Immunocompetent Adults," *Antimicrob Agents Chemother*, 1995, 39 (7):1546-53.

Bodsworth NJ, Crooks RJ, Borelli S, et al, "Valaciclovir Versus Aciclovir in Patients Initiated Treatment of Recurrent Genital Herpes: A Randomized, Double-Blind Clinical Trial. International Valaciclovir HSV Study Group," *Genitourin Med*, 1997, 73(2):110-6.

Grant DM, Mauskopf JA, Bell L, et al, "Comparison of Valacyclovir and Acyclovir for the Treatment of Herpes Zoster in Immunocompetent Patients Over 50 Years of Age: A Cost-Consequence Model," *Pharmacotherapy*, 1997, 17(2):333-41.

Patel R, Bodsworth NJ, Woolley P, et al, "Valaciclovir for the Suppression of Recurrent Genital HSV Infection: A Placebo Controlled Study of Once Daily Therapy. International Valaciclovir HSV Study Group," *Genitourin Med*, 1997, 73(2):105-9.

Perry CM and Faulds D, "Valaciclovir. A Review of Its Antiviral Activity, Pharmacokinetic Properties and Therapeutic Efficacy in Herpesvirus Infections," *Drugs*, 1996, 52(5):754-72.

Reitano M, Tyring S, Lang W, et al, "Valaciclovir for the Suppression of Recurrent Genital Herpes Simplex Virus Infection: A Large-Scale Dose Range-Finding Study. International Valaciclovir HSV Study Group," *J Infect Dis*, 1998, 178(3):603-10.

Tyring SK, Douglas JM Jr, Corey L, et al, "A Randomized, Placebo-Controlled Comparison of Oral Valacyclovir and Acyclovir in Immunocompetent Patients With Recurrent Genital Herpes Infections. The Valaciclovir International Study Group," *Arch Dermatol*, 1998, 134(2):185-91.

"Valacyclovir," *Med Lett Drugs Ther*, 1996, 38(965):3-4.

Weller S, Blum MR, Doucette M, et al, "Pharmacokinetics of the Acyclovir Prodrug Valaciclovir After Escalating Single- and Multiple-Dose Administration to Normal Volunteers," *Clin Pharmacol Ther*, 1993, 54(6):595-605.

◆ **Valacyclovir Hydrochloride** see Valacyclovir on page 1441

◆ **Valcyte®** see Valganciclovir on page 1443

Valganciclovir (val gan SYE kloh veer)

Medication Safety Issues
Sound-alike/look-alike issues:
Valcyte® may be confused with Valium®, Valtrex®
ValGANCIclovir may be confused with valACYclovir

U.S. Brand Names Valcyte®

Canadian Brand Names Valcyte®

Index Terms Valganciclovir Hydrochloride

Pharmacologic Category Antiviral Agent

Generic Available No

Use
Treatment of cytomegalovirus (CMV) retinitis in patients with acquired immunodeficiency syndrome (AIDS); prevention of CMV disease in high-risk patients (donor CMV positive/recipient CMV negative) undergoing kidney, heart, or kidney/pancreas transplantation

Mechanism of Action
Valganciclovir is rapidly converted to ganciclovir in the body. The bioavailability of ganciclovir from valganciclovir is increased 10-fold compared to oral ganciclovir. A dose of 900 mg achieved systemic exposure of ganciclovir comparable to that achieved with the recommended doses of intravenous ganciclovir of 5 mg/kg. Ganciclovir is phosphorylated to a substrate which competitively inhibits the binding of deoxyguanosine triphosphate to DNA polymerase resulting in inhibition of viral DNA synthesis.

Pharmacodynamics/Kinetics
Absorption: Well absorbed; high-fat meal increases AUC by 30%

Distribution: V_{dss}: Ganciclovir: 0.7 L/kg; widely to all tissue including CSF and ocular tissue

Protein binding: Ganciclovir: 1% to 2%

Metabolism: Converted to ganciclovir by intestinal mucosal cells and hepatocytes

Bioavailability: With food: 60%

Half-life elimination: Ganciclovir: 4.08 hours; prolonged with renal impairment; Severe renal impairment: Up to 68 hours

Time to peak: Ganciclovir: 1-3 hours

Excretion: Urine (primarily as ganciclovir)

Dosage Oral:
Children 4 months to 16 years: Prevention of CMV disease following kidney or heart transplantation: Dose (mg) = 7 x body surface area x creatinine clearance* once daily beginning within 10 days of transplantation; continue therapy until 100 days post-transplantation. Doses should be rounded to the nearest 25 mg increment; maximum dose: 900 mg/day.

*Cl_{cr} (mL/minute/1.73 m^2) = [k x Height (cm)] divided by serum creatinine (mg/dL)

Note: Calculated using *modified* Schwartz formula where k is as follows:
Patients <2 years: k = 0.45
Girls 2-16 years: k = 0.55
Boys 2 to <13 years: k = 0.55
Boys 13-16 years: k = 0.7

Children >16 years and Adults:
CMV retinitis:
Induction: 900 mg twice daily for 21 days
Maintenance: Following induction treatment, or for patients with inactive CMV retinitis who require maintenance therapy: 900 mg once daily
Prevention of CMV disease following transplantation: 900 mg once daily beginning within 10 days of transplantation; continue therapy until 100 days post-transplantation

Dosage adjustment in renal impairment:
Children 4 months to 16 years: No additional dosage adjustments required; calculation for all patients adjusts for renal function.

Children >16 years and Adults:
Induction dose:
Cl_{cr} 40-59 mL/minute: 450 mg twice daily
Cl_{cr} 25-39 mL/minute: 450 mg once daily
Cl_{cr} 10-24 mL/minute: 450 mg every 2 days

Maintenance dose:
Cl_{cr} 40-59 mL/minute: 450 mg once daily
Cl_{cr} 25-39 mL/minute: 450 mg every 2 days
Cl_{cr} 10-24 mL/minute: 450 mg twice weekly
Note: Valganciclovir is not recommended in patients receiving hemodialysis. For patients on hemodialysis (Cl_{cr} <10 mL/minute), it is recommended that ganciclovir be used (dose adjusted as specified for ganciclovir).

Stability

Oral solution: Store dry powder at 25°C (77°F); excursions permitted to 15°C to 30°C (59°F to 86°F). Prior to dispensing, prepare the oral solution by adding 91 mL of purified water to the bottle; shake well. Store oral solution under refrigeration at 2°C to 8°C (36°F to 46°F); do not freeze. Discard any unused medication after 49 days. A reconstituted 100 mL bottle will only provide 88 mL of solution for administration.

Tablet: Store at 25°C (77°F); excursions permitted to 15°C to 30°C (59°F to 86°F).

Administration Valganciclovir should be taken with meals. The preferred dosage form for pediatric patients is the oral solution; however, valganciclovir tablets may used so long as the calculated dose is within 10% of the available tablet strength (450 mg).

Due to the carcinogenic and mutagenic potential, avoid direct contact with broken or crushed tablets, powder for oral solution, and oral solution. Consideration should be given to handling and disposal according to guidelines issued for antineoplastic drugs. However, there is no consensus on the need for these precautions.

Monitoring Parameters Retinal exam (at least every 4-6 weeks), CBC, platelet counts, serum creatinine

Pregnancy Risk Factor C

Contraindications Hypersensitivity to valganciclovir, ganciclovir, or any component of the formulation; absolute neutrophil count <500/mm^3; platelet count <25,000/mm^3; hemoglobin <8 g/dL

Warnings/Precautions Hazardous agent - use appropriate precautions for handling and disposal. **[U.S. Boxed Warning]: May cause dose- or therapy-limiting granulocytopenia, anemia, and/or thrombocytopenia;** use caution in patients with impaired renal function (dose adjustment required). **[U.S. Boxed Warning]: Ganciclovir may be teratogenic, carcinogenic, and cause aspermatogenesis.** Due to its teratogenic potential, contraceptive precautions for female and male patients need to be followed during and for at least 90 days after therapy with the drug. Fertility may be temporarily or permanently impaired in males and females. Due to differences in bioavailability, valganciclovir tablets cannot be substituted for ganciclovir capsules on a one-to-one basis. The preferred dosage form for pediatric patients is the oral solution; however, valganciclovir tablets may used so long as the calculated dose is within 10% of the available tablet strength (450 mg). Not indicated for use in liver transplant patients (higher incidence of tissue-invasive CMV relative to oral ganciclovir was observed in trials). Use of valganciclovir for the treatment of congenital CMV disease has not been evaluated.

Adverse Reactions

>10%:
Cardiovascular: Hypertension (18%)
Central nervous system: Fever (13% to 31%), headache (9% to 22%), insomnia (16% to 20%)
Gastrointestinal: Diarrhea (16% to 41%), nausea (8% to 30%), vomiting (16% to 21%), abdominal pain (15%), constipation
Hematologic: Anemia (8% to 26%), neutropenia (11% to 19%)
Neuromuscular & skeletal: Tremor (28%)
Ocular: Retinal detachment (15%)
Respiratory: Cough, upper respiratory tract infection
5% to 10%:
Central nervous system: Peripheral neuropathy (9%), paresthesia (8%)
Hematologic: Thrombocytopenia (6%)
<5%:
Cardiovascular: Edema, hypotension, peripheral edema

Central nervous system: Agitation, confusion, depression, dizziness, fatigue, hallucination, pain, psychosis, seizure

Dermatologic: Acne, dermatitis, pruritus

Endocrine & metabolic: Dehydration, hyperglycemia, hyper-/hypokalemia, hypocalcemia, hypomagnesemia, hypophosphatemia

Gastrointestinal: Abdominal distention/pain, appetite (decreased), dyspepsia

Genitourinary: Urinary tract infection

Hematologic: Aplastic anemia, bleeding (potentially life-threatening due to thrombocytopenia), bone marrow depression, pancytopenia

Hepatic: Ascites

Neuromuscular & skeletal: Arthralgia, back pain, limb pain, muscle cramps, weakness

Renal: Creatinine clearance (decreased), dysuria, renal impairment

Respiratory: Dyspnea, nasopharyngitis, pharyngitis, pleural effusion, rhinorrhea

Miscellaneous: Allergic reaction, local and systemic infection (including sepsis)

<1% (Limited to important or life-threatening): Valganciclovir is expected to share the toxicities which may occur at a low incidence or due to idiosyncratic reactions which have been associated with ganciclovir

Drug Interactions

Avoid Concomitant Use There are no known interactions where it is recommended to avoid concomitant use.

Increased Effect/Toxicity

ValGANCIclovir may increase the levels/effects of: Mycophenolate; Reverse Transcriptase Inhibitors (Nucleoside); Tenofovir

The levels/effects of ValGANCIclovir may be increased by: Mycophenolate

Decreased Effect There are no known significant interactions involving a decrease in effect.

Ethanol/Nutrition/Herb Interactions Food: Coadministration with a high-fat meal increased AUC by 30%.

Dietary Considerations Should be taken with meals.

Product Availability

Valcyte® oral solution: FDA approved August 2009; availability expected January 2010

Dosage Forms Excipient information presented when available (limited, particularly for generics); consult specific product labeling.

Powder for suspension, oral:

Valcyte®: 50 mg/mL (100 mL) [contains sodium benzoate; tutti-frutti flavor]

Tablet, oral:

Valcyte®: 450 mg

◆ **Valganciclovir Hydrochloride** *see* Valganciclovir *on page 1443*

◆ **Valisone® Scalp Lotion (Can)** *see* Betamethasone *on page 186*

◆ **Valium®** *see* Diazepam *on page 409*

◆ **Valorin [OTC]** *see* Acetaminophen *on page 25*

◆ **Valorin Extra [OTC]** *see* Acetaminophen *on page 25*

◆ **Valproate Semisodium** *see* Valproic Acid and Derivatives *on page 1445*

◆ **Valproate Sodium** *see* Valproic Acid and Derivatives *on page 1445*

◆ **Valproic Acid** *see* Valproic Acid and Derivatives *on page 1445*

Valproic Acid and Derivatives (val PROE ik AS id & dah RIV ah tives)

Medication Safety Issues

Sound-alike/look-alike issues:

Depakene® may be confused with Depakote®

Depakote® may be confused with Depakene®, Depakote® ER, Senokot®

Depakote® ER may be confused with Depakote®, divalproex enteric coated

◀ **Related Information**

Chronic Pain Management *on page 1546*
Chronic Renal Failure *on page 1552*
Perioperative Management of Patients on Antiseizure Medication *on page 1577*
Porphyria: Safe and Unsafe Drugs *on page 1800*
Status Epilepticus *on page 1737*

U.S. Brand Names Depacon®; Depakene®; Depakote®; Depakote® ER; Depakote® Sprinkle; Stavzor™

Canadian Brand Names Alti-Divalproex; Apo-Divalproex®; Apo-Valproic®; Depakene®; Dom-Divalproex; Epival® I.V.; Gen-Divalproex; Mylan-Divalproex; Mylan-Valproic; Novo-Divalproex; Nu-Divalproex; PHL-Divalproex; PHL-Valproic Acid; PHL-Valproic Acid E.C.; PMS-Valproic Acid; PMS-Valproic Acid E.C.; ratio-Valproic; ratio-Valproic ECC; Rhoxal-valproic; Sandoz-Valproic

Index Terms 2-Propylpentanoic Acid; 2-Propylvaleric Acid; Dipropylacetic Acid; Divalproex Sodium; DPA; Valproate Semisodium; Valproate Sodium; Valproic Acid

Pharmacologic Category Anticonvulsant, Miscellaneous; Antimanic Agent; Histone Deacetylase Inhibitor

Generic Available Yes: Excludes capsule (softgel/delayed release)

Use

Depacon®, Depakene®, Depakote®, Depakote® ER, Depakote® Sprinkle, Stavzor™: Monotherapy and adjunctive therapy in the treatment of patients with complex partial seizures; monotherapy and adjunctive therapy of simple and complex absence seizures; adjunctive therapy in patients with multiple seizure types that include absence seizures

Depakote®, Depakote® ER, Stavzor™: Mania associated with bipolar disorder; migraine prophylaxis

Unlabeled/Investigational Use Status epilepticus

Mechanism of Action Causes increased availability of gamma-aminobutyric acid (GABA), an inhibitory neurotransmitter, to brain neurons or may enhance the action of GABA or mimic its action at postsynaptic receptor sites

Pharmacodynamics/Kinetics

Distribution: Total valproate: 11 L/1.73 m^2; free valproate 92 L/1.73 m^2

Protein binding (dose dependent): 80% to 90%; decreased in the elderly and with hepatic or renal dysfunction

Metabolism: Extensively hepatic via glucuronide conjugation and mitochondrial beta-oxidation. The relationship between dose and total valproate concentration is nonlinear; concentration does not increase proportionally with the dose, but increases to a lesser extent due to saturable plasma protein binding. The kinetics of unbound drug are linear.

Bioavailability: Depakote® ER: ~90% relative to I.V. dose and ~89% relative to delayed release formulation

Half-life elimination (increased in neonates and with liver disease): Children >2 months: 7-13 hours; Adults: 9-16 hours

Time to peak, serum: Depakote® tablet: ~4 hours; Depakote® ER: 4-17 hours; Stavzor™: 2 hours

Excretion: Urine (30% to 50% as glucuronide conjugate, 3% as unchanged drug)

Dosage

Seizure disorders: **Note:** Administer doses >250 mg/day in divided doses.

Oral:

Simple and complex absence seizures: Children and Adults: Initial: 15 mg/kg/day; increase by 5-10 mg/kg/day at weekly intervals until therapeutic levels are achieved; maximum: 60 mg/kg/day. Larger maintenance doses may be required in younger children.

Complex partial seizures: Children ≥10 years and Adults: Initial: 10-15 mg/kg/day; increase by 5-10 mg/kg/day at weekly intervals until therapeutic levels are achieved; maximum: 60 mg/kg/day. Larger maintenance doses may be required in younger children.

Note: Regular release and delayed release formulations are usually given in 2-4 divided doses/day; extended release formulation (Depakote® ER) is usually given once daily. Conversion to Depakote® ER from a stable dose of Depakote® may require an increase in the total daily dose between 8% and

20% to maintain similar serum concentrations. Depakote® ER is not recommended for use in children <10 years of age.

I.V.: Administer as a 60-minute infusion (≤20 mg/minute) with the same frequency as oral products; switch patient to oral products as soon as possible. Rapid infusions ≤45 mg/kg over 5-10 minutes (1.5-6 mg/kg/minute) were generally well tolerated in a clinical trial.

Rectal (unlabeled): Dilute syrup 1:1 with water for use as a retention enema; loading dose: 17-20 mg/kg one time; maintenance: 10-15 mg/kg/dose every 8 hours

Status epilepticus (unlabeled use): Adults:
Loading dose: I.V.: 15-45 mg/kg administered at ≤6 mg/kg/minute.
Maintenance dose: I.V. infusion: 1-4 mg/kg/hour; titrate dose as needed based upon patient response and evaluation of drug-drug interactions

Mania: Adults: Oral:
Depakote® tablet, Stavzor™: Initial: 750 mg/day in divided doses; dose should be adjusted as rapidly as possible to desired clinical effect; maximum recommended dosage: 60 mg/kg/day
Depakote® ER: Initial: 25 mg/kg/day given once daily; dose should be adjusted as rapidly as possible to desired clinical effect; maximum recommended dose: 60 mg/kg/day.

Migraine prophylaxis:
Children ≥12 years (Stavzor™): 250 mg twice daily; adjust dose based on patient response, up to 1000 mg/day
Children ≥16 years and Adults: Oral:
Depakote® tablet: 250 mg twice daily; adjust dose based on patient response, up to 1000 mg/day
Depakote® ER: 500 mg once daily for 7 days, then increase to 1000 mg once daily; adjust dose based on patient response; usual dosage range 500-1000 mg/day

Elderly: Elimination is decreased in the elderly. Studies of elderly patients with dementia show a high incidence of somnolence. In some patients, this was associated with weight loss. Starting doses should be lower and increases should be slow, with careful monitoring of nutritional intake and dehydration. Safety and efficacy for use in patients >65 years have not been studied for migraine prophylaxis.

Dosing adjustment in renal impairment: A 27% reduction in clearance of unbound valproate is seen in patients with Cl_{cr} <10 mL/minute. Hemodialysis reduces valproate concentrations by 20%, therefore no dose adjustment is needed in patients with renal failure. Protein binding is reduced, monitoring only total valproate concentrations may be misleading.

Dosing adjustment/comments in hepatic impairment: Reduce dose. Clearance is decreased with liver impairment. Hepatic disease is also associated with decreased albumin concentrations and 2- to 2.6-fold increase in the unbound fraction. Free concentrations of valproate may be elevated while total concentrations appear normal. Use is contraindicated in severe impairment.

Stability

Depakote® tablet, Depakene® solution: Store below 30°C (86°F).
Depakote® Sprinkles: Store below 25°C (77°F).
Depakote® ER, Stavzor™: Store at controlled room temperature of 25°C (77°F).
Depakene® capsule: Store at controlled room temperature of 15°C to 25°C (59°F to 77°F).
Depacon®: Store vial at room temperature of 15°C to 30°C (59°F to 86°F). Injection should be diluted in 50 mL of a compatible diluent. Stable in D_5W, NS, and LR for at least 24 hours when stored in glass or PVC.

Administration

Depakote® ER: Swallow whole; do not crush or chew. Patients who need dose adjustments smaller than 500 mg/day for migraine prophylaxis should be changed to Depakote® delayed release tablets.
Depakote® Sprinkle capsules may be swallowed whole or open capsule and sprinkle on small amount (1 teaspoonful) of soft food and use immediately (do not store or chew).

◀ Depacon®: Following dilution to final concentration, administer over 60 minutes at a rate ≤20 mg/minute. Alternatively, single doses up to 45 mg/kg have been administered as a rapid infusion over 5-10 minutes (1.5-6 mg/kg/minute).

Depakene® capsule, Stavzor™: Swallow whole; do not chew.

Monitoring Parameters Liver enzymes (at baseline and during therapy), CBC with platelets (baseline and periodic intervals), PT/PTT (especially prior to surgery), serum ammonia (with symptoms of lethargy, mental status change), serum valproate levels; suicidality (eg, suicidal thoughts, depression, behavioral changes)

Reference Range

Therapeutic:

Epilepsy: 50-100 mcg/mL (SI: 350-690 µmol/L)

Mania: 85-125 mcg/mL (SI: 350-860 µmol/L)

Toxic: Some laboratories may report >200 mcg/mL (SI: >1390 µmol/L) as a toxic threshold, although clinical toxicity can occur at lower concentrations. Probability of thrombocytopenia increases with total valproate levels ≥110 mcg/mL in females or ≥135 mcg/mL in males.

Seizure control: May improve at levels >100 mcg/mL (SI: 690 µmol/L), but toxicity may occur at levels of 100-150 mcg/mL (SI: 690-1040 µmol/L)

Mania: Clinical response seen with trough levels between 85-125 mcg/mL; risk of toxicity increases at levels >125 mcg/mL

Anesthesia and Critical Care Concerns/Other Considerations Evidence-Based Information: Valproic acid may be used in pharmacologic treatment of refractory status epilepticus (Limdi, 2005; Meierkord, 2006). Intravenous infusions are generally well tolerated (Limdi, 2006; Limdi, 2007).

Pregnancy Risk Factor D

Contraindications Hypersensitivity to valproic acid, derivatives, or any component of the formulation; hepatic disease or significant impairment; urea cycle disorders

Warnings/Precautions

[U.S. Boxed Warning]: Hepatic failure resulting in fatalities has occurred in patients; children <2 years of age are at considerable risk. Other risk factors include organic brain disease, mental retardation with severe seizure disorders, congenital metabolic disorders, and patients on multiple anticonvulsants. Hepatotoxicity has usually been reported within 6 months of therapy initiation. Monitor patients closely for appearance of malaise, weakness, facial edema, anorexia, jaundice, and vomiting; discontinue immediately with signs/symptom of significant or suspected impairment. Liver function tests should be performed at baseline and at regular intervals after initiation of therapy, especially within the first 6 months. Hepatic dysfunction may progress despite discontinuing treatment. Should only be used as monotherapy in children <2 years of age and patients at high risk for hepatotoxicity. Contraindicated with severe impairment.

[U.S. Boxed Warning]: Cases of life-threatening pancreatitis, occurring at the start of therapy or following years of use, have been reported in adults and children. Some cases have been hemorrhagic with rapid progression of initial symptoms to death. Promptly evaluate symptoms of abdominal pain, nausea, vomiting, and/or anorexia; should generally be discontinued if pancreatitis is diagnosed.

[U.S. Boxed Warning]: May cause teratogenic effects such as neural tube defects (eg, spina bifida). Use in women of childbearing potential requires that benefits of use in mother be weighed against the potential risk to fetus, especially when used for conditions not associated with permanent injury or risk of death (eg, migraine).

May cause severe thrombocytopenia, inhibition of platelet aggregation, and bleeding. Tremors may indicate overdosage; use with caution in patients receiving other anticonvulsants. Hypersensitivity reactions affecting multiple organs have been reported in association with valproic acid use; may include dermatologic and/or hematologic changes (eosinophilia, neutropenia, thrombocytopenia) or symptoms of organ dysfunction.

Hyperammonemia and/or encephalopathy, sometimes fatal, have been reported following the initiation of valproic acid therapy and may be present with normal transaminase levels. Ammonia levels should be measured in patients who develop unexplained lethargy and vomiting, changes in mental status, or in patients who present with hypothermia (unintentional drop in core body temperature to <35°C/95°F). Discontinue therapy if ammonia levels are increased and evaluate for possible urea cycle disorder (UCD); contraindicated in patients with UCD. Evaluation of UCD should be considered for the following patients prior to the start of therapy: History of unexplained encephalopathy or coma; encephalopathy associated with protein load; pregnancy or postpartum encephalopathy; unexplained mental retardation; history of elevated plasma ammonia or glutamine; history of cyclical vomiting and lethargy; episodic extreme irritability, ataxia; low BUN or protein avoidance; family history of UCD or unexplained infant deaths (particularly male); or signs or symptoms of UCD (hyperammonemia, encephalopathy, respiratory alkalosis). Hypothermia has been reported with valproic acid therapy; may or may not be associated with hyperammonemia; may also occur with concomitant topiramate therapy.

In vitro studies have suggested valproic acid stimulates the replication of HIV and CMV viruses under experimental conditions. The clinical consequence of this is unknown, but should be considered when monitoring affected patients.

Antiepileptics are associated with an increased risk of suicidal behavior/thoughts with use (regardless of indication); patients should be monitored for signs/symptoms of depression, suicidal tendencies, and other unusual behavior changes during therapy and instructed to inform their healthcare provider immediately if symptoms occur.

Use of Depacon® injection is not recommended for post-traumatic seizure prophylaxis following acute head trauma. Anticonvulsants should not be discontinued abruptly because of the possibility of increasing seizure frequency; valproic acid should be withdrawn gradually to minimize the potential of increased seizure frequency, unless safety concerns require a more rapid withdrawal. Concomitant use with carbapenem antibiotics may reduce valproic acid levels to subtherapeutic levels; monitor levels frequently and consider alternate therapy if levels drop significantly or lack of seizure control occurs. Concomitant use with clonazepam may induce absence status. Patients treated for bipolar disorder should be monitored closely for clinical worsening or suicidality; prescriptions should be written for the smallest quantity consistent with good patient care.

CNS depression may occur with valproic acid use. Patients must be cautioned about performing tasks which require mental alertness (operating machinery or driving). Effects with other sedative drugs or ethanol may be potentiated. Use with caution in the elderly.

Adverse Reactions

>10%:
  Central nervous system: Headache (≤31%), somnolence (≤30%), dizziness (12% to 25%), insomnia (>1% to 15%), nervousness (>1% to 11%), pain (1% to 11%)
  Dermatologic: Alopecia (>1% to 24%)
  Gastrointestinal: Nausea (15% to 48%), vomiting (7% to 27%), diarrhea (7% to 23%), abdominal pain (7% to 23%), dyspepsia (7% to 23%), anorexia (>1% to 12%)
  Hematologic: Thrombocytopenia (1% to 24%; dose related)
  Neuromuscular & skeletal: Tremor (≤57%), weakness (6% to 27%)
  Ocular: Diplopia (>1% to 16%), amblyopia/blurred vision (≤12%)
  Miscellaneous: Infection (≤20%), flu-like syndrome (12%)
1% to 10%:
  Cardiovascular: Peripheral edema (>1% to 8%), chest pain (>1% to <5%), edema (>1% to <5%), facial edema (>1% to <5%), hypertension (>1% to <5%), hypotension (>1% to <5%), palpitation (>1% to <5%), postural hypotension (>1% to <5%), tachycardia (>1% to <5%), vasodilation (>1% to <5%), arrhythmia
  Central nervous system: Ataxia (>1% to 8%), amnesia (>1% to 7%), emotional lability (>1% to 6%), fever (>1% to 6%), abnormal thinking (≤6%), depression (>1% to 5%), abnormal dreams (>1% to <5%), agitation (>1% to <5%), anxiety (>1% to <5%), catatonia (>1% to <5%), chills (>1% to <5%), confusion (>1% to <5%), coordination abnormal (>1% to <5%), hallucination (>1% to <5%),

malaise (>1% to <5%), personality disorder (>1% to <5%), speech disorder (>1% to <5%), tardive dyskinesia (>1% to <5%), vertigo (>1% to <5%), euphoria (1%), hypoesthesia (1%)

Dermatologic: Rash (>1% to 6%), bruising (>1% to 5%), discoid lupus erythematosus (>1% to <5%), dry skin (>1% to <5%), furunculosis (>1% to <5%), petechia (>1% to <5%), pruritus (>1% to <5%), seborrhea (>1% to <5%)

Endocrine & metabolic: Amenorrhea (>1% to <5%), dysmenorrhea (>1% to <5%), metrorrhagia (>1% to <5%), hypoproteinemia

Gastrointestinal: Weight gain (4% to 9%), weight loss (6%), appetite increased (≤6%), constipation (>1% to 5%), xerostomia (>1% to 5%), eructation (>1% to <5%), fecal incontinence (>1% to <5%), flatulence (>1% to <5%), gastro-enteritis (>1% to <5%), glossitis (>1% to <5%), hematemesis (>1% to <5%), pancreatitis (>1% to <5%), periodontal abscess (>1% to <5%), stomatitis (>1% to <5%), taste perversion (>1% to <5%), dysphagia, gum hemorrhage, mouth ulceration

Genitourinary: Cystitis (>1% to 5%), dysuria (>1% to 5%), urinary frequency (>1% to <5%), urinary incontinence (>1% to <5%), vaginal hemorrhage (>1% to 5%), vaginitis (>1% to <5%)

Hepatic: ALT increased (>1% to <5%), AST increased (>1% to <5%)

Local: Injection site pain (3%), injection site reaction (2%), injection site inflammation (1%)

Neuromuscular & skeletal: Back pain (≤8%), abnormal gait (>1% to <5%), arthralgia (>1% to <5%), arthrosis (>1% to <5%), dysarthria (>1% to <5%), hypertonia (>1% to <5%), hypokinesia (>1% to <5%), leg cramps (>1% to <5%), myalgia (>1% to <5%), myasthenia (>1% to <5%), neck pain (>1% to <5%), neck rigidity (>1% to <5%), paresthesia (>1% to <5%), reflex increased (>1% to <5%), twitching (>1% to <5%)

Ocular: Nystagmus (1% to 8%), dry eyes (>1% to 5%), eye pain (>1% to 5%), abnormal vision (>1% to <5%), conjunctivitis (>1% to <5%)

Otic: Tinnitus (1% to 7%), ear pain (>1% to 5%), deafness (>1% to <5%), otitis media (>1% to <5%)

Respiratory: Pharyngitis (2% to 8%), bronchitis (5%), rhinitis (>1% to 5%), dyspnea (1% to 5%), cough (>1% to <5%), epistaxis (>1% to <5%), pneumonia (>1% to <5%), sinusitis (>1% to <5%)

Miscellaneous: Diaphoresis (1%), hiccups

<1% (Limited to important and/or life-threatening): Aggression, agranulocytosis, allergic reaction, anaphylaxis, anemia, aplastic anemia, asterixis, behavioral deterioration, bilirubin increased, bleeding time altered, bone marrow suppression, bone pain, bradycardia, breast enlargement, cutaneous vasculitis, carnitine decreased, cerebral atrophy (reversible), coma (rare), dementia, encephalopathy (rare), enuresis, eosinophilia, erythema multiforme, Fanconi-like syndrome (rare, in children), galactorrhea, hematoma formation, hemor-rhage, hepatic failure, hepatotoxicity, hostility, hyperactivity, hyperammonemia, hyperammonemic encephalopathy (in patients with UCD), hyperglycinemia, hypersensitivity reactions (severe, with multiorgan dysfunction), hypofibrinoge-nemia, hyponatremia, hypothermia, inappropriate ADH secretion, intermittent porphyria, LDH increased, leukopenia, lupus, lymphocytosis, macrocytosis, menstrual irregularities, pancytopenia parkinsonism, parotid gland swelling, photosensitivity, platelet aggregation inhibited, polycystic ovary disease (rare), psychosis, seeing "spots before the eyes," Stevens-Johnson syndrome, suicidal behavior/ideation, thyroid function tests abnormal, toxic epidermal necrolysis (rare), urinary tract infection

Drug Interactions

Metabolism/Transport Effects For valproic acid: **Substrate** (minor) of CYP2A6, 2B6, 2C9, 2C19, 2E1; **Inhibits** CYP2C9 (weak), 2C19 (weak), 2D6 (weak), 3A4 (weak); **Induces** CYP2A6 (weak)

Avoid Concomitant Use There are no known interactions where it is recommended to avoid concomitant use.

Increased Effect/Toxicity

Valproic Acid and Derivatives may increase the levels/effects of: Barbiturates; Ethosuximide; LamoTRIgine; LORazepam; Paliperidone; Primidone; Risper-idone; Rufinamide; Temozolomide; Tricyclic Antidepressants; Vorinostat; Zidovudine

The levels/effects of Valproic Acid and Derivatives may be increased by: ChlorproMAZINE; Felbamate; Salicylates; Topiramate

Decreased Effect

Valproic Acid and Derivatives may decrease the levels/effects of: Amino-camptothecin; CarBAMazepine; OXcarbazepine; Phenytoin

The levels/effects of Valproic Acid and Derivatives may be decreased by: Barbiturates; CarBAMazepine; Carbapenems; Ethosuximide; Methylfolate; Phenytoin; Primidone; Protease Inhibitors; Rifampin

Ethanol/Nutrition/Herb Interactions

Ethanol: Avoid ethanol (may increase CNS depression).

Food: Food may delay but does not affect the extent of absorption. Valproic acid serum concentrations may be decreased if taken with food. Milk has no effect on absorption.

Herb/Nutraceutical: Avoid evening primrose (seizure threshold decreased).

Test Interactions False-positive result for urine ketones; accuracy of thyroid function tests

Dietary Considerations Valproic acid may cause GI upset; take with large amount of water or food to decrease GI upset. May need to split doses to avoid GI upset.

Depakote® Sprinkle capsule contents may be mixed with semisolid food (eg, applesauce or pudding) in patients having difficulty swallowing; particles should be swallowed and not chewed.

Valproate sodium oral solution will generate valproic acid in carbonated beverages and may cause mouth and throat irritation; do not mix valproate sodium oral solution with carbonated beverages.

Dosage Forms Excipient information presented when available (limited, particularly for generics); consult specific product labeling. **Note:** Strength expressed as valproic acid

Capsule, softgel, as valproic acid: 250 mg

Depakene®: 250 mg

Capsule, softgel, delayed release, as valproic acid:

Stavzor™: 125 mg, 250 mg, 500 mg

Capsule, sprinkles, as divalproex sodium: 125 mg

Depakote® Sprinkle: 125 mg

Injection, solution, as valproate sodium: 100 mg/mL (5 mL)

Depacon®: 100 mg/mL (5 mL) [contains edetate disodium]

Syrup, as valproic acid: 250 mg/5 mL (5 mL, 10 mL, 480 mL)

Depakene®: 250 mg/5 mL (480 mL)

Tablet, delayed release, as divalproex sodium: 125 mg, 250 mg, 500 mg

Depakote®: 125 mg, 250 mg, 500 mg

Tablet, extended release, as divalproex sodium: 250 mg, 500 mg

Depakote® ER: 250 mg, 500 mg

References

Chez MG, Hammer MS, Loeffel M, et al, "Clinical Experience of Three Pediatric and One Adult Case of Spike-and-Wave Status Epilepticus Treated With Injectable Valproic Acid," *J Child Neurol*, 1999, 14(4):239-42.

Hovinga CA, Chicella MF, Rose DF, et al, "Use of Intravenous Valproate in Three Pediatric Patients With Nonconvulsive or Convulsive Status Epilepticus," *Ann Pharmacother*, 1999, 33(5):579-84.

Limdi NA, Knowlton RK, Cofield SS, et al, "Safety of Rapid Intravenous Loading of Valproate," *Epilepsia*, 2007, 48(3):478-83.

Limdi NA, Shimpi AV, Faught E, et al, "Efficacy of Rapid I.V. Administration of Valproic Acid for Status Epilepticus," *Neurology*, 2005, 64(2):353-5.

Manno EM, "New Management Strategies in the Treatment of Status Epilepticus," *Mayo Clin Proc*, 2003, 78(4):508-18.

Mehta V, Singhi P, and Singhi S, "Intravenous Sodium Valproate Versus Diazepam Infusion for the Control of Refractory Status Epilepticus in Children: A Randomized Controlled Trial," *J Child Neurology*, 2007, 22(10):1191-7.

Meierkord H, Boon P, Engelsen B, et al, "EFNS Guideline on the Management of Status Epilepticus," *Eur J Neurol*, 2006, 13(5):445-50.

Sinha S and Naritoku DK, "Intravenous Valproate is Well Tolerated in Unstable Patients With Status Epilepticus," *Neurology*, 2000, 55(5):722-4.

Venkataraman V and Wheless JW, "Safety of Rapid Intravenous Infusion of Valproate Loading Doses in Epilepsy Patients," *Epilepsy Res*, 1999, 35(2):147-53.

Valsartan (val SAR tan)

Related Information
Angiotensin Agents *on page 1652*
Heart Failure (Systolic) *on page 1739*
Preoperative Evaluation of the Cardiac Patient for Noncardiac Surgery *on page 1598*

U.S. Brand Names Diovan®
Canadian Brand Names Diovan®
Pharmacologic Category Angiotensin II Receptor Blocker

Use Alone or in combination with other antihypertensive agents in the treatment of essential hypertension; reduction of cardiovascular mortality in patients with left ventricular dysfunction postmyocardial infarction; treatment of heart failure (NYHA Class II-IV)

Pharmacodynamics/Kinetics
Onset of action: ~2 hours
Duration: 24 hours
Distribution: V_d: 17 L (adults)
Protein binding: 95%, primarily albumin
Metabolism: To inactive metabolite
Bioavailability: Tablet: 25% (range 10% to 35%); suspension: ~40% (~1.6 times more than tablet)
Half-life elimination: ~6 hours
Time to peak, serum: 2-4 hours
Excretion: Feces (83%) and urine (13%) as unchanged drug

Dosage Oral:
Hypertension:
Children 6-16 years: Initial: 1.3 mg/kg once daily (maximum: 40 mg/day); dose may be increased to achieve desired effect; doses >2.7 mg/kg (maximum: 160 mg) have not been studied
Adults: Initial: 80 mg or 160 mg once daily (in patients who are not volume depleted); dose may be increased to achieve desired effect; maximum recommended dose: 320 mg/day
Heart failure: Adults: Initial: 40 mg twice daily; titrate dose to 80-160 mg twice daily, as tolerated; maximum daily dose: 320 mg
Left ventricular dysfunction after MI: Adults: Initial: 20 mg twice daily; titrate dose to target of 160 mg twice daily as tolerated; may initiate ≥12 hours following MI

Dosing adjustment in renal impairment:
Children: Use is not recommended if Cl_{cr} <30 mL/minute.
Adults: No dosage adjustment necessary if Cl_{cr} >10 mL/minute.
Dialysis: Not significantly removed
Dosing adjustment in hepatic impairment In mild-to-moderate liver disease no adjustment is needed. Use caution in patients with liver disease. Patients with mild-to-moderate chronic disease have twice the exposure as healthy volunteers.

Anesthesia and Critical Care Concerns/Other Considerations
Clinical Pearls/Comments: In patients on chronic angiotensin receptor blocker (ARB) therapy, intraoperative hypotension may occur with induction and maintenance of general anesthesia; however, discontinuation of therapy prior to surgery is controversial. If continued preoperatively, avoidance of hypotensive agents during surgery is prudent. Episodes of intraoperative hypotension may be managed by fluid administration and/or modest doses of alpha-adrenergic agents. Severe hypotension may occur in patients who are sodium- and/or volume-depleted; initiate lower doses and monitor closely when starting therapy in these patients. ARB therapy may elicit an increase in potassium and creatinine, especially when used in patients with bilateral renal artery stenosis. Concomitant NSAID therapy may attenuate blood pressure control; use of NSAIDs should be avoided or limited, with monitoring of blood pressure control. In the setting of heart failure, NSAID use may be associated with an increased risk for fluid accumulation and edema and therefore should be avoided.

Evidence-Based Information: The angiotensin II receptor antagonists have similar indications as ACE inhibitors. In heart failure, the angiotensin II antagonists are especially useful in providing an alternative therapy in those patients who have intractable cough due to ACE inhibitor therapy. Candesartan has been studied as an alternative therapy in chronic heart failure patients who cannot tolerate an ACE-I (CHARM-Alternative) and as an added therapy in heart failure patients who are maintained on an ACE-I (CHARM-Added). In both studies, the combined endpoint of cardiovascular death or heart failure hospitalizations was significantly improved over the placebo-treated group.

Additional Information Complete prescribing information for this medication should be consulted for additional detail.

Dosage Forms Excipient information presented when available (limited, particularly for generics); consult specific product labeling.
Tablet:
Diovan®: 40 mg [scored]
Diovan®: 80 mg, 160 mg, 320 mg

◆ **Valtrex®** *see* Valacyclovir *on page 1441*
◆ **Vancocin®** *see* Vancomycin *on page 1453*

Vancomycin (van koe MYE sin)

Medication Safety Issues
Sound-alike/look-alike issues:
I.V. vancomycin may be confused with Invanz®
Vancomycin may be confused with clindamycin, gentamicin, tobramycin, valACYclovir, vecuronium, Vibramycin®

High alert medication: The Institute for Safe Medication Practices (ISMP) includes this medication (intrathecal administration) among its list of drug classes which have a heightened risk of causing significant patient harm when used in error.

Related Information
Anesthesia for Patients With Liver Disease *on page 1537*
Chronic Renal Failure *on page 1552*
Desensitization Protocols *on page 1692*
Dosing Considerations for the Critically-Ill Patient With Morbid Obesity *on page 1561*
Prevention of Infective Endocarditis *on page 1718*
Prevention of Wound Infection and Sepsis in Surgical Patients *on page 1721*

U.S. Brand Names Vancocin®

Canadian Brand Names Vancocin®

Index Terms Vancomycin Hydrochloride

Pharmacologic Category Antibiotic, Miscellaneous

Generic Available Yes: Injection

Use Treatment of patients with infections caused by staphylococcal species and streptococcal species; used orally for staphylococcal enterocolitis or for antibiotic-associated pseudomembranous colitis produced by *C. difficile*

Unlabeled/Investigational Use Bacterial endophthalmitis; treatment of infections caused by gram-positive organisms in patients who have serious allergies to beta-lactam agents; treatment of beta-lactam resistant gram-positive infections

Mechanism of Action Inhibits bacterial cell wall synthesis by blocking glycopeptide polymerization through binding tightly to D-alanyl-D-alanine portion of cell wall precursor

Pharmacodynamics/Kinetics
Absorption: Oral: Poor; I.M.: Erratic; Intraperitoneal: ~38%
Distribution: V_d: 0.4-1 L/kg; Distributes widely in body tissue and fluids, except for CSF
Relative diffusion from blood into CSF: Good only with inflammation (exceeds usual MICs)
Uninflamed meninges: 0-4 mcg/mL; serum concentration dependent
Inflamed meninges: 6-11 mcg/mL; serum concentration dependent
CSF:blood level ratio: Normal meninges: Nil; Inflamed meninges: 20% to 30%
Protein binding: ~50%

◀ Half-life elimination: Biphasic: Terminal:

Newborns: 6-10 hours

Infants and Children 3 months to 4 years: 4 hours

Children >3 years: 2.2-3 hours

Adults: 5-11 hours; significantly prolonged with renal impairment

End-stage renal disease: 200-250 hours

Time to peak, serum: I.V.: Immediately after completion of infusion

Excretion: I.V.: Urine (80% to 90% as unchanged drug); Oral: Primarily feces

Dosage

Usual dosage range:

Infants >1 month and Children: I.V.: 10-15 mg/kg every 6 hours

Adults:

I.V.: 2-3 g/day (or 30-60 mg/kg/day) in divided doses every 8-12 hours (Rybak, 2009); **Note:** Dose requires adjustment in renal impairment

Oral: 500-1000 mg/day in divided doses every 6 hours

Indication-specific dosing:

Infants >1 month and Children:

Colitis *(C. difficile)*, enterocolitis *(S. aureus)*: Oral: 40 mg/kg/day in 3-4 divided doses added to fluids for 7-10 days (maximum: 2000 mg/day)

Meningitis/CNS infection:

I.V.: 15 mg/kg every 6 hours

Intrathecal: 5-20 mg/day

Prophylaxis against infective endocarditis: I.V.:

Dental, oral, or upper respiratory tract surgery: 20 mg/kg 1 hour prior to the procedure. **Note:** American Heart Association (AHA) guidelines now recommend prophylaxis only in patients undergoing invasive procedures and in whom underlying cardiac conditions may predispose to a higher risk of adverse outcomes should infection occur.

GI/GU procedure: 20 mg/kg plus gentamicin 2 mg/kg 1 hour prior to surgery. **Note:** As of April 2007, routine prophylaxis no longer recommended by the AHA.

Susceptible gram-positive infections: I.V.: 10 mg/kg every 6 hours

Adults: Initial intravenous dosing should be based on actual body weight; subsequent dosing adjusted based on serum trough vancomycin concentrations.

Complicated infections in seriously-ill patients (Rybak, 2009): I.V.: Loading dose: 25-30 mg/kg (based on actual body weight) may be used to rapidly achieve target concentration; then 15-20 mg/kg/dose every 8-12 hours.

Catheter-related infections: Antibiotic lock technique (Mermel, 2009): 2 mg/mL ± 10 units heparin/mL **or** 2.5 mg/mL ± 2500 **or** 5000 units heparin/mL **or** 5 mg/mL ± 5000 units heparin/mL (preferred regimen); instill into catheter port with a volume sufficient to fill the catheter (2-5 mL). **Note:** May use SWFI/NS or D_5W as diluents. Do not mix with any other solutions. Dwell times generally should not exceed 48 hours before renewal of lock solution. Remove lock solution prior to catheter use then replace.

Colitis *(C. difficile)*, enterocolitis *(S. aureus)*: Oral: 500-2000 mg/day in 3-4 divided doses for 7-10 days (usual dose: 125-250 mg every 6 hours)

Endophthalmitis (unlabeled use): Intravitreal: Usual dose: 1 mg/0.1 mL NS instilled into vitreum; may repeat administration if necessary in 3-4 days, usually in combination with ceftazidime or an aminoglycoside

Note: Some clinicians have recommended using a lower dose of 0.2 mg/0.1 mL, based on concerns for retinotoxicity.

Hospital-acquired pneumonia (HAP): I.V.: 15 mg/kg/dose every 12 hours (American Thoracic Society [ATS] 2005 guidelines)

Meningitis *(Pneumococcus* or *Staphylococcus)*:

I.V.: 30-60 mg/kg/day in divided doses every 8-12 hours (Rybak, 2009) **or** 500-750 mg every 6 hours (with third-generation cephalosporin for PCN-resistant *Streptococcus pneumoniae*)

Intrathecal: 5-20 mg/day

Prophylaxis against infective endocarditis: I.V.:

Dental, oral, or upper respiratory tract surgery: 1 g 1 hour before surgery. **Note:** AHA guidelines now recommend prophylaxis only in patients undergoing invasive procedures and in whom underlying cardiac conditions may predispose to a higher risk of adverse outcomes should infection occur

GI/GU procedure: 1 g plus 1.5 mg/kg gentamicin 1 hour prior to surgery. **Note:** As of April 2007, routine prophylaxis no longer recommended by the AHA.

Susceptible (MIC ≤1 mcg/mL; Rybak, 2009) gram-positive infections: I.V.: 15-20 mg/kg/dose (usual: 750-1500 mg) every 8-12 hours

Note: If MIC ≥2 mcg/mL, the targeted AUC:MIC >400 is not achievable with conventional dosing methods in patients with normal renal function and alternative therapies are recommended.

Dosing interval in renal impairment (vancomycin levels should be monitored in patients with any renal impairment):

Cl_{cr} >50 mL/minute: Start with 15-20 mg/kg/dose (usual: 750-1500 mg) every 8-12 hours

Cl_{cr} 20-49 mL/minute: Start with 15-20 mg/kg/dose (usual: 750-1500 mg) every 24 hours

Cl_{cr} <20 mL/minute: Will need longer intervals; determine by serum concentration monitoring

Note: In the critically-ill patient with renal insufficiency, the initial loading dose (25-30 mg/kg) should not be reduced. However, subsequent dosage adjustments should be made based on renal function and trough serum concentrations.

Dialysis: Variable, depending on method; poorly dialyzable by conventional hemodialysis (0% to 5%). Use of high-flux membranes and continuous renal replacement therapy (CRRT) increases vancomycin clearance, and generally requires replacement dosing.

Hemodialysis (HD): Following loading dose of 15-20 mg/kg, give 500 mg to 1 g after each dialysis session, depending on factors such as HD membrane type and flow rate; monitor levels closely.

Continuous ambulatory peritoneal dialysis (CAPD):

Administration via CAPD fluid: 15-30 mg/L (15-30 mcg/mL) of CAPD fluid

Systemic: 1 g loading dose, followed by 500 mg to 1 g every 48-72 hours with close monitoring of levels

Continuous renal replacement therapy (CRRT): Removal of vancomycin is highly dependent on the method of replacement, filter type, and flow rate. Appropriate dosing requires close monitoring of levels in relation to target trough. The following are general recommendations only (Trotman, 2005), and require consideration of the aforementioned parameters.

CVVH: Following loading dose of 15-20 mg/kg, give 1 g every 48 hours

CVVHD or CVVHDF: Following loading dose of 15-20 mg/kg, give 1 g every 24 hours

Trotman RL, Williamson JC, Shoemaker DM, et al, "Antibiotic Dosing in Critically Ill Adult Patients Receiving Continuous Renal Replacement Therapy," *Clin Infect Dis*, 2005, 41:1159-66.

Stability Reconstituted 500 mg and 1 g vials are stable at either room temperature or under refrigeration for 14 days. **Note:** Vials contain no bacteriostatic agent. Solutions diluted for administration in either D_5W or NS are stable under refrigeration for 14 days or at room temperature for 7 days. Reconstitute vials with 20 mL of SWFI for each 1 g of vancomycin (10 mL/500 mg vial; 20 mL/1 g vial; 100 mL/5 g vial; 200 mL/10 g vial). The reconstituted solution must be further diluted with at least 100 mL of a compatible diluent per 500 mg of vancomycin prior to parenteral administration.

Intrathecal: Vancomycin is available as a powder for injection and may be diluted to 1-5 mg/mL concentration in preservative free 0.9% sodium chloride for administration into the CSF.

Administration

Intravenous: Administer vancomycin with a final concentration not to exceed 5 mg/mL by I.V. intermittent infusion over at least 60 minutes (recommended infusion period of ≥30 minutes for every 500 mg administered).

If a maculopapular rash appears on the face, neck, trunk, and/or upper extremities (red man syndrome), slow the infusion rate to over 1¹/₂ to 2 hours and increase the dilution volume. Hypotension, shock, and cardiac arrest (rare) have also been reported with too rapid of infusion. Reactions are often treated with antihistamines and steroids.

Intrathecal: Vancomycin is available as a powder for injection and may be diluted to 1-5 mg/mL concentration in preservative free 0.9% sodium chloride for intrathecal administration.

Intravitreal: May be administered by intravitreal injection (unlabeled use).

Oral: May be administered with food. If patient cannot swallow capsules, the powder for injection may be reconstituted and diluted for oral administration.

Not for I.M. administration.

Extravasation treatment: Monitor I.V. site closely; extravasation will cause serious injury with possible necrosis and tissue sloughing. Rotate infusion site frequently.

Monitoring Parameters Periodic renal function tests, urinalysis, WBC; serum trough vancomycin concentrations in select patients (eg, aggressive dosing, unstable renal function, concurrent nephrotoxins, prolonged courses)

Frequency of trough vancomycin concentration monitoring (Rybak, 2009):

Hemodynamically stable patients: Draw trough concentrations at least once-weekly.

Hemodynamically unstable patients: Draw trough concentrations more frequently or in some instances daily.

Prolonged courses (>3-5 days): Draw at least one steady-state trough concentration; repeat as clinically appropriate.

Note: Drawing >1 trough concentration prior to the fourth dose for short course (<3 days) or lower intensity dosing (target trough concentrations <15 mcg/mL) is not recommended.

Reference Range

Timing of serum samples: Draw trough just before next dose at steady-state conditions (approximately after the fourth dose). Drawing peak concentrations is no longer recommended.

Therapeutic levels: Trough: ≥10 mcg/mL. For pathogens with an MIC ≤1 mcg/mL, the minimum trough concentration should be 15 mcg/mL to meet target AUC/MIC of ≥400 (see **"Note"**). For complicated infections (eg, bacteremia, endocarditis, osteomyelitis, meningitis, and hospital-acquired pneumonia caused by *S. aureus*), trough concentrations of 15-20 mcg/mL are recommended to improve penetration and improve clinical outcomes (Rybak, 2009). The American Thoracic Society (ATS) guidelines for hospital-acquired pneumonia and the Infectious Disease Society of America (IDSA) meningitis guidelines also recommend trough concentrations of 15-20 mcg/mL.

Note: Although AUC/MIC is the preferred pharmacokinetic-pharmacodynamic parameter used to determine clinical effectiveness, trough serum concentrations may be used as a surrogate marker for AUC and is recommended as the most accurate and practical method of vancomycin monitoring (Rybak, 2009).

Toxic: >80 mcg/mL (SI: >54 µmol/L)

Anesthesia and Critical Care Concerns/Other Considerations

Clinical Pearls/Comments: "Red man syndrome" (characterized by skin rash and hypotension) is not an allergic reaction, but rather is associated with infusion administered too rapidly. To alleviate or prevent the reaction, infuse vancomycin at a rate of ≥30 minutes for each 500 mg of drug being administered (eg, 1 g over ≥60 minutes; 1.5 g over ≥90 minutes). CVVHD clears vancomycin from the circulation while conventional hemodialysis does not.

Limitations which may contribute to clinical failure include poor lung penetration, slow bactericidal activity against *S. aureus*, limited CNS penetration, high-level resistance to enterococci and *S. aureus*, and limited activity against bacteria that coat prosthetic devices.

Pregnancy Risk Factor B (oral); C (injection)

Contraindications Hypersensitivity to vancomycin or any component of the formulation; avoid in patients with previous severe hearing loss

Warnings/Precautions May cause nephrotoxicity although limited data suggest direct causal relationship; usual risk factors include pre-existing renal impairment, concomitant nephrotoxic medications, advanced age, and dehydration. If multiple sequential (≥2) serum creatinine concentrations demonstrate an increase of 0.5 mg/dL or ≥50% increase from baseline (whichever is greater) in the absence of an alternative explanation, the patient should be identified as having vancomycin-induced nephrotoxicity (Rybak, 2009). Discontinue treatment if signs of nephrotoxicity occur; renal damage is usually reversible. May cause neurotoxicity; usual risk factors include pre-existing renal impairment, concomitant neuro-/nephrotoxic medications, advanced age, and dehydration. Ototoxicity, although rarely associated with monotherapy, is proportional to the amount of drug given and the duration of treatment. Tinnitus or vertigo may be indications of vestibular injury and impending bilateral irreversible damage. Discontinue treatment if signs of ototoxicity occur. Prolonged therapy (>1 week) or total doses exceeding 25 g may increase the risk of neutropenia; prompt reversal of neutropenia is expected after discontinuation of therapy. Prolonged use may result in fungal or bacterial superinfection, including *C. difficile*-associated diarrhea (CDAD) and pseudomembranous colitis; CDAD has been observed >2 months postantibiotic treatment. Use with caution in patients with renal impairment or those receiving other nephrotoxic or ototoxic drugs; dosage modification required in patients with impaired renal function (especially elderly). Rapid I.V. administration may result in hypotension, flushing, erythema, urticaria, and/or pruritus. Oral vancomycin is only indicated for the treatment of pseudomembranous colitis due to *C. difficile* and enterocolitis due to *S. aureus* and is not effective for systemic infections; parenteral vancomycin is not effective for the treatment of colitis due to *C. difficile* and enterocolitis due to *S. aureus*.

Adverse Reactions

Oral:

>10%: Gastrointestinal: Bitter taste, nausea, vomiting, stomatitis

1% to 10%:
 Central nervous system: Chills, drug fever
 Hematologic: Eosinophilia

<1% (Limited to important or life-threatening): Interstitial nephritis, ototoxicity, renal failure, skin rash, thrombocytopenia, vasculitis

Parenteral:

>10%:
 Cardiovascular: Hypotension accompanied by flushing
 Dermatologic: Erythematous rash on face and upper body (red neck or red man syndrome)

1% to 10%:
 Central nervous system: Chills, drug fever
 Hematologic: Eosinophilia, reversible neutropenia
 Local: Phlebitis

 <1% (Limited to important or life-threatening): Drug rash with eosinophilia and systemic symptoms (DRESS), ototoxicity (rare; use of other ototoxic agents may increase risk), renal failure (limited data suggesting direct relationship), Stevens-Johnson syndrome, thrombocytopenia, vasculitis

Drug Interactions

Avoid Concomitant Use

 Avoid concomitant use of Vancomycin with any of the following: Gallium Nitrate

Increased Effect/Toxicity

 Vancomycin may increase the levels/effects of: Aminoglycosides; Colistimethate; Gallium Nitrate; Neuromuscular-Blocking Agents

 The levels/effects of Vancomycin may be increased by: Nonsteroidal Anti-Inflammatory Agents

Decreased Effect

 Vancomycin may decrease the levels/effects of: Typhoid Vaccine

Dietary Considerations May be taken with food.

Dosage Forms Excipient information presented when available (limited, particularly for generics); consult specific product labeling.
 Capsule (Vancocin®): 125 mg, 250 mg

◀ Infusion [premixed in iso-osmotic dextrose] (Vancocin®): 500 mg (100 mL); 1 g (200 mL)

Injection, powder for reconstitution: 500 mg, 1 g, 5 g, 10 g

References

American Thoracic Society and Infectious Diseases Society of America, "Guidelines for the Management of Adults With Hospital-Acquired, Ventilator-Associated, and Healthcare-Associated Pneumonia," *Am J Respir Crit Care Med*, 2005, 171(4):388-416.

Gilbert DN, Moellering RC, Eliopoulos GM, et al, eds, *The Sanford Guide To Antimicrobial Therapy*, 2006, 36th ed, Hyde Park, VT: Antimicrobial Therapy, Inc, 2006, 6-7.

Joy MS, Matzke GR, Frye RF, et al, "Determinants of Vancomycin Clearance by Continuous Veno-Venous Hemofiltration and Continuous Veno-Venous Hemodialysis," *Am J Kidney Dis*, 1998, 31 (6):1019-27.

Murray BE, "Vancomycin-Resistant Enterococcal Infections," *N Engl J Med*, 2000, 342(10):710-21.

Trotman RL, Williamson JC, Shoemaker DM, et al, "Antibiotic Dosing in Critically Ill Adult Patients Receiving Continuous Renal Replacement Therapy," *Clin Infect Dis*, 2005, 41:1159-66.

Tunkel AR, Hartman BJ, Kaplan SL, et al, "Practice Guidelines for the Management of Bacterial Meningitis," *Clin Infect Dis*, 2004, 39(9):1267-84.

Wilson W, Taubert KA, Gewitz M, et al, "Prevention of Infective Endocarditis. Guidelines From the American Heart Association. A Guideline From the American Heart Association Rheumatic Fever, Endocarditis, and Kawasaki Disease Committee, Council on Cardiovascular Disease in the Young, and the Council on Clinical Cardiology, Council on Cardiovascular Surgery and Anesthesia, and the Quality of Care and Outcomes Research Interdisciplinary Working Group," *Circulation*, 2007, 115. Available at http://circ.ahajournals.org/cgi/reprint/CIRCULATIONAHA.106.183095v1; last accessed July 26, 2007.

◆ **Vancomycin Hydrochloride** *see* Vancomycin *on page 1453*

◆ **Vandazole®** *see* MetroNIDAZOLE *on page 928*

◆ **Vaprisol®** *see* Conivaptan *on page 349*

Vasopressin (vay soe PRES in)

Medication Safety Issues

Use care when prescribing and/or administering vasopressin solutions. Close attention should be given to concentration of solution, route of administration, dose, and rate of administration (units/minute, units/kg/minute, units/kg/hour).

Related Information

Anesthesia Considerations for Neurosurgery *on page 1514*
Hemodynamic Support, Intravenous *on page 1681*

U.S. Brand Names Pitressin®

Canadian Brand Names Pressyn®; Pressyn® AR

Index Terms 8-Arginine Vasopressin; ADH; Antidiuretic Hormone; AVP

Pharmacologic Category Antidiuretic Hormone Analog; Hormone, Posterior Pituitary

Generic Available Yes

Use Treatment of central diabetes insipidus; differential diagnosis of diabetes insipidus

Unlabeled/Investigational Use Adjunct in the treatment of GI hemorrhage and esophageal varices; pulseless arrest (ventricular tachycardia [VT]/ventricular fibrillation [VF], asystole/pulseless electrical activity [PEA]); vasodilatory shock (septic shock); donor management in brain-dead patients (hormone replacement therapy)

Mechanism of Action Increases cyclic adenosine monophosphate (cAMP) which increases water permeability at the renal tubule resulting in decreased urine volume and increased osmolality; causes peristalsis by directly stimulating the smooth muscle in the GI tract; direct vasoconstrictor without inotropic or chronotropic effects

Pharmacodynamics/Kinetics

Onset of action: Nasal: 1 hour

Duration: Nasal: 3-8 hours; I.M., SubQ: 2-8 hours

Metabolism: Nasal/Parenteral: Hepatic, renal

Half-life elimination: Nasal: 15 minutes; Parenteral: 10-20 minutes

Excretion: Nasal: Urine; SubQ: Urine (5% as unchanged drug) after 4 hours

Dosage

Central diabetes insipidus: **Note:** Dosage is highly variable; titrate based on serum and urine sodium and osmolality in addition to fluid balance and urine output. Use of vasopressin is impractical for chronic therapy.

I.M., SubQ:

Children: 2.5-10 units 2-4 times/day as needed

Adults: 5-10 units 2-4 times/day as needed

Continuous I.V. infusion (unlabeled route): **Note:** The optimum rate of infusion has not been well established; many protocols exist.

Children: Initial: 0.0005 units/kg/hour; increase dose by 0.0005 units/kg/hour increments every 5-10 minutes as needed to adequately reduce urine output (maximum dose: 0.01 unit/kg/hour) (Wise-Faberowski, 2004). **Note:** Although clinical trial titrated every 5-10 minutes, a reduced frequency of titration (eg, every 30 minutes) may be more appropriate given the half-life of vasopressin.

Adults: Continuous infusion has not been formally evaluated in the post-neurosurgical adult. However, some convert I.M./SubQ requirement to an hourly continuous I.V. infusion rate.

Central diabetes insipidus, post-traumatic (unlabeled use): Adults: I.V.: Initial: 2.5 units/hour; titrate to adequately reduce urine output (Levitt, 1984)

Donor management in brain-dead patients (hormone replacement therapy) (unlabeled use): Adults: I.V.: Initial: 1 unit bolus followed by 0.5-4 units/hour (UNOS Critical Pathway, 2002; Rosendale, 2003)

GI/variceal hemorrhage (unlabeled use): Continuous I.V. infusion: Dilute in NS or D_5W to 0.1-1 unit/mL. **Note:** Other therapies may be preferred.

GI hemorrhage (unlabeled use): Children: Initial I.V. bolus: 0.3 unit/kg (maximum: 20 units) may be given. Continuous I.V. infusion: 0.001-0.01 units/kg/minute; titrate dose as needed; maximum: 0.01 unit/kg/minute; if bleeding controlled for 12-24 hours, then taper off over 24-36 hours

Variceal hemorrhage (unlabeled use) [AASLD guidelines, 2007]: Adults: Initial: 0.2-0.4 units/minute, may titrate dose as needed to a maximum dose of 0.8 units/minute; maximum duration: 24 hours at highest effective dose continuously (to reduce incidence of adverse effects). Patient should also receive I.V. nitroglycerin concurrently to prevent myocardial ischemic complications; monitor closely for signs/symptoms of ischemia (myocardial, peripheral, bowel)

Pulseless arrest (unlabeled use) [ACLS, 2005]: Adults: I.V., I.O.: 40 units; may give 1 dose to replace first or second dose of epinephrine. I.V./I.O. drug administration is preferred, but if no access, may give endotracheally. ACLS guidelines do not recommend a specific endotracheal dose; however, may be given endotracheally using the same I.V. dose (Wenzel, 1997). Mix with 5-10 mL of water or normal saline, and administer down the endotracheal tube.

Vasodilatory shock/septic shock (unlabeled use): Adults: I.V.: 0.01-0.04 units/minute for the treatment of septic shock. Doses >0.04 units/minute may have more cardiovascular side effects. Most case reports have used 0.04 units/minute continuous infusion as a fixed dose.

Dosing adjustment in hepatic impairment: Some patients respond to much lower doses with cirrhosis

Stability Store injection at room temperature; do not freeze. Protect from heat. Use only clear solutions.

Administration

I.V.: Use extreme caution to avoid extravasation because of risk of necrosis and gangrene. In treatment of varices, infusions are often supplemented with nitroglycerin infusions to minimize cardiac effects.

Usual concentration: 100 units in 500 mL D_5W. **Note:** In one clinical trial with lower dosing (eg, 0.0005 units/kg/hour) in pediatric patients, a more dilute solution (eg, 20 units in 500 mL D_5W) was employed (Wise-Faberowski, 2004).

Vasodilatory shock: Administration through a central catheter is recommended.

Intranasal (topical administration on nasal mucosa): Administer injectable vasopressin on cotton plugs, as nasal spray, or by dropper. Should not be inhaled.

Endotracheal: If no I.V./I.O. access may give endotracheally. ACLS guidelines do not recommend a specific endotracheal dose; however, may be given endotracheally using the same I.V. dose (Wenzel, 1997). Mix with 5-10 mL of water or normal saline, and administer down the endotracheal tube.

Monitoring Parameters Serum and urine sodium, urine specific gravity, urine and serum osmolality; urine output, fluid input and output, blood pressure, heart rate

◄ **Reference Range** Plasma: 0-2 pg/mL (SI: 0-2 ng/L) if osmolality <285 mOsm/L; 2-12 pg/mL (SI: 2-12 ng/L) if osmolality >290 mOsm/L

Anesthesia and Critical Care Concerns/Other Considerations
Clinical Pearls/Comments:

Shock: Vasopressin binds to different receptors than the catecholamine pressors. Vasoconstrictor effects are through the V_1 vascular receptors. In clinical studies and case reports, vasopressin increased blood pressure, systemic vascular resistance, and urine output. Vasopressin may decrease heart rate and cardiac output, especially at higher doses. Vasopressin has been used in doses of 0.01-0.1 units/minute. Doses >0.04 units/minute may have more cardiovascular effects (decreased cardiac output, asystole, cardiac ischemia). Use caution in patients with underlying cardiac dysfunction. Vasoconstriction appears to remain effective in severe acidosis. When possible, low-dose vasopressin should be infused via central catheter for the management of vasodilatory shock; peripheral administration has been associated with skin necrosis.

Evidence-Based Information:

Septic Shock: A multicenter, double-blind, randomized study looked at the effect of vasopressin versus norepinephrine in the treatment of septic shock (Russell, 2008). Inclusion criteria included patients >16 years with septic shock who were resistant to fluid resuscitation or the requirement of vasopressor therapy. They excluded patients with unstable coronary syndrome, >24 hours since meeting study criteria, use of open-labeled vasopressin, malignancy, acute ischemia, NYHA class III or IV heart disease, severe hyponatremia, traumatic brain injury, Raynaud's phenomenon, pregnancy, and not committed to aggressive care. Vasopressin was started at 0.01 units/minute and titrated to a maximum of 0.03 units/minute. Norepinephrine was started at 5 mcg/minute and titrated to a maximum of 15 mcg/minute. The primary outcome was 28-day all cause mortality. Secondary outcomes included 90-day mortality; days alive and free of organ failure during the first 28 days; days alive and free of vasopressors, mechanical ventilation, or renal replacement therapy; days alive and free of SIRS; days alive and free of corticosteroids; and length of ICU and hospital stay. Seven hundred seventy-eight patients with septic shock were enrolled. There was no significant difference in 28-day mortality between the vasopressin group versus norepinephrine group (35.4% vs 39.3%, respectively; p=0.26). There were no significant differences in the rate of serious adverse effects between groups or the other secondary outcome measures. In a subgroup of patients who were defined as less severe septic shock (norepinephrine <15 mcg/minute), there was a possible mortality benefit of vasopressin versus norepinephrine at 28 days (26.5% vs 35.7%; p=0.05) and 90 days (35.8% vs 46.1%, p=0.04). However in the group with more severe septic shock (norepinephrine >15 mcg/minute), there was no mortality benefit. The authors concluded that low-dose vasopressin did not decrease mortality when compared to norepinephrine in septic shock patients.

The 2008 Surviving Sepsis Campaign guidelines (Dellinger, 2007) suggest vasopressin should not be administered as the initial vasopressor in septic shock. Vasopressin 0.03 units/minute may be added to norepinephrine with anticipation of an effect equivalent to norepinephrine alone (Grade 2C).

Cardiac Arrest:

Out-of-hospital cardiac arrest: A prospective, multicenter, double-blind randomized, controlled trial evaluated the efficacy of vasopressin or epinephrine when administered to adult patients who suffered an out-of-hospital cardiac arrest (Wenzel, 2004). For inclusions, patients presented with ventricular fibrillation, pulseless electrical activity, or asystole. They were excluded if they were successfully defibrillated without the administration of a vasopressor, had a terminal illness or had a "do not resuscitate" (DNR) order, a lack of intravenous access, hemorrhagic shock, pregnancy, cardiac arrest due to trauma, or were <18 years of age. Eligible patients were randomized to intravenous vasopressin (40 units, n=589) or epinephrine (1 mg, n=597). Each patient received an injection of the study drug, if spontaneous circulation was not restored in 3 minutes they received a second dose (same amount) of the same study drug. If there was no response, the managing physician had the option of giving epinephrine. Patients with ventricular fibrillation were randomized after the first three attempts at defibrillation failed; all others were randomized immediately. The primary endpoint was survival to hospital admission; the secondary endpoint was survival to hospital discharge. Five hundred and eighty-nine patients were randomized to vasopressin and five hundred and ninety-seven patients were randomized to epinephrine. There was no significant difference in the rate of hospital admission between the vasopressin group and the epinephrine group if they had ventricular fibrillation (46.2% vs 43% respectively, p: 0.48) or pulseless electrical activity (33.7% vs 30.5% respectively, p: 0.65). Patients with asystole responded significantly better to vasopressin; having higher rates of hospital admission (29% vs 20.3% in the epinephrine group, p: 0.02) and hospital discharge (4.7% vs 1.5% in the epinephrine group, p: 0.04). Patients who failed vasopressin therapy and received additional epinephrine had significant improvement in survival to hospital admission (25.7% vs 16.4% in the epinephrine group, p: 0.002) and discharge (6.2% vs 1.7%, p: 0.002). Similar patients who were randomized to epinephrine and failed to respond did not improve with additional epinephrine. Cerebral performance among all patients who survived to discharge was similar in both groups. In this trial, vasopressin was superior to epinephrine in patients with asystole. Vasopressin followed by epinephrine may be more effective than epinephrine alone in refractory out-of-hospital cardiac arrest.

There was no significant difference in the rate of hospital admission between the vasopressin group and the epinephrine group if they had ventricular fibrillation (46.2% vs 43% respectively, p=0.48) or pulseless electrical activity (33.7% vs 30.5% respectively, p=0.65). Patients with asystole responded significantly better to vasopressin; having higher rates of hospital admission (29% vs 20.3% in the epinephrine group, p=0.02) and hospital discharge (4.7% vs 1.5% in the epinephrine group, p=0.04). Patients who failed vasopressin therapy and received additional epinephrine had significant improvement in survival to hospital admission (25.7% vs 16.4% in the epinephrine group, p=0.002) and discharge (6.2% vs 1.7%, p=0.002). Similar patients who were randomized to epinephrine and failed to respond did not improve with additional epinephrine. Cerebral performance among all patients who survived to discharge was similar in both groups. In this trial, vasopressin was superior to epinephrine in patients with asystole. Vasopressin followed by epinephrine may be more effective than epinephrine alone in refractory out-of-hospital cardiac arrest.

More recently, Gueugniaud, et al (2008) evaluated the combination of vasopressin and epinephrine compared to epinephrine alone in the treatment of out-of-hospital cardiac arrest. This multicenter, double-blind, randomized, controlled trial enrolled 2894 adult patients with out-of-hospital cardiac arrest with either ventricular fibrillation, pulseless electrical activity, or asystole. Patients were excluded if <18 years of age, successfully defibrillated without vasopressors, traumatic cardiac arrest, pregnant, documented terminal illness, and DNR orders or irreversible cardiac arrest. Patients were randomized to either intravenous vasopressin (40 units) and epinephrine (1 mg) or epinephrine (1 mg) and a placebo. The medications/placebo were given within 10 seconds of each other and followed by a saline flush. Patients with ventricular fibrillation received defibrillation before the administration of study drug. The primary endpoint was survival to hospital admission; secondary endpoints were return of spontaneous circulation, survival to hospital discharge, good neurologic recovery, and 1-year survival. Similar to the previous study, there was no significant difference in the rate of hospital admission between the two groups (20.7% vs 21.3%, p=0.69). Also, return of spontaneous circulation, survival to hospital discharge, good neurologic recovery, and 1-year survival were all similar between groups. In contrast to the previous study, patients with asystole had no benefit from the combination of vasopressin and epinephrine when compared to epinephrine/placebo. In this study, asystole was the most common initial cardiac rhythm, presenting in 82.8% of the patients. Based on the results of the most recent study, it appears that vasopressin plus epinephrine has no benefit over epinephrine in out-of-hospital cardiopulmonary resuscitation.

In-hospital cardiac arrest: A small in-hospital cardiac arrest study evaluated the efficacy of vasopressin or epinephrine in 200 patients. These investigators did not find any differences between the two treatment groups with regard to survival, discharge, or cerebral performance (Stiell, 2001).

Pregnancy Risk Factor C

◀ **Contraindications** Hypersensitivity to vasopressin or any component of the formulation

Warnings/Precautions Use with caution in patients with seizure disorders, migraine, asthma, vascular disease, renal disease, cardiac disease; chronic nephritis with nitrogen retention, goiter with cardiac complications, or arteriosclerosis. I.V. infiltration may lead to severe vasoconstriction and localized tissue necrosis, gangrene of extremities, tongue, and ischemic colitis. May cause water intoxication; early signs include drowsiness, listlessness, and headache, these should be recognized to prevent coma and seizures. Elderly patients should be cautioned not to increase their fluid intake beyond that sufficient to satisfy their thirst in order to avoid water intoxication and hyponatremia; under experimental conditions, the elderly have shown to have a decreased responsiveness to vasopressin with respect to its effects on water homeostasis.

Adverse Reactions Frequency not defined.

Cardiovascular: Arrhythmia, asystole (>0.04 units/minute), blood pressure increased, cardiac output decreased (>0.04 units/minute), chest pain, MI, vasoconstriction (with higher doses), venous thrombosis

Central nervous system: Pounding in head, fever, vertigo

Dermatologic: Ischemic skin lesions, circumoral pallor, urticaria

Gastrointestinal: Abdominal cramps, flatulence, mesenteric ischemia, nausea, vomiting

Genitourinary: Uterine contraction

Neuromuscular & skeletal: Tremor

Respiratory: Bronchial constriction

Miscellaneous: Diaphoresis

Drug Interactions

Avoid Concomitant Use There are no known interactions where it is recommended to avoid concomitant use.

Increased Effect/Toxicity There are no known significant interactions involving an increase in effect.

Decreased Effect There are no known significant interactions involving a decrease in effect.

Ethanol/Nutrition/Herb Interactions Ethanol: Avoid ethanol (due to effects on ADH).

Dosage Forms Excipient information presented when available (limited, particularly for generics); consult specific product labeling.

Injection, solution: 20 units/mL (0.5 mL, 1 mL, 10 mL)

Pitressin®: 20 units/mL (1 mL)

References

"2005 American Heart Association Guidelines for Cardiopulmonary Resuscitation and Emergency Cardiovascular Care," *Circulation*, 2005, 112(24 Suppl): 1-211.

Aung K and Htay T, "Vasopressin for Cardiac Arrest: A Systematic Review and Meta-Analysis," *Arch Intern Med*, 2005, 165(1):17-24.

Dellinger RP, Levy MM, Carlet JM, et al, "Surviving Sepsis Campaign: International Guidelines for Management of Severe Sepsis and Septic Shock: 2008," *Intensive Care Med*, 2008, 34(1): 17-60. Available at http://www.survivingsepsis.org/system/files/images/2008_20International_20SSC_20-Guidelines_1_.pdf

Dunser MW, Mayr AJ, Ulmer H, et al, "The Effects of Vasopressin on Systemic Hemodynamics in Catecholamine-Resistant Septic and Postcardiotomy Shock: A Retrospective Analysis," *Anest Analg*, 2001, 93(1):7-13.

Gazmuri RJ and Shakeri SA, "Low-Dose Vasopressin for Reversing Vasodilation During Septic Shock," *Crit Care Med*, 2001, 29(3):673-5.

Gueugniaud PY, David JS, Chanzy E, et al, "Vasopressin and Epinephrine vs. Epinephrine Alone in Cardiopulmonary Resuscitation," *N Engl J Med*, 2008, 359(1):21-30.

Holmes CL, Walley KR, Chittock DR, et al, "The Effects of Vasopressin on Hemodynamics and Renal Function in Severe Septic Shock: A Case Series," *Inten Care Med*, 2001, 27(8):1416-21.

Kahn JM, Kress JP, and Hall JB, "Skin Necrosis After Extravasation of Low-Dose Vasopressin Administered for Septic Shock," *Crit Care Med*, 2002, 30(8):1899-901.

Landry DW, Levin HR, Gallant EM, et al, "Vasopressin Deficiency Contributes to the Vasodilation of Septic Shock," *Circulation*, 1997, 95(5):1122-5.

Malay MB, Ashton RC, Landry DW, et al, "Low-Dose Vasopressin in the Treatment of Vasodilatory Septic Shock," *J Trauma*, 1999, 47(4):699-705.

Reid IA, "Role of Vasopressin Deficiency in the Vasodilation of Septic Shock," *Circulation*, 1997, 95 (5):1108-10.

Rozenfeld V and Cheng JW, "The Role of Vasopressin in the Treatment of Vasodilation in Shock States," *Ann Pharmacother*, 2000, 34(2):250-4.

Russell JA, Walley KR, Singer J, et al, "Vasopressin Versus Norepinephrine Infusion in Patients With Septic Shock," *N Engl J Med*, 2008, 358(9):877-87.

Stiell IG, Hebert PC, Wells GA, et al, "Vasopressin Versus Epinephrine for in Hospital Cardiac Arrest: A Randomised Controlled Trial," *Lancet*, 2001, 358(9276):105-9.

Tsuneyoshi I, Yamada H, Kakihana Y, et al, "Hemodynamic and Metabolic Effects of Low-Dose Vasopressin Infusions in Vasodilatory Septic Shock," *Crit Care Med*, 2001, 29(3):487-93.

Tuggle DW, Bennett KG, Scott J, et al, "Intravenous Vasopressin and Gastrointestinal Hemorrhage in Children," *J Pediatr Surg*, 1988, 23(7):627-9.

Wenzel V, Krismer AC, Arntz HR, et al, "A Comparison of Vasopressin and Epinephrine for Out-of-Hospital Cardiopulmonary Resuscitation," *N Engl J Med*, 2004, 350(2):105-13.

◆ **Vasotec®** *see* Enalapril *on page 478*

◆ **Vasotec® I.V. (Can)** *see* Enalapril *on page 478*

Vecuronium (vek ue ROE nee um)

Medication Safety Issues
Sound-alike/look-alike issues:
Vecuronium may be confused with vancomycin
Norcuron® may be confused with Narcan®

High alert medication: The Institute for Safe Medication Practices (ISMP) includes this medication among its list of drugs which have a heightened risk of causing significant patient harm when used in error.

United States Pharmacopeia (USP) 2006: The Interdisciplinary Safe Medication Use Expert Committee of the USP has recommended the following:
- Hospitals, clinics, and other practice sites should institute special safeguards in the storage, labeling, and use of these agents and should include these safeguards in staff orientation and competency training.
- Healthcare professionals should be on high alert (especially vigilant) whenever a neuromuscular-blocking agent (NMBA) is stocked, ordered, prepared, or administered.

Related Information
Allergic Reactions *on page 1508*
Anesthesia Considerations for Neurosurgery *on page 1514*
Chronic Renal Failure *on page 1552*
Dosing Considerations for the Critically-Ill Patient With Morbid Obesity *on page 1561*
Neuromuscular-Blocking Agents *on page 1684*
Perioperative Management of Patients on Antiseizure Medication *on page 1577*

Canadian Brand Names Norcuron®

Index Terms Norcuron; ORG NC 45

Pharmacologic Category Neuromuscular Blocker Agent, Nondepolarizing

Generic Available Yes

Use To facilitate endotracheal intubation and to relax skeletal muscles during surgery; to facilitate mechanical ventilation in ICU patients; does not relieve pain or produce sedation

Mechanism of Action Blocks acetylcholine from binding to receptors on motor endplate inhibiting depolarization

Pharmacodynamics/Kinetics
Onset of action:
Good intubation conditions: Within 2.5-3 minutes
Maximum neuromuscular blockade: Within 3-5 minutes
Duration: Under balanced anesthesia (time to recovery to 25% of control): 25-40 minutes; recovery 95% complete ~45-65 minutes after injection of intubating dose
Distribution: V_d: 0.3-0.4 L/kg
Protein binding: 60% to 80%
Metabolism: Active metabolite: 3-desacetyl vecuronium ($1/2$ the activity of parent drug)
Half-life elimination: Healthy surgical patients and renal failure patients undergoing transplant surgery: 65-75 minutes; Late pregnancy: 35-40 minutes
Excretion: Primarily feces (40% to 75%); urine (30% as unchanged drug and metabolites)

◄ **Dosage** Administer I.V.; dose to effect; doses will vary due to interpatient variability:

Children: ICU paralysis (eg, facilitate mechanical ventilation) in selected adequately sedated patients (unlabeled; Martin, 1999): Initial bolus dose: 0.1-0.15 mg/kg, then a continuous I.V. infusion of 1-2.5 mcg/kg/minute; monitor depth of blockade using train-of-four (TOF) every 2-3 hours initially until stable dose, then every 8-12 hours

Intermittent bolus dosing (Eldadah, 1989): 0.1 mg/kg every 1 hour as needed when TOF count ≥1/4

Children ≥1 year and Adults: Surgical relaxation: **Note:** Children 1-10 years may require slightly higher initial doses and more frequent supplementation. For obese (≥130% of IBW) adult patients, may use ideal body weight (IBW) (Erstad, 2004; Schwartz, 1992; Weinstein, 1988); onset time may be slightly delayed using IBW.

Tracheal intubation: I.V.: Initial: 0.08-0.1 mg/kg. **Note:** If intubation is performed using succinylcholine (not preferred agent in pediatric patients), the initial dose of vecuronium may be reduced to 0.04-0.06 mg/kg with inhalation anesthesia and 0.05-0.06 mg/kg with balanced anesthesia. Inhaled anesthetic agents prolong the duration of action of vecuronium.

Pretreatment/priming: Adults: 10% of intubating dose given 3-5 minutes before intubating dose

Maintenance for continued surgical relaxation: Intermittent dosing (see **"Note"**): 0.01-0.015 mg/kg administered at 25% recovery of control T_1 or continuous infusion: Initial: 1 mcg/kg/minute only after early evidence of spontaneous recovery of neuromuscular function. Infusion rates range: 0.8-1.2 mcg/kg/minute.

Note: Use lower end of the dosing range when anesthesia is maintained with an inhaled anesthetic agent, with the redosing interval guided by monitoring with a peripheral nerve stimulator.

Adults:

ICU paralysis (eg, facilitate mechanical ventilation) in selected adequately sedated patients (Darrah, 1987; Murray, 2002; Rudis, 1997): Initial bolus dose: 0.08-0.1 mg/kg, then a continuous I.V. infusion of 0.8-1.7 mcg/kg/minute; monitor depth of blockade every 1-2 hours initially until stable dose, then every 8-12 hours

Dosage adjustment (Rudis, 1996; Rudis, 1997): Adjust rate of administration in increments of 0.3 mcg/kg/minute or by 50% reductions of previous dose according to peripheral nerve stimulation response (eg, train-of-four [TOF] count) or desired clinical response as long as TOF count >1/4 is present. If no response on TOF, discontinue infusion and reinitiate when TOF count ≥1/4 occurs.

Note: When possible, minimize depth and duration of paralysis. Stopping the infusion daily for some time until forced to restart based on patient condition is recommended to reduce post-paralytic complications (eg, acute quadriplegic myopathy syndrome [AQMS]) (Murray, 2002, Segredo, 1992).

Intermittent bolus dosing (Hunter, 1985): 0.1-0.2 mg/kg/dose; may be repeated when TOF count >1/4

Control of refractory shivering in adequately sedated patients during therapeutic hypothermia after cardiac arrest (unlabeled use; Bernard, 2002; Nolan, 2003; Polderman, 2009): I.V.: 8-12 mg; redose as needed to control shivering. **Note:** Duration of action prolonged in patients undergoing induced hypothermia. May also mask seizure activity.

Dosing adjustment in renal impairment: In general, patients with renal impairment do not experience clinically significant prolongation of neuromuscular blockade with vecuronium; however, in patients who are anephric, the clinical duration may be prolonged.

Dosing adjustment in hepatic impairment: Dose reductions are necessary in patients with cirrhosis or cholestasis

Stability Store intact vials of powder for injection at room temperature 20°C to 25°C (68°F to 77°F). Vials reconstituted with bacteriostatic water for injection (BWFI) may be stored for 5 days under refrigeration or at room temperature. Vials reconstituted with other compatible diluents (nonbacteriostatic) should be stored under refrigeration and used within 24 hours. Reconstitute with compatible solution for injection to final concentration of 1 mg/mL.

Administration Concentration of 1 mg/mL may be administered by rapid I.V. injection. May further dilute reconstituted vial to 0.1-0.2 mg/mL in a compatible solution for I.V. infusion. Concentration of 1 mg/mL may be used for I.V. infusion in fluid-restricted patients.

Monitoring Parameters Blood pressure, heart rate; peripheral nerve stimulation (eg, train-of-four [TOF] count)

Anesthesia and Critical Care Concerns/Other Considerations

Clinical Pearls/Comments: Classified as an intermediate duration neuro-muscular-blocking agent; produces minimal, if any, histamine release. Brady-cardia may occur with concurrent administration of a potent opioid.

Critically-Ill Adult Patients:

The 2008 Surviving Sepsis Campaign guidelines recommend avoiding use of neuromuscular blockers if at all possible in the septic patient due to the risk of prolonged neuromuscular blockade following discontinuation. If one is required, monitor the depth of blockade (Grade 1B).

The 2002 ACCM/SCCM/ASHP clinical practice guidelines for sustained neuro-muscular blockade in the adult critically-ill patient recommend:

Optimize sedatives and analgesics prior to initiation and monitor and adjust accordingly during course. Neuromuscular blockers do not relieve pain or produce sedation.

Protect patient's eyes from development of keratitis and corneal abrasion by administering ophthalmic ointment and taping eyelids closed or using eye patches. Reposition patient routinely to protect pressure points from break-down. Address DVT prophylaxis.

Concurrent use of a neuromuscular blocker and corticosteroids appear to increase the risk of certain ICU myopathies; avoid or administer the corticosteroid at the lowest dose possible. Reassess need for neuromuscular blocker daily.

Using daily drug holidays (stopping neuromuscular-blocking agent until patient requires it again) may decrease the incidence of acute quadriplegic myopathy syndrome.

Tachyphylaxis can develop; switch to another neuromuscular blocker (taking into consideration the patient's organ function) if paralysis is still necessary.

Monitor patients clinically and via "Train of Four" (TOF) testing with a goal of adjusting the degree of blockade to 1-2 twitches.

Pregnancy Risk Factor C

Contraindications Hypersensitivity to vecuronium or any component of the formulation

Warnings/Precautions Ventilation must be supported during neuromuscular blockade. Vecuronium does not relieve pain or produce sedation; use should include appropriate anesthesia, pain control, and sedation. In patients requiring long-term administration, use of a peripheral nerve stimulator to monitor drug effects is strongly recommended. Additional doses of vecuronium or any other neuromuscular-blocking agent should be avoided unless nerve stimulation response suggests inadequate neuromuscular blockade. Certain clinical conditions may result in potentiation or antagonism of neuromuscular blockade:

Antagonism: Alkalosis, hypercalcemia, demyelinating lesions, peripheral neuro-pathies, denervation, immobilization, infection, and muscle trauma

Potentiation: Electrolyte abnormalities, severe hyponatremia, severe hypocalce-mia, severe hypokalemia, hypermagnesemia, cachexia, neuromuscular diseases, acidosis, Eaton-Lambert syndrome, and myasthenia gravis

Resistance may occur in burn patients (>30% of body) for period of 5-70 days postinjury. Hypothermia may prolong the duration of action. Use with caution in patients with hepatic impairment; clinical duration may be prolonged. Use with caution in patients who are anephric; clinical duration may be prolonged. Use with caution in patients who have underlying respiratory disease. Some patients may experience delayed recovery of neuromuscular function after administration (especially after prolonged use). Other factors associated with delayed recovery should be considered (eg, corticosteroid use, disease-related conditions). Cross-sensitivity with other neuromuscular-blocking agents may occur; use extreme caution in patients with previous anaphylactic reactions. Use caution in the elderly. Children 1-10 years of age may require slightly higher initial doses and slightly more frequent supplementation. **[U.S. Boxed Warning]: Should be** ▶

administered by adequately trained individuals familiar with its use. Some dosage forms may contain benzyl alcohol which has been associated with "gasping syndrome" in neonates.

Adverse Reactions <1% (Limited to important or life-threatening): Acute quadriplegic myopathy syndrome (prolonged use), Bradycardia, circulatory collapse, edema, flushing; hypersensitivity reaction (hypotension, tachycardia, erythema, rash, urticaria); itching, myositis ossificans (prolonged use), rash

Drug Interactions

Avoid Concomitant Use

Avoid concomitant use of Vecuronium with any of the following: QuiNINE

Increased Effect/Toxicity

Vecuronium may increase the levels/effects of: Cardiac Glycosides; Corticosteroids (Systemic); OnabotulinumtoxinA; RimabotulinumtoxinB

The levels/effects of Vecuronium may be increased by: AbobotulinumtoxinA; Aminoglycosides; Calcium Channel Blockers; Capreomycin; Colistimethate; Inhalational Anesthetics; Ketorolac; Lincosamide Antibiotics; Lithium; Loop Diuretics; Magnesium Salts; Polymyxin B; Procainamide; QuiNIDine; QuiNINE; Spironolactone; Tetracycline Derivatives; Vancomycin

Decreased Effect

The levels/effects of Vecuronium may be decreased by: Acetylcholinesterase Inhibitors; CarBAMazepine; Loop Diuretics; Phenytoin

Dosage Forms Excipient information presented when available (limited, particularly for generics); consult specific product labeling.

Injection, powder for reconstitution, as bromide: 10 mg, 20 mg [may be supplied with diluent containing benzyl alcohol]

References

Dellinger RP, Levy MM, Carlet JM, et al, "Surviving Sepsis Campaign: International Guidelines for Management of Severe Sepsis and Septic Shock: 2008," *Intensive Care Med*, 2008, 34(1): 17-60. Available at http://www.survivingsepsis.org/system/files/images/2008_20International_20SSC_20-Guidelines_1_.pdf

Murray MJ, Cowen J, DeBlock H, et al, "Clinical Practice Guidelines for Sustained Neuromuscular Blockade in the Adult Critically Ill Patient. Task Force of the American College of Critical Care Medicine (ACCM) of the Society of Critical Care Medicine (SCCM), American Society of Health-System Pharmacists, American College of Chest Physicians," *Crit Care Med*, 2002, 30(1):142-56; viewable at http://www.sccm.org/pdf/NeuromuscularBlockade.pdf.

◆ **Velivet™** *see* Ethinyl Estradiol and Desogestrel *on page 544*

Venlafaxine (ven la FAX een)

Related Information

Antidepressant Agents *on page 1660*

Chronic Pain Management *on page 1546*

U.S. Brand Names Effexor XR®; Effexor®

Canadian Brand Names CO Venlafaxine XR; Effexor® XR; GEN-Venlafaxine XR; Mylan-Venlafaxine XR; Novo-Venlafaxine XR; PMS-Venlafaxine XR; ratio-Venlafaxine XR; Riva-Venlafaxine XR; Sandoz-Venlafaxine XR

Pharmacologic Category Antidepressant, Serotonin/Norepinephrine Reuptake Inhibitor

Use Treatment of major depressive disorder, generalized anxiety disorder (GAD), social anxiety disorder (social phobia), panic disorder

Unlabeled/Investigational Use Obsessive-compulsive disorder (OCD); hot flashes; neuropathic pain; attention-deficit/hyperactivity disorder (ADHD); post-traumatic stress disorder (PTSD)

Pharmacodynamics/Kinetics

Absorption: Oral: 92% to 100%; food has no significant effect on the absorption of venlafaxine or formation of the active metabolite O-desmethylvenlafaxine (ODV)

Distribution: At steady state: Venlafaxine 7.5 ± 3.7 L/kg, ODV 5.7 ± 1.8 L/Kg

Protein binding: Bound to human plasma protein: Venlafaxine 27%, ODV 30%

Metabolism: Hepatic via CYP2D6 to active metabolite, O-desmethylvenlafaxine (ODV); other metabolites include N-desmethylvenlafaxine and N,O-didesmethylvenlafaxine

Bioavailability: Absolute: ~45%

Half-life elimination: Venlafaxine: 3-7 hours; ODV: 9-13 hours; Steady-state, plasma: Venlafaxine/ODV: Within 3 days of multiple-dose therapy; prolonged with cirrhosis (Adults: Venlafaxine: ~30%, ODV: ~60%) and with dialysis (Adults: Venlafaxine: ~180%, ODV: ~142%)

Time to peak:

Immediate release: Venlafaxine: 2 hours, ODV: 3 hours

Extended release: Venlafaxine: 5.5 hours, ODV: 9 hours

Excretion: Urine (~87%, 5% as unchanged drug, 29% as unconjugated ODV, 26% as conjugated ODV, 27% as minor inactive metabolites) within 48 hours

Clearance at steady state: Venlafaxine: 1.3 ± 0.6 L/hour/kg, ODV: 0.4 ± 0.2 L/hour/kg

Clearance decreased with:

Cirrhosis: Adults: Venlafaxine: ~50%, ODV: ~30%

Severe cirrhosis: Adults: Venlafaxine: ~90%

Renal impairment (Cl_{cr} 10-70 mL/minute): Adults: Venlafaxine: ~24%

Dialysis: Adults: Venlafaxine: ~57%, ODV: ~56%; due to large volume of distribution, a significant amount of drug is not likely to be removed.

Dosage Oral:

Children and Adolescents:

Attention-deficit/hyperactivity disorder (unlabeled use): Initial: 12.5 mg/day

Children <40 kg: Increase by 12.5 mg/week to maximum of 50 mg/day in 2 divided doses

Children ≥40 kg: Increase by 25 mg/week to maximum of 75 mg/day in 3 divided doses.

Mean dose: 60 mg or 1.4 mg/kg administered in 2-3 divided doses

Adults:

Depression:

Immediate-release tablets: 75 mg/day, administered in 2 or 3 divided doses, taken with food; dose may be increased in 75 mg/day increments at intervals of at least 4 days, up to 225-375 mg/day

Extended-release capsules or tablets: 75 mg once daily taken with food; for some new patients, it may be desirable to start at 37.5 mg/day for 4-7 days before increasing to 75 mg once daily; dose may be increased by up to 75 mg/day increments every 4 days as tolerated, up to a recommended maximum of 225 mg/day

Generalized anxiety disorder: Extended-release capsules: 75 mg once daily taken with food; for some new patients, it may be desirable to start at 37.5 mg/day for 4-7 days before increasing to 75 mg once daily; dose may be increased by up to 75 mg/day increments every 4 days as tolerated, up to a maximum of 225 mg/day

Panic disorder: Extended-release capsules: 37.5 mg once daily for 1 week; may increase to 75 mg daily, with subsequent weekly increases of 75 mg/day up to a maximum of 225 mg/day.

Social anxiety disorder:

Extended-release capsules: 75 mg once daily taken with food; for some new patients, it may be desirable to start at 37.5 mg/day for 4-7 days before increasing to 75 mg once daily; dose may be increased by up to 75 mg/day increments every 4 days as tolerated, up to a maximum of 225 mg/day

Extended release tablets: 75 mg once daily taken with food (maximum: 75 mg/day); no evidence that doses >75 mg/day offer any additional benefit

Obsessive-compulsive disorder (unlabeled use): Titrate to usual dosage range of 150-300 mg/day; however, doses up to 375 mg daily have been used; response may be seen in 4 weeks

Neuropathic pain (unlabeled use): Dosages evaluated varied considerably based on etiology of chronic pain, but efficacy has been shown for many conditions in the range of 75-225 mg/day; onset of relief may occur in 1-2 weeks, or take up to 6 weeks for full benefit.

Hot flashes (unlabeled use): Doses of 37.5-75 mg/day have demonstrated significant improvement of vasomotor symptoms after 4-8 weeks of treatment; in one study, doses >75 mg/day offered no additional benefit; however, higher doses (225 mg/day) may be beneficial in patients with perimenopausal depression.

◀ Attention-deficit disorder (unlabeled use): Initial: Doses vary between 18.75 to 75 mg/day; may increase after 4 weeks to 150 mg/day; if tolerated, doses up to 225 mg/day have been used

Post-traumatic stress disorder (PTSD) (unlabeled use): Extended release formulation: 37.5-300 mg/day

Note: When discontinuing this medication after more than 1 week of treatment, it is generally recommended that the dose be tapered. If venlafaxine is used for 6 weeks or longer, the dose should be tapered over 2 weeks when discontinuing its use.

Elderly: Alzheimer's dementia-related depression:

Immediate-release tablets: Initial: 25 mg/day; may increase at weekly intervals to maximum of 375 mg/day in divided doses

Extended-release capsules: Initial: 37.5 mg/day; may increase at weekly intervals to maximum of 225 mg/day

Dosing adjustment in renal impairment: Cl_{cr} 10-70 mL/minute: Decrease dose by 25%; decrease total daily dose by 50% if dialysis patients; dialysis patients should receive dosing after completion of dialysis

Dosing adjustment in moderate hepatic impairment: Reduce total daily dosage by 50%

Additional Information Complete prescribing information for this medication should be consulted for additional detail.

Dosage Forms Excipient information presented when available (limited, particularly for generics); consult specific product labeling. [DSC] = Discontinued product

Capsule, extended release:

Effexor XR®: 37.5 mg, 75 mg, 150 mg

Tablet: 25 mg, 37.5 mg, 50 mg, 75 mg, 100 mg

Effexor®: 25 mg, 37.5 mg, 50 mg; 75 mg [DSC]; 100 mg [DSC]

Tablet, extended release: 37.5 mg, 75 mg, 150 mg, 225 mg

◆ **Ventavis®** *see* Iloprost *on page* 725

◆ **Ventolin® (Can)** *see* Albuterol *on page* 49

◆ **Ventolin® Diskus (Can)** *see* Albuterol *on page* 49

◆ **Ventolin® HFA** *see* Albuterol *on page* 49

◆ **Ventolin® I.V. Infusion (Can)** *see* Albuterol *on page* 49

◆ **Ventrodisk (Can)** *see* Albuterol *on page* 49

◆ **Veramyst®** *see* Fluticasone *on page* 620

Verapamil (ver AP a mil)

Medication Safety Issues

Sound-alike/look-alike issues:

Calan® may be confused with Colace®, diltiazem

Covera-HS® may be confused with Provera®

Isoptin® may be confused with Isopto® Tears

Verelan® may be confused with Virilon®, Voltaren®

High alert medication: The Institute for Safe Medication Practices (ISMP) includes this medication (I.V. formulation) among its list of drug classes which have a heightened risk of causing significant patient harm when used in error.

Significant differences exist between oral and I.V. dosing. Use caution when converting from one route of administration to another.

International issues:

Calan®: Brand name for vinpocetine in Japan

Related Information
Anesthesia for Patients With Liver Disease *on page 1537*
Antiarrhythmic Drugs *on page 1656*
Calcium Channel Blockers *on page 1672*
Dosing Considerations for the Critically-Ill Patient With Morbid Obesity *on page 1561*
Hypertension *on page 1754*
Inhalational Anesthetics *on page 1632*

U.S. Brand Names Calan®; Calan® SR; Covera-HS®; Isoptin® SR; Verelan®; Verelan® PM

Canadian Brand Names Apo-Verap®; Apo-Verap® SR; Calan®; Chronovera®; Covera-HS®; Covera®; Dom-Verapamil SR; Gen-Verapamil; Gen-Verapamil SR; Isoptin® SR; Med-Verapamil; Mylan-Verapamil; Mylan-Verapamil SR; Novo-Veramil; Novo-Veramil SR; Nu-Verap; Nu-Verap SR; PHL-Verapamil; PMS-Verapamil SR; PRO-Verapamil SR; Riva-Verapamil SR; Verapamil Hydrochloride Injection, USP; Verelan SRC; ZYM-Verapamil SR

Index Terms Iproveratril Hydrochloride; Verapamil Hydrochloride

Pharmacologic Category Antiarrhythmic Agent, Class IV; Calcium Channel Blocker; Calcium Channel Blocker, Nondihydropyridine

Generic Available Yes

Use Orally for treatment of angina pectoris (vasospastic, chronic stable, unstable) and hypertension; I.V. for supraventricular tachyarrhythmias (PSVT, atrial fibrillation, atrial flutter)

Unlabeled/Investigational Use Migraine; hypertrophic cardiomyopathy; bipolar disorder (manic manifestations)

Mechanism of Action Inhibits calcium ion from entering the "slow channels" or select voltage-sensitive areas of vascular smooth muscle and myocardium during depolarization; produces a relaxation of coronary vascular smooth muscle and coronary vasodilation; increases myocardial oxygen delivery in patients with vasospastic angina; slows automaticity and conduction of AV node.

Pharmacodynamics/Kinetics
Onset of action: Peak effect: Oral: Immediate release: 1-2 hours; I.V.: 1-5 minutes
Duration: Oral: Immediate release tablets: 6-8 hours; I.V.: 10-20 minutes
Absorption: Well absorbed
Distribution: V_d: 3.89 L/kg (Storstein, 1984)
Protein binding: 90%
Metabolism: Hepatic (extensive first-pass effect) via multiple CYP isoenzymes; primary metabolite is norverapamil (20% pharmacologic activity of verapamil)
Bioavailability: Oral: 20% to 35%
Half-life elimination: Infants: 4.4-6.9 hours; Adults: Single dose: 2-8 hours, Multiple doses: 4.5-12 hours; prolonged with hepatic cirrhosis
Time to peak, serum: Oral: Immediate release: 1-2 hours
Excretion: Urine (70%, 3% to 4% as unchanged drug); feces (16%)

Dosage
Children: SVT:
I.V.:
<1 year: 0.1-0.2 mg/kg over 2 minutes; repeat every 30 minutes as needed
1-15 years: 0.1-0.3 mg/kg over 2 minutes; maximum: 5 mg/dose, may repeat dose in 15 minutes if adequate response not achieved; maximum for second dose: 10 mg/dose
Oral (dose not well established):
1-5 years: 4-8 mg/kg/day in 3 divided doses **or** 40-80 mg every 8 hours
>5 years: 80 mg every 6-8 hours
Adults:
SVT: I.V.: 2.5-5 mg (over 2 minutes); second dose of 5-10 mg (~0.15 mg/kg) may be given 15-30 minutes after the initial dose if patient tolerates, but does not respond to initial dose; maximum total dose: 20 mg
Angina: Oral: Initial dose: 80-120 mg 3 times/day (elderly or small stature: 40 mg 3 times/day); range: 240-480 mg/day in 3-4 divided doses
Hypertension: Oral:
Immediate release: 80 mg 3 times/day; usual dose range (JNC 7): 80-320 mg/day in 2 divided doses

Sustained release: 240 mg/day; usual dose range (JNC 7): 120-360 mg/day in 1-2 divided doses; 120 mg/day in the elderly or small patients (no evidence of additional benefit in doses >360 mg/day).

Extended release:

Covera-HS®: Usual dose range (JNC 7): 120-360 mg once daily (once-daily dosing is recommended at bedtime)

Verelan® PM: Usual dose range: 200-400 mg once daily at bedtime

Dosing adjustment in renal impairment: Manufacturer recommends caution and additional ECG monitoring in patients with renal insufficiency. **Note:** A multiple dose study in adults suggests reduced renal clearance of verapamil and its metabolite (norverapamil) with advanced renal failure (Storstein, 1984). Additionally, several clinical papers report adverse effects of verapamil in patients with chronic renal failure receiving recommended doses of verapamil (Pritza, 1991; Váquez, 1996). In contrast, a number of single dose studies show no difference in verapamil (or norverapamil metabolite) disposition between chronic renal failure and control patients (Beyerlein, 1990; Hanyok, 1988; Mooy, 1985; Zachariah, 1991).

Dialysis: Not removed by hemodialysis (Mooy, 1985); supplemental dose is not necessary.

Dosing adjustment/comments in hepatic disease: In cirrhosis, reduce dose to 20% and 50% of normal for oral and intravenous administration, respectively, and monitor ECG (Somogyi, 1981).

Stability Store injection at room temperature; do not freeze. Protect from heat. Use only clear solutions. Physically compatible in solutions of pH of 3-6, but may precipitate in solutions having a pH ≥6. Protect I.V. solution from light.

Administration

Oral: Do not crush or chew sustained or extended release products.

Calan® SR, Isoptin® SR: Administer with food.

Verelan®, Verelan® PM: Capsules may be opened and the contents sprinkled on 1 tablespoonful of applesauce, then swallowed without chewing.

I.V.: Rate of infusion: Over 2 minutes.

Monitoring Parameters Monitor blood pressure closely

Reference Range Therapeutic: 50-200 ng/mL (SI: 100-410 nmol/L) for parent; under normal conditions, norverapamil concentration is the same as parent drug. Toxic: >90 mcg/mL

Anesthesia and Critical Care Concerns/Other Considerations

Clinical Pearls/Comments: I.V. administration, concomitant hypertrophic cardiomyopathy, sick sinus syndrome, or moderate-to-severe heart failure, and concomitant therapy with beta-blockers or digoxin can all increase incidence of adverse effects. Verapamil should be avoided in patients with left ventricular dysfunction, pulmonary congestion, or heart failure. Verapamil may be administered intravenously in the acute setting to attain ventricular rate control in patients with atrial fibrillation or flutter. Patients who respond, defined in general as at least a 20% decrease in ventricular response rate or attaining a rate <100 beats/minute, can be continued on oral therapy to maintain control. It is important to consider the potential drug interaction with digoxin, as these agents are both used in this setting.

Extemporaneously Prepared: To prepare a verapamil 50 mg/mL liquid, crush 75 verapamil hydrochloride 80 mg tablets into a fine powder. Add ~40 mL of either Ora-Sweet® and Ora-Plus® (1:1 preparation), or Ora-Sweet® SF and Ora-Plus® (1:1 preparation), or cherry syrup. Mix to a uniform paste. Continue to add the vehicle to bring the final volume to 120 mL. The preparation is stable for 60 days; shake well before using and protect from light.

Pregnancy Risk Factor C

Contraindications Hypersensitivity to verapamil or any component of the formulation; severe left ventricular dysfunction; hypotension (systolic pressure <90 mm Hg) or cardiogenic shock; sick sinus syndrome (except in patients with a functioning artificial pacemaker); second- or third-degree AV block (except in patients with a functioning artificial pacemaker); atrial flutter or fibrillation and an accessory bypass tract (WPW, Lown-Ganong-Levine syndrome)

Warnings/Precautions Increased angina and/or MI has occurred with initiation or dosage titration of calcium channel blockers. The most common side effect is peripheral edema; occurs within 2-3 weeks of starting therapy. Avoid use in heart failure; can exacerbate condition. Symptomatic hypotension with or without syncope can rarely occur; blood pressure must be lowered at a rate appropriate for the patient's clinical condition. Rare increases in liver function tests can be observed. Can cause first-degree AV block or sinus bradycardia. Other conduction abnormalities are rare. Use caution when using verapamil together with a beta-blocker. Avoid I.V. verapamil with an I.V. beta-blocker; can result in asystole. Use I.V. with caution in patients with hypertrophic subaortic stenosis (IHSS). Use I.V. with caution in patients with attenuated neuromuscular transmission (Duchenne's muscular dystrophy, myasthenia gravis). Use with caution in renal impairment; monitor hemodynamics and possibly ECG if severe impairment, particularly if concomitant hepatic impairment. Use with caution in patients with hepatic impairment; may require lower starting dose in cirrhosis or severe impairment. Verapamil significantly increases digoxin serum concentrations (adjust digoxin's dose). May prolong recovery from nondepolarizing neuromuscular-blocking agents.

Adverse Reactions
>10%: Gastrointestinal: Gingival hyperplasia (up to 19%), constipation (12% up to 42% in clinical trials)

1% to 10%:
Cardiovascular: Bradycardia (1.2 to 1.4%); first-, second-, or third-degree AV block (1.2%); CHF (1.8%); hypotension (2.5% to 3%); peripheral edema (1.9%), symptomatic hypotension (1.5% I.V.); severe tachycardia (1%)
Central nervous system: Dizziness (1.2% to 3.3%), fatigue (1.7%), headache (1.2% to 2.2%)
Dermatologic: Rash (1.2%)
Gastrointestinal: Nausea (0.9% to 2.7%)
Respiratory: Dyspnea (1.4%)

<1% (Limited to important or life-threatening): Alopecia, angina, arthralgia, asystole, atrioventricular dissociation, bronchial/laryngeal spasm, cerebrovascular accident, chest pain, claudication, confusion, diarrhea, dry mouth, ecchymosis, electrical mechanical dissociation (EMD), emotional depression, eosinophilia, equilibrium disorders, erythema multiforme, exanthema, exfoliative dermatitis, galactorrhea/hyperprolactinemia, GI obstruction, gingival hyperplasia, gynecomastia, hair color change, impotence, muscle cramps, MI, myoclonus, paresthesia, Parkinsonian syndrome, psychotic symptoms, purpura (vasculitis), rash, respiratory failure, rotary nystagmus, shakiness, shock, somnolence, Stevens-Johnson syndrome, syncope, urticaria, ventricular fibrillation, vertigo

Drug Interactions
Metabolism/Transport Effects Substrate of CYP1A2 (minor), 2B6 (minor), 2C9 (minor), 2C18 (minor), 2E1 (minor), 3A4 (major); **Inhibits** CYP1A2 (weak), 2C9 (weak), 2D6 (weak), 3A4 (moderate)

Avoid Concomitant Use
Avoid concomitant use of Verapamil with any of the following: Dabigatran Etexilate; Dofetilide; Everolimus; Ranolazine; Tolvaptan; Topotecan

Increased Effect/Toxicity
Verapamil may increase the levels/effects of: Alcohol (Ethyl); Amifostine; Amiodarone; Antihypertensives; Atorvastatin; Benzodiazepines (metabolized by oxidation); Beta-Blockers; BusPIRone; Calcium Channel Blockers (Dihydropyridine); CarBAMazepine; Cardiac Glycosides; Colchicine; Corticosteroids (Systemic); CycloSPORINE; CYP3A4 Substrates; Dabigatran Etexilate; Dofetilide; Dronedarone; Eletriptan; Eplerenone; Everolimus; Fexofenadine; Halofantrine; Hypotensive Agents; Lithium; Lovastatin; Magnesium Salts; Midodrine; Neuromuscular-Blocking Agents (Nondepolarizing); Nitroprusside; P-Glycoprotein Substrates; Phenytoin; Pimecrolimus; QuiNIDine; Ranolazine; Red Yeast Rice; Risperidone; RiTUXimab; Rivaroxaban; Salicylates; Salmeterol; Saxagliptin; Simvastatin; Tacrolimus; Tolvaptan; Topotecan

The levels/effects of Verapamil may be increased by: Alpha1-Blockers; Anilidopiperidine Opioids; Antifungal Agents (Azole Derivatives, Systemic); Atorvastatin; Cimetidine; CycloSPORINE; CYP3A4 Inhibitors (Moderate); CYP3A4 Inhibitors (Strong); Dasatinib; Diazoxide; Dronedarone; Everolimus; Fluconazole; Grapefruit Juice; Herbs (Hypotensive Properties); Macrolide

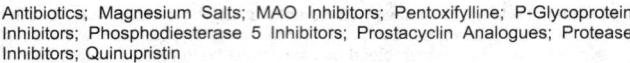

Antibiotics; Magnesium Salts; MAO Inhibitors; Pentoxifylline; P-Glycoprotein Inhibitors; Phosphodiesterase 5 Inhibitors; Prostacyclin Analogues; Protease Inhibitors; Quinupristin

Decreased Effect

Verapamil may decrease the levels/effects of: Clopidogrel

The levels/effects of Verapamil may be decreased by: Barbiturates; Calcium Salts; CarBAMazepine; CYP3A4 Inducers (Strong); Deferasirox; Herbs (CYP3A4 Inducers); Herbs (Hypertensive Properties); Methylphenidate; Nafcillin; P-Glycoprotein Inducers; Rifamycin Derivatives; Yohimbine

Ethanol/Nutrition/Herb Interactions

Ethanol: Avoid or limit ethanol (may increase ethanol levels).

Food: Grapefruit juice may increase the serum concentration of verapamil; avoid concurrent use.

Herb/Nutraceutical: St John's wort may decrease levels. Avoid dong quai if using for hypertension (has estrogenic activity). Avoid ephedra, yohimbe, ginseng (may worsen arrhythmia or hypertension). Avoid garlic (may have increased antihypertensive effect).

Dietary Considerations Calan® SR and Isoptin® SR products may be taken with food or milk, other formulations may be administered without regard to meals; sprinkling contents of Verelan® or Verelan® PM capsule onto applesauce does not affect oral absorption.

Dosage Forms Excipient information presented when available (limited, particularly for generics); consult specific product labeling. [DSC] = Discontinued product

Caplet, sustained release, as hydrochloride: 120 mg, 180 mg, 240 mg
　Calan® SR: 120 mg
　Calan® SR: 180 mg, 240 mg [scored]
Capsule, extended release, as hydrochloride: 120 mg, 180 mg, 240 mg
Capsule, extended release, controlled onset, as hydrochloride: 100 mg, 200 mg, 300 mg
　Verelan® PM: 100 mg, 200 mg, 300 mg
Capsule, sustained release, as hydrochloride: 120 mg, 180 mg, 240 mg, 360 mg
　Verelan®: 120 mg, 180 mg, 240 mg, 360 mg
Injection, solution, as hydrochloride: 2.5 mg/mL (2 mL, 4 mL)
Tablet, as hydrochloride: 40 mg, 80 mg, 120 mg
　Calan®: 40 mg [DSC]
　Calan®: 80 mg, 120 mg [scored]
Tablet, extended release, as hydrochloride: 120 mg, 180 mg, 240 mg
Tablet, extended release, controlled onset, as hydrochloride:
　Covera-HS®: 180 mg, 240 mg
Tablet, sustained release, as hydrochloride: 120 mg, 180 mg, 240 mg
　Isoptin® SR: 120 mg
　Isoptin® SR: 180 mg, 240 mg [scored]

◆ **Verapamil Hydrochloride** *see* Verapamil *on page 1468*

◆ **Verapamil Hydrochloride Injection, USP (Can)** *see* Verapamil *on page 1468*

◆ **Verelan®** *see* Verapamil *on page 1468*

◆ **Verelan® PM** *see* Verapamil *on page 1468*

◆ **Verelan SRC (Can)** *see* Verapamil *on page 1468*

◆ **Veripred™ 20** *see* PrednisoLONE *on page 1164*

◆ **Versed** *see* Midazolam *on page 935*

◆ **Versiclear™** *see* Sodium Thiosulfate *on page 1316*

◆ **VFEND®** *see* Voriconazole *on page 1474*

◆ **Viagra®** *see* Sildenafil *on page 1287*

◆ **Vibativ™** *see* Telavancin *on page 1353*

◆ **Vibramycin®** *see* Doxycycline *on page 456*

◆ **Vibra-Tabs®** *see* Doxycycline *on page 456*

◆ **Vicks® Sinex® Nasal Spray [OTC]** *see* Phenylephrine *on page 1114*

◆ **Vicks® Sinex® UltraFine Mist [OTC]** *see* Phenylephrine *on page 1114*

♦ **Vicodin®** *see* Hydrocodone and Acetaminophen *on page 697*

♦ **Vicodin® ES** *see* Hydrocodone and Acetaminophen *on page 697*

♦ **Vicodin® HP** *see* Hydrocodone and Acetaminophen *on page 697*

Vigabatrin (vye GA ba trin)

Related Information
Perioperative Management of Patients on Antiseizure Medication *on page 1577*
U.S. Brand Names Sabril®
Canadian Brand Names Sabril®
Pharmacologic Category Anticonvulsant, Miscellaneous
Restrictions Vigabatrin is only available in the U.S. under a special restricted distribution program (SHARE). Under the SHARE program, only prescribers and pharmacies registered with the program are able to prescribe and distribute vigabatrin. Vigabatrin may only be dispensed to patients who are enrolled in and meet all conditions of SHARE. Contact the SHARE program at 1-888-45-SHARE.
Use Treatment of infantile spasms; refractory complex partial seizures not controlled by usual treatments

Additional uses in Canadian labeling (not in U.S. labeling): Active management of partial or secondary generalized seizures not controlled by usual treatments
Unlabeled/Investigational Use Spasticity, tardive dyskinesias
Pharmacodynamics/Kinetics
Duration (rate of GABA-T resynthesis dependent): Variable (not strictly correlated to serum concentrations)
Absorption: Rapid
Distribution: V_d: 1.1 L/kg
Metabolism: Insignificant
Half-life elimination: Infants: 5.7 hours; Adults: 7.5 hours; Elderly: 12-13 hours
Time to peak: Infants: 2.5 hours; Children: 1 hour; Adults: 1 hour
Excretion: Urine (80%, as unchanged drug)
Dosage Oral:
Children 1 month to 2 years: Infantile spasms: Initial dosing: 50 mg/kg/day divided twice daily; may titrate upwards by 25-50 mg/kg/day every 3 days to a maximum of 150 mg/kg/day
Note: To taper, decrease dose by 25-50 mg/kg/day every 3-4 days
Children: Adjunctive treatment of seizures (Canadian labeling; not in U.S. labeling): Initial: 40 mg/kg/day divided twice daily; maintenance dosages based on patient weight:
10-15 kg: 0.5-1 g/day divided twice daily
16-30 kg: 1-1.5 g/day divided twice daily
31-50 kg: 1.5-3 g/day divided twice daily
>50 kg: 2-3 g/day divided twice daily
Adolescents ≥16 years and Adults: Refractory complex partial seizures: Initial: 500 mg twice daily; increase daily dose by 500 mg at weekly intervals based on response and tolerability. Recommended dose: 3 g/day
Note: To taper, decrease dose by 1 g/day on a weekly basis
Elderly: Refractory complex partial seizures: Initiate at low end of dosage range (refer to Adult dosing); monitor closely for sedation and confusion

Dosage adjustment in renal impairment:
Cl_{cr} >50-80 mL/minute: Decrease dose by 25%
Cl_{cr} >30-50 mL/minute: Decrease dose by 50%
Cl_{cr} >10-30 mL/minute: Decrease dose by 75%
Additional Information Not available in U.S. Complete prescribing information for this medication should be consulted for additional detail.
Dosage Forms Excipient information presented when available (limited, particularly for generics); consult specific product labeling. [CAN] = Canadian product
Powder for solution, oral:
Sabril®: 500 mg/packet (50s)
Powder for suspension, oral [sachets]:
Sabril® [CAN]: 0.5 g

Tablet, oral:
Sabril®: 500 mg

References

Bar-Oz B, Nulman I, Koren G, et al, "Anticonvulsants and Breast-Feeding: A Critical Review," *Paediatr Drugs*, 2000, 2(2):113-26.

Challier JC, Rey E, Bintein T, et al, "Passage of S(+) and R(-) Gamma-vinyl-GABA Across the Human Isolated Perfused Placenta," *Br J Clin Pharmacol*, 1992, 34(2):139-43.

Sabers A and Gram L, "Newer Anticonvulsants: Comparative Review of Drug Interactions and Adverse Effects," *Drugs*, 2000, 60(1):23-33.

Sabril® product monograph, Aventis Pharma Inc, Quebec, April 2001.

Tran A, O'Mahoney T, Rey E, et al, "Vigabatrin: Placental Transfer *in vivo* and Excretion Into Breast Milk of the Enantiomers," *Br J Clin Pharmacol*, 1998, 45(4):409-11.

- ◆ **Vigamox®** *see* Moxifloxacin *on page 961*
- ◆ **Vimpat®** *see* Lacosamide *on page 795*
- ◆ **Visicol®** *see* Sodium Phosphates *on page 1309*
- ◆ **Visken® (Can)** *see* Pindolol *on page 1130*
- ◆ **Vitamin B$_3$** *see* Niacin *on page 1001*
- ◆ **Vitamin B$_{12a}$** *see* Hydroxocobalamin *on page 711*
- ◆ **Vitamin K$_1$** *see* Phytonadione *on page 1128*
- ◆ **Vitrase®** *see* Hyaluronidase *on page 692*
- ◆ **Vitrasert®** *see* Ganciclovir *on page 654*
- ◆ **Vivarin® [OTC]** *see* Caffeine *on page 225*
- ◆ **Vivelle® [DSC]** *see* Estradiol *on page 531*
- ◆ **Vivelle-Dot®** *see* Estradiol *on page 531*
- ◆ **Vivitrol™** *see* Naltrexone *on page 985*
- ◆ **Voltaren®** *see* Diclofenac *on page 414*
- ◆ **Voltaren® Emulgel™ (Can)** *see* Diclofenac *on page 414*
- ◆ **Voltaren® Gel** *see* Diclofenac *on page 414*
- ◆ **Voltaren Ophtha® (Can)** *see* Diclofenac *on page 414*
- ◆ **Voltaren Ophthalmic®** *see* Diclofenac *on page 414*
- ◆ **Voltaren Rapide® (Can)** *see* Diclofenac *on page 414*
- ◆ **Voltaren SR® (Can)** *see* Diclofenac *on page 414*
- ◆ **Voltaren®-XR** *see* Diclofenac *on page 414*
- ◆ **Voluven®** *see* Hetastarch *on page 688*

Voriconazole (vor i KOE na zole)

Related Information
Antifungal Agents *on page 1664*
U.S. Brand Names VFEND®
Canadian Brand Names VFEND®
Index Terms UK109496
Pharmacologic Category Antifungal Agent, Oral; Antifungal Agent, Parenteral
Generic Available No

Use Treatment of invasive aspergillosis; treatment of esophageal candidiasis; treatment of candidemia (in non-neutropenic patients); treatment of disseminated *Candida* infections of the skin and viscera; treatment of serious fungal infections caused by *Scedosporium apiospermum* and *Fusarium* spp (including *Fusarium solani*) in patients intolerant of, or refractory to, other therapy

Unlabeled/Investigational Use
Fungal infection prophylaxis in intermediate or high risk neutropenic cancer patients with myelodysplastic syndrome (MDS) or acute myelogenous leukemia (AML), neutropenic allogeneic hematopoietic stem cell recipients, and patients with significant graft-versus-host disease; empiric antifungal therapy (second-line) for persistent neutropenic fever

Mechanism of Action Interferes with fungal cytochrome P450 activity (selectively inhibits 14-alpha-lanosterol demethylation), decreasing ergosterol synthesis (principal sterol in fungal cell membrane) and inhibiting fungal cell membrane formation.

Pharmacodynamics/Kinetics

Absorption: Well absorbed after oral administration; administration of crushed tablets is considered bioequivalent to whole tablets

Distribution: V_d: 4.6 L/kg

Protein binding: 58%

Metabolism: Hepatic, via CYP2C19 (major pathway) and CYP2C9 and CYP3A4 (less significant); saturable (may demonstrate nonlinearity)

Bioavailability: 96%

Half-life elimination: Variable, dose-dependent

Time to peak: Oral: 1-2 hours; 0.5 hours (crushed tablet)

Excretion: Urine (as inactive metabolites; <2% as unchanged drug)

Dosage

Usual dosage ranges:

Children <12 years: Dosage not established

Children ≥12 years and Adults:

Oral: 100-300 mg every 12 hours

I.V.: 6 mg/kg every 12 hours for 2 doses; followed by maintenance dose of 4 mg/kg every 12 hours

Indication-specific dosing: Children ≥12 years and Adults:

Aspergillosis, invasive, including disseminated and extrapulmonary infection: Duration of therapy should be a minimum of 6-12 weeks or throughout period of immunosuppression.

I.V.: Initial: Loading dose: 6 mg/kg every 12 hours for 2 doses; followed by maintenance dose of 4 mg/kg every 12 hours

Oral: May consider oral therapy in place of I.V. with dosing of 4 mg/kg (rounded up to convenient tablet dosage form) every 12 hours; however, I.V. administration is preferred in serious infections since comparative efficacy with the oral formulation has not been established.

Scedosporiosis, fusariosis: I.V.: Initial: Loading dose: 6 mg/kg every 12 hours for 2 doses; followed by maintenance dose of 4 mg/kg every 12 hours

Candidemia and other deep tissue *Candida* infections: I.V.: Initial: Loading dose 6 mg/kg every 12 hours for 2 doses; followed by maintenance dose of 3-4 mg/kg every 12 hours

Endophthalmitis, fungal (unlabeled use, Pappas, 2009): I.V.: 6 mg/kg every 12 hours for 2 doses, then 3-4 mg/kg every 12 hours

Esophageal candidiasis: Oral:

Patients <40 kg: 100 mg every 12 hours; maximum: 300 mg/day

Patients ≥40 kg: 200 mg every 12 hours; maximum: 600 mg/day

Note: Treatment should continue for a minimum of 14 days, and for at least 7 days following resolution of symptoms.

Conversion to oral dosing:

Patients <40 kg: 100 mg every 12 hours; increase to 150 mg every 12 hours in patients who fail to respond adequately

Patients ≥40 kg: 200 mg every 12 hours; increase to 300 mg every 12 hours in patients who fail to respond adequately

Dosage adjustment in patients unable to tolerate treatment:

I.V.: Dose may be reduced to 3 mg/kg every 12 hours

Oral: Dose may be reduced in 50 mg decrements to a minimum dosage of 200 mg every 12 hours in patients weighing ≥40 kg (100 mg every 12 hours in patients <40 kg)

Dosage adjustment in patients receiving concomitant CYP450 enzyme inducers or substrates:

Cyclosporine: Reduce cyclosporine dose by ¹/₂ and monitor closely.

Efavirenz: Oral: Increase maintenance dose of voriconazole to 400 mg every 12 hours and reduce efavirenz dose to 300 mg once daily

Phenytoin:

I.V.: Increase maintenance dosage to 5 mg/kg every 12 hours

Oral: Increase dose to 400 mg every 12 hours in patients ≥40 kg (200 mg every 12 hours in patients <40 kg)

◄ **Dosage adjustment in renal impairment:** In patients with Cl_{cr} <50 mL/minute, accumulation of the intravenous vehicle (cyclodextrin) occurs. After initial I.V. loading dose, oral voriconazole should be administered to these patients, unless an assessment of the benefit:risk to the patient justifies the use of I.V. voriconazole. Monitor serum creatinine and change to oral voriconazole therapy when possible.

Hemodialysis: Oral dosage adjustment not required; I.V. dosing not recommended since cyclodextrin vehicle is cleared at half the rate of voriconazole and may accumulate

Dosage adjustment in hepatic impairment:

Mild-to-moderate hepatic dysfunction (Child-Pugh class A and B): Following standard loading dose, reduce maintenance dosage by 50%

Severe hepatic impairment: Should only be used if benefit outweighs risk; monitor closely for toxicity

Stability

Powder for injection: Store at 15°C to 30°C (59°F to 86°F). Reconstitute 200 mg vial with 19 mL of sterile water for injection (use of automated syringe is not recommended). Resultant solution (20 mL) has a concentration of 10 mg/mL. Prior to infusion, must dilute to 0.5-5 mg/mL with NS, LR, D_5WLR, D_5W^1/2NS, D_5W, D_5W with KCl 20 mEq, ^{1}/2NS, or D_5WNS. Do not dilute with 4.2% sodium bicarbonate infusion. Reconstituted solutions are stable for up to 24 hours under refrigeration at 2°C to 8°C (36°F to 46°F).

Powder for oral suspension: Store at 2°C to 8°C (36°F to 46°F). Add 46 mL of water to the bottle to make 40 mg/mL suspension. Reconstituted oral suspension may be stored at 15°C to 30°C (59°F to 86°F). Discard after 14 days.

Tablets: Store at 15°C to 30°C (59°F to 86°F).

Administration

Oral: Administer 1 hour before or 1 hour after a meal.

I.V.: Infuse over 1-2 hours (rate not to exceed 3 mg/kg/hour). Do not infuse concomitantly into same line or cannula with other drug infusions, including TPN.

Monitoring Parameters Hepatic function at initiation and during course of treatment; renal function; serum electrolytes (particularly calcium, magnesium and potassium) prior to therapy initiation; visual function (visual acuity, visual field and color perception) if treatment course continues >28 days; may consider obtaining voriconazole trough level in patients failing therapy or exhibiting signs of toxicity; pancreatic function (in patients at risk for acute pancreatitis)

Anesthesia and Critical Care Concerns/Other Considerations

Clinical Pearls/Comments: Based on high oral bioavailability, switching between I.V. and oral administration is appropriate when clinically indicated. Infusions of blood products and any electrolyte supplementation must not occur simultaneously with intravenous voriconazole. Voriconazole I.V. must not be infused into the same line or cannula concomitantly with other drug infusions.

Pregnancy Risk Factor D

Contraindications Hypersensitivity to voriconazole or any component of the formulation (cross-reaction with other azole antifungal agents may occur but has not been established, use caution); coadministration of CYP3A4 substrates which may lead to QT_c prolongation (cisapride, pimozide, or quinidine); coadministration with barbiturates (long acting), carbamazepine, efavirenz (with standard [eg, not adjusted] voriconazole and efavirenz doses), ergot derivatives, rifampin, rifabutin, ritonavir (≥800 mg/day), sirolimus, St John's wort

Warnings/Precautions Visual changes, including blurred vision, changes in visual acuity, color perception, and photophobia, are commonly associated with treatment. Patients should be warned to avoid tasks which depend on vision, including operating machinery or driving. Changes are reversible on discontinuation following brief exposure/treatment regimens (≤28 days).

Serious hepatic reactions (including hepatitis, cholestasis, and fulminant hepatic failure) have occurred during treatment, primarily in patients with serious concomitant medical conditions. However, hepatotoxicity has occurred in patients with no identifiable risk factors. Use caution in patients with pre-existing hepatic impairment (dose adjustment or discontinuation may be required).

Voriconazole tablets contain lactose; avoid administration in hereditary galactose intolerance, Lapp lactase deficiency, or glucose-galactose malabsorption.

Suspension contains sucrose; use caution with fructose intolerance, sucrose-isomaltase deficiency, or glucose-galactose malabsorption. Avoid/limit use of intravenous formulation in patients with renal impairment; intravenous formulation contains excipient cyclodextrin (sulfobutyl ether beta-cyclodextrin), which may accumulate in renal insufficiency. Acute renal failure has been observed in severely ill patients; use with caution in patients receiving concomitant nephrotoxic medications. Anaphylactoid-type infusion-related reactions may occur with intravenous dosing. Consider discontinuation of infusion if reaction is severe.

Use caution in patients taking strong cytochrome P450 inducers, CYP2C9 inhibitors, and major 3A4 substrates (see Drug Interactions); consider alternative agents that avoid or lessen the potential for CYP-mediated interactions. QT interval prolongation has been associated with voriconazole use; rare cases of arrhythmia (including torsade de pointes), cardiac arrest, and sudden death have been reported, usually in seriously ill patients with comorbidities and/or risk factors (eg, prior cardiotoxic chemotherapy, cardiomyopathy, electrolyte imbalance, or concomitant QT_c-prolonging drugs). Use with caution in these patient populations; correct electrolyte abnormalities (eg, hypokalemia, hypomagnesemia, hypocalcemia) prior to initiating therapy. Do not infuse concomitantly with blood products or short-term concentrated electrolyte solutions, even if the two infusions are running in separate intravenous lines (or cannulas). Rarely, serious cutaneous reactions (including Stevens-Johnson syndrome) have been reported with treatment. Consider discontinuing in patients developing a rash. Avoid strong, direct exposure to sunlight; may cause photosensitivity, especially with long-term use. Monitor pancreatic function in patients (children and adults) at risk for acute pancreatitis (eg, recent chemotherapy or hematopoietic stem cell transplantation); there have been postmarketing reports of pancreatitis in children. Safety and efficacy have not been established in children <12 years of age.

Adverse Reactions
>10%:
- Central nervous system: Hallucinations (4% to 12%; auditory and/or visual and likely serum concentration-dependent)
- Ocular: Visual changes (dose related; photophobia, color changes, increased or decreased visual acuity, or blurred vision occur in ~21%)
- Renal: Creatinine increased (1% to 21%)

2% to 10%:
- Cardiovascular: Tachycardia (≤2%)
- Central nervous system: Fever (≤6%), chills (≤4%), headache (≤3%)
- Dermatologic: Rash (≤7%)
- Endocrine & metabolic: Hypokalemia (≤2%)
- Gastrointestinal: Nausea (1% to 5%), vomiting (1% to 4%)
- Hepatic: Alkaline phosphatase increased (4% to 5%), AST increased (2% to 4%), ALT increased (2% to 3%), cholestatic jaundice (1% to 2%)
- Ocular: Photophobia (2% to 3%)

<2% (Limited to important or life-threatening): Acute tubular necrosis, adrenal cortical insufficiency, agranulocytosis, allergic reaction, anaphylactoid reaction, anemia (aplastic, hemolytic, macrocytic, megaloblastic, or microcytic), angioedema, anuria, ascites, atrial arrhythmia, atrial fibrillation, AV block, bigeminy, bleeding time increased, bone marrow depression, bone necrosis, bradycardia, brain edema, bundle branch block, BUN increased, cardiac arrest, cardiomegaly, cardiomyopathy, cerebral hemorrhage/ischemia, cerebrovascular accident, chest pain, CHF, cholecystitis, cholelithiasis, chromatopsia, color blindness, coma, confusion, cyanosis, delirium, dementia, depersonalization, depression, diabetes insipidus, diarrhea, DIC, discoid lupus erythematosus, duodenal ulcer perforation, DVT, dyspnea, edema, encephalopathy, endocarditis, eosinophilia, erythema multiforme, exfoliative dermatitis, extrapyramidal symptoms, fixed drug eruption, fulminant hepatic failure, GI hemorrhage, GGT/LDH increased, glucose tolerance decreased, Guillain-Barré syndrome, hematemesis, hepatic coma, hepatic failure, hepatitis, hepatomegaly, hydronephrosis, hyper-/hypocalcemia, hyper-/hypoglycemia, hyper-/hypomagnesemia, hyper-/hyponatremia, hyper-/hypotension, hyper-/hypothyroidism, hyperbilirubinemia, hypercholesterolemia, hyperkalemia, hyperuricemia, hypophosphatemia, hypoxia, intestinal perforation, intracranial hypertension, jaundice, leukopenia, lung edema, ▶

◀ lymphadenopathy, lymphangitis, maculopapular rash, MI, multiorgan failure, myasthenia, myopathy, nephritis, nephrosis, neuropathy, night blindness, nodal arrhythmia, oculogyric crisis, optic atrophy, optic neuritis, osteomalacia, osteoporosis, palpitation, pancreatitis, pancytopenia, papilledema, paresthesia, peripheral edema, peritonitis, petechia, photosensitivity, pleural effusion, postural hypotension, pruritus, pseudomembraneous colitis, psychosis, pulmonary embolus, purpura, QT interval prolongation, renal dysfunction, renal failure (acute), respiratory distress syndrome, retinal hemorrhage, seizure, sepsis, spleen enlarged, Stevens-Johnson syndrome, suicidal ideation, supraventricular extrasystoles, supraventricular tachycardia, syncope, thrombocytopenia, thrombophlebitis, thrombotic thrombocytopenic purpura, tongue edema, torsade de pointes, toxic epidermal necrolysis, uremia, urinary retention, urticaria, uveitis, vasodilation, ventricular arrhythmia, ventricular fibrillation, ventricular tachycardia, visual field defect

Drug Interactions
Metabolism/Transport Effects **Substrate** of CYP2C9 (major), 2C19 (major), 3A4 (minor); **Inhibits** CYP2C9 (weak), 2C19 (weak), 3A4 (moderate)

Avoid Concomitant Use
Avoid concomitant use of Voriconazole with any of the following: Alfuzosin; Artemether; Barbiturates; CarBAMazepine; Cisapride; Conivaptan; Darunavir; Dofetilide; Dronedarone; Eplerenone; Ergot Derivatives; Everolimus; Halofantrine; Lopinavir; Lumefantrine; Nilotinib; Nisoldipine; Pimozide; QuiNIDine; QuiNINE; Ranolazine; Rifamycin Derivatives; Ritonavir; Rivaroxaban; Salmeterol; Silodosin; Sirolimus; St Johns Wort; Tetrabenazine; Thioridazine; Tolvaptan; Ziprasidone

Increased Effect/Toxicity
Voriconazole may increase the levels/effects of: Alfentanil; Alfuzosin; Almotriptan; Alosetron; Antineoplastic Agents (Vinca Alkaloids); Aprepitant; Benzodiazepines (metabolized by oxidation); Bosentan; BusPIRone; Busulfan; Calcium Channel Blockers; CarBAMazepine; Cardiac Glycosides; Ciclesonide; Cilostazol; Cinacalcet; Cisapride; Colchicine; Conivaptan; Corticosteroids (Orally Inhaled); Corticosteroids (Systemic); CycloSPORINE; CYP3A4 Substrates; Diclofenac; Docetaxel; Dofetilide; Dronedarone; Dutasteride; Eletriptan; Eplerenone; Ergot Derivatives; Erlotinib; Eszopiclone; Everolimus; FentaNYL; Fesoterodine; Fosaprepitant; Gefitinib; Halofantrine; HMG-CoA Reductase Inhibitors; Imatinib; Irinotecan; Ixabepilone; Losartan; Macrolide Antibiotics; Maraviroc; Methadone; Nilotinib; Nisoldipine; Oral Contraceptive (Estrogens); Oral Contraceptive (Progestins); Paricalcitol; Phenytoin; Phosphodiesterase 5 Inhibitors; Pimecrolimus; Pimozide; Protease Inhibitors; QTc-Prolonging Agents; QuiNIDine; QuiNINE; Ramelteon; Ranolazine; Repaglinide; Reverse Transcriptase Inhibitors (Non-Nucleoside); Rifamycin Derivatives; Rivaroxaban; Salmeterol; Saxagliptin; Silodosin; Sirolimus; Solifenacin; Sorafenib; Sunitinib; Tacrolimus; Tadalafil; Temsirolimus; Tetrabenazine; Thioridazine; Tolterodine; Tolvaptan; Trimetrexate; Venlafaxine; Vitamin K Antagonists; Ziprasidone; Zolpidem

The levels/effects of Voriconazole may be increased by: Alfuzosin; Artemether; Chloroquine; Ciprofloxacin; CYP2C9 Inhibitors (Moderate); CYP2C9 Inhibitors (Strong); Gadobutrol; Grapefruit Juice; Lumefantrine; Macrolide Antibiotics; Nilotinib; Oral Contraceptive (Estrogens); Oral Contraceptive (Progestins); Protease Inhibitors; Proton Pump Inhibitors; QuiNINE

Decreased Effect
Voriconazole may decrease the levels/effects of: Amphotericin B; Prasugrel; *Saccharomyces boulardii*

The levels/effects of Voriconazole may be decreased by: Barbiturates; CarBAMazepine; CYP2C19 Inducers (Strong); CYP2C9 Inducers (Highly Effective); Darunavir; Didanosine; Lopinavir; Peginterferon Alfa-2b; Phenytoin; Reverse Transcriptase Inhibitors (Non-Nucleoside); Rifamycin Derivatives; Ritonavir; St Johns Wort; Sucralfate

Ethanol/Nutrition/Herb Interactions
Food: May decrease voriconazole absorption. Voriconazole should be taken 1 hour before or 1 hour after a meal. Avoid grapefruit juice (may decrease voriconazole levels).

Herb/Nutraceutical: St John's wort may decrease voriconazole levels; concurrent use with voriconazole is contraindicated.

Dietary Considerations Oral: Should be taken 1 hour before or 1 hour after a meal. Voriconazole tablets contain lactose; avoid administration in hereditary galactose intolerance, Lapp lactase deficiency, or glucose-galactose malabsorption. Suspension contains sucrose; use caution with fructose intolerance, sucrose-isomaltase deficiency, or glucose-galactose malabsorption.

Dosage Forms Excipient information presented when available (limited, particularly for generics); consult specific product labeling.

Injection, powder for reconstitution:

VFEND®: 200 mg [contains cyclodextrin]

Powder for oral suspension:

VFEND®: 200 mg/5 mL (70 mL) [contains sodium benzoate and sucrose; orange flavor]

Tablet:

VFEND®: 50 mg, 200 mg

♦ **VoSpire ER®** *see* Albuterol *on page 49*

Warfarin (WAR far in)

Medication Safety Issues

Sound-alike/look-alike issues:

Coumadin® may be confused with Avandia®, Cardura®, Compazine®, Kemadrin®

Jantoven® may be confused with Janumet™, Januvia™

High alert medication: The Institute for Safe Medication Practices (ISMP) includes this medication among its list of drugs which have a heightened risk of causing significant patient harm when used in error.

2009 National Patient Safety Goals: The Joint Commission on Accreditation of Healthcare Organizations requires healthcare organizations that provide anticoagulant therapy to have a process in place to reduce the risk of anticoagulant-associated patient harm. Patients receiving anticoagulants should receive individualized care through a defined process that includes standardized ordering, dispensing, administration, monitoring and education. This does not apply to routine short-term use of anticoagulants for prevention of venous thromboembolism when the expectation is that the patient's laboratory values will remain within or close to normal values (NPSG.03.05.01).

Medication Guide An FDA-approved patient medication guide, which is available with the product information and at http://www.fda.gov/downloads/Drugs/DrugSafety/ucm088578.pdf, must be dispensed with this medication for each new outpatient prescription and refill.

Related Information

Anesthesia Considerations for Neurosurgery *on page 1514*

Anesthesia for Obstetric Patients in Nonobstetric Surgery *on page 1532*

Perioperative / Periprocedural Management of Anticoagulant and Antiplatelet Therapy *on page 1607*

Regional Anesthesia in Patients Receiving Anticoagulant and Antiplatelet Therapy *on page 1642*

U.S. Brand Names Coumadin®; Jantoven®

Canadian Brand Names Apo-Warfarin®; Coumadin®; Gen-Warfarin; Mylan-Warfarin; Novo-Warfarin; Taro-Warfarin

Index Terms Warfarin Sodium

Pharmacologic Category Anticoagulant, Coumarin Derivative; Vitamin K Antagonist

Generic Available Yes: Tablet

Use Prophylaxis and treatment of thromboembolic disorders (eg, venous, pulmonary) and embolic complications arising from atrial fibrillation or cardiac valve replacement; adjunct to reduce risk of systemic embolism (eg, recurrent MI, stroke) after myocardial infarction

Unlabeled/Investigational Use Prevention of recurrent transient ischemic attacks

▶

◄ **Mechanism of Action** Hepatic synthesis of coagulation factors II, VII, IX, and X, as well as proteins C and S, requires the presence of vitamin K. These clotting factors are biologically activated by the addition of carboxyl groups to key glutamic acid residues within the proteins' structure. In the process, "active" vitamin K is oxidatively converted to an "inactive" form, which is then subsequently re-activated by vitamin K epoxide reductase complex 1 (VKORC1). Warfarin competitively inhibits the subunit 1 of the multi-unit VKOR complex, thus depleting functional vitamin K reserves and hence reduces synthesis of active clotting factors.

Pharmacodynamics/Kinetics

Onset of action: Anticoagulation: Oral: 24-72 hours

Peak effect: Full therapeutic effect: 5-7 days; INR may increase in 36-72 hours

Duration: 2-5 days

Absorption: Oral: Rapid, complete

Distribution: 0.14 L/kg

Protein binding: 99%

Metabolism: Hepatic, primarily via CYP2C9; minor pathways include CYP2C8, 2C18, 2C19, 1A2, and 3A4

Genomic variants: Approximately 37% reduced clearance of S-warfarin in patients heterozygous for 2C9 (*1/*2 or *1/*3), and ~70% reduced in patients homozygous for reduced function alleles (*2/*2, *2/*3, or *3/*3)

Half-life elimination: 20-60 hours; Mean: 40 hours; highly variable among individuals

Time to peak, plasma: Oral: ~4 hours

Excretion: Urine (92%, primarily as metabolites)

Dosage Note: New labeling identifies genetic factors which may increase patient sensitivity to warfarin. Specifically, genetic variations in the proteins CYP2C9 and VKORC1, responsible for warfarin's primary metabolism and pharmacodynamic activity, respectively, have been identified as predisposing factors associated with decreased dose requirement and increased bleeding risk. A genotyping test is available, and may provide important guidance on initiation of anticoagulant therapy.

Oral:

Infants and Children (unlabeled use): Initial loading dose (if baseline INR is 1-1.3): 0.2 mg/kg (maximum: 10 mg/dose); adjust dose based on INR (reported ranges to maintain INR of 2-3: 0.09-0.33 mg/kg/day). Infants <12 months of age may require doses at or near the high end of this range; consistent anticoagulation may be difficult to maintain in children <5 years of age.

Adults: Initial dosing must be individualized. Consider the patient (hepatic function, cardiac function, age, nutritional status, concurrent therapy, risk of bleeding) in addition to prior dose response (if available) and the clinical situation. Start 2-5 mg daily for 2 days **or** 5-10 mg daily for 1-2 days (Ansell, 2008). Adjust dose according to INR results; usual maintenance dose ranges from 2-10 mg daily (individual patients may require loading and maintenance doses outside these general guidelines).

Note: Lower starting doses may be required for patients with hepatic impairment, poor nutrition, CHF, elderly, high risk of bleeding, or patients who are debilitated, or those with reduced function genomic variants of the catabolic enzymes CYP2C9 (*2 or *3 alleles) or VKORC1 (-1639 poly-morphism). Higher initial doses may be reasonable in selected patients (ie, receiving enzyme-inducing agents and with low risk of bleeding).

I.V.: Adults: 2-5 mg/day administered as a slow bolus injection

Dosing adjustment in renal disease: No adjustment required, however, patients with renal failure have an increased risk of bleeding complications. Monitor closely.

Dosing adjustment in hepatic disease: Monitor effect at usual doses; the response to oral anticoagulants may be markedly enhanced in obstructive jaundice (due to reduced vitamin K absorption) and also in hepatitis and cirrhosis (due to decreased production of vitamin K-dependent clotting factors); INR should be closely monitored

Stability

Injection: Prior to reconstitution, store at 15°C to 30°C (59°F to 86°F). Following reconstitution with 2.7 mL of sterile water (yields 2 mg/mL solution), stable for 4 hours at 15°C to 30°C (59°F to 86°F). Protect from light.

Tablet: Store at 15°C to 30°C (59°F to 86°F). Protect from light.

Administration

Oral: Administer with or without food. Take at the same time each day.

I.V.: Administer as a slow bolus injection over 1-2 minutes; avoid all I.M. injections

Monitoring Parameters Prothrombin time, hematocrit, INR; consider genotyping of CYP2C9 and VKORC1 prior to initiation of therapy, if available

Reference Range

INR = patient prothrombin time/mean normal prothrombin time

ISI = international sensitivity index

INR should be increased by 2-3.5 times depending upon indication. An INR >4 does not generally add additional therapeutic benefit and is associated with increased risk of bleeding. **Note:** To prevent gastrointestinal bleeding events in patients receiving the combination of warfarin, aspirin, and clopidogrel, an INR of 2-2.5 is recommended unless condition requires a higher INR target (eg, certain mechanical heart valves) (Bhatt, 2008).

Adult INR ranges based upon indication: See table.

Adult Target INR Ranges Based Upon Indication

Indication	Targeted INR	Targeted INR Range
Cardiac		
Acute myocardial infarction (high risk)[1]	2.5	2-3[2,3]
Atrial fibrillation or atrial flutter	2.5	2-3
Valvular		
Bileaflet or Medtronic Hall tilting disk mechanical aortic valve in normal sinus rhythm and normal LA size	2.5	2-3
Bileaflet or tilting disk mechanical mitral valve	3	2.5-3.5
Caged ball or caged disk mechanical valve	3	2.5-3.5
Mechanical prosthetic valve with systemic embolism despite adequate anticoagulation	3 or 3.5[4]	2.5-3.5[4] or 3-4[4]
Mechanical valve and risk factors for thromboembolism (eg, AF, MI[5], LA enlargement, hypercoagulable state, low EF) or history of atherosclerotic vascular disease	3	2.5-3.5[6]
Bioprosthetic mitral valve	2.5	2-3[7]
Bioprosthetic mitral or aortic valve with prior history of systemic embolism	2.5	2-3[7]
Bioprosthetic mitral or aortic valve with evidence of LA thrombus at surgery	2.5	2-3[8]
Bioprosthetic mitral or aortic valve with risk factors for thromboembolism (eg, AF, hypercoagulable state or low EF)	2.5	2-3[9]
Prosthetic mitral valve thrombosis (resolved)	4	3.5-4.5[3]
Prosthetic aortic valve thrombosis (resolved)	3.5	3-4[3]
Rheumatic mitral valve disease and normal sinus rhythm (LA diameter >5.5 cm), AF, previous systemic embolism, or LA thrombus	2.5	2-3
Thromboembolism Treatment		
Venous thromboembolism	2.5	2-3[10,11]
Thromboprophylaxis		
Chronic thromboembolic pulmonary hypertension (CTPH)	2.5	2-3
Idiopathic pulmonary artery hypertension (IPAH)[12]	2	1.5-2.5
Lupus inhibitor (no other risk factors)	2.5	2-3
Lupus inhibitor and recurrent thromboembolism	3	2.5-3.5
Major trauma patients with impaired mobility undergoing rehabilitation	2.5	2-3
Spinal cord injury (acute) undergoing rehabilitation	2.5	2-3
Total hip or knee replacement (elective) or hip fracture surgery	2.5	2-3[13]

Adult Target INR Ranges Based Upon Indication *(continued)*

Indication	Targeted INR	Targeted INR Range
Other Indications		
Cerebral venous sinus thrombosis	2.5	2-3[14]
Ischemic stroke due to AF	2.5	2-3

[1]High-risk includes large anterior MI, significant heart failure, intracardiac thrombus, atrial fibrillation, history of thromboembolism.

[2]Maintain anticoagulation for 3 months.

[3]Combine with aspirin 81 mg/day.

[4]Combine with aspirin 81 mg/day, if not previously receiving, **and/or** if previous target INR was 2.5, then new target INR should be 3 (2.5-3.5). If previous target INR was 3, then new target INR should be 3.5 (3-4).

[5]MI refers to anterior-apical ST-segment elevation myocardial infarction.

[6]Combine with aspirin 81 mg/day unless patient is at high risk of bleeding (eg, history of GI bleed, age >80 years).

[7]Maintain anticoagulation for 3 months after valve insertion then switch to aspirin 81 mg/day if no other indications for warfarin exist or clinically reassess need for warfarin in patients with prior history of systemic embolism.

[8]Maintain anticoagulation with warfarin until thrombus resolution.

[9]If patient has history of atherosclerotic vascular disease, combine with aspirin 81 mg/day unless patient is at high risk of bleeding (eg, history of GI bleed, age >80 years).

[10]Treat for 3 months in patients with VTE due to transient reversible risk factor. Treat for a minimum of 3 months in patients with unprovoked VTE and evaluate for long term therapy. Other risk groups (eg, cancer) may require >3 months of therapy.

[11]In patients with unprovoked VTE who prefer less frequent INR monitoring, low-intensity therapy (INR range: 1.5-1.9) with less frequent monitoring is recommended over stopping treatment.

[12]Recommendation from the ACCF/AHA 2009 Expert Consensus Document on Pulmonary Hypertension (McLaughlin, 2009)

[13]Continue for at least 10 days and up to 35 days after surgery.

[14]Continue for up to 12 months.

Warfarin levels are not used for monitoring degree of anticoagulation. They may be useful if a patient with unexplained coagulopathy is using the drug surreptitiously or if it is unclear whether clinical resistance is due to true drug resistance or lack of drug intake.

Normal prothrombin time (PT): 10.9-12.9 seconds. Healthy premature newborns have prolonged coagulation test screening results (eg, PT, aPTT, TT) which return to normal adult values at approximately 6 months of age. Healthy prematures, however, do not develop spontaneous hemorrhage or thrombotic complications because of a balance between procoagulants and inhibitors.

Anesthesia and Critical Care Concerns/Other Considerations

Clinical Pearls/Comments: Tube-feeding formulas are often a rich source of vitamin K.

Management of Oral Anticoagulation Prior to Surgery:

Patients with low risk of thromboembolism: Stop warfarin therapy approximately 4 days before surgery, allow the INR to return to a near normal level, briefly administer postoperative prophylaxis (if the intervention itself creates a higher risk of thrombosis) using low-dose heparin or LMWH, and simultaneously begin warfarin therapy after surgery.

Patients with intermediate risk of thromboembolism: Stop warfarin therapy approximately 4 days before surgery, allow the INR to fall. Initiate low-dose heparin or prophylactic dose of LMWH beginning 2 days before surgery. Then commence full-dose heparin or LMWH, and warfarin therapy after surgery.

Patients with high risk of thromboembolism (eg, a recent [<3 months] history of venous thromboembolism, a mechanical cardiac valve in the mitral position, or an old model of cardiac valve [ball/cage]): Stop warfarin therapy approximately 4 days before surgery, allow the INR to return to a normal level, begin therapy with full-dose heparin or full-dose LMWH as the INR falls (approximately 2 days before surgery). Heparin can be administered as a SubQ injection on an outpatient basis, can then be given as a continuous I.V. infusion after hospital admission in preparation for surgery, and can be discontinued 5 hours before surgery with the expectation that the anticoagulant effect will have worn off at the time of surgery. It is also possible to continue the administration of SubQ heparin or LMWH and to stop therapy 12-24 hours before surgery with the expectation that the anticoagulant effect will be very low or will have worn off by the time of surgery.

Patients with low risk of bleeding: Continue warfarin therapy at a lower dose and operate at an INR of 1.3-1.5, an intensity that has been shown to be safe in randomized trials of gynecologic and orthopedic surgical patients. The dose of warfarin can be lowered 4-5 days before surgery. Warfarin therapy then can be restarted after surgery and supplemented with low-dose heparin or LMWH if necessary.

Heparin-Induced Thrombocytopenia (HIT) or Heparin-Induced Thrombotic Thrombocytopenia Syndrome (HITTS): When a patient develops HIT/HITTS, warfarin monotherapy is contraindicated. Rather, a direct thrombin inhibitor should be initiated. Warfarin anticoagulation should be postponed in the patient with HIT until substantial recovery of the platelet count has occurred. When appropriate, initiating warfarin at low doses and overlapping with a direct thrombin inhibitor for at least 5 days and until the INR is therapeutic for at least 48 hours is suggested.

Evidence-Based Information:
Management of Intracerebral Hemorrhage (ICH) Due to Warfarin: Overall management of ICH is similar regardless of cause; however, iatrogenic spontaneous ICH may have specific treatments. According to the 2007 ACC/ASA Guidelines for the Management of Spontaneous Intracerebral Hemorrhage, warfarin-related ICH should be treated with I.V. vitamin K at a dose of 10 mg given slowly (not to exceed 1 mg/minute) (Class I recommendation). It is important to also administer fresh frozen plasma (FFP) since vitamin K may take several hours to normalize INR. Other options besides FFP include prothrombin complex concentrate (PCC) which contains high levels of vitamin K-dependent factors (II, VII, and X) and factor IX complex which contains factors II, VII, IX, and X (Class IIb recommendation). Use of rFVIIa has shown promise for this indication. Advantages to rFVIIa include faster onset of action compared to FFP and vitamin K and a 50% lower volume is required compared to FFP. Disadvantages include a short half-life (~2.6 hours) requiring multiple doses to maintain a normalized INR and an increased risk of thromboembolic complications. Dosing of rFVIIa ranges between 15-90 mcg/kg. The use of factor-containing products has a risk of thromboembolism.

Pregnancy Risk Factor X

Contraindications Hypersensitivity to warfarin or any component of the formulation; hemorrhagic tendencies (eg, patients bleeding from the GI, respiratory, or GU tract; aneurysm; cerebrovascular hemorrhage; following spinal puncture and other diagnostic or therapeutic procedures with potential for significant bleeding; history of bleeding diathesis); recent or potential surgery of the eye or CNS; major regional lumbar block anesthesia or surgery resulting in large, open surfaces; blood dyscrasias; severe uncontrolled or malignant hypertension; pericarditis or pericardial effusion; subacute bacterial endocarditis; history of warfarin-induced necrosis; an unreliable, noncompliant patient; alcoholism; patient who has a history of falls or is a significant fall risk; unsupervised senile or psychotic patient; eclampsia/pre-eclampsia, threatened abortion, pregnancy

Warnings/Precautions Use care in the selection of patients appropriate for this treatment. Ensure patient cooperation especially from the alcoholic, illicit drug user, demented, or psychotic patient; ability to comply with routine laboratory monitoring is essential. Use with caution in trauma, acute infection, moderate-severe renal insufficiency, prolonged dietary insufficiencies, moderate-severe hypertension, polycythemia vera, vasculitis, open wound, active TB, any disruption in normal GI flora, history of PUD, anaphylactic disorders, indwelling catheters, severe diabetes, thyroid disease, and menstruating and postpartum women. Use with caution in protein C deficiency. Use with caution in patients with heparin-induced thrombocytopenia and DVT. Warfarin monotherapy is contra-indicated in the initial treatment of active HIT. Reduced liver function, regardless of etiology, may impair synthesis of coagulation factors leading to increased warfarin sensitivity.

[U.S. Boxed Warning]: May cause major or fatal bleeding. Risk factors for bleeding include high intensity anticoagulation (INR >4), age (>65 years), variable

INRs, history of GI bleeding, hypertension, cerebrovascular disease, serious heart disease, anemia, malignancy, trauma, renal insufficiency, drug-drug interactions, long duration of therapy, or known genetic deficiency in CYP2C9 activity. Patient must be instructed to report bleeding, accidents, or falls. Unrecognized bleeding sites (eg, colon cancer) may be uncovered by anticoagulation. Patient must also report any new or discontinued medications, herbal or alternative products used, or significant changes in smoking or dietary habits. Necrosis or gangrene of the skin and other tissue can occur, usually in conjunction with protein C or S deficiency. "Purple toes syndrome," due to cholesterol microembolization, may rarely occur. Women may be at risk of developing ovarian hemorrhage at the time of ovulation. The elderly may be more sensitive to anticoagulant therapy. Safety and efficacy have not been established in children; monitor closely.

Presence of the CYP2C9*2 or *3 allele and/or polymorphism of the vitamin K oxidoreductase (VKORC1) gene may increase the risk of bleeding. Lower doses may be required in these patients; genetic testing may help determine appropriate dosing.

Adverse Reactions Bleeding is the major adverse effect of warfarin. Hemorrhage may occur at virtually any site. Risk is dependent on multiple variables, including the intensity of anticoagulation and patient susceptibility.

Cardiovascular: Angina, chest pain, edema, hemorrhagic shock, hypotension, pallor, syncope, vasculitis

Central nervous system: Coma, dizziness, fatigue, fever, headache, lethargy, malaise, pain, stroke

Dermatologic: Alopecia, bullous eruptions, dermatitis, rash, pruritus, urticaria

Gastrointestinal: Abdominal cramps, abdominal pain, anorexia, diarrhea, flatulence, gastrointestinal bleeding, mouth ulcers, nausea, taste disturbance, vomiting

Genitourinary: Hematuria, priapism

Hematologic: Agranulocytosis, anemia, leukopenia, retroperitoneal hematoma, unrecognized bleeding sites (eg, colon cancer) may be uncovered by anticoagulation

Hepatic: Cholestatic jaundice, hepatic injury, hepatitis, transaminases increased

Neuromuscular & skeletal: Joint pain, muscle pain, osteoporosis (potential association with long-term use), paralysis, paresthesia, weakness

Respiratory: Dyspnea, tracheobronchial calcification

Miscellaneous: Anaphylactic reaction, cold intolerance, hypersensitivity/allergic reactions, skin necrosis, gangrene, "purple toes" syndrome

Drug Interactions

Metabolism/Transport Effects Substrate of CYP1A2 (minor), 2C9 (major), 2C19 (minor), 3A4 (minor); **Inhibits** CYP2C9 (moderate), 2C19 (weak)

Avoid Concomitant Use

Avoid concomitant use of Warfarin with any of the following: Tamoxifen

Increased Effect/Toxicity

Warfarin may increase the levels/effects of: Anticoagulants; Carvedilol; CYP2C9 Substrates (High risk); Drotrecogin Alfa; Phenytoin

The levels/effects of Warfarin may be increased by: Acetaminophen; Allopurinol; Amiodarone; Androgens; Antineoplastic Agents; Antiplatelet Agents; Atazanavir; Bicalutamide; Capecitabine; Cephalosporins; Cimetidine; Clopidogrel; Corticosteroids (Systemic); Cranberry; CYP2C9 Inhibitors (Moderate); CYP2C9 Inhibitors (Strong); Dasatinib; Desvenlafaxine; Disulfiram; Dronedarone; Efavirenz; Esomeprazole; Etoposide; Fenofibrate; Fenofibric Acid; Fenugreek; Fibric Acid Derivatives; Fluconazole; Fluorouracil; Fosamprenavir; Gefitinib; Ginkgo Biloba; Glucagon; Green Tea; Herbs (Anticoagulant/Antiplatelet Properties); HMG-CoA Reductase Inhibitors; Ifosfamide; Imatinib; Itraconazole; Ivermectin; Ketoconazole; Lansoprazole; Leflunomide; Macrolide Antibiotics; MetroNIDAZOLE; Miconazole; Milnacipran; NSAID (COX-2 Inhibitor); NSAID (Non-selective); Omega-3-Acid Ethyl Esters; Omeprazole; Orlistat; Pentosan Polysulfate Sodium; Pentoxifylline; Phenytoin; Posaconazole; Propafenone; Propoxyphene; Prostacyclin Analogues; QuiNIDine; Quinolone Antibiotics; Ranitidine; Salicylates; Selective Serotonin Reuptake Inhibitors; Sitaxsentan; Sorafenib; Sulfinpyrazone [Off Market]; Sulfonamide Derivatives; Tamoxifen; Tetracycline Derivatives; Thrombolytic Agents; Thyroid Products; Tigecycline;

Tolterodine; Torsemide; Tricyclic Antidepressants; Venlafaxine; Vitamin A; Vitamin E; Voriconazole; Vorinostat; Zafirlukast; Zileuton

Decreased Effect

The levels/effects of Warfarin may be decreased by: Aminoglutethimide; Antineoplastic Agents; Antithyroid Agents; Aprepitant; AzaTHIOprine; Barbiturates; Bile Acid Sequestrants; Bosentan; CarBAMazepine; Coenzyme Q-10; Contraceptive (Progestins); CYP2C9 Inducers (Highly Effective); Darunavir; Dicloxacillin; Fosaprepitant; Ginseng (American); Glutethimide; Green Tea; Griseofulvin; Lopinavir; Mercaptopurine; Nafcillin; Oral Contraceptive (Estrogens); Peginterferon Alfa-2b; Phytonadione; Rifamycin Derivatives; Ritonavir; St Johns Wort; Sucralfate

Ethanol/Nutrition/Herb Interactions

Ethanol: Avoid ethanol. Acute ethanol ingestion (binge drinking) decreases the metabolism of warfarin and increases PT/INR. Chronic daily ethanol use increases the metabolism of warfarin and decreases PT/INR.

Food: The anticoagulant effects of warfarin may be decreased if taken with foods rich in vitamin K. Vitamin E may increase warfarin effect. Cranberry juice may increase warfarin effect.

Herb/Nutraceutical: Cranberry, fenugreek, ginkgo biloba, glucosamine, may enhance bleeding or increase warfarin's effect. Ginseng (American), coenzyme Q_{10}, and St John's wort may decrease warfarin levels and effects. Avoid alfalfa, anise, bilberry, bladderwrack, bromelain, cat's claw, celery, chamomile, coleus, cordyceps, dong quai, evening primrose oil, fenugreek, feverfew, garlic, ginger, ginkgo biloba, ginseng (American), ginseng (Panax), ginseng (Siberian), grapeseed, green tea, guggul, horse chestnut seed, horseradish, licorice, omega-3-acids, prickly ash, red clover, reishi, SAMe (s-adenosylmethionine), sweet clover, turmeric, and white willow (all have additional antiplatelet activity).

Dietary Considerations

Foods high in vitamin K (eg, beef liver, pork liver, green tea, and leafy green vegetables) inhibit anticoagulant effect. Do not change dietary habits once stabilized on warfarin therapy. A balanced diet with a consistent intake of vitamin K is essential. Avoid large amounts of alfalfa, asparagus, broccoli, Brussels sprouts, cabbage, cauliflower, green teas, kale, lettuce, spinach, turnip greens, and watercress; decreased efficacy of warfarin. It is recommended that the diet contain a CONSISTENT vitamin K content of 70-140 mcg/day. Check with healthcare provider before changing diet.

Dosage Forms

Excipient information presented when available (limited, particularly for generics); consult specific product labeling.

Injection, powder for reconstitution, as sodium:
Coumadin®: 5 mg

Tablet, as sodium: 1 mg, 2 mg, 2.5 mg, 3 mg, 4 mg, 5 mg, 6 mg, 7.5 mg, 10 mg
Coumadin®: 1 mg, 2 mg, 2.5 mg, 3 mg, 4 mg, 5 mg, 6 mg, 7.5 mg [scored]
Coumadin®: 10 mg [scored; dye free]
Jantoven®: 1 mg, 2 mg, 2.5 mg, 3 mg, 4 mg, 5 mg, 6 mg, 7.5 mg [scored]
Jantoven®: 10 mg [scored; dye free]

References

Albers GW, Amarenco P, Easton JD, et al, "Antithrombotic and Thrombolytic Therapy for Ischemic Stroke: The Seventh ACCP Conference on Antithrombotic and Thrombolytic Therapy," *Chest*, 2004, 126(3 Suppl):483-512.

Arepally GM and Ortel TL, "Heparin-Induced Thrombocytopenia," *N Engl J Med*, 2006, 355 (8):809-17.

Broderick J, Connolly S, Feldmann E, et al, "Guidelines for the Management of Spontaneous Intracerebral Hemorrhage in Adults: 2007 Update: A Guideline From the American Heart Association/American Stroke Association Stroke Council, High Blood Pressure Research Council, and the Quality of Care and Outcomes in Research Interdisciplinary Working Group," *Stroke*, 2007, 38(6):2001-23. Available at http://stroke.ahajournals.org/cgi/content/short/STROKEAHA.107.183689.

Dager WE and White RH, "Pharmacotherapy of Heparin-Induced Thrombocytopenia," *Expert Opin Pharmacother*, 2003, 4(6):919-40.

Dager WE, King JF, Regalia RC, et al, "Reversal of Elevated International Normalized Ratios and Bleeding With Low-Dose Recombinant Activated Factor VII in Patients Receiving Warfarin," *Pharmacotherapy*, 2006, 26(8):1091-8.

Hirsh J, Guyatt G, Albers GW, et al, "The Seventh ACCP Conference on Antithrombotic and Thrombolytic Therapy: Evidence-Based Guidelines," *Chest*, 2004, 126(3 Suppl):163S-608S.

◆ **Warfarin Sodium** *see* Warfarin *on page 1479*

◆ **4 Way® Fast Acting [OTC]** *see* Phenylephrine *on page 1114*

◆ **4 Way® Menthol [OTC]** *see* Phenylephrine *on page 1114*

- ◆ **4 Way® No Drip [OTC]** *see* Phenylephrine *on page 1114*
- ◆ **4-Way® Saline Moisturizing Mist [OTC]** *see* Sodium Chloride *on page 1304*
- ◆ **Wellbutrin®** *see* BuPROPion *on page 217*
- ◆ **Wellbutrin XL®** *see* BuPROPion *on page 217*
- ◆ **Wellbutrin SR®** *see* BuPROPion *on page 217*
- ◆ **Westcort®** *see* Hydrocortisone *on page 699*
- ◆ **Westhroid™** *see* Thyroid, Desiccated *on page 1379*
- ◆ **Winpred™ (Can)** *see* PredniSONE *on page 1166*
- ◆ **Wound Wash Saline™ [OTC]** *see* Sodium Chloride *on page 1304*
- ◆ **Xanax®** *see* ALPRAZolam *on page 64*
- ◆ **Xanax TS™ (Can)** *see* ALPRAZolam *on page 64*
- ◆ **Xanax XR®** *see* ALPRAZolam *on page 64*
- ◆ **Xarelto® (Can)** *see* Rivaroxaban *on page 1255*
- ◆ **Xigris®** *see* Drotrecogin Alfa *on page 466*
- ◆ **Xilep** *see* Rufinamide *on page 1271*
- ◆ **Xodol® 5/300** *see* Hydrocodone and Acetaminophen *on page 697*
- ◆ **Xodol® 7.5/300** *see* Hydrocodone and Acetaminophen *on page 697*
- ◆ **Xodol® 10/300** *see* Hydrocodone and Acetaminophen *on page 697*
- ◆ **Xolair®** *see* Omalizumab *on page 1046*
- ◆ **Xolegel®** *see* Ketoconazole *on page 780*
- ◆ **Xopenex®** *see* Levalbuterol *on page 813*
- ◆ **Xopenex HFA™** *see* Levalbuterol *on page 813*
- ◆ **Xylocaine®** *see* Lidocaine *on page 836*
- ◆ **Xylocaine® Dental** *see* Lidocaine *on page 836*
- ◆ **Xylocaine® MPF** *see* Lidocaine *on page 836*
- ◆ **Xylocaine® Viscous** *see* Lidocaine *on page 836*
- ◆ **Xylocard® (Can)** *see* Lidocaine *on page 836*
- ◆ **Xyntha™** *see* Antihemophilic Factor (Recombinant) *on page 124*
- ◆ **Yasmin®** *see* Ethinyl Estradiol and Drospirenone *on page 546*
- ◆ **Yaz®** *see* Ethinyl Estradiol and Drospirenone *on page 546*
- ◆ **YM087** *see* Conivaptan *on page 349*
- ◆ **Zamicet™** *see* Hydrocodone and Acetaminophen *on page 697*

Zanamivir (za NA mi veer)

Medication Safety Issues
Sound-alike/look-alike issues:
Relenza® may be confused with Albenza®, Aplenzin™

U.S. Brand Names Relenza®

Canadian Brand Names Relenza®

Pharmacologic Category Antiviral Agent; Neuraminidase Inhibitor

Restrictions Compassionate use protocol: There are limited supplies of zanamivir *aqueous solution* available via a compassionate use protocol for the treatment of serious influenza illness. Zanamivir aqueous solution intended for nebulization or intravenous (I.V.) use is **not** currently approved. Data on safety and efficacy via these routes of administration are limited. Relenza® *inhalation powder* is the only commercially available formulation of zanamivir and should only be administered via inhalation using the provided Diskhaler® delivery device. Prior to requesting zanamivir aqueous solution for compassionate use, clinicians should consider the following:
  - There is only a very limited supply available and supply can not be guaranteed.
  - Each request will be evaluated on a case-by-case basis by a member of the Food and Drug Administration (FDA) and a GlaxoSmithKline (GSK) physician.

Patients will be considered for therapy if all inclusion criteria are met:
1) Hospitalization with serious influenza illness in the setting of a pandemic threat
2) Laboratory confirmation of influenza (PCR, rapid assay or culture)
3) Unable to use other approved influenza medications or zanamivir aqueous solution is more appropriate

In addition, patients must be >6 months of age to receive I.V. zanamivir. Patients who are pregnant may not be eligible unless the benefits are expected to outweigh the risks.

Contact GSK or the FDA for more information regarding procurement, patient eligibility, dosing, and preparation, in the U.S. or Canada:

GSK:
Annie Cameron (1-919-483-6958 [office] or 1-919-632-9380 [mobile])
Vinne Lopez (1-919-315-4697 [office] or 1-919-601-0498 [mobile])

FDA:
Normal business hours (8:00 am - 4:30 pm EST): Call DAVP at 301-796-0824
After business hours (4:30 pm - 8:00 am EST): Call FDA at 301-796-9900 or 301-443-1240

Generic Available No

Use Treatment of uncomplicated acute illness due to influenza virus A and B in patients who have been symptomatic for no more than 2 days; prophylaxis against influenza virus A and B

The Advisory Committee on Immunization Practices (ACIP) recommends that **treatment** be considered for the following:
• Persons hospitalized with laboratory confirmed influenza (may also have benefit if started >48 hours after onset of illness).
• Persons with laboratory confirmed influenza pneumonia.
• Persons with laboratory confirmed influenza and bacterial infections.
• Persons with laboratory confirmed influenza and who are at higher risk for influenza complications.
• Persons presenting for care within 48 hours of laboratory confirmed influenza onset and who want to decrease duration and/or severity of their symptoms or decrease the risk of transmission to those at high risk for complications.

The ACIP recommends that **prophylaxis** be considered for the following:
• Persons at high risk for influenza infection during the first 2 weeks following vaccination (eg, children <9 years and not previously vaccinated) if the virus is circulating in the community.
• Persons at high risk for influenza infection, but the vaccination is contraindicated.
• Unvaccinated family members or healthcare providers with prolonged exposure to or close contact with high-risk persons, unvaccinated persons, or infants <6 months of age.
• Persons at high risk for influenza infection, their family members and close contacts, and healthcare workers when the circulating strain of influenza is not matched with the vaccine.
• Persons with immune deficiency or those who may not respond to vaccination.
• Unvaccinated staff and persons during response to an outbreak in a closed institutional setting that has patients at high risk for infection (eg, extended care facilities).

Unlabeled/Investigational Use Treatment and chemoprophylaxis of novel influenza A (H1N1) virus

Mechanism of Action Zanamivir inhibits influenza virus neuraminidase enzymes, potentially altering virus particle aggregation and release.

Pharmacodynamics/Kinetics
Absorption: Inhalation: ~4% to 17%
Protein binding, plasma: <10%
Metabolism: None
Half-life elimination, serum: 2.5-5.1 hours
Excretion: Urine (as unchanged drug); feces (unabsorbed drug)

◀ **Dosage** Oral inhalation:

Children ≥5 years and Adults: Prophylaxis (household setting): Two inhalations (10 mg) once daily for 10 days. Begin within 1½ days following onset of signs or symptoms of index case.

Children ≥7 years and Adults: Treatment: Two inhalations (10 mg total) twice daily for 5 days. Doses on first day should be separated by at least 2 hours; on subsequent days, doses should be spaced by ~12 hours. Begin within 2 days of signs or symptoms.

Adolescents and Adults: Prophylaxis (community outbreak): Two inhalations (10 mg) once daily for 28 days. Begin within 5 days of outbreak.

Stability Store at controlled room temperature 25°C (77°F). Do not puncture blister until taking a dose using the Diskhaler®.

Administration Inhalation: Must be used with Diskhaler® delivery device. The foil blister disk containing zanamivir inhalation powder should not be manipulated, solubilized, or administered via a nebulizer. Patients who are scheduled to use an inhaled bronchodilator should use their bronchodilator prior to zanamivir. With the exception of the initial dose when used for treatment, administer at the same time each day.

Anesthesia and Critical Care Concerns/Other Considerations Patients with asthma or COPD should be informed of the risk of bronchospasm and should have a fast-acting bronchodilator available when treated with zanamivir. Majority of patients included in clinical trials were infected with influenza A, however, a number of patients with influenza B infections were also enrolled. Patients with lower temperature or less severe symptoms appeared to derive less benefit from therapy. No consistent treatment benefit was demonstrated in patients with chronic underlying medical conditions.

Pregnancy Risk Factor C

Contraindications Hypersensitivity to zanamivir or any component of the formulation

Warnings/Precautions Allergic-like reactions, including anaphylaxis, oropharyngeal edema, and serious skin rashes have been reported. Rare occurrences of neuropsychiatric events (including confusion, delirium, hallucinations, and/or self-injury) have been reported from postmarketing surveillance; direct causation is difficult to establish (influenza infection may also be associated with behavioral and neurologic changes). Patients must be instructed in the use of the delivery system. No data are available to support the use of this drug in patients who begin use for treatment after 48 hours of symptoms. Effectiveness has not been established in patients with significant underlying medical conditions or for prophylaxis of influenza in nursing home patients. Not recommended for use in patients with underlying respiratory disease, such as asthma or COPD, due to lack of efficacy and risk of serious adverse effects. Bronchospasm, decreased lung function, and other serious adverse reactions, including those with fatal outcomes, have been reported in patients with and without airway disease; discontinue with bronchospasm or signs of decreased lung function. For a patient with an underlying airway disease where a medical decision has been made to use zanamivir, a fast-acting bronchodilator should be made available, and used prior to each dose. Not a substitute for annual flu vaccination; has not been shown to reduce risk of transmission of influenza to others. Consider primary or concomitant bacterial infections. Powder for oral inhalation contains lactose. The inhalation powder should only be administered via inhalation using the provided Diskhaler® delivery device. The commercially available formulation is **not** intended to be solubilized or administered via any nebulizer/mechanical ventilator; inappropriate administration has resulted in death. Safety and efficacy of repeated courses or use with severe renal impairment have not been established. Indicated for children ≥5 years of age (for influenza prophylaxis) and children ≥7 years of age (for influenza treatment); children ages 5-6 years may have inadequate inhalation (via Diskhaler®) for the treatment of influenza.

Adverse Reactions Most adverse reactions occurred at a frequency which was less than or equal to the control (lactose vehicle).

>10%:

Central nervous system: Headache (prophylaxis 13% to 24%; treatment 2%)

Gastrointestinal: Throat/tonsil discomfort/pain (prophylaxis 8% to 19%)

Respiratory: Nasal signs and symptoms (prophylaxis 12% to 20%; treatment 2%), cough (prophylaxis 7% to 17%; treatment ≤2%)

Miscellaneous: Viral infection (prophylaxis 3% to 13%)

1% to 10%:

Central nervous system: Fever/chills (prophylaxis 5% to 9%; treatment <1.5%), fatigue (prophylaxis 5% to 8%; treatment <1.5%), malaise (prophylaxis 5% to 8%; treatment <1.5%), dizziness (treatment 1% to 2%)

Dermatologic: Urticaria (treatment <1.5%)

Gastrointestinal: Anorexia/appetite decreased (prophylaxis 2% to 4%), appetite increased (prophylaxis 2% to 4%), nausea (prophylaxis 1% to 2%; treatment ≤3%), diarrhea (prophylaxis 2%; treatment 2% to 3%), vomiting (prophylaxis 1% to 2%; treatment 1% to 2%), abdominal pain (treatment <1.5%)

Neuromuscular & skeletal: Muscle pain (prophylaxis 3% to 8%), musculoskeletal pain (prophylaxis 6%), arthralgia/articular rheumatism (prophylaxis 2%), arthralgia (treatment <1.5%), myalgia (treatment <1.5%)

Respiratory: Infection (ear/nose/throat; prophylaxis 2%; treatment 1% to 5%), sinusitis (treatment 3%), bronchitis (treatment 2%), nasal inflammation (prophylaxis 1%)

<1% (Limited to important or life-threatening): Abnormal behavior, agitation, allergic or allergic-like reaction (including oropharyngeal edema), anxiety, arrhythmia, asthma, bronchospasm, consciousness altered, delusions, dyspnea, facial edema, hallucination, hemorrhage (ear/nose/throat), neuropsychiatric events (self-injury, confusion, delirium), nightmares, rash (including serious cutaneous reactions), seizure, syncope

Drug Interactions

Avoid Concomitant Use There are no known interactions where it is recommended to avoid concomitant use.

Increased Effect/Toxicity There are no known significant interactions involving an increase in effect.

Decreased Effect

Zanamivir may decrease the levels/effects of: Influenza Virus Vaccine

Dosage Forms Excipient information presented when available (limited, particularly for generics); consult specific product labeling.

Powder for oral inhalation:

Relenza®: 5 mg/blister (20s) [contains lactose 20 mg/blister; 4 blisters per Rotadisk® foil pack, 5 Rotadisk® per package; packaged with Diskhaler® inhalation device]

◆ **Zilactin® (Can)** *see* Lidocaine *on page 836*

◆ **Zilactin-L® [OTC]** *see* Lidocaine *on page 836*

◆ **Zinacef®** *see* Cefuroxime *on page 272*

◆ **Zingo™ [DSC]** *see* Lidocaine *on page 836*

Ziprasidone (zi PRAS i done)

U.S. Brand Names Geodon®

Canadian Brand Names Zeldox®

Index Terms Zeldox; Ziprasidone Hydrochloride; Ziprasidone Mesylate

Pharmacologic Category Antipsychotic Agent, Atypical

Generic Available No

Use Treatment of schizophrenia; treatment of acute manic or mixed episodes associated with bipolar disorder with or without psychosis; acute agitation in patients with schizophrenia

Unlabeled/Investigational Use Tourette's syndrome; psychosis/agitation related to Alzheimer's dementia

Mechanism of Action Ziprasidone is a benzylisothiazolylpiperazine antipsychotic. The exact mechanism of action is unknown. However, *in vitro* radioligand studies show that ziprasidone has high affinity for D_2, D_3, 5-HT_{2A}, 5-HT_{1A}, 5-HT_{2C}, 5-HT_{1D}, and $alpha_1$-adrenergic; moderate affinity for histamine H_1 receptors; and no appreciable affinity for $alpha_2$-adrenergic receptors, beta-adrenergic, 5-HT_3, 5-HT_4, cholinergic, mu, sigma, or benzodiazepine receptors. Ziprasidone functions as an antagonist at the D_2, 5-HT_{2A}, and 5-HT_{1D} receptors and as an agonist at the 5-HT_{1A} receptor. Ziprasidone moderately inhibits the reuptake of serotonin and norepinephrine.

Pharmacodynamics/Kinetics

Absorption: Well absorbed

Distribution: V_d: 1.5 L/kg

Protein binding: 99%, primarily to albumin and $alpha_1$-acid glycoprotein

Metabolism: Extensively hepatic, primarily via aldehyde oxidase; less than $1/3$ of total metabolism via CYP3A4 and CYP1A2 (minor)

Bioavailability: Oral (with food): 60% (up to twofold increase with food); I.M.: 100%

Half-life elimination: Oral: 7 hours; I.M.: 2-5 hours

Time to peak: Oral: 6-8 hours; I.M.: ≤60 minutes

Excretion: Feces (66%) and urine (20%) as metabolites; little as unchanged drug (1% urine, 4% feces)

Clearance: 7.5 mL/minute/kg

Dosage

Children and Adolescents: Tourette's syndrome (unlabeled use): Oral: 5-40 mg/day

Adults:

Bipolar mania: Oral: Initial: 40 mg twice daily (with food)

Adjustment: May increase to 60 or 80 mg twice daily on second day of treatment; average dose 40-80 mg twice daily

Schizophrenia: Oral: Initial: 20 mg twice daily (with food)

Adjustment: Increases (if indicated) should be made no more frequently than every 2 days; ordinarily patients should be observed for improvement over several weeks before adjusting the dose

Maintenance: Range 20-100 mg twice daily; however, dosages >80 mg twice daily are generally not recommended

Acute agitation (schizophrenia): I.M.: 10 mg every 2 hours **or** 20 mg every 4 hours; maximum: 40 mg/day; oral therapy should replace I.M. administration as soon as possible

Elderly: No dosage adjustment is recommended; consider initiating at a low end of the dosage range, with slower titration

Dosage adjustment in renal impairment:

Oral: No dosage adjustment is recommended

I.M.: Cyclodextrin, an excipient in the I.M. formulation, is cleared by renal filtration; use with caution.

Ziprasidone is not removed by hemodialysis.

Dosage adjustment in hepatic impairment: No dosage adjustment is recommended

Stability

Capsule: Store at controlled room temperature of 15°C to 30°C (59°F to 86°F).

Vials for injection: Store at controlled room temperature of 15°C to 30°C (59°F to 86°F). Protect from light. Each vial should be reconstituted with 1.2 mL SWI. Shake vigorously. Will form a pale, pink solution containing 20 mg/mL ziprasidone. Following reconstitution, injection may be stored at room temperature up to 24 hours or up to 7 days if refrigerated. Protect from light.

Administration

Oral: Administer with food.

Injection: For I.M. administration only.

Monitoring Parameters Vital signs; serum potassium and magnesium; fasting lipid profile and fasting blood glucose/Hgb A_{1c} (prior to treatment, at 3 months, then annually); BMI, personal/family history of obesity, waist circumference; blood pressure; mental status, abnormal involuntary movement scale (AIMS), extrapyramidal symptoms. Weight should be assessed prior to treatment, at 4 weeks, 8 weeks, 12 weeks, and then at quarterly intervals. Consider titrating to a different antipsychotic agent for a weight gain ≥5% of the initial weight. The value of routine ECG screening or monitoring has not been established.

Pregnancy Risk Factor C

Contraindications Hypersensitivity to ziprasidone or any component of the formulation; history (or current) prolonged QT; congenital long QT syndrome; recent myocardial infarction; history of arrhythmias; uncompensated heart failure; concurrent use of other QT_c-prolonging agents including amiodarone, arsenic trioxide, bretylium, chlorpromazine, cisapride, class Ia antiarrhythmics (quinidine, procainamide), dofetilide, dolasetron, droperidol, ibutilide, levomethadyl, mefloquine, mesoridazine, pentamidine, pimozide, probucol, some quinolone antibiotics (moxifloxacin), sotalol, tacrolimus, and thioridazine

Warnings/Precautions [U.S. Boxed Warning]: Elderly patients with dementia-related behavioral disorders treated with antipsychotics are at an increased risk of death compared to placebo. Most deaths appeared to be either cardiovascular (eg, heart failure, sudden death) or infectious (eg, pneumonia) in nature. Ziprasidone is not approved for the treatment of dementia-related psychosis.

May result in QT_c prolongation (dose related), which has been associated with the development of malignant ventricular arrhythmias (torsade de pointes) and sudden death. Note contraindications related to this effect. Observed prolongation was greater than with other atypical antipsychotic agents (risperidone, olanzapine, quetiapine), but less than with thioridazine. Avoid hypokalemia, hypomagnesemia. Use caution in patients with bradycardia. Discontinue in patients found to have persistent QT_c intervals >500 msec. Patients with symptoms of dizziness, palpitations, or syncope should receive further cardiac evaluation. May cause orthostatic hypotension. Use with caution in patients with cardiovascular disease, including prior myocardial infarction or unstable heart disease.

Leukopenia, neutropenia, and agranulocytosis (sometimes fatal) have been reported in clinical trials and postmarketing reports with antipsychotic use; presence of risk factors (eg, pre-existing low WBC or history of drug-induced leuko-/neutropenia) should prompt periodic blood count assessment. Discontinue therapy at first signs of blood dyscrasias or if absolute neutrophil count <1000/mm^3.

May cause extrapyramidal symptoms (EPS). Risk of dystonia (and probably other EPS) may be greater with increased doses, use of conventional antipsychotics, males, and younger patients. Impaired core body temperature regulation may occur; caution with strenuous exercise, heat exposure, dehydration, and concomitant medication possessing anticholinergic effects; not reported in premarketing trials of ziprasidone. Antipsychotic use may also be associated with neuroleptic malignant syndrome (NMS). Use with caution in patients at risk of seizures.

◄ Atypical antipsychotics have been associated with development of hyper-glycemia. There is limited documentation with ziprasidone and specific risk associated with this agent is not known. Use caution in patients with diabetes or other disorders of glucose regulation; monitor for worsening of glucose control. May increase prolactin levels; clinical significance of hyperprolactinemia in patients with breast cancer or other prolactin-dependent tumors is unknown.

Cognitive and/or motor impairment (sedation) is common with ziprasidone. Use with caution in disorders where CNS depression is a feature. Use with caution in Parkinson's disease. Antipsychotic use has been associated with esophageal dysmotility and aspiration; use with caution in patients at risk of pneumonia (ie, Alzheimer's disease). Use caution in hepatic impairment. Ziprasidone has been associated with a fairly high incidence of rash (5%). Significant weight gain has been observed with antipsychotic therapy; incidence varies with product. Monitor waist circumference and BMI. Rare cases of priapism have been reported. Use the intramuscular formulation with caution in patients with renal impairment; formulation contains cyclodextrin, an excipient which may accumulate in renal insufficiency. Safety and efficacy have not been established in pediatric patients.

The possibility of a suicide attempt is inherent in psychotic illness or bipolar disorder; use caution in high-risk patients during initiation of therapy. Prescriptions should be written for the smallest quantity consistent with good patient care.

Adverse Reactions Note: Although minor QT_c prolongation (mean: 10 msec at 160 mg/day) may occur more frequently (incidence not specified), clinically-relevant prolongation (>500 msec) was rare (0.06%) and less than placebo (0.23%).

>10%:
Central nervous system: Extrapyramidal symptoms (2% to 31%), somnolence (8% to 31%), headache (3% to 18%), dizziness (3% to 16%)
Gastrointestinal: Nausea (4% to 12%)

1% to 10%:
Cardiovascular: Chest pain (5%), postural hypotension (5%), hypertension (2% to 3%), bradycardia (2%), tachycardia (2%), vasodilation (1%), facial edema, orthostatic hypotension
Central nervous system: Akathisia (2% to 10%), anxiety (2% to 5%), insomnia (3%), agitation (2%), speech disorder (2%), personality disorder (2%), psychosis (1%), akinesia, amnesia, ataxia, chills, confusion, coordination abnormal, delirium, dystonia, fever, hostility, hypothermia, oculogyric crisis, vertigo
Dermatologic: Rash (4%), fungal dermatitis (2%)
Endocrine & metabolic: Dysmenorrhea (2%)
Gastrointestinal: Weight gain (10%), constipation (2% to 9%), dyspepsia (1% to 8%), diarrhea (3% to 5%), vomiting (3% to 5%), salivation increased (4%), xerostomia (1% to 5%), tongue edema (3%), abdominal pain (2%), anorexia (2%), dysphagia (2%), rectal hemorrhage (2%), tooth disorder (1%), buccoglossal syndrome
Genitourinary: Priapism (1%)
Local: Injection site pain (7% to 9%)
Neuromuscular & skeletal: Weakness (2% to 6%), hypoesthesia (2%), myalgia (2%), paresthesia (2%), back pain (1%), cogwheel rigidity (1%), hypertonia (1%), abnormal gait, choreoathetosis, dysarthria, dyskinesia, hyper-/hypoki-nesia, hypotonia, neuropathy, tremor, twitching
Ocular: Vision abnormal (3% to 6%), diplopia
Respiratory: Infection (8%), rhinitis (1% to 4%), cough (3%), pharyngitis (3%), dyspnea (2%)
Miscellaneous: Diaphoresis (2%), furunculosis (2%), flu-like syndrome (1%), photosensitivity reaction, withdrawal syndrome

<1% (Limited to important or life-threatening): Akinesia, allergic reaction, angina, atrial fibrillation, ataxia, AV block (first degree), bundle branch block, cerebral infarction, cholestatic jaundice, choreoathetosis, delirium, dysarthria, dysphagia, eosinophilia, exfoliative dermatitis, galactorrhea, gout, gynecomastia, hemor-rhage, hepatitis, jaundice, myocarditis, neuroleptic malignant syndrome, neuro-pathy, opisthotonos, photophobia, pneumonia, pulmonary embolism, QT_c prolongation >500 msec (0.06%), seizure (0.4%), sexual dysfunction (male

and female), stroke, syncope (0.6%), tardive dyskinesia, tenosynovitis, thrombocytopenia, thyroiditis, torsade de pointes, torticollis, urinary retention

Drug Interactions

Metabolism/Transport Effects Substrate (minor) of CYP1A2, 3A4; **Inhibits** CYP2D6 (weak), 3A4 (weak)

Avoid Concomitant Use

Avoid concomitant use of Ziprasidone with any of the following: Artemether; Dronedarone; Lumefantrine; Nilotinib; Pimozide; QTc-Prolonging Agents; QuiNINE; Tetrabenazine; Thioridazine

Increased Effect/Toxicity

Ziprasidone may increase the levels/effects of: Alcohol (Ethyl); CNS Depressants; Dronedarone; Pimozide; QTc-Prolonging Agents; QuiNINE; Tetrabenazine; Thioridazine

The levels/effects of Ziprasidone may be increased by: Acetylcholinesterase Inhibitors (Central); Alfuzosin; Antifungal Agents (Azole Derivatives, Systemic); Artemether; Chloroquine; Ciprofloxacin; Gadobutrol; Lithium formulations; Lumefantrine; Nilotinib; QTc-Prolonging Agents; QuiNINE; Tetrabenazine

Decreased Effect

Ziprasidone may decrease the levels/effects of: Amphetamines; Anti-Parkinson's Agents (Dopamine Agonist)

The levels/effects of Ziprasidone may be decreased by: CarBAMazepine; Lithium formulations

Ethanol/Nutrition/Herb Interactions

Ethanol: Avoid ethanol (may increase CNS depression).

Food: Administration with food increases serum levels twofold. Grapefruit juice may increase serum concentration of ziprasidone.

Herb/Nutraceutical: St John's wort may decrease serum levels of ziprasidone, due to a potential effect on CYP3A4. This has not been specifically studied. Avoid kava kava, chamomile (may increase CNS depression).

Test Interactions Increased cholesterol, triglycerides, eosinophils

Dosage Forms Excipient information presented when available (limited, particularly for generics); consult specific product labeling.

Capsule, as hydrochloride: 20 mg, 40 mg, 60 mg, 80 mg
Geodon®: 20 mg, 40 mg, 60 mg, 80 mg
Injection, powder for reconstitution, as mesylate: 20 mg [contains cyclodextrin]
Geodon®: 20 mg [contains cyclodextrin]

♦ **Ziprasidone Hydrochloride** *see* Ziprasidone *on page 1490*

♦ **Ziprasidone Mesylate** *see* Ziprasidone *on page 1490*

♦ **Zipsor™** *see* Diclofenac *on page 414*

♦ **Zirgan™** *see* Ganciclovir *on page 654*

♦ **Zithromax®** *see* Azithromycin *on page 169*

♦ **Zithromax® TRI-PAK™** *see* Azithromycin *on page 169*

♦ **Zithromax® Z-PAK®** *see* Azithromycin *on page 169*

♦ **Zmax®** *see* Azithromycin *on page 169*

♦ **Zocor®** *see* Simvastatin *on page 1293*

♦ **Zofran®** *see* Ondansetron *on page 1057*

♦ **Zofran® ODT** *see* Ondansetron *on page 1057*

Zolmitriptan (zohl mi TRIP tan)

U.S. Brand Names Zomig-ZMT®; Zomig®
Canadian Brand Names Zomig®; Zomig® Nasal Spray; Zomig® Rapimelt
Index Terms 311C90
Pharmacologic Category Antimigraine Agent; Serotonin 5-HT$_{1B, 1D}$ Receptor Agonist
Use Acute treatment of migraine with or without aura

Pharmacodynamics/Kinetics
Onset of action: 0.5-1 hour

Absorption: Well absorbed

Distribution: V_d: 7 L/kg

Protein binding: 25%

Metabolism: Converted to an active N-desmethyl metabolite (2-6 times more potent than zolmitriptan)

Bioavailability: 40%

Half-life elimination: 2.8-3.7 hours

Time to peak, serum: Tablet: 1.5 hours; Orally-disintegrating tablet and nasal spray: 3 hours

Excretion: Urine (~60% to 65% total dose); feces (30% to 40%)

Dosage Oral:
Children: Safety and efficacy have not been established

Adults: Migraine:

Tablet: Initial: ≤2.5 mg at the onset of migraine headache; may break 2.5 mg tablet in half

Orally-disintegrating tablet: Initial: 2.5 mg at the onset of migraine headache

Nasal spray: Initial: 1 spray (5 mg) at the onset of migraine headache

Note: Use the lowest possible dose to minimize adverse events. If the headache returns, the dose may be repeated after 2 hours; do not exceed 10 mg within a 24-hour period. Controlled trials have not established the effectiveness of a second dose if the initial one was ineffective.

Elderly: No dosage adjustment needed but elderly patients are more likely to have underlying cardiovascular disease and should have careful evaluation of cardiovascular system before prescribing.

Dosage adjustment in renal impairment: No dosage adjustment recommended. There is a 25% reduction in zolmitriptan's clearance in patients with severe renal impairment (Cl_{cr} 5-25 mL/minute).

Dosage adjustment in hepatic impairment: Administer with caution in patients with liver disease, generally using doses <2.5 mg (doses <5 mg can only be achieved using oral tablets). Patients with moderate-to-severe hepatic impairment may have decreased clearance of zolmitriptan, and significant elevation in blood pressure was observed in some patients.

Anesthesia and Critical Care Concerns/Other Considerations
Zolmitriptan should not be used in patients with a history of vasospastic disease, Prinzmetal's angina, or any critical vascular disease.

Additional Information
Complete prescribing information for this medication should be consulted for additional detail.

Dosage Forms
Excipient information presented when available (limited, particularly for generics); consult specific product labeling.

Solution, intranasal [spray]:

Zomig®: 5 mg/0.1 mL (0.1 mL)

Tablet:

Zomig®: 2.5 mg, 5 mg

Tablet, orally disintegrating:

Zomig-ZMT®: 2.5 mg [contains phenylalanine 2.81 mg/tablet; orange flavor]; 5 mg [contains phenylalanine 5.62 mg/tablet; orange flavor]

Zolpidem (zole PI dem)

Medication Safety Issues
Sound-alike/look-alike issues:

Ambien® may be confused with Abilify®, Ativan®, Ambi 10®

Zolpidem may be confused with lorazepam, zaleplon

Medication Guide An FDA-approved patient medication guide, which is available with the product information and at the following website locations, must be dispensed with this medication for each new outpatient prescription and refill:

Ambien®: http://www.fda.gov/downloads/Drugs/DrugSafety/ucm085906.pdf

Ambien CR®: http://www.fda.gov/downloads/Drugs/DrugSafety/ucm085908.pdf

Edluar™: http://www.fda.gov/downloads/Drugs/DrugSafety/UCM135937.pdf

Zolpidem: http://www.fda.gov/downloads/Drugs/DrugSafety/ucm089833.pdf

Zolpimist®: http://www.fda.gov/downloads/Drugs/DrugSafety/UCM143465.pdf

U.S. Brand Names Ambien CR®; Ambien®; Edluar™; Zolpimist®
Index Terms Zolpidem Tartrate
Pharmacologic Category Hypnotic, Nonbenzodiazepine
Restrictions C-IV
Generic Available Yes: Excludes extended release tablet, sublingual tablet
Use
Ambien®, Edluar™: Short-term treatment of insomnia (with difficulty of sleep onset)
Ambien CR®: Treatment of insomnia (with difficulty of sleep onset and/or sleep maintenance)
Mechanism of Action Zolpidem, an imidazopyridine hypnotic that is structurally dissimilar to benzodiazepines, enhances the activity of the inhibitory neurotransmitter, γ-aminobutyric acid (GABA), via selective agonism at the benzodiazepine-1 (BZ_1) receptor; the result is increased chloride conductance, neuronal hyperpolarization, inhibition of the action potential, and a decrease in neuronal excitability leading to sedative and hypnotic effects. Because of its selectivity for the BZ_1 receptor site over the BZ_2 receptor site, zolpidem exhibits minimal anxiolytic, myorelaxant, and anticonvulsant properties (effects largely attributed to agonism at the BZ_2 receptor site).
Pharmacodynamics/Kinetics
Onset of action: Immediate release: 30 minutes
Duration: Immediate release: 6-8 hours
Absorption: Rapid
Distribution: V_d: 0.54 L/kg
Protein binding: ~93%
Metabolism: Hepatic methylation and hydroxylation via CYP3A4 (~60%), CYP2C9 (~22%), CYP1A2 (~14%), CYP2D6 (~3%), and CYP2C19 (~3%) to three inactive metabolites
Bioavailability: 70%
Half-life elimination:
Immediate release, Extended release: ~2.5 hours (range 1.4-4.5 hours); Cirrhosis: Up to 9.9 hours; Elderly: Prolonged up to 32%
Sublingual: ~3 hours (range: 1.6-6.7 hours)
Time to peak, plasma:
Immediate release: 1.6 hours; 2.2 hours with food
Extended release: 1.5 hours; 4 hours with food
Sublingual: ~1.4 hours; ~1.8 hours with food
Excretion: Urine (48% to 67%, primarily as metabolites); feces (29% to 42%, primarily as metabolites)
Dosage Oral:
Adults:
Immediate release, Sublingual: 10 mg immediately before bedtime; maximum dose: 10 mg
Extended release: 12.5 mg immediately before bedtime
Elderly:
Immediate release, Sublingual: 5 mg immediately before bedtime
Extended release: 6.25 mg immediately before bedtime
Dosing adjustment in renal impairment: Dose adjustment not required; monitor closely
Hemodialysis: Not dialyzable
Dosing adjustment in hepatic impairment:
Immediate release, Sublingual: 5 mg
Extended release: 6.25 mg
Stability
Ambien®, Edluar™: Store at 20°C to 25°C (68°F to 77°F). Protect sublingual tablets from light and moisture.
Ambien CR®: Store at 15°C to 25°C (59°F to 77°F); limited excursions up to 30°C (86°F) permitted.
Administration Ingest immediately before bedtime due to rapid onset of action. Ambien CR® tablets should be swallowed whole; do not divide, crush, or chew. Edluar™ sublingual tablets should be placed under the tongue and allowed to disintegrate; do not swallow or administer with water.
Monitoring Parameters Daytime alertness; respiratory rate; behavior profile

◀ **Anesthesia and Critical Care Concerns/Other Considerations**
Clinical Pearls/Comments: Causes fewer disturbances in sleep stages as compared to benzodiazepines. Time spent in sleep stages 3 and 4 are maintained; zolpidem decreases sleep latency; should not be prescribed in quantities exceeding a 1-month supply.

Pregnancy Risk Factor C

Contraindications Hypersensitivity to zolpidem or any component of the formulation

Warnings/Precautions Should be used only after evaluation of potential causes of sleep disturbance. Failure of sleep disturbance to resolve after 7-10 days may indicate psychiatric or medical illness. Hypnotics/sedatives have been associated with abnormal thinking and behavior changes including decreased inhibition, aggression, bizarre behavior, agitation, hallucinations, and depersonalization. These changes may occur unpredictably and may indicate previously unrecognized psychiatric disorders; evaluate appropriately. Sedative/hypnotics may produce withdrawal symptoms following abrupt discontinuation. Use with caution in patients with depression; worsening of depression, including suicide or suicidal ideation has been reported with the use of hypnotics. Intentional overdose may be an issue in this population. The minimum dose that will effectively treat the individual patient should be used. Prescriptions should be written for the smallest quantity consistent with good patient care. Causes CNS depression, which may impair physical and mental capabilities. Zolpidem should only be administered when the patient is able to stay in bed a full night (7-8 hours) before being active again. Effects with other sedative drugs or ethanol may be potentiated.

Use caution in patients with myasthenia gravis. Use caution in the elderly; dose adjustment recommended. Closely monitor elderly or debilitated patients for impaired cognitive or motor performance. Avoid use in patients with sleep apnea or a history of sedative-hypnotic abuse. Postmarketing studies have indicated that the use of hypnotic/sedative agents for sleep has been associated with hypersensitivity reactions including anaphylaxis as well as angioedema. An increased risk for hazardous sleep-related activities such as sleep-driving; cooking and eating food, and making phone calls while asleep have also been noted; amnesia may also occur. Discontinue treatment in patients who report a sleep-driving episode.

Use caution with respiratory disease. Use caution with hepatic impairment; dose adjustment required. Because of the rapid onset of action, administer immediately prior to bedtime or after the patient has gone to bed and is having difficulty falling asleep. Safety and efficacy have not been established in pediatric patients.

Adverse Reactions Actual frequency may be dosage form, dose, and/or age dependent

>10%: Central nervous system: Dizziness, headache, somnolence

1% to 10%:
  Cardiovascular: Blood pressure increased, chest discomfort/pain, palpitation
  Central nervous system: Abnormal dreams, anxiety, apathy, amnesia, ataxia, attention disturbance, body temperature increased, confusion, depersonalization, depression, disinhibition, disorientation, drowsiness, drugged feeling, euphoria, fatigue, fever, hallucinations, hypoesthesia, insomnia, lethargy, lightheadedness, memory disorder, mood swings, sleep disorder, stress
  Dermatologic: Rash, urticaria, wrinkling
  Endocrine & metabolic: Menorrhagia
  Gastrointestinal: Abdominal discomfort, abdominal pain, abdominal tenderness, appetite disorder, constipation, diarrhea, dyspepsia, flatulence, gastroenteritis, gastroesophageal reflux, hiccup, nausea, vomiting, xerostomia
  Genitourinary: Urinary tract infection
  Neuromuscular & skeletal: Arthralgia, back pain, balance disorder, myalgia, neck pain, paresthesia, psychomotor retardation, tremor, weakness
  Ocular: Asthenopia, blurred vision, depth perception altered, diplopia, red eye, visual disturbance
  Otic: Labyrinthitis, tinnitus, vertigo
  Renal: Dysuria
  Respiratory: Pharyngitis, sinusitis, throat irritation, upper respiratory tract infection
  Miscellaneous: Allergy, binge eating, flu-like syndrome

<1% (Limited to important or life-threatening): Agitation, anaphylaxis, angioedema, anorexia, arthritis, bronchitis, cerebrovascular disorder, cognition decreased, complex sleep-related behavior (sleep-driving, cooking or eating food, making phone calls), concentrating difficulty, constipation, cough, cystitis, diaphoresis, dysarthria, dysphagia, dyspnea, edema, emotional lability, eye irritation, falling, hepatic function abnormalities, hyperglycemia, hyper-/hypotension, illusion, leg cramps, menstrual disorder, nervousness, pallor, paresthesia of the tongue (sublingual tablets), postural hypotension, pruritus, rhinitis, scleritis, somnambulism (sleepwalking), speech disorder, stupor, sublingual erythema (sublingual tablets), syncope, tachycardia, taste perversion, thirst, urinary incontinence, vaginitis

Drug Interactions

Metabolism/Transport Effects Substrate of CYP1A2 (minor), 2C9 (minor), 2C19 (minor), 2D6 (minor), 3A4 (major)

Avoid Concomitant Use There are no known interactions where it is recommended to avoid concomitant use.

Increased Effect/Toxicity

Zolpidem may increase the levels/effects of: Alcohol (Ethyl); CNS Depressants; Methotrimeprazine

The levels/effects of Zolpidem may be increased by: Antifungal Agents (Azole Derivatives, Systemic); CYP3A4 Inhibitors (Moderate); CYP3A4 Inhibitors (Strong); Dasatinib; Methotrimeprazine

Decreased Effect

The levels/effects of Zolpidem may be decreased by: CYP3A4 Inducers (Strong); Deferasirox; Flumazenil; Herbs (CYP3A4 Inducers); Peginterferon Alfa-2b; Rifamycin Derivatives

Ethanol/Nutrition/Herb Interactions

Ethanol: May enhance the adverse/toxic effects of zolpidem; avoid use.

Food: Maximum plasma concentration and bioavailability are decreased with food; time to peak plasma concentration is increased; half-life remains unchanged. Grapefruit juice may decrease the metabolism of zolpidem.

Herb/Nutraceutical: St John's wort may decrease the levels/effects of zolpidem; avoid concomitant use. In addition, concomitant use of valerian, kava kava, and gotu kola should be avoided due to the risk of increased CNS depression.

Dietary Considerations For faster sleep onset, do not administer with (or immediately after) a meal.

Product Availability Zolpimist® oral spray: FDA approved December, 2008; availability currently undetermined

Zolpimist® is an oral spray of zolpidem indicated for the short-term treatment of insomnia characterized by difficulties with sleep initiation.

Dosage Forms Excipient information presented when available (limited, particularly for generics); consult specific product labeling.

Tablet, oral, as tartrate: 5 mg, 10 mg
Ambien®: 5 mg, 10 mg

Tablet, extended release, oral, as tartrate:
Ambien CR®: 6.25 mg, 12.5 mg

Tablet, sublingual, as tartrate:
Edluar™: 5 mg, 10 mg

References

Garnier R, Guerault E, Muzard D, et al, "Acute Zolpidem Poisoning - Analysis of 344 Cases," *J Toxicol Clin Toxicol*, 1994, 32(4):391-404.

Zonisamide (zoe NIS a mide)

Related Information
Chronic Pain Management *on page 1546*
Perioperative Management of Patients on Antiseizure Medication *on page 1577*
U.S. Brand Names Zonegran®
Pharmacologic Category Anticonvulsant, Miscellaneous
Use Adjunct treatment of partial seizures in children >16 years of age and adults with epilepsy
Unlabeled/Investigational Use Bipolar disorder
Pharmacodynamics/Kinetics
Distribution: V_d: 1.45 L/kg
Protein binding: 40%
Metabolism: Hepatic via CYP3A4; forms N-acetyl zonisamide and 2-sulfamoyla-cetyl phenol (SMAP)
Half-life elimination: 63 hours
Time to peak: 2-6 hours
Excretion: Urine (62%, 35% as unchanged drug, 65% as metabolites); feces (3%)
Dosage Oral:
Children >16 years and Adults:
Adjunctive treatment of partial seizures: Initial: 100 mg/day; dose may be increased to 200 mg/day after 2 weeks. Further dosage increases to 300 mg/day and 400 mg/day can then be made with a minimum of 2 weeks between adjustments, in order to reach steady state at each dosage level. Doses of up to 600 mg/day have been studied, however, there is no evidence of increased response with doses above 400 mg/day.
Mania (unlabeled use): Initial: 100-200 mg/day; maximum: 600 mg/day (Kanba, 1994)
Elderly: Data from clinical trials is insufficient for patients >65 years; begin dosing at the low end of the dosing range.
Dosage adjustment in renal/hepatic impairment: Slower titration and frequent monitoring are indicated in patients with renal or hepatic disease. There is insufficient experience regarding dosing/toxicity in patients with estimated GFR <50 mL/minute. Marked renal impairment (Cl_{cr} <20 mL/minute) was associated with a 35% increase in AUC.
Additional Information Complete prescribing information for this medication should be consulted for additional detail.
Dosage Forms Excipient information presented when available (limited, particularly for generics); consult specific product labeling.
Capsule: 25 mg, 50 mg, 100 mg
Zonegran®: 25 mg, 100 mg

SPECIAL TOPICS / ISSUES
TABLE OF CONTENTS

ACUTE POSTOPERATIVE PAIN

Pain in a surgical patient can be due to pre-existing disease, the surgical procedure (surgical incision, related drains and tubes, body positioning, immobility, excessive stretching or trauma to a peripheral nerve, postoperative ileus), or a combination of pre-existing disease and procedure-related causes. Pain can occur at rest and/or with movement or physical activity. Effective postoperative pain management should provide subjective pain relief, minimize the risk for adverse effects, and allow the patient to return to normal daily activities as soon as possible. In addition, postoperative pain management should minimize the detrimental effects from unrelieved pain which include: Thromboembolic and pulmonary complications; impairment of immune function; unnecessary fear and/or anxiety; and development of chronic pain.

Preparation should begin before the surgical procedure by performing a pain history and physical exam; treating pre-existing pain and anxiety; and educating the patient about his or her role in reporting pain, reporting analgesic adverse effects, and properly using analgesic modalities (eg, patient controlled analgesia) and non-pharmacological techniques. Then, the pain management plan can be made.

It is now recommended to utilize a combination of analgesic agents and techniques that work by different mechanisms to provide postoperative analgesia (multimodal analgesia). Combining analgesics and analgesic techniques provides additive or synergistic analgesia with lower doses compared to monotherapy, potentially minimizing adverse effects and improving recovery and function. Furthermore, the use of multimodal analgesic techniques prior to surgery can reduce the number of patients developing chronic pain following surgery. Examples of multimodal analgesia include a nonsteroidal anti-inflammatory agent (NSAID) or acetaminophen combined with an opioid following surgery and a continuous femoral nerve block (using a local anesthetic) with an intravenous opioid following total knee arthroplasty. In some cases, therapy for postoperative pain management actually begins before surgery. Peroperative administration of epidural anagesia, local anesthetic wound infiltration, and/or an NSAID has been shown to significantly improved postoperative analgesia.

Analgesic drugs can be divided into opioid and nonpioid drugs. Examples of nonopioid analgesics commonly used to manage postoperative pain include NSAIDs, acetaminophen, and local anesthetics. Ketamine, gabapentin, and pregabalin are drugs that are used for other indications but have analgesic/antihyperalgesic properties. Opioids are the mainstay of analgesic therapy for moderate and severe pain. This chapter will review the commonly used drugs in the management of acute postoperative pain.

ACETAMINOPHEN

Acetaminophen, alone or in combination with an opioid or NSAID, is frequently used for treatment of mild-to-moderate postoperative pain. Acetaminophen most likely provides analgesia by inhibiting prostaglandin synthesis in the central nervous system, with no peripheral anti-inflammatory effects. Acetaminophen may improve analgesia and has been shown to have a morphine-sparing effect in the first 24-hours after surgery, but does not seem to be able to reduce opioid-related adverse effects. Acetaminophen is generally well tolerated when administered in a daily maximum dose of 4 grams for short-term pain management in adults with normal liver function. Acetaminophen is an excellent alternative analgesic in a patient who should not receive an NSAID (or celecoxib).

NONSTEROIDAL ANTI-INFLAMMATORY DRUGS (NSAIDs)

NSAIDs are commonly used for postoperative pain management. These agents are frequently the first-line therapy for mild to moderate postoperative pain. NSAIDs inhibit the production of prostaglandins by inhibiting cyclooxygenase. NSAIDs have both a peripheral and central effect, with their central effect providing a significant portion of the analgesia and their peripheral effect diminishing postinjury inflammation and the hyperalgesic state following surgical trauma. NSAIDs are known to reduce pain intensity, have a morphine-sparing effect and possibly postoperative nausea/vomiting and sedation from opioids.

The perioperative limitation of traditional nonselective NSAIDs is most often due to their potential to impair platelet aggregation, which can increase bleeding. Cases of gastrointestinal bleeding or ulceration have been reported. Under normal, euvolemic conditions, prostaglandins do not play a major role in the maintenance of renal blood flow and glomerular circulation. However, in chronic renal insufficiency, hypovolemia, hepatic cirrhosis, and heart failure, prostaglandin production increases to preserve renal perfusion. Recent data suggests that all NSAIDs (nonselective agents and celecoxib) could increase the risk of new onset hypertension, worsen pre-existing disease, and ultimately increase the risk of cardiovascular events. In the postoperative setting, NSAIDs can increase the risk of severe bleeding. Therefore, NSAIDs (nonselective agents and celecoxib) should not be administered to patients with a history of ischemic heart disease, stroke, heart failure, or to patients who have recently undergone coronary artery bypass grafting. All NSAIDs should be administered in the lowest effective dose for the shortest duration possible.

GABAPENTIN AND PREGABALIN

Gabapentin and pregabalin bind to the $\alpha_2\delta$ subunit of the voltage-dependent calcium channels preventing release of nociceptive pain neurotransmitters. In addition, these agents may have antihyperalgesic and anxiolytic effects. The most common adverse effects of gabapentin and pregabalin are sedation and dizziness, and with chronic use, peripheral edema.

KETAMINE

Ketamine, a NMDA-receptor antagonist, has antihyperalgesic effects when administered in low (0.15-0.25 mg/kg/hour I.V.) doses as an adjunct analgesic. In patients at high risk for opioid-resistant postoperative pain (eg, chronic opioid use, back surgery) or chronic pain syndrome following surgery (eg, patients undergoing mastectomy or thoracotomy), intra- and postoperative administration of low-dose ketamine may be considered. When these low doses of ketamine are used, sedation and psychomimetic adverse effects from ketamine are not a concern.

TRAMADOL

Tramadol provides analgesia by inhibiting reuptake of norepinephrine and serotonin, as well as binding to mu-opioid receptors. Similar to oral opioid-acetaminophen combination products, tramadol is effective for treating moderate pain. Adverse effects that can occur with tramadol include nausea, vomiting, dizziness, and seizures. Tramadol should be used with caution in patients with a history of seizure disorder or taking a selective serotonin reuptake inhibitor. Although tramadol is not classified as a controlled substance, physical dependence on tramadol has been reported.

Table 1. Acetaminophen and Select NSAIDs

Drug	Usual Dose for Adults >50 kg Body Weight	Usual Dose for Adults <50 kg Body Weight
Acetaminophen (Tylenol®)	650 mg q4h or 1000 mg q6h	10-15 mg/kg q4h maximum of 4 g/day
Ibuprofen (Motrin®, others)	400-600 mg q6h	10 mg/kg q6-8h
Ketorolac tromethamine tablets[1] (Toradol®)	10 mg q4-6h to a maximum of 40 mg/d	
Naproxen (Naprosyn®)	250-275 mg q6-8h	5 mg/kg q8h
Naproxen sodium (Anaprox®)	275 mg q6-8h	
Ketorolac tromethamine injection (Toradol®)	60 mg I.M. or 30 mg I.V. initially, then 30 mg q6h, not to exceed 5 days	30 mg I.M. or 15 mg I.V. initially, then 15 mg q6h, not to exceed 5 days

[1]For short-term use only.

Note: Only the above NSAIDs have FDA approval for use as simple analgesics, but clinical experience has been gained with other drugs as well. Doses are for patients with normal renal and hepatic function.

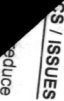

ainstay of treatment for moderate-to-severe postoperative pain ~y are commonly used as the initial analgesic agent in the >erative period and are continued postoperatively, for days to ate or severe pain. Opioids are administered by the oral, parenteral, ·, with the severity of pain and type of surgical procedure dictating the ~~~~~ which they are administered. Oral opioids, either alone or in combination with acetaminophen, are frequently administered for moderate pain. Parenteral and neuraxial opioids are usually administered for severe pain.

Opioids exert their effects by binding to central opioid receptors. The activity of the specific opioid depends on the actual agent and how well it binds to a given opioid receptor. Unlike NSAIDs and local anesthetics, opioids do not interrupt nociceptive transmission but rather decrease the ability to discern pain.

The patient's pain history, previous experience with opioids, and the extent of the injury are taken into consideration when selecting the initial opiod. Opioids differ in potency, safety, and patient characteristics. Propoxyphene, codeine, and hydro-codone are less potent opioids that are used in combination with acetaminophen. These combination products are indicated for moderate pain. Higher doses of these opioids would be required to treat severe pain and would cause significant adverse effects for the patient, including acetaminophen overdose. Morphine, hydro-morphone, and fentanyl are potent opioids that can be used alone in a dose that will treat moderate or severe pain. Oxycodone can be used for moderate or severe pain, depending upon the product formulation. When combined with acetaminophen or aspirin, the dose is limited by the amount of acetaminophen or aspirin in the product. Therefore, the dose of oxycodone needed to treat severe pain could not be provided with a combination product. Meperidine undergoes extensive first-pass metabolism, limiting its usefulness as an oral analgesic. High levels of its metabolite, normeperidine, can result in central nervous system excitation ranging from agitation to seizures. Meperidine also inhibits serotonin reuptake, raising concerns about development of the serotonin syndrome particularly if a second serotonergic agent (eg, selective serotonin reuptake inhibitor or SSRI) is concurrently administered. For safety, many hospitals limit the use of meperidine for analgesia. For patients with renal and/or hepatic insufficiency, the doses of most opioids should be reduced. Morphine, for example, has an active metabolite (morphine-6-glucuronide) that can accumulate in renal impairment. Table 2 represents the most frequently prescribed oral opioids for acute postoperative pain management.

Table 2. Oral Opioids for Acute Postoperative Pain

Drug	Equianalgesic Dose	Effective Adult Dosing[1]	Indication
Codeine[2]	180 mg	15-60 mg q4-6h	Moderate pain
Hydrocodone[2]	30 mg	5-10 mg q4-6h	Moderate pain
Oxycodone[2]	20 mg	5-10 mg q4-6h	Moderate pain
Tramadol	N/A	50-100 mg q4-6h[3]	Moderate pain

[1]For patients with normal renal and hepatic function.

[2]When combined with acetaminophen or aspirin.

[3]Not to exceed 400 mg/day in adults or 300 mg/day in patients ≥75 years of age.

Parenteral opioids remain an important component of any analgesic regimen for managing severe postoperative pain in the inpatient and ambulatory setting. Ambulatory surgery patients may receive short-acting parenteral analgesics (eg, fentanyl), or limited amounts of morphine, in intermittent bolus doses for treatment of severe pain. The intramuscular route of administration should be avoided if possible due to pain on injection, variability in absorption, and a longer time to peak effect (when compared to intravenous administration). Patient-controlled analgesia (PCA), the self-administered intermittent I.V. administration of an opioid, is the preferred method for administering intravenous (I.V.) opioids for managing postoperative pain. The advantage of PCA over traditional intermittent I.M. or I.V. administration is that once patient reaches his or her ideal level of analgesia (eg, following an opioid loading dose in the PACU), the patient should then have minimal fluctuation within the analgesic range and a feeling of control over his or her postoperative pain. The key to using PCA appropriately is assuring that an adequate initial bolus dose is administered, adequately educating the patient, and adjusting as needed. Appropriate patient selection is important. PCA is not indicated in a patient who is not able to understand the technique of PCA or press the PCA button, unwilling to assume control of his or her analgesia, or who is obtunded or sedated by his or her illness or medication. Table 3 represents the usual PCA doses of common opioids for the treatment of moderate or severe acute postoperative pain.

Table 3. Usual Adult PCA Opioid Dosing[1]

Drug	Equianalgesic Dose	Loading Dose[2]	Usual PCA Dose	Lockout Interval
Fentanyl	20 mcg	25-75 mcg	20-40 mcg	5-10 min
Hydromorphone (Dilaudid®)	0.2 mg	0.2-1 mg	0.2-0.4 mg	5-10 min
Morphine	1 mg	2-5 mg	1-2 mg	5-10 min

[1]In opioid-naïve patients with normal renal and hepatic function.

[2]Titrate in increments to desired level of analgesia or occurrence of excessive adverse effects.

Neuraxial opioid administration is another route that is used for management of moderate or severe acute postoperative pain. Neuraxial administration of opioids works by binding to opioid receptors on the spinal cord. This type of opioid administration can be used to provide analgesia for major abdominal, thoracic, and pelvic procedures. In these types of surgeries, epidural analgesia often provides better postoperative analgesia than parenteral opioids. Epidural administration of opioids is much more common than intrathecal administration for postoperative pain management. Table 4 represents neuraxial analgesic doses of opioid agonists for the treatment of moderate or severe acute postoperative pain.

Table 4. Usual Neuraxial Opioid Dosing in Adults

Agent	Epidural Bolus Dose	Epidural Continuous Infusion[1]	Intrathecal Bolus Dose
Fentanyl	25-100 mcg	8-100 mcg/h	5-25 mcg
Hydromorphone	1 mg	0.1-0.2 mg/h	–
Morphine	5 mg	0.1-1 mg/h	0.1-0.3 mg
Sufentanil	10-50 mcg	4-10 mcg/h	0.02-0.05 mcg/kg

[1]When combined with bupivacaine 0.05% to 0.125%

Adverse Effects

Adverse effects of oral, parenteral, and neuraxial opioid therapy for treatment of acute postoperative pain include sedation, dizziness, nausea, vomiting, pruritus, urinary retention, and respiratory depression. Risk factors for respiratory depression include large doses administered to an opioid-naive patient, pulmonary dysfunction (eg, asthma, obstructive sleep apnea), obesity, multiple comorbidities (eg, liver failure, renal failure), age >64, and concurrent medications that potentiate the respiratory depressant effect of the opioid (eg, benzodiazepines, sedating antiemetics, or antihistamines to treat opioid side effects). The potential for opioid-induced respiratory depression to occur is greatest in the first 24 hours following surgery, particularly when parenteral or neuroaxial opioids are administered. Frequent assessment of the patient's sedation level and respiratory status are critical to safe opioid administration. If increasing sedation is noted, reduce dose and monitor more frequently until sedation level is acceptable. Adding acetaminophen or an NSAID allows for lower opioid doses, which may result in fewer opioid adverse effects.

Another concern with the use of opioids (including short-term perioperative use) is the occurrence of opioid-induced hyperalgesia, which manifests as worsening pain despite increasing opioid doses and/or abnormal pain symptoms such as allodynia or dramatically increased sensitivity to pain. By using multimodal analgesia, opioid-induced enhancement of postoperative pain sensitivity could be reduced.

▶

◀ LOCAL ANESTHETICS

Local anesthetics provide effective postoperative analgesia. These agents can be administered by the intrathecal or epidural route, as a peripheral nerve block (PNB), or near the wound via infiltration. Peripheral nerve blocks of upper and lower extremities (eg, brachial plexus block, femoral nerve block) are often performed to provide intra- and postoperative anesthesia. A local anesthetic is injected near or around a nerve or nerve plexus to stop the pain impulses that originate from the surgical site. In addition to sensory fibers, motor and sympathetic fibers are also affected by injection of the local anesthetic solution. Patients undergoing more extensive, and therefore more painful, shoulder, elbow, knee, foot, or ankle surgeries are potential candidates for PNBs. These nerve blocks can be provided by a single injection and may be followed by a continuous infusion of a local anesthetic to provide postoperative analgesia. Local anesthetic wound infiltration (single injection or a continuous infusion) has been shown to decrease postoperative pain. However, in an experimental model, continuous intra-articular infusion of bupivacaine into a smaller joint produced significant chondrotoxic effects. The authors cautioned against the use of continuous infusion of local anesthetic into joints. Local anesthetics administered epidurally or intrathecally are frequently combined with opioids to provide "balanced analgesia" and avoid tachyphylaxis. The most common local anesthetic agents used for intra- and postoperative analgesia are lidocaine, mepivacaine, bupivacaine, and ropivacaine. (Table 5)

Table 5. Common Local Anesthetic Agents and Doses for Intra- and Postoperative Analgesia

Agent	Local Infiltration	Peripheral Nerve Block[1]	Continuous Peripheral Nerve Block	Continuous Epidural Analgesia
Lidocaine	0.5%-1%, 1-50 mL	1.5%-2%, 20 mL	–	
Bupivacaine	0.25%, 1-50 mL	0.25%-0.5%, 30 mL	0.1%-0.2% at 6-10 mL/h[2]	0.05%-0.125% at 4-10 mL/h[3]
Ropivacaine	0.5%, 1-40 mL	0.5%-0.75%, 30 mL	0.15%-0.2% at 6-10 mL/h[2]	0.1%-0.2% at 4-10 mL/h
Mepivacaine	0.5%-1%, 1-50 mL	1.5%-2%, 30 mL	–	–

[1]For a 70 kg patient; doses can vary with the type of block and should not exceed the maximum recommended dose.

[2]Patient-controlled regional anesthesia may be used; the concentration and rate of the local anesthetic solution may vary with the type of PNB and the patient's underlying medical condition.

[3]When administered in combination with fentanyl, sufentanil, hydromorphone, or morphine.

The adverse effects most commonly seen with analgesic doses of local anesthetics include hypotension (following intrathecal or epidural administration secondary to sympathetic blockade) and dose-related motor blockade. The potential for CNS and cardiovascular toxicity exists if a large amount of these agents is inadvertently administered systemically.

SUMMARY

The goal of acute postoperative pain management is to provide good analgesia with minimal adverse effects. Oftentimes, this is best accomplished with the use of a combination of analgesic agents and techniques that provide analgesia by different mechanisms.

REFERENCES AND RECOMMENDED READING

American Society of Anesthesiologists Task Force on Acute Pain Management, "Practice Guidelines for Acute Pain Management in the Perioperative Setting," *Anesthesiology*, 2004, 100(6):1573-81.

Boezaart AP, "Perineural Infusion of Local Anesthetics," *Anesthesiology*, 2006, 104(4):872-80.

Elia N, Lysakowski C, and Tramèr MR, "Does Multimodal Analgesia With Acetaminophen, Nonsteroidal Anti-inflammatory Drugs, or Selective Cyclooxygenase-2 Inhibitors and Patient-Controlled Analgesia Morphine Offer Advantages Over Morphine Alone? Meta-analyses of Randomized Trials," *Anesthesiology*, 2005, 103(6):1296-304.

Gajraj NM, "Pregabalin: Its Pharmacology and Use In Pain Management," *Anesth Analg*, 2007, 105 (6):1805-15.

Gornoll AH, Kang RW, Williams JM, et al, "Chondrolysis After Continuous Intra-Articular Bupivacaine Infusion: An Experimental Model Investigating Chondrotoxicity in the Rabbit Shoulder," *Arthroscopy*, 2006, 22(8):813-9.

Grass JA, "Patient-Controlled Analgesia," *Anesth Analg*, 2005, 101(5 Suppl):S44-61.

Himmelseher S and Durieux ME, "Ketamine For Perioperative Pain Management," *Anesthesiology*, 2005, 102(1):211-20.

Ong CK, Lirk P, Seymour RA, et al, "The Efficacy of Preemptive Analgesia For Acute Postoperative Pain Management: A Meta-Analysis," *Anesth Analg*, 2005, 100(3):757-73.

Pasero C, "Assessment of Sedation During Opioid Administration For Pain Management," *J Perianesth Nurs*, 2009, 24(3):186-90.

Remy C, Marret E, and Bonnet F, "Effects of Acetaminophen on Morphine Side-effects and Consumption After Major Surgery: Meta-Analysis of Randomized Controlled Trials," *Br J Anaesth*, 2005, 94(4):505-13.

Richman JM, Liu SS, Courpas G, et al, "Does Continuous Peripheral Nerve Block Provide Superior Pain Control to Opioids? A Meta-Analysis," *Anesth Analg*, 2006, 102(1):248-57.

ALLERGIC REACTIONS

An allergic drug reaction can be considered an adverse effect involving immunologic mechanisms. True allergic reactions are much less common than nonallergic responses such as side effects and drug-drug interactions. As a result, it is important to carefully evaluate patients who present with allergies to drugs. Patients frequently state an allergy to a drug when the reaction was a predictable side effect (eg, nausea/vomiting with codeine). If a patient presents a history of one or more of the following signs or symptoms after drug administration, an allergic reaction should be assumed until proven otherwise: Skin manifestations (pruritus with hives or flushing), facial or oral swelling, shortness of breath, choking, wheezing, and vascular collapse. In these situations, an alternate agent should be selected.

CLASSIFICATION OF ALLERGIC REACTIONS

Allergic reactions can be classified into one of four immunopathologic categories (types I through IV) using the Coombs and Gell Classification System. The following table summarizes the key characteristics of each type of reaction.

Type	Characteristics	Usual Onset	Examples
I - Anaphylactic (IgE mediated)	Requires the presence of IgE specific for drug antigen or other allergen; allergen binds to IgE on basophils and mast cells resulting in release of inflammatory mediators (eg, histamine, serotonin, proteases, bradykinin generating factor, eosinophil chemotactic factors, neutrophil chemotactic factor, leukotrienes, prostaglandins, thromboxanes)	Within 30 minutes	Immediate penicillin reaction Immediate latex reaction Blood products Vaccines Dextran Polypeptide hormones
II - Cytotoxic	Destruction of host cells; cell-associated antigen initiates cytolysis by antigen-specific antibody (IgG or IgM); most often involves blood elements (eg, erythrocytes, leukocytes, platelets)	Usually 5-12 hours	Penicillin, quinidine, phenylbutazone, thiouracils, sulfonamides, methyldopa
III - Immune complex	Antigen-antibody complexes form and deposit on blood vessel walls and activate complement. Result is a serum-sickness-like syndrome.	3-8 hours	Serum sickness; may be caused by penicillins, sulfonamides, I.V. contrast media, hydantoins
IV - Cell mediated (delayed)	Antigens cause activation of lymphocytes (T cells), which release inflammatory mediators	24-48 hours	Graft rejection Latex contact dermatitis Tuberculin reaction

DiPiro JT, "Allergic and Pseudoallergic Drug Reactions," *Pharmacotherapy: A Pathophysiologic Approach*, 7th ed, Dipiro JT, Talbert RL, Yee GC, et al, eds, New York, NY: McGraw-Hill, 2008, 1447-82.

ANESTHESIA-RELATED AGENTS ASSOCIATED WITH ALLERGY

Certain agents are most often responsible for allergic reactions in surgical patients. These include neuromuscular blocking agents, latex, antibiotics, colloids, hypnotics, opioids, local anesthetics, I.V. contrast media, and blood products. The antibiotics most commonly associated with allergic reactions are the sulfonamides, penicillins, and cephalosporins. There is high cross reactivity between penicillin and the carbapenems (eg, imipenem); carbapenems should be avoided in patients who have a penicillin allergy suggestive of a type I anaphylactic reaction. Propofol contains soybean oil and egg yolk components; propofol should be avoided in patients with allergies to these items. It should be noted that the sensitizing protein in the majority of patients with egg allergy is egg albumin which is found in the egg white. The ester-type local anesthetics can produce allergic reactions secondary to the metabolite para-aminobenzoic acid. The methylparaben preservative in amide-type local anesthetics may also produce an allergic reaction in patients sensitive to para-aminobenzoic acid. However, allergic reactions to local anesthetics are uncommon. Most of the adverse reactions reported are the result of inadvertent intravascular injections. Sulfites, which are used as preservatives in various drug products, can produce pulmonary complications in patients, occurring more frequently in asthmatics. Allergies to opioids are not common. If a patient is allergic to an opioid, an opioid with a different chemical structure (phenanthrene, phenylpiperidine, phenylheptane) should be selected to avoid the potential for cross sensitivity. Serious allergic reactions are more common in hyperosmolar, ionic, iodinated contrast media when compared to nonionic contrast. Special consideration should be given to a patient who presents a personal or family history of allergy to halothane or succinylcholine as this may actually represent an occurrence of malignant hyperthermia.

ANAPHYLAXIS

Anaphylaxis is the most severe form of allergic reaction. It can present as an acute, life-threatening reaction with multiple organ system involvement or it can be more localized in appearance. When antibodies are not involved in the process, the reaction is termed anaphylactoid. It is not possible through clinical observation to distinguish between anaphylactic and anaphylactoid reactions. Anaphylaxis can occur at any time during anesthesia. It has been estimated that 1 in every 13,000 to 1 in every 20,000 patients undergoing anesthesia (general and regional) experience drug-induced anaphylaxis. This number decreases to 1 in 6500 anesthetics for anaphylaxis to neuromuscular blocking agents. The incidence of anaphylactoid and anaphylactic reactions is greater in females when compared to males. In a survey examining the incidence of intraoperative anaphylaxis, 54% of the anaphylactic reactions were due to neuromuscular blocking agents, 22.3% due to latex, 14.7% due to antibiotics, 2.8% due to colloids, 2.4% due to opioids, 0.8% due to hypnotics, 0.6% due to local anesthetics, and 2.4% due to other agents (Mertes, 2004). Succinylcholine (37.6%) and rocuronium (26.2%) were the neuromuscular blocking agents most frequently implicated in anaphylaxis (Mertes, 2004). It has been suggested that succinylcholine and rocuronium should be considered to have a high risk of sensitization, with pancuronium and vecuronium a medium risk, and atracurium and cisatracurium a low risk. Cross-sensitization between one or more neuromuscular blocking agents was seen in 63.4% of the cases, with rocuronium and vecuronium having the highest rate of cross-reactivity (Mertes, 2004).

As already mentioned, anaphylactoid and anaphylactic reactions are not able to be differentiated based solely on clinical symptoms. However, if one looks at the severity of symptoms of the anaphylactic and anaphylactoid reactions occurring during anesthesia, anaphylactoid are usually less severe than anaphylactic (Mertes, 2004).

Severity Grade	Symptoms	Anaphylactoid Reactions	Anaphylactic Reactions
1	Cutaneous: Urticaria, erythema, angioedema	60%	13%
2	Measurable/nonlife-threatening: Tachycardia, cutaneous, hypotension, respiratory	26%	22%
3	Life-threatening: Bronchospasm, tachycardia, bradycardia, arrhythmias, cardiovascular collapse	15%	60%
4	Cardiac arrest, respiratory arrest, death	–	5%

Pathophysiology

Anaphylaxis is initiated by an antigen binding to IgE antibodies; however, prior exposure to the antigen or a substance with a similar structure is first required to sensitize the patient to the antigen. The binding of the antigen to the IgE antibodies on the surface of basophils and mast cells causes release of histamine and the chemotactic factors of anaphylaxis. Other chemical mediators (leukotrienes, prostaglandins, kinins) are also released in response to cellular activation. The liberated mediators produce bronchospasm, upper airway edema, vasodilation, increased capillary permeability, and urticaria. The effects of multiple mediators on the heart and peripheral vasculature cause the cardiovascular collapse seen during anaphylaxis. Antigenic challenge in a sensitized individual usually produces immediate clinical manifestations of anaphylaxis; however, the onset may be delayed by up to 30 minutes. The reaction can vary in severity, from minor clinical changes to acute cardiopulmonary collapse.

Signs / Symptoms of Anaphylactic Reaction

The following table lists the signs and symptoms that may indicate an anaphylactic reaction during anesthesia.

Systems	Symptoms	Signs
Cutaneous	Itching, burning	Urticaria (hives), flushing, perioral edema, periorbital edema
Respiratory	Dyspnea, chest tightness	Coughing, wheezing, sneezing, laryngeal edema, decreased pulmonary compliance, pulmonary edema, acute respiratory distress, bronchospasm
Cardiovascular	Dizziness, malaise, retrosternal oppression	Disorientation, diaphoresis, loss of consciousness, hypotension, tachycardia, dysrhythmias, decreased systemic vascular resistance, pulmonary hypertension, cardiovascular collapse

Levy JH, *Anaphylactic Reactions in Anesthesia and Intensive Care*, Stoneham, Butterworth-Heinemann, 1992.

Treatment of Anaphylactic Reaction

Treatment of a severe, life-threatening anaphylactic reaction must be immediate. Initial therapy should consist of: 1) stop administration of precipitating drug; 2) maintain airway and administer 100% oxygen; 3) discontinue all anesthetic agents; 4) intravascular volume expansion with crystalloid solution; and 5) epinephrine administration. Secondary therapy consists of administration of H_1 and H_2 receptor antagonists (eg, diphenhydramine, ranitidine), catecholamine infusions (eg, norepinephrine), inhaled bronchodilators (eg, albuterol) for bronchospasm, and corticosteroids (eg, hydrocortisone, methylprednisolone). Patients should be admitted to an ICU for at least 24 hours following an anaphylactic reaction because of the possibility of recurrent "late-phase" reactions.

REFERENCES AND RECOMMENDED READING

DiPiro JT, "Allergic and Pseudoallergic Drug Reactions," *Pharmacotherapy: A Pathophysiologic Approach*, 7th ed, Dipiro JT, Talbert RL, Yee GC, et al, eds, New York, NY: McGraw-Hill, 2008, 1447-82.

Golembiewski JA, "Allergic Reactions to Drugs: Implications for Perioperative Care," *J Perianesth Nurs*, 2002, 17(6):393-8.

Hepner DL and Castells MC, "Anaphylaxis During the Perioperative Period," *Anesth Analg*, 2003, 97 (5):1381-95.

Laxenaire MC, Mertes PM, and Moss M, "Identifying Anaphylactic and Anaphylactoid Reactions During Anesthesia," *Pharmacy Practice News*, 2005, 32(2):91-4.

Levy JH, "The Allergic Response," *Clinical Anesthesia*, 5th ed, Barash PG, et al, eds, Philadelphia, PA: Lippincott Williams and Wilkins, 2005, 1298-1312.

Mertes PM, Laxenaire MC, Alla F, et al, "Anaphylactic and Anaphylactoid Reactions Occurring During Anesthesia in France in 1999-2000," *Anesthesiology*, 2003, 99(3):536-45.

Mertes PM, Laxenaire MC, and GERAP, et al, "Anaphylactic and Anaphylactoid Reactions Occurring During Anaesthesia in France. Seventh Epidemiologic Survey (January 2001-December 2002)," *Ann Fr Anesth Reanim*, 2004, 23(12):1133-43.

LATEX ALLERGY

The incidence of clinically significant latex allergy is increasing. This increase has been suggested to be due in part to the implementation of universal precautions by the CDC in 1987 secondary to the AIDS epidemic. **Because of the increased incidence of latex allergy, all patients need a complete history including risk factor evaluation and previous evidence of clinical signs and symptoms suggesting contact dermatitis or urticaria.** For example, patients should be questioned about the presence of swelling or itching of the hands or other areas after contact with rubber gloves, condoms, diaphragms, toys, or other rubber products and about itching or swelling of the lips or mouth after dental exams, blowing up balloons, or after eating bananas, chestnuts, and avocados.

It is important today for health care institutions to have a comprehensive plan (including a perioperative component) in place for dealing with latex allergic patients and healthcare personnel. In cardiovascular medicine, the high proportion of procedures and imaging modalities heightens exposure to latex allergens, usually related to rubber gloves. This is a potentially life-threatening problem, both for the patient and healthcare personnel, in situations such as the cardiac catheterization laboratory. Some institutions have avoided use of latex products throughout the hospital environment.

Hypersensitivity Reactions Caused by Latex

Latex-containing products can produce type I and type IV hypersensitivity reactions.

The type I (IgE-mediated) hypersensitivity reaction is the true "allergic" reaction seen with latex products. Proteins found in the latex promote the production of an antibody of the IgE class which attaches to basophils and mast cells. When the antigen (protein) is encountered again, histamine and other physiologically active mediators are released from mast cells and basophils. The clinical manifestations can include single or multiple system involvement, be mild or severe, ranging from itching to edema, and from mild hypotension to shock. It has been estimated that 10% of the true anaphylactic reactions during anesthesia are due to latex allergy. These reactions are usually seen 5-30 minutes after induction of anesthesia and start of surgery. Seventy-nine percent of of type I patients previously had type IV symptoms.

In the type IV (delayed type) reaction, a contact dermatitis is seen. The preservatives, stabilizers, accelerators, and antioxidants used in the latex manufacturing process serve as the antigens for T-cell lymphocytes. The dermatitis produced can be uncomfortable but is not life-threatening and usually occurs over a 24-hour period; limited to site of contact. Not all patients with type IV symptoms will progress to type I reactivity.

Routes of Exposure to Latex Proteins

It is important to consider the route of exposure of the latex protein in allergic patients as this can be a determinant of the type of reaction produced. The following table summarizes major routes of exposure.

Type of Exposure	Reaction
Direct skin contact	Localized or generalized urticaria
Mucous membrane	Rhinitis, conjunctivitis, stomatitis, angioedema; severe anaphylactic reactions and death reported
Inhalation of airborne starch-protein particles	Wheezing, bronchospasm, reduced lung compliance, episodes of desaturation and/or severe hypoxemia
Intravascular absorption of water soluble latex particles from surgical gloves	Sudden tachycardia, severe hypotension, cardiorespiratory collapse

◀ **High-Risk Patients**

Several groups have been identified as "high-risk" for allergic reactions to latex. Special consideration should be given these individuals.

Patients having multiple surgical procedures (eg, spina bifida patients/patients with congenital urologic abnormalities). A 30% to 70% incidence of latex allergy has been reported for spina bifida patients. These patients are routinely exposed to latex-containing urinary catheters.

Healthcare providers. Latex sensitivity may be as high as 17%. Approximately 70% of adverse events reported to FDA regarding latex involve healthcare workers.

Workers with occupational exposure to natural rubber latex (eg, hairdressers, greenhouse workers, latex manufacturers).

Patients with a history of atopy, hay fever, rhinitis, asthma, or eczema. Atopy is one of the significant predisposing risk factors for latex allergy.

Patients with history of food allergy to tropical fruits (eg, avocado, kiwi, bananas), chestnuts, stone fruits, and additional specific foods. These plants contain several proteins similar/identical to those found in latex.

Individuals with severe or anaphylactic responses to latex should consider having an Epi-Pen® available at all times, and having a Medic-Alert® bracelet to alert healthcare workers to the potential for life-threatening allergic reactions.

Treatment of Anaphylactic Reaction

Management of an anaphylactic reaction which is thought to be due to latex allergy must be immediate. Initial therapy should consist of the following.

- Stop administration of offending agent.
- Removal of all latex products (switch to nonlatex gloves and latex-free intravenous tubing). Latex-free precautions must accompany the patient throughout the perioperative and hospital stay (PACU, ICU, general floor, and discharge unit).
- Discontinue all antibiotic and blood administration.
- Maintain airway with 100% oxygen.
- Intubate the trachea (as indicated).
- Intravascular volume expansion with crystalloid or colloid.
- Epinephrine administration (see Epinephrine monograph).
- Discontinue all anesthetic agents if appropriate.
- Consider use of Military Anti-Shock Trousers (MAST).
- Display prominent signs to identify latex allergy.
- When appropriate, administer antihistamines (eg, diphenhydramine), cortico-steroids (eg, hydrocortisone), catecholamine infusions (eg, norepinephrine), inhaled bronchodilators (eg, albuterol) for bronchospasm, and sodium bicarbonate (guided by arterial blood gas results). Patients should be admitted to the ICU for 24 hours following an anaphylactic reaction because of the possibility of recurrent "late-phase" reactions. To confirm a latex allergy, RAST or AlaSTAT test may be performed.
- Details of any allergic reaction should be clearly documented in the patient's chart and reported to FDA MedWatch program.
- Contact dermatitis and type IV reactions:
    - Avoid irritating skin cleansers.
    - Topical corticosteroids can be applied locally.

Perioperative Management of a Latex Allergic Patient

No evidence exists to demonstrate that prophylaxis before surgery prevents latex-induced anaphylactic reactions. In spite of this, prophylaxis has been used in patients with a positive history of allergy; one suggested regimen uses diphenhydramine P.O. or I.V. every 6 hours at 13, 7, and 1 hours before surgery, prednisone P.O. every 6 hours at 13, 7, and 1 hours before surgery (hydrocortisone I.V. may be substituted), and ranitidine P.O. or I.V. every 12 hours at 13 and 1 hours before surgery. This regimen is continued for 12 hours after surgery.

The key to the hospital management of the latex allergic patient is to provide a latex-free environment. To accomplish this, the following actions should be taken.

- Substitute all items with nonlatex alternatives when possible; if there is a question concerning the latex content of a product, the manufacturer should be called.
- Gloves made of neoprene or other polymers should be used.
- Latex-based adhesives should be eliminated.
- Stopcocks should be used for drug administration instead of injection ports on I.V. tubing.
- Syringes not containing rubber tips on the plunger should be used.
- Drug products in glass ampuls should be used whenever possible; if a vial must be used, utilize a vial stopper remover so the stopper does not have to be punctured or puncture only once.
- To reduce exposure to aerosolized glove powder which is a known carrier of latex proteins, schedule the surgery as the first case of the day. Some institutions have reserved an O.R. suite for latex allergic patients.

Testing for Latex Allergy

Testing for latex allergy is recommended for high-risk patients. Both *in vitro* and *in vivo* tests are available as seen in the following table.

Test	Type	Description
Skin prick (SPT)	*in vivo*	Sensitive method to confirm IgE-mediated latex hypersensitivity; correlates well with clinical presence of allergy; high sensitivity (100%), high specificity (99%)
Patch	*in vivo*	Test for type IV hypersensitivity reaction; test performed with 1 inch square of rubber glove; skin observed for contact dermatitis after 48 hours
Radioallergosorbent (RAST)	*in vitro*	Performed on the serum of patients with natural latex as the antigen; used to detect and quantify allergen specific IgE in patient's serum; positive RAST response correlates strongly with *in vivo* allergic response; sensitivity 67% to 82%
Enzymeallergosorbent (EAST)	*in vitro*	Enzyme-linked immunometric assay used to measure latex-specific IgE antibodies; can be false negatives

REFERENCES AND RECOMMENDED READING

Dakin MJ and Yentis SM, "Latex Allergy: A Strategy for Management," *Anaesthesia*, 1998, 53 (8):774-81.

Hancock DL, "Latex Allergy. Prevention and Treatment," *Anesthesiol Rev*, 1994, 21(5):153-63.

Katz JD, Holzman RS, Brown RH, et al, "Natural Rubber Latex Allergy: Considerations for Anesthesiologists," American Society of Anesthesiologists (ASA), 2005. Available at: http://www.asahq.org/publicationsAndServices/latexallergy.pdf. Last accessed December 6, 2007.

Senst BL and Johnson RA, "Latex Allergy," *Am J Health Syst Pharm*, 1997, 54(9):1071-5.

Steelman VM, "Latex Allergy Precautions. A Research-Based Protocol," *Nurs Clin North Am*, 1995, 30(3):475-93.

Sussman G and Gold M, "Guidelines for the Management of Latex Allergies and Safe Latex Use in Health Care Facilities." Available at: http://www.acaai.org/public/physicians/latex.htm.

ANESTHESIA CONSIDERATIONS FOR NEUROSURGERY

Various factors must be taken into account for the neurosurgical patient. These include the surgical procedure; the type of anesthesia; the need for special anesthetic techniques (eg, controlled hypotension, EEG monitoring); and the effects of the anesthetic agents on brain physiology (cerebral blood flow, cerebral metabolic requirements, and cerebral vasodilation). This section will review key aspects of the anesthetic management of neurosurgical patients.

PHYSIOLOGY

Cerebral Blood Flow

Cerebral blood flow (CBF) is equal to cerebral perfusion pressure (CPP) divided by the cerebral vascular resistance. Cerebral perfusion pressure is defined as the difference between mean arterial pressure (MABP) and the greater of intracranial pressure (ICP) or central venous pressure.

$$CPP = MAP - ICP$$

Autoregulation maintains CBF at a constant level (50 mL/100 g brain/minute) between the MABP (or CPP) of approximately 50 and 150 mm Hg (see Figure A). Various conditions and/or medications can attenuate or abolish autoregulation, making blood flow dependent on MABP. These include the volatile inhalation agents, hypoxia, hypercarbia, and cerebral ischemia. Hypoxia causes cerebral vasodilation and an increase in CBF when PaO_2 <50 mm Hg (see Figure B) while decreases in carbon dioxide concentration cause a linear decrease in CBF between $PaCO_2$ of 80 and 20 mm Hg (see Figure C).

Cerebral Metabolic Rate

Cerebral metabolic rate for oxygen ($CMRO_2$) and CBF are directly related; as $CMRO_2$ increases, so does CBF to ensure sufficient substrate is available for metabolic demand (see Figure D). This condition is called "coupling." Conditions and/or medications that influence $CMRO_2$ include seizures ($\uparrow$ $CMRO_2$), temperature (hypothermia $\downarrow$ $CMRO_2$), and various anesthetics (eg, volatile inhalation agents and most I.V. sedative drugs $\downarrow$ $CMRO_2$).

The Brain's Protective Mechanisms

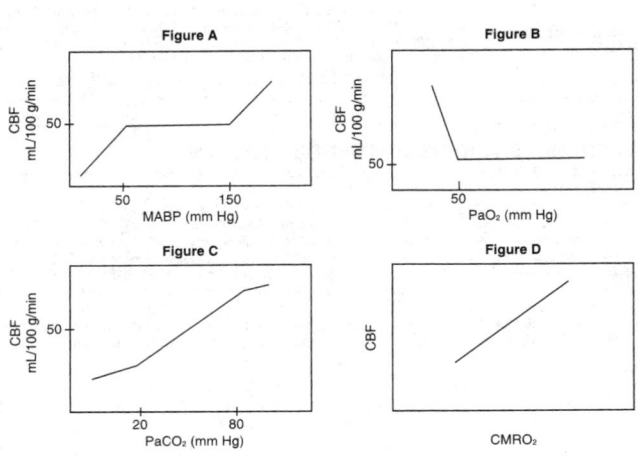

Intracranial Pressure

Normal ICP values are between 5 and 15 mm Hg (7-18 cm H_2O) and reflect the relationship between the volume of the cranial vault and intracranial contents. Since the cranial vault is rigid, the capacity of the intracranial contents to adjust to an increasing volume (compliance) will ultimately be exceeded, resulting in a marked increase in ICP with a small increase in volume. Signs and symptoms of increased ICP are found in Table 1. It must be kept in mind that a patient with an increased intracranial volume as a result of a tumor, for example, may be especially sensitive to volume increases produced by cerebral vasodilation caused by factors such as CO_2 retention or volatile inhalational anesthetic agents. Elevated ICP can be treated by reducing cerebral blood volume, reducing brain tissue volume, or reducing cerebrospinal fluid (CSF) volume (Table 2).

Table 1. Signs and Symptoms of Increased Intracranial Pressure

Headache

Nausea/vomiting

Decreased level of consciousness

Hypertension

Bradycardia

Irregular breathing

Oculomotor (third cranial) nerve palsy

Pupillary dilation

Abducens (sixth cranial) nerve palsy

Hemiparesis or hemiplegia

Coma

Respiratory arrest

Table 2. Treatment of Elevated Intracranial Pressure

Reduction of Cerebral Blood Volume

Avoid hypoxia and hypercarbia, as they cause cerebral vasodilation

Hyperventilate to a $PaCO_2$ of 25-30 mm Hg (produces cerebral vasoconstriction)

Promote venous drainage (eg, elevate head 30 degrees)

Treat severe hypertension

Treat seizures

Administer medications to produce cerebral vasoconstriction (eg, barbiturates, propofol, etomidate, benzodiazepines)

Reduction of Brain Tissue Volume

Increase serum osmolality to 305-320 mOsm/L with the administration of mannitol (0.2-1 g/kg I.V.), hypertonic saline 3% (5 mL/kg), 23.4% (30-60 mL over 30 min)

Administer furosemide (0.5-1 mg/kg I.V.); optimal results seen when combined with mannitol (↓ furosemide dose to 0.15-0.3 mg/kg I.V.)

Administer steroids (effective for tumors)

Resection of brain

Reduction of Cerebrospinal Fluid Volume

Drain CSF through lumbar subarachnoid or ventriculostomy catheter

Decrease CSF production (furosemide 0.5 mg/kg) and/or increase CSF reabsorption

Cerebrospinal Fluid

The CSF volume in an adult is approximately 150 mL. It is formed in the choroid plexus of the cerebral ventricles (0.35 mL/minute) by the transport of sodium, chloride, and bicarbonate with osmotic movement of water. CSF is absorbed into the venous system of the brain through arachnoid membrane villi. Furosemide and

◀ acetazolamide can reduce CSF formation by inhibiting the combined transport of sodium and chloride and by reducing bicarbonate transport, respectively.

EFFECTS OF MEDICATIONS ON BRAIN PHYSIOLOGY

Table 3 lists the effects of anesthetic agents on cerebral blood flow, cerebral metabolic oxygen requirements, and cerebral vasodilation. In general, inhalational anesthetics decrease cerebral metabolism and increase CBF whereas intravenous agents decrease both cerebral metabolism and blood flow. Of note, ketamine increases both oxygen demand and CBF, and as a result is not commonly used in neuroanesthesia. Isoflurane continues to be an excellent choice for a volatile inhalation agent. Its mild direct vasodilating action is partly offset by its ability to reduce cerebral metabolic rate and subsequently CBF, thereby limiting the net increase in CBF. The newer volatile inhalation agents desflurane and sevoflurane act similarly. Nondepolarizing neuromuscular blocking (NMB) agents have no direct effects on CBF and $CMRO_2$ as they do not cross the blood brain barrier; they may have an indirect effect secondary to their effects on heart rate (eg, pancuronium produces tachycardia) and blood pressure (eg, tubocurarine produces hypotension) if autoregulation has been abolished. Succinylcholine does increase CBF and $CMRO_2$, but this has minimal clinical impact. The vasopressors epinephrine, phenylephrine, and norepinephrine also have little to no direct cerebral effects but may indirectly increase CBF by increasing cerebral perfusion pressure. The vasodilators nitroglycerin, sodium nitroprusside, and hydralazine can increase CBF and ICP via direct cerebral vasodilation if arterial blood pressure is maintained. Beta-blockers (esmolol, labetalol) do not alter cerebral metabolism or vascular tone.

Table 3. Effects of Anesthetic Agents on Brain Physiology

Medication	Cerebral Blood Flow	Cerebral Metabolic Rate	Direct Cerebral Vasodilation
Inhalation Anesthetic Agents			
Desflurane	↑	↓↓	Yes
Enflurane	↑↑	↓	Yes
Halothane	↑↑↑	↓	Yes
Isoflurane	↑	↓↓	Yes
Nitrous oxide	↑↑/0	↑/0	Yes
Nitrous oxide with volatile inhalation agent	↑	↑/0	–
Nitrous oxide with intravenous anesthetic agent	0	0	–
Sevoflurane	↑	↓↓	Yes
Intravenous Anesthetic Agents			
Barbiturates	↓↓↓	↓↓↓	No
Etomidate	↓↓↓	↓↓↓	No
Fentanyl	↓/0	↓/0	No
Ketamine	↑↑	↑	Yes
Midazolam	↓	↓	No
Propofol	↓↓	↓↓	No

ELECTROPHYSIOLOGIC MONITORING

Electroencephalogram

The electroencephalogram (EEG) is used to monitor cerebral electrical activity and may allow early detection of ischemia before CBF is inadequate to maintain tissue viability. It can also be used for localization of epileptic foci. As a general rule, anesthetic effects on the EEG are global in nature in contrast to the focal changes seen with ischemia (see Table 4).

Table 4. EEG Rhythms

Wave Forms	Frequency	Activity
Delta	0-3 Hz	Deep sleep Deep anesthesia Ischemia
Theta	4-7 Hz	Light sleep Light anesthesia
Alpha	8-13 Hz	Resting and awake
Beta	14-30 Hz	Mental concentration Light sedation (ie, benzodiazepines)

Evoked Potentials

Evoked potentials monitor the functional integrity of ascending sensory pathways and descending motor pathways. Somato sensory evoked potentials (SSEP) are recorded from the cerebral cortex following peripheral (sensory nerve) stimulation. Transcranial motor evoked potentials (TcMEP) are recorded from peripheral muscle activity initiated by stimulation of the motor cortex. Evoked potentials are classified by the nerve tract being evaluated (somatosensory, auditory, visual, motor) (see Table 5). The type of evoked potential monitored depends on the area of CNS at risk for intraoperative injury. Evoked potentials are measured in terms of latency (how long it takes the stimulus to reach the recording device) and amplitude (the peak to trough height of the recorded waveform). An increase in latency time of 10% to 15% and/or a 40% to 50% decrease in amplitude is considered significant. Because anesthetic agents affect the latency and/or amplitude measurements (Table 6) it is important to obtain a baseline measurement after establishment of anesthesia. Thereafter, the anesthetic regimen should not be altered so that any subsequent decrease in amplitude or increase in latency reflects neuronal ischemia, not a change in depth of anesthesia. Maintaining an adequate depth of anesthesia when monitoring TcMEPs is difficult, especially since muscle relaxants must be used sparingly, if at all, to preserve the motor response. Other factors that can alter evoked potentials include hypotension, hypoxia, and hypothermia.

The reader is referred to any major anesthesia text for a further discussion of electrophysiologic monitoring.

Table 5. Evoked Potentials and the Neuronal Tracts They Monitor

Evoked Potential	CNS Tract	Surgical Procedures
SSEP (somatosensory evoked potential)	Sensory neural axis from peripheral nerves to brainstem and cortex	Spinal cord surgery (tumor, scoliosis), carotid endarterectomy, aortic surgery, cerebral aneurysm
BAER (brainstem auditory evoked response)	Brain stem	Acoustic neuroma, posterior fossa lesions, surgery involving cranial nerve VIII or auditory canal
VER (visual evoked response)	Retina, optic chiasm, optic radiation, occipital cortex	Orbit tumors, sphenoid wing meningiomas, supracellular/pituitary tumors, surgery around optic nerve or occipital cortex
TcMEP[1] (transcranial motor evoked potentials)	Motor cortex and descending motor tracts	Spinal cord surgery (tumor, scoliosis)

[1]Myogenic evoked motor potentials are monitored from the spinal cord and are relatively resistant to anesthetic-induced depression

Table 6. Drug Effects on Evoked Potentials

	Amplitude	Latency
I.V. Drugs		
Barbiturates	↓	↑
Benzodiazepines	↓	↑
Droperidol	↓	↑
Etomidate	↑,→	↑,→
Ketamine	↑	→
Narcotics	↓	↑,→
Propofol	↓	↑
Anesthetic Gases		
Inhalational agents (0.5 MAC)	→	→
Inhalational agents (>1 MAC)	↓	↑
Nitrous oxide	↓	→

STROKE

Stroke is the third leading cause of death. Approximately 700,000 new strokes occur per year in the United States, resulting in 160,000 deaths. Forty percent of primary stroke or transient ischemic attack (TIA) patients will experience a second event within 5 years, and 15% to 30% of stroke survivors are permanently disabled. The indirect annual cost is estimated at $57.9 billion. It is projected that in the United States the annual number of new and recurrent strokes/year will be nearly 1 million by 2050.

Modifiable risk factors include hypertension, smoking, excessive alcohol use, obesity, and lack of physical activity. Therapeutic treatment includes lifestyle modifications, drugs (anticoagulant and antiplatelet agents), and/or surgical (carotid artery surgery, angioplasty).

Nonmodifiable risk factors include age, gender, race/ethnicity, and family history. Additional factors include low birth weight (<2500 g), diabetes, sickle cell anemia, sleep apnea, metabolic syndrome, illicit drugs, and oral contraceptive use in female smokers. Infection, migraine, and inflammation are also emerging risk factors.

Table 7. Stroke Risk Factors and Goals

Hypertension	Weight loss, exercise, diet and drug therapy to keep blood pressure <120/80 mm Hg
Diabetes mellitus	Tight glucose control to hemoglobin A_{1c} <7%
Cholesterol	Diet, exercise, statins to achieve LDL <100 mg/dL
Smoking	Avoid both direct and second hand tobacco
Alcohol	Men: <2 drinks/day Women: <1 drink/day
Obesity	BMI: 18.5-24.9 kg/m^2 Waist: Men: <40 inches; Women: <35 inches
Physical activity	30 minutes of moderate-intensity exercise most days

Ischemic versus Hemorrhagic Stroke

The clinical presentation may aid in making the diagnosis of ischemic vs hemorrhagic stroke. Ischemic stroke frequently occurs with an early morning presentation, usually does not progress, and headache can occur but is not a major symptom. Hemorrhagic stroke usually presents as an acute focal neurologic deficit while the patient is active, progressing over minutes to hours. Subarachnoid hemorrhage usually has a sudden onset that is frequently associated with severe headache, vomiting, elevated blood pressure, and impaired consciousness. The amount of intracerebral hemorrhage and the Glasgow Coma Scale score are strong predictors of death within 30 days. Because of progressive bleeding, hemorrhagic stroke patients can rapidly deteriorate and need intensive care. Growth of the hematoma during the first several hours is associated with a 5-fold increase in poor outcome and/or death. Both CT and MRI are important in making the diagnosis. CT is better at demonstrating ventricular extension of hemorrhage while MRI can better detect underlying structural lesions, perihematoma edema, and herniation. Because many stroke patients cannot tolerate MRI, CT with contrast and CT angio are used to identify aneurysm, arteriovenous malformations (AVM), and tumor.

Treatment of Ischemic Stroke or TIA

Ischemic stroke caused by carotid stenosis: Several randomized, multicenter trials (NASCET, ECST, VA Cooperative study) have shown that patients with severe carotid artery stenosis (>70%) should have carotid endarterectomy (CEA) performed by a skilled surgeon with a perioperative morbidity/mortality <6%. Patients with symptomatic moderate stenosis (50% to 60%) should have CEA depending on other patient-specific factors (ie, age, health). If stenosis is <50% surgery is not indicated. Once diagnosed, surgery should not be delayed. For difficult cases (surgical access or patient concerns) carotid artery stenting should be performed.

Ischemic stroke: Patients diagnosed with an ischemic thrombotic stroke within 3 hours of onset of symptoms may be candidates for I.V. recombinant tPA therapy (ie, alteplase). The American Heart Association/American Stroke Association (AHA/ASA) now support administration of alteplase to patients presenting within 3 to 4.5 hours of symptom onset based on results of the ECASS-3 trial. Current guidelines also permit intra-arterial alteplase up to the 6th hour in patients with major stroke due to occlusion of the middle cerebral artery (MCA) or those who are not candidates for IV tPA, and current research is investigating the extention of this time frame in certain patients. Patients who have an ischemic stroke caused by cardiac emboli and atrial fibrillation, whether persistent or paroxysmal, should be treated with warfarin. Aspirin should be used for patients who cannot tolerate warfarin.

For ischemic stroke and TIA caused by less common conditions, AHA/ASA recommendations for treatment can be found in their guidelines (Adams, 2007; Adams, 2008).

Intracerebral Hemorrhagic (ICH) Stroke

Treatment of ICH involves slowing or stopping the hemorrhage, including potential removal of blood from the brain and/or ventricles to eliminate the mass effect and chemical factors that injure the brain; maintain adequate cerebral perfusion (MAP-ICP ≥60-70 mm Hg); manage/treat hyperglycemia, fever, nutrition, infection, DVT prophylaxis. Therapies that have not proven to be beneficial include steroids, hemodilution, and glycerol. Initial trials using recombinant activated factor VII have demonstrated a somewhat improved outcome despite an increase in thromboembolic events.

Guidelines for management of blood pressure, use of mannitol, and type of I.V. fluid therapy do not have strong research evidence to direct treatment. Elevation of the head of the bed with the patient's head in a neutral position enhances venous outflow. Management of hyperglycemia is recommended, but the target glucose range is still being evaluated. It is important to treat overt clinical seizures in addition to prophylactic antiseizure therapy. Infection needs to be diagnosed and treated; additionally, antipyretic medication should be used for febrile patients. Intermittent pneumatic leg compression devices have been shown to prevent venous thromboembolism. Studies comparing this proven method against SubQ heparin or low molecular weight heparin are pending.

◀ **Surgical Treatment**

Craniotomy to decompress the brain may or may not be helpful. Endoscopic aspiration (with or without thrombolytic therapy) is also being evaluated. The timing of surgery is uncertain, other than patients with cerebellar hemorrhage >3 cm and deteriorating, who have brain stem compression and/or hydrocephalus should be operated on as soon as possible. Delayed evacuation has little benefit.

ANESTHESIA CONCERNS FOR SOME NEURO-SURGICAL PROCEDURES

The following information should be considered when anesthetizing patients undergoing neurosurgical procedures.

Intracranial Tumors

- Assess fluid and electrolyte status. Hypovolemia, which is not uncommon in patients who have been at bedrest and/or treated with mannitol, can predispose the patient to hypotension during induction of anesthesia.

- Care should be taken in premedicating patients as they may be especially sensitive to central nervous system (CNS) depressant drugs; sedatives/analgesics are often not administered until the patient is monitored in the operating room.

- Monitoring may include measurement of arterial blood gases, intra-arterial blood pressure, central venous pressure, and urinary output in addition to the standard monitoring.

- Goals of anesthesia management: Avoid hypertension, hypotension, hypoxia, hypercarbia, and coughing; ICP should not be increased nor CBF compromised.

  - Thiopental, propofol, etomidate, or midazolam are all suitable induction agents.

  - An opioid can be administered to blunt the response to intubation.

  - A nondepolarizing muscle relaxant with minimal cardiovascular effects (eg, vecuronium, rocuronium) should be used if airway management is not considered problematic.

  - A deep level of anesthesia should be established before laryngoscopy/intubation and head pinning to minimize increases in blood pressure and ICP due to sympathetic stimulation.

  - Mannitol (0.25-1 g/kg) is used to decrease brain volume. Furosemide (10-20 mg) may be added.

  - Hyperventilation to a $PaCO_2$ of 25-30 mm Hg produces cerebral vasoconstriction and decreases intracranial pressure without producing cerebral ischemia.

  - $PaCO_2$ should be normalized near the end of surgery.

  - Long-acting agents should be avoided for the last 1-2 hours of surgery to prevent prolonged wake-up and allow a neurologic examination at the end of surgery.

  - Consider administering lidocaine (0.5-1 mg/kg I.V.) 90 seconds before suctioning/extubation to minimize coughing, straining, and hypertension.

  - Before extubation, the patient's ability to protect his/her airway and the adequacy of respiration should be assessed.

  - Hypertension should be treated to minimize bleeding, prevent brain edema, and hematoma; esmolol, sodium nitroprusside, nitroglycerin, nicardipine, and labetalol are suitable options.

  - A neurologic exam should be performed after the patient is extubated.

Pituitary Tumors

- ICP may be less of a concern if the tumor is small.
- Endocrine function should be assessed preoperatively.
- Supplemental, short-acting corticosteroid therapy may need to be administered perioperatively.

- With the transcranial approach, ICP may be a concern; measures to control ICP intraoperatively should be instituted.
- Hypertension, tachycardia, arrhythmias, and myocardial ischemia may be seen when phenylephrine, lidocaine with epinephrine, and/or cocaine are used to prepare the nares for the transphenoidal approach.
- At the end of transphenoidal surgery, nasal breathing will not be possible due to nasal packing; make sure the patient is fully conscious before extubation.
- Diabetes insipidus frequently occurs after surgery (within first 12 hours) requiring treatment with I.V. fluids and/or vasopressin (titrate dose based on serum/urine sodium and osmolality, fluid balance, urine output).

Intracranial Aneurysms

- Complications of subarachnoid hemorrhage include increased ICP, aneurysm rebleed, vasospasm, and hydrocephalus.
- Thiopental, propofol, opioids, and volatile inhalation agents can be used to induce/maintain anesthesia.
- Lidocaine, esmolol, or labetalol can be used during intubation to reduce the risk of hypertension and rupture of the aneurysm.
- Following induction, $PaCO_2$ should be maintained between 25-35 mm Hg to decrease cerebral blood volume while maintaining oxygen delivery.
- In addition to hyperventilation, osmotic diuresis (ie, mannitol) and CSF drainage may be used to provide a "slack" brain.
- Controlled hypotension may be considered during dissection of the aneurysm.
- Normotension or a slight increase in blood pressure may be employed with temporary "trapping" of the aneurysm.
- EEG or evoked potentials may be used to monitor the safety of temporary arterial occlusion.
- Although mild hypothermia (32°C to 34°C) has been shown to improve the brain's ability to tolerate ischemia in many laboratory studies, the IHAST study demonstrates that it did not improve neurologic outcome in ASA I-II patients with ruptured cerebral aneurysms.
- Treat hyperglycemia because ischemic damage is worse when it occurs with elevated blood glucose levels (>150-180 mg/dL).
- Minimize coughing, straining, hypertension at extubation.
- A neurologic exam should be performed in the operating room.

REFERENCES AND RECOMMENDED READING

Adams HP Jr, del Zoppo G, Alberts MJ, et al, "Guidelines for the Early Management of Adults With Ischemic Stroke: A Guideline From the American Heart Association/American Stroke Association Stroke Council, Clinical Cardiology Council, Cardiovascular Radiology and Intervention Council, and the Atherosclerotic Peripheral Vascular Disease and Quality of Care Outcomes in Research Interdisciplinary Working Groups: The American Academy of Neurology Affirms the Value of This Guideline as an Educational Tool for Neurologists," Stroke, 2007, 38(5):1655-711.

Adams RJ, Albers G, Alberts MJ, et al, "Update to the AHA/ASA Recommendations for the Prevention of Stroke in Patients With Stroke and Transient Ischemic Attack," Stroke, 2008, 39 (5):1647-52.

Albin MS, ed, Textbook of Neuroanesthesia With Neurosurgical and Neuroscience Perspectives, New York, NY: McGraw-Hill, 1997.

Barash PG, Cullen BF, and Stoelting RK, "Neurophysiology and Neuroanesthesia," Handbook of Clinical Anesthesia, 2nd ed, Philadelphia, PA: JB Lippincott, 1993, 256-76.

Bendo AA, Kass IS, Hartung J, et al. "Anesthesia for Neurosurgery," Barash PG, Cullen BF, Stoelting RK, eds, Clinical Anesthesia, 3rd ed, Philadelphia, PA: Lippincott-Raven, 1997, 699-745.

"Beneficial Effect of Carotid Endarterectomy in Symptomatic Patients With High-Grade Carotid Stenosis. North American Symptomatic Carotid Endarterectomy Trial Collaborators," N Engl J Med, 1991, 325(7):445-53.

Cottrell JE and Smith DS, Anesthesia and Neurosurgery, 3rd ed, St Louis, MO: Mosby Co, 1994.

Del Zoppo GJ, Saver JL, Jauch EC, et al, "Expansion of the Time Window for Treatment of Acute Ischemic Stroke With Intravenous Tissue Plasminogen Activator: A Science Advisory From the American Heart Association/American Stroke Association," Stroke, 2009, 40(8):2945-8.

Hacke W, Kaste M, Bluhmki E, et al, "Thrombolysis With Alteplase 3 to 4.5 Hours After Acute Ischemic Stroke," N Engl J Med, 2008, 359(13):1317-29.

Mayberg MR, Wilson SE, Yatsu F, et al, "Carotid Endarterectomy and Prevention of Cerebral Ischemia in Symptomatic Carotid Stenosis. Veterans Affairs Cooperative Studies Program 309 Trialist Group," *JAMA*, 1991, 266(23):3289-94.

Mayer SA, Brun NC, Broderick J, et al, "Recombinant Activated Factor VII for Acute Intracerebral Hemorrhage: US Phase IIA Trial," *Neurocrit Care*, 2006, 4(3):206-14.

"MRC European Carotid Surgery Trial: Interim Results for Symptomatic Patients With Severe (70% to 99%) or With Mild (0% to 29%) Carotid Stenosis. European Carotid Surgery Trialists' Collaborative Group," *Lancet*, 1991, 337(8752):1235-43.

Rozet I, Tontisirin N, Muangman S, et al, "Effect of Equiosmolar Solutions of Mannitol Versus Hypertonic Saline on Intraoperative Brain Relaxation and Electrolyte Balance," *Anesthesiology*, 2007, 107(5):697-704.

"Secondary Prevention in Non-Rheumatic Atrial Fibrillation After Transient Ischaemic Attack or Minor Stroke. EAFT (European Atrial Fibrillation Trial) Study Group," *Lancet*, 1993, 342(8882):1255-62.

Todd MM, Hindman BJ, Clarke WR, et al, "Mild Intraoperative Hypothermia During Surgery for Intracranial Aneurysm," *N Engl J Med*, 2005, 352(2):135-45.

ANESTHESIA FOR GERIATRIC PATIENTS

**"No skill or art is needed to grow old,
but the trick is to endure it." – Goethe**

In 1980, people 65 years of age and older made up 12% of the population in the United States but consumed 30% of the healthcare expenditures. By 2040, the elderly will make up about 25% of the population and account for 50% of healthcare costs. Because at least half will require surgery, understanding physiologic and pathologic changes in the geriatric population is important to reduce perioperative morbidity and mortality.

In 1961, the perioperative mortality rate in geriatric patients approached 20%. Because of increased understanding of the physiology of aging and improved perianesthetic monitoring, the mortality rate decreased to <5% by 1980, although the mortality associated with emergency surgery is 3-10 times greater than when the same surgery is performed on an elective basis. Improvements in preoperative evaluation, intraoperative management, and postoperative treatment have further reduced morbidity and mortality in geriatric patients.

As a general rule, older people have more pre-existing diseases than younger people do. In addition, geriatric patients have significant alterations in anatomy, physiology, pharmacokinetics, pharmacodynamics, recovery ability, and psycho-logical coping mechanisms. The purpose of this chapter is to identify those major changes which necessitate a modification in perioperative practice. A brief review of major organ systems highlights the natural aging process and the common disease processes that compromise the elderly person.

Figure 1: Changes in physiologic function with age in humans expressed as percentage of mean value at age 30 years.

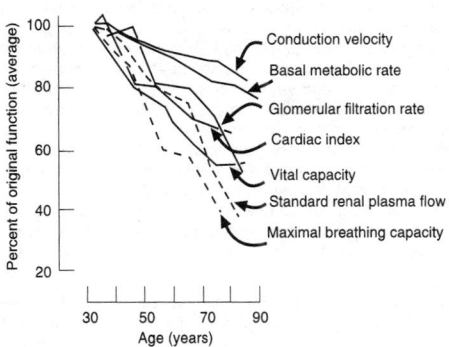

CARDIOVASCULAR SYSTEM

Hypertension and atherosclerotic cardiovascular disease occur in more than half of the elderly. Loss of elasticity in arterial walls increases vascular resistance leading to an increase in systolic blood pressure which, in time, produces left ventricular hypertrophy. With aging, the vascular muscular layer is replaced with fibrous tissue and plaque, which cannot stretch, exaggerating the blood pressure rise during systole and fall during diastole. This widened pulse pressure is a marker of compromised compliance in the vessel wall and is associated with increased risk of coronary events.

A decrease in adrenergic activity leads to a slower resting heart rate, a lower maximal heart rate, and a depressed baroreceptor reflex. These physiologic changes associated with aging impair a person's ability to respond to hypovolemia, hypotension, or hypoxemia by attenuating increases in heart rate and cardiac output. A slow circulation time, frequently found in geriatric patients, prolongs onset of action for I.V. drugs (eg, thiopental, propofol, fentanyl), while speeding the induction of anesthesia using inhalational agents (eg, sevoflurane, isoflurane).

Normal Physiologic Changes	Pathophysiologic Changes
Decreased elasticity	Atherosclerosis
Increased afterload	Coronary artery disease
Increased left ventricular hypertrophy	Hypertension
Increased systolic blood pressure	Congestive heart failure
Decreased diastolic blood pressure	Arrhythmias
Decreased adrenergic activity	
Decreased resting heart rate	
Decreased maximum heart rate	
Decreased baroreceptor reflex	
Slowed circulation time	

The development of atherosclerosis is a pathologic process which produces critical coronary stenosis. Congestive heart failure and myocardial ischemia compromise cardiac function, which influences other organ systems. Onset of arrhythmias reflects disease of the cardiac conduction system, with atrial fibrillation as the most common arrhythmia. Elderly patients frequently take nitrates, beta-blockers, calcium channel blockers, and ACE inhibitors/receptor blockers. Optimization of cardiac function preoperatively, continuing treatment with most chronic cardiac medications, and understanding drug interactions between anesthetics and perioperative medications is important. Knowledge of not only drug action but also physiologic reaction if chronic medications are discontinued is essential. For example, a person receiving beta-blockers following myocardial infarction or for treatment of hypertension may experience rebound hypertension and ventricular arrhythmias with abrupt discontinuation of this medication. The duration of antiplatelet therapy following coronary stenting is not completely understood, with reports of acute thrombosis following discontinuation of the drugs even after one year of administration. Current practice is to use clopidogrel and aspirin for at least 4-6 weeks following placement of bare metal stents and at least 1 year following insertion of drug eluting stents. Some cardiologists recommend life-long dosing of at least aspirin and possibly both drugs. The decision to continue or discontinue these medications may have serious consequences; the risk of operating on patients with concurrent antithrombotic therapy may be deadly.

Hypertension is another common cardiovascular disease. Therapy crosses many drug categories. Knowledge about the specific antihypertensive medications and their interactions with anesthetic drugs (eg, clonidine decreases anesthetic drug requirements and may cause arrhythmias if abruptly withdrawn) is important. Discontinuation of antihypertensive medication can produce preoperative hypertension, with enhanced hemodynamic instability. The decision to continue diuretic therapy preoperatively depends on the patient. Patients prone to congestive heart failure should be maintained on their diuretic therapy, whereas a chronic hypertensive patient receiving a bowel prep for GI surgery does not need additional loss of intravascular volume prior to surgery. Serum potassium may be low in patients taking a thiazide diuretic. This is especially important for people taking digitalis. Anesthesiologists, cardiologists, and intensivists have over the years expressed concern that maintenance of chronic drug therapy (ie, beta-blockers, calcium channel blockers, diuretics, ACE inhibitors, angiotensin receptor blockers [ARBs]) may produce significant hypotension, especially during induction of anesthesia. Current thinking is that maintaining the patient in his optimal state of preoperative hemodynamic control provides the best situation for perianesthetic management, although some anesthesiologists discontinue ACE inhibitors/ARBs and diuretics preoperatively. Recently, anesthesiologists echo cardiologists in suggesting that initiation of perioperative beta-blocker therapy for geriatric patients with cardiovascular disease decreases operative morbidity and mortality. Aging also leads to abnormal response to endothelium-dependent vasodilators (ie, acetylcholine) and decreased production of endothelial-derived vasodilator substances (nitric oxide). A poorly controlled hypertensive patient may have a reduced blood volume and will experience tremendous swings in blood pressure during anesthesia and surgery.

RESPIRATORY SYSTEM

A carefully performed history and physical examination can identify patients whose normal pulmonary aging changes have become a pathophysiologic risk. History of recurrent pulmonary infections, smoking, asthma, COPD, and emphysema place patients at high risk for pulmonary complications. Preoperative optimization of pulmonary function (treat infection, stop smoking, use of bronchodilators) and instruction in the use and importance of incentive spirometry can improve the perioperative pulmonary course. Pulmonary function tests add little to the preoperative evaluation, except for lung resection surgery.

Smoking is a serious problem for geriatric population because they have more years of tobacco exposure and more pulmonary damage. The TORCH trial demonstrated that in patients with a diagnosis of COPD, pulmonary disease caused more deaths than cardiovascular disease. Cessation of smoking the day before surgery does two things: a) decreases the level of carbon monoxide in the blood and therefore enhances oxygen carrying capacity, and b) increases bronchial reactivity to stimuli due to the acute withdrawal of nicotine. To improve pulmonary function, the patient must stop smoking at least 6 weeks before surgery. Anatomic and physiologic damage are not reversed; however, the rate of continuing organ dysfunction is reduced to reflect the normal aging process. Supplemental oxygen may be needed in the immediate postoperative period.

Normal Physiologic Changes	Pathophysiologic Changes
Decreased pulmonary elasticity	Emphysema
Decreased alveolar surface and FEV	Chronic bronchitis
Increased V_d, RV, FRC	Pneumonia
Increased closing capacity	Lung cancer
V/Q mismatching	Tuberculosis
Decreased PaO_2	
Increased chest wall rigidity	
Decreased cough	
Blunted response to hypercapnia/hypoxia	
Progressive kyphosis/scoliosis	
Decreased total lung capacity	

Reduction in elastic recoil of the lung and chest wall, in addition to a decrease in pulmonary blood flow, leads to changes in ventilation:perfusion ratio. Dead space (V_d) increases and small airway collapse occurs during tidal volume ventilation, resulting in decreased gas exchange. This leads to an increase in the alveolar/arterial oxygen gradient and a decrease in arterial oxygen tension. Residual volume (RV) and functional residual capacity (FRC) increase as lung elasticity decreases with a concomitant decrease in forced expiratory volume (FEV). A "rule of thumb" for the normal deterioration of pulmonary function to predict expected change in arterial oxygenation while breathing room air is:

PaO_2 (expected) = 100 - (age/4) **or** PaO_2 decreases 0.35 mm Hg per year

◀ CENTRAL NERVOUS SYSTEM

With aging, there is a progressive decrease in cerebral cortical mass and an increase in brain sensitivity to anesthetic agents. The MAC of inhalational anesthetics decreases 40% to 60% by 80 years of age. This occurs not only with inhalational anesthetic gases, but also with intravenous, intrathecal, and epidural drugs. For example, the induction dose of sodium thiopental decreases from 5 mg/kg to 2 mg/kg in the 70 year old patient.

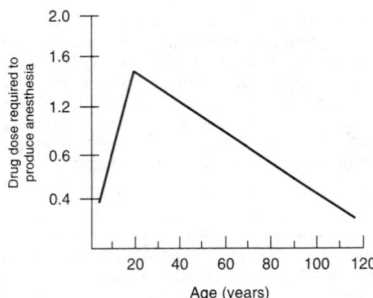

Figure 2: Refers to inhalation, intravenous, and spinal/epidural anesthetic doses

Therefore, it is easy to overdose elderly patients who do not have reserve capacity to overcome the profound side effects of "normal" anesthetic doses. The duration of anesthetics is also prolonged, slowing recovery and increasing postoperative confusion, often for days.

Approximately 60% of old patients experience postoperative delirium (POD) following surgery while some experience postoperative cognitive decline (POCD) and may never return to their preoperative state. POD may be related to inadequate sleep and pain control following surgery. POCD occurs most commonly following cardiac surgery (10% to 65%), but also appears after other operations (25% at one week, decreasing to 10% at 3 months). Risk factors appear to include advanced age, preexisting cognitive impairment, alcohol abuse, and severity of coexisting diseases. It is felt that the activation of a proinflammatory cytokine response (IL-1beta, TNF-alpha) may be a primary factor in the development of POCD.

Normal Physiologic Changes	Pathophysiologic Changes
Decreased cerebral cortex volume	Stroke
Decreased cerebral blood flow (CBF)	Dementia
Decreased cerebral metabolic rate (CMR O_2)	Alzheimer's disease
POCD	Memory impairment
POD	

The blood pressure of patients with cerebrovascular disease should be maintained in the patient's normal range during and after surgery. The head should be maintained in the neutral position to prevent occlusion of the carotid or vertebral circulation. Patients with Parkinsonism should continue taking levodopa up to the time of surgery. Drugs with antidopaminergic effects are to be avoided (ie, phenothiazines, butyrophenones). Surgery for patients with recent stroke should be delayed at least 6 weeks to allow for restabilization of the blood-brain barrier and resumption of cerebral autoregulation.

ENDOCRINE SYSTEM

Normal Physiologic Changes	Pathophysiologic Changes
Decreased insulin secretion	Obesity
Increased insulin resistance	Type 2 diabetes mellitus
Decreased thyroid function	Poor wound healing
	Decreased leukocyte function

Adult onset diabetes is a common geriatric disease. It affects approximately 35 million people in the United States and is predicted to increase 200% over the next several decades. The severity of the disease and success of glucose management predict end-organ damage. Historically, tight glucose control, the medical management goal for diabetes, was relaxed in the perioperative period. However, recently there is evidence that tight glucose control in the perioperative and ICU periods improves outcome. These studies show a striking increase in cardiovascular risk with even a mild increase in blood glucose concentration. Whether tight glucose control to <110 mg/dL is also important for outpatient or non-ICU surgical patients is not known. It is well known that hyperglycemia decreases wound healing and increases infection. Hyperglycemia will also increase the amount of cerebral injury should ischemia occur; however, hypoglycemia can cause cerebral and myocardial ischemia and death.

For the insulin-controlled diabetic, there is no ideal preoperative management protocol. Therapy ranges from withholding all insulin preoperatively vs administering a fraction of the usual dose vs initiation of a continuous dextrose/insulin infusion. Surgery is stressful and blood glucose increases. Without insulin an osmotic glucose diuresis can occur, producing dehydration. Some clinicians feel that the administration of exogenous insulin improves patient outcome by providing the body with a source of energy during this time of stress. The critical aspect of any management regimen is the frequent evaluation of blood glucose levels and appropriate treatment of hyper- or hypoglycemia.

UROLOGIC SYSTEM

Aging decreases renal function as reflected by a reduction in glomerular filtration rate and creatinine clearance. An increase in serum creatinine may not be evident on laboratory tests because total body muscle mass and creatinine production decrease with aging. However, BUN increases on an average of 0.2 mg/dL/year. Decreased ability to concentrate/dilute urine puts the geriatric patient at risk for dehydration/fluid overload. The patient's capacity to metabolize and excrete drugs is also affected.

Normal Physiologic Changes	Pathophysiologic Changes
Decreased renal blood flow	Diabetic nephropathy
Decreased kidney mass	Hypertensive nephropathy
Decreased tubular function	Prostatic enlargement

Elderly males with benign prostatic hypertrophy may experience bladder distention with loss of detrusor muscle tone leading to urinary retention. This can occur with general anesthesia, but is more common with spinal/epidural anesthesia. Neuraxial anesthesia decreases detrusor tone while increasing sphincter tone. Because neuraxial anesthesia produces a sympathectomy and a decrease in blood pressure, fluid administration to maintain normal blood pressure frequently complicates the situation by overdistending the urinary bladder.

Renal blood flow decreases with aging, with a 50% reduction by age 75. This places the geriatric patient at greater risk for perioperative renal damage/failure. Hypotension during anesthesia can further decrease renal perfusion, which can lead to additional renal damage. Maintenance of 0.5 mL/kg/hour urine output is recommended. A decrease in renal blood flow reduces clearance of many drugs, which can prolong drug action and may necessitate a reduction in drug dosage and/or frequency of administration.

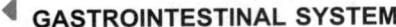

GASTROINTESTINAL SYSTEM

Hepatic blood flow decreases with age, as does hepatic protein synthesis and drug metabolism. Gastric emptying also slows, slowing absorption of orally administered drugs. Many drugs are highly protein bound, therefore a decrease in albumin concentration significantly increases the amount of free drug. Because many drugs are metabolized by the liver, clearance can be decreased. See Pharmacokinetic/ Pharmacodynamic section.

MUSCULOSKELETAL SYSTEM

Normal Physiologic Changes	Pathophysiologic Changes
Decreased muscle mass	Weakness
Decreased joint mobility	Arthritis
Decreased dentition	Airway management problems
Increased osteoporosis	Bone fractures

Changes in the musculoskeletal system pose significant problems in positioning elderly patients. Alterations in skin elasticity and perfusion put patients at risk for ischemic ulcers at pressure points. Restricted joint mobility compounds this problem.

Many geriatric patients are edentulous, which facilitates intubation; however, many others have poor dentition or only a few teeth left, which are critical in supporting their dental bridges. Poor dentition increases the risk of dental trauma. Loss of mandibular bone contour can complicate adequate mask fit, making positive pressure ventilation difficult. Cervical arthritis and temporomandibular problems are not uncommon, as are gastroesophageal reflux and hiatal hernia, which put the patient at risk for inadequate ventilation or aspiration.

Osteoporosis reduces bone density and produces skeletal fragility, especially in postmenopausal women (40% in white females). Hormone replacement therapy in addition to calcium, vitamin D, and exercise, lowers the likelihood of osteoporotic fractures by at least 25%. Estrogen blocks bone resorption by inhibiting cytokine signals necessary for recruitment of bone-resorbing osteoclasts, but has been associated with increased cardiovascular adverse events. Drug therapy (ie, alendronate) also interferes with bone resorption.

The initial dose of muscle relaxant drugs is unchanged, but elderly patients require a decrease in frequency of redosing (due to prolonged elimination). The exceptions to this general rule are drugs that are metabolized in the blood by Hoffman elimination or nonspecific esterases (atracurium, mivacurium, and cisatracurium).

HYPOTHERMIA

Geriatric patients experience more intraoperative hypothermia than younger patients do. The consequences of this include prolonged awakening, slower drug elimination, increased shivering, enhanced coagulation, and increased postoperative metabolic demand associated with increased catabolism. Oxygen demand is increased, and if pulmonary and cardiovascular systems are unable to handle this increased workload, the potential for myocardial ischemia increases. Myocardial oxygen consumption can increase up to 500% with postoperative shivering. Maintenance of intraoperative temperature has been associated with significantly improved wound healing, duration of hospital stay, and perioperative cardiac events. Early implementation of heat conserving measures (eg, forced air systems, warming the operation room) blunts intraoperative hypothermia.

PHARMACOKINETICS / PHARMACODYNAMICS

Figure 3: Example of effect of advancing
age on half-life (diazepam)

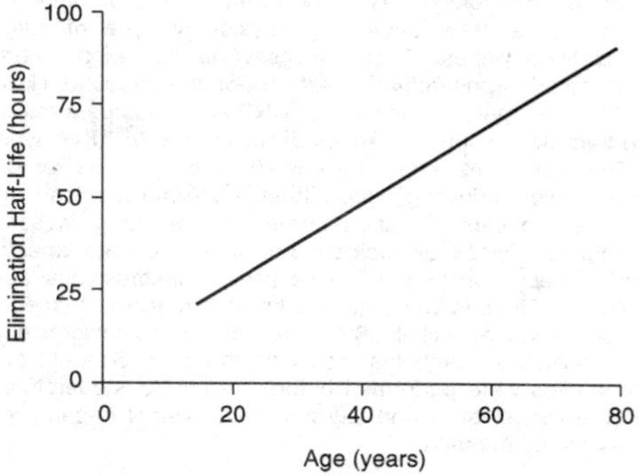

Gastrointestinal absorption of orally administered drugs is affected by aging. There are changes in gastric acidity, intestinal motility, and intestinal perfusion. Once a drug is absorbed, its pharmacologic action is altered by an age-related reduction of ~15% of total body water and by an increase of 50% to 100% of body fat concentration. Redistribution of drugs from the vessel-rich group is slowed, especially for highly lipid soluble drugs. Decreased hepatic perfusion and drug metabolism by liver microsomal enzymes combined with a reduced renal excretion of drug and/or metabolites can lead to an increased and prolonged drug effect. A decreased number of receptors leads to receptor saturation at substantially lower serum concentration. A decrease in both the amount of plasma protein (10% to 20% decrease in albumin) and the quality of drug-protein binding leads to an increase in free fraction of the drug.

Drug Dosing Adjustments in the Elderly

Drug	Action	Mechanism
Inhalational anesthetics	Decrease dose 40%	↑ sensitivity
I.V. induction drugs[1]	Decrease dose 50%	↑ sensitivity, ↓ clearance/half-life
Antibiotics		
Initial dose	No change	
Repeat doses	Decrease frequency	↓ clearance, ↑ half-life
Muscle relaxants[2]		
Initial bolus	No change	
Repeat bolus	Decrease frequency	↓ clearance, ↑ half-life
Infusion	Decrease dose	↓ clearance, ↑ half-life
Narcotics[3]		
Initial bolus	Decrease dose 50%	↑ sensitivity
Infusion	Decrease dose 30%	↓ clearance, ↑ half-life

[1]Sodium thiopental, propofol, midazolam, etomidate, methohexital.

[2]This does not include muscle relaxants that are metabolized by Hoffman elimination.

[3]This does not include remifentanil.

◀ # TYPE OF ANESTHESIA: GENERAL vs REGIONAL

The debate between regional vs general anesthesia continues to be a topic for discussion, for no single anesthetic technique has been shown to be better for either the young or the geriatric patient. The type of anesthesia depends on the patient, concurrent medical diseases, underlying physiology, type of surgery, and the patient's expectations/wishes. There are several surgeries where the above statement is debated: transurethral resection of the prostate (TURP), cataract extraction, and knee surgery. Traditionally, TURP surgery is performed with regional anesthesia so that mental status changes associated with TURP syndrome can be elicited early. This may be less important when 0.9 normal saline, rather than glycine, is used as the surgical irrigating fluid; although volume overload and pulmonary edema are still of concern. Cataract surgery is minimally invasive, with local ophthalmic analgesia (block or topical) providing adequate anesthesia for the procedure and thereby avoiding the physiologic transgressions associated with general anesthesia. Patients with hip and knee surgery performed with regional anesthesia experienced an initial 50% reduction in the incidence of deep vein thrombosis and pulmonary embolus; however, the 3- to 6-month outcomes were similar. These studies were performed before the intra/postoperative use of lower extremity compression sleeves and low molecular weight heparin. A modern day comparison has not been made.

Postoperative mental changes attributed to general anesthesia are not uncommon in the elderly; however, the use of heavy sedation during regional or local anesthesia can also produce a similar prolonged alteration of mental status. The incidence of postoperative cognitive decline (POCD) increases with advanced age. Recent studies suggest that long tern postoperative morbidity and mortality is associated with (1) extent of comorbidities, (2) duration of intraoperative hypotension, and (3) duration of deep general anesthesia. Drug metabolism and elimination are slowed, producing prolonged sedative effects. It has been proposed that outpatient surgery may disrupt daily habits less and the elderly may actually return to normal faster when in a familiar environment.

END OF LIFE ISSUES

Many geriatric patients have developed end of life plans which may include a DNR or Advanced Directive document. In the past, it was assumed that the DNR was automatically suspended when the patient came to the operating room, but this is no longer the case. Many of these documents prohibit activities that anesthesiologists routinely perform such as endotracheal intubation and use of pressor drugs to treat hypotension. Therefore the anesthesiologist needs to discuss with the patient and/or the family the importance of rescinding the DNR status or portions of it prior to surgery. This discussion needs to be documented in the patient's chart. If this is not done the anesthesiologist may be guilty of battery.

EDUCATION FOR GERIATRIC ANESTHESIA

The Anesthesiology Residency Review Committee has mandated that each program provide didactic instruction and clinical experience in managing the geriatric surgical population. The Society for the Advancement of Geriatric Anesthesia (SAGA, www.sagahq.org) was established in 2000 to improve the care of the older person having surgery. There is a joint project between the ASA Committee on Geriatric Anesthesiology (www.ASAhq.org/clinical/geriatrics/syllabus.htm), SAGA, and the American Geriatrics Society (AGS, www.americangeriatrics.org) to develop a curriculum for geriatric anesthesia education. These educational materials can be accessed via the internet.

SUMMARY

The aging process is a progressive alteration of normal physiology over time. This deterioration can significantly alter the patient's response to anesthetics and perioperative medications. Frequently, coexistent with this progressive depression of organ function are superimposed disease processes, which further impair organ function. Geriatric patients present a significant challenge to the physician.

REFERENCES AND RECOMMENDED READING

Calverley PM, Anderson JA, Celli B, et al, "Salmeterol and Fluticasone Propionate and Survival in Chronic Obstructive Pulmonary Disease," *N Engl J Med*, 2007, 356(8):775-89.

Frank SM, Fleisher LA, Breslow MJ, et al, "Perioperative Maintenance of Normothermia Reduces the Incidence of Morbid Cardiac Events. A Randomized Clinical Trial," *JAMA*, 1997, 277(14):1127-34.

Ganai S, Lee KF, Merrill A, et al, "Adverse Outcomes of Geriatric Patients Undergoing Abdominal Surgery Who Are at High Risk for Delirium," *Arch Surg*, 2007, 142(11):1072-8.

Gottlieb SS, McCarter RJ, and Vogel RA, "Effect of Beta-Blockade on Mortality Among High-Risk and Low-Risk Patients After Myocardial Infarction," *N Engl J Med*, 1998, 339(8):489-97.

Gu W, Pagel PS, Warltier DC, et al, "Modifying Cardiovascular Risk in Diabetes Mellitus," *Anesthesiology*, 2003, 98(3):774-9.

Hudetz JA, Iqbal Z, Gandhi SD, et al, "Postoperative Cognitive Dysfunction in Older Patients With a History of Alcohol Abuse," *Anesthesiology*, 2007, 106(3):423-30.

Jin F and Chung F, "Minimizing Perioperative Adverse Events in the Elderly," *Br J Anaesth*, 2001, 87 (4):608-24.

Kurz A, Sessler DI, and Lenhardt R, "Perioperative Normothermia to Reduce the Incidence of Surgical-Wound Infection and Shorten Hospitalization. Study of Wound Infection and Temperature Group," *N Engl J Med*, 1996, 334(19):1209-15.

Modig J, Borg T, Karlstrom G, et al, "Thromboembolism After Total Hip Replacement: Role of Epidural and General Anesthesia," *Anesth Analg*, 1983, 62(2):174-80.

Moller JT, Cluitmans P, Rasmussen LS, et al, "Long-Term Postoperative Cognitive "Dysfunction in the Elderly ISPOCD1 Study. ISPOCD Investigators. International Study of Post-Operative Cognitive Dysfunction," *Lancet*, 1998, 351(9106):857-61.

Monk TG, Saini V, Weldon BC, et al, "Anesthetic Management and One-Year Mortality After Noncardiac Surgery," *Anesth Analg*, 2005, 100(1):4-10.

Muravchick S, ed, *Geroanesthesia: Principles for Managment of the Elderly Patient*, St. Louis, MO: Mosby, 1997.

Newman S, Stygall J, Hirani S, et al, "Postoperative Cognitive Dysfunction After Noncardiac Surgery: A Systematic Review," *Anesthesiology*, 2007, 106(3):572-90.

Pittas AG, Siegel RD, and Lau J, "Insulin Therapy for Critically Ill Hospitalized Patients: A Meta-Analysis of Randomized Controlled Trials," *Arch Intern Med*, 2004, 164(18):2005-11.

Priebe HJ, "The Aged Cardiovascular Risk Patient," *Br J Anaesth*, 2000, 85(5):763-78.

Rivera R and Antognini JF, "Perioperative Drug Therapy in Elderly Patients," *Anesthesiology*, 2009, 110(5):1176-81.

Sessler DI, "Mild Perioperative Hypothermia," *N Engl J Med*, 1997, 336(24):1730-7.

Sieber F, *Geriatric Anesthesia*, McGraw-Hill Companies: New York, NY, 2007.

Silverstein JH, *Geriatric Anesthesiology*, 2nd ed, Springer: New York, NY, 2008.

Tuman KJ, McCarthy RJ, March RJ, et al, "Effects of Epidural Anesthesia and Analgesia on Coagulation and Outcome After Major Vascular Surgery," *Anesth Analg*, 1991, 73(6):696-704.

Wallace A, Layug B, Tateo I, et al, "Prophylactic Atenolol Reduces Postoperative Myocardial Ischemia. McSPI Research Group," *Anesthesiology*, 1998, 88(1):7-17

Wan Y, Xu J, Ma D, et al, "Postoperative Impairment of Cognitive Function in Rats: A Possible Role for Cytokine-Mediated Inflammation in the Hippocampus," *Anesthesiology*, 2007, 106(3):436-43.

ANESTHESIA FOR OBSTETRIC PATIENTS IN NONOBSTETRIC SURGERY

Every year 0.75% to 2% of pregnant women undergo a nonobstetric surgical procedure. The major indications for these approximately 75,000 anesthetics are trauma, ovarian cysts, appendicitis, breast tumors, and cervical incompetence. More serious procedures such as cardiac surgery and cerebral aneurysm clipping are not uncommon. Because of the advances in treating complex medical problems, the number of women dying from diseases exacerbated by pregnancy (ie, cardiac diseases and psychiatric problems) exceed those directly caused by pregnancy (ie, thromboembolism). Cardiomyopathy, myocardial infarction, aortic dissection, and pulmonary hypertension are leading causes of mortality in the pregnant patient. These patients need to be treated by a multidisciplinary team of physicians.

Preoperative, intraoperative, and postoperative care of the pregnant patient is unique because the physician must be concerned about two patients (the mother and the fetus), each with its own special needs. The physician must take into account the normal physiologic changes of pregnancy, and the possibility of pregnancy-related disease (eg, pre-eclampsia, HELLP, gestational hypertension, gestational diabetes). Two additional major concerns that must continually be attended to during nonobstetric surgery are the maintenance of uterine perfusion and the prevention of premature labor. In order to understand the importance of these factors, a brief review of the physiologic changes of pregnancy is required.

PHYSIOLOGY OF PREGNANCY

Cardiovascular

Intravascular volume and cardiac output begin to increase during the first trimester and become 30% to 40% above the nonpregnant state by 28 weeks gestational age. Despite this increase in intravascular volume, the mother and fetus are at risk for hypotension which is caused by the gravid uterus compressing the aorta and/or inferior vena cava. This significantly reduces venous return and is called the supine hypotension syndrome. It occurs starting at 18-20 weeks gestation. The reduction in venous return may or may not be evident as maternal hypotension and puts the fetus at substantial risk of inadequate uteroplacental perfusion even in the asymptomatic mother. The most effective therapy is uterine displacement (ie, lateral position or displace the uterus to the left manually or with a wedge under the right hip). Correct positioning of the pregnant woman is critically important in maintaining adequate uterine blood flow.

Pregnant women are anemic despite a 35% increase in red blood cell mass. This happens because plasma volume, and therefore total blood volume, increases by 50% to 55%, producing a condition called physiologic anemia of pregnancy. Leukocytosis is also present in pregnant women, making the diagnosis of infection more difficult.

Respiratory

During pregnancy, the female experiences a 20% decrease in functional residual capacity concurrent with a 60% increase in oxygen consumption. This places the pregnant female and her infant at risk for hypoxia. Minute ventilation normally increases 50%, with most of this due to an increase in tidal volume. Closing volume (the lung volume at which airways collapse) moves from functional residual capacity into tidal volume ventilation in 30% of parturients, further increasing the risk of hypoxia. Mild hyperventilation reduces $PaCO_2$ by 10 mm Hg with a compensatory decrease in bicarbonate, maintaining a normal pH; therefore, mechanical ventilation with a $PaCO_2$ of 40 mm Hg will produce respiratory acidosis. Positive pressure ventilation can decrease uterine blood flow 25% by reducing venous return. Therefore adequacy of uterine perfusion needs to be evaluated in pregnant women who are mechanically ventilated by monitoring fetal heart tones (eg, looking for loss of beat-to-beat variability, decelerations, fetal bradycardia).

Capillary engorgement increases the possibility of bleeding with the use of oral and nasal airways. The probability of a difficult intubation increases 8-fold during pregnancy; therefore, a smaller size endotracheal tube (6 or 6.5) should be used. Nasal intubations and nasogastric tubes should be avoided if possible.

Gastrointestinal

Pregnant women are at risk for aspiration after the first trimester because of increased gastric volume. Gastric emptying is similar in pregnant and nonpregnant patients. It is delayed only during labor, largely because of administration of narcotics. Pregnant patients are at risk for aspiration because of elevation of the stomach and rotation on its axis to the right by the gravid uterus. This leads to incompetence of the lower esophageal sphincter. Up to 80% of pregnant patients experience heartburn.

Use of an oral nonparticulate antacid (ie, sodium citrate, 30 mL) is recommended immediately prior to induction of general anesthesia. Histamine-2 receptor blocker (ie, cimetidine 300 mg I.V.; ranitidine 50 mg I.V.) should be given 60-90 minutes prior to induction of general anesthesia to decrease acid production. Metoclopramide (10 mg I.V.) is given to enhance gastric emptying. Intubation should be performed by rapid sequence with cricoid pressure to prevent regurgitation and aspiration.

Renal

Because pregnant females experience an increase in glomerular filtration rate (GFR), their blood urea nitrogen (BUN) and creatinine (Cr) levels are decreased. Therefore, a pregnant woman with high-normal values may have renal insufficiency.

Coagulation

Pregnant women are hypercoagulable with an increase in factors V, VII, VIII, IX, X, XII, and fibrinogen and a decrease in factor XI, XIII, and antithrombin III. Platelet turnover is also increased. They are at risk for deep vein thrombosis (DVT) and pulmonary embolism which accounts for 25% of maternal deaths in the United States annually.

Neurology

Pregnant women have an increased sensitivity to anesthetic agents and other sedative/hypnotic/analgesic drugs because of increased levels of endorphins. Minimum alveolar concentration (MAC) for inhalational anesthetics is decreased 40% and the dose of spinal/epidural drugs may need to be decreased by a similar amount because of engorgement of epidural veins. It is also thought that the elevated level of circulating progesterone increases neuronal sensitivity (both central and peripheral) to anesthetic/analgesic drugs.

The ability of anesthetics to affect central nervous system development is currently not only an exciting research topic but also a concern for practicing anesthesiologists. Laboratory studies using various models (rats, mice, monkeys, cell cultures) and anesthetic drugs/doses (ketamine, nitrous oxide, isoflurane – alone or in combination) have demonstrated enhanced neuronal apoptosis. Whether this is true in humans remains to be determined. It is difficult to translate these data to the human condition because brain developmental stages occur at different times in the various models. The current recommendation is to avoid surgery in the pregnant patient if at all possible.

TERATOGENICITY

The incidence of both major and minor anatomic birth defects ranges as high as 7% to 10%. Drug exposure accounts for 2% to 3% and genetic abnormalities for 25% of birth defects, while the etiology for the rest remains unknown. The fetus is most vulnerable to teratogenic drug effects from 2-13 weeks gestational age, when organogenesis is occurring. Unfortunately, many women do not know that they are pregnant during this period.

◀ Drugs are routinely tested in animal teratologic studies; however, there are many examples where extensive animal testing does not correlate with human results. For example, thalidomide was tested in both rats and mice and was not found to be teratogenic; however, the teratogenic effects in the human fetus are profound, especially since no signs of toxicity are present in the mother. Conversely, drugs that are teratogenic in certain animal models, such as steroid therapy, have not exhibited any significant effect on the human fetus. A general statement is that most drugs, at some dose, can be teratogenic in some animal model but few drugs have a proven, clinically significant, teratogenic potential. See FDA Pregnancy Categories on page 15.

Possible Teratogens

Alcohol: This teratogen produces fetal alcohol syndrome with an incidence of 2/1000 live births, which is probably an underestimate of the real number. There is a twofold increase in spontaneous abortion, which increases to 5% with heavy alcohol consumption. Gestational alcohol consumption is a leading cause of mental retardation, which exceeds that found with Down syndrome and cerebral palsy. Hyperactivity, speech, language, and hearing difficulties, microcephaly, and abnormal brain development are also common.

Anesthetics: Although there is great concern that anesthetic agents may injure the developing fetus, there is little solid evidence for this. Nitrous oxide inhibits methionine synthetase activity which is involved in thymidine production and subsequent DNA synthesis and cell division. However, recent human studies have shown no effect on fetal outcome. Despite these negative studies, it is still wise to postpone surgery or unnecessary drug therapy until after delivery if possible.

Anticonvulsants: The risk of birth defects increases to 7% in women taking antiepileptic drugs during pregnancy (vs 2% to 3% in controls). The incidence increases in mothers taking higher doses and/or multiple antiseizure drugs. The epoxide metabolites of these drugs appear to produce the fetal abnormalities; however, discontinuation of antiseizure drugs may also be dangerous if the fetus is exposed to hypoxia due to maternal seizures.

Benzodiazepines: Retrospective studies from the 1970s showed an increased incidence of cleft lip and palate in infants of mothers who were using benzodiazepines during pregnancy. However, recent epidemiologic studies have been unable to demonstrate this association.

Caffeine: There is no convincing data that caffeine is teratogenic in humans.

Cocaine: Cocaine and heroin exposure of both the mother and the father is associated with fetal microcephaly and other neurologic abnormalities.

Hyperglycemia: Diabetic mothers have a 4% to 12% incidence of major congenital anomalies, which can be significantly reduced to 1.2% when blood glucose levels are tightly controlled during pregnancy.

Marijuana: The placenta acts as a barrier to fetal marijuana exposure. Several studies have demonstrated maternal blood levels of marijuana with nondetectable drug concentration in the cord blood. Cannabinoids are also nonteratogenic in animals.

Retinoids (tretinoin, isotretinoin, etretinate): These drugs are used to treat acne, gram-negative folliculitis, hidradenitis suppurativa, and psoriasis. Teratogenic effects include CNS, cardiac, thymus, craniofacial abnormalities, and spontaneous abortion. Birth control must be practiced when using this class of drugs.

Tobacco: Cigarette smoking during pregnancy is associated with growth retardation. Reports of anencephaly, congenital heart defects, and orofacial clefts have not been confirmed.

Warfarin: Because of its small molecular weight, warfarin easily crosses the placenta. Administration between the 6th and 9th weeks of pregnancy can produce the warfarin embryopathy syndrome which consists of nasal hypoplasia, stippling of uncalcified epiphysis, shortened fingers with nail hypoplasia, low birth weight, and mental retardation in 13% of exposed fetuses.

GESTATIONAL PHARMACOKINETICS AND PHARMACODYNAMICS

Drugs cross the placenta by simple diffusion. Lipid soluble drugs with low molecular weight (ie, fentanyl, thiopental, isoflurane) cross easily while highly polar water soluble drugs (ie, succinylcholine, nondepolarizing-neuromuscular blocking agents, neostigmine, insulin) do not readily cross the placenta. Because fetal pH is lower than maternal pH, the ionized fraction of weak bases (ie, narcotics, local anesthetics) is higher in the fetus than in the mother. This is called "ion trapping." Ion trapping increases total fetal drug level, which will prolong clearance of the drug from the fetus. Ion trapping has been connected with lidocaine (a weak base) and fetal acidosis, leading to "floppy baby syndrome."

PRINCIPLES OF SURGICAL MANAGEMENT

1. The most important thing is to notify your hospital obstetrician about the case before starting it.
2. Postpone surgery until the second trimester or delay until after delivery, if possible.
3. Use a nonparticulate antacid preoperatively.
4. Maintain maternal oxygenation and blood pressure.
5. Document fetal heart tones before and after surgery.
6. Monitor for uterine contraction and fetal heart rate intraoperatively, if possible, when the gestational age is >24 weeks or institutional determined age of viability. Intraoperative monitoring is frequently not done when gestational age is <24 weeks (age of nonviability).
7. Use left uterine displacement during the entire perioperative period.
8. Consider the use of prophylactic tocolytic agents (note that inhalational anesthetic gases are tocolytics)
9. Nonsteroidal anti-inflammatory drugs should not be used after 32 weeks gestational age because of the concern that the ductus arteriosus may close.
10. Based on gestational age, the obstetrician may give betamethasone prior to surgery to promote fetal lung maturity in case of premature delivery.

The reason to monitor fetal heart tones and uterine contractions is to provide the physician with the opportunity to prevent/treat fetal hypoxia and early delivery. Monitoring fetal heart rate will allow the physician to optimize the fetal environment by augmenting oxygen delivery if fetal bradycardia or loss of heart rate variability occurs. Because most anesthetic drugs depress fetal beat-to-beat variability, this monitor of fetal well-being cannot be relied upon during and following surgery until the drug is cleared from the fetus.

Taking care of the pregnant patient for nonobstetric surgery requires recognition of the physiologic changes that accompany pregnancy and the need to treat two patients – the mother and the baby.

Physiologic Changes of Pregnancy

Cardiovascular	Increased cardiac output 50% Increased red blood cell mass 35% Increased plasma volume 55% Increased total blood volume 50% Physiologic anemia of pregnancy (Hgb ~10 mg/dL) Decreased systemic vascular resistance 20%
Pulmonary	Decreased functional reserve capacity (FRC) 20% Increased oxygen consumption (VO_2) 60% Increased minute ventilation (MV) 50% Increased respiratory rate (RR) 10% Increased tidal volume (V_T) 40% Decreased $PaCO_2$ by 10 mm Hg
Gastrointestinal	Increased gastric volume Decreased gastric pH Incompetent lower esophageal sphincter
Renal	Increased glomerular filtration rate (GFR) Decreased blood urea nitrogen (BUN) Decreased creatinine (Cr)
Coagulation	Increased factors V, VII, VIII, X, XII Increased fibrinogen Decreased factor XI, XIII, and antithrombin III Increased platelet turnover
Neurology	Decreased anesthesia/analgesia drug requirements (35% to 40%) Increased circulating endorphins

REFERENCES AND RECOMMENDED READING

Brodsky JB, Cohen EN, Brown BW Jr, et al, "Surgery During Pregnancy and Fetal Outcome," *Am J Obstet Gynecol*, 1980, 138(8):1165-7.

Bucklin BA, "Gerard W. Ostheimer - What's New in Obstetric Anesthesia − Lecture," Anesthesiology, 2006, 104(4):865-71.

Cohen EN, Bellville JW, and Brown BW Jr, "Anesthesia, Pregnancy, and Miscarriage: A Study of Operating Room Nurses and Anesthetists," *Anesthesiology*, 1971, 35(4):343-7.

Dewan DM and Hood DD, eds, "Anesthesia for Non-Birth Related Surgery During Pregnancy," *Practical Obstetric Anesthesia*, 1st ed, Chapter 20, Philadelphia, PA: WB Saunders Company, 1997, 309-20.

Kaneko M, Saito Y, Kirihara Y, et al, "Pregnancy Enhances the Antinociceptive Effects of Extradural Lignocaine in the Rat," *Br J Anaesth*, 1994, 72(6):657-61.

Lewis G, *Why Mothers Die 2000-2002: The Sixth Report of Confidential Enquiries into Maternal Deaths in the United Kingdom*, London, United Kingdom: RCOG Press, 2004.

Liu PL, Warren TM, Ostheimer GW, et al, "Foetal Monitoring in Parturients Undergoing Surgery Unrelated to Pregnancy," *Can Anaesth Soc J*, 1985, 32(5):525-32.

Mazze RI and Kallen B, "Reproductive Outcome After Anesthesia and Operation During Pregnancy: A Register Study of 5405 Cases," *Am J Obstet Gynecol*, 1989, 161(5):1178-85.

Medina VM, Dawson-Basoa ME, and Gintzler AR, "17 Beta-Estradiol and Progesterone Positively Modulate Spinal Cord Dynorphin: Relevance to the Analgesia of Pregnancy," *Neuroendocrinology*, 1993, 58(3):310-5.

Naughton NN and Cohen S, "Nonobstetric Surgery During Pregnancy," *Obstetric Anesthesia: Principles and Practice*, 3rd ed, Chapter 16, Chestnut DH, ed, Philadelphia, PA: Mosby, 2004, 255-74.

Niebyl JR, ed, *Drug Use in Pregnancy*, Philadelphia, PA; Lea & Febiger, 1988.

Palahniuk FJ, Schnider SM, and Eger EI 2nd, "Pregnancy Decreases the Requirement for Inhaled Anesthetic Agents," *Anesthesiology*, 1974, 41(1):82-3.

Pedersen H and Finster M, "Anesthetic Risk in the Pregnant Surgical Patient," *Anesthesiology*, 1979, 51(5):439-51.

Ray P, Murphy GJ, and Shutt LE, "Recognition and Management of Maternal Cardiac Disease in Pregnancy," *Br J Anaesth*, 2004, 93(3):428-39.

Rosenberg L, Mitchell AA, Parsells JL, et al, "Lack of Relation of Oral Clefts to Diazepam Use During Pregnancy," *N Engl J Med*, 1983, 309(21):1282-5.

ANESTHESIA FOR PATIENTS WITH LIVER DISEASE

Patients with liver disease pose a significant problem to the perioperative physician. Although the prevalence of clinically significant unsuspected liver disease is 1%, abnormal liver function tests may occur in 33% of screened patients. Additionally, the number of patients with hepatic injury coming for elective/nonelective surgery is increasing, in part due to the success of liver transplantation. All patients with liver disease are at greater risk undergoing anesthesia and surgery.

The liver is the largest gland in the body, receiving 25% of the cardiac output. While the hepatic artery supplies 25% of the blood flow (and 45% to 50% of the hepatic oxygen supply), the portal vein provides 75% of the blood flow (but only 50% of the oxygen delivery). This unique blood flow circuitry puts the liver at risk for ischemia since half of its oxygen supply is provided by venous blood. Oxygen delivery to this essential organ can be decreased by either an increase in oxygen extraction (reducing portal vein oxygen concentration) or a decrease in arterial blood pressure resulting in a decrease in hepatic artery blood flow.

FUNCTIONS OF THE LIVER

Glucose homeostasis
  Glycogen storage
  Gluconeogenesis
Fat metabolism (beta oxidation)
Protein synthesis
  Albumin, gamma globulin, alpha$_1$-glycoprotein
  Drug binding
  Coagulation factors
  Hydrolysis of ester linkage
Drug and hormone metabolism
Bilirubin formation and excretion
Phagocytize bacteria

PATHOPHYSIOLOGY OF LIVER INJURY

To simplify this presentation, liver disease is divided into two categories: 1) cholestatic disease and 2) parenchymal disease, including acute and chronic hepatitis and cirrhosis.

1. With cholestasis (obstructive jaundice), the liver is unable to secrete bile because of either hepatocellular dysfunction or extrahepatic obstruction. Bilirubin accumulation affects cellular respiration; heme biosynthesis; metabolism of lipids, amino acids, and proteins; and alteration of drug/albumin binding. Coagulation defects occur because of deficient production of vitamin K-dependent factors by the dysfunctional hepatocytes.

   Drugs/conditions that cause cholestasis:

   Primary biliary cirrhosis

   Estrogens

   Methyltestosterone

   Bile duct gallstones

   Bile duct stricture

   Pancreatic cancer obstructing bile duct

2. Hepatic parenchymal disease (ie, hepatitis, cirrhosis) is associated with a hyperdynamic cardiovascular state. Cardiac output increases due to arterio-venous fistulae which decrease systemic vascular resistance and lead to an increased intravascular volume. Patients who do not have this hyperdynamic circulatory pattern have worse perioperative outcomes. Blood pressure and heart rate remain normal but portal vein blood flow (and therefore oxygen delivery) to the liver is decreased. Hypoxemia occurs because of intrapulmonary shunting (hepatopulmonary syndrome [HPS]). Patients with Type I HPS (microvascular shunting) improve with the addition of inspired oxygen. Patients with Type II (macrovascular shunting) do not respond to increased oxygen delivery, and may not even improve after liver transplantation. Ascites can limit diaphragm excursion. The oxygen dissociation curve is shifted to the right and hypoxic pulmonary vasoconstriction is blunted. The patient is anemic due to increased plasma volume, GI bleeding, hemolysis, and malnutrition. Thrombo-cytopenia occurs from bone marrow depression and hypersplenism. The depressed synthetic function of the liver is manifested by decreased albumin production and prolonged PT and PTT due to decreased production of factors II, VII, IX, and X. The encephalopathy that appears with acute liver failure is probably due to cerebral edema, while chronic encephalopathy may be caused by decreased elimination of nitrogenous compounds (ie, ammonia). GI bleeding, infection, and excessive use of diuretics increases blood urea nitrogen (BUN). Ascites and peripheral edema are produced by hypoalbuminemia and renal reabsorption of urinary sodium. As hepatic dysfunction progresses, hepatorenal syndrome may develop in patients with portal hypertension and ascites. This is functional renal failure, with normal histology, and can only be cured by liver transplant.

SOME CAUSES OF HEPATIC INJURY

Viral	Infection
Drugs	NSAIDs
	Acetaminophen (high dose)
	ACE inhibitors
	Antifungal agents (eg, intraconazole)
	Sulfonamides
	Some diet drugs (?)
Other	Reye's syndrome
	Wilson's disease
	Fatty liver due to pregnancy, obesity, nonalcoholic steatohepatitis (NASH)
	Hemochromatosis
	Cystic fibrosis
	Alpha$_1$-antitrypsin deficiency
	Total parenteral nutrition

LIVER FUNCTION TESTS AND DIFFERENTIAL DIAGNOSIS

Diagnostic Factors	Cholestatic Intrahepatic	Cholestatic Extrahepatic	Parenchymal Hepatocellular
Symptom	Deep jaundice, dark urine, light stools, pruritus	Deep jaundice, dark urine, light stools, pruritus, biliary cholic, cholangitis	Nausea, vomit, fever, anorexia
Physical findings	Tender hepatomegaly	Hepatomegaly, palpable gallbladder	Tender hepatomegaly, ± splenomegaly
Bilirubin, total	>30 mg/dL	<30 mg/dL	↑ conjugated
Transaminases	2-5 fold ↑	>2-3 fold ↑	>5 fold ↑
Alkaline phosphatase	>3-5 fold ↑	<3-5 fold ↑	2-3 fold ↑
Prothrombin time	Prolonged	Prolonged	Prolonged
PT correct with vitamin K	Variable	Yes	No
Causes	Stones, sepsis	Hemolysis, hematoma reabsorption, bili overload from whole blood transfusion	Viral, drugs, sepsis, hypoxemia, cirrhosis

THE EFFECTS OF ANESTHESIA AND SURGERY ON LIVER FUNCTION

Preanesthesia Evaluation: Unless a patient has already been diagnosed with liver disease, the preoperative history should include questions that could suggest hepatic injury, such as prior blood transfusions, intravenous drug use, excessive alcohol use, easy bruising, and high risk sexual practices. Physical examination markers include pruritus, jaundice, hepatic tenderness, testicular atrophy, gynecomastia in males, palmer erythema, spider nevi, and ascites. Abnormal laboratory tests are difficult to interpret since they may not provide an assessment of the degree of hepatic dysfunction. That is, the elevated liver function test may indicate onset or resolution of a liver injury. Additionally, there are little data that quantify the operative risk or outcome of patients undergoing surgery with elevated liver tests. This does not mean that surgery should proceed if abnormal tests are encountered during the preoperative evaluation.

Presentation and Operation Decision

Abnormal liver function tests	Delay elective surgery and investigate
Acute hepatitis	Postpone surgery until active inflammation resolves
Chronic hepatitis (mild)	Proceed with surgery
Chronic hepatitis (severe)	Proceed with surgery if the procedure is to improve the clinical state
Cirrhosis	Delay nonemergent surgery to improve MELD score
Fatty liver	Probably alright to proceed

MELD = model for end-stage liver disease (numerical scale used in rating the patient's need for liver transplant)

Anesthesia Management: Liver injury can occur during surgery either from decreased hepatic oxygen delivery or direct drug toxicity. The most injurious conditions in the perioperative period are hypotension, hypoxemia, and hypovolemia, all of which decrease hepatic oxygen delivery. Surgical stress carries a high mortality in patients with severe liver disease, with the greatest insult to the liver occurring with

◀ upper abdominal surgery. Patient position and type of surgery are more important in compromising hepatic blood flow than the type of anesthesia.

Management of the patient with hepatic parenchymal injury requires maintenance of arterial blood pressure and cardiac output to assure adequate hepatic oxygen delivery. When blood flow decreases, the body extracts more oxygen to maintain adequate tissue oxygenation. In the normal person, when portal blood flow decreases, hepatic arterial blood flow increases, thereby ensuring adequate oxygen delivery. In the patient with severe hepatic dysfunction, this vascular autoregulation does not occur, leading to reduced hepatic oxygenation.

Both regional and general anesthesia can decrease hepatic blood flow if blood pressure decreases during surgery. Mechanical ventilation may decrease venous return, decrease cardiac output, and produce liver engorgement, all of which decrease hepatic blood flow. Conversely, hypoventilation (hypercapnia) can produce vasoconstriction, which decreases portal venous flow. Blood pressure management is more important than the type of anesthesia/drugs, as all anesthetics tend to produce a slight rise in transaminases or bilirubin. This is usually unimportant in normal patients but may be significant in patients with severe liver disease.

Anesthetic concerns with regional anesthesia include coagulopathy and hypotension. "Halothane hepatitis" is a concern with repeat halothane exposure, with multiple case reports implicating other inhalational anesthetics. "Halothane hepatitis" is an immune-mediated response which requires previous exposure and antibody formation against an oxidative trifluoroacetyl halide metabolite of halothane. Genetic susceptibility is probable and it can be fatal.

CLASSIFICATION OF SURGICAL RISK (BASED ON SEVERITY OF INJURY)

Child Classification	(A) Minimal	(B) Mild	(C) Severe
Bilirubin (mg/dL)	<2	2-3	>3
Albumin (g/dL)	>3.5	3-3.5	<3
Prothrombin time (sec prolonged)	1-4	4-6	>6
Encephalopathy	None	Moderate	Severe
Nutrition	Excellent	Good	Poor
Ascites	None	Moderate	Marked

Reference: Child CG and Turcotte JG, "Surgery and Portal Hypertension," *The Liver and Portal Hypertension*, Childs CG, ed, Philadelphia, PA: Saunders, 1964, 50.

MELD CLASSIFICATION SYSTEM

The newer MELD classification system (Model for End-Stage Liver Disease) is a numerical scale used to quantify a patient's risk of dying while waiting for a liver transplant. It is determined by objective and verifiable medical data. Serum creatinine measures renal function, bilirubin evaluates how effectively the liver excretes bile, and INR (prothrombin time) determines the liver's ability to make blood clotting factors. Based on these values the liver failure patient's status is scored from 6 (less ill) to 40 (gravely ill). Using this system patients are prioritized in their need for liver transplantation. This scoring system helps ensure that transplanted livers go to those in greatest need. For children <12 years old, the PELD scoring system is used. It includes bilirubin, INR, albumin, and growth failure.

PHARMACOKINETICS

There are significant changes in the pharmacokinetic profiles of many drugs in the patient with liver disease because the liver is important in metabolism and elimination of drugs. Multiple hepatic enzymes are responsible for drug metabolism, with the cytochrome P450 family of enzymes important in mixed function oxidative reactions.

Albumin is produced solely by the liver; therefore, a decrease in albumin concentration can indicate significant liver disease or malnutrition. Prothrombin time is considered a more sensitive indicator of liver disease than albumin because severe liver disease can affect hepatic synthetic function sufficiently to prolong prothrombin time within 24 hours.

Hepatic drug metabolism and elimination can be classified based on alterations in hepatic blood flow, volume of distribution, and protein binding.

Hepatic blood flow patterns change with hepatic injury. As the liver architecture changes with the development of cirrhosis, portal venous blood is shunted from the liver by collateral channels into the systemic circulation. This blood, along with orally administered drugs absorbed from the GI tract, avoids the hepatic first-pass effect preventing the initial drug metabolism and increasing the amount of drug presented to the central circulation. Blood that passes through the liver has decreased exposure to hepatocyte enzymes because of increased fibrosis and a decrease in number and size of loose endothelial junctions, which limits blood exposure to hepatocytes for drug metabolism. If clearance is high, then changes in hepatic blood flow will significantly alter drug elimination (flow limited drugs). Conversely, clearance ·is not affected by a decrease in hepatic blood flow for enzyme-limited drugs. The clearance of enzyme-limited drugs may either be protein-binding sensitive (>85% bound) or protein-binding insensitive (<50% bound).

Volume of distribution (V_d) is altered by the development of ascites (which increases the body's total fluid component) and altered hepatic production of plasma proteins. As the volume of distribution increases, drug concentration at steady state decreases. For example, V_d of propranolol and verapamil is doubled in patients with ascites. This condition may lead to an increase in drug half-life and a decrease in drug clearance.

Protein binding is altered with cirrhosis because of a decrease in serum albumin and an accumulation of substances that displace drugs from albumin-binding sites. In this circumstance, the availability of unbound drug increases, leading to greater drug effect. For example, phenytoin is 90% albumin bound. With hypoalbuminemia, the free fraction increases 20% to 30%, which can double or triple unbound active phenytoin, producing drug toxicity; however, this effect may be countered if there is an increase in volume of distribution (V_d) due to ascites. An increase in free unbound drug may also increase clearance, because more drug is available to be metabolized, which can shorten its half-life. The effect of altered protein binding on drug pharmacokinetics is difficult to predict. A simple rule of thumb is that a change in protein binding has a greater effect on drugs that are normally highly protein bound (>60%) compared to poorly bound drugs.

Drug Characteristics in Normal Subjects and Liver Failure Patients

Drug	Protein Binding (%)	Volume of Distribution (V_d) (L/kg)	Half-life (h)	Clearance (Cl) (mL/min)	Effect of Liver Disease on Drug Disposition	Adjustment of Dose
Antibiotics / Antiviral / Antifungal						
Ampicillin	30	0.28	1.0	340	Half-life ↑; V_d ↑; Cl →	None
Cefazolin	84	0.15	1.8	68	Half-life ↓; f_p ↑	None
Cefotetan	83	0.15	3.7	39.5	Negligible unless renal function decreased	None
Cefoxitin	73	0.12	1.0	98	Negligible unless renal function decreased	None
Clindamycin	79	0.58	2.0	160	Half-life slight ↑; V_d →; Cl ↓ 23%; f_p →	Decrease dose in severe cases
Erythromycin	80	0.77	1.6	600	Half-life ↑	Decrease dose in moderate or severe disease
Gentamicin	<5	0.25	2.0	100	Negligible unless renal function decreased	None
Nafcillin	90	0.4	1.0	580	Half-life ↑ but little change; V_d ↓; Cl ↓ 50% to 60%; f_p ?→	Decrease dose in moderate or severe disease
Vancomycin	55	0.4	5.0	80	Half-life ↑; V_d →; Cl ↓	Decrease dose
Analgesic						
Alfentanil	90	0.28	1.5	200	Half-life ↑; V_d →; Cl ↓; f_p ↑ (dose-dependent)	Decrease dose
Fentanyl	80	3.5	4.0	750	Half-life →; V_d →; Cl →	None
Hydromorphone	15	4	1.5	1500	Half-life ↑	Decrease dose
Methadone	80	4.0	28	150	Half-life ↑ with severe liver disease; Cl →	None or decrease
Morphine	35	3.7	2.0	1200	Half-life →; V_d →; Cl →; f_p →, by some reports f_p ↑	None, but avoid in severe liver disease
Remifentanil	70	0.1	0.12	3000	No effect	None

Drug Characteristics in Normal Subjects and Liver Failure Patients *continued*

Drug	Protein Binding (%)	Volume of Distribution (V_d) (L/kg)	Half-life (h)	Clearance (Cl) (mL/min)	Effect of Liver Disease on Drug Disposition	Adjustment of Dose
Sufentanil	92	3	2	1000	Half-life ↑	Decrease dose
Antiepileptic						
Phenytoin	92	0.65	15.0 nonlinear	40	AVH half-life →; Cl →; f_p ↑. Cirrhosis f_p ↑	Decrease dose in moderate to severe liver disease
Phenobarbital	50	0.8	100	8	Half-life ↑; presumed Cl ↓	Decrease with severe liver disease
Cardiovascular						
Digoxin	30	6.0	35	150	Appears negligible	None
Esmolol	55	1.2	0.15	310/kg	Negligible	None
Labetalol	50	11.5	3.0	1600	Half-life →; V_d ↓; Cl → or ↓; f_p ?, assume ↑	Decrease oral dose; decrease I.V. dose to much smaller extent
Lidocaine	65 nonlinear	1.1	2.0	1000	Half-life ↑; V_d ↑ or →; Cl ↓ ~50%; f_p ? Low therapeutic ratio; decrease in Cl depends on severity of disease	Decrease dose by 50% in severe liver disease
Metoprolol	10	3.2	4.0	800	Half-life ↑; V_d ↑ slightly; Cl ↓ 23%; f_p ?	Decrease dose slightly
Sedative / Hypnotic						
Diazepam	99	1.2	45	28	Half-life ↑; V_d ↑; Cl ↓ 50%; f_p ↑. AVH and cirrhosis increase half-life. Large therapeutic index — safe	Single dose, no change; chronic, decrease dose
Etomidate	76	4	2.6	1200	Negligible	Decrease dose
Lorazepam	90	1.3	12.0	53	Half-life ↑; V_d ↑; Cl→; f_p ↑. Neither AVH nor cirrhosis affects drug dosing	None

Drug Characteristics in Normal Subjects and Liver Failure Patients *continued*

Drug	Protein Binding (%)	Volume of Distribution (V_d) (L/kg)	Half-life (h)	Clearance (Cl) (mL/min)	Effect of Liver Disease on Drug Disposition	Adjustment of Dose
Methohexital	—	61	2.0	829	No data; assume Cl ↓, half-life↑	Probably decrease dose
Midazolam	—	1.3	1.6	624	Half-life ↑; V_d slightly ↑; Cl ↓	Decrease dose
Propofol	73	4	4	2500	Half-life ↑; Cl ↓	None
Thiopental	85	2.3	9.0	275	Half-life →; V_d →; Cl →; f_p ↑	Uncertain; may need to decrease dose
Muscle Relaxants						
Atracurium	—	0.16	0.33	385	Half-life →; V_d ↑; Cl →; long half-life of metabolite	Decrease dose if long-term use
Cisatracurium	—	0.15	0.5	350	Negligible	None
Rocuronium	30	0.25	1	280	Half-life ↑; V_d ↑; Cl →	Slight decrease
Vercuronium	70	0.4	1	280	Half-life ↑; Cl ↓	Slight decrease in dose

AVH = acute viral hepatitis; LD = liver disease; fp = fraction of unbound drug; Cl$_{int}$ = intrinsic clearance; ↑ = increased; ↓ = decreased; → = no change

REFERENCES AND RECOMMENDED READING

Child CG and Turcotte JG, "Surgery and Portal Hypertension," *The Liver and Portal Hypertension*, Childs CG, ed, Philadelphia, PA: Saunders, 1964, 50.

Farnsworth N, Fagan SP, Berger DH, et al, "Child-Turcotte-Pugh Versus MELD Score as a Predictor of Outcome After Elective and Emergent Surgery in Cirrhotic Patients," *Am J Surg*, 2004, 188 (5):580-3.

Gelman S, Dillard E, and Bradley EL Jr, "Hepatic Circulation During Surgical Stress and Anesthesia With Halothane, Isoflurane, or Fentanyl," *Anesth Anal*, 1987, 66(10):936-43.

Gelman S and Ernst EA, "Role of pH, PCO_2, and O_2 Content of Portal Blood in Hepatic Autoregulation," *Am J Physiol*, 1977, 233(4):E255-62.

Gelman S, "General Anesthesia and Hepatic Circulation," *Can J Physiol Pharmacol*, 1987, 65 (8):1762-79.

Jalan R and Hayes PC, "Hepatic Encephalopathy and Ascites," *Lancet*, 1997, 350(9087):1309-15.

Kamath PS, "Clinical Approach to the Patient With Abnormal Liver Test Results," *Mayo Clin Proc*, 1996, 71(11):1089-94.

Kaufman BS and Roccaforte JD, "Hepatic Anatomy, Function, and Physiology," *Clinical Anesthesia*, 6th ed, Barash PG, Cullen BF, Stoelting RK, et al, eds, Philadelphia, PA: Lippincott Williams and Wilkins, 2009, 1247-78.

Keegan MT and Plevak DJ, "Preoperative Assessment of the Patient With Liver Disease," *Am J Gastroenterol*, 2005, 100(9):2116-27.

Krowka MJ, Porayko MK, Plevak DJ, et al, "Hepatopulmonary Syndrome With Progressive Hypoxemia as an Indication for Liver Transplantation: Case Reports and Literature Review," *Mayo Clin Proc*, 1997, 72(1):44-53.

Kubisty CA, Arns RA, Wedlund PJ, et al, "Adjustment of Medication in Liver Failure," *The Pharmacologic Approach to the Critically Ill Patient*, Chernow B, ed, 3rd ed, Baltimore, MD: Williams & Wilkins, 1994, 95-113.

Neal E, Meffin PJ, Gregory PB, et al, "Enhanced Bioavailability and Decreased Clearance of Analgesics in Patients With Cirrhosis," *Gastroenterology*, 1979, 77(1):96-102.

Patel T, "Surgery in the Patient With Liver Disease," *Mayo Clin Proc*, 1999, 74(6):593-9.

Rizvon MK and Chou CL, "Surgery in the Patient With Liver Disease," *Med Clin North Am*, 2003, 87 (1):211-27.

Srikureja W, Kyulo NL, Runyon BA, et al, "MELD Score is a Better Prognostic Model Than Child-Turcotte-Pugh Score or Discriminant Function Score in Patients With Alcoholic Hepatitis," *J Hepatol*, 2005, 42(5):700-6.

Wiklund RA, "Preoperative Preparation of Patients With Advanced Liver Disease," *Crit Care Med*, 2004, 32(4 Suppl):S106-15.

Ziser A, Plevak DJ, Wiesner RH, et al, "Morbidity and Mortality in Cirrhotic Patients Undergoing Anesthesia and Surgery," *Anesthesiology*, 1999, 90(1):42-53.

CHRONIC PAIN MANAGEMENT

Chronic pain is a common problem that is considered one of the least effectively treated disease states in society today. Chronic pain is defined as pain that persists beyond the usual course of an acute disease or after a reasonable time for healing to occur (eg, months to years). Unlike acute pain, the source of the pain cannot always be identified. Chronic pain can be neuropathic, nociceptive, or mixed nociceptive and neuropathic in nature. Patients with chronic pain often have functional loss, psychological problems, and may interfere not only with their livelihood but also with normal activities of daily living. Therefore, the goal of chronic pain management is not to eliminate pain, but to control pain sufficiently to allow the patient to function and improve his or her quality of life.

Chronic pain is most successfully treated using a multidisciplinary, multimodal approach. The involvement of the anesthesiologist, as a pain specialist, in the management of chronic pain is becoming increasingly evident. Specifically, knowledge of the mechanism of action, pharmacologic effects, dosage, and side effects of the agents recommended for the treatment of chronic pain is necessary.

When treating chronic pain, many analgesic medications are used. These agents include nonsteroidal anti-inflammatory drugs (NSAIDs), antidepressants, anticonvulsants, local anesthetics, alpha$_2$-adrenergic agonist, and others. Such agents are preferable to opioids when chronic pain is not of a malignant origin. The initial choice of agent often depends upon the severity, pathophysiology, and etiology of the pain (nociceptive, neuropathic, psychogenic). When treating chronic pain that has a neuropathic component, it usually takes 1-3 weeks before beneficial effects from these agents are seen.

Opioids are used in the treatment of chronic pain when the pain is malignant or when other conservative or procedure-type approaches have failed and the pain is significantly affecting the patients' quality of life. With careful titration and monitoring, opioids can effectively manage many types of chronic pain without intolerable adverse effects.

This section will review the agents, doses, and dosage regimens of the nonopioid agents and the common opioids used for the treatment of chronic pain.

NONSTEROIDAL ANTI-INFLAMMATORY AGENTS

The nonsteroidal anti-inflammatory drugs (NSAIDs) have anti-inflammatory, analgesic, and antipyretic properties. NSAIDs work by inhibiting cyclooxygenase activity (peripherally and centrally) to prevent the formation of prostaglandins. NSAIDs are considered first-line agents for managing mild to moderate pain. Careful patient screening for age, cardiovascular disease, renal dysfunction, gastritis, gastric ulcers, or bleeding disorders due to platelet dysfunction and use of the lowest effective dose for the least amount of time is important for minimizing the risk of serious cardiovascular events and/or gastrointestinal bleeding. NSAIDs are contraindicated in patients who have experienced asthma, urticaria, or allergic-type reactions after taking aspirin or other NSAIDs.

Refer to the table Nonsteroidal Anti-Inflammatory Agents on page 1687.

ANTIDEPRESSANTS

Antidepressant agents have an analgesic effect that occurs at a dose lower than the dose needed for their antidepressant effect. It is theorized that antidepressants may work in the treatment of pain by altering a biochemical mechanism (through inhibition of norepinephrine and/or serotonin reuptake) that may be related to both depression and pain. Antidepressants may also enhance or modulate endogenous opioid analgesia.

Antidepressants are considered first- or second-line therapy for neuropathic pain. Tricyclic antidepressants (TCAs) effectively treat neuropathic pain, but their adverse effect profile can be problematic. Anticholinergic effects (dry mouth, constipation, blurred vision, sedation, dizziness, urinary retention) can occur, particularly when the tertiary amine amitriptyline is used. Secondary amines such as nortriptyline and desipramine cause less sedation and anticholinergic effects than amitriptyline, making them a better choice for older or debilitated patients. Cardiovascular effects of TCAs include orthostatic hypotension, conduction defects, and arrhythmias due to their quinidine-like effect. Cardiovascular effects may be most concerning when amitriptyline is used. Selective serotonin reuptake inhibitors (SSRIs) are better tolerated than TCAs but have not been shown to be as effective as TCAs for managing neuropathic pain symptoms in nondepressed patients.

Duloxetine, an antidepressant that acts by highly specific inhibition of serotonin and norepinephrine reuptake, has been shown to effectively manage painful diabetic neuropathy. Somnolence and constipation are its most common adverse effects.

Venlafaxine, a bicyclic antidepressant, inhibits the reuptake of serotonin at low doses and norepinephrine at moderate doses. Adverse effects are similar to that of SSRIs. Venlafaxine may be considered for neuropathic pain that does not respond to TCAs, duloxetine, or anticonvulsants. All of the antidepressants require anywhere from one (eg, duloxetine) to three weeks (eg, TCAs) for an adequate trial for managing neuropathic pain.

Antidepressants

Drug	Starting Dose (mg/day)	Dose Range (mg/day)	Adverse Effects
Amitriptyline (TCA)	10-25	75-150	Dry mouth, constipation, blurred vision, sedation, weight gain, sexual dysfunction, postural hypotension, QT abnormalities, arrhythmias[1]
Citalopram (SSRI)	10	20-60	Nausea, insomnia, anxiety, tremor
Desipramine (TCA)	25-50	75-200	Dry mouth, constipation, blurred vision, sedation, weight gain, sexual dysfunction, postural hypotension, QT abnormalities, arrhythmias[1]
Duloxetine (SNRI)	60	60-120	Somnolence, fatigue, loss of strength or energy, constipation, nausea, dry mouth, dizziness, sweating, decreased appetite
Fluoxetine (SSRI)	10	10-20	Insomnia, anxiety, restlessness, nervousness, gastrointestinal symptoms, sexual dysfunction
Nortriptyline (TCA)	10-25	75-150	Dry mouth, constipation, blurred vision, sedation, weight gain, sexual dysfunction, postural hypotension, QT abnormalities, arrhythmias[1]
Venlafaxine (SNRI)	37.5	150-375	Nausea, dizziness, insomnia, sedation, dry mouth, sweating, hypertension, impotence

[1]Use TCAs with caution in patients with cardiac risk factors. Amitriptyline, a tertiary amine, is more likely to cause these adverse effects than desipramine or nortriptyline (secondary amines).

Key: TCA = tricyclic antidepressant; SSRI = selective serotonin reuptake inhibitor; SNRI = serotonin and norepinephrine reuptake inhibitor

ANTICONVULSANTS

Anticonvulsant agents are another class of drugs that have been used for chronic pain management, specifically neuropathic pain and trigeminal neuralgia. Anticonvulsant agents may be used as a first- or second-line therapy for neuropathic pain, exerting their analgesic effects by decreasing spontaneous sensory nerve firing after nerve injury. These agents are usually used when other treatments, such as antidepressants, are unsuccessful. Gabapentin or pregabalin, however, may be administered as first-line therapy. When using anticonvulsants as an analgesic, efficacy does not correlate with therapeutic serum concentrations. Newer agents (gabapentin, pregabalin) are less toxic than the older agents (carbamazepine, phenytoin, and valproic acid) and are preferred. The adverse effects of gabapentin and pregabalin include sedation, dizziness, dry mouth, and peripheral edema. Carbamazepine can produce a rash, has a toxic epoxide metabolite (for which regular blood tests are warranted), has a negative effect on bone density, and has significant drug-drug interactions. It has also been associated with Stevens-Johnson syndrome and toxic epidermal necrosis. Topiramate, zonisamide, levetiracetam, and tiagabine may provide analgesia in patients unresponsive to more proven anticonvulsants. Lamotrigine, another second-line agent, also has antidepressant properties. Strict dose titration of lamotrigine is necessary to minimize the risk of serious adverse effects such as Stevens-Johnson Syndrome and toxic epidermal necrosis. Discontinue lamotrigine with the first sign of a rash. Clonazepam has been effectively used for trigeminal neuralgia, post-traumatic neuralgia, paroxysmal postlaminectomy pain, and lancinating phantom limb pain. Like other benzodiazepines, drowsiness is common and withdrawal symptoms may occur following abrupt discontinuation.

The following table lists the agents and doses of anticonvulsants used for chronic pain management.

Anticonvulsants

Drug	Starting Dose (mg/day)	Dose Range (mg/day)
Clonazepam	0.5	5-20
Gabapentin	900	1800-3600
Lamotrigine	50	200-600
Pregabalin	150	150-300
Tiagabine	4	12-60
Topiramate	25	100-400

OTHER ADJUVANTS

In patients with cancer, corticosteroids can be added to elevate mood, stimulate appetite, reduce nausea and vomiting, and reduce inflammation. Because of their potent anti-inflammatory effects, corticosteroids can be effective for pain caused by soft tissue infiltration, visceral distension, or increased intracranial pressure. Oral muscle relaxants (eg, cyclobenzaprine, carisoprodol, methocarbamol) exert their effects by depressing spinal polysynaptic pathways and producing sedation. These agents are most helpful in acute musculoskeletal conditions such as neck and back pain. Efficacy from long-term administration has not been demonstrated and abrupt discontinuation following prolonged administration can cause withdrawal symptoms. Tizanidine, a centrally-acting muscle relaxant, has been shown to have antinociceptive, anti-inflammatory, and alpha$_2$-agonist properties. Tizanidine requires gradual dose titration over 2–4 weeks and is best used to treat chronic muscle spasticity, such as that seen with multiple sclerosis. Baclofen, an agonist at the GABA$_B$ receptor, acts at the spinal end of the upper motor neurons to cause muscle relaxation. It has been used to treat trigeminal neuralgia and other neuropathic pain, as well as muscle spasms from conditions such as multiple sclerosis or spinal cord lesions. Adverse effects can be minimized by gradual dose titration over several days to weeks. Baclofen should be tapered and not abruptly discontinued because of the risk for serious withdrawal symptoms such as delirium and seizures. Clonidine, a centrally-acting alpha$_2$-agonist, provides analgesia by blocking transmission of noxious sensory information in the dorsal horn of the spinal cord. When administered transdermally, clonidine may also have a peripheral site of action. Tramadol provides analgesia by inhibiting reuptake of norepinephrine and serotonin within (central nervous system) pain pathways and is a weak mu-opioid receptor agonist. It has been effectively used for short-term (eg, flare-ups from osteoarthritis) and long-term (eg, low back, osteoarthritis, or cancer pain) treatment of chronic pain.

Other Adjuvants

Drug	Starting Dose (mg/day)	Dose Range (mg/day)	Adverse Effects
Baclofen	15	40-80	Nausea, constipation, weakness, confusion, dizziness, drowsiness
Clonidine (transdermal)	0.1	0.1-0.3	Drowsiness, dry mouth, fatigue, headache, local skin reaction, hypotension
Dexamethasone	1	2-8	Edema, hyperglycemia, immunosuppression, euphoria, depression, cognitive impairment
Prednisone	5	5-60	Edema, hyperglycemia, immunosuppression, euphoria, depression, cognitive impairment
Tizanidine	4	6-36	Drowsiness, insomnia, dizziness, fatigue, dry mouth, hypotension, elevated liver function tests
Tramadol	50 (100 mg extended-release formulation)	150-300	Nausea, dizziness, vomiting, drowsiness

TOPICAL AGENTS

When the pain is localized, topical agents can be effective for chronic conditions such as arthritic and neuropathic pain. Capsaicin initially releases substance P, which results in an initial burning sensation and heat hyperalgesia during the first few days of its use. After several weeks of continued application, substance P becomes depleted from the nerve terminals, C-fibers are desensitized (superficial fibers may be killed), and analgesia occurs. Studies evaluating its efficacy have not been overwhelmingly favorable, but patients with postherpetic neuralgia and diabetic neuropathy have reported modest pain relief from capsaicin. When administered topically, lidocaine acts directly at the local site through inhibition of sodium channels in nerve endings to reduce neuropathic pain transmission. Topical 5% lidocaine patches have been shown to effectively treat localized neuropathic pain syndromes.

Topical Agents

Drug	Starting Dose	Dose Range	Adverse Effects
Capsaicin	0.025% applied 3-4 times/day[1]	0.025% to 0.075% applied 3-4 times/day[1]	Burning, stinging, redness of the skin
Lidocaine	5% patch	Up to three patches for 12 hours daily[2]	Localized skin reaction, burning or abnormal sensation, skin discoloration, pruritus

[1] A minimum of 4 weeks is required to determine effectiveness.

[2] A minimum of 2 weeks is required to determine effectiveness.

OPIOIDS

Opioids are routinely used in the treatment of cancer pain. However, opioids can also be effective as a component of chronic noncancer pain management when other agents are not sufficient and even when the pain is neuropathic in nature. The primary care physician or pain specialist will decide whether an opioid could be successful for the chronic pain patient on a patient-specific basis.

Many opioid agents, formulations, and routes of administration are available for chronic pain management. Morphine, oxycodone, and hydromorphone are commonly used and available in short-acting formulations. Long-acting agents include sustained-release formulations of oxycodone and morphine, transdermal fentanyl, and methadone. Opioid therapy may be initiated using short-acting formulations to provide immediate pain relief and allow titration to a minimal effective dose, then switched to a long-acting agent to provide a longer duration of effective analgesia, minimize adverse effects, and improve compliance. For patients who are unable to take oral tablets, morphine can be administered as an oral liquid, rectally, or intravenously, whereas fentanyl can be administered transdermally or trans-mucosally. All opioids are metabolized by the liver (several to an active metabolite) and excreted in the urine. Meperidine is metabolized to normeperidine, a renally-eliminated metabolite that can cause anxiety, tremors, myoclonus, and seizures when the dose of meperidine is high and/or repeated doses are administered. Meperidine also has serotonergic activity which, when combined with other serotonin reuptake inhibitors (eg, MAOI, SSRI), can produce a serious serotonin toxicity reaction. Oral meperidine undergoes extensive first-pass metabolism, with significant amounts of normeperidine formed. For these reasons, meperidine has no place in chronic pain management. Propoxyphene is metabolized to norpropoxyphene, which has a long half-life, is renally eliminated, and may accumulate with chronic use. Propoxyphene is not recommended for older adults or patients with renal impairment.

Opioids

Drug	Approximate Equianalgesic Parenteral Dose	Approximate Equianalgesic Oral Dose	Usual Oral Starting Dose for Opioid-Naïve Adults
Morphine[1] (MS Contin®, others)	10 mg	30 mg	15-30 mg q3-6 hours
Hydromorphone[1] (Dilaudid®)	1.5 mg	7.5 mg	4-8 mg q3-6 hours
Methadone[2] (Dolophine®, others)	10 mg	Varies	2.5 mg q8-12 hours
Oxycodone (Roxicodone®, others)	Not available	20 mg	10-20 mg q3-6 hours

Combination Opioid Preparations[3]

Drug	Approximate Equianalgesic Oral Dose	Usual Oral Starting Dose for Opioid-Naïve Adults
Codeine (Tylenol® with codeine, others)	200 mg	60 mg q4-6 hours
Hydrocodone (Lorcet®, Lortab®, Norco®, Vicodin®, Vicoprofen®, others)	30 mg	10 mg q3-6 hours
Oxycodone (in Percocet®, Percodan®, Tylox®, others)	20 mg	10 mg q3-6 hours

Note: Tables vary in the suggested doses that are equianalgesic to morphine. Furthermore, when a patient has been taking a very large dose of an opioid for a long time, equianalgesic dosing may be quite different. Therefore, clinical response is the criterion that must be applied for each patient; titration to clinical response is necessary. Because there is incomplete cross tolerance between opioids, it may be better to use 25% to 30% less than the calculated equianalgesic dose when switching opioids and retitrate to desired response.

Caution: Recommended doses do not apply to patients with renal or hepatic insufficiency or other conditions affecting drug metabolism and pharmacokinetics.

[1] **Caution:** For morphine and hydromorphone, rectal administration is an alternate route for patients unable to take oral medications. Equianalgesic doses for rectal administration may differ from oral and parenteral doses because of pharmacokinetic differences. **Note:** A short-acting opioid should be used for initial therapy of moderate-severe pain, and then switched to a long-acting preparation once the optimal dose has been reached. Usual starting dose of morphine is NOT for the sustained-release formulation.

[2] Methadone is significantly more potent with repetitive dosing (due to its active metabolite). Ratios between oral morphine and oral methadone can range from 3:1 to 20:1, depending upon the current daily oral morphine dose.

[3] The maximum dose of these combination products is limited by the acetaminophen, aspirin, or ibuprofen in each tablet. For that reason, these combination products should not be used for severe pain.

REFERENCES AND RECOMMENDED READING

Ables AZ and Baughman OL 3rd, "Antidepressants: Update on New Agents and Indications," *Am Fam Physician*, 2003, 67(3):547-54.

Argoff CE, Backonja MM, Belgrade MJ, et al, "Consensus Guidelines: Treatment Planning and Options. Diabetic Peripheral Neuropathic Pain," *Mayo Clin Proc*, 2006, 81(4 Suppl):S12-25.

Backonja MM, "Use of Anticonvulsants for Treatment of Neuropathic Pain," *Neurology*, 2002, 59(5 Suppl 2):S14-7.

Beebe FA, Barkin RL, and Barkin S, "A Clinical and Pharmacologic Review of Skeletal Muscle Relaxants for Musculoskeletal Conditions," *Am J Ther*, 2005, 12(2):151-71.

Eisenberg E, McNicol ED, and Carr DB, "Efficacy and Safety of Opioid Agonists in the Treatment of Neuropathic Pain of Nonmalignant Origin: Systematic Review and Meta-Analysis of Randomized Controlled Trials," *JAMA*, 2005, 293(24):3043-52.

Gardner-Nix J, "Principles of Opioid Use in Chronic Noncancer Pain," *CMAJ*, 2003, 169(1):38-43.

Guay DR, "Adjunctive Agents in the Management of Chronic Pain," *Pharmacotherapy*, 2001, 21 (9):1070-81.

Irving GA, "Contemporary Assessment and Management of Neuropathic Pain," *Neurology*, 2005, 64 (12 Supp 3):S21-7.

Jackson KC 2nd and St. Onge EL, "Antidepressant Pharmacotherapy: Considerations for the Pain Clinician," *Pain Practice*, 2003, 3(2):135-43.

"Principles of Analgesic Use in the Treatment of Acute Pain and Cancer Pain," 6th ed, Glenview, IL: American Cancer Pain Society, 2008.

CHRONIC RENAL FAILURE

In chronic renal failure, there is a progressive loss of nephron function. Depending upon the extent of loss, signs, symptoms, and biochemical abnormalities may or may not be present. Signs of renal failure (eg, nocturia) begin to appear when the number of functioning nephrons decreases to 10% to 40%. This stage of renal failure is referred to as renal insufficiency. Patients at this stage have little or no renal reserve; the ability to metabolize and excrete certain drugs is impaired as is the ability to eliminate large quantities of protein catabolic products. Serum creatinine (Cr) and blood urea nitrogen (BUN) are increased. The loss of approximately 95% of functioning nephrons results in the uremic syndrome. Acid-base, hematologic, and electrolyte abnormalities (hyperkalemia, hyponatremia, hypercalcemia, hypocalcemia, hypermagnesemia, hyperphosphatemia) are routinely seen as is fluid overload, which can result in decompensated heart failure, hypertension, and left ventricular hypertrophy. Hyperkalemia is an important consideration because of its ability to precipitate fatal cardiac arrhythmias. Gastrointestinal disorders (eg, nausea, vomiting, anorexia, GI bleeding), chronic anemia, and an altered immune system are also present.

EFFECT ON DRUG DISPOSITION

Bioavailability

Several factors affect drug absorption in renal failure patients. Absorption of drugs can be decreased in uremic patients who have nausea, vomiting, diarrhea, gastritis, and pancreatitis. Uremia can result in an increase in gastric pH, thereby reducing the bioavailability of drugs requiring an acidic medium for absorption. An increase in gastric pH can also occur secondary to antacid use, which is often needed by renal failure patients. Antacids bind to other drugs, reducing their absorption. Gastric emptying time, gastric mobility, and intestinal motility can be decreased in the uremic patient, which can influence drug absorption.

Protein Binding

A drug's effect is produced by its free or unbound fraction. In renal failure patients, protein binding is reduced, which increases the amount of unbound drug. For example, this is seen with acidic drugs normally bound to albumin; since albumin is frequently decreased in renal failure, a greater free fraction of drug is seen. This effect is most important for drugs with high protein binding (>80%), such as phenytoin and valproic acid. The increase in free fraction can increase clearance of phenytoin since it is a low extraction ratio drug. Increased free drug can also result from the displacement of acidic drugs from albumin binding sites by acidic by-products seen in uremia and as a result of conformational changes in albumin which reduce the number/affinity of binding sites for drugs.

Metabolism

Renal failure significantly impacts on drug metabolism in a number of organs. The kidney houses the renal cytochrome P450 system which contributes to the metabolism of a number of drugs. Renal failure has been demonstrated to potentially increase, decrease, or have no effect on drug metabolism. Renal failure can also impact on drugs, which are metabolized by the liver to active metabolites. If these metabolites are renally eliminated, they accumulate in renal failure leading to increased activity and/or adverse effects. Meperidine (normeperidine), morphine (morphine-6-glucuronide), procainamide (N-acetylprocainamide), midazolam (1-hydroxymidazolam), and allopurinol (oxypurinol) are some examples of such drugs. Dosages of these drugs should be carefully titrated in renal failure patients, and potential toxic effects should be monitored.

Elimination

The degree of renal impairment and the percentage of drug normally excreted unchanged in the urine will determine the impact of renal failure on elimination. Drugs are eliminated by the kidney via either filtration or active secretion. Molecular size and protein binding will determine a drug's filterability; low protein bound and small drugs are filtered more easily. Renal secretion is dependent on the anionic and cationic pathways. Depending on the cause of the renal disease, alterations in secretion and filtration can occur independently of each other. Estimates of GFR such as creatinine clearance are generally used to estimate renal function. But estimates of GFR may not predict alterations in clearance due to tubular dysfunction and altered secretion. Therefore close monitoring for efficacy and toxicity of renally eliminated drugs is necessary even when appropriate dosage alterations based on estimates of creatinine clearance have been performed.

Renal Dosing

Individualized drug dosage regimens for patients with renal failure generally utilize a correlation between creatinine clearance and drug clearance. Creatinine clearance is best estimated from a stable serum creatinine in patients with normal muscle mass and weight. A number of equations to estimate creatinine clearance are available. Multiple methods of renal dosage modification may be available, and they generally include increasing the interval or decreasing the dose. Both of these methods maintain the same steady state serum concentrations. Increasing the interval maintains similar peaks and troughs as usual dosing. Decreasing the dose results in lower peaks and higher troughs. This method is useful for antibiotics such as cephalosporins where the lack of postantibiotic effect necessitates maintenance of serum concentrations above the MIC.

Drug Dosing in Renal Replacement Therapy

Drug removal by hemodialysis is impacted by numerous drug-related factors. Molecular weight less than 500 daltons is generally associated with drug removal by traditional hemodialysis methods. However, high-flux filters can remove drugs of 5,000 daltons or greater. Water soluble drugs are more likely to be removed than drugs of poor solubility in aqueous media. Protein binding is an additional significant factor, since only free drug is available to diffuse across the semipermeable membrane. Volume of distribution also correlates well, as drugs with smaller volumes of distribution are more likely to come in contact with the semipermeable membrane and are more significantly dialyzed than drugs with large volumes of distribution that are largely distributed to tissue.

Characteristics of the dialysis procedure also impact on the amount of drug removed. A variety of dialysis filters of various compositions are available. Significant differences in drug clearances with different dialysis membranes and filters have been described. In addition blood and dialysate flow rates vary along with the length of the dialysis session. Therefore, drug clearances can vary significantly based on the specific dialysis prescription.

The need for supplemental dosing after dialysis is based on the relative amount of drug removed by a typical dialysis session. When >25% to 30% of a dose is removed by a typical 4-hour dialysis session, it is generally recommended that a supplemental dose be administered. Use of high-flux membranes may necessitate more aggressive supplementation, especially for some drugs that are not removed by typical procedures (eg, vancomycin). Given the multitude of factors impacting the potential amount of drug removed, close monitoring for efficacy and toxicity is necessary.

PREOPERATIVE EVALUATION OF THE CHRONIC RENAL FAILURE PATIENT

Assessment of renal function should be part of the comprehensive preoperative evaluation of the chronic renal failure patient. Tests are used in an attempt to quantify renal function and include BUN, serum creatinine, measured creatinine clearance, and estimated creatinine clearance. The table on the next page lists the advantages and disadvantages for each test as well as their normal values.

Test	Normal Values	Advantages / Disadvantages
BUN	8-20 mg/dL	- Rapid, inexact estimate of creatinine clearance
		- BUN is increased by high protein intake, blood in GI tract, accelerated catabolism
		- Hepatic dysfunction decreases BUN concentration
		- Reabsorption of urea is greater when urinary flow is low
S_{cr}	0.5-1.2 mg/dL	- Rapid, inexact estimate of creatinine clearance
		- Creatinine is produced at a lower rate in elderly and in females; levels may fail to accurately reflect degree of nephron loss
		- Patients with muscle wasting from chronic disease may have low serum creatinine levels
		- Heavily muscled patients or acutely catabolic patients may have higher than normal serum creatinine levels secondary to more rapid muscle breakdown
Cl_{cr} (measured)	120 mL/minute	- Best overall indicator of GFR
		- Must accurately record urinary volume
		- Hydration can influence GFR determination
Cl_{cr} (estimated)	120 mL/minute	- Superior to BUN or serum creatinine for quantification of renal reserve
		- Same disadvantages as serum creatinine

Urinalysis assesses urinary pH as well as the presence of hematuria, pyuria, cellular casts, and proteinuria. The patient's cardiovascular status, hemoglobin concentration, and adequacy of dialysis therapy should also be assessed.

INTRAOPERATIVE MANAGEMENT OF THE CHRONIC RENAL FAILURE PATIENT

Monitoring

Intraoperative monitoring should include blood pressure, heart rate, EKG, oxygen saturation (via pulse oximeter), carbon dioxide (via capnometry), and degree of neuromuscular blockade (via a peripheral nerve stimulator). Invasive cardiovascular monitoring should be performed as needed.

Fluid Management

Fluid management must take into consideration the chronic renal failure patient's inability to excrete excess sodium and water. In those patients not requiring hemodialysis, a urine output >0.5 mL/kg/hour can usually be maintained by administration of a balanced salt solution at a rate of 3-5 mL/kg/hour. If necessary, the patient can be dialyzed postoperatively if intravascular volume is increased to an unsatisfactory level intraoperatively.

Selection of Anesthetic Agents

Knowledge of drug action in renal failure is important in determining an appropriate drug regimen (drug and dose). The reader is referred to the drugs' individual monographs to determine dosing in renal failure. Several examples follow.

I.V. anesthetic agents. Thiopental is highly bound to plasma proteins. Since protein binding is reduced in renal failure, a larger fraction of unbound thiopental is available. Further, a greater proportion of thiopental is found in the nonionized, unbound form secondary to the acidic pH seen in renal failure. Finally, uremia alters the blood-brain barrier, which results in an increased sensitivity to thiopental. Because of these factors, a lower induction dose of thiopental is needed for uremic patients.

Induction doses of ketamine and benzodiazepines require less reduction since they are less protein-bound than thiopental. Normal benzodiazepine doses, however, may show an exaggerated response in debilitated renal failure patients. Ketamine, because of its ability to increase blood pressure and cardiac output, may worsen the hypertension seen with renal failure.

Morphine's elimination half-life and clearance are not changed in renal failure. As already alluded to, its glucuronide metabolite accumulates in renal failure and can cause prolonged respiratory depression The synthetic opioids, fentanyl, sufentanil, and alfentanil are hepatically metabolized with their metabolites renally excreted. The rapid tissue redistribution seen with these agents after small doses should result in a short duration of action in both normal and renal failure patients. Sufentanil does, however, have an active metabolite which can accumulate in chronic renal failure patients. Remifentanil, because of its metabolism by nonspecific esterases in blood and tissue, is not affected by renal failure. Dosing remains the same as in normal patients.

Inhalational agents. The major route of elimination of these agents is via the lungs, not the kidneys. Metabolism of some of these agents can result in renally excreted metabolites. Enflurane and sevoflurane are metabolized to inorganic fluoride, which can accumulate in renal failure patients. Sevoflurane is currently not recommended for use in patients with a serum creatinine >1.5 mg/dL. An advantage of the volatile inhalation agents is that they produce neuromuscular blockade, which can reduce the dose of neuromuscular blocking agent required.

Neuromuscular-blocking agents. The depolarizing neuromuscular blocking agent succinylcholine causes a transient increase in serum potassium of approximately 0.5-1 mEq/L. This may become a problem in uremic patients who have an elevated serum potassium; the increase may be enough to produce cardiac arrhythmias. Plasma cholinesterase levels are sufficient in renal failure patients so that no clinically significant prolongation of succinylcholine's effect should be expected.

The elimination of nondepolarizing neuromuscular blocking agents is dependent to varying degrees on renal excretion. The following table lists the elimination profiles of the commercially available nondepolarizing agents. The elimination half-lives of agents primarily eliminated renally are increased in patients with renal failure. Atracurium and cisatracurium, because of their primarily nonrenal elimination, are ideal agents to use in renal failure patients. Both pancuronium and vecuronium have active metabolites that can accumulate in renal failure. Laudanosine, a metabolite of atracurium, can also accumulate in renal failure. Laudanosine has no neuromuscular blocking activity but has been shown to cause CNS excitation in animals; this effect has not been demonstrated in humans.

Agent	Renal	Hepatic	Biliary	Plasma
Atracurium	<5%	—	—	Hofmann elimination Ester hydrolysis
Cisatracurium	R/H <20%	R/H <20%	—	Hofmann elimination
Pancuronium	60% to 80%	15% to 40%	5% to 10%	—
Rocuronium	30%	—	50%	—
Vecuronium	30%	20% to 30%	40% to 75%	—

R/H = renal/hepatic metabolism.

Renal failure increases the duration of action of the anticholinesterase agents (neostigmine, pyridostigmine, edrophonium) commonly used to reverse the residual effects of neuromuscular blockade by 100% or more (secondary to their elimination primarily by the kidneys). This makes the possibility of recurarization unlikely. Other factors which influence reversal of neuromuscular blockade in the renal failure patient include acid-base status, electrolyte levels, concomitant use of potentiating drugs (eg, aminoglycosides), and temperature.

POSTOPERATIVE MANAGEMENT OF THE CHRONIC RENAL FAILURE PATIENT

Hypertension is frequently seen in the postoperative period. Vasodilators (eg, esmolol, fenoldopam, labetalol, nicardipine) may be useful as initial therapy. Nitroprusside can be used transiently, but large doses or prolonged use could be associated with thiocyanate toxicity in renal failure. If hypervolemia is the cause, dialysis can be used to remove excess fluid if it is an option. Supplemental oxygen should be considered if anemia is present, continuous monitoring of the EKG is warranted if arrhythmias are a concern in a hyperkalemic patient, and caution should be used when administering opioids for pain secondary to the potential for CNS depression and hypoventilation.

REFERENCES AND RECOMMENDED READING

Quan DJ and Aweeka FT, "Dosing of Drugs in Renal Failure," *Applied Therapeutics: The Clinical Use of Drugs*, Young LY and Koda-Kimble MA, eds, 8th ed, Vancouver, WA: Applied Therapeutics Inc, 2004, 32(1)-(26).

Matzke GR and Frye RF, "Drug Therapy Individualization for Patients With Renal Insufficiency," *Pharmacotherapy: A Pathophysiologic Approach*, DiPiro JT, Talbert RL, Yee GC, et al, eds, 7th ed, New York, NY: McGraw-Hill Companies, 2008, 833-44.

Stafford-Smith M, Shaw A, George R, et al, "The Renal System and Anesthesia for Urologic Surgery," *Clinical Anesthesia*, Barash PG, Cullen BF, Stoelting RK, eds, 6th ed, Philadelphia, PA: Lippincott Williams & Wilkins, 2009, 1346-74.

Stoelting RK and Dierdorf SF, "Renal Disease," *Anesthesia and Co-Existing Disease*, 3rd ed, New York, NY: Churchill Livingstone, 1993, 289-312.

CONTINUOUS RENAL REPLACEMENT THERAPY

Continuous renal replacement therapy (CRRT) has evolved over the last 25 years as a means of providing safe and effective renal replacement therapy to critically ill patients with fluid overload and/or renal failure who may not tolerate the hemodynamic disturbances that accompany traditional intermittent hemodialysis. CRRT provides additional benefits by decreasing fluid and electrolyte shifts, improving dialysis adequacy, and providing the potential for unlimited fluid administration to accommodate optimal nutrition. More recently, CRRT has also been investigated for removal of inflammatory substances or mediators in conditions such as acute respiratory distress syndrome or sepsis. Although CRRT has been found to remove these substances, its clinical impact has not yet been defined.

CRRT procedures utilize diffusion, filtration (convection), or combined diffusion/filtration techniques which assist in the management of fluid volume, electrolytes, and acid base status. Vascular access for these procedures can be either arterial or venous. Whereas arterial access utilizes the patient's own blood pressure for the maintenance of filtration pressure, venous access systems incorporating a blood pump are utilized more frequently as they result in higher solute clearance. Procedures offering only fluid volume control include slow continuous ultrafiltration (SCUF), and continuous arterio- and venovenous hemofiltration (CAVH and CVVH). Procedures which provide both solute and fluid volume control include continuous arterio- and venovenous hemodialysis (CAVHD and CVVHD), and continuous arterio- and venovenous hemodiafiltration (CAVHDF and CVVHDF). The method selected is determined by the patient's clinical needs.

Continuous Renal Replacement Therapies

Therapy	Abbreviation	Definition	Volume Control	Solute Control
Ultrafiltration	SCUF	Plasma water removal	Effective	Ineffective
Hemofiltration	CAVH CVVH	Convective process using semipermeable membrane	Effective	Ineffective
Hemodialysis	CAVHD CVVHD	Diffusion using dialysate and semipermeable membrane	Effective	Effective
Hemodiafiltration	CAVHDF CVVHDF	Diffusion and convection	Effective	Effective

ANTICOAGULATION IN CRRT

All hemodialysis procedures are prone to clotting of the blood lines and/or hemofilter due to platelet activation. Clotting is more likely to occur in an arteriovenous procedure since the blood flow rates are lower than in a venovenous one.

Numerous anticoagulation schemes are employed which provide safe and effective CRRT with filter survival times often >48 hours.

Systemic Anticoagulants Used In CRRT

Drug	Dose	Monitoring Goal
Heparin	500-1000 units bolus, then 5-10 units/kg/h	aPTT 35-45 seconds
Dalteparin	20 units/kg bolus, then 10 units/kg/h	
Prostacyclin (PGI$_2$, epoprostenol)	2-10 ng/kg/min	
Lepirudin (r-Hirudin)[1]	0.01 mg/kg bolus, then 0.005 mg/kg/h	
Argatroban	0.4-0.9 mcg/kg/min	aPTT 2-2.5 x normal

[1]Due to extensive renal elimination, lepirudin has been associated with hemorrhagic complications when used in patients requiring CRRT.

Unfractionated heparin is the most commonly used anticoagulant in CRRT procedures due to its lack of renal elimination and the low propensity for removal through dialysis. Critically ill patients are often at risk of bleeding due to concomitant organ failure and coagulopathies. Even with low dose regimens and monitoring, bleeding rates have been reported to be as high as 50%. Heparin-induced thrombocytopenia (HIT) is another potential complication of this therapy.

Low molecular weight heparins have been useful anticoagulants in chronic hemodialysis, and have been investigated in CRRT. Dalteparin provides comparable filter patency and bleeding rates to heparin, but has significant renal elimination, may accumulate in renal failure, and is not removed by filtration. Low molecular weight heparins may be associated with a higher incidence of bleeding than heparin due to their longer half-lives in renal failure and an inability to be predictably neutralized by protamine. Low molecular weight heparins should not be used in patients with HIT.

Prostacyclin (PGI$_2$ or epoprostenol) is an inhibitor of platelet aggregation and a vasodilator. It has been successfully employed both in combination with reduced doses of heparin and alone in patients felt to be at risk of bleeding due to coagulopathy. Hypotension, an expected side effect, is generally not observed due to 30% to 40% clearance by filtration. Cost is the most commonly cited factor limiting its use.

Lepirudin (r-Hirudin) is a recombinant polypeptide which directly inhibits thrombin. It is 90% renally eliminated and has at least a 100-fold increase in its half-life in renal failure. Limited information is available regarding lepirudin use in CRRT, and its use has been associated with hemorrhage. In addition, some patients develop antihirudin antibodies which further prolong the drug's elimination and complicate therapy. The aPTT does not correlate well with bleeding risk from lepirudin.

Argatroban, an alternative direct thrombin inhibitor, may be the most promising option for patients on CRRT who have HIT. Argatroban is hepatically eliminated and a very effective option for HIT in critically ill patients with renal failure. Very little data is available regarding its clinical use in CRRT. Lower doses of 0.4-0.6 mcg/kg/min have been used for patients with combined liver and renal failure.

Another option for anticoagulation for patients with HIT or at high risk of bleeding is regional citrate. Citrate chelates calcium, which is necessary for activity of a number of factors in the clotting cascade. Numerous citrate anticoagulant procedures have been described to provide effective anticoagulation with filter durations ranging from 1-4 days with minimal bleeding rates. Anticoagulant citrate dextrose (ACD-A) solution or 4% trisodium citrate are generally administered prefilter at a rate to achieve a postfilter ionized Ca concentration of 1-1.4 mg/dL (0.25-0.35 mmol/L). Specialized dialysate solutions used in these procedures are low sodium, low or calcium-free, and low or bicarbonate-free. One potential complication of citrate anticoagulation is systemic alkalosis, since citrate is metabolized to bicarbonate. Citrate toxicity may also be observed when citrate is ineffectively removed in patients with liver failure, or hypoperfusion. High ratios of total calcium to ionized calcium occur when the citrate-calcium complex accumulates. Despite the need for specialized dialysate solutions, the additional need for intensive monitoring of ionized calcium concentrations, and the potential for metabolic alkalosis, citrate anticoagulation is growing in popularity due to its ability to provide longer filter life with a low incidence of bleeding.

Regional (Prefilter) Citrate Anticoagulation

Drug	Dose	Monitoring Goal
Citrate (ACD-A or trisodium citrate 4%)	ACD-A[1]: Initial rate: 180 mL/hour (~1.5 x blood flow rate)[2] or 0.03 x blood flow rate[3] **or** Trisodium citrate 4%: Initial rate: 140-205 mL/hour[4]	Maintain circuit Ca^{++}: 1-1.4 mg/dL Maintain patient's serum Ca^{++}: 4.6-5.3 mg/dL[5]

[1]Contains dextrose 2.45 g/100 mL.

[2]Mount K, Vermillion B, Shidham G, et al, "Safety and Efficacy of Regional Citrate Anticoagulation in Continuous Renal Replacement Therapy," Crit Care Med, 2008, 36(12 Suppl):606.

[3]Burry LD, Tung DD, Hallett D, et al, "Regional Citrate Anticoagulation for PrismaFlex Continuous Renal Replacement Therapy," Ann Pharmacother, 2009, 43(9):1419-25.

[4]Must administer calcium (preferably calcium chloride) to maintain patient's serum ionized Ca^{++} between 4.6-5.3 mg/dL (1.15-1.33 mmol/L).

[5]Morgera S, Schneider M, Slowinski T, et al, "A Safe Citrate Anticoagulation Protocol With Variable Treatment Efficacy and Excellent Control of the Acid-Base Status," Crit Care Med, 2009, 37(6):2018-24.

CRRT in the absence of any anticoagulation is a final option. Saline flushes (100 mL/h) have provided filter patency for approximately 24 hours. This alternative may be an option for patients with bleeding risk, HIT, or liver failure.

DRUG DOSING IN CRRT

Many principles that apply to drug removal by traditional hemodialysis methods also apply to CRRT (refer to Chronic Renal Failure Chapter section on Dialysis Dosing). Similar drug (eg, molecular weight, protein binding, and volume of distribution) and procedure (eg, hemofilter) characteristics responsible for drug removal in intermittent dialysis are also important in CRRT. However, the large variety of procedures makes generalizations regarding removal of any individual drug difficult. In CRRT there is the possibility of more significant convection with or without diffusion, along with a variety of different dialysis membranes. In addition the dialysis/hemofiltration process is continual rather than for a limited time period. All of these factors make generalizations about the extent of drug removal by a specific type of CRRT procedure difficult to formulate. Nonrenal routes of elimination may become more important in renal failure. The amount of drug lost due to dialysis may be small compared to the amount cleared extrarenally. Some patients being treated with CRRT may have significant residual renal function, which may also contribute to drug clearance. Therefore, the patient's clinical status, liver and renal function, and the specific CRRT prescription should be closely evaluated when drug dosage recommendations are formulated.

During filtration processes such as CAVH and CVVH, the amount of drug removed is largely dependent on the filtration rate, the drug's protein binding characteristics, and the specific filter being utilized. Significant differences between filters have been documented with regard to the amount of drug removed by these procedures. The sieving coefficient is the ratio of drug found in ultrafiltrate to the prefilter plasma water concentration. The sieving coefficient often approximates the drug's free fraction in plasma. However, it can also vary with the specific filter used and as a result of altered plasma protein binding in renal disease or due to critical illness. Information regarding dosing alterations for filtration procedures is available for some drugs. When it is not available, the amount of drug removed during SCUF, CAVH, or CVVH can be estimated by the equation:

$$\text{Estimated amount removed}_{(CVVH/CAVH)} = \frac{(Q_f)\,(SC)\,(C_{pss})\,(\tau)}{(S)\,(F)}$$

where Q_f is the ultrafiltration rate, SC is the sieving coefficient, C_{pss} is the desired steady state plasma concentration, τ is the dosing interval, S is the salt form of the drug, and F is the fraction absorbed. When the sieving coefficient is unknown, f_{up} (free fraction in plasma) can be substituted. Once the amount of drug removed for a given interval can be estimated a clinical decision can be made with regard to the necessity of a supplemental dose or alteration in the dosage regimen. Typically dosage alterations are necessary when more than 25% to 30% of a dose is being removed over the specific interval.

For procedures that utilize diffusion (CVVHD and CAVHD), or both diffusion and convection (CVVHDF and CAVHDF), the amount of drug removed depends on the relative amounts of dialysis and filtration, along with the specific filter, and the drug's characteristics. The primary factor correlating with degree of drug removal is rate of dialysis, with ultrafiltration rate secondarily contributing. Drug dosage recommendations for these types of procedures are not widely available and uniform recommendations are difficult to formulate due to the large variety of potential combinations of dialysis rate, ultrafiltration rate and available filters. Case reports or studies are useful for assisting with development of dosing recommendations for individual patients undergoing these procedures. When dosing information is not available, the amount of drug removed during CVVHD/CAVHD or CVVHDF/CAVHDF can be estimated by the following equations:

$$\text{Estimated amount removed}_{(CVVHD/CAVHD)} = \frac{(Q_{dial})\,(f_{up})\,(C_{pss})\,(\tau)}{(S)\,(F)}$$

$$\text{Estimated amount removed}_{(CVVHDF/CAVHDF)} = \frac{(Q_{dial} + Q_f)\,(f_{up})\,(C_{pss})\,(\tau)}{(S)\,(F)}$$

where Q_{dial} is the dialysate flow rate. As above, if the amount of drug removed is significant, an alteration in the dosage regimen to account for lost drug is necessary.

Close attention to a patient's CRRT therapy is needed for a number of reasons. The dialysis prescription should be evaluated to verify the presence of dialysis and or ultrafiltration, since terminologies for the procedures are often misused in the clinical setting. The dialysis prescription (dialysate rate, ultrafiltration rate) often changes frequently in order to adequately manage the patient's fluid, electrolyte, and hemodynamic status. Patency of the extracorporeal unit and the ability to continue dialysis is another challenge. Therefore, repeated alterations in drug dosing may be needed in order to best individualize the patient's pharmacotherapeutic regimen. Given the paucity of available information regarding drug dosing in CRRT, close monitoring of drug efficacy and safety is essential.

REFERENCES AND RECOMMENDED READING

Davenport A, "Anticoagulation for Continuous Renal Replacement Therapy," *Contrib Nephrol*, 2004, 144:228-38.

Joy MS, Matzke GR, Armstrong DK, et al, "A Primer on Continuous Renal Replacement Therapy for Critically Ill Patients," *Ann Pharmacother*, 1998, 32(3):362-75.

Heintz BH, Matzke GR, and Dager WE, "Antimicrobial Dosing Concepts and Recommendations for Critically Ill Adult Patients Receiving Continuous Renal Replacement Therapy or Intermittent Hemodialysis," *Pharmacotherapy*, 2009, 29(5):562-77.

Matzke GR and Frye RF, "Drug Therapy Individualization for Patients With Renal Insufficiency," *Pharmacotherapy: A Pathophysiologic Approach*, DiPiro JT, Talbert RL, Yee GC, et al, eds, 7th ed, New York, NY: McGraw-Hill Companies, 2008, 833-844.

Mueller BA, Pasko DA, and Sowinski KM, "Higher Renal Replacement Therapy Dose Delivery Influences on Drug Therapy," *Artif Organs*, 2003, 27(9):808-14.

Paganini EP, "Continuous Renal Replacement Therapy," *Critical Care Medicine: Principles of Diagnosis and Management in the Adult*, Parillo JE and Dellinger RP, eds, 2nd ed, St Louis, MO: Mosby, 2002, 270-94.

Pea F, Viale P, Pavan F, et al, "Pharmacokinetic Considerations for Antimicrobial Therapy in Patients Receiving Continuous Renal Replacement Therapy," *Clin Pharmacokinet*, 2007, 46(12):997-1038.

Schetz M, "Drug Dosing in Continuous Renal Replacement Therapy: General Rules," *Curr Opin Crit Care*, 2007, 13(6):645-51.

Trotman RL, Williamson JC, Shoemaker DM, et al, "Antibiotic Dosing in Critically Ill Adult Patients Receiving Continuous Renal Replacement Therapy," *Clin Infect Dis*, 2005, 41(8):1159-66.

DOSING CONSIDERATIONS FOR THE CRITICALLY-ILL PATIENT WITH MORBID OBESITY

Most recent estimates from the World Health Organization (WHO) report that approximately 32% of the U.S. population is considered obese, defined as a body mass index (BMI) of ≥30 kg/m^2. Patients with morbid obesity (Obese class III), defined by the WHO as a BMI ≥40 kg/m^2, are challenging to care for especially when critically ill. Although obese class II (BMI 35 to <40 kg/m^2) are commonly encountered, patients with morbid obesity require dosage adjustment to achieve similar therapeutic results. Patients at the extremes of body weight are seldom included within clinical trials, forcing the clinician to use knowledge of pharmacokinetic principles (eg, volume of distribution) to properly dose the morbidly obese patient. Many drugs (eg, vasopressors, inotropes, neuromuscular blockers) used in the ICU are adjusted based on immediate measurable patient responses; however, many drugs (eg, antibiotics, drotrecogin alfa, LMWHs) do not have this advantage and inadequate dosing may lead to treatment failure. In the critical situation, the need to give the right dose to achieve an optimal clinical response is paramount.

Table 1. The International Classification of Adult Overweight and Obesity According to BMI

Classification	BMI (kg/m^2)
Normal range	18.5-24.99
Overweight	≥25
Pre-obese	25-29.99
Obese	≥30
Obese class I	30-34.99
Obese class II	35-39.99
Obese class III	≥40

BMI = Body mass index; defined as weight in kilograms divided by height in meters squared.

IMPORTANT PHARMACOKINETIC CONSIDERATIONS

Several pharmacokinetic parameters are altered in the morbidly obese patient due to increases in cardiac output, blood volume, organ mass, lean body mass, and adipose tissue mass. Three pharmacokinetic parameters are affected by obesity are distribution, metabolism, and excretion.

DISTRIBUTION

Distribution is altered due to a higher ratio of body fat to lean tissue and body water. This becomes important for drugs with lipophilic properties (eg, fentanyl, diazepam). Generally, as the octanol/water *log* partition coefficient (LPC) of the drug increases, distribution into adipose tissue increases. Exceptions to this include cyclosporine, digoxin, procainamide, and remifentanil. These agents may be highly lipophilic and have a high volume of distribution (V_d) but they are not significantly influenced by obesity. Therefore, it is not always possible to devise straightforward dosing schemes using volume of distribution alone. Clinical trials in obese and normal weight patients are necessary to determine whether or not the expected distribution for a particular drug actually occurs in the obese patient.

METABOLISM

Data on the relationship between obesity (especially morbid obesity) and alterations in drug metabolism/transport are inconclusive; however, evidence supports alterations in cytochrome P450 enzyme activity in the obese patient. CYP2E1 activity is increased and CYP3A4 and CYP1A activity may be decreased or unchanged. The effect of obesity on other CYP450 enzymes remains unclear. In general, increased glucuronidation and sulfation activity may occur with some drugs (eg, lorazepam) requiring more frequent administration of maintenance doses. Determinants of drug disposition may be altered in obesity, but the specific direction and magnitude of any such change is, at present, unclear. Increased monitoring seems prudent.

EXCRETION

Glomerular filtration rate (GFR) may be higher in patients who are obese compared to normal weight patients. It has been demonstrated that obese (BMI ≥30 kg/m^2) kidney donors have a significantly higher glomerular planar surface area compared to those kidneys of nonobese donors. Drugs dependant on GFR for excretion (eg, aminoglycosides) have been shown to have higher clearance rates in the obese patient. Therefore, maintenance dosing may be more frequent for agents which rely on glomerular filtration for excretion.

Although the Cockcroft-Gault formula used to estimate creatinine clearance (Cl_{Cr}) is the predominant equation used in clinical practice, choice of weight will often underestimate (eg, IBW) or overestimate (eg, TBW) Cl_{Cr}. The most precise formula estimation of Cl_{Cr} in the obese patient is the Salazar-Corcoran formula; however, this formula has not been validated in a large sample of obese subjects. The Modification of Diet in Renal Disease (MDRD) formula, although it does not incorporate weight, also has not been validated in a large sample of obese subjects. Of note, the result obtained with the MDRD equation may not correlate with Cl_{Cr} cutoffs for dosage adjustment for many drugs since evaluation of renal function for these agents used the Cockcroft-Gault formula to develop dosing regimens in patients with renal impairment. Use of a timed 24-hour urine collection may be a more accurate method to determine Cl_{Cr}. Recently, the three equations used to determine glomerular filtration (GFR)/Cl_{Cr} were compared to results obtained using a timed 24-hour urine collection in morbidly obese patients. Use of the MDRD and IBW in the Cockcroft-Gault equation both underestimated Cl_{Cr}. The Salazar-Corcoran equation and the use of TBW or adjusted body weight (AdjBW) in the Cockcroft-Gault equation overestimated Cl_{Cr}. The authors concluded that the use of a lean body weight (LBW) estimate (see Table 2) based on TBW and BMI incorporated into the Cockcroft-Gault equation provides a relatively precise and accurate estimate of 24-hour measured Cl_{Cr} in morbidly obese patients.

DOSING MODIFICATIONS IN THE OBESE PATIENT

The importance of achieving similar concentrations in the critically ill obese patient as compared to the normal weight patient is imperative. However, dosing agents is not straightforward and requires pharmacokinetic evaluations in this patient population to define the optimal dose or dosing weight that should be used to determine an optimal dose for a particular agent. Many evaluations of this kind have been done but more clinical trials still need to be done. A summary of recommendations from various sources has been devised to assist the clinician in determining the most appropriate dosing weight or dosing strategy for this patient population (see Table 3). Equations for different body weight calculations are noted below.

Table 2. Body Weight Calculations

Ideal Body Weight (IBW)[1]	Male: 50 + (2.3 x height in inches over 5 feet) Female: 45.5 + (2.3 x height in inches over 5 feet)
Lean Body Weight (LBW)[1,2]	Male: (9270 x TBW)/(6680 + 216 x BMI) Female: (9270 x TBW)/(8780 + 244 x BMI)
Adjusted Body Weight (AdjBW) or Dosing Weight (DW)[1,3]	AdjBW or DW = IBW + 0.4 (TBW − IBW)

BMI = body mass index in kg/m^2; TBW = total body weight

[1]IBW, LBW, AdjBW, and DW are in kilograms

[2]Janmahasatian S, Duffull SB, Ash S, et al, "Quantification of Lean Bodyweight," *Clin Pharmacokinet,* 2005, 44(10):1051-65.

[3]The difference between TBW and IBW is multiplied by a factor between 0.2-0.5. The factor most often used is 0.4; however, this may be modified for certain drugs (eg, ciprofloxacin).

Table 3. Selected Agents and Recommended Dosing Strategies in the Obese Patient

Drug	Recommendation for Dosing in Obese Patients	
	Loading Dose	**Maintenance Dose[1]**
Analgesics		
Fentanyl	Use TBW	Use: 0.8 x IBW; titrate to pain control
Morphine	Use IBW	Use IBW; titrate to pain control
Remifentanil	Use IBW	Use IBW; titrate to pain control
Sufentanil	Use TBW	Use: 0.8 x IBW; titrate to pain control
Antiarrhythmics		
Amiodarone	Use IBW or standard dose	IBW or standard dose
Lidocaine	Use TBW	IBW, standard infusion rate
Procainamide	Use IBW	Use IBW, standard infusion rate
Antibiotics		
Acyclovir	NA	IBW
Aminoglycosides[2]	Use IBW + 0.4 (TBW − IBW)	Use IBW + 0.4 (TBW − IBW)
Cefazolin	Surgical prophylaxis: 2 g prior to induction	Not established
Ciprofloxacin	NA	Use IBW + 0.45 (TBW − IBW) or 800 mg q12h
Daptomycin	NA	Use TBW; concentrations expected to be higher; monitor closely for skeletal muscle toxicity
Fluconazole	NA	Prudent to use higher doses; none established[3]
Flucytosine	NA	Use IBW
Linezolid	NA	Use standard dosing
Meropenem	NA	Use standard dosing[4]
Quinupristin / Dalfopristin	NA	Use TBW
Vancomycin	Use TBW	Use TBW; may require more frequent dosing
Anticoagulants		
Argatroban	NA	Use TBW (BMI <51 kg/m^2)
Enoxaparin (and other LMWHs)	Use TBW	Use TBW; monitor anti-Xa levels (if available) in patients >190 kg
Heparin	Not established	Not established; titrate to aPTT results
Antiepileptics		
Phenytoin	Use: DW = IBW + 1.33 x (TBW − IBW) or may give 14 mg/kg (IBW) + 19 mg/kg for weight in excess of IBW (maximum dose: 2 g)	Use IBW; monitor levels
Beta-Blockers		
Esmolol	Use IBW	Individualize
Labetalol	Use IBW or standard dose	Individualize
Metoprolol	Use IBW or standard dose	Individualize

Table 3. Selected Agents and Recommended Dosing Strategies in the Obese Patient (continued)

Drug	Recommendation for Dosing in Obese Patients	
	Loading Dose	Maintenance Dose[1]
Calcium Channel Blockers		
Diltiazem	Use TBW or standard dose	Individualize
Verapamil	Use TBW or standard dose	Individualize
Neuromuscular Blocking Agents[5]		
Atracurium	Use TBW	Use TBW
Rocuronium	Use IBW	Use IBW
Succinylcholine	Use TBW	NA
Vecuronium	Use IBW	Use IBW
Sedative / Hypnotic		
Etomidate	Use TBW	NA
Ketamine	Use IBW	Use IBW
Propofol	Use DW = IBW + 0.4 (TBW – IBW)	Use DW = IBW + 0.4 (TBW – IBW)
Thiopental	Use TBW	Use IBW
Other Agents		
Adenosine	Use IBW; standard dose	NA
Digoxin	Use IBW	NA
Drotrecogin alfa	NA	Use TBW
Rasburicase	NA	Use IBW

BMI = body mass index; DW = dosing weight; IBW = ideal body weight; NA = not applicable; TBW = total body weight.

[1]If therapeutic drug monitoring is available, it is recommended that this be done in all patients who are morbidly obese.

[2]Use once daily dosing regimens with caution in the morbidly obese patient as adequate studies have not been conducted in this patient population.

[3]It has been recommended that fluconazole be dosed using 6 mg/kg/day using TBW.

[4]May require higher doses for multi-drug resistant organisms.

[5]Monitor clinical effects, peripheral nerve stimulation.

REFERENCES

Arnold TM, Reuter JP, Delman BS, et al, "Use of Single-Dose Rasburicase in an Obese Female," *Ann Pharmacother*, 2004, 38(9):1428-31.

Bearden DT and Rodvold KA, "Dosage Adjustments for Antibacterials in Obese Patients: Applying Clinical Pharmacokinetics," *Clin Pharmacokinet*, 2000, 38(5):415-26.

Blouin RA, Bauer LA, Miller DD, et al, "Vancomycin Pharmacokinetics in Normal and Morbidly Obese Subjects," *Antimicrob Agents Chemother*, 1982, 21(4):575-80.

Blouin RA and Ensom MHH, "Special Pharmacokinetic Considerations in the Obese," *Applied Pharmacokinetics & Pharmacodynamics*, 4th ed, Burton ME, Shaw LE, Schentag JJ, et al, eds, Baltimore, MD: Lippincott Williams & Wilkins, 2006, 231-241.

Brunette DD, "Resuscitation of the Morbidly Obese Patient," *Am J Emerg Med*, 2004, 22(1):40-7.

Cheymol G, "Effects of Obesity on Pharmacokinetics Implications for Drug Therapy," *Clin Pharmacokinet*, 2000, 39(3):215-31.

Demirovic JA, Pai AB, and Pai MP, "Estimation of Creatinine Clearance in Morbidly Obese Patients," *Am J Health Syst Pharm*, 2009, 66(7):642-8.

Dvorchik BH and Damphousse D, "The Pharmacokinetics of Daptomycin in Moderately Obese, Morbidly Obese, and Matched Nonobese Subjects," *J Clin Pharmacol*, 2005, 45(1):48-56.

Erstad BL, "Dosing of Medications in Morbidly Obese Patients in the Intensive Care Unit Setting," *Intensive Care Med*, 2004, 30(1):18-32.

Galletti F, Fasano ML, Ferrara LA, et al, "Obesity and Beta-Blockers: Influence of Body Fat on Their Kinetics and Cardiovascular Effects," *J Clin Pharmacol*, 1989, 29(3):212-6.

Hernandez JO, Norstrom J, and Wysock G, "Acyclovir-Induced Renal Failure in an Obese Patient," *Am J Health Syst Pharm*, 2009, 66(14):1288-91.

Kotlyar M and Carson SW, "Effects of Obesity on the Cytochrome P450 Enzyme System," *Int J Clin Pharmacol Ther*, 1999, 37(1):8-19.

Levy H, Small D, Heiselman DE, et al, "Obesity Does Not Alter the Pharmacokinetics of Drotrecogin Alfa (Activated) in Severe Sepsis," *Ann Pharmacother*, 2005, 39(2):262-7.

Leykin Y, Pellis T, Lucca M, et al, "The Pharmacodynamic Effects of Rocuronium When Dosed According to Real Body Weight or Ideal Body Weight in Morbidly Obese Patients," *Anesth Analg*, 2004, 99(4):1086-9.

Meyhoff CS, Lund J, Jenstrup MT, et al, "Should Dosing of Rocuronium in Obese Patients be Based on Ideal or Corrected Body Weight?" *Anesth Analg*, 2009, 109(3):787-92.

Nutescu EA, Spinler SA, Wittkowsky A, et al, "Low-Molecular-Weight Heparins in Renal Impairment and Obesity: Available Evidence and Clinical Practice Recommendations Across Medical and Surgical Settings," *Ann Pharmacother*, 2009, 43(6):1064-83.

Pai MP and Bearden DT, "Antimicrobial Ddosing Considerations in Obese Adult Patients," *Pharmacotherapy*, 2007, 27(8):1081-91.

Penzak SR, Gubbins PO, Rodvold KA, et al, "Therapeutic Drug Monitoring of Vancomycin in a Morbidly Obese Patient," *Ther Drug Monit*, 1998, 20(3):261-5.

Rea DJ, Heimbach JK, Grande JP, et al, "Glomerular Volume and Renal Histology in Obese and Nonobese Living Kidney Donors," *Kidney Int*, 2006, 70(9):1636-41.

Rex JH, Bennett JE, Sugar AM, et al, "A Randomized Trial Comparing Fluconazole With Amphotericin B for the Treatment of Candidemia in Patients Without Neutropenia. Candidemia Study Group and the National Institute," *N Engl J Med*, 1994, 331(20):1325-30.

Rice L, Hursting MJ, Baillie GM, et al, "Argatroban Anticoagulation in Obese Versus Nonobese Patients: Implications for Treating Heparin-Induced Thrombocytopenia," *J Clin Pharmacol*, 2007, 47 (8):1028-34.

Roberts JA and Lipman J, "Pharmacokinetic Issues for Antibiotics in the Critically Ill Patient," *Crit Care Med*, 2009, 37(3):840-51.

Poirier P, Alpert MA, Fleisher LA, et al, "Cardiovascular Evaluation and Management of Severely Obese Patients Undergoing Surgery: A Science Advisory From the American Heart Association," *Circulation*, 2009, 120(1):86-95.

Salazar DE and Corcoran GB, "Predicting Creatinine Clearance and Renal Drug Clearance in Obese Patients From Estimated Fat-Free Body Mass," *Am J Med*, 1988, 84(6):1053-60.

Servin F, Farinotti R, Haberer JP, et al, "Propofol Infusion for Maintenance of Anesthesia in Morbidly Obese Patients Receiving Nitrous Oxide. A Clinical and Pharmacokinetic Study," *Anesthesiology*, 1993, 78(4):657-65.

Stein GE, Schooley SL, Peloquin CA, et al, "Pharmacokinetics and Pharmacodynamics of Linezolid in Obese Patients With Cellulitis," *Ann Pharmacother*, 2005, 39(3):427-32.

Vance-Bryan K, Guay DR, Gilliland SS, et al, "Effect of Obesity on Vancomycin Pharmacokinetic Parameters as Determined by Using a Bayesian Forecasting Technique," *Antimicrob Agents Chemother*, 1993, 37(3):436-40.

MODERATE SEDATION

The goal of moderate sedation is to produce a state where: 1) patients are able to tolerate and successfully complete unpleasant procedures; 2) adequate cardiorespiratory function is maintained; 3) patients are able to respond purposefully to verbal commands and/or tactile stimulation; 4) the risks of adverse events from the sedation and analgesia are minimal; and 5) there is a rapid return to a state of consciousness that allows for safe discharge. Progression from light sedation to general anesthesia is a continuum, with no clear division between levels. Nearly all drugs administered for moderate sedation could induce a state of deep sedation or general anesthesia (where protective airway reflexes are lost). This could occur when these drugs are administered in high doses, in combination with one another, or at a point during the procedure when drug effects are maximal but stimulation from the procedure has stopped.

Practitioners who are not anesthesia professionals (eg, licensed physicians, dentists, podiatrists) should have appropriate education and training before being permitted to supervise the administration of moderate sedation. The formal training program should include presedation evaluation, the safe use of sedative/analgesic drugs, appropriate monitoring so as to maintain the patient at the desired level of sedation, and techniques and methods for rescuing patients who experience adverse consequences of a deeper-than-intended level of sedation. Once licensure, training, and competency are demonstrated, medical staff privileges to administer and supervise moderate sedation can be granted. If the sedation practitioner is the person performing the procedure, he or she should not administer the sedation for the procedure. Instead, he or she should supervise a sedation professional (a licensed registered nurse, advanced practice nurse, or physician assistant) who has been trained to administer sedative/analgesic drugs, document, and monitor the patient.

PATIENT EVALUATION

A preprocedural evaluation, including a relevant patient history and pertinent physical exam to assess risks and comorbidities should be performed. The patient's preprocedural evaluation should also include a presedation evaluation and plan. Elements include:

- Chief complaint/present illness
- Relevant medical, surgical, family, and social history
- Medications
- Allergies
- Pregnancy status, if appropriate
- Previous sedation or anesthetics, including complications experienced
- Family history of anesthetic difficulties
- Time/nature of last oral intake (eg, clear liquids >2-3 hours, solids >6-8 hours)
- Weight and vital signs (pulse, blood pressure, respiratory rate, temperature, oxygen saturation)
- ASA classification
- Cardiopulmonary examination and examination of relevant body systems and any relevant findings
- Evaluation of the patient's airway, including assessing dentition, ability to open the mouth, and flex/extend the neck

The nonanesthesia sedation professional explains the options and risks of sedation and analgesia, then obtains informed consent. The practitioner must be able to recognize patients whose airway management and/or medical condition suggests that sedation should be provided by an anesthesia professional. If the sedation is being performed in an area where an individual with advanced life support skills (eg, code team) is not immediately (≤5 minutes) available, the nonanesthesia sedation profession should have Advanced Cardiac Life Support (ACLS) and, if appropriate, Pediatric Advanced Life Support (PALS) certification.

SEDATION AND ANALGESIA PLAN

A sedation and analgesia plan must be developed and communicated to the patient, family, and other healthcare providers involved with the procedure as well as be documented in the patient's medical record. The plan should be re-evaluated immediately prior to beginning sedation and analgesia.

MONITORING

Monitoring of the patient during moderate sedation is necessary to assure adequacy of oxygenation, circulation, and level of consciousness during the procedure. Monitoring and recognizing abnormalities of physiologic variables should include:

- Depth of sedation
- Blood pressure, heart rate, respiratory rate, and oxygen saturation
- Temperature, pre- and postprocedure
- ECG for ASA class III or IV patients
- Consider using capnography if moderate sedation is administered in a setting where the patients ventilatory function cannot be directly monitored

Minimally, the patient's hemodynamic variables (heart rate, blood pressure), ventilatory status (respiratory rate), and oxygenation status (pulse oximetry) should be obtained and documented before the administration of sedative/analgesic agents at regular intervals during the procedure and throughout recovery until discharge. All physiologic monitors should have appropriately set audible alarms that are used continuously during the sedation period. The drugs administered should be documented at regular intervals throughout the sedation period. Finally, the level of consciousness should be assessed and documented throughout the sedation and recovery period until the patient is no longer at risk for respiratory depression.

Signs and symptoms of toxicity associated with sedation/analgesia include deep sedation, somnolence, confusion, respiratory depression, apnea, respiratory arrest, hypotension, cardiac arrest, nausea and vomiting, diminished reflexes, impaired coordination, and severe changes in vital signs.

It is critical that an appropriately trained individual other than the person performing the procedure be present to continuously monitor the patient throughout the procedure and the recovery period.

EQUIPMENT REQUIREMENTS

The following equipment and supplies should be present or readily available (within or adjacent to the procedure room):

- Oxygen source and oxygen administration equipment of various types and sizes (eg, nasal cannula, facemask)
- Suction apparatus with vacuum capability
- Emergency airway equipment (variety of laryngoscope blades and handles, oral and nasal airways, and various sizes of endotracheal tubes with stylets)
- A self-inflating positive-pressure oxygen delivery system (eg, Ambu or other resuscitation bag)
- Emergency drugs for cardiopulmonary arrest (eg, drugs recommended in the current ACLS guidelines)
- Pharmacologic antagonists (eg, naloxone for opioids, flumazenil for benzodiazepines)
- Intravenous equipment; for patients receiving drugs intravenously, I.V. access should be maintained throughout the whole procedure and until the patient is not at risk for serious adverse events from the drugs administered (eg, cardiorespiratory depression)
- Pulse oximetry
- Noninvasive blood pressure equipment

- Electrocardiogram
- Thermometer or equivalent device for measuring temperature
- In areas credentialed for inhalational sedation with nitrous oxide: Inhalation delivery systems capable of delivering 100% oxygen and never less than 25% oxygen
- Telephone

AGENT SELECTION / DOSE TITRATION

Sedatives (eg, midazolam, chloral hydrate) are routinely used to decrease anxiety and promote somnolence. Analgesics (eg, morphine, fentanyl) are routinely used to relieve pain. Combinations of opioids and sedatives may increase the incidence of adverse effects.

When given intravenously, sedative/analgesic drugs should be administered in small, incremental doses until the desired effect is achieved (titrated to effect). Please refer to the individual drug monographs for appropriate dosing guidelines. Care must be taken to allow a sufficient time between doses to allow the effect of each dose to be seen. Dosage reductions are often required in the chronically ill or elderly as well as with the concomitant administration of an opioid and sedative agent (eg, benzodiazepine). Additional time should be allowed between doses when drugs are administered by nonintravenous routes (eg, oral, rectal, I.M.) secondary to the time required for drug absorption.

In selected centers, propofol may be approved for use in moderate sedation. Due to its potential for cardiorespiratory depression, propofol warrants special precautions for dosing and usage. Propofol's rapid onset and short duration of action often allow patients to wake up, recover, and return to baseline activities and diet sooner than some of the other sedation agents. However, profound changes in level of consciousness, as well as respiratory and hemodynamic status can occur quickly and without warning. Propofol should be administered for moderate sedation only by a person who is: 1) trained in administration of drugs that produce general anesthesia; 2) able to intubate the patient if necessary; and 3) not involved in performing the procedure itself.

RECOVERY

Patients may continue to be at risk for complications after the procedure and must be monitored (level of consciousness, vital signs, respiratory function) throughout the recovery period until meeting discharge criteria. If a reversal agent has been administered, an appropriate time (up to 2 hours) should have elapsed to ensure that resedation does not occur secondary to the reversal agent's short duration of action when compared to the sedation/analgesia agent's duration of action. Inpatients should be recovered adequately until they can safely return to their preprocedure level of care and monitoring. Outpatients must be discharged to the care of a responsible adult. The patient and accompanying adult should be given verbal and written postprocedural instructions.

QUALITY ASSURANCE

Any unanticipated or unintentional occurrences or adverse drug reactions should be reported via the quality assurance program in place for moderate sedation. These events should be monitored on a regular basis, with an independent expert review when necessary. Ongoing evaluation of sedation practitioner performances and patient outcomes is necessary for performance improvement and patient safety.

Agents for Moderate Sedation in Adults

Medication	Onset of Action	Duration of Action	Adult Dose	Reversal Agent	Comments
Dexmedetomidine	I.V.: 5-10 min	I.V.: 1-2 h (dose dependent)	I.V.: 0.5-1 mcg/kg over 10 min, then 0.2-1 mcg/kg/h	None	Hypertension, hypotension, bradycardia, arrhythmias
Diazepam	P.O.15-30 min I.V.: 3-10 min	P.O./I.V.: 6-8 h	P.O.: 10 mg I.V.: 2-5 mg Repeat dosage q10min prn; Max: 0.1-0.2 mg/kg (10 mg)	Flumazenil	
Fentanyl	I.V.: 1-2 min	I.V.: 30-60 min	I.V.: 25-50 mcg Repeat dosage q3-5min prn; Max: 500 mcg/4 h	Naloxone	
Flumazenil	I.V.: 1-2 min	I.V.: 1-2 h	I.V.: 0.2 mg Repeat dosage q1min prn; Max: 1 mg		Reversal agent for BZD
Lorazepam	I.V.: 5-10 min P.O.: 20-30 min	I.V.: 4-6 h P.O.: 6-8 h	Slow I.V.: 0.5-2 mg P.O.: 2 mg Repeat dosage q20min prn; Max: 4 mg	Flumazenil	Hypotension and bradycardia with fast injection
Methohexital	Immediate	I.V.: 10-20 min	50-120 mg Repeat 20-40 mg q4-7min prn	None	Use with caution if CV instability, severe liver disease, or asthma
Midazolam	I.V.: 1-5 min	I.V.: 30-120 min	<60 y: Slow I.V.: 1-2 mg Repeat dosage q2min prn; Max: 0.1 mg/kg (10 mg)/h >60 y or debilitated: I.V.: 0.5 mg Repeat dosage q3min prn; Max: 0.05 mg/kg (5 mg)/h	Flumazenil	Hypotension and bradycardia with fast injection
Morphine	I.V.: 5-10 min I.M.: 3-7 h	I.V.: 2-4 h	I.V.: 1-2 mg Repeat dosage q3-5min prn; Max: 20 mg	Naloxone	Hypotension due to histamine release
Naloxone	I.V.: 1-2 min	I.V.: 30-60 min	I.V.: 40-100 mcg Repeat dosage q2-3min prn; Max: 2 mg		Reversal agent for opioids

REFERENCES AND RECOMMENDED READING

American Academy of Pediatrics; American Academy of Pediatric Dentistry, Coté CJ, et al, "Guidelines for Monitoring and Management of Pediatric Patients During and After Sedation for Diagnostic and Therapeutic Procedures: An Update," *Pediatrics*, 2006, 118(6):2587-602.

American Society of Anesthesiologists, "Statement on Granting Privileges for Administration of Moderate Sedation to Practitioners Who Are Not Anesthesia Professionals, " 2006. Available at: http://www.asahq.org/publicationsAndServices/standards/40.pdf. Last accessed December 20, 2007.

Cravero JP and Blike GT, "Review of Pediatric Sedation," *Anesth Analg*, 2004, 99(5):1355-64.

Godwin SA, Caro DA, Wolf SJ, et al, "Clinical Policy: Procedural Sedation and Analgesia in the Emergency Department," *Ann Emerg Med*, 2005, 45(2):177-96.

Krauss B and Green SM, "Procedural Sedation and Analgesia in Children," *Lancet*, 2006, 367 (9512):766-80.

"Practice Guidelines for Sedation and Analgesia by Non-Anesthesiologists. An Updated Report by the American Society of Anesthesiologist Task Force on Sedation and Analgesia by Non-anesthesiologists," *Anesthesiology*, 2002, 96(4):1004-17.

MANAGEMENT OF POSTOPERATIVE ARRHYTHMIAS

Arrhythmias commonly occur in the postoperative setting and can contribute to patient morbidity and mortality. Postoperative supraventricular arrhythmias have been reported to occur in 3% to 13% of patients, depending on the surgical procedure. After cardiac surgery, atrial flutter and fibrillation occur in an even higher incidence (12% to 60%). Patients with structural heart disease are most likely to experience arrhythmias in the postoperative setting. The duration of the arrhythmia, ventricular response rate, and the patient's underlying cardiac function are several of the factors that contribute to the physiologic consequences of an arrhythmia.

CLASSIFICATION OF ARRHYTHMIAS

Arrhythmias can be broadly grouped into bradyarrhythmias and tachyarrhythmias. Tachyarrhythmias are further divided by anatomical origin as either supraventricular or ventricular. Table 1 lists common supraventricular and ventricular arrhythmias. Further classifying tachyarrhythmias into those that do and do not traverse the atrioventricular (AV) node (Table 1) is useful when determining appropriate treatment. For example, pharmacologic agents that slow AV node conduction can be used to control the ventricular response if the arrhythmia traverses the AV node.

Table 1. Common Supraventricular and Ventricular Arrhythmias

BRADYARRHYTHMIAS

    Sinus bradycardia

    Sinoatrial (SA) block

    Sinus pause

    Sinus arrest (slow junctional rhythm)

TACHYARRHYTHMIAS

Supraventricular Arrhythmias

    Sinus tachycardia[1]

    Atrial flutter[1]

    Atrial fibrillation[1]

    Automatic (ectopic) atrial tachycardia[1]

    Multifocal atrial tachycardia[1]

    Junctional tachycardia

    Atrioventricular nodal re-entrant tachycardias[1]

    Atrioventricular reciprocating tachycardias[1]

Ventricular Arrhythmias

    Premature ventricular beats

    Ventricular tachycardia

    Ventricular fibrillation

[1]Traverse the AV node.

PREDISPOSING FACTORS

Factors that predispose patients to postoperative arrhythmias can be found in Table 2. Risk factors for development of atrial fibrillation following open heart surgery include advanced age, obesity, previous cardiac surgery, history of atrial fibrillation, COPD, rheumatic heart disease, heart failure, absence of or discontinuation of preoperative beta-blocker therapy, preoperative use of digoxin, pulmonary vein venting, prolonged cross-clamp time, bicaval venous cannulation, and postoperative atrial pacing. In the postoperative setting, factors that decrease sympathetic or increase parasympathetic activity can lead to sinus bradycardia (Table 3). Severe hypoxemia, SA nodal ischemia, and sick sinus syndrome can also reduce sinus rate. Postoperative ventricular tachycardia or fibrillation usually reflects severe myocardial ischemia, systemic acidemia, or hypoxemia.

The genesis of arrhythmias can be multifactorial; caution should be taken not to attribute an arrhythmia to a single factor without fully considering the potential for multiple factors to be at play.

Table 2. Factors Predisposing Patients to Postoperative Arrhythmias

Myocardial ischemia	Acid-base imbalance
Endogenous or exogenous catecholamines	Electrolyte abnormalities
Hypoxemia	Mechanical factors
Hypercarbia	Administration of select medications
Preoperative arrhythmia (eg, atrial fibrillation)	

Table 3. Factors Predisposing Patients to Sinus Bradycardia

Decrease Sympathetic Activity

High epidural or spinal anesthesia

Severe acidemia/hypoxemia

Withdrawal of stimulus

Emptying bladder

Sympatholytic medications (eg, beta-blockers, opioids, local anesthetics)

Increase Parasympathetic Activity

Increased vagal tone

Carotid sinus massage

Valsalva maneuver

Gagging

Increased ocular pressure

Bladder distension

Pharyngeal stimulation

Anxiety/pain (centrally mediated response)

Surgery (eg, traction on peritoneum during vascular surgery)

Parasympathomimetic medications (eg, acetylcholinesterase inhibitors, alpha-adrenergic drugs, opioids, succinylcholine)

PRINCIPLES / GOALS OF TREATMENT

Several principles must be kept in mind when managing patients with postoperative arrhythmias. The most important is to treat the patient and not the electrocardiogram (EKG). Questions one should ask include whether an arrhythmia is truly present (vs an artifact) and whether the rhythm seen on the EKG can account for the patient's condition. The urgency for treatment should then be decided. Items such as the patient's pulse, blood pressure, peripheral perfusion, and the presence of myocardial ischemia and congestive heart failure should be evaluated. For example, prompt electrical cardioversion is indicated in a patient who becomes unconscious or hemodynamically unstable in the presence of a tachyarrhythmia (excluding sinus tachycardia). Treatment should also be instituted if the arrhythmia is a precursor of a more severe arrhythmia. The type of arrhythmia will dictate the goals of therapy. Foremost is the need to establish hemodynamic stability. For tachyarrhythmias, attention is first given to slowing the ventricular response whereas with bradyarrhythmias, the ventricular rate must be increased. Once the patient is hemodynamically stable, restoration of sinus rhythm becomes the goal. If this is not possible, the focus should shift to preventing complications from occurring. In patients without overt cardiac disease, therapy of self-terminating arrhythmias is often not needed.

TREATMENT

Table 4. Common Drugs Used for Postoperative Arrhythmias

Drug	Dose	Indications	Adverse Reactions
Adenosine	6 mg rapid IVP (over 1-2 seconds); if no response within 1-2 minutes then 12 mg IVP; may repeat 12 mg dose if needed	PSVT	Transient heart block, facial flushing, chest pain, hypotension
Amiodarone	150 mg I.V. over 10 minutes, then 1 mg/minute over 6 hours, then 0.5 mg/minute; VF/pulseless VT: 300 mg in 20-30 mL D_5W or NS IVP	VT or VF; rate control AF or A flutter	Hypotension, bradycardia, exacerbation of CHF, QT prolongation, AV nodal arrhythmias
Atropine	0.5-1 mg I.V. every 5 minutes, not to exceed a total of 3 mg or 0.04 mg/kg	Bradycardia or AV block	Excessive tachycardia, myocardial ischemia
Digoxin	Total digitalizing dose (TDD): 0.5-1 mg or 10-15 mcg/kg IBW; Give ½ of the TDD as the initial dose, then give ¼ of the TDD as two separate subsequent doses at 6- to 8-hour intervals	Rate control	Arrhythmias, nausea, vomiting
Diltiazem	0.25 mg/kg I.V. over 2 minutes (20 mg average adult dose); if inadequate response after 15 minutes, 0.35 mg/kg I.V. over 2 minutes (25 mg average adult dose); maintenance infusion: 5-15 mg/hour	Rate control	Hypotension, bradycardia, dizziness, exacerbation of CHF, headache
Esmolol	500 mcg/kg I.V. over 1 minute, followed by infusion of 50 mcg/kg/minute; if inadequate response, repeat bolus after 5 minutes and increase infusion by 50 mcg/kg/minute; infusion can be titrated to 300 mcg/kg/minute	Rapid rate control	Hypotension, nausea, dizziness, exacerbation of CHF, bronchospasm (dose >300 mcg/kg/minute)
Ibutilide	1 mg (0.01 mg/kg if <60 kg) I.V. over 10 minutes, may repeat 10 minutes after end of initial infusion	Conversion of AF	QT prolongation, torsade de pointes, headache, hypotension
Lidocaine	1-1.5 mg/kg IVP over 1-1.5 minutes followed by infusion of 1-4 mg/minute (15-50 mcg/kg/minute), repeat bolus of 0.5-1 mg/kg may be required 5-30 minutes after initial bolus	PVBs; VT or VF	CNS toxicity (eg, confusion, paresthesias, tremor, ataxia, seizures), sinus arrest
Metoprolol	5 mg IVP over 1 minute, repeat every 5 minutes for 3 doses	Rate control	Bronchospasm, hypotension, exacerbation of CHF
Procainamide	15-18 mg/kg (12 mg/kg in patients with severe renal insufficiency) (eg, Cl_{cr} <30 mL/minute) I.V. over 25-30 minutes or 100-200 mg/dose every 5 minutes as needed to a total dose of 1 g; maintenance infusion of 1-6 mg/minute	VT; ventricular premature beats; AF or A flutter	Hypotension, QT prolongation, torsade de pointes, headache

IVP = intravenous push; CHF = congestive heart failure; IBW = ideal body weight; AV = atrioventricular; PSVT = paroxysmal supraventricular tachycardia; AF = atrial fibrillation; A flutter = atrial flutter; VT = ventricular tachycardia; VF = ventricular fibrillation; PVB = premature ventricular beat; Cl_{cr} = creatinine clearance

Bradycardia

Treatment of bradycardia centers on the elimination of factors causing autonomic nervous system imbalance. For example, if bradycardia is due to increased vagal tone, the provoking stimulus should be discontinued. No treatment is necessary if the bradycardia is transient and not associated with hemodynamic compromise. If hypotension occurs, atropine or beta-mimetic medications should be used to restore sinus rhythm. Cardiac pacing may be necessary in some patients.

Heart Block

Treatment for first-degree heart block is not necessary in the absence of hypotension or severe bradycardia. Treatment for Mobitz type I block is necessary only if bundle branch block, bradycardia, or congestive heart failure occurs. Transvenous pacing may be required. The use of a pacemaker is required for a Mobitz type II block as it may progress to complete heart block. Postoperative patients with high grade second- or third-degree atrioventricular block persisting for >7-14 days should be considered for permanent pacemaker implantation.

Sinus Tachycardia

Sinus tachycardia is common postoperatively, is nearly always associated with a physiologic increase in sympathetic nervous system influence, and is usually harmless. Common causes in the postoperative setting include pain, fever, anxiety, hypovolemia, hypoxemia, anemia, and medications. Treatment should be directed at the underlying cause and not the rhythm. For example, I.V. fluids can be administered for hypovolemia, sedatives for anxiety, and analgesics for pain. If the tachycardia constitutes a risk for myocardial ischemia, continuous use of a beta-blocker may be indicated.

Paroxysmal Supraventricular Tachycardia

AV nodal reentry is the most common paroxysmal supraventricular tachycardia. Sinus rhythm may be restored with carotid sinus massage or other vagal maneuvers. Adenosine is the initial drug of choice for this condition secondary to its short half-life (3-10 seconds) which minimizes its side effect potential. In the presence of circulatory insufficiency, cardioversion may be necessary. Beta-blockers or calcium channel blockers can also be used for this arrhythmia. Caution should be used when administering beta-blockers or calcium channel blockers to patients with PSVT and wide complex or delta waves as they may be at risk for rapid ventricular response secondary to conduction down the accessory pathway.

Atrial Premature Beats

Atrial premature beats occur when ectopic foci in the atria fire before the next expected impulse from the sinus node. The presence of these beats is common, benign (do not cause hemodynamic compromise), and usually requires no treatment.

Atrial Fibrillation

Prophylaxis. A beta-blocker should be administered preoperatively and continued postoperatively for patients undergoing CABG surgery unless contraindicated. In patients at high risk for postoperative atrial fibrillation, the addition of amiodarone or sotalol may provide additional benefit. Evidence that these agents routinely reduce hospital length of stay and overall cost is currently lacking. However, one meta-analysis demonstrated a 1 ± 0.2 day overall decrease in hospital stay (p <0.001) (Zimmer, 2003).

Treatment. In postsurgical patients who are hemodynamically unstable, direct current cardioversion (DCC) should be performed. In hemodynamically stable patients, the ventricular rate should be controlled with pharmacologic agents; digoxin is appropriate for mildly symptomatic patients. An intravenous beta-blocker or diltiazem should be used when faster ventricular rate control is needed (eg, symptomatic patient). Digoxin is the least effective and beta-blockers are the most effective for controlling ventricular response during atrial fibrillation. If patient does not spontaneously convert to sinus rhythm in ≤48 hours, anticoagulation with heparin should be considered. Ibutilide can be used to pharmacologically convert the patient to normal sinus rhythm. If pharmacologic conversion is not successful, DCC should be performed; it is not necessary to have the post-CABG patient anticoagulated for 3 weeks prior to attempting DCC if done within 48 hours of onset.

Atrial Flutter

Atrial flutter is rare in postoperative patients. It is managed similar to atrial fibrillation, with some differences. Rapid atrial pacing may be effective in terminating the atrial flutter, especially when combined with a class IA antiarrhythmic agent. Care must be taken when using antiarrhythmic agents because sufficient slowing of the flutter rate may result in 1:1 conduction across the AV node.

Ventricular Premature Beats

Ventricular premature beats (VPBs) commonly occur in patients with or without cardiac disease. VPBs occurring in healthy individuals with no cardiac disease pose little, if any, risk and do not require treatment. Historically, lidocaine has been used for VPB suppression, specifically in the setting of acute myocardial infarction, as VPBs were felt to be a warning arrhythmia for ventricular fibrillation. However, warning arrhythmias are no more common in patients who experience ventricular fibrillation than in those who do not. Hence, treatment of the VPBs with an antiarrhythmic agent is not necessary beyond the routine use of beta-blockers. Beta-blockers are administered in the post-MI population for mortality reduction rather than VPB suppression.

Nonsustained Ventricular Tachycardia

Nonsustained ventricular tachycardia is a common arrhythmia encountered in the ICU and has been extensively studied in cardiac surgery patients. Treatment is usually not necessary in patients with good ventricular function and the arrhythmia is not predictive of adverse outcomes. Monitoring, however, is required as it may be indicative of an underlying problem such as hypoxia, ischemia, or acidosis. In patients with poor postoperative cardiac output or those who have undergone valve replacement and have thick, hypertrophic hearts, there is an increased risk that nonsustained ventricular tachycardia may progress to sustained ventricular tachycardia or to ventricular fibrillation. It is not certain whether antiarrhythmic agents are beneficial in this situation. Antiarrhythmic agents may be useful in patients with nonsustained ventricular tachycardia who are at very high risk due to poor left ventricles or from hemodynamic instability. Amiodarone is most frequently used. Lidocaine and procainamide may be considered.

Sustained Monomorphic Ventricular Tachycardia

This reentrant arrhythmia is commonly seen >48 hours after myocardial infarction. Management depends on its rate, duration, and extent of underlying cardiac disease. In hemodynamically stable patients felt to be at risk for imminent circulatory collapse, amiodarone, lidocaine, or procainamide can be started. Direct current cardioversion is indicated in hemodynamically unstable patients or those with angina.

Sustained Polymorphic Ventricular Tachycardia

This arrhythmia is most commonly seen in patients with myocardial ischemia or infarction. Most episodes of polymorphic ventricular tachycardia terminate spontaneously. They can, however, lead to hemodynamic instability. Treatment is similar to that seen with monomorphic ventricular tachycardia. Direct current cardioversion should be used in unstable patients while antiarrhythmic agents that do not prolong the QT interval should be employed for sustained episodes. In addition to the treatment employed for the arrhythmia, beta-blockers and I.V. nitroglycerin should be used for the coronary disease present.

Torsade de Pointes

This is a rapid form of polymorphic ventricular tachycardia associated with QT prolongation. QT prolongation can be seen with various electrolyte abnormalities (eg, hypomagnesemia, hypokalemia), drugs (eg, type IA or type III antiarrhythmic agents, erythromycin, azole antifungal agents), and conditions such as cerebrovascular accident and hypothyroidism. For an acute episode of torsade de pointes, most patients will require DCC. All patients with suspected torsade de pointes should receive I.V. magnesium (2-6 g I.V. over several minutes followed by continuous

◀ infusion of 3-20 mg/minute for 5-48 hours), which suppresses triggered activity, as the benefits of doing so far outweigh the risk associated with it. Patients may also benefit from a short-term isoproterenol infusion until a temporary pacemaker can be inserted to increase ventricular rate.

Ventricular Fibrillation

The presence of postoperative ventricular fibrillation usually indicates severe myocardial ischemia, acidosis, or hypoxemia. Please refer to the ACLS algorithm for the treatment of ventricular fibrillation on page 1767.

REFERENCES AND RECOMMENDED READING

Baker WL and White CM, "Post-Cardiothoracic Surgery Atrial Fibrillation: A Review of Preventive Strategies," *Ann Pharmacother*, 2007, 41(4):587-98.

Burgess DC, Kilborn MJ, and Keech AC, "Interventions for Prevention of Post-Operative Atrial Fibrillation and Its Complications After Cardiac Surgery: A Meta-Analysis," *Eur Heart J*, 2006, 27 (23):2846-57.

DiDomenico RJ and Massad MG, "Pharmacologic Strategies for Prevention of Atrial Fibrillation After Open Heart Surgery," *Ann Thorac Surg*, 2005, 79(2):728-40.

Fleisher LA, Beckman JA, Brown KA, et al, "ACC/AHA 2007 Guidelines on Perioperative Cardiovascular Evaluation and Care for Noncardiac Surgery: A Report of the American College of Cardiology/American Heart Association Task Force on Practice Guidelines (Writing Committee to Revise the 2002 Guidelines on Perioperative Cardiovascular Evaluation for Noncardiac Surgery): Developed in Collaboration With the American Society of Echocardiography, American Society of Nuclear Cardiology, Heart Rhythm Society, Society of Cardiovascular Anesthesiologists, Society for Cardiovascular Angiography and Interventions, Society for Vascular Medicine and Biology, and Society for Vascular Surgery," *Circulation*, 2007, 116(17):e418-99.

Fuster V, Rydén LE, Cannom DS, et al, "ACC/AHA/ESC 2006 Guidelines for the Management of Patients With Atrial Fibrillation: Full Text: A Report of the American College of Cardiology/American Heart Association Task Force on Practice Guidelines and the European Society of Cardiology Committee for Practice Guidelines (Writing Committee to Revise the 2001 Guidelines for the Management of Patients With Atrial Fibrillation) Developed in Collaboration With the European Heart Rhythm Association and the Heart Rhythm Society," *Europace*, 2006, 8(9):651-745.

Gomes JA, Ip J, Santoni-Rugiu F, et al, "Oral d,l Sotalol Reduces the Incidence of Postoperative Atrial Fibrillation in Coronary Artery Bypass Surgery Patients: A Randomized, Double-Blind, Placebo-Controlled Study," *J Am Coll Cardiol*, 1999, 34(2):334-9.

Guarnieri T, Nolan S, Gottlieb SO, et al, "Intravenous Amiodarone for the Prevention of Atrial Fibrillation After Open-Heart Surgery: The Amiodarone Reduction in Coronary Heart (ARCH) Trial," *J Am Coll Cardiol*, 1999, 34(2):343-7.

Hollenberg SM and Dellinger RP, "Noncardiac Surgery: Postoperative Arrhythmias," *Crit Care Med*, 2000, 28(10 Suppl):N145-50.

Kailasam R, Palin CA, and Hogue CW Jr, "Atrial Fibrillation After Cardiac Surgery: An Evidence-Based Approach to Prevention," *Semin Cardiothorac Vasc Anesth*, 2005, 9(1):77-85.

Napolitano C, Priori SG, and Schwartz PJ, "Torsade de Pointes. Mechanisms and Management," *Drugs*, 1994, 47(1):51-65.

Patel AA, White CM, Gillespie EL, et al, "Safety of Amiodarone in the Prevention of Postoperative Atrial Fibrillation: A Meta-Analysis," *Am J Health Syst Pharm*, 2006, 63(9):829-37.

Tisdale JE, Padhi ID, Goldberg AD, et al, "A Randomized, Double-Blind Comparison of Intravenous Diltiazem and Digoxin for Atrial Fibrillation After Coronary Artery Bypass Surgery," *Am Heart J*, 1998, 135(5 Pt 1):739-47.

VanderLugt JT, Mattioni T, Denker S, et al, "Efficacy and Safety of Ibutilide Fumarate for the Conversion of Atrial Arrhythmias After Cardiac Surgery," *Circulation*, 1999, 100(4):369-75.

White CM, Caron MF, Kalus JS, et al, "Intravenous Plus Oral Amiodarone, Atrial Septal Pacing, or Both Strategies to Prevent Post-Cardiothoracic Surgery Atrial Fibrillation: The Atrial Fibrillation Suppression Trial II (AFIST II)," *Circulation*, 2003, 108(Suppl 1):II200-6.

Zimmer J, Pezzullo J, Choucair W, et al, "Meta-Analysis of Antiarrhythmic Therapy in the Prevention of Postoperative Atrial Fibrillation and the Effect on Hospital Length of Stay, Costs, Cerebrovascular Accidents, and Mortality in Patients Undergoing Cardiac Surgery," *Am J Cardiol*, 2003, 91 (9):1137-40.

PERIOPERATIVE MANAGEMENT OF PATIENTS ON ANTISEIZURE MEDICATION

Approximately 40 million people worldwide have epilepsy. It is more common during childhood and after age 65, but can occur at any age. Some people experience only one or two seizures during their entire life. One must have repeated seizure activity to be diagnosed. The pathophysiologic conditions that produce seizure activation and the drugs used to treat or prevent it will be discussed in addition to the recommended perioperative management for these situations.

ETIOLOGY OF SEIZURES

Brain injury:	Trauma, surgery, subarachnoid hemorrhage (SAH)
Hypoxia/ischemia:	Stroke, cardiac arrest, shock, hypotension, hypoxemia, cerebral edema
Infection:	Meningitis, encephalitis, abscess
Metabolic:	Electrolyte abnormalities, hepatic or renal failure, hyperglycemia, hypoglycemia, genetic metabolic abnormalities
Drug toxicity:	Alcohol, cocaine, metrizamide
Pathologic states:	Drug withdrawal, eclampsia, cerebral tumor, AVM, cortical vein thrombosis, SAH
Idiopathic epilepsy:	Etiology unknown

TYPES OF SEIZURES

Seizures are recurrent, synchronous, rhythmic firings of cortical neurons. Seizures are classified into five major groups.

Classification of Seizures

1. Generalized seizures
   a. Excitatory (myoclonic, clonic/tonic) = grand mal
   b. Inhibitors (absence, atonic) = petit mal
2. Partial seizures
   a. Simple partial
   b. Complex partial
   c. Partial onset with generalization
3. Pseudoseizures
4. Status epilepticus
5. Unclassified seizures

Generalized Seizures

Excitatory seizures occur over the entire brain with no obvious focal onset. They may present with an aura followed by tonic-clonic motor activity. Loss of consciousness occurs along with loss of bladder and bowel sphincter tone. The patient becomes apneic with absence of respiratory effort. During the postictal period, the patient may be somnolent or confused. Seizure treatment is supportive, assuring ventilation/oxygenation and preventing the patient from becoming injured from the motor activity.

Inhibitory seizures include absence seizures (petit mal) and atonic seizures (person loses motor tone and falls down).

◀ **Partial Seizures**

Partial seizure activity has a focal onset and is frequently asymptomatic (aura or simple seizure). Intracranial EEG recordings are often necessary to identify this type of seizure. Seizure activity must be sustained for at least 10-30 seconds before a physical manifestation occurs. The clinical response depends on the area of the brain containing the seizure focus (ie, uncontrollable hand moving = precentral gyrus; laughing, crying, fear = limbic; visual light flashes = occipital). These complex seizures are frequently termed psychomotor or temporal lobe seizures. When the seizure activity spreads throughout the entire brain it is called secondary generalization which presents as either tonic or clonic seizures.

Pseudoseizures

Pseudoseizures have no EEG abnormality and are usually attributed to malingering or the psychiatric condition of conversion disorder.

Status Epilepticus

Seizures are usually short-lived; however, when they are prolonged or recur without the patient regaining consciousness, the condition is called status epilepticus. Over 60,000 cases of status epilepticus occur per year in the United States. The longer the episode of untreated or inadequately treated status epilepticus, the more difficult it is to control and the greater the risk of permanent brain damage. Ventilation may need to be controlled since most of the drugs used to treat this condition can produce respiratory insufficiency.

Recommended Acute Intravenous Drug Therapy for Status Epilepticus

1. Diazepam (0.2 mg/kg) or lorazepam (0.1-0.22 mg/kg) in adults. Watch for recurrence of seizures when the benzodiazepine redistributes from the brain, decreasing brain concentration.
   OR
2. Phenytoin (15-20 mg/kg in adults) and the prodrug fosphenytoin (15-20 mg/kg phenytoin equivalents [PE]) effectively treats 41% to 90% of patients. Phenytoin cannot be administered faster than 50 mg/minute without significant hypotension. Fosphenytoin can be administered up to a maximum rate of 150 mg PE/minute. It can be administered at a faster rate than phenytoin because it has fewer cardiovascular side effects.
   OR
3. Phenobarbital (20 mg/kg in adults) is also effective, however, this drug has a prolonged half-life and it is difficult to differentiate between drug-induced sedation vs postictal state vs other CNS concerns.

If these drug therapies are unsuccessful, general anesthesia using an inhalational agent (excluding enflurane, which has the potential to produce EEG seizure activity) can be used. Sevoflurane has also been reported to produce epileptiform EEG activity, but with no proven detrimental effect. The use of inhalational anesthetics is a temporizing measure, for upon withdrawal of the anesthetic gas the seizures may recommence.

Unclassified Seizures

Not all seizures are epileptic seizures, for example, alcohol withdrawal or toxic brain injury from liver failure. These seizures usually present with tonic/clonic activity.

SEIZURE CLASSIFICATION AND SUGGESTED DRUG THERAPY

Type	Clinical Features	Drug Therapy
Generalized		
Myoclonic	Clonic jerks	Valproic acid Phenobarbital Clonazepam Lamotrigine Levetiracetam Phenytoin Carbamazepine Topiramate
Absence	Brief loss of consciousness; staring; little or no motor activity	Valproic acid Ethosuximide Clonazepam
Partial		
Simple partial	Focal motor or sensory disturbances	Valproic acid Carbamazepine Gabapentin Phenytoin Fosphenytoin Lamotrigine Levetiracetam Pregabalin Topiramate Tiagabine Zonisamide
Complex partial	Aura; bizarre behavior with impaired consciousness	Valproic acid Carbamazepine Gabapentin Phenytoin Fosphenytoin Lamotrigine Levetiracetam Topiramate Tiagabine Zonisamide
Status epilepticus	Continual seizure activity	Diazepam Phenytoin Fosphenytoin Phenobarbital

PATHOPHYSIOLOGY OF SEIZURES

As the mechanisms that produce seizure activity become evident, the use of specific antiseizure drugs becomes more logical. It is thought that partial seizures result from a reduction of inhibitory or an increase of excitatory synaptic activity. High frequency neuronal firing also produces seizures. Inactivation of the inner gate of the sodium channel prolongs the time the channels are inactive and inhibits rapid firing. This is probably the mechanism of action for carbamazepine, phenytoin, and valproate.

Another mechanism of seizure modulation involves GABA (gamma amino butyric acid) mediated synaptic inhibition, which reduces neuronal excitability and raises the seizure threshold. Activation of the GABAa receptor inhibits the postsynaptic neuron whereas a decrease in GABA receptor number or activity allows the unopposed excitatory activity to dominate. Benzodiazepines and barbiturates activate GABA receptors. Vigabatrin and valproate reduce the metabolism of GABA, and gabapentin enhances release of GABA from presynaptic cells. All decrease neuronal excitability.

Generalized seizures arise from reciprocal firing between the thalamus and cortex. Thalamic stimulation produces the 3/second spike and wave EEG pattern of absence seizures. These seizures are produced by voltage-regulated calcium currents. Drugs such as ethosuximide, trimethadione, and valproic acid inhibit this low threshold current.

◀ PRINCIPLES OF SEIZURE THERAPY

Determine the cause of the seizure. Initiate therapy with a single drug. If this drug does not provide adequate control, another drug should be substituted. When discontinuing a drug, reduce the dosage gradually to prevent status epilepticus. Monitor for toxicity. The selection of epilepsy therapy should be individualized, based on efficacy, tolerability, cost, serious side effects, and the patient's concurrent medical concerns. For example, the SANAD study recommends lamotrigine as standard treatment for partial seizures and valproate for generalized seizure patients. However, these drugs should not be selected for patients with sleep disorders or a history of pancreatitis, respectively.

PERIOPERATIVE MANAGEMENT: THE PATIENT WITH EPILEPSY

For patients with epilepsy, it is important to maintain adequate antiseizure drug levels during the perioperative period. Since many seizure medications only exist as oral drugs, this needs to be taken into consideration, especially for long surgical procedures. Current intravenous drugs that can be used as antiseizure prophylaxis during brain surgery include diazepam, fosphenytoin, levetiracetam, midazolam, phenobarbital, phenytoin, and valproate. Patients receiving chronic phenytoin therapy are resistant to neuromuscular blocking agents, requiring both higher blood levels and more frequent dosing. Acute loading of phenytoin can enhance neuromuscular blockade because it blocks sodium channels.

Anesthetic management includes continuation of the anticonvulsant therapy and avoidance of drugs that stimulate seizure activity (enflurane, methohexital, sevoflurane). High-dose opioids and etomidate have been implicated in producing seizures; however, these drugs induce muscle hypertonus, producing a myoclonic action which can be mistaken for seizure activity. The only narcotic that has demonstrated seizure activity in humans is meperidine. Its metabolite normeperidine has a long half-life and is a known CNS stimulant. It has produced seizures in patients with renal failure and in patients receiving large doses of meperidine over a prolonged time. It is a central sympathetic stimulant, but it also blocks neuronal NMDA receptor activation. (NMDA receptors are activated by glutamate, the major brain excitatory neurotransmitter.) These drug recommendations are only recommendations.

PERIOPERATIVE MANAGEMENT: EXCISION OF SEIZURE FOCUS

When chronic medical therapy is unsuccessful in controlling epileptic seizures, patients may undergo craniotomy for resection of the epileptic foci. For these patients, their antiseizure medications are usually reduced or withdrawn prior to surgery to enhance identification of seizure prone tissue. Craniotomy may be performed under general anesthesia or local anesthesia with I.V. sedation, depending on the surgeon's preference, the patient's ability to cooperate, and the site of the seizure foci. The depth of anesthesia and/or sedation must be light enough not to mask seizure activity (ie, patients should not receive large doses of drugs that depress EEG activity or elevate the seizure threshold). Electrocorticography, or mapping the brain electrical activity using intraoperative cortical surface electrodes, identifies the target areas. Because anticonvulsant medications are discontinued preoperatively, there is a high possibility of stimulating generalized seizure activity, which needs to be treated so the sedated patient does not injure himself. For patients anesthetized with general anesthesia and muscle relaxants, the induced seizure activity may be less obvious. In either case, treatment is needed; however, large doses of long-acting anticonvulsants (eg, phenobarbital) may limit the sensitivity of additional electrocorticography.

PREGNANCY

Stillbirth and infant mortality are higher in epileptic mothers taking antiseizure medication during pregnancy. There is a significant correlation with multidrug therapy and higher blood drug levels. Teratogenicity is greatest for trimethadione. Valproate is associated with spina bifida and neural tube defects. Carbamazepine is associated with craniofacial defects, fingernail hypoplasia, and developmental delays. The formation of epoxide intermediates from carbamazepine and phenytoin metabolism is associated with fetal malformation. However, this does not mean that every epileptic female should discontinue her antiseizure medications. Pregnant women should continue their antiseizure medication if needed for their safety. The effect of hypoxemia on the fetus from seizure-induced respiratory depression is more dangerous than seizure medication. Recommendations are to keep the dosage as small as possible, administer drugs in divided doses to avoid peak blood levels, and limit therapy to only one drug if at all possible.

ECLAMPSIA

Pregnant women with pre-eclampsia routinely receive magnesium sulfate seizure prophylaxis treatment even though it is still debatable as to whether magnesium sulfate is an anticonvulsant. Because magnesium blocks calcium entry into myocytes, it causes smooth (vascular, uterine) muscle relaxation with a synergistic interaction with nondepolarizing muscle relaxants (ie, vecuronium, rocuronium). Magnesium is cleared via the kidney and must be given cautiously when renal function is decreased.

SUBARACHNOID HEMORRHAGE / HEAD TRAUMA

Seizures frequently occur with subarachnoid hemorrhage associated with rupture of a cerebral aneurysm, arteriovenous malformation (AVM), or with head trauma. It is routine clinical practice to prophylactically treat these patients with antiseizure medication (primarily phenytoin). The benefit of seizure prophylaxis needs to be weighed against the side effects of the drug therapy.

FEBRILE SEIZURES

Although 2% to 4% of children experience a seizure during a febrile illness, only 2% to 3% of them will develop epilepsy later in life. This is a sixfold higher risk than in the general population. Febrile seizures do not have an infectious or metabolic origin within the CNS (eg, not produced by meningitis/encephalitis). Factors associated with this increased risk are pre-existing neurologic disorder, a family history of epilepsy, or a complicated febrile seizure (ie, lasting longer than 15 minutes or followed by another seizure within 24 hours). Fever is usually >102°F. The more rapid the rise in temperature, the greater the likelihood for seizure development. The most common age is between 3 months and 5 years. Adults can also experience febrile seizures. The use of chronic prophylactic antiseizure therapy is questionable because of the drug side effects, especially with regards to cognitive function. Temporary prophylaxis may be useful in subsequent febrile episodes (diazepam 0.33 mg/kg every 8 hours during the fever).

MAJOR ANTISEIZURE DRUGS AND SIDE EFFECTS

Name	Dose-Related Side Effect	Toxic Effect
Carbamazepine	Double vision, lethargy, leukopenia, photosensitivity	Skin rash, blood dyscrasia, hepatic/renal dysfunction, acute intermittent porphyria, Stevens-Johnson syndrome
Diazepam	Depression, lethargy, nystagmus, muscle weakness	Hypotension, respiratory depression
Felbamate (not a first line drug)	GI symptoms, somnolence, headache	Aplastic anemia, liver failure
Gabapentin	Cognitive difficulties, somnolence, depression	Ataxia, tremors, amnesia
Lamotrigine	Somnolence, diplopia, ataxia, insomnia	Rash, nausea
Levetiracetam	Somnolence, headache, nervousness	Psychotic reactions, depression, suicide, ataxia
Midazolam	Depression, lethargy, nystagmus, muscle weakness	Hypotension, respiratory depression
Oxcarbazepine	Somnolence, cognitive difficulties, ataxia	Multiorgan hypersensitivity reaction, Stevens-Johnson syndrome, erythema multiforme, toxic epidermal necrosis
Phenobarbital	Irritability, lethargy, hallucinations, hepatic enzyme induction	Rash, respiratory depression, hypotension
Phenytoin, Fosphenytoin	Ataxia, gingival hyperplasia, hirsutism, nystagmus, rash, lethargy	Neuropathy, rash, lupus (Stevens-Johnson), blood dyscrasia, hypotension, bradycardia
Pregabalin	Peripheral edema, dizziness, somnolence	Angioedema, hypersensitivity reactions
Tiagabine	Dizziness, CNS depression, tremor, ataxia, myalgia	Hepatic/renal dysfunction
Topiramate	Psychomotor slowing, speech problems, somnolence, weight loss, kidney stones	Metabolic acidosis
Valproic acid	Tremor, somnolence, anorexia, alopecia	Hepatic failure, pancreatitis, neutropenia, thrombocytopenia
Vigabatrin (not a first line drug)	Behavioral changes, headache, fatigue	Neurotoxicity, ophthalmologic toxicity including vision loss
Zonisamide	Somnolence, dizziness, ataxia	Oligohydrosis, hepatic/renal dysfunction

PHARMACOKINETIC PRINCIPLES

1. Tight capillary endothelial junctions limit the passage of water soluble drugs (eg, phenytoin, carbamazepine) into the brain while permitting the rapid transit of lipid soluble drugs (benzodiazepines, barbiturates).

2. The therapeutic effect obtained from active drug concentration depends on drug absorption and bioavailability (ie, phenytoin binds to enteral feedings, which decrease drug absorption from the gastrointestinal tract).

3. Barbiturates enhance cytochrome P450 enzymes, which increase hepatic metabolism of antiseizure drugs.

4. Most antiseizure drugs are bound to plasma proteins. Therefore, a decrease in protein production in the severely ill patient can acutely increase the concentration of free active drug. Because alcohol and metoclopramide have greater plasma protein binding affinity, the benzodiazepine free fraction will increase with coadministration. It is recommended to assay for free drug rather than for total drug concentration for a better understanding of drug availability/activity.

5. Volume of distribution/redistribution. The first phase of distribution delivers antiseizure drugs directly to the brain for a rapid onset of action. During the second phase of distribution (called redistribution) the drug moves out of the brain and equilibrates with the total body's volume of distribution, thus decreasing brain concentration and diminishing the acute drug effect. During the third phase, the drug moves into adipose tissue and is slowly released into the circulation over time.

6. Metabolism of most antiepileptic drugs follows first order kinetics (ie, a constant rate is metabolized). Phenytoin demonstrates saturation kinetics. When the enzymes responsible for phenytoin metabolism become saturated, additional doses are not metabolized at the same rate and higher blood levels occur. This is important because the drug level increases exponentially after enzyme saturation occurs, which is at approximately 10 mcg/mL (total drug) and 1-2.5 mcg/mL (free drug) - the lower therapeutic level for phenytoin.

7. The therapeutic target drug level is the one at which the patient stops seizing. This is the level that provides the best protection from seizures; however, it may not be the best level regarding side effects.

REFERENCES AND RECOMMENDED READING

Litt B and Krauss GL, "Pharmacologic Approach to Acute Seizures and Antiepileptic Drugs P484-506," Chernow B, ed, The Pharmacologic Approach to the Critically Ill Patient, 3rd ed, Baltimore, MD: Williams & Wilkins, 1994, 484-506.

Marson AG, Al-Kharusi AM, Alwaidh M, et al, "The SANAD Study of Effectiveness of Carbamazepine, Gabapentin, Lamotrigine, Oxcarbazepine, or Topiramate for Treatment of Partial Epilepsy: An Unblinded Randomised Controlled Trial," Lancet, 2007, 369(9566):1000-15.

Marson AG, Al-Kharusi AM, Alwaidh M, et al, "The SANAD Study of Effectiveness of Valproate, Lamotrigine, or Topiramate for Generalised and Unclassifiable Epilepsy: An Unblinded Randomised Controlled Trial," Lancet, 2007, 369(9566):1016-26.

McNamara JO, "Drugs Effective in the Therapy of the Epilepsies," Gardman JG, Limbird LE, eds, Goodman & Gilman's The Pharmacological Basis of Therapeutics, 9th ed, New York, NY: McGraw Hill, 1996, 461-86.

Miller JW and Anderson HH, "The Effect of N-demethylation on Certain Pharmacologic Actions of Morphine, Codeine, and Meperidine in the Mouse," J Pharmacol Exp Ther, 1954, 112(2):191-6.

National Institute for Clinical Excellence, "Newer Drugs for Epilepsy in Adults," 2004. Available at: http://www.nice.org.uk/TA076guidance. Last accessed December 6, 2007.

Rosman NP, Colton T, Labazzo J, et al, "A Controlled Trial of Diazepam Administered During Febrile Illnesses to Prevent Recurrence of Febrile Seizures," N Engl J Med, 1993, 329(2):79-84.

Runge JW and Allen FH, "Emergency Treatment of Status Epilepticus," Neurology, 1996, 46(6 Suppl 1):S20-3.

Sadler M, "Lamotrigine Associated With Insomnia," Epilepsia, 1999, 40(3):322-5.

Szeto HH, Inturrisi CE, Houde R, et al, "Accumulation of Normeperidine, an Active Metabolite of Meperidine, in Patients With Renal Failure of Cancer," Ann Intern Med, 1977, 86(6):738-41.

PERIOPERATIVE MANAGEMENT OF THE DIABETIC PATIENT

Diabetes is the most common endocrine problem occurring in 10% of the U.S. population. It is characterized by abnormal carbohydrate metabolism, which causes hyperglycemia. It has become a major cause of early onset illness and increased mortality, occurring in 7% of the U.S. population, with an expected doubling by 2030. It is associated with increased health care utilization and costs. Diabetes is a disease that necessitates close consideration in the patient undergoing surgery due to the complexity of the disease and high risk of cardiovascular, neurologic, and/or renal complications. A review of the classification, associated diseases, risks and management of perioperative insulin, oral hypoglycemics, and postoperative management will be discussed.

CLASSIFICATION

Diabetes mellitus is classified as Type 1 (formerly, insulin-dependent diabetes mellitus) or Type 2 (formerly, noninsulin-dependent diabetes mellitus). The following table describes their general characteristics.

	Type 1 (Insulin-Dependent)	Type 2 (Noninsulin-Dependent)
Incidence	10%	90%
Age at onset	Juvenile	Adult
Insulin secretion	Very low	Normal or high
Physical characteristic	Lean	Obese
Pathophysiology	Absolute insulin deficiency due to autoimmune destruction of pancreatic beta cells	Relative insulin resistance associated with failure to secrete insulin
Response to insulin	Sensitive	Resistant
Ketosis likelihood	High	Low
Hereditary influence	Moderate	Great
Treatment	Insulin	Diet, oral agents, insulin

Characterizations are general; there may be overlap between the two types. Note that Type 2 diabetes may also be treated with insulin.

ASSOCIATED DISEASES AND PERIOPERATIVE RISKS

In the perioperative setting, mortality and morbidity are higher in both types of diabetes when compared to the nondiabetic patient. Diabetic patients undergoing major surgery will spend approximately 30% to 50% more time in the hospital, compared to a nondiabetic patient. Their mortality rate is significantly higher, usually associated with cardiac events.

The perioperative mortality rate of the diabetic patient ranges between 3.7% to 13%. The major causes are secondary to cardiovascular complications and postoperative infections. It is currently thought that the increased morbidity in the diabetic patient is secondary to the increase in fasting blood glucose levels, the hyperglycemic stress response, and the micro and macro vasculopathy caused by this disease. Recent studies propose that adipose tissue acts like an endocrine organ, producing hormones and inflammatory substances that suppress both insulin signaling and the immune system. Insulin has anabolic, anti-inflammatory, and antiapoptotic effects. It also improves dyslipidemias and prevents endothelial dysfunction and hypercoagulation.

ENDOCRINE AND METABOLIC RESPONSE TO SURGERY IN DIABETIC PATIENTS

Endocrine

- Increased secretion of counterregulatory hormones: Catecholamines, glucagon, cortisol (predominantly catabolic hormones), and growth hormone
- Decreased insulin secretion causes a loss of anticatabolic effects of insulin
- Decreased insulin action due to increased insulin resistance secondary to the counterregulatory hormones

Metabolic

- Increased hepatic glucose production leading to hyperglycemia
- Decreased glucose disposal (utilization)
- Increased glucose production secondary to glycogenolysis and gluconeogenesis
- Increased protein catabolism
- Variable increase in lipolysis with ketone body formation
- General increase in metabolic rate and catabolism

Immediate and Long-Term Effects

- Dehydration and hemodynamic instability due to osmotic diuresis and volume loss during surgery
- Loss of lean body mass, negative nitrogen balance, impaired wound healing, decreased resistance to infection
- Loss of adipose tissue and energy reserve from fatty acids
- Deficiency of essential amino acids, vitamins, and minerals

In addition to the above, the diabetic patient is predisposed to disease-state complications. These complications include macrovascular disease (coronary atherosclerosis, peripheral vascular disease), microvascular disease (nephropathy, retinopathy), distal polyneuropathies, and autonomic neuropathy (gastrointestinal, genitourinary, cardiovascular).

Many diabetic patients have coronary artery disease, autonomic neuropathy, and impaired renal function. Furthermore, diabetics may present with asymptomatic cardiac ischemia. They are more likely to experience an ischemic event during the perioperative time. Patients with autonomic neuropathy are more likely to experience hypotension during induction of anesthesia, arrhythmias during the surgical procedure, and respond inadequately to drugs such as atropine when used for treatment of bradycardia. In addition, many diabetic patients are predisposed to dehydration due to osmotic diuresis caused by glycosuria and electrolyte imbalance secondary to renal insufficiency, which can affect intraoperative and postoperative fluid management. It is for these reasons that comprehensive preoperative assessment is important.

PREOPERATIVE ASSESSMENT

A preoperative evaluation of the diabetic patient undergoing a surgical procedure should include the following:

Identification of Diabetes Type

- Type 1 – absolute need for continual insulin therapy
- Type 2 – associated with increased insulin needs (may or may not require insulin)

Determination of Level of Preceding Glycemic Control

- Self-monitoring of blood glucose levels – review blood glucose records
- Review glycosylated hemoglobin levels; goal = Hgb A_{1c} <7%
- Frequency, timing, and severity of hypoglycemia

◄ **Determination of Presence of Diabetic Complications**
- Nephropathy – fluid balance, hypotension, drug dosage
- Autonomic neuropathy – cardiovascular response (arrhythmias, postural hypotension), gastrointestinal (gastroparesis, postoperative nausea or vomiting), bladder dysfunction (urinary retention)
- Retinopathy
- Peripheral vascular disease
- Coronary artery disease

Assessment of Operative Risk
- Cardiovascular disease, hypertension, congestive heart failure
- Pulmonary
- Renal
- Hematologic

Pharmacological Glycemic Regimen
- Medication type (Oral, SubQ), dosage, and frequency

Anticipated Surgery
- Type of procedure
- Type of anesthesia
- Duration of procedure

Depending on the severity of the disease and the surgical procedure, complete blood count, electrolyte panel, renal function, and baseline electrocardiogram may be needed. A preoperative glucose level is required. If the diabetic patient experiences cardiovascular, autonomic, or renal complications preoperatively, the patient should be optimized before undergoing the surgical procedure. In addition, these conditions must be monitored closely throughout the surgical procedure to prevent increased morbidity/mortality.

PERIOPERATIVE INSULIN / GLUCOSE MANAGEMENT

Recently, strategies have evolved regarding glycemic control and insulin therapy. Because elevated glucose levels predispose patients to infection, decreased wound healing, and worsening neurologic/cardiac status during ischemia, the medical community was ready to modify perioperative glycemic management. One study showed that critically ill surgical patients treated with intensive insulin therapy (target glucose level between 80 and 110 mg/dL) had better outcomes, and intensive glycemic control became an accepted practice (Van den Berghe, 2001). However, subsequent studies on mainly medical ICU patients failed to show improvement in patients randomized to tight glucose control, while placing them at increased risk of hypoglycemia (Brunkhorst, 2008; Van den Berghe, 2006). Additional meta-analyses (Griesdale, 2009; Wiener, 2008) and the NICE-SUGAR study (Finfer, 2009) failed to demonstrate any benefit of tight glucose control, while increasing the incidence of hypoglycemia. Intraoperative hypoglycemia is difficult to detect and causes cerebral and myocardial morbidity and mortality. Based on these and other studies, intensive glucose control lost favor and has been replaced by a more liberal target glucose level of 120-180 mg/dL. The benefit of perioperative glucose control in outpatients or those undergoing short surgical procedures is unknown.

INSULIN-TREATED / INSULIN-REQUIRING PATIENTS

Major Surgery

There are two methods for administering insulin in the preoperative setting. The first is administration of 33% to 50% of the patient's normal intermediate-acting insulin dose (ie, NPH) the morning of surgery. This method is sometimes referred to as the "split-dose method." The insulin dose should be administered after arrival at the hospital, after the morning blood glucose level is checked, and after the intravenous line is started. If the patient becomes hypoglycemic (<80 mg/dL) or hyperglycemic (>150-180 mg/dL) dextrose (I.V.) or regular insulin (SubQ or I.V.) should be administered. If insulin is administered as an intravenous bolus, its duration of action is only 10-20 minutes; therefore requiring frequent glucose evaluations and repeat boluses or initiation of an insulin infusion.

Because of the potential for either hypoglycemia or hyperglycemia with subcutaneous administration method, it is rarely the method of choice for perioperative insulin administration in the patient requiring a lengthy major surgical procedure. There is additional concern about erratic absorption during surgery because of either vasoconstriction due to the cold operating room environment or vasodilatation due to active patient heating methodologies. Subcutaneous insulin, however, is still commonly used in the insulin-requiring diabetic undergoing minor surgical procedures.

The second method for perioperative insulin administration is the continuous infusion method. This is a recommended method and is preferred because it allows for a more predictable and accurate way of administering insulin. For the brittle diabetic patient and patients that will have changing insulin requirements (steroid administration, pancreatic transplant), it is advisable to use a separate insulin and dextrose infusion perioperatively. Single I.V. bolus doses of insulin can also be given, but the effect lasts only 10-20 minutes.

Guidelines for Perioperative Diabetes Management With a Separate Insulin Infusion

- Insulin: Regular 100 units in 100 mL of normal saline (1 unit/1mL)
- Flush insulin infusion through the I.V. tubing before connecting to patient to coat the tubing
- Piggyback insulin line to perioperative maintenance fluid line
- The recommendation that perioperative maintenance fluids contain 5% dextrose (rate: 100 mL/hour) to prevent hypoglycemia is debatable because the effect of an interoperative glucose infusion on blood glucose control has not been studied. This recommendation comes from ICU patients and may not apply to the surgical patient due to the surgical stress response.
- Monitor blood glucose intraoperatively at least every hour. There are several algorithms for insulin infusion rate. A reasonable estimate of insulin infusion rate (units/hour) is determined by dividing the blood glucose value by 150.
- If the blood glucose level is <120 mg/dL stop the insulin infusion.
- Insulin needs may be decreased in patients treated with diet or oral agents, who require <50 units insulin/day, or who have endocrinologic deficiencies
- Insulin needs may be increased by obesity, sepsis, steroid therapy, renal transplant, and during coronary artery bypass

For all patients receiving an insulin infusion for a major surgical procedure, blood glucose should be monitored every hour during and after the surgical procedure. Potassium levels should also be closely monitored because glucose/insulin will shift potassium intracellularly.

Minor Surgery

For Type 1 diabetic patients undergoing minor surgical procedures or invasive diagnostic procedures, the administration of insulin is similar to that of the major surgical procedures. The "split-dose" insulin administration method is commonly used in this setting. The blood glucose monitoring is, however, less intense. These patients should have their blood glucose monitored every 1-4 hours, which is in contrast to every 1 hour for the patient undergoing a major surgical procedure.

ORAL HYPOGLYCEMIC TREATMENT

Management of the diabetic patient taking an oral hypoglycemic agent depends on the length and type of surgical procedure. Most oral hypoglycemic agents are discontinued the day of surgery, with the exception of chlorpropamide (which has a 24-48 hour duration of action) and metformin (which has the potential for lactic acidosis and renal toxicity with radiocontrast dye).

◄ Diabetic patients taking an oral hypoglycemic drug and undergoing a prolonged major surgical procedure should be managed like the insulin-requiring diabetic patient perioperatively. For the diabetic patient taking an oral hypoglycemic agent undergoing minor surgical procedures, the goal is "no glucose - no insulin." These patients should not routinely receive dextrose-containing fluids or insulin, and must have their blood glucose checked before the surgical or invasive diagnostic procedure and again postoperatively. The patient can receive insulin if the blood glucose is elevated. See Insulin Products table on page 1682.

POSTOPERATIVE MANAGEMENT

The immediate postoperative management of the diabetic patient is as important as the intraoperative management. Continue intraoperative insulin infusion if the patient is going to an ICU. If the patient is admitted to the floor and able to eat, resume preoperative dosing. Monitor blood glucose level every 4-6 hours and use a rapid-acting insulin as needed. Insulin requirements may be greatest in the postsurgical period due to persistent stress, infection, pain, steroid therapy, or parenteral nutrition.

CONCLUSION

The above recommendations are only guidelines. It is important to realize that the physician must individualize diabetic treatment based on the patient's coexisting diseases, type of diabetes, hypoglycemic medication, and surgical procedure. The health care professional must also remember that the disease-state complications of the diabetic patient (ie, cardiac, renal, fluid/electrolyte abnormalities) are major concerns in the perioperative setting. The associated diseases should always be optimized preoperatively and monitored closely in the intraoperative and post-operative period. Goal should be the prevention of complications as a result of hyperglycemia in the surgical patient.

REFERENCES AND RECOMMENDED READING

Ahmed Z, Lockhart CH, Weiner M, et al, "Advances in Diabetic Management: Implications for Anesthesia," *Anesth Analg*, 2005 100(3):666-9.

Brunkhorst FM, Engel C, Bloos F, et al, "Intensive Insulin Therapy and Pentastarch Resuscitation in Severe Sepsis," *N Engl J Med*, 2008, 358(2):125-39.

Capes SE, Hunt D, Malmberg K, et al, "Stress Hyperglycemia and Prognosis of Stroke in Nondiabetic and Diabetic Patients: A Systematic Overview," *Stroke*, 2001, 32(10):2426-32.

Clement S, Braithwaite SS, Magee MF, et al, "Management of Diabetes and Hyperglycemia in Hospitals," *Diabetes Care*, 2004, 27(2):553-91.

Finney SJ, Zekveld C, Elia A, et al, "Glucose Control and Mortality in Critically Ill Patients," *JAMA*, 2003, 290(15):2041-7.

Finfer S, Chittock DR, Su SY, et al, "Intensive Versus Conventional Glucose Control in Critically Ill Patients," *N Engl J Med*, 2009, 360(13):1283-97.

Griesdale DE, de Souza RJ, van Dam RM, et al, "Intensive Insulin Therapy and Mortality Among Critically Ill Patients: A Meta-Analysis Including NICE-SUGAR Study Data," *CMAJ*, 2009, 180 (8):821-7.

Harrigan RA, Nathan MS, and Beattie P, "Oral Agents for the Treatment of Type 2 Diabetes Mellitus: Pharmacology, Toxicity, and Treatment," *Ann Emerg Med*, 2001, 38(1):68-78.

Krinsley JS, "Association Between Hyperglycemia and Increased Hospital Mortality in a Heterogeneous Population of Critically Ill Patients," *Mayo Clin Proc*, 2003, 78(12):1471-8.

Lazar MA, "How Obesity Causes Diabetes: Not a Tall Tale," *Science*, 2005, 307(5708):373-5.

McMahon GT and Dluhy RG, "Intention to Treat-Initiating Insulin and the 4-T Study," *N Engl J Med*, 2007, 357(17):1759-61.

Moghissi ES, Korytkowski MT, DiNardo M, et al, "American Association of Clinical Endocrinologists and American Diabetes Association Consensus Statement on Inpatient Glycemic Control," *Endocr Pract*, 2009, 15(4):353-69.

Moitra VK and Meiler SE, "The Diabetic Surgical Patient," *Curr Opin Anaesthesiol*, 2006, 19 (3):339-45.

Oiknine R, Bernbaum M, and Mooradian AD, "A Critical Appraisal of the Role of Insulin Analogues in the Management of Diabetes Mellitus," *Drugs*, 2005, 5(3):325-40.

Rhodes ET, Ferrari LR, and Wolfsdorf JI, "Perioperative Management of Pediatric Surgical Patients With Diabetes Mellitus," *Anesth Analg*, 2005, 101(4):986-99.

van den Berghe G, Wilmer A, Hermans G, et al, "Intensive Insulin Therapy in the Medical ICU," *N Engl J Med*, 2006, 354(5):449-61.

van den Berghe G, Wouters P, Weekers F, et al, "Intensive Insulin Therapy in the Critically Ill Patients," *N Engl J Med*, 2001, 345(19):1359-67.

Wiener RS, Wiener DC, and Larson RJ, "Benefits and Risks of Tight Glucose Control in Critically Ill Adults: A Meta-Analysis," *JAMA*, 2008, 300(8):933-44.

Wild S, Roglic G, Green A, et al, "Global Prevalence of Diabetes: Estimates for the Year 2000 and Projections for 2030," *Diabetes Care*, 2004, 27(5):1047-53.

Wilson M, Weinreb J, and Hoo GW, "Intensive Insulin Therapy in Critical Care: A Review of 12 Protocols," *Diabetes Care*, 2007, 30(4):1005-11.

POSTOPERATIVE HYPERTENSION

It has been estimated that the overall incidence of postoperative hypertension (HTN) is approximately 3%. More than 50% of patients who develop postoperative HTN in the postanesthesia care unit (PACU) have pre-existing hypertension. Patients who do not take/receive their antihypertensive medications on the day of surgery are especially prone to hypertension postoperatively. Therefore, it is important to counsel patients to take their antihypertensive medications up to and including the day of their surgical procedures.

In the PACU, a number of postoperative factors can either cause or worsen postoperative hypertension. These include pain, anxiety, bladder distension, hypercarbia, hypoxia, fluid overload, hypothermia, antihypertensive withdrawal, myocardial ischemia, hypovolemia, increased intracranial pressure, and pulmonary embolism. If after treatment, the hypertension has not resolved, antihypertensive drug therapy should be employed. Short-term injectable therapy is preferred in patients without pre-existing HTN as most postoperative HTN resolves within 4 hours. Patients whose hypertension was controlled prior to surgery should have their antihypertensive medication reinstated as soon as possible postoperatively.

A wide range of parenteral agents is now available for management of postoperative HTN when a patient is not yet tolerating the oral route of administration (Table 1). The drug of choice depends on each patient's circumstances. The dosages of antihypertensive agents are often titrated to attain a blood pressure value 10% above the patient's normal blood pressure to prevent overshooting the desired value. Unless the situation warrants an immediate reduction in blood pressure (eg, myocardial infarction, dissecting aortic aneurysm, malignant hypertension), the reduction can be achieved over a longer period of time.

Table 1. Select I.V. Agents Used in the Treatment of Postoperative Hypertension

Drug	Dose	Onset	Duration	Mechanism of Action	Potential Adverse Effects
Sodium nitroprusside (Nitropress®)	I.V. infusion: 0.25-0.5 mcg/kg/min initially, titrate every 1-2 min (maximum: 10 mcg/kg/min, limit to <10 min duration)	Immediate	1-2 min	Vasodilator (arterial and venous; nitric oxide donor)	Nausea, vomiting, muscle twitching, hypotension, sweating, cyanide or thiocyanate toxicity, elevated ICP, tachycardia, myocardial ischemia
Nitroglycerin (Tridil®, Nitro-Bid®)	I.V. infusion: 5 mcg/min initially, titrate every 3-5 min by 5-20 mcg/min increments	2-5 min	5-10 min	Vasodilator (venous; nitric oxide donor)	Headache, tachycardia, hypotension (especially in volume-depleted patients), tolerance, methemoglobinemia (high dose, prolonged infusion)
Nicardipine (Cardene®)	I.V. infusion: 5 mg/h initially, titrate every 5-15 min by 2.5 mg/h increments; maintenance: 3 mg/h once blood pressure goals have been met (maximum: 15 mg/h)	5-10 min	15-30 min, up to ≥4 h	Vasodilator (primarily arterial; dihydropyridine L-type calcium channel blocker)	Headache, tachycardia, flushing, phlebitis, hypotension, nausea, vomiting
Clevidipine (Cleviprex™)	I.V. infusion: Initially 1-2 mg/h; titrate every 90 seconds initially and then every 5-10 min as blood pressure goals are approached; maintenance: 4-6 mg/h once blood pressure goals have been met (recommended maximum: 21 mg/h); limited experience with doses >32 mg/h	2-4 min	5-15 min	Vasodilator (primarily arterial; dihydropyridine L-type calcium channel blocker)	Nausea, fever, insomnia, headache, acute renal failure
Enalaprilat (Vasotec®)	Intermittent I.V.: 0.625-1.25 mg every 6 h; use lower dose if hyponatremia, volume depletion, renal failure, or concurrent diuretic therapy in use (maximum: 20 mg/24 h period)	15-30 min	6-12 h	Vasodilator (angiotensin-converting enzyme inhibitor)	Renal dysfunction, hyperkalemia, angioedema

Table 1. Select I.V. Agents Used in the Treatment of Postoperative Hypertension *continued*

Drug	Dose	Onset	Duration	Mechanism of Action	Potential Adverse Effects
Hydralazine (Apresoline®)	Intermittent I.V.: 3-20 mg; use lower end of dosing range immediately postoperatively. Can dose every 20-60 min for desired response.	10-20 min	1-4 h	Vasodilator (arterial)	Headache, flushing, tachycardia, vomiting, aggravation of angina
Fenoldopam (Corlopam®)	I.V. infusion: 0.1-0.3 mcg/kg/min initially, titrate every 15 min by 0.1 mcg/kg/min (maximum: 1.6 mcg/kg/min)	<5 min	30 min	Vasodilator (dopamine-type 1 receptor agonist)	Headache, flushing, nausea, tachycardia, hypotension, dizziness, bradycardia
Labetalol (Normodyne®, Trandate®)	Intermittent I.V.: 10-20 mg over 2 min initially, repeat every 10 min (maximum single dose: 80 mg; maximum cumulative dose: 300 mg/day); higher doses may be well tolerated. I.V. infusion: 0.5-4 mg/min initially; titrate every 10 min until desired effect, toxicity, or a cumulative dose of 300 mg in a 24 h period	5-10 min	3-6 h	Alpha₁ and beta blocker	Bronchoconstriction, hypotension, bradycardia, conduction delays, left ventricular dysfunction
Esmolol (Brevibloc®)	I.V. infusion: 250-500 mcg/kg/min for 1 min initially, then 50-100 mcg/kg/min (maximum: 300 mcg/kg/min); can repeat bolus in 5 min and increase infusion by 50 mcg/kg/min	1-2 min	10-30 min	Beta blocker, beta₁ selective	Bronchoconstriction, hypotension, bradycardia, conduction delays, left ventricular dysfunction

REFERENCES AND RECOMMENDED READING

Chobanian AV, Bakris GI, Black HR, et al, "Seventh Report of the Joint National Committee on Prevention, Detection, Evaluation, and Treatment of High Blood Pressure," *Hypertension*, 2003, 42 (6):1206-52.

Erstad BL and Barletta JF, "Treatment of Hypertension in the Perioperative Patient," *Ann Pharmacother*, 2000, 34(1):66-79.

Feeley TW and Macario A, "The Postanesthesia Care Unit," *Miller's Anesthesia*, 6th ed, Miller RD, ed, New York, NY: Elsevier, 2005, 2703-28.

Haas CE and LeBlanc JM, "Acute Postoperative Hypertension: A Review of Therapeutic Options," *Am J Health Syst Pharm*, 2004, 61(16):1661-73.

Lewis KS, "Pharmacological Review of Postoperative Hypertension," *J Pharm Prac*, 2002, 15 (2):135-46.

Singla N, Warltier DC, Gandhi SD, et al, "Treatment of Acute Postoperative Hypertension in Cardiac Surgery Patients: An Efficacy Study of Clevidipine Assessing Its Postoperative Antihypertensive Effect in Cardiac Surgery-2 (ESCAPE-2), a Randomized, Double-Blind, Placebo-Controlled Trial," *Anesth Analg*, 2008, 107(1):59-67.

POSTOPERATIVE NAUSEA AND VOMITING

Postoperative nausea and vomiting (PONV) is a common postoperative problem, with an overall incidence of approximately 30%. PONV may continue for up to 3 days following surgery or discharge from an ambulatory surgery facility. In addition to causing distress for patients, uncontrolled vomiting can cause prolonged recovery room stay, unanticipated hospital admission, and can increase the risk for aspiration and suture dehiscence.

NEUROTRANSMITTERS INVOLVED IN THE DEVELOPMENT OF PONV

Nausea and vomiting may be triggered by multiple physiologic pathways. The vomiting center is located in the brainstem and includes the area postrema, the nucleus tractus solitarius, and the dorsal motor nucleus of the vagus nerve. Key neurotransmitters and receptors that are involved in the emetic response are located in the brainstem vomiting center. These include serotonin ($5-HT_3$) receptors, dopamine (D_2) receptors, histamine (H_1) receptors, muscarinic (M_1) receptors, and substance P (NK_1) receptors. Receptors in the gastrointestinal (GI) tract also contribute to the development of PONV. These receptors include $5-HT_3$ receptors, D_2 receptors, and NK_1 receptors. M_1 and H_1 receptors in the vestibular labyrinth of the inner ear, can also contribute to the development of PONV. Inhibition of one or more of these receptors are targets for antiemetic therapy for prevention and treatment of PONV.

RISK FACTORS

Risk factors for PONV in adults are listed below. These can be used to identify patients at a higher risk for PONV; such patients would benefit from prophylactic antiemetic administration.

Table 1. Risk Factors for PONV in Adults

Patient-Specific

- Female gender[1]
- Nonsmoking status[1]
- History of PONV/motion sickness[1]

Anesthetic

- Use of volatile anesthetics[1]
- Use of opioids (intra- and postop)[1]
- Nitrous oxide use[1]

Surgical

Duration of surgery	Maxillofacial surgery
Breast surgery	Neurosurgery
Laparoscopic surgery	Strabismus surgery
Laparotomy	Plastic surgery
Gynecological surgery	Ophthalmologic surgery
Abdominal surgery	Urologic surgery

[1]These are the most important risk factors.

ASSESSMENT OF RISK

Prophylaxis for PONV is not needed for every patient. The patient's level of risk (eg, low, moderate, high) for PONV is estimated, then an intervention(s) can be made to prevent PONV. For adults, Apfel's simplified risk score may be used, where one point is assigned for each of the following four risk factors: Female gender, history of PONV, nonsmoking status, and use of postoperative opioids. The PONV risk for adults with 0, 1, 2, 3, or 4 risk factors is approximately 10%, 20%, 40%, 60%, and 80% respectively. For children, Eberhart's simplified risk score for postoperative vomiting (POV) assigns one point for each of the following four risk factors: Surgery ≥30 minutes, age ≥3 years, strabismus surgery, history of POV or PONV in relatives. When 0, 1, 2, 3, or 4 risk factors are present, the risk for POV is approximately 10%, 10%, 30%, 55%, or 70%, respectively.

REDUCING BASELINE RISK FACTORS

Whenever possible, baseline risk factors should be reduced to decrease the likelihood of PONV.

Strategies to reduce baseline risk factors include use of propofol for induction and maintenance of anesthesia, use of regional anesthesia (to avoid general anesthesia with volatile anesthetics), and avoid or minimized the use of nitrous oxide, high-dose neostigmine, and postoperative opioids.

PONV PROPHYLAXIS

The patient's risk level for PONV will dictate whether prophylactic antiemetic therapy should be administered and, if so, how many agents are given to the patient. For example, a "wait and see" approach is taken with an adult patient at a low risk (0-1 risk factors in Apfel's model) for PONV unless vomiting would lead to complications postoperatively. For patients at moderate risk (1 or 2 risk factors in Apfel's model) for PONV, one or two antiemetic agents should be administered for prophylaxis. For patients at high risk (3 or 4 risk factors in Apfel's model) for PONV, at least two interventions (eg, propofol or regional anesthesia with one or more antiemetic agents) should be utilized. When administering more than one antiemetic agent, it is important that the agents have different mechanisms of action to optimize efficacy.

Antiemetics recommended for prophylaxis in adult patients at moderate-to-high risk for PONV include the serotonin antagonists (ondansetron, dolasetron, granisetron), butyrophenones (droperidol), dexamethasone, transdermal scopolamine, and aprepitant. Serotonin antagonists are most effective when administered at the end of surgery and they have a favorable side effect profile (see table). Prophylactic doses of droperidol (0.625–1.25 mg I.V.) are as effective as ondansetron (4 mg I.V.) for preventing PONV (Apfel, 2004; Fourtney, 1998). Droperidol, like the serotonin antagonists, is best administered at the end of surgery. Despite the FDA's "black box" warning, the risk of an arrhythmia or serious cardiac event from this low dose of droperidol is negligible (Charbit, 2005; Nuttall, 2007). Dexamethasone (4 mg I.V.) is best administered at induction, rather than the end of surgery, and has been shown to be as effective as ondansetron (4 mg I.V.) (Apfel, 2004). Transdermal scopolamine, when applied the evening before surgery or 4 hours before the end of anesthesia, effectively prevents PONV. Adverse effects are generally mild, with visual disturbances, dry mouth, and dizziness being the most common adverse effects. The NK_1 antagonist aprepitant (40 mg orally) is comparable to ondansetron (4 mg I.V.) in reducing nausea and the need for rescue in the first 24 hours following surgery. However, aprepitant is significantly better than ondansetron in preventing vomiting (Diemunsch, 2007; Gan, 2007).

In adult high-risk patients, combination therapy has been shown to have greater efficacy than one prophylactic for PONV prophylaxis (Apfel, 2004). When combination prophylactic therapy is indicated, drugs with different mechanisms of action should be used for optimal efficacy.

TREATMENT OF PONV

If a patient received no antiemetic prophylaxis and develops PONV, an appropriate antiemetic agent (eg, $5\text{-}HT_3$ receptor antagonist) should be administered. Dexamethasone and transdermal scopolamine are not recommended for the acute treatment of PONV secondary to their longer onset of action. If a patient received one or more prophylactic antiemetic agents and still develops PONV, a drug from a different class (different mechanism of action) should be administered for treatment. Treatment doses of the serotonin antagonists are lower than doses used for prophylaxis. Ondansetron 1 mg I.V. and granisetron 0.1 mg I.V. can be used for treatment; dolasetron doses <12.5 mg have not been studied. No drug should be readministered for treatment of PONV unless at least 6 hours have elapsed.

Antiemetic Agents

Antiemetic Drug	Proposed Receptor Site of Action	Usual Dose[1]	Duration of Action	Adverse Effects	Comments and Recommendations for Use
Butyrophenones					
Droperidol (Inapsine®)	D_2	**Adults:** I.V.: 0.625-1.25 mg **Pediatrics:** I.V.: 10-15 mcg/kg	12-24 h	Sedation, hypotension (especially in hypovolemic patients), EPS	Monitor ECG for QT prolongation/torsade de pointes; duration of action depends on size of dose
Phenothiazines					
Prochlorperazine (Compazine®)	D_2	**Adults:** I.V./I.M.: 5-10 mg P.R.: 25 mg **Pediatrics:** P.O.: 0.1 mg/kg I.M.: 0.13 mg/kg P.R.: 2.5 mg	4-6 h (12 h when given P.R.)	Sedation, hypotension (especially in hypovolemic patients), EPS	None
Antimuscarinics / Antihistamines					
Diphenhydramine (Benadryl®)	H_1, M_1	**Adults:** I.V./I.M.: 12.5-50 mg **Pediatrics:** P.O./I.V.: 1 mg/kg (max: 25 mg for <6 y old)	4-6 h	Sedation, dry mouth, blurred vision, urinary retention	None
Promethazine (Phenergan®)	D_2, H_1, M_1	**Adults:** I.V./I.M./P.R.: 6.25-25 mg **Pediatrics (>2 y):** I.V./I.M./P.R.: 0.25-0.5 mg/kg[3]	4 h	Sedation, hypotension (especially in hypovolemic patients), EPS	I.V. irritant: Dilute in 10-20 mL of saline, inject through a running I.V. and instruct patients to report I.V. site discomfort I.M.: Administer into deep muscle
Scopolamine (Transderm Scōp®)	M_1	**Adults:** 1.5 mg transdermal patch **Pediatrics:** N/A	72 h[3]	Dry mouth, visual disturbances, dizziness	Apply at least 2-4 hours before the end of surgery; wash hands after handling patch

Antiemetic Agents *continued*

Antiemetic Drug	Proposed Receptor Site of Action	Usual Dose[1]	Duration of Action	Adverse Effects	Comments and Recommendations for Use
Benzamides					
Metoclopramide (Reglan®)	D_2	**Adults:** I.V.: 10-25 mg **Pediatrics:** I.V.: 0.25 mg/kg	≤6 h	Sedation, hypotension, EPS	Consider for treatment if N/V may be due to gastric stasis; 10 mg dose is not effective for preventing PONV
Serotonin Antagonists					
Dolasetron (Anzemet®)	$5-HT_3$	**Adults:** I.V.: 12.5 mg **Pediatrics:** I.V.: 0.35 mg/kg	Up to 24 h	Headache, lightheadedness, elevated liver enzymes, constipation	Greater antivomiting than antinausea effect
Granisetron (Kytril®)	$5-HT_3$	**Adults:** I.V.: 0.35-1 mg **Pediatrics:** Not known	Up to 24 h	Headache, lightheadedness, elevated liver enzymes, constipation	Greater antivomiting than antinausea effect
Ondansetron (Zofran®)	$5-HT_3$	**Adults:** I.V.: 4 mg **Pediatrics:** I.V.: 0.05-0.1 mg/kg	Up to 24 h	Headache, lightheadedness, elevated liver enzymes, constipation	Greater antivomiting than antinausea effect
Other					
Dexamethasone (Decadron®)	None	**Adults:** I.V.: 4 mg **Pediatrics:** I.V.: 0.5-1 mg/kg	Up to 24 h	Genital itching, flushing	A single dose is well tolerated in healthy patients
Ephedrine	None	**Adults:** I.M.: 0.5 mg/kg **Pediatrics:** N/A	Up to 24 h	Transient elevations in blood pressure	Consider when postural hypotension is present
Propofol (Diprivan®)	None	**Adults:** I.V.: 10-20 mg **Pediatrics:** N/A	<10 minutes	Sedation	Very short acting; excessive sedation may be a concern

D_2 = dopamine type 2 receptor; H_1 = histamine type 1 receptor; M_1 = muscarinic cholinergic type 1 receptor; $5-HT_3$ = serotonin type 3 receptor; EPS = extrapyramidal symptoms such as motor restlessness or acute dystonia; N/A = not applicable; I.V. = intravenous; I.M. = intramuscular; P.R. = per rectum; P.O. = per os (by mouth); ECG = electrocardiogram; N/V = nausea and/or vomiting.

[1] Pediatric doses should not exceed the adult dose, unless otherwise indicated.

[2] Children >10 kg or 2 years of age only; change from I.M. to oral as soon as possible. When administering P.R., the dosing interval varies from 8-24 hours depending upon the child's weight.

[3] Remove after 24 hours. Instruct patients to wash the site where the patch was, as well as their hands, thoroughly.

NONPHARMACOLOGIC THERAPY

Stimulation of the P-6 acupuncture point has been shown to reduce the incidence of nausea, vomiting, and the need for rescue medications (Lee, 1999). When compared to ondansetron, P-6 stimulation was more effective in reducing the incidence and severity of nausea (Gan, 2004).

CONCLUSION

There are are independent predictors for developing PONV. For adults, the main predictors are female gender, nonsmoker, history of motion sickness or PONV, use of volatile anesthetics, use of nitrous oxide, and use of opioids. These factors can be classified as patient-specific and anesthesia-related. Casuality from other factors, such as the type and duration of surgery, has not been clearly established. A simplified risk score, such as Apfel's, is very effective for predicting PONV risk for an adult undergoing general inhalational anesthesia. For high-risk patients, a multimodal approach is best (using antiemetics from different classes and other interventions such as propofol or regional anesthesia). For rescue treatment, administer an antiemetic from a different class than the prophylactic antiemetic.

REFERENCES AND RECOMMENDED READING

Apfel CC, Korttila K, Abdalla M, et al, "A Factorial Trial of Six Interventions for the Prevention of Postoperative Nausea and Vomiting," N Engl J Med, 2004, 350(24):2441-51.

Apfel CC, Läärä E, Koivuranta M, et al, "A Simplified Risk Score for Predicting Postoperative Nausea and Vomiting: Conclusions From Cross-Validations Between Two Centers," Anesthesiology, 1999, 91(3):693-700.

Borgeat A, Wilder-Smith OH, Saiah M, et al, "Subhypnotic Doses of Propofol Possess Direct Antiemetic Properties," Anesth Analg, 1992, 74(4):539-41.

Charbit B, Albaladejo P, Funck-Brentano C, et al, "Prolongation of QT$_c$ Interval After Postoperative Nausea and Vomiting Treatment By Droperidol or Ondansetron," Anesthesiology, 2005, 102 (6):1094-100.

Diemunsch P, Gan TJ, Philip BK, et al, "Single-Dose Aprepitant Vs Ondansetron for the Prevention of Postoperative Nausea and Vomiting: A Randomized, Double-Blind Phase III Trial in Patients Undergoing Open Abdominal Surgery," Br J Anaesth, 2007, 99(2):202-11.

Domino KB, Anderson EA, Polissar NL, et al, "Comparative Efficacy and Safety of Ondansetron, Droperidol, and Metoclopramide for Preventing Postoperative Nausea and Vomiting: A Meta-Analysis," Anesth Analg, 1999, 88(6):1370-9.

Fortney JT, Gan TJ, Graczyk S, et al, "A Comparison of the Efficacy, Safety, and Patient Satisfaction of Ondansetron Versus Droperidol as Antiemetics for Elective Outpatient Surgical Procedures. S3A-409 and S3A-410 Study Groups," Anesth Analg, 1998, 86(4):731-8.

Gan TJ, Apfel CC, Kovac A, et al, "A Randomized, Double-Blind Comparison of the NK$_1$ Antagonist, Aprepitant, Versus Ondansetron for the Prevention of Postoperative Nausea and Vomiting," Anesth Analg, 2007, 104(5):1082-9.

Gan TJ, Jiao KR, Zenn M, et al, "A Randomized Controlled Comparison of Electro-Acupoint Stimulation or Ondansetron Versus Placebo for the Prevention of Postoperative Nausea and Vomiting," Anesth Analg, 2004, 99(4):1070-5.

Gan TJ, Meyer TA, Apfel CC, et al, "Society for Ambulatory Anesthesia Guidelines for the Management of Postoperative Nausea and Vomiting," Anesth Analg, 2007, 105(6):1615-28.

Lee A and Done ML, "The Use of Nonpharmacologic Techniques to Prevent Postoperative Nausea and Vomiting: A Meta-Analysis," Anesth Analg, 1999, 88(6):1362-9.

Nuttall GA, Eckerman KM, Jacob KA, et al, "Does Low-Dose Droperidol Administration Increase the Risk of Drug-Induced QT Prolongation and Torsade de Pointes in the General Surgical Population?" Anesthesiology, 2007, 107(4):531-6.

Wallenborn J, Gelbrich G, Bulst D, et al, "Prevention of Postoperative Nausea and Vomiting By Metoclopramide Combined With Dexamethasone: Randomised Double Blind Multicentre Trial," BMJ, 2006, 333(7563):324.

PREOPERATIVE EVALUATION OF THE CARDIAC PATIENT FOR NONCARDIAC SURGERY

As age increases, so does the prevalence of cardiac disease. Annually, 10% of the United States population has noncardiac surgery, with an overall cardiac morbidity/ mortality rate of less than 6% for patients older than 40 years of age undergoing major operations.[1,2] This risk is increased in older patients and those with cardiac disease. As the population ages, the number of patients older than 65 years old presenting for surgery will increase 25% to 35% over the next 30 years.

The purpose of this chapter is to identify those patients at high risk for postoperative cardiac complications. The preoperative evaluation should stratify patients with preexisting cardiac disease and recommend further workup for those at high risk, while avoiding additional testing for those patients with low potential for postoperative cardiac morbidity or mortality. Preoperative testing should be restricted to those patients in whom the results will change the surgical procedure, modify medical therapy and/or monitoring during and after surgery, or postpone surgery until the cardiac condition is corrected or stabilized.

HISTORY OF CARDIAC RISK ASSESSMENTS

Historically, coronary artery disease and congestive heart failure are two clinical conditions closely correlated with postoperative cardiac morbidity (Table 1). Classic teaching based on the works by Tarhan[3] and Steen[4] in the 1970s reported approximately 30% reinfarction/mortality risk in patients who had surgery within 3 months of their myocardial infarction, decreasing to about 15% if their surgery was within 4-6 months of their MI, and 6% if the surgery was delayed more than 6 months. By 1983, Rao et al reported a reduction in the risk of recurrent MI/cardiac mortality to 6% if operated on within 3 months of a prior MI and 2% if surgery occurred between 4-6 months.[5] Shah confirmed Rao's data of improved cardiac risk in 1990.[6] The purposed reasons for this improvement in risk included the intensive postoperative care/monitoring and tighter control of hemodynamic variables.

Table 1. Incidence of Perioperative Myocardial Reinfarction (1972-1990)

Time Elapsed Since Prior Myocardial Infarction (mo)	Tarhan, et al[1] (%)	Steen, et al[2] (%)	Rao, et al[3] (%)	Shah, et al[4] (%)
0-3	37	27	5.7	4.3
4-6	16	11	2.3	0
>6	5	6		5.7

[1]Tarhan S, Moffitt EA, Taylor WF, et al, "Myocardial Infarction After General Anesthesia," *JAMA*, 1972, 220(11):1451-4.

[2]Steen PA, Tinker JH, and Tarhan S, "Myocardial Infarction After Anesthesia and Surgery," *JAMA*, 1978, 239(24):2566-70.

[3]Rao TL, Jacobs KH, and El-Etr AA, "Reinfarction Following Anesthesia in Patients With Myocardial Infarction," *Anesthesiology*, 1983, 59(6):499-505.

[4]Shah KB, Kleinman BS, Sami H, et al, "Reevaluation of Perioperative Myocardial Infarction in Patients With Prior Myocardial Infarction Undergoing Noncardiac Operations," *Anesth Analg*, 1990, 71(3):231-5.

CARDIAC RISK INDEXES

In 1977, Goldman[2] identified nine independent correlates of perioperative cardiac events and assigned them relative value points (Table 2). This index stratified patients by cumulative points into four risk classes: Class 1 = 1-5 points (1% to 2% risk of death/major complications. Class II = 6-12 points (5% risk). Class III = 13-25 points (15% risk). Class IV = >25 points (56% risk).

Table 2. Goldman Cardiac Risk Index

Variable	Point Score
History	
Age >70 years	5
Preoperative MI within 6 months	10
Physical examination	
S3 gallop or increased JVP >12	11
Significant valvular aortic stenosis	3
EKG	
Rhythm other than sinus or atrial ectopy	7
PVCs >5/minute at any time	7
General medical status	3
PO_2 <60 or PCO_2 >59	
K^+ <3 or HCO_3 <20	
BUN >50 or creatinine >3	
Chronic liver disease or debilitation	
Operation	
Intraperitoneal, intrathoracic, or aortic	3
Emergency	4
Total possible points	53

Goldman L, Caldera DL, Nussbaum SR, et al, "Multifactorial Index of Cardiac Risk in Noncardiac Surgical Procedures," *N Engl J Med*, 1977, 297(16):845-50.

In 1999, Lee revised the Goldman Cardiac Risk Index to simplify risk assessment (using data from approximately 4500 patients) by identifying six independent predictors of cardiac complications (Table 3). Rates of major complications with 0, 1, 2, and 3+ of these factors were 0.4%, 0.9%, 7%, and 11% respectively.[7] Two other indexes focused primarily on high-risk patients. The Detsky risk index[8] added angina and pulmonary edema to Goldman's original criteria, and Eagle Criteria[9] looked at only patients undergoing major vascular surgery. These indexes were more specific to the high-risk population and not very sensitive to patients at the lower risk level.

Table 3. Revised Goldman Cardiac Risk Index

High risk type of surgery (major vascular, thoracic, abdominal, orthopedic)

Ischemic heart disease (prior MI, positive stress test, chest pain, Q waves)

Congestive heart failure (prior pulmonary edema, PND, peripheral edema, rales, S3, CXR with pulmonary vascular redistribution)

Cerebrovascular disease (history of TIA or stroke)

Preoperative treatment with insulin

Preoperative serum creatinine >2 mg/dL

Lee TH, Marcantonio ER, Mangione CM, et al, "Derivation and Prospective Validation of a Simple Index for Prediction of Cardiac Risk of Major Noncardiac Surgery," *Circulation*, 1999, 100(10):1043-9.

In 2002, the American College of Cardiology in association with the American Heart Association (AHA) published practice guidelines to assist anesthesiologists and cardiologists in the preoperative evaluation of the cardiac patient for noncardiac surgery.[10] In 2007 the ACC and AHA revised these guidelines based on recent studies that help direct "best practice" recommendations.

◀ ACC/AHA GUIDELINES - 2007[11]

The perioperative anesthesiologist needs to assess the severity and stability of the patient's cardiac status and determine if additional workup will provide important information prior to the proposed surgery. Following a thorough history and physical examination, the anesthesiologist needs to risk stratify the patient. The predictors of increased perioperative cardiovascular risk, which can lead to myocardial infarction, heart failure, and death, are **Clinical Risk Factors**, **Functional Capacity**, and **Risk of Surgical Procedure**.

Table 4: ACC/AHA Active Clinical Cardiac Conditions: These conditions mandate intervention/intensive care management and possible delay/cancellation of surgery.

1. Unstable coronary syndromes
   - Recent MI (>7 days and within 1 month)[1]
   - Unstable or severe angina
2. Decompensated heart failure
3. Significant arrhythmias
   - High grade AV block
   - Mobitz II AV block
   - 3rd degree AV block
   - Symptomatic ventricular arrhythmias
   - Supraventricular arrhythmias with uncontrolled HR >100 bpm
   - Symptomatic bradycardia
   - New ventricular tachycardia
4. Severe valvular disease
   - Severe aortic stenosis (gradient >40 mm Hg, valve area <1 cm^2)
   - Symptomatic mitral stenosis (progressive dyspnea on exertion, exertional presyncope, heart failure)
5. [1]An important change from the 2002 ACC/AHA recommendation is the definition of recent MI to <30 days. This emphasizes the importance of "recent" and eliminates the historical 3-month/6-month criteria.

Table 5: ACC/AHA Clinical Risk Factors

1. History of ischemic heart disease
2. History of compensated or prior heart failure
3. History of cerebrovascular disease
4. Diabetes mellitus
5. Renal insufficiency

Minor predictors are recognized as potential markers for cardiovascular disease; however, they have not been proven to be independent criteria for perioperative cardiac risk. Therefore, they are not incorporated into these recommendations: Age >70 years, abnormal ECG (LVH, LBBB, ST-T abnormalities), rhythm other than sinus, and uncontrolled hypertension.

Table 6: ACC/AHA Functional Capacity

1-4 METs	Able to do activities of daily living, walk 1-2 blocks on level ground, light housework (eg, dusting, washing dishes)
4-10 METs	Able to climb a flight of stairs, walk on level ground at 4 mph, do heavy housework, participate in physical activities like dancing, doubles tennis, golf
>10 METs	Strenuous sports (eg, swimming, football, basketball, skiing, singles tennis)

METs = metabolic equivalents

Perioperative cardiac and long-term risks are increased in patients unable to achieve 4-MET demand. For patients who have not had an exercise stress test, functional status is estimated by ability to perform activities of daily living. Resting basal metabolic rate of a 40 year old average size male is 3.5 mL oxygen consumed per minute or 1 MET. >10 METs = excellent, 7-10 METs = good, 4-7 METs = moderate, <4 METs = poor.[12,13,14]

Table 7: ACC/AHA Risk of Surgical Procedure

Risk Stratification	Procedure Examples
Vascular (cardiac risk >5%)	Aortic & major vascular surgery Peripheral vascular surgery
Intermediate (cardiac risk 1-5%)	Intraperitoneal and intrathoracic surgery Carotid endarterectomy Head and neck surgery Orthopedic surgery
Low (cardiac risk <1%)	Endoscopic procedures Superficial procedures Cataract surgery Breast surgery Ambulatory surgery

[1]Low risk procedures do not generally require further preoperative cardiac testing.

Summary: Five Step Approach to Perioperative Cardiac Assessment

Step 1:	Determine whether there is time for cardiac evaluation. If the patient needs emergency surgery, there may be no time for a cardiac evaluation. Careful management of blood pressure, heart rate, and volume status is required intraoperatively. The patient should be risk stratified in the postoperative period and additional cardiac workup performed as indicated.
Step 2:	Determine whether the patient has any cardiac condition that needs to have evaluation/treatment before surgery (Table 4) If the patient has had a coronary artery bypass operation within the past 5 years, or percutaneous coronary intervention between 6 months and 5 years ago, and the clinical status is stable with no ischemia, then additional workup is not needed because the risk of MI is very small.
Step 3:	If the patient is stable and undergoing low risk surgery (Table 7), then additional cardiac testing is not needed.
Step 4:	Does the patient have good functional capacity (Table 6) without symptoms? Functional capacity is a reliable predictor of perioperative cardiac evaluation. For patients with known cardiovascular disease or 1 clinical risk factor, perioperative heart rate control is appropriate.

Step 5:	If functional capacity is poor, then clinical risk factors (Table 5) determine the need for further workup:
	    0 clinical risk factors − proceed with surgery
	    1-2 clinical risk factors − surgery with heart rate control
	    3+ clinical risk factors − surgery specific risk is important (Table 7). For high risk surgery, consider testing if it will change management. For intermediate risk surgery, proceed with heart rate control. Only do noninvasive testing if the results will modify surgical or anesthesia management.

REVIEW OF SYSTEMS

Cardiac: With some patients coronary artery disease is obvious − angina, congestive heart failure, status post CABG, and/or stent placement. However, for many patients the diagnosis is more difficult. Angina may be silent or the patient's functional activity level unclear due to other limiting factors (eg, age, arthritis, muscle wasting). These patients may benefit from further workup (due to low *Functional Capacity*, see Table 6) − unless they are not candidates for myocardial revascularization.

Although age and gender are not independent risk factors, mortality increases with perioperative MI in both the aged and females.[9] Hypertension (systolic <180 mm Hg and diastolic <110 mm Hg) is not an independent risk factor for perioperative cardiovascular complications, and thus acceptable to proceed with surgery.[2,9] However, for greater hypertension, the benefits of delaying surgery for better blood pressure control need to be discussed. If surgery is performed these patients have a greater incidence of hypotension, which is associated with more cardiovascular and renal complications. Anesthesia associated hypotension has been reported more commonly in patients on diuretic therapy and angiotensin converting enzyme (ACE) inhibitor/angiotensin receptor blockers (ARBs).

Questions that should be addressed by cardiology consultation include:

How much myocardium at risk?

What is the ischemic threshold (ie, heart rate at ischemia)?

What is the ventricular function?

Is the patient optimized on current medical regimen?

Which noninvasive stress test can answer the above questions?

Does the patient need invasive cardiac testing?

Pulmonary: Obstructive or restrictive disease increases the risk of postoperative respiratory complications. Preoperative symptoms/signs include hypoxemia, hypercapnia, acidosis, increased work of breathing, wheezing, and pneumonia. Preoperative treatment with bronchodilators and steroids may improve pulmonary function and gas exchange. If infection is suspected, antibiotic treatment is essential. Encouragement to stop tobacco use can decrease carboxyhemoglobin and decrease the progression of pulmonary damage.

Diabetes mellitus: Cardiac disease is more common in diabetics, especially those who require insulin. Compounding the risk is the fact that cardiac ischemia symptoms are silent, often not unmasked until a catastrophic event occurs. Chronic tight glucose control (measured by a glycated hemoglobin A_{1c} level <7%) may decrease the severity and rapidity of vascular disease, which has a beneficial effect for critical organs such as brain, heart, lung, and kidney. Aggressive perioperative glucose control, which requires frequent intraoperative evaluation, can improve outcome in surgical ICU patients.[15] Recent literature has demonstrated a benefit in treating diabetic patients with ACE inhibitors and/or ARBs as demonstrated by a decrease in the incidence of heart failure and proteinuria.

Renal: Azotemia is associated with increased cardiovascular events. Treatment of CHF with fluid restriction and diuretics can produce further worsening of renal function by decrease in glomeruli perfusion. Although treatment with ACE inhibitors and ARBs can produce small increases in BUN and creatinine, they should not be discontinued because they have been shown to improve renal function and survival of diabetic patients. Volume status is complicated in dialysis patients, fluctuating from overloaded to hypovolemia, depending on frequency of dialysis. A large study has shown that preoperative creatinine >2 mg/dL is an independent predictor of postoperative cardiac complications after noncardiac surgery.[16]

Hematologic: Severe anemia provokes heart failure and myocardial infarction. Although concern for disease transmission via transfusion of blood products exists, a hematocrit <28% is associated with an increased incidence of complications.[17,18] Conditions that increase blood viscosity increase thrombosis. Thrombocytopenia and decreased coagulation factors promote bleeding.

Table 8: Supplemental Preoperative Evaluation

Assessment of Left Ventricular Function

Recommended	Patients with dyspnea of unknown origin Patients with heart failure and change in clinical status reassessment
Not established	Clinically stable patients with known cardiomyopathy
Not recommended	Routine perioperative evaluation

Noninvasive Stress Testing

Recommended	Patients with active cardiac conditions (Table 4)
Reasonable	Patients with 3 or more clinical risk factors and <4 METs functional capacity for vascular surgery, if it will change management
Consider	Patients with 1-2 clinical risk factors, <4 METs functional capacity for intermediate-risk surgery, if it will change management Patients with 1-2 clinical risk factors and good functional capacity for vascular surgery
Not recommended	Patients with no clinical risk factors for intermediate-risk surgery Patients for low-risk surgery

12 Lead ECG

Recommended	Patients with at least 1 clinical risk factor for vascular surgical procedures Patients with known heart disease, peripheral arterial disease, or cerebrovascular disease for intermediate-risk surgery
Reasonable	Patients with no clinical risk factors for vascular surgery Patients with at least 1 clinical risk factor for intermediate-risk surgery
Not recommended	Asymptomatic patients for low-risk surgery

Fleisher LA, Beckman JA, Brown KA, et al, "ACC/AHA 2007 Guidelines on Perioperative Cardiovascular Evaluation and Care for Noncardiac Surgery: A Report of the American College of Cardiology/American Heart Association Task Force on Practice Guidelines (Writing Committee to Revise the 2002 Guidelines on Perioperative Cardiovascular Evaluation for Noncardiac Surgery) Developed in Collaboration With the American Society of Echocardiography, American Society of Nuclear Cardiology, Heart Rhythm Society, Society of Cardiovascular Anesthesiologists, Society for Cardiovascular Angiography and Interventions, Society for Vascular Medicine and Biology, and Society for Vascular Surgery," *J Am Coll Cardiol*, 2007, 50(17):e159-241.

PERIOPERATIVE CARDIOPROTECTIVE DRUGS

Beta Blockade: There is evidence that the use of perioperative beta blocker therapy decreases risk of perioperative ischemic cardiac events and long-term mortality.[19, 20] This therapy is especially effective in reducing perioperative mortality in patients with diabetes, left ventricular hypertrophy, coronary artery disease, and renal insufficiency. It has also been shown to decrease the incidence of postoperative atrial fibrillation.[21] Despite evidence of their protective effects, they are currently underused in the perioperative period. Part of the reason may be that physicians are concerned about using beta blockers in patients with severe cardiomyopathy, A-V conduction delay, or obstructive pulmonary disease. Additionally, since most anesthesiologists do not direct patient care in the postoperative period, many feel uncomfortable about prescribing this drug category. Another concern is whether all beta blockers possess the same therapeutic profile. Neither the timing, dose, target heart rate, or duration of beta blockade is known. It was initially assumed that beta blockade was beneficial because it reduces heart rate and contractility. It also decreases shear stress and reduces inflammation by decreasing sympathetic tone.[22] The most recent ACC/AHA recommendations are:

Beta-blockers are recommended in patients having noncardiac surgery with a history of coronary artery disease, peripheral arterial disease, stroke, heart failure, and/or major vasular surgery.

Beta-blockers should be continued in patients undergoing surgery who are receiving them to treat angina, symptomatic arrhythmias, hypertension.

Beta-blockers should be given to patients undergoing vascular surgery who are at high cardiac risk (ischemia on preoperative test).

◀ Beta-blockers are probably recommended for patients undergoing vascular or intermediate risk surgery in whom preoperative assessment identifies coronary heart disease or 2 or more clinical risk factors.

It is uncertain whether beta-blockers are useful for patients who are undergoing intermediate or vascular procedures in whom preoperative evaluation identifies a single cardiac risk factor or in vascular surgery patients with no cardiac risk factors who are not currently on beta-blockers.

The POISE (PeriOperative Ischemic Evaluation) trial evaluated the ability of metoprolol (extended-release) to prevent heart attacks and death in patients with cardiac problems undergoing noncardiac surgery. It concluded that perioperative beta blockade prevents myocardial infarction, but increases the risk of death and stroke. This may be due to the metoprolol dose (200 mg/day) and/or the low heart rate and blood pressure limits before intervention.[23]

Angiotensin converting enzyme (ACE) inhibitors/angiotensin receptor blockers (ARBs): The perioperative use of these drugs is still debated. They have been shown to decrease the decline in renal function for patients with diabetes and to improve cardiac function in patients with congestive heart failure. There is some concern about reports of severe intraoperative hypotension with chronic drug administration[24] and several studies have reported increased cardiac and renal complications, although this has not been confirmed by additional studies.

Alpha$_2$-agonists (clonidine): Several studies have demonstrated improved outcomes with perioperative use of these drugs for vascular surgery. ACC/AHA recommends alpha$_2$-agonists may be considered for perioperative control of hypertension in patients who have coronary artery disease or at least one clinical risk factor.[25] The use of dexmedetomidine may also provide these benefits.[26,27]

HMG-CoA reductase inhibitors (statins): HMG-CoA reductase inhibitor therapy has been shown to prevent cardiac events in high risk patients with or without prior myocardial infarct. It has been shown to lower the incidence of MI, stroke, and death in both hypertensive and normotensive patients.[28,29] Statin therapy not only decreases lipid levels, it also improves endothelial function, reduces vascular inflammation, and stabilized atherosclerotic plaque. ACA/AHA recommendations:

Those patients currently taking HMG-CoA reductase inhibitors continue perioperatively.

HMG-CoA reductase inhibitor therapy is reasonable for patients undergoing vascular (high risk) surgery regardless of whether or not they have clinical risk factors.

HMG-CoA reductase inhibitor therapy can be considered for patients with at least 1 clinical risk who are undergoing intermediate risk surgical procedures.

Calcium channel blockers: Although a meta-analysis showed reduced ischemia and supraventricular tachycardia,[30] ACA/AHA concluded that additional data are necessary before making recommendations.

ACC/AHA PERIOPERATIVE CORONARY REVASCULARIZATION WITH CABG OR PERCUTANEOUS CORONARY INTERVENTION (PCI) RECOMMENDATIONS

Coronary revascularization is recommended for patients with high-risk unstable angina, non-ST segment elevation MI, and acute ST-elevation MI. It is considered useful for patients with stable angina and (a) left main disease, (b) 3-vessel disease, (c) 2-vessel disease with significant LAD stenosis, and either EF<0.50 or ischemia on noninvasive testing.[31]

PCI before noncardiac surgery is not superior to medical therapy in patients with 1-2 vessel disease. Angioplasty with stenting in asymptomatic patients may increase the risk for perioperative cardiovascular complications including myocardial infarction.

PCI with angioplasty and/or bare metal stents (BMS) is appropriate for patients with cardiac symptoms who need elective surgery within one year. They should receive a thienopyridine (ie, clopidogrel, prasugrel, or ticlopidine) for at least 1 month with aspirin indefinitely. Patients with placement of a drug eluting stent (DES) should receive antiplatelet therapy for at least 1 year with aspirin indefinitely. Elective noncardiac surgery should be postponed for at least 6 weeks after PCI and placement of a BMS[11,32] and for at least 1 year after PCI and placement of a DES.[11,33] When surgery is scheduled, the thienopyridine (if patient still receiving) should be stopped for as brief a time as possible with aspirin continued perioperatively if at all possible.[34]

SUMMARY

Preoperative evaluation of the cardiac patient involves careful analysis of the risk predictors (clinical risk factors, functional capacity, and risk of the surgical procedure). It also involves evaluation of the comorbid disease states that commonly coexist with cardiac dysfunction. The ACC/AHA Guidelines offer the preoperative physician a methodology for the evaluation of these patients. The readers are referred to this article for much greater detail and explanation.[11]

ACA/AHA recommended that it is the role of the anesthesiologist to integrate the laboratory reports, consultant evaluations, and patient preference into the anesthetic plan. This plan includes drug selection, monitors, temperature control, glucose management, arrhythmia management, postoperative monitoring, and pain control plan. The choice of anesthetic technique and intraoperative monitors is best left to the discretion of the anesthesia care team.

FOOTNOTES

[1]Goldman L, "Assessment of Perioperative Cardiac Risk," *N Engl J Med*, 1994, 330(10):707-9.

[2]Goldman L, Caldera DL, Nussbaum SR, et al, "Multifactorial Index of Cardiac Risk in Noncardiac Surgical Procedures," *N Engl J Med*, 1977, 297(16):845-50.

[3]Tarhan S, Moffitt EA, Taylor WF, et al, "Myocardial Infarction After General Anesthesia," *JAMA*, 1972, 220(11):1451-4.

[4]Steen PA, Tinker JH, and Tarhan S, "Myocardial Infarction After Anesthesia and Surgery," *JAMA*, 1978, 239(24):2566-70.

[5]Rao TL, Jacobs KH, and El-Etr AA, "Reinfarction Following Anesthesia in Patients With Myocardial Infarction," *Anesthesiology*, 1983, 59(6):499-505.

[6]Shah KB, Kleinman BS, Sami H, et al, "Reevaluation of Perioperative Myocardial Infarction in Patients With Prior Myocardial Infarction Undergoing Noncardiac Operations," *Anesth Analg*, 1990, 71(3):231-5.

[7]Lee TH, Marcantonio ER, Mangione CM, et al, "Derivation and Prospective Validation of a Simple Index for Prediction of Cardiac Risk of Major Noncardiac Surgery," *Circulation*, 1999, 100 (10):1043-9.

[8]Detsky AS, Abrams HB, Forbath N, et al, "Cardiac Assessment for Patients Undergoing Noncardiac Surgery. A Multifactorial Clinical Risk Index," *Arch Intern Med*, 1986, 146(11):2131-4.

[9]Eagle KA, Coley CM, Newell JB, et al, "Combining Clinical and Thallium Data Optimizes Preoperative Assessment of Cardiac Risk Before Major Vascular Surgery," *Ann Intern Med*, 1989, 110(11):859-66.

[10]Eagle KA, Berger PB, Calkins H, et al, "ACC/AHA Guideline Update for Perioperative Cardiovascular Evaluation for Noncardiac Surgery – Executive Summary: A Report of the American College of Cardiology/American Heart Association Task Force on Practice Guidelines (Committee to Update the 1996 Guidelines on Perioperative Cardiovascular Evaluation for Noncardiac Surgery)," *J Am Coll Cardiol*, 2002, 39(3):542-53.

[11]Fleisher LA, Beckman JA, Brown KA, et al, "ACC/AHA 2007 Guidelines on Perioperative Cardiovascular Evaluation and Care for Noncardiac Surgery: A Report of the American College of Cardiology/American Heart Association Task Force on Practice Guidelines (Writing Committee to Revise the 2002 Guidelines on Perioperative Cardiovascular Evaluation for Noncardiac Surgery) Developed in Collaboration With the American Society of Echocardiography, American Society of Nuclear Cardiology, Heart Rhythm Society, Society of Cardiovascular Anesthesiologists, Society for Cardiovascular Angiography and Interventions, Society for Vascular Medicine and Biology, and Society for Vascular Surgery," *J Am Coll Cardiol*, 2007, 50(17):e159-241.

[12]Hlatky MA, Boineau RE, Higginbotham MB, et al, "A Brief Self-Administered Questionnaire to Determine Functional Capacity (The Duke Activity Status Index)," *Am J Cardiol*, 1989, 64 (10):651-4.

[13]Fletcher GF, Blair SN, Blumenthal J, et al, "Statement on Exercise. Benefits and Recommendations for Physical Activity Programs for All Americans. A Statement for Health Professionals by the Committee on Exercise and Cardiac Rehabilitation of the Council on Clinical Cardiology, American Heart Association," *Circulation*, 1992, 86(1):340-4.

[14]Reilly DF, McNeely MJ, Doerner D, et al, "Self-Reported Exercise Tolerance and the Risk of Serious Perioperative Complications," *Arch Intern Med*, 1999, 159(18):2185-92.

[15]van den Berghe G, Wouters P, Weekers F, et al, "Intensive Insulin Therapy in the Critically Ill Patients," *N Engl J Med*, 2001, 345(19):1359-67.

[16]Plotkin JS, Benitez RM, Kuo PC, et al, "Dobutamine Stress Echocardiography for Preoperative Cardiac Risk Stratification in Patients Undergoing Orthotopic Liver Transplantation," *Liver Transpl Surg*, 1998, 4(4):253-7.

[17]Hogue CW Jr, Goodnough LT, and Monk TG, "Perioperative Myocardial Ischemic Episodes Are Related to Hematocrit Level in Patients Undergoing Radical Prostatectomy," *Transfusion*, 1998, 38 (10):924-31.

[18]Nelson AH, Fleisher LA, and Rosenbaum SH, "Relationship Between Postoperative Anemia and Cardiac Morbidity in High-Risk Vascular Patients in the Intensive Care Unit," *Crit Care Med*, 1993, 21(6):860-6.

[19]Fleisher LA, Beckman JA, Brown KA, et al, "ACC/AHA 2006 Guideline Update on Perioperative Cardiovascular Evaluation for Noncardiac Surgery: Focused Update on Perioperative Beta-Blocker Therapy: A Report of the American College of Cardiology/American Heart Association Task Force on Practice Guidelines (Writing Committee to Update the 2002 Guidelines on Perioperative Cardiovascular Evaluation for Noncardiac Surgery) Developed in Collaboration With the American Society of Echocardiography, American Society of Nuclear Cardiology, Heart Rhythm Society, Society of Cardiovascular Anesthesiologists, Society for Cardiovascular Angiography and Interventions, and Society for Vascular Medicine and Biology," *J Am Coll Cardiol*, 2006, 47 (11):2343-55.

[20]Mangano DT, Layug EL, Wallace A, et al, "Effect of Atenolol on Mortality and Cardiovascular Morbidity After Noncardiac Surgery. Multicenter Study of Perioperative Ischemia Research Group," *N Engl J Med*, 1996, 335(23):1713-20.

[21]Jakobsen CJ, Bille S, Ahlburg P, et al, "Perioperative Metoprolol Reduces the Frequency of Atrial Fibrillation After Thoracotomy for Lung Resection," *J Cardiothorac Vasc Anesth*, 1997, 11 (6):746-51.

[22]Ohtsuka T, Hamada M, Hiasa G, et al, "Effect of Beta-Blockers on Circulating Levels of Inflammatory and Anti-Inflammatory Cytokines in Patients With Dilated Cardiomyopathy," *J Am Coll Cardiol*, 2001, 37(2):412-7.

[23]POISE Study Group, Devereaux PJ, Yang H, et al, "Effects of Extended-Release Metoprolol Succinate in Patients Undergoing Noncardiac Surgery (POISE Trial): A Randomised Controlled Trial," *Lancet*, 2008, 371(9627):1839-47.

[24]Brabant SM, Bertrand M, Eyraud D, et al, "The Hemodynamic Effects of Anesthetic Induction in Vascular Surgical Patients Chronically Treated With Angiotensin II Receptor Antagonists," *Anesth Analg*, 1999, 89(6):1388-92.

[25]Wallace AW, Galindez D, Salahieh A, et al, "Effect of Clonidine on Cardiovascular Morbidity and Mortality After Noncardiac Surgery," *Anesthesiology*, 2004, 101(2):284-93.

[26]Talke P, Chen R, Thomas B, et al, "The Hemodynamic and Adrenergic Effects of Perioperative Dexmedetomidine Infusion After Vascular Surgery," *Anesth Analg*, 2000, 90(4):834-9.

[27]Talke P, Li J, Jain U, et al, "Effects of Perioperative Dexmedetomidine Infusion in Patients Undergoing Vascular Surgery. The Study of Perioperative Ischemia Research Group," *Anesthesiology*, 1995, 82(3):620-33.

[28]Hindler K, Shaw AD, Samuels J, et al, "Improved Postoperative Outcomes Associated With Preoperative Statin Therapy," *Anesthesiology*, 2006, 105(6):1260-72.

[29]Messerli FH, Pinto L, Tang SS, et al, "Impact of Systemic Hypertension on the Cardiovascular Benefits of Statin Therapy: A Meta-Analysis," *Am J Cardiol*, 2008, 101(3):319-25.

[30]Wijeysundera DN and Beattie WS, "Calcium Channel Blockers for Reducing Cardiac Morbidity After Noncardiac Surgery: A Meta-Analysis," *Anesth Analg*, 2003, 97(3):634-41.

[31]Eagle KA, Guyton RA, Davidoff R, et al, "ACC/AHA 2004 Guideline Update for Coronary Artery Bypass Graft Surgery: A Report of the American College of Cardiology/American Heart Association Task Force on Practice Guidelines (Committee to Update the 1999 Guidelines for Coronary Artery Bypass Graft Surgery)," *Circulation*, 2004, 110(14):e340-437.

[32]Grines CL, Bonow RO, Casey DE Jr, et al, "Prevention of Premature Discontinuation of Dual Antiplatelet Therapy in Patients With Coronary Artery Stents: A Science Advisory From the American Heart Association, American College of Cardiology, Society for Cardiovascular Angiography and Interventions, American College of Surgeons, and American Dental Association, With Representation From the American College of Physicians," *Circulation*, 2007, 115(6):813-8.

[33]Nuttall GA, Brown MJ, Stombaugh JW, et al, "Time and Cardiac Risk of Surgery After Bare-Metal Stent Percutaneous Coronary Intervention," *Anesthesiology*, 2008, 109(4):588-95.

[34]Rabbitts JA, Nuttall GA, Brown MJ, et al, "Cardiac Risk of Noncardiac Surgery After Percutaneous Coronary Intervention With Drug-Eluting Stents," *Anesthesiology*, 2008, 109(4):596-604.

PERIOPERATIVE / PERIPROCEDURAL MANAGEMENT OF ANTICOAGULANT AND ANTIPLATELET THERAPY

Risk of Perioperative Arterial or Venous Thromboembolism

Perioperative management of patients who may require temporary interruption of antithrombotic therapy is a common challenge in patient care. Interruption of antithrombotic therapy in some patients may cause devastating consequences (eg, MI, stroke, valve thrombosis). It is important to address two questions prior to interrupting antithrombotic therapy. First, is interruption in the perioperative period necessary? Secondly, if interruption is necessary, is bridging anticoagulation necessary? The answers to these questions are determined by the type of surgery or procedure and the risk of thrombosis if antithrombotic therapy is interrupted, respectively. Although a validated risk stratification tool does not exist, the following guidelines (see Table 1) may be helpful in identifying those patients who are at risk of arterial or venous thromboembolism. In patients with atrial fibrillation, the $CHADS_2$ (Cardiac failure-Hypertension-Age-Diabetes-Stroke [doubled]) score, which identifies those patients at higher risk of stroke, must be calculated (see Table 2) to determine level of risk for perioperative arterial or venous thromboembolism.

Table 1. Suggested Risk Stratification for Perioperative Arterial or Venous Thromboembolism (Douketis, 2008)

Indication for Warfarin	High Risk	Moderate Risk	Low Risk
Mechanical Heart Valve	Any mitral valve prosthesis; Older (caged-ball or tilting disc) aortic valve prosthesis Recent (within 6 months) stroke or TIA	Bileaflet aortic valve prosthesis and at least one of the following: • AF • Prior stroke or TIA • Hypertension • Diabetes • Heart failure • Age >75 years	Bileaflet aortic valve prosthesis without AF or other risk factors for stroke
Atrial Fibrillation[1]	$CHADS_2$ score of 5 or 6 Recent (within 3 months) stroke or TIA Rheumatic valvular heart disease	$CHADS_2$ score of 3 or 4	$CHADS_2$ score of 0-2 (no prior stroke or TIA)
Venous Thromboembolism (VTE)	Recent (within 3 months) VTE Protein C or S deficiency, antithrombin or antiphospholipid antibodies, or multiple thrombophilic abnormalities	VTE within in the past 3-12 months Heterozygous factor V Leiden or factor II mutation Recurrent VTE Cancer (active)	Single VTE occurring >12 months ago (no additional risk factors)

$CHADS_2$ = Cardiac failure-Hypertension-Age-Diabetes-Stroke (doubled), TIA = transient ischemic attack

[1]Calculate $CHADS_2$ score (see Table 2) to determine level of risk for perioperative thrombosis

Table 2. $CHADS_2$ Index: Stroke Risk in Patients with Nonvalvular AF Not Treated with Anticoagulation (Fuster, 2006)

$CHADS_2$ Risk Criteria	Point(s)
Prior stroke or TIA	2
Age >75 years	1
Hypertension	1
Diabetes mellitus	1
Heart failure	1

AF = atrial fibrillation; $CHADS_2$ = Cardiac failure-Hypertension-Age-Diabetes-Stroke (doubled); TIA = transient ischemic attack

Table 3. Perioperative / Periprocedural Management of Warfarin

Type of Surgery / Procedure / Patient Population	Action	Reinstitution	Comments
Urgent surgery/ procedures	Administer I.V. or oral vitamin K low-dose (2.5-5 mg)		Consider FFP or recombinant factor VIIa in addition to vitamin K; however, these effects are temporary and may not last as long as the vitamin K inhibition
Surgery/procedure requiring normalization of INR	Stop 5 days before surgery	12-24 hours **AFTER** surgery/procedure when adequate hemostasis achieved	Administer low-dose oral vitamin K (1-2 mg); if INR is still elevated (≥1.5) 1-2 days before surgery
Mechanical heart valve or AF or VTE at **HIGH** risk of thromboembolism	Bridge with therapeutic SubQ LMWH or I.V. UFH	*Minor surgery/ procedures:* Therapeutic SubQ LMWH - 24 hours **AFTER** surgery/ procedure when adequate hemostasis achieved *Major surgery/ procedures:* Delay initiation of LMWH/UFH for 48-72 hours **AFTER** surgery/procedure when adequate hemostasis achieved	Last dose of therapeutic SubQ LMWH should be given 24 hours PRIOR to surgery/procedure (may give half the dose); for therapeutic I.V. UFH, stop 4 hours **BEFORE** surgery/procedure *Major surgery/ procedures:* Always consider the anticipated bleeding risk prior to reinstitution of LMWH/ UFH instead of resuming at a fixed time.
Mechanical heart valve or AF or VTE at **MODERATE** risk of thromboembolism	Bridge with therapeutic SubQ LMWH or I.V. UFH or low-dose SubQ LMWH	*Minor surgery/ procedures:* Therapeutic SubQ LMWH, 24 hours **AFTER** surgery/ procedure when adequate hemostasis achieved *Major surgery/ procedures:* Either delay initiation of LMWH/UFH for 48-72 hours *AFTER* adequate hemostasis achieved; administer low-dose SubQ LMWH/UFH; or avoid completely	Therapeutic SubQ LMHW preferred over other options; last dose of therapeutic SubQ LMWH should be given 24 hours **PRIOR** to surgery/ procedure (may give half the dose); for therapeutic I.V. UFH, stop 4 hours **BEFORE** surgery/ procedure *Major surgery/ procedures:* Always consider the anticipated bleeding risk prior to reinstitution of LMWH/ UFH instead of resuming at a fixed time.
Mechanical heart valve or AF or VTE at **LOW** risk of thromboembolism	Low-dose SubQ LMWH or none		
Minor dental procedures	Continue and administer oral prohemostatic agent (eg, aminocaproic acid)		
Minor dermatologic procedures	Continue through procedure		

AF = atrial fibrillation; FFP = fresh frozen plasma; INR = international normalized ratio; LMWH = low molecular weight heparin; SubQ = Subcutaneous; UFH = unfractionated heparin; VTE = venous thromboembolism

Table 4. Perioperative/Periprocedural Management of Antiplatelet Therapy – Aspirin / Clopidogrel / Ticlopidine

Type of Surgery / Procedure / Patient Population	Action	Reinstitution	Comments
Urgent surgery/ procedures	Transfuse with platelets or administer other prohemostatic agents		
Surgery/procedure requiring temporary interruption of aspirin or clopidogrel	Stop 7-10 days **PRIOR** to surgery/procedure	24 hours **AFTER** surgery/ procedure when adequate hemostasis achieved	
Noncardiac surgery: **HIGH** risk of cardiac events (exclusive of coronary stents)	Aspirin: Continue through surgery Clopidogrel: Stop at least 5 days, preferably 10 days before surgery		
CABG	Aspirin: Continue through surgery Clopidogrel: Stop at least 5 days, preferably 10 days before surgery	Aspirin: If stopped, restart 6-48 hours **AFTER** CABG when adequate hemostasis achieved	
PCI	Aspirin: Continue through procedure Clopidogrel: Continue through procedure	Clopidogrel: If stopped, restart **AFTER** PCI with loading dose (300-600 mg)	
Bare metal coronary stent: Surgery within 6 weeks of stent placement	Continue aspirin and clopidogrel in the preoperative period		If antiplatelet agent is stopped, do not bridge with UFH, LMWH, direct thrombin inhibitor, or glycoprotein IIb/IIIa inhibitor; no efficacy or safety data to support If increased bleeding is anticipated or procedure is elective with a significant risk of bleeding, then antiplatelet regimen should be completed first (Grines, 2007).
Drug-eluting coronary stent: Surgery within 12 months of stent placement	Continue aspirin and clopidogrel in the preoperative period		If antiplatelet agent is stopped, do not bridge with UFH, LMWH, direct thrombin inhibitor, or glycoprotein IIb/IIIa inhibitor; no efficacy or safety data to support If increased bleeding is anticipated or procedure is elective with a significant risk of bleeding, then antiplatelet regimen should be completed first (Grines, 2007).
Minor dental and dermatologic procedures	Aspirin: Continue through procedure Clopidogrel: See above indications for stent		In patients receiving dual antiplatelet therapy for prevention of stent thrombosis, the American Heart Association and other organizations recommend that aspirin and clopidogrel be continued throughout the procedure. If increased bleeding is anticipated or procedure is elective with a significant risk of bleeding, then antiplatelet regimen should be completed first (Grines, 2007).
Regional/neuraxial anesthesia	Refer to Regional Anesthesia in Patients Receiving Anticoagulant and Antiplatelet Therapy on page 1642.	**AFTER** catheter removal	NSAIDs (including aspirin) do not appear to increase the risk of spinal hematoma. The actual risk of spinal hematoma with clopidogrel or ticlopidine is unknown.

ACS = Acute coronary syndrome; CABG = coronary artery bypass graft; LMWH = subcutaneous low molecular weight heparin; NSAIDs = nonsteroidal anti-inflammatory drugs; PCI = percutaneous coronary intervention; UFH = unfractionated heparin

◄ **Note:** If patient receiving antiplatelet regimen for prevention of stent thrombosis,
contact patient's cardiologist prior to discontinuation (Grines, 2007). Premature
interruption of therapy may result in stent thrombosis with subsequent fatal and
nonfatal MI. See Table 5 for duration of antiplatelet therapy according to current
practice guidelines.

**Table 5. Duration of Antiplatelet Therapy
According to Current Practice Guidelines**

Indication for Antiplatelet Therapy	Recommended Duration of Aspirin	Recommended Duration of Clopidogrel[1] or Ticlopidine
Acute Coronary Syndrome (ACS)		
NSTEMI	Indefinite	12 months
NSTEMI with subsequent CABG	Indefinite	9-12 months
STEMI with or without fibrinolysis	Indefinite	2-4 weeks
Percutaneous Coronary Intervention (PCI)		
BMS implantation following ACS	Indefinite	12 months[2]
BMS implantation without ongoing ACS	Indefinite	At least 1 month (ideally 12 months)
DES implantation with or without ongoing ACS	Indefinite	12 months[2,3]

BMS = Bare metal stent; CABG = Coronary artery bypass graft; DES = Drug eluting stent; NSTEMI =
Non ST-elevation myocardial infarction; STEMI = ST-elevation myocardial infarction

[1]Clopidogrel is the preferred thienopyridine due to its lower incidence of serious side effects (eg,
neutropenia) as compared to ticlopidine. **Note:** Prasugrel, a newer thienopyridine indicated for
patients with ACS managed with PCI, may also be used with the same durations.

[2]The optimal duration of therapy >1 year has not been established. Clinical predictors of late stent
thrombosis during this time period include stenting ostial or bifurcation lesions, prior brachytherapy,
advanced age, diabetes mellitus, renal failure, and others.

[3]The ACC/AHA/SCAI 2007 Focused guideline update for PCI recommends a minimum of 3 months
for a sirolimus DES and 6 months for a paclitaxel DES.

References

Douketis JD, Berger PB, Dunn AS, et al, "The Perioperative Management of Antithrombotic Therapy:
American College of Chest Physicians Evidence-Based Clinical Practice Guidelines (8th Edition),"
Chest, 2008, 133(6 Suppl):299S-339S.

Fuster V, Rydén LE, Cannom DS, et al, "ACC/AHA/ESC 2006 Guidelines for the Management of
Patients With Atrial Fibrillation–Executive Summary: A Report of the American College of
Cardiology/American Heart Association Task Force on Practice Guidelines and the European
Society of Cardiology Committee for Practice Guidelines (Writing Committee to Revise the 2001
Guidelines for the Management of Patients With Atrial Fibrillation)," *J Am Coll Cardiol*, 2006, 48
(4):854-906.

Grines CL, Bonow RO, Casey DE Jr, et al, "Prevention of Premature Discontinuation of Dual
Antiplatelet Therapy in Patients With Coronary Artery Stents: A Science Advisory From the
American Heart Association, American College of Cardiology, Society for Cardiovascular
Angiography and Interventions, and American College of Surgeons, and American Dental Association,
With Representation From the American College of Physicians," *Circulation*, 2007, 115(6):813-8.
Available at http://www.acc.org/qualityandscience/clinical/pdfs/Final_Dual_Antiplatelet_State-
ment_010507.pdf.

King SB 3rd, Smith SC Jr, Hirshfeld JW Jr, et al, "2007 Focused Update of the ACC/AHA/SCAI 2005
Guideline Update for Percutaneous Coronary Intervention: A Report of the American College of
Cardiology/American Heart Association Task Force on Practice Guidelines," *J Am Coll Cardiol*,
2008, 51(2):172-209.

Smith SC Jr, Feldman TE, Hirshfeld JW Jr, et al, "ACC/AHA/SCAI 2005 Guideline Update for
Percutaneous Coronary Intervention-Summary Article: A Report of the American College of
Cardiology/American Heart Association Task Force on Practice Guidelines (ACC/AHA/SCAI Writing
Committee to Update the 2001 Guidelines for Percutaneous Coronary Intervention)," *J Am Coll
Cardiol*, 2006, 47(1):216-35.

STRESS REPLACEMENT OF CORTICOSTEROIDS

Recommendations for stress replacement of corticosteroids vary due to the inconsistent data to predict adrenal suppression in patients receiving steroids. Because of the low risk involved with supplementation, some advocate administration of corticosteroids for any patient who has received steroids, including topical steroids, within a year. However, patients receiving 5 mg/day or less of prednisone maintain an intact HPA axis. Supplementation of corticosteroids during stress or acute illness may be required to prevent adrenal suppression. Furthermore in severe sepsis, supplementation of corticosteroids will reduce catecholamine vasopressor requirements and may lead to decreased mortality and morbidity in patients with relative adrenal insufficiency. However, recent data regarding the mortality benefit for steroids in sepsis are conflicting. Lastly, patients on concurrent medications (such as phenytoin, barbiturates, rifampin, etc) may require larger doses of steroids due to increased metabolism.

Corticosteroid Supplementation

Steroid Status	Prednisone Dose[1]	Severity of Surgery	Steroid Regimen
Taking steroids	<10 mg/d	Any surgery	Additional steroid coverage not required; assume normal HPA response
	>10 mg/d	Minor surgery	25 mg hydrocortisone at induction on day of induction only
		Moderate surgery	Hydrocortisone 25 mg at induction, **plus** 50-100 mg hydrocortisone per day for ~24 hours Taper quickly over 1-2 days to usual dose
		Major surgery	Hydrocortisone 25 mg at induction **plus** 100-150 mg hydrocortisone per day for 48-72 hours Taper quickly over 1-2 days to usual dose
	High-dose immunosuppression	Any surgery	Give usual immunosuppressive doses during perioperative period
Critically ill: Sepsis-induced hypotension or shock, after confirmation of relative adrenal insufficiency[2]			Hydrocortisone 50 mg every 6 hours for a total of 7-11 days; consider adding fludrocortisones 50 mcg every 24 hours **OR** Dexamethasone 4 mg every 12 hours[3]

[1]If patient receiving a different corticosteroid, please use the table below to convert to an equivalent prednisone dose.

[2]Relative adrenal insufficiency defined as an increase of cortisol <9 mcg/dL from the baseline cortisol level, measured at 30 or 60 minutes after the administration of 250 mcg of adrenocorticotropin hormone (ACTH). Some authors define adrenal insufficiency at a baseline cortisol level ≤15 mcg/dL in the critically ill.

[3]Dexamethasone will not interfere with the rapid ACTH stimulation test and may be given while determining the adrenal status of the patient.

Patients receiving prednisone ≤5 mg/day should receive normal dose of corticosteroid and should not need additional coverage.

Patients receiving prednisone >5 mg/day should receive regimen listed above based on surgical severity or stress, in addition to patient's maintenance therapy.

Steroid Status	Time Off Steroid	Comments
Not currently taking steroids	<3 months	Treat as if receiving steroids
	>3 months	No perioperative steroids necessary

Corticosteroid Potency and Equivalent Dose Conversion

Steroid	Relative Potency		Equivalent Dose (mg)
	Anti-inflammatory	Mineralocorticoid	
Short-Acting			
Cortisone	0.8	0.8	25
Hydrocortisone	1	1	20
Intermediate-Acting			
Prednisone	4	0.8	5
Prednisolone	4	0.8	5
Methylprednisolone	5	0.5	4
Triamcinolone	5	0	4
Long-Acting			
Dexamethasone	25	0	0.75
Betamethasone	25	0	0.6-0.75

REFERENCES AND RECOMMENDED READING

Annane D, Sebille V, Charpentier C, et al, "Effect of Treatment With Low Doses of Hydrocortisone and Fludrocortisone on Mortality in Patients with Septic Shock," *JAMA*, 2002, 288(7):862-71.

Cooper MS and Stewart PM, "Corticosteroid Insufficiency in Acutely Ill Patients," *N Engl J Med*, 2003, 348(8):727-34.

Coursin DB and Wood KE, "Corticosteroid Supplementation for Adrenal Insufficiency," *JAMA*, 2002, 287(2):236-40.

Henriques HF III and Lebovic D, "Defining and Focusing Perioperative Steroid Supplementation," *Am Surg*, 1995, 61(9):809-13.

Gonzalez H, Nardi O, and Annane D, "Relative Adrenal Failure in the ICU: An Identifiable Problem Requiring Treatment," *Crit Care Clin*, 2006, 22(1):105-18.

Marik PE and Zaloga GP, "Adrenal Insufficiency in the Critically Ill: A New Look at an Old Problem," *Chest*, 2002, 122(5):1784-96.

Marik PE, Pastores SM, Annane D, et al, "Recommendations for the Diagnosis and Management of Corticosteroid Insufficiency in Critically Ill Adult Patients: Consensus Statements From an International Task Force By The American College of Critical Care Medicine," *Crit Care Med*, 2008, 36(6):1937-49.

Nicholson G, Burrin JM, and Hall GM, "Perioperative Steroid Supplementation," *Anaesthesia*, 1998, 53(11):1091-104.

Salem M, Tainsh RE Jr, Bromberg J, et al, "Perioperative Glucocorticoid Coverage. A Reassessment 42 Years After Emergence of a Problem.," *Ann Surg*, 1994, 219(4):416-25.

Sprung CL, Annane D, Keh D, et al, "Hydrocortisone Therapy for Patients With Septic Shock," *N Engl J Med*, 2008, 358(2):111-24.

Thomas Z and Fraser GL, "An Update on the Diagnosis of Adrenal Insufficiency and the Use of Corticotherapy in Critical Illness," *Ann Pharmacother*, 2007, 41(9):1456-65.

ANESTHETIC CONSIDERATIONS IN THE SUBSTANCE-ABUSING PATIENT

Substance abuse is a problem that must be considered when evaluating a patient for surgery under general anesthesia. Many substances can potentially interfere with anesthetic and other agents administered in the perioperative setting. Substances of abuse such as ethanol, central nervous system depressants (opioids, benzodiazepines, barbiturates), and cocaine can all influence the type and the amount of anesthetic administered. Below are brief discussions referring to drugs of abuse and how to perioperatively manage those patients who are abusing the agents.

ETHANOL

Chronic ethanol abuse results in induction of the cytochrome P450 system which can affect anesthetic and other medications used perioperatively. Because of this liver enzyme induction, certain agents may need to be dosed more frequently to achieve the desired effect. Larger doses of anesthetic agents may be required in chronic alcohol abusers because of cross-tolerance.

Acute ethanol intoxication causes significant central nervous system (CNS) depression. For those individuals, including chronic alcoholics undergoing anesthesia while intoxicated, the anesthetic requirements may be reduced.

MARIJUANA

Marijuana is one of the most popular recreational drugs of abuse. When combined with alcohol or benzodiazepines, one can see an increase in sedative effects while an increase in stimulatory effects is seen when combined with cocaine or amphetamines. It is rare to see major anesthesia interactions from marijuana; however, one must keep in mind that it affects every organ system and its clinical effects are unpredictable. Tachycardia and increased cardiac output can be seen with low or moderate doses; this results from an increase in sympathetic activity with a reduction in parasympathetic activity. When high doses are taken, sympathetic activity is inhibited but not parasympathetic activity, resulting in possible bradycardia and hypotension. In terms of cardiac rhythm abnormalities, an increase in supraventricular or ventricular ectopic activity has been reported as has reversible ST-segment and T-wave abnormalities.

Central nervous system depression can be enhanced when marijuana is combined with other sedative hypnotic drugs. In addition, since marijuana use can result in myocardial depression and tachycardia, it may potentiate anesthetic drugs that affect heart rate and blood pressure. Increased myocardial depression may be seen when the effects of marijuana are combined with those of the potent inhalation agents (eg, desflurane, sevoflurane, isoflurane). Likewise, drugs increasing heart rate (eg, epinephrine, ketamine, pancuronium, atropine) should be avoided in patients with acute marijuana abuse.

Marijuana inhalation is associated with upper-airway irritability, impairment of airway epithelial function, and damage to bronchial tissue which can result in chronic cough, bronchitis, emphysema, and bronchospasm. In marijuana-smoking patients who have undergone general anesthesia, oropharyngitis and acute upper-airway edema and obstruction have been reported.

OPIOIDS

Opioids can be abused by the oral, subcutaneous, or intravenous routes. Opioids that have been reported as abused include heroin, morphine, fentanyl, meperidine, methadone, codeine, oxycodone, propoxyphene, and hydrocodone. In people abusing opioids, addiction can occur rapidly if increasing doses are taken on a daily basis. Opioid withdrawal can be seen as soon as 4-6 hours after the last dose and peaks between 48-72 hours. Maintaining adequate perioperative opioid dosing is paramount to preventing withdrawal.

Intraoperatively, patients on chronic opioids can have cross tolerance to other CNS depressants; anesthetic requirements may be increased. Postoperatively, patients on chronic opioids have higher pain scores and an increased requirement for opioids. Opioid antagonists and mixed agonist-antagonists must not be given to the patient addicted to opioids. Doing so can precipitate an acute withdrawal reaction.

CENTRAL NERVOUS SYSTEM DEPRESSANTS

Patients taking CNS depressants on a chronic basis will frequently need increased doses of certain anesthetic agents. Patients who are taking barbiturates chronically will have liver enzyme induction which increases the potential for drug interactions and may increase anesthetic requirements.

Rhohypnol (flunitrazepam) is a benzodiazepine that has been used as a "date rape" drug. It is not manufactured in the United States. Rhohypnol's effects are approximately 7-10 times those of diazepam. Onset of effects is seen within 30 minutes, peak effects in 1-2 hours, with an average duration of 8-10 hours. The anesthetic requirements of the acutely intoxicated patient will be decreased and respiratory depression can be seen in the presence of opioids.

γ-Hydroxybutyrate (GHB) is a metabolite of γ-hydroxybutyric acid (GABA). Onset of effect is within 10-20 minutes and can last from 3-6 hours. It is a CNS depressant and in large doses can result in respiratory depression, coma, and death.

COCAINE

Perioperative management of the suspected cocaine intoxicated patient should be aimed at cardiovascular stability. Cocaine can cause profound cardiovascular effects secondary to adrenergic stimulation from increased plasma catecholamines. Hypertension, tachycardia, and cardiac arrhythmias secondary to myocardial ischemia can be seen in cocaine-abusing patients undergoing general anesthesia. Severe hypertension resulting from direct laryngoscopy can also be seen in the cocaine-abusing patient.

To blunt this response, an antihypertensive agent can be administered prior to induction. Beta-blockers (eg, propranolol, esmolol, metoprolol) are contraindicated due to their potential to produce unopposed alpha-adrenergic stimulation and enhancement of cocaine-induced coronary vasoconstriction. Labetalol, an α- and β-blocker, has the advantages of a fast onset of action and the ability to reduce blood pressure without changes in heart rate; however, unopposed alpha-stimulation may still be seen with this agent due to the substantially lower α-blocking activity. Hydralazine is effective in reducing systemic vascular resistance as a result of its vasodilating properties; however, the reflex tachycardia that can be seen may not be optimal in the cocaine-abusing patient who may already be tachycardic. Benzodiazepines may be helpful in reducing heart rate and blood pressure. Nitroglycerin should be readily available.

Ketamine should be used with caution, if at all, since it may increase catecholamine levels and stimulate the central nervous system. One must also be careful when using etomidate in this patient population because of its ability to cause myoclonus, seizures, and hyper-reflexia. Propofol and thiopental have been demonstrated to be safe induction agents for cocaine-abusing patients.

Anesthetic management of the cocaine-intoxicated patient remains an unresolved issue. The anesthesiologist and the surgeon should consider the risk/benefit analysis of delaying the procedure. If the procedure is emergent and/or the patient is clinically nontoxic, it need not be postponed and the above precautions and techniques should be considered.

Routine urine toxicology screening for cocaine detects the parent compound and its metabolites. The metabolites of cocaine include egonine methyl ester (EME), benzoylecgonine, and norcocaine. These metabolites can render a urine toxicology screen for cocaine positive for up to 60 hours after cocaine intake. Yet, these metabolites do not produce cocaine-like cardiovascular stimulation and the patient may be clinically nontoxic. Some practitioners have stopped performing urine toxicology testing for cocaine. Instead, patients are screened on the day of surgery for signs of acute cocaine toxicity by evaluating mental status, heart rate, blood pressure, and ECG (eg, QT_c interval should be <500 msec).

AMPHETAMINES

Acutely, amphetamines can produce hypertensive effects that are similar to those seen with cocaine. It would be prudent to avoid beta-blockade in these patients Acute intoxication with amphetamines can increase anesthetic requirements, whereas chronic abuse of amphetamines reduce anesthetic requirements. Because catecholamine stores are depleted, hypotension should be treated with direct-acting vasopressors (eg, phenylephrine, epinephrine).

SOLVENTS

Toluene is the most frequently abused solvent. It can be found in glue, rubber cement, household paints, and various cleaning agents. Solvents are a favorite item of abuse for adolescents due to their ready accessibility. Cardiac arrhythmias, bronchial irritation, methemoglobinemia, pulmonary hypertension, and pulmonary edema have been reported with solvent inhalant abuse.

HALLUCINOGENS

Common hallucinogens include phencyclidine (PCP), lysergic acid diethylamide (LSD), mescaline, and psilocybin. People taking these drugs experience hallucinations (visual, tactile, auditory) with distortion of surroundings and body image, panic attacks, and anxiety. Abuse of these drugs does not result in physical dependence but psychological dependence and tolerance can be seen. Sympathetic nervous system activation occurs with the hallucinogens, resulting in hypertension and tachycardia. An increase in body temperature and pupil dilation can also be seen. When acutely ingested, the effects of theses drugs last for approximately 12 hours. Respiratory depression, seizures, coma, and death have been reported in overdose situations.

The anesthesia provider needs to be aware that there is high likelihood of autonomic dysregulation in these patients. It is important that blood pressure and heart rate be controlled. Vasopressors should be used with caution as an exaggerated response can often times be seen. Arrhythmias have been reported in this situation. Further, the analgesic and respiratory depressant effects of opioids may be prolonged by the hallucinogens. It has been suggested that PCP and LSD inhibit plasma cholinesterase activity with a resultant prolongation of the effects of succinylcholine.

MDMA (3,4-METHYLENEDIOXMETHAMPHETAMINE)

MDMA, commonly known as ecstasy, has both stimulant and hallucinogenic properties. Onset of effects usually occurs within 30 minutes, peaks at 2 hours, and lasts 3-6 hours. MDMA users may present with hypertension, tachycardia, hyperthermia, mydriasis, profound sweating, jaw clenching, and teeth grinding. Seizures have been reported as a result of hyponatremia and cerebral edema secondary to the large amount of water ingested by MDMA users. When used long term, cardiomyopathy can occur. Hepatitis and acute renal failure have also been seen in MDMA users. Profound hyperthermia appears to be a major factor in MDMA deaths. Caution should be used in patients predisposed to malignant hyperthermia (MH) who have taken MDMA as some postulate that MDMA may trigger MH.

The anesthesia provider, when presented with a patient with a history of MDMA use or currently taking MDMA, needs to evaluate and correct fluid and electrolyte abnormalities (eg, hyponatremia). In acutely intoxicated patients, autonomic dysregulation should be expected. For hyperthermia, supportive measures such as cooling intravenous fluids, hydration to establish urine output, and 100% oxygen may help. Since MDMA users may have hepatic dysfunction and renal failure, anesthetic medications that are eliminated via these routes may have prolonged effects. Avoid using succinylcholine or the volatile inhalation agents in MDMA patients with a history of hyperthermia.

◄ REFERENCES

Culver JL and Walker JR, "Anesthetic Implications of Illicit Drug Use," *J Perianesth Nurs*, 1999, 14 (2):82-90.

Hernandez M, Birnbach DJ, and Van Zundert AA, "Anesthetic Management of the Illicit-Substance-Using Patient," *Curr Opin Anaesthesiol*, 2005, 18(3):315-24.

Hill GE, Ogunnaike BO, and Johnson ER, "General Anaesthesia for the Cocaine Abusing Patient. Is It Safe?" *Br J Anaesth*, 2006, 97(5):654-7.

Klein M and Kramer F, "Rave Drugs: Pharmacological Considerations," *AANA J*, 2004, 72(1):61-7.

Mitra S and Sinatra RS, "Perioperative Management of Acute Pain in the Opioid-Dependent Patient," *Anesthesiology*, 2004, 101(1):212-27.

Steadman JL and Birnbach DJ, "Patients on Party Drugs Undergoing Anesthesia," *Curr Opin Anaesthiesiol*, 2003, 16(2):147-52.

APPENDIX TABLE OF CONTENTS

BODY SURFACE AREA OF ADULTS AND CHILDREN

Calculating Body Surface Area in Children

In a child of average size, find weight and corresponding surface area on the boxed scale to the left; or, use the nomogram to the right. Lay a straightedge on the correct height and weight points for the child, then read the intersecting point on the surface area scale. (**Note:** 2.2 lb = 1 kg)

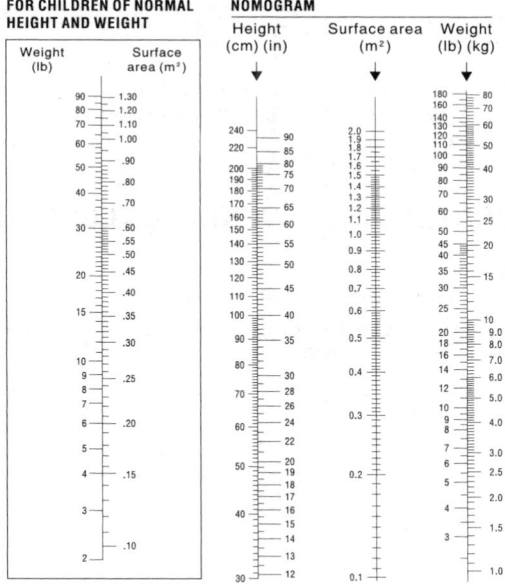

BODY SURFACE AREA FORMULA
(Adult and Pediatric)

$$\text{BSA (m}^2) = \sqrt{\frac{\text{Ht (in) x Wt (lb)}}{3131}} \text{ or, in metric: BSA (m}^2) = \sqrt{\frac{\text{Ht (cm) x Wt (kg)}}{3600}}$$

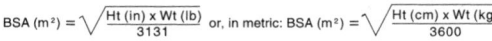

References

Lam TK and Leung DT, "More on Simplified Calculation of Body Surface Area," *N Engl J Med*, 1988, 318(17):1130 (Letter).
Mosteller RD, "Simplified Calculation of Body Surface Area", *N Engl J Med*, 1987, 317(17):1098 (Letter).

IDEAL BODY WEIGHT CALCULATION

Adults (18 years and older)

IBW (male) = 50 + (2.3 x height in inches over 5 feet)

IBW (female) = 45.5 + (2.3 x height in inches over 5 feet)

IBW is in kg.

Children

a. 1-18 years

$$IBW = \frac{(height^2 \times 1.65)}{1000}$$

IBW is in kg.

Height is in cm.

b. 5 feet and taller

IBW (male) = 39 + (2.27 x height in inches over 5 feet)

IBW (female) = 42.2 + (2.27 x height in inches over 5 feet)

IBW is in kg.

ADJUSTED BODY WEIGHT CALCULATION

Adults (18 years and older)

ABW = IBW + 0.4 (actual body weight − IBW)

Note: This calculation is used in dosing certain medications when patient weighs >20% of his/her IBW. ABW is in kg.

MILLIEQUIVALENT AND MILLIMOLE CALCULATIONS AND CONVERSIONS

DEFINITIONS AND CALCULATIONS

Definitions

mole	=	gram molecular weight of a substance (aka molar weight)
millimole (mM)	=	milligram molecular weight of a substance (a millimole is 1/1000 of a mole)
equivalent weight	=	gram weight of a substance which will combine with or replace 1 gram (1 mole) of hydrogen; an equivalent weight can be determined by dividing the molar weight of a substance by its ionic valence
milliequivalent (mEq)	=	milligram weight of a substance which will combine with or replace 1 milligram (1 millimole) of hydrogen (a milliequivalent is 1/1000 of an equivalent)

Calculations

moles	=	$\dfrac{\text{weight of a substance (grams)}}{\text{molecular weight of that substance (grams)}}$
millimoles	=	$\dfrac{\text{weight of a substance (milligrams)}}{\text{molecular weight of that substance (milligrams)}}$
equivalents	=	moles x valence of ion
milliequivalents	=	millimoles x valence of ion
moles	=	$\dfrac{\text{equivalents}}{\text{valence of ion}}$
millimoles	=	$\dfrac{\text{milliequivalents}}{\text{valence of ion}}$
millimoles	=	moles x 1000
milliequivalents	=	equivalents x 1000

Note: Use of equivalents and milliequivalents is valid only for those substances which have fixed ionic valences (eg, sodium, potassium, calcium, chlorine, magnesium bromine, etc). For substances with variable ionic valences (eg, phosphorous), a reliable equivalent value cannot be determined. In these instances, one should calculate millimoles (which are fixed and reliable) rather than milliequivalents.

MILLIEQUIVALENT CONVERSIONS

To convert mg/100 mL to mEq/L the following formula may be used:

$$\frac{(\text{mg/100 mL}) \times 10 \times \text{valence}}{\text{atomic weight}} = \text{mEq/L}$$

To convert mEq/L to mg/100 mL the following formula may be used:

$$\frac{(\text{mEq/L}) \times \text{atomic weight}}{10 \times \text{valence}} = \text{mg/100 mL}$$

To convert mEq/L to volume of percent of a gas the following formula may be used:

$$\frac{(\text{mEq/L}) \times 22.4}{10} = \text{volume percent}$$

Valences and Atomic Weights of Selected Ions

Substance	Electrolyte	Valence	Molecular Wt
Calcium	Ca^{++}	2	40
Chloride	Cl^-	1	35.5
Magnesium	Mg^{++}	2	24
Phosphate	HPO_4^{--} (80%)	1.8	96^1
pH = 7.4	$H_2PO_4^-$ (20%)	1.8	96^1
Potassium	K^+	1	39
Sodium	Na^+	1	23
Sulfate	SO_4^{--}	2	96^1

[1]The molecular weight of phosphorus only is 31, and sulfur only is 32.

Approximate Milliequivalents — Weights of Selected Ions

Salt	mEq/g Salt	mg Salt/mEq
Calcium carbonate [$CaCO_3$]	20	50
Calcium chloride [$CaCl_2 \cdot 2H_2O$]	14	74
Calcium gluceptate [$Ca(C_7H_{13}O_8)_2$]	4	245
Calcium gluconate [$Ca(C_6H_{11}O_7)_2 \cdot H_2O$]	5	224
Calcium lactate [$Ca(C_3H_5O_3)_2 \cdot 5H_2O$]	7	154
Magnesium gluconate [$Mg(C_6H_{11}O_7)_2 \cdot H_2O$]	5	216
Magnesium oxide [MgO]	50	20
Magnesium sulfate [$MgSO_4$]	17	60
Magnesium sulfate [$MgSO_4 \cdot 7H_2O$]	8	123
Potassium acetate [$K(C_2H_3O_2)$]	10	98
Potassium chloride [KCl]	13	75
Potassium citrate [$K_3(C_6H_5O_7) \cdot H_2O$]	9	108
Potassium iodide [KI]	6	166
Sodium acetate [$Na(C_2H_3O_2)$]	12	82
Sodium acetate [$Na(C_2H_3O_2) \cdot 3H_2O$]	7	136
Sodium bicarbonate [$NaHCO_3$]	12	84
Sodium chloride [$NaCl$]	17	58
Sodium citrate [$Na_3(C_6H_5O_7) \cdot 2H_2O$]	10	98
Sodium iodine [NaI]	7	150
Sodium lactate [$Na(C_3H_5O_3)$]	9	112
Zinc sulfate [$ZnSO_4 \cdot 7H_2O$]	7	144

CORRECTED SODIUM

Corrected Na^+ = measured Na^+ + [1.5 x (glucose − 150 divided by 100)]

Note: Do not correct for glucose <150.

WATER DEFICIT

Water deficit = 0.6 x body weight [1 − (140 divided by Na^+)]

Note: Body weight is estimated weight in kg when fully hydrated; **Na^+** is serum or plasma sodium. Use corrected Na^+ if necessary. Consult medical references for recommendations for replacement of deficit.

TOTAL SERUM CALCIUM CORRECTED FOR ALBUMIN LEVEL

[(Normal albumin – patient's albumin) x 0.8] + patient's measured total calcium

ACID-BASE ASSESSMENT

Henderson-Hasselbalch Equation

$pH = 6.1 + \log (HCO_3^- / (0.03)(pCO_2))$

Alveolar Gas Equation

PIO_2 = FiO_2 x (total atmospheric pressure – vapor pressure of H_2O at 37°C)

= FiO_2 x (760 mm Hg – 47 mm Hg)

PAO_2 = $PIO_2 - PACO_2 / R$

Alveolar/arterial oxygen gradient = $PAO_2 - PaO_2$

Normal ranges:

Children	15-20 mm Hg
Adults	20-25 mm Hg

where:

PIO_2	=	Oxygen partial pressure of inspired gas (mm Hg) (150 mm Hg in room air at sea level)
FiO_2	=	Fractional pressure of oxygen in inspired gas (0.21 in room air)
PAO_2	=	Alveolar oxygen partial pressure
$PACO_2$	=	Alveolar carbon dioxide partial pressure
PaO_2	=	Arterial oxygen partial pressure
R	=	Respiratory exchange quotient (typically 0.8, increases with high carbohydrate diet, decreases with high fat diet)

Acid-Base Disorders

Acute metabolic acidosis:
$PaCO_2$ expected = 1.5 (HCO_3^-) + 8 ± 2 **or**
Expected decrease in $PaCO_2$ = 1.3 (1-1.5) x decrease in HCO_3^-

Acute metabolic alkalosis:
Expected increase in $PaCO_2$ = 0.6 (0.5-1) x increase in HCO_3^-

Acute respiratory acidosis (<6 h duration):
For every $PaCO_2$ increase of 10 mm Hg, HCO_3 increases by 1 mEq/L

Chronic respiratory acidosis (>6 h duration):
For every $PaCO_2$ increase of 10 mm Hg, HCO_3 increases by 4 mEq/L

Acute respiratory alkalosis (<6 h duration):
For every $PaCO_2$ decrease of 10 mm Hg, HCO_3 decreases by 2 mEq/L

Chronic respiratory alkalosis (>6 h duration):
For every $PaCO_2$ decrease of 10 mm Hg, HCO_3 increases by 5 mEq/L

ACID-BASE EQUATION

H^+ (in mEq/L) = (24 x $PaCO_2$) divided by HCO_3^-

◀

Aa GRADIENT

Aa gradient $[(713)(FiO_2 - (PaCO_2 \text{ divided by } 0.8))] - PaO_2$

Aa gradient	=	alveolar-arterial oxygen gradient
FiO_2	=	inspired oxygen (expressed as a fraction)
$PaCO_2$	=	arterial partial pressure carbon dioxide (mm Hg)
PaO_2	=	arterial partial pressure oxygen (mm Hg)

OSMOLALITY

Definition: The summed concentrations of all osmotically active solute particles.

Predicted serum osmolality =

$$mOsm/L = (2 \times \text{serum } Na^{++}) + \frac{\text{serum glucose}}{18} + \frac{BUN}{2.8}$$

The normal range of serum osmolality is 285-295 mOsm/L.

Calculated Osm

Note: Osm is a term used to reconcile osmolality and osmolarity

Osmol gap = measured Osm − calculated Osm

0 to +10: Normal
>10: Abnormal
<0: Probable lab or calculation error

Drugs Causing Osmolar Gap

(by freezing-point depression, gap is >10 mOsm)
Ethanol
Ethylene glycol
Glycerol
Iodine (questionable)
Isopropanol (acetone)
Mannitol
Methanol
Sorbitol

BICARBONATE DEFICIT

HCO_3^- deficit = (0.4 x wt in kg) x (HCO_3^- desired − HCO_3^- measured)

Note: In clinical practice, the calculated quantity may differ markedly from the actual amount of bicarbonate needed or that which may be safely administered.

ANION GAP

Definition: The difference in concentration between unmeasured cation and anion equivalents in serum.

Anion gap = $Na^+ - (Cl^- + HCO_3^-)$
(The normal anion gap is 10-14 mEq/L)

Differential Diagnosis of Increased Anion Gap Acidosis

Organic anions
Lactate (sepsis, hypovolemia, seizures, large tumor burden)
Pyruvate
Uremia
Ketoacidosis (β-hydroxybutyrate and acetoacetate)
Amino acids and their metabolites
Other organic acids

Inorganic anions
  Hyperphosphatemia
  Sulfates
  Nitrates

Differential Diagnosis of Decreased Anion Gap

Organic cations
  Hypergammaglobulinemia

Inorganic cations
  Hyperkalemia
  Hypercalcemia
  Hypermagnesemia

Medications and toxins
  Lithium

Hypoalbuminemia

RETICULOCYTE INDEX

(% retic divided by 2) x (patient's Hct divided by normal Hct) **or**
(% retic divided by 2) x (patient's Hgb divided by normal Hgb)

Normal index: 1.0
Good marrow response: 2.0-6.0

POUNDS / KILOGRAMS CONVERSION

1 pound = 0.45359 kilograms
1 kilogram = 2.2 pounds

lb =	kg	lb =	kg	lb =	kg
1	0.45	70	31.75	140	63.50
5	2.27	75	34.02	145	65.77
10	4.54	80	36.29	150	68.04
15	6.80	85	38.56	155	70.31
20	9.07	90	40.82	160	72.58
25	11.34	95	43.09	165	74.84
30	13.61	100	45.36	170	77.11
35	15.88	105	47.63	175	79.38
40	18.14	110	49.90	180	81.65
45	20.41	115	52.16	185	83.92
50	22.68	120	54.43	190	86.18
55	24.95	125	56.70	195	88.45
60	27.22	130	58.91	200	90.72
65	29.48	135	61.24		

TEMPERATURE CONVERSION

Celsius to Fahrenheit = (°C x 9/5) + 32 = °F
Fahrenheit to Celsius = (°F - 32) x 5/9 = °C

°C =	°F	°C =	°F	°C =	°F
100.0	212.0	39.0	102.2	36.8	98.2
50.0	122.0	38.8	101.8	36.6	97.9
41.0	105.8	38.6	101.5	36.4	97.5
40.8	105.4	38.4	101.1	36.2	97.2
40.6	105.1	38.2	100.8	36.0	96.8
40.4	104.7	38.0	100.4	35.8	96.4
40.2	104.4	37.8	100.1	35.6	96.1
40.0	104.0	37.6	99.7	35.4	95.7
39.8	103.6	37.4	99.3	35.2	95.4
39.6	103.3	37.2	99.0	35.0	95.0
39.4	102.9	37.0	98.6	0	32.0
39.2	102.6				

ALDRETE SCORING SYSTEM

Activity	
Able to move 4 extremities voluntarily or on command	2
Able to move 2 extremities voluntarily or on command	1
Not able to move extremities voluntarily or on command	0
Respiration	
Able to deep breathe and cough freely	2
Dyspnea, shallow or limited breathing	1
Apneic	0
Circulation	
Blood pressure within 20% of preanesthesia level	2
Blood pressure 20% to 50% of preanesthesia level	1
Blood pressure within 50% of preanesthesia level	0
Consciousness	
Fully awake	2
Arousable on calling	1
Not responding	0
Oxygen saturation	
>92% breathing room air	2
Needs supplemental oxygen to maintain saturation >90%	1
<90% even with supplemental oxygen	0

Note: This scoring system is used to determine readiness of patient to be discharged to unit (if inpatient) or to phase II recovery (if outpatient); patients with a score of 9 or above are considered fit for discharge.

Adapted from Aldrete JA, "The Post-Anesthesia Recovery Score Revisited," *J Clin Anesth*, 1995, 7 (1):89-91.

AMERICAN SOCIETY OF ANESTHESIOLOGISTS (ASA) PHYSICAL STATUS CLASSIFICATION

Category	Description
P1	Normal, healthy patient
P2	Mild systemic disease — no functional limitation (eg, anemia, chronic bronchitis, controlled hypertension, extremes of age, mild diabetes mellitus, morbid obesity)
P3	Severe systemic disease — definite functional limitation (eg, angina pectoris, diabetes mellitus with vascular complications, history of prior myocardial infarction, obstructive pulmonary disease, poorly controlled hypertension)
P4	Severe systemic disease that is a constant threat to life (eg, advanced pulmonary or hepatic dysfunction, congestive heart failure, heart failure, renal failure)
P5	Moribund patient unlikely to survive 24 hours with or without operation
P6	A declared brain-dead patient whose organs are being removed for donor purposes

For procedures performed on an emergency basis, the letter " **E**" should be added to the ASA status.

ASA DIFFICULT AIRWAY ALGORITHM

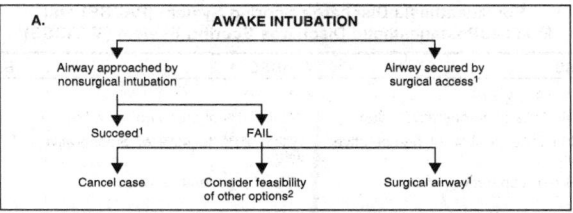

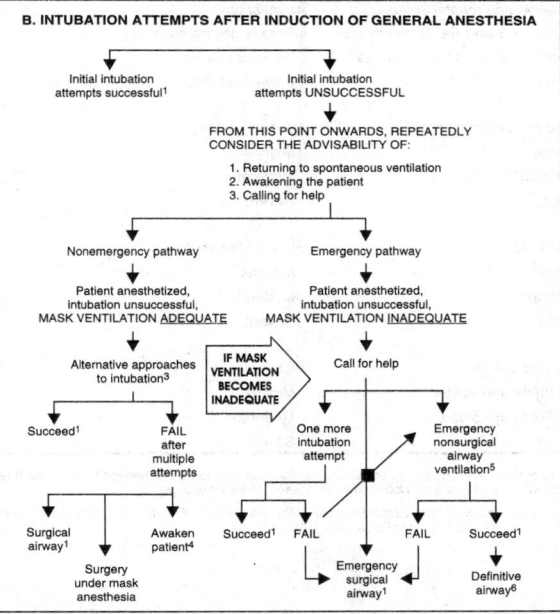

[1]Confirm intubation with exhaled CO_2.

[2]Other options include (but are not limited to): surgery under mask anesthesia, surgery under local anesthesia infiltration or regional nerve blockade, or intubation attempts after induction of general anesthesia.

[3]Alternative approaches to difficult intubation include (but are not limited to): use of different laryngoscope blades, awake intubation, blind oral or nasal intubation, fiberoptic intubation, intubating stylet or tube changer, light wand, retrograde intubation, and surgical airway access.

[4]See awake intubation.

[5]Options for emergency nonsurgical airway ventilation include (but are not limited to): transtracheal jet ventilation, laryngeal mask ventilation, or esophageal-tracheal combitube ventilation.

[6]Options for establishing a definitive airway include (but are not limited to): returning to awake state with spontaneous ventilation, tracheotomy, or endotracheal intubation.

Modified with permission from "Practice Guidelines for Management of the Difficult Airway. A Report by the ASA Task Force on Management in the Difficult Airway," *Anesthesiology*, 1993, 78:597-602.

AMBULATORY SURGERY DISCHARGE SCORING SYSTEMS

**Postanesthesia Discharge Scoring System (PADSS) and
ModifiedPostanesthetic Discharge Scoring System (MPADSS)[1]**

PADSS	MPADSS	Score
Vital signs	*Vital signs*	
Within 20% of preoperative value	Within 20% of preoperative value	2
Within 20% to 40% of preoperative value	Within 20% to 40% of preoperative value	1
40% of preoperative value	40% of preoperative value	0
Ambulation and mental status	*Ambulation*	
Oriented x 3 **and** has a steady gait	Steady gait/no dizziness	2
Oriented x 3 **or** has a steady gait	With assistance	1
Neither	None/dizziness	0
Pain or nausea/vomiting	*Nausea/vomiting*	
Minimal	Minimal	2
Moderate	Moderate	1
Severe	Severe	0
Surgical bleeding	*Surgical bleeding*	
Minimal	Minimal	2
Moderate	Moderate	1
Severe	Severe	0
Intake and output	*Pain*	
P.O. fluids **and** voided	Minimal	2
P.O. fluids **or** voided	Moderate	1
Neither	Severe	0

[1]Used to determine readiness of ambulatory surgery patient to be discharged from phase II recovery; patients with a score of 9 or above are considered fit for discharge.

Adapted from Chung F, "Discharge Process," *The Ambulatory Anesthesia Handbook*, Twersky RS, ed, New York, NY: Mosby-Year Book, Inc, 1995, 431-49.

CRITERIA FOR ASSESSING FAST-TRACK ELIGIBILITY IN OUTPATIENTS [ABILITY TO SKIP PHASE I (PACU) RECOVERY]

The patient must meet all the criteria below, when evaluated in the operating room, to be eligible to bypass phase I (PACU) recovery and in the judgment of the anesthesia provider, be capable of transfer to the step-down unit.

- Awake, alert, oriented, responsive (or return to baseline)
- Minimal pain
- Minimal nausea
- No vomiting
- No active bleeding
- Vital signs stable (not likely to require pharmacologic intervention)
- Patient can perform a 5-second head lift if a nondepolarizing neuromuscular blocking agent used
- Oxygen saturation of 94% on room air (3 minutes or longer) **or** return of oxygen saturation to baseline or higher

A minimal score of 12 (with no score <1 in any individual category) is required to bypass phase I (PACU) recovery

	Score
Level of consciousness	
Awake and oriented	2
Arousable with minimal stimulation	1
Responsive only to tactile stimulation	0
Physical activity	
Able to move all extremities on command	2
Some weakness in movement of extremities	1
Unable to voluntarily move extremities	0
Hemodynamic stability	
Blood pressure <15% of baseline mean arterial pressure (MAP)	2
Blood pressure 15% to 30% of baseline MAP	1
Blood pressure >30% below baseline MAP value	0
Respiratory stability	
Able to breathe deeply	2
Tachypnea with good cough	1
Dyspneic with weak cough	0
Oxygen saturation status	
Maintains value >90% on room air	2
Requires supplemental oxygen (nasal prongs)	1
Saturation <90% with supplemental oxygen	0
Postoperative pain assessment	
None or mild discomfort	2
Moderate to severe pain controlled with I.V. analgesics	1
Persistent severe pain	0
Postoperative emetic symptoms	
None or mild nausea with no active vomiting	2
Transient vomiting or retching	1
Persistent moderate to severe nausea and vomiting	0
Total score	**14**

References

Apfelbaum JL, "Current Controversies in Adult Outpatient Anesthesia," ASA Annual Refresher Course Lecture, Dallas, TX, 1999.

White PF and Song D, "New Criteria for Fast-Tracking After Outpatient Anesthesia: A Comparison With the Modified Aldrete's Scoring System," *Anesth Analg*, 1999, 88(5):1069-72.

INHALATIONAL ANESTHETICS

Factors Affecting Minimum Alveolar Concentration (MAC)

Variable	Effect on MAC
Age (young / elderly)	↑ / ↓
Alcohol (acute intoxication / chronic use)	↓ / ↑
Anemia Hematocrit <5 g/dL	↓
Blood pressure MABP <40 mm Hg	↓
Drugs	
Barbiturates	↓
Benzodiazepines	↓
Ketamine	↓
Etomidate	↓
Lithium	↓
Local anesthetics	↓
Opioids	↓
Propofol	↓
Alpha$_2$-agonist (clonidine / dexmedetomidine)	↓ / ↑
Sympathomimetics	
Amphetamine (acute / chronic)	↑ / ↓
Cocaine	↑
Ephedrine	↑
MAOI	↑
Verapamil	↓
Electrolytes	
Hypercalcemia	↓
Hypernatremia	↑
Hyponatremia	↓
PaO$_2$ <40 mm Hg	↓
PaCO$_2$ >95 mm Hg	↓
Pregnancy	↓
Temperature (>42°C / hypothermia)	↑ / ↓
Thyroid (hyperthyroid / hypothyroid)	No change

Modified from Stoelting RK and Miller RD, eds, *Basics of Anesthesia,* 5th ed, New York, NY: Churchill Livingstone, 2007.

Effects of Inhalational Anesthetics on Organ Systems

	Desflurane	Enflurane	Halothane	Isoflurane	Nitrous Oxide	Sevoflurane
MAC (%)[1]	6.0	1.68	0.74	1.2	105	2.6
Blood/Gas Partition Coefficient[2]	0.42	1.9	2.4	1.4	0.47	0.63
Cardiovascular						
Blood pressure	↓↓	↓↓	↓↓	↓↓	No change	↓↓
Cardiac output[3]	No change	↓↓	→	No change	No change	No change
Heart rate	↑	↑	→	↑	No change	No change
Systemic vascular resistance	↓↓	→	No change	↓↓	No change	→
Cerebral						
Blood flow	↑	↑	↑↑	↑	↑↑	↑
Intracranial pressure	↑	↑↑	↑↑	↑	↑	↑
Seizures	→	↑	→	→	→	↓ / ↑
Hepatic						
Blood flow	→	↓↓	↓↓	→	↑	→
Metabolism[4]	0.02%	2% to 5%	15% to 50%	0.2%	0.004%	3% to 5%
Neuromuscular						
Nondepolarizing blockade	↑↑↑	↑↑↑	↑↑	↑↑↑	No change	↑↑↑
Renal						
Glomerular filtration rate	?	↓↓	↓↓	↓↓	↓↓	?
Renal blood flow	→	↓↓	↓↓	↓↓	↓↓	→
Urinary output	?	↓↓	↓↓	↓↓	↓↓	?

Effects of Inhalational Anesthetics on Organ Systems *continued*

	Desflurane	Enflurane	Halothane	Isoflurane	Nitrous Oxide	Sevoflurane
Respiratory						
PaCO$_2$						
Resting	↑	↑↑	↑	↑	No change	↑
Challenge	↑	↑↑	↑	↑	↑	↑
Respiratory rate	↑	↑↑	↑↑	↑	↑	↑
Tidal volume	↓	↓	↓	↓	↓	↓

[1]Minimum alveolar concentration (MAC) = percentage of inspired concentration to prevent 50% of patients from moving to surgical stimulus (ED$_{50}$).

[2]Solubility of gas in blood at 37°C; less soluble gases have faster onset of action.

[3]Controlled ventilation.

[4]Metabolism = percentage of absorbed anesthetic undergoing metabolism.

Modified from Morgan GE and Mikhail MS, "Clinical Anesthesiology," New York, NY: Lange Medical Books/McGraw-Hill, 1996:138.

INTRAVENOUS ANESTHETIC AGENTS

Agent	Anesthesia Bolus	Anesthesia Maintenance	Sedation Bolus	Sedation Maintenance
Diazepam	0.3-0.6 mg/kg	—	0.04-0.2 mg/kg	—
Etomidate	0.2-0.5 mg/kg	10-20 mcg/kg/min	—	—
Ketamine	1-2 mg/kg	15-75 mcg/kg/min	0.5-1 mg/kg	—
Lorazepam	0.02-0.05 mg/kg	—	0.03-0.05 mg/kg	—
Methohexital	1-2 mg/kg	50-150mcg/kg/min	0.25-1 mg/kg	10-50 mcg/kg/min
Midazolam	0.2-0.6 mg/kg	0.25-2 mcg/kg/min	0.01-0.1 mg/kg	—
Propofol	1.5-2.5 mg/kg	100-200 mcg/kg/min	0.25-1 mg/kg	25-100 mcg/kg/min
Thiopental	3-5 mg/kg	30-200 mcg/kg/min	0.5-1.5 mg/kg	—

LOCAL ANESTHETICS

Amides – Use / Concentration

Agent	Use	Concentration
Bupivacaine	Infil, PNB, epid, spin	0.25% (infil); 0.25%, 0.5% (PNB); 0.25%, 0.5%, 0.75% (epid); 0.5%, 0.75% (spin)
Lidocaine	PNB, epid, infil, spin, topical, Bier	1%, 1.5%, 2% (PNB, epid); 5% (spin); 2%, 2.5%, 5% (topical); 0.5%, 1% (infil); 0.5% (Bier)
Mepivacaine	Infil, PNB, epid	1% (infil); 1%, 2% (PNB), 1%, 1.5%, 2% (epid)
Prilocaine	Infil, PNB. epid	1%, 2% (infil); 1%, 2%, 3% (PNB, epid)
Ropivacaine	Infil, PNB, epid, spin	0.5% (infil); 0.5% (PNB), 0.5%, 0.75% (epid)

epid = epidural; infil = infiltration; PNB = peripheral nerve block; spin = spinal.

Esters – Use / Concentration

Agent	Use	Concentration
Chloroprocaine	Epid, infil, PNB	1% (infil); 1%, 2% (PNB); 2%, 3% (epid, spin)
Cocaine	Anesthetize and constrict nasal mucosa prior to nasal intubation; nasal surgery; vasoconstriction properties	4% (topical)
Procaine	Infil, PNB, spin	1%, 2% (infil); 5% (spinal)
Tetracaine	Spinal, topical	0.1%, 0.5% (spinal); 2% (topical)

epid = epidural; infil = infiltration; PNB = peripheral nerve block; spin = spinal.

Pharmacodynamics / Kinetics, Maximum Dose, and Toxic Threshold Concentration

Agent	pKa	Protein Binding (%)	Onset	Duration[1] (h)	Maximum Dose (mg/kg)	Toxic Threshold Concentration (mcg/mL)
Bupivacaine	8.1	95	Intermediate	1.5-8.5	2.5	1.6
Chloroprocaine	9.2	<10	Rapid	0.5-1	12	—
Lidocaine	7.8	70-75	Rapid	1-4	5 w/o epi; 7 w/epi	5-6
Mepivacaine	7.6	75	Rapid	2-3	5 w/o epi; 7 w/epi	5-6
Prilocaine	7.8	50	Rapid	2-6	8	5-6
Procaine	8.9	<10	Slow	0.5-1	12	—
Ropivacaine	8.1	95	Intermediate	1.5-9	3	ND
Tetracaine	8.2	75-80	Slow	1-3 (topical)	3	—

[1]Duration of action depends on site of local anesthetic administration.

MALIGNANT HYPERTHERMIA

SIGNS AND SYMPTOMS

Tachycardia (unexplained)

Increased end-tidal carbon dioxide

Arrhythmias (ventricular, unexplained)

Acidosis (respiratory, metabolic)

Muscle rigidity

Tachypnea

Fever

Cyanosis

Hypoxemia

Hyperkalemia

Coagulopathy (eg, DIC)

Myoglobinuria

THERAPY FOR MALIGNANT HYPERTHERMIA (MH) EMERGENCY

CAUTION: This protocol may not apply to every patient and must of necessity be altered according to specific patient needs.

1. Immediately discontinue all inhalation anesthetics and succinylcholine. Hyperventilate with 100% oxygen at high gas flows (≥10 L/minute).

2. Halt the procedure as soon as possible; if emergent, continue with non-triggering anesthetic technique.

3. Dantrolene sodium should be obtained, mixed with 60 mL of sterile water for injection USP (without a bacteriostatic agent), and 2.5 mg/kg administered intravenously. At present, dantrolene is packaged as a lyophilized preparation that contains 20 mg of dantrolene and 3 g mannitol per vial.

4. In the absence of blood gas analysis, intravenous bicarbonate 1-2 mEq/kg should be administered.

5. Simultaneously, cooling should be started by all routes: surface, nasogastric lavage, intravenous cold solutions, wound, and rectally.

6. Arrhythmias will usually respond to treatment of acidosis and hyperkalemia. If they persist or are life-threatening, standard antiarrhythmic agents may be used, with the exception of calcium channel blockers, which may cause hyperkalemia or cardiac arrest in the presence of dantrolene.

7. Administer further doses of dantrolene as necessary titrated to heart rate, muscle rigidity, and temperature. Response to dantrolene should begin to occur in minutes; if not, more drug should be administered. Although the average successful dose of dantrolene is about 2.5 mg/kg, much higher doses may be needed (≥10 mg/kg). Fortunately, dantrolene does not produce significant myocardial depression at these doses.

8. Change anesthetic tubing.

9. Determine and monitor closely urine output, serum potassium, calcium, arterial blood gases, end tidal CO_2, and clotting studies. Hyperkalemia is common in the acute phase of MH and should be treated with intravenous calcium chloride, dextrose, and insulin.

10. Observe the patient in an ICU setting for at least 24 hours since recrudescence of MH may occur, particularly following a case that was difficult to treat.

11. Continue intravenous dantrolene 1 mg/kg every 4-6 hours or 0.25 mg/kg/hour as an infusion for at least 24 hours.

12. Follow CK, calcium, potassium, and clotting studies until such time as they return.

13. ECG should also be obtained and followed postoperatively.

14. Monitor body temperature closely since overvigorous treatment of MH may lead to hypothermia. Temperature instability may persist for several days after the acute episode. Body temperatures of 41°C to 42°C are compatible with survival and normal brain function if treated promptly.

15. Ensure urine output >1 mL/kg/hour. Consider CVP monitoring because of fluid shifts that may occur.

16. When the patient's condition has stabilized, convert from intravenous to oral dantrolene. Although data are not available regarding optimal doses and duration of treatment with dantrolene after an episode, the patient should probably receive a total dose of 4-8 mg/kg/day in 4 divided doses for 48 hours postoperatively.

17. Counsel the patient and family regarding MH and further precautions. Refer patient to the Malignant Hyperthermia Association of the United States (MHAUS).

18. Fill out and send in the Adverse Metabolic Reaction to Anesthesia (AMRA) form (www.mhreg.org) and notify the patient's physician. Refer patient to the nearest Biopsy Center for follow-up.

Once crisis is controlled, contact:

The Malignant Hyperthermia Hotline 1-800-644-9737

Or outside the U.S.: 1-315-464-7079

MALLAMPATI AIRWAY CLASSIFICATION

Mallampati Airway Classification[1,2]

Class	Description
1	Faucial pillars, soft palate, and uvula are visible
2	Faucial pillars and soft palate are visible, but uvula is masked by the base of the tongue
3	Only soft palate is visible

[1]Evaluation made with patient sitting upright, the mouth open, and the tongue protruded maximally.

[2]Intubation is predicted to be difficult in patients with class 3 airways.

OPIOIDS

Opioid Agonist-Antagonists

Agent	I.V.	I.M.	Oral	Epidural	Nasal
Buprenorphine	0.3 mg; 4-6 h	0.3 mg; 4-6 h	—	—	—
Butorphanol	0.5-2 mg; 3-4 h	1-4 mg; 3-4 h	—	2 mg	1 spray/nostril
Pentazocine	30 mg; 3-4 h	30-60 mg; 3-4 h	50 mg; 3-4 h	50 mg; 3-4 h	—

Analgesic Doses

Agent	PCA Load Dose	PCA Bolus Dose	PCA Lockout	Epidural Bolus Dose
Alfentanil	50-100 mcg	10-100 mcg	3-10 min	500-1000 mcg
Fentanyl	25-75 mcg	10-50 mcg	2-10 min	25-100 mcg
Hydromorphone	0.25 mg	0.05-0.4 mg	5-10 min	1-2 mg
Morphine	5-10 mg	0.5-3 mg	5-12 min	2-6 mg
Nalbuphine	2-5 mg	1-5 mg	5-15 min	1-10 mg
Sufentanil	2-5 mcg	2-10 mcg	2-10 min	10-60 mcg

Agent	Epidural Continuous Infusion	Intrathecal Bolus Dose	Intermittent I.M.	Intermittent I.V.
Alfentanil	200 mcg/h	—	—	—
Fentanyl	25-100 mcg/h	5-25 mcg	—	1-2 mcg/kg
Hydromorphone	0.1-0.2 mg/h	—	1.5 mg	1-2 mg
Morphine	0.1-1 mg/h	0.1-0.5 mg	2-10 mg	2-10 mg
Nalbuphine	0.5 mg/h	—	10 mg	5-10 mg
Sufentanil	5-30 mcg/h	0.02-0.05 mcg/kg	—	0.2-0.5 mcg/kg

REGIONAL ANESTHESIA IN PATIENTS RECEIVING ANTICOAGULANT AND ANTIPLATELET THERAPY

Drug	Recommendations
Heparin I.V.	Therapeutic anticoagulation with heparin may be performed at least 60 minutes after needle placement for spinal or epidural anesthesia.
	Monitor heparin effect closely; maintain aPTT within therapeutic range while catheter is in place.
	In patients with epidural catheters who are receiving I.V. heparin, removal of the catheter should occur at least 2-4 hours following discontinuation of heparin and assessment of anticoagulation status. Assess sensory/motor function in lower extremities for at least 12 hours after catheter removal. May reanticoagulate 1 hour after catheter removal.
Heparin SubQ (Low-dose prophylaxis)	Check platelet count in patients receiving heparin for >45 days prior to neuraxial block and epidural catheter removal.
	No contraindication to neuraxial block in presence of low-dose SubQ heparin. Consider delaying initiation of heparin for 1 hour after needle placement if technical difficulty is expected.
LMWH[1]	***Patients receiving LMWH preoperatively***[2]
	Thromboprophylaxis doses (eg, enoxaparin 30 mg every 12 hours or 40 mg once daily): Delay needle placement for at least 10-12 hours after the last dose of LMWH.
	Treatment doses (eg, enoxaparin 1 mg/kg every 12 hours or 1.5 mg/kg once daily): Delay needle placement for at least 24 hours after the last dose of LMWH.
	Avoid neuraxial techniques during peak anticoagulant activity (eg, general surgery patients who received LMWH 2 hours prior to surgery).
	Postoperative initiation of LMWH[3]
	First dose of LMWH should be given ≥24 hours postoperatively.
	When LMWH is dosed twice a day, the epidural catheter may remain overnight, removed the following day, and the first dose of LMWH given 2 hrs after catheter removal.
	When LMWH is dosed once a day, the epidural catheter removal should not be performed for 10-12 hours after the last dose of LMWH. The next dose of LMWH can be given ≥2 hours after catheter removal.
	Beginning LMWH in presence of indwelling catheter must be done with caution and patient's neurologic status monitored closely.
Warfarin	Discontinue warfarin 4-5 days prior to planned procedure with INR measured prior to initiation of neuraxial block; ensure INR is within normal limits.
	When warfarin is initiated in the presence of a continuous epidural catheter, monitor PT/INR daily and check before catheter removal. Catheter should be removed when INR <1.5. Routinely monitor sensory/motor function.
Antiplatelet agents[4]	*Clopidogrel or prasugrel:* Must be discontinued for at least 7 days prior to performing neuraxial block. May reinitiate after catheter removal.
	Ticlopidine: Must be discontinued for at least 14 days prior to performing neuraxial block. May reinitiate after catheter removal.

Drug	Recommendations
Glycoprotein IIb/IIIa inhibitors	Avoid neuraxial techniques until platelet function has recovered. Time to platelet function recovery is 24-48 hours for abciximab and 4-8 hours for eptifibatide and tirofiban.[5]

[1]Recommendations based on the assumption of normal renal function.

[2]Assume anticoagulation is altered. Single-dose spinal anesthetic may be safest technique in this patient population.

[3]Management is based on total daily dose of LMWH, timing of first postoperative dose, and dosing schedule. Single-dose or continuous catheter techniques can be used.

[4]NSAIDs (including aspirin) when used alone do not appear to increase the risk of spinal hematoma. The actual risk of spinal hematoma with clopidogrel or ticlopidine is unknown.

[5]Antiplatelet effects for both eptifibatide and tirofiban are prolonged with renal impairment.

Note: Drugs not considered to place the patient at risk when used alone (eg, aspirin) may increase the risk of spinal hematoma when combined with anticoagulants such as warfarin, heparin, or LMWH.

Monitor for early signs of cord compression in the perioperative period:

- progression of numbness/weakness
- bowel/bladder dysfunction
- severe back pain may or may not be present

Reference

Horlocker TT, Wedel DJ, Benzon H, et al, "Regional Anesthesia in the Anticoagulated Patient: Defining the Risks (The Second ASRA Consensus Conference on Neuraxial Anesthesia and Anticoagulation)," *Reg Anesth Pain Med*, 2003, 28(3):172-97.

SKIN DERMATOMES

A dermatome is defined as that area of the skin supplied by a single spinal nerve. The body, with the exception of the face, is supplied in sequence by dermatomes C2 through S5. Knowledge of the distribution of spinal nerves is helpful in interpreting the effects of epidural and spinal anesthesia.

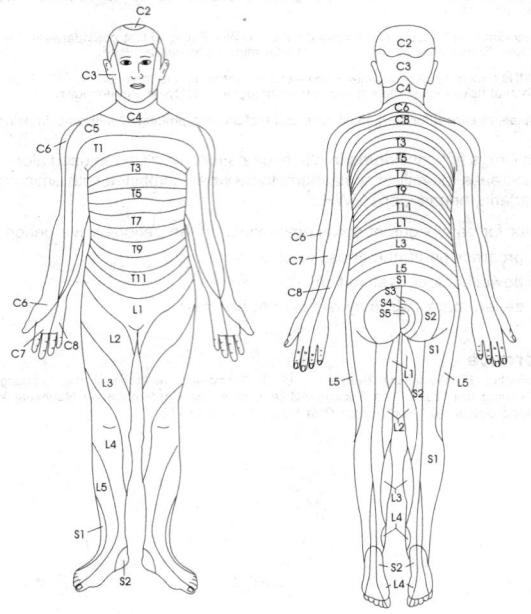

Skin dermatomes corresponding to respective sensory innervation by spinal nerves.

LIVER DISEASE

Pugh's Modification of Child's Classification for Severity

Parameter	Points for Increasing Abnormality		
	1	2	3
Encephalopathy	None	1 or 2	3 or 4
Ascites	Absent	Slight	Moderate
Bilirubin (mg/dL)	<2.9	2.9-5.8	>5.8
Albumin (g/dL)	>3.5	2.8-3.5	<2.8
Prothrombin time (seconds over control)	1-4	4-6	>6

Scores:

Mild hepatic impairment = <6 points.

Moderate hepatic impairment = 6-10 points.

Severe hepatic impairment = >10 points.

Considerations for Drug Dose Adjustment

Extent of Change in Drug Dose	Conditions or Requirements to Be Satisfied
No or minor change	Mild liver disease
	Extensive elimination of drug by kidneys and no renal dysfunction
	Elimination by pathways of metabolism spared by liver disease
	Drug is enzyme-limited and given acutely
	Drug is flow/enzyme-sensitive and only given acutely by I.V. route
	No alteration in drug sensitivity
Decrease in dose up to 25%	Elimination by the liver does not exceed 40% of the dose; no renal dysfunction
	Drug is flow-limited and given by I.V. route, with no large change in protein binding
	Drug is flow/enzyme-limited and given acutely by oral route
	Drug has a large therapeutic ratio
>25% decrease in dose	Drug metabolism is affected by liver disease; drug administered chronically
	Drug has a narrow therapeutic range; protein binding altered significantly
	Drug is flow-limited and given orally
	Drug is eliminated by kidneys and renal function severely affected
	Altered sensitivity to drug due to liver disease

Reference

Arns PA, Wedlund PJ, and Branch RA, "Adjustment of Medications in Liver Failure," *The Pharmacologic Approach to the Critically Ill Patient*, 2nd ed, Chernow B, ed, Baltimore, MD: Williams & Wilkins, 1988, 85-111.

CREATININE CLEARANCE ESTIMATING METHODS IN PATIENTS WITH STABLE RENAL FUNCTION

These formulas provide an acceptable estimate of the patient's creatinine clearance **except** in the following instances.

- Patient's serum creatinine is changing rapidly (either increasing or decreasing).
- Patient is markedly emaciated.

In above situations, certain assumptions have to be made.

- In a patient with rapidly rising serum creatinine (ie, >0.5-0.7 mg/dL/day), it is best to assume that the patient's creatinine clearance is probably <10 mL/minute.
- In an emaciated patient, although their actual creatinine clearance is less than their calculated creatinine clearance (because of decreased creatinine production), it is not possible to easily predict how much less.

INFANTS

Estimation of creatinine clearance using serum creatinine and body length (to be used when an adequate timed specimen cannot be obtained). **Note:** This formula may not provide an accurate estimation of creatinine clearance for infants younger than 6 months of age and for patients with severe starvation or muscle wasting.

$$Cl_{cr} = K \times L/S_{cr}$$

where:

Cl_{cr} = creatinine clearance in mL/minute/1.73 m^2
K = constant of proportionality that is age specific

Age	K
Low birth weight ≤1 y	0.33
Full-term ≤1 y	0.45
2-12 y	0.55
13-21 y female	0.55
13-21 y male	0.70

L = length in cm
S_{cr} = serum creatinine concentration in mg/dL

Reference
Schwartz GJ, Brion LP, and Spitzer A, "The Use of Plasma Creatinine Concentration for Estimating Glomerular Filtration Rate in Infants, Children and Adolescents," *Pediatr Clin North Am*, 1987, 34 (3):571-90.

CHILDREN (1-18 years)

Method 1: (Traub SL and Johnson CE, *Am J Hosp Pharm*, 1980, 37(2):195-201)

$$Cl_{cr} = 0.48 \times (height) / S_{cr}$$

where:

Cl_{cr} = creatinine clearance in mL/min/1.73 m^2
S_{cr} = serum creatinine in mg/dL
Height = height in cm

<u>Method 2</u>: Nomogram (Traub SL and Johnson CE, *Am J Hosp Pharm*, 1980, 37 (2):195-201)

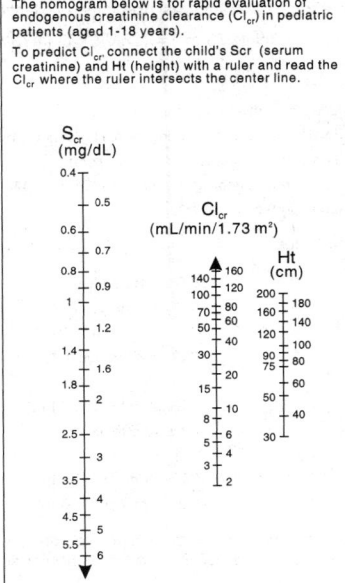

The nomogram below is for rapid evaluation of endogenous creatinine clearance (Cl_{cr}) in pediatric patients (aged 1-18 years).

To predict Cl_{cr} connect the child's Scr (serum creatinine) and Ht (height) with a ruler and read the Cl_{cr} where the ruler intersects the center line.

ADULTS (18 years and older)

<u>Method 1</u>: (Cockroft DW and Gault MH, *Nephron*, 1976, 16:31-41)

Estimated creatinine clearance (Cl_{cr}) (mL/min):

Male = (140 – age) x BW (kg) / 72 x S_{cr}
Female = male x 0.85

Note: Use of actual body weight (BW) in obese patients (and possibly patients with ascites) may significantly overestimate creatinine clearance. Some clinicians prefer to use an adjusted ideal body weight (IBW) in such cases [eg, IBW + 0.4(ABW-IBW)], especially when calculating dosages for aminoglycoside antibiotics.

<u>Method 2</u>: (Jelliffe RW, *Ann Intern Med*, 1973, 79:604)

Estimated creatinine clearance (Cl_{cr}) (mL/min/1.73 m^2):

Male = 98 – 0.8 (age – 20) / S_{cr}
Female = male x 0.90

RENAL FUNCTION TESTS

Endogenous Creatinine Clearance vs Age (timed collection)

Creatinine clearance (mL/min/1.73 m^2) = (Cr$_u$V/Cr$_s$T) (1.73/A)

where:

Cr$_u$	=	urine creatinine concentration (mg/dL)
V	=	total urine collected during sampling period (mL)
Cr$_s$	=	serum creatinine concentration (mg/dL)
T	=	duration of sampling period (min) (24 h = 1440 min)
A	=	body surface area (m^2)

Age-specific normal values

5-7 d	50.6 ± 5.8 mL/min/1.73 m^2
1-2 mo	64.6 ± 5.8 mL/min/1.73 m^2
5-8 mo	87.7 ± 11.9 mL/min/1.73 m^2
9-12 mo	86.9 ± 8.4 mL/min/1.73 m^2
≥18 mo	
male	124 ± 26 mL/min/1.73 m^2
female	109 ± 13.5 mL/min/1.73 m^2
Adults	
male	105 ± 14 mL/min/1.73 m^2
female	95 ± 18 mL/min/1.73 m^2

Note: In patients with renal failure (creatinine clearance <25 mL/min), creatinine clearance may be elevated over GFR because of tubular secretion of creatinine.

Calculation of Creatinine Clearance From a 24-Hour Urine Collection

Equation 1:

$$Cl_{cr} = \frac{U \times V}{P}$$

where:

Cl$_{cr}$	=	creatinine clearance
U	=	urine concentration of creatinine
V	=	total urine volume in the collection
P	=	plasma creatinine concentration

Equation 2:

$$Cl_{cr} = \frac{(\text{total urine volume [mL]}) \times (\text{urine Cr concentration [mg/dL]})}{(\text{serum creatinine [mg/dL]}) \times (\text{time of urine collection [minutes]})}$$

Occasionally, a patient will have a 12- or 24-hour urine collection done for direct calculation of creatinine clearance. Although a urine collection for 24 hours is best, it is difficult to do since many urine collections occur for a much shorter period. A 24-hour urine collection is the desired duration of urine collection because the urine excretion of creatinine is diurnal and thus the measured creatinine clearance will vary throughout the day as the creatinine in the urine varies. When the urine collection is less than 24 hours, the total excreted creatinine will be affected by the time of the day during which the collection is performed. A 24-hour urine collection is sufficient to be able to accurately average the diurnal creatinine excretion variations. If a patient has 24 hours of urine collected for creatinine clearance, equation 1 can be used for calculating the creatinine clearance. To use equation 1 to calculate the creatinine clearance, it will be necessary to know the duration of urine collection, the urine collection volume, the urine creatinine concentration, and the serum creatinine value that reflects the urine collection period. In most cases, a serum creatinine concentration is drawn anytime during the day, but it is best to have the value drawn halfway through the collection period.

Amylase:Creatinine Clearance Ratio

$$\frac{Amylase_u \times creatinine_p}{Amylase_p \times creatinine_u} \times 100$$

u = urine; p = plasma

Serum BUN:Serum Creatinine Ratio

Serum BUN (mg/dL:serum creatinine (mg/dL))

Normal BUN:creatinine ratio is 10-15

BUN:creatinine ratio >20 suggests prerenal azotemia (also seen with high urea-generation states such as GI bleeding)

BUN:creatinine ratio <5 may be seen with disorders affecting urea biosynthesis such as urea cycle enzyme deficiencies and with hepatitis.

Fractional Sodium Excretion

Fractional sodium secretion (FENa) = $Na_u Cr_s / Na_s Cr_u \times 100\%$

where:

Na_u	=	urine sodium (mEq/L)
Na_s	=	serum sodium (mEq/L)
Cr_u	=	urine creatinine (mg/dL)
Cr_s	=	serum creatinine (mg/dL)

FENa <1% suggests prerenal failure
FENa >2% suggest intrinsic renal failure (for newborns, normal FENa is approximately 2.5%)

Note: Disease states associated with a falsely elevated FENa include severe volume depletion (>10%), early acute tubular necrosis, and volume depletion in chronic renal disease. Disorders associated with a lowered FENa include acute glomerulonephritis, hemoglobinuric or myoglobinuric renal failure, nonoliguric acute tubular necrosis, and acute urinary tract obstruction. In addition, FENa may be <1% in patients with acute renal failure **and** a second condition predisposing to sodium retention (eg, burns, congestive heart failure, nephrotic syndrome).

Urine Calcium:Urine Creatinine Ratio (spot sample)

Urine calcium (mg/dL): urine creatinine (mg/dL)

Normal values <0.21 (mean values 0.08 males, 0.06 females)

Premature infants show wide variability of calcium:creatinine ratio, and tend to have lower thresholds for calcium loss than older children. Prematures without nephrolithiasis had mean Ca:Cr ratio of 0.75 ± 0.76. Infants with nephrolithiasis had mean Ca:Cr ratio of 1.32 ± 1.03 (Jacinto JS, Modanlou HD, Crade M, et al, "Renal Calcification Incidence in Very Low Birth Weight Infants," *Pediatrics*, 1988, 81:31.)

◀ **Urine Protein:Urine Creatinine Ratio (spot sample)**

P_u/Cr_u	Total Protein Excretion $(mg/m^2/d)$
0.1	80
1	800
10	8000

where:

P_u = urine protein concentration (mg/dL)
Cr_u = urine creatinine concentration (mg/dL)

ACETAMINOPHEN AND NSAIDS, DOSING IN THE MANAGEMENT OF PAIN

Drug	Usual Dose for Adults >50 kg Body Weight	Usual Dose for Adults[1] <50 kg Body Weight
Acetaminophen and Over-the-Counter NSAIDs		
Acetaminophen[2]	650 mg q4h	10-15 mg/kg q4h
	975 mg q6h	15-20 mg/kg q4h (rectal)
	1000 mg q4-6h (maximum dose: 4000 mg/24 hours)	
Aspirin[3]	650 mg q4h	10-15 mg/kg q4h
	975 mg q6h	15-20 mg/kg q4h (rectal)
Ibuprofen (Motrin®, others)	400-600 mg q6h	10 mg/kg q6-8h
Magnesium salicylate (Doan's®)	304 mg q4h	
Naproxen sodium (Aleve®)	220 mg q8-12h	
Prescription NSAIDs		
Celecoxib (Celebrex®)[4]	200 mg q12h	
Choline magnesium trisalicylate (Trilisate®)[4]	1000-1500 mg tid	25 mg/kg tid
Diclofenac (Cataflam®)	50 mg q8h	
Diflunisal (Dolobid®)[5]	500 mg q12h	
Etodolac (Lodine®)	200-400 mg q6-8h	≤20 mg/kg/day
Fenoprofen calcium (Nalfon®)	300-600 mg q6h	
Flurbiprofen (Ansaid®)	100 mg q12h	
Ketoprofen (Oruvail®)	100-300 mg q24h	
Ketorolac tromethamine (Toradol®)[6]	10 mg q4-6h to a maximum of 40 mg/d	
Meclofenamate sodium (Meclomen®)[7]	50-100 mg q6h	
Naproxen (Naprosyn®)	250-275 mg q6-8h	5 mg/kg q8h
Naproxen sodium (Anaprox®)	275 mg q6-8h	
Sulindac (Clinoril®)	200 mg q12h	
Parenteral NSAIDs		
Ibuprofen (Caldolor®)[8]	400-800 mg I.V. q6h	
Ketorolac tromethamine[7,9] (Toradol®)	60 mg I.M. or 30 mg I.V. initially, then 30 mg q6h, not to exceed 5 days	30 mg I.M. or 15 mg I.V. initially, then 15 mg q6h, not to exceed 5 days

[1] Acetaminophen and NSAID dosages for adults weighing <50 kg should be adjusted for weight.

[2] Acetaminophen lacks the peripheral anti-inflammatory and antiplatelet activities of the other NSAIDs

[3] The standard against which other NSAIDs are compared. May inhibit platelet aggregation for ≥1 week and may cause bleeding.

[4] May have minimal antiplatelet activity.

[5] Administration with antacids may decrease absorption

[6] For short-term use only.

[7] Coombs'-positive autoimmune hemolytic anemia has been associated with prolonged use.

[8] Must dilute prior to administration; hemolysis may occur if not diluted.

[9] Has the same GI toxicities as oral NSAIDs, dosing for patients with normal renal function.

Note: Only the above NSAIDs have FDA approval for use as simple analgesics, but clinical experience has been gained with other drugs as well.

ANGIOTENSIN AGENTS

Comparison of Indications and Adult Dosages

Drug	Hypertension	HF	Renal Dysfunction	Dialyzable	Strengths (mg)
ACE Inhibitors					
Benazepril (Lotensin®)	10-40 mg/day	Not FDA approved	Cl_{cr} <30 mL/min: 5 mg/day initially Maximum: 40 mg/day	Yes	Tablets 5, 10, 20, 40
Captopril (Capoten®)	25-100 mg/day bid-tid	6.25-100 mg tid Maximum: 450 mg/day	Cl_{cr} 10-50 mL/min: 75% of usual dose Cl_{cr} <10 mL/min: 50% of usual dose	Yes	Tablets 12.5, 25, 50, 100
Cilazapril (Inhibace®) Note: Not available in U.S.	2.5-10 mg/day	0.5-2.5 mg/day	Cl_{cr} 10-40 mL/min: Initial: 0.5 mg/day (0.25-0.5 mg/day for HF) (maximum: 2.5 mg/day) Cl_{cr} <10 mL/minute: 0.25-0.5 mg once or twice weekly	Yes	Tablets 1, 2.5, 5
Enalapril (Vasotec®)	2.5-40 mg/day qd-bid	2.5-20 mg bid Maximum: 20 mg bid	Cl_{cr} 30-80 mL/min: 5 mg/day initially Cl_{cr} <30 mL/min: 2.5 mg/day initially	Yes	Tablets 2.5, 5, 10, 20
Enalaprilat[1]	0.625 mg, 1.25 mg, 2.5 mg q6h Maximum: 5 mg q6h	Not FDA approved	Cl_{cr} <30 mL/min: 0.625 mg q6h	Yes	1.25 mg/mL (1 mL, 2 mL vials)
Fosinopril (Monopril®)	10-40 mg/day	10-40 mg/day	No dosage reduction necessary	Not well dialyzed	Tablets 10, 20, 40
Lisinopril (Prinivil®, Zestril®)	10-40 mg/day Maximum: 40 mg/day	5-40 mg/day	Cl_{cr} 10-30 mL/min: 5 mg/day initially Cl_{cr} <10 mL/min: 2.5 mg/day initially	Yes	Tablets 2.5, 5, 10, 20, 30, 40
Moexipril (Univasc®)	7.5-30 mg/day qd-bid Maximum: 30 mg/day	LV dysfunction (post-MI): 7.5-30 mg/day	Cl_{cr} <40 mL/min: 3.75 mg/day initially Maximum: 15 mg/day	Unknown	Tablets 7.5, 15
Perindopril (Aceon®)	4-8 mg/day	4-8 mg/day Maximum: 16 mg/day	Cl_{cr} 30-60 mL/min: 2 mg/day Cl_{cr} 15-29 mL/min: 2 mg qod Cl_{cr} <15 mL/min: 2 mg on dialysis days	Yes	Tablets 2, 4, 8
Quinapril (Accupril®)	10-40 mg/day qd-bid	5-20 mg bid	Cl_{cr} 30-60 mL/min: 5 mg/day initially Cl_{cr} <10-30 mL/min: 2.5 mg/day initially	Not well dialyzed	Tablets 5, 10, 20, 40

Comparison of Indications and Adult Dosages *continued*

Drug	Hypertension	HF	Renal Dysfunction	Dialyzable	Strengths (mg)
Ramipril (Altace®)	2.5-20 mg/day qd-bid	2.5-10 mg/day	Cl$_{cr}$ <40 mL/min: 25% of normal dose	Unknown	Capsules 1.25, 2.5, 5, 10
Trandolapril (Mavik®)	1-4 mg/day Maximum: 8 mg/day qd-bid	LV dysfunction (post-MI): 1-4 mg/day	Cl$_{cr}$ <30 mL/min: 0.5 mg/day initially	No	Tablets 1, 2, 4
Angiotensin II Receptor Blockers					
Candesartan (Atacand®)	8-32 mg/day	Target: 32 mg once daily	No dosage adjustment necessary	No	Tablets 4, 8, 16, 32
Eprosartan (Teveten®)	400-800 mg/day qd-bid	Not FDA approved	No dosage adjustment necessary	Unknown	Tablets 400, 600
Irbesartan (Avapro®)	150-300 mg/day	Not FDA approved	No dosage reduction necessary	No	Tablets 75, 150, 300
Losartan (Cozaar®)	25-100 mg qd or bid	Not FDA approved	No dosage adjustment necessary	No	Tablets 25, 50, 100
Olmesartan (Benicar®)	20-40 mg/day	Not FDA approved	No dosage adjustment necessary	Unknown	Tablets 5, 20, 40
Telmisartan (Micardis®)	20-80 mg/day	Not FDA approved	No dosage reduction necessary	No	Tablets 20, 40, 80
Valsartan (Diovan®)	80-320 mg/day	Target: 160 mg bid	Decrease dose only if Cl$_{cr}$ <10 mL/minute	No	Tablets 40, 80, 160, 320
Renin Inhibitors					
Aliskiren (Tekturna®)	150-300 mg once daily	Not FDA approved	No dosage adjustment necessary in mild-to-moderate impairment; not adequately studied in severe impairment	Unknown	Tablets 150, 300

Dosage is based on 70 kg adult with normal hepatic and renal function.

[†]Enalaprilat is the only available ACE inhibitor in a parenteral formulation.

ACE Inhibitors: Comparative Pharmacokinetics

Drug	Prodrug	Absorption (%)	Serum $t_{1/2}$ (h) Normal Renal Function	Serum Protein Binding (%)	Elimination	Onset of BP Lowering Action (h)	Peak BP Lowering Effects (h)	Duration of BP Lowering Effects (h)
Benazepril	Yes	37		~97	Renal (32%), biliary (~12%)	1	2-4	24
Benazeprilat			10-11 (effective)	~95%				
Captopril	No	60-75 (fasting)	1.9 (elimination)	25-30	Renal	0.25-0.5	1-1.5	~6
Enalapril	Yes	55-75	2	50-60	Renal (60%-80%), fecal	1	4-6	12-24
Enalaprilat			11 (effective)					
Fosinopril		36			Renal (~50%), biliary (~50%)	1		24
Fosinoprilat			12 (effective)	>99				
Lisinopril	No	25	11-12	25	Renal	1	6	24
Moexipril	Yes		1	90	Fecal (53%), renal (8%)		1-2	>24
Moexiprilat			2-10	50				
Perindopril	Yes		1.5-3	60	Renal		3-7	
Perindoprilat			3-10 (effective)	10-20				
Quinapril	Yes	>60	0.8	97	Renal (~60%) as metabolite, fecal	1	2-4	24
Quinaprilat			2					
Ramipril	Yes	50-60	1-2	73	Renal (60%), fecal (40%)	1-2	3-6	24
Ramiprilat			13-17 (effective)	56				
Trandolapril	Yes		6	80	Renal (33%), fecal (66%)	1-2	6	≥24
Trandolaprilat			10	65-94				

Angiotensin II Receptor Blockers and Renin Inhibitors: Comparative Pharmacokinetics

Drug	Prodrug	Time to Peak	Bioavailability	Food "Area-Under-the-Curve"	Elimination Half-Life	Elimination Altered in Renal Dysfunction	Precautions in Severe Renal Dysfunction	Elimination Altered in Hepatic Dysfunction	Precautions in Hepatic Dysfunction	Protein Binding
Angiotensin II Receptor Blockers										
Candesartan (Atacand®)	Yes[1]	3-4 h	15%	No effect	9 h	Yes[2]	Yes	No	Yes	>99%
Eprosartan (Teveten®)	No	1-2 h	13%	No effect	5-9 h	No	Yes	No	Yes	98%
Irbesartan (Avapro®)	No	1.5-2 h	60%-80%	No effect	11-15 h	No	Yes	No	No	90%
Losartan (Cozaar®)	Yes[3]	1 h / 3-4 h[3]	33%	9%-10%	1.5-2 h / 6-9 h[3]	No	Yes	Yes	Yes	~99%
Olmesartan (Benicar®)	Yes	1-2 h	26%	No effect	13 h	Yes	Yes	Yes	No	99%
Telmisartan (Micardis®)	No	0.5-1 h	42%-58%	9.6%-20%	24 h	No	Yes	Yes	Yes	>99.5%
Valsartan (Diovan®)	No	2-4 h	25%	9%-40%	6 h	No	Yes	Yes	Yes	95%
Renin Inhibitors										
Aliskiren (Tekturna®)	No	1-3 h	~3%	85% (high-fat meal)	16-32 h	Yes[4]	Yes	No	No	?

[1] Candesartan cilexetil: Active metabolite candesartan.

[2] Dosage adjustments are not necessary.

[3] Losartan: Active metabolite E-3174.

[4] No initial dosage adjustment in mild-to-moderate impairment.

ANTIARRHYTHMIC DRUGS

Vaughan Williams Classification of Antiarrhythmic Drugs Based on Cardiac Effects

Class	Drug(s)	Conduction Velocity[1]	Refractory Period	Automaticity
I				
Ia	Disopyramide Procainamide Quinidine	↓	↑	↓
Ib	Lidocaine Mexiletine	0/↓	↓	↓
Ic	Flecainide Propafenone[2]	↓↓	0	↓
II	Beta-blockers	0	0	↓
III	Amiodarone Dofetilide Ibutilide Sotalol[2]	0	↑↑	0
IV	Diltiazem Verapamil[3]	↓	↑	↓
Miscellaneous	Dronedarone[4]	↓	↑	↓

[1]Variables for normal tissue models in ventricular tissue.

[2]Also has type II, beta-blocking action.

[3]Variables for SA and AV nodal tissue only.

[4]Dronedarone has effects of all V-W classes similar to amiodarone; yet to be classified

Expected Electrocardiographic Changes of Antiarrhythmic Agents

Class	Drug(s)	PR Interval	QRS Duration	QT Interval
I				
Ia	Disopyramide Procainamide Quinidine	0/↑	↑	↑
Ib	Lidocaine Mexiletine	0	0	0
Ic	Flecainide	↑	↑	↑
	Propafenone	↑	↑	0
II	Beta-blockers	↑	0	0
III	Amiodarone	↑	0/↑	↑
	Dofetilide	0	0	↑↑
	Ibutilide	0	0	↑↑
	Sotalol	↑	0	↑
IV	Diltiazem Verapamil	↑↑	0	0
Miscellaneous	Dronedarone	↑	0	↑

Vaughan Williams Classification, Indications, and Adverse Effects of Antiarrhythmic Agents

Class	Drug(s)	Primary Uses	Route of Administration	Adverse Effects
I				
Ia	Disopyramide	AF, VT	P.O.	Anticholinergic effects, CHF
	Procainamide	AF, VT, WPW	P.O. (not available in U.S.)/I.V.	GI, CNS, lupus, fever, hematological, anticholinergic effects
	Quinidine	AF, PSVT, VT, WPW	P.O./I.V.	Hypotension, GI, thrombocytopenia, cinchonism
Ib	Lidocaine	VT, VF, PVC	I.V.	CNS, GI
	Mexiletine	VT	P.O.	GI, CNS
Ic	Flecainide	AF, PSVT, VT	P.O.	CHF, GI, CNS, blurred vision
	Propafenone	AF, PSVT, VT	P.O.	GI, blurred vision, dizziness
II	Esmolol	VT, SVT	I.V.	CHF, CNS, lupus-like syndrome, hypotension, bradycardia, bronchospasm
	Propranolol	SVT, VT, PVC	P.O./I.V.	CHF, bradycardia, hypotension, CNS, fatigue
III	Amiodarone	AF, SVT, VF, VT	P.O./I.V.	CNS, GI, thyroid, pulmonary fibrosis, liver, corneal deposits
	Dofetilide	AF	P.O.	Headache, dizziness, VT, torsade de pointes
	Ibutilide	AF	I.V.	Torsade de pointes, hypotension, bundle branch block, AV block
	Sotalol	AF, VT	P.O.	Bradycardia, hypotension, CHF, CNS, fatigue
IV	Diltiazem	AF, PSVT	P.O./I.V.	Hypotension, CHF, bradycardia
	Verapamil	AF, PSVT	P.O./I.V.	Hypotension, CHF, bradycardia, vertigo, constipation
Miscellaneous	Adenosine	SVT, PSVT	I.V.	Flushing, dizziness, bradycardia, syncope
	Digoxin	AF, PSVT	P.O./I.V.	GI, CNS, arrhythmias
	Dronedarone	AF	P.O.	Bradycardia, diarrhea, nausea
	Magnesium	VT, VF	I.V.	Hypotension, CNS, hypothermia, myocardial depression

AF = atrial fibrillation; PSVT = paroxysmal supraventricular tachycardia; VT = ventricular tachycardia; WPW = Wolf-Parkinson-White arrhythmias; VF = ventricular fibrillation; SVT = supraventricular tachycardia.

Comparative Pharmacokinetic Properties of Antiarrhythmic Agents

Class	Drug(s)	Bioavailability (%)	Primary Route of Elimination	Volume of Distribution (L/kg)	Protein Binding (%)	Half-Life	Therapeutic Range (mcg/mL)
I							
Ia	Disopyramide	60-83	Hepatic/renal	0.8-2	20-60	4-10 h	2-6
	Procainamide	80-90[1]	Hepatic/renal	2	15-20	PA: 2.5-5 h NAPA: 6-8 h	PA: 4-10 NAPA: 15-25
	Quinidine	70-80	Hepatic	2-3	80-90	6-8 h	2-6
Ib	Lidocaine	NA	Hepatic	1-2	60-80	Initial: 7-30 min Terminal: 90-120 min	1.5-5
	Mexiletine	80-95	Hepatic	5-7	50-60	10-14 h	0.8-2
Ic	Flecainide	85-90	Hepatic/renal	5-13	40-50	7-22 h	0.3-2.5
	Propafenone	3-11	Hepatic	2-5	85-95	PM: 10-32 h EM: 2-10 h	—
II	Esmolol			Refer to Beta-Blocker Comparison Chart			
	Propranolol			Refer to Beta-Blocker Comparison Chart			
III	Amiodarone	35-65	Hepatic	18-148	95-97	26-107 d	1-2.5[2]
	Dofetilide	>90%	Renal	3	60-70	10 h	—
	Ibutilide	NA	Hepatic	11	40	2-12 h	—
	Sotalol	90-100	Renal	1.2-2.4	Negligible	12-15 h	—
IV	Diltiazem	40	Hepatic	3-13	70-80	3-5 h	—
	Verapamil	20-35	Hepatic	4	90	2-12 h	—

Comparative Pharmacokinetic Properties of Antiarrhythmic Agents *continued*

Class	Drug(s)	Bioavailability (%)	Primary Route of Elimination	Volume of Distribution (L/kg)	Protein Binding (%)	Half-Life	Therapeutic Range (mcg/mL)
Miscellaneous	Adenosine	NA	—	—	—	<10 sec	—
	Digoxin	70-80	Renal	6-7	30	38-48 h	0.8-2 ng/mL[3]
	Dronedarone	4-15	Hepatic	~20	>98	13-19 h	—

DEA = desethylamiodarone; EM = extensive metabolizers; PA = procainamide; PM = poor metabolizers; NAPA = N-acetylprocainamide

[1]Oral formulation not available in the U.S.

[2]The active metabolite, desethylamiodarone (DEA) equates to levels of the parent compound. Poor correlation exists between level and therapeutic or toxic effects of amiodarone.

[3]Higher end of range may be necessary to control ventricular response; monitor closely for digoxin toxicity. Therapeutic range for patients with heart failure without atrial arrhythmia is 0.5-0.8 ng/mL.

ANTIDEPRESSANT AGENTS

Comparison of Usual Adult Dosage, Mechanism of Action, and Adverse Effects

Drug	Initial Adult Dose	Usual Adult Dosage (mg/d)	Dosage Forms	Adverse Effects						Comments
				ACH	Drowsiness	Orthostatic Hypotension	Conduction Abnormalities[1]	GI Distress	Weight Gain	
Tricyclic Antidepressants and Related Compounds[1]										
Amitriptyline	25–75 mg qhs	100–300	T, I	4+	4+	3+	3+	1+	4+	Also used in chronic pain, migraine, and as a hypnotic; contraindicated with cisapride
Amoxapine	50 mg bid	100–400	T	2+	2+	2+	2+	0	2+	May cause extrapyramidal symptom (EPS)
Clomipramine[2] (Anafranil®)	25–75 mg qhs	100–250	C	4+	4+	2+	3+	1+	4+	Approved for OCD
Desipramine (Norpramin®)	25–75 mg qhs	100–300	T	1+	2+	2+	2+	0	1+	Blood levels useful for therapeutic monitoring
Doxepin (Sinequan® [DSC], Zonalon®)	25–75 mg qhs	100–300	C, L	3+	4+	2+	2+	0	4+	
Imipramine (Tofranil®, Tofranil-PM®)	25–75 mg qhs	100–300	T, C	3+	3+	4+	3+	1+	4+	Blood levels useful for therapeutic monitoring
Maprotiline	25–75 mg qhs	100–225	T	2+	3+	2+	2+	0	2+	
Nortriptyline (Pamelor®)	25–50 mg qhs	50–150	C, L	2+	2+	1+	2+	0	1+	Blood levels useful for therapeutic monitoring
Protriptyline (Vivactil®)	15 mg qAM	15–60	T	2+	1+	2+	3+	1+	1+	
Trimipramine (Surmontil®)	25–75 mg qhs	100–300	C	4+	4+	3+	3+	0	4+	

Comparison of Usual Adult Dosage, Mechanism of Action, and Adverse Effects *continued*

Drug	Initial Adult Dose	Usual Adult Dosage (mg/d)	Dosage Forms	ACH	Drowsiness	Orthostatic Hypotension	Conduction Abnormalities[3]	GI Distress	Weight Gain	Comments
							Adverse Effects			
Selective Serotonin Reuptake Inhibitors[3]										
Citalopram (Celexa®)	20 mg qAM	20–60	T	0	0	0	0	$3+^4$	1+	
Escitalopram (Lexapro®)	10 mg qAM	10–20	T	0	0	0	0	3+	1+	S-enantiomer of citalopram
Fluoxetine (Prozac®, Prozac® Weekly™, Sarafem®, Selfemra™)	10–20 mg qAM	20–80	C, L, T	0	0	0	0	$3+^4$	1+	CYP2B6 and 2D6 inhibitor
Fluvoxamine[2] (Luvox® CR)	50 mg qhs	100–300	T	0	0	0	0	$3+^4$	1+	Contraindicated with pimozide, thioridazine, mesoridazine, CYP1A2, 2B6, 2C19, and 3A4 inhibitors
Paroxetine (Paxil®, Paxil CR®, Pexeva®)	10–20 mg qAM	20–50	T, L	1+	1+	0	0	$3+^4$	2+	CYP2B6 and 2D6 inhibitor
Sertraline (Zoloft®)	25–50 mg qAM	50–200	T	0	0	0	0	$3+^4$	1+	CYP2B6 and 2C19 inhibitor
Dopamine-Reuptake Blocking Compounds										
Bupropion (Aplenzin®, Budeprion SR®, Budeprion XL®, Wellbutrin®, Wellbutrin SR®, Wellbutrin XL®)	100 mg bid-tid IR[5] 150 mg qAM-bid SR[6]	300–450[7]	T	0	0	0	1+/0	1+	0	Contraindicated with seizures, bulimia, and anorexia; low incidence of sexual dysfunction IR: A 6-h interval between doses preferred SR: An 8-h interval between doses preferred

Comparison of Usual Adult Dosage, Mechanism of Action, and Adverse Effects *continued*

Drug	Initial Adult Dose	Usual Adult Dosage (mg/d)	Dosage Forms	ACH	Drowsiness	Orthostatic Hypotension	Conduction Abnormalities	GI Distress	Weight Gain	Comments
Serotonin / Norepinephrine Reuptake Inhibitors[8]										
Duloxetine (Cymbalta®)	40-60 mg/d	40-60	C	1+	1+	0	1+	3+	0	Useful for stress incontinence and chronic pain
Desvenlafaxine (Pristiq™)	50 mg/d	50-100	T/SR	0	1+	1+	0	3+[4]	0	
Venlafaxine (Effexor®, Effexor XR®)	25 mg bid-tid IR 37.5 mg qd XR	75-375	T	1+	1+	0	1+	3+[4]	0	High-dose is useful to treat refractory depression; frequency of hypertension increases with dosage >225 mg/d
5-HT₂ Receptor Antagonist Properties										
Nefazodone	100 mg bid	300-600	T	1+	1+	2+	1+	1+	0	Contraindicated with carbamazepine, pimozide, astemizole, cisapride, and terfenadine; caution with triazolam and alprazolam; low incidence of sexual dysfunction
Trazodone	50 mg tid	150-600	T	0	4+	3+	1+	1+	2+	
Noradrenergic Antagonist										
Mirtazapine (Remeron®, Remeron SolTab®)	15 mg qhs	15-45	T	1+	3+	1+	1+	0	3+	Dose >15 mg/d less sedating, low incidence of sexual dysfunction

Comparison of Usual Adult Dosage, Mechanism of Action, and Adverse Effects *continued*

Drug	Initial Adult Dose	Usual Adult Dosage (mg/d)	Dosage Forms	Adverse Effects							Comments
				ACH	Drowsiness	Orthostatic Hypotension	Conduction Abnormalities	GI Distress	Weight Gain		

Monoamine Oxidase Inhibitors

Drug	Initial Adult Dose	Usual Adult Dosage (mg/d)	Dosage Forms	ACH	Drowsiness	Orthostatic Hypotension	Conduction Abnormalities	GI Distress	Weight Gain	Comments
Isocarboxazid (Marplan®)	10 mg tid	10–30	T	2+	2+	2+	1+	1+	2+	Diet must be low in tyramine; contraindicated with sympathomimetics and other antidepressants
Phenelzine (Nardil®)	15 mg tid	15–90	T	2+	2+	2+	0	1+	3+	
Tranylcypromine (Parnate®)	10 mg bid	10–60	T	2+	1+	2+	1+	1+	2+	
Selegiline (EmSam®)	6 mg/d	6–12	Trans-dermal	2+	1+	2+	0	1+	0	Low tyramine diet not required for 6 mg/d dosage

ACH = anticholinergic effects (dry mouth, blurred vision, urinary retention, constipation); 0 - 4+ = absent or rare - relatively common. T = tablet, L = liquid, I = injectable, C = capsule; IR = immediate release, SR = sustained release.

[1] **Important note:** A 1-week supply taken all at once in a patient receiving the maximum dose can be fatal.

[2] Not approved by FDA for depression. Approved for OCD.

[3] Flat dose response curve, headache, nausea, and sexual dysfunction are common side effects for SSRIs.

[4] Nausea is usually mild and transient.

[5] IR: 100 mg bid, may be increased to 100 mg tid no sooner than 3 days after beginning therapy.

[6] SR: 150 mg qAM, may be increased to 150 mg bid as early as day 4 of dosing.

[7] To minimize seizure risk, do not exceed IR 150 mg/dose or SR 200 mg/dose.

[8] Do not use with sibutramine; relatively safe in overdose.

ANTIFUNGAL AGENTS

Activities of Various Agents Against Specific Fungi

Organisms	Amphotericin B[1]	Caspofungin	Fluconazole	Flucytosine
Aspergillus spp	FA	FA	N	?
Blastomyces dermatitidis	FA	?	A	N
Candida albicans	FA	FA	FA	FA
Candida glabrata	A	A	?	A
Candida krusei	FA	A	?	A
Candida tropicalis	FA	A	?	A
Coccidioides immitis	FA	?	A	N
Cryptococcus spp	FA	N	FA	FA
Dermatophytes	A	?	A	?
Fusarium spp	A	N	N	N
Histoplasma capsulatum	FA	A?	A	N
Penicillium spp	A	?	?	A
Pseudoallescheria boydii	?	A	N	N
Sporothrix schenckii	A	?	?	?
Zygomycetes (Mucor, Rhizopus)	A	N	N	N

Organisms	Griseofulvin	Itraconazole	Ketoconazole	Micafungin
Aspergillus spp	N	FA	N	A
Blastomyces dermatitidis	N	FA	FA	?
Candida albicans	N	FA	FA	FA
Candida glabrata	N	?	?	FA
Candida krusei	N	A	?	A
Candida tropicalis	N	?	?	A
Coccidioides immitis	N	A	FA	?
Cryptococcus spp	N	A	A	N
Dermatophytes	FA	A	A	?
Fusarium spp	N	N	N	?
Histoplasma capsulatum	N	FA	FA	?
Penicillium spp	N	?	N	?
Pseudoallescheria boydii	N	N	N	?
Sporothrix schenckii	N	?	N	?
Zygomycetes (Mucor, Rhizopus)	N	N	N	N

Organisms	Miconazole	Nystatin	Terbinafine	Voriconazole
Aspergillus spp	N	A	N	FA
Blastomyces dermatitidis	N	A	N	A
Candida albicans	FA	FA	A	A
Candida glabrata	?	A	?	A
Candida krusei	?	A	?	A
Candida tropicalis	?	A	?	A
Coccidioides immitis	A	N	N	A
Cryptococcus spp	A	N	N	A
Dermatophytes	N	N	FA	?
Fusarium spp	N	N	N	FA
Histoplasma capsulatum	N	N	N	A
Penicillium spp	N	N	N	?
Pseudoallescheria boydii	N	N	N	FA
Sporothrix schenckii	?	N	N	?
Zygomycetes (Mucor, Rhizopus)	N	N	N	N?

Organisms	Anidulafungin	Posaconazole
Aspergillus spp	A	FA
Blastomyces dermatitidis	N	A
Candida albicans	FA	FA
Candida glabrata	FA	A
Candida krusei	A	A
Candida tropicalis	FA	A
Coccidioides immitis	?	A
Cryptococcus spp	N	A
Dermatophytes	N?	A
Fusarium spp	N	A
Histoplasma capsulatum	?	A
Penicillium spp	A	A
Pseudoallescheria boydii	?	A
Sporothrix schenckii	?	A
Zygomycetes (Mucor, Rhizopus)	N?	A

FA = FDA approved indication. A = active. ? = unknown or questionable. N = not active.

[1]Various lipid products have differing indications, but all have activity against the same organisms.

References

Espinel-Ingroff A, "Comparison of *In Vitro* Activities of the New Triazole SCH56592 and the Echinocandins MK-0991 (L-743,872) and LY303366 Against Opportunistic Filamentous and Dimorphic Fungi and Yeasts," *J Clin Microbiol*, 1998, 36(10):2950-6.

Sabatelli F, Patel R, Mann PA, et al, "*In Vitro* Activities of Posaconazole, Fluconazole, Itraconazole, Voriconazole, and Amphotericin B Against a Large Collection of Clinically Important Molds and Yeasts," *Antimicrob Agents Chemother*, 2006, 50(6):2009-15.

Torres HA, Hachem RY, Chemaly RF, et al, "Posaconazole: A Broad-Spectrum Triazole Antifungal," *Lancet Infect Dis*, 2005, 5(12):775-85.

Vazquez JA, "Anidulafungin: A New Echinocandin With a Novel Profile," *Clin Ther*, 2005, 27 (6):657-73.

Zhanel GG, Karlowsky JA, Harding GA, et al, "*In Vitro* Activity of a New Semisynthetic Echinocandin, LY-303366, Against Systemic Isolates of *Candida* Species, *Cryptococcus neoformans*, *Blastomyces dermatitidis*, and *Aspergillus* Species," *Antimicrob Agents Chemother*, 1997, 41 (4):863-5.

BENZODIAZEPINES

Agent	FDA-Approved Indication	Dosage Forms	Relative Potency	Peak Blood Levels (oral) (h)	Protein Binding (%)	Volume of Distribution (L/kg)	Major Active Metabolite	Onset	Metabolism	Half-Life (parent) (h)	Half-Life[1] (metabolite) (h)	Elimination	Usual Initial Oral Dose	Adult Oral Dosage Range
						Anxiolytic								
Alprazolam (Alprazolam Intensol®, Niravam™, Xanax®, Xanax XR®)	Anxiety, anxiety associated with depression, panic disorder treatment	Sol, tab	0.5	IR: 1-2 XR: 9	80	0.9-1.2	No	Intermediate	Hepatic via CYP3A4	12-15	—	Urine	0.25-0.5 tid	0.75-4 mg/d
Chlordiazepoxide (Librium®)	Anxiety, EtOH withdrawal, adjunct to anesthesia (I.V.)	Cap, powd for inj	10	2-4	90-98	0.3	Yes	Intermediate	Hepatic via CYP3A4	5-30	24-96	Urine	5-25 mg tid-qid	15-100 mg/d
Diazepam (Diastat®, Diastat® AcuDial™, Diazepam Intensol™, Valium®)	Anxiety, EtOH withdrawal, adjunct to anesthesia (I.V.), anxiety/amnesiac during cardioversion (I.V.), anxiety/ amnesia in endoscopic procedures, convulsions/status epilepticus (I.V.), adjunct in epilepsy (rectal gel), skeletal muscle spasms	Gel, inj, sol, tab	5	0.5-2	98	1.1	Yes	Rapid	Hepatic via 2C19 and 3A4	20-80	50-100	Urine	2-10 mg bid-qid	4-40 mg/d
Lorazepam (Ativan®, Lorazepam Intensol™)[2]	Anxiety, anxiety associated with depression, adjunct to anesthesia (I.V.), convulsions/status epilepticus (I.V.)	Inj, sol, tab	1	1-6	88-92	1.3	No	Intermediate	Hepatic	10-20	—	Urine and feces (minimal)	0.5-2 mg tid-qid	2-4 mg/d
Oxazepam (Serax®)	Anxiety, anxiety associated with depression, EtOH withdrawal	Cap, tab	15-30	2-4	86-99	0.6-2	No	Slow	Hepatic via glucuronide conjugation	5-20	—	Urine as unchanged (50%) and glucuronide	10-30 mg tid-qid	30-120 mg/d

Agent	FDA-Approved Indication	Dosage Forms	Relative Potency	Peak Blood Levels (oral) (h)	Protein Binding (%)	Volume of Distribution (L/kg)	Major Active Metabolite	Onset	Metabolism	Half-Life (parent) (h)	Half-Life[1] (metabolite) (h)	Elimination	Usual Initial Oral Dose	Adult Oral Dosage Range
Sedative / Hypnotic														
Estazolam	Insomnia	Tab	0.3	2	93	—	No	Slow	Hepatic via CYP3A4	10-24	—	Urine	1 mg qhs	1-2 mg
Flurazepam (Dalmane® [DSC])	Insomnia	Cap	5	0.5-2	97	—	Yes	Rapid	Hepatic via CYP3A4	Not significant	40-114	Urine	15 mg qhs	15-60 mg
Quazepam (Doral®)	Insomnia	Tab	5	2	95	5	Yes	Intermediate	Hepatic via CYP3A4	25-41	28-114	Urine	15 mg qhs	7.5-15 mg
Temazepam (Restoril™)	Insomnia	Cap	5	2-3	96	1.4	No	Slow	Hepatic via CYP2B6, 2C8/9, 2C19, 3A4	10-40	—	Urine as inactive metabolites	15-30 mg qhs	15-30 mg
Triazolam (Halcion®)	Insomnia	Tab	0.1	1	89-94	0.8-1.3	No	Intermediate	Hepatic via CYP3A4	2.3	—	Urine as unchanged drug and metabolites	0.125-0.25 qhs	0.125-0.25 mg

Agent	FDA-Approved Indication	Dosage Forms	Relative Potency	Peak Blood Levels (oral) (h)	Protein Binding (%)	Volume of Distribution (L/kg)	Major Active Metabolite	Onset	Metabolism	Half-Life (parent) (h)	Half-Life[1] (metabolite) (h)	Elimination	Usual Initial Oral Dose	Adult Oral Dosage Range
						Miscellaneous								
Clonazepam (Klonopin®, Klonopin® Wafers)	Adjunct in Lennox-Gastuat syndrome, akinetic seizures, myoclonic seizures, adjunct in absence seizures, panic disorder treatment	Tab	0.25-0.5	1-2	86	1.8-4	No	Intermediate	Hepatic via glucoronide and sulfate conjugation	18-50	—	Urine as glucoronide or sulfate conjugate	0.5 mg tid	1.5-20 mg/d
Clorazepate (Tranxene® SD™, Tranxene® SD™ Half Strength, Tranxene® T-Tab®)	Anxiety, EtOH withdrawal, adjunct in partial seizures	Cap, tab	7.5	1-2	80-95	—	Yes	Rapid	Decarboxy-lated in acidic stomach prior to absorption and hepatic via CYP3A4	Not significant	50-100	Urine	7.5-15 mg bid-qid	15-60 mg
Midazolam	Adjunct to anesthesia, anxiety/amnesia during cardioversion, anxiety/amnesia in endoscopic procedures	Inj	NA	0.4-0.7[3]	95	0.8-6.6	Yes	Rapid	Hepatic via CYP3A4	2-5 h	12 h	Urine	NA	NA

IR = immediate release; XR = extended release; NA = not available.

Rapid = 15 minutes or less; intermediate = 15–30 minutes; slow = 30–60 minutes.

[1] Significant metabolite.

[2] Reliable bioavailability when given I.M.

[3] I.V. only.

BETA-BLOCKERS

Agent	Adrenergic Receptor Blocking Activity	Intrinsic Sympathomimetic Activity (ISA)	Lipid Solubility	Protein Bound (%)	Half-Life (h)	Bioavailability (%)	Primary Site of Metabolism	Primary (Secondary) Route of Elimination	Indications	Usual Dosage
Acebutolol (Sectral®)	$beta_1$	Yes	Low	15-25	3-4	40 7-fold[1]	Hepatic	Feces (renal)	Hypertension, arrhythmias	P.O.: 400-1200 mg/d
Atenolol (Tenormin®)	$beta_1$	No	Low	<5-10	6-9[2]	50-60 4-fold[1]	Hepatic (limited)	Feces (renal)	Hypertension, angina pectoris, acute MI	P.O.: 50-200 mg/d I.V. Acute MI: 5 mg x 2 doses
Betaxolol (Kerlone®)	$beta_1$	No	Low	50-55	14-22	84-94	Hepatic	Renal	Hypertension	P.O.: 5-20 mg/d
Bisoprolol (Zebeta®)	$beta_1$	No	Low	26-33	9-12	80	Hepatic	Renal	Hypertension, heart failure	P.O.: HF: 2.5-10 mg/d HTN: 2.5-20 mg/d
Carvedilol (Coreg®, Coreg CR®)	$alpha_1$, $beta_1$, $beta_2$	No	ND	98	7-10	25-35	Hepatic	Feces	Hypertension, heart failure (mild to severe)	P.O.: 3.125-25 mg twice daily
Esmolol (Brevibloc®)	$beta_1$	No	Low	55	0.15	NA 5-fold[1]	Red blood cell esterase	Renal	Supraventricular tachycardia, sinus tachycardia, atrial fibrillation/flutter, hypertension	I.V. infusion: 25-300 mcg/kg/min
Labetalol (Trandate®)	$alpha_1$, $beta_1$, $beta_2$	No	Moderate	50	5.5-8	18-30 10-fold[1]	Hepatic	Renal	Hypertension	P.O.: 200-2400 mg/d I.V.: 20-80 mg at 10-min intervals up to a maximum of 300 mg or continuous infusion of 2-6 mg/min

Agent	Adrenergic Receptor Blocking Activity	Intrinsic Sympathomimetic Activity (ISA)	Lipid Solubility	Protein Bound (%)	Half-Life (h)	Bioavailability (%)	Primary Site of Metabolism	Primary (Secondary) Route of Elimination	Indications	Usual Dosage
Metoprolol (Lopressor®, Toprol-XL®)	beta$_1$	No	Moderate	10-12	3-7	50 7- to 10-fold[1] (Toprol XL®: 77)	Hepatic	Renal	Hypertension, angina pectoris, acute MI, heart failure (mild to moderate; XL formulation only), atrial tachyarrhythmias (rate control)	P.O.: 100-450 mg/d HF. (Toprol-XL®): 12.5-200 mg/d I.V.: Acute MI: 5 mg q2 min x 3 doses AF (rate control): 2.5-5 mg q2-5 min (max total dose: 15 mg over 0-15 min)
Nadolol (Corgard®)	beta$_1$, beta$_2$	No	Low	25-30	20-24	30 5- to 8-fold[1]	None	Renal	Hypertension, angina pectoris	P.O.: 40-320 mg/d
Nebivolol (Bystolic®)	beta$_1$	No	High	98	10-12[4]	12[5]	Hepatic	Renal (feces)	Hypertension	P.O.: 5-40 mg/d
Penbutolol (Levatol®)	beta$_1$, beta$_2$	Yes	High	80-98	5	~100	Hepatic	Renal	Hypertension	P.O.: 20-80 mg/d
Pindolol	beta$_1$, beta$_2$	Yes	Moderate	57	3-4[2]	90 2- to 2.5-fold[1]	Hepatic	Renal (feces)	Hypertension	P.O.: 20-60 mg/d
Propranolol (Inderal®, various)	beta$_1$, beta$_2$	No	High	90	3-5[2]	25 2- to 3-fold[1]	Hepatic	Renal	Hypertension, angina pectoris, arrhythmias, prophylaxis (post-MI)	P.O.: 40-480 mg/d I.V.: Tachyarrhythmias: 1-3 mg q2-5 min (max: 5 mg)
Propranolol long-acting (Inderal-LA®, InnoPran XL™)	beta$_1$, beta$_2$	No	High	90	9-18	25 2- to 3-fold[1]	Hepatic	Renal	Hypertrophic cardiomyopathy with outflow tract obstruction, prophylaxis (post-MI)	P.O.: 180-240 mg/d

Agent	Adrenergic Receptor Blocking Activity	Intrinsic Sympathomimetic Activity (ISA)	Lipid Solubility	Protein Bound (%)	Half-Life (h)	Bioavailability (%)	Primary Site of Metabolism	Primary (Secondary) Route of Elimination	Indications	Usual Dosage
Sotalol (Betapace®, Betapace AF®, Sorine®)	beta$_1$ beta$_2$	No	Low	0	12	90-100	None	Renal[2]	Atrial and ventricular tachyarrhythmias	P.O. 160-320 mg/d
Timolol (Blocadren®)	beta$_1$ beta$_2$	No	Low to moderate	<10	4	75 7-fold[1]	Hepatic	Renal	Hypertension, prophylaxis (post-MI)	P.O.: 20-60 mg/d

Dosage is based on 70 kg adult with normal hepatic and renal function.

Note: All beta$_1$-selective agents will inhibit beta$_2$ receptors at higher doses.

[1] Interpatient variations in plasma levels.

[2] Primarily (>50%) as unchanged drug.

[3] Half-life increased to 16-27 hours in creatinine clearance of 15-35 mL/minute and >27 hours in creatinine clearance <15 mL/minute.

[4] Half-life increased to 19-32 hours in patients with poor CYP2D6 metabolism.

[5] Bioavailability increased to 96% in patients with poor CYP2D6 metabolism.

CALCIUM CHANNEL BLOCKERS

Comparative Pharmacokinetics

Agent	Bioavailability (%)	Protein Binding (%)	Onset of BP Effect (min)	Duration of BP Effect (h)	Half-Life (h)	Volume of Distribution	Route of Metabolism	Route of Excretion
Dihydropyridines								
Amlodipine (Norvasc®)	64-90	93-98	30-50	24	30-50	21 L/kg	Hepatic; inactive metabolites	Urine: 10% as parent
Clevidipine (Cleviprex™)		>99.5	2-4	5-15 min	1-15 min	0.17 L/kg	Blood and extravascular tissue esterases	Urine(63% to 74%; as metabolites); feces (7% to 22%)
Felodipine (Plendil®)	20	>99	2-5 h	24	11-16	10 L/kg	Hepatic; CYP3A4 substrate (major); inactive metabolites; extensive first pass	Urine (70%; as metabolites); feces 10%
Isradipine (DynaCirc® [DSC]) (immediate release)	15-24	95	20	>12	8	3 L/kg	Hepatic; CYP3A4 substrate (major); inactive metabolites; extensive first pass	Urine as metabolites
Nicardipine (Cardene®) (immediate release)	35	>95	30	≤8	2-4		Hepatic; CYP3A4 substrate (major); saturable first pass	Urine (60%; as metabolites); feces 35%
Nifedipine (Procardia®) (immediate release)	40-77	92-98	Within 20	2-5	2-5		Hepatic; CYP3A4 substrate (major); inactive metabolites	Urine as metabolites
Nimodipine (Nimotop®)	13	>95	ND	4-6	1-2		Hepatic; CYP3A4 substrate (major); metabolites inactive or less active than parent; extensive first pass	Urine (50%; as metabolites); feces 32%

Comparative Pharmacokinetics continued

Agent	Bioavailability (%)	Protein Binding (%)	Onset of BP Effect (min)	Duration of BP Effect (h)	Half-Life (h)	Volume of Distribution	Route of Metabolism	Route of Excretion
Phenylalkylamines								
Nisoldipine (Sular®)	5	>99	ND	6-12	7-12		Hepatic; CYP3A4 substrate (major); 1 active metabolite (10% of parent); extensive first pass	Urine as metabolites
Verapamil (Calan®) (immediate release)	20-35	90	30	6-8	4.5-12		Hepatic; CYP3A4 substrate (major); 1 active metabolite (20% of parent); extensive first pass	Urine (70%; 3%-4% as unchanged drug); feces 16%
Benzothiazepines								
Diltiazem (Cardizem®) (immediate release)	~40	70-80	30-60	6-8	3-4.5	3-13 L/kg	Hepatic; CYP3A4 substrate (major); 1 major metabolite (20%-50% of parent); extensive first pass	Urine as metabolites

COMPATIBILITY OF DRUGS

Drug Compatibility Guide

KEY
C = Compatible
X = Incompatible
Ø = Conflicting Reports
Blank = No information

	azithromycin	butorphanol	calcium gluconate	cefazolin	ciprofloxacin	cisatracurium	clindamycin	dobutamine	dopamine	drotrecogin alfa	fentanyl	fluconazole	furosemide	heparin	lansoprazole	levofloxacin	lorazepam	magnesium
azithromycin	■				X		X				X		X			X		
butorphanol		■				C									X			
calcium gluconate			■		C	C					C	X		C	X			
cefazolin				■		Ø					C	C		C	X			C
ciprofloxacin	X		C		■	C		C	C	X			X	X	X		C	X
cisatracurium		C	C	Ø	C	■	C	C	C	C	C	C	Ø	Ø			C	C
clindamycin	X					C	■	C		X	C	X		C	X	C		C
dobutamine					C	C	C	■		X	C	C		Ø	X	C		C
dopamine					C	C			■	X	C	C		C	X	C	C	
drotrecogin alfa					X	C	X	X	X	■		C	X	X		X		X
fentanyl	X		C	C		C	C	C	C		■		C	C	C	C	C	
fluconazole			X	C		C	X	C	C	C		■	X	C	C		C	
furosemide	X				X	Ø				X	C	X	■	C	X	X	C	
heparin			C	C	X	Ø	C	Ø	C	X	C	C	C	■	C	X	C	C
lansoprazole		X	X	X	X		X	X	X		C	C	X	C	■	X	X	X
levofloxacin	X						C	C	C	X	C		X	X	X	■	C	
lorazepam					C	C					C	C	C	C	X	C	■	
magnesium				C	X	C	C	C		X				C	X			■
methylprednisolone					X	Ø								Ø	X			
metronidazole					C	C				Ø	X	C	C		C	X	C	C
midazolam			C	C	C	C	C	C	Ø	C	X	C	C	X	C	X		
morphine	X			C		C		C		C			C	X	C	X	C	C
nesiritide								C	C		C		X	X				
nitroglycerin										C	C	C	X	Ø	X	X		
nitroprusside						Ø				X				C		X		
norepinephrine						C		C	X					C				
pantoprazole			X	X	X		X	Ø	X		X	X	X			X	X	Ø
piperacillin & tazobactam																		
potassium chloride	X		C		C	C			C	C	C		C			X	C	C
potassium phosphate					X					X					X			
prochlorperazine			Ø			C						C		C	X			
promethazine					C	C						C	X	C	X			
propofol		C	C	C	C		C	C	C		Ø	C	C	C			Ø	C
ranitidine				C	C	C		C	C	X		C		C	X		C	
sodium bicarbonate					Ø	Ø						C		C	X	C		
vancomycin					C					X	C	C		Ø	X	C	C	C

Note: Because the compatibility of two or more drugs in solution depends on several variables such as the solution itself, drug concentration and the method of mixing (bottle, syringe, or Y-site), this table is intended to be used solely as a guide to general drug compatibilities. Before mixing any drugs, the healthcare professional should ascertain if a potential incompatibility exists by referring to an appropriate information source.

Drug Compatibility Guide

KEY
C = Compatible
X = Incompatible
Ø = Conflicting Reports
Blank = No information

	methylprednisolone	metronidazole	midazolam	morphine	nesiritide	nitroglycerin	nitroprusside	norepinephrine	pantoprazole	piperacillin & tazobactam	potassium chloride	potassium phosphate	prochlorperazine	promethazine	propofol	ranitidine	sodium bicarbonate	vancomycin
azithromycin				X					X									
butorphanol															C			
calcium gluconate			C						X		C		Ø		C			
cefazolin			C	C					X						C	C		Ø
ciprofloxacin	X	C	C						X		C	X			C	C	C	Ø
cisatracurium	Ø	C	C	C		C	Ø	C			C		C	C		C	Ø	C
clindamycin			C	C					X						C			
dobutamine			Ø		C				Ø						C	C		
dopamine		Ø	C	C	C			C	X		C				C	C		
drotrecogin alfa		X	X			C	X	X			C	X				X		X
fentanyl		C	C		C	C			X		C				Ø		C	C
fluconazole		C	C	C		C			X				C	C	C	C		C
furosemide			X	X	X	X			X		C				X	C		
heparin	Ø	C	C	C	X	Ø	C	C	X		C		C	C	C	C	C	Ø
lansoprazole	X	X	X	X		X					X	X	X	X		X	X	X
levofloxacin		C		C		X	X		X								C	C
lorazepam		C							X		C				Ø	C		C
magnesium		C		C					Ø		C				C			C
methylprednisolone	■	C	X	C					X		X				X			
metronidazole	C	■	C	C					X									
midazolam	X	C	■	C		C	C	C	X		Ø				C	C	X	C
morphine	C	C	C	■	C		C	C	X		C				C			C
nesiritide				C	■	C	C	C										
nitroglycerin			C		C	■			X						C	C		
nitroprusside			C	C	C		■		X									
norepinephrine			C	C	C			■	X		C				C			
pantoprazole	X	X	X	X		X	X	X	■	X	C	X	X		X	X	X	C
piperacillin & tazobactam									X	■								
potassium chloride	X		Ø	C				C	C		■		C	C	C		C	
potassium phosphate									X			■						
prochlorperazine									X		C		■		C			
promethazine											C			■				
propofol	X		X	C		C		C	X		C		C		■	C	C	C
ranitidine		C				C			X						C	■		
sodium bicarbonate		X							X		C				C		■	
vancomycin			C	C					C						C			■

Chart created using the King Guide to Parental Admixtures, available through Lexi-Drugs Online www.lexi.com.

CORTICOSTEROIDS

Corticosteroids, Systemic Equivalencies

Glucocorticoid	Approximate Equivalent Dose (mg)	Routes of Administration	Relative Anti-inflammatory Potency	Relative Mineralocorticoid Potency	Protein Binding (%)	Half-life Plasma (min)	Half-life Biologic (h)
Short-Acting							
Cortisone	25	P.O., I.M.	0.8	2	90	30	8-12
Hydrocortisone	20	I.M., I.V.	1	2	90	80-118	8-12
Intermediate-Acting							
Methylprednisolone[1]	4	P.O., I.M., I.V.	5	0	—	78-188	18-36
Prednisolone	5	P.O., I.M., I.V., intra-articular, intradermal, soft tissue injection	4	1	90-95	115-212	18-36
Prednisone	5	P.O.	4	1	70	60	18-36
Triamcinolone[1]	4	P.O., I.M., intra-articular, intradermal, intrasynovial, soft tissue injection	5	0	—	200+	18-36
Long-Acting							
Betamethasone	0.6-0.75	P.O., I.M., intra-articular, intradermal, intrasynovial, soft tissue injection	25	0	64	300+	36-54
Dexamethasone	0.75	P.O., I.M., I.V., intra-articular, intradermal, soft tissue injection	25-30	0	—	110-210	36-54
Mineralocorticoids							
Fludrocortisone	—	P.O.	10	125	42	210+	18-36

[1]May contain propylene glycol as an excipient in injectable forms.

GUIDELINES FOR SELECTION AND USE OF TOPICAL CORTICOSTEROIDS

The quantity prescribed and the frequency of refills should be monitored to reduce the risk of adrenal suppression. In general, high or super-potency agents are preferable to prolonged use of low potency. After control is achieved, control should be maintained with a low potency preparation.

1. Low-to-medium potency agents are usually effective for treating thin, acute, inflammatory skin lesions; whereas, high or super-potent agents are often required for treating chronic, hyperkeratotic, or lichenified lesions.

2. Since the stratum corneum is thin on the face and intertriginous areas, low-potency agents are preferred but a higher potency agent may be used for 2 weeks.

3. Because the palms and soles have a thick stratum corneum, high or super-potent agents are frequently required.

4. Low potency agents are preferred for infants and the elderly. Infants have a high body surface area to weight ratio; elderly patients have thin, fragile skin.

5. The vehicle in which the topical corticosteroid is formulated influences the absorption and potency of the drug. Ointment bases are preferred for thick, lichenified lesions; they enhance penetration of the drug. Creams are preferred for acute and subacute dermatoses; they may be used on moist skin areas or intertriginous areas. Solutions, gels, and sprays are preferred for the scalp or for areas where a nonoil-based vehicle is needed.

6. In general, super-potent agents should not be used for longer than 2-3 weeks unless the lesion is limited to a small body area. Medium-to-high potency agents usually cause only rare adverse effects when treatment is limited to 3 months or less, and use on the face and intertriginous areas are avoided. If long-term treatment is needed, intermittent vs continued treatment is recommended.

7. Most preparations are applied once or twice daily. More frequent application may be necessary for the palms or soles because the preparation is easily removed by normal activity and penetration is poor due to a thick stratum corneum. Every-other-day or weekend-only application may be effective for treating some chronic conditions.

Corticosteroids, Topical

	Steroid	Vehicle
	Very High Potency	
0.05%	Betamethasone dipropionate, augmented	Lotion, ointment
0.05%	Clobetasol propionate	Cream, foam, gel, lotion, ointment, shampoo, spray
0.05%	Diflorasone diacetate	Ointment
0.05%	Halobetasol propionate	Cream, ointment
	High Potency	
0.1%	Amcinonide	Cream, ointment, lotion
0.05%	Betamethasone dipropionate, augmented	Cream
0.05%	Betamethasone dipropionate	Cream, ointment
0.1%	Betamethasone valerate	Ointment
0.05%	Desoximetasone	Gel
0.25%	Desoximetasone	Cream, ointment
0.05%	Diflorasone diacetate	Cream, ointment
0.05%	Fluocinonide	Cream, ointment, gel
0.1%	Halcinonide	Cream, ointment
0.5%	Triamcinolone acetonide	Cream

Corticosteroids, Topical *(continued)*

	Steroid	Vehicle
	Intermediate Potency	
0.05%	Betamethasone dipropionate	Lotion
0.1%	Betamethasone valerate	Cream
0.1%	Clocortolone pivalate	Cream
0.05%	Desoximetasone	Cream
0.025%	Fluocinolone acetonide	Cream, ointment
0.05%	Flurandrenolide	Cream, ointment, lotion, tape
0.005%	Fluticasone propionate	Ointment
0.05%	Fluticasone propionate	Cream
0.1%	Hydrocortisone butyrate[1]	Ointment, solution
0.2%	Hydrocortisone valerate[1]	Cream, ointment
0.1%	Mometasone furoate[1]	Cream, ointment, lotion
0.1%	Prednicarbate	Cream, ointment
0.025%	Triamcinolone acetonide	Cream, ointment, lotion
0.1%	Triamcinolone acetonide	Cream, ointment, lotion
	Low Potency	
0.05%	Alclometasone dipropionate[1]	Cream, ointment
0.05%	Desonide	Cream
0.01%	Fluocinolone acetonide	Cream, solution
0.5%	Hydrocortisone[1]	Cream, ointment, lotion
0.5%	Hydrocortisone acetate[1]	Cream, ointment
1%	Hydrocortisone acetate[1]	Cream, ointment
1%	Hydrocortisone[1]	Cream, ointment, lotion, solution
2.5%	Hydrocortisone[1]	Cream, ointment, lotion

[1]Not fluorinated.

CYCLOPLEGIC MYDRIATICS

Agent	Peak Mydriasis	Peak Cycloplegia	Time to Recovery
Atropine	30-40 min	1-3 h	>14 d
Cyclopentolate	25-75 min	25-75 min	24 h
Homatropine	30-90 min	30-90 min	6 h - 4 d
Scopolamine	20-30 min	30 min - 1 h	5-7 d
Tropicamide	20-40 min	20-35 min	1-6 h

DIURETICS, LOOP

Agent	Equivalent Potency	Usual Dose	Oral Bioavailability (%)	Duration of Action (h)
Bumetanide				
oral	1	0.5-2 mg qd	72-95	4-6
I.V. injection	1	0.5-1 mg qd	—	2-3
Ethacrynic acid				
oral	100	50-100 mg qd-bid	90-100	6-12
I.V. injection	100	50 mg[1]	—	2
Furosemide				
oral	40	20-80 mg bid	47-64	6-8
I.V. injection	40	1-5 mg q6h	—	2
Torsemide				
oral	10-20	5-10 mg qd	80-90	6
I.V. injection	10-20	10-20 mg qd	—	6

[1]Dilute in D_5W or NS to 1 mg/mL; infuse over several minutes. Repeat doses may be required based upon response to initial doses.

Dosage is based on 70 kg adult with normal hepatic and renal function.

HEMODYNAMIC SUPPORT, INTRAVENOUS

Drug	Dose	Hemodynamic Effects				
		HR	MAP	PAOP	CI	SVR
Dopamine	1-3 mcg/kg/min	↑	0	↓	0/↑	0/↓
	3-10 mcg/kg/min	↑	↑	0	↑	0
	>10-20 mcg/kg/min	↑↑	↑↑	0	↑	↑
Epinephrine	0.01-0.05 mcg/kg/min	↑	↑	0/↓	↑↑	0/↓
	>0.05 mcg/kg/min	↑↑	↑↑	↑	↑↑	↑↑
Norepinephrine	0.02-3 mcg/kg/min	0/↑	↑↑↑	↑↑	0/↓/↑	↑↑↑
Phenylephrine	0.5-9 mcg/kg/min	0/↓	↑	↑	0/↓/↑	↑↑↑
Vasopressin	0.04 units/min	0/↓	↑↑	↑	0/↓	↑↑
Dobutamine	2-10 mcg/kg/min	0/↑	↑	↓	↑	0/↓
	>10-20 mcg/kg/min	↑↑	↓/↑	↓	↑	↓
Milrinone	0.375-0.75 mcg/kg/min	↑↑	0/↓/↑	↓	↑	↓↓
Nesiritide	2 mcg/kg bolus 0.01-0.03 mcg/kg/min	0	↓	↓	0/↑	↓
Nitroglycerin	0.1-2 mcg/kg/min	0/↑	0/↓	↓	0/↑	↓
Nitroprusside	0.25-10 mcg/kg/min	0/↑	0/↓	↓	↑/↑↑↑	↓/↓↓

HR = heart rate; MAP = mean arterial pressure; PAOP = pulmonary artery occlusion pressure; CI = cardiac index; SVR = systemic vascular resistance.

↑ = increase; ↓ = decrease; 0 = no change.

Drug	Dose	Receptor Activity						
		α_1	α_2	β_1	β_2	DA_1	V_1	V_2
Dobutamine	2-10 mcg/kg/min	+	0	+++	++	0	0	0
	>10-20 mcg/kg/min	++	0	++++	+++	0	0	0
Dopamine	1-3 mcg/kg/min	0	0	+	0	++++	0	0
	3-10 mcg/kg/min	0/+	0	++++	++	++++	0	0
	>10-20 mcg/kg/min	+++	0	++++	+	0	0	0
Epinephrine	0.01-0.05 mcg/kg/min	++	++	++++	+++	0	0	0
	>0.05 mcg/kg/min	++++	++++	+++	+	0	0	0
Norepinephrine	0.02-3 mcg/kg/min	++++	++	++	0	0	0	0
Phenylephrine	0.5-9 mcg/kg/min	++++	+	0	0	0	0	0
Vasopressin	0.04 units/min	0	0	0	0	0	+++	+++

Activity ranges from no activity (0) or maximal activity (++++).

DA = dopaminergic; V = vasopressin

Reference
MacLaren R, Rudis MI, and Dasta JF, "Use of Vasopressors and Inotropes in the Pharmacotherapy of Shock," *Pharmacotherapy: A Pathophysiologic Approach*, 7th ed, Dipiro JT, Talbert RL, Yee GC, et al, eds, Stamford, CT: McGraw-Hill, 2008, 417-39.

INSULIN PRODUCTS

Types of Insulin	Onset (h)	Peak Glycemic Effect (h)	Duration (h)
Rapid-Acting			
Insulin lispro (Humalog®)	0.25-0.5	0.5-2.5	≤5
Insulin aspart (NovoLog®)	0.2-0.3	1-3	3-5
Insulin glulisine (Apidra®)	0.2-0.5	1.6-2.8	3-4
Short-Acting			
Insulin regular (Humulin® R, Novolin® R)	0.5	2.5-5	4-12
Intermediate-Acting			
Insulin NPH (isophane suspension) (Humulin® N, Novolin® N)	1-2	4-12	14-24
Intermediate- to Long-Acting			
Insulin detemir (Levemir®)	3-4	3-9	6-23
Long-Acting			
Insulin glargine (Lantus®)	3-4	*	≥24
Combinations			
Insulin aspart protamine suspension and insulin aspart (Novolog® Mix 70/30)	0.1-0.2	1-4	18-24
Insulin lispro protamine and insulin lispro (Humalog® Mix 75/25™)	0.25-0.5	1-6.5	14-24
Insulin NPH suspension and insulin regular solution (Novolin® 70/30)	0.5	2-12	18-24

*Insulin glargine has no pronounced peak.

LAXATIVES, CLASSIFICATION AND PROPERTIES

Laxative	Onset of Action	Site of Action	Mechanism of Action
Saline			
Magnesium citrate Magnesium hydroxide (Phillips'® Milk of Magnesia)	30 min to 3 h	Small and large intestine	Attract/retain water in intestinal lumen increasing intraluminal pressure; cholecystokinin release
Sodium phosphates (Fleet® Enema)	2-15 min	Colon	
Irritant / Stimulant			
Senna (Senokot®)	6-10 h	Colon	Direct action on intestinal mucosa; stimulate myenteric plexus; alter water and electrolyte secretion
Bisacodyl (Dulcolax®) tablets, suppositories	15 min to 1 h	Colon	
Castor oil	2-6 h	Small intestine	
Bulk-Producing			
Methylcellulose (Citrucel®) Psyllium (Metamucil®)	12-24 h (up to 72 h)	Small and large intestine	Holds water in stool; mechanical distention; malt soup extract reduces fecal pH
Lubricant			
Mineral oil	6-8 h	Colon	Lubricates intestine; retards colonic absorption of fecal water; softens stool
Surfactants / Stool Softener			
Docusate sodium (Colace®) Docusate calcium (Surfak®)	24-72 h	Small and large intestine	Detergent activity; facilitates admixture of fat and water to soften stool
Miscellaneous and Combination Laxatives			
Glycerin suppository	15-30 min	Colon	Local irritation; hyperosmotic action
Lactulose	24-48 h	Colon	Delivers osmotically active molecules to colon
Lubiprostone (Amitiza®)	24-48 h	Apical membrane of the GI epithelium	Activates intestinal chloride channels increasing intestinal fluid
Docusate/senna (Peri-Colace®)	8-12 h	Small and large intestine	Senna – mild irritant; docusate – stool softener
Polyethylene glycol 3350 (GlycoLax™, MiraLax™)	48 h	Small and large intestine	Nonabsorbable solution which acts as an osmotic agent
Sorbitol 70%	24-48 h	Colon	Delivers osmotically active molecules to colon

NEUROMUSCULAR-BLOCKING AGENTS

Suggested Dosing Guidelines for the Use of Neuromuscular-Blocking Agents in the Intensive Care Unit

Agent	Intermittent Injection	Continuous Infusion
Intermediate Duration		
Atracurium	0.4-0.5 mg/kg every 25-35 minutes	0.4-1 mg/kg/h
Cisatracurium (Nimbex®)	0.15-0.2 mg/kg every 40-60 minutes	0.03-0.6 mg/kg/h
Rocuronium (Zemuron®)	0.6 mg/kg every 30 minutes	0.6 mg/kg/h
Vecuronium	0.1 mg/kg every 35-45 minutes	0.05-0.1 mg/kg/h
Long Duration		
Pancuronium	0.1 mg/kg every 90-100 minutes	0.05-0.1 mg/kg/h

Pharmacokinetic and Pharmacodynamic Properties of Neuromuscular Blocking Agents

Agent	Clearance (mL/kg/min)	V_{dss} (L/kg)	Half-life (min)	ED95[1] (mg/kg)	Initial Adult Dose[2,3] (mg/kg)	Onset (min)	Clinical Duration of Action of Initial Dose (min)	Administration as an Intraoperative Infusion (mcg/kg/min)
Ultra-Short Duration								
Succinylcholine	Unknown	Unknown	Unknown	0.2	1-1.5	0.5-1	4-6	10-100
Intermediate Duration								
Atracurium	5-7	0.2	20	0.2	0.4-0.5	2-3	60-70 (dose dependent)	4-12
Cisatracurium	4.6	0.15	22-29	0.05	0.15-0.2	2-3	25-93	1-3
Rocuronium	4	0.17-0.29	60-70	0.3	0.6-1.2	1-1.5	~30	4-16
Vecuronium	4.5	0.16-0.27	51-80	0.05	0.08-0.1	2-3	20-40	0.8-2
Long Duration								
Pancuronium	1-2	0.18-0.26	107-169	0.07	0.08-0.1	3-5	60-100	n/a

[1] ED95: Effective dose causing 95% blockade.

[2] Initial dose (intubation dose) is usually 2 x ED95 with the exception of cisatracurium where the recommended initial dose is 3-4 x ED95.

[3] Prior administration of succinylcholine generally enhances the magnitude and duration of nondepolarizing NMB agents; initial doses should be lower.

NITRATES

Nitrates[1]	Dosage Form	Onset (min)	Duration
Nitroglycerin	I.V.	1-2	3-5 min
	Sublingual	1-3	30-60 min
	Translingual spray	2	30-60 min
	Oral, sustained release	40	4-8 h
	Topical ointment	20-60	2-12 h
	Transdermal	40-60	18-24 h
Isosorbide dinitrate	Sublingual and chewable	2-5	1-2 h
	Oral	20-40	4-6 h
	Oral, sustained release	Slow	8-12 h
Isosorbide mononitrate	Oral	60-120	5-12 h

[1]Hemodynamic and antianginal tolerance often develops within 24-48 hours of continuous nitrate administration.

Adapted from Corwin S and Reiffel JA, "Nitrate Therapy for Angina Pectoris," *Arch Intern Med*, 1985, 145:538-43 and Franciosa JA, "Nitroglycerin and Nitrates in Congestive Heart Failure," *Heart and Lung*, 1980, 9(5):873-82.

NONSTEROIDAL ANTI-INFLAMMATORY AGENTS

Comparative Dosages and Pharmacokinetics

Drug	Maximum Recommended Daily Dose (mg)	Time to Peak Levels[1] (h)	Half-life (h)
Acetic Acids			
Diclofenac potassium immediate release (Cataflam®)	200	1	1-2
Diclofenac sodium delayed release (Voltaren®)	225	2-3	1-2
Etodolac	1200	1-2	7.3
Indomethacin (Indocin®)	200	1-2	4.5
Indomethacin sustained release (Indocin® SR)	150	2-4	4.5-6
Ketorolac (Toradol®)	I.M.: 120[2] P.O.: 40	0.5-1	3.8-8.6
Sulindac (Clinoril®)	400	2-4	7.8 (16.4)[3]
Tolmetin (Tolectin®)	2000	0.5-1	1-1.5
Fenamates (Anthranilic Acids)			
Meclofenamate	400	0.5-1	2 (3.3)[4]
Mefenamic acid (Ponstel®)	1000	2-4	2-4
Propionic Acids			
Fenoprofen (Nalfon®)	3200	1-2	2-3
Flurbiprofen	300	1.5	5.7
Ibuprofen (various)	3200	1-2	1.8-2.5
Ketoprofen	300	0.5-2	2-4
Naproxen (Naprosyn®)	1500	2-4	12-15
Naproxen sodium (Anaprox®, others)	1375	1-2	12-13
Oxaprozin (Daypro®)	1800	3-5	42-50
Nonacidic Agent			
Nabumetone	2000	3-6	24
Salicylic Acid Derivative			
Diflunisal	1500	2-3	8-12
Salsalate	3000	2-3	7-8
COX-2 Inhibitor			
Celecoxib (Celebrex®)	400	3	11
Oxicam			
Meloxicam (Mobic®)	15	4-5	15-20
Piroxicam (Feldene®)	20	3-5	30-86

Dosage is based on 70 kg adult with normal hepatic and renal function.

[1]Food decreases the rate of absorption and may delay the time to peak levels.

[2]150 mg on the first day.

[3]Half-life of active sulfide metabolite.

[4]Half-life with multiple doses.

OPIOID ANALGESICS

This table serves as a general guide to opioid conversion. Utilization of a direct conversion without a detailed patients and medication assessment is not recommended and may result in over- or underdosing. Chronic administration may alter pharmacokinetics and change parental:oral ratio.

Opioid Analgesics – Initial Oral Dosing Commonly Used for Severe Pain

Drug	Equianalgesic Dose (mg)		Initial Oral Dose	
	Oral[1]	Parenteral[2]	Children[3] (mg/kg)	Adults (mg)
Buprenorphine	—	0.4	—	—
Butorphanol	—	2	—	—
Fentanyl	—	0.1	—	—
Hydromorphone	7.5	1.5	0.06	2-4
Levorphanol	Acute: 4 Chronic: 1	Acute: 2 Chronic: 1	0.04	2-4
Meperidine[4]	300	75	Not recommended	
Methadone[5]	Acute: 10 Chronic: Varies depending upon opioid dose[5]	Acute: 5	0.2	5-10
Morphine	30	10	0.3	15-30
Nalbuphine	—	10	—	—
Pentazocine	50	30	—	—
Oxycodone	20	—	0.2	10-20
Oxymorphone	10	1	—	5-10

[1]Elderly: Starting dose should be lower for this population group.

[2]Standard parenteral doses for acute pain in adults; can be used to doses for I.V. infusions and repeated small I.V. boluses. Single I.V. boluses, use half the I.M. dose.

[3]The pharmacokinetics of opioids in children and infants >6 months old are similar to adults but infants <6 months old, especially premature or physically compromised ones, are at risk of apnea.

[4]Not recommended for routine use.

[5]Conversion of higher doses may be guided by the following (consult a pain or palliative care specialist if unfamiliar with methadone prescribing): As the total daily dose of morphine increases, the equianalgesic dose ratio (methadone:morphine) increases in adults with ongoing cancer pain. (American Pain Society, 2008; National Comprehensive Cancer Network, 2009). Applicability to pediatric patients is unknown.

References

National Cancer Institute, "Pain (PDQ®)," Last Modified 5/7/09. Available at http://www.cancer.gov/cancertopics/pdq/supportivecare/pain/HealthProfessional/page1.

National Comprehensive Cancer Network® (NCCN), "Clinical Practice Guidelines in Oncology™: Adult Cancer Pain," Version 1, 2009. Available at http://www.nccn.org/professionals/physician_gls/PDF/pain.pdf.

Patanwala AE, Duby J, Waters D, et al, "Opioid Conversions in Acute Care," *Ann Pharmacother*, 2007, 41(2):255-66.

Principles of Analgesic Use in the Treatment of Acute Pain and Cancer Pain, 6th ed, Glenview, IL: American Pain Society, 2008.

Comparative Pharmacology

Drug	Analgesic	Antitussive	Constipation	Respiratory Depression	Sedation	Emesis
Phenanthrenes						
Codeine	+	+++	+	+	+	+
Hydrocodone	++	+++				
Hydromorphone	++	++	+	++	+	+
Levorphanol	++	++		++	++	+
Morphine	++	++	++	++	++	++
Oxycodone	++	+++	++	++	++	++
Oxymorphone	++	+	+++	+++		+++
Phenylpiperidines						
Meperidine	++		+	++	+	
Diphenylheptanes						
Methadone	++	++	+	++	+	+
Propoxyphene	+			+	+	+
Agonist / Antagonist						
Pentazocine	++		+	++	++ or stimulation	++

Adapted from Catalano RB, "The Medical Approach to Management of Pain Caused by Cancer," *Semin Oncol*, 1975, 2(4):379-92.

SEDATIVE AGENTS IN THE INTENSIVE CARE UNIT

Comparative Dosages of Sedative Agents

Drug	Recommended Pediatric Dosage	Recommended Adult Dosage	Continuous Infusion Dosage
Benzodiazepines			
Diazepam	P.O.: 0.12-0.8 mg/kg/day in divided doses q6-8h I.M./I.V.: 0.04-0.3 mg/kg/dose q2-4h to a maximum of 0.6 mg/kg/8 h period	I.V.: 0.03-0.1 mg q0.5-6h	**Not recommended** due to poor stability
Lorazepam	I.M./P.O.: 0.05 mg/kg/dose (maximum: 2 mg/dose) q4-8h prn; range: 0.02-0.1 mg/kg	Intermittent I.V. dose: 0.02-0.06 mg/kg q2-6h	0.01-0.1 mg/kg/h **Note:** Propylene glycol (vehicle may accumulate with high dose and/or long infusion durations. Watch solution for precipitation.
Midazolam	P.O.: ≤5 y: 0.25-0.5 mg/kg/dose; higher doses (<1 mg/kg/dose) may be required >5 y: 0.425-0.5 mg/kg/dose Usual duration: 2 h I.M.: 0.1-0.15 mg/kg/dose I.V.: ≤5 y: 0.05-0.1 mg/kg/dose; may repeat up to a total dose of 0.6 mg/kg (6 mg) >5 y: 0.025-0.05 mg/kg/dose; may repeat up to a total dose of 0.4 mg/kg (10 mg) Intranasal: 0.2-0.3 mg/kg by needleleless syringe to nares over 15 sec; may repeat in 5-15 min	Acute agitation: I.V.: 2-5 mg q5-15min until controlled Intermittent I.V. dose: 0.02-0.08 mg/kg q0.5-2h	Children: Loading dose: 0.05-0.2 mg/kg, followed by 1-2 mcg/kg/min titrated to desired effect (usual range 0.4-6 mcg/kg/min Adults: 0.04-0.2 mg/kg/h **Note:** Midazolam/1-hydroxymidazolam may accumulate with long infusion durations and/or renal failure.

Comparative Dosages of Sedative Agents *continued*

Drug	Recommended Pediatric Dosage	Recommended Adult Dosage	Continuous Infusion Dosage
		Other Agents	
Haloperidol	Limited Data	I.M./I.V.: Mild agitation: 0.5-2 mg Moderate agitation: 2-5 mg Severe agitation: 10-20 mg Repeat dose after 30 minutes; double dose and administer after another 30 minutes and continue until calm achieved; may repeat additional doses at 6- to 12-hour intervals Acute delirium: I.V.: 2-10 mg q15-30 min until controlled, then 25% loading dose every 4-6 h Intermittent I.V. dose: 0.03-0.15 mg/kg q0.5-6h	Infusion rates of 3-25 mg/h for treatment durations of 2-12 days have been reported **Note:** Monitor QT_c interval especially with high doses. May produce extrapyramidal symptoms (EPS).
Propofol	Limited Data	–	Adults: 5-80 mcg/kg/min (0.3-4.8 mg/kg/h)
Dexmedetomidine	–	–	Children (limited data): Loading dose: 0.5-1 mcg/kg; followed by 0.1-0.7 mcg/kg/h Adults: Loading dose: 0.5-1 mcg/kg; followed by 0.2-1.5 mcg/kg/h **Note:** Loading dose is optional in critically-ill mechanically ventilated patients.

SELECTED REFERENCES

American College of Critical Care Medicine of the Society of Critical Care Medicine, American Society of Health-System Pharmacists, and American College of Chest Physicians, "Clinical Practice Guidelines for the Sustained Use of Sedatives and Analgesics in the Critically Ill Adult," *Am J Health Syst Pharm*, 2002, 59(2):150-78.

Buck ML and Willson DF, "Use of Dexmedetomidine in the Pediatric Intensive Care Unit," *Pharmacotherapy*, 2008, 28(1):51-7.

Pandharipande PP, Pun BT, Herr DL, et al, "Effect of Sedation With Dexmedetomidine Vs Lorazepam on Acute Brain Dysfunction in Mechanically Ventilated Patients: The MENDS Randomized Controlled Trial," *JAMA*, 2007, 298(22):2644-53.

Playfor S, Jenkins I, Boyles C, et al, "Consensus Guidelines on Sedation and Analgesia in Critically Ill Children," *Intensive Care Med*, 2006, 32(8):1125-36.

Riker RR, Shehabi Y, Bokesch PM, et al, "Dexmedetomidine Vs Midazolam for Sedation of Critically Ill Patients: A Randomized Trial," *JAMA*, 2009, 301(5):489-99.

DESENSITIZATION PROTOCOLS

PENICILLIN DESENSITIZATION PROTOCOL: MUST BE DONE BY PHYSICIAN!

Acute penicillin desensitization should only be performed in an intensive care setting. Any remedial risk factor should be corrected. All β-adrenergic antagonists such as propranolol or even timolol ophthalmic drops should be discontinued. Asthmatic patients should be under optimal control. An intravenous line should be established, baseline electrocardiogram (ECG) and spirometry should be performed, and continuous ECG monitoring should be instituted. Premedication with antihistamines or steroids is not recommended, as these drugs have not proven effective in suppressing severe reactions but may mask early signs of reactivity that would otherwise result in a modification of the protocol.

Protocols have been developed for penicillin desensitization using both the oral and parenteral route. As of 1987 there were 93 reported cases of oral desensitization, 74 of which were done by Sullivan and his collaborators. Of these 74 patients, 32% experienced a transient allergic reaction either during desensitization (one-third) or during penicillin treatment after desensitization (two-thirds). These reactions were usually mild and self-limited in nature. Only one IgE-mediated reaction (wheezing and bronchospasm) required discontinuation of the procedure before desensitization could be completed. It has been argued that oral desensitization may be safer than parenteral desensitization, but most patients can also be safely desensitized by parenteral route.

During desensitization any dose that causes mild systemic reactions such as pruritus, fleeting urticaria, rhinitis, or mild wheezing should be repeated until the patient tolerates the dose without systemic symptoms or signs. More serious reactions such as hypotension, laryngeal edema, or asthma require appropriate treatment, and if desensitization is continued, the dose should be decreased by at least 10-fold and withheld until the patient is stable.

Once desensitized, the patient's treatment with penicillin must not lapse or the risk of an allergic reaction increases. If the patient requires a β-lactam antibiotic in the future and still remains skin test-positive to penicillin reagents, desensitization would be required again.

Several patients have been maintained on long-term, low-dose penicillin therapy (usually bid-tid) to sustain a chronic state of desensitization. Such individuals usually require chronic desensitization because of continuous occupationally related exposure to β-lactam drugs.

Order for placement/availability at the bedside in the event of a hypersensitivity reaction during scratch/skin testing and desensitization:
Hydrocortisone: 100 mg IVP
Diphenhydramine: 50 mg IVP
Epinephrine: 1:1000 SubQ

Several investigators have demonstrated that penicillin can be administered to history positive, skin test positive patients if initially small but gradually increasing doses are given. However, patients with a history of exfoliative dermatitis secondary to penicillin should not be re-exposed to the drug, even by desensitization.

Desensitization is a potentially dangerous procedure and should be only performed in an area where immediate access to emergency drugs and equipment can be assured.

Begin between 8-10 AM in the morning.

Follow desensitization as indicated for penicillin G or ampicillin.

AMPICILLIN
Oral Desensitization Protocol

1. Begin 0.03 mg of ampicillin
2. Double the dose administered every 30 minutes until complete
3. Example of oral dosing regimen:

Dose #	Ampicillin (mg)
1	0.03
2	0.06
3	0.12
4	0.23
5	0.47
6	0.94
7	1.87
8	3.75
9	7.5
10	15
11	30
12	60
13	125
14	250
15	500

PENICILLIN G
Parenteral Desensitization Protocol: Typical Schedule

Injection No.	Benzylpenicillin Concentration (units/mL)	Volume and Route (mL)[1]
1[2]	100	0.1 I.D.
2	↓	0.2 SubQ
3		0.4 SubQ
4		0.8 SubQ
5[2]	1000	0.1 I.D.
6	↓	0.3 SubQ
7		0.6 SubQ
8[2]	10,000	0.1 I.D.
9	↓	0.2 SubQ
10		0.4 SubQ
11		0.8 SubQ
12[2]	100,000	0.1 I.D.
13	↓	0.3 SubQ
14		0.6 SubQ
15[2]	1,000,000	0.1 I.D.
16	↓	0.2 SubQ
17		0.2 I.M.
18		0.4 I.M.
19	Continuous I.V. infusion (1,000,000 units/h)	

[1]Administer progressive doses at intervals of not less than 20 minutes.

[2]Observe and record skin wheal and flare response to intradermal dose.

Abbreviations: I.D. = intradermal, SubQ = subcutaneous, I.M. = intramuscular, I.V. = intravenous.

PENICILLIN
Oral Desensitization Protocol

Step[1]	Phenoxymethyl Penicillin (units/mL)	Amount (mL)	Dose (units)	Cumulative Dosage (units)
1	1000	0.1	100	100
2	1000	0.2	200	300
3	1000	0.4	400	700
4	1000	0.8	800	1500
5	1000	1.6	1600	3100
6	1000	3.2	3200	6300
7	1000	6.4	6400	12,700
8	10,000	1.2	12,000	24,700
9	10,000	2.4	24,000	48,700
10	10,000	4.8	48,000	96,700
11	80,000	1	80,000	176,700
12	80,000	2	160,000	336,700
13	80,000	4	320,000	656,700
14	80,000	8	640,000	1,296,700
Observe patient for 30 minutes				
Change to benzylpenicillin G I.V.				
15	500,000	0.25	125,000	
16	500,000	0.50	250,000	
17	500,000	1	500,000	
18	500,000	2.25	1,125,000	

[1]Interval between steps, 15 min

ALLOPURINOL
Successful Desensitization for Treatment of a Fixed Drug Eruption

	Oral Dose of Allopurinol
Days 1-3	50 mcg/day
Days 4-6	100 mcg/day
Days 7-9	200 mcg/day
Days 10-12	500 mcg/day
Days 13-15	1 mg/day
Days 16-18	5 mg/day
Days 19-21	10 mg/day
Days 22-24	25 mg/day
Days 25-27	50 mg/day
Day 28	100 mg/day
Prednisone 10 mg/day through desensitization and 1 month after reaching dose of 100 mg allopurinol	

Modified from *J Allergy Clin Immunol*, 1996, 97:1171-2.

AMPHOTERICIN B
Challenge and Desensitization Protocol

1.   Procedure supervised by physician
2.   Epinephrine, 1:1000 wt/vol, multidose vial at bedside
3.   Premixed albutenol solution at bedside for nebulization
4.   Endotracheal intubation supplies at bedside with anesthesiologist on standby
5.   Continuous cardiac telemetry with electronic monitoring of blood pressure
6.   Continuous pulse oximetry
7.   Premedication with methylprednisolone, 60 mg, I.V. and diphenhydramine, 25 mg I.V.
8.   Amphotericin B (Fungizone®)[1] administration schedule

   a. 10^{-6}, infused over 10 minutes

   b. 10^{-5}, infused over 10 minutes

   c. 10^{-4}, infused over 10 minutes

   d. 10^{-3}, infused over 10 minutes

   e. 10^{-2}, infused over 10 minutes

   f. 10^{-1} (1 mg), infused over 30 minutes

   g.   30 mg in 250 mL 5% dextrose, infused over 4 hours

[1]Mixtures were prepared in 10 mL 5% dextrose by hospital intensive care unit pharmacy, unless otherwise noted.

From Kemp SF and Lockey RF, "Amphotericin B: Emergency Challenge in a Neutropenic, Asthmatic Patient With Fungal Sepsis," *J Allergy Clin Immunol*, 1995, 96(3):425-7.

BACTRIM™
Oral Desensitization Protocol

(Adapted from Gluckstein D and Ruskin J, "Rapid Oral Desensitization to Trimethoprim-Sulfamethoxazole (TMP-SMZ): Use in Prophylaxis for *Pneumocystis carinii* Pneumonia in Patients With AIDS Who Were Previously Intolerant to TMP-SMZ," *Clin Infect Dis*, 1995, 20:849-53.)

Please read the directions carefully before starting the protocol!

1.   There must be a clear cut need for a sulfa drug or a sulfa drug combination product such as Bactrim™. The decision to use sulfa must be made prior to skin testing.
2.   Informed consent from the patient or an appropriate relative must have been obtained.
3.   A trained individual, physician, nurse, or aide, **must be with the patient** at all times.
4.   A physician **must** be on the floor at all times.
5.   Injectable epinephrine 0.3 mL 1:1000, diphenhydramine (Benadryl®) 50 mg, corticosteroids and oral ibuprofen 400 mg solution should be drawn up and available at the bedside.
6.   Appropriate resuscitative equipment must be available.
7.   All dilution of oral Bactrim™ should be made up prior to beginning procedure.
8.   Patient should drink 180 mL of water after each Bactrim™ dose.

Dilution for Bactrim™ Desensitization

Final Concentration	Bottle #	Procedure
Oral Bactrim™ 40/200 mg/5 mL	A	Conventional oral Bactrim™ suspension 5 mL = 40/200 mg
Oral Bactrim™ 0.4/2 mg/mL	B	1. Add 5 mL conventional oral Bactrim™ suspension or A (concentration = 40/200 mg/5 mL) to 95 mL of sterile water 2. Shake well. This will give 100 mL of 40/200 mg Bactrim™; each mL = 0.4/2 mg Bactrim™. 3. Dispense 20 mL for use
Oral Bactrim™ 0.004/0.02 mg/mL	C	1. Add 1 mL of the 0.4/2 mg/mL Bactrim™ or B to 99 mL of sterile water 2. Shake well. This will give 100 mL of 0.4/2 mg Bactrim™; each mL = 0.004/0.02 mg Bactrim™. 3. Dispense 20 mL for use

Adverse Reactions and Response During the Protocol

Types of Reactions	Alteration of Protocol
Mild reactions (rash, fever, nausea)	I.V. diphenhydramine (Benadryl®) 50 mg and oral ibuprofen suspension 400 mg
Urticaria, dyspnea, severe vomiting, or hypotension	**STOP** the protocol IMMEDIATELY

- If patient tolerates up to Bactrim™ DS, he/she is desensitized.
- Assuming that there were no complications, the procedure will take up to 6 hours.

Sample Bactrim™ Desensitization Flow Sheet

Patient Name _____

Diagnosis _____ Physician _____

Age _____ Gender _____ Pager _____ Hospital # _____

History of sulfa reaction _____

# Hour	Actual Time	Suggested Dose	Form	Suggested Volume	Actual Dose	Form	Actual Volume	Reaction / Notes	Initial
0		Bactrim™ 0.004/0.02 mg (use **0.004/0.02 mg/mL** bottle or bottle C)	Susp (C)	1 mL					
1		Bactrim™ 0.04/0.2 mg (use 0.004/0.02 mg/mL bottle or bottle C)	Susp (C)	10 mL					
2		Bactrim™ 0.4/2 mg (use **0.4/2 mg/mL bottle** or bottle B)	Susp (B)	1 mL					
3		Bactrim™ 4/20 mg (use 0.4/2 mg/mL bottle or bottle B)	Susp (B)	10 mL					
4		Bactrim™ 40/200 mg (use **40/200 mg/5 mL unit dose** Bactrim™ or A)	Susp (A)	5 mL					
5		Bactrim™ 80/400 mg (use 40/200 mg/5 mL unit dose Bactrim™ or A)	Susp (A)	10 mL					
6		Bactrim™ DS tablet	Tablet	1 DS pill					

Note: Drink 180 mL of water after each Bactrim™ dose.

◀

ALTERNATIVE BACTRIM™ PROTOCOL

Adapted from Leoung GS, Stanford JF, Giordano MF, et al, "Trimethoprim-Sulfamethoxazole (TMP-SMZ) Dose Escalation Versus Direct Rechallenge for *Pneumocystis carinii* Pneumonia, Prophylaxis in Human Immunodeficiency Virus-Infected Patients With Previous Adverse Reaction to TMP-SMZ," *J Infect Dis*, 2001, 184(8):992-7.

Trimethoprim-Sulfamethoxazole (TMP-SMZ) Dose-Escalation Regimen in Human Immunodeficiency Virus-Infected Patients With Previous Mild-to-Moderate Treatment-Limiting Rash and/or Fever

Dosing Level	Portion of Single-Strength TMP-SMZ (%)	Amount (Frequency) of Pediatric Suspension (mL)	Total TMP Dose (mg)	Total SMZ Dose (mg)
1	12.5	1.25 qd	10	50
2	25	1.25 bid	20	100
3	37.5	1.25 tid	30	150
4	50	2.5 bid	40	200
5	75	2.5 tid	60	300
6	100	1 single-strength tablet	80	400

Note: Each dosing level is a daily dose. For successful completion of the reintroduction phase, patients must have taken each dose level at least once. Patients were permitted to repeat dose levels once; dose levels were completed in increasing increments, and the level 6 dose was taken no later than day 13 of the reintroduction phase. Patients were permitted to withhold study drug for 2 days during the reintroduction phase (withholding study drug for >2 days during reintroduction resulted in permanent discontinuation). Patients were required to take an antihistamine during dose escalation.

VANCOMYCIN DESENSITIZATION PROTOCOL

(Adapted from Wong JT, Ripple RE, MacLean JA, et al, "Vancomycin Hypersensitivity: Synergism with Narcotics and Desensitization by a Rapid Continuous Intravenous Protocol," *J Allergy Clin Immunol*, 1994, 94(2 Pt 1):189-94.)

Please read the directions carefully before starting the protocol!

1. Vancomycin desensitization is indicated only for cases with a definitive need for vancomycin and persistent allergic reaction despite slowing of infusion rate and the addition of Benadryl® or cases with reported vancomycin anaphylactic reactions.

2. Informed consent from the patient or an appropriate relative must have been obtained.

3. A trained individual, physician, nurse, or aide, **must be with the patient** at all times.

4. A physician **must** be on the floor at all times.

5. Injectable epinephrine 0.3 mL 1:1000, diphenhydramine (Benadryl®) 50 mg, corticosteroids and oral ibuprofen 400 mg solution should be drawn up and available at the bedside.

6. Appropriate resuscitative equipment must be available.

7. All dilution of I.V. vancomycin should be made up prior to beginning procedure.

8. All patients are pretreated with 25-50 mg Benadryl®.

9. Infusion rates are to be tightly regulated with **syringe pump**.

Dilution for Vancomycin Desensitization

Final Concentration	Bottle #	Procedure
10 mg/mL	A	1. Dilute 1 g of vancomycin in 10 mL of sterile water 2. Shake well until the drug is completely dissolved 3. Add 2 mL of solution to 18 mL of 0.9% normal saline 4. Mix well 5. This will give 20 mL of 10 mg/mL concentration of vancomycin or (Bottle A) 6. Dispense 10-15 mL in a syringe for syringe pump. Label the syringe as "SYR A: conc = 10 mg/mL" with patient's name, ID, room number, date, and dispensor's initial/pharmacist's initial.
1 mg/mL	B	1. Add 2 mL of bottle A vancomycin (10 mg/mL) to 18 mL of 0.9% normal saline 2. Mix well 3. This will give 20 mL of 1 mg/mL concentration vancomycin or (Bottle B) 4. Dispense 10-15 mL in a syringe for syringe pump. Label the syringe as "SYR B: conc = 1 mg/mL" with patient's name, ID, room number, date, and dispensor's initial/pharmacist's initial.
0.1 mg/mL	C	1. Add 2 mL of Bottle B vancomycin (1 mg/mL) to 18 mL of 0.9% normal saline 2. Mix well 3. This will give 20 mL of 0.1 mg/mL concentration vancomycin or (Bottle C) 4. Dispense 10-15 mL in a syringe for syringe pump. Label the syringe as "SYR C: conc = 0.1 mg/mL" with patient's name, ID, room number, date, and dispensor's initial/pharmacist's initial.
0.01 mg/mL	D	1. Add 2 mL of Bottle C vancomycin (0.1 mg/mL) to 18 mL of 0.9% normal saline 2. Mix well 3. This will give 20 mL of 0.01 mg/mL concentration vancomycin or (Bottle D) 4. Dispense 10-15 mL in a syringe for syringe pump. Label the syringe as "SYR D: conc = 0.01 mg/mL" with patient's name, ID, room number, date, and dispensor's initial/pharmacist's initial.
0.001 mg/mL	E	1. Add 2 mL of Bottle D vancomycin (0.01 mg/mL) to 18 mL of 0.9% normal saline 2. Mix well 3. This will give 20 mL of 0.001 mg/mL concentration vancomycin or (Bottle E) 4. Dispense 10-15 mL in a syringe for syringe pump. Label the syringe as "SYR E: conc = 0.001 mg/mL" with patient's name, ID, room number, date, and dispensor's initial/pharmacist's initial.
0.0001 mg/mL	F	1. Add 2 mL of Bottle E vancomycin (0.001 mg/mL) to 18 mL of 0.9% normal saline 2. Mix well 3. This will give 20 mL of 0.0001 mg/mL concentration vancomycin or (Bottle F) 4. Dispense 10-15 mL in a syringe for syringe pump. Label the syringe as "SYR F: conc = 0.0001 mg/mL" with patient's name, ID, room number, date, and dispensor's initial/pharmacist's initial.

Sample Vancomycin Desensitization Flow Sheet

Patient Name _____   Age _____   Gender _____   Hospital # _____

Diagnosis _____   Physician _____   Pager _____   History of vancomycin reaction _____

Time (h/min)	Actual Time	Vancomycin Concentration (mg/mL)	Syr #	Fluid Infusion Rate (mL/min)	VIR (mg/min)	Actual Concentration (mg/mL)	Syr #	Infusion Rate (mL/min)	Reaction / Notes	Initial
0:00		0.0001	F	1	0.0001					
0:10		0.001	E	0.33	0.00033					
0:20		0.001	E	1.0	0.001					
0:30		0.01	D	0.33	0.0033					
0:40		0.01	D	1.0	0.010					
0:50		0.1	C	0.33	0.033					
1:00		0.1	C	0.33	0.033					
1:10		1.0	B	0.33	0.33					
1:20		1.0	B	1	1					
1:30		10.0	A	0.22	2.2^1					
1:30		10.0	A	0.44	4.4^1					

[1] After a VIR of 2.2-4.4 mg/min is achieved, full dose of vancomycin can be administered at the VIR for the first day. The rate can be gradually advanced over the next few days as tolerated.

Patients in whom a VIR of 2.2-4.4 mg/min can **not** be achieved, continue to receive vancomycin at the highest tolerated infusion rate for the first day. The rate is to be gradually advanced over the next few days as tolerated.

ALTERNATIVE VANCOMYCIN PROTOCOL

Adapted from Wazny LD and Daghigh B, "Desensitization Protocols for Vancomycin Hypersensitivity," *Ann Pharmacother*, 2001, 35(11):1458-64.

Rapid Vancomycin Desensitization Protocol (Lerner and Dwyer)

Premedication

Diphenhydramine 50 mg I.V. and hydrocortisone 100 mg I.V. 15 minutes prior to initiation of protocol, then q6h throughout protocol.

Infusion No.	Dilution	Vancomycin Dose (mg)	Concentration (mg/mL)
1	1:10,000	0.02	0.0002
2	1:1000	0.20	0.002
3	1:100	2	0.02
4	1:10	20	0.2
5	Standard	500	2

Preparation

1. Prepare a standard bag of 500 mg vancomycin in 250 mL NS or D_5W; label as infusion no. 5, vancomycin 2 mg/mL.
2. Draw up 10 mL of the standard vancomycin 2 mg/mL preparation and place in 100 mL bag of NS or D_5W; label as infusion no. 4, vancomycin 0.2 mg/mL.
3. Draw up 10 mL of the 0.2 mg/mL solution and place in a 100 mL bag of NS or D_5W; label as infusion no. 3, vancomycin 0.02 mg/mL.
4. Draw up 10 mL of the 0.02 mg/mL solution and place in a 100 mL bag of NS or D_5W; label as infusion no. 2, vancomycin 0.002 mg/mL.
5. Draw up 10 mL of the 0.002 mg/mL solution and place in a 100 mL bag of NS or D_5W; label as infusion no. 1, vancomycin 0.0002 mg/mL.

Infusion Rate Directions

Initiate infusion rate at 0.5 mL/min (30 mL/h) and increase by 0.5 mL/min (30 mL/h) as tolerated every 5 minutes to a maximum rate of 5 mL/min (300 mL/h). If pruritus, hypotension, rash, or difficulty breathing occurs, stop infusion and reinfuse the previously tolerated infusion at the highest tolerated rate. This step may be repeated up to three times for any given concentration.

Upon completion of infusion no. 5, immediately administer the required dose of vancomycin in the usual dilution of NS or D_5W over 2 hours. Decrease rate if patient becomes symptomatic or, alternatively, increase rate if patient tolerates dose. Administer diphenhydramine 50 mg P.O. 60 minutes prior to each dose.

CEFTRIAXONE DESENSITIZATION PROTOCOL

Dose	Concentration (mg/mL)	Volume (mL)	Dose (mg)
Subcutaneous Route: 15-minute intervals between all doses			
1	0.2	0.5	0.1
2	0.2	1	0.2
3	2	0.25	0.5
4	2	0.5	1
5	2	1	2
6	16	0.25	4
7	16	0.5	8
8	16	1	16
Intravenous Route: Infuse over 20-30 minutes; 15 minutes between doses			
9	20	1.5 mL qs to 50 mL	30 mg/50 mL
10	20	3 mL qs to 50 mL	60 mg/50 mL
11	20	6 mL qs to 50 mL	120 mg/50 mL
12	20	12.5 mL qs to 50 mL	250 mg/50 mL
13	–	–	1 g/50 mL

Pharmacy Admixture Instructions

1. Mix ceftriaxone 1 g/50 mL NS (concentration 20 mg/mL); label **Bag A**.
2. Remove 1 mL from Bag A and add 99 mL NS (concentration 0.2 mg/mL); label **Bag B**.
3. Use **Bag B** to make doses 1 and 2.
4. Remove 1 mL from Bag A and add 9 mL NS (concentration 2 mg/mL); label **Bag C**.
5. Use Bag C to make doses 3, 4, and 5.
6. Remove 1 mL from Bag A and add 0.25 mL NS (concentration 16 mg/mL); label **Bag D**.
7. Use Bag D to make doses 6 and 7.
8. Repeat step 6 to make dose 8 (step 6 only makes 1.25 mL; therefore need to repeat to make dose 8).
9. Take a 50 mL bag of NS and remove overfill plus 1.5 mL; add 1.5 mL from Bag A to NS bag (30 mg/50 mL); this is dose 9.
10. Take a 50 mL bag of NS and remove overfill plus 3 mL; add 3 mL from Bag A to NS bag (60 mg/50 mL); this is dose 10.
11. Take a 50 mL bag of NS and remove overfill plus 6 mL; add 6 mL from Bag A to NS bag (120 mg/50 mL); this is dose 11.
12. Take a 50 mL bag of NS and remove overfill plus 12.5 mL; add 12.5 mL from Bag A to NS bag (250 mg/50 mL); this is dose 12.
13. Dispense 1 g/50 mL for dose 13.

CIPROFLOXACIN

Modified from *J Allergy Clin Immunol*, 1996, 97:1426-7.

Premedicated with diphenhydramine hydrochloride, ranitidine, and prednisone 1 hour before the desensitization.

The individual doses were administered at 15-minute intervals. Because the patient was intubated in the intensive care unit, vital signs were continually monitored. The patient's skin was inspected for development of urticaria, and his chest was auscultated for wheezing every 10 minutes. No rash, hypotension, or wheezing developed during desensitization. The procedure took 4 hours, and once finished, the patient had received an equivalent to his first scheduled dose (400 mg twice daily). The second dose was given 4 hours later, followed by routine administration of 400 mg every 12 hours, with a small dose (25 mg intravenously) between therapeutic doses to maintain a drug level in the blood. The patient subsequently received 4 weeks of ciprofloxacin treatment without difficulty.

Desensitization Regimen for Ciprofloxacin

Ciprofloxacin Concentration (mg/mL)	Volume Given (mL)	Absolute Amount (mg)	Cumulative Total Dose (mg)
0.1	0.1	0.01	0.01
0.1	0.2	0.02	0.03
0.1	0.4	0.04	0.07
0.1	0.8	0.08	0.15
1	0.16	0.16	0.31
1	0.32	0.32	0.63
1	0.64	0.64	1.27
2	0.6	1.2	2.47
2	1.2	2.4	4.87
2	2.4	4.8	9.67
2	5	10	19.67
2	10	20	39.67
2	20	40	79.67
2	40	80	159.67
2	120	240	399.67

Drug volumes <1 mL were mixed with normal saline solution to a final volume of 3 mL and then slowly infused; the other doses were administered over 10 minutes, except the last dose (240 mg in 120 mL), which was given with an infusion pump over 20 minutes.

IMIPENEM DESENSITIZATION PROTOCOL

Adapted from Saxon A, Adelman DC, Patel A, et al, "Imipenem Cross-Reactivity With Penicillin in Humans," *J Allergy Clin Immunol*, 1988, 82(2):213-7.

Indication: Need for imipenem in the setting of anaphylactic potential to penicillin. Cross-reactivity between imipenem and penicillin is high.

Subcutaneous Route: 15-minute intervals between all doses

Dose	Solution No.	Concentration (mg/mL)	SubQ Injections q15min	
			Volume (mL)	Dosage (mg)
1	3	0.05	0.5	0.025
2		0.05	1	0.05
3	2	0.5	0.2	0.1
4		0.5	0.4	0.2
5		0.5	0.8	0.4
6	1	5	0.12	0.6
7		5	0.25	1.25
8		5	0.5	2.5
9		5	1	5

———— Wait 30 minutes ————

Intravenous Route: Infuse over 20-30 minutes; 15 minutes between doses

Dose	Solution No.	I.V. Imipenem Dose (using 50 mL NSS)	Concentration (mg/mL)	Total Dosage (mg)
10	1	2 mL in 50 mL NSS	10 mg/50 mL	10
11		4 mL in 50 mL NSS	20 mg/50 mL	20
12		8 mL in 50 mL NSS	40 mg/50 mL	40
13		12 mL in 50 mL NSS	60 mg/50 mL	60
	Add 10 mL NSS to 500 mg vial Primaxin®			
14		2.5 mL in 50 mL NSS	125 mg/50 mL	125
15		5 mL in 50 mL NSS	250 mg/50 mL	250

INSULIN

Lilly's appropriate diluting fluid, sterile saline, or distilled water, to which 1 mL of the patient's blood or the addition of 1 mL of 1% serum albumin (making a 0.1% solution) for each 10 mL of stock diluent, is a satisfactory diluent. The albumin in the blood or serum albumin solution is necessary to retain the integrity of the higher dilutions by preventing adsorption to glass or plastic. Dilution is stable 30 days under refrigeration or room temperature, but should be used within 24 hours due to a lack of preservative.

1. Make a 1:1 dilution of single species (beef, pork, or human) insulin (50 units/mL).
2. Add 0.5 mL of the above dilution to 4.5 mL of diluent (5 units/mL).
3. Add 0.5 mL of the 5 units/mL dilution to 4.5 mL of diluent (0.5 unit/mL).
4. Add 0.5 mL of the 0.5 unit/mL dilution to 4.5 mL of diluent (0.05 unit/mL).
5. Add 0.5 mL of the 0.05 unit/mL dilution to 4.5 mL of diluent (0.005 unit/mL).

The 5 vials containing 50, 5, 0.5, 0.05, and 0.005 unit/mL are ready for skin testing or desensitization procedures.

One may start desensitization by giving 0.02 mL of 0.05 unit/mL concentration (1/1000 unit) intradermally. If no reaction occurs, administer 0.04 and 0.08 mL of the same concentration at 30-minute intervals.

The procedure continues proceeding to the next greater concentration (0.5 unit/mL) and giving 0.02, 0.04, and 0.08 mL at 30-minute intervals.

In the same manner proceed through the 5 units/mL and 50 units/mL concentrations with the exception that these injections should be given subcutaneously.

Note: If a reaction is noted, back up 2 steps and try to proceed forward again.

If the patient reacts to the initial injection, it will be necessary to utilize the lower concentration (0.005 unit/mL) to initiate the procedure.

It is essential that manifestations of allergic reactions not be obscured. Therefore, antihistamines or steroids should not be used during desensitization except to treat severe allergic reactions. The use of these agents may obscure mild to moderate reactions to the lower doses and result in more severe reactions as doses increase, leading to failure of the desensitization program.

NELFINAVIR DESENSITIZATION PROTOCOL

Adapted from Abraham PE, Sorensen SJ, Baker WH, et al, "Nelfinavir Desensitization," *Ann Pharmacother*, 2001, 35(5):553-6.

Step	Time (min)	Nelfinavir Dose (mg)	
		q30min	Total
1	0	0.5	0.5
2	30	1	1.5
3	60	2	3.5
4	90	5	8.5
5	120	10	18.5
6	150	20	38.5
7	180	40	78.5
8	210	80	158.5
9	240	160	318.5
10	270	250	568.5
11	300	500	1068.5
12	330	750	1818.5
Observe patient in ICU for 2 hours before discharge			

RIFAMPIN and ETHAMBUTOL
Oral Desensitization in Mycobacterial Disease

Time from Start (h:min)	Rifampin (mg)	Ethambutol (mg)
0	0.1	0.1
00:45	0.5	0.5
01:30	1	1
02:15	2	2
03:00	4	4
03:45	8	8
04:30	16	16
05:15	32	32
06:00	50	50
06:45	100	100
07:30	150	200
11:00	300	400
Next day		
6:30 AM	300 mg twice daily	400 mg 3 times/day

From *Am J Respir Crit Care Med*, 1994, 149:815-7.

SKIN TESTS

PENICILLIN ALLERGY

The recommended battery of major and minor determinants used in penicillin skin testing will disclose those individuals with circulating IgE antibodies. This procedure is therefore useful to identify patients at risk for immediate or accelerated reactions. Skin tests are of no value in predicting the occurrence of non-IgE-mediated hypersensitivity reactions to penicillin such as delayed exanthem, drug fever, hemolytic anemia, interstitial nephritis, or exfoliative dermatitis. Based on large scale trials, skin testing solutions have been standardized.

Antihistamines, tricyclic antidepressants, and adrenergic drugs, all of which may inhibit skin test results, should be discontinued at least 24 hours prior to skin testing. Antihistamines with long half-lives (hydroxyzine, terfenadine, astemizole, etc) may attenuate skin test results up to a week, or longer after discontinuation.

When properly performed with due consideration for preliminary scratch tests and appropriate dilutions, skin testing with penicillin reagents can almost always be safely accomplished. Systemic reactions accompany about 1% of positive skin tests; these are usually mild but can be serious. **Therefore skin tests should be done in the presence of a physician and with immediate access to medications and equipment needed to treat anaphylaxis.**

History of Penicillin Allergy

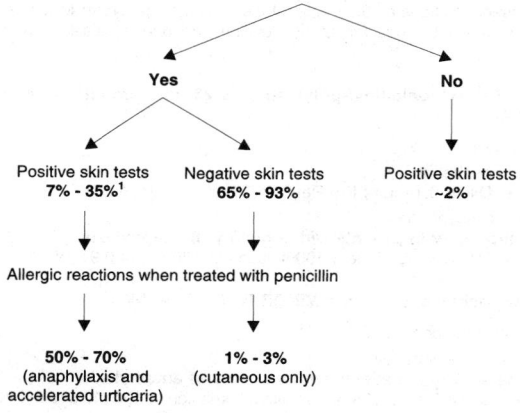

[1] One study found 65% positive.
Prevalence of positive and negative skin tests and subsequent allergic reactions in patients treated with penicilin (based on studies using both penicilloyl-polylysine and minor determinant mixture as skin test reagents).

Penicillin Skin Testing Protocol

Skin tests evaluate the patient for the presence of penicillin IgE – sensitive mast cells which are responsible for anaphylaxis and other immediate hypersensitivity reactions. Local or systemic allergic reactions rarely occur due to skin testing, therefore, a tourniquet, I.V., and epinephrine should be at the bedside. The breakdown products of penicillin provide the antigen which is responsible for the allergy. Testing is performed with benzylpenicilloyl-polylysine (Pre-Pen®), the major determinant, penicillin G which provides the minor determinants and the actual penicillin which will be administered.

Controls are important if the patient is extremely ill or is taking antihistamines, codeine, or morphine. Normal saline is the negative control. Morphine sulfate, a mast cell degranulator, can be used as a positive control, if the patient is not on morphine or codeine. Histamine is the preferred positive control, however, is not manufactured in a pharmaceutical formulation anymore. A false-positive or false-negative will make further skin testing invalid.

Control Solutions

Normal saline = negative control
Morphine sulfate (10 mg/100 mL 0.9% NaCl, 0.1 mg/mL) = positive control

Test Solutions

Order the necessary solutions as 0.5 mL in a tuberculin syringe. **Note:** May need to order 2 syringes of each – one for scratch testing and one for intradermal skin testing.

I. **Pre-Pen®: Benzylpenicilloyl-polylysine (0.25 mL ampul) = MAJOR DETERMINANT**

    A. Undiluted Pre-Pen®
    B. 1:100 concentration
        To make: Dilute 0.1 mL of Pre-Pen® in 10 mL of 0.9% NaCl
    C. 1:10,000 concentration
        (Only necessary in patients with a history of anaphylaxis)
        To make: Dilute 1 mL of the 1:100 solution in 100 mL of 0.9% NaCl

II. **Penicillin G sodium/potassium = MINOR DETERMINANT**

    A. 5000 units/mL concentration
    B. 5 units/mL concentration
        (Only necessary in patients with a history of anaphylaxis)
        To make: Dilute 0.1 mL of a 5000 units/mL solution in 100 mL of 0.9% NaCl

III. **Penicillin product to be administered — if not penicillin G**

    A. **Ampicillin** 2.5 mg/mL concentration

        To make: Dilute 250 mg in 100 mL of 0.9% NaCl
    B. **Nafcillin** 2.5 mg/mL concentration
        To make: Dilute 250 mg in 100 mL of 0.9% NaCl

Order for placement/availability at the bedside in the event of a hypersensitivity reaction during scratch/skin testing and desensitization:

Hydrocortisone: 100 mg IVP
Diphenhydramine: 50 mg IVP
Epinephrine: 1:1000 SubQ

Scratch / Skin Testing Protocol: Must Be Done by Physician!

1. Begin with the control solutions (ie, normal saline and morphine).

2. Administer **scratch tests** in the following order (beginning with the most dilute solution):

Pre-Pen®	Syringes: C,B,A
Penicillin G	Syringes: E,D
Ampicillin/Nafcillin	Syringe: F

The inner volar surface of the forearm is usually used.

A nonbleeding scratch of 3-5 mm in length is made in the epidermis with a 20-gauge needle.

If bleeding occurs, another site should be selected and another scratch made using less pressure.

A small drop of the test solution is then applied and rubbed gently into the scratch using an applicator, toothpick, or the side of the needle.

The scratch test site should be observed for the appearance of a wheal, erythema, and pruritus.

A positive reaction is signified by the appearance within 15 minutes of a pale wheal (usually with pseudopods) ranging from 5-15 mm or more in diameter.

As soon as a positive response is elicited, or 15 minutes has elapsed, the solution should be wiped off the scratch.

If the scratch test is negative or equivocal (ie, a wheal of <5 mm in diameter with little or no erythema or itching appears), an intradermal test may be performed.

If significant reaction, treat and proceed to desensitization.

3. Administer **intradermal tests** in the following order (beginning with the most dilute solution):

Pre-Pen®	Syringes: C,B,A
Penicillin G	Syringes: E,D
Ampicillin/Nafcillin	Syringe: F

Intradermal tests are usually performed on a sterilized area of the upper outer arm at a sufficient distance below the deltoid muscle to permit proximal application of a tourniquet if a severe reaction occurs.

Using a tuberculin syringe with a $3/8$- $5/8$ inch 26- to 30-gauge needle, an amount of each test solution sufficient to raise the smallest perceptible bleb (usually 0.01-0.02 mL) is injected immediately under the surface of the skin.

A separate needle and syringe must be used for each solution.

Each test and control site should be at least 15 cm apart.

Positive reactions are manifested as a wheal at the test site with a diameter at least 5 mm larger than the saline control, often accompanied by itching and a marked increase in the size of the bleb.

Skin responses to penicillin testing will develop within 15 minutes.

If no significant reaction, may challenge patient with reduced dosage of the penicillin to be administered.

Physician should be at the bedside during this challenge dose!

If significant reaction, treat and begin desensitization.

◀

Delayed Hypersensitivity (Anergy)

Delayed cutaneous hypersensitivity (DCH) is a cell-mediated immunological response which has been used diagnostically to assess previous infection (eg, purified protein derivative (PPD) and coccidioidin) or as an indicator of the status of the immune system by using mumps, *Candida*, tetanus toxoid, or trichophyton to test for anergy. Anergy is a defect in cell-mediated immunity that is characterized by an impaired response, or lack of a response to DCH testing with injected antigens. Anergy has been associated with several disease states, malnutrition, and immunosuppressive therapy, and has been correlated with increased risk of infection, morbidity, and mortality.

Many of the skin test antigens have not been approved by the FDA as tests for anergy, and so the directions for use and interpretation of reactions to these products may differ from that of the product labeling. There is also disagreement in the published literature as to the selection and interpretation of these tests for anergy assessment, leading to different recommendations for use of these products.

General Guidelines

Read these guidelines before using any skin test.

Administration

1. Use a separate sterile TB syringe for each antigen. Immediately after the antigen is drawn up, make the injection intradermally in the flexor surface of the forearm.
2. A small bleb 6-10 mm in diameter will form if the injection is made at the correct depth. If a bleb does not form or if the antigen solution leaks from the site, the injection must be repeated.
3. When applying more than one skin test, make the injections at least 5 cm apart.
4. Do any serologic blood tests before testing or wait 48-96 hours.

Reading

1. Read all tests at 24, 48, and 72 hours. Reactions occurring before 24 hours are indicative of an immediate rather than a delayed hypersensitivity.
2. Measure the diameter of the induration in two directions (at right angles) with a ruler and record each diameter in millimeters. Ballpoint pen method of measurement is the most accurate.
3. Test results should be recorded by the nurse in the Physician's Progress Notes section of the chart, and should include the millimeters of induration present, and a picture of the arm showing the location of the test(s).

Factors Causing False-Negative Reactions

1. Improper administration, interpretation, or use of outdated antigen
2. Test is applied too soon after exposure to the antigen (DCH takes 2-20 weeks to develop)
3. Concurrent viral illnesses (eg, rubeola, influenza, mumps, and probably others) or recent administration of live attenuated virus vaccines (eg, measles)
4. Anergy may be associated with:
   a. Immune suppressing chronic illnesses such as diabetes, uremia, sarcoidosis, metastatic carcinomas, Hodgkin's, acute lymphocytic leukemia, hypothyroidism, chronic hepatitis, and cirrhosis.
   b. Some antineoplastic agents, radiation therapy, and corticosteroids. If possible, discontinue steroids at least 48 hours prior to DCH skin testing.
   c. Congenital immune deficiencies.
   d. Malnutrition, shock, severe burns, and trauma.
   e. Severe disseminated infections (miliary or cavitary TB, cocci granuloma, and other disseminated mycotic infections, gram-negative bacillary septicemia).
   f. Leukocytosis (>15,000 cells/mm^3).

Factors Causing False-Positive Reactions

1. Improper interpretation
2. Patient sensitivity to minor ingredients in the antigen solutions such as the phenol or thimerosal preservatives
3. Cross-reactions between similar antigens

Candida 1:1000
Dose = 0.1 mL intradermally (30% of children <18 months of age and 50% >18 months of age respond)
Can be used as a control antigen

Coccidioidin 1:1000
Dose = 0.1 mL intradermally (apply with PPD **and** a control antigen)
Mercury derivative used as a preservative for Spherulin®.

Multitest CMI (Candida, diphtheria toxoid, tetanus toxoid, Streptococcus, old tuberculin, Trichophyton, Proteus antigen, and negative control)
Press loaded unit into the skin with sufficient pressure to puncture the skin and allow adequate penetration of all points.

Mumps 40 cfu/mL
Dose = 0.1 mL intradermally (contraindicated in patients allergic to eggs, egg products, or thimerosal)

Dosage as Part of Disease Diagnosis

Tuberculin Testing
Purified Protein Derivative (PPD)

Preparation	Dilution	Units/0.1 mL
First strength	1:10,000	1
Intermediate strength	1:2000	5
Second strength	1:100	250

The usual initial dose is 0.1 mL of the intermediate strength. The first strength should be used in the individuals suspected of being highly sensitive. The second strength is used only for individuals who fail to respond to a previous injection of the first or intermediate strengths.

A positive reaction is ≥10 mm induration except in HIV-infected individuals where a positive reaction is ≥5 mm of induration.

Adverse Reactions

In patients who are highly sensitive, or when higher than recommended doses are used, exaggerated local reactions may occur, including erythema, pain, blisters, necrosis, and scarring. Although systemic reactions are rare, a few cases of lymph node enlargement, fever, malaise, and fatigue have been reported.

To prevent severe local reactions, never use second test strengths as the initial agent. Use diluted first strengths in patients with known or suspected hypersensitivity to the antigen.

Have epinephrine and antihistamines on hand to treat severe allergic reactions that may occur.

Treatment of Adverse Reactions

Severe reactions to intradermal skin tests are rare and treatment consists of symptomatic care.

◀ **Skin Testing**

All skin tests are given intradermally into the flexor surface of one arm.

Purified protein derivative (PPD) is used most often in the diagnosis of tuberculosis. *Candida*, *Trichophyton*, and mumps skin tests are used most often as controls for anergy.

Dose: The usual skin test dose is as follows:

Antigen		Standard Dose	Concentration
PPD	1 TU	0.1 mL	1 TU − highly sensitive patients
	5 TU	0.1 mL	5 TU − standard dose
	250 TU	0.1 mL	250 TU − anergic patients in whom TB is suspected
Candida		0.02 mL	
Mumps		0.1 mL	
Trichophyton		0.02 mL	

Interpretation:

Skin Test	Reading Time	Positive Reaction
PPD	48-72 h	**≥5 mm considered positive for:** • close contacts to an infectious case • persons with abnormal chest x-ray indicating old healed TB • persons with known or suspected HIV infection **≥10 mm considered positive for:** • other medical risk factors • foreign born from high prevalence areas • medically underserved, low income populations • alcoholics and intravenous drug users • residents of long-term care facilities (including correctional facilities and nursing homes) • staff in settings where disease would pose a hazard to large number of susceptible persons **≥15 mm considered positive for:** • persons without risk factors for TB
Candida	24-72 h	≥5 mm induration
Mumps	24-36 h	≥5 mm
Trichophyton	24-72 h	≥5 mm induration

Recommended Interpretation of Skin Test Reactions

Reaction	Local Reaction	
	After Intradermal Injections of Antigens	After Dinitrochlorobenzene
1+	Erythema >10 mm and/or induration >1-5 mm	Erythema and/or induration covering <½ area of dose site
2+	Induration 6-10 mm	Induration covering >½ area of dose site
3+	Induration 11-20 mm	Vesiculation and induration at dose site or spontaneous flare at days 7-14 at the site
4+	Induration >20 mm	Bulla or ulceration at dose site or spontaneous flare at days 7-14 at the site

COMMONLY USED HERBAL MEDICINES

The use of herbal medicines by the general population continues to increase. In 1988, retail sales of herbal products was approximately $200 million with this number increasing to $5.1 billion in 1997. If the current trend in herbal medicine use continues, annual sales of $25 billion are expected by the year 2010. A survey of surgical patients performed in 1999 revealed that 17.4% reported taking herbals or nutrachemicals. In this survey, the most common herbs taken were gingko (32.4%), garlic (26.5%), ginger (26.5%), ginseng (14%), and St John's wort (14%). A major problem with herbal medicine use is that patients frequently do not report this use to their healthcare providers. This results in the potential for adverse interactions between the patient's prescription medications and herbal products. Further, the use of herbal medicine may cause problems not anticipated by the healthcare provider (eg, increased bleeding potential) if its use is not communicated. Hence, it is critical that all healthcare providers question patients about herbal use as part of their routine medication history. One may also want to consider having the patient stop taking select herbal medicines up to 2 weeks prior to surgery, if possible, secondary to their potential effects on coagulation (eg, feverfew, garlic, ginger, ginkgo, horse chestnut seed, kava-kava). Although there are hundreds of herbal products available on the market, a relatively small number (10-20) account for the majority of sales. The table that follows lists some of the most commonly used herbal medicines, their traditional uses, and cautions and contraindications with regard to their use. Keep in mind that there are few well-designed studies assessing these products, as they are considered dietary supplements, and as such, are not held to the rigid FDA testing standards for drugs.

Herb	Use(s)	Cautions and Contraindications
Cat's claw *(Unacaria tomentosa)*	– Treatment of allergies, arthritis – Adjunct therapy for AIDS – Adjunct agent for cancer therapy – Immune stimulant – Postradiation therapy – Antiparasitic	– Should not be taken when pregnant, nursing, or by transplant recipients – May see diarrhea or changes in bowel movement – Use with caution in conjunction with anticoagulants (may increase risk of bleeding due to platelet activating factor inhibition) – Use with caution with NSAIDs (may increase risk of GI bleeding)
Cayenne *(Capsicum annuum)*	– **External:** Muscle spasm or soreness, shingles, diabetic neuropathy, cluster headache, osteoarthritis, rheumatoid arthritis – **Internal:** GI tract disorders	– **External:** Potential for skin ulceration and blistering with >2 days' use – **Internal:** Overdose may cause severe hypothermia
Echinacea *(Echinacea purpurea)*	– Prevention and treatment of colds and flu, allergies, infections, tonsillitis, sore throat – Chronic skin complaints	– Should not be administered with immunosuppressants – People with chronic suppressed immunity should not take for extended periods of time (>10-14 days)

Herb	Use(s)	Cautions and Contraindications
Ephedra *(Ephedra sinica)*	– Over-the-counter diet aids – Antitussive – Enhance athletic performance (CNS stimulant)	– Active constituent is ephedrine – Intraoperative hemodymanic instability – Palpitations and increased blood pressure can be seen with its use – Potential for increased blood pressure when combined with caffeine-containing botanicals (eg, Metabolife™, Formula One™) – Enhanced sympathomimetic effects with guanethedine and MAOIs – Hypertension when given with oxytocin – Arrhythmias with halothane or cardiac glycosides – Higher doses produce euphoria – Misuse has resulted in death
Evening primrose oil *(Oenothera biennis)*	– Reduce cholesterol – Allergic/inflammatory conditions – Treatment of PMS	– Reduces platelet aggregation (monitor bleeding times and PT in patients on antiplatelet drugs, warfarin, or other anticoagulant drugs)
Feverfew *(Tanacetum parthenium)*	– Treatment of arthritis – Migraine prophylaxis/treatment – Antipyretic	– Can inhibit platelet activity and increase bleeding; avoid use in patients on warfarin or other anticoagulants or antiplatelet drugs – Rebound headache with sudden cessation – Avoid in pregnant women (uterine stimulant) – Users may develop aphthous ulcers or GI tract irritation (5% to 15%) – Use with caution when administering with drugs that increase serotonin (eg, fluoxetine, sumatriptan) secondary to increased risk of serotonin syndrome
Garlic *(Allium sativum)*	– Lower cholesterol and blood pressure – Has antiplatelet, antioxidant, and antithrombotic qualities – Prevent infections	– Reduces platelet aggregation and increases fibrinolytic activity; monitor bleeding times and PT in patients on antiplatelet drugs and warfarin – Monitor blood glucose (decreased blood glucose secondary to increased serum insulin levels) – May potentiate antihypertensives – Vasodilator properties
Ginger *(Zingiber officinale)*	– Antinauseant – Antispasmodic	– Potent inhibitor of thromboxane synthetase; may increase bleeding time – May interact with anticoagulant and antiplatelet drugs to increase risk of bleeding – May alter effects of calcium channel blockers (ginger increases calcium uptake by the heart)

Herb	Use(s)	Cautions and Contraindications
Ginkgo *(Ginkgo biloba)*	– Treatment of dementia associated with Alzheimer's disease or other conditions associated with cerebral vascular insufficiency – Treatment of vertigo, headache, tinnitus, depression, peripheral vascular disease, Raynaud's disease	– Ginkgolides inhibit platelet activating factor and antagonize thrombus formation; may enhance bleeding in patients on anticoagulant or antithrombotic therapy
Ginseng *(Panax schinseng)*	– Enhance mental and physical performance – Increase energy, decrease stress – Improve immune function – Adaptogen – Antioxidant	– Use caution in patients on digoxin therapy – Hypoglycemic effect – Ginsenosides inhibit platelet aggregation and enhance fibrinolysis; may interact with warfarin or antiplatelet drugs to increase risk of bleeding – Should not be used in pregnancy or acute infection – May potentiate action of MAOIs
Goldenseal *(Hydrastis canadensis)*	– Diuretic – Hemostatic – Anti-inflammatory – Laxative	– High doses may induce paralysis – Should not be taken during pregnancy or while nursing – Functions as an aquaretic – Functions as an oxytocic
Grape seed extract *(Vitis vinifera)*	– Treatment of allergies, asthma – Improve peripheral circulation – Decrease platelet aggregation, capillary fragility – Improve general circulation – Antioxidant	– Monitor bleeding times and PT in patients on antiplatelet drugs and warfarin
Green tea leaf *(Camellia sinensis)*	– Antioxidant/free radical scavenger – Preventative for cancer and cardiovascular disease – Preventative for atherosclerosis and hypertension – Antibacterial – Lower cholesterol – Platelet inhibition actions	– Use with caution in patients on anticoagulant therapy
Hawthorn *(Crataegus oxyacantha)*	– Treatment for angina, arrhythmias, tachycardia, hypo-/hypertension, irregular heartbeat, peripheral vascular disorders, vascular spasms – Lower cholesterol	– May potentiate digoxin and ACE inhibitors
Horse chestnut seed *(Aesculus hippocastanum)*	– Treatment of varicose veins, hemorrhoids, venous insufficiencies	– Contains coumarin and aescin constituents; use with caution in patients on anticoagulant or antiplatelet therapy (can cause severe bleeding or bruising)

Herb	Use(s)	Cautions and Contraindications
Kava-kava *(Piper methysticum)*	– Anxiolytic – Analgesic – Antidepressant – Insomnia	– Kava lactones (active constituents of kava-kava) potentiate the effects of other CNS depressants such as barbiturates, benzodiazepines, opioids, and anesthetics – Can potentiate ethanol effects – Avoid in endogenous depression – May worsen symptoms of Parkinson's disease (kava-kava antagonizes dopamine)
Licorice root *(Glycyrrhiza glabra)*	– Gastric and duodenal ulcers – Adrenal insufficiency – Expectorant and antitussive	– Contraindicated in many chronic liver conditions, severe kidney insufficiency, hypertension, cardiac disease, hypokalemia – Contraindicated in pregnancy and diabetes – Glycyrrhizic acid in licorice may cause high blood pressure, hypokalemia, and edema
Passionflower vine *(Passiflora incarnata)*	– Sedative and hypnotic – In combination with valerian to produce restful sleep	– May potentiate sedative actions of pharmaceuticals – Use with caution in patients on MAOI therapy – Use with caution with consumption of alcohol
Saw palmetto *(Serenoa repens)*	– Benign prostatic hypertrophy	– Antiestrogen effect (avoid during pregnancy and in patients with breast cancer) – Can cause hypertension and GI disturbances
St John's wort *(Hypericum perforatum)*	– **External:** Herpes simplex 1, minor – **Internal:** Treatment for depression, nervousness, anxiety	– May prolong effects of anesthesia – Photosensitivity in large doses in light-skinned people – Serotonin syndrome that is reversed by decreasing dose – May be prudent to avoid SSRIs, MAOIs, and meperidine – Increases metabolism of many perioperative drugs
Turmeric *(Curcuma longa)*	– Antioxidant – Anti-inflammatory – Antirheumatic – Lower blood lipid levels	– Use with caution if currently taking anticoagulant medications – Use with caution if peptic ulceration is present – Do not use if biliary obstruction is present
Valerian *(Valeriana officinalis)*	– Mild sedative and anxiolytic	– May potentiate the effects of CNS depressants (eg, barbiturates, anesthetics) and anxiolytics – May decrease symptoms of benzodiazepine withdrawal – Many extracts contain alcohol; potential to interact with disulfiram

References

American Society of Anesthesiologists, "Considerations for Anesthesiologists: What You Should Know About Your Patients' Use of Herbal Medicines," 1999 (brochure).

Ang-Lee MK, Moss J, and Yuan CS, "Herbal Medicines and Perioperative Care," *JAMA*, 2001, 286 (2):208-16.

Blumenthal M, *The Complete German Commission E Monographs. Therapeutic Guide to Herbal Medicines*, Austin, Texas: American Botanical Council, 1998.

DerMarderosian A, *The Review of Natural Products*, St Louis, MO: Facts and Comparisons, 1999.

Eisenberg DM, Davis RB, Ettner SL, et al, "Trends in Alternative Medicine Use in the United States, 1990-1997: Results of a Follow-up National Survey," *JAMA*, 1998, 280(18):1569-75.

Klepser TB and Klepser ME, "Unsafe and Potentially Safe Herbal Therapies," *Am J Health Syst Pharm*, 1999, 56(2):125-38.

LaValle JB, "Phytotherapy: A Guide to the Safe and Effective Use of Medicinal Herbs," *Pharmacy Practice News*, 1999, 26(11):57-61.

Mahady GB, "Herbal Medicine and Pharmacy Education," *J Amer Pharm Assoc*, 1998, 38:274.

McDermott JH, "Herbal Chart for Healthcare Professionals," *Pharmacy Today*, 1999, 5(8) (centerfold poster).

McLeskey CH, Meyer TA, Baisden CE, et al, "The Incidence of Herbal and Selected Nutrachemical Use in Surgical Patients," *Anesthesiology*, 1999, 91:A1168.

Miller LG, "Herbal Medicinals: Selected Clinical Considerations Focusing on Known or Potential Drug-Herb Interactions," *Arch Intern Med*, 1998, 158(20):2200-11.

Murphy JM, "Preoperative Considerations With Herbal Medicines," *AORN J*, 1999, 69(1):173-5, 177-8, 180-3.

Murray M, *The Healing Power of Herbs: The Enlightened Person's Guide to the Wonders of Medicinal Plants*, Rocklin, CA: Prima Publishing, 1995.

Newall CA, Anderson LA, and Phillipson JD, *Herbal Medicines: A Guide for Health Care Professionals*, London, England: The Pharmaceutical Press, 1996.

Schulz V, Hansel R, and Tyler VE, *Rational Phytotherapy, A Physician's Guide to Herbal Medicine*, New York, NY: Springer, 1998.

Zaglaniczny KL, "An Introduction to Herbal Medicine and Anesthetic Considerations," *Nurse Anesthetist, Forum*, 1999, 2(3):4-5,11.

PREVENTION OF INFECTIVE ENDOCARDITIS

Recommendations by the American Heart Association
(*Circulation*, 2007, 116(15):1736-54.)

Consensus Process – The recommendations were formulated by a writing group under the auspices of the American Heart Association (AHA), and included representation from the Infectious Diseases Society of America (IDSA), the American Academy of Pediatrics (AAP), and the American Dental Association (ADA). Additionally, input was received from both national and international experts on infective endocarditis (IE). These guidelines are based on expert interpretation and review of scientific literature from 1950 through 2006. The consensus statement was subsequently reviewed by outside experts not affiliated with the writing group and by the Science Advisory and Coordinating Committee of the American Heart Association. These guidelines are meant to aid practitioners but are not intended as the standard of care or as a substitute for clinical judgment.

Significant change from the previous 1997 guidelines – The previously published guidelines identified a broad range of cardiac conditions thought to predispose patients to a higher risk of IE. The document stratified these conditions into high-, moderate-, and low-risk categories, based on the likelihood of developing IE. The subsequent recommendations for prophylaxis were based on this classification, in conjunction with specification of numerous invasive procedures which were assumed to confer a higher risk of bacteremia, and therefore a higher risk of endocarditis. However, it is the consensus of the current writing group that existing data fail to show a clear link between many of these procedures, preexisting cardiovascular condition and IE. In the case of dental procedures, it was determined that the cumulative lifetime risk of developing bacteremia as a result of normal hygiene measures (eg, teeth brushing, flossing) vastly exceeded the risk associated with many of the procedures for which prophylaxis was previously recommended. Similarly, the writing group estimated that the absolute risk of developing IE as a result of dental procedures in patients with preexisting cardiac conditions was quite low, and there was little evidence to support the value of prophylactic antimicrobial efficacy in these cases.

In a major departure from the former recommendations, the current guidelines have been greatly simplified to place a much greater emphasis on a very limited number of underlying cardiac conditions (see below). These specific conditions have been associated with the highest risk of adverse outcomes due to IE. Patients should receive IE prophylaxis only if they are undergoing certain invasive procedures (see Table 1) and have one of the underlying cardiovascular conditions specified below.

Common situations for which routine prophylaxis was previously, but no longer recommended, include mitral valve prolapse, general dental cleanings and local anesthetic administration (noninfected tissue), and bronchoscopy (see Table 1).

Specific cardiac conditions for which IE antibiotic prophylaxis is recommended:

- Previous infective endocarditis
- Prosthetic cardiac valve or prosthetic material used for cardiac valve repair
- Cardiac transplantation patients who develop valvulopathy
- Congenital heart disease (CHD), only under the following conditions:
    - Unrepaired cyanotic CHD, including palliative shunts and conduits
    - Completely repaired defects (with prosthetic materials/devices), regardless of method of repair, within the first 6 months after the procedure
    - Repaired CHD with residual defects at or adjacent to the site of repair

Table 1. Guidance for Use of Prophylactic Antibiotic Therapy Based on Procedure or Condition[1]

Location of Procedure	Prophylaxis Recommended	Prophylaxis NOT Recommended
Dental	All invasive manipulations of the gingival or periapical region or perforation of oral mucosa	Anesthetic injections (through noninfected tissue), radiographs, placement/adjustment/removal prosthodontic/orthodontic appliances or brackets, shedding of deciduous teeth, trauma-induced bleeding from lips, gums, or oral mucosa
Respiratory tract	Biopsy/incision of respiratory mucosa (eg, tonsillectomy/adenoidectomy); drainage of abscess or empyema[2]	Bronchoscopy (unless incision of mucosa required)
Gastrointestinal (GI) or genitourinary (GU) tract	Established GI/GU infection or prevention of infectious sequelae[3]; elective cystoscopy or other urinary tract procedure with established enterococci infection/colonization[3,4]	Routine diagnostic procedures, including esophagogastroduodenoscopy or colonoscopy in the absence of active infection; vaginal delivery and hysterectomy
Skin, skin structure, or musculoskeletal	Any surgical procedure involving infected tissue	Procedures conducted in noninfected tissue; tattoos and ear/body piercing

[1]Patients should receive prophylactic antibiotic therapy if they meet the criteria for a specified procedure/condition in this table and they have a high-risk cardiovascular condition listed in the preceding text.

[2]If treating an infection of known staphylococcal origin, consider antistaphylococcal penicillin or cephalosporin, or vancomycin in beta-lactam-sensitive patients.

[3]Alternative agents with activity against enterococci to consider: Vancomycin (for beta-lactam-sensitive patients) or piperacillin.

[4]Eradication of enterococci from the urinary tract should be considered.

◀ **Table 2. Prophylactic Regimens for Oral / Dental, Respiratory Tract, Genitoruinary Tract, or Esophageal Procedures**

Situation	Agent	Regimen to Be Given 30-60 Minutes Before Procedure	
		Adults	Children[1]
Standard general prophylaxis	Amoxicillin	2 g P.O.	50 mg/kg P.O.
Unable to take oral medications	Ampicillin **or**	2 g I.M./I.V.	50 mg/kg I.M./I.V.
	Cefazolin or ceftriaxone	1 g I.M./I.V.	50 mg/kg I.M./I.V.
Allergic to penicillin	Clindamycin **or**	600 mg P.O.	20 mg/kg P.O.
	Cephalexin[2] or other dose-equivalent first/second generation cephalosporin **or**	2 g P.O	50 mg/kg P.O.
	Azithromycin or clarithromycin	500 mg P.O.	15 mg/kg P.O.
Allergic to penicillin and unable to take oral medications	Clindamycin **or**	600 mg I.V.	20 mg/kg I.V.
	Cefazolin or ceftriaxone[2]	1 g I.M./I.V.	50 mg/kg I.M./I.V.

[1]Total children's dose should not exceed adult dose.

[2]Cephalosporins should not be used in individuals with immediate-type hypersensitivity reaction (urticaria, angioedema, or anaphylaxis) to penicillins.

Reference

Wilson W, Taubert KA, Gewitz M, et al, "Prevention of Infective Endocarditis. Guidelines From the American Heart Association. A Guideline From the American Heart Association Rheumatic Fever, Endocarditis, and Kawasaki Disease Committee, Council on Cardiovascular Disease in the Young, and the Council on Clinical Cardiology, Council on Cardiovascular Surgery and Anesthesia, and the Quality of Care and Outcomes Research Interdisciplinary Working Group," *Circulation*, 2007, 116 (15):1736-54.

PREVENTION OF WOUND INFECTION AND SEPSIS IN SURGICAL PATIENTS

Nature of Operation	Likely Pathogens	Recommended Drugs	Adult Dosage Before Surgery[1]
Cardiac	S. aureus, S. epidermidis	Cefazolin or cefuroxime or vancomycin[3]	1-2 g I.V.[2] 1.5 g I.V.[2] 1 g I.V.
Gastrointestinal			
Esophageal, gastroduodenal	Enteric gram-negative bacilli, gram-positive cocci	High risk[4] only: Cefazolin[5]	1-2 g I.V.
Biliary tract	Enteric gram-negative bacilli, enterococci, clostridia	High risk[6] only: Cefazolin[5]	1-2 g I.V.
Colorectal	Enteric gram-negative bacilli, anaerobes, enterococci	Oral: Neomycin + erythromycin base[7] or neomycin + metronidazole[7]	1 g of each x 3 doses 2 g of each x 2 doses
		Parenteral:	
		Cefoxitin[5] or cefazolin[5] + metronidazole[5]	1-2 g I.V. 1-2 g I.V. 0.5-1 g I.V.
Appendectomy, nonperforated	Enteric gram-negative bacilli, anaerobes, enterococci	Cefoxitin[5] or cefazolin[5] + metronidazole or ampicillin/ sulbactam	1-2 g I.V. 1-2 g I.V. 0.5 g I.V. 3 g I.V.
Ruptured viscus	Enteric gram-negative bacilli, anaerobes, enterococci	Cefoxitin ± gentamicin[5,8]	1-2 g I.V. q6h 1.5 mg/kg I.V. q8h
Genitourinary	Enteric gram-negative bacilli, enterococci	High risk[9] only: Ciprofloxacin	500 mg P.O. or 400 mg I.V.
Gynecologic and Obstetric			
Vaginal, abdominal, or laparoscopic hysterectomy	Enteric gram-negative bacilli, anaerobes, group B streptococci, enterococci	Cefoxitin[5] or cefazolin[5] or ampicillin/ sulbactam[5]	1-2 g I.V. 1-2 g I.V. 3 g I.V.
Cesarean section	Same as for hysterectomy	Cefazolin[5]	1-2 g I.V. after cord clamping
Abortion	Same as for hysterectomy	First trimester, high-risk[10]:	
		Aqueous penicillin G or doxycycline	2 mill units I.V. or 300 mg P.O.[11]
		Second trimester:	
		Cefazolin[5]	1-2 g I.V.
Head and Neck			
Incisions through oral or pharyngeal mucosa	Anaerobes, enteric gram-negative bacilli, S. aureus	Clindamycin + gentamicin or cefazolin	600-900 mg I.V. 1.5 mg/kg I.V. 1-2 g I.V.
Neurosurgery	S. aureus, S. epidermidis	Cefazolin or vancomycin[3]	1-2 g I.V. 1 g I.V.

PREVENTION OF WOUND INFECTION AND SEPSIS IN SURGICAL PATIENTS

Nature of Operation	Likely Pathogens	Recommended Drugs	Adult Dosage Before Surgery[1]
Ophthalmic	S. epidermidis, S. aureus, streptococci, enteric gram-negative bacilli, Pseudomonas	Gentamicin, tobramycin, ciprofloxacin, levofloxacin, moxifloxacin, ofloxacin, or neomycin- gramicidin- polymyxin B	Multiple drops topically over 2-24 hours
		Cefazolin	100 mg subconjunctivally
Orthopedic	S. aureus, S. epidermidis	Cefazolin[12] or cefuroxime[12] or vancomycin[3,12]	1-2 g I.V. 1.5 g I.V. 1 g I.V.
Thoracic (Noncardiac)	S. aureus, S. epidermidis, streptococci, enteric gram-negative bacilli	Cefazolin or cefuroxime or vancomycin[3]	1-2 g I.V. 1.5 g I.V. 1 g I.V.
Vascular			
Arterial surgery involving a prosthesis, the abdominal aorta, or a groin incision	S. aureus, S. epidermidis, enteric gram-negative bacilli	Cefazolin or vancomycin[3]	1-2 g I.V. 1 g I.V.
Lower extremity amputation for ischemia	S. aureus, S. epidermidis, enteric gram-negative bacilli, clostridia	Cefazolin or vancomycin[3]	1-2 g I.V. 1 g I.V.

[1]Parenteral prophylactic antimicrobials can be given as a single I.V. dose begun 60 minutes or less before the operation. For prolonged operations, additional intraoperative doses should be given at intervals 1-2 times the half-life of the drug for the duration of the procedure. If vancomycin or a fluoroquinolone is used, the infusion should be started 60-120 minutes before incision in order to minimize the possibility of an infusion reaction close to the time of induction of anesthesia and to have adequate tissue levels at the time of incision.

[2]Some consultants recommend an additional dose when patients are removed from bypass during open-heart surgery.

[3]For hospitals in which methicillin-resistant S. aureus and S. epidermidis are a frequent cause of postoperative wound infection, for patients previously colonized with MRSA, or for patients allergic to penicillins or cephalosporin. Rapid I.V. administration may cause hypotension, which could be especially dangerous during induction of anesthesia. Even if the drug is given over 60 minutes, hypotension may occur; treatment with diphenhydramine (Benadryl® and others) and further slowing of the infusion rate may be helpful. For procedures in which enteric gram-negative bacilli are likely pathogens, such as vascular surgery involving a groin incision, cefazolin or cefuroxime should be included in the prophylaxis regimen for patients not allergic to cephalosporins; ciprofloxacin, levofloxacin (750 mg), gentamicin, or aztreonam, each one in combination with vancomycin, can be used in patients who cannot tolerate a cephalosporin.

[4]Morbid obesity, esophageal obstruction, decreased gastric acidity, or gastrointestinal motility.

[5]For patients allergic to cephalosporins, clindamycin with either gentamicin, ciprofloxacin, levofloxacin (750 mg), or aztreonam is a reasonable alternative.

[6]Age >70 years, acute cholecystitis, nonfunctioning gallbladder, obstructive jaundice, or common duct stones.

[7]After appropriate diet and catharsis, 1 g of neomycin plus 1 g of erythromycin at 1 PM, 2 PM, and 11 PM the day before an 8 AM operation or 2 g of neomycin plus 2 g of metronidazole at 7 PM and 11 PM the day before an 8 AM operation.

[8]Therapy is often continued for about 5 days. Ruptured viscus in postoperative setting (dehiscence) requires antibacterials to include coverage of nosocomial pathogens.

[9]Urine culture positive or unavailable, preoperative catheter, transrectal prostatic biopsy, placement of prosthetic material.

[10]Patients with previous pelvic inflammatory disease, previous gonorrhea, or multiple sex partners.

[11]Divided into 100 mg 1 hour before the abortion and 200 mg 30 minutes after.

[12]If a tourniquet is to be used in the procedure, the entire dose of antibiotic must be infused prior to its inflation.

References

Adapted with permission from "Antimicrobial Prophylaxis for Surgery," *Treatment Guidelines From The Medical Letter®*, 2006, 4(52):83-8.

Bratzler DW, Houck PM, Surgical Infection Prevention Guidelines Writers Workgroup, et al, "Antimicrobial Prophylaxis for Surgery: An Advisory Statement From the National Surgical Infection Prevention Project," *Clin Infect Dis*, 2004, 38(12):1706-15.

REFERENCE VALUES FOR ADULTS

CHEMISTRY

Test	Values	Remarks
Serum / Plasma		
Acetone	Negative	
Albumin	3.2-5 g/dL	
Alcohol, ethyl	Negative	
Aldolase	1.2-7.6 IU/L	
Ammonia	20-70 mcg/dL	Specimen to be placed on ice as soon as collected.
Amylase	30-110 units/L	
Bilirubin, direct	0-0.3 mg/dL	
Bilirubin, total	0.1-1.2 mg/dL	
Calcium	8.6-10.3 mg/dL	
Calcium, ionized	2.24-2.46 mEq/L	
Chloride	95-108 mEq/L	
Cholesterol, total	≤200 mg/dL	Fasted blood required – normal value affected by dietary habits. This reference range is for a general adult population.
HDL cholesterol	40-60 mg/dL	Fasted blood required – normal value affected by dietary habits.
LDL cholesterol	<160 mg/dL	If triglyceride is >400 mg/dL, LDL cannot be calculated accurately (Friedewald equation). Target LDL-C depends on patient's risk factors.
CO_2	23-30 mEq/L	
Creatine kinase (CK) isoenzymes		
CK-BB	0%	
CK-MB (cardiac)	0%-3.9%	
CK-MM (muscle)	96%-100%	

CK-MB levels must be both ≥4% and 10 IU/L to meet diagnostic criteria for CK-MB positive result consistent with myocardial injury.

Test	Values	Remarks
Creatine phosphokinase (CPK)	8-150 IU/L	
Creatinine	0.5-1.4 mg/dL	
Ferritin	13-300 ng/mL	
Folate	3.6-20 ng/dL	
GGT (gamma-glutamyltranspeptidase)		
male	11-63 IU/L	
female	8-35 IU/L	
GLDH	To be determined	
Glucose (preprandial)	<115 mg/dL	Goals different for diabetics.
Glucose, fasting	60-110 mg/dL	Goals different for diabetics.
Glucose, nonfasting (2-h postprandial)	<120 mg/dL	Goals different for diabetics.

CHEMISTRY *(continued)*

Test	Values	Remarks
Hemoglobin A_{1c}	<8	
Hemoglobin, plasma free	<2.5 mg/100 mL	
Hemoglobin, total glycosolated (Hb A_1)	4%-8%	
Iron	65-150 mcg/dL	
Iron binding capacity, total (TIBC)	250-420 mcg/dL	
Lactic acid	0.7-2.1 mEq/L	Specimen to be kept on ice and sent to lab as soon as possible.
Lactate dehydrogenase (LDH)	56-194 IU/L	
Lactate dehydrogenase (LDH) isoenzymes		
LD_1	20%-34%	
LD_2	29%-41%	
LD_3	15%-25%	
LD_4	1%-12%	
LD_5	1%-15%	

Flipped LD_1/LD_2 ratios (>1 may be consistent with myocardial injury) particularly when considered in combination with a recent CK-MB positive result.

Test	Values	Remarks
Lipase	23-208 units/L	
Magnesium	1.6-2.5 mg/dL	Increased by slight hemolysis.
Osmolality	289-308 mOsm/kg	
Phosphatase, alkaline		
adults 25-60 y	33-131 IU/L	
adults ≥61 y	51-153 IU/L	
infancy-adolescence	Values range up to 3-5 times higher than adults	
Phosphate, inorganic	2.8-4.2 mg/dL	
Potassium	3.5-5.2 mEq/L	Increased by slight hemolysis.
Prealbumin	>15 mg/dL	
Protein, total	6.5-7.9 g/dL	
AST	<35 IU/L (20-48)	
ALT (10-35)	<35 IU/L	
Sodium	134-149 mEq/L	
Thyroid stimulating hormone (TSH)		
adults ≤20 y	0.7-6.4 mIU/L	
21-54 y	0.4-4.2 mIU/L	
55-87 y	0.5-8.9 mIU/L	
Transferrin	>200 mg/dL	
Triglycerides	45-155 mg/dL	Fasted blood required.
Troponin I	<1.5 ng/mL	
Urea nitrogen (BUN)	7-20 mg/dL	
Uric acid		
male	2-8 mg/dL	
female	2-7.5 mg/dL	

CHEMISTRY *(continued)*

Test	Values	Remarks
Cerebrospinal Fluid		
Glucose	50-70 mg/dL	
Protein	15-45 mg/dL	CSF obtained by lumbar puncture.

Note: Bloody specimen gives erroneously high value due to contamination with blood proteins

Urine
(24-hour specimen is required for all these tests unless specified)

Test	Values	Remarks
Amylase	32-641 units/L	The value is in units/L and **not** calculated for total volume.
Amylase, fluid (random samples)		Interpretation of value left for physician, depends on the nature of fluid.
Calcium	Depends upon dietary intake	
Creatine		
male	150 mg/24 h	Higher value on children and during pregnancy.
female	250 mg/24 h	
Creatinine	1000-2000 mg/24 h	
Creatinine clearance (endogenous)		
male	85-125 mL/min	A blood sample must accompany urine specimen.
female	75-115 mL/min	
Glucose	1 g/24 h	
5-hydroxyindoleacetic acid	2-8 mg/24 h	
Iron	0.15 mg/24 h	Acid washed container required.
Magnesium	146-209 mg/24 h	
Osmolality	500-800 mOsm/kg	With normal fluid intake.
Oxalate	10-40 mg/24 h	
Phosphate	400-1300 mg/24 h	
Potassium	25-120 mEq/24 h	Varies with diet; the interpretation of urine electrolytes and osmolality should be left for the physician.
Sodium	40-220 mEq/24 h	
Porphobilinogen, qualitative	Negative	
Porphyrins, qualitative	Negative	
Proteins	0.05-0.1 g/24 h	
Salicylate	Negative	
Urea clearance	60-95 mL/min	A blood sample must accompany specimen.
Urea N	10-40 g/24 h	Dependent on protein intake.
Uric acid	250-750 mg/24 h	Dependent on diet and therapy.
Urobilinogen	0.5-3.5 mg/24 h	For qualitative determination on random urine, send sample to urinalysis section in Hematology Lab.
Xylose absorption test		
children	16%-33% of ingested xylose	

◀ **CHEMISTRY** (continued)

Test	Values	Remarks
Feces		
Fat, 3-day collection	<5 g/d	Value depends on fat intake of 100 g/d for 3 days preceding and during collection.
Gastric Acidity		
Acidity, total, 12 h	10-60 mEq/L	Titrated at pH 7.

Blood Gases

	Arterial	Capillary	Venous
pH	7.35-7.45	7.35-7.45	7.32-7.42
pCO_2 (mm Hg)	35-45	35-45	38-52
pO_2 (mm Hg)	70-100	60-80	24-48
HCO_3 (mEq/L)	19-25	19-25	19-25
TCO_2 (mEq/L)	19-29	19-29	23-33
O_2 saturation (%)	90-95	90-95	40-70
Base excess (mEq/L)	-5 to +5	-5 to +5	-5 to +5

HEMATOLOGY

Complete Blood Count

Age	Hgb (g/dL)	Hct (%)	RBC (mill/mm^3)	RDW
0-3 d	15.0-20.0	45-61	4.0-5.9	<18
1-2 wk	12.5-18.5	39-57	3.6-5.5	<17
1-6 mo	10.0-13.0	29-42	3.1-4.3	<16.5
7 mo to 2 y	10.5-13.0	33-38	3.7-4.9	<16
2-5 y	11.5-13.0	34-39	3.9-5.0	<15
5-8 y	11.5-14.5	35-42	4.0-4.9	<15
13-18 y	12.0-15.2	36-47	4.5-5.1	<14.5
Adult male	13.5-16.5	41-50	4.5-5.5	<14.5
Adult female	12.0-15.0	36-44	4.0-4.9	<14.5

Age	MCV (fL)	MCH (pg)	MCHC (%)	Plts (x 10^3/mm^3)
0-3 d	95-115	31-37	29-37	250-450
1-2 wk	86-110	28-36	28-38	250-450
1-6 mo	74-96	25-35	30-36	300-700
7 mo to 2 y	70-84	23-30	31-37	250-600
2-5 y	75-87	24-30	31-37	250-550
5-8 y	77-95	25-33	31-37	250-550
13-18 y	78-96	25-35	31-37	150-450
Adult male	80-100	26-34	31-37	150-450
Adult female	80-100	26-34	31-37	150-450

WBC and Differential

Age	WBC (x 10^3/mm^3)	Segs	Bands	Lymphs	Monos
0-3 d	9.0-35.0	32-62	10-18	19-29	5-7
1-2 wk	5.0-20.0	14-34	6-14	36-45	6-10
1-6 mo	6.0-17.5	13-33	4-12	41-71	4-7
7 mo to 2 y	6.0-17.0	15-35	5-11	45-76	3-6
2-5 y	5.5-15.5	23-45	5-11	35-65	3-6
5-8 y	5.0-14.5	32-54	5-11	28-48	3-6
13-18 y	4.5-13.0	34-64	5-11	25-45	3-6
Adults	4.5-11.0	35-66	5-11	24-44	3-6

Age	Eosinophils	Basophils	Atypical Lymphs	No. of NRBCs
0-3 d	0-2	0-1	0-8	0-2
1-2 wk	0-2	0-1	0-8	0
1-6 mo	0-3	0-1	0-8	0
7 mo to 2 y	0-3	0-1	0-8	0
2-5 y	0-3	0-1	0-8	0
5-8 y	0-3	0-1	0-8	0
13-18 y	0-3	0-1	0-8	0
Adults	0-3	0-1	0-8	0

Segs = segmented neutrophils.

Bands = band neutrophils.

Lymphs = lymphocytes.

Monos = monocytes.

Erythrocyte Sedimentation Rates and Reticulocyte Counts

Sedimentation rate, Westergren

Children	0-20 mm/h
Adult male	0-15 mm/h
Adult female	0-20 mm/h

Sedimentation rate, Wintrobe

Children	0-13 mm/h
Adult male	0-10 mm/h
Adult female	0-15 mm/h

Reticulocyte count

Newborns	2%-6%
1-6 mo	0%-2.8%
Adults	0.5%-1.5%

ASTHMA

MANAGEMENT OF ASTHMA IN ADULTS AND CHILDREN

Goals of Asthma Treatment

- Prevent chronic and troublesome symptoms: Minimal or no chronic symptoms day or night
- No limitations on activities; no school/work missed
- Minimal use of inhaled short-acting beta$_2$-agonist (≤2 days/week, <1 canister/month) (not including prevention of exercise induced asthma)
- Minimal or no adverse effects from medications
- Maintain (near) normal pulmonary function
- Prevent recurrent exacerbations (ie, trips to emergency department or hospitalizations)

All Patients

- Short-acting bronchodilator: **Inhaled beta$_2$-agonists** as needed for symptoms.
- Intensity of treatment will depend on severity of exacerbation; see "Management of Asthma Exacerbations".
- Use of short-acting inhaled beta$_2$-agonists on a daily basis, or increasing use, indicates the need to initiate or titrate long-term control therapy.

Education

- Teach self-management.
- Teach about controlling environmental factors (avoidance of allergens or other factors that contribute to asthma severity).
- Review administration technique and compliance with patient.
- Use a written action plan to help educate.

Stepwise Approach for Managing Asthma in Adults and Children ≥12 Years of Age

Symptoms	Lung Function	Daily Medications
STEP 6: Severe Asthma		
Day: Throughout the day Night: Often 7 times/week SABA use: Several times/day	FEV$_1$ <60% predicted FEV$_1$/FVC reduced 5%	**Preferred:** High dose ICS plus LABA plus oral corticosteroid AND Consider: Omalizumab (in those with allergies)[1]
STEP 5: Severe Asthma		
Day: Throughout the day Night: Often 7 times/week SABA use: Several times/day	FEV$_1$ <60% predicted FEV$_1$/FVC reduced 5%	**Preferred:** High dose ICS plus LABA AND Consider: Omalizumab (in those with allergies)[1]
STEP 4: Severe Asthma		
Day: Throughout the day Night: Often 7 times/week SABA use: Several times/day	FEV$_1$ <60% predicted FEV$_1$/FVC reduced 5%	**Preferred:** Medium dose ICS plus LABA **Alternatives[2]:** Medium dose ICS plus either LTRA, theophylline, or zileuton[3]

Stepwise Approach for Managing Asthma
in Adults and Children ≥12 Years of Age *(continued)*

Symptoms	Lung Function	Daily Medications
STEP 3: Moderate Asthma		
Day: Daily Night: >1 night/week (not nightly) SABA use: Daily	FEV_1 >60%, <80% predicted FEV_1/FVC reduced 5%	**Preferred:** Low dose ICS plus LABA OR Medium dose ICS **Alternatives[2]:** Low dose ICS plus either LTRA, theophylline, or zileuton[3]
STEP 2: Mild Asthma		
Day: >2 days/week (not daily) Night: 3-4 times/month SABA use: >2 days/week, no more than once per day (not daily)	FEV_1 <80% FEV_1/FVC normal	**Preferred:** Low dose ICS **Alternatives[2]:** Cromolyn, LTRA, nedocromil, or theophylline
STEP 1: Intermittent Asthma		
Day: ≤2 days/week Night: ≤2 nights/month SABA use: ≤2 days/week	FEV_1 normal between exacerbations FEV_1 >80% predicted FEV_1/FVC normal	Preferred: SABA as needed

Note: Treatment options within each step are listed in alphabetical order.

Steps 2-4: Consider subcutaneous allergen immunotherapy for patients with allergic asthma.[1]

Consult with asthma specialist if Step 4 or higher care is needed.

FEV_1 = forced expiratory volume in 1 second; FVC = forced vital capacity; ICS = inhaled corticosteroid; LABA = long-acting inhaled beta$_2$-agonist; SABA = short-acting inhaled beta$_2$-agonist; LTRA = leukotriene receptor antagonist.

[1]When using immunotherapy or omalizumab, clinicians should be prepared to identify and treat anaphylaxis in the event it occurs.

[2]If alternative treatment is used and response is inadequate, discontinue it and use preferred treatment before stepping up.

[3]Zileuton is less desirable alternative due to limited studies and need to monitor liver function.

Notes:

- **The stepwise approach presents general guidelines to assist clinical decision making; it is not intended to be a specific prescription. Asthma is highly variable; clinicians should tailor specific medication plans to the needs and circumstances of individual patients.**

- Gain control as quickly as possible; then decrease treatment to the least medication necessary to maintain control.

- A rescue course of systemic corticosteroids may be needed at any time and at any step.

- Some patients with intermittent asthma experience severe and life-threatening exacerbations separated by long periods of normal lung function and no symptoms. This may be especially common with exacerbations provoked by respiratory infections.

- At each step, patient education, environmental control, management of comorbidities emphasized.

- Antibiotics are not recommended for treatment of acute asthma exacerbations except where there is evidence or suspicion of bacterial infection.

- Consultation with an asthma specialist is recommended for moderate or severe persistent asthma.

- Peak flow monitoring for patients with moderate-severe persistent asthma and patients who have a history of severe exacerbations should be considered.

MANAGEMENT OF ASTHMA IN INFANTS AND YOUNG CHILDREN (<12 YEARS OF AGE)

Stepwise Approach for Managing Asthma in Children 0-4 Years of Age

Symptoms	Daily Medications[1]
STEP 6: Severe Asthma	
Day: Throughout the day Night: >1 time/week SABA use: Several times/ day	**Preferred:** High dose ICS plus either LABA or montelukast Oral systemic corticosteroids
STEP 5: Severe Asthma	
Day: Throughout the day Night: >1 time/week SABA use: Daily	**Preferred:** High dose ICS plus either LABA or montelukast
STEP 4: Moderate Asthma	
Day: Daily Night: 3-4 times/month SABA use: Daily	**Preferred:** Medium dose ICS plus either LABA or montelukast
STEP 3: Moderate Asthma	
Day: Daily Night: 3-4 times/month SABA use: Daily	**Preferred:** Medium dose ICS
STEP 2: Mild Asthma	
Day: >2 days/week (not daily) Night: 1-2 times/month SABA use: >2 days/week, no more than once per day (not daily)	**Preferred:** Low dose ICS **Alternatives[2]:** Cromolyn, montelukast
STEP 1: Intermittent Asthma	
Day: ≤2 days/week Night: No symptoms SABA use: ≤2 days/week	SABA as needed

Consult with asthma specialist if Step 3 or higher care is needed.

FEV_1 = forced expiratory volume in 1 second; FVC = forced vital capacity; ICS = inhaled corticosteroid; LABA = long-acting inhaled beta$_2$-agonist; SABA = short-acting inhaled beta$_2$-agonist.

[1]Studies on children 0-4 years old are limited. Many recommendations are based on expert opinion and extrapolation from studies of older children.

[2]If alternative treatment is used and response is inadequate, discontinue it and use preferred treatment before stepping up.

Stepwise Approach for Managing Asthma in Children 5-11 Years

Symptoms	Lung Function	Daily Medications
STEP 6: Severe Asthma		
Day: Throughout the day Night: Often 7 times/week SABA use: Several times/ day	FEV$_1$ <60% predicted FEV$_1$/FVC <75%	**Preferred:** High dose ICS plus LABA plus oral corticosteroid **Alternative[1]:** High dose ICS plus either LTRA or theophylline[2] plus oral systemic corticosteroid
STEP 5: Severe Asthma		
Day: Throughout the day Night: Often 7 times/week SABA use: Several times/ day	FEV$_1$ <60% predicted FEV$_1$/FVC <75%	**Preferred:** High dose ICS plus LABA **Alternative[1]:** High dose ICS plus either LTRA or theophylline[2]
STEP 4: Severe Asthma		
Day: Throughout the day Night: Often 7 times/week SABA use: Several times/ day	FEV$_1$ <60% predicted FEV$_1$/FVC <75%	**Preferred:** Medium dose ICS plus LABA **Alternative[1]:** Medium dose ICS plus either LTRA or theophylline[2]
STEP 3: Moderate Asthma		
Day: Daily Night: >1 time/week (not nightly) SABA use: Daily	FEV$_1$ 60% to 80% predicted FEV$_1$/FVC 75% to 80%	**Preferred:** Low dose ICS plus either LABA, LTRA, or theophylline[2] OR Medium dose ICS
STEP 2: Mild Asthma		
Day: >2 days/week (not daily) Night: 3-4 times/month SABA use: >2 days/week, no more than once per day (not daily)	FEV$_1$ ≥80% predicted FEV$_1$/FVC >80%	**Preferred:** Low dose ICS **Alternatives[1]:** Cromolyn, LTRA, nedocromil, or theophylline[2]
STEP 1: Intermittent Asthma		
Day: ≤2 days/week Night: ≤2 times/month SABA use: ≤2 days/week	FEV$_1$ normal between exacerbations FEV$_1$ >80% predicted FEV$_1$/FVC >85%	SABA as needed

Steps 2-4: Consider subcutaneous allergen immunotherapy for patients with allergic asthma.[3]

Consult with asthma specialist if Step 4 or higher care is needed.

FEV$_1$ = forced expiratory volume in 1 second; FVC = forced vital capacity; ICS = inhaled corticosteroid; LABA = long-acting inhaled beta$_2$-agonist; SABA = short-acting inhaled beta$_2$-agonist; LTRA = leukotriene receptor antagonist.

[1]If alternative treatment is used and response is inadequate, discontinue it and use preferred treatment before stepping up.

[2]Theophylline is a less desirable alternative due monitoring required.

[3]When using immunotherapy, clinicians should be prepared to identify and treat anaphylaxis in the event it occurs.

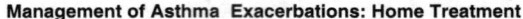

Management of Asthma Exacerbations: Home Treatment

Assess Severity

- **Patients at high risk for a fatal attack require immediate medical attention after initial treatment.**

- Symptoms and signs suggestive of a more serious exacerbation such as marked breathlessness, inability to speak more than short phrases, use of accessory muscles, or drowsiness should result in initial treatment while immediately consulting with a clinician.

- If available, measure PEF—values of 50% to 79% predicted or personal best indicate the need for quick-relief mediation. Depending on the response to treatment, contact with a clinician may also be indicated. Values below 50% indicate the need for immediate medical care.

Initial Treatment

- Inhaled SABA: Up to two treatments 20 minutes apart of 2–6 puffs by metered-dose inhaler (MDI) or nebulizer treatments.

- Note: Medication delivery is highly variable. Children and individuals who have exacerbations of lesser severity may need fewer puffs than suggested above.

Good Response	**Incomplete Response**	**Poor Response**
No wheezing or dyspnea (assess tachypnea in young children).	Persistent wheezing and dyspnea (tachypnea).	Marked wheezing and dyspnea.
PEF ≥80% predicted or personal best.	PEF 50% to 79% predicted or personal best.	PEF <50% predicted or personal best.

• Contact clinician for followup instructions and further management.
• May continue inhaled SABA every 3–4 hours for 24–48 hours.
• Consider short course of oral systemic corticosteroids.
	• Add oral systemic corticosteroid.
	• Continue inhaled SABA.
	• Contact clinician urgently (this day) for further instruction.
		• Add oral systemic corticosteroid
		• Repeat inhaled SABA immediately.
		• If distress is severe and nonresponsive to initial treatment:
		  – Call your doctor AND
		  – **PROCEED TO EMERGENCY DEPARTMENT**;
		  – Consider calling 911 (ambulance transport).

- To emergency department.

MDI: Metered-dose inhaler; PEF: Peak expiratory flow; SABA: Short-acting beta$_2$-agonist (quick relief inhaler)

Management of Asthma Exacerbations: Emergency Department and Hospital-Based Care

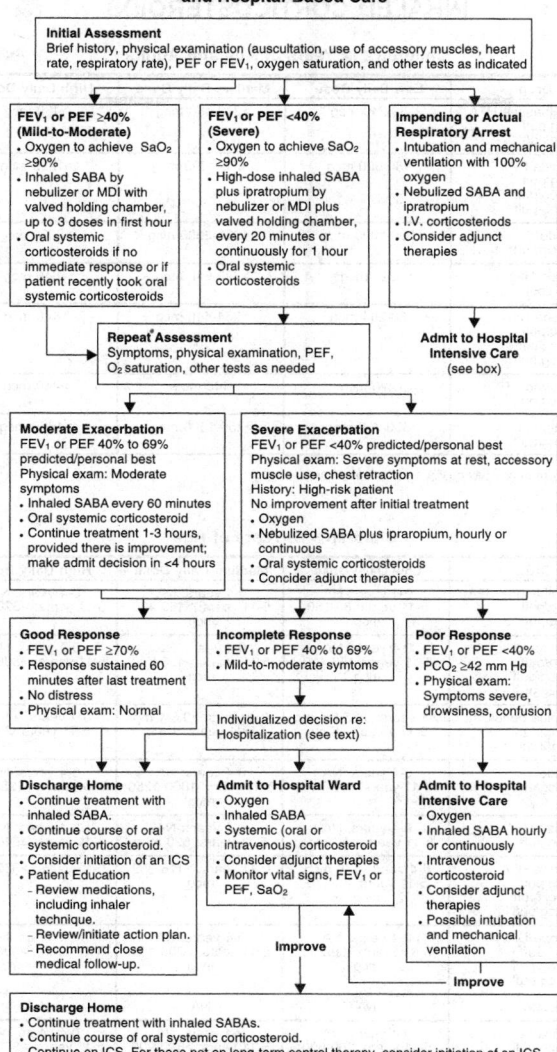

Initial Assessment
Brief history, physical examination (auscultation, use of accessory muscles, heart rate, respiratory rate), PEF or FEV$_1$, oxygen saturation, and other tests as indicated

FEV$_1$ or PEF ≥40% (Mild-to-Moderate)
- Oxygen to achieve SaO$_2$ ≥90%
- Inhaled SABA by nebulizer or MDI with valved holding chamber, up to 3 doses in first hour
- Oral systemic corticosteroids if no immediate response or if patient recently took oral systemic corticosteroids

FEV$_1$ or PEF <40% (Severe)
- Oxygen to achieve SaO$_2$ ≥90%
- High-dose inhaled SABA plus ipratropium by nebulizer or MDI plus valved holding chamber, every 20 minutes or continuously for 1 hour
- Oral systemic corticosteroids

Impending or Actual Respiratory Arrest
- Intubation and mechanical ventilation with 100% oxygen
- Nebulized SABA and ipratropium
- I.V. corticosteroids
- Consider adjunct therapies

Repeat Assessment
Symptoms, physical examination, PEF, O$_2$ saturation, other tests as needed

Admit to Hospital Intensive Care
(see box)

Moderate Exacerbation
FEV$_1$ or PEF 40% to 69% predicted/personal best
Physical exam: Moderate symptoms
- Inhaled SABA every 60 minutes
- Oral systemic corticosteroid
- Continue treatment 1-3 hours, provided there is improvement; make admit decision in <4 hours

Severe Exacerbation
FEV$_1$ or PEF <40% predicted/personal best
Physical exam: Severe symptoms at rest, accessory muscle use, chest retraction
History: High-risk patient
No improvement after initial treatment
- Oxygen
- Nebulized SABA plus ipraropium, hourly or continuous
- Oral systemic corticosteroids
- Concider adjunct therapies

Good Response
- FEV$_1$ or PEF ≥70%
- Response sustained 60 minutes after last treatment
- No distress
- Physical exam: Normal

Incomplete Response
- FEV$_1$ or PEF 40% to 69%
- Mild-to-moderate symtoms

Individualized decision re: Hospitalization (see text)

Poor Response
- FEV$_1$ or PEF <40%
- PCO$_2$ ≥42 mm Hg
- Physical exam: Symptoms severe, drowsiness, confusion

Discharge Home
- Continue treatment with inhaled SABA.
- Continue course of oral systemic corticosteroid.
- Consider initiation of an ICS.
- Patient Education
  - Review medications, including inhaler technique.
  - Review/initiate action plan.
  - Recommend close medical follow-up.

Admit to Hospital Ward
- Oxygen
- Inhaled SABA
- Systemic (oral or intravenous) corticosteroid
- Consider adjunct therapies
- Monitor vital signs, FEV$_1$ or PEF, SaO$_2$

Improve

Admit to Hospital Intensive Care
- Oxygen
- Inhaled SABA hourly or continuously
- Intravenous corticosteroid
- Consider adjunct therapies
- Possible intubation and mechanical ventilation

Improve

Discharge Home
- Continue treatment with inhaled SABAs.
- Continue course of oral systemic corticosteroid.
- Continue on ICS. For those not on long-term control therapy, consider initiation of an ICS.
- Patient education (eg, review medications, including inhaler technique and, whenever possible, environmental control measures; review/initiate action plan; recommend close medical follow-up).
- Before discharge, schedule follow-up appointment with primary care provider and/or asthma specialist in 1-4 weeks.

FEV$_1$ = forced expiratory volume in 1 second; ICS = inhaled corticosteroid; MDI = metered dose inhaler; PCO$_2$ = partial pressure carbon dioxide; PEF = peak expiratory flow; SABA = short-acting beta$_2$-agonist; SaO$_2$ = oxygen saturation

ESTIMATED COMPARATIVE <u>DAILY</u> DOSAGES FOR INHALED CORTICOSTEROIDS

Children ≥12 Years of Age and Adults

Drug	Low Daily Dose	Medium Daily Dose	High Daily Dose
Beclomethasone HFA 40 mcg/puff 80 mcg/puff	80-240 mcg	>240-480 mcg	>480 mcg
Budesonide DPI 90 mcg/puff 180 mcg/puff 200 mcg/puff	180-600 mcg	>600-1200 mcg	>1200 mcg
Flunisolide 250 mcg/puff	500-1000 mcg	>1000-2000 mcg	>2000 mcg
Flunisolide HFA 80 mcg/puff	320 mcg	>320-640 mcg	>640 mcg
Fluticasone HFA 44 mcg/puff 110 mcg/puff 220 mcg/puff	88-264 mcg	>264-440 mcg	>440 mcg
Mometasone DPI 220 mcg/puff	220 mcg	440 mcg	>440 mcg
Triamcinolone 100 mcg/puff	300-750 mcg	>750-1500 mcg	>1500 mcg

DPI = dry powder inhaler; HFA = hydrofluoroalkane.

Children <12 Years of Age

Drug	Low Daily Dose	Medium Daily Dose	High Daily Dose
Beclomethasone HFA 40 mcg/puff 80 mcg/puff	0-4 years: NA 5-11 years: 80-160 mcg	0-4 years: NA 5-11 years: >160-320 mcg	0-4 years: NA 5-11 years: >320 mcg
Budesonide DPI 90 mcg/puff 180 mcg/puff 200 mcg/puff	0-4 years: NA 5-11 years: 180-400 mcg	0-4 years: NA 5-11 years: >400-800 mcg	0-4 years: NA 5-11 years: >800 mcg
Budesonide nebulized 0.25 mg/2 mL 0.5 mg/2 mL	0-4 years: 0.25-0.5 mg 5-11 years: 0.5 mg	0-4 years: >0.5-1 mg 5-11 years: 1 mg	0-4 years: >1 mg 5-11 years: 2 mg
Flunisolide 250 mcg/puff	0-4 years: NA 5-11 years: 500-750 mcg	0-4 years: NA 5-11 years: 1000-1250 mcg	0-4 years: NA 5-11 years: >1250 mcg
Flunisolide HFA 80 mcg/puff	0-4 years: NA 5-11 years: 160 mcg	0-4 years: NA 5-11 years: 320 mcg	0-4 years: NA 5-11 years: ≥640 mcg
Fluticasone HFA 44 mcg/puff 110 mcg/puff 220 mcg/puff	0-4 years: 176 mcg 5-11 years: 88-176 mcg	0-11 years: >176-352 mcg	0-11 years: >352 mcg
Fluticasone DPI 50 mcg/puff 100 mcg/puff 250 mcg/puff	0-4 years: NA 5-11 years: 100-200 mcg	0-4 years: NA 5-11 years: >200-400 mcg	0-4 years: NA 5-11 years: >400 mcg
Mometasone	NA	NA	NA
Triamcinolone 100 mcg/puff	0-4 years: NA 5-11 years: 300-600 mcg	0-4 years: NA 5-11 years: >600-900 mcg	0-4 years: NA 5-11 years: >900 mcg

DPI = dry powder inhaler; HFA = hydrofluoroalkane.

NA = not approved for use in this age group or no data available.

Reference

Expert Panel Report 3, "Guidelines for the Diagnosis and Management of Asthma," *Clinical Practice Guidelines*, National Institutes of Health, National Heart, Lung, and Blood Institute, NIH Publication No. 08-4051, prepublication 2007. Available at http://www.nhlbi.nih.gov/guidelines/asthma/asthgdln.htm.

CONTRAST MEDIA REACTIONS, PREMEDICATION FOR PROPHYLAXIS

It is estimated that approximately 5% to 10% of patients will experience adverse reactions to administration of contrast dye (less for nonionic contrast). In approximately 1000-2000 administrations, a life-threatening reaction will occur.

A variety of premedication regimens have been proposed, both for pretreatment of "at risk" patients who require contrast media and before the routine administration of the intravenous high osmolar contrast media (HOCM). Such regimens have been shown in clinical trials to decrease the frequency of all forms of contrast medium reactions. Pretreatment with a 2-dose regimen of methylprednisolone 32 mg, 12 and 2 hours prior to intravenous administration of HOCM (ionic), has been shown to decrease mild, moderate, and severe reactions in patients at increased risk and perhaps in patients without risk factors. Logistical and feasibility problems may preclude adequate premedication with this or any regimen for all patients. It is unclear at this time that steroid pretreatment prior to administration of ionic contrast media reduces the incidence of reactions to the same extent or less than that achieved with the use of nonionic contrast media alone. Information about the efficacy of nonionic contrast media combined with a premedication strategy, including steroids, is preliminary or not yet currently available. For high-risk patients (ie, previous contrast reactors), the combination of a pretreatment regimen with nonionic contrast media has empirical merit and may warrant consideration. Oral administration of steroids appears preferable to intravascular routes, and the drug may be prednisone or methylprednisolone. Supplemental administration of H_1 and H_2 antihistamine therapies, orally or intravenously, may reduce the frequency of urticaria, angioedema, and respiratory symptoms. Additionally, ephedrine administration has been suggested to decrease the frequency of contrast reactions, but caution is advised in patients with cardiac disease, hypertension, or hyperthyroidism. No premedication strategy should be a substitute for the ABC approach to preadministration preparedness listed above. Contrast reactions do occur despite any and all premedication prophylaxis. The incidence can be decreased, however, in some categories of "at risk" patients receiving HOCM plus a medication regimen. For patients with previous contrast medium reactions, there is a slight chance that recurrence may be more severe or the same as the prior reaction, however, it is more likely that there will be no recurrence.

A general premedication regimen is

Methylprednisolone	32 mg orally 12 and 2 hours prior to procedure
Diphenhydramine	50 mg orally 1 hour prior to the procedure

An alternative premedication regimen is

Prednisone	50 mg orally 13, 7, and 1 hour before the procedure
Diphenhydramine	50 mg orally 1 hour before the procedure
Ephedrine	25 mg orally 1 hour before the procedure (except when contraindicated)

Indications for Nonionic Contrast

- Previous reaction to contrast – premedicate. **Note:** For life-threatening reactions (throat swelling, laryngeal edema, etc), consider omitting the intravenous contrast
- Known allergy to iodine or shellfish
- Asthma, especially if on medication
- Myocardial instability or HF
- Risk for aspiration or severe nausea and vomiting

- Difficulty communicating or inability to give history
- Patients taking beta-blockers
- Small children at risk for electrolyte imbalance or extravasation
- Renal failure with diabetes, sickle cell disease, or myeloma
- At physician or patient request

Contrast Induced Nephrotoxicity (CIN)

CIN is a common complication after exposure to intravenous radio-contrast agents. In the literature, CIN is defined as a rise in serum creatinine concentration of at least 0.5 mg/dL or an increase of 25% compared to baseline occurring after exposure to contrast medium. Most of the time, this increase in serum creatinine is transient; however, in some cases, the impairment may be permanent with some patients requiring dialysis. Many agents have been evaluated for prevention of this adverse event; however, only N-acetylcysteine, sodium bicarbonate, and sodium chloride have been shown to be of benefit.

Risk Factors for CIN:

- Pre-existing renal impairment
- Diabetes nephropathy
- Age >70 years
- Hypovolemia
- Anemia
- Heart failure
- Hypotension
- Concomitant nephrotoxins (eg, aminoglycosides)
- Large contrast medium doses (eg, ≥140 mL)
- Type of contrast agent uses (high-osmolar contrast media > low-osmolar contrast media)

Strategies for the Prevention of CIN

N-acetylcysteine, P.O.	600 mg orally twice daily on the day before and the day of the scan in addition to hydration with 0.45% saline intravenously
N-acetylcysteine, I.V./P.O.[1]	1200 mg I.V. over 5-10 minutes prior to cardiac catheterization, followed by 1200 mg **orally** twice daily for 48 hours; hydrate with 1 mL/kg/hour for 12 hours after procedure (may use 0.5 mL/kg/hour in patients with overt heart failure)
Sodium Bicarbonate I.V.	3 mL/kg/hour for 1 hour prior to contrast injection, then 1 mL/kg/hour during contrast exposure and for 6 hours after procedure
Sodium Chloride 0.45% or 0.9%, I.V.	1 mL/kg/hour for 12 hours prior to and for 12 hours after procedure

[1]This regimen has only been evaluated in patients with acute MI requiring primary angioplasty (Marenzi, 2006).

References

American College of Radiology, "Manual on Contrast Media, Version 6.0," 2008. Available at http://www.acr.org/SecondaryMainMenuCategories/quality_safety/contrast_manual.aspx

Marenzi G, Assanelli E, Marana I, et al, "N-acetylcysteine and Contrast-Induced Nephropathy in Primary Angioplasty," N Engl J Med, 2006, 354(26):2773-82.

Massicotte A, "Contrast Medium-Induced Nephropathy: Strategies for Prevention," Pharmacotherapy, 2008, 28(9):1140-50.

Merten GJ, Burgess WP, Gray LV, et al, "Prevention of Contrast-Induced Nephropathy With Sodium Bicarbonate: A Randomized Controlled Trial," JAMA, 2004, 291(19):2328-34.

STATUS EPILEPTICUS

CONVULSIVE STATUS EPILEPTICUS

Treatment Guidelines

Convulsive status epilepticus is an emergency that is associated with high morbidity and mortality. The outcome largely depends on etiology, but prompt and appropriate pharmacological therapy can reduce morbidity and mortality. Etiology varies in children and adults and reflects the distribution of disease in these age groups. Antiepileptic drug administration should be initiated whenever a seizure has lasted 5-10 minutes. Immediate concerns include supporting respiration, maintaining blood pressure, gaining intravenous access, and identifying and treating the underlying cause. Initial therapeutic and diagnostic measures are conducted simultaneously. The goal of therapy is rapid termination of clinical and electrical seizure activity; the longer a seizure continues, the greater the likelihood of an adverse outcome. Several drug protocols now in use will terminate status epilepticus. Common to all patients is the need for a clear plan, prompt administration of appropriate drugs in adequate doses, and attention to the possibility of apnea, hypoventilation, or other metabolic abnormalities.

Management of Status Epilepticus

Time Since Seizure Onset	Drug Treatment		Evaluations / Actions
	Adults	**Children**	
Prolonged Seizure: Premonitory Stage (Out-of-Hospital)			
5 min	Diazepam 10 mg rectally	Diazepam 0.5 mg/kg rectally	• Airway/breathing • Monitor vital signs • Establish I.V. access • Blood glucose determination
If seizures continue ↓			
Early Status Epilepticus: First Stage (Out-of-Hospital or Inpatient)			
5-30 min	Lorazepam 4 mg I.V. bolus (≤2 mg/min) **or** Diazepam 5-10 mg I.V. (≤5 mg/min; maximum dose: 30 mg) May repeat dose after 5-10 minutes	Lorazepam 0.05-0.1 mg/kg I.V. (≤2 mg/min; maximum dose: 4 mg) **or** Diazepam 0.1-0.3 mg/kg I.V. (≤5 mg/min; maximum dose: 10 mg) May repeat dose after 5-10 minutes	• ABGs, oxygen/ventilation • CBC, electrolytes, renal/hepatic status • Cardiac monitoring, ECG • Neurologic assessment toxicology screen • Consider I.V. dextrose ± thiamine • AED concentrations
If seizures continue ↓			
Established Status Epilepticus: Second Stage			
30-60 min	Fosphenytoin 15-20 mg PE/kg I.V. (maximum rate: 150 mg/min) **or** Phenytoin 15-20 mg/kg I.V. (maximum rate: 50 mg/min)	Fosphenytoin 15-20 mg PE/kg I.V. (maximum rate: 150 mg/min) **or** Phenytoin 20 mg/kg I.V. (maximum rate: 50 mg/min) **or** Phenobarbital 15-20 mg/kg I.V. (maximum rate: <100 mg/min[1])	• Intubation/mechanical ventilation • Cardiorespiratory function • Vasopressors if needed • Neurologic: CT, CSF, EEG

Management of Status Epilepticus *(continued)*

Time Since Seizure Onset	Drug Treatment		Evaluations / Actions
	Adults	**Children**	
	If seizures continue ↓ **Refractory Status Epilepticus: Third Stage**		
>60 min	Phenobarbital 10-20 mg/kg I.V. (maximum: 100 mg/min[1]) **or** Pentobarbital 10-20 mg/kg I.V. (maximum: 100 mg/min[1]), then 0.5-3 mg/kg/h **or** Midazolam 0.2 mg/kg bolus, then continuous infusion of 0.05-0.6 mg/kg/h **or** Propofol 1-2 mg/kg bolus, then continuous infusion of 1.5-10 mg/kg/h	Phenobarbital 15-20 mg/kg I.V. (maximum: <100 mg/min[1]) **or** Pentobarbital 5-15 mg/kg I.V., then 0.5-5 mg/kg/h[1] **or** Midazolam 0.15 mg/kg bolus, then continuous infusion of 0.06 mg/kg/h	• ICU admission • Anesthesia monitoring/ hemodynamics • Therapeutic AED monitoring

AED = antiepileptic drug.

[1]May induce hypotension; consider alternative agents in hemodynamically unstable patients. Monitor closely and reduce rate if hypotension develops. Fluids and/or vasopressors may be necessary to control significant hypotension.

References

Hanhan UA, Fiallos MR, and Orlowski JP, "Status Epilepticus," *Pediatr Clin North Am*, 2001, 48 (3):683-94.

Kälviäinen R, "Status Epilepticus Treatment Guidelines," *Epilepsia*, 2007, 48(Suppl 8):99-102.

Kälviäinen R, Eriksson K, and Parviainen I, "Refractory Generalised Convulsive Status Epilepticus: A Guide to Treatment," *CNS Drugs*, 2005, 19(9):759-68.

Lowenstein DH, "Treatment Options for Status Epilepticus," *Curr Opin Pharmacol*, 2005, 5(3):334-9.

Meierkord H, Boon P, Engelsen B, et al, "EFNS Guideline on the Management of Status Epilepticus," *Eur J Neurol*, 2006, 13(5):445-50.

HEART FAILURE (SYSTOLIC)

INTRODUCTORY COMMENTS

This summarizes the pharmacotherapy of patients with systolic heart failure with respect to treating mild-to-moderate exacerbations and chronic therapy. A more detailed discussion is available at: http://content.onlinejacc.org/cgi/content/full/j.jacc.2008.11.013.

It should be recognized that the most common cause for exacerbations of patients' heart failure is poor adherence to therapy (medications and diet restriction). Healthcare providers need to educate patients about the importance of adherence to medical regimens.

For many years, therapy of heart failure focused on correcting the hemodynamic imbalances that occurred in heart failure. It is now recognized that heart failure triggers the release of several neurohormones that, in the short-run, help the patient; but, in the long-run, are detrimental. Newer pharmacotherapeutic approaches address counteracting the actions of these harmful neurohormones as well as address hemodynamic issues.

Diuretics

Although data have yet to demonstrate that diuretics reduce the mortality associated with heart failure, they relieve symptoms seen in heart failure. Diuretics should only be used in patients experiencing congestion with their heart failure. Although not usually the case, some patients do have heart failure without any congestion. In such rare instances, diuretic therapy is not indicated since they further stimulate the deleterious neurohormonal responses seen.

Although some heart failure patients with congestion can be controlled with thiazide diuretics, most will require the more potent loop diuretics, either because a strong diuretic effect is needed or the renal function of the patients is compromised (thus limiting the effectiveness of the thiazide diuretic). When patients with heart failure are discovered to have mild-to-moderate worsening congestion, they often can be controlled by adjusting their oral loop diuretic dose or, if applicable, initiating a loop diuretic regimen. If a more aggressive diuresis is indicated, especially if the patient is suffering from pulmonary congestion, intravenous loop diuretics would be indicated. When loop diuretics are given intravenously, before any diuretic effect occurs, they benefit the patient by dilating veins and reducing preload, thus relieving pulmonary congestion. Intravenous loop diuresis may also be considered in a patient where concerns exist about the ability of the patient to absorb the orally administered medication.

If already on an oral loop diuretic, the dosage should be increased (generally, 1.5-2 times their current regimen) in an effort for the patient to lose about 1-1.5 liters of fluid per day (about equivalent to 1-1.5 kg of weight per day). If the patient had yet to be started on a diuretic or was previously receiving a thiazide diuretic, initiating furosemide at 20-40 mg once or twice daily is a reasonable consideration. If the initial increase (or initiation) in dosage fails to induce a diuretic response, the dosage may be increased. If the initial increase (or initiation) does induce a diuretic response but the patient fails to lose weight or is not losing more fluids than taking in, the frequency of giving the loop diuretic can be increased. When an effective regimen is achieved, this regimen should be continued until the patient achieves a goal "dry" weight. Once this weight is attained, a decision needs to be made on how to continue the patient on diuretic therapy. If the patient had not been on a diuretic at home, continuation of the loop diuretic at a reduced dose is a worthy consideration. If the exacerbation was related to noncompliance with the diuretic or diet, the previous home dose might be continued with education on compliance. If the exacerbation was caused by an inadequate pharmacotherapeutic regimen (such as vasodilator was not being use), the previous home dose might be continued in conjunction with a more complete pharmacotherapeutic regimen. If the patient was compliant and on an acceptable pharmacotherapeutic regimen, the patient's original diuretic dose would be increased to some dosage greater than their home regimen, yet generally less than what was just used to achieve their dry weight.

The use of loop diuretics can lead to hypokalemia and/or hypomagnesemia. Electrolyte disturbances can predispose a patient to serious cardiac arrhythmias particularly if the patient is concurrently receiving digoxin. Fluid depletion, hypotension, and azotemia can also result from excessive use of diuretics. In contrast to thiazide diuretics, a loop diuretic can also lower serum calcium concentrations. For some patients, despite higher doses of loop diuretic treatment, an adequate diuretic response cannot be attained. Diuretic resistance can usually be overcome by intravenous administration (including continuous infusion), the use of 2 diuretics together (eg, furosemide and metolazone), or the use of a diuretic with a positive inotropic agent. When such combinations are used, serum electrolytes need to be monitored even more closely.

When loop diuretics are used in patients with renal dysfunction, to achieve the desired diuretic response, dosages typically will need to be greater than what is used in patients with normal renal function.

Due to its long existence and inexpensive price, furosemide tends to be the loop diuretic most commonly used. Bumetanide is now available as a generic and its use has been increasing consequently. The oral bioavailability of bumetanide and torsemide are nearly 100%; whereas, furosemide's oral bioavailability averages about 50%. A useful rule of thumb for conversion of intravenous loop diuretics is 40 mg of furosemide is equal to 1 mg bumetanide is equal to 15 mg torsemide. A few patients have allergies to diuretics because many contain a sulfur element. The only loop diuretic that lacks a sulfur element is ethacrynic acid.

Vasodilators

Vasodilator therapy, specifically the combination of hydralazine and isosorbide dinitrate, was the first pharmacotherapeutic treatment demonstrated to enhance survival of heart failure patients. The use of hydralazine 75 mg (which reduces afterload) and isosorbide dinitrate 40 mg 4 times a day (which reduces preload) demonstrated enhanced survival compared to placebo and prazosin. Unfortunately, many patients were unable to tolerate this regimen (primarily due to headaches and gastrointestinal disturbances) and the magnitude of benefit in survival dissipated with time.

Later, a series of investigations demonstrated that enalapril (which reduces both afterload and preload) enhances the survival of heart failure patients. Dosages used in these trials averaged about 10 mg twice daily. Since these trials, other ACE inhibitors were proven to benefit heart failure patients.

ACE Inhibitors

This led to the question, which is superior, ACE inhibitor or the combination of hydralazine and isosorbide dinitrate? In a comparative trial, using doses described above, enalapril was superior to the combination of hydralazine and isosorbide dinitrate, making an ACE inhibitor the vasodilator of choice in heart failure patients. An ACE inhibitor can alleviate symptoms, improve clinical status, and enhance a patient's quality of life. In addition an ACE inhibitor can reduce the risk of death and the combined risk of death or hospitalization.

Adverse effects associated with ACE inhibitors include hyperkalemia, rash, dysgeusia, dry cough, and (rarely) angioedema. Patients sometime develop renal dysfunction with the initiation of ACE inhibitors. This is not due to direct nephrotoxicity of the kidney but related to the ACE inhibitor dilating the efferent renal artery of the kidney, thus shunting blood away from being filtered in the glomerulus. The risk for renal dysfunction is increased when the ACE inhibitor is introduced to a patient who is hypovolemic, is being aggressively diuresed, is on an NSAID, or has bilateral renal artery stenosis (unilateral if only one kidney is present). Avoid NSAIDs in heart failure patients. ACE inhibitors should be avoided in patients with known renal artery stenosis. Monitor renal function and serum potassium within 1-2 weeks of initiation of therapy and routinely thereafter especially in patients with pre-existing hypotension, hyponatremia, diabetes, azotemia, or in those taking potassium supplements. Some patients will have an exaggerated hypotensive response following the initial doses (especially the first dose) of an ACE inhibitor.

A major limitation to using ACE inhibitors treatment in heart failure can be the dry cough that some patients develop. Lowering the ACE inhibitor dose sometimes can control it, but this may limit the effectiveness of the ACE inhibitor treatment. The development of angiotensin receptor blockers (ARBs) has helped address this issue. ARBs were demonstrated to enhance survival of heart failure patients. Although they are not the vasodilator of first choice in heart failure, they are a reasonable alternative in patients who cannot tolerate an ACE inhibitor due to the cough or some other adverse effect (with the exception of hyperkalemia and renal dysfunction; ARBs can induce as well). ARBs do not cause an accumulation of kinins as ACE inhibitors do.

Can ARBs be used in patients who suffer angioedema with ACE inhibitors? Reports are available in the literature describing patients who experienced angioedema with both ACE inhibitors and ARBs. These cases do not indicate the safety of an ARB when used in a patient who has experienced an ACE inhibitor-induced angioedema. The CHARM-Alternative trial confirmed that only one of 39 patients (~2.6%) who experienced angioedema with an ACE inhibitors also experienced it with an ARB.

Concurrent Use of an ACE Inhibitor and an ARB

In Val-HeFT, valsartan added to conventional treatment (included ACE inhibitor treatment) did not impact survival but did reduce morbidity. Of note, a subgroup analysis of this trial suggested the combination of valsartan and an ACE inhibitor may be detrimental to patients also receiving a beta-blocker. In CHARM-Added, candesartan added to ACE inhibitor therapy was of benefit to heart failure patients (modest reduction in hospitalization; increased risk of hyperkalemia and renal dysfunction), even for those receiving a beta-blocker. As a result, the recently released ACC/AHA Practice Guidelines do not speak against using the combination of ACE inhibitors and ARBs. However, few patients in these trials were receiving an aldosterone blocker (such as spironolactone), which is now known to be of benefit to heart failure patients. Since there is enhanced risk for hyperkalemia and outcome data are currently unknown, the ACC/AHA Practice Guidelines for heart failure do not advocate the combined use of ACE inhibitors, ARBs, and an aldosterone inhibitor.

In summary, vasodilator therapy should initially consist of an ACE inhibitor. If such therapy cannot be tolerated due to renal failure or hyperkalemia, the combination of hydralazine and isosorbide dinitrate may be considered as ARBs can also cause renal failure and hyperkalemia. If the ACE inhibitor cannot be tolerated due to adverse effects such as dry cough, an ARB may be considered. If an ACE inhibitor and beta-blocker have been maximized yet heart failure symptoms persist, consider adding hydralazine and isosorbide dinitrate. This approach, in fact, has been demonstrated to enhance the survival of African-American patients with heart failure. Another approach may be to add an ARB to the ACE inhibitor; but caution should occur, due to the risk of hyperkalemia.

Beta-Blockers

Despite being negative inotropes, beta-blockers have been demonstrated to enhance the survival of systolic heart failure patients. Their benefit is attributed to their ability to protect the myocardium from the "bombardment" of catecholamines present in heart failure that can lead to ventricular remodeling. Bisoprolol, metoprolol succinate (extended release), and carvedilol have been demonstrated in trials to improve survival. At present, superiority of one agent over another has not been definitively demonstrated. For patients to be able to tolerate this therapy, beta-blocker treatment needs to be initiated at low doses and titrated slowly (generally, the dose is double every two weeks). Following the initiation of treatment and the increase in dosage, patients may feel that their disease is worsening but this should dissipate after a few days. If this ill feeling continues beyond a few days, consideration should be given to regimen adjustments. If the patient is congested, increase the diuretic dosage. If the patient's discomfort is related to hypotension, staggering the beta-blocker dose with the vasodilator dose and/or lowering the vasodilator dosage may be helpful. If these approaches are ineffective or cannot explain the patient's ill feeling, consideration should be given to lowering the beta-blocker dosage and attempt a dose titration increase later on. Sometimes, a patient may not be able to tolerate "goal" doses of both beta-blockers and concurrent vasodilator treatment due to hypotension. It is the consensus opinion that a reduced dose of each agent is better than a goal dose of just one agent. Beta-blockers are not necessarily contraindicated but need to be used cautiously in patients with bronchospastic disease, peripheral artery disease, or diabetes mellitus.

Aldosterone Blockers

Of the pharmacotherapeutic treatments of heart failure demonstrated to benefit patients, the use of aldosterone blockers is the newest. It has been demonstrated, especially in the more severe forms of heart failure, that spironolactone, at an average dose of 25 mg daily, enhances the survival of heart failure patients. In patients who suffer hyperkalemia at this relatively low dosage, lowering the dose to 25 mg every other day may be attempted. In patients who remain symptomatic with their heart failure and have maximized the other proven treatments of heart failure and whose potassium concentrations can tolerate increases, the spironolactone dose may be increased to 50 mg daily.

Obviously, hyperkalemia is a concern with this treatment, especially since patients generally will also be receiving an ACE inhibitor or ARB. It has been demonstrated that the number of emergency visits related to hyperkalemia in heart failure has increased with the introduction of aldosterone blocking therapy in treating heart failure. About 10% of patients will experience endocrinological effects with spironolactone. In men, breast tenderness and gynecomastia may occur. In women, menstrual irregularities may be seen. In such instances, the use of eplerenone may be considered. Eplerenone is less apt to induce endocrinological effects but it is more expensive. A typical dose is 25-50 mg daily. Eplerenone has been demonstrated to enhance survival of post-MI patients with reduced ejection fractions. Spironolactone has not been studied in this patient group.

These medications should not be started in patients with renal insufficiency. These medications should be avoided if the serum creatinine exceeds 2.5 mg/dL in men (2 mg/dL in women) or if baseline potassium ≥5 mEq/L.

Digoxin

The value of digoxin in heart failure has crossed the spectrum. In the late 1980s, further investigation with digoxin suggested that indeed it may have a role in heart failure treatment, but the methods of these trials were not ideal (digoxin was taken away from stabilized patients to see if the condition of patients worsened – it did). Finally, digoxin was studied in a prospective manner where patients were on known optimal heart failure treatment at the time and randomized to placebo or digoxin. The digoxin dosage used resulted in digoxin steady-state concentrations of 1 mcg/L. This trial revealed that digoxin did not impact survival but reduced the number of patient hospitalizations, suggesting digoxin has a morbidity benefit. Many are of the opinion that digoxin's benefit is unrelated to its positive inotropic activity but related to inhibiting neurohormal activity. Healthcare providers may consider adding digoxin in patients with persistent heart failure symptoms as a fourth line agent.

Digoxin is primarily renally eliminated; therefore, renal function of patients should be closely monitored and the dose adjusted. Digoxin does become difficult to use in patients whose renal function is unstable. In the DIG trial, effective digoxin steady-state concentrations ranged between 0.7-1 mcg/L. Concentrations much beyond 1 mcg/L were associated with worsened outcomes, especially in women. Since digoxin's benefit is long-term, a loading dose is not necessary. When checking a digoxin serum concentration, the sample should not be obtained until 12 hours after a dose, especially if it was oral, since digoxin has a relatively long distribution phase. It should also be assured that the patient is at steady-state (recall that the half-life of digoxin in a patient with normal renal function is approximately 36 hours and that patients with heart failure generally have worsened renal function).

Hypokalemia, hypomagnesia, hypercalcemia, and hypothyroidism can precipitate digoxin toxicity in the presence of a therapeutic digoxin concentration. This toxicity can be alleviated by correcting the electrolyte abnormality. In acute digoxin overdoses, hyperkalemia can occur since digoxin inhibits the sodium-potassium ATPase pump. For this reason, one should not assume potassium is given to just **any** patient with digoxin toxicity. Digoxin toxicity can present as bradyarrhythmias, heart blocks, ventricular tachyarrhythmias, and atrial tachyarrhythmias (PAT with block is pathognomic). Other toxic manifestations include visual disturbances (including greenish-yellowish vision and halos around lights), gastrointestinal disturbances, anorexia, and altered mental status. Many medications elevate digoxin concentrations and a patient's regimen should be assessed for potential interactions.

Other Heart Failure Therapeutic Considerations

- If a calcium channel blocker is desired, amlodipine and felodipine are preferred choices.
- To treat arrhythmias, amiodarone and dofetilide are best documented to lack significant proarrhythmic propensity in heart failure patients. Dronedarone, a newer antiarrhythmic agent structurally similar to amiodarone, is contraindicated in patients with NYHA Class IV heart failure or Class II-III heart failure with recent decompensation requiring hospitalization or referral to a specialized heart failure clinic.
- In heart failure patients with diabetes mellitus, metformin should not be used and "glitazones" should not be used in severe heart failure (NYHA III and IV) and used cautiously, if at all, in mild-to-moderate heart failure.
- The use of cilostazol, because it has type III phosphodiesterase-inhibiting properties, is contraindicated in heart failure. This is because the chronic use of oral milrinone and inamrinone, also type III phosphodiesterase inhibitors, resulted in enhanced mortality in heart failure patients (and therefore, these two agents were never FDA-approved for oral use).
- NSAID use should be avoided or used minimally as these agents antagonize the effects of diuretics and ACE inhibitors.
- Retrospective data suggests that daily aspirin may also negate the effects of ACE inhibitors but this has yet to be definitively proven in prospective trials. Using the lowest possible aspirin dose with the highest possible ACE inhibitor dose has been suggested as a way to best circumvent this issue.
- Routine intermittent infusions of positive inotropes are not recommended; can be used as palliation in end-stage disease.

Class I Recommendations for the Hospitalized Patient With Acute Decompensated Heart Failure

- Patients presenting to the hospital with fluid overload should be treated immediately with intravenous loop diuretics (eg, furosemide) since earlier treatment may be associated with better outcomes. If chronically receiving oral loop diuretic therapy, the initial intravenous dose should equal or exceed their chronic oral daily dose and titrated to relieve symptoms and reduce fluid excess. If this is inadequate, use of higher doses of loop diuretics, adding a second diuretic (eg, intravenous chlorothiazide), or a continuous infusion of the loop diuretic may improve diuresis.
- If evidence of hypotension with associated hypoperfusion and elevated cardiac filling pressures (eg, increase JVP) exists, intravenous inotropic support (eg, dobutamine) or vasopressor drugs (eg, dopamine) should be administered. Use of intravenous inotropes in patients without evidence of hypoperfusion is not recommended.
- In the absence of hemodynamic instability or contraindications, the use of therapies known to improve outcomes (eg, ACE inhibitors or ARBs, and beta-blockers) should be continued during the hospital stay. When appropriate, these agents should be initiated or reinitiated to stabilized patients prior to hospital discharge. Beta-blockers should only be initiated upon successful discontinuation of intravenous diuretics, vasodilators, and inotropic agents in the stabilized patient; initiate at a low dose and use caution in those patients who required inotropic support during their hospital course.

Dosing of ACE Inhibitors in Heart Failure[1]

ACEI	Initial Dose	Maximum Dose
Captopril	6.25 mg tid	50 mg tid
Enalapril	2.5 mg bid	10-20 mg bid
Fosinopril	5-10 mg daily	40 mg daily
Lisinopril	2.5-5 mg daily	20-40 mg daily
Perindopril	2 mg daily	8-16 mg daily
Quinapril	5 mg bid	20 mg bid
Ramipril	1.25-2.5 mg daily	10 mg daily
Trandolapril	1 mg daily	4 mg daily

[1]From ACC/AHA Guidelines.

Dosing of ARBs in Heart Failure[1]

ARB	Initial Dose	Maximum Dose
Candesartan	4-8 mg daily	32 mg daily
Losartan	25-50 mg daily	50-100 mg daily
Valsartan	20-40 mg bid	160 mg bid

[1]From ACC/AHA Guidelines.

Initial and Target Doses for Beta-Blocker Therapy in Heart Failure[1]

Beta-Blocker	Starting Dose	Target Dose	Comment
Bisoprolol	1.25 mg daily	10 mg daily	β_1-Selective blocker Inconvenient dosage forms for initial dose titration
Carvedilol	3.125 mg bid	25 mg bid (≤85 kg) 50 mg bid (>85 kg)	β-Nonselective blocker α_1-Blocking properties
Carvedilol phosphate, extended release	10 mg daily	80 mg daily[2]	
Metoprolol succinate, extended release	12.5-25 mg daily	200 mg daily	β_1-Selective blocker

[1]From ACC/AHA Guidelines.

[2]Equivalent to carvedilol immediate release 25 mg twice daily

Conversion From Immediate Release to Extended Release Carvedilol (Coreg CR®)

Carvedilol Immediate Release Dose	Carvedilol Phosphate Extended Release Dose
3.125 mg twice daily	10 mg once daily
6.25 mg twice daily	20 mg once daily
12.5 mg twice daily	40 mg once daily
25 mg twice daily	80 mg once daily

References

Brater DC, "Diuretic Therapy," *N Engl J Med*, 1998, 339(6):387-95.

Granger CB, McMurray JJ, Yusuf S, et al, "Effects of Candesartan in Patients With Chronic Heart Failure and Reduced Left-Ventricular Systolic Function Intolerant to Angiotensin-Converting-Enzyme Inhibitors: The CHARM-Alternative Trial," *Lancet*, 2003, 362(9386):772-6.

Hunt SA, Abraham WT, Chin MH, et al, "2009 Focused Update Incorporated Into the ACC/AHA 2005 Guidelines for the Diagnosis and Management of Heart Failure in Adults A Report of the American College of Cardiology Foundation/American Heart Association Task Force on Practice Guidelines Developed in Collaboration With the International Society for Heart and Lung Transplantation," *J Am Coll Cardiol*, 2009, 53(15):e1-e90.

McMurray JJ, Ostergren J, Swedberg K, et al, "Effects of Candesartan in Patients With Chronic Heart Failure and Reduced Left-Ventricular Systolic Function Taking Angiotensin-Converting-Enzyme Inhibitors: The CHARM-Added Trial," *Lancet*, 2003, 362(9386):767-71.

Taylor AL, Ziesche S, Yancy C, et al, "Combination of Isosorbide Dinitrate and Hydralazine in Blacks With Heart Failure," *N Engl J Med*, 2004, 351(20):2049-57.

HELICOBACTER PYLORI TREATMENT

Multiple Drug Regimens for the Treatment of *H. pylori* Infection

Drug	Dosages	Duration of Therapy
H₂-receptor antagonist[1]	Any one given at appropriate dose	4 weeks
plus		
Bismuth subsalicylate	525 mg 4 times/day	2 weeks
plus		
Metronidazole	250 mg 4 times/day	2 weeks
plus		
Tetracycline	500 mg 4 times/day	2 weeks
Proton pump inhibitor[1]	Esomeprazole 40 mg once daily	10 days
plus		
Clarithromycin	500 mg twice daily	10 days
plus		
Amoxicillin	1000 mg twice daily	10 days
Proton pump inhibitor[1]	Lansoprazole 30 mg twice daily or Omeprazole 20 mg twice daily	10-14 days
plus		
Clarithromycin	500 mg twice daily	10-14 days
plus		
Amoxicillin	1000 mg twice daily	10-14 days
Proton pump inhibitor[1]	Rabeprazole 20 mg twice daily	7 days
plus		
Clarithromycin	500 mg twice daily	7 days
plus		
Amoxicillin	1000 mg twice daily	7 days
Proton pump inhibitor	Lansoprazole 30 mg twice daily or Omeprazole 20 mg twice daily	2 weeks
plus		
Clarithromycin	500 mg twice daily	2 weeks
plus		
Metronidazole	500 mg twice daily	2 weeks
Proton pump inhibitor	Lansoprazole 30 mg once daily or Omeprazole 20 mg once daily	2 weeks
plus		
Bismuth	525 mg 4 times/day	2 weeks
plus		
Metronidazole	500 mg 3 times/day	2 weeks
plus		
Tetracycline	500 mg 4 times/day	2 weeks

[1]FDA-approved regimen

Modified from Howden CS and Hunt RH, "Guidelines for the Management of *Helicobacter pylori* Infection," *AJG*, 1998, 93:2336.

HYPERLIPIDEMIA MANAGEMENT

MORTALITY

There is a strong link between serum cholesterol and cardiovascular mortality. This association becomes stronger in patients with established coronary artery disease. Lipid-lowering trials show that reductions in LDL cholesterol are followed by reductions in mortality. In general, each 1% fall in LDL cholesterol confers a 2% reduction in cardiovascular events. The aim of therapy for hyperlipidemia is to decrease cardiovascular morbidity and mortality by lowering cholesterol to a target level using safe and cost-effective treatment modalities. The target LDL cholesterol is determined by the number of patient risk factors (see the following Risk Factors and Goal LDL Cholesterol tables). The goal is achieved through diet, lifestyle modification, and drug therapy. The basis for these recommendations is provided by longitudinal interventional studies, demonstrating that lipid-lowering in patients with prior cardiovascular events (secondary prevention) and in patients with hyperlipidemia but no prior cardiac event (primary prevention) lowers the occurrence of future cardiovascular events, including stroke.

Major Risk Factors That Modify LDL Goals

Positive risk factors	Male ≥45 years
	Female ≥55 years
	Family history of premature coronary heart disease, defined as CHD in male first-degree relative <55 years; CHD in female first-degree relative <65 years
	Cigarette smoking
	Hypertension (blood pressure ≥140/90 mm Hg) or taking antihypertensive medication
	Low HDL (<40 mg/dL [1.03 mmol/L])
Negative risk factors	High HDL (≥60 mg/dL [1.6 mmol/L])[1]

[1] If HDL is ≥60 mg/dL, may subtract one positive risk factor.

Adult Treatment Panel (ATP) III LDL-C Goals and Cutpoints for Therapeutic Lifestyle Changes (TLC) and Drug Therapy in Different Risk Categories

Risk Category	LDL-C Goal	Initiate TLC	Consider Drug Therapy[1]
High risk: CHD[2] or CHD risk equivalents[3] (10-year risk >20%)	<100 mg/dL (optional goal: <70 mg/dL)[4]	≥100 mg/dL[5]	≥100 mg/dL[6] (<100 mg/dL: Consider drug options)[1]
Moderately high risk: ≥2 risk factors[7] (10-year risk 10% to 20%)[8]	<130 mg/dL[9]	≥130 mg/dL[5]	≥130 mg/dL (100-120 mg/dL: Consider drug options)[10]
Moderate risk: ≥2 risk factors[7] (10-year risk <10%)[8]	<130 mg/dL	≥130 mg/dL	≥160 mg/dL
Lower risk: 0-1 risk factor[11]	<160 mg/dL	≥160 mg/dL	≥190 mg/dL (160-189 mg/dL: LDL-lowering drug optional)

[1] When LDL-lowering drug therapy is employed, it is advised that intensity of therapy be sufficient to achieve at least a 30% to 40% reduction in LDL-C levels.

[2] CHD includes history of myocardial infarction, unstable angina, stable angina, coronary artery procedures (angioplasty or bypass surgery), or evidence of clinically significant myocardial ischemia.

[3] CHD risk equivalents include clinical manifestations of noncoronary forms of atherosclerotic disease (peripheral arterial disease, abdominal aortic aneurysm, and carotid artery disease [transient ischemic attacks or stroke of carotid origin or >50% obstruction of a carotid artery]), diabetes, and 2+ risk factors with 10-year risk for hard CHD >20%.

[4] Very high risk favors the optional LDL-C goal of <70 mg/dL, and in patients with high triglycerides, non-HDL-C <100 mg/dL.

[5]Any person at high risk or moderately high risk who has lifestyle-related risk factors (eg, obesity, physical inactivity, elevated triglyceride, low HDL-C, or metabolic syndrome) is a candidate for therapeutic lifestyle changes to modify these risk factors regardless of LDL-C level.

[6]If baseline LDL-C is <100 mg/dL, institution of an LDL-lowering drug is a therapeutic option on the basis of available clinical trial results. If a high-risk person has high triglycerides or low HDL-C, combining a fibrate or nicotinic acid with an LDL-lowering drug can be considered.

[7]Risk factors include cigarette smoking, hypertension (BP ≥140/90 mm Hg or on antihypertensive medication), low HDL cholesterol (<40 mg/dL), family history of premature CHD (CHD in male first-degree relative <55 years of age; CHD in female first-degree relative <65 years of age), and age (men ≥45 years; women ≥55 years).

[8]Electronic 10-year risk calculators are available at www.nhlbi.nih.gov/guidelines/cholesterol.

[9]Optional LDL-C goal <100 mg/dL.

[10]For moderately high-risk persons, when LDL-C level is 100-129 mg/dL, at baseline or on lifestyle therapy, initiation of an LDL-lowering drug to achieve an LDL-C level <100 mg/dL is a therapeutic option on the basis of available clinical trial results.

[11]Almost all people with zero or 1 risk factor have a 10-year risk <10%, and 10-year risk assessment in people with zero or 1 risk factor thus not necessary.

Any person with elevated LDL cholesterol or other form of hyperlipidemia should undergo evaluation to rule out secondary dyslipidemia. Causes of secondary dyslipidemia include diabetes, hypothyroidism, obstructive liver disease, chronic renal failure, and drugs that increase LDL and decrease HDL (progestins, anabolic steroids, corticosteroids).

Elevated Serum Triglyceride Levels

Elevated serum triglyceride levels may be an independent risk factor for coronary heart disease. Factors that contribute to hypertriglyceridemia include obesity, inactivity, cigarette smoking, excess alcohol intake, high carbohydrate diets (>60% of energy intake), type 2 diabetes, chronic renal failure, nephrotic syndrome, certain medications (corticosteroids, estrogens, retinoids, higher doses of beta-blockers), and genetic disorders. Non-HDL cholesterol (total cholesterol minus HDL cholesterol) is a secondary focus for clinicians treating patients with high serum triglyceride levels (≥200 mg/dL). The goal for non-HDL cholesterol in patients with high serum triglyceride levels can be set 30 mg/dL higher than usual LDL cholesterol goals. Patients with serum triglyceride levels <200 mg/dL should aim for the target LDL cholesterol goal.

ATP classification of serum triglyceride levels:
- Normal triglycerides: <150 mg/dL
- Borderline-high: 150-199 mg/dL
- High: 200-499 mg/dL
- Very high: ≥500 mg/dL

NONDRUG THERAPY

Dietary therapy and lifestyle modifications should be individualized for each patient. A total lifestyle change is recommended for all patients. Dietary and lifestyle modifications should be tried for 3 months, if deemed appropriate. Nondrug and drug therapy should be initiated simultaneously in patients with highly elevated cholesterol (see LDL Cholesterol Goals and Cutpoints for Therapeutic Lifestyle Changes and Drug Therapy in Different Risk Categories table). Increasing physical activity and smoking cessation will aid in the treatment of hyperlipidemia and improve cardiovascular health.

Note: Refer to the National Cholesterol Education Program reference for details concerning the calculation of 10-year risk of CHD using Framingham risk scoring. Risk assessment tool is available on-line at http://hin.nhlbi.nih.gov/atpiii/calculator. asp?usertype=prof, last accessed March 14, 2002.

Total Lifestyle Change (TLC) Diet

	Recommended Intake
Total fat	25%-35% of total calories
Saturated fat[1]	<7% of total calories
Polyunsaturated fat	≤10% of total calories
Monounsaturated fat	≤20% of total calories
Carbohydrates[2]	50%-60% of total calories
Fiber	20-30 g/day
Protein	~15% of total calories
Cholesterol	<200 mg/day
Total calories[3]	Balance energy intake and expenditure to maintain desirable body weight/prevent weight gain

[1] *Trans* fatty acids (partially hydrogenated oils) intake should be kept low. These are found in potato chips, other snack foods, margarines and shortenings, and fast-foods.

[2] Complex carbohydrates including grains (especially whole grains, fruits, and vegetables).

[3] Daily energy expenditure should include at least moderate physical activity.

DRUG THERAPY

Drug therapy should be selected based on the patient's lipid profile, concomitant disease states, and the cost of therapy. The following table lists specific advantages and disadvantages for various classes of lipid-lowering medications. The expected reduction in lipids with therapy is listed in the Lipid-Lowering Agents table. Refer to individual drug monographs for detailed information.

Advantages and Disadvantages of Specific Lipid-Lowering Therapies

	Advantages	Disadvantages
Bile acid sequestrants	Good choice for ↑ LDL, especially when combined with a statin (↓ LDL ≤50%); low potential for systemic side effects; good choice for younger patients	May increase triglycerides; higher incidence of adverse effects; moderately expensive; drug interactions; inconvenient dosing
Niacin	Good choice for almost any lipid abnormality; inexpensive; greatest increase in HDL	High incidence of adverse effects; may adversely affect type 2 DM (with high dose >1.5 g/day) and gout; sustained release niacin may decrease the incidence of flushing and circumvent the need for multiple daily dosing; sustained release niacin may not increase HDL cholesterol or decrease triglycerides as well as immediate release niacin .
HMG-CoA reductase inhibitors	Produces greatest ↓ in LDL; generally well-tolerated; convenient once-daily dosing; proven decrease in mortality	Expensive
Fibric acid derivatives	Good choice in patients with ↑ triglycerides where niacin is contraindicated or not well-tolerated	Variable effects on LDL
Ezetimibe	Additional cholesterol-lowering effects when combined with HMG-CoA reductase inhibitors	Effects similar to bile acid sequestrants

Lipid-Lowering Agents

Drug	Dose / Day	Effect on LDL (%)	Effect on HDL (%)	Effect on TG (%)
HMG-CoA Reductase Inhibitors				
Atorvastatin	10 mg	-39	+6	-19
	20 mg	-43	+9	-26
	40 mg	-50	+6	-29
	80 mg	-60	+5	-37
Fluvastatin	20 mg	-22	+3	-12
	40 mg	-25	+4	-14
	80 mg	-36	+6	-18
Lovastatin	10 mg	-21	+5	-10
	20 mg	-27	+6	-8
	40 mg	-31	+5	-8
	80 mg	-40	+9.5	-19
Pitavastatin	1 mg	-32	+8	-15
	2 mg	-39	+7	-27
	4 mg	-45	+7	-28
Pravastatin	10 mg	-22	+7	-15
	20 mg	-32	+2	-11
	40 mg	-34	+12	-24
	80 mg	-37	+3	-19
Rosuvastatin	5 mg	-45	+13	-35
	10 mg	-52	+14	-10
	20 mg	-55	+8	-23
	40 mg	-63	+10	-28
Simvastatin	5 mg	-26	+10	-12
	10 mg	-30	+12	-15
	20 mg	-38	+8	-19
	40 mg	-41	+13	-28
	80 mg	-47	+16	-33
Bile Acid Sequestrants				
Cholestyramine	4-24 g	-15 to -30	+3 to +5	+0 to +20
Colestipol	7-30 g	-15 to -30	+3 to +5	+0 to +20
Colesevelam	6 tablets	-15	+3	+10
	7 tablets	-18	+3	+9
Fibric Acid Derivatives				
Fenofibrate	67-200 mg	-20 to -25	+1 to +20	-30 to -50
Gemfibrozil	600 mg twice daily	-5 to -10[1]	+10 to +20	-40 to -60
Niacin	1.5-6 g	-21 to -27	+10 to +35	-10 to -50
2-Azetidinone				
Ezetimibe	10 mg	-18	+1	-8
Omega-3-Acid Ethyl Esters	4 g	+44.5	+9.1	-44.9
Combination Products				
Ezetimibe and simvastatin	10/10 mg	-45	+8	-23
	10/20 mg	-52	+10	-24
	10/40 mg	-55	+6	-23
	10/80 mg	-60	+6	-31
Niacin and lovastatin	1000/20 mg	-30	+20	-32
	1000/40 mg	-36	+20	-39
	1500/40 mg	-37	+27	-44
	2000/40 mg	-42	+30	-44
Niacin and simvastatin	1000/20 mg	-12	+21	-27
	1000/40 mg	-7	+15	-23
	2000/20 mg	-14	+29	-38
	2000/40 mg	-5	+24	-32

[1]May increase LDL in some patients.

Recommended Liver Function Monitoring for HMG-CoA Reductase Inhibitors

Agent	Initial and After Elevation in Dose	6 Weeks[1]	12 Weeks[1]	Periodically
Atorvastatin (Lipitor®)	x		x	x
Fluvastatin (Lescol®)	x		x	x
Lovastatin (Mevacor®)	x	x	x	x
Pitavastatin (Livalo®)	x		x	x
Pravastatin (Pravachol®)	x			x
Rosuvastatin (Crestor®)	x		x	x
Simvastatin (Zocor®)	x			x

[1]After initiation of therapy or any elevation in dose.

Progression of Drug Therapy in Primary Prevention

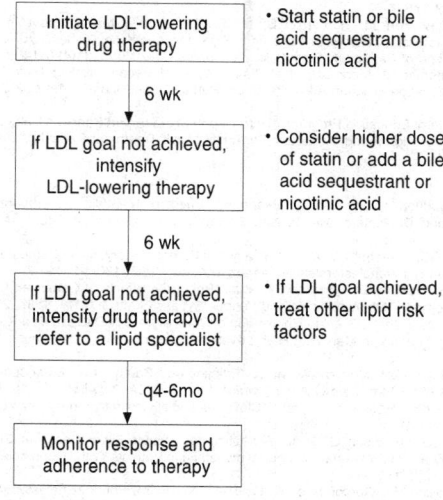

Initiate LDL-lowering drug therapy
- Start statin or bile acid sequestrant or nicotinic acid

↓ 6 wk

If LDL goal not achieved, intensify LDL-lowering therapy
- Consider higher dose of statin or add a bile acid sequestrant or nicotinic acid

↓ 6 wk

If LDL goal not achieved, intensify drug therapy or refer to a lipid specialist
- If LDL goal achieved, treat other lipid risk factors

↓ q4-6mo

Monitor response and adherence to therapy

DRUG SELECTION

Lipid Profile	Monotherapy	Combination Therapies
Increased LDL with normal HDL and triglycerides (TG)	Resin Niacin[1] Statin	Resin plus niacin[1] or statin Statin plus niacin[1,2]
Increased LDL and increased TG (200-499 mg/dL)[2]	Intensify LDL-lowering therapy	Statin plus niacin[1,3] Statin plus fibrate[3]
Increased LDL and increased TG (≥500 mg/dL)[2]	Consider combination therapy (niacin,[1] fibrates, statin)	
Increased TG	Niacin[1] Fibrates	Niacin[1] plus fibrates
Increased LDL and low HDL	Niacin[1] Statin	Statin plus niacin[1,2]

[1]Avoid in diabetics.

[2]Emphasize weight reduction and increased physical activity.

[3]Risk of myopathy with combination.

Resins = bile acid sequestrants; statins = HMG-CoA reductase inhibitors; fibrates = fibric acid derivatives (eg, gemfibrozil, fenofibrate).

COMBINATION DRUG THERAPY

If after at least 6 weeks of therapy at the maximum recommended or tolerated dose, the patient's LDL cholesterol is not at target, consider optimizing nondrug measures, prescribing a higher dose of current lipid-lowering drug, or adding another lipid-lowering medication to the current therapy. Successful drug combinations include statin and niacin, statin and bile acid sequestrant, or niacin and bile acid sequestrant. At maximum recommended doses, LDL cholesterol may be decreased by 50% to 60% with combination therapy. This is the same reduction achieved by atorvastatin 40 mg twice daily. If a bile acid sequestrant is used with other lipid-lowering agents, space doses 1 hour before or 4 hours after the bile acid sequestrant administration. Statins combined with either fenofibrate, gemfibrozil, or niacin increase the risk of rhabdomyolysis. In this situation, patient education (muscle pain/weakness) and careful follow-up are warranted.

References

Guidelines

American Diabetes Association, "Standards of Medical Care in Diabetes - 2008," *Diabetes Care*, 2008, 31(Suppl 1):S12-54.

Brunzell JD, Davidson M, Furberg CD, et al, "Lipoprotein Management in Patients With Cardiometabolic Risk: Consensus Statement From the American Diabetes Association and the American College of Cardiology Foundation," *Diabetes Care*, 2008, 31(4):811-22.

Grundy SM, Cleeman JI, Merz CN, et al, "Implications of Recent Clinical Trials for the National Cholesterol Education Program Adult Treatment Panel III Guidelines," *J Am Coll Cardiol*, 2004, 44 (3):720-32.

National Cholesterol Education Program, "Third Report of the Expert Panel on Detection, Evaluation, and Treatment of High Blood Cholesterol in Adults (Adult Treatment Panel III)," *JAMA*, 2001, 285 (19):2486-97.

Others

Berthold HK, Sudhop T, and von Bergmann K, "Effect of a Garlic Oil Preparation on Serum Lipoproteins and Cholesterol Metabolism: A Randomized Controlled Trial," *JAMA*, 1998, 279 (23):1900-2.

Bertolini S, Bon GB, Campbell LM, et al, "Efficacy and Safety of Atorvastatin Compared to Pravastatin in Patients With Hypercholesterolemia," *Atherosclerosis*, 1997, 130(1-2):191-7.

Blankenhorn DH, Nessim SA, Johnson RL, et al, "Beneficial Effects of Combined Colestipol-Niacin Therapy on Coronary Atherosclerosis and Venous Bypass Grafts," *JAMA*, 1987, 257(23):3233-40.

Brown G, Albers JJ, Fisher LD, et al, "Regression of Coronary Artery Disease as a Result of Intensive Lipid-Lowering Therapy in Men With High Levels of Apolipoprotein B," *N Engl J Med*, 1990, 323 (19):1289-98.

Capuzzi DM, Guyton JR, Morgan JM, et al, "Efficacy and Safety of an Extended-Release Niacin (Niaspan®): A Long-Term Study," *Am J Cardiol*, 1998, 82(12A):74U-81U.

Coronary Drug Project Research Program, "Clofibrate and Niacin in Coronary Heart Disease," *JAMA*, 1975, 231(4):360-81.

Dart A, Jerums G, Nicholson G, et al, "A Multicenter, Double-Blind, One-Year Study Comparing Safety and Efficacy of Atorvastatin Versus Simvastatin in Patients With Hypercholesterolemia," *Am J Cardiol*, 1997, 80(1):39-44.

Davidson MH, Dillon MA, Gordon B, et al, "Colesevelam Hydrochloride (Cholestagel): A New Potent Bile Acid Sequestrant Associated With a Low Incidence of Gastrointestinal Side Effects," *Arch Intern Med*, 1999, 159(16):1893-900.

Davidson M, McKenney J, Stein E, et al, "Comparison of One-Year Efficacy and Safety of Atorvastatin Versus Lovastatin in Primary Hypercholesterolemia," *Am J Cardiol*, 1997, 79 (11):1475-81.

Frick MH, Heinonen OP, Huttunen JK, et al, "Helsinki Heart Study: Primary-Prevention Trial With Gemfibrozil in Middle-Aged Men With Dyslipidemia," *N Engl J Med*, 1987, 317(20):1237-45.

Garber AM, Browner WS, and Hulley SB, "Clinical Guideline, Part 2: Cholesterol Screening in Asymptomatic Adults, Revisited," *Ann Intern Med*, 1995, 124(5):518-31.

Johannesson M, Jonsson B, Kjekshus J, et al, "Cost-Effectiveness of Simvastatin Treatment to Lower Cholesterol Levels in Patients With Coronary Heart Disease. Scandinavian Simvastatin Survival Study Group," *N Engl N Med*, 1997, 336(5):332-6.

Jones P, Kafonek S, Laurora I, et al, "Comparative Dose Efficacy Study of Atorvastatin Versus Simvastatin, Pravastatin, Lovastatin, and Fluvastatin in Patients With Hypercholesterolemia," *Am J Cardiol*, 1998, 81(5):582-7.

Kasiske BL, Ma JZ, Kalil RS, et al, "Effects of Antihypertensive Therapy on Serum Lipids," *Ann Intern Med*, 1995, 122(2):133-41.

Lipid Research Clinics Program, "The Lipid Research Clinics Coronary Primary Prevention Trial Results: I. Reduction in Incidence of Coronary Heart Disease," *JAMA*, 1984, 251(3):351-64.

Mauro VF and Tuckerman CE, "Ezetimibe for Management of Hypercholesterolemia," *Ann Pharmacother*, 2003, 37(6):839-48.

Multiple Risk Factor Intervention Trial Research Group, "Multiple Risk Factor Intervention Trial: Risk Factor Changes and Mortality Results," *JAMA*, 1982, 248(12):1465-77.

Pitt B, Waters D, Brown WV, et al, "Aggressive Lipid-Lowering Therapy Compared With Angioplasty in Stable Coronary Artery Disease. Atorvastatin Versus Revascularization Treatment Investigators," *N Engl J Med*, 1999, 341(2):70-6.

Ross SD, Allen IE, Connelly JE, et al, "Clinical Outcomes in Statin Treatment Trials: A Meta-Analysis," *Arch Intern Med*, 1999, 159(15):1793-802.

Sacks FM, Pfeffer MA, Moye LA, et al, "The Effect of Pravastatin on Coronary Events After Myocardial Infarction in Patients With Average Cholesterol Levels," *N Engl J Med*, 1996, 335 (14):1001-9.

Scandinavian Simvastatin Survival Study, "Randomized Trial of Cholesterol Lowering in 4444 Patients With Coronary Heart Disease: The Scandinavian Simvastatin Survival Study (4S)," *Lancet*, 1994, 344(8934):1383-9.

Schrott HG, Bittner V, Vittinghoff E, et al, "Adherence to National Cholesterol Education Program Treatment Goals in Postmenopausal Women With Heart Disease. The Heart and Estrogen/Progestin Replacement Study (HERS)," *JAMA*, 1997, 277(16):1281-6.

Shepherd J, Cobbe SM, Ford I, et al, "Prevention of Coronary Heart Disease With Pravastatin in Men With Hypercholesterolemia, The West of Scotland Coronary Prevention Study Group," *N Engl J Med*, 1995, 333(20):1301-7.

Stein EA, Davidson MH, Dobs AS, et al, "Efficacy and Safety of Simvastatin 80 mg/day in Hypercholesterolemic Patients. The Expanded Dose Simvastatin U.S. Study Group," *Am J Cardiol*, 1998, 82(3):311-6.

HYPERTENSION

The optimal blood pressure for adults is <120/80 mm Hg. Consistent systolic pressure ≥140 mm Hg or a diastolic pressure ≥90 mm Hg, in the absence of a secondary cause, defines hypertension. Hypertension affects approximately 25% (50 million people) in the United States. Of those patients on antihypertensive medication, only one in three have their blood pressure controlled (<140/90 mm Hg).

Controlling systolic hypertension has been much more difficult than controlling diastolic hypertension. Educating patients in lifestyle management, cardiovascular risk reduction, and drug therapy aids in improving the morbidity and mortality of patients with hypertension.

The Seventh Report of the Joint National Committee (JNC VII) is an excellent reference and guide for the treatment of hypertension (Chobanian AV, Bakris GL, Black HR, et al, "The Seventh Report of the Joint National Committee on Prevention, Detection, Evaluation, and Treatment of High Blood Pressure: The JNC 7 Report," *JAMA*, 2003, 289(19):2560-71. For adults, hypertension is classified in stages (see following table).

Adult Classification of Blood Pressure

Category	Systolic (mm Hg)		Diastolic (mm Hg)
Normal	<120	and	<80
Prehypertension	120-139	or	80-89
Hypertension			
Stage 1	140-159	or	90-99
Stage 2	≥160	or	≥100

Adapted from Chobanian AV, Bakris GL, Black HR, et al, "The Seventh Report of the Joint National Committee on Prevention, Detection, Evaluation, and Treatment of High Blood Pressure: The JNC 7 Report," *JAMA*, 2003, 289(19):2560-71.

Normal Blood Pressure in Children

Age (y)	Girls' SBP / DBP (mm Hg)		Boys' SBP / DBP (mm Hg)	
	50th Percentile for Height	75th Percentile for Height	50th Percentile for Height	75th Percentile for Height
1	104/58	105/59	102/57	104/58
6	111/73	112/73	114/74	115/75
12	123/80	124/81	123/81	125/82
17	129/84	130/85	136/87	138/88

SBP = systolic blood pressure.

DBP = diastolic blood pressure.

Adapted from the report by the NHBPEP Working Group on Hypertension Control in Children and Adolescents, *Pediatrics*, 1996, 98(4 Pt 1):649-58.

PATIENT ASSESSMENT

- **Cardiovascular Risk Factors:** <u>Hypertension</u>, cigarette smoking, <u>obesity</u> (BMI ≥30), inactive lifestyle, <u>dyslipidemia</u>, <u>diabetes mellitus</u>, microalbuminuria or estimated GFR <60 mL/minute, age (>55 years for men, >65 years for women), family history of premature cardiovascular disease (men <55 years or women >65 years).

  Components of metabolic syndrome include <u>hypertension</u>, <u>obesity</u>, <u>dyslipidemia</u>, <u>diabetes mellitus</u>.
- Identify causes of high BP.
- Assess target-organ damage and CVD.

Target-Organ Disease

Organ System	Manifestation
Cardiac	Clinical, ECG, or radiologic evidence of coronary artery disease; prior MI, angina, post-CABG; left ventricular hypertrophy (LVH); left ventricular dysfunction or cardiac failure, prior coronary revascularization
Cerebrovascular	Transient ischemic attack or stroke
Peripheral vascular	Absence of pulses in extremities (except dorsalis pedis), claudication, aneurysm, peripheral arterial disease
Renal	Serum creatinine ≥130 µmol/L (1.5 mg/dL); proteinuria (≥1+); microalbuminuria, chronic kidney disease
Eye	Hemorrhages or exudates, with or without papilledema; retinopathy

Adapted from Chobanian AV, Bakris GL, Black HR, et al, "The Seventh Report of the Joint National Committee on Prevention, Detection, Evaluation, and Treatment of High Blood Pressure: The JNC 7 Report," *JAMA*, 2003, 289(19):2560-71.

BLOOD PRESSURE MEASUREMENT

At an office visit, patients should be seated quietly for ≥5 minutes in a chair with feet on the floor and arm supported at heart level. At least two measurements should be made. Patients should be given their results and their goal BP.

Ambulatory BP monitoring is useful in evaluating "white coat hypertension" (no end-organ damage), drug resistance, hypotensive symptoms, episodic hypertension, and autonomic dysfunction. Ambulatory BP monitoring correlates better with end-organ damage than office measurements.

Having patients monitor their own BP helps to improve compliance and provides information on response to therapeutic interventions.

Based on these initial assessments, treatment strategies for patients with hypertension are stratified based on their blood pressure and comorbidities (compelling indications).

Management of Blood Pressure

BP Classification	Management: Based upon highest BP category		
	Lifestyle Modification	Initial Therapy Without Compelling Indication	Initial Therapy With Compelling Indication[1]
Normal	Encourage	None	None
Prehypertensive	Yes	None	Treat patients with chronic kidney disease or diabetes to BP goal of <130/80 mm Hg
Hypertension			
Stage 1	Yes	Thiazide-type diuretic for most; consider ACEI, ARB, β-blocker, CCB, or combination	Drugs for the compelling indications; other antihypertensives as needed
Stage 2	Yes	Two drug combos (typically a thiazide-type diuretic and ACEI or ARB or β-blocker or CCB). Use combo cautiously in patients at risk for orthostasis.	Drugs for the compelling indications; other antihypertensives as needed

[1]Compelling Indication: Conditions for which specific classes of antihypertensive drugs have proven beneficial.

Adapted from Chobanian AV, Bakris GL, Black HR, et al, "The Seventh Report of the Joint National Committee on Prevention, Detection, Evaluation, and Treatment of High Blood Pressure: The JNC 7 Report," *JAMA*, 2003, 289(19):2560-71.

◀ ACHIEVING BLOOD PRESSURE CONTROL

Treatment of hypertension should be individualized. Lower blood pressure (goal <130/80 mm Hg) should be achieved in patients with diabetes or chronic renal disease. The following Hypertension Treatment Algorithm may be used to select specific antihypertensives based on compelling indications.

Special consideration for starting combination therapy should be made in each patient.

Starting drug therapy at a low dose and titrating upward if blood pressure is not controlled is recommended.

Most patients with hypertension will require two or more drugs to achieve their BP goals.

Adding a second drug from a different class will help when a single drug at reasonable doses has failed to achieve the goal.

If the untreated BP is >20/10 mm Hg away from the goal, consider initiating therapy with two drugs. Use caution in those at risk for orthostasis (eg, diabetics, geriatrics, and those with autonomic dysfunction).

Low-dose aspirin therapy should be considered when BP is controlled; use in uncontrolled hypertension can increase the risk of hemorrhagic stroke.

Lifestyle modification and risk reduction should always be reviewed and reinforced.

MONITORING THERAPY

Generally, monthly follow-up is recommended until BP control is reached.

More frequent monitoring is required for those patients with Stage 2 hypertension or those with complications.

Serum potassium and serum creatinine should be monitored at least twice yearly.

When BP is at goal and stable, follow-up can be maintained every 3-6 months. Treat other cardiovascular risk factors if present.

Hypertension Treatment Algorithm

> **Begin or continue lifestyle modifications**

↓

> **Not at goal blood pressure** (<140/90 mm Hg or <130/80 mm Hg for patients with diabetes or chronic renal disease)

↓

Initial Drug Choice

Hypertension

<u>Stage I</u>
Thiazide-type diuretic for most. Consider ACEI, ARB, β-blocker, CCB, or combo.

<u>Stage 2</u>
Two-drug combo for most (typically thiazide-type diuretic + ACEI or ARB or β-blocker or CCB)

Compelling Indications

Chronic kidney disease
- ACEI
- ARB

Diabetes mellitus
- ACEI
- ARB
- β-blocker
- CCB
- Diuretic

Heart failure
- ACEI
- Aldosterone blocker
- ARB
- β-blocker
- Diuretic

High coronary risk
- ACEI
- β-blocker
- CCB
- Diuretic

Myocardial infarction
- ACEI
- Aldosterone blocker
- β-blocker

Recurrent stroke prevention
- ACEI
- Diuretic

↓

> **Not at goal blood pressure**

↓   ↓

Optimize dosages or add additional drugs until goal BP achieved.

Consider consultation with hypertension specialist.

Additional Considerations for Specific Therapies

Indication	Drug Therapy
Atrial tachyarrhythmias	β-blocker, CCB (non-DHP)
Chronic kidney disease	
Cl_{cr} <60 mL/min or albuminuria	ACEI or ARB
Cl_{cr} <30 mL/min	Increase loop diuretic
Diabetes	Thiazide diuretic, β-blocker, ACEI, ARB, CCB
Nephropathy	ACEI, ARB
Essential tremor	β-blocker (noncardioselective)
Heart failure	
Ventricular dysfunction (asymptomatic)	ACEI, β-blocker
Ventricular dysfunction (symptomatic)	ACEI, β-blocker, ARB, aldosterone blocker, loop diuretic
Hypertensive women who are pregnant	Methyldopa, β-blocker, vasodilator
Ischemic heart disease	
Angina	β-blocker, CCB (long-acting)
Acute coronary syndromes	β-blocker, ACEI
Migraine	β-blocker (noncardioselective), CCB (long-acting, non-DHP)
Osteoporosis	Thiazide diuretic
Perioperative hypertension	β-blocker
Prostatism (BPH)	Alpha-adrenergic blocking agent
Raynaud syndrome	CCB
Thyrotoxicosis	β-blocker

Note: ACEI = angiotensin-converting enzyme inhibitor; ARB = angiotensin receptor blocker; CCB = calcium channel blocker; DHP = dihydropyridine.

May Have Unfavorable Effects on Comorbid Conditions

Condition	Drug Therapy to Avoid
Angioedema	ACEI
Bronchospastic disease	β-blocker
Gout	Thiazide diuretic
Heart block (second or third degree)	β-blocker, CCB (non-DHP)
Hyponatremia	Thiazide diuretic
Potassium >5 mEq/L before treatment	Potassium sparing diuretic, aldosterone antagonist
Pregnancy or those likely to become pregnant	ACEI, ARB

Note: ACEI = angiotensin-converting enzyme inhibitor; ARB = angiotensin receptor blocker; CCB = calcium channel blocker; DHP = dihydropyridine.

HYPERTENSIVE EMERGENCIES AND URGENCIES

General Treatment Principles in the Treatment of Hypertensive Emergencies

Principle	Considerations
Admit the patient to the hospital, preferably in the ICU. Monitor vital signs appropriately.	Establish I.V. access and place patient on a cardiac monitor. Place a femoral intra-arterial line and pulmonary arterial catheter, if indicated, to assess cardiopulmonary function and intravascular volume status.
Perform rapid but thorough history and physical examination.	Determine cause of, or precipitating factors to, hypertensive crisis if possible (remember to obtain a medication history including Rx, OTC, and illicit drugs). Obtain details regarding any prior history of hypertension (severity, duration, treatment), as well as other coexisting illnesses. Assess the extent of hypertensive end organ damage. Determine if a hypertensive urgency or emergency exists.
Determine goal blood pressure based on premorbid level, duration, severity and rapidity of increase of blood pressure, concomitant medical conditions, race, and age.	Acute decreases in blood pressure to normal or subnormal levels during the initial treatment period may reduce perfusion to the brain, heart, and kidneys, and must be avoided except in specific instances (ie, dissecting aortic aneurysm). Gradually establish a normal (or reasonable) blood pressure over the next 1-2 weeks.
Select an appropriate antihypertensive depending on the individual patient and clinical setting.	Initiate a controlled decrease in blood pressure. Avoid concomitant administration of multiple agents that may cause precipitous falls in blood pressure. Select the agent with the best hemodynamic profile based on the primary treatment goal. Avoid diuretics and sodium restriction during the initial treatment period unless there is a clear clinical indication (ie, CHF, pulmonary edema). Avoid sedating antihypertensives in patients with hypertensive encephalopathy, CVA, or other CNS disorders in whom mental status must be monitored. Use caution with direct vasodilating agents that induce reflex tachycardia or increase cardiac output in patients with coronary heart disease, history of angina or myocardial infarction, or dissecting aortic aneurysm. Preferably choose an agent that does not adversely affect glomerular filtration rate or renal blood flow and also agents that have favorable effects on cerebral blood flow and its autoregulation, especially for patients with hypertensive encephalopathy or CVAs. Select the most efficacious agent with the fewest adverse effects based on the underlying cause of the hypertensive crisis and other individual patient factors.
Initiate a chronic antihypertensive regimen after the patient's blood pressure is stabilized	Begin oral antihypertensive therapy once goal blood pressure is achieved before gradually tapering parenteral medications. Select the best oral regimen based on cost, ease of administration, adverse effect profile, and concomitant medical conditions.

Oral Agents Used in the Treatment of Hypertensive Urgencies

Drug	Dose	Onset	Cautions
Captopril[1]	P.O.: 25 mg, repeat as required	15-30 min	Hypotension, renal failure in bilateral renal artery stenosis
Clonidine	P.O.: 0.1-0.2 mg, repeated every hour as needed to a total dose of 0.6 mg	30-60 min	Hypotension, drowsiness, dry mouth
Labetalol	P.O.: 200-400 mg, repeat every 2-3 h	30 min to 2 h	Bronchoconstriction, heart block, orthostatic hypotension

[1]There is no clearly defined clinical advantage in the use of sublingual over oral routes of administration with these agents.

Recommendations for the Use of Intravenous Antihypertensive Drugs in Selected Hypertensive Emergencies

Condition	Agent(s) of Choice	Agent(s) to Avoid or Use With Caution	General Treatment Principles
Hypertensive encephalopathy	Nitroprusside, labetalol	Methyldopa, reserpine	Avoid drugs with CNS-sedating effects.
Acute intracranial or subarachnoid hemorrhage	Nicardipine,[1] nitroprusside	β-blocker	Careful titration with a short-acting agent.
Cerebral infarction	Nicardipine,[1] nitroprusside, labetalol	β-blocker, minoxidil	Careful titration with a short-acting agent. Avoid agents that may decrease cerebral blood flow.
Head trauma	Esmolol, labetalol	Methyldopa, reserpine, nitroprusside, nitroglycerin, hydralazine	Avoid drugs with CNS-sedating effects, or those that may increase intracranial pressure.
Acute myocardial infarction, myocardial ischemia	Nitroglycerin, nicardipine[1] (calcium channel blocker), labetalol	Hydralazine, minoxidil	Avoid drugs which cause reflex tachycardia and increased myocardial oxygen consumption.
Acute pulmonary edema	Nitroprusside, nitroglycerin, loop diuretics	β-blocker (labetalol), minoxidil, methyldopa	Avoid drugs which may cause sodium and water retention and edema exacerbation.
Renal dysfunction	Hydralazine, calcium channel blocker	Nitroprusside, ACE inhibitors, β-blocker (labetalol)	Avoid drugs with increased toxicity in renal failure and those that may cause decreased renal blood flow.
Eclampsia	Hydralazine, labetalol, nitroprusside[2]	Diuretics	Avoid drugs that may cause adverse fetal effects, compromise placental circulation, or decrease cardiac output.
Pheochromo- cytoma	Phentolamine, nitroprusside, β-blocker (eg, esmolol) only after alpha blockade (phentolamine)	β-blocker in the absence of alpha blockade, methyldopa, minoxidil	Use drugs of proven efficacy and specificity. Unopposed beta-blockade may exacerbate hypertension.
Dissecting aortic aneurysm	Nitroprusside and beta-blockade	Hydralazine, minoxidil	Avoid drugs which may increase cardiac output.
Postoperative hypertension	Nitroprusside, nicardipine,[1] labetalol, clevidipine		Avoid drugs which may exacerbate postoperative ileus.

[1]The use of nicardipine in these situations is by the recommendation of the author based on a review of the literature.

[2]Reserve nitroprusside for eclamptic patients with life-threatening hypertension unresponsive to other agents due to the potential risk to the fetus (cyanide and thiocyanate metabolites may cross the placenta).

Selected Intravenous Agents for Hypertensive Emergencies

Drug	Dose[1]	Onset of Action	Duration of Action	Adverse Effects[2]	Special Indications
Vasodilators					
Sodium nitroprusside	0.25-10 mcg/kg/min as I.V. infusion[3] (max: 10 min only)	Immediate	1-2 min	Nausea, vomiting, muscle twitching, sweating, thiocyanate and cyanide intoxication	Most hypertensive emergencies; caution with high intracranial pressure or azotemia
Nicardipine hydrochloride	5-15 mg/h I.V.	5-10 min	1-4 h	Tachycardia, headache, flushing, local phlebitis	Most hypertensive emergencies except acute heart failure; caution with coronary ischemia
Clevidipine butyrate	1-21 mg/h I.V.	2-4 min	5-15 min	Atrial fibrillation, nausea, insomnia, fever	Most hypertensive emergencies; caution with lipid disorder
Fenoldopam mesylate	0.1-0.3 mcg/kg/min as I.V. infusion	<5 min	30 min	Tachycardia, headache, nausea, flushing	Most hypertensive emergencies; caution with glaucoma
Nitroglycerin	5-100 mcg/min as I.V. infusion[3]	2-5 min	3-5 min	Headache, vomiting, methemoglobinemia, tolerance with prolonged use	Coronary ischemia
Enalaprilat	1.25-5 mg every 6 hours I.V.	15-30 min	6 h	Precipitous fall in pressure in high-renin states; response variable	Acute left ventricular failure; avoid in acute myocardial infarction
Hydralazine hydrochloride	10-20 mg I.V. 10-50 mg I.M.	10-20 min 20-30 min	3-8 h	Tachycardia, flushing, headache, vomiting, aggravation of angina	Eclampsia
Adrenergic Inhibitors					
Labetalol hydrochloride	20-80 mg I.V. bolus every 10 min; 0.5-2 mg/min as I.V. infusion	5-10 min	3-6 h	Vomiting, scalp tingling, burning in throat, dizziness, nausea, heart block, orthostatic hypotension	Most hypertensive emergencies except acute heart failure
Esmolol hydrochloride	250-500 mcg/kg/min for 1 min, then 50-100 mcg/kg/min for 4 min; may repeat	1-2 min	10-20 min	Hypotension, nausea	Aortic dissection, perioperative
Phentolamine	5-15 mg I.V.	1-2 min	3-10 min	Tachycardia, flushing, headache	Catecholamine excess

[1]These doses may vary from those in the *Physicians' Desk Reference* (51st edition).

[2]Hypotension may occur with all agents.

[3]Require special delivery system.

References

Guidelines

"1999 World Health Organization-International Society of Hypertension Guidelines for the Management of Hypertension. Guidelines Subcommittee," *J Hypertens*, 1999, 17(2):151-83.

Chobanian AV, Bakris GL, Black HR, et al, "The Seventh Report of the Joint National Committee on Prevention, Detection, Evaluation, and Treatment of High Blood Pressure: The JNC 7 Report," *JAMA*, 2003, 289(19):2560-72.

National High Blood Pressure Education Program Working Group on Hypertension Control in Children and Adolescents, "Update on the 1987 Task Force Report on High Blood Pressure in Children and Adolescents: A Working Group Report From the National High Blood Pressure Education Program," *Pediatrics*, 1996, 98(4 Pt 1):649-58.

National High Blood Pressure Education Program Working Group, "1995 Update of the Working Group Reports on Chronic Renal Failure and Renovascular Hypertension," *Arch Intern Med*, 1996, 156(17):1938-47.

"The Sixth Report of the National Committee on Detection, Evaluation, and Treatment of High Blood Pressure (JNC-VI)," *Arch Intern Med*, 1997, 157(21):2413-46.

Others

Appel LJ, Moore TJ, Obarzanek E, et al, "A Clinical Trial of the Effect of Dietary Patterns on Blood Pressure. The DASH Collaborative Research Group," *N Engl J Med*, 1997, 336(16):1117-24.

Epstein M and Bakris G, "Newer Approaches to Antihypertensive Therapy: Use of Fixed-Dose Combination Therapy," *Arch Intern Med*, 1996, 156(17):1969-78.

Estacio RO and Schrier RW, "Antihypertensive Therapy in Type II Diabetes: Implications of the Appropriate Blood Pressure Control in Diabetes (ABCD) Trial," *Am J Cardiol*, 1998, 82(9B):9R-14R.

Flack JM, Neaton J, Grimm RJ, et al, "Blood Pressure and Mortality Among Men With Prior Myocardial Infarction. The Multiple Risk Factor Intervention Trial Research Group," *Circulation*, 1995, 92(9):2437-45.

Frishman WH, Bryzinski BS, Coulson LR, et al, "A Multifactorial Trial Design to Assess Combination Therapy in Hypertension: Treatment With Bisoprolol and Hydrochlorothiazide," *Arch Intern Med*, 1994, 154(13):1461-8.

Furberg CD, Psaty BM, and Meyer JV, "Nifedipine: Dose-Related Increase in Mortality in Patients With Coronary Heart Disease," *Circulation*, 1995, 92(5):1326-31.

Glynn RJ, Brock DB, Harris T, et al, "Use of Antihypertensive Drugs and Trends in Blood Pressure in the Elderly," *Arch Intern Med*, 1995, 155:1855-60.

Gradman AH, Cutler NR, Davis PJ, et al, "Combined Enalapril and Felodipine Extended Release (ER) for Systemic Hypertension. The Enalapril-Felodipine ER Factorial Study Group," *Am J Cardiol*, 1997, 79(4):431-5.

Grimm RH Jr, Flack JM, Grandits GA, et al, "Long-Term Effects on Plasma Lipids of Diet and Drugs to Treat Hypertension. The Treatment of Mild Hypertension Study (TOMHS) Research Group," *JAMA*, 1996, 275(20):1549-56.

Grimm RH Jr, Grandits GA, Cutler JA, et al, "Relationships of Quality-of-Life Measures to Long-Term Lifestyle and Drug Treatment in the Treatment of Mild Hypertension Study. The TOMHS Research Group," *Arch Intern Med*, 1997, 157(6):638-48.

Grossman E, Messerli FH, Grodzicki T, et al, "Should a Moratorium Be Placed on Sublingual Nifedipine Capsules Given for Hypertensive Emergencies and Pseudoemergencies?" *JAMA*, 1996, 276(16):1328-31.

Hansson L, Zanchetti A, Carruthers SG, et al, "Effects of Intensive Blood Pressure Lowering and Low-Dose Aspirin in Patients With Hypertension: Principal Results of the Hypertension Optimal Treatment (HOT) Randomized Trial. HOT Study Group," *Lancet*, 1998, 351(9118):1755-62.

Kaplan NM and Gifford RW Jr, "Choice of Initial Therapy for Hypertension," *JAMA*, 1996, 275(20):1577-80.

Kasiske BL, Ma JZ, Kalil RSN, et al, "Effects of Antihypertensive Therapy in Serum Lipids," *Ann Intern Med*, 1995, 122(2):133-41.

Kostis JB, Davis BR, Cutler J, et al, "Prevention of Heart Failure by Antihypertensive Drug Treatment in Older Persons With Isolated Systolic Hypertension. SHEP Cooperative Research Group," *JAMA*, 1997, 278(3):212-6.

Lazarus JM, Bourgoignie JJ, Buckalew VM, et al, "Achievement and Safety of a Low Blood Pressure Goal in Chronic Renal Disease: The Modification of Diet in Renal Disease Study Group," *Hypertension*, 1997, 29(2):641-50.

Lindheimer MD, "Hypertension in Pregnancy," *Hypertension*, 1993, 22(1):127-37.

Materson BJ, Reda DJ, Cushman WC, et al, "Single-Drug Therapy for Hypertension in Men: A Comparison of Six Antihypertensive Agents With Placebo. The Department of Veterans Affairs Cooperative Study Group on Antihypertensive Agents," *N Engl J Med*, 1993, 328(13):914-21.

Miller NH, Hill M, Kottke T, et al, "The Multi-Level Compliance Challenge: Recommendations for a Call to Action; A Statement for Healthcare Professionals," *Circulation*, 1997, 95(4):1085-90.

Neaton JD and Wentworth D, "Serum Cholesterol, Blood Pressure, Cigarette Smoking, and Death From Coronary Heart Disease: Overall Findings and Differences by Age for 316,099 White Men. The Multiple Risk Factor Intervention Trial Research Group," *Arch Intern Med*, 1992, 152(1):56-64.

Neaton JD, Grim RH, Prineas RJ, et al, "Treatment of Mild Hypertension Study. Final Results. Treatment of Mild Hypertension Study Research Group," *JAMA*, 1993, 270(6):713-24.

Oparil S, Levine JH, Zuschke CA, et al, "Effects of Candesartan Cilexetil in Patients With Severe Systemic Hypertension," *Am J Cardiol*, 1999, 84(3):289-93.

Peacock WF, Varon J, Garrison N, et al, "I.V. Clevidipine for Hypertension: Safety, Efficacy, and Transition to Oral Therapy," *Ann Emerg Med*, 2007, 50(3 Suppl):S8-9.

Perloff D, Grim C, Flack J, et al, "Human Blood Pressure Determination by Sphygmomanometry," *Circulation*, 1993, 88(5 Pt 1):2460-7.

Perry HM Jr, Bingham S, Horney A, et al, "Antihypertensive Efficacy of Treatment Regimens Used in Veterans Administration Hypertension Clinics. Department of Veterans Affairs Cooperative Study Group on Antihypertensive Agents," *Hypertension*, 1998, 31(3):771-9.

Preston RA, Materson BJ, Reda DJ, et al, "Age-Race Subgroup Compared With Renin Profile as Predictors of Blood Pressure Response to Antihypertensive Therapy," *JAMA*, 1998, 280 (13):1168-72.

Psaty BM, Smith NL, Siscovick DS, et al, "Health Outcomes Associated With Antihypertensive Therapies Used as First-Line Agents. A Systemic Review and Meta-analysis," *JAMA*, 1997, 277 (9):739-45.

Radevski IV, Valtchanova SP, Candy GP, et al, "Comparison of Acebutolol With and Without Hydrochlorothiazide Versus Carvedilol With and Without Hydrochlorothiazide in Black Patients With Mild to Moderate Systemic Hypertension," *Am J Cardiol*, 1999, 84(1):70-5.

Setaro JF and Black HR, "Refractory Hypertension," *N Engl J Med*, 1992, 327(8):543-7.

SHEP Cooperative Research Group, "Prevention of Stroke by Antihypertensive Drug Treatment in Older Persons With Isolated Systolic Hypertension: Final Results of the Systolic Hypertension in the Elderly Program (SHEP)," *JAMA*, 1991, 265(24):3255-64.

Sibai BM, "Treatment of Hypertension in Pregnant Women," *N Engl J Med*, 1996, 335(4):257-65.

Singla N, Warltier DC, Gandhi SD, et al, "Treatment of Acute Postoperative Hypertension in Cardiac Surgery Patients: An Efficacy Study of Clevidipine Assessing Its Postoperative Antihypertensive Effect in Cardiac Surgery-2 (ESCAPE-2), a Randomized, Double-Blind, Placebo-Controlled Trial," *Anesth Analg*, 2008, 107(1):59-67.

Sowers JR, "Comorbidity of Hypertension and Diabetes: The Fosinopril Versus Amlodipine Cardiovascular Events Trial," *Am J Cardiol*, 1998, 82(9B):15R-19R.

Sternberg H, Rosenthal T, Shamiss A, et al, "Altered Circadian Rhythm of Blood Pressure in Shift Workers," *J Hum Hypertens*, 1995, 9(5):349-53.

"The Hypertension Prevention Trial: Three-Year Effects of Dietary Changes on Blood Pressure. Hypertension Prevention Trial Research Group," *Arch Intern Med*, 1990, 150(1):153-62.

Trials of Hypertension Prevention Collaborative Research Group, "Effects of Weight Loss and Sodium Reduction Intervention on Blood Pressure and Hypertension Incidence in Overweight People With High-Normal Blood Pressure: The Trials of Hypertension Prevention, Phase II," *Arch Intern Med*, 1997, 157(6):657-67.

Tuomilehto J, Rastenyte D, Birkenhager WH, et al, "Effects of Calcium Channel Blockade in Older Patients With Diabetes and Systolic Hypertension," *N Engl J Med*, 1999, 340(9):677-84.

Veelken R and Schmieder RE, "Overview of Alpha-1 Adrenoceptor Antagonism and Recent Advances in Hypertensive Therapy," *Am J Hypertens*, 1996, 9(11):139S-49S.

White WB, Black HR, Weber MA, et al, "Comparison of Effects of Controlled Onset Extended Release Verapamil at Bedtime and Nifedipine Gastrointestinal Therapeutic System on Arising on Early Morning Blood Pressure, Heart Rate, and the Heart Rate-Blood Pressure Product," *Am J Cardiol*, 1998, 81(4):424-31.

PEDIATRIC ALS ALGORITHMS

PALS Bradycardia Algorithm

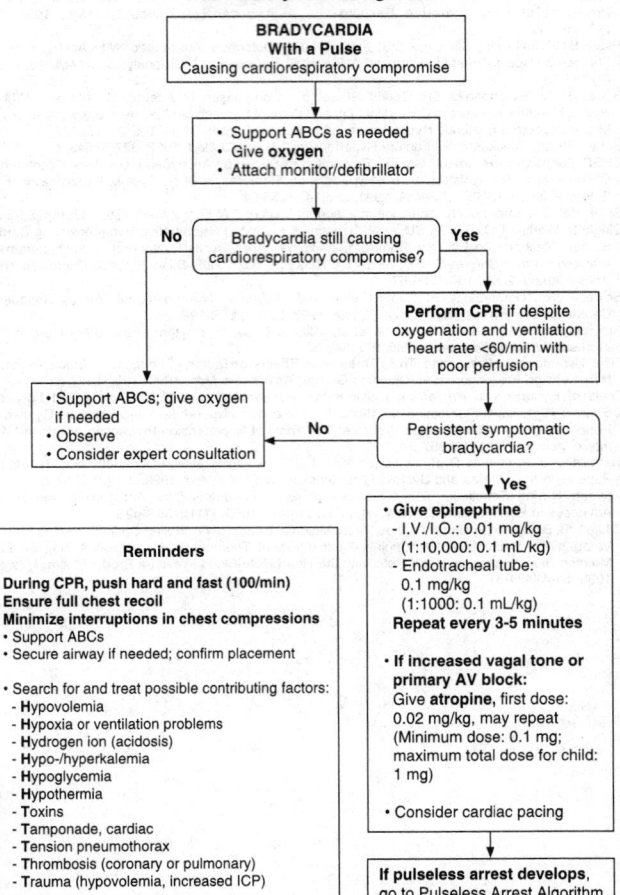

BRADYCARDIA
With a Pulse
Causing cardiorespiratory compromise

- Support ABCs as needed
- Give **oxygen**
- Attach monitor/defibrillator

No ← Bradycardia still causing cardiorespiratory compromise? → **Yes**

Perform CPR if despite oxygenation and ventilation heart rate <60/min with poor perfusion

- Support ABCs; give oxygen if needed
- Observe
- Consider expert consultation

No ← Persistent symptomatic bradycardia?

↓ **Yes**

- **Give epinephrine**
  - I.V./I.O.: 0.01 mg/kg (1:10,000: 0.1 mL/kg)
  - Endotracheal tube: 0.1 mg/kg (1:1000: 0.1 mL/kg)
  Repeat every 3-5 minutes

- **If increased vagal tone or primary AV block:**
  Give **atropine**, first dose: 0.02 mg/kg, may repeat (Minimum dose: 0.1 mg; maximum total dose for child: 1 mg)

- Consider cardiac pacing

If pulseless arrest develops, go to Pulseless Arrest Algorithm

Reminders

During CPR, push hard and fast (100/min)
Ensure full chest recoil
Minimize interruptions in chest compressions
- Support ABCs
- Secure airway if needed; confirm placement

- Search for and treat possible contributing factors:
  - Hypovolemia
  - Hypoxia or ventilation problems
  - Hydrogen ion (acidosis)
  - Hypo-/hyperkalemia
  - Hypoglycemia
  - Hypothermia
  - Toxins
  - Tamponade, cardiac
  - Tension pneumothorax
  - Thrombosis (coronary or pulmonary)
  - Trauma (hypovolemia, increased ICP)

PALS Pulseless Arrest Algorithm

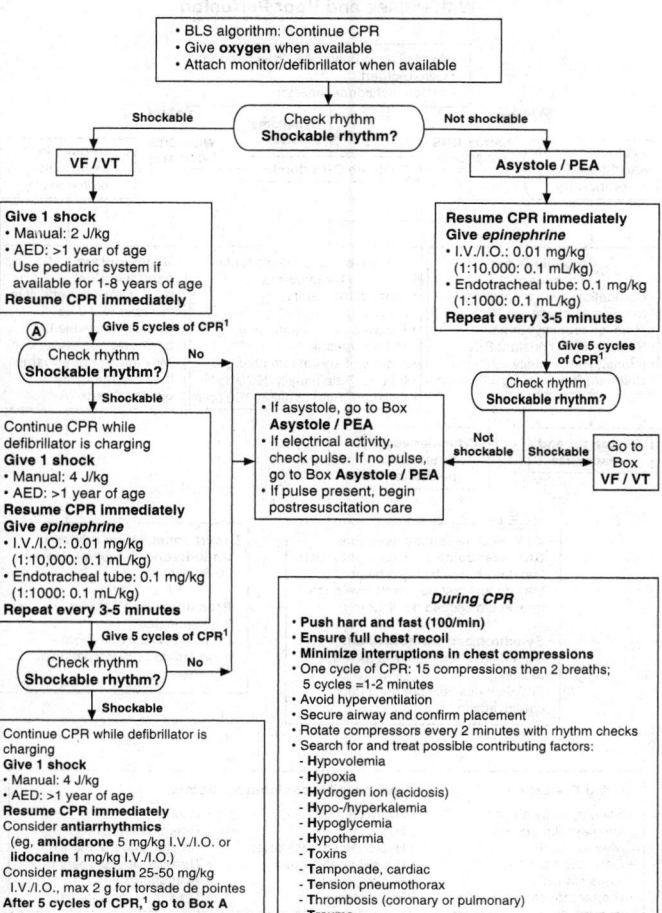

- BLS algorithm: Continue CPR
- Give **oxygen** when available
- Attach monitor/defibrillator when available

Check rhythm
Shockable rhythm?

Shockable → **VF / VT**

Not shockable → **Asystole / PEA**

VF / VT

Give 1 shock
- Manual: 2 J/kg
- AED: >1 year of age
 Use pediatric system if
 available for 1-8 years of age
Resume CPR immediately

(A) Give 5 cycles of CPR[1]

Check rhythm
Shockable rhythm? No

Shockable

Continue CPR while
defibrillator is charging
Give 1 shock
- Manual: 4 J/kg
- AED: >1 year of age
Resume CPR immediately
Give *epinephrine*
- I.V./I.O.: 0.01 mg/kg
 (1:10,000: 0.1 mL/kg)
- Endotracheal tube: 0.1 mg/kg
 (1:1000: 0.1 mL/kg)
Repeat every 3-5 minutes

Give 5 cycles of CPR[1]

Check rhythm
Shockable rhythm? No

Shockable

Continue CPR while defibrillator is
charging
Give 1 shock
- Manual: 4 J/kg
- AED: >1 year of age
Resume CPR immediately
Consider **antiarrhythmics**
 (eg, **amiodarone** 5 mg/kg I.V./I.O. or
 lidocaine 1 mg/kg I.V./I.O.)
Consider **magnesium** 25-50 mg/kg
I.V./I.O., max 2 g for torsade de pointes
**After 5 cycles of CPR,[1] go to Box A
above**

Asystole / PEA

Resume CPR immediately
Give *epinephrine*
- I.V./I.O.: 0.01 mg/kg
 (1:10,000: 0.1 mL/kg)
- Endotracheal tube: 0.1 mg/kg
 (1:1000: 0.1 mL/kg)
Repeat every 3-5 minutes

Give 5 cycles
of CPR[1]

Check rhythm
Shockable rhythm?

**Not
shockable** | **Shockable** → Go to
Box
VF / VT

- If asystole, go to Box
 Asystole / PEA
- If electrical activity,
 check pulse. If no pulse,
 go to Box **Asystole / PEA**
- If pulse present, begin
 postresuscitation care

During CPR

- **Push hard and fast (100/min)**
- **Ensure full chest recoil**
- **Minimize interruptions in chest compressions**
- One cycle of CPR: 15 compressions then 2 breaths;
 5 cycles =1-2 minutes
- Avoid hyperventilation
- Secure airway and confirm placement
- Rotate compressors every 2 minutes with rhythm checks
- Search for and treat possible contributing factors:
 - Hypovolemia
 - Hypoxia
 - Hydrogen ion (acidosis)
 - Hypo-/hyperkalemia
 - Hypoglycemia
 - Hypothermia
 - Toxins
 - Tamponade, cardiac
 - Tension pneumothorax
 - Thrombosis (coronary or pulmonary)
 - Trauma

VF = ventricular fibrillation; VT = ventricular tachycardia; PEA = pulseless electrical activity; AED = automated external defibrillator.

[1]After an advanced airway is placed, rescuers no longer deliver "cycles" of CPR. Give continuous chest compressions without pauses for breaths. Give 8-10 breaths/min. Check rhythm every 2 minutes.

Reproduced With Permission, "2005 American Heart Association Guidelines for Cardiopulmonary Resuscitation and Emergency Cardiovascular Care," *Circulation*, 2005, 112(24 Suppl):IV1-203. ©2005, American Heart Association.

PALS Tachycardia Algorithm
With Pulses and Poor Perfusion

- Assess and support ABCs as needed
- Give **oxygen**
- Attach monitor/defibrillator

Evaluate rhythm with 12-lead ECG or monitor

← Narrow QRS (≤0.08 sec) ←

Symptoms persist

Evaluate QRS duration

→ Wide QRS (>0.08 sec) →

Possible ventricular tachycardia

Probable Sinus Tachycardia
- Compatible history consistent with known cause
- P waves present/normal
- Variable R-R; constant P-R
- Infants: Rate usually <220 bpm
- Children: Rate usually <180 bpm

Probable Supraventricular Tachycardia
- Compatible history (vague, nonspecific)
- P waves absent/abnormal
- HR not variable
- History of abrupt rate changes
- Infants: Rate usually ≥220 bpm
- Children: Rate usually ≥180 bpm

- **Synchronized cardioversion:** 0.5-1 J/kg; if not effective, increase to 2 J/kg Sedate if possible but don't delay cardioversion
- May attempt **adenosine** if it does not delay electrical cardioversion

Search for and treat cause

Consider vagal maneuvers (no delays)

- **If I.V. access readily available:** Give adenosine 0.1 mg/kg (maximum first dose 6 mg) by rapid bolus May double first dose and give once (maximum second dose 12 mg)
  or
- **Synchronized cardioversion:** 0.5-1 J/kg; if not effective, increase to 2 J/kg Sedate if possible but don't delay cardioversion

Expert consultation advised
- **Amiodarone:** 5 mg/kg I.V. over 20-60 minutes
  or
- **Procainamide** 15 mg/kg I.V. over 30-60 minutes *Do not routinely administer amiodarone and procainamide together*

During Evaluation	*Treat possible contributing factors:*	
• Secure, verify airway and vascular access when possible	• **H**ypovolemia	• **T**oxins
• Consider expert consultation	• **H**ypoxia	• **T**amponade, cardiac
• Prepare for cardioversion	• **H**ydrogen ion (acidosis)	• **T**ension pneumothorax
	• **H**ypo-/hyperkalemia	• **T**hrombosis (coronary or pulmonary)
	• **H**ypoglycemia	• **T**rauma (hypovolemia)
	• **H**ypothermia	

ADULT ACLS ALGORITHMS

Bradycardia Algorithm

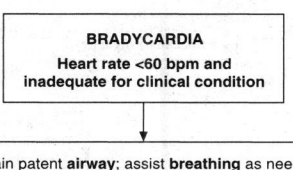

> **BRADYCARDIA**
> Heart rate <60 bpm and
> inadequate for clinical condition

⬇

- Maintain patent **airway**; assist **breathing** as needed
- Give **oxygen**
- Monitor ECG (identify rhythm), blood pressure, oximetry
- Establish I.V. access

⬇

Signs or symptoms of poor perfusion caused by the bradycardia?
(eg, acute altered mental status, ongoing chest pain, hypotension, or other signs of shock)

Adequate Perfusion → Observe / Monitor

Poor Perfusion →

- **Prepare for transcutaneous pacing;** use without delay for high-degree block (type II second-degree block or third-degree AV block)
- Consider **atropine** 0.5 mg I.V. while awaiting pacer. May repeat to a total dose of 3 mg. If ineffective, begin pacing.
- Consider **epinephrine** (2-10 mcg/min) or **dopamine** (2-10 mcg/kg/min) infusion while awaiting pacer or if pacing ineffective

⬇

- Prepare for **transvenous pacing**
- Treat contributing causes
- Consider expert consultation

Reminders

- If pulseless arrest develops, *see* Pulseless Arrest Algorithm
- Search for and treat possible contributing factors:
  - **H**ypovolemia
  - **H**ypoxia
  - **H**ydrogen ion (acidosis)
  - **H**ypo-/hyperkalemia
  - **H**ypoglycemia
  - **H**ypothermia
  - **T**oxins
  - **T**amponade, cardiac
  - **T**ension pneumothorax
  - **T**hrombosis (coronary or pulmonary)
  - **T**rauma (hypovolemia, increased ICP)

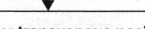

ACLS Pulseless Arrest Algorithm

- BLS algorithm: Call for help, give CPR
- Give **oxygen** when available
- Attach monitor/defibrillator when available

Check rhythm
Shockable rhythm?

Shockable → **VF / VT**

Not shockable → **Asystole / PEA**

VF / VT

Give 1 shock
- Manual biphasic: Device specific (typically 120-200 J)
  Note: If unknown, use 200 J
- AED: Device specific
- Monophasic: 360 J
Resume CPR immediately

(A) Give 5 cycles of CPR[1]

Check rhythm
Shockable rhythm? — No

Shockable

Continue CPR while defibrillator is charging
Give 1 shock
- Manual biphasic: Device specific (same as first shock or higher dose)
  Note: If unknown, use 200 J
- AED: Device specific
- Monophasic: 360 J
Resume CPR immediately after the shock. When I.V./I.O. available, give vasopressor during CPR (before or after the shock)
- **Epinephrine** 1 mg I.V./I.O.
  Repeat every 3-5 minutes *or*
- May give 1 dose of **vasopressin** 40 units I.V./I.O. to replace first or second dose of **epinephrine**

Give 5 cycles of CPR[1]

Check rhythm
Shockable rhythm? — No

Shockable

Continue CPR while defibrillator is charging
Give 1 shock
- Manual biphasic: Device specific (same as first shock or higher dose)
  Note: If unknown, use 200 J
- AED: Device specific
- Monophasic: 360 J
Resume CPR immediately after the shock.
Consider **antiarrhythmics;** give during CPR (before or after the shock) **amiodarone** (300 mg I.V./I.O. once, then consider additional 150 mg I.V./I.O. once) or **lidocaine** (1-1.5 mg/kg first dose, then 0.5-0.75 mg/kg I.V./I.O., maximum 3 doses or 3 mg/kg)
Consider **magnesium,** loading dose 1-2 g I.V./I.O. for torsade de pointes
After 5 cycles of CPR,[1] go to Box A above

Asystole / PEA

Resume CPR immediately for 5 cycles.
When I.V./I.O. available, give vasopressor.
- **Epinephrine** 1 mg I.V./I.O.
  Repeat every 3-5 minutes *or*
- May give 1 dose of **vasopressin** 40 units I.V./I.O. to replace first or second dose of **epinephrine**
Consider **atropine** 1 mg I.V./I.O. for asystole or slow PEA rate
Repeat every 3-5 min (up to 3 doses)

Give 5 cycles of CPR[1]

Check rhythm
Shockable rhythm?

Not shockable | Shockable → Go to Box VF / VT

- If asystole, go to Box **Asystole / PEA**
- If electrical activity, check pulse. If no pulse, go to Box **Asystole / PEA.**
- If pulse present, begin postresuscitation care

During CPR
- **Push hard and fast (100/min)**
- **Ensure full chest recoil**
- **Minimize interruptions in chest compressions**
- One cycle of CPR: 30 compressions then 2 breaths; 5 cycles = 2 minutes
- Avoid hyperventilation
- Secure airway and confirm placement
- Rotate compressors every 2 minutes with rhythm checks
- Search for and treat possible contributing factors:
  - Hypovolemia
  - Hypoxia
  - Hydrogen ion (acidosis)
  - Hypo-/hyperkalemia
  - Hypoglycemia
  - Hypothermia
  - Toxins
  - Tamponade, cardiac
  - Tension pneumothorax
  - Thrombosis (coronary or pulmonary)
  - Trauma

[1] After an advanced airway is placed, rescuers no longer deliver "cycles" of CPR. Give continuous chest compressions without pauses for breaths. Give 8-10 breaths/min. Check rhythm every 2 minutes.

VF = ventricular fibrillation; VT = ventricular tachycardia; PEA = pulseless electrical activity; AED = automated external defibrillator.

ACLS Tachycardia Algorithm
With Pulses

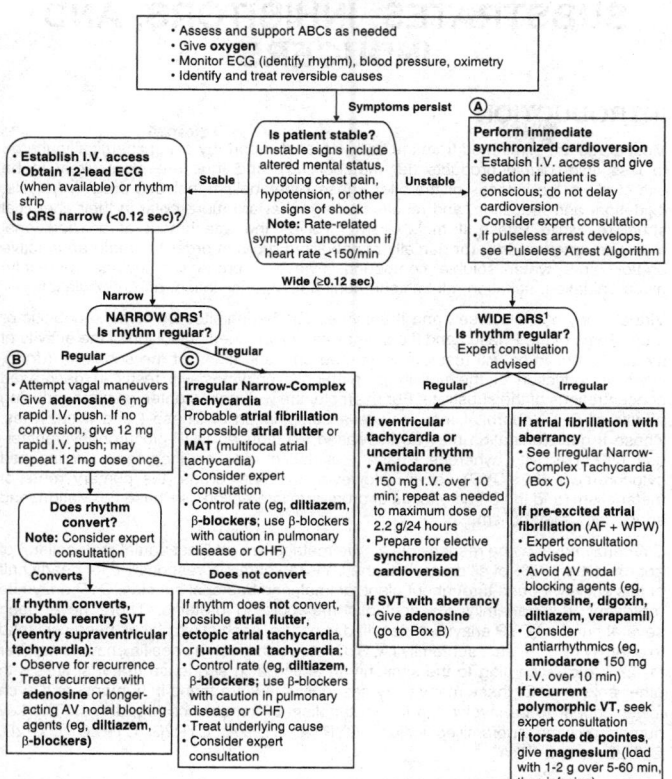

- Assess and support ABCs as needed
- Give **oxygen**
- Monitor ECG (identify rhythm), blood pressure, oximetry
- Identify and treat reversible causes

Symptoms persist **(A)**

Is patient stable?
Unstable signs include altered mental status, ongoing chest pain, hypotension, or other signs of shock
Note: Rate-related symptoms uncommon if heart rate <150/min

Perform immediate synchronized cardioversion
- Establish I.V. access and give sedation if patient is conscious; do not delay cardioversion
- Consider expert consultation
- If pulseless arrest develops, see Pulseless Arrest Algorithm

Stable / Unstable

- **Establish I.V. access**
- **Obtain 12-lead ECG** (when available) or rhythm strip
Is QRS narrow (<0.12 sec)?

Narrow / Wide (≥0.12 sec)

NARROW QRS¹
Is rhythm regular?

WIDE QRS¹
Is rhythm regular?
Expert consultation advised

(B) Regular / **(C)** Irregular

Regular / Irregular

- Attempt vagal maneuvers
- Give **adenosine** 6 mg rapid I.V. push. If no conversion, give 12 mg rapid I.V. push; may repeat 12 mg dose once.

Irregular Narrow-Complex Tachycardia
Probable **atrial fibrillation** or possible **atrial flutter** or **MAT** (multifocal atrial tachycardia)
- Consider expert consultation
- Control rate (eg, **diltiazem**, β-blockers; use β-blockers with caution in pulmonary disease or CHF)

If ventricular tachycardia or uncertain rhythm
- **Amiodarone** 150 mg I.V. over 10 min; repeat as needed to maximum dose of 2.2 g/24 hours
- Prepare for elective **synchronized cardioversion**

If SVT with aberrancy
- Give **adenosine** (go to Box B)

If atrial fibrillation with aberrancy
- See Irregular Narrow-Complex Tachycardia (Box C)

If pre-excited atrial fibrillation (AF + WPW)
- Expert consultation advised
- Avoid AV nodal blocking agents (eg, **adenosine, digoxin, diltiazem, verapamil**)
- Consider antiarrhythmics (eg, **amiodarone** 150 mg I.V. over 10 min)

If recurrent polymorphic VT, seek expert consultation

If torsade de pointes, give **magnesium** (load with 1-2 g over 5-60 min, then infusion)

Does rhythm convert?
Note: Consider expert consultation

Converts / Does not convert

If rhythm converts, probable reentry SVT (reentry supraventricular tachycardia):
- Observe for recurrence
- Treat recurrence with **adenosine** or longer-acting AV nodal blocking agents (eg, **diltiazem**, β-blockers)

If rhythm does **not** convert, possible **atrial flutter, ectopic atrial tachycardia**, or **junctional tachycardia**:
- Control rate (eg, **diltiazem**, β-blockers; use β-blockers with caution in pulmonary disease or CHF)
- Treat underlying cause
- Consider expert consultation

During Evaluation	**Treat possible contributing factors:**	
• Secure, verify airway and vascular access when possible	• Hypovolemia	• Toxins
• Consider expert consultation	• Hypoxia	• Tamponade, cardiac
• Prepare for cardioversion	• Hydrogen ion (acidosis)	• Tension pneumothorax
	• Hypo-/hyperkalemia	• Thrombosis (coronary or pulmonary)
	• Hypoglycemia	• Trauma (hypovolemia)
	• Hypothermia	

SVT = supraventricular tachycardia; VT = ventricular tachycardia.
¹If patient becomes unstable, go to Box A.

CYTOCHROME P450 ENZYMES: SUBSTRATES, INHIBITORS, AND INDUCERS

INTRODUCTION

Most drugs are eliminated from the body, at least in part, by being chemically altered to less lipid-soluble products (ie, metabolized), and thus are more likely to be excreted via the kidneys or the bile. Phase I metabolism includes drug hydrolysis, oxidation, and reduction, and results in drugs that are more polar in their chemical structure, while Phase II metabolism involves the attachment of an additional molecule onto the drug (or partially metabolized drug) in order to create an inactive and/or more water soluble compound. Phase II processes include (primarily) glucuronidation, sulfation, glutathione conjugation, acetylation, and methylation.

Virtually any of the Phase I and II enzymes can be inhibited by some xenobiotic or drug. Some of the Phase I and II enzymes can be induced. Inhibition of the activity of metabolic enzymes will result in increased concentrations of the substrate (drug), whereas induction of the activity of metabolic enzymes will result in decreased concentrations of the substrate. For example, the well-documented enzyme-inducing effects of PHENobarbital may include a combination of Phase I and II enzymes. Phase II glucuronidation may be increased via induced UDP-glucuronosyltransferase (UGT) activity, whereas Phase I oxidation may be increased via induced cytochrome P450 (CYP) activity. However, for most drugs, the primary route of metabolism (and the primary focus of drug-drug interaction) is Phase I oxidation, and specifically, metabolism.

CYP enzymes may be responsible for the metabolism (at least partial metabolism) of approximately 75% of all drugs, with the CYP3A subfamily responsible for nearly half of this activity. Found throughout plant, animal, and bacterial species, CYP enzymes represent a superfamily of xenobiotic metabolizing proteins. There have been several hundred CYP enzymes identified in nature, each of which has been assigned to a family (1, 2, 3, etc), subfamily (A, B, C, etc), and given a specific enzyme number (1, 2, 3, etc) according to the similarity in amino acid sequence that it shares with other enzymes. Of these many enzymes, only a few are found in humans, and even fewer appear to be involved in the metabolism of xenobiotics (eg, drugs). The key human enzyme subfamilies include CYP1A, CYP2A, CYP2B, CYP2C, CYP2D, CYP2E, and CYP3A.

CYP enzymes are found in the endoplasmic reticulum of cells in a variety of human tissues (eg, skin, kidneys, brain, lungs), but their predominant sites of concentration and activity are the liver and intestine. Though the abundance of CYP enzymes throughout the body is relatively equally distributed among the various subfamilies, the relative contribution to drug metabolism is (in decreasing order of magnitude) CYP3A4 (nearly 50%), CYP2D6 (nearly 25%), CYP2C8/9 (nearly 15%), then CYP1A2, CYP2C19, CYP2A6, and CYP2E1. Owing to their potential for numerous drug-drug interactions, those drugs that are identified in preclinical studies as substrates of CYP3A enzymes are often given a lower priority for continued research and development in favor of drugs that appear to be less affected by (or less likely to affect) this enzyme subfamily.

Each enzyme subfamily possesses unique selectivity toward potential substrates. For example, CYP1A2 preferentially binds medium-sized, planar, lipophilic molecules, while CYP2D6 preferentially binds molecules that possess a basic nitrogen atom. Some CYP subfamilies exhibit polymorphism (ie, multiple allelic variants that manifest differing catalytic properties). The best described polymorphisms involve CYP2C9, CYP2C19, and CYP2D6. Individuals possessing "wild type" gene alleles exhibit normal functioning CYP capacity. Others, however, possess allelic variants that leave the person with a subnormal level of catalytic potential (so called "poor metabolizers"). Poor metabolizers would be more likely to experience toxicity from drugs metabolized by the affected enzymes (or less effects if the enzyme is responsible for converting a prodrug to it's active form as in the case of codeine). The percentage of people classified as poor metabolizers varies by enzyme and population group. As an example, approximately 7% of Caucasians and only about 1% of Orientals appear to be CYP2D6 poor metabolizers.

CYP enzymes can be both inhibited and induced by other drugs, leading to increased or decreased serum concentrations (along with the associated effects), respectively. Induction occurs when a drug causes an increase in the amount of smooth endoplasmic reticulum, secondary to increasing the amount of the affected CYP enzymes in the tissues. This "revving up" of the CYP enzyme system may take several days to reach peak activity, and likewise, may take several days, even months, to return to normal following discontinuation of the inducing agent.

CYP inhibition occurs via several potential mechanisms. Most commonly, a CYP inhibitor competitively (and reversibly) binds to the active site on the enzyme, thus preventing the substrate from binding to the same site, and preventing the substrate from being metabolized. The affinity of an inhibitor for an enzyme may be expressed by an inhibition constant (Ki) or IC50 (defined as the concentration of the inhibitor required to cause 50% inhibition under a given set of conditions). In addition to reversible competition for an enzyme site, drugs may inhibit enzyme activity by binding to sites on the enzyme other than that to which the substrate would bind, and thereby cause a change in the functionality or physical structure of the enzyme. A drug may also bind to the enzyme in an irreversible (ie, "suicide") fashion. In such a case, it is not the concentration of drug at the enzyme site that is important (constantly binding and releasing), but the number of molecules available for binding (once bound, always bound).

Although an inhibitor or inducer may be known to affect a variety of CYP subfamilies, it may only inhibit one or two in a clinically important fashion. Likewise, although a substrate is known to be at least partially metabolized by a variety of CYP enzymes, only one or two enzymes may contribute significantly enough to its overall metabolism to warrant concern when used with potential inducers or inhibitors. Therefore, when attempting to predict the level of risk of using two drugs that may affect each other via altered CYP function, it is important to identify the relative effectiveness of the inhibiting/inducing drug on the CYP subfamilies that significantly contribute to the metabolism of the substrate. The contribution of a specific CYP pathway to substrate metabolism should be considered not only in light of other known CYP pathways, but also other nonoxidative pathways for substrate metabolism (eg, glucuronidation) and transporter proteins (eg, P-glycoprotein) that may affect the presentation of a substrate to a metabolic pathway.

HOW TO USE THE TABLES

The following CYP SUBSTRATES, INHIBITORS, and INDUCERS tables provide a clinically relevant perspective on drugs that are affected by, or affect, cytochrome P450 (CYP) enzymes. Not all human, drug-metabolizing CYP enzymes are specifically (or separately) included in the tables. Some enzymes have been excluded because they do not appear to significantly contribute to the metabolism of marketed drugs (eg, CYP2C18). In the case of CYP3A4, the industry routinely uses this single enzyme designation to represent all enzymes in the CYP3A subfamily. CYP3A7 is present in fetal livers. It is effectively absent from adult livers. CYP3A4 (adult) and CYP3A7 (fetal) appear to share similar properties in their respective hosts. The impact of CYP3A7 in fetal and neonatal drug interactions has not been investigated.

The **CYP Substrates table** contains a list of drugs reported to be metabolized, at least in part, by one or more CYP enzymes. An enzyme that appears to play a clinically significant (major) role in a drug's metabolism is indicated by "•", and an enzyme whose role appears to be clinically insignificant (minor) is indicated by "○". A clinically significant designation is the result of a two-phase review. The first phase considered the contribution of each CYP enzyme to the overall metabolism of the drug. The enzyme pathway was considered potentially clinically relevant if it was responsible for at least 30% of the metabolism of the drug. If so, the drug was subjected to a second phase. The second phase considered the clinical relevance of a substrate's concentration being increased twofold, or decreased by one-half (such as might be observed if combined with an effective CYP inhibitor or inducer, respectively). If either of these changes was considered to present a clinically significant concern, the CYP pathway for the drug was designated "major." If neither change would appear to present a clinically significant concern, or if the CYP enzyme was responsible for a smaller portion of the overall metabolism (ie, <30%), the pathway was designated "minor."

The **CYP Inhibitors table** contains a list of drugs that are reported to inhibit one or more CYP enzymes. Enzymes that are strongly inhibited by a drug are indicated by "●". Enzymes that are moderately inhibited are indicated by "□". Enzymes that are weakly inhibited are indicated by "○". The designations are the result of a review of published clinical reports, available Ki data, and assessments published by other experts in the field. As it pertains to Ki values set in a ratio with achievable serum drug concentrations ([I]) under normal dosing conditions, the following parameters were employed: [I]/Ki ≥1 = strong; [I]/Ki 0.1-1 = moderate; [I]/Ki <0.1 = weak.

The **CYP Inducers table** contains a list of drugs that are reported to induce one or more CYP enzymes. Enzymes that appear to be effectively induced by a drug are indicated by "●", and enzymes that do not appear to be effectively induced are indicated by "○". The designations are the result of a review of published clinical reports and assessments published by experts in the field.

In general, clinically significant interactions are more likely to occur between substrates and either inhibitors or inducers of the same enzyme(s), all of which have been indicated by "●". However, these assessments possess a degree of subjectivity, at times based on limited indications regarding the significance of CYP effects of particular agents. An attempt has been made to balance a conservative, clinically-sensitive presentation of the data with a desire to avoid the numbing effect of a "beware of everything" approach. Even so, other potential interactions (ie, those involving enzymes indicated by "○") may warrant consideration in some cases. It is important to note that information related to CYP metabolism of drugs is expanding at a rapid pace, and thus, the contents of this table should only be considered to represent a "snapshot" of the information available at the time of publication.

Selected Readings

Bjornsson TD, Callaghan JT, Einolf HJ, et al, "The Conduct of *in vitro* and *in vivo* Drug-Drug Interaction Studies: A PhRMA Perspective," *J Clin Pharmacol*, 2003, 43(5):443-69.

Drug-Drug Interactions, Rodrigues AD, ed, New York, NY: Marcel Dekker, Inc, 2002.

Levy RH, Thummel KE, Trager WF, et al, eds, *Metabolic Drug Interactions*, Philadelphia, PA: Lippincott Williams & Wilkins, 2000.

Michalets EL, "Update: Clinically Significant Cytochrome P-450 Drug Interactions," *Pharmacotherapy*, 1998, 18(1):84-112.

Thummel KE and Wilkinson GR, " *In vitro* and *in vivo* Drug Interactions Involving Human CYP3A," *Annu Rev Pharmacol Toxicol*, 1998, 38:389-430.

Zhang Y and Benet LZ, "The Gut as a Barrier to Drug Absorption: Combined Role of Cytochrome P450 3A and P-Glycoprotein," *Clin Pharmacokinet*, 2001, 40(3):159-68.

Selected Websites

http://www.gentest.com
http://www.imm.ki.se/CYPalleles
http://medicine.iupui.edu/flockhart
http://www.mhc.com/Cytochromes

CYP Substrates

● = major substrate; ○ = minor substrate

Drug	1A2	2A6	2B6	2C8	2C9	2C19	2D6	2E1	3A4
Acenocoumarol	●				●	○			
Acetaminophen	○	○			○		○	○	○
Albendazole	○								○
Alfentanil									●
Alfuzosin									●
Aliskiren									○
Almotriptan							○		○
Alosetron	●				○				○

CYP Substrates (continued)

Drug	1A2	2A6	2B6	2C8	2C9	2C19	2D6	2E1	3A4
ALPRAZolam									●
Ambrisentan						●			●
Aminophylline	●							○	○
Amiodarone	○			●		○	○		●
Amitriptyline	○		○		○	○	●		○
AmLODIPine									●
Amoxapine							●		
Amprenavir					○				●
Anagrelide	○								
Apomorphine	○					○			○
Aprepitant	○					○			●
Arformoterol						○	○		
Argatroban									○
Aripiprazole							●		●
Armodafinil									●
Aspirin					○				
Atazanavir									●
Atomoxetine						○	●		
Atorvastatin									●
Azelastine	○					○	○		○
Azithromycin									○
Benzphetamine			○						●
Benztropine							○		
Benzydamine	○					○	○		○
Betaxolol	●						●		
Bexarotene									○
Bezafibrate									○
Bisoprolol							○		●
Bortezomib	○				○	●	○		●
Bosentan					●				●
Brinzolamide									○
Bromazepam									●
Bromocriptine									●
Budesonide									●
Bupivacaine	○					○	○		○
Buprenorphine									●
BuPROPion	○	○	●		○		○	○	○
BusPIRone							○		●
Busulfan									●
Caffeine	●				○		○	○	○
Candesartan					○				
Capsaicin								○	
Captopril							●		
CarBAMazepine				○					●
Carisoprodol						●			
Carteolol							○		

CYP Substrates *(continued)*

Drug	1A2	2A6	2B6	2C8	2C9	2C19	2D6	2E1	3A4
Carvedilol	o				•		•	o	o
Celecoxib					•				o
Cetirizine									o
Cevimeline							o		o
ChlordiazePOXIDE									•
Chloroquine							•		•
Chlorpheniramine							o		•
ChlorproMAZINE	o						•		o
ChlorproPAMIDE					o				
Chlorzoxazone	o	o					o	•	o
Ciclesonide	.						o		•
Cilostazol	o					o	o		•
Cisapride	o	o	o		o	o			•
Citalopram						•	o		•
Clarithromycin									•
Clobazam						•			•
ClomiPRAMINE	•					•	•		o
ClonazePAM									•
Clopidogrel	o								o
Clorazepate									•
Clozapine	•	o			o	o	o		o
Cocaine									•
Codeine[1]							•		o
Colchicine									•
Conivaptan									•
Cyclobenzaprine	•						o		o
Cyclophosphamide[2]		o	•		o	o			•
CycloSPORINE									•
Dacarbazine	•							•	
Dantrolene									•
Dapsone			o	•	o			o	•
Darifenacin							o		•
Darunavir									•
Dasatinib									•
Delavirdine							o		•
Desipramine	o						•		
Desogestrel						•			
Desvenlafaxine									o
Dexamethasone									o
Dexmedetomidine		•							
Dextromethorphan			o		o	o	•	o	o
Diazepam	o		o		o	•			•
Diclofenac	o		o	o	o	o	o		o
Digoxin									o
Dihydrocodeine[1]							o		
Dihydroergotamine									•

CYP Substrates (continued)

Drug	1A2	2A6	2B6	2C8	2C9	2C19	2D6	2E1	3A4
Diltiazem					o		o		•
Disopyramide									•
Disulfiram	o	o	o				o	o	o
Docetaxel									•
Dofetilide									o
Dolasetron					o				o
Domperidone									o
Donepezil							o		o
Dorzolamide					o				o
Doxepin	•						•		•
DOXOrubicin							•		•
Drospirenone									o
DULoxetine	•						•		
Dutasteride									o
Efavirenz			•						•
Eletriptan									•
Enalapril									o
Enflurane								•	
Eplerenone									•
Ergoloid mesylates									•
Ergonovine									•
Ergotamine									•
Erlotinib	o								•
Erythromycin			o						•
Escitalopram						•			•
Esomeprazole						•			•
Estazolam									o
Estradiol	•	o	o		o	o	o	o	•
Estrogens, conjugated A/synthetic	•	o	o		o	o	o	o	•
Estrogens, conjugated equine	•	o	o		o	o	o	o	•
Estrogens, conjugated esterified	•		o		o			o	•
Estropipate	•		o		o			o	•
Eszopiclone								o	•
Ethinyl estradiol					o				•
Ethosuximide									•
Etonogestrel									o
Etoposide	o							o	•
Exemestane									•
Felbamate								o	•
Felodipine									•
Fenofibrate									o
FentaNYL									•
Fexofenadine									o
Finasteride									o
Flecainide	o						•		

CYP Substrates *(continued)*

Drug	1A2	2A6	2B6	2C8	2C9	2C19	2D6	2E1	3A4
Flunisolide									●
FLUoxetine	○		○		●	○	●	○	○
Fluphenazine							●		
Flurazepam									●
Flurbiprofen					○				
Flutamide	●								●
Fluticasone									●
Fluvastatin				○	●		○		○
Fluvoxamine	●						●		
Formoterol		○			○	○	○		
Fosamprenavir (as amprenavir)					○				●
Fosaprepitant	○					○			●
Fosphenytoin (as phenytoin)					●	●			○
Frovatriptan	○								
Fulvestrant									○
Galantamine							○		○
Gefitinib									●
Gemfibrozil									○
Glimepiride					●				
GlipiZIDE					●				
Granisetron									○
Guanabenz	●								
Haloperidol	○						●		●
Halothane		○	○		○		○	●	○
HYDROcodone[1]							●		
Hydrocortisone									○
Ibuprofen					○	○			
Ifosfamide[3]		●	○	○	○	●			●
Imatinib	○				○	○	○		●
Imipramine	○		○			●	●		○
Imiquimod	○								○
Indinavir							○		●
Indomethacin					○	○			
Irbesartan					○				
Irinotecan			●						●
Isoflurane								●	
Isoniazid								●	
Isosorbide									●
Isosorbide dinitrate									●
Isosorbide mononitrate									●
Isradipine									●
Itraconazole									●
Ivermectin									○
Ixabepilone									●
Ketamine			●		●				●
Ketoconazole									●

CYP Substrates *(continued)*

Drug	1A2	2A6	2B6	2C8	2C9	2C19	2D6	2E1	3A4
Lansoprazole					o	●			●
Lapatinib				o					●
Letrozole		o							o
Levobupivacaine	o								o
Levonorgestrel									●
Lidocaine	o	o	o		o		●		●
Lomustine							●		
Loperamide			o						
Lopinavir									●
Loratadine							o		o
Losartan					●				●
Lovastatin									●
Maprotiline							●		
Maraviroc									●
MedroxyPROGESTERone									●
Mefenamic acid					o				
Mefloquine									●
Meloxicam					o				o
Meperidine			o			o			o
Mephobarbital			o		o	●			
Mestranol[4]					●				●
Methadone					o	o	o		●
Methamphetamine							●		
Methoxsalen		o							
Methsuximide						●			
Methylergonovine									●
MethylPREDNISolone									●
Metoclopramide	o						o		
Metoprolol						o	●		
Mexiletine	●						●		
Micafungin									o
Miconazole									●
Midazolam			o						●
Mifepristone									o
Mirtazapine	●				o		●		●
Moclobemide						●	●		
Modafinil									●
Mometasone									o
Montelukast					●				●
Moricizine									●
Morphine sulfate							o		
Naproxen	o				o				
Nateglinide					●				●
Nebivolol							●		
Nefazodone							●		●
Nelfinavir					o	●	o		●

CYP Substrates (continued)

Drug	1A2	2A6	2B6	2C8	2C9	2C19	2D6	2E1	3A4
Nevirapine			o				o		•
NiCARdipine	o				o		o	o	•
Nicotine	o	o	o		o	o	o	o	o
NIFEdipine							o		•
Nilotinib									•
Nilutamide						•			
NiMODipine									•
Nisoldipine									•
Norelgestromin									o
Norethindrone									•
Norgestrel									•
Nortriptyline	o					o	•		o
OLANZapine	•						o		
Omeprazole		o			o	•	o		•
Ondansetron	o				o		o	o	•
Orphenadrine	o		o				o		o
Oxybutynin									o
OxyCODONE[1]							•		
Paclitaxel				•	•				•
Palonosetron	o						o		o
Pantoprazole					o	•	o		o
Paricalcitol									•
PARoxetine							•		
Pentamidine						•			
Perphenazine	o				o	o	•		o
PHENobarbital					o	•		o	
Phenytoin					•	•			o
Pimecrolimus									o
Pimozide	•								•
Pindolol							•		
Pioglitazone				•					o
Piroxicam					o				
Pravastatin									o
PrednisoLONE									o
PredniSONE									o
Primaquine									•
Procainamide							•		
Progesterone	o	o			o	•	o		•
Proguanil	o					o			o
Promethazine			•				•		
Propafenone	o						•		o
Propofol	o	o	•		•	o	o	o	o
Propranolol	•					o	•		o
Protriptyline							•		
Quazepam						•			•
QUEtiapine							o		•

CYP Substrates *(continued)*

Drug	1A2	2A6	2B6	2C8	2C9	2C19	2D6	2E1	3A4
QuiNIDine					○			○	●
QuiNINE	○					○			●
Rabeprazole						●			●
Ramelteon	●								○
Ranitidine	○					○	○		
Ranolazine							○		●
Rasagiline	●								
Repaglinide				●					●
Rifabutin									●
Riluzole	●								
Risperidone							●		○
Ritonavir	○		○				●		●
Ropinirole	●								○
Ropivacaine	●		○				○		○
Rosiglitazone				●	○				
Rosuvastatin					○				○
Salmeterol									●
Saquinavir							○		●
Selegiline	○	○	●	○		○	○		○
Sertraline			○		○	●	●		○
Sevoflurane		○	○					●	○
Sibutramine									●
Sildenafil					○				●
Simvastatin									●
Sirolimus									●
SitaGLIPtin				○					○
Sitaxsentan					○				○
Solifenacin									●
Sorafenib									○
Spiramycin									●
SUFentanil									●
SulfaDIAZINE					●			○	○
Sulfamethoxazole					●				○
SulfiSOXAZOLE					●				
Sunitinib									●
Tacrine	●								
Tacrolimus									●
Tadalafil									●
Tamoxifen		○	○		●		●	○	●
Tamsulosin							●		●
Telithromycin	○								●
Temazepam			○		○	○			○
Temsirolimus									●
Teniposide									●
Terbinafine	○				○	○			○
Testosterone			○		○	○			○

CYP Substrates (continued)

Drug	1A2	2A6	2B6	2C8	2C9	2C19	2D6	2E1	3A4
Tetracycline									●
Theophylline	●				○		○	●	●
Thiabendazole	○								
Thioridazine						○	●		
Thiothixene	●								
TiaGABine									●
Ticlopidine									●
Timolol							●		
Tinidazole			○						●
Tiotropium							○		○
Tipranavir									●
TiZANidine	●								
TOLBUTamide					●	○			
Tolcapone					○				
Tolterodine					○	○	●		●
Toremifene	○								●
Torsemide				○	●				
TraMADol[1]							●		●
TraZODone							○		●
Tretinoin		○	○	●	○				
Triazolam									●
Trifluoperazine	●								
Trimethoprim					●				●
Trimipramine						●	●		●
Valproic acid		○	○		○	○		○	
Vardenafil									●
Venlafaxine					○	○	●		●
Verapamil	○		○		○			○	●
VinBLAStine							○		●
VinCRIStine									●
Vinorelbine							○		●
Voriconazole					●	●			○
Warfarin	○				●	○			○
Yohimbine							○		
Zafirlukast					●				
Zaleplon									○
Zidovudine		○			○	○			○
Zileuton	○				○				○
Ziprasidone	○								○
Zolmitriptan	○								
Zolpidem	○				○	○	○		●
Zonisamide						○			●

CYP Substrates *(continued)*

Drug	1A2	2A6	2B6	2C8	2C9	2C19	2D6	2E1	3A4
Zopiclone						●			●
Zuclopenthixol							●		

[1]This opioid analgesic is bioactivated *in vivo* via CYP2D6. Inhibiting this enzyme would decrease the effects of the analgesic. The active metabolite might also affect, or be affected by, CYP enzymes.

[2]Cyclophosphamide is bioactivated *in vivo* to acrolein via CYP2B6 and 3A4. Inhibiting these enzymes would decrease the effects of cyclophosphamide.

[3]Ifosfamide is bioactivated *in vivo* to acrolein via CYP3A4. Inhibiting this enzyme would decrease the effects of ifosfamide.

[4]Mestranol is bioactivated *in vivo* to ethinyl estradiol via CYP2C8/9. See Ethinyl Estradiol for additional CYP information.

CYP Inhibitors

● = strong inhibitor; □ = moderate inhibitor; o = weak inhibitor

Drug	1A2	2A6	2B6	2C8	2C9	2C19	2D6	2E1	3A4
Acebutolol							o		
Acetaminophen									o
AcetaZOLAMIDE									o
Albendazole	o								
Alosetron	o							o	
Amiodarone	o	□	o		□	o	□		□
Amitriptyline	o				o	o	o	o	
AmLODIPine	□	o	o	o	o		o		o
Amphetamine							o		
Amprenavir						o			●
Anastrozole	o			o	o				o
Apomorphine	o						o		
Aprepitant					o	o			□
Armodafinil						□			
Atazanavir	o			●	o				●
Atorvastatin									o
Azelastine			o		o	o	o		o
Azithromycin									o
Betamethasone									o
Betaxolol							o		
Bortezomib	o				o	□	o		o
Bromazepam							o		
Bromocriptine	o								o
Buprenorphine	o	o				o	o		
BuPROPion							o		
Caffeine	o								□
Candesartan				o	o				
Celecoxib				□			o		
Chloramphenicol					o				o
Chloroquine							□		
Chlorpheniramine							o		
ChlorproMAZINE							●	o	
Chlorzoxazone								o	o

CYP Inhibitors *(continued)*

Drug	1A2	2A6	2B6	2C8	2C9	2C19	2D6	2E1	3A4
Cholecalciferol					○	○	○		
Cimetidine	□				○	□	□	○	□
Cinacalcet							●		
Ciprofloxacin	●								○
Cisapride							○		○
Citalopram	○		○			○	○		
Clarithromycin	○								●
Clemastine							○		○
ClomiPRAMINE							□		
Clopidogrel					○				
Clotrimazole	○	○	○	○	○	○	○	○	□
Clozapine	○				○	○	□	○	○
Cocaine							●		○
Codeine							○		
Conivaptan									●
Cyclophosphamide									○
CycloSPORINE					○				□
Danazol									○
Darifenacin							□		○
Dasatinib									○
Delavirdine	○				●	●	●		●
Desipramine		□	□				□	○	□
Desvenlafaxine									○
Dexmedetomidine	○				○		●		○
Dextromethorphan							○		
Diazepam						○			○
Diclofenac	□				○			○	○
Dihydroergotamine									○
Diltiazem					○		○		□
DiphenhydrAMINE							□		
Disulfiram	○	○	○		○		○	●	○
Docetaxel									○
Dolasetron							○		
DOXOrubicin			□				○		○
Doxycycline									□
Drospirenone	○				○	○			○
DULoxetine							□		
Econazole								○	
Efavirenz					□	□			□
Entacapone	○	○			○	○	○	○	○
Eprosartan					○				
Ergotamine									○
Erythromycin	○								□
Escitalopram							○		
Esomeprazole						□			
Estradiol	○			○					

CYP Inhibitors *(continued)*

Drug	1A2	2A6	2B6	2C8	2C9	2C19	2D6	2E1	3A4
Estrogens, conjugated A/synthetic	o								
Estrogens, conjugated equine	o			o					
Ethinyl estradiol	o		o	o		o			o
Ethotoin						o			
Etoposide					o				o
Felbamate						o			
Felodipine				□	o		o		o
Fenofibrate		o		o	o	o			
FentaNYL									o
Fexofenadine							o		
Flavocoxid	o				o	o	o		o
Flecainide							o		
Fluconazole	o				●	●			□
FLUoxetine	□		o		o	□	●		o
Fluphenazine	o				o		o	o	
Flurazepam								o	
Flurbiprofen					●				
Flutamide	o								
Fluvastatin	o			o	□		o		o
Fluvoxamine	●		o		o	●	o		o
Fosamprenavir (as amprenavir)						o			●
Fosaprepitant					o	o			□
Gefitinib							o	o	
Gemfibrozil	□			●	●	●			
GlyBURIDE				o					o
Haloperidol							□		□
HydrALAZINE									o
HydrOXYzine							o		
Ibuprofen					●				
Ifosfamide									o
Imatinib					o		□		●
Imipramine	o					o	□	o	
Indinavir					o	o	o		●
Indomethacin					●	o			
Interferon alfa-2a	o								
Interferon alfa-2b	o								
Interferon gamma-1b	o							o	
Irbesartan				□	□		o		o
Isoflurane			o						
Isoniazid	o	□			o	●	□	□	●
Isradipine									o
Itraconazole									●
Ketoconazole	●	□	o	o	●	□	□		●
Ketoprofen					o				
Lansoprazole					o	□	o		o

CYP Inhibitors (continued)

Drug	1A2	2A6	2B6	2C8	2C9	2C19	2D6	2E1	3A4
Leflunomide					○				
Letrozole		●				○			
Lidocaine	●						□		□
Lomustine							○		○
Loratadine				○		□	○		
Losartan	○			□	□	○			○
Lovastatin					○		○		○
Mefenamic acid					●				
Mefloquine							○		○
Meloxicam					○				
Mephobarbital						○			
Mestranol	○		○			○			○
Methadone							□		○
Methimazole	○	○	○		○	○	□	○	○
Methotrimeprazine							○		
Methoxsalen	●	●			○	○	○	○	○
Methsuximide						○			
Methylnaltrexone							○		
Methylphenidate							○		
MethylPREDNISolone				○					○
Metoclopramide							○		
Metoprolol							○		
MetroNIDAZOLE					○				□
Metyrapone		○							
Mexiletine	●								
Micafungin									○
Miconazole	□	●	○		●	●	●	□	●
Midazolam				○	○				○
Mifepristone							○		○
Mirtazapine	○								○
Mitoxantrone									○
Moclobemide	○					○	○		
Modafinil	○	○			○	●		○	○
Montelukast				○	○				
Nateglinide					○				
Nefazodone	○		○	○			○		●
Nelfinavir	○		○		○	○	○		●
Nevirapine	○						○		○
NiCARdipine					●	□	□		●
Nicotine		○						○	
NIFEdipine	□				○		○		○
Nilutamide						○			
Nisoldipine	○								○
Nizatidine									○
Norfloxacin	●								□
Nortriptyline							○	○	

CYP Inhibitors (continued)

Drug	1A2	2A6	2B6	2C8	2C9	2C19	2D6	2E1	3A4
Ofloxacin	●								
OLANZapine	o				o	o	o		o
Omeprazole	o				□	●	o		o
Ondansetron	o				o		o		
Orphenadrine	o	o	o		o	o	o	o	o
OXcarbazepine						o			
Oxprenolol							o		
Oxybutynin				o			o		o
Pantoprazole						o			
PARoxetine	o		□		o	o	●		o
Peginterferon alfa-2a	o								
Peginterferon alfa-2b	o								
Pentamidine				o	o	o	o		o
Pentoxifylline	o								
Perphenazine	o						o		
Pilocarpine		o						o	o
Pimozide						o	o	o	o
Pindolol							o		
Pioglitazone				□	o	o	□		
Piroxicam					●				
Posaconazole									●
Pravastatin					o		o		o
Praziquantel							o		
PrednisoLONE									o
Primaquine	●						o		o
Probenecid						o			
Progesterone					o	o			o
Promethazine							o		
Propafenone	o						o		
Propofol	□				o	□	o	o	●
Propoxyphene					o		o		o
Propranolol	o						o		
Pyrimethamine					□		□		
QuiNIDine					o		●		●
QuiNINE				□	□		□		o
Quinupristin									o
Rabeprazole				□		□	o		o
Ranitidine	o						o		
Ranolazine							□		o
Risperidone							o		o
Ritonavir				●	o	o	●	o	●
Ropinirole	o								
Rosiglitazone				□	o	o	o		
Saquinavir					o	o	o		□
Selegiline	o	o			o	o	o	o	o
Sertraline	o		□	o	o	□	□		□

CYP Inhibitors *(continued)*

Drug	1A2	2A6	2B6	2C8	2C9	2C19	2D6	2E1	3A4
Sildenafil	o				o	o	o	o	o
Simvastatin			o		o		o		
Sirolimus									o
Sitaxsentan					●	●			□
Sorafenib			□	●	□				
Sulconazole	o	o			o	o	o	o	o
SulfaDIAZINE					●				
Sulfamethoxazole					□				
SulfiSOXAZOLE					●				
Tacrine	o								
Tacrolimus									o
Tamoxifen			o	□	o				o
Telithromycin							o		●
Telmisartan					o				
Temsirolimus							o		o
Teniposide					o				o
Tenofovir	o								
Terbinafine							●		
Testosterone									o
Tetracycline									□
Theophylline	o								
Thiabendazole	●								
Thioridazine	o				o		□	o	
Thiotepa			●						
Thiothixene							o		
Ticlopidine	o				o	●	□	o	o
Timolol							o		
Tioconazole	o	o			o	o	o	o	
Tocainide	o								
TOLBUTamide				o	●				
Tolcapone					o				
Topiramate						o			
Torsemide						o			
Tranylcypromine	□	●		o	o	□	□	o	o
TraZODone							□		o
Tretinoin					o				
Triazolam				o	o				
Trimethoprim				□	□				
Triprolidine							o		
Valproic acid					o	o	o		o
Valsartan					o				
Venlafaxine			o				o		o
Verapamil	o				o		o		□
VinBLAStine							o		o
VinCRIStine									o
Vinorelbine							o		o

CYP Inhibitors *(continued)*

Drug	1A2	2A6	2B6	2C8	2C9	2C19	2D6	2E1	3A4
Voriconazole					o	o			□
Warfarin					□	o			
Yohimbine							o		
Zafirlukast	o			o	□	o	o		o
Zileuton	□								
Ziprasidone							o		o

CYP Inducers

● = effectively induced; o = not effectively induced

Drug	1A2	2A6	2B6	2C8	2C9	2C19	2D6	2E1	3A4
Aminoglutethimide	●					●			●
Amobarbital		●							
Aprepitant					o				o
Armodafinil	o								o
Bexarotene									o
Bosentan					●				●
Calcitriol									o
CarBAMazepine	●		●	●	●	●			●
Colchicine				o	o			o	o
Cyclophosphamide			o	o	o				
Dexamethasone		o	o	o	o				●
Dicloxacillin									o
Efavirenz (in liver only)			o						●
Estradiol									o
Estrogens, conjugated A/ synthetic									o
Estrogens, conjugated equine									o
Felbamate									o
Fosaprepitant					o				o
Fosphenytoin (as phenytoin)			●	●	●	●			●
Griseofulvin	o			o	o				o
Hydrocortisone									o
Ifosfamide				o	o				
Insulin preparations	o								
Isoniazid (after D/C)								o	
Lansoprazole	o								
MedroxyPROGESTERone									o
Mephobarbital		o							
Metyrapone									o
Modafinil	o		o						o
Moricizine	o								o
Nafcillin									●
Nevirapine			●						●
Norethindrone						o			
Omeprazole	o								

CYP Inducers (continued)

Drug	1A2	2A6	2B6	2C8	2C9	2C19	2D6	2E1	3A4
OXcarbazepine									●
Paclitaxel									○
Pantoprazole	○								○
PENTobarbital		●							●
PHENobarbital	●	●	●	●	●				●
Phenytoin			●	●	●	●			●
Pioglitazone									○
PredniSONE						○			○
Primaquine	○								
Primidone[1]	●		●	●	●				●
Rifabutin									●
Rifampin	●	●	●	●	●	●			●
Rifapentine			●		●				●
Rifaximin									○
Ritonavir (long-term)	○			○	○				○
Secobarbital		●		●	●				
Terbinafine									○
Topiramate									○
Tretinoin								○	
Valproic acid		○							

[1]Primidone is partially metabolized to PHENobarbital. See PHENobarbital for additional CYP information.

EXTRAVASATION TREATMENT OF DRUGS

Medication Extravasated	Cold / Warm Pack	Antidote
Vasopressors		
Dopamine Epinephrine Norepinephrine Phenylephrine	None	Phentolamine (Regitine®) Mix 5 mg with 9 mL of NS Inject a small amount of this dilution into extravasated area. Blanching should reverse immediately. Monitor site. If blanching should recur, additional injections of phentolamine may be needed.
I.V. Fluids and Other Medications		
Aminophylline Calcium Dextrose, 10% Electrolyte solutions Esmolol Magnesium sulfate Metoprolol Nafcillin Parenteral nutrition preparations Phenytoin Potassium Radiocontrast media Sodium solutions	Cold	

ORAL MEDICATIONS THAT SHOULD NOT BE CRUSHED OR ALTERED

There are a variety of reasons for crushing tablets or capsule contents prior to administering to the patient. Patients may have nasogastric tubes which do not permit the administration of tablets or capsules; an oral solution for a particular medication may not be available from the manufacturer or readily prepared by pharmacy; patients may have difficulty swallowing capsules or tablets; or mixing of powdered medication with food or drink may make the drug more palatable.

Generally, medications which should not be crushed fall into one of the following categories.

- **Extended-Release Products.** The formulation of some tablets is specialized as to allow the medication within it to be slowly released into the body. This is sometimes accomplished by centering the drug within the core of the tablet, with a subsequent shedding of multiple layers around the core. Wax melts in the GI tract. Slow-K® is an example of this. Capsules may contain beads which have multiple layers which are slowly dissolved with time.

Common Abbreviations for Extended-Release Products

CD	Controlled dose
CR	Controlled release
CRT	Controlled-release tablet
LA	Long-acting
SR	Sustained release
TR	Timed release
TD	Time delay
SA	Sustained action
XL	Extended release
XR	Extended release

- **Medications Which Are Irritating to the Stomach.** Tablets which are irritating to the stomach may be enteric-coated which delays release of the drug until the time when it reaches the small intestine. Enteric-coated aspirin is an example of this.
- **Foul-Tasting Medication.** Some drugs are quite unpleasant to taste so the manufacturer coats the tablet in a sugar coating to increase its palatability. By crushing the tablet, this sugar coating is lost and the patient tastes the unpleasant tasting medication.
- **Sublingual Medication.** Medication intended for use under the tongue should not be crushed. While it appears to be obvious, it is not always easy to determine if a medication is to be used sublingually. Sublingual medications should indicate on the package that they are intended for sublingual use.
- **Effervescent Tablets.** These are tablets which, when dropped into a liquid, quickly dissolve to yield a solution. Many effervescent tablets, when crushed, lose their ability to quickly dissolve.

RECOMMENDATIONS

1. It is not advisable to crush certain medications.
2. Consult individual monographs prior to crushing capsule or tablet.
3. If crushing a tablet or capsule is contraindicated, consult with your pharmacist to determine whether an oral solution exists or can be compounded.

Drug Product	Dosage Form	Dosage Reasons / Comments
Accuhist®	Tablet	Slow release[8]
Accutane®	Capsule	Mucous membrane irritant
Aciphex®	Tablet	Slow release
Actiq®	Lozenge	Slow release. This lollipop delivery system requires the patient to dissolve it slowly.
Actonel®	Tablet	Irritant. Chewed, crushed, or sucked tablets may cause oropharyngeal irritation.
Adalat® CC	Tablet	Slow release
Adderall XR™	Capsule	Slow release[1]
Advicor®	Tablet	Slow release
AeroHist Plus™	Tablet	Slow release[8]
Afeditab™ CR	Tablet	Slow release
Afinitor®	Tablet	Mucous membrane irritant
Aggrenox®	Capsule	Slow release. Capsule may be opened; contents include an aspirin tablet that may be chewed and dipyridamole pellets that may be sprinkled on applesauce.
Alavert™ Allergy Sinus 12 Hour	Tablet	Slow release
Allegra-D®	Tablet	Slow release
Allfen Jr	Tablet	Slow release
Alprazolam ER	Tablet	Slow release
Altocor™	Tablet	Slow release
Altoprev®	Tablet	Slow release
Ambien CR™	Tablet	Slow release
Amitiza®	Capsule	Slow release
Amrix®	Capsule	Slow release
Aplenzin™	Tablet	Slow release
Aptivus®	Capsule	Taste. Oil emulsion within spheres
Arthrotec®	Tablet	Enteric-coated
Asacol®	Tablet	Slow release
Ascriptin® A/D	Tablet	Enteric-coated
Augmentin XR®	Tablet	Slow release[2, 8]
Avinza™	Capsule	Slow release[1] (applesauce)
Avodart™	Capsule	Teratogenic potential
Azulfidine® EN-tabs®	Tablet	Enteric-coated
Bayer® Aspirin EC	Caplet	Enteric-coated
Bayer® Aspirin, Low Adult 81 mg	Tablet	Enteric-coated
Bayer® Aspirin, Regular Strength 325 mg	Caplet	Enteric-coated
Biaxin® XL	Tablet	Slow release
Bidhist	Tablet	Slow release
Biltricide®	Tablet	Taste[8]
Bisac-Evac™	Tablet	Enteric-coated[3]
Bisacodyl	Tablet	Enteric-coated[3]

ORAL MEDICATIONS THAT SHOULD NOT BE CRUSHED OR ALTERED

Drug Product	Dosage Form	Dosage Reasons / Comments
Boniva®	Tablet	Irritant. Chewed, crushed, or sucked tablets may cause oropharyngeal irritation.
Bontril® Slow-Release	Capsule	Slow release
Bromfed®	Capsule	Slow release
Bromfed®-PD	Capsule	Slow release
Budeprion™ SR, XL	Tablet	Slow release
Buproban™	Tablet	Slow release
Bupropion SR	Tablet	Slow release
Calan® SR	Tablet	Slow release[8]
Carbatrol®	Capsule	Slow release[1]
Cardene® SR	Capsule	Slow release
Cardizem®	Tablet	Not described as slow release but releases drug over 3 hours.
Cardizem® CD	Capsule	Slow release
Cardizem® LA	Tablet	Slow release
Cardura® XL	Tablet	Slow release
Cartia® XT	Capsule	Slow release
Cefaclor extended release	Tablet	Slow release
Ceftin®	Tablet	Taste[2]. Use suspension for children.
Cefuroxime	Tablet	Taste[2]. Use suspension for children.
CellCept®	Capsule, tablet	Teratogenic potential[9]
Charcoal Plus®	Tablet	Enteric-coated
Chlor-Trimeton® 12-Hour	Tablet	Slow release[2]
Cipro® XR	Tablet	Slow release
Claritin-D® 12-Hour	Tablet	Slow release
Claritin-D® 24-Hour	Tablet	Slow release
Colace®	Capsule	Taste[5]
Colestid®	Tablet	Slow release
Commit™	Lozenge	Integrity compromised by chewing or crushing.
Concerta®	Tablet	Slow release
Coreg CR™	Capsule	Slow release[1]
Cotazym-S®	Capsule	Enteric-coated[1]
Covera-HS™	Tablet	Slow release
Creon® 5, 10, 20	Capsule	Slow release[1]
Crixivan®	Capsule	Taste. Capsule may be opened and mixed with fruit puree (eg, banana).
Cymbalta®	Capsule	Enteric-coated
Cytovene®	Capsule	Skin irritant
Cytoxan®	Tablet	Drug may be crushed, but manufacturer recommends using injection.
Dallergy®	Caplet	Slow release[2,8]
Deconamine® SR	Capsule	Slow release[2]

Drug Product	Dosage Form	Dosage Reasons / Comments
Depakene®	Capsule	Slow release; mucous membrane irritant[2]
Depakote®	Tablet	Slow release
Depakote® ER	Tablet	Slow release
Detrol® LA	Capsule	Slow release
Dexedrine® Spansule®	Capsule	Slow release
Diamox® Sequels®	Capsule	Slow release
Dilacor® XR	Capsule	Slow release
Dilatrate-SR®	Capsule	Slow release
Dilt-CD	Capsule	Slow release
Dilt-XR	Capsule	Slow release
Diltia XT®	Capsule	Slow release
Ditropan® XL	Tablet	Slow release
Divalproex ER	Tablet	Slow release
Donnatal® Extentab®	Tablet	Slow release[2]
Doxidan®	Tablet	Enteric-coated[3]
Drisdol®	Capsule	Liquid filled[4]
Drixoral® Cold and Allergy	Tablet	Slow release
Droxia®	Capsule	May be opened; wear gloves to handle.
Dulcolax®	Capsule	Liquid-filled
Dulcolax®	Tablet	Enteric-coated[3]
DuraHist™	Tablet	Slow release[8]
Duraphen™ II DM	Tablet	Slow release[8]
Duraphen™ Forte	Tablet	Slow release[8]
Duratuss®	Tablet	Slow release[8]
DynaCirc® CR	Tablet	Slow release
Easprin®	Tablet	Enteric-coated
EC-Naprosyn®	Tablet	Enteric-coated
Ecotrin® Adult Low Strength	Tablet	Enteric-coated
Ecotrin® Maximum Strength	Tablet	Enteric-coated
Ecotrin® Regular Strength	Tablet	Enteric-coated
Ed A-Hist™	Caplet	Slow release[2]
E.E.S.® 400	Tablet	Enteric-coated[2]
Effer-K™	Tablet	Effervescent tablet[6]
Effervescent Potassium	Tablet	Effervescent tablet[6]
Effexor® XR	Capsule	Slow release
Efidac/24® Pseudoephedrine	Tablet	Slow release
Efidac® 24	Tablet	Slow release
E-Mycin®	Tablet	Enteric-coated
Enablex®	Tablet	Slow release
Entex® LA	Capsule	Slow release[2]
Entex® PSE	Capsule	Slow release
Entocort® EC	Capsule	Enteric-coated[1]
Equetro™	Capsule	Slow release[1]

Drug Product	Dosage Form	Dosage Reasons / Comments
Ergomar®	Tablet	Sublingual form[7]
Ery-Tab®	Tablet	Enteric-coated
Erythrocin Stearate	Tablet	Enteric-coated
Erythromycin Base	Tablet	Enteric-coated
Erythromycin Delayed-Release	Capsule	Enteric-coated pellets[1]
Evista®	Tablet	Taste; teratogenic potential[9]
ExeFen-PD	Tablet	Slow release[8]
Extendryl JR	Capsule	Slow release
Extendryl SR	Capsule	Slow release[2]
Feldene®	Capsule	Mucous membrane irritant
Fentora™	Tablet	Buccal tablet
Feosol®	Tablet	Enteric-coated[2]
Feratab®	Tablet	Enteric-coated[2]
Fergon®	Tablet	Enteric-coated
Fero-Grad 500®	Tablet	Slow release
Ferro-Sequels®	Tablet	Slow release
Flagyl ER®	Tablet	Slow release
Flomax®	Capsule	Slow release
Focalin® XR	Capsule	Slow release[1]
Fosamax®	Tablet	Mucous membrane irritant
Fosamax Plus D™	Tablet	Mucous membrane irritant
Gleevec®	Tablet	Taste[8]. May be dissolved in water or apple juice.
Glipizide	Tablet	Slow release
Glucophage® XR	Tablet	Slow release
Glucotrol® XL	Tablet	Slow release
Glumetza™	Tablet	Slow release
Guaifed®	Capsule	Slow release
Guaifed®-PD	Capsule	Slow release
Guaifenex® DM	Tablet	Slow release[8]
Guaifenex® PSE	Tablet	Slow release[8]
Guaimax-D®	Tablet	Slow release[8]
Halfprin®	Tablet	Enteric coated
Hista-Vent® DA	Tablet	Slow release[8]
Hydrea®	Capsule	Can be opened and mixed with water; wear gloves to handle.
Imdur™	Tablet	Slow release[8]
Inderal® LA	Capsule	Slow release
Indocin® SR	Capsule	Slow release[1,2]
InnoPran XL™	Capsule	Slow release
Intelence™	Tablet	Tablet should be swallowed whole and not crushed; tablet may be dispersed in water
Invega™	Tablet	Slow release
Ionamin®	Capsule	Slow release
Isochron™	Tablet	Slow release

Drug Product	Dosage Form	Dosage Reasons / Comments
Isoptin® SR	Tablet	Slow release[8]
Isordil® Sublingual	Tablet	Sublingual form[7]
Isosorbide Dinitrate Sublingual	Tablet	Sublingual form[7]
Isosorbide SR	Tablet	Slow release
Kadian®	Capsule	Slow release[1]. Do not give via NG tubes.
Kaletra®	Tablet	Film coated
Kaon-Cl®	Tablet	Slow release[2]
Kapidex™	Capsule	Slow release[1]
K-Dur®	Tablet	Slow release
Keppra®	Tablet	Taste[2]
Ketek®	Tablet	Slow release
Klor-Con®	Tablet	Slow release[2]
Klor-Con® M	Tablet	Slow release[2]; some strengths are scored
Klotrix®	Tablet	Slow release[2]
K-Lyte®	Tablet	Effervescent tablet[6]
K-Lyte/Cl®	Tablet	Effervescent tablet[6]
K-Lyte DS®	Tablet	Effervescent tablet[6]
K-Tab®	Tablet	Slow release[2]
Lescol® XL	Tablet	Slow release
Letairis™	Tablet	Film coated
Levbid®	Tablet	Slow release[8]
Levsinex® Timecaps®	Capsule	Slow release
Lexxel®	Tablet	Slow release
Lialda™	Tablet	Delayed release, enteric coated
Lipram 4500	Capsule	Enteric-coated[1]
Lipram-PN	Capsule	Slow release[1]
Lipram-UL	Capsule	Slow release[1]
Liquibid-D®	Tablet	Slow release
Lithobid®	Tablet	Slow release
Lodrane® 24	Capsule	Slow release
Lodrane® 24D	Capsule	Slow release
LoHist 12D	Tablet	Slow release
Lovaza®	Capsule	Contents of capsule may erode walls of styrofoam or plastic materials
Luvox® CR	Capsule	Slow release
Mag-Tab® SR	Tablet	Slow release
Maxifed DM	Tablet	Slow release[8]
Maxifed DMX	Tablet	Slow release[8]
Maxifed-G®	Tablet	Slow release
Maxiphen DM	Tablet	Slow release[8]
Medent-DM	Tablet	Slow release
Mestinon® Timespan®	Tablet	Slow release[2]
Metadate® CD	Capsule	Slow release[1]

ORAL MEDICATIONS THAT SHOULD NOT BE CRUSHED OR ALTERED

Drug Product	Dosage Form	Dosage Reasons / Comments
Metadate™ ER	Tablet	Slow release
Methylin™ ER	Tablet	Slow release
Metoprolol ER	Tablet	Slow release
MicroK®	Capsule	Slow release[1,2]
Morphine sulfate extended-release	Tablet	Slow release
Motrin®	Tablet	Taste[5]
Moxatag™	Tablet	Slow release
MS Contin®	Tablet	Slow release[2]
Mucinex®	Tablet	Slow release
Mucinex® DM	Tablet	Slow release[2]
Myfortic®	Tablet	Slow release
Naprelan®	Tablet	Slow release
Nasatab® LA	Tablet	Slow release[8]
Nexium®	Capsule	Slow release[1]
Niaspan®	Tablet	Slow release
Nicotinic Acid	Capsule, Tablet	Slow release[8]
Nifediac™ CC	Tablet	Slow release
Nifedical™ XL	Tablet	Slow release
Nifedipine ER	Tablet	Slow release
Nitrostat®	Tablet	Sublingual route[7]
Norflex™	Tablet	Slow release
Norpace® CR	Capsule	Slow release
Opana® ER	Tablet	Slow release
Oracea™	Capsule	Slow release
Oramorph SR®	Tablet	Slow release[2]
OxyContin®	Tablet	Slow release
Pancrease®	Capsule	Enteric-coated[1]
Pancrecarb MS®	Capsule	Enteric-coated[1]
Pancrelipase	Capsule	Enteric-coated[1]
Panocaps	Capsule	Enteric-coated[1]
Papaverine Sustained Action	Capsule	Slow release
Paxil CR™	Tablet	Slow release
Pentasa®	Capsule	Slow release
PhenaVent™ D	Tablet	Slow release
PhenaVent™ LA	Capsule	Slow release
Plendil®	Tablet	Slow release
Prevacid®	Capsule	Slow release[1]
Prevacid®	Suspension	Slow release. Not for use in NG tubes.
Prevacid® SoluTab™	Tablet	Orally disintegrating. Do not swallow; dissolve in water only and dispense via dosing syringe or NG tube.
Prilosec®	Capsule	Slow release
Prilosec OTC™	Tablet	Slow release
Procardia XL®	Tablet	Slow release

Drug Product	Dosage Form	Dosage Reasons / Comments
Profen II®	Tablet	Slow release[8]
Profen II DM®	Tablet	Slow release[8]
Profen Forte™ DM	Tablet	Slow release
Propecia®	Tablet	**Note:** Women who are, or may become, pregnant, should not handle crushed or broken tablets.
Proquin® XR	Tablet	Slow release
Proscar®	Tablet	Teratogenic potential[9]
Protonix®	Tablet	Slow release
Prozac® Weekly™	Capsule	Enteric coated
Pseudovent™	Capsule	Slow release
Pseudovent™-Ped	Capsule	Slow release
QDALL® AR	Capsule	Slow release
Ralix	Tablet	Slow release
Ranexa®	Tablet	Slow release
Razadyne™ ER	Capsule	Slow release
Renagel®	Tablet	Expands in liquid if broken/crushed.
Rescon®	Tablet	Slow release
Rescon-Jr	Tablet	Slow release
Rescon® MX	Tablet	Slow release[8]
Rescriptor®	Tablet	If unable to swallow, may dissolve 100 mg tablets in water and drink; 200 mg tablets must be swallowed whole
Respa®-1st	Tablet	Slow release[2,8]
Respa-DM®	Tablet	Slow release[2,8]
Respahist®	Capsule	Slow release[2,8]
Respaire®-60 SR/-120 SR	Capsule	Slow release[2]
Resperdal® M-Tab	Tablet	Orally disintegrating. Do not chew or break tablet; after dissolving under tongue, tablet may be swallowed
Revlimid®	Capsule	Teratogenic potential[9]
Ritalin® LA	Capsule	Slow release[1]
Ritalin-SR®	Tablet	Slow release
R-Tanna	Tablet	Slow release
Rythmol® SR	Capsule	Slow release
Seroquel® XR	Tablet	Slow release
Sinemet® CR	Tablet	Slow release
SINUvent® PE	Tablet	Slow release[8]
Slo-Niacin®	Tablet	Slow release[8]
Slow-Mag®	Tablet	Slow release
Solodyn™	Tablet	Slow release
Somnote™	Capsule	Liquid filled
Sprycel®	Tablet	Film coated[9]
Strattera®	Capsule	Capsule contents can cause ocular irritation.
Sudafed® 12-Hour	Capsule	Slow release[2]

Drug Product	Dosage Form	Dosage Reasons / Comments
Sudafed® 24-Hour	Capsule	Slow release[2]
Sulfazine EC	Tablet	Delayed release, enteric coated
Sular®	Tablet	Slow release
Sustiva®	Tablet	Tablets should not be broken (capsules should be used if dosage adjustment needed)
Symax SR	Tablet	Slow release
Taztia XT™	Capsule	Slow release[1]
Tegretol®-XR	Tablet	Slow release
Temodar®	Capsule	**Note:** If capsules are accidentally opened or damaged, rigorous precautions should be taken to avoid inhalation or contact of contents with the skin or mucous membranes[9].
Tessalon®	Capsule	Swallow whole; pharmacologic action may cause choking if chewed or opened and swallowed.
Theo-24®	Tablet	Slow release[2]
Theochron™	Tablet	Slow release[2]
Tiazac®	Capsule	Slow release[1]
Topamax®	Capsule	Taste[1]
Topamax®	Tablet	Taste
Toprol XL®	Tablet	Slow release[8]
Touro™ CC/CC-LD	Caplet	Slow release[2,8]
Touro LA®	Caplet	Slow release
Toviaz™	Tablet	Slow release
Tracleer®	Tablet	Teratogenic potential[9]
Trental®	Tablet	Slow release
Tylenol® Arthritis Pain	Caplet	Slow release
Tylenol® 8 Hour	Caplet	Slow release
Ultram® ER	Tablet	Slow release. Tablet disruption my cause a potentially fatal overdose.
Ultrase®	Capsule	Enteric-coated[1]
Ultrase® MT	Capsule	Enteric-coated[1]
Uniphyl®	Tablet	Slow release
Urocit®-K	Tablet	Wax-coated
Uroxatral®	Tablet	Slow release
Valcyte™	Tablet	Teratogenic potential[9]
Verapamil SR	Tablet	Slow release[8]
Verelan®	Capsule	Slow release[1]
Verelan® PM	Capsule	Slow release[1]
VESIcare®	Tablet	Enteric-coated
Videx® EC	Capsule	Slow release
Voltaren®-XR	Tablet	Slow release
VoSpire ER™	Tablet	Slow release
Wellbutrin SR®	Tablet	Slow release
Wellbutrin XL™	Tablet	Slow release

Drug Product	Dosage Form	Dosage Reasons / Comments
Xanax XR®	Tablet	Slow release
Zonlinza™	Capsule	Use gloves to handle.
ZORprin®	Tablet	Slow release
Zyban®	Tablet	Slow release
Zyflo CR™	Tablet	Slow release
Zyrtec-D® Allergy & Congestion	Tablet	Slow release

[1]Capsule may be opened and the contents taken without crushing or chewing; soft food such as applesauce or pudding may facilitate administration; contents may generally be administered via nasogastric tube using an appropriate fluid, provided entire contents are washed down the tube.

[2]Liquid dosage forms of the product are available; however, dose, frequency of administration, and manufacturers may differ from that of the solid dosage form.

[3]Antacids and/or milk may prematurely dissolve the coating of the tablet.

[4]Capsule may be opened and the liquid contents removed for administration.

[5]The taste of this product in a liquid form would likely be unacceptable to the patient; administration via nasogastric tube should be acceptable.

[6]Effervescent tablets must be dissolved in the amount of diluent recommended by the manufacturer.

[7]Tablets are made to disintegrate under the tongue.

[8]Tablet is scored and may be broken in half without affecting release characteristics.

[9]Women who are or may become pregnant should not handle medication especially if crushed or broken; avoid direct contact.

Mitchell JF, "Oral Dosage Forms That Should Not Be Crushed." Available at: http://www.ismp.org/tools/DoNotCrush.pdf. Last accessed May 11, 2009.

PORPHYRIA: SAFE AND UNSAFE DRUGS

Categories of Safe and Unsafe Drugs in Acute Intermittent Porphyria, Hereditary Coproporphyria, and Variegate Porphyria

Unsafe	Safe
Alcohol	Acetaminophen
Aminolevulinic acid	Aspirin
Barbiturates	Atropine
Carbamazepine	Bromides
Carisoprodol	Glucocorticoids
Danazol	Insulin
Ergots	Narcotic analgesics
Ethchlorvynol	Penicillin and derivatives
Glutethimide	Phenothiazines
Griseofulvin	Streptomycin
Mephenytoin	
Meprobamate	
Methyprylon	
Mifepristone	
Phenytoin	
Porfimer	
Pyrazolones	
Succinimides	
Sulfonamide antibiotics	
Synthetic estrogens and progestins	
Valproic acid	
Verteporfin	

PHARMACOLOGIC CATEGORY INDEX

NOTES

NOTES

NOTES

NOTES

Other Products Offered by Lexi-Comp

Drug Information Handbook

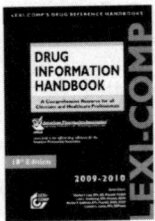

This easy-to-use drug reference is for the pharmacist, physician, or other healthcare professional requiring fast access to comprehensive drug information.

Over 1400 drug monographs are detailed with up to 34 fields of information per monograph. A valuable appendix includes hundreds of charts and reviews of special topics such as guidelines for treatment and therapy recommendations. A pharmacologic category index is also provided.

Drug Information Handbook with International Trade Names Index

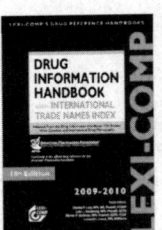

The *Drug International Handbook with Trade Names Index* includes the content of our Drug Information Handbook, plus international drug monographs for use worldwide! This easy-to-use reference is complied especially for the pharmacist, physician, or other healthcare professional seeking quick access to comprehensive drug information.

Drug Information Handbook for Advanced Practice Nursing

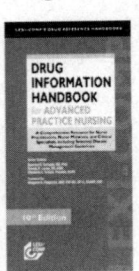

Designed to assist the advanced practice nurse with prescribing, monitoring and educating patients.

Includes: Over 4800 generic and brand names cross-referenced by page number; Generic drug names and cross-references highlighted in RED; Labeled and Investigational indications; Adult, Geriatric, and Pediatric dosing; and up to 60 fields of information per monograph, including Patient Education and Physical Assessment.

Drug Information Handbook for Nursing

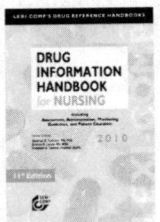

Designed for registered professional nurses and upper-division nursing students requiring dosing, administration, monitoring and patient education information.

Includes: Over 4800 generic and brand name drugs, cross-referenced by page number; drug names and specific nursing fields highlighted in RED for easy reference, Nursing Actions field includes Physical Assessment and Patient Education guidelines.

Other Products Offered by Lexi-Comp

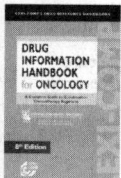
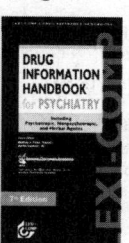
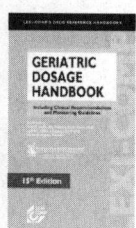
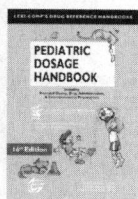

Other Products Offered by Lexi-Comp

Pediatric Dosage Handbook with International Trade Names Index

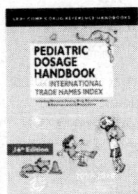

The *Pediatric Dosage Handbook with International Trade Names Index* is the trusted pediatric drug resource of medical professionals worldwide. The International Edition contains all the content of the Lexi-Comp's *Pediatric Dosage Handbook,* plus an International Trade Names Index including trade names from over 100 countries.

Pharmacogenomics Handbook

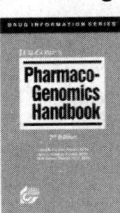

Ideal for any healthcare professional or student wishing to gain insight into the emerging field of pharmacogenomics.

Includes: Information concerning key genetic variations to may influence drug disposition and/or sensitivity; brief introductions to fundamental concepts in genetics and genomics. A foundation for all clinicians who will be called on to integrate rapid-expanding genomics knowledge into the management of drug therapy.

Rating Scales for Mental Health

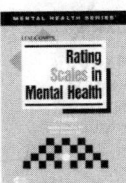

Ideal for clinicians as well as administrators, this book provides an overview of over 100 recommended rating scales for mental assessment.

Includes: Rating scales for conditions such as General Anxiety, Social/Family Functioning, Eating Disorders, and Sleep Disorders; Monograph format covering such topics as Overview of Scale, General Applications, Psychometric Properties, and References.

Other Products Offered by Lexi-Comp

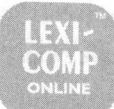

Lexi-Comp ONLINE

Lexi-Comp® ONLINE™ integrates industry-leading databases and enhanced searching technology to bring you time-sensitive clinical information at the point-of-care. Our easy-to-use interface and concise information eliminate the need to navigate through multiple pages or make unnecessary mouse clicks.

Lexi-Comp ONLINE includes multiple databases and modules covering the following topic areas:

- Core drug information with specialty fields
- Pediatrics and Geriatrics
- Interaction Analysis
- Pharmacogenomics
- Infectious Diseases
- Laboratory Tests and Diagnostic Procedures
- Natural Products
- Patient Education
- Drug Identification
- Calculations
- I.V. Compatibility: *King® Guide to Parenteral Admixtures®*
- Toxicology

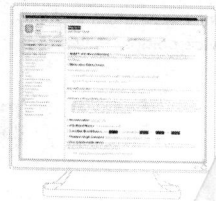

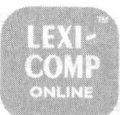
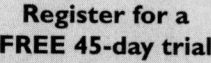
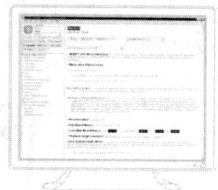

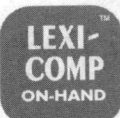
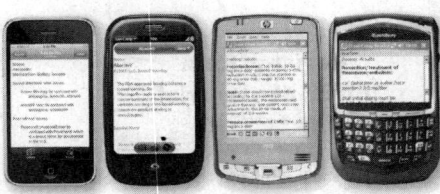